INTERNAL MEDICINE
FOR DENTISTRY

INTERNAL MEDICINE FOR DENTISTRY

LOUIS F. ROSE, D.D.S., M.D.

Professor of Periodontics,
University of Pennsylvania, School of Dental Medicine;
Professor of Medicine and Surgery,
Chief, Division of Dental Medicine,
Medical College of Pennsylvania,
Philadelphia, Pennsylvania

DONALD KAYE, M.D.

Professor and Chairman, Department of Medicine,
Medical College of Pennsylvania,
Philadelphia, Pennsylvania

with **284** illustrations

The C. V. Mosby Company

ST. LOUIS • TORONTO • LONDON   1983

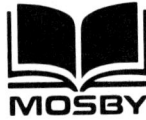

A TRADITION OF PUBLISHING EXCELLENCE

Editor: Darlene Warfel
Assistant editor: Melba Steube
Editing supervisor: Peggy Fagen
Book design: Susan Trail
Cover design: Suzanne Oberholtzer
Production: Carol O'Leary, Barbara Merritt

Copyright © 1983 by The C.V. Mosby Company

All rights reserved. No part of this publication may be reproduced, stored in a retrieval system, or transmitted, in any form or by any means, electronic, mechanical, photocopying, recording, or otherwise, without prior written permission from the publisher.

Printed in the United States of America

The C.V. Mosby Company
11830 Westline Industrial Drive, St. Louis, Missouri 63146

Library of Congress Cataloging in Publication Data
Main entry under title:

Internal medicine for dentistry.

   Includes bibliographies and index.
   1. Internal medicine. 2. Dentists. I. Rose, Louis F.
II. Kaye, Donald. [DNLM: 1. Internal medicine.
2. Oral manifestations. WB 115 I6107]
RC46.I524   1983   616   82-25881
ISBN 0-8016-4200-0

C/VH/VH 9 8 7 6 5 4   01/B/060

SECTION EDITORS

DORIS G. BARTUSKA, M.D.
Professor of Medicine and Chief, Division of Endocrinology and Metabolism, The Medical College of Pennsylvania, Philadelphia, Pennsylvania

ROSALIE A. BURNS, M.D.
Professor and Chairman, Department of Neurology, The Medical College of Pennsylvania, Philadelphia, Pennsylvania

TOBY R. ENGEL, M.D.
Professor of Medicine, The Medical College of Pennsylvania, Philadelphia, Pennsylvania

HARVEY M. FRIEDMAN, M.D.
Associate Professor of Medicine, University of Pennsylvania School of Medicine; Director, Diagnostic Virology Laboratory, The Children's Hospital of Philadelphia, Philadelphia, Pennsylvania

ROSALINE R. JOSEPH, M.D.
Professor of Medicine and Chief, Division of Hematology and Oncology, The Medical College of Pennsylvania, Philadelphia, Pennsylvania

WARREN A. KATZ, M.D.
Clinical Professor of Medicine and Chief, Division of Rheumatology, The Medical College of Pennsylvania; Attending Physician, Moss Rehabilitation Hospital, Philadelphia, Pennsylvania

DONALD KAYE, M.D.
Professor and Chairman, Department of Medicine, The Medical College of Pennsylvania; Chief of Medicine, The Hospital of the Medical College of Pennsylvania, Philadelphia, Pennsylvania

BERNARD A. KIRSHBAUM, M.D.
Clinical Professor of Medicine and Chief, Division of Dermatology, The Medical College of Pennsylvania, Philadelphia, Pennsylvania

SANDRA P. LEVISON, M.D.
Professor of Medicine and Chief, Division of Nephrology and Hypertension, The Medical College of Pennsylvania, Philadelphia, Pennsylvania

WILLIAM L. MORRISSEY, M.D.
Associate Professor of Medicine and Chief, Division of Pulmonary Diseases, The Medical College of Pennsylvania, Philadelphia, Pennsylvania

LOUIS F. ROSE, D.D.S., M.D.
Professor of Periodontics, University of Pennsylvania, School of Dental Medicine; Professor of Medicine and Surgery, Chief of Dental Medicine, Medical College of Pennsylvania, Philadelphia, Pennsylvania

WALTER RUBIN, M.D.
Professor of Medicine and Anatomy and Chief, Division of Gastroenterology, The Medical College of Pennsylvania, Philadelphia, Pennsylvania

CONSULTING EDITOR OF DENTAL MEDICINE

MARTIN S. GREENBERG, D.D.S.
Professor of Oral Medicine, University of Pennsylvania, School of Dental Medicine; Chairman, Department of Dental Medicine, Hospital of the University of Pennsylvania, Philadelphia, Pennsylvania

CONTRIBUTORS

ELIAS ABRUTYN, M.D.
Associate Professor of Medicine, The Medical College of Pennsylvania; Chief, Infectious Diseases, and Assistant Chief of Medical Service, Philadelphia Veterans Administration Medical Center; Adjunct Associate Professor of Medicine, University of Pennsylvania School of Medicine, Philadelphia, Pennsylvania

BRAJESH AGARWAL, M.D.
Professor of Medicine, Thomas Jefferson University Medical School, Philadelphia, Pennsylvania; Chief of Medical Services, Veterans Administration Medical and Regional Center, Wilmington, Delaware

PASHA AGARWAL, M.D.
Assistant Professor of Pathology, The Medical College of Pennsylvania, Philadelphia, Pennsylvania

STANLEY L. ALTSCHULER, M.D.
Clinical Assistant Professor of Medicine, The Medical College of Pennsylvania, Philadelphia, Pennsylvania

EZRA A. AMSTERDAM, M.D.
Professor of Medicine and Chief, Coronary Care Unit, University of California–Davis School of Medicine and Medical Center, Davis, California

JAMES T. AMSTERDAM, D.M.D., M.D.
Clinical Instructor, Department of Surgery, Division of Dental Medicine, The Medical College of Pennsylvania, Philadelphia, Pennsylvania

KARL E. ANDERSON, M.D.
Associate Professor, The Rockefeller University Hospital, New York, New York

ALLAN M. ARBETER, M.D.
Assistant Professor, University of Pennsylvania School of Medicine, Philadelphia, Pennsylvania

ROBERT N. ARM, B.A., D.M.D.
Director, Department of Dentistry, and Educational Coordinator, General Practice Residency Program, Wilmington Medical Center; Consultant and Educational Coordinator, General Practice Residency Program, Delaware State Hospital; Coordinator, Oral Pathology, Delaware Technical and Community College, Wilmington, Delaware

BALU H. ATHREYA, M.D.
Clinical Director, Children's Seashore House; Chief of Rheumatology, The Children's Hospital of Philadelphia; Associate Professor of Pediatrics, University of Pennsylvania School of Medicine, Philadelphia, Pennsylvania

FRANK BARCH, M.D.
Clinical Assistant Professor of Medicine, The Medical College of Pennsylvania, Philadelphia, Pennsylvania

MICHAEL J. BARRETT, M.D.
Associate Professor of Medicine and Director, Non-Invasive Laboratory, The Medical College of Pennsylvania, Philadelphia, Pennsylvania

WILLIAM E. BARRY, M.D.
Professor of Medicine, Section of Hematology-Oncology, Temple University Health Sciences Center, Philadelphia, Pennsylvania

CHRISTINE P. BASTL, M.D.
Associate Professor of Medicine, Temple University Health Sciences Center, Philadelphia, Pennsylvania

ROBERT W. BEIDEMAN, D.M.D.
Associate Professor, Director of Radiology, University of Pennsylvania, School of Dental Medicine, Philadelphia, Pennsylvania

ANTHONY V. BENEDETTO, D.O.
Clinical Assistant Professor of Medicine (Dermatology), The Medical College of Pennsylvania, Philadelphia, Pennsylvania

JOHN E. BENNETT, M.D.
Head, Clinical Mycology Section, National Institute of Allergy and Infectious Diseases, National Institutes of Health, Bethesda, Maryland

EMMANUEL C. BESA, M.D.
Associate Professor of Medicine, The Medical College of Pennsylvania, Philadelphia, Pennsylvania

CONTRIBUTORS

IAIN F.S. BLACK, M.D.

Professor, Department of Pediatrics, Temple University School of Medicine; Chief, Section of Cardiology, St. Christopher's Hospital for Children, Philadelphia, Pennsylvania

RANDOLPH C. BLODGETT, Jr., M.D.

Director, Clinical Investigation—U.S., Clinical Research and Development, Smith Kline & French Laboratories; Clinical Professor of Medicine, The Medical College of Pennsylvania, Philadelphia, Pennsylvania

GUENTHER BODEN, M.D.

Professor of Medicine and Chief, Division of Diabetes/Metabolism, Temple University School of Medicine, Philadelphia, Pennsylvania

JEROME A. BOSCIA, M.D.

Assistant Professor of Medicine, The Medical College of Pennsylvania, Philadelphia, Pennsylvania

VERNON J. BRIGHTMAN, D.M.D., M.D.Sc., Ph.D.

Professor of Oral Medicine, University of Pennsylvania, School of Dental Medicine; Attending in Oral Medicine, Hospital of the University of Pennsylvania, Philadelphia, Pennsylvania

JEROME I. BRODY, M.D.

Professor of Medicine, The Medical College of Pennsylvania, Philadelphia, Pennsylvania

SHIRLEY BROWN, D.M.D.

Assistant Professor of Surgery, Division of Dental Medicine, The Medical College of Pennsylvania; Adjunct Assistant Professor of Oral Medicine, University of Pennsylvania, School of Dental Medicine, Philadelphia, Pennsylvania

R. MICHAEL BUCKLEY, Jr., M.D.

Clinical Assistant Professor of Medicine, University of Pennsylvania School of Medicine; Infectious Disease Section, Pennsylvania Hospital, Philadelphia, Pennsylvania

BERNADINE HEALY BULKLEY, M.D.

Associate Professor of Medicine, Assistant Professor of Pathology, and Assistant Dean, Postdoctoral Program and Faculty Development, Johns Hopkins University School of Medicine, Baltimore, Maryland

CHARLES A. BUSH, M.D.

Associate Professor of Medicine, Division of Cardiology, and Director, Cardiac Catheterization Laboratories, Ohio State University College of Medicine, Columbus, Ohio

†LEOPOLD CANALES, M.D.

Associate Professor of Neurology, The Medical College of Pennsylvania; Chief of Neurology, Philadelphia Veterans Administration Medical Center, Philadelphia, Pennsylvania

DAVID M. CAPUZZI, M.D., Ph.D.

Chairman of Research, The Lankenau Medical Research Center; Associate Professor of Medicine, The Medical College of Pennsylvania; Associate Professor of Medicine (Adjunct), University of Pennsylvania, Philadelphia, Pennsylvania

HUGH J. CARROLL, M.D.

Professor of Medicine and Director, Electrolyte and Hypertension Division, State University of New York, Downstate Medical Center, Brooklyn, New York

PATRICIA M. CATALANO, M.D.

Clinical Assistant Professor of Medicine, Thomas Jefferson University Medical School, Philadelphia, Pennsylvania

S. GARY COHEN, D.M.D.

Director, General Practice Residency and Attending in Dental Medicine, Hospital of the University of Pennsylvania; Attending Oral Medicine and Dental Research, Albert Einstein Medical Center; Clinical Associate in Oral Medicine, University of Pennsylvania, School of Dental Medicine, Philadelphia, Pennsylvania

ANTHONY N. DeMARIA, M.D.

Professor of Medicine and Chief, Cardiology Division, University of Kentucky School of Medicine, Lexington, Kentucky

B. KYLE DeMARTINO, B.A., D.D.S., F.A.D.S.A.

Clinical Assistant Professor of Oral Surgery and Anesthesiology, University of Pennsylvania, School of Dental Medicine; Clinical Assistant Professor of Dental Medicine, The Medical College of Pennsylvania, Philadelphia, Pennsylvania

SANDEEP DHAND, M.D.

Clinical Assistant Professor of Medicine, The Medical College of Pennsylvania, Philadelphia, Pennsylvania

VASANT DHOPESH, M.D.

Associate Professor, Department of Neurology, The Medical College of Pennsylvania, Philadelphia, Pennsylvania

NIKOLAY V. DIMITROV, M.D.

Professor of Medicine, Department of Medicine, College of Human Medicine, Michigan State University, East Lansing, Michigan

---

† Deceased.

GERALD R. DONOWITZ, M.D.

Assistant Professor of Medicine, University of Virginia School of Medicine, Charlottesville, Virginia

MARY B. DRATMAN, M.D.

Professor, Department of Medicine, The Medical College of Pennsylvania; Medical Investigator, Veterans Administration Medical Center, Philadelphia, Pennsylvania

W. BRUCE DUNKMAN, M.D.

Chief, Clinical Cardiology Service, Veterans Administration Medical Center; Assistant Professor of Medicine, University of Pennsylvania School of Medicine, Philadelphia, Pennsylvania

DAVID DUNN, M.D.

Associate Professor of Neurology and Anatomic Pathology, The Medical College of Pennsylvania, Philadelphia, Pennsylvania

ROGER DUVOISIN, M.D.

Professor and Chairman, Department of Neurology, University of Medicine and Dentistry of New Jersey, Rutgers Medical School; Director, Neurology Service, Middlesex General Hospital, New Brunswick, New Jersey

NORMAN H. ERTEL, M.D.

Chief, Medical Service, Veterans Administration Medical Center, East Orange, New Jersey; Professor of Medicine, College of Medicine and Dentistry of New Jersey, New Jersey Medical School, Newark, New Jersey

GERALD H. ESCOVITZ, M.D.

Associate Professor of Medicine, The Medical College of Pennsylvania, Philadelphia, Pennsylvania

CALVIN EZRIN, M.D.

Clinical Professor of Medicine, Cedars-Sinai Medical Center, University of California–Los Angeles, Los Angeles, California

ANTHONY S. FAUCI, M.D.

Chief, Laboratory of Immunoregulation, National Institute of Allergy and Infectious Diseases, National Institutes of Health, Bethesda, Maryland

PEDRO C. FERNANDEZ, M.D.

Director, Hemodialysis Unit, Philadelphia Veterans Administration Medical Center; Associate Professor of Medicine, The Medical College of Pennsylvania, Philadelphia, Pennsylvania

JAMES O. FINNEGAN, M.D.

Associate Professor of Surgery and Chief, Division of Cardiothoracic Surgery, The Medical College of Pennsylvania, Philadelphia, Pennsylvania

STUART L. FISCHMAN, D.M.D., F.I.C.D., F.A.C.D.

Professor of Oral Medicine, State University of New York at Buffalo, School of Dentistry; Director of Dentistry, Erie County Medical Center, Buffalo, New York

GARY R. FLEISHER, M.D.

Assistant Professor of Pediatrics, University of Pennsylvania School of Medicine; Division of Infectious Diseases, The Children's Hospital of Philadelphia, Philadelphia, Pennsylvania

JOSEPH A. FRANCIOSA, M.D.

Professor of Medicine and Chief, Cardiovascular Division, University of Arkansas for Medical Sciences, Little Rock, Arkansas

WILLIAM O. FRANK, M.D.

Assistant Professor of Medicine, The Medical College of Pennsylvania; Staff Physician, Philadelphia Veterans Administration Medical Center, Philadelphia, Pennsylvania

ROBERT D. FRIEDMAN, D.D.S., M.A., Ph.D.

Assistant Professor of Oral Medicine, University of Pennsylvania, School of Dental Medicine, Philadelphia, Pennsylvania

FRANK H. GARDNER, M.D.

Professor of Medicine and Director, Division of Hematology-Oncology, University of Texas Medical Branch, Galveston, Texas

ADI A. GARFUNKEL, D.M.D.

Associate Professor of Oral Medicine, Chairman, Hospital Oral Medicine Service, Hadassah-Hebrew University School of Dental Medicine, Jerusalem, Israel; Adjunct Associate Professor, University of Pennsylvania, School of Dental Medicine, Philadelphia, Pennsylvania

ELAINE GERMAN, M.D.

Director of Medicine, United Hospitals of Newark; Clinical Professor of Medicine, New Jersey College of Medicine, Newark, New Jersey

LEONARD S. GIRSH, M.D.

Clinical Associate Professor of Medicine and Chief, Division of Allergy and Clinical Immunology, The Medical College of Pennsylvania, Philadelphia, Pennsylvania

STEPHEN J. GLUCKMAN, M.D.

Chief, Infectious Disease Section, Pennsylvania Hospital; Clinical Assistant Professor of Medicine, University of Pennsylvania School of Medicine, Philadelphia, Pennsylvania

PHILIP M. GODFREY, D.M.D., M.D.

Staff, Department of General Surgery, Hartford Hospital, Hartford, Connecticut

ERNEST M. GOLD, M.D.
Executive Associate Dean and Professor of Internal Medicine, University of California–Davis School of Medicine, Davis, California

BURTON H. GOLDSTEIN, D.M.D., M.S.
Associate Professor and Chairman, Department of Oral and Maxillofacial Surgery, University of British Columbia, Faculty of Dentistry, Vancouver, British Columbia, Canada

ROBERT H. GORDON, M.D.
Clinical Assistant Professor of Medicine, The Medical College of Pennsylvania, Philadelphia, Pennsylvania

TERRY S. GOTTHELF, D.D.S., M.S.
Assistant Professor of Dental Medicine, The Medical College of Pennsylvania, Philadelphia, Pennsylvania

HARRY GOTTLIEB, M.D.
Clinical Professor of Medicine and Chief, Subsection of Diabetes and Metabolic Diseases, The Medical College of Pennsylvania, Philadelphia, Pennsylvania

MARTIN S. GREENBERG, D.D.S.
Professor of Oral Medicine, University of Pennsylvania, School of Dental Medicine; Chairman, Department of Dental Medicine, Hospital of the University of Pennsylvania, Philadelphia, Pennsylvania

ROBERT A. GROSSMAN, M.D.
Associate Professor of Medicine, University of Pennsylvania School of Medicine, Philadelphia, Pennsylvania

BARRY H. HENDLER, D.D.S., M.D.
Associate Professor of Surgery, Division of Dental Medicine, Director of Oral and Maxillofacial Surgery, Medical College of Pennsylvania; Associate Professor and Acting Chairman, Department of Oral and Maxillofacial Surgery, University of Pennsylvania, School of Dental Medicine, Philadelphia, Pennsylvania

LINDA B. HINER, M.D.
Associate Professor of Pediatrics, The Medical College of Pennsylvania, Philadelphia, Pennsylvania

ROBERT D. HOELDTKE, M.D., Ph.D.
Assistant Professor of Medicine, Division of Metabolism, Temple University School of Medicine, Philadelphia, Pennsylvania

BRUCE I. HOFFMAN, M.D.
Clinical Assistant Professor of Medicine, The Medical College of Pennsylvania, Philadelphia, Pennsylvania

WILLIAM A. HORTON, M.D.
Associate Professor of Medicine and Pediatrics, University of Kansas School of Medicine, Kansas City, Kansas

LEONORE C. HUPPERT, M.D.
Assistant Professor of Obstetrics and Gynecology, The Medical College of Pennsylvania, Philadelphia, Pennsylvania

GRAHAM H. JEFFRIES, M.B., Ch.B., D.Phil.
Professor and Chairman, Department of Medicine, The Pennsylvania State University College of Medicine, Hershey, Pennsylvania

SERGIO A. JIMENEZ, M.D.
Director, Collagen Research Laboratories, and Associate Professor of Medicine, Rheumatology Section, Department of Medicine, University of Pennsylvania School of Medicine, Philadelphia, Pennsylvania

THOMAS C. JONES, M.D.
Professor of Medicine and Chief, Division of International Medicine, Cornell University Medical College, New York, New York

JAMES A. JOYE, M.D.
Assistant Professor of Internal Medicine, University of California–Davis School of Medicine, Davis, California

ATTALLAH KAPPAS, M.D.
Professor and Physician-in-Chief, The Rockefeller University Hospital, New York, New York

JOHN H. KARAM, M.D.
Associate Professor of Medicine and Chief, Clinical Endocrinology, Moffitt Hospital, University of California–San Francisco School of Medicine, San Francisco, California

JULIAN KATZ, M.D.
Clinical Professor of Medicine, Lecturer in Biochemistry and Physiology, The Medical College of Pennsylvania, Philadelphia, Pennsylvania

LOIS ANNE KATZ, M.D.
Associate Chief, Nephrology, and Associate Chief of Staff for Ambulatory Care, New York Veterans Administration Medical Center; Associate Professor of Clinical Medicine, New York University School of Medicine, New York, New York

PAUL KATZ, M.D.
Assistant Professor of Medicine, Division of Clinical Immunology, University of Florida College of Medicine, Gainesville, Florida

JUNE F. KLINGHOFFER, M.D.
Professor of Medicine, The Medical College of Pennsylvania, Philadelphia, Pennsylvania

OKSANA M. KORZENIOWSKI, M.D.
Assistant Professor of Medicine, The Medical College of Pennsylvania; Department of Medicine, Philadelphia Veterans Administration Medical Center, Philadelphia, Pennsylvania

PAUL J. KOVNAT, M.D.
Associate Clinical Professor of Medicine, The University of New Mexico School of Medicine, Albuquerque, New Mexico

SAMUEL T. KUNA, M.D.
Assistant Professor of Medicine, University of Texas Medical School of Galveston, Galveston, Texas

ELIZABETH D. LABOVITZ, M.D.
Associate Professor of Medicine, Division of Nephrology and Hypertension, The Medical College of Pennsylvania, Philadelphia, Pennsylvania

SALLY D. LANE, M.D.
Clinical Assistant Professor of Medicine, The Medical College of Pennsylvania, Philadelphia, Pennsylvania

ROBERT L. LAVINE, M.D.
Associate Professor of Medicine and Associate Director, Division of Endocrinology and Metabolism, Hahnemann Medical College and Hospital of Philadelphia, Philadelphia, Pennsylvania

GEOFFREY LEFFERTS, M.D.
Associate Professor of Medicine and Chief, Division of General Medicine, The Medical College of Pennsylvania, Philadelphia, Pennsylvania

HARVEY B. LEFTON, M.D.
Clinical Associate Professor of Medicine, The Medical College of Pennsylvania, Philadelphia, Pennsylvania

CARL V. LEIER, M.D.
Associate Professor of Medicine and Pharmacology, Division of Cardiology, Department of Medicine, Ohio State University College of Medicine, Columbus, Ohio

GREGORY S. LENCHNER, M.D.
Clinical Assistant Professor of Medicine, Hahnemann Medical College and Hospital, Philadelphia, Pennsylvania

SANFORD LEVINE, M.D.
Chief, Pulmonary Diseases Section, Veterans Administration Medical Center; Associate Professor of Medicine, The Medical College of Pennsylvania; Adjunct Associate Professor of Medicine, University of Pennsylvania School of Medicine, Philadelphia, Pennsylvania

MATTHEW E. LEVISON, M.D.
Professor of Medicine and Chief, Division of Infectious Diseases, Department of Medicine, The Medical College of Pennsylvania, Philadelphia, Pennsylvania

DONALD H. LIEBERMAN, M.D.
Clinical Assistant Professor of Medicine, The Medical College of Pennsylvania, Philadelphia, Pennsylvania

KAREN LIPINSKI, M.D.
Assistant Dermatologist to the Outpatient Clinic, Bryn Mawr Hospital, Bryn Mawr, Pennsylvania

SAL A. LOFARO, M.D.
Attending Physician, Delaware County Memorial Hospital, Drexel Hill, Pennsylvania

REGINALD I. LOW, M.D.
Assistant Professor of Medicine, Section of Cardiovascular Medicine, University of California–Davis School of Medicine, University of California–Davis Medical Center, Davis, California

ROBERT J. LUCHI, M.D.
Professor and Vice-Chairman, Department of Medicine, Baylor College of Medicine; Chief, Medical Service, Veterans Administration Medical Center, Houston, Texas

JERRY C. LUCK, M.D.
Assistant Professor of Medicine, Baylor College of Medicine, Houston, Texas

DAVID T. LUSH, M.D.
Assistant Professor of Medicine, The Medical College of Pennsylvania, Philadelphia, Pennsylvania

MALCOLM W. MacNAB, M.D., Ph.D.
Instructor, Department of Medicine, The Medical College of Pennsylvania, Philadelphia, Pennsylvania

GERALD L. MANDELL, M.D.
Professor of Medicine and Head, Division of Infectious Disease, University of Virginia School of Medicine, Charlottesville, Virginia

CLARENCE MARTIN, M.D.
Instructor in Medicine, The Medical College of Pennsylvania, Philadelphia, Pennsylvania

DEAN T. MASON, M.D.
Professor of Medicine and Physiology, University of California–Davis School of Medicine, University of California–Davis Medical Center; Editor-in-Chief, American Heart Journal, Davis, California

DEBORAH MAYER, C.R.N.P.
Head Nurse, Biological Response Modifiers Program, National Cancer Institute, Frederick, Maryland

MARIAN F. McNAMARA, M.D.
Associate Professor of Surgery and Head of the Division of Vascular Surgery, The Medical College of Pennsylvania, Philadelphia, Pennsylvania

STEVEN G. MEISTER, M.D.
Professor of Medicine and Chief, Cardiology Division, The Medical College of Pennsylvania, Philadelphia, Pennsylvania

HIROSHI MITSUMOTO, M.D.
Assistant Professor of Neurology and Neuropathology, Veterans Administration Medical Center and Case Western Reserve University School of Medicine, Cleveland, Ohio

THEODORE L. MUNSAT, M.D.
Professor and Chairman, Department of Neurology, and Neurologist-in-Chief, Tufts–New England Medical Center, Boston, Massachusetts

DAVID M.F. MURPHY, M.B., M.R.C.P. (U.K.)
Assistant Professor of Medicine and Director of the Pulmonary Function Laboratory, Hospital of the University of Pennsylvania, Philadelphia, Pennsylvania

RALPH M. MYERSON, M.D.
Clinical Professor of Medicine, The Medical College of Pennsylvania; Group Director, Smith Kline & French Laboratories, Philadelphia, Pennsylvania

ROBERT G. NARINS, M.D.
Professor of Medicine and Chief, Renal Section, Temple University Health Sciences Center, Philadelphia, Pennsylvania

THOMAS F. NIKOLAI, M.D.
Clinical Associate Professor of Medicine, University of Wisconsin Medical School; Staff Physician, Department of Internal Medicine, Section of Endocrinology, Marshfield Clinic, Marshfield, Wisconsin

STEVEN NUSSBAUM, M.D.
Clinical Assistant Professor of Medicine, The Medical College of Pennsylvania, Philadelphia, Pennsylvania

MAN S. OH, M.D.
Associate Professor of Medicine and Co-Director, Electrolyte and Hypertension Division, State University of New York Downstate Medical Center, Brooklyn, New York

GEORGE A. OMURA, M.D.
Professor of Medicine, University of Alabama in Birmingham, Birmingham, Alabama

OLIVER OWEN, M.D.
Professor of Medicine, Temple University School of Medicine, Philadelphia, Pennsylvania

GEORGE PAULSON, M.D.
Clinical Professor of Neurology, Ohio State University College of Medicine; Program Director, Neurology, Riverside Methodist Hospital, Columbus, Ohio

STEVEN J. PEITZMAN, M.D.
Associate Professor of Medicine, The Medical College of Pennsylvania, Philadelphia, Pennsylvania

LEWIS PERELMUTTER, Ph.D.
Chief, Immunology, Bureau of Medical Biochemistry, Laboratory Center for Disease Control; Senior Lecturer in Immunology, Department of Medicine, University of Ottawa, Ottawa, Ontario, Canada

GEORGE A. POPORAD, M.D.
Assistant Professor of Medicine, The Medical College of Pennsylvania, Philadelphia, Pennsylvania

T.K.S. RAO, M.D.
Associate Professor of Medicine, State University of New York Downstate Medical Center, Brooklyn, New York

HOWARD RASMUSSEN, M.D., Ph.D.
Professor of Medicine, Physiology, and Cell Biology and Chief, Division of Endocrinology, Yale University School of Medicine, New Haven, Connecticut

MICHAEL F. REIN, M.D.
Associate Professor of Medicine, Division of Infectious Disease, University of Virginia School of Medicine, Charlottesville, Virginia

LESLIE I. ROSE, M.D.
Professor of Medicine and Director of the Section of Endocrinology-Metabolism, Hahnemann Medical College and Hospital, Philadelphia, Pennsylvania

LOUIS F. ROSE, D.D.S., M.D.
Professor of Periodontics, University of Pennsylvania, School of Dental Medicine; Professor of Medicine and Surgery, Chief of Dental Medicine, Medical College of Pennsylvania, Philadelphia, Pennsylvania

MARC ROSENSHEIN, M.D.
Clinical Assistant Professor of Medicine, University of Washington School of Medicine, Seattle, Washington

MORTON RUBENSTEIN, M.D.
Clinical Assistant Professor of Medicine, Pennsylvania State University College of Medicine, Hershey, Pennsylvania; Associate Medical Director, Department of Respiratory Services, Harrisburg Hospital, Harrisburg, Pennsylvania

DONALD H. RUBIN, M.D.
Assistant Professor of Medicine, Departments of Medicine and Microbiology, University of Pennsylvania School of Medicine, Philadelphia, Pennsylvania

MICHAEL R. RUDNICK, M.D.
Associate Professor of Medicine and Director of Hemodialysis, Temple University Health Sciences Center, Philadelphia, Pennsylvania

MERLE A. SANDE, M.D.
Professor and Vice Chairman, Department of Medicine, University of California–San Francisco; Chief of Medical Services, San Francisco General Hospital, San Francisco, California

JEROME SANTORO, M.D.
Clinical Assistant Professor of Medicine, The Medical College of Pennsylvania, Philadelphia, Pennsylvania

SHIGERU SASSA, M.D., Ph.D.
Associate Professor, The Rockefeller University Hospital, New York, New York

W. MICHAEL SCHELD, M.D.
Assistant Professor of Internal Medicine, Infectious Diseases and Neurosurgery, University of Virginia School of Medicine, Charlottesville, Virginia

PAUL L. SCHRAEDER, M.D.
Associate Professor of Neurology and Director, Epilepsy Treatment Program, The Medical College of Pennsylvania, Philadelphia, Pennsylvania

I. ROBERT SCHWARTZ, M.D.
Director, Blood Bank, Albert Einstein Medical Center, Northern Division; Clinical Associate Professor of Medicine, Schools of Medicine and Dentistry, Temple University, Philadelphia, Pennsylvania

RICHARD K. SHADDUCK, M.D.
Professor of Medicine, University of Pittsburgh School of Medicine; Head, Hematology-Oncology Unit, Montefiore Hospital, Pittsburgh, Pennsylvania

CHARLES R. SHUMAN, M.D.
Professor of Medicine, Temple University School of Medicine, Philadelphia, Pennsylvania

PAUL D. SIEGEL, M.D.
Clinical Professor of Medicine, The Medical College of Pennsylvania, Philadelphia, Pennsylvania

SURENDER SINGH, M.D.
Assistant Professor of Medicine, The Medical College of Pennsylvania, Philadelphia, Pennsylvania

GREGORY W. SISKIND, M.D.
Professor of Medicine and Head of the Division of Allergy and Immunology, Department of Medicine, The New York Hospital–Cornell Medical Center, New York, New York

RICHARD V. SMALLEY, M.D.
Chief, Biologic Resources Branch, Biologic Response Modifiers Program, National Cancer Institute, Frederick, Maryland

RICHARD SNEPAR, M.D.
Formerly Instructor in Medicine, The Medical College of Pennsylvania, Philadelphia, Pennsylvania

JACK D. SOBEL, M.D., F.C.P.(S.A.), M.R.C.P.(U.K.)
Associate Professor of Medicine, Department of Medicine, Division of Infectious Diseases, The Medical College of Pennsylvania, Philadelphia, Pennsylvania

ROGER D. SOLOWAY, M.D.
Professor of Medicine, University of Pennsylvania School of Medicine, Philadelphia, Pennsylvania

†MAURICE SONES, M.D.
Clinical Professor of Medicine, The Medical College of Pennsylvania, Philadelphia, Pennsylvania

---

† Deceased

PHILIP S. SPRINGER, D.M.D.

Attending Staff, Department of Dental Medicine, Hospital of the University of Pennsylvania; Clinical Associate in Oral Medicine, University of Pennsylvania, School of Dental Medicine, Philadelphia, Pennsylvania

JOHN M. STANG, M.D.

Assistant Professor of Medicine, Division of Cardiology, and Director, Coronary Care, Ohio State University College of Medicine, Columbus, Ohio

STUART E. STARR, M.D.

Assistant Professor of Pediatrics, University of Pennsylvania School of Medicine, Philadelphia, Pennsylvania

BARBARA J. STEINBERG, D.D.S.

Associate Professor, Department of Surgery, Medical College of Pennsylvania; Assistant Professor, Department of Oral Medicine, University of Pennsylvania, School of Dental Medicine, Philadelphia, Pennsylvania

RAY E. STEWART, D.M.D., M.S.

Associate Professor of Pediatrics and Medical Genetics, Harbor General Hospital, University of California, Los Angeles Medical Center, Torrance, California

MARY CATHERINE STOM, M.D.

Assistant Professor of Medicine, Renal Section, Temple University Health Sciences Center, Philadephia, Pennsylvania

JOSEPH U. TOGLIA, M.D.

Professor of Neurology and Director of Electrodiagnostic Laboratories, Temple University Hospital and School of Medicine, Philadelphia, Pennsylvania

KATHLEEN E. TOOMEY, M.D.

Assistant Professor, Child Health and Development, George Washington University, Children's Hospital National Medical Center, Washington, D.C.

WALLACE W. TOURTELLOTTE, M.D., Ph.D.

Chief of Neurology, Veterans Administration Medical Center–Wadsworth; Professor and Vice-Chairman, Department of Neurology, University of California–Los Angeles School of Medicine, Los Angeles, California

MICHAEL J. WALSH, M.B., B.Ch.

Assistant Professor, Department of Neurology, University of California–Los Angeles School of Medicine, Los Angeles, California

PAUL B. WEISBERG, M.D.

Clinical Assistant Professor of Medicine, The Medical College of Pennsylvania, Philadelphia, Pennsylvania

GARY B. WEISS, M.D., Ph.D.

Assistant Professor of Medicine, Division of Hematology-Oncology, University of Texas Medical Branch, Galveston, Texas

WILLIAM WEISS, M.D.

Professor of Medicine and Director, Division of Occupational Medicine, Hahnemann Medical College and Hospital, Philadelphia, Pennsylvania

NELSON N. WOLF, M.D.

Associate Professor of Medicine and Director, Cardiac Catheterization Laboratory, The Medical College of Pennsylvania, Philadelphia, Pennsylvania

CLINTON W. YOUNG, M.D.

Assistant Professor of Medicine, University of California–San Francisco Medical School; Associate Director of Medical Education and Director, Medical Clinics, Presbyterian Hospital, San Francisco, California

JAMES B. YOUNG, M.D.

Associate Director of Cardiology, Ben Taub General Hospital; Assistant Professor of Medicine, Baylor College of Medicine, Houston, Texas

PREFACE

Dental education has been remiss in adequately preparing the dentist to evaluate the general health status of a patient. Today, more than ever before, when one considers the revolutionary advances that are occurring in medicine and the fact that a rapidly growing segment of the population consists of geriatric and medically compromised patients, the importance of medicine and its relationship to dental practice becomes clear. One area of special neglect is the failure to correlate internal medicine to dental practice. Unfortunately, many of the concepts of medical management of the dental patient are lost once the student is thrust into an intensive course in the technical principles of dentistry.

Recent dental graduates, although far more sophisticated in many ways than their predecessors, may not possess a sufficient understanding regarding the mechanisms of the disease processes in order to deal intelligently with the dental problems of such patients. *Internal Medicine for Dentistry* has been written for both the dental student and the dental practitioner.

This textbook describes the basic mechanisms involved in the various disease processes included in internal medicine, the symptoms they produce, and the manner in which they are diagnosed and managed. The information available in the field of internal medicine is enormous, and we believed that a complete yet concise textbook specifically designed for dentistry was needed. We have attempted to organize and present dental considerations in a succinct fashion at the end of each organ system. The exceptions to this format are microbial diseases, skin diseases and manifestations of systemic diseases, and genetics and metabolism. In these sections, the dental information is an integral part of the body of the medical text. The book provides all the necessary information relevant to internal medicine, but even more important to the dental professional, it discusses, where appropriate, the oral manifestations and dental management of patients with medical disorders.

Since we did not restrict the contributing authors by imposing rigid boundaries that might have limited their freedom to provide broad coverage of their subject, inevitably there is some overlap. However, we tried to minimize duplication by the use of cross-referencing and indexing, to exclude highly speculative material, and to avoid extensive bibliographies. The bibliographies at the end of the chapters are for the most part limited to reviews and monographs that contain comprehensive bibliographies. The text was kept current by rapid processing of the manuscript with review and modification just before publication. All the chapters were written by experts in their fields who have considerable clinical experience.

The textbook has been arranged by organ systems with a description of the disease entities affecting each system. To minimize repetition, it was necessary to arbitrarily classify a disease within a specific system. For example, gout is discussed in the section "Rheumatic and Granulomatous Diseases," but it could just as properly have been classified as a metabolic or renal disease. When such multisystem diseases are described primarily under one system, cross-references to the major description are included.

We would like to thank our wives, Claire Rose and Janet Kaye, and our children, David and Michael Rose and Kenneth, Karen, Kendra, and Keith Kaye, for their patience. Those who have never taken part in a project such as this cannot possibly appreciate the enormity of the task and the many hundreds of hours required that we might otherwise have spent with our families. Special thanks are due the section editors, who took much of the load off our shoulders and without whom we could never have completed this book. We also thank our office staff who were so helpful in the preparation of the book: Janet Mintzer, Margaret Nyalka, Faith Shoemaker, and Beverly Kravitz. Finally, we wish to thank the staff at The C.V. Mosby Company, whose expert and accurate editing, prompt processing, and encouragement allowed the rapid publication of this text.

Louis F. Rose
Donald Kaye

To my wife
Claire
my children
David and **Michael**
and my parents and grandmother
with love

L.F.R.

To my wife
Janet
my children
Kenneth, Karen, Kendra, and **Keith**
and my parents
with love

D.K.

CONTENTS

Section One
APPROACH TO EVALUATION OF THE PATIENT
edited by Donald Kaye

Introduction, 1
David T. Lush, Geoffrey Lefferts, Louis F. Rose, and Barry H. Hendler

1 History, 5
David T. Lush, Geoffrey Lefferts, Louis F. Rose, and Barry H. Hendler

Patient identification, 5
Source of information, 5
Chief complaint, 5
Present illness, 5
Past history, 5
Review of systems, 5
Social history, 7
Family history, 7

2 Physical examination, 7
David T. Lush, Geoffrey Lefferts, Louis F. Rose, and Barry H. Hendler

Methods, 7
Preliminaries, 7
Specific areas, 8

Section Two
IMMUNOLOGIC AND ALLERGIC DISEASES
edited by Warren A. Katz and Donald Kaye

3 Immunologic principles, 15
Donald Kaye and Warren A. Katz

Lymphocytic system, 15
Immunoglobulins, 16
Phagocytic system, 17
Complement system, 17
Types of immunologic reactions, 18
  Type I reactions, 18
  Type II reactions, 18
  Type III reactions, 18
  Type IV reactions, 19
Autoimmunity, 19
Immune-complex disease, 19
Graft-versus-host disease, 19

4 Atopic disease, 19
Gregory W. Siskind

Rhinitis, 20
Asthma of allergic etiology, 23

5 Urticaria and angioedema, 25
Leonard S. Girsh and Lewis Perelmutter

Urticaria pigmentosa (systemic mastocytosis), 26
Hereditary angioedema, 26

6 Serum sickness, 26
Leonard S. Girsh and Lewis Perelmutter

7 Contact dermatitis, 27
Leonard S. Girsh and Lewis Perelmutter

8 Drug allergy, 27
Leonard S. Girsh and Lewis Perelmutter

Dental correlations, 29
Martin S. Greenberg

9 Immunodeficiency diseases, 31
Leonard S. Girsh and Lewis Perelmutter

Disorders of B lymphocytes, 31
Disorders of T lymphocytes, 31
Disorders of polymorphonuclear leukocytes, 31
Defects in the complement system, 31
Evaluation of immunity, 31
  B-cell function, 31
  T-cell function, 32
  Complement, 32
  Leukocytes, 32
Classification, 32
  Defects in B-cell function (antibody production), 32
  Defects in T-cell function (cellular immunity), 33
  Defects in both B- and T-cell function, 33
Management, 34

Dental correlations, 34
Martin S. Greenberg

xvii

Section Three
RHEUMATIC AND GRANULOMATOUS DISEASES
edited by Warren A. Katz

10 Rheumatoid arthritis, 35
Warren A. Katz

Sjögren's syndrome, 36

11 Juvenile rheumatoid arthritis, 43
Balu H. Athreya

12 Ankylosing spondylitis, 48
Randolph C. Blodgett, Jr.

13 Psoriatic arthritis, 50
Warren A. Katz

14 Reiter's syndrome, 52
Warren A. Katz

15 Intermittent rheumatic diseases, 53
Randolph C. Blodgett, Jr.

Behçet's syndrome, 53

16 Systemic lupus erythematosus, 53
June F. Klinghoffer

Drug-induced connective tissue disease (CTD) (drug-induced lupus), 57
Chronic discoid lupus erythematosus, 57

17 Systemic sclerosis, 58
Sergio Jimenez

18 Raynaud's phenomenon, 62
Warren A. Katz

19 Polymyositis and dermatomyositis, 64
Donald H. Lieberman

20 Vasculitis, 66
Paul Katz and Anthony S. Fauci

21 Schönlein-Henoch purpura, 70
Warren A. Katz

22 Wegener's granulomatosis and midline granuloma, 70
Paul Katz and Anthony S. Fauci

Wegener's granulomatosis, 70
Midline granuloma, 73

23 Polymyalgia rheumatica and temporal arteritis, 74
June F. Klinghoffer

24 Sarcoidosis, 75
Warren A. Katz

25 Weber-Christian disease, 78
Robert H. Gordon

26 Infectious arthritis, 79
Bruce I. Hoffman

Pyogenic arthritis, 79
 Gonococcal arthritis, 79
 Nongonococcal septic arthritis, 79
Tuberculous and fungal arthritis, 81
 Arthritis caused by *Mycobacterium tuberculosis*, 81
 Arthritis caused by other mycobacteria, 81
 Arthritis caused by fungi, 81
Arthritis caused by viruses, 81

27 Osteomyelitis, 82
Bruce I. Hoffman

28 Osteoarthritis, 83
Donald H. Lieberman

Primary osteoarthritis, 83
Variants of osteoarthritis, 86
 Erosive osteoarthritis, 86
 Neuropathic arthropathy, 86
 Diffuse idiopathic skeletal hyperostosis, 86

29 Paget's disease (osteitis deformans), 86
Donald H. Lieberman

30 Osteoporosis, 88
Donald H. Lieberman

31 Gout and pseudogout, 89
Warren A. Katz

Gout, 89
Pseudogout, 94
Other crystal deposition disease, 95

32 Nonarticular rheumatism, 96
Robert H. Gordon

Fibrositis, 96
Regional and local nonarticular syndromes, 97
 Myofascial syndromes, 97
 Nerve entrapments, 98
 Bursitis, 98
 Tendinitis, 99
 Miscellaneous nonarticular syndromes, 100

33 Miscellaneous rheumatic disorders, 102
Warren A. Katz

Relapsing polychondritis, 102
Hypertrophic osteoarthropathy, 103

Fibrous dysplasia, 104
Avascular necrosis, 104
Hemarthrosis, 104

34 Fibrosing syndromes, 105
Jerome A. Boscia and Donald Kaye

Dental correlations, 105

Rheumatoid arthritis, 105
Martin S. Greenberg

Psoriatic arthritis of the temporomandibular joint, 106
Martin S. Greenberg

Osteoarthritis of the temporomandibular joint, 107
Martin S. Greenberg

Synovial chondromatosis of the temporomandibular joint (chondrometaplasia), 108
Martin S. Greenberg

Septic arthritis of the temporomandibular joint, 108
Martin S. Greenberg

Gouty arthritis of the temporomandibular joint, 108
Martin S. Greenberg

Myofascial pain dysfunction syndrome of the temporomandibular joint, 109
Martin S. Greenberg

Reiter's syndrome, 110
Philip Springer

Behçet's syndrome, 110
Martin S. Greenberg

Lupus erythematosus, 111
Philip Springer

Systemic sclerosis, 112
Philip Springer

Polymyositis-dermatomyositis, 112
Philip Springer

Wegener's granulomatosis, 113
Philip Springer

Midline granuloma, 113
Philip Springer

Sarcoidosis, 113
Philip Springer

Paget's disease of the jaws, 114
Philip Springer

Osteoporosis, 115
Philip Springer

Fibrous dysplasia of the jaws, 115
Martin S. Greenberg

Osteomyelitis of the jaws, 116
Philip Springer

Section Four
MICROBIAL DISEASES
edited by **Donald Kaye**

35 Introduction to microbial diseases, 118
Donald Kaye

Fever and chills, 118
Diagnosis of microbial diseases, 118
Laboratory evaluation, 118
Management, 119
Fever of unknown origin, 119
  Laboratory approach, 120

Unit A
VIRAL DISEASES
edited by **Harvey M. Friedman**

36 Introduction, classification, and laboratory diagnosis, 121
Harvey M. Friedman

37 Diseases caused by viruses, 125

Viral infections of the fetus and newborn, 125
Stuart E. Starr

Herpesviruses, 127
Gary R. Fleisher

Herpes simplex virus, 128
Varicella-zoster virus, 129
Cytomegalovirus, 130
Epstein-Barr virus, 131

Viral infections of the central nervous system, 134
Stephen Gluckman

Herpes simplex, 135
Enteroviruses, 136
Mumps, 137
Other childhood infections, 138
  Measles, 138
  Varicella-zoster, 138
Lymphocytic choriomeningitis virus, 138
Rabies, 138
Treatable causes of "aseptic meningoencephalitis," 139
Evaluation of the patient with aseptic meningitis or viral encephalitis, 139

Mumps, 139
Donald Kaye

Viral respiratory infections, 140
Michael Buckley

Influenza, 140
Respiratory syncytial virus, 141
Parainfluenza viruses, 142
Adenoviruses, 143
Picornaviruses, 144
Rhinoviruses, 144

Enteroviruses, 144
Coronaviruses, 144

Exanthems of viral or presumed viral origin, 145
Allan M. Arbeter

Measles (rubeola), 145
Rubella (German measles), 146
Roseola (exanthema subitum), 147
Erythema infectiosum (fifth disease), 147
Kawasaki disease, 147
Adenovirus exanthems, 148
Enterovirus exanthems, 148

Viral gastroenteritis, 149
Donald H. Rubin

Rotaviruses, 149
27-nm Norwalk-like agents, 150
Other agents, 150
Diagnosis, 150
Management, 150

Cat-scratch fever, 151
Allan M. Arbeter

38 Prevention and treatment with vaccines and antiviral agents
Harvey M. Friedman

Viral vaccines in general use, 151
  Poliovirus, 151
  Rubella virus, 152
  Measles virus, 152
  Mumps virus, 152
Viral vaccines for special circumstances, 152
  Influenza viruses, 152
  Rabies virus, 153
Antiviral agents, 153
  Amantadine, 154
  Vidarabine (adenine arabinoside), 154
  Acyclovir (acycloguanosine), 154
  Interferons, 154

Unit B
BACTERIAL DISEASES

39 Use of antimicrobial agents, 155
Donald Kaye

Determination of susceptibility of microorganisms, 155
Significance of a bacteriostatic versus bactericidal activity, 155
Activity of agent at site of infection, 156
Pharmacology, 157
  Route of administration, 157
  Plasma (serum) concentrations, 157
  Excretion or inactivation, 158
Modification of dosages, 158
Duration of therapy, 158
Toxicity of antimicrobial agents, 158
Failure of therapy with antimicrobial agents, 158
  Delay of therapy, 158
  Incorrect diagnosis, 159
  Microbial resistance, 159
  Failure to deliver the agent to the site of infection in antimicrobial concentrations, 159
  Adverse conditions at the site of infection, 159
  Infection in the immunocompromised host, 159
  Apparent failure related to drug fever, 159
Specific antimicrobial agents, 159
  Penicillins, 159
  Cephalosporins, 164
  Aminoglycosides, 165
  Vancomycin, 167
  Erythromycin, lincomycin, and clindamycin, 167
  Tetracyclines, 168
  Chloramphenicol, 168
  Polymyxins, 169
  Sulfonamides, 169
  Trimethoprim-sulfamethoxazole, 170
  Trimethoprim, 170
  Spectinomycin, 170
  Metronidazole, 170
  Nitrofurantoin, 170
  Nalidixic acid, 171
  Methenamine mandelate and methenamine hippurate, 171

40 Infections of specific anatomic sites, 171

Bacterial pneumonia, 171
Gerald R. Donowitz and Gerald L. Mandell

Pneumonia syndromes, 173
  Syndrome of acute community-acquired pneumonia, 173
  Nosocomial gram-negative bacillus pneumonia syndrome, 176
  Atypical pneumonia syndrome, 177
  Aspiration (anaerobic organism) pneumonia syndrome, 177

Infective endocarditis, 178
Donald Kaye

Bacterial infections of the central nervous system, 186
Merle A. Sande and W. Michael Scheld

Bacterial meningitis, 186
Parameningeal and epidural infections, 191
  Brain abscess, 191
  Subdural empyema, 193
  Epidural abscess, 193
  Transverse myelitis or myelopathy, 194

Urinary tract infection and perinephric abscess, 195
Donald Kaye

Perinephric abscess, 199

41 Diseases spread through food and water, 199
Matthew E. Levison

Botulism, 204

Cholera, 204

Shigellosis, 205

Salmonelloses, 206

Salmonella gastroenteritis, 206
Enteric (typhoid) fever, 207
Salmonella bacteremia and localized infection, 208

42 Diseases caused by rickettsiae, 209
Oksana M. Korzeniowski

Rocky Mountain spotted fever, 210
Rickettsialpox, 211
Louse-borne (epidemic) typhus fever, 212
Murine (flea-borne) typhus fever, 212
Q fever, 213

43 Diseases caused by chlamydiae, 214
Michael F. Rein

Chlamydia trachomatis, 214
    Trachoma, 214
    Genital infections and complications, 214
    Lymphogranuloma venereum, 216
Chlamydia psittaci, 216
    Psittacosis, 216

44 Diseases caused by mycoplasmas, 217
Gerald R. Donowitz and Gerald L. Mandell

Mycoplasmal pneumonia, 217
Genital mycoplasmas, 218

45 Diseases caused by gram-positive cocci, 218

Staphylococcal infections, 218
Gerald R. Donowitz and Gerald L. Mandell

Staphylococcal osteomyelitis, 221

Streptococcal infections and rheumatic fever, 222
Jerome Santoro

Group A streptococci, 223
    Acute streptococcal pharyngitis, 223
    Streptococcal skin infections, 225
    Other group A streptococcal infections, 226
Group B streptococci, 227
Group C and G streptococci, 227
Group D streptococci, 227
Viridans streptococci, 228
Anaerobic streptococci, 228
Acute rheumatic fever, 228

46 Diseases caused by gram-negative cocci, 230

Gonococcal infections, 230
Donald Kaye

Meningococcal infections, 233
Merle A. Sande and W. Michael Scheld

47 Diseases caused by gram-negative bacilli, 235

***Haemophilus influenzae* infections,** 235
Jerome Santoro

Pertussis (whooping cough), 237
Jerome Santoro

Donovanosis (granuloma inguinale), 238
Michael F. Rein

Chancroid, 238
Michael F. Rein

Gram-negative bacillary bacteremia, 239
George A. Poporad and Jaime Carrizosa

Plague, 242
Elias Abrutyn

Tularemia, 242
Oksana M. Korzeniowski

Brucellosis, 243
Jerome Santoro

48 Diseases caused by gram-positive bacilli, 245

Anthrax, 245
Elias Abrutyn

Listeriosis, 246
Jaime Carrizosa

Erysipeloid, 246
Jaime Carrizosa

Actinomycosis, 247
John E. Bennett

Nocardiosis, 247
John E. Bennett

Diphtheria, 247
Oksana M. Korzeniowski

49 Diseases caused by anaerobic bacteria, 249

Infections caused by nonsporeforming anaerobes, 249
Matthew E. Levison

Clostridial infection, 251
Matthew E. Levison

Tetanus, 251
Clostridial soft tissue infection (gas gangrene and clostridial cellulitis), 252

50 Diseases caused by mycobacteria, 254
Elias Abrutyn

Tuberculosis, 254
Nontuberculous mycobacterial infections, 261
Leprosy, 261

51 Diseases caused by spirochetes, 264

Syphilis, 264
Michael F. Rein

Rat-bite fever, 272
Merle A. Sande

Streptobacillary rat-bite fever, 272
Spirillary rat-bite fever, 272

Leptospirosis, 273
Merle A. Sande

Unit C
FUNGAL DISEASES

52 Diseases caused by fungi, 274
John E. Bennett

Histoplasmosis, 274
Coccidioidomycosis, 275
Blastomycosis, 275
Cryptococcosis, 275
Sporotrichosis, 276
Candidiasis, 276
Aspergillosis, 276
Mucormycosis, 277
Mycetoma, 277
Chromomycosis, 277

53 Agents used in treatment of mycotic infections, 278
Donald Kaye

Treatment of deep mycoses, 278
Treatment of superficial mycoses, 278

Unit D
PROTOZOAL DISEASES

54 Diseases caused by protozoa, 279
Thomas C. Jones

Malaria, 279
Diseases caused by amebae, 281
 Amebiasis, 281
 Diseases caused by free-living amebae, 283
Giardiasis, 283
Toxoplasmosis, 284
Trichomoniasis, 286
Trypanosomiasis, 286
Pneumocystosis, 287
Babesiosis, 288

Unit E
HELMINTHIC DISEASES

55 Diseases caused by nematodes (roundworms), 289
Donald Kaye

Enterobiasis, 289
Trichuriasis, 290
Ascariasis, 290
Visceral larva migrans, 290
Anisakiasis, 291
Hookworm disease, 291
Cutaneous larva migrans, 291
Strongyloidiasis, 291
Trichinosis, 292
Bancroftian and Malayan filariasis, 292

56 Diseases caused by cestodes (tapeworms), 292
Jaime Carrizosa

Taeniasis saginata, 293
Taeniasis solium, 293
 Human cysticercosis, 293
Diphyllobothriasis, 293
Treatment of *Taenia saginata, Taenia solium,* and *Diphyllobothrium latum* infection, 294
Echinococcosis (hydatid disease), 294

57 Diseases caused by trematodes (flukes), 294
Jaime Carrizosa

Schistosomiasis (bilharziasis), 294

Unit F
MISCELLANEOUS MICROBIAL DISEASES

58 Diseases of presumed microbial origin, 297

Lyme disease, 297
George A. Poporad and Donald Kaye

Toxic shock syndrome, 298
Jerome A. Boscia and Donald Kaye

Dental correlations, 298
Adi Garfunkel, Jack Sobel, and Louis F. Rose

Viral infection, 298
 Herpes simplex, 298
 Varicella-zoster virus infection, 299
 Cytomegalovirus, 300
 Epstein-Barr virus (EBV), 300
 Measles (rubeola), 300
 Rubella (German measles), 300
 Hand-foot-and-mouth disease, 300
 Cat-scratch disease, 300
 Herpangina (Coxsackie A virus infection), 301
 Mumps, 301
Bacterial infections, 301
 Infective endocarditis, 301
 Gonococcal stomatitis, 302
 Lymphogranuloma venereum (LGV), 302
 Fusospirochetal infections, 302
 Syphilis, 302
 Bacterial infections of the central nervous system, 303
 Tuberculosis, 304
 Leprosy, 304
 Actinomycosis, 305
 Tularemia, 305
 Diphtheria, 305
 Anthrax, 305

Staphylococcal oral lesions, 306
Gram-negative oral lesions, 306
Fungal infections, 306
Histoplasmosis, 306
Candidiasis, 307
Mucormycosis, 308

Section Five
HEMATOLOGIC DISORDERS
edited by **Rosaline R. Joseph**

59 Introduction to hematologic disorders, 310
Rosaline R. Joseph

Unit A
DISORDERS OF RED BLOOD CELL PRODUCTION AND IRON METABOLISM

60 Introduction to anemia and approach to patients with anemia, 311
Emmanuel C. Besa

Normal red blood cell production and pathology, 311
Approach to the anemic patient, 312

61 Megaloblastic anemia, 316
Emmanuel C. Besa

62 Bone marrow failure, sideroblastic anemia, and myelophthisic anemia, 318
Emmanuel C. Besa

Aplastic anemia, 319
Primary refractory anemia (preleukemic and myelodysplastic syndromes), 320
Sideroblastic anemia, 321
Myelophthisis and secondary forms of myelofibrosis, 322

63 Acute posthemorrhagic anemia, 323
William E. Barry

64 Iron deficiency anemia, 323
William E. Barry

65 Other hypochromic microcytic anemias, 325
William E. Barry

66 Anemia of chronic disease, 325
William E. Barry

67 Anemias caused by red cell destruction, 326
Jerome I. Brody

Congenital hemolytic anemias, 328
Membrane defects, 328
Deficiencies within the hexose monophosphate (HMP) shunt, 329
Disorders of hemoglobin, 331

Hemolysis caused by acquired abnormalities, 337
Immunohemolytic anemias, 337
Traumatic hemolytic anemias and red cell fragmentation syndromes, 340
Paroxysmal nocturnal hemoglobinuria, 341
Hemolytic anemias caused by drugs, 342
Hemolysis resulting from other causes, 342

68 Abnormal hemoglobin pigments, 343
Jerome I. Brody

Methemoglobinemia, 343
Acquired methemoglobinemia, 343
Hereditary methemoglobinemias, 344
Other pigments, 344
Sulfhemoglobinemia, 344
Carboxyhemoglobinemia, 344

69 Hemochromatosis, 345
William E. Barry

70 Principles of blood banking and transfusion therapy, 346
I. Robert Schwartz

Procurement and collection, 346
Fitness and safety, 347
Transmissible diseases, 347
Compatibility, 348
Principles of transfusion therapy, 349
Transfusion reactions, 351

71 Polycythemia, 352
Frank H. Gardner and Gary B. Weiss

Polycythemia vera, 352
Secondary polycythemia, 353
Hypoxia, 353
Familial polycythemia, 354
Polycythemia related to abnormal hemoglobin, 354
Polycythemia related to tumor, 354
Polycythemia related to local hypoxia, 354
Relative polycythemia, 354

Unit B
WHITE BLOOD CELL DISORDERS

72 Qualitative and quantitative neutrophil disorders, 355
Richard K. Shadduck

Neutrophil kinetics, 355
Neutrophil dysfunction syndromes, 356
Defects in chemotaxis, 356
Defects in phagocytosis, 357
Defects in microbicidal activity, 357
Neutropenia—agranulocytosis, 358
Production defects, 358
Destructive defects, 359
Congenital neutropenia, 359

Chronic idiopathic neutropenic syndromes, 360
Drug-induced neutropenia, 360
General approach to the neutropenic patient, 361
Management, 361
Leukemoid reactions, 361
Monocytosis, 362
Eosinophilia, 362

73 The leukemias, 363
George A. Omura

Acute leukemias, 364
Chronic myelogenous leukemia, 369
Chronic lymphocytic leukemia, 370

74 The eosinophil and eosinophilic syndromes, 372
Richard Snepar and Donald Kaye

75 Myeloproliferative disease, 373
Frank H. Gardner and Gary B. Weiss

Chronic granulocytic leukemia, 373
Essential thrombocythemia, 373
Agnogenic myeloid metaplasia (myelofibrosis with myeloid metaplasia), 374

76 Plasma cell disorders, 376
Nikolay V. Dimitrov

Multiple myeloma, 378
Waldenström's macroglobulinemia, 382
Heavy-chain disease, 384

Amyloidosis, 385
Malcolm W. MacNab

77 Hodgkin's disease and non-Hodgkin's lymphoma, 387
Deborah Mayer and Richard V. Smalley

Hodgkin's disease, 387
Non-Hodgkin's lymphoma, 391
Extranodal disease, 394

78 Diseases of the spleen and reticuloendothelial system, 394
Sally D. Lane

Evaluation of the patient with splenomegaly, 395
Functional disorders, 395
Hyposplenism, 395
Hypersplenism, 395
Extramedullary hematopoiesis, 396
The lipidoses, 396
Gaucher's disease, 396
Niemann-Pick disease, 397
Chédiak-Higashi syndrome, 397
Proliferative disorders, 397
Idiopathic histiocytosis, 397
Histiocytic medullary reticulosis (malignant histiocytosis), 398
Miscellaneous disorders, 398

Unit C
HEMOSTATIC DISORDERS

79 Introduction to hemostasis, 399
Patricia M. Catalano

80 Platelet and vascular disorders, 400
Patricia M. Catalano

Thrombocytopenia, 400
Thrombocytopenias caused by decreased platelet production, 401
Thrombocytopenias caused by increased platelet destruction, 402
Disorders of distribution, 404
Thrombocytosis, 404
Primary thrombocytosis, 404
Secondary thrombocytosis, 404
Qualitative platelet abnormalities, 405
Congenital disorders of platelet function, 405
Acquired disorders of platelet function, 405
Vascular purpuras, 406
Cushing's syndrome, 406
Amyloidosis, 406
Vitamin C deficiency, 406
Autoerythrocyte sensitization, 406
Schönlein-Henoch purpura, 406
Osler-Weber-Rendu syndrome, 407
Various connective tissue disorders, 407
Other purpuric disorders, 407
Von Willebrand's disease, 407

81 Disorders of the coagulation mechanism, 408
Marc Rosenshein

Inherited disorders of coagulation, 409
Hemophilia A, 409
Hemophilia B, 410
Von Willebrand's disease, 410
Other hereditary coagulation disorders, 411
Acquired disorders of coagulation, 411
Vitamin K deficiency, 411
Liver disease, 411
Acquired anticoagulants, 411
Disseminated intravascular coagulation, 412
Fibrinolytic states, 413
Anticoagulant therapy, 413
Heparin, 413
Coumarin anticoagulants, 414

Dental correlations, 414

Anemias and deficiency states, 414

Pernicious anemia, 414
S. Gary Cohen

Folic acid deficiency, 415
S. Gary Cohen

Aplastic anemia, 415
S. Gary Cohen

Iron deficiency anemia, 416
S. Gary Cohen

Plummer-Vinson syndrome, 416
S. Gary Cohen

Sickle cell anemia, 416
S. Gary Cohen

Hemolytic disease of the newborn (erythroblastosis fetalis), 418
S. Gary Cohen

Cold agglutinin disease, 418
S. Gary Cohen

Enzyme deficiency anemias, 418
S. Gary Cohen

Glucose-6-phosphate dehydrogenase deficiency, 418
S. Gary Cohen

Thalassemia, 418
S. Gary Cohen

Polycythemia vera, 419
S. Gary Cohen

Neutrophil dysfunction syndromes, 420
Martin S. Greenberg

Leukemia, 420
Martin S. Greenberg

Multiple myeloma, 422
Martin S. Greenberg

Macroglobulinemia, 423
Martin S. Greenberg

Amyloidosis, 423
Martin S. Greenberg

Lymphoma, 424
Martin S. Greenberg

Histiocytosis X, 425
Martin S. Greenberg

Gaucher's disease, 425
Martin S. Greenberg

Platelet disorders, 425

Thrombocytopenia, 425
S. Gary Cohen

Thrombocytosis, 426
S. Gary Cohen

Thrombasthenia, 426
 Bleeding secondary to aspirin, 426
Von Willebrand's disease, 426

Hemophilia, 427
S. Gary Cohen

Factor deficiencies, 428
S. Gary Cohen

  Hemophilia B—factor IX deficiency, 428

  Factor XI deficiency, 429
  Factor V, VII, and X deficiency, 429
  Afibrinogenemia, 429
  Disseminated intravascular coagulopathy (DIC), 429
S. Gary Cohen

Anticoagulant therapy, 429
S. Gary Cohen

  Heparin, 429
  Coumarin, 429

Section Six
NEOPLASTIC DISEASES
edited by **Rosaline R. Joseph**

82 Introduction to medical oncology, 431
Rosaline R. Joseph

83 An overview of neoplasia, 431
Rosaline R. Joseph

Carcinogenesis, 431
 Environmental carcinogenesis, 431
 Genetic factors in carcinogenesis, 433
 Viral oncogenesis, 433
 Immune factors in carcinogenesis, 433
Detection, diagnosis, and staging of cancer, 434
 Detection, 434
 Diagnosis, 434
 Staging of tumors, 435
Clinical manifestations, 436
 Obstruction and compression, 436
 Loss or alteration of organ function, 437
 Tumor secretion, 437
 Miscellaneous paraneoplastic syndromes, 437
Complications of therapy, 438

84 Principles of systemic cancer therapy, 438
Rosaline R. Joseph

Treatment of localized or regional disease, 438
Treatment of disseminated malignancies, 439
 Chemotherapy, 439
 Hormonal manipulation, 443
 Immunotherapy, 444
 Interferon, 445
 Supportive care, 445
Management of specific malignancies, 447
 Carcinoma of the lung, 447
 Gastrointestinal cancer, 447
 Breast cancer, 448
 Genitourinary tumors, 449
 Gynecologic cancers, 449
 Head and neck cancer, 449
 Sarcomas, 449
 Malignant melanoma, 450
 Endocrine tumors, 450

Dental correlations, 450

Chemotherapy, 450
Martin S. Greenberg

Section Seven
CARDIOVASCULAR DISEASES
edited by **Toby R. Engel**

85 Introduction to cardiovascular disease, 452
Toby R. Engel

86 Congestive heart failure, 452
Joseph A. Franciosa and W. Bruce Dunkman

87 Systemic hypertension, 465
Surender Singh

88 Shock, 475
Carl V. Leier

89 Diagnostic procedures in cardiology, 479
James A. Joye, Reginald I. Low, Anthony N. DeMaria, Ezra A. Amsterdam, and Dean T. Mason

Electrocardiography, 479
  Cardiac electrophysiology, 479
  Lead systems and recording, 480
  Normal electrocardiogram, 480
  Abnormalities of the electrocardiogram, 484
Echocardiography, 485
  Normal echocardiogram, 486
Cardiac catheterization, 487
  Indications, 487
  Right-sided heart catheterization, 488
  Left-sided heart catheterization, 488
  Angiocardiography, 488
Nuclear cardiology, 489

90 Pulmonary embolism, 489
Steven G. Meister and Toby R. Engel

91 Thrombophlebitis, 494
Steven G. Meister

92 Primary pulmonary hypertension, 496
Nelson M. Wolf

93 Congenital heart disease, 497
Iain F.S. Black

Hemodynamics of congenital heart disease, 498
The pediatric electrocardiogram, 499
Pediatric arrhythmias, 500
  Tachycardias, 500
  Blocks, 500
  Preexcitation patterns: Wolff-Parkinson-White (WPW) syndrome, 500
  Sinus node disorders, 501
The chest roentgenogram in congenital heart disease, 501
Cardiac catheterization, 501
Noninvasive studies, 502
Specific congenital heart lesions, 502
  Acyanotic heart lesions with left-to-right shunts, 502
  Acyanotic heart disease with obstructive lesions, 505
  Cyanotic heart lesions, 506
Myocardial failure in congenital heart disease, 508
Surgical management of congenital heart disease, 509

94 Valvular heart disease, 510
Michael J. Barrett

Mitral regurgitation, 510
Mitral valve prolapse, 511
Mitral stenosis, 512
Aortic stenosis, 514
Aortic regurgitation, 515
Tricuspid and pulmonic valve disease, 516

95 Primary muscle diseases of the heart, 517
Bernadine Healy Bulkley

Idiopathic hypertrophic cardiomyopathy and asymmetric septal hypertrophy, 517
Idiopathic dilated congestive cardiomyopathies, 520
Idiopathic restrictive cardiomyopathies, 522
Secondary cardiomyopathies, 522
  Secondary hypertrophic cardiomyopathies (glycogen storage disease, hypertension, aortic stenosis), 522
  Secondary congestive cardiomyopathies (sarcoidosis, scleroderma, ischemic heart disease), 522
  Secondary restrictive cardiomyopathies (amyloidosis, hemochromatosis), 523
  Metabolic or nutritional cardiomyopathies, 523

96 Coronary heart disease, 524
James B. Young and Robert J. Luchi

Coronary artery anatomy and myocardial perfusion, 524
Epidemiology and prevention of coronary heart disease, 526
Angina pectoris, 527
  Unstable angina, 532
  Prinzmetal's variant angina, 533
  Angina with normal coronary arteries, 533
Acute myocardial infarction, 533
Sudden death, 538

97 Cardiac arrhythmias, 541
Jerry C. Luck and Toby R. Engel

Normal conduction and rhythm, 541
Tachycardias, 542
  Sinus tachycardia, 542
  Mechanisms of ectopic tachycardias, 542
  Atrial tachycardia, 542
  Atrial flutter and fibrillation, 543
  AV junctional tachycardia, 545
  Ventricular tachycardia, 545
  Ventricular flutter and fibrillation, 546
Bradycardias and heart block, 546
  Sinus bradycardia and sick sinus syndrome, 546
  AV block, 547
Ventricular ectopic beats (VEBs), 548

Wolff-Parkinson-White (WPW) syndrome, 548
Cardioversion, 549

98 Pericarditis, 550
Charles A. Bush and John M. Stang

Acute pericarditis, 550
Constrictive pericarditis, 551
Effusive pericarditis, 553
Other pericardial diseases, 555

99 Diseases of the thoracic aorta, 555
James O. Finnegan

Anatomy of the aorta, 555
  Ascending aorta, 555
  Arch of the aorta, 556
  Descending aorta, 556
Congenital anomalies of the thoracic aorta, 556
  Patent ductus arteriosus, 556
  Coarctation of the aorta, 557
Thoracic aneurysms, 557
  Aneurysms of the sinuses of Valsalva, 558
  Aneurysms of the ascending aorta, 558
  Aneurysms of the aortic arch, 559
  Aneurysms of the descending aorta, 559
Aortic dissection, 560
Aortic arch syndrome, 562
  Subclavian steal syndrome, 563
  Takayasu's arteritis, 563
  Syphilitic aortitis, 563

100 Diseases of the distal aorta and branches of the aorta, 564
Marian F. McNamara

Cerebrovascular disease, 564
Aneurysms, 565
  Elective aneurysm resection, 566
  Ruptured abdominal aortic aneurysms, 567
  Popliteal artery aneurysms, 567
Acute arterial insufficiency, 567
  Emboli, 568
Chronic arterial diseases of the aorta and its branches, 568
  Leriche's syndrome (aortoiliac disease), 569
  Superficial femoral occlusion, 570
  Buerger's disease (thromboangiitis obliterans), 570

Dental correlations, 571
Louis F. Rose, Philip Godfrey, and Barbara J. Steinberg

Congestive heart failure, 571
Hypertension, 572
Shock, 575
  Septic and hypovolemic shock, 575
  Anaphylactic shock, 576
  Cardiogenic shock, 576
  Vasovagal syncope, 576
Pulmonary embolism, 577
Primary pulmonary hypertension, 578
Congenital heart disease, 578
Valvular heart disease, 579
  Endocarditis, 581
Cardiomyopathy, 582
Coronary heart disease, 582
Arrhythmia, 584
Pericarditis, 585
Disease of the aorta and its branches, 586

Section Eight
DISEASES OF THE KIDNEY AND DISTURBANCES IN ELECTROLYTE AND ACID BASE METABOLISM
edited by Sandra P. Levison

101 Introduction, 588
Sandra P. Levison

Determining the site of injury, 588
Hematuria, 588
Proteinuria, 589
Pyuria, 590

102 Structure and function of the kidney, 590
Pedro C. Fernandez

Renal blood flow and glomerular filtration, 590
Renal handling of sodium and water, 591
Role of the kidney in acid-base homeostasis, 592
Renal handling of potassium, 593

103 Disturbances in fluid, electrolyte, and acid-base metabolism, 593
Hugh J. Carroll and Man S. Oh

Sodium and water metabolism, 593
  Hyponatremia, 594
  Hypernatremia, 595
  Volume depletion states, 596
  Edema, 597
Potassium metabolism, 597
  Hypokalemia, 597
  Hyperkalemia, 598
Acid-base balance, 599
  Metabolic acidosis, 599
  Metabolic alkalosis, 600
  Respiratory acidosis, 600
  Respiratory alkalosis, 601
  Mixed acid-base disorders, 601

104 Investigation of renal function and structure, 603
Pedro C. Fernandez

Clinical assessment of renal function, 603
  Clearance measurements, 603
  Measurements of renal concentrating ability, 604
  Urinalysis, 604
  Assessment of proteinuria, 605
Roentgenographic and ultrasonographic examination of the kidneys, 605
  Intravenous urography, 606

Retrograde pyelography, 606
Antegrade pyelography, 607
Renal angiography, 607
Computed tomography, 607
Renal ultrasonography, 607
Radioisotope imaging, 607
Renal biopsy, 608

105 Primary glomerular disease, 608
Pasha Agarwal and Brajesh Agarwal

Asymptomatic urinary abnormalities, 609
Nephritic syndrome, 609
   Acute poststreptococcal glomerulonephritis, 609
   Rapidly progressive glomerulonephritis, 610
   Goodpasture's syndrome, 611
   Focal glomerulonephritis, 611
   Glomerulonephritis associated with bacterial endocarditis and ventriculoatrial shunt infection, 611
   Hereditary nephritis (Alport's syndrome), 611
Nephrotic syndrome, 612
   Primary glomerular diseases resulting in the nephrotic syndrome, 613

106 Renal lesions in systemic disease, 615
Brajesh Agarwal and Pasha Agarwal

Collagen-vascular diseases, 615
   Systemic lupus erythematosus, 615
   Scleroderma, 615
   Polyarteritis nodosa, 616
   Wegener's granulomatosis, 616
   Schönlein-Henoch purpura, 616
   Hemolytic-uremic syndrome and thrombotic thrombocytopenic purpura, 617
Metabolic and other systemic diseases, 617
   Diabetes mellitus, 617
   Renal amyloidosis, 617
   Multiple myeloma, 617
   Waldenström's macroglobulinemia, 618
   Essential cryoglobulinemia, 618
   Sickle cell disease, 618
   Sarcoidosis, 618

107 Interstitial nephritis, 619
Paul J. Kovnat

Hyperoxaluria, 620
Analgesic abuse nephropathy, 621

108 Other renal diseases, 621
Steven J. Peitzman

Nephrogenic diabetes insipidus, 621
Hypokalemic nephropathy, 622
Hypercalcemic nephropathy, 622
Uric acid nephropathy, 622
Renal tubular acidosis, 622
Hyporeninemic hypoaldosteronism, 623

109 Toxic nephropathy, 624
Michael R. Rudnick, Christine P. Bastl, and Robert G. Narins

Pathogenesis, 624
Clinical syndromes associated with nephrotoxicity, 625
   Acute renal failure, 625
   Chronic renal failure, 626
   Glomerulopathies, 626
   Tubular disorders, 626
   Interstitial disorders, 626
   Vascular disorders, 626
   Obstruction, 627
Specific nephrotoxins, 627
   Heavy metals, 627
   Roentgenographic dyes, 628
   Antibiotics, 628
   Analgesics, nonsteroidal anti-inflammatory agents, and drug abuse, 629
   Hydrocarbons and glycols, 629
   Pigments, 629
   Miscellaneous toxins, 629

110 Acute renal failure, 630
T.K.S. Rao

111 Chronic renal failure, 635
T.K.S. Rao

112 Treatment of irreversible renal failure by dialysis, 640
Lois Anne Katz

Peritoneal dialysis, 640
Hemodialysis, 641
New developments, 642
Complications, 642

113 Renal transplantation, 642
Robert A. Grossman

Patient selection and preparation, 643
   Histocompatibility determination, 643
   Cadaver donors, 644
Surgical procedure, 644
Immunosuppressive therapy, 644
Complications, 644
   Rejection reactions, 644
   Graft nonfunction, 645
   Infection, 645
   Hypertension, 645
   Recurrent disease, 645
   Malignancy, 645
   Other complications, 645
Outcome, 646

114 Nephrolithiasis, 646
Mary Catherine Stom and Elizabeth D. Labovitz

Calcium stones, 646
   Hypercalciuria, 647

Hyperuricosuric, calcium oxalate nephrolithiasis, 648
Hyperoxaluria, 648
Idiopathic calcium stones, 648
Struvite stones, 648
Uric acid stones, 649
Cystine stones, 649
Management of acute urolithiasis, 649

115 Malformations of the urinary tract, 649
Linda B. Hiner

Renal anomalies, 649
Renal agenesis, 649
Renal hypoplasia, 649
Renal dysplasia, 650
Anomalies of renal position, 650
Ureteral anomalies, 650
Bladder anomalies, 651
Urethral anomalies, 651

116 Renal cysts and cystic diseases of the kidney, 651
Linda B. Hiner

Simple cysts, 651
Polycystic disease, 651
Adult polycystic disease, 652
Infantile polycystic disease, 652
Medullary cystic disease (nephronophthisis), 653
Medullary sponge kidney, 653

117 Obstructive uropathy, 653
Clarence Martin and **Sandra P. Levison**

118 Neoplasms of the urinary tract, 656
Linda B. Hiner

Renal neoplasms, 656
Renal cell carcinoma, 656
Nephroblastoma (Wilms' tumor), 658
Urothelial tumors of the kidney, 658
Bladder neoplasms, 659
Papillary tumors, 659
Solid carcinomas, 659
Prostatic carcinoma, 659

119 Vascular disorders of the kidney, 660
Sal A. Lofaro and **Sandra P. Levison**

Renal artery stenosis, 660
Renal vein thrombosis, 662

120 Renal disease in pregnancy, 663
Sal A. Lofaro and **Sandra P. Levison**

Changes in renal physiology associated with normal pregnancy, 663
Acute renal failure, 664
Glomerulonephritis, 664
Postpartum renal failure, 664
Nephrotic syndrome, 664
Toxemia, 665
Pyelonephritis, 666
Systemic lupus erythematosus and other collagen-vascular diseases, 666

Dental correlations, 666
Burton H. Goldstein
edited by **James T. Amsterdam**

Summary, 670

Section Nine
RESPIRATORY DISEASES
edited by **William L. Morrissey**

121 Introduction to the respiratory system, 672
Sanford Levine and **Samuel T. Kuna**

Definitions, 672
Overview of respiration, 672
Total ventilation versus alveolar ventilation, 673
Alveolar ventilation and arterial carbon dioxide tension, 673
Composition of alveolar gas and arterial oxygen tension, 673
Calculation of mean P_{AO_2}, 673
Pulmonary perfusion, 673
Relationship between alveolar ventilation and pulmonary capillary blood flow, 674
Distribution of pulmonary capillary blood flow, 674
Distribution of alveolar ventilation, 674
Matching of alveolar ventilation and pulmonary capillary blood flow, 674
Effects of $\dot{V}a/\dot{Q}c$ abnormalities on Pa_{CO_2}, 674
Effects of ventilation-perfusion abnormalities on Pa_{O_2}, 676
Role of diffusion in alveolar-capillary gas transfer, 676
Measurements of diffusing capacity, 676
Clinical relevance of D_{LCO}, 676
Control of ventilation, 676
Evaluation of pulmonary performance, 677
Measurement of lung volumes and capacities, 677
Measurement of the forced expiratory vital capacity, 677
Measurement of functional residual capacity, 679
Exercise testing, 679
Airway resistance, 680
Categorization of lung disease, 680
Restrictive ventilatory disorders, 680
Obstructive ventilatory disorders, 680
Initial evaluation of arterial blood gas measurements, 681
Arterial hypercapnia, 681
Acute versus chronic arterial hypercapnia, 681
Physical signs of hypercapnia, 681
Therapy for acute symptomatic hypercapnia, 681
Relationship of arterial hypercapnia to lung disease, 681

Arterial hypoxemia, 681
  Inspiring air (or a gas mixture) with a low P_{O_2}, 681
  Alveolar hypoventilation, 682
  Diffusion, 682
  Ventilation-perfusion mismatch, 682
  Right-to-left shunt, 682

122 Respiratory diagnostic procedures, 683
Samuel T. Kuna and **Sanford Levine**

Specialized aspects of the physical examination of the respiratory system, 683
  Examination of nonthoracic areas, 683
  Examination of the thorax, 684
Chest roentgenographic examination, 685
  Posteroanterior and lateral chest views, 685
  Special views, 686
Sputum examination, 686
Radionuclide scans, 687
  Perfusion scan, 687
  Ventilation scan, 687
  Use of radionuclide scans in the diagnosis of pulmonary emboli, 687
  Use of perfusion lung scans in the preoperative assessment of patients undergoing lung resection, 687
Ultrasonography, 687
Thoracentesis, 687
  Methodology and complications, 687
  Pleural fluid analysis, 688
  Transudative effusions, 688
  Exudative effusions, 688
Bronchoscopy, 688
Bronchography, 689
Percutaneous needle aspiration, 689
Open lung biopsy, 689
Mediastinoscopy and mediastinotomy, 689
Pulmonary angiography, 689

123 Chronic bronchitis and emphysema, 690
Paul D. Siegel and **Frank Barch**

Chronic bronchitis, 691
Emphysema, 693

124 Pulmonary hypertension and cor pulmonale, 696
William L. Morrissey

125 Bronchiectasis, 696
Paul D. Siegel and **Frank Barch**

126 Lung abscess, 698
Donald Kaye

127 Cystic fibrosis, 700
Paul D. Siegel and **Frank Barch**

128 Bullous emphysema and lung cysts, 700
Paul D. Siegel and **Frank Barch**

Bullous emphysema, 700
Lung cysts, 701

129 Atelectasis, 702
Paul D. Seigel and **Frank Barch**

Middle lobe syndrome, 703

130 Asthma, 704
Gregory S. Lenchner

131 Respiratory failure, 707
Sandeep Dhand

Oxygen transport, 707
Carbon dioxide transport, 708
Hypoxemia and its mechanisms, 708
Classification of respiratory failure, 708
Adult respiratory distress syndrome (ARDS), 708
Pulmonary edema, 710
Chronic obstructive disease and asthma, 710
Respiratory failure with normal lungs, 711
  Abnormal respiratory control, 711
  Chest bellows disease, 712
  Upper airway obstruction, 713

132 Diffuse lung diseases, 713
Morton Rubenstein

Pulmonary fibrosis, 713
  Idiopathic pulmonary fibrosis, 713
  Lymphocytic interstitial pneumonitis, 715
  Systemic lupus erythematosus, 715
  Scleroderma (progressive systemic sclerosis), 715
  Rheumatoid arthritis, 715
  Polymyositis-dermatomyositis, 716
  Mixed connective tissue disease (overlap syndrome), 716
  Sjögren's syndrome, 716
  Ankylosing spondylitis, 716
Interstitial diseases of unknown cause, 716
  Sarcoidosis, 716
  Histiocytosis X, 718
  Amyloid, 719
Pulmonary vasculitides, 719
  Polyarteritis nodosa and related vasculitides, 719
  Wegener's granulomatosis, 719
Diffuse hemorrhagic lung disease and pulmonary hemosiderosis, 720
  Goodpasture's syndrome, 720
  Idiopathic pulmonary hemosiderosis, 720
Eosinophilic diseases, 721
  Pulmonary infiltrates with eosinophilia (PIE syndrome), 721
Familial diseases, 721
  Gaucher's disease, 721
  Niemann-Pick disease, 721

Familial interstitial pneumonitis, 721
Neurofibromatosis, 721
Tuberous sclerosis, 721
Drug-induced disease, 721
Radiation pneumonitis and fibrosis, 722

133 Environmental (occupational) lung disease, 723
David M.F. Murphy

Silicosis, 723
Coal workers' pneumoconiosis, 725
Asbestos-related disorders, 725
Pleural plaques, 726
Asbestosis, 726
Malignant mesothelioma, 726
Bronchogenic carcinoma, 727
Hypersensitivity pneumonitis, 727
Occupational asthma, 728
Lung disease caused by inhaled gases and vapors, 728
Smoke inhalation, 729
Oxygen toxicity, 729

134 Diseases of the pleura, 730
Maurice Sones

Pleuritis, 730
Pleural effusion, 731
Pneumothorax, 733
Pleural tumors, 734

135 Diseases of the mediastinum, diaphragm, and chest wall, 734
Stanley L. Altschuler

Mediastinal disease, 734
Mediastinitis, 734
Pneumomediastinum, 735
Anterior mediastinal masses, 735
Middle mediastinal masses, 735
Posterior mediastinal masses, 736
Diaphragmatic disease, 736
Abnormalities of motion, 736
Eventration, 736
Herniation, 736
Miscellaneous conditions, 736
Chest wall disease, 737
Rib lesions, 737
Sternal abnormalities, 737
Thoracic spinal abnormalities, 737
Ankylosing spondylitis, 737

136 Primary malignancies of the lung, 738
William Weiss

137 Tumors of the lung other than bronchogenic carcinoma, 743
William L. Morrissey

Bronchial adenoma, 743
Lymphoma and lymphoproliferative disorders, 743

Benign tumors, 743
Metastatic tumors, 743
Solitary pulmonary nodule, 744

Dental correlations, 744
B. Kyle DeMartino and **Stuart Fischman**

Chronic bronchitis, 745
Pulmonary emphysema, 746
Bronchiectasis, 746
Lung abscess, 746
Cystic fibrosis, 747
Bullous emphysema and lung cysts, 747
Asthma, 747
Diffuse lung disease, 747
Environmental diseases, 747

Section Ten
ENVIRONMENTAL INJURIES
edited by **Donald Kaye**

138 Chemical and environmental injuries, 749
Geoffrey Lefferts and **David T. Lush**

Radiation injury, 749
Dental radiation dosage, 751
Robert Beiderman

Electrical injury, 751
Poisonings, 752
Heavy metal toxicity, 752
Other common poisons, 754
Abnormalities of temperature regulation, 755
Heat syndromes, 755
Hypothermia, 756

Section Eleven
NEUROLOGIC DISEASES
edited by **Rosalie A. Burns**

139 Introduction to neurology, 757
Rosalie A. Burns

Neurologic lesions, 757
Lesions of the frontal lobe, 757
Lesions of the parietal lobe, 758
Lesions of the temporal lobe, 759
Lesions of the occipital lobe, 759
Lesions of basal ganglia, 759
Lesions of corticospinal pathways, 759
Lesions of the thalamus, 759
Lesions of the cerebellum, 759
Lesions of the brainstem, 760
Lesions of the spinal cord, 760
Lesions of nerve roots, peripheral nerves, neuromuscular junction, and muscle, 761
Diagnostic tests, 761

140 Alterations in consciousness, 762
Leopold Canales

Stupor and coma, 763
Pathophysiology of unconsciousness, 764
Initial physical and neurologic examination of the patient in coma, 765
Lesions producing unconsciousness, 767
  Supratentorial mass lesions, 767
  Infratentorial lesions, 767
  Metabolic encephalopathies, 768
Laboratory data in the diagnosis of unconsciousness, 768

141 Sleep disorders, 769
Leopold Canales

142 Disorders of cognition, 770
Leopold Canales

Information processing and focal hemispheric lesions, 770
Information processing deficit and diffuse hemispheric pathology (dementia), 773

143 Central nervous system intoxications, 775
Paul L. Schraeder

CNS depressants, 775
CNS stimulants, 777
Other commonly abused drugs, 778
Neurologic effects of commonly prescribed drugs, 779

144 Syncope, 780
Paul L. Schraeder

145 Epilepsy (seizure disorders), 781
Paul L. Schraeder

146 Headache and face pain, 788
Vasant Dhopesh

Vascular headache, 788
  Migraine, 788
  Cluster headache, 789
Muscle contraction (tension) headache, 789
Other forms of headache, 789
  Posttraumatic headache, 789
  Hypertensive headache, 789
  Headache in temporal arteritis, 789
  Headache from sinus or eye disease, 790
  Traction headache, 790
  Lumbar puncture headache, 790
  Headache in pseudotumor cerebri, 790
  Headache in subarachnoid hemorrhage, 790
  Headache in meningitis, 790
Trigeminal neuralgia, 790
Atypical facial neuralgia, 791
Carotidynia, 791

147 Vertigo, dizziness, and hearing loss, 792
Joseph U. Toglia

Vertigo, 792
  Diseases causing vertigo, 792
  Vascular diseases, 793
Dizziness, 794
Hearing loss, 794
  Conductive hearing loss, 795
  Sensorineural hearing loss, 795
  Central hearing loss, 795

148 Demyelinating, degenerative, and heredofamilial diseases of the central nervous system, 796
Michael J. Walsh and Wallace W. Tourtellotte

Diseases of white matter, 796
  Demyelinating diseases, 796
  Dysmyelinating diseases, 801
Degenerative disorders, 803
  Motor neuron disease, 803
Syndromes of progressive hereditary ataxia, 805
Syringomyelia, 807
Combined system disease (vitamin B_{12} deficiency), 808
Neurocutaneous syndromes, 808
  Neurofibromatosis (von Recklinghausen's disease), 808
  Von Hippel-Lindau disease, 809
  Ataxia-telangiectasia, 809
  Sturge-Weber syndrome, 810
  Tuberous sclerosis (Bourneville's disease), 810
  Incontinentia pigmenti (Bloch-Sulzberger syndrome), 810

149 Abnormalities of the craniovertebral junction, 810
Paul L. Schraeder

Platybasia and basilar impression, 811
Arnold-Chiari malformations, 811
Klippel-Feil syndrome, 811

150 Basal ganglia disorders and related conditions, 812
Roger Duvoisin

Parkinsonism, 812
Essential tremor, 815
Chorea, 816
  Huntington's chorea, 816
  Hemichorea, 818
  Sydenham's chorea, 818
Torsion dystonias, 819
  Spasmodic torticollis, 819
  Dystonia musculorum deformans, 820
  Writer's cramp, 821
  Oromandibular dystonia, 821
Gilles de la Tourette's syndrome, 821

Wilson's disease, 822
Idiopathic orthostatic hypotension, 823

151 Viral and slow viral infections of the central nervous system, 824
David P. Dunn

Aseptic meningitis, 824
Encephalitis, 825
    Arbovirus encephalitis, 825
    Herpes simplex encephalitis, 825
    Cytomegalovirus, 826
    Rabies, 826
Poliomyelitis, 826
Herpes zoster (shingles), 826
Reye's syndrome, 827
Postinfectious encephalomyelitis and postvaccinal encephalomyelitis (acute disseminated encephalomyelitis), 827
Slow viral infections of the central nervous system, 828
    Kuru, 828
    Creutzfeldt-Jakob disease, 828
    Subacute sclerosing panencephalitis, 828
    Progressive multifocal leukoencephalopathy, 828

152 Vascular diseases of the central nervous system, 829
Rosalie A. Burns

Anatomy and physiology of the cerebral circulation, 829
Infarction of the brain, 830
    Syndromes of the cerebral arteries, 832
    Syndromes of the basilar artery and its branches, 833
    Syndromes of the vertebral arteries, 835
    Lacunar syndromes, 835
Infarction of the spinal cord, 835
Transient ischemic attacks, 836
Cerebral hemorrhage, 838
Subarachnoid hemorrhage and other manifestations of vascular anomalies, 839
    Aneurysms, 839
    Arteriovenous malformations, 840
    Arteriovenous fistulas, 840
Spinal cord hemorrhage, 840
Venous thrombosis, 840
Hypertensive encephalopathy, 841
Uncommon vascular diseases of the central nervous system, 841

153 Effects of primary and metastatic tumors on the central nervous system, and pseudotumor cerebri, 843
George Paulson

Brain tumors, 843
Neurologic complications of cancer therapy, 847
Effects of remote tumors on the nervous system, 847
Pseudotumor cerebri, or benign intracranial hypertension, 848

154 Nutritional disorders of the nervous system, 849
David P. Dunn

Peripheral neuropathy, 849
Wernicke's encephalopathy and Korsakoff's psychosis, 849
Nutritional amblyopia, 850
Pellagra, 850
Cerebellar cortical degeneration, 850
Vitamin B_{12} deficiency (pernicious anemia), 851

155 Problems of nerve and muscle, 851
Hiroshi Mitsumoto and **Theodore L. Munsat**

Structure and function, 851
Signs and symptoms, 852
Pathophysiology, 852
    Pathology, 852
    Electrophysiology, 852
    Clinical enzymology, 853
Peripheral neuropathies, 853
    Nutritional deficiencies, 853
    Toxic and metabolic neuropathies, 853
    Systemic disorders, 854
    Infectious and parainfectious neuropathies, 854
    Hereditary neuropathies, 855
    Carcinomatous (paraneoplastic) neuropathies, 855
Neuromuscular junction disorders, 855
    Myasthenia gravis, 855
    Eaton-Lambert (myasthenic) syndrome, 856
    Botulism, 856
Disorders of muscle, 856
    Muscular dystrophies, 856
    Inflammatory myopathies, 858
    Metabolic myopathies, 858
    Myotonic disorders, 859
    Congenital myopathies, 859
    Myoglobinuria, 859
Disorders of the spinal roots, brachial plexus, and spinal cord, 860
    General signs and symptoms, 860
    Specific disorders, 860

Dental correlations, 861
Vernon J. Brightman

Sleep disorders, 861
    Nocturnal bruxism, 861
    Sleep apnea syndrome, 861
    Sleep disturbance associated with depression, 861
Alcoholism and drug abuse, 862
Syncope, 864
Patient with a history of epilepsy, 864
    History, 865
    Examination, 865
    Medical consultation, 865
    Phenytoin-induced gingival hyperplasia, 865
    Anesthesia, 866
    Removable appliances, 866
    Managing a patient having a seizure, 866

Aural symptoms associated with temporomandibular joint dysfunction, odontogenic dizziness, and the otomandibular syndrome, 867
Demyelinating, degenerative, and heredofamilial diseases of the central nervous system, 868
  Demyelinating and degenerative diseases of the CNS possibly associated with transmissible agents, 868
  Syringomyelia, 869
  Vitamin B_{12} deficiency, 869
  Phakomatoses, 869
Tremors and other abnormal involuntary jaw movements, 870
Stroke, 871
Problems of nerve and muscle, 873
  Neuromuscular disease, 873
  Peripheral neuropathy, 874
  Myasthenia gravis, 874
  Inflammatory myopathies, 874
  Malignant hyperthermia, 875

Section Twelve
SKIN DISEASES AND THEIR ORAL MANIFESTATIONS
edited by **Bernard A. Kirshbaum** and **Robert N. Arm**

Oral management overview, 876

156 Congenital diseases, 876
Robert N. Arm, Bernard A. Kirshbaum, Anthony V. Benedetto, and **Karen Lipinski**

Anhidrotic ecotodermal dysplasia, 876
Epidermolysis bullosa dystrophica, 877
Neurofibromatosis (von Recklinghausen's disease), 878
Tuberous sclerosis; adenoma sebaceum; epiloia (Bourneville-Pringle syndrome), 880
Sturge-Weber syndrome (encephalotrigeminal angiomatosis), 881
Bloom's syndrome, 882
Basal cell nevus syndrome (nevoid basalioma syndrome; nevoid basal cell carcinoma syndrome), 883
Pseudoxanthoma elasticum (Grönblad-Strandberg syndrome), 884

157 Endocrine and metabolic disorders, 884
Bernard A. Kirshbaum, Anthony V. Benedetto, Karen Lipinski, and **Robert N. Arm**

Diabetes mellitus, 884
Thyroid disease, 886
  Hyperthyroidism, 886
  Hypothyroidism, 886
Acromegaly, 886
Adrenal insufficiency (Addison's disease), 886
Adrenal cortical hyperplasia (Cushing's syndrome), 887
Acanthosis nigricans, 887
Porphyria, 888
Hyperlipidemias, 889
Hemochromatosis, 890

158 Gastrointestinal disorders with cutaneous lesions, 891
Bernard A. Kirshbaum, Anthony V. Benedetto, Karen Lipinski, and **Robert N. Arm**

Gardner's syndrome, 891
Peutz-Jeghers syndrome (melanosis-polyposis), 891
Cronkhite-Canada syndrome, 891
Ulcerative colitis with pyoderma gangrenosum and pyostomatitis vegetans, 892
Regional enteritis (Crohn's disease), 892
Dermatitis herpetiformis, 892
Malignant atrophic papulosis (Degos' disease), 893
Hereditary hemorrhagic telangiectasis (Weber-Osler-Rendu disease), 894
Acrodermatitis enteropathica, 894

159 Liver disorders, 896
Bernard A. Kirshbaum, Anthony V. Benedetto, and **Karen Lipinski**

160 Renal disorders, 896
Bernard A. Kirshbaum, Anthony V. Benedetto, and **Karen Lipinski**

161 Hematologic disorders, 897
Bernard A. Kirshbaum, Anthony V. Benedetto, and **Karen Lipinski**

Polycythemia vera, 897
Sickle cell disease, 898
Thrombocytopenia and other platelet abnormalities, 898
Leukemias, 898
  Specific lesions, 898
  Nonspecific lesions, 899
Multiple myeloma, 899
Malignant lymphoma, 899
Mycosis fungoides, 900

162 Connective tissue disorders, 902
Bernard A. Kirshbaum, Anthony V. Benedetto, Karen Lipinski, and **Robert N. Arm**

Lupus erythematosus, 902
Scleroderma, 903
  Morphea (circumscribed scleroderma), 903
  Progressive systemic sclerosis, 903
Dermatomyositis, 904
Mixed connective tissue disease (overlap syndrome), 906
Rheumatoid arthritis, 906
Wegener's and lymphomatoid granulomatosis, 906
  Wegener's granulomatosis, 906
Behçet's disease, 906
Reiter's syndrome, 907

163 Miscellaneous skin disorders, 909
Bernard A. Kirshbaum, Anthony V. Benedetto, Karen Lipinski, and **Robert N. Arm**

Mastocytosis, 909
  Urticaria pigmentosa, 909
  Mastocytoma, 909

Telangiectasia macularis eruptiva perstans, 909
Diffuse mastocytosis, 909
Systemic mastocytosis, 909
Sarcoidosis, 910
Angiokeratoma corporis diffusum (Fabry's disease), 911

164 Cutaneous signs of internal malignancy, 912
Bernard A. Kirshbaum, Anthony V. Benedetto, and Karen Lipinski

165 Neoplasms of the skin, 913
Robert N. Arm, Bernard A. Kirshbaum, Anthony V. Benedetto, and Karen Lipinski

Seborrheic keratosis, 913
Premalignant lesions—actinic keratosis and Bowen's disease, 914
Malignant neoplasms, 914
   Squamous cell carcinoma, 915
   Basal cell carcinoma, 915
   Malignant melanoma, 916
   Neoplasms of the mouth, 918
   Kaposi's hemorrhagic sarcoma, 920

166 Erythemas, 922
Robert N. Arm, Bernard A. Kirshbaum, Anthony V. Benedetto, and Karen Lipinski

Erythema multiforme, 922
Erythema nodosum, 924
Erythema chronicum migrans, 925

167 Infections, 926
Bernard A. Kirshbaum, Anthony V. Benedetto, and Karen Lipinski

Viral infections, 926
   Herpes simplex, 926
   Herpes zoster, 927
   Warts, 927
   Molluscum contagiosum, 927
Fungal infections, 928
Yeast *(Candida)* infections, 929

168 Skin diseases, 931
Bernard A. Kirshbaum, Robert N. Arm, Anthony V. Benedetto, and Karen Lipinski

Toxic epidermal necrolysis (Lyell's disease), 931
   Adult disease, 931
   Staphylococcal scalded skin syndrome, 932
Pemphigus and pemphigoid, 932
   Pemphigus, 932
   Pemphigoid, 935
Psoriasis, 936
Erythema migrans, 938
Lichen planus, 938

Section Thirteen
DISORDERS OF THE DIGESTIVE SYSTEM
edited by **Walter Rubin**

169 The structure and function of the digestive system, 940
Walter Rubin

Overview, 940
Esophagus and swallowing, 942
Stomach, 942
Small intestine, pancreas, and liver, 945
Digestion, absorption, and motility in the small intestine, 946
Large intestine, 947
Splanchnic blood flow, 948

170 Manifestations of disorders of the digestive system, 949
Walter Rubin

Nature and symptoms of digestive disorders and approach to evaluating patients, 949
Pain, 950
Diarrhea, 952
Constipation, 955
Nausea and vomiting, 956
Gastrointestinal bleeding, 957
Gaseousness, 960
Other manifestations of gastrointestinal disorders, 961

171 Special techniques for diagnosing disorders of the digestive system, 961
William O. Frank

Esophagus, 961
   Bernstein test, 961
   Esophageal manometry, 962
   pH probe test for reflux, 962
   Gastroesophageal scintigram, 962
   Esophagoscopy, 962
Stomach, 962
   Endoscopy, 962
   Gastric motility studies, 963
   Scintigraphic technique to measure enterogastric reflux, 964
Small bowel, 964
   Small bowel biopsy, 964
Colon, 964
   Colonoscopy, 965
   Fiberoptic sigmoidoscopy, 965
Liver, 965
   Transthoracic liver biopsy, 965
   Laparoscopy, 966
   Hepatic radionuclide imaging, 966
Hepatobiliary tree, 967
   Transhepatic cholangiography with the Chiba needle, 968
   Endoscopic retrograde cannulation of the pancreaticobiliary tree, 968
   HIDA and PIPIDA imaging, 969

Pancreas, 969
  Endoscopic retrograde cannulation of the pancreaticobiliary tree, 969
  Pancreatic biopsy, 969
Other diagnostic methods, 969
  Abdominal ultrasonography, 969
  Computed tomography, 971
  Visceral angiography, 971

172 Disorders of the esophagus, 972
Steven Nussbaum

Anatomy and physiology of the esophagus, 972
Symptoms of esophageal disease, 974
  Dysphagia, 974
  Heartburn, 974
  Odynophagia, 975
  Esophageal spasm, 975
  Hematemesis, 975
Disorders of esophageal motility, 975
  Disorders of striated muscle, 975
  Disorders of smooth muscle, 976
  Motility disorders of the esophagus in systemic diseases, 981
Gastroesophageal reflux disease and hiatus hernia, 982
Tumors of the esophagus, 985
Esophagitis resulting from infectious and physical agents, 985
  Infectious diseases, 985
  Physical agents, 985
Laceration and perforation of the esophagus, 986
  Mallory-Weiss syndrome, 986

173 Acid-peptic diseases, 987
Walter Rubin

Peptic ulcer disease, 987
Zollinger-Ellison syndrome, 994
Stress erosions, 995
Gastritis, 996
Other gastric disorders, 997
  Acute gastric dilation, 997
  Adult hypertrophic pyloric stenosis, 997
  Gastric volvulus, 998
  Gastric diverticula, 998
  Bezoars, 998

174 Disorders of absorption—the malabsorption syndrome, 998
Gerald H. Escovitz

Normal physiology, 998
Pathophysiology, 999
Clinical presentation, 1000
Clinical approach, 1000
Specific disorders causing malabsorption, 1001
  Pancreatic insufficiency, 1001
  Mucosal disease, 1001
  Disorders of lymphatic transport, 1003
  Miscellaneous causes of malabsorption, 1003
Disorders of carbohydrate absorption, 1004
  Normal physiology, 1004
  Lactose intolerance (lactase deficiency), 1004

175 Inflammatory diseases of the intestines, 1005
Harvey B. Lefton

Inflammatory bowel disease, 1005
  Chronic ulcerative colitis, 1007
  Crohn's disease, 1011
Appendicitis and appendiceal abscess, 1015
Diverticular disease of the colon, 1017
Pseudomembranous enterocolitis and antibiotic-induced diarrhea, 1018
Radiation enteritis, 1018
Intestinal ulcer, 1019

176 Vascular diseases of the gut, 1020
Ralph M. Myerson

Occlusive vascular disease of the gut, 1020
Nonocclusive vascular disease of the gut, 1020
Ischemic colitis, 1021
Venous thrombosis, 1021
Other vascular disorders, 1022
  Vasculitis, 1022
  Arteriovenous malformations, 1022
  Hereditary hemorrhagic telangiectasia, 1023

177 Intestinal obstruction, 1024
Steven Nussbaum

Mechanical obstruction and ileus, 1024
Megacolon, 1026

178 Functional bowel disease, 1027
Julian Katz

179 Anorectal disorders, 1029
Harvey B. Lefton

Skin disorders, 1030
Hemorrhoids, 1030
Fissures, 1031
Fistulas, 1031
Tumors, 1031

180 Tumors of the gut, 1031
Paul B. Weisberg

Esophageal neoplasms, 1031
  Benign tumors, 1031
  Malignant tumors, 1032
Gastric neoplasms, 1033
  Benign tumors, 1033
  Malignant tumors, 1035
Small bowel neoplasms, 1037
  Benign tumors, 1037
  Malignant tumors, 1037
Colonic and rectal neoplasms, 1038
  Benign tumors, 1038

Malignant tumors, 1039
Other malignancies, 1041
Gastrointestinal polyposis syndromes, 1042
Familial polyposis coli, 1042
Gardner's syndrome, 1042
Peutz-Jeghers syndrome, 1042
Juvenile polyposis, 1042

181 Diseases of the peritoneum and mesentery, 1043
William O. Frank

Anatomy and physiology, 1043
Diagnosis of peritoneal diseases, 1043
Ascites, 1044
Infections of the peritoneum, 1046
Tuberculous peritonitis, 1046
Intra-abdominal abscess, 1047
Neoplasms of the peritoneum, 1047
Primary mesothelioma, 1047
Secondary carcinomatosis, 1047
Familial paroxysmal polyserositis, 1048
Other diseases of the peritoneum, 1048
Peritoneal vasculitis, 1048
Granulomatous peritonitis, 1048
Diseases of the mesentery and omentum, 1048
Mesenteric inflammatory disease, 1048
Mesenteric cysts, 1049
Mesenteric tumors, 1049
Mesenteric hernias, 1049
Omental torsion and infarction, 1049

182 Disorders of the pancreas, 1049
Ralph M. Myerson

Disorders of the pancreas, 1050
Congenital abnormalities, 1050
Acute pancreatitis, 1051
Relapsing acute pancreatitis, 1055
Chronic pancreatitis, 1055
Tumors of the pancreas, 1056

183 Diseases of the liver, 1057
Graham H. Jeffries

Clinical manifestations of hepatic disease, 1057
Jaundice, 1057
Cutaneous manifestations, 1058
Oral manifestations, 1059
Changes in liver size or consistency, 1059
Portal hypertension, 1060
Hepatic coma and precoma, 1061
Impaired hepatic detoxification, 1061
Changes in nutrition and metabolism, 1062
Hematologic abnormalities, 1063
Immunologic manifestations, 1064
Circulatory and renal manifestations, 1064
Clinical and laboratory assessment of patients, 1064
Assessment of liver function, 1064
Assessment for occult liver disease, 1066
Assessment of the patient with jaundice, 1066

Diseases of the liver, 1067
Disorders of bilirubin metabolism, 1067
Acute viral hepatitis, 1068
Bacterial infection and liver disease, 1074
Pyogenic liver abscess, 1074
Toxic and drug-induced liver disease, 1075
Fatty liver, 1077
Liver disease resulting from hepatic congestion and/or decreased perfusion, 1077
Chronic active hepatitis, 1078
Cirrhosis of the liver, 1079
Granulomatous and infiltrative diseases, 1084
Neoplastic diseases, 1084

184 Diseases of the biliary tract, 1085
Roger D. Soloway

Bile secretion and composition, 1085
Cholelithiasis and cholecystitis, 1086
Cholesterol stones, 1086
Neoplastic disease, 1089
Carcinoma of the gallbladder and extrahepatic biliary ducts, 1089
Carcinoma of the ampulla of Vater, 1090

Dental correlations, 1090
Barry H. Hendler, Barbara J. Steinberg, and Shirley Brown

Diseases of the esophagus, 1091
Acid peptic disease, 1092
Tumors and vascular and inflammatory diseases of the gastrointestinal tract, 1092
Tumors of the gut, 1093
Adenocarcinoma of the stomach, 1093
Adenocarcinoma of the colon and rectum, 1093
Gastrointestinal polyposis syndromes, 1093
Vascular disease of the gut, 1095
Hereditary hemorrhagic telangiectasia, 1095
Inflammatory bowel disease, 1095
Ulcerative colitis, 1095
Crohn's disease, 1096
Diseases of the liver, 1097
Chronic liver disease, 1098
Spontaneous or postsurgical bleeding, 1098
Viral hepatitis, 1098
Diseases of the pancreas, 1101
Cystic fibrosis, 1101
Nutritional disorders, 1102
General malnutrition, 1102
Specific nutritional deficiencies, 1104
Nutritional therapy, 1111

Section Fourteen
ENDOCRINOLOGY
edited by Doris G. Bartuska

185 Introduction to the diseases of the endocrine system and the mechanism of action of hormones, 1114
Mary B. Dratman

186 Hypothalamic and pituitary disorders, 1116
Calvin Ezrin

Endocrine hypothalamus, 1116
Control of anterior pituitary secretion, 1116
    Thyrotropin, or thyroid-stimulating hormone (TSH), 1116
    Corticotropin, or adrenocorticotropic hormone (ACTH), 1117
    Gonadotrophic hormones—follicle-stimulating hormone (FSH) and luteinizing hormone (LH), 1118
    Prolactin, 1118
    Somatotropin, or growth hormone, 1118
Clinical pituitary disorders, 1118
    Hyperpituitary syndromes, 1119
    Anterior pituitary insufficiency, 1121
    General investigation of pituitary problems, 1123
    Treatment of patients undergoing pituitary surgery, 1124
    Conditions simulating hypopituitarism, 1124
    Diseases of the posterior pituitary—diabetes insipidus, 1125
Pineal gland, 1126

187 The thyroid gland, 1126
Thomas F. Nikolai

Anatomy, 1126
Histology, 1128
Chemistry, 1128
    Extrathyroidal iodine metabolism, 1128
    Synthesis of thyroid hormones, 1128
    Storage and secretion of thyroid hormones, 1130
    Peripheral binding, metabolism, and physiologic effects of thyroid hormones, 1131
Tests of thyroid function and concentration and binding of thyroid hormones, 1133
Clinical assessment of thyroid function, 1136
    Hypothyroidism, 1136
    Hyperthyroidism, 1140
    Nontoxic goiter, 1148
    Thyroiditis, 1149
    Adenomas, 1150
    Carcinoma of the thyroid, 1150

188 The adrenal cortex, 1153
Ernest M. Gold

Structure and function, 1153
Glucocorticoid deficiency syndromes (Addison's disease), 1155
Glucocorticoid excess syndromes (Cushing's syndrome), 1157
Mineralocorticoid deficiency syndromes, 1159
Mineralocorticoid excess syndromes (aldosteronism), 1160
Congenital adrenal hyperplasias, 1162

189 Pheochromocytoma, 1164
Norman H. Ertel

190 The testes, 1168
Elaine German and **Leslie I. Rose**

Embryonic development, 1168
Hypogonadism, 1170
    Primary hypogonadism, 1170
    Secondary hypogonadism, 1172
    Evaluation and management, 1173
Hypergonadism, 1173
Testicular tumors, 1173

191 The ovary, 1173
Leonore C. Huppert

Histology and embryology, 1173
Follicular growth and development, 1174
Endocrine events of the menstrual cycle, 1174
Control mechanisms of the hypothalamic-pituitary-ovarian axis, 1175
Pituitary-ovarian relationships from birth to menopause, 1175
The abnormal ovary, 1176
    Functional disorders—amenorrhea, 1176
    Ovarian neoplasm, 1177

192 Humoral syndromes associated with neoplasms, 1178
Doris G. Bartuska

Hypercalcemia and neoplasms, 1179
Cushing's syndrome, 1180
Inappropriate antidiuresis, 1181
Hypoglycemia, 1181
Ectopic gonadotropins, 1181

193 Mineral metabolism and metabolic bone disease, 1181
Howard Rasmussen

Physiology of bone, 1181
    Structure and turnover of bone, 1181
    Mineral metabolism, 1183
Primary disorders of mineral homeostasis, 1189
    Hypercalcemia, 1189
    Hypocalcemia, 1195
    Hypoparathyroidism, 1196
    Pseudohypoparathyroidism, 1197
    Medullary carcinoma, 1197
Disorders of skeletal and mineral homeostasis, 1198
    Osteomalacia, 1198
    Inherited disorders of vitamin D metabolism, 1200
    Hypophosphatasia, 1200
    Renal osteodystrophy, 1200
Primary disorders of skeletal homeostasis, 1201
    Osteoporosis, 1201
    Osteogenesis imperfecta, 1203
    Osteopetrosis, 1203

Dental correlations
Barbara J. Steinberg and **Louis F. Rose**

Disorders of pituitary, 1204
    Hypopituitarism, 1204

Disorders of thyroid gland, 1205
   Hyperthyroidism, 1205
   Hypothyroidism, 1205
Disorders of adrenal gland, 1206
   Hyperadrenocorticism—Cushing's syndrome, 1206
   Hypoadrenocorticism—Addison's disease (primary adrenal insufficiency), 1207
Pheochromocytoma, 1207
Mineral metabolic and metabolic bone disease, 1207

   Hyperparathyroidism, 1207
   S. Gary Cohen

   Hypoparathyroidism, 1208
   S. Gary Cohen

   Hypophosphatasia, 1209
   Osteomalacia, 1209
   Osteoporosis, 1210
Sex hormonal alterations, 1210
   Ovaries, 1210
   Testes, 1214

Section Fifteen
GENETICS AND METABOLISM
edited by **Doris G. Bartuska**

194 Human genetics, 1216
Kathleen Toomey

Basic principles, 1216
   Gene concept and single gene inheritance, 1216
   Chromosome structure and abnormalities, 1220
   Multifactorial inheritance, 1222
Clinical genetics, 1223
   Pedigree construction and analysis, 1223
   Clinical cytogenetic disorders, 1224
   Single gene disorders, 1226
   Complex genetic syndromes, 1227
   Multifactorial disease, 1228
   The human gene map, linkage, and association, 1228
   Prenatal diagnosis, 1229

195 Inherited metabolic disorders, 1230
William A. Horton and **Robert D. Friedman**

Disorders of lysosomal storage, 1230
   Glycosphingolipidoses, 1230
   Mucopolysaccharidoses, 1233
   Mucolipidoses, 1235
Aminoacidopathies, 1236
   Aromatic amino acid disorders, 1236
   Sulfur-containing amino acid disorders, 1237
   Branched-chain amino acid disorders, 1237
Urea cycle disorders, 1238
Disorders of nucleic acid metabolism, 1239
Disorders of mineral metabolism, 1240
Connective tissue disorders, 1240

196 The porphyrias, 1246
Karl E. Anderson, Shigeru Sassa, and **Attallah Kappas**

Heme biosynthetic pathway, 1247
Classification and diagnosis of the human porphyrias, 1248
   Congenital erythropoietic porphyria, 1248
   Erythropoietic protoporphyria, 1250
   Acute intermittent porphyria, 1250
   Hereditary coproporphyria, 1252
   Variegate porphyria, 1253
   Porphyria cutanea tarda, 1253
   Porphyria associated with other disorders, 1254

197 Metabolic and direct toxic effects of alcohol, 1255
Ralph Myerson

Alcohol metabolism, 1255
Metabolic effects of alcohol, 1256
Direct toxic effects of alcohol, 1257

198 Pathogenesis and diagnosis of diabetes mellitus, 1259
Oliver E. Owen, Charles R. Shuman, Guenther Boden, and **Robert D. Hoeldtke**

199 Treatment of diabetes mellitus, 1264
Harry Gottlieb

Diet, 1265
Oral hypoglycemic agents, 1266
Insulin therapy, 1267
   Insulin management in special situations, 1268
Diabetic ketoacidosis, 1269
Hyperglycemic, hyperosmolar, nonketotic coma, 1270
Alcoholic ketoacidosis, 1270
Combined ketoacidosis and lactic acidosis, 1271
Diabetes in pregnancy, 1271

200 Chronic complications of diabetes mellitus, 1272
Robert L. Lavine

Arteriosclerotic complications, 1272
   Coronary artery disease, 1272
   Cerebrovascular disease, 1272
   Peripheral vascular disease, 1273
The "diabetic foot," 1273
Eye complications—cataracts and retinopathy, 1273
Nephropathy, 1274
Neuropathy, 1274
   Peripheral neuropathy, 1275
   Mononeuropathy, 1275
   Radiculopathy, 1275
   Amyotrophy, 1275
   Autonomic neuropathy, 1275
   Diabetic pseudotabes, 1276
Dermopathy, 1276

201 Hypoglycemia and hypoglycemic disorders, 1276
Clinton W. Young and John H. Karam

202 Disorders of lipoprotein metabolism, 1280
David M. Capuzzi

Plasma lipoproteins, 1280
Plasma apolipoproteins, 1280
Dynamics of lipid transport by lipoproteins, 1282
Pathophysiology of lipid transport, 1284
    Overproduction of triglyceride-rich lipoproteins, 1284
    Delayed clearance of triglyceride-rich lipoproteins, 1284
    Defective catabolism of triglyceride-rich lipoprotein remnants, 1285
    Defective catabolism of LDL, 1285
    Liver disease and lipoprotein metabolism, 1286
Classifiction of hyperlipoproteinemia, 1286
    Genetic hyperlipoproteinemias, 1286
Evaluation of patients, 1287
    Clinical assessment, 1287
    Plasma lipid and lipoprotein sampling, 1288
Management of hyperlipidemia, 1289
    Drug therapy, 1290
    Innovative forms of therapy, 1291
Familial lipoprotein deficiency disorders, 1291
    Abetalipoproteinemia, 1291
    Hypobetalipoproteinemia, 1292
    Tangier disease, 1292
    Familial LCAT deficiency, 1292

Dental correlations, 1294

Diabetes mellitus, 1294
Terry S. Gotthelf and **Louis F. Rose**

Disorders of lipoprotein metabolism, 1296
Barbara J. Steinberg and **Barry H. Hendler**

    Fabry-Anderson syndrome, 1296
    Gaucher's disease, 1296
    Urbach-Wiethe disease, 1296
    Type V hyperlipoproteinemia, 1296

Alcoholism, 1296
Barbara J. Steinberg and **Barry H. Hendler**

Porphyria, 1298
Barbara J. Steinberg and **Barry H. Hendler**

Section Sixteen
CRANIOFACIAL MALFORMATIONS
edited by **Louis F. Rose**

203 Malformations of the craniofacial complex: an overview, 1300
Ray E. Stewart

Definitions and nomenclature, 1301
Etiology of craniofacial malformations, 1301
    Rubella syndrome, 1303
    Aminopterin and methotrexate syndrome, 1303
    Fetal warfarin syndrome, 1303
    Fetal phenytoin syndrome, 1303
    Fetal alcohol syndrome, 1303
Prenatal craniofacial development, 1304
Pathogenesis and classification of craniofacial malformations, 1308
    Otocraniofacial syndromes, 1309
    Craniosynostosis syndromes, 1312
    Midface syndromes, 1316
    Craniofacial clefts, 1318
    Clefts of the primary and secondary palates, 1320

Section One

APPROACH TO EVALUATION OF THE PATIENT

edited by **Donald Kaye**

INTRODUCTION

David T. Lush and Geoffrey Lefferts
Louis F. Rose and Barry H. Hendler

The history and physical examination are a comprehensive evaluation of the patient's medical status. A standard method of performing and recording this evaluation has evolved.

While the history and physical examination are appropriately treated in this section in mechanical fashion, the examiner must remember that this is a significant event for most patients, and the examiner must display a personal as well as a professional attitude for the proper rapport to develop. Enlisting the patient's cooperation is an important aspect of an accurate, comprehensive examination.

It is the responsibility of every practicing dentist and the auxiliary staff to identify patients who may be a potential medical risk by securing a comprehensive pretreatment physical evaluation.

In their article on the significance of physical diagnosis, patient history, data, and medical screening in the dental office, Little and King summarize the reasons for physical evaluation as follows:

1. To identify patients with undetected systemic disease that could be a serious threat to the life of the patient or that could be complicated by dental treatment
2. To identify patients who are taking drugs or medication that could be potentiated by drugs prescribed by the dentist, that would complicate dental therapy, or that may serve as a clue to an underlying systemic disease that the patient has omitted from the history
3. To allow the dentist to modify the treatment plan for the patient in light of any systemic disease the patient may have or drugs he may be taking
4. To protect the patient and the dentist from commitment (or allegations thereof) of any malpractice
5. To enable the dentist to select and communicate with a medical consultant concerning a patient's possible systemic problems
6. To help establish a good patient/doctor relationship by showing the patients that the dentist is interested in them as individuals and that the dentist is concerned about their overall well-being

In fact, the data obtained from a history and physical examination may even prevent the occurrence of a medical emergency. A well-conceived total physical evaluation involves (1) medical history, (2) physical examination, (3) laboratory studies (if indicated), and (4) medical/dental consultation or referral.

Two basic methods for obtaining a medical history are the questionnaire and personal dialogue interview. A personal history elicited by dialogue allows for observation of the way the patient reacts to questions and provides the practitioner with an opportunity to evaluate the patient's mental status in a nonthreatening atmosphere. The patient who is uninterested or evasive may respond quite differently from one who is anxious to provide the best information he can. The questionnaire is a legitimate method of securing data if used in conjunction with a dialogue. It may help a patient recall frequently used medications or various symptoms of disease.

The questionnaire (Fig. 1) component can also assist the dentist in ascertaining which areas in the dialogue history to emphasize and further explore. More importantly, a completed and dated form, signed by the patient, may be utilized as evidence in any possible malpractice litigation.

Obviously, a dialogue medical history (Fig. 2) helps the dentist evaluate the present health status of a patient, past medical history, allergies, medications, and the like. Here the focus shifts from one of intensive diagnostic effort to a procedure that must effectively determine the physical and emotional ability of a patient to tolerate dental treatment. Though evaluation in an outpatient setting may be somewhat less detailed, the information obtained should adequately identify any condition that might compromise the patient's well-being during therapy. In essence, an abbreviated outpatient evaluation must assure the dentist that treatment may be carried out with relative safety; if this is not the case, medical consultation must be obtained before instituting any treatment.

It is evident that any total physical evaluation actually

DENTAL HEALTH QUESTIONNAIRE

Name _____

Date _____ Referred by _____

Previous Dentist _____

Address _____

Physician _____

Address _____

Reason for appointment _____

DIRECTIONS TO PATIENTS:

Answers to these questions will help the dentist decide how to best treat your dental problems. Try to check each answer "yes" or "no." If you have no idea of the answer to the question, do not check either answer.

Medical history   Yes No

1. Have you been treated by a physician or been in the   ___ ___
   hospital in the past year?

2. Has there been any change in your general health in   ___ ___
   the past year?

3. List all the medications or drugs you are taking at
   the present time:

   Medications   Dosage
   _____   _____
   _____   _____
   _____   _____
   _____   _____
   _____   _____

4. Have you ever been told you had a thyroid problem?   ___ ___

5. Have you ever been told you had sugar diabetes?   ___ ___

6. Have you taken daily cortisone medication (Prednisone)   ___ ___
   in the past year?

7. Have you ever had persistent pain or difficulty swallowing? ___ ___

8. Have you ever had jaundice, hepatitis, or some other   ___ ___
   liver problem?

Fig. 1. Dental health questionnaire.

9. Do you get short of breath on mild exertion or when you lie down?

10. Have you ever had TB (tuberculosis) or lived with anyone who had TB?

11. Have you ever had asthma?

12. Have you ever been told you had:
    Rheumatic fever
    Heart murmur
    Heart attack or coronary
    Angina
    Heart surgery
    High or low blood pressure

13. Have you ever had prolonged bleeding (more than is normal for you) for a cut, injury, or tooth extraction?

14. Have you ever had hemophilia or some other bleeding disorder?

15. Have you ever had anemia, low blood, or thin blood?

16. Have you ever had gonorrhea, syphilis, bad blood, or venereal disease?

17. Are you pregnant or think you are pregnant?

18. Are you now taking birth control pills?

19. Have you ever had troublesome pain in your jaw joint?

20. Have you ever had fits, seizures, convulsions, or epilepsy?

21. Have you ever had a stroke?

22. Have you been treated for some allergic condition?

23. Are you allergic to penicillin?

24. Has anyone ever told you not to take a particular drug (aspirin, novocaine, sulfa, etc.)?

25. Are there any medications that make you sick or ill?

Fig. 1, cont'd. Dental health questionnaire.

```
Name _____ Tel. home _____ Date _____
Address_____ Tel. bus. _____ Date of birth _____
Referred by_____

DENTAL HISTORY:
Dentist_____ Telephone _____ Last visit _____
Chief complaint:

History of present illness:

Past dental history:

MEDICAL HISTORY:
Physician_____ Telephone _____ Last visit _____
Present health status

Hospitalizations

Illnesses
Allergies _____ ASA _____ LA _____ PCN _____
Meds_____ OC _____
Review of systems
    Skin _____
    EENT _____
    Respiratory _____
    Cardiac_____ RhF _____ RhHD _____ M _____
    Gastrointestinal _____
    Genitourinary _____
    Menstrual Hx _____ Pregnancy _____ Children _____
    Endocrine _____ Diabetes _____
    Extremities _____
    Nervous_____ Psychiatric _____
    Hematopoietic _____

Family history
    Diabetes _____ Hypertension _____ Cardiac _____
    Epilepsy_____ Other_____
Social history
    Occupation _____ Smoking _____ Alcohol _____ Other _____

REGIONAL EXAMINATION
1. Face _____ 5. Floor _____ 9. Gingiva _____
2. Lips _____ 6. Palate hard_____
3. Buccal mucosa _____ 7. Palate soft_____ 10. Lymph nodes_____
4. Tongue _____ 8. Pharynx _____ VITAL SIGNS  BP _____ P__

MEDICAL SUMMARY:


RECOMMENDATIONS:
```

Fig. 2. Comprehensive dialogue medical history.

can be elicited in two ways. The first is a systemic approach to history and physical examination suitable for contact with the hospital inpatient, and the second is a physical evaluation of the patient in an ambulatory care facility, such as the dental office. Of necessity, all practitioners must know and utilize the more comprehensive format as basis for the less comprehensive second approach. The text that follows offers the essential information required in performing the most comprehensive and diagnostic type of inpatient history and physical examination.

1 • HISTORY

David T. Lush and Geoffrey Lefferts
Louis F. Rose and Barry H. Hendler

PATIENT IDENTIFICATION

Before recording the examination, note the patient's full name, age and date of birth, sex, race, and marital status. When pertinent, occupation, place of birth, or religion should be included, otherwise they may be considered later as a part of the social history.

SOURCE OF INFORMATION

Be sure to include the sources of information used in compiling the history. The patient, a friend or relative, previous medical charts, or a referral letter from a physician or institution are usual sources. Include also an assessment of the reliability of this information.

CHIEF COMPLAINT

Ascertain the principal reason the patient is seeking medical attention. This is best recorded as a simple phrase stating the complaint and its duration. There is no obligation to use the patient's own words, although they may be enlightening.

An example of how a typical chief complaint may be written follows:
1. Abdominal pain for 1 month
2. Vomiting blood for 1 day

PRESENT ILLNESS

Question the patient in detail concerning his complaints and record the history in chronological order. Unlike the chief complaint, the description of the present illness should be written in paragraph form. Make inquiries about all symptoms pertaining to the chief complaint as listed in the discussion of the review of systems. The patient must be questioned regarding all other potentially relevant information, especially the presence or absence of symptoms classically associated with diseases known to cause similar complaints. Mention of "pertinent negatives" is a fundamental and essential part of a thorough present illness evaluation. Include laboratory tests performed during the course of the present illness workup and the results of previous attempts at therapy. Lastly, the patient's current medications must be completely reviewed.

PAST HISTORY

Check the following areas in this section.
1. General: previous illnesses and response to therapy, known active medical problems, previous hospitalizations and surgery
2. Medication allergies: drugs, contrast media
3. Immunizations: tetanus, diphtheria, pneumonia, and influenza, poliomyelitis, measles, rubella, mumps
4. Trauma: significant injuries, blood transfusions

REVIEW OF SYSTEMS

When reviewing the systems as part of the medical history, present each major symptom to the patient and ask if he is experiencing or has experienced any of them. The purpose is to uncover symptoms that may aid in identifying the process responsible for the patient's chief complaint and to identify any possible unrelated coexisting disease. At the same time, asking about previous symptoms serves as a check on the accuracy and completeness of the patient's past history.

When symptoms pertinent to the present illness are discovered during the review of systems, they are, of course, incorporated into the present illness portion of the history when the examination is put into writing. Most examiners then record only positives and related pertinent negatives in the review of systems.

Following is a list of the symptoms to be reviewed in this section of the history.
1. General: fever, chills, perspiration, weakness, fatigue, change in weight
2. Skin: rash, itch, pigmentation, bruising, scars; *nails*—change in shape, brittleness, pitting; *hair*—excessive loss, change in texture or distribution
3. Head: headache, trauma
4. Eyes: double vision, blurry vision, transient or permanent loss of vision, spots, pain, redness, tearing, discharge, sensitivity to light, use of glasses or contact lenses, cataracts, most recent examination for glaucoma
5. Ears: hearing loss, ringing, dizziness associated with subjective feeling of rotation, pain, discharge
6. Nose and sinuses: bleeding, discharge, obstruction, colds, change in sense of smell, facial pain
7. Mouth: pain, lesions, dryness; *tongue*—soreness, lesions or coating, enlargement, problems with taste; *teeth*—pain, extractions, most recent dental examination; *gums*—bleeding, lesions, discoloration; *throat*—frequent sore throats or tonsillitis, hoarseness, problems with swallowing
8. Neck: pain, stiffness, swelling, lumps, limitation of motion, thyroid enlargement
9. Breasts: lumps, tenderness, discharge, change in nipple, changes on self-examination

---

REVIEW OF SYSTEMS

1. Skin: itching, rash, ulcers, changes in hair, hair loss.

2. Eyes: vision, diplopia, blurring.

3. Ears, nose, throat: hearing, earache, epistaxis, sore throat, hoarseness, sinus pain.

4. Respiratory: cough, sputum (describe quantity, color, odor, blood) wheezing, infections, exposure to tuberculosis.

5. Cardiac: chest pain on exertion, palpitation, dyspnea, orthopnea, swelling of ankles. History of rheumatic fever, rheumatic heart disease, "heart attack," high blood pressure, murmur.

6. Gastrointestinal: appetite, nausea, vomiting, dysphagia, heartburn,, indigestion, food intolerance, abdominal pain, jaundice.

7. Genito-urinary: dysuria, nocturia, polyuria, hematuria, frequency, difficulty starting stream; venereal disease and treatment, kidney infection.
   FOR WOMEN:

   a. *Menstrual history:* last menstrual period and previous menstrual period; dysmenorrhea

   b. *Menopause:* age of occurrence, hot flushes

   c. *Obstetrical history:* pregnancies, miscarriages, living children

8. Extremities:
   a. Vascular: varicose veins, phlebitis
   b. Joints: pain, stiffness, swelling of joints
   c. Muscles: weakness, pain, tenderness, cramps

9. Nervous system: syncope, convulsions, headache, vertigo, tremor, paralysis, paresthesias, anesthesias.

10. Hematopoietic: bleeding tendency, excessive bruising, anemia, known exposure to radiation or toxic agents.

11. Psychiatric: "nervousness," irritability, depressions, history of previous "nervous breakdown."

Fig. 1-1. Information that should be obtained regarding each body system.

10. Respiratory system: cough, sputum, coughing up blood, night sweats, shortness of breath, wheezing, pain with breathing, exposure to tuberculosis (TB), most recent TB skin test and chest roentgenogram
11. Heart: chest pain, shortness of breath with exertion or when lying down, swelling in legs or feet, chest pounding, irregular or rapid heartbeats, heart murmur, high blood pressure
12. Vascular system: lower extremity pain with exertion, leg cramps, blood clots, varicose veins, coldness or change in color of extremity
13. Gastrointestinal tract: poor appetite, food intolerance, regurgitation, chest pain or fullness after eating or when lying down, pain or problems with swallowing, belching, nausea, vomiting, vomiting blood, abdominal pain, diarrhea, constipation, change in bowel habits or in color or character of stool, hemorrhoids, anal itch, gallstones, yellow color to eyes or skin, abdominal swelling, liver disease or hepatitis
14. Urinary tract: pain on urination; frequent, urgent, repeated, or nocturnal need to void; bloody urine; loss of urine on clothes or bed; difficulty starting

or stopping stream; change in size of stream or color of urine; kidney stones; infections, flank pain
15. Genitoreproductive system:
    a. Female: *menses*—age of onset, frequency, duration, pain, amount of flow, presence of clots, date of most recent period; *menopause*—age, associated symptoms, bleeding since menopause; vaginal pain, itch, discharge, and odor; date of most recent pelvic examination and Pap smear; venereal diseases; *pregnancy*—number, outcome, use of diethylstilbestrol by patient or mother; contraceptive history
    b. Male: penile lesions, discharge, and pain; ability to achieve and maintain erection; scrotal or testicular pain, swelling, and lumps; venereal diseases
16. Joints: pain, redness, warmth, swelling, stiffness, limitation of motion, deformities
17. Lymph nodes: enlargement, pain, tenderness
18. Blood: anemia, easy bruising or bleeding, blood transfusions
19. Endocrine system: thyroid enlargement or malfunction; heat or cold intolerance; change in skin or hair texture; diabetes; excessive eating, drinking, or urinating; change in skin pigmentation or hair distribution
20. Allergies: hives, hay fever, allergic rashes, asthma, nonmedication allergies
21. Neurology: *cerebral*—seizures, loss of consciousness, fainting, memory loss, confusion, speech impairment; cranial nerves (covered in review of head and neck systems); *motor*—loss of strength, local paralysis, involuntary movements, loss of coordination; *sensory*—numbness, tingling, pain
22. Psychiatric considerations: depression; anxiety; worries; problems with family, friends, job, or financial matters; difficulty in sleeping

NOTE: The review of body systems is actually the main component of the interview approach to history taking. Fig. 1-1 is an abbreviated form that can be utilized in the dental office.

SOCIAL HISTORY

Developing the social history involves the patient's interactions in three major areas:
1. Environment: present and previous residences, occupations, and climatic exposures
2. Society: education; religion; marital status; living arrangements; financial situation; hours of work, sleep, and daily exercise
3. Drugs: coffee, tea, alcohol, cigarettes, illegal drugs

FAMILY HISTORY

Inquire about the age, medical problems, and, if applicable, cause of death of parents, spouse, siblings, and children. Then ask specifically about the presence in the family of cancer, high blood pressure, heart disease, diabetes, tuberculosis, anemia, bleeding disorders, migraine headaches, seizures, kidney disease, psychiatric problems, allergies, alcoholism, glaucoma, blindness, arthritis, ulcers, or strokes.

2 • PHYSICAL EXAMINATION

David T. Lush and **Geoffrey Lefferts**
Louis F. Rose and **Barry H. Hendler**

The areas covered in the physical examination of the patient are presented in this chapter, and the methods of performing specific parts of the examination are described where appropriate. The material is listed in a systems approach. Some parts of one system may be best examined in the supine position, while other parts of the same system may require the sitting or standing position for adequate analysis. Therefore, in the interests of efficiency for the examiner and convenience for the patient, the examination is not performed in a strictly systems manner. The examiner must be prepared to perform the examination with minimal position change of the patient. This is especially important with the incapacitated patient.

METHODS

Four methods of examination are available:

INSPECTION. This encompasses observing the total patient and then visualizing various areas of the body more closely. It is performed with the patient at rest and during certain maneuvers.

PALPATION. This method involves the use of fingertips for touch, the metacarpophalangeal area of the palms for vibration, and the dorsal aspect of the hand for temperature.

PERCUSSION. Indirect percussion consists of striking the distal interphalangeal joint of the middle finger of one hand with the tip of the middle finger of the other hand. This is used to define the position of certain organs and to analyze the density of tissues. The examiner must be able to distinguish tympany (stomach bubble), hyperresonance (emphysematous lung), resonance (normal lung), dullness (normal liver), and flatness (normal thigh). Direct percussion—tapping the patient directly with the finger—is much less frequently used.

AUSCULTATION. In most instances, auscultation involves listening through the stethoscope. High-pitched sounds are best heard with the diaphragm, and low-pitched sounds with the bellpiece.

PRELIMINARIES

For the purpose of standardization, the examiner should consistently use the patient's right side in performing the examination.

The recording of the physical examination should begin with a brief description of the patient's overall appearance, including references to his general state of health and nutrition and to any distress. Gross abnormalities of posture, facial expression, personal hygiene, and mental status should be noted. This description might be stated as follows: Mr. Jones is a well-developed but moderately obese white male who appears to be in no distress.

SPECIFIC AREAS

VITAL SIGNS. Check blood pressure, pulse, respiration rate, and temperature and record height and weight.

SKIN. Observe turgor, texture (cool, wet), pigmentation, lesions (distribution, configuration, morphology), scars, hair distribution, and nails. Measure turgor by squeezing some skin between the thumb and index finger. When released, the skin should return promptly to its usual place. This is customarily done over the sternum.

HEAD. Check size, shape, lumps, depressions, and hair distribution.

EYES. Examine position, color vision, and visual acuity. Check vision with standard pocket or wall charts.

Visual fields. Position yourself facing the patient at a distance of about 50 cm. Have the patient stare into your left eye with his right eye. Both of you should close the other eye. Bring a target object in from the periphery at different angles, and have the patient tell you when it comes into view. Compare his performance with your own.

Lids. Check motion, swelling, and lesions.

Sclera and conjunctiva. Examine for injection, hemorrhage, or icterus.

Cornea and lens. Check for arcus senilis and for abrasions or opacities.

Pupils. Test equality, roundness, regularity, reaction to light (direct and consensual), and accommodation. Shine a light obliquely into a pupil. Observe for constriction in the same (direct) and opposite (consensual) pupil. Repeat on the other pupil. With the patient looking into the distance, test accommodation by having him change his focus to your finger, which is held about 5 cm from his nose. The normal response is convergence of the eyes and pupillary constriction.

Extraocular movements. Have the patient fixate on your finger as it traces an "H" in the air.

Nystagmus. Observe the eyes in primary position and with some lateral gaze for repetitive movements.

Strabismus. Cover, then uncover, each eye while the patient maintains fixation on an object in the distance. Movement to take up fixation indicates strabismus.

Ophthalmoscopic examination (Fig. 2-1). Check pupil and lens (red reflex, opacities), disc (margins, size of physiologic cup), vessels (size, crossing changes), retina (hemorrhage, exudate), and macula (hemorrhage, exudate). With the ophthalmoscopic lens set at 0 diopters, darken the room and have the patient stare straight into the distance. Examine the patient's right eye with your right eye and with your right hand on the ophthalmoscope, reversing the procedure for his left eye. Beginning at a distance of about 30 cm, find the red reflex, and move slowly closer to the patient's eye. Then adjust the lens setting until the retinal structures come into focus. Find the optic disc. The margins should be distinct, although there may

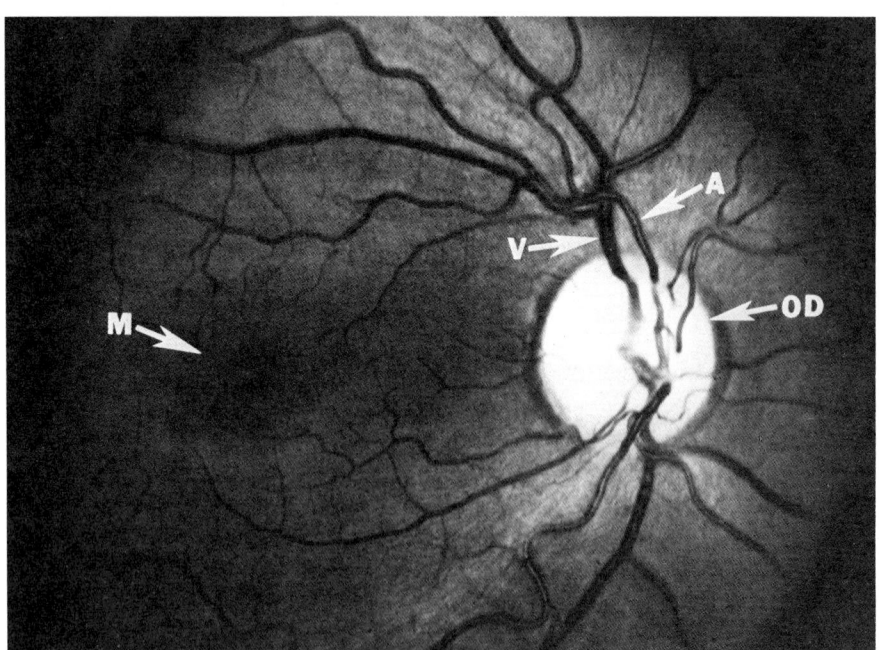

Fig. 2-1. Retina. Note optic disc, *OD*, artery, *A*, vein, *V*, and macula, *M*. Fovea centralis can be seen in center of macula. (Courtesy of W. Tasman, M.D.)

be slight blurring medially. The physiologic cup is a pale area within the disc but on its lateral side. Note its size in relation to the disc as a whole. Next, follow the course of each major vessel from its emergence in the disc, through the disc margin (it should remain in focus), then distally as far as possible. An artery and vein should run together, the vein being larger and darker red. Compare the relative size of the vessels and record this as vein/artery ratio (usually about 5 : 4). Note any focal vessel spasm. Inspect the arteriovenous crossings for any humping, banking, tapering, or nicking. As you follow the course of the vessels, also notice any hemorrhages or exudates in that area of the retina. The location and size of any abnormalities observed can most conveniently be expressed in terms of disc diameters. The macula is located about 2 to 3 disc diameters lateral to the disc. It appears as a small, dark red spot with a central point light reflex. Always examine this area for hemorrhages and exudates. If opacities are noted on initial viewing of the red reflex, the lens can be examined by changing the ophthalmoscope to the short focal-length settings, usually about +12 diopters.

EARS

External. Check deformities and if pain occurs with mild pressure or movement.

Meatus. Examine for cerumen and any discharge, swelling, redness, masses, or foreign bodies.

Otoscopic examination (Fig. 2-2). Assess light reflex, malleus, and drum perforation, bulging, or retraction. When examining the patient's right ear, grip the otoscope in your right hand. With your left hand gently pull the auricle upward and backward. Using the largest one the patient's canal will comfortably accommodate, insert the speculum at a slightly anterior and downward angle. It will eventually be necessary to tilt or rotate the speculum slightly to see as much of the drum and middle ear structures as possible.

Hearing tests. *Spoken and whispered voice:* Testing each ear separately, occlude the other with your finger or the patient's. Test hearing using high-pitch (whisper—512-cycle-per-second [cps] tuning fork) and low-pitch (spoken voice) sounds. Note that the 512-cps fork is used in the ear examination, and the 125-cps fork is used to test vibration sense. *Weber's test:* touch the handle of the vibrating tuning fork against the patient's forehead. The sound should be heard with equal intensity in both ears. *Rinne test:* touch the handle of the vibrating tuning fork to the patient's mastoid process. When the patient can no longer hear this sound, hold the vibrating end near the ear. This air-conducted sound should still be audible, although the bone-conducted sound is not.

NOSE. Check deformities and patency of nostrils. Note mucosal color or swelling, septal deviation or perforation, turbinate swelling or polyps, and sinus tenderness. Compress each nostril and have the patient breathe through the other. The internal structures of the nose are best examined with a nasal speculum, but an otoscope with a short, wide nasal attachment can be used.

MOUTH

Lips. Check color and lesions.

Teeth. Examine for missing or loose teeth, caries, and fillings and check shape and tenderness.

Gums. Note any retraction, discoloration, bleeding, swelling, or inflammation.

Buccal mucosa. Assess color, lesions, and duct openings.

Tongue (dorsum and undersurface). Check color, size, papilla, coating, tremors, lesions, and masses.

Palate. Note color, masses, and petechiae.

Tonsils. Examine pillars, size, and exudate.

Pharynx. Check color, exudate, masses, and gag reflex.

Procedure. Dentures should be removed to allow complete examination of the mouth. Examine the undersurface of the tongue with special care. Have the patient raise his tongue against the roof of his mouth while you inspect anteriorly. Then, with his tongue behind his lower teeth, insert a tongue blade between the lower teeth and push the tongue medially, inspecting this gutter area as far back as the tonsillar pillar.

NECK. Check position, symmetry, and masses.

Muscles. Examine for hypertrophy, atrophy, and tenderness.

Nodes. Assess size, mobility, and tenderness (Fig. 2-

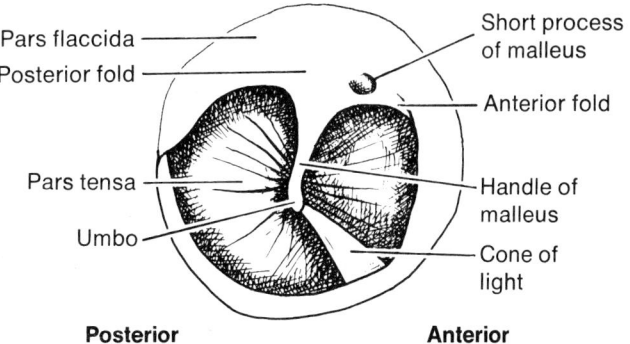

Fig. 2-2. Otoscopic view of tympanic membrane and middle ear structures.

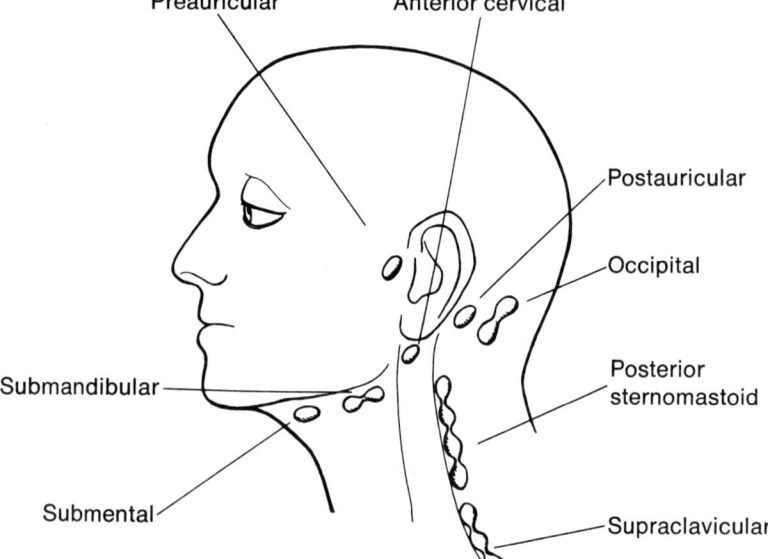

Fig. 2-3. Superficial lymph nodes of neck. (Redrawn from DeGowin, E.L., and DeGowin, R.L.: Bedside diagnostic examination, ed. 2, New York, 1969, Macmillan, Inc.)

3). Palpate the entire neck area for nodes, paying special attention to the area in front of and behind the ear, at the base of the skull, in front of (especially superiorly), under, and behind the sternomastoid muscle, along the underside of the mandible, and behind the head of the clavicle.

Trachea. Check position.

Thyroid gland. Note size, shape, symmetry, nodules, tenderness, and bruits (Fig. 2-4). With the thumb and index finger, begin at the base of the thyroid cartilage and palpate downward until the thyroid isthmus is detected. Ask the patient to swallow and feel the thyroid rise against your fingers. Facing the patient with the index and middle fingers behind his sternomastoid muscle and the thumb anterior to it, palpate the thyroid gland as the thumb of your other hand pushes the thyroid cartilage toward the side being examined.

Jugular venous distention (Fig. 2-5). Observe the external jugular vessels as the patient's position is changed from the sitting to the supine position. Stop at the point where the venous column is visible a few centimeters above the clavicle. The internal jugular pulse is even more reliable but is clinically more difficult to evaluate. The central venous pressure is the distance from the top of the venous column to the right atrium, which is estimated to be at the midpoint of a line drawn from the anterior fourth intercostal space through the back.

Carotid arteries. The carotid pulse should be palpated during head and neck examination, for its importance in assessing cardiac rate and rhythm during a medical emergency is readily apparent. The patient's head should be turned slightly toward the side being examined. One side should be palpated at a time, with the examiner's index and middle fingers at the medial edge of sternocleidomastoid muscle, pressing gently on the carotid artery in the lower half of the neck. Rate and rhythm can be noted as well as amplitude, which is graded on a 0 to 4+ scale. Decreased or absent carotid pulse suggests arterial narrow-

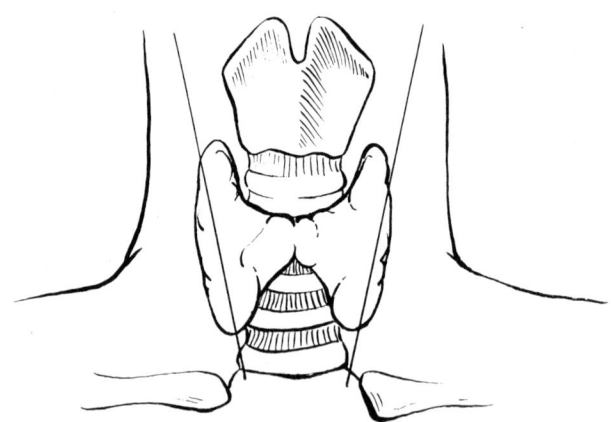

Fig. 2-4. Thyroid gland.

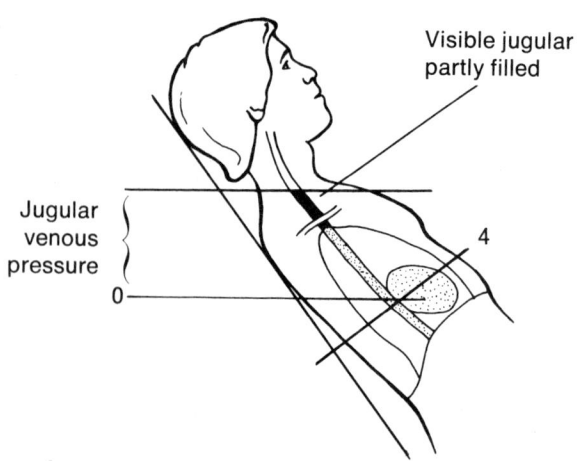

Fig. 2-5. Jugular venous distention (see text). (Redrawn from DeGowin, E.L., and DeGowin, R.L.: Bedside diagnostic examination, ed. 2, New York, 1969, Macmillan, Inc.)

```
                    REGIONAL EXAMINATION

    VITAL SIGNS          BP_____ P_____ R_____

    HEAD AND NECK

    Face—color, expression, lesions, eyes

    Trachea—midline

    Thyroid—enlarged, tender

    Carotids—patent, prominence

    Jugular veins—prominence

    Lymph nodes—palpable

    ORAL CAVITY

    Lips

    Buccal mucosa

    Gingiva

    Floor of mouth

    Tongue

    Hard palate

    Soft palate

    Pharynx

    Gag reflex

    Other
```

Fig. 2-6. Regional examination of head, neck, and oral cavity; baseline readings of vital signs.

ing or occlusion, principally by atherosclerotic plaques.

NOTE: In outpatient dental practice the emphasis of physical examination is often placed on a regional examination of the head, neck, and oral cavity (Fig. 2-6). In addition, every patient who enters the dental office should have baseline vital signs recorded. Without these parameters, the evaluation of a medical emergency would be most perplexing and management could be inappropriate and ineffective.

BREASTS. Assess size, symmetry, venous pattern, tenderness, and masses. With the patient sitting, observe the breasts for retraction or asymmetry, both at rest and while she performs specific maneuvers. Have the patient raise her arms above her head, push her hands firmly against her hips, and lean forward. Then have the patient assume the supine position, with the hand on the side of the breast to be examined behind the head. Examine each quadrant by pressing the breast against the chest wall with the tips of the fingers. It may be necessary to place one hand on the lateral side of the breast for stabilization. Then repeat the examination, this time squeezing the breast between your thumb and index finger. Use your other hand to support the remainder of the breast during this procedure.

Nipple and areola. Check color, lesions, retraction, discharge, and fissures. Squeeze the nipples and observe for discharge.

AXILLAE. Note any lesions, lumps, or nodes. Examine the patient's right axilla with your right hand, controlling the patient's arm position with your left hand on the patient's right wrist. Push your hand deep into the axilla and then let the patient's arm drop lightly over your hand. Use your fingertips to compress axillary contents against ribs.

THORAX. Assess chest size and shape, rib deformities, and any tenderness.

LUNGS

Inspection. Check respiratory rate and rhythm, retraction of interspaces with inspiration, accessory muscles of respiration, and respiratory excursions.

Palpation. Examine for tactile fremitus. The patient should be in the sitting position. Since vibration is being measured, use the metacarpophalangeal area of the palm. Ask the patient to repeat the words "ninety-nine." Using only one hand, begin at the top and compare symmetric areas of the chest as you descend.

Percussion. Check lung resonance, lower borders, and diaphragmatic movement. Percuss symmetric areas of the chest and compare the sounds.

Auscultation. *Breath sounds*—note intensity and inspiratory/expiratory ratio. *Adventitious sounds*—note location, timing, pitch, and persistence after coughing. *Voice sounds*—note loudness, distinctness, and symmetry. Listen to the breath sounds as the patient breathes deeply through his mouth. The inspiratory phase is normally longer than the expiratory phase, except in the area over the manubrium and in the upper interscapular region where the two phases may be about equal. Again, ask the patient to repeat the words "ninety-nine," comparing this time the sounds heard through the stethoscope. Test with both spoken and whispered voice. The sounds should be equal bilaterally and very indistinct. Some abnormalities, such as consolidation, may make these sounds more distinct, while others, such as pleural effusion, make the sounds more distant.

HEART

Inspection. Check apical impulse and other impulses. With the patient in the supine position, look for the apical impulse. This is visibly present in about one fifth of the normal population and is usually located about 1 cm medial to the midclavicular line on the left side in the fifth intercostal space. Then inspect the remainder of the chest wall for other impulses. Impulses medial to the apical impulse in the third to fifth intercostal spaces are from the right ventricle. Note whether the impulse is visible only in the interspaces or if the lower sternum also moves.

Palpation. Note apical impulse, abnormal impulses, palpable heart sounds or rubs, and thrills. Use the palms to palpate over the heart, since findings through vibration more than through touch are being sought. Palpate over visible impulses first. The normal location of the apical impulse, described earlier, is often palpable despite not being visible in the majority of people. Then palpate over the remainder of the precordium. The presence of the right ventricular impulse (location already described) or pulsations over the base of the heart is abnormal. Note the difference between pulsations and vibrations. Vibrations representing palpable murmurs are called thrills. Note their timing by comparing them to the apical impulse or carotid pulse.

Auscultation. Check rate, rhythm, heart sounds, gallops, and murmurs. Auscultation of the heart is also usually performed with the patient in the supine position; changing to other positions brings out specific abnormalities, such as sitting and leaning forward to check for aortic disorders and assuming the left lateral decubitus position for mitral disorders. Listen first over the apex for rate and rhythm. Then sequentially auscultate over the entire precordium for normal heart sounds, then extra heart sounds, and finally murmurs. Move the stethoscope in short steps beginning in the aortic area (right second intercostal space), moving toward the pulmonic area (left second intercostal space), Erb's point (third intercostal space at left sternal border), tricuspid area (fifth intercostal space at left sternal border), mitral area (left fifth intercostal space in midclavicular line), and finally toward the axilla. Repeat this procedure as necessary, evaluating each sound or murmur individually. The apical impulse or the carotid pulse can be used to identify which of the sounds is the first heart sound. Note especially the splitting of the second sound with inspiration in the second left intercostal space. Clearly identify the heart sounds before pursuing other sounds. Distinguish between extra heart sounds (S_3, S_4, click) and murmurs or rubs. Note the timing, location, and pitch of extra sounds. Evaluate murmurs for timing, location, pattern (decrescendo, crescendo, diamond shaped), pitch, quality (blowing, rumbling), radiation, and effect of position change (standing, squatting), and Valsalva maneuver. Intensity is graded on a scale of 1 to 6. The subjectivity of this scale can be minimized by following these guidelines:

Grade 1—very faint and heard only when paying close attention

Grade 2—faint, but unmistakably present

Grade 3—clearly louder than "faint," but not associated with a thrill

Grade 4—loud and associated with a thrill

Grade 5—very loud but requiring the stethoscope partly on the chest

Grade 6—able to be heard with the stethoscope off the chest

ABDOMEN

Inspection. Check contour, pulsations, venous dilation, peristalsis, scars, and masses. With the patient in the supine position, inspect the abdomen from the side, your head at a level only slightly above that of the abdominal surface.

Auscultation. Assess bowel sounds, bruits, and friction rubs. Note that in the abdominal examination, auscultation should precede palpation and percussion.

Palpation. Examine for muscle spasm, tenderness, normal organs, organomegaly, masses, and aorta. Using the fingertips of the right hand, press lightly over all regions of the abdomen. This will help relax the anxious patient and will localize tender areas. Then repeat the examination using deeper palpation. Examine from lower to upper abdomen to avoid missing the liver or spleen edge. Examine the left side first unless it has a history of pain or is tender on light palpation. The quadrant in which symptoms exist should be examined last; if palpation there causes pain, it will be difficult for the patient to relax for palpation of the other abdominal areas. If tenderness is elicited, check for rebound tenderness by pushing in slowly then quickly letting go.

Since the spleen should not be palpated on routine deep palpation, pull up on the patient's left lower thorax with the left hand while pushing the right hand under his lower ribs on the left as the patient inspires deeply. If the spleen is not palpated, feel for the spleen on deep inspiration, with the patient in the right lateral decubitus position with his left knee bent and his right leg straight. Examine the middle upper abdomen for the aortic pulse. Assess the aortic diameter by simultaneously feeling the aorta's left border with the left hand and its right border with the right hand. Put the left hand under the patient at the level of the lower right ribs and pull lightly while the right hand is pressed under the lower right ribs, just lateral to the rectus muscles. As the patient inspires deeply, the liver will descend toward the examining hand. Masses should be evaluated for location, size, shape, consistency, mobility, pulsations, and tenderness.

Percussion. Estimate liver size. Note that liver palpation does not provide any information regarding the location of the upper border of the liver. Therefore percussion is essential to estimate liver size. Percuss the right chest in the midclavicular line from the upper part downward. Identify the site of liver dullness in expiration and mark the chest. Then percuss upward from the right lower quadrant, also in the midclavicular line, making sure to start in an area of unequivocal tympany. Identify the lower border of liver dullness in expiration. The liver normally measures 6 to 12 cm along the midclavicular line.

MALE GENITALIA

Penis. Examine circumcision status, lesions, urethral orifice, and any discharge. Be sure to retract foreskin if the patient is uncircumcised. Squeeze the tip of the penis to try to express discharge.

Scrotum. Check skin lesions, testicular size, tenderness or lumps, nontesticular masses, and hernia. Examine the testes simultaneously between thumb and index finger, then use both hands to examine each testicle individually. The normal adult testicle measures about 5 cm in diameter. If masses are detected, touch your penlight to the posterior surface of the scrotum and observe for transillumination. Follow the course of the spermatic cord superiorly, checking for masses along its path. Have the patient stand and instruct him to bear down. Observe the inguinal area for any bulges. Push the gloved index finger of the right hand through the scrotal skin posterior to the testicle into the right inguinal ring area. Have the patient bear down and note any masses descending to touch the finger. Examine the left side with the left hand.

RECTAL AREA. Check for hemorrhoids, lesions, sphincter tone, anal and rectal wall masses, tenderness, and induration. Also examine prostate size, consistency, or lumps; stool color; and occult blood. The rectal examination is usually performed with the patient in the left lateral decubitus position with his hips flexed. The examination can also be performed with the patient standing and resting his chest on the examining table. The disadvantage of those positions is that abdominal masses tend to fall away from the examining finger; these positions should not be used if there is any reason to suspect an abdominal mass. The supine position is best for detecting abdominal masses.

Insert the gloved index finger into the patient's rectum with the flexor surface facing posteriorly. Examine 90 degrees in each direction and then rotate your position so that the flexor surface of the finger faces anteriorly; then examine that side of the bowel wall. After examining the anterior bowel wall, focus your attention on the prostate gland. The median furrow should be identified; it separates the lateral lobes. The finger should be able to identify the uppermost extent of the prostate. Palpate carefully the entire surface of the gland.

PERIPHERAL VASCULAR SYSTEM. Check for the presence of carotid, radial, femoral, dorsalis pedis, and posterior tibial pulses. Examine their equality, contour, rhythm, and for volume changes and bruits. Grading the strength of pulses is necessarily arbitrary. This is most simply done by designating them normal, diminished, or absent. Examine the carotid pulse in the lower half of the neck so as not to stimulate the carotid sinus.

EXTREMITIES. Check venous pattern, lesions, hair distribution, nails, redness, cyanosis, edema, temperature, and nodes. Check the patient's lower extremities for edema by pressing the thumb firmly over the dorsum of the foot and over the tibia at midankle. If edema is found, check at higher levels as well. If the patient has been supine, check also over the sacrum. Estimate the depth of pitting in millimeters

SPINE. Examine for kyphosis, scoliosis, and lordosis; check range of motion, spinal process tenderness, and local muscle spasm. Test cervical range of motion by observing the patient's ability to extend his neck and to touch ear to shoulder, chin to shoulder, and chin to chest. Evaluate the thoracic spine with trunk rotation and lateral bending. Have the patient attempt to touch his toes to assess lumbar spine motion.

PERIPHERAL JOINTS. Check for redness, swelling, active range of motion, deformity, local muscle atrophy, tenderness, passive range of motion, warmth, and crepitation. Examine each joint individually.

NEUROLOGY

Cranial nerves. Note that the evaluation of the cranial nerves involves many maneuvers already described. Evaluate these nerves by assessing the following functions related to the separate nerves:

I—smell
II—visual acuity, color vision, visual fields
III, IV, VI—extraocular movements, pupil reactions
V—motor; masseter muscle strength, lip tremor (Have the patient bite down while you palpate the masseter muscle for strength and symmetry.)
V—sensory; sensation over face; corneal reflex (Touching the cornea with a piece of gauze should cause blinking.)
VII—motor; asymmetry, tics (Have the patient perform several facial movements, such as exposing the teeth, puffing the cheeks, closing the eyes tightly, and raising the eyebrows, and check for asymmetry.)
VII—sensory; taste
VIII—cochlear; hearing
VIII—vestibular; nystagmus
IX, X—uvula movement, gag reflex
XI—trapezius and sternocleidomastoid strength (Have the patient force his head from the side toward the midline against the resistance of your hand. Note the force generated and use your other hand to feel the tension in the sternocleidomastoid muscle.)
XII—tongue movement, tremor, atrophy

Motor nerves. Check for atrophy, symmetry, and abnormal movements. Assess strength of proximal and distal muscle groups of upper and lower extremities. Strength is measured using an arbitrary scale of 0 to 5:
0—no motion or muscle contraction
1—slight muscle contraction but no joint motion
2—motion without gravity
3—motion against gravity
4—motion against some resistance
5—motion against significant resistance (normal)

Screen for proximal muscle weakness by having the patient hold his arms straight out laterally from the shoulder while you attempt to push his arm down. With the patient lying down, have him flex and then extend his hip against the resistance of your hand. Screen distal muscle strength by having the patient squeeze your hands. Have him flex and then extend his feet against the resistance of your hand.

Sensory nerves. Assess superficial pain, touch, proprioception, vibration, and stereognosis. *Superficial pain*—test ability to distinguish the sharp from the dull end of a safety pin in symmetrical areas. *Touch*—check ability to detect cotton or gauze stimulation. *Proprioception*—holding a finger or toe by its sides (to avoid stimulating pressure sensation), see if the patient can differentiate the flexed from the extended position. *Vibration*—using a 125-cps fork, compare symmetry and sensation (by comparison with yourself) of vibratory sense over superficial bones. *Stereognosis*—place common small objects in the patient's hand (coin, keys, pen) and have him identify them by touch alone.

Deep tendon reflexes. Routine testing should include biceps, triceps, knee, and ankle reflexes. Reflexes can be arbitrarily graded as:
0—no response
1—decreased
2—normal
3—increased
4—clonus

Superficial reflexes. Check abdominal and cremasteric (male) reflexes. *Abdominal reflex*—with the patient in the supine position, stroke his abdomen with a moderately sharp object, such as a key or a reflex hammer handle, from the lateral side toward the midline. There should normally be abdominal muscle contraction on the side of the stimulation, with movement of the umbilicus toward the stimulus. Test both sides, above and below the umbilicus. This reflex may be difficult to elicit in obese patients.

Pathologic reflexes. Test Babinski's sign also with the patient in the supine position and using a moderately sharp stimulus. Lightly stroke the lateral aspect of the sole of the foot vertically from heel to the base of the toes. As you approach the toes, change the course of the stimulation to a medially directed path along the base of the toes toward the great toe. The normal response is plantar flexion of the toes. Be careful not to confuse an abnormal response (dorsiflexion of the great toe, fanning of the other toes, dorsiflexion of the ankle, flexing of the knee and thigh) with a simple withdrawal response.

Brainstem reflexes. Test with the cranial nerves.

Coordination. Observe the patient's gait and his ability to perform rapid alternating movements.

MENTAL STATUS. Assess by noting the following:
Appearance—dress, grooming
Motor behavior—facial expression, posture, poise
Verbal behavior—voice (pitch, intensity), relevance, vocabulary
Mood—emotion, tones
Thought processes—delusions, hallucinations
Cognitive functions—orientation (person, place, time), memory (immediate, distant), general knowledge (name of presidents, large cities), abstraction (proverb interpretation, similarities), calculations (serial sevens), judgment (test questions)

BIBLIOGRAPHY FOR SECTION ONE

Bates, B.: A guide to physical examination, ed. 2, Philadelphia, 1979, J.B. Lippincott Co.

DeGowin, E.L., and DeGowin, R.L.: Bedside diagnostic examination, ed. 2, New York, 1969, Macmillan, Inc.

Delp, M.H., and Manning, R.T.: Physical diagnosis, ed. 8, Philadelphia, 1975, W.B. Saunders Co.

Little, J.W., and King, O.R.: The significance of physical diagnosis, patient history, data, and medical screening in the dental office, Ann. Dent. **3**:31, 42-55, Fall 1972.

Rose, L.F., and Hendler, B.H., editors: Medical emergencies in dental practice, Chicago, 1981, Quintessence Publishing Co.

Section Two
IMMUNOLOGIC AND ALLERGIC DISEASES
edited by **Warren A. Katz** and **Donald Kaye**

3 • IMMUNOLOGIC PRINCIPLES
Donald Kaye and Warren A. Katz

Immunologic reactions are the result of an immune response after exposure to an antigen to which the host has become sensitized. After exposure to an antigen, the host responds by producing antibodies in the form of immunoglobulins and/or by developing cellular (cell-mediated) immunity. Delayed hypersensitivity, such as skin test reactivity to such antigens as tuberculoprotein, is one expression of cellular immunity and is useful in screening for integrity of cellular immune responses. After sensitization, reexposure to the antigen evoking the immune response elicits an inflammatory reaction and tissue injury—the immunologic reaction. The key cell in these responses is the lymphocyte.

The elements of the immune system include the lymphocytic, the phagocytic, and the complement systems. This chapter describes these systems, along with various immunoglobulins and immunologic reactions.

LYMPHOCYTIC SYSTEM

Lymphocytes are derived from the pluripotent bone marrow stem cell and develop into two major cell types. One type originates in the bone marrow but leaves the marrow for the thymus, where it completes its development. After maturing and multiplying in the thymus under the influence of the thymic environment and thymic hormones such as thymopoietin and tymosin, the thymus-derived lymphocyte, or *T cell*, disseminates throughout the body. The other major type of lymphocyte also originates in the marrow; it matures in the marrow and perhaps in other sites and is called a *B cell*.

T lymphocytes mediate cellular immunity, which is important in defense against mycobacteria, viruses, and fungi and is responsible for tumor immunity and homograft rejection. For T cell activation to occur, macrophages must first interact with antigen. Contact of the macrophage, which has antigen on its surface, with T lymphocytes containing the surface receptors for the antigen results in activation of the T cells and proliferation into (1) T cells called *killer T cells* that are cytotoxic and can react with the antigen, such as a tumor cell or a cell containing virus particles, and can destroy the target cell; (2) T cells called *helper T cells* that can release factors that together with the antigen can affect B lymphocytes and cause them to produce antibodies; (3) T cells that after interacting with antigen produce substances called *lymphokines*, which enhance the host response and mediate delayed hypersensitivity (see box); and (4) cells called *suppressor T cells* that down-regulate the immune response and can decrease the response of both T and B lymphocytes.

There is increasing evidence that in order for an antigen to stimulate an immune response, it must be presented to T cells and perhaps also B cells as a complex with (or at least in close proximity to) surface molecules on macrophages that are coded for by genes in the major histocompatibility complex.

In addition, factors secreted by macrophages appear to be important in bringing about normal proliferation of T cells in response to antigens. Thus in recent years an increasingly important role for the macrophage in the afferent limb of the immune response has been envisioned.

B cells are responsible for humoral immunity mediated by antibodies produced by these cells. For B cells to react to an antigen, the antigen must first be "processed" by a macrophage that interacts with helper T cells. When helper factor (released by helper T cells) plus antigen (perhaps on the surfaces of macrophages) interact with mature B cells that have specific surface receptors for

---

Some of the lymphokines produced by activated lymphocytes

migration inhibition factor (MIF)—inhibits migration of macrophages away from the antigen or site of injury; also activates macrophages to make them microbicidal

interferon—prevents infection of noninfected cells by viruses

chemotactic factors—for macrophages, neutrophils, eosinophils, and basophils

mitogenic factors—stimulate lymphocytes

cytotoxic factors—kill cells

transfer factor—transfer delayed (cellular) immunity to an antigen from a sensitive individual to a nonsensitized person; for example, tuberculin reactivity the antigen, the B cells are stimulated to differentiate and multiply to yield an expanded clone of specific B cells, some of which further differentiate into plasma cells that produce large amounts of antibody specific for the offending immunogen. Exposure of a B lymphocyte to an antigen is unlikely to result in development of antibody-producing cells unless there is also interaction with a helper T cell or a macrophage or both. The responses to different antigens vary in their degree of requirement for helper T-cell activity. Thus some antigens are referred to as thymic (T-cell) dependent and others as thymic independent. These should be understood to be relative rather than absolute distinctions. Antibodies may act in a variety of ways. They may neutralize an antigen, such as viruses; they may coat the antigen to promote phagocytosis (opsonization); or they may bind complement, markedly augmenting phagocytosis. Binding of complement may also lyse the antigen. Furthermore, the interaction with complement generates pharmacologically active fragments of complement that dilate blood vessels, increase vascular permeability, and attract polymorphonuclear leukocytes. In this way an acute inflammatory reaction is produced, and the killing of bacteria proceeds efficiently.

B and T cells cannot be distinguished microscopically. However, B cells, which constitute 10% to 15% of the circulating lymphocyte population, can be shown to have immunoglobulin on their surfaces and to possess receptors for the Fc portion of immunoglobulin of the IgG class and for C3b, a fragment of one of the elements of the complement system. T cells, which form about 85% of the circulating lymphocyte population, have little or no demonstrable surface membrane immunoglobulin or receptor for complement, but some have receptors for the Fc portion of IgM (mainly helper T cells) or IgG (mainly suppressor T cells). Moreover, T cells, but not B cells, form rosettes with sheep red blood cells, a useful distinguishing characteristic. Lymphocytes that have no immunoglobulin on the surface and do not form rosettes are called *null cells*. B and T cells react differently during in vitro tests to various mitogens derived from plant proteins, such as pokeweed mitogen, concanavalin A, and phytohemagglutinin. The in vitro blastogenic responses to these stimulants and to specific antigens are useful in assessing the functional integrity of immune responses.

IMMUNOGLOBULINS

The immunoglobulins produced by B cells may be divided into five major classes: IgG, IgM, IgA, IgD, and IgE. IgG can be further divided into four subclasses: IgG1, IgG2, IgG3, and IgG4. The basic structure of the immunoglobulins is shown in Fig. 3-1. There are two heavy (H) polypeptide chains and two light (L) polypeptide chains, which are held together by disulfide bonds. The H chain is about twice as long as the L chain. One end of the H and L chains (Fab) is highly variable in amino acid sequence

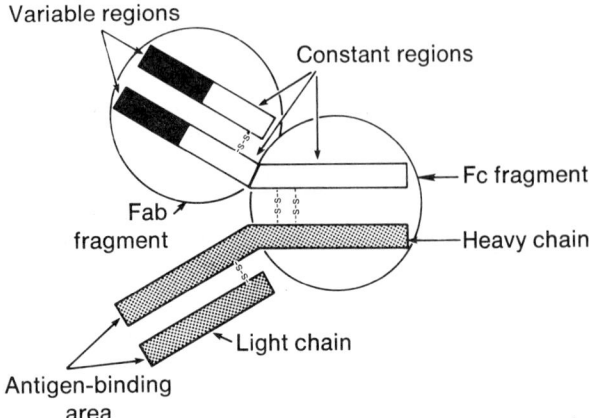

Fig. 3-1. Basic four-chain molecule of immunoglobulins (see text).

and combines with antigen. The extreme variability in structure undoubtedly accounts for the ability to respond with specific immunoglobulin production to an enormous number of different antigens. The other end of the chains (Fc) is constant in structure and does not directly participate in antigen binding; rather it participates in attachment of the antigen-antibody complex to the cell membrane, complement activation, and transfer across the placenta. Light chains are of two types: κ and λ. The heavy chains are specific for the five immunoglobulin classes. The four-chain basic structure can be split enzymatically into one Fc and two Fab fragments. The Fab fragments contain the antigen-combining sites, and the Fc fragment is active in complement fixation and binding to cell membranes.

IgG (and probably IgD and IgE) appears as a four-chain molecule (Fig. 3-1) and is a 7S protein. IgM also has a basic four-chain structure and is polymerized into a macroglobulin of five such four-chain units, forming a 19S protein (Fig. 3-2). IgA is either a four-chain 7S molecule or a polymer of larger size. Polymerized immunoglobulins are held together with J chains. IgG crosses the placenta, whereas IgM and IgA do not.

IgG constitutes about 75% of the serum immunoglobulins. It is the only immunoglobulin that crosses the placenta. It can fix complement, and the Fc fragment of IgG will bind to phagocytic cells. It is a major defense against invading organisms by virtue of its opsonizing and complement-fixing activities.

IgM accounts for about 10% of serum immunoglobulins. It is extremely efficient in fixing complement. IgM production predominates early in response to antigenic stimulation. Later, IgG production predominates. This difference in host response is often helpful in distinguishing recent from more distant infection. IgM is a major defense against invading microorganisms and is also an important cell surface antigen receptor on B lymphocytes. Anti-A or anti-B blood group antibody is IgM. It has been suggested that IgG antibody inhibits formation of IgM through mechanisms not yet clearly defined.

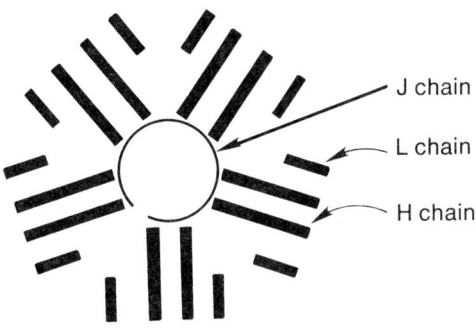

Fig. 3-2. IgM molecule composed of five four-chain immunoglobulin molecules polymerized into a macroglobulin. Four-chain molecules are held together by a J chain.

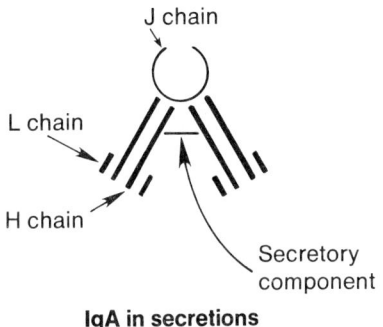

IgA in secretions

Fig. 3-3. IgA molecule composed of two four-chain molecules held together by a J chain and another molecule called secretory component, which is found only in secretions.

IgA constitutes about 15% of serum immunoglobulins. It is the predominant antibody in secretions, consisting of two four-chain units and attached to a protein called secretory component, which is produced by epithelial cells (Fig. 3-3). It probably coats viruses and bacteria and prevents attachment to mucosal surfaces so that penetration cannot occur.

IgD is found in serum only in small amounts, representing 0.2% of immunoglobulins. It is probably important as an antigen receptor on B lymphocytes.

IgE, called reagin, is also found in serum in only trace amounts. It binds to tissue mast cells and basophils. When mast cell–bound IgE combines with an antigen, the mast cell releases histamine and other vasoactive substances. This mechanism is responsible for many allergic reactions. Both IgA and IgE are synthesized locally in tissues.

PHAGOCYTIC SYSTEM

The phagocytic system includes polymorphonuclear leukocytes and the monocyte-macrophage system. These cells mobilize to the site of injury or microbial invasion, then ingest and degrade or destroy antigen. They also elaborate materials, such as enzymes, that participate in the inflammatory response. Fixed macrophages in the liver, spleen, lung, and other sites (the reticuloendothelial system) are also part of the phagocytic system. They phagocytize antigen present in the blood or alveoli. Macrophages also process antigen in the development of both humoral and cellular immunity.

COMPLEMENT SYSTEM

The complement system is composed of circulating blood proteins (C1 to C9) that react in a specific sequence, or cascade, when activated. Activation of the complement system can result in direct destruction of cells (bacteria, viruses, erythrocytes), attraction of white blood cells (chemotaxis), release of histamine (anaphylatoxin activity), and kinin activity, which causes increased vascular permeability and smooth muscle contraction.

There are two pathways by which the complement system can be activated: the *classic pathway* and the *alternative pathway,* or properdin pathway. The two pathways differ in the sequence leading to activation of C3; thereafter the sequence is the same (Fig. 3-4).

The *classic pathway* is activated by antigen-antibody (IgG1, IgG2, IgG3, or IgM) complexes, trypsinlike enzymes, and staphylococcal protein A. Activation of C1, composed of the three proteins C1q, C1r, C1s, results in the formation of serine esterase, an enzyme that acts on C2 and C4 to form a complex proteolytic enzyme, $\overline{C1,4,2}$ (the bar indicates enzymatic activity), that adheres to the cell membrane. $\overline{C1,4,2}$ then cleaves C3 into C3a and C3b; the latter forms enzyme $\overline{C1,4,2,3b}$ on the membrane. C3b has an affinity for receptors on phagocytes.

The *alternative pathway* may be activated by IgA, possibly IgE, and occasionally IgG. It can also be activated by trypsinlike enzymes, polysaccharides, lipopolysaccharides (endotoxin, part of the cell wall of gram-negative bacilli), and cobra venom. In this pathway C3 is activated directly to C3b, some of which complexes with proteins (different from those in the classic pathway) and is fixed on the cell membrane. This complex then activates more C3 (amplification system).

The next step in both pathways is activation of C5. C5 is cleaved by $\overline{C1,4,2,3b}$ (the classic pathway) or the $\overline{C3b}$ complex (the alternative pathway), resulting in formation of C5a and C5b. C5b binds C6 and C7, forming $\overline{C5b,6,7}$. Thereafter C8 and C9 are bound, resulting in $\overline{C5b,6,7,8,9}$, which lyses the membrane.

Natural inhibitors of activation exist at many stages of the cascade, such as $\overline{C1}$ esterase inhibitor and C3b inactivator. The well-known $\overline{C1}$ esterase inhibitor is absent in patients with hereditary angioedema.

C3a and C5a are products of the reaction sequence and cause release of histamine from mast cells (anaphylatoxin activity). C3a has kinin activity, C5a causes release of enzymes from lysosomes, and C5a has chemotactic activity, attracting leukocytes, particularly polymorphonuclear ones. $\overline{C5b,6,7}$ also has chemotactic activity.

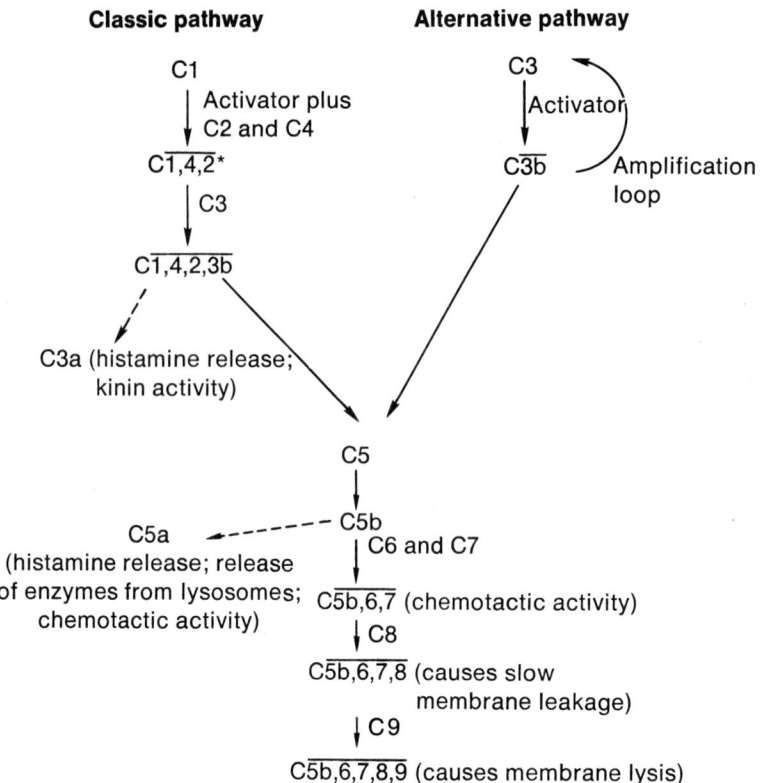

Fig. 3-4. Complement system can be activated by classic pathway or alternative pathway (see text). *Bar indicates activated substance with enzymatic activity.

TYPES OF IMMUNOLOGIC REACTIONS

According to the Gell and Coombs classification, there are four types of immunologic tissue damage. This classification, although useful, is somewhat arbitrary. In most situations complex combinations of mechanisms are operative.

Type I reactions

Type I reactions, also called immediate or anaphylactic hypersensitivity reactions, occur within minutes after exposure to an allergen. Allergic rhinitis, hay fever, asthma, urticaria, and generalized anaphylaxis fall into this group. In this reaction antibodies (usually IgE) become fixed to basophils and tissue mast cells by the Fc fragment. When the antibodies combine with antigen, these cells release chemical mediators, which cause the clinical manifestations. The allergic reaction follows combination of the cell-associated or cytotropic IgE (reagin) with the specific allergen (for example, ragweed pollen). Some of the mediators released are histamine, serotonin, kinins, eosinophil chemotactic factor, slow-reacting substance of anaphylaxis (SRS-A), and platelet activating factor. These mediators act on the shock organs, producing the clinical manifestations. There is evidence that eosinophils, which are attracted to sites of IgE-mediated reactions by eosinophil chemotactic factor released from mast cells, serve to down-regulate the reaction. Thus eosinophils release histaminase that destroys histamine, arylsulfatase that destroys SRS-A, and phospholipase that destroys platelet activating factor.

Type II reactions

Type II reactions, or cytotoxic reactions, involve combination of IgG or IgM antibody with antigenic constituents on cell membranes, either as a part of the cell membrane or as an antigen fixed to the cell. Cytotoxicity may be mediated either via complement fixation (with destruction of the cell) or via phagocytosis (when leukocytes become bound to the Fc portion of the antibody). Examples of type II reactions are immune hemolytic anemias, idiopathic thrombocytopenia, and acute kidney graft rejection.

Type III reactions

Type III reactions result from localization of antigen-antibody complexes in vessels or tissues, causing vasculitis or other tissue damage. Complement is fixed and phagocytes are attracted. There is release of vasoactive amines, an increase of vascular permeability, and release of lysosomal enzymes from leukocytes, all resulting in tissue damage. Examples of type III reactions include types of immune-complex reactions, such as the Arthus reaction (local swelling at the site of antigen injection occurring several hours later), serum sickness, autoimmune glomerulonephritis, and lupus nephritis. In these conditions antibody combines with an often unknown antigen intravascularly and the immune complex is deposited in blood vessels, provoking the inflammatory reaction and tissue injury.

Type IV reactions

Type IV reactions, or cell-mediated immune reactions (the delayed type of hypersensitivity), occur when T cells and macrophages produce direct cellular injury. Neither antibody nor complement is involved. Type IV reactions include the delayed skin test (develops over 24 to 48 hours), contact dermatitis, tumor immunity, aspects of graft-versus-host disease, and homograft rejection. In this reaction antigen is bound to T cells with the appropriate specific antigen receptors. Lymphokines are released from the T cells, which attract phagocytes, induce mitogenesis in lymphocytes, and activate macrophages. The result is inflammation and tissue injury at the site of the antigen. The clinical reaction does not begin for several hours and peaks at 2 to 3 days.

Sensitive patients may exhibit any combination of the four types of reactions. For example, immunologic reactions to penicillin can produce anaphylaxis (type I), hemolytic anemia (type II), a serum sickness–like illness (type III), and delayed hypersensitivity (type IV).

• • •

Other reactions that do not produce tissue damage occur when antibodies interact with hormones or other biologically active molecules or with receptors for these molecules and either activate or block a process. Examples include long-acting thyroid stimulator (LATS), which is an antibody to the thyrotropin receptor in thyroid disease, antibodies to intrinsic factor in pernicious anemia, anti–acetylcholine receptor antibody in myasthenia gravis, anti-insulin antibody or antibodies to the insulin receptor in some diabetics, antibodies to the β-adrenergic receptor in some patients with asthma, and blocking antibodies that inhibit the interaction of the antigen with antibodies of a different class (for example, IgG antibody blocking IgE interaction with an allergen).

AUTOIMMUNITY

Some people develop antibodies against autologous antigens. These antibodies may cause little or no observable injury or may result in disease. Some examples of autoantibodies are antiplatelet antibody in idiopathic thrombocytopenic purpura, anti–red cell antibody in acquired hemolytic anemia, anti–acetylcholine receptor antibody in myasthenia gravis, antithyroid antibody in Hashimoto's disease, anti-γ-globulin antibody (rheumatoid factor) in rheumatoid arthritis, and anti-DNA and antinuclear antibodies in systemic lupus erythematosus. Autoimmune diseases affect mainly young adults with a preponderance of women. This is in contrast to the incidence of autoantibodies, which increases in the aged in the absence of apparent autoimmune disease. Thus the diagnostic significance of detecting autoantibodies is very different in old and young subjects. It must be emphasized that the mere presence of autoantibodies does not mean that they are causing pathologic consequences such as autoimmune disease.

IMMUNE-COMPLEX DISEASE

Deposition of antibody-antigen complexes in blood vessels produces a type III reaction in the organ. This is the main mechanism of disease production in lupus nephritis and poststreptococcal glomerulonephritis. Many of the manifestations of infective endocarditis are thought to occur on an immune-complex basis, such as glomerulonephritis, petechiae, and arthritis. Patients who have persistent antigenemia with the surface antigen of hepatitis B virus may develop a polyarteritis-like syndrome related to circulating immune complexes.

GRAFT-VERSUS-HOST DISEASE

In animals graft-versus-host disease occurs when immunocompetent foreign lymphoid cells are transplanted into a genetically dissimilar immunoincompetent host. This syndrome may occur in persons who have received bone marrow grafts or in immunodeficient patients who have received transfusions of fresh blood. Skin lesions (ulceration, thickening, and loss of hair), edema, cardiac disease, hepatic lesions, joint lesions, and hemolytic anemia have all been described in relation to this disease.

BIBLIOGRAPHY

Bellanti, J.A.: Immunology, ed. 2, Philadelphia, 1978, W.B. Saunders Co.
Fudenberg, H.H., and others, editors: Basic and clinical immunology, Los Altos, Calif., 1980, Lange Medical Publications.
Gell, P.G.H., Coombs, R.R.A., and Lachmann, P.J., editors: Clinical aspects of immunology, ed. 3, Oxford, 1975, Blackwell Scientific Publications.
Katz, D.H.: Lymphocyte differentiation, recognition and regulation, New York, 1977, Academic Press, Inc.
Samter, M., editor: Immunological diseases, ed. 3, Boston, 1978, Little, Brown & Co.
Stobo, J.D.: Basic mechanisms of immunity, Hosp. Med., July 1980, p.22.

4 • ATOPIC DISEASE

Gregory W. Siskind

The term "atopy" refers to a predisposition to develop IgE-mediated allergic reactions to environmental antigens (often referred to as allergens). This predisposition to allergies affects roughly 15% of the population and appears to have a genetic basis, although no simple inheritance pattern has been identified. The tendency to manufacture

IgE in response to environmental allergens is most often manifested clinically as rhinitis (hay fever), asthma, or urticaria. The nature of the manifestation (that is, asthma or hay fever) also appears to be influenced by genetic factors, since familial clustering of symptom patterns has been described. IgE-mediated allergic reactions are clearly not the only cause of rhinitis, asthma, and urticaria; they are the sole etiologic factor in only a minority of cases. When IgE-mediated allergic reactions are involved, the mechanism for generating symptoms is the type I reaction described in Chapter 3. It must be remembered that other immunologic mechanisms can also cause urticaria and asthma.

Childhood (atopic) eczema is a characteristic feature of the atopic state. Nearly half the children with atopic eczema have asthma with or without other allergies as they grow older. Many atopic adults have a history of eczema in infancy and childhood. Children with atopic eczema have high serum IgE levels and often have multiple food allergies. In addition, several metabolic abnormalities have been demonstrated in these patients. Elimination of foods to which a patient appears to be allergic results in improvement of symptoms in childhood atopic eczema. However, the condition is usually not completely controlled by rigorous dietary regulation. As the child grows older, he is often able to tolerate foods to which he previously appeared to be allergic. The mechanism for this change in clinical sensitivity is unknown, but it may be related to changes in absorption or digestion of foods. The relationship between atopic eczema and the IgE-mediated manifestations of the atopic state is not fully understood, but the association is unequivocal. In the adult there is no convincing evidence that eczema is caused by an IgE-mediated mechanism.

The predisposition to produce IgE antibodies manifested by atopic persons appears to be related mainly to antigens presented repeatedly, usually in relatively low concentration, across a mucosal membrane (nasal, tracheobronchial, or gastrointestinal). It is not clear whether such patients have an increased tendency to produce IgE antibodies to parenterally administered allergens. Observations have suggested that atopic persons are no more likely to develop IgE antibodies to penicillin than are nonatopic persons.

RHINITIS

CLINICAL MANIFESTATIONS, CLASSIFICATION, AND PATHOGENESIS. Rhinitis is characterized by nasal congestion and rhinorrhea. The patients complain of stuffiness or running of the nose. Rhinitis may be associated with sneezing, itching of the nose and sometimes also of the eyes, throat, and ears, conjunctivitis that is usually mild, postnasal drip, and signs and symptoms of sinusitis. The physical findings include swollen nasal mucosa that may be pale, grayish, or inflamed and increased nasal secretions that vary from clear and watery to frankly purulent. Rhinitis can be classified as allergic, vasomotor, infectious, or medicamentosum.

Allergic rhinitis. In allergic rhinitis the pathogenetic mechanism is a type I, IgE-mediated, immunologic reaction to inhaled organic substances (see Chapter 3). The allergens commonly involved are animal danders (epithelial flakes), tree, grass, weed, or other pollens, and mold spores. The severity of the symptoms presumably depends on a large number of poorly understood factors including the concentration and affinity of the allergen-specific IgE, IgG, and IgA antibodies, the extent of transport of antibodies of different isotypes (classes) from serum to nasal secretions, the concentration and isotype of locally produced antibodies, the number of allergens to which the patient has IgE antibodies and to which the patient is simultaneously exposed, the structure of the nasal passages as it influences airflow patterns, the permeability of the nasal mucosa, the baseline rate of production and the consistency of the nasal secretions, and the physiologic state (responsiveness to stimuli) of the nasal vasculature and mucus-secreting cells. Other factors affecting the severity of symptoms include the concentration of allergens to which the patient is exposed, which is influenced by both the concentration of allergens in the environment and the patient's breathing pattern; the number of allergens to which the patient is exposed simultaneously; the frequency of exposure to an allergen; and simultaneous exposure to an allergen and any of numerous irritants such as perfume, smoke, or organic solvents. With frequent exposure, as occurs during a normal pollen season, the patient's sensitivity changes and the concentration of allergen required to elicit a given degree of symptoms decreases.

Vasomotor rhinitis. Vasomotor rhinitis occurs in a large group of patients whose symptoms appear to reflect hyperresponsiveness of their nasal mucosa to a wide variety of chemical and physical irritants. Sudden changes in temperature (as occur when going from the cold outdoors into a heated room) and numerous irritants such as dust, perfumes, smoke, strong odors, organic solvents, gas vapors, soap powders, and ammonia bring on nasal congestion, paroxysmal sneezing, and watery nasal discharge. The symptoms may be essentially continuous with exacerbation following exposure to irritants, or they may occur only after exposure to irritants. Vasomotor rhinitis appears to represent an unusually vigorous response of a normal host defense mechanism, aimed at removing a noxious agent or preventing it from entering the nasal passages. At a high enough concentration most substances that elicit vasomotor rhinitis cause the same symptoms in all persons. Patients who manifest vasomotor rhinitis appear to have a more vigorous response to these substances, which occurs at concentrations of the irritant that are too low to affect the average person. In some cases the release of mediators from mast cells by poorly understood nonallergic mechanisms appears to underlie the generation of symptoms.

Infectious rhinitis. In infectious rhinitis patients have hyperplastic sinusitis, purulent nasal secretions, infiltrates of neutrophils in their nasal mucosa, and a variety of organisms (most often staphylococci, streptococci, or pneumococci) detected in culture specimens of their nasal membranes and sinuses. It has been suggested that rhinitis in these patients is caused by a chronic bacterial infection of the nasal membranes, perhaps complicated by an allergic reaction to products of the infecting bacteria. There is, however, no adequate evidence to support this concept. Autogenous and stock bacterial vaccines have not been shown to be efficacious in treatment of these patients, and the role of infection in causing chronic rhinitis is still unclear.

Rhinitis medicamentosum. Rhinitis medicamentosum results from the irritant effects of nasal medications, usually nose drops. It is most often seen in patients who have had rhinitis of allergic, vasomotor, or infectious origin and have treated it with nose drops. The palliative effect of the nose drops is often followed by a rebound in which greater congestion occurs, the patient uses more nose drops, and a vicious circle of increasing symptoms and increasing use of nose drops is established.

DIAGNOSIS. The diagnosis of rhinitis is based primarily on a detailed history of the conditions associated with the symptoms. A seasonal history or symptoms occurring after exposure to a particular species of animal such as a cat or dog suggest an allergic basis. The seasonal distribution of symptoms provides clues as to the probable offending allergen (such as ragweed hay fever in the fall). The time of appearance of different pollens and the nature of the dominant allergenic pollens vary from place to place. Sneezing, conjunctival symptoms, and itching of the nose, throat, and eyes occur more commonly in allergic rhinitis. Patients with allergic rhinitis have a greater incidence of other allergic manifestations such as food allergies and childhood eczema. A family history of allergies is also useful in diagnosing allergic rhinitis. Perennial symptoms, without seasonal exacerbation, and an association of symptoms with exposure to the types of irritants previously noted suggest vasomotor rhinitis. However, certain allergens such as dog dander may be present throughout the year and can therefore induce perennial symptoms. Rhinitis medicamentosum is diagnosed on the basis of a history of nose drop abuse or habitual use of some other local medication or drug. Infectious rhinitis is suggested by the presence of an inflamed nasal mucosa and purulent nasal secretions.

LABORATORY FINDINGS. Laboratory tests are of limited value in confirming the diagnosis of rhinitis. Moderate eosinophilia and an abundance of eosinophils in the nasal secretions suggests an allergic basis. However, similar findings are often present in vasomotor rhinitis. An elevated serum IgE level suggests that the patient is atopic and makes an allergic basis for the rhinitis more likely but does not prove that the symptoms have an allergic origin. In many patients with rhinitis, multiple mechanisms are involved in the generation of symptoms. For example, a patient with perennial vasomotor rhinitis may have an exacerbation of symptoms in the spring or fall because of a superimposed allergic reaction to pollens.

If allergic rhinitis is suggested by the patient's history, the specific allergens involved can be identified by skin tests or by the radioallergosorbent test (RAST). Other types of tests are sometimes employed, including scratch, prick, and provocative intranasal challenge; since the overall significance of these procedures is similar to that of the more common intradermal skin test, they will not be discussed here. Skin testing is most often performed by injecting approximately 0.02 ml of a low concentration of the suspected allergen intradermally, generally into the outer aspect of the upper arm. After 15 to 20 minutes the diameter of any wheal formed at the site of injection is measured. A wheal 5 mm or greater in diameter is generally regarded as a positive reaction. A positive skin test indicates the presence of IgE antibodies specific for antigens in the skin test preparation. It should be emphasized that positive results of a skin test can be seen in persons who have no symptoms after exposure to the allergen in question. Therefore, the presence of IgE antibodies does not in itself mean that symptoms will occur following exposure to the allergen under the usual conditions. This is why the diagnosis of a specific allergy is based on the patient's history rather than on skin test results. Skin tests should be regarded as merely confirmatory and not diagnostic. Their primary importance is in patients who are candidates for immunotherapy (hyposensitization) (see "Management"), and patients who are not being considered for immunotherapy should not be subjected to extensive skin testing. When the history does not provide a definitive diagnosis, especially in patients who seem to have combined vasomotor and allergic rhinitis, skin tests may be helpful diagnostically because multiple positive reactions make an allergic origin more likely.

The RAST, a radioimmunoassay for specific IgE antibodies, has recently become popular. The significance of a positive assay is essentially identical to that of a positive skin test; the RAST provides no more diagnostic information than does a skin test. The advantages of the RAST over the routine skin test are the following:

1. *Ease of performance.* The RAST requires no technical skill because it is performed by a commercial laboratory on a serum sample.
2. *Patient comfort.* Multiple intradermal injections are unnecessary, which is especially important with young children.
3. *Special patient problems.* The RAST is useful for patients with disseminated skin lesions who lack sites for intradermal testing and for patients whose

skin fails to form a wheal in response to histamine. (These patients can be identified during skin testing because they have a negative reaction to a skin test with histamine; this occurs very rarely and many such patients have normal skin reactions to specific allergens.)

4. *Safety.* There is an extremely small possibility of an anaphylactic reaction in response to the intradermally injected allergen.

The advantages of the skin test over the RAST are the following:

1. *Sensitivity.* The skin test is more sensitive than the RAST, which more often yields false negative results.
2. *Specificity.* Available allergen preparations are generally crude extracts that vary quantitatively from lot to lot. A positive result of a skin test indicates that the patient has antibody to an allergen in the preparation used, whereas a positive RAST indicates that the patient has antibody to something in the laboratory's preparation but does not indicate if that allergen is actually present in significant amounts in the skin test preparation. This could have negative implications for immunotherapy if the skin test preparation is used.
3. *Cost.* If multiple tests are to be performed, skin testing is significantly less expensive.

It is probable that the best test is an inhalation challenge with an appropriate allergen preparation and observation for the appearance of symptoms, but to perform such challenges properly is difficult, time consuming, and expensive. They are therefore rarely used except for research purposes. Skin testing is preferred in all but a few cases.

Some comment should be made regarding tests for food allergies, even though such allergies are more germane to a discussion of urticaria (see Chapter 5). Skin tests for food allergies have proved unreliable; there is a high incidence of false positive reactions, and perhaps false negative reactions also occur. The false positive reactions may be caused by the presence of nonspecific irritants in the crude extracts used for testing or to the presence of IgE antibodies in the patient that are not clinically significant. The false negative results probably occur when extracts used for testing do not contain the same allergens the patient absorbs after cooking and digesting food.

Cytotoxicity testing, which involves observing a change in the microscopic morphology of leukocytes following exposure to an allergen, has not proved to be a reproducible procedure.

MANAGEMENT

Allergic rhinitis. Eliminating or reducing the concentration of the offending allergen leads to marked improvement, but this approach is often not practical.

The primary treatment of allergic rhinitis is antihistamine medication. The main side effect of these medications is sedation. Although some generalizations can be made (for example, diphenhydramine [Benadryl] is highly sedative, whereas chlorpheniramine maleate [Chlor-Trimeton] causes little sedation), individual responses differ widely; a trial with a variety of antihistamines ultimately determines the best one for a given patient. Some patients are effectively treated with occasional use of antihistamines when their symptoms are severe; however, most patients seem to do best with continuous use of antihistamines throughout their "allergy season."

Corticosteroids are highly effective in eliminating symptoms of allergic rhinitis. The serious side effects of these medications, when administered systemically, make teir use in this relatively benign disease undesirable. However, when symptoms are extremely severe and of short duration such as 1 month, a brief course of systemic steroids can occasionally be justified. Administration of steroids locally by nasal spray (for example, Turbinaire Decadron) is also effective and reduces some of the complications of systemic steroids. Steroids are, however, absorbed across the nasal mucosa and can have systemic effects. Recently steroid preparations that are absorbed to a lesser extent or are degraded rapidly after absorption have become available for nasal administration.

Immunotherapy (also referred to as hyposensitization) is useful for patients whose symptoms are severe and cannot be controlled by antihistamines. The procedure involves weekly injections of allergen in increasing doses. After a high dosage is achieved, the interval between injections is extended gradually until treatment is given once a month. If improvement is to occur, it usually does so within 2 years. However, some patients do not improve for up to 4 to 5 years. Therapy is discontinued after improvement and then 3 years of minimal or no symptoms or after 5 years with no improvement. Following successful immunotherapy, symptoms often do not recur or recur only mildly, and no further treatment is required. If symptoms return and are severe enough to warrant therapy, immunotherapy can be reinstituted. Double-blind studies have documented the efficacy of immunotherapy in the treatment of allergies to pollens. The degree of improvement varies, and rarely are symptoms totally eliminated. There is currently no way of predicting which patients will benefit. Immunotherapy is ineffective in the treatment of food allergies. Allergies to the dander (epithelial flakes) of household pets are a common problem. Immunotherapy for this condition has not generally proved effective in improving symptoms, probably because the concentration of allergen in the home environment is so high.

The mechanism of hyposensitization has been extensively studied but is still incompletely understood. At least two factors appear to be involved: (1) the stimulation of specific suppressor T cells that depress the IgE response to the offending allergen, and (2) the stimulation of production of IgG antibodies specific for the offending allergen. These so-called blocking antibodies appear to act by two mechanisms: (1) they compete with IgE antibodies on mast cells for available antigen, thereby preventing the elicitation of symptoms, and (2) they bind antigen, thus blocking it from stimulating further IgE antibody production and preventing the usual seasonal boost in specific IgE antibodies.

Eliminating the allergen from the environment or reducing its concentration is generally the most effective method of alleviating symptoms. Often, however, this is not a practical approach. Drug therapy with antihistamines and steroids is next in order of effectiveness. Immunotherapy is, in general, the least effective of the routinely employed approaches to the treatment of allergic rhinitis.

Vasomotor rhinitis. The treatment of vasomotor rhinitis generally relies on antihistamines and avoidance, if possible, of the inciting irritants. In view of the chronicity of the symptoms, systemic steroids should usually not be administered, although the use of local steroids may at times be justified. Similarly, the use of nose drops should usually be avoided since, although they provide temporary relief, their habitual use tends to be locally irritating, thereby exacerbating the problem.

Infectious rhinitis. The approach to infectious rhinitis is similar to that used for allergic rhinitis, but antibiotic therapy is often administered in addition. The effectiveness of the antibiotics has been difficult to evaluate.

Rhinitis medicamentosum. Rhinitis medicamentosum is treated by terminating the regular use of nose drops. A short course (7 to 10 days) of local steroid treatment is useful to control symptoms while nose drops are being discontinued.

ASTHMA OF ALLERGIC ETIOLOGY

Asthma is a common disorder, affecting nearly 5% of the population. The term "asthma" refers to a group of diseases characterized by wheezing, coughing, and dyspnea. The cause is narrowing of the air passages as a consequence of bronchoconstriction, mucosal edema, increased thick bronchial secretions, or some combination of these factors. A number of different etiologic factors and pathogenetic mechanisms can lead to airway narrowing with signs and symptoms of asthma.

CLINICAL MANIFESTATIONS, CLASSIFICATION, AND PATHOGENESIS. The major symptom of asthma is wheezing. In addition, the patient may complain of a heaviness in the chest, shortness of breath, especially on exertion, cough with or without sputum production, and a sense of anxiety or air hunger. A conventional but not completely satisfactory classification of asthma divides it into intrinsic and extrinsic forms. Extrinsic asthma is considered to be IgE mediated and caused purely by allergic reactions to substances in the environment. Intrinsic asthma includes asthma caused by all other (nonallergic) mechanisms and is discussed in Chapter 130. The majority of patients with asthma appear to have multiple etiologic factors combining to cause symptoms. Factors that may be involved include allergies, infection (bronchitis), hyperresponsiveness of bronchi to nonspecific irritants or to cold, increased vagal tone, relative β-adrenergic blockade, alterations in the cyclic AMP system, and psychologic factors. Allergic factors appear to predominate in a relatively small proportion of asthma patients, although they may contribute to the disease process in a somewhat larger group. Immunologic mechanisms also play major causative roles in occupational asthma, hypersensitivity pneumonitis, and bronchopulmonary aspergillosis. These conditions are discussed in Chapters 130 and 132.

The pathogenesis of allergic asthma is a type I mechanism similar to that of allergic rhinitis except that the site of reaction is the bronchi and bronchioles.

Some patients exhibit symptoms only during exercise or have symptoms exacerbated by exercise. This exercise-induced asthma most commonly occurs in children and young adults. It may be present as an isolated finding or may complicate asthma caused by other factors. This symptom reflects a hyperreactivity of the bronchi to cooling. With exercise, an increase airflow causes an increased evaporation of water from the mucosa of the tracheobronchial tree leading to cooling and reflex bronchoconstriction. It is important to note that not all forms of exercise (at equivalent levels of work performed) have the same tendency to induce asthma in susceptible individuals. Swimming is far better tolerated than are other forms of exercise because the ambient air during swimming is saturated with water vapor; evaporation from mucous membranes is reduced and cooling does not occur.

Psychologic factors appear to contribute to the generation of symptoms in many asthmatic patients. However, they are unlikely to be the sole etiologic factor in the disease. Often the patients are aware of a relationship between exacerbation of their symptoms and acute stress. More complex psychosomatic theories of asthma have thus far not been supported by unambiguous evidence. The efficacy of psychotherapy in the treatment of asthma has not yet been adequately documented, and in a disease such as asthma that is characterized by remissions and exacerbations, such documentation is extremely difficult to obtain. A patient who is unaware of a relationship between acute stress and the onset or exacerbation of symptoms should not be told that his disease is due to psychologic factors, since such a conclusion would be likely to be incorrect.

A clinical triad of asthma (generally intrinsic), nasal polyps, and aspirin sensitivity has been described. It is important to be aware of this relationship because aspirin ingestion by these patients may lead to marked exacerbation of asthmatic symptoms. This sensitivity to aspirin can be thought of as an idiosyncratic drug reaction. It is clearly not IgE mediated. Aspirin-sensitive patients are often also sensitive to aminopyrine, mefenamic acid, dextropropoxyphene, pentazocine, indomethacin, and some other nonsteroidal anti-inflammatory drugs. A small percentage of aspirin-sensitive patients also react to tartrazine dyes, which are common additives in foods and medications. Aspirin-sensitive patients can generally tolerate sodium salicylate, acetaminophen, and propoxyphene. Aspirin-induced asthma is believed to be related to the effects of the incriminated drugs on prostaglandin production because these drugs are inhibitors of the cyclo-oxygenase pathway of prostaglandin synthesis.

DIAGNOSIS. The diagnosis of asthma is based primarily on a detailed patient's history. Allergic (extrinsic) asthma is distinguished from other forms of asthma by a tendency for onset at an earlier age (usually in childhood); association of symptoms with exposure to some allergen; a tendency for patients to have other allergic manifestations such as childhood eczema, food allergies, or hay fever; a family history of allergy; complete absence of symptoms when the patient is not exposed to the allergen; and absence of a chronic cough or the production of purulent sputum. Allergies to pollens may induce seasonal symptoms, and allergies to household pets may induce perennial symptoms. The role of allergies to dust or mold spores must also be considered.

Physical findings during an attack include a prolongation of the expiratory phase of the respiratory cycle and wheezing that is usually more pronounced during expiration. Rhonchi may be present as a result of increased mucus secretion. The chest may be hyperresonant, and the diaphragms may be low. In severe cases breath sounds may be markedly decreased and the patient uses the accessory muscles of respiration. The patient may be cyanotic, mainly as a consequence of a ventilation-perfusion imbalance caused by mucus plugging of small airways and airway narrowing caused by bronchoconstriction.

Laboratory studies are useful in diagnosis. Moderate eosinophilia is somewhat more common in extrinsic asthma, although marked eosinophilia is sometimes seen in intrinsic asthma, especially in aspirin-sensitive patients. Elevated serum IgE levels and positive results of IgE-mediated skin tests to environmental allergens suggest an allergic cause. If a patient is atopic and has multiple allergies, an allergic cause for the asthma is more likely. Pulmonary function studies are of value in confirming the diagnosis of asthma and documenting its course but are of no help in establishing its cause. It is important to determine whether the airway obstruction is improved with bronchodilators. Irreversibility suggests that factors other than or in addition to bronchoconstriction are involved, including excessive mucus production, thick viscous mucus, or infection (bronchitis). Details of pulmonary function testing are discussed in Chapter 122. Studies of patients after an acute asthmatic attack have shown that symptoms clear first but physical findings of bronchoconstriction often persist for several weeks after symptoms disappear. Careful testing may show that pulmonary function abnormalities persist for weeks. It appears that after an acute attack of asthma the bronchi are particularly sensitive to both allergens and irritants for a relatively prolonged period. This provides the rationale for continuing therapy after symptoms subside. During an acute attack of asthma, arterial blood gas studies (P_{O_2}, P_{CO_2}, and pH) may be useful for evaluating the severity of the attack. A low P_{O_2} and a normal or low P_{CO_2} are commonly observed. An increased P_{CO_2} is a particularly ominous sign.

It should be pointed out that many patients with asthma, both intrinsic and extrinsic, have "hyperirritable" bronchi. That is, in response to agents such as methacholine that cause bronchoconstriction in all persons, their bronchi constrict at concentrations that are considerably lower than those required to induce bronchoconstriction in nonasthmatic subjects. This bronchial hyperreactivity may play an important role in both intrinsic and extrinsic asthma. Many asthmatic patients find their symptoms exacerbated by exposure to smoke, dust, paint fumes, and other irritants. These reactions are generally not allergic but rather reflect the hyperreactivity of these subjects' bronchi to a variety of irritants.

MANAGEMENT. In general the medical treatment of allergic asthma is similar to the treatment of asthma of other causes. β-Adrenergic agonists and theophylline derivatives are the mainstay for management of the routine case of asthma (see Chapter 130).

In severe cases corticosteroids are extremely valuable. Inhaled steroid preparations can be used to minimize the undesirable systemic side effects of long-term steroid therapy, but inhaled steroids are ineffective in acutely ill patients. Therefore therapy is usually initiated with parenteral or oral medication, and after symptoms are controlled, inhaled steroids are initiated. The dosage of oral steroids is then gradually decreased if possible, and the patient is maintained with inhaled steroids. The majority of patients with asthma can be treated successfully without the use of steroids.

As noted previously, for several months after an acute asthmatic attack a patient may be particularly prone to the triggering of bronchoconstriction by irritants, allergens, or other factors. This leads to the common clinical situation of a patient whose asthmatic attack is treated in the emergency room and who is discharged symptom free without medication only to return a day or two later with repeated attacks of increasing severity. When such a pattern is observed, more prolonged therapy should be undertaken even though the patient is symptom free. When a patient has had frequent severe asthmatic attacks, it is therefore logical to maintain steroid therapy for a long time and then reduce the dosage slowly to a level sufficient to maintain the patient without signs and symptoms. In some cases, after symptoms are controlled, the patient can be given alternate-day steroid therapy or inhaled steroids to minimize systemic side effects. After the patient has done well for several months, steroid therapy should be terminated if possible.

Cromolyn sodium has been used by inhalation with considerable success in some patients (particularly children) with asthma. The drug acts locally to inhibit the release of pharmacologically active mediators from mast cells. It is generally recommended for patients with extrinsic asthma. However, since some patients with intrinsic asthma may benefit from cromolyn, a trial of this drug in these patients is reasonable if their disease is not otherwise controlled. In some severe cases its use will permit the reduction of steroid dosage required for maintenance. It should be emphasized that cromolyn is used only prophylactically. It is not a bronchodilator and has no efficacy in treating an acute asthmatic attack. Cromolyn is particularly useful in preventing exercise-induced asthma.

Several aspects of therapy are specifically related to allergic asthma. (1) Environmental manipulation is directed toward eliminating environmental substances to which the patient is allergic, including removal of pets from the home, extensive cleaning to remove dust, redecorating to eliminate dust-promoting factors such as rugs and draperies, use of electrostatic air filters, use of foam rubber rather than feather pillows, use of mattress and blanket covers, and so forth. A cold water humidifier is sometimes helpful, but it must be cleaned meticulously every day to prevent the growth of molds that in themselves can be a significant cause of allergic asthma. (2) In patients who have symptoms that can be attributed to specific allergens on the basis of the history and skin test findings, immunotherapy (hyposensitization) appears appropriate. Although the efficacy of immunotherapy in asthma has not been definitely established, its use in *clearly* allergic patients with severe disease seems reasonable in view of the low toxicity of the therapy, the logic of the therapy, and the existence of data suggesting its beneficial effects. A trial of 3 to 5 years seems appropriate. After that time the physician should discontinue therapy and attempt a clinical judgment as to whether the therapy was beneficial. If the patient's symptoms seem worse without therapy, injections can be reinstituted. It should be emphasized that, as in the treatment of allergic rhinitis, immunotherapy is generally ineffective in treating asthma caused by allergic reactions to the dander of household pets.

BIBLIOGRAPHY

Bellanti, J.A.: Immunology, ed. 2, Philadelphia, 1978, W.B. Saunders Co.
Middleton, E., Reed, C., and Ellis, E., editors: Allergy: principles and practice (2 vols.), St. Louis, 1978, The C.V. Mosby Co.
Norins, A.L.: Atopic dermatitis, Pediatr. Clin. North Am. **18**:801, 1971.
Patterson, R., editor: Allergic diseases: diagnosis and management, Philadelphia, 1972, J.B. Lippincott Co.
Patterson, R.: Rhinitis, Med. Clin. North Am. **58**:43, 1974.
Sheldon, J.M., Lovell, R.G., and Mathews, K.P.: A manual of clinical allergy, ed. 2, Philadelphia, 1967, W.B. Saunders Co.

5 • URTICARIA AND ANGIOEDEMA

Leonard S. Girsh and **Lewis Perelmutter**

Urticaria and angioedema are type I allergic reactions that develop when the skin is the shock organ. These reactions may be acute or chronic (recurrent). Urticaria, or hives, are elevated, erythematous wheals that are intensely pruritic. Angioedema (angioneurotic edema) is allergic swelling of an entire anatomic part, such as the thumb, hand, lip, eyelid, or buttock; it is not painful or pruritic. Angioedema is urticaria involving the subcutaneous or submucosal tissues rather than the skin.

ETIOLOGY AND PATHOGENESIS. Allergic urticaria and allergic angioedema are most commonly produced by foods or drugs against which the patient has IgE antibody. Eggs, seafood, and nuts are among the foods most often implicated in IgE-mediated allergic reactions manifested as urticaria or angioedema. Some examples of food-induced urticaria may be due to the presence in food (such as strawberries) of substances that act directly on mast cells to cause histamine release, rather than to an IgE-mediated reaction. Penicillin is the agent most often implicated in IgE-mediated allergic reactions to drugs. Sulfonamides and aspirin are often associated with urticaria, but the mechanisms involved are not well understood. The combination of circulating antigen with IgE fixed to mast cells in the skin results in hives (urticaria) or subcutaneous or submucosal edema (angioedema). Lesions can also occur from infection with parasites, bacteria, fungi, and viruses, as a result of *Hymenoptera* stings, and in patients with neoplasms (especially lymphoma) or connective tissue diseases. The interaction of antigen and IgE directed against the antigen results in release of mediators such as histamine, kinins, and slow-reacting substance of anaphylaxis (SRS-A) from mast cells. This results in capillary leakage, edema, and urticaria or angioedema. Onset of lesions is usually within minutes after exposure to the allergen.

Urticaria can also occur on an apparently nonimmunologic basis, although the mediators of the reaction are probably the same—histamine, kinins, and SRS-A. Some of the nonimmunologic causes are heat, cold, emotions, exercise, and drugs that can cause release of mediators by direct action on mast cells, such as morphine, hydralazine, quinine, and organic iodides. Cold urticaria may also occur in underlying diseases such as syphilis and cryoglobulinemia.

Recurrent (chronic) urticaria occasionally may be due to drug or food allergy but in most cases is not of allergic origin. Malignancy (especially lymphoma), thyroid disease, the collagen-vascular group of diseases, vasculitis, and circulating antigen-antibody complexes are all associated with chronic urticaria. However, in the majority of cases no underlying cause can be identified.

CLINICAL MANIFESTATIONS. The urticarial lesion is usually a 1- to 5-cm irregular wheal with a pale center surrounded by erythema. Lesions are often intensely pruritic and usually appear and fade rapidly. They tend to occur at pressure points. Urticaria is most often disseminated.

Angioedema is seen as a painless, usually nonpruritic swelling of an area (finger, hand, foot, lip, eyelid, penis) and tends to last for several days. There is a syndrome of angioedema, asthma, and nasal polyps that is associated with aspirin ingestion. Laryngeal involvement represents an uncommon but severe complication of allergic angioedema.

PREVENTION AND MANAGEMENT. Avoidance of the identified etiologic agents is the key to prevention. Allergic urticaria or angioedema is treated with antihistamines, for example, 50 mg diphenhydramine hydrochloride or 25 to 100 mg hydroxyzine four times daily. If the patient is acutely ill, epinephrine in a dose of 0.3 ml of a 1:1000 solution administered subcutaneously will usually give relief. Prednisone, 40 to 60 mg daily, is reserved for severe cases.

Patients with chronic recurrent urticaria should be evaluated for underlying diseases, such as malignancies or connective tissue disease. Chronic urticaria frequently responds to hydroxyzine therapy. After prolonged treatment, the drug can often be gradually discontinued without a recurrence of symptoms.

Dietary causes of urticaria may be apparent to the patient; when not apparent, a dietary trial for 3 to 4 weeks may be helpful. Foods of high allergic potential (listed in the previous section on etiology and pathogenesis), as well as dyes and preservatives, are eliminated from the diet. One new food is then added every 5 to 7 days to determine which is the inciting agent. The treatment of food allergies is strictly dependent on avoiding the offending allergen. Hyposensitization therapy is not effective therapeutically. Skin testing and the radioallergosorbent test (RAST) have a high incidence of false positive and false negative reactions and are therefore not usually helpful.

Urticaria pigmentosa (systemic mastocytosis)

Urticaria pigmentosa is a malignancy of the mast cells; it is associated with hyperpigmentation in spots that represent mast cell infiltrates. When these frecklelike lesions are stroked, histamine is released and an urticarial lesion develops.

Hereditary angioedema

Patients with a hereditary defect of $\overline{C1}$ esterase inhibitor are prone to develop recurrent attacks of nonpruritic angioedema on a nonimmunologic basis. The skin, viscera, and larynx are often involved.

Most patients are young women. Presenting complaints may be either episodes of angioedema, often involving the face, or a nonspecific gastrointestinal disturbance including abdominal pain, nausea, vomiting, and diarrhea. Death commonly occurs as a result of laryngeal edema. The disease has two forms: one in which no $\overline{C1}$ esterase inhibitor is produced, and one that is less common in which an inactive $\overline{C1}$ esterase inhibitor protein is present. The two forms are clinically identical and are treated in the same manner. However, the usual assay for $\overline{C1}$ esterase inhibitor, which measures the protein immunologically, gives a false normal value in patients who have the functionally inactive protein. Thus if a normal test result is obtained for a patient with a history suggestive of the disease, more sophisticated assays of inhibitor activity are needed.

Hereditary angioedema usually responds poorly to antihistamines, epinephrine, and steroids. Administration of nonmasculinizing androgens such as danazol, 200 mg three times a day, has resulted in increased levels of $\overline{C1}$ esterase inhibitor in serum and marked clinical improvement.

BIBLIOGRAPHY

Fudenberg, H.H., and others, editors: Basic and clinical immunology, ed. 3, Los Altos, Calif., 1980, Lange Medical Publications.

Gelfand, J.A., and others: Treatment of hereditary angioedema with danazol: reversal of clinical and biochemical abnormalities, N. Engl. J. Med. **295:**1444, 1976.

Matthews, K.P.: A current view of urticaria, Med. Clin. North Am. **58:**185, 1974.

NIAD Task Force Report: Asthma and the other allergic diseases, NIH Pub. No. 79-387, Washington, D.C., 1979, U.S. Department of Health and Human Services, U.S. Public Health Service.

6 • SERUM SICKNESS

Leonard S. Girsh and Lewis Perelmutter

Serum sickness (a type III and perhaps type I immunologic reaction) refers to the syndrome that may occur following injection of foreign serum. A similar syndrome can be produced by drug allergy, although the precise mechanism may be somewhat different. The disease is characterized by fever, arthralgias or arthritis, and urticaria or other rashes. Lymphadenopathy may be present.

ETIOLOGY AND EPIDEMIOLOGY. Before the development of antibiotics, several types of bacterial infections in man were prevented or treated by injecting patients with a large volume of antiserum prepared in horses or rabbits. Heterologous antisera are now used much less in medicine; for example, tetanus antitoxin is mainly derived from human instead of horse serum. Currently, serum sickness–like reactions most commonly occur as allergic reactions to penicillin or other drugs.

Historically, serum sickness has occurred in about 5% of those receiving equine tetanus antitoxin and in 15% of those receiving equine rabies antitoxin. The probability of serum sickness is increased with larger volumes of serum; the incidence and severity are greater in adults than in children.

PATHOGENESIS. Serum sickness is a generalized allergic reaction believed to be caused by deposition of antigen-antibody complexes in blood vessels. The induction or incubation period for serum sickness is dependent on the period of sensitization, usually 3 to 12 days. During this incubation period, heterologous serum continues to circulate (or the drug is continued) as the host becomes sensitized to the injected foreign material and produces antibody. The allergic reaction occurs when circulating antibody combines with the circulating antigen to produce antigen-antibody complexes. These complexes are deposited in the walls of blood vessels at various sites. IgG and IgM complexes fix complement and attract polymorphonuclear leukocytes, producing injury that may result in thrombosis and hemorrhage. IgE complexes cause release of vasoactive substances from mast cells, such as histamine, kinins, serotonin, and the slow-reacting substance of anaphylaxis, with production of edema (for example, urticaria). Drugs causing serum sickness usually must combine with host protein to produce a protein-drug antigen (the drug is a hapten) against which the antibody is produced. In rabbits renal disease (immune complex nephritis) is common, but this manifestation is rare in humans.

Removal of the immune complexes by the cells of the reticuloendothelial system ultimately ends the disease. However, as long as circulating antibody remains, readministration of the antigen will reproduce the manifestations of the disease with a shorter incubation period.

CLINICAL MANIFESTATIONS. Serum sickness includes four symptom complexes: fever; enlarged lymph nodes and/or spleen; erythematous, petechial, or urticarial rashes; and arthralgia or arthritis. The disease is self-limited and subsides within a few days to weeks.

Other manifestations include abdominal pain, carditis, and neurologic disease.

LABORATORY FINDINGS. Testing reveals that eosinophilia is uncommon and the erythrocyte sedimentation rate is often normal. Circulating immune complexes can be detected by various techniques not commonly available except in specialized reference laboratories. Serum complement levels are decreased. Occasionally, circulating plasma cells are seen.

MANAGEMENT. Antihistamines are used in mild forms of serum sickness, but corticosteroids are required in severe cases. Response to steroids is prompt; 40 to 60 mg prednisone daily for 4 to 5 days is usually sufficient.

PREVENTION. Human serum products rather than foreign serum should be used when possible. In the United States today it is rarely, if ever, necessary to use horse serum.

BIBLIOGRAPHY

Bellanti, J.A.: Immunology, ed. 2, Philadelphia, 1978, W.B. Saunders Co.

Fudenberg, H.H., and others, editors: Basic and clinical immunology, ed. 3, Los Altos, Calif., 1980, Lange Medical Publications.

7 • CONTACT DERMATITIS

Leonard S. Girsh and Lewis Perelmutter

Contact dermatitis, typified by poison ivy, is a type IV (cell-mediated) reaction. Specific T cells interact with the antigen and secrete a series of pharmacologically active protein mediators (lymphokines) that collectively bring about local changes characteristic of a chronic inflammatory reaction. Other incitants include soap, detergents, nickel, dyes in fabrics, and drugs. Substances that cause contact sensitivity reactions are generally chemically reactive haptens that combine with host proteins to yield complete antigens.

The skin lesions are erythematous with vesicles. Characteristic of contact dermatitis is the presence of lesions on exposed areas; lesions limited to clothed areas suggest a reaction to laundry detergents or to a particular fabric. History taking and patch testing with common allergens usually reveal the diagnosis. Avoidance is the primary approach to prevention.

Poison ivy is a self-limited disease, and mild cases do not require treatment. In severe cases local or systemic steroids, given in moderate doses for 7 to 10 days, are usually effective in eliminating symptoms. When large areas of skin are involved, systemic steroids are probably preferable because they are more convenient to use and are usually more effective. Furthermore, when local steroids are applied to large areas of inflamed skin, a sufficient amount is absorbed to produce systemic effects, thus eliminating one of the major advantages of local application.

BIBLIOGRAPHY

Fisher, A.A.: Contact dermatitis, Philadelphia, 1974, Lea & Febiger.

8 • DRUG ALLERGY

Leonard S. Girsh and Lewis Perelmutter

''Drug allergy'' refers to a reaction to a drug that is mediated by an immunologic mechanism. The term does not include toxic reactions to drugs that are not immunologic in origin, such as tremor and syncope with use of epinephrine or diarrhea with the use of tetracycline. Drug allergy does not include idiosyncratic reactions that have no immune basis, such as aplastic anemia from chloramphenicol, which is probably related to peculiarities of drug metabolism in the individual. Similarly, the organic iodides, such as contrast media, may cause an idiosyncratic release of mediators from mast cells, producing an anaphylactoid reaction that is clinically indistinguishable from an IgE-mediated anaphylactic reaction, although it is not immunologically mediated.

ETIOLOGY AND EPIDEMIOLOGY. Any drug may produce an allergic reaction; drugs may be of high or low allergic potential. Drugs of high allergic potential include penicillins and cephalosporins, which may cross-react with one another. Drugs of low allergic potential include erythromycin, tetracycline, lidocaine, digitalis derivatives, and acetaminophen. Sulfonamides, dyes, para-aminobenzines such as the "-caine" drugs, barbiturates, and narcotics often cause drug reactions. However, the precise mechanisms are uncertain in most cases.

The risk of drug allergy depends not only on the composition of the drug but also on degree of exposure, route of administration, and patient susceptibility. Intermittent exposure seems to heighten the risk of developing an allergic reaction. Topical application also increases the risk, whereas oral administration lessens the risk. The risk of drug reaction is greater in adults than in children. Drug hypersensitivity reactions are probably more common in patients with prior drug reactions. States characterized by hyperactive immune responses, such as lupus erythematosus, are thought to be associated with an increased risk of drug reaction.

PATHOGENESIS. Allergic drug reactions occur as a result of sensitization, particularly after repeated exposure to drugs of high allergic potential, whether administered topically, orally, or by injection. The allergen in drug allergy is usually composed of a protein-drug complex (a bond is formed between the low-molecular-weight drug or metabolic degradative product of the drug and plasma or tissue protein). The drug or a product derived from it acts as a hapten, and the host protein is the carrier. Drugs, or their metabolites, that readily form covalent bonds with proteins are most apt to cause drug allergy. All types of immunologic tissue damage may result from drugs. A type I reaction results when a drug-protein complex reacts with IgE antibody bound to mast cells. This interaction causes release of mediators from the mast cells and can result in generalized anaphylaxis or localized urticaria (Chapter 5). Type II reactions occur when the drug binds to a host cell such as an RBC or a platelet. IgG or IgM antibodies interact with the drug bound to the host cell and cause rapid destruction of the cell, leading to anemia or thrombocytopenia. Complement may or may not be bound to the antibody-drug-cell complex. This mechanism of tissue damage is most often seen when large doses of a drug are being administered. Serum sickness–like reactions (type III mechanism) can also result from drugs (Chapter 6).

Local application of drugs can result in a type IV reaction following interaction of drug-protein complexes with sensitized T lymphocytes. This delayed hypersensitivity reaction produces contact dermatitis (Chapter 7).

CLINICAL MANIFESTATIONS. Although a drug reaction may be seen as pure urticaria or serum sickness, many reactions have mixed features. The nature of the drug reaction depends on many factors such as drug dose, specificity of the antibodies produced, class (isotype) and subclass of the antibodies produced, distribution of the drug, and its interaction with different host constituents.

Generalized anaphylaxis. Generalized anaphylaxis (a type I reaction) is the systemic reaction generally resulting from release of vasoactive mediators, such as histamine and slow-reacting substance of anaphylaxis from mast cells following an antigen-IgE reaction. Alternatively, the complement system may be activated through a variety of mechanisms, with release of C3a and C5a, both of which have anaphylatoxin activity; however, this does not appear to be a common mechanism in human anaphylaxis. The result is vasodilation, increased vascular permeability, and contraction of smooth muscle. Multiple organ systems are involved simultaneously, and death may ensue. Although drugs are the most common cause of generalized anaphylaxis, foods and insect stings are also causes.

Shortly after exposure to an allergen, one or more of the following systems are involved: cardiovascular, respiratory, skin, and gastrointestinal. Shock may result secondary to generalized vasodilation and increased vascular permeability leading to decreased blood volume from leakage of plasma into extravascular sites. Nasal obstruction, rhinorrhea, laryngeal edema, and bronchospasm may all occur. Urticaria, angioedema, and severe pruritus may affect the skin. Gastrointestinal involvement can cause abdominal pain, vomiting, and diarrhea. There is evidence that cardiac arrhythmias may occur. A severe anaphylactic reaction can lead to death within a few minutes.

Drug fever. Fever, which may be very high and accompanied by shaking chills, may be the only manifestation of a drug reaction or may be accompanied by arthralgia or arthritis, rash, and eosinophilia. The fever probably has an immunologic origin and generally disappears within several days after stopping the drug.

Allergic rash. Rashes, most of which are probably caused by hypersensitivity vasculitis, may be maculopapular, erythematous (measleslike), urticarial, eczematoid (contact dermatitis), petechial, or even exfoliative. Erythema nodosum or erythema multiforme may occur.

Erythema nodosum. Erythema nodosum is often associated with drug reactions, especially involving penicillins and sulfonamides, but other common causes are sarcoidosis, streptococcal pharyngitis, and acute coccidioidomycosis. It also occurs in tuberculosis, leprosy, viral infections, other fungal infections, and inflammatory bowel disease. The rash usually appears as bilateral tender erythematous nodules on the pretibial area and occasionally on the extensor surfaces of the arms. It is associated with fever and arthralgia or arthritis. It usually lasts several weeks, but recurrent episodes (relapses) may occur.

Erythema multiforme. Erythema multiforme is a rash consisting of erythematous patches that tend to be sharply outlined and have central clearing. These evolve into concentric rings, the so-called target lesion. While drugs are a common cause, the rash may occur with viral or mycoplasmal infection, with malignancy, and with no apparent cause. The rash may be accompanied by high fever and extensive bullous lesions. In its most severe form, in which there is mucosal involvement, it is called the Stevens-Johnson syndrome. There are ulcerations in the mouth, vagina, conjunctivae, and gastrointestinal tract. Pneumonia and nephritis may also occur.

Photosensitivity. Certain drugs (tetracycline derivatives, sulfonamides, thiazides) can increase the tendency to sunburn on the exposed parts of the body. Some of these reactions may be allergic.

Disseminated vasculitis. As a part of a drug reaction, vasculitis can involve essentially any organ. For example, a polyarteritis nodosa–like syndrome may be produced by sulfonamides. Penicillins, especially methicillin, may produce nephritis, commonly associated with hematuria, rash, and eosinophilia. Procainamide, hydralazine, and other agents can cause a syndrome similar to systemic lupus erythematosus. The liver, central nervous system, and gastrointestinal tract can all be involved in the vasculitis from drug allergy.

Hematologic disorders. Drugs may produce hemolytic anemia (penicillins, methyldopa), thrombocytopenia (penicillins, quinine, quinidine), or leukopenia (penicillins, cephalosporins, sulfonamides). Eosinophilia may appear without other manifestations or with rash or fever.

DIAGNOSIS. Any unexpected occurrence in a patient receiving a drug should suggest a drug reaction. This includes aspirin, cathartics, sleeping pills, and any other self-medication the patient may be taking. Patients must be questioned carefully as to drug history.

There is no certain way of proving that a reaction is caused by a drug other than rechallenging with the drug and observing for the same reaction. Occult reactions, such as drug fever, are virtually impossible to prove as a drug reaction without rechallenge. However, rechallenge is often unwise, unnecessary, and may be dangerous. While eosinophilia may suggest a drug reaction, it is often absent. Furthermore, eosinophilia per se does not indicate that the observed reaction is caused by the drug. Many patients who are prone to allergies normally have eosinophilia or may develop eosinophilia secondary to drugs with no other clinical manifestations.

MANAGEMENT. Discontinuation of the causative agent is the major approach to treating drug reactions. However, it is also important to recognize that environmental contamination with drugs is common, such as penicillin in milk products.

Generalized anaphylaxis is a medical emergency and requires immediate therapy. The drug of choice is 0.2 to 0.5 ml of 1:1000 aqueous epinephrine subcutaneously, repeated every 15 minutes as required; the cardiac rate and blood pressure must be monitored. If anaphylaxis occurs after injection of a drug, a tourniquet should be placed proximal to the site of injection and 0.2 ml of 1:1000 aqueous epinephrine injected at the drug injection site to slow absorption of the drug. The shock seen in anaphylaxis is due to hypovolemia. Therefore lack of a prompt response to epinephrine indicates the need for expansion of blood volume with saline or other volume expanders. Although steroids and antihistamines are often administered, these agents are clearly of secondary importance to epinephrine and volume replacement. Vasopressors, such as levarterenol bitartrate, are sometimes used when the response of shock to other measures is insufficient; however, these vasopressors tend to be ineffective if the blood volume is not expanded and unnecessary once an adequate intravascular volume is achieved with appropriate volume expanders. An endotracheal tube may be necessary.

Antihistamines, such as 50 mg diphenhydramine hydrochloride or 25 to 100 mg hydroxyzine four times daily, may be used in milder allergic reactions involving the skin. More severe reactions, such as the Stevens-Johnson syndrome and severe disseminated vasculitis, should be treated with 60 mg prednisone daily, with rapid tapering after control of the reaction.

BIBLIOGRAPHY

Austen, K.F.: Systemic anaphylaxis in the human being, N. Engl. J. Med. **291**:661, 1974.

Dash, C.H., and Jones, H.E.H.: Mechanisms in drug allergy, Baltimore, 1972, The Williams & Wilkins Co.

Parker, C.W.: Drug therapy: drug allergy I, N. Engl. J. Med. **292**:511, 1975.

Parker, C.W.: Drug therapy: drug allergy II, N. Engl. J. Med. **292**:732, 1975.

Parker, C.W.: Drug therapy: drug allergy III, N. Engl. J. Med. **292**:957, 1975.

Dental correlations

Martin S. Greenberg

The field of allergy has direct application to dental practice in two major circumstances: the differential diagnosis of a patient presenting with ulcerative or vesiculobullous lesions of the oral mucosa, and the evaluation of a patient with a history of allergy to medication or materials used by a dentist. Many patients, as well as some clinicians, use the term "allergy" to describe all adverse reactions. This broad, unfortunate use of the term causes difficulty for the patient and the dentist. All too frequently, patients who feel dizzy or nauseous or who have heart palpitations from a psychic or toxic reaction after a local anesthetic injection are labeled "allergic." Such patients then inform each succeeding dentist and physician of the "allergy," unnecessarily complicating treatment. It is the dentist's responsibility to use the term "allergic reaction" carefully so that the patient is not denied the use of a medication or a material that will be helpful for successful management. It is important to be capable of distinguishing between true allergic reactions and toxic or psychic reactions. When a true allergic reaction occurs to a local anesthetic, the dentist should inform the patient regarding the class of local anesthetic that caused the allergic reaction. For example, patients allergic to the amide group may frequently be able to take the para-aminobenzoic acid group safely.

CLINICAL MANIFESTATIONS. Anaphylactic (type I) allergic reactions or cell-mediated (type IV) allergic reactions have been ascribed to a wide variety of substances used in dental practice. Contact allergy to dental amalgam is most frequently caused by mercury released during condensation. Dermatitis and stomatitis developing from mercury have been described. Investigations have demonstrated an increasing level of allergy to mercury in a group of dental students as they progressed through school. At the beginning of the freshman year 2% of the dental students had a positive reaction to mercury. This is consistent with the level of mercury allergy in the general population. During their senior year, 11% of the students had positive reactions to mercury. All reactions were from mercury itself and not to condensed amalgam, which is a much less common cause of allergy. Dentists, for their own protection, must be careful to follow good mercury hygiene not only to eliminate the known toxic effects of the substance but also to reduce allergic reactions.

Allergy to properly condensed amalgam occurs rarely. A case of generalized gingival inflammation occurring in a patient with multiple amalgam fillings has been reported. The skin test was positive to condensed amalgam. The amalgam fillings were replaced with gold and the inflammation resolved.

Most reactions to acrylic are caused by contact with the free monomer. The number of allergic reactions to acrylic can be greatly reduced by avoiding use of uncured acrylic directly in the mouth. There have been reported cases of severe allergic dermatitis, stomatitis, and bronchospasm occurring after contact with a bench-cured acrylic temporary bridge. An erythema multiforme reaction after contact with uncured acrylic has been noted. The lesions resolved after the acrylic bridge was heat cured to remove the free monomer. An allergic reaction to heat-cured acrylic is very rare. Allergic reactions have also been occasionally reported to composite resin, nickel in chrome, cobalt prostheses, cinnamon oil in chewing gum, and epimine-containing impression materials.

Hypersensitivity reactions not caused by dental materials may also affect the oral region. One major example is angioneurotic edema of the lips or tongue. This is a type I allergic reaction caused by IgE bound to mast cells, which release mediators such as histamine, causing edema. This disfiguring disorder may be life-threatening if it compromises the airway by involving the posterior tongue or larynx.

Erythema multiforme is a symptom complex involving the skin and mucous membranes; it may be caused by reactions to microorganisms, food, drugs, radiotherapy, or malignancy. The drugs most commonly related to an erythema multiforme reaction are antibiotics, barbiturates, phenylbutazone, and carbamazepine (Tegretol). Particularly interesting are the reports of erythema multiforme related to recurrent herpes labialis. Shelly reported that 15% of the cases of recurrent erythema multiforme have a preceding recurrent herpes simplex infection as the precipitating factor. The majority of cases of erythema multiforme have no related allergy or disease and are labeled idiopathic. Erythema multiforme most frequently occurs in children and young adults and has an acute onset. The most common cutaneous lesions are found on the hands, feet, and extensor surfaces of the elbows and knees. The face and neck are also commonly involved but only severe cases will affect the trunk. Oral lesions appear along with the cutaneous manifestations but in some cases the oral lesions are the predominant or only sign of the disease. The skin lesions may take many forms but the target lesion is the pathognomonic sign and should be searched for in each case. The target lesion consists of a central bulla surrounded by edema with concentric bands of erythema. The oral lesions begin as bullae on an erythematous base, but these break rapidly into large irregular lesions. In full-blown cases the lips are extensively eroded and large portions of the oral mucosa are denuded of epithelium. Treatment of erythema multiforme consists of supportive care for mild cases. In severe cases, systemic corticosteroids should be used.

DENTAL MANAGEMENT. Treatment of contact or type IV allergic reactions of the oral mucosa can be treated successfully by eliminating the allergen and using topical corticosteroids and diphenhydramine (Benadryl). Anaphylactic or type I reaction can be treated with 0.5 ml of 1:1000 epinephrine subcutaneously when a life-threatening reaction occurs. Hives are not life threatening and can be treated successfully with Benadryl.

BIBLIOGRAPHY

Catsakis, L.H., and Sulica, V.I.: Allergy to silver amalgams, Oral Surg. **46:**371, 1978.

Duxbury, A.J., Turner, E.P., and Watts, D.C.: Hypersensitivity to epimine containing dental materials, Br. Dent. J. **147:**331, 1979.

Eversole, L.R.: Allergic stomatitides, J. Oral. Med. **34:**93, 1979.

Nathanson, D., and Lockhart, P.: Delayed extraoral hypersensitivity to dental composite material, Oral Surg. **47:**329, 1979.

Rickles, N.H.: Allergy in surface lesions of the oral mucosa, Oral Surg. **33:**744, 1972.

Sturgis, T.L., and Fink, J.N.: Hypersensitivity to acrylic resin, J. Prosth. Dent. **22:**425, 1969.

White, R.R., and Brandt, R.L.: Development of mercury hypersensitivity among dental students, J. Am. Dent. Assoc. **92:**1204, 1976.

Wood, J.F.L.: Mucosal reaction to cobalt-chromium alloy, Br. Dent. J. **136:**423, 1974.

9 • IMMUNODEFICIENCY DISEASES

Leonard S. Girsh and **Lewis Perelmutter**

Immunodeficiency diseases are characterized by increased susceptibility of patients to infection; the types of infection may suggest the type of deficiency. These patients may also have an increased tendency to develop malignancies, particularly lymphomas. The defects may be severe or mild and may involve the phagocytic system, the complement system, or the immunologic system itself (B and/or T lymphocytes). Clinical manifestations will thus vary in nature and severity.

DISORDERS OF B LYMPHOCYTES

Patients with disorders of the B-lymphocyte arm have a defect in antibody production, resulting in agammaglobulinemia or hypogammaglobulinemia. This defect primarily predisposes to infection with encapsulated organisms requiring opsonins in order for phagocytosis by leukocytes to occur. Infections are most commonly caused by *Streptococcus pneumoniae* and *Haemophilus influenzae*. Other organisms sometimes implicated are group A β-hemolytic streptococci and meningococci. Viral illnesses are usually handled normally, but recurrences tend to appear, as in multiple episodes of measles. One exception to the absence of increased severity in viral illness occurs with hepatitis B; there is an increased frequency of chronic carriers of hepatitic B antigen and an increased frequency of fulminant hepatitis B. The types of infection commonly seen are recurrent pneumonia, sinusitis, otitis media, bacteremia, and meningitis. *Giardia lamblia* infections are common in patients with no IgA in intestinal secretions.

DISORDERS OF T LYMPHOCYTES

Patients with disorders of the T-lymphocyte arm have decreased cellular immunity. The infections noted most often are those caused by intracellular parasites. In particular, these patients are more likely to develop the following infections and have a more severe form: bacterial infections (tuberculosis, *Listeria monocytogenes* infections), herpesvirus infections (herpes simplex, herpes zoster with dissemination, cytomegalovirus infection), fungal infections (cryptococcal meningitis, mucocutaneous and/or disseminated *Candida* infection), and protozoan infections (*Pneumocystis carinii* pneumonia, severe toxoplasmosis). Graft-versus-host reactions can occur following blood transfusion because of the survival of donor lymphocytes.

Patients with T-lymphocyte abnormalities also may have variable defects in antibody production, which result from the loss of the normal modulating effect of T cells on antibody production.

DISORDERS OF POLYMORPHONUCLEAR LEUKOCYTES

In patients with leukopenia, infections are most often caused by gram-negative bacilli (*Escherichia coli, Klebsiella-Enterobacter, Proteus, Pseudomonas*) and *Staphylococcus aureus*. For polymorphonuclear and other phagocytic cells to function normally in host defense, they must be capable of three distinct processes: (1) directed movement toward the site of the foreign organism (chemotaxis); (2) binding and internalizing the foreign organism (phagocytosis); and (3) performing a series of chemical reactions that generate substances toxic for the foreign organism. Defects in all three of these essential functions have been described and can be responsible for an increased susceptibility to the infections just listed.

DEFECTS IN THE COMPLEMENT SYSTEM

Defects in the complement system have also been associated with increased susceptibility to bacterial infection. C3 deficiency or low C3 secondary to absent C3b inactivator (resulting in consumption of C3) predisposes to *S. aureus* and gram-negative bacillary infections. Deficiencies of C6, C7, and C8 have been associated with recurrent meningococcal and gonococcal bacteremia.

Complement deficiencies have been associated with autoimmune disease, particularly a syndrome resembling systemic lupus erythematosus.

The basis of hereditary angioedema is a deficiency of $\overline{C1}$ esterase inhibitor.

EVALUATION OF IMMUNITY

Evaluation of the status of the immune system involves a careful history and a series of laboratory tests. The types of infection may suggest whether the defect is one of antibody production, cellular immunity, phagocytic function, or the complement system. A number of tests can be performed to evaluate defense mechanisms. Many of these tests are widely available, but others require specialized laboratories.

B-cell function

Measurement of serum immunoglobins determines if any are present in insufficient concentrations. Lower limits of normal in adults are 550 mg/dl for IgG, 45 mg/dl for IgM, and 60 mg/dl for IgA. If borderline values are found or if there is a question as to ability to make antibodies, existing or induced antibodies can be measured. Measurement of anti-A and anti-B blood group antibodies and determination of anti-O and anti-H antibodies after typhoid immunization or of antibodies against influenza virus after influenza vaccination are particularly helpful. Other studies requiring special laboratories include determination of IgA in secretions, examination of lymph node biopsies for plasma cells by histologic and immunofluorescent methods, measurement of the four IgG subclasses, staining and enumeration of blood lymphocytes for surface immunoglobulins, and in vitro induction of B-cell proliferation or immunoglobulin secretion by pokeweed or other mitogens.

T-cell function

Delayed hypersensitivity skin tests such as *Candida*, mumps, and *Trichophyton*, which are positive in a large proportion of the normal population, are helpful in screening for defects. The ability to develop delayed hypersensitivity to a new antigen can be determined by using an effective sensitizing antigen, dinitrochlorobenzene. A sensitizing dose is applied to the skin and a patch test is applied 2 weeks later at another site. Other studies requiring specialized laboratories are enumeration of circulating T cells using specific antiserum or the sheep-cell rosette technique; in vitro stimulation of T cells by phytohemagglutinin, concanavalin A, or antigens such as purified protein derivative (of tuberculin) (PPD); measurement of the production of macrophage inhibition factor or other lymphokines by activated T cells; and assay of T-cell subsets using appropriate antisera.

Complement

Total hemolytic complement, C2, C4, $\overline{C1}$ esterase inhibitor protein, and C3 measurements are available in most hospital laboratories. Measurement of the other components is available only in specialized laboratories.

Leukocytes

A white blood count and differential smear will determine whether adequate mature polymorphonuclear leukocytes are present and if abnormal forms are present, such as the giant granules of Chédiak-Higashi syndrome. Studies for leukocyte function, such as reduction of nitroblue tetrazolium (for chronic granulomatous disease), chemotactic response, and phagocytic, metabolic, and bactericidal activity, are available only in specialized laboratories.

CLASSIFICATION

Immunodeficiency diseases may be primary or secondary to an underlying disease. The primary diseases are discussed in this chapter. The diseases that secondarily produce immunodeficiencies are discussed in the appropriate chapters. Examples of secondary immune deficiencies include defects in antibody production in chronic lymphatic leukemia, in multiple myeloma, and in protein-losing enteropathies and defects in cellular immunity in Hodgkin's disease and from use of immunosuppressant agents. Corticosteroids decrease leukocytic adherence and migration and interfere with cellular immunity.

The primary immunodeficiency diseases are usually congenital and are classified by whether the defect involves B-cell function (antibody production), T-cell function (cellular immunity), or both. In fact, most T-cell immunodeficiency diseases also affect B-cell function, and an apparent B-cell defect may actually be related to abnormalities in T cells (helper or suppressor function).

Defects in B-cell function (antibody production)

X-LINKED AGAMMAGLOBULINEMIA (BRUTON TYPE). Bruton-type X-linked agammaglobulinemia (or hypogammaglobulinemia) represents an inherited failure in the development of the B lymphoid system. There are no fully developed B lymphocytes or plasma cells. Affected patients show an isolated defect in humoral immunity with little or no production of antibody and low levels of all immunoglobulins in serum. It is transmitted as an X-linked recessive trait and occurs almost exclusively in males. Because of the transplacental transfer of maternal IgG antibodies, individuals with this disorder do not become symptomatic until the end of the first year of life. They develop severe and recurrent infections caused by encapsulated bacteria, such as *S. pneumoniae* and *H. influenzae*. As a result of recurrent pulmonary infections, these individuals frequently develop chronic pulmonary disease and respiratory failure. Some patients develop arthritis resembling rheumatoid arthritis. Management consists of prompt therapy of infections and injections of γ-globulin every 2 weeks to maintain serum IgG at 100 to 300 mg/dl as a preventive measure.

X-LINKED IMMUNODEFICIENCY WITH HYPER-IgM. In this defect IgM is elevated with decreases in serum IgG and IgA. Infections and management are similar to those for X-linked agammaglobulinemia.

SELECTIVE DEFICIENCIES OF IMMUNOGLOBULIN

IgA deficiency. The most common immunoglobulin deficiency is that of IgA, involving both serum and secretory IgA and affecting 1 in every 600 people. About half are symptomatic, and symptoms may not appear until late in life. Recurrent "low-grade" respiratory infections are common. Severe infections such as those seen in agammaglobulinemia are uncommon. Patients have an increased tendency to develop an allergic diathesis (such as asthma and other atopic diseases), chronic diarrhea, and autoimmune disorders and connective tissue diseases (particularly rheumatoid arthritis and systemic lupus erythematosus). *G. lamblia* infection is common in IgA-deficient patients.

Patients may develop anaphylaxis from blood transfusions, since they are capable of developing antibody against IgA. No treatment is available for IgA deficiency. Administration of γ-globulin is contraindicated; it is not effective and is dangerous because the IgA present may stimulate an immune response leading to allergic manifestations when γ-globulin or a transfusion is subsequently required. Transfusions, if required, should be from IgA-deficient donors.

Other isotype deficiencies. Isolated deficiency of IgM or of one or more of the IgG subclasses has rarely been reported. Infections and management are similar to those for X-linked agammaglobulinemia.

COMMON VARIABLE (UNCLASSIFIABLE) IMMUNODEFICIENCY (ACQUIRED AGAMMAGLOBULINEMIA). Common variable immunodeficiency is a mixed group of defects (familial or acquired) with the common manifestation of agammaglobulinemia (or hypogammaglobulinemia). It is not linked to sex, and symptoms usually do not appear until after age 15. Sinopulmonary infections and infections caused by pneumococci and *H. influenzae* are common. Autoimmune diseases and diarrhea with malabsorption are frequent manifestations. Lymphoid nodular hyperplasia and splenomegaly are common in acquired agammaglobulinemia but are absent in X-linked agammaglobulinemia.

Plasma cells are absent in lymph nodes, and there is little or no antibody response. Cell-mediated immunity is usually normal but may be depressed. Therapy is the same as for X-linked agammaglobulinemia.

Common variable immunodeficiency is a large group of disorders that are classified together because their detailed pathogenesis is unknown. It has recently been shown that a small subset of patients with these conditions (5% or less) have increased nonspecific suppressor T-cell activity as the mechanism of their disease. Nonspecific suppressor macrophages appear to be present in some patients, and a defect in helper T-cell activity has been reported in one patient. The mechanisms involved in most of these patients, however, remain undefined.

WISKOTT-ALDRICH SYNDROME. Wiskott-Aldrich syndrome, an X-linked recessive disease, consists of eczema, thrombocytopenia, and recurrent infections caused by pneumococci, *H. influenzae,* meningococci, and viral organisms. Affected individuals show a low concentration of IgM, normal IgG and IgA levels, and high IgE concentrations. There is a poor response to polysaccharide antigens. Although T-cell function seems to be intact in vitro, anergy is frequent. Patients are predisposed to develop lymphoproliferative neoplasms. The major approach to therapy is prompt treatment of infections. Injection of transfer factor, a lymphokine, has resulted in improvement in some patients. Bone marrow transplantation has been successful in a few patients.

IMMUNODEFICIENCY WITH THYMOMA. Patients with agammaglobulinemia may have a thymoma. Myasthenia gravis, aplastic anemia, granulocytopenia, and thrombocytopenia may also be present. Some patients have deficient T-cell function. Removal of the thymoma does not result in improvement of the immunodeficiency.

Defects in T-cell function (cellular immunity)

DiGEORGE's SYNDROME. DiGeorge's syndrome is a developmental abnormality that results from a failure in the embryologic development of the third and fourth pharyngeal pouches. As a result, both the parathyroid glands and the thymus fail to develop; the T lymphoid system is thus deficient. It does not appear to have a hereditary basis. Hypocalcemic tetany often occurs in the neonatal period. Cardiac defects are also common. Children with this disorder commonly experience recurrent infections with viruses, fungi, protozoa, and certain bacteria. Immunoglobins may be normal or selectively decreased. Patients usually do not survive beyond age 2 without transplantation of fetal thymus. With transplantation, prolonged survival has been reported.

ATAXIA-TELANGIECTASIA. Ataxia-telangiectasia, an autosomal recessive inherited disease, is characterized by progressive degeneration of the cerebellum with ataxia, cutaneous and ocular telangiectasia, recurrent sinopulmonary infections, and immunologic deficiencies. Ataxia begins in infancy and is progressive; patients also show an increased susceptibility to lymphomas. The thymus does not develop, and T-cell function is poor. IgA, IgE, and sometimes IgG in serum are decreased, probably secondary to poor T-cell function. Death is usually secondary to malignancy or chronic pulmonary disease.

CHRONIC MUCOCUTANEOUS CANDIDIASIS. Recurrent, protracted superficial *Candida* infections may involve the skin, nails, and oral and vaginal mucous membranes. Hypoparathyroidism and hypoadrenalism can occur. Anergy to *Candida* and frequently other antigens is present, but humoral immunity is usually intact. Except for the skin infection, serious infection is uncommon. Administration of agents active against *Candida* is the major approach to therapy. Transfer factor has been used successfully in some patients. This syndrome probably reflects several distinct but as yet poorly differentiated diseases.

Defects in both B- and T-cell function

COMBINED SYSTEMS DISEASE. Combined systems disease represents the most severe form of immunodeficiency. Affected infants show marked impairment in development of both the B and T lymphoid systems. Autosomal recessive and X-linked (Swiss-type agammaglobulinemia) types have been described. Clinical manifestations usually appear shortly after birth as profound failure in normal growth and development. Many types of severe infection occur. Diarrhea and generalized unremitting dermatitis are present; these infants suffer severe and sustained infections. Survival beyond age 2 is rare. There have been reports of successful bone marrow transplants with restoration of immunity. About half of those with autosomal recessive disease have associated absence of adenosine deaminase or nucleoside phosphorylase in red blood cells and other cells. Transfusion with red cells containing normal amounts of adenosine deaminase in those with a deficiency of this enzyme can lead to a transient remission of the disease. Some patients have been successfully treated with bone marrow, fetal liver, or fetal thymus transplants.

A number of patients have been reported with combined system disease associated with thymoma. As with other immunodeficiencies, removal of the tumor does not correct the defect.

MANAGEMENT

Therapy for the immunodeficiency diseases mainly involves replacement of γ-globulins in patients with agammaglobulinemia and use of transfer factor or bone marrow, fetal liver, or fetal thymus transplants in those with T-cell defects. γ-Globulin is contraindicated in patients with selective IgA deficiency. Prompt therapy of infection and proper bronchopulmonary care, chest physiotherapy, and postural drainage in patients with chronic pulmonary infections are essential.

BIBLIOGRAPHY

Cooper, M.D., and others: Wiskott-Aldrich syndrome: immunologic deficiency disease involving the afferent limb of immunity, Am. J. Med. **44:**489, 1968.

DiGeorge, A.M.: Congenital absence of the thymus and its immunologic consequences: concurrence with congenital hypoparathyroidism. In Bergsma, D., and McKusick, F.A., editors: Immunologic deficiency diseases in man, National Foundation–March of Dimes original article series, Baltimore, 1968, The Williams & Wilkins Co.

Hermans, P.E., Diaz-Buxo, J.A., and Stobo, J.D.: Idiopathic late-onset immunoglobulin deficiency: clinical observations in 50 patients, Am. J. Med. **61:**221, 1976.

Hirschhorn, R., and Martin, D.W.: Enzyme defects in immunodeficiency diseases, Semin. Immunopathol. **1:**299, 1978.

Hitzig, W.H.: Congenital thymic and lymphocytic deficiency disorders. In Stiehm, E.R., and Fulginiti, V., editors: Immunologic disorders in infants and children, Philadelphia, 1973, W.B. Saunders Co.

Kirkpatrick, C.H., Rich, R.R., and Bennett, J.E.: Chronic mucocutaneous candidiasis: model building in cellular immunity, Ann. Intern. Med. **74:**955, 1971.

Petersen, B.H., and others: *Neisseria meningitidis* and *Neisseria gonorrhoeae* bacteremia associated with C6, C7, or C8 deficiency, Ann. Intern. Med. **90:**917, 1979

Peterson, R.D.A., Cooper, M.D., and Good, R.A.: Lymphoid tissue abnormalities asociated with ataxia–telangiectasia, Am. J. Med. **41:**342, 1966.

Rosen, F.S., and Janeway, C.A.: The gammaglobulins. III. The antibody deficiency syndromes, N. Engl. J. Med. **275:**709, 1966.

Dental correlations

Martin S. Greenberg

CLINICAL MANIFESTATION. Oral signs are common in patients with T-lymphocyte disorders. The most prominent oral sign in this group of patients is chronic oral candidiasis. These lesions are widespread and deep seated. They are not easily scraped off the mucosa, and biopsies demonstrate yeast deep into the epithelium. The dentist should consider the possibility of impaired T-lymphocyte function in patients with chronic oral candidiasis that does not respond permanently to standard antifungal medication.

Herpes simplex virus infections are often commonly seen in patients with T-lymphocyte disorders. The patients may have severe primary herpes infections or extensive recurrent herpes infections that may be localized to the mouth or become disseminated and potentially lethal.

Recently, there has been significant interest in the relationship of the immune response to periodontal disease, oral ulcers, and dental caries. A recent study evaluated 23 patients with primary immune deficiencies and compared them with normal controls. The patients with immune deficiencies had decreased gingival inflammation, due to a decreased inflammatory response, but there was no difference noted in the extent of periodontal breakdown. Also noted was a decreased caries rate in the immune-deficient group.

DENTAL MANAGEMENT. Patients with T-lymphocyte abnormalities will have a decrease in the levels of circulating immunoglobulins. Dental treatment should not be performed on these patients unless the γ-globulin level is at least 20 mg/dl. When oral surgery is necessary, an extra dose of γ-globulin should be administered the day before surgery at a dose between 100 and 200 mg/kg body weight. This dose should be administered intramuscularly rather than intravenously to decrease the risk of transfusion reaction.

Transfusion reactions are common in patients with the primary immunodeficiency diseases since the missing immunoglobulin is a foreign protein and may cause an allergic response. Therefore patients with a selective immunoglobulin deficiency must be given blood with the missing immunoglobulin depleted. A second problem that may occur in patients with primary immunodeficiency is a development of graft-versus-host disease. The lymphocytes in the transfused blood will react against the tissues of the immunodeficient recipient. Only fresh blood in which the immunocompetent lymphocytes have been destroyed can be used.

BIBLIOGRAPHY

Barreckman, R.W., and others: Gingivitis in hypogammaglobulinemia, J. Periodontol. **44:**171, 1973.

Robert, W.R., and Walker, D.M.: The periodontal management of a patient with a profound immunodeficiency disorder, J. Clin. Periodontol. **3:**186, 1976.

Robertson, P.B., and others: Periodontal status of patients with abnormalities of the immune system, J. Periodont. Res. **13:**37, 1978.

Section Three
RHEUMATIC AND GRANULOMATOUS DISEASES

edited by **Warren A. Katz**

Few subspecialties of internal medicine have engendered more confusing terminology than the field of rheumatology. For example, arthritis in its narrowest sense implies inflammation of the joint, yet the term "arthritis" is usually interpreted more broadly. Arthritis is sometimes used interchangeably with rheumatoid arthritis or osteoarthritis. It has been used to describe forms of nonarticular rheumatism, such as fibromyositis, even when the joints are not involved.

Arthritis is often confused with the term "rheumatic disease" when used to describe any acute or chronic affliction of the joints and other musculoskeletal problems, with the exception of fractures or congenital abnormalities. Arthritis is only one type of rheumatic disease. Connective tissue disorders, also rheumatic diseases, refer to those diseases that affect not only the musculoskeletal system but the skin and internal organs of the body as well. These disorders tend to be more severe than most primary forms of arthritis and may be fatal. Major connective tissue diseases include rheumatoid arthritis, rheumatic fever, systemic lupus erythematosus, systemic sclerosis (scleroderma), dermatomyositis or polymyositis, vasculitis, and Sjögren's syndrome. Some features from two or more of these entities may coexist in the same patient in a variety of ways. Under these circumstances the term "overlap," "undifferentiated," or "mixed" connective tissue disease is applied. Noninfectious granulomatous diseases such as sarcoidosis share the tendency toward multiorgan involvement, musculoskeletal system manifestations, and a variety of immunologic phenomena. Immune complexes may be detected in the sera of many rheumatic patients.

More than 30 million Americans suffer from one or more rheumatic diseases. Fibromyositis and other forms of nonarticular rheumatism are the most common rheumatic diseases seen in office practice. Osteoarthritis is the most prevalent type of arthritis; almost all people over age 60 display at least roentgenographic evidence of the disease. Some types of arthritis are peculiar to certain age groups: rheumatic fever is basically a disease of children, gonococcal arthritis is most apt to be found in young adults, and rheumatoid arthritis is primarily a disease of young to middle-aged women. Gout usually strikes middle-aged and older men, whereas polymyalgia rheumatica and pseudogout are almost always confined to the elderly.

Patients with rheumatoid arthritis and other joint diseases complain of pain as the major symptom. Stiffness, muscle weakness, disability, swelling, tenderness, redness, heat, and deformity are other clinical features of rheumatic disease. A variety of biochemical and immunologic blood studies, as well as various roentgenographic procedures, enable more precise diagnosis, but these ancillary features rarely in themselves are diagnostic. Few forms of rheumatic diseases are curable, but most can be treated to the point that the patient is relatively asymptomatic. In some instances precise therapy will be lifesaving. As in all diseases, proper management depends on proper diagnosis, so development of a basic understanding of various arthritic, connective tissue, and granulomatous diseases is a requisite for sound medical practice.

10 • RHEUMATOID ARTHRITIS
Warren A. Katz

Although rheumatoid arthritis is a prototype of chronic destructive joint disease, the inflammatory process extends not only to the articular and tendon synovium but to many organs of the body. Rheumatoid arthritis is a protean disease that appears in many different forms. Some patients exhibit mild evanescent arthritis, whereas others experience unrelenting joint inflammation with ultimate crippling that confines them to bed. Most develop slowly progressive, moderately painful polyarthritis. Yet, patients with rheumatoid arthritis usually manage to function, although with difficulty.

Rheumatoid arthritis appears to be a disease of modern times, with no descriptions of it apparent in the literature prior to the 1800s. Innumerable research studies and new medical technical advances have not brought a cure but have enabled physicians to render most patients relatively symptom free and functional.

PATHOGENESIS/PATHOLOGY. The cause of rheumatoid arthritis is not known, but many investigators have suspected infectious, genetic, and endocrine factors. The current theory is that the genetically predisposed host, subjected to a foreign, offensive agent such as infection or trauma, undergoes unique immunologic changes that result in a perpetuating inflammatory process within the joints. Normally, in response to insult, the body mobilizes its immune defenses. IgG antibodies form in response to antigenic stimulation but somehow become altered or aggregated in patients with rheumatoid arthritis so that the body no longer recognizes IgG as "self." Rheumatoid factor (RF) is an antibody against this altered IgG antibody, and molecules of RF can link to one another to form "self-associated rheumatoid factor complexes" that in effect generate inflammation. One theory is that the offending agents in rheumatoid arthritis are bacterial cell-wall peptidoglycans that act as a chronic immunogenic stimulus. Furthermore, once destructive change in the joints takes place, altered cartilage components (proteoglycans) evoke additional immune responses, perpetuating inflammation. In the process the complement cascade is activated and polymorphonuclear leukocytes are attracted that ingest immune complexes. These eventually trigger the release of multiple mediators of inflammation that include prostaglandins, lysosomal enzymes, and collagenase, all of which aid in joint destruction. How and why the rheumatoid process is self-propagating are poorly understood.

CLINICAL MANIFESTATIONS. Rheumatoid arthritis can strike at any age, but usually bimodal distribution peaks are seen at the ages of 40 and 60. Women are 2½ times more likely to develop the disease than men. Rheumatoid arthritis may develop without any apparent associated phenomenon. In some cases emotional stress, trauma, and exposure to infections seem to predispose to rheumatoid arthritis.

Onset. Rheumatoid arthritis may develop at any time and in many ways. The usual mode of onset is that of indolent polyarthralgias, sometimes preceded by fatigue and muscle aches. The hands, feet, elbows, shoulders, and knees may, in additive fashion, become involved. Prolonged morning stiffness and clumsiness may be relatively early symptoms. Within weeks the symmetric polyarthritis characterized by tenderness and swelling becomes apparent. Less frequently, arthritis begins episodically in only one joint or causes excessive morning stiffness without appreciable joint pain. In other cases there is a marked systemic component, characterized by low-grade fever, malaise, anorexia, and weight loss. Rarely, explosive polyarthritis may be associated with high fever. At times there is relatively asymptomatic progressive swelling of the joints, particularly in the knees. Generalized weakness may accompany any presentation of arthritis.

Joint manifestations. Physical findings may be sparse in early rheumatoid arthritis. Ultimately, well-established patterns of involvement are noted, usually characterized by tenderness, swelling, and heat. Redness, except in very acute forms, is usually absent. Metacarpal phalangeal joints, proximal interphalangeal joints, metatarsal phalangeal joints, wrists, knees, shoulders, hips, elbows, ankles, tarsal joints, cervical spine, and temporomandibular joints are all prone to develop arthritis (Table 10-1). The lower spine and distal interphalangeal joints are usually spared. Painless tenosynovitis, particularly of the extensor carpi ulnaris tendon, may be one of the earliest signs of rheumatoid arthritis. There is evidence of autonomic dysfunction in the hands and feet, such as palmar erythema, increased sweating, generalized edema, and a mottled appearance to the skin.

The most diagnostic changes of rheumatoid arthritis are noted in the hands and wrists. Dorsal interosseous muscle atrophy frequently occurs. Swan-neck or boutonniére deformities of the hand are late findings (Fig. 10-1). The metacarpal phalangeal joints may be subluxed and deviated in an ulnar direction. Elbows become swollen and contracted. Limitation of motion is noted at the shoulders; with chronic progressive disease, the distal clavicles may erode and resorb.

One of the most ominous of all rheumatoid changes is subluxation of the first cervical vertebra on the second caused by weakening of the transverse ligament. Although most patients with a C1-2 subluxation are asymptomatic from a neurologic point of view, occipital headaches, weakness, and digital paresthesias should alert one to the diagnosis. Sudden snapping of the neck or undue mobilization during anesthetic or dental procedures may cause further dislocation if caution is not taken.

Temporomandibular arthritis is not uncommon in the rheumatoid process. Jaw pain, especially when chewing, is the major symptom. Overt inflammation may be noted just anterior to the ear. Opening the mouth may cause a snap or click. Occasionally, crepitus and hypermobility of the jaw develop. Extensive resorption of the mandibular condyles may cause recession of the chin, resembling the "Andy Gump" caricature.

Extra-articular manifestations. In about one third of the patients with progressive rheumatoid arthritis, several extra-articular manifestations may be noted. These include subcutaneous rheumatoid nodules in areas of pressure, cardiopulmonary lesions, peripheral neuritis, vasculitis, skin ulcerations, myositis, lymphadenopathy, and osteoporosis. Felty's syndrome is a complex of chronic rheumatoid arthritis, splenomegaly, anemia, thrombocytopenia, and neutropenia. Infections, leg ulcerations, and cutaneous pigmentation may be present with this disease.

Sjögren's syndrome

Although Sjögren's syndrome is a separate entity, it is most often associated with rheumatoid arthritis. Sjögren's syndrome, seen predominantly in women, is a chronic inflammation of the salivary, lacrimal, and other secreting glands characterized primarily by keratoconjunctivitis sicca

Table 10-1. Distribution of joint involvement in adult rheumatoid arthritis

Usual	Unusual	Rare
Ankles	Carpometacarpal joints	Distal interphalangeal joints
Cervical spine	Cricoarytenoid joints	Dorsal spine
Elbows	Sacroiliac joints	Lumbar spine
Hips	Sternoclavicular joints	
knees		
Metacarpal phalangeal joints		
Metatarsal phalangeal joints		
Proximal interphalangeal joints		
Shoulders		
Tarsal joints		
Temporomandibular joints		
Wrists		

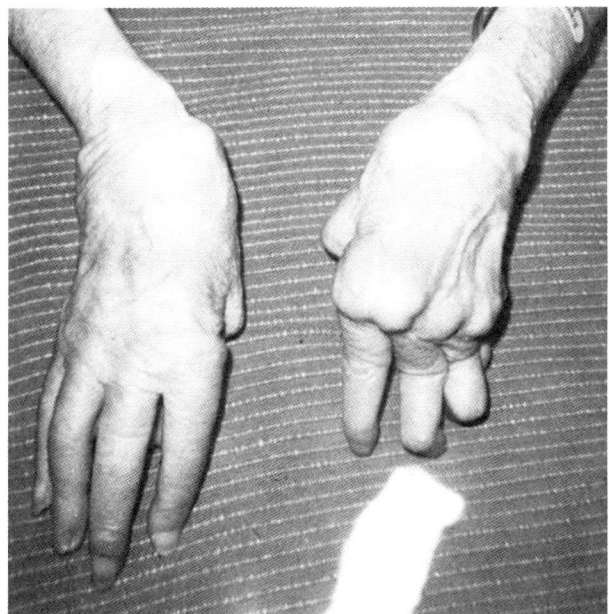

Fig. 10-1. Swan-neck deformity, ulnar deviation, dorsal interosseous muscle atrophy, and swelling of wrist–characteristics of rheumatoid arthritis.

and xerostomia. Dryness of the mouth, nose, eyes, tracheobronchial tree, rectum, and vagina may be profound. Patients complain of the tongue sticking to the roof of the mouth. The tongue is characteristically cracked, dry, and red. Salivary glands may be enlarged. Salivary flow rates are diminished or absent, and radioisotopic scintigraphy studies reveal glandular dysfunction. Diagnosis is confirmed by a lip biopsy. Antisalivary-duct antibody is detected in approximately 70% of these patients. Renal tubular acidosis, nonthrombocytopenic purpura, polymyopathy, neuritis, chronic liver disease, lymphoma, interstitial lung disease, hyperviscosity, and other plasma-cell dyscrasias may be noted.

LABORATORY FINDINGS

Laboratory studies. None of the multiple blood, synovial fluid, and biopsy studies in rheumatoid arthritis is specific for the disease. Almost all patients exhibit an elevated erythrocyte sedimentation rate during active phases, but this is nonspecific. Yet, a normal sedimentation rate should cause one to look on the diagnosis with some degree of suspicion. About 25% of patients with rheumatoid arthritis have some degree of anemia. This is usually a result of failure of iron utilization rather than direct iron loss through gastrointestinal blood loss.

Antinuclear antibody (ANA) is detectable in about 50% of patients with rheumatoid arthritis but has no diagnostic specificity because many other connective tissue diseases are characterized by high titers of ANA.

About 80% of patients with classic or definite rheumatoid arthritis exhibit significant elevations of RF, which are not, however, diagnostic. The higher the titer of RF, the more likely is the presence of rheumatoid arthritis, particularly when the titers are greater than 1:1280. The physician should bear in mind that RF does not parallel disease activity, although it is more likely to be present in high levels in patients with more advanced stages of the disease. High titers of RF, particularly when they appear early, seem to serve as indicators of a poor prognosis.

Rheumatoid synovial fluid is cloudy and often tinged green (Fig. 10-2). It forms a poor clot when acetic acid is added (Ropes test). The white cell counts may vary from 5000 to 60,000; the cells are predominantly polymorphonuclear leukocytes. White cells that have engulfed immune complexes are sometimes noted in rheumatoid synovial fluid in high numbers. These cytoplasmic inclusions in leukocytes are called *ragocytes*. Rheumatoid fluid is watery because of the breakdown of the viscous protein hyaluronate. Glucose in rheumatoid synovial and pleural fluids is appreciably lower than in serum. Rheumatoid nodules often give a characteristic pathologic picture on biopsy, but histologic evaluation of synovium, muscle, or

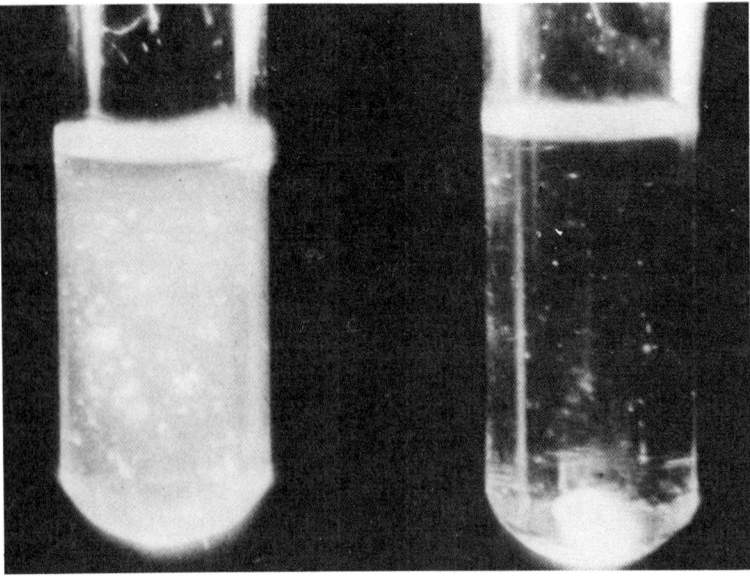

Fig. 10-2. Rheumatoid synovial fluid is cloudy and exhibits poor clotting when acetic acid is added *(left)*, compared to the tight clump formed in osteoarthritic fluid *(right)*. (From the Revised Clinical Slide Collection on the Rheumatic Diseases. Copyright 1981 by the Arthritis Foundation.)

other tissue mainly serves to rule out other confusing diseases.

Roentgenographic findings. Soft tissue swelling, subchondral osteopenia, marginal erosions, and joint space narrowing and deformity are the most common rheumatoid changes on roentgenograms, especially when symmetric (Fig. 10-3). Cervical spine roentgenograms may indicate a C1-2 subluxation that is recognized on the flexion-extension views as a widening of the interval between the odontoid process and the anterior ramus of the atlas (Fig. 10-4). Subluxation with a "staircase" appearance may be noted in lower cervical vertebrae.

Temporomandibular joint narrowing, erosion, subluxation, limitation of motion, and flattening of the condylar heads are apparent rheumatoid findings. Tomography is sometimes indicated to detect these changes.

DIAGNOSIS. The diagnosis of rheumatoid arthritis is based on a carefully obtained history, a diligent physical examination to uncover subtle signs of inflammation, and appropriate use of ancillary studies. By the time advanced deformities have taken place, the diagnosis is clear-cut. The art of medicine in rheumatoid arthritis is to detect the disease as early as possible in an effort to prevent crippling changes.

The American Rheumatism Association's diagnostic criteria aid in clinical diagnosis but were primarily designed for research and literary purposes (see box on pp. 40 and 41).

Differential diagnosis includes ankylosing spondylitis, rheumatic fever, psoriatic arthritis, Reiter's syndrome, arthritis of chronic inflammatory bowel disease, infectious arthritis, chronic tophaceous gout, pseudogout, polytendinitis, osteoarthritis, sympathetic reflex dystrophy, sarcoidosis, and hypertrophic pulmonary arthropathy. Other connective tissue diseases, such as systemic lupus erythematosus, polymyositis, and systemic sclerosis, may mimic the disease. In older people polymyalgia rheumatica, characterized by symmetric polyarthralgias in association with a marked elevated sedimentation rate, poses a formidable differential diagnosis. Fibromyalgia syndrome is a relatively benign condition in terms of crippling; patients experience multiple joint pain, but there are no constitutional symptoms. The erythrocyte sedimentation rate is normal, and the test for RF is usually negative. Roentgenograms of the involved joints are normal. Some of these patients complain of jaw pain and clicking that may imitate arthritis of the temporomandibular joint.

MANAGEMENT. Clearly the success of managing rheumatoid arthritis lies in a comprehensive, multidisciplinary approach. Systemically administered drugs, local injections of corticosteroids, physical therapy, occupational therapy, psychosocial support, patient education, family involvement, surgical intervention, and vocational rehabilitation are all part of the daily management program of patients with rheumatoid arthritis.

In general patients should be fully and honestly indoctrinated concerning their disease and the advantages of proper therapy and should be assured of a favorable outcome in terms of crippling if the management program is followed. Families are frequently helpful in motivating patients, aiding them in taking their medications, and assisting in physical and occupational therapy. Patients with rheumatoid arthritis require a balance of rest and exercise.

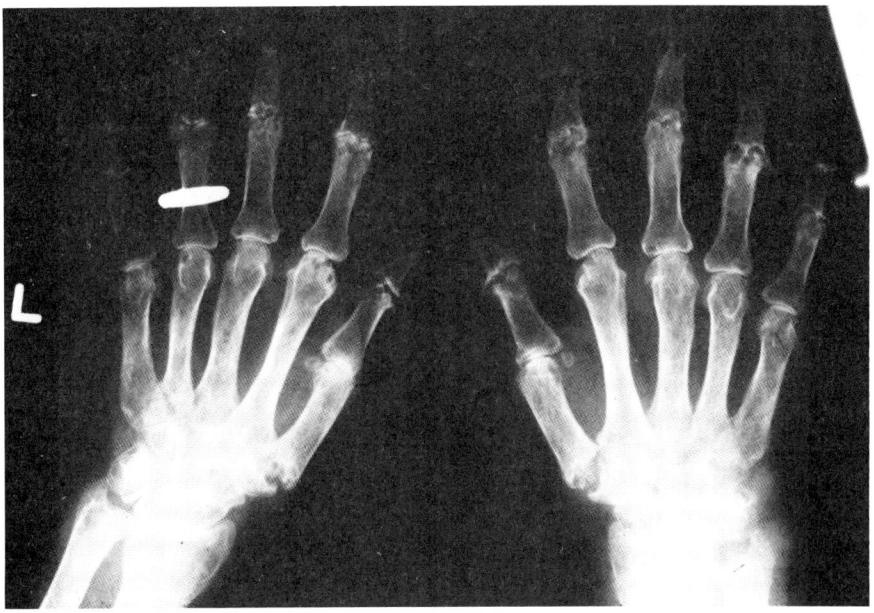

Fig. 10-3. Typical roentgenographic changes in hands of patient with rheumatoid arthritis. Note osteopenia, joint-space narrowing, and erosions. (From Katz, W.A.: Rheumatic diseases: diagnosis and management, Philadelphia, 1977, J.B. Lippincott Co.)

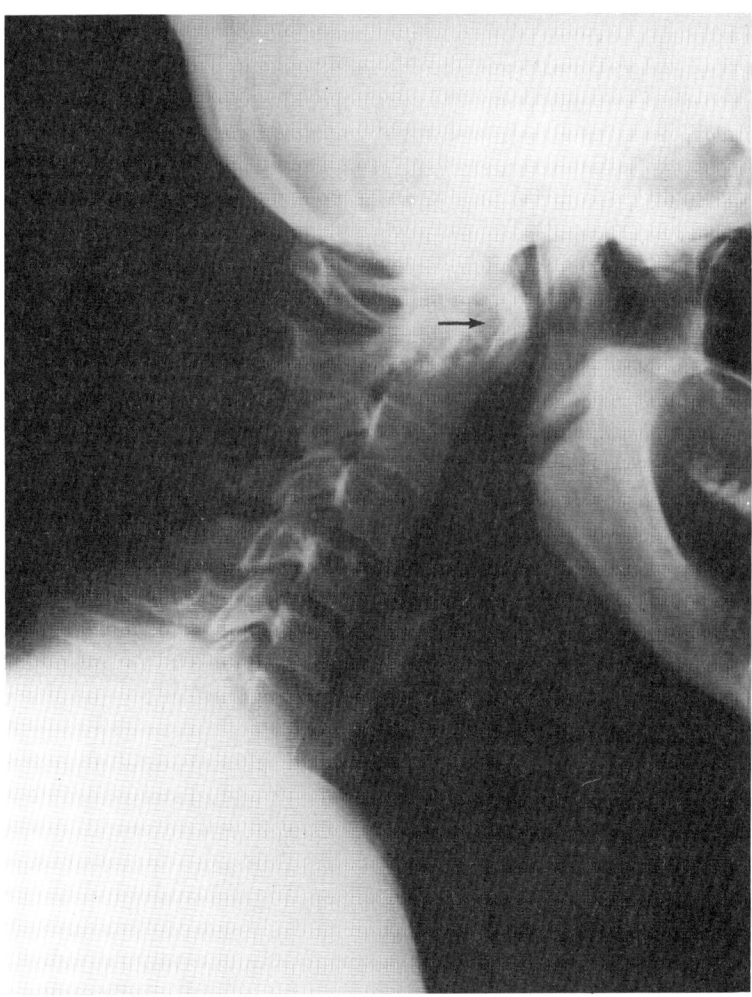

Fig. 10-4. C1-2 subluxation in rheumatoid arthritis. Arrow points to space between odontoid process and anterior arch of atlas.

American Rheumatism Association Criteria for the Diagnosis of Rheumatoid Arthritis

A. *Classical rheumatoid arthritis*

This diagnosis requires seven of the following criteria. In criteria 1 through 5 the joint signs or symptoms must be continuous for at least six weeks. (Any one of the features listed under "Exclusions" will exclude a patient from this and all categories.)
   1. Morning stiffness.
   2. Pain on motion or tenderness in at least one joint (observed by a physician).
   3. Swelling (soft tissue thickening or fluid, not bony overgrowth alone) in at least one joint (observed by a physician).
   4. Swelling (observed by a physician) of at least one other joint (any interval free of joint symptoms between the two joint involvements may not be more than 3 months).
   5. Symmetrical joint swelling (observed by a physician) with simultaneous involvement of the same joint on both sides of the body (bilateral involvement of proximal interphalangeal, metacarpophalangeal, or metatarsophalangeal joints is acceptable without absolute symmetry). Terminal phalangeal joint involvement will not satisfy this criterion.
   6. Subcutaneous nodules (observed by a physician) over bony prominences, on extensor surfaces, or in juxta-articular regions.
   7. Roentgenographic changes typical of rheumatoid arthritis (which must include at least bony decalcification localized to or most marked adjacent to the involved joints and not just degenerative changes). Degenerative changes do not exclude patients from any group classified as rheumatoid arthritis.
   8. Positive agglutination test—demonstration of the "rheumatoid factor" by any method which, in two laboratories, has been positive in not over 5% of normal controls—or positive streptococcal agglutination test. (The latter is now obsolete).
   9. Poor mucin precipitate from synovial fluid (with shreds and cloudy solution).
   10. Characteristic histologic changes in synovium with three or more of the following: marked villous hypertrophy; proliferation of superficial synovial cells often with palisading; marked infiltration of chronic inflammatory cells (lymphocytes or plasma cells predominating) with tendency to form "lymphoid nodules": deposition of compact fibrin either on surface or interstitially; foci of necrosis.
   11. Characteristic histologic changes in nodules showgranulomatous foci with central zones of cell necrosis, surrounded by a palisade of proliferated macrophages, and peripheral fibrosis and chronic inflammatory cell infiltration, predominantly perivascular.

B. *Definite rheumatoid arthritis*

This diagnosis requires five of the above criteria. In criteria 1 through 5 the joint signs or symptoms must be continuous for at least six weeks.

C. *Probably rheumatoid arthritis*

This diagnosis requires three of the above criteria. In at least one of 1 through 5 the joint signs or symptoms must be continuous for at least six weeks.

D. *Possible rheumatoid arthritis*

This diagnosis requires two of the following criteria and total duration of joint symptoms must be at least three weeks.
   1. Morning stiffness.
   2. Tenderness or pain on motion (observed by a physician) with history of recurrence or persistence for three weeks.

Copyright 1981 by the Arthritis Foundation.

American Rheumatism Association Criteria for the Diagnosis of Rheumatoid Arthritis—cont'd

    3. History or observation of joint swelling.
    4. Subcutaneous nodules (observed by a physician).
    5. Elevated sedimentation rate or C-reactive protein.
    6. Iritis (of dubious value as a criterion except in the case of juvenile rheumatoid arthritis).

E. *Exclusions*
    1. The typical rash of systemic lupus erythematosus (with butterfly distribution, follicle plugging, and areas of atrophy).
    2. High concentration of lupus erythematosus cells (four or more in two smears prepared from heparinized blood incubated not over two hours or other clearcut evidence of systemic lupus erythematosus).
    3. Histologic evidence of periarteritis nodosa with segmental necrosis of arteries associated with nodular leukocytic infiltration extending perivascularly and tending to include many eosinophils.
    4. Weakness of neck, trunk, and pharyngeal muscles or persistent muscle swelling or dermatomyositis.
    5. Definite scleroderma (not limited to the fingers). (The latter is an arguable point.)
    6. A clinical picture characteristic of rheumatic fever with migratory joint involvement and evidence of endocarditis, especially if accompanied by subcutaneous nodules or erythema marginatum or chorea. (An elevated antistreptolysin titer will not rule out the diagnosis of rheumatoid arthritis.)
    7. A clinical picture characteristic of gouty arthritis with acute attacks of swelling, redness, and pain in one or more joints, especially if relieved by colchicine.
    8. Tophi.
    9. A clinical picture characteristic of acute infectious arthritis of bacterial or viral origin with an acute focus of infection or in close association with a disease of known infectious origin: chills; fever; and an acute joint involvement, usually migratory initially (especially if there are organisms in the joint fluid or response to antibiotic therapy).
   10. Tubercle bacilli in the joints or histologic evidence of joint tuberculosis.
   11. A clinical picture characteristic of Reiter's syndrome with urethritis and conjunctivitis associated with acute joint involvement, usually migratory initially.
   12. A clinical picture characteristic of the shoulder-hand syndrome with unilateral involvement of shoulder and hand, with diffuse swelling of the hand followed by atrophy and contractures.
   13. A clinical picture characteristic of hypertrophic osteoarthropathy with clubbing of fingers and/or hypertrophic periostitis along the shafts of the long bones especially if an intrapulmonary lesion (or other appropriate underlying disorder) is present.
   14. A clinical picture characteristic of neuroarthropathy with condensation and destruction of bones of involved joints and with associated neurologic findings.
   15. Homogentisic acid in the urine, detectable grossly with alkalinization.
   16. Histologic evidence of sarcoid or positive Kveim test.
   17. Multiple myeloma as evidenced by marked increase in plasma cells in the bone marrow, or Bence-Jones protein in the urine.
   18. Characteristic skin lesions of erythema nodosum.
   19. Leukemia or lymphoma with characteristic cells in peripheral blood, bone marrow, or tissue.
   20. Agammaglobulinemia.

*

---

*EDITOR'S NOTE: Psoriatic arthritis, ankylosing spondylitis, and enteropathic arthropathy would be reasonable additions to this list.

Although certain vitamins and diets appear to be effective in some patients with rheumatoid arthritis, none has been proved to be better than the expected placebo response. More investigation is certainly required before diet and vitamin therapy can be recommended to the exclusion of other modalities of therapy.

Drugs. The pharmaceutical agents used against rheumatoid arthritis include analgesics, nonsteroidal anti-inflammatory drugs (NSAIDs), corticosteroids, remittive agents, and immunosuppressive drugs. NSAIDs (Table 10-2), whether aspirin or the more potent, more expensive drugs, serve to reduce inflammation and then pain. There is great patient individuality in terms of response to the NSAIDs, and each should be given an adequate trial before abandoning this type of therapy. These drugs as a general class tend to cause gastrointestinal irritation and fluid retention. Skin rash and mouth ulcers may occur.

Systemic corticosteroids are reserved for certain unusual cases of rheumatoid arthritis when other forms of therapy fail to stem a progressive, disabling, consumptive course. In all instances the dose of prednisone should be minimized.

On the other hand, local injections of corticosteroids, particularly after aspiration of one or two inflamed joints, may be extremely valuable and render the patient in some instances completely asymptomatic. At the very least, corticosteroid injections are adjunctive to systemic agents.

Available disease-modifying remittive agents include gold salts, antimalarial drugs, and penicillamine (Table 10-3). With long-term administration these drugs stand the best chance of inducing remission or at least effecting a long-term suppression of symptoms. None of these drugs works well in all patients with rheumatoid arthritis, but those who respond tend to respond well. Significant alleviation of symptoms, however, is not to be expected before 6 weeks. Penicillamine is gradually increased over several months. Major toxicity to gold consists of mouth ulcerations and skin rashes, but usually the drug can be recontinued after the side effects have cleared. Auranofin causes diarrhea. Antimalarial agents are apt to cause gastrointestinal upset and changes in vision. Penicillamine may precipitate mouth ulcers, renal toxicity, and gastrointestinal upset; a rash may be noted by some patients. Bone marrow suppression may occur. A peculiar side effect is loss of taste, although smell usually remains intact.

Azathioprine has been approved by the Food and Drug Administration for the treatment of chronic, recalcitrant forms of rheumatoid arthritis. The other immunosuppressive drugs still must be considered investigational. The side effects vary, and these agents tend to be toxic. Hematologic and hepatic manifestations must be closely observed. Some immunosuppressive drugs are capable of producing mouth ulcerations during treatment.

Tranquilizers, antidepressants, and muscle relaxants may be prescribed for certain patients with rheumatoid arthritis. The physician must bear in mind that other illnesses that call for specific therapy may affect the rheumatoid patient.

Physical and occupational therapy. Pain relief and reduction of inflammation can be achieved through applications of heat and ice; the form used is a matter of personal preference. Range of motion exercises to all joints helps prevent restriction of joints. Splints of various types help immobilize the joint, reduce inflammation, and alleviate the pain.

Surgery. Various operations are now performed on patients with rheumatoid arthritis. Persistent synovitis, despite conservative but intensive medical therapy, may call for a synovectomy. By the time surgery is performed in most cases, moderate to marked destructive changes are noted so that the surgeon is required to perform an arthroplasty in addition to a synovectomy. When the joint space is destroyed and the patient is rendered either bedridden or in severe pain because of joint destruction, total joint re-

Table 10-2. Nonsteroidal anti-inflammatory drugs used in the treatment of rheumatoid arthritis

Drug	Usual daily dose
Aspirin	900 mg q.i.d.
Fenoprofen	300-600 mg q.i.d.
Ibuprofen	400-600 mg q.i.d.
Indomethacin	25-50 mg q.i.d.
Meclofenamic acid	50-100 mg t.i.d.
Naproxen	200-375 mg b.i.d.
Sulindac	150-200 mg b.i.d.
Tolmetin	200-400 mg q.i.d.

Table 10-3. Remittive drugs used in the treatment of rheumatoid arthritis

Drug	Usual dose
Antimalarials (chloroquine, 250 mg, or hydroxychloroquine, 200 mg)	One tablet b.i.d.
Gold parenterally (sodium aurothiomalate or aurothioglucose)	Test dose 10 mg, then 25-50 mg weekly for 4-6 mo, then every 2 wk, then every 3 wk; maintenance dose 50 mg monthly as tolerated
Gold orally (auranofin, 3 mg)	One tablet twice a day
Penicillamine (125-250 mg)	Initial dose 250 mg daily, raised by 125-mg increments every 6-8 wk as tolerated if active arthritis persists; maximum daily dose 1500 mg

placement, such as a total knee or total hip arthroplasty, is considered.

Psychosocial-sexual problems. Psychologic ramifications of rheumatoid arthritis are unlimited. Some cases of rheumatoid arthritis arise from stressful situations; in others the rheumatoid arthritis itself creates the stress. It is almost impossible to treat patients with chronic rheumatoid arthritis without dealing with their problems of stress and other psychologic situations. Rheumatoid arthritis, by causing persistent pain and limitation of motion in key joints, presents sexual difficulties. Families, friends, and employers are often drawn into the therapeutic interaction.

Hospitalization. Most patients with rheumatoid arthritis do not require hospitalization, but removing the patient from his usual environment often fosters a remission of disease activity.

Other advantages of hospitalization include facilitation of the indoctrination period when rheumatoid arthritis is recent, intensive physical and occupational therapy, assurance that medication and other therapies are carried out, administration of potent drugs that need monitoring, and joint surgery in the setting of a comprehensive team approach.

PROGNOSIS. Patients with rheumatoid arthritis usually advance to chronicity, but progressive disabling deformities are not inevitable. Most patients will have flare-ups and exacerbations for many years, yet with proper management and encouragement, they can work and function well in activities of daily living.

The prognosis is worse in females, when onset is insidious and when active arthritis persists. The presence of multiple effusions, early constitutional symptoms, rheumatoid nodules, and high levels of RF in serum adversely affect the prognosis.

BIBLIOGRAPHY

Bennett, J.C.: The infectious etiology of rheumatoid arthritis: new considerations, Arthritis Rheum. **21:**531, 1978.

Bluestone, R., and Bacon, P.A.: Extraarticular manifestations of rheumatoid arthritis, Clin. Rheum. Dis. **3:**385, 1973.

Bunch, T.W., and O'Duffy, J.D.: Disease-modifying drugs for progressive rheumatoid arthritis, Mayo Clin. Proc. **55:**161, 1980.

Harris, E.D., Jr.: Recent insights into the pathogenesis of the proliferative lesion in rheumatoid arthritis, Arthritis Rheum. **19:**68, 1966.

Jaffe, I.A.: D-Penicillamine, Bull. Rheum. Dis. **28:**948, 1977–1978.

Johnson, P.M., and Faulk, W.P.: Rheumatoid factor: its nature, specificity, and production in rheumatoid arthritis, Clin. Immunol. Immunopathol. **6:**414, 1976.

Mason, M., and Currey, H.L.F.: Clinical rheumatology, Philadelphia, 1970, J.B. Lippincott Co.

McMichael, A.J., and others: Increased frequency of HLA-Cw3 and HLA-D24 in rheumatoid arthritis, Arthritis Rheum. **20:**1037, 1980.

11 • JUVENILE RHEUMATOID ARTHRITIS

Balu H. Athreya

Juvenile rheumatoid arthritis (JRA) is a disease characterized by chronic synovitis, with or without extra-articular manifestations. It is also known as Still's disease, juvenile chronic polyarthritis, and chronic childhood arthritis; the preferred term in the United States is JRA.

There are approximately 100,000 to 200,000 children with JRA in the United States. The ratio of JRA compared to adult rheumatoid arthritis is approximately 1:20. JRA has been reported from tropical, subtropical, and temperate climates.

JRA is not a single disease; it is probably a group of diseases. There are least five recognized subgroups, each with a fairly characteristic clinical course and prognosis. Whether splitting JRA into subgroups will lead to better understanding of the cause or pathogenesis remains to be seen.

JRA is a *chronic* disease. Since there are no diagnostic laboratory tests, it is diagnosed *clinically* after *exclusion* of other diseases.

ETIOLOGY. The etiology of JRA is unknown. A history of recent systemic infection or trauma is obtained in many patients with JRA. Exacerbations of the disease may follow intercurrent infections, trauma, or psychologic stress. Usually there is no family history of rheumatoid arthritis. Association between HLA (histocompatibility) antigens (DR5 and DR8) and JRA has been reported. There is a subset of JRA (pauciarticular with sacroiliitis) in which HLA-B27 is usually present.

The proposed etiologic mechanisms and pathology are similar to those in adults, but there are many differences in the clinical syndromes (Chapter 10). Even rheumatoid factor (RF), which is present in over 80% of adults with rheumatoid arthritis, is found in less than 20% of children with JRA. It is also interesting to note that children with agammaglobulinemia and IgA deficiency may develop chronic polyarthritis indistinguishable from JRA.

CLINICAL MANIFESTATIONS OF VARIOUS SUBTYPES (TABLE 11-1)

Polyarticular (RF positive) JRA. Polyarticular (RF positive) JRA occurs in approximately 10% of children with JRA. As the name implies, these children have RF in the serum, and the disease course resembles adult-onset arthritis. Girls are more often affected. The onset is usually in the preadolescent age group and is characterized by symmetric and polyarticular involvement of both large and small joints. Characteristic swelling of small joints of the fingers is common (Fig. 11-1). The cervical spine is involved in approximately 30% of the children, as evidenced by neck pain, torticollis, and limitation of range of move-

Table 11-1. Subgroups of JRA

Subgroup	Sex ratio	Age at onset	Joints affected	Serologic and genetic tests*	Extra-articular manifestations	Prognosis
RF positive, polyarticular	80% girls	Late childhood	Any joints	ANA 75% RF 100%	Low-grade fever, anemia, malaise, rheumatoid nodules	>50% severe arthritis
RF negative, polyarticular	90% girls	Any age	Any joints	ANA 5% RF negative	Low-grade fever, mild anemia, malaise, growth retardation	10%-15% severe arthritis
Pauciarticular (type 1) with chronic iridocyclitis	80% girls	Early childhood	A few large joints (hips and sacroiliac joints spared)	ANA 50% RF negative	Few constitutional complaints, chronic iridocyclitis in 50%	Severe arthritis uncommon, 10%-20% ocular damage from iridocyclitis
Pauciarticular (type 2) with sacroiliitis	90% boys	Late childhood	A few large joints (hip and sacroiliac involvement common)	ANA negative RF negative HLA-B27 75%	Few constitutional complaints, acute iridocyclitis in 5%-10% during childhood	Some have ankylosing spondylitis at follow-up
Systemic onset	60% boys	Any age	Any joints	ANA negative RF negative	High fever, rash, organomegaly, polyserositis, leukocytosis, growth retardation	25% severe arthritis

Modified and reprinted by permission of the publisher from The spectrum of juvenile rheumatoid arthritis by J.G. Schaller. In Franklin, E.C., editor: Clinical immunology update. Copyright 1979 by Elsevier Science Publishing Co., Inc.
*ANA, antinuclear antibody; RF, rheumatoid factor; HLA-B27, histocompatibility antigen-B27.

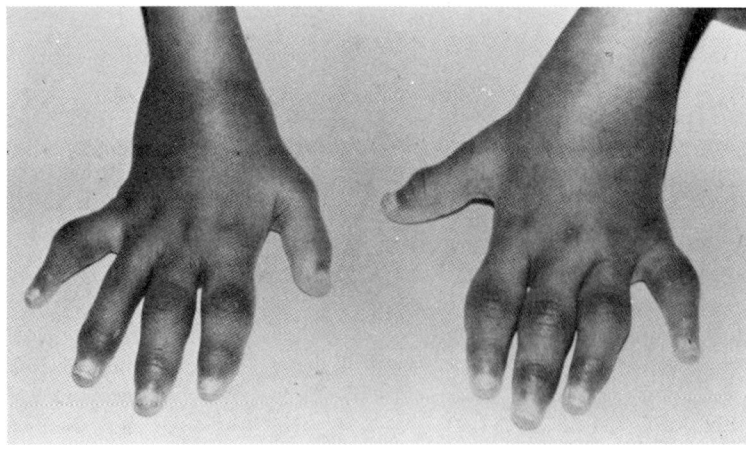

Fig. 11-1. Hands of child with severe JRA. Note bilateral involvement of wrists and small joints of fingers.

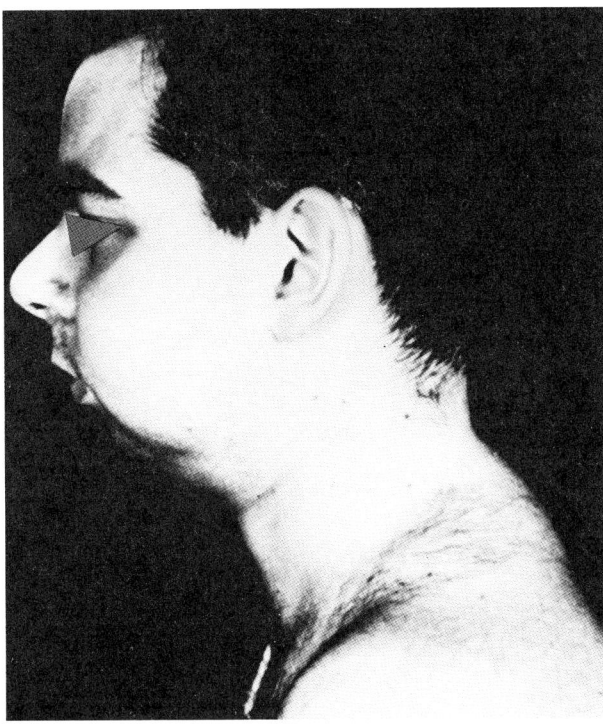

Fig. 11-2. Micrognathia of JRA. (From the Revised Clinical Slide Collection on the Rheumatic Diseases. Copyright 1981 by the Arthritis Foundation.)

ment of the neck. Subluxation of the atlantoaxial joint is a serious consequence of cervical spine involvement. This is an important point to remember, since careless manipulation of the neck during anesthesia in the presence of atlantoaxial subluxation may be fatal.

Temporomandibular joint (TMJ) involvement is also common in this group. The involvement may be unilateral or bilateral with such symptoms as pain at the joint, ear pain, pain during eating, and inability to open the mouth. Micrognathia (Fig. 11-2) is also a common feature in children with severe polyarticular disease.

Other findings include low-grade fever, loss of weight, anemia, and growth retardation. Morning stiffness is very common and often disabling. Rheumatoid nodules occur most commonly in this group and are seen often over the extensor aspect of the joints and behind the ear. Sjögren's syndrome and rheumatoid vasculitis may also develop in this age group. All these patients have RF in the serum, and almost 75% have antinuclear antibody (ANA).

Polyarticular (RF negative) JRA. Polyarticular (RF negative) JRA occurs in almost 30% of patients with JRA. It affects mostly girls, and the clinical characteristics are similar to those of polyarticular (RF positive) disease. The major differences are (1) RF is absent in the serum, (2) onset is common at any age, (3) prognosis is more favorable (Table 11-1), and (4) rheumatoid vasculitis does not occur. About 5% of these patients have ANA in the serum.

Pauciarticular JRA (type 1). Pauciarticular JRA (type 1) with chronic iridocyclitis occurs predominantly in girls under age 5. It accounts for almost 25% of patients with JRA. The term "pauciarticular" denotes that these children have less than four joints affected during the first 6 months of the disease. Usually large joints are affected, although not to the exclusion of the temporomandibular joints, cervical spine, and small joints of the fingers. Even though these children may have chronic or recurrent bouts of arthritis, serious disability rarely occurs.

Children in this particular group, however, are at high risk for developing chronic iridocyclitis. The iridocyclitis can occur before, during, or after the onset of arthritis. It is usually unilateral and insidious in onset (unlike acute iridocyclitis of ankylosing spondylitis).

Pauciarticular JRA (type 2). Pauciarticular JRA (type 2) is seen in almost 15% of children with JRA. These are mostly boys in the preadolescent age group. They do not have RF or ANA in the serum. Although they are classified clinically as having JRA at the time of diagnosis, the condition of many will probably evolve into ankylosing spondylitis or Reiter's syndrome. About 75% of the children in this group carry HLA-B27 antigen. Sacroiliitis is common in this age group. They tend to develop acute rather than chronic iridocyclitis.

Systemic-onset JRA. Systemic-onset JRA, also known as the febrile form of Still's disease, occurs in 20% of

Table 11-2. Drug treatment of JRA

Drug	Initial dose range	Side effects
Acetylsalicylic acid (aspirin, ASA)	Initial dose 75-90 mg/kg/day, increase gradually to 120 mg/kg/day, aim for serum salicylate level of 20-30 mg/dl	Gastric irritation, hepatotoxicity, hyperpnea, platelet problems
Nonsteroidal anti-inflammatory drugs (NSAID)	Alternative to aspirin	
Tolmetin (Tolectin), FDA approved for pediatric use	Initial dose 15 mg/kg/day, increase to 30 mg/kg/day, maximum dose 1800 mg/day	Gastric irritation, headache, hematuria
Indomethacin (Indocin), not approved by FDA	Initial dose 0.5 mg/kg/day, increase gradually to 2.5 mg/kg/day or a maximum of 100 mg/day	Gastric irritation, headache, hematuria
Ibuprofen (Motrin), not approved by FDA	Dose not established for children, up to 40 mg/kg/day has been used	Transient rash, gastric irritation, thrombocytopenia, hematuria
Naproxen (Naprosyn), not approved by FDA	10 mg/kg/day in two divided doses	Gastric irritation, rash, headache
Slow-acting antirheumatic drugs (SAARD)	Administered with aspirin or one of the NSAID	
Gold (Myochrysine or Solganal)	Weekly injections for 20-24 wk: test dose is 2 mg for infants, 5 mg for older children, 10 mg for adolescents	Rash, bone marrow depression, renal toxicity
	If no anaphylactoid reaction to test dose, increase weekly dose gradually, with 0.25 mg/kg on wk 1, 0.5 mg/kg on wk 2, 0.75 mg/kg on wk 3; maintain on 1 mg/kg/wk with maximum single weekly dose of 25 mg for older children and 50 mg for adolescents; after 20-24 wk, if no response, discontinue; with response, continue at same dose but only once monthly	
Chloroquine (Aralen)	4-5 mg/kg/day, maximum 250 mg/day	Toxicity to retina, corneal deposits, bleaching of hair, light sensitivity
Hydrochloroquine (Plaquenil)	7-8 mg/kg/day, maximum 400 mg/day	
Penicillamine (Cuprimine, Depen)	Initial dose 3 mg/kg/day, after 1 mo increase to 6 mg/kg/day, after 3 mo increase to 9 mg/kg/day	Skin rash, renal toxicity, bone marrow depression
Steroids	Use sparingly and for as short a time as possible; intra-articular steroids for persistently active single joint disease, topical use for iridocyclitis	Many side effects include growth retardation, osteoporosis, hypertension

children with JRA. This is most common in children under age 5, although it is now being recognized later in life as adult-onset Still's disease. It occurs in both boys and girls. The onset is characterized by high fevers, up to 104° F (40° C), which should initially alert physicians to exclude various infectious diseases. These children get an evanescent, macular pink rash that appears during the height of fever. It is seen mostly on the trunk and upper arm and is nonpruritic. Generalized lymphadenopathy and hepatosplenomegaly are common; therefore, leukemia and neuroblastoma have to be considered in the differential diagnosis and excluded. Pleuritis and pericarditis may be heralded by chest pain. In the early stages these children may have arthralgia, muscle spasm, and morning stiffness but no true synovitis. After 1 or 2 years, fever episodes subside, but polyarticular arthritis remains as the major problem. RF or ANA are not detected in the serum.

LABORATORY FINDINGS. Mild to moderate anemia and leukocytosis (up to 50,000/mm^3) are common, particularly in systemic JRA. Platelet counts, when elevated in the systemic and polyarticular varieties, often indicate poor prognosis for full recovery. Urinalysis is normal. Acute phase reactants, such as erythrocyte sedimentation rate (ESR), C-reactive protein, haptoglobin, and C3 complement, are elevated, even in the pauciarticular variety. Serum proteins are often abnormal with elevated alpha-2 and gammaglobulins. RF factor (>1:40) is demonstrated in the serum of all patients with the special RF-positive subtype described earlier, but it is present in only 10% to 20% of the entire group. ANA may be present in the sera of patients with polyarticular arthritis (both types) and pauciarticular arthritis (type 1) but not in pauciarticular arthritis (type 2) and systemic forms.

Synovial fluid analysis is often essential in the diagnosis of pauciarticular arthritis. The fluid appears cloudy, with an increased number of cells (up to 100,000/mm^3), most of which are polymorphonuclear. Glucose levels are normal, cultures are negative, and levels of C3 and C4 may be low.

Early roentgenographic findings of affected joints include swelling of soft tissue, effusion, and periostitis. Later, osteoporosis and accelerated bone growth may be seen. In long-standing arthritis, subchondral erosions, narrowing of joint space, bone destruction, and fusion may develop. In roentgenograms of the temporomandibular joint, erosion, flattening, and rarefaction of the condyle are seen. The glenoid fossa is often shallow.

DIFFERENTIAL DIAGNOSIS. Since JRA is a diagnosis of exclusion and there are many subgroups, the differential diagnostic process should continue throughout follow-up. A male child with pauciarticular arthritis may develop clinical features of ankylosing spondylitis in later life. A child with the systemic type of JRA may later develop features of scleroderma or systemic lupus erythematosus.

In the systemic form, infections, leukemia, and neuroblastoma have to be ruled out. In the monoarticular variety, however, local causes of joint disease, such as infectious arthritis, aseptic necrosis, and pigmented villonodular synovitis, must be considered. In the differential diagnosis of early stages of polyarticular arthritis, the following diseases have to be considered: acute rheumatic fever, systemic lupus erythematosus, gonococcal arthritis-dermatitis syndrome, and scleroderma. The differential diagnosis of pauciarticular arthritis includes ankylosing spondylitis, Reiter's syndrome, and arthritis of inflammatory bowel disease.

MANAGEMENT. Since JRA carries a reasonably good prognosis and is not life-threatening, the goals of treatment should be (1) to treat with drugs less dangerous than the disease, (2) to preserve joint function, and (3) to educate the family and the child so that the child is encouraged to lead as normal a life as possible. This requires a comprehensive management program supervised by a primary physician. Teamwork involving the primary physician, rheumatologist, child, family, orthopedic surgeon, physical therapist, occupational therapist, school teacher, school gym teacher, and orthodontist is ideal.

Bed rest is not of proven value, particularly in the pediatric age group, except in the presence of pericarditis. Local rest, best provided with a splint, is indicated for severely inflamed joints. Proper nutrition is obviously needed. A list of drugs commonly used in this disease is given in Table 11-2. Of these drugs, acetylsalicylic acid (aspirin, ASA) is the safest, simplest, and most economic and is adequate to control the disease in over 80% of cases. One of the nonsteroidal anti-inflammatory drugs (NSAID) may be used in the place of ASA, but none of them is more effective than ASA. Of these drugs, only tolmetin is approved for use in children. This drug is used when the child is allergic to ASA or develops gastric or hepatic complications with ASA. After a trial with one of these drugs (ASA or NSAID) for 6 to 12 weeks in adequate dosages with no response, one of the drugs from the slow-acting antirheumatic group (SAARD), such as gold, is added to the treatment program. Steroids are used only for pericarditis, severe systemic forms of JRA unresponsive to therapy, or severe iridocyclitis. Local steroids are used for less severe eye disease and for intra-articular injections of single joints with severe inflammation.

Simple measures to alleviate morning stiffness include sleeping in a sleeping bag and taking warm tub baths in the morning. Physical therapy and occupational therapy programs should be tailored to the child's age and developmental needs and the family's problems. Simple activities such as tricycling, bicycling, and swimming are more likely to be followed than formal therapy programs. Children with severe deformities and active disease may need intensive therapy programs.

Children with severe TMJ pain may have to be fed liquids with a straw to maintain nutrition. Fortunately, this is needed for only 1 or 2 days during an acute flare-up. The best physical therapy program for TMJ, in my experience, is chewing gum.

In the pediatric age group, orthopedic surgery is infrequently indicated. Soft tissue surgery to release contractures is likely to be needed more often than synovectomy or joint replacement. Total hip replacements, however, have been performed successfully in teenagers.

Iridocyclitis needs urgent, expert care. All children with JRA require yearly slit-lamp examinations. Children with pauciarticular arthritis (type 1) should have their eyes checked every 3 months during the active stage of the disease and every 6 months after the arthritis is controlled.

PROGNOSIS. With proper total care, most children with JRA should be able to lead active lives. Although there is no "cure" for this disease, it is not a "killing disease," and prognosis is good for most patients. About 80% of children recover fully without residual deformities. About 15% recover with mild to moderate deformities. Less than 5% are left with severe deformities. The mortality rate is less than 1%. The prognosis is worse for children with systemic and polyarticular (RF positive) varieties of JRA. For children with pauciarticular (type 1) JRA, the major problems are related to the eyes.

BIBLIOGRAPHY

Calabro, J.J., and others: Juvenile rheumatoid arthritis: a general review and report of 100 patients observed for 15 years, Semin. Arthritis Rheum. **5:**257, 1976.

Proceedings of the ARA conference on the rheumatic diseases of childhood, Arthritis Rheum. **20**(Suppl. 2), 1977.

Schaller, J.G.: The spectrum of juvenile rheumatoid arthritis. In Franklin, E.C., editor: Clinical immunology update, New York, 1979, Elsevier Publishing Co.

12 • ANKYLOSING SPONDYLITIS
Randolph C. Blodgett, Jr.

Ankylosing spondylitis is the preferred term to describe a connective tissue inflammation involving the sacroiliac and apophyseal joints of the vertebrae and associated articulations that may progress to bony fusion of the axial skeleton. Inflammation may also involve the central and peripheral joints. There is general agreement that ankylosing spondylitis is distinct from rheumatoid arthritis, although both diseases share common features. Synonyms include Marie-Strümpell disease, Bechterew's disease, and rheumatoid spondylitis.

EPIDEMIOLOGY. Ankylosing spondylitis is more common in males than females by a ratio of 9:1. Careful history taking suggests a familial prevalence. More recently, tissue histocompatibility typing has indicated a 90% occurrence of HLA-B27 antigen in a population of white patients with ankylosing spondylitis, compared with a 7% incidence of HLA-B27 antigen in an apparently normal white population. The variability between ethnic groups supports the concept of a hereditary factor.

The HLA-B27 antigen has become a potential marker for ankylosing spondylitis susceptibility, but care should be exercised not to invoke the tissue histocompatibility marker as a diagnostic test. The incidence of HLA-B27 antigen is also increased in other connective tissue diseases, such as Reiter's syndrome and psoriatic arthritis.

Ankylosing spondylitis usually becomes symptomatic in late adolescence or early adulthood, from ages 15 to 35.

PATHOGENESIS. The cause of ankylosing spondylitis is unknown. This inflammatory disease process involves primarily the axial skeleton, including the sacroiliac, apophyseal, and central joints (temporomandibular, symphysis pubis, sternomanubrium, acromioclavicular). Peripheral synovial joint inflammation is more common in the large joints, such as hips, shoulders, and knees, than in the distal joints of the extremities.

With progression of the inflammatory process, there is more synovitis, granulation, and fibroblast activity leading to fibrosis of the joint capsule and the periarticular structures. This may lead to calcification of the ligaments, anulus fibrosus, and even the joints themselves. Syndesmophytes are calcified bridges from vertebra to vertebra.

Extra-articular manifestations of ankylosing spondylitis include aortitis, which can result in aortic insufficiency, and inflammation of the uveal tract (uveitis) that occurs in about 25% of patients.

CLINICAL MANIFESTATIONS
Symptoms. Early symptoms of ankylosing spondylitis are most often localized to the lower back and sacroiliac region and less commonly to the shoulders, hips, peripheral joints, and thoracic cage.

The onset of symptoms is insidious in about 75% of patients with ankylosing spondylitis. Even when abrupt, the *initial* symptoms are usually intermittent and may be so mild that they are minimized by the patient unless he is intensely questioned. The tendency for the early symptoms to be intermittent may help in the diagnosis, even when the symptoms have become more persistent later in the course of the disease. Patients with lower back distress often relate their symptoms to assumed trauma; however, trauma is not an etiologic factor in ankylosing spondylitis.

Pain is of a deep, boring quality in various portions of the pelvic girdle. Sciatica-like pain radiating into the posterior thighs is a common complaint, but careful inquiry will often disclose intermittent, *alternating* or bilateral buttock discomfort—a useful clue differentiating this pain from a lumbar disc syndrome. Nocturnal pain usually involves the lower back or pelvic girdle with occasional radiation into the leg. This characteristically appears in the early morning after 2 to 4 hours of sleep, mimicking the time pattern of fibrositic stiffness. Thoracic cage pain related to the spine or costochondral joints is a complaint in more advanced stages of the disease.

Stiffness commonly occurs in the lower back following rest or immobilization. It is characteristically worse in the morning on arising and may be so severe that the patient must "roll out of bed" rather than sit up normally. This stiffness is typically relieved by heat or activity and recurs with relative immobility.

Physical examination. Findings will vary with exacerbations and remissions of disease activity. In the early stages of ankylosing spondylitis, the history provides more diagnostic clues than the physical examination. Paravertebral muscle spasm may be an early finding, especially during an exacerbation of clinical symptoms. These areas of spasm will be tender to percussion. Postural changes may be evident early. The lumbar spine may flatten (loss of normal lordosis), yet the patient may maintain full range of motion. Early limitation of motion is intermittent. Early evidence of these functional losses will be noted only with careful examination of the back for posture and range of motion. Increasing thoracic kyphosis and cervical flexion may be associated with a loss of height and stooped-over, "hangdog" specter. The classic "poker spine" suggests a late or advanced stage of ankylosing spondylitis. Rigidity of the entire spine and hips may prohibit any flexion whatsoever of the axial skeleton.

The temporomandibular joints may be involved in ankylosing spondylitis in a manner identical to rheumatoid arthritis. Mandibular and cephalic pain are characteristic symptoms. The C1 and C2 vertebrae may dislocate. The spine once fused is subject to fracture. Restriction of chest expansion usually occurs later in the disease, with involvement of the thoracic portion of the spine and the costovertebral articulations. Peripheral joint involvement develops most often in the large or proximal joints. It may be clinically indistinguishable from rheumatoid arthritis.

Iritis and aortic regurgitation secondary to aortitis are important extra-articular manifestations that can be overlooked on a cursory physical examination.

LABORATORY FINDINGS. Routine laboratory tests are of little diagnostic support in uncovering ankylosing spondylitis. The erythrocyte sedimentation rate (ESR) is elevated in 75% to 80% of patients and may be helpful in following the course of disease activity. Anemia and leukocytosis, when present, are nonspecific; the rheumatoid factor is generally negative.

Although there is no diagnostic laboratory test for ankylosing spondylitis, the recent introduction of tissue histocompatibility testing (see discussion of epidemiology) has provided a screening technique for patients with lower back symptoms by indicating those who require more intensive evaluation or observation for rheumatic disease. The HLA-B27 antigen is present in about 90% of patients with ankylosing spondylitis, yet detectable in only 7% of healthy control subjects. A positive test is not diagnostic because HLA-B27 is not peculiar to ankylosing spondylitis and is positive in a variety of other diseases, including the seronegative arthropathies, such as psoriatic arthritis, Reiter's syndrome, and arthritis of inflammatory bowel disease. Nevertheless, a negative HLA-B27 antigen test indicates a low probability of ankylosing spondylitis in a patient with back pain.

Roentgenographic findings. In early ankylosing spondylitis the roentgenograms of the sacroiliac joints and spine may be normal. There may not even be demonstrable changes for several years after the onset of symptoms, until the disease process has caused sufficient cartilage and subchondral bone destruction to be visualized by roentgenographic examination.

Sacroiliac joint involvement occurs in 98% of patients with well-developed ankylosing spondylitis. Blurry, irregular margins and joint-space widening are early manifestations in the sacroiliac joints. Subsequently, there will be varying degrees of marginal sclerosis on both sides of the

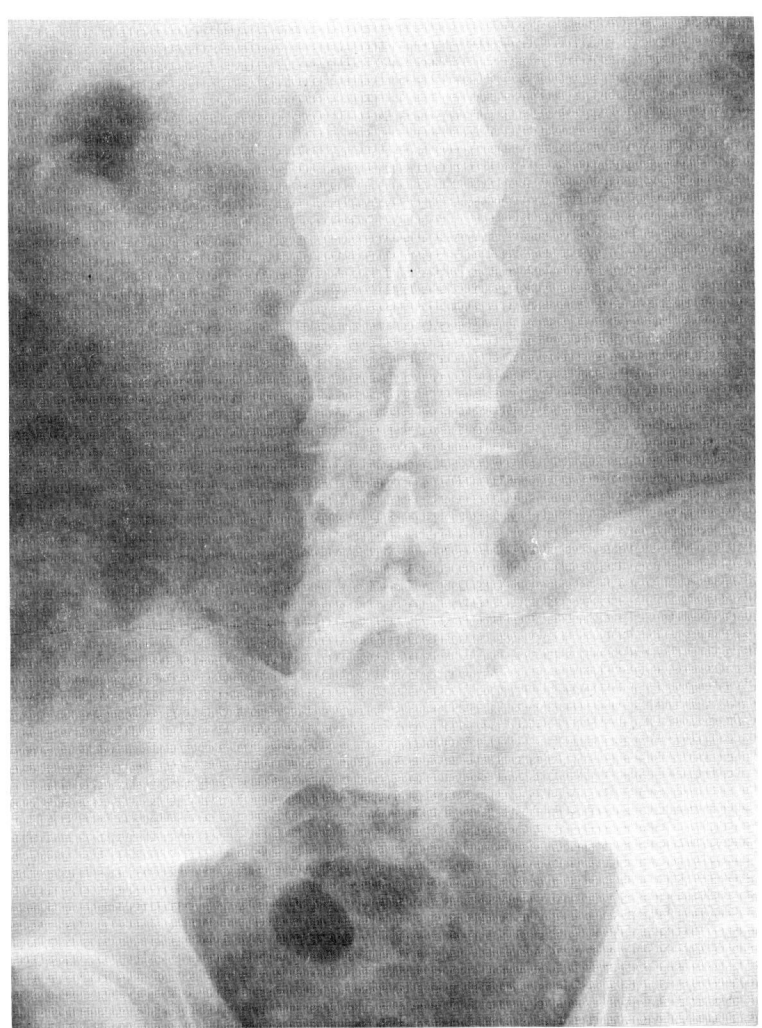

Fig. 12-1. Typical "bamboo spine" of advanced ankylosing spondylitis. Note absence of sacroiliac joints.

joint, with narrowing of the joint space. This process may lead to complete ankylosis. It is uncommon to have normal sacroiliac joints in established ankylosing spondylitis.

An early clue in diagnosing ankylosing spondylitis is the loss of concavity on the anterior aspect of the vertebrae or "squaring" of the vertebrae, giving a blocklike appearance on the lateral view of the dorsal and lumbar spine. Later changes are progressive calcification of the anulus fibrosus, longitudinal ligaments, and the other paravertebral ligaments. Linear calcification along the vertebral bodies develops into syndesmophytes, which are bridges between the vertebrae. The progressive calcification of these tissues produces the classic "bamboo spine," which is seen in late or advanced ankylosing spondylitis (Fig. 12-1).

DIAGNOSIS. Lower back pain is a very common complaint. Obviously, few patients with back pain actually have ankylosing spondylitis. The diagnosis is not merely one of exclusion; ankylosing spondylitis should be suspected on the basis of characteristic historic clues and physical findings.

Ankylosing spondylitis must be distinguished from an intervertebral disc syndrome. Disc problems may occur in both sexes at any age, but ankylosing spondylitis is prevalent in 15- to 35-year-old males. A history of trauma favors a herniated disc. Degenerative changes on a roentgenogram, with normal sacroiliac joints, are of differential value. If symptoms are acute, it may be difficult to differentiate between a disc syndrome and ankylosing spondylitis. Bilateral or alternating sciatica favors ankylosing spondylitis, whereas a disc tends to produce unilateral sciatica, except in the uncommon occurrence of a midline protrusion.

A formidable differential diagnosis in older patients with more advanced symptoms is diffuse idiopathic skeletal hyperostosis (DISH), a degenerative rather than inflammatory disease, also primarily affecting men. Although these patients have pain with stiffness of the spine and roentgenographic evidence of a "bamboo spine," the disc spaces are well maintained and the sacroiliac joints uninvolved.

Other conditions to be aware of include osteoarthritis of the spine, osteoporosis, vertebral epiphysitis (in adolescents), spondylolisthesis, and the chronic infections (tuberculosis, fungus, brucella).

MANAGEMENT AND PROGNOSIS. Treatment of ankylosing spondylitis is best accomplished through the medium of an excellent physician-patient relationship. Education of the patient concerning the disease and what to anticipate during its progression and treatment is fundamental.

Physical therapy includes a program of rest, posture, and exercise. As fatigue is common with ankylosing spondylitis, extra rest may be necessary during periods of increased disease activity. Constant attention to posture is mandatory to avoid thoracic kyphosis or fixed flexion of the neck. This includes good sleeping habits, with an extrafirm mattress and no pillows under the head and knees. Exercises are required to maintain range of motion and are performed better under the tutelage of a physical therapist.

The armamentarium of effective medications is small. Salicylates, with their analgesic anti-inflammatory effects in therapeutic dosage, may be quite helpful, especially in early or mild cases. When a greater anti-inflammatory effect is necessary, a nonsteroidal anti-inflammatory drug (NSAID) may be useful. Historically, phenylbutazone and indomethacin have been effective. Some of the newer NSAIDs may also be employed.

Corticosteroids are less frequently used in treating ankylosing spondylitis, mainly because they are not uniformly effective. The disease-modifying antirheumatic drugs (DMARD), such as gold and the antimalarials, have not been helpful in treating ankylosing spondylitis.

Patients with any stage of the disease usually manage to be employed and active. Some 40% will exhibit an insidious, slowly progressive course. Others are relatively symptom free, despite extreme roentgenographic changes.

BIBLIOGRAPHY

Calin, A., and others: Clinical history as a screening test for ankylosing spondylitis, J.A.M.A. **237:**2613, 1977.
Constantz, R., and Bluestone, R.: Diagnosis of the seronegative spondyloarthropathies: HLA-B27 testing as an aid to diagnosis, Contemp. Orthop. **2:**141, 1980.
Katz, W.A.: Ankylosing spondylitis. In Katz, W.A., editor: Rheumatic diseases: diagnosis and management, Philadelphia, 1977, J.B. Lippincott Co.
Namey, T.C., and others: Nucleographic studies of axial spondyloarthrotides. I. Quantitative sacroiliac scintigraphy in early HLA-B27 associated scroiliitis, Arthritis Rheum. **20:**1058, 1977.

13 • PSORIATIC ARTHRITIS
Warren A. Katz

Various types of arthritis may be found in patients with psoriasis—a fairly common, chronic, erythematous, scaling lesion of the skin. Psoriasis tends to appear over the elbows, knees, and scalp but may be found on any part of the body. The silver-scaled lesions sometimes cover all cutaneous surfaces; at other times they must be sought as minute, localized plaques. Nail changes in psoriasis consist of pitting, hyperkeratosis, brownish discoloration, or even total destruction. It was once thought that joint inflammation in association with psoriasis was really rheumatoid arthritis; however, there are enough distinctive features that psoriatic arthritis is now recognized as a separate entity. The cause of psoriasis or psoriatic arthritis is generally not known, but a hereditary predisposition is apparent in some families. The incidence of the histocompatibility antigen HLA-B27 is especially high in psoriatic spondylitis (arthritis of the spine).

CLINICAL MANIFESTATIONS. In about 75% of patients with psoriatic arthritis, the most common presentation is asymmetric oligoarthritis, with one or few joints involved at a time. Characteristically, a sausagelike swelling of either the fingers or toes is found and may herald the disease, even in the asymptomatic patient. Most patients, however, complain of pain of varying degree; sometimes there is tenderness, redness, and even heat. Few joints are spared, but the feet, knees, hands, and (in contrast to rheumatoid arthritis) the distal interphalangeal (DIP) joints, are frequently involved (Fig. 13-1). Digital flexor tenosynovitis, often painful, may dominate the arthritis picture. Attacks of psoriatic arthritis tend to appear more abruptly and disappear more rapidly than those in rheumatoid arthritis. Despite having active arthritis, most patients are able to function.

Less often, psoriatic arthritis is confined to the DIP joints. Signs of inflammation may be subtle. Multiple DIP joint involvement with simultaneous nail psoriasis is a striking picture. About 15% of all patients have symmetric polyarthritis that is similar to rheumatoid arthritis. Such patients, however, are seronegative for rheumatoid factor (RF); the types of deformities developed are identical to those of rheumatoid arthritis. Actually, extensive destruction to the point of resorption of the joint is more common in psoriatic arthritis. The telescoping digit has been referred to as "main en lorgnette" (opera-glass hand); fortunately, this catastrophe is uncommon.

Sacroiliac joint and spinal inflammation may be similar to that of ankylosing spondylitis. In contrast, unilateral sacroiliitis is more common in psoriasis. The patient with HLA-B27 antigen is predisposed to both ankylosing and psoriatic spondylosis.

An acute monarticular presentation of psoriatic arthritis resembles gout. Indeed, it has been suggested that gout is more common in these patients; a search for urate crystals in synovial fluid should differentiate the two.

In some cases psoriasis and arthritis flare concomitantly; however, in most patients skin manifestations antedate those of joints by many years. In the few cases in which the arthritis precedes the psoriatic skin lesions, diagnosis is a challenge. Psoriatic arthritis occasionally has been associated with Sjögren's syndrome.

LABORATORY FINDINGS. There are no characteristic laboratory tests for psoriatic arthritis. Diagnosis is based on clinical grounds. The erythrocyte sedimentation rate (ESR) is elevated during the flare-ups of the disease and tends to fall to normal between episodes. This is in contrast to rheumatoid arthritis, where the ESR may remain elevated even though the patient feels better. Tests for RF are normal. Synovial fluid analysis usually shows the same changes as in rheumatoid arthritis.

Roentgenograms of patients with psoriatic arthritis, although rarely diagnostic, may provide important clues in advanced cases. The characteristic sausagelike soft tissue swelling may be evident. Marginal erosions along the phalangeal shaft may produce a scalloped appearance despite the maintenance of the joint space. The distal phalanx of both fingers and toes may become whittled and actually resorbed. There may be bone overgrowth at the site of tendon insertions, producing a pencil-in-cup deformity.

DIAGNOSIS. The following are features that suggest psoriatic arthritis rather than rheumatoid or other types:
1. Psoriasis, with the tendency for nail lesions
2. A predisposition for DIP joints
3. Sausagelike swelling of fingers and toes
4. Asymmetric pauciarticular arthritis
5. Unilateral sacroiliitis with "skip" involvement of the lumbar and dorsal spine
6. Concomitant flaring of arthritis and psoriasis
7. More abrupt exacerbations and more complete remissions
8. Absence of subcutaneous nodules
9. Seronegativity for RF
10. HLA-B27 in psoriatic patients with back pain
11. Characteristic resorptive roentgenographic changes with periostitis

Rheumatoid arthritis, Reiter's syndrome, ankylosing spondylitis, gout, sarcoidosis, and primary generalized osteoarthritis are the major differential diagnoses.

MANAGEMENT. Psoriatic arthritis is managed in a manner similar to rheumatoid arthritis, with the focus on drug therapy, patient education, physical modalities, and even surgery. Patients with psoriatic arthritis tend to respond well to aspirin and the other nonsteroidal anti-inflammatory agents. Some with psoriatic arthritis react exceedingly well to small doses of systemic corticosteroids. There seems to be little justification for the prolonged use of high-dose corticosteroids. Remittive agents such as gold

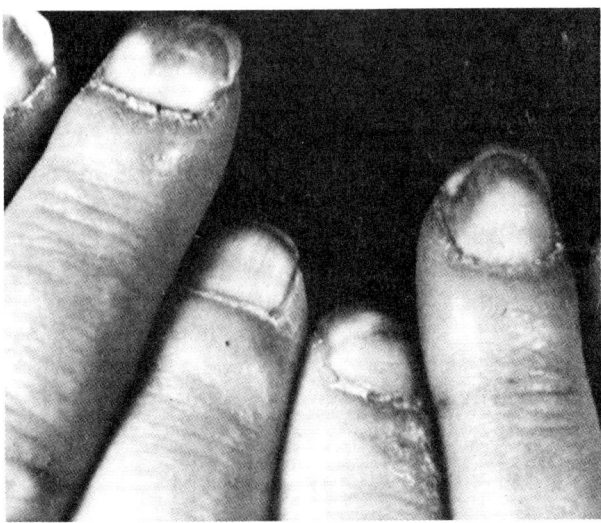

Fig. 13-1. Distal interphalangeal involvement and nail and skin changes in psoriatic arthritis.

have been used successfully in patients with psoriatic arthritis, but penicillamine and antimalarial drugs are not indicated. Immunosuppressive drugs, notably methotrexate, have been used with outstanding success in many patients with extensive psoriatic skin lesions and arthritis. Because there is a moderate incidence of hepatotoxicity and hematologic abnormalities, careful follow-up is essential. Liver biopsy is often necessary to assess the adverse effects of methotrexate; stomatitis may be profound.

It is not surprising that pain, extensive joint destruction, and unsightly skin changes may produce emotional problems in some patients with the disease. The physician plays an important role in implementing a psychosocial program.

BIBLIOGRAPHY

Eastmond, C.J., and Woodrow, J.C.: The HLA system and the arthropathies associated with psoriasis, Ann. Rheum. Dis. **36**:112, 1977.

Lassus, A., and Karvonen, J.: Reactive arthritis, Reiter's disease and psoriatic arthritis, Clin. Rheum. **3**:281, 1977.

Moll, J.M.H., and Wright, V.: Psoriatic arthritis, Semin. Arthritis Rheum. **3**:55, 1973.

Wright, V.: Seronegative polyarthritis: a unified concept, Arthritis Rheum. **21**:619, 1978.

14 • REITER'S SYNDROME

Warren A. Katz

Reiter's syndrome, classically referred to as the triad of polyarthritis, conjunctivitis, and urethritis, has now been expanded to include mucosal ulcerations, keratodermia blennorrhagicum, and balanitis circinata. In addition, involvement of the heart and central nervous system may occur infrequently.

PATHOGENESIS AND PATHOLOGY. The etiology of Reiter's syndrome is unknown, but the nature of the illness, particularly occasionally apparent venereal transmission, suggests an infectious cause. *Mycoplasma* and *Chlamydia* have been suspected as etiologic agents. The finding of HLA-B27 tissue type in more than 75% of patients with Reiter's syndrome suggests a hereditary predisposition to the disease. The term "Reiter's syndrome" may now be passé; some or all of its manifestations can be seen in the genetically predisposed person following infections with *Yersinia, Shigella,* and other agents. These manifestations have been referred to as reactive arthritis. Pathology of the involved synovial membrane shows hyperemia without the pannus found in rheumatoid arthritis. Late in the course of the disease there may be osteolysis.

CLINICAL MANIFESTATIONS. Reiter's syndrome, as it is known now, almost always affects young males. It may affect women more often than believed, going undetected. It frequently begins with nongonococcal urethritis following sexual intercourse. There may then develop, sequentially or simultaneously, arthritis, conjunctivitis, and other signs. Most patients are not seriously ill, although considerable fatigue, weight loss, hectic fever, lymphadenopathy, or splenomegaly has been seen. Arthritis is generally acute, asymmetric, and pauciarticular. The small joints of the feet, ankles, and knees and the sacroiliac joints may be involved. Reiter's syndrome infrequently resembles ankylosing spondylitis clinically. Achilles tendinitis and heel tenderness secondary to calcaneal bursitis ("lover's heel") may be striking. Residual joint deformity resembling rheumatoid arthritis is unusual.

Conjunctivitis is the most common ocular manifestation of Reiter's syndrome, occurring in at least one third of cases. Iritis is more apt to develop later in the disease than during the first attack. Urethritis produces a frankly purulent or watery discharge. Digital prostatic massage may yield pus in otherwise asymptomatic patients. Keratodermia blennorrhagicum is a peculiar skin lesion suggested by macular, hyperkeratotic lesions on the hands and soles of the feet. Subungual lesions resembling psoriasis may occur with the other skin manifestations or as an isolated finding. Weeping or dry ulcerations and scaling of the penis (balanitis) may be noted in some patients with Reiter's syndrome. Asymptomatic mucosal ulcerations of the buccal or palatal mucosa are found in approximately 10% of patients. If these lesions are painful, another diagnosis should be sought.

Cardiac lesions, unusual but varied, include aortis insufficiency, conduction defects, and pericarditis. Neurologic sequelae include neuritis, seizures, and hemiplegia.

LABORATORY FINDINGS. There are no diagnostic tests for Reiter's syndrome. The erythrocyte sedimentation rate is usually elevated during an acute attack, and in more chronic cases there is often anemia. The urethral discharge frequently contains large numbers of leukocytes. Synovial fluid analysis may show a granulocyte count as high as 100,000/mm^3. Large macrophages that have phagocytized many polymorphonuclear leukocytes (Reiter's cells) occasionally are noted.

Roentgenographs of involved joints variably show isolated osteoporosis, periarticular erosive changes, "fluffy" periostitis, calcaneal spurs, sacroiliitis, or nonmarginal osteophytes along the spine. Early in the disease there are usually no changes.

DIAGNOSIS. In any young man with a rather abrupt onset of asymmetric polyarthritis, Reiter's syndrome or reactive arthritis should be suspected. The concomitant or sequential development of urethritis, conjunctivitis, or the other stigmata help confirm the diagnosis. Ancillary studies that suggest Reiter's syndrome include the presence of HLA-B27, a negative test for rheumatoid factor, Reiter's cells in synovial fluid, and the aforementioned roentgenographic findings.

Differential diagnosis includes gonorrhea, another condition that causes arthritis, urethritis, and conjunctivitis in young men. The rapid response to penicillin suggests this disease, whereas the presence of keratodermia blennorrhagicum, asymptomatic mucosal ulcers, and balanitis circinata is evidence in favor of Reiter's disease. The problem here is further confused by Reiter's syndrome possibly coexisting with or following bona fide cases of gonorrhea. Psoriatic arthritis is also confused with Reiter's syndrome because of the skin, nail, and spondylitic changes. It, too, may coexist with Reiter's syndrome. Balanitis, urethritis, and mucosal lesions are not found in psoriasis; the arthritis is usually less destructive in Reiter's disease. Rheumatoid arthritis or ankylosing spondylitis may be mimicked by Reiter's syndrome, particularly that of the chronic variety. Behçet's syndrome causes recurrent iritis, genital ulcers, stomatitis, polyarthritis, neurologic manifestations, aortic root lesions, and pustular skin lesions that may closely resemble Reiter's syndrome. The incidence of vascular lesions is increased in Behçet's syndrome. Oral mucosal lesions are painful in Behçet's syndrome, which is of contrasting significance.

MANAGEMENT AND PROGNOSIS. Most patients with Reiter's syndrome respond to a combination of nonsteroidal anti-inflammatory drugs, joint aspiration, and intra-articular corticosteroids (Chapter 10). Tetracycline or similar antibiotics seemingly have no effect on the arthritis, but there is circumstantial evidence that some cases of urethritis do respond.

If there is a marked systemic component to Reiter's syndrome, then initial bed rest is indicated. Patients should be properly educated as to the nature of the disease and the generally favorable prognosis, since chronic disability resulting from destructive, deforming changes in the joints is unusual. Some patients may have recurrent acute or subacute polyarthritis for several years.

ENTERIC AND REACTIVE ARTHRITIDES. Reactive arthritis that follows certain enteric bacterial infections in genetically predisposed hosts represents one of the most obvious associations between specific microbial organisms and HLA antigens. A syndrome resembling Reiter's syndrome may follow infection with *Yersinia, Salmonella,* and *Shigella* in patients positive for HLA-B27. The knee, ankle, and wrist are most frequently involved. A migratory pattern is common. The term "reactive arthritis" has been used for these arthritides and for arthritis associated with ulcerative colitis, regional enteritis, and intestinal bypass surgery in the broad category of enteric arthropathy.

Patients with ulcerative colitis or regional enteritis may have subacute asymmetric polyarthritis or spondylitis either alone or with flare-ups of diarrhea, mucous stools, and abdominal pain. Erythemanodosum and oral ulcerations are other extraintestinal manifestations. Most patients with enteric spondylitis have detectable HLA-B27 antigen.

Arthritis and arthralgias complicate jejunocolic bypass surgery in 20% to 30% of patients. Joint symptoms usually remit spontaneously over several weeks, but chronic, recurrent cases have been reported.

It is clear that ankylosing spondylitis is the prototype of a group of seronegative spondyloarthropathies that also include psoriatic arthritis, Reiter's syndrome, and enteric arthritis. Common to each is (1) a negative test for rheumatoid factor; (2) absence of rheumatoid nodules; (3) inflammatory peripheral arthritis; (4) roentgenographic sacroiliitis with or without spondylitis; (5) mucocutaneous, ocular, genital, or gastrointestinal manifestations; (6) association with HLA-B27; and (7) tendency for familial clustering.

BIBLIOGRAPHY

Bluestone, R., editor: Symposium on seronegative spondyloarthropathies, Clin. Orthop. **143**:1, 1979.

Calin, A., and Fries, J.F.: "Experimental" epidemic of Reiter's syndrome revisited, Ann. Intern. Med. **84**:564, 1976.

Good, A.E.: Reiter's disease: a review with special attention to cardiovascular and neurologic sequelae, Semin. Arthritis Rheum. **3**:253, 1974.

McClusky, O.E., Lorden, R.E., and Arnett, K.C.: HLA-B27 in Reiter's syndrome and psoriatic arthritis: a genetic factor in disease susceptibility and expression, J. Rheumatol. **1**:263, 1974.

Utsinger, P.D.: Bypass disease: a bacterial antigen-antibody systemic immune complex disease (abstract), Arthritis Rheum. **23**:758, 1980.

15 • INTERMITTENT RHEUMATIC DISEASES
Randolph C. Blodgett, Jr.

BEHÇET'S SYNDROME

See dental correlations.

16 • SYSTEMIC LUPUS ERYTHEMATOSUS
June F. Klinghoffer

Systemic lupus erythematosus (SLE) is a chronic disease of unknown cause. It characteristically involves several organ systems, has a striking predilection to affect young adult women, and shows an impressive number of immunologic abnormalities. It is regarded as the prototype of autoimmune disease because of the wide array of autoantibodies found in patients. It may more aptly be termed an immune-complex disease; tissue damage is secondary to the deposition of immune complexes formed by the autoantibodies and host antigens. The clinical picture may be exceedingly varied, but the most commonly encountered manifestations are skin rashes, joint pain, fever, pleurisy, and nephritis.

Prior to 1948, SLE was considered a rare and grave

disease. The recognition of the lupus erythematosus (LE) cell phenomenon by Hargraves in that year provided the first specific diagnostic test for SLE and ushered in a new era of understanding concerning the disease and immunologic mechanisms. A marked apparent increase in incidence of SLE has occurred in the past 30 years; the availability of more sensitive diagnostic tests has led to the recognition of earlier and milder cases, and SLE is now considered fairly common and compatible with long survival.

A recent epidemiologic study in a large prepaid health clinic in San Francisco found the incidence of new cases of SLE to be 7.6 per 100,000 persons. The overall prevalence was 1 case in 1969 persons; in women aged 15 to 64 it was 1 in 700; and in black women of the same age it was 1 in 245.

Women are affected 5 to 10 times more frequently than men, and blacks are affected more frequently than whites. Onset of symptoms is most frequent between the ages of 15 and 40, but the disease may occur in both children and the elderly.

ETIOLOGY AND PATHOGENESIS. The serologic hallmark of SLE is the presence of multiple autoantibodies. Those antibodies directed against nuclear material are known as antinuclear antibodies (ANA). Other autoantibodies to cytoplasmic material, blood proteins, and cell membranes may be present. Some of these latter antibodies may have a direct pathogenetic role in such manifestations as hemolytic anemia, leukopenia, or thrombocytopenia. The major pathology, however, is mediated via immune complex formation and deposition in such sites as blood vessel walls, glomerular basement membrane, skin, and other areas. These complexes are formed by nuclear antigens and ANA, especially DNA/anti-DNA. The complexes activate the complement system, causing the release of chemotactic factors and subsequent release of lysosmal enzymes that directly attack and damage the various tissue sites.

The basic etiologic or initiating factors are not known. Evidence pointing to the importance of genetic factors includes the increased incidence of clinical SLE or serologic positivity in family members, increased concordance of SLE in identical twins, and increased incidence in persons with congenital deficiency of certain components of complement (especially C2).

Exogenous factors, such as sun exposure, infections, and drug ingestion, appear operative in some patients. The possible role of a specific infectious agent such as a virus is speculative at this time.

Three factors may thus be involved in the pathogenesis of SLE: (1) genetic predisposition, (2) abnormal host immune reaction, and (3) latent viral infection.

PATHOLOGY. Few characteristic lesions are seen grossly or by routine light microscopy. Fibrinoid deposits may be seen on serosal surfaces and in blood vessel walls. Vasculitis involves the small arteries. "Onion-skin" lesions and concentric perivascular fibrosis are seen in the spleen; nonbacterial vegetations are occasionally seen on the heart valves. The kidneys may show focal glomerulitis, diffuse proliferative nephritis, or membranous nephritis. Thickening of the basement membrane of the glomeruli may produce the characteristic "wire-loop" lesion. Hematoxylin bodies, similar in appearance to the inclusions within LE cells, are infrequently seen in the various tissues but are considered pathognomonic. The mesangial lesion, present in all patients with SLE, is characterized by proliferation of glomerular mesangial cells and deposition of immune complexes that may be detected by immunofluorescence.

During acute SLE of the skin, histologic examination of skin shows hyperkeratosis of the epidermis and follicular plugging. More chronic events include hypertrophy of the periphery of the lesion and central fibrosis. Immunofluorescent staining is demonstrated at the dermal-epidermal junction (lupus band test). Even clinically uninvolved skin may show a positive band test in SLE.

CLINICAL MANIFESTATIONS. The clinical picture may range from a mild, indolent disorder manifested chiefly by recurrent arthralgias or skin rash to a fulminant life-threatening illness with renal failure. Onset may be abrupt but more usually is insidious. The course is most often one of exacerbations and remissions over many years. The initial complaints are usually joint pain or skin rash. Constitutional symptoms such as fatigue, malaise, and fever are common.

Musculoskeletal manifestations. Almost all patients have joint involvement at some time during the disease, often at the onset. They may have polyarthralgias or actual arthritis with objective signs of swelling and inflammation. The small joints of the fingers, hands, and wrists are most frequently involved, but knees, ankles, and elbows are also affected. Swelling of the proximal interphalangeal and metacarpophalangeal joints may be highly suggestive of rheumatoid arthritis. Minor deformities such as swan-neck fingers may develop; these appear to be caused by soft tissue laxity. No bone erosions are seen on roentgenograms.

Avascular necrosis of bone develops in a small percent of patients, especially those on prolonged high-dose corticosteroid therapy. The femoral head is most frequently involved.

Proximal muscle pain or weakness is occasionally seen and reflects accompanying myositis.

Mucocutaneous manifestations. Between 75% and 85% of patients will have signs or symptoms involving the skin, mucous membranes, or hair. The classic butterfly rash over the cheeks and bridge of the nose is seen in about 50% of patients and will range from a faint malar flush to a more extensive scaly, maculopapular, erythematous rash (Fig. 16-1). About one third will exhibit photosensitivity, with the rash appearing only after sun exposure. Skin rashes are most common on the face, neck, and upper

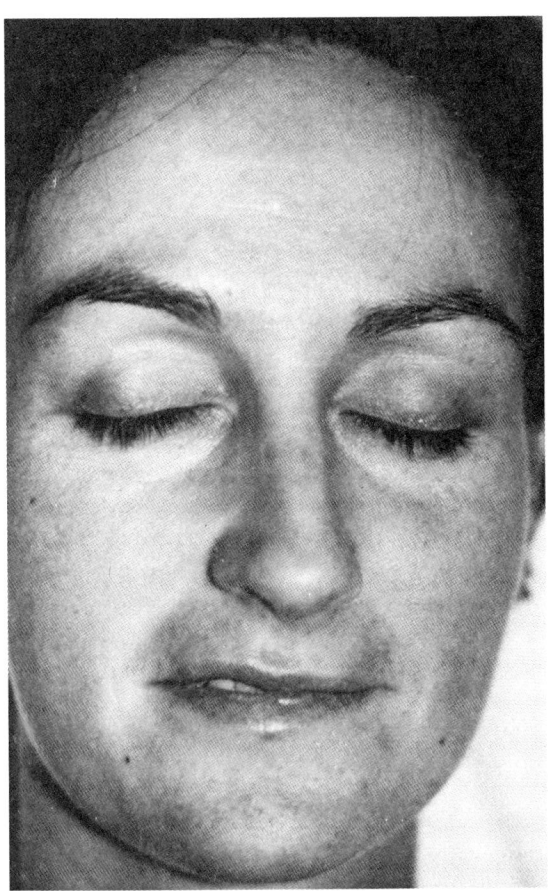

Fig. 16-1. Facial rash over bridge of nose, upper lip, and chin in patient with active SLE.

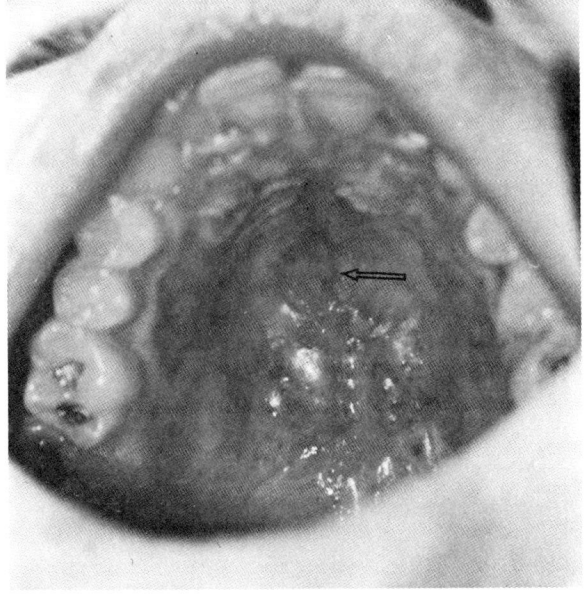

Fig. 16-2. Palatal mouth ulcer *(arrow)* in acutely ill patient.

chest but may appear elsewhere, especially on sun-exposed areas such as the extremities and scalp. Vasculitic lesions are commonly seen on the palms of the hands and on the distal finger pads. Raynaud's phenomenon occurs in about 20% of patients. Telangiectasia, livedo reticularis, periungual erythema, petechiae, purpura, bullae, and urticaria have all been described. Areas of hyperpigmentation and vitiligo are quite common.

Mucosal ulcerative lesions occur in approximately 40% of patients. Since these ulcers are frequently painless, they must be actively sought through the history and examination. The ulcers characteristically occur on the hard or soft palate but may also involve the buccal and gingival mucosa and resemble the common aphthous ulcer (Fig. 16-2). They occur most frequently in those patients with active skin lesions or during flare-ups of SLE. Ulcers may also involve the nasal mucosa and may lead to septal perforation.

Alopecia is an important but frequently overlooked diagnostic sign. The hair loss may be diffuse or patchy; the patient may merely be aware of the hair thinning or of an unusual amount of hair coming out on combing. Alopecia often signals a flare-up in the disease and is reversible.

Serositis. Pleurisy or painless pleural effusion is common. Less frequently, pulmonary infiltrates or patchy areas of atelectasis may be seen on roentgenograms. Pericarditis with or without effusion is also fairly common. Nonbacterial verrucous endocarditis (Libman-Sacks endocarditis) may be seen at autopsy but is not commonly recognized clinically. Sterile peritonitis occasionally occurs.

Renal disease. More than 50% of patients show evidence of renal involvement. This may be clinically expressed as the nephrotic syndrome with marked proteinuria and edema, or as nephritis with hematuria, hypertension, and progressive impairment of renal function with eventual uremia. This is the most serious complication of SLE and is the leading cause of death. Fortunately, most patients show only a mild to moderate proteinuria. A rising blood urea nitrogen (BUN) and creatinine is an ominous sign. Renal biopsy with immunofluorescence may help to assess the presence and extent of renal changes.

Nervous system. There has been increasing recognition of the significant incidence of both neurologic and psychiatric manifestations. Seizures, psychosis, and organic brain syndrome are the major manifestations. Also seen are coma, hemiparesis, chorea, cranial nerve palsies, aphasia, and peripheral neuropathy. It is often difficult to differentiate between organic psychosis secondary to the disease and steroid psychosis. Depression and anxiety are common. A brain scan may show a diffuse abnormality.

Other manifestations. Lymph nodes may be enlarged but are not tender. Splenomegaly may occur in 10% to 15% of cases but is usually of a slight degree. The liver is normal in size. Abdominal pain may be secondary to peritonitis, pancreatitis, mesenteric lymphadenopathy, or mesenteric arteritis. Parotid gland enlargement may occur and sometimes reflects an accompanying Sjögren's syndrome. "Cotton wool" exudates or "cytoid bodies" may be seen on the retina.

LABORATORY FINDINGS. Mild to moderate normochromic anemia is common. The Coombs' test may be positive, with or without accompanying hemolytic anemia. Leukopenia occurs in 50% of patients, usually with significant lymphopenia. Thrombocytopenia is usually of a mild degree and in most cases not clinically significant; occasionally frank thrombocytopenic purpura may be the initial manifestation of SLE. A circulating anticoagulant is sometimes demonstrable. The erythrocyte sedimentation rate is rapid. With renal involvement, the urine may show protein, red and white blood cells, and casts.

Immunologic abnormalities abound. The most significant from the standpoint of diagnosis and monitoring response to therapy are positive LE cell test (70% to 80% of patients), ANA (95% to 100%), rheumatoid factor (20%), false positive serology for syphilis (20%), anti-DNA antibodies (70%), increased gamma globulin, decreased serum complement, and cryoglobulins.

A positive fluorescent test for ANA (FANA) is found in virtually all cases, and thus a negative test weighs against the diagnosis of SLE. A positive test is not diagnostic, since it occurs in rheumatoid arthritis and other connective tissue diseases. Four patterns of fluorescent staining are recognized: (1) homogenous, or diffuse; (2) peripheral, or rim; (3) speckled; and (4) nucleolar. The diffuse pattern is produced by antibody binding to nucleoprotein (the LE factor); the peripheral pattern results from antibody binding to DNA and is more specific, especially if in high titer (Fig. 16-3). Rising titer of anti-DNA antibody and decreasing levels of serum complement are indicative of acute activity and highly suggestive of lupus nephritis. Serum complement may be profoundly depressed with active SLE. Cryoglobulins indicate the presence of circulating immune complexes.

Biopsy of skin or kidney may be of value in determining the presence or extent of characteristic lupus lesions (see discussion of pathology).

The detection of LE cells (Fig. 16-4) by special techniques in blood, synovial fluid, and pleural fluid represents one of the major diagnostic criteria (see discussion of diagnosis).

DIAGNOSIS. The following 14 criteria have been proposed by the American Rheumatism Association. The presence of any four of these either serially or simulta-

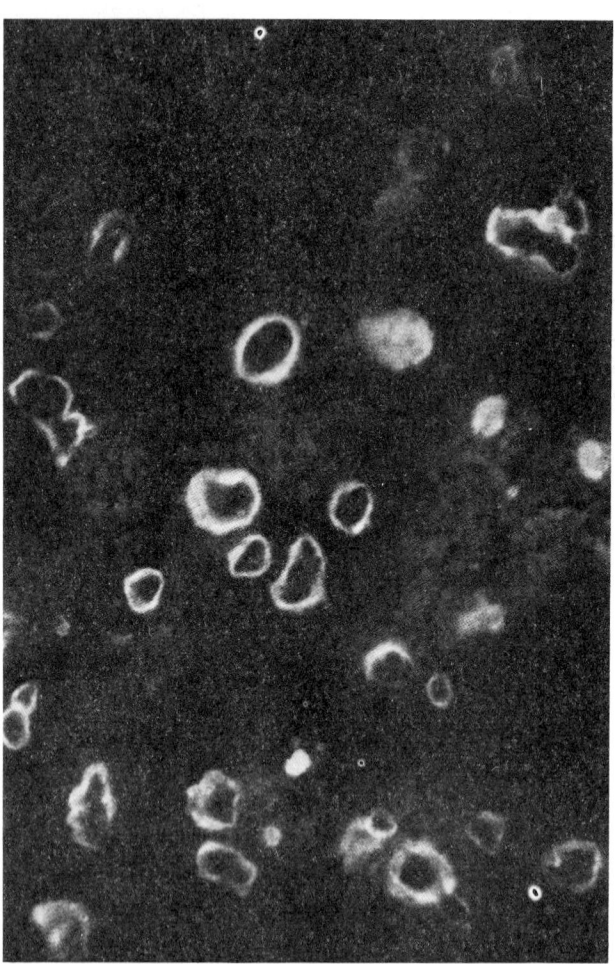

Fig. 16-3. Typical peripheral (ring) pattern of ANA fluorescence.

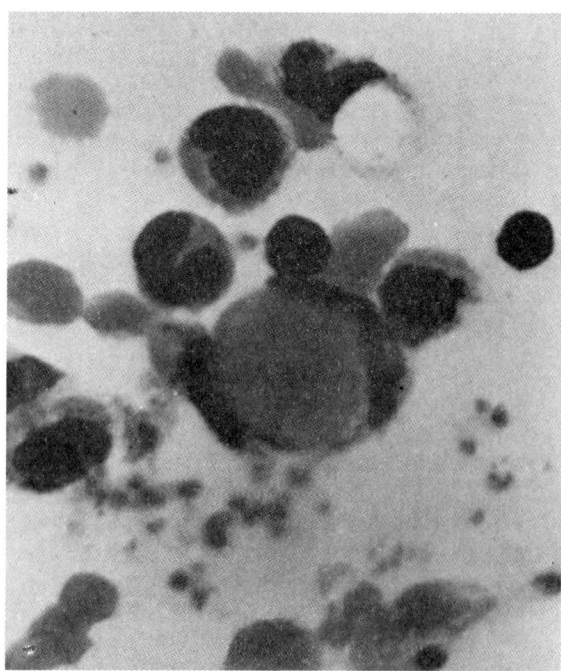

Fig. 16-4. LE cell preparation demonstrating polymorphonuclear leukocyte that has phagocytized homogeneous nuclear material.

neously is highly suggestive of but not necessarily diagnostic of SLE:

1. Facial erythema
2. Discoid lupus
3. Raynaud's phenomenon
4. Alopecia
5. Photosensitivity
6. Oral or nasopharyngeal ulceration
7. Arthritis without deformity
8. LE cells
9. Chronic false positive serology for syphilis
10. Proteinuria greater than 3.5 g daily
11. Cellular casts
12. Pleuritis and/or pericarditis
13. Psychosis and/or convulsions
14. One or more: hemolytic anemia, leukopenia (less than 4000/mm^3), and thrombocytopenia (less than 100,000/mm^3).

Differential diagnostic problems are most apt to occur with rheumatoid arthritis, the overlap syndromes, and in those cases with a single manifestation such as convulsions or pericarditis. The diagnosis must always be considered in women in their childbearing years, especially when symptoms appear in the early postpartum period or following unusual sun exposure.

The most sensitive diagnostic screening test is the FANA. The most specific diagnostic findings are a high titer of anti-DNA antibodies and decreased serum complement levels.

PROGNOSIS. Survival figures have shown dramatic improvement. Five-year survival now approximates 95% and 10-year survival 85%. The chief causes of death are intercurrent infection, renal failure, and central nervous system (CNS) involvement.

MANAGEMENT. Many patients do well on simple supportive measures. All should be advised to avoid sun exposure, guard against infections, avoid drugs such as sulfonamides or oral contraceptives that often precipitate exacerbations of SLE, and avoid overfatigue. Topical sunscreen preparations are useful in patients with marked photosensitivity.

Arthralgias and arthritis usually respond well to salicylates or one of the nonsteroidal anti-inflammatory drugs. Hydroxychloroquine, an antimalarial drug, is effective in controlling skin lesions and arthritis at a dose of 200 mg daily. Periodic ophthalmologic evaluations every 6 months are necessary when this drug is used because of the danger of retinal damage. Topical corticosteroids are effective for cutaneous lesions. Sunscreens may prevent them.

Systemic corticosteroid therapy is indicated for renal and CNS disease, pericarditis, pulmonary disease, and hematologic complications such as hemolytic anemia or thrombocytopenia. Such therapy may also be required in patients with fever, arthritis, and skin lesions that do not respond to other measures. Dosage varies widely. Renal and CNS disease may require 100 to 200 mg of prednisone daily. Other manifestations will usually respond to a dose of 40 to 60 mg daily. Dosage is tapered as early as possible to avoid complications, such as avascular necrosis of bone, osteoporosis, and fluid retention. Alternate day therapy is used when possible. Immunosuppresive drugs such as azathioprine and cyclophosphamide are occasionally used in addition to prednisone for lupus nephritis. Recent therapeutic approaches under investigation include "pulse therapy" for lupus nephritis, consisting of intravenous bolus doses of 1 g of methylprednisolone daily for 3 days and plasmapheresis in an attempt to remove immune complexes.

DRUG-INDUCED CONNECTIVE TISSUE DISEASE (CTD) (DRUG-INDUCED LUPUS)

Many drugs are capable of triggering exacerbations of SLE. Others are capable of inducing the formation of ANA, including the LE cell. A smaller group of drugs produces a clinical lupuslike syndrome. Procainamide, a drug widely used in the treatment of cardiac arrhythmias, is the major cause of drug-induced CTD at this time. Three fourths of patients receiving the drug develop ANA and LE cells; a much smaller percent develop the clinical syndrome.

Characteristics of drug-induced CTD are increased incidence in males and older patients, absence of renal and CNS involvement, normal serum complement, and absence of antibodies to native DNA. The most frequent manifestations are arthralgias, fever, and pleural and pericardial effusions. Symptoms usually disappear when the drug is stopped, but FANA may persist for months to several years.

Other implicated drugs are hydralazine, isoniazid, the anticonvulsants, the thiouracils, phenothiazine compounds, penicillamine, sulfonamides, and oral contraceptives.

CHRONIC DISCOID LUPUS ERYTHEMATOSUS

Skin lesions of chronic discoid lupus erythematosus (CDLE) may occur in a small percent of patients with SLE but generally represent an independent entity. The typical CDLE lesion starts as a papular eruption that spreads and yields to erythema, edema, induration, and ultimately fibrosis with central atrophy and depression. The lesions are usually found on the scalp and face. Hair loss and loss of pigmentation may ensue.

BIBLIOGRAPHY

Baldwin, D.S., and others: Lupus nephritis, Am. J. Med. **62**:12, 1977.

Cathcart, E.S., and others: Beneficial effects of methylprednisolone "pulse" therapy in diffuse proliferative nephritis, Lancet **1**:163, 1976.

Dubois, E.L.: Lupus erythematosus, ed. 2, Los Angeles, 1974, University of Southern California Press.

Feinglass, E.J., Arnett, F.C., and Dorsch, C.A.: Neuropsychiatric manifestations of systemic lupus erythematosus, Medicine **55**:323, 1976.

Fessel, W.J.: Systemic lupus erythematosus in the community, Arch. Intern. Med. **134:**1027, 1974.

Fries, J.F., and Holman, H.R.: Systemic lupus erythematosus: a clinical analysis. In Smith, L.H., editor: Major problems in internal medicine, vol. VI, Philadelphia, 1975, W.B. Saunders Co.

Lee, S.L., and Chase, H.P.: Drug-induced lupus erythematosus: a critical review, Semin. Arthritis Rheum. **5:**83, 1975.

Phillips, P.E.: The virus hypothesis in systemic lupus erythematosus, Ann. Intern. Med. **83:**709, 1975.

Rothfield, N.F.: Systemic lupus erythematosus. In Katz, W.A.: Rheumatic diseases: diagnosis and management, Philadelphia, 1977, J.B. Lippincott Co.

Rothfield, N.F.: Systemic lupus erythematosus. In McCarthy, D.J., editor: Arthritis and allied conditions, ed. 9, Philadelphia, 1979, Lea & Febiger.

Urman, J.D., and others: Oral mucosal ulceration in systemic lupus erythematosus, Arthritis Rheum. **21:**58, 1978.

Diseases with skin changes resembling scleroderma

Mixed connective tissue disease
Eosinophilic fasciitis
Scleredema
Scleromyxedema
Diseases caused by vinyl chloride
Silica-induced diseases
Graft-versus-host reaction
Vibration-induced diseases

Carcinoid syndrome
Phenylketonuria
Werner's syndrome
Progeria
Acromegaly
Primary amyloidosis
Porphyria cutanea tarda
Congenital porphyria

---

17 • SYSTEMIC SCLEROSIS

Sergio Jimenez

Systemic sclerosis is a disease of unknown origin characterized by excessive deposition of collagen and other connective tissue components in skin and multiple internal organs. It is associated with prominent and often severe alterations in the microvasculature and the autonomic nervous system. Because of the frequent presence of immunologic abnormalities, systemic sclerosis has been included in the group of autoimmune diseases.

The disease is relatively uncommon; it has been stated that from four to 12 new cases per 1 million population are diagnosed in the United States each year, but this is probably an underestimation. Systemic sclerosis affects women three to four times more frequently than men, and there is no racial predilection. The initial symptoms usually appear in the third to fifth decade of life, although the disease has been described in children and the elderly. Systemic sclerosis is a complex and clinically heterogeneous disease with clinical forms ranging from localized skin involvement with minimal systemic alterations to forms with severe internal organ disease and a fulminant course.

In many cases skin involvement is confined to the digits and the dorsum of the hands and feet (acrosclerosis), and progression of the sclerotic process is relatively slow. This form of disease is frequently associated with calcinosis, long-standing Raynaud's phenomenon, sclerodactyly, and telangiectasia, and has been termed CRST syndrome. Although the distinction between CRST syndrome and more fulminant visceral scleroderma is often clear-cut, in many instances it is difficult to make a distinct separation because the clinical manifestations overlap markedly.

In another group of patients there are classic clinical features of systemic sclerosis overlapping manifestations of the other connective tissue diseases, such as systemic lupus erythematosus and dermatomyositis/polymyositis. Recently, one subgroup of these patients, with a more specific entity called mixed connective tissue disease (see later in this chapter), has been identified based on the presence of a specific antiribonucleoprotein antibody in the sera.

New syndromes resembling systemic sclerosis include chemically induced sclerosis, graft-versus-host disease of bone marrow transplants, and the severe fasciitis associated with eosinophilia (see box above). Pseudoscleroderma embraces a variety of genetic and acquired diseases that should be excluded whenever the possibility of systemic scleroderma is considered.

PATHOGENESIS. Although the exact pathogenetic mechanisms in systemic sclerosis are not understood, it is clear that many of the clinical manifestations of the disease, as already stated, are caused by the accumulation of excessive collagen and other connective tissue components in the affected organs. Experimental evidence has recently appeared indicating a marked increase in the rate of collagen synthesis in scleroderma that may result from a somatic mutation of sclerodermatous fibroblasts. Because alterations in the microvasculature are frequently found in scleroderma and in many instances precede clinical manifestations, it has been suggested that they may be responsible for increased fibroblast activity.

Finally, immunologic factors can be implicated because lymphocytes seem capable of regulating connective tissue synthesis by fibroblasts.

PATHOLOGY. The pathologic changes in systemic sclerosis represent variable stages of progression and development of at least three major processes occurring in the affected tissues:

1. Connective tissue alterations, with fibroblast proliferation, fibrosis, and increased ground substance
2. Inflammation, occurring predominantly in the early stages of disease and characterized by infiltration with large numbers of mononuclear cells, predominantly lymphocytes
3. Vascular disease, characterized by intimal prolifer-

ation, concentric subendothelial deposition of collagen and mucinous material, and narrowing of the vessel lumen and thrombosis

Some less frequent pathologic changes include classic vasculitic lesions, with necrotic disruption and inflammatory infiltration of vessel walls, and deposition of calcific material in the subcutaneous and periarticular tissues.

Progression of the vascular and fibrotic reactions and decrease in the inflammatory component lead to the final stage of atrophic changes in the affected organs. Skin changes include a marked decrease in the thickness of the epidermis, flattening of the rete pegs, and replacement of sebaceous and sweat glands, as well as hair follicles, by dense fibrous tissue. In the lungs there is fibrotic infiltration of the alveolocapillary membrane, with atrophy of the alveolar lining and finally complete disruption of the architecture of the lung. In rare cases malignant proliferation of alveolar cells may lead to alveolar cell carcinomas. In the heart and other areas there is replacement with dense connective tissue, cellular atrophy, and tissue fibrosis.

CLINICAL MANIFESTATIONS. The most impressive clinical features of systemic sclerosis are related to the generalized thickening and infiltration of the skin, but some degree of multiple organ involvement is almost always present. The skin is affected in almost all cases, but rarely, classic visceral involvement can be demonstrated without clinical evidence of skin disease.

Skin. Sclerosis and thickening of the skin are present in almost all patients. The affected areas are firmly matted and bound to the subcutaneous tissue. Because of the marked dermal infiltration with collagen, the skin thickness is almost always increased. Subsequently, there is atrophy of the normal cutaneous structures, with disappearance of hair follicles and sweat glands. The skin over the hands is most frequently affected, but as the disease progresses, the sclerotic changes extend to the entire upper extremity, face, neck, trunk, and abdomen. The lower extremities, however, are sometimes spared the infiltrative process.

Skin ulceration, usually localized to fingertips or areas of pressure, is present in about 30% of cases (Fig. 17-1). Ulceration of nostrils and of ear lobes is less common.

Pigmentary changes are frequent and characterized by diffuse darkening associated with localized areas of depigmentation that often assume a punctate appearance (Fig. 17-1). Intense pruritus may precede pigmentary changes. Nonpitting edema localized to hands and feet is usually an early manifestation.

The telangiectases, present in about 20% of cases, are commonly periungual or mucosal, although they can occur on palms, face, chest, neck, or elsewhere. Calcinosis, most commonly found in fingertips and periarticular tissues, can be a clue to the diagnosis of systemic sclerosis. In many cases large, calcified masses promote ulceration of the skin, with development of draining sinus tracts.

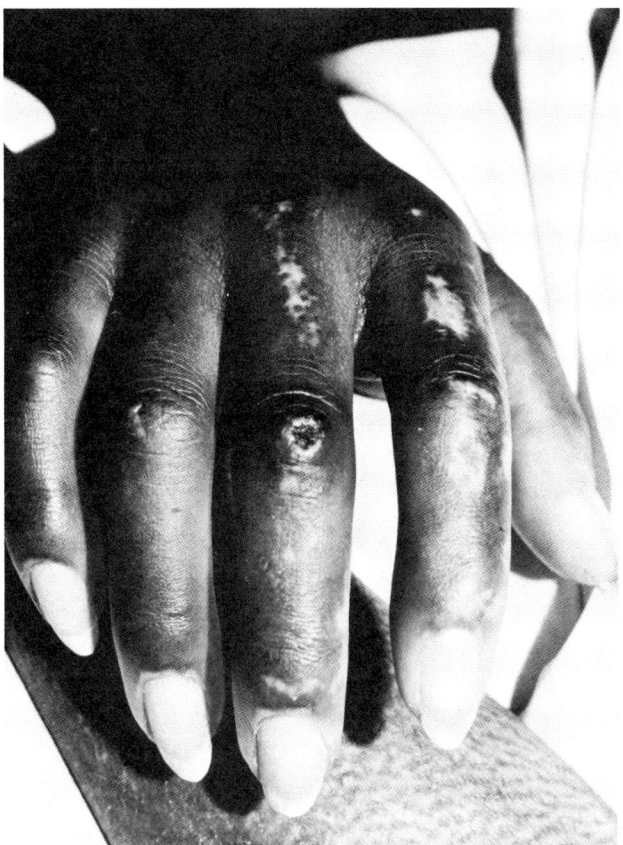

Fig. 17-1. Hand of 29-year-old woman with systemic sclerosis demonstrating digital sclerosis, pigmentary changes, cutaneous ulcers, and joint flexion contractures.

Vessels. Raynaud's phenomenon is the second most common manifestation of systemic sclerosis, present in more than 85% of patients. It usually appears simultaneously with other manifestations, but may antedate them by several years. Raynaud's phenomenon is usually triggered by cold exposure and occasionally by stressful circumstances. Episodes are often painful and are characterized by a triphasic reaction involving fingers, toes, and occasionally the face. Initial vasoconstriction and blanching are followed by a dusky cyanosis. With return of blood flow, there is reactive erythema. In many patients there is a decrease in the number of skin capillary loops, which is readily demonstrated by capillaroscopy at the nail folds and in the skin over the distal phalanges. Often marked dilation and distortion of the remaining capillaries are observed. In some cases larger blood vessels are affected, and luminal narrowing and occlusion, which may be demonstrated by angiographic studies, can result in ischemic necrosis of the extremities or internal organs.

Musculoskeletal system. Musculoskeletal symptoms, present in about 30% of patients, are often the initial manifestations of disease. Symptoms vary from mild polyarthralgias to severe arthritis sometimes indistinguishable from that of rheumatoid arthritis. Severe flexion contractures result from thickening and induration of periarticular tissues. Terminal phalangeal atrophy and resorption of digital tufts may lead to total disappearance of the phalanx. An early sign of the disease is the presence of a leathery rub heard on movement of various tendons. Many patients frequently complain of myalgia and weakness; at times there may be muscle tenderness and objective weakness, but more often, physical examination is negative. Determination of serum enzymes, particularly aldolase, or electromyographic or histologic examination may be necessary to document the presence of muscle involvement. Synovitis with effusion may be found; characteristically, the aspirated synovial fluid is mildly inflammatory.

Gastrointestinal tract. The gastrointestinal tract is the most common internal organ system involved in scleroderma. Esophageal symptoms are present in approximately 40% of patients. When more sensitive methods such as cineradiography and manometric study are used, however, esophageal abnormalities can be detected in about 90%. Early symptoms are characterized by midchest pain, fullness, heartburn, and regurgitation of food, especially in the recumbent position. In severe cases chronic peptic esophagitis can lead to stricture and dysphagia. Poor gastric emptying and involvement of the small intestine may cause abdominal distention, bloating, nausea, and pain. In many cases bacterial overgrowth with deconjugation of bile salts and secondary vitamin deficiency, malabsorption, diarrhea, and weight loss have been described. Occasionally, obstipation associated with abnormalities in colonic motility can occur.

Lungs. The most prominent symptoms in the lungs are tachypnea and exertional dyspnea usually secondary to pulmonary fibrosis. Less often, there is chronic nonproductive cough and pleuritic chest pain. Many patients remain asymptomatic despite evidence of severe fibrotic involvement of the parenchyma.

Heart. Pericardial involvement may appear as acute or chronic pericarditis but usually is asymptomatic. Pericardial effusions, however, are found by echocardiography or autopsy examination in about one half of patients. Anginal pain, arrhythmias (including various degrees of heart block), myocardiopathy with left ventricular or biventricular insufficiency, and cor pulmonale may be found in patients with systemic sclerosis.

Kidneys. Renal disease is the most serious internal organ involvement in systemic sclerosis, and it is responsible for nearly one half of all deaths in patients with this disorder. It is typically characterized by abrupt development of highly malignant arterial hypertension and irreversible renal insufficiency. The onset of arterial hypertension has been occasionally linked with corticosteroid therapy.

In most cases renal disease appears in patients with rapidly progressive systemic sclerosis and only rarely in individuals with the CRST syndrome. The development of hypertension is often heralded by severe headache, visual symptoms resulting from severe hypertensive retinopathy, seizures and other central nervous system symptoms, or sudden left ventricular failure. Within a few days or weeks there is evidence of severe renal disease, with appearance of proteinuria and rapidly increasing azotemia terminating in oliguria, anuria, and uremia. The blood pressure rarely remains within normal limits, but severe hypertension associated with extremely high plasma renin levels is the rule. In the past, patients died 3 to 6 months after the onset of this most feared complication, but recently a more aggressive approach has resulted in improved prognosis for these patients.

Nervous system. Peripheral neuropathy and trigeminal neuralgia have been reported but are rarely apparent clinically. In contrast with direct involvement of the nervous system, entrapment neuropathies are relatively common, especially carpal tunnel syndrome.

Liver. Primary disease of the liver is unusual in systemic sclerosis, but recently the occurrence of primary biliary cirrhosis in a number of patients with the CRST syndrome has been documented. In these patients jaundice, pruritus, and hepatomegaly develop; laboratory tests show marked elevation of serum alkaline phosphatase and high titers of antimitochondrial antibodies.

LABORATORY FINDINGS. Hematologic studies show mild anemia, usually normochromic and normocytic, in one third of patients. Elevation of the erythrocyte sedimentation rate (ESR) is not common; when present, it is usually related to rapid disease activity or to the presence of synovitis. Serum globulins are often elevated, especially IgM, and sometimes there is hypoalbuminemia. Circulating cryoglobulins have been detected in almost one half of patients studied and may be associated with rheumatoid factor. Antinuclear antibodies (ANA) are found in almost all cases and are usually of a course, speckled pattern. Less frequently, a distinctive nucleolar pattern relatively specific for systemic sclerosis can be demonstrated. Lupus erythematosus cells are rarely seen.

Some laboratory tests may provide a clue to involvement of different organ systems. Proteinuria or azotemia almost invariably precedes the development of severe renal disease. Elevations of creatinine phosphokinase and aldolase indicate the presence of myositis. Lactic acid dehydrogenase and glutamic oxaloacetic transaminase elevations may result from both muscular and pulmonary involvement. Urinary hydroxyproline, an amino acid present exclusively in collagen, has been used as an index of activity and progression of the disease.

The most common abnormality found on musculoskeletal roentgenographic examination is erosion and resorption of the tufts of the terminal digital phalanges, frequently accompanied by periarticular and subcutaneous calcinosis. Alterations in the joints are generally confined to thickening of the periarticular soft tissues and juxta-articular osteoporosis. These features are helpful in differentiating the articular involvement in systemic sclerosis from that of other inflammatory arthritides, particularly rheumatoid arthritis.

Roentgenographic examination of the gastrointestinal tract shows the characteristic findings of hypomotility and dilation of the distal esophagus; gastroesophageal reflux and frequently diaphragmatic hernias occur even in asymptomatic patients. Other findings include gastric dilation and poor emptying, small intestinal dilation (especially of the duodenum), slow transit time throughout the bowel, and distinctive widemouthed sacculations of the colon.

The classic finding from chest roentgenograms is fine, fibronodular interstitial fibrosis, most prominent at the lung bases. In early stages an alveolar pattern may also be present, suggesting an inflammatory component. Pleural effusions are occasionally seen. In advanced cases fine honeycombing can be seen, and even changes suggestive of bibasilar emphysema have been described.

Manometric determinations to detect lower-third esophageal dysfunction are even more sensitive than cineradiographs, showing abnormalities in about 90% of sclerosis patients. The classic findings are decreased or absent peristalsis in the lower esophagus and decreased lower esophageal sphincter pressure. The upper esophagus in systemic sclerosis is normal, a feature helpful in differentiating it from polymyositis/dermatomyositis.

Pulmonary function tests usually show decreased diffusing capacity early in the disease, even in the absence of any clinical findings. Somewhat later a restrictive picture resulting from interstitial, pleural, and chest wall fibrosis can be found.

Electrocardiograms and cardiac catheterization usually show evidence of rhythm abnormalities, cardiac hypertrophy, pericarditis, pulmonary hypertension, and conduction defects.

DIAGNOSIS. Recently, the American Rheumatism Association has established preliminary criteria for the diagnosis and classification of systemic sclerosis. These criteria are useful for epidemiologic investigational studies and for moderately advanced cases. Skin sclerosis, involving parts of the body proximal to the metacarpophalangeal or metatarsophalangeal joints or truncal and facial skin, constitutes the single major criterion for systemic sclerosis. Minor criteria are sclerodactyly, digital pitting, scars of fingertips or loss of substance of the distal finger pads, and bibasilar pulmonary fibrosis. The major or two minor criteria were found in 97% of patients with definite systemic sclerosis but in only 2% of patients with systemic lupus erythematosus, polymyositis/dermatomyositis, or Raynaud's phenomenon not associated with connective tissue disease.

The diagnosis of systemic sclerosis is not as difficult in patients with Raynaud's phenomenon and characteristic hidebound skin as in those with Raynaud's phenomenon alone. Raynaud's phenomenon may be present in other rheumatic diseases, in cryoglobulinemia and serum hyperviscosity syndromes, in association with obliterative vascular disorders, and with occupational use of vibrating instruments. It is important to search for evidence of visceral scleroderma, such as esophageal hypomotility, abnormalities in pulmonary function tests, and elevations of the muscle enzymes, that serve as clues even in asymptomatic patients.

A number of disease entities with cutaneous features resembling the skin involvement in systemic sclerosis should be considered in the differential diagnosis.

MANAGEMENT. At present there is no specific treatment for systemic sclerosis and its variants; in most cases the disease progresses relentlessly despite therapy with currently available drugs. Steroids and cytotoxic agents have proved remarkably ineffective in the treatment of this disease. Because excessive collagen deposition is responsible for many of the clinical manifestations, drugs capable of inhibiting collagen accumulation may prove to be of benefit in controlling some of the most disabling manifestations. One such compound is penicillamine, which has been shown to interfere with normal collagen maturation by preventing the formation of stable collagen cross-links, but this form of therapy is still experimental.

In some cases of systemic sclerosis, the connective tissue alterations may result from a defect in normal collagen degradation. A rational therapeutic approach would thus involve the administration of compounds that increase collagen breakdown, such as colchicine, which may stimulate synthesis of collagenase and decrease collagen secretion by the fibroblasts. Colchicine use in treatment of systemic sclerosis is still controversial, and further investigations are needed.

The treatment of Raynaud's phenomenon is often disappointing. Vaodilating drugs in high doses may increase the threshold for initiation of vasospasm. Reserpine has been frequently used in doses ranging from 0.25 to 1 mg daily. Other recommended agents include guanethidine, methylodopa, and tolazoline. Since the response is clearly dose related, these drugs should be slowly increased to the maximum tolerance, especially during heavy exposure to cold or unusual stress. The role of intra-arterial reserpine requires more study.

Since exposure to cold is an important factor in determining the persistence and frequency of vasospastic episodes, patients should be advised to avoid exposure to cold, to dress warmly, and to wear heavy gloves, especially during winter. In extreme cases, when peripheral gangrene and occlusion of medium-sized and small vessels has been documented by arteriographic studies, intravascular platelet thrombosis may contribute to the symptoms; therefore, antiplatelet therapy may be beneficial. In the most severe cases dipyridamole can be used to potentiate the antiplatelet effect of aspirin.

Symptomatic esophageal hypomotility may be managed with the same measures used to treat gastroesophageal reflux from other causes. Avoidance of the recumbent position after meals, elevation of the head of the bed, and use of antacid preparations are helpful in the treatment of peptic esophagitis. Cimetidine has been used effectively to decrease gastric acid production. Metoclopramide has been reported effective in improving esophageal sphincter pressure. Symptoms of intestinal bacterial overgrowth can be ameliorated with the cyclic use of broad-spectrum antibiotics such as tetracycline. Occasionally, low-residue diets and medium-chain triglyceride food may be necessary. In severe cases of generalized gastrointestinal atony, intravenous hyperalimentation may be required.

Arthritis and arthralgia often require treatment with high doses of aspirin or other anti-inflammatory agents. The myopathy of scleroderma does not require corticosteroid therapy unless severe muscle destruction is demonstrated by laboratory findings. Severe and painful calcinosis may require treatment with diphosphonates or probenecid.

Therapy for sclerodermatous lung disease includes antibiotic treatment of superimposed infections, chest expansion exercises, and administration of oxygen when necessary.

Treatment of sclerodermatous and hypertensive cardiomyopathy is difficult, since patients are extremely prone to digitalis toxicity. These patients should be carefully managed with digitalis therapy, salt restriction, and diuretics. If pericardial constriction occurs, surgical decompression should be performed.

Kidney involvement is the most significant and serious complication of progressive scleroderma and usually appears abruptly. It was previously believed that development of kidney disease in scleroderma was irreversible and invariably lethal; however, it has been shown that a combination of aggressive antihypertensive therapy with chronic hemodialysis can result in prolonged survival of these patients, especially if instituted early. The combination of hydralazine (also a potent inhibitor of collagen synthesis), methyldopa, and propanolol usually results in satisfactory blood pressure control. Because the renin-angiotensin system may play an important role in sclerodermatous hypertensive renal disease, therapy with captopril, a specific inhibitor of angiotensin-converting enzyme may be extremely effective for patients with renal crisis in scleroderma.

PROGNOSIS. The prognosis of systemic sclerosis and its variants is as heterogeneous as the clinical manifestations; it depends primarily on the type and extent of internal organ involvement and secondarily on the rapidity and progression of skin changes. A recent study correlated the extent of specific organ involvement with prognosis employing life-table analysis. In this series the 7-year cumulative survival rate for patients with systemic sclerosis was only 35% from the time of diagnosis. Approximately 50% of patients were dead in 5 years. Extent and type of visceral involvement dramatically influenced the survival rates. All patients with azotemic renal involvement were dead within 10 months. Cardiac involvement was the second most common cause of death. When pulmonary involvement was the only visceral complication, there was a 45% survival after 5 years. Gastrointestinal involvement apparently did not affect the survival data.

These results indicate that although systemic sclerosis is a serious and often lethal disease, not all patients necessarily progress and some seem to improve spontaneously. Physicians should be aware that systemic sclerosis cannot be cured with therapeutic measures available today; this should be emphasized early in the management of the patient, since patients have a tendency to search from doctor to doctor for a miraculous cure. Many patients are treated with empiric modes of therapy or receive unapproved medications and may develop complications. The role of physicians in counseling the patient and his family, explaining the complications and prognosis of scleroderma, and attempting to convey a clear understanding of the goals in management of systemic sclerosis is of paramount importance.

BIBLIOGRAPHY

Campbell, P.M., and LeRoy, E.C.: Pathogenesis of systemic sclerosis: a vascular hypothesis, Semin. Arthritis Rheum. **4**:351, 1975.

D'Angelo, W.A., and others: Pathologic observations in systemic sclerosis (scleroderma), Am. J. Med. **46**:428, 1969.

Fleischmajer, R.: The pathophysiology of scleroderma, Int. J. Dermatol. **16**:310, 1977.

Jimenez, S.A.: General management and prognosis of scleroderma, Clinical conference, Cohen, S., moderator, Gastroenterology **79**:163, 1980.

Rodman, G.P.: Progressive systemic sclerosis, Clin. Rheum. Dis. **5**:49, 1979.

Sackner, M.A.: Scleroderma (monograph), New York, 1966, Grune & Stratton, Inc.

18 • RAYNAUD'S PHENOMENON

Warren A. Katz

Raynaud's phenomenon is characterized by periodic attacks of bilateral digital pallor followed by cyanosis, usually on exposure to cold. Raynaud's phenomenon most often begins in women between the ages of 18 and 40 years. The ischemic changes in the fingers and toes are caused by vasoconstriction of the digital and palmar or plantar arteries. Early in the attack the small cutaneous vessels are constricted, causing pallor; later the capillaries and venules dilate and the slow blood flow causes cyanosis. Following relief of vasoconstriction, the blood supply increases considerably and there is a red color (rubor). Pathologically, the vessels are normal in the early stages of Raynaud's phenomenon, but later intimal proliferation of the vessel wall and hypertrophy of the muscle layer become evident. If the vessels thrombose, focal gangrene of the tips of the fingers and toes develops.

CLINICAL MANIFESTATIONS. Clinical manifestations in the typical patient with Raynaud's phenomenon consist of pain, paresthesias, and stiffness in the fingers and toes on exposure to refrigerator air, cold wind, air conditioning, or other low-temperature settings. Three sequential stages of Raynaud's phenomenon are recognized: pallor (vasoconstriction), cyanosis (poorly oxygenated blood in dilated capillaries and venules), and rubor (reactive hyperemia). The digits are cold and numb during vasoconstriction and painful during hyperemia. Not all stages may be prominent during each attack of Raynaud's phenomenon. In addition to the fingers and toes, the earlobes, nose, cheeks, and chin may exhibit ischemic changes. Besides exposure to cold, emotional tension and trauma may precipitate Raynaud's phenomenon.

Most cases are accompanied by one or more of a variety of conditions. Raynaud's phenomenon often heralds rheumatic disorders such as systemic sclerosis and mixed connective tissue disease by months or several years. Systemic lupus erythematosus, polymyositis, and rheumatoid arthritis are less often associated with Raynaud's phenomenon. The condition is rare in polyarteritis and giant cell arteritis. Raynaud's phenomenon may be associated with the following factors:

Connective tissue disorders
    Systemic sclerosis
    Mixed connective tissue disease
    Systemic lupus erythematosus
    Rheumatoid arthritis
    Dermatomyositis and polymyositis
Peripheral arterial disease
    Thromboangiitis obliterans (Buerger's disease)
    Arteriosclerosis obliterans
    Arteritis
Neurovascular compression syndromes
    Thoracic outlet syndrome
Hematologic abnormalities
    Cryoproteinemia
    Paraproteinemia
    Polycythemia vera
Occupational exposures
    Vibratory tool workers (pneumatic hammer operators)
    Percussion instrument workers (pianists, typists)
    Acro-osteolysis (resorption of digital tips) caused by polyvinylchloride
    Traumatic occlusive arterial disease
Drugs and toxins
    Ergot compounds
    β-Adrenergic blockers
    Sympathomimetic drugs
    Oral contraceptives
    Methysergide
    Heavy metals

Raynaud's disease is the term applied if there are no apparent associated conditions after at least 2 years of observation. In contrast to Raynaud's phenomenon, Raynaud's disease is not usually attended by digital necrosis, cutaneous atrophy, or calcinosis. Angiography generally reveals no structural changes in the vessels. Laboratory evaluations for connective tissue and other diseases are unremarkable.

The course of Raynaud's phenomenon is variable. It may recur at irregular intervals but is usually worse in the winter. Some patients improve spontaneously, but most have recurring mild to severe symptoms. With long-standing Raynaud's phenomenon, atrophic changes of the fingers characterized by tapering and flattening of the digital pulp may develop. Sometimes the skin over the proximal interphalangeal joints becomes taut and shiny (sclerodactyly).

DIAGNOSIS. Raynaud's phenomenon is suspected when pain, paresthesias, pallor, or cyanosis of the fingers and toes develops following the patient's exposure to cold. The workup is designed to differentiate Raynaud's phenomenon from Raynaud's disease and also to establish any of the usual causes of Raynaud's phenomenon listed previously. It must be recognized, however, that Raynaud's phenomenon may precede any of the associated diseases. The minimal ancillary evaluation includes a complete blood count, erythrocyte sedimentation rate, rheumatoid factor, antinuclear antibody, cryoglobulins, serum protein electrophoresis, and muscle enzyme determinations. Raynaud's phenomenon may be differentiated from acrocyanosis (persistent cyanosis aggravated by exposure to cold) and occlusive vascular disease by the sequential color changes, intermittency, and localization of gangrene to the digital tips in Raynaud's phenomenon.

MANAGEMENT. Proper management of Raynaud's phenomenon usually diminishes digital ischemia, alleviates symptoms once they develop, and prevents dystrophic alterations in the extremities. Because emotional stress in itself may trigger Raynaud's phenomenon, patients generally respond to the reassurance that the overall prognosis is good and that, although there is no cure, the condition can be treated. As with other forms of peripheral vascular disease, patients with Raynaud's phenomenon should be discouraged from smoking. The hands must be kept warm during the winter months by avoiding cold when possible and wearing heavy gloves and outerwear when such exposure cannot be avoided. Patients should be careful about touching cold doorknobs, reaching into the refrigerator for cold bottles, and swimming in cold pools. Sores and ulcers, once having developed, may be slow to heal, so whenever possible patients should wear protective gloves while indulging in activities, such as gardening or carpentry, that may cause trauma to the hands. Seemingly, keeping the hands well lubricated will prevent chafing and cracking.

Drug therapy may decrease peripheral vasoconstriction. Reserpine, guanethidine, methyldopa, and prazosin may be partially successful in relieving or preventing Raynaud's phenomenon.

Sympathectomy to eliminate vasoconstricting impulses is successful in some cases of Raynaud's phenomenon. The procedure is of no benefit in patients with scleroderma. Treating the underlying cause of Raynaud's phenomenon may be the most important aspect of therapy when such treatment is available.

BIBLIOGRAPHY

Coffman, J.D., and Davies, E.T.: Vasospastic diseases: a review, Prog. Cardiovasc. Dis. **18:**123, 1975.

19 • POLYMYOSITIS AND DERMATOMYOSITIS

Donald H. Lieberman

Polymyositis is an inflammatory disorder of striated muscle associated with symmetric proximal weakness and atrophy. When accompanied by characteristic skin lesions, the disease is referred to as dermatomyositis. The cause is unknown, but recent evidence incriminates abnormalities in cellular immunity. It is more common in women (2:1) and has a peak incidence in the sixth and seventh decades. The childhood disease resembles the adult form but has distinct characteristics that will be discussed separately. The following classification provides a useful framework for discussion:

Type I—polymyositis in adults
Type II—typical dermatomyositis in adults
Type III—inflammatory myositis associated with malignant disease
Type IV—childhood myositis
Type V—myositis associated with an overlap syndrome (for example, scleroderma or systemic lupus erythematosus)

"Pure" polymyositis and dermatomyositis (types I and II) comprise more than half of the cases in this classification.

Polymyositis may be mimicked by other connective tissue diseases or muscular dystrophy.

CLINICAL MANIFESTATIONS. The constant feature in all types of polymyositis regardless of other associations is weakness of proximal muscles. The onset of the disease is variable, and the initial diagnosis may be missed when the disease has an insidious onset. The pelvic and shoulder girdles seem to be affected most often. Patients may complain of difficulty ascending stairs, getting on a bus, or merely rising from a chair. Later they may find it difficult to reach overhead. The flexors of the neck and the pharyngeal muscles often become involved. Severe dysphagia and dysphonia can result. If the respiratory muscles become involved in a rapidly progressive or advanced case, the patient may have a life-threatening or fatal respiratory insufficiency.

Skin. When the myositis is accompanied by a rash, the disease is referred to as dermatomyositis. The rash consists of a purplish, dusky, erythematous eruption chiefly involving the face, neck, upper arms, and trunk. A violaceous discoloration of the eyelids has been called a "heliotrope" rash and is a characteristic sign of dermatomyositis. A rash may also be seen on the extensor surfaces of the forearms, knees, elbows, and knuckles. These lesions may become scaly and plaquelike with disease progression.

Raynaud's phenomenon. Raynaud's phenomenon is relatively uncommon unless patients have an overlap with another connective tissue disease, most commonly scleroderma or systemic lupus erythematosus. When it does occur, it is usually mild and does not result in digital ulceration or necrosis.

Other clinical manifestation. When patients do not have an overlap form of myositis, involvement outside the skeletal muscle is uncommon. Mild arthralgias or arthritis can occur and may be accompanied by joint effusions. Joint destruction is rare, and the arthritis responds well to corticosteroid therapy. Pulmonary involvement as a primary finding (as opposed to that caused by aspiration) is uncommon. When it occurs, interstitial pneumonitis with a nonproductive cough, dyspnea, and hypoxemia characterize the clinical picture. The chest roentgenogram demonstrates interstitial infiltrates with a predilection for the lung bases. Most cases respond favorably to corticosteroids. When cardiac muscle is involved, conduction abnormalities and nonspecific electrocardiographic changes result. Purely neurologic symptoms do not occur. The other clinical features seen with overlap forms are characteristic of the disease in concert with the myositis. There may be periorbital edema.

ASSOCIATION WITH MALIGNANCY. The association of malignancy with polymyositis and dermatomyositis remains a controversial subject. Some studies suggest an association with malignancy in 6% to 35% of cases of polymyositis. A recent study at the University of California at Los Angeles and a critical review of the literature place the figure in both dermatomyositis and polymyositis at approximately 8% to 9%. The male to female ratio for disease associated with malignancy is equal; however, the average age for these patients is higher than for those without malignancy. The tumors are most commonly found in the breast, lung, ovary, stomach, colon, and uterus. There are no clinical manifestations that seem to be specifically associated with patients with malignancy. Most tumors are discovered within 1 year of the onset of myopathy; conversely, when myositis develops after the discovery of the malignancy, it usually does so within 1 year. There are anecdotal reports of amelioration of myositis after treatment of the associated malignancy, but the improvement is usually only temporary, and the patients eventually die as a result of the malignancy.

DERMATOMYOSITIS OF CHILDHOOD. When myositis occurs in childhood, the rash of dermatomyositis is seen in the majority of patients. The other features resemble those seen in adults. Proximal muscle weakness predominates. Some children have a benign course, whereas others have severe atrophy and muscle shortening with resultant crippling contractures. The erythematous patches seen over the knuckles in some adults are particularly characteristic of the disease in childhood. Abdominal pain, sometimes accompanied by gastrointestinal bleeding, is a feature unique to the disease in the young. Vasculitis involving the gastrointestinal tract is responsible for this severe complication. Vasculitis may also be present in the skeletal muscles, and in many children marked subcutaneous calcifications develop when dermatomyositis is of long standing.

LABORATORY FINDINGS. Routine "connective tissue screening" tests are not very helpful in the diagnosis of polymyositis. The erythrocyte sedimentation rate may be elevated, but this is an inconsistent finding; it may be normal even in the presence of active disease. Tests for antinuclear antibodies, rheumatoid factor, and alteration of the erythrocyte sedimentation rate lend little help in diagnosis. These tests are useful, however, in assessing the possibility of disease overlap with the other connective tissue disorders.

Muscle enzymes. Necrosis of muscle during the course of myositis results in the release of enzymes into the serum. Evaluation of the enzyme levels is helpful not only diagnostically but also prognostically as a guide to therapy. The determination of creatine phosphokinase (CPK), aldolase, and lactic dehydrogenase levels is of greatest use, since the levels of these enzymes decline rapidly with treatment.

PM-1 and antitoxoplasma antibodies. A new precipitin reaction has been observed between calf thymus nuclear extract and polymyositis sera. The antibody involved, called PM-1 antibody, seems to be a specific for polymyositis. These antibody studies are not widely available.

The prevalence of antitoxoplasma antibodies has been reported to be greater in patients with polymyositis than in patients with other inflammatory muscle diseases or systemic diseases that do not involve the musculature. The significance of this finding remains unclear.

Electromyogram. The triad of spontaneous fibrillation, polyphasic action potentials, and pseudomyotonic discharges is said to be almost pathognomonic of polymyositis.

Pulmonary function tests. The early evaluation of pulmonary function is helpful in detecting intercostal muscle involvement, which is especially prevalent in children. There may be defects in vital capacity and oxygen diffusion.

Muscle biopsy. Proximal muscles are preferred for biopsy. The electromyogram (EMG) may be helpful in the selection of a biopsy site. A common practice is to obtain the biopsy from the side of the body opposite that in which the EMG was done to avoid changes caused by needle insertion. The classic biopsy shows widespread degeneration of muscle fibers, basophilia with central positioning of nuclei (evidence of regeneration), a chronic inflammatory cell infiltrate (especially lymphocytes), variation in cross-sectional fiber diameter (partial regeneration), and fibrosis.

MANAGEMENT. It is now accepted that all patients with polymyositis or dermatomyositis should be treated with corticosteroids. The usual starting dose is 60 mg of prednisone daily. Response to steroids means increased muscle strength but not necessarily a decrease in enzyme levels, which may precede a return of strength or may occur with little or no clinical improvement in some cases. Once strength returns, the dose of steroids should be slowly tapered and increased if any "flare-up" is detected. Rare patients can be completely weaned from corticosteroids, but most patients require persistent maintenance therapy with doses of 7.5 to 20 mg daily.

It must be kept in mind that there has never been a carefully controlled study to determine if steroids have an influence on ultimate mortality in this disease. One investigation found that, although morbidity was greatly improved, corticosteroids did not appear to affect the eventual outcome. In patients in whom the response is poor or the disease becomes life threatening, immunosuppressive agents such as methotrexate have been used with reported success.

PROGNOSIS. When not accompanied by a malignancy, polymyositis and dermatomyositis have a good prognosis. Most patients have an impressive return of muscle strength and live fairly normal lives. As previously mentioned, low doses of maintenance corticosteroids are required in the majority of patients to suppress disease.

BIBLIOGRAPHY

Barnes, B.E,: Dermatomyositis and malignancy: a review of the literature, Ann. Intern. Med. **84:**68, 1976.

Bohan, A., and others: A computerized analysis of 153 patients with polymyositis and dermatomyositis, Medicine **56:**255, 1977.

Kagen, L.J., Kimball, A.C., and Chrisitan, C.L.: Serologic evidence of toxoplasmosis among patients with polymyositis, Am. J. Med. **56:**186, 1974.

Schumacher, H.R., and others: Articular manifestations of polymyositis and dermatomyositis, Am. J. Med. **67:**287, 1979.

Schwarz, M.I., and others: Interstitial lung disease in polymyositis and dermatomyositis: analysis of six cases and a review of the literature, Medicine **55:**89, 1976.

Winkleman, R.K., and others: Course of dermatomyositis-polymyositis: comparison of untreated and cortisone treated patients, Mayo Clin. Proc. **43:**545, 1968.

Wolfe, J.F., Adelstein, E., and Sharp, G.C.: Antinuclear antibody with distinct specificity for polymyositis, J. Clin. Invest. **59:**176, 1976.

20 • VASCULITIS

Paul Katz and **Anthony S. Fauci**

Vasculitis encompasses a broad range of heterogeneous syndromes characterized by inflammation and necrosis of blood vessels. This clinicopathologic process may be the primary manifestation of a particular disease or it may exist merely as an accessory finding of another underlying disease. One of the major problems in discussing the vasculitides involves the proper delineation of specific disease syndromes. Previous attempts at classification have resulted in the oversimplification of complicated processes or the creation of cumbersome and often artificial categories in which little allowance for disease overlap was made. We propose the following revised scheme for the classification of the vasculitides:

>Polyarteritis nodosa group of systemic necrotizing vasculitis
>>Classic polyarteritis nodosa
>>Allergic angiitis and granulomatosis
>>Systemic necrotizing vasculitis—"overlap syndrome"
>
>Hypersensitivity vasculitis
>>Serum sickness and serum sickness–like reactions
>>Schönlein-Henoch purpura
>>Essential mixed cryoglobulinemia with vasculitis
>>Vasculitis associated with malignancies
>>Vasculitis associated with other primary disorders
>
>Wegener's granulomatosis
>Lymphomatoid granulomatosis
>Giant cell arteritides
>>Temporal arteritis
>>Takayasu's arteritis
>
>Miscellaneous vasculitides
>>Thromboangiitis obliterans (Buerger's disease)
>>Mucocutaneous lymph node syndrome

From this basic outline we will direct our attention to the pathogenesis, immunologic mechanisms, clinical manifestations, and therapeutic approach to this heterogeneous group of disorders as a whole and to certain specific disease states.

PATHOGENESIS. It has become increasingly apparent that most, if not all, of the vasculitides are initiated by immunopathogenic mechanisms. Although in the majority of cases a definite offending agent or antigen cannot be identified, the histologic and clinical aspects of the vasculitides suggest that they are mediated by immunologic events. At the present time the predominant theory is that these disorders are initiated by the deposition of immune complexes in blood vessel walls. Experimental data suggest that, after exposure to antigen, soluble antigen-antibody complexes in a state of antigen excess are formed in the circulation. If these are not cleared by the reticuloendothelial system, they are deposited in blood vessel walls. This deposition is aided by increased vascular permeability resulting from the release of vasoactive amines from platelets and basophils. The deposited complexes activate the complement cascade, resulting in the generation of factors chemotactic for neutrophils. After migration into the vessel wall, these cells release their lysosomal enzymes, which cause damage and eventual necrosis of the involved blood vessel. Secondarily, thrombosis, occlusion, hemorrhage, and tissue ischemic changes may ensue. Even in such situations with presumed immune complex origins, circulating or tissue antigen-antibody complexes are often not demonstrable. In all likelihood the lack of detectable circulating complexes is due to rapid clearance from the circulation. Furthermore, in animals tissue immune complexes have been shown to disappear from tissue sites 24 to 48 hours following deposition.

In addition to immune complex mediation, cell-mediated immune reactions may play a role in the development of vascular damage.

CLINICAL MANIFESTATIONS. The original description of systemic vasculitis was that of a case of classic polyarteritis nodosa by Kussmaul and Maier in 1866. Subsequently, as additional cases of similar but not identical systemic vasculitides appeared, they were grouped into the single category of polyarteritis nodosa. As it became apparent that further categorization of these processes was mandatory, numerous and often oversimplified classifications appeared. We have devised a classification of the systemic vasculitides based on the etiologic, pathologic, clinical, and therapeutic differences within this group (see the preceding outline). Although certain of these disorders have distinct clinicopathologic features that render them easily distinguishable, others lack this clarity. With this in mind, we have found this classification to be useful not as an artificial separator of often similar syndromes, but rather as a guide to the systematic approach to these disorders.

Systemic necrotizing vasculitis. Systemic necrotizing vasculitis is a rather large group encompassing classic polyarteritis nodosa, allergic angiitis and granulomatosis and what we refer to as the overlap syndrome.

Classic polyarteritis nodosa as originally described is a systemic necrotizing vasculitis of small and medium-sized arteries. Vessel involvement tends to be segmental with a propensity for bifurcations and branches. Vascular lesions in all stages of development may be seen, and the type and degree of clinical findings reflect the location and severity of vessel involvement. The following are typical findings of classic polyarteritis nodosa:

>Necrotizing vasculitis of small and medium-sized muscular arteries
>Eosinophilia and granulomata not characteristic
>Allergic history uncommon
>Renal involvement
>>Related to vasculitis (80%)
>>Glomerulitis (30%)

Hypertension

Gastrointestinal—infarction of viscera

Hepatic—subclinical disease caused by chronic active hepatitis in patients with hepatitis B antigenemia; liver disease related to vasculitis (up to 50%)

Coronary arteritis—particularly in children

Neurologic—mononeuritis multiplex

Lung and spleen characteristically uninvolved

Cutaneous—uncommon; usually subcutaneous nodules, livedo reticularis

Genitourinary—testes, bladder, epididymis, ovary involved

Arthralgias common; arthritis rare

These features are important to remember, since they aid in distinguishing classic polyarteritis nodosa from other syndromes in the systemic necrotizing vasculitis group.

Allergic angiitis and granulomatosis is a disorder similar in many respects to classic polyarteritis nodosa, except that the hallmark of this disease is pulmonary involvement. It is frequently characterized by a previous history of asthma and allergies. The exact incidence of allergic granulomatosis is uncertain, but it appears to be relatively rare. Pulmonary symptoms, usually in the form of asthma, dominate the clinical picture. Granulomatous tissue reactions with eosinophilic infiltration are typically seen, and peripheral eosinophilia is seen in one half of patients. With the exception of the pulmonary manifestations, the clinical characteristics of allergic angiitis and granulomatosis may be virtually identical to those of classic polyarteritis nodosa.

We refer to the third syndrome in this group as the overlap syndrome, since it is manifested by features of both classic polyarteritis nodosa and allergic angiitis and granulomatosis. This is a multisystem vasculitis with variable clinical manifestations. Patients may or may not have atopic histories, peripheral eosinophilia, eosinophilic tissue infiltration, granulomatous inflammation, and lung involvement accompanying necrotizing vasculitis of the small vessels (arterioles, capillaries, and venules) and small and medium-sized arteries (Fig. 20-1).

Hypersensitivity vasculitis. Hypersensitivity vasculitis is a large and heterogeneous group comprising syndromes with predominantly small vessel involvement. The term evolved from the fact that in many cases this syndrome could be traced to offending antigens such as drugs or microorganisms. Recently it has been shown that endogenous "self"-antigens such as autologous proteins or tumor antigens could incite antibody production. Immune complexes have been postulated as the pathogenetic bases for these syndromes. Typically, the skin is the most frequently involved system, usually in the form of leukocytoclastic vasculitis of the postcapillary venules. Skin lesions may be present as palpable purpura, papules, nodules, vesicles, bullae, or ulcers. Although virtually any organ system may be involved in varying degrees, the cutaneous involvement dominates the clinical picture. In this regard this group differs from the systemic necrotizing vasculitides, in which extracutaneous disease generally prevails (Fig. 20-2). Within this large group of disorders exist many distinct identifiable syndromes.

Lymphomatoid granulomatosis. Lymphomatoid granulomatosis is an unusual form of vasculitis hallmarked by angiotrophic and angiodestructive tissue infiltration with atypical cells in combination with a granulomatous reaction. Cellular infiltrates in this disease are polymorphic and composed of normal lymphoid cells with atypical lymphocytoid, plasmacytoid, and reticuloendothelial cells. These cells often have mitotic figures, giving them the appear-

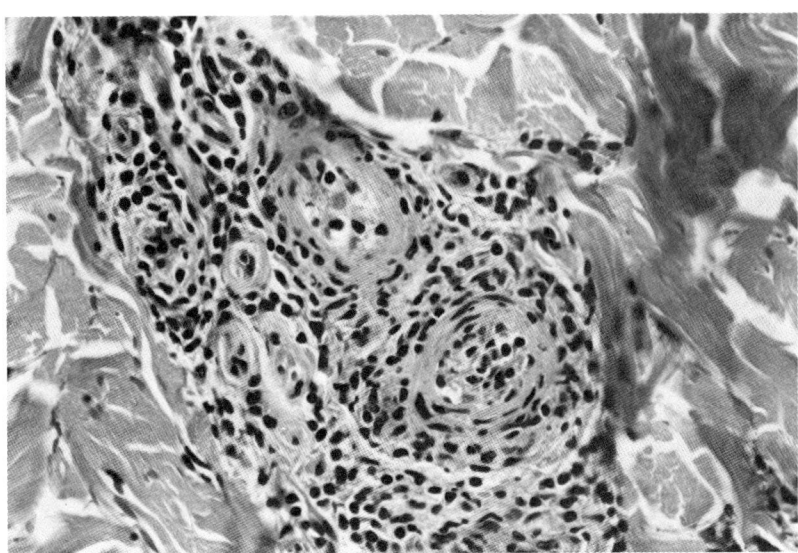

Fig. 20-1. Small vessel vasculitis of subcutaneous tissue (×100).

68 Section Three • RHEUMATIC AND GRANULOMATOUS DISEASES

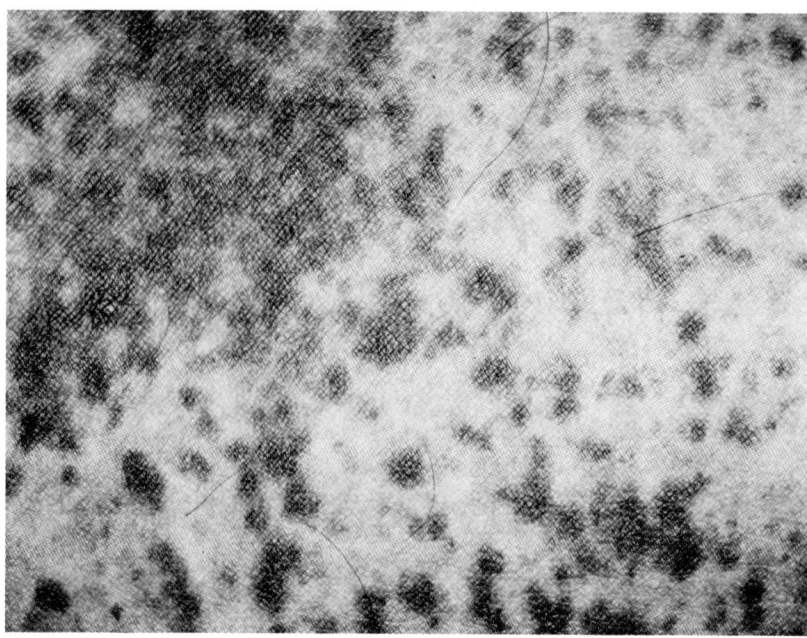

Fig. 20-2. Close-up view of palpable purpura in patient with hypersensitivity vasculitis.

Table 20-1. Characteristics of the giant cell arteritides

	Temporal arteritis	**Takayasu's arteritis**
Patients	Disease of the elderly; women more than men	More prevalent in young women; more common in the Orient, but neither racially nor geographically restricted
Blood vessels	Characteristically involves branches of carotid artery (temporal artery), but is a systemic arteritis and may involve any medium-sized or large artery	Large and medium-sized arteries with predilection for aortic arch and its branches; may involve pulmonary artery
Histopathology	Panarteritis; inflammatory mononuclear cell infiltrates; frequent giant cell formation within vessel wall; fragmentation of internal elastic lamina; proliferation of intima	Panarteritis; inflammatory mononuclear cell infiltrates; intimal proliferation and fibrosis; scarring and vascularization of media; disruption and degeneration of elastic lamina
Manifestations	Classic complex of fever, anemia, high erythrocyte sedimentation rate, muscle aches in an elderly person; headache may be present; strongly associated with polymyalgia rheumatica syndrome	Generalized systemic symptoms; local signs and symptoms related to involved vessels; occlusive phase
Complications	Ocular (sudden blindness)	Related to distribution of involved vessels; death usually occurs from congestive heart failure or cerebrovascular accident
Diagnosis	Temporal artery biopsy; lesions may be segmental; multiple sections, arteriography, and bilateral biopsy may aid in diagnosis	Arteriography; biopsy of involved vessel
Treatment	Corticosteroids highly effective	Corticosteroids not of proven efficacy; cytotoxic agents untried

Adapted from Fauci, A.S., Haynes, B.F., and Katz, P.: Ann. Intern. Med. **89**:660, 1978.

ance of a lymphoproliferative disease. In the past this disorder was often confused with Wegener's granulomatosis because of the presence of granulomatous vasculitis. However, in lymphomatoid granulomatosis granulomata are fewer in number and less distinct and the "vasculitis" is characterized by an infiltration of blood vessels of various sizes with atypical mononuclear cells.

Giant cell arteritides. The giant cell arteritides are temporal arteritis and Takayasu's arteritis (Table 20-1). Both disorders are panarteritides with involvement of medium-sized and large arteries, although they differ in the age of onset, location of vessel involvement, and response to therapy. Their causes are uncertain, but immunologic mechanisms are postulated for both.

Temporal arteritis is often accompanied by the polymyalgia rheumatica syndrome of stiffness and pain of the neck, shoulder, lower back, hip, and thigh muscles (see Chapter 23). The clinical picture of temporal arteritis is usually well circumscribed. It consists of fever, anemia, headache, myalgias, and a high erythrocyte sedimentation rate in older people. The diagnosis is confirmed by the finding of panarteritis in temporal artery biopsy specimens. One of the most serious complications of temporal arteritis is sudden blindness caused by ophthalmic arteritis. As will be described, it is important to be attentive to symptomatology in this disorder, since ocular involvement can usually be prevented by corticosteroid therapy.

Takayasu's arteritis, or pulseless disease, is a less common disorder with characteristics clearly different from those of temporal arteritis (Table 20-1). This disease may have complex and varied symptoms ranging from generalized, nonspecific complaints to local signs resulting from compromised blood flow to the extremities or other organs. Most commonly, this is manifested as absent pulses or bruits. Clinically, the course of this disease is variable, but generally a gradual deterioration is seen. Because of this variability with a tendency toward remissions and exacerbations, the evaluation of appropriate therapy has been difficult. However, compared to temporal arteritis, Takayasu's arteritis is much less responsive to corticosteroid therapy. Death is usually caused by congestive heart failure or a cerebrovascular accident.

Other vasculitides. Other, less common vasculitic syndromes include thromboangiitis obliterans (Buerger's disease) and the mucocutaneous lymph node syndrome (Kawasaki disease).

Thromboangiitis obliterans. Thromboangiitis obliterans is an inflammatory occlusive peripheral vascular disease of arteries and veins. There is a male predominance, and the age of onset is usually 20 to 40 years. The vasculitis segmentally involves veins and small to medium-sized arteries. The inflammatory stage of the disease is almost always associated with a thrombus. The cause of Buerger's disease is unknown, but almost uniformly it is associated with heavy smoking. Evidence implying immunologic mediation is lacking. Patients show signs of vascular insufficiency in the extremities. The disease follows an indolent course characterized by recurrences and leading finally to amputation unless interrupted by the therapy of choice, cessation of tobacco use.

Mucocutaneous lymph node syndrome. The mucocutaneous lymph node syndrome is an acute febrile illness of children and young adults characterized by nonsuppurative cervical lymphadenopathy, erythema of the oropharynx, desquamative skin rash, and unresponsiveness to antibiotics. Although it is usually self-limited, a small percentage of patients (approximately 2%) die suddenly from coronary arteritis. This syndrome was first believed to be restricted to Japan, but cases have now been well documented throughout the continental United States. The cause of the disease is uncertain, and to date no therapy has proved to be of value in the prevention of coronary involvement.

MANAGEMENT. Much of the difficulty in developing treatment protocols for the vasculitides has been related to problems with their classification. Using the categories described in this chapter, we have developed a therapeutic approach. The prototype disorder for our pharmacologic regimen is Wegener's granulomatosis. Because this disease is uniformly fatal and usually fails to respond to corticosteroids, cyclophosphamide has been employed.

Because of the success with the regimen for Wegener's granulomatosis, it has been employed for the treatment of lymphomatoid granulomatosis and systemic necrotizing vasculitis. Patients with lymphomatoid granulomatosis, if left untreated, have a fulminant, usually fatal course, often characterized by the development of an aggressive lymphoproliferative disorder. Similarly, without therapy patients with systemic necrotizing vasculitis have a poor prognosis. Thus both diseases in the past had a dismal prognosis even with the use of various cytotoxic regimens. Using cyclophosphamide alone or in combination with corticosteroids, in the same manner as in Wegener's granulomatosis, we have seen a significant reduction in the morbidity and mortality from these two diseases. It is imperative, however, that therapy be instituted early in the course of these entities before irreversible end-organ damage has occurred.

In the hypersensitivity vasculitides in which an offending antigen or an underlying disorder can be identified, therapy is aimed at removal of the antigen or treatment of the primary illness. When such causes are suspected but cannot be proved or when the process appears to be self-limited, a brief course of corticosteroids may be warranted to hasten resolution of the process.

As described previously, giant cell arteritis is usually extremely responsive to corticosteroids. Initial high-dose therapy of 40 to 60 mg of prednisone a day is gradually tapered to a daily maintenance dose of 7.5 to 10 mg. Therapy probably should be continued for 1 to 2 years. With this regimen, the prognosis is generally good and complete remission is usually attained. In Takayasu's arteritis corticosteroid therapy has proved to be of variable efficacy, but it does not appear that these agents prolong life. Experience with cytotoxic agents in this disease is at present only anecdotal, and no firm conclusions can yet be drawn regarding the efficacy of these agents.

In all types of vasculitis treatment of underlying or associated conditions such as connective tissue disease or infection is imperative. Management depends in large part on which organs are primarily involved (for example, myocardial infarction, ischemic bowel, or digital gangrene).

BIBLIOGRAPHY

Churg, J., and Strauss, L.: Allergic granulomatosis, allergic angiitis, and periarteritis nodosa, Am. J. Pathol. **27**:227, 1951.
Fauci, A.S.: Granulomatous vasculitis: Distinct but related, Ann. Intern. Med. **87**:782, 1977.
Fauci, A.S., and Wolff, S.M.: Wegener's granulomatosis: studies in eighteen patients and a review of the literature, Medicine **52**:535, 1973.
Fauci, A.S., Haynes, B.F., and Katz, P.: The spectrum of vasculitis: Clinical, pathologic, immunologic, and therapeutic consideration, Ann. Intern. Med. **89**:660, 1978.
Fauci, A.S., and others: Cyclophosphamide therapy of severe systemic necrotizing vasculitis, N. Engl. J. Med. **301**:235, 1979.
Rose, G.A., and Spencer, H.: Polyarteritis nodosa, Q. J. Med. **26**:43, 1957.

21 • SCHÖNLEIN-HENOCH PURPURA

Warren A. Katz

Schönlein-Henoch purpura is a vasculitic syndrome closely related to hypersensitivity angiitis. It usually follows streptococcal infections in children, but occasionally it may be caused by a drug or food allergy. Most typically it consists of a clinical tetrad of purpura, arthralgias, abdominal pain, and glomerulonephritis. Cutaneous manifestations are invariable and consist of raised purpuric or ecchymotic lesions, most often on the extensor surface of the lower extremities. The lesions may appear hemorrhagic or urticarial. The rash may involve the face.

Rheumatic manifestations include polyarthralgia and sometimes overt arthritis, particularly of the knees and ankles. Deformities do not develop. Hemorrhage within the gastrointestinal wall may cause colicky abdominal pain, hematemesis, and melena. Hematuria is the most common manifestation of glomerulonephritis; some patients have chronic nephritis with uremia. The most characteristic finding is a leukocytoclastic angiitis seen on skin biopsy with IgG and C3 deposits on immunofluorescence studies.

The disease is usually self-limited, particularly in young people. The systemic administration of corticosteroids may be required for acutely ill patients.

BIBLIOGRAPHY

Cream, J.J., Gumpel, J.M., and Peachey, R.D.: Schönlein-Henoch purpura in the adult: a study of 77 adults with anaphylactoid or Schönlein-Henoch purpura, Q. J. Med. **34**:461, 1970.

22 • WEGENER'S GRANULOMATOSIS AND MIDLINE GRANULOMA

Paul Katz and **Anthony S. Fauci**

Wegener's granulomatosis (WG) and midline granuloma (MLG) are uncommon diseases of unknown cause. Although these disorders are clinically distinct, they may be confused because of their propensity to involve the upper airways. As will be described, WG is a systemic disease with glomerulonephritis and necrotizing granulomatous vasculitis of the upper and lower respiratory tracts. Upper airway disease in WG rarely causes the palatal perforation and facial erosion characteristic of MLG. Conversely, MLG is a localized process of the nasal and oropharyngeal area that infrequently manifests true vasculitis. Additionally, these diseases differ in their response to cytotoxic therapy. The following discussion will highlight the important points of both diseases and compare and contrast the clinical, pathologic, and therapeutic aspects of each.

WEGENER'S GRANULOMATOSIS

WG is a disseminated granulomatous necrotizing vasculitis of the small vessels of the upper and lower respiratory tracts. In the generalized form, glomerulonephritis is an important component of the disease process. Although a localized, limited form confined to the airways has been described, this likely represents an early stage of generalized disease before the development of detectable renal disease.

PATHOGENESIS. The immunopathogenic mechanisms responsible for the development of WG remain largely unknown. Circulating and tissue immune complex-like material are demonstrable in some individuals with this disease. Theoretically, these complexes could activate the complement cascade with the resultant generation of factors chemotactic for neutrophils. Sensitized lymphocytes could likewise react with the offending antigen(s), which would result in the release of lymphokines important in the initiation of granulomatous inflammation. Furthermore, immune complexes can potentially directly trigger monocyte-macrophages to form granulomata. It must be emphasized that in many patients immune complex mediation can only be assumed and not conclusively proved. The identity and nature of the antigen or antigens responsible for initiating the inflammatory processes are unknown.

PATHOLOGY. The histologic features characteristic of WG include necrotizing vasculitis of small arteries and veins with coexistent granuloma formation. Disease of the upper airway is manifested by paranasal sinus and nasopharyngeal necrotizing granulomata in the presence or absence of vasculitis. This may be accompanied by pansinusitis, bony erosion, septal perforation, and in some cases saddle nose deformity. Lung lesions are usually present roentgenographically as multiple, bilateral nodular infiltrates with a tendency to cavitate. Histologically, involved lung tissue manifests the classic necrotizing vasculitis and associated granulomata (Fig. 22-1). Renal disease in WG is characterized by focal and segmental glomerulonephritis with accompanying crescent formation. Depending on the stage of kidney involvement at the time of biopsy, renal disease may range from mild focal glomerulitis to fulminant proliferative glomerulonephritis to fibrosed and sclerosed end-stage glomeruli. Organ systems other than the lungs and kidneys may display vasculitis or granulomata or both.

CLINICAL MANIFESTATIONS. The mean age at onset of WG is 40 years, and the male to female ratio is 3:2. Early in the disease the clinical picture is dominated by upper respiratory tract signs, including rhinorrhea, paranasal sinus pain, sinusitis, nasal ulcerations, purulent or bloody nasal discharge, septal perforation, saddle nose deformity, and otitis media. However, virtually any manifestation of the disease may be seen at the time of presentation. Nonspecific pulmonary complaints may include cough, hemoptysis, chest discomfort, and shortness of breath. It is not uncommon for asymptomatic pulmonary infiltrates to be seen on roentgenograms of the chest.

Renal disease as the sole presenting manifestation of WG is rare without demonstrable airway disease. The development of renal disease may be insidious, with only smoldering low-level activity, or may be acute and rapidly progressive, with ultimate progression to end-stage kidney failure.

Virtually any organ system may be involved in WG, but these manifestations are usually less dramatic in comparison to the respiratory tract and renal disease (Table 22-1). However, certain important manifestations are worth mentioning. Peripheral or central nervous system disease occurs in 25% to 50% of the patients, with peripheral involvement more common. Neuropathy induced by vasculitis of the vasa nervorum is manifested as cranial neuritis or mononeuritis multiplex. The rarer central nervous system involvement is caused by cerebral vasculitis or space-occupying granulomata that directly extend from paranasal sinuses or form in situ. Cardiac disease is seen as pericarditis or coronary artery vasculitis in one third of the patients. Skin disease results from vasculitis with or without granuloma formation and is manifested in up to 50% of the patients as petechiae, palpable purpura, papules, vesicles, ulcerations, or subcutaneous nodules. Oral and other mucosal membrane ulcerations can also occur (Fig. 22-2). One half of the patients have eye disease ranging from mild conjunctivitis to episcleritis, sclerouveitis, or scleromalacia perforans. Vasculitic compromise of the optic nerve may lead to sudden blindness, and retro-orbital granuloma formation may cause proptosis.

LABORATORY FINDINGS. There are no specific laboratory tests diagnostic of WG. However, there are several nonspecific laboratory abnormalities, including the invariably elevated erythrocyte sedimentation rate, mild anemia, leukocytosis, and thrombocytosis. Low-titer rheumatoid

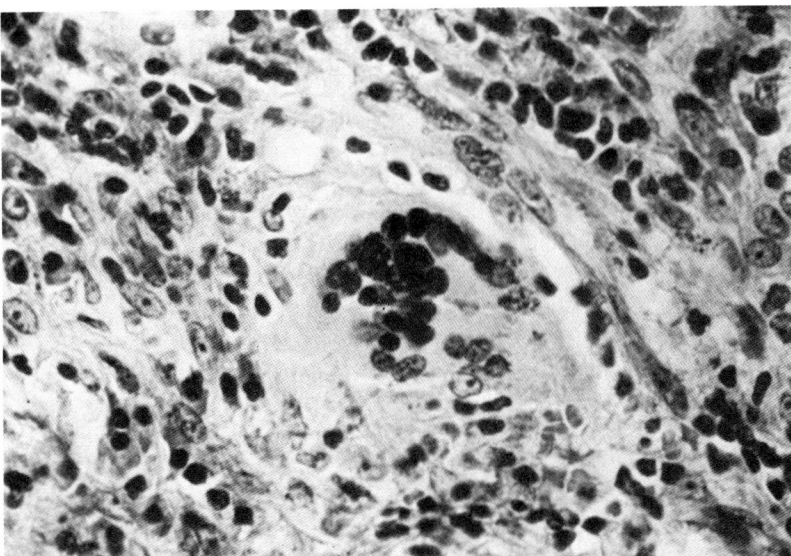

Fig. 22-1. Lung biopsy specimen from patient with Wegener's granulomatosis showing granulomatous inflammation and presence of multinucleated giant cells (×100).

Table 22-1. Characteristic features of organ system involvement in Wegener's granulomatosis

Organ system	Approximate frequency (%)	Typical features
Nasopharynx	75	Necrotizing granuloma with mucosal ulceration; saddle nose deformity
Paranasal sinuses	90	Pansinusitis; necrotizing granuloma; secondary bacterial infection
Eyes	60	Keratoconjunctivitis; granulomatous sclerouveitis
Ears	35	Serous otitis media; secondary bacterial infection
Lungs	95	Multiple nodular cavitary infiltrates; necrotizing granulomatous vasculitis
Kidneys	85	Focal and segmental glomerulitis; necrotizing glomerulonephritis later in course
Heart	15	Coronary vasculitis; pericarditis
Nervous system	20	Mononeuritis multiplex; cranial neuritis
Skin	40	Dermal vasculitis with secondary ulcerations
Joints	50	Polyarthralgias

Adapted from Fauci, A.S., Haynes, B.F., and Katz, P.: Ann. Intern. Med. **89**:660, 1978.

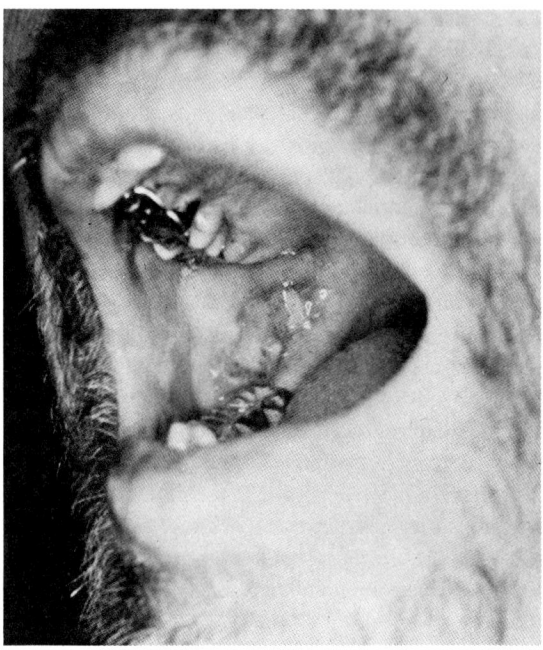

Fig. 22-2. Oral mucosal membrane ulcerations in patient with Wegener's granulomatosis.

factor, mild elevations of serum immunoglobulins, particularly IgA, and positive tests for circulating immune complexes are frequently seen. HLA-B8, a histocompatibility antigen often associated with "autoimmune diseases," occurs with increased frequency in these patients.

DIAGNOSIS. The diagnosis of WG can be clinically suspected in an individual with the classic triad of upper and lower respiratory tract disease and coexistent renal involvement. Histologic diagnosis is mandatory and can be confirmed by the presence of necrotizing granulomatous vasculitis in involved tissue. Lung parenchyma is the source with the highest yield and is usually best approached via open thoracotomy. Percutaneous renal biopsy is advisable not only to confirm the diagnosis but also to assess the extent of involvement.

The clinical triad in combination with the characteristic histopathologic findings usually makes the diagnosis reasonably straightforward. Included in the differential diagnosis are the other vasculitides, infectious and noninfectious granulomatous diseases, collagen vascular diseases, and neoplasms of the upper and lower airways. Goodpasture's syndrome may be differentiated by the presence of circulating or tissue anti–glomerular basement membrane antibody. The distinction from idiopathic midline granuloma, which will be discussed later in the chapter, can be made on the basis of clinical and pathologic criteria.

Lymphomatoid granulomatosis (see Chapter 20) is a type of vasculitis with many characteristics of a lymphoma involving the skin, lungs, kidney, and central nervous system. The vasculitis is unlike WG in that there is angiocentric and angiodestructive inflammation with atypical lymphocytoid and plasmacytoid cells. Additionally, renal involvement in lymphomatoid granulomatosis is due to nodular infiltration with clusters of these atypical cells rather than a true glomerulonephritis.

MANAGEMENT AND PROGNOSIS. Before the advent of cytotoxic therapy, WG was uniformly fatal within several months following the onset of renal involvement. Corticosteroids produced a transient clinical improvement but alone were ineffective in prolonging life. Approximately 10 years ago we began a treatment protocol with cyclophosphamide in an oral dose of 1 to 2 mg/kg/day. Therapy in fulminant cases may be initiated with 4 to 5 mg/kg/day of drug intavenously for 3 to 4 days followed by conversion to the lower oral maintenance dose. After therapy is begun, the dose is carefully adjusted to maintain the total leukocyte count in a range of 3000 to 4000 cells/mm^3 with an absolute neutrophil count of 1000 to 1500 cells/mm^3. In this range life-threatening infection resulting from neutropenia is avoided. In subjects unable or unwilling to take cyclophosphamide because of leukopenia, hemorrhagic cystitis, or potential gonadal damage, azathioprine in similar doses may be substituted. It should be remembered, however, that this agent is clearly less effective in inducing remissions than cyclophosphamide.

Corticosteroids, usually 1 mg/kg/day of prednisone, are used early in the course of the disease until cyclophosphamide becomes effective, that is, about 2 to 3 weeks. At that time prednisone is converted to an alternate-day regimen, then tapered, and finally discontinued. Longer courses of daily or alternate-day prednisone should be reserved for patients with ocular disease, central nervous system involvement, or symptomatic serosal inflammation. The erythrocyte sedimentation rate is the most sensitive indicator of disease activity and should be normal for at least 1 year before cyclophosphamide is tapered and ultimately discontinued. With this treatment protocol, several patients have had prolonged remissions following cessation of cytotoxic therapy.

Besides drugs, maintenance of a patent airway by tracheostomy, if required, control of complicating infection, monitoring of fluids and electrolytes, and advice regarding activities of daily living are important features of the management program.

MIDLINE GRANULOMA

Midline granuloma (MLG) is a locally destructive, progressive process of the nose, paranasal sinuses, and palate, often with erosion through the face and orbit. An uncommon disease, it can occur in all age groups, although most patients are in the fifth and sixth decades of life. There is a slight female predominance.

PATHOGENESIS AND PATHOLOGY. The cause of idiopathic MLG is unknown. Because of the presence of granulomatous inflammation suggestive of a hypersensitivity or cell-mediated immune reaction, it has been postulated that the disease represents a localized hypersensitivity reaction to unidentified antigen(s). It may be that certain susceptible individuals hyperreact to this antigenic stimulus, resulting in the chronic inflammation characteristic of this entity. Certain tumors can produce a clinical and histologic picture so similar to MLG as to camouflage the underlying neoplastic process. Likewise, certain infectious processes can induce similar upper airway destruction. However, in true idiopathic MLG no underlying neoplasm or microbial agent can be identified even with careful histologic study of multiple tissue specimens, meticulous culturing of involved tissue, and searches for disease outside the facial area.

The histologic diagnosis of MLG is complicated by the nonspecificity of the pathologic changes. The usual features include necrosis accompanying acute and chronic inflammation. The tissue is infiltrated with neutrophils, lymphocytes, monocytes, plasma cells, and in some cases eosinophils. As indicated by its name, MLG is characterized by granuloma formation (with or without Langhans' giant cells), although in many cases this may be obscured by the massive amounts of tissue necrosis. Vascular involvement in the form of small vessel thrombosis and perivascular cellular infiltration may occur, but true vasculitis is rare.

CLINICAL MANIFESTATIONS. Although the presentation is variable, most patients develop rhinorrhea and nasal congestion early in the course of the disease. These symptoms become progressive, and the nasal discharge may become purulent because of infection. Nonhealing ulcerations and perforation of the nasal septum frequently occur. Disease initially confined to the orpharynx may be present as ulcerations of the buccal mucosa, gums, and hard and soft palates. On occasion ocular complaints develop first. Regardless of location, the disease process is always progressive with destruction of soft tissue, cartilage, and bone. In most patients destructive lesions of the palate, the nasal septum, and in some cases the entire nose eventually develop. With erosion and mutilation of the facial architecture, necrotic tissue frequently becomes superinfected, usually with *Staphylococcus aureus*. In addition to the idiopathic form in which no underlying or neoplastic process can be identified, MLG may occur as a manifestation of a local upper airway neoplasm. These localized neoplasms can usually be diagnosed through a careful study of adequate histologic sections and a complete search for sites of tumor involvement elsewhere.

LABORATORY FINDINGS. There are no characteristic laboratory features of MLG that aid in its diagnosis. With chronic inflammation, leukocytosis, an elevated erythrocyte sedimentation rate, mild anemia caused by chronic disease, and hypergammaglobulinemia may be observed. Laboratory evidence of disease activity outside the upper airways necessitates the search for a different disease. Roentgenography of the sinuses reveals pansinusitis with varying degrees of destruction of bone and cartilage.

DIAGNOSIS. The diagnosis rests on the histopathologic findings in concert with a compatible clinical picture. It cannot be emphasized too strongly that other diseases with similar presentations and features must be ruled out before the diagnosis of idiopathic MLG is made. The most difficult distinction is between idiopathic MLG and neoplasms of the upper airways, particularly midline malignant reticulosis and certain lymphomas. This difficulty in diagnosis is due to the similarity in inflammatory and destructive histopathologic changes that can obscure the true malignant character of the underlying tumor. It is therefore imperative in all cases of suspected idiopathic MLG that a meticulous search for disseminated malignancy be made. This should be combined with a careful microscopic review of adequate biopsy specimens. Infectious diseases included in the differential diagnosis are syphilis, tuberculosis, histoplasmosis, lepromatous leprosy, blastomycosis, coccidioidomycosis, mucocutaneous leishmaniasis, rhinoscleroma caused by *Klebsiella rhinoscleromatis*, and orbital pseu-

Table 22-2. Differences between Wegener's granulomatosis and midline granuloma

	Wegener's granulomatosis	Midline granuloma
Organ systems involved	Systemic disease with upper and lower respiratory tracts and kidneys primarily involved	Local disease of upper respiratory tract exclusively
Nature of upper airway lesions	Palatal perforation and facial erosion virtually never occur	Palatal perforation and facial erosion common
Pathologic findings	Necrotizing granulomatous vasculitis	Nonspecific inflammation with or without granulomata
Response to cytotoxic agents	Good	Poor

dotumor. Wegener's granulomatosis can cause similar upper airway findings. The distinction can be made on the basis of the clinical and pathologic findings listed in Table 22-2.

MANAGEMENT AND PROGNOSIS. Although the course may vary in the rapidity of its progression, the disease is uniformly fatal if untreated. Death usually results from systemic infection, inanition, erosion into blood vessels with exsanguination, or erosion into the central nervous system.

Earlier attempts at surgical therapy of idiopathic MLG often resulted in an acceleration of the disease process without effecting a beneficial response. Corticosteroids and cytotoxic agents have likewise proved to be of little benefit unless the disease was misdiagnosed. We have had good success with local, high-dose (5000 rad) radiation in the involved areas. With this therapy a remission rate of greater than 70% has been achieved, often with remissions lasting 10 years or more. The side effects and complications of therapy may be profound, but they are obviously worth the risk considering the otherwise fatal outcome. Once remission has been achieved, reconstructive plastic surgery and prosthetic placement can be performed to correct much of the disfigurement.

BIBLIOGRAPHY

Fauci, A.S., and Wolff, S.M.: Wegener's granulomatosis: studies in eighteen patients and a review of the literature, Medicine **52**:535, 1973.

Fauci, A.S., Haynes, B.F., and Katz, P.: The spectrum of vasculitis: clinical, pathologic, immunologic, and therapeutic considerations, Ann. Intern. Med. **89**:660, 1978.

Fauci, A.S., Johnson, R.E., and Wolff, S.M.: Radiation therapy of midline granuloma, Ann. Intern. Med. **84**:140, 1976.

Friedmann, I.: Midline granuloma, Proc. R. Soc. Med. **57**:289, 1964.

Stewart, J.P.: Progressive lethal granulomatous ulceration of the nose, J. Laryngol. **48**:657, 1933.

Wolff, S.M., and others: Wegener's granulomatosis, Ann. Intern. Med. **81**:513, 1974.

23 • POLYMYALGIA RHEUMATICA AND TEMPORAL ARTERITIS

June F. Klinghoffer

Polymyalgia rheumatica (PMR) is a clinical syndrome of unknown cause, seen primarily in older patients, and characterized by pain and stiffness in the muscles of the shoulder, neck, low back, and pelvic girdle and by a very rapid erythrocyte sedimentation rate.

Giant cell arteritis is a granulomatous form of arteritis that involves large and medium-sized arteries. The cause is unknown. The major branches coming off the aortic arch, especially the cranial arteries, are most characteristically involved. By common usage, the term "temporal arteritis" includes giant cell arteritis of any of the cranial arteries, such as the temporal, facial, ophthalmic, and occipital arteries.

PMR and temporal arteritis are closely associated. The myalgic syndrome often precedes or appears simultaneously with evidence of temporal arteritis. Conversely, clinical or histologic evidence of temporal arteritis is found in 20% to 40% of cases of PMR. It is thus not clear whether PMR is a distinct, separate entity or whether it is always a clinical manifestation of underlying vasculitis.

EPIDEMIOLOGY. Some authors have estimated the prevalence of PMR to be similar or equal to that of gout or systemic lupus erythematosus. It occurs primarily in persons over the age of 55 and is rare in those under 50. Women are affected somewhat more frequently than men, and it is uncommon in blacks.

CLINICAL MANIFESTATIONS. The onset of PMR may be insidious or acute. Many patients can give a specific date on which their illness began. They may describe a flulike syndrome at the onset or refer to waking sore and stiff one morning as if they had engaged in vigorous physical exertion the previous day. There is muscle pain and stiffness involving the shoulders, upper arms, and neck. Patients may complain of inability to lift the arms and difficulty in combing the hair or dressing. There may also be pain in the hips, buttocks, groin, and thighs and difficulty in walking up stairs or getting up from a chair.

The limitation of movement may be misinterpreted as weakness, but physical examination rules out both muscle weakness and joint disease. Muscle atrophy is not usually seen. There may be some muscle tenderness. Morning stiffness is often so severe that the patient requires help in getting out of bed. Nocturnal discomfort interferes with sleep.

Constitutional symptoms are frequent and may be misleading. The common findings are low-grade fever, night sweats, fatigue, malaise, anorexia, weight loss, and depression. Giant cell arteritis may be a cause of fever of unknown origin. An increased incidence of the carpal tunnel syndrome has recently been reported.

The clinical manifestations of associated temporal arteritis are:

1. Unilateral or bilateral temporal headache
2. Tenderness over the temporal artery, thickening or nodularity of the temporal artery, and/or absence of pulsation
3. Visual disturbances or actual blindness
4. Scalp tenderness
5. Jaw pain on chewing or talking (masseter claudication)

Other, less common manifestations are trismus (masseter spasm), difficulty in swallowing, recurrent blanching or actual gangrene of the tongue, facial pain, earache, toothache, and loss of taste sensation. Masseter claudication is considered a pathognomonic sign of giant cell arteritis. Histologic evidence of temporal arteritis may be found even in the absence of clinical symptoms.

LABORATORY FINDINGS. The most striking finding is a very rapid erythrocyte sedimentation rate—almost always over 50 mm/hr (Westergren method) and often in the range of 80 to 120 mm/hr. A mild hypochromic or normochromic anemia is common. Alpha-2 globulin and fibrinogen may be elevated. Recent reports document a high incidence of elevated alkaline phosphatase and occasional elevations of the other liver enzymes.

Other laboratory studies, including muscle enzymes, are normal. The muscle biopsy is usually normal, as are electromyographic studies. Tests for rheumatoid factor, antinuclear antibodies, and complement are normal.

Biopsy of the superficial temporal artery may reveal the classic picture of giant cell arteritis, but false-negative results are possible because of the patchy nature of the vascular involvement.

DIAGNOSIS. A carefully detailed clinical history is most important for diagnosis. Proximal symmetric muscle pain and stiffness in older patients, a rapid sedimentation rate, absence of intrinsic muscle weakness or objective arthropathy, normal muscle enzymes, and the presence of constitutional symptoms comprise the classic clinical picture. Symptoms suggestive of associated temporal arteritis must be actively sought.

The diagnosis of temporal arteritis can be confirmed by positive biopsy of the temporal artery; it cannot be excluded on the basis of a negative biopsy because of the segmental nature of giant cell arteritis. Diagnoses to be excluded are polymyositis, rheumatoid arthritis, fibrositis, occult neoplasms (especially multiple myeloma), and occult infection. Confirmation of the diagnosis is provided by a therapeutic test with small doses of prednisone.

COURSE AND PROGNOSIS. PMR is considered a self-limited illness that runs its course in 1 to 5 years. In the absence of associated giant cell arteritis there is no increase in mortality, but severe incapacity may occur in untreated persons with the disease. In the presence of arteritis the gravest threat is blindness, and early adequate therapy is essential. Complications arising from systemic giant cell arteritis such as cerebrovascular accident, myocardial infarction, claudication of the extremities, and other ischemic manifestations are occasionally seen.

MANAGEMENT. Few if any illnesses show as rapid and gratifying a response to low-dose steroids as PMR. Complete relief of symptoms occurs within 4 or 5 days (often within 1 to 2 days) with a daily dose of 10 to 20 mg of prednisone. This experience has enabled some physicians to use a 10-day trial of steroids as a diagnostic aid. The sedimentation rate falls to normal, and the anemia is corrected within 2 weeks. The prednisone dosage is tapered, using the patient's clinical status and sedimentation rate as guides. The average patient can be maintained without symptoms with 5 to 7.5 mg of prednisone daily for 1 to 2 years. Alternate-day steroid therapy is ineffective.

In the presence of clinical or histologic evidence of temporal arteritis, higher prednisone dosage is necessary; 60 mg daily should be started immediately. Tapering of dosage is usually possible after approximately 1 month.

BIBLIOGRAPHY

Desser, E.J.: Miosis, trismus, and dysphagia: an unusual presentation of temporal arteritis, Ann. Intern. Med. **71**:961, 1969.

Goodman, B.W.: Temporal arteritis, Am. J. Med. **67**:839, 1979.

Hamilton, C.R., Jr., Shelley, W.M., and Tumulty, P.A.: Giant cell arteritis: including temporal arteritis and polymyalgia rheumatica, Medicine **50**:1, 1971.

Healey, L.A., and Wilske, K.R.: Manifestations of giant cell arteritis, Med. Clin. North Am. **61**:261, 1977.

Hunder, G.G., and Allen, G.L.: Giant cell arteritis: a review, Bull. Rheum. Dis. **29**:980, 1979.

24 • SARCOIDOSIS

Warren A. Katz

Sarcoidosis is a systemic disease of unknown cause that is characterized pathologically by the presence of noncaseating giant cell granulomata in multiple organs. Granulomatous lesions are found in lymph nodes, lungs, liver, skin, and synovial membrane. Bones, subcutaneous tissues, muscle, bursae, tendon sheaths, eyes, and the viscera may be sites of sarcoid infiltration.

PATHOGENESIS AND PATHOLOGY. Although the cause of sarcoidosis is unknown, various organisms have been claimed to have caused the disease, including mycobacteria and viruses. The occurrence of sarcoidosis in family lines suggests a mode of inheritance in some people. Indeed, a high incidence of HLA-B8 tissue type has been noted in patients who have sarcoidosis with erythema nodosum and arthritis. Pine cone pollen, clay dust, peanut dust, and pine pitch have all been implicated in the etiology. Foreign body reactions to beryllium, talc, silica, zirconium, and fungi form sarcoidlike noncaseating granulomata. One theory for the pathogenesis of sarcoidosis presupposes that an antigenic insult triggers a T-cell and B-cell immunologic response and that through a variety of possible mechanisms, including transformation, inhibition, and cell interaction, T cells become depleted. This theory would explain the depressed delayed reactivity to skin tests and depressed lymphocyte transformation observed in sarcoidosis. Unopposed B-cell lymphoproliferation would result in an increase in circulating immunoglobulins and histologically in granuloma formation, both seen in sarcoidosis. In addition, circulating immune complexes may be present in erythema nodosum with hilar adenopathy in sarcoidosis. Histologically, the granulomata are composed of discrete hyperplastic tubercles consisting primarily of epithelioid cells containing Langhans-type giant cells with cytoplasmic inclusions.

CLINICAL MANIFESTATIONS. Two types of sarcoidosis with differences in onset, physical manifestations, ancillary phenomena, prognosis, and treatment are apparent. The acute (or abortive) form is more common than the chronic form worldwide (Table 24-1).

Chronic sarcoidosis. Chronic sarcoidosis is the more common form of sarcoidosis recognized in the United States. It is mainly a disease of blacks. Although it frequently begins in young adults, it often is not detected until after the age of 40.

Chronic sarcoidosis is characterized by respiratory symptoms, manifestations of extrathoracic involvement, constitutional symptoms of fever, malaise, and weight loss, or may be seen as asymptomatic bilateral hilar adenopathy detected on chest roentgenography. Pulmonary symptoms usually include dyspnea, cough, nonpleuritic chest pain, or rarely hemoptysis. Even though only 60% of patients with chronic sarcoidosis actually have a respiratory presentation, some abnormality on the chest roentgenogram is present in 92%. Early in the course of the disease the chest roentgenogram is negative, but later mediastinal adenopathy becomes apparent. With advancing disease, pulmonary parenchymal infiltrates may appear on the roentgenogram as discrete fluffy nodules, confluent infiltrates, or linear interstitial fibrosis. At this stage dyspnea becomes apparent even on mild exercise. Patients with pulmonary parenchymal disease do not usually have subsequent hilar adenopathy, although the reverse may be true. In the later stages there is extensive parenchymal involvement with marked fibrosis characterized clinically by chronic dyspnea even at rest. Bronchiectasis may result from compression of the bronchi.

Hemoptysis, sometimes massive, may be associated with bronchiectasis. Pulmonary function studies correlate with the degree of pulmonary involvement. The diffusion capacity, vital capacity, and maximal midexpiratory flow rate are markedly diminished. The defect in gas exchange is the first abnormality to be detected on pulmonary function studies.

Granulomatous lesions of the nose, nasopharynx, and larynx may occasionally develop. This presentation is far more common in women than in men and occurs particularly in the third decade of life. The degree of destruction may resemble that of midline granuloma.

Sarcoid skin lesions may be of several types, including

Table 24-1. Differentiation between acute and chronic sarcoidosis

Parameter	Acute	Chronic
Onset	Abrupt	Insidious
Age	Under 40 years	Over 40 years
Race	Predominantly whites	Predominantly blacks
Erythema nodosum	Usually present	Usually absent
Respiratory symptoms	Usually absent	Usually present
Duration of arthritis	Transient	Persistent
Distribution in joints	Polyarthritis	Pauciarthritis
Periarthritis of ankles	Usually present	Absent
Digital swelling	Usually absent	Often present
Joint deformity	Never	Somtimes
Roentgenograms of joints	Soft tissue swelling	Bone lesions somtimes
Synovial biopsy	Mild, nonspecific inflammation	Noncaseating granuloma
Roentgenogram of chest	Bilateral hilar adenopathy	Hilar adenopathy and parenchymal infiltration
Hypercalcemia	Usually absent	Sometimes present
Angiotensin-converting enzyme	Increased	Increased unless burned out
Urinary hydroxyproline	Increased	Normal
Spontaneous remission	Usual	Unusual

maculopapular rashes, plaques, subcutaneous nodules, and scars. Most of these lesions, when biopsied, show a typical sarcoid reaction.

Uveitis can be detected in 25% of the patients with chronic sarcoidosis; in addition, conjunctival lesions, keratoconjunctivitis, scleral plaques, retinal vasculitis, papilledema, and even cataracts may be present. Glaucoma may result from ocular sarcoidosis. Heerfordt's disease consists of uveitis in association with parotid gland enlargement, seventh nerve palsy, and fever. Salivary gland enlargement, unilateral or bilateral, may be present; sometimes there is Sjögren's syndrome consisting of keratoconjunctivitis sicca.

Chronic sarcoidosis may also cause hepatosplenomegaly, peripheral and central nervous system lesions (including diabetes insipidus), cardiomyopathy, and renal disease. Peripheral lymphadenopathy may be evident in any part of the body, notably the supraclavicular fossa.

Chronic sarcoidosis of bone is most often characterized by pain in the hands or feet caused by punched-out bony lesions or destruction of the joint surfaces. Multiple joints may be painful and swollen because the synovium is infiltrated with noncaseating granulomata. Ankles, knees, elbows, wrists, and the small joints of the hand are most commonly affected. Flexion contractures of the fingers may develop, but these pose minimal discomfort to the patient. Tenosynovitis of the wrist may occur, and the fingers may become irregularly swollen and deformed, taking on a rheumatoid appearance. Usually, however, chronic sarcoid arthritis is nondestructive. Granulomata may infiltrate muscle, causing proximal muscle weakness and pain.

Abortive or acute sarcoidosis. Acute sarcoidosis most commonly manifests itself as the so-called Löfgren's syndrome, characterized by polyarthritis, erythema nodosum, and bilateral hilar adenopathy. The disease is abrupt in onset, strikes people generally under the age of 40, and is most prevalent in Sweden. It develops mostly in the spring and summer. Most patients seek medical attention because of articular manifestations, but constitutional symptoms of fatigue, malaise, weakness, anorexia, weight loss, minor chills, and low-grade fever may actually antedate arthritis by several weeks. Acute transient sarcoid arthritis does not cause symptoms secondary to sarcoid involvement of the joint. Rather, the synovitis is nonspecific.

Lymph node enlargement including bilateral hilar adenopathy, erythema nodosum, sarcoid skin lesions, uveitis, and even sialadenitis may be evident; however, bone cysts and chronic arthritis are not seen in this form of the disease.

Articular manifestations of acute sarcoidosis may be profound, characterized by stiffness and pain in several joints. Initially arthralgias are migratory, but then overt inflammation persists in one or more joints. The most dramatic articular finding is inflammation, predominantly in tissues around the ankle (periarthritis); the joint seems to move well with minimal pain on motion, but there is marked periarticular tenderness, redness, and swelling (Fig. 24-1). Periarthritis, commonly mistaken for gout, is a manifestation of erythema nodosum.

LABORATORY FINDINGS. Whether sarcoidosis is acute or chronic, the diagnosis can be established by histologic examination of affected tissue, notably the skin, lymph nodes, and liver. To be certain of the diagnosis, it is useful to demonstrate sarcoid lesions in at least two separate organs. Liver biopsy is helpful to detect sarcoidosis in the liver (about 70% positive). Sarcoidosis is the most common cause of hepatic granulomata. Bronchial or lung tissue obtained through a fiberoptic bronchoscope is positive for granulomata in 80% of the cases, particularly if hilar adenopathy is present. Gastrocnemius biopsy may show granulomata even in the absence of muscle symptoms. The Kveim-Siltzbach skin test is positive in 80% to 90% of patients with acute or chronic sarcoidosis. In abortive sarcoidosis, synovium, periarticular tissues of the ankle, and the lesions of erythema nodosum fail to show noncaseating granulomata.

In both forms of the disease, the erythrocyte sedimentation rate is elevated, and the latex fixation test for rheumatoid factor may be positive in low titer. Purified protein derivative (PPD) anergy is the rule.

The serum angiotensin-converting enzyme (ACE) is elevated in the majority of patients with active disease but is normal in burned-out sarcoidosis, lymphoma, leukemia,

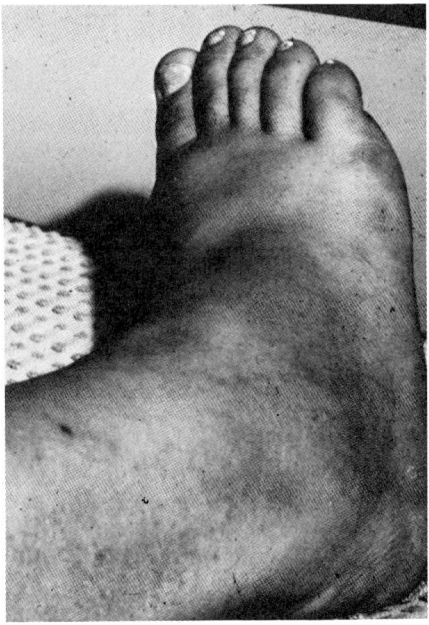

Fig. 24-1. Swelling of ankle in patient with acute sarcoidosis. Darkened skin areas are sites of erythema.

and other pulmonary conditions that mimic sarcoidosis, such as tuberculosis. Increased levels of urine hydroxyproline may be found in patients with acute sarcoidosis. On the other hand, hypercalcemia and increased alkaline phosphatase are peculiar to the chronic type, appearing in 15% of the patients.

Roentgenograms of the chest are valuable in the diagnosis of both forms. Almost all patients exhibit bilateral hilar adenopathy either before or after the onset of other manifestations of sarcoidosis. In the chronic form pulmonary infiltration predominates, and pleural effusions are rare. Roentgenograms of bones and joints in chronic sarcoidosis show mottled radiolucent areas and "punched-out" lesions, usually in the phalanges. No changes such as these are noted in the abortive form.

DIAGNOSIS. Polyarthritis, periarticular inflammation of the ankles, erythema nodosum, and bilateral hilar adenopathy (Löfgren's syndrome) comprise a symptom complex so distinctive that the diagnosis of acute (abortive) sarcoidosis should not be difficult. Indeed, any young person with polyarthritis and erythema nodosum should be suspected of having sarcoidosis, which can be confirmed by sequential chest roentgenograms. Elevations of serum ACE and hydroxyprolinuria provide additional ancillary evidence. There is usually concern that hilar adenopathy may represent lymphoma, but erythema nodosum coexisting with asymptomatic bilateral adenopathy is extremely strong evidence against a malignancy.

The chronic forms of sarcoidosis may present difficulties in diagnosis. The presence of pulmonary findings with multisystem disease, particularly if the eyes are involved, should raise suspicion. Sarcoidosis can be distinguished from other granulomatous diseases by the Kveim-Siltzbach skin test and by appropriate biopsies.

Articular manifestations of sarcoidosis may mimic rheumatoid arthritis, rheumatic fever, lymphoma, gout, psoriatic arthritis, infection, and a variety of other conditions.

MANAGEMENT AND PROGNOSIS. Mild sarcoidosis, particularly of the abortive type, may be managed by salicylates. Colchicine has been shown to be effective in some cases of acute sarcoid arthritis, and small doses of corticosteroids (such as prednisone, 5 mg daily) may be administered if fatigue is profound. Articular manifestations disappear within several weeks with or without treatment. Higher doses (such as prednisone, 40 to 60 mg daily) may be needed for chronic sarcoidosis, especially if there are uveitis, progression of pulmonary manifestations, marked hypercalciuria, extremely disfiguring skin lesions, progressive arthritis, and hypersplenism. If corticosteroids fail, azathioprine has been shown to be useful in certain cases.

Acute sarcoidosis usually resolves within several weeks except for adenopathy, which may last up to 1 year. In the chronic type lifelong disease, particularly pulmonary fibrosis, can be expected in many cases. Fortunately, the mortality rate is low; death usually results from respiratory failure, myocarditis, or renal failure caused by nephrocalcinosis.

BIBLIOGRAPHY

James, D.G., Neville, E., and Walker, A.N.: Immunology of sarcoidosis, Am. J. Med. **59**:388, 1975.
Lieberman, J.: Serum angiotensin-converting enzyme and sarcoidosis, Am. J. Med. **59**:365, 1975.
Siltzbach, L.E., editor: Seventh International Conference on Sarcoidosis and Other Granulomatous Disorders, Ann. N.Y. Acad. Sci. **278**:1, 1976.
Spilberg, I., Siltzbach, L.E., and McEwen, C.: The arthritis of sarcoidosis, Arthritis Rheum. **12**:126, 1969.
Winterbauer, R.H., Belic, N., and Moores, K.D.: A clinical interpretation of bilateral hilar adenopathy, Ann. Intern. Med. **78**:65, 1973.

25 • WEBER-CHRISTIAN DISEASE
Robert H. Gordon

Weber-Christian disease is characterized by an acute, febrile, recurrent, nodular inflammation of adipose tissue (panniculitis) involving the subcutaneous fat and, less often, adipose tissue elsewhere in the body (systemic Weber-Christian disease).

EPIDEMIOLOGY. The term "Weber-Christian disease" in the past encompassed a heterogeneous group of disorders. It is now applied only when panniculitis is the primary pathologic finding and after other underlying diseases have been ruled out. This disorder is uncommon and generally affects adults of either sex between the ages of 20 and 60, although cases in children as young as newborns have been reported. It does not appear to have any distinct familial, racial, or geographic associations.

PATHOGENESIS AND PATHOLOGY. The cause of Weber-Christian disease is unknown. Local pressure and trauma sometimes play a role. Hypersensitivity to drugs such as bromides, iodides, and some antibiotics or to bacterial and viral antigens following infection or immunization has been implicated. Cultures of the lesions are sterile. Other suggested causes have included disordered fat metabolism, alpha-1-antitrypsin deficiency, and autoimmunity. Immunoglobulins have not been identified in the lesions. One case report has described an infant who had a remission of his disease when T lymphocytes were depleted. This finding raised the possibility of altered cellular immunity. Pancreatic enzymes have been elevated in some patients.

The histopathologic picture is nonspecific; it can occur in any condition causing acute panniculitis. Three stages have been noted: (1) infiltration of fat lobules by polymorphonuclear cells, often accompanied by fat cell degeneration, (2) mononuclear and histiocytic infiltration of the panniculus with variable fat cell necrosis and phagocytosis of fatty debris with formation of lipophages, and (3) fibroblastic proliferation with subsequent fibrosis. The inflammatory process usually spares the epidermis and dermis. Blood vessels are affected by circumferential spread only.

CLINICAL MANIFESTATIONS. The characteristic finding of nodules in Weber-Christian disease is important in establishing the diagnosis. These can be few or many in number and located in one area or all over the body. The thighs, buttocks, and breasts may be particularly affected. The nodules range in size from 0.5 to 8 cm. They are tender and occasionally erythematous, and some may suppurate, draining an oily material. At first they are slightly mobile, but later they become adherent to the skin; this results in cutaneous dimpling or a central depression.

The systemic features depend on the sites of involvement. The lungs (parenchymal infiltrates, effusions), heart (pericarditis), liver (hepatomegaly), spleen (splenomegaly), kidneys, gastrointestinal tract (abdominal pain, perforation), retroperitoneum, mediastinum, and even the bone marrow can be involved. Musculoskeletal complaints include arthralgias, myalgias, and occasional joint effusions. Retroperitoneal and mediastinal fibrosis has been associated with Weber-Christian disease.

LABORATORY FINDINGS. No laboratory tests are diagnostic. The sedimentation rate may be elevated. Anemia, leukocytosis, and rarely eosinophilia have been reported. Serum, urine, or tissue levels of amylase and lipase are sometimes elevated without documentable pancreatic disease. Cryoglobulinemia and normal serum complement are also reported.

DIAGNOSIS. Weber-Christian disease should be considered in the evaluation of subcutaneous nodules that show evidence of recent or healed panniculitis on biopsy. Neither finding is pathognomonic for the disease. Therefore patients need a thorough evaluation to rule out other underlying conditions.

Erythema nodosum is one of the most common disorders giving rise to painful subcutaneous nodules on the legs and occasionally on the arms and face. The nodules are limited to subcutaneous tissue and are not found elsewhere. This syndrome is associated with many nonrelated diseases and is believed to be a hypersensitivity response. Polyarteritis, erythema induratum, lupus profundus, metastatic fat necrosis from pancreatitis or carcinoma of the pancreas, morphea, and a rare syndrome called subcutaneous fat necrosis of the newborn need also be considered. However, in an effort to diagnose exotic disease, common causes of painful panniculitis should not be overlooked. These include trauma, infection, bites, local fat atrophy from insulin injections, drug abuse, and self-inflicted wounds.

MANAGEMENT. Many treatments have been tried through the years, including potassium iodide, antibiotics, antituberculous drugs, antihistamines, antimalarials, hormones, vitamins, sulphones, heavy metals, antirheumatics, blood transfusions, and even radiation therapy. None of these has proved successful. Corticosteroids offer the best symptomatic relief, but the basic pathologic process may continue.

COURSE AND PROGNOSIS. The course is variable. Although each nodule may last between 2 and 6 weeks, the disease itself may persist for 8 months to several years. Morbidity and mortality are related to visceral complications.

BIBLIOGRAPHY

Forstrom, L., and Winkleman, R.K.: Acute panniculitis: a clinical and histopathologic study of 34 cases, Arch. Dermatol. **113**:909, 1977.

Milner, R.D.G., and Mitchinson, M.J.: Systemic Weber-Christian disease, J. Clin. Pathol. **18**:150, 1965.

26 • INFECTIOUS ARTHRITIS
Bruce I. Hoffman

Infectious arthritis occurs when microbial agents (bacteria, mycobacteria, fungi, or viruses) are introduced into the synovium, overwhelm the normal clearance mechanisms, and multiply. In most instances organisms are introduced hematogenously from an extra-articular focus. However, infection may be caused by direct introduction from trauma, intra-articular injection, surgery, or a para-articular focus. Infectious arthritis may be classified as (1) pyogenic arthritis (gonococcal and nongonococcal septic arthritis), (2) tuberculous and fungal arthritis, and (3) arthritis caused by viruses. The presentation, course, and therapy are sufficiently different that each syndrome will be discussed separately.

PYOGENIC ARTHRITIS

Pyogenic infections are those caused by gonococcal or nongonococcal bacteria. The bacteria that cause septic arthritis tend to differ with the age and condition of the patient. Gram-positive organisms, particularly *Staphylococcus aureus*, are most important in the causation of septic arthritis in all ages except adolescence and young adulthood. Of particular importance is the vast predominance of *Neisseria gonorrhoeae* in adolescents and young adults. In infants *Haemophilus infuenzae* causes a significant number of infections of the joints as it does at other sites. A minority of cases are produced by gram-negative bacilli; however, this number has increased, particularly in older, debilitated adults. In general, septic arthritis produces joints more painful than in any other entity except gout.

Gonococcal arthritis

See discussion of "Gonococcal infections" in Chapter 46.

Nongonococcal septic arthritis

Septic arthritis caused by pyogenic bacteria other than *N. gonorrhoeae* is uncommon, but its potential for rapid joint destruction and mortality gives it an important position in the differential diagnosis of acute monarticular and pauciarticular arthritis.

PATHOGENESIS. Gram-positive organisms, particularly *S. aureus, Streptococcus pyogenes,* and *S. pneumoniae,* predominate as causes of nongonococcal septic arthritis. In adults gram-negative enteric bacillary infections have become more prevalent, especially after urinary tract operative procedures. A wide variety of other bacteria have caused septic arthritis less frequently.

PATHOLOGY. After organisms become established and multiply, an intense inflammatory response is provoked. Enzymes that cause the degradation of articular cartilage are released. It appears that the bacteria can cause an immunogenic arthritis that can continue after the organisms have been eradicated. As infection progresses, bone is invaded and osteomyelitis ensues. Why joints are damaged so rapidly in comparison to noninfectious diseases such as gout in which an equally intense response occurs is unknown.

CLINICAL MANIFESTATIONS. Nongonococcal septic arthritis (NGSA) rapidly progresses to severe pain, swelling, warmth, and erythema over 24 to 72 hours. It is generally a monarticular disease, but patients may have two to five joints simultaneously involved. Fever, tachypnea, and rigors may be intense. Infection is most common in large joints, including in order of frequency the knees, hips, shoulders, elbows, wrists, and ankles. Small joints such as the sternoclavicular or sacroiliac joints may be affected.

Factors that predispose individuals to the development of septic arthritis include (1) an extra-articular focus, (2) debilitating illness, (3) immunosuppressive therapy, (4) previous joint damage, and (5) intravenous drug abuse. Not surprisingly, in many patients an extra-articular focus in the skin, lungs, genitourinary system, or gastrointestinal tract can be identified. Unlike gonococcal arthritis, in which the hosts are otherwise healthy, NGSA tends to strike debilitated individuals. Patients often have diabetes mellitus, malignancies, or cirrhosis. They may be receiving immunosuppressive drugs or corticosteroids. Perhaps most importantly, NGSA affects previously damaged joints. Patients with rheumatoid arthritis comprise as much as 30% of those with NGSA. The propensity to joint infections is related to impaired local defenses against infection and intra-articular injection of corticosteroids. In intravenous drug abusers septic arthritis develops in unusual locations such as sternoclavicular and sacroiliac joints and with unusual organisms such as *Pseudomonas aeruginosa* and *Serratia marcescens.*

LABORATORY FINDINGS. Patients with NGSA generally have peripheral leukocytosis. Synovial fluid examination usually shows 80,000 to 100,000 white blood cells/mm^3, of which greater than 90% are polymorphonuclear leukocytes. The synovial fluid glucose level is less than 40 mg/dl. Gram stain of the synovial fluid is positive in 50% to 80%, whereas a culture is nearly always positive unless antibiotics have been administered previously. Organisms grow in blood cultures in approximately 50% of the patients.

Early in the course the joint appears normal on roentgenographic examination. Osteoporosis subsequently develops. The joint space narrows as cartilage is eroded. Ultimately, total joint destruction, fusion, and osteomyelitis may be seen.

DIAGNOSIS. NGSA is rare in young or middle-aged healthy adults. In the usual older age range of NGSA, gout and pseudogout are the most common entities associated with acute inflammatory monarticular arthritis. Monarticular inflammation in a patient with preexisting rheumatoid arthritis often signals a flare of the disease but may also indicate pyogenic arthritis. In patients with rheumatoid arthritis any joint involved out of proportion to the others should be aspirated and cultured.

MANAGEMENT. The principles of treatment are the same as those in any closed-space infection. They include adequate antibiotics, drainage, and physical measures to protect the joint and preserve function.

When the identity and sensitivity of the infecting organism are known, parenteral administration of high doses of minimally toxic bactericidal agents is indicated. Treatment should not be delayed while awaiting cultures and should be based on Gram stain (Table 26-1). Therapy is continued for 2 to 4 weeks.

Table 26-1. Treatment of pyogenic arthritis based on Gram stain

Gram stain finding	Therapy First choice	Alternative
Gram-positive cocci		
Clusters, single cocci, or diplococci	Penicillinase-resistant penicillin or cephalosporin for *S. aureus*	Vancomycin
Chains	Penicillin G for streptococci	Erythromycin
Gram-negative cocci	See Chapter 46 for *N. gonorrhoeae*	
Gram-negative bacilli	Carbenicillin or ticarcillin plus gentamicin or tobramycin	
Gram-negative coccobacilli	Ampicillin for *H. influenzae*	Chloramphenicol
Gram stain negative		
In young patients	Treatment for gonococcal infection	
In older or debilitated patients	Penicillinase-resistant penicillin and aminoglycoside	

Involved joints should be drained by arthrocentesis at least daily. If there is no response in 5 to 7 days (that is, there is continued fever, failure to sterilize the joint, purulent exudate, or development of joint destruction), surgical drainage procedures are advised. Surgery is also indicated in all septic hips and when adequate drainage cannot be accomplished with a needle.

Joints should be splinted until inflammation subsides. They should be put through a passive range of motion several times a day as soon as pain permits.

PROGNOSIS. Even with appropriate therapy, the outcome of NGSA is unsatisfactory. The most important factor is early diagnosis, because patients treated less than 7 days from the beginning of symptoms fare better. The outcome is poor, as shown by ankylosis, recurrence, osteomyelitis, or death in 50% of *S. aureus* infections, 20% of streptococcal infections, 5% of pneumococcal infections, and 75% of gram-negative bacillary infections. Younger, healthier patients have a better prognosis.

TUBERCULOUS AND FUNGAL ARTHRITIS
Arthritis caused by *Mycobacterium tuberculosis*

The incidence of tuberculosis in the United States has dramatically declined over the past 40 years. Arthritis caused by *M. tuberculosis*, never common, is now rare. The diagnosis of bone and joint infection is often delayed. During primary dissemination foci of infection develop by direct extension or secondary hematogenous spread, and they later reactivate. At the time of presentation 10% to 50% of the patients have active pulmonary disease. Commonly there is no evidence of previous tuberculosis.

CLINICAL MANIFESTATIONS. Bone and joint tuberculosis takes two general forms: osteomyelitis and synovitis. Tuberculous osteomyelitis classically affects the thoracic spine (Pott's disease). The infection destroys the disc space and occasionally the vertebral bodies. The patients have back pain, spasm, and root pain. Complications include kyphosis from collapse of the disc space or vertebral body, cold (tuberculous) abscesses, and neurologic sequelae from cord compression. Other sites of involvement are the ribs and sacroiliac joints.

Tuberculosis of the joints generally occurs as a monarticular arthritis. The hip and knee are involved most frequently, but other joints and tendon sheaths are also affected. The patients have slowly progressive pain, stiffness, and swelling.

LABORATORY FINDINGS. The synovial fluid white cell count has a wide range, generally 10,000 to 20,000/mm^3, of which most are polymorphonuclear leukocytes. The glucose level is often reduced. Roentgenograms may be normal initially, but later there are osteoporosis, marginal erosions, and finally joint destruction with little reactive bone. When there is concurrent osteomyelitis, oval lucencies are seen beneath the articular cartilage.

DIAGNOSIS. An intermediate-strength purified protein derivative (PPD) skin test should be performed. The results are positive except with advanced disease and in debilitated or immunosuppressed hosts. Synovial fluid cultures are positive in 80% of the cases. Biopsy of the synovium should be done in every suspected case. The histologic finding is granulomatous synovitis. The combination of histology and culture permits a precise diagnosis in greater than 90% of the patients.

MANAGEMENT. Effective therapy requires adequate chemotherapy and occasionally surgery (see Chapter 50). Surgery is performed for debridement of osteomyelitis, synovectomy, or joint fusion. Successful total hip replacement is done routinely in previously affected hips once the infection is controlled. Fusion of spinal lesions is occasionally performed.

Arthritis caused by other mycobacteria

Mycobacteria other than *M. tuberculosis* can cause bone and joint infection, sometimes involving multiple joints. Infections caused by *M. kansasii*, *M. marinum*, *M. intracellularis*, and *M. scrofulaceum* have been reported. These infections are often more difficult to treat (see "Nontuberculous mycobacterial infections" in Chapter 50).

Arthritis caused by fungi

Arthritis caused by mycotic infection is rare. Coccidioidomycosis is most prevalent in the southwestern United States. The primary infection is usually a self-limited pulmonary disease. During this phase arthritis is accompanied by erythema nodosum. With disseminated disease, monarthritis of the knee, ankle, or other joints and tenosynovitis may occur. There may be eventual joint destruction. Osteomyelitis with multiple lytic lesions is a complication. The diagnosis is by culture; synovial biopsy shows granulomata. The therapy is with amphotericin B.

Sporotrichosis occurs after skin inoculation and is usually limited. When it is disseminated, a monarticular or pauciarticular arthritis may occur. The diagnosis is by culture, and the treatment is with amphotericin B.

Arthritis is rarely seen with blastomycosis, histoplasmosis, cryptococcosis, or disseminated *Candida* infection.

ARTHRITIS CAUSED BY VIRUSES

Viruses frequently cause self-limited arthritis and are perhaps involved in the pathogenesis of rheumatoid arthritis and systemic lupus erythematosus.

Hepatitis B is associated with arthralgia and arthritis during the incubation period in approximately 50% of the cases. Patients have a variety of skin lesions, usually urticarial. The arthritis is polyarticular and symmetric. It generally subsides with the onset of jaundice. These manifestations are probably caused by circulating immune complexes. The diagnosis is made by demonstration of hepatitis B surface antigen in the blood. The treatment is symptomatic with salicylates.

Rubella (German measles) is associated with symmetric polyarthritis lasting 1 to 7 days and usually associated with the rash. It is much more common in adults than in children. Rubella vaccination has also been associated with arthritis, again much more frequently in adults.

Lyme disease, probably caused by an arthopod-borne virus, can lead to arthritis in association with the rash of erythema chronicum migrans (see discussion of "Lyme disease" in Chapter 58).

Clinicians often witness transient monarthritis or polyarthritis as part of an obvious viral clinical picture, but specific diagnoses are rarely made. Treatment of the various viral arthritides is supportive only.

BIBLIOGRAPHY

Berney, S., Goldstein, M., and Bisko, F.: Clinical and diagnostic features of tuberculous arthritis, Am. J. Med. **53**:36, 1972.
Brandt, R.D., Cathcart, E.S., and Cohen, A.S.: Gonococcal arthritis: clinical features correlated with blood, synovial fluid and genitourinary cultures, Arthritis Rheum. **17**:503, 1974.
Goldberg, D.L., and Cohen, A.S.: Acute infectious arthritis: a review of patients with non-gonococcal joint infections (with emphasis on therapy and prognosis), Am. J. Med. **60**:369, 1976.
Handsfield, H.H., Wiesner, P.J., and Holmes, K.K.: Treatment of the gonococcal arthritis-dermatitis syndrome, Ann. Intern. Med. **84**:661, 1976.
Rosenthal, J., Bole, G.G., and Robinson, W.D.: Acute nongonococcal infectious arthritis: evaluation of risk factors, therapy and outcome, Arthritis Rheum. **23**:889, 1980.
Schmid, F.R.: Infectious arthritis. In Katz, W.A., editor: Rheumatic diseases: diagnosis and management, Philadelphia, 1977, J.B. Lippincott Co.

27 • OSTEOMYELITIS

Bruce I. Hoffman

Osteomyelitis is infection of bone by microorganisms. Usually these are bacterial infections; however, mycobacteria and fungi also cause osteomyelitis when they invade the skeleton.

EPIDEMIOLOGY. Osteomyelitis is more common in men than in women and is usually confined to bones of the lower extremities. Several factors predispose an individual to the development of osteomyelitis: diabetes with vascular insufficiency of the lower extremities, genitourinary infection, neoplasms, intravenous drug abuse, and sickle cell anemia.

PATHOLOGY. There are three routes by which bone becomes infected: hematogenously, by contiguous infection, or directly as during surgery. These types of infection often are caused by different bacteria and have a different clinical spectrum.

Before puberty infection occurs at the metaphysis of long bones because of slow blood flow in this area and the absence of phagocytic cells. When infection is established in children or adults, regardless of route, pus spreads along haversian and Volkmann's canals until it reaches the periosteum. As pressure increases, ischemic necrosis of bone forms a sequestrum of necrotic bone. At this point the infection is considered chronic.

CLINICAL MANIFESTATIONS. The clinical picture and causative-bacteria vary according to the route and site of infection and the age of the patient. Acute hematogenous osteomyelitis usually seeds the long bones of children or vertebral discs of adults. Most cases are caused by *Staphylococcus aureus* in both children and adults, but the incidence of gram-negative bacillary infection increases in adults. In drug abusers *Pseudomonas aeruginosa* is particularly important. In patients with sickle cell hemoglobinopathy there is a propensity toward *Salmonella* osteomyelitis.

Children generally have high fever and local symptoms at the site of infection. In adults symptoms are usually insidious in onset with low-grade fever, and the diagnosis is often delayed.

Infection from a contiguous focus is a sequela of surgery, soft tissue infections, or oral infections. The infections are often polybacterial, although *S. aureus* still predominates. Fever with local pain, erythema, and swelling is the characteristic finding in osteomyelitis.

Vascular insufficiency, especially caused by diabetes mellitus, is particularly important in the development of osteomyelitis in the older age group. Most commonly, osteomyelitis occurs in the feet at the site of a diabetic ulcer and is polybacterial. There is often a neuropathy with the plantar ulceration but few systemic symptoms.

Once osteomyelitis is established and there is bone necrosis, the disease becomes chronic and difficult to treat and tends to recur.

LABORATORY FINDINGS AND DIAGNOSIS. Early in the course, osteomyelitis may be difficult to diagnose. The only useful laboratory study is the erythrocyte sedimentation rate, which is almost always elevated. An important exception is sickle cell anemia, in which the sedimentation rate may be normal.

Roentgenographic findings are most specific. First there is elevation of the periosteum followed by the development of a lucent area in the underlying bone and finally the formation of a sequestrum. These findings are often delayed. Bone scanning offers an opportunity to make an early diagnosis. Technetium or gallium scanning is usually positive within the first few days. The definitive diagnosis is by bone biopsy, which allows the infecting organism to be clearly identified. Cultures of sinus drainage are less exact because the sinus tract may contain organisms not found in the bone. Blood cultures are positive in 50% of those with hematogenously spread disease.

MANAGEMENT. Osteomyelitis is treated with antibiotics appropriate to the infecting organism. This should be prolonged, often for months. Therapy is given by the parenteral route usually for 4 to 6 weeks and then continued with orally administered agents. When chronic osteomyelitis ensues, surgical debridement is often essential.

PROGNOSIS. The prognosis of acute osteomyelitis is excellent when treatment starts within the first few days. When osteomyelitis becomes chronic, the prognosis is much worse; patients are often left with recurring draining sinuses. In some patients generalized amyloidosis develops in response to chronic osteomyelitis.

BIBLIOGRAPHY

Norden, C.W.: Osteomyelitis. In Mandell, G.L., Douglas, R.G., Jr., and Bennett, J.E., editors: Principles and practice of infectious diseases, New York, 1979, John Wiley & Sons, Inc.

Waldvogel, F.A., Modoff, G., and Swartz, M.N.: Osteomyelitis: a review of clinical features, therapeutic considerations and unusual aspects, I., N. Engl. J. Med. **282:**198, 1970.

Waldvogel, F.A., Modoff, G., and Swartz, M.N.: Osteomyelitis: a review of clinical features, therapeutic considerations and unusual aspects, II., N. Engl. J. Med. **282:**260, 1970.

Waldvogel, F.A., Modoff, G., and Swartz, M.N.: Osteomyelitis: a review of clinical features, therapeutic considerations and unusual aspects, III., Osteomyelitis associated with vascular insufficiency, N. Engl. J. Med. **282:**316, 1970.

28 • OSTEOARTHRITIS

Donald H. Lieberman

With age, certain degenerative changes affect the joints. Whether these changes should "physiologically" accompany the passage of years or should be construed as pathologic is debatable. The result is pain, stiffness, and eventual loss of motion. Degenerative joint disease and osteoarthrosis have been used as alternative terms for osteoarthritis and have been considered by some to be preferable, since osteoarthritis seems to imply an inflammatory disorder. Although mild to moderate synovitis may accompany the disease, it may progress without inflammation.

Osteoarthritis is the most common form of arthritis. Although the earliest changes begin in the third decade of life, clinical effects are not usually apparent until many years later. In most cases the disease is mild, causing little or no disability. Because osteoarthritis is so widespread, however, the number of people with severe disability is significant.

Osteoarthritis is usually classified into primary (idiopathic) and secondary forms. This artificial classification underscores the lack of knowledge concerning the basic pathologic mechanisms.

PRIMARY OSTEOARTHRITIS

Although a number of hypotheses have been suggested, no definitive cause has been proved in primary osteoarthritis. There seems to be a genetic predisposition. The disease is more prevalent in younger men and older women, with more generalized and severe disease in women. The joints most frequently involved are the distal interphalangeal (DIP) joints of the fingers, proximal interphalangeal (PIP) joints, first carpometacarpal joint, hips, knees, first metatarsophalangeal joint, and cervical and lower lumbar vertebrae. It is common to see patients with enlargement of the DIP joints resulting from bony proliferation leading to spur formation. These changes are termed Heberden's nodes (Fig. 28-1). Generalized primary osteoarthritis accompanied by Heberden's nodes is determined by a single autosomal gene, dominant in females and recessive in males. Generalized osteoarthritis unaccompanied by Heberden's nodes appears to have a polygenic mode of inheritance.

Certain joints seem to be spared in osteoarthritis. It is uncommon for advanced involvement of the metacarpophalangeal joints, wrists, elbows, shoulders, or ankles to

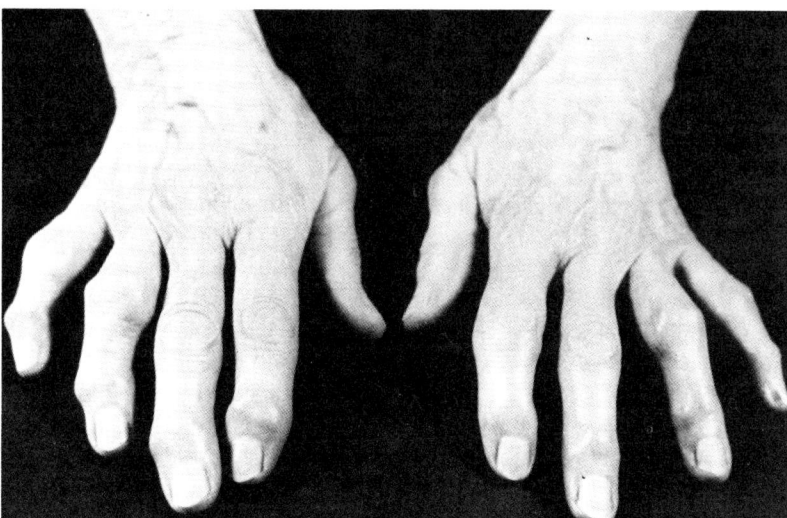

Fig. 28-1. Bony enlargement of distal interphalangeal (Heberden's nodes) and proximal interphalangeal (Bouchard's nodes) joints in osteoarthritis. Note lateral deviation of these joints.

occur. Trauma to the joint, as might occur in the knee of a football player or the elbow of a baseball pitcher, causes an earlier onset of osteoarthritis. Either a single major insult or repeated minor injuries may have this effect. Obesity also predisposes an individual to an earlier onset in weight-bearing joints.

CLINICAL MANIFESTATIONS. In most cases osteoarthritis involves only one or a limited number of joints. The patient is commonly over 50 years of age. The presenting symptom is usually pain described as an annoying or a dull ache, which increases with activity and is relieved by rest. There is generally a feeling of stiffness after rest and difficulty in "getting started." This is usually short lived in contrast to the prolonged stiffness, especially in the morning, associated with rheumatoid arthritis. As the process progresses, the pain becomes more constant; eventually there is loss of movement.

Hands. Heberden's nodes are 10 times more frequent in women than in men. In some patients they go unnoticed and cause little concern. Other patients have great anxiety over the nodes' appearance and are concerned that they are only the beginning of a "crippling disease." Similar swellings may be seen in the PIP joints where they are called Bouchard's nodes. Both Heberden's and Bouchard's nodes may be single at the onset, but eventually they involve multiple fingers. The fingers often become deviated in either the ulnar or the radial direction. Diagnostic difficulty occasionally arises when synovitis accompanies the degenerative process and neither Heberden's nor Bouchard's nodes form. In this situation the patient's clinical appearance may mimic mild or early rheumatoid arthritis. Conversely, the diagnosis of rheumatoid arthritis may be obscured in a patient with marked "nodal" disease.

First carpometacarpal joint. Involvement of the first carpometacarpal joint results in pain and tenderness over the joint between the trapezium, and the first metacarpal. The thumb may become adducted, and together with subluxation of the base of the metacarpal this produces squaring of the base of the thumb.

Shoulders, elbows, and wrists. The shoulders (except in the elderly), elbows, and wrists are rarely involved.

Feet. The first metatarsophalangeal joint is a common site of osteoarthritis. An explanation for this might be that no joint in the body carries more weight.

Knees. Osteoarthritis of the knees is an important cause of disability. Tenderness, effusion, osteophytes, and mild inflammation may be found. When effusions are large, they may cause a swelling in the posterior aspect of the knee known as a Baker's or popliteal cyst. Occasionally there is extensive degeneration of either the medial or the lateral compartment of the knee, leading to genu varum or genu valgum.

Hips. Osteoarthritis of the hip is usually seen in older patients unless there has been a predisposing cause such as congenital dislocation or trauma. It occurs more frequently in males. Pain may cause limping and an awkward gait. The pain may be referred to the buttocks, groin, sciatic region, or knee. Muscle wasting is common as the disease progresses.

Spine. Involvement of the spine is common in osteoarthritis. Once again a problem in semantics arises. The term "spondylosis" has been used in reference to changes that involve the intervertebral discs and vertebral bodies. The intervertebral disc articulations are nonsynovial. However, the posterior intervertebral articulations are synovial (apophyseal joints), and degenerative changes here are similar to changes in the other "true joints." Since changes in these structures are usually seen together, the terms "spondylosis" and "spinal osteoarthritis" are used synonymously. Pain syndromes arising from changes in the cervical and lumbar spine are common. Changes in the cervical spine can produce localized pain and may cause radicular pain down the arm as a result of nerve root impingement. Lumbar involvement can cause backache and radicular pain down the leg, commonly called sciatica.

The spinal cord can become involved through compression. An important example of this in the cervical spine is vertebrobasilar insufficiency caused by compression of the vertebral artery, which can result in episodic dizziness, headaches, ataxia, and visual problems.

LABORATORY FINDINGS. Characteristically, all laboratory tests are normal in osteoarthritis. The disease, unlike rheumatoid arthritis, is limited to the joints. When effusions are present, examination of the synovial fluid reveals it to be clear, viscous, and almost acellular.

The most useful diagnostic procedure is roentgenographic evaluation of the involved areas. It must be kept in mind that (1) pain may be present before roentgenographic changes and (2) roentgenographic changes may be present but not responsible for pain or disability. Typical roentgenographic features include bony sclerosis, hypertrophic spur formation, and joint space narrowing. Weight-bearing roentgenograms are helpful in emphasizing these changes in the knees.

MANAGEMENT. Treatment of osteoarthritis depends on the severity of the condition. Patients should be told what to expect. When a patient sees deformity of the hands, it may produce anxiety even if the changes are not accompanied by symptoms. This type of patient and similar patients with minimal disease usually need nothing more than reassurance that they do not have a progressive crippling disorder. When weight-bearing joints are involved, patients should be encouraged to lose weight. Periods of rest should be recommended, and walking aids such as a cane or walker may be beneficial if the patient's pride can accept them. Exercises aimed at preserving motion and strengthening muscles are helpful. The use of heat is beneficial for some people, but in others it seems to aggravate the situation. When heat fails, some physicians advise a short trial of cold.

Analgesic and anti-inflammatory drugs are useful in the treatment of osteoarthritis, but they rarely bring about the dramatic relief often seen in rheumatoid arthritis. Aspirin has been the traditional first drug of choice. With the development of the new nonsteroidal anti-inflammatory drugs (NSAIDs), physicians have a choice of agents depending on the patient's drug compliance, sensitivity to aspirin, and concurrent drug therapy. When aspirin is used, the starting dosage is two aspirin tablets (650 mg) four times a day. This dosage can be increased if relief is not obtained. Acetaminophen in the same dosage may suffice for some patients. Indomethacin has been available for many years and remains useful. Starting dosage is 25 mg three times a day; this may be increased to 200 mg daily.

The rationale behind the use of the newer anti-inflammatory drugs is twofold. First, although osteoarthritis is primarily a degenerative disease, synovitis is frequently found. Second, some of the drugs have analgesic properties in addition to the anti-inflammatory effect. The newer drugs and their dosages are listed in Table 10-2.

The oral administration of steroids is contraindicated in the treatment of osteoarthritis. There is controversy concerning the intra-articular use of steroids in osteoarthritis. Some clinicians believe that they have no role, whereas others try them in a "refractory" joint. Some patients claim weeks or even months of relief after an injection into a joint that was "flaring." In no instance should repeated injections be given at frequent intervals, since damage may result from the effects of corticosteroids on cartilage and from repeated trauma associated with the procedure.

Surgery is reserved for patients in whom destruction has taken place and restoration will create greater mobility. Occasionally procedures are done to relieve pain even with less severe roentgenographic changes. The development and use of prostheses that have a long life and restore function to severely damaged joints have radically changed the lives of many patients who would otherwise have permanent disability.

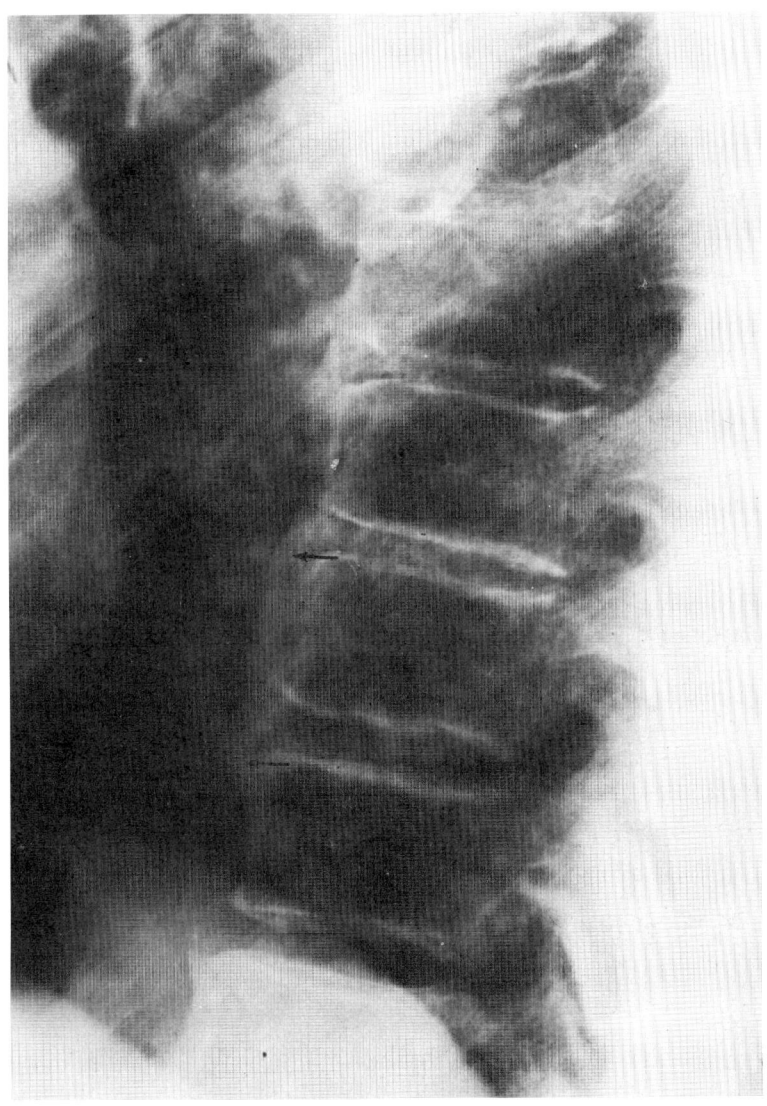

Fig. 28-2. Ligamentous calcification flowing along anterolateral border of lumbar spine in patient with DISH.

VARIANTS OF OSTEOARTHRITIS
Erosive osteoarthritis

Erosive osteoarthritis is a variant of primary osteoarthritis in which juxta-articular erosions are prominent. This form involves the DIP and PIP joints of the hands and occasionally the hip joints. Middle-aged and postmenopausal women are typically affected. The disease is characterized by flares of activity lasting from months to years with eventual quiescence. Erosive osteoarthritis may be only a phase of more severe osteoarthritis to follow.

Neuropathic arthropathy

Markedly advanced osteoarthropathy with dramatic distortion of articular architecture may develop slowly in patients who have loss of proprioception or pain sensation. This has been referred to as Charcot's joint disease. It may be seen in syphilis, diabetes mellitus, syringomyelia, congenital insensitivity to pain, and other chronic neurologic diseases. Physical examination shows a large, distorted joint. Other than bracing, there is no successful treatment.

Diffuse idiopathic skeletal hyperostosis

Diffuse idiopathic skeletal hyperostosis (DISH) is a recently proposed name for a disorder that has been recognized for several decades as Forestier's disease. It closely resembles degenerative joint disease because hypertrophic new bone is layered onto the vertebral bodies and at ligamentous attachments to bone. The origin of DISH is not known other than it appears to be an ossifying diathesis. DISH tends to develop in response to surgery, in diabetes mellitus, and in rheumatoid arthritis. Most patients are over 55 years of age.

Patients complain of profound musculoskeletal stiffness and moderate pain in the axial and, less often, extraaxial skeleton. Dysphagia has been noted when hypertrophic cervical spurs compress the esophagus.

Diagnosis is dependent on the detection of characteristic roentgenographic signs. These include linear calcification flowing along the anterolateral aspect of the spine (Fig. 28-2), bumpy spinal contour, a radiolucent zone between the bony deposition and subjacent vertebrae, and anterior bony bridging between vertebrae particularly in the cervical spine. The intervertebral disc spaces are usually intact. Neither the sacroiliac nor apophyseal joints are involved. Extraspinal characteristics are bony excrescences at tendon and ligament attachments to bone (for example, elbow, ischial tuberosity, iliac crest, and patella). Furthermore, hypertrophic spurs at the articular margins are prominent and the iliolumbar and sacrotuberous ligaments may ossify. There are no appreciable laboratory abnormalities.

Management consists of nonsteroidal anti-inflammatory drugs and physical therapy.

BIBLIOGRAPHY

Howell, D.S., and others: The pathogenesis of osteoarthritis, Semin. Arthritis Rheum. **5**:384, 1976.

Moskowitz, R.W.: Osteoarthritis and traumatic conditions. In Katz, W.A., editor: Rheumatic diseases: diagnosis and management, Philadelphia, 1977, J.B. Lippincott Co.

Peter, J.B., Pearson, C.M., and Marmor, L.: Erosive osteoarthritis of the hands, Arthritis Rheum. **9**:365, 1966.

Resnick, D., and others: Diffuse idiopathic skeletal hyperostosis (DISH) (ankylosing hyperostosis of Forestier and Rates-Querol), Semin. Arthritis Rheum. **7**:153, 1978.

29 • PAGET'S DISEASE (OSTEITIS DEFORMANS)
Donald H. Lieberman

Paget's disease of bone is a common chronic disease characterized by excessive osteoblastic and osteoclastic activity that results in poorly mineralized, distorted bones. Most cases are clinically inapparent. Pagetic bones usually produce typical roentgenographic changes, and the diagnosis is often made when roentgenograms are taken during the workup of another problem. The incidence of disease rises with age, and men have a slight predominance. There are some reports of familial clustering.

ETIOLOGY. The cause of Paget's disease is unknown. Recently a "slow viral" origin has been proposed. The intranuclear inclusions seen in slow viral disease such as subacute sclerosing panencephalitis (SSPE) resemble intranuclear inclusions described in the osteoclasts in Paget's disease. No virus has been isolated to date; even if isolation is achieved, it will have to be established whether the virus is responsible for the pathologic changes or is merely an innocent bystander. Other possible causes of Paget's disease are hormonal deficiency or excess, neoplasm, autoimmune disease, inherited abnormality of connective tissue, and vascular disturbance.

CLINICAL MANIFESTATIONS. Pain is the most common complaint in symptomatic Paget's disease. It may be present before roentgenographic changes, and the diagnosis at that time is often missed. The pain is aggravated by weight bearing if the lower extremity or spine is involved.

Headaches, dizziness, and reduced hearing may result from disease in the skull. Cranial enlargement may develop over many years. With marked involvement of the skull, patients may have cranial nerve compression. Other skeletal deformities can include distortion of the clavicles, multiple compression fractures of pagetic vertebrae resulting in severe kyphosis, bowing and elongation of the tibia and fibula, and unsuspected pathologic fractures.

Radionuclide bone scanning has added much to the delineation of the disease, and the following anatomic distribution has been reported: pelvis, 78%; spine, 63%; skull,

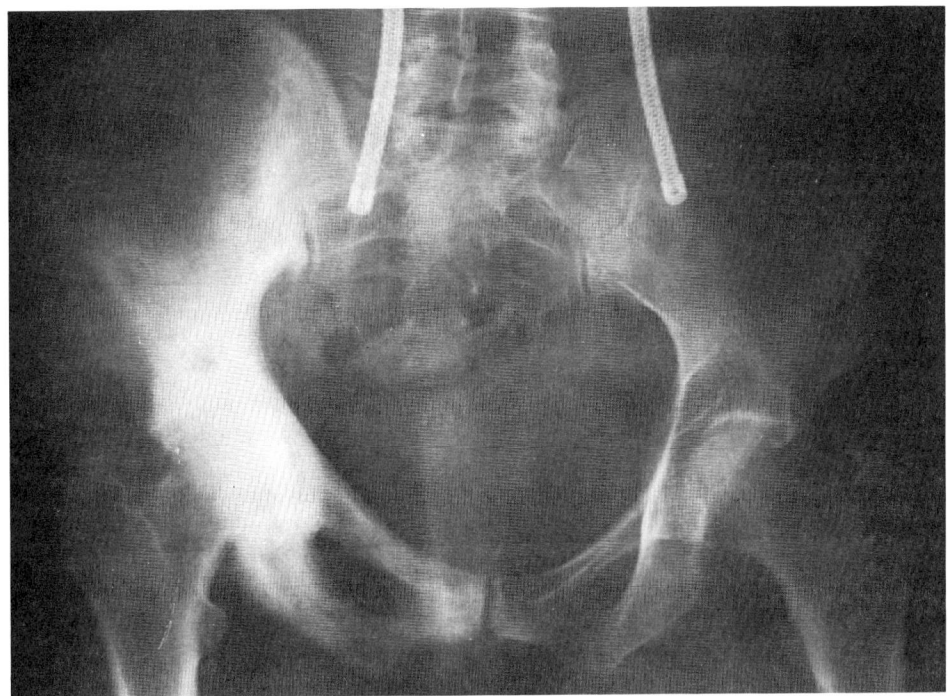

Fig. 29-1. Paget's disease of right pelvis and femur. Note thickening of bone and coarse trabecular pattern.

48%; femur, 48%; scapula, 37%; tibia, 22%; humerus, 17%; and lesser amounts in other bones. Patients who have one third or more of the skeleton involved can have increased cardiac output owing to increased vascularity of the bone lesions. This can lead to congestive heart failure.

On physical examination, bowing of one or both lower extremities may be observed. The tibia is generally more involved than the femur. Shortening of the involved leg occurs, and painful osteoarthritis may develop in the opposite limb as it bears more stress. Juxtalesional joints, especially the hip and knee, may show marked degenerative arthritis with loss of range of motion. Because of the increased vascularity of bone often found, the skin over the involved area may be much warmer than the contralateral side.

Angioid streaks may be seen around the optic discs; these appear as gray "cracks" in the retina. Angioid streaks are not pathognomonic signs of Paget's disease.

DIAGNOSIS. Roentgenographic evaluation of the skull and long bones remains the primary means of diagnosing Paget's disease (Fig. 29-1). The roentgenographic appearance includes a mottled increase in bone density, incomplete fractures or pseudofractures, localized areas of demineralization of the skull (osteoporosis circumscripta), thickening of the cortex, and coarse trabeculae. In some instances it is difficult to distinguish advanced Paget's disease from metastatic disease. The use of bone scanning has increased the ability to make an earlier diagnosis. It is employed when pain is present without roentgenographic change and is also helpful in determining if particular lesions are active.

LABORATORY FINDINGS. Both serum alkaline phosphatase and urinary hydroxyproline excretion are elevated. The latter is most helpful diagnostically when other concomitant disease may elevate the alkaline phosphatase. Serum calcium and phosphorus are usually normal. Occasional patients who are immobilized may have elevated calcium levels. If patients have an unusual presenting location and the diagnosis is in question, a bone biopsy is useful. Findings on the specimen depend on the stage of disease present and require an experienced pathologist. Biopsy is also used to diagnose the rare complication of osteogenic sarcoma.

The typical roentgenographic findings and an elevated serum alkaline phosphatase are usually sufficient for diagnosis. Major concerns in differential diagnosis are the presence of osteosarcoma or carcinoma that has metastasized to bone, especially from the prostate. Bone biopsy may be needed for confirmation, particularly if pain has been a salient feature. The acid phosphatase is usually elevated in prostatic carcinoma.

MANAGEMENT. Only patients with symptomatic disease require treatment. Mildly symptomatic disease can be treated with analgesics or anti-inflammatory drugs. With more severe disease, therapeutic decisions become more

difficult. The following criteria for the more vigorous treatment of Paget's disease have been proposed:
1. Disabling pain unrelieved by analgesics and anti-inflammatory agents
2. Progression of the skeletal aspects of the disease as indicated by increasing deformity, increased head or appendicular bone enlargement, frequent fractures, vertebral compression, or acetabular protrusion
3. Neurologic complications
4. Rapidly increasing deafness
5. High-output congestive heart failure
6. A greatly increased serum alkaline phosphatase and/or urinary hydroxyproline excretion (four or more times the normal in symptomatic patients)

The most promising drugs now employed in the treatment of Paget's disease are the calcitonins and diphosphonates. Calcitonin inhibits bone resorption. The patient response is extremely variable. The recommended dosage is 50 to 100 MRC units per day or every other day either subcutaneously or intramuscularly. If no improvement is noted after 3 months, the drug is usually stopped. The side effects include nausea, malaise, and flushing. The treatment need not be discontinued because of the side effects, which usually decrease with continued therapy.

Diphosphonates are the newest class of drugs available for the treatment of Paget's disease. Etidronate disodium is the agent most frequently used. The current recommended dosage is 5 mg/kg/day, although higher doses have been used with more severe disease. This medicine is taken orally and is active in suppressing both osteoblastic and osteoclastic activity.

Intra-articular injection of steroids in the knee and hip has been helpful in local disease. When severe hip disease is present, total joint replacement may become necessary.

BIBLIOGRAPHY

Nagant de Deuxchaisnes, C., and Krane, S.M.: Paget's disease of bone: clinical and metabolic observations, Medicine **43**:233, 1964.

Shirazi, P.H., Ryan, W.G., and Fordham, E.W.: Bone scanning in evaluation of Paget's disease of bone, CRC Crit. Rev. Clin. Radiol. Nucl. Med.. **5**:523, 1974.

Wallach, S., and others: Paget's disease of bone, Phoenix, Ariz., 1979, Armour Pharmaceutical Co.

30 • OSTEOPOROSIS

Donald H. Lieberman

Osteoporosis is the most common metabolic bone disorder and the most common cause of osteopenia in the elderly. It represents a disease state of skeletal metabolism in which the rate of bone matrix formation is depressed and unable to compensate for the excessive resorption. Ossification is normal, but there is inadequate matrix to ossify. It is known that loss of bone mass accompanies normal physiologic aging, but in osteoporosis the rate of atrophy is accelerated well beyond the usual 1% per year. Clinical osteoporosis, characterized by bone pain and pathologic fractures, develops when 30% or greater of the bone mass is lost. The rate of loss determines the age at which the disease is clinically apparent. Osteoporosis must be differentiated from osteomalacia, a condition in which there is a failure to mineralize the organic matrix of bone. In osteoporosis the ratio of mineralized bone to unmineralized matrix is normal, but there is a decreased mass per unit volume of bone.

Although osteoporosis usually occurs as a primary disorder associated with aging, the presence of underlying disease must be evaluated. The following is a useful classification:

Association with aging
    Postmenopausal
    Senile
Association with endocrine disturbances (not necessarily causative)
    Hypogonadism
    Thyrotoxicosis
    Hyperadrenocorticism
    Diabetes mellitus
    Acromegaly
Nutritional deficiency
    General malnutrition
    Calcium deficiency
    Scurvy
    Malabsorption syndrome
Heritable disorders
    Ehlers-Danlos syndrome
    Osteogenesis imperfecta
    Marfan's syndrome
States involving chronic inanition
    Rheumatoid arthritis and related disorders
    Malignant tumors
    Alcoholism
    Epilepsy
    Chronic obstructive pulmonary disease
Iatrogenic conditions
    Immobilization
    Prolonged heparin use
    Excessive antacid intake
    Prolonged corticosteroid therapy
Miscellaneous
    Idiopathic osteoporosis of children and adults
    Trauma

In many of these disease states a pathophysiologic explanation exists for the decreased skeletal mass. Many of the conditions, however, have an increased frequency of incidence of osteoporosis without explanation.

Osteoporosis is uncommon in black women and extremely rare in black men. Among whites it occurs more frequently in women.

CLINICAL MANIFESTATIONS. Osteoporosis is a generalized disorder that affects trabecular bone more commonly than cortical bone. The vertebrae and ends of long bones are therefore more likely to become involved. Mild trauma may result in fractures, with the midthoracic, low thoracic, and lumbar spine, and the femoral neck most commonly involved. Patients may relate the sudden onset of pain to minor stress such as lifting a child. The pain of a vertebral fracture may follow a segmental distribution corresponding to the distribution of the affected nerve rootlets. It becomes extremely difficult to find a comfortable position; coughing and sneezing can produce severe pain. Weeks to months may pass before the symptoms subside. Some patients continue to have pain even after healing of bone. Many patients have multiple similar episodes. Fortunately, cord compression is rare. Decrease of body height may ensue with forward bending leading to dorsal kyphosis. As height continues to diminish with successive fractures, skin folds may develop along the base of the thoracic cage, and in some patients there is virtually no distance between the pelvis and rib cage.

LABORATORY FINDINGS. Routine roentgenographic examinations are of little value in detecting early osteoporosis because the skeletal mass must be reduced by 30% before the loss is roentgenographically apparent. Most findings on the plain film are nonspecific. The vertebral bodies may become biconcave because of the pressure of the intervertebral discs. This produces the so-called codfish vertebrae. Localized disc herniations into softened vertebrae are called Schmorl's nodes. Fractures of end-plates and flattening of vertebral bodies are most prominently seen in the anterior portion. Loss of striation and decrease in cortical thickness may be noted in the proximal femur. If destructive lesions or cortical discontinuity is detected, a search for an underlying disorder should ensue.

Serum and urinary calcium and phosphorus determinations are usually normal in primary osteoporosis. Alkaline phosphorus in not elevated.

MANAGEMENT. The most important therapeutic consideration is not to miss another disorder underlying or mimicking osteoporosis. A careful review of the patient's record is often helpful in considering differential diagnoses. Secondary forms of osteoporosis should be sought so they can be optimally treated.

Once the diagnosis of senile osteoporosis is fairly certain, the physician must decide which therapeutic course to follow. Analgesics are helpful in relieving the pain of vertebral fractures. Some patients may require narcotics, but habituation is common and must be avoided. Braces are poorly tolerated by most patients, but they provide comfort to some. Although initial bed rest is required following acute vertebral fracture, excessive inactivity promotes more osteopenia.

Four drug types have been employed in the treatment of osteoporosis: sodium fluoride, estrogens, anabolic steroids, and calcitonin. All are predominantly inhibitors of bone resorption. Calcium and vitamin D supplements may also be useful.

Some authors suggest that sodium fluoride may work by increasing new bone formation, but it probably works largely as an inhibitor of bone resorption. In either case it is an unduly emphasized drug in the treatment of osteoporosis.

There is evidence that estrogens prevent age-related bone atrophy in women who take them after menopause. Pysicians are reluctant to prescribe estrogen because of the increased risk of endometrial carcinoma; estrogen therapy should therefore be short term.

Preliminary studies indicate that anabolic androgens may increase bone mass, but benefits in clinical osteoporosis are still controversial. Adverse effects include virilization, nausea, hepatic toxicity, and salt and water retention. The dosage depends on the preparation used.

Calcitonin (see Chapter 29) has been advocated for use in osteoporosis because it inhibits bone resorption. Controlled studies are needed to support this hypothesis.

BIBLIOGRAPHY

Avioli, A.V.: Osteoporosis: pathogenesis and therapy. In Avioli, L.V., and Krane, S.M., editors: Metabolic bone disease, vol. 1, New York, 1977, Academic Press, Inc.

Howell, D.S.: Metabolic bone disease. In McCarty, D.J., editor: Arthritis and allied conditions, Philadelphia, 1979, Lea & Febiger.

Wallach, S.: Management of osteoporosis, Hosp. Practice 13:91, 1978.

31 • GOUT AND PSEUDOGOUT

Warren A. Katz

GOUT

Gout is a metabolic disorder characterized by hyperuricemia, recurrent attacks of acute arthritis, deposition of sodium urate in and around joints, and formation of urinary uric acid calculi in some cases. The hereditary nature of gout has been recognized since earliest times. Gout rarely occurs in females. It was previously thought that gout was a disease of the wealthy or of geniuses, but present-day knowledge has altered the significance of the social status of gout, even though some reports find elevated levels of uric acid in college professors, business executives, and other high achievers.

Secondary gout refers to gout developing in lymphoproliferative and myeloproliferative diseases, starvation, and hypertriglyceridemia and following administration of certain drugs.

PATHOGENESIS AND PATHOLOGY. The pathogenesis of gout is conveniently described in three phases: hyperuricemia, urate deposition, and inflammation induced by urate crystals.

Hyperuricemia. Normal serum urate levels vary from

one laboratory to another. The upper limits of normal are 6.0 to 8.8 mg/dl depending on the testing method used. Women have slightly lower values that by menopause approach the levels found in men. Hyperuricemia may be defined as excessive levels of uric acid in serum. Not all patients with hyperuricemia develop gout. More than 5% of the normal adult population have hyperuricemia, yet gout develops in only a small minority of these. Although not all patients with bona fide gout have hyperuricemia, all those with untreated gout have excess quantities of urate in the extracellular tissues. The average patient with gout has a serum urate level of 9 to 10 mg/dl; the value is considerably higher in secondary forms of gout caused by blood dyscrasias.

Normally, uric acid is a breakdown product of purine that is formed de novo in the biosynthesis of nucleic acids. Some purines are derived from the diet, and others may be traced to tissue breakdown. Adenine and guanine are the usual sources of uric acid through a complicated metabolic pathway. Uric acid in the form of monosodium urate exists in most body fluids that are slightly alkaline. About two thirds of uric acid formed is eliminated through the kidney and the remainder through the gastrointestinal tract. Because uric acid is degraded by intestinal bacteria, only minimal amounts of it may be found in the feces. All the uric acid that is presented to the kidneys is filtered through the glomerulus, and almost all of it is immediately reabsorbed in the proximal tubules. The uric acid in the urine (350 to 500 mg/24 hr) is derived from active tubular secretion at the distal tubules. The amount of uric acid found in urine depends on several factors, including the rate of de novo synthesis, the degree of tissue breakdown, the amount of ingested purine, and renal function.

Hyperuricemia usually results from excessive de novo synthesis, failure of renal elimination of uric acid, or a combination of these factors. Some mechanisms of primary hyperuricemia have been clearly defined and usually result from specific enzyme defects.

Since approximately one third of patients with primary gout exhibit no evidence of overproduction of uric acid, it is assumed that disorders of renal tubular function result in decreased uric acid clearance and thus cause hyperuricemia. Indeed, it can be shown that patients with renal gout do have diminished clearances of uric acid. A variety of drugs, especially the thiazide diuretics, and certain metabolites (lactic acid) diminish urate clearance in the kidney and may be responsible for hyperuricemia in some patients with gout.

Urate deposition. In most patients with hyperuricemia, gout or uric acid stones never develop. The higher the serum uric acid and the longer it persists, the more likely that the predisposed patient will have clinical manifestations of gout.

Despite a recent focus of attention on the urate deposition phenomenon, its cause is still unknown. Several theories involving urate concentration, sodium flux, avascularity, and diminished permeability of urate in the synovium have been proposed to explain urate crystallization in the joint.

Urates tend to be deposited in the articular cartilage of patients with gout, but they may also be found in tendon sheaths, synovium, synovial fluid, and subcutaneous tissues. Urates rarely are found in parenchymal organs such as the brain, liver, or spleen. It has recently been proposed that urates have an affinity for connective tissue proteoglycans. Probably proteoglycans entrap urate molecules, rendering them supersaturated in hyperuricemic subjects and therefore preventing the deposition of urates. When the normal metabolic turnover of connective tissue is accelerated under the influence of lysosomal and other proteolytic enzymes, the proteoglycans so digested can no longer solubilize urates. Therefore urate deposition results just as crystallization would take place from supersaturated solutions of proteoglycans with urate if similar enzymes were added. Indeed, the breakdown product of proteoglycans (glycosaminoglycans) is found to be elevated in serum of most patients with proven gout but not in normal individuals or hyperuricemic individuals without gout. Selective nocturnal water resorption from traumatic joint effusions may lead to increased urate concentrations.

Acute gouty attack. Monosodium urate is sparingly soluble in plasma and other body fluids. Once urates are deposited, for whatever reason, they may or may not be phagocytized to set off an intense inflammatory reaction. Neither the initial mechanism of urate crystallization nor the mechanism of the initial urate inflammatory stimulating effect is known. Microcrystals of monosodium urate are coated with plasma proteins, including immunoglobulins. The presence of IgG is believed to promote phagocytosis by polymorphonuclear leukocytes that carry immunoglobulin (Fc) receptor sites on their surfaces. Phagocytosis having been achieved, the microcrystals become incorporated into phagolysosomes, leading to the formation of chemotactic factor that mobilizes additional leukocytes. Almost immediately after crystal phagocytosis, there is rapid degranulation and disintegration of the cells with the release of the lysosomal enzymes that induce inflammation. In addition, lysosomal enzymes degrade articular cartilage and ultimately destroy it (Fig. 31-1).

CLINICAL MANIFESTATIONS

Acute gouty arthritis. Acute arthritis is the major clinical expression of gout. Podagra, or involvement of the first metatarsophalangeal joint, occurs during the first attack in about 75% of the cases (Fig. 31-2). Sydenham's initial description in 1683 is so clear and dramatic that it remains the classic description of acute gouty arthritis:

> The victim goes to bed and sleeps in good health. About two o'clock in the morning he is awakened by severe pain in the great toe; more rarely in the heel, ankle or instep. This pain like that of a dislocation, and yet the parts feel as if cold water were

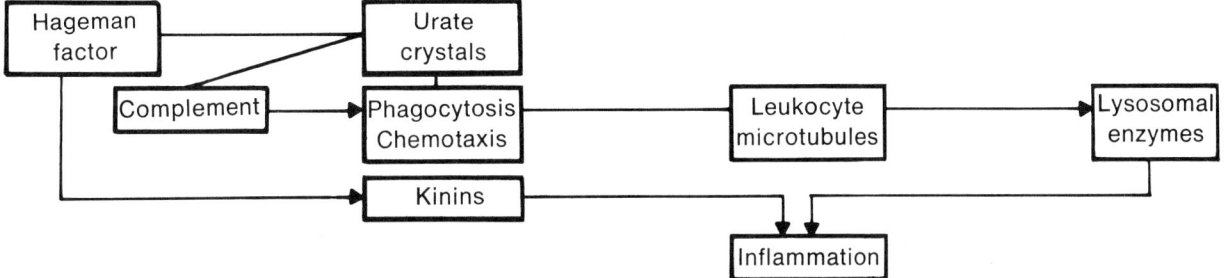

Fig. 31-1. Postulated schema for urate crystal–induced inflammation in gout. Once deposited in joint, urate crystals evoke foreign body–like reaction that causes chemotaxis of leukocytes and then phagocytosis of crystals through leukocyte microtubule mechanism. Hageman factor, complement, and kinins are released, and these factors plus lysosomal enzymes released from leukocytes immediately after phagocytosis produce inflammatory reaction. (Modified from Katz, W.A.: Rheumatic diseases: diagnosis and management, Philadelphia, 1977, J.B. Lippincott Co.)

poured over them. Then follows chills and shivers, and a little fever. The pain, which was at first moderate, becomes more intense. With its intensity, the chills and shivers increase. After a time, this comes to its height, accommodating itself to the bones and ligaments of the tarsus and metatarsus. Now it is a violent stretching and tearing of the ligaments—now it is a gnawing pain, and now a pressure and tightening. So exquisite and lively meanwhile is the part affected, that it cannot bear the weight of the bed clothes nor the jar of a person walking in the room. Night is passed in torture, sleeplessness, turning of the part affected, and perpetual change of posture.

Examination shows the toe or adjacent area to be swollen, shiny, and red or sometimes even violaceous. The overlying skin frequently becomes desquamated as the attack resolves. If untreated, a gouty attack lasts for several days but may persist longer. Complete resolution is the rule.

The other small joints of the feet and the ankles, knees, elbows, and wrists are frequently involved with acute gouty arthritis. Less commonly the finger joints and rarely the shoulders, hips, and sacroiliac joints are affected.

Acute arthritis of one joint is most typical, but polyarthritis may be seen even during the first attack. Under these circumstances the joint distribution is asymmetric and confined mostly to the lower extremities.

Acute gouty attacks tend to recur in unpredictable and episodic fashion. About 60% of those with gout have a second attack within a year, especially if they are untreated. Many patients report minor attacks of joint inflammation even in the absence of the more florid typical attacks.

It is not always clear what precipitates the acute attack of gout in the predisposed hyperuricemic patient or for that matter in the nonhyperuricemic patient. The association with wine and gluttony dates back to ancient times. Indeed, about half of the patients with gout are significantly overweight, and about 75% have hypertriglyceridemia. It is possible, but not proven, that excessive caloric intake, par-

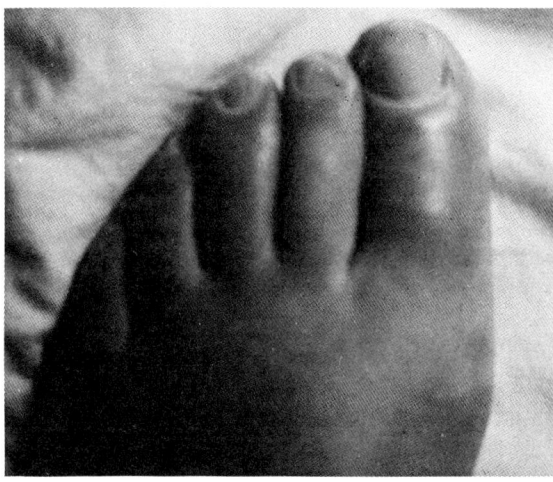

Fig. 31-2. Typical inflamed first metatarsophalangeal joint and adjacent tissues during acute gout. Note sheen of dorsum of toe and loss of normal wrinkles.

ticularly of certain foods, makes PRPP more readily available and thus stimulates the metabolic pathway. Heavy alcoholic intake may raise the concentration of blood lactate to a point at which it interferes with the renal excretion of urates so that a rapid rise in uric acid concentration results. Dramatic fluctuations in serum urate induced by fasting, heavy consumption of alcoholic beverages, and certain foods are often followed by flares in gouty arthritis. Identical swings may be noted during treatment with uric acid–lowering drugs such as allopurinol or probenecid or with drugs that affect renal handling of uric acid such as the thiazide diuretics. Trauma, surgery, and associated illnesses may predispose an individual to gouty arthritis.

Hematologic diseases, neoplastic diseases, hypertension, coronary artery disease, diabetes mellitus, glycogen storage disease, lead intoxication, and intrinsic renal disease are all associated with gout and hyperuricemia. Hy-

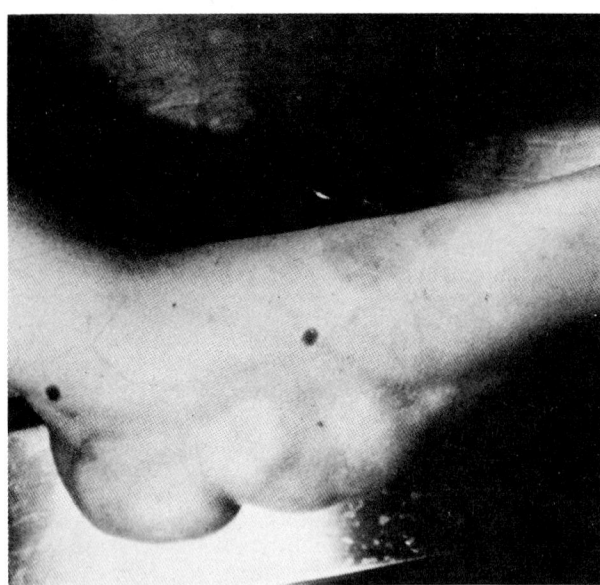

Fig. 31-3. Gouty tophus of olecranon bursa.

peruricemia may be also induced by ethacrynic acid, furosemide, acetazolamide, pyrazinamide, low-dose salicylates, and certain other drugs.

Chronic tophaceous gout. Early in the course of gout, asymptomatic intervals are usually prolonged. As attacks become more frequent, symptom-free periods become shorter; ultimately, in the untreated individual, tophaceous deposits with secondary degenerative changes will leave permanent arthralgias and stiffness. Extensive tophaceous gout may be just as disabling and crippling as advanced rheumatoid arthritis. Tophi may cause similar deformity, entrap nerves, and cause draining, infected sinus tracts.

Tophi are usually seen in the first metatarsophalangeal joint, olecranon, articular synovium, and tendon sheaths of the hand (Fig. 31-3). The development of tophi in predisposed individuals is directly related to the duration and degree of hyperuricemia.

Uric acid lithiasis. In the general population 10% of all renal stones are composed of uric acid. Nephrolithiasis develops in about 20% to 25% of the patients with primary gout, as compared with about 50% of those with secondary gout. In more than one third of the patients with primary gout, renal lithiasis precedes the first attack of acute gouty arthritis. The prevalence of uric acid lithiasis is related to the serum and urinary uric acid output. This association, however, is not as strong as once believed.

LABORATORY FINDINGS. Most, but not all, patients with gout exhibit hyperuricemia either during or after the acute attack. However, the serum uric acid level cannot be used as a diagnostic tool because hyperuricemia is so variable, fluctuates from day to day, is not universal in patients with gout, and affects so many otherwise healthy people.

Estimation of the 24-hour urine uric acid is not diagnostic either; however, it does help to predict whether or not a patient is a candidate for uric acid stones. Extremely high levels of urine uric acid, especially when greater than 1 g daily, make the patient with gout particularly vulnerable to nephrolithiasis.

The identification, under the light of a polarized microscope, of monosodium urate crystals in the synovial fluid from an acute gouty joint definitely establishes the diagnosis (Fig. 31-4). The needlelike crystals frequently may be found piercing the leukocytes during an acute attack. Monosodium urate crystals can also be detected in aspirates from tophi or biopsy material.

Roentgenographic findings. It is unusual to find roentgenographic abnormalities during the first attack of gout. However, some patients have gouty episodes of such lowgrade intensity that they may be missed, yet many years later characteristic tophaceous lesions may be found in the joints, notably in the feet. For this reason roentgenograms of the feet should be obtained when there is a diagnostic dilemma. Typical lesions are sharply defined. Marginal erosions of subchondral bone may appear at the periphery as a thin shell with an overhanging edge. These changes are particularly seen at the first metatarsophalangeal joint; although they are highly suggestive, they are not diagnostic of gout.

DIAGNOSIS. In the typical case of acute podagra developing in a susceptible patient the diagnosis of gout usually is correctly suspected. Nonetheless, synovial fluid analysis for urate crystals is a necessary confirmatory test. Since gout rarely develops in premenopausal women, in this age group other causes of acute arthritis should be sought. Uric acid crystals are not always obtainable from joint fluid. Under these circumstances the diagnosis must rely heavily on a history of repeated attacks of acute arthritis that peak within 1 day and are associated with redness and exquisite tenderness, particularly in the first metatarsophalangeal joint. In the early stages (first 24 to 48 hours) of acute gouty arthritis, colchicine given orally or intravenously induces a dramatic therapeutic response not usually seen in other rheumatic diseases.

The differential diagnosis of gout includes pseudogout, rheumatoid arthritis, rheumatoid variants, osteoarthritis, sarcoid arthritis, psoriatic arthritis, infectious arthritis, palindromic rheumatism, cellulitis, acute bursitis, acute rheumatic fever, and local trauma.

MANAGEMENT. With the development of highly effective drugs, dietary restriction of purines and alcohol is not as important in treating gout as it once was. However, in patients whose gout is difficult to control, a diet relatively free of purines may be recommended at least temporarily. A well-balanced diet somewhat lower in calories and proteins is desirable. Obese patients should make every attempt to lose weight gradually, since starvation usually causes ketone-induced hyperuricemia and susceptibility to the acute gouty attack.

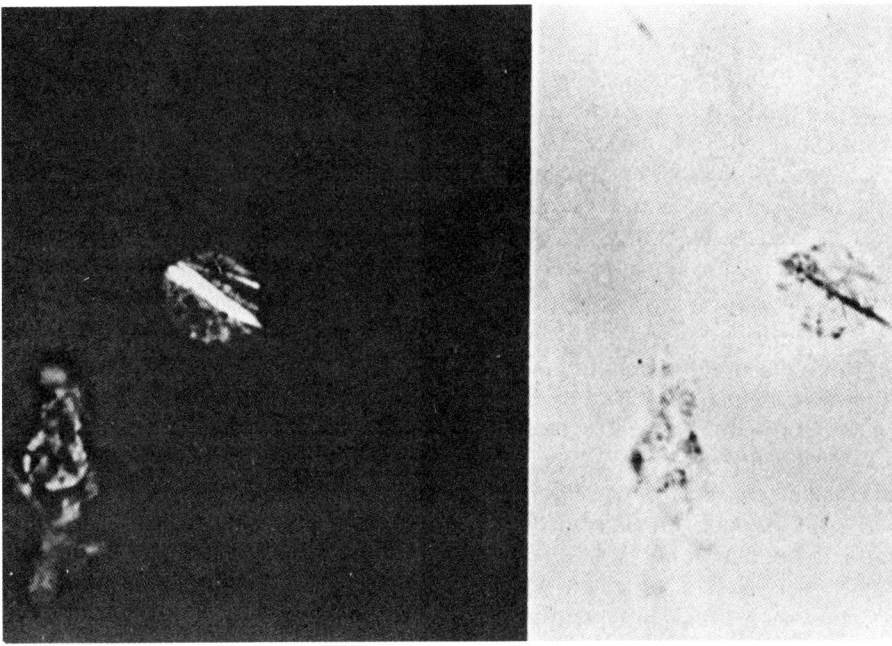

Fig. 31-4. Monosodium urate crystal under light *(right)* and polarized *(left)* microscopy. Note that crystal has pointed ends and pierces polymorphonuclear leukocyte. (Reproduced from the Revised Clinical Slide Collection on the Rheumatic Diseases. Copyright 1981 by the Arthritis Foundation.)

The management of acute gouty arthritis is fairly standard, although treatment of asymptomatic hyperuricemia, intercritical gout (asymptomatic intervals), and tophaceous gout remains somewhat controversial.

Acute gouty arthritis. Acute attacks of gout can be treated with colchicine, nonsteroidal anti-inflammatory drugs, adrenocorticotropic hormone (ACTH), and local injections of corticosteroids.

Because of colchicine's effectiveness and relative specificity, it has the advantage of facilitating the diagnosis of gout. The sooner colchicine is administered during the acute attack, the more effective it will be. Colchicine is effective in about 75% of the patients. Gastrointestinal toxic reactions in the form of cramps, diarrhea, and nausea may appear within 12 hours of initiating therapy. Colchicine can be administered intravenously to avoid gastrointestinal side effects. The major risk of intravenous administration of colchicine is extravasation of the drug with local tissue damage.

Phenylbutazone, oxyphenbutazone, indomethacin, sulindac, and a number of other nonsteroidal anti-inflammatory drugs have been advocated in the treatment of acute gout. Each is effective and may be continued during the first few days of therapy until the attack subsides completely.

Aspiration of crystals from the joint, local administration of corticosteroids, or parenteral administration of ACTH also is advocated for patients who cannot take drugs by mouth or who are intolerant of the agents usually given to treat the acute attack of gout. Warm soaks, ice application, immobilization, and hydration provide additional nondrug therapy.

Asymptomatic hyperuricemia. Few patients with asymptomatic hyperuricemia require treatment. Most such patients have uric acid levels just a milligram or two greater than normal and therefore are at minimal risk of ever having an acute attack of gout. Patients with significantly higher levels of uric acid might be at greater risk of having gouty arthritis and even uric acid stones, but the incidence and ultimate morbidity would be so small that prophylactic treatment is unwise. There is no strong evidence to indicate that significant, irreversible renal damage develops in patients with asymptomatic hyperuricemia.

Intercritical gout. No drug therapy is needed in patients whose attacks of arthritis occur at wide intervals, but they should be assessed periodically. If gouty episodes are becoming frequent and prolonged, colchicine will prevent almost all attacks regardless of serum uric acid levels. If the patient cannot tolerate higher levels of colchicine, if recurrent attacks develop during colchicine therapy, or if roentgenographic changes are taking place, uric acid–lowering drugs should be slowly introduced.

Chronic tophaceous gout. A very large tophus may be surgically removed providing it has not become an integral part of bone mass. Most patients with chronic tophaceous gout are treated with uric acid–lowering drugs such as uricosuric agents (probenecid or sulfinpyrazone) or allopurinol, a xanthine oxidase inhibitor.

Uric acid stones. Whether or not uric acid stones occur in association with gouty arthritis, a large daily fluid intake is required to prevent stone formation. In most instances alkalinization of the urine with sodium citrate or bicarbonate to maintain a pH greater than 6 is desired. This increases the solubility of urates. Allopurinol is a more specific method of preventing uric acid stones.

PSEUDOGOUT

Pseudogout is a crystal-induced disease characterized by acute arthritis that mimics gout caused by urate crystals. Chronic joint inflammation may develop, mimicking rheumatoid arthritis and osteoarthritis. Pseudogout has been referred to as chondrocalcinosis, pyrophosphate arthropathy, and calcium pyrophosphate crystal disease. The disorder represents a distinct clinical entity caused by the deposition of calcium pyrophosphate dihydrate (CPPD) crystals in joints. Pseudogout is the clinical state, whereas "chondrocalcinosis" merely refers to calcification of cartilage whether or not the patient is symptomatic. Although many cases of pseudogout are undoubtedly missed diagnostically, gout is still a much more common disease. Familial aggregations of pseudogout have been noted in Czechoslovakia and Chile; a dominant pattern of transmission is suggested.

PATHOLOGY AND PATHOGENESIS. The metabolic basis for CPPD deposition is unknown. Deficiency of pyrophosphatases in cartilage and other connective tissues has been considered. The initial site of CPPD crystal formation is most likely in the articular cartilage, and indeed CPPD crystals are frequently found in these sites. It is not clear how the crystals precipitate. Somehow they are shed into the joint space and evoke acute inflammation similar to that of gout. The role of trauma, metabolic disorders, and concomitant medical illnesses remains to be clarified. The degree of degenerative change in the joint resembling osteoarthritis varies from quite mild to marked destruction akin to that of Charcot's joints.

CLINICAL MANIFESTATIONS. Pseudogout has several presentations. Acute inflammation of one or a few joints is the hallmark of the disease. The inflammation is intense and sometimes associated with low-grade fever. Pseudogout is slightly more prevalent in women than in men. Most patients are in their sixties during the first attack. Those in a younger age group usually inherit the disease. Larger joints, especially the knees, are most prone to involvement. Wrists, elbows, ankles, and even shoulders and hips are frequently affected. Smaller joints of the fingers and toes are less likely to be inflamed. The first metatarsophalangeal joint is not usually involved in pseudogout.

The duration of the acute attack of pseudogout varies from several days to several weeks, certainly lasting longer than the typical untreated attack of gout. As in gout, the joint becomes red, hot, swollen, and limited in motion. Attacks tend to cluster in a given extremity. The intercritical period is variable and may last from days to years.

McCarty lists the following primary types of pseudogout:

1. In type A, pseudogout, there are typical intermittent acute attacks with asymptomatic intervals.
2. In type B, pseudorheumatoid arthritis, patients may have multiple-joint involvement with subacute attacks lasting for several weeks to months. Because of prolonged morning stiffness, fatigue, and synovial thickening with an elevated erythrocyte sedimentation rate, these patients are often thought to have rheumatoid arthritis.
3. In types C and D, pseudo-osteoarthritis, progressive degeneration of multiple joints occurs. In contrast to typical osteoarthritis, the wrists, metatarsophalangeal joints, shoulders, elbows, and ankles are frequently involved. Patients with type C have superimposed acute attacks, whereas those with type D have no apparent inflammatory component.
4. Type E is lanthanic (asymptomatic CPPD crystal deposition).
5. In type F, pseudoneuropathic joints, patients have Charcot's arthropathy, sometimes without neurologic deficit but with evidence of chondrocalcinosis.

Associated diseases. A true association exists between CPPD crystal deposition disease and hyperparathyroidism, hemochromatosis, hemosiderosis, hypophosphatasia, hypomagnesemia, hypothyroidism, gout, neuropathic joints, and aging. A less clear-cut association is noted between CPPD and hyperthyroidism, calcium renal stones, ankylosing hyperostosis, ochronosis, Wilson's disease, and hemophilic arthropathy. In spite of previous statements to the contrary, it is unlikely that there is a true association with diabetes mellitus, hypertension, mild azotemia, hyperuricemia, gynecomastia, inflammatory bowel disease, rheumatoid arthritis, Paget's disease, and acromegaly.

LABORATORY FINDINGS. Synovial fluid analysis provides the most important diagnostic determination of pseudogout. A single drop is all that is needed to detect the typical crystals, which vary in morphology but generally are irregular, rhomboid, or parallelepiped (Fig. 31-5). During an acute attack crystals are usually seen in leukocytes. They also may be rod shaped, and as such they resemble urate crystals except that the ends are blunted. The cell counts in synovial fluid may be very high as in infectious arthritis, but cell counts of 21,000/mm^3 are the average.

Synovial biopsy may be necessary to establish the disease if synovial fluid is unavailable for diagnosis. High-power microscopy and sometimes electron microscopy are required for identification of crystals.

Roentgenographically, CPPD crystal deposition is noted in fibrocartilaginous structures, articular cartilage, ligaments, and joint capsules. The radiodensity may be

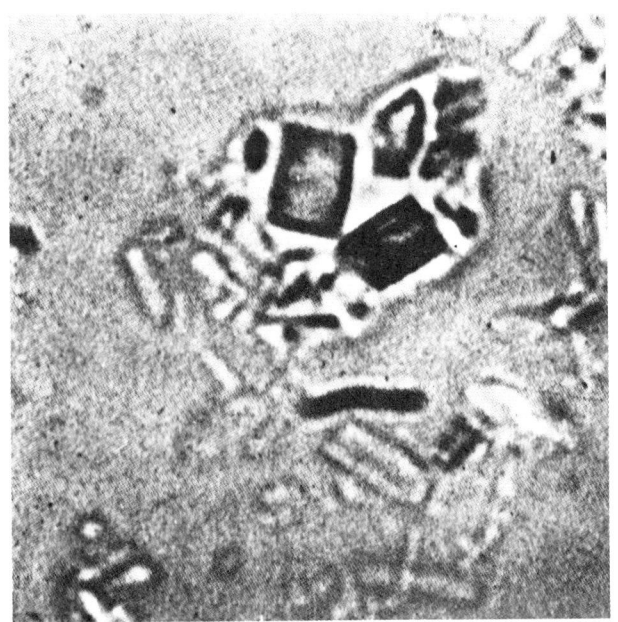

Fig. 31-5. Microscopic appearance of irregular, rhomboid, calcium pyrophosphate dihydrate crystals in synovial fluid from patient with pseudogout.

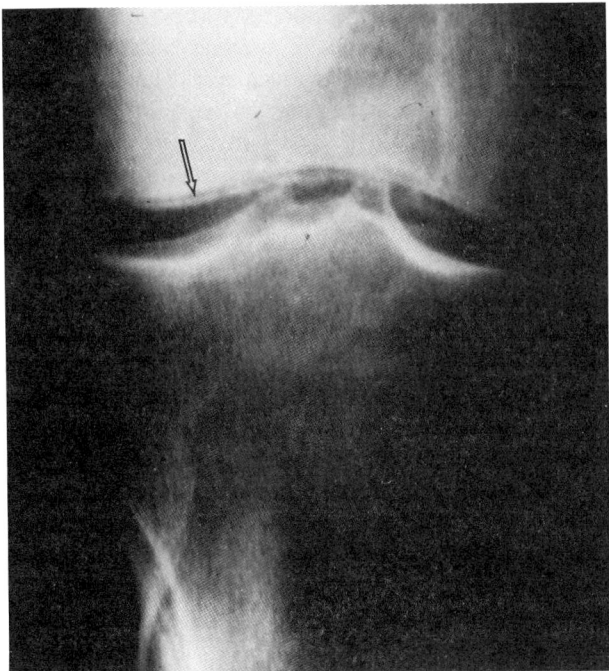

Fig. 31-6. Linear calcification of cartilage of knee (chondrocalcinosis) in patient with pseudogout.

linear or punctate, particularly in the meniscus and articular cartilage of the knees (Fig. 31-6). The articular disc of the distal radial ulnar joint, the symphysis pubis, the acetabular and glenoid fossae, and the anulus fibrosus of the intervertebral disc may calcify.

DIAGNOSIS. Pseudogout is suspected whenever acute or pauciarticular arthritis develops in an elderly person, especially if there are concomitant associated diseases. Discovery of the characteristic CPPD crystals when phagocytized in synovial fluid and the typical linear calcifications on the roentgenogram are additional evidence for the existence of this disease. Septic arthritis, gouty arthritis, palindromic rheumatism, intermittent hydrarthrosis, osteoarthritis, and rheumatoid arthritis are the usual differential diagnoses.

MANAGEMENT. Acute attacks of pseudogout are treated by thorough aspiration and perhaps even lavage of the involved joint, followed by local instillation of corticosteroids. Phenylbutazone, indomethacin, and other nonsteroidal anti-inflammatory drugs are usually effective. Colchicine seems to abort some attacks of pseudogout, but its effectiveness is unpredictable. There is no reliable way of preventing pseudogout.

OTHER CRYSTAL DEPOSITION DISEASE

Calcium hydroxyapatite crystals have been seen in calcific periarthritis for many years. Recently, these crystals were detected in synovial fluid from patients with previously undiagnosed acute arthritis and exacerbations of osteoarthritis. Calcium hydroxyapatite crystals may induce synovitis similar to that caused by urate crystals in gout and pyrophosphate crystals in pseudogout. Detection of these crystals by light microscopy is difficult. Purple-staining cytoplasmic inclusions or extracellular globules may suggest clumps of calcium crystals, but electron microscopic and roentgenographic differential techniques, not readily available in most laboratories, are needed to confirm their presence.

A peculiar type of hydroxyapatite crystal–induced arthritis may affect the shoulders in the elderly, usually women (Milwaukee shoulder). The joints may become acutely or subacutely painful and swollen. Shoulder motion is limited. Rotator cuff tears can usually be demonstrated by arthroscopy. These patients usually have osteoarthritis and chondrocalcinosis in other joints. Temporary relief can be obtained from aspiration of the joint, instillation of corticosteroids, nonsteroidal anti-inflammatory drugs, rest, and range of motion exercises.

BIBLIOGRAPHY

Fessel, W.J.: Renal outcomes of gout and hyperuricemia, Am. J. Med. 67:74, 1979.

Kelley, W.N., and Weiner, I.M.: Uric acid: handbook of experimental pharmacology, Berlin, 1978, Springer-Verlag.

McCarty, D.J.: Calcium pyrophosphate crystal deposition disease (pseudogout; articular chondrocalcinosis). In McCarty, D.J.: Arthritis and allied conditions, Philadelphia, 1979, Lea & Febiger.

McCarty, D.J., and others: "Milwaukee shoulder"—association of microspheroids containing hydroxyapatite crystals, active collagenase, and neutral protease with rotator cuff defects. I. Clinical aspects, Arthritis Rheum. **24**:464, 1981.

Schumacher, H.R., Jr., and others: Arthritis associated with apatite crystals, Ann. Intern. Med. **87**:411, 1977.

Wyngaarden, J.B., and Kelley, W.N.: Gout and hyperuricemia, New York, 1976, Grune & Stratton, Inc.

Yu, T.-F.: Milestones in the treatment of gout, Am. J. Med. **56**:767, 1974.

Yu, T.-F., and Katz, W.A.: Gout and pseudogout. In Katz, W.A.: Rheumatic diseases: diagnosis and management, Philadelphia, 1977, J.B. Lippincott Co.

32 • NONARTICULAR RHEUMATISM

Robert H. Gordon

The term "nonarticular (soft tissue) rheumatism" encompasses a variety of musculoskeletal complaints that do not arise directly from disease in the joints. Pain in these conditions is attributed to dysfunction or inflammation of connective tissues such as muscle, tendons, ligaments, and bursae. In some conditions the intercellular matrix, the supporting ground substance of connective tissue, may be involved, although the exact nature of the involvement is unknown.

Some of the disorders of nonarticular rheumatism have signs and symptoms that are well localized and quite specific. For these, successful treatment can be offered. However, other forms are marked by vague complaints of diffuse pain that the physician cannot easily attribute to local pathology. These conditions are distressing for both the patient and the physician because the diagnosis is difficult and the results of treatment are sometimes less than satisfactory.

Laboratory studies are usually of little help in making or supporting these diagnoses. The erythrocyte sedimentation rate is most often normal despite the intensity of symptoms. Other routine blood studies are also normal or, when not, should suggest the presence of other underlying disease. The correct diagnosis is therefore usually made on the basis of the clinical history and physical findings.

FIBROSITIS

Fibrositis, also known as myofascitis, fibromyositis, or fibromyalgia, refers to a muscle pain amplification syndrome. Fibrositis has been a general term for pain complaints that failed to fit any other diagnosis. It is still a mysterious, inconsistent, controversial clinical entity, but fortunately, recent studies have done much to clear the confusion and define the syndrome.

PATHOGENESIS. Relatively little is known about the pathogenesis of fibrositis. Attempts to define the disease by muscle biopsy or electromyography have been unsuccessful.

Sleep studies have focused on the relationship between non–rapid eye movement (non-REM) sleep disturbances and fibrositic complaints. Some fibrositic patients showed abnormal electroencephalograms characterized by non-REM sleep disturbances. Normal subjects whose sleep was interrupted during the same non-REM phase also complained of morning fatigue and other musculoskeletal symptoms suggestive of fibrositis. Further studies have tested the effects of chlorpromazine, a drug that had been reported to facilitate slow-wave non-REM sleep. Some amelioration of symptoms was noted. Tricyclic antidepressants may also be of benefit by inducing a similar normalization of this stage of sleep.

CLINICAL MANIFESTATIONS. Two groups of patients with fibrositis are described. Those with primary fibrositis have no known underlying disease. Secondary fibrositis is associated with other recognized diseases such a rheumatoid arthritis. Both groups have similar presentations.

Pain, the chief complaint, is diffuse, aching, and especially pronounced about the neck, shoulders, low back, and pelvis. The trunk and extremities may also be involved. Stiffness and fatigue when present are often worse on wakening, typically after a restless sleep. Muscle strength is generally maintained. Some patients think that their muscles are swollen, but usually the apparent enlargement represents muscle spasm.

Tension, anxiety, cold, fatigue, and prolonged immobility exacerbate the problem, whereas heat, relaxation, and gentle exercises tend to alleviate it. The onset of the disease is often dated to a stressful life situation, family upheaval, or accident. It is noteworthy that these patients are frequently described as perfectionists, overdemanding of themselves and others, and unable to relax.

The physical examination initially may appear to be normal. Muscle strength is preserved, and the patient seems to be in good health. However, more detailed evaluation will elicit trigger points, specific sites of tenderness that when palpated reproduce the pain. Patients are frequently unaware of these areas and are often relieved to know that the physician is able to find the source of their pain. Fourteen characteristic sites have been described (Fig. 32-1). It is important to appreciate that these areas are often tender in normal individuals. It is the *degree* of the tenderness that marks the patient with fibrositis. Excessive cutaneous blanching followed by hyperemia is often noted after these areas are palpated. The muscles may be in spasm.

LABORATORY FINDINGS. Roentgenographic and laboratory studies are of no help in diagnosing primary fibrositis. Despite extreme muscle tenderness, muscle enzymes and the sedimentation rate are normal. Other laboratory studies, including tests for rheumatoid factor and autoantibodies, are negative. The muscle biopsy is normal. If any of these are abnormal, other diseases or conditions associated with secondary fibrositis should be considered.

DIAGNOSIS. Several criteria have been proposed to support the diagnosis of fibrositis. These include (1) widespread aching of more than 3 months' duration, (2) local tenderness at 12 of the 14 sites (Fig. 32-1), (3) diffuse tenderness in the upper scapular region, (4) disturbed sleep with morning fatigue and stiffness, and (5) normal sedimentation rate, rheumatoid factor, antinuclear antibody, muscle enzymes, and other laboratory studies. The last criterion is necessary in ruling out conditions that can mimic fibrositis but have different causes and treatment.

MANAGEMENT. It is important to assure the patient that the disease is not crippling, that the prognosis is good, that significant disability is rare, and that a productive life-style can be maintained. Patients should be encouraged to maintain good muscle tone through graded programs of exercise, but overexercise can worsen symptoms. Back or neck supports may be helpful. Rest and relaxation are important and should be encouraged for overanxious or overworked individuals. Physical therapy using heat packs, ultrasound, massage, and whirlpool is beneficial. Anti-inflammatory drugs including aspirin and the newer nonsteroidal agents can be tried, but their efficacy has not been determined by controlled tests. Sometimes injections of local anesthetics are helpful for specific trigger points; whether local injections of corticosteroids provide additional benefits is a moot point. The disturbed sleep pattern may be helped by small to moderate doses of tricyclic antidepressant medications (such as imipramine, 25 to 100 mg) before bedtime. Counseling regarding marital, occupational, or other problems is critical to successful therapy in some fibrositic patients.

REGIONAL AND LOCAL NONARTICULAR SYNDROMES
Myofascial syndromes

HEAD AND NECK. Several specific myofascial pain syndromes can be identified in the head and neck on careful evaluation (Fig. 32-2). Tenderness and spasm can be detected over trigger points in one or more of the following muscles: temporalis, masseter, external pterygoid (Fig. 32-3), internal pterygoid, sternocleidomastoid, and splenius capitis. Myofascial pain dysfunction syndrome of the

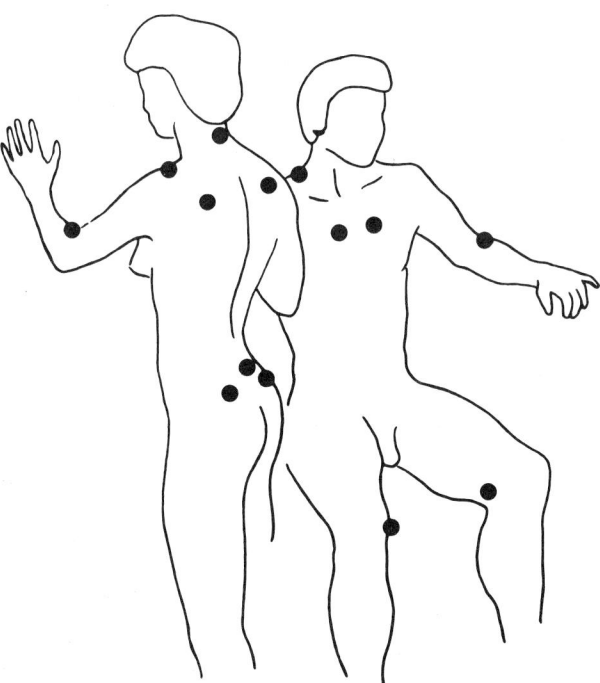

Fig. 32-1. Location of 14 sites of deep tenderness in fibrositis. (From Smythe, H.A., and Moldofsky, H.: Bull. Rheum. Dis. **28:**928, 1977-1978.)

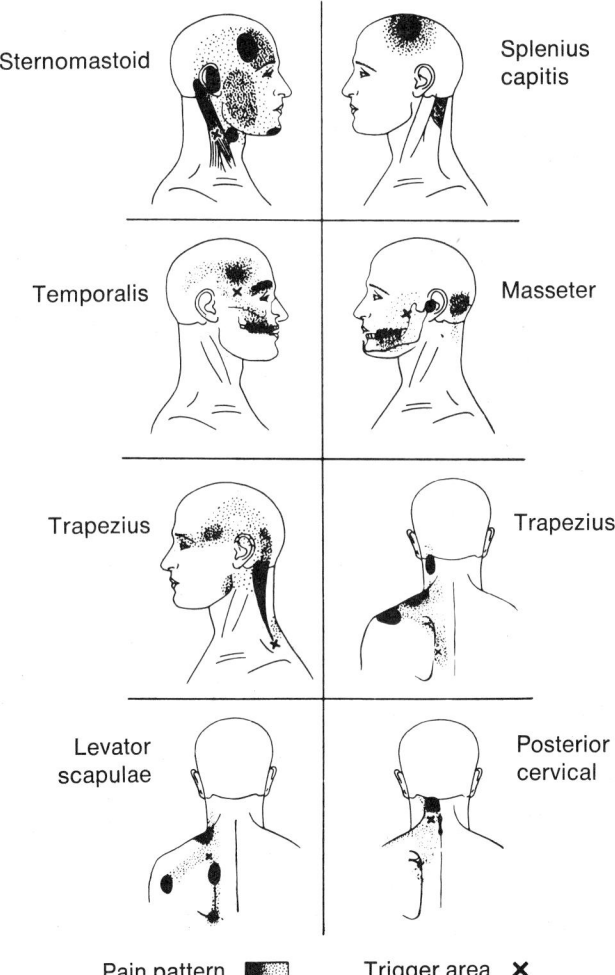

Fig. 32-2. Myofascial syndromes of head and neck. (From Travell, J., and Rinzler, S.H.: Postgrad. Med. **11:**425, 1952.)

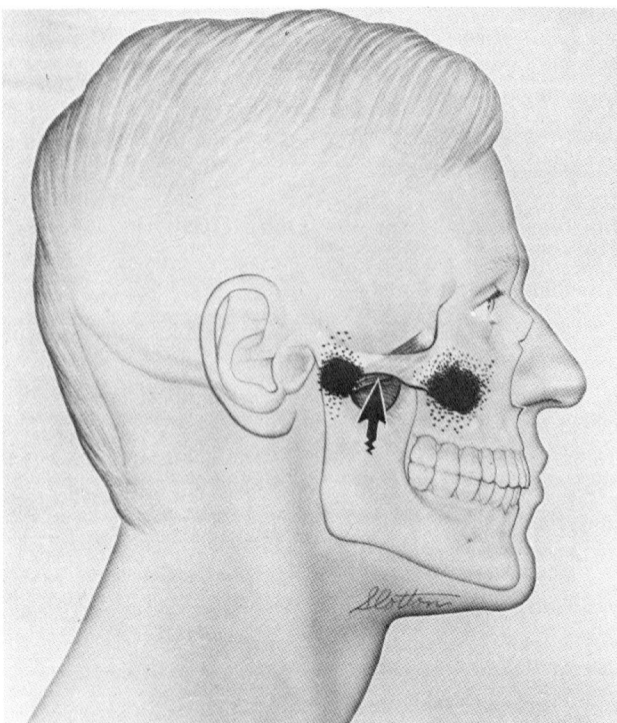

Fig. 32-3. External pterygoid trigger point. (From Shaber, E.P.: Considerations in the treatment of muscle spasm. In Morgan, D.H., Hall, W.P., and Vamvas, S.J.: Diseases of the temporomandibular apparatus, St. Louis, 1977, The C.V. Mosby Co.)

temporomandibular joint is discussed in the Dental Correlations section of this chapter.

SHOULDER, UPPER ARMS, AND CHEST. As in the head and neck, several important muscle syndromes can cause significant pain and disability in the shoulder, upper arm, and chest. The *supraspinatus muscle* frequently causes radiation of pain from the muscle body into the deltoid and upper outer portions of the upper arm. The *subscapularis muscle* can give rise to pain felt maximally at the posterior aspect of the shoulder and over the scapula. Other not infrequent syndromes involve the *infraspinatus, scaleni, deltoid, trapezius,* and *pectoral muscles.*

BACK AND LEG. Specific muscle pain syndromes can be found on examination of the painful back or leg. Frequently these can mimic lumbar disc disease with radicular pain, and their identification may save the patient from unnecessary diagnostic or therapeutic procedures. Spasm of the gluteus medius and minimus muscles is particularly likely to be misdiagnosed as true sciatica.

Nerve entrapments

CARPAL TUNNEL SYNDROME. Carpal tunnel syndrome is the most common cause of pain and paresthesia in the first three fingers of the hand. Occasionally the pain radiates proximally into the forearm and even into the shoulder. The symptoms are due to compression of the median nerve at the proximal volar wrist underneath the tight transverse carpal ligament. Patients frequently complain of waking during the night with a numb and painful hand relieved only by vigorous shaking. The condition may be worsened by prolonged wrist flexion (Phalen's sign) or by tapping the nerve at the wrist (Tinel's sign). The syndrome is seen in any condition that causes pressure on the nerve, such as trauma, tenosynovitis, and connective tissue diseases (for example, rheumatoid arthritis). Diabetes mellitus, pregnancy, myxedema, acromegaly, and amyloidosis are other associated conditions. Nerve conduction studies document median nerve injury. Treating the primary disease may relieve the compression. Wrist splints to hold the wrist in slight extension, corticosteroid injections, or surgical release of the nerve may be necessary.

MERALGIA PARESTHETICA. Meralgia paresthetica is a syndrome produced by compression of the lateral femoral cutaneous nerve beneath the inguinal ligament medial to the anterior-superior iliac spine. Paresthesias are noted in the lateral thigh. Pregnancy, obesity, or a tightly fitted corset may be associated factors. Gradual weight loss and proper posture are usually corrective. Local injections of corticosteroids may be tried. Transcutaneous electrical nerve stimulators have been helpful for this and other localized pain syndromes.

TARSAL TUNNEL SYNDROME. Tarsal tunnel syndrome is produced by entrapment of the posterior tibial nerve as it passes beneath the medial malleolus. It is associated with a burning pain and numbness of the toes and sole of the foot. It can be traumatic in origin, although it has also been associated with rheumatoid arthritis, ankylosing spondylitis, and leprosy. Neuromas and ganglia in the area may also entrap the nerve. The treatment is similar to that for carpal tunnel syndrome.

Bursitis

SUBDELTOID BURSITIS. Subdeltoid bursitis (Fig. 32-4) causes pain that in many instances is difficult to distinguish from that of rotator cuff injuries (discussed later in chapter). Pain is felt about the shoulder and down the upper third of the arm. Often this condition coexists with rotator cuff injuries. The treatment involves rest, physical therapy, analgesics, and anti-inflammatory agents. Aspiration of calcified material and local injection of corticosteroids are helpful in acute episodes.

OLECRANON BURSITIS. Olecranon bursitis is an inflammatory condition of the bursa overlying the olecranon at the tip of the elbow. The bursa is swollen, usually warm, and tender, although occasionally remarkably asymptomatic. Causes include trauma, infection, and systemic disease such as rheumatoid arthritis and gout. The treatment is by oral administration of anti-inflammatory drugs along with aspiration of the bursa and local injection of corticosteroids. Antibiotics are used when appropriate.

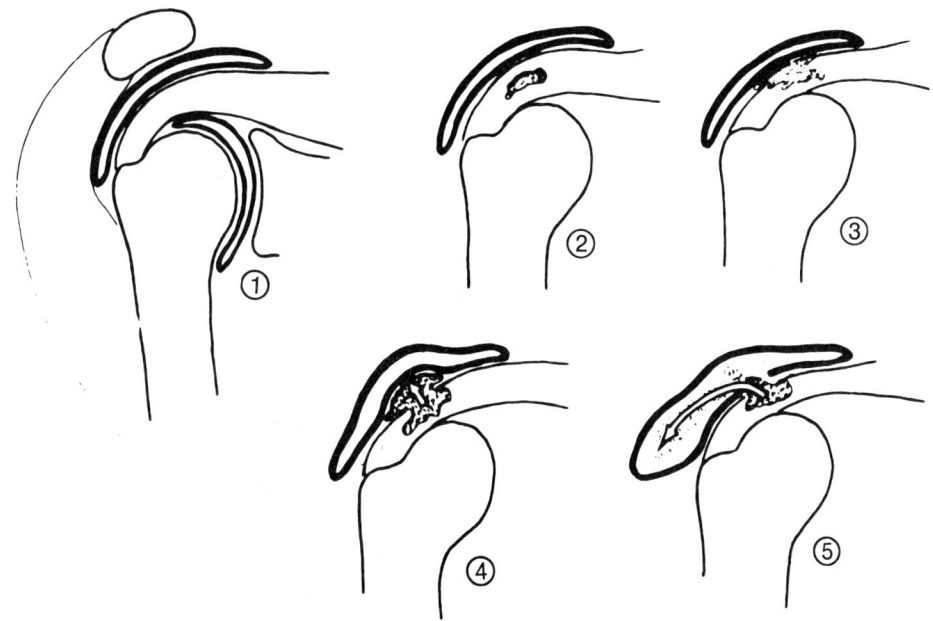

Fig. 32-4. Subdeltoid bursitis. Sequential changes showing deposition of calcium *(2)*, rupture through rotator cuff *(3)*, pressure on overlying bursa *(4)*, and rupture into bursa *(5)*. (From Cailliet, R.: Neck and arm pain, Philadelphia, 1964, F.A. Davis Co.)

BURSITIS IN THE LOWER EXTREMITIES. Bursitis is a common cause of pain in the leg. *Ischial bursitis* is an inflammation of the bursa that separates the gluteus maximus muscle from the ischial tuberosity. It is exposed and irritated when the patient is in a sitting position, and thus this condition is sometimes called weaver's bottom. Chronic inflammation in this area may be associated with calcification seen on roentgenographic examination. *Trochanteric bursitis* frequently causes pain over the lateral aspect of the thigh with radiation down the leg. Pressure over the greater trochanter will reproduce the patient's pain. *Prepatellar bursitis* or what was once called housemaid's knee is a tender, usually warm swelling just over the patella. It is most commonly caused by repeated local trauma as occurs in carpet layers, but it can also be associated with other connective tissue diseases. *Anserine bursitis*, an inflammation of the sartorius bursa located inferomedial to the patella, is frequently misdiagnosed as an intra-articular pathologic condition. Injection therapy, systemic administration of nonsteroidal anti-inflammatory agents, and physical therapy as described for subdeltoid and olecranon bursitis are helpful.

Tendinitis

CALCIFIC TENDINITIS. Calcific tendinitis is marked by tendon inflammation with calcium deposits seen on roentgenogram. The supraspinatus tendon is most frequently involved. Many cases are related to degenerative changes within the tendon from trauma or arthritis, but others have no known predisposing cause. The treatment involves rest, physical therapy, analgesics, anti-inflammatory agents such as indomethacin, and local injection of adrenocorticosteroids.

BICIPITAL TENDINITIS. Bicipital tendinitis is a common condition caused by inflammation of the tendon sheath as it passes through the bicipital groove of the humeral head. Pain is felt at the anterior aspect of the shoulder and is produced by forced supination of the hand with the elbow flexed. Bicipital tendinitis may also be associated with rotator cuff injuries (discussed later in the chapter). The therapy is as for calcific tendinitis.

FLEXOR TENOSYNOVITIS. Flexor tenosynovitis (trigger fingers) refers to inflammation of the flexor tendon sheaths of the hand. There is impediment to free movement of the tendons within the sheaths. The patient feels a snapping sensation in the palm when the fingers are flexed and may be unable to reextend the fingers. Deep message to break adhesions and local injection of corticosteroids are useful. Surgery may be needed.

DeQUERVAIN'S DISEASE. DeQuervain's disease is a tenosynovitis of the extensor pollicis brevis and abductor pollicis longus tendons at the radial wrist below the base of the thumb. It is more common in women and may be related to trauma, although the cause is usually unknown. The treatment is with anti-inflammatory drugs, injections, splinting, and occasionally surgical tendon release.

LATERAL EPICONDYLITIS. *Tennis elbow* is the common term for inflammation of the wrist extensor tendons at their origins on the lateral epicondyle. The condition is induced by forceful wrist extensions. It is often seen in tennis players, although any activity requiring repetitive wrist extension may cause it. Similarly, pain at the medial epicondyle of the elbow may be related to repetitive forceful wrist flexions. The treatment for both includes avoidance of activities that exacerbate the pain until the inflammation subsides, splinting, local application of heat, anti-inflammatory drugs, and local corticosteroid injections. Exercise to strengthen the forearm extensor and flexor muscles is helpful in preventing recurrence.

Miscellaneous nonarticular syndromes

DISORDERS OF THE HEAD AND NECK

Tension headache and cervical tension state. The most common cause of cephalic pain is the common tension headache. The pain is described as a tight or pressurelike sensation, usually bilateral, localizing in the frontal or occipital-nuchal area. It can be unrelenting, lasting several days, and is noted even when the patient wakes briefly during the night.

The causes are numerous. All tend to produce prolonged voluntary or involuntary spasm of the cranial and cervical musculature. Anxiety and chronic tension states are frequent culprits. Poor posture, osteoarthritis of the cervical spine with intervertebral disc degeneration or herniation, spur formation, and apophyseal joint disease all may play a role by inducing secondary muscle spasm or nerve root irritation. Intracranial lesions, visual problems, severe hypertension, and metabolic and other disorders must also be considered.

Temporomandibular joint syndrome (Costen's syndrome).* Pain in the area of the temporomandibular joint can be due to abnormal joint mechanics with secondary muscle strain and spasm or actual damage within the joint. Patients often complain of a clicking sensation on opening the mouth and pain radiating into the scalp. Crepitation and local muscle tenderness are often elicited. The treatment consists of alleviating the underlying condition, exercises to help coordinate joint motion, intra-articular injections, reassurance, and, infrequently, surgical correction.

DISORDERS OF THE SHOULDER, UPPER ARM, AND CHEST

Reflex sympathetic dystrophy (shoulder-hand syndrome). In reflex sympathetic dystrophy, also known as causalgia or Sudeck's atrophy, the shoulder is painful and motion is limited. The extremity may be edematous, cool, and tender. Patients complain of painful paresthesias. Causative factors include fracture, nerve injury, cerebrovascular accident, heart attack, cervical osteoarthritis, and some drugs. In one third of patients the syndrome develops without a known cause. Most of those affected are over the age of 50. This syndrome can affect the legs. Without treatment, the shoulder and hand become stiff, atrophied, and contracted. Roentgenograms may show patchy demineralization. Once this syndrome is recognized, it should be promptly treated. Physical therapy with remobilization exercises and local application of heat is extremely helpful. Orally administered or locally injected corticosteroids and nerve blocks may also be used.

Costochondritis or Tietze's syndrome. Costochondritis or Tietze's syndrome is a painful nodular tenderness at the costochondral junctions of the anterior ribs that is made worse by pressure or motion of the chest. It can involve any of the costochondral junctions, but most frequently the second and third are affected. Local inflammatory signs such as redness or heat are rare. Swelling is caused by cartilaginous hypertrophy and can easily be palpated. The cause is unknown, but local trauma may play a role. The treatment first includes reassurance that the pain is not cardiac in origin, then local application of heat, oral administration of anti-inflammatory or analgesic drugs, and if necessary local injections of anesthetics or corticosteroids.

Intercostal neuritis and *intercostal myalgia* are additional common causes of anterior chest discomfort.

Thoracic outlet syndromes. The term "thoracic outlet syndromes" is used to describe several neurovascular syndromes that produce symptoms in the shoulder and upper arm. The thoracic outlet is the region through which the neurovascular supply of the arm leaves the neck and thorax to enter the axilla. It represents an area of narrowed and fixed passages, and thus the exiting structures are subject to compression. The symptoms are variable and intermittent and may be felt as a burning or ache associated with numbness and paresthesia in the shoulder and down the arm into the fingers. The physical examination may show weakness or muscle atrophy. Depending on the structures involved, neural or vascular, there may be diminished sensation or changes in color and temperature. Raynaud's phenomenon and edema in the involved extremities may also be found.

The *scalenus anticus syndrome* is caused by a change from normal in the size, shape, or insertion of the scalenus anticus muscle (Fig. 32-5). Spasm may be a contributing cause. Compression of the subclavian artery or vein and the brachial plexus can occur between the muscle and first rib. Pain radiates into the arm and hand, usually on the ulnar side. The symptoms depend on relative neural, arterial, or venous impairment. Procedures useful in making the diagnosis include applying direct pressure to the muscle or using the Adson maneuver, which is performed by palpating the radial pulse on the side of involvement while the patient takes a deep breath, holds it, and extends and turns the head to the involved side. In a positive test the pulse is lost and the patient experiences a reproduction of the symptoms. This test is useful but not diagnostic. A systolic bruit can be heard below the midclavicle during the maneuver in some patients.

---

*Discussed in detail on p. 109 under Dental Correlations.

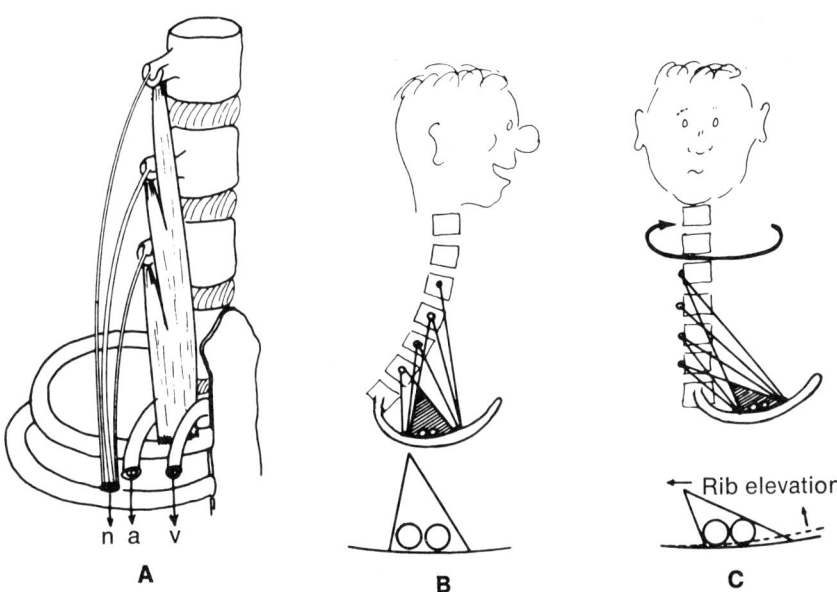

Fig. 32-5. A, Scalenus anticus syndrome. *n,* Brachial plexus; *a,* subclavian artery; *v,* subclavian vein. Scalenus anterior muscle lies between subclavian artery and vein. **B** and **C,** Rotating head and neck can place pressure on nerve, artery, or vein. Additionally, rib elevation as occurs by scalene action in deep inspiration can further compress neurovascular bundle. (From Cailliet, R.: Neck and arm pain, Philadelphia, 1964, F.A. Davis Co.)

Cervical ribs, which rise from the seventh cervical vertebra, are present in less than 1% of the population. The symptoms are due to compression of neurovascular structures between the rib and the scalenus anticus muscle. The diagnosis is supported by roentgenographic findings.

The *costoclavicular syndrome* results from compression of the vein, artery, and nerve between the clavicle and first rib when the shoulders are braced backward and downward. As in the scalenus anticus syndrome, the radial pulse may be decreased and a subclavian bruit may be heard. Backpackers whose backpack straps place excessive weight on the shoulders can have this syndrome.

The *hyperabduction* or *pectoralis minor syndrome* results from neurovascular compression between the pectoralis minor muscle, coracoid process, clavicle, and first rib. The symptoms are brought on by abducting and externally rotating the arms above the head. This can occur during sleep when the arms are folded under the head or as an occupational hazard in auto mechanics, painters, and ballet dancers.

Therapy of the thoracic outlet syndromes is directed at relieving the obstruction. If muscle spasm is present, deep heat as by ultrasound or local anesthetic injection can be tried. Exercises are helpful, but persistent symptoms may indicate the need for surgical resection of the first rib or scalenus anticus muscle.

Rotator cuff injury. The *rotator cuff* at the shoulder represents a conjoining of the tendons from the supraspinatus, infraspinatus, teres minor, and subscapularis muscles. Tears of the rotator cuff are common, especially on the dominant side. The lesions are divided into partial and complete tears. Both may produce acute pain and inability to fully abduct the arms, but patients with complete tears are demonstrably weak on abduction even when the pain is controlled. The treatment includes rest, physical therapy, analgesics, and anti-inflammatory drugs. Exercise is important once the inflammation has subsided. Surgery may be indicated for some acute complete tears.

Adhesive capsulitis. Adhesive capsulitis or *frozen shoulder* refers to shoulder pain that follows immobilization resulting from a fracture, wearing a cast, or other conditions facilitating disuse. The treatment is directed at remobilizing the shoulder through exercises that stretch the shoulder capsule. Intracapsular corticosteroid-anesthetic injections and anti-inflammatory drugs may be needed.

DISORDERS OF THE ELBOW, WRIST, AND HAND

Dupuytren's contracture. Dupuytren's contracture refers to a tightening and contracture of the palmar fascia. The cause is unknown. The condition is more common in men past the fourth decade and can affect the plantar fascia. Occasionally it has been associated with diseases such as diabetes mellitus and alcoholism. The fourth and fifth fingers are particularly affected and may become permanently flexed into the palm. The treatment for advanced contracture is surgical.

Synovial cysts. Synovial cysts or *ganglia* are cystic swellings containing a thick mucinous material that are found along tendon sheaths or joint capsules. They are especially common at the dorsum of the wrist, are usually slow growing, and are not painful. Simple aspiration of the cyst and injection of corticosteroids may be effective, although some require excision.

DISORDERS OF THE BACK AND LEGS

Fibrofatty nodules. Fibrofatty nodules may occur in subcutaneous tissue along the iliac crest and over the sacroiliac joints. They appear to be herniated adipose tissue and can be very tender. Biopsy shows mild cellular infiltration about blood vessels. The treatment is by injection of corticosteroids or surgical excision.

Shin splints. Shin splints is the common term for pain felt usually over the distal third of the tibia. Jogging is a common cause. Muscle-strengthening exercises may be helpful in relieving the problem.

DISORDERS OF THE FOOT AND ANKLE

Calcaneal spurs (plantar fasciitis). Calcaneal spurs are common causes of pain in the sole of the foot. Spurs may form at the origin of the plantar fascia as a result of constant strain applied to the calcaneus. These conditions are often traumatic in origin, and athletes are frequently affected. Connective tissue diseases such as ankylosing spondylitis, psoriatic arthritis, and Reiter's syndrome can cause spur formation. The treatment is aimed at reducing local pressure by supplying well-fitted shoes, heel cups, and sometimes strapping. Ultrasound and local injections of corticosteroids are useful.

Heel neuromas. Heel neuromas can form just below the calcaneus and cause a great deal of pain on walking. Orthoses are helpful in alleviating local pressure.

Pes planus. Pes planus or flat feet may be associated with an aching discomfort in the lower legs. This condition may be the result of peroneal muscle spasm, improper shoes, overweight, or most commonly a developmental abnormality. It is often corrected by properly fitted shoes.

BIBLIOGRAPHY

Cailliet, R.: Soft tissue pain and disability, Philadelphia, 1977, F.A. Davis Co.

Hench, P.K.: Nonarticular rheumatism. In Katz, W.A.: Rheumatic diseases: diagnosis and management, Philadelphia, 1977, J.B. Lippincott Co.

Moldofsky, H., and Scarisbrick, P.: Induction of neurasthenic musculoskeletal pain syndrome by selective sleep stage deprivation, Psychosom. Med. **38:**35, 1976.

Moldofsky, H., and others: Musculoskeletal symptoms and non-REM sleep disturbance in patients with "fibrositis syndrome" and healthy subjects, Psychosom. Med. **37:**341, 1975.

Norris, C.W., and Eakins, K.: Head and neck pain: temporomandibular joint syndrome, Laryngoscope **84:**1466, 1974.

Simons, D.G.: Muscle pain syndromes. I., Am. J. Phys. Med. **54:**289, 1975.

Simons, D.G.: Muscle pain syndromes. II., Am. J. Phys. Med. **55:**15, 1976.

Smythe, H.A., and Moldofsky, H.: Two contributions to understanding of the "fibrositis" syndrome, Bull. Rheum. Dis. **28:**928, 1977-1978.

Sola, A.E., and Williams, R.L.: Myofascial pain syndromes, Neurology **6:**91, 1956.

33 • MISCELLANEOUS RHEUMATIC DISORDERS

Warren A. Katz

RELAPSING POLYCHONDRITIS

Relapsing polychondritis is characterized by inflammation of cartilage and other tissues, such as the joints, ears, nose, and trachea, that contain large amounts of glycosaminoglycans. In about one third of the cases the disease may coexist with other rheumatic and immunologic diseases. There may be inflammation of the synovium and eyes, auditory disturbance, cardiovascular abnormalities, and fever. The disease tends to remit for varying periods of time lasting up to several years. The majority of patients are between the ages of 20 and 60, although infants and the very elderly may be affected.

PATHOGENESIS AND PATHOLOGY. The cause of relapsing polychondritis is unknown; however, the disease is thought to be immunologically mediated because delayed hypersensitivity and antibodies to cartilage have been demonstrated in many patients. Examination of diseased cartilage shows aggregates of plasma cells and lymphocytes. With progressive destruction of cartilage, granulation tissue develops but the cartilage does not show evidence of regeneration. Similar changes are noted in the aorta.

CLINICAL MANIFESTATIONS. Usually one or both ears suddenly become inflamed (Fig. 33-1). They are red, hot, and swollen, although the noncartilaginous portions such as the lobe are spared. Arthralgias, sometimes intense, are generally evident; occasionally there is overt arthritis. Most often, like other aspects of the disease, the arthritis is migratory and intermittently acute. Infrequently, the destructive changes are so severe that peripheral arthritis closely resembles rheumatoid arthritis or spinal involvement resembles ankylosing spondylitis. Chest pain may result from costrochondritis.

Less often, neck pain caused by laryngotracheitis may be detected. The larynx and trachea are tender. Some patients complain of cough and dyspnea when the cartilaginous tracheal rings collapse. Cartilage destruction in the nose may lead to a saddle deformity.

Ocular inflammation is usually in the form of episcleritis, but iritis, conjunctivitis, keratitis, keratoconjunctivitis sicca, exophthalmos, ophthalmoplegia, and retinal exudation may be apparent. Narrowing of the external auditory meatus by edematous tissues may cause hearing defects.

About 25% of the patients with relapsing polychondritis exhibit some cardiovascular manifestations, including valvular insufficiency caused by a prolapsed mitral valve or involvement of the aortic ring, aneurysmal dilation of the thoracid or abdominal aorta and its branches (occasionally with dissection and rupture), conduction defects, and cardiomegaly.

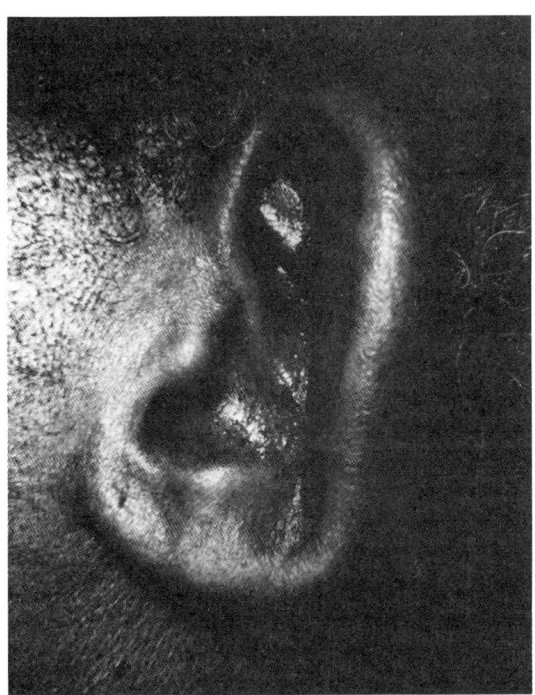

Fig. 33-1. Redness and swelling of entire ear in patient with relapsing polychondritis. (Courtesy of June F. Klinghoffer, M.D.)

LABORATORY FINDINGS. Cartilage biopsy is the most definitive procedure in diagnosing relapsing polychondritis. The ear, when affected, is the most accessible cartilaginous tissue. Detection of anticartilage antibodies in serum may be helpful, but this is still investigational. The erythrocyte sedimentation rate is elevated during the acute attack and tends to return to normal with remission. Roentgenographic evaluation may demonstrate collapse of tracheal cartilage and calcification of the ears.

DIFFERENTIAL DIAGNOSIS. When relapsing polychondritis appears with two or more cartilaginous sites involved, the diagnosis is relatively easy. When arthritis is extensive, rheumatoid arthritis should be suspected; however, ear, nose, and laryngotracheal cartilaginous involvement would not be expected with rheumatoid arthritis. Chondrodynia costosternalis, a variant of Tietze's syndrome, can resemble relapsing polychondritis but tends to be isolated to the anterior aspect of the chest. Wegener's granulomatosis, midline granuloma, sarcoidosis, syphilis, and tuberculosis all may cause destructive changes of the nose. Aural calcification may be caused by Addison's disease, hypervitaminosis A, hypoparathyroidism, and trauma. The diagnosis of relapsing polychondritis becomes most difficult when it is associated with other rheumatic diseases such as systemic lupus erythematosus, rheumatoid arthritis, vasculitis, ankylosing spondylitis, ulcerative colitis with arthritis, Reiter's syndrome, and Sjögren's syndrome.

MANAGEMENT AND PROGNOSIS. The treatment of relapsing polychondritis depends on systemic administration of corticosteroids, usually in relatively large doses. The clinical manifestations are usually rapidly suppressed; however, if protracted therapy is needed, corticosteroids should slowly be reduced to a minimum. Nonsteroidal anti-inflammatory drugs such as indomethacin have been found to be useful by some observers and will probably exert a corticosteroid-sparing effect. Immunosuppressive agents such as azathioprine or cyclophosphamide may be helpful when corticosteroids are not.

Tracheostomy, if tracheal collapse is imminent or has recently taken place, and aspiration of secretions may be lifesaving. Replacement of the aortic and mitral valves may be necessary, and aneurysmal dilations of the aorta may require repair. Most deaths result from cardiovascular or pulmonary complications.

HYPERTROPHIC OSTEOARTHROPATHY

Hypertrophic osteoarthropathy is a syndrome characterized by digital clubbing of the fingers and toes, periostitis of distal long bones, polyarthritis, and evidence of autonomic disturbance such as profuse sweating, flushing, and blanching of the hands and feet. The syndrome is usually associated with pulmonary neoplasms—hence the name hypertrophic pulmonary osteoarthropathy (HPO). However, osteoarthropathy may be associated with other types of malignancies and diseases. In addition, it may be hereditary or may occur without any apparent association.

The cause of HPO is unknown. Postulated mechanisms include autonomic reflex stimulation, excessive arteriolar pulse pressure, toxins or osteoblastic-stimulating agents released by tumors, pulmonary arteriovenous shunts, and growth hormone production by tumors.

The typical pathologic changes are found at the distal ends of the metacarpals, metatarsals, and long bones of the legs and arms. Other bones may be involved with advanced disease. Histologic changes are nonspecific and are characterized by round cell infiltration and periosteal edema. The synovial membrane, articular capsule, and surrounding periarticular structures are similarly affected. In acute cases pannuslike arthritis may result in cartilage destruction, matrix loss, and bony ankylosis.

Secondary hypertrophic osteoarthropathy may be associated not only with pulmonary neoplasms but also with diseases such as bronchiectasis, pulmonary abscess, cystic fibrosis, biliary cirrhosis, inflammatory bowel disease, sprue syndromes, and cardiac disorders such as subacute bacterial endocarditis, cyanotic heart disease, and atrial myxoma.

Patients may have an aching pain in the fingers aggravated by dependency of the limb. The clubbing that develops insidiously consists of widening of the distal fingers and toes, much like a drumstick. A loss of the normal 15-degree angle between the dorsal surface of the phalanx and the proximal portion of the nail is an early sign of clubbing.

Autonomic dysfunction is evidence by excessive sweating of the hands and feet and warmth of the fingertips. Gynecomastia may occur in some patients.

The erythrocyte sedimentation rate may be elevated. Other laboratory tests are unremarkable. Roentgenograms of involved joints may show symmetric subperiosteal newbone formation, typically at the distal diaphyseal regions of long bones.

The treatment of pulmonary hyperosteoarthropathy is directed toward removal of the primary causative factor, if possible. In the interim patients can be treated with salicylates and other nonsteroidal anti-inflammatory drugs, local injections of corticosteroids, and if required, systemic administration of corticosteroids. The prognosis of the disease varies with the primary cause.

FIBROUS DYSPLASIA

Fibrous dysplasia is a developmental disease of bone mesenchyme characterized by replacement of bone by cellular fibrous tissue. Histologically, numerous immature bone spicules resembling those of osteitis fibrosa are visible on roentgenographic examination. However, islands of cartilage are seen in fibrous dysplasia but not in osteitis fibrosa.

Although fibrous dysplasia is generally a localized disease, widespread involvement may be seen. In almost all cases there is insidious invasion of bone, often beginning in infancy but not becoming clinically apparent until the age of 5 or 10, when deformities such as bowing or pathologic fractures develop. At that time roentgenograms indicate the diagnosis. Typically they show cystlike lesions of the metaphysis with an expansion of adjacent cortex. Sometimes there is complete destruction of bone architecture. Areas of increased density may give way to a groundglass appearance over a period of years. Serum calcium and phosphorus levels are normal; with severe disease the alkaline phosphatase may be variably elevated.

In some young women fibrous dysplasia is associated with precocious puberty and a brownish pigmentation of the skin (Albright's syndrome). With extensive invasion of the skull, neurologic symptoms may appear because of nerve impingement. Some patients have concomitant osteomalacia, vitamin D–resistant rickets, or myositis ossificans.

There is no specific treatment for fibrous dysplasia. Calcitonin therapy has been tried but needs further investigation. Supportive measures such as splints, braces, and exercises may be suited to individual cases.

AVASCULAR NECROSIS

Avascular necrosis (osteonecrosis) is a consequence of disrupted blood supply to bone (most commonly the femoral head) with resultant pain and disability. Trauma from dislocation, fracture, or occasionally thermal injury or radiation is the usual cause. Avascular necrosis may be associated with a variety of hematologic disorders including hypercoagulability states, polycythemia vera, and hemoglobinopathies. Caisson disease is avascular necrosis caused by a nitrogen embolus in divers who fail to decompress themselves adequately. Sometimes avascular necrosis is seen in association with systemic lupus erythematosus, prolonged adrenocorticosteroid therapy, renal transplantation, hepatic cirrhosis, pancreatitis, alcoholism, hyperuricemia, and Gaucher's disease. In many instances, such as avascular necrosis in the femoral head in children (Legg-Calvé-Perthes disease), there is no associated cause. Similar types of osteonecrosis may be noted in other joints.

Pain and dysfunction resulting from involvement of a specific joint are the major complaints. Roentgenograms characteristically show areas of bone resorption adjacent to areas of increased bone density with fragmentation. The surface of the joint becomes flattened, and in the hip there is an area of radiolucency just below the joint surface, giving a thin eggshell appearance in early cases. Radioisotopic scanning may show increased uptake over affected joints, sometimes before roentgenographic changes appear.

Management depends on the specific joint involved, the age of the patient, and the underlying disorder. In most instances treatment consists of rest, physical therapy, and avoidance of overuse or misuse of the joint by means of canes, crutches, and other assistive weight-bearing devices. Analgesic agents and nonsteroidal anti-inflammatory drugs may be beneficial. In the early cases, before destructive changes have taken place, intramedullary bone grafting can be performed. Later, however, total joint replacement is the treatment of choice.

HEMARTHROSIS

Hemarthrosis, bloody effusion into one or more joints, may be caused by a variety of situations. Most often blunt trauma with or without associated fracture will result in pain, swelling, and, if the blood remains in the joint for a long enough time, even synovitis with heat and redness. Hemophilia, an inherited sex-linked recessive disorder of coagulation resulting from a deficiency of clotting factor VIII or IX, is responsible in some cases. Repeated hemorrhage into the joint causes arthritis of varying severity, depending on the adequacy of treatment, the number of bleeding episodes, and the duration of the blood in the joint. Villous hypertrophy of the synovium similar to that in rheumatoid arthritis may develop because of the irritant effect of blood on the synovium. Cartilage exposed to blood may actually be destroyed. Furthermore, bleeding within muscles surrounding joints causes "pseudotumors" because of the expanding hematomas. Patients with hemophilia have a great deal of joint pain and dysfunction. The disability may be profound and may result in a wheelchair- or bed-bound existence.

Intra-articular bleeding infrequently follows anticoagulation therapy. Hemorrhagic synovial fluid may also be found in association with pigmented villonodular synovitis, synovioma, neuropathic arthropathy, hemangioma, Ehlers-Danlos syndrome, and scurvy.

Initially, roentgenograms show soft tissue swelling indicative of the effusion. Later, large cyst formation, irregularity of the joint surface resulting from cartilage destruction, and even complete obliteration of the joint space may be found with repeated hemarthroses.

Management is directed toward aspiration of blood from the joint and elimination if possible of the precipitating factors. Initial mobilization of involved joints and assistive walking devices are also necessary. In more advanced cases, particularly of hemophilic arthropathy, extensive physical rehabilitation is required and in some instances even total joint arthroplasty is performed. Replacement of clotting factors is a requisite in the management of hemophilic arthropathy.

BIBLIOGRAPHY

Arnold, W.D., and Hildpartner, M.W.: Hemophilic arthropathy: current concept of pathogenesis and management, J. Bone Joint Surg. **59**:287, 1977.

Firat, D., and Stultzman, L.: Fibrous dysplasia of the bone, Am. J. Med. **44**:421, 1968.

Hammarstein, J.F., and O'Leary, J.: The features and significance of hypertrophic osteoarthropathy, Arch. Intern. Med. **99**:431, 1957.

McAdam, L.P., and others: Relapsing polychondritis: prospective study of 23 patients and a review of the literature, Medicine **55**:193, 1976.

Schumacher, H.R.: Articular manifestations of hypertrophic osteoarthropathy in bronchogenic carcinoma: a clinical and pathologic study, Arthritis Rheum. **19**:629, 1976.

34 • FIBROSING SYNDROMES

Jerome A. Boscia and Donald Kaye

The fibrosing syndromes are a group of rare disorders characterized by anatomic areas of chronic low-grade inflammatory processes progressing to scar tissue, which causes clinical manifestations by encasing, constricting, and limiting the movement of nearby structures. Usually these syndromes are reported as separate disease entities and are either idiopathic or caused by an underlying insult. Occasionally, two or more of these conditions have been observed in the same individual, suggesting a common process with multiple-system involvement, which has been termed multifocal fibrosclerosis.

Retroperitoneal fibrosis is idiopathic in about 70% of the cases. Another 20% are associated with methysergide therapy or malignancy. The disorder most commonly affects men in their sixth decade who have low back pain and may develop obstructive uropathy. An intravenous pyelogram reveals hydroureteronephrosis and medial displacement of the ureters. Laparotomy is usually indicated to relieve ureteral obstruction by ureterolysis and to exclude malignancy. Steroid therapy is controversial as an adjuvant to surgery, but it is worthwhile for patients who are not surgical candidates or who have recurrences. The prognosis is good if there is no associated malignancy.

Fibrosing mediastinitis is usually a result of granulomatous disease, particularly histoplasmosis, but it may be idiopathic. The clinical manifestations include cough, wheezing, and hemoptysis resulting from bronchial involvement. Obstruction of the superior vena cava usually progresses slowly, allowing collateral circulation to develop and therefore causing minimal morbidity and mortality. Mediastinoscopy or mediastinotomy may be required to establish the diagnosis and exclude malignancy. Antibiotic therapy is probably indicated for any underlying infectious process; steroids do not appear helpful.

Sclerosing cholangitis may be associated with ulcerative colitis, but usually the cause is unknown. Patients have jaundice, pruritus, and occasionally right upper quadrant discomfort. Liver function tests are compatible with extrahepatic biliary tract obstruction. Endoscopic retrograde cholangiography usually reveals the lesion, and laparotomy confirms the diagnosis and excludes malignancy. Prolonged T-tube or internal biliary tract drainage appears palliative. Steroids rarely seem useful. The prognosis is determined by the development of secondary biliary cirrhosis and its complications.

Practolol peritonitis is fibrotic encasement of the small intestine caused by the β-adrenergic blocking drug practolol. The disease is manifested by small bowel obstruction for which surgery is indicated. *Riedel's thyroiditis* is a fibrotic process of the thyroid and surrounding structures. Surgery is required to exclude malignancy and may be necessary to relieve pressure symptoms. Other fibrosing lesions include *Peyronie's disease,* which affects the corpora cavernosa of the penis, and *pseudotumor of the orbit,* which causes exophthalmos and must be differentiated from malignancy.

BIBLIOGRAPHY

Danzi, J.T., Makipour, H., and Farmer, R.G.: Primary sclerosing cholangitis: a report of nine cases and clinical review, Am. J. Gastroenterol. **65**:109, 1976.

Dines, D.E., and others: Mediastinal granuloma and fibrosing mediastinitis, Chest **75**:320, 1979.

Koep, L., and Zuidema, G.D.: The clinical significance of retroperitoneal fibrosis, Surgery **81**:250, 1977.

DENTAL CORRELATIONS

RHEUMATOID ARTHRITIS
Martin S. Greenberg

Involvement of the temporomandibular joint (TMJ) in rheumatoid arthritis results from granulomatous involvement of the articular surface of the synovial membrane leading to destruction of the underlying bone. The literature is inconsistent regarding the incidence of TMJ involvement in patients with rheumatoid arthritis due to the varied criteria used by investigators to diagnose arthritis of the joint. The majority of patients with rheumatoid arthritis have involvement of the temporomandibular joint sometime during the course of their disease, but only a small percentage of these patients will experience permanent, serious disability. A recent study analyzed 50 adults both clinically and radiographically for TMJ involvement. Thirty-one of these patients had symptoms of TMJ disease, with 21 having positive radiographic signs. Signs of rheumatoid arthritis of the temporomandibular joint appeared in 21 of the 28 patients who had rheumatoid arthritis for over 10 years. In another study TMJ involvement was noted in 62 patients with rheumatoid arthritis. Sixty-one percent of these patients had clinical evidence of TMJ disease and 79% had radiographic changes.

CLINICAL MANIFESTIONS. Common symptoms of rheumatoid arthritis of the temporomandibular joint include bilateral stiffness, crepitus, tenderness, and swelling over the region of the joints. Pain appears to be present only in the acute phase of the disorder, although destruction will often cause permanent limitation of opening. This decrease in mandibular opening, while apparent on clinical examination, is not clinically significant in many cases. Patients with juvenile rheumatoid arthritis with involvement of the joint often experience a decreased growth of the mandible resulting in micrognathia and anterior open bite. Occasional ankylosis is often seen in patients with juvenile rheumatoid arthritis requiring surgery.

Radiographic changes noted include narrowed joint space, flattened condyles, erosions, subchondral cysts, and osteoporosis.

DENTAL MANAGEMENT. It is unusual for arthritis itself to interfere with dental treatment unless fibrosis or ankylosis of the temporomandibular joint causes a decreased oral opening. One exception occurs in patients with Felty's syndrome. These patients may have neutropenia or thrombocytopenia. When treating a patient with a history of rheumatoid arthritis the dentist should determine whether or not the disease process is affecting the hematologic system.

Although arthritis is rarely a contraindication to dental treatment, the medications used to treat arthritis are a more common cause of complications. The dentist treating a patient with a history of arthritis must take a careful drug history. Some patients are taking high doses of aspirin, resulting in disorders of platelet function. Therefore the dentist should consider evaluation of platelet function before extensive surgical procedures. The bleeding time using the Ivy method is a good screening test for platelet function.

Others with arthritis may be taking gold salts or phenylbutazone. Either of these medications may cause blood dyscrasias including neutropenia or aplastic anemia. Patients taking these medications should have a routine complete blood count every other week. Indomethacin or ibuprofen is a rare cause of thrombocytopenia or granulocytopenia.

Since the discovery of these nonsteroidal anti-inflammatory agents, there has been a dramatic decrease in the use of long-term systemic corticosteroids for the treatment of rheumatoid arthritis. However, some patients with severe forms of rheumatoid arthritis not responding to nonsteroidal anti-inflammatory agents or gold will still be treated with systemic corticosteroids. The dentist must consider the possibility of adrenocortical suppression and increased susceptibility to infection.

Treatment depends on the severity of the signs and symptoms observed. Since rheumatoid arthritic patients rarely have involvement of the temporomandibular joint alone, they are usually given anti-inflammatory drugs, which effectively treat all involved joints. During acute exacerbation the patient should be restricted to a soft diet. In the past intermaxillary fixation has been used to manage patients experiencing acute exacerbations. This should be avoided because of the risk of fibrous ankylosis. The patient should begin a exercise program as soon as possible after the acute symptoms subside. When patients have severe symptoms, the use of intra-articular steroids should be considered. Intra-articular steroids should not be used more than once every 6 months, since localized osteoporosis may result. Patients who develop ankylosis will benefit from surgery. Surgery is to be avoided, however, during the acute phases of the disease since range of motion will improve after the acute inflammation subsides.

BIBLIOGRAPHY

Chalmers, I.M., and Blair, G.W.: Rheumatoid arthritis of the temporomandibular joint, Q. J. Med. **42**:369, 1973.

Kreutziger, K.L., and Mahan, P.L.: Temporomandibular degenerative joint disease: Part I. Anatomy, pathophysiology and clinical description, Oral Surg. **40**:165, 1975.

Kreutziger, K.L., and Mahan, P.L.: Temporomandibular degenerative joint disease: Part II. Diagnostic procedure and comprehensive management, Oral. Surg. **40**:297, 1975.

Ogus, H.: Rheumatoid arthritis of the temporomandibular joint, Br. J. Oral Surg. **12**:275, 1975.

Scott, A.S., and Frew, A.L.: Bilateral enlargement of the mandibular coronoid processes in a patient with rheumatoid arthritis of the temporomandibular joints, J. Oral Surg. **33**:787, 1975.

Seymour, R.L., Crouse, D.L., and Irby, W.: Temporomandibular ankylosis secondary to rheumatoid arthritis: report of case, Oral Surg. **40**:584, 1975.

Trenwith, J.A., and Beale, G.: Rheumatoid arthritis in the temporomandibular joint, N.Z. Dent. J. **72**:195, 1977.

PSORIATIC ARTHRITIS OF THE TEMPOROMANDIBULAR JOINT
Martin S. Greenberg

Psoriatic arthritis is a rare cause of TMJ disease. When it occurs, patients have symptoms similar to those seen in rheumatoid arthritis but the pain is most frequently unilateral. Symptoms include pain on opening the jaw, limitation of movement, deviation to the side of the pain, and tenderness directly over the joint. Radiographic findings are not specific and are similar to those seen in rheumatoid arthritis, including erosion of the condyle surface, flattening of the condyle, and proliferative changes. Diagnosis is based on arthritis occurring in a patient who has psoriasis and a negative rheumatoid factor. Case reports of psoriatic arthritis of the temporomandibular joint have noted improvement with conservative treatment including diathermy, physical therapy, exercise, and salicylates.

BIBLIOGRAPHY

Blair, G.S.: Psoriatic arthritis and the temporomandibular joint, J. Dent. **4:**123, 1976.

Franks, A.S.T.: Temporomandibular joint arthrosis associated with psoriasis, Oral Surg. **19:**301, 1965.

Lowry, J.C.: Psoriatic arthritis involving the temporomandibular joint, J. Oral Surg. **33:**206, 1975.

Sanders, B., and Halliday, R.: Psoriasis and rheumatoid arthritis: their relationship in temporomandibular joint ankylosis, J. Oral Med. **34:**4, 1979.

OSTEOARTHRITIS OF THE TEMPOROMANDIBULAR JOINT
Martin S. Greenberg

The most common intracapsular disorder of the temporomandibular joint is degenerative joint disease. The evaluation of the temporomandibular joints from 400 cadavers revealed degenerative changes in 40% of the joints from patients over 40. These changes, however, were usually seen in individuals who had no history of complaints relative to TMJ disease. Therefore clinicians must be careful when evaluating the cause of facial pain. Degenerative changes in the temporomandibular joint found on roentgenographic examination may be an incidental finding and not responsible for the symptoms. When one considers degenerative joint disease as a cause of pain in the region of the temporomandibular joint, the incidence of the disorder decreases dramatically. In another study 1500 patients with pain around the area of the temporomandibular joint were evaluated: the incidence of degenerative joint disease was found to be only 8%.

Some workers divide degenerative joint disease into primary and secondary arthritis. Primary arthritis refers to asymptomatic osteoarthritis of unknown cause while secondary osteoarthritis results from trauma, infection, or other forms of stress placed on the joint. Patients with generalized degenerative joint disease rarely have involvement of the temporomandibular joint as an important clinical finding. In one study 39 patients with a diagnosis of primary degenerative joint disease and 44 control patients were evaluated clinically and with circular tomography of the joint. No significant difference was found in the incidence of TMJ involvement between the two groups, and researchers concluded that primary osteoarthritis does not affect the temporomandibular joint.

CLINICAL MANIFESTATIONS. Major symptoms of degenerative joint disease of the temporomandibular joint include unilateral pain directly over the condyle, a decreased range of motion of the mandible, particularly limitation of opening, crepitus, and a feeling of stiffness after a period of inactivity. Examination will reveal pain on palpation with deviation of the jaw toward the affected side. This is in contrast to myofascial pain dysfunction syndrome, where the jaw deviates to the side opposite the pain because of spasm of the lateral pterygoid muscle.

Roentgenographic findings in osteoarthritis include loss of lamina dura of the condyle, particularly at the point of articular contact, narrowing of the joint space, irregular joint space, flattening of the articular surface, osteophyte formation, marginal lipping, and so-called elys cysts. In distinguishing radiographic changes found in degenerative joint disease from those changes noted in rheumatoid arthritis, one researcher noted that in degenerative joint disease degenerative changes begin at the center of the condyle, causing flattening, while in rheumatoid arthritis the joint destruction begins in the periphery, causing a spike.

DENTAL MANAGEMENT. Degenerative joint diseases of the temporomandibular joint can be managed conservatively in the majority of cases. Toller noted a significant improvement of many cases after 9 months and also noted a burning out of many cases by the end of 1 year. It seems prudent to manage a patient conservatively for a year before considering surgery. Conservative management includes soft diet, treatment of secondary myofascial pain dysfunction syndrome, and use of nonsteroidal anti-inflammatory drugs. Intra-articular steroids can be used once a year during acute episodes, but repeated injections may cause degenerative bony changes. Ankylosis is rare in degenerative joint disease but in some cases the pain and disability are so severe that surgery may be indicated. In the case of localized osteophyte formation in areas easily accessible to surgery, shaving of the condyle may help to relieve the symptoms. In other cases where involvement is more generalized, a high condylotomy should be performed.

BIBLIOGRAPHY

Blackwood, H.J.J.: Arthritis of the mandibular joint, Br. Dent. J. **115:**317, 1963.

Chalmers, I.M., and Blair, G.S.: Is the temporomandibular joint involved in primary osteoarthrosis? Oral Surg. **38:**75, 1974.

Hecker, R., and others: Symptomatic osteoarthritis of the temporomandibular joint: report of a case, J. Oral Surg. **33:**780, 1975.

Kopp, S.: Subjective symptoms in temporomandibular joint osteoarthrosis, Acta Odontol. Scand. **35:**207, 1977.

Nickerson, J.W., Grafft, M.L., and Sasima, H.J.: Bilateral coronoid process enlargement: report of case, J. Oral Surg. **27:**885, 1969.

Rowe, N.L.: Bilateral developmental hyperplasia of the mandibular coronoid process: report of two cases, Br. J. Oral Surg. **1:**90, 1963.

Toller, P.A.: Osteoarthrosis of the mandibular condyle, Br. Dent. J. **134:**223, 1973.

SYNOVIAL CHONDROMATOSIS OF THE TEMPOROMANDIBULAR JOINT (CHONDROMETAPLASIA)
Martin S. Greenberg

Synovial chondromatosis is metaplasia of the synovial membrane resulting in the formation of small foci of hyaline cartilage. In this disorder, cartilage develops from the connective tissue in the synovial membrane. Pieces of the cartilage are pinched off and released into the joint space, causing a secondary degenerative joint disease. The most common joint involved with synovial chondromatosis is the knee, but there have been several reports of this disorder in the temporomandibular joint. In one case a 61-year-old female had been complaining of swelling and crepitus in the temporomandibular joint region. Initially this swelling was confused with a parotid tumor. Radiographs showed calcified nodules in the joint. Several cases have been reported from the Mayo Clinic. The patients ranged in age from 40 to 60, and there was an increased incidence in women. Symptoms included pain, limitation of opening, deviation to the affected side, crepitus, and swelling. The presence of swelling helps to distinguish the disorder from degenerative joint disease. Radiographic findings include an irregular joint surface and the presence of loose calcified cartilage in the region of the joint. In addition, sclerosis of the glenoid fossa and mandibular condyle has been reported. Proper treatment of this disorder is surgical removal of the metaplastic tissue.

BIBLIOGRAPHY

Brooke, R.I.: Secondary osteoarthrosis (osteoarthritis) of the temporomandibular joint, Dent. J. **43**:325, 1977.

Guralnick, W., and others: Temporomandibular joint afflictions, N. Engl. J. Med. **298**:1263, 1978.

Marbach, J.J.: Arthritis of the temporomandibular joints and facial pain, Bull. Rheum. Dis. **27**:918, 1976.

Miller, A.S., Harwick, R.D., and Daley, D.J.: Temporomandibular joint synovial chondromatosis: report of case, J. Oral. Surg. **36**:467, 1978.

Noyek, A.M., and others: The radiologic findings in synovial chondromatosis of the temporomandibular joint, J. Otolaryngol. **6**:45, 1977.

Ronald, J.B., Keller, E.E., and Welland, L.H.: Synovial chondromatosis of the temporomandibular joint, J. Oral Surg. **36**:13, 1978.

Rosen, P.S., and others: Synovial chondromatosis affecting the temporomandibular joint: case report and literature review, Arthritis Rheum. **20**:736, 1977.

SEPTIC ARTHRITIS OF THE TEMPOROMANDIBULAR JOINT
Martin S. Greenberg

Septic arthritis of the temporomandibular joint most commonly results from blood-borne bacterial infection but may also result from trauma directly to the joint or extension of infection from adjacent sites such as the middle ear, maxillary molars, and parotid gland. Gonococci cause a majority of cases of septic arthritis of the temporomandibular joint. Other bacterial infections that have been reported include those with streptococci, staphylococci, and pneumococci. Cases have been reported of temporomandibular joint arthritis resulting from infection with viruses, particularly measles and influenza.

CLINICAL MANIFESTATIONS. Symptoms of septic arthritis of the temporomandibular joint include severe pain on movement and an inability to occlude the teeth due to presence of infection in the joint space. Examination reveals redness and swelling in the region of the involved joint. Large tender cervical nodes are frequently present on the side of the infection. This helps to distinguish septic arthritis from more common types of temporomandibular joint disorders. In some cases the swelling may be fluctuent and extend well beyond the region of the joint. Septic arthritis of the temporomandibular joint may result in serious sequelae including ankylosis or involvement of growth centers in children, resulting in facial asymmetry. In a review of 185 cases of ankylosis of the temporomandibular joint, 73 of the 185 cases resulted from infection. The most common sites of origin of the infections were the middle ear, teeth, and hematologic spread of gonorrhea. Evaluation of patients with suspected septic arthritis must include an evaluation for signs and symptoms of gonorrhea such as purulent urethral discharge or dysuria. The affected temporomandibular joint should be aspirated and fluid gram stained and cultured. If gram-negative diplococci are seen in the Gram stain or clinical symptoms and signs indicate the possibility of gonorrhea, cultures for *N. gonorrhoeae* should be obtained on special media and placed in an atmosphere containing carbon dioxide.

DENTAL MANAGEMENT. Treatment consists of surgical drainage and appropriate antibiotic coverage. Occasionally, immobilization may be temporarily performed during the acute stage when severe pain is present, but physical therapy should be started as soon as the acute symptoms subside.

BIBLIOGRAPHY

Bradley, P.: Actinomycosis of the temporomandibular joint, Br. J. Oral Surg. **9**:54, 1971.

Chue, P.W.: Gonococcal arthritis of the temporomandibular joint, Oral Surg. **39**:592, 1975.

Keffer, C.S., and Spink, W.W.: Gonococcal arthritis: pathogenesis, mechanism of recovery and treatment, J.A.M.A. **109**:1448, 1937.

Shapiro, L., and Gorlin, R.J.: Disorders of the temporomandibular joint. In Gorlin, R.J., and Goldman, H.M., editors: Thoma's oral pathology, vol. 2, St. Louis, 1970, The C.V. Mosby Co., p. 577.

Winters, S.E.: Staphylococcus infection of the temporomandibular joint, Oral Surg. **8**:148, 1955.

GOUTY ARTHRITIS OF THE TEMPOROMANDIBULAR JOINT
Martin S. Greenberg

Gouty arthritis involving the temporomandibular joint has rarely been reported in the American and European literature. Some authors have suggested that gout does not affect the temporomandibular joint. Three cases have been reported of pain in the TMJ region occurring during periods of hyperuricemia. The pain resolved with antigout medications, but no attempt was made to confirm the diagnosis by aspirating monosodium urate crystals from the synovial fluid of the temporomandibular joint. It has been suggested that clinicians should suspect gouty arthritis as a cause of TMJ pain in Filipinos, Chinese, and Japanese, who are said to be susceptible to this condition.

BIBLIOGRAPHY

Cacioppi, J.T., Morrissey, J.B., and Bacon, A.S.: Condyle destruction concomitant with advanced gout and rheumatoid arthritis, Oral Surg. **25**:919, 1968.

Chun, H.: Temporomandibular joint gout, J.A.M.A. **226**:353, 1973.

Kleinman, H.Z., and Eubank, R.L.: Gout of the temporomandibular joint, Oral Surg. **27**:281, 1969.

MYOFASCIAL PAIN DYSFUNCTION SYNDROME OF THE TEMPOROMANDIBULAR JOINT
Martin S. Greenberg

Significant confusion exists in both the medical and the dental literature as well as among clinicians regarding "temporomandibular joint disorders." A majority of complaints centering around the area of the temporomandibular joint do not originate from the joint itself but are caused by spasm of the muscles of mastication around the joint. Tenderness, spasm, and dysfunction of these muscles is known as myofascial pain dysfunction syndrome (MPD). Schwartz in his pioneering work was the first investigator to distinguish myofascial pain from other causes of discomfort in the region of the temporomandibular joint. Schwartz's work was also important in determining that malocclusion was not the most important cause of this disease. Studies by Laskin and others have confirmed and enlarged upon much of the work done by Schwartz.

The majority of cases of myofascial pain dysfunction are caused by oral habits such as clenching or grinding the teeth, which can be precipitated by stress. Patients with myofascial pain dysfunction have been shown to have difficulties in interpersonal relationships and social adjustment as well as increased anxiety levels. These may appear in otherwise normal individuals going through periods of stress as well as patients with severe psychiatric disturbances.

The symptoms of myofascial pain dysfunction are related to the severity of the spasm and the muscles of mastication involved. Common symptoms include pain in the temporal, preauricular, and masseteric regions that is made worse by eating or speaking, limitation of mandibular movement, deviation of the mandible on opening, and clicking or popping sounds in the temporomandibular joint. Patients with spasm of the muscles of mastication may also have pain and spasm of other muscles, most commonly the trapezius and sternocleidomastoid muscles. This has led some clinicians to speculate that back pain is caused by disorders of the temporomandibular joint. No evidence exists, however, to substantiate this claim. It is reasonable to assume that patients with spasm in one group of muscles are more prone to a similar problem in another group.

CLINICAL MANIFESTATIONS. Careful questioning will often reveal a patient with a history of habitual clenching or grinding of the teeth. If the patient clenches during sleep the most severe pain will be experienced in the morning. If the habit is the result of activities of daily living, the patient may awake asymptomatic but experience increased symptoms as the day progresses. Occasionally patients with myofascial pain dysfunction will have pain triggered by faulty dental restorations.

Examination of patients with suspected myofascial pain dysfunction must include careful palpation of each of the muscles of mastication. The muscles most commonly involved are the lateral pterygoid, which can be palpated posterior and lateral to the maxillary tuberosity or the masseter muscle. Pain and spasm of the lateral pterygoid muscle are often referred to the region of the joint itself and mistaken for evidence of temporomandibular joint disease. Spasm of the temporalis muscle may also occur either at its attachment on the skull or on the coronoid process, which must be palpated intraorally. Tenderness and spasm of the medial pterygoid muscle are observed less frequently. Other signs include decreased interincisal opening, which can easily be measured on a millimeter ruler, and deviation of the jaw on opening. Deviation is caused by muscle spasm, causing the patient to appear to have an abnormal occlusion. This sign of the disease has led some clinicians to regard occlusion as the primary cause and attempt treatment by adjusting the occlusion either with grinding or with prosthetics.

DENTAL MANAGEMENT. Treatment of myofascial pain dysfunction must be individualized according to the underlying cause as well as the severity of the symptoms. Some patients require nothing more than counseling consisting of an explanation of the cause of their pain and a method to help them decrease the clenching of their teeth. Patients with acute spasms of the muscles can be treated by a combination of injection of local anesthetic into the area of the spasm, use of ultrasound, and, when indicated, prescriptions for muscle-relaxing medication such as diazepam (Valium). Use of aspirin or nonsteroidal anti-inflammatory drugs will also be helpful. The treatment of chronic pain is much more difficult and demanding. Some patients will respond to moist heat and phsyiotherapy. Use of occlusal appliances such as maxillary Hawley with an anterior bite plane and night guards will be helpful, although the therapeutic effect of bite-altering appliances has not been supported with controlled studies.

BIBLIOGRAPHY

Cohen, E.S., and Hillis, R.E.: The use of hypnosis in treating the temporomandibular joint pain dysfunction syndrome, Oral Surg. **48**:193, 1979.

Kotani, H., and others: Quantitative electromyographic diagnosis of myofascial pain-dysfunction syndrome, J. Prosth. Dent. **43**:450, 1980.

Kydd, W.: Psychosomatic aspects of temporomandibular joint pain, J. Am. Dent. Assoc. **59**:31, 1959.

Laskin, D.M.: Etiology of the pain-dysfunction syndrome, J. Am. Dent. Assoc. **79**:147, 1969.

Schwartz, L.: Pain associated with the temporomandibular joint, J. Am. Dent. Assoc. **51**:594, 1955.

Weinberg, L.A.: The etiology, diagnosis, and treatment of temporomandibular joint dysfunction-pain syndrome: Part II. Differential diagnosis, J. Prosth. Dent. **43**:58, 1980.

Weinberg, L.A.: The etiology, diagnosis, and treatment of temporomandibular joint dysfunction-pain syndrome: Part III. Treatment, J. Prosth. Dent. **43**:186, 1980.

REITER'S SYNDROME
Philip Springer

CLINICAL MANIFESTATIONS. The reported incidence of oral lesions associated with Reiter's syndrome has been variable. As high as 85% of the patients diagnosed as having Reiter's syndrome may exhibit oral changes. The oral lesions may not consistently be noted because of their painless nature.

The oral lesions in Reiter's syndrome may affect the palate, tongue, gingiva, buccal mucosa, lips, tonsillar pillars, and pharynx. Involvement of the buccal mucosa, gingiva, and lips has been described as red, papular lesions measuring 1 mm to 1 cm in diameter and surrounded by a whitish circinate line. Frank ulcerations may develop. The tongue lesions appear similar to geographic tongue and are characterized by areas of superficial erosion. Multiple, small, bright red macules that later blend to form a darker area may be apparent when the palate is affected. Small opaque vesicles and areas of glistening erythema with a granular surface have also been reported as oral manifestations of Reiter's syndrome.

Histologically, these oral lesions exhibit parakeratosis, acanthosis, and elongation of the rete pegs. Intraepithelial microabscesses with a polymorphonuclear leukocyte infiltration may be apparent. A mixed inflammatory cell infiltrate is usually discernible in the connective tissue.

Striking clinical and histopathologic similarities have been noted between the oral lesions seen in Reiter's syndrome and those found in intraoral psoriasis, benign migratory glossitis, and "ectopic geographic tongue" of the buccal mucosa. These lesions have been grouped together and termed psoriatiform. However, it is unknown whether these conditions are related.

It is necessary to include erythema multiforme and Behçet's syndrome in the differential diagnosis of the introral lesions of Reiter's syndrome. Erythema multiforme is characterized by greater involvement of the lips and the presence of target lesions on the skin. The lesions of Behçet's syndrome are painful aphthous ulcerations.

DENTAL MANAGEMENT. The oral lesions associated with Reiter's syndrome usually do not require treatment because they are painless and self-limiting.

BIBLIOGRAPHY

Arnet, G.F.: Reiter's syndrome: report of a case, J. Oral Surg. **38**(5):382, 1976.

Pendborg, J.J., Gorlin, R.J., and Ashoc-Hansen, G.: Reiter's syndrome, Oral Surg. **16**:551, 1963.

Weathers, D.R., and others: Psoriasiform lesions of the oral mucosa (with emphasis on "ectopic geographic tongue"), Oral Surg. **37**(6):872, 1974.

BEHÇET'S SYNDROME
Martin S. Greenberg

CLINICAL MANIFESTATIONS. Behçet's syndrome is a disease of unknown cause that has been classically described as a triad of oral ulcers, genital ulcers, and inflammatory disease of the eye. Vasculitis is the predominant pathologic lesion, and involvement of multiple organ systems including the joints, the blood vessels, and the gastrointestinal tract have been reported frequently. The incidence of the disease is highest in Japan and the Middle East, but cases have been found worldwide, including Great Britain and North America.

The reports of involvement of multiple organ systems has led to confusion regarding the diagnosis of Behçet's syndrome. To alleviate this confusion, Mason and Barnes have listed the major and minor manifestations of the disease. The major manifestations include oral ulcerations, genital ulcerations, and ocular involvement. Minor manifestations include arthritis, thrombophlebitis, and gastrointestinal lesions. Diagnosis is based on the presence of three major manifestations or two major and two minor manifestations.

The most common site involved in Behçet's syndrome is the oral mucosa, with 90% of the patients reporting recurring oral ulcerations. The severity of the oral involvement varies considerably from patient to patient and may resemble the small lesions of recurring aphthous stomatitis or the large, scarring, disabling lesions of major aphthous ulcers (Sutton's disease). The characteristic skin lesion is a pustule that may occur spontaneously or be precipitated by trauma. One diagnostic feature of the disease is the formation within 1 day of a pustule at the site of a needle stick.

Involvement of the eye may take many forms. The lesions may include conjunctivitis or uveitis, involvement of the retinal vessels, or glaucoma. These lesions may be reversible or lead to permanent blindness.

Arthritis most frequently involves the large joints, which clinically appear to be red and swollen. The arthritis is reversible and rarely leads to permanent disability. Ulcerative colitis may appear as a manifestation of the disease, and involvement of the blood vessels can cause thrombophlebitis, aneurysms, or gangrene. A particularly distressing sign of Behçet's syndrome is the involvement of the central nervous system, which can include cranial nerve damage, spinal cord involvement, meningeal and spinal encephalitis leading to paralysis, psychiatric disease, and death.

DENTAL MANAGEMENT. Treatment of Behçet's syndrome depends on the severity of the disease. Minor oral ulcers may be treated with topical or intralesional corticosteroids. Severe disease is most frequently treated with a combination of systemic corticosteroids and immunosuppressive drug therapy. Some workers have reported beneficial results from use of transfer factor or fibrinolytic agents. These reports, however, have been equivocal. Recent reports have encouraged the use of colchicine for the treatment of Behçet syndrome. Colchicine, the commonly used antigout medication, inhibits the function of leukocytes, particularly the adhesiveness, motility, and hemotaxis of polymorphonuclear leukocytes. Complete resolution of Behçet's syndrome during colchicine treatment has been reported. Relief of symptoms and resolution of eye disorders occurred in 7 of the 12 patients with Behçet syndrome after treatment with colchicine.

BIBLIOGRAPHY

Hazen, P.G., and Michel, B.: Management of necrotizing vasculitis with colchicine, Arch. Dermatol. **115**:1303, 1979.

James, D.W., Walker, J.R., and Smith, M.J.H.: Abnormal polymorpholeucocyte chemotaxis in Behçet's syndrome, Ann. Rheum. Dis. **38**:219, 1979.

Ketch, L.L., and Buerk, C.A.: Surgical implications of Behçet's disease, Arch. Surg. **115**:759, 1980.

Mason, R.M., and Barnes, C.G.: Behçet's syndrome with arthritis, Ann. Rheum. Dis. **28**:95, 1969.

Matsumura, N., and Mizushima, Y.: Leucocyte movement and colchicine treatment in Behçet's disease, Lancet **2**:813, 1975.

LUPUS ERYTHEMATOSUS
Philip Springer

CHART MANIFESTATIONS

Chronic discoid lupus erythematosus. Oral manifestations of chronic discoid lupus erythematosus are apparent in approximately 25% of patients. The vermilion border of the lower lip and the buccal mucosa are the sites most often involved.

Lip lesions are initially erythematous but gradually become keratotic and scaly. An atrophic, red area or crusted ulcer surrounded by a keratotic border ultimately develops.

The lesion of chronic discoid lupus affecting the oral mucosa typically appears as a central red, slightly depressed atrophic area surrounded by a 2- to 4-mm wide white elevated zone of keratinization. A hyperemic area is often observed encircling the keratotic zone. Unlike lesions that form on the skin and at the vermilion border of the lip, scale formation rarely occurs in lesions of the oral mucosa. The central area may ulcerate, causing the lesion to become painful. This frequently occurs bilaterally in lesions of the buccal musosa located in the molar region. In most cases, however, the lesions remain asymptomatic.

Discoid lupus involvement of the tongue is characterized by atrophy of the papillae and occasional deep fissuring. The palatal and gingival tissues are also commonly affected. Ulcerated areas tend to heal by scar formation.

Lichen planus is clinically and histologically similar to chronic discoid lupus erythematosus (CDLE), and it is often difficult to make a differentiation. This is especially true in very early lesions. The most significant differences are the sawtooth configuration of the rete pegs in lichen planus and the pseudoepitheliomatous hyperplasia alternating with atrophy seen in chronic discoid lupus. Direct and indirect immunofluorescence may be helpful in diagnosing oral lesions of both chronic discoid and systemic lupus erythematosus.

Systemic lupus erythematosus. The typical oral lesion of systemic lupus erythematosus, as in chronic discoid lupus erythematosus, is a central atrophic area surrounded by a keratotic border. These are apparent in between 20% and 40% of patients. Increased hyperemia, edema, and peripheral spreading are seen in the oral lesions of systemic as compared to chronic discoid lupus erythematosus. There is also a greater tendency for the lesions to ulcerate and bleed. Lesions may involve the lips, hard palate, buccal mucosa, and tongue. An increase in oral lesions is observed during exacerbations of the systemic disease.

Other oral manifestations include petechiae, especially evident on the hard palate, and small superficial ulcerations surrounded by a red halo. The presence of petechiae may be attributable to the thrombocytopenia associated with the disease.

DENTAL MANAGEMENT

Chronic discoid lupus erythematosus. If the oral lesions of chronic discoid lupus erythematosus are painful, they can be treated by topical steroids under an occlusive dressing. Intralesional or systemic administration of steroids is also beneficial.

Systemic lupus erythematosus. The dental management of patients with systemic lupus erythematosus must take into consideration the systemic complications associated with the disease process in addition to problems attributable to steroid therapy.

Basic laboratory tests can aid the dentist in assessing the severity of systemic involvement. These include a complete blood count with differential to determine the extent of hemolytic anemia and leukopenia. A platelet count should be ordered because of the possibility of thrombocytopenia. Kidney function should be evaluated by BUN and creatinine levels.

The leukopenia, the decreased phagocytic ability of leukocytes, and the immunosuppressive action of high-dose systemic steroid therapy cause these patients to be more susceptible to infection. It is therefore advantageous to prophylactically administer antibiotics before an oral surgery procedure.

Systemic steroid therapy may lead to adrenal suppression. In order to prevent stress crisis, it is advisable to supplement the steroid dosage for oral surgery and other stress-producing dental procedures.

Bleeding problems are usually related to a thrombocytopenia. If more than 50,000 platelets/mm are present, it is usually safe to perform routine dental procedures, including extractions.

BIBLIOGRAPHY

Andreasen, J.O.: Oral manifestations in discoid and systemic lupus erythematosus—clinical investigation, Acta Odontol. Scand. **22**(3):295, 1964.

Mesa, M.: Oral discoid lupus erythematosus—a case report and review of the literature, J. Periodontal. **50**(2):90, 1974.

Nisengard, R.J., and others: Diagnostic importance of immunofluorescence in oral bullous diseases and lupus erythematosus, Oral Surg. **40**(3):365, 1975.

Samuelson, S.J., Friedlander, A.H., and Swerdloff, M.: Systemic lupus erythematosus, J. Am. Dent. Assoc, **100**:553, 1980.

Schiødt, M., and Pindborg, J.J.: Histologic differential diagnostic problems for oral discoid lupus erythematosus, Int. J. Oral Surg. **5**(5):250, 1976.

SYSTEMIC SCLEROSIS
Philip Springer

CLINICAL MANIFESTATIONS. The most common dental findings in systemic sclerosis are rigidity and thinness of the lips. In addition to contributing to the masklike, expressionless appearance of patients with the disease, the circumoral fibrosis causes puckering and pallor when an attempt is made to open the mouth wide. The collagenization may progress to produce a microstomia. This inability of the patient to open his mouth may hinder oral hygiene, mastication, speech, and placement of prostheses.

The diffuse hyperpigmentation of the skin commonly seen in systemic sclerosis rarely involves the oral mucous membrane. The mucous membrane may become ulcerated by the teeth as pressure intensifies. Inhibition of the reparative process following trauma to the oral mucosa has been reported.

Involvement of the tongue in systemic sclerosis may cause a decrease in mobility and diminished size.

A radiographic finding that has been classically associated with systemic sclerosis is widening of the periodontal ligament spaces, usually in posterior teeth. This finding, however, appears to be highly variable. One report noted thickening of the periodontal ligament in only 7% of 127 cases, whereas another found it in 37% of 35 patients studied. The investigators in the latter study theorized that the much higher incidence they noted may have resulted from the use of different criteria or the increased severity of the disease process in the patient population they studied. The first study also noted a decrease in the lamina dura of affected teeth whereas the second usually did not. Teeth in patients with systemic sclerosis who had thickening of the periodontal ligament tend to remain firm.

Additional radiographic changes that have been reported include resorption of the angle of the mandible, the condyle, and the coronoid process. These osseous changes apparently are related to pressure atrophy or ischemia and are associated with the advanced stages of systemic sclerosis. Pathologic fractures of the mandible may result from progression of the osseous resorption.

Telangiectasias, a common manifestation of several forms of systemic sclerosis, are often found on the lips and in the mouth. They are histologically identical to the lesions of hereditary hemorrhagic telangiectasia. A distinction can usually be made by the additional presence of Raynaud's phenomenon and a lack of family history.

MANAGEMENT. The most common complication encountered in attempting to perform routine dentistry on patients with systemic sclerosis is the lack of access to the oral cavity because of microstomia. An attempt should therefore be made to improve the oral hygiene of the patient to prevent oral problems. The inability to open, however, may limit even basic oral cleansing.

Techniques have been devised using a sectional tray technique to permit the taking of impressions for oral prostheses.

A bilateral commissurotomy should be considered when the overall disease process appears controlled and the limitation of opening significantly interferes in mastication, speech, or insertion of oral prostheses.

Practitioners performing surgical procedures should be cognizant of the serious bleeding problem that can occur when oral telangiectasias are inadvertently involved.

BIBLIOGRAPHY

Brown, A.E.: The CRST syndrome (calcinosis, Raynaud's phenomenon, sclerodactyly and telangiectasias), Br. J. Oral Surg. **14**(2):137, 1976.

Caplan, H.I., and Benny, R.A.: Total osteolysis of the mandibular condyle in progressive systemic sclerosis, Oral Surg. **46**(3):362, 1978.

Green, D.: Scleroderma and its oral manifestations, Oral Surg. **15**:1312, 1962.

Sanders, B., McKelvy, B., and Cruickshank, G.: Correction of microstomia secondary to sclerodermatomyositis, J. Oral Surg. **35**:57, 1977.

Seifert, M.H., Stergerwald, J.C., and Cliff, M.M.: Bone resorption of the mandible in progressive systemic sclerosis, Arthritis Rheum. **18**:507, 1975.

Smith, D.B.: Scleroderma: its oral manifestations, Oral Surg. **11**:865, 1958.

Stafne, E.C., and Austin, L.T.: A characteristic dental finding in acrosclerosis and diffuse scleroderma, Am. J. Orthod. **30**:25, 1944.

Uthman, A.A., Winkler, S., and Scott, D.J.: The scleroderma patient, J. Oral Med. **33**(2):65, 1978.

White, S.C., and others: Oral radiographic changes in patients with progressive systemic sclerosis, J. Am. Dent. Assoc. **94**:1178, 1977.

POLYMYOSITIS-DERMATOMYOSITIS
Philip Springer

CLINICAL MANIFESTATIONS. Weakness of the posterior pharyngeal muscles and tongue may cause dysphagia, dysphonia, and occasionally dysarthria in patients with dermatomyositis. In addition, difficulty chewing can result from weakness of the muscles of mastication and facial muscles.

A generalized stomatitis, including a gingivitis and glossitis, has been observed in dermatomyositis in approximately one third of patients. A diffuse erythema of the mucous membranes with occasional telangiectasias has been reported. The tongue sometimes appears denuded of papillae. Vesicles surrounded by an erythematous halo, similar to aphthous ulcerations, may be seen involving the palate, gingiva, and tongue. The lips and palate may be affected by erosive areas that heal by scar formation. Eating and swallowing may become increasingly difficult in dermatomyositis when the painful stomatitis occurs in patients already complaining of dysphagia related to muscle weakness.

DENTAL MANAGEMENT. Adrenal suppression secondary to steroid therapy is the primary complication that needs to be considered before treating a patient with dermatomyositis. Augmentation of the steroid dose may be required for stress-producing oral surgery and dental procedures. An increased risk of infection must also be given attention in cases where cytotoxic agents such as methotrexate are administered.

BIBLIOGRAPHY

Keil, H.: The manifestations in the skin and mucous membranes in dermatomyositis with special reference to the differential diagnosis from systemic lupus erythematosus, Ann. Intern. Med. **16**:828, 1942.

Metheny, J.A.: Dermatomyositis: a vocal and swallowing disease entity, Laryngoscope **88**(Pt. 1):147, 1978.

Pearson, C.M., and Bohan, A.: The spectrum of polymyositis and dermatomyositis, Med. Clin. North Am. **61**(2):439, 1977.

WEGENER'S GRANULOMATOSIS
Philip Springer

Oral complications are commonly associated with Wegener's granulomatosis. In addition to inflammation and ulceration of the oral mucosa, a characteristic hyperplastic gingivitis has been reported. This has been described as red, friable, and granulomatous. An appearance similar to an over-ripe strawberry has been noted. Alveolar bone loss has been mentioned in several case reports. The gingival involvement diminishes following cytotoxic therapy in responsive patients.

The dentist may play an important role in the early detection of Wegener's granulomatosis by associating the oral manifestations with the systemic changes of mild anemia, leukocytosis, thrombocytosis, and elevated erythrocyte sedimentation rate.

BIBLIOGRAPHY

Israelson, H., Binnie, W.H., and Hurt, W.C.: The hyperplastic gingivitis of Wegener's granulomatosis, J. Periodontol. **52**(2):81, 1981.

Kakehasi, S., and others: Wegener's granulomatosis—Report of a case involving the gingiva, Oral Surg. **19**:120, 1965.

Scoth, J., and Finch, L.D.: Wegener's granulomatosis presenting as gingivitis: review of the clinical and pathologic features and report of a case, Oral Surg. **34**:920, 1972.

MIDLINE GRANULOMA
Philip Springer

The oral presentation of midline granuloma has been described as a progressive ulceration and sloughing of soft tissue with osseous destruction. A fetid odor is characteristic and pain is usually not a major complaint.

The nonhealing granulomatosis frequently involves the hard palate as the lesion spreads from the maxillary sinus or floor of the nose. Midline granuloma has also been reported affecting the gingiva, buccal mucosa, tongue, and pharynx.

Cases of midline granuloma have first been recognized following tooth extraction. This may be related to an apparent acceleration of the lesion's destructive process after trauma or surgery.

BIBLIOGRAPHY

Fechner, R.E., and Lamppin, D.W.: Midline malignant reticulosis: a clinicopathologic entity, Arch. Otolaryngol. **95**: 467, 1972.

Jarrett, J.E., and Lehman, R.H.: Lethal midline granuloma: a review of the literature, Rocky Mt. Med. J. **68**:40, 1971.

MacKinnon, D.M.: Lethal midline granuloma of the face and larynx, J. Laryngol. Otol. **84**:1193, 1970.

SARCOIDOSIS
Philip Springer

CLINICAL MANIFESTATIONS. The most commonly reported involvement of structures associated with the oral cavity in patients with sarcoidosis include asymptomatic cervical lymphadenopathy and parotid gland enlargement. In a postmortem study of 31 confirmed cases of sarcoidosis, cervical lymphadenopathy was evident in 78% and unilateral or bilateral parotid gland swelling existed in 35% of the subjects.

Parotid gland enlargement, uveitis, seventh nerve palsy, malaise, and fever delineate the clinical picture of sarcoidosis associated with Heerfordt's syndrome. The granulomatous lesions in salivary glands may lead to xerostomia.

The occurrence of intraoral sarcoid lesions is generally considered to be rare. However, some investigators believe that these lesions are actually not uncommon but that they remain undiagnosed and unreported. The distinction between oral lesions that are simply isolated local sarcoid reactions and those that are associated with systemic sarcoidosis has been stressed by some researchers who have emphasized that corroborative clinical, radiographic, and laboratory studies are required before a diagnosis of systemic sarcoidosis can be rendered.

The lesions of the gingiva, tongue, and oral mucosa have variably been described as nodular, papular, ulcerated with elevated margins, plaquelike, or scaly. Involvement of the tongue may lead to gross enlargement, pain, and difficulty in speech and swallowing.

Sarcoid involvement of the maxilla and mandible has also been reported. Punched-out radiolucencies have been noted radiographically. Increased tooth mobility and failure of extraction sites to heal have been attributed to intrabony sarcoid lesions.

Biopsy of normal-appearing oral tissue as an aid in confirming the diagnosis of sarcoidosis has been espoused. Cahn and his associates performed punch biopsies of normal-appearing palatal tissue. In 10 of the 23 samples they noted the characteristic nodules indicative of sarcoid and in 56% of the cases a degenerative change was noted in the minor salivary glands. Tarpley and co-workers similarly biopsied the normal-appearing mucosal surface of the lower lip and noted changes in the minor salivary glands in 3 of 5 samples consistent with sarcoidosis.

DENTAL MANAGEMENT. The clinical dental management of patients with sarcoidosis is usually unremarkable. Adrenal suppression may need to be assessed in those patients being treated with steroids. A saliva substitute may be beneficial in cases of xerostomia related to sarcoid involvement of the salivary glands. Intraoral lesions are usually excised, especially if their presence interferes with speech, mastication, or deglutition.

BIBLIOGRAPHY

Cahn, L.R., and others: Biopsies of normal appearing palates in patients with known sarcoidosis, Oral Surg. **18:**342, 1964.
Gold, R.S., and Sager, E.: Oral sarcoidosis: review of the literature, J. Oral Surg. **34:**237, 1976.
Greer, R.O., and Sanger, R.G.: Primary intraoral sarcoidosis, J. Oral Surg. **35:**507, 1977.
Hamner, J.E., and Scofield, H.H.: Cervical lymphadenopathy and parotid gland swelling in sarcoidosis: a study of 31 cases, J. Am. Dent. Assoc. **74**(5):1224, 1967.
Hoggins, G.J., and Allan, D.: Sarcoidosis of the maxillary region, Oral Surg. **28:**623, 1969.
Orlian, A.I., and Birnbaum, M.: Intraoral localized sarcoid lesion, Oral Surg. **49**(4):341, 1980.
Tarpley, T.M., and others: Minor salivary gland involvement in sarcoidosis: report of 3 cases with positive lip biopsies, Oral Surg. **33:**755, 1972.
Thomas, R.F., Merkow, L., and White, N.S.: Sarcoidosis with involvement of the mandibular condyle, J. Oral Surg. **34:**1026, 1976.
Tillman, H.H.: Sarcoidosis with unsuspected oral manifestations: report of a case, Oral Surg. **18:**130, 1964.
Tillman, H.H., Taylor, R.G., and Carchidi, J.E.: Sarcoidosis of the tongue: report of a case, Oral Surg. **21:**190, 1966.
Watts, K.D.: Sarcoid of the gingivae: a case report, Br. J. Oral Surg. **6:**108, 1968.

PAGET'S DISEASE OF THE JAWS
Philip Springer

CLINICAL MANIFESTATION. Jaw involvement in Paget's disease is common. In a review of 138 patients with polyostotic osteitis deformans, 23 cases, a 16.6% incidence, were observed in which lesions of the jaws were apparent. Of the 23 cases, 20 occurred in the maxilla and three in the mandible. The increased frequency of the disease affecting the maxilla has subsequently been confirmed by other investigators. Jaw involvement is usually symmetric, although unilateral lesions have been reported.

The characteristic osteolytic, osteoblastic, and combined phases are evident in Paget's disease of the jaws. The initial demineralization is reflected by an increased trabeculation and ground-glass appearance of bone. Radiolucent, ill-defined demineralized areas may also be apparent. The osteoblastic and combined phases produce the well-known cotton-wool appearance associated with the disease. Bone during the final "burnt-out" stage is extremely dense and radiopaque.

A gradual encroachment by Paget's bone on the teeth may occur. Radiographic changes include a gradual loss of lamina dura, hypercementosis, and occasional calcification of pulp chambers. Increased periapical radiopacities have been noted associated with involved teeth, with little or no differentiation between tooth and bone. A case of Paget's disease of the mandible has been reported in which three teeth required extraction because of progressive resorption of the roots by the disease process.

The early osseous changes typical of Paget's disease may be apparent during a routine dental radiographic examination, and the dentist may therefore frequently be the first practitioner capable of detecting the disease. Similarly, dentists can play an important role in the diagnosis of unrecognized skeletal disease. Among the early presenting complaints of patients with osteitis deformans are changes interfering with wearing of dentures, spreading of teeth, and bone pain simulating facial neuralgia.

The primary oral manifestation of Paget's disease is a gradual enlargement of the maxilla and mandible. This osseous enlargement in the edentulous patient often causes an inability to wear existing dentures. In patients with teeth, the expansion of the jaws results in spreading and flaring of the dentition and the production of an abnormal occlusal pattern. The palate typically appears flattened. Surgical alveolectomy may be performed to recontour the expanded jaws in selected cases.

The new bone that is laid down during the osteoblastic stage is soft and extremely vascular. The overlying mucosa in affected areas tends to feel warmer than in normal regions because of extensive arteriovenous communications.

DENTAL MANAGEMENT. Bleeding is the most important complication encountered in performing oral surgery during the early stage of Paget's disease. Nonhealing extraction sites, bone exposure, and osteomyelitis commonly occur during the late stages of the disease. The use of antibiotics before, during, and after surgical procedures has been advocated to minimize the risk of osteomyelitis. Excision has been recommended if sequestration should occur.

An interesting observation has been made that enlargement of the jaws appears to be inhibited when the freeway space becomes obliterated. It has been hypothesized that accurate dentures, worn all the time, may be able to contain jaw expansion.

BIBLIOGRAPHY

Akin, R.K., Barton, K., and Walters, P.J.: Paget's disease of bone: a case report, Oral Surg. **39**(5):707, 1975.

Kirby, J.W., and Robinson, M.E.: Osteitis deformans of the maxilla: report of atypical case, J. Oral Surg. **31**:64, 1973.

McGowan, D.A.: Clinical problems in Paget's disease affecting the jaws, Br. J. Oral Surg. **11**:230, 1974.

Murphy, J.B., Segelman, A., and Doku, C.: Osteitis deformans: report of a long-standing case with extensive oral involvement, Oral Surg. **46**:(6):765, 1978.

Ripp, G.A.: A complication after extractions in a patient with advanced Paget's disease, Oral Surg. **33**:35, 1972.

Smith, N.H.H.: Monostotic Paget's disease of the mandible presenting with progressive resorption of the teeth, Oral Surg. **46**(2):247, 1978.

Spika, C.J., and Callahan, K.R.: A review of the differential diagnosis of the oral manifestations in early osteitis deformans, Oral Surg. **11**:809, 1958.

Stafne, E.C., and Austin, L.T.: A study of dental roentgenograms in cases of Paget's disease (osteitis deformans), osteitis fibrosa, cystica, and osteoma, J. Am. Dent. Assoc. **25**:1202, 1938.

Tillman, H.H.: Paget's disease of bone: a clinical radiographic and histopathologic study of twenty-four cases involving the jaws, Oral Surg. **15**:1225, 1962.

OSTEOPOROSIS
Philip Springer

CLINICAL MANIFESTATIONS. The mandible, in addition to the long bones and vertebrae, may exhibit changes related to generalized osteoporosis. Although most patients with osteoporosis do not suffer from an underlying systemic disease, certain disorders cause a decrease in mineral density that may become apparent in the mandible and alveolar bone. For this reason, changes in the mandible and alveolar bone can be an important means of recognizing disease states.

Osteoporosis of the mandible is usually manifested by a decrease in trabeculation. However, a decrease in mineral content of between 30% and 50% is required before diminished bone density becomes apparent on dental radiographs.

It has been shown that the densities of the mandible and radius are similarly affected by age; both show a comparable decrease in mineral density with increasing age.

Most of the systemic disorders causing secondary osteoporosis produce in the mandible, as in other bones, a decrease in trabeculation. The demineralization associated with hyperparathyroidism may cause a ground-glass appearance of bone and a loss of lamina dura.

The effect of osteoporosis on alveolar bone has been investigated. Ward and Manson noted no correlation between the amount of alveolar bone loss and the extent of osteoporosis as measured by the metacarpal index. Driezen found that steroid-induced osteoporosis involved the alveolar bone as well as the vertebral and appendicular skeleton. Carranza observed marked osteoporosis with decreased trabeculation in interradicular bone in animals fed a protein-deficient diet.

DENTAL MANAGEMENT. Periodic, routine dental radiographs provide a means to compare density changes in the mandible over a period of time. Further investigation is required when precipitous osteoporosis occurs that cannot be correlated with the aging process. A detailed review of systems is essential in following up on suspicious changes. A complete blood count with differential and serum calcium, phosphorus, and alkaline phosphatase levels should be determined to rule out endocrine, metabolic, or hematologic disorders. A bone biopsy may be helpful.

BIBLIOGRAPHY

Carranza, F.A., and others: Histometric analysis of interradicular bone in protein deficient animals, J. Periodont. Res. **4**:292, 1969.

Dreizen, S., Levy, B., and Bernick, S.: Studies on the biology of the periodontium of marmosets: cortisone induced periodontal and skeletal changes in adult cotton top marmosets, J. Periodontol. **42**:217, 1971.

Hemikson, P., and Wallenius, K.: The mandible and osteoporosis, J. Oral Rehab. **1**:67, 1974.

Ward, V.J., and Manson, J.D.: Alveolar bone loss in periodontal disease and the metacarpal index, J. Periodontol. **44**:763, 1973.

Warman, R.: Osteoporosis, J. Oral Med. **32**(4):113, 1977.

FIBROUS DYSPLASIA OF THE JAWS
Martin S. Greenberg

CLINICAL MANIFESTATIONS. Fibrous dysplasia involving the jaws has long been a controversial topic and many conflicting classification systems exist because of various theories of causation. The major reason for controversy is the fact that lesions may originate from dental and periodontal structures as well as from bone. Fibro-osseous lesions of the jaw have been divided into two categories: those originating from the periodontal membrane and those originating from medullary bone. Periodontal membrane lesions include cementoma and ossifying fibroma. Medullary bone lesions include cherubism, giant cell tumor, Paget's disease of bone, and fibrous dysplasia.

There is great clinical variability in the presentation of fibrous dysplasia of the jaws. Lesions occur more frequently in the maxilla than in the mandible. Most mandibular lesions occur in the angle of the jaw. Monostotic fibrous dysplasia lesions occur 20 times more frequently in the jaws than the polyostotic form of the disease. Clinical signs are related to a slow expansion of the jaw, usually on the buccal surface. Lesions may cause movement of teeth and resorption of roots. Approximately 1% of fibrous dysplasia lesions undergo malignant transformation. This is significantly higher if the lesion was treated with radiation.

Radiographic findings depend on the proportion of fibrous tissue to osseous tissue in the particular lesion encountered. Therefore radiographic findings may range from a cystlike appearance to diffuse sclerotic bone. Many lesions have a mixture of both radiolucency and radiopacity. Diagnosis is based on a combination of clinical, radiographic, and histologic findings. Suspected lesions of fibrous dysplasia should be biopsied.

Treatment of fibrous dysplasia of the jaw varies according to the severity. If there is minimal deformity no treatment is indicated, since the lesion may regress after puberty. In the case of deforming lesions, surgery is indicated. The type of surgery will depend on the histologic stage of the lesion. Curettage is indicated for osteolytic lesions while a superficial cosmetic recontouring or "shave" is usually performed for the solid osseous lesions. Radiotherapy is contraindicated because of the increased incidence of malignant transformation.

DENTAL MANAGEMENT. Dental management of patients with monostotic fibrous dysplasia provides no particular problem for restorative dentistry. However, the dentist should contact the patient's physician in cases of polyostotic dysplasia since this form of the disease may be associated with endocrinopathies, particularly hyperthyroidism or Cushing's syndrome.

BIBLIOGRAPHY

El Deeb, M., and others: Fibrous dysplasia of the jaws: report of five cases, Oral Surg. **47:**312, 1979.

El Deeb, M., Waite, D.E., and Gorlin, R.J.: Congenital monostotic fibrous dysplasia—a new possibly autosomal recessive disorder, J. Oral Surg. **37:**520, 1979.

Hamner, J.E., Scofield, H.H., and Cornyn, J.: Benign fibro-osseous jaw lesions of periodontal membrane origin: an analysis of 249 cases, Cancer **22:**861, 1968.

Obisesan, A.A., and others: The radiologic features of fibrous dysplasia of the craniofacial bone, Oral Surg. **44:**949, 1977.

Waldon, C.A., and Giansanti, J.S.: Benign fibro-osseous lesions of the jaws: a clinical-radiologic-histologic review of sixty-five cases. II. Benign fibro-osseous lesions of periodontal ligament origin, Oral Surg. **35:**340, 1973.

Zimmerman, D.C., Dahlen, D.C., and Stafne, E.C.: Fibrous dysplasia of the maxilla and mandible, Oral Surg. **11:**55, 1958.

OSTEOMYELITIS OF THE JAWS
Philip Springer

The inflammation of bone and marrow associated with osteomyelitis of the jaws usually occurs secondary to a bacterial dental infection. *Staphylococcus aureus, S. albus,* and varieties of *Streptococcus* are the microorganisms most commonly isolated from the involved bone. Both the maxilla and the mandible can be affected by osteomyelitis, but the mandible is more susceptible because of its discrete blood supply.

Osteomyelitis may be acute or chronic and produce suppurative, sclerosing, or proliferative responses in the jaws. The response that is seen depends on the pathogenicity of the organism, the extent of the infection, and the resistance of the patient.

Although osteomyelitis of the maxilla and mandible usually occurs in otherwise healthy individuals, certain patients may be more prone to its occurrence. Individuals with sickle cell disease, diabetes, and the bone disorders of osteopetrosis and Paget's disease are more susceptible. In addition, patients who have undergone radiation therapy for head and neck malignancies increasingly risk the occurrence of osteomyelitis of the mandible because of the severely compromised blood supply. Steroids and immunosuppressive drugs may also increase susceptibility to osteomyelitis by decreasing the ability of the host to limit infection.

The acute suppurative form of osteomyelitis of the mandible and maxilla is usually accompanied by severe pain, increased body temperature, soft tissue swelling, cervical lymphadenopathy, and an increase in white blood cells. Paresthesia of the area innervated by the mental nerve is a common finding in acute osteomyelitis of the mandible. The paresthesia is probably caused by a compression of the neurovascular bundle.

DENTAL MANAGEMENT. Chronic varieties of osteomyelitis are usually associated with milder symptoms or may be totally asymptomatic. Acute exacerbations may occur.

Treatment of acute osteomyelitis of the jaws usually involves drainage, debridement of necrotic bone when indicated, and antibiotic therapy. Cephalosporins have become popular in the treatment of osteomyelitis because of their broad-spectrum coverage and excellent penetrance. Antibiotics are usually continued at least 4 to 6 weeks after the patient becomes asymptomatic.

The recent use of hyperbaric oxygen therapy in conjunction with antibiotics has proved to be extremely beneficial in treating chronic cases of osteomyelitis of the mandible and maxilla. Several patients who had chronic diffuse sclerosing osteomyelitis were treated with prednisone and achieved excellent resolution of symptoms.

BIBLIOGRAPHY

Austin, G., Deasy, M., and Walsh, R.F.: Osteomyelitis associated with routine endodontic and periodontal therapy: a case report, J. Oral Med. **33**(4):120, 1978.

Barnard, J.D.: Osteomyelitis of the jaws as a sequel to dental local anaesthetic injections, Br. J. Oral Surg. **13**(3):264, 1976.

Ellis, D.J., Winslow, J.R., and Indovina, A.A.: Garre's osteomyelitis of the mandible: report of a case, Oral Surg. **44**(2):183, 1977.

Gallo, W.J., Shapiro, D.N., and Moss, M.: Suppurative candidiosis: review of the literature and report of case, J. Am. Dent. Assoc., 1976.

Girasole, R.V., and Lyon, E.D.: Sickle cell osteomyelitis of the mandible: report of three cases, J. Oral Surg. **35:**231, 1977.

Goldstein, B.H., Byrne, J.E., and Miller, A.S.: Chronic sclerosing osteomyelitis—Part I, J. Oral Surg. **37:**52, 1979.

Goldstein, B.H., Byrne, J.E., and Miller, A.S.: Chronic sclerosing osteomyelitis—Part 2, J. Oral Surg. **37:**101, 1979.

Goupil, M.T., and others: Hyperbaric oxygen in the adjunctive treatment of chronic osteomyelitis of the mandible: report of a case, J. Oral Surg. **36**(2):138, 1978.

Jacobsson, S., and Hollender, L.: Treatment and prognosis of diffuse sclerosing osteomyelitis (DSO) of the mandible, Oral Surg. **49**(1):7, 1980.

Jacobsson, S., and others: Chronic sclerosing osteomyelitis of the mandible, Oral Surg. **45**(2):167, 1978.

Nakajima, T., and others: Surgical treatment of chronic osteomyelitis of the mandible resistant to intraarterial infusion of antibiotics: report of case, J. Oral Surg. **35**:823, 1977.

Rabe, W.C., Angelillo, J.C., and Leipert, D.W.: Chronic sclerosing osteomyelitis: treatment considerations in an atypical case, Oral Surg. **49**(2):117, 1980.

Sanders, B.: Current concepts in the management of osteomyelitis of the mandible, J. Oral Med. **33**(2):40, 1978.

Sanders, B., McKelvy, B., and Adams, D.: Aseptic osteomyelitis and necrosis of the mandibular condylar head after intracapsular fracture, Oral Surg. **43**(5):665, 1977.

Shafer, W.G., Hine, M.K., and Levy, B.M.: A textbook of oral pathology, Philadelphia, 1974, W.B. Saunders Co.

Young, J., and Bump, R.: Hyperbaric oxygenation: prosthodontic responsibilities, J. Prosth. Dent. **39**(1):100, 1978.

Section Four

MICROBIAL DISEASES

edited by **Donald Kaye**

35 • INTRODUCTION TO MICROBIAL DISEASES

Donald Kaye

Infections can be categorized both by type of organism producing the infection (for example, virus, bacteria, protozoa) and by site of infection (for example, pneumonia, meningitis, urinary tract infection). This section uses both a microorganism and a site of infection approach.

FEVER AND CHILLS

Fever is the most common manifestation of infection, but fever can be produced by many other conditions such as vascular events (for example, pulmonary embolus and myocardial infarction), diseases of immunity (for example, drug fever and connective tissue disorders), neoplasms (especially lymphomas and solid tumors), trauma, and metabolic diseases (for example, thyroid crisis and an acute gouty attack).

Shaking chills occur with wide swings in temperature and precede the rises in temperature. Chills occur more often in bacterial than viral infections, but they also occur in fevers unrelated to infection. Aspirin and other antipyretics tend to precipitate chills by causing a sudden drop in temperature, which is followed by a sudden rise in temperature. Fever may be accompanied by symptoms such as myalgias or arthralgias, or it may be asymptomatic and go unnoticed by the patient.

Fever is ordinarily harmless to the patient and does not require therapy. Exceptions are temperatures over 106° F (41°C), fever in patients with borderline cardiac compensation, fever that causes delirium, fever in patients with thrombocytopenia, and fever that produces seizures. In these circumstances the body temperature should be reduced by using cool body baths, a cooling blanket, antipyretics such as aspirin, or, if necessary, corticosteroids. Antipyretics and corticosteroids must be used cautiously in the presence of very high fever, since the rapid drop in temperature can cause hypotension.

Fever may be of several different characteristic types: sustained (seen in typhoid fever and pneumococcal pneumonia); intermittent or spiking, with wide swings of temperature reaching normal each day (seen in abscesses and miliary tuberculosis); remittent, with a return toward normal but not reaching normal each day (seen in many febrile illnesses); and relapsing, in which the temperature becomes normal for 1 or more days between episodes of fever (seen in malaria, tick- or louse-borne relapsing fever, and Pel-Ebstein fever in Hodgkin's disease).

Patients with infection may be afebrile or even hypothermic. Chronic or indolent infections may not be associated with fever. Shock and hypothermia may be seen in acute life-threatening infections (for example, bacteremia caused by gram-negative bacilli); this is most likely to occur in infants, the elderly, and the immunocompromised host. Patients with renal failure tend to be hypothermic. Although the temperature rises with infection, it may not reach "febrile" levels.

DIAGNOSIS OF MICROBIAL DISEASES

The history and physical examination usually lead to a presumptive diagnosis. For example, cough, rales, and signs of pulmonic consolidation together suggest pneumonia. However, laboratory studies are needed to confirm the diagnosis (by direct isolation or by indirect demonstration of the presence of the pathogen) and, at times, may be the only clues to diagnosis (for example, positive blood cultures in fever from infective endocarditis with no abnormal physical findings).

LABORATORY EVALUATION

Some of the laboratory tests commonly available for diagnosis of microbial infections are listed below:
1. Complete blood count with examination of the smear
2. Erythrocyte sedimentation rate
3. Urinalysis with Gram stain
4. Microscopic examination with cell counts and/or smears of any exudate, effusions, indicated body fluid, lesion, or stool. Occasionally biopsies are necessary. Smears may be unstained as for *Treponema pallidum* (darkfield), Gram stained for bacteria, acid-fast stained for mycobacteria, stained

with fluorescent antibody, or stained with other special stains.
5. Cultures of blood, exudate, lesion, effusion, indicated body fluids, or occasionally mucosal surface (for example, group A streptococcal pharyngitis or gonorrhea); biopsies occasionally necessary for material to culture
6. Acute and convalescent serum specimens for study for a change in antibody titer to suspected infecting organisms; serologic test for syphilis
7. Antigen detection by counter immunoelectrophoresis or other techniques (for example, for *Haemophilus influenzae,* pneumococci, meningococci, or cryptococci in spinal fluid)
8. Skin tests (for example, tuberculosis)
9. Chest roentgenogram and other roentgenography and scans (radioactive, ultrasound, computed tomography) as determined by localized findings
10. Liver chemistries

The use of these tests will be directed by the findings on history and physical examination and by the course of the disease. The tests and their interpretation are discussed in the appropriate sections. However, some general comments are made here.

A blood count may be helpful in suggesting bacterial, viral, or helminthic infection. Leukocytosis with a shift to the left of the white cell series suggests bacterial infection; the presence of atypical lymphocytes suggests viral infection; and eosinophilia suggests helminthic infection. However, the white count may be normal (or there may even be leukopenia) in bacterial infection, and leukocytosis may occur in viral infections. The blood smear may show parasites in red cells (malaria) or bacteria in white cells (overwhelming meningococcemia or pneumococcemia). The erythrocyte sedimentation rate (ESR) serves as a screening test for inflammation; it is usually elevated in bacterial infections and often normal in viral illnesses. However, a normal ESR does not rule out bacterial infection nor does an elevated ESR rule out viral illness.

The major laboratory tools are microscopic examination of smears, cultures, and serologic studies for the etiologic agent. Exudates, effusions, lesions, body fluids, and so forth are studied as determined by the history and physical findings (for example, examination of sputum in a patient with cough or examination of fluid from a vesicle in a patient with vesicles). It is best to obtain specimens for smear and culture from closed spaces such as a joint or deep abscess rather than from an open surface where contamination is likely.

Appropriate media must be used for culture; special media and culture techniques are required for many bacteria (for example, chocolate agar with increased CO_2 for *Neisseria gonorrhoeae*). Urine should be cultured quantitatively. Anaerobic cultures should not be obtained on specimens that have been in contact with mucosal, skin, or sinus tract surfaces (for example, a draining sinus of osteomyelitis), because these surfaces can contain large numbers of anaerobes. For example, transtracheal aspirates rather than sputum and cul de sac puncture specimens rather than vaginal specimens should be submitted for anaerobic cultures. In general, anaerobic bacteria play an important role in infections in the abdomen and pelvis, in areas contiguous with the mucosa of the mouth and nose, and in aspiration pneumonia.

Testing of serologic specimens must be directed at specific diseases. It is inappropriate to ask for "viral antibody studies," since the laboratory must know which viruses to test for. The expense and quantity of serum necessary to test for antibodies to all viruses are prohibitive. A two-dilution (fourfold or greater) rise in titer early in the disease or an equivalent fall in titer late in the disease is strongly suggestive of infection with that agent. However, usually at least 1 to 2 weeks must elapse between titers, and by that time most patients have recovered spontaneously or have been treated.

Isolation of an organism or demonstration of a high titer of antibody to that organism does *not* unequivocally indicate that the agent was responsible for the observed clinical syndrome. The laboratory findings must be interpreted in light of the history, physical findings, and course of the disease. For example, the organism isolated may be part of the patient's normal flora or may be a contaminant, and a single high titer may reflect past infection.

Skin tests may be useful for determining past exposure to an antigen but are useless in determining the presence of infection. A negative test is not evidence against present or past infection. Skin tests for mumps, *Trichophyton,* and *Candida* are positive in most normal hosts and are therefore useful in evaluating for anergy.

MANAGEMENT

Many microbial diseases (for example, most viral illnesses) are self-limited, and therapy is often not indicated. In some infections (for example, chronic osteomyelitis and asymptomatic urinary tract infection) therapy should await specific bacteriologic diagnosis. However, life-threatening infections such as pneumonia, meningitis, or bacteremia should be treated before a specific diagnosis is made. The general rule is to direct therapy at the likely pathogens based on the history, physical examination, and laboratory tests that are immediately available (for example, Gram stains and chest roentgenograms).

FEVER OF UNKNOWN ORIGIN

When the temperature reaches at least 101° F (38.3° C) for at least 2 to 3 weeks and no diagnosis is obvious after an initial hospital evaluation, the patient is considered to have a fever of unknown origin (FUO). The use of these criteria will eliminate most viral illnesses and many infections (such as pneumonia and urinary tract infection) that are diagnosable by history, physical examination, simple roentgenograms, and laboratory examinations. The most common cause of febrile illness is viral infection. Since these infections are usually self-limited and the expense and morbidity of an FUO evaluation are great, the above criteria should be met to exclude common viral illnesses before embarking on an FUO workup. The usual course of such illness is less than 2 weeks of fever; exceptions are infectious mononucleosis, cytomegalovirus infection, and hepatitis.

Many of the causes of FUO are listed below:
1. Infections
    a. Miliary tuberculosis
    b. Intra-abdominal and pelvic bacterial infections
    c. Bacteremias, including bacterial endocarditis, brucellosis, meningococcemia, and salmonella bacteremia
    d. Viral infections such as hepatitis, infectious mononucleosis, and cytomegalovirus infections
    e. Rickettsial infections such as Q fever and psittacosis
    f. Parasitic infections such as trichinosis, visceral larva migrans, strongyloidiasis, malaria, and amebiasis
2. Neoplasms
    a. Solid tumors such as those of kidney, liver, and pancreas
    b. Metastatic tumors
    c. Lymphomas, sarcomas, and leukemias
    d. Atrial myxoma
3. Connective tissue disorders such as polyarteritis, lupus erythematosus, and temporal arteritis
4. Inflammatory bowel disease such as regional enteritis and ulcerative colitis
5. Granulomatous hepatitis
6. Sarcoidosis
7. Multiple pulmonary emboli
8. Familial Mediterranean fever and other periodic fevers
9. Diseases of the central nervous system (tumor, cerebrovascular accident, hypothalamic disease, and so forth)
10. Drug fever
11. Factitious fever

The vast majority of FUOs are caused by infections (the most common are miliary tuberculosis and intra-abdominal or pelvic infections), neoplasms (most commonly lymphomas), and connective tissue disorders. Drug and factitious fevers must always be excluded.

The evaluation of an FUO involves (1) a systematic evaluation beginning with a careful history and physical examination (including a pelvic and rectal examination) followed by progressive laboratory evaluation for the statistically most likely causes and (2) a directed approach when a localized finding suggests a direct route to diagnosis. Non-invasive tests are generally performed first and invasive tests reserved for later. For example, a history of potential exposure to an infectious disease (such as skinning a rabbit [tularemia] or working as a butcher or farmer [brucellosis or Q fever]) would suggest specific studies for these infections; a very high erythrocyte sedimentation rate plus tenderness over a temporal artery would suggest early biopsy of the artery to diagnose giant cell arteritis; abnormal liver chemistries would suggest early liver biopsy to attempt a histologic diagnosis.

Laboratory approach

Some of the tests that might be required either to reach a diagnosis or to suggest a localized area of disease that could be studied further include the following:

Initial studies

1. Complete blood count with examination of the smear
2. Urinalysis
3. Microscopic examination and cultures of exudates, effusions, and indicated body fluids and excreta; blood cultures
4. Erythrocyte sedimentation rate
5. Liver chemistries
6. Serologic studies for possible infectious diseases (for example, infectious mononucleosis, cytomegalovirus infection, toxoplasmosis, brucellosis) and for connective tissue disorders (for example, antinuclear antibody and rheumatoid factor)
7. Chest roentgenogram
8. Ultrasound of the abdomen and heart valves
9. Liver-speen scan
10. Skin tests for presence or absence of delayed hypersensitivity (PPD, *Tricophyton, Candida*)
11. Stool examination for occult blood

Subsequent studies

1. Computed tomography of the abdomen, lung, and brain
2. Roentgenograms—intravenous pyelogram, cholcystogram, barium enema, upper gastrointestinal and small bowel roentgenograms, bone roentgenograms
3. Sigmoidoscopy
4. Scans—bone scan, gallium scan, lung scan, renal scan
5. Biopsies (with cultures where indicated)—liver, bone marrow, lymph node (preferably not an inguinal node), skin and muscle, any abnormal mass or lesion, and temporal artery (only in the elderly)

Other studies

1. Abdominal aortography
2. Lymphangiogram
3. Exploratory laparotomy with biopsies and cultures

The recent availability of computed tomography of the abdomen has often helped define intra-abdominal lesions early in a workup, leading to a direct surgical approach and eliminating the need for many of the tests in the preceeding outline. Blind exploratory laparotomy with no localizing findings is usually not rewarding and is no longer considered a reasonable approach to diagnosis of FUO.

Therapeutic trials are never definitive. Lysis of fever may be fortuitous and unrelated to the drug administered. However, therapeutic trials may be justified when no diagnosis can be made or when the patient is moribund and therapy cannot await a diagnosis. Regimens should be as specific as possible for the suspected pathogen. Examples are the administration of isoniazid and ethambutol to patients who may have occult tuberculosis or the administration of penicillin plus an aminoglycoside (streptomycin or gentamicin) when endocarditis is suspected.

After a complete evaluation, up to 10% of patients with FUO remain undiagnosed. Some of these patients recover spontaneously, and others continue to be febrile without a diagnosis. In some who continue to have fever, an explanation is found on subsequent evaluation or at autopsy; others remain undiagnosed even by autopsy.

BIBLIOGRAPHY

Jacoby, G.A., and Swartz, M.N.: Fever of undetermined origin. N. Engl. J. Med. **289**:1407, 1973.

Mandell, G.L., Douglas, R.G., and Bennett, J.E.: Principles and practice of infectious diseases, New York, 1979, John Wiley & Sons, Inc.

Petersdorf, R.G., and Beeson, P.B.: Fever of unexplained origin: report of 100 cases. Medicine **40**:1, 1961.

Unit A • VIRAL DISEASES

edited by **Harvey M. Friedman**

36 • INTRODUCTION, CLASSIFICATION, AND LABORATORY DIAGNOSIS

Harvey M. Friedman

Viruses are among the most common infecting organisms of humans. They range in size from 17 nm to over 300 nm and, except for certain slow viruses, contain DNA or RNA but not both. The nucleic acid is surrounded by a protein shell termed a *capsid* that is arranged in either icosahedral (cubic) or helical symmetry. Those with cubic symmetry assume the shape of regular polyhedrons with 20 triangular surfaces and 12 corners. All viruses with helical symmetry are surrounded by a lipid *envelope,* whereas some viruses with cubic symmetry are enveloped but most are *naked.* The envelop is derived in part from host cells but also contains virus-specific proteins composing both the inner membrane layer and the glycoprotein spikes that protrude from the surface. Viruses multiple only within living cells and have sufficient nucleic acid to code from 2 to approximately 50 proteins. Several steps occur preceding replication, including attachment of viruses to host cells, penetration into the cells, and uncoating to expose the viral nucleic acid. For DNA viruses the nucleic acid serves as a template for production of messenger RNA, whereas for RNA viruses single-stranded RNA serves as its own messenger. Some RNA tumor viruses of animals contain reverse transcriptase, an enzyme capable of catalyzing synthesis of DNA from an RNA template. Once formed, messenger RNA codes for viral protein using host cell polysomes. Generally, synthesis of host cell proteins is suppressed to a variable degree during viral replication. Synthesis of viral daughter nucleic acid from parental templates occurs after early viral protein synthesis. Intact *virions* are then assembled and released from the cell by lysis or by budding. During extrusion, a lipid membrane may envelop the virus and form its outer coat.

Some viruses have the ability to remain latent within host cells following infection and subsequently reappear. An example is varicella virus, which is manifested as chickenpox during the primary infection and as shingles during a recurrence. Similarly, relapsing herpes lip and genital lesions represent latent infection with exacerbations of herpes simplex virus. The mechanisms of initiating and maintaining viral latency are incompletely understood but involve complex interactions among the virus, the infected host cells, and the immune system.

Transmission of viral infections may occur by aerosal spread, direct contact, fecal-oral contamination, food- and waterborne routes, and insect or animal bites. Once introduced, viruses spread to different organs by contiguous spread, by dissemination in blood or lymphatics, or by ascension in neural tissue. For some viruses (for example, cytomegalovirus) subclinical infection is the rule, whereas for others (for example, chickenpox and measles viruses), clinical illness is the usual result. The type of virus, the titer of the inoculum, the previous immune experience of the host, and the adequacy of the immune response are all determinants of the eventual outcome of the infection.

The immune system is beneficial to the host in terminating viral infections and preventing reinfections; however, in some circumstances the immune response may also be detrimental. For example, some chronic carriers of hepatitis B virus surface antigen have circulating immune complexes composed of surface antigen and antibody to this antigen. These complexes can be deposited in glomeruli, dermal vessels, and medium-sized arteries, producing glomerulonephritis and vasculitis.

A detailed discussion of the role of the immune response to viral infections is beyond the scope of this chapter. It is likely that a complex interaction of many components of the immune system is involved in control of most if not all viral infections. For some viruses, such as enteroviruses, humoral immunity appears to be of major importance for control of infection; whereas for others, including those in the herpes family, termination of viral shedding correlates closely with the development of cellular immunity. Interferon production in vesicle fluid appears to be important in preventing dissemination of varicella-zoster virus in patients with lymphoma. In addition, several viruses have been noted to activate the complement sequence in the absence of antibody, an event that may be an important early host response to the invading virus.

Over 300 antigenically distinct viruses causing at least 50 different clinical syndromes in humans have been identified. Viruses can be classified by chemical and physical characteristics or by the diseases they produce. For the clinician the latter is probably more useful. A classification of viruses commonly associated with various types of infections is shown in Table 36-1, and a classification based on viral nucleic acid content is presented in Table 36-2. The virology chapters in this book are prepared from a clinical perspective, discussing disease syndromes and the viruses that produce them.

Attempts at specific viral diagnosis are performed for a variety of reasons, ranging from etiologic diagnosis of an acute illness to retrospective serologic surveys. In some instances the diagnosis may influence patient management; in others the ultimate benefit may be to the community at large. In recent years technical improvements have permitted the emergence of methods for rapid viral diagnosis, which have become particularly important with the advent of antiviral chemotherapies.

The four major methods for the diagnosis of viral infections include (1) microscopy of tissues or exfoliated cells, examining for viral inclusions or other changes characteristic of certain viruses; (2) isolation and identification of viruses from infected tissues; (3) serologic studies to measure virus-specific antibodies in a patient's serum; and (4) tests to detect viruses or viral antigens directly in clinical specimens without requiring cultivation of the agents in the laboratory.

Microscopic examination of fixed and stained tissues or of exfoliated cells is usually performed by pathology or cytology laboratories. These methods are rapid and useful for establishing with high probability that a particular illness is caused by a virus. However, they do not permit

Table 36-1. Viruses associated with various types of infections

Type of infection	Common viral causes
Respiratory tract	
Upper respiratory infection	Rhinoviruses
	Coronaviruses
	Respiratory syncytial virus
	Adenoviruses
	Parainfluenza viruses types 1-3
	Influenza viruses types A and B
Croup, bronchiolitis	Respiratory syncytial virus
	Parainfluenza viruses types 1-3
Pneumonia (adults)	Influenza viruses types A and B
	Cytomegalovirus
	Adenoviruses
Pneumonia (children)	Respiratory syncytial virus
	Parainfluenza viruses types 1-3
	Influenza viruses types A and B
Eye	
Conjunctivitis	Adenoviruses
	Herpes simplex virus
Central nervous system	
Aseptic meningitis	Enteroviruses
	Mumps virus
Encephalitis	St. Louis encephalitis virus
	California encephalitis virus
	Western equine encephalitis virus
	Eastern equine encephalitis virus
	Herpes simplex viruses types 1 and 2
	Mumps virus
Skin and mucous membrane	
Mouth ulcers	Herpes simplex virus type 1
	Group A coxsackieviruses
Genital ulcers	Herpes simplex virus type 2
Maculopapular rash	Measles virus
	Rubella virus
	Enteroviruses
Vesicular rash	Herpes simplex viruses types 1 and 2
	Varicella-zoster virus
Gastrointestinal tract	
Gastroenteritis	Rotaviruses
	Norwalk agent group
Hepatitis	Hepatitis A, B, non A/B
	Epstein-Barr virus
	Cytomegalovirus
Congenital infection	
Microcephaly, hepato-splenomegaly	Cytomegalovirus
	Rubella virus
	Herpes simplex viruses

Table 36-2. Classification and common clinical manifestations of viruses

Virus group	Members	Common clinical manifestations
DNA viruses		
Adenoviruses	Types 1-31	Pharyngitis, pharyngoconjunctival fever, pneumonia
Herpesviruses	Herpes simplex types 1 and 2	Gingivostomatitis (type 1), vulvovaginitis (type 2), recurrent mucocutaneous eruption (types 1, 2), keratoconjunctivitis, generalized infection of newborn, encephalitis, esophagitis
	Varicella-zoster	Chickenpox, localized and disseminated zoster
	Cytomegalovirus	Congenital infection, mononucleosis syndrome, prolonged fever, and pneumonia in immunosuppressed patients
	Epstein-Barr virus	Infectious mononucleosis, encephalomyelitis, Guillain-Barré syndrome
Poxviruses	Smallpox (variola)	Smallpox
	Vaccinia	Complications of vaccination including disseminated vaccinia and encephalitis
	Cowpox, orf	Skin lesions in humans who handle infected cows (cowpox) or sheep (orf)
	Molluscum contagiosum	Pearly white 2-mm skin nodules
Papovaviruses	Papillomavirus	Human warts
	SV40, JC virus	Progressive multifocal leukoencephalopathy
	BK virus	Undetermined
RNA viruses		
Orthomyxoviruses	Influenza A, B, C	Influenza
Paramyxoviruses	Parainfluenza 1-4	Upper respiratory infections, pharyngitis, croup, laryngitis, pneumonia
	Mumps	Mumps, aseptic meningitis, encephalitis
	Measles	Measles, encephalitis
	Respiratory syncytial virus	Bronchiolitis, pneumonia, upper respiratory infections
Picornaviruses	Rhinoviruses, over 100 types	Upper respiratory infections

	Enteroviruses
	  Polioviruses 1-3
	  Coxsackieviruses A 1-24 and B 1-6
	  Echoviruses, over 30 types
		Aseptic meningitis, myocarditis, herpangina, fever with or without maculopapular rash, paralysis (poliomyelitis)

Rhabdovirus	Rabies	Rabies
Coronaviruses	229E, OC43, B814, OC16, OC37, OC48	Upper respiratory infections
Togaviruses	Rubella	Rubella, congenital infection
	Alphavirus, flavivirus (formerly arboviruses)	Encephalitis, yellow fever, dengue, hemorrhagic fever
Arenaviruses	Lymphocytic choriomeningitis	Aseptic meningitis
	Lassa fever	Lassa fever
	Junin, Machupo	Hemorrhagic fever
Reoviruses	Reovirus	Undetermined
	Orbivirus	Colorado tick fever
	Rotaviruses	Gastroenteritis

specific identification of the agent involved. Many different organisms can demonstrate viral inclusions. In particular, the characteristic changes produced in the brain by herpes simplex and rabies viruses, in skin vesicles by varicella-zoster and herpes simplex, in cervical cells by herpes simplex, and in lung tissue by cytomegalovirus are valuable diagnostic aids.

The isolation of viruses requires living host systems and is the cornerstone of diagnostic virology. Growth and identification of viruses usually take longer than their counterparts in bacteriology, ranging from 1 day to 6 weeks. A wide variety of host systems can be used for viral isolation, including embryonated eggs, tissue culture cells, and animals. Since many of these require expensive equipment and facilities, the range of methods available depends in part on the size of the laboratory. The most widely used method involves tissue culture isolation, in which clinical specimens are inoculated into cell cultures that are then observed for changes indicative of viral growth.

Deciding which specimens to select for viral cultures depends in part on which organs are involved and which

Table 36-3. Selection of specimens for viral isolation

Clinical syndrome	Type of specimen
Upper respiratory infection, laryngitis, croup, pneumonia	Nasopharyngeal aspirate, throat swab, or sputum
Meningitis	Cerebrospinal fluid, throat swab, stool or rectal swab
Congenital infection	Throat swab, urine
Vesicular lesions including oral and genital ulcers	Swab of base of lesion
Maculopapular rash	Throat or nasopharyngeal swab

viral agents are suspected. Some suggested specimens for viral isolation are shown in Table 36-3. In general, specimens taken from diseased organs are most useful, for example, spinal fluid in meningitis cases or respiratory secretions from patients with pneumonia. Several aspects of specimen collection require emphasis:

1. All swabs must be kept moist (in transport media).
2. Body fluids such as urine, pleural fluid, and spinal fluid can be transported to the laboratory without any special transport medium.
3. A specimen should be transported to the laboratory quickly, since once outside the body most viruses have a short survival time.
4. While waiting for transport, specimens keep best if stored at 39° F (4° C).

Specimens that are commonly contaminated with bacteria such as stool, urine, or respiratory secretions are treated with broad-spectrum antibiotics before inoculation onto tissue culture monolayers. To indicate the presence of a virus, cultures are observed for alterations in cell morphology (cytopathic effect, CPE). Alternatively some viruses can be detected by attachment of erythrocytes to infected cells in monolayers (hemadsorption) or by the interference with growth of other viruses in the infected monolayers. Based on the changes noted in the cell monolayer, a presumptive identification of the type of virus can be made. Specific immunologic methods are needed to identify definitively the isolated agent. A wide variety of tests are available for definitive identification, all of which employ antisera of known titer and specificity.

Isolation of a virus indicates that the patient is infected with that agent. Whether the virus is also causing the clinical illness requires consideration of several factors. It is important to realize that viruses often cause asymptomatic infection and that some viruses persist for extended periods in the body after infection. The site from which an isolate is obtained and the recognized capacity of the virus isolated to cause disease are important considerations in assigning significance to a particular isolate. Failure to recover virus from a patient does not mean that the illness is not caused by a virus, since some human viruses are noncultivatable. More commonly, a negative result reflects improper collection methods, the obtaining of specimens too late in the illness, poor transport, or incorrect storage of the specimens.

Serology is a useful tool to define, retrospectively, the incidence of viral infections in communities; to elucidate the need for, and efficacy of, immunization programs; and to monitor for recent infection. For the last, generally two serum samples are required, one in the acute phase taken as early as possible after the onset of illness and the other in the convalescent period drawn 1 to 3 weeks later. By comparing antibody titers in the two sera, which must be tested simultaneously, a diagnosis of recent infection can be established if there is a fourfold or greater rise in antibody titers. High antibody titers alone are not a reliable guide to recent infection, but often experience permits a presumptive diagnosis to be made on the basis of a single high titer in convalescent-phase serum. A more confident diagnosis can be made by measuring virus-specific IgM antibodies in convalescent-phase serum. However, at present few clinical laboratories can measure IgM responses to a wide variety of viruses.

For antibody testing, serum is the correct sample to obtain. Blood should not be frozen, since the ensuing red blood cell lysis interferes with serologic testing. Whole blood or the separated serum can be transported to the laboratory at room temperature; however, if there is a lag between collection and transport, the sample should be refrigerated at 39° F (4° C).

A wide variety of serologic assays are available. The complement fixation (CF) test is the most widely used because of its applicability to the vast majority of viruses and because reagents are commercially available. Other common assay methods include hemagglutination, neutralization, immunofluorescence, enzyme immunoassay, and radioimmunoassay. A serologic diagnosis requires the use of known viral antigens and therefore cannot supplant virus isolation as a means of discovering new viruses.

Detection of viral antigens in clinical specimens before inoculation of tissue culture monolayers has received wide attention in recent years. This permits rapid diagnosis of infection but requires viral antigens to be present in relatively high concentrations. Electron microscopy using negative staining methods is useful for detecting viruses in stool specimens (hepatitis A, rotavirus, Norwalk agent virus), in vesicle fluids (smallpox, chickenpox, herpes simplex viruses), and in urine (cytomegalovirus). Immunologic assays using ^{125}I-radiolabeled immunoglobulins have been successfully used to detect hepatitis B surface antigen in serum. Recently viral antigens in stool, respiratory secretions, and urine have been detected using enzyme immunoassays. Perhaps the most widely used technique for rapid viral diagnosis is immunofluorescence. Cells from infected tissues are spread on glass slides and examined for virus by direct or indirect immunofluorescence using virus-specific immune reagents.

Clinical laboratories skilled in diagnostic virology are becoming more numerous. In a survey of medical schools, over 80% indicated that they perform some virologic testing. The spectrum of services offered varied from testing antibodies to a select group of viruses, to broad-scale serologic and isolation studies. With the advent of effective antiviral agents, the need for accurate, rapid, and specific viral diagnosis is apparent. Clinicians involved in the care of acutely ill patients will likely find themselves requesting viral studies with increasing frequency in the future.

BIBLIOGRAPHY

Drew, W.L.: Basic virology: classification and general concepts. In Drew, W.L., editor: Viral infections: a clinical approach, Philadelphia, 1976, F.A. Davis Co.

Gardner, P.S., and McQuillin, J., editors: Rapid virus diagnosis: application of immunofluorescence, Woburn, Mass., 1974, Butterworth, Inc.

Hawkes, R.A.: General principles underlying laboratory diagnosis of viral infections. In Lennette, E.H., and Schmidt, N.J., editors: Diagnostic procedures for viral, rickettsial and chlamydial infections, Washington, D.C., 1979, American Public Health Association.

Herrmann, E.C., Jr., and Herrmann, J.A.: Laboratory diagnosis of viral disease. In Drew, W.L., editor: Viral infections: a clinical approach, Philadelphia, 1976, F.A. Davis Co.

Luria, S.E., and others: Animal viruses: adsorption and entry into the cell, multiplication of RNA viruses, multiplication of DNA viruses and retroviruses. In Luria, S.E., and others: General virology, New York, 1978, John Wiley & Sons, Inc.

Melnick, J.L.: Taxonomy of viruses, Prog. Med. Virol. **25:**160, 1979.

Menegus, M.A., and Douglas, R.G., Jr.: Viruses, rickettsiae, chlamydiae and mycoplasmas. In Mandel, G.L., Gordon, R.G., and Bennett, J.E., editors: Principles and practice of infectious diseases, New York, 1979, John Wiley & Sons, Inc.

37 • DISEASES CAUSED BY VIRUSES

Viral infections of the fetus and newborn

Stuart E. Starr

Possible consequences of viral infections of the fetus include abortions, stillbirths, and congenital malformations. Symptomatic live-born infants may die within the first few months of life, and survivors of infection are frequently left with neurologic and other sequelae. Infected neonates who appear undamaged at birth may later develop deficits of varying severity. The spectrum of viral infections acquired at the time of birth ranges from asymptomatic to severe and life threatening.

DEFINITION. A congenital infection is one that is present at the time of birth. Natal infections are acquired at the time of birth, most commonly from maternal cervicovaginal or stool flora, whereas postnatal infections are acquired after birth. The term ''perinatal infection'' is an inclusive one designating infections occurring before, during, or shortly after the time of birth.

ETIOLOGY. Several viruses can cause infection of the fetus and newborn. Those most commonly responsible are cytomegalovirus, herpes simplex types 1 and 2, rubella, coxsackievirus B, hepatitis B, and varicella-zoster.

EPIDEMIOLOGY. Congenital rubella may occur in epidemic fashion; the last outbreak in the United States took place in 1964 and was associated with an estimated 20,000 cases. Other viruses that commonly affect the fetus or newborn are endemic in human populations. The incidence of congenital or natal infection depends on a number of factors, including maternal age and, to some extent, socioeconomic status. Postnatal infections may be acquired as a result of exposure to breast milk or blood products or as a result of contact with infected individuals, including health personnel. Seasonal variation has been noted only for coxsackievirus B infections, which tend to occur during summer months.

PATHOGENESIS. Congenital infection is thought to occur usually as a result of maternal viremia and transplacental spread of the virus to the fetus. Several effects of virus infection, including inhibition of cell division, tissue necrosis, and vasculitis, may result in fetal damage. In the congenital rubella syndrome and rarely with varicella-zoster and herpes simplex infections, pathologic changes may cause congenital malformations. The timing of the maternal infection appears to be crucial in that damage tends to be more severe when the fetus is infected during the first trimester. Possible late manifestations of tissue damage include fibrosis and calcification. Persistent infection with rubella or cytomegalovirus during the first few years of life may result in further damage to certain organs.

Possible portals of entry for natal and postnatal virus infections include the skin, eyes, and gastrointestinal tract. Acquired infections may remain localized or may disseminate to involve multiple organs. The relative immaturity of neonatal immune defense mechanisms may contribute to the severity of some infections.

CLINICAL MANIFESTATIONS

Cytomegalovirus. From 0.5% to 2.5% of all newborns are congenitally infected with cytomegalovirus, making this virus the most common known cause of congenital infection. Only around 5% of congenitally infected neonates are symptomatic at the time of birth. Possible manifestations include intrauterine growth retardation, jaundice, hepatosplenomegaly, petechial skin rash, chorioretinitis, and intracranial calcifications. Microcephaly may be present at birth or develop during the first year of life. Most infants who have clinically apparent disease during the neonatal period survive, but they are left with sequelae that may include mental retardation, spasticity, seizure disorders, and visual or hearing deficits. Hearing deficits can be detected in 15% to 20% of congenitally infected neonates who are asymptomatic at the time of birth, making cytomegalovirus an important cause of deafness.

Cytomegalovirus infection can also be acquired at the time of birth from maternal cervical secretions. Neonates infected in this fashion begin to excrete the virus at 3 to 12 weeks of age. These infections are usually asymptomatic, but occasional infants have an interstitial pneumonitis that may take several weeks to resolve. Asymptomatic postnatal infection may also occur as a result of ingestion of breast milk containing cytomegalovirus. In premature infants who acquire infection as a result of blood transfusions, encephalitis, pneumonitis, hepatosplenomegaly, and thrombocytopenia may develop.

Herpes simplex virus. The incidence of neonatal herpetic infection is estimated at 1 per 2000 to 10,000 live births. The infection is generally acquired at the time of birth from the maternal genital tract and usually results from herpes simplex type 2, the virus type responsible for most genital herpetic infections. In most instances the maternal herpetic infection is not diagnosed because of the absence of specific findings. Vesicular skin lesions usually appear 2 to 12 days after birth; however, in around 20% of the cases of neonatal herpes, cutaneous lesions do not appear and the diagnosis is unsuspected. Rarely infants are born with herpetic lesions as a result of ascending or transplacental infection. In approximately 15% of the cases of neonatal herpes, infection remains localized to the skin or eyes. Isolated encephalitis occurs in 15% of the cases; in 70% of the cases disseminated infection develops with involvement of the liver, adrenal glands, lungs, and other organs. Possible clinical manifestations include vesicular skin rash, keratoconjunctivitis, hepatosplenomegaly, chorioretinitis, seizures, and bleeding caused by disseminated intravascular coagulation. Disseminated infections are fatal 80% to 90% of the time. Two thirds of neonates with localized encephalitis die, and around half of those that survive have neurologic damage. Neonates with infection limited to the skin have a better prognosis, but some of them will also have neurologic sequelae, presumably as a result of undetected encephalitis. Involvement of the eyes may result in visual impairment.

Rubella virus (German measles). Congenital rubella has become uncommon in the United States since the introduction of rubella vaccine. Clinical findings in neonates with congenital rubella include jaundice, hepatosplenomegaly, thrombocytopenic purpura, glaucoma, cataracts, bone lesions consisting of areas of radiolucency in the metaphyses of long bones, and congenital heart disease. The most common cardiac lesions are patent ductus arteriosus, pulmonary artery stenosis, and pulmonary valvular stenosis. Deafness is the most common consequence of congenital rubella and may occur in the absence of other findings. Possible neurologic sequelae include mental retardation, behavioral disorders, and autism. Other possible late manifestations are hypogammaglobulinemia, diabetes, and progressive panencephalitis.

Hepatitis B virus. Neonates are at highest risk of acquiring hepatitis B infection if their mothers are actively infected with the virus at the time of birth. Neonates whose mothers are chronic carriers of hepatitis B virus can also acquire infection. Carrier mothers who are e antigen positive are more likely to transmit the virus to their offspring. Most neonates who become infected remain asymptomatic, but some become chronic carriers of the virus. Mild elevations of liver enzymes and pathologic changes in liver biopsy specimens have been detected in some of these infants. Occasionally acute icteric hepatitis occurs at around 3 to 4 months of age. Fulminant hepatitis leading to early death from cirrhosis has rarely been observed.

Coxsackievirus B. In neonates with coxsackievirus B infection, symptoms usually develop 3 to 5 days after birth. Clinical findings include pneumonitis, seizures, hepatosplenomegaly, myocarditis, and heart failure. Severe infections may result in death, whereas less severely involved neonates usually recover completely.

Varicella-zoster virus (chickenpox). Transmission of varicella-zoster infection to the fetus is uncommon, since most pregnant women are immune. A rare syndrome of congenital varicella has occurred following first-trimester maternal varicella. Possible manifestations include hypoplastic extremities, atrophic digits, chorioretinitis, cataracts, optic atrophy, encephalitis, and severe psychomotor retardation.

Neonatal varicella can occur if varicella develops in a pregnant woman around the time of delivery. If maternal varicella appears within 5 days before delivery, the neonate may have typical vesicular skin lesions 5 to 10 days after birth. Fatal disseminated infection with pneumonitis, hepatitis, and encephalitis may develop. If maternal infection appears more than 5 days before delivery, neonatal varicella tends to be mild.

LABORATORY FINDINGS. Routine laboratory tests are useful to define the extent and follow the course of perinatal infections. Hemolytic anemia and thrombocytopenia are commonly detected. Elevations of direct bilirubin and liver enzymes indicate liver involvement. Cerebrospinal fluid pleocytosis and elevated protein content may be detected if encephalitis is present. Elevated levels of IgM in cord blood or sera collected during the first few days of life suggest congenital infection, since maternal IgM does not usually cross the placenta and the fetus does not produce IgM unless it is antigenically stimulated. Not all congenitally infected neonates, however, have elevated IgM levels. Possible roentgenographic findings include abnormalities in the metaphyses of long bones, pneumonitis, and calcifications of brain or liver.

DIAGNOSIS. Perinatal virus infection cannot be diagnosed on the basis of clinical findings and routine laboratory studies alone. Bacterial or fungal infections, toxoplasmosis, and noninfectious conditions such as erythroblastosis fetalis and autoimmune thrombocytopenia may be initially seen with similar findings. Certain manifestations do suggest a viral origin: for example, the presence of skin vesicles or keratoconjunctivitis suggests herpes simplex infection, whereas congenital cytomegalovirus infection should be suspected when periventricular intracranial calcifications are detected.

Viral infections can be identified on the basis of morphologic, virologic, and serologic findings. Characteristic histopathologic changes may be found in autopsy or biopsy specimens. Inclusion-bearing cells can be found in the urine of about 30% of neonates with symptomatic cytomegalovirus infection. Scrapings of skin or conjunctival lesions of neonates with herpes simplex or varicella-zoster infections frequently reveal multinucleated giant cells with intranuclear inclusions. In congenital cytomegalovirus infection, virus particles can be detected in the urine by electron microscopy. Definitive diagnosis is accomplished by isolation of the virus from throat, nasopharyngeal, urine, stool, skin, eye, buffy coat, or cerebrospinal fluid specimens.

Serologic tests are also available for the diagnosis of neonatal infections but must be interpreted with caution. The detection of antibodies in a neonate's serum may only reflect transplacental passage of maternal antibodies. The presence of IgM antibodies to a particular virus suggests congenital infection, since IgM antibodies do not usually cross the placenta; however, reliable tests for specific IgM antibodies are available in only a few laboratories. The serologic diagnosis of congenital infection can also be based on the persistence of specific antibodies in an infant, since transplacentally acquired maternal antibodies decline with time.

MANAGEMENT. Appropriate isolation procedures should be instituted whenever perinatal virus infection is suspected. Neonates with possible herpes simplex or varicella-zoster infections should be strictly isolated, and those with possible cytomegalovirus or rubella infections should be kept away from pregnant women. Blood precautions should be instituted for neonates exposed to maternal hepatitis B infection.

For symptomatic neonates, supportive measures such as blood and platelet transfusions, anticonvulsant therapy, and ventilatory assistance may be required. Effective antiviral therapy is unavailable for most of the viruses that can infect the newborn. An investigational drug, adenine arabinoside, has been reported to be of some benefit for neonates with herpetic infections. Further controlled clinical trials are in progress. Children who survive perinatal virus infections should receive careful follow-up study, including tests for hearing, vision, and neurologic function. Clinicians caring for such children must be alert for possible late manifestations.

PREVENTION. Prevention of perinatal viral infections is highly desirable in view of the associated morbidity and mortality. Congenital rubella is theoretically completely preventable with the availability of rubella vaccine. In fact, since the introduction of rubella vaccine, the number of cases in the United States has fallen markedly. Unfortunately, vaccines against other viruses that cause perinatal infections are not currently available.

Occasionally primary infection as a result of rubella or cytomegalovirus is documented in a pregnant woman. In this situation termination of the pregnancy to prevent possible congenital infection becomes an option.

Other possible preventive measures for pregnant women include avoidance of close contact with patients who are know to be infected with rubella or cytomegalovirus and, insofar as possible, avoidance of blood transfusions, which may transmit cytomegalovirus and hepatitis B. Delivery by cesarean section is advised for prevention of neonatal herpes when active genital herpes is documented in a pregnant woman close to the time of delivery.

Passive immunization of neonates may prevent varicella and hepatitis B infections. It is currently recommended that zoster immune globulin be given to neonates in whose mothers varicella developed less than 5 days before delivery. Neonates whose mothers either are actively infected with hepatitis B or are chronic carriers of this virus should be given hepatitis B immune globulin within 72 hours of birth and 6 weeks later.

BIBLIOGRAPHY

Hanshaw, J.B., and Dudgeion, J.A.: Viral diseases of the fetus and newborn, Philadelphia, 1978, W.B. Saunders Co.

Krugman, S., and Gershon, A.A., editors: Infections of the fetus and the newborn infant, New York, 1975, Allan R. Liss, Inc.

Nahmias, A., Visintine, A., and Starr, S.E.: Viral infection of the fetus and newborn. In Drew, L., editor: Viral infections: a clinical approach, Philadelphia, 1976, F.A. Davis Co.

Remington, J.S., and Klein, J.O.: Infectious diseases of the fetus and newborn infant, Philadelphia, 1976, W.B. Saunders Co.

Starr, S.E.: Cytomegalovirus, Pediatr. Clin. North Am. **16:**283, 1979.

Herpesviruses

Gary R. Fleisher

There are four members of the human herpesvirus family: herpes simplex virus (HSV or herpesvirus hominis), varicella-zoster virus (VZV or herpesvirus varicellae), cytomegalovirus (CMV), and Epstein-Barr virus (EBV). These relatively large viruses are comprised of a DNA core, an icosahedral protein capsid, and an outer lipid envelope. They are worldwide in distribution and produce disease at any age from the fetal period to the geriatric years. The infections vary in severity from trivial to fatal, with the most serious infections occurring in the immunocompromised host. Following the primary infection, a persistent viral carrier state is established.

Each of the herpesviruses will be discussed individually. Infections in the fetus and newborn are described in the preceding section.

HERPES SIMPLEX VIRUS

EPIDEMIOLOGY. There are two strains of herpes simplex virus (HSV) that differ in their antigenicity and anatomic distribution. HSV-1 more frequently causes oral lesions, and HSV-2 is usually isolated from the genital area. Both strains are found throughout the world. Large-scale epidemics do not occur, but small outbreaks are seen.

The initial infection with HSV is asymptomatic in 80% to 90% of the patients. Serologic surveys have established antibody prevalence rates among adults of 50% to 100%, depending on socioeconomic status. In children the majority of infections are caused by HSV-1, which is transmitted nonvenereally. HSV-2 is increasingly common after puberty, primarily as a result of spread by the genital route.

PATHOGENESIS. After inoculation at the primary site on the skin or mucosa, HSV replicates locally. In the intact host viremia has been infrequently observed; however, despite an immune response, the virus spreads to local ganglion cells via ascension along the neurons. Humoral antibodies achieve detectable levels in 1 to 3 weeks, and cell-mediated immunity can be demonstrated concurrently. Various local and systemic insults such as trauma or fever can produce reactivation of the latent virus.

Pathologically, the lesions of HSV are characterized by intranuclear inclusions and multinucleated giant cells. Degeneration of epithelial cells leads to interstitial edema and vesicle formation. Subsequently, polymorphonuclear leukocytes invade the area.

In the severely malnourished or immunocompromised host, viremia may result in visceral dissemination. Characteristic lesions, as described previously, are seen in the involved organs.

CLINICAL MANIFESTATIONS. The incubation period ranges from 2 to 20 days, with the average being 1 week. Primary infections produce clinically apparent lesions on the skin or mucosa in only 10% to 20% of cases. Acute gingivostomatitis is the most common manifestation in childhood, and it is increasingly seen among young seronegative adults with lower socioeconomic backgrounds. The illness begins with fever and inflammation of the oral mucosa. Over the next 1 to 2 days painful vesicular lesions appear in the mouth, usually anteriorly. The regional lymph nodes swell and become tender. Ulceration of the vesicles occurs rapidly, but complete resolution requires up to 14 days.

Primary infections also occur at sites of cutaneous trauma. In wrestlers this manifestation is referred to as herpes gladiatorum. Patients with extensive atopic dermatitis or burns are susceptible to widespread skin involvement. Rarely the eye may be the site of a primary infection. Primary genital infections have become increasingly prevalent. In some veneral disease clinics herpes simplex is the most common cause of genital ulcerations. There are two clinical syndromes of primary infection in the central nervous system. A benign aseptic meningitis is associated with HSV-2, and an extremely severe encephalitis is associated with HSV-1 (see discussion of "Viral infections of the central nervous system").

Recurrent infections are more common than primary infections, particularly after the age of 30 years. Herpes labialis is the most frequent and well-known manifestation, but vesicles may reappear at any site of initial infection.

LABORATORY FINDINGS. There are no characteristic laboratory findings with skin or mucous membrane infection. A mononuclear pleocytosis in the cerebrospinal fluid generally accompanies central nervous system involvement. Encephalitis caused by HSV is manifested as a focal lesion by radionuclide or computed tomographic scanning.

DIAGNOSIS. Histologic evidence of intranuclear inclusions and multinucleated giant cells at the base of a vesicle or in tissue is suggestive of an HSV infection. Immunofluorescent staining of brain biopsy specimens has proved useful clinically. A definitive diagnosis is made by isolation of the virus. Inoculation of tissue cultures produces cytopathic changes rapidly, often in 48 hours. Acute and convalescent sera can be tested for antibodies using a complement fixation, immunofluorescent, or neutralization assay. A fourfold rise in titer points to a recent infection.

The differential diagnosis of gingivostomatitis includes herpangina as a result of group A coxsackieviruses (see discussion of "Exanthems of viral or presumed viral origin") and thrush caused by *Candida* species. The lesions in herpes simplex are located predominantly in the anterior portion of the mouth, whereas those resulting from coxsackievirus are seen in the posterior oropharynx. Also the duration of illness is longer with herpes simplex virus. Genital herpetic lesions may be confused with chancroid or syphilis. Herpes encephalitis may be initially seen as a mass lesion or resemble disease caused by the arboviruses.

COURSE. In the normal host, primary herpetic infections resolve spontaneously in 1 to 2 weeks. Persistence should prompt an investigation for immunodeficiency. Gingivostomatitis may lead to dehydration as a result of limitation of oral intake by painful mouth lesions. Bacterial superinfection occurs occasionally. The widespread cutaneous disease seen with extensive disruption of the integument has a more complicated course and may be fatal. Recurrent infections are generally mild and of short duration.

Immunocompromised patients have more frequent and longer lasting mucocutaneous infections than the general population. However, visceral dissemination is reported only rarely. In one study 10 deaths occurred during remission in 476 leukemic children, all caused by nonbacterial agents other than HSV. Among renal transplant recipients in another report, 66% of the seropositive patients shed virus postoperatively. Although the vast majority had mucocutaneous disease, none showed evidence of visceral dissemination.

MANAGEMENT. The treatment of mucocutaneous disease

is supportive. Topical anesthetics and systemic analgesics provide some relief from pain. Young children with gingivostomatitis occasionally require intravenous hydration.

Ocular involvement mandates ophthalmologic consultation. Steroids are contraindicated. Both idoxuridine and vidarabine (adenine arabinoside) are effective locally. Topical use of acycloguanosine, a new agent with potent antiviral properties in vitro, has been promising in preliminary studies.

In encephalitis vidarabine has proved to be efficacious in reducing the mortality. It is possible to prevent reactivation of herpes simplex infection after operation on the trigeminal root with human leukocyte interferon. Additionally, acycloguanosine is currently undergoing clinical trials.

PREVENTION. Patients who have extensive skin disease or who are immunocompromised should avoid contact with patients who have active skin lesions. Sexual contact should be avoided during the active phase of genital herpes. In Scandinavian countries the use of condoms has markedly reduced the incidence of primary genital herpes infection. Attempts at prevention with passive immunization have been ineffective, but trials of active immunization using a subunit herpes simplex vaccine have recently begun.

VARICELLA-ZOSTER VIRUS

EPIDEMIOLOGY. Herpesvirus varicellae, the cause of both zoster and varicella (chickenpox), has a worldwide distribution. Varicella is endemic in industrialized countries and occurs in epidemics among clustered subgroups of susceptible children in setting such as classrooms or hospital wards. The prevalence of this disease reaches its highest levels during the winter and spring.

Varicella occurs predominantly in children between 2 and 10 years of age. Although transplacental passage of antibodies has been demonstrated, they do not confer protection against infection with the same reliability observed in many other childhood diseases. Thus occasional cases are seen in the first few months of life. Sporadic episodes also occur in susceptible adults. Most adults are seropositive from childhood exposures, since the attack rate within households is 90%. Seroepidemiologic surveys using the complement fixation technique have detected antibodies in 70% of the 10- to 20-year-old population in the United States; however, this is an underestimate of immunity, since these antibodies frequently decline to undetectable levels, with patients still being protected against infection.

Transmission is by airborne droplets and direct contact with infectious lesions. An individual is considered contagious from the day before the eruption until all the lesions are crusted, usually 6 to 7 days after eruption. However, infectivity decreases markedly after the first 3 days of illness.

In contrast to varicella, zoster occurs predominantly in older adults. More than 60% of episodes are in individuals over 45 years of age, although the disease is seen occasionally in childhood. There is an increased incidence of zoster in the immunocompromised host. In one study of patients with Hodgkin's disease, zoster developed in 22%.

Since a reactivation of latent virus is the antecedent of the eruption in zoster, an individual does not acquire this disease from an exogenous source. A susceptible individual may, however, have varicella after exposure to the lesions of zoster. Viral shedding occurs until all lesions are crusted, usually after 7 to 10 days in the normal host.

PATHOGENESIS. Entry of the virus, probably through the oropharynx, is followed in the susceptible host first by local replication and then by dissemination via the blood or lymphatics. Presumably, viremia occurs after exposure to the virus and before the onset of the exanthem, but this has not been demonstrated. However, investigators have recovered virus from the blood of immunocompromised patients with progressive disease. Specific humoral and cellular immune responses terminate the viremic stage, but enlargement of cutaneous lesions continues for several days. These intraepidermal vesicles become pustular after invasion by polymorphonuclear leukocytes. Multinucleated giant cells are located at the base of the vesicles.

It is postulated that during an episode of varicella, virus invades sensory nerve endings and ascends along the nerve fibers to the dorsal root ganglion where it becomes latent. Zoster represents reactivation of this latent virus, which then migrates along the nerve to the skin. Occasional vesicle formation outside a single dermatome occurs in 25% of healthy individuals with zoster, probably caused by viremia. In some immunosuppressed patients extensive disease can occur outside a dermatome and virus can be isolated from the blood.

CLINICAL MANIFESTATIONS. In the normal individual the incubation period of varicella is 10 to 21 days, with an average of 14 days. A mild 1- to 3-day prodrome of fever and malaise frequently precedes the exanthem; however, the presence of the rash is often the first sign of illness. In children the fever seldom exceeds 103.1° F (39.5° C) and accompanies the rash for 2 to 3 days. The fever and malaise are more pronounced in adults.

The exanthem appears initially on the trunk or face and spreads centripetally in contradistinction to smallpox, which begins on the periphery. The individual lesions are pruritic and evolve from erythematous macules and papules to vesicles and then pustules. This transition may occur rapidly over 6 to 8 hours. Early vesicles are 2 to 4 mm in diameter and have a "dewdroplike" appearance. Successive crops of new lesions erupt for 2 to 4 days and involve the mucosa of the oropharynx and vagina. Resolution occurs by rupture of the pustules and crusting. Characteristically there are lesions at all stages in any one area of the body. The severity of the cutaneous involvement in varicella is quite variable in that the total number of lesions may vary from one or two to several hundred.

Fever may or may not be present with zoster. The eruptions are often preceded by neuralgia, which is generally more severe in adults. Aside from confinement to a single dermatome in zoster, the appearance and evolution of the lesions are identical in both zoster and varicella. Regional lymph nodes are generally enlarged.

LABORATORY FINDINGS. There are no significant laboratory findings in uncomplicated varicella or zoster. In most cases the white blood cell count is within the normal range. If dissemination occurs, there may be leukocytosis, marked elevation of liver enzymes, pleocytosis in the cerebrospinal fluid, and infiltrates on the chest roentgenogram.

DIAGNOSIS. The typical case of varicella or zoster is diagnosed on the basis of clinical features, but laboratory confirmation is available. A Giemsa-stained smear from the base of a vesicle shows multinucleated giant cells. Varicella virus may be isolated from vesicular fluid obtained early in the course. Serologic tests include complement fixation (CF), fluorescent antibody to membrane antigen (FAMA), immune adherence hemagglutination (IAHA), and neutralization.

The differential diagnosis of varicella includes smallpox, eczema herpeticum, dermatitis herpetiformis, insect bites, scabies, and impetigo. Smallpox that has been modified by vaccination may be clinically indistinguishable from varicella. Zoster may be confused at times with herpes simplex. In the preeruptive phase the pain may resemble that of pleural, cardiac, or peritoneal origin.

COURSE. In the normal host varicella is a mild disease, although adults often experience more pronounced malaise. The lesions develop crusts by the end of a week and resolve in another 4 to 7 days. Secondary bacterial infection of the skin is the most common complication and may rarely lead to distant septic foci. Encephalitis occurs in less than 1 of every 1000 cases (see discussion of "Viral infections of the central nervous system"). The central nervous system involvement is often limited to cerebellar ataxia, but mortality rates as high as 27% have been reported. Pneumonia occurs mainly in adults. Other rare complications include hepatitis, uveitis, orchitis, glomerulonephritis, arthritis, and hemorrhagic diathesis. About 7% of the cases of Reye's syndrome follow a varicella infection.

In immunosuppressed patients, particularly with lymphoreticular malignancies, varicella is a serious infection. In addition to the complications just listed, visceral dissemination occurs in 25% to 33% of the cases. The lungs, liver, and central nervous system are frequently involved, leading to a mortality rate of 5% to 10%.

The eruption in zoster follows a course similar to that of varicella, but the duration of lesions and time to healing are often slightly longer. Postherpetic neuralgia and secondary bacterial infection may follow zoster in any location. The former is more frequent in adults. Other complications depend on the segmental localization. Ocular lesions occur in up to 50% of trigeminal nerve cases and may lead to visual impairment. Zoster of the seventh cranial nerve may produce facial palsy (Hunt's syndrome), and with involvement of cervical ganglia, diaphragmatic paralysis has been reported. Zoster may also disseminate viscerally in the immunocompromised patient, but this is not a frequent occurence. As in varicella, the organs involved include the liver, lungs, and brain. Cutaneous dissemination may occur with or without visceral disease.

MANAGEMENT. In the normal host with varicella or zoster, symptomatic treatment alone is provided in the form of analgesics and antipruritics. Ocular involvement in zoster demands the attention of an ophthalmologist and may require the instillation of topical steriods and antibiotics.

The role of systemic antiviral chemotherapy in the immunocompromised host has not yet been fully defined. Both adenosine arabinoside and interferon have shown some effectiveness in selected clinical situations as discussed in Chapter 38.

A new antiviral agent, acycloguanosine, has more activity in vitro than adenosine arabinoside. Clinical trials are currently under way.

PREVENTION. Epidemiologic measures, as well as both passive and active immunization, play a role in the prevention of varicella. Patients with lesions are isolated until crusting occurs, and susceptible individuals exposed to the disease should be excluded from critical areas such as hospitals. Zoster immune globulin (ZIG), a γ-globulin preparation with a high titer of antibodies to varicella-zoster virus, has been demonstrated to be effective in preventing the disease if administered within 72 hours of exposure. This therapy is indicated in patients with neoplasms or primary immunodeficiency and those undergoing immunosuppressive therapy, but not the normal host. Preliminary trials with an attenuated vaccine have shown the development of an immune response following inoculation.

CYTOMEGALOVIRUS

EPIDEMIOLOGY. Cytomegalovirus (CMV) has a worldwide distribution. It is found endemically and has no seasonal pattern. Of infants in the United States 1% to 2% acquire this infection in utero and another 10% during the first 3 months of life. By the age of 70 years, 80% to 90% of the population is seropositive.

The mode of acquisition of CMV remains to be definitively established, but it appears that intimate contact is necessary for the spread of natural infection. Both blood transfusions and organ transplantation may also transmit CMV. Following a primary infection, the virus persists in a latent state. Conditions such as neoplasia and pregnancy or the use of immunosuppressive medications often induce a reactivation of endogenous infection leading to excretion of virus.

In the normal host the vast majority of illnesses caused

by CMV after the newborn period are asymptomatic. Serious, often fatal, infections do occur with frequency in immuncompromised patients.

PATHOGENESIS. The pathogenesis of postnatally acquired CMV in humans remains uncertain. Viremia has been demonstrated during primary infection. Almost any organ system can be affected during this phase. The liver, kidneys, and salivary glands are frequently involved. A primary CMV infection evokes both humoral and cellmediated immune responses that contain the infection. Histologically, CMV disease is characterized by enlarged cells that contain intranuclear inclusions. Focal areas of necrosis occur, and there is an infiltration of mononuclear cells.

CLINICAL MANIFESTATIONS. The incubation period of naturally acquired CMV is unknown; however, symptoms begin 3 weeks after the transfusion of infected blood and a mean of 6 weeks after renal transplantation. The majority of immunologically normal children and adults with antibody to CMV remain asymptomatic or have a mild, nonspecific illness. In probably 1% or fewer an infectious mononucleosis—like (IM-like) syndrome, hepatitis, or pneumonia develops. The IM-like syndrome is characterized by 2 to 6 weeks of fever, mild adenopathy, minimal pharyngitis, and hepatitis. This syndrome has been observed in 10% of patients following open heart surgery with extracorporeal circulation. Hepatitis caused by CMV is generally mild. Neurologic syndromes described in association with this virus include encephalitis and the Guillain-Barré syndrome.

Both exogenous and endogenous CMV infections represent a serious threat to the immunocompromised host. A syndrome of severe respiratory distress and hepatomegaly during early infancy has been described. In childhood leukemia up to 25% of the patients excrete CMV when followed longitudinally, and pathologic evidence of disseminated disease is seen in 2% to 3% at autopsy. CMV infection occurs in as many as 75% of renal allograft recipients. Approximately one half are asymptomatic. The rest have prolonged fever, leukopenia, thrombocytopenia, pneumonia, or hepatitis. CMV pneumonia occurs in 30% of individuals receiving a bone marrow transplant.

CMV infection is common in male homosexuals, and an association has been noted relating male homosexuality, CMV infection, Kaposi's sarcoma, and infection with opportunistic pathogens such as *Pneumocystis carinii*.

LABORATORY FINDINGS. In CMV mononucleosis and the postperfusion syndrome there is significant lymphocytosis. As many as 25% of the mononuclear cells may be atypical. Although mild to moderate elevation of the liver enzymes occurs frequently, significant hyperbilirubinemia is rare.

DIAGNOSIS. The diagnosis of CMV infection may be suggested pathologically by the presence of intranuclear inclusions in biopsy material or in exfoliated cells in the urine. They are present in less than one half of the confirmed cases. Electron microscopy, when available, rapidly provides a presumptive identification in patients with congenital infection. The virus can be routinely cultured in several cell strains, but a cytopathic effect may not develop for 3 to 6 weeks. Serologic testing is available by many methods including complement fixation, indirect immunofluorescence, and neutralization. It is often difficult, however, to distinguish a primary infection from reactivation, even with specific serology and recovery of the virus, unless a preillness serum sample has no measurable antibodies. A fluorescent test to detect and IgM response and measurement of antibodies to early antigens currently suffers from technical difficulties and limited availability.

The differential diagnosis of acquired CMV includes hepatitis, toxoplasmosis, and other IM-like syndromes (see discussion of "Epstein-Barr virus").

COURSE. Most infections with CMV, whether asymptomatic or clinically evident, resolve without complications in the immunologically intact host beyond the neonatal period. Immunocompromised patients experience more severe infections with this virus. CMV infections requiring hospitalization occur in 75% of seronegative and 25% of seropositive renal transplant recipients. The rate of graft rejection is significantly increased in these patients. In bone marrow transplants CMV is the most commonly identified cause of interstitial pneumonia and has a fatality rate of 60% to 90%.

MANAGEMENT. No antiviral agent has yet demonstrated any clinical effect on the course of CMV infection. Trials are currently under way with acycloguanosine, which has activity against CMV in vitro.

PREVENTION. In a double-blind, placebo-controlled prophylactic trial, human leukocyte interferon delayed, but did not prevent, viral excretion in renal transplant recipients. Trials of passive immunization with high-titer CMV immunoglobulin are currently under way in high-risk patients. A live attenuated vaccine with demonstrated safety and immunogenicity in normal individuals and renal transplant patients has been developed. Studies of vaccine efficacy are now being conducted.

EPSTEIN-BARR VIRUS

EPIDEMIOLOGY. The Epstein-Barr virus (EBV) causes infectious mononucleosis (IM) and is etiologically associated with Burkitt's lymphoma (BL) and nasopharyngeal carcinoma (NPC). Infections with EBV have been detected serologically in all parts of the world. Based on these antibody surveys, primary EBV infection generally occurs in early childhood in underdeveloped countries under conditions of crowding and poor hygiene. Infants in the first 6 months are spared because of protection by maternal antibodies. A survey in Ghana, Africa, found a seroconversion rate of 85% by age 2 years. In economically advanced countries, however, nearly half of the more affluent individuals escape infection until late adolescence. Among college students, there is then a seroconversion rate of 10% to 15% yearly. In contrast to young infants (who remain asymptomatic) 33% to 50% of adolescents and young adults undergoing a primary EBV infection manifest the clinical picture of infectious mononucleosis. In school-age children there are sporadic cases of IM, but the majority of EBV infections are thought to be asymptomatic. Occasional episodes of clinical disease are described in adults even in the seventh and eighth decades. In the United States 90% of the population have antibodies at age 30 years.

Intimate salivary contact appears to be the most frequent mode of transmission of IM. This has led to the name "kissing disease." Although airborne spread has been postulated as an explanation for one outbreak of IM, there is not an increased incidence of disease among college roommates or classmates of clinically ill individuals.

The Epstein-Barr virus, in addition to causing IM, has been linked with two forms of cancer, Burkitt's lymphoma and nasopharyngeal carcinoma. EBV was initially discovered in a lymphocyte culture from a child with BL. This lymphoma occurs predominantly in Africa, and virtually all African children with BL have very high titers of antibodies to EBV. Additionally, EBV genomes have been demonstrated in BL cells. However, in other parts of the world many cases are not EBV associated. Nasopharyngeal carcinoma occurs frequently in southern China and northern Africa. Again, there are high titers of antibodies to EBV almost universally, and the genome is found in the tumor cells. Although several lines of evidence implicate EBV as a causal agent, it does not appear to act alone, since the vast majority of infected individuals remain free of these neoplasms.

PATHOGENESIS. The pathogenesis of IM remains speculative. Presumably the virus enters via the oropharynx, invading either epithelial or, more likely, lymphoid cells. Although the infection may be somewhat contained in asymptomatic cases, spread to circulating B lymphocytes and lymph nodes occurs in symptomatic IM. Both an antibody and a cellular immune response develop to the virus. The atypical lymphocytes seen on peripheral smear are primarily activated T cells responding to neoantigens on transformed B lymphocytes.

There is extensive hyperplasia of the lymphoid tissues in IM. The lymph nodes retain their follicular appearance, but the sinuses are invaded by macrophages and atypical lymphocytes. Infiltration of mononuclear cells may be noted in almost every organ.

CLINICAL MANIFESTATIONS. Following an incubation period of 4 to 6 weeks, the usual patient with IM has the triad of fever, sore throat, and extensive adenopathy. Malaise is a prominent early symptom that may persist for several months. The fever varies but may be as high as 102° to 104° F (30° to 40° C) and remain elevated 3 or 4 weeks. The pharynx is usually intensively inflamed, at times with exudate. Lymph nodes in any region may enlarge. Although anterior cervical adenopathy accompanies pharyngitis of any cause, posterior cervical involvement is very suggestive of IM. Nodal enlargement in the inguinal and axillary areas is common. Mediastinal widening has been described in IM as a result of lymphoid hyperplasia at the hilum. The spleen is enlarged in 50% to 60% of the cases, and the liver is enlarged in 10% to 20% of the cases. Additional findings include periorbital edema and an occasional maculopapular rash. Petechiae may occur at the junction of the hard and soft palates.

LABORATORY FINDINGS. The white blood cell count in most cases is 10,000 to 15,000/mm^3, but a leukocytosis of up to 30,000/mm^3 is not unusual. There is an absolute lymphocytosis, frequently 70% to 80%, and many of the lymphocytes appear atypical. Heterophil antibodies to sheep or horse red blood cells are detectable in 90% of adolescents but less frequently in younger children by routine assays. If followed serially, liver enzymes are significantly elevated in over 95% of the patients. Hyperbilirubinemia, however, is minimal and less frequent. Anemia and thrombocytopenia occur at times.

DIAGNOSIS. Usually the diagnosis of IM is made on the basis of the clinical and hematologic features in association with a significantly elevated heterophil antibody titer. As mentioned, these antibodies to sheep or horse red cells appear in 90% of the cases among adolescents. The specificity of the heterophil antibody response can be established by differential absorption with beef red cells and guinea pig kidney. The IM-specific antibodies are absorbed by the former but not the latter.

In heterophil-negative IM or in atypical EBV infections the diagnosis is made by assay of virus-specific antibodies. Antibodies are directed against viral capsid antigen (VCA), early antigens (EA), and EBV-associated nuclear antigen (EBNA). Each of these antibodies has a different chronology in relation to the time of EBV infection (Fig. 37-1). The IgM anti-VCA and IgG anti-VCA appear early in the course. Whereas the IgM response disappears in 4 to 6 weeks, the IgG anti-VCA response merely declines to lower levels that persist for life. About 80% of the patients with IM show a transient response to the diffuse (D) component of the early antigen complex, whereas antibodies to the restricted (R) component often develop in individuals with asymptomatic infections. In contrast to the antibodies just mentioned, those to EBNA appear, with few exceptions, weeks to months after the onset of illness. Viral culture is not a useful diagnostic tool, since it does not distinguish between past infection and recent infection. During the course of a primary EBV infection, the presence of virus can be demonstrated in oropharyngeal secretions (Fig. 37-1). The addition of this material to cord blood lymphocytes will produce transformation in a large percentage of cases. However, there is intermittent excretion of virus in the oropharynx for many years after the primary infection.

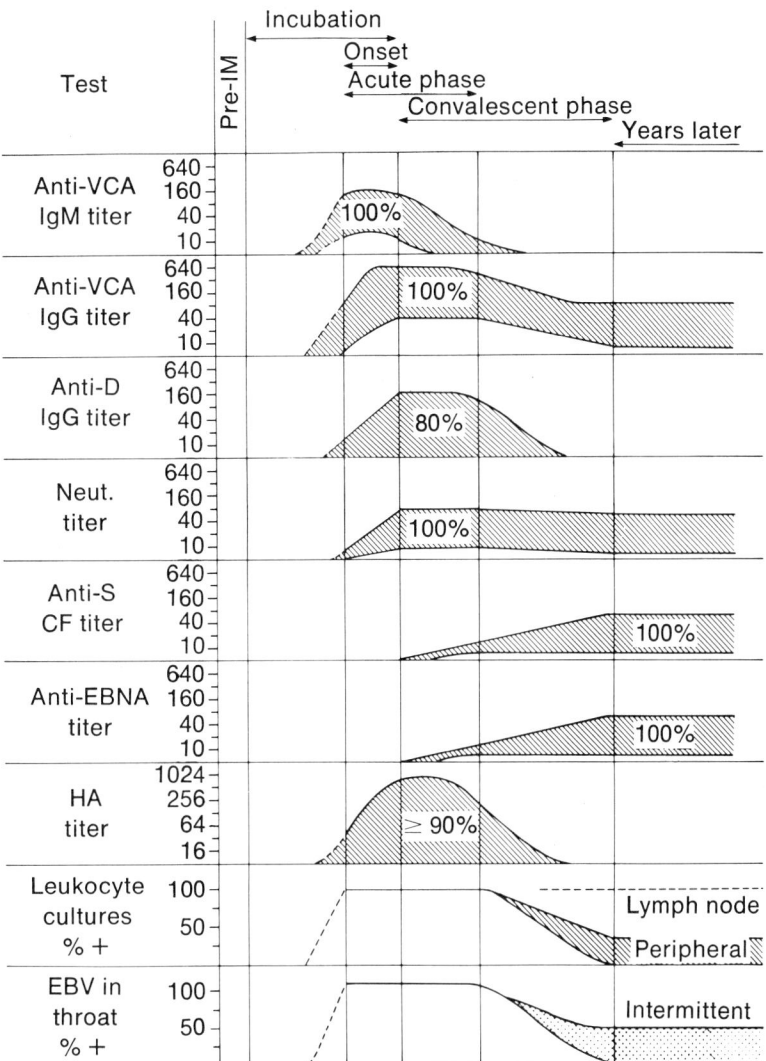

Fig. 37-1. Scheme of antibody response, leukocyte cultures, and EBV assays in throat washings during course of infectious mononucleosis. *IM,* Infectious mononucleosis; *Anti-VCA,* antibody against viral capsid antigen; *Anti-D,* antibody against diffuse component of early antigen complex; *Neut.,* neutralizing; *Anti-S,* antibody against soluble antigen; *Anti-EBNA,* antibody against EB virus–associated nuclear antigen; *HA,* hemagglutination antibody; *EBV,* EB virus. (From Henle, W., Henle, G., and Horwitz, C.A.: Hum. Pathol. **5:**551, 1974.)

Several organisms produce an IM-like syndrome and thus enter into the differential diagnosis. Those most frequently responsible include cytomegalovirus and *Toxoplasma*. Serum sickness and drug reactions may also lead to a similar clinical picture.

COURSE. Most infections with EBV are asymptomatic, and these generally resolve without complications. Occasionally IM is a brief illness, but the usual course is 4 to 6 weeks. Lymphadenopathy may persist for 3 months or longer.

Complications, although infrequent, may involve almost any organ in both symptomatic and asymptomatic infections. Lymphoid hyperplasia leads occasionally to significant respiratory obstruction by the tonsils and stretches the capsule of the spleen, predisposing it to rupture with even minor trauma. Neurologic involvement includes encephalitis, Guillain-Barré syndrome, and peripheral neuropathy. Hemolytic anemia and thrombocytopenia are at times clinically significant. Uveitis, myocarditis, pneumonia, nephritis, and Reye's syndrome have all been reported in association with IM. Unlike the other herpesviruses, EBV does not cause particularly severe disease in immunosuppressed patients other than those with Duncan's syndrome, a rare X-linked immunodeficiency disease.

MANAGEMENT. No specific antiviral therapy is available. The treatment is directed at alleviation of the symptoms. The malaise and fatigue mandate a period of decreased activity, the duration being determined by the severity of the illness. Because of the potential for splenic rupture, the patient should be cautioned to avoid contact sports for at least 6 weeks. Aspirin or acetaminophen is frequently sufficient for analgesia, but orally administered corticosteroids (up to 60 mg prednisone each day) may be necessary for patients with a more toxic condition. The lympholytic property of the steroids also makes these agents useful in the therapy of complications clearly resulting from lymphoid hyperplasia such as airway obstruction by large tonsils. An occasional patient requires hospitalization and intravenous hydration.

PREVENTION. The patient with IM should avoid intimate oral contact while virus excretion in the saliva is heaviest during the period of clinical illness. No isolation measures are indicated. Neither passive nor active immunization has been studied in humans. However, viral antigens have been purified as the first step in the preparation of a vaccine.

BIBLIOGRAPHY
Herpes simplex virus

Glezen, W.P., Fernald, G.W., and Cohn, J.N.: Acute respiratory disease of university students with special reference to the etiologic role of herpesvirus hominis, Am. J. Epidemiol. **101:**111, 1975.

Nahmias, A.J., and Roizman, B.: Infection with herpes simplex viruses 1 and 2 (in three parts), N. Engl. J. Med. **289:**667, 719, 781, 1973.

Rawls, W.E., and others: Measurement of antibodies to herpesvirus types 1 and 2 in human sera, J. Immunol. **117:**728, 1976.

Whitley, R.J., and others: Adenine arabinoside therapy of biopsy-proved herpes simplex encephalitis, N. Engl. J. Med. **297:**289, 1977.

Varicella-zoster virus

Asano, Y., and Takahashi, M.: Clinical and serological testing of a live varicella vaccine and two-year follow-up for immunity of the vaccinated children, Pediatrics **60:**810, 1977.

Feldman, S., and Cysp, E.: Isolation of varicella zoster virus from blood. J. Pediatr. **88:**265, 1976.

Gershon, A.A., and Krugman, S.: Seroepidemiologic survey of varicella: value of specific fluorescent antibody test, Pediatrics **56:**1005, 1975.

Gershon, A.A., Steinberg, S., and Bruxmell, P.A.: Zoster immune globulin: a further assessment, N. Engl. J. Med. **290:**243, 1974.

Cytomegalovirus

Abdallah, D.S., Mark, J.B., and Merigan, T.C.: Diagnosis of cytomegalovirus pneumonia in compromised host, Am. J. Med. **61:**326, 1976.

Armstrong, D., and others: Cytomegalovirus infections with viremia following renal transplantation, Arch. Intern. Med. **127:**111, 1971.

Hanshaw, J.B.: Congenital cytomegalovirus infection: a fifteen year perspective, J. Infect. Dis. **123:**555, 1971.

Plotkin, S.A., and others: Prevention and treatment of cytomegalovirus infection. In Nahmias, A.J., Dowdle, W.R., and Schinazi, R.F., editors: The human herpesviruses, New York, 1981, Elsevier.

Weller, T.H.: The cytomegaloviruses: ubiquitous agents with protean clinical manifestations, N. Engl. J. Med. **285:**203, 267, 1971.

Epstein-Barr virus

Henle, W.: The association of Epstein-Barr virus with Burkitt's lymphoma. In Osato, T., editor: Epstein-Barr oncogenesis, Sapporo, Japan, 1979, Hokkaido University School of Medicine.

Henle, W., and Henle, G.E.: Seroepidemiology of the virus. In Epstein, M., and Achang, B., editors: The Epstein-Barr virus, Berlin, 1979, Springer-Verlag.

Henle, W., Henle, G.E., and Horwitz, C.A.: Epstein-Barr virus specific diagnostic tests in infectious mononucleosis, Hum. Pathol. **5:**551, 1974.

Klein, G.: The relationship of the virus to nasopharyngeal carcinoma. In Epstein, M., and Achang, B., editors: The Epstein-Barr virus, Berlin, 1979, Springer-Verlag.

Viral infections of the central nervous system

Stephen Gluckman

(See also Chapter 151.)

Acute viral infections of the central nervous system (CNS) are more frequent than reported data would indicate. Some diagnosed infections are unreported, many more presumed viral infections are unproven, and probably still more are not even suspected. Recent statistics compiled by the Centers for Disease Control in Atlanta, Georgia describe about 4500 cases of acute viral CNS infections each year in the United States. About one third are encephalitis, and the remainder are aseptic meningitis. A discussion of the major causes of acute viral CNS infections will be included here. It must be stressed at the outset that the clinical syndromes and cerebrospinal fluid (CSF) findings are rarely specific for viral infections; therefore nonviral causes that are often treatable must be considered and recognized.

DEFINITIONS. The distinction between aseptic meningitis and encephalitis is determined by clinical features, although the syndromes can overlap. Although some organisms are more likely to cause one syndrome than the other, in general, infection with an organism may produce either syndrome. Aseptic meningitis implies meningeal inflammation. Although patients may be lethargic, their CNS function remains normal. In encephalitis there are signs of CNS functional impairment that may be manifest as altered mental status, motor or sensory deficits, or movement disorders. In most patients with encephalitis there are also findings of meningeal inflammation, and hence the term "meningoencephalitis" is properly used.

Encephalitis may be either primary or postinfectious. In the former there is invasion of the CNS by the pathogen. Histologically, neuronal involvement is found. The virus can often be cultured from the tissue, and inclusion bodies on light microscopy or viral particles on electron microscopy may be seen. In postinfectious encephalitis the virus cannot be seen or recovered and the neurons are spared; however, perivascular infiltrates and demyelination are present. It occurs after an infectious illness or the administration of certain vaccines. The pathogenesis of this disease has not been clearly established, but it is presumed to have a hypersensitivity basis. Infections with certain viruses may result in either syndrome.

ETIOLOGY. The following are major causes of aseptic meningitis and encephalitis in the United States:

Primary infections

Herpes simplex viruses types 1 and 2
Enteroviruses
    Coxsackievirus A
    Coxsackievirus B
    Echovirus
    Poliovirus
Arboviruses
    California encephalitis virus
    Eastern equine encephalitis virus
    Western equine encephalitis virus
    St. Louis encephalitis virus
    Venezuelan equine encephalitis virus
Childhood infections
    Mumps virus
    Measles virus
    Varicella-zoster virus
Other
    Cytomegaloviruses
    Epstein-Barr virus
    Lymphycytic choriomeningitis virus
    Adenoviruses
    Rabies virus
    Influenza virus

Postinfectious

Measles, mumps, varicella, rubella, influenza
Vaccine associated: vaccinia, yellow fever, rabies (duck embryo vaccine), pertussis

Several generalizations can help in approaching the specific origin of viral CNS infections. Of the proven causes of aseptic meningitis, the vast majority are associated with enteroviruses or with mumps: the former occur primarily in the summer and fall and the latter in the winter and spring. Other causes are rarely found. Similarly, the majority of proven encephalitis cases are caused by arboviruses, childhood infections, or herpes simplex type 1. Arboviruses predominate in the summer and fall. Childhood infections are most common in the winter and spring but like herpes virus can occur throughout the year. By merely using these few facts, most of the provable cases can be identified. The most common causes of aseptic meningitis and encephalitis where a cause is defined are as follows:

    Aseptic meningitis
        Summer-fall: enteroviruses
        Winter-spring: mumps
    Encephalitis
        Summer-fall: arboviruses
        Winter-spring: mumps
        Throughout year: herpes simplex

CLINICAL MANIFESTATIONS. The clinical presentation of aseptic meningitis is generally nonspecific, with fever and headache. Physical examination usually detects signs of meningeal irritation, but unless there are findings related to the specific virus (for example, swollen parotid glands with mumps, skin rash with enteroviruses), there are no other abnormalities. Encephalitis may have a a similar presentation, but in addition, there is altered mental status ranging from a subtle inability to calculate to complete unresponsiveness. Seizures are common, and focal abnormalities such as hemiparesis may develop. Hypothalamic involvement may result in either diabetes insipidus or the syndrome of inappropriate antidiuretic hormone (ADH) secretion. In the encephalitis of herpes simplex there are characteristically bizarre behavior, olfactory hallucinations, and aphasia, suggesting temporal lobe localization.

Examination of the cerebrospinal fluid (CSF), although not diagnostic, confirms the presence of CNS disease. The CSF protein is generally elevated, usually this is only to modestly high levels (that is, less than 150 mg/dl). The CSF glucose is usually normal (greater than 50% of the simultaneous blood glucose). However, infections with herpes simplex type 1, mumps, some enteroviruses, and lymphocytic choriomeningitis can result in hypoglycorrhachia. The CSF glucose is usually not at the extremely low levels seen with pyogenic bacteria, but such values should raise the possibility of other diagnoses, including tuberculosis, cryptococcosis, or meningeal spread of tumor. The CSF white blood cell count is typically elevated. However, levels of greater than $1000/mm^3$ are unusual and should prompt concern for other, nonviral causes. In general, lymphocytes predominate, but early in the course there may be a predominance of polymorphonuclear leukocytes. A repeat CSF cell count in 8 hours should show a clear shift from polymorphonuclear leukocytes to lymphocytes in 90% of those with viral disease.

In a patient with viral encephalitis the presence of red blood cells in the CSF that are not the result of a traumatic lumbar puncture should suggest herpes simplex.

HERPES SIMPLEX

Herpes simplex type 2 is traditionally associated with genital infections. It can, however, produce CNS disease. In newborns it is responsible for severe, usually fatal disseminated disease with encephalitis. In adults, however, the illness is characteristically an aseptic meningitis rather than encephalitis.

In contrast to type 2, herpes simplex type 1 CNS infections in adults usually result in encephalitis. Specific diagnosis is established only if brain tissue is obtained for viral studies by biopsy, a procedure that might be selected for the most severe forms of the disease. Perhaps for this reason it is an uncommonly reported disease, with fewer than 100 cases recognized annually. Nonetheless, it remains the most common cause of sporadic encephalitis in the United States, comprising approximately 10% of the cases for which a specific cause is determined. Untreated, biopsy-proven cases have a mortality of about 70%, and over 50% of the survivors are left with significant sequelae. The availability of antiviral therapy with vidarabine has changed these statistics as discussed in the following and in Chapter 38.

The disease can occur with primary infection or with reactivation of the latent organism. There is no seasonal predilection, and it is not associated with community outbreaks. It can affect persons of any age. Of the encephalitides, herpes simplex seems most likely to result in focal disease. On pathologic examination extensive necrosis with hemorrhage is characteristic. Cowdry type A intranuclear inclusions are often seen in the neurons.

CLINICAL MANIFESTATIONS. The onset may be acute or have a vague, subacute prodrome consisting of frontal headache and malaise lasting several days or weeks. Changes in mentation are often the first indication that the CNS is involved. When initially seen, herpes simplex encephalitis may not be distinguishable from other causes, but certain features if present are characteristic. Evidence of focal disease, particularly that of temporal lobe involvement, is typical. Symptoms of bizarre behavior, speech disorders, and gustatory or olfactory hallucinations are particularly suggestive of herpes simplex infection.

The focal involvement can occasionally occur elsewhere in the CNS, including the brainstem. Ninety percent of the patients have fever, often as high as 103° to 106° F (39.4° to 41.1° C). During the course of untreated illness in biopsy-proven cases, 85% become comatose, 20% have aphasia, and 40% to 60% have seizures. Cutaneous herpes is seen in less than 10% of the cases. Furthermore, the appearance of herpetic skin lesions can be a nonspecific concomitant of many febrile illnesses. Therefore the presence or absence of cutaneous herpes is of no diagnostic importance.

Standard laboratory tests are of limited value in diagnosis. CNS findings are nonspecific, although when present the findings of several hundred red cells and a low glucose level should suggest herpes simplex. The EEG, brain scan, and computed tomography (CT) scan are useful in confirming the locality of the disease and especially in confirming temporal lobe involvement if present. However, none of these tests establishes a specific etiologic diagnosis. Because of the localized illness, space-occupying lesions, such as a brain abscess, tumor, or intracerebral bleeding, are frequent differential diagnostic considerations.

In the laboratory, confirmation of herpes encephalitis can be established only by examination of brain tissue. Immunofluorescent staining of the tissue with fluorescein-labeled anti–herpes simplex antibody is sensitive (about 75% to 85%) and specific and can be performed in a few hours. Demonstration of typical Cowdry type A intranuclear inclusions by histologic stains is strongly suggestive of herpes simplex in acute encephalitis. The virus can usually be grown from brain tissue in 1 to 5 days. However, it has been cultured from lumbar CSF on only a few occasions. Serologic tests demonstrating significant antibody titer rises in serum are not specific for CNS disease, since they may reflect active virus infection elsewhere in the body (for example, reactivation of mouth lesions). A recent study suggests that the ratio of CSF antibodies to serum antibodies may be useful in diagnosis, but these changes develop fairly late after the onset of infection and are of little value in establishing an early diagnosis.

Vidarabine is the accepted therapy for herpes simplex encephalitis, although this regimen is derived from only a single, small, randomized trial. The standard course is 15 mg/kg/day for 10 days. In the study both the mortality and the long-term residua were significantly reduced with the use of the drug if it was given before there was a major alteration in the patient's level of consciousness; treating a patient who was already comatose was of no benefit. Although surprisingly nontoxic, the drug has been associated with bone marrow suppression and mild liver function abnormalities. When used in other contexts, there have been several reports of neurologic deterioration, which may be more common in patients with renal failure and masked in the presence of encephalitis. A potential problem with vidarabine is its low solubility, necessitating administration in a large volume of fluid. This can be a cause for some concern when the physician is trying to combat cerebral edema or an inappropriate ADH syndrome.

The exact role of brain biopsy versus empiric therapy in approaching suspected herpes encephalitis has been a source of recent debate. The following factors should be considered: (1) herpes simplex is a devastating illness; (2) vidarabine appears to be moderately effective if used *early* in the disease; (3) vidarabine is a potentially toxic drug; and (4) diagnosis of herpes encephalitis cannot be established by clinical evaluation or basic laboratory tests but requires brain biopsy and culture. At present, early biopsy rather than empiric therapy appears to be the best approach.

ENTEROVIRUSES

Although enteroviruses can be associated with a variety of neurologic syndromes, symptomatic CNS infections with these agents generally are manifested as aseptic meningitis. The enteroviruses are 20- to 30-nm icosahedral RNA viruses; they include over 70 serotypes that are grouped into the echoviruses, group A and B coxsackieviruses, and polioviruses. Many of the different viral serotypes can be responsible for CNS illness. Most frequently implicated are echoviruses 4, 6, 9, 11, 16, and 30; group A coxsackieviruses 7 and 9; and group B coxsackieviruses 1 to 5. These organisms are widespread and highly contagious. Serologic studies have revealed that infections in household contacts are frequent, although often asymptomatic. Infections with enteroviruses may result in a variety of different illnesses including febrile exanthems, herpangina, pleurodynia, myopericarditis, orchitis, and respiratory tract infections. The presence of these types of illnesses in the household or community of a patient with CNS infection is a useful epidemiologic suggestion that the causative agent is an enterovirus. Infections peak in the summer and fall, and most occur in children or young adults. They are spread via the fecal-oral route.

CLINICAL MANIFESTATIONS. Although aseptic meningitis is most frequent, neurologic illness can be manifested in a variety of less common ways, including encephalitis, cerebellar ataxia, radiculitis, and muscle weakness or paralysis such as that classically described in poliomyelitis. After an incubation period of 2 to 12 days, the onset may be subacute or acute, with increased temperatures, chilliness, myalgias, and headache being the predominant symptoms. Nausea and vomiting may occur. Meningeal signs are present on physical examination, and occasionally an erythematous maculopapular rash suggestive of an enterovirus may be seen. The disease on occasion is diphasic, beginning with a nonspecific febrile illness that lasts a few days. This is followed by 2 to 10 days of improvement that is terminated by the reappearance of fever, this time accompanied by meningeal signs. Patients who have had several remissions or relapses of enterovirus aseptic meningitis have been described.

Poliomyelitis infections are usually subclinical; however, an estimated 0.1% result in paralysis as a result of damage to anterior horn cells of the spinal cord or motor nuclei of the pons and medulla. Poliomyelitis has a usual incubation period of 9 to 12 days. Some patients have a nonspecific prodromal "minor illness" (fever, headache, sore throat) lasting 1 to 3 days, followed by a 2- to 5-day period of well-being. There is then onset of typical aseptic meningitis "major illness" (fever, headache, malaise, and meningeal signs). In some patients this is followed by muscle stiffness, pain, and progressive symmetric paralysis, most often involving the lower extremities, that develops over a period of days. Transient fasciculations may be noted in the involved muscles. There is no sensory loss. Bulbar palsy, often affecting the ninth and tenth cranial nerves, and autonomic dysfunction (hypertension, excessive sweating, urinary retention) may occur. Recovery of muscle strength may be noted for up to 1 year after the illness.

With enterovirus infection, routine laboratory tests are usually normal. CSF findings are abnormal but nonspecific. The CSF cell count generally ranges from 5 to 300/mm^3, with a predominance of lymphocytes. (As described previously, polymorphonuclear leukocytes may be seen early in the illness.) The CSF glucose is generally normal, and the protein is normal or mildly elevated.

Specific virologic diagnosis can be achieved by viral isolation from the CSF and by serologic testing. Coxsackievirus and echovirus can often be recovered from the CSF during the first several days of the illness. Throat and rectal swabs have a higher yield than CSF cultures, and the virus persists for a longer time, but isolation from these areas can only be suggestive of the etiologic agent because of the possibility of asymptomatic carriage of the enterovirus. This is especially likely in an epidemic setting. There is no group-specific serologic test. Because there are many enteroviruses, serologic screening is impractical. However, the clinical significance of a throat or rectal isolate can be confirmed by demonstrating a fourfold or greater rise in serotype-specific antibody titer to that isolate.

Treatment for all enteroviral infections is symptomatic, since there is no specific therapy. In fact, in epidemic situations when a patient is not severely ill and has a typical history, hospitalization may not be necessary. The prognosis for most enteroviral CNS infections is excellent, with the exception of paralytic poliomyelitis and infections in infants during the first year of life. Other than poliovirus vaccines, there are no specific preventive measures. Enteric precautions are suggested in hospitalized patients.

MUMPS

Despite the introduction of live attenuated vaccine in 1967, mumps virus continues to be a commonly diagnosed viral cause of CNS disease reported in the United States. Since the 1960s the incidence has decreased. However, mumps virus is still responsible for about 10% of encephalitis cases and 6% of aseptic meningitis cases for which an etiologic agent is determined.

CLINICAL MANIFESTATIONS. Mumps infections occur most frequently in the winter and spring months. These are seasons in which arboviral and enteroviral activity is virtually absent. Because of its contagious nature, an inquiry about exposure to a case of parotitis should be sought when considering this diagnosis in a patient.

CNS disease is the most common extrasalivary manifestation of mumps. Typically, CNS infection results in aseptic meningitis or encephalitis; rare cases of transverse myelitis, Guillain-Barré syndrome, facial palsy, cerebellar ataxia, and a poliomyelitis-like paralysis have been reported in association with mumps virus. In addition, deafness that is usually transient has been associated with mumps virus infection. Abnormalities of the CSF have been found in up to half of the patients with mumps parotitis. Clinical CNS disease, however, occurs in approximately 1%. On the other hand, at least one third of the patients with proven mumps CNS infection do not have parotitis. If both parotitis and CNS disease do occur, the CNS symptoms may be seen before, during, or up to 2 weeks after the parotid gland swelling.

Mumps meningitis or encephalitis is clinically indistinguishable from those caused by other viruses unless parotitis is present. However, the CSF leukocyte count is often particularly elevated for viral infection (occasionally greater than 1000/mm^3), and the shift from polymorphonuclear leukocytes to lymphocytes may be delayed for several days. In addition, a mild hypoglycorrhachia may occur. These findings make the consideration of other causes of the illness such as bacterial, mycobacterial, or fungal infection more urgent.

The diagnosis cannot be made with certainty on clinical grounds. However, in a susceptible person a history of exposure suggests the disease, and associated parotitis makes mumps quite likely. The diagnosis can be confirmed both by culture and by serology. Mumps virus can be grown from the pharynx and CSF for several days after the onset of illness and from the urine for several weeks. Complement-fixing antibodies directed against the soluble (S) antigen appear early in the illness and stay elevated for several months, whereas those directed against the viral (V) antigen appear after 2 to 4 weeks and stay elevated for years. Therefore a diagnosis of recent infection can be made from a single serum specimen if the titers are increased to S antigen and negative or increased to V antigen. Past infection is suggested by a negative S but an increased V titer.

There is no specific treatment. Complete recovery is the rule, although sequelae of mental retardation, permanent deafness, and seizure disorders can occur. The live virus vaccine is quite effective in preventing mumps (see Chapter 38). It is usually administered to children at 15 months of age as part of the measles-mumps-rubella (MMR) vaccine. Postexposure passive prophylaxis with immune serum globulin (ISG) or hyperimmune globulin has not been proved effective.

OTHER CHILDHOOD INFECTIONS
Measles

Encephalitis is a relatively common complication of measles, occurring in about 1 in 1000 cases. It typically is seen initially as fever, headache, and altered mental status 1 to 2 weeks after the appearance of the rash. The pathogenetic mechanism, primary or postinfectious, has not been clearly delineated.

Measles encephalitis can range from mild to severe, but generally it is a serious illness with a mortality rate of 10% and with permanent neurologic sequelae in 10% to 60% of the cases. Subacute sclerosing panencephalitis (SSPE), a late CNS complication of measles, is not included in these numbers.

Although the virus can be cultured, isolation procedures are difficult. Therefore measles is generally confirmed by demonstrating a fourfold or greater rise in serum antibody titers. Because the diagnosis can usually be suspected clinically, antibody measurement is often unnecessary.

There is no specific therapy. The live attenuated vaccine is very effective in preventing measles and is usually given at age 15 months along with mumps and rubella. ISG may be given as postexposure prophylaxis but is indicated only for susceptible persons at high risk of serious disease, that is, immunocompromised hosts.

Varicella-zoster

CNS disease can be a complication of varicella infections. It generally develops toward the end of the first week of the exanthem, although there have been cases in which the CNS involvement preceded the rash. The most frequent manifestation is a self-limited, acute cerebellar ataxia. Aseptic meningitis, encephalitis, transverse myelitis, and Guillain-Barré syndrome have all been reported.

CNS involvement may also be associated with zoster infection. Encephalitis can occur without cutaneous dissemination and with cutaneous involvement limited to noncranial dermatomes. As with varicella, symptoms usually appear toward the end of the first week of the rash and are more likely to develop in the immunocompromised host. Guillain-Barré syndrome, transverse myelitis, Bell's palsy, and Hunt's syndrome have all been associated with zoster infections. Finally, 7% of patients with Reye's syndrome have had a preceding varicella infection.

The diagnosis is suspected based on clinical features and can be confirmed by vesicular culture or by immunofluorescent staining of material scraped from the vesicular base. Histologic stains of such material can demonstrate herpesvirus inclusions and syncytial formation but do not permit distinction between herpes simplex and varicella-zoster viruses. There is no effective treatment once encephalitis has developed. Vidarabine may be beneficial in preventing dissemination of zoster infections in immunologically impaired patients (see Chapter 38). In similar patients zoster immune globulin is effective in attenuating varicella and preventing serious sequelae if given to susceptible individuals within 3 days of exposure.

LYMPHOCYTIC CHORIOMENINGITIS VIRUS

Lymphocytic choriomeningitis virus (LCM) is an arenavirus that is endemic in small rodents. Infections in humans occur in persons with close exposure to such animals as hamsters and mice. Most cases have been reported in laboratory workers. The illness is generally a self-limited aseptic meningitis, but fatal cases have been reported. The diagnosis is made by serologic testing and is generally suspected only in persons with a history of contact with rodents. There is no specific therapy.

RABIES

Rabies in humans has decreased to fewer than five cases per year in the United States. Cases in domestic animals have similarly decreased; 122 rabid dogs and cats were reported to the Centers for Disease Control in 1978. Therefore bites of wild animals have taken on a proportionately larger role as a source of infection in humans. Skunks, bats, foxes, and raccoons are the most frequently infected animals.

After an incubation period (usually 2 weeks to 2 months), half or more of the patients complain of pain or paresthesias at the site of the bite. However, initial symptoms may be nonspecific. Furthermore, early intubation and artificial ventilation may obscure the characteristic signs of hydrophobia and periods of hyperactivity interrupted by intervals of lucidity. Therefore the clinical diagnosis may be overlooked. It is important to consider the diagnosis of rabies in every undiagnosed case of encephalitis because of the potential public health implications. Diagnosis can be established by immunofluorescent staining of corneal impression smears, skin biopsies from the back of the neck or brain tissue, and assay for rabies antibody. There is no specific therapy. The disease is generally fatal. Considerations as to who should receive postexposure prophylaxis with rabies vaccine are discussed in Chapter 38.

TREATABLE CAUSES OF "ASEPTIC MENINGOENCEPHALITIS"

With the exception of herpes simplex type 1 encephalitis, no viral infections of the CNS are treatable with specific agents. Because of this, because the clinical presentations are usually relatively nonspecific, and because the CSF findings are not diagnostic, possible nonviral causes for the patient's illness must always be kept in mind. Generally, these causes have specific therapies. A partial list of diseases that may mimic CSF findings in viral meningitis and encephalitis follows:

Tuberculosis
Fungal infection (cryptococcosis, coccidioidomycosis)
Listeriosis
Partially treated bacterial meningitis
Falciparum malaria
Syphilis
Amoeba infection
Toxoplasmosis
Parameningeal infection (brain abscess, epidural and subdural infections)
Rocky Mountain spotted fever
Vasculitis
Behçet's disease
Sarcoidosis
Carcinomatous and lymphomatous meningitis

EVALUATION OF THE PATIENT WITH ASEPTIC MENINGITIS OR VIRAL ENCEPHALITIS

After deciding that a viral CNS infection is most likely, the physician is confronted with the problem of proving which agent is responsible. The approach to this problem should include the following steps:

1. Consider the age of the patient and the season of the year.
2. Obtain travel and exposure history.
3. Look for clues associated with specific viruses during the general physical examination.
4. Obtain viral cultures. Culture the CSF for enteroviruses, herpesviruses, and mumps; culture the throat for enteroviruses and mumps; and culture the stool for enteroviruses.
5. Obtain serologic tests. A single specimen may be employed to diagnose mumps and Epstein-Barr virus infection. Paired sera are required for other viruses.
6. If the clinical situation suggests herpes simplex, consider a brain biopsy and vidarabine therapy.
7. Always consider nonviral causes and obtain appropriate studies to evaluate these diseases.

BIBLIOGRAPHY

Barza, M., and Pauker, S.G.: The decision to biopsy, treat or wait in suspected herpes simplex encephalitis, Ann. Intern. Med. **92**:641, 1980.

Centers for Disease Control: Aseptic meningitis surveillance, Annual Summary, Atlanta, 1976.

Centers for Disease Control: Encephalitis surveillance, Atlanta, 1977.

Ehrenkranz, N.J., and Ventura, A.K.: Venezuelan equine encephalitis virus infection in man, Annu. Rev. Med. **25**:9, 1974.

Feigin, R.D., and Shackelford, P.G.: Value of repeat lumbar puncture in the differential diagnosis of meningitis, N. Engl. J. Med. **289**:571, 1973.

Levine, D.P., Lauter, C.B., and Lerner, A.M.: Simultaneous serum and cerebrospinal fluid antibodies in herpes simplex virus encephalitis, J.A.M.A. **240**:356, 1978.

Plotkin, S.A., and Koprowski, H.: Phobia of hydrophobia justified, N. Engl. J. Med. **300**:620, 1979.

Southern, P.M., Jr., and others: Clinical and laboratory features of epidemic St. Louis encephalitis, Ann. Intern. Med. **71**:681, 1969.

Vanzee, B.E., and others: Lymphocytic choriomeningitis in university hospital personnel, Am. J. Med. **58**:803, 1975.

Mumps

Donald Kaye

Mumps is an RNA virus that infects only humans. Most cases occur between 5 and 15 years of age. Transmission is by direct contact or by contact with droplets of saliva that contain virus several days before and up to 1 week after swelling of the parotid gland appears. Organs involved include the salivary glands, pancreas, testes, and central nervous system (see discussion of "Viral infections of the central nervous system"). Inapparent infection is common and results in lifetime immunity.

After an incubation period of 14 to 21 days, fever develops and is accompanied by swelling and tenderness of one or both parotid glands. Infection of other salivary glands, one or both testicles (rare before puberty), and meningocencephalitis may occur. The last may develop in patients who do not have parotitis. Clinical pancreatitis is uncommon.

The diagnosis is proved by isolation of the virus from saliva or by serologic means (see discussion of "Viral infections of the central nervous system"). There is no specific therapy. Analgesics and corticosteroids have been used to relieve the pain of orchitis, but they do not prevent atrophy. However, sterility is a rare consequence of mumps orchitis.

BIBLIOGRAPHY

Mandell, G.L., Douglas, R.G., and Bennett, J.E.: Principles and practice of infectious diseases, New York, 1979, John Wiley & Sons, Inc.

Viral respiratory infections

Michael Buckley

Over 60,000 deaths annually in the United States are attributable to respiratory illness, and over one half the visits to primary care physicians are related to respiratory infections. An estimated 80% of acute respiratory illnesses are viral in origin, indicating the major importance of respiratory viruses to clinician and investigator alike. More than 150 viruses have been associated with respiratory illnesses; however, distinct clinical features often permit a presumptive etiologic diagnosis and enable viral illnesses to be distinguished from bacterial infections. This latter point is important, since antibiotics are of no benefit in the treatment of viral diseases. The concentration here will be on the clinical characteristics of the common viral respiratory pathogens that are listed below:

Influenza viruses
Respiratory syncytial virus
Parainfluenza viruses
Adenoviruses
Picornaviruses
    Rhinoviruses
    Enteroviruses
Other viruses
    Cytomegalovirus
    Coronaviruses
    Varicella-zoster virus
    Measles virus

INFLUENZA

Influenza is an acute respiratory tract infection caused by influenza viruses. It occurs in localized outbreaks, epidemics, or pandemics (that is, epidemics of worldwide scope) and is associated with high morbidity and occasionally high mortality. Since 1580, 31 pandemics have been described, the greatest being the swine influenza pandemic of 1918-1919, which accounted for 21 million deaths worldwide and over 500,000 in the United States.

Three distinct types of influenza viruses exist; types A, B, and C. Minor outbreaks and epidemics have been associated with types A and B virus infections; however, to date pandemics have been recorded only with influenza A strains. Type C rarely causes detectable disease, although serologic surveys indicate that a large proportion of the population have evidence of past infection. The success of the influenza virus as a major respiratory pathogen is primarily related to two properties of the virus. The first is the highly contagious nature of the virus, enabling it to spread through communities. The second is related to changes in viral antigenicity. Strains of influenza A virus and, to a lesser extent, influenza B virus have the remarkable ability to change their genetic composition radically. Minor changes in influenza A strain (antigen drifts) generally occur every 1 to 4 years, whereas major changes (antigen shifts) develop approximately every 10 to 15 years (since 1918). To date, only antigen drifts have been detected in influenza B strains. The effect of these changes is that individuals who may have been immune to a previous influenza strain are now partially or totally susceptible to the new virus strain.

ETIOLOGY. Influenza viruses are 90-nm RNA viruses; they have helical symmetry and an envelope coat. Spikes composed of two antigenically and anatomically distinct glycoproteins protrude from the lipid envelope. These are the viral hemagglutinin and neuraminidase. Antibodies against hemagglutinin assume a central role in protection against infection, whereas antibodies against neuraminidase appear less protective.

These viruses are typed A, B, or C according to their nucleocapsid proteins. All type A strains share a common nucleocapsid antigen that is distinct from the common antigens shared by B viruses or C viruses. Within each type (A, B, C) strain differences are detected by antigenic variations in the hemagglutinin and neuraminidase. The present nomenclature of influenza viruses takes into account the viral type, the geographic location where first isolated, the strain number, the year when first isolated, and the antigenic composition of the hemagglutinin and neuraminidase. Thus one of the influenza A viruses isolated in England in the 1972 epidemic was termed A/England/42/72 (H3N2).

EPIDEMIOLOGY. Influenza viruses are spread by transmission of respiratory secretions, predominantly in the form of small-particle (<10 μm) aerosols.

The age-related attack rate of influenza tends to vary from one epidemic to another; however, generally the highest incidence occurs in children 5 to 9 years of age, whereas the most severe manifestations occur in elderly patients or those with complicating underlying disease. A typical outbreak of influenza is characterized by abrupt onset, a high attack rate in the population (often up to 30% to 50%), and rapid spread. Outbreaks often peak in 3 to 4 weeks and then subside over the next month. The severity of disease in a given outbreak depends on many factors, including strain virulence and prior immunity in the population.

The severity of an outbreak can be estimated from the increased incidence of school absenteeism, emergency room visits for respiratory illnesses, and deaths caused by pneumonia.

PATHOGENESIS AND PATHOLOGY. The influenza virus

hemagglutinin probably attaches to receptors on the surface of ciliated respiratory epithelial cells. Virus penetration and replication then follow, leading to degeneration and desquamation of respiratory cells and a mononuclear cell infiltrate. The alveolar walls become thickened, and hyaline membrane formation may occur.

CLINICAL MANIFESTATIONS. The clinical syndromes of influenza A and B viruses are indistinguishable and classically consist of onset of fever, dry cough, myalgias, and headache after an incubation period of 1 to 3 days. Often chills, nasal discharge, and painful eyes are also present. While fever need not be high, prostration may be marked. Nausea and vomiting may be present initially, but a predominance of these symptoms should lead to a different diagnosis. Fever lasts approximately 3 days, but the cough, nasal discharge, and malaise often persist for 1 to 2 weeks. Infection with influenza C does not produce this syndrome; rather, it causes afebrile common colds.

On physical examination the patient appears ill, and the temperature is generally elevated to 100° to 104° F (38° to 40° C). Expiratory wheezes and rhonchi may be detected even if the chest roentgenogram is normal. Clear nasal discharge, conjunctivitis, and injected throat may be present.

Laboratory parameters are nonspecific. The white blood cell count is often elevated initially and then falls, with a predominance of lymphocytes. Liver function studies are usually normal. The electrocardiogram can show some nonspecific T wave changes but usually shows only a persistent tachycardia. The chest roentgenogram, when abnormal, is indicative of either influenzal lower respiratory tract infection or secondary bacterial pneumonia. The former is usually a patchy interstitial infiltrate, and the latter is more consolidated. Gram stain of expectorated sputum examined for polymorphonuclear leukocytes and bacteria is particularly helpful in distinguishing between the two.

The major cause of excess mortality is development of pulmonary complications. Patients with underlying diseases such as chronic obstructive pulmonary disease, mitral stenosis, and other cardiovascular diseases are particularly prone to pneumonia, either primary influenza viral pneumonia (a high-mortality disease), which usually develops shortly after the onset of infection, or secondary bacterial pneumonia, which typically begins in the second week after a period of improvement from the initial symptoms. The bacteria most commonly associated with this entity are the pneumococcus, *Staphylococcus aureus*, and *Haemophilus influenzae*. Less common but potentially serious complications of influenza include myocarditis, encephalopathy, and Reye's syndrome. The last has been described chiefly in children and most often follows influenza B infection. The pathogenesis of this syndrome is unknown. The syndrome is characterized by nausea and vomiting and progression to lethargy, coma, and seizures. Laboratory tests reveal abnormal liver function tests, hypoglycemia, and, most commonly, an increase in blood ammonia. The mortality rate is approximately 20% to 40%. Minor complications of influenza include otitis media and sinusitis.

DIAGNOSIS. Once influenza virus has been isolated in the community, the diagnosis can generally be made based on the clinical syndrome. Some laboratories can perform immunofluorescence for rapid identification of the virus in respiratory secretions. The diagnosis is usually established by viral isolation from respiratory secretions. A fourfold rise in antibody titer from the acute to the convalescent specimen also confirms the diagnosis of recent influenza infection.

MANAGEMENT AND PREVENTION. In uncomplicated influenza, antipyretics, analgesics, rest, and oral fluids help to relieve symptoms. Antibiotics are not indicated. If pneumonia develops. Gram stains of expectorated sputum are important to distinguish viral from bacterial infection. Antibiotics should be used to treat otitis media, sinusitis, or bacterial pneumonia. Amantadine hydrochloride (Symmetrel) is useful against type A influenza viruses, mainly as a prophylactic drug but also as a therapeutic agent (see Chapter 38). For vaccines see Chapter 38.

RESPIRATORY SYNCYTIAL VIRUS

Respiratory syncytial virus (RSV) is a major cause of life-threatening lower respiratory infection in infants and an important pathogen worldwide. So effective is its spread that essentially all become infected by a young age. Unfortunately, immunity is incomplete and reinfections are common. Although RSV is primarily a pathogen of children, it causes upper respiratory infections in adults and can cause severe lower respiratory illness in aged individuals and immunocompromised hosts.

ETIOLOGY. RSV is a member of the paramyxovirus group, along with mumps, parainfluenza, and measles. It has an RNA-containing nucleocapsid, and in contrast to influenza only one antigenic variety is known. The virus derives its name from the fact that it forms large syncytia on primary inoculation of certain cell monolayers.

EPIDEMIOLOGY. The virus is probably transmitted by the airborne route or by contact with infected secretions. Its spread is rapid and extensive and occurs predominantly in midwinter and early spring. Outbreaks develop yearly, mainly affecting infants and children under 5 years of age.

PATHOGENESIS. After inoculation into the eye, nose, or mouth, the virus incubates for 2 to 8 days, with a mean of 5 days. Infection is generally confined to the respiratory tract. In bronchiolitis a lymphocytic peribronchiolar infiltrate develops with subsequent necrosis of bronchiolar epithelium. The small airway lumina become obstructed, airflow is impeded, and hyperinflation and air trapping ensue. Some patients have pneumonia characterized by mononuclear infiltrates, edema, and necrosis. Recovery is generally complete; however, morphologic alteration may persist indefinitely.

The mechanisms by which RSV induces these pathologic changes are unclear. Circulating humoral and cellular immunity is not totally protective; moreover, immunologic mechanisms may actually contribute to the pathogenesis of disease. This observation is supported by the severity of RSV infection in young infants in the presence of passive maternal antibody. In addition, children with high levels of humoral and cellular immunity induced by inactivated RSV vaccine may have severe disease on reinfection.

CLINICAL MANIFESTATIONS. The clinical syndromes of respiratory syncytial virus infection are somewhat age dependent. Infants and children under 5 years of age have a higher incidence of pneumonia, bronchiolitis, and otitis media than older children, in whom upper respiratory tract infection or tracheobronchitis is common. Adults have a "common cold" syndrome with a prolonged course compared with common colds of other causes. RSV can produce an acute exacerbation of bronchitis, and in immunosuppressed individuals bronchopneumonia may appear.

The typical picture of bronchiolitis is a child less than 1 year old who has a febrile upper respiratory infection and a cough, mucus production, expiratory wheezing, dyspnea, rib retraction, poor oral intake, and air hunger. On the chest roentgenogram diffuse hyperaeration and scattered infiltrates are seen. The infiltrates are caused by atelectasis but may be difficult to distinguish from changes seen in pneumonia. In the child or adult with bronchopneumonia rales can be heard on examination of the chest. The roentgenogram shows patchy or consolidated infiltrate, and the sputum is nonpurulent. The upper respiratory syndrome is nonspecific, with fever, cough, rhinitis, and mild pharyngitis.

DIAGNOSIS. In children the diagnosis is often suspected based on the seasonal presentation of a typical syndrome, bronchiolitis, or bronchopneumonia. Specific virologic diagnosis can best be made by culturing the virus from respiratory secretions, especially nasopharyngeal aspirates. Rapid diagnostic methods employing immunofluorescent techniques have been developed.

MANAGEMENT. There is no specific therapy. Antibiotics should be used only for treatment of suspected or proven bacterial superinfections such as otitis media or pneumonia.

PREVENTION. There is at present no effective vaccine.

PARAINFLUENZA VIRUSES

Parainfluenza viruses are a subgroup of the paramyxoviruses and are second only to respiratory syncytial virus as a cause of respiratory disease in infants and young children. They are the major identifiable cause of the croup syndrome. Like RSV, however, they cause a spectrum of disease ranging from a mild upper respiratory infection to pneumonia. Immunity after parainfluenza infection is incomplete, and most infections in older children and adults represent reinfection.

ETIOLOGY. Parainfluenza viruses are pleomorphic, contain a single-stranded RNA nucleocapsid, and possess an outer membrane with a hemagglutinin on the surface. Four antigenic types (1, 2, 3, 4), which have remained antigenically stable, have been identified. Typing is based on complement-fixing and hemagglutinating antigens.

EPIDEMIOLOGY. The distribution of all four types is worldwide. The virus is capable of rapid spread, especially among children in large confined groups. Like most respiratory viruses, an increase is often noted in the fall and winter months, although some disease activity occurs throughout the year. The clinical syndromes caused by the parainfluenza viruses are somewhat type specific. Type 4 virus appears to cause subclinical or mild clinical illness, which is not particularly well characterized yet. Types 1 and 2 are the most frequent causes of croup, accounting for about one third of the cases. Type 3 predominantly causes lower respiratory infections, including bronchiolitis and pneumonia, in very young infants. Although types 1 and 2 often alternate year to year as causes of respiratory illness in a given community, the level of type 3 activity remains relatively constant.

PATHOGENESIS. Parainfluenza viruses are transmitted from person to person quite readily, probably by direct contact and large droplet aerosols. The target cells of the respiratory tract seem to be ciliated epithelial cells. The mechanism for the subglottic involvement in laryngotracheobronchitis (the croup syndrome) is not understood.

CLINICAL MANIFESTATIONS. The spectrum of clinical illness caused by parainfluenza viruses ranges from the "common cold" to life-threatening lower respiratory infections. The syndromes are best discussed in relation to the age of those affected.

In children there are three major syndromes. The mildest is a typical respiratory infection with a sore throat, nasal discharge, and low-grade fever. The best-recognized childhood illness caused by parainfluenza viruses is the croup syndrome. This begins as a febrile upper respiratory infection and progresses to a characteristic barking spasmodic cough, hoarseness, and in severe cases inspiratory stridor. The last finding appears to be more common in children less than 4 years of age, and croup in general appears to be more severe when caused by parainfluenza viruses in contrast to other viral causes. Despite the stridor observed in some cases, the epiglottis is normal. The third syndrome in children usually associated with type 3 infection is lower respiratory infection, in which bronchitis, bronchiolitis, or pneumonia may occur. It is difficult to distinguish lower respiratory infections caused by parainfluenza viruses from those caused by respiratory syncytial virus except that the former are usually less severe. Bacterial superinfection is also less common after parainfluenza virus infections.

In adults the disease is commonly manifested as a mild upper respiratory infection. However, occasionally prostration may be severe, suggesting influenza infection. Parainfluenza virus infections in older children and adults are frequently accompanied by hoarseness, moderately severe sore throat, and low-grade fever. As with other viral respiratory infections, immunocompromised patients may have a more severe course.

DIAGNOSIS. The diagnosis is suspected in a child with croup or an adult with an upper respiratory infection if hoarseness is prominent. Rapid immunofluorescent techniques can be used to identify parainfluenza viruses in respiratory secretions. A fourfold rise in complement-fixing or hemagglutinating antibody is also diagnostic of recent infection.

MANAGEMENT. There is no specific antiviral chemotherapy. Symptomatic therapy is sufficient for upper respiratory illness. In mild cases management of the croup syndrome includes sedation and humidified air. If laryngeal obstruction supervenes, this constitutes a medical emergency. Intubation or tracheostomy may occasionally be required, but fortunately this is infrequent following parainfluenza infections. There is no convincing evidence that steroids are effective in croup.

PREVENTION. Reinfection with parainfluenza viruses is common even in the presence of antibody. Nevertheless, it has been observed that reinfection, especially in the presence of high antibody titer, is clinically milder than primary infection, and viral shedding occurs for a shorter period. Therefore there is great interest in the future development of vaccines against parainfluenza viruses.

ADENOVIRUSES

Adenoviruses are clinically important causes of conjunctivitis and acute respiratory infections. As with most respiratory viruses, they have diverse clinical manifestations. Although there is overlap, the clinical syndromes are somewhat type specific.

ETIOLOGY. Adenoviruses contain double-stranded DNA and have a protein or capsid coat. Over 30 types have been detected, certain ones of which are associated with common disease syndromes.

EPIDEMIOLOGY. Adenoviruses are worldwide in distribution. Infection spreads by aerosol and occurs with increasing frequency if crowding exists. In contrast to respiratory syncytial virus, infection before the age of 6 months is unusual; however, most children have been infected by age 10. Infection becomes uncommon after age 15 except in the military. The type of adenovirus causing infection and the resulting clinical syndrome are somewhat age dependent.

Types 1, 2, 5, and 6 are frequently isolated from tonsils and adenoids of children with upper respiratory tract infections. Types 3, 4, and 7 are often isolated from young adults with upper and lower respiratory tract diseases. Type 8 has frequently been isolated from the conjunctiva in adults. Type 4 has caused an acute respiratory disease in military recruits.

PATHOGENESIS. Adenoviruses can produce persistent or latent infection of tonsillar lymphoid tissue, lytic infection of respiratory epithelium, and oncogenic transformation of several in vitro cell strains. Most acute respiratory infections caused by adenoviruses are probably the result of host cell lysis produced during viral replication.

CLINICAL MANIFESTATIONS. The illnesses produced by adenoviruses are generally age related and fall into five major clinical syndromes: a mild upper respiratory infection, acute respiratory disease, pneumonia, pharyngoconjunctival fever, and keratoconjunctivitis. The last occurs in epidemics or as sporadic cases, usually involves adults, and consists of conjunctivitis of 1 to 4 weeks' duration, preauricular adenopathy, and keratitis that appears as the conjunctivitis wanes. The age-related syndromes are discussed in the following.

In contrast to RSV and parainfluenza viruses, infants are usually asymptomatic following adenovirus infections or have a mild coryza and pharyngitis. Rarely a fulminant bronchiolitis or pneumonia may be seen. Children generally have either pharyngoconjunctival fever or an upper respiratory infection with a mild tracheitis indistinguishable from other viral infections. The former occurs predominantly in school-age children, most often in the summer, and is characterized by conjunctivitis that is usually unilateral, pharyngitis, rhinitis, cervical adenitis, and fever. The infection is abrupt in onset and lasts 3 to 5 days. Bacterial superinfection or eye damage is rare. Adenovirus has also been isolated from children in association with whooping cough, but its precise role in this syndrome is not well defined.

In young adults, especially military recruits, the major syndromes are acute respiratory disease (ARD) and pneumonia, the latter being clinically indistinguishable from other viral pneumonias except on an epidemiologic basis. ARD is an epidemic disease of military recruits with cough, fever, pharyngitis, and rhinorrhea. Viral pneumonia appears to complicate ARD in approximately 10% of recruits. The moribidity is significant, but the mortality is low.

Adenoviruses can cause hemorrhagic cystitis in children (usually girls).

DIAGNOSIS. The diagnosis is often made clinically by recognizing one of the characteristic syndromes, such as ARD in military recruits. The virus may be isolated from respiratory secretions or demonstrated by immunofluorescent staining of exfoliated cells. Serology can be helpful in some cases.

MANAGEMENT AND PREVENTION. There is no specific chemotherapy currently available. Oral vaccines consisting of live type 4 and 7 viruses in enteric-coated capsules have been developed for use in military recruits. These are not attenuated viruses but do not produce disease when introduced by the gastrointestinal route. They have been effective in reducing the frequency of ARD in recruits.

PICORNAVIRUSES

The picornavirus group of RNA viruses has two major subgroups, the rhinoviruses and the enteroviruses. This is the largest group of viruses causing respiratory disease, although the respiratory illnesses are for the most part quite mild. The rhinoviruses are associated with the common cold syndrome, and the enteroviruses are associated with multiorgan disease, including infection of the respiratory tract.

RHINOVIRUSES

ETIOLOGY. There are more than 90 serotypes of rhinoviruses currently known. Since they do not share a common antigen, immunity appears to be largely type specific. The virus is small, has an RNA core, and exhibits cubic symmetry.

EPIDEMIOLOGY. The rhinoviruses are worldwide in distribution, infect adults more often than children, and occur year round but mainly in autumn and spring. They account for 30% of adult respiratory infections. Transmission may be by hand transfer and by the airborne route.

CLINICAL MANIFESTATIONS. The common cold caused by rhinovirus is an afebrile upper respiratory infection with nasal stuffiness, sneezing, and a scratchy throat. There is often an inflamed nasopharynx and a postnasal drip that leads to a cough. There is an extremely low complication rate. The incubation period is 1 to 3 days.

DIAGNOSIS AND MANAGEMENT. The diagnosis is easily suspected by the clinical syndrome. Although isolation of the virus and serologic confirmation are possible, the mild nature of the illness makes them impractical other than in research settings. No specific therapy is available.

PREVENTION. The common cold is caused by many antigenically unrelated viruses. Prevention by vaccination would therefore be difficult.

ENTEROVIRUSES

The enteroviruses include polioviruses, coxsackieviruses, and echoviruses. Certain coxsackieviruses and echoviruses cause a small percentage of respiratory infections, especially in the summer and fall months. They are, however, better known as causes of meningitis (see discussion of ''Viral infections of the central nervous system''), myopericarditis, and febrile illnesses with or without exanthems (see discussion of ''Exanthems of viral or presumed viral origin'').

CLINICAL MANIFESTATIONS. Herpangina, caused by group A coxsackieviruses, is characterized by fever, sore throat, and generally two to six papular lesions that progress to painful ulcers on the soft palate, tonsillar pillars, tonsils, pharynx, or tongue. Groups A and B coxsackieviruses also cause lymphonodular pharyngitis.

Group B coxsackieviruses cause epidemic pleurodynia (devil's grippe), which is characterized by the abrupt onset of pleuritic or abdominal pain, often paroxysmal and spasmodic, ranging from mild to severe. Cough is notably absent. The illness lasts approximately 5 days, and the pain gradually lessens over this period of time.

Echoviruses are occasionally isolated from children with fevers and sore throats. Bronchiolitis has been reported with echoviruses, and rarely lower respiratory infections may occur.

DIAGNOSIS. Presumptive diagnosis is made on the basis of the clinical syndrome, but definitive diagnosis requires isolation of the virus from respiratory secretions, stool, or spinal fluid (in cases of aseptic meningitis).

MANAGEMENT AND PREVENTION. There is no specific therapy. Poliomyelitis prevention is discussed in Chapter 38. The large number of serotypes and the generally mild illnesses make the development of vaccines unlikely.

CORONAVIRUSES

Coronaviruses derive their name from their crownlike external structure. They have an RNA core, but the internal structure and the antigenic relationships among the various coronaviruses are incompletely understood.

Clinical illness produced by these agents resembles the common cold syndrome caused by rhinoviruses. Occasionally lower respiratory infection develops. Illness usually occurs in adults. Diagnosis on clinical grounds is impossible, and most strains grow in vitro only in organ cultures of human embryonic tracheal or nasal epithelium. Serologic diagnosis can be performed using a complement fixation test. Neither specific therapy nor vaccines are available.

• • •

A large number of viruses cause acute respiratory illness. The more common causes of isolated respiratory illnesses are shown in Table 37-1.

It is important to remember that most upper respiratory infections are caused by viruses, with group A β-hemolytic streptococci being the only cause of acute pharyngitis and tonsillitis requiring antibiotics. On clinical grounds it is often difficult to distinguish group A streptococcal infection from viral pharyngitis, and a bacterial throat culture is required. With lower respiratory illness the distinction between viral and bacterial infection can be even more difficult. The clinical syndrome, seasonal occurrence, and, if available, examination of expectorated sputum by Gram stain are useful distinguishing features. The presence of polymorphonuclear leukocytes favors a bacterial cause. Of great value is information obtained from a regional diagnostic virology laboratory as to which viruses are present in the community. This input and working knowledge of the various clinical syndromes allow physicians to make educated clinical decisions and enable proper use of antibiotics.

Table 37-1. Common viral causes of various respiratory illnesses

Clinical syndromes	Common viral causes
Upper respiratory infections	
Common cold	Rhinoviruses, coronaviruses, respiratory syncytial virus, parainfluenza viruses
Tonsillitis, pharyngitis	Adenoviruses, Epstein-Barr virus, influenza viruses, parainfluenza viruses, respiratory syncytial virus, enteroviruses
Lower respiratory infections	
Group (hoarseness, barking cough, inspiratory stridor)	Parainfluenza viruses, respiratory syncytial virus
Tracheobronchitis (cough, rhonchi)	Respiratory syncytial virus, influenza viruses, parainfluenza viruses
Bronchiolitis (air trapping, expiratory wheezing)	Respiratory syncytial virus, parainfluenza viruses
Pneumonia (rales, infiltrate on roentgenogram)	Respiratory syncytial virus, influenza viruses, adenoviruses, parainfluenza viruses, cytomegalovirus

BIBLIOGRAPHY

Burrows, B., Knudson, R.J., and Lebowitz, M.D.: The relationship of childhood respiratory illness to adult obstructive airway disease, Am. Rev. Respir. Dis. **115:**751, 1977.

Fiala, M., and Guze, L.B.: The rhinoviruses of man, Calif. Med. **112:**1, 1970.

Glezen, W.P.: Respiratory viruses and mycoplasma pneumonia. In Drew, W.L., editor: Viral infections: a clinical approach, Philadelphia, 1976, F.A. Davis Co.

Glezen, W.P., and Denny, F.W.: Epidemiology of acute respiratory diseases in children, N. Engl. J. Med. **288:**498, 1973.

Jackson, G.G., and Muldoon, R.L.: Viruses causing common respiratory infections in man, J. Infect. Dis. **127:**328, 1973.

Jackson, G.G., and Muldoon, R.L.: Viruses causing common respiratory infections in man. II. Enteroviruses and paramyxoviruses. J. Infect. Dis. **128:**387, 1973.

Jackson, G.G., and Muldoon, R.L.: Viruses causing common respiratory infections in man. III. Respiratory syncytial viruses and coronaviruses, J. Infect. Dis. **128:**674, 1973.

Jackson, G.G., and Muldoon, R.L.: Viruses causing common respiratory infections in man. IV. Reoviruses and adenoviruses. J. Infect. Dis. **128:**811, 1973.

Knight, V., editor: Viral and mycoplasma infections of the respiratory tract, Philadelphia, 1973, Lea & Febiger.

Knight, V., and others: Amantadine therapy of epidemic influenza A2 (Hong Kong), Infect. Immun. **1:**220, 1970.

Mandell, G.L., Douglas, R.G., and Bennett, J.E., editors: Principles and practice of infectious diseases, New York, 1979, John Wiley & Sons, Inc.

Exanthems of viral or presumed viral origin

Allan M. Arbeter

MEASLES (RUBEOLA)

Measles is an acute respiratory infection associated with a 3- to 5-day prodrome and a characteristic maculopapular rash that lasts 5 to 7 days.

Measles virus is an enveloped RNA paramyxovirus with a diameter of 120 to 350 nm. The envelope contains surface hemagglutinin and hemolysin antigens. Antibody against the hemagglutinin correlates with protection against reinfection.

Measles occurs in young and school-age children worldwide. In countries where the vaccine for measles is in use, the number of cases in young children has declined dramatically but an increased incidence of the disease has occurred in older children and teenagers. The number of cases in a current "epidemic" year is less than 15% of the cases that occurred in the prevaccine era.

Measles virus initially infects the respiratory epithelium and is followed by viremia within leukocytes. Infection develops within reticuloendothelial cells, virus is released and reinvades leukocytes, and a secondary viremia occurs. During this phase extensive respiratory mucosal and skin infection develops. Respiratory manifestations may consist of cough, coryza, bronchopneumonia, and croup. The rash coincides with the development of an immune response and appears to be mediated by a delayed hypersensitivity reaction to the virus in the skin.

The incubation period is 10 to 14 days in children but may be as long as 21 days in adults. This is followed by a 3- to 5-day prodrome of increasing severity, consisting of cough, conjunctivitis, fever, malaise, loss of appetite, and coryza. At this time the disease may be indistinguishable from other severe upper respiratory illnesses except for the presence of Koplik's spots. These are multiple 0.25- to 1-mm whitish blue spots on a red base found in clusters on the buccal mucosa, usually opposite the second molars. These lesions represent sites of virus replication. A characteristic intense maculopapular rash then develops on the face and neck and spreads in a descending pattern to reach the hands and feet 3 to 5 days later. As the rash spreads, prior areas of involvement become confluent. Desquamation may occur. Complications of measles include viral pneumonia, secondary bacterial pneumonia, otitis media, laryngotracheal bronchitis, and encephalitis. The encephalitis may be fatal or leave the patient with permanent neurologic sequelae. Subacute sclerosing panencephalitis is a rare chronic sequela of measles virus infection when measles occurs early in life.

Unusual forms of measles include *modified measles* and *atypical measles*. Modified measles, which is very mild measles, occurs when the patient has received gamma globulin within 3 days of exposure. Modified measles has also been described in patients who previously had vaccine-induced immunity. Atypical measles is a distinct clinical syndrome occurring in patients previously immunized with killed measles vaccine. The illness includes high fever, maculopapular or purpuric rash of the extremities, and severe pneumonitis. The illness may resemble Rocky Mountain spotted fever or meningococcemia. When measles occurs in patients with deficiencies in cellular immunity, a severe giant cell pneumonia (Hecht's pneumonia) without rash can occur. This disease is frequently fatal in immunosuppressed patients, especially leukemic children undergoing chemotherapy.

Measles can be diagnosed by examination of mucosal cells, virus isolation, and antibody tests. Scraped cells from the conjunctiva, nasopharynx, or Koplik's spots demonstrate multinucleated giant cells and cells containing eosinophilic cytoplasmic inclusions. Direct immunofluorescent staining of exfoliated cells or skin biopsy material with measles virus–specific antisera can demonstrate viral antigen. Because the virus is difficult to grow in the laboratory, the diagnosis is usually made by serologic testing using either a complement fixation or a hemagglutination inhibition assay. When paired sera samples are tested, a fourfold or greater antibody rise is diagnostic of recent infection.

There is no specific therapy for measles virus infection.

Active immunization with live attenuated measles vaccine has been highly successful in reducing measles infection. The immunization when given at or after 15 months of age is expected to produce lifelong immunity.

Measles can also be prevented by giving exposed normal children the live vaccine within 3 days of exposure. Live measles vaccine should not be given to immunosuppressed patients. Measles can be modified and sometimes prevented by giving immune serum globulin. However, this does not provide permanent immunity.

RUBELLA (GERMAN MEASLES)

Rubella is a mild respiratory virus infection associated with an exanthem. Of major importance is the fetal damage that develops following transplacental infection (see discussion of "Viral infections of the fetus and newborn"). Infection occurring before 12 weeks' gestation may lead to abortions; severe birth defects, including micrencephaly; and cardiac anomalies. Infection later in pregnancy may lead to hepatitis, jaundice, thrombocytopenia, lymphadenopathy, and pneumonitis. Some infected infants are born without anomalies but may have progressive mental retardation and spastic diplegia.

Rubella virus contains an RNA nucleoprotein and a lipid envelope, has a diameter of 60 nm, and is classified as a togavirus. Antigens useful for serologic tests include nucleoprotein (complement fixation) and envelope (hemagglutinin) antigens.

Rubella occurs predominantly in the spring and early summer. The agent is highly contagious by the respiratory route. The incidence of rubella has decreased since the introduction of vaccine. However, because of poor compliance with immunization programs, local outbreaks continue to occur.

The virus is spread by respiratory secretions. Although heaviest viral shedding occurs at the time of the rash, rubella virus can be isolated several days before and after onset of the eruption. As with measles, primary and secondary viremia develop. The rash occurs at the end of the secondary viremia and coincides with the development of the immune response, suggesting that immune mechanisms may participate in the pathogenesis of the rash.

Postnatally acquired rubella is generally a benign disease in children and adults. The incubation period is 14 to 21 days. The rash may occur in a typical pattern or be nonspecific. The typical rash appears as a maculopapular eruption on the face and neck and is preceded by or associated with posterior cervical adenopathy. The rash descends from head to foot over 2 to 3 days, fading above as it appears below, and does not become confluent. An enanthem may develop simultaneously with the rash and consists chiefly of petechial lesions on the soft palate (Forscheimer spots). Fever is present for 1 to 2 days at the onset of the rash. In 30% to 40% of adult women with rubella, arthritis or arthralgias of the fingers, wrists, and knees develop.

A severe postinfectious encephalitis can occur with rubella but is uncommon. In several patients with congenital rubella a subacute sclerosing panencephalitis–like illness has developed in subsequent years.

The manifestations of rubella may be sufficiently mild (for example, nonspecific or absent rash) that many cases go undiagnosed. In addition, several other viruses can produce similar-appearing rashes. Therefore a clinical history of rubella cannot be relied on to indicate immunity. In nonvaccinated women of childbearing age the immune status should be evaluated by antibody testing.

Specific diagnosis of rubella is made by virus isolation or serologic tests. The virus can be cultured from throat samples and from urine in infants with congenital infection. The most widely used antibody test is the hemagglutination inhibition assay. Detecting recent infection is particularly important in pregnant women, since a positive result could lead to a therapeutic abortion. In paired serum samples a fourfold or greater rise in rubella antibody is diagnostic of recent infection. If only a convalescent serum sample is available, a rubella-specific IgM antibody assay can be performed; this is a useful diagnostic aid during pregnancy.

There is no treatment for rubella.

Since 1969, live attenuated rubella vaccines have been available. The currently available strain is RA 27/3, which is given subcutaneously. Prepubertal children and seronegative nonpregnant women are the main targets for vaccination.

Immune serum globulin is ineffective in preventing viremia and intrauterine infection, although it may modify the clinical illness.

ROSEOLA (EXANTHEMA SUBITUM)

Roseola is an acute illness of undefined origin. The diagnosis is established by the characteristic clinical syndrome. The disease occurs in infants and young children predominantly between 6 months and 3 years of age. It does not recur, suggesting that it is caused by a single serotype with persistent immunity. Illness occurs year round with a springtime peak. Secondary cases are usually limited to children of similar age rather than to siblings. The incubation period is 10 to 15 days.

The disease usually begins without a prodrome. There is a sudden onset of high temperature, commonly 104° F (40° C), malaise, irritability, and anorexia. The pharynx may be injected, anterior and posterior cervical adenopathy is often present, and on days 3 to 5 a maculopapular rash develops. The rash characteristically appears as the fever is declining or has disappeared. Rash is rarely found on the face or extremities but is located on the chest, abdomen, and neck and lasts 6 hours to 2 days. The diagnosis is made by the typical clinical manifestations. Laboratory tests are not helpful. The white blood cell count may be decreased, normal, or elevated.

Febrile convulsions may occur because of rapid onset of fever in young children. Since the rash is not present at the onset of fever, a lumbar spinal puncture for suspected meningitis is performed in many children. The cerebrospinal fluid is normal.

There is no specific therapy for this illness. Temperature control is recommended to prevent seizures. Since the etiologic agent has not been identified, no vaccine is available.

ERYTHEMA INFECTIOSUM (FIFTH DISEASE)

The etiologic agent of fifth disease has not been identified. The disease is categorized as an infection, probably viral, because of the seasonal occurrence, predominantly winter, and the clustering of cases separated by a 5- to 10-day incubation period. It most often affects children and is unusual in adults.

The clinical manifestations of erythema infectiosum are variable. The rash may be preceded by a mild prodrome of fever and coryza lasting 1 to 2 days. A marked erythema of the cheeks (so-called slapped cheeks) follows. Either simultaneously or shortly thereafter a red macular rash develops on the extremities, sparing the palms and soles. The rash, involving the face and extremities, is frequently sufficiently characteristic to enable a diagnosis. Circumoral pallor is common. On the extremities the rash has been described as lacy and includes a pattern of red blotches, some of which are confluent, circular, or annular. The rash may fade and reappear for several weeks. Additional features include high fever, pharyngitis, vomiting and diarrhea, adenopathy, and joint complaints. In adults there are more frequent complaints of arthritis.

The diagnosis of erythema infectiosum is based on the constellation of clinical features. When the clinical pattern is unusual, other illnesses must be considered, including erythema multiforme, infectious mononucleosis, rubella, and measles. There are no laboratory tests that confirm the diagnosis, and no specific treatments or preventive therapies are available.

KAWASAKI DISEASE

Kawasaki disease, also termed mucocutaneous lymph node syndrome, is an acute febrile disease of children with a reported 1% to 2% fatality rate, worldwide distribution, and unknown origin. The disease was originally described in Japan, where over 10,000 cases have been recorded, but has been diagnosed throughout North America as well. Several etiologic agents have been associated with specific outbreaks or individual cases, including rickettsiae, streptococci, and respiratory viruses. However, a specific etiologic agent for this syndrome has not been confirmed.

Fever occurs in almost 100% of the cases and lasts for a minimum of 1 week but may persist for 2 to 4 weeks, reaching daily spikes of 102° to 104° F (39° to 40° C). During the first week conjunctivitis, stomatitis, diffuse adenopathy, and a rash of the trunk and extremities develop. The conjunctivitis is predominantly bulbar and may be mild or severe. The discharge is thin and white, if present. The lips are bright red, fissured, and painful. The tongue is frequently desquamated, exposing the papillae and resembling the strawberry tongue of scarlet fever. The extremity rash can include a papular eruption of the arms and legs, but most striking are the edema and redness of the palms and soles. This blanching erythema may continue for 1 to 2 weeks before desquamation of the skin and hands occurs. Desquamation occurs in sheets, taking several days. In mild cases the peeling occurs only on the edges of the nails. The truncal rash may be a nonspecific papular rash reminiscent of measles, scarlet fever, or infectious mononucleosis. Nonsuppurative adenopathy, which is usually cervical but occasionally diffuse, may occur. Other clinical manifestations include gastrointestinal complaints, joint symptoms, and aseptic meningitis.

The major complication of Kawasaki disease is coronary arteritis early in the course and eventuating as coronary artery aneurysms. In addition, there may be a carditis affecting the conduction systems and papillary muscles. Death as a result of arrhythmias, coronary artery obstruction, and rupture or thrombosis of a coronary artery aneurysm may occur suddenly at any time from the acute illness to years later. The carditis is similar to that described as infantile polyarteritis nodosa, which may be the same disease.

Laboratory studies may support the clinical diagnosis. Findings include a leukocytosis with a shift toward immature forms, a marked thrombocytosis, sometimes exceeding 10^6 platelets/mm^3, and an elevated erythrocyte sedimentation rate. Serum IgE is elevated in the majority of cases. The electrocardiogram may show abnormalities in conduction and repolarization. If heart disease is suspected, further evaluation for carditis and aneurysms is indicated.

Beyond fever control, there is no immediate therapy for the acute illness. Aspirin and steroids have been proposed for the prevention and treatment of arteritis, but efficacy and safety have not yet been determined. No preventive therapies are available.

ADENOVIRUS EXANTHEMS

The adenoviruses are 70-nm double-stranded DNA viruses that cause frequent infections in humans. The diseases produced include conjunctivitis, pharyngitis, laryngitis, laryngotracheal bronchitis, pneumonitis, adenitis, and hemorrhagic cystitis (see discussion of "Viral respiratory infections"). Any of the clinical syndromes of adenovirus infection may be accompanied by rash. Although over 30 serotypes of adenoviruses exist, disease is most commonly produced by types 1 to 8.

The rash is nonspecific. It may vary from a very diffuse macular disease to a heavy, confluent maculopapular disease with involvement of the face, neck, trunk, and extremities. The rash may be present for 1 day or mimic measles, occurring after a prodrome and remaining for 5 to 7 days. Rarely the rash becomes vesicular. The nonspecific nature of the rash makes diagnosis more difficult; however, the presence of conjunctivitis, pharyngitis, and adenitis indicates a probable adenovirus infection.

Routine laboratory studies are nonspecific. Adenoviruses can be isolated on tissue culture cells. Viral serology, using the complement fixation method, will confirm recent infection if a fourfold or greater rise in antibody is noted.

There is no specific therapy for adenovirus infections. Prevention has been demonstrated after inoculation with live virus and inactivated vaccines. However, these vaccines are not in general use.

ENTEROVIRUS EXANTHEMS

The enteroviruses are members of the picornavirus family. These small RNA viruses lack a lipoprotein envelope. Those that cause exanthems include group A and B coxsackieviruses and the echoviruses. These viruses cause disease worldwide in infants, children, and adults. More than 70 serologically different enteroviruses have been detected.

Enterovirus infections result in a large number of clinical syndromes. Illnesses include nonspecific febrile diseases, stomatitis, tonsillitis, pharyngitis, aseptic meningitis, encephalitis, gastroenteritis, pneumonitis, pleurodynia, pericarditis, myocarditis, and exanthems.

The exanthems may be of a specific character (hand-foot-and-mouth disease) or of a variety of nonspecific types. The nonspecific rashes can include manifestations and clinical syndromes similar to measles, rubella, roseola, erythema infectiosum, and herpes simplex. The eruptions can occur with fever alone or in combination with any of the other enteroviral syndromes.

One of the characteristic exanthems of enteroviruses is hand-foot-and-mouth disease. This mild illness includes fever and oral vesicles followed by vesicles on the hands, feet, fingers, toes, soles, palms, and extensor surfaces of the arms and legs. These papulovesicular lesions can be painful and may last over 1 week. Virus can be isolated from the lesions. Coxsackieviruses A5, A10, A16, B2, and B5 have all been associated with hand-foot-and-mouth disease.

An additional characteristic exanthem is caused by coxsackievirus A9. This virus produces a papulovesicular rash that occurs with the onset of fever. Like chickenpox, the rash is heaviest on the trunk, neck, and head, but it differs because the lesion remains vesicular without pustulating or crusting. There is usually no enanthem.

Enteroviruses, particularly group A coxsackieviruses, may cause a vesicular enanthem of the fauces and soft palate termed herpangina. Fever, sore throat, and pain on swallowing are frequent symptoms. The throat is erythematous, and the tonsils may contain a mild exudate. Two to six, but rarely more, painful lesions are located on the soft palate, frequently at the free-hanging margin between the tonsils and uvula. Occasionally the tonsils, posterior pharyngeal wall, or buccal mucosa is involved. Lesions begin as small macules and over 24 hours evolve into 2- to 4-mm erythematous papules, which then centrally vesiculate. Fever lasts 2 to 4 days, and mouth lesions persist for up to 1 week.

Since enteroviral disease usually appears in epidemic form during the summer or fall months, the diagnosis is aided by knowledge of the local epidemiology.

Standard laboratory tests are generally not helpful. Cultures of throat and stool for viral isolation are the main methods for establishing a specific diagnosis. Group B coxsackieviruses and echoviruses will grow on cell culture, but group A coxsackieviruses may require suckling mouse inoculation for isolation. Serologic confirmation of enterovirus infection is not routinely done unless a specific enterovirus is suspected. The lack of a group-specific antigen common to all serotypes limits the use of antibody testing.

No specific antiviral treatment is available for enterovirus infections. An inactivated parenteral vaccine and an attenuated oral vaccine have been prepared for polioviruses (see Chapter 38); however, vaccines for other enteroviruses are not available.

For exanthems associated with herpesviruses see the discussion "Herpesviruses."

BIBLIOGRAPHY

Cherry, J.D.: Newer viral exanthems, Adv. Pediatr. **16**:233, 1969.

Evans, A.S.: Viral infections of humans: epidemiology and control, New York, 1976, Plenum Publishing Corp.

Krugman, S., and Katz, S.L.: Infectious diseases of children, ed. 7, St. Louis, 1980, The C.V. Mosby Co.

Mandell, G.L., Douglas, R.G., and Bennett, J.E.: Principles and practice of infectious diseases, New York, 1979, John Wiley & Sons, Inc.

Morens, D.M., Anderson, L.J., and Hurwitz, E.S.: National surveillance of Kawasaki's disease, Pediatrics **65**:21, 1980.

Vaughan, V.C., III, McKay, R.J., and Behrman, R.: Nelson's textbook of pediatrics, ed. 11, Philadelphia, 1979, W.B. Saunders Co.

Viral gastroenteritis

Donald H. Rubin

Symptoms of gastroenteritis consist of abdominal pain, nausea, vomiting, diarrhea, and fever, although not all features are present in each case. In a large study in Cleveland over a 10-year period, viral enteritis was the second most frequent disease encountered among families, second only to the common cold. The severity of viral-induced gastroenteritis depends in part on the host. In young children, the old, and the debilitated, viral enteritis can be lethal. The viral agents causing enteritis have a worldwide distribution and pose a major health problem.

The techniques of immune electron microscopy of stool and electron microscopy of infected intestinal mucosa have defined two major viral groups that cause gastroenteritis: the rotaviruses and the Norwalk-like, or 27-nm, agents (Table 37-2). Other viruses have also been seen by electron microscopy of stool; however, their role in gastroenteritis is not clearly defined. Traditionally, picornaviruses (poliovirus, echovirus, and coxsackievirus) have been considered "enteric" viruses (Table 37-2), yet only certain echovirus serotypes are definitely believed to be associated with enteritis. Most picornaviruses enter through the intestine to produce their major impact in organs outside the gastrointestinal tract, for example, in the central nervous system. These viral agents are considered elsewhere in more detail (see discussions of "Viral infections of the central nervous system" and "Exanthems of viral or presumed viral origin"). Rotaviruses and 27-nm Norwalk-like agents will be considered separately, since they produce unique syndromes.

ROTAVIRUSES

The rotaviruses are the most common agents causing sporadic and epidemic outbreaks of enteritis in infants and young children worldwide. Previously the rotaviruses were referred to as duoviruses, orbivirus-like agents, and infantile gastroenteritis virus. In temperate climates 50% of pediatric hospitalizations resulting from gastroenteritis are

Table 37-2. Agents believed to be responsible for gastroenteritis in man

Virus	Known serotypes or classifications	Diagnostic tests — Viral detection	Diagnostic tests — Antibody assay
Rotavirus	Types 1 and 2	Electron microscopy Enzyme immunoassay (ELISA) Radioimmunoassay Counter immunoelectrophoresis	Complement fixation Immunofluorescence Enzyme immunoassay (ELISA)
Norwalk-like agents	Norwalk Hawaii Montgomery County Ditchling "W" Cockle Parramatta	Electron microscopy	Immune electron microscopy Immune adherence hemagglutination Radioimmunoassay
Adenovirus		Electron microscopy Immunofluorescence of tissue culture cells Counter immunoelectrophoresis	
Coronavirus		Electron microscopy	
Minircovirus		Electron microscopy	
Astrovirus		Electron microscopy	
Picornavirus	Echovirus types 11, 14, and 18	Tissue culture isolation	
Hepatitis A		Electron microscopy	Radioimmunoassay Immune adherence hemagglutination

caused by rotaviruses. Symptomatic disease occurs primarily in the 6- to 24-month age group. Neonates and adults can, on occasion, develop symptomatic illness, but subclinical infection is more common. Illness tends to be milder in adults than in children. The peak incidence of symptomatic infection occurs in the winter months. Transmission is by the fecal-oral route. Nosocomial spread in the form of hospital epidemics in pediatric wards has occurred.

The major symptom is diarrhea; dehydration is the main cause for admission to pediatric wards. The incubation period is 24 to 48 hours, and symptoms peak in the following 1 to 3 days. Vomiting, when it occurs, develops early. Fever is present in 75% of the patients. Two serotypes are currently recognized in the United States. Serotype 2 is associated more often with clinical expression of disease, whereas serotype 1 infection is more frequently asymptomatic. Death is a rare sequela and occurs when dehydration is inadequately treated.

The pathogenesis of the disease is incompletely understood. The virus appears primarily in the small bowel, and virus is visualized in intestinal epithelial cells within the villi tips. Villi are shortened, crypts are hyperplastic, and an inflammatory cell infiltrate appears in the lamina propria. Abnormalities of carbohydrate metabolism are present, as evidenced by impaired D-xylose absorption.

Diagnosis is dependent on identification of the virus by electron microscopy or by immunologic assays as listed in Table 37-2. Several tests are available to detect antibody titer rises (Table 37-2). The presence of antibody to one serotype does not provide protection to the other rotavirus serotype. Serum antibody correlates poorly with protection, and specific local IgA may be required for immunity.

27-NM NORWALK-LIKE AGENTS

The 27-nm Norwalk-like agents have been responsible for an explosive self-limited illness that occurs epidemically. The diseases have variously been called viral diarrhea, epidemic diarrhea and vomiting, winter vomiting disease, epidemic collapse, and acute infectious nonbacterial gastroenteritis. Several agents have been detected, and some are named after the region where the epidemics occurred. The agents include Norwalk, Hawaii, Montgomery County, Ditchling, "W," Cockle, and Parramatta. Outbreaks are more frequent from September to March and have involved schools, families, and communities.

Symptoms usually start within 24 hours after exposure and last 1 to 2 days. In volunteers an attack rate of 66% was observed following exposure to the virus. In naturally acquired disease the attack rates have been 50% to 60%.

Symptoms include vomiting and diarrhea of varying severity. Vomiting is thought to be caused by delayed gastric emptying. Other symptoms are abdominal cramps, headache, malaise, nausea, myalgias, and low-grade fever. The laboratory tests are usually normal, except for mild leukocytosis.

The pathologic lesions caused by the 27-nm Norwalk-like agents are similar to those described with rotaviruses. Shortening of villi, altered mucosal architecture, and hyperplasia of crypts are encountered in the small intestine. Virus particles have not been seen on electron microscopic examination of the small intestine. Alterations in fat and carbohydrate metabolism occur. Adenyl cyclase activity appears normal in infected patients, and the exact mechanism for diarrhea is still unclear.

The 27-nm Norwalk-like agents have not been successfully adopted to tissue culture, and no animal model is available. To date, electron microscopy is the only method for detecting the viruses, although antibody responses can be measured by several assays (Table 37-5). Virus excretion in the stool correlates with the onset of symptomatic disease. The protective role of local gut immunity and systemic immunity is not well established.

OTHER AGENTS

Other viruses have been described as causes of symptomatic gastroenteritis. The adenoviruses are respiratory and enteric viruses. Nosocomial and community-acquired enteritis resulting from adenoviruses has been reported in children. The coronaviruses are likely to be an important cause of enteritis, since they are recognized to cause severe enteritis in numerous animal species. Although outbreaks of enteritis have been reported with recovery of coronarvirus in humans, the virus can also be recovered in persons without gastroenteritis and patients with tropical sprue. The role of the coronavirus as a pathogen in humans is still in doubt.

Astrovirus and minireovirus have both been detected by electron microscopy in diarrheal stool from infants and small children. The astroviruses and minireoviruses share morphologic features with the 27-nm Norwalk-like agents and the reoviruses, respectively. Further work is needed to define their role in nonbacterial gastroenteritis.

DIAGNOSIS

The diagnosis of viral gastroenteritis depends in part on eliminating other known causes of gastroenteritis, especially bacterial agents. A methylene blue stain of a fresh stool sample is used to determine whether leukocytes are present. Viral infections do not cause a polymorphonuclear leukocytosis in the stool, and their presence is sufficient reason for a thorough diagnostic evaluation. Specific viral diagnosis is indicated in severely ill patients. If available, electron microscopy is the procedure of choice, since it is rapid and sensitive. Serologic diagnostic procedures can confirm a diagnostic impression but are not positive during the acute illness.

MANAGEMENT

The treatment of viral enteritis is symptomatic. Oral therapy with glucose and electrolyte-rich solutions is recommended. Dehydration is of major concern, especially in young children, the elderly, and debilitated patients. Hospitalization may be required in dehydrated patients with severe vomiting or diarrhea to monitor fluid and electrolyte balance.

BIBLIOGRAPHY

Bishop, R.F., and others: Virus particles in epithelial cells of duodenal mucosa from children with acute nonbacterial gastroenteritis, Lancet **1**:149, 1974.

Kapikian, A.Z., and others: Human reovirus-like agent as the major pathogen associated with "winter" gastroenteritis in hospitalized infants and children, N. Engl. J. Med. **294**:965, 1976.

Kapikian, A.Z., and others: Prevalence of antibody to the Norwalk agent by a newly developed immune adherence hemagglutination assay, J. Med. Virol. **2**:281, 1978.

Schreiber, D.S., Blacklow, N.R., and Trier, J.S.: The mucosal lesion of the proximal small intestine in acute infectious nonbacterial gastroenteritis, N. Engl. J. Med. **288**:1318, 1973.

Thornhill, T.S., and others: Detection by immune electron microscopy of 26-27 nm virus-like particles associated with two family outbreaks of gastroenteritis, J. Infect. Dis. **135**:20, 1977.

Wenman, W., and others: Rotavirus infection in adults, N. Engl. J. Med. **301**:302, 1979.

Yolken, R.H., and others: Epidemiology of human rotavirus type 1 and 2 as studied by enzyme linked immunosorbent assay, N. Engl. J. Med. **299**:1156, 1978.

Cat-scratch fever

Allan M. Arbeter

Cat-scratch fever is a presumed viral infection contracted from cats. The disease has been reported in temperate climates but may occur worldwide. The majority of cases occur in the autumn and early winter, predominantly in young adults and children. A history of exposure to cats is present in virtually all the individuals, but demonstrable cat scratches may be lacking at the time of clinical illness.

The initial lesion is usually at the site of a scratch and occurs from 1 to 4 weeks after the scratch. A 0.5- to 1-cm nodular erythematous lesion develops that pustulates directly from the nodule. Lesions heal within 2 weeks. At that time regional lymph node involvement appears, but the onset may be as late as 2 to 3 months after the primary lesion. Lymphadenopathy is predominantly regional and often axillary but may include cervical or groin nodes. The usual clinical course is self-limited, with the nodes regressing spontaneously in 2 months. Suppuration of the lymph nodes may occur, requiring needle aspiration or excision. Malaise and fever occur in 30% to 60% of the patients. Other evidence of systemic involvement includes a nonspecific maculopapular rash, pneumonitis, headache, encephalitis, hepatosplenomegaly, thrombocytopenia, and osteolytic bone lesions. Occasionally a preauricular node will enlarge, confusing the diagnosis with mumps or streptococcal pharyngitis.

The diagnosis is usually made on clinical grounds. Histologic examination of a resected lymph node may show one or more features consistent with the diagnosis. These include hyperplastic elements, granulomatous areas, and suppuration. If all three are present, the diagnosis is reasonably certain.

Skin test material can be prepared from an inactivated filtrate of the pus from another individual's lesion. The skin test (which is intradermal and read at 48 hours) is positive in 90% of patients and about 20% of family members. However, the skin test reagent is not commercially available. Since there is concern regarding the presence of extraneous infectious or oncogenic agents, the skin test is indicated only in extremely ill patients where a confirmation of the diagnosis is essential.

BIBLIOGRAPHY

Warwick, W.J.: The cat scratch syndrome: many diseases or one disease? Prog. Med. Virol. **9**:256, 1967.

38 • PREVENTION AND TREATMENT WITH VACCINES AND ANTIVIRAL AGENTS

Harvey M. Friedman

VIRAL VACCINES IN GENERAL USE
Poliovirus

Both inactivated and live attenuated poliovirus vaccines have been effective in controlling paralytic poliomyelitis. Since 1969 trivalent oral poliovirus vaccine has been used almost exclusively in the United States. However, in countries such as Holland, Finland, and Sweden, which have used inactivated poliomyelitis vaccines, the decline in paralytic poliomyelitis has paralleled the response in the United States. The principal disadvantages of the inactivated vaccine are the need for multiple injections and boosters, the stringent production controls to ensure complete inactivation, and in some vaccine lots inadequate antigenic potency. The main disadvantage of live poliovirus vaccines is the risk of paralytic infection in vaccines or their contacts. The risk is highest for unimmunized young adults who are household contacts of vaccinated children, immunodeficient children, and adults undergoing initial vaccination.

The currently recommended immunization schedule for infants is three doses of trivalent oral poliovirus vaccine given at 2, 4, and 6 months of age. A fourth dose is given at 18 months, and a booster dose is advised in 10- to 12-year-old children to protect them in later years. Because of the risk of vaccine-associated paralysis, live vaccine is not routinely recommended for previously unimmunized adults. Unimmunized adults at increased risk of acquiring poliomyelitis, such as some health-care workers, persons traveling to endemic areas, and those living in an epidemic focus, should receive immunization. If a rapid immune response is required, trivalent live vaccine is recommended, whereas if time permits, a series of inactivated vaccinations is preferred. The inactivated vaccine is also recommended for immunodeficient children.

In the United States only 60% to 70% of the population have received three doses of oral poliovirus vaccine, and approximately 10% have received none at all. The live virus trivalent vaccine confers substantial immunity in even a single dose, and nonvaccinated persons may become immunized by contact infection. Despite the poor vaccination record, the almost total elimination of poliomyelitis from the United States argues strongly for the efficacy of the live vaccine.

Rubella virus

Live attenuated vaccine was licensed in the United States in 1969. The rationale for its use is to prevent congenital rubella infection. The vaccine is recommended mainly for children and susceptible postpubertal females. Vaccination of children protects them against rubella and prevents them from spreading infection to susceptible females, and vaccination of postpubertal females confers individual protection against rubella-induced fetal injury. The vaccine, given as a single subcutaneous injection, is produced in monovalent form and in combinations: measles-rubella or measles-mumps-rubella. The vaccine is recommended for use at 12 months of age unless given with measles vaccine, in which case it is administered at 15 months or older. The vaccine induces antibodies in approximately 95% of susceptible persons. Reinfection without illness can occur in individuals with low levels of naturally acquired or vaccine-induced antibody. However, viremia and significant pharyngeal excretion have not been detected after reinfection, which therefore poses little risk to susceptible contacts and fetuses.

Since the vaccine may cause viremia and can cross the placenta, women of childbearing age should receive vaccine only if they are not pregnant and they should not become pregnant for 3 months following vaccination. No infant has had the congenital rubella syndrome because of vaccination during pregnancy; however, virus has been isolated from fetal tissue and placenta following vaccination inadvertently given during pregnancy. Complications of vaccination are more common in adults than in children and are most common in women over 25 years of age. Side effects including rash, adenopathy, arthralgias, and occasionally arthritis can occur in up to 40% of adults. Joint symptoms generally begin 2 to 10 weeks after vaccination and persist for 1 to 3 days. Vaccination of children whose mothers are pregnant and susceptible to rubella does not pose a significant risk to the fetus.

Measles virus

Live and killed measles virus vaccines were licensed in the United States in 1963. The killed vaccine was withdrawn in 1968 because atypical measles infections occurred in vaccine recipients after exposure to natural virus (see "Exanthems of viral or presumed viral origin" in Chapter 37). The initial live virus vaccine (Edmonston B strain) was associated with a high incidence of side effects. To modify this, the vaccine was often administered with immune serum globulin. The development of better attenuated vaccines has reduced the incidence of reactions, and concomitant administration of immune serum globulin is no longer indicated. Passive immunization with immune serum globulin (0.5 mg/kg intramuscularly and 0.25 mg/kg below 1 year of age) is recommended for susceptible individuals who have been exposed and are at high risk of severe or fatal measles. These include children less than 1 year of age and children and adults with malignant diseases or defects in cellular immunity. To be effective, passive immunization should be given within 3 days of exposure.

It is currently recommended that live measles vaccine be given to all healthy children at 15 months of age. Approximately 95% manifest an antibody response. Children immunized before 12 months of age, with killed vaccine, or with concomitant administration of immune serum globulin should be reimmunized with live measles vaccine. No deleterious effects of reimmunization have been noted. The vaccine should not be used in pregnant women or in patients with defects in cellular immunity.

Mumps virus

Live attenuated mumps virus vaccine became available in the United States in 1967. A single subcutaneous inoculation produces mumps antibody in more than 95% of vaccinees. Adverse reactions to the vaccine are uncommon. The vaccine should be administered to all children over the age of 12 months. If it is given with measles vaccine, it should be administered at 15 months. Immunization can also be given to susceptible male adolescents and adults, especially medical personnel, to prevent orchitis, which occasionally is complicated by sterility. The vaccine is contraindicated in pregnancy and should not be given to patients undergoing immunosuppressive therapy or those with malignancies or immunodeficiency states.

VIRAL VACCINES FOR SPECIAL CIRCUMSTANCES
Influenza viruses

Inactivated influenza virus vaccines were first used in the United States in the 1940s. The composition of the vaccines varies from year to year, but generally they contain both influenza A and B viruses of types isolated during the previous influenza season. The viruses are grown in allantoic fluid of embryonated hen's eggs, are formalin inactivated, and are purified to remove egg proteins. Some preparations are treated with lipid solvents to produce split-product or subunit vaccines. Minor discomfort at the inoculation site occurs in approximately 25% of vaccinees within 24 hours of vaccination. Myalgias and fever develop in only 1% to 2% of adults but in up to 40% of children. During the 1976 national immunization program against swine influenza, an excess rate of Guillain-Barré syndrome occurred 2 to 6 weeks after vaccination. The estimated risk of neurologic disease was 1 in 100,000. Approximately 5% of these patients died, and an additional 5% to 10% had residual neurologic abnormalities. Since 1976 no increased incidence of Guillain-Barré syndrome has been detected among recipients of influenza vaccines.

The vaccine is contraindicated only in persons allergic to eggs. If a person can eat eggs or egg products, the vaccine is generally safe. The vaccine is indicated for those at increased risk of death from pulmonary complications of influenza. This includes all persons above 65 years of age and those with chronic diseases of the heart, lung, or kidney; chronic anemia or diabetes mellitus; or impaired host defenses because of immunosuppressive therapy or malignancies that alter host defense. Patients receiving chemotherapy should not be vaccinated simultaneously with chemotherapy administration because this tends to decrease the antibody response. Vaccination during pregnancy is recommended only in women with chronic diseases. Healthy persons below the age of 65 should be considered for vaccination if they provide essential community services.

Rabies virus

POSTEXPOSURE PROPHYLAXIS. Deciding which patients should receive prophylactic vaccination against rabies requies consideration of the species of the biting animal, the type of exposure, and the circumstances of the biting incident. Carnivorous wild animals such as skunks, raccoons, foxes, coyotes, and bobcats are much more likely to be infected with rabies virus than rodents such as squirrels, hamsters, guinea pigs, gerbils, chipmunks, rats, mice, rabbits, and hares. Prophylaxis should be initiated following the bite of or salivary exposure to a carnivorous animal, unless it is tested and shown not to be rabid, whereas rodent bites rarely call for antirabies prophylaxis. The likelihood of rabies in dogs and cats varies from region to region. In many cases the state or local health department should be consulted before initiating postexposure prophylaxis.

Rabies is transmitted only by introducing the virus into open wounds or mucous membranes. Accordingly, any bite penetration of skin and any contamination of scratches, wounds, or mucous membranes by saliva or other potentially infectious material (such as brain) should be considered significant exposure. An unprovoked attack is more likely to indicate that the animal is rabid than a provoked attack. Wild animals and stray dogs or cats that bite or scratch should be killed, and the head should be removed and tested for rabies antigen by immunofluorescence at the local or state health department. Domestic dogs and cats should be confined and observed for illness for 10 days. Any illness should be evaluated by a veterinarian, and if signs suggest rabies, the animal should be killed and the brain evaluated for rabies.

The essential components of postexposure prophylaxis are thorough washing of all bites, wounds, and scratches with soap and water and initiation of immunization as soon as possible. Immunization is both passive and active and includes human rabies immune globulin (20 units/kg), or if unavailable, equine antirabies serum (40 units/kg), which is given with the first dose of killed virus vaccine. Up to half the dose of rabies immune globulin should be infiltrated in the areas around the wound, and the rest is administered intramuscularly. The human diploid cell vaccine is now the vaccine of choice. Five doses, the first given with immune globulin, are administered intramuscularly on days 0 (the day treatment begins), 3, 7, 14, and 28. The antibody level should be checked on day 28 or 2 to 3 weeks after the last dose. If it is inadequate, a booster dose is given and the titers are rechecked. If the human diploid vaccine is unavailable, duck embryo vaccine should be given subcutaneously in 21 doses over 14 to 21 days, followed by doses 10 and 20 days after the twenty-first dose. Antibodies should be checked at the time of the last dose, and if no antibodies are present, three doses of the human diploid cell vaccine are given.

PREEXPOSURE IMMUNIZATION. Preexposure vaccination should be considered in certain high-risk groups such as veterinarians, animal handlers, some laboratory workers, and people living in countries where rabies is a constant threat. Although preexposure vaccination does not eliminate the need for additional therapy after rabies exposure, it does eliminate the need for globulin and decrease the number of vaccine doses required. The human diploid cell vaccine is preferred and should be given intramuscularly on days 0 (first day of treatment), 7, 21, and 28. A serum sample should be tested for rabies antibodies 2 to 3 weeks after the last injection. Individuals at continuous risk should receive a booster every 2 years or have serum titers checked and shown to be adequate. When a person with previously demonstrated rabies antibody is exposed to rabies, two doses of the human diploid cell vaccine (days 0 and 3) or five daily doses of duck embryo vaccine followed by a booster dose 20 days later are indicated.

ANTIVIRAL AGENTS

For many years the replication of viruses and the functioning of host cells were thought to require identical metabolic machinery. However, intracellular molecular events unique to virus replication are now recognized and can be used in defining virus-specific targets for new antiviral drugs. Rapid viral diagnosis is of major importance as a guide to the proper use of antiviral agents, since the toxic manifestations and narrow spectrum of the drugs indicate the need for cautious administration.

Amantadine

Amantadine was initially licensed for prophylactic use against Asian influenza (H2N2) infections in 1966. In 1976 it was licensed for use against all strains of influenza A viruses. It is ineffective against influenza B viruses. Although the mechanism of action is not fully known, it may interfere with the ability of the virus to penetrate the cell. It blocks uncoating of the virus and subsequent release of nucleic acid from the virus into the cell. The drug is rapidly absorbed after oral administration, it has a serum half-life of 9 to 37 hours (mean of 24 hours), and 90% is excreted unchanged in urine. Approximately 5% of healthy adults have side effects consisting of confusion, light-headedness, hallucinations, anxiety, and insomnia. These usually occur shortly after the start of therapy, are reversible if the drug is discontinued, and cease even if therapy is continued.

Controlled trials of amantadine (100 mg twice a day) as a prophylactic agent indicate protection against clinical illness in over 60% of the patients and protection against subclinical infection (measured by seroconversion) in about 50%. Amantadine used to treat influenza in the same dosage has caused an approximate 50% reduction in fever duration and a shortened course of illness. The drug must be administered within 24 to 48 hours of the onset of symptoms. Its value for influenzal pneumonia or other complications of influenza remains to be established.

Vidarabine (adenine arabinoside)

Initially vidarabine was developed as a potential anticancer agent. However, several human herpesviruses were found to be sensitive to it, and its therapeutic/toxic ratio was better than those noted for previous purine and pyrimidine analogs such as idoxuridine and cytosine arabinoside. Vidarabine inhibits DNA synthesis, with a preferential effect on viral, rather than cellular, DNA synthesis. In serum the drug is converted to arabinosyl hypoxanthine, a metabolite with diminished antiviral activity. The serum half-life of vidarabine is 4 hours, and 60% is excreted in the urine, principally as the hypoxanthine derivative. Levels in CSF are approximately half those in serum. Toxic effects are in part dose dependent and include nausea, vomiting, diarrhea, tremors, thrombocytopenia, leukopenia, and bone marrow megaloblastosis. The drug should be used with caution and should be avoided in patients with renal failure.

Vidarabine has been evaluated in immunocompromised patients with herpes zoster. Because of the crossover design of the study, only early events could be evaluated. The drug was effective in relieving pain, clearing the virus from vesicles, preventing new vesicle formation, and promoting vesicle healing. Its role in preventing disseminated infection and postzoster neuralgia or treating visceral infection remains to be established.

In a double-blind study of 28 biopsy-proven cases of herpes simplex encephalitis, vidarabine in doses of 15 mg/kg/day for 10 days reduced mortality from 70% to 28%. Survival was enhanced if the treatment was begun while the patient was still conscious. About 40% of survivors were able to resume normal activites. Controlled studies of vidarabine (15 mg/kg/day for 10 days) in neonatal herpes simplex infections also indicate a beneficial effect. This drug has been used to treat cytomegalovirus chorioretinitis in transplant patients and other impaired hosts.

Topical use of adenine arabinoside and idoxuridine is effective in treating herpes simplex corneal ulcers but does not reduce the frequency of recurrences. Topical preparations of antivirals have not yet proved useful in labial or genital forms of herpes simplex virus infection.

Acyclovir (acycloguanosine)

Acyclovir is an experimental agent with excellent in vitro activity against herpes simplex virus types 1 and 2. It is somewhat less effective against varicella-zoster and Epstein-Barr viruses-in vitro. Favorable results have been obtained in immunocompromised patients with herpes simplex or varicella-zoster infections.

Interferons

Interferons are not specific for a single virus but are capable of inhibiting a variety of DNA and RNA viruses. Type I interferon (virus-induced human interferon) has been used in most clinical trials, since it is available in greater quantities than type 2 (interferon produced by lymphocytes during immune responses). Interferons act by inhibiting the translation of viral messenger RNA into viral proteins and by modulating the immune response, thus enhancing the activity of natural killer cells and macrophages.

Clinical trials in immunocompromised patients with herpes zoster have shown that interferon decreased cutaneous spread, prevented dissemination, diminished the acute pain and severity of postherpetic neuralgia, and decreased visceral complications compared with placebo-treated controls. Treatment with interferon also diminished the visceral spread of virus following chickenpox infection in children with neoplasia.

Interferon has been evaluated as a prophylactic agent. Renal transplant recipients were treated twice weekly for 6 weeks in an attempt to prevent cytomegalovirus infection. Excretion of cytomegalovirus was delayed but not prevented, and cytomegalovirus viremia was reduced in the interferon group compared with controls. The prophylactic effects of interferon on herpes simplex infection have also been studies in patients undergoing microsurgical decompression of the trigeminal sensory root for treatment of trigeminal neuralgia. The incidence of herpesvirus shedding and herpes labialis was reduced in interferon recipients compared with controls. The eventual importance of interferons as antiviral agents remains to be determined.

BIBLIOGRAPHY

Couch, R.B., and Jackson, G.G.: Antiviral agents in influenza: summary of Influenza Workshop VIII, J. Infect. Dis. **134**:516, 1976.

Health information for international travelers, M.M.W.R. **27** (suppl.):1, 1978.

Hirsch. M.S., and Swartz, M.N.: Drug therapy: antiviral agents (in two parts), N. Engl. J. Med. **302**:903, 949, 1980.

Merigan, T.C., and others: Human leukocyte interferon for the treatment of herpes zoster in patients with cancer, N. Engl. J. Med. **298**:981, 1978.

Report of the Committee on Infectious Diseases. In American Academy of Pediatrics: Red Book, 1977, ed. 18, Evanston, Ill., 1977.

Whitley, R.J., and others: Adenine arabinoside therapy of herpes zoster in the immunosuppressed: NIAID Collaborative Antiviral Study, N. Engl. J. Med. **294**:1193, 1976.

Whitley, R.J., and others: Adenine arabinoside therapy of biopsy-proved herpes simplex encephalitis: NIAID Collaborative Antiviral Study, N. Engl. J. Med. **297**:289, 1977.

Unit B • BACTERIAL DISEASES

39 • USE OF ANTIMICROBIAL AGENTS
Donald Kaye

About one third of all hospitalized patients receive antimicrobial agents, and over half of these are treated improperly (wrong agent or dosage). Appropriate use of antimicrobial agents is critical in the patient who is seriously ill with an infection. Use of agents that are not needed exposes patients to unnecessary side effects (allergic and toxic reactions) and the risk of superinfection and encourages the emergence of resistant organisms.

Appropriate use of antimicrobial agents requires a bacteriologic diagnosis (either tentative or proven); knowledge of the susceptibility patterns of the likely infecting organism (that is, the antimicrobial spectra of different antimicrobial agents); knowledge of the pharmacology of the agents (absorption, distribution, levels, protein binding, sites and rate of excretion or metabolism, and toxicity); knowledge of how to alter doses when excretion is impaired; and knowledge of drug interactions with other agents. Before describing specific agents, certain of these principles of antimicrobial therapy will be discussed.

DETERMINATION OF SUSCEPTIBILITY OF MICROORGANISMS

Some organisms are uniformly susceptible to certain antimicrobial agents. For example, virtually all group A streptococci and meningococci are susceptible to penicillin G. However, these observations will not necessarily be true in the future, since susceptibility patterns are continually changing. For example, pneumococci *(Streptococcus pneumoniae)* were uniformly highly susceptible to penicillin G until resistant strains appeared in the past few years. In the majority of serious infections the infecting microorganisms are not uniformly susceptible to any single antimicrobial agent. Therefore it is often necessary to choose the agent(s) most likely to be active and to perform susceptibility tests as soon as the organism is isolated. The usual pattern of activity of an antimicrobial agent against microorganisms is known as its *spectrum of activity*.

The major methods of testing antimicrobial susceptibility are *agar diffusion* and *broth* or *agar dilution* methods, and these have been applied primarily to testing of bacteria. In the agar diffusion method a paper disk containing a standard amount of antimicrobial agent is placed on an agar plate containing a standardized inoculum of the microorganism. After incubation for 24 hours the zone size of inhibition is measured and results are reported as susceptible, resistant, or intermediate. An intermediate size zone indicates the need for high doses of the antimicrobial agent unless the therapy is for urinary tract infection (since very high concentrations of drug are usually achieved in urine). The zone size is inversely proportional to the minimal inhibitory concentration (MIC) of antimicrobial, that is, the minimal amount required to prevent growth.

The broth and agar dilution methods require dilution of the antimicrobial agent in broth or agar, addition of a standard inoculum of the microorganism, and incubation (for 24 hours with most bacteria). The MIC is the lowest concentration of antimicrobial agent that prevents growth in broth or agar.

Broth dilution methods allow determination of bactericidal activity of antimicrobial agents. After incubation for 24 hours the number of organisms remaining is determined by streaking on a plate. A 99.9% kill (1000-fold decrease in the number of organisms) is considered to be the criterion for bactericidal activity. The minimal concentration of antimicrobial required to achieve a bactericidal effect (99.9% kill) is the minimal bactericidal concentration (MBC).

SIGNIFICANCE OF A BACTERIOSTATIC VERSUS BACTERICIDAL ACTIVITY

Agents may be divided into those that are bactericidal at or near the MIC and those that have an MBC much higher (for example, 16-fold or greater) than the MIC. The former are considered bactericidal and the latter bacteriostatic. Penicillins, cephalosporins, vancomycin, aminoglycosides, and polymyxins are generally considered bactericidal, whereas erythromycin, tetracyclines, chloramphenicol, clindamycin, lincomycin, and sulfonamides are generally bacteriostatic. However, this division is not absolute, since bactericidal agents may be bacteriostatic against certain microorganisms and vice versa. For example, chloramphenicol is bactericidal against pneumococci, and penicillin has poor bactericidal activity against enterococci.

In certain infections bactericidal activity is necessary for a high cure rate. It appears that in these infections host defense mechanisms are at least partially lacking either at the local site or systemically. These infections are endocarditis, meningitis, serious staphylococcal infection, and perhaps serious gram-negative bacillary infection in the leukopenic patient. In such infections better results are obtained with agents that result in bactericidal activity than with those that have bacteriostatic activity. The outcome in endocarditis treated with bacteriostatic agents such as erythromycin, clindamycin, tetracycline, or chloramphenicol is poor. Penicillin, a bactericidal drug, will usually not cure enterococcal endocarditis unless an aminoglycoside is added to achieve a greater bactericidal effect. Chloramphenicol results in high cure rates in *Haemophilus influenzae,* memingococcal, and pneumococcal meningitis; it is bactericidal against these organisms. However, the failure rate is high in *Escherichia coli* meningitis despite bacteriostatic spinal fluid levels; chloramphenicol is not bactericidal against *E. coli*. The failure rate in *Staphylococcus aureus* pneumonia or bacteremia treated with bacteriostatic agents is high. Much better results are achieved with penicillins, cephalosporins, and vancomycin. The leukopenic patient with serious gram-negative bacillary infection also seems to fare better with bactericidal therapy such as penicillins, cephalosporins, and/or aminoglycosides.

In most infections, including pneumococcal pneumonia and urinary tract infection, there seems to be no advantage of bactericidal over bacteriostatic agents.

Combinations of antimicrobial agents are often necessary in serious infections before the infecting organism's antimicrobial susceptibility pattern is known in order to guarantee antimicrobial activity against the organism. Combinations are also frequently required in mixed infections. When antimicrobial agents are used in combination, certain in vitro observations can be made. In comparison to the effect of one of the agents alone, there may be more rapid or more complete bactericidal activity *(synergism)*, no change in bactericidal activity *(indifference)*, or less bactericidal activity *(antagonism)*.

In general, synergism is seen when combinations of bactericidal agents are used, indifference occurs with combinations of bacteriostatic agents, and antagonism occurs when a bacteriostatic agent is added to a bactericidal agent. However, these interactions are not totally predictable, and in vitro testing is necessary to determine the true interaction.

Antagonism has been shown to be of clinical significance in very few situations. Pneumococcal meningitis treated with penicillin (a bactericidal agent) plus tetracycline (a bacteriostatic agent) has a higher mortality rate than when treated with penicillin alone. It is likely that if a bacteriostatic agent were added to a bactericidal agent in treating endocarditis, the results would also be poor. In these infections host defenses at the site of infection are poor and sterilization of the site by the antimicrobial agent is necessary.

Synergism has also been shown to be of importance in relatively few infections. One is enterococcal endocarditis, in which an aminoglycoside must be added to penicillin to produce good in vitro bactericidal activity. Without the addition of an aminoglycoside, the relapse rate is very high. It is likely that snyergism is also important in leukopenic patients with serious *Pseudomonas aeruginosa* infection, since in these patients an aminoglycoside such as tobramycin plus a penicillin such as ticarcillin may give better results than either agent alone.

ACTIVITY OF AGENT AT SITE OF INFECTION

Results of therapy will not be satisfactory unless the antimicrobial agent is present in effective concentrations at the site of infection. It is important to remember in this regard that bacteremia is a manifestation of tissue infection, with organisms secondarily found in the blood; therapy *must* be directed at the tissue site.

In considering the site of infection, it is necessary to take into account the local conditions and the penetration, protein binding, and blood levels of the antimicrobial agent. In general, all agents other than the polymyxins penetrate well into inflamed joints and other body cavities such as the pleural and peritoneal spaces, but not necessarily into the cerebrospinal fluid (CSF). Therefore there is no advantage in instilling these agents into body cavities.

Less agent will reach an area with a poor blood supply, such as necrotic tissue. Many agents, including penicillins, pass through the blood-brain barrier poorly, resulting in low CSF concentrations as compared to serum concentrations, although higher CSF concentrations are usually achieved in the presence of inflammation. Therefore high doses of penicillins are required in meningitis. Some agents such as chloramphenicol, sulfonamides, and rifampin achieve adequate CSF levels with normal doses. The vegetation of endocarditis is also probably an area where penetration of some antimicrobials is impaired; therefore large doses are required. In contrast, urinary levels of most antibiotics are very high in patients with normal renal function. Since the results of therapy in urinary tract infections are related to urinary levels of antimicrobial agent, relatively low doses can be used. Most agents also achieve therapeutic levels in bile. However, with obstruction of the biliary or urinary tracts, levels are low in bile and urine.

The pH at the local site can have a major effect on therapy. For example, aminoglycosides and erythromycin are much less active at an acid pH (as in an abscess or infected body fluid) or the usual pH of urine. Sulfonamides are relatively inactive in abscesses because of the presence of large concentrations of para-aminobenzoic acid. Drainage of pus and removal of foreign bodies are essential for cure or even response of many infections. In addition to the low pH and poor blood supply of an abscess or a foreign body, there are other local factors. These areas are anaerobic, and aminoglycosides are not active against anaerobically metabolizing bacteria. Host defenses seem not to operate well at these sites. Furthermore, the bacteria may be metabolically altered so that even if effective concentrations of agents are reached, they may not be antimicrobial.

Protein binding may be important in determining tissue concentrations of an agent. The antibacterial activity is determined by concentrations of free agent. Although binding is reversible, with highly protein-bound agents, relatively small concentrations may be available for diffusion to a tissue site. In general, with agents having protein binding of less than 75%, impairment of diffusion is not a major factor. Such agents include penicillin G, methicillin, cephalothin, cephalexin, chloramphenicol, and aminoglycosides. With agents having higher protein binding, such as nafcillin, oxacillin, cloxacillin, and dicloxacillin, it is necessary to give doses large enough to compensate for protein binding.

The goal of antimicrobial therapy is to deliver to the site of infection an amount of free antimicrobial agent that exceeds the MIC of the infecting organism, taking local conditions into consideration. This concentration must be achieved often enough to prevent microorganisms from multiplying between doses.

PHARMACOLOGY
Route of administration

The drug must be administered in a manner to give antimicrobial activity at the site of infection. Some agents such as the aminoglycosides and vancomycin are not absorbed orally, and some such as methicillin are destroyed by gastric acid. For systemic infections these agents must be given by injection. Some agents (for example, cephalexin, doxycycline, chloramphenicol, and rifampin) are absorbed as well orally as by injection. However, with all oral agents there is the possibility of food or drugs binding to or in some other way interfering with absorption of the agent. It is prudent to give oral agents when the patient is in the fasting state, preferably 1 to 2 hours before meals. The intramuscular injection of some agents (such as penicillin G in large doses, tetracycline, and erythromycin) is painful, and these agents must be given intravenously when injection is required.

With serious infections, the effort is usually to achieve free antibacterial concentrations in serum (see discussion of protein binding under "Activity of agent at site of infection") that are active against the infecting organism. In infective endocarditis it is generally necessary to achieve serum bactericidal activity at a one-eighth dilution of serum (see discussion of "Infective endocarditis" in Chapter 40). In meningitis, serum concentrations must be high enough to guarantee adequate CSF concentrations. In urinary tract infection without bacteremia, serum concentrations are not important; only urinary concentrations are significant. This explains why agents such as nitrofurantoin are effective in urinary tract infection without achieving antibacterial activity in serum.

Plasma (serum) concentrations

The plasma concentration after the initial dose is determined by rate of absorption, rate of administration if given intravenously, size of dose, size of the individual, body habitus (that is, obese or lean), rate of excretion or inactivation, and volume of distribution in the body.

Volume of distribution refers to the body compartments in which the drug is distributed. The major compartments are the intravascular or plasma, the interstitial fluid, and the intracellular fluid compartments. Some antimicrobial agents are distributed mainly in the intravascular space, some in intravascular and interstitial spaces, and some even intracellularly. Some agents may be sequestered in various tissues (such as nafcillin in the liver).

With rapid intravenous injection of an agent, the drug is initially found mostly in the plasma compartment. After about 30 minutes intravascular drug equilibrates with the concentrations in the extravascular compartments. Subsequently, most drugs are eliminated from the body as a first-order process (that is, at a constant rate). With slow intravenous infusion, intramuscular injection, or oral administration, equilibration (and also excretion) take place simultaneously with absorption. Therefore peak plasma levels are higher with rapid intravenous injection than with the other routes of administration.

If not all the agent is eliminated before the next dose is given, the drug accumulates, giving higher plasma levels until a steady state is eventually reached. In general, accumulation does not occur if the maintenance dose is given every 3 to 4 plasma half-lives (see the following).

In serious infections, agents should be given intravenously or intramuscularly to guarantee rapid achievement of effective serum levels. With hypotension, the intravenous route must be used, since poor perfusion at the site of injection may slow absorption from the muscle. Sufficiently large doses should be given to guarantee adequate serum concentrations. Doses of toxic agents such as the aminoglycosides are usually given on the basis of milligrams per kilogram of body weight. Dosage based on body surface area is an alternative method commonly used in pediatrics. With relatively nontoxic agents such as the penicillins and cephalosporins, standard dosages can be used in adults.

Body habitus is important when administering the aminoglycosides. Aminoglycosides are not lipid soluble, and little reaches the adipose tissue. Therefore dosage should be based on lean body weight to avoid overdosage.

Excretion or inactivation

The rate of excretion or inactivation of an agent will help determine its duration of activity in serum and at other sites and its peak serum concentrations with repeated doses. (With retention of the agent, each dose will add to existing levels.) The excretion or inactivation rate also plays a role in determining the serum concentration with the initial dose when the antimicrobial agent is relatively slowly absorbed, as with oral, intramuscular, or slow intravenous routes.

Most antimicrobial agents, including most penicillins, cephalosporins, aminoglycosides, tetracyclines, vancomycin, and polymyxins, are excreted by the kidneys. Many penicillins and cephalosporins are excreted by tubular secretion as well as by glomerular filtration; probenecid has a marked effect in reducing the rate of excretion of these drugs by blocking tubular secretion. The aminoglycosides, most tetracyclines, vancomycin, sulfonamides, and polymyxins are excreted mainly by glomerular filtration. Erythromycin, lincomycin, clindamycin, rifampin, and nafcillin (a penicillin) are excreted mainly in the bile. Doxycycline is excreted mainly in the stool. Some agents are inactivated before excretion; cephalothin and certain other cephalosporins are deacetylated, chloramphenicol is conjugated by glucuronyl transferase, and isoniazid is acetylated in the liver. The rate of acetylation of isoniazid varies according to genetic composition; individuals may be rapid or slow acetylators.

A useful concept for describing the duration of antimicrobial activity in the blood is the plasma (or serum) halflife. This means the time required for the blood plasma level to fall by one half. The rate of fall is constant after equilibrium has been reached with the different fluid compartments. Elimination of drug is virtually complete (90% or more) after 3 to 4 half-lives.

MODIFICATION OF DOSAGES

When excretion of an agent is impaired, plasma levels may be higher or more prolonged than desired. In this situation, following a normal loading dose, subsequent doses must be decreased or the time between the doses increased.

It is necessary to monitor renal or hepatic function in patients receiving antimicrobial agents that are excreted or inactivated by the kidney or liver. When renal function is impaired, it is essential to modify dosage regimens of aminoglycosides, vancomycin, polymyxins, tetracyclines (other than doxycycline), sulfonamides, and flucytosine. When large doses of penicillins or cephalosporins are being used, it is also prudent to lower the dosage. With impairment of liver function it may be necessary to decrease doses of erythromycin, lincomycin, clindamycin, chloramphenicol, and nafcillin.

Although nomograms are available for modification of dosage regimens in the presence of renal insufficiency, they are not reliable. Determinations of serum concentrations are required for dosage modification, especially when toxic agents such as the aminoglycosides are being used.

DURATION OF THERAPY

The recommended duration of therapy for most infections is empiric. The majority of infections are treated for 7 to 14 days. Infective endocarditis and serious staphylococcal infections usually require at least 4 weeks of treatment. With suppuration (lung abscess, liver abscess, and so on) and osteomyelitis, longer therapy is usally needed. Mycobacterial and deep fungal disease may require a year or more of therapy. Specific recommendations are discussed under the disease entities.

TOXICITY OF ANTIMICROBIAL AGENTS

All agents have side effects. The side effects may be local such as pain or phlebitis at the site of administration, allergic such as rash or anaphylaxis, metabolic such as sodium loading and hypokalemic alkalosis from carbenicillin, or organ toxicity such as nephrotoxicity from aminoglycosides. Allergic reactions are not dose related, whereas metabolic reactions and organ toxicity are.

Toxicity may be related to the patient's age, renal function, or pregnancy or to interaction with another drug. For example, nephrotoxic and ototoxic agents such as aminoglycosides are more likely to cause toxic reactions in the elderly and in patients with renal insufficiency. Tetracyclines can cause damage to the teeth in the fetus when used in pregnancy or in the child when taken before age 8. Sulfonamides can cause kernicterus in the newborn by displacement of bilirubin from serum albumin, and chloramphenicol can cause the lethal "gray baby syndrome" in the newborn. Side effects are discussed with the specific agents.

FAILURE OF THERAPY WITH ANTIMICROBIAL AGENTS

The reasons for failure of therapy may be related to many factors.

Delay of therapy

In all serious infections there is a point of no return beyond which therapy is not effective. This is true even in infections with organisms that are highly susceptible to antibiotics (such as pneumococcal pneumonia). It is important to start therapy promptly in the seriously ill patient.

Incorrect diagnosis

If the patient does not have an infection, antimicrobial agents cannot be expected to have an effect.

Microbial resistance

An antimicrobial agent will not be effective when the organism is resistant. This can occur from lack of recognition of the infecting organism (for example, treatment of an intra-abdominal abscess containing aerobes and anaerobes with antibiotics active only against the aerobes). Resistance can be present and not recognized unless special tests are used. Such tests may include incubation at reduced temperatures such as 86° F (30° C) or use of a large inoculum for *S. aureus* resistant to methicillin. Resistance can develop in vivo as the patient is being treated, or superinfection with a new resistant organism can occur.

Failure to deliver the agent to the site of infection in antimicrobial concentrations

In the presence of an obstruction (such as biliary or urinary), effective antimicrobial levels may not be achieved in urine or bile. Many agents (for example, clindamycin and aminoglycosides) when given parenterally will not reach sufficient concentrations in the central nervous system to be effective. Many agents will not reach adequate concentrations in necrotic tissue or in an abscess. High blood levels of an agent are required for diffusion into a vegetation in infective endocarditis.

Adverse conditions at the site of infection

Antimicrobial agents will not work well in an area of necrosis, foreign body, or pus. For example, aminoglycosides are not very active at an acid pH as in pus or acid urine, and penicillin will not kill bacteria that are not multiplying as in pus. Pus and necrotic tissue must be drained and foreign bodies removed.

Infection in the immunocompromised host

In the severely immunocompromised patient (such as one with severe leukopenia) results of therapy are not as good as in the nonimmunocompromised patient. Even with use of optimal bactericidal therapy, host defense mechanisms are important.

Apparent failure related to drug fever

Fever caused by the antimicrobial agent may develop after the initial response. This is most likely to occur with penicillins, cephalosporins, vancomycin, and amphotericin B. If the drug is critically important, it should be continued despite the fever. However, a search for other causes of fever such as microbial resistance or superinfection should be made. If the drug is not critical, discontinuance with or without substitution of another agent will elucidate the problem, since the fever will usually disappear over a period of 1 to 3 days.

SPECIFIC ANTIMICROBIAL AGENTS

The important antibacterial agents are reviewed in this section. Table 39-1 lists the usual doses in adults with normal renal function and dosage regimens with creatinine clearances of less than 10 ml/min, 30 to 50 ml/min, and 75 ml/min. Table 39-2 lists some important infecting organisms and the appropriate antimicrobial agents used in therapy. Agents used in the treatment of tuberculosis (isoniazid, rifampin, ethambutol, and so on) are reviewed in the discussion of Antituberculosis drugs'' in Chapter 50. Agents used in the treatment of fungal diseases (such as amphotericin B and flucytosine) are reviewed in Chapter 53.

Penicillins

Penicillins are bactericidal antibiotics that work by inhibiting bacterial cell wall synthesis. The penicillins are relatively nontoxic, and to ensure adequate therapy, they are generally given in doses considerably larger than needed.

PENICILLINASE-SENSITIVE PENICILLINS. Penicillin G (benzyl penicillin) is active in relatively low concentrations against essentially all gram-positive cocci and bacilli (including anaerobes) with the exception of penicillinase-producing *S. aureus,* many strains of *S. epidermidis,* and rare strains of pneumococci. All meningococci and many gonococci are susceptible to relatively low concentrations of penicillin G.

Although penicillin G is active in much higher concentrations against many strains of *H. influenzae, E. coli, Proteus mirabilis,* and *Salmonella,* the tendency is to use ''broad-spectrum'' penicillins such as ampicillin for infections caused by these organisms. In high concentrations, penicillin G is also active against many anaerobic gram-negative bacilli. Penicillin G is available as aqueous penicillin G, procaine penicillin G, and benzathine penicillin G.

Aqueous penicillin G is usually given intravenously because intramuscular injection is painful. The intravenous form is used when high serum concentrations are required and large amounts must be given, as in meningitis or endocarditis. The standard dosage in adults is 5 to 20 million units each day either by continuous intravenous drip or in divided doses every 2 to 4 hours, since the half-life in the blood is only 30 minutes.

Procaine penicillin G is well tolerated intramuscularly but results in relatively low serum concentrations of penicillin. Because of slow release from the muscle, blood levels are prolonged and doses can be given every 6 to 24 hours. Procaine penicillin G is used in therapy for pneumococcal and group A streptococcal infections other than meningitis and in gonorrhea, syphilis, and endocarditis

Table 39-1. Doses of some commonly used antimicrobial agents

Agent	Usual total daily dose in adults	Dose interval	Route	Daily dose with creatine clearance (ml/min)		
				<10	30-50	≥75
Penicillinase-sensitive penicillins						
Aqueous penicillin G	5-20 million units	Continuous IV or q2-4h	IM, IV	1-2 million units q6h	NC*	NC
Procaine penicillin G	600,000-4.8 million units	q6-24h	IM	NC	NC	NC
Benzathine penicillin G	600,000-2.4 million units	Every 4 wk	IM	NC	NC	NC
Phenoxymethyl penicillin (penicillin V)	1-2 g	q6h	PO	250 mg q6h	NC	NC
Broad-spectrum penicillins						
Amoxicillin	0.75-3 g	q8h	PO	500 mg q12h	NC	NC
Ampicillin	1-4 g	q6h	PO	500 mg q12h	NC	NC
	4-12 g	q4-6h	IM, IV	1 g q8h	NC	NC
Carbenicillin (in serious infection)	500 mg/kg	q4h	IV	2 g q8h	2.5 g q4h	NC
Carbenicillin indanyl sodium	2-4 g	q6h	PO	Avoid use	NC	NC
Ticarcillin, mezlocillin, piperacillin	250-500 mg/kg	q4h	IV	1 g q6h	1 g q4h	NC
Penicillinase-resistant penicillins						
Cloxacillin	1-2 g	q6h	PO	NC	NC	NC
Dicloxacillin	1-2 g	q6h	PO	NC	NC	NC
Methicillin, nafcillin, oxacillin	6-12 g	q4h	IM, IV	1 g q4h	NC	NC
Cephalosporins						
Cephalothin, cephapirin	6-12 g	q4h	IV	1 g q8h	1 g q4-6h	NC
Cefazolin	2-6 g	q6-8h	IM, IV	0.5 g/day	0.5 g q6-12h	NC
Cefamandole, cefoxitin	6-12 g	q4h	IV	0.5 g q8h	1 g q6h	NC
Cephalexin, cephradine	1-2 g	q6h	PO	0.25 g/day	0.25 g q6h	NC
Cefactor	750 mg-1.5 g	q8h	PO	NC	NC	NC
Cefotaxime	4-12 g	q4-6h	IM, IV	1-2 g q8h	NC	NC

39 • Use of antimicrobial agents

Drug	Dose	Interval	Route	Notes
Aminoglycosides				
Amikacin	15 mg/kg	q12h	IM, IV	See text—measurement of serum levels is essential
Gentamicin, tobramycin	5 mg/kg	q8h	IM, IV	See text—measurement of serum levels is essential
Streptomycin	1-2 g	q12h	IM	0.5 g q3days	0.25 g q12-24h	NC
Vancomycin	2 g	q6h	IV	See text—measurement of serum levels is essential	NC
Erythromycin	1-2 g	q6h	PO	NC	NC	NC
Clindamycin	1-4 g	q6h	PO, IV	NC	NC	NC
	0.6-2.4 g	q6-8h	PO, IM, IV	NC	NC	NC
Tetracyclines						
Tetracycline	1-2 g	q6h	PO	Avoid use	Avoid use	NC
Doxycycline	1 g	q12h	IV	Avoid use	Avoid use	NC
Chloramphenicol	200 mg	q12h	PO, IV	NC	NC	NC
	50-100 mg/kg	q6h	PO, IV	NC	NC	NC
Sulfonamides						
Sulfisoxazole	4 g	q6h	PO	Avoid use	1 g q12h	NC
Sulfamethoxazole	2 g	q12h	PO	Avoid use	0.5 g q12h	NC
Trimethoprim-sulfamethoxazole[†]	320 mg trimethoprim and 1.6 g sulfamethoxazole (2 tablets q12h)	q12h	PO	Avoid use	1 tablet q12h	NC
Trimethoprim	200 mg	q12h	PO	Avoid use	50 mg q12h	NC
Metronidazole	750 mg-2.25 g	q6-8h	PO	NC	NC	NC
	30 mg/kg	q6h	IV	NC	NC	NC
Nitrofurantoin	200-400 mg	q6h	PO	Avoid use	Avoid use	NC
Nalidixic acid	4 g	q6h	PO	NC	NC	NC
Oxolinic acid	1.5 g	q12h	PO	NC	NC	NC
Methenamine mandelate	4 g	q6h	PO	Avoid use	Avoid use	NC
Methenamine hippurate	2 g	q12h	PO	Avoid use	Avoid use	NC

*NC, no change from usual total daily dose.
[†]For *Pneumocystis carinii*, 20 mg/kg trimethoprim and 100 mg/kg sulfamethoxazole daily IV or PO in divided doses q6h.

Table 39-2. Commonly used antibiotic regimens for selected infections (adult doses)

Bacteria	Infection	Regimen for adult patients with normal renal function
Mycoplasma pneumoniae	Pneumonia	Erythromycin or tetracycline, 500 mg PO q.i.d. × 7 days
Chlamydia trachomatis	Urethritis, cervicitis, salpingitis, proctitis, epididymitis	Tetracycline, 500 mg PO q.i.d. × 7 days
Streptococcus pneumoniae (pneumococcus)	Pneumonia	Procaine penicillin G, 600,000 units q12h × 7 days[1,2]
	Meningitis	Aqueous penicillin G, 20 million units/day IV × 10 days[3]
	Endocarditis	Aqueous penicillin G, 20 million units/day IV × 4 wk[2,4]
Group A Streptococcus	Pharyngitis	Penicillin V, 250 mg PO q.i.d. × 10 days[1]
	Cellulitis	Procaine penicillin G, 600,000 units/day IM × 10 days or as for pharyngitis[1]
Staphylococcus aureus	Soft tissue infection	Cloxacillin or cephalexin, 500 mg PO q.i.d. × 10 days, or nafcillin, 1.5 g IV q4h × 10 days
	Pneumonia	Nafcillin, 1.5 g IV q4h × 14 days[2,4]
	Bacteremia or endocarditis	Nafcillin, 1.5 g IV q4h × 4-6 wk[2,4]
Neisseria gonorrhoeae	Urethritis, cervicitis, proctitis, pharyngitis	Procaine penicillin G, 4.8 million units IM, plus probenicid, 1 g PO; or tetracycline, 0.5 g PO q.i.d. × 4 days; or ampicillin, 3.5 g PO, plus probenicid, 1 g PO; or spectinomycin, 2 g IM (ampicillin and spectinomycin not effective in gonococcal pharyngitis)
	Arthritis, bacteremia with skin lesions	Aqueous penicillin G, 10 million units/days IV until improvement, then ampicillin, 0.5 g PO q.i.d. × 7 days
	Salpingitis	Aqueous penicillin G, 20 million units/day IV until improvement, then ampicillin, 0.5 g PO q.i.d. × 10 days
Neisseria meningitidis	Meningitis	Aqueous penicillin G, 20 million units/day IV × 10 days[3]
Haemophilus influenzae	Bronchitis in patient with chronic obstructive pulmonary disease	Ampicillin, 1 g PO q.i.d.; or amoxicillin, 1 g PO t.i.d.; or tetracycline, 250 mg PO q.i.d.; all × 3-7 days
	Pneumonia	Ampicillin (if susceptible), 2 g IV q4h; or cefamandole, 2 g IV q4h; or chloramphenicol, 12.5 mg/kg PO or IV q6h; all × 7-10 days
	Meningitis	Chloramphenicol, 12.5-25 mg/kg IV q6h; or ampicillin (if susceptible), 50 mg/kg IV q4h; both × 7-10 days
Escherichia coli	Urinary tract infection without bacteremia	Lower tract: Oral therapy with one dose of 3 g amoxicillin or 320 mg trimethoprim plus 1.6 g sulfamethoxazole; or 1-3 days of sulfisoxazole, 1 g q.i.d., ampicillin, 500 mg q.i.d., cephalexin, 500 mg q.i.d., tetracycline, 250 mg q.i.d., or nitrofurantoin, 50-100 mg q.i.d.
		Upper tract: Two weeks of oral therapy with sulfisoxazole, 1 g q.i.d., ampicillin, 500 mg q.i.d., amoxicillin, 500 mg t.i.d., cephalexin, 500 mg q.i.d., tetracycline, 250 mg q.i.d., trimethoprim-sulfamethoxazole (160 mg and 800 mg respectively) q12h, or nitrofurantoin, 50-100 mg q.i.d.
	Bacteremia	Ampicillin, 2 g q4h IV, or cephalothin or cefazolin,[2] and/or gentamicin or tobramycin, 1.7 mg/kg q8h IM or IV, all × 7-10 days[5-7]
Klebsiella pneumoniae	Urinary tract infection without bacteremia	Lower tract: Cephalexin, 500 mg q.i.d. × 1-3 days Upper tract: Cephalexin, 500 mg q.i.d. × 14 days
	Pneumonia, bacteremia	Cephalothin, 2 g IV q4h, or cefazolin, 1-2 g IV or IM q6-8h, and/or gentamicin or tobramycin, 1.7 mg/kg IM or IV q8h × 14 days for pneumonia and 7-10 days for bacteremia[5-7]

[1]When penicillin cannot be used, erythromycin, 500 mg q.i.d., can be substituted.
[2]Cephalothin, 2 g IV q4h, or cefazolin, 1-2 g IM or IV q6-8h, can be administered.
[3]When penicillin cannot be used, chloramphenicol, 12.5-25 mg/kg IV q6h, can be given.
[4]Vancomycin, 500 mg IV q6h, should be used when a penicillin or cephalosporin cannot be given.
[5]If organism is resistant to gentamicin or tobramycin, amikacin, 7.5 mg/kg IM or IV q12h, can be administered.
[6]Cefotaxime, 2 g IV q4h, or other third-generation cephalosporins may be used if there is in vitro susceptibility with resistance to other cephalosporins.
[7]Ampicillin, a cephalosporin, carbenicillin, or ticarcillin is often used together with gentamicin or tobramycin in serious gram-negative bacillary infection.

Table 39-2 Commonly used antibiotic regimens for selected infections (adult doses)—cont'd

Bacteria	Infection	Regimen for adult patients with normal renal function
Enterobacter species	Urinary tract infection without bacteremia	Lower tract: Carbenicillin indanyl sodium, 1 g PO q.i.d. × 1-3 days
		Upper tract: Carbenicillin indanyl sodium, 1 g PO q.i.d. × 14 days
	Bacteremia	Gentamicin or tobramycin, 1.7 mg/kg IM or IV q8h, and/or ticarcillin, 40 mg/kg IV q4h × 7-10 days; cefamandole, 2 g IV q4h, may be used if the organism is sensitive[5-8]
Proteus mirabilis	Urinary tract infection without bacteremia	Lower tract: One dose of 3 g amoxicillin PO or ampicillin, 500 mg PO q.i.d. × 1-3 days, or cephalexin, 500 mg PO q.i.d. × 1-3 days
		Upper tract: Two weeks of oral therapy with ampicillin, 500 mg q.i.d., amoxicillin, 500 mg t.i.d., or cephalexin, 500 mg q.i.d.
	Bacteremia	As for E. coli bacteremia
Indole-positive Proteus	Urinary tract infection without bacteremia	Lower tract: As for Enterobacter urinary tract infection
		Upper tract: As for Enterobacter urinary tract infection
	Bacteremia	Gentamicin or tobramycin, 1.7 mg/kg IM or IV q8h, and/or ticarcillin, 40 mg/kg IV q4h × 7-10 days; cefoxitin, 2 g IV q4h may be used if the organism is sensitive[5-8]
Pseudomonas aeruginosa	Urinary tract infection	Lower tract: As for Enterobacter urinary tract infection
		Upper tract: As for Enterobacter urinary tract infection
	Bacteremia	Tobramycin, 1.7 mg/kg IM or IV q8h, plus ticarcillin, 40-80 mg/kg IV q4h × 7-10 days[5,8]
Bacteroides fragilis	Abscess or bacteremia	Clindamycin, 600 mg IV q6-8h, or chloramphenicol, 12.5 mg/kg IV q6h, or metronidazole, 7.5 mg/kg IV q6h as long as necessary[9]
Salmonella species	Typhoid fever	Ampicillin, 1 g IV q4h × 14 days, or chloramphenicol, 12.5 mg/kg PO or IV q6h × 14 days
	Bacteremia	Ampicillin, 2 g IV q4h × 2-4 wk, or chloramphenicol, 12.5 mg/kg PO or IV q6h × 2-4 wk
Shigella species	Colitis	Tetracycline 2.5 g PO in one dose, or ampicillin, 0.5-1 g PO q.i.d., or trimethoprim-sulfamethoxazole (160 mg and 800 mg, respectively) b.i.d. × 5 days

[8]Piperacillin or mezlocillin may replace carbenicillin and ticarcillin.
[9]Abscesses must be surgically drained. Aerobes are often present in abscesses and appropriate therapy must be included. Clindamycin cannot be used in central nervous system infection.

caused by highly susceptible organisms. The dosage is 600,000 to 1.2 million units intramuscularly every 12 to 24 hours. In endocarditis 1.2 million units every 6 hours is used.

Benzathine penicillin G is used intramuscularly and is released over a period of weeks. It provides very low blood levels of penicillin G that are adequate only for treatment of pneumococcal and group A streptococcal infections (excluding meningitis and endocarditis) and syphilis and for prophylaxis of rheumatic fever. One injection of 1.2 million units provides therapy for pneumococcal or streptococcal infection. For prophylaxis of rheumatic fever, monthly injections are given. The regimen in syphilis depends on the stage (see discussion of "Syphilis" in Chapter 51).

Penicillin G can be used orally, but it is unstable in the presence of gastric acid and absorption is unreliable. Therefore acid-stable analogs such as *phenoxymethyl penicillin (penicillin V)* have been developed. This agent is useful only in the treatment of nonserious gram-positive coccal infections such as pneumococcal pneumonia after response to parenteral penicillin or group A streptococcal phyaryngitis. The usual therapeutic dose is 250 to 500 mg four times a day.

BROAD-SPECTRUM PENICILLINS. *Ampicillin* has the same spectrum as penicillin G (it is also destroyed by staphylococcal penicillinase) but is more active against *H. influenzae, E. coli, P. mirabilis, Salmonella,* and *Shigella*. The injectable form can be used intramuscularly or intravenously. In serious infections the usual dosage is 12 g daily intravenously in divided doses every 4 to 6 hours. The oral form is useful in urinary tract infection, shigellosis, and respiratory tract infections in a dose of 250 mg to 1 g every 6 hours. In gonococcal urethritis a single does of 3.5 g together with 1 g of probenecid is administered. *Bacampicillin* is an oral ester of ampicillin that gives ampicillin levels in blood over twice those achieved with oral ampicillin. *Hetacillin,* another preparation, has no advantages over ampicillin.

Amoxicillin is very similar to ampicillin but is given only orally. It is much better absorbed than ampicillin, producing serum levels that are at least double. It can be substituted for ampicillin except in shigellosis, where it is far less effective.

Carbenicillin and *ticarcillin* have a spectrum of activity similar to that of ampicillin. They have less activity against gram-positive cocci, equivalent activity against the gram-negative bacilli *E. coli* and *P. mirabilis,* and much greater activity against the other gram-negative bacilli. They are also active against *Enterobacter* species, *P. aeruginosa,* and indole-positive *Proteus* species (that is, those other than *P. mirabilis*). *Klebsiella* and *Serratia* species are resistant to these agents. In general they should be reserved for use in proven or suspected *P. aeruginosa* or to a lesser degree in *Enterobacter* or indole-positive *Proteus* infections, since there is a potential problem of the emergence of resistant *P. aeruginosa.*

Minimal inhibitory concentrations of carbenicillin required to inhibit a majority of *P. aeruginosa* are 75 to 150 µg/ml. Therefore very high serum concentrations requiring high doses are needed to achieve therapeutic efficacy in serious infections. The dosage of carbenicillin in serious infections is 500 mg/kg body weight/day in divided doses every 4 hours by the intravenous route. Ticarcillin is twice as active as carbenicillin against *P. aeruginosa* and can be used in a dosage of 250 to 500 mg/kg/day in divided doses every 4 hours. Carbenicillin indanyl sodium, an oral form of carbenicillin, is useful only in urinary tract infection and chronic bacterial prostatitis. The dosage is 0.5 to 1 g every 6 hours. *Piperacillin, azlocillin,* and *mezlocillin,* the newer broad-spectrum penicillins, have greater activity than ticarcillin against many gram-negative bacilli. In addition, they are active against *Klebsiella* and *Serratia* species.

PENICILLINASE-RESISTANT PENICILLINS. *Methicillin, nafcillin,* and *oxacillin* parenterally and *cloxacillin* and *dicloxacillin* orally are the penicillins resistant to degradation by staphylococcal penicillinase. These agents have a narrow spectrum and are used primarily for the treatment of *S. aureus* infection. However, they also constitute adequate treatment for pneumococcal, group A streptococcal, and susceptible *S. epidermidis* infections. Injectable forms (methicillin, nafcillin, and oxacillin) must be used in serious infection and are given intravenously, 6 to 12 g a day in divided doses every 4 hours.

The oral agents cloxacillin and dicloxacillin are used in the treatment of nonserious *S. aureus* infection, such as soft tissue infections, in doses of 250 to 500 mg every 6 hours.

EXCRETION AND SIDE EFFECTS. All the penicillins with the exception of nafcillin are excreted primarily by the kidneys, both by tubular secretion and by glomerular filtration. Nafcillin is excreted mainly by the liver. Although it is advisable to decrease the doses of penicillins administered to patients with renal insufficiency, these modifications are often not critical.

All penicillins can cause hypersensitivity reactions, and there is cross-sensitivity among the different penicillins. There are two types of reaction: (1) immediate, including anaphylaxis, urticaria, and anigoneurotic edema, and (2) delayed, including morbilliform eruption and serum sickness. About 5% of patients given penicillins have hypersensitivity reactions, the most common of which is morbilliform rash. Drug fever may also be a result of hypersensitivity. Ampicillin causes a rash in the majority of patients with infectious mononucleosis; this rash is not related to hypersensitivity and has no negative implications for future use of the drug.

All penicillins can cause nephritis as the result of an immune reaction, but methicillin is most likely to cause this syndrome. All penicillins can cause leukopenia, but nafcillin is the most likely to produce this side effect. Coombs' positive hemolytic anemia and thrombocytopenia may result from the use of any penicillin.

With very high doses of penicillins as used in meningitis, especially in the presence of renal insufficiency, myoclonus and generalized seizures may be observed. Carbenicillin and ticarcillin in high doses, especially in patients with renal insufficiency, interfere with platelet function and can contribute to a bleeding diathesis.

Potassium penicillin G contains 1.6 mEq of potassium per 1 million units, and carbenicillin and ticarcillin contain about 5 mEq of sodium per gram. Large doses of these compounds in patients with renal insufficiency or heart failure, respectively, can cause a significant ion overload. In addition, hypokalemia and alkalosis may result from the use of carbenicillin or ticarcillin.

Cephalosporins

The cephalosporins are bactericidal agents with both a gram-positive and a gram-negative spectrum of activity. They work by inhibiting bacterial cell wall synthesis. They are relatively nontoxic, and to ensure adequate therapy, they are generally given in doses considerably larger than needed.

Cephalothin, a parenterally administered cephalosporin, is active against most gram-positive cocci and bacilli (including anaerobes). However, enterococci are resistant. Cephalothin is also active against *E. coli, Klebsiella,* and *P. mirabilis. Enterobacter,* indole-positive *Proteus, Pseudomonas,* and many anaerobic gram-negative bacilli (especially *Bacteroides fragilis*) are resistant. In serious infections 2 g is given every 4 hours intravenously. *Cephapirin* can be used interchangeably with cephalothin.

Cefazolin, a parenterally administered cephalosporin, has activity similar to that of cephalothin but does not cause as much pain when given intramuscularly. It results in higher blood levels that persist longer. The usual dose in serious infections is 1 to 2 g every 6 to 8 hours intramuscularly or intravenously.

Cephaloridine, which has activity similar to that of the cephalosporins previously discussed, is the only nephrotoxic cephalosporin and therefore should not be used.

The orally administered cephalosporins have a spectrum of activity similar to cephalothin and are used in urinary tract infection, soft tissue infection, and other non-life-threatening infections.

Cephalexin, cephradine, and *cefaclor* are the most commonly used oral cephalosporins and are given in doses of 250 to 500 mg every 6 hours for cephalexin and cephradine and every 8 hours for cefaclor. Cefaclor has better activity against *H. influenzae* than the other oral cephalosporins and is used in otitis media and other infections caused by *H. influenzae.*

Cefamandole and *cefoxitin* are parenterally administered cephalosporins with an antimicrobial spectrum somewhat greater than that of cephalothin. In addition to having the spectrum of cephalothin, cefamandole has much better activity against *H. influenzae* and some *Enterobacter* strains, and cefoxitin has much better activity against indole-positive *Proteus* strains, *Serratia* species, anaerobic gram-negative bacilli (including *B fragilis*), and some *E. coli, Klebsiella,* and *P. mirabilis* strains that are resistant to cephalothin. In serious infections 2 g is given intravenously every 4 hours. Neither of these agents has activity against *P. aeruginosa.* They are more expensive than cephalothin and cefazolin and should be used only in the relatively few situations where they have a real advantage.

THIRD-GENERATION CEPHALOSPORINS. Despite their collective title, the third-generation cephalosporins are not all cephalosporins in the strict sense. These newly developed agents (some of which have been recently marketed) have a considerably broadened spectrum of activity and increased potency against gram-negative bacilli. They also have some additional potential uses. Some of these agents are *cefotaxime, cefoperazone, moxalactam, cefsulodin, ceftazidime, ceftriaxone,* and *ceftizoxime.* In general they have greater activity against *E. coli, Klebsiella, Enterobacter, P. mirabilis,* indole-positive *Proteus* species, and *Serratia* species than the older cephalosporins. Their activity against *P. aeruginosa* is comparable to or better than that of ticarcillin. Their gram-positive activity is poor.

Although the earlier cephalosporins were not effective in meningitis, these new agents look promising in gram-negative bacillary meningitis because of the CSF levels achieved and their much greater antimicrobial activity. Cefotaxime is used in doses of 2 g every 4 hours intravenously in serious infections, and moxalactam and cefoperazone are used in doses of 2 g every 8 to 12 hours intravenously. These agents are expensive and are needed in relatively few situations.

EXCRETION AND SIDE EFFECTS. The cephalosporins are relatively nontoxic with the exception of the nephrotoxicity of cephaloridine. As with the penicillins, the doses used are generally much larger than needed. Most of the cephalosporins are excreted primarily in the urine, by glomerular filtration and some also by tubular secretion. Cefoperazone is excreted mainly by the liver. Although it is advisable to decrease doses in the presence of renal insufficiency, such decreases are often not of critical importance except with cephaloridine.

Hypersensitivity reactions (rash, urticaria, and anaphylaxis) occur less commonly with cephalosporins than with penicillins. Cross-sensitivity between penicillins and cephalosporins is probably uncommon. Cephalosporins can be administered cautiously to patients with a history of a delayed hypersensitivity reaction to penicillins. However, they should not be used if there is a history of an immediate reaction to a penicillin. Drug fever probably occurs as frequently with cephalosporins as with penicillins.

Thrombophlebitis is common with intravenous use of cephalothin, cephapirin, and some of the other cephalosporins. Cephaloridine is the only nephrotoxic cephalosporin. However, cephalothin used in combination with gentamicin has been shown to result in more nephrotoxicity than gentamicin alone. A positive Coombs' test, thrombocytopenia, and leukopenia may be seen following the use of cephalosporins.

Some of the cephalosporins such as cefamandole, moxalactam, and cefoperazone have a disulfiram-like effect and will cause nausea and vomiting with ingestion of alcohol. Some of the third-generation cephalosporins such as moxalactam and cefoperazone can cause elevations in the prothrombin time and partial thromboplastin time, requiring vitamin K therapy.

Aminoglycosides

The aminoglycosides are bactericidal and work by binding to the 30S ribosome and thus inhibiting bacterial protein synthesis. They include streptomycin, neomycin, kanamycin, gentamicin, tobramycin, and amikacin, none of which is absorbed orally. With the exception of streptomycin, which has a limited antimicrobial spectrum, all have good activity against gram-negative aerobic bacilli but lack activity against anaerobes. Neomycin and kanamycin have no activity against *P. aeruginosa,* whereas gentamicin, tobramycin, and amikacin have good activity against these organisms. The aminoglycosides are active against staphylococci but lack activity against streptococci, including pneumococci.

Streptomycin has specific, limited uses because of the development of resistance of many bacteria. It is employed as a companion drug with isoniazid or rifampin in the treatment of tuberculosis and with penicillin or vancomycin in the treatment or prophylaxis of streptococcal endocarditis. It is also used in the therapy for brucellosis, tularemia, and plague. The usual adult dose is 0.5 to 1 g every 12 hours intramuscularly. In tuberculosis 1 g is usually given once daily for several months and thereafter three times a week.

Neomycin and *kanamycin* were at one time used parenterally. Currently their use should be limited to oral or topical (eye, ear) application because of toxicity and the development of bacterial resistance. These agents are active against most *E. coli, Klebsiella, Enterobacter,* and *Proteus* strains but lack activity against *P. aeruginosa.* When they are used for bowel preparation before surgery or in the treatment of hepatic coma to reduce bacterial populations and therefore absorption of ammonia, the oral dosage is 4 to 8 g daily in divided doses every 6 hours. Topical use should be restricted to small amounts of areas, since absorption and toxicity can occur. Use on skin is generally not of value.

Gentamicin and *tobramycin* should be used only in the treatment of serious gram-negative bacillary infection. An additional use for gentamicin is as a companion drug with a penicillin or vancomycin in the treatment of enterococcal or *S. aureus* endocarditis or in prophylaxis of enterococcal endocarditis. These two agents are very similar in antimicrobial activity with only two significant differences. Tobramycin is about four times as active as gentamicin against *P. aeruginosa,* and gentamicin is more active than tobramycin against *S. marcescens.* The dosage of gentamicin or tobramycin in patients with normal renal function and serious infection is 5 mg/kg/day in divided doses every 8 hours intravenously (by slow infusion over at least 20 to 30 minutes) or intramuscularly.

Resistance of gram-negative bacilli to gentamicin and tobramycin has occurred in some hospitals, and hospital-acquired infections in those institutions cannot be treated with these agents. The resistance is most commonly due to a plasmid-mediated enzymatic alteration of the aminoglycoside.

Amikacin has the same spectrum of activity as gentamicin and tobramycin but is less susceptible to enzymatic inactivation. Therefore amikacin has great value in the management of serious infections caused by gram-negative bacilli that are resistant to gentamicin and tobramycin. Amikacin should be reserved for use in these infections or in gram-negative bacillary infections acquired in hospitals where organisms are known to be commonly resistant to gentamicin and tobramycin.

In patients with normal renal function the dosage of amikacin is 7.5 mg/kg body weight by slow intravenous infusion over at least 20 to 30 minutes or intramuscularly every 12 hours. Some use 5 mg/kg every 8 hours. Amikacin must be given in higher doses (15 mg/kg/day) than gentamicin or tobramycin (5 mg/kg/day) because higher plasma levels are needed (peaks of about 20 μg/ml for amikacin as compared to about 6 μg/ml for the other agents) to produce the higher concentrations of amikacin required to inhibit gram-negative bacilli.

Sisomicin and *netilmicin* are newer aminoglycosides not yet available in the United States. They seem to have no advantages over the already available agents.

EXCRETION AND SIDE EFFECTS. All aminoglycosides are excreted by glomerular filtration. They are toxic agents, and toxicity increases as blood levels increase. Therefore the principle in the use of these agents is to give doses large enough to yield therapeutic levels but no larger.

It is important to be cautious even in the topical use of the aminoglycosides, since they are absorbed from areas of denuded skin such as burns. They are absorbed well from the peritoneum, pleural cavity, and joints and should never be instilled in these cavities. Furthermore, there is no need to inject aminoglycosides into these spaces, since therapeutic levels are easily achieved following parenteral administration. However, intrathecal injection (5 mg gentamicin every 24 hours) is necessary in gram-negative bacillary meningitis because penetration into the CSF is poor.

Some aminoglycosides are slowly inactivated by high concentrations of carbenicillin and ticarcillin (and probably other penicillins and cephalosporins), and these agents should never be mixed with aminoglycosides in infusion bottles. Inactivation can occur in patients with renal failure when there are high blood levels of carbenicillin or ticarcillin and the aminoglycoside is given with long intervals between doses.

All aminoglycosides are nephrotoxic and ototoxic. Neomycin and kanamycin, which should no longer be used parenterally, are probably more toxic than the other aminoglycosides discussed here. Streptomycin has very little nephrotoxicity. Gentamicin is probably more nephrotoxic than tobramycin and amikacin. Nephrotoxicity is reversible and is more likely to occur with larger doses, higher blood levels, or longer duration of therapy and in elderly patients, those with preexisting renal disease, and those receiving furosemide, ethacrynic acid, or cephalothin.

Streptomycin and gentamicin are more likely to produce vestibular damage than hearing loss, whereas tobramycin and amikacin are more likely to produce hearing loss than vestibular damage. The eighth nerve toxicity is often irreversible. It is more likely to occur with larger doses, higher blood levels, or longer duration of therapy and in elderly patients, those with renal insufficiency, and those receiving ethacrynic acid.

To minimize the possiblity of ototoxic and nephrotoxic reactions, doses should be decreased in patients with impaired renal function. Following a normal loading dose (1.7 mg/kg body weight for gentamicin or tobramycin or 7.5 mg/kg for amikacin), smaller doses can be given at the customary intervals or normal doses can be given at increased intervals. It is best to give decreased doses at normal or somewhat increased intervals to avoid long periods of time with subtherapeutic blood levels. Although nomograms are available to calculate doses based on serum creatinine or creatinine clearance values, they are inaccurate, and with changing renal function they are absolutely worthless. When a nomogram must be used, the simplest method is to give the loading dose and then as a maintenance dose to give the loading dose divided by the serum creatinine value (assuming a stable creatinine) at the usual intervals. Another way to calculate the maintenance dose is to multiply the loading dose by the creatinine clearance, express this amount as a percentage, and add 5% to 10%. For example, with a creatinine clearance of 20 ml/min, give 25% to 30% of the loading dose at the usual intervals.

The best approach is to give a normal loading dose and then a second dose estimated on the basis of a nomogram. Serum concentrations should be measured just before ("trough") and 60 minutes after the second and subsequent intramuscular doses or 30 minutes after the second and subsequent intramuscular doses or 30 minutes after the second and subsequent 30-minute infusions of drug. The level 60 minutes after an intramuscular injection is the "peak" and is equivalent to the level 30 minutes after a 30-minute infusion. Doses are adjusted to give serum peak levels of 4 to 8 μg/ml for gentamicin and tobramycin and 16 to 25 μg/ml for amikacin. Troughs above 2 μg/ml for gentamicin and tobramycin and above 5 μg/ml for amikacin indicate retention of drug and a greater chance of toxicity. However, therapy must be aimed at achieving adequate peak levels every 8 hours for gentamicin and tobramycin and every 12 hours for amikacin. Serum concentrations can be measured by bioassay, enzymatic assay, or radioimmunoassay. When doses are adjusted and levels are stable, levels can be measured once a day or once every other day.

Intravenous injections of aminoglycosides should never be rapid and these agents should never be instilled into a body cavity, since neuromuscular blockade with respiratory arrest can occur. This is especially likely in patients with myasthenia gravis or receiving curare-like drugs. It is reversible with neostigmine or intravenous administration of calcium. Paresthesias and peripheral neuropathy may occur rarely. Hypersensitivity reactions may occasionally be observed.

Vancomycin

Vancomycin is a bactericidal agent that acts by inhibiting cell wall synthesis. It is active against all gram-positive cocci and bacilli, including *S. aureus* and *S. epidermidis* strains that are resistant to all penicillins and cephalosporins. It is the agent of choice in treating serious infections caused by these organisms, as well as serious staphylococcal infection and endocarditis caused by viridans streptococci or enterococci when penicillins or cephalosporins cannot be used because of drug allergy. All gram-negative bacilli are resistant to vancomycin.

Vancomycin is not absorbed orally and must be given intravenously for treatment of systemic illness. The dose is 500 mg intravenously every 6 hours in a slow infusion lasting over an hour.

Vancomycin is used orally in the treatment of *Clostridium difficile* colitis (antibiotic-associated colitis) and *S. aureus* enterocolitis. The dose is 250 to 500 mg every 6 hours.

EXCRETION AND SIDE EFFECTS. Common side effects with vancomycin are phlebitis and chills and fever during the infusion. Rash may be seen. Nephrotoxicity occurs occasionally, and deafness may be associated with very high blood levels, usually in patients with renal insufficiency. Since vancomycin is excreted by glomerular filtration, it is retained in the presence of renal insufficiency. Therefore serum concentrations must be measured and doses are accordingly decreased in patients with decreased renal function. The absence of excretion in patients with renal failure can be used to advantage in treating infection in patients requiring dialysis, since 0.5 to 1 g of vancomycin given every 7 days provides therapeutic serum levels.

Erythromycin, lincomycin, and clindamycin

Erythromycin, lincomycin, and clindamycin are primarily bacteriostic agents that work by binding to the 50*S* ribosome and thus inhibiting bacterial protein synthesis. These agents have a similar spectrum of activity against bacteria and are absorbed when given orally; they can also be administered parenterally.

Erythromycin is active against gram-positive cocci (including anaerobes) with the exception of enterococci. However, many *S. aureus* strains are now resistant to erythromycin. It is also active against *Mycoplasma pneumoniae, Chalmydia trachomatis,* the bacillus of Legionnaires' disease *(Legionella pneumophila)* and related organisms, *Corynebacterium diphtheriae,* and *Treponema pallidum.* It is the substitute of choice in group A streptococcal and pneumococcal infections (except meningitis) when penicillin cannot be used. It is the drug of choice in *M. pneumoniae* and *L. pneumophila* (and related organism) infection and in *C. diphtheriae* carriers. Erythromycin should not be used in serious *S. aureus* infection. Although erythromycin is active against anaerobic gram-negative bacilli, its activity is much less than that of clindamycin. It has, however, been used orally in combination with an oral aminoglycoside as a bowel preparation before gastrointestinal tract surgery.

Erythromycin base, estolate, proprionate, and stearate can all be given orally in doses of 250 mg to 1 g every 6 hours. Parenteral therapy is rarely required, but when necessary (as in severe Legionnaires' disease), the intravenous routine should be used.

Lincomycin is similar to clindamycin. It has no advantages over clindamycin, which is more active in vitro, is better absorbed orally, and therefore is a preferable drug.

Clindamycin has a spectrum of activity similar to erythromycin except that its activity against *Mycoplasma* is poor. As with erythromycin, clindamycin is not a reliable drug in serious. *S. aureus* infection. The major advantage of clindamycin over erythromycin is its much greater activity against anaerobic bacteria, especially *Bacterioides* species (including *B. fragilis*), which are often resistant to penicillins and cephalosporins. The principal use of clindamycin is in serious infections caused by anaerobic microorganisms, particularly when *B. fragilis* is likely to be present. However, clindamycin cannot be used in central nervous system infection because penetration through the blood-brain barrier is poor.

The usual dose is 150 to 300 mg every 6 hours orally or 300 to 600 mg every 6 to 8 hours intramuscularly or intravenously.

EXCRETION AND SIDE EFFECTS. Erythromycin, lincomycin, and clindamycin are excreted mainly in the bile, and little if any adjustment in dosage is required in the presence of renal insufficiency.

Common side effects of erythromycin are gastrointestinal tract disturbances, including nausea, vomiting, and diarrhea. Cholestatic jaundice can occur with the use of erythromycin estolate (and to a lesser degree other erythromycins); it usually appears after 10 days of therapy but can occur earlier if the agent has been given previously. Erythromycin cannot be used intramuscularly because of pain on administration, and it causes severe phlebitis when used intravenously. Hypersensitivity reactions are rare.

Oral and parenteral administration of clindamycin and lincomycin can cause diarrhea, which is sometimes severe. Pseudomembranous colitis may result. It has been recognized that the type of colitis caused by lincomycin and clindamycin can also result from administration of many other antibiotics such as ampicillin and cephalosporins. The cause of the colitis is *C. difficile,* which produces a toxin in the colon. The colitis responds to treatment with oral vancomycin. Hypersensitivity reactions may occur with lincomycin and clindamycin.

Tetracyclines

The tetracyclines are bacteriostatic agents that work by binding to the 30S ribosome and thus inhibiting bacterial protein synthesis. These agents are active against *Rickettsia, Mycoplasma, Chlamydia, T. pallidum,* and many gram-positive and gram-negative bacteria. However, many bacteria formerly sensitive to the tetracyclines have now become resistant. Over 5% of pneumococci, more than 20% of group A streptococci, most *S. aureus,* and many strains of gram-negative bacilli are currently resistant to tetracyclines.

At present the primary uses for the tetracyclines are in treating urinary tract infection, rickettsial infections, chlamydial infections, *Mycoplasma* infections, chronic bronchitis, shigellosis, brucellosis, granuloma inguinale, and chancroid and as alternative therapy to penicillin in gonorrhea and syphilis.

Tetracycline, chlortetracycline, and *oxytetracycline* are all equivalent, but tetracycline is by far the most commonly used. It is usually given orally in doses of 250 to 500 mg every 6 hours. Intramuscular administration is too painful, but tetracycline can be given intravenously in doses of 0.5 g (rarely 1g) every 12 hours.

Demethylchlortetracycline (demeclocycline), methacycline, doxycycline, and *minocycline* are long-acting tetracyclines for oral use. Their excretion is very slow, and therefore they can be given every 12 to 14 hours they have no therapeutic advantages except the need for fewer daily doses. The disadvantages are higher price, lower urine levels (in fact they may be subtherapeutic in some urinary tract infections), and more toxicity (see "Excretion and side effects" below).

In patients with renal insufficiency, doxycycline is the only tetracycline that can be used without accumulation and higher blood levels; however, there is rarely a circumstance in which a tetracycline must be used in the presence of renal insufficiency. The dose is 100 mg every 12 hours.

Minocycline is one of three agents (the others are rifampin and sulfonamides) that can eradicate meningococci from the nasopharynx. Presumably this is because of its high concentration owing to high lipid solubility. However, because of minocycline's tendency to cause vertigo, rifampin or a sulfonamide (if the meningococcus is susceptible to sulfonamides) is preferred.

EXCRETION AND SIDE EFFECTS. All the tetracyclines except doxycycline are excreted primarily in the urine by glomerular filtration, and in the presence of renal insufficiency blood levels increase with all tetracyclines other than doxycyline. All tetracyclines produce gastrointestinal side effects such as nausea, vomiting, and diarrhea with oral use and thrombophlebitis with intravenous use. Staining of teeth, hypoplasia of dental enamel, and abnormal bone growth can occur in the fetuses of pregnant women given tetracyclines or in children under 8 years given these agents. In infants, pseudotumor cerebri with increased intracranial pressure and bulging fontanelles may develop.

All tetracyclines have an antimetabolic effect and increase protein breakdown. In patients with renal insufficiency this can result in worsening of the uremic state by increasing the urea and acid load to the kidney. Outdated tetracyclines can degenerate and cause Fanconi's syndrome.

With excessive blood levels resulting from large doses, intravenous use, or renal insufficiency, fatal acute fatty degeneration of the liver may occur. This is especially likely during pregnancy.

The long-acting tetracyclines (especially demethylchlortetracycline) cause photosensitivity. Demethylchlortetracycline also can cause nephrogenic diabetes insipidus. Minocycline commonly causes vertigo.

Chloramphenicol

Chloramphenicol is bacteriostatic and works by binding to the 50S ribosome and thus inhibiting bacterial protein synthesis. It has a wide spectrum of activity against gram-positive and gram-negative cocci and bacilli (including anaerobes), *Rickettsia, Mycoplasma,* and *Chlamydia.* The major reason for restricting its use is the rare but lethal complication of aplastic anemia.

Chloramphenicol is the drug (or one of the drugs) of

choice in the following infections: (1) typhoid fever and other serious *Salmonella* infections; (2) meningitis caused by *H. influenzae* resistant to ampicillin or when ampicillin cannot be used with sensitive strains; (3) meningococcal or pneumococcal meningitis when a penicillin cannot be used: (4) serious infection caused by *B. fragilis* (including central nervous system infection); and (5) rickettsial infection not responding to tetracycline or in which tetracycline cannot be used. Chloramphenicol is well absorbed orally. The usual dosage is 50 mg/kg/day in four evenly divided doses: 100 mg/kg/day is often used in central nervous system infection. It is not absorbed well intramuscularly, and parenteral therapy should be by the intravenous route in the same dose regimen as orally.

EXCRETION AND SIDE EFFECTS. Chloramphenicol is metabolized by the liver, and therefore doses are not altered in the presence of renal insufficiency.

Two types of bone marrow depression may be caused by chloramphenicol. There is a dose-related reversible interference with iron metabolism and an irreversible idiosyncratic from the aplastic anemia. The reversible form occurs during therapy, particularly with high doses or a prolonged course and especially in patients with liver disease. It is manifested by increased serum iron, increased saturation of iron-binding capacity, decreased reticulocytes, vacuolization of red cell precursors, anemia, leukopenia, and thrombocytopenia.

Irreversible idiosyncratic aplastic anemia occurs in fewer than 1 in 25,000 patients given chloramphenicol. The onset may be delayed until after therapy has been discontinued.

The "gray baby syndrome" (pallor and listlessness), which is often fatal, can occur in neonates given chloramphenicol. It is related to very high blood levels resulting from an inability of the immature liver to metabolize chloramphenicol. Optic neuritis and peripheral neuropathy may be seen with prolonged use of chloramphenicol.

Polymyxins

Polymyxin B and *polymyxin E (colistin)* are polypeptide antibiotics that are bactericidal against most gram-negative bacilli (including *P. aeruginosa*) with the exception of *Proteus* species. They work by disrupting the bacterial cell membrane. They are not absorbed orally. Their major use has been in the treatment of *P. aeruginosa* infection. However, because the aminoglycosides are less toxic and probably more effective, they are more frequently used by the parenteral route for this purpose than the polymyxins. Polymyxin B is used topically for ear and eye infections.

When given parenterally, polymyxin B is administered intramuscularly every 8 hours or by continuous intravenous infusion in doses up to 2.5 mg/kg/day. Colistin is given in the form of colistimethate sodium, 3 to 5 mg/kg/day intramuscularly or intravenously in divided doses every 6 hours.

EXCRETION AND TOXICITY. The polymyxins are excreted by glomerular filtration. Higher blood levels are associated with increased toxicity, and therefore doses must be decreased in patients with impaired renal function.

The major toxic side effects are nephrotoxicity, which is usually reversible, and neurotoxicity. Nonserious neurotoxicity in the form of circumoral and fingertip paresthesias is common. With toxic blood levels, respiratory paralysis may occur; this is reversible with intravenously adminstered calcium but not with neostigmine. Hypersensitivity reactions may also be seen.

Sulfonamides

The sulfonamides are bacteriostatic and work by competitive inhibition of para-aminobenzoic acid. They are well absorbed orally. Sulfonamides are currently used in very few circumstances. These are (1) urinary tract infection (especially caused by *E. coli*); (2) nocardiosis where they are the agents of choice; (3) in combination with pyrimethamine in the treatment of toxoplasmosis; (4) as a substitute for penicillin in prophylaxis of rheumatic fever; (5) as prophylaxis against susceptible meningococcal strains; (6) in the form of sulfasalazine in ulcerative colitis; (7) in the form of silver sulfadiazine or mafenide in burns; (8) in chloroquine-resistant *Plasmodium falciparum* infection; (9) for dermatitis herpetiformis; and (10) in combination with trimethoprim for certain indications (see "Trimethoprim-sulfamethoxazole" in the following).

Sulfisoxazole and *sulfamethorazole* are the major agents used for urinary tract infection. *Sulfadiazine* is rarely used because of the danger of crystalluria. Combinations of three sulfonamides (trisulfapyrimidines) are also used because of their great solubility and low danger of crystalluria. The dosages are usually 1 g four times a day for sulfisoxazole and 1 g every 12 hours for sulfamethoxazole.

Long-acting sulfonamides such as sulfamethoxypyridazine and sulfadimethoxine are more toxic than shorter-acting sulfonamides and should not be used.

Nonabsorbable sulfonamides such as sulfasuxidine have been used as preparation for bowel surgery but have not been shown to be of value.

EXCRETION AND SIDE EFFECTS. The sulfonamides are excreted by glomerular filtration. They should not be used in the presence of renal insufficiency. One side effect is crystalluria, which can result in urinary obstruction or renal tubular necrosis. It is unlikely to occur with sulfisoxazole or sulfamethoxazole, and the risk can be diminished with the other sulfonamides by increasing fluid intake and by alkalinizing the urine to increase their solubility. Hypersensitivity reactions with fever and rash are common; vasculitis may occur. Activation of quiescent lupus erythematosus has been reported. Photosensitivity, hepatitis, and aplastic anemia are all complications of sulfonamide therapy. Administration of sulfonamides to the mother at term or to the newborn can cause kernicterus in the newborn by displacement of bilirubin from albumin. When patients with glucose-6-phosphate dehydrogenase deficiency are given sulfonamides, hemolytic anemia may result. Long-acting sulfonamides are more likely to cause Stevens-Johnson syndrome or myocarditis than the short-acting preparations.

Trimethoprim-sulfamethoxazole

Trimethoprim-sulfamethoxazole (co-trimoxazole) is a fixed combination of trimethoprim and sulfamethoxazole. Both drugs act to block the folic acid metabolism cycle of bacteria, and they are often much more active together than either agent alone would be. Sulfonamides competitively inhibit the incorporation of para-aminobenzoic acid, and trimethoprim prevents the reduction of dihydrofolate to tetrahydrofolate. The combined agent is bacteriostatic.

Trimethoprim-sulfamethoxazole is active in urinary tract infections. It will cure a minority of patients with chronic bacterial prostatitis caused by susceptible bacteria when given for 12 weeks. It is also effective in the prophylaxis of urinary tract infection in women who have multiple reinfections. Trimethoprim-sulfamethoxazole is the drug of choice for treatment of *Pneumocystis carinii* pneumonia and is also effective in prophylaxis of this infection in children with malignancies. It is the best agent for the treatment of typhoid fever when ampicillin and chloramphenicol cannot be used. It is effective in shigellosis, otitis media, gonorrhea, and acute exacerbations of chronic bronchitis.

The usual dose is two tablets (160 mg trimethoprim and 800 mg sulfamethoxazole) twice a day. Much higher doses (20 mg/kg/day trimethoprim and 100 mg/kg/day sulfamethoxazole in four divided doses) are used in the treatment of *P. carinii* pneumonia. Much lower doses (40 mg trimethoprim and 200 mg sulfamethoxazole each night) are used in the prophylaxis of urinary tract infection.

EXCRETION AND SIDE EFFECTS. Both trimethoprim and sulfamethoxazole are excreted in the urine. The side effects are those already listed for sulfonamides. Trimethoprim is less likely to cause side effects but can cause nausea, vomiting, rash, and folate deficiency resulting in macrocytic anemia. Nephrotoxicity can occur in patients with impaired renal function.

Trimethoprim

Trimethoprim alone is available for patients allergic to sulfonamides. It has been used mainly in the treatment of chronic bacterial prostatitis and urinary tract infection and the prophylaxis of urinary tract infection. The dose is 100 mg every 12 hours. The side effects are listed under "Trimethoprim-sulfamethoxazole."

Spectinomycin

Spectinomycin is a bactericidal antibiotic that works by binding to the 30S ribosome and thus inhibiting bacterial protein synthesis. It is approved for and used only in the treatment of gonococcal infections. It should be reserved for patients allergic to penicillin, for the treatment of infections caused by *N. gonorrhoeae* that produce pencillinase, and for patients who fail to respond to therapy with penicillin, ampicillin, or tetracycline. Spectinomycin is not effective in gonococcal pharyngitis.

A single dose of 2 g is given intramuscularly for gonococcal urethritis, cervicitis, and proctitis.

EXCRETION AND SIDE EFFECTS. Spectinomycin is excreted by glomerular filtration. Side effects other than hypersensitivity reactions and fever are rare with the dose used.

Metronidazole

Metronidazole is a microbicidal agent that has activity only against strictly anaerobic bacteria and protozoa, such as *Giardia lamblia, Entamoeba histolytica,* and *Trichomonas vaginalis*. It is not active against aerobic or even microaerophilic bacteria. Its major use is in the treatment of protozoal infections and in serious infections caused by anaerobes, particularly when *B. fragilis* is likely to be present (since this is the anaerobe most likely to be resistant to penicillins and cephalosporins). The major use in infections caused by anaerobes, therefore, is in intra-abdominal and pelvic infections. Because of poor activity against microaerophilic gram-positive cocci, it is not very effective in lung abscess where these organisms play an important role. Metronidazole penetrates the CSF in high concentrations, making it an effective drug in the treatment of meningitis or brain abscess caused by susceptible anaerobes. It has also been used for prophylaxis of infections associated with bowel surgery.

Metronidazole is absorbed well when given orally. The dose is 250 mg three times a day for 10 days in *Trichomonas* or *Giardia* infection and 750 mg three times a day for 5 to 10 days in amebiasis. A single 2-g dose is also effective in trichomoniasis. In serious infections caused by anaerobes the agent should be given intravenously in a dose of 15 mg/kg body weight followed by 7.5 mg/kg every 6 hours. A does of 500 mg every 6 hours can be given orally when the infection is less serious.

EXCRETION AND SIDE EFFECTS. Metronidazole is metabolized and the metabolites and some unmetabolized metronidazole are excreted mainly in the urine. The side effects are nausea, vomiting, headache, seizures, syncope, other central nervous system reactions, and peripheral neuropathy. Rush, fever, and reversible neutropenia have been reported. Metronidazole has caused cancer in mice and rats, but the risk to humans is unknown. A disulfiram-like reaction may occur if alcohol is ingested.

Nitrofurantoin

Nitrofurantoin is used orally, and the only indication is the treatment or prophylaxis of urinary tract infection. It is active against *E. coli* and *Klebsiella-Enterobacter* species. *Pseudomonas* and many strains of *Proteus* are resistant.

The dose is 50 to 100 mg four times a day for the treatment of urinary tract infection and 50 to 100 mg each night for prophylaxis in women who have multiple reinfections. Emergence of resistant organisms is not a major problem. Nitrofurantoin is excreted in the urine; it does not give antibacterial blood levels, but urinary levels are high.

Nitrofurantoin is contraindicated in the presence of renal insufficiency, since serious toxicity is a possibility. Its side effects are nausea and vomiting, which are less likely with the macrocystalline form (Macrodantin). Hypersensitivity reactions including fever, rash, and hypersensitivity pneumonitis may be observed. In addition, progressive pulmonary interstitial fibrosis may occur. Paresthesias, followed by a severe polyneuropathy if the drug is not discontinued, can result, especially when serum levels rise as in renal failure. Hemolytic anemia can occur in patients with glucose-6-phosphate dehydrogenase deficiency. Leukopenia and hepatotoxicity have also been reported.

Nalidixic acid

Nalidixic acid is an oral antimicrobial agent used only in the treatment of urinary tract infection. It is active against *E. coli, Klebsiella-Enterobacter,* and *Proteus* but not *Pseudomonas*. However, bacteria tend to become rapidly resistant. Nalidixic acid is excreted in the urine, giving very low blood levels but antibacterial urinary concentrations. It should not be used in the presence of renal insufficiency.

The dose is 1 g four times a day. The side effects are nausea, vomiting, rash, fever, headache, psychosis, and seizures. Papilledema may occur with the headache in children. Another very similar agent is *oxolinic acid*.

Methenamine mandelate and methenamine hippurate

Methenamine mandelate and methenamine hippurate are oral agents used only for the suppression or prophylaxis of urinary tract infection. They are excreted into the urine in high concentrations. At a pH of 5.5 or less, mandelic and hippuric acids are antibacterial and methenamine is converted to formaldehyde, which is antibacterial. These agents are active against *E. coli* and to a lesser extent against other bacilli.

To reduce the urinary pH to 5.5 or less, it is often necessary to add an acidifying agent such as methionine or ascorbic acid. When *Proteus* infections occur, these agents are usually not helpful because *Proteus* organisms produce urease and alkalinize the urine.

The usual dose is 1 g of methenamine mandelate four times a day and 1 g of the hippurate twice a day. The side effects are nausea, vomiting, rash, dysuria (especially with high doses), and metabolic acidosis, especially with the addition of acidifying agents in the presence of renal insufficiency. These agents should not be used in cases of renal insufficiency.

BIBLIOGRAPHY

Bennett, W.M., and others: Drug therapy in renal failure: dosing guidelines for adults, Ann. Intern. Med. **93**:62, 1980.

Goodman, L.S., and Gilman, A.: The pharmacological basis of therapeutics, ed. 5, New York, 1975, Macmillan, Inc.

Handbook of antimicrobial therapy. The Medical Letter on Drugs and Therapeutics (revised ed.), New Rochelle, N.Y., 1980.

Mandell, G.L., Douglas, R.G., and Bennett, J.E.: Principles and practice of infectious diseases, New York, 1979, John Wiley & Sons, Inc.

Sanford, M.P.: Guide to antimicrobial therapy, West Bethesda, Md., 1981, J.P. Sanford, M.D.

40 • INFECTIONS OF SPECIFIC ANATOMIC SITES

Bacterial pneumonia

Gerald R. Donowitz and Gerald L. Mandell

Pneumonia may be defined as parenchymal infection of the lung. The identification of the etiologic agent involved is of the utmost importance. The dangers and expense of "broad-spectrum," shotgun therapy and the impossibility of including all possible causes of pneumonia with empiric therapy make presumptive or, preferably, specific etiologic diagnosis a prerequisite for proper therapy. The following are the major etiologic agents of pneumonia:

I. Bacterial
  A. Common
     1. *Streptococcus pneumoniae*
     2. *Staphylococcus aureus*
     3. *Haemophilus influenzae*
     4. Mixed anareobic bacteria (aspiration)
     5. *Kiebsiella pneumoniae*
  B. Uncommon
     1. *Actinomyces* and *Arachnia* species
     2. *Bacillus anthracis*
     3. Enterobacteriaceae
        a. *Escherichia coli*
        b. *Salmonella* species
        c. *Enterobacter* species
        d. *Serratia* species
        e. *Proteus* species
        f. *Yersinia pestis*
     4. *Francisella tularensis*
     5. *Legionella pneumophila*
     6. *Neisseria meningitidis*
     7. *Nocardia*
     8. *Pasteurella multocida*
     9. *Pseudomonas aeruginosa*
     10. *Pseudomonas pseudomallei*
     11. *Streptococcus pyogenes*
     12. *Legionella micdadei* (Tatlock agent, Hcba agent, Pittsburgh pneumonia agent)
     13. *Legionella bozemanii* (Wiga)
II. Viral
  A. Children
     1. Common
        a. Respiratory syncytial virus

b. Parainfluenza virus types 1, 2, and 3
c. Influenza A virus
2. Uncommon
a. Adenovirus types 1, 2, 3, and 5
b. Influenza B virus
c. Rhinovirus
d. Coxsackievirus
e. Echovirus
f. Measles virus
B. Adults
1. Common
a. Influenza A virus
b. Influenza B virus
c. Adenovirus types 4 and 7 (in military recruits)
2. Rare
a. Rhinovirus
b. Adenovirus types 1, 2, 3, and 5
c. Enteroviruses
(1) Echovirus
(2) Coxsackievirus
(3) Poliovirus
d. Epstein-Barr virus
e. Varicella
III. Fungal
1. *Aspergillus* species
2. *Candida* species
3. *Coccidioides immitis*
4. *Cryptococcus neoformans*
5. *Histoplasma capsulatum*
6. Agents of mucormycosis

IV. Rickettsial
1. *Coxiella burnetti*
V. Bacteria-like agents
1. *Mycoplasma pneumoniae*
2. *Chlamydia* species
VI. Mycobacterial
1. *Mycobacterium tuberculosis*
2. Atypical mycobacteria
VII. Parasitic
1. *Ascaris lumbricoides*
2. *Ancylostoma duodenale*
3. *Echinococcus granulosus*
4. *Pneumocystis carinii*
5. *Schistosoma* species
6. *Strongyloides stercoralis*
7. *Toxoplasma gondii*
8. *Trichinella spiralis*

PATHOGENESIS. Defense mechanisms exist throughout the respiratory tract, and in the absence of disease they serve to maintain essentially sterile infralaryngeal airways and lung parenchyma. Lung defense mechanisms important in preventing infection include (1) filtration and humidification of inspired air through the upper airways; (2) intact reflexes including epiglottic and cough reflexes; (3) tracheobronchial secretions containing antibacterial substances such as α-1-antitrypsin, lysozyme, and lactoferrin; (4) mucociliary transport via the ciliated epithelium; (5) cell-mediated immunity (alveolar macrophages. T lympho-

Table 40-1. Pneumonia syndromes

Syndrome	Onset	Clinical manifestations	Laboratory findings	Roentgenographic findings	Etiologic agent
Community-acquired pneumonia	Acute (hours)	Fever, chills, pleuritic chest pain, productive cough, localized pulmonary findings	WBC elevated; sputum Gram stain shows many PMNs with predominant organism	Bronchopneumonia or lobar consolidation	*Streptococcus pneumoniae, Haemophilus influenzae, Staphylococcus aureus*
Nosocomial gram-negative bacillus pneumonia	Acute (hours)	Fever, chills, pleuritic chest pain, productive cough, localized pulmonary findings	WBC elevated; sputum Gram stain shows many PMNs with predominant organism	Lower lobe most commonly involved; pleural effusion and cavitites may be seen	*Pseudomonas, Klebsiella, Escherichia coli*
Atypical pneumonia	Subacute (3-4 days)	Predominantly constitutional symptoms; variably productive cough; pleuritic chest pains uncommon; respiratory findings minimal	WBC normal; sputum Gram stain shows few organisms or PMNs	Patchy, diffuse infiltrates in lower lobes; consolidation rare	*Mycoplasma pneumoniae, Legionella pneumophila, Coxiella burnetii* (Q fever), *Chlamydia* (psittacosis)
Aspiration pneumonia	Acute (hours) or indolent (weeks-months)	Fever, weight loss, productive cough, foul-smelling sputum	WBC elevated; foul sputum; Gram stain shows many PMNs with mixed population of microbes	Necrotizing pneumonia, lung abscess, empyema	Mixed aerobic-anaerobic pathogens including *Bacteroides*, streptococci, and fusobacteria

cytes); (6) humoral immunity (B lymphocytes, immunoglobulin, complement); and (7) polymorphonuclear leukocytes. The development of pneumonia implies a defect in normal lung defense mechanisms, a challenge by a particularly virulent organism, or an overwhelming inoculation. Inhalation of aerosolized material and aspiration of oropharyngeal contents represent the most common means of entry of pathogens into the lung. Less commonly, pneumonia may result from hematogenous spread of bacteria to the lung.

PNEUMONIA SYNDROMES

Because of the wide variety of organisms involved in causing pneumonia, the recognition of pneumonia syndromes and their likely causes aids in guiding diagnostic maneuvers and selecting specific antimicrobial therapy (Table 40-1). The major pneumonia syndromes caused by bacteria will be reviewed here.

Syndrome of acute community-acquired pneumonia

Most patients with acute community-acquired pneumonia are in the sixth decade of life and have one or more chronic underlying diseases such as chronic obstructive pulmonary disease, cardiovascular disease, diabetes, or alcoholism. The disease usually occurs in midwinter or early spring. The onset of pneumonia is acute and may be marked by the development of a sudden chill. Sustained temperature elevations of approximately 104° F (40° C), cough productive of mucopurulent sputum, and pleuritic chest pain follow. On physical examination the patient is febrile, tachycardic, and tachypneic. Localized pulmonary abnormalities are present, with rales noted early in the disease. There may be increased transmission of breath sounds, dullness to percussion, whispered pectoriloquy, and "E to A" changes. In the presence of a pleural effusion, dullness to percussion and decreased breath sounds may be noted.

White blood cell counts are in the range of 15,000 to 35,000 cells/mm^3 with an increased number of juvenile forms. The hematocrit is usually normal, suggesting an acute rather than a chronic process. Chest roentgenography reveals areas of parenchymal involvement, either in a bronchopneumonic pattern or less frequently in a dense lobar consolidation (Fig. 40-1). Arterial blood gas studies reveal moderate degrees of hypoxemia caused by ventilation-perfusion abnormalities. There are many polymorphonuclear leukocytes in the sputum, and causative organism may be identified by Gram stain and culture of expectorated sputum, transtracheal aspirate, pleural fluid, or blood.

The overwhelming majority (70% to 90%) of cases of community-acquired pneumonia are due to *S. pneumoniae, S. aureus,* and *H. influenzae.* Although many other agents (for example, *K. pneumoniae*) may be involved in causing community-acquired pneumonia, they do so rarely.

PNEUMOCOCCAL PNEUMONIA

Etiology. The pneumococcus *(S. pneumoniae)* is a gram-positive, lancet-shaped coccus usually appearing as paired diplococci but occasionally appearing as short chains or single cocci. Virulent strains of the organism are encapsulated, which inhibits phagocytosis by host neutrophils and thereby increases the organism's pathogenicity.

Epidemiology. The pneumococcus may be found in the oropharynx of normal individuals. Carriage rates have been shown to be highest in children (29% to 35%) and in adults who have preschool-age children in their families (18%). Patients with a history of chronic bronchitis have a higher incidence of upper airway colonization with the pneumococcus. These organisms may serve as a reservoir for exacerbation of chronic bronchitis and development of pneumonia.

Clinical manifestations. There is little to differentiate the onset of pneumococcal pneumonia from that of pneumonia caused by other pathogens. As noted previously, the sudden onset of chills followed by fever, pleuritic chest pain, and productive cough, which marks the onset of bacterial pneumonia in general, is characteristic of pneumococcal pneumonia.

Bacteremia occurs in 25% to 30% of the patients and has been associated with an increased mortality. Pleural effusion occurs in approximately 25% of the patients and represents the most common complication of pneumococcal pneumonia. Usually the effusions are exudative, with no demonstrable organisms on Gram stain or culture. The presence of true empyema is noted in about 1% of the patients. Lung abscess and pericarditis have occurred in association with pneumococcal pneumonia but are rare.

Diagnosis. The examination and culture of expectorated sputum remain the most valuable tools in the diagnosis of pneumococcal pneumonia. With the use of strict criteria for sputum Gram stain positivity, that is, a predominant flora, or more than 10 gram-positive, lancet-shaped diplococci per oil immersion field, or both, the specificity of the Gram stain has been shown to be 85% with a sensitivity of 62%. The diagnostic yield of the sputum examination may be enhanced by use of the quellung reaction, in which pneumococcal capsular antiserum reacts with capsular polysaccharide and produces a clearly outlined capsule. An 89% correlation between culture positivity and a positive quellung test has been reported.

Course. With adequate therapy fever usually resolves promptly. This may occur as quickly as 24 hours after the beginning of therapy or may take several days. The normalization of physical findings and roentgenographic changes may be much slower. Abnormal physical findings may persist for a week or more. Roentgenographic changes may be much slower. Abnormal physical findings may persist for a week or more. Roentgenographic changes may persist from 4 to 6 weeks until complete clearing is noted. Failure to respond suggests the presence

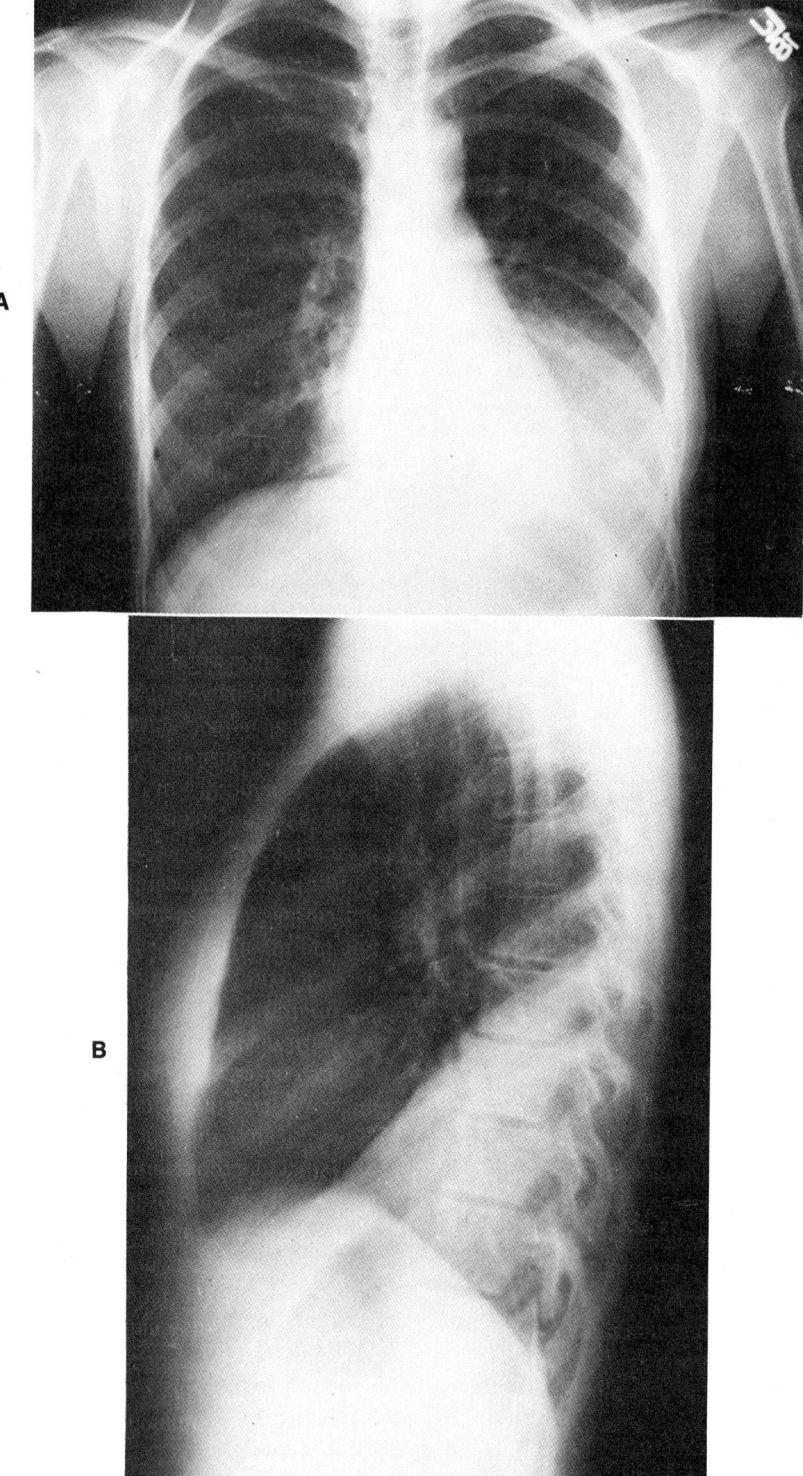

Fig. 40-1. A, PA and, **B,** lateral roentgenograms of patient with pneumococcal pneumonia. Dense lobar consolidation in left lower lobe is consistent with diagnosis but is less commonly seen than bronchopneumonic pattern. (From Mandell, G.L., Douglas, R.G., Jr., and Bennett, J.E., editors: Principles and practice of infectious disease, New York, 1979, John Wiley & Sons, Inc.)

of focal complications such as lung abscess, empyema, or pericarditis.

Patients with sickle cell disease or splenectomy may have a more accelerated disease course and a rapidly fatal outcome. Patients with agammaglobulinemia, lymphoma, myeloma, or lymphocytic leukemia are also at risk of more severe disease.

Management. Penicillin G remains the antibiotic of choice for pneumococcal pneumonia in non-penicillin-allergic patients. Patients with uncomplicated pneumococcal pneumonia should be treated with aqueous procaine penicillin G, 600,000 units given intramuscularly twice a day for 7 to 10 days. In pneumonia complicated by empyema, intravenous administration of 20 million units of penicillin daily is indicated, as well as drainage of the fluid. The decision to treat a patient with pneumonia as an outpatient involves judgmental decisions concerning the severity of the disease, the clinical stability of the patient, and the potential for close clinical monitoring. In these cases intramuscular administration of 600,000 units of procaine penicillin G may be followed by penicillin V, 500 mg orally four times a day for 10 days. In penicillin-allergic patients erythromycin or a cephalosporin may be used. Although penicillin-resistant strains of pneumococci have been noted elsewhere in the world, they are rare in the United States.

Prevention. A polyvalent antipneumococcal vaccine has been developed. Patients with underlying chronic renal, pulmonary, or cardiovascular disease, diabetic patients, elderly patients in general, and patients over 2 years of age with splenectomy (either functional or actual) should receive the vaccine. Children under 2 years of age do not respond as well with antibody titers as those in older age groups.

STAPHYLOCOCCUS AUREUS PNEUMONIA

Epidemiology. *S. aureus* pneumonia accounts for less than 5% of all community-acquired pneumonia. Infants, patients with cystic fibrosis, immunosuppressed patients, and those with or recovering from influenza are at particular risk. The importance of staphylococcal pneumonia in adults during outbreaks of influenza should be stressed. Although streptococcal *(S. pneumoniae)* pneumonia still accounts for the bulk of cases of postinfluenzal pneumonia, staphylococcal pneumonia is seen in about 25% of cases. Hematogenous spread of staphylococci to the lungs may occur in patients with endocarditis or other diseases associated with staphylococcal bacteremia.

Clinical manifestations. Patients with staphylococcal pneumonia are usually toxic with fever, multiple chills, and cough productive of markedly purulent sputum. Localized signs of consolidation are usually found on lung examination. Roentgenographically, early abscess formation, pleural effusions, or empyema is characteristic. Thin-walled cavities (pneumatoceles) are more often seen in children but may be seen in adults.

In patients with postinfluenzal staphylococcal pneumonia, symptoms of influenza initially appear to resolve. After a variable time period, usually 2 to 14 days, respiratory symptoms and systemic toxicity suddenly reappear.

Diagnosis. An elevated white blood cell count with a marked shift to the left may be noted. Staphylococcal pneumonia may be diagnosed by culturing the organism from sputum, blood, or pleural fluid. Sputum Gram stain reveals numerous neutrophils and gram-positive cocci in clumps.

Course. Even with adequate therapy, response is slow, and there is a 15% to 20% case fatality rate. A 3- to 4-week convalescent period is not unusual.

Management. The therapy of choice for staphylococcal pneumonia is a parenterally administered, penicillinase-resistant penicillin such as nafcillin, 1.5 to 2 g intravenously every 4 hours for 14 days. A cephalosporin or vancomycin may be used in penicillin-allergic patients.

GROUP A β-HEMOLYTIC STREPTOCOCCUS (STREPTOCOCCUS PYOGENES)

Epidemiology. Streptococcal pneumonia is relatively rare. Epidemics have been reported in populations of military recruits. An increased incidence is noted after previous upper respiratory tract infections and episodes of influenza. Increased nasopharyngeal carriage of the organism is also an important risk factor for the development of disease.

Clinical manifestations. Streptococcal pneumonia is marked by the development of fever, chills, pleuritic chest pain, and cough productive of purulent sputum. An associated streptococcal pharyngitis may occur in 30% of the patients. In 30% to 40% of the patients there is an associated exudative pleural effusion, which occurs early in the course of the disease. Bacteremia is noted in approximately 10% to 15% of the patients. Extrapulmonary complications are unusual but include mediastinitis and pericarditis. Nonsuppurative complications of streptococcal disease such as rheumatic fever and glomerulonephritis have been noted, albeit rarely.

Diagnosis. Isolation of streptococci from sputum, pleural fluid, or blood is a useful diagnostic test. Serologic tests for antibodies to streptococcal antigens may be positive after several days.

Course. Prolonged fever, even in the presence of adequate therapy, is characteristic of streptococcal pneumonia. In one series over 60% of the patients had persistent fever of a week or more, with only 4% of the patients having a fever as briefly as 1 to 2 days. As noted previously, persistence of fever may indicate the presence of localized infection such as empyema.

Management. Penicillin is the treatment of choice. If empyema is present, adequate drainage is also necessary.

HAEMOPHILUS INFLUENZAE PNEUMONIA

Etiology. *Haemophilus* species are small, gram-negative rods that may appear as coccobacillary forms on Gram stain of clinical material. *H. influenzae* is a somewhat fastidious organism, requiring the presence of two blood-associated factors (X and V) for growth.

Epidemiology. *H. influenzae* pneumonia usually occurs in the setting of chronic disease, most commonly chronic obstructive pulmonary disease, cardiovascular disease, and alcoholism. The upper airways of patients with chronic pulmonary disease are frequently colonized with this organism, and this may serve as a source of lower respiratory tract infections. Encapsulated type B organisms are responsible for most cases of pneumonia with bacteremia.

Clinical manifestations. The onset of *H. influenzae* pneumonia is similar to that of pneumonia caused by the other common bacterial pathogens. Pleural involvement with either demonstrable pleural fluid or pleuritic chest pain may be seen in up to 50% of the patients. Lower lobe involvement is noted most commonly, with more than one lobe involved in over two thirds of the patients.

Diagnosis. Definitive diagnosis of *H. influenzae* pneumonia is difficult. In cases of bacteremic pneumonia, sputum culture has been found positive in only 50% to 75% of the patients. Sputum Gram stains may often be misread, and the presence of *H. influenzae* may be overlooked. Since the organism may colonize the upper airways, its presence in sputum does not necessarily indicate that it is the cause of pneumonia.

Management. Ampicillin is the therapy of choice for pneumonia caused by sensitive strains of *H. influenzae*. Ampicillin-resistant strains of *H. influenzae* have been isolated from clinical material with variable frequency (5% to 30%). Cefamandole or chloramphenicol may be used as therapy for ampicillin-resistant strains or for pneumonia in penicillin-allergic patients.

KLEBSIELLA PNEUMONIAE **PNEUMONIA (FRIEDLÄNDER'S PNEUMONIA).** *Klebsiella* pneumonia, a rare form of community-acquired pneumonia, is usually seen in alcoholic men or chronically ill, debilitated patients. The *Klebsiella* organisms are heavily encapsulated and produce a necrotizing pneumonia.

The presentation resembles those of other bacterial pneumonias, but the sputum if often extremely viscous and has a brick-red color (currant jelly sputum). Multilobar involvement is common. Gram stain of the sputum shows large, encapsulated, gram-negative bacilli. The chest roentgenogram may demonstrate a bulging fissure. Cavitation and empyema are common.

The mortality rate is significant (up to 50%) even with appropriate therapy, which consists of cephalothin, 2 g every 4 hours intravenously, plus gentamicin, 1.7 mg/kg every 8 hours intravenously. If the organism is susceptible to cephalothin, the gentamicin may be discontinued.

Nosocomial gram-negative bacillus pneumonia syndrome

EPIDEMIOLOGY. Unlike *S. pneumoniae* and *H. influenzae*, gram-negative enteric organisms are relatively uncommon causes of community-acquired pneumonia, accounting for 2% to 11% of pneumonias in the outpatient setting. When gram-negative bacillus pneumonia does occur, chronic obstructive pulmonary disease, chronic cardiovascular disease, and alcoholism are important underlying factors.

Gram-negative organisms are important etiologic agents of pneumonia in hospitalized patients and immunosuppressed hosts. Within 24 to 48 hours after admission, colonization of the upper respiratory tract by enteric gram-negative rods has been shown to occur in patients in intensive care units. An increased incidence of gram-negative bacillus pneumonia has been associated with this colonization. Contaminated nebulizers have been demonstrated to be an important cause of hospital-acquired gram-negative bacillus pneumonia. Gram-negative rod pneumonia accounts for 21% of infectious episodes in patients with leukemia. Furthermore, the lungs serve as a source for bacteremia in over 60% of these patients. Tracheostomy sites frequently become infected with gram-negative bacilli.

CLINICAL MANIFESTATIONS. Patients frequently have severe underlying disease and are often on respirators. The signs and symptoms of gram-negative bacillus pneumonia are not distinctive. Fever, chills, and productive cough are usually seen.

Lower lobe disease is most common, with multilobar involvement occurring in 40% of the patients. Cavitation, microabscesses, and pleural effusion may occur. There is no characteristic roentgenographic picture that can differentiate one gram-negative organism from another.

DIAGNOSIS. Pleural fluid, sputum, and blood should be examined and cultured to establish a cause. Since upper airway colonization takes place in hospitalized patients, transtracheal aspiration is of help in differentiating upper airway colonization from lower airway infection, provided there is no tracheal tube in place. In immunosuppressed hosts pneumonic infiltrates are often assumed to be caused by gram-negative rods and are treated accordingly until a definitive diagnosis is made.

COURSE. Even with appropriate antibiotic therapy, the mortality from gram-negative bacillus pneumonia is about 50%. The debilitated condition of the host accounts for these high figures. Even with adequate therapy, signs and symptoms may persist for weeks.

MANAGEMENT. The treatment of gram-negative bacillus pneumonia depends on the antimicrobial sensitivites of the specific etiologic agent involved. Dual drug regimens have been used in certain instances to achieve antibiotic synergy. Recommended regimens of therapy include a cephalosporin plus an aminoglycoside for *Klebsiella* pneumonia and an aminoglycoside plus carbenicillin or ticarcillin for *Pseudomonas* pneumonia.

Atypical pneumonia syndrome

The atypical pneumonia syndrome is a symptom complex associated most commonly with *M. pneumoniae* (see Chapter 44). Unlike the acute bacterial pneumonias described previously, atypical pneumonias develop over a 3- to 4-day period. Constitutional symptoms predominate over specific respiratory symptoms. Fever, malaise, coryza, headache, and cough are the major symptoms. Pleuritic chest pain and respiratory distress are not usually seen. Sputum production is variable, and although sputum is purulent in one third of the patients, polymorphonuclear leukocytes are absent in most patients, and Gram stain and culture usually reveal only sparse normal flora. Roentgenographic findings most commonly include a patchy or diffuse infiltrate without lobar consolidation. White blood cell counts are usually less than 10,000/mm^3. Other etiologic agents that may cause the atypical pneumonia syndrome include parainfluenza virus, Epstein-Barr virus, respiratory syncytial virus, and adenovirus. Q fever and psittacosis are rare causes of atypical pneumonia. Legionnaires' disease may cause a rather severe atypical pneumonia.

LEGIONNAIRES' DISEASE

Etiology. *Legionella pneumophila* is a newly described, fastidious, gram-negative bacillus.

Epidemiology. Legionnaires' disease has been described in all age groups. Most commonly patients with the disease are in their midfifties and have chronic underlying diseases such as chronic obstructive pulmonary disease, cardiovascular disease, alcoholism, or diabetes. Epidemics most often occur in the summer months, although sporadic cases of disease have been noted to occur throughout the year. The disease is spread via the airborne route. Epidemics have been associated with contaminated air-conditioning and air treatment systems. Recently disturbed soil and excavation and construction sites have been suspected as the sources of the organism. Person-to-person transmission of the disease has not been proved.

Pathogenesis. *Legionella* can grow in human monocytes. Infection causes a fibrinopurulent pneumonia, often with diffuse alveolar damage. Bronchi appear to be spared. The inflammatory exudate consists of neutrophils and large numbers of macrophages. Focal necrosis appears to be more extensive than that noted in more common bacterial pneumonias.

Clinical manifestations. A prodrome of malaise, myalgia, and headache is often described. Within 48 hours fever and chills develop. Nausea, vomiting, and diarrhea may be seen in the early stages of the disease. Cough generally develops several days after the onset of symptoms and is usually nonproductive, although hemoptysis may occur. Pleuritic chest pain is seen in 30% to 40% of the patients. Confusion and delirium may develop. There is usually a moderately elevated leukocyte count with a shift to the left. Microscopic hematuria, proteinuria, elevations of liver transaminases, hypophosphatemia, and hyponatremia have been described. With progression of disease, hypoxemia and hypocapnia develop. Gram stain of expectorated sputum or transtracheal aspirates is unrevealing. Chest roentgenograms most commonly show either a patchy infiltrate or consolidation. Although most patients initially have unilateral involvement, bilateral, multilobar involvement usually develops. Cavitation has not been reported, and pleural effusions are uncommon.

Legionella may also be responsible for nonpneumonic disease. Diagnostic rises in antibody titer have been associated with a mild, febrile illness without signs of pneumonia (Pontiac fever).

Diagnosis. Legionnaires' disease must be differentiated from other causes of atypical pneumonia. The prodromal symptoms of diarrhea, confusion out of proportion to fever, nonproductive cough, and lack of pathogens noted on Gram stains of sputum or transtracheal aspirates should suggest this diagnosis. Elevation of liver enzymes, changes in mental status, and rapid progression of roentgenographic signs of disease are more suggestive of *Legionella* than of other agents involved in sporadic pneumonia.

The diagnosis of Legionnaires' disease can be made by demonstrating a rise in antibody titer; by culturing the organisms from lung tissue, pleural fluid, or sputum; and by demonstrating the presence of the organisms in lung tissue with fluorescent antibody staining or the Dieterle silver stain. Given the specialized nature of these diagnostic techniques, presumptive diagnosis is usually made on clinical grounds and therapy is started before the presence of *Legionella* is definitively documented.

Course. Without therapy Legionnaires' disease often runs a fulminant course. A 15% mortality is noted with a rapid progression of disease over 5 to 6 days. Respiratory failure and shock are usually terminal events. In nonpneumonic disease gradual spontaneous clearing of symptoms occurs.

Management. Erythromycin in doses of 0.5 to 1 g every 6 hours for 3 weeks is the therapy of choice. It is given intravenously to seriously ill patients.

Aspiration (anaerobic organism) pneumonia syndrome

ETIOLOGY. Anaerobic organism pneumonia is most commonly associated with organisms of the oropharynx. Pneumonia may be caused by anerobic bacteria alone (45% to 58% of the cases) or by anaerobes in conjunction with aerobic organisms (41% to 46% of the cases). The most commonly isolated anaerobes include the anaerobic or microaerophilic streptococci, *Fusobacterium*, and *Bac-*

teroides species *(melaninogenicus, fragilis,* and *oralis)*. In its chronic form anaerobic organism pneumonia is often classified as lung abscess.

EPIDEMIOLOGY. Anaerobic infections of the lung most commonly occur when aspiration of oropharyngeal contents has taken place. Conditions that compromise the normal gag and cough reflexes, such as sedative overdose, seizures, alcoholism, or loss of consciousness, predispose patients to aspiration and the development of anaerobic organism pneumonia. Lung damage from other causes such as tumor or bronchiectasis may create conditions in which anaerobic organisms can flourish. Poor dentition plays a major role in providing a source of anaerobes. Periodontal disease, heavy tartar deposition, and carious teeth are commonly found in patients with anaerobic organism disease. Anaerobic organism infection is uncommon in edentulous patients.

CLINICAL MANIFESTATIONS. The three major syndromes recognized as a consequence of aspiration are chemical pneumonitis, bronchial obstruction caused by aspiration of particulate matter, and bacterial aspiration pneumonia. Chemical pneumonitis and mechanical obstruction usually cause acute symptoms. In contrast, bacterial aspiration pneumonia is more insidious. Symptoms develop gradually several days to weeks after the initial episode of aspiration. Pneumonitis, necrotizing pneumonia, abscess, and empyema are the most common manifestations of anaerobic organism pneumonia. Symptoms of fever, weight loss, and productive cough may be present for several weeks before the patient seeks medical care. Putrid sputum is produced in 50% of the cases. Anemia and elevated white blood cell counts are frequently associated findings. Anemia suggests the presence of a chronic disease rather than the sudden change of health noted in the community-acquired pneumonia syndrome. Roentgenographic changes include necrotizing pneumonia, cavitation, or the presence of pleural effusion or empyema. Aspiration pneumonia most commonly involves either the posterior segment of the upper lobe or the superior or basilar segment of the lower lobe, depending on whether aspiration occurs in the reclining or upright position. Chronic aspiration most frequently results in a bilateral lower lobe pneumonia, although one side may be more involved than the other.

DIAGNOSIS. The presence of foul-smelling sputum in a patient with necrotizing or cavitary pneumonia suggests aspiration pneumonia. The isolation of anaerobic organisms from blood or pleural fluid requires special processing of samples. Cultural confirmation is rarely necessary, but if sputum is cultured, transtracheal aspiration should be carried out to bypass the oral anaerobic flora. Gram-stained empyema fluid, sputum samples, or transtracheal aspirates reveal numerous polymorphonuclear leukocytes with a mixed population of organisms.

COURSE. Even with the appropriate therapy, a slow resolution of symptoms is common with anaerobic lung infection. Residual pulmonary disease with bronchiectasis, pulmonary fibrosis, or chronic effusions occurs in 10% of the patients. A mortality rate of 15% to 19% has been noted.

MANAGEMENT. Penicillin is considered the therapy of choice for anaerobic organism lung infections. Intravenous administration of 20 million units daily is recommended initially. After response, penicillin V, 500 mg orally every 6 hours, can be given for 2 weeks or more until stabilization of the chest roentgenogram. Lung abscesses may require up to 6 weeks of therapy. If empyema exists, adequate drainage is mandatory. For cavitary lung disease appropriate postural drainage is important. Clindamycin and chloramphenicol have been successful alternative drugs in penicillin-allergic patients. If *B. fragilis* is isolated from blood or pleural fluid or if response to penicillin is inadequate, clindamycin or chloramphenicol should be given along with penicillin.

BIBLIOGRAPHY

Bartlett, J.G., and Finegold, S.M.: Anaerobic pleuropulmonary infections, Medicine **51:**413, 1972.

Bartlett, J.G., and Finegold, S.M.: Anaerobic infections of the lung and pleural space, Am. Rev. Respir. Dis. **110:**56, 1974.

Chang, H.Y., and others: Causes of death in adults with acute leukemia, Medicine **55:**259, 1976.

Fekety, F.R., and others: Bacteria, viruses, and mycoplasmas in acute pneumonia in adults, Am. Rev. Respir. Dis. **104:**449, 1971.

Hendley, J.O., and others: Spread of *Streptococcus pneumoniae* in families. I. Carriage rates and distribution of types, J. Infect. Dis. **132:**55, 1975.

Johanson, W.G., and others: Nosocomial respiratory infections with gram negative bacilli: the significance of colonization of the respiratory tract, Ann. Intern. Med. **77:**701, 1972.

Merrill, C., and others: Rapid identification of pneumococci, N. Engl. J. Med. **288:**510, 1973.

Newhouse, M., Sanchis, J., and Bienenstock, J.: Lung defense mechanisms, N. Engl. J. Med. **295:**990, 1976.

Rein, M.F., and others: Accuracy of the Gram stain in identifying pneumococci in sputum, J.A.M.A. **230:**2671, 1978.

Schwarzmann, S.W., and others: Bacterial pneumonia during the Hong Kong influenza epidemic of 1968-1969, Arch. Intern. Med. **127:**1037, 1971.

Sprunt, S.: Infection in chronic lung disease, Bull. N.Y. Acad. Med. **48:**698, 1972.

Swartz, M.N.: Clinical aspects of Legionnaires' disease, Ann. Intern. Med. **90:**492, 1979.

Unger, J.D., Rose, H.D., and Unger, G.F.: Gram-negative pneumonia, Radiology **107:**283, 1973.

Infective endocarditis

Donald Kaye

DEFINITION. Infective endocarditis is an infection on the endocardium and may involve a heart valve, a septal defect, or mural endocardium. It may be classified into acute and subacute disease. Acute endocarditis is most frequently caused by *Staphylococcus aureus;* it often occurs on a normal heart valve and results in rapid severe destruction. Metastatic foci of infection are common. If untreated, the infection will kill in days to weeks.

Subacute endocarditis is usually caused by streptococci of the viridans group and occurs on already damaged valves, producing additional damage slowly. Metastatic foci of infection are rare. Without therapy the infection will take 6 or more weeks or even years to kill. However, streptococci of the viridans group can occasionally cause endocarditis with an acute course on a normal valve, and S. aureus can cause subacute disease.

It is more important to classify endocarditis by infecting organism (for example, enterococcal endocarditis). The identity of the organism has implications for the course (that is, acute or subacute), but more importantly, it has therapeutic implications for the antimicrobial regimen.

Endarteritis, infection in an artery (for example, on a coarctation of the aorta), produces a syndrome indistinguishable from endocarditis.

ETIOLOGY. Almost any species of bacteria is capable of producing infective endocarditis. However, streptococci and staphylococci account for the vast majority of cases.

Streptococci. Streptococci are the causative microorganisms in 40% to 80% of the cases of endocarditis. Viridans streptococci account for about 50% of the cases of streptococcal endocarditis, S. bovis cause about 25%, enterococci cause about 10%, and the remaining streptococci (microaerophilic and anaerobic streptococci, nonhemolytic streptococci, and group A β-hemolytic streptococci) are isolated in the remainder of the cases.

Enterococci and group A β-hemolytic streptococci can attack normal or previously damaged heart valves and may cause rapid destruction. The other streptococci are much more likely to produce endocarditis on already damaged heart valves and rarely cause rapid destruction.

Staphylococci. Staphylococci are the causative microorganisms in 10% to 30% of the cases of infective endocarditis. S. aureus is isolated much more frequently than S. epidermidis.

S. aureus attacks either normal or previously damaged heart valves and causes rapid destruction. The course if often fulminant, leading to death from overwhelming bacteremia within days or from heart failure within weeks. Abscesses are common at multiple sites (for example, kidneys, lungs, brain, and heart). S. epidermidis usually attacks abnormal heart valves without causing rapid destruction.

Other bacteria. Almost all species of bacteria are reported as occasionally causing endocarditis, including the enteric gram-negative bacilli, gonococci, pneumococci, *Salmonella, Bacteroides, Haemophilus, Listeria,* and even diphtheroids. Gram-negative bacilli account for less than 5% of the cases of endocarditis but are common causes in drug addicts and patients with prosthetic heart valves.

Fungi. *Candida, Aspergillus,* and *Histoplasma* species are the most common causes of fungal endocarditis, with *Candida* endocarditis occurring most frequently. Fungal endocarditis is common in narcotic addicts *(Candida)* and in patients following cardiac surgery *(Candida* and *Aspergillus).*

The course of fungal endocarditis is usually subacute. Large, friable vegetations are common and give rise to large emboli, often in the lower extremities. In patients with prosthetic cardiac valves, malfunction of the valve may occur because of the size of the vegetations.

Other microorganisms. Spirochetes (such as *Spirillum minus*), cell wall-deficient bacteria, rickettsiae *(Coxiella burnetii),* and the psittacosis agent have all been reported as rare causes of endocarditis.

EPIDEMIOLOGY. Mean ages in most series range from the midforties to the midfifties. Endocarditis is uncommon in children. *Rheumatic valvular disease,* most often involving the mitral or aortic valves or both, is the underlying cardiac disease in about 25% to 60% of the patients with infective endocarditis, and the frequency seems to be decreasing.

Congenital heart disease is the underlying lesion in about 10% to 20% of the patients with endocarditis. Some predisposing lesions are patent ductus arteriosus, ventricular septal defect, tetralogy of Fallot, coarctation of the aorta, pulmonary stenosis, and bicuspid aortic valve. In contrast, atrial septal defects of the secundum type rarely serve as an underlying lesion.

Mitral valve prolapse is the underlying cardiac lesion in about 10% of the cases of endocarditis, and the frequency seems to be increasing.

Degenerative heart disease (for example, valves with degenerative changes and calcific aortic stenosis resulting from degenerative aortic valve disease or a bicuspid aortic valve) can be a predisposing cardiac lesion in endocarditis. Infective endocarditis has also been reported in patients with *asymmetric septal hypertrophy, Marfan's syndrome,* and *syphilitic aortic valve disease.*

A new and important cardiac lesion that serves as an underlying abnormality for production of endocarditis is the *prosthetic cardiac valve.* Similarly, intravascular sutures, pacemaker wires, and Teflon-Silastic tubes are predisposing factors to the development of endocarditis or endarteritis. Arterioarterial or arteriovenous fistulas also predispose individuals to endocarditis. Up to 10% of the cases of endocarditis occur in people who abuse drugs intravenously.

In 20% to 40% of the patients with infective endocarditis no underlying heart disease can be recognized.

PATHOGENESIS AND PATHOLOGY. The characteristic lesions of infective endocarditis are vegetations on the valve leaflets or elsewhere on the endocardium. The disease usually arises following localization of microorganisms on a sterile thrombotic vegetation (termed nonbacterial thrombotic endocarditis). This may form as a result of trauma to the endothelial cells or over a subendothelial inflammatory reaction, as in acute rheumatic fever or myocardial infarction.

When bacteremia occurs, the surface of the vegetation can become secondarily infected and converted to the typical vegetation of infective endocarditis. This results from deposition of platelets and fibrin over the bacteria. The vegetation then becomes a "protected site," which phagocytic cells penetrate poorly.

Hydrodynamic forces. The sites of involvement suggest an important role for hydrodynamic forces. Endocarditis occurs downstream from where blood flows through a narrow orifice at a high velocity from a high- to a low-pressure chamber. For example, endocarditis is found immediately distal to the constriction in coarctation of the aorta and on the pulmonary artery immediately beyond the junction with the ductus in patent ductus arteriosus.

Endocarditis does not usually occur when there is only a small pressure gradient, as in atrial septal defects. Valvular endocarditis occurs more frequently in valvular incompetence than in pure stenosis and is characteristically on the atrial side of the incompetent mitral valve and the ventricular surface of the incompetent aortic valve. A high-velocity stream of blood can produce satellite infected lesions at distant points of impact.

Invasion of circulation. Organisms must gain access to the circulation in sufficient numbers for a sufficient interval for endocarditis to result. Invasion of the bloodstream occurs in many infections (for example, pneumococcal pneumonia).

Transient bacteremia is common during traumatic procedures involving the epithelial surfaces normally laden with an indigenous bacterial flora (oropharynx, genitourinary and gastrointestinal tracts, and skin). Surgical incision of the skin, which is ordinarily inhabited by staphylococci and diphtheroids, is often associated with bacteremia, usually staphylococcal (either *S. aureus* or *S. epidermidis*). Bacteremia occurs in about 25% of patients after toothbrushing, chewing hard candy, or using an oral irrigation device. After trauma to the tissues of the mouth, streptococci of the viridans groups are the bacteria most commonly isolated from the blood, either alone or more often mixed with other bacteria. The frequency of bacteremia following dental procedures is related to the degree of periodontal disease and the amount of trauma.

Portal of entry. Although the portal of entry for the initiating episode of bacteremia in endocarditis is often inapparent, oral cavity infection or operative or manipulative dental procedures appear to be the most common clinically apparent portals of entry, especially in endocarditis caused by viridans streptococci. Endocarditis caused by viridans streptococci has also occurred in edentulous patients in association with oral ulcers from poorly fitting dentures.

Bacteremia occurs in up to one third of patients after transurethral prostatic resection, cystoscopy, urethral dilation, and urethral catheterization. The organisms are usually enterococci and gram-negative bacilli.

Mechanisms of production of lesions. The pathogenesis of the manifestations of endocarditis is both a result of the vegetations themselves and an immune reaction to the infection. The vegetations may become so extensive, especially in fungal endocarditis, that the valve orifice is occluded. There may be rapid, massive destruction of tissue with consequent valvular insufficiency, especially in *S. aureus* endocarditis. Areas of healing may cause scar formation and consequent valvular stenosis or insufficiency. Infection may extend into the myocardium, producing burrowing abscesses. Conduction abnormalities, fistulas, or rupture of the chordae, a papillary muscle, or the ventricular septum may result.

The vegetations are friable, and pieces embolize to the heart itself and to the brain, kidneys, spleen, extremities, and lungs (in endocarditis of the right side of the heart). Infarcts and perhaps abscesses (with *S. aureus* endocarditis) result at these sites. Septic embolization to the vasa vasorum or direct bacterial invasion of the arterial wall may result in the formation of mycotic aneurysms that may rupture. They most often develop in the cerebral arteries, aorta, sinus of Valsalva, ligated ductus arteriosus, and superior mesenteric, splenic, coronary, and pulmonary arteries. Vessels in the head are involved in about 50% of the patients, vessels in the abdomen and chest in about 40%, and vessels in the limbs in about 10%.

In addition, vasculitis on an immunologic basis is thought to contribute to the findings. Patients with infective endocarditis usually have high circulating antibody titers against the infecting microorganism. This contributes to the formation of circulating immune complexes. Diffuse glomerulonephritis, focal embolic glomerulitis, Roth's spots, petechiae, and Osler's nodes are thought usually to be due to allergic vasculitis caused by deposition of immune complexes. In contrast, Janeway's lesions are thought to have an embolic basis.

CLINICAL MANIFESTATIONS. A history of a dental procedure can be elicited in only 15% to 20% of the patients with endocarditis caused by streptococci of the viridans group. About 50% of the patients with enterococcal endocarditis have had a preceding urologic or genital tract procedure, and about 35% of the patients with staphylococcal endocarditis have a history of a preceding staphylococcal infection. Symptoms of endocarditis generally start within 2 or 3 weeks of the procedure. The onset is usually gradual, with mild fever and malaise in cases of endocarditis caused by streptococci of the viridans group and other organisms of low pathogenicity. With *S. aureus,* pneumococci, and other organisms of high pathogenicity, the onset is often acute with high fever.

Fever is present in almost all patients during the course of endocarditis. Most exceptions are elderly patients or patients with renal-failure, congestive heart failure, or severe debility. The temperature is usually low grade (less than 103° F [39.4° C]) except with acute disease. *Cardiac murmurs* are almost always present except with acute endocarditis or in intravenous narcotic addicts. Addicts often have vegetations on the tricuspid valve, and murmurs are frequently absent. True changes in murmurs or the appearance of a new murmur is uncommon except in acute endocarditis in which a new murmur (particularly aortic insufficiency) is a frequent occurrence.

Splenomegaly is present in about 30% of the reported cases of endocarditis and is most common in disease of long duration. *Petechiae* are present in 20% to 40% of the patients, most commonly those with more prolonged illness. Petechiae are most frequently found in the conjunctivae, palate, buccal mucosa, and extremities.

Splinter hemorrhages are subungual, linear, dark-red streaks that may appear in endocarditis but are also often the result of local trauma. What are commonly called *Roth's spots* are oval, retinal hemorrhages with a clear, pale center. These are seen in less than 5% of patients with endocarditis and may also occur in collagen vascular diseases and severe anemia. *Osler's nodes* are small, tender nodules, most frequently found on the finger or toe pads, which persist for hours to days. They are found in 10% to 25% of the patients with endocarditis, but they also occur in other diseases such as typhoid fever and collagen vascular disease; they are uncommon in acute endocarditis. *Clubbing of the fingers* is present in some patients, usually those with longstanding disease. *Janeway's lesions* are nontender, macular, hemorrhagic areas on the palms and soles, most commonly seen in acute endocarditis.

Clinically apparent embolic episodes are recognized in about one third of the patients with endocarditis and may occur as the first symptom or late (after successful therapy). *Mycotic aneurysms* occur in about 10% of the patients with infective endocarditis. These lesions can rupture at any time before, during, or even years after therapy for endocarditis.

Neurologic manifestations are present in about one third of the patients with endocarditis. Major cerebral emboli are not infrequent and usually involve the middle cerebral artery system. Mycotic aneurysms also most often involve this system. Toxic encephalopathy or personality changes or both can occur in patients with endocarditis. Brain abscess and purulent meningitis are most common with *S. aureus* endocarditis.

Congestive heart failure is a frequent complication of endocarditis and may occur at any time during the course of the disease, including long after cure. Some factors that contribute to heart failure are valve destruction, myocarditis from vasculitis, coronary artery emboli with infarction, and myocardial abscesses.

Renal disease is present in most patients with infective endocarditis. Up to 50% of the patients with endocarditis have microscopic hematuria, and proteinuria is even more common. These findings may be due to renal emboli, focal embolic glomerulitis, or diffuse glomerulonephritis. Renal insufficiency may occur in diffuse glomerulonephritis but is rare as a consequence of emboli or focal embolic glomerulitis.

SPECIAL SYNDROMES

Enterococcal endocarditis. Enterococci are streptococci that are normal inhabitants of the human gastrointestinal tract, the anterior urethra, and occasionally the mouth. All enterococci are in Lancefield's group D, although not all organisms in group D are enterococci.

The average age for men with enterococcal endocarditis is near 60 years, whereas in women it is just under 40 years. This age distribution is probably closely related to the suspected genitourinary tract portal of entry of the organism. About 50% of the patients give a history of recent genitourinary tract manipulation. For men this usually means instrumentation involving the prostate, thus explaining the older age in males. For women the genitourinary factors are abortion, pregnancy, cesarean section, and urethral catheterization, which occur mainly during the childbearing years. This explains the lower age of female patients.

***Streptococcus bovis* endocarditis.** Two other group D streptococci, *S. bovis* and *S. equinus,* should be considered separately from the enterococci because endocarditis caused by these two species can be treated like endocarditis caused by viridans streptococci. For all practical purposes *S. bovis* and *S. equinus* can be demonstrated not to be enterococci by the fact that they are highly susceptible to penicillin G (inhibited by 0.1 μ/ml), whereas enterococci are much more resistant. *S. bovis* endocarditis or bacteremia occurs in the elderly (80% over 60 years of age) and has a striking relationship to abnormalities in the gastrointestinal tract. One third to one half of the patients with this infection have gastrointestinal malignancies (usually of the colon) or villous adenomas or polyps of the colon.

Endocarditis in drug abusers. Infective endocarditis is a complication of parenteral narcotic addiction. *S. aureus* is responsible for over 50% of the cases, and fungi (mainly *Candida*) and gram-negative bacilli (most of which are *Pseudomonas* species) cause most of the remaining cases. Viridans streptococci are uncommon infecting agents in endocarditis in addicts.

The tricuspid valve is infected in over 50% of addicts with endocarditis, the aortic valve in 25%, and the mitral valve in about 20%. There is a striking association of *S. aureus* endocarditis with tricuspid valve involvement; over 75% of the patients with *S. aureus* infection have endocarditis on the tricuspid valve.

Signs and symptoms of pulmonary emboli or pneumonia related to septic pulmonary emboli are common presentations in addicts with tricuspid valve endocarditis, and murmurs are frequently absent.

Prosthetic valve endocarditis. An intracardiac prosthesis predisposes a patient to the development of endocarditis and makes eradication of the infection extremely difficult.

Endocarditis has been reported to occur in 1% to 3% of patients, with prosthetic valves.

Prosthetic valve endocarditis is usually divided into early endocarditis (onset within 2 months of valve replacement) and late endocarditis (onset after 2 months). Early endocarditis is a consequence of contamination during the perioperative period, whereas late endocarditis is related to bacteremia from dental, skin, and genitourinary tract trauma.

About one third of both early and late endocarditis episodes are caused by staphylococci, with *S. epidermidis* occurring more frequently than *S. aureus*. Gram-negative bacilli cause up to 25% of the early cases and are less common in late endocarditis. Fungi (most commonly *Candida*) are responsible for up to 10% of the early cases and are much less common in late endocarditis. Streptococci are the most frequent single causes of late endocarditis (about 40% of the cases) but are uncommon infecting organisms in early endocarditis. Diphtheroids have been the infecting organisms in up to 20% of the early cases and are less common in late endocarditis.

Early prosthetic valve endocarditis is often associated with valve dysfunction or dehiscence and a fulminant course. Although late endocarditis may have a similar clinical course, it is commonly characterized by a clinical syndrome indistinguishable from that occurring in patients without prosthetic valves.

LABORATORY FINDINGS. A normocytic and normochromic anemia is an almost constant finding in infective endocarditis except in acute cases. Most patients have normal white blood cell and differential counts. However, in acute disease leukocytosis may be present. Proteinuria or gross or microscopic hematuria or both are present in most patients. The erythrocyte sedimentation rate is almost always elevated. In those with severe renal complications (usually diffuse glomerulonephritis), the blood urea nitrogen or serum creatinine may be elevated.

About 50% of the patients with endocarditis of at least several weeks' duration have a positive serum test for rheumatoid factor, and circulating immune complexes have been demonstrated in the sera of a great majority of patients with endocarditis. These tend to disappear with cure of endocarditis. The serum complement may be decreased, especially in patients with glomerulonephritis. Bacteria can be seen inside leukocytes in buffy coat preparations of blood in about 50% of the patients with bacterial endocarditis.

The single most important finding in patients with endocarditis is bacteremia or fungemia. Blood cultures should be obtained promptly in anyone with suspected endocarditis and are positive in over 90% of the patients. The bacteremia of endocarditis is constant; if any cultures are positive, it is likely that all will be positive.

In patients with subacute disease who have not received previous antimicrobial therapy, five blood cultures should be obtained over a period of 12 hours and therapy should be initiated. If previous therapy has been given, treatment may be expeditiously delayed in an attempt to obtain positive blood cultures. In general, in acute disease therapy should not be delayed for more than 2 to 3 hours while cultures are obtained. In selected patients (especially those who have received previous antimicrobial therapy), cultures in hypertonic media may be helpful in an attempt to isolate cell wall–deficient forms. The addition of pyridoxal hydrochloride or cysteine to the media will improve the chances of isolating nutritionally variant streptococci.

Blood cultures have usually been negative in the rare cases of endocarditis caused by *Aspergillus, Histoplasma,* and *Coxiella burnetti*. In fungal endocarditis large emboli to the lower extremities are common, necessitating embolectomy. Histologic examination and culture of the embolus may be diagnostic.

Echocardiograms may suggest the location of a vegetation. Serial phonocardiography and cineradiography are useful for evaluating valve dysfunction or dehiscence in patients with prosthetic valve endocarditis. The disappearance of an opening or closing click suggests the presence of a vegetation on the valve; this is especially likely to occur with large vegetations, as are seen in fungal endocarditis. Cineradiography of the valve will show abnormal motion if the sutures are pulling out.

DIFFERENTIAL DIAGNOSIS. Infective endocarditis should be suspected in any patient with a heart murmur and unexplained fever present for at least 1 week. A definitive diagnosis can be made only in the presence of positive blood cultures. In the small percentage of patients with sterile blood cultures, the differential diagnosis can be very difficult.

Two clinical entities that can exactly duplicate the syndrome of infective endocarditis (including fever, murmur, and emboli) are atrial myxoma and nonbacterial thrombotic endocarditis. Acute rheumatic fever, lupus erythematous, and sickle cell disease can also produce fever and heart murmur. Fever related to another illness can develop in any patient with an existing heart murmur. Therefore in the absence of positive blood cultures a search must be made for other causes of fever.

Even in the absence of fever, murmur, or other signs of endocarditis, sustained bacteremia with ordinarily nonpathogenic bacteria (such as viridans streptococci, coagulase-negative staphylococci, or diphtheroids) is strongly suggestive of intravascular infection, usually endocarditis.

MANAGEMENT

Principles of therapy. To achieve cure of infective endocarditis, it is necessary to sterilize the vegetation. Therefore bactericidal drug regimens are required in the therapy of endocarditis, and treatment must be continued long enough to achieve sterilization of the vegetation. Available evidence indicates that if peak serum concentrations are bactericidal for the infecting microorganism at a 1:8 dilution in normal serum, therapy is probably adequate.

Specific antimicrobial regimens. The initial treatment of subacute infective endocarditis while awaiting culture results should be directed at the enterococcus. However, if the course is acute, the patient has an intracardiac foreign body, or the patient is a parenteral drug abuser, therapy for staphylococcal endocarditis must be added. Once the infecting organism is isolated, the regimen should promptly be altered.

Streptococcal endocarditis

STREPTOCOCCI INHIBITED BY 0.2 µg/ml PENICILLIN G. Streptococci inhibited by 0.2 µg/ml penicillin G are classified as penicillin susceptible and include over 90% of viridans streptococci but no enterococci. For these streptococci three regimens have been widely used: (1) penicillin G alone for 4 weeks in doses of 10 to 20 million units intravenously daily; (2) penicillin G, 10 to 20 million units intravenously daily, or procaine penicillin, 1.2 million units intramuscularly every 6 hours, plus streptomycin, 0.5 g intramuscularly every 12 hours for 2 weeks; or (3) penicillin plus streptomycin for 2 weeks with penicillin therapy extended another 2 weeks. I prefer the third regimen. If penicillin is contraindicated because of hypersensitivity, cephalothin, 2 g every 4 hours intravenously, or cefazolin, 1 g every 6 hours intravenously or intramuscularly, can be given for 4 weeks with or without streptomycin for the first 2 weeks. Patients who are hypersensitive to penicillin may also be hypersensitive to the cephalosporins. If neither penicillin nor a cephalosporin can be used, vancomycin can be given intravenously in a dose of 0.5 g every 6 hours for 4 weeks, with or without streptomycin for the first 2 weeks.

In these regimens streptomycin should be discontinued if vestibular toxic effects occur and should not be used if renal insufficiency is present.

STREPTOCOCCI RESISTANT TO 0.2 µg/ml PENICILLIN G. Streptococci resistant to 0.2 µg/ml penicillin G are classified as relatively resistant to penicillin and include all enterococci and 5% to 10% of viridans streptococci. Penicillin or ampicillin alone is inadequate therapy for enterococcal endocarditis. In vitro, streptomycin combined with penicillin provides a more rapid and complete bactericidal effect than penicillin alone against the majority of strains of enterococci. Some strains of enterococci do not demonstrate this in vitro effect with penicillin and streptomycin but do with penicillin and gentamicin.

The therapy recommended for enterococcal endocarditis is aqueous penicillin G, 20 million units daily intravenously by continuous drip, plus streptomycin, 0.5 g every 12 hours intramuscularly, or gentamicin, 1 mg/kg intramuscularly or intravenously every 8 hours for 4 to 6 weeks. Four weeks of therapy are probably adequate for most cases. The peak serum antibacterial activity should be determined, and if a 1:8 dilution does not kill the infecting enterococcus, the dose of penicillin should be doubled. It seems reasonable to use penicillin plus gentamicin until in vitro tests are completed. If the enterococcus is inhibited by 2000 µg/ml streptomycin, streptomycin can be used. Otherwise the gentamicin should be continued.

In patients with renal insufficiency, serum levels of streptomycin or gentamicin should be measured and the doses adjusted to maintain streptomycin peak levels of 10 to 15 µg/ml and gentamicin peaks of 3 to 5 µg/ml.

Enterococci are highly resistant to cephalosporins in vitro, and the clinical results with these agents have been unsatisfactory. No alternative drug has been extensively tested for efficacy in the treatment of enterococcal endocarditis. Therefore an effort should be made to use penicillin in most patients who have a history of delayed skin rash to penicillin or in those who have minor reactions during the course of therapy.

Patients with a history of anaphylaxis to penicillin or those who have severe reactions can be treated with vancomycin in a dose of 0.5 g intravenously every 6 hours for 4 to 6 weeks. Streptomycin or gentamicin should be included in the therapeutic program.

Endocarditis caused by nonenterococcal streptococci that are relatively resistant, that is, not inhibited by 0.2 µg/ml penicillin G in vitro, should be managed with 20 million units penicillin intravenously daily for 4 weeks and 0.5 g streptomycin intramuscularly every 12 hours for 2 to 4 weeks. Vancomycin should be substituted for penicillin in penicillin-allergic patients. However, with these nonenterococcal, relatively penicillin-resistant streptococci, a cephalosporin can often be used in penicillin-allergic patients, provided that adequate serum bactericidal activity is achieved.

Staphylococcal endocarditis. S. aureus endocarditis should be suspected when endocarditis occurs in narcotic addicts, after the insertion of prosthetic heart valves, or in the presence of the clinical syndrome of acute endocarditis. Only penicillinase-resistant penicillins (nafcillin, methicillin, or oxacillin) or cephalosporins may be relied on in the initial treatment of staphylococcal endocarditis. Therapy must be given for 4 to 6 weeks. The doses are 2 g of nafcillin, methicillin, oxacillin, or cephalothin intravenously every 4 hours or 1 to 2 g of cefazolin intramuscularly or intravenously every 6 hours. Only when staphylococci are inhibited by 0.1 µg/ml can penicillin G be used and then only in high doses (for example, 20 million units daily). If a penicillin or a cephalosporin cannot be used, vancomycin, 0.5 g intravenously every 6 hours, is the drug of choice.

Penicillins and gentamicin have been shown in vitro and in animal studies to result in a more rapid bactericidal effect against S. aureus than penicillins alone, and some investigators have recommended the use of the combination in endocarditis in humans. At present there is no evidence that the combination has any advantage over penicillin or a cephalosporin alone. Rifampin, 300 mg orally every 12 hours, has been added to penicillin, cephalosporin, or vancomycin in some reported cases when the clinical response was inadequate. The addition of rifampin resulted in an increase in serum bactericidal activity and a better clinical response in most reports.

Resistance of *S. aureus* to methicillin has been noted elsewhere in the world, but it is not a major problem in the United States. Methicillin-resistant strains of *S. aureus* are resistant to other penicillinase-resistant penicillins and to the cephalosporins as well. Endocarditis caused by methicillin-resistant *S. aureus* requires vancomycin therapy.

S. epidermidis endocarditis, which is often associated with prosthetic valves, should initially be treated with vancomycin. These organisms are often resistant to penicillin G and occasionally to methicillin. Endocarditis caused by methicillin-resistant strains of *S. epidermidis* requires therapy with vancomycin, since it may not respond well to therapy with cephalosporins despite apparent in vitro susceptibility. Many authorities are now adding rifampin (with or without gentamicin) to the vancomycin because of bad results with single-agent therapy. Endocarditis caused by methicillin-sensitive strains can be treated with a penicillinase-resistant penicillin with or without rifampin or gentamicin. If the organism is sensitive to penicillin G, this agent is probably the drug of choice.

Endocarditis caused by other organisms. Pneumococcal, gonococcal, and meningococcal endocarditis should be treated with 20 million units of penicillin G intravenously daily for 4 weeks.

The therapy for endocarditis caused by other organisms (including gram-negative bacilli) must consist of bactericidal antimicrobials, preferably a penicillin or cephalosporin with or without an aminoglycoside, and must be given in sufficient doses to achieve peak concentrations in the serum that are bactericidal for the infecting organism at a 1:8 dilution. If the organism is resistant to all penicillins and cephalosporins, vancomycin with (or without) an aminoglycoside should be used if in vitro studies indicate susceptibility. If the organism is resistant to penicillins, cephalosporins, and vancomycin, therapy will probably be unsuccessful. Under these circumstances treatment should be initiated with the bactericidal drug grouping that demonstrates the best activity in vitro; if the patient does not respond or if relapse occurs after 4 to 6 weeks of therapy, antimicrobial therapy plus cardiac surgery to remove the vegetation and replace the valve will probably be necessary.

Results of therapy of fungal endocarditis have been disappointing. Amphotericin B, the only fungicidal agent available for parenteral use, is very toxic and difficult to use. Another agent, flucytosine, is fungistatic but may increase the fungicidal activity of amphotericin B in vitro. Amphotericin B is generally administered intravenously in a dose of 0.5 mg/kg/day; flucytosine is given orally in a dose of 75 to 150 mg/kg/day. Although some cures have been reported with antifungal therapy alone, surgical intervention with valve replacement is usually necessary to achieve a cure.

Endocarditis with sterile blood cultures. Most experts favor treating patients with endocarditis and sterile blood cultures as they would patients with enterococcal endocarditis. If there is no clinical response to the penicillin-plus-aminoglycoside regimen within 3 to 5 days, the dose of penicillin should be doubled to 40 million units daily. When the course is acute and fulminant, antistaphylococcal therapy with a penicillinase-resistant penicillin or cephalosporin should be added.

Endocarditis on intracardiac prostheses or sutures. Patients with endocarditis on prostheses or sutures probably require longer courses of therapy than patients without intravascular foreign bodies. Treatment is usually continued for at least 6 weeks for streptococci inhibited by 0.2 μg/ml of penicillin and 8 weeks for all other microorganisms. With the exception of streptococcal endocarditis, results of medical therapy for prosthetic valve endocarditis have been poor. Therefore, in patients with endocarditis caused by organisms other than streptococci, valve replacement should be carefully considered.

Surgery in the management of endocarditis. When appropriate microbicidal therapy is unavailable and positive blood cultures continue during therapy or relapse occurs after therapy is discontinued, removal of the vegetation and replacement of the valve with a prosthesis should be considered. The surgical repair should ideally be performed after several days or more of the best available antimicrobial therapy. The therapy should then be continued for 2 weeks or longer in the case of organisms that tend to produce metastatic foci. Immediate valve replacement (even after only hours of therapy) is essential if congestive heart failure develops as a result of severe valvular insufficiency.

Current evidence indicates that to achieve cure in fungal endocarditis, surgical intervention is almost always required in addition to treatment with antifungal agents.

Patients with prosthetic valve endocarditis often require valve replacement for cure. The indications for valve replacement are valve dysfunction, heart failure, continuation of embolization, organisms resistant to bactericidal antimicrobials, fungal infection, and continuing bacteremia during or relapses after an appropriate course of therapy. Surgery is usually required in early prosthetic valve endocarditis both because of the microorganisms involved and because of valve dysfunction. Surgery is often required in nonstreptococcal prosthetic valve endocarditis.

Response to therapy. Defervescence and an increased sense of well-being usually occur within several days to a week after the initiation of appropriate antimicrobial therapy. Lack of response of fever may be associated with myocardial or metastatic abscess formation (especially in *S. aureus* endocarditis), but the most common cause of persistent or recurrent fever during therapy with an appropriate drug regimen is a reaction to the antimicrobial agents. Superinfection of a heart valve, although rare, is especially likely when intravascular plastic catheters are used for infusions.

Heart failure may occur at any time during or after therapy and is a poor prognostic sign. Heart failure is especially likely to develop in patients with aortic insufficiency, and these patients have a high mortality. In addition to valvular insufficiency, vegetations (especially in fungal endocarditis) may become large enough to cause obstruction of the valvular orifice.

The vast majority of relapses can be detected with blood cultures obtained 1, 2, and 4 weeks after discontinuation of therapy.

PROGNOSIS. The factors that tend to make the prognosis relatively bad are (1) nonstreptococcal disease, (2) development of heart failure, (3) aortic valve involvement, (4) prosthetic valve, and (5) old age. The cure rate in streptococcal endocarditis is about 90%. Most failures are due not to uncontrolled infection but to death from heart failure, an embolus, rupture of a mycotic aneurysm, or renal failure. The cure rate in nonaddicts with *S. aureus* endocarditis is about 50%, with most deaths caused by early overwhelming infection or heart failure. The cure rate in addicts with *S. aureus* endocarditis is much higher. Results in endocarditis caused by fungi and gram-negative bacilli have been poor. Early cardiac surgery for heart failure or for cases refractory to antimicrobial therapy should improve these results.

PREVENTION. An apparent portal of entry for the infecting organism can be demonstrated in only a minority of patients with infective endocarditis. However, it seems clear that the oropharynx serves as the site of origin for most patients, with the genitourinary tract next. It is obvious that oral hygiene should be optimal in patients with underlying cardiac lesions that predipose them to endocarditis, especially those who are to have prosthetic cardiac valves implanted.

Although the risk of endocarditis is small and there is no proof of efficacy, antimicrobial prophylaxis is recommended for patients with predisposing cardiac lesions who are to undergo procedures known to result in transient bacteremia. The cardiac conditions for which prophylaxis is recommended are valvular or congenital heart disease (except for uncomplicated atrial septal defect), intracardiac prostheses, and a previous episode of infective endocarditis. The antimicrobial therapy is directed at the bacteria that lodge at an endocardial site and therefore is analogous to the treatment of very early endocarditis.

Dental manipulations and other procedures in the mouth, nose, or throat. Prophylaxis is directed against viridans streptococci and is recommended for all procedures likely to cause gingival bleeding and for tonsillectomy and bronchoscopy. The regimens recommended by the American Heart Association are (1) aqueous penicillin G, 1 million units. mixed with procaine penicillin, 600,000 units, plus streptomycin, 1 g, both intramuscularly 30 minutes before the procedure; (2) aqueous penicillin G, 1 million units, mixed with procaine penicillin, 600,000 units, intramuscularly 30 minutes before the procedure; (3) vancomycin, 1 g intravenously over a 30- to 60-minute period starting 30 to 60 minutes before the procedure; (4) penicillin V, 2 g orally 30 minutes before the procedure; or (5) erythromycin, 1 g orally 1½ hours before the procedure. Regimens 1, 2, and 4 are followed by penicillin V, 0.5 g orally every 6 hours for eight doses. Regimens 3 and 5 are followed by erythromycin, 500 mg every 6 hours for eight doses. The penicillin-plus-streptomycin regimen is preferred for patients with prosthetic heart valves, and vancomycin or erythromycin should be used in patients who are hypersensitive to penicillin. The erythromycin regimen is probably the least effective. It is likely that only the first 24 hours of each regimen are necessary for effective prophylaxis.

Genitourinary and gastrointestinal tract procedures or surgery. Prophylaxis is directed against enterococci and is recommended for procedures that cause significant trauma to the genitourinary or gastrointestinal tracts (for example, urethral catheterization, prostatic surgery, and colonic or gallbladder surgery). Regimens recommended by the American Heart Association are (1) ampicillin, 1 g intramuscularly or intravenously, plus gentamicin, 1.5 mg/kg intramuscularly or intravenously, or streptomycin, 1 g intramuscularly, 30 minutes before the procedure, and then two additional doses every 8 hours for ampicillin plus gentamicin or every 12 hours for ampicillin plus streptomycin; or (2) in patients who are hypersensitive to penicillin, vancomycin, 1 g intravenously over a 30- to 60-minute period starting 30 to 60 minutes before the procedure, plus streptomycin, 1 g intramuscularly 30 to 60 minutes before the procedure.

BIBLIOGRAPHY

A.H.A. Committee Report: Prevention of bacterial endocarditis, Circulation **56**:139A, 1977.

Garvey, G.J., and Neu, H.C.: Infective endocarditis—an evolving disease: a review of endocarditis at the Columbia-Presbyterian Medical Center, Medicine **57**:105, 1978.

Karchmer, A.W., and others: Late prosthetic valve endocarditis: clinical features influencing therapy, Am. J. Med. **64**:199, 1978.

Kaye, D.: Infective endocarditis, Baltimore, 1976, University Park Press.

Kaye, D.: Antibiotic treatment of streptococcal endocarditis, Am. J. Med. **69**:650, 1980.

Reisberg, B.E.: Infective endocarditis in the narcotic addict, Prog. Cardiovasc. Dis. **22**:193, 1979.

Richardson, J.V., and others: Treatment of infective endocarditis: a 10-year comparative analysis, Circulation **58**:589, 1978.

Sande, M.A., and Scheld. W.M.: Combination antibiotic therapy of bacterial endocarditis, Ann. Intern. Med. **92**:390, 1980.

Tompsett, R., and Berman, W.: Enterococcal endocarditis: duration and mode of treatment, Trans. Am. Clin. Climatol. Assoc. **89**:49, 1977.

Bacterial infections of the central nervous system
Merle A. Sande and W. Michael Scheld

BACTERIAL MENINGITIS

DEFINITION AND PATHOLOGY. Bacterial meningitis is an infection involving the leptomeninges, the fine lining structures of the brain and spinal cord. These include the arachnoid, the pia mater, and the space between filled with the cerebrospinal fluid (CSF). The inflammatory process produces a purulent exudate that usually extends throughout the subarachnoid space initially involving the basal cisterns, around the cerebellum, then over the cerebral hemispheres. Ventriculitis is frequently present. There is usually no direct bacterial invasion of brain tissue or abscess formation, but leukocytes are found occasionally in the outer cortical layers. Associated cortical thrombophlebitis and cortical edema with herniation and cranial nerve damage may occur.

ETIOLOGY AND PATHOGENESIS. The bacteria responsible for meningitis all possess important virulence factors that provide a selective advantage in gaining access to and surviving within the CSF. The exact mechanisms by which meningitis is produced are obscure, however. The disease appears to develop when several unique conditions occur simultaneously. These include (1) recent acquisition of or colonization with an encapsulated organism to which the patient lacks bactericidal antibody, (2) dissemination of the bacteria into the bloodstream, usually from the nasopharynx or lungs, and (3) penetration into the subarachnoid space through an area of damage in the blood-brain barrier. Invasion of the CSF may also occur directly from the nasopharynx through the cribriform plate or as a result of extension from suppurative sinusitis or mastoiditis. In the CSF the organisms must initially withstand phagocytosis, multiply, and induce an inflammatory response. Meningitis is rarely caused by bacteria when the host possesses specific bactericidal or opsonizing antibody. Thus to a great extent the age of the patient dictates the likely infecting pathogen (Table 40-2). Neonates have protective maternal antibodies against most common pathogens but may be traumatized and heavily colonized during normal delivery with pathogenic group B streptococci, *Escherichia coli,* or other enteric bacilli. For example, 70% of neonates born from mothers vaginally colonized with group B streptococci *(S. agalactiae)* acquire the organism during birth. In instances where meningitis occurred, neither mother nor child had opsonizing antibody to the typical type III capsular polysaccharide, the serotype that usually produces disease. Approximately 75% of *E. coli* strains that produce neonatal meningitis carry the K1 antigen (compared with 36% of strains that invade the bloodstream but do not produce meningitis). The K1 antigen is an acidic polysaccharide (one of more than 100 *E. coli* antigens) and is antigenically related to the capsular polysaccharides of group B. *Neisseria meningitidis* and type III group B streptococci. The exact mechanism by which K1 antigen increases the propensity of these strains to produce meningitis is unknown, but it seems to be related to their ability to colonize the intestinal epithelium of the neonate and produce hematogenous dissemination. This important virulence characteristic has been confirmed in experimental infant animals fed *E. coli* with K1 antigen intragastrically.

The three most common etiologic agents of meningitis after the first month of age are *Haemophilus influenzae* (type B), *N. meningitidis,* and *S. pneumoniae.* All three possess polysaccharide capsules that protect them from phagocytosis. All are known to colonize the nasopharynx and produce disease in patients not possessing anticapsular antibody. The incidence of meningitis produced by *H. influenzae* falls dramatically after the first 6 years of life. This correlates with the appearance of antibody primarily directed against polyribose ribitol phosphate (PRP), the unique ribitol phosphate component of the type B polysaccharide capsule. These antibodies promote complement-mediated phagocytosis and bacteriolysis and are protective against type B disease in experimental animals and humans. The antibodies result from exposure not only to *H. influenzae* but also to other bacteria containing immunologically cross-reactive surface antigens. Other, less well-recognized protective antibodies that are directed against the so-called outer membrane (OM) antigens of *H. influenzae* have also been described.

The meningococcus produces meningitis in either epidemics or sporadic outbreaks, predominantly in children and young adults. The incidence of disease falls dramatically after the age of 40. The incidence is inversely proportional to the percentage of persons with bactericidal antibody against the various capsular polysaccharides (see discussion of "Meningococcal infections" in Chapter 46).

The pneumococcus produces meningitis throughout life, a characteristic that may be related to the large num-

Table 40-2. Approximate incidence, by age, of organisms causing bacterial meningitis

Organism	Age (%)		
	≤1 mo	1 mo-6 yr	≥6 yr
Haemophilus influenzae	0-1	40-50	5
Streptococcus pneumoniae	1-3	15-20	40-50
Neisseria meningitidis	0-1	25-30	30-40
S. agalactiae (group B)	30-40	1-4	1-5
Escherichia coli (and other gram-negative bacilli)	50-60	1-2	10
Listeria monocytogenes	2-10	1-2	5
Staphylococci	3-5	1-2	5-10
Others plus unidentified	10	10	10

ber (84) of antigenically distinct capsular polysaccharide types and the prevalence of this organism as a respiratory tract pathogen. Specific opsonizing antibody develops following infection with each type and rarely after infection from selected cross-reacting types.

Listeria monocytogenes produces meningitis predominantly in patients with impaired cellular immunity such as very young patients (neonates), patients with Hodgkin's disease, or individuals receiving corticosteroids or other immunosuppressive therapy. *Staphylococcus aureus* occasionally produces a meningitis-cerebritis syndrome associated with an overwhelming staphylococcal infection including endocarditis. Staphylococci and various gram-negative bacilli infect the meninges following accidental or neurosurgical traumatic disruption of the subarachnoid space. *S. epidermidis* is the most common cause of meningitis complicating the insertion of intracranial foreign bodies (such as CSF shunts). Anaerobic bacteria can be isolated from CSF following rupture of a brain abscess into the ventricles or the subarachnoid space. "Primary" anaerobic organism meningitis is quite rare.

EPIDEMIOLOGY. The setting in which meningitis occurs may give significant clues as to the causative agent. Group B streptococcal and *E. coli* septicemia and meningitis are frequently associated with prematurity or follow maternal complications at delivery such as premature rupture of the membranes. The meningococcus has been a common cause of meningitis epidemics in military recruit camps where crowding and introduction of new serogroups from widely disseminated regions occur. These outbreaks frequently follow spring epidemics of adenovirus infections and are preceded by a marked increase in the meningococcal carrier state. Susceptible close family contacts, especially sleeping partners of patients with either meningococcal or *H. influenzae* meningitis, are at increased risk of disease. *H. influenzae* meningitis also is frequently preceded by or accompanies an upper respiratory tract infection, especially otitis media or acute sinusitis.

Pneumococcal meningitis is frequently associated with acute otitis media and mastoiditis (30%), pneumonia (25%), and occasionally acute sinusitis. Significant head injury with or without skull fracture precedes pneumococcal meningitis in about 10% of the cases. The pneumococcus accounts for the vast majority of meningitis associated with a CSF leak (either otorrhea or rhinorrhea) and is by far the most common cause of recurrent episodes of meningitis. Meningitis occurring in the presence of immunodeficiency states (reduced levels of immunoglobulins), sickle cell disease, asplenism, or other conditions, including alcoholism, that reduce bacterial clearance from the bloodstream is usually caused by the pneumococcus. Meningococcal meningitis has been reported in complement deficiency states, especially when the terminal components of the complement cascade are absent.

CLINICAL MANIFESTATIONS. Early recognition of meningitis and prompt specific therapy are vital for survival from this disease. Thus it is critical to appreciate the setting and initial manifestations. The classic presentation of bacterial meningitis consists of the triad of fever, headache, and a stiff neck, usually in the setting of a preceding upper respiratory tract infection (rhinitis, sinusitis, otitis, or mastoiditis) and occasionally accompanied by pneumonia. Patients may have nausea and vomiting, especially when increased intracranial pressure is present. Generalized weakness and photophobia are common. With meningococcal disease severe myalgias, backache, and painful extremities (hyperalgesia) may occur. The level of consciousness is nearly always altered. Patients may be initially lethargic but can progress rapidly to coma. Seizures (either generalized or focal) accompany acute bacterial meningitis in 20% to 30% of the patients and cranial nerve palsies in 10% to 20%. The more rapid the onset of disease, the worse the prognosis. In approximately 10% of the patients symptoms leading to coma develop in less than 24 hours, and these patients have a mortality rate of at least 50%. Most patients have a more insidious onset, with symptoms developing over several days to a week. They have a mortality rate of less than 25%. Unfortunately, classic signs and symptoms are frequently obscure in neonates and the elderly. These patients may have only fever with irritability, lassitude, or confusion. Poor feeding in infants or an abrupt change in personality in the elderly may be the only manifestation of disease. In impaired hosts the presence of fever with confusion should suggest meningitis.

In most patients the physical examination reveals evidence of meningeal irritation (pain on flexion of the neck). A stiff neck may be absent very early in the disease, in neonates, or in obtunded elderly patients. Bulging fontanelles in infants are helpful diagnostically when present but are usually a late finding.

Cranial nerve abnormalities, especially of the third, fourth, sixth, and seventh cranial nerves, and focal cerebral signs including hemiparesis, dysphasia, and visual field abnormalities are not unusual early manifestations, especially in pneumococcal meningitis. Evidence of cerebral edema or increased intracranial pressure may accompany severe disease and should be promptly recognized. This may be manifested by third nerve dysfunction, corticospinal tract signs (abnormal reflexes), coma, hypertension, bradycardia, or abnormal respiration. Papilledema is unusual in bacterial meningitis, and when it is present, a mass lesion such as a brain abscess or epidural or subdural hematoma or abscess should be excluded before lumbar puncture.

The presence of rash (maculopapules, petechiae, or purpura) in a patient with meningeal signs usually indicates meningococcal sepsis and meningitis and occurs in approximately 50% of such cases. This clinical presentation also rarely results from echovirus (especially type 9) infection, in asplenic patients with pneumococcal sepsis, and in meningitis in patients with endocarditis caused by *S. aureus*.

LABORATORY FINDINGS. Immediate CSF examination is important when meningitis is suspected. When the patient is severely ill, treatment should be initiated before or while lumbar puncture is being performed. The opening pressure is almost always elevated (average 200 to 300 mm H_2O), although extremely high pressures (such as 600 mm H_2O) may be seen, as with cerebral edema. A low pressure may indicate a CSF block.

CSF pleocytosis is the hallmark of bacterial meningitis, and leukocyte counts usually range from 100 to 10,000/mm^3 with an average of 500 to 2000. Very high counts (greater than 50,000/mm^3) should alert the physician to the possibility of a ruptured intracranial abscess. Polymorphonuclear leukocytes predominate early in the disease (usually greater than 80%) with a gradual shift to mononuclear forms following successful therapy. Early in overwhelming bacterial meningitis, CSF white blood cell counts may be very low, even though the organism can be found on Gram stain of the CSF and cultures are positive.

CSF protein concentrations are elevated in over 90% of the cases, usually above 100 mg/dl. The CSF glucose is classically depressed to less than 40 mg/dl or less than 40% of simultaneous blood sugar (if the latter is less than 250 mg/dl). Hypoglycorrhachia is not diagnostic of bacterial infection, since a low CSF glucose may also be found in some cases of lymphocytic choriomeningitis virus infection, sarcoidosis, tuberculosis, fungal infection, meningeal carcinoma, or subarachnoid hemorrhage. In addition, patients with bacterial meningitis may have CSF glucose concentrations in the normal range.

The Gram stain of a spun specimen of CSF reveals the organism in up to 80% of the cases. However, errors in interpretation by inexperienced observers are common, since overdecolorized pneumococci may look like *H. influenzae*, *H. influenzae* may demonstrate bipolar staining and be confused with pneumococci, stain artifact may resemble gram-positive cocci, and intracellular meningococci may be confused with nuclear debris. Concomitant use of the quellung reaction (with omnisera) conclusively identifies the pneumococcus. Gram stains are positive in 60% of partially treated cases. When Gram stains are negative, cryptococci and mycobacteria should always be sought with india ink preparations and acid-fast (Ziehl-Neelsen) stains of CSF sediment. Cultures are positive in 70% to 90% of the cases of bacterial meningitis but may be negative if the patient has received prior antibiotic therapy. Cultures almost always remain positive in partially treated cases of *H. influenzae* meningitis.

New rapid techniques have recently become available to detect bacterial antigens in CSF. The most widely used is the counter immunoelectrophoresis (CIE) technique, which is positive in up to 80% of the cases of type B *H. influenzae*, meningococcal, or pneumococcal meningitis. Detection of CSF endotoxin by the Limulus lysate assay is possible in meningitis caused by gram-negative bacteria (including *H. influenzae* and the meningococcus). These methods are particularly helpful in cases in which the Gram stain is negative. Cryptococcal antigen detection in CSF is a sensitive and specific method for diagnosing cryptococcal meningitis. Elevated CSF lactate levels (greater than 35 mg/dl) may be of value in distinguishing purulent bacterial meningitis from aseptic meningitis.

Blood cultures should always be obtained, since they may reveal the infecting organism when CSF cultures are negative. Blood cultures are positive in the majority of patients with *H. influenzae* meningitis, about half of those with pneumococcal meningitis, and 40% of those with meningococcal meningitis. The serum sodium concentration should be measured because inappropriate ADH secretion may accompany meningitis and result in lethargy and seizures unless water is restricted during management. Clotting parameters may be abnormal, especially in meningococcal infection, in which disseminated intravascular coagulation may be a fatal complication. A peripheral leukocytosis with a shift to the left (early band forms) is common in bacterial meningitis and may be of value in distinguishing it from viral infections.

Roentgenographic evaluation of the chest, skull, mastoid processes, and sinuses is indicated early in the hospital course to elicit potentially inapparent areas of infection or fractures that may require medical or surgical attention. When evidence of elevated intracranial pressure is suspected during physical examination (and certainly if papilledema is present), a computed tomographic (CT) scan is necessary to exclude a mass lesion, that is, a brain abscess or subdural empyema.

DIAGNOSIS. The diagnosis of bacterial meningitis should be suspected in every patient with fever, alteration in mental status (lethargy, confusion, coma), headache, and a stiff neck. Initial evaluation should proceed immediately. If examination reveals no papilledema or focal neurologic signs that support the diagnosis of a mass lesion or impending herniation, a lumbar puncture should be performed. Antibiotic therapy should be initiated immediately after the lumbar puncture if the disease is acute (less than 24 hours' duration) or severe or if suspicion of meningitis is high. A meticulous examination of the CSF will only waste precious minutes. Therapy can be altered following such an examination.

If a mass is suspected, therapy should be initiated and a CT scan or other available procedures should be performed. In the vast majority of cases of bacterial meningitis no evidence for a mass lesion will be present and lumbar puncture can then be performed safely.

If the presentation is subacute, careful evaluation of the CSF is indicated. Therapy should be instituted if any of the following are present: (1) a CSF pleocytosis with a predominance of polymorphonuclear leukocytes; (2) positive Gram stain; (3) hypoglycorrhachia (less than 40% of the blood sugar level without another obvious explanation); or (4) a positive CIE or limulus lysate assay.

Although the diagnosis is usually readily apparent in the typical case, it may be less obvious in elderly obtunded patients, confused alcoholics with delirium tremens or hepatic encephalopathy, and irritable neonates or infants that fail to thrive. In these cases there must be a low threshold for examination of the CSF.

DIFFERENTIAL DIAGNOSIS. Other conditions that can mimic bacterial meningitis include aseptic meningitis, parameningeal infections, tuberculous meningitis, fungal meningitis, and amebic meningitis.

Aseptic meningitis. Aseptic meningitis is caused predominantly by the enteroviruses. The presentation is often similar with fever, headache, and meningeal signs. These cases generally occur in clusters in the late summer or early fall, and they are not usually associated with peripheral leukocytosis. Although CSF examination may reveal pleocytosis with a predominance of polymorphonuclear leukocytes early in the disease, the degree of pleocytosis is typically low (fewer than 500 cells/mm^3) and the CSF glucose is normal. Mumps meningitis may be associated with a CSF glucose in the 40 mg/dl range but is usually associated with parotitis, orchitis, or pancreatitis. Other viral causes include lymphocytic choriomeningitis virus, herpes simplex virus, and adenovirus. Leptospirosis may also produce an aseptic meningitis syndrome with the same CSF findings as viral meningitis.

Parameningeal infections. Parameningeal infections may cause CSF pleocytosis and neurologic symptoms including brain abscess, epidural abscess, subdural empyema, and septic venous sinus phlebitis. These conditions should be considered when the neurologic manifestations precede the onset of meningeal signs and symptoms or when obvious suppurative infections are present in the sinuses, mastoid processes, or lungs.

Tuberculous meningitis. Tuberculous meningitis usually produces lymphocytic pleocytosis (generally fewer than 500 cells/mm^3) in the CSF and a subacute to chronic course. However, occasionally it is clinically indistinguishable from acute bacterial meningitis with CSF pleocytosis consisting of predominantly polymorphonuclear leukocytes, hypoglycorrhachia, and a marked elevation in CSF protein. Careful examination of the CSF with Ziehl-Neelsen or fluorochrome stains may reveal the organism in up to 50% of the cases. The disease usually occurs in the course of miliary tuberculosis resulting from rupture of a leptomeningeal granuloma. Tuberculous foci of infection are usually evident elsewhere. This disease should always be considered when CSF pleocytosis is present, CSF glucose is depressed, but Gram stains and cultures for routine bacteria are negative. CSF cultures are positive in 40% to 88% of the cases of tuberculous meningitis.

Fungal meningitis. Fungal meningitis is usually chronic but (like tuberculous disease) may also produce an acute form. *Cryptococcus neoformans* accounts for the vast majority of cases and should be suspected in patients who have an impairment in cellular immune responses (as in Hodgkin's disease or corticosteroid therapy). The CSF typically exhibits a mononuclear pleocytosis with fewer than 400 cells/mm^3, elevated protein, and usually a decreased CSF sugar. India ink preparations are positive in over 50% of the cases, and the yield is increased with multiple examinations and centrifugation of large volumes (for example, 10 to 20 ml) of CSF. Cryptococcal antigens can be detected in CSF or serum in up to 95% of the cases. Coccidioidal meningitis should be considered in patients who have lived in or visited the southwest region of the United States. The diagnosis can be established by culture or detection of coccidioidal antigen (by complement fixation techniques) in CSF. *Candida* species occasionally produce meningitis in patients with disseminated candidiasis. Candidal meningitis may occur in patients receiving hyperalimentation and broad-spectrum antibiotics for prolonged periods of time.

Amebic meningitis. Amebic meningitis is a rare form of disease produced by free-living genera such as *Naegleria* and *Acanthamoeba*. Most patients give a history of swimming or diving in warm, shallow, freshwater lakes where these organisms may reach very high concentrations. They are motile and may be observed on wet mounts of unspun CSF.

Other forms. Other forms of culture-negative meningitis include meningeal carcinomatosis and sarcoidosis, which are often associated with marked hypoglycorrhachia; chemical meningitis from spinal anesthesics, roentgenographic contrast material, or other iatrogenically induced material; Behçet's syndrome, which is associated with recurrent oral and genital ulcers; Mollaret's recurrent meningitis (usually less acute and rare in the United States); systemic lupus erythematosus; and syphilitic meningitis.

MANAGEMENT. Bacterial meningitis constitutes a medical emergency, and antimicrobial treatment should be instituted promptly on recognition or suspicion. Since an etiologic agent is frequently not definitely established, selection must be aimed at the most likely possibilities based on available clinical clues such as age and setting (recruit camp, recent neurosurgical procedure, rash, and so forth). Ideal therapy includes the administration of bactericidal antibiotics in adequate dosages to achieve activity within the CSF. The following is suggested as initial therapy:

1. *Adults with suspected bacterial meningitis or with proven pneumococcal, meningococcal, or listerial meningitis:* Aqueous penicillin G, 12 to 20 million units intravenously each day either by constant infusion or in four to six divided doses. In patients with inflamed meninges this

dose should ensure up to 1 μg/ml of penicillin in the CSF, which is bactericidal for all strains of meningococci and all but the very rare penicillin-resistant strains of *S. pneumoniae*. Large (≥5 million units), rapid, intravenous bolus administration of penicillin should be avoided, since penicillin neurotoxicity (lethargy, multifocal myoclonus, and seizures) may occur when CSF concentrations exceed 10 μg/ml.

2. *Adults with allergy to penicillin and suspected bacterial meningitis or proven pneumococcal, meningococcal, or listerial meningitis:* Chloramphenicol, 4 to 6 g intravenously each day in four divided doses or 25 mg/kg every 6 hours, appears to be a suitable alternative. Other drugs used in penicillin-allergic patients, such as the cephalosporins and clindamycin, should probably not be given because of poor penetration into the CSF.

3. *Children greater than 6 weeks of age with suspected bacterial meningitis or proven H. influenzae meningitis:* A combination of chloramphenicol, 25 mg/kg intravenously every 6 hours, and ampicillin, 50 mg/kg intravenously every 4 hours, is currently recommended until cultural confirmation and in vitro sensitivity testing can be completed. Up to 25% of strains of *H. influenzae* are ampicillin resistant (β-lactamase producing). If the infecting organism (*H. influenzae, S. pneumoniae, N. meningitidis,* or another organism) is found to be sensitive to ampicillin, chloramphenicol should be discontinued. If the infecting organism proves to be an ampicillin-resistant strain of *H. influenzae,* the patient should continue treatment with chloramphenicol alone.

4. *Neonatal meningitis (less than 6 weeks of age):* Therapy must be directed against *E. coli,* group B streptococci, and *L. monocytogenes.* Therefore it should include ampicillin, 100 mg/kg intravenously every 8 hours, and an aminoglycoside, usually gentamicin, 1.5 mg/kg intravenously every 8 hours. At the present time intrathecal administration of aminoglycosides is not recommended in neonatal *E. coli* meningitis, although if follow-up lumbar puncture reveals persistence of infection, it may be necessary.

5. *Gram-negative bacillary meningitis (other than neonatal age group):* A combination of parenteral and intrathecal aminoglycosides is currently recommended. Most experience has been with gentamicin, 1.5 mg/kg every 8 hours intravenously or intramuscularly plus 5 to 10 mg administered intrathecally every 24 hours until cultures are sterile. Some patients with coexisting ventriculitis (up to 80% of the cases in some series) may not respond to this regimen and may require intraventricular administration via an Ommaya or a Rickham reservoir. The final drug selection should be based on in vitro sensitivity testing. Since gentamicin resistance has emerged as a significant problem in some hospitals, amikacin therapy may be necessary. For *Pseudomonas aeruginosa* infections, tobramycin intravenously and intrathecally (same dosages as gentamicin) plus carbenicillin, 500 mg/kg/day in divided doses every 4 hours, is recommended. Parenteral therapy should be continued for at least 3 weeks to prevent relapses. Some of the new third-generation cephalosporins including moxalactam have excellent activity in vitro and are proving effective in meningitis caused by gram-negative bacilli other than *Pseudomonas* species.

6. *S. aureus meningitis-cerebritis syndrome:* Nafcillin or another penicillinase-resistant penicillin should be administered at a dosage of 9 g intravenously each day in four to six divided doses. In patients allergic to penicillin, vancomycin, 1 g every 6 hours intravenously, can be used. In both instances CSF cultures should be monitored carefully, since intrathecal drug administration may be required in some cases. The penicillin, however, should not be given intrathecally.

COURSE. Therapy should be continued at full doses for 10 to 14 days or for 5 to 7 days after the patient becomes afebrile. Repeated CSF examinations are not indicated for the common forms of meningitis unless the patient remains febrile or fever recurs. A single follow-up lumbar puncture obtained 3 to 4 days after therapy is initiated should reveal sterile CSF, a return toward a normal CSF glucose level, and a shift from a predominantly polymorphonuclear leukocyte pleocytosis to mononuclear cells. Prolonged fever may indicate persistent meningitis or subdural effusions, other areas of hidden infection (sinusitis, mastoiditis, empyema, and so on), sinus thrombosis, drug fever, phlebitis, or other nonbacterial diseases listed previously under "Differential diagnosis." Meningococcal disease may be associated with a syndrome of sterile polyserositis (pericarditis, arthritis), resulting in prolonged fever that initially appears 6 to 10 days following the onset of infection.

ADJUVANT THERAPY. Even with aggressive antimicrobial therapy, the mortality from bacterial meningitis remains at approximately 5% to 10% for *H. influenzae* or meningococcal meningitis and 25% for pneumococcal meningitis. Permanent neurologic sequelae may result in up to 50% of the children with *H. influenzae* meningitis. Many deaths that occur early in the course of disease are a result of cerebral edema and temporal lobe or cerebellar herniation. When cerebral edema is suspected, aggressive monitoring of intracranial pressure is indicated, and elevated pressures are treated with hyperventilation, intravenous administration of mannitol, high doses of dexamethasone, or all of these. Anticonvulsant therapy should be used when seizures occur. Patients with meningococcal disease and disseminated intravascular coagulation may require heparin therapy if bleeding occurs.

PREVENTION. Both chemoprophylaxis and immunization have been used to prevent bacterial meningitis. When proven cases of meningococcal meningitis are identified, chemoprophylaxis is recommended for intimate contacts of the index case. This includes close household family members or roommates and persons with oral contact such as kissing or mouth-to-mouth resuscitation. Unless such intimate contact has occurred, prophylaxis is usually not recommended in a population such as schoolroom classmates or hospital personnel. The drug of choice is currently rifampin, 600 mg (two tablets), given orally twice a day for 2 days for adults, two doses of 10 mg/kg/day for 2 days for children over 1 year of age, and 5 mg/kg/day for 2 days for children less than 1 year of age. Although secondary cases of *H. influenzae* meningitis in close contacts have been identified, prophylaxis is not currently routinely recommended, but it is under active investigation.

Immunization is available for meningococcal (serogroups A and C) and pneumococcal (14 serotypes) infections. The use of meningococcal vaccine has markedly reduced the incidence of epidemics in recruit camps and has effectively abated epidemics in Brazil and other areas. Patients entering highly endemic or epidemic areas of disease should be vaccinated. Pneumococcal vaccine is recommended for patients with a high risk of pneumococcal disease, that is, those with recurrent meningitis or CSF rhinorrhea, sickle cell disease, asplenism, or chronic debilitating diseases.

PARAMENINGEAL AND EPIDURAL INFECTIONS

Suppurative infections may be found within the cranial vault under specific clinical conditions in three locations: (1) within the brain parenchyma (brain abscess), (2) between the dura and the arachnoid membrane (subdural empyema), and (3) between the dura and the cranium (epidural or extradural abscess). Each process has unique predisposing conditions, pathogenesis, clinical presentation, and specific therapy. They must be recognized early and distinguished from each other, since each is associated with significant morbidity and mortality.

Brain abscess

DEFINITION. A brain abscess is a focal collection of pus within the parenchyma of the brain. It is approximately one sixth as common as bacterial meningitis.

ETIOLOGY AND PATHOGENESIS. The brain is remarkably resistant to infection, and it is impossible to produce an abscess in experimental animals unless there is associated tissue damage (infarction) or foreign material injected with the microorganism. In humans brain abscesses are produced either by contiguous spread from extracranial suppurative foci or by hematogenous dissemination from distant infections. Most brain abscesses result from extension of infection from chronic middle ear, mastoid, or sinus infections. The bacteria invade either directly through bone, dura mater, and across subdural and subarachnoid spaces to the brain or along venous channels by extension of a septic thrombophlebitis. Otic suppuration accounts for one third to one half of all brain abscesses and produces disease either in the ipsilateral cerebellar hemisphere (especially in children) or in the temporal lobe. Extension from frontal sinusitis may produce disease in the anteroinferior aspect of the frontal lobes. Sphenoidal sinusitis extends to the frontal or temporal lobes and ethmoid sinusitis to the frontal lobes. An exacerbation of otitis, mastoiditis, or sinusitis commonly precedes extension of the infection into the brain. Compound fractures, osteomyelitis of the skull, and penetrating head wounds also can lead to brain abscesses or hematogenous spread. Metastatic infections account for the minority of brain abscesses, and in most cases a primary suppurative focus can be found elsewhere. The most common site is the lung (bronchiectasis, lung abscess, empyema), but dental, tonsillar, and uterine sources have also been implicated. Endocarditis is a rare predisposing cause (2% to 5% of cases). Right-to-left cardiac shunts are a particularly common associated finding in approximately 2% of all patients with cyanotic congenital heart disease. It has been suggested that the polycythemia associated with these congenital defects leads to areas of brain ischemia and necrosis that are more susceptible to hematogenously disseminated bacteria. Shunting of venous-borne bacteria around the pulmonary clearance mechanisms may also deliver a higher inoculum (mostly anaerobic organisms) to the brain. Most hematogenous abscesses are multiple and tend to occur in the white matter, especially distally in areas perfused by the middle cerebral artery.

The organisms most commonly isolated from brain abscesses are anaerobic and microaerophilic streptococci, followed by the various *Bacteroides, Fusobacterium,* and *Veillonella* species. These organisms are particularly common when the abscess is associated with suppurative infections of the lungs. *S. pneumoniae* is rarely found today, although it was common in the preantibiotic era. The anaerobic bacteria (especially *B. fragilis*) may also be found in combination with aerobic Enterobacteriaceae (*E. coli, Klebsiella,* and *Proteus* species), especially with otic infection. *S. aureus* is the isolate most frequently associated with penetrating wounds or endocarditis. Less commonly, *Actinomyces* species or *Nocardia asteroides* is found to be associated with pulmonary infections. Pulmonary infections with *Nocardia* are uniquely prevalent in compromised hosts and patients with pulmonary alveolar proteinosis. Disseminated fungal infections, including aspergillosis, mucormycosis, and candidiasis, may also result in brain abscesses in patients with impaired host resistance.

PATHOLOGY. A brain abscess evolves through several pathologic steps in its maturation. Initially after bacterial implantation there is a localized but poorly demarcated area of cerebritis or encephalitis. This is characterized by local edema, leukocyte infiltration, hyperemia, and parenchymal softening. Within days to several weeks central liquefaction and necrosis occur. Intense fibroblastic activity results in formation of granulation tissue and collagen, leading to an abscess wall that matures over weeks to months into a thick capsule. The abscess may penetrate the white matter and rupture into the ventricles, usually with catastrophic results. Infiltration of the leptomeninges near the abscess with polymorphonuclear leukocytes is common and may lead to a low-grade CSF pleocytosis without abscess rupture.

CLINICAL MANIFESTATIONS. Brain abscess typically shows signs and symptoms of an expanding mass lesion of the brain. Systemic signs of infection are frequently absent. Fever is present in only 50% of the patients and is usually at least 101° F (38.3° C). One third of the patients never have fever. Since specific predisposing conditions are associated with brain abscesses, their presence should immediately suggest the disease. Severe headache is the most common single symptom, occurring in 70% or more of the cases. Therefore, when an unexplained headache occurs in a patient with chronic otitis, sinusitis, mastoiditis, pulmonary infection, prior (even in the distant past) skull fractures or penetrating wound to the skull, or a right-to-left intracardiac shunt, a brain abscess should be considered. Alterations in the level of consciousness (lethargy, irritability, confusion, or coma) occur in most patients. Nausea and vomiting are present in at least half the patients and usually reflect increased intracranial pressure. Papilledema, however, is often a late finding and is reported in only one fourth of patients. Seizures, either generalized or focal, occur in 30%, and evidence of nuchal rigidity is present in 25%.

Focal neurologic signs are found in over 50% of the patients and reflect the location of the abscess. Abscesses in the temporal lobes (approximately 30% of all brain abscesses) are manifested by a selective aphasia (inability to name objects, read, write, or understand the spoken word). In some patients visual field cuts (homonymous upper quadrantic or hemianopic defects) or occasionally weakness of the lower face develops. Cerebellar abscesses account for 15% to 20% of the total and usually run a rapid course. Patients typically have ataxia, nystagmus, incoordination of the extremities, and occasionally an intention tremor. Frontal lobe abscesses (30% of all brain abscesses) may be inapparent with absent neurologic signs except for drowsiness or mild impairment of mental function. Hemiparesis, dysphasia, and seizures may develop during the course. Parietal lobe abscesses are unusual and may result in typical parietal lobe signs (impaired two-point discrimination, altered position sense, and astereognosis with anterior involvement and homonymous hemianopia, visual inattention, and impaired opticokinetic nystagmus with posterior lesions).

LABORATORY FINDINGS. Routine blood tests are of little help in the diagnosis of brain abscess. Lumbar puncture is contraindicated when a brain abscess is suspected, since this procedure may precipitate herniation when intracranial pressure is elevated.

Roentgenograms of the skull, sinuses, mastoid processes, and chest are recommended to locate possible associated suppurative processes. Electroencephalograms locate the lesion in over 50% of the cases, but this test is less sensitive than brain scan or CT scan. Radionuclide brain scan is a very accurate and sensitive technique for detecting brain abscesses 1 cm or larger. This test is positive in up to 95% of the cases. It is especially sensitive in the early cerebritis state when localized alterations in permeability of the blood-brain barrier may be visualized. CT scan is of greatest value when the abscesses are well formed and encapsulated and provides a more detailed view (for example, ventricular size, midline displacement) than the radionuclide scan. If the CT scan is negative, radionuclide scanning should still be performed if a high suspicion for brain abscess exists and symptoms are of short duration.

Carotid arteriography is of value in locating temporal lobe abscesses, and posterior circulation angiography may be necessary for detection of cerebellar abscesses. These invasive techniques are usually performed preoperatively.

DIAGNOSIS. In the presence of a demonstrated source of infection (ears, sinuses, lungs) or right-to-left cardiac shunt, evidence of increased intracranial pressure, focal neurologic signs, and a consistent CT or radionuclide scan, the diagnosis is easily established. When no signs of infection or other predisposing conditions are present, the differential diagnosis of an intracranial mass lesion includes neoplasm, hematoma, focal encephalitis, and subdural hematoma. When both the noninvasive and invasive techniques are inconclusive, surgical exploration must be performed to secure the diagnosis.

MANAGEMENT. Effective treatment usually requires a combination of antimicrobial agents and surgical drainage. The recommended antimicrobial regimen is a combination of penicillin G (20 million units each day intravenously) and chloramphenicol (4 to 6 g each day intravenously). This provides wide antimicrobial coverage for the major proportion of the infecting organisms commonly implicated in brain abscess. However, if *S. aureus* is a serious consideration, as in endocarditis or a penetrating wound, a semisynthetic pencillinase-resistant penicillin such as nafcillin should be added. Metronidazole is active against many anaerobic bacteria (especially *B. fragilis*) and penetrates well into brain tissue. It may have a valuable role in the treatment of brain abscess but should probably be used in combination with penicillin.

The timing of surgical drainage is controversial. If the lesion is treated early with appropriate antibiotics while still in the cerebritis stage or if the abscess is small, surgery may be avoided and the patient should be followed carefully with serial CT scans. Some patients have responded to antibiotics alone. Antibiotics should be given for at least 6 weeks. Surgery is urgent when the level of consciousness deteriorates or neurologic deficits increase during therapy. Drainage may be accomplished with either aspiration or complete excision and evacuation, depending on the site of the lesion. The latter procedure is preferred if possible. Mannitol, corticosteroids, or both can be used to reduce brain edema temporarily before surgery. Regardless of the therapeutic approach, mortality remains high, approaching 30% to 50% with residual neurologic deficits or seizures in 30% of the survivors.

Subdural empyema

DEFINITION AND PATHOLOGY. A subdural empyema is a collection of pus in the space between the dura and the arachnoid membrane. It varies in size from a few milliters to over 200 ml and is restricted to one cerebral hemisphere in three fourths of the cases. The space is limited above by the falx, laterally by the tentorium, and inferiorly by the foramen magnum and the anterior spinal canal. The major collection is usually over the frontal hemisphere; the posterior fossa is rarely involved.

PATHOGENESIS AND ETIOLOGY. Approximately 50% to 80% of cases result from an extension of infection from the frontal or ethmoid sinuses, with an additional 10% to 20% arising from middle ear or mastoid foci of disease. The infection traverses the bone and dura either by direct extension (with osteomyelitis of the frontal bone or an epidural abscess; one or both of these associated infections occur in 50% of subdural empyemas) or by emissary veins directly into the subdural space. Occasionally (5% of cases) the infection may arise hematogenously, usually from the lung. Surgical or accidental trauma may also be complicated by a subdural empyema, and rarely a subdural hematoma becomes secondarily infected.

The bacteria responsible for subdural empyema include the same spectrum that produces brain abscess. Streptococci, either anaerobic or microaerophilic, are found in up to 50% of cases, *S. aureus* in 10% (again usually associated with penetrating wounds), and a wide variety of gram-negative bacilli make up the remainder.

CLINICAL MANIFESTATIONS. Subdural empyemas usually occur in adults, and males predominate. The vast majority of patients have chronic sinusitis or otitis, and subdural empyema typically occurs after a flare-up of the chronic disease (that is, an increase in purulent nasal or otic discharge and pain). The first signs of intracranial infection may be obscured by the underlying process, which produces erythema, swelling, and percussion tenderness. Headache, initially mild and localized, becomes generalized and severe. Fever is usually present and is associated with chills, nausea, and vomiting. Nuchal rigidity may be present. Approximately half of the patients manifest changes in mental status early in the disease and may pass rapidly from lethargy to obtundation or coma within 48 to 72 hours. Focal or generalized seizures occur in 50% of the patients, and neurologic signs including hemiparesis, aphasia, sensory defects, or visual field cuts are common. Death caused by temporal lobe herniation usually occurs within 2 days following the onset of focal neurologic signs in untreated persons. Since increased intracranial pressure occurs relatively late in the disease, papilledema develops in less than 50% of the patients. The neurologic signs and symptoms result either from the mass lesion effect with compression of a single cerebral hemisphere or from the commonly associated thrombosis and phlebitis of the cortical veins, with secondary ischemic necrosis of the superficial layers of the cortex.

DIAGNOSIS. The diagnosis of subdural empyema should be considered in any patient with meningeal signs and focal neurologic deficits that are particularly localized to one cerebral hemisphere, especially if chronic sinusitis is present. A lumbar puncture should not be performed if evidence of increased intracranial presure is present.

Skull roentgenograms show sinusitis, otitis, or mastoiditis in two thirds of the cases and may show a pineal shift. The diagnostic procedure of choice is either the CT scan, which shows a collection of pus, or cerebral arteriography, which demonstrates separation of cerebral vessels from the cranium. In some cases burr holes drilled through the skull are necessary for diagnosis.

MANAGEMENT. A subdural empyema constitutes a true neurosurgical emergency, since death usually occurs rapidly once neurologic findings have appeared. Mannitol, hyperventilation, or corticosteroids may temporarily reduce cerebral edema and allow time to organize a surgical procedure, but immediate surgical drainage is essential.

Antibiotic coverage should include penicillin G in high doses (20 million units daily intravenously) and chloramphenicol (4 to 6 g daily intravenously).

Epidural abscess

CEREBRAL EPIDURAL ABSCESS. A cerebral epidural abscess usually results from extension of infection from osteomyelitis of the skull or chronic infection of the ear or paranasal sinuses. Since the dura forms the intracranial periosteum of the skull, an abscess can develop only by stripping this membrane from bone. Thus an epidural abscess is usually well confined in extent. It is difficult to diagnose, since the features of the more external infection dominate the clinical picture. Patients are not as ill as with subdural empyema but usually have pain. As the abscess enlarges, neurologic signs may develop with evidence of increased intracranial pressure. The pathogenesis and bacteriologic findings are similar to those of subdural empyema, and these conditions may be viewed as a continuum. The diagnosis is best made with a CT scan. When detected, these abscesses should be surgically drained to prevent progression to a subdural empyema. Antibotic therapy includes a combination of penicillin in high doses and chloramphenicol, as for subdural empyema and brain abscess.

SPINAL EPIDURAL ABSCESS

Definition. Within the spinal canal an epidural space

filled with fat and vascular tissue separates the dura from the vertebral bodies. An infection established in this space encounters little resistance to longitudinal spread, and because outward expansion is rigidly limited by the vertebral column, small volumes of pus can produce serious spinal cord compression and necrosis.

Etiology and pathogenesis. The spinal epidural space can be infected via the hematogenous metastatic route from a distant site (most cases), by direct extension from vertebral osteomyelitis (less common except with tuberculosis), or by an invasion from a decubitus or perispinal abscess. Cases have been associated with back surgery, lumbar puncture, and epidural spinal anesthesia. Up to 30% of the patients give a history of antecedent back trauma. Underlying conditions such as diabetes mellitus, intravenous drug use, and rarely pregnancy may predispose a patient to epidural abscesses.

S. aureus accounts for the majority (60% to 80%) of cases. The most common concurrent infections are cutaneous furuncles, boils, ulcers, and wound infections. Respiratory tract and genitourinary tract infections have also been implicated. Streptococci (anaerobic and aerobic) account for approximately 20%, and gram-negative aerobic rods (*E. coli, Pseudomonas, Salmonella, Klebsiella,* and others) cause approximately 10%. Ten percent of cultures are mixed. Tuberculosis is common in highly endemic areas. Various fungi have also rarely been implicated.

Pathology. Most abscesses are localized to the posterior portion of the spinal canal but spread to involve four to six vertebral bodies and occasionally the entire spine. The thoracic spine is most commonly involved (two thirds of cases), followed by lumbar areas (one fourth) and cervical areas (one fifth). Vertebral osteomyelitis is present in less than 20% of acute cases but in more than half of chronic cases.

Clinical manifestations. The clinical presentation of a spinal epidural abscess has been divided into four distinct phases. However, since this disease can present a very acute course, these artificial phases may fuse with each other. Initially there is focal pain or "spinal ache" and percussion tenderness over the involved area. Systemic symptoms (fever) are usually prominent, and spine stiffness and scoliosis may develop. The next phase is characterized by radicular or root pain. Meningeal signs become prominent, hyperalgesia or depressed reflexes may appear in the involved segments, and most patients have headache. The diagnosis may be readily made during this phase. Next, distinct neurologic deficits including motor loss (weakness), sensory loss (below the level of the lesion), or loss of sphincter tone (incontinence, urgency, retention) appear. Pain and nuchal rigidity become more severe. Within hours to several days paralysis that may be severe or even total occurs. If the lesion is not drained and paralysis remains for more than several hours, it is usually permanent.

The course is most rapid when hematogenous dissemination occurs and is accompanied by prominent systemic toxic effects and severe focal pain. When the abscess results from vertebral osteomyelitis, the initial phases may be prolonged (2 to 3 weeks); however, once radicular pain develops, the progression to paralysis is often rapid. Spinal epidural abscess can be mimicked by acute myelitis of various causes (although back pain is not usually as severe), progressive adhesive arachnoiditis, and in the chronic state malignant tumors, especially lymphomas.

Diagnosis. The diagnosis is still best established by myelogram, although CT scanning looks promising. Lumbar puncture should be done with care, and the spinal needle should be inserted either above or below the suspected lesion. The needle is advanced slowly, and repeated aspirations are attempted. If pus is not located, the needle (with the stylet in) is advanced into the subarachnoid space, CSF is obtained, and a myelogram is performed. The CSF is characteristically xanthochromic with few leukocytes. The glucose level is usually normal, but the protein level may be quite elevated (200 to 2000 mg/dl).

Management. Immediate neurosurgical exploration and drainage are required. A semisynthetic penicillinase-resistant penicillin should be administered to cover *S. aureus* and the streptococci. This should be altered or expanded if the Gram stain of the surgical specimen demonstrates other pathogens such as gram-negative bacilli.

Transverse myelitis or myelopathy

Transverse myelitis is a rare clinical syndrome with multiple causes that produces impaired neurologic function below well-delineated spinal cord segments. Pathologically, the lesion is an area of destruction commonly affecting both white and gray matter and may be characterized by demyelination, necrosis, and occasionally an inflammatory reaction. The conditions associated with this unusual disease are numerous and include viral infections, particularly enterovirus, herpes zoster, and Epstein-Barr virus; rabies and B virus myelitis; inflammatory diseases of the meninges (syphilis, pyogenic infections, tuberculosis, parasitic or fungal infections, and chronic adhesive arachnoiditis); and various vascular and nutritional abnormalities. In many cases (acute multiple sclerosis, postinfectious or necrotizing myelitis) the cause is unknown.

The clinical course usually begins with abrupt onset, occasionally in a setting of viral illness or minor trauma. The neurologic findings are variable, as are the characteristics of the CSF. It is imperative to rule out a correctable lesion or one requiring treatment (such as an epidural abscess). Most patients improve with supportive care.

BIBLIOGRAPHY

Baker, A.S., and others: Spinal epidural abscess, N. Engl. J. Med. **293:**463, 1975.

Carpenter, R.R., and Petersdorf, R.G.: The clinical spectrum of bacterial meningitis, Am. J. Med. **33:**262, 1962.

deLouvois, J.: The bacteriology and chemotherapy of brain abscess, J. Antimicrob. Chemother. **4:**395, 1978.

Feignin, R.D., and Dodge, P.R.: Bacterial meningitis: newer concepts of pathophysiology and neurologic sequelae, Pediatr. Clin. North Am. **23:**541, 1976.

Fothergill, L.D., and Wright, J.: Influenza meningitis: the relation of age incidence to the bactericidal power of blood against the causal organism, J. Immunol. **24:**273, 1933.

Handel, S.F., and others: Intracranial epidural abscess, Radiology **111:**117, 1974.

Kaufmann, D.M., and others: Subdural empyema: analysis of 17 recent cases and review of the literature, Medicine **54:**485, 1975.

Levin, S., and others: Bacterial meningitis. In Vinken, P.J., and Bruyn, G.W., editors: Handbook of clinical neurology, vol. 34, Amsterdam, 1979, Elsevier North-Holland Biomedical Press.

Meyer, H.M., and others: Central nervous system syndromes of "viral" etiology: a study of 713 cases, Am. J. Med. **29:**334, 1960.

Rosenblum, M.L., and others: Nonoperative treatment of brain abscesses in selected high-risk patients, J. Neurosurg. **52:**217, 1980.

Sampson, D.S., and Clark. L.: A current review of brain abscess, Am. J. Med. **54:**201, 1973.

Swartz, M.N., and Dodge, P.R.: Bacterial meningitis: a review of selected aspects. I. General clinical features, special problems and unusual meningeal reactions mimicking bacterial meningitis, N. Engl. J. Med. **272:**725, 779, 842, 898, 954, 1003, 1965.

Underman, A.E., Overturf, G.D., and Leedom, J.M.: Bacterial meningitis—1978, D.M. **24:**1, 1978.

Weisberg, L.A.: Computed tomography in the diagnosis of intracranial disease, Ann. Intern. Med. **91:**87, 1979.

Urinary tract infection and perinephric abscess

Donald Kaye

DEFINITIONS. *Significant bacteriuria* describes the numbers of bacteria in voided urine that exceed the numbers usually caused by contamination from the anterior urethra (that is, $\geq 10^5$ bacteria/ml). *Asymptomatic bacteriuria* refers to significant bacteriuria in a patient without symptoms. The term "cystitis" has been used to describe the syndrome involving dysuria, frequency, urgency, and occasionally suprapubic tenderness. However, these symptoms may be related to lower tract inflammation without bacterial infection and can be caused by urethritis (for example, gonorrhea or chlamydial urethritis). Furthermore, the presence of symptoms of lower tract infection without upper tract symptoms by no means excludes upper tract infection, which is also often present.

Acute pyelonephritis describes the clinical syndrome characterized by flank pain and tenderness and fever, often associated with dysuria, urgency, and frequency.

Urinary tract infection may occur de novo or may be a recurrent infection. Recurrences may be either *relapses* or *reinfections*. Relapse of bacteriuria refers to recurrence of bacteriuria with the *same* infecting microorganism that was present before therapy was started. This is due to persistence of the organism in the urinary tract. Reinfection is a recurrence of bacteriuria with a microorganism different from the original infecting bacterium. It is a new infection.

Occasionally reinfection may occur with the same microorganism, which may have persisted in the vagina or feces. This can be mistaken for a relapse.

The term "chronic pyelonephritis" means different things to different authors. To some, chronic pyelonephritis refers to pathologic changes in the kidney caused by infection only. However, identical pathologic alterations are found in several other entities such as chronic urinary tract obstruction, analgesic nephropathy, hypokalemic nephropathy, vascular disease, and uric acid nephropathy.

ETIOLOGY. *Escherichia coli* is the cause of the majority of cases of urinary tract infection. In patients with recurrent infections, structural abnormalities of the urinary tract, or hospital-acquired infections the frequency of infection caused by *Proteus, Klebsiella-Enterobacter, Pseudomonas,* enterococci, and staphylococci increases. Anaerobic organisms rarely cause urinary tract infection.

EPIDEMIOLOGY. Urinary tract infection is rare in men in the absence of instrumentation or structural abnormalities of the urinary tract. There is less than a 0.1% prevalence of infection in men until the age when prostatic disease occurs, at which time it increases to about 4%. The prevalence of bacteriuria is 1% to 3% in young adult women and rises with age (10% to 15% in elderly women). In the very old (men and women), the prevalence of bacteriuria is even higher. Each year bacteriuria clears in about 25% of bacteriuric women, and they are replaced by an equal number who have become infected (often women who have had urinary infection previously). At least 10% to 20% of the female population have a urinary tract infection at some time during their lives.

The prevalence of bacteriuria in pregnancy is 3% to 7% and increases with greater parity and a lower socioeconomic status. About 20% of the patients with bacteriuria early in gestation have acute pyelonephritis later in pregnancy. In contrast, less than 1% of the patients whose urine is uninfected early in gestation have acute infection. Over 75% of the cases of acute pyelonephritis can be prevented by eliminating asymptomatic bacteriuria in the early stages of pregnancy.

PATHOGENESIS. Although some renal infections occur via the hematogenous route (for example, staphylococcal abscesses resulting from staphylococcal bacteremia), classic urinary tract infection rarely if ever occurs this way. The vast majority of urinary tract infection occurs by the ascending route either spontaneously or following catheterization or instrumentation of the urinary tract. The vaginal introitus occasionally becomes colonized by gram-negative enteric bacilli, and this predisposes the woman to infection. The proximity of the vagina to the rectum and the short urethra of women undoubtedly increase the susceptibility of women to infection and help explain their much greater frequency of infection.

Obstruction, incomplete emptying of the bladder, and calculi have all been associated with infection. Vesicoureteral reflux tends to spread infection from the bladder to the kidney.

Certain virulence factors have been identified in bacteria (such as pili on *Proteus mirabilis* and *E. coli* and K antigen on *E. coli*).

CLINICAL MANIFESTATIONS. Most patients with either lower or upper urinary tract infection are asymptomatic. The symptoms of lower tract infection when present are dysuria, frequency, and urgency; fever is usually absent. However, up to 50% of the patients with these symptoms do not have significant bacteriuria. Some of these episodes (up to one half) are associated with low titers of Enterobacteriaceae (for example, 10^3/ml) in bladder urine. Others are caused by urethritis from trauma, gonorrhea, or *Chlaymdia*.

Symptoms of upper tract infection are flank pain, flank tenderness, and fever, which are often associated with lower tract symptoms.

DIAGNOSIS. Pyuria is usually present in symptomatic urinary infection but is often absent with asymptomatic bacteriuria. White cell casts in the urine indicate upper tract involvement. Many patients without infection have pyuria owing to other processes. Proteinuria is common in infection, and hematuria may occur.

Blood cultures are occasionally positive in patients with acute pyelonephritis. The most definitive diagnosis of urinary tract infection is based on finding $\geq 10^5$ bacteria/ml urine on a culture of a clean-catch, midstream urine specimen. One positive culture is adequate in the presence of symptoms, but two confirmatory cultures are necessary in asymptomatic patients. One positive culture gives only an 80% probability of infection in an asymptomatic patient; two positive cultures raise the probability to 95%. Visualization of more than one organism per 400 × microscopic field in a midstream, Gram-stained, uncentrifuged urine specimen correlates highly with a titer of $\geq 10^5$ bacteria/ml. A titer of $\geq 10^5$ bacteria/ml of catheterized urine or any growth from a suprapubic aspirate of urine is highly suggestive of infection. Cultures containing gram-negative bacilli in titers of 10^4 to 10^5/ml should be repeated. Gram-positive cocci do not grow well in urine, and infections with these organisms may often give titers of 10^4 to 10^5/ml.

Many different techniques have been developed to localize the site of infection. Loss of ability to concentrate urine and production of circulating antibody have been found to correlate with upper tract infection. More reliable but invasive methods involve (1) direct catheterization of the ureters with quantitative cultures of urine or (2) washout of the bladder with a solution containing antibiotic and enzymes to sterilize the bladder, and then immediate collection and quantitative culture of newly formed urine. (Presumably if the bacteria are found, they come from the ureters.)

Recently it has been determined that bacteria in urine of renal origin are coated with antibody. Thus the antibody-coated bacteria (ACB) test has been developed in which fluorescein-conjugated antihuman globulin added to bacteriuric urine is examined under a fluorescent microscope. Fluorescence indicates upper tract infection. False positive results may be observed in men with a prostatic focus of infection, and false negative results may occur in very early upper tract infection.

Patients at relatively high risk of urologic abnormalities (especially obstruction) should have an intravenous pyelogram and a postevacuation view of the bladder to evaluate for residual urine. This includes children, males of any age, patients who relapse after appropriate therapy, and those with bacteremia. It is unnecessary to obtain roentgenographic studies on adult women with their first urinary tract infection. After three or four reinfections evaluation is indicated.

Vesicoureteral reflux is particularly important in preschool-age children and predisposes them to renal scarring. Therefore all preschool children with proven urinary tract infection probably should be evaluated with a voiding cystourethrogram to detect reflux. This procedure is rarely indicated in older children and adults.

COURSE. Bacteremia may occur with pyelonephritis (especially in the presence of obstruction) and can be fatal. With or without treatment, symptoms of infection are self-limited and subside. Many infections spontaneously disappear. Recurrence is common in the form of either relapse after treatment (infection never eradicated) or reinfection (new infection). Reinfections are common in women but unusual in men unless catheterized.

In children, especially in the presence of vesicoureteral reflux (which is common in young children), infection can seriously damage the kidneys. In adults, in the absence of obstruction it is questionable if urinary tract infection ever is the major factor leading to renal insufficiency. Similarly, there is no clear-cut relationship between urinary tract infection and hypertension.

There is a definite association between acute pyelonephritis of pregnancy and premature delivery. The rate of prematurity can be as high as 20% to 50%. Prematurity also seems to be increased in patients with asymptomatic bacteriuria. Because of the implications for both mother and fetus, screening for and treatment of bacteriuria at the first prenatal visit seem justified. Treatment of bacteriuria during pregnancy has little effect on the long-term course of the mother.

MANAGEMENT. Since the prognosis of urinary tract infection in nonpregnant adult women seems to be quite good and reinfection is common, therapy probably makes little contribution to the patient's well-being other than eradicating symptoms. Urinary tract infection is very common in the elderly, and a higher frequency of side effects from chemotherapy would be expected in the older age group because of preexisting renal, auditory, and other diseases. Considering the usual absence of progressive renal impairment, the large numbers of patients involved, and the fact that intensive antimicrobial therapy may lead to an unwarranted financial burden and the danger of drug toxicity, such treatment may do more harm than good in elderly patients.

In contrast, bacteriuria in preschool-age children with vesicoureteral reflux can result in stunted growth of the kidney, scar formation, and rarely renal failure. Bacteriuria in pregnancy may also have serious implications. Treatment of children and pregnant women is most likely to be beneficial. Furthermore, it is feasible to treat all of these patients, since the prevalence of bacteriuria is relatively low in these groups.

It is usually necessary to treat symptomatic patients regardless of age, even when infection is likely to recur. Some patients have such frequent symptomatic episodes (either relapses or reinfections) that they are almost chronically incapacitated. In these patients it may be necessary to give prolonged therapy or prophylaxis to prevent recurrent symptoms.

Although there are theoretic reasons for (as well as against) forcing fluids in the management of urinary tract infection, these measures are not indicated in modern antimicrobial therapy. Urinary analgesics such as phenazopyridine hydrochloride (Pyridium) also have little place in the routine management of symptomatic infections. The dysuria of urinary tract infection usually responds rapidly to antibacterial therapy and requires no local analgesia.

Disappearance of bacteriuria is closely correlated with the sensitivity of the microorganism to the concentration of the antimicrobial agent achieved in the urine. Although blood levels of antimicrobials do not seem to be important in the treatment of urinary tract infection, they may be critical in patients with bacteremia.

In patients with renal insufficiency, dosage modifications are necessary for agents that are excreted primarily by the kidneys and cannot be cleared by any other mechanism. In renal failure the kidney may not be able to concentrate an antimicrobial agent in the urine, and difficulty in eradicating bacteriuria may occur.

There are four patterns of response of bacteriuria to antimicrobial therapy: cure, persistence, relapse, and reinfection. Quantitative bacterial counts in urine should decrease within 48 hours after initiation of an antimicrobial agent to which the microorganism is sensitive in vitro. If titers do not decrease within this time *(persistence)*, the therapy being given will be unsuccessful.

Relapse usually occurs within 2 weeks after cessation of chemotherapy and is often associated with renal infection, structural abnormalities of the urinary tract, or chronic bacterial prostatitis. Relapse indicates that the infecting microorganism has persisted in the urinary tract during therapy. However, an apparent relapse can be related to reinfection (new infection) with the same microorganism.

After initial sterilization of the urine, *reinfection* may occur during administration of chemotherapy or at any time thereafter. Reinfection is easy to identify when there is a change in bacterial species. However, there may be reinfection with a different serotype of the same species (usually *E. coli*) or even the same serotype.

Symptomatic urinary tract infection. The majority of patients with symptomatic urinary tract infection are women, usually of childbearing age. The onset of symptoms is frequently related to sexual intercourse. Although no one chemotherapeutic agent is unequivocally the drug of choice, a short-acting oral sulfonamide such as sulfisoxazole (Gantrisin), 1 g four times a day in adults, is preferred by some authorities. Equally effective are ampicillin, amoxicillin, cephalexin, cephradine, nitrofurantoin, tetracycline, and trimethoprim-sulfamethoxazole. The adult doses are ampicillin and amoxicillin, 500 mg to 1 g four times a day; cephalexin or cephradine, 250 to 500 mg four times a day; nitrofurantoin, 100 mg four times a day; tetracycline, 250 to 500 mg four times a day; and trimethoprim-sulfamethoxazole, two tablets twice a day.

In patients with lower tract infection, 1 day of therapy or, in fact, only one dose (for example, 3 g of amoxicillin or four tablets of trimethoprim-sulfamethoxazole) is usually sufficient for cure. It therefore seems reasonable to treat patients with lower tract symptoms only (that is, no fever, flank pain, or flank tenderness) with such short-term therapy.

In contrast to lower tract infection, patients with upper tract infection require at least 2 weeks of treatment. In these patients, urine cultures or microscopic examination of the urine for significant bacteriuria should be obtained after 3 or 4 days of therapy. If bacteriologic response has not occurred, the therapy is changed to one of the alternative drugs on the basis of sensitivity tests.

The antibody-coated bacteria test can help determine if upper tract infection is likely in the patient with only lower tract symptoms. With a positive test, the initial course of therapy should be 2 weeks.

If gram-negative bacillary bacteremia is suspected to be complicating urinary tract infection because of symptoms of high fever, shaking chills, and hypotension, chemotherapy should be directed at the life-threatening bacteremia (see Chapter 47).

A follow-up urine culture should be obtained 1 to 2 weeks after the discontinuance of therapy to detect relapses. In children additional follow-up cultures should be obtained at 6 weeks and 6 months to detect reinfections.

Asymptomatic bacteriuria. Most patients with asymptomatic bacteriuria are women, usually in the older age group. Although cure may result following treatment, relapse and especially reinfection are common. Although all children should be treated, therapy of asymptomatic bacteriuria in adults is by no means mandatory in the absence of obstruction. These patients can be treated providing that a nontoxic antimicrobial agent is used. If the infecting microorganism is resistant to all but toxic agents, treatment should not be instituted in nonobstructed, nonpregnant adults. It is reasonable to use single-dose therapy as a first approach. If the antibody-coated bacteria test is positive, therapy should be extended for 2 weeks.

Relapsing urinary tract infection. A patient who suffers a relapse after single-dose therapy should receive a standard 2-week course. A patient who relapses after a 2-week course most likely has (1) renal involvement, (2) a structural abnormality of the urinary tract (for example, calculi), or (3) chronic bacterial prostatitis.

Relapses, especially in the absence of structural abnormalities, may be related to renal infection that requires a longer duration of therapy (3 to 6 weeks or even longer). Urinary tract infection in the presence of obstruction is likely to be associated with renal involvement and a tendency for renal functional impairment and bacteremia. Calculi may be a cause of relapse of urinary tract infection. The ultimate success of chemotherapy depends on the removal of stones. Only carefully selected patients such as children, adults who have continuous symptoms, or adults who are at high risk of developing progressive renal damage (for example, those with obstruction not amenable to surgery) should be considered for long courses of therapy. Some of the agents that can be used for long-term therapy are ampicillin, amoxicillin, sulfisoxazole, cephalexin, cephradine, and trimethoprim-sulfamethoxazole in the usual doses already described; nitrofurantoin in full dosage for 1 week and then half the usual dose; nalidixic acid (1 g four times daily in adults); carbenicillin indanyl sodium (two tablets four times daily in adults); and methenamine mandelate (1 g four times daily in adults) with methionine or ascorbic acid to acidify the urine.

Patients receiving methenamine mandelate (or hippurate) are instructed to avoid alkalinizing foods such as milk, all fruit juices other than cranberry juice, and bicarbonate of soda. In addition, they are given nitrazine paper to test their urine several times a day to regulate the dosage of methionine or ascorbic acid so that the urinary pH is maintained at 5.5 or below. This increases the effectiveness of the antimicrobial agent. Urine cultures should be obtained at least monthly to determine the effectiveness of therapy.

Probably the most common cause of relapses of urinary tract infection in males is *chronic bacterial prostatitis*. Patients with this entity usually have no symptoms or signs related to the prostate but have a nidus of infection in the gland. Rectal examination is usually unremarkable. Periodically, urinary tract infection occurs when enough bacteria reach the bladder to overwhelm its normal defense mechanisms. The diagnosis is proved by means of a quantitative bacterial localization technique.

This study should be done at a time when the patient does not have significant bacteriuria. If bacteriuria is present, ampicillin, cephalexin, or nitrofurantoin should be given for 2 to 3 days to sterilize the urine; these agents do not affect bacterial counts in the prostate in chronic bacterial prostatitis. Because bacteria present in the urethra can contaminate prostatic secretions obtained by prostatic massage, accurate diagnosis requires simultaneous quantitative cultures of (1) urethral or first-voided urine (VB_1); (2) midstream urine (VB_2); (3) prostatic secretions expressed by massage (EPS); and (4) the urine voided after massage (VB_3). An ejaculate is probably preferable to the EPS.

The specimens must be cultured immediately after collection, and methods of quantitating small numbers of bacteria must be used. If chronic bacterial prostatitis is present, the number of bacteria in the EPS or ejaculate will exceed those in VB_1 or VB_2 urine by at least 10-fold. If no EPS or ejaculate can be obtained, the bacterial counts in the VB_3 specimen should be at least 10-fold higher than the VB_1 or VB_2 samples.

Trimethoprim-sulfamethoxazole appears to be the most effective therapy available for chronic bacterial prostatitis. Approximately one third of patients can be cured with prolonged therapy with this agent (that is, two tablets given twice daily for 12 weeks). Oral carbenicillin indanyl sodium may also be useful when given for long periods. If cure is not obtained, the patient should be managed either with treatment of acute exacerbations of urinary tract infection or with long-term suppressive therapy using low daily doses (for example, half normal doses) of an antimicrobial agent.

Reinfection of the urinary tract. Patients with reinfection can generally be divided into two groups: (1) those who have relatively infrequent reinfections, perhaps only once every 2 or 3 years to several times a year, and (2) those who have frequent reinfections. With infrequent reinfections, each episode can be approached with a course of therapy as if it were a new episode of either symptomatic or asymptomatic infection.

Many patients with frequent reinfections after therapy are middle-aged or elderly women in whom infection is limited to the lower urinary tract. Most asymptomatic reinfections in this group should not be treated because the frequent use of antimicrobial agents is apt to result in toxic side effects and because progressive destruction of the kidneys is rare. If, however, the episodes are symptomatic or the likelihood of renal damage is increased, these patients should be treated.

Occasionally patients of any age have symptomatic reinfection so frequently that they can be incapacitated. In some women these symptomatic reinfections are associated with sexual activity. Voiding immediately after intercourse may help prevent reinfection. However, single-dose prophylactic chemotherapy taken after sexual intercourse is a more effective method of decreasing episodes.

In other patients with frequent symptomatic reinfections, no precipitating event is apparent; in these patients, long-term chemoprophylaxis may be instituted when symptoms are severe. Although these courses seem to decrease the incidence of reinfections and symptoms in most patients, it is impossible to prevent reinfection completely in many patients. When reinfection occurs during chemoprophylaxis, the prophylactic agent must be changed.

Long-term chemoprophylaxis should be considered for asymptomatic patients who are reinfected frequently and are at risk of developing renal parenchymal damage with each reinfection (for example, young children with vesicoureteral reflux and children and adults with obstructive uropathy). Keeping patients in these groups abacteriuric will help protect the kidneys. Trimethoprim-sulfamethoxazole and nitrofurantoin are particularly useful for long-term prophylaxis because these drugs are unlikely to allow the emergence of antimicrobial-resistant bacteria with prolonged use. One 100-mg tablet of nitrofurantoin or one-half tablet of trimethoprim-sulfamethoxazole nightly will suffice.

Patients receiving long-term prophylaxis should be followed closely, with urine cultures at least monthly or more often if interim symptomatic episodes develop. Therapy is continued with the same agent as long as patients remain abacteriuric. If bacteriuria persists or recurs during administration of an antimicrobial agent, therapy is altered using the response of bacteriuria as a parameter of adequacy of therapy. Long-term prophylaxis can be undertaken only if urine cultures are obtained frequently, and therapy is altered if bacteriuria recurs.

PREVENTION. Catheterization of the urinary bladder should be avoided if possible. The risk of infection after a single catheterization is about 1% but is higher in elderly or debilitated patients, patients with urologic abnormalities, and pregnant women. Individuals with indwelling catheters have a much greater risk of infection. Essentially all patients with an open drainage system develop infection within 4 days. The use of a triple-lumen catheter with a neomycin-plus-polymyxin B continuous rinse or the use of a sterile drainage system delays the development of bacteriuria to beyond 10 days in most patients.

PERINEPHRIC ABSCESS

Perinephric abscess is an uncommon complication of urinary tract infection. It usually occurs as a result of obstruction of an infected kidney or calyx or occasionally as a result of bacteremia. The infecting bacteria are usually gram-negative enteric bacilli and occasionally gram-positive cocci when the infection is of hematogenous origin.

The patients have a syndrome suggestive of acute pyelonephritis with fever, abdominal and flank pain (usually unilateral), and often symptoms of lower urinary tract infection. The patients have often been ill for 2 or more weeks. The diagnosis of perinephric abscess should be strongly considered in any patient with a febrile illness and unilateral flank pain who does not respond to therapy for acute pyelonephritis. A palpable mass may or may not be present. About half of the patients have an abnormal plain film of the abdomen (such as an abdominal mass, a calculus, or a poorly defined renal shadow), and most have abnormal intravenous pyelograms.

Perinephric abscess is treated with surgical drainage after first starting parenteral antimicrobial therapy directed against the infecting organism isolated from the urine.

BIBLIOGRAPHY

Brocklehurst, J.C., and others: The prevalence and symptomatology of urinary infection in an aged population, Gerontol. Clin. **10**:242, 1968.

Fang, L.S.T., Tolokoff-Rubin, N.E., and Rubin, R.H.: Efficacy of single-dose and conventional amoxicillin therapy in urinary-tract infection localized by the antibody-coated bacteria technic, N. Engl. J. Med. **298**:413, 1978.

Harding, G.K.M., and Ronald, A.R.: A controlled study of antimicrobial prophylaxis of recurrent urinary infection in women, N. Engl. J. Med. **291**:597, 1974.

Jones, S.R., Smith, J.W., and Sanford, J.P.: Localization of urinary tract infections by detection of antibody-coated bacteria in urine sediment, N. Engl. J. Med. **290**:591, 1974.

Kaye, D., and Santoro, J.: Urinary tract infection. In Mandell, G.L., Douglas, R.G., Jr., and Bennett, J.E., editors: Principles and practice of infectious diseases, New York, 1979, John Wiley & Sons, Inc.

Kraft, J.K., and Stamey, T.A.: The natural history of symptomatic recurrent bacteriuria in women, Medicine **56**:55, 1977.

Kunin, C.M.: Detection, prevention and treatment of urinary tract infections, ed. 2, Philadelphia, 1974, Lea & Febiger.

Meares, E.M.: Long-term therapy of chronic bacterial prostatitis with trimethoprim-sulfamethoxazole, Can. Med. Assoc. J. **112**:225, 1975.

Sourander, L.B., and Kasanen, A.: A 5-year follow-up of bacteriuria in the aged, Gerontol. Clin. **14**:274, 1972.

Stamey, T.A., Condy, M., and Mihara, G.: Prophylactic efficacy of nitro-furantoin macrocrystals and trimethoprim-sulfamethoxazole in urinary infection, N. Engl. J. Med. **296**:780, 1977.

Stamey, T.A., and others: Serum versus urinary antimicrobial concentrations in cure of urinary-tract infections, N. Engl. J. Med. **291**:1159, 1974.

Stamm, W.E.: Guidelines for prevention of catheter-associated urinary tract infections, Ann. Intern. Med. **82**:386, 1975.

Stamm, W.E., and others: Antimicrobial prophylaxis of recurrent urinary tract infections, Ann. Intern. Med. **92**:770, 1980.

Stamm, W.E., and others: Causes of the acute urethral syndrome in women, N. Engl. J. Med. **303**:409, 1980.

41 • DISEASES SPREAD THROUGH FOOD AND WATER

Matthew E. Levison

DEFINITION. Food or water can produce illness by being toxic itself or by being contaminated with (1) chemical toxins (Table 41-1) or (2) infectious agents (Tables 41-2 to 41-4). Two types of microbial water- or foodborne illness are recognized: (1) intoxications following the ingestion of a preformed microbial toxin, examples of which

Table 41-1. Chemical food poisoning

Etiology	Incriminated foods	Incubation period	Clinical features	Duration of illness	Diagnosis	Therapy
Ciguatera fish poisoning: heat-stable ciguatoxin	Liver, other viscera, and muscle of large fish such as barracuda, red snapper, amberjack, and grouper (Hawaii and Florida)	1-6 hr	Paresthesias of lips, tongue, and throat, visual disturbances, vomiting, watery diarrhea; in more severe cases, sinus bradycardia, respiratory paralysis, hypotension	Few days-weeks	Detection of ciguatoxin in food	Symptomatic: cleansing of GI tract to remove unabsorbed toxin; ventilatory assistance
Scombroid fish poisoning: bacterial decomposition of fish flesh	Tuna, mackerel, bonito, shipjack	Few minutes-1 hr	Flushing, headache, abdominal cramps, nausea, vomiting, diarrhea, urticaria, and pruritus (symptoms are those of a histamine reaction); in more severe cases, bronchospasm	Few hours	Detection of toxic levels of histamine in food	Symptomatic—antihistamines, bronchodilators
Paralytic shellfish poisoning: ingestion of toxic heat-stable neurotoxin of dinoflagellates by shellfish	Bivalve mollusks: mussels, clams, oysters, scallops (June-October) (Pacific Coast and New England)	<30 min (few hours-days)	Paresthesias of mouth, lips, face, and extremities, visual disturbances, nausea, vomiting, diarrhea; in more severe cases, respiratory paralysis, muscle weakness, and paralysis	Few hours-days	Detection of toxin in shellfish; detection of dinoflagellates in water where shellfish were gathered	Symptomatic; cleansing of GI tract; ventilatory assistance
Neurotoxic shellfish poisoning: ingestion of toxic dinoflagellates by shellfish	Shellfish (Florida)	Few minutes-few hours	Paresthesias, nausea, vomiting, diarrhea, ataxia	Hours-days		Symptomatic
Heavy metal: tin, copper, zinc	Acidic liquids—fruit juices, carbonated beverages stored in metal containers	≤1 hr	Nausea, vomiting, diarrhea, abdominal cramping	Hours-days	Detection of metal in food	Symptomatic
Chinese restaurant syndrome	Chinese foods	≤1 hr	Paresthesias, headache	≤2 hours	Heavy concentration of monosodium glutamate in food	Symptomatic
Mushroom poisoning						
Mushroom species containing ibotenic acid and muscimol	Mushrooms	2-3 hr	Abdominal cramps, sweating, salivation, miosis, and bradycardia	Hours-few days	Detection of toxin in food	Symptomatic: remove unabsorbed toxin from GI tract; atropine
Mushroom species containing amatoxins	Mushrooms	6-12 hr	Abdominal pain, vomiting, diarrhea, confusion, paralysis, hepatic and renal failure	Days-weeks	Detection of toxin in food	Symptomatic

Table 41-2. Waterborne and foodborne illnesses resulting from bacterial toxins

Etiology	Incriminated foods	Incubation period	Clinical features	Duration of illness	Diagnosis	Therapy
Preformed toxins						
Staphylococcus aureus	Meat, dairy products	1-6 hr	Afebrile, nausea, vomiting, retching, abdominal cramping, diarrhea	6-8 hr	Detection of toxin or organism in food	Symptomatic
Clostridium botulinum	Vegetables (usually home-processed)	12-26 hr	Afebrile, dry mouth, pharyngeal pain, cranial nerve palsies, respiratory paralysis, nausea, vomiting, abdominal distention	Weeks	Detection by mouse inoculation of toxin in serum, stool, food*; culture of food for *C. botulinum*	Cleanse GI tract, administer trivalent (ABE) antitoxin*†; supportive care; measure vital capacity; guanidine HCl, 50 mg/kg/day‡
Bacillus cereus (emetic form)	Fried rice	1-6 hr	Vomiting, abdominal cramping	8-10 hr	Isolation of 10^5 organisms/g of food	Symptomatic
Endogenously produced toxins						
Clostridium perfringens, type A	Reheated meat dishes	8-24 hr	Diarrhea, abdominal cramping	<24 hr	Isolation of organism from food, stool	Symptomatic
Enterotoxigenic *Escherichia coli* (major cause of traveler's diarrhea)	Raw vegetables, water	8-14 hr	Watery diarrhea, abdominal cramping	48 hr	Detection of enterotoxin-producing strain in stool	Symptomatic, Pepto-Bismol
Vibrio cholerae	Water, fruits, vegetables	1-6 days	Watery diarrhea, vomiting, muscle cramps	1-7 days	Isolation of *V. cholerae* from stool—use TCBS agar	Symptomatic; volume replacement; tetracycline, 40 mg/kg/day PO × 2 days
Bacillus cereus (diarrheal form)	Meat, vegetables	6-14 hr	Watery diarrhea, abdominal cramps	24-36 hr	Isolation of *B. cereus* from food	Symptomatic
Infant botulism	Honey	?	Constipation, cranial nerve palsies, generalized weakness, especially of neck muscles—"floppy infants"		Isolation of *C. botulinum* from feces; demonstration of toxin in stool: EMG	Supportive

*Obtain from Centers for Disease Control, Atlanta, Ga. 30333; 404-329-3753 (day) or 404-329-3644 (night).
†Initial skin test for horse serum sensitivity.
‡Investigational.

are given in Table 41-2 (botulism, an example of this type of disease, is described in more detail in a subsequent section); and (2) true infections following the ingestion of viable microorganisms (Tables 41-2 to 41-4). Some of these intestinal pathogens only superficially colonize the mucosal surface, for example, enterotoxigenic *Escherichia coli* or *Vibrio cholerae* (Table 41-2). In these cases disease results from elaboration of various enterotoxins once mucosal colonization is established. Cholera, an example of this type of infection, is described in more detail in a subsequent section. Other intestinal pathogens invade the bowel wall, and disease results from the subsequent inflammatory reaction (Tables 41-3 and 41-4).

DIAGNOSIS. The types of food ingested can frequently suggest the diagnosis. For example, foodborne outbreaks caused by chemical toxins usually involve fish, mush-

Table 41-3. Waterborne and foodborne bacterial illnesses accompanied by fever

Etiology	Incriminated foods	Incubation period	Clinical features	Duration of illness	Diagnosis	Therapy
Superficial invasion						
Shigella	Water, poultry, dairy products	1-4 days	Watery diarrhea followed at times by dysentery with headache, nausea, abdominal pain, tenesmus	1-2 wk	Isolation of Shigella from stool	Ampicillin, 2g/day PO × 5 days or tetracycline, 2.5 g as a single dose in adults; symptomatic
Escherichia coli	Water	8-24 hr	Same as shigellosis	1-2 wk	Isolation of invasive E. coli from stool	Symptomatic—may treat like shigellosis
Deep invasion						
Salmonella						
Gastroenteritis	Water, poultry, eggs	8-48 hr	Nausea, vomiting, abdominal pain, diarrhea	2-5 days	Isolation of Salmonella from stool	Symptomatic
Enteric (typhoid) fever	Water, food	1-2 wk	Headache, cough, abdominal pain, constipation or diarrhea	3-4 wk	Isolation from blood, stool, urine	Chloramphenicol or ampicillin
Bacteremia	Same as Salmonella gastroenteritis	?	Fever, chills, no intestinal symptoms—metastatic foci	Weeks	Isolation of organism from blood	Same as typhoid fever
Vibrio parahaemolyticus	Seafoods	12-24 hr	Nausea, vomiting, abdominal pain, diarrhea	2-5 days	Isolation of organism from stool or vomitus, peptone water enrichment medium with 3% NaCl; TCBS agar	Symptomatic
Yersinia enterocolitica	Dairy products	?	Abdominal pain, tenderness, diarrhea, erythema nodosum, polyarthritis	Days to weeks	Serologic response (Yersinia agglutinins); isolation of organism from stool (cold enrichment of fecal specimens)	Symptomatic; tetracycline
Campylobacter fetus	Poultry, water	2-11 days	Abdominal pain, diarrhea, dysentery, or metastatic foci	10-14 days	Isolation from stool and/or blood	Supportive; antibiotics, for example, erythromycin

rooms, Chinese food, and beverages (Table 41-1), whereas foodborne outbreaks caused by bacteria involve beef, poultry, ham, desserts, and salads. Exceptions are smoked fish and mushrooms, which have caused botulism, and Chinese food, which has caused *Bacillus cereus* intoxication.

An intoxication, either from the food itself or from chemical or microbial contaminants, is suggested by an incubation period of less than several hours' duration (with the exception of botulism and some types of mushroom poisoning, which may have longer incubation periods).

Slightly longer incubation periods (hours to a few days) are associated with (1) diseases that require an initial bacterial proliferation in the intestinal tract and subsequent

Table 41-4. Miscellaneous waterborne and foodborne illnesses

Etiology	Incriminated foods	Incubation period	Clinical features	Duration of illness	Diagnosis	Therapy
Giardia lamblia	Water, vegetables, or fruit	9-15 days	Abdominal distention, flatulence, and diarrhea	Days-months	Identification of cyst in stool or trophozoite in stool or duodenal aspirate	Metronidazole,*† 250 mg PO t.i.d. × 10 days, or quinacrine, 100 mg PO t.i.d. × 7 days
Trichinella spiralis	Undercooked meats, mainly pork	7-14 days	Diarrhea followed by fever, myalgias, periorbital edema, subungual hemorrhages, encephalopathy, urticarial rash, myocarditis, and pneumonitis	4-8 wk	Serology (bentonite flocculation and immunofluorescent test); demonstration of larvae in muscle biopsy after 2 wk of illness; eosinophilia (up to 70%)	Symptomatic; bed rest; analgesics; corticosteroids if signs of CNS, pulmonary, or cardiac involvement are present; thiabendazole, 50 mg/kg/day × 5-7 days
Hepatitis A virus	Improperly cooked shellfish, water	15-40 days	Fever, myalgias, headache, abdominal pain, nausea, anorexia, jaundice, tender hepatomegaly, adenopathy	2-3 wk	Liver function abnormalities; hepatitis A antibody	Symptomatic
Amebiasis	Water, raw vegetables	1 wk	Diarrhea with blood-streaked mucus, abdominal pain	Weeks to months	Trophozoite or cyst in stool, serology	Metronidazole,† 750 mg PO t.i.d. × 5-10 days, with or without diiodohydroxyquin, 650 mg PO t.i.d. × 21 days
Reovirus	?	2 days	Diarrhea, vomiting, fever during winter in patients 6 mo to 2 yr old	2-4 days	Virus detection in stool by radioimmunoassay, ELISA, or electron microscopy	Symptomatic

*This use of metronidazole is not listed in the manufacturer's official directive.
†Metronidazole has teratogenic potential and should be avoided in pregnancy.

invasion, as listed in Table 41-3, and (2) diseases resulting from intraluminal production of an exterotoxin following colonization of the small bowel, as listed under "Endogenously produced toxins" in Table 41-2. Parasitic infections and illnesses caused by certain viruses become clinically manifest days to weeks following exposure (Table 41-4).

The presence of neurologic signs suggests chemical intoxication or botulism. An elevated temperature indicates tissue invasion caused by the organisms in Tables 41-3 and 41-4. A search for fecal leukocytes, using methylene blue stain, should be done in any patient with fever or bloody diarrhea. Fecal polymorphonuclear leukocytes in such a patient indicate invasive disease as in Table 41-3. (Note that fecal leukocytes may be sparse or absent in *Salmonella* gastroenteritis.)

PROGNOSIS. Fortunately, most water- and foodborne illness is acute and self-limited and requires only symptomatic therapy, such as oral electrolyte and fluid therapy. In cases of shigellosis, typhoid fever, and *Salmonella* bacteremia and localized infection, specific antibiotic therapy is indicated. Therapy may be helpful in *Yersinia* or *Campylobacter* infections. It is only patients with chronic, debilitating diseases, those at the extremes of age, or those with severe chemical food poisoning or botulism who die from these diseases.

Botulism

Botulism is an acute intoxication following ingestion of food containing a heat-labile neurotoxin elaborated by *Clostridium botulinum*. Neuromuscular disturbances occur. Similar manifestations can be seen when the neurotoxin is released in wounds infected with *C. botulinum* (wound botulism) or when exotoxin is released within the bowel lumen colonized by *C. botulinum* (infant botulism).

ETIOLOGY. *C. botulinum,* a sporeforming, gram-positive, anaerobic rod, can produce one of seven antigenically different types of neurotoxin, A to G. Disease is usually caused by types A, B, or E.

EPIDEMIOLOGY. The spores of *C. botulinum* are highly heat resistant; in water their destruction requires 5 hours at 212° F (100° C) or 6 minutes at 248° F (120° C). In improperly prepared food, spores may germinate and neurotoxin may be released when the food is preserved in an anaerobic environment (canned or vacuum-packed foods). Heating the food at 176° F (80° C) for 30 minutes or boiling for 10 minutes readily destroys the neurotoxin, but eating the food without prior cooking sufficient to destroy the neurotoxin may result in botulism. Since multiplication of *C. botulinum* is inhibited in acid media, alkaline-preserved foods are most commonly involved. These include home- or commercially preserved vegetables such as mushrooms, string beans, or corn; canned fruits; smoked fish; or pork and beef products. Widespread illness occurs as a result of national distribution of commercially prepared food, which may be marketed under several different brand names. Recent outbreaks have involved canned tuna fish, canned vichyssoise, and vacuum-packed smoked whitefish. Type E is frequently found in fish from the Great Lakes. Type E spores are relatively heat sensitive but survive smoking or light cooking.

PATHOGENESIS. Once ingested, even in extremely small amounts, the neurotoxin, which is resistant to gastric acidity, is rapidly absorbed from the intestinal tract. The toxin blocks neural conduction by preventing acetylcholine release.

CLINICAL MANIFESTATIONS. After an incubation period of 12 to 36 hours (range of 4 hours to 8 days), symptoms of weakness, blurred or double vision, difficulty swallowing and speaking, and dry mouth appear, accompanied by nausea, vomiting, and abdominal distention in some patients. Weakness spreads to involve the neck, trunk, and proximal limb muscle groups and the muscles of respiration. Nasal regurgitation and aspiration pneumonia may occur. Urinary retention and constipation are common. Sensory function, deep tendon reflexes, and level of consciousness are unimpaired.

DIAGNOSIS. The clinical manifestations may suggest botulism, but the diagnosis may not be obvious unless several patients are seen simultaneously with characteristic manifestations following ingestion of the same meal. Confirmation is obtained by demonstration of the toxin or *C. botulinum* in the suspected food and occasionally by the demonstration of the toxin in the blood and feces of the patient. Electromyography (EMG) may show diminished response to a single stimulus but facilitation of action potentials with repeated nerve stimulation.

PROGNOSIS. Mortality may be as high as 70% for type A, 10% to 30% for type B, and 30% to 50% for type E botulism. Death usually results from respiratory paralysis and aspiration pneumonia. In those who survive, recovery is complete but may be slow. If patients are supported by assisted ventilation during the acute phase of the illness, mortality should be considerably reduced.

MANAGEMENT. Specific horse antitoxin is probably most efficacious in type E botulism but is used for all types because of the possibility of the continued presence of circulating toxin. Multivalent antitoxin is used unless the type of botulism is definitely known. After testing for sensitivity to horse serum, two vials of trivalent (A, B, and E) serum are given intravenously and repeated in 2 to 4 hours. Guanidine (15 to 50 mg/kg/day via nasogastric tube) may improve nerve conduction. Catharsis may aid elimination of the toxin from the intestinal tract.

Measures to support respiration are most important in the treatment of botulism. Respiratory paralysis is best treated by using a cuffed tracheostomy and mechanically assisted ventilation.

PREVENTION. Prevention depends on proper home and commercial preservation of food and adequate heating of food before serving.

Cholera

DEFINITION. Cholera is an acute intoxication of the small bowel mucosa caused by an enterotoxin produced by *Vibrio cholerae,* which have colonized the epithelial surface of the small bowel. Profuse, watery diarrhea occurs and is accompanied by muscle cramps, dehydration, circulatory collapse, and renal failure.

ETIOLOGY. *V. cholerae* are short, motile, slightly curved, gram-negative bacilli. Two biotypes exist, the classic biotype and the El Tor variety. El Tor is distinguished by resistance to polymyxin B.

EPIDEMIOLOGY. Cholera has been endemic in the delta regions of the Ganges (Calcutta) and Brahmaputra rivers from which the disease has spread sporadically to become worldwide. The latest pandemic reached peak levels in 1971. In endemic areas cholera is a disease of children, but in epidemics people of all ages are affected.

PATHOGENESIS. Humans are the only known reservoir of infection. Vibrios are passed in the stool during the illness, for a variable period (usually for less than 1 month) during convalescence, in asymptomatic transient carriers, and perhaps in a small number of chronic gallbladder carriers. Cholera is spread by ingestion of water contaminated by feces, improperly prepared shellfish from contaminated seawater, or food directly contaminated with infected stool or night soil.

When large numbers (10^{10}) of relatively acid-susceptible vibrios are ingested, some may survive gastric acidity to colonize the mucosal surface of the small bowel and elaborate an enterotoxin. This toxin irreversibly binds to the epithelial surface and stimulates adenyl cyclase production. As a result, rapid excretion of isotonic alkaline fluid into the small bowel lumen occurs. Structural damage or inflammation in the bowel is not present.

CLINICAL MANIFESTATIONS. The disease starts, after an incubation period of about 1 to 6 days, with an abrupt onset of a variable amount of watery stool. Up to 1 L of stool is lost per hour during the first 24 hours with loss of sphincter control. There is no fever, severe abdominal cramping, or tenesmus. In severe cases muscle cramps and prostration develop. Stools that resemble rice water may be produced. If fluid loss is sufficiently severe and is not replaced rapidly enough, hypovolemic shock, metabolic acidosis, and renal failure develop. In children neurologic complications (seizures and decreased level of consciousness) may be seen.

DIAGNOSIS. Cholera should be suspected in an afebrile patient with an acute onset of painless, voluminous, watery diarrhea in an epidemic or endemic area. A similar illness may also be produced by other enterotoxin-producing organisms such as *Escherichia coli* or *Bacillus cereus,* but if there is equally severe fluid loss, these illnesses would require similar therapy. Examination of stool reveals no blood or pus, which are characteristic of shigellosis or dysentery produced by invasive strains of *E. coli*. The vibrios may be isolated from stool by cultivation on thiosulfate citrate bile salts sucrose (TCBS) agar and produce opaque yellow colonies in 18 hours.

MANAGEMENT. Rapid replacement of fluid and electrolytes is the most important means of treatment. A solution that is prepared by the addition of 4 g of sodium chloride, 6.5 g of sodium acetate, 1 g of potassium chloride, and 10 g of glucose to 1 L of sterile distilled water or lactated Ringer's solution may be given intravenously at a rate equal to gastrointestinal losses or to maintain a strong pulse and normal skin turgor. Oral replacement with a solution that contains 20 g of glucose, 3.5 g of sodium chloride, 2.5 g of sodium bicarbonate, and 1.5 g of potassium chloride per liter of drinking water can be given in mild cholera or after initial intravenous correction of hypovolemia. Tetracycline, 40 mg/kg/day for 2 days orally, can eradicate vibrios from stool and decrease the duration and volume of the diarrhea.

PROGNOSIS. In inadequately treated patients the mortality rate can exceed 50%, but almost all properly treated patients should survive.

PREVENTION. Immunization against cholera with either toxoid or killed bacterial vaccine confers only about 70% protection, which lasts for 3 to 6 months. The best protection in endemic or epidemic regions is the use of boiled water for drinking and the avoidance of uncooked vegetables or unpeeled, uncooked fruits. Eating improperly cooked shellfish from the Gulf of Mexico has posed a problem in the United States recently.

Shigellosis

DEFINITION. Shigellosis is an acute superficial infection of the distal large bowel caused by *Shigella*. Patients have frequent passage of stools containing blood, pus, and mucus, accompanied by abdominal cramps, tenesmus, and fever.

ETIOLOGY. Shigellae are members of the Enterobacteriaceae family. They are nonmotile, gram-negative bacilli that usually do not ferment lactose or produce gas when grown anaerobically. There are four species—*S. sonnei, S. flexneri, S. dysenteriae,* and *S. boydii*— and 39 serotypes. The frequency of isolation of the different species of shigellae varies geographically. *S. sonnei* and, to a lesser extent, *S. flexneri* produce disease in the United States. In other countries *S. dysenteriae* (Central America) and *S. boydii* are more frequent isolates, and these species may be imported into the United States by travelers from endemic areas.

EPIDEMIOLOGY. Man is the only known reservoir of infection. The source is the stool of infected individuals during illness or during a variable time in the convalescent period. There is no known chronic intestinal carriage of these bacteria. Because of the relatively few organisms sufficient to produce illness after ingestion (100 shigellae are sufficient to cause disease in 50% of exposed individuals), the disease is produced not only by contaminated food or water but also by direct person-to-person spread via the fecal-oral route. The conditions for person-to-person transmission are primarily related to poor personal hygiene and are most evident in the young, in the institutionalized retarded, and among the poor in crowded urban ghettos and underdeveloped countries. Shigellosis may be seen more frequently in homosexual men because of oral-anal sexual contact.

PATHOGENESIS. The few relatively acid-resistant shigellae ingested may survive gastric acidity and pass into the colon, where the organisms attach and colonize the epithelial surface (about 10^6 to 10^{10}/g of stool). They then invade epithelial cells to cause superficial ulcerations in the tips of the villi, which are covered by an exudate of polymorphonuclear leukocytes. An acute inflammatory reaction occurs in the lamina propria. Bacteremia and metastatic infection are rare. Certain strains produce an enterotoxin of unknown clinical significance that experimentally results in fluid and electrolyte loss from the small bowel.

CLINICAL MANIFESTATIONS. Shigellae may cause asymptomatic infection or, after an incubation period of 1 to 4 days, may produce a febrile illness of varying severity with either watery diarrhea or dysentery (tenesmus and frequent passage of blood, pus, and mucus in small-volume stools). A biphasic illness with watery diarrhea followed by dysentery may occur. Neurologic findings (irritability, lethargy, nuchal rigidity, or convulsions) are rare in adults, but they are quite common in children 1 to 4 years of age. Usually the symptoms subside in 1 to 2 weeks. Nonseptic arthritis may rarely complicate the illness in the convalescent period.

DIAGNOSIS. Diarrheal illness accompanied by fever, frequent tenesmus, and passage of stools with mucus, blood, and pus can be presumed to be shigellosis. Organisms that produce enterotoxin *(E. coli* or *V. cholerae)* cause an illness characterized by watery diarrhea and by the absence of fever or fecal purulence. Illness produced by more deeply invasive microorganisms such as salmonellae is characterized by fever but is unaccompanied by markedly purulent stool. Sigmoidoscopy in salmonellosis reveals diffuse erythema and edema without the superficial ulcerations of the mucosa seen in shigellosis. The definitive diagnosis depends on isolation of shigellae from stool but may require more than one specimen to yield a positive culture.

MANAGEMENT. Correction of fluid and electrolyte losses may be critical, especially in the watery diarrheal type of illness with signs of severe volume and electrolyte depletion that occurs in the very young and very old.

The use of agents that decrease bowel motility has been associated with more prolonged fever, diarrhea, and fecal excretion of shigellae and therefore should be avoided. Appropriate antimicrobial therapy shortens the illness and duration of excretion of shigellae. Shigellosis can be treated with orally administered ampicillin, 500 mg four times daily in adults (100 mg/kg/day in four divided doses in children) for 5 days; tetracycline, 2.5 to 3 g as a single dose in adults; or trimethoprim-sulfamethoxazole double strength, one tablet four times daily for 5 days, depending on antimicrobial susceptibility of strains. Although active in vitro, amoxicillin and aminoglycosides are not as effective clinically.

PROGNOSIS. *S. dysenteriae* produces the most severe infections, associated with mortality rates of 10% to 20% in untreated individuals, although adequate supportive and specific antimicrobial therapy undoubtedly would lower these rates. *S. sonnei* usually produces mild illness with a mortality rate of less than 1%.

PREVENTION. Good personal hygiene and the avoidance of potentially contaminated food and water are important in the prevention of shigellosis. Patients should avoid preparing food until three stool cultures are negative on consecutive days after discontinuation of antimicrobial therapy.

Salmonelloses

Salmonellae are Enterobacteriaceae that can cause asymptomatic infection or several different types of diseases: enteric fever, gastroenteritis, bacteremia, and localized metastatic infection at any site. There are over 1700 serotypes of salmonellae.

SALMONELLA GASTROENTERITIS

DEFINITION. *Salmonella* gastroenteritis is an acute gastroenteritis of variable severity that follows ingestion of food or water contaminated with salmonellae.

ETIOLOGY. *S. typhimurium* is the most common species isolated in cases of *Salmonella* gastroenteritis. Other common isolates are *S. newport, S. enteritidis,* and *S. heidelberg.*

EPIDEMIOLOGY. Salmonellae are found in many domestic animals (poultry, cattle, pigs, sheep). Salmonellae in meats may contaminate equipment in the processing plant, market, or kitchen and be carelessly transferred to other food from these items. If the contaminated food is allowed to stand at room temperature or is only minimally rewarmed before serving, it may become heavily contaminated as a result of growth of salmonellae. Cooking may not always eliminate these organisms. For example, cooking temperatures in the center of a stuffed turkey may be just right for optimal proliferation rather than for sterilization of the salmonellae. Other sources of food contamination include household pets such as dogs, cats, birds, and even turtles that are fed contaminated products of the meat processing industry.

Because enormous numbers of the relatively acid-sensitive salmonellae must be ingested for a few to survive gastric acidity and result in gastroenteritis, usually food in which the salmonellae have proliferated acts as the source for infection. Person-to-person spread is unusual except in especially susceptible individuals such as infants, the very elderly, those with achlorhydria, and homosexuals who have direct oral-anal contact. Homosexuals with oral-anal contact have been similarly shown to be at risk of other infections spread by the fecal-oral route such as giardiasis, shigellosis, hepatitis A, and amebiasis.

PATHOGENESIS. A few of the large numbers of ingested salmonellae survive gastric acidity, enter the small bowel, invade the lamina propria of the mucosa, and produce a deep inflammatory reaction, at times associated with transient bacteremia. There is little superficial ulceration.

CLINICAL MANIFESTATIONS. After an incubation period of ½ to 2 days, there is abrupt onset with chills, fever up to 105° F (40.5° C), headache, and myalgias accompanied by nausea, vomiting, abdominal cramps, and diarrhea of variable severity. This usually lasts from 2 to 5 days, and recovery is generally complete. Rarely do patients have metastatic infection from the early, transient bacteremia. Metastatic infection is usually seen in patients with hemolytic states such as sickle hemoglobinopathies, malaria, or bartonellosis. In sickle hemoglobinopathies salmonellae usually infect bone infarcts and result in septic arthritis or osteomyelitis.

DIAGNOSIS. If the illness develops in a group of patients who become ill at about the same time, a single exposure to a certain food can usually be defined by a careful food history. The food usually involves poultry products that have been improperly prepared. The food, if still available, may appear normal but may grow salmonellae on culture. The stool of patients contains few if any pus cells, but salmonellae can be grown from the stool during the illness and may persist in stool for several weeks after the illness. Blood cultures taken during the acute illness rarely grow the organism. Agglutination tests (febrile agglutinins) are too nonspecific to be of diagnostic importance.

PROGNOSIS. The illness is usually transient and is rarely (less than 1%) severe enough to cause death except in infants, the very elderly, or the severely debilitated, who die as a result of dehydration.

MANAGEMENT. Replacement of fluid and electrolyte losses should be instituted. Agents that slow bowel motility are theoretically not indicated, but they have been commonly used in the past to relieve abdominal discomfort without reported untoward effects. Apparently antimicrobials do not alleviate *Salmonella* gastroenteritis clinically or bacteriologically, and in fact, when these agents are given during the illness, they may prolong fecal shedding of the organism during convalescence.

PREVENTION. Prevention of *Salmonella* gastroenteritis involves care in the processing of food, especially food known to be frequently contaminated, such as poultry products. Professional food handlers may shed salmonellae on occasion in their stool as a result of constant occupational exposure. Attention to proper handwashing is essential in this group. Patients with acute illness should be isolated, and convalescent carriers should not prepare food for others unless three consecutive stool cultures obtained when the patient is not taking antibiotics are negative for salmonellae.

ENTERIC (TYPHOID) FEVER

DEFINITION AND ETIOLOGY. Enteric fever is an acute generalized infection caused by *S. typhi* and characterized by fever, prostration, relative bradycardia, a rose-colored exanthem, abdominal pain, hypoactive bowel sounds, and splenomegaly. A similar illness, although milder, can be produced by other salmonellae, usually *S. paratyphi* A or B. Of more than 1700 serotypes of *Salmonella*, only *S. typhi* is a pathogen restricted to humans.

EPIDEMIOLOGY. The source of infection is feces or urine from patients and asymptomatic carriers. (Two percent to 5% of patients may become chronic carriers, that is, have positive stool cultures for more than 1 year after illness.) Water or food becomes contaminated from these infectious materials. In the United States about 500 cases occur each year either in recent travelers from endemic areas or in those who have eaten food contaminated by a human carrier. Chronic carriers, when discovered, are registered with health authorities.

PATHOGENESIS. Following ingestion of large numbers of salmonellae, those that survive gastric acidity enter the small bowel, penetrate the mucosa, then invade the mesenteric nodes and subsequently the bloodstream. *S. typhi* parasitize mononuclear macrophages of the reticuloendothelial system. The macrophages fail to kill these organisms, which multiply and then are discharged into the bloodstream. Hypertrophy of the reticuloendothelial system occurs in the liver (micronodular areas of necrosis surrounded by macrophages and lymphocytes), spleen, and Peyer's patches in the gut. Enlarged lymphoid tissue in the terminal ilium and cecum may erode a blood vessel, resulting in intestinal hemorrhage, or may rupture into the bowel lumen, resulting in areas predisposed to perforation.

CLINICAL MANIFESTATIONS. The incubation period is 1 to 2 weeks, depending to some extent on the number of organisms ingested. There is a gradual onset of increasingly higher fever, chills, malaise, headache, myalgias, and abdominal pain, usually in the right lower quadrant. This is accompanied by constipation and cough or sore throat. After about 1 week the fever becomes sustained between 103° F (39.4° C) and 105° F (40.6° C) and diarrhea develops. Physical examination frequently reveals relative bradycardia, rose-colored exanthem ("rose spots") on the anterior trunk, splenomegaly, abdominal distention, and hypoactive bowel sounds. Because of the sustained fever, patients may become severely debilitated. In some patients the temperature may remain around 106° F (41.1° C) with delirium. Intestinal hemorrhage of varying severity or perforation may complicate the illness in the second to third weeks. Gradual recovery begins to occur in the fourth week of illness in untreated individuals. Granulocytopenia, thrombocytopenia, and anemia are commonly noted. Metastatic infection may occur in the lungs, kidneys, bones, joints, and gallbladder. Rarely alopecia, myocarditis, parotitis, and peripheral neuritis occur. Some patients, usually older women with preexisting gallbladder disease, become lifetime (chronic) gallbladder carriers. The infected bile in these patients discharges large numbers of salmonellae into the bowel lumen without local or systemic symptoms.

DIAGNOSIS. The diagnosis depends on the cultivation of the typhoid bacillus. Blood cultures are positive for *S. typhi* in the first week of illness in most patients; stool cultures and, in some patients, blood cultures are positive in the second week of illness; and urine and stool cultures are positive in the third week of illness. Because of frequent nonspecific rises in titer of agglutinins against O and H antigens of *S. typhi* (Widal's test), a diagnosis based on these tests alone is not dependable.

PROGNOSIS. Relapse occurs in about 10% of untreated cases and 20% of treated cases, and the frequency of relapse has been noted to be greater with early institution of antibiotic therapy. Untreated individuals have a mortality rate of 10% to 15%. Death occurs in less than 1% of antibiotic-treated patients. Severe intestinal hemorrhage or perforation carries about a 25% mortality and is the usual cause of death in typhoid fever.

MANAGEMENT. Typhoid fever can be treated with either chloramphenicol, 50 mg/kg/day intravenously or orally, or ampicillin, 200 mg/kg/day intravenously, if the organism is susceptible in vitro. Antimicrobial therapy is given for 2 weeks. In areas where plasmid-mediated resistance (R factor) to chloramphenicol and ampicillin is a problem, trimethoprim-sulfamethoxazole is the drug of choice. Relapse may be successfully treated by another 2-week course of the same drug that was used initially. Corticosteroids may be given for severe toxicity, and the dose can be rapidly tapered in 3 to 4 days. Antipyretics and ice blankets cause chilling, which may make the patient more uncomfortable. A too rapid fall in temperature may be associated with hypotension. Intestinal perforation is managed by nasogastric suction, antibiotics, and, only if necessary, surgery.

About one half to two thirds of chronic gallbladder carriers (primarily those without gallstones) can be cured with 1.5 g ampicillin and 500 mg probenecid every 6 hours orally for 6 weeks. In those who fail to respond to this regimen (especially those with cholelithiasis), cholecystectomy may be considered, but this procedure carries an operative risk and may not cure about 15% of the patients.

PREVENTION. Chronic carriers should avoid preparation of food for others, and travelers should avoid drinking unboiled water or eating uncooked vegetables and unpeeled fruits in areas where sanitation is not optimal. Hospitalized patients should be treated with enteric precautions. Vaccination against *S. typhi* will prevent typhoid fever from developing in about 70% of those vaccinated and should be repeated every 3 years for travelers in endemic regions. Because the immunity afforded by vaccination can be overcome by ingestion of large numbers of *S. typhi*, the best protection for travelers is to avoid potentially contaminated food and beverages. Vaccine against *S. paratyphi* A or B is of no value.

SALMONELLA BACTEREMIA AND LOCALIZED INFECTION

DEFINITION. A clinical syndrome identical to bacteremia produced by other facultative gram-negative bacilli is also produced by salmonellae and is characterized by repeated episodes of shaking chills, hectic fever followed by drenching sweats, and, in some patients, signs of localized infection.

ETIOLOGY. Although almost any serotype is capable of producing bacteremia or metastatic localized infection, *S. choleraesuis* and *S. typhimurium* are the most common causes.

EPIDEMIOLOGY AND PATHOGENESIS. About one third to one half of patients with *Salmonella* bacteremia have a severe underlying illness, for example, cancer, cirrhosis, systemic lupus erythematosus, or hemolytic conditions such as sickle cell anemia, bartonellosis, or malaria. In addition, persistent *Salmonella* bacteremia has been described in patients with schistosomiasis, probably as a result of salmonella parasitism of the schistosome.

Bacteremia results from invasion of the intestinal tract after ingestion of a sufficient number of organisms. Some bacteremias may be associated with an initial phase of gastroenteritis, but more commonly there is no history of gastroenteritis.

Salmonellae tend to localize at sites of preexisting disease such as bone infarcts in patients with sickle hemoglobinopathies, areas of degenerative arthritis, tumors, hematomas, or aneurysms. In fact, salmonellae rather than *Staphylococcus aureus* are the most common cause of osteomyelitis in patients with sickle hemoglobinopathies.

CLINICAL MANIFESTATIONS. Patients with *Salmonella* bacteremia have hectic fever. Unlike those with enteric fever, they do not have sustained fever, cough, rose spots, splenomegaly, and hypoactive bowel sounds. Localized infection may occur at almost any site and result in pneumonia, empyema, endarteritis, endocarditis, pyelonephritis, osteomyelitis, arthritis, or meningitis.

DIAGNOSIS. Diagnosis depends on isolation of the salmonellae from blood or from pus in localized infections. Agglutination reactions ("febrile agglutinins") are too nonspecific to be of diagnostic importance.

MANAGEMENT. Chloramphenicol (50 mg/kg/day in four divided doses) or ampicillin (12 g intravenously each day) for at least 2 weeks is the drug of choice for *Salmonella* bacteremia or localized infection, except for *Salmonella* endarteritis or endocarditis. Surgical drainage and a more prolonged course of antibiotic therapy (4 to 6 weeks) may be necessary for localized infection. In endarteritis or endocarditis bactericidal therapy is essential for cure, and ampicillin is the drug of choice if the *Salmonella* strain is susceptible. Ampicillin is also preferred for more prolonged courses of antibotic therapy because of problems with reversible bone marrow suppression seen with chloramphenicol. Some non-*typhi* salmonellae, however, are resistant to ampicillin.

PROGNOSIS. The morbidity of localized infection may be considerable, and the mortality rate of *S. choleraesuis* bacteremia may approach 20%. Therefore, when these infections are suspected, they should be treated early and appropriately, especially in patients at greater risk of *Salmonella* bacteremia and metastatic infection (for example, in those with sickle hemoglobinopathies).

BIBLIOGRAPHY

Black, R.E., and others: Epidemic *Yersinia enterocolitica* infection due to contaminated chocolate milk, N. Engl. J. Med. **298**:76, 1978.

Bolen, J.L., Zamiska, S.A., and Greenough, W.B., III: Clinical features in enteritis due to *Vibrio parahemolyticus*, Am. J. Med. **57**:638, 1974.

Bradford, W.D., Noce, P.S., and Gutman, L.T.: Pathologic features of enteric infection with *Yersinia enterocolitica*, Arch. Pathol. **98**:7, 1974.

Davidson, G.P., and others: Importance of a new virus in acute sporadic enteritis in children, Lancet **1**:242, 1975.
Ericsson, C.D., and others: Bismuth subsalicylate inhibits activity of crude toxins of *Escherichia coli* and *Vibrio cholerae*, J. Infect. Dis. **136**:693, 1977.
Gorbach, S.L., and others: Traveler's diarrhea and toxigenic *E. coli*, N. Engl. J. Med. **292**:933, 1975.
Guerrant, R.L., and others: Campylobacteriosis in man: pathogenic mechanisms and review of 91 bloodstream infections, Am. J. Med. **65**:584, 1978.
Hughes, J.M., and Merson, M.H.: Current concepts: fish and shellfish poisoning, N. Engl. J. Med. **295**:1117, 1976.
Hughes, J.M., and others: Foodborne disease outbreaks of chemical etiology in the United States, 1970-1974, Am. J. Epidemiol. **105**:233, 1977.
Loewenstein, M.S.: Epidemiology of *Clostridium perfringens* food poisoning, N. Engl. J. Med. **286**:1026, 1972.
Rosenberg, M.L., and others: Epidemic diarrhea at Crater Lake from enterotoxigenic *Escherichia coli*: a large, waterborne outbreak, Ann. Intern. Med. **86**:714, 1977.
Terranova, W., and Blake, P.A.: *Bacillus cereus* food poisoning, N. Engl. J. Med. **298**:143, 1978.
Wolfe, M.S.: Current concepts in parasitology: giardiasis, N. Engl. J. Med. **298**:319, 1978.

Botulism

Koenig, M.G., and others: Clinical and laboratory observations on type E botulism in man, Medicine **43**:517, 1964.
Koenig, M.G., and others: Type B botulism in man, Am. J. Med. **42**:208, 1967.
Merson, M.H., and Dowell, V.R.: Epidemiologic, clinical and laboratory aspects of wound botulism, N. Engl. J. Med. **289**:1005, 1973.
Pickett, J., and others: Syndrome of botulism in infancy: clinical and electrophysiologic study, N. Engl. J. Med. **295**:770, 1976.

Cholera

Barua, D., and Burrows, W., editors: Cholera, Philadelphia, 1975, W.B. Saunders Co.
Woodward, W.E., and Mosley, W.H.: The spectrum of cholera in rural Bangladesh. II. Comparison of El Tor, Ogawa and classical Inaba infection, Am. J. Epidemiol. **96**:342, 1971.

Shigellosis

DuPont, H., and Hornick, R.: Adverse effects of Lomotil therapy in shigellosis, J.A.M.A. **226**:1525, 1973.
DuPont, H., and Hornick, R.: Clinical approach to infectious diarrheas, Medicine **52**:265, 1973.
DuPont, H., and others: The response of man to virulent *Shigella flexneri* 2a, J. Infect. Dis. **119**:296, 1969.
Nelson, J.D., and others: Trimethoprim sulfamethoxazole therapy of shigellosis, J.A.M.A. **235**:1239, 1976.
Pickering, L.K., DuPont, H.L., and Olarte, J.: Single-dose tetracycline therapy for shigellosis in adults, J.A.M.A. **239**:853, 1978.

Salmonelloses

Bennett, I.L., Jr., and Hook, E.W.: Infectious disease (some aspects of salmonellosis), Annu. Rev. Med. **10**:1, 1957.
Black, P.H., Kunz, L.J., and Swartz, M.N.: Salmonellosis—a review of some unusual aspects, N. Engl. J. Med. **262**:811, 864, 921, 1960.
Hoffman, T.A., and others: Waterborne typhoid fever in Dade County, Florida: clinical and therapeutic evaluation of 105 bacteremic patients, Am. J. Med. **59**:481, 1975.
Hornick, R.B., and others: Typhoid fever: pathogenesis and immunologic control, N. Engl. J. Med. **283**:686, 739, 1970.
Mandal, B.K., and Mani, V.: Colonic involvement in salmonellosis, Lancet **1**:887, 1976.
Rubin, R.H., and Weinstein, L.: Salmonellosis: microbiologic, pathologic and clinical features, New York, 1977, Thieme-Stratton Inc.
Saphria, I., and Wasserman, M.: *Salmonella choleraesuis*: a clinical and epidemiological evaluation of 329 infections identified between 1940 and 1954 in the New York Salmonella Center, Am. J. Med. Sci. **228**:525, 1954.
Saphria, I., and Winter, J.W.: Clinical manifestations of salmonellosis in man: an evaluation of 7779 human infections identified at the New York Salmonella Center, N. Engl. J. Med. **256**:1128, 1957.
Stuart, B.M., and Pullen, R.L.: Typhoid: clinical analysis of three hundred and sixty cases, Arch. Intern. Med. **78**:629, 1946.
Walker, W.: The Aberdeen typhoid outbreak of 1964, Scott. Med. J. **10**:466, 1965.

42 • DISEASES CAUSED BY RICKETTSIAE

Oksana M. Korzeniowski

DEFINITION. Rickettsial diseases of humans include a variety of clinical entities caused by intracellular bacteria of the family Rickettsiaceae. With the exception of Q fever (caused by *Coxiella burnetii*), all share common clinical and pathologic features and require an insect vector for the transmission of infection to man.

ETIOLOGY. Rickettsiae are small, pleomorphic coccobacilli approximately 0.3 μm in diameter and 1 to 2μm in length. They stain poorly with aniline dyes and are best demonstrated in tissues by Giemsa or Gimenez stains. With the exception of *Rochalimaea quintana*, the agent of trench fever, all rickettsiae are obligate intracellular parasites. They are clearly bacterial in origin and possess independent metabolic activity and well-defined multilamellar cell walls. With the exception of *C. burnetii* and *R. quintana*, rickettsiae survive only briefly outside the host. Isolation can be achieved by infection of tissue culture monolayers, by subculture of host monocytes, by passage in embryonated eggs, or by animal inoculation. However, such methods are hazardous and should be performed only in reference laboratories skilled in handling rickettsiae.

The family of Rickettsiaceae contains three genera: *Rickettsia*, *Coxiella*, and *Rochalimaea*. The members of the genus *Rickettsia* have been broadly divided into the spotted fever and typhus groups on the basis of antigenic similarities and intracellular growth characteristics. The spotted fever group includes *R. rickettsii* (Rocky Mountain spotted fever), *R. conorii* (boutonneuse fever), *R. australis* (Queensland tick typhus), *R. sibirica* (North Asian tick typhus), and *R. akari* (rickettsialpox). The typhus group consists of *R. prowazekii* (epidemic and recrudescent typhus or Brill-Zinsser disease), *R. typhi* (murine typhus), and *R. tsutsugamushi* (scrub typhus). The genus *Coxiella* contains only one species, *C. burnetii*. This organism is unique in its resistance to desiccation, heat, and sunlight and its transmissibility by the airborne route without need for an intermediate vector. *Rochalimaea quintana,* formerly *Rickettsia quintana,* also merits a separate genus because of its extracellular development in an arthropod host and its cultivation in cell-free media.

EPIDEMIOLOGY. Rickettsiae are maintained in nature in reservoirs involving mammals and arthropod vectors. Each of the rickettsiae pathogenic for humans is capable of multiplying in one or more arthropods and in several mammals, usually small rodents or cattle. Except for louse-borne typhus and trench fever, in which man is the principal reservoir, man is an incidental host and is not needed to propagate the organism.

Rickettsial diseases are found in all areas of the world. In the United States, Rocky Mountain spotted fever (RMSF), murine typhus, and Q fever are endemic; rickettsialpox occurs but is infrequently recognized. Brill-Zinsser disease (recrudescent typhus) still occurs, predominantly in post–World War II Eastern European immigrants.

PATHOGENESIS. Infection with rickettsiae occurs through the skin or the respiratory tract. Ticks and mites, which transmit agents of the spotted fever group and scrub typhus, inoculated rickettsiae directly into the skin. Local lesions at the site of entry of rickettsiae appear with regularity only in scrub typhus, rickettsialpox, and spotted fevers of the Eastern Hemisphere. The louse and flea, vectors of epidemic typhus, trench fever, and murine typhus, deposit infected feces on the skin. Infection occurs when organisms are rubbed into the puncture wound produced by the arthropod. Inhalation of infected dust in Q fever deposits and rickettsial organisms in the lungs and results in pneumonitis.

Rickettsiae of the spotted fever and typhus groups invade endothelial cells of small arteries, veins, and capillaries, causing swelling, proliferation, and degeneration of involved endothelium. Fibrin-platelet thrombi may form. Perivascular cuffing with mononuclear cell infiltration is characteristic. Such foci of infection involve primarily skin but also brain, lungs, heart, and kidneys and can account for the clinical and pathophysiologic abnormalities seen in these infections, that is, rash, edema, increased extravascular fluid space, hypotension, gangrene, and clotting abnormalities.

CLINICAL MANIFESTATIONS AND LABORATORY FINDINGS. At the onset the signs and symptoms of rickettsial diseases are those common to many acute infectious processes. Exposure history in an endemic area is critical to early consideration of the diagnosis. In classic form rickettsial diseases display many common clinical features that vary in degree and detail: fever, cough, headaches, prostration, rash, altered mental state, and hypotension.

Laboratory features are nonspecific and include a low to normal white blood cell count, hyponatremia, renal insufficiency, and thrombocytopenia with or without other parameters of disseminated intravascular clotting.

DIAGNOSIS. Because isolation techniques for rickettsiae are cumbersome and hazardous, diagnosis is confirmed most often by serologic means. The Weil-Felix reaction, based on the agglutination of suspensions of rough strains of *Proteus* species (OX-2, OX-19, and OX-K) by serum from patients with spotted fever and typhus infections, has been widely applied. Complement fixation tests are more specific and can differentiate infections with rickettsia producing similar Weil-Felix reactions. A direct immunofluorescent test of skin biopsies has recently become available for RMSF. Other serologic tests are still experimental.

COURSE. The course and outcome of rickettsial infections are dependent on the infecting organism, the inoculum, and the institution of appropriate therapy. Rickettsialpox and trench fever are mild, uniformly nonfatal disorders, whereas untreated RMSF and epidemic typhus can result in high mortality. Relapses can occur even with appropriate antimicrobial therapy.

MANAGEMENT. Tetracycline and chloramphenicol are the antimicrobial agents of choice for the treatment of rickettsial diseases. Both drugs shorten the duration of symptoms and reduce mortality rates virtually to zero except in complicated cases. Since neither drug is rickettsicidal, ultimate clinical response and freedom from relapse depend on an adequate immune response of the patient. Both oral (tetracycline, 25 to 50 mg/kg/day in four divided doses: chloramphenicol, 50 to 75 mg/kg/day in four divided doses) and parenteral (tetracycline, 0.5 g every 6 hours intravenously; chloramphenicol succinate, 1 g every 8 to 12 hours intravenously) routes are effective. Antibiotics should be administered until the patient is afebrile and 10 to 14 days have elapsed from the day of onset of illness.

ROCKY MOUNTAIN SPOTTED FEVER

DEFINITION. RMSF, or tick-borne typhus, caused by *R. rickettsii,* is characterized by fever, headache, and rash originating on the extremities. Ticks capable of transmitting the disease to man are limited to the Western Hemisphere (United States, Mexico, Brazil).

ETIOLOGY. *R. rickettsii* shares group antigens with other members of the spotted fever group. It is unique in its ability to penetrate and multiply in the cytoplasm and nucleus of the host cell. An exotoxin has been identified, but its role in the pathogenesis of the disease is unclear. Although other species of spotted fever rickettsiae have been isolated from ticks in the United States, they have not been implicated in infections of man.

EPIDEMIOLOGY. The main vectors for transmission of *R. rickettsii* to man are hard (Ixodidae) ticks: *Dermacentor variabilis,* the dog tick, primarily distributed in the southern United States, and *D. andersoni,* the wood tick, found in the western United States. Other species serve as vectors in Central and South America. Rickettsiae multiply in salivary glands of infected ticks without causing vector death and are transmitted transovarially to all progeny. The reservoir for *R. rickettsii* in nature is a zoonotic cycle between infected ticks and small mammals, principally rodents. Illness is produced only in man, a dead-end host who intrudes into the zoonotic cycle by occupational or recreational exposure to tick-infested wooded areas or dogs. All ages are susceptible, but the disease is most common in children under age 15. The peak incidence of RMSF in the United States, from mid-April to mid-September, corresponds to the peak feeding and reproductive season of ticks.

PATHOGENESIS. Rickettsiae are directly inoculated into skin by a tick bite. Tick attachment of 4 to 6 hours appears critical. Ocular contamination with infected tick blood may also result in illness. A transient rickettsemia deposits the organism in vascular endothelial cells and produces a systemic angiitis. The virulence of *R. rickettsii* resides in its capacity to penetrate cells beyond the endothelium, thus producing pronounced thrombosis and necrosis of muscular layers of involved vessels. Microinfarction of organs such as skin, brain, heart, and kidneys is characteristic. Rickettsial action on tissue cell membranes produces a pronounced shift of water and electrolytes from intracellular to extracellular spaces.

CLINICAL MANIFESTATIONS. A history of tick exposure may be obtained from the majority of patients, but the site of the tick bite is frequently inapparent. The incubation period is dependent on the inoculum of rickettsiae and may range from 1 to 10 or more days (median 5.5 days). Clinical presentation is more severe after short incubation periods.

The onset is usually sudden with a severe frontal headache, chills, fever to 102.2° to 104° F (39° to 40° C), myalgia (especially in the legs), conjunctival injection, photophobia, periorbital edema, nausea, and prostration. The characteristic rash appears on the third to fifth day but occasionally may be present as early as the first day of illness. Four percent of confirmed cases never develop a rash.

The initial lesions are macular and blanching, 1 to 4 mm in diameter, and distributed primarily over the ankles and wrists. Rapid spread involves the palms, soles, trunk, face, and occasionally mucous membranes. In the absence of treatment the lesions become petechial, then purpuric, and finally coalesce. In fulminant or untreated cases shock, aztemia, peripheral gangrene, and skin infarction and gastrointestinal hemorrhage may occur. Adult respiratory distress syndrome may supervene. Central nervous system involvement manifested by delirium and stupor is common. Coma, focal neurologic findings, and seizures may ensue. Splenomegaly is common.

LABORATORY FINDINGS. The total white blood cell count is frequently normal or slightly depressed. Thrombocytopenia and disturbed clotting parameters may indicate disseminated intravascular coagulation. Hyponatremia from increased production of antidiuretic hormone is particularly common in children. Oliguria and azotemia are common in severe cases. The cerebrospinal fluid is usually normal but may contain a few mononuclear cells and elevated protein levels.

DIAGNOSIS. An acute febrile illness accompanied by a rash occurring during the appropriate season in a person with a history of exposure to ticks should alert the physician to the possiblity of RMSF. Serologic confirmation by the Weil-Felix reaction (elevated serum antibody titers to *Proteus* OX-2 and OX-19) or complement fixation test rarely yields results early enough for efficient management. Antibody rises are first detected 7 to 14 days after infection and may be delayed by antimicrobial treatment. The most promising early diagnostic technique is direct immunofluorescent detection of rickettsiae in skin biopsies.

COURSE AND MANAGEMENT. Overall mortality for RMSF remains between 3% and 10% (20% in untreated cases). Prognosis depends in part on the severity of the infection and the age of the host. The single most critical factor is early institution of appropriate antirickettsial treatment with tetracycline or chloramphenicol. In uncomplicated cases treated before the fifth day of illness, the residual morbidity and mortality are nil. In severe or complicated cases defervescence is by slow lysis and convalescence may take months. Death in nonfulminant cases usually occurs after 10 days and results from cardiac or respiratory failure.

PREVENTION. Prophylactic measures are aimed primarily at prevention of tick attachment or early tick removal. Effective vaccines are still in the experimental phase. Chemoprophylaxis only delays the onset of the disease.

RICKETTSIALPOX

DEFINITION. Rickettsialpox is a mild, self-limited rickettsial disease transmitted by rodent mites. It is characterized by an initial eschar and papulovesicular rash.

ETIOLOGY. The agent of rickettsialpox is *R. akari*, a member of the spotted fever group.

EPIDEMIOLOGY. *R. akari*, isolated in the United States, Soviet Union, and Korea, is maintained in nature in a zoonotic cycle involving house mice, voles, and the rodent mite *Allodermanyssus sanguineus*. Transovarial transmission of rickettsiae occurs in mites. Man is an incidental host parasitized by mites distributed by rodents proliferating in urban areas.

PATHOLOGY. Infection with *R. akari* produces the vascular lesions typical of other rickettsial infections; however, such lesions are limited to the epidermis and do not result in frank arteritis or hemorrhage. Necrosis of the superficial epithelium in the skin leads to formation of fluid-filled vesicles.

CLINICAL MANIFESTATIONS. An eschar develops at the site of rickettsial inoculation 7 to 10 days after a painless mite bite. The lesion progresses from an erythematous papule to a vesicle to a black encrusted lesion 1 to 2 cm in diameter that heals with scarring. Tender regional lymphadenopathy is common. Constitutional symptoms appear suddenly 1 week after the initial skin lesion develops and consist of intermittent fever, chills, headache, lassitude, myalgia, and photophobia. A sparse, generalized vesicular eruption, sparing the palms and soles, appears 1 to 4 days after the onset of fever.

LABORATORY FINDINGS AND DIAGNOSIS. Diagnosis is made primarily on clinical grounds; chickenpox must be excluded. Laboratory findings are not distinctive. Complement-fixing antibody titers peak 2 to 4 weeks after infection, but the Weil-Felix reaction is negative.

COURSE AND MANAGEMENT. In the absence of specific therapy the course of rickettsialpox remains benign; defervescence occurs in 1 week and the vesicles heal by desquamation without scarring. No deaths have been recorded. Antimicrobial therapy reduces the severity and duration of illness. Tetracycline is most effective.

PREVENTION. No vaccines are available. Rodent control is the definitive preventive measure, but effective miticides exist.

LOUSE-BORNE (EPIDEMIC) TYPHUS FEVER

DEFINITION. Classic typhus fever, a man-adapted acute rickettsial infection, is transmitted in epidemics by the human body louse. It is characterized by a sustained high fever, altered mental state, and a macular rash. Brill-Zinsser disease is a generally milder recurrent or recrudescent form of primary typhus.

ETIOLOGY. *R. prowazekii* has been isolated from patients with primary and recrudescent typhus. It is related antigenically to the agent of murine typhus.

EPIDEMIOLOGY. Louse-borne typhus occurs wherever living conditions predispose to the transfer of body lice among people. Man is the only definite interepidemic reservoir of *R. prowazekii,* although the organism has recently been isolated from flying squirrels in the United States. Rickettsiae from a person with primary or recrudescent typhus are ingested during a blood meal and multiply in the midgut of the body louse. Before its death from intestinal obstruction, the insect vector excretes large numbers of rickettsiae in its feces; there is no transovarian infection. Human disease is acquired by contamination of the louse bite site with crushed infective lice or lice feces or by inhalation of airborne infective lice feces. Primary louse-borne typhus no longer occurs in the United States. Recently, however, primary infections caused by *R. prowazekii* have been confirmed serologically in residents of the eastern United States who have the exposure to flying squirrels. The recrudescent form of the illness continues to surface in European immigrants who acquired the primary disease during World War II.

PATHOGENESIS. Histopathologically, classic typhus produces the systemic vasculitis of small vessels and capillaries typical of other rickettsial diseases. Skin, heart, muscle, brain, and kidneys are primary sites of involvement. Virulent, unmodified *R. prowazekii* can survive in tissues of an immune host for months to years. Rickettsemic recrudescene is believed to result from waning immunity.

CLINICAL MANIFESTATIONS. Abrupt onset of fever, chills, severe headache, myalgias, and mental clouding occurs 7 to 12 days after an inapparent louse bite. Photophobia, deafness, tinnitus, and vertigo are prominent features. Relative bradycardia and a nonproductive cough with minimal physical findings are present in the majority of patients. On approximately the fifth day a maculopapular rash begins on the trunk and in axillary folds and spreads to involve the extremities. The face, palms, and soles are spared. In severe cases the rash may become petechial and varying degrees of skin necrosis may occur. In classic untreated typhus hypotension, cyanosis, azotemia, progressive neurologic dysfunction with selective cranial nerve involvement and hemiplegia from vascular thrombosis, and gangrene of extremities may develop. Bacterial superinfection is common.

DIAGNOSIS. The Weil-Felix reaction yields positive results against *Proteus* OX-2 and OX-19 but does not distinguish among primary typhus, RMSF, and murine typhus. Complement fixation tests exclude RMSF. Indirect immunofluorescent techniques using serum selectively absorbed with *R. prowazekii* or *R. typhi* (murine typhus) can differentiate classic and murine typhus. The Weil-Felix reaction is negative in Brill-Zinsser disease. Detection of complement-fixing antibody of the IgG class separates recrudescent from primary (IgM) typhus.

COURSE. Death or recovery in primary classic typhus occurs between the ninth and the eighteenth days of illness. Mortality in untreated cases has ranged from 10% to 60%. Poor prognostic factors include advanced age, poor nutrition, concurrent diseases, hypotension, and deep coma. Antimicrobial treatment with tetracycline before the moribund state virtually eliminates fatal illness, but relapse may occur if treatment is begun very early after the onset of symptoms. Mortality is negligible in patients with prior vaccination or recrudescent disease.

PREVENTION. A heat-killed vaccine is available and attenuates the severity and mortality of the disease. Decontamination and delousing of the infected patient and the population at risk are of paramount importance in epidemic situations. Quarantine measures are unnecessary.

MURINE (FLEA-BORNE) TYPHUS FEVER

DEFINITION. Murine typhus, a sporadic rickettsial disease transmitted from rodent hosts to man by a rat-flea vector, resembles a mild form of classic epidemic typhus.

ETIOLOGY. *R. Typhi* (formerly *R. mooseri*) closely resembles the agent of classic typhus and confers cross-immunity after infection but not after vaccination.

EPIDEMIOLOGY. Murine typhus is found all over the world and is transmitted to man by fecal contamination of flea bites acquired during periods of abundance of vector fleas. The fleas normally coexist with rats and other small mammals, the amplifying hosts and reservoirs for murine typhus in nature. Rickettsiae multiply in and are shed from the guts of infected fleas without injuring the host.

PATHOLOGY. The lesions of murine typhus resemble those of louse-borne typhus.

COURSE AND DIAGNOSIS. Clinically, murine typhus closely resembles louse-borne typhus, but the manifestations are milder, the duration is shorter, and complication and mortality rates (<5%) are lower. Response to antirickettsial therapy is prompt. Serologic differentiation from classic typhus is based on indirect immunofluorescent techniques.

PREVENTION. Preventive measures are aimed at control of rodent and flea populations and prevention of flea infestation by repellent treatment of clothing.

Q FEVER

DEFINITION. Q fever is a rickettsial disease of man with three unique features: (1) it is acquired by inhalation and requires no arthropod vector, (2) it frequently produces a pneumonitis, and (3) it does not produce a rash.

ETIOLOGY. *C. burnetii,* the agent of Q fever, is resistant to desiccation and can survive for prolonged periods in dust and soil, on clothing, and in animal hides. In the host it multiplies in cytoplasmic vacuoles of endothelial cells and serosal cells. Two antigenic phases have been identified: phase I, or host-adapted, organisms are obtained from tissues of infected animals; phase II, or egg-adapted, organisms are recovered after serial passage in embryonated eggs.

EPIDEMIOLOGY. The true incidence of Q fever in man is unknown. Worldwide serologic evidence of animal and human exposure to *C. burnetii* suggests frequent occurrence of inapparent infections that remain undiagnosed.

Two major patterns of transmission are known: a first cycle involves wild animals, in which rickettsiae are transmitted by a tick vector, and a second cycle involves domesticated animals (cattle, sheep, goats), in which the principal mode of transmission is by an infectious aerosol of rickettsiae. Human beings acquire the disease by inhalation of dust contaminated by rickettsiae derived from birth tissues or excreta of infected animals, by processing infected animal products, or by ingestion of contaminated milk.

PATHOGENESIS. Pulmonary involvement in Q fever resembles a viral or chlamydial pneumonia, with alveolar and bronchial necrosis and mononuclear cell infiltration. Granulomata and/or inflammatory foci showing hepatocellular necrosis with macrophage infiltration are present in liver biopsy specimens. Myocarditis, pericarditis, or subacute endocarditis of the aortic and mitral valves may complicate the course of this disease.

CLINICAL MANIFESTATIONS AND COURSE. In patients with overt infections fever, chills, drenching sweats, myalgias, headache, and prostration develop abruptly after an incubation period of 9 to 28 days. A nonproductive cough and roentgenographic evidence of pneumonitis are present in approximately 50% of patients. Anicteric hepatitis with hepatomegaly and abnormalities of hepatic function is common. Defervescence usually occurs in 2 to 3 weeks, although fever may occasionally persist for several months. Convalescence is prolonged and relapse may occur. Mortality is less than 1%, even in untreated patients. Rarely, chronic disease in the form of micronodular cirrhosis or subacute endocarditis may appear years after the acute attack.

DIAGNOSIS. Diagnosis is based on occupational exposure to domestic animals and on serologic methods. Elevated complement-fixing antibody titers to phase II antigen and specific for an acute infection or prior exposure to *C. burnetii.* Reactions with phase I antigen indicate chronic disease, that is, endocarditis or hepatitis. Agglutination tests are also available in reference laboratories.

MANAGEMENT. Q fever is less clinically responsive to antimicrobial treatment than are the other rickettsioses. Tetracycline shortens the course of the acute disease only if administered within the first 3 days of illness. Q fever endocarditis is particularly resistant to antibiotics and requires prolonged drug therapy and possible value replacement to effect a cure.

PREVENTION. Commercial vaccines are not available, although several forms of live and killed preparations are under investigation in man and domestic animals. Current control measures are limited to pasteurization of milk and prompt destruction of infected placentas. Person-to-person transmission is rare, but isolation of patients with pneumonitis is recommended.

BIBLIOGRAPHY
Rocky Mountain spotted fever

Ascher, M.S., and others: Initial clinical evaluation of a new Rocky Mountain spotted fever vaccine of tissue culture origin, J. Infect. Dis. **138**:217, 1978.

Hattwick, M.A.W., O'Brien, R.J., and Hanson, B.F.: RMSF: epidemiology of an increasing problem, Ann. Intern. Med. **84**:732, 1976.

Hattwick, M.A.W., and others: Fatal RMSF, J.A.M.A. **240**:1499, 1978.

Miller, J.O., and Price, T.R.: Involvement of the brain in RMSF, South Med. J. **65**:437, 1972.

Riley, H.D.: RMSF, Hosp. Practice **12**:51, 1977.

Wilson, L.B., and Chowning, W.M.: Studies on pyroplasmosis hominis: "Spotted fever" or "tick fever" of the Rocky Mountains, Rev. Infect. Dis. **1**:540, 1979.

Woodward, T.E., and others: Prompt confirmation of RMSF: identification of rickettsiae in skin tissues, J. Infect. Dis. **134**:297, 1976.

Rickettsialpox

Rose, H.M.: The clinical manifestations and laboratory diagnosis of rickettsial pox, Ann. Intern. Med. **131**:871, 1949.

Wong, B., and others: Rickettsial pox, J.A.M.A. **242**:1998, 1979.

Louse-borne (epidemic) typhus fever

Murray, E.S., and others: Brill's disease. I. Clinical and laboratory diagnosis, J.A.M.A. **142**:1059, 1950.

Snyder, J.C.: Typhus fever rickettsiae. In Horsfall, F.L., Jr., and Tamm, I.: Viral and rickettsial infections of man, ed. 4, Philadelphia, 1965, J.B. Lippincott Co.

Woodward, T.E.: Rickettsial diseases in the United States, Med. Clin. North Am. **43**:1507, 1959.

Murine (flea-borne) typhus fever

Murine typhus: clinical conference at the Johns Hopkins Hospital, Johns Hopkins Med. J. **141**:303, 1977.

Q fever

Clark, W.H., and others: Q fever in California, Arch. Intern. Med. **88**:155, 1951.

Derrick, E.H.: The course of infection with *Coxiella burnetii*, Med. J. Aust. **1**:1051, 1973.

43 • DISEASES CAUSED BY CHLAMYDIAE

Michael F. Rein

Chlamydiae were described in the first decade of the twentieth century and have been known by a variety of names, including *Bedsonia, Miyagawanella,* psittacosis-lymphogranuloma-trachoma (PLT) agents, and trachoma-inclusion conjunctivitis (TRIC) agents. They have a biphasic life cycle. Elementary bodies are nonreproducing, infectious, 300-nm particles that are taken up by host cells. They then differentiate into reticulate bodies, approximately 1000 nm in size, which divide by binary fission through several generations and form one or more cytoplasmic inclusions that may displace the nucleus of the host cell. Each inclusion is actually a microcolony of reticulate bodies that change back into elementary bodies and burst forth from the cell to infect its neighbors. The reproductive cycle requires approximately 24 hours and depends on the ability of the host cell to generate metabolic energy. Because they are obligate intracellular parasites, chlamydiae have been confused with viruses and can only be isolated in tissue culture systems, which are not available to the majority of practitioners. Unlike the viruses, however, they reproduce by binary fission rather than subunit assembly, possess both DNA and RNA, and most importantly from the clinical standpoint, are susceptible to a variety of antimicrobial agents. They cause disease in a variety of birds and mammals, but only two species are pathogenic for man: *Chlamydia trachomatis* and *Chlamydia psittaci.*

CHLAMYDIA TRACHOMATIS

C. trachomatis is characterized by its sensitivity to sulfonamides, tetracyclines, and erythromycins and its limited sensitivity to penicillins. Intracellular inclusions stain with iodine. The species can be subdivided into serotypes A to C, which cause trachoma; D to K, associated with genital infections and their complications; and L_1 to L_3, which cause lymphogranuloma venereum (LGV).

Trachoma

The major single cause of blindness worldwide, trachoma is most prevalent in the Middle East and North Africa. In the 1950s there was a recrudescence of cases among Indians in the southwestern United States. Chlamydiae are thought to reach the conjunctiva by personal contact or on the feet of flies. The disease may begin abruptly with inflammation of the conjunctiva. Within a few weeks the patient develops hypertrophic follicles on the palpebral conjunctiva and microscopic ulcerations on the cornea. It is believed that initial infections may heal spontaneously at this point without significantly impairing vision. In endemic areas, however, reinfection is common and experimental evidence indicates that with each reinfection the disease becomes more severe, suggesting that an immune response may contribute to pathogenesis. Patients have vascularization of the cornea and scarring of the conjunctiva that result in a turning in of the lid and chronic irritation of the cornea by the lashes. Intercurrent bacterial infections may also be a problem. Typical chlamydial inclusions may be demonstrated by Giemsa stain or direct immunofluorescence of conjunctival scrapings, and chlamydial antibody is detectable in tears. Oral therapy with sulfonamide, tetracycline, or erythromycin can eradicate the infection, but surgery may be required to correct scarring.

Genital infections and complications

At least 95% of men with acute nongonococcal urethritis (NGU) are said to have nonspecific urethritis (NSU) because until recently the etiologic agents were unknown. *C. trachomatis* causes 30% to 50% of such infections. The agents responsible for chlamydiae-negative NSU have not been completely identified but probably include *Ureaplasma urealyticum.* Chlamydial urethritis tends to manifest somewhat differently from gonococcal urethritis, but there is considerable clinical overlap. The incubation period for chlamydial urethritis is typically described as lasting 7 to 14 days, but in one study almost 50% of the infected men had urethral symptoms within 4 days of infection. The urethral discharge is purulent in about one third of men with chlamydial infection and mucopurulent in about one half. A completely clear discharge may be seen in 10% of infected men. Dysuria is noted by 50% to 75% of patients with chlamydial urethritis and is generally less severe than with gonococcal infection. The symptoms of chlamydial urethritis may increase gradually over several days and may even resolve for brief periods. In women symptoms of urethritis include dysuria, frequency, urgency, and nocturia, resembling those of cystitis. Symptomatic women whose urine cultures fail to reveal standard bacterial pathogens are said to have the urethral syndrome; some of these cases are clearly chlamydial urethritis and respond to treatment with tetracycline. Frank urethral discharge is noticed by relatively few women.

So great are the clinical overlaps between chlamydial and gonococcal urethritis that differential diagnosis should not be made on clinical grounds along. Initial management should include examination of a Gram-stained smear of urethral discharge. The smear will reveal typical, gram-negative diplococci in about 95% of cases of gonococcal urethritis, but these will be present in less than 2% of symptomatic men who cannot be shown to have gonorrhea by culture. The observation of gram-negative diplococci lying between the cells predicts gonorrhea correctly only about 25% to 75% of the time. Urethral smears from patients with chlamydial urethritis generally show polymorphonuclear neutrophils and normal urethral flora. Patients with smears diagnostic of gonorrhea should be treated for that infection. Patients with smears suggesting NSU should be cultured for gonococci because the smear will miss 5% of gonococcal infections, but such patients may be started immediately on therapy directed against chlamydiae. Tetracycline, 500 mg orally four times daily for at least 7 days, is the treatment of choice for uncomplicated genital infection in men and nonpregnant women. Erythromycin stearate, ethylsuccinate, or a base in the same doses is an effective alternative in pregnancy; this avoids the risk of staining or dysplasia of fetal bones and teeth with tetracycline.

Direct proximal extension of urethral infection can involve the prostate or the epididymis. *C. trachomatis* is a major cause of acute epididymitis in young, sexually active men. About 75% of such patients have a urethral discharge, and a similar number note inguinal pain. Scrotal edema and erythema are more suggestive of other causes.

Chlamydiae may be transferred from the genitalia to the conjunctiva on the fingers and cause an oculogenital syndrome. Ocular findings resemble those of early trachoma, with hypertrophy of conjunctival follicles. Chlamydial urethritis can apparently incite Reiter's syndrome, consisting of NSU, conjunctivitis, arthritis, and dermatitis, but in this case the multisystem involvement probably results from an altered immune reponse rather than disseminated infection.

Chlamydiae have been recovered from the pharynx but have not clearly been associated with a specific pharyngitis syndrome. They are also cultured from the rectum, and although most of this carriage is asymptomatic, they may cause some cases of infectious proctitis in homosexual men.

Neisseria gonorrhoeae and *C. trachomatis* are sometimes acquired from the same sexual exposure. In this setting symptoms of gonococcal urethritis usually appear first. If the patient is treated with a penicillin, his gonorrhea will be cured and he may feel better for several days before a recurrence of milder urethral symptoms is seen. This syndrome of postgonococcal urethritis reflects the generally longer incubation period and relative resistance to penicillins of chlamydial infection. The physician must rule out the possibilities of reinfection with gonorrhea or true treatment failure. Postgonococcal urethritis is treated like NSU.

C. trachomatis can be recovered from the endocervix of 60% to 90% of the sexual partners of men with chlamydial NSU. Although such women are usually asymptomatic, the organism is far from benign, and the sexual contacts of infected men should be routinely treated. Cervical abnormalities, often mild, are seen in 80% of chlamydial carriers attending venereal disease clinics. *N. gonorrhoeae* and herpes simplex can also cause cervicitis and are part of the differential diagnosis. Chlamydial infection has, however, been specifically associated with hypertrophic cervicitis, manifesting as a friable, often asymmetric, edematous erosion usually accompanied by a purulent or mucopurulent cervical discharge. After appropriate treatment with tetracycline, the hypertrophic erosion generally diminishes to a "simple erosion" and the purulent discharge and friable, congested appearance resolve.

Chlamydiae can spread from the endocervix to the fallopian tubes, resulting in nongonococcal pelvic inflammatory disease (PID). The frequency with which PID follows chlamydial infection of the cervix has yet to be defined. Clinical features of chlamydial and gonococcal PID are similar—principally, lower abdominal pain that may be accompanied by vaginal discharge, dysuria, and fever. The pain is often dull or occasionally cramping and frequently begins or is exacerbated at the time of menstruation. Mild vaginal discharge occurs in more than one half of infected women and menstrual irregularities in about one third. Adnexal tenderness is detected in about 90% of such women, and pain on movement of the cervix is common, Peritonitis and perihepatitis may complicate chlamydial PID. Antibiotic therapy should be extended to 14 days.

Cervical infection is frequently transmitted to the baby during the birth process. Approximately 70% of babies vaginally delivered of infected women will be colonized with chlamydiae at the conjunctiva, pharynx, or rectum. Between 40% and 50% of such infants will go on to develop chlamydial ophthalmia neonatorum, and silver nitrate prophylaxis seems to have little effect on the incidence of this disease. Symptoms generally develop at about 8 days and include conjunctival infection, edema of the lids, and purulent discharge. Conjunctival follicular hypertrophy, characteristic of infection in adults, is not observed in neonates. Once again, the clinical overlap with gonococcal disease is extensive; differential diagnosis cannot be made on clinical grounds alone but must depend on microscopic examination and culture of the conjunctival discharge. Standard treatment for chlamydial eye disease has consisted of conjunctival sulfonamides. Recent work, however, has suggested that infected children might better be treated with systemic antibiotics such as erythromycin, which would also eliminate organisms from other sites of colonization. Tetracyclines should be avoided in children under the age of 8 because they may cause staining and dysplasia of bones and teeth.

Nasopharyngeal carriage of chlamydia has been associated with the subsequent development of pneumonia. Symptoms appear between 4 and 8 weeks of age and consist of paroxysms of coughing without the inspiratory whoop of the pertussis syndrome. Affected babies are usually afebrile, although they may become significantly hypoxic. About 50% have an accompanying or preceding conjunctivitis, and 75% manifest circulating eosinophilia. Chest roentgenograms reveal diffuse infiltrates and usually some degree of hyperinflation. Treatment with erythromycin ameliorates the condition.

Lymphogranuloma venereum

Fewer than 500 cases of LGV are reported annually in the United States, but the disease is considerably more prevalent in Southeast Asia and parts of Africa and South America. LGV is acquired principally through sexual contact, and the incubation period ranges from 3 days to 3 weeks. The initial genital lesion—a small, soft papule that may ulcerate—goes unnoticed by 70% to 95% of patients. Inguinal adenopathy is the most common initial complaint. It is unilateral in 70% of cases and is often initially noted as stiffness or aching in the groin 2 to 6 weeks after the infecting sexual contact. The nodes become matted and attached to the overlying skin, which sometimes develops a purplish color. Involved nodes are often painful and frequently suppurate and rupture; chronic lymphadenopathy develops in about 5% of patients. Inguinal adenopathy above and below Poupart's ligament often looks like a single lymphoid mass bisected by a groove. This phenomenon is observed in only 15% to 30% of patients with LGV but is highly suggestive of the diagnosis.

Primary inoculation into the oral or conjunctival mucosa has been reported. In these cases anterior and posterior cervical and preauricular adenopathy may result.

Fever, chills, headache, meningism, anorexia, and myalgias are common. Late involvement of the rectum may result from direct inoculation of patients practicing receptive anal intercourse or possibly by extension along lymphatics from a primary genital source. A colitis syndrome with a bloody, purulent discharge sometimes occurs, and stenosis, fissuring, and even perforation of the colon may eventuate. Rectal complications can develop a decade after the initial manifestations of disease. Obstructive scarring of the regional lymphatics occasionally causes lymphedema of the genitalia or lower extremities.

Diagnosis is generally based on complement fixation or microimmunofluorescent tests. A significant rise in antibody titer is observed in 95% of cases but may also occur in patients with other chlamydial infections.

LGV can be treated with tetracycline, 500 mg; erythromycin, 500 mg; or sulfisoxazole, 1 g; each administered orally four times daily for 3 weeks.

CHLAMYDIA PSITTACI

C. psittaci differs from *C. trachomatis* in that its intracellular inclusions do not contain glycogen. The organism is resistant to sulfonamides but is sensitive to tetracyclines and erythromycin. An economically important cause of illness in a variety of birds, it is transmitted to man following inhalation of dust contaminated with droppings. Sporadic cases have been associated with psittacine birds (parrots) but also with canaries, ducks, and pigeons. Psittacosis is also referred to as ornithosis, recognizing its acquisition from nonpsittacine birds. Recent epidemics have followed occupational exposure to turkeys, and rare acquisition from mammals has also been described. About 50 human cases are reported each year, and the decline in human incidence may be related to incorporation of tetracycline into animal feeds.

Psittacosis

After an incubation period of 7 to 14 days psittacosis usually starts abruptly with fever. The pulse rate may be slower than expected, but this pulse-temperature deficit occurs in a variety of other infections, including mycoplasmal pneumonia. About 50% of infected patients complain of a persistent and usually nonproductive cough, although small amounts of mucoid sputum, sometimes blood-tinged, may be seen; about 25% of those infected describe chills, headache, chest pain, or myalgias. Rarely, patients have meningitic manifestations or fever in the absence of any localizing symptoms.

Examination reveals rales but usually not consolidation. Roentgenographic changes are often considerably more extensive than expected on the basis of physical examination. Splenomegaly has been reported in up to 75% of infected patients, a finding suggestive of psittacosis.

The diagnosis is generally suspected on clinical grounds but may be confirmed using the chlamydial serologic tests already described. Major differential diagnoses include mycoplasmal pneumonia in young people and Legionnaires' disease in older populations. Treatment with tetracycline, 500 mg orally four times daily for at least 14 days, is effective.

BIBLIOGRAPHY

Alexander, E.R.: *Chlamydia:* the organism and neonatal infection, Hosp. Practice, July 1979, p. 63.

Hobson, D., and Holmes, K.K., editors: Nongonococcal urethritis and related infections, Washington, D.C., 1977, American Society of Microbiology.

Jacobs, N.F., and Kraus, S.J.: Gonococcal and nongonococcal urethritis in men: clinical and laboratory differentiation, Ann. Intern. Med. **82:**712, 1975.

Schachter, J.: Chlamydial infections, N. Engl. J. Med. **298:**428, 490, 540, 1978.

Schachter, J., and Dawson, C.R.: Human chlamydial infections, Littleton, Mass., 1978, PSG Publishing Co.

44 • DISEASES CAUSED BY MYCOPLASMAS

Gerald R. Donowitz and Gerald L. Mandell

Mycoplasmas are bacteria-like organisms that lack cell walls. They may exist as intracellular parasites or as saprophytes. Three species of mycoplasma cause disease in man. *Mycoplasma pneumoniae* causes a range of respiratory illnesses, including atypical pneumonia, tracheobronchitis, pharyngitis, otitis media, and bullous myringitis. The organism has been suspected of playing an etiologic role in pericarditis, myocarditis, and erythema multiforme. *Ureaplasma urealyticum* (T-strain mycoplasma) and *Mycoplasma hominis* causes urogenital infections. *U. urealyticum* may cause nonspecific urethritis (NSU) and chorioamnionitis. Both agents have been associated with pelvic inflammatory disease (PID), puerperal sepsis, and postpartum fever, although the association with *M. hominis* has been more clearly established.

MYCOPLASMAL PNEUMONIA

EPIDEMIOLOGY. Mycoplasmal pneumonia occurs in only 3% to 10% of patients infected with *M. pneumoniae*. Infections occur throughout the year, with a relative increase in disease in late summer and early fall. The disease affects older children, adolescents, and young adults. An increased incidence of the disease and true epidemics have been noted in enclosed populations, such as military bases, colleges, and boarding schools.

PATHOGENESIS. *M. pneumoniae* organisms appear to adhere to the surface epithelium of the respiratory tract. Disease is thought to be caused by both local effects of the organism and the host immune response to the organism. Infections are associated with changes in normal ciliary activity. Alveolar exudate with mononuclear cells and an interstitial infiltrate with plasma cells are noted. The bronchial epithelium remains intact, although mononuclear cell infiltration of the bronchial walls occurs. The rare involvement of other systems (central nervous, hematopoietic, skin, cardiovascular) is believed to result from immunologic phenomena. Recent data suggest that some central nervous system syndromes may result from direct infections.

CLINICAL MANIFESTATIONS. Constitutional symptoms usually predominate initially, with fever, malaise, and headache being major features. Cough develops several days later and become a prominent symptom. Specific respiratory tract signs and symptoms—shortness of breath, pleuritic chest pain, and splinting—are usually absent. Rhonchi, wheezing, or rales may be heard on physical examination, although evidence of consolidation is unusual. Sputum production is quite variable; purulent sputum has been noted in approximately one third of cases. Skin rash, pharyngitis, tender cervical lymphadenopathy, and myringitis may be associated findings. White blood cell counts are usually less than 10,000 cells/mm^3, with higher counts noted in only 20% of patients. Chest roentgenograms often reveal more extensive disease than would have been expected from the history or physical examination. Patchy infiltrates are most common, usually involving the lower lobes in a bronchial or peribronchial distribution. Upper lobe involvement and pleural effusions have been described but are unusual. Gram stain and culture of sputum, if any is present, reveal sparse mouth flora only. There are few polymorphonuclear leukocytes in the sputum smear.

COURSE. The course of mycoplasmal pneumonia is usually benign. Without therapy symtoms may persist for several weeks, with grandual normalization. Recurrences and progression of infiltrates, even with appropriate therapy, may occur. Rare complications include intravascular hemolysis, Raynaud's phenomenon, disseminated intravascular coagulation, meningoencephalitis, cerebellar ataxia, Guillain-Barré syndrome, myocarditis, pericarditis, Stevens-Johnson syndrome, hepatitis, and pancreatitis.

DIAGNOSIS. Definitive diagnosis of mycoplasmal pneumonia requires isolation of the organism. This is not routinely attempted by most microbiology laboratories. A diagnostic rise in complement fixation antibodies may be found in 80% of cases. Cold erythrocyte agglutinins in titers of greater than 1:64 appear in approximately 50% of cases. Other diseases that may cause a similar syndrome include psittacosis, viral pneumonia, Q fever, and Legionnaires' disease.

MANAGEMENT. The therapy of choice for mycoplasmal pneumonia is oral erythromycin, 500 mg every 6 to 8 hours, or tetracycline, 250 mg every 6 hours, for 2 to 3 weeks.

OTHER SYNDROMES

Tracheobronchitis and pharyngitis. Tracheobronchitis and pharyngitis may occur with mycoplasmal pneumonia or may appear as the sole manifestation of disease. Tracheobronchitis is the most common clinical manifestation of *M. pneumoniae* infection. The clinical presentation is much like that of mycoplasmal pneumonia, with constitutional symptoms predominating. Chest roentgenograms are normal. Pharyngitis caused by mycoplasma is indistinguishable from that caused by *Streptococcus pyogenes,* or respiratory viruses. An erythematous palate and posterior pharyngeal and tonsillar exudates are noted, along with tender cervical adenopathy. In both tracheobronchitis and pharyngitis, definitive diagnosis requires the isolation of the organism or a rise in specific antibody titer. No specific therapy is recommended, since the disease is self-limited.

Bullous myringitis and otitis. Bullous myringitis, otitis externa, and otitis media occur in association with mycoplasmal pneumonia and as isolated disease entities. Drainage of any fluid behind the tympanic membrane together with 7 to 10 days of erythromycin or tetracycline therapy is recommended.

GENITAL MYCOPLASMAS

M. hominis and *U. urealyticum* are known as the genital mycoplasmas and cause disease in both males and females.

EPIDEMIOLOGY. Both of these mycoplasmas have been isolated frequently from the genitourinary tract of sexually active men and women. In most cases patients with a positive culture have been asymptomatic, indicating a high rate of colonization but a rather low predilection for true infection. Lower socioeconomic status and increased sexual activity have been associated with a higher incidence of carriage. Infants may be colonized with genital mycoplasmas as they pass through an infected or colonized birth canal.

PATHOGENESIS. The genital mycoplasmas are associated with the epithelial lining of the genitourinary tract. The mechanism of cell destruction and the means by which disease symptoms are caused are not known. The production of toxins by the organisms has been postulated but not proved.

CLINICAL MANIFESTATIONS

Nongonococcal urethritis. NGU is a symptom complex of dysuria, frequency, urgency, and urethral discharge. The discharge associated with NGU is usually nonpurulent, containing relatively few polymorphonuclear leukocytes with no gonorrhea-like organisms on Gram stain. Postgonococcal urethritis is a related syndrome in which symptoms of urethritis persist after adequate therapy for proven gonorrhea. Chlamydiae are the cause of most cases of nongonococcal and postgonococcal urethritis. *U. urealyticum* appears to cause 20% to 30% of such cases.

Pelvic inflammatory disease. Both *M. hominis* and *U. urealyticum* have been isolated from patients with salpingitis, tubo-ovarian abscesses, and pelvic abscesses. In most cases fever, lower abdominal pain, and a cervix that is tender on palpation and movement have been characteristic features. In one series genital mycoplasmas were isolated via laparoscopy from the fallopian tubes in approximately 10% of cases of salpingitis. *M. hominis* has been more commonly associated with this syndrome than *U. urealyticum*.

Septic abortion and puerperal infections. *M. hominus* has been isolated from the blood in 7.8% of women undergoing febrile abortions. In one series 50% of women showed a rise in antibody titers to one or more strains of *M. hominis*. *U. urealyticum* has only rarely been associated with this syndrome. Postpartum fever without abdominal signs has also been associated with the isolation of both organisms.

Spontaneous abortion and low-birth-weight infants. Although no definitive data exist, there is at least a suggestion that cervical colonization with the genital mycoplasmas, especially *M. hominis*, is associated with spontaneous abortion and low-birth-weight infants and infertility.

DIAGNOSIS. The genital mycoplasmas are difficult to culture and are not routinely sought by most microbiologic laboratories. The clinical picture is therefore of great importance in making a diagnosis.

MANAGEMENT. Tetracycline, 250 mg orally every 6 hours for 7 to 10 days, is the therapy of choice for disease caused by the genital mycoplasmas. *M. hominis* is resistant to erythromycin, although *U. urealyticum* is not. Specific therapy for septic abortion and puerperal infections associated with *M. hominis* has not been shown to be effective.

BIBLIOGRAPHY

George, R.B., and others: Roentgenographic appearance of viral and mycoplasma pneumonias, Am. Rev. Respir. Dis. **96**:1144, 1967.

Jacobs, N.F., and Kraus, S.J.: Gonococcal and nongonococcal urethritis in men: clinical and laboratory differentiations, Ann. Intern. Med. **82**:712, 1975.

Levine, D.P., and Lerner, A.M.: The clinical spectrum of mycoplasma pneumonia infection, Med. Clin, North Am. **62**:961, 1978.

McCormack, W.M., Braun, P., and Lee, Y.H.: The genital mycoplasmas, N. Engl. J. Med. **288**:78, 1973.

Murray, H.W., and others: The protean manifestations of mycoplasma pneumonia in adults, Am. J. Med. **58**:229, 1975.

Robinson, D.T., and McCormack, W.M.: The genital mycoplasmas, N. Engl. J. Med. **302**:1003, 1980.

45 • DISEASES CAUSED BY GRAM-POSITIVE COCCI

Staphylococcal infections

Gerald R. Donowitz and Gerald L. Mandell

Staphylococci cause a wide range of diseases affecting all age groups. The majority of infections involve *Staphylococcus aureus*, but *S. epidermidis* has been involved in cerebrospinal and vascular shunt infections and prosthetic valve endocarditis, and *S. saprophyticus* has been implicated in urinary tract infections.

ETIOLOGY. Staphylococci are gram-positive cocci that occur in grapelike clusters in clinical and culture material. *S. aureus* can be separated from the other staphylococci by its production of coagulase. *S. aureus* also produces a range of extracellular products that serve as virulence factors. These include *lipolytic enzymes*, which aid the organism in resisting bactericidal lipids in the skin: *hemolysins*, which injure leukocytes, red blood cells, and platelets and cause smooth muscle spasm; *enterotoxins*, which may cause nausea, vomiting, and diarrhea; and *epidermolytic toxins*, which are involved in scalded skin syndrome.

EPIDEMOLOGY. A staphylococcal carrier state and subsequent person-to-person spread of the organism are the main epidemiologic factors involved in *S. aureus* disease. Between 20% and 40% of adults may be nasally colonized with staphylococci. In newborn populations the umbilicus, perineum, and stool may be colonized. Health care professionals have higher carriage rates than does the general population. While previously healthy people may be infected with staphylococci, patients with severe underlying disease and with abnormal host defense mechanisms represent specific populations at high risk. The presence of foreign bodies, such as intravenous catheters, vascular or cerebrospinal fluid shunts, and prosthetic devices, also represent a major risk factor.

CLINICAL SYNDROMES (OTHER THAN OSTEOMYELITIS)

Skin infections. In most cases skin infection with staphylococi is associated with nasal carriage of the organism or in some cases perineal carriage. Skin diseases associated with *S. aureus* are reviewed in Table 45-1. Three of the most important syndromes will be discussed.

Furuncles. Furuncles, or boils, are localized, deep-seated, cutaneous abscesses in and around hair follicles. They usually occur as a result of self-inoculation of staphylococci. Lesions occur on the neck, thighs, buttocks, axillae, groin, and legs. Furuncles begin as erythematous, pruritic nodules at the base of a hair follicle. Increased swelling and erythema occur and the overlying skin becomes painful and tense; a yellow head is formed and the center of the lesion becomes necrotic. Furuncles may appear singly or in crops, over a period of weeks to months, and then spontaneously resolve. Recurrences may occur several months or years later. Chronic recurrence has been associated with immunologic disorders and diabetes but is most commonly associated with nasal carriage of the organism by the patient or by family members. Spontaneous rupture of furuncles or surgical drainage usually results in rapid relief of symptoms.

Impetigo. Impetigo is a slowly evolving pustular eruption commonly seen in young children. The disease may be caused by *Streptococcus pyogenes* (group A streptococcus) or *S. aureus* or both. The disease usually begins with one or more superficial vesicles on the face that evolve into pustules with surrounding erythema. A thick, yellow crust develops, which leaves a moist, weeping lesion if re-

Table 45-1. Skin diseases caused by *S. aureus*

Disease	Age	Clinical characteristics	Other	Therapy
Bullous impetigo	Newborns, children	Localized form of scalded skin syndrome		Systemic antibiotics with penicillinase-resistant penicillin
Carbuncles	All ages	Resembling furuncles but more extensive Lesions may coalesce with multiple draining sinuses May become necrotic Bacteremia in 25% of patients	May be associated with underlying disease, especially diabetes or uremia	Incision, drainage Systemic antibiotics with penicillinase-resistant penicillin
Cellulitis	All ages	May be confused clinically with erysipelas, with well-delineated margins Induration, inflammation over affected site Fever, chills Lymphangitis may be present	Disease underlying cellulitis (infectious arthritis, osteomyelitis) to be considered	Systemic antibiotics with penicillinase-resistant penicillin
Furuncles	All ages	Infection around hair follicles Appears as nodule with fluctuant center Neck, thigh, buttocks affected in males Axillae, perineum affected in females	Associated with nasal or perineal carriage of *S. aureus*	Local therapy—moist heat Incision, drainage Identification, treatment of carrier state
Impetigo	Preschool age	Slowly evolving pustular eruption, usually on face Thick, yellow crust; weeping lesions	Often associated with streptococcal impetigo	Erythromycin Oral penicillinase-resistant penicillin
Scalded skin syndrome	Newborns, children < age 5, occasionally adults	Painful rash with formation of flaccid blisters Occurs over face, groin, axillae first, then becomes generalized	*S. aureus* type 2 associated with toxin production Disease may be associated with *S. aureus* infection elsewhere	Systemic antibiotics with penicillinase-resistant penicillin

moved. The lesions are contagious and may be spread via direct contact or via fomites (clothing, towels, bed linens).

Staphylococcal scalded skin syndrome. The staphylococcal scalded skin syndrome represents a form of toxic epidermal necrolysis associated with toxin production by staphylococci of phage group 2. The infection is usually at a site other than where the skin lesions appear.

While isolated cases have been reported in adults, most cases occur in children less than age 5. The disease is caused by an epidermolysin that cleaves the epidermis beneath the stratum granulosum. The central area of the face, neck, axillae, and groin are most commonly affected. Cutaneous tenderness and the demonstration of Nikolsky's sign (normal skin that easily separates from the deeper layers if rubbed) are characteristic findings. Within 24 to 48 hours after the onset of symptoms, a progression from a scarlantiniform rash to generalized spontaneous skin separation occurs, resulting in the formation of large, flaccid bullae. Recovery occurs in 5 to 7 days and is associated with a generalized postinflammatory desquamation. Although recover is common, sepsis, cellulitis, and pneumonia may occur, especially in newborns. Increased morbidity and mortality have been described in patients treated with steroids.

Gastrointestinal syndromes. *S. aureus* causes two major syndromes involving the gastrointestinal tract, acute food poisoning and enterocolitis.

Staphylococcal food poisoning. Staphyloccal food poisoning is caused by the ingestion of a heat-stable, acid-stable toxin. High-protein foods that have been allowed to remain at temperatures that permit bacterial growth and elaboration of toxin are most commonly involved. These include beef, pork, milk products, mayonnaise, and potato salad. Approximately 17% of confirmed cases of food poisoning are caused by staphylococcal enterotoxin.

The clinical presentation of staphylococcal food poisoning is quite characteristic. Anorexia, malaise, increased salivation, nausea, and vomiting develop, usually 2 to 7 hours after eating. In some cases diarrhea and abdominal distention may be present without any other symptoms. In more severe cases diarrhea accompanies nausea and vomiting. Fever is usually absent but may occur with more severe forms of the disease. Hypotension and electrolyte imbalances may follow more fulminant presentations.

Staphylococcal food poisoning is self-limited, with gradual resolution of symptoms over 24 to 48 hours. The disease is diagnosed by finding greater than 10^5 staphylococci per gram of food in the proper epidemiologic setting. Therapy involves supportive measures only.

Staphylococcal enterocolitis. Staphylococcal enterocolitis, now rarely seen, is a syndrome presumably produced by staphylococcal infection of the gut. The use of broad-spectrum antibiotics, usually before abdominal surgery, has been the most commonly identified predisposing factor. Outbreaks of enterocolitis in nurseries have occurred that are often associated with staphylococcal skin infections. In some cases a pseudomembrane may be produced, leading to diagnostic confusion with drug-induced pseudomembranous colitis.

Diarrhea is the most common manifestation. The production of profuse amounts of watery, foul-smelling stool is also characteristic; fever is commonly noted. Nausea and vomiting occur in about 10% of cases. Hypotension, shock, and renal failure may occur because of marked volume depletion. An elevated white cell count with a shift to the left is often noted.

The diagnosis is made by the presence of large numbers of gram-positive cocci on stool Gram stain and stool cultures positive for staphylococci. Therapy consists of oral vancomycin with or without a parenteral penicillinase-resistant penicillin. Supportive fluid and electrolyte therapy may also be indicated.

Staphylococcal bacteremia. Staphylococcal bacteremia may occur with any localized staphylococcal infection but is most commonly associated with skin infections, infected intravenous catheters, intravascular shunts and prosthetic devices, postoperative wound infections, endocarditis, and osteomyelitis. Neonates, the immunosuppressed, and the elderly are particularly at high risk. Spiking fevers, multiple rigors, and marked systemic toxicity are characteristic clinical findings. Depending on the source and duration of bacteremia, metastatic foci of infection may develop in the kidneys, lungs, bones, brain, and heart.

Staphylococcal bacteremia, even when treated appropriately, may be associated with a 20% to 30% mortality. The development of metastatic foci is the most serious complication. Controversy exists concerning both the frequency of endocarditis following staphylococcal bacteremia and the most efficient preventive therapy. When a removable source such as an intravascular catheter has been identified and removed, therapy has been started promptly with rapid disappearance of bacteremia and all signs of infection, and no sign of metastatic infection or underlying cardiac disease exists, 2 weeks of intravenous therapy with a penicillinase-resistant penicillin would appear to be adequate therapy. During this time the patient should be closely monitored for cardiac and peripheral signs of endocarditis. In patients with underlying cardiac diseases, prolonged bacteremia, or a bacteremia that has no identifiable source, the presumptive diagnosis should be endocarditis; 4 to 6 weeks of therapy with a penicillinase-resistant penicillin should be given.

The presence of teichoic acid antibody in high titer (appearing within 2 weeks of the bacteremia) has been associated with chronic deep infection and may aid in making the distinction between "transient" bacteremia and bacteremia associated with endocarditis or osteomyelitis.

MANAGEMENT (OTHER THAN FOR OSTEOMYELITIS). Minor staphylococcal skin infections such as furuncles are treated with only incision and drainage. More extensive skin disease or skin disease associated with signs of systemic toxicity requires systemic antibiotics for 5 to 10 days. Impetigo may be treated with oral antibiotics, but severe cellulitis and scalded skin syndrome require parenteral drugs. The presence of systemic staphylococcal disease, such as bacteremia, endocarditis, pneumonia, and enterocolitis, requires therapy with parenteral antibiotics.

From 60% to 80% of staphylococcal infections are caused by organisms that produce penicillinase and are therefore resistant to penicillin. Penicillinase-resistant penicillins, such as nafcillin, methicillin, or oxacillin, are the parenteral drugs of choice; our preference is nafcillin, 1.5 to 2 g intravenously every 4 hours. The oral penicillinase-resistant penicillins are nafcillin, oxacillin, cloxacillin, and dicloxacillin; our preference is cloxacillin, 500 mg every 6 hours. Penicillin G is more active than the penicillinase-resistant penicillins against staphylococci that are *not* penicillinase producers; it can be used in infections caused by susceptible strains of staphylococci.

For the patient allergic to penicillin, cephalosporins (which should be used with caution) and vancomycin are suitable alternative antibiotics. Cephalexin, 250 to 500 mg every 6 hours orally, or cephalothin, 2 g every 4 hours intravenously, are appropriate cephalosporins. Vancomycin, 500 mg every 6 hours intravenously, is the drug of choice for strains of staphylococci that are resistant to both penicillin G and the penicillinase-resistant penicillins. Tolerant staphylococci are those strains inhibited by usual levels of β-lactam antibiotics, such as nafcillin, but requiring high levels for bactericidal effect. The clinical significance and the therapeutic implications of this phenomenon have not been clearly defined.

STAPHYLOCOCCAL OSTEOMYELITIS

S. aureus in the most common cause of acute osteomyelitis in both pediatric and adult patients.

PATHOGENSIS. Three basic mechanisms spread disease to bone. By far the most common is hematogenous spread. Bacteremia is often produced by an inapparent infection; bacteria are carried to the metaphyseal area of long bones where blood flow is slow and phagocytic cells are few. Since the blood supply in these areas is nonanastomotic, obstruction to flow via thrombosis or bacterial plugging allows for microinfarction, devitalization of bone, and the production of an excellent area for bacterial growth. In children rapidly growing long bones are most commonly involved, with bones of the lower extremity (tibia, femur) predominating. In adults the vertebrae are often involved, an anatomic predilection that remains unexplained. Lumbar vertebrae are more commonly involved than thoracic vertebrae, and cervical vertebrae are least commonly involved. The body of the vertebrae is the part usually infected. Disease spreads easily to adjacent vertebrae via venous anastomoses, and at the time the patient is seen two vertebrae are usually simultaneously involved. Patients with a history of intravenous drug abuse may develop osteomyelitis of the clavicle.

The second mechanism by which staphylococci may be carried to bone is by spread from a contiguous focus of infection. This occurs most commonly postoperatively or in the presence of soft tissue infection. Osteomyelitis of the skull may occur after craniotomy or in association with infection of the sinuses and mastoid processes. Osteomyelitis of the fingers and toes is usually secondary to continguous soft tissue infection. Osteomyelitis of the mandible has been associated with dental infections. Several peripheral vascular disease predisposes to osteomyelitis of the toes and small bones of the foot.

Osteomyelitis resulting from traumatic contamination of bone is the third pathogenic mechanism and occurs when organisms are driven into bone or tissue close to the bone. Organisms involved tend to represent those found on the skin including *S. aureus*.

CLINICAL MANIFESTATIONS. In acute hematogenous osteomyelitis in children, localized pain, swelling, and limitation of movement occur in the infected limb and are accompanied by fever, rigors, and marked systemic toxicity. A history of trauma may be elicited in up to 30% of patients, although the etiologic importance of this finding is not clear. In adults symptoms may be confined to the infected limb. Draining sinus tracts are uncommon in acute osteomyelitis.

The onset of vertebral osteomyelitis is usually insidious, with a gradual development of back or neck pain that is slowly progressive over several weeks to months. Limitation of movement of the involved vertebrae with spasm of the paravertebral muscles is commonly noted, but spiking fevers, rigors, and systemic toxicity are uncommon.

Chronic osteomyelitis is not usually associated with systemic toxicity. Development of draining sinus tracts in the area of involvement may be the major manifestation of disease.

The earliest roentgenographic signs of osteomyelitis are localized areas of deep, soft tissue swelling in the metaphyseal area of infected long bones. This may occur as early as 3 days after onset of symptoms. Swelling of muscles and obliteration of radiolucent planes between muscles appear next. Bone changes consistent with osteomyelitis may not be seen for at least 10 days after the onset of symptoms and may be delayed for up to 1 month. Lytic bone lesions are not roentgenographically visible until 30% to 50% of bone is demineralized. Periosteal elevation usually occurs at the same time that lytic lesions are seen. Bone sclerosis and new bone formation are usually noted later, and their presence on x-ray film suggests that the disease has been present for longer than 1 month. In addition to lytic lesions, periosteal elevation, and new bone formation, cortical irregularity and sequestrum formation are other roentgenographic signs of osteomyelitis. In vertebral osteomyelitis, disc space narrowing, erosion of vertebrae, and new bone formation bridging vertebral disc spaces are characteristic roentgenographic signs.

The use of technetium bone scans and gallium scans may aid in the diagnosis of osteomyelitis. Positive bone scans indicate an increased blood supply or increased bone turnover in the involved area. Gallium collects in the area of inflammation or tumor. Scans have been shown to be positive as early as 3 days after the onset of symptoms, often before any roentgenographic changes occur.

Establishing a specific microbiologic etiology for osteomyelitis depends on the isolation of the offending organism from blood, bone, or joint fluid. Cultures of draining sinus tracts in chronic osteomyelitis do not reflect the etiology of bone disease except when S. aureus of mycobacteria are isolated. In most cases bone biopsy for culture and a histologic examination are needed for definitive diagnosis.

COURSE. If acute osteomyelitis is treated appropriately and quickly, usually within 3 to 5 days after the onset of symptoms, most cases resolve without sequelae. Delay in diagnosis and improper therapy with an inadequate drug or inadequate duration of therapy may allow the development of chronic osteomyelitis. Once chronic osteomyelitis occurs, therapy becomes much more difficult, requiring both surgical and medical intervention. Even with such intervention, a failure rate of 23% to 42% has been noted. In vertebral osteomyelitis, spinal compression, meningitis, and paravertebral abscess may occur. Cervical osteomyelitis may lead to retropharyngeal abscess. Osteomyelitis of the thoracic vertebrae may cause mediastinitis or mediastinal abscess. Secondary amyloidosis and nephrotic syndrome have been described as rare complications of chronic osteomyelitis.

MANAGEMENT. A major goal in the management of acute osteomyelitis is to prevent chronic osteomyelitis. In children less than 3 weeks of therapy is associated with an unacceptably high failure rate; 4 weeks of therapy with parenteral penicillins or cephalosporins is the therapy of choice. In adults 6 weeks of therapy with parenteral penicillins or cephalosporins is recommended because the onset is usually less acute. See ''Management (other than for osteomyelitis)'' earlier in this chapter for doses and agents. Therapy for chronic osteomyelitis should include a combined medical and surgical approach consisting of 6 weeks of parenteral antibiotics in association with surgical removal of devitalized bone. In addition, oral antibiotic therapy is given for another 2 to 6 months.

BIBLIOGRAPHY

Beaty, H.N.: *Staphylococcus aureus* bacteremia. In Remington, J.S., and Swartz, M.N., editors: Current clinical topics in infectious diseases, New York, 1980, McGraw-Hill Book Co.

Capitanio, M.A., and Kirkpatrick, J.A.: Early roentgen observations in acute osteomyelitis, Am. J. Roentgenol. Radium Ther. Nucl. Med. **108**:488, 1970.

Causey, W.A.: Staphylococcal and streptococcal infection of the skin, Primary Care **6**:127, 1979.

Dearing, W.H., and Needham, G.M.: Hospitalized patients with *Staphylococcus aureus* in the intestine, J.A.M.A. **174**:125, 1960.

Dich, V.Q., Nelson, J.D., and Haltalin, K.C.: Osteomyelitis in infants and children, Am. J. Dis. Child. **129**:1273, 1975.

Elias, P.M., Fritsch, P., and Epstein, E.H.: Staphylococcal scalded skin syndrome, Arch. Dermatol. **113**:207, 1977.

Horwitz, M.A.: Specific diagnosis of food borne disease, Gastroenterology **73**:375, 1977.

Mackowiak, P.A., Jones, S.R., and Smith, J.W.: Diagnostic value of sinus-tract cultures in chronic osteomyelitis, J.A.M.A. **239**:2772, 1978.

Waldvogel, F.A., Medoff, G., and Swartz, M.N.: Osteomyelitis: a review of clinical features, therapeutic considerations, and unusual aspects, N. Engl. J. Med. **282**:198, 1970.

Waldvogel, F.A., Medoff, G., and Swartz, M.N.: Osteomyelitis: a review of clinical features, therapeutic considerations, and unusual aspects. 2. N. Engl. J. Med. **282**:260, 1970.

Waldvogel, F.A., Medoff, G., and Swartz, M.N.: Osteomyelitis: a review of clinical features, therapeutic consideratins, and unusual aspects. 3. Osteomyelitis associated with vascular insufficiency, N. Engl. J. Med. **282**:316, 1970

West, W.F., Kelly, P.J., and Martin, W.J.: Chronic osteomyelitis. I. Factors affecting the results of treatment in 186 patients, J.A.M.A. **213**:1837, 1970.

Streptococcal infections and rheumatic fever

Jerome Santoro

The streptococci constitute a large group of gram-positive bacteria that are among the most frequent microbial pathogens infecting man. They cause several disease syndromes, including pharyngeal infections, skin infections, bacteremia, neonatal infections, puerperal sepsis, urinary tract infections, endocarditis, and others. *Streptococcus pyogenes,* the most important pathogen in the group, in addition to causing serious bacterial infection, is responsible for the so-called nonsuppurative sequelae of acute glomerulonephritis and rheumatic fever.

CLASSIFICATION. The streptococci are widely found in nature and are also among the normal bacterial flora of man. The organisms are catalase-negative, nonsporeforming gram-positive cocci that are facultatively anaerobic or in some instances strictly anaerobic. Streptocci are classified by either the pattern of hemolysis they produce when forming 1- to 2-mm nonpigmented colonies on blood agar or the antigenic composition of their cell wall carbohydrate. Three types of hemolytic reactions are noted: (1) α, or partial, hemolysis produces a greenish pigment around the colonies. Organisms that produce greening reactions are frequently designated viridans streptococci or *S. viridans;* these organisms tend to be less invasive and are part of the upper respiratory tract flora (2) β, or complete, hemolysis refers to total clearing of the blood agar. Strains that produce β hemolysis are often among the more virulent pathogens for man, such as *S. pyogenes* and *S. agalactiae.* (3) γ-Hemolytic streptococci are nonhemolytic.

A more precise method of classifying streptococci

originally described by Lancefield is based on the antigenic differences in their cell wall carbohydrates. Identification is made by precipitin reactions with group-specific antiserum. By this method organisms are designated group A to H or K to T. The majority of β-hemolytic streptococci, which tend to be more virulent pathogens, belong to groups A through D, F, and G. Some but not all α- and γ-streptococci have group antigens. Group D organisms, which can be β-hemolytic but frequently show α- or γ-reactions, are important pathogens for man.

Anaerobic and microaerophilic streptococci, including peptostreptococci, exhibit variable hemolysis and are classified separately. These organisms are part of the normal flora of the upper respiratory, gastrointestinal, and female genital tracts.

GROUP A STREPTOCOCCI

ETIOLOGY. The group A β-hemolytic streptococcus, *S. pyogenes,* is one of the most important bacterial pathogens for man. This organism is identified by its β reaction and the inhibition of its growth by low concentrations of bacitracin impregnated in a paper disk (A disk). Alternatively, the group carbohydrate can be identified using a fluorescent antibody technique.

S. pyogenes is a structurally complicated organism. There is a hyaluronic acid capsule that is not antigenic because of the similarity to the hyaluronic acid found in humans. The cell wall has three components: the group-specific carbohydrate, structural proteins, and mucopeptides. The group-specific carbohydrate is a polymer of rhamnose and *N*-acetyl glocosamine. The most important cell wall proteins is the *M protein*. The M protein resists phagocytosis by polymorphonuclear leukocytes and is thus an important virulence factor, and strains that produce more abundant M protein tend to be more virulent. Antibodies to the M protein promote opsonization and are protective. However, more than 60 M types are known, so repeated group A streptococcal infections may occur. Two other structural proteins, R and T, are important for epidemiologic purposes but are not virulence factors. The mucopeptide, which consists of alternating units of *N*-acetyl glucosamine and *N*-acetyl muramic acid, can produce carditis in rabbits, but its importance in the pathogenesis of rheumatic fever remains unclear. The cell membrane of group A streptococci has antigens that cross-react with human cardiac muscle, but the importance of this phenomenon is also unknown. Lipoteichoic acid (LTA), another component of the cell wall found in other streptococci and staphylococci as well, is important for adherence to host mucosal cells.

As group A streptococci grow, they produce a number of extracellular products. *Erythrogenic toxin* is responsible for the rash of scarlet fever. A particular strain of *S. pyogenes* acquires the ability to produce erythrogenic toxin via lysogeny with a bacteriophage. Streptolysin O, which is inhibited by oxygen and thus induces subsurface hemolysis on blood agar plates, is produced by all group A organisms as well by some group C and G organisms. This substance is highly immunogenic, and detection of antibody to streptolysin O (ASO titer) is an important laboratory tool used to detect recent streptococcal infection. Streptolysin S is responsible for surface hemolysis on blood agar plants but does not evoke an antibody response. However, both toxins are thought to be damaging to host cells. Other extracellular products, which may act by liquefying pus (streptokinase, deoxyribonucleases [DNases] A to D), facilitating spread of infection through tissue planes (hyaluronidase), or interfering with leukocytes (nicotinamide-adenine dinucleotodase [NADase]), also can promote antibody responses that may be useful in retrospective diagnosis.

EPIDEMIOLOGY. Streptococcal pharyngitis and pyoderma (impetigo) are quantitatively the most common infections caused by group A organisms. However, these two infections have very different epidemiologies. Upper respiratory tract infections from streptococci occur most frequently among children 5 to 15 years old in the winter in colder climates. The major mode of spread is by droplet nuclei, but foodborne epidemics (from milk) have been described. Children with streptococcal pharyngitis are highly infectious and can transmit disease within a household to the majority of siblings and even to some adults. Streptococcal carriers are not nearly as infectious as individuals with the disease. Organisms that cause pharyngitis tend to be low M types (such as 1 to 24).

In contrast, impetigo is most often seen during the summer or in tropical climates among preschool children, Under these circumstances the skin of the extremities and other areas of the body is likely to be exposed and subjected to minor trauma, such as scratches or insect bites. Presumably, these breaks in the skin barrier predispose to secondary invasion by bacteria. However, infection of normal skin probably occurs. Once impetigo is established, it can be spread from one part of the body to another by autoinoculation or to other individuals. Strains causing pyoderma frequently are high M types or nontypable. With both pharyngitis and pyoderma, epidemics occur when person-to-person spread is likely because of crowded conditions. as among lower socioeconomic groups or in the military. Other streptococcal skin infections, such as erysipelas, are acquired much like pyoderma. Nosocomial streptococcal skin infections are also recognized. These infections can occur post partum or postoperatively. Rectal or vaginal carriage of group A organisms by hospital personnel has been implicated in some institutional outbreaks.

Acute streptococcal pharyngitis

The pharynx and tonsillar regions are the most common sites of streptococcal infection in man. However, the accurate diagnosis of "strep throat" in the nonepidemic setting can be difficult. In the winter pharyngeal carriage of *S. pyogenes* in children can exceed 30%; many will go on to develop pharyngitis, but only about 50% will exhibit a significant rise in streptococcal antibodies. If one assumes that antibody production distinguishes infection from carriage, the isolation of group A β-hemolytic streptococci from a child with pharyngitis can have a false positive rate of infection that approaches 50%.

The patient's clinical picture, although suggestive, can also be misleading. In a typical case (observed in the older child or adult) there is an incubation period of 2 to 4 days followed by the sudden onset of fever (greater than 101° F [38.3° C]), headache, and severe sore throat with dysphagia. Anorexia and occasionally abdominal pain with nausea and vomiting (in younger children) may be present. On physical examination a beef-red pharynx with or without exudate and tender cervical adenopathy is seen. Cough, coryza, and hoarseness are not characteristic of streptococcal infection except in infants and should suggest a different diagnosis. It has been shown that most of these signs and symptoms are nonspecific, and viral illnesses such as that caused by adenovirus can reproduce them exactly. The only totally reliable sign is the presence of the rash of scarlet fever (see next section), which is encountered relatively infrequently. The presence of cervical adenopathy seems to be somewhat helpful but is found in only about 50% of the cases. In adults, however, the correlation of signs and symptoms with true infection is much better but by no means absolute. Infants with streptococcal upper respiratory tract infection do not have pharyngitis. In fact, pharyngitis in children less than age 3 is rarely streptococcal in origin. Infants display low-grade fever, rhinorrhea, and excoriation of the anterior nares. The illness in infants tends to be protracted, as opposed to 3 to 5 days' duration in older individuals.

The best approach to diagnosis is to combine clinical, epidemiologic, and bacteriologic information. In patients with equivocal findings, it is best to withhold therapy until culture results are available. If the epidemiologic data dictate, as with an infected sibling or a community epidemic, or in an adult with impressive findings, therapy can be started immediately.

Throat cultures are not difficult to obtain and can be performed in the office. Patients with bona fide streptococcal pharyngitis generally harbor large numbers of organisms in the throat, and this is reflected by heavy growth on the agar plate. On the other hand, the isolation of a few β-hemolytic colonies is more characteristic of the carrier state. However, when the clinical syndrome is compatible, especially when there is a previous history of rheumatic fever, it is best to err in favor of treatment. Streptococcal pharyngitis can be diagnosed retrospectively by measuring the host's antibody response to the organisms' extracellular products, such as streptolysin O, DNase, and hyaluronidase. However, such tests are much more helpful in establishing preexistent infection in a patient who is suspected of having poststreptococcal glomerulonephritis or rheumatic fever and lend little to the everyday management of streptococcal disease.

The differential diagnosis of acute streptococcal pharyngitis includes diphtheria, Vincent's angina, and viral pharyngitides, especially those caused by Epstein-Barr virus and adenovirus. The latter can appear identical to streptococcal pharyngitis and can only be differentiated accurately with the use of throat cultures.

COMPLICATIONS. The complications of streptococcal pharyngitis include scarlet fever and suppurative and nonsuppurative sequelae.

The incidence of scarlet fever has declined dramatically since the antibiotic era began. The initial symptoms of scarlet fever are identical to those of uncomplicated streptococcal pharyngitis. Within 1 to 5 days a characteristic fine "sandpaper" eruption appears, beginning on the chest and then spreading to other parts of the body. The tongue and buccal mucosa are usually involved, but the perioral area tends to be spared (circumoral pallor). The tongue initially is coated with bright-red papillae protruding through a white coating (strawberry tongue). Later the coating disappears and a beef-red tongue is noted (raspberry tongue). The rash is caused by capillary damage produced by erythrogenic toxin. In areas of trauma, such as the antecubital fossae, petechial hemorrhages called Pastia's lines are seen. These reflect the overall capillary fragility, which can be further demonstrated by the application of a tourniquet to the arm for 5 minutes (Rumpel-Leede sign). The latter maneuver produces extensive petechiae distal to the occlusion. Following recovery, desquamation is common.

The suppurative complications of streptococcal pharyngitis include peritonsillar abscess (quinsy), otitis media, sinusitis, acute cervical adenitis, and impetigo. Most of these entities are unusual in the antibiotic era and frequently occur (with the exception of peritonsillar abscess) in untreated preschool children.

Peritonsillar abscess begins with abrupt onset of increased soreness and swelling on the involved side. Initially, the tonsils and the involved anterior pillar are edematous, and the tonsil moves toward the midline of the throat. The involved cervical lymph nodes also enlarge and become more tender. A large, fluctuant mass eventually results. Infection may spread through tissue planes in the neck, or suppurative thrombophlebitis may occur. Interestingly, the organisms cultured from a peritonsillar abscess are not usually group A streptococci but the anaerobic flora of the upper respiratory tract. It is thought that the initial streptococcal infection somehow allows the normal upper airway bacteria to invade the pharyngeal lymphoid tissue.

Direct spread of hemolytic streptococci from the throat to the sinuses, mastoid processes, middle ear, and cervical lymph glands is responsible for infection of these organs.

The clinical presentation of these syndromes is identical to those produced by other organisms infecting these structures. Streptococci can be found in the throat of many children with clinical evidence of skin infection. However, obvious pharyngitis is the exception rather than the rule, and these organisms probably reach the pharynx after the skin is colonized.

Bacteremia with metastatic infection to such areas as bones, joints, and meninges is now a practically unheard of occurrence. Treatment of the suppurative complications of streptococcal pharyngitis consists of antimicrobial therapy (see next section) and surgical drainage when indicated.

The nonsuppurative complications are acute rheumatic fever and acute glomerulonephritis; both may follow all types of respiratory tract infections caused by group A β-hemolytic streptococci. Rheumatic fever (discussed later in this chapter) can occur in up to 3% of cases of severe epidemic pharyngitis, but the incidence in routine outbreaks is less than 0.1%. Glomerulonephritis occurs in 10% to 15% of patients when the infecting strain is nephritogenic. Unlike glomerulonephritis following impetigo (discussed later), penicillin treatment of pharyngitis dramatically reduces the incidence of rheumatic fever. The diagnosis of rheumatic fever and poststreptococcal glomerulonephritis is based on the presence of a compatible clinical picture and the demonstration of recent antecedent streptococcal infection by the use of serum antibody studies. It is important to remember that antibody response varies with the type of infection. For example, ASO and anti-NADase titers may not rise at all or by only weakly positive after impetigo. Since the history of previous infection cannot always be obtained, a combination of tests may be necessary (ASO, anti-DNase B, antihyaluronidase). The "streptozyme" test combines several streptococcal antigens fixed to red blood cells but has a higher false positive rate than a battery of individual antibody determinations. However, this test is very sensitive and, when negative, recent antecedent streptococcal infection can be considered unlikely.

MANAGEMENT. Treatment has relatively little effect on the course of pharyngitis per se. Patients who receive antibiotics have only a slightly shorter clinical course than those who do not. Thus the major reasons for treating "strep throat" are to reduce the incidence of nonsuppurative complications, especially rheumatic fever, and perhaps to prevent other problems, such as otitis media or peritonsillar abscess. Rheumatic fever can be prevented even if therapy is begun 9 days after infection, so there is no harm in waiting for culture results to begin therapy. However, to consistently eradicate *S. pyogenes* from the throat, penicillin levels must be present in pharyngeal secretions for at least 10 days. This can be accomplished in two ways: penicillin V, 125 to 250 mg orally every 6 hours for 10 days; or benzathine penicillin, 300,000 to 600,000 units for infants and children less than 30 kg (66 pounds), 900,000 units for older children, and 1.2 million units for adults intramuscularly as one does. The latter mode of therapy has been shown to be much more effective, especially among lower socioeconomic groups, because patient compliance is not a factor. Patients allergic to penicillin should receive erythromycin, 30 to 50 mg/kg/day in three or four divided doses. These dosage regimens can be applied to cases of streptococcal otitis media and sinusitis, but benzathine penicillin should be avoided. Peritonsillar abscesses can be treated with either intramuscular procaine penicillin G or intravenous penicillin G, 2 to 4 million units daily. Streptococci are variably resistant to tetracyclines, and these drugs should be avoided in all streptococcal infections.

Streptococcal skin infections

PYODERMA (IMPETIGO). The lesions of streptococcal impetigo begin as small papules that are rapidly transformed into 2- to 3-mm serous fluid-filled vesicles surrounded by a thin, erythematous margin. Fluid aspirated from these vesicles will frequently grow group A streptococci in pure culture. However, the vesicular phase is transient and easily missed. Lesions quickly become pustules, which rupture and form thick, amber-colored crusts. At this point cultures of lesions may yeild both *S. pyogenes* and *S. aureus*. *S. aureus* has thus been implicated in the origin of this type of pyoderma. However, prospective studies have shown that group A streptococci are the primary pathogens responsible for the vast majority of cases of *nonbullous* pyoderma, which is characterized by thick, amber crusts. *S. aureus*, on the other hand, is playing a secondary, noninfectious role of colonization under these circumstances. This concept is further supported by the changing over time of phage type of the *S. aureus* isolates as serial cultures are obtained. Whereas streptococcal pyoderma is characterized by small vesicles, persistent, often large bullae are seen with staphylococcal impetigo. Crusting occurs with staphylococcal disease, but the crusts are thin and white to gray in color. When there is difficulty in distinguishing streptococcal and staphylococcal impetigo, a Gram stain of vesicular or bullous fluid may aid in differentiating the two entities.

In contrast to streptococcal pharyngitis, impetigo is a slowly developing, insidious disease that is rarely, if ever, accompanied by fever, erythema, pain, or constitutional symptoms. Also in contradistinction to pharyngeal infection, rheumatic fever is *not* a sequela of pyodema. However, when nephritogenic strains cause impetigo, acute glomerulonephritis can develop in as many as 15% of cases. Because the infection involves only the most superficial dermis, scarring does not occur.

Untreated streptococcal impetigo is a mild, indolent, and occasionally self-limited illness. Local measures, such as the removal of crusts and washing with antiseptic soap, seem to promote healing of lesions. However, impetigo not treated with antimicrobial agents can lead to local and distant foci of infection. Antimicrobial therapy can thus be justified to prevent such complications. There is no good evidence to indicate that treatment will prevent glomerulonephritis following impetigo, as is the case for rheumatic fever following pharyngitis and perhaps for glomerulonephritis following pharyngitis.

Thus the proper treatment of streptococcal impetigo consists of the use of local measures and either local or systemic antimicrobial agents. Gentle but thorough debridement and removal of crusts are accomplished by washing with warm soap and water several times a day. If the lesions are well localized and few in number, bacitracin ointment can be tried. Oral or parenteral penicillin therapy is generally more efficacious and should always be used when lesions are extensive. Benzathine penicillin, 300,000 to 600,000 units for infants and children less than 30 kg (66 pounds), 900,000 units for older children, and 1.2 million units for adults, can be given intramuscularly as one dose. Intramuscular penicillin circumvents the problem of patient compliance, but nonsuppurative complications are not as great a consideration in this instance; an oral penicillin preparation such as penicillin V, 125 to 250 mg every 6 hours for 7 to 10 days, is quite acceptable. In patients with penicillin allergy, erythromycin, 30 to 50 mg/kg/day in three or four divided doses, is the alternative agent of choice. It should be pointed out that during epidemics of pyoderma, prophylactic intramuscular benzathine pencillin will reduce the number of new cases. Measures of this type become important when the infecting strain is nephritogenic and glomerulonephritis is occurring in epidemic proportions.

OTHER STREPTOCOCCAL SKIN INFECTIONS. Streptococci can invade lacerations, burns, and surgical wounds. When wounds and lacerations are involved, infection may remain localized or result in cellulitis as well (see next section). Infected burns appear inflamed and edematous and are characterized by marked weeping. In this situation severe systemic symptoms may be present. Lacerations can sometimes be managed with local measures, such as debridement and antibiotic ointment, and in some instances with oral antibiotics. Infected burns and wounds require parenteral therapy.

Steptococcal cellulitis (erysipelas) frequently follows minor, often unnoticed trauma. It is also common among patients with chronic dermatitis or venous stasis. In a typical case there is intense erythema, warmth, and brawny thickening of the skin clearly demarcated from the as yet uninvolved dermis. This border advances rapidly as infection spreads, and an occasion-streptococci can be isolated from the advancing margin; lymphangitis and bullae may be seen.

Erysipelas of the face was only a common infection but is now encountered infrequently. It characteristically begins near the nose and spreads laterally to involve the face in a "butterfly" distribution. On resolution of cellulitis of all types, desquamation is common.

Cellulitis is often a serious disease that can cause high fever, toxicity, and prostration; bacteremia is not uncommon and shock can occur. Erysipelas of the face tends to cause milder systemic signs and symptoms. The spread of cellulitis can be extremely rapid. For these reasons treatment must be prompt. In cases in which more than just a small area of skin is involved and systemic symptoms and toxicity are present, parenteral administration of antibiotics and hospitalization are often indicated.

Staphylococci are capable of producing cellulitis that can be similar to streptococcal disease. However, the area of involvement tends to remain more localized and lymphangitis is less common. Because of the difficulty in delineating these two enties, it is advisable to treat cellulitis with a parenteral pencillinase-resistant semisynthetic pencillin or cephalosporin, such as intramuscular or intravenous cefazolin, 2 to 4 g daily in three or four divided doses; or intravenous nafcillin, oxacillin, or cephalothin, 6 to 12 g daily in four to six divided doses. When neither a penicillin nor a cephalosporin can be administered, vancomycin is the drug of choice, 2 g intravenously in four divided doses daily.

Streptococcal cellulitis has the propensity to become recurrent and involve the same areas of the body. Prophylactic antimicrobials have been advocated under these circumstances but are of unproven efficacy.

Other group A streptococcal infections

BACTEREMIA. Group A streptococcal bacteremia usually occurs as a result of skin and soft tissue infection. Uncomplicated pharyngeal infection rarely causes bacteremia. Septic arthritis, osteomyelitis, meningitis, and endocarditis are potential complications of bacteremia. The clinical course of streptococcal septicemia may be fulminant, with shock, disseminated intravascular coagulation, and high mortality.

PNEUMONIA. Bacterial pneumonia caused by group A streptococci is uncommon. It is seen most often after viral respiratory infections, such as influenza, measles, pertussis, and varicella. It also occurs in epidemic form in the military. Streptococcal pneumonia is characterized by a 60% incidence of pleural involvement with bloody empyema. Treatment consists of penicillin therapy, 4 to 6 million units every 24 hours, and drainage of the pleural space by either thoracentesis or chest tube.

BONE AND JOINT INFECTION. *S. pyogenes* is a relatively common cause of osteomyelitis and septic arthritis. These infections are clinically similar to bone and joint infections caused by other bacteria.

PUERPERAL INFECTION. Puerperal infection (childbed fever) occurs when streptococci invade the endometrium. There is the abrupt onset of fever, chills, toxicity, with abdominal or pelvic pain usually within 24 to 48 hours after delivery. Serosanguineous, odorless vaginal discharge is noted. If not treated quickly, infection may result in pelvic cellulitis, septic pelvic thrombophlebitis, peritonitis, and pelvic abscess. A similar syndrome may be caused by group B streptococci and anerobic streptococci as well (see next section).

GROUP B STREPTOCOCCI

S. agalactiae was first recognized in association with bovine mastitis. However, these organisms are now clearly recognized as important pathogens for humans. Most group B streptococci exhibit β hemolysis and are resistant to bacitracin. They can be further distinguished from group A organisms by their ability to hydrolyse sodium hippurate. Group B organisms are divided into five antigenic subgroups: Ia, Ib, Ic, II, and III.

Group B streptococci have emerged as an extremely important cause of neonatal sepsis, and the incidence of group B infection rivals that of *Escherichia coli* as the most common organism. The bacteria colonize the birth canal, and neonates can acquire infection at the time of delivery. Alternatively, nosocomial transmission occurs in nurseries. The incidence of maternal carriage may be as high as 25%, and transmission to the neonate may also be quite high. Fortunately, the incidence of disease is low, about 2 cases for every 1000 births. This may be related to some degree, especially for type III organisms, to the transmission of maternal antibody to the neonate. Antibiotics have not been successful in eliminating maternal carriage.

Two syndromes of neonatal infection have been described. Early-onset infection begins in the first 10 days of life and is more common with prematurity and prolonged rupture of the membranes. However, infection can occur after uncomplicated term deliveries as well. The early-onset syndrome consists of fulminating bacteremia and shock. Pneumonia and/or meningitis are found in almost 50% of cases; despite antimicrobial therapy the mortality rate exceeds 50%. The late-onset syndrome, appearing after 10 days of life, is not correlated with obstetric complications and most often is seen as meningitis. The prognosis for the late-onset syndrome is somewhat better, with a mortality less than 30%. Whereas all subtypes of group B organisms may be encountered in the early syndrome, type III dominates with the late-onset presentation.

Group B streptococci cause a broad range of infections in adults. Patients are frequently women of childbearing age who develop infection in conjunction with delivery or gynecologic disorders. Elderly patients with genitourinary problems, diabetes, or other chronic diseases are also prone to these infections. In fact, about 2% of all bacteremias and about 8% of all streptococcal bacteremias in adults are caused by group B organisms. Infections caused by group B streptococci include pyelonephritis, endometritis, meningitis, endocarditis, pulmonary infections, and soft tissue infections.

Group B streptococci are sensitive to penicillin, but the minimum inhibitory concentrations (MIC) are somewhat higher when compared to *S. pyogenes*. Cephalosporins, erythromycin, clindamycin, and vancomycin are also active agents. Antimicrobial therapy for adults with serious infections from group B streptococci consists of high-dose intravenous penicillin, 10 to 20 million units every 24 hours.

GROUP C AND G STREPTOCOCCI

Group C and G streptococci are less commonly isolated in human streptococcal disease than group A organisms, with which they have many features in common. For example, most strains are β-hemolytic and some are even sensitive to bacitracin. Both groups also produce similar enzymes and toxins to those of group A streptococci, such as streptolysin O, streptokinase, DNase, NADase, hyaluronidase, and erythrogenic toxin. The group C carbohydrate is also similar to that of group A, and cross-reacting cell-membrane antigens can be demonstrated among groups A, C, and G.

These organisms are recognized as part of the normal throat, skin, and genitourinary flora. However, they have also been implicated as a cause of skin and wound infections, puerperal sepsis, bacteremia, and endocarditis. Purulent pharyngitis also sometimes occurs with scarlatiniform eruptions. Following these infections, elevations of the ASO titer and other antibodies to other extracellular products can frequently be demonstrated. Both group C and G organisms are sensitive to penicillin and erythromycin, and treatment regimens for group A streptococci can be employed for similar clinical situations.

GROUP D STREPTOCOCCI

Group D streptococci are divided into two major groups. Organisms that grow on bile and in 6.5% NaCl are designated *enterococci*, which include *S. faecalis* and other species. These organisms can be α-, β-, or γ-hemolytic. Organisms that grow on bile but not in 6.5% NaCl and that are nearly always α-hemolytic are called *nonenterococcal* group D streptococci and include *S. bovis* and *S. equinus*. Both groups are part of the normal gastrointestinal and genitourinary flora and are frequently isolated from patients with infections involving these areas. Both groups are also commonly the cause of bacterial endocarditis, and in this light their differences become important. Enterococci are the only members of the streptococci family that are consistently resistant to penicillin. Although ampicillin may be sufficient for urinary tract infections or other minor infections caused by these organisms, therapy for more serious processes, such as bacteremia or endocarditis, requires the synergistic combination of penicillin and an aminoglycoside (see Chapter 40). The patient who is allergic to penicillin often requires vanocomycin with an aminoglycoside or penicillin desensitization. Enterococci are resistant to cephalosporins, which should not be used.

S. equinus rarely causes infections in man. On the other hand, *S. bovis* is a very common cause of endocarditis. *S. bovis* is sensitive to penicillin, and treatment of endocarditis caused by this organism is similar to endovascular infection from *S. viridans*. Perhaps more importantly, an association between *S. bovis* bacteremia and endocarditis with colon carcinoma and perhaps other gastrointestinal tumors has been elucidated. Thus any patient with *S. bovis* isolated from the blood requires a thorough search for gastrointestinal (especially colon) neoplasia.

VIRIDANS STREPTOCOCCI

Viridans streptococci (by definition α-hemolytic) are members of the normal upper respiratory tract flora. They are still the most common cause of subacute bacterial endocarditis. Their classification is confusing in that some species are groupable and others are not. Five major species have been described: *S. salivarius, S. mitior, S. milleri, S. sanguis,* and *S. mutans*. For the most part viridans streptococci are noninvasive and cause infection on damaged heart valves after transient bacteremia. However, *S. milleri* is capable of causing serious pyogenic processes such as brain abscess, empyema, liver abscess, and peritonitis. *S. milleri* is frequently classified as microaerophilic; its behavior is similar to that of the anaerobic streptococci (see next section). Metastatic infection is also more likely to occur when *S. milleri* causes endocarditis when compared to other viridans streptococci.

These organisms are sensitive to penicillin but not to the degree of group A streptococci. Parenteral penicillin therapy, often with an aminoglycoside, is required for viridans streptococcal endocarditis (see Chapter 40).

ANAEROBIC STREPTOCOCCI

Anaerobic and microaerophilic streptococcal species reside in the pharynx, gastrointestinal tract, and genitourinary tract. These organisms are capable of causing several types of infection, including necrotizing pneumonia, lung abscess, empyema, sinusitis, brain abscess, and skin and wound infections. They are often found along with other anaerobic or aerobic bacteria. Foul-smelling pus and gas in the soft tissues are characteristic of these infections. The anaerobic streptococci are sensitive to penicillin. High-dose parenteral therapy is generally required.

ACUTE RHEUMATIC FEVER

EPIDEMIOLOGY. Because the diagnosis of acute rheumatic fever (ARF) is largely clinical and there is no specific diagnostic test, the exact incidence of this disorder is unknown. However, ARF seems to be much less common now than years ago, probably because of better living conditions, the advent of antimicrobial agents, and perhaps decreased "rheumatogenicity" of the streptococci themselves. When it occurs, ARF is most commonly seen in patients of lower socioeconomic strata, between ages 5 and 16. During epidemics of severe streptococcal pharyngitis in closed populations such as the military, the incidence of ARF may approach 2% to 3% among the untreated. On the other hand, with milder sporadic pharyngitis, the incidence is much lower. Other factors that seem to be related to the attack rate of ARF are the duration of carriage of group A streptococci in the throat and the magnitude of the individual's immune response to streptococcal antigens. Patients who suffer one attack of rheumatic fever are clearly at high risk for recurrence after subsequent group A streptococcal upper respiratory tract infections.

PATHOGENESIS. The exact mechanism by which group A streptococci precipitate tissue damage is still unproved. However, much experimental work and various clinical observations have provoked many theories in this regard. It appears both host and bacterial factors play important roles. For instance, since pyoderma does not precipitate ARF, investigators postulate that access to the rich lymphoid tissues of the pharynx that have connections with the heart may be needed to produce the disease. Other differences between strains that produce only pharyngitis and those that produce both pyoderma and pharyngitis have been pointed out. For example, strains producing pyoderma evoke a weak ASO response. These strains are also less "rheumatogenic"—they differ from those streptococcal strains that lack a serum opacity factor (SOR-negative) and seem to elicit high antibody levels as well as being capable of causing ARF. Certain streptococcal products such as streptolysin O have been shown to have direct cardiotoxic effects in animals. Some streptococcal antigens seem to have common components with cardiac tissue. In this regard, antibodies directed at the streptococcal antigens could cross-react with heart tissue and cause damage. Circulating heart antibodies have been demonstrated in high titers in the sera of patients with rheumatic fever. However, it is unclear whether these antibodies are the cause of the damage or the result of previous heart tissue destruction from some other insult. Another theory, which also emphasizes the role of humoral immunity, is the possibility of immune complex deposition causing the disease. Finally, there is also some experimental evidence linking streptococcal antigens to a nonspecific mitogenic response of delayed hypersensitivity. The latter would then precipitate T-cell cytotoxicity to cardiac cells.

PATHOLOGY. The lesions of ARF are found throughout the body. Focal lesions that consist of fibrinoid necrosis of connective tissue surrounded by inflammatory cells (Aschoff's bodies) are seen around small blood vessels in the heart. These eventually disappear, leaving fibrosis. Endothelial lesions heal with fibrous thickening, which may result in valvular dysfunction, turbulent blood flow, and further valvular damage.

CLINICAL MANIFESTATIONS. The severity of ARF tends to differ with the age of the patient. In children carditis seems to be more predominant, whereas in older children and adults joint manifestations are most prominent.

There are five major clinical features of ARF. *Acute migratory arthritis* occurs early in about 70% to 80% of cases and involves the large joints of the extremities. Arthralgia is seen in most of the remaining patients. The rash of ARF, *erythema marginatum,* is a nonpainful, nonpruritic, evanescent eruption that appears on the trunk and extremities. The rash is salmon-colored with serpiginous borders (smoke-ring-like). Lesions enlarge with central pallor and then disappear. Erythema marginatum is found in fewer than 5% of cases. *Sydenham's chorea* (St. Vitus' dance) is also a relatively uncommon feature of ARF. It is seen several months after the streptococcal infection, which usually has occurred without subsequent arthritic symptoms. Chorea is characterized by purposeless, involuntary movements that disappear with sleep, slurred speech, and emotional lability. The disorder usually clears without residual effects. Freely movable, painless *subcutaneous nodules* are found on extensor surfaces over tendons and over bony prominences such as the occiput. Nodules are found in severe disease, frequently with serious carditis. All of the manifestations just mentioned are seen only in ARF, and no permanent damage occurs. The one exception is Jaccoud's arthritis, which is seen in patients with repeated episodes of rheumatic fever. It is characterized by ulnar deviation and flexion of the metacarpophalangeal joints without pain.

The most important manifestation of ARF is *carditis*. It is the only manifestation that has the potential for causing long-term disability or death. Heart involvement in ARF can be pancarditis, causing an endocarditis, myocarditis, and pericarditis. No cardiac involvement or any combination of cardiac lesions may be present in the patient with ARF. In the absence of pericarditis or congestive heart failure, carditis may be silent. The clinical signs of carditis may include new heart murmur(s) (such as mitral or aortic regurgitation, but not stenosis), cardiac enlargement, congestive heart failure, and pericardial friction rub. Prolongation of the PR interval is frequently found but is not diagnostic of ARF.

DIAGNOSIS. Because there is no specific laboratory test for rheumatic fever and the clinical features are so diverse, the accurate diagnosis of ARF may be difficult. Obviously, the need for a precise diagnosis is critical to prevent subsequent attacks.

To avoid misdiagnosis, the modified criteria of Jones have been used (Table 45-2). However, this system is not foolproof, especially when arthritis is the sole major manifestation present. Thus, in addition to satisfying Jones' criteria, one must be able to verify that there has been a recent streptococcal infection. The latter is best documented either by a history of scarlet fever or antibody evidence of recent experience with group A streptococci, such as elevated ASO, DNase, antihyaluronidase, or positive streptozyme test. A history of recent pharyngitis or a positive throat culture, while suggestive, is not specific. Many patients with ARF give no history of recent sore throat, and the incidence of streptococcal carriage in the general population can be quite high.

COURSE. Acute disease usually subsides within a few weeks, and in most patients evidence of active inflammation is gone in 90 days. Less than 5% of patients may remain ill for 6 months or more. Valvular lesions may heal completely or may progress. In the preantibiotic era, more than 50% of patients had at least one recurrence and the risk of permanent valvular damage became more likely with each new attack. However, if carditis was absent during the initial bout, it was unlikely carditis would develop with recurrences.

MANAGEMENT. The goals of therapy in ARF are to decrease fever and toxicity, alleviate inflammation, and control congestive heart failure. The cornerstones of treatment are salicylates and corticosteroids. However, neither of

Table 45-2. Revised Jones' criteria* for diagnosis of ARF

Major manifestations	Minor manifestations	Supporting evidence
Carditis	Clinical	Elevated streptococcal antibodies
Polyarthritis	Previous rheumatic fever or rheumatic heart disease	Recent scarlet fever
Chorea	Arthralgia	Positive throat culture for group A streptococcus
Erythema marginatum	Fever	
Subcutaneous nodules	Laboratory	
	Elevated erythrocyte sedimentation rate	
	C-reactive protein	
	Leukocytosis	
	Prolonged PR interval	

Adapted from the recommendations of the Rheumatic Fever Committee of The American Heart Association (Circulation **32**:664, 1965).
*The presence of two major criteria, or one major and two minor criteria with supporting evidence of recent group A streptococcal infection, indicates high probability of rheumatic fever. The absence of the latter makes the diagnosis doubtful, except in instances of a long period of latency between infection and symptoms, as with Sydenham's chorea or low-grade carditis.

these agents prevent or modify the development of chronic rheumatic heart disease. Patients with joint manifestations and mild carditis (not congestive heart failure) can be managed with aspirin, 90 to 100 mg/kg/day, with modification of dose to achieve a therapeutic salicylate level. Although the use of steroids remains somewhat controversial, most experts use steroids (the equivalent of 40 to 60 mg/daily of prednisone orally or intravenously) when heart failure is present. The treatment of heart failure does not differ from the management of failure caused by other forms of organic heart disease. Bed rest for 3 weeks is recommended when carditis is absent. The period is extended to 1 month after subsidence of symptoms in mild cases of carditis, and longer periods are recommended when heart failure and cardiac enlargement are present. If streptococci are detected in throat cultures, therapy as for streptococcal pharyngitis should be undertaken.

PREVENTION. Primary prevention consists of eradicating streptococci from the pharynx when the initial infection is detected. Prevention of subsequent bouts of rheumatic fever requires the use of antimicrobial prophylaxis. Clinical studies have indicated that monthly intramuscular benzathine penicillin, 1.2 million units, is the most effective method. Alternate, but less reliable, methods include the use of oral penicillin G, 125 mg twice daily, or sulfisoxazole, 1 g daily or 500 mg daily for small children. When carefully adhered to, antimicrobial prophylaxis is extremely effective in protecting against acquisition of group A streptococci and therefore against rheumatic fever. At one time it was recommended that prophylaxis be continued for life. However, many experts now believe that it is safe to discontinue prophylaxis in adults who do not have intimate contact with school-age children and have not had an attack of rheumatic fever since childhood.

BIBLIOGRAPHY

Baker, C.J., and Kasper, D.L.: Correlation of maternal antibody deficiency with susceptibility to neonatal group B streptococcal infection, N. Engl. J. Med. **294:**752, 1976.

Bisno, A.L., and Ofek, I.: Serologic diagnosis of streptococcal infection: comparison of a rapid hemagglutination technique with conventional antibody tests, Am. J. Dis. Child. **127:**676, 1974.

Kaplan, E.L., and others: Diagnosis of streptococcal pharyngitis: differentiation of active infection from the carrier state in the symptomatic child, J. Infect. Dis. **123:**490, 1971.

Klein, R.S., and others: *Streptococcus bovis* septicemia and carcinoma of the colon, Ann. Intern. Med. **91:**560, 1979.

Lerner, P.I., and others: Group B streptococcus (*S. agalactiae*) bacteremia in adults: analysis of 32 cases and review of the literature, Medicine **56:**457, 1977.

McDonald, E.C., and Weisman, M.H.: Articular manifestations of rheumatic fever in adults, Ann. Intern. Med. **89:**917, 1978.

Murray, H.W., and others: Serious infections caused by *Streptococcus milleri*, Am. J. Med. **64:**759, 1978.

Reinarz, J.A., and Sanford, J.P.: Human infections caused by nongroup A streptococci, Medicine **44:**81, 1965.

Rheumatic Fever Committee, American Heart Association: Prevention of rheumatic fever, Circulation 55-S1, 1977.

Stollerman, G.H.: Rheumatic fever and streptococcal infection, New York, 1975, Grune & Stratton, Inc.

Wannamaker, L.W., and Ferrieri, P.: Streptococcal infections—updated, D.M., October 1975.

Wells, C.R.E.: Rheumatic fever. In Katz, W.A., editor: Rheumatic diseases: diagnosis and management, Philadelphia, 1977, J.B. Lippincott Co.

46 • DISEASES CAUSED BY GRAM-NEGATIVE COCCI

Gonococcal infections

Donald Kaye

DEFINITION AND ETIOLOGY. Gonorrhea is an infection of the mucous membranes of the urethra and genital tract caused by *Neisseria gonorrhoeae*. Involvement of the pharynx and anal canal is common. Infection is almost always the result of sexual contact. After invasion of mucosal sites, gonococci may spread and cause infections such as arthritis, tenosynovitis, perihepatitis, endocarditis, and meningitis.

Primary isolation of the gonococcus is difficult. Chocolate agar or special commercial media must be used. Most strains require an atmosphere of 2% to 10% carbon dioxide.

Thayer-Martin selective medium, containing a mixture of antimicrobials, permits growth of *N. meningitidis* and *N. gonorrhoeae* but inhibits growth of many other bacteria frequently found in specimens from the urethra, cervix, anal canal, and pharynx.

EPIDEMIOLOGY. Although gonorrhea is almost always acquired from sexual contact, exceptions are gonococcal conjunctivitis, which occurs primarily in infants, and vulvovaginitis. Conjunctivitis results either from passage of the infant through an infected genital tract (ophthalmia neonatorum) or from contamination after birth. Vulvovaginitis is an infection of the genital tract of infants and preadolescent girls that results from direct contact with infected adults or, rarely, from contact with contaminated towels or linens.

Repeated attacks of gonorrhea are common; therefore, individual attacks seem to confer little or no immunity. After an episode of acute gonorrhea, *N. gonorrhoeae* may remain in the genital tract for months. Chronic asymptomatic carriers of the gonococcus are important in the epidemiology of gonorrhea because they are difficult to detect and therefore are rarely treated. Most women with gonorrhea are relatively asymptomatic, and 5% to 10% of males with urethral gonorrhea are asymptomatic. It has been estimated that more than 2 million new cases of gonorrhea occur annually in the United States.

PATHOGENESIS AND PATHOLOGY. In males the urethra is

attacked first, resulting in purulent urethritis and involvement of the urethral glands. Direct spread of infection may result in prostatitis, epididymitis, or seminal vesiculitis (all rare). During healing, stricture formation may occur. Gonococcal proctitis in the male is almost always the result of rectal intercourse.

In the female urethritis is mild and transient. Bartholin's and Skene's glands and glands of the cervix may become infected with or without involvement of the urethra. Contiguous spread of infection can cause acute salpingitis, which occurs in about 10% of women. Proctitis may result from contiguous spread or rectal intercourse. Gonococcal salpingitis is usually bilateral and may cause pyosalpinx and formation of a tubo-ovarian abscess. The inflammation tends to heal with fibrosis and adhesions that may produce obstruction of the fallopian tubes and sterility.

Gonococcal infection of the pharynx is common and results from orogenital contact. Gonococcal pharyngeal infection has been demonstrated in up to 20% of homosexual men and 20% of women practicing fellatio who had gonococcal infection at any site.

Occasionally invasion of the blood occurs, and *N. gonorrhoeae* may disseminate and produce infection at distant foci. Joints are the most frequent extragenital sites of localization, but tenosynovitis, endocarditis, meningitis, skin lesions, and infection at other foci may also occur.

Dissemination of gonococcal infection is more common in women than in men and more common in homosexual males than in heterosexual males. The source for dissemination may be the genital trract, rectum, or pharynx.

CLINICAL MANIFESTATIONS

Gonorrhea in the male. The incubation period of gonococcal urethritis in the male is usually 2 to 8 days. There is sudden onset of dysuria, urgency, and frequency associated with mucoid urethral discharge that rapidly becomes purulent and profuse. Gonococcal urethritis usually does not cause fever.

Gonorrhea in the female. The disease may begin in the female with dysuria, urgency, and frequency after an incubation period of 2 to 8 days. However, the urethritis is frequently of short duration and often is mild or completely asymptomatic. Cervicitis gives rise to a mucopurulent discharge. Involvement of Skene's ducts or Bartholin's glands is common. Gonococci can be isolated from the anal canal in 20% to 50% of women with gonorrhea and occasionally can produce symptomatic proctitis. In 5% of women with gonococcal infection only the anorectal culture contains gonococci.

Salpingitis is manifested by acute onset of fever and lower abdominal pain. Physical examination usually reveals lower abdominal tenderness, pain on movement of the cervix, and tenderness of the adnexa (with or without palpable masses).

Extragenital gonococcal infection

Proctitis. Gonococcal proctitis is usually asymptomatic but may be manifested by anal discharge, burning rectal pain, blood and pus in the stools, and pain on defecation.

Pharyngitis. Gonococcal infection in the oropharynx can probably cause symptomatic pharyngitis, tonsillitis, and gingivitis but is usually asymptomatic.

Arthritis. Arthritis, the most common form of clinically recognized disseminated gonococcal infection, usually occurs within 1 to 3 weeks after initial infection in the genital tract or may follow pharyngeal or rectal infection. Onset may be gradual, with migratory polyarthralgias leading to frank arthritis in one or more joints, or it may be sudden, with hot, swollen, and extremely painful joints. Fever and leukocytosis are usually present. More than 75% of patients have polyarthritis. The joints most commonly involved are the knees, ankles, and wrists, but any joint may be affected. *Tenosynovitis,* which is rarely observed in other types of pyogenic arthritis, is common in gonococcal arthritis and most often occurs around the wrists and ankles. The skin lesions associated with gonococcal bacteremia are also frequently present. *N. gonorrhoeae* can be isolated from joint fluid in only 25% to 50% of cases. The fluid ranges from serous to frankly purulent, has the protein content of an exudate, and usually contains increased numbers of leukocytes that are mainly polymorphonuclear.

Gonococcal bacteremia. Gonococcal bacteremia can produce a syndrome with recurrent episodes of fever, skin lesions, tenosynovitis, arthralgia or arthritis, and intermittently positive blood cultures. This syndrome occurs with infection in the genital tract, anal canal, or pharynx, and, if untreated, can recur over months or even years. The rash usually appears during the first day of symptoms and may recur with each episode of fever. The rash is found on the distal part of the extremities and consists of scanty, pinpoint erythematous macules that rapidly become maculopapular, vesiculopustular, and frequently hemorrhagic. Gram-negative cocci can often be seen in stains of fluid from the lesions, but cultures for *N. gonorrhoeae* are usually negative. Immunofluorescent studies on the exudate from the pustules demonstrate *N. gonorrhoeae* in a high percentage of patients.

Perihepatitis (Fitz-Hugh–Curtis syndrome). Perihepatitis, a rare complication in women with gonococcal pelvic inflammatory disease, results from direct spread of gonococci from the pelvis to the upper abdomen. It is manifested by fever, upper quadrant pain (usually right), tenderness and spasm of the abdominal wall, and occasionally a friction rub over the liver. *N. gonorrhoeae* can frequently be found in the cervical or vaginal discharge.

The untreated disease subsides after 1 to 4 weeks, leaving "violin-string" adhesions between the anterior surface of the liver and the anterior abdominal wall.

DIAGNOSIS. In the male the presence of intracellular

gram-negative diplococci in smears of exudate from the urethra is strongly indicative of gonorrhea. Confirmation is obtained by culture or, if available, fluorescent antibody studies. Cultures of the anal canal should be obtained in homosexual males.

In a routine screening cervical cultures will detect the majority of females with asymptomatic gonorrhea. In the female with suspected gonorrhea, cultures of exudate from the cervix and anal canal should be obtained in addition to urethral cultures.

Pharyngeal cultures of *N. gonorrhoeae* should be obtained from homosexual males and females practicing fellatio. In all patients with suspected disseminated gonococcal infections, cultures of the pharynx and anal canal should be obtained in addition to genital tract cultures.

Exudates should be inoculated as soon as possible on Thayer-Martin medium or on a suitable transport medium for *N. gonorrhoeae* such as Transgrow, which is available commercially.

A substantial portion of the cases of urethritis in men in the United States today are nongonococcal. Many of these are caused by *Chlamydia trachomatis* and probably by *Ureaplasma urealyticum*.

Salpingitis. Acute salpingitis must be differentiated from appendicitis and tubal pregnancy. The presence of bilateral tenderness in the adnexa, a history of recent sexual intercourse followed by urethritis or vaginal discharge, and demonstration of gonococci in the cervical exudate are strongly suggestive of gonococcal salpingitis.

Arthritis; bloodborne lesions. Isolation of *N. gonorrhoeae* from the genital tract, rectum, or pharynx is supportive evidence in a patient with suspected disseminated gonococcal infection, and demonstration of gonococci in skin lesions, blood, or joint fluid is confirmatory.

When stains and cultures of joint fluid are negative for gonococci, as found in 50% to 75% of cases, it is frequently difficult to differentiate gonococcal arthritis from Reiter's syndrome (nonbacterial urethritis, conjunctivitis, and arthritis). Urethritis and arthritis in a female suggest gonococcal arthritis because this disease is more common in females, whereas Reiter's syndrome is rare in females. The presence of tenosynovitis and response to antimicrobial therapy strongly imply gonococcal arthritis.

MANAGEMENT. The recommendations of the Venereal Diseases Branch of the Centers for Disease Control for treatment of uncomplicated gonorrhea (urethral, cervical, pharyngeal, or anal canal) or for patients with known exposure to gonorrhea follow: aqueous procaine penicillin, 4.8 million units intramuscularly at one visit (two sites of injection), together with 1 g of oral probenecid; tetracycline hydrochloride, 0.5 g orally four times a day for 5 days; or ampicillin (3.5 g) or amoxicillin (3 g) orally, together with 1 g of probenecid. Patients who are allergic to penicillin should receive tetracycline; such patients who also cannot take tetracycline should receive a single intramuscular injection of 2 g of spectinomycin.

Pharyngeal infection should be treated with the procaine-penicillin or tetracycline regimens because of unacceptable failure rates with ampicillin and spectinomycin. The procaine-penicillin regimen is preferred in men with anorectal infection. All of these regimens except spectinomycin are likely to cure incubating (seronegative) syphilis. The tetracycline regimen will usually prevent postgonococcal urethritis in males.

In pregnancy tetracycline cannot be given, and the procaine-penicillin or the ampicillin or amoxicillin regimens should be used. In the penicillin-allergic, pregnant patient spectinomycin is the agent of choice.

A persistent discharge, despite elimination of gonococci, is frequently caused by nongonococcal (chlamydial) urethritis acquired at the same time as the gonorrhea. To evaluate cure of gonorrhea, a culture should be obtained 7 days after completion of therapy. In homosexual males and in females, anorectal cultures should be obtained as well as cervical cultures.

Patients in whom treatment has failed and those with uncomplicated gonorrhea known or suspected to be caused by a penicillinase-producing gonococcus should be treated with the spectinomycin regimen. Some treatment failures are caused by organisms relatively resistant to penicillin and some by totally resistant gonococci (penicillinase producers). All of these gonococci tend to be relatively resistant to tetracycline. Infection with penicillinase-producing gonococci should be suspected in patients acquiring their infection in the Far East, which is a large reservoir of these organisms. If a penicillinase-producing gonococcus is resistant to spectinomycin, cefoxitin, 2 g intramuscularly, together with probenecid, 1 g orally, can be used.

Gonococcal salpingitis is treated in the hospital with aqueous penicillin G, 20 million units intravenously daily, until improvement, followed by ampicillin, 0.5 g orally four times a day. Alternate therapy is tetracycline, 0.25 g intravenously four times a day until improvement, followed by 0.5 g orally four times a day. Outpatients can receive either tetracycline, 0.5 g orally four times a day, or the procaine penicillin or the ampicillin- or amoxicillin-plus-probenecid regimens for uncomplicated gonorrhea followed by ampicillin or amoxicillin, 0.5 g orally four times a day. Therapy for salpingitis is administered for 10 days.

Epididymitis is treated in a fashion similar to salpingitis. If gonococci are not seen on Gram stain, tetracycline should be used because of the possibility of chlamydial infection.

Gonococcal arthritis or the bacteremia syndrome can be treated with any of the regimens listed for salpingitis, and therapy should be continued for 7 days.

If deep or disseminated infection is caused by penicillinase-producing gonococci, spectinomycin, 2 g intramuscularly twice a day for 3 days, or erythromycin, 0.5 g orally four times a day, can be used.

In gonococcal arthritis pus should be aspirated by needle when possible. With the exception of the hip, open drainage of the joint is rarely necessary. Injection of penicillin into the joint is not indicated.

Serologic tests for syphilis should be performed prior to initiation of therapy in all patients treated for gonococcal infections. If the serologic test is positive, therapy for syphilis must be initiated.

PREVENTION. Use of a condom provides a high degree of protection for the uninfected partner. Sexual partners of patients with gonorrhea should be identified and treated as quickly as possible to prevent further spread of disease.

The instillation of 1% silver nitrate or an antimicrobial drug into the eyes of the newborn has largely eradicated gonococcal ophthalmia neonatorum.

BIBLIOGRAPHY

Blankenship, R.M., Holmes, R.K., and Sanford, S.P.: Treatment of disseminated gonococcal infection, N. Engl. J. Med. **290**:267, 1974.

Culliton, B.J.: Penicillin-resistant gonorrhea: new strain spreading worldwide, Science **194**:1395, 1976.

Danielsson, D., Juhlin, L., and Mardh, P.: Genital infections and their complications, Stockholm, 1975, Almqvist & Wiksell International.

Eschenbach, D.A., and others: Polymicrobial etiology of acute pelvic inflammatory disease, N. Engl. J. Med. **293**:166, 1975.

Handsfield, H.H., Wiesner, P.J., and Holmes, K.K.: Treatment of the gonococcal arthritis-dermatitis syndrome, Ann. Intern. Med. **84**:661, 1976.

Handsfield, H.H., and others: Asymptomatic gonorrhea in men: diagnosis, natural course, prevalence and significance, N. Engl. J. Med. **290**:117, 1974.

Klein, E. J., and others: Anorectal gonococcal infection, Ann. Intern. Med. **86**:340, 1977.

Kraus, S.J.: Incidence and therapy of gonococcal pharyngitis, Sex. Transm. Dis. **25**(suppl.):143, 1979.

McCormack, W.M., and others: Clinical spectrum of gonococcal infection in women, Lancet **1**:1182, 1977.

Wiesner, P.J., and others: Gonococcal diseases, D.M. **26**:1, 1980.

Meningococcal infections

Merle A. Sande and W. Michael Scheld

DEFINITION. The meningococcus is a virulent organism that has been responsible for some of the most notorious epidemics in modern history. Recent studies have advanced our understanding of the spread, immunity, and pathophysiology of the diseases produced by this organism. However, identification of an isolated case of meningococcal disease in the community continues to elicit considerable alarm among medical and lay persons.

Neisseria meningitidis is a gram-negative coccus that is characteristically found in diplococcus form, with flattened adjacent edges producing the so-called biscuit shape. It is easily grown on media enriched with 10% blood or serum and grows best at 95° to 98.6° F (35° to 37° C) in a 5% to 10% CO_2 environment. Chocolate agar in a candle jar serves as an excellent culture environment. This organism is very susceptible to drying or chilling. It is definitively identified by various sugar fermentation steps and a positive "oxidase" reaction.

Meningococci are divided into distinct serogroups on the basis of chemical and antigenic differences in their polysaccharide capsules. Currently recognized types are A, B, C, D, X, Y, Z, W-135, and 29E. A, B, C, and Y account for the majority of human disease.

EPIDEMIOLOGY. The only known reservoir for meningococcus is the human nasopharynx, and carrier rates vary from 2% to 15% in a normal population but increase to 40% when sporadic cases are identified and up to approximately 100% during epidemics. The carrier state lasts for weeks to months; one series had a median of 9.6 months.

The organism probably spreads by the respiratory droplet route, and spread is maximized in crowded environments. Most disease occurs during the late winter and early spring and may follow outbreaks of other respiratory viral infections. Attack rates are highest in children over 6 months of age, with a second peak occurring in adolescence. Close household contacts of index cases have a high attack rate of between 2.5% and 4%. Military recruits are particularly susceptible to epidemics, but in recent years civilian populations in Brazil, Finland, and Alaska have been similarly affected. Alcoholics, especially those living in unhealthy conditions, seem to be especially susceptible.

Historically, most epidemics have been produced by serogroup A; however, in 1963 serogroup B emerged as a predominant pathogen, and in 1969 to 1972 serogroup C was the prevalent epidemic-producing strain. In recent years a shift back toward serogroup B predominance and outbreaks of serogroup Y (mostly of pneumonia) have occurred. The epidemic in Brazil in 1971 began as predominantly group C but changed to group A in 1973 and finally faded out in 1976 after a massive immunization program.

PATHOGENESIS AND IMMUNITY. Meningococcal disease apparently occurs when the organism disseminates from the nasopharynx, producing generalized meningococcemia or metastatic infections in the meninges, joints, heart, pericardium, or skin. The factors that produce dissemination are not understood, but there is no doubt that the presence of bactericidal antibody is a strong deterrent. The peak attack rate of disease occurs in children between 6 and 12 months of age, when antibody titers are at the nadir. In a prospective study of military recruits it was found that only 3 of 54 subjects who developed meningococcal disease had preexisting type-specific bactericidal serum antibody compared to 440 of 550 matched controls who did not develop disease during an epidemic; 38.5% of recruits without antibody who acquired the epidemic strain developed meningococcal disease. These and other studies formed the basis for development of a vaccine containing type A and C polysaccharide, which has successfully aborted epidemics worldwide and has recently nearly eliminated these serogroups from vaccinated military recruits in the United States. Antibody develops naturally approximately 2 weeks following acquisition of the organism in the nasopharynx, and protective cross-reacting antibodies appear following colonization with avirulent, nongroupable *Neisseria* and other related species.

Following dissemination, the organism may produce a number of clinical syndromes, ranging from a transient benign bacteremia to overwhelming meningococcemia with shock. The meningococcus primarily affects blood vessels, with endothelial damage, inflammation, necrosis, thrombosis, and hemorrhage. Thus most involved organs will exhibit evidence of vasculitis. The mediator of these pathologic changes is primarily the lipopolysaccharide endotoxin, similar to that found in gram-negative bacilli. Endotoxin may also directly produce disseminated intravascular coagulation by activation of the clotting cascade. It may also be directly responsible for the pathologic changes in the adrenal glands and kidneys seen in the Waterhouse-Friderichsen syndrome. This process resembles that found in an experimentally induced, generalized Swartzman reaction.

CLINICAL MANIFESTATIONS. Infection confined to the nasopharynx is the most common and is usually asymptomatic, although many patients with meningococcal disease report antecedent nasopharyngitis.

Meningococcemia without meningitis. A mild form of meningococcemia is the most common form of illness. Following a nondescript prodrome with cough, headache, and sore throat, the patient typically develops spiking fever and chills associated with arthralgias and occasionally frank arthritis. Severe muscle pains are common in the back and lower extremities. At least 75% of patients develop rash. Early in the disease the rash may have a pink, macular appearance that disappears within 2 days. Most patients develop the typical petechial rash, which varies in presentation from a few crops, often located on the conjunctiva, wrists, or ankles, to a generalized rash spreading across the trunk and lower body. Ecchymosis may develop and in severe cases can lead to extensive subcutaneous hemorrhage. Vesicular or pustular lesions may appear on a hemorrhagic base. Purpuric lesions with irregular borders have also been described. Gram stains of scrapings of the petechial lesions may reveal the causative organism in 50% to 70% of cases.

Symptoms may regress, remit, or persist as the disease progresses. Diagnosis is definitively established by identification of the organisms on smear or culture from petechiae or blood cultures. Some patients with mild disease spontaneously recover in several weeks.

Approximately 10% to 20% of patients with meningococcemia develop acute fulminant meningococcemia (Waterhouse-Friderichsen syndrome). This condition is usually more abrupt in onset than the milder form and proceeds to severe prostration within hours. Typically, the patient exhibits shaking chills, severe headache, and dizziness associated with severe-orthostatic hypotension; shock rapidly supervenes. Patients are usually vasoconstricted, cyanotic, and pale with cold extremities but may be lucid. Most will exhibit extreme evidence of subcutaneous ecchymosis and bleeding indicative of disseminated intravascular coagulation (DIC). Bleeding around needle puncture sites may be profuse. Untreated, the patients rapidly progress to vascular collapse, with decreased cardiac output, oliguria, congestive heart failure, coma, and death.

Laboratory studies during the course of fulminant meningococcemia may reveal either leukocytosis or leukopenia, and organisms can frequently be seen within polymorphonuclear leukocytes in the peripheral blood (an indication of the high level of bacteremia). A metabolic acidosis with hypoxemia is usually present, and lactate levels are elevated in severe forms of the disease. Measurements of central venous or pulmonary wedge pressures usually reflect a low filling pressure initially, indicative of a decreased effective blood volume. As myocardial failure ensues, the filling pressure will rise without a concomitant increase in cardiac output. Pulmonary edema secondary to cardiac failure or the adult respiratory distress syndrome from endotoxemia or shock can frequently be detected clinically or by roentgenographic examination. Evidence of DIC with an elevated prothrombin time, partial thromboplastin time, and fibrin-split products with a reduced platelet count is common.

Therapy is aimed at correction of the metabolic, electrolyte, cardiovascular, pulmonary, and clotting abnormalities while eliminating the infection with penicillin, 20 million units intravenously daily. Meticulous attention to correction of each abnormality and close continuous monitoring is paramount to success in these extremely ill patients. Shifts in electrolyte and fluid balance occur quicly as the acid-base abnormalities develop, and abnormalities in cardiac function occur. Cardiotonic drugs such as dopamine are frequently necessary to maintain output. Acidosis must be corrected with sodium bicarbonate, which also increases the sodium load. Oxygen should be administered. Heparin may be indicated with fulminant DIC and clinical bleeding, but complications are common. The role of corticosteroids remains controversial. Even with the best of care, mortality is high and necrosis of limbs with gangrene is common in patients who survive.

Meningitis. More than 50% of patients with documented meningococcemia develop infection within the cerebrospinal fluid. The features of meningococcal meningitis are described under ''Bacterial infections of the central nervous system'' in Chapter 40.

Pneumonia. The meningococcus has been recognized as a potential lower respiratory tract pathogen for many years but only in the last decade has the importance of this disease been recognized. Most cases are produced by serogroup Y, and most reported series have originated from military camps. Presentation of the disease is similar to that seen with pneumococcal pneumonia, and since it responds well to penicillin, most cases probably go unrecognized. It is estimated that 1% to 2% of all cases of community-acquired pneumonia may be caused by the meningococcus. There are no typical clinical features that allow distinction between pneumonia caused by *Streptococcus pneumoniae* and that caused by the meningococcus.

COMPLICATIONS

Arthritis. Up to 10% of patients with meningococcemia develop monarticular or polyarticular arthritis. This may be a late occurrence, following the onset of bacteremia by 1 to 2 weeks. Cultures of the synovial fluid are usually sterile, and the pathogenesis of the disease may in part be an immunologic reaction to the organism. The development of arthritis may cause a persistent low-grade fever in the patient who has been adequately treated for his infection. These patients usually respond to recurrent aspirations of the affected joint and treatment with anti-inflammatory drugs.

Pericarditis. Between 5% and 20% of patients with meningococcemia will develop a friction rub and/or ECG evidence of pericarditis late in the course of the disease (up to 20 days after bacteremia). The typical clinical features of pericarditis may be present, with sharp anterior chest pain that changes with the position of the patient. This complication has led to cardiac tamponade.

Myocarditis. Myocarditis develops in the majority of fatal cases of overwhelming meningococcemia and usually occurs within the first or second day of disease. It is manifested by the appearance of cardiomegaly, an S_3 gallop, and increased pulmonary wedge pressure; these may result in congestive heart failure. Although the pathogenesis is unclear, myocarditis probably results from the endotoxemia or associated vasculitis.

MANAGEMENT AND PREVENTION.
Therapy and prevention of meningococcal meningitis are discussed under "Bacterial infections of the central nervous system" in Chapter 40.

BIBLIOGRAPHY

Ansari, B.M., and others: A comparative study of adverse factors in meningococcemia and meningococcal meningitis, Postgrad. Med. J. **55**:780, 1979.

Feldman, H.A.: Meningococcal infections, Adv. Intern. Med. **18**:177, 1972.

Goldschneider, I., and others: Human immunity to the meningococcus. I. The role of humoral antibody, J. Exp. Med. **129**:1307, 1969.

Koppes, G.M., and others: Group Y meningococcal disease in United States Air Force recruits, Am. J. Med. **62**:661, 1977.

Peltola, H., and others: Clinical efficacy of meningococcus group A capsular polysaccharide vaccine in children three months to five years of age, N. Engl. J. Med. **297**:686, 1977.

Pierce, I., and Cooper, E.: Meningococcal pericarditis: clinical features and therapy in five patients, Arch. Intern. Med. **129**:918, 1972.

47 • DISEASES CAUSED BY GRAM-NEGATIVE BACILLI

Haemophilus influenzae infections

Jerome Santoro

DEFINITION. *Haemophilus influenzae* is a small, facultative gram-negative rod that is pathogenic only for man. The organism is an important cause of respiratory and systemic infections in preschool children and occasionally infects adults.

ETIOLOGY. *H. influenzae* is distinguished from other *Haemophilus* species by its aerobic growth requirements for heat-labile nicotinamide-adenine dinucleotide (NAD) (V factor) and heat-stable hematin (X factor). Growth of the organism is accelerated by facilitating the release of these factors from red blood cells in the medium by either using chocolate agar or culturing the organism with *Staphylococcus aureus* (satellism). Growth is also promoted under 10% CO_2 (candle jar). Organisms obtained from agar plates examined by Gram stain are small, uniform gram-negative coccobacilli. However, in smears of clinical specimens the morphology of *H. influenzae* can vary from typical organisms to filamentous forms and even chains. In addition, organisms in stained clinical material may not take up dye properly and be missed.

H. influenzae are found among the upper respiratory tract flora of up to 80% of individuals. Most of these strains are nonencapsulated. Six encapsulated species (A to F) have been recognized. Type B is the most commonly isolated encapsulated strain and is responsible for virtually all cases of serious disease. The capsular polymer of type B contains polyribose ribitol phosphate (PRP), which is antigenically cross-reactive with the cell wall and capsular constituents of certain gram-positive organisms and enteric bacilli.

EPIDEMIOLOGY. Disease caused by *H. influenzae* is worldwide and is endemic among children 3 months to 5 years of age. Epidemiologic data seem to indicate that *H. influenzae* infections are occurring more frequently. Serious infections tend to be more common in certain families and among poor rural populations. Patients with splenectomy, sickle cell anemia, agammaglobulinemia, treated Hodgkin's lymphoma, and alcoholism are also more susceptible to infection.

PATHOGENESIS AND IMMUNITY. *H. influenzae*, usually unencapsulated strains, can cause disease by contiguous spread to respiratory tract structures such as the paranasal sinuses, middle ear, and bronchial tree (as in chronic obstructive pulmonary disease). The events that change asymptomatic infection, or carriage, into disease are not precisely known, but experimental evidence exists supporting a synergistic role for respiratory tract viruses. Bacteremia and deep tissue infections (pneumonia, cellulitis, epiglottitis) are caused solely by encapsulated strains that are virtually always type B. In this regard, the capsule of the organism is thought to protect it from phagocytosis by polymorphonuclear leukocytes, explaining why patients with defects in nonspecific opsonizing ability (splenectomy, sickle cell disease) are prone to infection with type B. However, the reason why type B and not other encapsulated strains tends to cause infection is unknown.

The antibody response to naturally acquired *H. influenzae* infection is complex and variable. Factors such as age, genetic makeup, and type of infection influence the production of one or several antibodies directed against components of the organism, such as PRP, outer membrane antigens, and lipopolysaccharides. These antibodies alone or in combination provide protection against further infection unless events in later life (chemotherapy, splenectomy) again place the individual at risk.

CLINICAL MANIFESTATIONS. Nonencapsulated strains of *H. influenzae* are a relatively frequent cause of otitis media in preschool children and sinusitis and bronchitis in all age groups. The clinical manifestations of these infections are not unique and mimic similar syndromes caused by other bacteria.

Type B organisms are responsible for more serious infections, of which *meningitis* is the most common. The clinical picture is that of typical bacterial meningitis (see discussion of "Bacterial infections of the central nervous system" in Chapter 40), but very young children may have nonspecific symptoms, such as fever, lethargy, and poor feeding. The mortality, despite therapy, is about 5% to 10%, and more than one third of survivors will develop significant neurologic residua. Meningitis may be seen in adults with basilar skull defects, alcoholism, and altered immunocompetence.

Epiglottitis is an extremely serious manifestation of *H. influenzae* infection. The disease begins with fever, malaise, and severe dysphagia, frequently without obvious pharyngitis or external swelling. This is followed by anxiety, evidence of upper airway obstruction, and drooling from inability to swallow oral secretions. Direct visualization of the epiglottis, which should only be done in the process of placing an airway, reveals a swollen and inflamed "cherry-red" structure.

Pneumonia caused by *H. influenzae* may be bronchial or lobar. Children with haemophilus pneumonia may develop empyema or pericarditis. *H. influenzae* is being recognized with greater frequency as a cause of pneumonia in elderly adults who may have underlying pulmonary disease or alcoholism.

H. influenzae cellulitis in children usually occurs on the cheek or the periorbital area and is characterized by a bluish hue. *H. influenzae bacteremia* may complicate pneumonia, epiglottitis, and cellulitis or occur without an obvious source in compromised individuals. Presumably, transient bacteremia (either symptomatic or asymptomatic) can lead to *septic arthritis* and less commonly *osteomyelitis*, as well as *bacterial endocardtis*.

DIAGNOSIS. Diagnosis of *H. influenzae* infection is most readily established with the acquisition of body fluids (spinal, pleural, joint) for Gram stain and subsequent cultures. Obviously isolation of the organism from blood is also diagnostic. Epiglottitis and facial cellulitis are distinctive enough to be diagnosed without culture confirmation. However, blood cultures may be positive in these two entities, and organisms can sometimes be isolated from an aspirate of the cellulitic margin. When Gram stains are negative or equivocal, the detection of PRP in cerebrospinal fluid, blood, and urine by various methods has proved useful in early diagnosis of haemophilus disease. However, as previously mentioned, PRP may cross-react with other bacterial antigens and false positive results, although infrequent, may occur. The diagnosis of *H. influenzae* pneumonia in adults without bacteremia may depend on the sputum Gram stain, since the presence or absence of organisms in the sputum culture is not helpful.

MANAGEMENT. The treatment of serious systemic *H. influenzae* infection has been complicated in recent years by the emergence of strains that produce β-lactamase and are thereby resistant to ampicillin. The incidence of resistance varies geographically and approaches 5% to 25% in some areas. Until the etiologic organism is shown to be sensitive to ampicillin, serious systemic illness caused by *H. influenzae* should be treated with chloramphenicol, 100 mg/kg/day intravenously in four divided doses at 6-hour intervals. Some experts recommend that ampicillin, 200 to 400 mg/kg/day intravenously in six divided doses at 4-hour intervals, be used initially as well. When the infecting strain is found to be sensitive to ampicillin, chloramphenicol is discontinued and ampicillin is either started or continued. Chloramphenicol is used alone for a full course when the patient is allergic to penicillin. Treatment is continued for 10 to 14 days when meningitis is present. The length of therapy for other syndromes is dictated by the clinical response or the disease process; for example, longer courses will be required for endocarditis or osteomyelitis. Oral ampicllin or amoxicillin or trimethorprim-sulfamethoxazole is used for ambulatory therapy of less serious disease. Because of the problem of β-lactamase production, it is reasonable to use trimethoprim-sulfamethoxazole as initial therapy. Other measures, such as drainage of empyema fluid, arthrocentesis for joint infection, maintenance of a patent airway in epiglottitis, and supportive care for patients with meningitis, are of obvious but paramount importance.

PREVENTION. Attempts at preventing *H. influenzae* infection with a vaccine composed of PRP have not been successful in children less than 18 months of age—those most frequently affected by these infections. New vaccines and nonvirulent bacteria with antigens that cross-react with the type B capsule are being evaluated experimentally. Rifampin has been used to eliminate the carrier state in intimate contacts of children with *H. influenzae* type B meningitis.

Pertussis (whooping cough)
Jerome Santoro

DEFINITION. Whooping cough is an acute respiratory tract infection that is seen primarily in infants and young children. The illness is characterized by paroxysms of cough followed by prolonged inspiratory stridor.

ETIOLOGY. The genus *Bordetella* is made up of three species: *B. pertussis, B. parapertussis,* and *B. bronchiseptica.* The latter organism causes infection in animals but rarely in man. *B. pertussis* and *B. parapertussis* are minute, gram-negative coccobacilli that have complex growth requirements that are met by Bordet-Gengou culture medium. These organisms were at one time classified with *Haemophilus* species, but the *Bordetella* group has no strict requirement for X and V factors and is antigenically distinct. Primary isolates of *B. pertussis* will not grow on conventional media, are designated phase I or S organisms, and are virulent. With passage, organisms can be induced to grow on standard media and change through phases II, III, and IV or R. Each phase is less virulent and only killed phase I organisms can be used as immunizing agents. *B. parapertussis* occasionally causes disease in man that is generally milder than that caused by *B. pertussis*.

EPIDEMIOLOGY. Pertussis is a disease of infants and young children with worldwide distribution. It is spread by droplet nuclei and has an attack rate of 70% to 90%. Among nonimmune populations, neither disease nor immunization produces lifelong protection and disease can be seen in adults. The incidence of pertussis, about 3000 cases a year in the United States, has fallen greatly because of several factors, such as improved living conditions and, most importantly, vaccination. The mortality rate has also dropped, probably as a result of better supportive care. The majority of deaths, about 70%, occur in individuals less than 1 year of age, and most of these are children less than 6 months of age.

PATHOLOGY AND PATHOGENESIS. Killed phase I organisms cause histamine and serotonin sensitivity and increased susceptibility to anaphylaxis, encephalomyelitis, lymphocytosis, and other effects when injected into animals. The significance of these properties is not clear in human carriers of the disease. *B. pertussis* attaches to the epithelium of the bronchi and bronchioles, where it multiples but does not invade the lung tissue or blood. Local bronchial and peribronchial inflammation with inspissation of mucus and debris results in atelectasis, localized emphysema, and interstitial pneumonitis. These effects can be extremely devastating in infants and children because of their small airways. Proposed mechanisms for the neurologic manifestations of pertussis are hypoxia from respiratory disease or the action of a bacterial neurotoxin.

CLINICAL MANIFESTATIONS. Illness begins after an incubation period of 7 to 10 days. Pertussis has classically been divided into three clinical phases: catarrhal, paroxysmal, and convalescent.

The catarrhal stage is characterized by nonspecific symptoms resembling a typical viral upper respiratory infection. Symptoms include malaise, anorexia, rhinorrhea and sneezing, conjunctivitis, and sometimes mild fever. During this stage the disease is highly contagious. Late in the catarrhal stage a nonproductive cough appears and a lymphocytosis is first noted.

After 1 to 2 weeks the paroxysmal stage begins. At this time the illness is characterized by as many as 40 to 50 periods of severe coughing daily. During paroxysms there may be venous engorgement and even cyanosis. The paroxysm is terminated by air drawn in forcibly through the glottis—the whoop. The whoop is often followed by vomiting, which is said to aid in the removal of the thick, tenacious mucus. Between paroxysms the patient is quiet but apprehensive. Fever is absent but lymphocytic leukocytosis is present, with counts as high as 100,000 consisting almost totally of small, typical lymphocytes. When fever and polymorphonuclear leukocytosis are present, bacterial superinfection should be suspected.

The convalescent stage begins within 4 weeks, when the frequency and severity of paroxysms decrease. Interestingly, patients experiencing respiratory tract infections several months after a bout of pertussis may again have symptoms similar to whooping cough.

The possible complications of pertussis are legion. Small children develop dehydration, malnutrition, and electrolyte and acid-base disturbances from vomiting and inability to eat or drink. Rarely, cerebral complications such as seizures and hemorrhage can result from anoxia or perhaps from elevated venous pressure. Epistaxis, petechiae, and scleral and conjunctival hemorrhages with periorbital edema are common. In the lung atelectasis and localized emphysema are frequently found; pneumothorax and pneumomediastinum are less commonly seen. Secondary bacterial otitis media occasionally occurs. The major causes of death in pertussis are bacterial superinfection of the lung and probably neurologic complications. Residual bronchiectasis is now less common, perhaps because of the availability of effective antimicrobial agents.

LABORATORY FINDINGS AND DIAGNOSIS. Unfortunately, because of the nonspecific findings, pertussis is very difficult to diagnose in the catarrhal stage, when it is most contagious and when the pending paroxysmal phase could possibly be modified. The differential diagnosis of whooping cough in the paroxysmal stage includes viral tracheobronchitis, *Mycoplasma pneumoniae* infection, and in infants chlamydial pneumonia. A syndrome caused by adenovirus that is very similar to pertussis has been described. When present, the marked lymphocytosis previously described is helpful in differentiating these syndromes.

B. pertussis and *B. parapertussis* can be cultured by immediately plating material obtained by nasopharyngeal swab onto Bordet-Gengou medium containing penicillin. The yield is 80% to 90% during the catarrhal stage but 50% or less in the paroxysmal stage. Cough plates have been abandoned because the yield is too low. A fluorescent antibody test can detect *B. pertussis* in nasopharyngeal smears but has a very high false positive rate. The test is perhaps more helpful in rapidly identifying organisms already isolated. Serologic tests are of little value.

MANAGEMENT. Treatment of pertussis with antimicrobial agents in the catarrhal stage can decrease and shorten the severity of the paroxysmal stage. However, initiation of therapy in the paroxysmal stage has no effect. Nevertheless, antimicrobial therapy is justified to prevent spread of infection. The drug of choice is erythromycin, 50 mg/kg daily in children and 2 g daily in adults in four divided doses for 5 to 10 days. Corticosteroids equivalent to hydrocortisone, 30 mg/kg/24 hours for 2 days, have been shown to shorten the duration and severity of the illness even when begun in the paroxysmal state. However, it is probably wise to reserve this therapy for severe cases. Hyperimmune human globulin is available but is not recommended routinely. Its use in severely ill infants and small children remains controversial.

Supportive therapy in the form of good nursing care, proper fluid and electrolyte balance, maintenance of adequate nutrition, and antimicrobial therapy of superinfection is of paramount importance, especially among the very young.

PREVENTION. Susceptible individuals who are exposed to pertussis should receive erythromycin for a few days as prophylaxis. Those less than 4 years old should be given booster doses of vaccine. Pertussis vaccine is generally not administered to individuals over 6 years of age because of the high risk of side effects, but small doses have been given to adults, such as hospital personnel, without much difficulty. Active immunization is begun at 6 to 12 weeks of age, in combination with alum-precipitated diphtheria and tetanus toxoid vaccines (DPT). The dose is repeated twice at 1-to 2-month intervals and again at 1 and 5 years of age. Vaccine does not confer complete or prolonged immunity, and after 10 years most individuals are again susceptible to disease. Because of this and documented outbreaks among adults, immunization practices may have to be reevaluated in the future.

BIBLIOGRAPHY
Haemophilus influenzae infections

American Academy of Pediatrics Committee on Infectious Diseases: Ampicillin-resistant strains of *Hemophilus influenzae* type B, Pediatrics **55**:145, 1975.

Norden, C.W.: *Hemophilus influenzae* infections in adults, Med. Clin. North Am. **62**:1037, 1978.
Todd, J.K., and Bruhn, F.W.: Severe *Haemophilus influenzae* infections, Am. J. Dis. Child. **129**:607, 1975.

Pertussis

Bassili, W.R., and Stewart, G.T.: Epidemiological evaluation of immunisation and other factors in the control of whooping cough, Lancet **1**:471, 1976.
Olson, L.C.: Pertussis, Medicine **54**:427, 1975.

Donovanosis (granuloma inguinale)
Michael F. Rein

Donovanosis, also referred to as granuloma inguinale, is a sexually transmitted infection caused by *Calymmatobacterium granulomatis,* a gram-negative bacterium possibly related to *Klebsiella* that can be cultured only with great difficulty. Fewer than 50 infections are reported annually in the United States, but the disease is prevalent in New Guinea, India, and parts of Australia, Africa, and South America. Infectivity is low, and prolonged or repeated contact may be necessary for transmission of the infection. About 50% of patients will have symptoms within 4 weeks of infection, but incubation periods of 3 months have been reported. The initial lesion is a papule, which erodes to form a gradually enlarging ulcer, usually in the genital area. A typical lesion has a heaped-up edge and a base consisting of beefy granulation tissue that becomes exuberantly hypertrophic in about 20% of patients. Extensive destruction of involved sites may result if treatment is delayed. Lesions have occurred in the mouth following orogenital contact. Infection may spread by autoinoculation, via the lymphatics to form subcutaneous granulomas in the groin, or, rarely, via the bloodstream to bone or the liver. The organism multiplies within host macrophages. Biopsy shows an infiltrate with polymorphonuclear neutrophils and macrophages and the capillary proliferation typical of granulation tissue. Diagnosis is best made by crushing a small biopsy specimen between glass slides. Wright's stain will reveal macrophages loaded with the organisms (Donovan bodies) in about 80% of cases, but the usual H and E sections are positive less than 10% of the time. Oral treatment with tetracycline, 500 mg four times a day, is generally successful, and gentamicin or chloramphenicol has also been used. Some studies have suggested an association between donovanosis and the subsequent development of genital carcinoma.

Chancroid
Michael F. Rein

Chancroid is a sexually transmitted infection caused by *Haemophilus ducreyi.* The disease is relatively rare in the United States but is much more prevalent in the Far East.

Although the incubation period may range from 24 hours to 3 weeks, symptoms generally develop 2 to 5 days after infection. Symptomatic infections are 10 times more common in men than in women. The initial lesion is a papule, which becomes pustular and then ulcerated and painful. About 70% of patients have a single ulcer at the time they seek medical attention, but multiple ulcerations are characteristic of untreated disease. These ulcers may vary considerably in size, which differentiates them from those of herpes genitalis, which are usually rather uniform. The ulcers are ragged with an undermined edge and a necrotic base. They have an erythematous border, but induration is unusual and should suggest a diagnosis of syphilis. Lesions may develop on the thighs by autoinoculation from lesions on the penis. About 1 week following the appearance of skin lesions, 25% to 60% of patients develop tender inguinal adenopathy, usually unilateral, with periadenitis and some erythema of the overlying skin. If untreated, these nodes become fluctuant and may rupture. The disease is usually diagnosed clinically, but care should be taken to avoid confusion with herpes genitalis, which is many times more common in the United States and also is seen as multiple, painful, genital ulcerations. A smear from the undermined edge of a lesion may reveal chains of gram-negative streptobacilli but will be negative in at least 30% of cases. The organism is cultured with difficulty from a lesion or an aspirate of the enlarged inguinal nodes. Treatment with sulfisoxazole, 1 g orally four times daily, or tetracycline, 500 mg orally four times daily, for 10 days is usually successful, but aminoglycosides or cephalosporins have been required for some resistant cases reported in the Far East.

BIBLIOGRAPHY
Donovanosis
Maddocks, I., Anders, E.M., and Dennis, E.: Donovanosis in Papua, New Guinea, Br. J. Vener. Dis. **52**:190, 1976.
Rao, M.S., and others: Oral lesions of granuloma inguinale, J. Oral Surg. **34**:1112, 1976.

Chancroid
Gaisin, A., and Heaton, C.L.: Chancroid: alias the soft chancre, Int. J. Dermatol. **14**:188, 1975.

Gram-negative bacillary bacteremia
George A. Poporad and Jaime Carrizosa

Bacteremia caused by gram-negative bacilli has been found with increasing frequency in the adult hospital population and accounts for many of the hospital-acquired (nosocomial) infections. An episode of bacteremia may be asymptomatic or may occur as a syndrome of sepsis in which the patient appears toxic, generally with fever and rigors. Shock and death may be the ultimate outcome in a high proportion of patients.

ETIOLOGY. Between 70% and 90% of gram-negative bacillary (GNB) bacteremias are nosocomial. The typical setting involves an elderly hospitalized patient with an underlying disease that predisposes him to bacteremic episodes.

The genitourinary tract is the most common source of bacteremia (60% of patients). Common predisposing factors are urinary tract obstruction, instrumentation, surgery, and an indwelling urinary catheter. The female genital tract can be a source following delivery, abortion, or gynecologic surgery. In approximately 25% of the cases of bacteremia the gastrointestinal tract is implicated as the source, usually in patients who have had some insult to their bowel integrity. Common predisposing factors are surgery, bowel obstruction or infarction, and neoplasms. Acute intra-abdominal infections, such as diverticulitis, appendicitis, cholecystitis, and infection following penetrating abdominal wounds, are also common clinical settings. In 5% of cases the skin appears to be the source of bacteremia. Common predisposing factors are operative wound infections, indwelling vascular catheters, and extensive damage to the skin, as in burns or exfoliative dermatitis. When these occur, the damaged skin becomes rapidly colonized with gram-negative organisms that may gain access to the bloodstream.

The respiratory tract is not a common source of GNB bacteremia. However, in cases of pneumonia secondary to contaminated aerosols or in patients with infected tracheostomies, GNB bacteremia may occur.

Certain systemic diseases are often associated with bacteremia. Patients with hematologic malignancies (leukemia, lymphoma, multiple myeloma) or agranulocytosis or patients receiving corticosteroids show alterations of host defense mechanisms, predisposing them to the development of GNB bacteremia. Patients with diabetes mellitus and severe liver disease also appear to have significant predisposition to GNB bacteremia.

The most common organisms responsible for bacteremia belong to the family Enterobacteriaceae. This is expected because this group of organisms makes up an important part of the bowel flora and is the major cause of urinary tract infections. *Escherichia coli* accounts for about 40% of the infections. *Klebsiella-Enterobacter* and *Proteus* species follow in importance. *Bacteroides fragilis*, a gram-negative anaerobic rod and a predominant organism in bowel flora, is becoming increasingly important as a cause of bacteremia. Bacteremia caused by *Pseudomonas* species has increased because of increasing numbers of leukopenic patients. *Pseudomonas* bacteremia rarely occurs in the absence of leukopenia (<1000 mature polymorphonuclear leukocytes/mm^3), or denudation of the skin, as in burns or exfoliative dermatitis.

PATHOGENESIS OF SEPTIC SHOCK. The pathophysiology of shock resulting from GNB bacteremia is not completely understood. The basic phenomena seen in bacteremia and subsequent shock appear to be related to the toxic effects of endotoxin, a complex lipopolysaccharide that is part of the bacterial cell wall of gram-negative bacilli. However, gram-positive organisms and fungi that lack endotoxin are also able to produce the septic shock syndrome; therefore, other mechanisms play a role in infections with these organisms. The effects of endotoxin include fever, major hemodynamic changes secondary to release of vasoactive amines, and direct cellular injury. These effects are mediated through the activation of several interrelated systems: the complement system, the coagulation system, the fibrinolytic system, and the kinin system. The hemodynamic consequences follow a pattern of an initial decrease in peripheral resistance, probably because of arteriovenous shunting. There is also peripheral pooling in the capillary beds. Cardiac output increases to maintain the blood pressure. The central and pulmonary venous pressures are low because of decreased venous return to the right side of the heart. As pooling increases and venous return to the heart decreases, the blood pressure drops secondary to decreased cardiac output. Later in the shock syndrome stagnant anoxia in the capillary cells causes release of lysozomal enzymes that, together with endotoxin, cause cell damage, resulting in leakage of plasma into the interstitial spaces. The blood pressure drops further and vasoconstriction leads to increased peripheral resistance. When the syndrome reaches this stage, the shock is usually irreversible.

Disseminated intravascular coagulation (DIC) may accompany the shock syndrome. Endotoxin activates the coagulation system by its activity on platelets and Hageman factor (factor XII). In intravascular coagulation there is consumption of clotting factors II, V, and VIII, fibrinogen, and platelets. Deposition of fibrin thrombi in capillaries is important in the pathogenesis of the adult respiratory distress syndrome and of renal failure during sepsis.

Endotoxin can activate the alternate complement pathway with subsequent granulocyte aggregation by C5a. Leukoembolization of these aggregates to the lungs can result in pulmonary endothelial damage. The lung is also susceptible to the direct effect of endotoxin, resulting in endothelial damage, capillary thrombosis, and leakage of plasma. Clinical manifestations of lung damage are severe hypoxia and pulmonary edmema.

DIAGNOSIS. GNB bacteremia is a clinical diagnosis that should be considered in febrile patients with a known predisposing condition.

Classically, the onset of bacteremia is usually manifested by a shaking chill preceding the fever spike. The temperature usually ranges from 101° to 105° F (37.2° to 40.5° C). Sepsis, however, may be manifested as circulatory collapse or shock in 20% to 30% of patients; in some, especially the elderly or debilitated, fever may be absent. Patients receiving steroids, patients with renal failure, and those who are in deep shock may be hypothermic. Patients with the syndrome of sepsis are generally restless, apprehensive, disoriented, tachypneic, and tachycardic. The shock syndrome can initially be "warm shock" (with warm, dry hands), reflecting early hemodynamic alterations producing vasodilation and decreased peripheral resistance, or "cold shock" (with cold, clammy hands), reflecting a stage characterized by intense vasoconstriction. When the initial manifestation is warm shock, progression to cold shock follows unless therapy is initiated. When the shock progresses, increasing mental confusion, oliguria and anuria, and respiratory distress with cyanosis develop.

Laboratory abnormalities include initial leukopenia followed by leukocytosis with neutrophilia. Continuing leukopenia may be associated with overwhelming sepsis. Initially, arterial blood gases show a respiratory alkalosis associated with tachypnea and hyperventilation. Subsequently, metabolic acidosis and hypoxia supervene. No roentgenographic changes in the chest are seen in initial stages of shock, but in the later stages a pattern typical of pulmonary edema ("shock lung") may develop.

Leukopenic patients with GNB bacteremia, particularly with *Pseudomonas* infection, may develop the skin lesions of ecthyma gangrenosum. This is a tender vesicle that ulcerates and becomes necrotic. The pathogenesis is bacterial invasion of blood vessel walls with thrombosis. Cultures of the lesions are positive.

MANAGEMENT. In patients suspected of having GNB bacteremia, blood cultures, both aerobic and anaerobic, should be obtained. Changes in the stage of consciousness, blood pressure, and hourly urine output allow proper assessment of perfusion to vital organs. An alert sensorium, a stable blood pressure, and a urine output of 30 ml an hour indicate adequate perfusion. Measurements of the central venous or pulmonary wedge pressures permit assessment of intravascular fluid volume and cardiac performance and alert to possible heart failure. Arterial blood gases are necessary for the evaluation of the respiratory and metabolic status of the patient. Determinations of the serum creatinine measure renal function. Evaluation of possible coagulation abnormalities include measurements of the platelet count, prothrombin time, partial thromboplastin time, fibrinogen level, and fibrin split products.

The first priority in the treatment of septic shock is the restoration and expansion of the blood volume. This is accomplished by the rapid infusion of blood, normal saline, dextran, or any other volume expander to raise the blood pressure and increase tissue perfusion. Rapid volume expansion should be continued until the central venous pressure reaches 12 cm H_2O or the pulmonary wedge pressure rises to 18 mm Hg. If these pressures rise or are elevated from the start and hypotension persists, dopamine is indicated.

Administration of dopamine results in increases in cardiac output, blood pressure, and urine output. Thus infusion of dopamine is titrated upward until the desired hemodynamic and renal responses are obtained. It is recommended that low infusion rates (2 to 5 µg/kg/min intravenously) be used as initial therapy in patients with moderate hypotension and oliguria. In patients with more severe degrees of shock it may be necessary to start at higher initial doses. Most patients, however, respond to rates less than 20 µg/kg/min. Doses greater than 40 µg/kg/min produce vasoconstriction and are to be avoided if possible. Since dopamine and other sympathomimetic drugs do not exert their full effect in the presence of acidosis, hypoxia and acidosis must be corrected.

Specific antibiotic therapy depends on the evaluation of the most likely etiologic microorganism. Initial examination of the patient and review of the laboratory studies may suggest the source of the infection and the identity of the bacteria. The aminoglycoside antibiotics provide the most extensive coverage of the possible etiologic organisms. The aminoglycosides, however, are unreliable in terms of achieving antibacterial serum and tissue levels and are not active against pneumococci and streptococci, which can also produce a syndrome indistinguishable from GNB bactermia. Thus a cephalosporin antibiotic or ampicillin is usually added to the aminoglycoside. The aminoglycosides gentamicin or tobramycin, 1.7 mg/kg every 8 hours intramuscularly or intravenously, and cephalothin or ampicillin, 2 g intravenously every 4 hours, are drugs typically administered. Amikacin, 7.5 mg/kg every 12 hours, is used as the aminoglycoside in hospitals where gentamicin-resistant gram-negative bacilli commonly cause infection. Cefazolin, 1 to 2 g every 6 hours, may be used instead of cephalothin. Third-generation cephalosporins such as cefotaxime, moxalactam, and cefoperazone are useful when infecting organisms are resistant to older cephalosporins. Further studies may indicate that these agents can be used alone (without aminoglycosides) in the initial treatment of GNB bacteremia.

When an intra-abdominal or pelvic source is likely, coverage for anaerobic gram-negative rods *(Bacteroides fragilis)* is necessary and the addition of clindamycin, 600 mg intravenously every 8 hours, is recommended. In patients with significant neutropenia (<1000 mature polymorphonuclear leukocytes/mm^3) or extensive burns, *Pseudomonas* bacteremia should be suspected and carbenicillin or ticarcillin, 500 mg/kg/day intravenously in divided doses every 4 hours, is added to the aminoglycoside rather than a cephalosporin or ampicillin. Mezlocillin or piperacillin will probably replace carbenicillin and ticarcillin in this situation. Following identification and sensitivity studies of the pathogen, antibiotic coverage is appropriately tailored and continued for at least 7 to 10 days.

The role of steroids in the treatment of septic shock remains controversial. Animal studies indicate that steroids in high doses improve the cardiac index and perfusion in the microcirculation. They have recently been shown to be of benefit in preventing the pulmonary manifestations of "shock lung" by preventing leukoagglutination in the lung. If steroids are to be used, pharmacologic doses are necessary; methyl prednisolone, in an intravenous bolus of 30 mg/kg, is recommended.

Recently naloxone, an opiate antagonist, has been shown to increase systolic blood pressure and improve mental status in bacteremic hypotensive patients. Presumably, endogenous opiates (endorphins) are released during the stress of bacteremia and contribute to the hypotension. Naloxone appears to reverse this effect in some patients.

Leukocyte transfusions may be helpful in leukopenic patients with bacteremia not responding to antibiotic therapy. Heparin therapy is rarely indicated as treatment for DIC. The key to therapy of the DIC is elimination of shock.

PROGNOSIS. The prognosis is related to the infecting organism (such as a higher mortality rate with *Pseudomonas aeruginosa* than with *E. coli*), whether or not shock develops, and the underlying disease. With rapidly fatal diseases such as acute leukemia the mortality is much higher than with nonfatal diseases such as bacteremia after prostatectomy.

PREVENTION. In view of the high mortality associated with GNB bacteremia, special consideration should be given to its prevention. Potential causes of infection are the urinary catheter, the intravenous catheter, and contaminated respiratory equipment. Indwelling urinary catheters should be avoided if possible, and if they are necessary, sterile drainage systems should be used. Intravascular catheters should also be avoided; if they are essential, they should be handled aseptically and removed as soon as possible, certainly within 48 hours. Respiratory equipment should be cleaned daily and nebulization reservoirs sterilized each day.

BIBLIOGRAPHY

Christy, J.H.: Treatment of gram negative shock, Am. J. Med. **50:**77, 1971.

Jacob, H.S., and others: Complement-induced granulocyte aggregation, an unsuspected mechanism of disease, N. Engl. J. Med. **302:**789, 1980.

McHenry, M.C., and Hawk, W.A.: Bacteremia caused by gram negative bacilli, Med. Clin. North Am. **58:**623, 1974.

Peters, W.P., and others: Pressor effect of naloxone in septic shock, Lancet, **1:**529, 1981.

Schumer, W.: Steroids in the treatment of clinical septic shock, Ann. Surg. **184:**333, 1976.

Winslow, E.J., and others: Hemodynamic studies and results of therapy in fifty patients with bacteremic shock, Am. J. Med. **54:**421, 1973.

Young, L.S., and others: Gram negative rod bacteremia: microbiologic, immunologic and therapeutic considerations, Ann. Intern. Med. **86:**456, 1977.

Plague

Elias Abrutyn

DEFINITION. Plague, an endemic and epidemic infection of animals, is occasionally transmitted to man, most commonly causing bubonic plague but also septicemia, meningitis, and pneumonia.

ETIOLOGY. *Yersinia pestis,* formerly *Pasteurella pestis,* is a pleomorphic, aerobic, nonmotile, nonsporeforming gram-negative rod that grows well, but slowly, on most culture media. The characteristic bipolar or safety-pin appearance is best demonstrated with Wayson's or Giemsa stain; the Gram stain is less reliable. Virulence, although not completely understood, appears in part related to a lipopolysaccharide endotoxin and to a capsular antigen that inhibits phagocytosis.

EPIDEMIOLOGY. Infected wild rodents and mammals (sylvatic plague) form a large, usually inapparent natural reservoir of infection. Transmission is maintained primarily by infected fleas, and spread of fleas to the domestic rat (urban or rat plague) provides the setting for major outbreaks of human disease. Plague in humans is acquired from the bite of an infected flea or by direct contact with contaminated animal tissues. Nonreservoir hosts such as dogs, cats, and other carnivores have also been implicated as an occasional source for human infection. Asymptomatic pharyngeal carriage in man has been reported, but its role in transmission is unknown.

In the United States animal plague is prevalent in the 15 western states, and human plague is reported most frequently in New Mexico, Arizona, Colorado, and Utah. During the summer months cases are usually related to fleas, whereas during the winter cases are usually related to hunting and direct contact. Rat plague has been virtually eliminated in the United States.

PATHOGENESIS AND PATHOLOGY. During feeding, fleas whose foregut has been blocked by a mass of organisms regurgitate thousands of bacteria into the host. The bacilli travel via the lymphatics to the regional lymph nodes, where they multiply. The nodes become hyperplastic, necrotic, and contain masses of bacteria; edema with or without hemorrhage surrounds the involved nodes. Although polymorphonuclear leukocytes ingest and kill the bacteria, the organisms survive in monocytes and elaborate a capsule that enables them to resist further phagocytosis. Bacteremia commonly occurs and can result in metastatic infection, including involvement of the meninges and lungs.

CLINICAL MANIFESTATIONS. The incubation period for bubonic plague is 2 to 6 days. Fever, constitutional symptoms, and excruciatingly painful lymphadenopathy (bubo) are characteristic. In descending order of frequency, the nodes involved are the inguinal-femoral, axillary, cervical, and epitrochlear; multiple areas of nodal involvement occasionally occur. Rarely, a pustule or papule develops at the flea bite site. Septicemic plague differs from bubonic plague in that nodal involvement is not apparent. Bacteremia, which can complicate either form, may result in meningitis or pneumonia (secondary plague pneumonia). The latter complication has special public health significance because such infected persons may be the source for airborne spread of pneumonia to contacts (primary plague pneumonia), resulting in a highly contagious, fulminant, often fatal disease. Untreated patients may develop shock, convulsions, and disseminated intravascular coagulation with bleeding or necrosis of peripheral tissues.

DIAGNOSIS. The disease needs to be differentiated from other causes of regional lymphadenitis, and a diagnosis is most readily made in persons who have had known contact with infected animals or their ectoparasites. Fluid from buboes, blood, and other body fluids should be stained, examined microscopically, and cultured. Material stained using the fluorescent antibody technique may provide a rapid presumptive diagnosis verified by culture, phage lysis, agglutination tests, and animal inoculation. Specific antibody may be detected in convalescent-phase serum, but serologic tests are not diagnostic during the acute phase.

MANAGEMENT. Streptomycin and tetracycline are preferred in drug therapy against plague. Streptomycin, 30 mg/kg/day in divided doses, or tetracycline, 30 to 50 mg/kg/day in divided doses, should be administered for 7 to 10 days. Chloramphenicol is highly active and is the preferred agent for treating meningitis and pregnant women. Trimethoprim-sulfamethoxazole, kanamycin, and sulfonamides have also been effective.

PROGNOSIS. When treated, bubonic plague has an excellent prognosis. The other forms respond well if recognized and treated early, but positive blood cultures or bacilli on blood smears are bad prognostic signs.

PREVENTION. Control measures include education of persons in endemic areas, surveillance for plague activity in reservoir animals or carnivores, rat control, and immunization of persons at high risk of exposure. Chemoprophylaxis may be indicated for contacts of patients with plague pneumonia and for household contacts of cases acquired from fleas and consists of tetracycline, 1 g daily, or sulfadiazine, 2 to 3 g daily, for 7 days. Quarantine may be necessary and strict isolation procedures are mandatory for hospitalized patients.

BIBLIOGRAPHY

Reed, W.P., and others: Bubonic plague in the Southwestern United States: a review of recent experience, Medicine **49**:465, 1970.

Tularemia

Oksana M. Korzeniowski

DEFINITION. Tularemia is a zoonotic bacterial infection acquired by man from mammals or arthropods. The various portals of entry determine the clinical variant of the disease.

ETIOLOGY. *Francisella tularensis* is a nonmotile, pleomorphic gram-negative rod. It does not grow on routine culture media, but aerobic cultivation on blood glucose-cystine agar yields colonies in 2 to 4 days. Two antigenically identical variants differing in a few biochemical reactions and in virulence for man and rabbits have been identified.

EPIDEMIOLOGY. Tularemia occurs in the Northern Hemisphere: America, Europe, and Asia. Many species of wild and domestic mammals, birds, amphibians, and arthropods harbor the organism. In the United States the main reservoirs are rabbits, hares, and ticks found in Arkansas, Illinois, Tennessee, Missouri, Texas, and Virginia. Man is highly susceptible to infection and acquires the disease through skin contact with tissues or body fluids of infected animals, arthropod bites, inhalation of infectious aerosols, or ingestion of contaminated water or inadequately cooked meat of infected animals. Ten to 50 bacilli inhaled or inoculated into minimally abraded skin can produce disease, but 10^8 organisms are needed to produce disease following oral challenge.

PATHOGENESIS. An ulcerated lesion develops at the site of bacterial inoculation in 75% of patients. Bacteremia results in entrapment of the organism within macrophages of the reticuloendothelial system, where it may survive for prolonged periods. The early lesions in affected organs (lymph nodes, liver, spleen, lung) demonstrate focal necrosis surrounded by polymorphonuclear leukocytes and macrophages. Later, granulomas with central caseation or small local abscesses can be found.

CLINICAL MANIFESTATIONS. The incubation period is 2 to 10 days. Constitutional symptoms of fever, malaise, and headache, frequently preceded by a rigor, are nonspecific. Hepatomegaly is common. Ulceroglandular tularemia acquired by skin inoculation is the most common variant, occurring in 80% to 90% of reported cases. A reddish papule that ulcerates is usually located on the fingers, hands, or lower extremities. Painful regional lymph node enlargement progresses to fluctuation. Early incision of fluctuant nodes produces bacteremia and toxemia. Pneumonic tularemia, found in 20% to 30% of cases, can result from inhalation or from hematogenous spread of organisms from ulceroglandular tularemia. Laboratory accidents are the most common cause of primary pulmonary involvement. Symptoms include cough, which may be productive of mucoid or bloody sputum, substernal tightness, pleuritic chest pain, and respiratory distress. Physical findings of consolidation are scant but pleural effusions are common. Roentgenographs demonstrate patchy, ill-defined infiltrates and hilar node enlargement. Typhoidal tularemia, occurring in 15% of patients, results from ingestion of organisms and may resemble typhoid fever, abdominal pain and fever are predominant symptoms, and cervical lymph node enlargement may be prominent. Oculoglandular tularemia, found in less than 1% of patients, is a unilateral, painful purulent conjunctivitis with ulceration of the conjunctivae or cornea; it occurs after contamination of the eye with infected animal or tick fluids. Preauricular or cervical lymph nodes are enlarged. Loss of vision may occur in untreated cases.

DIAGNOSIS. Gram stains of sputum or exudates frequently do not demonstrate presence of the organism. Cultivation of the bacillus is usually not attempted in hospital laboratories because of the hazard of aerosolization. Diagnosis most frequently is made serologically. A rise in agglutinins may be detected 8 to 10 days after the onset of illness. An intradermal test of the delayed sensitivity type that utilizes a purified killed suspension of *F. tularensis* is highly specific and becomes positive in the first week of illness.

COURSE. Untreated tularemia may produce significant prolonged morbidity and a mortality of 5% to 30%. Antimicrobial therapy results in prompt defervescence and constitutional improvement. Lifelong immunity usually develops, although a few reinfections have been documented.

MANAGEMENT. Streptomycin, 15 to 20 mg/kg/day for 7 to 10 days, is the preferred antimicrobial agent for the treatment of tularemia. Chloramphenicol and tetracycline are effective in producing a clinical response, but they may fail to eradicate the organism and relapse may occur.

PREVENTION. The risks of acquiring tularemia may be minimized by wearing gloves when processing potentially infected animals, by thorough cooking of suspected meat, and by avoidance of tick infestation. A vaccine prepared from an attenuated strain of *F. tularensis* provides partial protection and is available for laboratory workers and others who may have frequent exposure to infected animals.

BIBLIOGRAPHY

Miller, R.P., and Bates, J.H.: Pleuropulmonary tularemia: a review of 29 patients, Am. Rev. Respir. Dis. **99**:31, 1967.

Overholt, E.L., and others: An analysis of forty-two cases of laboratory acquired tularemia: treatment with broad spectrum antibiotics, Am. J. Med. **30**:785, 1961.

Pullen, R.L., and Stuart, B.M.: Tularemia: analysis of 225 cases, J.A.M.A. **129**:495, 1945.

Brucellosis

Jerome Santoro

DEFINITION. Brucellosis is an infectious disease characterized by fever, malaise, and weight loss that is caused by bacteria of the genus *Brucella*. It is acquired by man from infected animals through either occupational or food contact.

ETIOLOGY. The brucellae are small, nonmotile, nonsporeforming, aerobic gram-negative bacilli. Three of the six recognized species—*B. abortus* (cattle), *B. suis* (hogs), and *B. melitensis* (goats)—are responsible for the majority of human infections. *B. canis* (dogs) has occasionally caused illness in humans. Human infection occurs through contact of infected animal tissues with breaks in the skin or less commonly via conjunctival contact and inhalation. Infection from ingestion of contaminated milk, cheese, or meat is now less frequent because of pasteurization and refrigeration. *B. abortus* strain 19, an attenuated strain used to vaccinate animals, causes infections among veterinarians.

EPIDEMIOLOGY. Brucellosis in the United States is chiefly an occupational disease of abattoir workers, livestock raisers, farmers, and veterinarians. About 200 to 300 cases are reported each year. *B. melitensis* is the most common cause of disease worldwide, but in the United States *B. wuis* and *B. abortus* are isolated most frequently. Most cases are seen in recent slaughterhouse employees and younger veterinarians, which implies that immunity is acquired through long-term exposure. Studies have confirmed the existence of brucella antibodies in chronically exposed persons. Interestingly, most of these individuals have no history of clinical illness, illustrating that asymptomatic infection is more common than overt disease.

PATHOGENESIS. After invasion of epithelial cells of the oropharynx or skin, brucellae are taken up by cells in the reticuloendothelial system (lymph nodes, liver, spleen, bone marrow). At this time the infection can presumably be controlled by the killing of bacteria by macrophages. Alternatively, organisms may multiply intracellularly; in response the host forms epithelioid granulomas. Eventually bacteria escape from their intracellular habitat and enter the bloodstream. If this process is allowed to continue, infection can occur in virtually any organ in the body, including bones, joints, lungs, the genitourinary tract, and the cardiovascular system. Granulomas eventually coalesce and may suppurate in any organ or tissue affected. *B. suis* and *B. melitensis* tend to be more virulent and cause more severe infection than *B. abortus;* strain 19 disease tends to be quite mild.

CLINICAL MANIFESTATIONS AND COURSE. After an incubation period of 1 to 3 weeks the illness begins either insidiously or, less commonly, acutely (chills, fever, prostration). The signs and symptoms of bruellosis are for the most part nonspecific. Often such diseases as influenza, typhoid fever, infectious mononucleosis, endocarditis, and nonspecific viral illnesses are suspected until a history of animal exposure is elicited. Most patients typically have fever, sweating, weakness, and malaise, and more than 50% have anorexia, weight loss, and headache. The physical examination is usually not helpful. Findings such as lymphadenopathy, hepatosplenomegaly, and orchitis are seen in severe and often long-standing forms of the disease.

The complications of brucellosis are many. Infection may develop in various tissues and organ systems, such as bones and joints (especially the vertebrae), the genitourinary system (orchitis, epididymitis, cystitis, pyelitis), lungs, pleural spaces, heart valves, and the gallbladder.

Abscesses can be found in liver, spleen, kidneys, and other areas. Sometimes there are nervous system and ophthalmic manifestations that cannot always be explained by invasion of the organism, such as aseptic meningitis, encephalitis, retinitis, optic neuritis, keratitis, and uveitis. Enlargement of the spleen and perhaps chronic infection involving the bone marrow may result in pancytopenia. In short, brucellosis can resemble other chronic granulomatous infections caused by such organisms as mycobacteria and various fungi.

In the preantibiotic era most patients attained permanent remission within 3 to 6 months after the initial symptoms. A small percent of patients may relapse even with therapy. Chronic brucellosis is difficult to define. There is no doubt that a very small minority of patients can develop bacteriologically proven disease that lasts for years. However, many patients with nonspecific neuropsychiatric complaints have a diagnosis of chronic brucellosis made on the basis of meager evidence, such as a skin test or misinterpreted agglutinin test (see next section) or may actually have reinfection.

Most individuals, asymptomatic or symptomatic, who acquire brucellosis are probably at least partially protected from further infection, but reinfections surely occur. Veterinarians previously exposed to brucella sometimes develop an acute local inflammatory response accompanied by high fever and malaise in response to skin contact with infected material or vaccine; the latter quickly responds to corticosteroids.

DIAGNOSIS AND LABORATORY FINDINGS. Routine laboratory studies, including white blood cell count, erythrocyte sedimentation rate, and urinalysis, are not helpful in making a precise diagnosis of brucellosis. The diagnosis is best secured by the isolation of the organism. Blood cultures, which may take up to 3 weeks of incubation for growth, are positive early in the illness in more than 50% of cases. Later, cultures of lymph nodes, liver, and especially bone marrow may be more fruitful than blood cultures. However, most cases of brucellosis in the United States are not diagnosed by isolation of the organism but by the *Brucella agglutination test,* which measures both IgG and IgM antibodies. Early in primary disease, from weeks 1 to 3, IgM antibody is detected, and later, both IgG and IgM are found. Thus the demonstration of a fourfold or greater rise in agglutinin titer is good evidence for brucellosis, provided infectious diseases caused by agents with cross-reacting antibodies are not being considered, such as *Vibrio* species, *Yersinia* species, and *Francisella tularensis*. In addition, when high titers of antibody circulate, blocking antibodies may be formed and titers may be falsely negative. This problem, called "prozone," can be ruled out if all tests are carried out to high dilution, greater than or equal to 1:1280. As infection resolves, IgG antibody disappears, but IgM may continue to circulate. With persistent, relapsing, or new infection IgG titers remain elevated or again rise. Therefore a simple positive agglutinin test may not be accurate for diagnosis in the latter situations because of possible persistence of IgM antibody. This problem can be circumvented by measuring IgG antibody alone, after mercaptoethanol precipitation of IgM. Titers of 1:160 or greater are said to make active or ongoing disease likely. Conversely, a "negative" test in a patient with prolonged symptoms makes the possibility of active brucellosis remote.

The *Brucella* skin test has no diagnostic worth and should not be used because of interference with serologic studies.

MANAGEMENT. The course of brucellosis is shortened and complications are prevented by antimicrobial therapy. Tetracycline, 500 mg orally four times daily for at least 3 weeks in adults, is the best single agent and has the lowest relapse rate. The addition of streptomycin, 500 mg intramuscularly every 12 hours, further reduces the risk of relapse. Patients with severe disease should usually receive both drugs. Most relapses occur within 3 months of terminating therapy. For patients who are extremely debilitated with severe anorexia, adrenocorticosteroids such as prednisone, 40 to 60 mg daily for 72 hours, can be used.

PREVENTION. The most important aspect of prevention of brucellosis is the ongoing surveillance, prevention (vaccine), and elimination of the disease in domestic animals. No vaccine for man is available in the United States. Individuals at risk should carefully cover lacerated skin and wear gloves, wear protective goggles to avoid splashes, and avoid unpasteurized milk.

BIBLIOGRAPHY

Buchanan, T.M., and others: Brucellosis in the United States, 1960-1972: an abattoir-associated disease, Medicine **53**:403, 1974.

Fox, M., and Kaufman, A.F.: Brucellosis in the United States, 1965-1974, J. Infect. Dis. **136**:312, 1977.

48 • DISEASES CAUSED BY GRAM-POSITIVE BACILLI

Anthrax

Elias Abrutyn

DEFINITION. Anthrax, a disease of animals, occurs in man in three forms: cutaneous, inhalational, and gastrointestinal. Bacteremia and meningitis may complicate any form.

ETIOLOGY. *Bacillus anthracis* is a large, gram-positive, aerobic, sporeforming organism. In clinical specimens the organism occurs singly or in chains of two or three square-ended bacilli. The organism is surrounded by a capsule that has antiphagocytic properties; it produces a toxin that has several properties, including the ability to produce edema. Spores that survive in soil or on animal products for years are important in the persistence of the disease.

EPIDEMIOLOGY. In the United States anthrax occurs primarily after industrial exposure to imported contaminated animal products, such as hides, goat hair, wool, and bone, and to a lesser extent after agricultural exposure to diseased animals, such as horses and cattle; three or four cases are reported annually.

PATHOLOGY AND PATHOGENESIS. Cutaneous and gastrointestinal anthrax follow dermal inoculation or ingestion of spores. In inhalation anthrax spores are deposited in the lung and are transported to the mediastinal lymph nodes, where they germinate and multiply. Histologically, edema, necrosis, hemorrhage, and inflammatory cells are seen.

CLINICAL MANIFESTATIONS. Cutaneous anthrax, the most common form, frequently involves exposed areas. The lesion begins as a papule that becomes vesicular and then ulcerates. Eventually, the characteristic black eschar is formed. Nonpitting edema that surrounds the lesion may be quite prominent. Pain is rare, but pruritus occurs. Constitutional symptoms are infrequent. Pharyngeal anthrax has been reported but is exceedingly rare.

After an initial stage resembling a mild respiratory illness, severe respiratory distress, hemorrhagic mediastinitis, and disseminated disease including hemorrhagic meningitis develop in patients with inhalation anthrax. Gastrointestinal anthrax is characterized by anorexia, nausea, vomiting, acute abdominal pain, bloody diarrhea, toxemia, and shock.

DIAGNOSIS. Anthrax is most readily diagnosed in persons with occupational exposure to infected animals or their products. Gram smears and cultures of fluid from skin and other body fluids are usually positive. Serologic tests are useful in epidemiologic studies but not in the diagnosis of acute disease.

PROGNOSIS. Cutaneous anthrax has an excellent prognosis, but inhalation and gastrointestinal forms of the disease are usually fatal.

MANAGEMENT. In uncomplicated mild cutaneous anthrax penicillin V, 500 mg orally every 6 hours for 5 to 7 days, may be administered. More severe cases may require procaine penicillin, 600,000 units intramuscularly twice daily. Inhalation and gastrointestinal anthrax require high-dose intravenous penicillin, 18 to 24 million units daily. Tetracycline, erythromycin, and chloramphenicol are effective alternatives.

PREVENTION. Control depends on proper handling of infected animals and their products. Vaccination is recommended for those with a high risk of exposure.

BIBLIOGRAPHY

Gold, H.: Treatment of anthrax, Fed. Proc. **67**:1563, 1967.

Nalin, D.R., and others: Survival of a patient with gastrointestinal anthrax, Am. J. Med. **62**:130, 1977.

Plotkin, S.A., and others: An epidemic of inhalation anthrax: the first in the twentieth century, Am. J. Med. **29**:992, 1960.

Listeriosis
Jaime Carrizosa

Listeriosis is an infectious disease caused by *Listeria monocytogenes,* a gram-positive, nonsporeforming, aerobic bacillus. The organism, found worldwide, causes infection in man and domestic animals. The infection may be acquired by direct contact, inhalation, or ingestion. Transmission from the pregnant woman to her offspring also occurs.

Listeriosis is primarily a disease of infants, immunocompromised hosts, and the elderly. The disease has been recently reported with increasing frequency in healthy individuals.

Several clinical pictures are associated with the disease. Meningitis, the most common clinical presentation, appears abruptly or may have an insidious course. Its clinical manifestations include headache, fever, nausea, vomiting, and nuchal rigidity. Cranial nerve involvement and other focal findings, as well as a diffuse encephalitic syndrome, may also be seen. The cerebrospinal fluid shows a cellular response that is initially mainly granulocytes but later can become predominantly mononuclear cells. The protein is high, and the sugar is low.

In the neonate the disease ranges from meningitis to a disseminated infection with a papular skin rash, hepatosplenomegaly, respiratory distress syndrome, and circulatory collapse. Diffuse organ involvement characterized by development of microabscesses and granulomatous formation resembling miliary tuberculosis may be found. Disseminated listeriosis has also been seen in children and adults, particularly in patients with cancer or debilitating diseases or in those receiving steroids or immunosuppressive agents.

Other clinical presentations include pharyngitis associated with diffuse lymphadenopathy simulating infectious mononucleosis, endocarditis, and a purulent conjunctivitis also associated with lymphadenopathy.

The diagnosis of listeriosis is based on the isolation and identification of the organism from cultures. Since the isolation of a gram-positive bacillus usually receives the label of a diphtheroid, special measures should be taken to provide appropriate identification. Serologic tests to detect agglutinins have low specificity and are not diagnostic. Leukocytosis with neutrophilia is common in all acute forms of the disease; monocytosis is uncommon.

L. monocytogenes is sensitive to many antibiotics in vitro, including penicillin, erythromycin, tetracyclines, chloramphenicol, and sulfonamides. The drug of choice for the treatment of meningitis, endocarditis, or disseminated disease is intravenous penicillin G or ampicillin. Penicillin G, 20 million units intravenously in adults daily and 200,000 units/kg/day in children in divided doses every 4 hours, is recommended. In severe disseminated disease the addition of an aminoglycoside has been suggested because of the synergistic activity of this combination. Pharyngitis or conjunctivitis can be treated with oral erythromycin, 500 mg every 6 hours or 30 mg/kg/day in four divided doses for 2 weeks.

The prognosis of appropriately treated *Listeria* infections is good. However, meningitis may be associated with residual damage or with normal pressure hydrocephalus that may require decompression. Severe cases of disseminated listeriosis carry a significant mortality rate.

Erysipeloid
Jaime Carrizosa

Erysipeloid is an infection caused by a gram-positive, nonsporeforming aerobic bacillus, *Erysipelothrix rhusiopathiae*. The infection is usually acquired by contact through a break in the skin and is usually restricted to individuals who handle dead animals or animal products. It is worldwide in distribution.

The clinical manifestations of the disease are a severely edematous but relatively nontender violaceous lesion of the hand or fingers resembling severe cellulitis; the lesion is not accompanied by suppurative lymphangitis or satellite adenopathy. It rarely extends above the wrist. The adjacent joints may be stiff and moderately painful. The area of involvement has a slow progression, primarily in a proximal direction. The disease heals spontaneously in about 3 to 4 weeks, but relapses are frequent. Systemic symptoms and signs such as fever are uncommon.

The infection occasionally progresses to a generalized form characterized by polyarthritis and additional skin lesions with erythema, swelling, and pruritus. The most serious form of the disease is *Erysipelothrix* endocarditis. The organism affects normal as well as previously damaged valves. Most patients are young men with a typical occupational history and classical manifestations of endocarditis.

The diagnosis of erysipeloid is made on the basis of the clinical picture and the isolation of the organism from a skin biopsy at the margin of the lesion, body fluids, or blood cultures.

The organism is susceptible to many antibiotics, such as penicillin, tetracycline, erythromycin, clindamycin, cephalosporins, and chloramphenicol. The drug of choice is benzathine penicillin G in a single intramuscular dose of 1.2 million units. Systemic infection is treated with 20 million units of penicillin G intravenously each day for 4 to 6 weeks.

BIBLIOGRAPHY
Listeriosis

Moore, R.M., and Zehmer, R.B.: Listeriosis in the United States, J. Infect. Dis. **127**:610, 1973.

Erysipeloid

Borchardt, K.A.: *Erysipelothrix rhusiopathiae* endocarditis, West. J. Med. **127**:149, 1977.

Nelson, E.: Five hundred cases of erysipeloid, Rocky Mt. Med. J. **52**:40, 1955.

Actinomycosis

John E. Bennett

Actinomycosis is the name of a clinical syndrome caused by a closely related group of organisms that are all anaerobic or microaerophilic branching higher bacteria. *Actinomyces israelii* is the most common microbe. All the etiologic agents are normal inhabitants of the human mouth and gastrointestinal tract. The microbes grow in tissue as tightly packed clusters called sulfur granules. These pale yellow, firm granules (a few millimeters in diameter) are found in the pus of abscesses or draining sinuses caused by the infection. Resected tonsils sometimes show a sulfur granule in a tonsillar crypt that does not cause disease. Illness comes when the microbe penetrates deeper tissue. Infection usually begins in the cervicofacial, thoracic, or ileocecal area. The portal of entry for cervicofacial infection may be dental caries, dental abscess, tooth extraction, or penetrating trauma. An indolent indurated mass forms in the submandibular area, cheek, or anterior cervical triangle. Tenderness may be only slight; fever is typically absent. Draining sinuses intermittently discharge pus.

Pulmonary actinomycosis presumably results from aspiration of normal oral flora. A chronic pneumonia results and tends to extend to contiguous structures, such as the chest wall and thoracic spine. Abdominal actinomycosis most often originates in the appendix. Draining sinuses may extend outside the abdominal wall. Pelvic actinomycosis may result from long-term use of an intrauterine contraceptive device. Hematogenous dissemination can result from any site, with resulting abscesses in liver, brain, bone, or other organs.

Diagnosis of actinomycosis depends heavily on the demonstration of sulfur granules in pus. Granules may be found by examining the dressing covering a wound or by close inspection of pus in aspirates or biopsied tissue. Suspected sulfur granules should be Gram stained to demonstrate the branching, gram-positive hyphae. Washing the granules in sterile saline before culture may diminish the number of associated bacteria in the pus. Reliance on histologic section to demonstrate sulfur granules is unwise because the granules are present only in scattered areas. Culture of *A. israelii* from the mouth, stool, or sputum is of no diagnostic value.

Antibiotic therapy of actinomycosis often must be prolonged for 6 to 12 months to prevent relapse. Milder cases may be treated with tetracycline, 2 g/day, oral penicillin V, 3 to 4 g/day, or erythromycin, 1 to 2 g/day. More severe cases may require initial therapy with intravenous penicillin, 20 million units each day.

Nocardiosis

John E. Bennett

Nocardia are aerobic, branching, higher bacteria that normally live in soil. When introduced into subcutaneous tissue by minor trauma, they grow in pus as grains, causing mycetoma (see Chapter 52). When no grains are formed, the infection is called nocardiosis. Nocardiosis usually begins as pneumonia but has a marked tendency to spread hematogenously to the brain and other organs. Therapy with adrenal corticosteroids, the presence of Cushing's disease, and hematologic malignancies predispose to nocardiosis. Diagnosis is suspected by the demonstration of gram-positive, weakly acid-fast, branching bacteria in pus or sputum. Confirmation of the diagnosis is by culture.

Infection may be subacute or chronic, but fatal progression occurs in the absence of appropriate therapy. Sulfonamides are the drugs of choice. The initial dose is usually 6 to 9 g daily, and therapy is usually continued for 12 months.

BIBLIOGRAPHY

Actinomycosis

Weese, E.C., and Smith, I.M.: A study of 57 cases of actinomycosis over a 36-year period, Arch. Intern. Med. **135**:1562, 1975.

Nocardiosis

Palmer, D.L., Harvey, R.L., and Wheeler, J.K.: Diagnostic and therapeutic considerations in *Nocardia asteroides* infection, Medicine **53**:391, 1974.

Diphtheria

Oksana M. Korzeniowski

DEFINITION. Diphtheria, caused by *Corynebacterium diphtheriae,* is an acute infectious disease that may be symptomless or may be seen as a rapidly fatal hypertoxic disease characterized by a local inflammatory lesion in the upper airway or skin and by remote effects produced by an exotoxin elaborated by the organism.

ETIOLOGY. *C. diphtheriae* is an aerobic, gram-positive, pleomorphic, nonsporeforming, nonmotile organism. In stained preparations it appears club shaped, contains metachromatic granules, and aligns in palisades resembling Chinese characters. Media containing tellurite promote growth and impart a characteristic black pigment to the isolates. The diphtheria bacillus has been classified by in vitro characteristics into three stable types: gravis, intermedius, and mitis. Each type can cause epidemic diphtheria. Virulence resides in the production of an exotoxin (conferred by lysogeny with a bacteriophage) and of other biologically active extracellular products such as spreading factor (hyaluronidase). Spreading factor promotes tissue invasion and may account for the occurrence of diphtheria in well-immunized individuals or in individuals infected with nontoxigenic strains.

EPIDEMIOLOGY. Diphtheria is primarily a disease of nonimmunized low-income urban populations residing in crowded conditions. It is worldwide in distribution, and epidemics still occur in the United States. Intimate contact is required for spread of diphtheria. Transmission occurs by infected droplets generated from nasopharyngeal secretions or by exudates from infected skin lesions; fomites, milk, and dust may have a minor role. Asymptomatic carriers harboring toxin-producing strains in the nasopharynx or skin constitute the reservoir from which disease spreads to susceptible individuals. Immunity against diphtheria does not prevent nasopharyngeal carriage or the development of local disease but does attenuate or abort the distant toxic effects. The highest attack rates, morbidity, and mortality in diphtheria occur in nonimmunized children under age 14. Highly contagious skin infections may be important in maintaining the endemicity of diphtheria by increasing the rates of acquisition and transmission of the organism and thus expanding the potential reservoir.

PATHOGENESIS. The membrane, the primary local manifestation of diphtheria, is composed of bacteria, necrotic epithelium, fibrin, and phagocytes. The painless, thick, leathery, blue-white membrane is usually located in the upper airway, where it firmly adheres to underlying tissues. Other sites, such as conjunctivae, vagina, or ear, may also be involved. Forcible removal of the membrane causes bleeding.

Exotoxin is elaborated and absorbed at the primary lesion. Rapidly distributed hematogenously, it binds to specific receptors on susceptible cells (primarily nerve, myocardium, and kidney) and penetrates into the cytoplasm, where it inactivates the "elongation factor," a critical protein moiety required for the translocation of tRNA during protein synthesis. Arrest of protein synthesis results in fatty degeneration of muscle and of medullary sheets of motor nerves (and to a lesser degree of sensory nerves), as well as enlargement and cloudy swelling of the kidney.

CLINICAL MANIFESTATIONS. The primary determinants of the clinical manifestation of diphtheria are the patient's immune status, the virulence and toxicity of the infecting strain, and the anatomic location of infection. Strains that do not produce toxin cause only local disease.

The incubation period is 2 to 6 days. A copious, thick, serosanguineous discharge in nasal diphtheria produces local irritation but rarely results in intoxication. Pharyngeal diphtheria confined to the tonsils may cause only local discomfort (pharyngitis) and mild systemic symptoms of fever and headache. Spread of the membrane to the uvula, soft palate, and pharyngeal wall enlarges the surface area for toxin absorption; signs of toxemia, such as listlessness, tachycardia, and weakness, are common. Local edema of submandibular areas and the anterior neck imparts a characteristic "bull-neck" appearance. Airway occlusion, as well as severe toxic manifestations, occurs in laryngeal, tracheal, and bronchial diphtheria. Cutaneous diphtheria, which occurs primarily in the tropics, develops as a shallow, nonhealing ulcer covered by a grayish membrane.

Conduction abnormalities and arrhythmias appearing in the first or second week of illness are indicative of diphtheritic myocarditis. Circulatory collapse is an ominous sign. Cranial and peripheral motor nerve palsies develop after 2 to 6 weeks. Respiratory insufficiency may result from paralysis of the diaphragm. Encephalitis is a rare toxic complication.

DIAGNOSIS. A provisional diagnosis of diphtheria should be made on clinical grounds and treatment instituted immediately. Specific diagnosis by bacteriologic confirmation, strain identification, and detection of toxin elaboration by precipitin reactions with antiserum (Elek test) is important for epidemiologic reasons but should not delay therapy.

COURSE. Nontoxic diphtheria is a self-limited disease, although chronic carriage of the bacillus may ensue. Prior to the use of antitoxin, diphtheria of moderate severity (that is, accompanied by toxemia) and laryngeal diphtheria carried mortality rates of 35% and 90%, respectively. Currently, overall mortality in the United States remains between 4% and 10%. Myocarditis, paralysis, and death occur primarily in nonimmunized, very young, or very old persons. Myocardial damage (fibrosis) and neurologic deficits may persist in survivors.

MANAGEMENT. Patients with diphtheria require isolation and strict bed rest. Early use of diphtheria horse serum anti-toxin, 20,000 to 100,000 units, depending on the extent of the disease, is the most important specific treatment for the prevention of toxic complications. Rapid binding of the toxin to susceptible tissue sites may render antitoxin ineffective if it is administered more than 48 hours after the onset of illness. Sensitivity to horse serum must be determined, with desensitization performed if necessary. Antibiotics are used to terminate the carrier state. Erythromycin, 500 mg four times a day for 7 days, is the drug of choice, but procaine penicillin is an effective alternative. Control of epidemic outbreaks requires early treatment of carriers and active immunization of susceptible individuals.

PREVENTION. Diphtheria is preventable with active immunization. Diphtheria-pertussis-tetanus (DPT) vaccines should be administered in three (in infants) and two (in children) doses of 0.5 ml each at 4- to 6-week intervals. Boosters should be given after 1 year and just before entry into school. Adult primary immunization follows the same schedule, but adult-type diphtheria-tetanus (dT) vaccine, which contains less diphtheria toxoid, should be used. Booster immunization should be administered every 5 to

10 years, depending on occupational exposure. An intradermal injection of highly purified diphtheria toxin (Schick test) may be useful in determining immune status. A local reaction indicates lack of antibody and therefore lack of immunity.

BIBLIOGRAPHY

McCloskey, R.W., and others: The 1970 epidemic of diphtheria in San Antonio, Ann. Intern. Med. **75**:495, 1971.

Pappenheimer, A.M., Jr., and Gill, D.M.: Diphtheria: recent studies have clarified the molecular mechanisms involved in its pathogenesis, Science **182**:353, 1973.

Scheid, W.: Diphtherial paralysis, J. Nerv. Ment. Dis. **116**:1095, 1952.

49 • DISEASES CAUSED BY ANAEROBIC BACTERIA

Infections caused by nonsporeforming anaerobes

Matthew E. Levison

DEFINITION. Obligate anaerobic bacteria are those that require an anaerobic environment for survival and growth.

Sporeforming obligate anaerobes are called clostridia. Pathogenic sporeless obligate anaerobes are either species of *Fusobacterium* or *Bacteroides* (gram-negative bacilli); *Propionibacterium, Lactobacillus, Actinomyces, Bifidobacterium,* or *Eubacterium* (gram-positive bacilli); *Peptococcus* or *Peptostreptococcus* (gram-positive cocci); or *Veillonella* or *Acidaminococcus* (gram-negative cocci). The obligate anaerobes are the predominant members of the normal microflora on the skin and adjacent mucous membranes, that is, gingival crevice, lower intestinal tract, vagina, or distal third of the urethra. In the gingival crevice and colon there are 10^{10} to 10^{11}/ml, and in the vagina there are 10^8 to 10^9/ml. At each site there is a characteristic flora composed of a distinctive number of species, including more than 100 in the gingival crevice or colon but only about five in the vagina, and a distinctive type of species, such as *Bacteroides melaninogenicus* in the gingival crevice, *B. thetaiotaomicron* and *B. fragilis* in the colon, and *Lactobacillus* and anaerobic gram-positive cocci in the vagina.

PATHOGENESIS. Infections caused by anaerobes are usually endogenous in origin; they are caused by the microflora on the skin and mucous membranes. These infections are primarily dependent on defects in local host defense mechanisms (defects in the mucosal barrier and presence of necrotic tissue as a consequence of trauma, neoplasia, or ischemia) at sites that normally have a microflora. Most intra-abdominal and pelvic infections and infections in and about the mouth contain anaerobes. However, of the numerous species found in the microflora, only a few are frequently isolated from clinical specimens. Of the anaerobic species involved, the more commonly found are those containing virulence factors, such as polysaccharide capsules (*B. fragilis, B. asaccharolyticus*) or endotoxin (*Fusobacterium nucleatum*). Other virulence factors include production of proteolytic enzymes, gas, or heparinase, which promote further tissue necrosis, local spread, or hematogenous dissemination. In addition, the anaerobes isolated from clinical specimens tend to be characteristic of the microflora normally found at that site, such as *B. fragilis* if the infection is colonic in origin or *B. asaccharolyticus* if it is oral in origin. These infections are characteristically polymicrobial; about 5 species (range 3 to 10) are usually isolated. The anaerobes are at times mixed with aerobic or faculative species. The aerobic or facultative component of these polymicrobial infections also reflects the microflora at the site of the defect in host defenses, such as *Escherichia coli* or enterococci if the infection is colonic in origin or various streptococci if it is oral in origin. Alterations of microflora on skin or mucosal surface due to a primary disease process will also be reflected in the type of pathogens isolated from the clinical specimen. For example, vaginal microflora after normal delivery, abortion, gynecologic surgery, or with trichomoniasis may be composed of colonic-type microorganisms, such as *B. fragilis, E. coli,* or enterococci, and infections in these situations will reflect the change in microflora.

CLINICAL MANIFESTATIONS. Certain findings suggest an anaerobic bacterial origin. The location of anaerobic infections is usually at or near sites that contain a predominantly anaerobic microflora. There is usually associated tumor; vascular obstruction (such as that caused by atherosclerosis or diabetes mellitus), or trauma that has resulted in tissue necrosis. The obstruction of a paranasal sinus or of the lower respiratory airway by a tumor or foreign body may be associated with anaerobic infection in the poorly ventilated and poorly drained areas. The aspiration of the contents of the oral cavity into the lower respiratory tract may result in anaerobic pleuropulmonary infection. Anaerobic bacteria usually produce a foul odor in purulent material, unlike most aerobic or facultative pathogens; the absence of such an odor, however, does not exclude the presence of anaerobic pathogens. Gas is frequently produced in tissues, resulting in crepitation. Anaerobic infection in the female genital tract may be complicated by suppurative thrombophlebitis of the pelvic veins, with septic embolization to the lung; anaerobic infection in the intestinal tract may be complicated by thrombophlebitis in the portal system, with septic embolization to the liver. Bacteremia may also result in endocarditis or metastatic infection in any organ, such as the brain, bones, joints, spleen, and liver.

Infection by the anaerobic microflora may also result from an animal or human bite or accidental subcutaneous or intravenous self-inoculation of saliva or feces.

DIAGNOSIS. The presence of anaerobes should be suspected in the appropriate clinical setting as described previously. Gram stain is important in identifying the anaerobes that may have a characteristic morphology, such as *Actinomyces,* and in detecting the presence of a polymicrobial infection. Bacteriologic confirmation depends on avoidance of contamination, even by minute amounts of secretions that contain skin or mucosal microflora, such as upper respiratory tract, intestinal, vaginal, or urethral secretions. These secretions contain enormous numbers of microorganisms that may or may not be identical to the organisms causing the disease.

To obtain lower respiratory tract material for anaerobic culture, an invasive procedure such as transtracheal aspiration or percutaneous lung puncture is involved. Frequently, these invasive and risky procedures are not performed if the clinical diagnostic features (for example, community-acquired putrid lung abscess) are sufficiently apparent. Blood and pleural, synovial, or peritoneal fluid should be obtained for anaerobic culture depending on the clinical situation.

Anaerobes are frequently fastidious and will not grow at optimal rates when handled by methods that are routinely used for facultative organisms. These organisms must be transported to the laboratory as quickly as possible in an anaerobic environment (for example, aspirated purulent material transported to the laboratory in a "corked" syringe) and placed on enriched solid and liquid media as soon as they arrive in the laboratory. The media should then be incubated in an anaerobic environment for at least 48 to 72 hours before being discarded. If the Gram stain of the purulent material initially revealed a polymicrobial infection but few of the organisms or only the facultative organism were recovered on culture, the more fastidious anaerobes can be presumed to have been lost in the laboratory processing.

MANAGEMENT. Surgery is the primary mode of therapy, except for lung abscess or endometritis. The aims of surgery are (1) to stop further contamination; (2) to remove all gross foreign material, such as necrotic tissue, feces, and blood, since virulence is enhanced by the presence of these substances; (3) to eliminate anaerobic conditions; (4) to reduce the bacterial count to a minimum; and (5) to provide drainage of purulent material. At times, surgical drainage alone may be all that is necessary for a well-localized abscess, such as a surgical wound abscess.

The role of antimicrobial therapy in the outcome of infection caused by anaerobes is extremely difficult to assess. This is primarily because of the often dramatic response to surgical drainage and debridement alone when there is localized infection. Nevertheless, appropriate antimicrobial therapy has been shown to significantly reduce mortality among patients with bacteremic infections caused by Bacteroidaceae or Enterobacteriaceae. Antimicrobial drugs are expected to control bacteremia and early metastatic foci of infection, to reduce suppurative complications if administered early, and to prevent local spread of existing infection. However, once suppuration has occurred, unless abscesses are quite small, antimicrobial drugs without surgical drainage and debridement cannot be expected to eliminate the infection.

Antimicrobial therapy should be started immediately after appropriate specimens such as blood and purulent material are obtained for culture. This means that antimicrobial therapy is often started prior to completion of in vitro antimicrobial sensitivity testing of the specific facultative pathogens. Rapid isolation and identification of anaerobes, in contrast to the testing of facultative pathogens, are often not possible in many community hospitals. In addition, in vitro sensitivity testing by the conventional disk diffusion technique has not been standardized for anaerobes. Therefore, initial chemotherapy is usually empiric, based on the most reliable and least toxic antimicrobial agents for the most probable anaerobic and facultative pathogens.

Because these infections are commonly polymicrobial, a broad spectrum of antimicrobial activity is required. Drugs active against anaerobic bacteria may be quite inactive against the accompanying aerobic or facultative pathogens in the mixed infections and vice versa. For this reason, combinations of usually two or three drugs may have to be used. These combinations of antimicrobial agents are selected for their activity against most of the more virulent pathogens expected to be present in the infective mixture (such as in infection caused by colonic microflora, the Enterobacteriaceae, and *B. fragilis*).

Infection caused by oral anaerobes can usually be adequately treated with the penicillins or cephalosporins because oral microflora are usually sensitive to these antibiotics. *B. fragilis,* which produces a β-lactamase, and Enterobacteriaceae are usually not involved in these infections.

Chloramphenicol, clindamycin, and metronidazole are the most active antibiotics against *B. fragilis*. Infection caused by colonic microflora (intra-abdominal, pelvic, perineal) can best be initially treated with (1) chloramphenicol, 50 to 100 mg/kg/day orally or intravenously in four divided doses, and gentamicin (or tobramycin), 1.7 mg/kg intravenously or intramuscularly every 8 hours (if renal function is normal); (2) clindamycin, 600 mg intravenously or intramuscularly every 6 to 8 hours, and gentamicin (or tobramycin); or (3) metronidazole, 15 mg/kg intravenously followed by 7.5 mg/kg intravenously or orally every 6 hours, gentamicin (or tobramycin), and a penicillin or cephalosporin. Amikacin is the aminoglycoside of choice if resistant gram-negative facultative bacilli are suspected. Some physicians add ampicillin because of the frequent presence of enterococci, but this antibiotic does not always seem to be necessary despite the presence of this organism. An appropriate β-lactam antibiotic such as a cephalosporin or penicillin should be subsequently substituted for the aminoglycoside if indicated by results of in vitro disk susceptibility tests on the facultative isolates. No reliable disk sensitivity tests are available for anaerobes. The duration of therapy is usually prolonged to prevent relapse because host defenses cannot be relied on to completely eradicate the pathogens from sequestered areas of extensive tissue necrosis and abscess formation, many of which are not accessible to adequate surgical drainage. Antibiotic therapy should be given before, during, and after surgery to ensure tissue and blood levels that will combat local and metastatic spread of the infection.

PROGNOSIS. Morbidity is unusually prolonged in patients with anaerobic infection. The presence of residual infection as a result of inadequate surgical management (more common in patients with multiple abscesses); extensive tissue necrosis caused by malignancy, ischemia, or trauma: or continued contamination is associated with significantly greater morbidity or mortality.

PREVENTION. Anaerobic infection can be prevented by adequate management of conditions that predispose to invasion by surface microflora. For example, prevention of postoperative wound infection and peritonitis requires avoiding contamination of the peritoneum with gastrointestinal or vaginal secretions during abdominal or pelvic surgery. In addition to good surgical technique, the complex gastrointestinal or vaginal flora can be reduced prior to surgery. Mechanical cleansing of the bowel with a low-residue diet followed by a liquid diet, cathartics, and enemas can reduce the total fecal mass. Preoperative oral antibiotics to reduce the bacterial concentration in the colon are also commonly used.

Parenteral antibiotics have also been used in gastrointestinal and gynecologic surgery prophylactically when there is a chance of contamination with normal microflora at the operative site ("clean, contaminated surgery"). These types of operations involve, for example, cutting through the large bowel without significant spillage; compromising the blood supply of the large bowel; cutting through the stomach or small bowel when there is anticipated intraluminal bacterial overgrowth; appendectomy for appendicitis without rupture; penetrating wounds of the abdomen; gallbladder surgery in the elderly; cesarean section following rupture of the membranes and labor; vaginal hysterectomy in the premenopausal woman; and radical pelvic surgery for gynecologic malignancy. Several studies have shown significant reduction in the frequency of postoperative infection from about 20% to 30% to about 4% to 8% following prophylactic antibiotics in clean, contaminated surgery.

The basic principle of antibiotic prophylaxis is to provide adequate tissue levels at the site of contamination and adequate blood levels during the procedure and for about 24 hours following the procedure. Prophylaxis is started within 1 to 2 hours prior to the procedure and continued for about 24 hours. Early treatment of a primary infection can also reduce postoperative infection. For example, in one study the rate of wound infection in patients with a perforated appendix was greater than 50% if no chemotherapy was used and 15% in the group given appropriate antibiotic therapy.

Clostridial infection
Matthew E. Levison

Clostridia are anaerobic sporeforming gram-positive (occasionally gram-negative) bacilli normally found in the intestinal tract of man and animals and in the soil. Most disease is produced by *Clostridium perfringens,* but other pathogenic species include *C. novyi, C. septicum, C. sordellii, C. histolyticum,* and *C. difficile.* These organisms produce a diverse variety of diseases that are found worldwide, including wound infection, spreading cellulitis, myonecrosis, transient bacteremia, septicemia, metastatic infection (as in the lung, pleura, and meninges), enterotoxigenic enteritis or colitis, tetanus, and botulism.

TETANUS

DEFINITION. Tetanus is an acute infectious disease characterized by tonic spasm of voluntary muscles with episodic tonic convulsions and autonomic nervous dysfunction, caused by a potent neurotoxin elaborated in tissues by *C. tetani.*

ETIOLOGY. Tetanus is caused by an exotoxin produced by *C. tetani,* a motile gram-positive anaerobic sporeforming bacillus. Terminal spores, larger in diameter than the width of the vegatative cell, distend the ends of the rod (drumstick shape). The spores are found in soil and in human and animal feces; they survive for many years in dried earth.

EPIDEMIOLOGY. Spores may contaminate wounds caused by nail punctures, hypodermic injections of addicts, gunshots, compound fractures, and accidents to agricultural or construction workers. Occasionally, the postpartum uterus or umbilical cord is contaminated. Because spores may remain dormant in wounds for prolonged periods, the site of entry may not be obvious.

PATHOGENESIS. The presence in the wound of calcium salts, tissue anoxia, or increased acidity caused by infection with other soil bacteria (and the activity of granulocytes) facilitate germination of *C. tetani* spores. Subsequently, a potent neurotoxin is produced that acts on motor end-plates and also on the anterior horn cells of the spinal cord and brainstem, causing spasm. Generalized tonic spasticity occurs with intermittent tonic convulsions.

CLINICAL MANIFESTATIONS. There are three forms of tetanus: localized, cephalic, and generalized.

The localized form is characterized by spasticity of a group of muscles close to the site of injury. The spasticity may persist for several months and usually resolves gradually without residual findings. Some patients, however, may develop generalized tetanus.

Cephalic tetanus usually occurs 1 or 2 days following injury to the head or otitis media. It is characterized by involvement of the cranial motor nerves, primarily the seventh cranial nerve, and has a poor prognosis.

Generalized tetanus usually affects the body in a descending manner, beginning with trismus and ultimately involving the extremities. Less than 1 week between the occurrence of the wound and the first symptoms of generalized tetanus and less than 48 hours between the first symptoms and the first generalized spasm is associated with more severe disease. The initial complaint is stiffness of the jaw, followed by difficulty swallowing and opening the jaw (trismus), spasm of the facial muscles (risus sardonicus), and rigidity and painful spasms of the anterior abdominal wall and of neck and back muscles (opisthotonos). There is usually diffuse sweating. Painful tonic convulsions are precipitated by minor stimulation. Other findings include a moderate fever, rapid shallow respirations, rapid pulse rate, and widely fluctuating blood pressure. Hyperpyrexia may occur in the absence of infection, a result of continuous heat production from muscle contractions and cutaneous vasoconstriction. Because of spasm of the glottis and respiratory muscles, the patient may develop respiratory insufficiency. Difficulty in swallowing secretions may result in aspiration. Constipation and urinary retention result from spasm of the respective sphincters.

DIAGNOSIS. The history and clincal findings suggest the diagnosis. Tetanus must be differentiated from trismus caused by dental infections, nuchal rigidity caused by meningitis (in which trismus is absent), and strychnine or phenothiazine intoxication.

PROGNOSIS. Mortality may exceed 50% with inadequate treatment. In severe cases the prognosis is related to the ability to support the patient's respirations and to prevent dehydration and aspiration pneumonia for up to 2 weeks. In patients who survive, recovery is complete except for some muscle stiffness that may persist for months.

MANAGEMENT. Human antitoxin, 3000 to 10,000 units intravenously, should be administered as early as possible and before exploration of the wound to inactivate toxin released during surgery. The wound, if present, should be incised, foreign bodies should be removed, and the wound thoroughly cleansed. Penicillin, 10 million units intravenously, or tetracycline should be administered to eradicate vegetative clostridia present in wounds.

An attack of tetanus does not confer immunity, since a fatal dose of toxin is probably less than that required to stimulate an immune response. Therefore patients should be immunized with absorbed toxoid, the full course being completed during the recovery period (for example, three doses of toxoid no less than 1 month apart).

To minimize respiratory problems in patients with difficulty swallowing secretions or with laryngeal spasm, tracheal intubation with a cuffed tube should be initiated, followed by elective tracheostomy with a cuffed tube. Muscle spasms can be controlled to some extent with diazepam, 10 mg every 4 hours orally or parenterally. Muscle spasms complicated by drug-induced sedation may lead to hypoventilation; patients may then require total muscle paralysis with curare and mechanically assisted ventilation. After 1 to 4 weeks of therapy in severely affected patients, curare and diazepam requirements gradually decrease.

As a result of excessive sweating and increased insensible fluid loss, dehydration may occur if intravenous fluid replacement is not carefully maintained.

Marked muscle spasms, cyanosis, cardiac arrhythmias, and hypertension may occur as a result of stimulation such as tracheal suction. β-Adrenergic blocking agents such as propranolol have been used to control some of these problems, which are thought to result from sympathetic autonomic overreactivity.

PREVENTION. Active immunization should be given to children as part of a mixed diphtheria-pertussis-tetanus (DPT) vaccine program in infancy, on entry to school, and subsequently at 10-year intervals. Booster injections should be administered after injury if the last injection was given more than 5 to 10 years previously, depending on the type of wound; in addition, human tetanus antitoxin, 250 units intramuscularly, is recommended for dirty wounds untreated for more than 24 hours.

CLOSTRIDIAL SOFT TISSUE INFECTION (GAS GANGRENE AND CLOSTRIDIAL CELLULITIS)

DEFINITION. Clostridial soft tissue infection is a rapidly spreading infection of soft tissue caused by *Clostridium,* usually *C. perfringens*. If myonecrosis, or gas gangrene, occurs as a result of bacterial exotoxins, the disease is accompanied by toxemia and prostration.

ETIOLOGY. Several species of *Clostridium* may be associated with gas gangrene or clostridial cellulitis. The most commonly encountered are *C. histolyticum, C. perfringens, C. novyi,* and *C. septicum*. Each alone can cause the disease, but wounds may often contain two or more species. *C. perfringens* are large, gram-positive or gram-negative rods, frequently surrounded by a capsule. Abundant gas and volatile organic acid production during fermentation is typical of many clostridia.

EPIDEMIOLOGY AND PATHOGENESIS. Infection is usually the result of contamination of a wound with clostridia or their spores. Severe wounds acquired in military combat, automobile or industrial accidents, criminal abortions, surgery or hypodermic injections in the hip or thigh, or any wounds grossly contaminated with soil or fecal matter are particularly likely to contain clostridial spores. Severity of infection may vary from simple contamination or mild cellulitis to gas gangrene. Conditions that facilitate germination of clostridial spores are the low redox potential and acidity of devitalized tissue and concomitant growth of facultative organisms inoculated into the wound at the same time as the clostridia. As a result, the clostridia proliferate and elaborate potent exotoxins that cause further tissue necrosis. The exotoxins of *C. perfringens* include alpha toxin (a lecithinase and hemolysin), collagenase, hyaluronidase, and deoxyribonuclease. Since lecithin is present in membranes of many different kinds of cells, the alpha toxin can cause extensive damage. The resulting edema and gas (hydrogen and carbon dioxide) in tissues and fascial sheaths tend to spread the infection and increase tissue pressure, further impairing blood supply. Gas gangrene is accompanied by severe prostration and terminal shock. Clostridia may also be found in localized collections of foul-smelling pus in wounds (Welch's abscess).

CLINICAL MANIFESTATIONS. The incubation period for clostridial cellulitis is usually more than 3 days after wounding. Its onset is gradual with only slight toxicity and little local pain, swelling, or change in skin color. A dark, thin, foul-smelling discharge is produced, showing short, wide, gram-positive rods and a variable number of polymorphonuclear leukocytes on Gram stain. Extensive gas production is characteristic and causes spreading crepitus; muscles are not involved. A similar clinical presentation is also caused by other organisms, usually a mixed flora consisting of *Bacteroides,* anaerobic gram-positive cocci, and Enterobacteriaceae.

In contrast to clostridial cellulitis, gas gangrene is characterized by an incubation of less than 3 days, sudden onset, severe local pain, and swelling. Initially blanched, the skin becomes dark. Blebs appear and are filled with a dark, thin fluid containing many clostridia and few polymorphonuclear leukocytes. Gas production is usually not extensive and may be obscured by the edema. Exploration of the wound will reveal necrotic muscle that fails to contract on stimulation. Although patients with gas gangrene are severely toxic, the syndrome of *C. perfringens* septicemia (hemolytic anemia, hemoglobinemia, and hemoglobinuria) is rarely seen in gas gangrene unless the uterus is involved.

Clostridial uterine myonecrosis is characterized by fever, bacteremia, rapidly developing severe intravascular hemolysis, hemoglobinuria and hemoglobinemia, shock, and renal failure. Gas may be evident in the uterine wall on roentgenograms and at surgery.

After penetrating wounds, clostridia can infect the traumatized organ (for example, the brain, lung, or eye) or cause hematogenous infection (for example, of the pleura, endocardium, or meninges). Clostridia may also cause cholecystitis or transient, benign bacteremia.

DIAGNOSIS. Gas gangrene is evident by clinical presentation, by roentgenography (which may show gas bubbles in muscle), and by the presence of myonecrosis on surgical exploration. Blood cultures are generally negative unless the uterus is involved. Myonecrosis caused by anaerobic gram-positive cocci develops insidiously 3 to 4 days after wounding, with swelling and a purulent exudate in which many polymorphonuclear leukocytes and chains of gram-positive cocci are found; pain follows. This disease has been seen in addicts who administer drugs intramuscularly.

PROGNOSIS AND MANAGEMENT. Gas gangrene is a uniformly fatal disease if not treated early and aggressively. Clostridial cellulitis has a lower mortality. All necrotic tissue and foreign bodies—materials conducive to growth of clostridia—must be removed in both clostridial cellulitis and gas gangrene. Amputation of an involved extremity or hysterectomy may be necessary in myonecrosis. The incised area is left open with drains in place to allow free drainage and to increase the partial pressure of oxygen locally.

Hyperbaric oxygen at 3 atm has been used in therapy of gas gangrene. In this treatment, a patient breathes oxygen at a markedly increased Po_2 and potentially increasing tissue oxygen. The reports of use of hyperbaric oxygen in clostridial myonecrosis seem promising. Therefore, if adequate hyperbaric oxygen facilites are available (hyperbaric chambers large enough for medical personnel to attend the patient), the patient with clostridial myonecrosis should be transported immediately to these facilities. Hyperbaric oxygen *does not* eliminate the need for surgical removal of necrotic muscle or treatment with antimicrobial agents. Both cellulitis and myonecrosis are treated with penicillin, 20 million units intravenously daily, or cephalothin, 12 g intravenously daily. Antimicrobial therapy for gas gangrene can be administered in hyperbaric chambers. The efficacy of clostridial polyvalent antitoxin for clostridial myonecrosis or bacteremia is unclear, and anaphylaxis and serum sickness are complications of its use.

PREVENTION. Careful and prompt cleansing and surgical care of dirty wounds to remove all devitalized tissue and foreign material is essential: vascular obstruction from tight casts or tourniquets should be avoided.

BIBLIOGRAPHY
Infections caused by nonsporeforming anaerobes
Attebery, H.R., Sutter, V.L., and Finegold, S.M.: Effect of a partially chemically defined diet on normal human fecal flora, Am. J. Clin. Nutr. **25**:1391, 1972.

Fingold, S.M.: Anaerobic bacteria in human disease, New York, 1977, Academic Press, Inc.

Rosenblatt, J.E., Fallon, A., and Finegold, S.M.: Comparison of methods for isolation of anaerobic bacteria from clinical specimens, Appl. Microbiol. **25**:77, 1973.

Tally, F.P., and others: Oxygen tolerance of fresh clinical anaerobic bacteria, J. Clin. Microbiol. **1**:161, 1975.

Tetanus
Buchanan, T.M., and others: Tetanus in the United States, 1968 and 1969, J. Infect. Dis. **122**:564, 1970.

Faust, R.A., Vickers, O.R., and Cohn, I.: Tetanus: 2449 cases in 68 years at Charity Hospital, J. Trauma **16**:704, 1976.

Kanarek, D.J., Kaufman, B., and Zwi, S.: Severe sympathetic hyperactivity associated with tetanus. Arch. Intern. Med. **132:**602, 1973.

Weinstein, L.: Tetanus, N. Engl. J. Med. **289:**1293, 1973.

Clostridial soft tissue infection

Altemeier, W.A., and Culbertson, W.R.: Acute non-clostridial crepitant cellulitis, Surg. Gynecol. Obstet. **87:**206, 1948.

Finegold, S.M.: Anaerobic bacteria in human disease, New York, 1977, Academic Press, Inc.

MacLennan, J.D.: The histotoxic clostridial infections of man, Bacteriol. Rev. **26:**232, 1962.

50 • DISEASES CAUSED BY MYCOBACTERIA

Elias Abrutyn

TUBERCULOSIS

DEFINITION. Tuberculosis is a chronic bacterial infection of the lungs and other organs caused by the tubercle bacilli: *Mycobacterium tuberculosis* and *M. bovis*. In the United States disease caused by *M. bovis* is rare.

ETIOLOGY. *M. tuberculosis* is an aerobic, nonmotile, nonsporeforming bacillus approximately 1 to 4 μm in length and 0.3 to 0.5 μm in width. The organism is acid fast, that is, markedly resistant to decolorization with acid-alcohol solution. Although this characteristic is typical of *M. tuberculosis,* it is nonspecific. It appears to be related to certain lipid constituents and is most pronounced in intact cells.

M. tuberculosis is an obligate aerobe and grows best in oxygen concentrations approximating that found in alveolar air (140 mm Hg), a factor that may account for the frequent appearance of infection in organs with a high oxygen content (kidneys, bones, and the apices of the lungs). Because the doubling time is long, about 12 to 18 hours, growth is slow in cultures and colonies first become visible after 3 to 4 weeks. The organism has a distinctive spiral-like pattern of growth that results in colonies with an appearance resembling cords. This characteristic is related to a lipid called cording factor. The presence of colonies demonstrating cording permits presumptive identification of an isolate as *M. tuberculosis*. Other characteristics useful in identifying *M. tuberculosis* include optimal growth at 95° to 102° F (35° to 39° C), absence of pigment production, ability to synthesize niacin and reduce nitrates, and loss of catalase activity at 154° F (68° C).

EPIDEMIOLOGY. Since the early 1900s the case and death rates for tuberculosis have declined dramatically, changes attributed in part to an improved standard of living. These declines have been further accelerated by the introduction of effective chemotherapy. Despite the decreases, tuberculosis remains a common problem. In 1980, for example, 27,749 cases and 1770 deaths (provisionally caused by tuberculosis) were recorded in the United States, giving case and death rates of 12.3 and 0.8 per 100,000 population, respectively.

Associated with these decreases has been a change in the age at first infection. In the early 1900s infection at a young age was common; today infection among school-age children is rare. For the population in general the annual estimated incidence of new infection is 1 per 5000 to 10,000, an attack rate so low as to be difficult to measure. The risk of infection is highest in those in close contact (such as household contact) to persons with untreated, sputum-positive tuberculosis. The risk of clinical disease developing is highest in the first 5 years after infection but remains present lifelong. In the United States the case rates are higher in males, in the older age groups, in races other than white, in large cities, in the Southeast, and along the Mexican border.

PATHOGENESIS AND PATHOLOGY. Tuberculosis is virtually always acquired by inhalation of airborne droplet nuclei containing tubercle bacilli; inoculation and ingestion also occur but are rare. Droplet nuclei are small (1- to 5-μm) particles that are generated and dispersed by persons with active pulmonary disease during coughing, sneezing, singing, or talking. Their small size imparts two characteristics important in the acquisition and spread of tuberculosis: they remain suspended in air for long periods, and they are small enough to escape deposition on the nasal hairs or mucociliary blanket and to enter the terminal airways, respiratory bronchioles, alveolar ducts, and alveoli. These particles are commonly deposited in the lower portions of the lung where ventilation is best. After deposition the bacteria multiply, and a nonspecific inflammatory response occurs. Despite the presence of phagocytes, multiplication continues, and the bacteria spread via the lymphatic system to the regional lymph nodes and then into the bloodstream. The invasion of the blood leads to widespread dissemination throughout the body including other parts of the lung and is the critical factor responsible for the later development of pulmonary or extrapulmonary disease. After several weeks specific cell-mediated immunity, which effects localization and control of the infection, and the characteristic tissue reaction, the granuloma, develop. The granuloma is characterized by epithelioid cells. Langhan's giant cells, lymphocytes, and a particular form of necrosis called caseation necrosis, a name derived from the macroscopic appearance, which resembles cheese. Cavities formed after liquefaction and drainage of the caseous material into the bronchial tree are particularly important because they are associated with large populations of bacteria and are thus associated with a high likelihood of spread to others.

In most patients cell-mediated immunity controls the infection and the lesions heal by resolution, fibrosis, and calcification; bacilli, however, may survive in a dormant state in the lung or other sites, providing a nidus for possible reactivation at a later date. In other patients the cell-mediated immune responses fail to arrest the infection and progressive disease occurs (progressive primary tuberculosis).

The sequence of events—(1) primary pulmonary infection; (2) lymphohematogenous spread; and (3) host response (producing usually dormant infection)—must be understood to comprehend the varied clinical presentations of tuberculosis. These events explain clinical disease developing in the lung or at other sites with the initial infection or disease developing in any of these sites at a later date after reactivation of a focus that has been quiescent.

CLINICAL MANIFESTATIONS. Recent initial infection most often produces no symptoms. When present, the symptoms are nonspecific and can include fever, cough, and malaise. With the development of cell-mediated immunity, they usually subside. Rarely the initial pulmonary infection is uncontrolled and infection progresses, producing primary pulmonary tuberculosis. Infection at sites infected during the bacteremia is also usually controlled by cell-mediated immunity, but occasionally infection progresses, producing clinical disease. For example, the bacteremia may result in tuberculous meningitis or in a debilitating generalized acute infection called miliary tuberculosis because the appearance of the lesions resembles millet seeds. The bacteremia may also result in tuberculous pleurisy or lymphadenitis. In young children enlarged hilar nodes may produce bronchial obstruction and collapse of a portion of the lung, or they may become necrotic and discharge bacilli into the lung, producing tuberculous pneumonia, a diffuse, particularly severe form of pneumonia. Occasionally the initial infection is accompanied by allergic manifestations including erythema nodosum or phlyctenular conjunctivitis, which appears as small vesicles at the junction of the cornea and conjunctiva. The risk of certain manifestations appears in part to be age dependent; miliary and meningeal forms of tuberculosis are common in young children, and progressive primary disease and pleural disease are common in young adults.

Pulmonary tuberculosis. Pulmonary tuberculosis may evolve either from the initial infection or after a variable period by reactivation of a dormant focus, usually in the lung apex.

The onset is usually insidious. Nonspecific constitutional symptoms are common and include fever, fatigue, malaise, weakness, anorexia, and weight loss. The temperature may rise in the afternoon or evening and fall at night; drenching perspiration (night sweats) may accompany the fall in temperature. Cough occurs and may be accompanied by production of sputum that is occasionally blood streaked; massive hemoptysis occurs rarely. Chest pain may be present if the infection extends to the pleura. Wheezing, shortness of breath, and shaking chills are rare.

The physical examination often underestimates the extent of disease demonstrable roentgenographically, and the two must be correlated. Rales may be heard over diseased areas, particularly when a full expiration and then a cough precede a full inspiration (posttussive rales). Dullness, increased fremitus, and other signs of consolidation may be present but are uncommon. The destructive and reparative processes producing cavitation and fibrosis may lead to a variety of findings including tracheal deviation, decreased mobility and volume of the affected hemithorax, apical dullness, and amphoric or bronchial breath sounds. Extrapulmonary findings that suggest previous tuberculous infection but are insignificant in gauging activity of disease include choroid tubercles in the retina and nodules in the epididymis. Erythema nodosum and phlyctenular conjunctivitis are allergic manifestations that suggest active disease.

Pulmonary tuberculosis may lead to involvement of the pleura, bronchi, trachea, and larynx. Inflammation of the pleura overlying a parenchymal lesion may give rise to pleuritic chest pain, so-called dry pleurisy. Erosion of a parenchymal lesion through the pleura and discharge of the caseous material into the pleural space evoke a vigorous inflammatory response and formation of large amounts of pleural fluid (tuberculous pleural effusion). Such effusions are usually unilateral and may be accompanied by fever, cough, pleuritic pain, and shortness of breath. The fluid is exudative in character and has a pH less than 7.2. It contains protein in excess of 3 g/100 ml, and elevated lactic dehydrogenase, and between 300 and 3000 white blood cells/mm^3, predominantly lymphocytes. The glucose concentration may be decreased. The diagnosis of pulmonary tuberculosis should be considered strongly in young adults with an unexplained pleural effusion. The diagnosis must occasionally be made on clinical grounds because the confirmatory tests can be negative. Tuberculous empyema, a rare, occasionally fatal complication resulting from massive contamination, can be differentiated from tuberculous pleural effusion because the fluid more closely resembles pus and smears are usually positive for the organisms. Pneumothorax and bronchopleural fistula may also complicate pulmonary tuberculosis.

The bronchial mucosa bathed in secretions from tuberculous lesions may become infected. Endobronchial tuberculosis almost always appears near cavitary lesions because such lesions have a high bacterial population. Endobronchial spread may also be responsible for the development of lesions remote from the main area of active infection such as in dependent regions or the contralateral lung. The lesions are ulcerative and may bleed, producing blood-streaked sputum; massive hemoptysis results from erosion of a branch of the pulmonary artery. Large endobronchial lesions, particularly in the prechemotherapy era, produced bronchial obstruction and collapse of a segment or lobe. Bronchial distortion often occurs in areas involved in the tuberculous process. Bronchiectatic lesions in the upper lobes are rarely of consequence, but secondary bacterial infection of lesions in the lower lobes can cause chronic cough and sputum production. Tuberculosis of the larynx may develop through direct contamination with infected bronchial secretions, or it may result from bloodborne spread of tubercle bacilli. Hoarseness and pain are common symptoms. Laryngeal tuberculosis, although rare, is of special importance because contagiousness is high owing to ready generation of contaminated aerosols by the vibrating vocal cords.

Tuberculosis in other organs. Tuberculosis in organs other than the lungs may be accompanied by concurrent active pulmonary disease. Whenever extrapulmonary tuberculosis is found, an evaluation for active pulmonary tuberculosis is required.

Cervical nodes (scrofula). Tuberculosis may involve the cervical nodes as well as the hilar nodes. The spread is usually hematogenous, but it may result from lymphatic drainage of a primary pulmonary focus or rarely from direct cervical lymphatic drainage of a local oropharyngeal infection. Clinically, there is usually unilateral painless enlargement without signs of acute inflammation. The nodes are soft, and systemic manifestations are commonly absent. If untreated, the nodes may rupture and discharge caseous material. The response to therapy is excellent. Bacteriologic confirmation is required because scrofula is commonly caused by other mycobacteria that are more resistant to drugs and require surgery for cure. Years ago, milk contaminated with *M. bovis* was a frequent cause of cervical lymphadenitis, but control of bovine tuberculosis and pasteurization of milk have made disease caused by *M. bovis* rare.

Pericardium. The pericardium becomes involved by spread of organisms from a focus in a contiguous lymph node or the lung or rarely by hematogenous dissemination. As in the pleura and other serosal surfaces, infection stimulates an intense inflammatory reaction and accumulation of fluid with characteristics of an exudate, and with resolution there may be fibrosis. During the exudative phase the clinical picture is that of fever and chest pain with or without cardiac tamponade. Dyspnea, cough, ankle swelling, cervical venous distention, and apparent cardiac enlargement may be present. With fibrosis the findings are those of constrictive pericarditis.

Peritoneum. The peritoneum may become involved during hematogenous dissemination or directly by spread from a focus in the intestine, the female genital tract, or a mesenteric lymph node. Fever, abdominal pain, and unexplained ascites may be present, accompanied by weight loss, anorexia, and night sweats. Abdominal tenderness may occur, but rebound may be absent. A "doughy" abdomen is now a rare finding. Recognition in cirrhotic patients who have ascites may be difficult.

Kidneys. The kidneys become infected by hematogenous spread of tubercle bacilli early in the primary pulmonary infection. Clinical disease usually develops after reactivation of dormant foci that undergo caseation, form cavities, and discharge bacilli into the collecting ducts, the ureters, the bladder, and, in males, the genital tract. Because spread is bloodborne, both kidneys are usually infected, although disease may be evident on only one side.

Symptoms are highly variable and may be absent. Common symptoms are frequency, dysuria, nocturia, urgency, and hematuria. Fever and other signs common to acute bacterial infection of the kidneys may be absent. The diagnosis should be suspected when pyuria with or without hermaturia is noted in a patient who has negative urine cultures by standard techniques (sterile pyuria). Intravenous pyelography and cystoscopy may reveal parenchymal calcification of cavitation, papillary necrosis, calyceal dilation, ureteral strictures, and structural defects of the ureteral orifices.

Male genitalia. The prostate, epididymis, vas deferens, seminal vesicles, and rarely the testes may become involved either from hematogenous spread or from active or previously active renal tuberculosis. Epididymitis, a common form of male genital tuberculosis, appears as a painless nodule or as a tender mass that may drain. Tenderness and swelling may also be found with active infection in the other genital organs.

Female genitalia. Female genital tuberculosis begins in the fallopian tube after hematogenous dissemination and spreads to the ovary, the peritoneum, the endometrium, or rarely the cervix. The symptoms are mild and include abdominal pain, vaginal discharge, and menstrual disorders. Constitutional signs are often absent, but a tubal mass may be found. Tubal scarring may lead to infertility or ectopic pregnancy.

Bones and joints. In children infection of the skeleton results from hematogenous spread and commonly involves the long bones and vertebrae. Involvement of these areas may be related to a high oxygen concentration in the growth plates, which are highly vascular. In adults infection results from hematogenous seeding or by spread from adjacent infected paravertebral lymph nodes; the anterior portions of the lower thoracic and lumbar vertebrae are commonly involved (Pott's disease). Pain with or without limitation of motion or constitutional symptoms may be found. Roentgenographically, the earliest finding is narrowing of the intravertebral disc space. Later, destruction is evident in both vertebrae adjacent to the involved disc (Fig. 50-1). Severe destruction leads to scoliosis and kyphosis, which when marked cause severe anterior flexion of the spine with protrusion of the spine posteriorly (hunchback deformity of gibbus formation).

Tuberculous arthritis occurs as a chronic monarticular arthritis involving the hips, knees, elbows, shoulders, and other joints. Tuberculosis may also involve the costochondral junctions of the ribs or the bursae.

Meningitis. Tuberculous meningitis occurs by extension from an adjacent focus such as a subependymal or

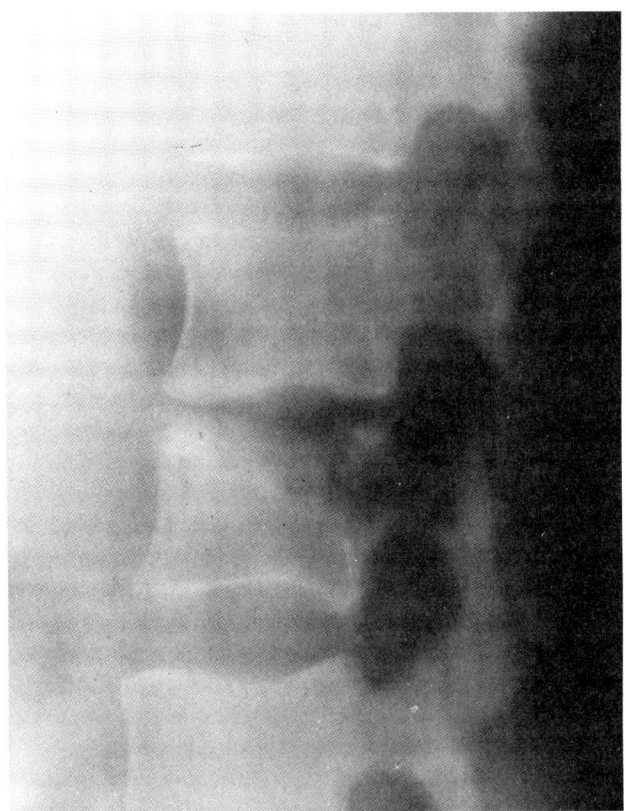

Fig. 50-1. Tomogram of spine of patient with tuberculosis of L2 and L3. There is destruction of vertebral bodies and of disc between L2 and L3.

parameningeal tubercle, or it can complicate miliary tuberculosis. The onset is usually subacute but may be more abrupt or slow, and the clinical findings are nonspecific, resembling those found in meningitis from any cause. The spinal fluid pressure is elevated and the cerebrospinal fluid typically contains an elevated protein content, depressed sugar concentration, and a cell count below 1000/mm^3 with a predominance of lymphocytes. A cerebrospinal fluid containing predominantly lymphocytes and a low glucose concentration should always lead to consideration of this diagnosis, even though other conditions can produce the same findings. The complications are related to the inflammatory process and the thick exudate at the base of the brain and include cranial nerve palsies, hydrocephalus, blindness, and optic atrophy. Therapy should be instituted promptly when the diagnosis of tuberculous meningitis is considered highly likely because death is almost inevitable if the condition is untreated and bacteriologic confirmation, even if positive, requires several weeks.

Disseminated (miliary) tuberculosis. Miliary tuberculosis results from widespread bloodborne dissemination of the tubercle bacillus from a focus in the lungs or other organs, causing infection in many organs throughout the body. This complication, dreaded because of the high mortality it produces if untreated, may occur during the initial infection or years later after reactivation of a dormant focus. The disease may be acute and overwhelming or more chronic in nature. The acute form appears as a severe, prostrating illness with fever, night sweats, anorexia, and headache. There may be abdominal pain with or without peritonitis, pleuritis, and meningitis. The presence of "miliary" lesions on chest roentgenogram should suggest the diagnosis, but they may be absent. The chronic form is similar but more indolent, and destructive lesions may be identified in bones, kidneys, or other organs. The nonspecific protean nature of the findings mandates consideration of this diagnosis whenever a persistent, unexplained febrile illness is present.

Rare forms of tuberculosis. Gastrointestinal tuberculosis occurs as a complication of pulmonary disease or from ingestion of contaminated milk. Tuberculosis may involve the oropharynx, esophagus, small and large intestines, and rectum. The lesions are ulcerative or hyperplastic or both and may lead to bleeding, obstruction, or perforation. The diagnosis is usually made at surgery. Addison's disease resulting from tuberculosis is now rare. Involvement of other organs including the eye, ear, thyroid, pancreas, and breast occasionally occurs.

DIAGNOSIS AND LABORATORY FINDINGS

Tuberculin skin test. The preferred test is the intracutaneous (Mantoux) test employing as antigen 0.1 ml of a solution containing 5 tuberculin units (TU) of purified protein derivative (PPD), the so-called intermediate-strength PPD. In 48 to 72 hours after the antigen is injected into the dermis on the volar surface of the forearm, the diameter of induration around the injection site is measured; erythema is disregarded. A positive test, that is, induration of 10 mm or more, denotes previous infection with *M. tuberculosis*. A doubtful reaction, 5 to 9 mm, signifies probable prior infection with other related mycobacteria, but previous infection with *M. tuberculosis* is also possible. A negative test, 0 to 4 mm, means that previous tuberculous infection or infection with other organisms is unlikely.

If the "intermediate" skin test is negative and tuberculosis remains a likely possibility, repeat testing with 250 TU (second-strength PPD) is indicated. Other skin test antigens (*Candida,* mumps, *Trichophyton,* and so forth) are frequently applied simultaneously to determine whether or not the patient is anergic. A negative response to all skin test antigens means that the person is anergic and that tuberculosis should remain a diagnostic possibility. A positive second-strength test irrespective of the other tests means that infection with either *M. tuberculosis* or other mycobacteria has occurred and that the patient is not anergic. A negative second-strength test in a person responding to at least one other antigen means that anergy is not present and prior infection with *M. tuberculosis* is most unlikely.

A first-strength skin test employing 1 TU as antigen is

available for use in patients likely to develop large necrotic lesions at the injection site, but it is rarely used.

Roentgenography. The chest roentgenogram never provides an etiologic diagnosis, but the findings are often sufficient to make the diagnosis highly likely. The chest film is also useful in monitoring response to therapy. The initial lesions appear as a parenchymal infiltrate in any portion of the lung in association with hilar adenopathy. With healing, these lesions may calcify and remain identifiable as the "Ghon complex." In reactivation tuberculosis involving the lung, the type most commonly found in adults, the roentgenogram usually shows parenchymal infiltrates with or without cavitation or fibrosis in the apical-posterior area(s) of the upper lobe(s) (Fig. 50-2). Occasionally the predominant lesions is found in the superior segment of the lower lobe. In contrast to lung abscess, cavities in tuberculosis usually contain no fluid. Discrete, fluffy infiltrates in other areas of the lung indicate bronchogenic spread. Healed inactive disease may appear as apical pleural scars, fibrosis with loss of volume in affected areas, or calcified areas. Tuberculous pneumonia resembles other bacterial pneumonias, and in miliary tuberculosis fine, discrete nodules may be found distributed throughout both lungs. Evidence of pleural or pericardial effusion may also be found. Other roentgenographic studies such as intravenous pyelography and bone roentgenograms may be useful in demonstrating destructive or fibrotic lesions consistent with tuberculosis.

Bacteriology. Definitive diagnosis requires isolation and speciation of the organism from body fluids or tissue, a process that takes several weeks because the organism grows slowly. A presumptive diagnosis, however, can be made when smears stained for examination by fluorescent microscopy or by conventional methods (Ziehl-Neelsen or Kinyoun stain) are positive.

Sputum is the material most frequently examined. Multiple specimens, preferably those obtained in the early morning, should be examined. If the patient fails to produce sputum spontaneously, sputum production can be induced by having the patient breathe an aerosol of heated saline. Occasionally sputum is obtained by bronchial washing and brushing during bronchoscopy; postbronchoscopy sputum specimens may be positive when other specimens are negative. Gastric aspiration to obtain swallowed bronchial secretions is sometimes helpful. Although cultures of this material may be positive, smears are unreliable because nontuberculous mycobacteria are frequently present. Urine smears are unreliable for the same reason. Smears of other body fluids (pleural, pericardial, peritoneal, cerebrospinal, synovial, and pus) should always be performed because a positive result in highly suggestive, but the yield is usually low.

Histology. A presumptive diagnosis may also be made when granulomata with or without caseation or organisms are seen in histologic secretions, although granuloma formation is not specific for tuberculosis. Histologic examination of tissue is particularly useful when the pleural, pericardial, peritoneal, or synovial membranes appear involved because cultures of the respective body fluids and tissues themselves are often negative. Examination of biopsy material from the liver and bone marrow is helpful in miliary tuberculosis, and biopsy may be useful in diagnosing disease in other sites, including the lymph nodes and the genital tract.

Other laboratory tests. Routine laboratory tests are of little value. The hemoglobin and hematocrit may be normal or show anemia of chronic disease. The white cell count may be normal, but a leukemoid reaction is occasionally seen. The serum sodium may be low from inappropriate secretion of antidiuretic hormone or rarely from Addison's disease. Sterile pyuria or hematuria suggests renal involvement. Exudative pleural, peritoneal, pericardial, or synovial effusion, with lymphocytes as the predominant cell type, should suggest tuberculosis, as should lymphocytosis in the cerebrospinal fluid.

MANAGEMENT. The treatment of tuberculosis no longer requires institutionalization, prolonged bed rest, or deforming chest surgery, but it does require prolonged antituberculous chemotherapy. Hospitalization, although not required, facilitates performance of diagnostic procedures and permits evaluation of the response to and tolerance of chemotherapy.

The treatment of tuberculosis necessitates rigid adherence to certain principles. First, bactericidal drugs (isoniazid and rifampin) are preferred, and at least one should be included in the therapeutic regimen if possible. Second, two drugs active against the infecting organism should al-

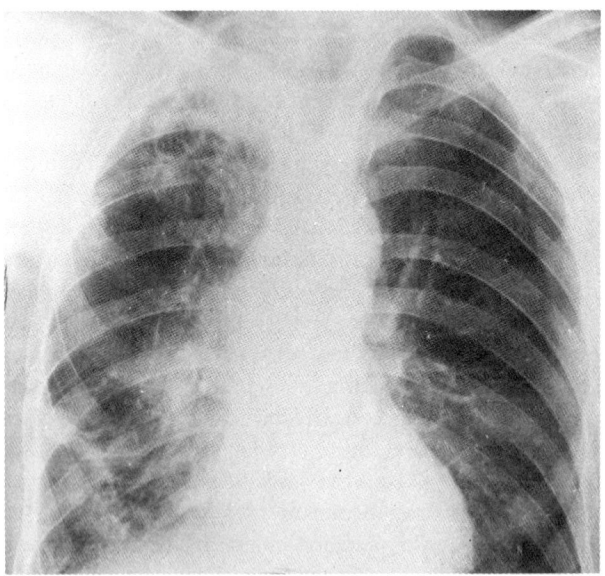

Fig. 50-2. Pulmonary tuberculosis with right upper lobe cavity and spillage of disease to middle and lower lobes.

ways be used to treat active disease because resistance is likely to emerge during therapy when only one drug is employed. Third, chemotherapy should be continued sufficiently long to eradicate the organism; a major reason for failure of therapy is noncompliance with the prescribed regimen. Fourth, retreatment requires a regimen containing two drugs not previously used in the therapy or at least two drugs known to be active. Last, chemotherapy should not be withheld from ill persons pending culture results because the morbidity and mortality rates of untreated disease are high. Rather, treatment should be begun when the results of diagnostic tests (smears, roentgenograms, histologic tests, and so on) indicate that tuberculosis is the most likely diagnosis.

Antituberculosis drugs. The major drugs used in treatment are isoniazid, rifampin, ethambutol, and streptomycin. Supplemental drugs include pyrazinamide, ethionamide, cycloserine, para-aminosalicylic acid, capreomycin, and kanamycin.

Isoniazid. Isoniazid (INH), the most useful chemotherapeutic agent, is tuberculocidal, effective when given orally, and relatively nontoxic. The prevalence of INH resistance among untreated cases in the United States is low. In the Far East INH resistance is common. In adults the dosage is usually 5 to 10 mg/kg or 300 mg once daily orally. The drug diffuses into tissues well. It is acetylated in the liver and excreted by the kidneys. Individuals vary in their ability to acetylate INH, but the response to chemotherapy with the regimens in common use is not altered because of this. The toxic effects include peripheral neuritis, which can be prevented or treated with pyridoxine; hypersensitivity reactions: and liver damage. About 10% of the patients have transient elevations in serum transaminase levels, which often resolve despite continued administration of the drug. A more severe, occasionally fatal form of hepatitis with nausea, vomiting, and jaundice also occurs. The frequency is low but is increased in older age groups. Treatment requires stopping INH; resolution usually follows. INH increases the toxic potential of phenytoin (Dilantin). Pryidoxine, 50 mg daily, is often given to prevent neuropathy and is recommended when the daily dose of INH exceeds 300 mg.

Rifampin. The introduction of rifampin (RIF) has revolutionized the treatment of tuberculosis by permitting the development of regimens requiring shorter courses of therapy. The drug is bactericidal, absorbed from the gastrointestinal tract, widely distributed in tissues, and of low toxicity, but it is more expensive than INH. It interferes with protein synthesis by inhibiting RNA polymerase. In adults the dose of 10 mg/kg or 600 mg is administered once daily. RIF causes hepatitis, gastrointestinal reactions, and hypersensitivity reactions including a flulike syndrome, hemolytic anemia, thrombocytopenia, and renal failure. When high doses are given intermittently, hypersensitivity reactions are common, but with doses of 450 to 600 mg they are rare. RIF decreases the effectiveness of warfarin sodium and birth control pills, and it turns the urine orange-red. It has shown immunosuppressive activity, but this appears clinically unimportant.

Ethambutol. Ethambutol (EMB) is a bacteriostatic agent widely used as a companion drug in conventional long-term treatment regimens, as substitution therapy when resistance or a toxic reaction to another drug develops, and as a component of some short-treatment regimens. The dose of 15 to 25 mg/kg is administered once daily orally and is well tolerated. Optic toxicity manifested by changes in visual acuity, color vision, and visual fields is dose dependent and usually reversible. Hyperuricemia has been reported.

Streptomycin. Streptomycin (SM), an aminoglycoside antibiotic that inhibits protein synthesis, is administered parenterally. It is used in some long- and short-course treatment regimens and for those unable to ingest medication. It is also used for poorly compliant patients in intermittent treatment regimens fully supervised by medical personnel. The dose of SM during the first few months is 1 g daily intramuscularly in one injection and thereafter 1 g three times a week. Eighth cranial nerve toxicity may occur in the form of vertigo; nephrotoxicity is extremely rare. Dose reduction is appropriate for persons with renal failure and for the elderly.

Pyrazinamide. Pyrazinamide (PZA) is generally used for retreatment, particularly when multiple drug resistance is present. Hepatotoxicity is the most troublesome side effect, and hyperuricemia occurs. The dose of 20 to 35 mg/kg, usually 1.5 to 2 g, may be given once daily orally. The combination of PZA and SM has excellent antituberculosis activity.

Ethionamide. Ethionamide (ETH), related in structure to INH but less effective, is used primarily in retreatment, especially when multiple drug resistance is present. Gastrointestinal intolerance (manifested by metallic taste, anorexia, and vomiting) or liver injury limits use. The total daily dosage of 750 to 1000 mg is given in three or four doses of 250 mg orally after meals.

Cycloserine. Cycloserine (CS), a toxic, relatively ineffective agent that inhibits cell wall synthesis, is used in retreatment. Seizures, depression, psychotic behavior, and other central nervous system symptoms occur; the drug is contraindicated in epileptic patients and persons with psychosis. The total daily dosage of 750 to 1000 mg is given in two equally divided doses by mouth.

Para-aminosalicylic acid. Para-aminosalicylic acid (PAS) is rarely used today; previously it was a major drug. Gastrointestinal intolerance is frequent, and hypersensitivity reactions occur. PAS preparations with bentonite as the excipient may inhibit the absorption of RIF. The usual daily dosage of 12 to 15 g (150 to 200 mg/kg) is given orally in three or four equally divided portions.

Capreomycin. Capreomycin (CM) resembles streptomycin in activity, dosage, and side effects. It is used intramuscularly in retreatment.

Kanamycin. Kanamycin (KM), a nephrotoxic and ototoxic aminoglycoside antibiotic, is primarily reserved for retreatment regimens. It is given intramuscularly.

Choice of regimen. Short-course chemotherapy, recently recommended for use in the United States, is likely to become the preferred mode of therapy for newly diagnosed cases of pulmonary tuberculosis. The regimen recommended for adult use consists of INH (300 mg) and RIF (600 mg) given during the initial phase of treatment, which may range from 2 weeks to 2 months. Thereafter treatment with INH and RIF is continued daily if self-administered. An alternative for noncompliant patients is fully supervised, twice-weekly therapy using a dose of 15 mg/ INH and 600 mg RIF on each treatment day. Treatment continues for at least 9 months but longer if necessary; at least 6 months should elapse from conversion of the sputum to culture negativity before therapy is stopped. If the patient has resided in or emigrated from an area with a high level of drug resistance (for example, the Far East) or has been treated before, EMB (15 mg/kg daily) should be added until the results of drug susceptibility tests are known. At present short-course therapy is not recommended for patients with extrapulmonary tuberculosis or those with certain special medical conditions (silicosis, diabetes, or immunosuppressed states) because the effectiveness in these situations has not been evaluated.

Conventional therapy consisting of at least two drugs active against the infecting organism for 18 months is used when patients do not qualify for short-course chemotherapy or when drug toxicity precludes continuation of short-course treatment. A regimen in wide use is INH (300 mg daily) and EMB (15 to 15 mg/kg dialy for the first 2 or 3 months and 15 mg/kg daily thereafter). When the population of bacteria is considered high, for example, when sputum smears are positive, RIF (600 mg daily) or ST (0.75 to 1 g each day) is often added for the first few months of treatment.

In addition to the short-course intermittent regimen, other fully supervised intermittent regimens are available. Such therapy should be used for persons who cannot or will not comply with other regimens.

Retreatment of persons given inadequate initial therapy, those failing to complete a prescribed regimen, or those with relapse after apparently successful therapy requires great skill, and expert advice should be sought. In such cases drug susceptibility testing is mandatory, and if treatment is begun before the results are available, the regimen must include at least two drugs not used previously.

Additional measures. Corticosteriods are occasionally used in the treatment of patients seriously ill or moribund from overwhelming disease. They are also employed in tuberculous meningitis when cranial nerve palsies are present and to reduce elevated intracranial pressure. In tuberculous pericarditis and pleuritis they may increase the rate of resolution of the exudate. Their efficacy in preventing or retarding the development of residual fibrosis and the complications thereof remains unproven. The routine use of corticosteriods is not advised, but when they are used, concurrent chemotherapy is mandatory.

Surgery is now used infrequently because chemotherapy is effective. Surgery may be required for massive hemoptysis, bronchopleural fistula, pneumothorax, tuberculous empyema, bronchiectasis, pericardial tamponade, constrictive pericarditis, intestinal obstruction, ureteral obstruction, or abscess. In cases of spinal tuberculosis, surgery or immobilization with casts is rarely if ever necessary.

PREVENTION AND CONTROL

Preventive chemotherapy. The risk of reactivating dormant tuberculosis can be reduced by administering INH at a dose of 300 mg (5 to 10 mg/kg in children) once daily for 12 months. In recommending preventive therapy, the risk of disease must be balanced against the risk of INH hepatitis.

Household and other close contacts of patients with newly discovered tuberculosis are at special risk and should be examined for active disease, which, if present, should be treated accordingly. Skin test–positive contacts (that is, positive intermediate-strength PPD) without disease should receive preventive therapy. Skin test–negative contacts may also be started on INH (children are always treated), but they should have a repeat skin test at 3 months. If the repeat test is positive, therapy is either continued or started; if the test is negative, no treatment is required.

Other candidates for preventive therapy are (1) patients with positive skin tests and chest roentgenographic findings consistent with nonprogressive tuberculosis; (2) patients with a past history of tuberculosis never treated adequately with chemotherapy; (3) newly infected persons, that is, those whose skin test has converted within the previous 2 years; and (4) patients with special conditions associated with a high risk of reactivation, including prolonged steroid therapy, immunosuppressive therapy, malignancy such as Hodgkin's disease, diabetes mellitus, silicosis, and previous gastrectomy. Finally, tuberculin reactors under 35 years old should be treated even in the absence of risk factors associated with reactivation. Those over 35 years old should be considered for therapy only if they are contacts or converters or have a special condition enhancing the risk for reactivation, because their risk of INH hepatitis is high. Preventive therapy for pregnant patients is generally begun after delivery.

Vaccination. Bacille Calmette Guérin (BCG) is a live attenuated strain of *M. bovis* used as a vaccine. Vaccination may not reduce the risk of infection but does reduce the risk of serious forms of the disease such as miliary tuberculosis or meningitis. The efficacy of vaccination remains a controversial issue, and in the United States its use is restricted to unifected persons who have repeated exposure to infectious cases and who could not obtain or accept treatment if they were to become ill. Adverse reactions include severe or prolonged ulceration at the vaccination site, lymphadenitis, osteomyelitis, disseminated infection, and death. Pregnancy and impaired immunity preclude vaccination.

PROGNOSIS. With adequate chemotherapy, the prognosis of tuberculosis is excellent.

NONTUBERCULOUS MYCOBACTERIAL INFECTIONS

DEFINITION. Many mycobacteria other than *M. tuberculosis* and *M. leprae* have been identified, some of which cause disease. In the past these organisms were called atypical or anonymous mycobacteria, but today they are referred to by the specific species name.

ETIOLOGY. In 1959 Runyon grouped the mycobacteria according to colonial morphology, pigmentation, and rate of growth. The relationship between the Runyon classification and the various species is as follows. The group I organisms, the photochromogens, grow slowly, produce pigment only after exposure to light, and include *M. kansasii, M. marimum,* and *M. simiae.* Group II organisms, the scotochromogens, also grow slowly but produce pigment only in the dark: *M. scrofulaceum* and *M. szulgai* are in this group. Group III, the nonchromogens, grow slowly, produce no pigment, and include the *M. avium-intracellulare* complex, *M. xenopi,* and *M. ulcerans.* Group IV, the rapid growers, grow quickly, produce no pigment, and include *M. chelonei* and *M. fortuitum*. In the United States *M. kansasii,* the *M. avium-intracellulare* complex, and *M. scrofulaceum* are the predominant agents of human disease. Other species of mycobacteria have also been identified but are generally considered nonpathogenic.

EPIDEMIOLOGY. Disease caused by the nontuberculous mycobacteria occurs worldwide. Several species are present in the environment, and isolates of some have been recovered from food, water, animals, soil, and house dust. They have also been recovered from persons without recognizable evidence of disease. Multiple cases in families are rare, and evidence of person-to-person transmission is lacking.

Results of skin tests with antigens from several species reveal that there is wide cross-reactivity among the various species and to *M. tuberculosis,* that skin tests are not generally helpful in diagnosing infection in the individual patient, and that many healthy individuals have had infection with these organisms.

PATHOGENESIS AND PATHOLOGY. The exact mode of transmission is unknown, but inhalation, ingestion, and inoculation may account for pulmonary disease, cervical lymphadenitis, and dermal infection, respectively. Histologically, the lesions are granulomatous, resembling tuberculosis, but suppuration is occasionally present.

CLINICAL MANIFESTATIONS

Pulmonary disease. Pulmonary disease clinically indistinguishable from tuberculosis may be caused by *M. kansasii*, the *M. avium-intracellulare* complex, and, less commonly, other species. Chronic obstructive pulmonary disease is frequently present. The diagnosis requires isolation of the organism from multiple specimens because these mycobacteria may occur as saprophytes. Antibiotic susceptibility testing is required because susceptibility varies among the different species and resistance is common. *M. kansasii* generally responds well to a combination of isoniazid, rifampin, and ethambutol given for 2 years in the same doses as for tuberculosis. The other species are more resistant, and four or more antituberculosis drugs are often used in initial therapy. Surgery is occasionally required.

Lymphadenitis. Painless, unilateral cervical lymphadenitis may be seen, particularly in children. *M. scrofulaceum* is frequently isolated, but other species may also be incriminated. Total excision of the involved nodes is required for cure.

Skin and subcutaneous infection. *M. marinum,* the cause of "swimming pool granuloma," has been isolated from swimming pools, fish tanks, and natural bodies of water. After entering the skin through abrasions or cuts, the organism produces verrucous or ulcerating lesions that remain localized because the organism grows poorly, if at all, at body temperature. Rifampin and ethambutol given for 6 weeks in the same doses as for tuberculosis are effective; tetracycline, 500 mg every 6 hours, or minocycline, 100 mg twice a day, may also be useful.

M. ulcerans produces deep, mutilating ulceration involving the skin, subcutaneous tissue, and muscle. The disease occurs in tropical areas. Excisional surgery is required.

Other infections. Local abscess after injection with contaminated needles, bone and joint disease, genitourinary infection, sternal wound infection after cardiac surgery, and eye infection have occurred. Disseminated disease, particularly in immunosuppressed hosts, and endocarditis have also been described. Surgery may be required for cure.

LEPROSY

DEFINITION. Leprosy is a chronic granulomatous disease affecting the skin and peripheral nerves. The disease is highly variable, and different forms that have prognostic and therapeutic significance have been defined. The major types, listed in order from limited to widespread disease, are tuberculoid, borderline, and lepromatous leprosy. An indeterminate form that may evolve into one of the other forms is also seen.

ETIOLOGY. *M. leprae* is an intracellular, acid-fast bacillus that has never been grown in vitro. A relationship to other mycobacteria has been established on the basis of the presence of mycolic acids, multiple cross-reacting antigens, and similar filamentous surface structures. *M. leprae* can be readily transmitted to animals. In the mouse foot pad it produces a distinctive growth curve with an unusually slow generation time of 11 to 13 days, and in armadillos it causes a lepromatous leprosy–like illness. These animal models have provided a means to study immunotherapy and chemotherapy and sufficient antigen for biochemical and metabolic analyses and for vaccine development. The ability of *M. leprae* to infect peripheral nerves is unique, providing a marker distinct for this disease. Temperature may be an important factor in growth, since disease occurs in cooler areas of the skin.

The lepromin skin test uses heat-killed *M. leprae* from tissues of lepromatous patients or armadillos as an antigen. Intradermal injection may elicit a tuberculin-like reaction (Fernandez reaction) at 48 hours or a papular reaction (Mitsuda reaction) at 3 to 4 weeks. The latter reaction aids in classifying patients because it is negative in lepromatous leprosy and positive in tuberculoid leprosy. However, the skin test is not useful in diagnosis because normal adults are frequently positive.

EPIDEMIOLOGY. Leprosy affects 10 to 20 million persons worldwide and is found in most tropical and temperate regions. In the United States the disease is reported frequently from Florida, Texas, California, Hawaii, Louisiana, New York, and Puerto Rico. Although many cases are indigenous, most are imported, often from Mexico, the Philippines, and American Samoa.

The mode of transmission is unknown but had been assumed to be direct skin-to-skin contact. Recently the respiratory route has been considered the likely major mode of transmission because the number of organisms shed from the skin is low and in untreated lepromatous individuals shedding from the nose is high. Contagiousness appears to be related to the number of viable bacilli shed from the nose and is highest in lepromatous leprosy; tuberculoid leprosy is probably not contagious. Study of transmission is most difficult because of the long incubation period, estimated to average 3 to 5 years. Prolonged contact appears to be important in the acquisition of disease; casual contacts are at low risk.

PATHOLOGY AND PATHOGENESIS. The pathogenesis is poorly understood, but bacteremia is thought to be important in the development and perhaps the progression of the disease. Defects in cellular immunity in all types of leprosy have been described and are most severe in the more generalized forms. The ability of the host to generate an immune response to *M. leprae* after infection may determine the subsequent course of the disease.

Histologically, the lesions in tuberculoid leprosy are characterized by epithelioid cells, lymphocytes, giant cells, and rare bacilli. In lepromatous leprosy foamy his-

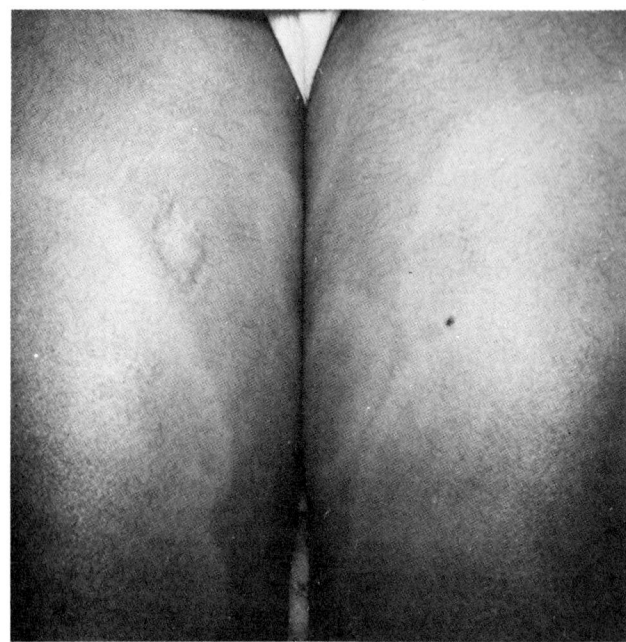

Fig. 50-3. Tuberculoid leprosy showing two large, well-demarcated plaques on thighs with hypopigmented centers.

tiocytes, occasional lymphocytes, and many intracellular bacilli are seen. Borderline lesions have features of both types. Nerve involvement is found in all forms of the disease and is most severe in tuberculoid leprosy.

CLINICAL MANIFESTATIONS. In tuberculoid leprosy one (occasionally two or three) large, well-demarcated plaque that has a raised erythematous edge and a flat, hypopigmented, hairless, dry center is found (Fig. 50-3). Nerves (commonly the ulnar, radial, median, great auricular, or superficial peroneal) in the area of the plaque are often visibly or palpably enlarged. The area is anesthetic and therefore susceptible to infection or trauma. Muscle atrophy and contractures may occur as complications.

The lesions of lepromatous leprosy are bilaterally symmetric, diffuse, and poorly demarcated. They appear as macules, nodules, or plaques commonly involving the face, wrists, buttocks, knees, or skin over other bony prominences, but they can occur anywhere on the body. Nasal involvement producing complaints of nasal "stuffiness" occurs early, and lesions involving the gums, buccal mucosa, tongue, palate, tonsillar pillars, and posterior pharyngeal wall may be seen. Infiltration and thickening of the skin progress slowly and can produce loss of eyebrows, the classic leonine facies, or pendulous earlobes (Fig. 50-4). Septal and palatal perforation, nasal collapse, atrophy of the maxillary alveolar process, laryngitis, blindness, gynecomastia, and sterility may occur late in the course. Nerve involvement, although diffuse, is less severe than in tuberculoid disease. Nerve thickening is not marked, and sensory loss is patchy.

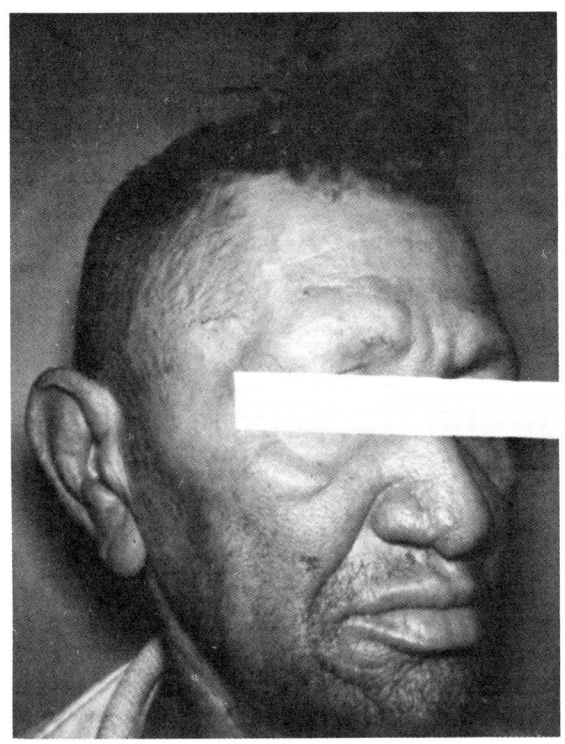

Fig. 50-4. Lepromatous leprosy showing loss of eyebrows, pendulous earlobes, and leonine facies with prominence of eyebrow ridge.

The course of patients with leprosy may be complicated by a variety of acute episodes called reactions. Erythema nodosum leprosum (ENL), one reaction form, occurs in lepromatous leprosy, often during the first year of therapy. Tender, inflamed, subcutaneous nodules appear. Histologically, the lesions resemble an Arthus reaction, and bacterial viability may be reduced. There may also be fever, arthritis, lymphadenopathy, iridocyclitis, and glomerulonephritis. Reversal reactions occur in borderline cases; existing lesions become erythematous and indurated, and new lesions may occur. The histologic findings may shift toward either the tuberculoid or the lepromatous type.

DIAGNOSIS. The peripheral nerve involvement in leprosy distinguishes it from other skin diseases with a similar appearance. The diagnosis is best confirmed by skin biopsy. The finding of acid-fast bacilli in smears of material obtained by scraping the cut surface of a fresh skin incision is highly suggestive.

MANAGEMENT. Dapsone, the drug of choice, is administered to adults in doses of 50 to 100 mg daily for about 2 to 4 years in indeterminate and tuberculoid leprosy and for 10 years to life in lepromatous disease. Combined therapy is recommended for lepromatous leprosy because dapsone resistance occurs and dapsone-sensitive organisms may persist in tissues despite years of therapy. Rifampin, the companion drug of choice, is bactericidal but expensive. It is used for 3 to 6 months in daily doses of 600 mg. Rifampin resistance occurs. Clofazimine, another major drug, is employed most often incombination to treat drug-resistant cases, but its use is limited because it discolors the skin. The choice of one or two drugs for the treatment of borderline leprosy depends on the severity of the disease. ENL and reversal reactions may require antipyretics, anti-inflammatory agents, or steroids. Thalidomide, a teratogenic compound contraindicated in pregnancy, is remarkably effective in ENL but not in reversal reactions. The does is 300 mg a day tapered to 100 mg a day. Immunotherapy with transfer factor or transfusion of allogeneic leukocytes remains experimental. In addition to specific chemotherapy, plastic surgery, vocational training, education, and physiotherapy are important.

PREVENTION. New cases of leprosy should be reported to public health authorities, and household contacts should be examined for active disease. Preventive chemotherapy and periodic examinations may be indicated for some contacts, and guidance in these matters should be sought from experts. The efficacy of BCG in preventing cases has been evaluated, but the results are variable. The U.S. Public Health Service, which has a mandate to maintain facilities for treating leprosy, can provide assistance.

PROGNOSIS. Patients with indeterminate or tuberculoid leprosy may undergo spontaneous cure, but progressive disease is common with the other types. Amyloidosis is a late complication. With therapy, the prognosis is excellent, but relapses occur.

BIBLIOGRAPHY
Tuberculosis

American Thoracic Society: Preventive therapy of tuberculosis infection, Am. Rev. Respir. Dis. **110:**371, 1974.

American Thoracic Society: Treatment of mycobacterial disease, Am. Rev. Respir. Dis. **115:**185, 1977.

American Thoracic Society and the Centers for Disease Control: Guidelines for short course tuberculosis chemotherapy, M.M.W.R. **29:**97, 1980.

Barksdale, L., and Kim, K.: Mycobacterium, Bacteriol Rev. **41:**217, 1977.

Bernstein, R.E.: Isoniazid hepatotoxicity and acetylation during tuberculosis chemoprophylaxis, Am. Rev. Respir. Dis. **118:**429, 1980.

First International Conference on Tuberculosis, sponsored by the Pittsfield, Massachusetts, Antituberculous Association, the American College of Chest Physicians, and the North American Region of the International Union Against Tuberculosis. Chest **76**(suppl. 6):737, 1979.

Johnston, R.F., and Wildrick, K.H.: The impact of chemotherapy on the care of patients with tuberculosis, Am. Rev. Respir. Dis. **109:**636. 1974.

Mayock, R.L., and MacGregor. R.R.: Diagnosis, prevention and early therapy of tuberculosis, D.M. **22:**1, 1976.

Sbarbaro, J.A., Catlin, B.J., and Iseman, M.: Long-term effectiveness of intermittent therapy of tuberculosis: final report of three Denver studies, Am. Rev. Respir. Dis. **121:**172, 1980.

Stead, W.W., and Dutt, A.K., editors: Clinics in Chest Medicine **1:**165, 1980.

Tuberculosis prevention trial: trial of BCG vaccines in south India for tuberculosis prevention: first report, Bull. WHO **57:**819, 1979.

Youmans, G.P.: Tuberculosis, Philadelphia, 1979, W.B. Saunders Co.

Nontuberculous mycobacterial infections

Izumi, A.K., Hanke, W., and Higaki, M.: *Mycobacterium marinum* infections treated with tetracycline, Arch. Dermatol. **113:**1067, 1977.

Wolinsky, E.: Non-tuberculous mycobacteria and associated diseases, Am. Rev. Respir. Dis. **119:**107, 1979.

Leprosy

Bullock, W.E.: The immunobiology of leprosy. In Nahmias, A., and O'Reilly, R., editors: Immunology of human infections. Part I. Mycoplasmae, chlamydiae, and fungi. Vol. 8 in the series Comprehensive immunology, edited by Good, R.A., and Day, S.B, New York, Plenum Publishing Co. (In press.)

Felice, G.A., and Fraser, D.W.: Management of household contacts of leprosy patients, Ann. Intern. Med. **88:**538, 1978.

Fifth report of the WHO Expert Committee on Leprosy, WHO Tech. Rep. Ser. No. 607, p. 3, 1977.

Girdhar, B.K., and Deskian, K.V.: A clinical study of the mouth in untreated lepromatous patients, Lepr. Rev. **50:**25, 1979.

Sansonetti, P., and Lagrange, P.H.: The immunology of leprosy: speculations on the leprosy spectrum, Rev. Infect. Dis. **3:**422, 1981.

51 • DISEASES CAUSED BY SPIROCHETES

Syphilis

Michael F. Rein

Syphilis is a specific infection with the spirochete *Treponema pallidum*. The disease is chronic with subacute symptomatic periods and asymptomatic intervals during which the diagnosis can be made only serologically. Because of its ability to involve all organ systems and the variability of its clinical presentations, syphilis has been called "the great imitator." Sir William Osler commented that "he who knows syphilis, knows medicine." The infection is acquired almost entirely by sexual contact, although it must be recognized that this term encompasses far more than coitus.

ETIOLOGY. The genus *Treponema* includes at least three species pathogenic for man: *T. carateum,* the agent of pinta; *T. pertenue,* the agent of yaws; and *T. pallidum,* the agent of syphilis. Bejel, a nonvenereal infection, is caused by an organism that is indistinguishable from *T. pallidum* and is usually referred to as a variant. Some believe that *T. pallidum* evolved as the cause of venereal syphilis from the older organisms responsible for the nonvenereal treponematoses. Infection with any of these agents elicits reactive serologic tests for syphilis.

T. pallidum is a fine spiral organism approximately 0.15 μm wide and 6 to 15 μm long. The organism is poorly visualized with routine microbiologic and histologic stains, but it may be seen in tissue with a variety of silver stains and is identified by darkfield microscopy in fluid recovered from lesions or lymph nodes. When observed in the living state, the organism displays 6 to 14 regular spirals that are maintained during its movements. *T. pallidum* has a characteristic motility that helps differentiate it from other spirochetes. The organism is seen to rotate in corkscrew fashion around the long axis of the cylinder formed by its spirals. It moves forward and backward along this axis and is sometimes observed to bend at its midpoint.

T. pallidum has a trilaminar outer membrane similar to that seen in gram-negative bacteria. Unlike these, however, *T. pallidum* has not been shown to possess a biologically active endotoxin.

The spirochete is microaerophilic and survives poorly in atmospheric oxygen. This, in addition to its sensitivity to drying and to extremes of temperature, explains in part its almost exclusively venereal mode of transmission. At present it has not been cultured on artificial media, although its viability and virulence can be maintained by serial passage in susceptible animals, principally rabbits. The inability to culture the organism has increased dependence on clinical, microscopic, and serologic diagnosis.

Fortunately, *T. pallidum* has remained sensitive to the antibiotics used for the treatment of syphilis. The organism appears to be killed with first-order kinetics; a maximal rate of killings occurs at 0.1 μg/ml of penicillin. Exposing organisms to higher concentrations of penicillin does not increase the rate at which they are killed. Thus syphilis can be cured by treatments that present the spirochete with very low levels of penicillin. On the other hand, a relatively long course of therapy is required to eradicate the infecting organisms, since the rate of killing is for the most part uninfluenced by increasing the dose of antibiotic administered.

EPIDEMIOLOGY. The venereal nature of syphilis is clearly established and was recognized in its earliest descriptions. As one would expect, the disease is prevalent among the sexual partners of infected patients. Syphilis appears to develop in approximately 30% of these people, but some will have had many exposures to the infected partner while others will have had only a single sexual contact. Thus, although the 30% figure represents an average prevalence, the risks to an individual cannot be quantitated. There is no estimate of the risk of acquiring syphilis from a single sexual exposure to an infected partner; this clearly depends on the type of exposure and the specific condition of the active lesions. The 30% prevalence, however, is considered sufficiently high to indicate a need for "epidemiologic treatment." Persons who within the past 90 days have been the sexual partners of patients with infectious syphilis should be treated even before their infections have been confirmed in the laboratory. This approach undoubtedly results in the treatment of uninfected people, but it eliminates the risk of losing infected individuals to follow-up, prevents the development of infectious lesions and further spread of disease, and often prevents the development of seroreactivity. Epidemiologic treatment has been a cornerstone of syphilis control in the United States.

Syphilis is most prevalent in sexually active populations and age groups. The highest age-adjusted rates for early syphilis reported in the United States are found in 20- to 24-year-old men and women. Syphilis is also particularly prevalent among 24- to 34-year-old men. Interestingly, syphilis is prevalent in a somewhat older age group than gonorrhea. As with other sexually transmitted diseases, syphilis is more common in larger cities. The prevalence of infection is also increased in homosexual men; more than half of the cases in larger cities are reported in homosexual populations. More than one third of infected men are exclusively homosexual or bisexual, and overall the disease is three times more common in men than in women.

Other sexually transmitted diseases are prevalent among patients with syphilis, although the exact coincidence figures probably vary markedly among populations. In 1946, for example, gonorrhea was found in 23% of the patients with early syphilis, and syphilis was diagnosed in 8.4% of the patients with gonorrhea. The frequency with which gonorrhea and incubating syphilis occur in the same patient today is unknown but probably very low. This possibility previously served as one of the bases for regarding aqueous procaine penicillin G as the treatment of choice for uncomplicated gonococcal infection, since such treatment would also presumably abort the incubating syphilis. Although this therapeutic consideration may no longer be valid because the prevalence of syphilis among patients with gonorrhea is now low, patients with syphilis should still be carefully screened for other sexually transmitted diseases.

About 80,000 cases of syphilis are reported annually among American civilians. Of these, 25,000 are early syphilis, so defined because the patients are still potentially contagious. Estimates of underdiagnosis and underreporting suggest that 80,000 Americans acquire syphilis annually. The number of reported cases of syphilis diminished rapidly after the introduction of penicillin in the late 1940s and reached a nadir in 1955. Although the prevalence of late syphilis has continued to decrease dramatically since the introduction of penicillin, the incidence of early syphilis initially rose and since the early 1960s has been relatively stable. This is in marked contrast to the 15% annual increase in incidence of gonorrhea over the same period. Part of the explanation for this discrepancy may lie in the continued sensitivity of *T. pallidum* to antibiotics at a time when the resistance of the gonococcus was increasing. It may be that syphilis is in part controlled by the inadvertent treatment of unsuspected cases with antibiotics administered for other purposes.

About one fifth of the patients with primary and secondary syphilis are identified serologically. Another two thirds of these patients present themselves for examination because they have noticed symptoms of illness or because they have been advised by sexual partners to seek medical attention. Finally, about one sixth of these patients are brought to treatment through the efforts of public health workers performing careful contact tracing. It is this last category that makes it particularly important to report cases of syphilis to the appropriate public health facility so that individuals with unsuspected infection may be diagnosed and treated.

Nonvenereal transmission. Syphilis can be spread by kissing a syphilitic individual with active oral lesions. Digital chancres have occasionally been noted to develop in dentists coming in contact with such lesions. Acquisition by transfusion is no longer a significant problem because serologic tests for syphilis are routinely performed on donated blood and because *T. pallidum* does not survive some of the current methods of prolonged blood storage. The disease has been acquired from contaminated needles, but this is an extraordinarily rare occurrence.

Syphilis may be contracted from intimate but nonvenereal contact with an infected person. Cases of children acquiring syphilis by sharing a bed with an infected parent have been reported. However, acquired syphilis in a child should raise the question of child abuse in the mind of the examiner, and the possibility should be discreetly but thoroughly investigated.

The most important nonvenereal mode of acquisition occurs in utero. Congenital infection begins with maternal spirochetemia, which usually occurs early in infection. Thus the risk of congenital syphilis is increased if syphilis is acquired during pregnancy. Penicillin administered to pregnant women in doses appropriate to cure their syphilis will also eradicate the infection in the fetus. Babies vaginally delivered of mothers with active genital lesions may acquire syphilis during the birth process, and a typical primary chancre may develop.

PATHOGENESIS. *T. pallidum* can penetrate intact mucous membranes or infect via tiny cuts or abrasions in cornified epithelium. The minimal infecting dose in experimental syphilis is two spirochetes injected intradermally. The organism divides every 30 to 33 hours, and lesions appear when the organisms have attained a concentration of approximately 10^7/g of tissue. Very early in infection, well before the first lesion appears or the blood test becomes reactive, spirochetes enter the blood and lymphatic system and widely disseminate.

Two relatively nonspecific pathologic lesions characterize syphilis. The first is an obliterative endarteritis manifested as endothelial proliferation and perivascular infiltration primarily with mononuclear cells. This process may impair blood flow. Involvement of blood vessels in the central nervous system (CNS) gives rise to many of the neurologic sequelae of late syphilis, and involvement of the vasa vasorum may damage large blood vessels and lead to the syndromes of cardiovascular syphilis.

The second characteristic lesion of syphilis is a granulomatous reaction called a gumma. The granuloma is nonspecific and invites confusion with other chronic infections and granulomatous diseases of unknown origin including sarcoidosis and Crohn's disease. Gummas may occur in any organ, and when they involve the skin, they give rise to the characteristic lesions of late "benign" syphilis.

Immunologic processes contribute to the pathogenesis. Work with experimental human syphilis suggests that the gumma is a manifestation of delayed hypersensitivity in the immune host. For many years it was believed that a fetus of less than 16 weeks' gestation would not be invaded by spirochetes. This conclusion was based on the consistent lack of pathologic evidence of congenital syphilis in early abortuses. Recent work, however, has shown that spirochetes do indeed cross the placenta early in gestation but that before 16 weeks the fetus fails to mount an inflammatory reaction to the microorganisms and the infection remains clinically inapparent. Thus immune processes appear to be of great significance in the pathogenesis of congenital syphilis.

Antigen-antibody complexes have been detected in the blood of patients with secondary syphilis. These complexes are responsible for the glomerulonephritis and nephrotic syndrome that occasionally accompany this stage. Treatment of primary or secondary syphilis often results in an acute, febrile response known as the Jarisch-Herxheimer reaction. Although the pathogenesis of this reaction remains incompletely defined, one attractive explanation is that it results from the rapid lysis of spirochetes with the subsequent release of bacterial antigen and exacerbation of immune-complex disease.

Patients with syphilis develop antibodies directed against a variety of lipids. These antibodies are detected by the standard nontreponemal tests for syphilis. Lipids cross-reacting with these antibodies are found in the liver, heart, brain, and mitochondria and raise the possibility that some manifestations of syphilis may have an autoimmune basis. The pathogenic role of such antibodies, however, is speculative at present.

CLINICAL MANIFESTATIONS. In the early nineteenth century the natural history of syphilis was divided into stages. After acquiring the organism but before clinical or serologic manifestations develop, patients are said to have incubating syphilis. Spirochetemia occurs early, and such patients may be able to transmit syphilis via blood transfusion or transplacentally.

Primary syphilis. The incubation period for syphilis can range from 10 to 90 days but generally lasts about 3 weeks. At that time a lesion, the chancre, develops at the point of initial inoculation of the spirochete. The chancre typically begins as a papule that subsequently erodes to form a gradually enlarging ulcer with a clean base and an indurated edge (Fig. 51-1). The chancre may be slightly tender, but severe pain is extremely rare. Although the classic chancre of primary syphilis is a single lesion, in recent series almost half of the patients with proven pri-

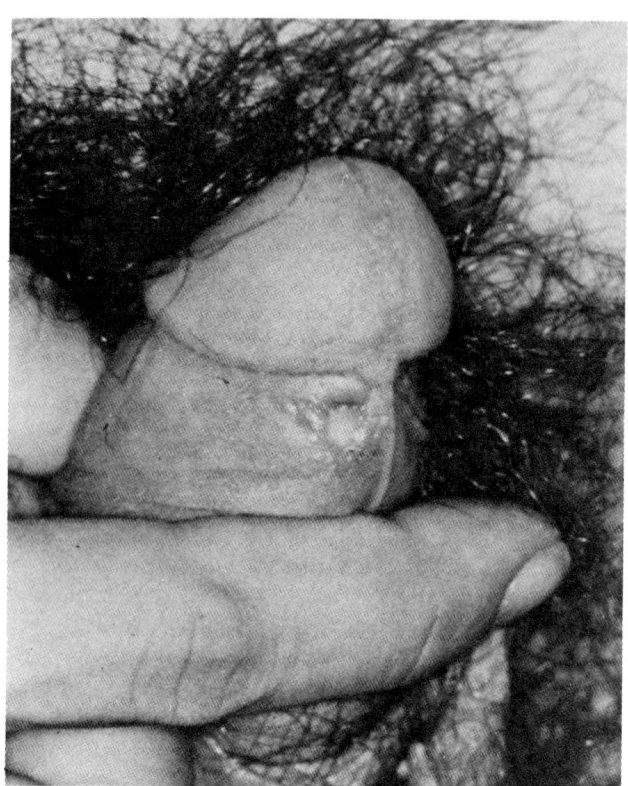

Fig. 51-1. Penile chancre.

mary syphilis had more than one penile ulcer. If the infected patient's normal skin comes in contact with the chancre, autoinoculation may produce additional lesions. Although most chancres appear on the genitalia, the clinician must always bear in mind the possible syphilitic origin of sores on other parts of the body. Chancres of the gum, throat and tonsil, lip, nipple, hand, and a variety of other anatomic sites are well described.

The morphology of chancres is highly variable, and the differential diagnosis of ulcerative lesions of the genitalia may be difficult. Herpes genitalis usually occurs initially as grouped, umbilicated vesicles on an erythematous base that subsequently ulcerate to form groups of painful lesions. Chancroid may produce multiple painful ulcers that are usually ragged and have necrotic bases. Lymphogranuloma venereum often produces a tiny primary ulceration that goes unnoticed by 70% of the infected men and almost all infected women. Tularemia and Behçet's syndrome are discussed in Chapters 47 and 15, respectively.

Relatively painless, usually bilateral, inguinal adenopathy (satellite bubo) appears in 50% to 70% of the patients with primary syphilis of the genitalia. Since the cervix and the proximal portion of the vagina are drained by deep inguinal nodes, satellite bubo does not occur in women with chancres at these sites. Regional adenopathy may, however, accompany primary inoculation at other sites. The patient with an oral, gingival, tonsillar, or pharyngeal chancre often manifests anterior cervical adenopathy. Sometimes the chancre may go completely unnoticed, and the patient appears to have isolated adenopathy. Affected nodes generally become enlarged about 7 days after the appearance of the chancre. They usually occur as a chain and are discrete, firm, and freely movable.

Primary syphilis may go unnoticed by the patient, particularly if the chancre appears in an area not routinely examined. Subcurative doses of antibiotics may modify or almost entirely eliminate the chancre. Primary syphilis per se does not occur in patients with congenital syphilis in which organisms are introduced directly into the bloodstream.

Even without treatment, the chancre heals completely within about 4 to 6 weeks and the regional adenopathy resolves.

Secondary syphilis. In 2 to 8 weeks after the appearance of the chancre, the manifestations of secondary syphilis may develop. The actual time course is highly variable and may range from 2 weeks to 6 months. In most cases the chancre will already have healed by the time secondary syphilis appears, but sometimes primary and secondary syphilis overlap. Secondary syphilis is a generalized illness that often begins as a syndrome suggesting a viral infection. Headache, sore throat, and low-grade fever are common, and some workers have described a nasal discharge as part of the syndrome. Mild leukocytosis with a relative lymphocytosis frequently occurs, but atypical lymphocytes are not seen, a feature that may help to differentiate the syndrome from infectious mononucleosis.

The hallmarks of secondary syphilis are lymphadenopathy and lesions of the skin and mucous membranes. Adenopathy, often generalized, is described in 75% of the affected patients. The nodal groups most commonly involved are the inguinal, suboccipital, posterior auricular, and cervical, particularly the posterior cervical chains. Epitrochlear adenopathy is seen frequently and should raise suspicions of secondary syphilis, although it also occurs with other conditions causing generalized lymphadenopathy, particularly infectious mononucleosis, sarcoidosis, and lymphoma. Affected nodes are usually discrete, relatively nontender, firm, and freely movable. Suppuration is extremely uncommon, and periadenitis and lymphangitis are very rare.

Skin lesions are found in 80% of the infected patients, but they are highly variable, and diligent examination is often required. The lesions are protean and have contributed much to the status of syphilis as the great imitator. Macular lesions are seen in about one third of the patients, primarily over the flanks, abdomen, shoulders, and back. They are generally bilaterally symmetric, tend to follow lines of skin cleavage, and have a coppery or boiled ham color. The lesions are only mildly if at all pruritic, and significant pruritus argues against a diagnosis of secondary

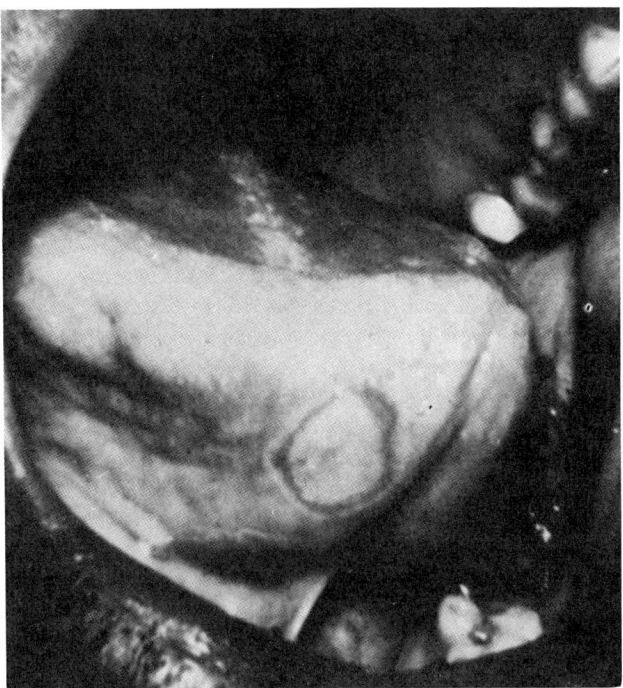

Fig. 51-2. Mucous patch in patient with secondary syphilis. (Courtesy of Department of Health and Human Services, Centers for Disease Control, Atlanta, Ga.)

syphilis. The rash almost invariably involves the genitalia, and when generalized it is frequently prominent on the palms and soles, a distribution highly suggestive of syphilis. Maculopapular lesions are also commonly seen, and follicular lesions may be particularly prevalent on the back and extensor surfaces of the extremities. Somewhat less common skin lesions include annular lesions appearing principally around the face and pustular lesions, which are seen in only about 2% of the patients. Vesicles or bullae are rare in secondary syphilis in adults, although they may be seen in congenital syphilis.

The mucous membranes are involved in more than half of the cases of secondary syphilis. Here again, however, the lesions may be sufficiently subtle to avoid detection by casual examination. It is important to use a tongue blade and to examine the buccal mucosa and the undersurface of the tongue completely. Mucous patches develop in about one third of the patients. These are painless, oval ulcerations usually covered with a grayish or yellowish membrane (Fig. 51-2). Split papules may be observed at the corners of the mouth.

Condylomata lata are flat, hypertrophic lesions resembling warts that develop in moist areas. They are frequently found around the anus or vagina and occasionally in the axilla or under the breasts. They do not reflect areas of inoculation with *T. pallidum* but are manifestations of hematogenous dissemination.

The moist lesions of secondary syphilis (mucous patches, condylomata lata) contain large numbers of spirochetes and must be considered potentially contagious. Dry lesions may reveal spirochetes if vigorously abraded, but their potential for spreading infection is considerably lower. This discrepancy further supports the venereal nature of infectious syphilis.

Patchy, nonpruritic alopecia may involve the scalp, the beard, or even the eyebrows and is suggestive of secondary syphilis.

The clinical overlap between secondary syphilis and a variety of other dermatologic and generalized diseases is very high. Therefore the clinician should have a low threshold of suspicion for secondary syphilis and should be willing to order nontreponemal tests (such as the VDRL test) to confirm or rule out the diagnosis. It is important to remember that about one fifth of men and almost one half of women with secondary syphilis do not give a history of a specific primary lesion.

Although CNS symptoms accompany only about 2% of the cases of secondary syphilis, asymptomatic involvement of the CNS occurs in about one third of the patients and may be manifested by pleocytosis, elevated protein, and reactive nontreponemal tests for syphilis in the cerebrospinal fluid (CSF). Asymptomatic CNS involvement does not require special therapy but responds to standard regimens effective for secondary syphilis. Because the results may be confusing, it is probably inadvisable to examine the CSF of asymptomatic patients with secondary syphilis. Symptomatic involvement of the CNS, however, occurs in approximately 2% of the affected patients, and in many of these acute syphilitic meningitis develops. In such a case the CSF may contain 500 white cells/mm^3, principally mononuclear cells. CSF protein is frequently in excess of 100 mg/ml. The symptoms are those of basilar meningitis, with meningeal signs and cranial nerve involvement in more than half of the patients. Such patients should probably be treated with penicillin intravenously in high doses that are effective for pneumococcal and meningococcal meningitis as well.

Hepatitis is occasionally described in secondary syphilis, but splenomegaly is quite rare. Nephritis and even a nephrotic syndrome develop in some patients because of antigen-antibody complex deposition in the glomeruli. Uveitis and osteitis are occasionally observed.

Secondary syphilis usually resolves within 2 to 6 weeks even in the absence of therapy, although some of the lesions may heal with scarring.

Latent syphilis. With the disappearance of the stigmata of secondary syphilis, patients enter a stage of latency in which the diagnosis can be made only serologically. This stage is usually divided into early latency (within 2 to 4 years of infection) and late latency (thereafter). The distinction is important because during early latency at least 25% of the patients have one or more mucocutaneous relapses during which the dermatologic and systemic manifestations of secondary syphilis reappear. At these times patients once again become infectious to sexual partners and, if pregnant, may transmit infection to the fetus. Most of these relapses occur within the first year following the acquisition of syphilis, and they are extremely rare after 4 years of latency. Thus after 4 years patients are no longer public health hazards.

About one third of the patients who enter latency are spontaneously cured of their disease with a gradual return of nontreponemal serologic tests to nonreactive. Another one third of the patients remain seroreactive and presumably infected but never have further clinical manifestations of disease. Late syphilis develops in the remaining one third of the patients. Thus latent syphilis is likely to lead to significant clinical disease in a sizable minority of affected patients. Attempts to detect unsuspected latent syphilis by serologic screening constitute the majority of the 38 million serologic tests for syphilis performed in the United States annually.

Late syphilis. Late benign syphilis is the term applied to granulomatous (gummatous) involvement, which may affect about 15% of untreated syphilitic individuals and appears many years after acquisition of the disease. The granulomata have a destructive effect on surrounding tissue, but their rate of progression and the degree of inflammation may be low. Gummas of the skin display a variety of clinical features. Small numbers of solitary or grouped lesions, distributed asymmetrically about the body, are often indurated and indolent. An arciform configuration with the borders of lesions forming segments of circles is suggestive of syphilis. Lesions may be serpiginous, healing in one area while advancing in another area. Active lesions usually have a sharp margin, and ulcers may have a punched-out appearance with peripheral hyperpigmentation. Gummas often heal with atrophic, superficial scarring, but their destructive clinical picture may invite confusion with malignancy. The biopsy is nonspecific, revealing granulomata. Organisms are rarely seen.

Gummas may also involve the viscera, resulting in gastrointestinal or hepatic disease. Bones are frequently involved, with periostitis characterized by thickening and with localized increases in bone density and destructive lesions surrounded by sclerosis. The tibia is involved in about half of the patients and the clavicle, skull, or fibula in about one fourth each.

In about 10% of persons with untreated syphilis late cardiovascular manifestations develop. The mean age at diagnosis is 65 years, and the disease is almost twice as common in men (about 14% of all cases) as in women (8%). These observations have led to the theory that prolonged cardiac strain, perhaps related to a lifetime of manual labor or diastolic hypertension, might contribute to the pathogenesis. *T. pallidum* may directly affect the aortic endothelium, and the involved aorta shows a characteristic irregularity of the intima reminiscent of tree bark. The aortic valve cusps themselves may be involved, with rolling and thickening leading to aortic insufficiency, to which weakening and dilation of the aortic valve ring may contribute. Aortic insufficiency decreases coronary perfusion, and the coronary arteries may themselves be directly involved in the endarteritic process leading to coronary occlusion. Endarteritis of the vasa vasorum causes ischemia and weakening of the aortic media, and an aortic aneurysm that is more commonly saccular than fusiform may then develop. About half of syphilitic aneurysms occur in the arotic arch, and another 40% involve other parts of the thoracic aorta. The abdominal aorta is involved in only 10% of syphilitic aneurysms.

Patients with cardiovascular syphilis may be asymptomatic for long periods of time. Early clues to the diagnosis include the observation of localized aortic bulging on chest roentgenogram; an altered aortic second sound, sometimes described as having a tambour quality; an aortic systolic murmur in a young person without hypertension; and precordial chest pain in a young person without other predisposing factors. Clinical or serologic evidence of syphilis of course supports the diagnosis. Later, symptoms of aortic insufficiency develop. Aortic insufficiency murmurs having a peak intensity at the third and fourth intercostal space at the *right* sternal border predict syphilitic disease about 50% of the time. Symptoms of congestive heart failure or angina generally develop, but dissection of an aortic aneurysm is uncommon. The value of antisyphilis therapy remains controversial; treatment certainly does not reverse existing cardiac damage. There is some suggestion, however, that appropriate therapy may slow the progression of the disease.

In about 8% of untreated persons late syphilis involves the CNS. CNS involvement has been detected in 15% to 40% of the patients with cardiovascular syphilis, although in this setting it is usually mild. CNS involvement is initially asymptomatic and in this stage can be detected only by examination of the CSF. Thus CSF should be examined in all patients being treated for syphilis of more than 1 year's duration or whose disease is of unknown duration. The CSF should also be examined in patients who have had a suboptimal serologic response to therapy for early syphilis, since unsuspected, asymptomatic neurosyphilis may account for a small percentage of "treatment failures."

In untreated persons symptoms of neurosyphilis may develop. Meningovascular syphilis results from syphilitic endarteritis and is usually manifested as seizures or cerebrovascular accident. Symptoms may develop 5 to 10 years after the acquisition of syphilis, and a cerebrovascular accident in a young person with no history of hypertension should prompt evaluation for meningovascular syphilis. In occasional patients meningeal signs predominate, and symptoms suggesting a basilar meningitis may develop. These patients usually have a lymphocytic pleocytosis and increased protein in the CSF. The VDRL test of spinal fluid (see "Serologic tests") is almost always positive and should be regarded as diagnostic of this form of syphilis because false positive reactions in the CSF are very rare.

Spirochetes also involve the substance of the brain directly. Within 15 to 20 years after acquiring syphilis, general paresis may develop, usually as a disorder of higher cerebral functions. The patients may suffer personality changes and dementia. Delusional states are common and have been frequently portrayed in song and story. Sometimes the patients have the Argyll Robertson pupil, which is small and further constricts with accommodation but does not react to light, a finding highly suggestive of neurosyphilis. Some series suggest that the CSF is always abnormal, and the serologic tests for syphilis on serum and CSF are invariably reactive. The concept is misleading, however, and depends on the fact that since dementia has multiple causes, the diagnosis of paresis is usually dependent on positive serologic tests.

Tabes dorsalis resulting from involvement of the posterior columns and dorsal roots of the spinal cord usually develops somewhat later, often 30 years after acquiring syphilis. Affected individuals often manifest loss of vibration sense and proprioception resulting in a characteristic broad-based gait. Patients also complain of severe, sharp pains (lightning pains) that may affect any part of the body. Impotence and bladder dysfunction are relatively common. Optic atrophy may be seen in one fourth of the affected patients, and Argyll Robertson pupils are more common than in paresis. The syndrome of tabes dorsalis accounts for somewhat less than half of all cases of neurosyphilis. It is considered sufficiently characteristic that it may be diagnosed clinically. Thus it is not surprising that some patients with tabes have normal CSF and some have nonreactive nontreponemal tests for syphilis on serum and CSF.

Congenital syphilis. Spirochetemia during pregnancy may result in syphilitic placentitis and subsequent infusion of spirochetes into the fetus via the umbilical vein. Babies with congenital syphilis may be completely asymptomatic at birth but often have highly suggestive stigmata. Disseminated lesions of the skin and mucous membranes may develop in affected children. The nasal mucous membranes are particularly susceptible, and syphilitic involvement results in snuffles, a persistent, mucopurulent nasal discharge containing large numbers of spirochetes. Hemorrhagic rhinitis eventuates in severe cases and is almost pathognomonic of congenital syphilis. Condylomata lata, which are frequently seen in secondary syphilis in adults, occur in moist areas, often around the anus or vagina in babies, and contain large numbers of spirochetes. Roentgenographic evidence of bone involvement is seen in almost all babies with congenital syphilis. The long bones show a characteristic area of provisional calcification at the epiphysis that surmounts an area of rarefaction. Proximally, there is moth-eaten calcification of the metaphysis with tongues of calcium protruding into the area of rarefaction. Periostitis may result in concentric layers of subperiosteal bone formation, giving a layered appearance to the shafts of long bones. Wimberger's sign (bilateral rarefaction of the medial tibial metaphyses) is highly suggestive of congenital syphilis. Skeletal involvement may create pain on movement resulting in voluntary splinting of an extremity, the pseudoparalysis of Parrot.

Many other signs are relatively common in congenital syphilis but are less specific. Neonatal hepatosplenomegaly and jaundice are seen in about one fifth of the infected patients. Skin lesions may be diffuse and involve the palms and soles. They are often, however, associated with a diaper rash distribution. The lesions may closely resemble those of secondary syphilis in adults, but bullous lesions are considerably more common in congenital syphilis.

Approximately 75% to 90% of cases of congenital syphilis are diagnosed in patients over 10 years old. This distressing finding indicates the flaws in the neonatal health care delivery system and also suggests the need for clinicians to be aware of the late manifestations of congenital syphilis. The hutchinsonian triad is traditionally associated with late congenital syphilis. One element, Hutchinson's teeth, is generally recognized only after the eruption of the permanent central and lateral incisors at 7 years of age (Fig. 51-3). The affected teeth are shorter and narrower than normal. The middle third of the tooth is principally affected, resulting in the appearance of a semilunar notch in the center of the edge. The central third of the tooth may also be discolored because of an incomplete enamel covering. Hutchinson's teeth have been diagnosed before eruption on the basis of dental roentgenograms. The six-year molar may also be affected, with distortion of the cusps yielding a mulberry-like appearance. A second element of the triad is interstitial keratitis, usually appearing between 5 and 20 years of age. The inflammation is manifested by photophobia, eye pain, blurred vision, and tearing; it may be chronic. Spirochetes are not found in the eye in this setting, and the mechanism is incompletely understood. Nerve deafness completes the triad. Characteristic fissures around the mouth and anus, called rhagades, are rare, and the mechanism is unknown. Skeletal lesions may be hypertrophic with new-bone formation resulting in anterior bowing of the tibia (saber shins) or enlargement of the medial end of the clavicle. Erosive lesions occasionally result in perforation of the palate, and syphilis was once its most common cause. Collapse of the nasal bones may produce a saddle nose deformity.

LABORATORY FINDINGS. Syphilis is most convincingly diagnosed by demonstrating typically motile spirochetes in a lesion. Because of its small size and poor staining characteristics, *T. pallidum* is best observed by darkfield microscopy in which the organisms are visualized with reflected rather than transmitted light. Chancres, mucous patches, and condylomata lata are usually positive for the organism, but difficulties may be experienced in differentiating *T. pallidum* from normal spirochetal flora of the mouth or vagina. Dry skin lesions of secondary syphilis are occasionally darkfield positive. Proper preparation of the lesion is crucial and involves cleaning its surface and lightly abrading it so that relatively blood-free tissue fluid can be collected and examined as a wet mount. Darkfield

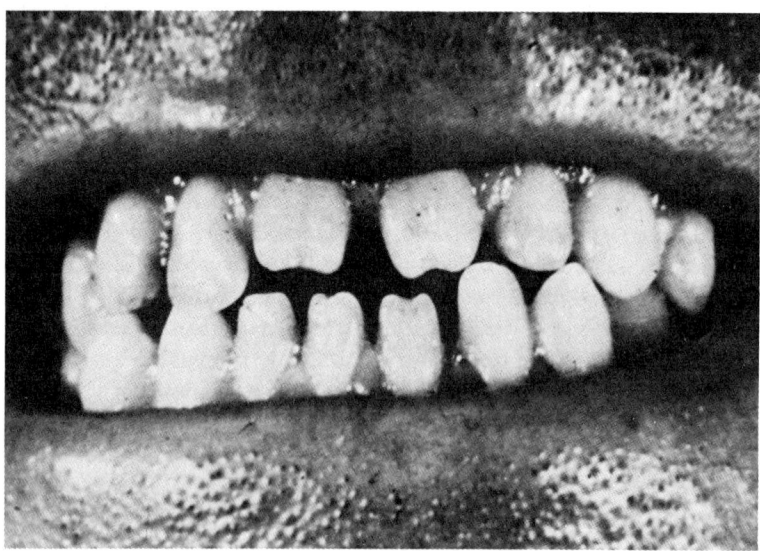

Fig. 51-3. Hutchinson's teeth in patient with late congenital syphilis. (Courtesy of Department of Health and Human Services. Centers for Disease Control, Atlanta, Ga.)

diagnosis can be difficult and is best left to clinicians with previous experience.

Serologic tests. Patients with syphilis usually have antibodies directed against a poorly defined lipid that may be a component of the spirochete. Cross-reacting lipids are found in a variety of normal tissues and serve as the basis for the nontreponemal tests for syphilis, which employ a lipid extracted from beef heart (cardiolipin) as an antigen. The antigen is mixed with patients' serum, and clumping of the antigen particles is observed by a variety of techniques that vary with the tests. Nontreponemal tests are inexpensive and technically easy to perform. A number of such tests have been developed in the past, but those commonly in use today are the Veneral Disease Research Laboratories (VDRL) test, the Rapid Plasma Reagin (RPR) test, and the Automated Reagin Test (ART). All of these tests may be positive in a variety of other diseases, including acute viral illnesses such as varicella, hepatitis, and infectious mononucleosis; bacterial infections such as leprosy, tuberculosis, and leptospirosis; and disease associated with the formation of unusual immunoglobulins such as intravenous drug addiction and collagen vascular diseases.

Nontreponemal tests can be quantitated, and the results are usually expressed as the highest dilution of serum yielding a positive reaction. The clinician should be cautioned, however, that the RPR and ART may yield titers twofold to eightfold higher than those obtained with the VDRL on the same serum. Since rising or falling titers may have great clinical significance, patients followed over a period of time should be studied with the same nontreponemal test.

Patients with syphilis also have antitreponemal antibodies that can be detected by a variety of procedures using *T. pallidum* as the antigen. The principal treponemal test in current use is the fluorescent treponemal antibody absorption (FTA-ABS) test in which antitreponemal antibody is detected by an indirect fluorescence method using spirochetes attached to a slide. Although the FTA-ABS test requires a fluorescence microscope and is more technically demanding than the nontreponemal tests, it is the current standard for the diagnosis of syphilis. The microhemagglutination test for *T. pallidum* (MHA-TP) uses treponemal antigens attached to the surface of erythrocytes, which will agglutinate when mixed with the serum from patients with syphilis. This test is considerably easier to perform than the FTA-ABS and is now coming into increased use. It is, however, somewhat less sensitive than the FTA-ABS. Treponemal tests are generally used to confirm the diagnosis of syphilis in patients with reactive nontreponemal tests.

The interpretation of serologic tests for syphilis has resulted in some confusion. Certain facts should be borne in mind. Both the treponemal and nontreponemal tests may be nonreactive in the patient who has just developed a chancre. Thus a nonreactive test for syphilis does not rule out the diagnosis in the patient whose lesion has just appeared. In this setting about 10% of the patients have a nonreactive nontreponemal test but a reactive treponemal test for syphilis. In secondary syphilis essentially all of the serologic tests are reactive. This is particularly useful because the clinical diagnosis of secondary syphilis may be difficult. Thus a negative nontreponemal serologic test for syphilis essentially rules out secondary syphilis. Unfortunately, nontreponemal tests for syphilis frequently become nonreactive in patients with late syphilis. Fully 50% of patients diagnosed as having tabes dorsalis have a nonreactive nontreponemal test for syphilis. Patients being evaluated for late syphilis should have an FTA-ABS test performed even if the nontreponemal tests are nonreactive because many of these patients will be diagnosed only by the more sensitive treponemal tests. Following adquate treatment of syphilis, the titer of the nontreponemal tests should drop at least fourfold (for example, from 1:32 before treatment to 1:8 or less after treatment), but such reductions may require several months. Within 2 years of adequate treatment, the VDRL returns to nonreactive in about 95% of the patients with primary syphilis and 75% of those with secondary syphilis. Patients with syphilis of longer than 2 years duration may have a persistently positive nontreponemal test for syphilis. The FTA-ABS test remains positive for many years (possibly for life) even after adequate treatment of syphilis. Thus a persistently positive FTA-ABS is not an indication for retreating patients with a prior history of adquate therapy. A rise in titer of the nontreponemal tests, however, may indicate relapse or reinfection and indeed may indicate a need for retreating patients previously thought to have been adequately treated.

Serodiagnosis of neonatal congenital syphilis poses special problems because it may be difficult to differentiate fetal antibody synthesized in response to in utero infection from transplacentally acquired maternal antibody. Tests based on the identification of IgM antibody that does not cross the placenta are beset by an apparent lack of sensitivity and specificity.

MANAGEMENT. Penicillin G remains the treatment of choice for all stages of syphilis in patients who are not hypersensitive to the drug. Duration of therapy is important, and treatment for early syphilis is usually based on the administration of benzathine penicillin G, which produces very low serum levels persisting for 3 weeks following a single intramuscular injection. Early syphilis (up to 1 year) can be adequately treated with a single administration of 2.4 million units of benzathine penicillin G. Syphilis of more than 1 year's duration, with the possible exception of neurosyphilis, can be adequately treated with three or four weekly injections of the same dose of benzathine penicillin G. The therapy of neurosyphilis remains somewhat controversial because of the relatively poor penetration of penicillin into the CSF. Therefore syphilis of the CNS might better be treated with regimens producing considerably higher levels, such as aqueous penicillin G by continuous intravenous administration at a rate of 20 million units a day for a leats 10 days. Congenital syphilis that has spared the CNS can be treated with benzathine penicillin G, but if the CNS is involved, a penicillin regimen yielding higher serum levels should be used.

Patients allergic to penicillin may be treated with erythromycin or tetracycline (500 mg orally every 6 hours) to which the spirochete is sensitive. These regimens generally involve taking the medication for 2 weeks for syphilis of less than 1 year's duration and for 4 weeks in all other circumstances. They require considerable patient compliance. The overall efficacy of drugs other than penicillin in the treatment of syphilis has been less well established, and the history of penicillin allergy should be carefully investigated in patients requiring treatment for syphilis.

More than half of the patients treated for early syphilis with penicillin have a Jarisch-Herxheimer reaction, usually beginning within 6 hours of treatment. The reaction consists of fever, a transient exacerbation of skin lesions or adenopathy, occasional arthralgias, and, rarely, transient hypotension. The reaction is usually mild and abates in less than 24 hours. It can be managed with aspirin and reassurance.

BIBLIOGRAPHY

Chapel, T.A.: The variability of syphilitic chancres, Sex. Transm. Dis. **5**:68, 1978.
Fiumara, N.J., and others: The incidence of prenatal syphilis at the Boston City Hospital, N. Engl. J. Med. **247**:48, 1952.
Jaffe, H.W.: The laboratory diagnosis of syphilis: new concepts, Ann. Intern. Med. **83**:846, 1975.
Kampmeier, R.H.: The late manifestations of syphilis: skeletal, visceral, and cardiovascular, Med. Clin, North Am. **48**:667, 1964.
Krolls, S.O., and others: Oral manifestations of syphilis, Hosp. Med. **8**:14, 1972.
Sparling, P.F.: Diagnosis and treatment of syphilis, N. Engl. J. Med. **284**:642, 1977.
Stokes, J.H., Beerman, H., and Ingraham, N.R.: Modern clinical syphiliology, Philadelphia, 1944, W.B. Saunders Co.
Syphilis: a synopsis, Washington, D.C., 1968, U.S.P.H.S. Pub. no. 1660.
Syphilotherapy 1976: position papers for the current U.S.P.H.S. recommendation, J. Am. Vener. Dis. Assoc. **3**:98, 1976.

Rat-bite fever

Merle A. Sande

Rat-bite fever is a term used to describe two distinct types of febrile illnesses that usually follow the bite of a rat, mouse, or other rodent. The more common in the United States is caused by *Streptobacillus moniliformis* and has become predominantly a disease of laboratory workers. The second is caused by a spirochete, *Spirillum minus*.

STREPTOBACILLARY RAT-BITE FEVER

S. moniliformis is a pleomorphic, gram-negative bacillus found in the oropharynx of over 50% of healthy rats. It may cause pneumonia, conjunctivitis, or other infections in rats, mice, turkeys, and guinea pigs. It usually causes disease in humans following an animal bite, but contact with dead rodents and ingestion of contaminated milk (Haverhill fever) have been implicated in human outbreaks. Disease occurs most commonly in persons having contact with rats (laboratory workers, children, slum dwellers) and has a worldwide distribution.

CLINICAL MANIFESTATIONS. Usually within 10 days following the animal bite, fever and shaking chills; headache; severe myalgias, especially in the back; weakness; and vomiting develop. These symptoms are followed in several days by arthralgias and frank arthritis usually involving multiple large joints, especially the wrists and elbows. On the third day of illness a morbilliform or petechial rash appears in over 90% of the cases. The initial bite heals well. Symptoms typically remit after 2 to 5 days but may relapse at irregular intervals for weeks to months. Endocarditis and pericarditis have been reported and may lead to death.

LABORATORY FINDINGS. Leukocytosis is common, with white blood cell counts ranging from 6000 to 30,000/mm^3. Biologically false serologic tests for syphilis have been reported in 25% of the cases. The diagnosis is established by isolating the bacteria from blood or joint fluid. The organism grows well in ordinary nutrient media (trypticase soy broth or agar), particularly when supplemented with 20% horse serum and incubated in 5% to 10% CO_2. Growth may be slow, and cultures should be held for several weeks if this diagnosis is suspected.

DIFFERENTIAL DIAGNOSIS. Streptobacillary fever should be considered in any patient (especially a laboratory worker) who has been exposed to rats and has fever, arthritis, and rash. Other infections that should be ruled out include several viral diseases (rubella, hepatitis B. dengue, and the various arboviruses). Rocky Mountain spotted fever, disseminated gonococcal disease, meningococcemia, and leptospirosis.

MANAGEMENT. Either penicillin V or tetracycline administered orally, 500 mg every 6 hours, or procaine penicillin, 600,000 units intramuscularly every 12 hours for 10 days, is effective in reducing the duration of fever. The organism is also sensitive to many other antimicrobial drugs.

SPIRILLARY RAT-BITE FEVER

S. minus is a thick, tightly coiled, flagellated, gram-negative spirochete that is 2 to 5 μm in length and contains two to five spirals. It can be recognized in wet mounts of infected tissue by its rapid, darting motion. The organism produces an ocular infection in rats.

The disease in humans usually occurs at least 10 days

after a rat bite. The primary site initially heals but then becomes inflamed, suppurates, and may ulcerate. Fever and regional adenitis develop and last for 3 to 5 days. An urticarial rash may occur but is usually less prominent than that seen in streptobacillary fever. Arthritis is rare. Recurrence of symptoms in several days is common.

The diagnosis is established by darkfield examination of aspirated material from the primary infected site or an involved lymph node. The organism has not been cultured. Treatment with either penicillin or streptomycin is effective.

Leptospirosis
Merle A. Sande

ETIOLOGY AND EPIDEMIOLOGY. Leptospirosis is a term used to identify several clinical entities caused by a single species of spirochete, *Leptospira interrogans*. Although documented relatively rarely (fewer than 100 cases per year reported in the United States), it probably accounts for a much higher number of cases of undiagnosed aseptic meningitis. *L. interrogans* is a primary pathogen for wild animals (foxes, skunks, opposums, rats) and domestic animals (cattle, dogs, cats) throughout the United States. It occasionally causes disease in animals. The organism commonly invades the renal tubules, where it may be asymptomatically excreted in the urine for years. Under optimal conditions it remains viable in soil or water for weeks. Humans are usually infected following contact with the contaminated environment. The spirochete penetrates mucous membranes or abrasions in the skin and rapidly and widely disseminates hematogenously. Most cases occur in the summer and fall, and the disease affects predominantly children, teenagers, and housewives. It also has been found in people who have swum in rivers or freshwater ponds, farmers, abbatoir workers, veterinarians, coal miners, and sewer workers. Since cross-infection between wild and domestic animal species may occur, household pets (even though vaccinated) may acquire and secrete the organism in their urine. Rats are the most common source of disease throughout the world except in the United States, where transmission is usually from dogs, livestock, and cats.

Over 130 serotypes have been identified and grouped into 16 serogroups. Some of the more common of these are *L. pomona, L. canicola, L. icterohaemorrhagiae, L. autumnalis,* and *L. grippotyphosa*. There seems to be little relationship between these serogroups and the clinical syndrome, although historically *L. icterohaemorrhagiae* has been associated with the more severe form of the disease (Weil's disease).

CLINICAL MANIFESTATIONS. Most cases of leptospirosis are probably asymptomatic, as judged by the relatively high rate of seropositivity in persons with a high exposure to animals. In addition, over 90% of those with clinical disease have a relatively mild form. The typical illness is characterized by a biphasic pattern. Following a 1- to 2-week incubation period, the first or septicemic phase begins abruptly with high fever (102° F [39° C]), chills, frontal or generalized headache, severe muscle pains, malaise, prostration, conjunctival suffusion, and frequently cough or chest pain. Nausea, vomiting, and abdominal pain are common, and diarrhea may also occur. A rash may be present on the trunk. During this phase, which usually lasts 4 to 7 days, spirochetes can be isolated from the blood and cerebrospinal fluid (CSF). Symptoms then disappear as the leptospires are cleared from the bloodstream, and in many instances this signals the end of the illness.

The second or immune phase, which begins after 1 to 3 symptom-free days, may simulate the first phase except fever is usually mild and short lived or absent. Myalgias again dominate the clinical picture and are typically localized to the back and calves. The frontal or bitemporal headache is usually severe and constant and signifies the presence of aseptic meningitis. Nausea, vomiting, and abdominal pain are usually present. Examination of the CSF reveals pleocytosis (fewer than 1000 white blood cells/mm^3), mainly with lymphocytes, although polymorphonuclear leukocytes may predominate in the early phases. The CSF protein is elevated, and the glucose is normal. This disease is self-limited and almost never fatal. Mild delirium may occur, but other signs of CNS dysfunction are rare.

A small proportion (5% to 10%) of patients have the severe form of disease (Weil's disease), which is characterized by jaundice of the intrahepatic obstructive type without significant hepatic destruction and by renal failure with acute tubular necrosis and associated azotemia, proteinuria, pyuria, and hematuria. Alterations in mental function usually follow. Vascular collapse, severe hemorrhage, and death occur in 5% to 10% of these cases. The death rate is significantly increased in the older age group. Myocarditis is common in the fatal disease. Leukocytosis is usually present, and hemolytic anemia and thrombocytopenia may occur. The initial stages of Weil's disease are similar to the less severe forms of leptospirosis, but high persistent fever, sometimes lasting several weeks, generally accompanies the second phase of the disease. The resolution of disease is usually complete, with occasional mild residual impairment of renal function.

DIAGNOSIS. The diagnosis is usually established retrospectively by serologic methods. The macroscopic slide agglutination is an excellent screening test, and the microscopic agglutination is more specific and used for confirmation. Antibodies against the *Leptospira* antigens usually appear during the second week of illness and reach peak titers in the third or fourth week. A fourfold rise in agglutinating antibody is diagnostic of leptospirosis. A single titer of greater than 1:100 by the microscopic agglutination test or a positive slide agglutination test is presumptive evidence when combined with a compatible clinical course. Rarely, patients remain seronegative.

During the first or septicemic phase of illness (first week) organisms can be cultured from blood and CSF, and they then may be found in the urine for months following the clinical disease. Whole blood or CSF should be cultured on a semisolid medium such as Fletcher medium or the new Tween 80-albumin medium. Organisms also survive up to 11 days in noncitrated anticoagulated blood. Blood can then be sent to either state laboratories or the Centers for Disease Control for culture of the organisms if local facilities are unavailable.

Most cases of leptospirosis undoubtedly go undiagnosed because of the physician's failure to consider this organism in the differential diagnosis. It should be at least considered in any patient with a high fever and severe muscle pains, conjunctival suffusion, clinical symptoms of a biphasic temporal character, aseptic meningitis, or an ill-defined febrile illness with a history of contact with animals.

MANAGEMENT. The efficacy of antimicrobial therapy for leptospirosis is open to question. Some studies suggest that either penicillin G or tetracycline may shorten the duration of fever or reduce the incidence of complications but only if given before the fifth day of illness. Thus in the vast majority of diagnosed cases the therapy is probably instituted after any benefit could be expected.

BIBLIOGRAPHY
Rat-bite fever

Cole, J.S., Stoll, R.W., and Bulger, R.J.: Rat bite fever: report of three cases, Ann. Intern. Med. **71**:979, 1969.

Gill, F.A.: Rat bite fever. In Mandell, G.L., Douglas, R.G., and Bennett, J.E., editors: Principles and practice of infectious diseases, New York, 1979, John Wiley & Sons, Inc.

Roughgarden, J.W.: Antimicrobial therapy of rat bite fever, Arch. Intern. Med. **116**:39, 1965.

Leptospirosis

Farrar, W.E.: *Leptospira* species. In Mandell, G.L., Douglas, R.G., Jr., and Bennett, J.E., editors: Principles and practice of infectious diseases, New York, 1979, John Wiley & Sons, Inc.

Feigin, R.D., and Anderson, D.C.: Human leptospirosis, CRC Crit. Rev. Clin. Lab. Sci. **5**:413, 1975.

Unit C • FUNGAL DISEASES

52 • DISEASES CAUSED BY FUNGI
John E. Bennett

HISTOPLASMOSIS

Histoplasmosis is the infection caused by *Histoplasma capsulatum*. This fungus is encountered in many parts of the world, living in bat guano and in rich, moist soil, particularly soil enriched with bird droppings. The fungus grows as a mold in nature, and its spores reach the lung by inhalation. In the lung the fungus changes to a small budding yeast. The resulting pneumonia is usually self-limited and causes only a few days of fever, dry cough, and chest ache. These mild cases are detectable as persistent positive skin test reactivity to histoplasmin. In highly endemic areas of the central and mid-Atlantic United States, up to 80% of the adults are skin test positive. Patients with more severe cases (also usually self-limited) may have up to 2 weeks of high fever, cyanosis, and prostration. Chest roentgenography reveals one or more areas of infiltration. Death is rare, but the disease may leave one or numerous areas of calcification in the lung and hilar nodes. Enlarged hilar nodes may cause bronchial compression and atelectasis. The slowly resolving pulmonary granuloma may resemble carcinoma roentgenographically and may lead to an unnecessary thoracotomy.

More serious complications occur in less than 1% of infections and are usually not preceded by severe primary pneumonia. Chronic fibrocavitary pulmonary infection, closely resembling tuberculosis, tends to occur in 30- to 50-year-old men who have a long history of cigarette smoking. The illness progresses insidiously and variably, but the untreated disease usually leads to death by bacterial pulmonary superinfection or cor pulmonale within several years.

Dissemination beyond the lung and hilar nodes can occur in self-limited primary pulmonary infection. Progressive extrapulmonary dissemination is a rare but highly lethal form of the disease. Many patients are either young children or immunosuppressed adults, but previously normal adults can also acquire the disease. The clinical manifestations are extremely variable, depending on which organs are involved. Hepatomegaly, splenomegaly, lymphadenopathy, chronic meningitis, endocarditis, adrenal insufficiency, pancytopenia, or granulomatous hepatitis may develop. Ulcerations of the upper airway occur in one fourth of the adults with disseminated histoplasmosis. Methenamine silver stain of the biopsy shows numerous small yeast cells in the submucosa.

H. capsulatum can be cultured from the sputum of patients with chronic fibrocavitary disease and from the mucosal lesions, blood, bone marrow, liver, lymph nodes, or urine of many patients with disseminated disease.

A complement fixation or agar gel diffusion test can be used to detect serum antibody to the fungus. These tests can suggest the possibility of infection but are too insensitive and nonspecific to make or exclude the diagnosis. Skin testing is not helpful in diagnosis except when conversion from negative to positive is observed in acute infection.

Intravenous administration of amphotericin B is very effective in curing fibrocavitary pulmonary or progressive disseminated infection. The drug is too toxic to warrant its use in self-limited pulmonary disease. Ketoconazole, a recently marketed oral drug, appears in early trials to have some efficacy in treating chronic pulmonary and disseminated histoplasmosis. (See Chapter 53 for a discussion of these agents.)

COCCIDIOIDOMYCOSIS

Coccidioidomycosis is the infection caused by *Coccidioides immitis*. The fungus lives as a mold in the soil of certain hot, dry portions of the southwestern United States, Mexico, and Central and South America. Spores of this fungus are very resistant to heat and desiccation. When airborne, they can be inhaled into the lung and cause pneumonia. The resulting infection may pass unnoticed or be a self-limited influenza-like illness with cough, fever, and chest pain. Within the lung the fungus is transformed into a rounded form (spherule) that does not bud like a yeast but reproduces by endosporulation. Tiny spores form inside a ''mother'' cell that ruptures, releasing them. Each spore grows into a mature spherule, and the process is repeated. Depending on the stage of maturation, the structures may be much smaller than a human erythrocyte or several times that size.

Initial pulmonary infection may be associated with arthralgia, erythema nodosum, or erythema multiforme. Mild eosinophilia is common. The fever often subsides within 2 weeks, but roentgenographic resolution of the pneumonia is slow. Easy fatigability may persist for many weeks. The diagnosis may be suspected when there has been exposure to desert dust, as in construction, rock collecting, or digging for archeologic artifacts. Seroconversion of the complement fixation or agar gel test for *Coccidioides* is helpful for diagnosis but may require several weeks from the onset of illness.

The resolving pulmonary infiltrate may be rounded and suggest carcinoma. The round lesion may cavitate and persist as a thin-walled cavity for months or years. Such cavities may be a source of hemoptysis.

Dissemination beyond the lung and hilar nodes is a rare but frequently lethal complication. This complication is more likely when the patient is black, Filipino, pregnant, or immunosuppressed. Dissemination may be manifested by chronic meningitis, one or more areas of indolent osteomyelitis, skin lesions, or subcutaneous abscesses. Spread beyond the lung is most likely to be recognized at the time of primary infection rather than years later. Clues to dissemination include continuation beyond the initial illness of the fever, elevated erythrocyte sedimentation rate, and eosinophilia, as well as a negative skin test with coccidioidin and elevation of the complement fixation titer to *Coccidioides* antigen beyond a level of roughly 1:16. The fungus may be recovered from pus, urine, cerebrospinal fluid (CSF), or rarely blood.

Amphotericin B provides amelioration of the infection, although relapse of disseminated infection is usual. Ketoconazole has resulted in improvement in some patients with chronic disseminated coccidioidomycosis. (For use of these agents see Chapter 53.) Persistent thin-walled cavities are best treated by observation or lobectomy.

BLASTOMYCOSIS

Blastomycosis is the infection caused by *Blastomyces dermatitidis*. The majority of cases occur in the United States and Canada, but occasional cases occur in Mexico, Africa, Central America, and northern South America. The portal of entry is the lung. A few cases of acute, self-limited pneumonitis have been recognized, but most cases occur as pneumonia of indolent onset and slow progression. Alternatively, the pneumonia may cause so few symptoms that on initial examination the patient has metastatic lesions in the skin, bones, prostate, epididymis, or other sites. Rarely, painless nodular or plaquelike lesions occur in the mouth, larynx, or nose. The fungus can be seen as a budding yeast in methenamine silver–stained biopsy tissue or can be cultured from sputum, pus, urine, or tissue samples from infected sites. Skin tests and serologic tests are not helpful. Intravenous administration of amphotericin B is usually curative.

CRYPTOCOCCOSIS

Cryptococcosis is the mycosis caused by *Cryptococcus neoformans*, an encapsulated, budding, yeastlike fungus. The infection is infrequent but worldwide. It is rare in children but more common in patients with corticosteroid therapy, lymphoma, or sarcoidosis. The portal of entry is the lungs. The most common presentation is as chronic meningitis, with headache, nausea, vomiting, and unsteady gait. The CSF may demonstrate decreased glucose, lymphocytic pleocytosis, and elevated protein. If untreated, the infection is fatal in a few weeks to a year. Less commonly infection is seen as a chronic pneumonia or lesions in the skin, bones, or other organs. The diagnosis can be made by culturing the fungus from CSF, blood, urine, or pus. In about half the cases of meningitis the fungus can be seen in an india ink smear of CSF. Latex agglutination tests of serum and CSF detect the capsular antigen in about 94% of the patients with meningitis and in the serum of a lesser proportion of nonmeningeal cases. The treatment of choice is intravenously administered amphotericin B given either alone or in combination with oral flucytosine (see Chapter 53).

SPOROTRICHOSIS

Sporotrichosis is the mycosis caused by *Sporothrix schenckii*. The infection is worldwide but infrequent. The fungus lives on certain plants and enters the skin following minor injury, such as by rose thorns. Within subcutaneous tissue the fungus grows in a budding, yeastlike form. A small, slightly tender pimple forms and may discharge small amounts of pus intermittently. The lesion persists, and over the ensuring weeks other nodules form in the same extremity along proximal lymphatic channels. Infection beginning in the skin is chronic but not life threatening. Uncommonly, infection begins in the lung. Hematogenous dissemination to bones and joints can occur, albeit rarely, from the lung or from an occult portal of entry. The diagnosis is best made by culturing the fungus from pus. The fungus may be difficult to see or identify in histologic section. Cutaneous disease responds well to oral administration of saturated potassium iodide. The adult dosage is 2 ml three times a day with meals, increasing gradually as tolerated to 3 to 4 ml three times a day. Hematogenously disseminated disease requires therapy with amphotericin B.

CANDIDIASIS

Candidiasis, also called moniliasis or candidosis, is an infection by species of *Candida,* a yeastlike fungus. By far the most common species is *C. albicans,* a normal inhabitant of the human mouth, vagina, and intestinal tract. Superficial invasion of the mucous membranes and skin by *Candida* is called thrush. In the mouth thrush most commonly occurs as a white, adherent plaque on the buccal mucosa. Scraping up an edge of the leathery plaque reveals a bleeding base. Plaques also may be present on the inner aspect of the lips or on the gums, palate, or tongue. Thrush under an upper denture may be erythematous without a distinct membrane. Oral thrush is relatively painless except for fissuring at the corners of the mouth (angular chelitis), which is usually painful.

Vaginal thrush causes discharge, burning, and dyspareunia. Cutaneous thrush occurs as erythema of moist areas, such as diaper rash and rash under pendulous breasts and in intergluteal clefts of obese patients. Perianal thrush may cause pruritus ani. Onychomycosis may occur when hands are exposed frequently to water, as in cannery workers or bartenders.

Systemic factors also contribute to thrush. Newborn infants are prone to this condition, as are patients with diabetes mellitus or those receiving adrenal corticosteroids or broad-spectrum antibiotics. Women taking oral contraceptives or in the third trimester of pregnancy are predisposed to vaginal thrush. Children with certain immuno-deficiency states and adults with thymoma may acquire chronic mucocutaneous candidiasis. These patients have heaped-up skin lesions in addition to thrush of the mouth, vagina, and nails.

The diagnosis of thrush is best made by demonstrating pseudohyphae in wet smears of scrapings from the lesions. Gram stain is less helpful. Culture can confirm the diagnosis but is not diagnostic alone because *Candida* is a frequent commensal in the same sites.

Oral thrush is treated with nystatin suspension. The adult dosage is 500,000 units four times daily, amply swished around the mouth before swallowing. The treatment is continued for 48 hours after the lesions have disappeared. Painting the mouth with gentian violet is messy and not more effective. Vaginal thrush and skin lesions can be treated with a variety of drugs, but miconazole cream is as good as or better than other preparations. Ketoconazole is very effective in chronic mucocutaneous candidiasis.

Disseminated candidiasis results from a break in the integument when there is either a foreign body (such as an intravascular catheter) at the site or impaired host defense. Patients receiving hyperalimentation are particularly prone to *Candida* sepsis. The fungus passes from the skin to a deep vein along the plastic intravenous catheter. Patients with neutropenia resulting from acute leukemia and its treatment are at special risk of gastrointestinal candidiasis, which then can disseminate. The most common sign of disseminated candidiasis is fever. Focal findings are often absent but include symptoms and signs of endophthalmitis, endocarditis, renal abscess, hepatitis, meningitis, embolic skin lesions, and osteomyelitis. The diagnosis can be made by culture of blood, CSF, or biopsy material. Appearance of the fungus in methenamine silver–stained tissue is also diagnostic. Serologic tests are not of proven value. The treatment is with intravenously administered amphotericin B, with or without orally administered flucytosine.

For use of agents in treatment of *Candida* infections see Chapter 53.

ASPERGILLOSIS

As currently used, aspergillosis is a broad term referring to infection, allergy, or colonization with species of *Aspergillus*. This extremely common mold lives on decaying vegetation and grain the world over. Most normal individuals are highly resistant to infection. Infection occurs in patients who are severely immunosuppressed, particularly those with acute leukemia. Infection begins as a dense pneumonia that is prone to hematogenous dissemination. Vascular invasion by fungal hyphae leads to infarction of tissue. Positive sputum cultures are not usually helpful, since they do not necessarily indicate tissue invasion. The diagnosis is made by demonstrating the narrow, septate hyphae in biopsied tissue. Death often occurs within 2 weeks of onset. Patients whose immunosuppression is lessened dramatically may respond to intravenous administration of amphotericin B.

Patients with chronic lung disease and impaired bronchopulmonary clearance mechanisms may have *Aspergillus* growing in their bronchi. Plugs of fungal hyphae may be expectorated. Preexisting cavities or cysts in the lung may fill with hyphae, creating a so-called fungus ball. No tissue invasion occurs under most circumstances. Repeated hemoptysis demonstrated to be from a fungus ball may require surgical excision. Antifungal therapy is ineffective.

Allergic bronchopulmonary aspergillosis is a syndrome in which patients exhibit asthma, IgE and frequently IgG antibody to *Aspergillus*, and intermittent bronchial plugging. Eosinophilia and elevated serum IgE are usual.

MUCORMYCOSIS

Mucormycosis is infection caused by fungi of the order Mucorales. These fungi are common saprophytes in nature. There are two principal forms of the disease: craniofacial infection in patients with diabetes mellitus and pneumonia in patients with immunosuppression. Craniofacial mucormycosis, which is caused most often by species of *Rhizopus*, usually begins in the maxillary sinus. The symptoms resemble those of bacterial sinusitis for the first few days, but the infection progresses to contiguous structures such as the orbit, nose, hard palate, face, and eventually the brain. The fungus invades blood vessels, causing infarction and necrosis of tissue. Proptosis, ophthalmoplegia, coma, and necrotic lesions of the palate or nasal mucous membranes are common findings. The diagnosis is made by demonstrating the distinctive hyphae in biopsied tissue. If mucormycosis is untreated, death ensures in a week or two. Approximately half the patients are cured by rigorous control of the diabetes mellitus, radical surgical exenteration of infected tissue, and intravenous administration of amphotericin B.

Pulmonary mucormycosis is most often caused by species of *Mucor*. Infection occurs in patients with severe immunosuppression. They are usually severely neutropenic and are also receiving adrenal corticosteroids or cytotoxic drugs. The infection is seen most often as a rapidly fatal pneumonia. The diagnosis requires demonstrating the broad nonseptate fungi in lung biopsy specimen. Amphotericin B is the drug of choice, but recovery is rare.

MYCETOMA

Mycetoma, or maduromycosis, is a chronic, suppurative infection of the subcutaneous tissue. The causative agent can be any one of a large number of fungi or aerobic higher bacteria called actinomycetes. These organisms live in soil or vegetation in many tropical and subtropical areas of the world and enter the feet or other unprotected areas of the body through minor trauma. The microbe lives in pus as a colony or grain a few millimeters in diameter. Extensive fibrosis, swelling, draining sinuses, destruction of underlying bone, and extension to contiguous soft tissues mark the slow progression of the lesion. Antibiotic therapy benefits actinomycete mycetoma. Fungal mycetoma usually requires amputation.

CHROMOMYCOSIS

Chromomycosis is a chronic mycotic infection of the skin and subcutaneous tissue. Certain fungi growing on soil or vegetation enter the skin during minor trauma. These fungi grow in the subcutaneous tissue as brownish round cells. One or more verrucous plaques form during the ensuing months or years and may become papillary. There is no pain or bony destruction. The diagnosis is made by culture and histology of the lesion. Excision of small lesions and oral flucytosine therapy are helpful. For extensive chronic lesions, intravenously administered amphotericin B plus oral flucytosine may be preferable because drug resistance tends to develop with flucytosine alone.

BIBLIOGRAPHY
Histoplasmosis

Goodwin, R.A., Jr., and others: Chronic pulmonary histoplasmosis, Medicine **55**:413, 1976.

Smith, J.W., and Utz, J.P.: Progressive disseminated histoplasmosis, Ann. Intern. Med. **76**:557, 1972.

Coccidioidomycosis

Drutz, D.J., and Catanzaro, A.: Coccidioidomycosis, Am. Rev. Respir. Dis. **117**:559, 1978.

Fiese, M.J.: Coccidioidomycosis, Springfield, Ill., 1958, Charles C Thomas, Publisher.

Stevens, D., editor: Coccidioidomycosis: a text, New York, 1979, Plenum Publishing Corp.

Blastomycosis

Emmons, C.W., and others: Medical mycology. ed. 3, Philadelphia, 1977, Lea & Febiger.

Cryptococcosis

Diamond, R.D.: *Cryptococcus neoformans*. In Mandell, G.L., Douglas, R.G., and Bennett, J.E., editors: Principles and practice of infectious diseases, New York, 1979, John Wiley & Sons, Inc.

Sporotrichosis

Wilson, D.E., and others: Clinical features of extracutaneous sporotrichosis, Medicine **46**:265, 1967.

Candidiasis

Cawson, R.A., and Lehner, T.: Chronic hyperplastic candidiasis—candidal leukoplakia, Br. J. Dermatol. **80**:9, 1968.

Gaines, J.D., and Remington, J.S.: Disseminated candidiasis in the surgical patient, Surgery **72**:730, 1972.

Kirkpatrick, C.H., and Smith, T.K.: Chronic mucocutaneous candidiasis: immunologic and antibiotic therapy, Ann. Intern. Med. **80**:310, 1974.

Odds, F.C.: *Candida* and candidosis, Baltimore, 1979, University Park Press.

Aspergillosis

Bennett, J.E.: *Aspergillus* species. In Mandell, G.L., Douglas, R.G., and Bennett, J.E., editors: Principles and practice of infectious diseases, New York, 1979, John Wiley & Sons, Inc.

Mucormycosis

Meyer, R.D., Rosen, P., and Armstrong, D.: Phycomycosis complicating leukemia and lymphoma, Ann. Intern. Med. **77:**871, 1972.

Meyers, B.R., and others: Rhinocerebral mucormycosis: premortem diagnosis and therapy, Arch. Intern. Med. **139:**557, 1979.

Mycetoma

Mahgoub, E.S., and Murray, I.G.: Mycetoma, London, 1973, William Heinemann.

Chromomycosis

Rippon, J.W.: Medical mycology, Philadelphia, 1974, W.B. Saunders Co.

53 • AGENTS USED IN TREATMENT OF MYCOTIC INFECTIONS

Donald Kaye

TREATMENT OF DEEP MYCOSES

Amphotericin B is the primary agent used in the therapy of systemic fungal infections. It is degraded in the body, and serum levels are unaffected by renal or hepatic failure.

Amphotericin B is a very toxic drug and must be given intravenously. It regularly produces nephrotoxicity, some of which is irreversible. It results in hypokalemia (caused by renal loss of potassium) and a normocytic, normochromic anemia. Patients frequently have fever, chills, nausea, and vomiting while the drug is being administered, and phlebitis is common.

The dose is usually 0.3 to 0.5 mg/kg intravenously daily or 1 mg/kg every other day. Doses are given over 2 to 4 hours in 5% glucose in water. When therapy is started, a test dose of 1 mg is given to assess its pyrogenicity in the patient. Gradually increasing doses over 3 to 4 days are then given followed by full dosage. In a critically ill patient, 1 mg, 10 mg, 20 mg, and so on can be given 8 hours apart followed by full dosage. The duration of therapy is 6 to 12 weeks for most systemic fungal infections.

Cryptococcal meningitis can be treated with intravenous administration of amphotericin B for 10 weeks. With the addition of orally administered *flucytosine* (150 mg/kg/day in four divided doses), doses of amphotericin B should be decreased to 0.3 mg/kg/day and a duration of therapy of 6 weeks is often adequate. Flucytosine may be synergistic or additive in action with amphotericin B against other fungi such as *Candida* and *Aspergillus,* but clinical trials are inconclusive. Although relatively nontoxic in patients with normal renal function, flucytosine has bone marrow toxicity when excessive blood levels are achieved. This occurs in the presence of renal insufficiency. Flucytosine also may demonstrate a dose-related gastrointestinal toxicity with nausea, abdominal pain, and diarrhea. Abnormal liver chemistries and rash may also occur.

In meningitis caused by *Coccidioides,* in addition to parenteral therapy, amphotericin B is given intrathecally in doses of 0.5 mg three times a week. Therapy is usually prolonged for months.

Miconazole and *ketoconazole* are recently developed imidazoles that are active in vitro against many fungi. Miconazole is not absorbed orally and is given intravenously in deep mycotic infections. However, effective blood levels are difficult to maintain. Ketoconazole is absorbed orally, and effective blood levels are more easily achieved and maintained. Both agents are metabolized in the body and are relatively nontoxic. The doses are not changed in patients with renal insufficiency.

Miconazole is given intravenously in a dose of 200 mg to 1.2 g (usually 1 g) every 8 hours over a 1- to 2-hour period. Responses have been obtained in patients with certain disseminated mycoses including coccidioidomycosis and paracoccidioidomycosis. Therapy is continued for weeks to months depending on the infection. Miconazole does not penetrate well into the cerebrospinal fluid nor are effective urinary levels achieved; intrathecal or bladder instillation is necessary for infections at these sites. Side effects are rash, phlebitis, pruritus, nausea, vomiting, fever, hyponatremia, and hyperlipidemia (from the infusion fluid). The dose is not altered with renal insufficiency. Miconazole does not seem to be the therapy of choice for any deep mycosis.

Ketoconazole is given orally in a recommended dose of 200 to 400 mg once daily; the use of higher doses is currently being explored. The presence of gastric acid is required for absorption. Ketoconazole is effective in chronic mucocutaneous candidiasis, in which it is probably the drug of choice. It is also effective in griseofulvin-resistant dermatomycoses. A limited experience suggests that it may be useful in paracoccidioidomycosis, coccidioidomycosis, and histoplasmosis. Therapy is continued for weeks to months depending on the infection (at least 6 months for systemic mycoses). Chronic mucocutaneous candidiasis requires maintenance therapy. Ketoconazole does not penetrate well into the cerebrospinal fluid. Side effects include nausea, vomiting, abdominal pain, pruritus, rash, heacache, somnolence, and abnormal liver chemistries.

Ketoconazole must be evaluated further before it can be recommended as primary therapy in any deep mycosis.

TREATMENT OF SUPERFICIAL MYCOSES

(See the discussion of fungal and yeast infections in Chapter 167.)

A number of agents are useful by local application for the treatment of superficial mycoses.

Nystatin is available for local use in oral and vaginal candidiasis. *Miconazole* and *clotrimazole* are imidazoles that are effective against *Candida* and dermatophytes *(Trichophyton, Microsporum,* and *Epidermophyton)* that cause tinea infections.

Undecylenic acid, haloprogin, and *tolnaftate* are topical antifungal agents that are active against dermatophytes but not *Candida.* They are not as effective as the imidazoles.

Griseofulvin is an oral agent that is active against the dermatophytes but not *Candida.* The dose is 500 mg once a day for 4 weeks; for infection of the nail 4 to 6 months of treatment is necessary. Griseofulvin is not effective against deep mycoses, and it should not be used in patients with porphyria. Side effects are photosensitivity, hypersensitivity reactions, nausea, vomiting, diarrhea, headache, fatigue, confusion, and leukopenia. It can cause a disulfiram-like reaction when taken with alcohol. It also increases the dosage of coumarin drugs needed for anticoagulation.

BIBLIOGRAPHY

First International Symposium on Ketoconazole, Rev. Infect. Dis. **2**:519, 1980.

Goodman, L.S., and Gilman, A.: The pharmacological basis of therapeutics, ed. 5, New York, 1975, Macmillan, Inc.

Handbook of antimicrobial therapy. The Medical Letter on Drugs and Therapeutics (revised ed.), New Rochelle, N.Y., 1980.

Mandell, G.L., Douglas, R.G., and Bennett, J.E.: Principles and practice of infectious diseases, New York, 1979, John Wiley & Sons, Inc.

Sanford, J.P.: Guide to antimicrobial therapy, West Bethesda, Md., 1981, J.P. Sanford, M.D.

Unit D • PROTOZOAL DISEASES

54 • DISEASES CAUSED BY PROTOZOA

Thomas C. Jones

Protozoa are single-cell eukaryotic microbes. They form a diverse group of organisms that are divided on the basis of morphologic and functional characteristics into flagellates, amebae, sporozoa, and ciliates. Protozoa such as the trypanosomes or the malaria parasites reside primarily in the tissue, whereas those such as trichomonads, *Giardia,* or amebae reside on the mucosal surfaces. Some organisms such as amebae and *Giardia* are transmitted to humans by ingestion of food or water contaminated with human feces. Other organisms are transmitted to humans by insect vectors of disease such as those that transmit malaria and leishmaniasis.

This chapter will emphasize six protozoal diseases of humans: malaria, amebiasis, giardiasis, toxoplasmosis, trichomoniasis, and leishmaniasis. In addition, the diseases African trypanosomiasis, South American trypanosomiasis, pneumocystosis, and babesiosis will be discussed. The diagnosis of protozoal diseases depends on smears of body secretions when the protozoa are lumen-dwelling microbes such as those causing amebiasis, giardiasis, and trichomoniasis; smears of peripheral blood in cases of malaria, babesiosis, and trypanosomiasis; smears of tissue specimens from affected areas in leishmaniasis and pneumocystosis; and serologic antibody testing in cases of toxoplasmosis, hepatic amebiasis, and South American trypanosomiasis.

Protozoal infections are sufficiently distinct from one another that the commonly used phrase "rule out parasitic disease" is both unhelpful and unnecessary. The following descriptions of each of the protozoal diseases should provide the background for making a clinical diagnosis and supporting that diagnosis by appropriate laboratory testing.

MALARIA

Malaria in nonimmune individuals is an acute febrile illness associated with vigorous shaking chills, prostration, splenomegaly, and anemia. In partially immune patients who live in an area endemic for malaria, the illness is characterized by splenomegaly, anemia, intermittent fever, and occasionally immune-complex glomerulonephritis.

EPIDEMIOLOGY. Malaria occurs throughout the tropics and subtropics and even in temperate climates where inadequate treatment of patients with marlari and inadequate control of the mosquito vectors of malaria exist. The incidence of malaria is increasing throughout Africa, Asia, and Central and South America. Approximately 100 million cases of malaria occur each year. The mortality rate associated with malaria is variable, depending on the *Plasmodium* species prevalent in the area, the availability of medical care, and the level of immunity in the population. Mortality may be over 10% in areas where *P. falciparum* occurs.

LIFE CYCLE OF THE ORGANISM. The protozoa plasmodia are part of the subphylum Sporozoa. This class of microbes has two cycles: a sexual cycle termed sporogony, which occurs in the female *Anopheles* mosquito vector, and an asexual cycle, schizogony, which occurs in the human host. For a human to be infected during the mosquito bite, the mosquito must have taken up the blood of an infected human 2 weeks previously. The blood meal contains the male and female gametocytes, which are necessary for the initiation of the sexual cycle in the mosquito. After ingestion of the blood meal, the gametocytes are liberated in the stomach of the mosquito, the male gametocyte fertilizes the female, and a zygote is formed. This transforms into a motile ookinete that migrates through the stomach wall, encysts in the tissue of the stomach wall, and replicates. The cyst then ruptures, releasing sporozoites that migrate to the salivary gland of the mosquito, where they remain until the time of the next mosquito feeding. At the time of the bite the sporozoites in the salivary juices of the mosquito are inoculated into the vascular system of the human host. The sporozoites circulate for less than half an hour and then enter the cells of the liver. At this point they are said to initiate the pre-erythrocytic stage of malaria infection. After a period lasting from 5 to 16 days, depending on the species of *Plasmodium,* the parasites rupture the hepatic cells, enter the vascular system, and, now termed merozoites, enter circulating red blood cells. This initiates the erythrocytic cycle of malaria. During this cycle they replicate in the red cells by the process termed schizogony and are called schizonts. After 48 to 72 hours, depending on the species, the cycle is complete and the red cells rupture, releasing the merozoites to infect additional red cells. During this process some of the merozoites become male and female gametocytes. These then circulate along with the schizonts of malaria, awaiting ingestion with the next blood meal of a mosquito and the continuation of the cycle. Patients can also be infected by transfusions or communal use of a needle as occurs among drug addicts. Although there are over 100 different species of *Plasmodium* that can infect various mammals, birds, and reptiles, only four of these species—*P. falciparum, P. vivax, P. ovale,* and *P. malariae*—infect humans.

PATHOLOGY. The pathologic changes that are seen in malaria occur at the time the merozoites enter and replicate within the red blood cells. During this process the red cells are changed dramatically. Under the electron microscope, for example, the membranes of erythrocytes appear to have electron-dense knoblike projections; the cells take on unusual shapes and are no longer as deformable as red cells from uninfected persons. Most importantly, they become adhesive to vascular endothelium and to each other, and they demonstrate an increase in osmotic fragility. As a result of these changes and the rupture of the red cells during the cycle of schizogony, the patient demonstrates changes of intravascular hemolysis, progressive anemia, and occlusion of blood vessels. This leads to generalized tissue anoxia, which is noted in falciparum malaria most prominently as cerebral and renal anoxia. Patients with severe forms of malaria may also have hepatitis and pulmonary edema. Patients also have evidence of bone marrow impairment and the syndrome of disseminated intravascular coagulation. Some patients have such impressive hemolysis that they are described as having "blackwater fever," a complication of malaria caused by rapid hemolysis with hemoglobin damage to the kidneys resulting in acute renal failure. Patients with more prolonged malaria may have immune complex damage to the glomeruli of the kidney, resulting in a nephrotic syndrome. Others with chronic malaria may demonstrate the syndrome of tropical splenomegaly caused by repeated malaria attacks and an exaggerated immune response. Some patients are resistant to malaria because of hemoglobinopathies that interfere with replication of the malaria parasite in the red cell. For example, *P. falciparum* multiplies poorly in red cells containing sickle hemoglobin. Some patients are resistant because they lack the blood groups on the surface of the red cell that are necessary for attachment of the malaria parasite, a requirement for entry into the cells. For example, one of the blood group substances called the Duffy blood group is essential for the attachment of *P. vivax* to red cells. Patients without the Duffy blood group substance are resistant to vivax malaria. Blacks frequently lack Duffy substance.

CLINICAL MANIFESTATIONS. Patients with malaria have shaking chills, fever, headache, and myalgias. During the early stages of the infection the fever may occur daily, but within a few days a synchronous pattern emerges. This has been referred to as tertian or quartan malaria, depending on whether the malaria fevers are occurring at 48- or 72-hour intervals. With *P. vivax* and *P. ovale,* fever occurs every 48 hours; with *P. malariae,* fever occurs every 72 hours; and with *P. falciparum,* fever tends to be continuous or irregular. A characteristic attack is preceded by a shaking chill, and then the temperature increases to 104° F (40° C). This followed by malaise and headache lasting several hours. The attack is terminated by profuse sweating and a fall in the temperature. The patient may then feel well for 1 to 2 days before the fever recurs. Malaria is associated with a number of nonspecific symptoms such as cough, abdominal pains, nausea, vomiting, and diarrhea. These symptoms mislead physicians to make other diagnoses such as upper respiratory illness or gastroenteritis. Occasionally liver dysfunction is a prominent feature of malaria, and the disease may be misdiagnosed as hepatitis. Enlargement of the spleen is common in vivax and ovale malaria but is less frequently seen during the early stages of falciparum malaria. Laboratory tests reveal the anemia and thrombocytopenia associated with malaria. Eosinophilia is not a feature of malaria. Liver dysfunction is often evidenced by elevation of serum transaminase levels and the appearance of bile in the urine. The complications of malaria are those associated with severe anoxia to the brain, kidneys, and lungs and severe hemolytic anemia.

DIAGNOSIS. The diagnosis of malaria is made by first suspecting the disease in any symptomatic patient who has been to a malarious area, has received a blood transfusion, or is a drug addict. The clinical suspicion of malaria is confirmed by taking thin and thick smears of the patient's blood, staining them with Giemsa stain, and examining them microscopically for evidence of *Plasmodium*-infected red blood cells. The falciparum malaria parasite appears as a delicate ring of blue cytoplasm with a purple dot, which resembles a signet ring. This is called the "ring form" of malaria. The red cells are normal in size, and there are no red dots in the erythrocyte characteristic of other forms of malaria. Since the maturation of this form of malaria does not occur in the peripheral blood, mature-stage schizogony is not seen in *P. falciparum* infection. In contrast to other types of malaria, parasitemia may reach high levels (over 10%). The gametocyte of *P. falciparum* is characteristic and is shaped like a banana or crescent. *P. vivax* can be readily distinguished from falciparum ring forms. Unlike other types of malaria, the red cells are larger than uninfected red cells and contain red dots referred to as Schuffner's dots. In addition, the blue cytoplasm of *P. vavax* is much larger and more diffusely distributed throughout the red cell. Since vivax malaria parasites mature in the peripheral blood (unlike *P. falciparum*), developmental forms of schizogony, including the mature schizont that contains 12 to 24 chromatin dots, can be seen. *P. malariae* and *P. ovale* also mature in the peripheral blood. *P. malariae* may be recognized by the band form in which the mature schizont stretches in a band across the red cell. Malaria parasites are present in the peripheral blood throughout the period of malaria infection, although they may be present in larger numbers a few hours after the patient's chills and fever begin. Antibodies appear in the peripheral blood; however, serologic tests are not useful in diagnosing the acute illness. They are of value for screening blood donors when transfusion malaria has occurred and for determining the prevalence of malaria in the population.

MANAGEMENT. The therapy of malaria is directed at eradicating *Plasmodium* during the erythrocytic stage of the infection. This is done primarily by the use of chloroquine, which interferes with nucleic acid synthesis of the developing parasite. Over a period of 2 days 1.5 g of base is given (600 mg base initially followed by 300 mg base at 6, 24, and 48 hours). Administration is oral or if necessary parenteral. When patients are infected with species of *Plasmodium* such as vivax and ovale that have prolonged hepatic stages of infection, primaquine must be added to eradicate the tissue phase. Primaquine is given orally as one tablet (15 mg of base) daily for 14 days.

In some parts of the world, such as Southeast Asia and the central regions of South America, *P. falciparum* malaria is resistant to chloroquine. Malaria acquired in these regions requires use of the time-honored drug against malaria, quinine, in combination with pyrimethamine and a sulfa drug such as sulfadiazine. The quinine is given in a dose of 650 mg every 8 hours for 7 days, and the pyrimethamine (50 mg each day) and sulfa (for example, sulfadiazine, 1 g every 6 hours) are given for 3 and 5 days, respectively. This combination will eradicate parasitemia and prevent the recrudescence of the malaria. The patient with severe malaria must be provided with important supportive therapy, such as management of coma when the patient is unconscious, to prevent aspiration pneumonia and pressure ulcerations. In addition, acute renal failure may require dialysis, and anemia may necessitate the transfusion of red blood cells.

PREVENTION. Malaria can be prevented only by decreasing the contact with infected mosquitoes through appropriate use of mosquito netting and insect repellents and by taking drugs prophylactically against the erythrocytic stage. Chloroquine, 300 mg base orally once a week for adults, is used in areas where the malaria is still sensitive to the drug. This treatment should be started 1 week before arriving in the endemic area and should be continued during the stay and for at least 6 weeks after leaving the endemic area. In areas where chloroquine resistance occurs, a tablet combining pyrimethamine and sulfadoxine is taken in a similar fashion once a week. This product is now available in the United States. When patients return from areas heavily infected with vivax or ovale, they should be given a 2-week course of primaquine (15 mg base daily orally) to prevent relapse of their malaria. At the present time no vaccine is available for preventing malaria; however, active investigation in this area makes it a likely possibility in the near future. Control of malaria in a community depends primarily on controlling the insect vector by draining areas of insect development and residual insecticide spraying.

DISEASES CAUSED BY AMEBAE
Amebiasis

Amebiasis is an infection of the human colon yielding a spectrum of illness from asymptomatic to severe invasive inflammatory bowel disease. In addition, it may cause extraintestinal disease, particularly liver abscess. The infection is acquired by the ingestion of water or food contaminated with human feces.

EPIDEMIOLOGY. The pathogenic organism that causes amebiasis, *Entamoeba histolytica,* is distributed widely throughout the tropics, subtropics, and temperate climates. It is most common where proper disposal of human feces is not provided, including all of the developing countries of the world, and where fecal contamination is common for sociologic reasons, as among the homosexual community. In many areas of the tropics over 40% of the population is infected. Epidemics of amebiasis have occurred where ameba-contaminated stool has gained access to water supply systems. The disease associated with amebiasis appears to be more severe in some parts of the world than in others. This may be associated with variations in strains of *E. histolytica.*

LIFE CYCLE OF THE ORGANISM. *E. histolytica* exists in two stages: an encysted stage in which the organism can persist in nature for long periods of time and a trophozoite stage in which the organism exists in the human bowel under appropriate environmental conditions. An infected person may pass either the cyst or the trophozoite in the stool. However, the trophozoite must encyst shortly after passage to survive in the conditions outside the human gastrointestinal tract. During conversion of the trophozoite to the cyst, the trophozoite first develops a wall around itself, then a glycogen vacuole and a chromatoid body. The nuclear material of the newly encysted trophozoite then divides twice, forming a cyst containing four nuclei. This encysted structure can persist in water or moist soil for weeks to months. When this form is ingested, the organism can successfully pass the low pH of the stomach and then emerge from the cyst in the environment of the upper small intestine. If conditions are proper in the colon, it may persist in the lumen for long periods or invade the mucosa of the bowel. Trophozoites are facultative anaerobes and can survive and replicate only under complex conditions, such as the presence of other bacteria in the environment, low oxygen tension, and the availability of carbohydrates. These conditions determine the degree of virulence of the ameba and also lead to the wide spectrum of symptoms seen in patients infected with the same ameba. Some patients, for example, are completely asymptomatic, with infection documented only by the identification of the ameba in the stool. Others may have a progressive, even fatal, disease associated with the invasion of the ameba into tissue.

PATHOLOGY. The ameba gains access to the submucosa of the large bowel by excreting a material that allows it to pass between the mucosal cells. Once in the submucosal environment, the organism releases substances that contribute to tissue anoxia, necrosis, and changes in the environment that render it ideal for replication of the ameba. The ameba then ingests host tissue, particularly red blood cells, to maintain its growth. During this process an ulcer is formed in the submucosa. Since the ulcer is much larger at the base of the submucosa than at the mucosal surface, it appears flask shaped. Depending on the degree of inflammatory changes in the bowel, a few punctate lesions may be associated with the bowel infection or there may be generalized and marked inflammatory changes. Marked inflammation often follows loss of mucosal integrity after significant submucosal tissue destruction by the ameba. This then leads to secondary bacterial infection. Ulceration of the bowel may extend through the serosal surface and lead to peritonitis.

During the submucosal infection two other complications may result. The first is a local marked inflammatory reaction to the combination of amebae and bacteria. This causes an intestinal mass called an ameboma. The second, and most common complication of amebiasis is invasion of the vascular system of the bowel, which allows amebae to be transported to the liver. Amebic infection of the liver results in progressive necrosis of liver substance in the region where amebae are replicating. This appears pathologically as a gradually expanding necrotic lesion referred to as amebic liver abscess. The central region of the abscess is filled with debris and the end products of liver necrosis. The liquid has a reddish brown, anchovy paste-like appearance. Under the microscope the amebae are seen at the periphery of the abscess at the edge of normal liver tissue. It should be pointed out that this lesion, although referred to as an abscess, is not a typical inflammatory abscess that requires surgical drainage but rather an area of liver necrosis. Occasionally this enlarging area of liver necrosis may rupture into the peritoneum, through the diaphragm into the pleural cavity, or into the pericardial space. This rupture is a serious and often fatal complication of amebiasis. Rarely, amebae may gain access to other sites such as the brain or skin.

CLINICAL MANIFESTATIONS. Amebiasis can be divided into two distinct clinical entities: intestinal amebiasis and extraintestinal amebiasis. Patients with intestinal amebiasis show signs and symptoms of colonic irritation, including abdominal pain with mucus and occasionally blood in the stools. When the colonic involvement becomes severe, the patient may present all the signs and symptoms of an acute abdominal condition, including abdominal distention, absence of bowel sounds, and vomiting. A patient with an ameboma may have subtle clinical manifestations, and the ameboma may be identified during barium enema examination. It is often confused with a colonic carcinoma. A distinguishing feature is that the serologic test for amebae is positive if the lesion is due to ameboma. Some patients have a chronic irritative bowel syndrome associated with amebic colitis, which may be indistinguishable from that of ulcerative colitis.

Extraintestinal amebiasis may be present without any history of or association with gastrointestinal signs or symptoms. The patient with hepatic amebiasis usually has fever, pain in the right upper quadrant and epigastrium, right shoulder pain caused by irritation of the diaphragm, and a palpable liver. The patient may have a history of rapid weight loss of 20 to 30 pounds over several weeks. The hepatic lesions of amebiasis are more often in the right lobe of the liver. Point tenderness over that part of the chest and abdomen is an important sign in identifying amebic liver abscess. Laboratory testing in amebic abscess reveals anemia, leukocytosis without eosinophilia, an elevated diaphragm on chest roentgenogram, and abnormal liver function tests. The leukocytosis associated with amebic liver abscess may lead some physicians to consider a diagnosis of pyogenic infection of the liver, but leukocytosis is a common feature of amebiasis. Jaundice may or may not be present. When rupture of amebic abscess occurs, it is a catastrophic illness causing severe impairment in function at the site of the rupture. If the rupture occurs, for instance, into the pleural space, pulmonary signs and symptoms are prominent; with rupture into the pericardial space, cardiac tamponade may be an impressive feature of the illness.

DIAGNOSIS. Intestinal amebiasis is diagnosed by identifying the ameba, *E. histolytica,* in microscopic examination of stool specimens. The diagnosis is confirmed by finding either trophozoites or cysts. The physician can do this during sigmoidoscopy by placing a small aspirate of liquid from a colonic lesion on a glass slide and looking for the characteristic motility of the ameba. When specimens are sent to the laboratory, the technician examines a specimen directly and then a concentration of the stool looking for cysts. Some laboratories culture the fluid for the ameba. Since the shedding of amebae in mild infections may be intermittent, several stools over a period of days may be necessary to exclude the diagnosis of amebiasis. In addition, purging to obtain multiple stool samples has been suggested as a means for diagnosis of amebiasis. Serologic tests are of limited value in the diagnosis of intestinal amebiasis. However, they should be obtained because of the possibility of invasive disease such as ameboma and amebic liver abscess. The diagnosis of extraintestinal amebiasis relies on demonstrating antibodies against the ameba in the peripheral blood and on obtaining tissue from the site of the inflamed bowel or fluid from an amebic liver abscess. Findings that are characteristic of amebic liver abscess include elevation of the right diaphragm on chest roentgenogram, leukocytosis, and liver function abnormalities. Radioisotopic scanning and computed tomography of the liver are helpful in the diagnosis of amebic liver abscess. The stool examination shows amebae in only one third of those cases with documented amebic abscess of the liver. The clinical signs and symptoms of extraintestinal amebiasis resolve promptly after therapy against amebiasis is initiated, and this has been suggested as a reasonable and noninvasive diagnostic test.

MANAGEMENT. The treatment of amebiasis varies depending on whether the site of the inflammation is in the colon or the liver. The treatment of intestinal amebiasis depends on whether it is asymptomatic or evidence of invasive disease is present. If there is no evidence of invasive disease, drugs directed at the luminal phase of the infection are used. These include paromomycin, diiodohydroxyquin, and diloxanide furoate (available from the Centers for Disease Control*). The nitroimidazoles are the most effective drugs against the invasive form of the disease. Metronidazole is the only drug in this group available in the United States. The dosage is 2.25 g daily in three divided doses for 5 to 10 days. Metronidazole may cause some side effects such as nausea and abdominal discomfort. In addition, drinking alcohol during treatment with this drug may make the patient very ill.

Extraintestinal amebiasis is also treated with metronidazole in the same doses. Some physicians add chloroquine, 500 mg a day, as an adjunct to the therapy of amebic liver abscess. If a patient with amebic liver abscess does not respond during the first few days of metronidazole therapy, aspiration of the abscess site is indicated. This can be done either by needle aspiration or by open drainage, depending on the patient's clinical course. If amebic peritonitis is a complication of intestinal amebiasis, laparotomy should be avoided if possible because the bowel is almost impossible to resuture. Supportive measures such as maintaining fluid and electrolyte balance are essential when patients with amebic liver abscess and peritonitis are seriously ill.

PREVENTION. Amebiasis is prevented by interrupting the contamination of food and water with human feces. The most commonly contaminated foods are vegetables grown near the ground such as lettuce, celery, tomatoes, and cucumbers. In addition, water is a frequent vehicle for the transmission of amebiasis. Both fresh, uncooked food and water should be avoided in any developing country because of the danger of contamination with amebae. Chlorine treatment is not completely effective in preventing infection by amebae. Boiling water for 10 minutes, on the other hand, kills both trophozoites and cysts. Improvement in waste disposal and water purification is the most important factor in ultimately reducing the risk of acquiring amebic disease.

Diseases caused by free-living amebae

There are free-living amebae that live in fresh water and the soil as well as in the oral cavity of humans. Recently one genus, *Naegleria,* has been associated with amebic meningoencephalitis in humans. This disease occurs when amebae in fresh water are forced under pressure through the nasal mucosa covering the cribriform plate and into the brain tissue. This occurs during diving and water-skiing in contaminated freshwater lakes. Another ameba, *Acanthamoeba,* has been found as a normal inhabitant of the human mouth. It has been associated recently with progressive inflammatory lesions in the eye and granulomatous lesions in the brain. There is no known disease of the oral cavity associated with the *Acanthamoeba.* Treatment is ineffective in both of these illnesses, although amphotericin B has been successful in two cases in the treatment of *Naegleria* meningoencephalitis. The infection of the eye with *Acanthamoeba* is usually associated with other organisms that contribute to the ulcerative lesion.

GIARDIASIS

Giardia lamblia is a flagellate that resides in the lumen of the upper gastrointestinal tract and may cause inflam-

---

*Parasitic Disease Drug Service, Center for Infectious Diseases, Centers for Disease Control, Atlanta, Ga. 30333. Telephone: days, 404-329-3670, nights and weekends, 404-329-3644.

matory changes in the mucosa leading to enteritis and malabsorption.

EPIDEMIOLOGY. *Giardia* are distributed throughout the world in both temperate and tropical climates. Because of the resistance of the cyst stage of the organism in water, the occurrence of giardiasis is one of the first signs of a break in the water purification system. The disease is both endemic and epidemic. For example, in Colorado there is a high prevalence of infection among citizens in rural towns, and the disease has occurred in epidemics among skiers at ski lodges during the winter months. These epidemics undoubtedly result from overtaxing of waste disposal and water purification facilities by large numbers of people. The organism is a common cause of infection throughout the developing countries because of incomplete management of human waste disposal. Recently strains of *Giardia* that can infect humans have been identified in animal reservoirs such as beavers, further complicating the epidemiology and efforts to control the spread of infection. Immunodeficient patients have a much higher prevalence of giardiasis than normal individuals even though they have not traveled to recognized endemic areas.

LIFE CYCLE OF THE ORGANISM. *Giardia* exists in two stages: the cyst and the trophozoite. The cyst stage is the mechanism by which the *Giardia* is able to persist in water for long periods. The cyst is oval shaped, approximately 14 μm long and 8 μm wide. It has two to four nuclei and a characteristic central rodlike structure called an axostyle. When the cyst is ingested, it can pass through the stomach to the upper duodenum, where excystation occurs. The second stage is the trophozoite. This organism has two nuclei and four pairs of flagella that contribute to its active motility. The trophozoite resides on the mucosal surface of the upper intestinal tract. For unknown reasons this association produces impaired absorption and inflammatory changes leading to the signs and symptoms of giardiasis.

CLINICAL MANIFESTATIONS. The main symptoms of giardiasis include abdominal pain, distention, increased sensations of bowel activity, nausea, and intermittent watery diarrhea. During chronic infections anorexia, intolerance of certain foods, and weight loss are characteristic. The diagnosis is made by identifying either the cysts or the trophozoites of *Giardia* on microscopic examination of stool specimens. Occasionally the presence of *Giardia* cannot be detected in the stool, and the organism must be sought in specimens from the upper intestinal tract. This is done by microscopic examination of a string that has been passed into the upper intestinal tract. An aspirate of duodenal contents will also reveal the organisms.

MANAGEMENT. Treatment of giardiasis is accomplished by one of two drugs: quinacrine, 100 mg three times a day for 7 days, or metronidazole, one tablet (250 mg) three times a day for 5 to 10 days. Either will eradicate the infection in the majority of patients. If patients have a recurrence of their illness, retreatment is indicated.

PREVENTION. The prevention of giardiasis is accomplished only by ensuring that water purification systems are complete. The cysts are resistant to chlorination alone; therefore purification systems that rely entirely on this mechanism are not safe. Boiling water for 10 to 15 minutes and sophisticated water purification systems such as aeration, sedimentation, filtration, and chlorination will prevent spread of the infection.

TOXOPLASMOSIS

Infection with the protozoan *Toxoplasma gondii* is common in all mammals and birds. Human infection often occurs without symptoms; however, there may be transient lymphadenopathy and fever in immunologically normal adults and a severe progressive disease in individuals with impaired immune responsiveness. Recurrent inflammatory disease of the eye is also a manifestation of toxoplasmosis. The organism is acquired by ingesting undercooked meat that contains the viable organisms or by contact with the infectious oocyst stage in the feces of cats.

EPIDEMIOLOGY. *T. gondii* is the most common single species that infects all mammals. Its prevalence rate is extremely high in some parts of the world, such as Tahiti and some Caribbean islands, where infection approaches 100% in humans. In most parts of the world the prevalence ranges from 30% to 60%, depending on the disposal facilities for cat feces and the propensity of the population to eat undercooked meats such as mutton, pork, or beef. Only in very dry or extremely cold areas in the world is the infection of low prevalence. A few islands in the Pacific where cats have never been introduced remain free of toxoplasmosis. The most common means of the spread of disease among humans in the United States is by ingesting meat contaminated with *Toxoplasma* cysts. Because of this, 1% of the 15- to 50-year-old population is infected each year. Once infected, a person remains infected for life, although symptoms of the infection may be absent or only transient in nature.

LIFE CYCLE OF THE ORGANISM. When a mammal eats meat containing the cyst, the cyst passes into the intestine and liberates hundreds or thousands of trophozoites, the obligate intracellular form. The trophozoites, which are 7 μm long and 3 to 4 μm wide, enter the mucosal cells of the gastrointestinal tract. They then divide with a generation time of 5 to 10 hours, rupture the cells, and infect adjacent cells. During this process they enter cells that gain access to the vascular system and are distributed throughout the body. During the immune response the generation time of the parasite lengthens and a firm wall forms around the *Toxoplasma* organism. The encysted parasite persists in muscle and brain tissue throughout the lifetime of the host. When another mammal ingests this tissue, the life cycle is continued. This is referred to as the asexual cycle of toxoplasmosis.

When a cat ingests the infectious form of *Toxoplasma*,

an additional process occurs. A sexual cycle is initiated in the intestinal mucosa of members of the feline family. The penetrating trophozoites develop into macrogametocytes or microgametocytes. After cross-fertilization a zygote is formed and matures into an infective oocyst. The excreted cat feces containing the infective oocysts then contaminate the environment. Cattle, sheep, and pigs are usually infected by ingesting these oocysts. These two mechanisms are responsible for the high prevalence of infection in nature.

PATHOLOGY. After *Toxoplasma* has entered the cell, divided, and caused the rupture of the cell, an acute inflammatory response occurs in the presence of this progressive tissue necrosis. If the human has no immune responsiveness, as in a fetus, a progressive severe necrotic process results throughout the body. However, in immunologically normal adults an immune response against the organism occurs. This is first manifested by fever and enlargement of lymph nodes. At this time the invasion of muscle tissue by *Toxoplasma* organisms leads to limited myositis. If the immune response is complete, the encysted *Toxoplasma* causes no further damage to the infected tissue after the initial invasion period. Intermittently, a cyst may rupture and is then rapidly controlled by an intense delayed hypersensitivity inflammatory response to the organism. This prevents spread of the infection once the patient is immune, even though living organisms persist in the tissue for life. In very sensitive areas, such as the retina of the eye, this well-localized inflammatory reaction can cause signs and symptoms such as retinochoroiditis. If an illness associated with immunosuppression develops, toxoplasmosis can reactivate and lead to progressive necrosis. This often occurs in the central nervous system and the patient exhibits signs of encephalitis.

CLINICAL MANIFESTATIONS. Toxoplasmosis can be divided into four clinical patterns of disease: acquired lymphatic toxoplasmosis, congenital toxoplasmosis, toxoplasmic retinochoroiditis, and the syndrome of toxoplasmosis in the altered host. Those with acquired toxoplasmosis, when symptomatic, usually have lymph node enlargement, most commonly of the cervical lymph nodes. Approximately half of these patients also have fever, myalgias, malaise, and fatigue. The lymph nodes are usually nontender and rubbery in consistency. These symptoms last for 1 to 2 weeks; however, in most patients the lymphadenopathy persists for months. Rarely, symptoms of severe myocarditis or myositis occur at the time of acute infection in an otherwise healthy adult. Laboratory tests of patients with acquired toxoplasmosis demonstrate a slight monocytosis or lymphocytosis. Atypical lymphocytes, which are seen in infectious mononucleosis, are not present in large numbers. There may be slight changes in liver function tests during the first few days or weeks of the illness. The blood counts are usually normal. Biopsy of the lymph node shows a typical pattern of hyperplasia of histiocytes.

Neonates with congenital toxoplasmosis have severe inflammatory changes in the organs. The manifestations may be microphthalmia, hydrocephalus, hepatosplenomegaly, pneumonitis, and fever. The brain lesions may lead to calcification that can be identified roentgenographically several months after infection. Some neonates may not show the full picture of congenital toxoplasmosis at birth, and there may be a progressive inflammatory disease during the first months of life. In addition, some infants infected late in the pregnancy may have only mild signs or symptoms at birth but may demonstrate subtle changes in the central nervous system such as seizures or retinochoroiditis later in life.

The onset of toxoplasmic retinochoroiditis most often occurs during the second or third decade of life, even though infection commonly occurs during intrauterine life. This is therefore a later sequela of infection associated with a hypersensitivity response to the organisms. This illness is often recurrent with intermittent episodes of loss of vision and pain in the eye and resulting scar formation. Systemic signs of *Toxoplasma* infection are not present during this local inflammatory reaction.

Toxoplasmosis in the altered host usually occurs as a disseminated disease in a patient with altered cellular immune responsiveness such as Hodgkin's disease. Patients often have fever and progressive signs of encephalitis. Disseminated signs and symptoms such as those seen in congenital toxoplasmosis may also be present. Patients with less severe immunosuppression may have recurrent lymphadenopathy associated with toxoplasmosis or with progressive polymyositis as evidence of impaired ability to control the replication of the *Toxoplasma* organisms.

DIAGNOSIS. The diagnosis of toxoplasmosis rests on three standard procedures: first, the isolation of the protozoan from infected tissue; second, histopathologic identification of the organism in tissue; and third, interpretation of the changing serologic pattern associated with infection.

Since the organism is an obligate intracellular parasite, isolation techniques require the use of animal inoculation or cell culture systems. In most laboratories animal inoculation is used. The tissue for examination is made into a suspension and inoculated into the peritoneal cavity of mice. Several weeks after the inoculation the mice are examined for the presence of developing *Toxoplasma* organisms. *Toxoplasma* organisms can be identified in tissue by routine staining procedures. It must be recognized that identification of *Toxoplasma* cysts in muscle or brain tissue may have no pathologic significance because these will be present in the tissue of any person with antibodies against the organism. On the other hand, identification of clusters of organisms in muscle or brain associated with inflammatory cells is good evidence for an association of the pathologic process and the microbe.

Usually the diagnosis of toxoplasmosis rests on noninvasive testing such as serologic evaluation. Four different serologic tests are used in toxoplasmosis. The classic test, the Sabin-Feldman dye test, is one of the most specific antibody tests in medicine; a positive test indicates previous infection. However, since infection with *T. gondii* is so common, it may not be helpful in distinguishing the recently infected, diseased patient from the patient infected many years before. The indirect fluorescent antibody (IFA) test measures the same antibody as the Sabin-Feldman dye test and can be substituted for that test, since it is simpler to perform and less expensive. Laboratories using the IFA test must be aware that it depends on appropriate standardization of the reagents. To document recent exposure to *T. gondii*, the IgM-fluorescent antibody test and the soluble-antigen complement fixation test are available. High or changing antibody titers of these tests are consistent with recent infection. A hemagglutination test is also used in toxoplasmosis. Like the Sabin-Feldman dye test, it is helpful in documenting past *Toxoplasma* infection; however, it is unreliable for determining recent infection.

The four main clinical presentations of toxoplasmosis have separate differential diagnoses. Adult-acquired toxoplasmosis must be distinguished from infectious mononucleosis and lymphoma. Congenital toxoplasmosis must be distinguished from cytomegalovirus infection, viral encephalitis, and the rubella syndrome. Toxoplasmic retinochoroiditis must be distinguished from other causes of inflammation of the retina such as tuberculosis, histoplasmosis, and sarcoidosis. Toxoplasmosis in the altered host requires differentiation from the other disseminated infectious diseases occurring in immunosuppressed patients. These include viral encephalitis, cryptococcosis, and progression of the underlying disease.

MANAGEMENT. Toxoplasmosis is treated with a combination of drugs directed at inhibiting folate metabolism. The most effective combination at the present time is a combination of pyrimethamine and sulfadiazine. Pyrimethamine is given in doses of 75 mg the first day and 25 mg each day thereafter for 1 to 2 months depending on the illness. Sulfadiazine is given as 4 g a day in four divided doses. Folinic acid is administered intramuscularly along with these medicines to prevent bone marrow toxicity.

Patients with mild forms of adult-acquired toxoplasmosis do not require therapy. However, those with severe toxoplasmosis, toxoplasmic retinochoroiditis, and congenital toxoplasmosis may benefit from therapy against *Toxoplasma*. In addition, retinochoroiditis is treated with corticosteroids to inhibit the inflammatory response that leads to much of the eye damage.

PREVENTION. Prevention of toxoplasmosis is accomplished by appropriate cooking of all meats. This means that meat should be cooked to a temperature of at least 140° F (60° C) throughout for 15 minutes. Exposure to oocysts from cat feces can be limited by having little contact with scavenger cats and their environment, changing cat litter boxes daily, and using gloves for gardening and work in sandboxes. Pregnant women and immunosuppressed patients should be particularly cautious and should avoid exposure to either of the two means of acquiring toxoplasmosis.

TRICHOMONIASIS

One of the most common protozoal infections in temperate climates is caused by the venerally spread protozoan *Trichomonas vaginalis*. The organism is a flagellate, 10 to 20 μm in size with a single nucleus, a central structure called an axostyle, and an undulating membrane. It moves in exudative material by a jerky, rotating motion. Unlike *Giardia* or amebae, the trichomonad has no vegetative stage, and infection requires direct contact with infected surfaces. The organism may persist for long periods in endocervical or urethral glands and less commonly in other sites of the genitourinary system without causing inflammation. It is sensitive to pH changes and does not survive well at a pH below 5. Under ideal conditions for protozoal replication it induces marked inflammation of the mucosal surfaces of the vagina, urethra, urinary bladder, or prostate. Patients usually have symptoms of vaginal itching, burning, and a yellow, blood-tinged discharge. If the urethra is involved, the symptoms of inflammation include dysuria and frequency of urination.

The diagnosis is made by observing the motile organisms in fresh vaginal or urethral material. A drop of the material is mixed with saline and a small amount of methylene blue and examined under the low or medium power of the microscope.

Treatment of *T. vaginalis* is accomplished by a single dose of metronidazole. Either 1 or 2 g has been recommended. If this is ineffective, the more traditional, longer duration therapy with 250 mg three times a day for 10 days can be used. The most important point in the management of trichomoniasis is that all sexual partners must be treated to prevent reinfection. Rarely the infection can be transmitted to infants during birth and among individuals in institutions where personal hygiene is poor.

Two other *Trichomonas* species, *T. tenax* and *T. hominis,* exist in humans but are considered nonpathogens.

TRYPANOSOMIASIS

There are two main types of trypanosomes that infect humans. The first is organisms in the *Trypanosoma brucei* complex, which cause African trypanosomiasis. The second is *T. cruzi*, the cause of American trypanosomiasis. These two diseases are distinct clinically and geographically. Their geographic distribution is determined by their different vectors. African trypanosomiasis, also called sleeping sickness, is transmitted from person to person or animal to human by the tsetse fly. American trypanosomiasis is transmitted during the feeding of the reduviid bug.

African trypanosomiasis, because of the distribution of the vector, is confined to tropical regions of Africa. The pathologic response during African trypanosomiasis includes an initial immune response with lymph node and spleen enlargement while the flagellated protozoa are circulating in the peripheral blood. Following the vascular phase, invasion of the central nervous system occurs, causing central nervous system vasculitis and encephalitis. The cellular response includes infiltration of mononuclear cells around the blood vessels of the brain. During the immune response to trypanosomiasis large amounts of IgM antibody are produced. Continued variation in the antigens on the surface of the trypanosome is believed to allow persistence of the organism in the host until death occurs. The clinical features of African trypanosomiasis include high fever and lymphadenopathy in the early phase of the illness. During central nervous system invasion there is initially a phase of sleeplessness, then a progression to somnolence and coma. In this phase the lack of attention to proper eating and aspiration leads to death of the patient as a result of malnutrition and secondary infection. The diagnosis is made by identifying the flagellated protozoa in the peripheral blood or spinal fluid. Serologic tests may be helpful in confirming the diagnosis. The treatment is complex and includes the use of arsenicals and the polysulfated drug suramin. Prevention of the infection depends mainly on avoiding the bite of an infected tsetse fly. Chemoprophylaxis is not recommended.

American trypanosomiasis, or Chagas' disease, occurs throughout South America. During the bite of the reduviid bug, which feeds at night while the subject is sleeping, the contaminated feces of the bug are inoculated into the wound. At this site a trypanosomal chancre occurs, and if it is in the eye, a unilateral conjunctivitis referred to as Romana's sign is seen. Shortly after inoculation of the protozoa there is a period of parasitemia. The microbes then enter the muscle cells of the myocardium and also induce damage in the parasympathetic ganglia (particularly Auerbach's plexus in the esophagus). Damage to these organs produces the late complications of Chagas' disease, including dysfunction of the myocardium and abnormal function of the intestinal tract. The clinical presentation of Chagas' disease includes an initial acute-phase illness and a subsequent chronic phase. The acute illness is characterized by high fever and myocarditis. The initial illness may have as a hallmark the appearance of a skin lesion at the inoculation site or unilateral conjunctivitis. Some patients are asymptomatic during this initial infection. The diagnosis is made by observation of parasitemia. Many years later persistence of the organism in the myocardium and nerve tissue leads to signs of congestive myocardiopathy and/or the so-called mega-syndromes, that is, megaesophagus caused by dysfunction of esophageal motility or megacolon caused by dysfunction of the colon. A patient with congestive myocardiopathy may also have complications of intermittent arrhythmias and thrombi on the inner surface of the myocardium. Pulmonary emboli or fatal arrhythmias are the common causes of death in Chagas' heart disease. The diagnosis in this chronic phase is made by serologic tests or xenodiagnosis. The acute phase of the illness is treated with nifurtimox or benzimidazole (available from the Centers for Disease Control*). The chronic form of the disease does not respond to antiprotozoal therapy, and careful management of arrhythmias and thrombotic complications is indicated. Prevention of the disease is accomplished only by avoiding the bite of the reduviid bug, which resides especially in and around houses constructed of mud and sticks. In addition, the disease may be transmitted by the transfusion of improperly treated blood.

PNEUMOCYSTOSIS

Pneumocystosis is an acute infection of the lungs characterized by fever, shortness of breath, and cyanosis. It occurs in patients who are immunodeficient as a result of malnutrition, malignancy, or immunosuppressive therapy. The causative organism, *Pneumocystis* species, is of uncertain classification but is probably a protozoan. It is presumed to cause frequent but asymptomatic infection in healthy mammalian hosts.

EPIDEMIOLOGY. Different species of *Pneumocystis* are widely distributed throughout the animal kingdom. However, pneumocystosis is not a zoonosis because the organisms are species specific. Therefore humans are infected only from other human reservoirs, not from other animals. It is thought that the disease is spread by respiratory droplet spray from an infected individual. The epidemiologic data suggest that the organism is quite infectious but of low pathogenicity. The disease occurs most commonly in patients who are agammaglobulinemic or are receiving corticosteroids or antimetabolites.

LIFE CYCLE OF THE ORGANISM. *Pneumocystis* occurs in two stages in the lung of the infected host. The first stage is referred to as the trophozoite. In the second stage the trophozoite evolves into a cyst, apparently by converting an inner membrane into a germinal surface from which oval bodies called sporozoites develop. Six to eight sporozoites develop within the cyst, which is surrounded by a thick, polysaccharide-containing wall. The cyst then ruptures, releasing sporozoites to initiate other cysts. After release the sporozoites are termed trophozoites. It is also believed that some form of division of trophozoites can lead to a trophozoite-trophozoite cycle. The trophozoite forms can be stained with Giemsa stain; however, the cyst requires staining with special stains for the cyst wall such as the Gram-Weigert and methenamine silver stains.

PATHOLOGY. When patients are immunosuppressed, the *Pneumocystis* organisms divide in the alveolar spaces of

---

*Parasitic Disease Drug Service, Center for Infectious Diseases, Centers for Disease Control, Atlanta, Ga. 30333. Telephone: days, 404-329-3670, nights and weekends, 404-329-3644.

the lung. This initiates an inflammatory response characterized by mononuclear cells, in some cases including plasma cells. The alveoli become filled with a proteinaceous material and clumps of *Pneumocystis* organisms. The interstitial spaces of the alveoli are filled with inflammatory cells. This process leads to decreased oxygen exchange and the signs and symptoms of respiratory insufficiency.

CLINICAL MANIFESTATIONS. The major symptoms of pneumocystosis are shortness of breath and a nonproductive cough. Fever may be present. In some patients the symptoms are insidious in onset, whereas in others they are more rapid. The patient may progress to a moribund state caused by the anoxia resulting from poor oxygen exchange. Physical examination indicates respiratory distress and cyanosis. The lungs may reveal diffuse scattered rales and rhonchi. Diagnostic laboratory tests detect abnormalities in blood gas exchange, and chest roentgenography shows diffuse alveolar and interstitial pneumonitis.

DIAGNOSIS. The diagnosis of pneumocystosis is made by biopsy of infected lung and appropriate staining for the cysts. In immunosuppressed patients this biopsy is necessary to exclude other causes of pulmonary inflammation. An immunofluorescent antibody test is also available; however, it should not be relied on for definite diagnosis, since it may not always be positive in immunosuppressed patients.

MANAGEMENT. Pneumocystosis is treated with the combination drug trimethoprim-sulfamethoxazole, 20 mg/kg/day of trimethoprim and 100 mg/kg/day of sulfamethoxazole in four divided doses. This therapy has reduced mortality from nearly 100% to below 50%. Supportive therapy for respiration is essential. In addition, reduction in doses of corticosteroids should be attempted. However, the symptoms may require a transient increase in the dose.

PREVENTION. Pneumocystosis can be prevented by interfering with the transmission of the organism among immunosuppressed patients. Therefore patients with the disease should be managed with respiratory precautions. In addition, crowding among patients who are potentially immunosuppressed, as in wards devoted to patients with malignancies or in clinics, should be avoided. Early detection, rapid treatment, and isolation of infected patients can also diminish the spread of the disease.

Prophylaxis of pneumocystosis has been achieved in selected high-risk populations (such as children with acute lymphocytic leukemia) by giving maintenance trimethoprim-sulfamethoxazole.

BABESIOSIS

Babesiosis is an acute febrile disease characterized by fever, myalgias, and hemolytic anemia. It is caused by the intraerythrocytic protozoan microbe *Babesia*, which is transmitted to humans by infected ticks.

EPIDEMIOLOGY. *Babesia* organisms are distributed throughout nature and infect numerous animals, including cattle, dogs, horses, and rodents. In the past, infection of humans was confined to those who were immunosuppressed, such as by splenectomy, and who had exposure to farm animals infected with *Babesia*. Recently, however, epidemics have occurred on the northeastern coast of the United States, where transmission of *B. microti* from rodents to humans has occurred.

PATHOLOGY. In human infection with *Babesia* the organism enters and destroys red blood cells, which leads to hemolytic anemia and obstruction of capillary blood flow with secondary tissue anoxia. The infection is usually controlled by immune responses in the normal host. However, infection with *B. microti* occurs in patients over the age of 45 years who are immunologically normal. Patients who have had splenectomy are susceptible to severe and progressive disease.

CLINICAL MANIFESTATIONS. The clinical manifestations of babesiosis include high fever, drenching sweats, and chills, as well as marked lethargy and muscle discomfort. The illness usually begins 1 to 6 weeks after the tick bite transmits the infection to the patient. The patient may appear very toxic. In addition, nausea, vomiting, and abdominal pain have been reported. Laboratory tests demonstrate thrombocytopenia, anemia, and proteinuria. Liver function may be slightly abnormal. The diagnosis of babesiosis is made by examination of a blood smear stained with Giemsa or Wright's stain, which demonstrates the intracellular *Babesia* organisms in 1% to 10% of red blood cells. The diagnosis can be confirmed by inoculating the patient's blood into animals and performing serologic tests for the presence of *Babesia*.

MANAGEMENT. The treatment is with pentamidine (available from the Centers for Disease Control*), 4mg/kg/day intramuscularly until symptomatic improvement occurs 5 to 10 days after the initiation of therapy. In some patients exchange transfusion has been necessary to reverse progressive deterioration. Some patients can be managed successfully with analgesics alone.

PREVENTION. The prevention of babesiosis is accomplished by avoiding tick-infested areas and using appropriate tick repellents. Splenectomized patients should not vacation or work during the summer months in areas of heavy tick infestation.

---

*Parasitic Disease Drug Service, Center for Infectious Diseases, Centers for Disease Control, Atlanta, Ga. 30333. Telephone: days, 404-329-3670, nights and weekends, 404-329-3644.

BIBLIOGRAPHY

Malaria

Hall, A.P.: The treatment of malaria, Br. Med. J. **1**:323, 1976.

Jeffrey, G.M.: Malaria control in the twentieth century, Am. J. Trop. Med. Hyg. **25**:361, 1976.

Maegraith, B., and Fletcher, A.: The pathogenesis of mammalian malaria, Adv. Parasitol. **10**:49, 1972.

Neva, F.A., and others: Malaria: host-defense mechanisms and complications, Ann. Intern. Med. **73**:295, 1970.

World Health Organization: Chemotherapy of malaria and resistance to antimalarials, WHO Tech. Rep. Ser. No. 529, p. 1, 1973.

Amebiasis

Adams, E.B., and MacLeod, I.N.: Invasive amebiasis. I. Amebic dysentery and its complications, Medicine **56**:315, 1977.

Adams, E.B., and MacLeod, I.N.: Invasive amebiasis. II. Amebic liver abscess and its complications, Medicine **56**:325, 1977.

Barbour, G.L., and Juniper, K., Jr.: A clinical comparison of amebic and pyogenic abscess of the liver in sixty-six patients, Am. J. Med. **53**:323, 1972.

Elsdon-Dew, R.: The epidemiology of amoebiasis, Adv. Parasitol. **1**:62, 1968.

Kean, B.H.: The treatment of amebiasis, J.A.M.A. **235**:501, 1976.

Powell, S.J., and Elsdon-Dew, R.: Some new nitroimidazole derivatives: clinical trials in amebic liver abscess, Am. J. Trop. Med. Hyg. **21**:518, 1972.

Nagington, J., and others: Amoebic infection of the eye, Lancet **2**:1537, 1974.

Neva, F.A.: Amebic meningoencephalitis: a new disease, N. Engl. J. Med. **282**:450, 1970.

Wang, S.S., and Feldman, H.A.: Isolation of *Hartmanella* species from human throats, N. Engl. J. Med. **277**:1174, 1967.

Giardiasis

Hoskins, L.C., and others: Clinical giardiasis and intestinal malabsorption, Gastroenterology **53**:265, 1967.

Knight, R.: Giardiasis, isosporiasis, and balantidiasis, Clin. Gastroenterol. **7**:31, 1978.

Yardley, J.H., Takano, J., and Hendrix, T.B.: Epithelial and other mucosal lesions of the jejunum in giardiasis: jejunal biopsy studies, Bull. Hopkins Hosp. **115**:389, 1964.

Toxoplasmosis

Beverley, J.K.A.: Toxoplasmosis, Br. Med. J. **2**:475, 1973.

Frenkel, J.K.: Toxoplasma in and around us, Bio. Science **26**:343, 1973.

Remington, J.S.: Toxoplasmosis: recent developments, Annu. Rev. Med. **21**:201, 1970.

Ruskin, J., and Remington, J.S.: Toxoplasmosis in the compromised host, Ann. Intern. Med. **84**:193, 1976.

Welch, P.C., and others: The serologic diagnosis of acute lymphadenopathic toxoplasmosis, J. Infect. Dis. **142**:256, 1980.

Trichomoniasis

Dykers, J.R.: Single dose metronidazole for trichomonal vaginitis: a follow-up, N. Engl. J. Med. **295**:395, 1976.

Trussell, R.E.: *Trichomonas vaginalis* and trichomoniasis, Springfield, Ill., 1947, Charles C Thomas, Publisher.

Trypanosomiasis

American trypanosomiasis research, PAHO Scientific Publication 318, 1975.

Andrade, Z., and Andrade, S.G.: Chagas' disease (American trypanosomiasis). In Marcial-Rojas, R.A., editor: Pathology of protozoal and helminthic diseases, Baltimore, 1971, The William & Wilkins Co.

Pneumocystosis

Burke, B.A., and Good, R.A.: *Pneumocystis carinii* infection, Medicine **52**:23, 1973.

Walzer, P.D., and others: *Pneumocystis carinii* pneumonia in the United States: epidemiologic, diagnostic, and clinical features, Ann. Intern. Med. **80**:83, 1974.

Babesiosis

Healy, G.R., Spielman, A., and Gleason, N.: Human babesiosis: reservoir of infection on Nantucket Island, Science **192**:479, 1976.

Ruebush, R.K., II, and others: Human babesiosis on Nantucket Island, Ann. Intern. Med. **86**:6, 1977.

Unit E • HELMINTHIC DISEASES

The parasitic worms that infect humans can be divided into the nematodes (roundworms), cestodes (tapeworms), and trematodes (flukes). All helminthic infections are capable of producing eosinophilia. The more invasive the worm or the stage of the disease, the higher the eosinophilia. Large worm burdens in close contact with tissue such as occur in strongyloidiasis, visceral larva migrans, and trichinosis are particularly prone to cause high eosinophilia. Eosinophilia caused by parasitic infection must be differentiated from that occurring in polyarteritis nodosa, eosinophilic leukemia, lymphoma, and allergic conditions.

55 • DISEASES CAUSED BY NEMATODES (ROUNDWORMS)

Donald Kaye

ENTEROBIASIS

Enterobius vermicularis (pinworm) is found worldwide in all socioeconomic groups and infects mainly children. The adult female is about 10 mm long and lives with the smaller male in the large bowel. At night the females migrate to the anus where they deposit eggs. The eggs and the migrating females cause pruritus ani. The eggs can be transmitted to the mouth via the hands or can contaminate the bedclothes and then be carried to the mouth on the hands. If swallowed, the eggs can develop into adult worms and perpetuate the infection. Appendicitis and vaginitis are occasional complications related to migration of the worms.

The diagnosis is best made by demonstrating eggs in the perianal area. On arising in the morning, before washing, the patient folds cellophane tape sticky side out over over the finger or a tongue depressor and applies it against the anal margins. The tape is then folded on itself or stuck on a slide and examined for the characteristic eggs, which a 50 μm long and flattened on one side. Adult worms may occasionally be found in the feces or in the perianal area. Examination of the stool for ova is not a reliable way to make the diagnosis of pinworm. It is common for more than one member of the family to be affected, and all should be examined. Eosinophilia is rare.

The therapy is with one 100-mg tablet of mebendazole, which should be repeated in 2 weeks. Pyrantel pamoate, 11 mg/kg body weight (maximum dose 1 g), can also be used and should be repeated in 2 weeks. All bedclothes and undergarments should be cleaned during the 2 weeks between treatments.

TRICHURIASIS

Trichuris trichura (whipworm) is found all over the world but most frequently in the tropics. The worms are 30 to 50 mm long with a thin anterior (the whip) buried in the mucosa of the colon and a thicker posterior (the whip handle) projecting into the colon. Eggs passed in the feces become infective after 3 weeks in the soil and are ingested following contamination of food and water. Adult worms develop and survive in the large bowel for at least 3 years.

Although the vast majority of patients are asymptomatic, heavy worm loads may cause colic, diarrhea, bleeding, and iron deficiency anemia. Large rectal worm loads can cause rectal prolapse (coconut cake rectum). Migrating worms can result in appendicitis. Eosinophilia is mild if present.

The diagnosis is made by finding the characteristic eggs, which are 50 μm long with bipolar plugs, in the feces. The treatment is with mebendazole, 100 mg twice a day for 3 days. Prevention depends on sanitary disposal of human feces and avoidance of fecal contamination of food.

ASCARIASIS

Ascaris lumbricoides is found worldwide but most often in the tropics. The adult is 15 to 30 cm long and lives in the small intestine. The worms stay in place by bridging themselves across the lumen of the gut. The life span of *Ascaris* is 1 to 2 years.

Eggs passed in the feces become infective after about 10 days. After ingestion the eggs hatch in the small intestine, and larvae penetrate the intestinal mucosa. They are borne in the lymphatic system and bloodstream to the lung where they rupture into the airways, are carried up the respiratory passages via ciliated epithelium, and are reswallowed. The adult worms then develop in the small intestine.

Light infections are usually asymptomatic. During the pulmonary phase of larval migration, fever, cough, bronchospasm, and hemoptysis may occur. There may be peripheral and sputum eosinophilia. Intestinal infection with the large, muscular worms may result in colic, perforation with peritonitis, obstructive (from large masses of worms) or appendicitis, bile duct obstruction, or pancreatic duct obstruction (from migration of the worms). Worms may be vomited up and aspirated.

The diagnosis is made by finding the characteristic eggs, which are rough and 50 μm long, in the feces. The worms may be seen after a barium meal, since barium appears in the *Ascaris* intestine.

The therapy is with mebendazole, 100 mg twice a day for 3 days, or pyrantel pamoate, 11 mg/kg body weight in one dose (maximum dose 1 g). Prevention depends on sanitary disposal of human feces and avoidance of fecal contamination of food.

VISCERAL LARVA MIGRANS

Visceral larva migrans, an infection primarily of children, results from human infection with the dog or cat *Ascaris* and is found all over the world. *Toxocara canis* (dog *Ascaris*) and *T. cati* (cat *Ascaris*) eggs become infective 2 weeks after being passed in the feces of the host animal (usually a puppy). If ingested by humans, larvae penetrate the wall of the intestine as in *A. lumbricoides* infection. However, the cycle is not completed, and the larvae migrate to the liver and other organs such as the eye, where they become trapped.

The symptoms are fever and high eosinophilia (50% or more). Tender hepatomegaly, endophthalmitis, pneumonitis, cerebritis, myositis, and other manifestations of local organ involvement can result. Symptoms can persist for over a year.

Isoagglutinin titers (anti-A and anti-B) are usually elevated in visceral larva migrans as are other antibody titers (for example, indirect hemagglutination or precipitins against the worm), but these are nonspecific. The diagnosis may be suggested by serologic tests, but biopsy of an affected organ showing larvae is the only definitive method of diagnosis.

Diethylcarbamazine, thiabendazole, and steroids have all been used in therapy. Thiabendazole, 50 mg/kg/day for 1 to 2 weeks, is probably the treatment of choice. In life-threatening infections 20 to 40 mg of prednisone daily is added. Prevention depends on worming pets and teaching children to wash their hands before putting them in their mouths.

ANISAKIASIS

Anisakiasis is caused by larvae of *Anisakis marina,* an ascarid of sea mammals (porpoises, dolphins, seals, and whales). The disease occurs in humans when the 2- to 4-cm-long larval form is ingested while eating raw or pickled squid, cod, salmon, or most often herring. The larvae may be vomited up, or they can burrow into the mucosa of the stomach or intestine and produce eosinophilic granulomatous tumors. The lesion can be mistaken for carcinoma or inflammatory bowel disease. The larvae can also penetrate the bowel wall and cause lesions in other organs.

There may be an acute syndrome (most common in Japan) in which epigastric pain and vomiting occur within a few hours of ingesting the larvae and are due to larvae penetrating the wall of the stomach. In Europe the small intestine is most often involved and there may be an acute abdominal condition with fever, pain, and tenderness, requiring surgery. This is usually more delayed and occurs 1 week or longer after the larvae have been ingested.

Eosinophilia may or may not occur. The diagnosis can be made only by seeing larvae through an endoscope or by histologic means in tissue. Therapy is conservative unless surgery for intestinal perforation or obstruction becomes necessary. The larvae can be killed by cooking fish or storing it at $-4°$ F $(-20°$ C) for 24 hours.

HOOKWORM DISEASE

Ancylostoma duodenale and *Necator americanus* are the two hookworms that infect humans. They are found all over the world, mainly in warm climates. The worms are about 1 cm long and live in the small intestine where they attach and suck blood.

The eggs are passed in the feces and hatch into rhabditi-form larvae that molt into filariform larvae. Filariform larvae can survive in warm soil for months and can rapidly penetrate intact skin. After they penetrate the skin, the cycle is much like that of *A. lumbricoides.* Larvae travel in the lymphatic system and the bloodstream to the lungs where they break out into the airways. They are carried up the trachea by ciliated epithelium, are swallowed, and develop into adults in the small intestine.

Light infection is asymptomatic. A pruritic rash may develop at the site of entry of the larva. As with *A. lumbricoides* infection, eosinophilia and pulmonary symptoms may occur during the pulmonary phase. With a heavy worm load, iron deficiency anemia and associated symptoms of anemia may develop.

The diagnosis is made by demonstrating characterstic eggs in the stool; they are 60 μm by 40 μm and have a clear shell.

Mebendazole, 100 mg twice a day for 3 days, or pyrantel pamoate, 11 mg/kg body weight in one dose (maximum dose 1 g), is the treatment of choice. The anemia should be treated with ferrous sulfate. Prevention depends on sanitary disposal of human feces and wearing of shoes.

CUTANEOUS LARVA MIGRANS

The usual cause of cutaneous larva migrans (creeping eruption) is *Ancylostoma braziliense,* a hookworm of dogs and cats. The disease is found in warm climates (including the southern United States) where the soil supports development of the larvae.

The larvae of *A. braziliense* develop in soil and penetrate the skin in a fashion similar to hookworms. However, the cycle is not completed, and the larvae migrate in the skin at a speed of 1 to 2 cm per day. They produce an erythematous, serpiginous, intensely pruritic burrow in the skin. The burrowing can continue for up to a year.

The treatment is with thiabendazole, 25 mg/kg body weight twice a day for 2 days. Wearing of shoes helps prevent the infection.

STRONGYLOIDIASIS

Strongyloides stercoralis is about 2 mm long and lives in the mucosa of the small intestine. It is found worldwide but is most common in tropical climates.

The eggs produced by the worms hatch into larvae in the intestine and can (1) invade the bowel mucosa directly; (2) invade soiled perianal skin after defecation; or (3) invade skin that contacts larvae deposited in the soil. A free-living form that develops in the soil can keep soil infected for long periods of time.

After invasion of the skin or mucosa, the cycle is similar to the *Ascaris* and hookworm cycles. Larvae are carried to the lungs and up the airways. They are then swallowed and develop in the small intestine, where they burrow into the mucosa.

A pruritic, urticarial rash may occur at the site of invasion (often on the buttocks). The pulmonary phase may be associated with cough, hemoptysis, pneumonia, or bronchospasm. The infection is usually asymptomatic, but because of the possibility of unchecked autoinfection, the potential for lethal overwhelming infection exists. The potentially lethal hyperinfective syndrome tends to occur in patients who are debilitated or receiving corticosteroids or immunosuppressive agents.

The hyperinfective syndrome may result in intensely inflamed bowel mucosa, intestinal hemorrhage, and malabsorption. Larvae become trapped in the liver, lungs, and other organs. *Escherichia coli* bacteremia may occur because of bowel ulceration.

Abdominal pain, tenderness, diarrhea, and vomiting occur with marked intestinal involvement. With the hyperinfective syndrome, marked eosinophilia is usually present and symptoms can result from multiple-organ involvement. Bacterial infection frequently contributes to death. Unexplained eosinophilia should suggest the possibility of strongyloidiasis. On the other hand, eosinophilia may not occur even with heavy infections in immunosuppressed patients. The diagnosis is made by finding larvae in fresh stool or a duodenal aspirate. A serologic test may be helpful in making the diagnosis.

All patients with *S. stercoralis* infection should be treated with thiabendazole, 25 mg/kg body weight twice daily for 3 days. Prevention depends on sanitary disposal of human feces and wearing of shoes.

TRICHINOSIS

Trichinosis is found all over the world among meat-eating populations. *Trichinella spiralis* infection is acquired when infected meat of a carnivorous animal (such as a pig or bear) is ingested. The larvae develop into adults within a week in the small intestine. The adult females release larvae for 4 to 8 weeks. The larvae penetrate the mucosa and are carried to organs all over the body. They encyst in striated muscle where they persist. In other organs such as the heart, brain, and eye the larvae degenerate, provoking an inflammatory reaction such as myocarditis, cerebritis, or retinitis.

Many patients with trichinosis are asymptomatic. With heavy infection there may be mild intestinal symptoms during the first week while the adult worms develop. Subsequently there are fever, high eosinophilia (over 50%), muscle pain, and periorbital edema lasting 4 to 8 weeks. Myocarditis may cause heart failure, and cerebritis may lead to coma. Death may result.

The diagnosis of trichinosis should be suspected when there is high eosinophilia. Muscle pain and tenderness with elevated serum muscle enzymes in a patient with eosinophilia are suggestive. Although serologic tests may be helpful, a muscle biopsy demonstrating larvae in the deltoid or gastrocnemius muscle is the preferred diagnostic test.

Severe infection should be treated with corticosteroids and thiabendazole, 25 mg/kg body weight twice daily for 5 days. Prevention depends on adequately cooking the meat of pigs and other carnivorous animals.

BANCROFTIAN AND MALAYAN FILARIASIS

Wuchereria bancrofti and *Brugia malayi* are filariae found in Africa, Asia, and South America. The adult worms are 5 to 10 cm long and live for many years in the lymphatic system (often in the inguinal region). The females release microfilariae (larval forms) found in the peripheral circulation, often only at night. The infection is acquired by the bite of a mosquito, which injects larval forms. The mosquito becomes infected by aspirating microfilariae when drinking a blood meal.

Light infections are usually asymptomatic. Inflammation and fibrosis in the lymphatic system may lead to lymphadenopathy, lymphatic obstruction, and edema.

Rarely, marked edema of the lower extremities, scrotum, or arms may occur. The end result may be gigantic, deformed, hyperkeratotic limbs (elephantiasis). Lymphatic obstruction may result in chyluria from either the kidneys or the urinary bladder. Streptococcal cellulitis is common in edematous areas and may make the edema worse by damaging the lymphatic system.

The diagnosis is made by observing microfilariae on a blood smear (usually at night). Microfilariae are usually absent in late stages of the disease. Eosinophilia is generally low grade or absent. A positive complement-fixing antibody test indicates only infection with one of the filarial group but is suggestive of *W. bancrofti* or *B. malayi* infection in a patient with unexplained edema.

Lymphangiograms demonstrate the extent of lymphatic obstruction, and roentgenograms may reveal dead calcified worms. Involved lymph nodes should not be resected, since this may further compromise lymphatic drainage.

The treatment of choice is diethylcarbamazine, 6 mg/kg body weight orally in three divided doses (after meals) each day for 14 days.

BIBLIOGRAPHY

Brown, H.W.: Basic clinical parasitology, ed. 4, New York, 1975, Appleton-Century-Crofts.
Drugs for parasitic infections, Med. Lett. Drugs Ther. 20:17, 1978.
Marsden, P.D.: Other nematodes, Clin. Gastroenterol. 7:219, 1978.
Neva, F.A.: Parasitic diseases of the gastrointestinal tract in the United States, D.M. 18:1, 1972.

56 • DISEASES CAUSED BY CESTODES (TAPEWORMS)

Jaime Carrizosa

The cestodes are flatworms that in their adult stage live in the gastrointestinal tract of vertebrates. The infected vertebrate becomes the definitive host of the parasite. The adult tapeworm is composed of a scolex or head that possesses organs that allow attachment to the intestinal mucosa; the neck; and the strobila composed of many segments or proglottids, each containing one or more sets of reproductive organs. A proglottid can copulate with itself or with other proglottids of the same or other worms. After fertilization the gravid proglottid, full of eggs, reaches the end of the strobila, detaches, and passes into the feces or disintegrates, releasing eggs that may be visualized in the stool. When eggs are ingested by an intermediate host, they hatch and larvae are released. The larva penetrates the gut wall and develops into the cysticercus, which is the head of the future tapeworm in a cyst. Development of the larva varies in the different species, and this leads to different clinical syndromes. Ingestion of larvae in uncooked meat results in digestion of the cyst wall, release of the head, and maturation into an adult worm. The ingestion of eggs leads to the development of cysticercosis.

TAENIASIS SAGINATA

Infection with *Taenia saginata,* the beef tapeworm, is acquired by the ingestion of cysticercus forms in poorly cooked or raw beef. Humans are the definitive hosts of the worm. The worm matures in about 2 months, reaching lengths of 5 to 10 m with over 1000 proglottids. The scolex is characterized by the presence of four suckers and has no hooklets. Proglottids, which can be passed intact, contain over 12 uterine branches. This distinguishes them from the proglottids of *T. solium,* the pork tapeworm. Eggs found in the stool have a thick, brown, radially striated shell and contain a full embryo. When the eggs are ingested by cattle or other herbivores, the embryo released in the intestine traverses the intestinal wall and is carried by the circulation into the muscles of the limbs, diaphragm, and tongue. In striated muscles the embryo develops into a cysticercus that remains viable for 1 to 3 years.

The infection is found all over the world. However, it is most frequent in the Middle East, Kenya, Ethiopia, and Yugoslavia. The clinical manifestations are mild, nonspecific abdominal pain and diarrhea. Mild eosinophilia may be present. There may be passage of motile proglottids through the anal sphincter. The diagnosis of *T. saginata* infection is made by identification of the proglottids or the eggs in the stool. Thorough cooking of beef prevents the infection.

TAENIASIS SOLIUM

Infection with *Taenia solium,* the pork tapeworm, is acquired by ingestion of pork containing cysticercus forms. As with *T. saginata,* humans are the definitive hosts of the worm. However, unlike *T. saginata,* cysticercosis, the intermediate form of the infection, can also develop in humans.

After ingestion the cysticercus is digested and the worm is released in the small bowel, where it establishes habitat and matures to a full size of 2 to 4 m. *T. solium* is differentiated from *T. saginata* by the presence of four suckers and two rows of hooklets on the scolex and fewer than 12 uterine branches in the gravid proglottid. The eggs of *T. solium* and *T. saginata* are indistinguishable.

The clinical manifestations of *T. solium* infection are similar to those of *T. saginata* infection. The diagnosis is made by examining the feces for the proglottids and eggs of *T. solium.* When the scolex is available, the diagnosis is more reliable. Mild eosinophilia may be seen in both *T. saginata* and *T. solium* infection. Thorough cooking of pork prevents the infection.

Human cysticercosis

Human infection caused by the ingestion of eggs of *T. solium* is known as cysticercosis. After ingestion the larva penetrates the intestinal wall and invades the tissues. Commonly involved organs are the subcutaneous tissue, central nervous system, muscle, heart, liver, and lung. Infection of the brain is associated with headaches, signs of increased intracranial pressure, and seizures. The diagnosis of cysticercosis is based on the identification of multiple space-occupying lesions by electroencephalography, computed tomography, arteriography, and simple skull films, since the cysticercus calcifies after its death. However, the diagnosis is made frequently by identification of the cyst at surgery. A serologic test that detects the presence of antibodies to the cysticercus is valuable in confirming the diagnosis.

The treatment of cysticercosis is usually surgical. Symptomatic treatment consists of antiepileptic drugs and steroids to reduce inflammation and edema. Mebendazole in very large doses has been shown to kill the larvae in vitro, but its effectiveness in vivo has not been established and may be limited, since the parasite is not usually viable when the manifestations appear.

DIPHYLLOBOTHRIASIS

Infection with *Diphyllobothrium latum,* the fish tapeworm, is acquired by eating raw or undercooked fish. Humans are the definitive hosts of the tapeworm, but other fish-eating animals also serve as final hosts. The adult worm is the largest tapeworm, reaching lengths of up to 10 to 15 m. Eggs released from an infected host reach the water, embryonate, and release a ciliated larva (coracidium). The coracidium, when eaten by a freshwater flea, develops into a procercoid. In turn, when the flea is eaten by a freshwater fish, the procercoid further develops into a plerocercoid. When infected raw fish is eaten by a human or a fish-eating mammal, the plerocercoid develops into an adult worm. The infection is common in the Scandinavian countries, the Baltic Sea area, Canada, Alaska, the northern United States, and Florida. The clinical manifestations of the disease are minimal, but complications of the infection produce important symptoms. The tapeworm splits vitamin B_{12} from its complex with intrinsic factor and utilizes it. The result may be a vitamin B_{12} deficiency with megaloblastic anemia and associated neurologic symptoms.

The diagnosis of *D. latum* infection is made by the identification of the eggs in the stool. The eggs, usually found in large numbers, are yellowish and operculated. The infection is prevented by thorough cooking of fresh fish; freezing for more than 24 hours also kills the larvae.

TREATMENT OF TAENIA SAGINATA, TAENIA SOLIUM, AND DIPHYLLOBOTHRIUM LATUM INFECTION

Niclosamide (available from the Centers for Disease Control*) is the drug of choice in the treatment of *T. saginata, T. solium,* and *D. latum* infections. One oral dose of 2 g (four tablets) kills the worm on contact; during expulsion the worm is digested, and it is not possible to identify it in the stool. The stool should be examined at 3 and 6 months to verify the effectiveness of the treatment. Quinacrine (Atabrine) and paromomycin (Humatin) have been used as alternative therapies.

ECHINOCOCCOSIS (HYDATID DISEASE)

Echinococcosis is an infection produced by the larvae of *Echinococcus granulosus* or *E. multilocularis,* tapeworms that have as definitive hosts the dog and other canines such as the wolf, the fox, and the jackal. Humans and other mammals such as sheep and cattle serve as intermediate hosts. When eggs of *Echinococcus* are ingested, they hatch and release embryos that penetrate the small bowel wall and enter the portal circulation. They lodge primarily in the liver and lung but may reach other organs such as the brain, kidney, or bone. By a very slow process of growth, the larva (oncosphere) develops into a cystic structure that can reach the size of a human head and is lined by an outer hard layer and an inner germinal layer. The latter gives origin to the daughter cysts, each filled with scolices, that produce infection when eaten by the definitive host. Residua from the cyst layers and released scolices from cyst sediment are known as hydatid sand.

Hydatid disease can occur anywhere but is seen more frequently in countries with predominant sheep- and cattle-raising economies such as Australia, New Zealand, Argentina, and Wales. Most of the infections diagnosed in the United States have been contracted outside the country.

The clinical manifestations of the infection result from progressive enlargement of the hydatid cyst, and many cases are diagnosed during routine examinations of asymptomatic individuals. The most common location of hydatid cysts is the right lobe of the liver. The enlarging cyst causes diffuse pain, cholestasis, and atrophy of the adjacent tissues. Occasionally the cyst ruptures, causing acute complications. Rupture or just leakage of the fluid may cause anaphylactic reactions and seeding of the peritoneal cavity with formation of new cysts; moreover, the cysts may become secondarily infected and produce a liver or lung abscess. Rupture of a lung cyst may cause chest pain, bronchospasm, and hemoptysis. Rupture into the biliary tract may resemble acute cholecystitis. Hydatid cysts of the brain present symptoms of space-occupying lesions, those in the kidney cause hematuria and flank pain, and those in bone result in a destructive process with the development of a pathologic fracture. The diagnosis is established by the demonstration of the cysts with ultrasonic scanning, radioisotope scanning, and arteriography. On roentgenograms of the abdomen, the cysts may show a small rim of calcification, which suggests the diagnosis. Several serologic tests are available to detect antibodies against the *Echinococcus*. The indirect hemagglutination test and the bentonite flocculation test are frequently used. Casoni's test, a skin test that uses cyst fluid, is usually positive in cases of echinococcosis, but it has not been standardized and thus is unreliable. Eosinophilia may occur.

Surgery with complete removal of the intact cyst is the preferred treatment. When the cyst cannot be removed marsupialization and sterilization of the cyst with a solution of 10% formalin, 1% iodine, or hypertonic (30%) saline should be attempted. Aspiration of the cyst should never be attempted because of the danger of rupture and spillage of the cyst fluid. A new method of treatment using high doses of mebendazole has been tried in patients in whom surgery cannot be performed. Although therapeutic trials have shown good results, more information is necessary before the treatment is accepted. High doses of the drug may cause bone marrow depression.

The disease can be prevented by avoiding contamination with feces of infected animals and by proper disposal of organs containing cysts from infected sheep and cattle to prevent the disease in the definitive hosts.

BIBLIOGRAPHY

Jones, T.C.: Cestodes, Clin. Gastroenterol. 7:105, 1978.
Katz, A.M., and Pan, C.: *Echinococcus* disease in the United States, Am. J. Med. 25:759, 1958.
Most, H.: Drug therapy: common parasitic infections of man, N. Engl. J. Med. 287:495, 1972.
Pawlowski, Z., and Schultz, M.E.: Taeniasis and cysticercosis *(Taenia saginata),* Adv. Parasitol. 10:296, 1972.
Schmidt, G.D., and Roberts, L.S.: Foundations of parasitology, St. Louis, 1977, The C.V. Mosby Co.
Williams, J.F., and others: Current prevalence and distribution of hydatidosis with special reference to the Americas, Am. J. Trop. Med. Hyg. 20:224, 1971.

57 • DISEASES CAUSED BY TREMATODES (FLUKES)

Jaime Carrizosa

SCHISTOSOMIASIS (BILHARZIASIS)

Schistosomiasis is a chronic infection caused by three different trematodes (flukes), *Schistosoma mansoni, S. haematobium,* and *S. japonicum.* The disease affects peo-

---

*Parasitic Disease Drug Service, Center for Infectious Diseases, Centers for Disease Control, Atlanta, Ga. 30333. Telephone: days, 404-329-3670, nights and weekends, 404-329-3644.

ple living in tropical and subtropical areas of the world. The infection is acquired by repeated immersion in fresh water contaminated with cercariae, the infecting forms of the schistosome, which penetrate the skin, develop into adult worms in the circulatory system, and settle into a permanent habitat in the veins of the intestine or the urinary bladder. The disease is produced by the severe inflammatory reaction resulting from the presence of ova released by mature parasites into the adjacent tissues or the bloodstream. The characteristics of schistosomiasis depend on the type of infecting schistosome, the specific organ involved, the degree of infestation, and the duration of the illness.

ETIOLOGY. As just discussed, three species of schistosomes are known to parasitize humans: *S. mansoni, S. haematobium,* and *S. japonicum.* The males are shorter than the females and have a ventral longitudinal groove, the gynecophoral canal, where the female resides. The worms absorb metabolites through the intestine and integument and have a rapid metabolic rate dependent on energy obtained from the anaerobic oxidation of carbohydrates. The adult worms live in the veins that drain organs of the abdominal cavity. Each species has specific preferences: *S. haematobium* lives in the veins of the urinary bladder plexus, *S. mansoni* lives in the veins of the colon, and *S. japonicum* lives primarily in the veins of the small intestine. The eggs are distinctive for each species. The egg of *S. haematobium* is ellipsoidal with a terminal spine, the egg of *S. mansoni* is ellipsoidal but has a lateral spine, and the egg of *S. japonicum* is oval, almost spherical, with only a rudimentary spine. Once the eggs are laid, some traverse the venule wall and pass through the tissues, producing significant inflammatory reaction, until they reach the bladder or gut lumen and are excreted from the body in the urine or stool. Many eggs never reach the lumen but remain in the tissues or bloodstream and are carried to other organs such as the liver or lungs.

The life cycle of the schistosome begins when the eggs hatch following exposure to fresh water. The miracidium develops and emerges from the egg to seek its snail host. It then penetrates the snail and develops into a sporocyst. Two weeks later the mother sporocyst gives birth to daughter sporocysts that migrate to the organs of the snail. In 2 to 3 weeks the snail begins to shed fork-tailed cercariae into the water where they remain alive for 1 to 3 days but lose their infectivity by 20 hours. When they come in contact with the skin of a prospective host, they attach to and penetrate the epidermis, losing their tails in the process. Within 24 hours after penetration, the altered cercariae, now called schistosomula, enter the peripheral circulation and reach the pulmonary vessels, where they remain several days before they enter the systemic circulation and are carried into the liver. After reaching maturity in the liver, the worms migrate to their final organ of infestation where they copulate and begin producing eggs, thus completing the life cycle. The life span of a schistosome is 5 to 10 years.

EPIDEMIOLOGY. It is estimated that schistosomiasis affects over 200 million people in tropical and subtropical areas of the world. The disease is not found in the continental United States owing to the lack of the appropriate snail, but it is endemic in Puerto Rico.

In the Western Hemisphere infection is caused by species of *S. mansoni,* most probably brought to America by African slaves. The infection is found in Brazil, Venzuela, Surinam, and some Caribbean islands (Dominican Republic, Martinique, St. Lucia, Antigua, Guadeloupe, and Puerto Rico). Infection with both *S. mansoni* and *S. haematobium* is widespread in Africa. *S. japonicum* is endemic in the Orient (Japan, China, the Philippines, and Southeast Asia).

The single most important epidemiologic factor in schistosomiasis is the deposition of human waste in water containing the appropriate intermediate snail host. The species of snail prevalent in the area will determine the specific infecting schistosome. The disease frequently occurs in children who bathe, wade, or play in water contaminated with cercariae. Reinfection occurs every time there is contact with contaminated water. The best measures for the control of schistosomiasis are based on the proper disposal of excreta, appropriate provision of water supplies, education of the population concerning the methods of acquisition of the infection, and availability of treatment programs. Programs for extermination of the intermediary hosts (snails) have not been highly successful.

PATHOGENESIS AND CLINICAL MANIFESTATIONS. The characteristics of schistosomiasis depend on the degree of infection and the species of schistosome. Initial manifestations of the infection occur within 1 day following the penetration of the cercariae and are characterized by a papular, pruritic rash known as swimmers' itch. The rash develops as a result of the death of some of the cercariae following penetration of the skin. All cercariae of schistosomes nonpathogenic to humans die after penetration, causing the most severe rashes. The dermatitis appears to be a sensitization phenomenon characterized by infiltration of the dermis and epidermis with round cells as seen in delayed hypersensitivity reactions.

Katayama fever. Katayama fever is a syndrome of schistosomiasis characterized by fever, chills, profuse diaphoresis, cough, wheezing, headache, and diarrhea and associated with hepatosplenomegaly, lymphadenopathy, and urticaria. The clinical picture is most frequently seen 20 to 60 days after infection with *S. japonicum,* but it can occur with very heavy infestations of *S. mansoni.* The syndrome may last up to 12 weeks, and occasional deaths have been reported. The symptoms appear to be caused by a severe hypersensitivity reaction to a large antigenic load of ova and parasites.

Intermediate phase of schistosomiasis. The changes seen

in the intermediate phase of the disease result from the deposition of a large number of eggs in the venules of the infected organs. Eggs may be finally excreted in the stool or urine, may be carried in the bloodstream to the liver or lungs, or may remain in the adjacent tissues. At this stage the infection is characterized by a severe tissue reaction to the deposited eggs. Manifestations of bowel invasion range from mild diarrhea and congestion to fibrosis, ulceration, bleeding, or formation of inflammatory polyps. Manifestations of bladder invasion are ulceration, fibrosis, hematuria, polyps, and calcification.

Hepatosplenic schistosomiasis. Deposition of eggs in the liver initiates a granulomatous reaction that results in intrahepatic blocking of portal blood flow with subsequent development of portal hypertension, usually over a period of many years. The clinical manifestations are hepatosplenomegaly, development of collateral circulation, esophageal varices, and hematemesis. Patients with hepatic schistosomiasis have relatively normal liver function, and hepatic insufficiency is rarely seen. Bacteremia caused by *Salmonella* and *Escherichia coli* is a frequent complication of hepatic schistosomiasis. Other manifestations of the disease are anemia, moderate eosinophilia, and pancytopenia resulting from hypersplenism.

Pulmonary schistosomiasis. Schistosomal eggs reach the pulmonary capillaries through collateral veins developed because of portal hypertension or by passage of eggs from the vesical plexus into the inferior vena cava. The presence of eggs in the pulmonary capillaries produces marked inflammation and fibrosis with development of pulmonary hypertension and cor pulmonale.

Urinary tract schistosomiasis. Urinary tract involvement in *S. haematobium* infection is initially manifested by hematuria and ureteral obstruction caused by granuloma formation. Bladder involvement results in fibrosis and calcification. Obstructive uropathy and renal insufficiency may complicate the infection. In countries with a high prevalence or urinary schistosomiasis, a significant association with bladder carcinoma and urinary carriage of *Salmonella* has been noted.

Central nervous system schistosomiasis. Schistosomal eggs carried into the central nervous system can result in seizure activity and in focal damage suggestive of space-occupying lesions. Spinal cord lesions such as transverse myelitis have been reported in cases of *S. mansoni* and *S. haematobium* infection.

DIAGNOSIS AND LABORATORY FINDINGS. The diagnosis of schistosomiasis is established by the presence of ova in the stool, urine, or biopsy specimens. Concentration techniques may be necessary to establish the presence of eggs in the stool. The Kato thick smear provides a method to estimate egg output and severity of the infection. Determination of eggs in urine specimens is made by examining the sediment in samples obtained at noon. Rectal biopsy is one of the preferred methods in cases of *S. mansoni* or *S. japonicum* infection. Several specimens are taken from the valves of Houston, pressed between glass slides, and examined for eggs under the microscope. Since dead eggs may persist in the tissues for prolonged periods of time, a hatching test performed by incubating eggs in water and observing them for the emergence of miracidia is necessary to rule out burned-out or successfully treated disease. Eosinophilia is characteristic of schistosomiasis, and its presence provides additional laboratory support.

Several serologic tests to detect antischistosomal antibodies (complement fixation, precipitin, indirect fluorescent antibody, and counter immunoelectrophoresis) are available but lack sensitivity and specificity. The intradermal skin test for schistosomiasis has epidemiologic value but should not be used as a diagnostic tool.

In cases of *S. mansoni* and *S. japonicum* infection, liver biopsy and roentgenographic evaluation of the gastrointestinal tract are helpful in determining the extent of the disease. In *S. haematobium* infection, cystoscopy and intravenous pyelogram may help confirm the diagnosis.

MANAGEMENT. Several factors should be taken into account when the treatment of a case of schistosomiasis is considered: (1) Schistosomal dermatitis is treated symptomatically. Specific treatment is not available. (2) In cases of light infection (egg counts of fewer than 50/g of stool) therapy is not required. Appropriate follow-up examination is necessary to verify the intensity of the infection. (3) In cases of heavy infection, schistosomicidal drugs are required. However, all available agents are highly toxic and require appropriate administration and close control. The most commonly used agents are the antimony compounds tartar emetic, stibocaptate (Astiban), and niridazole (Ambilhar).

Niridazole, 25 mg/kg/day orally in two divided doses for 7 days, or stibocaptate, 8 mg/kg intramuscularly once a week for 5 weeks, is preferred, and both drugs are available from the Centers for Disease Control.* If symptoms of liver or cerebral disease are present, stibocaptate should be used. Toxic manifestations of the antimony compounds are hepatitis, electrocardiographic changes suggestive of myocarditis, cardiac arrhythmias, and even sudden death. Niridazole should not be used in patients with hepatosplenomegaly and collateral circulation, since it predisposes them to a higher incidence of central nervous system complications. Niridazole also should not be used in patients wih a history of seizures.

Patients with severe hepatosplenic schistosomiasis have portal hypertension and frequently bleeding from esophageal varices. Surgical treatment is not recommended unless there are repeated episodes of bleeding because patients have good hepatic function and hepatic encephalopathy

---

*Parasitic Disease Drug Service, Center for Infectious Diseases, Centers for Disease Control, Atlanta, Ga. 30333. Telephone: days, 404-329-3670, nights and weekends, 404-329-3644.

rarely develops. If shunting becomes absolutely necessary, splenorenal shunt is preferred and antischistosomal treatment is recommended to prevent passage of the eggs into the caval circulation with seeding of the lungs and development of pulmonary fibrosis, hypertension, and cor pulmonale.

PROGNOSIS. Many patients with schistosomiasis are asymptomatic; only patients with heavy infections have symptoms and complications and may die of the disease. Treatment results in symptomatic improvement, prevention of organ damage, and perhaps even gradual regression of lesions. The overall prognosis of the disease is good.

BIBLIOGRAPHY

Clark, W.D., and others: Acute schistosomiasis mansoni in 10 boys: an outbreak in Caguas, Puerto Rico, Ann. Intern. Med. **73**:379, 1970.

Jones, E.A., and others: Massive infection with *Fasciola hepatica* in man, Am. J. Med. **63**:842, 1977.

Mahmoud, A.A.: Current concepts—schistosomiasis, N. Engl. J. Med. **297**:1329, 1977.

Prata, A.: Schistosomiasis mansoni, Clin. Gastroenterol. **7**:49, 1978.

Sadum, E.H., and Buck, A.A.: Paragonimiasis in South Korea: immunodiagnostic, epidemiologic, clinical, roentgenologic and therapeutic studies, Am. J. Trop. Med. Hyg. **9**:562, 1960.

Seah, S.K.K.: Digenetic trematodes. Clin. Gastroenterol. **7**:871, 1978.

Unit F • MISCELLANEOUS MICROBIAL DISEASES

58 • DISEASES OF PRESUMED MICROBIAL ORIGIN

Lyme disease

George A. Poporad and Donald Kaye

Lyme disease (named for Lyme, Connecticut) is a syndrome that includes a characteristic skin rash, monarticular or oligoarticular arthritis, and neurologic and cardiac abnormalities.

EPIDEMIOLOGY AND ETIOLOGY. Cases have been described along the northeast shore of the United States (Cape Cod, Rhode Island, Connecticut, Long Island), in the Midwest (Wisconsin), and in the West (California, Oregon). The origin of the disease remains uncertain, but there is evidence for transmission of a causative agent by a tick vector *(Ixodes dammini)*.

CLINICAL MANIFESTATIONS. Lyme disease typically occurs in summer or fall. Initially the patient has a characteristic skin lesion called erythema chronicum migrans, which begins as an erythematous papule and develops into an expanding, red, flat, annular lesion usually with partial central clearing. The lesion (occasionally multiple) is often on the proximal part of an extremity of on the trunk and may grow to be as large as 20 to 50 cm in diameter. It may itch or burn. Malaise, fatigue, fever, vomiting, headache, stiff neck, malar rash, sore throat, lymphadenopathy, and splenomegaly can occur with the rash or precede it by a few days. Some patients recall being bitten by a tick 4 days to 3 weeks before onset of the rash. Typically the rash lasts 1 to 5 weeks, but evanescent lesions may recur.

Arthritis may appear within days of the onset of the rash or in some instances more than 2 years later. Intermittent, recurrent attacks of arthritis in several large joints, particularly the knee, are characteristic. Occasionally chronic arthritis develops. Fever, myalgias, headache, stiff neck, and the rash may occur with or precede the attacks of arthritis.

A small percentage of patients may have neurologic abnormalities that appear while the rash is still present or 1 to 6 months later. The usual pattern is one of recurrent attacks of meningoencephalitis with superimposed cranial and peripheral radiculoneuropathy. The patient may have weeks of illness alternating with weeks of well-being. Neurologic abnormalities such as facial paralysis, oculomotor weakness, peripheral motor weakness, radicular pain, cerebellar ataxia, and chorea have been reported. Recovery generally occurs in 2 to 8 months.

Rarely, cardiac abnormalities may develop from 4 days to several months after the onset of erythema chronicum migrans. Most commonly these are fluctuating degrees of AV block, but ST-T wave changes or pericarditis may also occur.

LABORATORY FINDINGS. The white blood count may be slightly elevated with a mild left shift of the differential count. The erythrocyte sedimentation rate is usually elevated. Elevated levels of serum IgM and cryoglobulins are found in most patients with erythema chronicum migrans who later develop arthritis but rarely in those who do not. Patients with cardiac involvement may have an elevated serum glutamic-oxaloacetic transaminase. A spinal fluid lymphocytic pleocytosis of up to 450 cells/mm^3 with elevated protein and normal glucose may occur in patients with neurologic involvement. Patients with arthritis may have a joint fluid white cell count of 20,000 to 75,000/mm^3, mainly granulocytes.

DIAGNOSIS. Skin, joint, and presumably nervous system or cardiac involvement may occur separately. Without the classic rash or a history of tick bite, the diagnosis of Lyme disease is extremely difficult. The presence of elevated serum levels of IgM and cryoglobulins may be helpful. Onset in summer and occurrence in a geographic area where erythema chronicum migrans has been reported are important clues to the diagnosis.

MANAGEMENT. Oral administration of penicillin, 250,000 units four times a day, or tetracycline, 250 mg four times a day for 7 to 10 days, shortens the duration of the rash and associated symptoms. Although treatment also seems to prevent or attenuate arthritis, it appears to have no effect on the development of neurologic or cardiac disease.

The presence of cryoglobulins in the serum and immune complexes in serum and synovial fluid suggests that a host immune response plays a role in joint, cardiac, and nervous system manifestations. Prednisone, 20 mg/day for children and 40 to 60 mg/day for adults, is recommended for meningoencephalitis. Cardiac abnormalities may be treated with aspirin, prednisone, and/or a pacemaker depending on their severity. Joint manifestations respond to aspirin or, if necessary, prednisone.

BIBLIOGRAPHY

Reik, L., and others: Neurologic abnormalities of Lyme disease, Medicine **58**:281, 1979.

Steere, A.C., and others: Erythema chronicum migrans and Lyme arthritis: the enlarging clinical spectrum, Ann. Intern. Med. **86**:685, 1977.

Steere, A.C., and others: Antibiotic therapy in Lyme disease, Ann. Intern. Med. **93**:1, 1980.

Steere, A.C., and others: Lyme carditis: cardiac abnormalities of Lyme disease, Ann. Intern. Med. **93**:8, 1980.

Toxic shock syndrome

Jerome A. Boscia and **Donald Kaye**

Toxic shock syndrome (TSS) is a recently recognized, serious disease characterized by the sudden onset of high fever, vomiting, and diarrhea, followed by dehydration, hypotension, and in severe cases shock. These manifestations are accompanied by a diffuse, macular, erythematous rash that desquamates during the recovery phase, particularly on the palms and soles. Complications may include adult respiratory distress syndrome, acute renal failure, and disseminated intravascular coagulation, with mortality approximating 8%.

Approximately 95% of the cases occur in young women during a menstrual period, and there is a significant association between tampon use, especially continuous use throughout menstruation, and the development of the disease. *Staphylococcus aureus*, which has been cultured from the vaginas of about 7% of healthy menstruating women, has been isolated from the vaginas of 73% to 98% of menstruating women with TSS. In the rare cases in men and nonmenstruating women *S. aureus* has been cultured from skin (abscesses), bone (osteomyelitis), and lung (pneumonia and empyema). *S. aureus* has not been isolated from blood or unused tampons in patients with the disease. The clinical manifestations may be associated with a toxin produced by *S. aureus*, and tampons might introduce the organism into the vagina during insertion, favor the growth of the organism in the vagina, and/or facilitate production and absorption of toxin by the vagina.

Therapy for TSS includes aggressive hydration and supportive care. β-lactamase-resistant antistaphylococcal antibiotics do not appear to alter the disease but are indicated, since they seem to prevent recurrences, which occur in about 30% of untreated cases. It is recommended that women who have had the disease discontinue using tampons (at least until *S. aureus* has been eradicated from the vagina). Women in general can significantly reduce the small risk of acquiring the disease by eliminating tampon use or by using them intermittently during menstruation.

BIBLIOGRAPHY

Todd, J., and others: Toxic shock syndrome associated with phage-group 1 staphylococci, Lancet **2**:1116, 1978.

Toxic shock syndrome, M.M.W.R. **29**:229, 297, 441, 1980.

DENTAL CORRELATIONS

Adi Garfunkel, Jack Sobel, and **Louis F. Rose**

VIRAL INFECTION
Herpes simplex

Acute herpetic gingivostomatitis is a common primary infection with herpes simplex virus, usually type 1 but occasionally type 2. The renewed interest in this disease arises from the recognition that it attacks not only infants and young children but also adults in their second and third decades.

ORAL MANIFESTATIONS. The oral manifestations are dominated by small vesicles that rupture easily and lead to the formation of shallow ulcers with smooth margins surrounded by a red halo. The lesions occur on all areas of the mouth, with the most dramatic signs on the lips and gingivae. The lip ulcers, which penetrate into the subepithelium, induce bleeding with formation of crusts. The gingiva shows signs of acute inflammation due to the viral infection, which is further aggravated by accumulation of dental plaque, due to poor oral hygiene and the interruption of masticatory function. Superinfection by the normal oral flora may further complicate the picture. Ulcers develop on the gingival tissues and bleeding from the marginal gingiva is not uncommon. Severe pain with marked difficulty in chewing, talking, and swallowing is the chief complaint of patients with primary herpetic gingivostomatitis and as a direct result, saliva drooling is apparent. In infants lack of food and fluid ingestion may result in dehydration, requiring hospitalization and parenteral fluid administration. Swollen, tender regional lymph nodes are frequently observed. The ulcerations heal in approximately 14 days, although the gingival inflammation may take longer to resolve. Herpesvirus sialadenitis is rare although the virus has been cultured from saliva and gingival crevicular fluid.

A clue to the diagnosis may be rapidly obtained by cytologic examination of material from the base of the vesicle or ulcer, which shows multinucleated cells with nuclear inclusion bodies and ballooning of the nucleus. Definitive diagnosis is by isolation of the virus from the vesicular fluid and culture of the virus in tissue cell culture systems. Both vesicles and oral secretions yield positive cultures in the acute symptomatic phase and for several weeks after the acute disease. A fourfold rise in antibody titer comparing acute and convalescent sera points to a recent infection but is not helpful in the initial clinical presentation. When primary herpetic gingivostomatitis occurs during the first trimester of pregnancy, as a result of viremia, the herpes virus may cross the placental barrier and infect the fetus, resulting in severe congenital malformations. If the oral infection is diagnosed close to delivery, a pelvic examination is indicated and if vaginal or cervical involvement coexists a cesarean section must be considered. Both primary and reactivation herpetic oral lesions in immunocompromised hosts are characterized by their severity and intensity of local complications.

DENTAL MANAGEMENT. Treatment of acute herpetic gingivostomatitis is mainly supportive, in order to alleviate the pain and reduce the chance of secondary infection. Mouthrinses with a 2% lidocaine viscous solution are beneficial and facilitate drinking, eating of soft foods, and oral hygiene. A milder anesthetic action may be obtained by the use of a 5% aqueous diphenhydramine (Benadryl) solution. An ice cube containing 1 ml may be held in the mouth; it should not be swallowed but rather spit out as it melts. Abundant bicarbonate or saline solution mouthwashes will provide mechanical cleansing. Antibiotics are of no benefit. In severe cases, secondary monilial infection occurs and is treated with antimycotic agents such as nystatin suspension, 100,000 U/ml, or amphotericin B lozenges, four to six times a day.

Use of antiviral agents. Idoxuridine, Vidarabine, and vidarabine monophosphate have not shown convincing efficacy in treating oral lesions and are cytotoxic due to their indiscriminate action on normal as well as on herpes virus-infected cells.

A recently introduced agent, acyclovir, selectively inhibits the replication of virus without affecting noninfected cells. Acyclovir (ACV, 9-[2-Hydro-xyethoxymethyl] guanine, acycloguanosine) inhibits herpes simplex virus types 1 and 2, varicella-zoster virus, and cytomegalovirus in vitro. In its activated form, acyclovir blocks the replication of the virus by inhibiting viral DNA polymerase activity. Used as a 5% ointment for primary herpes genitalis, acyclovir has been shown to significantly reduce the duration of viral shedding and shorten the period of pain, discomfort, and healing. In spite of this encouraging information, acyclovir is not currently recommended for primary or recurrent herpetic stomatitis or labialis in normal hosts but should be considered for localized mucocutaneous manifestations in immunocompromised hosts.

RECURRENT HERPES SIMPLEX VIRUS INFECTION

Herpesvirus in a latent form may continuously infect sensory ganglia in patients who recover from the primary infection. Following infection in the oral and circumoral areas, the latent virus may be cultured from the trigeminal ganglia.

Recurrent herpes labialis (the common coldsore or fever blister) is not the only form of recurrent oral infection; it may also be present in an intraoral form. The latter develops as small but painful vesicles and ulcers on heavily keratinized mucosa. They appear in clusters, have regular borders, are shallow (intraepithelial vesicles), and are surrounded by an inflammatory halo. Intraoral herpesvirus infection has to be differentiated from recurrent aphthous ulcerations, a condition that is nonviral in origin.

Herpes simplex labialis develops on the vermilion border, which is considered a "locus minoris resistentiae." The lesions then spread to the adjacent skin and clusters of deep-seated vesicles form. The surrounding lip tissue is swollen as with an allergic reaction. An itching sensation generally precedes the appearance of the lesions, and experienced patients can easily predict a new attack. This endogenous infection is reactivated by stimuli such as fever, sunlight, stressful situations, hormonal imbalance, or surgical resection of the trigeminal ganglion in cases of trigeminal neuralgia.

In healthy people the treatment of recurrent herpes infections of the lip is palliative. In patients with debilitating diseases, more aggressive treatment measures are being sought.

Varicella-zoster virus infection

The primary infection causes varicella (chickenpox) chiefly in children, and reactivation of the virus results in herpes zoster (shingles) mainly in adults. Oral lesions occur in herpes zoster only when the trigeminal nerve is involved. The increased frequency of zoster virus infections in patients with malignant diseases and disease involving the immune system has been substantiated in clinical studies, particularly with regard to severity of the local manifestations and tendency to systemic dissemination.

The symptoms include severe pain, described as stabbing, burning, or aching. The pain may appear during the prodromal stage and persist during healing or even after the mucocutaneous lesions disappear. Persistent neuralgia is one of the severe sequelae of the disease. There are reports of tooth exfoliation and osteonecrosis of the jaw following herpes zoster infection, possibly secondary to avascular bone necrosis in patients with diminished local resistance. Treatment of oral lesions is usually symptomatic and is similar to that of herpes simplex virus infection.

Cytomegalovirus

The cytomegalovirus appears to have sialadenotropism, which for the most part remains asymptomatic. In addition to the systemic manifestations, inclusion bodies of cytomegalic disease are often found in the salivary glands. In adults, symptomatic disease is rare and usually affects the submandibular gland. In infants and children the parotid gland is most often affected. The developing sialadenitis resembles other virus-induced diseases of the salivary glands. However, the cytomegalovirus is excreted in saliva for weeks or months, resulting in environmental contamination.

When leukopenia and thrombocytopenia are present, the oral lesions are dominated by petechiae covering most of the mucosa. Oral involvement must be differentiated from that of infectious mononucleosis, although in contrast to Epstein-Barr virus infection pharyngitis and cervical lymphadenitis are uncommon.

There is no specific treatment for oral or salivary gland involvement in cytomegalovirus disease. Elective dental treatment should be postponed during the period the virus is present in the oral tissues and fluids.

Epstein-Barr virus (EBV)

Infectious mononucleosis is caused by the EBV and in this disease a variety of oral lesions may occur, depending on the severity of the disease. Petechiae and erythema may involve the oral mucosa, with a predilection for the palate. Ulcerations have been described in cases with a reduced polymorphonuclear leukocyte count. In infectious mononucleosis there may be extensive lymphocytic or monocytic infiltration of the stroma of salivary glands. Since EBV is found to be invariably present in a cell-free form in saliva but not in the cells of the oropharynx, it is suggested that the salivary glands are the site of EBV reproduction in the oropharynx.

Epstein-Barr virus is also linked with Burkitt's lymphoma, a tumor developing in young children and involving mainly the lower jaw adjacent to developing tooth buds. The jaw lesions are characteristic and may be the reason patients seek medical attention. The gingiva is heavily infiltrated with Burkitt's lymphoma cells, causing swelling, redness, pain, and spontaneous bleeding. Secondary infection with anaerobic organisms residing in the gingival sulcus produces necrotizing ulcerations with crater formation in the interdental papillae area.

The lymphomatous cell infiltration may involve the mental nerve leading to paresthesia of the lip and lack of signs of vitality in anterior lower teeth. Malignant cell infiltrates into the periodontal ligament cause a widening of this space and seem to be characteristic of the disease. Alveolar bone resorption with disappearance of the alveolar crests and furcation involvement further aggravates the picture.

Measles (rubeola)

Oral manifestations during the full-blown picture of the disease are characterized by stomatitis and exanthems localized to the buccal mucosa, pharynx, and tonsillar fauces. On the palate, the mucous glands are inflamed with pinpointed white orifices. Two to three days before the exanthem, Koplik's spots appear and are considered pathognomonic for measles. They have been described throughout the mouth but the buccal mucosal lesions predominate. Koplik's spots are small, bluish, and surrounded by an erythematous halo. At times they induce some discomfort accompanied by a burning sensation. It is unclear whether Koplik's spots represent sites of inflammation of the mucous glands only or in addition are the site of virus replication.

As in other stomatitides of viral origin, treatment is symptomatic.

Rubella (German measles)

Tooth defects ranging from enamel hypoplasia and pitting to total aplasia have been described in a high percentage of children whose mothers suffered from rubella during the first trimester of pregnancy. Retarded eruption may also be present. Oral abnormalities include cleft lip and palate.

The oral manifestations of rubella virus infection contracted in childhood or young adulthood include small red petechial spots on the soft palate.

Hand-foot-and-mouth disease

Coxsackievirus A16 (less commonly other strains) is the etiologic agent of a distinctive vesicular eruption known as hand-foot-and-mouth disease. The illness is mild and lasts for 1 week or less. Most children complain of sore throat or sore mouth and refuse to eat. Fever of 38° to 39° C lasts 1 to 2 days and is accompanied by vesicles in the oral cavity. These occur chiefly on the buccal mucosa and tongue. Several lesions may coalesce to form bullae that frequently ulcerate. Swelling of the lips and tongue is frequent. Clinically the lesions resemble those of herpes simplex, herpangina, and other coxsackievirus strains, but the characteristic exanthems on the hands and feet usually permit definitive diagnosis.

Cat-scratch disease

Children with cervical lymphadenopathy suspected of having cat-scratch disease are referred for dental examination in order to exclude oral infection as the reason for the lymph node involvement. Shklar described one patient with laboratory confirmation of cat-scratch disease in whom oral vesicular lesions appeared and ruptured to form ulcers.

Herpangina (Coxsackie A virus infection)

Herpangina, unlike herpesvirus oral infection, involves the posterior half of the mouth, pharynx, and tonsils. The gingivae, buccal mucosa, floor of the mouth, and lips are involved less frequently. The lesions consists of small vesicles surrounded by an erythematous area. Up to 20 vesicles are present. The vesicles rupture shortly after they are formed, leaving small ulcerated areas. The oral symptoms of herpangina tend to be milder than those of herpesvirus infection; however, the throat pain is quite severe. Lesions of herpangina in the pharynx and on the tongue make drinking, chewing, and talking difficult. Herpangina may occasionally be associated with bilateral parotitis.

Bacterial pharyngitis, acute herpetic gingivostomatitis, and aphthous stomatitis must be considered in the differential diagnosis. As with other viral diseases there is no specific therapy for herpangina. Symptomatic relief with anesthetic mouthwashes and/or analgesic medication is recommended.

Mumps

Parotid salivary gland swelling is the major sign of mumps or epidemic parotitis. Submandibular and sublingual glands may also become involved, either unilaterally or bilaterally. Parotid gland viral adenitis presents with swelling in the preauricular area extending down to the mandibular angle. When the patient is examined from behind, a characteristic rise of the earlobe is observed. The area is very tender to palpation and may be somewhat warm and reddened.

Submandibular gland swelling is observed parallel to the lower border of the mandibular body. Occasionally blockage of the secretion of the submandibular gland induces formation of a ranula (*rana,* frog) on the floor of the mouth. This distention of the salivary gland duct is produced by the accumulation of saliva. The tongue may be elevated. Considerable pain and discomfort are present.

Spontaneous drainage is at times achieved with fistula formation. Because of the severe inflammatory process the margins of the salivary duct fistula become indurated and raised with apparent undermined borders, a picture that may resemble malignancy. When parotitis is present, Stenson's duct orifice is often inflamed and accompanied by impaired saliva secretion and variable xerostomia. In most cases, the clinical examination and the disease history are sufficient to establish the diagnosis of mumps. Neither sialography nor scintigraphy are indicated during the acute phase of the disease. The virus is detectable in the saliva 2 to 4 days before the clinical manifestation and for about 1 week thereafter. With the onset of clinical symptoms, a rise of serum amylase may be observed.

BIBLIOGRAPHY

Check, W.A.: Acyclovir for herpes: no clinical payoff yet (news), J.A.M.A. **244:**2021, 1980.

Cooper, J.C.: Tooth exfoliation and osteonecrosis of the jaw following herpes zoster, Br. Dent. J. **143:**297, 1977.

Guinan, M.E., and others: Topical ether and herpes simplex labialis, J.A.M.A. **243:**1059, 1980.

Morgan, D.G., and others: Site of Epstein-Barr virus replication in the oropharynx, Lancet **2:**1154, 1979.

O'Meara, A., and others: Acyclovir for treatment of mucocutaneous herpes infection in a child with leukemia (letter), Lancet **2**(8153):1196, 1979.

BACTERIAL INFECTIONS
Infective endocarditis

Bacteremia following dental treatment occurs frequently in all individuals, however, in persons suffering from valvular and other structural defects in the heart, this bacteremia may cause bacterial endocarditis.

Certain dental procedures have been associated with the production of bacteremia: extraction, toothbrushing, use of dental floss, and pressure from inserting amalgam dental extractions. Bacteremia secondary to dental treatment was demonstrated in 18% to 85% of the cases, the percentage varying in accordance with the technique and sensitivity of the tests used.

Epidemiologic data indicate that patients most prone to endocarditis belong to the following categories:

1. Patients with congenital heart disease (excluding atrial septal defect, secundum type)
2. Patients with acquired valvular disease—includes cases of rheumatic heart disease, calcified valvulitis, and syphilitic heart disease
3. Patients with a prosthetic heart valve
4. Patients who have undergone open heart surgery for correction of an intracardiac defect or closure of patient ductus arteriosus within 6 months prior to the dental treatment
5. Patients with a history of bacterial endocarditis
6. Patients with prolapse of mitral valve

Not included in these high-risk categories are the following:

1. Patients who have suffered acute myocardial infarctions
2. Patients with angina pectoris or arteriosclerotic cardiovascular diseases
3. Patients who have undergone coronary bypass surgery
4. Patients with a functional heart murmur
5. Patients who have had a heart pacemaker implanted.

The regimens currently recommended by the American Heart Association as prophylaxis directed against *Streptococcus viridans* are described in the chapter on infective endocarditis. When considering the prophylactic administration of antibiotics in dental patients prone to bacterial endocarditis, certain factors should be considered. Prophylaxis should not begin until shortly before dental treatment is initiated and should continue for at least 24 hours after the procedure and in general should be continued for a total of 48 hours. Patients with prosthetic heart valves have the greatest risk, and the dental surgeon must be aware of the specific antibiotic regimens recommended. Patients on long-term daily penicillin prophylaxis for rheumatic fever have been found to acquire resistant oral streptococcal strains. These organisms are capable of causing bacterial endocarditis unless additional prophylactic antibiotic treatment is instituted. In this situation either the penicillin plus streptomycin regimen, vancomycin, or erythromycin is suggested. The bacterial inoculum penetrating mouth tissue and gaining access to blood vessels during dental procedures may be reduced by the use of mouthrinse shortly before treatment. Chlorhexidine aqueous solution, 0.2% in a 5 ml mouthrinse for 30 seconds before intervention, was shown to fulfill these requirements.

In spite of the broad coverage given to infective endocarditis, the American Heart Association recognizes that its recommendations, revised in 1977, are necessarily *protective*. Over 30 cases of infective endocarditis have resulted from apparent prophylaxis failure raising important medical and legal questions. A registry to record such cases was established and case reports have been solicited.

Instruction in proper oral hygiene for this specific group of patients is also of significance. Simple oral hygiene measures such as toothbrushing, flossing, and mouthrinses do prevent accumulation of dental plaque. In the gingival crevice of a normal adult there are approximately 1.8×10^{10} anaerobes and 2.2×10^{10} aerobes per gram net weight. The most commonly isolated organisms are aerobic streptococci and anaerobic organisms including *Actinomyces, Corynebacterium, Lactobacillus, Veillonella, Bacteroides, Fusobacterium,* and *Peptostreptococcus*. Species from among these bacteria are the usual pathogens in odontogenic infections. Staphylococci are associated with perioral skin and nasal mucosa infections. Recently, *Capnocytophaga* isolated from periodontal pockets have received much attention because of their possible role in systemic leukocyte dysfunction.

In conclusion, the importance of removal of these microorganisms in patients prone to infection cannot be overemphasized.

Gonococcal stomatitis

Gonococcal infection of the oral cavity is uncommon and occurs mainly in adults. The incubation period of *Neisseria gonorrhoeae* in the oral cavity varies from 1 day to 2 weeks. Oral lesions in adults result from orogenital contact or contamination through the hands. In newborns, gonococcal stomatitis is acquired during contact with the involved mother's vaginal mucosa.

The appearance of oral lesions is nonspecific. Superficial ulcers with a yellow-white slough or pseudomembrane may develop on the gingiva, tongue, and soft palate. The gingivae are generally inflamed and resemble necrotizing ulcerative gingivitis. If the stomatitis becomes generalized, the entire oral mucosa appears red or inflamed. Alternatively and most commonly infection is asymptomatic or present as pharyngitis. Gonococci can also invade the salivary glands and lead to parotitis.

Therapy of gonococcal lesions of the oral mucosa, although similar to that of genital gonorrhea, differs in that antibiotic failures have been seen with ampicillin and tetracycline, hence parenteral procaine penicillin is the method of choice.

Lymphogranuloma venereum (LGV)

Rarely lymphogranuloma venereum may involve the oropharynx and occur as a result of orogenital sex.

In oral infection with *Chlamydia trachomatis,* the tongue is most often affected and a blisterlike lesion develops. The lesion is painless and the tongue is involved with areas of acute inflammation and depapillation, leading to sensitivity to spicy foods. The affected tongue generally shows signs of inflammation for long periods of time. Prominent submandibular lymphadenopathy develops that may progress to fluctuant buboes.

Fusospirochetal infections

Oral fusopirochetal infections, notably acute necrotizing ulcerative gingivitis (ANUG), occurs when predisposing factors are present. Local factors such as lack of oral hygiene, teeth with faulty contact or ill-designed restorations, and pericoronitis around wisdom teeth are the most common causes. However, a severe form of the oral disease is precipitated in the presence of debilitating medical conditions. Stress, extreme fatigue, and malnutrition are considered by most authors as contributory. Hematologic malignancies may also be accompanied by fusospirochetal infections of the gingiva or oral mucosa. The disease is characterized by tissue necrosis.

Treatment consists of local debridement, a vigorous oral hygiene regimen, and removal of the superficial necrotic tissues. In most cases pain is quite severe and preperiodontal treatment with anesthetic mouthrinses are necessary. Hydrogen peroxide (5%) mouthrinses have an inhibitory effect on the anaerobic organisms.

Signs of the spread of infection with lymphadenopathy and fever require antibiotic therapy. Penicillin is the most widely used antibiotic in the treatment of ANUG. The regular adult dose given in tablets is 1 to 2 g day. Recently, metronidazole (flagyl) has been suggested as the drug of choice in the chemotherapy of strictly anaerobic infections.

Syphilis

Oral manifestations of syphilis are found in both congenital and acquired syphilis and continue to be seen in the primary and secondary stages of active syphilis.

In primary syphilis a chancre can develop on the lips

(vermilion border or commissural area), the tip of the tongue, the tonsils, or the gingiva. Significant regional lympadenopathy is observed unilaterally and facilitates the diagnosis. The chancre, as well as the lymph nodes, abound with *Treponema pallidum*. Intraoral chancres tend to be infected by other commensal oral spirochetes as well. Accordingly darkfield examination of intraoral syphilitic lesions may be unreliable.

In secondary syphilis the oral lesions are protean in nature, including the characteristic intraoral mucous patches that resemble the macular and maculopapular skin lesions of secondary syphilis. The mucous patches are raised on the mucosal surface and appear inflamed with an area of central erosion covered by a grayish white membrane. Upon removal of the membrane a clear, flat, erythematous base is seen. The patches are found on the tongue, buccal mucosa, oropharynx, and the inner aspect of the lips but are rarely seen on the gingival surface. Syphilitic, mucous patches are highly contagious, and during this phase infected saliva droplets can easily transmit the disease.

Maculopapular lesions may develop on the palate. When present at the corners of the mouth they are called "split papules." They form a painless fissure between the upper and lower lip. These lesions must be differentiated from angular cheilosis such as caused by riboflavin deficiency. Papular lesions of the hard or soft palate may break down, resulting in snail-track ulcers.

Relapses of oropharyngeal mucosal involvement may interrupt the early latent stage of syphilis.

Gummatous infiltration of oral tissue and diffuse glossitis are manifestations of tertiary syphilis. Gummas are painless granulomas that become necrotic. They develop on the lips, oral mucosa, salivary glands, palate, and jawbone. Proliferative changes and necrosis accompany the pathologic process, leading to the formation of punched-out ulcers. Involvement of the palate will eventually be followed by its perforation. Gummas on the tongue will produce lingua lobulata. Ulcerations and fibrosis will induce surface irregularities of the tongue.

Clinical and histologic diagnosis is difficult, since such lesions are similar to those found in tuberculosis, leishmaniasis, sarcoidosis, or leprosy or mycotic granulomas. Malignancy of the tongue cannot be ruled out without a biopsy.

Atrophy of the tongue secondary to the resulting ischemia is the next stage, together with a smooth surface and shrinkage in the musculature. Leukoplakia often accompanies these changes, which result from the chronic irritation of depapillated, unprotected tongue surface. This leukoplakic area may undergo malignant changes.

The hutchinsonian triad is a result of spirochetemia during the development of the embryo. The dental deformities are caused by hypoplasia following spirochetemia. The timing of hypoplasia corresponds with the attack on the middle mamelon of the central incisors, resulting in an increased anteroposterior diameter, with a narrow incisal dimension. Only the permanent teeth are affected, and among them only those in which the calcification started in the first year of life, for example, upper central incisors and all first molars. The first molars have a narrow crown with multiple small, underdeveloped cusps and are called "mulberry molars." It was estimated that about 45% of patients with congenital syphilis had typical syphilitic incisors and 22% had characteristic syphilitic molars. These dental changes can be prevented if appropriate antimicrobial therapy is initiated before the fourth month of fetal development. Perioral rhagades are present in perhaps 15% of patients with congenital syphilis. These linear lesions are found around the oral and anal orifices and are the result of luetic skin involvement. The rhagades appear at first as red or copper-colored linear areas covered with a crust. They are radially arranged, as if starting from the vermilion border. These cracks are considered pathognomonic for congenital syphilis.

BIBLIOGRAPHY

Fiumara, N.J., and others: Papular secondary syphilis of the tongue: report of a case, Oral Surg. **45**(4):540, 1978.

Bacterial infections of the central nervous system

Oral and dental infections may be complicated by acute bacterial infections of the brain and meninges, often with fatal outcome. Microorganisms isolated from these infections include *Fusobacterium* species and anaerobic gram-positive cocci. Although dental infection may spread spontaneously, not infrequently complications follow extraction of infected teeth.

The propagated infection from dental foci may take a direct route via openings in the cranial bones, such openings being found mostly in the temporal bone. Another route may be the venous system via emissary veins connecting the extracranial and intracranial venous systems. The most important of these emissary veins is the one leading from the facial to the ophthalmic vein. The ophthalmic vein directly communicates with the cavernous sinus.

Cavernous sinus thrombosis is a rare but grave complication of dental infection. The common clinical picture of this condition presents with unilateral or bilateral proptosis, periorbital and conjunctival edema, ophthalmoplegia, and fever. The involved teeth are sensitive to percussion and in most of the cases radiographic evidence is present as radiolucent areas of chronic dental infection. Nerve involvement of the trigeminal nerve, ophthalmic division, and trochlear and abducens nerves can be observed, resulting in paralysis, ptosis, dilated pupils, and abolition of corneal reflexes. The antibiotic treatment is directed at streptococcal, staphylococcal, and anaerobic organisms. Massive doses of parenteral penicillin, chloramiphenicol, and a penicillinase-resistant beta lactam antibiotic is recommended. In the presence of a fluctuating oral abscess, incision and drainage should be undertaken and extraction of the involved tooth should be considered.

Meningitis, encephalitis, and brain abscesses are discussed in the chapter on bacterial infections of the central nervous system.

Tuberculosis

Tubercular infection of oral tissues may arise from either an exogenous or an endogenous source of microorganisms. It appears that direct primary infection of oral tissues is rarer than seeding of tuberculous microorganisms via hematogenous or lymphatic routes. The prevalence of oral tuberculosis according to the literature ranges from 0.05% to 1.44%.

ORAL MANIFESTATIONS

Tuberculous ulceration. Tuberculous ulceration is irregular with a typically undermined border. The ulcer base is covered with a purulent exudate; the surrounding tissue is indurated. Tuberculous proliferative lesions may be seen singly or concomitantly with ulcerative ones.

Tuberculous granulomas. Tuberculous granulomas have been misdiagnosed as periapical dental lesions when seen radiographically. The only clinical manifestation is increased mobility of the involved teeth.

Orofacial tuberculosis. Oral mucosal tuberculous lesions are typically found near the mucocutaneous junction. In addition, the tongue, buccal mucosa, palate, and gingiva may be the site of infection. Lesions result from autoinoculation of tubercle bacilli emanating from underlying advanced pulmonary tuberculosis, although occasionally they may represent the primary lesion.

Tubercular lesions of the lips usually begin as swellings that later develop into ulcers. The ulcers are extremely painful and characterized by prolonged healing time that may take months to complete. The adjacent facial skin may exhibit various manifestations including plaque-like verrucous and nodular lesions. Occasionally, tuberculous erythematous nodular gingivitis occurs. The organisms may enter the alveolar bone through the teeth and form a periapical granuloma or even osteomyelitis.

Tuberculous osteomyelitis of the jaws. Although rare, tuberculous osteomyelitis of the mandibular and maxillary bones has been encountered. In tuberculous lesions of the jaw bones some swelling occurs over the involved area, as a result of subperiosteal new bone formation. Bone destruction is characteristic, and sequestra develop. With time, the swelling ruptures and secreting fistulas are evident.

The radiologic picture of tuberculous osteomyelitis reveals blurring of bone detail and erosion of the cortical plate. When tuberculosis affects the periodontal tissues the radiologic signs may be the same as those of destructive periodontal disease.

Tuberculosis of the salivary glands. Fewer than 100 cases of tuberculosis of the salivary glands have been described in the literature. Tuberculosis mainly affects the parotid glands of young adults. Two types of lesions were described, including a chronic encapsulated form as well as an acute diffuse inflammatory process. The chronic lesions are present as small swellings that are usually freely movable when palpated.

Tuberculous cervical lymphadenitis (scrofulosis). Enlargement of the submandibular and cervical lymph nodes is not always present in association with oral mucosal tuberculous disease and often is only the consequence of secondary bacterial infection. Nevertheless the presenting manifestation of oral tuberculosis includes progressive enlargement of regional lymph nodes.

Tuberculous cervical lymphadenitis may also occur in the absence of visible oropharyngeal tuberculosis. Formerly a common disease in children, it has become infrequent. It usually represents breakdown of prior cervical node tuberculosis, either acquired by ingestion of infected milk (bovine tuberculosis) or more commonly by lymphohematogenous spread of infection from a primary pulmonary focus. In the United States scrofula in young children is now most frequently caused by atypical mycobacteria, particularly *M. scrofulaceum*.

Treatment. In cases of oral involvement in tuberculosis the systemic treatment is supplemented with local palliative measures. Causes of trauma, such as sharp broken teeth, ill-fitted dentures, or massive dental calculus, should be eliminated. Mouthrinses should be instituted in copious amounts to prevent secondary infection of the existing specific ulcers.

BIBLIOGRAPHY

De Lathouwer, L., and others: A rare and complex case of multifocal mucocutaneous lupus tuberculosis with isolated lesion of the tongue, Oral Surg. **39** (2):211, 1975.

Fujibayashi, T., and others: Tuberculosis of the tongue: a case report with immunologic study, Oral Surg. **47** (5):427, 1979.

Garber, H.T., and others: Tuberculous osteomyelitis of the mandible with pathologic fracture, J. Oral Surg. **36** (2):144, 1978.

Prabhu, S.R., and others: Tuberculous ulcer of the tongue: report of a case, J. Oral Surg. **36** (5):384, 1978.

Rauch, M.D., and others: Systemic tuberculosis initially seen as an oral ulceration: report of a case, J. Oral Surg. **36**:384, 1978.

Turbiner, S., and others: Orificial tuberculosis of the lip, J. Oral Surg. **33** (6):443, 1975.

Leprosy

Facial and oral manifestations of leprosy continue to be seen, particularly in endemic areas in both hemispheres. The clinical manifestations depend on both the histopathologic type and the duration of leprosy.

Facial involvement results in a "leonine" facies including loss of eyebrows and sagging of facial skin. Deformity of the ears is common, and lesions of the oral mucosa and tongue have been reported in 20% to 60% of patients. Early manifestations of oral leprosy include the formation of nodules or lepromas, which may be yellowish red, soft or hard, sessile, and often ulcerated. Healing tissues are usually fibrotic, which tends to add to the physical disfigurement. Although all oral structures may be involved, the incisive papilla, premaxilla, hard and soft palate, uvula, and tongue are most commonly involved. Granulomatous bone involvement leads to destruction of the premaxilla and loss of the front teeth. Chronic gingivitis and periodontitis with loss of alveolar bone, although frequently observed, are not specific for leprosy.

Dental changes are described as odontodysplasia leprosa. Tooth diameters are concentrically reduced and roots are shortened and tapered. Enamel and cement hypoplasia has been found in osteoarcheologic material.

Both sensory and motor peripheral nerve fibers of the cranial nerves are commonly involved. Hence bilateral facial nerve paralysis occurs in about 25% of patients with tuberculoid leprosy and trigeminal neuralgia may develop, the most commonly affected branch being the maxillary division.

BIBLIOGRAPHY
Reichart, P.: Facial and oral manifestations in leprosy: an evaluation of seventy cases. Oral Surg. **41** (3):385, 1976.

Actinomycosis

CERVICOFACIAL MANIFESTATIONS. *Actinomyces israelii,* a normal inhabitant of the oral cavity, has been isolated from dental plaque, calculus, salivary calculus, necrotic dental pulps, and tonsils. In spite of its prevalence, clinical infection from *Actinomyces* is relatively rare.

Poor oral hygiene is one of the contributory factors in oral actinomycosis. The infection extends from the necrotic tooth pulp to the periapical area and alveolar bone and penetrates through the periosteum into the muscles. The infection becomes apparent as sinus tracts on the skin. Cases have been described in which the infection ascended along the mandibular ramus and penetrated the middle cranial fossa, causing intracranial infection.

In typical cases, the mandibular area is involved, a condition known as "lumpy jaw." Involvement of the gums, oral mucosa, floor of the mouth, and palate may follow localized infection. Ascending infection of the salivary glands is possible through their ducts. Further spread of the disease may involve the muscles of mastication, resulting in severe trismus.

Actinomycosis of the tongue is rare. It involves the anterior third of the tongue as an indurated nodule that is deep seated, painful to palpation, and adherent to the musculature. The absence of regional lymphadenopathy is a striking feature.

The prognosis of cervicofacial actinomycosis is relatively good, except in the presence of chronic osteomyelitis. Therapy consists of prolonged parenteral penicillin administration.

BIBLIOGRAPHY
Kuepper, R.S., and Harrigan, W.T.: Actinomycosis of the tongue: report of case, J. Oral Surg. **37** (2):123, 1979.

Tularemia

Sporadic cases of oral involvement by *Francisella tularensis* have been reported. Solitary, painful necrotic ulcers of the labial, lingual, and palatal mucosa are described. The ulcers are covered with a whitish pseudomembrane, and rarely generalized stomatitis has been reported. Oral manifestations are invariably accompanied by other typical clinical manifestations including conjunctivitis, regional lymphadenopathy, headache, chills, and fever.

Diphtheria

In the recent literature there are few reports of diphtheritic involvement of the oral tissues. This is the direct result of effective worldwide immunization; however, sporadic cases are still seen in many countries when immunization is absent or incomplete.

Diphtheria pseudomembrane may cover the entire oral mucosa. Involvement of the lower lip, the gums around erupting primary teeth, and the corners of the mouth and tongue have been reported in young children. Lowender and Squires described a case of diphthertic involvement of the lip following the extraction of two loosened anterior teeth. Cultures obtained from the sockets indicated the presence of the diphtheria bacillus, most likely due to direct infection or contamination from the saliva.

Cervial lymphadenopathy accompanies oral and pharyngeal lesions.

BIBLIOGRAPHY
Diphtheritic involvement of the lips with absence of signs in the nose and throat, J.A.M.A. **111**:915, 1938.

Anthrax

Infection with *Bacillus anthracis* limited to the oral cavity is an uncommon condition. A typical case was described by Burnett and associates as being caused by a toothbrush contaminated with anthrax spores. The hard palate was first involved, was severely swollen, and discharged a "straw-colored" fluid. The infectious process spread to the bone, destroying the palate and alveolar bone. Overeruption of the teeth was apparent. On the mucosal surface pustules with bright-red bases appeared and developed into vesicles that broke, scabbed, and later healed. The treatment recommended in this case was antianthrax serum.

The perioral and intraoral types of anthrax are particularly dangerous because of the possibility that they may spread to the oropharynx. Edema of the glottis is also possible. Involvement of the lips and tongue has been encountered in workers from industries in which there is a risk of exposure to anthrax. This anthrax infection is most frequently the edematous type, characterized by cinnabar to black-red edema of doughy consistency. The tongue, lips, and eyelids become severely enlarged. Anthrax of the face, mouth, or throat has a much graver prognosis than that of the skin.

BIBLIOGRAPHY

Anthrax of the oral cavity, J. Am. Dent. Assoc. **36:**119, 1948.

Staphylococcal oral lesions

In large population studies staphylococci are frequently found in the oral cavity. In the gingival sulcus they constituted 2% of the viable count and about 6.5% on the dorsum of the tongue. However, they were rarely found in dental plaque.

Staphylococcus aureus was found in low counts in saliva of about half of the subjects examined. However, the proportion of carriers increased to about three quarters when the nose, throat, and mouth were cultured. In spite of the prevalence of this organism, oral mucosal lesions caused by *Staphylococcus aureus* are rare. In toxic epidermal necrolysis induced by this organism, bullae are formed, involving the lips and the oral mucosa, followed by desquamation of the epithelium.

FURUNCLES. Furuncles resulting from staphylococcal infection of the face and mainly of the upper lip may present a serious danger to the patient because of possible spread of the infection from the facial region. The most common pathway involves the superior labial veins to the external nasal veins and subsequently to angular veins to the inferior and superior ophthalmic veins, reaching the cavernous sinus. The infection may result in cavernous sinus thrombosis, meningitis, and encephalitis.

Gram-negative oral lesions
ORAL MANIFESTATIONS

Pseudomonas aeruginosa infections. *Pseudomonas* species were cultured in more than 50% of patients with acute leukemia. The infections observed were mainly septicemia and cellulitis. Oral lesions developed in the perioral skin, lips, and mucosa. The lesions were characterised by a central black area of necrosis surrounded by a red halo. There was no pus formation or exudate present and the lesions were dry and gangrenous.

Patients complain of discomfort on eating, drinking, or talking.

Serratia. Patients with hematologic malignancies develop infections with *Serratia* species following the use of broad-spectrum antibiotics. The oral lesions are white, well-circumscribed papules that become darker and ulcerate. They are observed at the commissures of the lips and other sites of tissue trauma.

Klebsiella. *Klebsiella* species infection are common in patients with acute leukemia. *Klebsiella* species constitute a substantial percentage of fatal infection.

The intraoral lesions are "creamy white," raised, glistening, spreading, and superficially erosive on the reddened base. They are painful and the lack of pus is a frequent observation. Lesions occur on the gingiva, lips, tongue, and palatal mucosa. The gingival lesions must be differentiated from those found in acute necrotizing gingivitis.

Enterobacter. Oral lesions with *Enterobacter* present as peritonsillar abscess, tongue ulcers, and diffuse involvement of the oral mucosa. Their clinical appearance is similar to that of *Klebsiella* infection. They are extremely painful, erosive, and ulcerative. The gingival lesions resemble acute necrotizing gingivitis.

Escherichia coli **and** *Proteus* **species.** Oral infections caused by *Escherichia coli* and *proteus* species in patients with acute leukemia are manifested as gingivitis, mucositis, and osteomyelitis. The oral mucosal lesions are grayish white or yellow with a slight exudate and surrounded by a red halo. They vary in size from 2 to 5 mm in diameter. Pain is the chief complaint of patients with *E. coli* infection of the tongue.

DENTAL MANAGEMENT. Early diagnosis and treatment of oral lesions produced by gram-negative bacilli are imperative because of the precipitous course following these infections in leukemic patients. Antibiotic therapy administered according to sensitivity studies must be initiated immediately.

The importance of aggressive treatment of even innocent looking gram-negative oral lesions cannot be overemphasized. Carbenicillin plus aminoglycosides are indicated for *Pseudomonas* infections, and cephalosporins and gentamicin are effective in eliminating the infection of the remaining gram-negative organisms.

BIBLIOGRAPHY

American Heart Association Committee on Rheumatic Fever and Bacterial Endocarditis: Prevention of bacterial endocarditis, Circulation **56:**139A, 1977.

Palank, E.A., and others: Fatal acute bacterial endocarditis after dentoalveolar abscess, Am. J. Cardiol. **43** (6):1238, 1979.

Pyrexia of dental origin (editorial), Lancet **1** (8179):1175, 1980.

Sanchez, C.S., and others: Occurrence of staphylococcus in periodontal pockets of diabetic and nondiabetic adults, J. Periodontol. **50:**109, 1979.

Stenhouse, D., and others: Staphylococcal submandibular lymphadenitis in childhood, Br. J. Oral Surg. **16:**73, 1978.

Those venerable notions (editorial), N. Engl. J. Med. **301** (16):888, 1979.

FUNGAL INFECTIONS
Histoplasmosis

About one third of patients with progressive disseminated histoplasmosis develop oral lesions. Ulcers and granulomas are the dominant manifestations in the oral cavity. Cases have been described in which primary lesions were diagnosed in the mouth.

Extreme destruction of the palate, pharynx, and nasal septum is known to follow the infection of these respective areas. Histoplasmosis of the jawbone will induce mobility of the teeth in the area and possible oroantral fistulas. Radiographs show diffuse osteolysis of the alveolus without subperiosteal new bone formation.

The diagnostic process requires a biopsy and culture. Microscopic examination reveals a granuloma with enlarged histiocytes containing spores of *Histoplasma*.

As in the case of systemic histoplasmosis, the treatment of choice for oral involvement is amphotericin B. Miconazole has been utilized with varying success.

BIBLIOGRAPHY

Daramola, J.O., and others: Maxillary African histoplasmosis mimicking malignant jaw tumour, Br. J. Oral Surg. **16** (3):241, 1979.

Mace, M.C.: Oral African histoplasmosis resembling Burkitt's lymphoma, Oral Sug. **46** (3):407, 1978.

Yusuf, H., and others: Disseminated histoplasmosis presenting with oral lesions: report of a case, Br. J. Oral Surg. **16** (3):234, 1979.

Candidiasis

Oral candidiasis (moniliasis) is a well-recognized common fungal infection, mainly associated with extremes of age, debilitation, immunodeficiency, and prolonged antimicrobial therapy. Specifically the principal defects in the immune system that predispose to oral candidiasis are granulocytopenia and depressed cell-mediated immunity. Chronic mucocutaneous candidiasis may be associated with hypoparathyroidism, hypoadrenalism, and mental retardation.

ORAL MANIFESTATIONS. The typical oral *Candida* lesion is pearly and blush white and covers any part or all of the oral mucosa. The patches of candidiasis resembling "milk curds" and extending to the mouth corners are called "perleche." The white plaques are attached to the underlying mucosa and when scraped leave erythematous mucosa with bleeding spots. The creamy whitish material is almost pure *Candida albicans* culture. In the absence of the white lesions, an erythematous, atrophic, acute and chronic form is also seen, particularly on dental-bearing mucosa.

Pain is the most common symptom encountered, although it is not invariably present and tends to be most severe in the acute atrophic form. Other frequent complaints include a burning sensation of oral mucosa, especially the tongue, a loss of taste, and the onset of a metallic taste in the mouth. Painful dysphagia develops dramatically when *Candida* lesions involve the throat and extend to cause *Candida* esophagitis. In spite of the not inconsiderable suffering the patient remains afebrile.

PREDISPOSING FACTORS. In the vast majority of cases, oral candidiasis is superimposed on the background of underlying medical disease. The most common predisposing factors are:

1. Prematurity in infants
2. Debilitation
   a. Postoperative, multiple trauma
   b. Underlying malignancy
   c. Stress-induced conditions such as necrotizing ulcerative gingivitis
3. Immunosuppression
   a. Hematologic disease (acute leukemia and advanced lymphoma, granulocytopenia)
   b. Drug-induced (Corticosteroids, azathioprim, etc.), chemotherapy of neoplasia
4. Radiotherapy of head and neck.
5. Prolonged antibiotic treatment
6. Diabetes (brittle, insulin dependent)
7. Oral contraceptives
8. Endocrinopathy, hypoparathyroidism, hypoadrenalism
9. Chronic irritants
   a. Denture stomatitis (combined with poor oral hygiene)
   b. Heavy smoking
10. Xerostomia secondary to salivary gland disease

Different species of *Candida* have been cultured from the mouths of patients who are considered asymptomatic carriers and from patients with frank oral candidiasis. *Candida albicans* is the most commonly isolated fungal pathogen in oral thrush. *Candida* yeast are frequently found as normal oral inhabitants in the general population and are considered noncontagious and of low virulence. The above-mentioned predisposing factors have to be present to permit or facilitate *Candida* overgrowth and the development of symptomatic disease. Hence oral candidasis is considered an opportunistic infection. Furthermore, in severely immunocompromised patients, the dangers of oral candidiasis are not limited to the local disease manifestations; in addition, candidemia and systemic metastatic dissemination of fungi occur, resulting in life-threatening sequelae, including *Candida* endophthalmitis, meningitis, osteomyelitis, and renal abscesses.

CHRONIC MUCOCUTANEOUS CANDIDIASIS. This rare congenital syndrome is characterized by chronic and relapsing *Candida* infection of the oral mucosa, lips, perioral skin, and nails. In vitro studies have identified a specific defect in cell-mediated immunity (CMI) in relation to *Candida* antigen while T cell function in response to other antigens is normal. The clinical manifestations tend to be severe, unrelenting, and hypertrophic or atrophic in nature, yet systemic manifestations and visceral spread are extremely rare.

Another clinical syndrome characterized by chronic oral *Candida* yeast infection has been noted to be associated with familial hypoparathyroidism, mental retardation, and often additional hypoadrenalism. The finding of chronic or recurrent oral *Candida* infections in otherwise healthy patients should alert the dental practitioner to the possibility of undiagnosed endocrinopathy or defective immunity, justifying further investigation.

ASYMPTOMATIC CARRIERS. In healthy dentate adult subjects the prevalence of oral carriers of *Candida albicans* varies from 29.6% to 44.4%, depending on the culture method used. Smokers have higher rates than nonsmokers, and women are more frequent carriers than men. The highest frequency of *C. albicans* isolation occurs from the posterior half of the tongue. As such, the tongue is considered a primary reservoir from which the rest of the oral tissues are colonized. It follows, therefore, that in the absence of typical mucosal lesions showing yeast and pseudohyphae on Gram stain, the finding of *Candida* on oral or pharyngeal cultures does not prove complicity in causing symptoms.

TREATMENT. Where possible, the eradication of predisposing factors should be attempted and sometimes may be sufficient to control and cure the oral candidiasis. In the acute symptomatic phase, however, treatment is justified.

Nystatin. One milliliters of *nystatin* in suspension (100,000 to 200,000 units/ml) is held in the mouth for at least 5 minutes and then swallowed. This treatment should be repeated four times a day while the disease is still active (hyphae are present) and for several days after the symptoms and signs have improved. Nystatin is not absorbed from the mucous membranes. When it is taken orally, practically all the drug is excreted in the feces.

The direct contact needed between the drug and the yeast or fungus is better achieved when a nystatin ointment is used. A custom plastic tray fitting the upper jaw of the patient is built. On its inner surface, nystatin, 100,000 units/ml, is applied and worn for about 2 hours. This treatment is repeated four times a day. This ensures the prolonged presence of a high concentration of the agent in the oral cavity. Another advantage of this method is that the plastic cover protects ulcers that develop on the hard palate or gums in patients suffering from leukemia or agranulocytosis as well as patients undergoing irradiation.

In edentulous patients wearing full dentures, the dentures can be used as drug carriers when indicated.

Regular nystatin tablets are *not* effective for treatment of oral moniliasis, because their dissolving time is slow and the bitter taste is not tolerated by patients. They are used only in cases of intestinal candidiasis.

Vaginal nystatin tablets (pessaries), however, *can* be used for treatment of oral moniliasis. They are taken four times a day and allowed to dissolve in the mouth. There is no known resistance of *Candida albicans* to this drug, even after prolonged use.

Amphotericin B. *Amphotericin B* is closely related to nystatin and is highly effective against *Candida albicans*, although it is poorly absorbed from the gastrointestinal tract and oral mucosa. Amphotericin B lozenges are available in several countries and can be used for oral candidiasis. One should be taken four times daily. The lozenge is held in the mouth until it dissolves. Parenteral use of amphotericin B requires hospitalization. Amphotericin B is still the drug of choice in cases of serious *Candida* infection. At present it is not licensed in the United States for oral topical therapy.

Imidazole derivatives. A number of imidazole derivatives have been shown to be effective in topical therapy of oral thrush. Both clotrimazole and miconazole are efficacious and are not absorbed via the gastrointestinal tract. Recently ketoconazole, 200 to 400 mg daily, has become available as oral systemic therapy for oropharyngeal *Candida* infections with excellent results, even in immunocompromised hosts.

Miconazole nitrate gel is a substituted phenylethylimidazole derivative active against bacteria and fungi. The drug is not absorbable following topical application. A 5 ml solution kept in the mouth for 5 minutes, four times daily, leads to improvement of oral candidiasis in a short period of time.

In general the use of these drugs for prevention of oral candidiasis is not very effective. However, anti-fungal medications can be used on a continuous basis in immunosuppressed or leukemic patients prone to developing oral candidiasis.

Mucormycosis

Oral infection with Mucorales fungi is rare but its outcome may be fatal. Patients at risk include those with diabetes (who are prone to ketoacidosis), leukemia, granulocytopenia, and uremia.

The involved mucosa, whether palatal or nasal, becomes dark, magenta black colored and necrotic. Ulceration of these areas will eventually be followed by perforation. Ipsilateral facial and other cranial nerve palsy develops with intracerebral mucormycosis. Anesthesia of the areas supplied by the ophthalmic and maxillary branches of the trigeminal nerve is a common finding.

BIBLIOGRAPHY

Arondor, T.M., and Walker, D.M.: The prevalence and intraoral distribution of *Candida albicans* in man, Arch. Oral Biol. **25**:1, 1980.

Kirkpatrick, C.H., and Alling, D.W.: Treatment of chronic oral candidiasis with clotrimazole troches: a controlled clinical trial, N. Engl. J. Med. **299**:1201, 1978.

Neisel, P., and Taylor, D. S.: Chronic mucocutaneous candidiasis: treatment of the oral lesion with miconazole, Br. J. Oral Surg. **18**:51, 1980.

Pisanty S., and Garfunkel, A.: Familial hypopatathyroidism with candidiasis and mental retardation, Oral Surg. **44**:374, 1977.

BIBLIOGRAPHY FOR SECTION FOUR

Altman, E.G.: Rational use of metromidazole, Aust. Dent. J. **25**:135, 1980.

Brown, L.R., and others: Comparison of the plaque microflora in immunodeficient and immunocompetent dental patients, J. Dent. Res. **58**:2344, 1979.

Burnett, G.W., and Schester, G.S.: Oral microbiology and infectious disease, Baltimore, 1978, The Williams & Wilkins Co.

Gorlin, R.J., and Goldman, H.M.: Thoma's oral pathology, ed. 6, St. Louis, 1970, The C. V. Mosby Co.

Greenberg, R.N., and others: Microbiologic and antibiotic aspects of infections in the oral and maxillofacial region, J. Oral Surg. **37:**873, 1979.

Levinson, S.L., and others: Occult dental infection as a cause of fever of obscure origin, Am. J. Med. **66:**463, 1979.

Lynch, M.A.: Burket's oral medicine: diagnosis and treatment, ed. 7, Philadelphia, 1977, J.B. Lippincott Co.

McCarthy, P.L., and Shklar, G.: Disease of the oral mucosa, ed. 2, Philadelphia, 1980, Lea and Febiger.

Van Palenstein-Helderman, W.H.: Longitudinal microbial changes in developing human supragingival and subgingival dental plaque, Arch. Oral Biol. **26:**7, 1980.

Section Five
HEMATOLOGIC DISORDERS
edited by **Rosaline R. Joseph**

59 • INTRODUCTION TO HEMATOLOGIC DISORDERS
Rosaline R. Joseph

A wide variety of diseases are considered within the realm of hematology, including not only disturbances of the hematopoietic organs and the cellular elements of the peripheral blood but also abnormalities of the lymphoreticular and hemostatic mechanisms. The latter represents a complex interaction among the blood vessels, the platelets, and the plasma coagulation factors.

The cardinal symptoms and signs associated with hematologic disease are those resulting from underproduction to overproduction of red blood cells (anemia or erythrocytosis), leukocytes (leukopenia or leukocytosis), or platelets (thrombocytopenia or thrombocytosis); defective hemostasis (hemorrhage or intravascular coagulation); or neoplasia of the lymphoreticular system (lymphomas, reticuloendothelioses, or plasma cell dyscrasias). The disturbance in hematologic parameters may represent a primary hematologic disorder or may be caused by an underlying disease. However, in both situations the signs and symptoms are the same. It is extremely important to differentiate between primary and secondary disorders. Anemia caused by bleeding from a gastrointestinal neoplasm, leukocytosis caused by an infection, bleeding tendency resulting from a vitamin K deficiency caused by biliary obstruction, or splenomegaly resulting from malaria is of vastly different significance from a morphologically similar anemia associated with a thalassemia trait, a similar degree of leukocytosis from chronic granulocytic leukemia, bleeding caused by a congenital factor deficiency, or splenomegaly from Hodgkin's disease. Frequently it is the careful evaluation of an apparent hematologic abnormality that leads to the diagnosis of a previously unsuspected primary disorder.

Proper laboratory investigation of hematologic abnormalities should follow a logical sequence. Often a few simple, inexpensive, but crucial studies provide more information than a whole battery of more costly, frequently unnecessary or inappropriate tests. For instance, a reticulocyte count will generally distinguish the anemias associated with marrow dysfunction from the hemolytic anemias associated with the increased red blood cell destruction. Careful attention to red blood cell morphology on a well-stained peripheral blood smear can yield a wealth of data on the pathophysiologic basis of an anemia. Assessment of the size (microcytic, normocytic, or macrocytic) and degree of hemoglobinization (hypochromic, normochromic) of the red blood cell is important in narrowing the diagnostic possibilities in a given case. The degree of variability in size (anisocytosis) and shape (poikilocytosis) provides a measure of the severity of the process. Finally, discovery of specific red blood cell morphologic abnormalities, such as sickle cells, target cells, teardrop cells, and basophilic stippling, on the peripheral smear is of major diagnostic importance. Differential white blood counts and examination of white cell morphology on the peripheral smear give invaluable information in evaluating leukocytic disorders.

In the investigation of bleeding disorders, an initial screening consisting of prothrombin time, partial thromboplastin time, platelet count, and bleeding time will categorize the abnormalities into intrinsic, extrinsic, common pathway, or platelet-vascular disorders. Further studies may then be directed to the specific pathway or pathways concerned. For the diagnosis of hematologic malignancy, examination of tissue is essential. Bone marrow aspiration, biopsy, or both are imperative in all cases of unexplained leukopenia, leukocytosis, anemia, or thrombocytopenia. A diagnosis of lymphoma cannot be made without histologic examination of an involved area, most often a lymph node. In all of these situations further studies may be necessary to pinpoint the exact diagnosis, but expense and inconvenience to the patient are minimized by appropriate initial screening.

The treatment of hematologic disorders should, whenever possible, be directed to the correction of a specific defect. Proper evaluation of a hypochromic microcytic anemia will avoid unnecessary, prolonged, and even harmful iron therapy for situations other than iron deficiency. Indiscriminate use of "shotgun" hematinic combinations should be condemned, and cyanocobalamin should not be administered unless a vitamin B_{12} deficiency has been documented. Use of corticosteroids should be confined to situations in which there is a rational indication for their use, such as autoimmune hemolytic anemia. Use of specific blood components for specific clinical needs should be emphasized. This practice not only maximizes the efficient use of whole blood but also minimizes the risks to the patient of unnecessary transfusion. The availability of factor VIII concentrates has vastly improved the lot of the patient with classic hemophilia, and patients who require repeated platelet transfusions can receive HLA-typed, matched platelets.

The treatment of hematologic malignancies is an area of constant change and improvement. In no branch of medicine has there been greater progress recently in treating heretofore fatal disease. The availability of successful chemotherapy and radiotherapy together with sophisticated support systems has changed the outlook for many patients with acute leukemia or lymphoma.

Unit A • DISORDERS OF RED BLOOD CELL PRODUCTION AND IRON METABOLISM

60 • INTRODUCTION TO ANEMIA AND APPROACH TO PATIENTS WITH ANEMIA

Emmanuel C. Besa

Anemia is usually discovered accidentally, since this clinical condition presents vague, nonspecific symptoms and commonly occurs in such a slow, chronic fashion that the patient may not realize that he or she is unwell. However, once the anemia is discovered, the physician should determine the underlying disease process. There is no correlation between the degree of anemia and the severity of the underlying disease. A patient often needs several uncomfortable and expensive laboratory tests to find the cause of the anemia. Thus the physician must decide when these tests are necessary to rule out a serious disorder such as an early occult malignancy. However, the physician should practice restraint in subjecting a young woman with iron deficiency probably caused by menstrual loss to unnecessary testing.

Anemia is usually defined as a significant decrease in red corpuscles or hemoglobin. The laboratory measurements generally used to determine the presence or absence of anemia are the packed red cell volume or hematocrit and the hemoglobin concentration of the peripheral blood.

Any hemoglobin or hematocrit value below the lower limits of normal is worthy of investigation. The normal hemoglobin value in men is 15.5 g/dl of blood with a range from 13.3 to 17.7 g/dl. In women the average is 13.7 g/dl with a range from 11.7 to 15.7 g/dl. A drop in hemoglobin is suspicious even if the level is still within the normal range.

The normal value for the hematocrit in men is 46 ml/dl of blood with a range of 39.8 to 52.2 ml/dl. In women the normal value is 40.9 ml/dl with a range of 34.9 to 46.9 ml/dl. These measurements merely reflect the ratio of red cells to plasma. The degree or severity of an anemia may be accentuated or masked by conditions that alter the plasma volume. For example, dehydration will increase the hematocrit by decreasing the plasma volume, whereas abnormal serum proteins such as those in multiple myeloma expand the plasma volume, producing the opposite effect and accentuating a mild anemia. Acute bleeding with equal amounts of red cell and plasma loss may not change the hematocrit for the first 12 to 24 hours even when severe. Since the more accurate blood volume measurements are often not readily available, the physician must depend on hematocrit and hemoglobin measurements. These tests are adequate for evaluation of the anemia if the physician understands the limitations of the measurements and correlates them with the clinical picture. The plasma volume is altered by fluid depletion, electrolyte imbalances, and abnormal serum proteins. The presence of any of these conditions should influence the interpretations of the laboratory results and aid in the evaluation of the severity of the anemia.

NORMAL RED BLOOD CELL PRODUCTION AND PATHOLOGY (FIG. 60-1)

The normal red blood cell (RBC) survival time is approximately 120 days. Old red cells are removed from the circulation by the reticuloendothelial cells in the spleen and liver. The old cells are replaced by reticulated young RBCs called reticulocytes, which are released from the bone marrow. A sensitive oxygen sensor in the kidney informs the bone marrow to increase or decrease the rate of maturation of young RBCs. The amount of oxygen delivered to the kidney is altered by changes in oxygen diffusion from the lung, the amount of hemoglobin available, the affinity or ability of the hemoglobin to release the oxygen to the cells, and the adequacy of the circulation of the kidney. Any hypoxic stimulus systemically or locally in the kidney results in the release of erythropoietin from the kidney and perhaps from the liver. This hormone in-

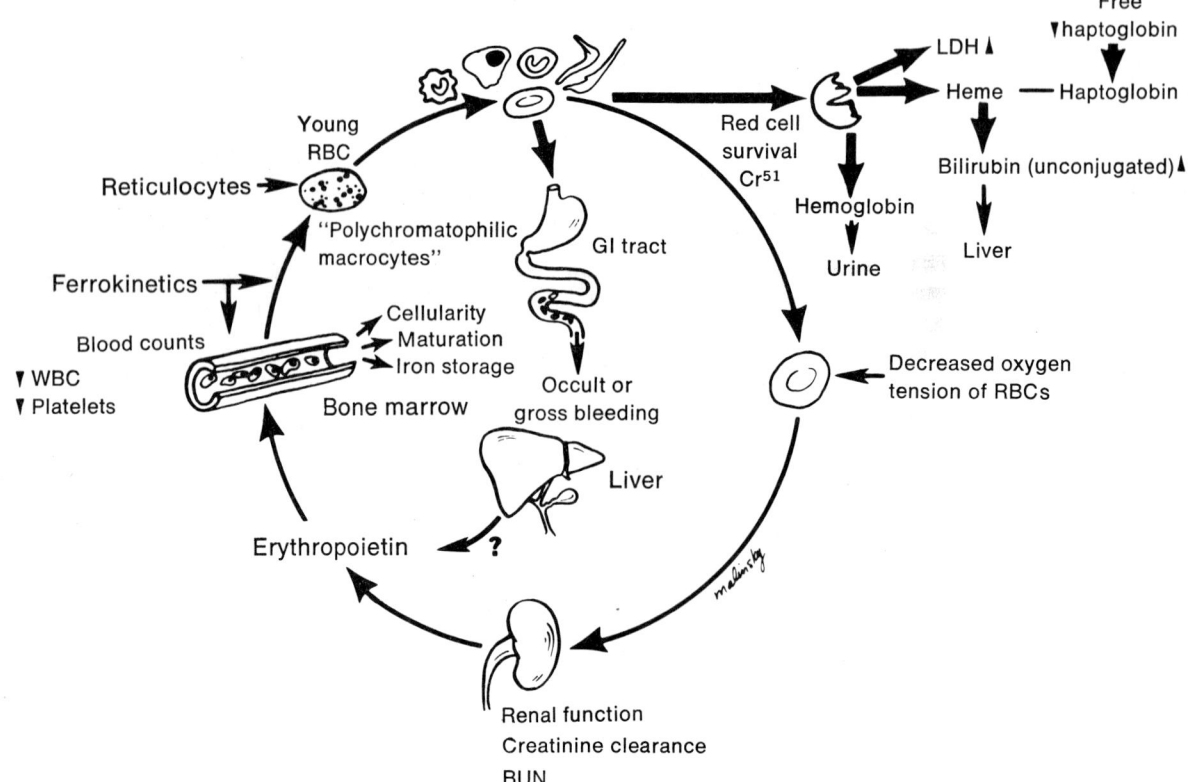

Fig. 60-1. Different tests used in defining cause of anemia are shown in relation to normal mechanism of red blood cell production. Evaluation of blood smear is direct study of finished product in which defective red cells are most likely to be uncovered. Testing stools for blood is used to search for obscure bleeding source. Increased blood levels of LDH, free hemoglobin, or decreased haptoglobin reflect hemolysis. Hemoglobin may eventually be excreted in urine or increase unconjugated bilirubin in serum. Severe renal dysfunction eventually affects ability of kidney to release regulatory hormone erythropoietin and excrete waste products inhibitory to bone marrow function. Liver may be another source of erythropoietin but is unable to compensate for diseased kidney. Finally, source of cells may be involved and can be studied either by direct examination of bone marrow or its ability to compensate for anemia by rate of release of young red cells or reticulocytes. Cellular marrow with red cell precursors may be unable to produce viable RBCs (called ineffective erythropoiesis). Rate of red cell production and release can be studied by tracing radioactive iron as it is taken up by bone marrow and its appearance in circulation (called ferrokinetics). Presence or absence of iron or cells in bone marrow reflects nature of functional failure of blood production.

duces proliferation of the red cell precursors in the bone marrow and shortens the time of maturation so that more RBCs can be released more quickly into the circulation.

Anemia may result from any disturbance or breakdown in the normal mechanism of red cell production. The causes of anemia fall into the following groups: (1) decreased red cell production owing to bone marrow failure or deficiency of "building blocks," (2) increased red cell destruction or blood loss, and (3) low erythropoietin levels in severe renal failure.

One or more of these categories are generally involved in the pathophysiology of the usual forms of anemia. Decreased red cell production owing to bone marrow failure or aplasia may also produce defective red cells that do not survive long enough to be released into the circulation. This is referred to as "ineffective erythropoiesis."

APPROACH TO THE ANEMIC PATIENT

HISTORY AND PHYSICAL EXAMINATION. After detection of the anemia, the physician may benefit by reviewing the history and physical examination as a check for information that was missed during the initial evaluation. It is often necessary to inquire about a family history of anemia, jaundice, splenectomy, bleeding, and abnormal hemoglobin. The patient may have had occupational exposure to chemicals, drugs, or radiation.

The patient frequently neglects to mention taking aspirin or other nonsteroidal anti-inflammatory agents that can give rise to gastric mucosal damage and gastrointestinal bleeding. The patient should be asked specifically about the use of these agents. The dietary history is often omitted and may be deliberately hidden from the physician owing to embarrassment on the part of the patient.

Although iron deficiency is rarely due to dietary deficiency in adults, it remains fairly common cause in infants, especially premature infants. The possibility of an underlying chronic disease should be explored by a meticulous review of systems. A careful examination should be performed with special attention to adenopathy, organ enlargement, bleeding in the skin and mucous membranes, nail changes, and neurologic abnormalities. An important component of the examination is the rectal examination and a test of the stool for occult blood. The importance of a carefully done and complete physical examination in the evaluation of a patient's anemia cannot be overemphasized.

DIAGNOSTIC PROCEDURES. A logical and orderly approach to a patient with anemia is shown in Fig. 60-2. With the advent of electronic counting devices, values used for computing the indices have become more consistent and reproducible. Most reports of blood counts include computer values for the RBC indices. The physician, however, cannot rely on the technician's ability to interpret peripheral blood smears and should examine the blood smear to avoid missing valuable clues and information.

Normal RBC indices (Coulter counter) are as follows:

RBC indices	Formula	Normal values
Mean corpuscular or cell volume (MCV)	$\dfrac{Hct}{RBC}$	$92 \pm 10 \ \mu m^3$
Mean corpuscular or cell hemoglobin (MCH)	$\dfrac{Hgb}{RBC}$	30 ± 3 pg
Mean corpuscular or cell hemoglobin concentration (MCHC)	$\dfrac{Hgb}{Hct}$	33 ± 2 g/dl or %

EXAMINATION OF THE SMEAR. Certain changes in the size or shape of the red cells and the presence of certain inclusion bodies may give the physician information to pursue the diagnosis in a more systematic fashion. Table 60-1 lists these RBC changes and the particular conditions in which they are frequently observed. The morphologic RBC changes may reflect the pathophysiology of the underlying disease or cause of the anemia. Examination of the smears also gives the physician an opportunity to observe abnormalities in the white blood cells and platelets, which are often affected when the bone marrow is involved in the disease process.

Reticulocyte count. The reticulocyte count is one of the most neglected parts of the blood count. Since this test is done using in vivo staining with methylene blue, fresh blood is necessary; fixed smears of the peripheral blood cannot be used. The test is inexpensive and can be performed as an office procedure. Because the counts are reported in a percentage as the number of reticulated cells per 100 RBCs, the degree of anemia may falsely elevate a low or normal reticulocyte count. The correction factor is calculated as follows:

Corrected reticulocyte count =
$$\dfrac{\text{Reported reticulocyte count (\%)} \times \text{Hct (\%)}}{\text{Normal Hct (40\%-45\%)}}$$

A normal value is 0.5% to 1.5%. Elevation of the reticulocyte count indicates that the bone marrow is producing more RBCs than in the normal steady state and thus usually implies a hemorrhagic episode, a hemolytic process, or a response to an appropriately treated anemia. An elevation in the reticulocyte count also indicates the ability of the bone marrow to respond to erythropoietin. Low counts often reflect bone marrow hypoplasia or dysplasia, or failure of the kidney to release erythropoietin. The information provided by the reticulocyte count may not be very specific but often leads to a systematic evaluation of an obscure anemia.

Serum chemistries. Other helpful serologic tests and findings include (1) elevated LDH, low haptoglobin, and increased unconjugated bilirubin, which reflect RBC hemolysis (Fig. 60-1); (2) serum iron, iron-binding capacity, and percentage of saturation of iron-binding protein (to detect iron deficiency); vitamin B_{12} and folate serum level to detect vitamin deficiency; (3) liver, endocrine, and renal function tests where indicated (may reflect other system dysfunction); and (4) serum ferritin levels, which have recently been advocated to replace bone marrow in the evaluation of iron stores. The serum ferritin seems to correlate well with the amount of iron stores; that is, when ferritin levels are low or absent, iron stores are low, and when serum ferritin is markedly elevated, iron stores are increased. However, normal serum ferritin levels may be found in some patients with iron deficiency who also have liver damage. This test needs further evaluation to determine its clinical applicability.

Special procedures. A bone marrow aspiration is indicated (1) to evaluate the marrow cellular elements, (2) to evaluate iron stores, (3) to evaluate maturation of cellular elements, and (4) to look for the presence of abnormal cells or infection. Bone marrow biopsy is indicated (1) to judge accurately the cellularity of the marrow, (2) to look for malignancies or granulomata, and (3) when aspiration is "dry" or inadequate for evaluation.

Other special procedures such as red cell survival and ferrokinetics are performed in complicated and mixed-type anemias. The patient's RBCs are tagged with ^{51}Cr to determine how long they stay in the circulation. Information about splenic sequestration or occult intermittent gastrointestinal bleeding may be gathered by scanning the spleen and measuring radioactivity of ^{51}Cr in the stools respectively. In patients with refractory anemia the alterations in red cell production may be elucidated by ferrokinetic studies. ^{59}Fe is given intravenously, and the time for the patient to clear the ^{59}Fe from the plasma indicates the activity

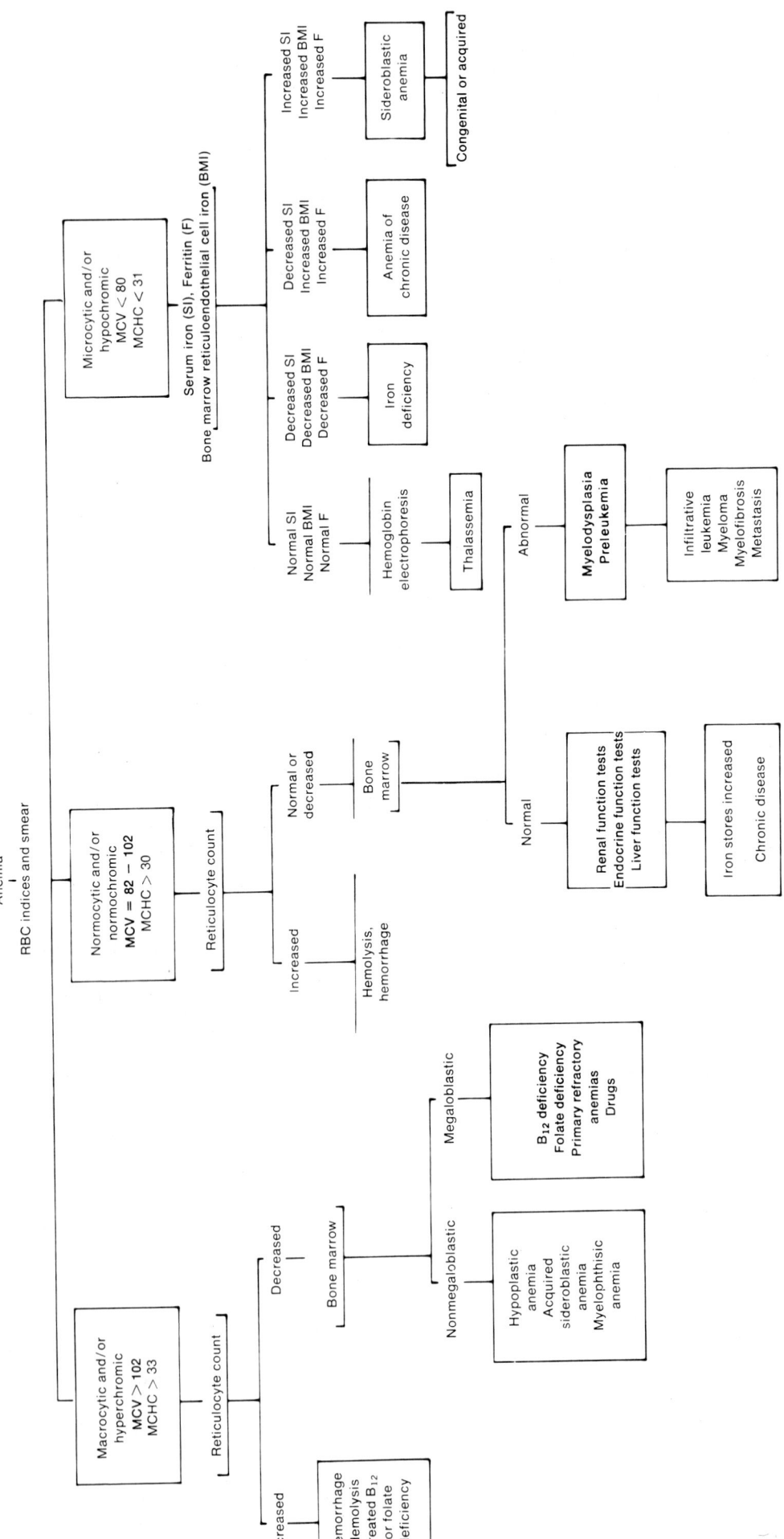

Fig. 60-2. Logical and systematic decision tree illustrates successive steps in differential diagnosis of anemia. Good history, physical examination, blood smear examination, and determination of red cell indices may make subsequent steps unnecessary in some cases. (From Besa, E.C.: Current topics, vol. 2, Philadelphia, 1978, Medical College of Pennsylvania.)

Table 60-1. Evaluation of RBCs in the examination of the blood smear

Name of cell or inclusion	Description	Disease entity
Abnormal shapes		
Acanthocyte ("spur cells" or "burr cells")	Spicules on cell	Abetalipoproteinemia, cirrhosis and other liver diseases, uremia
Dacryocyte	Teardrop shape	Most commonly myelofibrosis but also Heinz body anemia, thalassemia, hemolytic anemia
Drepanocyte	Sickle shape	Sickle cell anemia (trait after deoxygenation), other rare hemoglobinopathies
Schistocyte	Helmet form, RBC fragments	Intravascular coagulation, fibrin deposits in blood vessels, vascular or valve prostheses, malignant hypertension
Spherocyte	Spheroid	Hereditary or acquired hemolytic anemia
Stomatocyte	Slitlike area of central pallor	Hereditary or acquired hemolytic anemia
Target cell	Target form	Hemoglobin C or E, liver disease, obstructive jaundice, thalassemia, postsplenectomy
Inclusion bodies		
Nucleated RBC	Pyknotic nucleus	Acute hemorrhage, acute anoxemia with congestive heart failure, severe hemolytic anemia, leukemia, myelofibrosis, bone marrow metastasis, normal asplenic individuals
Basophilic stippling	Punctate basophilia	Lead intoxication, sideroblastic anemias, disordered erythropoiesis associated with myeloproliferative syndrome
Howell-Jolly bodies	Small round bodies	Most commonly asplenic individuals or functional asplenia but also hemolytic anemias
Cabot rings	Rings or figures-of-eight	Severe anemias, dyserythropoiesis

of the bone marrow. Patients with iron deficiency and hemolytic anemias have a rapid clearance, whereas in aplastic anemia and other bone marrow failure states the plasma ^{59}Fe clearance is prolonged. The true measure of effective red cell production is ^{59}Fe incorporation into the circulating RBC; 80% to 100% of the radioactive dose is incorporated 10 to 14 days after administration in normal individuals. In patients with bone marrow failure or ineffective erythropoiesis this value is decreased below normal depending on the severity of the anemia.

Electrophoretic analysis of the patient's hemoglobin is indicated in characterizing the different hemoglobinopathies and their combinations. It is also used in the differential diagnosis of hypochromic microcytic anemia when iron deficiency has been ruled out (Fig. 60-2).

Patients with occult iron deficiency anemia should receive a thorough gastrointestinal workup including a barium enema, an upper gastrointestinal series, and sigmoidoscopy.

MANAGEMENT. There are numerous specific therapies for different types of anemia (once the cause is identified by the physician) that will be discussed in subsequent chapters. However, supportive therapy such as blood transfusion is often erroneously given, modifying the clinical picture so that establishment of the diagnosis becomes more difficult.

Emergency blood transfusions are indicated only in life-threatening situations such as when anemia is accompanied by severe coronary artery disease, congestive heart failure, or severe hypoxia. The physician should try to obtain most of the diagnostic tests before transfusion. Freezing serum samples and keeping unstained smears for examination at a later date are always good practices.

Most chronic anemias are compensated by increments of RBC 2,3-diphosphoglycerate, which increases the ability of hemoglobin to release oxygen to the tissue. Most anemic patients with normal cardiac function and deficiency anemia can tolerate a hematologic workup and will recover by replacement therapy without needing a blood transfusion. Circulatory overload and pulmonary edema are risks of transfusion in severely anemic patients with borderline or poor cardiac function. Transfusion of packed RBCs and the use of rapid-acting diuretics are often necessary in this situation.

The use of hematinic drugs containing combinations of iron, folate, vitamin B_{12}, and other vitamins and minerals without first identifying the type and cause of the anemia should be condemned. This type of therapy should be differentiated from properly supervised therapeutic trials, which may be necessary when mixed types of anemia complicate the clinical and laboratory picture. Under these circumstances baseline studies of the blood counts are performed and repeated at intervals to determine a response. The drugs or vitamins are prescribed individually, using optimal doses so that the response can be identified. "Shotgun" therapy or indiscriminate use of these drugs without careful follow-up should be conscientiously avoided.

61 • MEGALOBLASTIC ANEMIA

Emmanuel C. Besa

DEFINITIONS. The term "megaloblast" describes the large erythroid precursors, which have morphologically immature nuclei associated with normally hemoglobinized cytoplasm. This dissociation of maturation between nuclei and cytoplasm is not limited to the erythroid precursors but may be observed in all cell lines in the bone marrow. Macrocytosis, the presence of large red blood cells in the peripheral blood, is characterized by an increased mean corpuscular volume (MCV). Mild to moderate degrees of macrocytosis may be seen with an increase in reticulocytes or in liver disease without a megaloblastic bone marrow. Macrocytosis greater than 10% (MCV of 115 μm^3 or greater) or even in the absence of anemia should be pursued, since early vitamin B_{12} or folate deficiency, liver disease, or neoplasm may be found.

ETIOLOGY. A state of unbalanced growth in the hematopoietic cells of the bone marrow is due to abnormal DNA synthesis with a delay in nuclear maturation while protein synthesis in the cytoplasm proceeds at a normal rate. This "cytonuclear dissociation" results from impairment of conversion of deoxyuridylate to thymidylate, which is necessary for DNA synthesis. The exact mechanism of the resulting anemia is unclear, but evidence points to an early destruction of the hematopoietic cells before their release into the circulation. The ineffective erythropoiesis is not confined to the red cells but involves all cell lines in hematopoiesis and other cells with a rapid cellular turnover rate such as those of the intestinal mucosa.

In the majority of patients megaloblastic anemia is due to folate or vitamin B_{12} deficiency. A small number of cases may be caused by a disturbance in hematopoiesis unrelated to either deficiency, for example, erythroleukemia, Lesch-Nyhan syndrome, or congenital abnormalities such as orotic aciduria.

Vitamin B_{12} and folate are closely interrelated, as evidenced by clinical and biochemical studies. High doses of folate can correct the anemia of vitamin B_{12} deficiency but exacerbate the neurologic symptoms, and high doses of vitamin B_{12} can cause reticulocytosis in folate deficiency. Serum levels of folate are reduced in vitamin B_{12} deficiency, and depressed vitamin B_{12} serum levels accompany folate deficiency.

FOLATE METABOLISM. Folates are widely distributed in a variety of foods, and the normal daily diet contains 600 to 700 μg of folate. Since folates are water soluble and heat labile, excessive heating or boiling of food substantially decreases dietary folate content. This loss of folate may be important in patients with malabsorption or with increased requirement for the vitamin as in pregnancy or hemolytic anemia. Folate is best absorbed in the proximal jejunum and duodenum. Approximately 50 to 100 μg is required daily to balance the fecal and urinary losses. Liver and other tissues store small amounts (5 to 20 mg) of folate. This usually takes 5 weeks to 4 months to exhaust in the absence of dietary folate intake.

FOLATE DEFICIENCY. The following are some clinical causes of folate deficiency:

Dietary deficiency
    Water and toast diet
Malabsorption
    Sprue
    Jejunal resection
Drugs
    Alcohol
    Phenytoin
    Methotrexate
    Triamterene
    Trimethoprim
Increased requirement
    Pregnancy
    Chronic hemolytic anemia
    Hyperthyroidism
    Neoplasms
    Exfoliative dermatitis
    Long-term hemodialysis

A dietary lack of folate leads to megaloblastic anemia in a few months. Lack of absorption caused by diseases involving the proximal small intestine such as celiac disease (gluten enteropathy) frequently results in a deficient state. Increased DNA synthesis, as in pregnancy, hemolysis, hyperthyroidism, malignancies, agnogenic myeloid metaplasia, and chronic exfoliative dermatitis, increases the folate requirement and may cause mild to moderate folate deficiency. Folate and other dialyzable vitamins must be replaced in patients undergoing long-term hemodialysis.

One common cause of folate deficiency is alcoholism. The anemia of alcoholism is due to diverse etiologic mechanisms of which folate deficiency is only one. Drugs such as phenytoin, methotrexate, triamterene, and trimethoprim have been associated with folate deficiency anemia. The mechanisms implicated in this relationship are poor absorption owing to drug effects on intestinal cells, competitive interaction between folate coenzymes and the drug, increased catabolism of folate by the liver induced by the drug, and displacement of folate from serum binding proteins.

VITAMIN B_{12} METABOLISM. The main source of vitamin B_{12} in the human diet is bacterially synthesized vitamin B_{12} in animal tissues. In vegetarians a mild megaloblastic anemia may eventually develop. The average diet contains 5 to 30 μg of vitamin B_{12}. The daily requirement is 1 to 3 μg. Since large amount (2 to 4 mg) of the vitamin are stored in the liver, malabsorption of vitamin B_{12} does not cause megaloblastic anemia until 2 to 5 years after the effective absorption of the vitamin ceases.

Only about 1% of vitamin B_{12} is absorbed throughout the small intestine by the passive route. Vitamin B_{12} is actively absorbed in the distal ileum. Active absorption of the vitamin depends on the presence of a glycoprotein, intrinsic factor (IF), secreted by the parietal cells in the fundus of the stomach.

VITAMIN B_{12} DEFICIENCY (PERNICIOUS ANEMIA). The causes of vitamin B_{12} deficiency include the following:

Lack of intrinsic factor
    Pernicious anemia
    Gastrectomy
Dietary deficiency
    Strict vegetarians
Biologic competition
    Small bowel bacterial overgrowth
        Diverticulosis
        Anastomosis and fistulas
        Blind loops and strictures
        Scleroderma
    Fish tapeworm
Impaired absorption
    Regional ileitis, ileal resection
    Sprue (tropical)
    Drugs such as alcohol, neomycin, colchicine, and para-aminosalicylic acid

The most common and classic form of vitamin B_{12} deficiency is pernicious anemia (PA) caused by malabsorption owing to the absence of IF secretion. This usually occurs in middle-aged and elderly persons with an associated genetic susceptibility and age-related chronic atrophic gastritis. PA has been described most frequently in patients of Northern European ancestry. Recent studies in the United States demonstrate that PA is found with equal frequency in the black population and in white patients of all origins. PA occurs at a younger age in black women and is associated with a greater prevalence of circulating antibodies against IF.

The origin of the impairment in the production of IF in PA is poorly understood. An autoimmune process has been implicated, since most patients with PA have antibodies directed against IF and parietal cells in the serum and gastric juice.

The association of PA and other autoimmune disorders such as Hashimoto's thyroiditis and Graves' disease has strengthened the concept that PA is an autoimmune disease. A cause-and-effect relationship between the antibodies and the disease process has not been proved, and current evidence suggests that a cell-mediated immune mechanism, rather than the abnormal circulating antibodies, may be responsible for the atrophic gastritis in PA.

Dietary deficiency of vitamin B_{12} is rare and is limited to strict vegetarians who do not eat dairy products.

Poor absorption of vitamin B_{12} can result form the destruction of the absorption site at the distal ileum or of the vitamin B_{12} en route to the ileum. The mucosa of the distal ileum may be damaged in diseases such as regional ileitis or by drugs such as alcohol, neomycin, colchicine, or para-aminosalicylic acid. The vitamin B_{12} may not reach the ileum because of utilization by bacteria in intestinal diverticula or in "blind loops." The fish tapeworm *(Diphyllobothrium latum),* frequently found in Scandinavian countries, also utilizes vitamin B_{12}.

CLINICAL MANIFESTATIONS. The history and physical examination often provide important clues for differentiating folate deficiency and vitamin B_{12} deficiency, the two most common causes of megaloblastic anemia. A positive family history may be found in a third of the cases of PA. The dietary history is essential and usually is normal in PA. Vegetarians who do not eat any food of animal origin may become vitamin B_{12} deficient. Folate deficiency is usually due to a poor or bizarre diet. Knowledge of previous gastric or intestinal resection and symptoms of malabsorption may help identify a patient's particular deficiency. Information concerning medications and drugs is essential in the history of patients with megaloblastic anemia.

Neurologic abnormalities are associated mainly with vitamin B_{12} deficiency (see Chapter 148). Paresthesias, abnormalities in gait and fine coordination, and overt psychoses (megaloblastic madness) are often described as part of PA. Neurologic abnormalities referable to subacute combined degeneration involving the posterior and lateral columns of the spinal cord are manifested by impairment of vibratory and position sense, increases in deep tendon reflexes, ataxic or spastic gait, and impairment of bowel and bladder functions. These changes may occur in PA without anemia in 1 to 500 cases, usually in patients taking folates or in vegetarians eating a high-folate diet. A recent study of patients with severe folate deficiency in a general hospital revealed a significant increase in organic brain syndrome and pyramidal tract damage. These findings were independent of the degree of anemia or presence of alcoholism, suggesting that severe folate deficiency per se may cause neurologic deficits.

Physical findings include a smooth tongue with absent papillation, pallor, mild icterus, and minimal splenomegaly. Weight loss, anorexia, and bowel disturbances indicate megaloblastic changes in the gastrointestinal tract. Palmar hyperpigmentation has been observed in black patients with PA. This finding reverses with vitamin B_{12} therapy.

LABORATORY FINDINGS. Macrocytosis can easily be

identified with the use of electronic erythrocyte sizing equipment. When the MCV is 115 μm^3 or greater, the chances of having a deficiency of folate or vitamin B_{12} or both are significant. The peripheral blood smear confirms the presence of large red cells and poikilocytosis. The platelets may be large, and the polymorphonuclear leukocytes are hypersegmented. Hypersegmentation refers to the presence of six or more lobes in a significant number of neutrophils. Varying degrees of anemia, thrombocytopenia, neutropenia, or pancytopenia may be found.

The bone marrow is usually hypercellular with an increase in mitotic figures. The typical cytonuclear dissociation is manifested morphologically in all the hematopoietic cell lines. The red cell precursors demonstrate an immature, nonpyknotic nucleus with open chromatin material and a normally hemoglobinized cytoplasm. The myeloid series shows large metamyelocytes and bands with huge "horseshoe" nuclei and hypersegmented neutrophils. Megakaryocyte nuclei have been described to be multilobulated with an absence of normal connections between the lobes. The increase in cellularity may be confused with a malignant or preleukemic state.

The diagnostic tests differentiating the cause of the megaloblastic anemia are the measurements of the serum and red cell folate levels and the serum vitamin B_{12} level.

The serum levels of folate and vitamin B_{12} can be determined by microbiologic methods or by radioimmunoassay. The advantages of the latter technique are rapidity in obtaining the results and lack of influence by drugs such as folate antagonists or antibiotics.

Once a deficiency of vitamin B_{12} is found in the serum, the Schilling test or vitamin B_{12} absorption test is performed to differentiate PA from vitamin B_{12} malabsorption of intestinal origin.

Gastric achlorhydria is present in virtually all patients with PA. They do not demonstrate any response when maximally stimulated with histamine.

In therapeutic trials with vitamin B_{12} or folate given in physiologic doses for 10 days, the patient is observed for a reticulocyte response, which should occur within 7 days. The diet during the therapeutic trial must be low in vitamin B_{12} and folate. The demonstration of circulating antibodies to IF is strong evidence in favor of PA.

MANAGEMENT. Patients with documented folate deficiency respond well to small doses of folic acid given orally even in the presence of small bowel disease. Since most of the larger doses of folate are lost in the urine and such doses may exacerbate the neurologic symptoms in PA, the maximal recommended dose of folate is 1 mg of folic acid a day. After the body stores are replenished in 2 weeks, lower doses of 0.1 to 0.15 mg daily can be given as maintenance or supplements. Alcoholic patients will respond to these doses even if they continue to imbibe alcohol. Folate therapy can be given during anticonvulsant therapy without the need to withdraw the anticonvulsant. Preventive or prophylactic doses are required in pregnancy, hemolytic anemias, tropical sprue, and patients undergoing hemodialysis.

Vitamin B_{12} deficiency often requires parenteral administration of cyanocobalamin, except perhaps in vegetarians, who can be given oral preparations. Hydroxycobalamin, the preferred preparation, is given intramuscularly on a schedule of six weekly doses of 1000 μg to build body stores of about 3 mg. Then a maintenance dose of 1000 μg every 3 months should provide adequate vitamin B_{12} levels. The widespread use of vitamin B_{12} shots as a tonic or placebo is deplorable.

Blood transfusions are not required unless the patient is elderly or critically ill. Packed RBCs given slowly with or without diuretics may be necessary to prevent the precipitation of congestive heart failure.

BIBLIOGRAPHY

Carmel, R., and Johnson, C.S.: Racial patterns in pernicious anemia: early age at onset and increased frequency of intrinsic-factor antibody in black women, N. Engl. J. Med. **298**:647, 1978.

Doscherholmen, A., and Ripley, D.: Plasma absorption of cyanocobalamin Co 57: diagnostic value in vitamin B_{12} malabsorption sites, Arch. Intern. Med. **134**:1019, 1974.

Erbe, R.W.: Inborn errors of folate metabolism, N. Engl. J. Med. **293**:753, 1975.

Goldberg, L.S., and others: Human autoimmunity, with pernicious anemia as a model, Ann. Intern. Med. **81**:372, 1974.

Lindenbaum, J., Pezzimenti, J.F., and Shea, N.: Small-intestinal function in vitamin B_{12} deficiency, Ann. Intern. Med. **80**:326, 1974.

McPhedran, P., and others: Interpretation of electronically determined macrocytosis, Ann. Intern. Med. **78**:677, 1973.

62 • BONE MARROW FAILURE, SIDEROBLASTIC ANEMIA, AND MYELOPHTHISIC ANEMIA

Emmanuel C. Besa

Bone marrow failure may occur with a reduction in one, two, or all three formed elements of the blood—the red cells, leukocytes, and platelets. The mechanisms involved are not fully understood. The following conditions lead to bone marrow failure:

Hypoplasia or aplasia of marrow
    Aplastic anemia, idiopathic or caused by drugs, chemicals, ionizing radiation, or viral infections
    Fanconi's constitutional anemia, Diamond-Blackfan anemia
    Paroxysmal nocturnal hemoglobinuria
    Immune mechanisms
Normocellular or hypercellular states of marrow
    Myelodysplastic syndromes
    Refractory anemia, preleukemia
    Sideroblastic anemia
Infiltrating lesions in marrow
    Myelophthisic anemia
    Primary myelofibrosis, myelosclerosis
    Agnogenic myeloid metaplasia

Direct injury to the marrow by toxins and drugs or infiltration and destruction by malignant tissue with reactive fibrosis will result in a decrease in marrow cellularity. In such instances the bone marrow study is diagnostic. However, since some patients with peripheral cytopenia may have a normal or hypercellular marrow, peripheral sequestration or destruction of cells in a hypertrophied and overreactive reticuloendothelial system must be considered as a type of "marrow failure." Ineffective hematopoiesis has been inferred in patients with pancytopenia and normal or hypercellular marrows, indicating formation of defective cells that are rapidly removed from the circulation or death within the marrow. Patients with no obvious cause for bone marrow failure should be investigated for marrow cellularity and extent of cytopenia. Some individual clinical syndromes reflecting these mechanisms, such as aplastic anemia, the primary refractory anemias (preleukemic syndromes), sideroblastic anemia, and myelophthisic anemia, will be discussed in this chapter.

APLASTIC ANEMIA

The term "aplastic anemia" usually refers to a condition characterized by abnormally low red cell, neutrophil, and platelet counts in the peripheral blood and by a hypocellular or aplastic bone marrow. Since a single bone marrow aspiration may not represent the total marrow cellularity, it is often difficult to classify patients with one study if a cellular marrow was obtained. Repeat bone marrow aspirations performed at other sites will often confirm the overall hypocellularity of the marrow despite the fact that localized areas of the marrow may remain cellular. Patients with pancytopenia and a hypercellular marrow fall into the broad category of primary refractory anemia. Even if the term "aplastic anemia" is restricted to the hypocellular marrow group, it has become evident that aplastic or hypoplastic anemia is not a single clinical entity.

ETIOLOGY. The following factors may be involved in the aplastic anemia:

Genetic factors
    Fanconi's anemia, Diamond-Blackfan anemia
    Chloramphenicol sensitivity
Agents
    Drugs (antineoplastic, chemotherapeutic, chloramphenicol)
    Chemicals (benzene)
    Ionizing irradiation
    Viral infection (hepatitis)
Immune mechanisms
    Pure red cell aplasia
    Systemic lupus erythematosus
Paroxysmal nocturnal hemoglobinuria

Most cases can be divided into two general groups: (1) those associated with exposure to some toxic agent and (2) those that develop with no identifiable bone marrow insult, that is, idiopathic aplastic anemia (IAA).

The toxic agents can be divided into those that regularly induce bone marrow suppression and those that cause "idiosyncratic" reactions in a few patients. Chemotherapeutic drugs used in cancer treatment produce a predictable dose-related marrow suppression that is usually followed by recovery after withdrawal of the drug. However, a drug such as chloramphenicol may cause either of the two types of bone marrow toxicity. Current evidence indicates a lack of relationship between the reversible suppression and the irreversible aplastic anemia associated with chloramphenicol. The reversible bone marrow suppression is due to mitochondrial injury with profound inhibition of protein synthesis, whereas the aplastic anemia induced by chloramphenicol may be due to a genetic predisposition, as evidence by studies of DNA synthesis in marrows from patients and their relatives.

Transient bone marrow failure may occur during a viral infection. This may lead to mild depression of blood counts with no clinical consequences. In patients with sickle cell anemia and other hereditary hemolytic anemias, a viral infection may induce an aplastic crisis needing supportive care during this transient period. These patients ultimately recover. The aplastic anemia developing after viral hepatitis, however, is a more severe form of bone marrow failure and is often fatal.

PATHOGENESIS. The current concept of hematopoiesis proposes that blood cells originate from pluripotential stem cells that give rise to unipotential committed cells and differentiate into the mature cellular blood elements under the influence or presence of appropriate stimulating substances, among which erythropoietin is the best characterized. These cells have been studied in vitro and defined by their ability to form colonies of mature cells. Bone marrow culture studies in both humans and animals have suggested several possible pathologic sites in aplastic anemia.

The defect in aplastic anemia may be any of the following:

1. *Quantitative or qualitative abnormalities of hematopoietic stem cells.*

2. *Abnormal humoral or cellular control of hematopoiesis.*

3. *Abnormal or hostile hematopoietic microenvironment such as "stromal" abnormalities and immune suppression of hematopoiesis.*

The majority of cases represent a stem cell defect with low colony growth from the bone marrow and successful therapy by transplanting normal marrow from an identical twin or HLA-compatible donor. Providing normal hematopoietic stem cells to these patients may correct the hematologic defect.

It appears that aplastic anemia will prove to be several diseases that share common clinical and morphologic features. With greater use of bone marrow culture techniques, it may be possible to differentiate subgroups of patients and help determine the best possible therapy for each group.

CLINICAL MANIFESTATIONS. The usual symptoms of anemia may bring the patient to a physician, but in most instances the clinical course is insidious. When pancytopenia occurs, the patient has symptoms of bleeding, fever, and/or severe infection (often gram-negative bacillary bacteremia). It may be difficult to distinguish between disseminated intravascular coagulopathy and the underlying thrombocytopenia as the cause of hemorrhage. Not infrequently, petechiae, purpura, or gum bleeding occurs. The physical examination may be unremarkable except for pallor and petechiae. The spleen is not usually enlarged but may become palpable in the final stages of the disease. It is unusual for hepatomegaly or lymphadenopathy to be present in these patients. Patients who have had multiple transfusions may have signs and symptoms of hemosiderosis or hemochromatosis.

LABORATORY FINDINGS. Pancytopenia is an invariable finding in aplastic anemia, with varying degrees of severity in the individual erythrocyte, leukocyte, and platelet counts. The anemia is usually normochromic and normocytic but may occasionally be macrocytic. Reticulocytopenia is usually found, but counts may vary from none to 5%. The total granulocyte count is low and is responsible for the leukopenia, but the absolute lymphocyte count is often decreased as well. Coagulation tests are normal except for the increased bleeding time and poor clot retraction, which reflect the underlying thrombocytopenia. The plasma iron level is normal or slightly increased with a normal iron-binding capacity. Erythropoietin levels are increased in proportion to the degree of anemia, and the fetal hemoglobin level may be elevated in some patients.

The bone marrow may be cellular or markedly hypocellular. When it is cellular, another site is aspirated and biopsied, since focal areas of hyperplasia may occur and may not reflect the total marrow activity. Marked hypocellularity will cause bone marrow aspiration to be "dry," indicating the importance of performing a core biopsy. The biopsy may also reveal other causes, for example, granulomata or malignancy such as metastatic carcinoma or aleukemic leukemia. Iron stores are usually increased unless there was a chronic bleeding problem before the onset of the disease.

It is essential to rule out the other possible causes of pancytopenia listed on p. 319.

COURSE AND PROGNOSIS. The course of aplastic anemia may be short and rapidly fatal, evolving in a few months, or chronic and prolonged, lasting for many years.

The prognosis appears to be better when a bone marrow toxin is evident than in the idiopathic type. Aplastic anemia after viral hepatitis carries a poor prognosis in most instances. When the disease process demonstrates a steady progression, it is invariably fatal. Of patients with a protracted course, a third may go into remission, another third will continue to have a tolerable but low platelet (and sometimes leukocyte) count, and the remaining third will continue to depend on steroids or androgens.

MANAGEMENT. Supportive therapy is necessary to maintain patients with aplastic anemia, and recent developments in blood component separation have made it possible to administer specific cells as required. An ambulatory, asymptomatic patient should be maintained without transfusions, since serious complications such as iron overload, development of platelet antibodies, and serum hepatitis often accompany multiple, long-term transfusions. The value of granulocyte transfusions is still questionable, and they should be reserved for serious infection with a poor response to antibiotic therapy. Iron overload may be prevented by the early administration of desferrioxamine. HLA-matched platelets may benefit patients who are sensitized to previous random-donor platelet transfusions. Specific antibiotics are indicated for different types of infections. Splenectomy is of questionable value and should be avoided unless there is evidence of shortened RBC or platelet survival owing to hypersplenism.

Androgen therapy alone or with corticosteroids may be of value in some patients. A 50% response rate has been observed, but this has been questioned because there are a significant number of spontaneous remissions. The oral forms of androgen have a high incidence of liver toxicity, and all these preparations are virilizing. The grave prognosis of aplastic anemia, however, merits a clinical trial of androgens for 3 months.

In the severe type of aplastic anemia, patients less than 40 years old and their relatives should have tissue typing. If an identical twin or HLA-compatible donor is available, bone marrow transplantation in a center where there are existing facilities and expertise should be attempted. A 50% survival up to 6 years has been reported in patients who received successful grafts in a major medical center.

PRIMARY REFRACTORY ANEMIA (PRELEUKEMIC AND MYELODYSPLASTIC SYNDROMES)

Refractory anemia is a group of bone marrow failure syndromes characterized by varying degrees of anemia, leukopenia, and thrombocytopenia. Bone marrow studies reveal normal or increased cellularity, which distinguishes the syndrome from aplastic anemia. The exclusion of disorders resulting in increased peripheral destruction, known nutritional deficiencies, and acute leukemias is required. The term "refractory" refers to the usual unresponsive course of these syndromes to vitamins, iron, or hormonal therapy.

This heterogeneous group of syndromes has been given several descriptive names such as megaloblastic refractory anemia, aregenerative anemia, chronic marrow failure, preleukemia, and, more recently, the myelodysplastic syndromes. These syndromes should be distinguished from distinct disease entities that predispose patients to the development of acute leukemia, such as Fanconi's anemia.

ETIOLOGY. The abnormal maturation in the myelodysplastic syndromes or refractory anemia results in ineffective erythropoiesis, granulocytopoiesis, and thrombocytopoiesis. The cause of this disorder is frequently undetermined or idiopathic, and it often evolves into an acute myeloblastic or myelomonocytic leukemia. For this reason it has been called preleukemia or smoldering acute leukemia. These terms should be avoided, since leukemia is not an inevitable outcome.

PATHOGENESIS. A dysplasia is a derangement of the development of cells and tissues resulting in a defect in cellular size growth and maturation. If the inciting cause can be identified and removed, the anemia may be reversible. In refractory anemia the dysplasia may be a consequence of both qualitative and quantitative defects in the hematopoietic stem cells. A role of the microenvironment and suppressor cells similar to that in the aplastic anemia syndrome has been suggested. The cytogenetic changes imply an evolution to an abnormal clone in the hematopoietic stem cells and may be a result of marrow injury.

CLINICAL MANIFESTATIONS. The course of refractory anemia is similar to that of aplastic anemia, but patients may have a decrease in one or two cell lines rather than pancytopenia.

LABORATORY FINDINGS. The anemia in this disorder is usually normochromic and normocytic. A slight macrocytosis with red cells demonstrating anisopoikilocytosis may be found in most cases. The reticulocytes are decreased, and neutropenia is common. Platelet counts may vary from normal to mild or moderate thrombocytopenia. Platelets are large and hypogranular. Neutrophils demonstrate poor granulation with an occasional Pelger-Huët-like anomaly (increased numbers of band forms).

The bone marrow is often cellular to hypercellular, and maturational defects are seen in all three cell lines. "Megaloblastoid" changes in the red cell precursors with vacuolation of cytoplasm are observed, and sideroblasts are frequent.

DIAGNOSIS. Refractory anemia with accompanying leukopenia or thrombocytopenia is often accompanied by a cellular marrow with a slight increase in blasts and megaloblastic changes indicating a maturational defect. This must be differentiated from aleukemic leukemia, nutritional deficiency anemia, or erythroleukemia. Secondary causes must be ruled out, since most of these are reversible.

COURSE. The duration of the hematologic disorder before the development of an acute and fatal type of leukemia may vary from 6 months to 1 to 2 years. A few patients have a prolonged course of up to 20 years. Since these patients frequently die from other illness such as congestive heart failure or from the complications of their cytopenias, the incidence of leukemic transformation is at best speculative, but it is probably 10% to 50%.

MANAGEMENT. The treatment of refractory anemia remains difficult, since there are no existing methods to distinguish the patients in whom leukemia will develop within the next few weeks from those who will have a chronic course of 5 to 10 years or longer. Aggressive antileukemic therapy has not been shown to be of benefit until an overt form of leukemia becomes evident.

Supportive therapy such as periodic blood transfusions for the existing cytopenias remains the mainstay of treatment. Attempts to stimulate the bone marrow with pharmacologic doses of cyanocobalamin, folate, pyridoxine, pyridoxal phosphate, androgens, and corticosteroids have been of limited success. Splenectomy is usually ineffective, although an occasional patient may show a decrease in neutropenia or thrombocytopenia.

SIDEROBLASTIC ANEMIA

Sideroblastic anemia is another form of bone marrow failure. Anemia, the most prominent feature, is associated with an increase in red cell precursors called ringed sideroblasts that contain excess stainable iron granules around the cell nucleus. Electron microscopy of these cells demonstrates the abnormal accumulation of iron in the mitochondria. This hematologic disorder may be either hereditary or acquired and is observed in association with a heterogeneous etiologic background.

ETIOLOGY. Familial forms of sideroblastic anemia may or may not respond to high doses of pyridoxine and may have an X-linked or autosomal form of inheritance (see Chapter 65). The acquired form of this syndrome may be idiopathic or secondary to a toxin. Drugs such as chloramphenicol, pyrazinamide, and isoniazid and toxins such as alcohol and lead have been observed to cause a reversible form of sideroblastic anemia that responds favorably to the administration of pyridoxine and the withdrawal of the causative agent. The idiopathic refractory form does not respond to such treatment and carries a risk of leukemic transformation. The syndrome may be another form or manifestation of a hematopoietic stem cell mutation similar to preleukemia. An immunologic cause has been implicated in some cases, and association with lupus erythematosus, autoimmune hemolytic anemia, and monoclonal gammopathy with lymphoma has been reported. An IgG antibody–mediated acquired sideroblastic anemia has been shown to respond to immunosuppressive therapy.

PATHOGENESIS. The basic defect in sideroblastic anemia is an impairment of the heme biosynthetic pathway at the iron and protoporphyrin step resulting in the accumulation of mitochondrial iron and lack of heme synthesis. Deficiency or abnormalities in the enzyme activities of aminolevulinic acid (ALA) synthetase, uroporphyrinogen decarboxylase, or heme synthetase have been observed in these patients. A deficiency in pyridoxine or a defect in the conversion of pyridoxin to pyridoxal-5-phosphate, the active moiety for the ALA synthetase, may lead to sideroblastic anemia. These abnormalities will lead to lack of protoporphyrin and iron accumulation in the mitochondria. Iron loading of the mitochondria will eventually cause peroxidation of the lipids, swelling and disintegration of these organelles, and eventual cell death resulting in ineffective erythropoiesis.

CLINICAL MANIFESTATIONS. Idiopathic refractory sideroblastic anemia usually occurs equally in men and women in their sixth decade. Most of these patients have symptoms referable to the anemia. Skin and mucosal pallor is the most prominent physical finding. Less than half of the patients have hepatosplenomegaly.

LABORATORY FINDINGS. The acquired idiopathic type of sideroblastic anemia is usually associated with a macrocytic, hypochromic type of anemia. The reticulocyte count is usually normal or increased, and the peripheral blood smear shows a dimorphic population with both normal appearing red blood cells and large hypochromic cells with basophilic stippling. The white cell and platelet counts are usually normal. The bone marrow is hypercellular with a characteristic erythroid hyperplasia and increased iron stores. Chromosomal aberrations similar to those described in preleukemia have been observed.

DIAGNOSIS. The important diagnostic feature is the demonstration of characteristic ringed sideroblasts in the bone marrow. Although the red cell indices indicate hypochromia, the peripheral red cells tend to be macrocytic rather than microcytic, in contrast to iron deficiency, thalassemia, and the pyridoxine-responsive sideroblastic anemias. It is important to eliminate secondary causes in the history; occasionally serum lead levels may reveal an occult lead poisoning. Megaloblastic changes in the red cell precursor may also require differentiation from disorders of vitamin B_{12} and folate metabolism. Differentiation from the preleukemic patient can be the most difficult problem. It is suggested that chromosomal aberration and the presence of elevated levels of hemoglobin F indicate a poor prognosis whereas thrombocytosis may indicate a benign course. The appearance of sideroblasts in the bone marrow of patients taking alkylating agents usually indicates an early stage of leukemic transformation.

COURSE. Hereditary forms of sideroblastic anemia are heterogeneous and may or may not respond to pyridoxine. The pyridoxine-responsive anemias require maintenance therapy. The acquired idiopathic form may have a chronic, protracted course or may terminate in acute leukemia. Reports have suggested that half of the patients are preleukemic or at an early stage of DiGuglielmo syndrome. However, a recent larger study indicates that the majority of cases have a prolonged course with a median survival of 10 years and that only about 7% to 10% undergo leukemic transformation.

MANAGEMENT. Most patients with sideroblastic anemia are refractory to all forms of therapy and require maintenance transfusions. The use of iron chelators may be necessary to avoid iron overload. Every patient should have a therapeutic trial of pyridoxine and folic acid. Steroids and androgens for 3 months may reduce the transfusion requirements in a few patients. Immunosuppression by cyclophosphamide has been successful in documented immune-mediated sideroblastic anemia. Aggressive chemotherapy may be indicated at the time of leukemic transformation, but the outcome is usually unfavorable.

MYELOPHTHISIS AND SECONDARY FORMS OF MYELOFIBROSIS

The term "myelophthisis" refers to the association of marrow invasion or injury by abnormal cells and/or fibrosis with characteristic "leukoerythroblastic" peripheral blood changes.

ETIOLOGY. The following are some causes of myelophthisic anemia:

Hematologic neoplasm
    Leukemia
        Chronic myelocytic leukemia
        Acute myeloblastic leukemia
    Multiple myeloma
    Hodgkins's disease
    Lymphosarcoma
    Reticulum cell sarcoma
Other tumors
    Prostatic carcinoma
    Breast carcinoma
    Stomach adenocarcinoma
    Lung carcinoma, primarily oat cell carcinoma
Infection
    Tuberculosis
    Osteomyelitis (focal fibrosis)
Other diseases
    Agnogenic myeloid metaplasia, polycythemia vera
    Marble bone disease
    Paget's disease
    Gaucher's disease
    Amyloidosis

The majority of the hematologic malignancies such as leukemias, lymphomas, and multiple myeloma involve infiltration of the marrow by abnormal cells, resulting in failure of normal hematopoiesis. Malignant tumors from other organs such as the prostate, breast, and lungs often metastasize to the marrow. Tuberculosis and fungal infections may involve the marrow and cause myelophthisic anemia. Inherited enzymatic defects such as Gaucher's disease may be associated with abnormal cells in the bone marrow, but the hematologic abnormality in these diseases usually results from hypersplenism.

PATHOGENESIS. The marrow is usually replaced by tumor cells and myelofibrosis. The mechanism involved in the resulting cytopenia, release of the hematopoietic precursor cells into the circulation, and myelofibrosis is unknown. Tumor cells are not always demonstrated in the marrow with myelofibrosis, but reversal of the fibrosis is associated with response of the primary disease to antitumor therapy in Hodgkin's disease and carcinomas of the prostate and breast.

CLINICAL MANIFESTATIONS AND LABORATORY FINDINGS.

The most striking finds in this entity or syndrome are the laboratory test results. The clinical manifestations are attributable to the primary disease but occasionally may include symptoms referable to the pancytopenia such as infection, bleeding, or severe anemia. Hepatosplenomegaly is prominent if hypersplenism is present. The leukoerythroblastic blood picture consists of nucleated red cells and the presence of myeloid precursor cells.

Bone marrow aspiration and biopsy are usually diagnostic for the primary disease if performed in the involved area. The bone scan may be helpful in determining which iliac crest to biopsy if the marrow is involved in localized areas. In disseminated metastasis or miliary tuberculosis the marrow examination can be performed in any of the usual sites of bone marrow examination.

MANAGEMENT. Myelophthisis is managed with supportive therapy for the hematologic abnormalities and specific treatment of the underlying disease.

BIBLIOGRAPHY

Camitta, B.M., and others: A prospective study of androgens and bone marrow transplantation for treatment of severe aplastic anemia, Blood **53**:504, 1979.

Cartwright, G.E., and Deiss, A.: Sideroblasts, siderocytes, and sideroblastic anemia, N. Engl. J. Med. **292**:185, 1975.

Chang, D.S., Kushner, J.P., and Wintrobe, M.M.: Idiopathic refractory sideroblastic anemia: incidence and risk factors for leukemic transformation, Cancer **44**:724, 1979.

Fitchen, J.H., and Cline, M.J.: Recent developments in understanding the pathogenesis of aplastic anemia, Am. J. Hematol. **5**:365, 1978.

Kushner, J.P., and others: Idiopathic refractory sideroblastic anemia: clinical and laboratory investigation of 17 patients and review of the literature, Medicine **50**:139, 1971.

Linman, J.W., and Saarni, M.I.: The preleukemic syndrome, Semin. Hematol. **11**:93, 1974.

Piere, R.V.: Preleukemic states, Semin. Hematol. **11**:73, 1974.

Speck, B., and others: Immunologic aspects of aplasia, Transplant. Proc. **10**:131, 1978.

Wintrobe, M.M., and others: Clinical hematology, ed. 7, Philadelphia, 1974, Lea & Febiger.

63 • ACUTE POSTHEMORRHAGIC ANEMIA

William E. Barry

Acute posthemorrhagic anemia results from the rapid loss of whole blood. It may occur from trauma (including surgery), rupture or erosion of blood vessels, or defects in hemostasis. It is usually apparent, except when it occurs in body tissues (muscle, retroperitoneal space), body cavities (pleural, pericardial, or peritoneal), or transiently in the gastrointestinal tract.

CLINICAL MANIFESTATIONS. The clinical manifestations vary with the amount, rate, and location of the hemorrhage, as well as with the patient's general state of health and the presence of disease in critical organ systems. The early effects of hemorrhage involve changes in blood volume and organ perfusion. Following cessation of hemorrhage, compensatory or reparative functions related to red cell production become apparent. In the healthy young adult the rapid loss of 500 to 1000 ml of blood (10% to 20% of blood volume) is usually tolerated without symptoms. Some, however, may have weakness, sweating, nausea, bradycardia, and hypotension. Occasionally syncope occurs. The rapid loss of 1000 to 1500 ml of blood (20% to 30% of blood volume) may cause symptoms only in the upright position or with exertion. The rapid loss of 1500 to 2000 ml (30% to 40% of blood volume) usually results in hypovolemic shock, which may be irreversible if the blood loss exceeds 2000 to 2500 ml (40% to 50% of blood volume).

LABORATORY FINDINGS. Following hemorrhage there is no immediate change in the hemoglobin or hematocrit level, since plasma and red cells are lost proportionately. Within hours an increase in white blood cells and platelets is seen. The restoration of plasma volume begins quickly, but its magnitude is such that dilutional changes in the hemoglobin and hematocrit continue over a period of 2 to 3 days. Thus the magnitude of the blood loss cannot be appreciated in the first few hours, perhaps not even for 24 hours, by which time the maximal rate of plasma volume restoration is achieved. Further decline in the hemoglobin and hematocrit levels continues slowly over the next 48 to 72 hours but is less significant than the decline at 24 hours.

Evidence of active red blood cell regeneration, manifested by an increase in reticulocytes, begins after about 3 days, reaching a maximum (rarely higher than 15%) in 5 to 10 days. Acute blood loss in the presence of normal iron sources does not usually result in a hypochromic anemia. Chronic blood loss with exhaustion of iron stores is necessary to produce the hypochromic anemia of iron deficiency.

MANAGEMENT. The immediate treatment of posthemorrhagic anemia is directed toward restoration of blood volume, preferably with whole blood. If whole blood is not immediately available, albumin, plasma, plasma volume expanders, or even saline solutions can be given intravenously.

BIBLIOGRAPHY

Wintrobe, M.M., and others: Clinical hematology, ed. 7, Philadelphia, 1974, Lea & Febiger.

64 • IRON DEFICIENCY ANEMIA

William E. Barry

On a worldwide basis, iron deficiency is the most common cause of anemia encountered in epidemiologic studies and clinical practice. About 10% to 15% of women in the reproductive years have been noted to have iron deficiency anemia. Even in women without overt anemia, body iron depletion, that is, absent or diminished iron stores, is very common. Pregnancy, infancy, and adolescence represent other critical periods of life when body iron deficiency and iron deficiency anemia are frequent. The importance of iron deficiency anemia can scarcely be overestimated, not only because it is such a common and universally occurring health problem but also because of the tragic implications for the individual patient in whom iron deficiency anemia is caused by blood loss from an unrecognized and hence neglected gastrointestinal neoplasm.

ETIOLOGY. The most important cause of iron deficiency anemia in adults is *blood loss*. Most often this is due to gastrointestinal tract lesions such as peptic ulcer, hemorrhoids, colonic neoplasms, gastritis from long-term aspirin ingestion, hiatus hernia, and diverticulosis.

In women menstrual blood loss accounts for most instances of iron deficiency anemia. Rare causes in both sexes include mechanical hemolytic anemia with persistent urinary hemoglobin loss, excessive blood donation, idiopathic pulmonary hemosiderosis, and hereditary hemorrhagic telangiectasia.

Dietary lack of iron is an important cause of iron deficiency anemia *only* in children under age 3. This is especially true when body iron stores are deficient at birth, as in premature infants, twins, and those with late clamping of the umbilical cord. A prolonged milk diet in infancy, containing little iron, is perhaps the most frequent cause of iron deficiency anemia in such children. The early introduction to solid foods and iron fortification of infant formulas serve to reduce the frequency of this problem. Even in this age group gastrointestinal blood loss from a Meckel's diverticulum or from mucosal bleeding caused by milk intolerance is occasionally seen. The growth spurt of adolescence, although less rapid than that occuring in the first year of life, may cause a transient discrepancy between iron supply and body iron requirements, resulting in iron deficiency but rarely in overt iron deficiency anemia.

Pregnancy causes a net iron loss to the mother of about 680 mg and a temporary "loss" of another 450 mg to her expanded red cell mass. This exceeds a woman's usual iron stores. Further, most of the iron drain occurs in the last trimester and cannot be made up rapidly enough from dietary sources despite increased absorption of iron from food. Hence, iron supplementation is needed to prevent overt iron deficiency anemia in most pregnant women. The problem is aggravated if a women enters pregnancy with depleted or absent iron stores owing to previous menstrual blood loss.

PATHOGENESIS. Iron deficiency anemia results, ultimately, from an inadequate supply of iron for normal hemoglobin synthesis in developing erythroid cells in the bone marrow. Understanding how this comes about requires an appreciation of certain aspects of normal iron metabolism.

CLINICAL MANIFESTATIONS. The symptoms of iron deficiency anemia vary in severity, depending on the degree of anemia, the rapidity of its onset, and the presence of disease in other organ systems. In older patients symptoms of dyspnea, palpitations, or angina pectoris may occur, reflecting the frequency of coexisting organic heart disease. In younger patients the symptoms may be vague and nonspecific and may include fatigue, lassitude, and anorexia.

Physical findings include pallor of the skin and mucous membranes. Loss of papillae on the lateral aspect of the tongue frequently occurs, and occasionally cracking at the corners of the mouth is seen. Hemic (flow) murmurs are commonly heard. A palpable spleen has been reported in up to 10% of the patients. Rarely, retinal hemorrhages and even papilledema are seen with severe anemia. Spoon-shaped nails are characteristic but not pathognomonic of severe iron deficiency anemia.

LABORATORY FINDINGS. A hypochromic microcytic anemia is characteristic of iron deficiency anemia. In cases where the anemia is only slight, the red cell indices may be normal. The serum iron level is low, and the total iron-binding capacity is usually increased. A variety of abnormal red blood cell shapes may be seen in the stained blood smear. The reticulocyte count is normal or low, and the platelet count may be increased.

The bone marrow is usually cellular. Erythroid hyperplasia is sometimes seen. The nucleated red blood cells are hemoglobin poor, with scanty cytoplasm. No stainable iron is visible in the marrow fragment or the nucleated erythroid cells. The serum ferritin level is low. The level of protoporphyrin in mature red cells is elevated.

DIAGNOSIS. The diagnosis of iron deficiency anemia is made by finding the characteristic hypochromic microcytic red cell indices with a low serum iron level and elevated total iron-binding capacity. In doubtful cases the diagnosis of iron deficiency is confirmed by the lack of stainable marrow iron.

Iron deficiency anemia can be confused with the thalassemia trait, or the two may occasionally coexist. The β-thalassemia trait is associated with an elevated percentage of hemoglobin A_2. Patients with the α-thalassemia trait have normal levels of hemoglobin A_2, and family studies are needed to establish the diagnosis.

Anemia of chronic disease usually has normocytic normochromic red blood cell indices, but occasionally the red blood cells are hypochromic. In this disorder the serum iron level is low, similar to iron deficiency, but the total iron-binding capacity is low rather than high. In addition, stainable iron is present in the marrow in RE cells. Rarely, iron deficiency may coexist with anemia of chronic disease and defy precise diagnosis.

When iron deficiency anemia is confirmed, it is imperative to determine the cause, which almost always is blood loss. It is particularly important to exclude a gastrointestinal neoplasm by appropriate studies.

COURSE. Iron deficiency anemia often pursues an insidious course owing to adaptive mechanisms that limit the impact on the patient despite significantly low levels of hemoglobin. These adaptive mechanisms include an increase in red blood cell production and an increase in the level of 2,3-diphosphoglycerate (2,3-DPG) in the mature erythrocyte. The increase in 2,3-DPG, a product of glycolysis, causes a shift in the oxygen dissociation curve of hemoglobin, enabling oxygen to be more readily released to tissues. Despite these adaptive mechanisms, and possibly because iron deficiency may affect intracellular enzyme function in a way not yet clearly defined, the symptoms eventually assume proportions sufficient to cause the patient to seek help. Alternatively, the asymptomatic state may prevail, and the diagnosis is made by a routine blood count in the course of evaluating an unrelated disorder.

Once the diagnosis is defined accurately, treatment with iron usually results in a satisfactory improvement in the symptoms and the hemoglobin level. Anemia may recur if the cause is not permanently removed. Thus any source of chronic blood loss may be important in the failure to correct, completely or permanently, iron deficiency anemia despite appropriate therapy.

MANAGEMENT. The treatment of iron deficiency anemia is usually simple, effective, and inexpensive. Ferrous sulfate, 300 mg orally three times a day, is the treatment of choice. About 10% of the patients complain of unacceptable gastrointestinal intolerance and may require parenteral therapy. Delayed-release forms of orally administered iron, although well tolerated, may be ineffective owing to relatively poor absorption of iron beyond the duodenum.

In an otherwise uncomplicated case a complete response is achieved by 4 to 8 weeks. If a response is not achieved by that time, reevaluation is indicated regarding (1) accuracy of the diagnosis, (2) patient compliance with the prescribed dose of iron, (3) continued blood loss, or (4) (rarely) malabsorption of orally administered iron.

BIBLIOGRAPHY

Finch, C.A., and others: Ferrokinetics in man, Medicine **49**:17, 1970.
Hallberg, L., Harwerth, H.-G., and Vannotti, A., editors: Iron deficiency: pathogenesis, clinical aspects, therapy, New York, 1970, Academic Press, Inc.
Hillman, R.S., and Finch, C.A.: Red cell manual, Philadelphia, 1974, F.A. Davis Co.

65 • OTHER HYPOCHROMIC MICROCYTIC ANEMIAS

William E. Barry

In addition to iron deficiency, other disorders may result in inadequate hemoglobin synthesis in the erythrocyte. Three principal mechanisms usually account for this: (1) inadequate porphyrin synthesis, (2) a defect in coupling of iron to protoporphyrin to form heme, and (3) a defect in globin synthesis. Compared with iron deficiency, these disorders are rare.

Inadequate porphyrin synthesis occurs in *pyridoxine-responsive anemia*. Pyridoxal phosphate is required as a cofactor in the first step in porphyrin synthesis, the formation of δ-aminolevulinic acid from glycine and coenzyme A. Since large amounts of pyridoxine are necessary for therapy, it appears that the anemia is not due to an absolute deficiency of pyridoxine. A similar anemia may occur if there is interference with the activity of pyridoxine by drugs such as isoniazid. Lead poisoning interferes with porphyrin synthesis at several steps resulting in a net deficiency of hemoglobin, among other effects of lead on protein synthesis and membrane function. Lead poisoning characteristically causes basophilic stippling in the erythrocyte. Other laboratory features of lead poisoning include elevated blood and urine levels and increased excretion of porphyrins in urine. Defects in enzymatic coupling of iron to protoporphyrin to form heme have been implicated rarely as a cause of hypochromic anemia.

"Ringed" sideroblasts, resulting from the perinuclear mitochondrial accumulation of iron not utilized in heme synthesis, may be seen in these hypochromic anemias. The presence of ringed sideroblasts is characteristic of the sideroblastic anemias, some of which result from identifiable defects in heme synthesis as just noted. In others (the hereditary or acquired "idiopathic" types), the exact mechanisms have not been defined. These are discussed in Chapter 62.

The thalassemias are examples of inadequate synthesis of α- or β-globin chains. Since heme synthesis is unaffected, ringed sideroblasts do not occur.

A rare cause of hypochromic anemia is atransferrinemia, wherein iron cannot be transported to the erythroblast but is deposited in excess amounts in other organs. A rare disorder has also been described in which transferrin iron, although present in increased amount, cannot enter the erythroblast, possibly because of an abnormality in the transferrin receptor site on the erythroblast membrane.

BIBLIOGRAPHY

Anemias characterized by deficient hemoglobin synthesis and impaired iron metabolism. In Wintrobe, M.M., and others, editors: Clinical hematology, ed. 7, Philadelphia, 1974, Lea & Febiger.

66 • ANEMIA OF CHRONIC DISEASE

William E. Barry

DEFINITION. The anemia of chronic disease is the most common anemia seen in hospitalized patients. Many terms, such as anemia of infection, anemia of malignancy, and simple chronic anemia, are used to describe this disorder.

ETIOLOGY. Systemic illnesses, especially those characterized by chronic inflammation, frequently are associated with the anemia of chronic disease. These include lung abscess, osteomyelitis, pneumonia, bacterial endocarditis, and a variety of other chronic inflammatory processes. Rheumatoid arthritis and metastatic malignancy are other typical diseases characterized by this secondary form of anemia. The anemia is not confined to these illnesses, however, and occasionally is found in the absence of any identifiable underlying disease.

PATHOGENESIS. The anemia of chronic disease is characterized by (1) a hemolytic component manifested by a slight shortening of red cell survival, (2) inadequate marrow compensatory response to this shortened red cell survival, and (3) low serum iron level and decreased total iron-binding capacity.

The mechanism of the shortened red cell survival has not been clearly defined. Immunoglobulins are not detected on the red cell membrane, nor are there identified abnormalities of the red cell itself. It has been suggested that the phagocytic function of the reticuloendothelial (RE) system is "hyperactive" for both circulating red cells and developing erythroblasts in the marrow.

The mechanism for the functional marrow inadequacy has been the subject of recent investigation. The evidence is conflicting, but it appears that an inappropriately low synthesis of erythropoietin or a defect in marrow response to erythropoietin is the most likely explanation. Whether the inadequate response is related to an insufficient usable marrow supply or iron has not been definitely proved. Nevertheless, the characteristically low serum iron level is an essential marker of the anemia and is related to a block in RE cell release of iron to plasma transferrin. It has been suggested that the RE cell, during the processing of hemoglobin from senescent red cells, shunts iron preferentially into ferritin within the cell rather than dispersing it rapidly out of the cell to plasma transferrin, resulting in a low serum iron level.

CLINICAL MANIFESTATIONS. The anemia of chronic disease is usually of little clinical consequence. The underlying disease responsible for the anemia dominates the clinical picture. Occasionally, however, the anemia is severe enough to cause symptoms and may require red cell transfusions.

The anemia develops slowly as a rule, only occasionally occurring in illnesses lasting less than 3 to 6 weeks. Thus acute infections are not usually associated with anemia unless additional mechanisms, such as an autoimmune hemolytic process, or an underlying illness is already present.

LABORATORY FINDINGS. The anemia of chronic disease, with hemoglobin levels between 9 and 11 g/dl, is typically normochromic and normocytic, but on occasion a hypochromic picture is noted. The reticulocyte count is low. The most characteristic feature is a low serum iron level accompanied (unlike iron deficiency) by a low total iron-binding capacity. The serum ferritin level is usually modestly elevated.

Bone marrow examination discloses no morphologic abnormalities, except for the iron stain, which shows stainable iron in RE cells but reduced iron in developing red blood cells.

DIAGNOSIS. The finding of a mild normocytic normochromic anemia in a patient with a chronic illness, accompanied by a low serum iron level and a low total iron-binding capacity, is enough to establish a diagnosis of anemia of chronic disease. The most important differential diagnosis is between mild iron deficiency anemia and anemia of chronic disease. When the serum iron changes are equivocal, determination of the serum ferritin level or, more reliably, a sample of bone marrow stained for iron is necessary to distinguish between the two disorders.

COURSE AND MANAGEMENT. The course of anemia of chronic disease varies with the progress of the underlying illness. There is no useful treatment available for the anemia, and it responds only to successful treatment of the underlying disease. Packed red cell transfusions are sometimes of temporary benefit if the anemia is severe or compromises cardiovascular function. Iron therapy is ineffective.

BIBLIOGRAPHY

Cartwright, G.: The anemia of chronic disorders, Semin. Hematol. 3:351, 1966.

67 • ANEMIAS CAUSED BY RED CELL DESTRUCTION

Jerome I. Brody

Hemolytic anemia is the clinical state or condition in which there is a reduction in the life span (normally about 120 days) of the circulating red blood cell associated with failure of the bone marrow to restore completely the quantity of erythrocytes prematurely eliminated from the peripheral blood. Normally, erythropoiesis maintains a dynamic state in which the rate of red blood cell production equals the rate of destruction. These processes are balanced, so that in a 70-kg person 1% of the total red cell mass or 25 ml of red cells is replaced daily. If red cell destruction exceeds the bone marrow's capacity to increase red blood cell output (the usual maximum is six to eight times normal), the hemolysis is uncompensated and anemia results. On the other hand, if the marrow can meet the peripheral demands, hemolysis may be ongoing but is compensated and anemia does not occur.

There are certain similarities and differences between the events of normal red cell clearance and those sequences occurring during inappropriate hemolysis. Whereas gross red cell membrane injury, such as that caused by a mismatched transfusion, may lead to intravascular hemolysis, the alterations associated with red cell aging are more delicate. Physiologic erythrocyte removal takes place within the reticuloendothelial system, especially the spleen and liver, and less importantly in the bone marrow and lungs. Most abnormal and excessive red cell destruction also occurs extravascularly.

The exact signal that identifies the effete red cell and the precise and detailed mechanism for its removal are unknown. Conceivably, subtle changes in shape and biophysical characteristics indicate senescence and recognition for elimination. Because of its microanatomy and vascular structure, the spleen is admirably suited to mechanical trapping of red cells as they course through the splenic arterioles into the sinuses of the red pulp. The liver also participates in red cell removal but clears erythrocytes having comparatively more severe biochemical, physical, and immunogenic injury or abnormalities.

Within the reticuloendothelial macrophages, red cell hemoglobin degradation begins by cleavage of heme protoporphyrin to produce biliverdin, which is promply reduced to bilirubin. After conjugation in the liver the bilirubin is excreted into the bile and reduced in the colon to urobilinogen by anaerobic bacteria. In a healthy, 70-kg person, the 6.25 g of hemoglobin derived daily from the 25 ml of aged erythrocytes is metabolized easily by the liver. Unconjugated hyperbilirubinemia may occur if there is a twofold increase in bilirubin turnover of a 50% reduction in hepatic bilirubin clearance. Such changes result in a doubling of the plasma bilirubin concentration. However, even when the maximal daily rate of bilirubin production of 40 mg/kg, about eight times the upper limit of normal, is reached, such overproduction will elevate the plasma unconjugated bilirubin concentration no higher than 3.5 to 4 mg/dl. Therefore a plasma unconjugated bilirubin concentration persistently in excess of 4 mg/dl implies abnormal hepatic function irrespective of hemolysis.

If intravascular hemolysis rather than extravascular red cell removal occurs, hemoglobinemia and hemoglobinuria may be detected. When the plasma haptoglobin binding capacity for hemoglobin and the proximal renal tubular reabsorption ability are exceeded, free hemoglobin passes into the glomerular filtrate, resulting in hemoglobinuria. The hemoglobin may be absorbed by the renal tubular cells, degraded to hemosiderin in situ by heme oxygenase, and later excreted, resulting in hemosiderinuria. A portion of the intervascular hemoglobin may also be oxidized to methemoglobin, which then dissociates to free hemin and globin.

The diagnosis of hemolytic anemia may be suspected because of the ethnic, racial, and familial background of the patient; prior anemia; ingestion of drugs known to cause hemolysis; presence of certain systemic disorders; special events such as previous surgery for valvular heart disease; and specific patient complaints involving organ systems frequently associated with excess red blood cell destruction.

The symptoms of hemolytic anemia are those of anemia in general. Their severity depends on how the hemoglobin and packed cell volume levels are, the rate at which these levels have been reached, the degree of shift in the oxygen dissociation curve, the compensatory capacity of the cardiovascular and pulmonary systems, and, finally, whether the anemia is stable, progressive, or episodic. General complaints may vary and may include early fatigue, lassitude, decreased exercise tolerance, palpitations, dyspnea, tachypnea, dizziness, headache, and tinnitus. Some symptoms may be more specific and directed toward a particular organ system. Physical findings depend on the specific disease present and may include pallor, tachycardia, icterus, lymphadenopathy, hepatomegaly, splenomegaly, bony tenderness, and neurologic abnormalities.

The following outline classifies the causes of hemolytic anemia:

I. Congenital hemolytic anemias
   A. Membrane defects
      1. Hereditary spherocytosis
      2. Hereditary elliptocytosis
      3. Hereditary stomatocytosis
      4. Lipid abnormalities
   B. Enzyme deficiencies
      1. Defects of the Embden-Meyerhof pathway
      2. Deficiencies in the hexose monophosphate shunt and glutathione metabolism
      3. Other enzyme defects
   C. Disorders of hemoglobin
      1. Single amino acid substitutions
         a. β-Chain (hemoglobins S, C, D, and so on)
         b. α-Chain
         c. γ-Chain
         d. δ-Chain
      2. Two amino acid substitutions in the subunit (hemoglobin C_{Harlem})
      3. Unbalanced subunit synthesis (quantitatively deficient globin chain synthesis)
         a. β-Thalassemia
         b. α-Thalassemia and so on
      4. Errors in subunit termination (nucleoside base substitution in terminal codon)
         a. α-Chain (hemoglobin Constant Spring)
         b. β-Chain (hemoglobin Tak)
      5. Fusion hemoglobins (hemoglobins Lepore, Miyada, Kenya)
      6. Amino acid deletions (many unstable hemoglobins)
      7. Frame shift mutation (deletion of one or two codon nucleoside bases; hemoglobin Wayne)
      8. Other abnormal hemoglobins
II. Acquired hemolytic anemias
   A. Immunohemolytic anemias
      1. Alloimmune
         a. Incompatible blood transfusions
         b. Hemolytic disease of the newborn

2. Autoimmune
   a. Warm-reacting antibodies
   b. Cold-reacting antibodies
B. Traumatic hemolytic anemia
   1. Prosthetic valves and other vascular abnormalities
   2. Microangiopathic hemolysis
   3. March hemoglobinuria
C. Paroxysmal nocturnal hemoglobinuria (PNH; membrane dysplasia)
D. Drug-induced anemia
   1. Immunocytolytic
   2. Nonimmune
      a. Enzyme deficiencies
      b. Unstable hemoglobins
      c. Others
E. Hemolysis owing to other causes
   1. Chemical and physical agents
   2. Metabolic defects
   3. Infectious agents
F. Sequestration hemolysis
   1. Hypersplenism
   2. Reticuloendothelioses

The degree of anemia and reticulocytosis may be inconstant. The level of reticulocytosis is a function of the bone marrow's attempt to compensate for the reduced peripheral red cell mass. Reticulocytosis should be comparatively higher as the anemia becomes more severe, providing the bone marrow is competent and sufficient hematinics are available. Depending on the dynamics, degree, and type of the anemia, methemoglobinemia, hemoglobinemia, hemoglobinuria, and hemosiderinuria may or may not be present.

The definitive diagnostic test for excessive erythrocyte destruction is the evaluation of the red cell life span. For clinical purposes this is usually done by labeling red cells with ^{51}Cr and calculating their survival from the radioactivity in sequential blood samples using the dilution principle. Normal survival as measured by this method is 60 rather than 120 days, with results expressed as the chromium half-life activity ($T_{\frac{1}{2}}$). Normally this is 28 to 32 days. If gastrointestinal bleeding is a clinical consideration in addition to hemolysis, simultaneous assay of fecal radioactivity is necessary to avoid misinterpretation of the data provided by this technique.

CONGENITAL HEMOLYTIC ANEMIAS
Membrane defects
HEREDITARY SPHEROCYTOSIS

DEFINITION AND PATHOGENESIS. Hereditary spherocytosis (HS), also called congenital hemolytic jaundice, is a congenital hemolytic anemia transmitted as an autosomal dominant trait. In this condition an abnormality within the red cell membrane leads to a gradual loss of membrane surface area during the life span of the erythrocyte, so that instead of remaining a flexible biconcave disk it becomes a tight sphere. The primary lesion has not been identified precisely. Whatever the ultimate defect, it increases the glycolytic rate, augments the entry of sodium and water to the cell, and alters the shape of the cell. The change in shape and reduced cell deformability are the pivotal factors that permit the spleen, with its low-velocity blood flow and acidic environment, to become the selective and focal organ for red cell sequestration and destruction.

EPIDEMIOLOGY AND CLINICAL MANIFESTATIONS. HS occurs worldwide but is most common in Northern Europeans. It is the most frequently observed congenital hemolytic anemia in whites.

The clinical manifestations of HS may be remarkably diverse and may vary from one patient to another and from family to family. Its mode of presentation may be age dependent. It can be mild and go completely unnoticed in childhood until a systemic infection intervenes, provoking either an aplastic or a hemolytic crisis. In adults HS may surface first as cholelithiasis or cholecystitis, found in 43% to 80% of the patients. Physical findings may include intermittent, variable jaundice. The spleen is commonly enlarged, and it is unusual to find it impalpable. It may produce hypersplenism, especially during active infection. Chronic leg ulcerations are present in 10% to 15% of the patients.

LABORATORY FINDINGS. The anemia may be variable with hemoglobin levels usually at 9 to 12 g/dl. Depending on the ability of the marrow to increase erythropoiesis, compensation for hemolysis may be complete or partial. During a crisis the hemoglobin may fall rapidly and leukocytosis may occur. Lymphocytosis and basophilia have been described with chronic, steady anemia. A reticulocyte count of 5% to 20% is common, and during hemolytic crises it may rise as high as 50% to 90%. Reticulocytopenia may follow aplastic episodes.

The peripheral blood smear may show the characteristic small, dark, spheroidal red cells without a central area of pallor. Polychromasia and nucleated red cells also may be present. There is inconstant indirect hyperbilirubinemia of 1 to 4 mg/dl, the haptoglobin level may be low even though the hemolysis is mainly extravascular, the fecal urobilinogen level may be elevated, and thrombocytopenia with or without leukopenia and caused by hypersplenism may be detected. The bone marrow shows erythroid hyperplasia, but during an aplastic crisis, compensation is transiently interrupted, producing erythroid hypoplasia and bone marrow failure.

DIAGNOSIS. HS should be suspected when the mean corpuscular hemoglobin concentration (MCHC) rises above 36% in association with the preceding clinical and laboratory data. The diagnosis is confirmed by the osmotic fragility test in which red blood cells are suspended in saline solutions of varying tonicity, producing a greater hemoglobin leak in spherocytes than in normal, control red cells. The concentration of hemoglobin appearing in the suspension supernatants can be measured spectrophotometrically, and a curve can be plotted using these values. For the test to be positive, at least 1% to 2% of the red cell population must be spherocytic. Therefore in mild disease this assay may be normal. The occult red cell defect is uncovered by the incubated osmotic fragility test in which whole blood is held at 98.6° F (37° C) for 24 hours and then the procedure just described is repeated. Another examination is the autohemolysis test performed by suspending red cells in a glucose-free medium, which results in 10% to 50% spontaneous hemolysis of spherocytes. The Coombs' test is negative in HS.

MANAGEMENT. The treatment is by splenectomy when the disease is active. This increases the red cell survival almost but not quite to normal because the primary red cell defect persists. Splenectomy markedly increases susceptibility to infections caused by pneumococci, meningococci, and *Haemophilus influenzae*. Since susceptibility is greatest below age 6, it is best to postpone surgery until the patient is older. Immunization with the pneumococcal vaccine before surgery seems prudent.

Blood transfusions are rarely necessary except in aplastic crises, which are sometimes due to folate deficiency, occur most frequently in childhood, and are usually provoked by infection. Because of the ongoing hemolysis and increased hematinic needs, 1 mg of folic acid daily probably should be administered.

DEFICIENCIES WITHIN THE HEXOSE MONOPHOSPHATE (HMP) SHUNT

GLUCOSE-6-PHOSPHATE DEHYDROGENASE DEFICIENCY. The HMP shunt forms pentose from glucose and, more importantly, serves as the sole mechanism that prevents oxidative denaturation of intracellular and membrane components of the erythrocyte. Glucose-6-phosphate dehydrogenase (G-6-PD) is a crucial enzyme because it initiates the first reaction in the shunt pathway and generates NADPH required as a cofactor in the maintenance of glutathione (GSH). The latter compound protects hemoglobin sulfhydryls (—SH) and —SH-containing enzymes against oxidation and destruction. In the face of G-6-PD deficiency the NADPH reductive processes and maintenance of GSH are impaired, leading to deleterious biochemical and physical changes in the red blood cell and its premature removal from the circulation.

G-6-PD deficiency causes a hereditary, sex-linked hemolytic anemia apparent mainly during certain stressful situations. The defect is due to a coded gene on the X chromosome and is completely expressed in male hemizygotes, observed in rare female homozygotes, and minimally overt in female heterozygotes. The deficiency has been shown to have a worldwide distribution but is most common among people living in tropical and subtropical areas. About 10% of American blacks and 8% to 20% of West African blacks harbor the deficiency.

Although over 100 forms of G-6-PD already have been discovered, the majority are mainly of theoretic and biochemical interest. Only a few require special mention. The genotypic symbol for the enzyme is Gd. The normal enzyme, designated GdB+, represents the comparative enzyme standard, with the plus sign indicating full-level enzyme activity. It is the most commonly observed form in all population groups, being present in almost all whites and approximately 70% of normal blacks. GdA+, another normal variant, is prevalent in 30% of normal blacks. On electrophoresis this form is seen to migrate more rapidly than GdB+. The next type, GdA−, is the most frequent, clinically significant abnormal form in blacks. The minus sign denotes enzyme activity reduced to less than 25% of the normal counterpart, GdA+. Electrophoretic migration of GdA− is identical to that of GdA+, but the former is less active, possibly because it is relatively unstable and its activity diminishes as the red cell ages.

The most common abnormal variant in white people is Gd Mediterranean. The intracellular enzyme concentration is less than 1% of normal, in contrast to the usual 5% to 15% enzyme level observed in the GdA− form. Mild subclinical hemolysis with a minimal reduction of the erythrocyte life span is always present in the red cells with Gd Mediterranean deficiency. The defect is not restricted to the red blood cell, as with GdA−, but extends to the leukocytes and platelets as well.

Hemolysis in G-6-PD deficiency is overt only under the following circumstances.

Drug-induced hemolysis. These compounds induce hemolysis in persons with G-6-PD deficiency:

Antibacterials
    Chloramphenicol*
    Isoniazid
    Para-aminosalicylic acid
    Nalidixic acid
Antipyretics and analgesics
    Acetanilid
    Aspirin
    Acetophenetidin (phenacetin)
    Antipyrine†
    Aminopyrine†
Antimalarials
    Chloroquine
    Primaquine
    Pamaquine
    Pentaquine
    Quinocide
    Quinacrine (Atabrine)
    Quinine†
Sulfonamides
    Sulfanilamide
    Sulfapyridine

---

*Hemolytic in persons with G-6-PD Mediterranean deficiency.
†Hemolytic in whites, not in GdA− blacks.

Salicylazosulfapyridine (Azulfidine)
Sulfamethoxypyridazine (Kynex)
Sulfacetamide
N_2-Acetylsulfanilamide
2-Amino-5-sulfanilylthiazole
Sulfisoxazole (Gantrisin)
Sulfones
  Thiazolsulfone (Promizole)
  Diaminodiphenylsulfone (DDS)
  Sulfoxone* (dapsone)
Nitrofurans
  Nitrofurantoin (Furadantin)
  Furazolidone (Furoxone)
  Nitrofurazone (Furacin)
Miscellaneous compounds
  Naphthalene (mothballs)
  Probenecid (Benemid)
  Vitamin K (water-soluble analogs)
  Phenylhydrazine
  Trinitrotoluene
  Methylene blue
  Dimercaprol (BAL)
  Quinidine†
  Fava beans†
  Ascorbic acid‡

The mechanism by which these drugs produce oxidative degradation of hemoglobin is not entirely clear. These agents, or their active derivatives, interact with oxyhemoglobin, resulting in either the formation of free radicals or the generation of hydrogen peroxide, which oxidizes and precipitates globin recognizable as Heinz bodies after incubation with supravital stains. These damaged erythrocytes are removed by the spleen.

The typical hemolytic episode may occur from 1 to 3 days after drug administration and may last 7 to 12 days. With GdA−, hemolysis usually occurs 24 to 36 hours after exposure. Hemoglobinemia, hemoglobinuria, and jaundice are usual; the resultant anemia is moderate with the hemoglobin level rarely less than 8 g/dl. Hemolysis is self-limited, and the anemia reaches its nadir at 8 to 12 days. Recovery occurs even during continued drug administration because the younger cells leaving the bone marrow contain the more active enzyme resistant to oxidant stress. In the Gd Mediterranean defect hemolysis may occur earlier, within 3 to 24 hours of drug ingestion. Hemoglobinuria and jaundice are constant concurrents, hemolysis may not be self-limited, and the hemoglobin may drop to an extremely low level. Because massive intravascular hemolysis can cause severe hypotension and renal failure, these episodes may be fatal. Usually, however, clinical recovery is the rule, and the hemoglobin and hematocrit levels return to normal by approximately 5 weeks.

---

*Slightly hemolytic in large doses only in GdA− persons.
†Hemolytic in whites, not in GdA− persons.
‡Hemolytic in massive doses.

Infection. Hemolysis also may be induced during viral or bacterial infection, perhaps by hydrogen peroxide evolving during phagocytosis by neutrophils. The vulnerability of the erythrocyte to destruction in this case is analogous to that produced by drug contact. Anemia caused by infection is mild, and jaundice usually is absent. Reticulocytosis may not be observed because infection per se may suppress erythropoiesis. Recovery from the anemia therefore may be delayed until the infection has disappeared. The mechanism of injury, in addition to peroxide generation, also may be attributed to the infectious organism itself and its toxic metabolic products. Shock, hypotension, decreased renal function, and death have been described in the Gd Mediterranean form of deficiency when hemolysis has been associated with the hepatitis virus. Red cell destruction may be massive, jaundice extreme, and hyperbilirubinemia striking.

Favism. Hemolysis is induced by fresh or dried fava beans only in those with the Gd Mediterranean defect and may be sudden, occurring within a few hours after plant pollen inhalation or within 2 days after the vegetable is eaten. It is produced mainly, but not solely, in male children between the ages of 2 and 5 years. The resultant anemia may reach hemoglobin levels of 2 g/dl with lethal clinical consequences. Favism is not to be taken lightly as a clinical entity. Not all G-6-PD-deficient patients have hemolysis when exposed to the fava bean, suggesting that additional, possibly nonenzymatic factors may provoke susceptibility. On the other hand, favism affects only individuals who are G-6-PD deficient.

Neonatal jaundice. The premature, white, G-6-PD-deficient infant is especially prone to excessive hemolysis, jaundice, and hyperbilirubinemia without evidence of immunologic incompatibility and unrelated to drugs given to either the mother or her infant. This syndrome is seen in babies with the Gd Mediterranean variant and is rare among black infants with GdA− deficiency. The jaundice that follows may be severe enough to require exchange transfusions to prevent kernicterus.

Hereditary nonspherocytic hemolytic anemia. Hemolysis without drug ingestion occurs in certain rare types of G-6-PD deficiency, usually when the enzyme is unstable or its level is very low. This form of anemia generally is observed in whites, may begin in early infancy, and is mild, with limited or negligible transfusion needs. Exacerbations may be caused by fever, infection, and drugs. Splenomegaly is common. Rarely, when the anemia is severe, splenectomy has been clinically helpful in treatment.

Other causes. In addition to hereditary nonspherocytic hemolytic anemia, hemolysis may be provoked without drug contact in the presence of acidosis, renal disease, uremia, and diabetic coma. The features of red cell destruction in these instances resemble those of infection-related hemolysis.

The erythrocyte in G-6-PD deficiency usually looks normal on the peripheral blood smear between hemolytic episodes. During active hemolysis, however, polychromasia, spherocytes, schistocytes, and Heinz bodies all may appear. The level of the reticulocytosis will depend on the severity of the stress. Hyperbilirubinemia of varying levels may be observed.

The diagnosis of G-6-PD deficiency depends on the demonstration of enzyme deficiency through either screening tests or quantitative enzyme assay. The former methods are visual, more easily available, and sufficient for clinical purposes. They include the ascorbate-cyanide test and the reduction of certain dyes such as brilliant cresyl blue (BCB) or methylene blue (MB). Actual spectrophotometric, quantitative measurement of enzyme activity in red cell hemolysates is rarely necessary but may be useful when the Gd variant is unusual or escapes detection by simpler means. Since hemolysis induced by drugs may occur in the presence of unstable hemoglobins, tests for these hemoglobin forms also should be considered.

Usually no active treatment is needed for G-6-PD deficiency other than the avoidance of drugs known to initiate hemolysis. When red cell destruction is particularly severe, as with the Gd Mediterranean defect (especially when associated with viral hepatitis), the episode should be treated like any other hemolytic anemia in which renal failure and anuria are potential sequelae.

Disorders of hemoglobin

Abnormalities of hemoglobin may be classified as caused either by departures from the usual structural organization of this iron-containing protein or by the absence or reduced synthesis of one or more of the normal globin polypeptides necessary for complete integrity of the hemoglobin molecule. Hemoglobinopathy is the term applied to the former category, and the thalassemias represent the latter group.

In adults there are three physiologic hemoglobins. The first is hemoglobin A (Hb A), constituting approximately 97% of the total hemoglobin complement. It consists of four polypeptide chains, two α-chains, each with 141 amino acids, and two β-chains, each with 146 amino acids. The whole molecule is designated $\alpha_2\beta_2$. An iron-containing heme group is attached to each polypeptide. This tetrameric structure provides for cooperative binding of four oxygen molecules and establishes normal hemoglobin's affinity for oxygen. A minor adult component is hemoglobin A_2 (Hb A_2), consisting of two α- and two δ-chains ($\alpha_2\delta_2$). The final normal adult component is hemoglobin F (Hb F), fetal hemoglobin, which is present in concentrations of less than 1%, is composed of two pairs of α- and two pairs of γ-polypeptides, and is designated $\alpha_2\gamma_2$. Hemoglobin F is the major fetal and newborn hemoglobin component. During the neonatal period a switch occurs to Hb A synthesis, and γ-chain production is considerably reduced.

The capability of hemoglobin to function as a respiratory protein depends on its inherent molecular structure and three major interdependent properties. The first is oxygen affinity, generally expressed in terms of oxygen tension when the hemoglobin is 50% saturated (P_{50}). Oxygen affinity of normal hemoglobin rises with its increasing saturation. Oxygen affinity is influenced by and inversely proportional to the intracellular concentration of 2,3-DPG. The presence of 2,3,-DPG facilitates oxygen unloading to the tissues by shifting the oxygen dissociation curve to the right. This is a major advantage under circumstances such as anemia, high altitude, and chronic hypoxia.

The next important characteristic of hemoglobin is its cooperative interactions, which produce a sigmoid-shaped oxygen dissociation curve. The sigmoidal oxygen dissociation curve reflects the successive binding of oxygen to each of the four iron atoms within the hemoglobin molecule and progressive affinity for this gas. The physiologic benefit of this curve form is obvious. For example, at the plateau portion of the curve, Po_2 levels from 70 to 100 mm Hg all result in nearly complete hemoglobin saturation, even at the lower oxygen partial pressures. Therefore maximal oxygen delivery occurs with a minimal change in oxygen tension.

The final salient feature of hemoglobin is the Bohr effect, the change in oxygen affinity with altered pH. As acidity increases, oxygen affinity is reduced, so that oxygen release is enhanced in the tissues with dropping pH and rising carbon dioxide or lactate levels. Conversely, within the lungs the increased pH that follows carbon dioxide excretion increases oxygen affinity and uptake.

In addition to the genetically determined, hereditary disorders of hemoglobin, analogous abnormalities also may be required. These deviations are hemoglobin A_1, a glycosylated, posttranslation hemoglobin observed in poorly controlled diabetes mellitus, iron deficiency, and azotemia, in which a hexose is bound to the amino terminal valine of the β-chains; increased Hb F in pregnancy, leukemia, aplastic anemia, and certain of the myeloproliferative disorders; elevated Hb A_2 in megaloblastic anemias; and lowered Hb A_2 in iron deficiency. Finally, hemoglobin H, a β-tetramer (β_4), may rise progressively during the evolution of erythroleukemia.

HEMOGLOBINOPATHIES

Hemoglobinopathies, of which sickle cell anemia is the first and prime example, are inherited as autosomal codominants. Heterozygotes called carriers have a proportionately greater concentration of normal hemoglobin but also have the abnormal hemoglobin present in each red cell. The simplest example of this is sickle cell trait, designated Hb AS. Since the genes that determine the structure of each hemoglobin polypeptide chain are alleles, a patient with sickle cell–Hb C disease, to cite another instance, acquires the sickle hemoglobin gene from one parent and the gene for Hb C from the other. The genotype for Hb S-C, then, would be written $\alpha^A\beta^S/\alpha^A\beta^C$, recognizing that both Hb S and Hb C are β-chain abnormalities. This is a double form of heterozygosity. A mixed heterozygote is one in which different, rather than the same, polypeptide chains are abnormal.

SICKLE CELL ANEMIA

Definition and pathogenesis. Sickle cell anemia (SCA) is a homozygous, genetically determined hemolytic anemia caused by a mutation at a single point in the DNA codon that results in an mRNA coding for valine rather than the glutamic acid usually placed in the sixth position of the β-globin polypeptide. This genetic change leads to the synthesis of Hb S. The amino acid substitution forms the molecular basis for sickling observed when, at a PO_2 of 50 to 60 mm Hg, deoxyhemoglobin S first begins to undergo molecular alignment into spirally arranged, insoluble, fibrillar polymers, also called tactoids, that cause the hemoglobin to gel. This hemoglobin rearrangement distorts the red cell shape, increases cellular rigidity, and causes membrane damage with potentially irreversible sickling.

Such a sequence provokes a vicious circle of sickling, erythrostasis, increased blood viscosity, reduced blood flow velocity, hypoxia, and further sickling. These events are compounded by the inherent diminished oxygen affinity of deoxyhemoglobin S, which itself augments sickling, and the local change to an acid pH, which also lowers oxygen affinity. All of these further advance gelation and sickling. The ability of the sickled red cell to pass through the microvasculature is impaired, producing vasocclusion, the protean manifestations of sickle cell anemia, and its long-term and widespread organ damage. The recent demonstration that the sickled erythrocyte is more adherent than normal red cells to the vascular endothelium suggests an additional mechanism for vascular obstruction.

Epidemiology and clinical manifestations. In Africa the Hb S gene is distributed in a broad equatorial belt and may reach an incidence of 40% in some mid-African tribes. In the United States the homozygous state producing a hemolytic anemia occurs in 1 of 600 blacks. The characteristic clinical features of sickle cell anemia are the crises, which are acute, episodic manifestations superimposed on a chronic hemolytic state. These incidents add a new series of usually transient signs and symptoms. Crises may be classified as follows.

The first and most common is the *symptomatic, vasocclusive,* or *infarctive crisis.* This usually begins de novo or occasionally, as in children, may be provoked by an upper respiratory or other type of infection. It is the clinical outcome of the sickling phenomenon previously described and results from blood vessel obstruction by the rigid, tangled, and sickled red blood cells. The major symptom is pain, sometimes excruciating to the point of immobility. The patient may be jaundiced with fever, tachycardia, tachypnea, occasional hypertension, and abdominal tenderness with or without rigidity.

The next and less frequent crisis is the *hematopoietic crisis,* which may be *hemolytic* or *aplastic.* The former may be associated fortuitously with G-6-PD deficiency, may be provoked by infection, and may lead to active intravascular red cell destruction with all the clinical and laboratory features of abrupt diminution in the red cell mass. The aplastic or hypoplastic crisis is marked by sudden cessation of marrow function, worsening of the anemia, and reticulocytopenia.

The last type of crisis is the *sequestration syndrome,* seen mainly in children and expressed as sudden, massive, painful enlargement of the liver and spleen and an acute fall in the hemoglobin level. This is a serious complication with a high morbidity and mortality.

Although not actually considered a form of crisis, in children a singular abnormality called the hand-foot syndrome or sickle cell dactylitis may develop, with painful, swollen, hot, tender hands and feet. It may be associated with fever, leukocytosis, and roentgenographic evidence of periostitis and osteolysis.

Symptoms of SCA usually begin during the second half of the first year of life as the amount of hemoglobin F progressively is reduced and supplanted by Hb S. SCA truly is a systemic disease. There is scarcely an organ system or body focus that is not touched by this hemoglobinopathy.

The central nervous system is damaged by thromboses that occur in the capillaries and the small and large arteries and veins and can produce hemiplegia, convulsions, decreased consciousness, and visual disturbances. Intracranial and subarachnoid hemorrhage and spinal cord infarctions also occur. Conjunctival vessel tortuosity, vitreous hemorrhages, retinal detachment, microaneurysms, and chorioretinal infarction all may appear as ocular sequelae.

Cardiovascular involvement manifested as dyspnea, palpitations, and decreased exercise tolerance is not unusual. Precordial murmurs are heard frequently and may mimic those of mitral valve disease. These physical findings are in accord with roentgenographically demonstrable biventricular enlargement, prominence of the pulmonary artery conus, and electrocardiographic evidence of abnormalities in the right and left ventricles. Congestive heart failure may occur with aging.

Significant pulmonary disease and pulmonary hypertension evolve mainly because of infarction resulting from vasocclusion. Infection caused by the pneumococcus is common. Infarction and infection may occur separately or in combination and at times are hard to differentiate from one another, especially during a symptomatic crisis when patients are febrile and complain of chest pain. Gas exchange may be abnormal, and there may be ventilation-perfusion disparity as a result of intrapulmonary shunting.

Episodic abdominal pain is common and is related to microinfarction of the gastrointestinal tract. Gallbladder disease is often present in patients with SCA; 30% to 60%

of the patients have cholelithiasis with radiolucent stones, but only 10% to 15% have signs and symptoms related to this abnormality. Elective cholecystectomy is not recommended, but the possibility of cholecystitis should always be considered in patients with SCA who enter the hospital with abdominal pain.

Hepatomegaly and liver dysfunction are extremely common. Liver enlargement is moderate and is seen in about 55% of the patients. Elevated liver enzymes, alkaline phosphatase, and bilirubin levels reflect the microinfarction, destruction, and regeneration of the hepatic parenchyma. These events actually are continuous even when the patients are in the supposed stable state without an overt crisis. Hepatitis and hemosiderosis, which may follow repeated blood transfusion, also contribute to liver damage.

Splenomegaly, sometimes with tenderness, is seen in 50% of the younger patients and is particularly prominent in the childhood sequestration crises described previously. As the disease continues, repetitive infarction and thrombosis diminish the size of the spleen, and it ultimately atrophies. Splenic hypofunction is not uncommon in adolescents and adults with SCA, as demonstrated by the presence of Howell-Jolly bodies in the peripheral blood. A consequence of reduced splenic activity is an increased tendency toward infection, In febrile adolescents and young adults an impalpable spleen may suddenly become enlarged, suggesting the presence of bacteremia and sepsis.

Renal disease has diverse presentations in SCA. These include hyposthenuria (the most common renal defect), hematuria, papillary necrosis, renal infarcts, the nephrotic syndrome, occasionally renal vein thrombosis, and inability to acidify the urine. The frequency of pyelonephritis may also be increased. In spite of functional impairment, end-stage renal failure is an unusual cause of death.

An additional urinary tract abnormality is priapism resulting from engorgement of the corpora cavernosa. Repeated microthromboses leading to fibrosis of the arteriovenous mechanism of penile erection may prevent detumescence.

Leg ulcerations, most commonly around the medial malleolus, are observed in 10% to 12% of the patients, mainly those who are younger. Lymphadenopathy occurs in a large proportion of patients with SCA and may be detected by careful examination.

Joint abnormalities in SCA include hemarthroses with or without hemosiderosis, gout, and avascular (aseptic) necrosis of the humerus and femur. Finger clubbing resulting from chronic anemia occurs in approximately 8% of the individuals with SCA. Bony infarcts caused by vascular obstruction are largely responsible for the pain in the symptomatic crises. The infarcts may be demonstrated by roentgenograms or radionuclide tracer studies. Bone marrow erythroid hyperplasia eventuates in widening of the diploë, frontal bossing, occasional maxillary overgrowth, and compression of the vertebrae with a central concavity leading to the fish-mouth appearance.

Pregnancy and SCA may interact. During the last trimester and the immediate postpartum period, congestive heart failure, thrombophlebitis, and pulmonary infarction or infection all may be observed. There is an increased incidence of toxemia, endometritis, spontaneous abortions, stillbirths, prematurity, and decreased infant viability.

Laboratory findings. The hemoglobin level ranges from 5 to 13 g/dl and does not change in the usual symptomatic crisis. The anemia is mainly normocytic and normochromic, but the mean corpuscular volume (MCV) may be diminished. During infection and aplasia the anemia may become more severe. The peripheral smear may show marked and diverse morphologic distortions. Basophilic stippling, nucleated red cells, polychromasia. Howell-Jolly bodies, Cabot's rings, and Pappenheimer bodies (granules of hemosiderin) all may be present. Reticulocytosis usually is sustained, and the reticulocyte count averages 5% to 10%. Reticulocytopenia may develop during infection or sepsis associated with an aplastic crisis. A constant leukocytosis of 12,000 to 15,000 cells/mm^3 is common; this increases during a crisis to above 20,000 cells/mm^3. The platelet level is often elevated; however, immediately before crises it may decrease. The bone marrow shows marked erythroid hyperplasia. Megaloblastosis also may appear because of an increased need for folic acid.

Diagnosis. SCA may be suspected in anemic patients with the proper racial background and sickled cells seen in the peripheral blood smear. The presumption should be supported by a screening test using sodium metabisulfite or the newer commercially available reagents. The definitive identification of the abnormal hemoglobin is made by hemoglobin electrophoresis.

Management and prognosis. Since there is no specific treatment for SCA, major attention should be given to managing the many complications of each organ injury, such as congestive heart failure. Anticoagulants are not routinely recommended for pulmonary infarcts. Infections in SCA should be treated aggressively with appropriate antibiotics based on bacteriologic culture data. Regardless of the number of times a patient has been admitted for what appears to be a febrile symptomatic crisis, a search for infection must never be neglected. Organisms producing disease with special frequency in SCA are *Streptococcus pneumoniae,* perhaps resulting from decreased serum opsonins and a defective alternate complement pathway, and *Salmonella.* The most common infections are bacteremia, pneumonia, meningitis, and osteomyelitis. *Salmonella* is the most common cause of osteomyelitis in SCA.

A variety of experimental agents have been used in attempts to modify the biochemical and biophysical abnormalities that augment sickling. The most recent ones have been urea and cyanates, neither of which has been ultimately shown to be clinically effective. Unfortunately, treatment still remains symptomatic, with pain controlled by the judicious use of narcotics. Patients given this type of therapy are potential drug addicts. Ordinary hydration to maintain adequate fluid balance and administration of oxygen are appropriate during crises. Folic acid, 1 mg daily, particularly in children, may prevent worsening of the anemia but does not raise the hemoglobin level beyond that dictated by the genetic code. Pneumococcal vaccine should be given as prophylaxis. Regular and continuing blood transfusions, as employed in thalassemia major, usually are not required. When a symptomatic crises is extended, narcotic requirements are rising, or pain relief does not occur, limited isovolemic exchange transfusion usually will terminate a particular episode. Although previously patients with sickle cell disease often died in childhood, they are currently living longer.

SICKLE CELL TRAIT. Individuals heterozygous for Hb S have sickle cell trait. They have inherited one gene for the abnormal Hb S β-polypeptide and one determinant for the normal Hb A β-chain. Heterozygosity is seen in 8% to 10% of blacks in the Western Hemisphere. This carrier state is innocuous except in the following circumstances. With marked reduction in oxygen tension, as may occur in the renal medulla, in vivo sickling of trait erythrocytes occurs. This may explain the renal abnormalities of hyposthenuria, spontaneous hematuria, and renal papillary necrosis. Most recently, von Willebrand's disease has been discovered in some of these patients and has been suggested as an auxiliary basis for their hematuria. Asymptomatic bacteriuria seems to be more frequent in women with sickle cell trait than in the general population. Aseptic necrosis rarely occurs in patients with sickle cell trait.

SICKLE CELL–HEMOGLOBIN C DISEASE. Sickle cell–hemoglobin C or Hb S-C disease is a doubly heterozygous state in which the red cells contain a mixture of Hb S and Hb C resulting from the inheritance of the S gene from one parent and the C gene from the other. Clinically, the disease may be so mild as to be virtually asymptomatic and may be discovered only during routine screening procedures or physical examination. On the other hand, the presentation may be that of a mild form of sickle cell anemia. About half of the patients with symptomatic disease are detected during childhood, and the remainder are diagnosed as growth and development proceed through adolescence into adulthood.

General physical and sexual development is nearly normal. The most common complaint is focal or diffuse bone pain, with any portion of the skeleton involved. Of particular importance is the development of aseptic necrosis of the femoral head in a high proportion of these patients. Splenomegaly is detected in approximately two thirds of adults and may result in splenic infarction and the sequestration syndrome. Hepatomegaly, usually without clinical evidence of jaundice, is present in 40% of the cases. Proliferative retinal vascular disease and acute pulmonary infarction are frequently observed. Leg ulceration in 20% of the patients and hematuria also occur.

The hemoglobin level rarely is less than 10 g/dl, and reticulocytosis is modest. The red cells generally are normocytic and normochromic, but the peripheral smear contains many target cells, rare sickle cells, and a variety of bizarrely shaped erythrocytes. The diagnosis is made by hemoglobin electrophoresis.

HEMOGLOBIN C DISEASE. In the Hb C defect, lysine replaces glutamic acid in the sixth position of the β-chain polypeptide. About 1 of 6000 American blacks has Hb C disease. Patients may be completely asymptomatic or complain of mild, intermittent abdominal pain and occasional arthralgia with periodic mild jaundice and occasional hematuria. Splenomegaly is fairly common. Cholelithiasis is not unusual. The hemoglobin level in Hb C disease may vary from 8 to 12 g/dl. Reticulocytosis, marrow erythroid hyperplasia, and a modest reduction in the red cell life span all are part of the clinical complex. The peripheral red blood cells are strikingly abnormal with a large proportion of target cells, microspherocytes, and occasional cells with intraerythrocytic crystals. Specific therapy is neither available nor required.

THALASSEMIAS

The thalassemic syndromes are a group of hereditary hemoglobin disorders in which synthesis of one or more of the normal hemoglobin polypeptides is either totally absent or reduced, causing decreased hemoglobinization of the erythrocytes, microcythemia, and hypochromia. Continued unbalanced synthesis of the normal globin chain, however, leads to its intracellular precipitation, altered flow characteristics of the red cells, and their premature destruction. The last provides a significant hemolytic component to this group of red cell abnormalities. The thalassemias are classified according to the type of globin chain that is absent or present in decreased amount. Each thalassemia may occur in the homozygous or heterozygous form. The thalassemias and their principal features are listed in Tables 67-1 and 67-2.

β-THALASSEMIAS

Homozygous β-thalassemia. The homozygous β-thalassemia syndromes are observed most frequently within the Mediterranean basin, Middle East, Southeast Asia, India, Pakistan, and foci in West and North Africa. Actually, however, their distribution is worldwide, and they may appear sporadically in all racial groups, including whites of Northern European ancestry. The symbol β° in Table 67-1 denotes that protein synthesis from this affected genetic locus is totally absent, so that there is no Hb A in these patients' red blood cells. Erythropoiesis is ineffective, leading to the severe disease known as Cooley's anemia or

Table 67-1. Classification of β-thalassemias

Type of thalassemia	Parental genotype	Hemoglobin findings	Molecular defect	Clinical designation and features
Homozygous				
β^0-Thalassemia	Both β^0/β	Hb F, 10%-95%; Hb A_2, variable	Absent or mutant nonfunctional βmRNA	Thalassemia major (Cooley's anemia); pallor, jaundice, bony deformities, abnormal facies, hepatosplenomegaly; transfusion dependent; severe anemia with markedly abnormal red cell morphology
β^+-Thalassemia	Both β^+/β	Hb A, present but reduced; Hb F, 46%-80%; Hb A_2, variable	Marked decrease of βmRNA: structurally unstable βmRNA	Thalassemia major (Cooley's anemia); pallor, hepatosplenomegaly, jaundice, anemia, and morphologic changes moderate; transfusions usually not required; in blacks may be less severe and resemble thalassemia intermedia
$\delta\beta$-Thalassemia (high F)	Both $\delta\beta^0/\delta\beta$	Absent Hb A and Hb A_2; Hb F, 100%	Absent δ and βmRNA*	Thalassemia intermedia; mild jaundice, hepatosplenomegaly, anemia mild to moderate; moderate morphologic distortions; usually survival without transfusion
Hb Lepore	Both Hb Lepore/β	Absent Hb A and Hb A_2; Hb F, 75%; Hb Lepore, 25%	Reduced β-like mRNA; unstable $\delta\beta$mRNA†	Thalassemia major (Cooley's anemia)
Heterozygous				
β^0-Thalassemia	β^0/β, normal	Hb A_2, 3.5%–7.5%; Hb F, 1%-6%	Deficient βmRNA	Ordinary or high Hb A_2 thalassemia (thalassemia minor); most common type; perhaps mild icterus and splenomegaly; anemia mild to moderate; microcythemia and hypochromia
β^+-Thalassemia	β^+/β, normal	As above	Deficient or nonfunctional βmRNA	Thalassemia minor; physical findings usually absent; anemia absent to mild; microcythemia and hypochromia
$\delta\beta^0$-Thalassemia	$\delta\beta^0/\delta\beta$, normal	Hb A_2, normal or low; Hb F, 5%-20%	Some deficiency of β and δmRNA	Thalassemia minor; physical findings usually absent; anemia absent to mild; microcythemia and hypochromia
Hb Lepore	Hb Lepore/β, normal	Hb A, low or normal; Hb F, slightly elevated; Hb Lepore, 6%-15%	Unstable $\delta\beta$mRNA (?)	Thalassemia minor; resembles ordinary high Hb A_2 thalassemia

*δ and probably β genes deleted.
†Fusion genes present only.

thalassemia major. Infants appear normal at birth, but anemia occurs during the first few months of life and becomes progressively more severe. Physical growth and development are impaired. The physical features of prominent frontal bossing and cheekbones, maxillary overgrowth, and mongoloid facies all appear with time. Gallstones, leg ulcers, and skin pigmentation also are frequent complications. In addition to delayed sexual maturation, other endocrine disturbances such as hypoparathyroidism and hypoadrenalism develop. Later, diabetes mellitus and pigmentary infiltration of the myocardium and pericardium occur, resembling the changes of hemochromatosis. Intellectual development is not retarded.

Anemia is severe, with the hemoglobin level falling as

Table 67-2. Classification of α-thalassemias

Type of thalassemia	Parental genotype	Hemoglobin findings	Molecular defects	Clinical designation and features
Homozygous α-thalassemia	Both α-thalassemia$_1$	Hb Bart's, 80%; rest Hb H and Hb Portland (an embryonic hemoglobin)	All α genes deleted; absent αmRNA	Lethal hydrops fetalis; hepatosplenomegaly, heart failure, stillbirth, or death within 24 hours; red cell hypochromia, anisopoikilocytosis, severe anemia
Hb H disease	α-Thalassemia trait/ silent carrier	Hb H, 4%-30% in adults; Hb Bart's, 25% in cord blood	Three of four genes gone, marked deficiency of α-chain synthesis	Variable severity; thalassemia intermedia; microcythemia and hypochromia
	α-Thalassemia trait/Hb CS* heterozygote	When CS gene present, 2%-3% Hb CS	Two of four genes gone; one normal, one Hb CS gene	
Heterozygous α-thalassemia	α-Thalassemia trait/ normal	Normal in adults; Hb Bart's, 5%-15% in newborn	Two of four genes gone on same chromosome	Clinically mild; very mild in blacks†
Silent carrier	Silent carrier/normal	Normal in adults; Hb Bart's 1%-2% in newborn	One of four genes gone	Neither anemia nor red cell morphologic abnormalities
Heterozygous Hb CS	Hb CS* heterozygote/ normal	Hb CS, 1%	Three of four genes present; one Hb CS gene	Silent

*Hemoglobin Constant Spring.
†See text.

low as 2 to 3 g/dl. The peripheral blood film shows anisopoikilocytosis, target cells, microcythemia, hypochromia, polychromasia, and basophilic stippling. Poorly hemoglobinized normoblasts are seen in the peripheral blood with their number increasing markedly after splenectomy. Even when the anemia is severe, the reticulocyte count may not be very high because of ineffective erythropoiesis and massive intramedullary red cell death. The bone marrow is very hypercellular with marked erythroid hyperplasia. Poorly hemoglobinized normoblasts appear as micronormoblasts. Occasionally, storage cells resembling Gaucher's cells are observed. If the bone marrow is examined under phase microscopy or stained with methyl violet, α-chain aggregates are visible as inclusion bodies in normoblasts. This may be used as a diagnostic test for homozygous β-thalassemia. Increased indirect hyperbilirubinemia and other evidence of hemolysis may be present. The total white blood cell and platelet counts may be mildly elevated unless hypersplenism has intervened. The hemoglobin pattern is described in Table 67-1.

In vitro data relative to the pathophysiology of β-thalassemia show that α-chain synthesis alone exceeds that of β, γ, and δ together. This leads to polypeptide imbalance and excess free α-chains that are present as inclusion bodies and are responsible for altered membrane behavior. Heme synthesis also is defective, probably as a result of diminished globin formation. Consequently, increased amounts of intracellular and mitochondrial iron are deposited, suppressing ATP regeneration. All the foregoing factors compound the ineffective erythropoiesis. There is an attempt to raise the hemoglobin level by the compensatory γ-chain synthesis, but this is never quite sufficient. The Hb F thus produced is distributed heterogenously in the red cells. In addition to inherently increased iron absorption, tissue iron storage is augmented further by autologous iron recycling resulting from hemolysis and by the repeated blood transfusions that are the mainstay of therapy in patients with thalassemia.

Roentgenographic changes consist of widening of the diploë, the "hair-on-end" appearance of the cranial vault, and increased trabeculation of the long bones and phalanges. All of these reflect medullary expansion that may lead to bony fractures. Additional complicating aspects of this disease are extramedullary hematopoiesis occurring as paraspinal or mediastinal masses, splenomegaly leading ultimately to hypersplenism, and bleeding, occasionally uncontrollable, resulting from hepatic dysfunction. Finally, deposition of iron in the myocardium and pericardium, which ultimately leads to congestive cardiomyopathy and heart failure, plays a major role in the decreased longevity of these patients.

Another form of homozygous thalassemia is designated in Table 67-1 by the symbol β+. This denotes that, in contrast to the previously described thalassemia in which β-chain production is totally absent, some synthesis of β-polypeptides does occur in this form of thalassemia. The capacity for β-chain synthesis is stable within families but shows a family-to-family variation. Thus the molecular defect in β+-thalassemia demonstrates considerable heterogeneity. The clinical expression of β+-thalassemia is somewhat less severe than classic thalassemia major or Cooley's anemia, but it may, nevertheless, resemble the latter. β+-Thalassemia may be appreciably less destructive in blacks than in whites and may be considered a form of thalassemia intermedia. The features of this syndrome are shown in Table 67-1.

Heterozygous thalassemias. Table 67-1 indicates that the thalassemias also may be present in the heterozygous form. This occurs when only a single β-thalassemia mutation is inherited, resulting clinically in the thalassemic trait or thalassemia minor. In this instance hemoglobin synthesis depends largely on the compensatory capacity of the normal β-globin gene in the trans position, that is, on the noninvolved, opposite chromosome. Usually it is capable of a limited, increased output of β-chains, and developing red cells accumulate approximately 75% of the normal amount of Hb A. However, the marrow responds to this reduction in Hb A synthesis by producing a larger number of smaller-than-normal red cells. This is observed as the classic hypochromia and microcythemia of the β-thalassemia trait. Since δ-chain synthesis also is relatively, and sometimes absolutely, increased, the percentage of Hb A_2 is elevated unless the gene is deleted or abnormal.

COMPLICATIONS AND MANAGEMENT OF THE THALASSEMIAS.
The thalassemic syndromes are preventable by genetic counseling of documented heterozygous prospective parents and antenatal study of fetuses. Active treatment is necessary mainly in homozygous and severe heterozygous forms and is basically supportive, since specific therapy does not exist.

One line of therapy is regular blood transfusion to produce hematocrit levels between 33% and 35%, which helps normalize patient growth and development, suppresses ineffective erythropoiesis, reduces iron absorption, and helps prevent bony abnormalities. However, this therapy has the disadvantage of organ iron loading, which is only partially ameliorated by desferrioxamine chelation. Repeated blood transfusions also may produce bleeding syndromes caused by hepatic dysfunction, endocrinopathies, and progressive splenomegaly with hypersplenism. Increasing splenic enlargement may aggravate the anemia, actually augment the transfusion requirements by causing sequestration of transfused red cells, and produce pancytopenia. Splenectomy may eliminate these adverse transfusion effects. Because splenectomy promotes the hazard of infection, particularly in young children, it is prudent to delay this operation at least until the patient is older than 5 years of age. The availability of the pneumococcal vaccine makes this surgery somewhat less worrisome.

HEREDITARY PERSISTENCE OF FETAL HEMOGLOBIN

In hereditary persistence of fetal hemoglobin (HPFH) the synthesis of relatively large amounts of fetal hemoglobin persists into adult life without major hematologic abnormalities. HPFH is a heterogeneous entity expressing itself with some diversity in several ethnic groups. It is inherited as a single autosomal codominant, closely linked or allelic to the gene determining the structure of the β-chain itself in the β-thalassemia gene. In black homozygotes who are clinically well, 100% of the hemoglobin is Hb F, distributed homogeneously in the small, poorly hemoglobinized peripheral erythrocyte, with total absence of β- and δ-polypeptide synthesis. In black heterozygotes Hb F ranges from 20% to 35%. Additional patterns are observed in the Greek, Swiss, and English variants.

HEMOLYSIS CAUSED BY ACQUIRED ABNORMALITIES
Immunohemolytic anemias

Red cell destruction in the immunohemolytic anemias is immunogenic. If the anemia is caused by specific red cell antibodies, as seen in transfusion reactions and hemolytic disease of the newborn (HDN), it is called *isoimmune* or *alloimmune*. If the anemia is due to the selective deposition of certain self-produced immunoglobulins and complement on the red cell, the anemia is considered autoimmune. Transfusion reactions are discussed in Chapter 70.

HEMOLYTIC DISEASE OF THE NEWBORN

DEFINITION AND PATHOGENESIS.
HDN is caused by the transplacental entry of IgG antibodies into the fetal circulation following isoimmunization of the mother against the infant's red cells, which contain an antigen foreign to her. This results in the coating of the fetal erythrocytes with antibody and thereby hemolysis in the infant. In Rh hemolytic disease the most common offender is the Rh_0 (D) antigen. Incompatibilities provoked by C, E, and Kell antigens also occur. Immunization by the ABO antigen group, although more common than Rh hemolytic disease of the newborn, is not as important clinically because it results in disease of far less severity.

Initial maternal immunization takes place most commonly during the last half of pregnancy and at delivery as small numbers of fetal red cells escape through the placenta and enter the mother's bloodstream. A prior blood transfusion with Rh-positive red cells or an abortion may serve the same immunizing purpose. A later challenge as small as 0.1 ml of red cells produces anamnestic antibody that becomes available to react against fetal red cells during subsequent gestations.

CLINICAL MANIFESTATIONS.
Hepatosplenomegaly, jaundice, generalized edema (hydrops fetalis), congestive heart failure, bone marrow erythroid hyperplasia, the release of nucleated red cells into the peripheral blood, and progressive anemia if destruction exceeds marrow compensation

all may occur, depending on the level of maternal immunization. However, the principal danger to the live-born neonate lies in the accumulation of unconjugated bilirubin, which occurs because the protective effect of the placenta, the organ responsible for removing excess bilirubin, is no longer present. The neonatal liver is not able to conjugate and excrete bilirubin effectively. When the amount of unconjugated bilirubin exceeds the albumin-binding capacity, the unbound, unconjugated bilirubin diffuses into the central nervous system. Kernicterus that often is fatal or produces permanent brain damage results.

LABORATORY FINDINGS. Babies with HDN look well at birth when the cord hemoglobin level may be only at the lower limits of normal (14 g/dl). Icterus usually develops during the first 24 hours of life. Bilirubin levels above 4 mg/dl suggest severe disease, and levels up to 40 to 50 mg/dl may be reached. The hemoglobin level begins to fall during the first 24 hours of life and thereafter may drop at a rate of 3 g/day. Microcythemia and polychromasia are marked. The reticulocyte count may be as high as 60%. There is a great increase in peripheral blood nucleated red cells, hence the term "erythroblastosis." Leukocytosis may be pronounced, and counts in excess of 30,000/mm^3, especially in severely affected infants, have been reported. The platelet level is usually normal but may be depressed in severe disease.

DIAGNOSIS. Laboratory investigation of suspected HDN should begin with antenatal titers of the mother's blood for anti-Rh antibodies. A baseline titer should be measured at 16 weeks' gestation, followed by a second titer at 28 to 32 weeks, and subsequent assays at intervals of 1 to 4 weeks, depending on the rate of increase. If the titer rise shows evidence of possible HDN in utero, the suspicion may be verified by antenatal examination of the amniotic fluid spectrophotometrically for levels of bilirubin-like catabolic products.

The immediate diagnosis of anti-Rh HDN at birth is by a positive direct Coombs' test of cord red blood cells using an anti-IgG reagent. Most infants also show a positive indirect Coombs' reaction.

MANAGEMENT. If there is risk of hydrops fetalis, the standard procedure is intrauterine and intraperitoneal transfusions followed by induced labor at 34 weeks. For a baby with documented and overt HDN, exchange transfusion using blood compatible with the mother's serum is the proper treatment. Guidelines for this are a hemoglobin level of 13 g/dl or less and a serum bilirubin level higher than 4 mg/dl. An alternative form of management, especially in ABO incompatibility, is phototherapy using a blue light that converts indirect bilirubin into water-soluble products excreted in the bile and urine. Finally, IgG anti-D antibody should be given at delivery to Rh-negative mothers who deliver Rh-positive infants and to all Rh-negative women who have abortions unless the father of the fetus is known to be Rh negative.

AUTOIMMUNE HEMOLYTIC ANEMIAS

The autoimmune hemolytic anemias (AIHA) may be divided into those caused by warm-reacting antibodies, usually involving IgG (and sometimes complement), and those caused by cold-reacting antibodies, invariably mediated by IgM and complement.

WARM-REACTING AUTOIMMUNE HEMOLYTIC ANEMIA

Etiology and pathogenesis. Incomplete antibodies of many different specificities, functional at 98.6° F (37° C) or close to this physiologic thermal point, have been incriminated in the pathogenesis of warm-reacting AIHA. Red cell destruction is the hallmark of this disease. Premature red cell removal may be generated, in part, by the attachment of the IgG to the red cell. This occurs with the Fc portion of the immunoglobulin molecule protruding outward from the cell surface, an arrangement permitting the splenic and the liver macrophage to hold the coated red cell and ultimately to destroy it. Complement (C3) probably also is present on the red cell perimeter and may be a stronger attractant for the monocyte and macrophage receptor than the IgG itself.

This form of hemolytic anemia is recognized under three primary circumstances. First is its de novo occurrence in approximately 25% to 30% of the patients, especially young women, without any obvious predisposing cause. The second and more common presentation (about 50% of instances) results from the lymphoproliferative disorders, mainly chronic lymphocytic leukemia. The remaining patients with warm-reacting AIHA are those with the connective tissue disorders, especially systemic lupus erythematosus. AIHA may also be found associated with immunodeficiency disorders, drug reactions, other malignant tumors, inflammatory bowel syndromes, and liver diseases.

Clinical manifestations. The clinical characteristics depend on the underlying disease provoking the inappropriate, mainly extravascular red cell destruction and the level of anemia. Jaundice and pallor may be evident on physical examination. Splenomegaly occurs in more than half of the patients, and hepatomegaly also may occur.

Laboratory findings and diagnosis. The degree of anemia and reticulocytosis is variable. The peripheral smear shows macrocytes, polychromasia, anisopoikilocytosis, microspherocytes, and nucleated red cells in differing proportions and combinations. A mild leukocytosis also may be observed. There is predominantly indirect hyperbilirubinemia with levels between 2.5 and 5 mg/dl. Although the hemolysis is mainly extravascular, the serum haptoglobin level may be depressed. The bone marrow demonstrates erythroid hyperplasia.

The diagnosis is made by a positive direct Coombs' reaction obtained first with broad-spectrum screening and thereafter with a more specific reagent. The immunoreactant coating the red cell may reflect the primary disease with which the anemia is associated. The differing disorders produce certain characteristic serologic reactivity patterns. The Coombs' test in idiopathic AIHA and that caused by the lymphoproliferative disorders is positive for IgG with or without complement and rarely for complement alone. On the other hand, the Coombs' test in systemic lupus erythematosus is never positive only against IgG but is reactive with complement alone or combined with the immunoglobulin.

Management. Warm-reacting AIHA is treated first with 1 mg/kg prednisone in three or four divided daily doses because single doses are ineffective under acute circumstances. Initial improvement, signaled by reduced reticulocytosis and a rising hemoglobin level, will occur within the first 2 weeks in approximately 50% of the patients with de novo or connective tissue–related hemolysis. After 3 to 4 weeks the steroids are reduced gradually over a similar period to avoid recurrence. Treatment of a specific disease is an obvious concurrent necessity. Transfusions are used during the acute hemolytic episode only in a life-threatening emergency because of the difficulty in obtaining complete cross-match compatibility.

Patients who do not show a response to prednisone and do not have a treatable underlying disease are considered for splenectomy. If surgery also is unsuccessful, immunosuppressive agents such as azathioprine or cyclophosphamide may be tried. However, these drugs are teratogenic and oncogenic, and their efficacy is erratic and unpredictable.

COLD-REACTING AUTOIMMUNE HEMOLYTIC ANEMIA. Immunohemolytic anemias caused by cold-reacting antibodies are those in which the humoral reactants are characterized by their ability to coat red blood cells at temperatures below 98.6° F (37° C), their dissociation from the binding site when the temperature rises to that of the body, and their production of agglutination and/or hemolysis. Cold agglutinins cause two major clinical disorders, the cold agglutinin syndrome and paroxysmal cold hemoglobinuria.

Cold-agglutinin syndromes. Cold agglutinins originate in association with certain infections, most commonly those caused by *Mycoplasma pneumoniae,* cytomegalovirus, and Epstein-Barr virus. These antibodies are polyclonal, most frequently of the IgM and rarely of the IgA or IgG class, with specificity directed against the I-i and Pr groups of red cell antigens. Monoclonal cold agglutinins with I-i specificity may be found in patients with malignant diseases such as the lymphoproliferative disorders and gastric and ovarian carcinomas. Finally, IgM monoclonal cold agglutinins may arise de novo without obvious cause, leading to the chronic, idiopathic cold agglutinin syndrome.

Cold agglutinins do not react with red cells at temperatures of 89.7° F (32° C) or higher but may induce injury within the range of 50° to 89.7° F (10° to 32° C). Subsequent red cell destruction may evolve in more than one way. The first occurs when the IgM antibody attaches to the red cell at lower temperatures and simultaneously fixes complement (C) to the cell membrane. At higher temperatures, which the erythrocyte meets as it comes from distal body sites (nose, fingers, and toes) and enters the core circulation, IgM is disengaged and C fixation occurs with potential activation of the complement attack unit (C5 through C9). If this sequence is completed and there is enough complement on the red cell surface, intravascular hemolysis follows. Usually this does not occur, because there is complement adequate only for red cell sequestration via the C3b receptor in the reticuloendothelial system. This produces rapid removal by Kupffer's cells and the extravascular means for reduction of red cell longevity. Red cells also are phagocytized by the spleen.

The red cell, however, may be held only transiently by the macrophage and released by serum C3 inactivator. This protects the red cell mass from progressive destruction and additional phagocytosis. These immunologic features partially explain the comparative benignity of the cold agglutinins.

Clinical manifestations. The signs and symptoms frequently are those of the underlying disease. With infection, clinically overt hemolysis is most unusual despite the high cold agglutinin titers that peak at about 2 to 3 weeks after the onset of the illness. Cold-related hemolysis is not ordinarily a major manifestation of lymphoid neoplasms.

Chronic idiopathic cold agglutinin disease produces a chronic hemolytic anemia that occurs predominantly in the sixth through the eighth decades, although it may occur in patients in their twenties and thirties. The disorder is accompanied by mild hepatosplenomegaly, mild jaundice, and, predominantly, circulatory changes of acrocyanosis. This phenomenon is caused by intravascular red cell agglutination taking place in the cooler distal body parts. These may turn purple and be painful, with rapid reversion to normal on rewarming. Repetitive episodes may lead to local tissue destruction and necrosis. With sudden exposure to severe chilling, fever, chills, hemoglobinemia, hemoglobinuria, and renal failure may occur.

Laboratory findings. The degree of anemia varies, with hemoglobin levels infrequently below 7 g/dl. The total serum bilirubin rarely exceeds 3 g/dl. Serum complement may be decreased, especially if hemolysis is acute and severe. Serum cold agglutinin titers, which normally are measurable up to a 1:64 dilution, may vary from 1:1000 to 1:1,000,000. Coombs' test specific for complement components is positive.

Management. Treatment of acute cold agglutinin disease rarely is necessary, since the disease is usually self-limited. Occasionally, with excessive hemolysis, transfusions with washed red cells are needed. Problems in typing and cross-matching may be encountered. In unusual situations when hemolysis is fulminant, exchange transfusion is applied.

Splenectomy and the administration of adrenal corticosteroids have little value. Alkylating agents, theoretically the most rational approach to suppress antibody synthesis, have been successful mainly during the treatment of lymphoid malignancies. Idiopathic chronic cold agglutinin disease is treated primarily by avoiding exposure to low temperatures.

Paroxysmal cold hemoglobinuria. The rarest form of immunohemolytic anemia, paroxysmal cold hemoglobinuria (PCH), is characterized by sudden, episodic hemoglobinuria occurring after local or general body exposure to the cold. The cause of this syndrome is the Donath-Landsteiner (D-L) antibody identified as an IgG antibody, which acts as an extremely potent hemolysin, sometimes even in relatively low concentrations. The antibody is described classically as biphasic because it unites avidly with red cells at lower temperatures (32° to 59° F [0° to 15° C]), and then hemolyzes them when the temperature of the reacting mixture moves closer to or reaches that of the body. The hemolytic sequence in the peripheral circulation consists of sensitization of the red cell with IgG and complement at low temperature, elution of IgG on warming, and hemolysis following activation of the entire complement cascade. The IgG also may cause red cell agglutination.

Previously the disease was thought to be associated primarily with congenital or teritary syphilis, but this seems rare nowadays. More commonly, it occurs during the course of acute viral infections, especially in children with measles or mumps, or may arise without any apparent preceding disease or event.

Clinical manifestations. The syndrome, usually mild, may be life threatening, particularly in children after viral infections. There is striking passage of dark-brown or black urine after local or general exposure to cold. Lethargy, pallor, and fatigue may follow the acute attack, and icterus may be clinically apparent. Hepatosplenomegaly also may be present. The disease may become chronic in patients who are continually exposed to cold, and a persistent hemolytic anemia may evolve thereafter.

Laboratory findings and diagnosis. A massive hemolytic episode may cause hemoglobinuria and hemoglobinemia. Other pigments resulting from intravascular hemolysis, such as methemalbumin, and moderate, indirect hyperbilirubinemia also may be detectable. The red cells appear normal on peripheral blood smear. Occasionally, erythrophagocytosis and immature leukocytes are visible in the peripheral blood.

During an acute attack the direct Coombs' test with a complement-specific reagent is positive. The diagnosis is established by demonstrating supernatant hemolysis in red cell suspensions that have been chilled in ice and subsequently warmed to 98.6° F (37° C).

Management. Aside from treating syphilis, specific therapy is unavailable. Acute hemolytic episodes during infections are self-limited. In chronic PCH, avoidance of exposure to cold is the most prudent and practical approach. Adrenal corticosteroids have not been beneficial, and immunosuppressive agents are both toxic and relatively untried.

Traumatic hemolytic anemias and red cell fragmentation syndromes

When red cells are subjected to excessive physical trauma within the cardiovascular system, they may undergo premature fragmentation and lysis because undue shear stress is placed on them and the elastic limits of their membranes are exceeded. In an abnormal environment progressive membrane deformation leads to eventual membrane rupture. Syndromes produced as the result of these events are fragmentation hemolysis associated with abnormalities of the heart and great vessels and red cell destruction related to small-vessel disease, so-called microangiopathic hemolytic anemia.

CARDIOVASCULAR ANOMALIES

Hemolysis may be produced by many types of valvular prostheses; valvular heart disease per se, especially aortic valve abnormalities; arteriovenous fistulas; and aortic coarctation. Early red cell death is due mainly to turbulence and secondarily to direct trauma to the erythrocyte caused by impact on an abnormal natural or artificial vascular structure. Hemolysis rises as patient activity and the cardiac output increase. A vicious circle of greater hemolysis, more severe anemia, augmented cardiac hyperkinesis, and progressive anemia is the outcome.

The severity of the anemia varies. The peripheral red cells usually are normocytic and normochromic, although microcythemia and polychromasia with brisk reticulocytosis may be seen if the hemolysis is active. Morphologic evidence of trauma with a variety of bizarre red cell forms also may be observed. With prolonged hemolysis, hemosiderinuria and hypochromia resulting from iron deficiency may develop. Elevations of bilirubin, LDH, and methemalbumin and decreased serum haptoglobin also are found.

If the anemia is stable and tolerated by the patient and the bone marrow provides an acceptable degree of compensation, the treatment may be with iron and other hematinics such as folic acid. Otherwise, management may require valve replacement or other appropirate operative procedures, since these syndromes usually do not improve spontaneously. Rarely hypersplenism develops, and splenectomy may be necessary.

MICROANGIOPATHIC HEMOLYSIS

Hemolysis resulting from irregularities in the microcirculation is associated with thrombotic thrombocytopenic purpura (TTP); the hemolytic-uremic syndrome; disseminated intravascular coagulation (DIC); pregnancy with eclampsia, preeclampsia, and the postpartum hemolytic syndrome; immunogenic vasculitides, as are present in the collagen disorders; renal homograft rejection and glomerulonephritis; vascular anomalies such as the giant cavernous hemangiomas (Kasabach-Merrit syndrome); disseminated carcinomatosis; oral contraceptives; and malignant hypertension.

The adverse effects in microangiopathic hemolytic anemia are related to changes in the red cells as they course through a fibrin mesh network under applied pressure, which leads to their incisional sectioning and ultimate fragmentation. Release of abnormally shaped residual elements follows. A second mechanism operates when there is a direct vascular lesion. Red cell fragmentation then is thought to result from shearing stress applied to the erythrocytes by the forceful column of arterial blood as it moves past red cells attached to an inflamed, proliferative, and distorted endothelium.

The manifestations of and suspicion for a microangiopathic hemolytic anemia depend on the underlying process responsible for the patient's clinical presentation. Diagnostic support is provided by demonstrating schistocytes and other red cell irregularities in the peripheral blood. The treatment depends largely on the management of the basic disease.

MARCH HEMOGLOBINURIA

March hemoglobinuria is a hemolytic disorder caused by injury to normal red cells within the microcirculation of certain body parts as they forcefully strike hard surfaces. It is detected in marathon runners, karate experts, pelota players, bongo drummers, and patients who hit their heads repeatedly during unusual emotional behavior. It is most probably due to mechanical disruption of the circulating red cells, producing intravascular hemolysis and resulting hemoglobinuria.

The clinical findings usually are insignificant. Transient hemoglobinuria after exertion is the only complaint. Mild jaundice may be present. Nausea and muscle aching may occur early in the episode.

Anemia is very uncommon. The peripheral blood smear shows only polychromasia with a mild reticulocytosis. The serum bilirubin level does not exceed 2 mg/dl, although the serum LDH level may be elevated. Albuminuria and abnormalities of the urinary sediment occasionally have been noted, but chronic renal disease is rare. The disorder is most frequent at the beginning of an exercise program and more often than not remits spontaneously despite continuance of activity.

Paroxysmal nocturnal hemoglobinuria

DEFINITION. Paroxysmal nocturnal hemoglobinuria (PNH; Marchiafava-Micheli syndrome) is an uncommon, acquired intrinsic disorder of the erythrocyte membrane characterized by chronic hemolysis, intermittent but persistent hemoglobinuria and hemosiderinuria, thrombotic phenomena, and bone marrow hypoplasia.

ETIOLOGY AND PATHOGENESIS. This disease supposedly evolves from a defective bone marrow stem cell clone producing several red cell populations that vary in their sensitivity to activated complement components. This diverse vulnerability permits division of the disease into three clinical subgroups, with progressive severity depending on the inherent hemolytic features of the erythrocyte. Increased complement susceptibility, greatest among the youngest circulating erythrocytes, occurs via the classic, antibody-activated, C1-dependent pathway, as well as through the alternate, properdin-dependent complement route in an acidified medium.

CLINICAL MANIFESTATIONS. PNH may be benign or aggressive and debilitating. In its classic form it is hemolytic anemia of insidious onset without racial, familial, or sexual predilection, most frequently surfacing in the third and fourth decades but occasionally manifesting first during childhood. Rather than beginning abruptly with nocturnal hemoglobinuria, the disease may initially be indicated by general signs and symptoms of anemia. Episodic hemoglobinuria actually occurs in only 25% of instances. It is sleep related, since the hemolytic pattern is reversible if the patient sleeps by day rather than during the night. The nocturnal exacerbations, followed by morning excretion of dark urine, may be related to mild reduction of blood pH. Hemolysis, however, also may follow infection, strenuous exercise, or other events such as surgery, menstruation, blood transfusion, and therapeutic ingestion of iron. Symptoms that may be associated with hemolysis are bone and muscle aching, malaise, and fever.

The tendency toward spontaneous intravascular thromboses, perhaps caused by the release of red cell thromboplastins, may produce abdominal pain with obstruction of the mesenteric, portal, or hepatic veins. Obstruction in the last site, which is especially frequent, is associated with sudden hepatomegaly and ascites and may be fatal. Headache caused by cerebrovascular occlusions is a common complaint. Infections are relatively frequent and may be ascribed to qualitative and quantitative neutrophil abnormalities. Additional findings during the patient's clinical course are pallor, jaundice, bronzing of the skin, and splenomegaly.

PNH or a variant may be associated with aplastic anemia, preleukemia, myeloproliferative disorders, and overt leukemia. These combinations support the perception that PNH is one of several myelodysplastic syndromes.

LABORATORY FINDINGS. The anemia may be severe with hemoglobin levels of 6 g/dl or less. Anisocytosis is observed with hypochromia and microcythemia caused by prolonged hemosiderinuria. A relative reticulocytosis, which actually is low in absolute terms, may be present. The bone marrow most often is hyperplastic, but hypoplasia and even aplasia evolve during some stage of the disease. The serum LDH level may be elevated, and the haptoglobin level may be reduced. Hemosiderinuria is detected easily, a process that leads to renal tubular iron deposition and proximal tubular dysfunction.

DIAGNOSIS. The diagnosis, which should be considered in any patient with a puzzling hemolytic anemia, iron deficiency, pancytopenia, splenomegaly, and thrombotic episodes, is based on special tests that challenge the red cell resistance to small amounts of complement.

MANAGEMENT. Since there is no specific treatment, management is symptomatic. If blood transfusions become necessary, saline-washed or, better still, thawed frozen deglycerolized packed red blood cells should be used, since fresh donor plasma may accelerate hemolysis. Therapeutic administration of iron may precipitate hemolysis by causing membrane peroxidation or the release of young, susceptible red cells into the circulation. It should be given after transfusion-suppressed erythropoiesis. Androgens also have been recommended. Heparin and the coumarin-type anticoagulants may be useful on a limited, short-term basis during surgery, parturition, or acute episodes when progressive diffuse hepatic thrombosis is suspected. Adrenal corticosteroids have modified hemolysis in a few patients, particularly in those rare instances associated with a positive Coombs' test. They should be given to patients with otherwise unmanageable signs and symptoms. Splenectomy carries a high morbidity and postoperative mortality. Bone marrow transplantation may become an option in the future.

Hemolytic anemias caused by drugs
IMMUNE HEMOLYSIS

Drug-related immune hemolytic anemias fall into three major categories. In the first type the drugs act as antigens only when bound to plasma proteins and stimulate antibodies mainly of the IgM class. Antigen-antibody (immune) complexes form and adsorb to the red cell surface while simultaneously fixing and activating complement. Drugs frequently associated with this innocent bystander reaction are quinidine, quinine, thorazine, phenacetin, chlorpropamide, para-aminosalicylic acid, and stibophen. The patient need take only a small quantity of the drug for acute intravascular hemolysis, hemoglobinemia, hemoglobinuria, and renal failure to occur. Thrombocytopenia may also be observed occasionally. The direct Coombs' test is positive as a result of the presence of surface complement components. The immune complex does not bind very firmly to the red cells, usually dissociates, and becomes free to react with other cells and extend hemolysis.

In the second form of drug-related hemolysis, caused mainly by penicillin, the drug forms a hapten with the red cell itself, resulting in elaboration of a high-titer IgG antibody directed against the erythrocyte-penicillin complex. Typically, hemolysis develops only in patients receiving very large intravenous doses of penicillin, at least 10 million units daily, for more than 1 week. The anemia commonly is less acute in onset than that caused by drugs of the prior group, red cell destruction is mainly extravascular, and complement is not a major, active ingredient. Although this form of anemia is comparatively benign, it may be lethal if the hemolytic episode goes unrecognized and drug administration is continued. The direct gamma (IgG) Coombs' test is strongly positive. Complete recovery usually follows drug withdrawal, but hemolysis of decreasing severity may persist for several weeks thereafter.

The third type of drug-related hemolytic anemia involves an IgG antibody resembling that of warm-reacting autoimmune hemolytic anemias. The direct IgG Coombs' test is positive in 5% to 15% of the patients taking methyldopa (Aldomet), with the highest incidence in whites, lower frequency in Orientals, and the reaction almost absent in blacks. The anemia appears after 3 to 6 months of treatment, with the positive Coombs' test showing dose dependence. Approximately three times more patients taking more than 2 g of the drug daily have a positive Coombs test compared with patients receiving less than 1 g. Similar antibodies have been observed in patients taking levodopa and mefenamic acid. Splenomegaly may occur. The frequency of overt hemolysis in those receiving methyldopa varies from none to 5%, with the general average approximately 0.8%. The anemia resolves spontaneously after the drug is discontinued. The Coombs' test may remain positive for up to a year after the drug is discontinued and during resolution of the anemia and hemolysis.

NONIMMUNE HEMOLYSIS

In addition to hemolysis generated by oxidant and immune injury and hemoglobin dissociation, as described earlier, certain substances may be toxic by membrane injury or destruction. These include alcohols, steroids, general anesthetics, nonionic detergents, antihistamines, antimalarials, tranquilizers, neuroleptics, antidepressants, local anesthetics, organic and acidic compounds such as phenytoin, barbiturates, and fatty acids. They may produce stomatocytes and acanthocytes. Anthracyclines such as doxorubicin may provoke red cell injury indirectly through the generation of superoxide.

Hemolysis resulting from other causes
TOXINS, CHEMICALS, AND POISONS

Phospholipase in snake and spider venoms may cause hemolysis by releasing membrane phospholipids. Heavy metals such as copper may produce the hemolytic anemia in Wilson's disease by binding to sulfhydryl membrane groups. Zinc and chloramines also have been implicated in hemolysis.

METABOLIC AND RELATED ABNORMALITIES

Hemolysis may occur in liver failure and with alcoholism. The latter may result from the altered membrane cholesterol/phospholipid ratio, as in spur cell anemia. Premature red cell destruction may also be observed in renal failure and in hypophosphatemia. Low serum phosphate levels may reduce red cell ATP synthesis and cause increased membrane rigidity.

INFECTIONS

Red cell injury and removal from the circulation may follow infection caused by microorganisms such as gram-positive cocci, gram-negative bacilli, clostridia, and protozoa (plasmodia, *Babesia, Leishmania,* and *Toxoplasma*). The effects are probably caused by direct membrane injury.

BIBLIOGRAPHY
Congenital hemolytic anemias

Beutler, E.: Red cell enzyme defects as nondiseases and diseases, Blood **54**:1, 1979.

Brody, J.I., Levison, S.P., and Jung, C.J.: Sickle cell trait and hematuria associated with von Willebrand syndromes, Ann. Intern. Med. **86**:529, 1977.

Brody, J.I., and others: Sickle cell crisis treated by limited exchange transfusion, Ann. Intern. Med. **72**:327, 1970.

Dean, J., and Schechter, A.N.: Sickle cell anemia: molecular and cellular basis of therapeutic approaches, N. Engl. J. Med. **299**:752, 804, 863, 1978.

Forget, B.G.: Molecular genetics of human hemoglobin synthesis, Ann. Intern. Med. **91**:605, 1979.

Huisman, T.H.J.: Sickle cell anemia as a syndrome: a review of diagnostic features, Am. J. Hematol. **6**:173, 1979.

Huntsman, R.G., and Lehmann, H.: Treatment of sickle-cell disease, Br. J. Haematol, **25**:437, 1974.

Miwa, S.: Significance of the determination of red cell enzyme activities, Am. J. Hematol. **6**:163, 1979.

Orkin, S.H., and Nathan, D.G.: Current concepts in genetics: the thalassemias, N. Engl. J. Med. **295**:710, 1976.

Palek, J.S., Liu, S.C., and Snyder, L.M.: Metabolic dependence of protein arrangement in human erythrocyte membranes. I. Analysis of spectin-rich complexes in ATP-depleted red cells, Blood **51**:385, 1978.

Valentine, W.N.: The Stratton lecture: hemolytic anemia and inborn errors of metabolism, Blood **54**:549, 1979.

Hemolysis caused by acquired abnormalities

Brown, D.L.: The immune interaction between red cells and leukocytes and the pathogenesis of spherocytosis, Br. J. Haematol. **25**:691, 1973.

Engelfriet, C.P.: Autoantibodies in hematological disorders, Clin. Immunobiol. **3**:345, 1976.

Frank, M.M., Atkinson, J.P., and Gadek, J.: Cold agglutinins and cold-agglutinin disease, Annu. Rev. Med. **28**:291, 1977.

Frank, M.M., and others: Pathophysiology of immune hemolytic anemia, Ann. Intern. Med. **87**:210, 1977.

Garratty, G., and Petz, L.D.: Drug-induced immune hemolytic anemia, Am. J. Med. **58**:398, 1975.

68 • ABNORMAL HEMOGLOBIN PIGMENTS
Jerome I. Brody

METHEMOGLOBINEMIA

Methemoglobinemia is a clinical condition in which there is greater than the normal 1% level of methemoglobin, an oxidation product of hemoglobin, present in the circulation. It may be acquired or hereditary.

Acquired methemoglobinemia

Various therapeutic agents, industrial compounds, materials used in the home, food, and well water can cause methemoglobinemia when they either oxidize circulating hemoglobin directly or facilitate its coupled oxidation by molecular oxygen. Although methemoglobin is constantly present in vivo, its excess formation is prevented by a hemoglobin conversion system in the red cell with the major pathway involving nucleotide adenine diphosphate (NADH)-methemoglobin reductase (diaphorase). This enzyme catalyzes methemoglobin reduction via cytochrome b_5, using NADH as a hydrogen donor. The reduced cytochrome reduces methemoglobin to hemoglobin.

The symptoms of methemoglobinemia vary in intensity depending on the offending compound's rate of entry into the circulation, its metabolism and conversion to various intermediate forms, its excretion, and the capacity of the erythrocyte to reduce the oxidized pigment. Generally, a 10% to 25% methemoglobin level produces cyanosis but is tolerated without illness. At a 35% to 40% methemoglobin level, slight exertional dyspnea, headache, fatigue, vertigo, and tachycardia may be observed. However, if methemoglobinemia develops very quickly, symptoms may occur at the somewhat lower concentration of 20% to 30%. At a 55% to 60% level of methemoglobin, lethargy and stupor result. The 70% methemoglobin level is lethal. Levels above 50% do not occur in hereditary methemoglobinemia (see following discussion), and toxic symptoms are most uncommon in this form of pigment disorder. Symptoms are caused largely by the inability of methemoglobin to transport oxygen and by increased oxygen affinity of the residual unaltered hemoglobin.

The diagnosis should be suspected if the clinical situation warrants it and the presence of cyanosis defies a common explanation. The specific diagnosis is confirmed spectrophotometrically by the presence of a hemolysate absorption band at 502 and 632 nm that disappears on the addition of a cyanide. If the oxidant stress is especially severe, supravital dye staining may show Heinz bodies in the peripheral blood, and overt hemolysis may take place.

Methemoglobinemia with levels of 20% to 30% disappears spontaneously 24 to 72 hours after the inducing agent is removed, and therefore treatment usually is unnecessary. When exposure has been great and signs and symptoms are severe, treatment with methylene blue is appropriate. A 1% solution in a dosage of 1 mg/kg may be injected intravenously over a 5-minute period. This promptly activates the hexose monophosphate shunt, and conversion of methemoglobin begins. If cyanosis has not disappeared within the hour, a second dose of 2 mg/kg may be given. It is unwise to exceed a total dose of 7 mg/kg because methylene blue itself is toxic.

Hereditary methemoglobinemias

Hereditary methemoglobinemias are caused by structurally altered hemoglobins and also by an enzyme variant. The precise location and nature of the abnormal amino acid substitutions in the altered hemoglobins are shown in Table 68-1. The miscoded amino acid replacements in the primary hemoglobin structure lead to an increased oxidation tendency of the heme iron or prevent reduction of methemoglobin. Only heterozygotes have been identified, since the homozygous condition probably is incompatible with life. The abnormal hemoglobin concentration does not exceed 25% to 30%, the hemoglobin M is heterogeneously distributed among the erythrocytes, and the older red cells contain comparatively more abnormal pigment. Hemoglobin M_{Iwate} probably is the most important hemoglobinopathy in Japan and is called hereditary nigremia because of the peculiar color of the blood pigment.

A second form of hereditary methemoglobinemia is due to NADH-methemoglobin reductase (diaphorase) deficiency. In homozygotes the enzyme is completely absent. No clinical or laboratory abnormality is detectable in heterozygotes because the red cell's reducing capability exceeds its oxidizing capacity by 250 times.

Cyanosis usually is the sole clinical manifestation in patients with the M hemoglobins. The diagnosis may be suspected clinically and confirmed by spectrophotometric examination of acid methemoglobin hemolysates at wavelengths between 500 and 600 nm and also by electrophoresis.

Patients with the enzyme defect are not ill. The most striking clinical feature is their cyanotic slate-gray, gray-brown, or violet skin color, with these changes particularly conspicuous on the lips, oral mucous membranes, tongue, palate, nose, and ears. Clubbing and other evidence of cardiopulmonary disease are absent.

Methemoglobin is present at a level of 20% to 50%. Most of the methemoglobin is in the minor, aging red cell population, possibly because the protection provided by ancillary (glutathione) pathways is reduced as the red cell becomes senescent. The decreased oxygen-carrying capacity of the abnormal pigment may inconstantly lead to mild erythrocytosis. The red cell life span is normal. The initial diagnosis of the enzyme disorder may be made with a rapid screening test using the disappearance of fluorescence during formation of NADH as an endpoint. Treatment is not required for the hemoglobin variants, and it is given for the enzyme deficiency only for cosmetic reasons. Methylene blue, 100 to 300 mg a day orally to reduce the methemoglobin concentration to 10%, has been recommended. A less effective alternative is oral ascorbic acid.

OTHER PIGMENTS
Sulfhemoglobinemia

Sulfhemoglobin (SH) is an irreversibly denatured, further oxidized form of hemoglobin defined by its solubility and its spectral absorption band at 620 nm, which does not disappear with the addition of cyanide. SH is associated with drugs similar to those producing methemoglobinemia. Why methemoglobin develops in certain patients and SH in others under identical circumstances is unclear. The clinical symptoms resemble those of methemoglobinemia. Since sulfhemoglobin cannot be reconverted to hemoglobin, there is no treatment other than waiting for the abnormal red cells to disappear.

Carboxyhemoglobinemia

Carbon monoxide (CO) binds reversibly to hemoglobin when the iron is in the reduced state to produce carboxyhemoglobin. Its adverse effects are negligible at the normal endogenous level of 0.3% to 0.7%. The toxicity of CO is related to its high affinity for heme, which is 210 times greater than that of oxygen. At a 20% concentration of carboxyhemoglobin a healthy person will complain of headache, nausea, vomiting, and loss of manual dexterity. When a 50% carboxyhemoglobin level is reached in normal persons, convulsions and coma occur. The lethal level of this pigment is 70%. Patients with heart disease may be symptomatic at lower CO concentrations.

After acute CO exposure the gas remains tightly bound to hemoglobin for 4 hours, causing a left shift of the oxygen dissociation curve and relative homogeneous red cell distribution of CO. The treatment of choice remains exposure to the highest possible concentration of inspired oxygen. The half-life of carboxyhemoglobin while the subject is breathing room air is approximately 240 minutes. At 100% oxygen ventilation the half-life decreases to 40 minutes.

BIBLIOGRAPHY

Jackson, D.L., and Menges, H.: Accidental carbon monoxide poisoning, J.A.M.A. **243**:772, 1980.

Table 68-1. Hemoglobin M variants

Hemoglobin	Amino acid change
Hb M_{Boston}	($\alpha_2$58 His → Tyr β_2)
Hb M_{Iwate}	($\alpha_2$87 His → Try β_2)
Hb $M_{Saskatoon}$	($\alpha_2\beta_2$63 His → Tyr)
Hb $M_{Hyde\ Park}$	($\alpha_2\beta_2$92 His → Tyr)
Hb $M_{Milwaukee_1}$	($\alpha_2\beta_2$ Val → Glu)

69 • HEMOCHROMATOSIS

William E. Barry

DEFINITION. Hemochromatosis is a syndrome characterized by increased deposition of iron in body tissues, frequently accompanied by organ damage.

ETIOLOGY. Body iron overload occurs in several disorders. Refractory anemia with multiple transfusions (100 or more), prolonged excess dietary iron (as in Bantu siderosis) or medicinal iron, and other environmental sources of iron such as certain forms of alcoholic beverages consumed by patients with alcoholic cirrhosis cause typical varieties of "secondary" hemochromatosis. In the absence of an underlying disease or an identifiable source of excess iron, hemochromatosis is termed "primary" or "idiopathic." There is compelling evidence that idiopathic hemochromatosis is a genetically determined disorder of iron absorption.

PATHOGENESIS. The amount of iron absorbed from the diet is controlled within narrow limits by poorly understood mechanisms and normally amounts to about 1 mg a day. Physiologic iron loss exactly balances absorption but cannot be increased significantly; hence increments in total body iron reflect changes in absorption. Since there are limits to iron absorption even when intake is very high, it takes many years to accumulate the enormous amounts of body iron found in hemochromatosis, unless the iron excess occurs by blood transfusions or parenteral administration of iron. An excess of only 2 mg of absorbed iron daily over 60 years will result in over 40 g of excess body iron, an amount common in patients with hemochromatosis.

It is not difficult to understand how excess environmental iron over many years can lead to large increases in total body iron. When there is no increase in environmental iron, as in idiopathic hemochromatosis, it seems clear that the iron absorption process is enhanced. The precise defect has not yet been established. Genetic determination is supported by the familial occurrence of the disease and the recently noted association with certain HLA markers.

The mechanism of organ damage associated with iron overload is not well understood. The liver parenchyma is most commonly involved by iron overload in primary hemochromatosis; eventually fibrosis occurs with cirrhosis as the result. Iron deposition in advanced disease also occurs frequently in the pancreas, endocrine glands, and myocardium. Skin pigmentation commonly results from increased melanin deposition; iron in skin is often lacking or present in only small amounts.

Parenteral iron, or iron derived from multiple transfusions, is deposited initially in reticuloendothelial cells and does not appear to result in organ damage. Redistribution to parenchymal cells eventually occurs, however, and the clinical and pathologic features of primary hemochromatosis may be seen in some patients with secondary hemochromatosis.

CLINICAL MANIFESTATIONS. Hemochromatosis is found most commonly in men and postmenopausal women. The classic clinical findings of increased skin pigmentation, cirrhosis, and diabetes are seen in advanced disease. There is much variation in individual patients. Skin pigmentation may be minimal or lacking, and diabetes mellitus may or may not be present. Family members of patients with hemochromatosis and diabetes have a higher incidence of diabetes than the general population. Congestive heart failure is not confined to older patients but seems to be less common than in earlier reports.

Cirrhosis of the liver is the dominating clinical feature, with the usual findings of spider angiomata, palmar erythema, gynecomastia, and testicular atrophy. The liver is usually enlarged, and splenomegaly may be present. Hepatoma is said to be a more frequent complication in hemochromatosis than in alcoholic cirrhosis.

Arthritis is present in many patients at some time in the course of their disease. Chondrocalcinosis is frequent, and occasionally iron deposits are found in synovial membranes.

LABORATORY FINDINGS. Anemia is not a typical feature of hemochromatosis but may occur as a manifestation of the accompanying cirrhosis or dietary folate deficiency. Liver function abnormalities may be relatively mild. The most consistent laboratory feature is an elevated serum iron level, often with near saturation of transferrin. An increased serum ferritin level is seen. Depending on the extent of other organ dysfunction, abnormalities in the blood sugar, hormone levels, or electrocardiogram may be found.

DIAGNOSIS. The diagnosis is not difficult when the clinical triad of increased skin pigmentation, diabetes mellitus, and hepatic cirrhosis is present. Confirmation is best made by liver biopsy, which demonstrates iron overload accompanying the histologic features of cirrhosis. Support for a diagnosis of idiopathic hemochromatosis rests on (1) excluding a source of excess iron and (2) family studies documenting idiopathic iron overload. HLA typing may prove to be a useful means of identifying family members who warrant particular attention. Simpler measures such as the determination of serum iron and ferritin levels are readily available screening tests for family members, especially those in younger age groups, who may have only moderate degrees of iron overload and hepatic damage. Family studies, although tedious and time consuming, are important to identify members in the precirrhotic stage, who may clearly benefit from the removal of excess iron by periodic phlebotomies.

COURSE. Improvement in overall survival since the institution of phlebotomy therapy in hemochromatosis has been documented. The most common causes of death are hepatoma, liver failure, and congestive heart failure. Improvement in liver function and decreased insulin requirements in the diabetic may occur following successful phlebotomy therapy, but such therapy may not prevent the development of hepatoma nor the severity of the arthritis that may accompany hemochromatosis.

MANAGEMENT. The treatment of choice in primary hemochromatosis is phlebotomy therapy to eliminate iron overload. This can often be done at weekly intervals and is surprisingly well tolerated. Since each 500 ml of blood removed by phlebotomy contains about 250 mg of iron, it may take several years to remove the often enormous amounts of iron (40 to 60 g) present. Iron-chelating agents are not generally used owing to their relative inefficiency compared with phlebotomy, the need for parenteral injection, their cost, and their uncertain long-term adverse effects.

In secondary hemochromatosis resulting from transfusions for refractory anemia, phlebotomies have little place. In these patients iron-chelating agents may prove beneficial, but experience with this therapy is still limited.

BIBLIOGRAPHY

Crosby, W.H.: Hemochromatosis: the unsolved problems, Semin. Hematol. 14:135, 1977.

Fairbanks, V.F., Fahey, J.L., and Beutler, E.: Hemosiderosis and hemochromatosis. In Fairbanks, V.F., Fahey, J.L., and Beutler, E., editors: Clinical disorders of iron metabolism, ed. 2, New York, 1971, Grune & Stratton, Inc.

Finch, S.C., and Finch, C.A.: Idiopathic hemochromatosis: an iron storage disease, Medicine 34:381, 1955.

Jacobs, A.: Iron overload: clinical and pathologic aspects, Semin. Hematol. 14:89, 1977.

70 • PRINCIPLES OF BLOOD BANKING AND TRANSFUSION THERAPY

I. Robert Schwartz

Much of the recent progress in medicine and surgery would not have been possible without concurrent advances in blood transfusion therapy. Blood transfusions now exceed 5 million a year in the United States alone and tend to be regarded as commonplace and routine. However, as with many boons to mankind, blood transfusion is fraught with dangers and pitfalls. Those whose job it is to prescribe blood for transfusions must have adequate knowledge of this complex subject to maximize benefits while minimizing risks. The amount of information, with its detailed specifics, has become so voluminous that only a specialist in this field can hope to maintain scientific and clinical mastery. Physicians who order blood should at least be conversant with the principles of transfusion therapy, so that they can provide rational therapy for their patients and cooperate intelligently with those in the blood transfusion service. All involved should be committed to safety in transfusion therapy. The work of the blood bank extends to every aspect of transfusion therapy, and a discussion of its activities will serve as a framework for the introduction of the essential principles and practice of transfusion therapy.

PROCUREMENT AND COLLECTION

Improvements in the technique for the collection of blood have led to increased versatility and flexibility in its use. The most noteworthy advances include the use of plastic containers rather than glass bottles, the use of improved anticoagulant-storage solutions, the development of automated blood cell separators, and the permanent storage of frozen glycerolized red cells.

Plastic containers provide ease in transferring plasma and other components to satellite bags without breaking sterility. Thus blood can readily be fractionated into its component parts: plasma, red cells, platelet concentrates, and cryoprecipitates. Unwanted components such as white cells can be removed. This has led to the present era of component therapy, in which only the specific component required is transfused. An additional benefit, the salvage of the remaining components of whole blood, makes the system efficient in the conservation of this valuable resource.

Automated cell separators are machines that instantly separate blood into its component parts as it flows from the donor and strikes the wall of a spinning centrifuge bowl. These machines are of two types. In the continuous flow method the separator operates continuously from beginning to end of the donation, simultaneously returning the red cells to the donor. The intermittent flow method accomplishes the same purpose, with short interruptions of flow for the return of red cells to the donor. Large quantities of plasma (plasmapheresis), white cells (leukapheresis), or platelets (plateletpheresis) may be removed from a donor very rapidly. Fractionation may also be carried out without the benefit of an automated separator by drawing whole blood into a plastic container, centrifuging it, separating the plasma, white cells, or platelets, and then returning the red cells to the donor. This method does not require expensive equipment, but it is tedious and time consuming and exposes the donor to the risk of receiving the wrong red cells in return. In certain diseases plasma exchange has been shown to be useful in the removal of undesirable constituents from the blood. The removed plasma is replaced partially with saline and partially with normal plasma, serum albumin, or plasma protein fraction.

Cell separators can be used for plasma exchange to correct the hyperviscosity syndrome seen in Waldenström's macroglobulinemia. Immune-complex disease and diseases of excessive antibody formation are also being treated experimentally in this way. Examples of such diseases are systemic lupus erythematosus, Goodpasture's syndrome, and myasthenia gravis. Cell separators are also used to collect single-donor platelets and white cells for transfusion. However, most platelet concentrates are made from whole blood drawn into plastic bags and then centrifuged gently to produce platelet-rich plasma. This then is transferred to a satellite bag and centrifuged rapidly, yielding a platelet concentrate and a supernatant of platelet-poor plasma. The platelet-poor plasma is removed to be used for fresh-frozen plasma or for the production of cryoprecipitate. Patients requiring platelet transfusions generally receive 6 to 10 such preparations at one time, each concentrate coming from a different donor. Antibodies against foreign platelets develop within several weeks of such transfusions, and transfusions of random platelets are then useless because of the rapid destruction of the platelets by alloantibodies. However, the platelets of a donor who has the same HLA antigens as the patient may survive normally in the patient's circulation. The problem is to obtain a yield of platelets from the single matched donor equal to the amount derived from 6 to 10 random donors. The cell separator can do this efficiently, and it is in such instances that it finds its best present-day use in the area of platelet transfusion. White cell transfusions are still somewhat controversial, but most authorities agree that such transfusions are useful as part of the total care of the patient with a temporary marrow aplasia. In acute nonlymphatic leukemia, after induction of remission with aplasia-producing drugs, white cell transfusions may be useful in infections refractory to antimicrobial therapy.

Cell processors can produce white cells fairly efficiently if hydroxyethyl starch (a red cell sedimenting agent) is used to facilitate cell separation and if corticosteroids are given to raise the donor's granulocyte count. All processors can achieve clinically significant yields (about 10^{10} white cells).

The freezing of blood for prolonged storage has become a practical reality. However, because of the relatively high cost of the process (about two to three times the cost of storage in the liquid form), it has not become routine. Its best application is in the stockpiling of bloods of rare types for use in patients who have antibodies against most donor red cells. This provides rapid availability of blood for such patients, avoiding the search for suitable ambulatory donors on short notice. In addition, nonanemic patients with rare antibodies may donate their own blood for storage in the frozen state in anticipation of future transfusion needs (autologous transfusion). Glycerol is added to the blood before freezing, and the blood is stored at $-136°$ F ($-80°$ C) or lower. After thawing but before transfusion, the glycerol must be removed from the red cells or hemolysis will occur on contact with plasma. A continuous automated method for deglycerolization using wash solutions during centrifugation simplifies the procedure. Since only laboratories equipped for cryopreservation can provide the services necessary, frozen blood is generally available only in hospitals with such facilities or through a community blood center. Frozen blood cells are virtually free of plasma, white cells, and platelets as a result of the deglycerolizing process. Therefore thawed cells for transfusion are useful in avoiding sensitization to leukocyte transplantation antigens in patients who are to have organ transplants.

Frozen red blood cells have some important specialized applications but are unsuitable for routine use because of two factors: the high cost and the need to use them within 24 hours of thawing to avoid bacterial contamination. Although it was once believed that serum hepatitis from blood transfusion might be eliminated by using frozen blood, more recent experience has not borne this out.

FITNESS AND SAFETY

The safe use of blood transfusions depends on the quality of the blood itself, as well as its compatibility with the recipient's blood.

Transmissible diseases

Certain diseases may be transmitted by blood transfusions. The most significant of these are hepatitis, syphilis, and malaria. Exclusion of these diseases from blood depends in large part on careful donor selection. Each donor must be asked a series of questions to uncover possible infection or exposure to these diseases. Blood obtained from voluntary donors is far less frequently involved in the transmission of disease than blood from paid donors. This is especially true of serum hepatitis, which is transmitted about 10 times more frequently by blood drawn from paid donors than by blood from voluntary donors. The use of blood from paid donors should be avoided whenever possible. The reasons for the difference are unknown but probably have to do with the reliability of the donor history and the increased prevalence of hepatitis in the less affluent paid donor population. Tests for hepatitis-associated antigen are now mandatory for every unit of blood for transfusion. The most common method for detecting the hepatitis B surface antigen (HB_sAg) is the radioimmunoassay. This procedure has dramatically reduced the transmission of hepatitis B. There is still considerable transmission of non A/non B hepatitis, for which there is not yet a reliable test.

Even when all precautions have been taken, there remains a significant unavoidable risk of transmitting hepatitis. Therefore the administration of blood and all of its products capable of transmitting hepatitis should be regarded as potentially harmful and life threatening. No transfusion should be ordered without good justification. Blood should be used to correct the adverse effects of anemia when there is no other way to accomplish this. It should never be used capriciously, cosmetically, or carelessly.

Transfusion-transmitted syphilis is now rare with serologic testing and refrigeration of blood, which in most cases destroys the spirochete in about 3 days.

Blood containing malarial parasites may remain infective after a week of refrigerated storage. Donors who may have malaria must be screened by a careful history, which should include the donor's past involvement with malaria, recent malarial attacks, antimalarial medication, and sojourn or travel in a malarial area. Definite rules for blood donation and donor rejection are prescribed for these conditions.

Cytomegalovirus infection may occur after the transfusion of large amounts of blood, especially after heart surgery. This produces a disorder resembling infectious mononucleosis, with fever, splenomegaly, and leukopenia (postperfusion syndrome). Infectious mononucleosis may occasionally be transmitted by blood transfusions. Other diseases reported to be transmitted in this manner are brucellosis, Chagas' disease, sleeping sickness (trypanosomiasis), kala-azar (leishmaniasis), filariasis, and possibly toxoplasmosis.

Compatibility

Before blood may be safely transfused into a patient, the possibility of immunologic incompatibility between donor and recipient must be investigated. Such an incompatibility may result in the rapid destruction of the transfused red cells with immediate consequences to the recipient or in the delayed sensitization of the recipient to donor cells with production of antibodies. Sensitization may jeopardize the safety of future transfusions or pregnancies. When blood is transfused, the greatest potential mischief lies in the donor red cells, which contain antigens foreign to the recipient. The donor plasma is far less likely to produce serious problems, since plasma antibodies usually are rendered harmless by dilution in the recipient's plasma before they can interact with the recipient's cells. Exceptions to this are the transfusion of massive amounts of plasma and also of plasma with very high titers of antibody. Occasionally anaphylactoid reactions develop in IgA-deficient recipients following transfusions as a result of the action of the recipient's antibodies (anti-IgA) against IgA immunoglobulins in the donor plasma.

Since there are in excess of 20 known blood group systems and 389 red cell antigens, it is impossible to test for donor-recipient compatibility in all of these systems. Fortunately, it is unnecessary to do so. Although there are many blood groups, they are not all of equal clinical importance.

The most important systems by far are the ABO and Rh systems because (1) almost everyone (AB individuals excepted) has naturally occurring alloantibodies against blood group antigens A or B; (2) 15% of the population is Rh negative and 70% of these will produce antibodies if the Rh antigen is introduced into their blood; and (3) all of these antibodies are capable of producing severe hemolytic reactions. The rest of the blood group systems are of lesser importance, some being very rarely involved in transfusion reactions.

Most red cell antibodies are formed in response to the transfusion or injection of red cells or as a result of pregnancy with the fetus carrying the sensitizing antigen. When antibodies form without sensitizing antigenic exposure, they are said to be naturally occurring. In the ABO system the absence of an antigen from an individual's phenotype is always associated with the development of naturally occurring antibodies against that antigen. In some other blood group systems naturally occurring antibodies sometimes form, and in still others antibodies never occur naturally but only in response to specific antigenic exposure via transfusions or pregnancy.

The discovery of the ABO system opened the way to the clinical use of blood transfusions. For each phenotypic antigen, A, B, and O, there is a corresponding gene, *A, B,* and *O.* Each individual inherits one gene from each parent, resulting in the following possible combinations:

Genotype	Phenotype	Antigen present A	B
AA	A	+	−
AO	A	+	−
BB	B	−	+
BO	B	−	+
OO	O	−	−
AB	AB	+	+

It can be seen that there is no recognizable antigen as a result of having *O* genes. Individuals produce antibodies against A and B antigens when they are lacking. Therefore antibodies are formed as follows:

Phenotype of red cell	Alloantibody in the plasma
A	Anti-B
B	Anti-A
O	Anti-A and anti-B
AB	None

The prevalence of the various phenotypes in the American population is as follows:

Phenotype	West European descent	African descent
A	45%	29%
B	8%	17%
O	43%	50%
AB	4%	4%

With the use of antiserum known to be specific against A or B antigen, the presence of these phenotypes can be detected in donor and recipient blood. Naturally occurring antibodies against A or B are of the IgM type and will agglutinate red cells in a saline medium at room temperature. They are complete antibodies and do not require incubation or special techniques to produce agglutination. Further confirmation of the blood group is carried out by reverse grouping, which employs red cells of known blood groups. The test serum is checked against these red cells to see if it contains the corroborative antibodies.

When the patient's blood group is known, donor blood of the same group is chosen for further testing. When group-specific blood is unavailable, group-compatible blood may be used. Compatible blood contains no red cell antigens for which there are specific antibodies in the recipient plasma but may contain antibodies against the recipient's red cells. Therefore, when many units of nonidentical blood are to be given, it is important to use blood with the plasma removed (packed red cells) or whole blood with a low titer of antibody in the plasma. The following are examples of group-compatible blood:

Recipient's group	Compatible donor group
A	O
B	O
O	—
AB	O, A, B

In an immunologic reaction resulting from direct exposure to red cells of group A or B, a different class of antibodies is formed. These are of the IgG type and are termed hyperimmune. They may cross the placenta to produce erythroblastosis. They are also incomplete antibodies and can be distinguished in the laboratory from naturally occurring antibodies.

When choosing blood for cross-matching purposes, both the ABO and the Rh systems are taken into account. In the Rh system the blood is specifically tested for the antigen called Rh_0 or D. It is by far the most immunogenic of the Rh antigens and is therefore the most significant clinically. Because it is so immunogenic, the donor and recipient should be matched for it whenever possible, but occasionally it is necessary to give Rh-positive blood to an Rh_0-negative recipient when there is a life-threatening emergency and no Rh-negative blood can be obtained. This can be done only if the recipient has no anti-Rh_0 antibodies. Rh-positive transfusions will expose the recipient to Rh_0 sensitization and may affect the recipient's future transfusability with Rh-positive blood. Transfusions of Rh-positive blood in young Rh-negative patients, especially girls and women of childbearing age, should be avoided because of the danger of Rh sensitization with possible future hemolytic disease of the newborn (HDN). Rh-negative women who have been pregnant may have formed antibodies against Rh_0 as a result of fetal sensitization. These patients would almost certainly have a severe hemolytic transfusion reaction if given a transfusion of Rh-positive blood by error. Rh sensitization may be prevented in most cases if adequate amounts of anti-D (Rh_0) immune globulin are administered shortly after exposure to the Rh_0 antigen as a result of either childbirth or the transfusion of Rh-positive blood. The administered Rh immune globulin combines with the Rh_0 antigen, rendering it nonimmunogenic. Maternal sensitization may therefore be avoided and transfusions of unmatched blood (by mistake or intention) may be made harmless if treated promptly.

About 15% of whites and 2% of blacks are Rh negative. This low frequency sometimes leads to the problem of short supply of Rh-negative blood for transfusions.

Testing for the other antigens in the Rh system (C, c, E, e) is not routinely performed because they cause sensitization much less frequently. This also holds true for all other blood group antigens. Nevertheless, any one of these antigens may be a potential source of trouble in a given case. The solution to this problem is to depend on the cross-match test between the recipient's serum and the donor's cells. If an incompatibility is found, attempts should be made to identify the irregular antibody or antibodies present. This may be done by the use of a "panel" of test cells that has been carefully constructed to yield a specific reaction pattern for each antigen included in the panel. According to the pattern of reactions produced by a given antibody, the corresponding antigen can be identified. It then becomes a matter of screening many units of blood with the specific antiserum to find compatible units that lack the antigen in question and therefore are not reactive with the recipient's serum.

In emergency transfusions there may not be time to identify an antibody causing incompatible cross-matches. In this case many units of blood are cross matched in the hope of finding a sufficient number of compatible units by chance alone. The decision to use such "compatible" blood must be based on the relative risk of waiting for proper antibody identification versus the risk of proceeding with transfusion in the face of an unidentified antibody or antibodies. In such circumstances reliance on the cross-match alone for donor selection is risky. Although the amount of antibody present in the recipient's serum may be sufficient to detect incompatible donor units with red cells homozygous for the offending antigen, it may be insufficient to detect those units with heterozygous red cells. The final decision must be made by the attending physician in consultation with the director of the transfusion service.

Compatibility testing is the foundation of the blood bank's safety procedure. It is the final common pathway of the blood bank's activities leading to the release of blood for transfusion. It is the last in a series of steps to find possible immunologic discrepancies, the ultimate check for possible technical errors previously committed, and the final seal of approval placed on the blood by those performing the testing. Nevertheless, in rare instances cross-matching will be unable to detect certain problems such as potential delayed transfusion reactions.

Cross-matching or compatibility testing is carried out by mixing donor red cells with patient serum to detect antibodies against donor red cell antigens as manifested by red cell agglutination or hemolysis.

PRINCIPLES OF TRANSFUSION THERAPY

Blood transfusion should be used only when other, less dangerous methods of correcting anemia are not applicable. Whenever a timely and safe correction can be achieved by using hematinics such as iron or cyanocobalamin, this course is preferable. However, there are times when these alternatives are ineffective or take too long to be useful and safe. Some examples are refractory chronic anemias, anemia in patients with ischemic heart disease, anemia severe enough to be life threatening, and anemia in a patient being prepared for nonelective surgery. With today's availability of component therapy, the deficiencies that need to be corrected in any given case should be determined, and only the required components should be used. The practice of using whole blood for blood transfusion has been largely overcome through educational efforts and by making whole blood much less available than it was previously. Most large regional blood centers remove the plasma from the majority of blood drawn. This plasma is used for the preparation of other blood components and derivatives such as cryoprecipitates, serum albumin, and clotting factor concentrates. Red blood cells have the following advantages over whole blood in transfusion therapy: (1) less fluid volume; (2) less citrate; (3) less storage waste products such as potassium and ammonia; and (4) less donor antibodies. The major advantage is volume reduction, which may be essential for safe transfusions in patients with actual or borderline cardiac decompensation. In massive transfusion the advantages of less citrate and less storage waste products take on considerably more importance. Since it is now more difficult to obtain whole blood than red blood cells, the clinician is forced to think of red blood cells as the routine way to use blood and must have indications for selecting whole blood. Most authorities agree that these indications are few.

Most transfusions are used to correct the inadequate oxygen-carrying power of the blood resulting from anemia, and red blood cells are needed for this purpose. The problem arises in the treatment of shock and massive hemorrhage, when the circulatory volume must be restored. However, even under these circumstances whole blood should be used sparingly and not in every case. A number of plasma substitutes, used alone or in conjunction with red blood cells, will provide optimal management of such patients. These plasma substitutes are colloid solutions of dextran and starch, albumin, and plasma protein derivative. Also, plasma itself may be used as a separate component to provide the volume of fluid to be replaced. In the initial treatment of shock, crystalloids (saline, Ringer's lactate, and so forth) have been found useful and can be administered immediately without waiting for preparation of blood, thawing of plasma, or reconstitution of powdered materials. In cases of massive hemorrhage, blood can be replaced with red blood cells, adding additional volume in the form of colloids or solutions of plasma proteins as required. When the amount of blood loss exceeds 40% of the patient's blood volume, whole blood transfusion can justifiably be employed. Even under these circumstances it is probably best to alternate each unit of whole blood with 1 unit of red blood cells. If additional fluid volume is required (as judged by the central venous pressure), it can be given in the form of colloids or plasma protein solution.

There is no need for whole blood during routine blood replacement at surgery. The blood volume, as judged by the vital signs, may be maintained easily with intravenous solutions, and the oxygen-carrying capacity may be maintained with red blood cell transfusions based on estimated blood loss.

Massive blood loss requires massive replacement transfusion, which may produce problems of its own. Stored blood undergoes changes that generally do not cause clinical problems if transfusions are given in usual amounts over suitable periods of time. However, these abnormalities may become significant when massive transfusions (more than 10 units in 24 hours) are given. The transfused blood is cold and acidic; has no ionized calcium but a high sodium and potassium content; has decreased ability to deliver oxygen to tissues (low 2,3-diphosphoglycerate); contains potential microemboli in the form of microaggregates of platelets, leukocytes, and fibrinogen; and has low levels of labile coagulation factors. Furthermore, the blood contains large amounts of citrate, which if given rapidly may produce serious toxic effects such as cardiac arrhythmias because of a reduction in the ionized calcium level. This may require correction with intravenous calcium solution. Impaired liver function makes the patient much more susceptible to citrate toxicity. Patients with advanced liver disease present a special problem, since they are more likely to have clinical emergencies requiring massive transfusions, such as esophageal varices, peptic ulcer, and coagulation defects. Ice-cold blood may also produce cardiac arrhythmias when given rapidly. Blood should be prewarmed when rapid transfusion is required. In posttransfusion studies of patients receiving massive amounts of blood, it was found that the serum sodium level did not rise, and the serum potassium level actually fell in spite of high levels in the transfused blood. A suggested explanation was the loss of potassium through hemorrhage. In some cases it was even necessary to administer additional potassium after massive transfusions. Microaggregates may be filtered out using special micropore filters, but these may reduce the maximal rate at which blood can be administered. Furthermore, there is no definite proof that these microaggregates are capable of causing pulmonary insufficiency, and there is no consensus favoring the usefulness of the filters. Platelet transfusions may be given if the posttransfusion platelet count falls to levels (below $20,000/mm^3$) that may give rise to spontaneous bleeding or cause a perpetuation of preexisting bleeding. Fresh-frozen plasma is useful to correct deficiencies of labile clotting factors. An acceptable routine to be employed for massive blood replacement is (1) to use a blood warmer after the administration of 3 units of bank blood; (2) to administer one ampule of sodium bicarbonate (44.6 mEq) for every 5 units of blood transfused; and (3) to give 2 units of fresh-frozen plasma for every 10 units of blood transfused. If red blood cells are being transfused, the serum albumin level should be checked and electrolyte administration should be carefully monitored. When there is impaired liver function, evidence of citrate toxicity should be sought, and if present it should be treated with judicious amounts of intravenous calcium. Electrocardiographic monitoring should be a part of the total care of these patients whenever possible.

TRANSFUSION REACTIONS

Blood group incompatibilities cause the most serious transfusion reactions, usually producing intravascular hemolysis. This should be a rare event, but it may occur when procedure is not followed. Errors in the blood bank laboratory may come from attempting to set up more than one cross-match at a time or from careless labeling of cross-matched blood. There is more danger to be found in patient-care areas because many more people are involved, responsibility is more diffuse, and constant supervision is nearly impossible. The major concern here is the incorrect identification of the patient or the patient's blood specimen. The blood bank cannot detect an erroneously labeled specimen from a patient new to the blood bank. If previous records are available in the blood bank, they must be consulted every time a new specimen is received. When no records exist, the patient receives whatever blood is compatible with the blood in the submitted specimen tube. Some safeguards can be taken. It may be advisable at the bedside to recheck the recipient's blood type on a fresh specimen before starting a first transfusion. This is especially useful in the operating and delivery rooms, where signs of blood transfusion reactions are likely to be masked as a result of general anesthesia. Emphasis on rigid identification procedures can prevent possible labeling errors when specimens are drawn for typing and cross-matching and when blood transfusions are started. Although such procedures may be tedious and difficult to follow at times, uncompromising insistence on adherence to exact performance is the only effective safeguard against errors in identification.

If a hemolytic transfusion reaction should occur, it will usually be heralded by chills, fever, and back pain. The patient should be warned to signal for help immediately if any of these symptoms appears. On discovery of such a reaction, the first step is to stop the blood transfusion and to keep the needle open with a saline drip. An immediate check for a possible error in identification should be made. Specimens of blood and urine should be sent to the laboratory for immediate examination, including tests for free hemoglobin, retyping, re-cross-matching, evidence of antigen-antibody reactions, and bacterial contamination. The blood bag, even if empty, should also be returned to the blood bank.

The patient should be observed carefully for decreased urinary output and evidence of hemolysis. If either is present, mannitol or furosemide should be given intravenously to promote urinary flow. A nephrology consultation should be obtained as soon as possible. Hypovolemic shock should be treated promptly with appropriate solutions. After a cross-match for compatibility, type O red blood cells may be used in cases of severe anemia. The patient should be observed for possible intravascular coagulation. Urinary output must be monitored hourly for the next several days. In the case of persistent uremia, renal dialysis is necessary. Other reactions to blood may be dealt with according to their specific nature. Initially they may mimic hemolytic transfusion reactions.

Allergic reactions are fairly common and not often serious. They may be controlled with parenteral administration of antihistamines or corticosteroids. Severe reactions such as anaphylactoid reactions or angioneurotic edema may require epinephrine. Whether to continue the blood transfusion cautiously is a decision that must be individualized in each case. Premedication may prevent subsequent allergic reactions in many instances.

Antileukocyte antibodies arising from previous transfusions or pregnancies sometimes cause febrile transfusion reactions. Such reactions may be prevented by removing leukocytes from the donor blood. This may be done by filtration, centrifugation, batch washing, the addition of sedimenting agents, or a combination of these procedures. Also, frozen and thawed red cells are leukocyte free and may be used for transfusion in this case.

Bacterial contamination of donor blood is extremely uncommon, but if sepsis is produced in this way, it should be treated promptly with appropriate antibiotics.

Antibodies against IgA are occasionally found in blood recipients who are IgA deficient, and these may incite anaphylactic reactions to plasma protein. These reactions can be severe even with the administration of very small amounts (2 to 3 ml) of plasma. Prompt and vigorous treatment for anaphylaxis should be given immediately after the transfusion has been stopped. Future transfusions should be taken from donors with IgA deficiency, or transmembrane-washed red cells (as in deglycerolizing) should be used. A small amount of blood should be injected as a test dose before further blood transfusion is given after a previous reaction.

BIBLIOGRAPHY

Greenwalt, T.J.: General principles of blood transfusion, ed. 3, Chicago, 1977, American Medical Association.

Issitt, P.D., and Issitt, C.H.: Applied blood group serology, Oxnard, Calif., 1975, Spectra Biologicals.

Mollison, P.L.: Blood transfusion in clinical medicine, Oxford, 1979, Blackwell Scientific Publications.

Race, R.R., and Sanger, R.: Blood groups in man, Oxford, 1975, Blackwell Scientific Publications.

Technical manual of the American Association of Blood Banks, ed. 7, Philadelphia, 1977, J.B. Lippincott Co.

71 • POLYCYTHEMIA

Frank H. Gardner and **Gary B. Weiss**

In past years the diagnosis of polycythemia (defined as an increased number of circulating red cells) has been made by an interpretation of peripheral blood measurements reflecting changes in the red cell, hemoglobin, and hematocrit values. With more accurate isotopic measurements of red cell and plasma volumes, it can now be appreciated that there may be misinterpretation of the peripheral blood measurement, since a reduced plasma volume elevates the hematocrit and hemoglobin values. Although polycythemia vera is the classic disorder that initiated the study of erythrocytosis, the most commonly seen form of elevated hemoglobin is *stress polycythemia* or erythocythemia. This is 10 times more frequent than polycythemia vera.

The rate of red cell production in the normal individual is carefully regulated and involves the response of the committed stem cell compartment to the predominantly kidney-elaborated hormone erythropoietin. It is believed that minimal changes in oxygen diffusion activate the release of erythropoietin from the kidney. The hormone, depending on the concentration, interacts with the committed erythroid stem cell to increase red cell maturation. When there is a marked increase in erythropoietin that can react with the committed stem cell, there will be an increased production of red cells with concurrent elevation of the peripheral hematocrit and hemoglobin values. Hence, any stimulus that increases erythropoietin production eventually could elevate the total red blood cell volume. Such changes in *secondary polycythemia* have been noted with the physiologic adaptation to hypoxia and with inappropriate erythropoietin production by kidney, liver, and lung tumors. A classification of the various types of polycythemia is outlined below:

I. Polycythemia vera
II. Secondary polycythemia
   A. Generalized hypoxia
      1. High altitude
      2. Chronic obstructive pulmonary disease
      3. Cardiovascular shunt (right to left)
      4. Pickwickian syndrome (massive obesity)
      5. High–oxygen affinity hemoglobin
      6. Smoking
   B. Localized hypoxia
      1. Renal cysts
      2. Hydronephrosis
      3. Renal artery stenosis
   C. Autonomous erythropoietin production
      1. Tumor
         a. Renal carcinoma
         b. Hepatoma
         c. Cerebellar hemangioblastoma
         d. Uterine fibroid tumors
         e. Miscellaneous
      2. Recessive familial polycythemia
III. Relative polycythemia
   A. Acute
   B. Chronic (stress)

POLYCYTHEMIA VERA

Polycythemia vera is a relatively uncommon disorder diagnosed most frequently after the age of 50. The disease is slightly more frequent in men and is seen more often in Jews of Eastern European ancestry; it is rare in blacks and Latin Americans. It traditionally has been classified as a myeloproliferative disorder, implying that there is an autonomous production of all cell lines, erythrocytes, granulocytes, and platelets, with a rare chance of transformation into myelofibrosis or acute leukemia.

Recent studies have indicated that polycythemia vera is a specific clonal proliferation of a marrow population. Hence, when the various stem cell components can be identified by glucose-6-phosphate dehydrogenase (G-6-PD) enzyme classification (in women heterozygous for G-6-PD enzymes), there is evidence that all of the proliferating cells observed in polycythemia vera have only a single enzyme component. This demonstrates transformation to a generalized proliferation of a single clone of cells. A second (normal) clone of cells remains relatively inactive in the marrow and is overshadowed by the transformed polycythemia vera clone. The autonomous abnormal clone has no response in vitro to erythropoietin. Serum concentrations of erythropoietin are usually low in the untreated patient owing to inhibition of production by erythrocytosis.

CLINICAL MANIFESTATIONS. Polycythemia vera may be an insidious clinical illness that is undiagnosed for years. Patients may ignore the predominant symptoms of headache, weakness, dizziness, and sweating for a long period. The diagnosis is often considered because of physical findings of plethora (67%), conjunctival engorgement (59%), splenomegaly (70%), and hepatomegaly (40%). However, most often the diagnosis begins with identification of an elevated hematocrit and/or hemoglobin level. A hemoglobin value greater than 17.5 g/dl for men or 16 g/dl for women (hematocrit of 55% and 50% at sea level, respectively) is abnormal and requires further diagnostic study.

As noted, early measurement of the red cell mass is most critical for diagnosis, and this procedure is usually carried out by labeling a known amount of red cells with ^{51}Cr and determining the radioactivity in the blood samples after reinjection. Some laboratories also perform a plasma volume determination by injecting ^{131}I-labeled albumin. A red cell mass greater than 36 ml/kg for men or 32 ml/kg for women is abnormal and can be considered diagnostic of polycythemia. Bone marrow studies show hyperplasia of all precursors with a decreased amount of marrow fat. A variety of abnormal chromosome patterns have been described in these patients before therapy. However, in the past decade these abnormalities have not been helpful in defining the response to therapy or determining survival.

Bone marrow studies may be useful for this type of data collection but do not contribute to the diagnosis.

The first steps in the study of these patients are to obtain a careful medical history and to perform a physical examination to note if the findings just listed are present. Careful attention must be paid to the history of smoking, symptoms of pulmonary disease, and the presence or absence of a palpable spleen. Clues to secondary polycythemia in the history or physical examination may shorten the laboratory workup and allow an earlier diagnosis.

The causes of secondary polycythemia include high-altitude acclimatization, pulmonary disease, cardiovascular disease with arteriovenous shunts, alveolar hypoventilation, defective oxygen transport, and elevated carbon monoxide levels in tobacco smokers. In essence, this group of causes for secondary polycythemia represents a physiologic response to hypoxia with an elevation of erythropoietin. The remaining causes of secondary polycythemia are also related to increased production of erythropoietin and include erythrocytosis resulting from renal vascular impairment, renal cyst, or hydronephrosis. Other sources of abnormal erythropoietin production are hypernephromas, uterine myomas, cerebellar hemangiomas, hepatomas, and endocrine disorders associated with increased androgen production. A small but important group of patients have a rare hereditary overproduction of erythropoietin associated with erythrocytosis from early childhood. Because of the rarity of some of these diagnoses, many hematologists limit the screening laboratory tests to arterial blood oxygen saturation, hemoglobin electrophoresis or determination of the hemoglobin-oxygen dissociation curve, and intravenous pyelogram. The type of secondary polycythemia usually can be identified on the basis of the results of these tests.

In the absence of a cause for secondary polycythemia, the Polycythemia Vera Study Group (PVSG) has established the following widely accepted criteria for the diagnosis of polycythemia vera: an increased red cell mass, a normal arterial oxygen saturation (greater than or equal to 92%), and splenomegaly. In the absence of splenomegaly, two of the following abnormalities must be present: (1) thrombocytosis (platelet count greater than 400,000/mm^3); (2) leukocytosis (white count greater than 12,000/mm^3 in the absence of fever or infection); (3) elevated leukocyte alkaline phosphatase score (greater than 100 in the absence of fever or infection); and (4) elevated serum vitamin B_{12} (greater than 900 pg/ml) or an unbound vitamin B_{12}–binding capacity greater than 2200 pg/ml.

Patients with polycythemia vera have an increased tendency toward thrombotic episodes (such as cerebrovascular thrombosis) and bleeding (such as gastrointestinal hemorrhage). Both tendencies generally normalize with correction of the hematocrit to normal. Patients with polycythemia vera also have an increased risk of acute myeloblastic leukemia.

MANAGEMENT. The PVSG has been evaluating treatment programs for the past 15 years. This cooperative group has noted a marked increase in the transition to acute myeloblastic leukemia in patients receiving alkylating drugs such as chlorambucil. The more accepted therapy with radioactive phosphorus (^{32}P) has about half the incidence of leukemia, and a regular program of phlebotomies has the lowest incidence of leukemia. In the initial years of treatment with phlebotomy this therapy carried an increased risk of cerebrovascular accident. This has made optimal choice of therapies somewhat complicated. In future years the PVSG will compare ^{32}P treatment with phlebotomy therapy in which the patients take aspirin and dipyridamole orally to alter platelet aggregation. The hematocrit should be maintained at levels between 40% to 42% for ideal control of the disease. It has been shown in recent years that falsely high microhematocrits may be observed when the spun hematocrit is compared with that derived from calculation using the red cell count and the mean corpuscular volume (MCV). This is attributed to trapping of the plasma in the direct centrifuge measurements. The difference is exaggerated when the MCV is low, as it often is in iron-deficient phlebotomized patients with polycythemia. Therefore it is suggested that in patients with polycythemia vera, hematocrits be determined with automated equipment and hemoglobin levels be determined spectrophotometrically. Bleeding problems, especially at surgery, are common in untreated persons with polycythemia. All elective surgery, including dental extractions, should be delayed until treatment has normalized the hematocrit.

SECONDARY POLYCYTHEMIA
Hypoxia

The majority of patients with secondary polycythemia have an increased red cell mass attributable to hypoxia. Significant elevations of red cell mass do not occur unless the arterial oxygen saturation falls below 92% and the Po_2 is less than 65 mm Hg. Polycythemia may be present in patients with chronic hypoxemia even in the absence of dyspnea, and it is not rare for polycythemia rather than dyspnea to be the abnormality that first brings the hypoxemic patient to medical attention. It must be emphasized that the peripheral blood values are not always as elevated as would be expected for the degree of hypoxia because of an inappropriate response of the marrow to erythropoietin in the presence of a persistent pulmonary infection (chronic bronchitis). In some patients there is a low Po_2 and an arterial oxygen saturation of less than 90%, but the hematocrit remains in the 55% to 60% range because of an increased plasma volume.

All types of cardiac shunts that allow mixing of venous with arterial blood result in decreased oxygen saturation and secondary polycythemia. The patient with severe cardiac disease may have a hematocrit of 75% to 85%. This is associated with a marked increase in the red cell mass and a very diminished plasma volume. These patients should be protected from dehydration at all times, since enhanced viscosity from fever may cause sludging and infarction in the cerebral circulation. It should be noted that patients with cyanotic secondary polycythemia may also have thrombocytopenia. The cause of the low platelet count has not been defined completely but may be related to decreased plasma volume or low-grade disseminated intravascular coagulopathy.

MANAGEMENT. There is no agreement on a specific therapy program. Treatment, if possible, should be aimed at the cause. Many patients have felt better when the hematocrit was lowered to about 60% by a regular phlebotomy program, but symptomatic relief is more important than laboratory values, and each patient must be titrated to obtain optimal results. Some clinics reinfuse equal amounts of colloid or plasma substitutes to replace the volume of blood removed. Patients with cardiac disease have improved exercise tolerance and variable increments in the platelet count, probably as a result of expansion of the plasma volume with the phlebotomy program. The patients are iron depleted by the frequent phlebotomies. If there are symptoms of glossitis, skin irritation, or fatigue, small doses of iron may be given orally with subjective improvement. Oral folate should be prescribed if there is any doubt about adequate dietary intake. At all times the physiologic abnormalities require attention, such as correction of pulmonary infection or surgical repair of an arteriovenous shunt. Many patients are unable to have surgical procedures, and the phlebotomy program must be continued indefinitely.

Familial polycythemia

In recent years the clinical measurement of erythropoietin has defined a small group of patients who have an increased red cell mass resulting from elevated serum erythropoietin levels. These patients have a genetic abnormality of increased erythropoietin with the onset of erythrocytosis in childhood. Hematocrit values vary in the range of 70% to 80%. The diagnosis is more likely if the patient had elevated hematocrit values in childhood. The diagnosis in part must be related to (1) the exclusion of other forms of secondary polycythemia that also have elevated erythropoietin values, (2) the presence of elevated hematocrit values in other family members, usually siblings, and (3) measurements of erythropoietin. There is no specific therapy other than phlebotomy to reduce the hematocrit to approximately 60% and to obtain maximal subjective improvement, as in hypoxic polycythemia.

Polycythemia related to abnormal hemoglobin

A variety of abnormal hemoglobins associated with erythrocytosis have been reported in the past 15 years. The erythrocytosis is related to a shift in the oxygen dissociation curve to the left of the normal pattern. This shift causes a slower release of oxygen for tissue utilization and thus mild hypoxia. Since the initial description of hemoglobin Chesapeake, 18 abnormal hemoglobins have been described, with expectations of additional types in the future. The inherited abnormality is ascribed to deranged function of oxygen release from the heme molecule. The increased affinity of oxygen to the heme molecule induces impaired oxygen release to varying degrees. There is a wide spectrum of oxygen dissociation curves with these hemoglobin mutants, and rarely a determination of the dissociation curve may be required in the patient's evaluation. Again we emphasize that these patients have only the expected response to erythropoietin, namely erythroid hyperplasia but no leukocytosis, thrombocytosis, or splenomegaly.

Polycythemia related to tumor

Some tumors have been found to excrete erythropoietin, resulting in polycythemia. This is most common with renal (hypernephroma), liver (hepatoma), and cerebellar tumors but can occur with other tumors as well. Treatment of the malignancy, if possible, may control the polycythemia.

Polycythemia related to local hypoxia

The kidney is the normal site of erythropoietin production. When the oxygen supply to one kidney is decreased by renal arterial stenosis, a cyst, or ureteral obstruction, polycythemia can develop. These conditions are amenable to surgical therapy.

RELATIVE POLYCYTHEMIA

A decreased plasma volume may be the reason for increased hemoglobin or hematocrit values in patients whose red cell mass is not elevated, as determined by isotopic measurements. The plasma volume should be obtained simultaneously with the red cell volume to confirm that it is decreased. This condition is called relative polycythemia. Although such plasma volume changes may rarely be associated with the use of a diuretic, vomiting, diarrhea, excess sweating, or high capillary pressure (increased catecholamines or heart failure), these conditions are rare and the initial cause usually is easily recognized.

The chronic forms of relative polycythemia have been called *spurious polycythemia, pseudopolycythemia, stress polycythemia, benign polycythemia,* or *Gaisböck's syndrome.* Most patients with this disorder are middle-aged white men, often tense or under physiologic stress, mildly overweight, hypertensive, and frequently heavy smokers. Indeed, almost all of the studies refer to smoking as a contributory cause or do not report the smoking data.

It is estimated that 3% of the 50 million adults who smoke have an elevated hematocrit value. The inhalation of carbon monoxide by smokers may elevate carboxyhemoglobin levels 4% to 30% with a mean of 10%. Since most of these patients have the same clinical manifestations as those with stress polycythemia, we have included smokers' polycythemia under the general classification of stress polycythemia, although it is actually a form of secondary polycythemia.

Aside from the elevated hematocrit and hemoglobin values and decreased plasma volume levels in stress polycythemia, laboratory findings are generally normal, although an increased incidence of elevated serum uric acid and lipid levels has been noted. The cause of the decreased plasma volume is unknown, but altered venous tone from increased catecholamine secretion induced by carbon monoxide has been suggested as an explanation. Although this disorder has been considered a benign form of polycythemia and does not represent a hematologic malignancy, stress polycythemia carries a poor prognosis. Recent studies have demonstrated an increased incidence of cardiovascular accidents in these patients. Since stress polycythemia represents the most common cause of elevated hematocrit and hemoglobin, its detection is most important.

MANAGEMENT. The major goal of treatment of stress polycythemia is to lower the elevated level of carboxyhemoglobin that causes inefficient oxygen transport. Smoking should not be permitted. The patient should also initiate a weight reduction program to an ideal body weight based on nomogram measurements. If hypertension is present, treatment should preferably be with minimal use of diuretics, which might reduce the plasma volume. The results of treatment can be impressive, with the hematocrit returning to the normal range in 6 to 8 months after weight reduction and cessation of smoking.

Treatment may be much more important for these patients than for those with polycythemia vera. Only in the past decade have the high morbidity and mortality of stress polycythemia been appreciated. The patients were previously looked on as having only an abnormal laboratory measurement, and until recent years reassurance was the main therapy, with occasional participation in regular phlebotomy programs. Patients with stress and/or smokers' polycythemia require the most careful supervision.

BIBLIOGRAPHY

Berlin, N.I.: Diagnosis and classification of the polycythemias, Semin. Hematol. **12**:339, 1975.

Bessman, J.D.: Microcytic polycythemia: frequency of nonthalassemic causes, J.A.M.A. **238**:2391, 1977.

Burge, P.S., Johnson, W.S., and Prankerd, T.A.J.: Morbidity and mortality in pseudopolycythemia, Lancet **1**:1266, 1975.

Smith, J.R., and Landaw, S.A.: Smokers' polycythemia, N. Engl. J. Med. **298**:6, 1978.

Wasserman, L.R.: The treatment of polycythemia vera, Semin. Hamatol. **13**:57, 1976.

Unit B • WHITE BLOOD CELL DISORDERS

72 • QUALITATIVE AND QUANTITATIVE NEUTROPHIL DISORDERS

Richard K. Shadduck

NEUTROPHIL KINETICS

The production of mature polymorphonuclear neutrophils or neutrophilic granulocytes represents an orderly process wherein various stem cell compartments provide a continuous supply of precursor cells in the bone marrow. Such stem cells have not been recognized morphologically but have been assayed by various experimental techniques. From transplantation studies in animals, it is clear that virtually all hematopoietic cells arise from a common pluripotential stem cell that is responsible for erythroid, granulocytic, and megakaryocytic production. This cell appears to differentiate into three classes of unipotential or committed stem cells, each of which is restricted to a single line of differentiation, that is, erythroid, granulocytic, or megakaryocytic. These unipotential cells seem to respond to humoral stimuli that induce the further growth and maturation of specific precursor cells in the marrow. It is well established that erythropoietin is a humoral substance responsible for erythroblast maturation; however, granulopoietic control mechanisms are less well defined.

In vitro studies suggest that the production of mature granulocytes and macrophages may be governed by the action of one or a series of glycoprotein materials termed colony-stimulating factors. These substances are derived from macrophages, fibroblasts, stimulated lymphocytes, and endothelial cells and can be detected in the serum and urine. When added to suspensions of bone marrow cells in semisolid gels, they induce committed stem cells to differentiate into myeloblasts and subsequently to generate large individual colonies of granulocytes and macrophages. The colony-forming cells are present in low concentrations representing about 0.1% of the total marrow cellularity. Colony assays have been useful in helping to define the reduction in numbers or proliferative defect in committed stem cells in disorders such as aplastic anemia and acute leukemia.

Many investigators believe that colony-stimulating factor is a specific substance responsible for granulocyte and macrophage differentiation. Although levels of colony-stimulating factor are increased in neutropenic states, the marked lability of the neutrophil system has thus far precluded definitive in vivo studies. In addition to this positive stimulus for cell production, a number of inhibitory substances have been described. These materials, which are extracted from mature neutrophils, markedly reduce the growth of granulocytic colonies in vitro. The best-characterized inhibitor is lactoferrin, an iron-binding glycoprotein found in neutrophil granules, which is active in extremely low concentrations. As yet, it is uncertain whether this or other inhibitory materials participate in the regulation of granulopoiesis.

The identifiable granulocytic precursor cells in the marrow are classified as (1) the proliferative compartment, which includes myeloblasts, promyelocytes, and myelocytes, and (2) a maturation and storage pool of nonproliferative metamyelocytes, band cells, and segmented neutrophils. These cells are readily identified by the appearance of granules seen only in the neutrophilic series. Large red-purple (on Wright stain) or primary granules that contain myeloperoxidase and other enzymes initially develop in the promyelocyte. Specific or secondary granules form in the myelocyte stage. Both types of granules persist throughout development to the mature neutrophil, where they function in the process of bacterial killing.

The transit time through the bone marrow requires about 9 to 12 days, of which 4 to 6 days are spent in the proliferative compartment. The storage pool of band and segmented cells is approximately 10 times the size of the peripheral blood granulocyte pool and can be readily mobilized in response to peripheral demand. In times of increased need, as with severe infection, band cells and mature neutrophils are immediately released from the marrow into the circulation. This appears to result from the action of another serum factor termed neutrophil releasing factor, which is rapidly produced in response to bacterial endotoxins. This material is believed to be responsible for the early neutrophilia seen with infection but probably is not involved in the basal level of granulocyte production. A similar response is noted after injection of etiocholanolone, which is the basis of an experimental test for neutrophil reserves in patients with various types of neutropenia.

Once released into the circulation, mature neutrophils are equally divided between the circulating and marginal pools. The latter consists of cells loosely adherent to the blood vessels in the lungs, spleen, and elsewhere, which are immediately available in response to stress. Injection of epinephrine causes a transitory increase in the neutrophil count owing to rapid demargination of these cells. This stress reaction probably explains the neutrophilia seen in acutely agitated patients, particularly in the pediatric age group. In some instances infusion of epinephrine may be used to document neutropenic syndromes that are characterized by excessive sequestration rather than destruction of neutrophils.

The half-life of circulating neutrophils is relatively short with a $T_{\frac{1}{2}}$ of 6 to 7 hours. The intravascular life span is frequently shortened to several hours in the neutropenic state and prolonged with neutrophilia. For instance, neutrophils in patients with uncontrolled chronic myelogenous leukemia may circulate for up to 3 days; half-lives return to normal values with appropriate therapy. The short intravascular life span limits the use of therapeutic white cell transfusions in the treatment of acute infections in patients with reversible agranulocytosis.

Neutrophils leave the circulation by traversing the endothelium of capillaries, usually in response to chemotactic factors generated by bacterial growth. Materials such as endotoxin, bradykinin, activated components of complement, and antigen-antibody complexes induce a positive stimulus for neutrophil migration into the tissues. It is believed that the extravascular life span may exceed the time in the circulation by several days. Eventual loss occurs by destruction in the reticuloendothelial system, shedding into the respiratory, genital, or gastrointestinal tracts, or more likely by cell dissolution following phagocytosis and bacterial killing.

NEUTROPHIL DYSFUNCTION SYNDROMES

In response to chemotactic stimuli, neutrophils migrate to the site of infection where they ingest bacteria by phagocytosis. This process is augmented in the presence of opsonizing materials such as immunoglobulins and complement components, which coat the bacterial cell wall. The opsonized bacteria are engulfed and carried to the interior of the cell in a phagocytic vacuole, which is lined by the invaginated cell membrane. This process leads to a sequence of events that includes degranulation with discharge of granule contents into the vacuole and a series of metabolic events termed the respiratory burst. Oxygen consumption rises, and oxygen is converted to superoxide and then to hydrogen peroxide. This is accompanied by a marked increase in activity of the hexose monophosphate shunt.

Although superoxide and hydrogen peroxide have modest bactericidal properties, the major degree of cell killing requires interaction with chloride or other halide ions. Myeloperoxidase released from primary granules catalyzes the reaction of chloride ion with hydrogen peroxide to form hypochlorite, which directly kills the invading organisms.

A number of defects in bacterial killing by neutrophils have been described. The most common serious defect is neutropenia or a lack of neutrophils (see "Neutropenia—agranulocytosis"). There may also be defects in chemotaxis, phagocytosis, and microbicidal activity.

Defects in chemotaxis

Neutropenia results in inadequate accumulation of leukocytes in areas of inflammation. In addition, alcohol and corticosteroids interfere with adherence of neutrophils to endothelial cells, which impairs mobilization to the site of injury. Defects in the complement system can interfere with the production of chemotactic factors, resulting in poor chemotaxis. These may be seen on a congenital basis as well as in newborns and diabetics. A cellular defect in chemotaxis has been described in newborns and patients with diabetes, rheumatoid arthritis, hypophosphatemia, Chédiak-Higashi syndrome, Job's syndrome, and the lazy leukocyte syndrome.

Job's syndrome is characterized by recurrent indolent staphylococcal skin abscesses, eczema, and high serum IgE levels. The neutrophils manifest a cellular defect in chemotaxis.

The *lazy leukocyte syndrome* is a syndrome of neutropenia in association with certain forms of periodontitis and otitis media. There is a cellular defect in chemotaxis.

Defects in phagocytosis

Defects in phagocytosis can result from agammaglobulinemia or from poor opsonization of microorganisms as a result of congenital or acquired defects in the complement system. Opsonins are defective in some newborns and in some patients with lupus erythematosus and cirrhosis. The lack of opsonins for pneumococci may contribute to the association of sickle cell anemia with severe pneumococcal infections.

Cellular defects in phagocytosis have been described in some patients with diabetes, rheumatoid arthritis, systemic lupus erythematosus, and hypophosphatemia.

Defects in microbicidal activity

A number of syndromes associated with known defects in neutrophil microbicidal activity have been described.

CHRONIC GRANULOMATOUS DISEASE. The best-characterized disorder of neutrophil (and monocyte) microbicidal function is a condition termed chronic granulomatous disease (CGD), in which infants have repeated severe pyogenic infections with *Staphylococcus aureus* and gram-negative bacteria. The infections are slow to heal and invariably lead to multiple granulomatous abscesses. The most common form is X linked, with male inheritance and an asymptomatic carrier state in females. Multiple abscesses in the skin, lymph nodes, bone, liver, spleen, and lungs are the hallmark of the disease. Recent infections show an extensive neutrophilic infiltration, and established abscesses consolidate into granulomata.

Patients with CGD have normal or elevated neutrophil counts, immunoglobulin levels, and delayed hypersensitivity. The chemotactic and phagocytic responses are normal. CGD results from an inability of the neutrophil to produce hydrogen peroxide, which is necessary for cell killing. The deficient enzyme is usually NADPH oxidase, but other enzymes may be deficient in variants of CGD. CGD neutrophils effectively kill organisms that elaborate hydrogen peroxide, such as streptococci and pneumococci, by providing substrate for the myeloperoxidase reaction.

The diagnosis is readily established by documenting an impaired respiratory burst activity in response to bacterial exposure. One common test employs the ability of normal neutrophils to reduce nitroblue tetrazolium (NBT) dye to blue formazan. All neutrophils of patients with CGD and a portion of the neutrophils of female carriers are unable to reduce NBT dye. Another in vitro test involves measurement of the rate at which neutrophils kill *S. aureus;* CGD neutrophils kill at a much slower rate than normal neutrophils, and CGD carriers have neutrophils of a mixed population that kill at an intermediate rate.

Chronic lymphadenitis with extensive and diffuse lymphadenopathy is the most common feature of the disease. Severe eczematoid dermatitis, pneumonitis, and hepatosplenomegaly are regularly observed. Subphrenic abscesses, osteomyelitis, and perianal abscesses are frequent features. Thus far, treatment is confined to antibiotic therapy and surgical drainage of the abscesses. Continuous prophylactic antibiotic therapy may be of use in some patients; granulocyte transfusions may be required in severe, life-threatening infection.

CHÉDIAK-HIGASHI SYNDROME. Chédiak-Higashi syndrome is an autosomal recessive disorder that is usually discovered during childhood and consists of partial albinism, increased susceptibility to infection, and morphologic and functional abnormalities of leukocytes. The cytoplasm of the neutrophils, monocytes, and lymphocytes contains giant granules readily seen on routine Wright-Giemsa stains. Functional abnormalities of the neutrophils include decreased chemotaxis and slow degranulation resulting in delayed microbial killing. An "accelerated phase" with pancytopenia; lymphohistiocytic infiltration in the liver, spleen, and bone marrow; unexplained fever; peripheral neuropathy; and frequent bacterial and viral infection is usually fatal.

The treatment consists of appropriate antibiotic therapy. Corticosteroids and vincristine have been used in the treatment of the accelerated phase, but results have been inconsistent.

MYELOPEROXIDASE DEFICIENCY. Myeloperoxidase deficiency in neutrophils may be hereditary or acquired. There may be increased susceptibility to infection, especially with *Candida*. A defect can be demonstrated in bactericidal and fungicidal activity of neutrophils in vitro.

SEVERE DEFICIENCY OF GLUCOSE-6-PHOSPHATE DEHYDROGENASE. With leukocyte glucose-6-phosphate dehydrogenase deficiency 5% of normal or lower, there is neutrophil dysfunction and increased susceptibility to infection.

LIPOCHROME HISTIOCYTOSIS. Lipochrome histiocytosis is a rare familial disease in which there are many large, pigmented, lipid-laden histiocytes in numerous tissues. The neutrophils have a microbicidal defect similar to that in CGD.

NEUTROPENIA—AGRANULOCYTOSIS

Blood leukocyte counts normally range between 5000 and 10,000 cells/mm^3 with a predominance of neutrophils. Although a reduction in circulating neutrophils usually leads to a decline in the total leukocyte count, such values are not meaningful unless a differential count is performed and the absolute numbers of each cell type are calculated. In healthy individuals total neutrophil counts range between 1800 and 7200 cells/mm^3, with slightly lower values in the black population. Thus neutropenia is defined as a decrease in the neutrophil count below 1800 cells/mm^3, with the reservation that certain blacks may have values as low as 1200 to 1500 cells/mm^3 with no detectable disease process.

Neutropenia may occur as an isolated finding or may be associated with a variety of underlying disorders, which may cause anemia and thrombocytopenia as well. In general, neutropenia associated with some definable disease process results from marrow production defects or excessive cellular destruction.

Production defects

APLASIA OR HYPOPLASIA. The most common form of reversible bone marrow hypoplasia results from the use of cytotoxic drug regimens for the treatment of neoplastic disease. Many of the combination therapies include alkylating agents, which induce acute neutropenia and thrombocytopenia that persist 1 to 2 weeks. Exceptions are noted with the nitrosourea agents, which generally manifest a delayed reaction with variable degrees of neutropenia 3 to 4 weeks after therapy.

Ionizing irradiation in doses of 2000 to 4000 rad causes a near total ablation of myelopoiesis in the areas of irradiated bone marrow. The injury is biphasic, with a transient loss of cell production resulting from ablation of the hematopoietic stem cells. Cellularity returns for several months but eventually ceases owing to a permanent defect in the microcirculation. If the extent of the irradiation field is sufficiently wide, some patients may have a permanent depression in cell production with borderline neutrophil counts. In evaluating neutropenia in this situation, it is important to obtain bone marrow samples outside the previous treatment field, since irradiated sites show severe degrees of aplasia.

Severe acquired aplastic anemia usually affects all three major cell lines, resulting in neutropenia, thrombocytopenia, and severe anemia. The disease generally has an abrupt onset owing to infection or widespread mucosal bleeding caused by low numbers of platelets. In most instances this disorder is thought to result from a quantitative reduction in hematopoietic stem cells, since marrow aspirates and biopsy specimens show only scattered foci of lymphocytes and plasma cells. However, a small percentage of cases may be due to immunologic suppression of the marrow or to a basic defect in the marrow stroma.

Paroxysmal nocturnal hemoglobinuria may represent a variant form of bone marrow aplasia. It is believed that spontaneous recovery from aplasia may result in an aberrant stem cell that yields mature cells with abnormal membrane characteristics. The red cells are unduly sensitive to pH change, which is the basis for the acid hemolysis test. Recently membrane abnormalities have been detected in the neutrophils and platelets as well. In the absence of significant hemolysis, this disorder is characterized primarily by neutropenia and splenomegaly. In some cases further stem cell mutation may occur with conversion to acute myeloblastic leukemia.

INFILTRATIVE DISORDERS OF THE BONE MARROW. Infiltration of the marrow with foreign cells may result in a myelophthisic process with a disruption of the usual orderly release of mature cells. The peripheral blood may show leukopenia, thrombocytopenia, and anemia with a leukoerythroblastic picture (variable numbers of myelocytes, metamyelocytes, and nucleated red cell precursors). This often results from hematologic neoplasms such as the leukemias, non-Hodgkin's lymphomas, and multiple myeloma. The presence of bone pain or the finding of marked bony tenderness over the involved areas may be the major clue to the diagnosis.

A variety of carcinomas may also diffusely infiltrate the marrow cavity and produce a similar clinical picture. The neoplasms that most commonly "seed" in the marrow arise from the breast, lung, kidney, prostate, and thyroid. At times the primary tumor may be undetectable, and multiple diagnostic tests may be required to document the site of origin. The marrow may also be infiltrated or largely replaced by fibroblasts, granulomata, or storage cells. Idiopathic myelofibrosis may be suggested by the presence of marked hepatosplenomegaly and numerous teardrop poikilocytes in the peripheral blood smear. Attempts at bone marrow aspiration usually result in a "dry tap"; core biopsy of the marrow reveals a dense collagen fibrosis. On occasion, diffuse hematogenous spread of tuberculosis may mimic the picture of idiopathic myelofibrosis with hepatosplenomegaly, anemia, thrombocytopenia, and variable changes in neutrophil counts. The diagnosis of tuberculosis or other granulomatous processes may be established by biopsy of the bone marrow or the liver.

Various types of lipid storage abnormalities are characterized by lipid-filled macrophages throughout the reticuloendothelial system. Infants with Gaucher's, Tay-Sachs, or Niemann-Pick disease may have variable degrees of neutropenia as a result of the marrow infiltration. In contrast, the adult form of Gaucher's disease is usually characterized by hypersplenic destruction of platelets and neutrophils with some improvement following splenectomy.

METABOLIC DISORDERS. In addition to the well-known megaloblastic anemias, deficiencies of vitamin B_{12} and folic acid may cause decreases in neutrophil counts. These deficiencies are characterized by glossitis, gastrointestinal disturbances, mild hyperbilirubinemia, and, in pernicious anemia, associated neurologic defects. Peripheral blood smears show macrocytosis with oval cells, high red cell mean corpuscular volumes, and numerous hypersegmented neutrophils. Although five-lobed neutrophils may be seen occasionally in the normal smear, the finding of six- or seven-lobed cells is virtually diagnostic of a megaloblastic process. Marrow aspirates are hypercellular with increased numbers of granulocytic precursors, many of which are twice the normal size. Kinetically this form of neutropenia is characterized by excess intramedullary destruction of the precursor cells. Neutrophil counts promptly return to normal levels with appropriate therapy.

INFECTIOUS DISEASES. Acute viral infections such as influenza and infectious mononucleosis are often associated with modest degrees of neutropenia. Although most bacterial infections lead to neutrophilia, typhoid fever is frequently associated with a depression in circulating neutrophils. The exact mechanism has not been defined, but with many viral infections there is a related depression in platelet counts and red cell production, particularly in patients with severe chronic hemolytic anemias. It seems likely that these changes result from an acute suppression of bone marrow function. The neutropenia is of modest degree, with recovery of normal counts within 1 to 2 weeks of diagnosis.

This form of neutropenia must be distinguished from that seen in acute overwhelming bacterial infections. Occasional patients with extensive pneumonitis, diffuse skin infections resulting from exfoliative dermatitis, or severe sepsis have virtually no circulating neutrophils. Bone marrow aspirates show increased numbers of proliferative cells but few metamyelocyte, band, or segmented neutrophils. This is due to depletion of the marrow storage pool with exudation of the cells into the site of infection. Such patients require vigorous therapy with bactericidal antibiotics, since 4 to 5 days may elapse before a new wave of mature cells is generated.

Destructive defects

Increased neutrophil destruction may result from hypersplenism or from the presence of antibodies directed against mature neutrophils.

HYPERSPLENISM. Hypersplenism is suggested by the finding of variable degrees of neutropenia, thrombocytopenia, and a mild hemolytic anemia in association with splenomegaly. In the peripheral blood smear the ratio of band to segmented cells is increased, and marrow aspirates show hyperplasia of proliferative cells. The marrow storage pool is reduced as a reflection of the increased rate of cellular release into the peripheral blood. Although the exact mechanism has not been defined, it seems likely that the hyperplastic reticuloendothelial cells of the splenic sinusoids are responsible for the neutrophil destruction.

Hypersplenism usually results from congestive splenomegaly that accompanies long-standing hepatic cirrhosis, but it may be seen with portal vein thrombosis, with chronic infections involving the reticuloendothelial system (such as brucellosis), or occasionally with chronic lymphocytic leukemia. Splenectomy usually resolves the neutropenia but is rarely indicated.

Rheumatoid arthritis may lead to the development of splenomegaly and neutropenia *(Felty's syndrome)*. This usually occurs in patients with long-standing disease with rheumatoid nodules and high rheumatoid factor titers. Frequently, the arthritis is relatively inactive; indeed, the major problem may be that of indolent leg ulcers. It is assumed that Felty's syndrome is due to splenic sequestration or to antineutrophil antibodies; however, multiple mechanisms may be operative. Some patients show increased neutrophil production, whereas others have an associated marrow defect. Splenectomy has been variably successful but should be attempted only in patients with repeated episodes of infection.

ANTINEUTROPHIL ANTIBODIES. Certain neonatal forms of neutropenia are due to transplacental passage of leukoagglutinins from the mother to the fetus. This results from maternal immunization to specific neutrophil antigens of the fetus by virtue of previous pregnancies or prior blood transfusions. The disorder persists for several months until the maternal antibody is gradually consumed.

Only a few cases of autoimmune neutropenia have been described in adults. It is likely that this mechanism occurs in association with rheumatoid arthritis, systemic lupus erythematosus, and other connective tissue diseases; however, documentation has been hampered by the difficulties inherent in the antibody assays. Leukoagglutinins occur in the sera of many individuals without a corresponding abnormality in leukocyte production. Serum inhibitors have been detected by the colony-forming assays, but such determinations are often plagued by nonspecific inhibitory materials, particularly when assayed against bone marrows from unrelated donors. In the absence of a specific assay system, autoimmune neutropenia can be inferred only by the absence of splenomegaly and the finding of granulocytic hyperplasia of the marrow in the appropriate clinical setting. Therapy with corticosteroids may occasionally reduce the accelerated cell destruction and increase the numbers of circulating neutrophils. Such treatment may also be somewhat hazardous, since corticosteroids block the egress of neutrophils into inflammatory exudates.

Congenital neutropenia

Various forms of congenital neutropenia have been defined. Many show a dominant inheritance pattern, but the mechanisms of neutropenia are widely disparate. Granulocytic stem cells have been increased in some types, reduced in others, and virtually absent from the marrow in one variant. In most instances the defect is mild, with neutrophil counts in the range of 500 to 1000 cells/mm^3 and only modest infections. Some patients with severe neutropenia may show a compensatory increase in monocytes, which appears to reduce the likelihood of infections. One congenital defect *(Kostman's syndrome)* is characterized by increased marrow stem cells and early granulocytic precursors but a virtual absence of myelocytes and further granulocytic cells. The severity of the neutropenia is sufficiently great that most patients die of an infection before age 20.

Chronic idiopathic neutropenic syndromes

After appropriate evaluation to exclude other causes, there remains a group of adult patients with variable degrees of neutropenia and normal myeloid cellularity in the bone marrow. In one series of 41 patients studied over a 6-year period, infection occurred in 27%. The majority of these had fewer than 500 circulating neutrophils/mm^3. Most patients had normal or increased numbers of granulocytic stem cells in the marrow and appeared to respond to the neutropenic stress with an increased proportion of these colony-forming cells in DNA synthesis. The only defect that has been identified is a reduction in colony-stimulating factor production by marrow cells themselves, suggesting that this form of neutropenia may result from insufficient medullary production of this regulator of granulopoiesis.

Some patients with chronic neutropenia may have a period of oscillatory cell production. This "cyclic neutropenia" does not represent a distinct clinical syndrome but rather reflects a markedly reduced pluripotential stem cell compartment. Neutrophil counts vary cyclically from none to approximately 2000 cells/mm^3 every 2 to 3 weeks, with frequent infections during the severely neutropenic intervals. The reticulocyte and platelet counts frequently oscillate out of cycle with the neutrophils, which suggests that stem cell competition may be responsible for this unique phenomenon. On occasion the oscillation may disappear with normalization of the blood counts later in life.

Drug-induced neutropenia

Aside from the cytotoxic drugs used in cancer chemotherapy, a wide variety of agents can cause a severe reversible neutropenia. This symptom complex, which has been termed agranulocytosis, arises as an idiosyncratic reaction, usually within 4 to 8 weeks of instituting therapy. The most severe reactions produce a clinical picture of fever, pharyngitis with gray necrotic oral ulcers, and a virtual absence of circulating neutrophils. Without prompt recognition and therapy, the course is complicated by hyperpyrexia, stupor, and death from generalized sepsis.

The reaction to some agents such as aminopyrine is characterized by the development of drug-dependent antibodies. The drug may act as a hapten attached to a leukocyte protein. The initial reaction leads to agranulocytosis, fever, and infection. Although the peripheral blood and bone marrow are devoid of mature cells, increased numbers of neutrophil precursors such as myeloblasts, promyelocytes, and myelocytes are observed in the marrow. Discontinuance of the offending drug usually leads to recovery in 5 to 6 days. On reexposure the patient has shaking chills and a disappearance of circulating neutrophils within hours of drug ingestion. In volunteers who receive an infusion of the patient's plasma, a similar immediate neutropenia develops following a single drug exposure.

In contrast, drugs of the phenothiazine group produce agranulocytosis by inhibiting cell production. Although the clinical picture is indistinguishable from that seen with aminopyrine, the bone marrow is characterized by selective granulocytic aplasia. This inhibition of cell production leads to a prolonged agranulocytosis for intervals up to 2 weeks. Studies have shown that patients with agranulocytosis as a result of phenothiazines have a defect in DNA synthesis in their myeloid precursors, as measured by thymidine incorporation. Moreover, even in the absence of phenothiazines, their marrow cells show a lower labeling index than those of normal controls. Modest quantities of chlorpromazine inhibit normal cell growth in vitro, whereas even minute doses of this agent are inhibitory to granulocyte colonies from susceptible individuals.

Although idiosyncratic reactions to phenothiazines are relatively uncommon, a mild stable neutropenia develops in many patients during the course of therapy. Bone marrow studies show only a slight generalized reduction in granulocytic cells. If necessary, drug therapy may be continued, since most such patients do not have the severe idiosyncratic suppression of granulopoiesis.

Many drugs have been implicated as causative factors in agranulocytosis. These are listed below:

Analgesics
  Aminopyrine
Antibiotics
  Chloramphenicol
  Methicillin
  Nafcillin
Anticonvulsants
  Phenytoin
  Trimethadione
Anti-inflammatory drugs
  Gold salts
  Indomethacin
  Phenylbutazone
Antithyroid compounds
  Methimazole
  Propylthiouracil
Diuretics
  Acetazolamide
  Thiazides
  Mercurials
Hypoglycemic agents
Phenothiazines
  Chlorpromazine
Sulfonamides

Although most of these appear to act by inhibiting cell production, occasional reports have suggested that antithyroid compounds, gold salts, phenylbutazone, and sulfonamides may also serve as haptens to induce drug-dependent antibodies.

General approach to the neutropenic patient

Frequently, a careful history reveals drug ingestion, toxin exposure, or symptoms suggestive of a generalized hematologic disorder. The findings of adenopathy and splenomegaly may indicate an underlying lymphoproliferative disease, whereas petechiae and sternal tenderness raise the suspicion of acute leukemia. In most cases careful study of the peripheral blood and bone marrow is sufficient to establish the diagnosis. If the marrow aspirate shows a reduction in the normal myeloid/erythroid ratio and the biopsy specimen is hypocellular, it is reasonably clear that the neutropenia is due to a production defect. In contrast, increased cellularity with a "left shift" or an increased proportion of early granulocytic cells is presumptive evidence of increased neutrophil destruction.

In general, a reduction in circulating neutrophils to 500 to 1000 cells/mm^3 is associated with a modest increase in the risk of infection. Values below 500 cells/mm^3 frequently lead to life-threatening sepsis. However, it must be emphasized that these generalizations are derived from patients with severe production defects such as acute leukemia or aplastic anemia. Occasional individuals with severe hypersplenism or Felty's syndrome tolerate circulating neutrophil levels of 100 to 200 cells/mm^3 without an increased frequency or severity of infection. In all likelihood such patients have a redistribution phenomenon with an increase in marginated cells. Thus the marginal blood granulocyte pool may exceed circulating levels by threefold to fivefold and may be readily mobilized on demand.

When infection develops in patients with neutropenia, the organisms involved are most often gram-negative bacilli (particularly *Pseudomonas aeruginosa*) and *S. aureus*.

Management

The treatment of neutropenia is highly dependent on the causative factor. Leukemia, lymphoma, myeloma, and other responsive neoplasms are best managed by appropriate drug regimens. Aplastic anemia may be cured by transplantation with HLA-compatible bone marrow or in some instances by treatment with antithymocyte globulin, since recent evidence suggests an immune origin in a small proportion of cases. Although androgens and corticosteroids are widely used in the treatment of bone marrow failure, most controlled studies show no substantial benefit. Indeed, corticosteroids may worsen the infection by reducing neutrophil egress into the site of infection. Lithium therapy increases the production of colony-stimulating factor and, in hematologically normal individuals treated for manic depressive psychosis, causes a modest neutrophilia. Preliminary studies suggest that lithium therapy may shorten the neutropenic interval after chemotherapy, but no substantial benefit has been noted in patients with stable neutropenic disorders. Splenectomy is rarely indicated except in certain patients with Felty's syndrome.

The acutely infected neutropenic patient should have cultures taken of blood, urine, sputum, and any suspected portal of entry. Prompt therapy with combinations of antibiotics such as cephalothin, carbenicillin, and gentamicin should be promptly instituted. Careful attention should be paid to skin, oral, and anal hygiene. If the patient remains febrile and acutely ill for 24 to 48 hours after antibiotics are instituted, white cell transfusions may be of short-term benefit. Daily infusions of approximately 10^{10} fresh normal leukocytes do not lead to an appreciable increase in circulating neutrophils, but such therapy markedly reduces the mortality from sepsis. Since leukocyte transfusions are beneficial only over short intervals, their use should be confined to patients with acute reversible neutropenia such as that following therapy for acute leukemia. In some centers isolation of neutropenic patients in sterile "life islands" or laminar airflow environments has further reduced the mortality from acute sepsis. However, such techniques are costly, create problems with patient management, and may induce psychologic disturbances from the prolonged periods of isolation.

LEUKEMOID REACTIONS

Although the original description of leukemoid blood pictures included patients with both increased and decreased total leukocyte counts, present usage refers to a reactive leukocytosis not readily explained by acute bacterial infection. The term "leukemoid reaction" usually refers to a marked increase in circulating mature neutrophils, whereas specific designations such as lymphocytosis, monocytosis, or eosinophilia are used to describe marked elevations in other normal cell types.

Acute bacterial infections are usually accompanied by a twofold to fivefold increase in neutrophil counts with a left shift, that is, increased numbers of band cells in the blood. After control of the infection by appropriate therapy, neutrophil counts promptly return to baseline levels. Frequently, older patients or those with compromised bone marrow function do not show increases in the total count; indeed, the only clue to an infectious process may be an alteration in the band cell/segmented cell ratio, with greater than 450 band cells/mm^3 of blood. Other conditions that acutely increase the neutrophil count include severe hemorrhage, hemolysis, and corticosteroid therapy.

In contrast, leukemoid reactions are characterized by a marked elevation in the total leukocyte count, frequently in excess of 50,000 cells/mm^3, with a predominance of mature neutrophils. The cells appear relatively normal but may show increased azurophilic granules (toxic granulation) or pale blue inclusions in the cytoplasm (Döhle's bodies). These reactions are usually due to a chronic pyogenic infection, tissue necrosis, or an underlying neoplasm. Leukemoid reactions are differentiated from myeloproliferative syndromes or leukemia by the absence of red cell or platelet abnormalities, the absence of organ infiltration, and the finding of a high neutrophil alkaline phosphatase level. Bone marrow samples are hypercellular with increased granulocytic precursors but are not diagnostic of this condition. Leukemoid reactions may mimic chronic myelogenous leukemia (CML) but can be differentiated from this condition by the absence of splenomegaly, anemia, and thrombocytosis. Furthermore, leukemoid reactions are not associated with the Philadelphia chromosome in marrow cells nor with a depression in neutrophil alkaline phosphatase, both of which characterize CML.

Marked leukemoid reactions are occasionally seen in association with acute bacterial infections as well as bacterial endocarditis, severe disseminated tuberculosis, and chronic perforation of the bowel wall with localized abscess formation. Although recognition and treatment of the underlying disorder generally lead to a prompt reduction in the marked neutrophilia, reactions associated with tuberculosis may take many months to subside.

Tissue necrosis such as that seen following major surgery may also induce an acute leukemoid reaction. Similar findings are often seen with severe burns or extensive gangrene. It has been postulated that some of the leukemoid reactions seen with malignancies may result from extensive tumor necrosis.

A variety of neoplasms such as carcinomas of the lung, kidney, and genitourinary tract have produced marked leukemoid reactions with neutrophil counts in excess of 150,000 cells/mm^3. On occasion widespread Hodgkin's disease may also lead to an extensive neutrophilic leukocytosis. In the past it was believed that tumor-associated reactions were due either to extensive tumor necrosis or to metastasis to the bone marrow with alterations in the normal mechanisms of cellular release. Recent evidence suggests that tumor neutrophilia may instead be due to a humoral mechanism with extensive uncontrolled production of colony-stimulating factor.

Occasional individuals may have a stable chronic neutrophilia for years without detection of an underlying cause or other hematologic abnormality. This condition, which has been termed *chronic idiopathic leukocytosis,* probably represents a mild aberration in normal feedback control mechanisms. Leukemoid reactions should also be differentiated from a distinctly unusual myeloproliferative syndrome known as *chronic neutrophilic leukemia.* This disease is characterized by splenomegaly and marked neutrophilia but differs from CML in that the cells are mature, platelet counts are normal, neutrophil alkaline phosphatase values are high, and the Philadelphia chromosome is lacking. This form of neutrophilic leukemia is characterized by extensive infiltration of the liver, spleen, and lymph nodes with mature neutrophils and by a bleeding tendency.

MONOCYTOSIS

Monocytes are produced in the bone marrow by the action of a specific "macrophage" subclass of colony-stimulating factor, which acts on stem cells with bipotential capabilities for either granulocyte or macrophage differentiation. The cells pass through the monoblast and promonocyte stage to emerge into the peripheral blood as mature monocytes. The differentiation pathway is more rapid than that of the granulocytic series. This explains the early monocytosis, which, after granulocytic aplasia, frequently precedes neutrophil recovery by 48 to 72 hours. Monocytes leave the blood with a half-life of 8 hours and lodge in the liver, spleen, bone marrow, and lung to mature into tissue macrophages. These cells, which are an integral part of the reticuloendothelial system, may persist for many weeks in the tissues. Both monocytes and macrophages actively phagocytize bacteria and fungi, but they have a predilection for dealing with intracellular organisms such as mycobacteria and *Brucella.*

Monocytosis is a frequent finding in patients with malignant tumors. In one study 62% of patients with solid tumors had greater than 500 monocytes/mm^3. Additional disease processes that are believed to be autoimmune in nature, such as rheumatoid arthritis, systemic lupus erythematosus, regional enteritis, and ulcerative colitis, account for approximately 15% of all patients with monocytosis. Infections such as tuberculosis, brucellosis, and subacute bacterial endocarditis may also produce this blood picture. On occasion, extensive carcinomas and widely disseminated tuberculosis may be associated with extreme monocytosis with counts as high as 100,000 cells/mm^3. These marked reactions have often been termed monocytic leukemoid reactions. Gradual improvement of the monocytic reaction generally occurs with effective treatment of the underlying condition.

EOSINOPHILIA

Eosinophils are produced in the bone marrow in much the same way as neutrophilic granulocytes. A separate stem cell is acted on by a specific eosinophilic type of colony-stimulating factor to induce cellular differentiation. Eosinophilic precursors are first recognized at the promyelocyte stage by the presence of large orange-red granules in the cytoplasm. Over a period of approximately 9 days, the precursor cells differentiate into eosinophils, and these mature cells are released into the blood where they disappear rapidly with a half-life of less than 1 hour. The life span of eosinophils in the tissues is relatively long, with some mature cells persisting for 7 to 10 days. Surveys have yielded different values for normal blood eosinophil counts, with ranges of none to 450 cells/mm^3 in one study and none to 700 cells/mm^3 in another.

Eosinophilia is observed in patients with certain parasitic infections, allergic diseases, drug reactions, and dermatoses such as pemphigus, pemphigoid, and atopic dermatitis (see Chapter 74).

Numerous pulmonary disorders with lung infiltrates and eosinophilia have been recognized. Löffler's syndrome is characterized by cough, pulmonary infiltrates, and large numbers of eosinophils in the sputum and peripheral blood. This disorder is presumed to represent a hypersensitivity reaction to inhaled antigens, to drugs, or to pulmonary migration by the larval forms of certain parasites. Generally the clinical manifestations are transient, with recovery in 3 to 4 weeks.

Pulmonary infiltration with eosinophilia (PIE syndrome) is a more chronic relapsing illness with fever, cough, and dyspnea. Pulmonary infiltrates recur with persistent symptoms for many months. This entity may be associated with chronic infections, drug hypersensitivity, parasitic infestations, collagen vascular disorders, or various neoplasms such as Hodgkin's disease. The manifestations of lung involvement frequently improve with corticosteroid therapy if the underlying condition does not prevent their use.

Although periarteritis nodosa is not usually associated with eosinophilia, patients with severe asthma and pulmonary involvement have marked elevations of circulating eosinophils. In most of these patients severe neurologic deficits develop by virtue of central nervous system or peripheral nerve involvement, and frequently patients die of the disease in 1 to 2 months.

Marked hypereosinophilia or leukemoid blood pictures occur in association with severe tissue infiltration by eosinophils, with eosinophilic leukemia, or with large necrotic tumors. In many cases of hypereosinophilic syndromes there are signs and symptoms of organ involvement with hepatosplenomegaly, central nervous system damage, and pulmonary fibrosis. The greatest degree of tissue damage occurs in the heart with a marked eosinophilic infiltration, development of mural thrombi, and endocardial and myocardial fibrosis. Differentiation from a leukemic process is difficult, but eosinophilic leukemia is generally characterized by circulating blast cells, severe anemia, thrombocytopenia, and organ infiltration by immature cells. The prognosis in such disorders is grave with survival times of less than 1 year.

BIBLIOGRAPHY

Babior, B.M.: Oxygen-dependent killing by phagocytes, N. Engl. J. Med. **298**:659, 721, 1978.

Beeson, P.B., and Bass, D.A.: The eosinophil. In Smith, L.H., Jr.: Major problems in internal medicine, vol. 14, Philadelphia, 1977, W.B. Saunders Co.

Blume, R.S., and Wolff, S.M.: The Chédiak-Higashi syndrome: studies in four patients and a review of the literature, Medicine **51**:247, 1972.

Boggs, D.R.: The kinetics of neutrophilic leukocytes in health and disease, Semin. Hematol. **4**:359, 1967.

Boxer, L.A., and others: Autoimmune neutropenia, N. Engl. J. Med. **293**:748, 1975.

Burlington, H., and others: Colony stimulating activity in cultures of granulocytosis inducing tumor, Proc. Soc. Exp. Biol. Med. **154**:86, 1977.

Dale, D.C., and others: Chronic neutropenia, Medicine **58**:128, 1979.

Finch, S.C.: Granulocytopenia. In Williams, W.J., editor: Hematology, ed. 2, New York, 1977, McGraw-Hill Book Co.

Greenberg, P.L., and others: The chronic idiopathic neutropenia syndrome: correlation of clinical features with in vitro parameters of granulocytopoiesis, Blood **55**:915, 1980.

Metcalf, D.: Regulation of granulocyte and monocyte-macrophage proliferation by colony stimulating factor (CSF): a review, Exp. Hematol. **1**:185, 1973.

Pisciotta, A.V.: Immune and toxic mechanisms in drug-induced agranulocytosis, Semin. Hematol. **10**:279, 1973.

Ward, P.C.J.: The myeloid leukocytoses, Postgrad. Med. **67**:219, 1980.

73 • THE LEUKEMIAS

George A. Omura

The leukemias are cancers of the hematopoietic tissues characterized by infiltration of peripheral blood, bone marrow, and other tissues by cells of a particular line, usually lymphoid or myeloid. The involved cells may be immature in appearance, in which case the process is called "acute," or they may be mature looking, in which case the process is "chronic." Originally, the morphologic distinction correlated well with the prognosis, but progress in the treatment of acute leukemia has been so great, especially relative to the chronic leukemias, that the terms "acute" and "chronic" have become less meaningful. Although the leukemias have much in common, there are sufficient differences regarding symptoms, physical examination, hematologic findings, prognosis, and response to various treatments that acute leukemias, chronic myelogenous (or granulocytic) leukemias (CML), and chronic lymphocytic leukemia (CLL) should be considered separately. There are several other uncommon varieties of acute and chronic leukemias that are not included in this chapter because of their rarity, lack of effective treatment, and failure to illustrate principles not otherwise covered.

There are currently about 22,000 new cases of leukemia each year in the United States, with a slightly higher incidence in males. Almost half of the cases are acute, whereas about 30% are CLL, 20% CML, and the rest uncommon types of leukemia.

There are marked variations with age; acute lymphoblastic leukemia (ALL) comprises about 80% of childhood leukemias, whereas acute myelogenous leukemia (AML) is the usual type of adult acute leukemia. In children CML is uncommon and CLL virtually unknown.

Progress in understanding the cause and treatment of leukemia has had and will have relevance to the management of other types of cancer. Parallel with the goal of cure is the need to identify minimal residual disease. Minute amounts of residual leukemia may represent thousands, millions, or billions of malignant cells remaining after treatment, more than enough to reproduce the disease. Thus a breakthrough in treatment may not be recognized with any confidence until a breakthrough also occurs in identifying, with immunologic, biochemical, or other techniques, minimal residual disease. The identification of leukemia-associated antigens is very promising. In the meantime, progress in diagnosis, treatment, and supportive care is occurring in a stepwise fashion, although progress is sometimes hard to recognize without time-consuming, large-scale clinical trials and lengthy follow-up.

ACUTE LEUKEMIAS

DEFINITION. Acute leukemias are cancers of the blood-forming organs causing marrow failure and infiltration of various organs and tissues by blast cells. If the disease is untreated, death ensues in a few weeks to several months.

ETIOLOGY. The cause of human acute leukemia remains uncertain, but of the many possible causes that have been suggested, ionizing radiation, certain chemicals, and viruses have received the most attention. Radiation exposure from atomic bomb blasts, radiation therapy, or inadequate shielding of radiologists has been associated with an increased incidence of AML and CML. Chronic benzene exposure, chloramphenicol, and certain anticancer drugs such as alkylating agents have also been implicated. It seems highly likely, but is still unproven, that certain viruses may cause some human leukemias. Circumstantial evidence includes the observation that animal leukemias, including some in primates, are of viral causation. RNA-dependent DNA polymerase characteristic of certain RNA tumor viruses has been found in some human leukemias. Patients with Down's syndrome (trisomy 21) or Fanconi's anemia and the identical twins of leukemic children have an increased incidence of leukemia, suggesting a role for genetic and hereditary factors.

PATHOGENESIS. Once the leukemic process is initiated, there is a progressive, but not necessarily rapid, expansion of the leukemic population. In particular, there is an increase in the population of leukemic stem cells (that is, cells that retain their ability to multiply in the future). This process is associated with a maturation defect (the acute leukemic cells mature very little beyond the blast stage), so that mature functional cells capable of fighting infection (and having a limited life span) are not produced. Although leukemic, the abnormal cells may respond at least partially to normal regulatory mechanisms. For example, there is a decrease in "growth fraction" with increase in population density, as in normal tissues. The presence of leukemic cells in the marrow inhibits production of normal blood cells; this seems to be caused not only by the space-occupying effect of the leukemic infiltrate but also by inhibitory effects on normal cell growth at population densities that would not be expected to interfere on a physical or mechanical basis. In cases where a marker of the acute leukemic clone is present (such as an abnormal karyotype), this marker is not detectable during remission and reappears in relapse, indicating that the leukemic population is in fact a separate clone and that normal marrow elements persist that are capable of repopulating the marrow. This is in contrast to CML in which the marker chromosome seldom disappears during "remission."

CLINICAL MANIFESTATIONS. The signs and symptoms of acute leukemia are caused by marrow failure (anemia, granulocytopenia, and thrombocytopenia from decreased production) and by infiltration of the blood and other organs and tissues by leukemic cells. The severity of manifestations is quite variable, as is the duration of symptoms before diagnosis; symptoms may have been present for less than a week or for many months. Easy fatigability, dyspnea, palpitations, and other symptoms of anemia may be present. Fever with or without demonstrable infection is very common. Bleeding or easy bruising or both may occur. Bone or joint pain may be prominent, especially in children. The physical examination may be negative or may show fever, pallor, petechiae or purpura, enlargement of cervical and other peripheral lymph nodes, splenomegaly, and sometimes hepatomegaly. Signs of an infection may be present, although typical findings of a purulent infection or inflammatory response may be muted in patients with severe granulocytopenia. Other signs of tissue and organ infiltration by the leukemia may include striking gum hypertrophy, especially in monocytic variants of AML; a mediastinal mass in T-cell ALL; tonsillar enlargement; or skin infiltrates. Discrete tumor masses (chloromas) may occur in various tissues in AML. Tenderness over the sternum or other marrow-containing bones is frequently present. If the circulating blast count is markedly elevated (blast crisis), the patient may be obtunded, short of breath, or both from impaired cerebral or pulmonary circulation. A variety of neurologic signs and symptoms may occur during the course of the disease, especially meningeal leukemia, but these are not usually overt at the time of initial diagnosis.

LABORATORY FINDINGS. Anemia of variable severity is almost always present and is usually normochromic and normocytic. The reticulocyte count may be normal but is inappropriately low in relation to the anemia, indicating decreased production of erythrocytes. The platelet count is usually low; when it is extremely low (5000 to 10,000), especially in conjunction with generalized bleeding, the possibility of disseminated intravascular clotting (DIC), usually associated with the promyelocytic variant of AML, should be considered. A high platelet count raises the possibility that the patient had a previously undiagnosed "chronic myeloproliferative disorder" that has now transformed into an acute leukemic phase.

Although the term "leukemia" was originally coined to emphasize the elevated white blood count, normal or low counts are not uncommon. The terms "subleukemic" and "aleukemic" leukemia have been used, but the disease process is basically the same; in fact, cases with high white counts might be viewed as very advanced stage disease. The differential count in the peripheral blood includes a variable percentage, usually reduced in absolute number, of mature neutrophils. In most cases at least a few abnormal cells are present; these are usually blast forms with large nuclei, one or more nucleoli, and no cytoplasmic inclusions. Additional features and special stains (see below) may indicate that they are lymphoblasts or myeloblasts. In some cases monocytes (in AML) or lymphocytes of varying maturity may be part or most of the leukemic population. Abnormal promyelocytes may be seen in AML, but it is unusual for granulocytes of intermediate differentiation (myelocytes and metamyelocytes) to be part of the blood picture; this gives rise to the "hiatus leukemicus" or gap (mature and immature cells, but not intermediate forms) seen in the differential count in acute leukemia as opposed to the complete spectrum of maturation seen in CML. The two major types of acute leukemia should be distinguished whenever possible, since management and prognosis differ substantially.

In ALL on routine staining, lymphoblasts have a relatively large round or oval nucleus that occupies most of the cell. Only one or two nucleoli are usually seen, although this may vary with the stain. Cytoplasmic granules are rare or absent; Auer's bodies (see below) are not expected. The periodic acid–Schiff (PAS) stain is positive, whereas Sudan black and peroxidase stains are negative. Although the "common" case shows a very uniform population of cells in size and appearance, some patients have more pleomorphic populations, and a few patients have large cells with striking cytoplasmic vacuoles (Burkitt's cell type lymphoma). Immunologic studies may be very helpful; although the usual case has no cell surface markers, about one fourth of the cases have "T-cell" markers and the Burkitt type frequently has "B-cell" markers. Recently some cases previously called "null cell" have been shown to have a proliferation of "pre-B" cells. The null-cell and pre-B-cell types tend to have a better prognosis. Another distinctive feature of null cell and T lymphoblasts is the presence of large amounts of terminal deoxynucleotidyltransferase, an enzyme not expected in myeloblasts. The presence of glucocorticoid receptors may be of diagnostic and therapeutic significance.

Although ALL may have several subtypes, AML is even more heterogeneous. Included in this group are myeloblastic, promyelocytic, myelomonocytic, monocytic, and erythroleukemic variants. The myeloblast tends to be larger than the lymphoblast with a more abundant and variably shaped margin of cytoplasm around the nucleus. Multiple nucleoli and a finely granular nuclear chromatin pattern are frequent, although the stain may modify these details. Cytoplasmic granules may be present; distinctive inclusions known as Auer's bodies are sometimes seen. These needlelike structures apparently represent the abnormal development of lysosomal granules and are virtually pathognomonic of AML. Some cases show a mixed population of blasts plus promyelocytes, blasts plus monocytes, or blasts plus megaloblastoid erythroid precursors.

Myeloblasts usually give positive reactions with peroxidase and Sudan black stains but not with PAS. Esterase stains may be helpful in identifying monocytes. Lysozyme (muramidase) may be increased in the serum and urine in monocytic leukemia. An area of current investigation is the identification of "leukemia-associated antigens" characteristic of different types of leukemia; this approach may be helpful not only in classification but especially in the recognition of minimal residual disease.

On chromosome analysis abnormalities are seen in about half the patients both with AML and with ALL, but there is no consistent finding except in promyelocytic leukemia, in which a 15 to 17 translocation is common, and in B-cell ALL, which has been associated with an abnormal number 14 chromosome. AML patients with grossly abnormal karyotypes have a significantly shorter survival than those with chromosomally normal cells.

The bone marrow aspirate is usually hypercellular with a profusion of leukemic cells. Normal marrow elements are moderately to markedly depleted. In ALL virtually all the cells are abnormal, giving a monotonous appearance, whereas in AML less complete replacement of the marrow is common so that a more pleomorphic appearance may be noted.

Some cases of acute leukemia are not readily or consistently classified by the preceding techniques and may be referred to as acute undifferentiated leukemia. In addition, there are rare cases in which another cell line is involved in the abnormal proliferation.

Sometimes no marrow can be aspirated (dry tap) because the marrow cavity is "packed" with leukemic cells. This can be misinterpreted as an empty marrow (that is, aplastic anemia), but the confusion is quickly resolved by a needle biopsy of the marrow; "touch" preparations are made from the core of marrow to visualize cellular detail, and sections of the biopsy show diffuse infiltration of the marrow with primitive round cells. Occasionally the marrow in AML is surprisingly hypocellular despite a predominance of blasts; this raises the possibilities that the leukemia has developed in the setting of a previously undiagnosed aplastic anemia or that the process will behave in a somewhat indolent fashion (smoldering leukemia).

DIAGNOSIS. Although the diagnosis is not difficult in the average case and major progress has been made in treatment, the diagnosis of acute leukemia is still a devastating one that should not be made in haste. On occasion other disorders including benign ones can cause confusion. Most patients can be carried with supportive measures for a few days while any residual doubt is resolved. Two exceptions occur when the process represents a medical emergency: the patient with disseminated intravascular clotting complicating the leukemia and the leukostasis syndrome in which the cerebral or pulmonary circulation is compromised. In those situations correct diagnosis and treatment must be rendered on an urgent basis.

One of the most troubling problems in morphologic diagnosis is the regenerating marrow after a toxic injury, the cause of which may be readily apparent or quite obscure. For example, a normal recovering marrow, after a large dose of cytotoxic chemotherapy, may transiently show a relatively synchronized population of immature blast cells indistinguishable from acute leukemia. Within a few days to a week at least some of the cells mature, the blood counts normalize, and the confusion resolves.

The patient with anemia, thrombocytopenia, granulocytopenia, and a profusion of blast forms infiltrating the blood and marrow usually presents little difficulty in diagnosis, even though subclassification may be a problem. However, when the patient first comes to medical attention, the various signs and symptoms may suggest an upper respiratory infection, mononucleosis or other viral syndromes, a bleeding disorder, or even rheumatic fever. Once the blood counts are known, aplastic anemia, lymphoma, carcinoma or fibrosis in the marrow, or megaloblastic anemias (pernicious anemia or folate deficiency) may be suspected if pancytopenia is present. If the white count is high, the possibility of a leukemoid reaction is raised. However, leukemoid reactions with a predominance of blast cells are uncommon; severe anemia and thrombocytopenia are not expected as features and there should be an underlying process (for example, severe infection or metastatic carcinoma) demonstrable. Finally, splenomegaly or other evidence of tissue infiltration from the leukemoid reaction is not expected. Depending on the morphology and extent of maturation of leukemic cells, confusion with the chronic leukemias may occur, but this is not usually troublesome. There are instances in which the acute phase of CML is seen without an antecedent chronic phase or in which a preexisting hematologic disorder may cause confusion.

MANAGEMENT. In the late 1940s drugs that had striking, albeit temporary, effects on acute leukemia began to be available; a patient on the brink of death from infectious or bleeding complications might have a complete resolution of all signs, symptoms, and laboratory evidence of leukemia, yet within a few months full relapse of the disease was apparent. Considerable progress has been made in preventing relapse, so that relapse is now uncommon in the null-cell type of childhood ALL; a small but increasing number of adults with AML also remain in prolonged remission.

Before summarizing treatment, it is appropriate to define remission and comment on the "arithmetic" of leukemia. A complete remission exists when there is no evidence of leukemia by current testing capabilities. Symptoms of the disease should disappear; splenomegaly, adenopathy, and other evidence of tissue infiltration should resolve; the blood counts should normalize; and the bone marrow should appear normal. When the patient is in complete remission, the quality of life should be excellent; at this point there might be no remaining leukemic cells in the body (cure) or there might be as many as several billion. (In a mouse leukemia model, one transplanted leukemic cell can reproduce the disease.)

These billions of cells may not be recognized because (1) it is normal to have a few (0.3% to 5%) blast cells in a healthy marrow and (2) the leukemic cells are usually not sufficiently distinctive to be recognizable as such in the midst of normal marrow elements. If the normal marrow weighs 500 to 1000 g and if a million cells (10^6) weigh roughly 1 mg, 1% blast cells in the marrow would represent 5 to 10 billion cells throughout the body. With a trillion cells (10^{12}) present at the time of diagnosis, a 3 log reduction (to 10^9) will produce a complete remission. If the generation time is 5 days, 10 doublings will increase the leukemic population from 10^9 back to 10^{12} in 50 days. It should not be surprising that a partial remission is significantly inferior to a complete remission in prolonging survival, since the "cell kill" is apt to be far less.

A treatment strategy has evolved in which the first step is "remission induction" with a follow-up phase (or phases) of "cytoreduction" to reduce the leukemic cell burden still further below the level currently detectable as residual disease. This second step is frequently divided into an earlier phase of "consolidation" of the remission and then "remission maintenance," although some regimens emphasize a lengthy consolidation phase while others use an intensive maintenance program. The point is that the leukemic cells develop resistance to particular classes of anticancer drugs, which is frequently relative rather than absolute; moreover, sanctuaries exist where adequate drug concentrations are not achieved after systemic administration. The latter finding has led to a major advance in the management of ALL, "prophylactic" central nervous system therapy (intrathecal administration of methotrexate with or without cranial irradiation) to irradicate occult foci of leukemia that are not adequately treated by systemic drugs.

Drug dosages will not be given here because dose and drug regimens are still evolving, and the use of these regimens should be restricted to leukemia experts.

Childhood ALL. There are at least eight classes of drugs with activity in childhood ALL, including corticosteroids (prednisone), the plant alkaloid vincristine, folic acid analogs (methotrexate), purine analogs (6-mercaptopurine, thioguanine), alkylating agents (cyclophosphamide), the enzyme asparaginase, the pyrimidine nucleoside analog arabinosyl cytosine, and the anthracycline antibiotics (daunorubicin, doxorubicin). Remission can be accomplished in about 90% of children with a combination of prednisone and vincristine (some programs also include asparaginase, an anthracycline, or methotrexate).

In contrast to the temporary enhancement of marrow failure caused by the type of induction therapy required in AML, this regimen does not exacerbate marrow dysfunction. It rapidly causes regression of lymphoblastic leukemia so that in 1 or 2 weeks the hematologic status is usually improved, and by 3 or 4 weeks many patients are in remission. If this regimen is continued on a long-term basis, however, not only are steroid side effects and neurotoxicity from vincristine increasingly troublesome, but resistance rapidly develops leading to early relapse. Thus there is a need in the postremission cytoreductive phase to change to other active drugs, usually in combinations designed to reduce the likelihood of resistance while attacking multiple biochemical sites in the leukemic cells. Longterm administration of two or three drugs such as 6-mercaptopurine and methotrexate with or without cyclophosphamide has been used as has a rapidly rotating schedule of multiple drugs. Increasing the number of drugs may, however, increase the frequency of severe or life-threatening immunosuppressive complications. Periodic reinforcement or inducer dosing with prednisone and vincristine is sometimes used, although the need for it is disputed. Early in remission, a series of intrathecal injections of methotrexate is given; this is frequently coupled with a fractionated course of supravoltage irradiation of the cranial contents designed to encompass all the extensions of the meninges. Late effects of irradiation on mentation in long-term survivors have been reported; thus long-term intrathecal methotrexate maintenance therapy without cranial irradiation has its proponents. The optimal duration of combination chemotherapy is unclear; up to 3 years of treatment have been given in some trials, in the hope of eradicating leukemic cells that may be in a prolonged resting phase in which they are less sensitive to chemotherapy than actively growing cells. Late relapse in the testis is an occasional problem. Although very late hematologic relapses (or possible reinduction of the disease by the causative agent) may occur, the current results of comprehensive treatment are sufficiently impressive that the burden of proof would seem to be on those who doubt the curability of childhood ALL.

Treatment is still evolving, partly to reduce the short-term and long-term toxicity of these complex regimens in the highly responsive "common" ALL and partly to develop more intensive regimens tailored to subsets of patients such as those with T-cell ALL in which the remission rate and duration are unsatisfactory.

In patients who have relapsed, remission can frequently be reinduced, but sustained second remissions are rare; remission duration tends to become shorter and shorter with retreatment to the point at which neither standard nor investigational drugs are effective and fatal infections or bleeding supervene.

Adult ALL. Adults with ALL have a lower remission rate and shorter remission duration and survival compared with children given the same treatment. Sustained remissions are uncommon. Three-drug induction regimens are usually successful in inducing remission (80% overall, 90% in teenagers); multidrug consolidation and maintenance are used in an effort to improve remission duration. Central nervous system (CNS) prophylaxis has decreased the incidence of overt CNS leukemia. It is likely that some of the adult ALLs actually are poorly differentiated lymphomas. Current clinical trials are attempting to identify, by immunologic and biochemical means, subsets of patients who are curable with current treatment and those whose disease requires new approaches.

Adult AML. In contrast to ALL the spectrum of drugs useful in systemic treatment of AML is markedly constricted; only two classes of drugs have significant activity: cytidine analogs, especially arabinosyl cytosine (cytosine arabinoside, ara-C) and anthracycline antibiotics such as daunorubicin and doxorubicin. The other six classes of drugs previously noted have only marginal activity. Regimens including daunorubicin or doxorubicin (Adriamycin) plus ara-C with or without other drugs are capable of inducing complete remission in at least half of AML patients; with careful selection and skillful management, most younger adults can achieve remission. Older patients tend to fare poorly, but this may be largely because of the multisystem diseases to which they are prone rather than an intrinsic difference in the disease. On the other hand, some older adults have atypical features to their leukemia and may have an indolent course without specific treatment. Special care should be used in selecting them for antileukemic treatment.

With three doses of an anthracycline and a 7-day infusion of ara-C, the peripheral blood blast count usually falls dramatically; by the end of the infusion about 85% of the patients will have severely hypocellular or aplastic marrows. Over the next 2 or 3 weeks normal precursors appear in the marrow, the peripheral platelet count and reticulocyte count rise, and granulocytes reappear in the blood. Some patients require repeated courses of treatment to achieve remission, whereas a few are completely refractory to current drugs. Until remission occurs, intensive support care is essential (see below).

The optimal consolidation strategy is unclear but may involve one or both of the highly active agents in combination with other drugs. The intensity and duration of consolidation treatment are somewhat limited by the restriction on total accumulated dose of anthracyclines, which are cardiotoxic; by the isoimmunization that frequently develops to transfused platelets and thus interferes with supportive care; by the reduced tolerance of the normal marrow to chemotherapy while normal marrow elements are rapidly regenerating; by the physical toll of sustained therapy, repeated courses of nephrotoxic antibiotics, and malnutrition, which is sometimes correctable only by hyperalimentation; and by the psychologic burden of prolonged hospitalization. Despite all these problems, it may be possible to give three or more courses of combined therapy, for example, with thioguanine, cytosine arabinoside, and daunorubicin over a 9- or 10-week period. Although very early relapses occur, the majority of patients remain in remission through the consolidation period.

It is customary to continue treatment beyond the consolidation phase, although the best type of maintenance treatment and its duration are uncertain. Unfortunately, the value of maintenance regimens is not routinely tested by comparison with no maintenance; at the same time it must be said that it is essential, if possible, to prevent relapse. To the extent that maintenance therapy actually accomplishes that, it should be used. Repeated courses of ara-C combinations are usually employed.

Childhood AML. About 15% of children with acute leukemia have AML; the complete remission rate (56% to 66%) and remission duration (10 to 21 months) in various series are markedly inferior to results in ALL. The spectrum of active drugs appears to be broader than in adult AML, but the results to date are not clearly better. The strategy for treatment of these children continues to evolve.

Immunotherapy. Spontaneous remissions of acute leukemia occur on rare occasions, suggesting that host factors may be important in combating the disease. Moreover, some studies have indicated a correlation between immunocompetence and prognosis. Several clinical trials have been carried out using active nonspecific stimulation of the immune system with agents such as bacille Calmette-Guérin, sometimes along with allogeneic irradiated leukemic cells, as an adjunct to chemotherapy for acute leukemia. The results have been variable, with lengthened survival in some studies. This approach remains experimental.

Transplantation. Patients who have a healthy identical twin should undergo marrow transplantation. Others who have an HLA-compatible sibling should be considered for transplantation once they are in chemotherapy-induced remission, since the interim results of this procedure appear superior in remission duration and survival to what has been accomplished so far with chemotherapy. It should be mentioned, however, that an appropriately controlled trial comparing these approaches has not been done. Many problems are encountered in transplant patients, such as graft-versus-host disease, interstitial pneumonitis, and, despite preparation of the patient with total body irradiation and high-dose chemotherapy, recurrence of the leukemia in some cases.

COMPLICATIONS AND SUPPORTIVE CARE. Infections are a major and recurrent problem while the acute leukemia is in relapse and are the usual cause of death. Because of leukopenia, the usual infecting organisms are gram-negative bacilli and *Staphylococcus aureus*. Gram-negative bacillary pneumonias and septicemias, especially caused by *Pseudomonas* and *Escherichia coli*, are particularly common as are perirectal abscesses and urinary tract infections. Dental infections and thrush may be troublesome.

Systemic fungal infections are not common early but become more likely later in the course. Fevers usually result from infection that, because of neutropenia, rapidly becomes fulminant despite only minimal signs and symptoms. Prompt broad-spectrum antibiotic coverage (along with appropriate diagnostic studies) is essential. *Pneumocystis carinii* infections require specific treatment with trimetho-prim-sulfamethoxazole (see Chapter 54). Strict reverse isolation techniques may be helpful in reducing the incidence of infections but interfere with frequent examination of the patient and incur a psychologic burden; use of a private room, limiting the traffic in the room, and handwashing before touching the patient may be an acceptable compromise. Prophylaxis with trimethoprim-sulfamethoxazole during consolidation has been advocated. Granulocyte transfusions may be a useful adjunct for documented infections occurring while the patient is severely leukopenic.

Cutaneous, gingival, and nasal bleeding are common. Gastrointestinal and pulmonary bleeding are life threatening; intracranial bleeding is usually progressive and fatal. Prophylactic platelet transfusions are given when the platelet count is precipitously falling or is below 20,000. Menses should be suppressed with a progestin while a young female patient is in relapse, since endometrial bleeding is occasionally uncontrollable. Heparin and replacement of consumable clotting factors may be helpful if DIC is demonstrated. Extreme elevation of the peripheral blast count may result in occlusion and perivascular infiltration of cerebral and pulmonary vessels; cerebral hemorrhage is a common sequela. In addition to urgent initiation of chemotherapy, the use of hydroxyurea, leukapheresis, or both may be helpful in promptly reducing the cell count.

The rapid breakdown of tumor tissue can elevate serum uric acid and result in acute renal failure from marked deposition of urate in the kidneys or ureters. The use of allopurinol prophylactically for the first 2 or 3 weeks of treatment is indicated, but vigorous hydration for the first few days, within the patient's tolerance, should also be used, since xanthine nephropathy has been described in patients given allopurinol without adequate hydration. Alkalinization of the urine is sometimes indicated, and rarely dialysis is required.

Leukemic meningitis occurs in the majority of children and increasing numbers of adults with ALL if the central nervous system is not specifically treated. Since this process, once overt, is very difficult to eradicate and is a source of reseeding the marrow with leukemic cells, "prophylaxis" is indicated. This complication is not sufficiently common at present in adult AML to warrant prophylaxis, but the incidence may increase as more patients achieve prolonged hematologic remission.

Anemia should be at least partially corrected with packed red cell transfusions to relieve symptoms and to provide a margin in the event of sudden hemorrhage.

PROGNOSIS. Without treatment or if treatment does not result in a complete remission, the median survival for acute leukemia is about 3 months. On the other hand, half of the properly treated children with ALL survive without evidence of recurrent leukemia and are probably cured. The prognosis for adult ALL is much less favorable; in one series the median remission duration was 19 months and survival 26 months for adult ALL patients receiving CNS prophylaxis. Longer median remission durations have been reported but not consistently. In adult AML, a median remission duration of 8 to 14 months and median survival of about 2 years have been observed for those in complete remission. Sustained remissions are seen in a few cases; the percentage may be increasing in recent trials. Promyelocytic leukemia patients may have a longer survival and monocytic leukemia patients a shorter survival. Thus, although still one of the most feared diseases, acute leukemia is no longer invariably hopeless, and depending on the specific type, cure may be a realistic goal of current management.

CHRONIC MYELOGENOUS LEUKEMIA

DEFINITION. Chronic myelogenous leukemia (CML) or granulocytic leukemia is a disorder of the bone marrow, spleen, and other blood-forming organs in which myeloid elements, especially granulocytes and sometimes megakaryocytes and erythroid precursors, proliferate inappropriately. After a variable period of time ranging from months to years, most cases terminate in a refractory acute leukemic process.

ETIOLOGY. In most cases the cause is unclear, but ionizing radiation or long-term benzene exposure has been associated with some cases.

PATHOGENESIS. Proliferation kinetic studies show increased production as well as longer survival of granulocytes in CML. There is also an appreciable spontaneous death rate of the leukemic cells. There is usually an increased number of colony-forming cells in the marrow and a marked increase in these cells in the circulation as shown by in vitro agar culture techniques. There is an active exchange of leukemic cells among the bone marrow, blood, and spleen. In some cases spontaneous oscillations of the white blood count occur, suggesting some residual feedback control.

CLINICAL MANIFESTATIONS. CML is typically a disease of young to middle-aged adults but can occur at any age. Fatigue, sweating, indigestion, and left upper quadrant discomfort are common presenting complaints, but sometimes there are no symptoms. Occasionally, abdominal pain (from splenic infarction), symptoms of anemia, an attack of secondary gout, or bleeding manifestations (related to platelet dysfunction) following a dental procedure will first bring the patient to medical attention. Moderate to marked splenomegaly is usually present, but adenopathy is not expected in the chronic phase; if present, adenopathy may indicate that the blastic phase (see below) has already started or that a second disorder exists. However, it should be kept in mind that granulocytic infiltration of lymph nodes may be mistaken on biopsy for lymphoma. Hepatomegaly and bone tenderness may be present. Fever is uncommon.

LABORATORY FINDINGS. The peripheral white blood count is usually over 50,000 and may reach several hundred thousand. There is a profusion of neutrophils, band cells, metamyelocytes, and myelocytes, with relatively few promyelocytes and blasts in the chronic phase. Eosinophils and basophils are increased, sometimes so strikingly as to justify calling a case eosinophilic leukemia or basophilic leukemia. The platelet count may be high, low, or normal. In some cases thrombocytosis is the most significant management problem, causing bleeding or clotting complications. The hematocrit may be normal, slightly increased, or decreased. Anemia if present is usually normochromic and normocytic. The bone marrow is hypercellular with a spectrum of granulocytic elements; megakaryocytes may be strikingly increased as well. A marrow biopsy may show variable amounts of fibrous tissue. A characteristic finding demonstrable in about 85% of cases in marrow preparations and in immature granulocytes from peripheral blood is the Philadelphia chromosome, a deletion of one of the long arms of a number 22 chromosome. The missing arm is usually translocated to a number 9 chromosome. Although present in granulocytes, erythroid precursors, and megakaryocytes, this lesion is not found in lymphocytes, skin fibroblasts, or buccal mucosa cells, indicating that it is an acquired rather than inherited abnormality. Curiously, patients without this abnormality tend to fare worse. Another distinctive finding in most patients with CML is a low or zero leukocyte (neutrophil) alkaline phosphatase (LAP) score. With treatment or with secondary infections the LAP score in CML may increase into the normal range; old neutrophils tend to have less enzyme than young ones. The pretreatment serum uric acid is frequently increased as is the serum vitamin B_{12} level, the latter as a consequence of an increase in transcobalamin I, one of the B_{12}-binding proteins. These increases result from the increased turnover of white blood cells in this disorder. In contrast to acute leukemia and chronic lymphocytic leukemia, the leukemic cells in CML are functional, thus accounting for the low incidence of infection and the relatively benign course of the chronic phase.

DIAGNOSIS. In the typical middle-aged patient with splenomegaly, a white blood count of 200,000, including a spectrum of mature and immature granulocytes, and a low LAP score, the diagnosis is not difficult. Nevertheless, a chromosome analysis should be performed, since it is of diagnostic (if positive) and prognostic (if negative) value.

A bone marrow biopsy may be helpful in demonstrating extreme hyperplasia and fibrosis. The major sources of confusion are myelofibrosis with myeloid metaplasia (MMM) and leukemoid reactions. Rarely, polycythemia vera and other myeloproliferative disorders are troublesome. Patients with MMM tend to have lower white cell counts but truly massive splenomegaly, more extensive marrow fibrosis, and higher LAP scores; no consistent chromosome abnormalities are found. A leukemoid reaction should be in response to some underlying process such as an infection or a carcinoma, does not itself produce organomegaly or marrow changes other than hyperplasia, and should be associated with a normal chromosome analysis and a high LAP score. Occasionally none of the initial findings is clear-cut, in which case careful observation rather than a hasty diagnosis is appropriate.

COURSE AND PROGNOSIS. The typical patient responds well to intermittent therapy for 3 or 4 years, at which point it becomes more and more difficult to control the white blood cell count, platelet count, or recurrent left upper quadrant pain (splenic infarctions). Serial karyotypes may become increasingly bizarre. Fever, skin infiltrates, or adenopathy may herald the onset of the blastic phase, which is largely indistinguishable from acute leukemia, except that it is usually refractory to treatment. The acute phase lasts weeks or months. A fulminating "blastic crisis" with extreme leukocytosis, cerebrovascular accident, or pulmonary insufficiency is much less common than a gradual metamorphosis or transformation evolving over several months. A few patients die of marrow failure with extensive marrow fibrosis, drug toxicity, or other causes without entering an acute phase, but most patients have a blastic transformation sooner or later. In fact, occasional patients who appear to have de novo acute leukemia are found on chromosome analysis to be Philadelphia chromosome positive, suggesting that the chronic phase of the disease was asymptomatic and undiagnosed.

MANAGEMENT. Drug dosages will not be given because dose and drug regimens are still evolving, and the use of these regimens should be restricted to leukemia experts.

Alkylating agents, especially busulfan (Myler101), are the current treatment of choice for CML. It has been difficult to find a more effective agent, and the chronic phase of CML may be managed with deceptive ease using busulfan. Even patients who denied symptoms often feel better after treatment is started. Nevertheless, patients should be undertreated with this drug. On a short-term basis, busulfan is treacherous because of its prolonged marrow toxicity; the hematologic toxicity may be slow in onset (weeks or months), but once established, may be life threatening and is very slow to resolve. During the period of daily treatment, frequent reduction of dose is essential as the patient responds; treatment should be stopped before the blood counts normalize so as not to overshoot and cause marrow aplasia. On a long-term basis, pulmonary fibrosis, cytologic atypia (?carcinogenesis), and an addisonian-like syndrome of weakness, hypotension, and hyperpigmentation may occur. More importantly, survival is not significantly prolonged, although the quality of life is frequently improved. Intermittent treatment with busulfan when leukocytosis and splenomegaly recur is recommended in most cases; only in selected instances or later in the course is long-term maintenance therapy indicated. Hydroxyurea has a very rapid effect that is also rapidly dissipated; this is useful in rapidly lowering blood counts but requires frequent monitoring to adjust the dose. Thioguanine is occasionally useful. Splenic irradiation may cause a hematologic remission by an "abscopal" or remote effect that is not well understood. Intravenous radioactive phosphorus has also been used. Even though the blood counts, marrow hypercellularity, and splenomegaly may be dramatically improved by treatment, repeat chromosome analysis of the marrow in Philadelphia chromosome-positive cases shows this leukemic cell marker in abundance; thus the magnitude of leukemic cell kill has been minimal (from 10^{12} to perhaps 10^{11}) despite the appearance of remission, which might better be called "pseudoremission." Moreover, the onset of the blastic or "malignant" phase is not delayed. Since a true complete remission is not achieved and the accelerated phase is unaltered, it is not surprising that survival has not been lengthened. Recently some clinical trials have been directed at trying to eradicate the abnormal clone of Philadelphia chromosome-positive cells. This presupposes that there is a residue of normal cells to subsequently repopulate the marrow. With a combined approach of aggressive chemotherapy, splenic irradiation, and splenectomy, a few patients have had a marked, but usually temporary, reduction or disappearance of the abnormal clone. Whether such vigorous treatment might be curative for some patients is unclear. Once the patient is in the blastic phase, the leukemia is usually quite resistant to the type of therapy used in AML. A minority of patients, however, show a temporary response to prednisone and vincristine combinations. This largely corresponds to the curious observation that about 30% of blastic CMLs have cell characteristics (surface markers, terminal transferase, corticoid receptors, morphologic or staining characteristics) of lymphoblasts rather than myeloblasts. Presumably, the leukemic transformation in these cases is occurring in primitive cells that antedate differentiation into myeloid and lymphoid lines. Splenectomy in the blastic phase (for cytopenia or recurrent splenic infarcts) is occasionally useful but has a high complication rate in some series. There is controversy about its value in the chronic phase.

CHRONIC LYMPHOCYTIC LEUKEMIA

DEFINITION. Chronic lymphocytic leukemia (CLL) is a monoclonal proliferation of mature-looking, long-lived lymphocytes that accumulate in the bone marrow, blood, and lymphoid tissues of some older adults. It usually, but not invariably, shortens life expectancy. Less than 30% of leukemias in the United States are of this type.

ETIOLOGY. The cause of CLL is unknown. In contrast

to the myeloid leukemias, neither irradiation nor chemicals have been implicated. A viral causation has not been shown. Familial occurrence has been reported but is rare. Immune defects may play a role.

PATHOLOGY. A profusion of lymphocytes may be seen infiltrating the marrow, nodes, spleen, and liver, but the extent of infiltration at the time of diagnosis is variable. Other tissues may be affected, but virtually never the central nervous system. The histologic appearance is that of a well-differentiated lymphocytic lymphoma; sometimes transitions between these two disorders are seen.

CLINICAL MANIFESTATIONS. The typical patient is a 60-year-old man complaining of fatigue and perhaps painless lumps in the neck, armpits, or groin. On examination, symmetrically enlarged, firm, nontender lymph nodes are usually felt in most or all node-bearing areas. The spleen is frequently enlarged, but not massively. The liver may also be enlarged. However, a few patients have no signs or symptoms and are recognized by an absolute lymphocytosis found at the time of a routine blood count. Occasionally, symptoms of anemia, bleeding, or recurrent infection bring the patient to medical attention. Fever, if present, is rarely attributable to the disease process; secondary infection is usually the cause. Skin lesions of specific (infiltrative) and nonspecific types are sometimes seen.

Infections with encapsulated bacteria (pneumococci, *Haemophilus influenzae,* and group A streptococci) are common, presumably because of the patient's inability to produce antibody.

LABORATORY FINDINGS. In a normal adult, the absolute lymphocyte count (percentage of lymphocytes × total white blood count) is less than 4500. When the lymphocyte count is 100,000 to 200,000, the abnormality is readily apparent, but minimal elevations, for example, a white blood count of 10,000 with 60% lymphocytes, are troublesome unless the monoclonal nature of the lymphocyte population or tissue infiltration can be shown. The percentage of mature neutrophils in the differential count is often very low, but the absolute neutrophil count may be normal except in advanced disease or as a result of treatment. The platelet count is usually normal or slightly decreased; severe anemia may result from an associated autoimmune (Coombs'-positive) hemolysis, bleeding, or very advanced disease. The serum uric acid is usually normal before treatment but may increase significantly with treatment. Bone marrow examination is largely confirmatory rather than essential for diagnosis; a profusion of lymphocytes, mostly mature looking, is seen. Marrow cellularity may be normal but is sometimes "packed" with a lymphocytic infiltrate. There is no consistent chromosome abnormality. Serum immunoglobulin levels are frequently low and the circulating antibody response to vaccines is impaired, but delayed hypersensitivity reactions to recall antigens are usually intact. In vitro lymphocyte transformation after stimulation with mitogens is impaired. Most cases have cell surface characteristics of a single clone of "B" lymphocytes. Cases with "T" lymphocyte characteristics have also been described. Hilar, mediastinal, or retroperitoneal adenopathy may be demonstrated with appropriate roentgenograms and scans. An abnormal serum paraprotein or cryoglobulin may be found.

DIAGNOSIS. An adult with a markedly elevated lymphocyte count, especially in association with generalized adenopathy and splenomegaly, usually presents no problem in diagnosis. Other causes of lymphocytosis such as pertussis, infectious mononucleosis, and infectious lymphocytosis occur largely in childhood or adolescence. A slight lymphocytosis may be seen in tuberculosis, thyrotoxicosis, and Addison's disease, but the associated features should be distinctive. In all of these nonneoplastic disorders the lymphocyte proliferation should be polyclonal. When there is uncertainty, especially with a modest lymphocytosis, lymphocyte typing should be done. Confusion may arise in differentiating CLL from a well-differentiated lymphocytic lymphoma when there is a minimal increase in circulating lymphocytes, but current management is similar. Variants of CLL such as chronic lymphosarcoma cell leukemia and prolymphocytic leukemia have been described.

MANAGEMENT. Several treatments of modest value are available, including corticosteroids, alkylating agents such as chlorambucil, and ionizing radiation. There is considerable controversy, however, about whether asymptomatic patients should be treated, since they often have a benign course over months or years, since treatment may have side effects and complications, and since survival is not predictably improved. Recently a clinical staging system ranging from stage 0 to stage IV has been proposed. Stage 0 is lymphocytosis alone; stage I is lymphocytosis plus adenopathy; stage II adds splenomegaly and/or hepatomegaly. In stage III anemia is present and in stage IV thrombocytopenia. There is a significant difference in survival of early-stage and late-stage patients. Current efforts are focused on treating advanced disease, since the prognosis for such cases with casual treatment is relatively poor. It is possible, using chlorambucil plus prednisone, to achieve a complete response in a minority of patients; most patients show at least some response. Patients with complete remission have a significant improvement in survival, and current studies are directed toward improving remission rates. Total body radiotherapy in conjunction with chemotherapy is being investigated. Bulky masses of nodes may regress dramatically after localized radiotherapy when the response to systemic treatment is inadequate. A variety of dosage schedules of chlorambucil and prednisone have been advocated; typically, chlorambucil is given on a long-term daily basis, but a fortnightly bolus of the drug has been used with promising results. Several intermittent schedules of prednisone are currently used. It is important to avoid a long-term daily dose if possible because of the well-known complications of long-term steroid therapy, especially in a group of patients who already have multiple defects of immunocompetence. At present, treatment is not recommended for early-stage asymptomatic patients. High lymphocyte counts are not associated per se with the acute leukostasis problem seen in acute leukemia, but extreme leukocytosis (several hundred thousand cells per cubic millimeter) may be an indication for treatment. Patients with progressive, symptomatic, or advanced stage disease should have a trial of systemic therapy for at least 6 months. The maximal response may require many months. The optimal duration of treatment is unclear, but indefinite therapy must be tempered by the potential carcinogenic effects of alkylating agent treatment. Patients whose leukemia progresses after an unmaintained remission may respond again, although resistance to standard agents ultimately develops. Other drugs have generally been disappointing after failure with chlorambucil and prednisone. As better methods of subclassifying CLL are developed, the selection of subsets of patients for treatment should be simpler.

SUPPORTIVE CARE. Before treatment is started, allopurinal and vigorous hydration should be used to decrease the risk of uric acid nephropathy. Fever should always be assumed to result from infection rather than the leukemia, although other causes such as drugs may be apparent. Prompt diagnosis and treatment of infections are essential. Prophylactic antibiotics or γ-globulin injections have been advocated but are not recommended for routine use. Splenectomy may be useful for autoimmune hemolysis or thrombocytopenia unresponsive to steroids and for "hypersplenism."

COURSE AND PROGNOSIS. CLL may be indolent or progress rapidly over several months with hematologic deterioration and recurrent, ultimately fatal infections. Blastic transformation has been reported but is very rare. The incidence of second malignancies is increased.

The prognosis depends on the stage of the disease and the quality of the response to treatment. Longevity may range from 19 months in stage IV to over 12 years in stage 0. Some patients with CLL may achieve normal life expectancy (cure), whereas for others CLL may be more malignant than acute leukemia.

BIBLIOGRAPHY
Acute leukemias
Cline, M.J., and others: Acute leukemia: biology and treatment, Ann. Intern. Med. **91:**758, 1979.
Gale, R.P.: Advances in the treatment of acute myelogenous leukemia, N. Engl. J. Med. **300:**1189, 1979.
Mauer, A.M.: Treatment of acute leukemia in children, Clin. Haematol. **7:**245, 1978.
Omura, G.A., and others: Combination chemotherapy of adult acute lymphoblastic leukemia with randomized central nervous system prophylaxis, Blood **55:**199, 1980.

Chronic myelogenous leukemia
Barton, J.C., and Conrad, M.E.: Current status of blastic transformation in chronic myelogenous leukemia, Am. J. Hematol. **4:**281, 1978.

Moloney, W.C.: Chronic myelogenous leukemia, Cancer **42:**865, 1978.
Strychmans, P.A.: Treatment of chronic myeloid leukemia, Annu. Rev. Med. **31:**159, 1980.

Chronic lymphocytic leukemia
Huguley, C.M.: Treatment of chronic lymphocytic leukemia, Cancer Treat. Rev. **4:**261, 1977.
Rai, K.R., and others: Clinical staging of chronic lymphocytic leukemia, Blood **46:**219, 1975.

74 • THE EOSINOPHIL AND EOSINOPHILIC SYNDROMES
Richard Snepar and Donald Kaye

The finding of increased numbers of eosinophils in the peripheral blood is abnormal and may represent one of a number of diverse pathologic conditions. Blood eosinophilia rarely occurs as an isolated event and is usually associated with other sites of organ infiltration.

Eosinophils are produced in the bone marrow, but their cell of origin remains unknown. In the peripheral blood "normal" ranges for eosinophils vary depending on how they are expressed. As a percentage of the total leukocyte count, up to 4% is considered normal. A more accurate expression is the number of eosinophils per cubic millimeter. Counted in this manner, the range of normal is approximately 0 to 700/mm^3, with a mean normal value of 120/mm^3 in adults.

The eosinophil is distinct from other leukocytes; most have bilobed nuclei, and the granules stain orange to deep red with Wright's or Giemsa stains. The granules elaborate numerous enzymes including eosinophil arylsulfatase, which can inactivate both slow-reacting substance of anaphylaxis and eosinophil chemotactic factor of anaphylaxis in vitro. The role of the eosinophil in the host response may be to modulate the inflammatory reaction and to aid in the defense against multicellular parasites (worms).

There are certain conditions that are frequently associated with a rise in circulating eosinophils. Parasitic infection is a prominent cause. While most helminthic infections can cause a mild rise in circulating eosinophils, those associated with tissue invasion cause the most marked elevations. *Trichinella*, *Strongyloides*, and *Toxocara canis* and *cati* are notorious causes of high peripheral blood eosinophil counts. Alternatively, protozoan infections (other than *Pneumocystis carinii*) rarely cause a significant eosinophilia.

The eosinophilic pulmonary syndromes (see Chapter 132) are (1) *Löffler's syndrome*, a 3- to 4-week illness consisting of peripheral blood eosinophilia, eosinophils in the sputum, and transient fluffy pulmonary infiltrates, which is often caused by drugs, inhaled antigens, or parasitic infections and is responsive to steroid therapy; (2) *pulmonary infiltrates with eosinophilia* (PIE), an illness of longer duration characterized by peripheral and apical pulmonary infiltration, fever, and dyspnea often caused by drugs, parasites, connective tissue disorders, or neoplasms and frequently responsive to steroids; and (3) *tropical pulmonary eosinophilia*, a syndrome of fever, pulmonary infiltrates, and bronchospasm caused by occult microfilarial infection. The last usually responds to diethylcarbamazine.

The *hypereosinophilic syndrome* represents a group of conditions characterized by persistent marked eosinophilia and diffuse organ infiltration with eosinophils. These conditions lack evidence of a known cause of eosinophilia. They range from prolonged benign eosinophilia to eosinophilic leukemia. The cardiovascular system is nearly always involved, generally in the form of myocarditis and endocardial fibrosis with congestive heart failure (presumably caused by a direct effect of the eosinophil), and marrow eosinophilia and leukocytosis are consistently noted. The lung (interstitial infiltrates), skin (rash), kidney, and liver are frequently involved.

Eosinophilia is also seen in association with asthma, polyarteritis nodosa, allergic rhinitis, drug allergy, and skin diseases, notably pemphigus and pemphigoid. Less frequently, eosinophilia may be associated with lymphoma and disseminated carcinoma, immune deficiency states, graft-versus-host reactions, and inflammatory bowel disease.

There is a group of pathologic conditions involving specific organ infiltration with eosinophils with or without blood eosinophilia. Eosinophilic gastroenteritis is characterized by eosinophilic infiltration of the stomach and small intestine (see Chapter 125). Eosinophilic fasciitis refers to eosinophilic infiltration and thickening of the fascia clinically resembling dermatomyositis (see Chapter 17). Eosinophilic cholecystitis, cystitis, and prostatitis have also been described. Eosinophilic granulomata, aggregates of histiocytes and eosinophils, may be found in bone or soft tissues (see Chapter 78).

BIBLIOGRAPHY

Beeson, P., and Bass, D.A.: The eosinophil, Philadelphia, 1977, W.B. Saunders Co.

Chusid, M.J., and others: The hypereosinophilic syndrome, Medicine **54**:1, 1975.

75 • MYELOPROLIFERATIVE DISEASE

Frank H. Gardner and Gary B. Weiss

The term "myeloproliferative disorders" has been used to characterize a group of clinical neoplastic and non-neoplastic proliferations of all bone marrow precursor elements. The encompassing term has been useful in emphasizing that proliferation of the primordial stem cell can

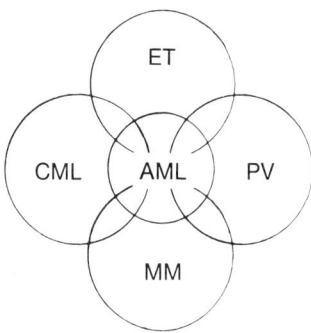

Fig. 75-1. Schematic concept of interaction of different types of myeloproliferative disease. Lower overlaps of circles indicate relationship of myeloid metaplasia, *MM*, with chronic granulocytic leukemia. *CML*, and polycythemia vera, *PV*. Upper overlaps of circles reflect transitions of essential thrombocythemia, *ET*, into CML and PV. In a small number of patients any of these disorders can evolve into acute myeloblastic leukemia, *AML*.

have an abnormal response in any of the committed cell compartments. Fig. 75-1 outlines a schematic concept that has been developed in the past three decades regarding the overlapping definitions of these various disorders. The proliferation of the committed stem cell is self-perpetuating and in this regard appears to be a neoplastic disease. Indeed, the transition may be a preneoplastic disorder for years or through the lifetime observation of the patient. In this group of diseases we include chronic granulocytic leukemia, polycythemia vera, agnogenic myeloid metaplasia with myelofibrosis, and essential thrombocythemia. A schematic relationship of the transition among these different types of proliferative disorders is represented in Fig. 75-1.

In all instances the stimulation of one committed stem cell is associated with a generalized marrow hyperplasia, implying that there is general activation of all the committed stem cell compartments. With this proliferative activity, reticulin fibers are increased to suggest that bone marrow fibroblasts also have increased activity.

CHRONIC GRANULOCYTIC LEUKEMIA

As with polycythemia vera, current data indicate that chronic granulocytic leukemia or chronic myelogenous leukemia (CML) also is an abnormal clonal malignancy. CML is discussed in Chapter 73, and polycythemia vera is discussed in Chapter 71.

ESSENTIAL THROMBOCYTHEMIA

Essential thrombocythemia is defined as an elevation of the platelet count above 400,000/mm^3, associated with a bone marrow megakaryocytic hyperplasia and a mild neutrophilic leukocytosis. It is seen with increased frequency in middle-aged women. The disease usually is diagnosed because of spontaneous subcutaneous bleeding that may occur for months or years. It is known for the frequency of gastrointestinal bleeding and associated hypochromic iron deficiency anemia. On physical examination the patient may have evidence of superficial phlebitis, and splenomegaly is found in more than three fourths of the patients. The spleens are not massive but usually weigh 500 to 600 g.

Laboratory examination may be diagnostic with a platelet count ranging from 500,000 to several million; the platelets are enlarged, abnormal in size, and are found in large clumps on examination of the peripheral blood film. In many instances the abnormal platelet morphology is associated with impaired platelet function as measured by platelet aggregation techniques and prolonged bleeding time. Abnormal chromosome patterns are rarely found with essential thrombocythemia.

The presence of thrombocytosis should alert the physician to associated myeloproliferative disorders. Platelet counts are usually not as high in chronic leukemia, myeloid metaplasia, or polycythemia vera.

The disease is not treated unless the patient is symptomatic. If there is evidence of bleeding as demonstrated by ecchymoses or abnormal venous coagulation with thrombophlebitis or by hypochromic anemia with chronic gastrointestinal bleeding, the patient should be treated with either an alkylating agent (L-phenylalanine mustard) or radioactive phosphorus. From current observations both therapies appear to reduce the platelet count satisfactorily. Both modalities are associated with an increased frequency of acute leukemia if therapy is continued over many years. Hence, it is the usual policy to treat the patient only until the platelet count is in the range of 200,000 to 400,000/mm^3. Thereafter, retreatment is not planned until there is evidence of abnormal platelet function with symptoms as described in the preceding.

AGNOGENIC MYELOID METAPLASIA (MYELOFIBROSIS WITH MYELOID METAPLASIA)

DEFINITION. The term "agnogenic myeloid metaplasia" has been used to describe a group of middle-aged patients (50 to 70 years predominantly) who have fibrosis of the bone marrow (myelofibrosis) and bone marrow precursors circulating in the blood and found outside sites of normal adult marrow, especially in the liver and spleen. Since the fibrosis is the predominant pathologic finding without explanation, the term "agnogenic," for an unknown mechanism, has been preferred.

It is thought that myelofibrosis is the end stage of polycythemia vera in possibly 10% of such patients. In past years there have been repeated references to myelofibrosis associated with toxicity from solvents, especially benzene. This was much more frequent 30 years ago, especially in the shoe industry with the use of rubber cement, than it is today. Following the atomic bomb episode in Japan, increased myeloid metaplasia has been described, suggesting that ionizing radiation also may be a factor. Although estrogens may induce an alteration like myelofibrosis in many animals, there has been no correlation made in humans. The disorder is associated with abnormal chromosomes in hematopoietic cells in 40% to 50% of the patients, but there has been no adequate documentation that the bone marrow fibroblasts have the same chromosome abnormality.

PATHOGENESIS. With the abnormal proliferation of bone marrow–committed stem cells in extramedullary areas, there is progressive enlargement of the spleen and liver and ultimately the lymph nodes, as well as increased fibrosis in the marrow cavity. There is a concurrent osteosclerosis. There may be transition to an acute leukemic process as with other myeloproliferative disorders, and a blastic crisis develops in 5% to 10% of patients with myeloid metaplasia.

CLINICAL MANIFESTATIONS. Although the disease is primarily one of middle to old age (over 95%), with men affected slightly more frequently than women, this disorder may occur in a small group of younger patients between 20 and 40 years of age, who have a tendency for a more rapid progression and complications. The clinical manifestations are protean and vary from the asymptomatic patient who is discovered to have splenomegaly on routine examination, with evidence of a mild leukocytosis and a rare normoblast on the peripheral blood film, to other patients who may have numerous symptoms. Seventy-five percent of patients complain of marked fatigue, which may or may not be associated with anemia. In over half of the patients there is a weight loss, which has been attributed to an increased metabolic rate and to distortion of the alimentary tract with impaired nutrition because of the massive splenomegaly. Indeed, some patients may be seen in a terminal cachectic state related to the weight loss. Abnormal abdominal pressure and signs of distention because of the splenomegaly are noted in two thirds of the patients.

It should be emphasized that over half of the patients may have prolonged intervals of low-grade fever associated with the organ enlargement. Often it is difficult to distinguish this fever from the fever of infection. About one fourth of the patients have bone pain, which can be a diagnostic problem to the physician and the patient. Usually such patients have roentgenographic evidence of osteosclerosis (Fig. 75-2). The pain has a chronic aching pattern, characteristically in the humeri and femora. In some instances the patient may have swollen joints suggestive of rheumatoid arthritis. Indeed, with a marked hyperuricemia, the physician may interpret this to be a gouty attack.

With the abnormal proliferation of marrow elements, often there are complications of impaired platelet function. Patients may initially have symptoms similar to those of essential thrombocythemia because of platelet abnormalities.

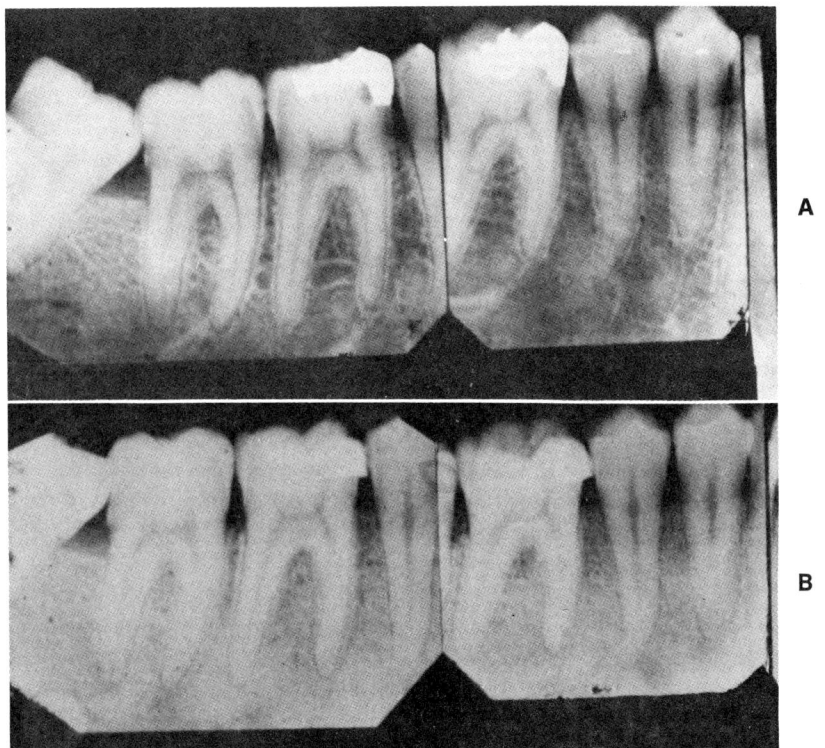

Fig. 75-2. Roentgenograms of 26-year-old man with myeloid metaplasia. He complained of diffuse aching of entire mandible. Radiologic studies, **B**, revealed osteosclerosis with distinct loss of alveolar bone with crestal deficiency reaching level of molar bifurcation. Similar view taken 2 years previously, **A**, was available to show progressive osteosclerosis, **B**, from normal pattern.

Although the spleen is usually grossly enlarged, in a few instances the splenomegaly may not be palpable and may be demonstrable only by radioisotope scanning. There is some correlation between the duration of the disease and the size of the spleen.

LABORATORY FINDINGS. The peripheral blood smear in myeloid metaplasia characteristically contains tear-shaped red cells. Polychromatophilia, stippling, and nucleated red cells are required by some clinicians for a well-defined diagnosis. Reticulocytosis usually is insignificant and ranges from 2% to 7% in the classic case. The leukoerythroblastic response demonstrates all stages of granulocyte precursors with variable numbers of myeloblasts (2% to 20%) and nucleated red blood cells. It should be emphasized that the morphology of the red cells may be helpful in the differential diagnosis from chronic granulocytic leukemia.

The degree of anemia varies somewhat with the duration and severity of the disease. Leukocyte counts can range from normal to values above 80,000/mm^3. Platelet counts exceeding 1 million with abnormal platelet morphology and function are seen, but most often the platelet count is in the range of 200,000 to 400,000/mm^3. Leukocyte alkaline phosphatase (LAP) scores initially were thought to be useful, but in large series the scores may be found to range from low to high. A high score is helpful in excluding chronic granulocytic leukemia. In all instances the scores are above those seen in CML. Hyperuricemia with occasional gouty attacks occurs in 25% to 50% of the cases. About one fourth of the patients have abnormal serum protein electrophoretic patterns of either a monoclonal or polyclonal type. With the elevated levels of early granulocytes, the histamine blood levels are always elevated.

In recent years the cytogenetic abnormalities on bone marrow study have been of special interest in myeloid metaplasia, since about half of the patients have a variety of duplications or translocations, most frequently in the C group. There is no evidence that the Philadelphia chromosome is found in this disorder.

Roentgenographic studies demonstrate the generalized increase in bone density with a mottled appearance of the bones, especially vertebrae and long bones. Bone marrow biopsy is often the most important diagnostic study in demonstrating the increased thickness of trabecular patterns along with marrow fibrosis. These changes are best demonstrated by 2- to 3-cm long cores obtained from the posterior iliac crest. The degree of fibrosis varies markedly from only increased reticulin fibers to more than two thirds of the marrow replaced by collagen. In the early stages of the fibrotic phase, megakaryocytes appear to be increased, but there has not been an exact way to quantitate them. It should be noted that aspirations are often unsuccessful (dry tap).

Extramedullary hematopoiesis in the spleen and liver can be demonstrated by radioiron isotopic studies. In such instances uptake and release of iron from the spleen imply extramedullary production of red cells. There has been an increased frequency of complications from needle aspiration biopsies of the liver in this disorder, and in most instances it should not be performed. Gastrointestinal roentgenograms may reveal an increased incidence of asymptomatic esophageal varices, possibly related to the disproportion of blood flow from the enlarged spleen into the portal circulation. A few patients have had serious bleeding complications requiring a portacaval shunt. Radioisotope scanning techniques may demonstrate large areas of opacity in the spleen from repeated splenic infarcts.

PROGNOSIS. Patients with myeloid metaplasia usually survive 4 to 5 years from the time of diagnosis. The major causes of death are hemorrhage and infection. Leukemic transformation probably occurs in 10% of the cases. Current data suggest that patients with myeloid metaplasia who have an abnormal chromosome have a shorter survival of about 2 years compared to 5 years in patients without a cytogenetic abnormality. A rare variety called acute myelofibrosis is characterized by a rapidly fatal course with pancytopenia and diffuse marrow fibrosis. This may be a transitional form of acute myeloblastic leukemia.

MANAGEMENT. There is no available literature that demonstrates an improvement in survival with the various therapies at the present time. Androgens in high doses (testosterone or nandrolone, 200 to 400 mg weekly) have increased hemoglobin levels and red cell mass and decreased the need for red cell transfusions. Patients with abnormal chromosome patterns have not responded satisfactorily to any type of androgen treatment. Androgen therapy is well tolerated by men but is distressful to women because of masculinization. It should be emphasized that all androgens used orally to treat these disorders are associated with abnormal liver function tests.

Patients with excessive hemolysis, thrombocytopenia, or painful massive spleens have tolerated splenectomy with marked improvement. Large painful spleens become intolerable to some patients. Patients with high white blood cell counts and no significant anemia may tolerate irradiation of the spleen to decrease the size and to improve alimentary nutrition. Some patients who have marked leukocytosis may benefit from judicious use of alkylating agents such as L-phenylalanine mustard or busulfan. Patients with massive splenomegaly and thrombocytosis who receive splenectomy have been treated with cytosine arabinoside or hydroxyurea to decrease platelet counts in the postsplenectomy period. Some patients with massive hemolysis have responded to corticosteroids, but the therapy for the most part is distressing because of the complications of adrenal steroids and is therefore not advised unless necessary.

BIBLIOGRAPHY

Gardner, F.H., and Nathan, D.G.: Androgens and erythropoiesis. III. Further evaluation of testosterone treatment of myelofibrosis, N. Engl. J. Med. **274:**420, 1966.

Silverstein, M.N.: Agnogenic myeloid metaplasia, Acton, Mass., 1975, Publishing Sciences Group, Inc.

Ward, H.P., and Block, M.H.: The natural history of agnogenic myeloid metaplasia (AMM) and a critical evaluation of its relationship with the myeloproliferative syndrome, Medicine **50:**357, 1971.

76 • PLASMA CELL DISORDERS
Nikolay V. Dimitrov

The immune system includes two major components, cellular immunity and humoral immunity. These components develop along separate but interrelated pathways of differentiation. The lymphocyte is considered to be the central cell involved in the physiology and pathophysiology of the immune system. Studies of various membrane markers of lymphocytes and their functional activities have provided tools for identification of two major populations of lymphocytes. Thymus-derived cells (T cells) are responsible for cell-mediated immune responses. Bone marrow-derived cells (B cells) are the precursors of the plasma cell line and are responsible for antibody production. B cells can be readily identified by immunoglobulin determinants present on their surface. These cells constitute about 30% to 40% of the circulating lymphocytes and have relatively short life spans. They are found in the lymphoid follicles and medullary cords of lymph nodes, in the peripheral white pulp and red pulp of the spleen, and in the lymphoid follicles adjacent to the mucosa of the gastrointestinal and respiratory tracts. Although the circulating antibodies are produced by lymphocytes and plasma cells, which are progeny of B cells, the participation of T suppressor and helper cells in regulation of the antibody response is essential (Fig. 76-1). This chapter will discuss disorders of plasma cell and B lymphocytes that share the common characteristics of production of excessive or abnormal monoclonal immunoglobulins. This occurs as a result of uncontrolled proliferation of cells normally involved in antibody production. Thus the plasma cell disorders arise when a malignantly transformed B lymphocyte enters uncontrolled proliferation, forming a clone of abnormal cells. The growth of the malignant clone may be unrestrained, producing a systemic malignant disease as in multiple myeloma, Waldenström's macroglobulinemia, and some types of heavy-chain disease. In other disorders such as benign monoclonal gammopathy, the malignant

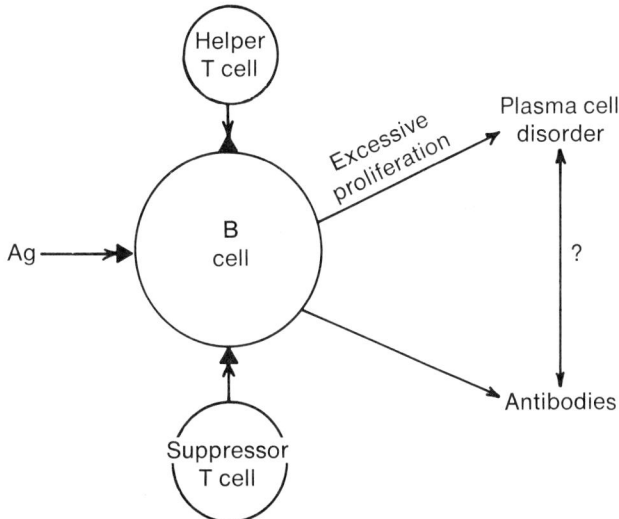

Fig. 76-1. Schematic presentation of factors affecting B-lymphocyte function. Antigen, *Ag*, interacts with B cells that proliferate to form plasma cells. B lymphocytes and plasma cells produce antibodies; antibody production is modulated by helper and suppressor T cells. Excessive proliferation of abnormal B cells and plasma cells leads to plasma cell malignancies. Relationship between normal production of antibodies and abnormal plasma cells is unclear.

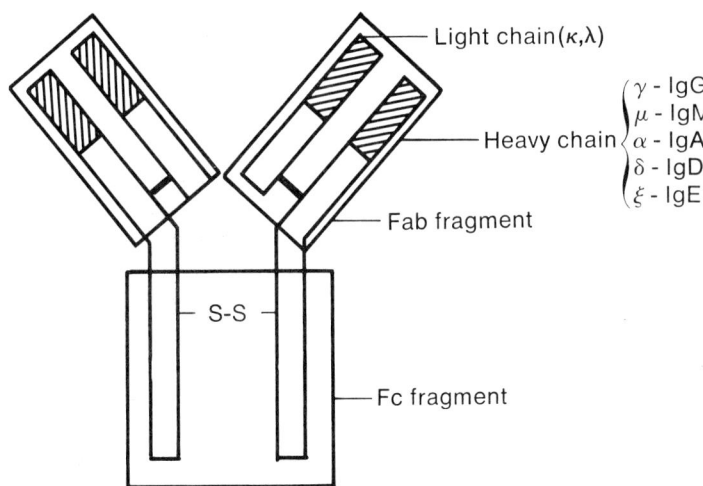

Fig. 76-2. Schematic representation of immunoglobulin molecule, showing two heavy (H) and two light (L) chains. Papain digestion cleaves molecule into Fc fragment (two portions of heavy chains) and two Fab fragments consisting of light chain and portion of heavy chain.

clone may grow to a certain extent and then become controlled with stabilization of the proliferation. Rarely in both instances the clone may regress.

Since plasma cell disorders are associated with anomalous production of proteins, the accurate diagnosis of these disorders requires identification and quantitation of the abnormal monoclonal immunoglobulins (IgG, IgA, IgM, IgD, IgE). Some authors use the term "M protein," which refers to the electrophoretically homogeneous components in the serum or urine and means "malignant," "myeloma," or more recently, "monoclonal." "Monoclonal" should be used.

The structure of immunoglobulin molecules is a multichain assembly consisting of two heavy and two light polypeptide chains. The arrangements of IgG molecules are presented in Fig. 76-2. Various enzymes are capable of splitting the heavy chains, thus forming two fragments: the Fab fragment consisting of a light chain joined to a portion of the heavy chain and the Fc fragment consisting of portions of the two heavy chains (square portions on Fig. 76-2).

Protein electrophoresis is a routine test that in the majority of cases appears to be sufficient for detecting a monoclonal protein in the serum or urine (Fig. 76-3). For

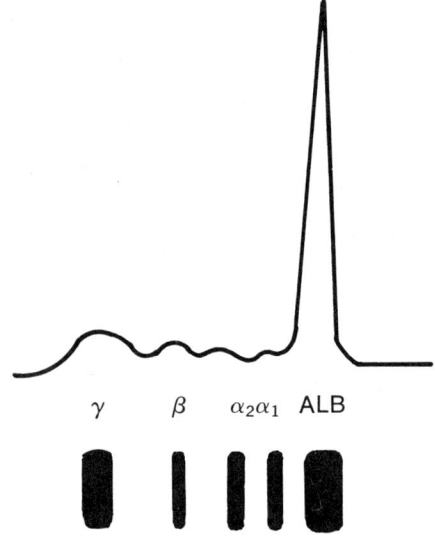

Fig. 76-3. Pattern of normal protein electrophoresis.

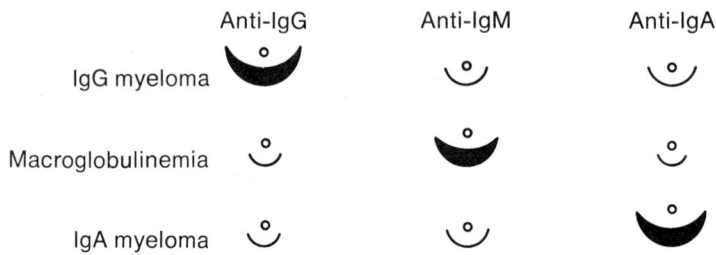

Fig. 76-4. Precipitation arcs resulting from exposure of patient's serum after electrophoresis to specific antisera. Patterns of IgG myeloma, IgA myeloma, and macroglobulinemia are illustrated.

further identification of the monoclonal protein components, immunoelectrophoresis should be used. This method employs protein electrophoresis for separation of the major components and immunodiffusion using specific antisera for identification of the abnormal monoclonal immunoglobulin (Fig. 76-4). Quantitation of monoclonal immunoglobulin in the serum or of light chains in the urine provides a marker of malignant cell activity. Serial studies are useful as an evaluation procedure for changes that occur during the treatment or in the course of observation.

For practical purposes these three methods for identification and quantitation of monoclonal protein are sufficient. With the development of modern immunology many other methods for identification of numerous subclasses of immunoglobulins are available, but at this time their value lies mostly in research.

Although the information from the monoclonal protein studies appears quite specific, the approach to diagnosis and treatment of plasma cell disorders should rely on a combination of clinical, morphologic, and laboratory considerations.

MULTIPLE MYELOMA

Multiple myeloma is a malignant disorder of plasma cells with clinical manifestations characterized by the formation of a tumor, bone marrow dysfunction associated with marrow replacement by abnormal plasma cells, bony lesions, renal disease, and abnormal synthesis of immunoglobulins.

ETIOLOGY. Multiple myeloma shares some of the general aspects of the origin of the neoplastic diseases. The exact cause of multiple myeloma is unknown. Some clinical and experimental observations suggest that chronic stimulation of the reticuloendothelial system may play a role in the development of plasma cell disorders. This has been supported by the development of plasma cell tumors in mice following injections of mineral oil, Freund adjuvant, and plastics. In humans, plasma cell disorders have been found in association with chronic diseases such as tuberculosis, chronic osteomyelitis, pyelonephritis, chronic hepatitis, and rheumatoid arthritis.

A viral cause has been suggested by experiments in mice using transmissible viral agents that induce the development of plasmacytomas containing viruslike particles. This has been associated with the presence of monoclonal protein and excretion of Bence Jones proteins in some of the animals.

The importance of genetic factors has been suggested by observation of some familial aggregations of multiple myeloma, particularly those occurring in siblings.

PATHOGENESIS. The pathophysiologic manifestations in multiple myeloma are closely related to the abnormal proliferation of immature and mature plasma cells, bone marrow dysfunction, and protein abnormalities. The abnormal proliferation of plasma cells occurs in the bone marrow with the formation of solitary osseous tumors. Isolated extraskeletal myeloma tumors can be found occasionally. These pathologic findings are considered to be a cause for transient or permanent skeletal pain and diffuse or local skeletal demineralization. Extensive involvement of the skeleton frequently leads to pathologic fractures. Destruction of the bones may result in increased serum and urine calcium.

The abnormal proliferation of the plasma cells in the bone marrow appears to impair its function. The exact mechanism for the decreased bone marrow function is unknown, but the extent of the plasma cell infiltration seems to play an important role. Impairment of bone marrow function is usually proportional to the number of plasma cells in the marrow. Mainly the erythroid elements are affected, resulting in the development of anemia, but thrombopoietic and leukopoietic function may also be impaired with the development of thrombocytopenia and leukopenia.

Myeloma cells are responsible for the production of abnormal proteins found in the serum and urine of patients with the disease. These proteins play an important role in the diagnosis of multiple myeloma and related disorders. Most patients with plasma cell disorders have increased concentrations of homogeneous proteins called "M" (monoclonal) components in the serum. These components can be IgG, IgM, IgA, IgD, or IgE. In addition, either κ or λ light chains may be present in urine. In other cases free κ or λ light chains or fragments of heavy chains in the urine may be the only abnormality detected.

It has been generally accepted that the precipitation of the light chain (Bence Jones) proteins in the renal tubule may result in a unique kidney disease, sometimes designated "myeloma kidney."

Although the γ-globulin level is increased, synthesis of antibodies appears to be defective. This, together with a decreased number of granulocytes, increased catabolism of γ-globulin, and the immunosuppressive effect of chemotherapy, leads to increased susceptibility to infection, which is the major problem in the management of this disorder. The infections are most commonly caused by encapsulated organisms (pneumococci, *Haemophilus influenzae,* and group A streptococci) and occur because of lack of antibody. There is also an increased incidence of herpes zoster, which is also more likely to generalize.

CLINICAL MANIFESTATIONS. Multiple myeloma is a disease predominantly of middle and old age. Almost 90% of the patients are over the age of 45. Men appear to be affected more often than women.

The onset may be preceded by an asymptomatic period that is variable in length. The most common presenting symptom is pain, which is related to bone involvement and pressure on the adjacent nerves. Pathologic fractures are a common complication that can lead to spinal cord or nerve root compression. Invasion of the nerve roots by myeloma cells or symmetric peripheral neuropathy unrelated to invasion has been reported. However, intracranial and cranial nerve involvement is considered a rare finding, even though the skull bones are a common site of myeloma lesions.

The roentgenographic abnormalities vary from patient to patient. The dominant pattern is generalized osteoporosis, occurring in 90% of the patients. Scattered osteolytic lesions may be found in about 75%. The most common sites of osteolytic lesions are the skull, mandible, ribs, clavicles, spine, pelvis, and sternum. The characteristic roentgenographic findings are described as "punched-out" lesions without osteoblastic reaction (Fig. 76-5). This indicates that roentgenograms are the method of choice for radiologic diagnosis of multiple myeloma. Bone scans have no practical value for the evaluation of patients with this disease. Solitary skeletal lesions can be found on roentgenograms in a small percentage of patients, mostly localized in the vertebra, pelvis, or femur. In such cases thorough investigation may reveal protein abnormalities or even distant bone marrow involvement. In a patient with solitary lesions disseminated disease usually develops after several months or years.

The presence of bone destruction frequently is associated with hypercalcemia. Patients with restricted physical activity are prone to hypercalcemia, which is aggravated by dehydration and oliguria. These patients have nausea, vomiting, drowsiness, and general weakness.

As a result of bone marrow impairment, anemia of variable severity is present in nearly all patients with multiple myeloma. In certain cases blood loss and shortened red cell survival may contribute to this abnormality. Most often anemia is moderate and has a normocytic and normochromic pattern. Examination of the peripheral blood smear shows formation of rouleaux, which is attributed to increased plasma protein concentration.

Abnormal bleeding can be a major problem for the clinician and surgeon. Besides thrombocytopenia, 2% to 5% of patients with multiple myeloma have hyperviscosity as a result of elevated serum levels of a monoclonal immunoglobulin. The presence of this abnormal protein affects several of the coagulation factors and the function of the platelets, resulting in hemorrhagic disturbances such as ep-

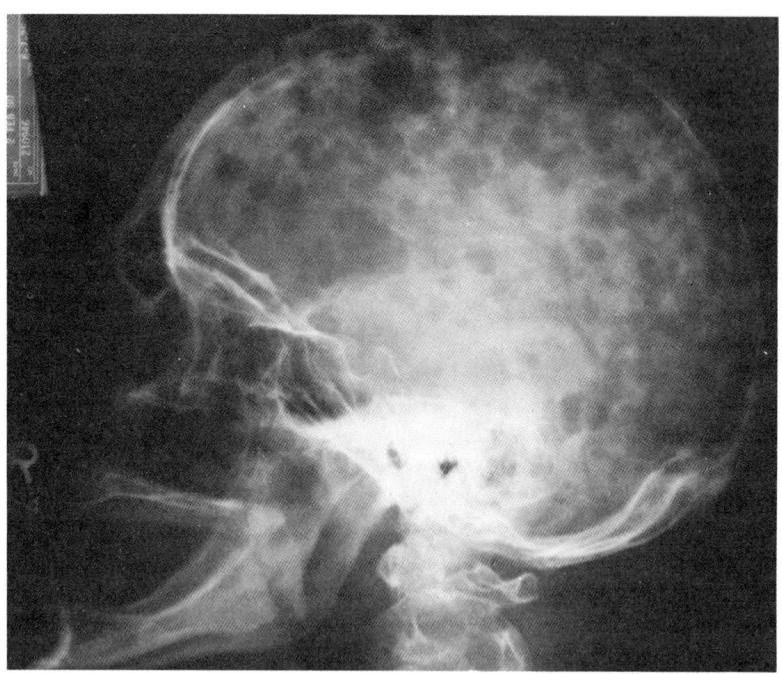

Fig. 76-5. Multiple myeloma. Roentgenogram of skull and mandible shows multiple lytic lesions ("punched-out" lesions).

istaxis, gum bleeding, gastrointestinal bleeding, purpura, ecchymoses, and hemorrhage in the eye grounds. Patients with multiple myeloma who are scheduled for any kind of surgery, including tooth extraction, require a thorough hematologic evaluation. Hyperviscosity can interfere with blood circulation in the central nervous system, causing changing neurologic findings (paresis, impaired consciousness, and deafness). Heart failure and pulmonary insufficiency may also occur as a result of hyperviscosity.

The relationship between protein abnormalities in multiple myeloma and the formation of amyloid is well established. In some patients the occurrence of congestive heart failure, arthropathy, nephrotic syndrome, or peripheral neuropathy may be associated with amyloidosis. Occasionally patients with multiple myeloma may have increased cryoglobulins in the serum that can be responsible for aggravation of the clinical picture on exposure to cold.

Chronic renal failure is a frequent complication of the disease. The clinical picture is related to the extent of renal involvement and varies from slight insufficiency to advanced irreversible azotemia. The presence of the nephrotic syndrome is usually associated with amyloidosis.

LABORATORY FINDINGS. The diagnosis of multiple myeloma always requires thorough examination of the bone marrow. In most cases the aspirate is sufficient for diagnostic purposes, but if a dry aspiration is obtained because the marrow is packed with plasma cells, biopsy is indicated. Increased numbers of atypical plasma cells are present in almost all of the patients with multiple myeloma (Fig. 76-6). The number of such cells should exceed at least 15% of the total marrow cells. Plasmacytosis of bone marrow may be encountered in chronic infections and various neoplastic diseases. Plasma cells seen in multiple myeloma vary in size and shape, possess polychromasia, may contain a large nucleolus, and frequently have cytoplasmic and intranuclear inclusion bodies. The terms "Russell's bodies," "Mott cells," "morular cells," and "grape cells" refer to the presence of cytoplasmic spherules that appear to all be of the same origin. The increased numbers of plasma cells in the marrow usually suppress the erythroid, myeloid, and megakaryocyte function to a variable extent.

Protein abnormalities are the most important findings for documentation of the diagnosis. The serum globulin level is elevated in most cases. The exceptions are patients who overproduce only light chains that are lost in the urine. Serum protein electrophoresis typically shows a prominent monoclonal spike (Fig. 76-7). Immunoelectrophoresis identifies the involvement of specific immunoglobulin (Fig. 76-4). Quantitation is important for diagnosis and follow-up. Some characteristics of various types of immunoglobulins are presented in Table 76-1. Patients with plasma cells producing only κ or λ chains (light-chain disease) frequently have agammaglobulinemia.

Bence Jones proteins are found in the urine of most patients with multiple myeloma, with κ and λ chains being equally distributed. The detection of these proteins in the urine requires the presence of a protein concentration above 0.1 to 0.2 g/dl.

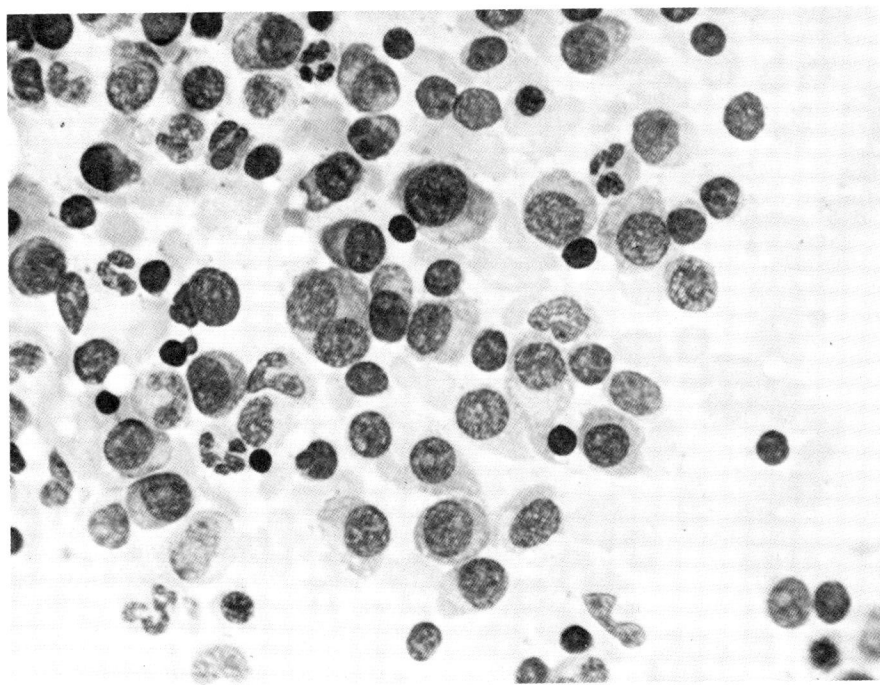

Fig. 76-6. Multiple myeloma. Bone marrow shows atypical mononuclear and binucleated plasma cells with pleomorphism.

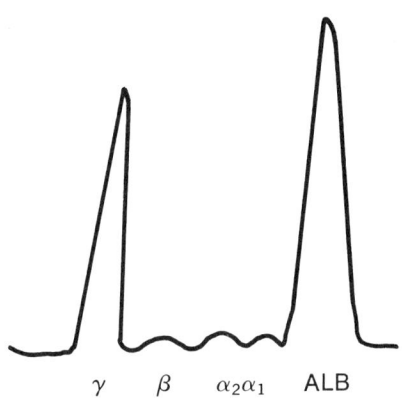

Fig. 76-7. Electrophoretic pattern of serum protein from patient with multiple myeloma (IgG).

Table 76-1. Some characteristics of immunoglobulins

Type	IgG	IgM	IgA	IgD	IgE
Molecular weight (approximate)	150,000	900,000	160,000	180,000	190,000
Serum concentration (mg/dl)	600-1600	50-150	60-330	2-5	0.01-0.04
Subclasses	$IgG_{1,2,3,4}$	$IgM_{1,2}$	$IgA_{1,2}$	—	—
Transport across placenta	+	—	—	—	—
Survival—$T_{\frac{1}{2}}$ (average days)	20	5	5	3	2

Changes in the biochemical profile are related to the extent of the disease. Hypercalcemia is the most common complication that is frequently associated with hyperuricemia. If the kidneys are involved, elevated BUN and creatinine levels may be found. In some cases the serum alkaline phosphatase level is slightly elevated.

DIAGNOSIS. The clinical presentation does not have a characteristic pattern, and diagnosis requires laboratory studies such as bone marrow examination, detailed studies of the serum and urinary proteins, and roentgenographic bone survey. The occurrence of atypical plasmacytosis in the marrow is strongly suggestive of the diagnosis of multiple myeloma. This should be verified by finding abnormal immunoglobulins in the serum and/or light chains in the urine. Osteolytic skeletal lesions are compatible with the diagnosis of multiple myeloma in the presence of the findings just described.

COURSE. Multiple myeloma is a fatal disease with an average median survival time of 3 years from the onset of symptoms. However, the survival may be very prolonged with repeated exacerbations and remissions. Kidney involvement is the most unfavorable factor influencing the prognosis. Recent developments in the management of myeloma patients, including supportive therapy, have contributed substantially to prolongation of their survival time.

MANAGEMENT. Severe pain is a common and almost permanent problem that must be addressed in the management of the patient with myeloma. Most of the time it is due to localized osteolytic lesions that usually respond well to radiotherapy. Orthopedic supports, physical therapy, and immobilization are additional approaches to the treatment of local pain.

Drugs are used to suppress plasma cell growth. Among them, alkylating agents (cyclophosphamide, L-phenylalanine mustard) and adrenocorticosteroids are the most commonly used. A variety of other antineoplastic agents have been used as well.

A variety of androgenic steroids have been tried to stimulate erythropoiesis. In cases of extreme granulocytopenia and progressive infection, leukocyte transfusions are used as supportive therapy.

Physical therapy, anabolic steroids, fluoride, calcium, and vitamin D have been recommended to promote bone remineralization. However, their effects appear to be quite limited.

In cases of hypercalcemia, hydration and corticosteroids (prednisone) are usually sufficient. The use of mithramycin or chelation is reserved for resistant cases. Hyperuricemia requires hydration and administration of the xanthine oxidase inhibitor allopurinol for the reduction of serum and urinary uric acid levels. Hyperviscosity is best treated by plasmapheresis.

WALDENSTRÖM'S MACROGLOBULINEMIA

Increased concentrations of macroglobulins have been observed in a number of clinical conditions such as connective tissue disorders, chronic infections, viral infections, a variety of neoplastic diseases, and "benign monoclonal gammopathy," which is considered to be a stable serologic abnormality in the absence of other underlying disease. The levels of macroglobulins in these conditions are usually slightly to moderately elevated.

In Waldenström's macroglobulinemia there is lymphoid hyperplasia and marked elevation of the serum macroglobulins. The origin and pathogenesis of this disorder do not differ from that described in multiple myeloma. The pathophysiologic mechanism involved in macroglobulinemia is related to the high intrinsic viscosity of the macroglobulins, resulting in serum hyperviscosity. This can cause impaired circulation in the central nervous system, resulting in vascular insufficiency syndromes (intermittent paresis, impaired consciousness, deafness, and so forth). Hyperviscosity can also produce heart failure and pulmonary insufficiency.

CLINICAL MANIFESTATIONS. Waldenström's macroglobulinemia is more common in men than in women and occurs mostly in patients over 50 years of age. In most cases the overt clinical picture is preceded by an asymptomatic or presymptomatic period of many years. The most common presenting symptoms are fatigue, weakness, weight loss, bleeding, neurologic disturbances, visual disturbances, and sometimes cold sensitivity, cold urticaria, and Raynaud's phenomenon. The most frequent physical findings are hepatosplenomegaly, ocular changes (as described in the following paragraph), enlarged lymph nodes, neurologic abnormalities, purpura, and rarely symptoms of congestive heart failure. Mikulicz's syndrome (enlargement of salivary and lacrimal glands) may be observed in some patients. In most cases with gradual development of lymphadenopathy, splenomegaly, and hepatomegaly the clinical pattern closely resembles that of malignant lymphoma or chronic lymphocytic leukemia. In contrast to multiple myeloma, skeletal lesions, bone pain, and frequent infections are not prominent features of Waldenström's macroglobulinemia. Renal disease and amyloidosis may occur but are much less common than in multiple myeloma. Although osteoporosis has been frequently observed, no direct association with macroglobulinemia has been established.

The examination of the eye grounds reveals characteristic findings caused by hyperviscosity. The retinal veins present "sausage effects," consisting of alternating bulges and constrictions. This may be accompanied by exudates, hemorrhages, and visual impairment.

LABORATORY FINDINGS. A normocytic and normochromic anemia is the most common finding. In some cases the anemia may be profound with hemoglobin levels in the range of 6 to 8 g/dl. Several factors are responsible for this complication. The involvement of the bone marrow contributes to the decreased erythropoiesis, but hemolysis and blood loss may play a substantial role in the pathogenesis of anemia. The expanded plasma volume results in hemodilution, which contributes to the low hemoglobin concentration in patients with macroglobulinemia. Coating of the erythrocytes with IgM is considered a cause for erythrocyte rouleaux formation in the peripheral blood smear, positive Coomb's tests, autoagglutinins, and crossmatching problems encountered in many patients with this disease.

There may be neutropenia with a normal lymphocyte count. Eosinophilia is occasionally seen. In some cases lymphocytosis is observed. The morphologic characteristics of the lymphocytes in the peripheral blood may be changed in the terminal phase of the disease and resemble the lymphoid cells seen in the bone marrow. The circulating lymphocytes have monoclonal IgM on their surface; and some lymphocytes may show intracytoplasmic IgM.

Thrombocytopenia is present in about 10% of the patients and contributes to the bleeding diathesis, which is a result of several factors. Coating of the platelets with macroglobulins appears to interfere with their function and particularly with the release of platelet factor.

The pathogenesis of the bleeding diathesis includes changes of the vessels and slowing of the blood flow with increase of the lateral pressure in small vessels. This leads to dilation, tortuosity, and thrombosis with extravasation. This pattern is a result of the hyperviscosity in patients with macroglobulinemia. Formation of complexes between the macroglobulins and certain clotting factors also contributes to the bleeding diathesis.

The erythrocyte sedimentation rate is usually very high. The Sia test, which is based on the insolubility of the macroglobulins in water, is frequently positive. About 25% of patients with Waldenström's macroglobulinemia have Bence Jones proteins in the urine. Serum viscosity is elevated in the majority of the patients. In 49% of the patients the viscosity is above 4 (normal is 1.4 to 1.8).

Bone marrow examination reveals a preponderance of "plasmacytoid" cells that also possess the characteristics of the lymphocyte and the plasma cell. In addition, varying numbers of small lymphocytes, plasma cells, and reticulum cells are seen. Another characteristic feature of the bone marrow finding is an increased number of basophils and tissue mast cells. The cytologic picture of lymph node aspirates or imprints is similar to that described for the bone marrow.

The precise diagnosis of Waldenström's macroglobulinemia rests on the information obtained from protein studies. The serum electrophoresis reveals a homogeneous spike (M component) with mobility between β- and γ-fractions (Fig. 76-8). This mobility suggests IgM protein, but immunoelectrophoresis is the definitive study that determines that IgM identity of the spike (Fig. 76-4). Ultracentrifugation of the serum demonstrates a homogeneous protein with a sedimentation coefficient of 19S. In addition to the macroglobulin, in about 40% of the patients serum cryoglobulins are demonstrated. This may precipitate symptoms of cold hypersensitivity, which is one of the

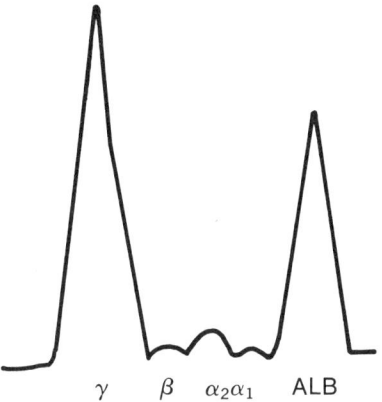

Fig. 76-8. Electrophoretic pattern of serum protein from patient with Waldenström's macroglobulinemia.

clinical features of this disease (Raynaud's phenomenon).

DIAGNOSIS AND COURSE. The clinical presentation is dominated mostly by symptoms resulting from hyperviscosity, lymphadenopathy, hepatosplenomegaly, and anemia. The diagnosis is supported by bone marrow examination, revealing a proliferation of lymphocytic and plasma cell forms with many intermediate and transitional cell types. Hyperproteinemia with large quantities of monoclonal IgM confirms the diagnosis of Waldenström's macroglobulinemia. The presence of symptoms precipitated by cold is sustained by the demonstration of cryoglobulins.

The course of the disease varies from protracted in the majority of cases to fulminant in complicated cases. Uncontrolled hyperviscosity and severe hemorrhages are usually the causes for rapid deterioration of the patient's condition.

MANAGEMENT. The results of treatment of Waldenström's macroglobulinemia are erratic. Since the disease is relatively rare, organized randomized studies appear to be difficult. Treatment should be individualized. Asymptomatic patients and those with a mild clinical picture should not be treated but should be closely observed. Disease progression is an indication for therapeutic intervention.

The most effective drugs in the treatment of Waldenström's macroglobulinemia are the alkylating agents. Chlorambucil or possibly cyclophosphamide or L-phenylalanine mustard (melphalan) may produce objective responses in this disease. Addition of corticosteroids to the alkylating agent appears to be beneficial for some patients. In patients with a significant hyperviscosity syndrome the use of plasmapheresis should be considered as a temporary measure for control of symptoms. This procedure should be followed by chemotherapy. Use of chelating agents has also been of some benefit. These agents can reduce the disulfide bonds of the protein molecule, which may result in dissociation of macroglobulin aggregates. This treatment is also considered as an addition to chemotherapy.

Since the natural course of the disease varies substantially, the therapeutic response appears to follow similar patterns. Patients resistant to treatment will have a short survival time, whereas those who respond may survive a decade or longer.

HEAVY-CHAIN DISEASE

Heavy-chain diseases are proliferative disorders of B lymphocytes distinguished by the presence in the serum of a population of immunoglobulin molecules consisting of incomplete heavy chains belonging to a given class and devoid of light chains. Thus, α, γ, or μ chain disease may be recognized by the presence of heavy chains from IgA, IgG, or IgM, respectively. The origin of this group of diseases is unknown, but there is an association with chronic infections, granulomata, autoimmune disorders, malignancies, and viral infections.

CLINICAL MANIFESTATIONS. More than 150 cases of heavy-chain disease with predominance of an α type have been reported. The disease affects young and old equally; the α type appears to have predilection for a younger age, including children. The majority of the patients with γ type are over the age of 50. Type μ heavy-chain disease is the rarest among the three groups, and only a few cases have been reported. Most of the cases of this type appear to have close association with long-standing underlying disease such as chronic lymphocytic leukemia or malignant lymphoma. The major clinical and laboratory features of the heavy-chain diseases are presented in Table 76-2.

The onset of the disease is gradual, but acute cases have been reported. The most common symptoms are generalized lymphadenopathy, fever, hepatosplenomegaly, and anemia. Palatal erythema and edema may result in respiratory difficulties of mechanical origin. This finding is considered to be a result of lymphadenopathy of the nodes composing Waldeyer's ring. In patients with α-type heavy-chain disease, diarrhea and a malabsorption syndrome are characteristic clinical features. This is a result of infiltration of the intestine by plasma cells, lymphocytes, and reticulum cells. Occasionally pulmonary symptoms also develop.

In some cases roentgenograms of the bones may reveal lesions similar to those seen in multiple myeloma. The suppressed immune system in these patients is a predisposing factor for repeated bacterial infections, which are the most common cause of death.

LABORATORY FINDINGS. All patients have normocytic and normochromic anemia. The majority have leukopenia with a decreased number of granulocytes and eosinophilia. Atypical lymphocytes or plasma cells may be present in the peripheral blood smear. The platelet count is decreased in half of the patients.

Bone marrow examination reveals an increased number of reticulum cells, plasma cells, lymphocytes, and eosinophils. Some of these cells possess neoplastic features. In patients with μ heavy-chain disease and chronic lymphocytic leukemia, the presence of vacuolated plasma cells in the marrow is a characteristic finding.

The serum protein level may be elevated, and an abnormal protein migrating from the β to γ region may be found on electrophoresis. The same protein may be detected in the urine. Immunochemical studies for detection of heavy-chain fragments in the serum are necessary for confirmation of the diagnosis.

In patients with α heavy-chain disease a small bowel biopsy reveals characteristic cellular infiltrates comprised of plasma cells, lymphocytes, and reticulum cells in the lamina propria of the intestine.

DIAGNOSIS AND COURSE. The diagnosis of heavy-chain disease is suggested by clinicopathologic and hematologic findings that resemble those of malignant lymphoma and is confirmed by immunochemical studies. Additional studies such as bone marrow examination and small bowel biopsy may be helpful.

The course of the disease depends on its extent, the frequency and type of infections, and the presence of underlying malignant disease. Survival varies from several months to several years. Various therapeutic attempts have failed to provide a successful treatment for these disorders.

Table 76-2. Features of heavy-chain disease

	γ	α	μ
Age (predilection)	Above 50	Below 40	Above 50
Underlying disease	—	—	Chronic lymphocytic leukemia, lymphoma
Palatal edema	Yes	—	—
Bowel lesions	—	Yes	—
Bony lesions	Rare	—	Rare
Hepatosplenomegaly	Yes	—	Yes
Peripheral lymphadenopathy	Yes	Rare	Yes
Bone marrow	Eosinophilia, plasmacytosis	—	Lymphocytosis
γ-Globulin	Reduced	Normal or reduced	Reduced
Urinary protein	γ Chain	α Chain	μ Chain

BIBLIOGRAPHY

Azur, H.A., and Potter, M.: Multiple myeloma and related disorders, vol. 1, New York, 1973, Harper & Row Publishers, Inc.

Bergsagel, D.E.: Plasma cell myeloma. In Williams, W.J., and others, editors: Hematology, New York, 1977, McGraw-Hill Book Co.

Bloch, K.J., and Maki, D.G.: Hyperviscosity syndromes associated with immunoglobulin abnormalities, Semin. Hematol. **10**:113, 1973.

Frangione, B., and Franklin, E.C.: Heavy chain disease: clinical features and molecular significance of the disordered immunoglobulin structure, Semin. Hematol. **10**:35, 1973.

Franklin, E.C., and Buxbaum, J.: Immunoglobulin structure, synthesis, secretion and relations to neoplasms of B cells, Clin. Haematol. **6**:503, 1977.

Lackner, H.: Hemostatic abnormalities associated with dysproteinemias, Semin. Hematol. **10**:125, 1973.

MacKenzie, M.R., and Fudenberg, H.H.: Macroglobulinemia: an analysis of forty patients, Blood **39**:874, 1972.

Natvig, J.B., and Kunkel, H.G.: Human immunoglobulins: classes, subclasses, genetic variations and idiotypes, Adv. Immunol. **16**:1, 1973.

Waldenström, J.G.: Macroglobulinemia, Adv. Metab. Disord. **2**:115, 1965.

Wintrobe, M.M.: Clinical hematology; plasma cell dyscrasia: multiple myeloma, Philadelphia, 1974, Lea & Febiger.

Amyloidosis
Malcolm W. MacNab

The term "amyloidosis" refers to amyloid, the extracellular tissue infiltrate that characterizes this group of diseases. Amyloid has a characteristic emerald-green birefringence as seen by polarized microscopy on Congo red–stained tissues. The deposition may be diffuse and is composed of proteinaceous fibrils of a β-pleated structure, a specific protein conformation not normally found in mammalian tissues. The nature of each specific protein is different and is used as a form of classification, but the unifying characteristic is the twisted β-pleated sheet fibrils of all amyloid deposits.

CLASSIFICATION. There is great diversity to amyloidosis, and it should not be considered one disease. The classification is based on differences in clinical syndromes and amyloid proteins. The types include primary amyloidosis in which there is no evidence of underlying systemic disease and the secondary form that occurs in association with chronic inflammation or infection such as rheumatoid arthritis and osteomyelitis.

Amyloid deposits are also associated with plasma cell dyscrasias and aging. There are heredofamilial amyloid syndromes, and amyloidosis is associated with familial Mediterranean fever. Localized deposition without evidence of systemic involvement has been reported. Since the clinical and pathologic syndrome of primary amyloidosis is similar to that associated with multiple myeloma and other plasma cell dyscrasias, it has been suggested that these amyloid diseases be classified together as "immunocyte dyscrasias with amyloidosis." Because the amyloid in these cases is actually "secondary" to the immunocyte abnormality, it may be best to discard the term "secondary amyloidosis." What was formerly called secondary amyloidosis (that is, secondary to other diseases such as tuberculosis) should now be called "reactive systemic amyloidosis" (Table 76-3).

PROTEINS. The fibril materials of primary and myeloma-associated amyloid (immunocyte dyscrasias with amyloidosis) have the same protein component, which is an N-terminal fragment of an immunoglobulin light chain termed AL (amyloid light chain). AL chains range from

Table 76-3. Classification of amyloidosis

Classification	Disease	Fibril protein*
Acquired systemic amyloidosis		
Primary and myeloma associated or immunocyte dyscrasias with amyloidosis	Myeloma	AL
	Monoclonal gammopathy	AL
	Macroglobulinemia	AL
	Heavy-chain disease	AL
	Agammaglobulinemia	AL
Secondary or reactive systemic amyloidosis	Chronic infections (TB)	AA
	Chronic inflammation (rheumatoid arthritis)	AA
	Hodgkin's disease	AA
	Nonlymphoid tumors (hypernephroma)	X
Heredofamilial systemic amyloidosis	Neuropathic forms	
	Portuguese	AFp
	Other	X
	Nonneuropathic forms	
	Familial Mediterranean fever	AA
	Other	X
Organ limited		
Cardiovascular ("senile")		ASc
Cerebral plaques		X
Cutaneous (lichenoid)		X
Immunocyte derived	Respiratory tract, urinary tract, bone marrow, and lymphoid	AL
Localized deposition		
Endocrine organ associated	Medullary carcinoma of the thyroid	AEt
	Insulinoma	X
	Pituitary, intestinal, and pancreatic tumors	X
Plasmacytoma		AL
Conjunctival		X
Renal casts in "myeloma nephrosis"		AL
Nonlymphoid solid tumors		X
Hereditary deposits		X
Concretions (prostate, lung, liver)		X
Aged persons		X

Adapted from Glenner, C.: N. Engl. J. Med. **302**:1333,1980.
*X, Structure not confirmed.

5000 to 25,000 daltons. Primary and myeloma-associated amyloidosis is the most common type of the disease, and it is of interest that a plasma cell dyscrasia develops in some patients with this type.

In contrast, the amyloid protein of the secondary form (reactive systemic amyloidosis) and of familial Mediterranean fever is unrelated to any known immunoglobulin and is termed amyloid A (AA). It has a molecular weight of about 8500 daltons. Most likely the AA protein is a fragment of a normal serum component (SAA) whose function is unknown. SAA is an acute-phase reactant that is increased in infection, inflammation, cancer, all types of amyloidosis, multiple myeloma, lymphomas, and pregnancy, making SAA measurement not very useful in differentiating the types of amyloidosis. The amyloidosis of familial Mediterranean fever results from the presence of AA protein, whereas the remaining heredofamilial types result from the presence of other proteins such as AFp, which is found in familial Portuguese polyneuropathy (type I).

Localized amyloid deposits have been associated with endocrine neoplasms. These amyloid fibrils are composed of peptide hormone fragments and are termed AE. An example is AEt, a fibril from medullary thyroid carcinoma with fragments of thyrocalcitonin. ASc represents the particular amyloid fibril of cardiac "senile" amyloidosis. There are many other forms of local amyloidosis, but the nature of these amyloid fibrils has not been well defined (see Table 76-3).

Fibrils are not the only components of the amyloid deposits. All types of amyloid also contain a pentagonal substance known as the P component. P component has an amino acid sequence different from that of amyloid fibrils and is found in normal serum with no relationship to the presence or absence of any type of amyloidosis. It is closely related to C-reactive protein. P component's role in the disease process is unclear, but it may act as a template for the amyloid-fibril proteins.

The pathogenesis of abnormal fibril production is unknown, but the destruction caused by the deposits can be significant, since the fibrils are nonimmunogenic and resist normal defense mechanisms. β-Pleated sheet fibrils have been produced in vitro from Bence Jones protein by proteolytic action. This may also occur in vivo by proteolytic cleavage of light chains. Similar proteolytic action producing AA fibrils may occur on SAA produced by the liver, on the surface of monocytes, or in phagocytic lysosomes.

CLINICAL MANIFESTATIONS. In primary or immunocyte dyscrasias with amyloidosis (AL amyloid fibrils) the sites of infiltration are widely dispersed. A restrictive cardiomyopathy is observed in this type of amyloidosis but is also seen in heredofamilial and "senile" types. There is direct infiltration of muscle, and macroglossia may result. Amyloid material in the glenohumeral joint results in the "shoulder-pad" sign of amyloidosis, and patients may have the carpal tunnel syndrome. In about 50% of patients with AL amyloidosis, renal disease and eventually the nephrotic syndrome develop. Gastrointestinal infiltration is also observed and may be manifested by diarrhea, malabsorption, or any one of multiple complaints. Sensory motor and autonomic neuropathies may occur. Dermatologic manifestations include purpura, waxy cutaneous papules, alopecia, and scleroderma-like infiltration. Small vessel infiltrates cause purpura, and bleeding may be aggravated by a deficiency of procoagulant factor X. Pulmonary tissue, as well as the liver and spleen, may be involved in primary immunocyte dyscrasias.

In secondary or reactive systemic amyloidosis (AA amyloid-fibril) the infiltrates are not as widely dispersed. Infiltration occurs primarily in the kidneys, spleen, liver, and adrenal glands and rarely in the cardiac, musculoskeletal, and gastrointestinal systems. The nephrotic syndrome develops in most patients with this form of amyloidosis. Hepatosplenomegaly may be marked. Carpal tunnel syndrome is uncommon, as are macroglossia, purpura, and peripheral neuropathies. Reactive amyloidosis is generally asymptomatic when it involves the gastrointestinal tract.

In several types of amyloidosis and localized amyloidosis the clinical presentation is limited to a specific organ. Lichenoid amyloid is a common local cutaneous type. This is a separate entity and should be distinguished from the lesions of systemic primary or immunocytic amyloidosis. Amyloid deposits are found in the cerebrum and heart of older people, with the incidence increasing with age.

DIAGNOSIS AND MANAGEMENT. The diagnosis requires histologic confirmation, with the biopsy site dependent on the clinical presentation. Material should be stained with Congo red and examined under a polarizing microscope. If a bone marrow biopsy is performed in the evaluation of an associated plasma cell dyscrasia, the diagnosis may be confirmed from the specimen, but if this examination is negative, a rectal biopsy should be performed, since 75% to 80% of cases of generalized amyloidosis show rectal deposition. It is important to include a small blood vessel because involvement is frequently limited to the vessels. A gingival biopsy may also be helpful, but a liver biopsy is contraindicated because of an increased risk of bleeding in the amyloid-involved liver.

There is no established treatment for amyloidosis, and therapeutic measures should be directed toward any associated diseases. Cytotoxic drugs used in the treatment of monoclonal gammopathies have resulted in a decrease in levels of the immunoglobulin without changes in the amyloidosis. Colchicine therapy can decrease the febrile attacks of familial Mediterranean fever and prevent the progression of amyloidosis in this disease, but it has been ineffective in other types of amyloidosis. Dimethyl sulfoxide, an amyloid-fibril denaturing agent, is now being evaluated in amyloidosis and may be shown to have clinical value.

BIBLIOGRAPHY

Franklin, E.: Immunopathology of amyloid disease, Hosp. Pract. **15**:70, 1980.

Franklin, E.C., and Zucker-Franklin, D.: Current concepts of amyloid, Adv. Immunol. **15**:249, 1972.

Glenner, G.: Amyloid deposits and amyloidosis: the beta-fibrilloses (in two parts), N. Engl. J. Med. **302**:1283, 1333, 1980.

Glenner, G., Costa, P., and Frietas, F., editors: Amyloid and amyloidosis: international congress series, vol. 497, New York, 1980, Elsevier/Excerpta Medica.

Lavie, G., Zucker-Franklin, D., and Franklin, E.C.: Degradation of serum amyloid A protein by surface-associated enzymes of human blood monocytes, J. Exp. Med. **148**:1020, 1978.

77 • HODGKIN'S DISEASE AND NON-HODGKIN'S LYMPHOMA

Deborah Mayer and Richard V. Smalley

HODGKIN'S DISEASE

Hodgkin's disease, accounting for 40% of all lymphomas, has been recognized as a neoplastic entity since 1832. This disease, which was usually considered fatal one or two decades ago, now can be cured in a majority of patients. These significant advances are a result of a better understanding of the histology and clinical behavior and of interdisciplinary cooperation in disease management.

According to American Cancer Society estimates there were 7100 new cases and 1900 deaths in the United States in 1980 from Hodgkin's disease, with an expected overall 5-year survival of 50% to 60%. A bimodal incidence has been noted with a peak in adolescence and young adulthood and a second sustained increase in later life. The characteristics may vary depending on the age at onset. In younger patients there is an equal male/female ratio, a predominance of the nodular sclerosis histologic subtype, frequent mediastinal involvement, and in general a more benign clinical course. In older patients the mixed cellular histologic subtype, which is associated with a more aggressive clinical course, predominates. The overall male/female ratio is 1.4:1.

EPIDEMIOLOGY. There have been many studies exploring possible infectious, genetic, and environmental origins of this disease. Much effort has been placed in evaluating the occasional time-space case clusterings reported, but to date no lead has proved significant. There is the suggestion of an increased incidence of Hodgkin's disease following infectious mononucleosis, which raises the possibility of an association with the Epstein-Barr virus.

In developing countries the lower age peak of Hodgkin's disease is seen in adolescence, whereas in the United States it is during the twenties, proportional to the level of socioeconomic development. This pattern is similar to that of poliomyelitis. Although the cause of Hodgkin's disease remains unknown, both genetic and environmental factors appear to be involved.

IMMUNITY. The majority of patients with Hodgkin's disease display decreased or defective cellular immunity, and in most there is demonstrable cutaneous anergy. This decreased T-lymphocyte function may be due to increased suppressor cell activity. The immunologic deficiency increases with both advancing disease and increasingly aggressive therapy, with the most pronounced effect noted in patients receiving both chemotherapy and radiotherapy. Because of their defective immune state, patients with Hodgkin's disease are at higher risk for infections caused by microorganisms and parasites that produce intracellular infection. These include bacteria such as *Mycobacterium tuberculosis* and *Listeria,* fungi such as *Cryptococcus,* viruses such as herpes zoster, and protozoa such as *Pneumocystis.*

CLINICAL MANIFESTATIONS. Patients with Hodgkin's disease generally have painless, asymmetric, "rubbery" lymphadenopathy, most commonly (60% to 80%) in the cervical area (Fig. 77-1). One fourth to one third of the patients also have associated symptoms of unexplained weight loss ($\geq$10% in 6 months), fever (>100.4° F [38° C]), and sweats. Malaise and pruritus may be present. Splenomegaly is noted in 50% to 70% of the patients, but despite being enlarged, the spleen may not be involved histologically. Other constitutional symptoms related to the site of nodal involvement include dry cough and dysphagia with mediastinal involvement and lower extremity edema or organ obstruction with abdominal involvement. It is said that rarely ingestion of alcohol causes pain at Hodgkin's disease sites. A mild normocytic and normochromic anemia with or without eosinophilia, neutrophilic leukocytosis, and autoimmune hemolytic anemia is present in 30% to 50% of the patients. The erythrocyte sedimentation rate and serum copper levels may be elevated and can be used as indicators of disease activity to monitor the effects of therapy.

Other disorders to be considered with this type of clinical presentation include infectious mononucleosis, phenytoin-reactive hyperplasia, and other infections that may cause reactive inflammatory changes. The diagnosis must be established by biopsy.

PATHOLOGY. The diagnosis and histologic subtype are established by pathologic examination of involved tissue, usually an enlarged lymph node. The Rye classification, established in 1966, is universally used by pathologists today. The presence of the Reed-Sternberg (R-S) cell, which has a macrophage derivation, is required but is not pathognomonic for the diagnosis of Hodgkin's disease. Morphologically, this cell has a large diameter, either a binucleated or a deeply indented lobate nucleus, one or more prominent acidophilic nucleoli, and a clear perinuclear area. Generally, the prognosis is worse when a large num-

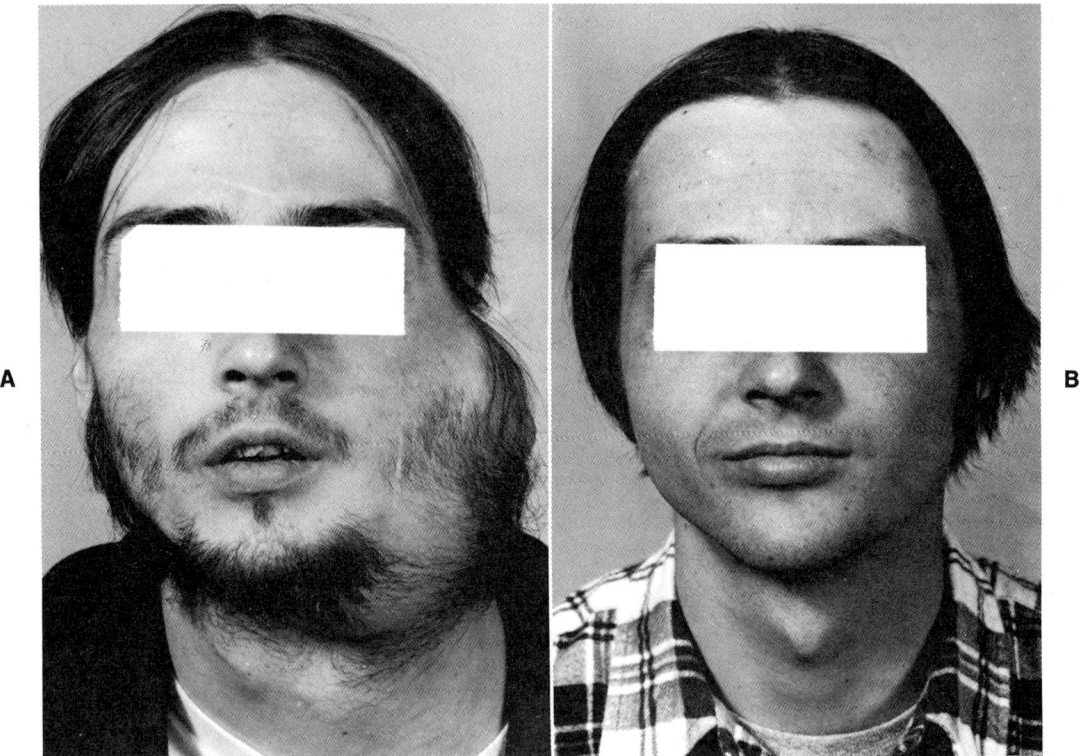

Fig. 77-1. A, Cervical lymphadenopathy in patient before treatment. **B,** Complete resolution after 6 months of combination chemotherapy.

ber of R-S cells are present. The following histologic subtypes are recognized.

Lymphocyte predominance. In lymphocyte predominance (LP), normal mature lymphocytes predominate with only an occasional R-S cell noted. As in all histologic subtypes, the normal lymph node architecture is destroyed by the cellular infiltrate. LP accounts for about 10% of all cases of Hodgkin's disease, and it occurs more commonly in younger patients. There is a slight male predominance. Patients with this subtype tend to have localized disease (75% are stage I or II) and therefore usually have an excellent prognosis.

Mixed cellularity. In mixed cellularity (MC) there is a pleomorphic infiltrate of normal-appearing plasma cells, eosinophils, neutrophils, and lymphocytes in addition to R-S cells. This subtype accounts for up to 35% to 40% of cases. Patients tend to have more extensive disease and are more commonly symptomatic (>50% stages III and IV). Therefore they have an intermediate prognosis.

Lymphocyte depletion. Lymphocyte depletion (LD) accounts for 10% to 15% of all cases, and patients with this subtype usually have the poorest prognosis. There generally are large numbers of R-S cells with few lymphocytes or other white cells. LD is more commonly seen in older patients and is usually extensive on initial examination (80% stages III and IV).

Nodular sclerosis. In nodular sclerosis (NS) the tumor infiltrate forms multiple nodules divided by bands of reticulin that are easily demonstrable, usually by hematoxylin-eosin stain and always by reticulin stain. The nodules generally are visible with the unassisted eye. In addition, "lacunar cells," atypical R-S cells with clear spaces surrounding the cytoplasm, are characteristically noted. This subtype is more predominant in women and in the younger age group and carries almost as good a prognosis as LP because the patients usually have limited disease. It accounts for 50% to 60% of the cases.

DIAGNOSIS

Staging. Staging at the time of diagnosis is the single most important prognostic variable and the determinant of initial therapy. The Ann Arbor staging classification of patients with Hodgkin's and non-Hodgkin's lymphoma (below) was established in 1970 and is universally used by clinicians.

Stage	Definition
I	Involvement of a single lymph node region (I) or of a single extralymphatic* organ or site (I_E)
II	Involvement of two or more lymph node regions on the same side of the diaphragm (II) or involvement of a

---

*Extralymphatic may include sites in the lung, bone, bone marrow, liver, or brain. Each stage is subclassified by the presence (B) or absence (A) of one or more of the following unexplained symptoms: weight loss >10% over 6 months, fever >100.4° F (38° C), night sweats.

contiguous extralymphatic organ or site and one or more lymph node regions on the same side of the diaphragm (II$_E$)

III Involvement of lymph nodes on both sides of the diaphragm (III), which may be accompanied by localized involvement of a contiguous extralymphatic organ or site (III$_E$), involvement of the spleen (III$_S$), or both (III$_{SE}$)

IV Diffuse or disseminated involvement of one or more extralymphatic organs or tissues, with or without associated lymph node involvement

It has become apparent that Hodgkin's disease most often arises as a single focus and spreads in a predictable manner from nodal group to contiguous nodal group. Parenchymal organ involvement may subsequently occur either by direct extension, that is, the lung contiguous to mediastinal involvement, or by hematogenous dissemination. The staging evaluation should be carried out in a logical manner, taking into account both "prior probabilities" (the probability of a patient having a greater or lesser clinical involvement as related to the histologic subtype) and benefit versus risk factors. Patients with Hodgkin's disease infrequently have extranodal disease (<5% with bone marrow, skeletal, liver, or brain involvement). Because of this, routine bone, brain, or liver scans should not be obtained unless there are specific clinical indications.

Initial staging should begin with a thorough history and physical examination, with particular attention to weight loss, fever, sweats, lymphadenopathy, and abdominal organomegaly. The presence of any of the three so-called B symptoms (weight loss >10% of body weight, fever >100.4° F [38° C], and profuse night sweats) is associated with a poor prognosis. Patients with one or more of these symptoms are considered to be "symptomatic" according to the Ann Arbor classification and are subclassed "B." Patients without any of these symptoms have a better prognosis, are considered to be "asymptomatic" (regardless of other symptomatology), and are classified "A."

Baseline blood studies should include a complete blood count, erythrocyte sedimentation rate, and biochemistry profile. A chest roentgenogram is adequate for demonstrating mediastinal or hilar lymphadenopathy, which is present in 25% of the patients (Fig. 77-2). Pulmonary parenchymal involvement is rare, although a relatively large percentage of patients probably have nondemonstrable contiguous pulmonary involvement in association with bulky mediastinal disease. Gallium scanning and ultrasonography are used to evaluate intra-abdominal disease. Hodgkin's disease is a "gallium-avid" tumor, but this technique is less sensitive in detecting infradiaphragmatic involvement than supradiaphragmatic involvement. In conjunction with ultrasonography there is a greater than 80% accuracy in detecting infradiaphragmatic nodes larger than 2 cm; however, both false positive and false negative findings occur. Lymphangiography is useful for documenting para-aortic

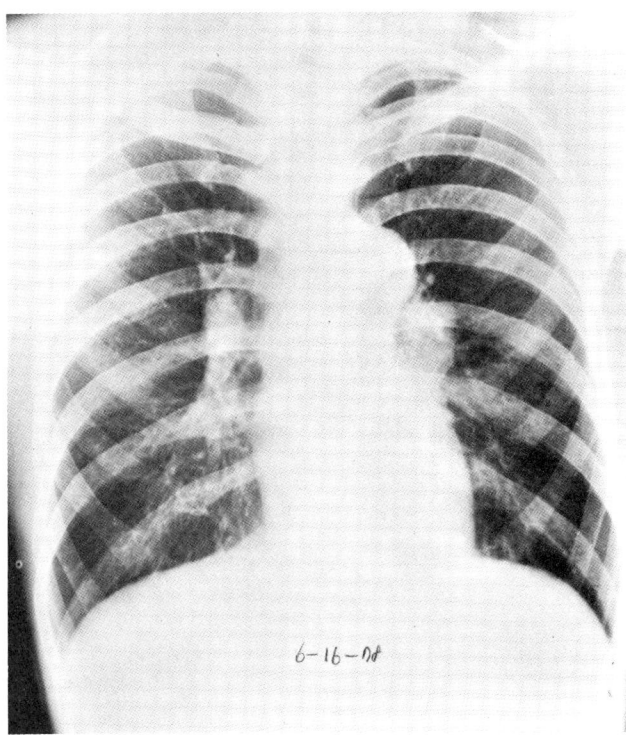

Fig. 77-2. Pronounced mediastinal and hilar adenopathy noted on chest roentgenogram of patient in Fig. 77-1.

and retroperitoneal involvement (Fig. 77-3). Nodes less than 2 cm in size may be histologically involved, and lymphangiography is helpful in these circumstances. It is not useful in the evaluation of celiac, mesenteric, or splenic hilar nodes. Potential complications from this procedure include pulmonary dye embolism (especially in older patients with compromised pulmonary function) and cellulitis at the cutdown site. Each of these studies is frequently used to confirm the others. Other studies such as bone marrow biopsy are of such low yield in asymptomatic patients that they are not generally or routinely used. The role of computed tomography in staging is currently being evaluated.

Laparotomy. Despite the value of the procedures just described, surgical staging (laparotomy) is frequently indicated as a final definitive procedure. Patients with unequivocal stage IIIB or IV disease as determined by the preceding studies do not require laparotomy. It should be performed in patients with clinical stage I to IIIA disease in whom positive laparotomy findings would change therapy.

MANAGEMENT. The selection of treatment for patients with Hodgkin's disease is closely correlated with the stage of disease rather than the histologic subclassification. Hodgkin's disease is radiosensitive, and 4000 to 4500 rad given in 20 to 25 daily fractions effectively "sterilizes" and permanently controls nearly all disease within the

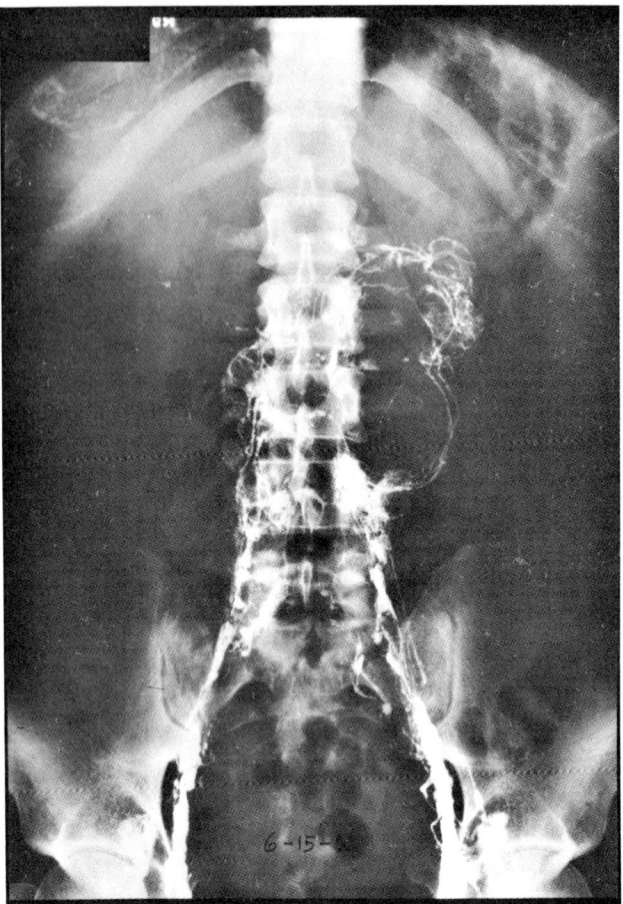

Fig. 77-3. Positive lymphangiogram with extensive para-aortic involvement. Wide deviation of left para-aortic lymphatics indicates collateral flow around enlarged nodes that have been replaced by tumor. Several right para-aortic nodes are also enlarged and foamy, suggestive of tumor involvement.

Table 77-1. Cytotoxic combinations useful in treating Hodgkin's disease

MOPP *(each cycle repeated every 28 days)*	
Nitrogen mustard (Mustargen)	6mg/m² IV days 1, 8
Vincristine (Oncovin)	1.4 mg/m² IV days 1, 8 (max—2 mg)
Prednisone	100 mg/m² PO days 1-14
Procarbazine (Matulane)	100 mg/m² PO days 1-14
BCVPP *(each cycle repeated every 28 days)*	
BCNU (carmustine)	100 mg/m² IV day 1
Cyclophosphamide (Cytoxan)	600 mg/m² IV day 1
Vinblastine (Velban)	5 mg/m² IV day 1
Procarbazine	100 mg/m² PO days 1-10
Prednisone	60 mg/m² PO days 1-10
ABVD *(each cycle repeated every 28 days)*	
Hydroxydaunomycin or doxorubicin (Adriamycin)	25 mg/m² IV days, 1, 14
Bleomycin (Blenoxane)	10 mg/m² IV days 1, 14
Vinblastine	6 mg/m² IV days 1, 14
Imidazole carboxamide (DTIC, dacarbazine)	150 mg/m² IV days 1-5

treatment area. Patients with stage IA or IIA disease may thus anticipate a complete response and a prolonged disease-free survival following either involved field irradiation (treatment of disease-bearing areas only) or subtotal nodal irradiation (SNI). The latter technique delivers treatment to the mantle area (mediastinal, cervical, axillary, and supraclavicular areas bilaterally) and to the para-aortic nodes. It has not been adequately determined whether SNI is more valuable than involved field irradiation. Several series have demonstrated a disease-free survival of at least 2½ to 10 years in 85% to 90% of pathologically staged IA or IIA patients following radiotherapy.

Patients with stage IIB disease (true stage IB disease may be nonexistent) may do well (85% to 90% prolonged survival) with a combined modality approach using SNI or total nodal irradiation (TNI—treatment of all axial node-bearing areas), either followed by 6 months of combination chemotherapy (Table 77-1). Another approach is TNI followed by chemotherapy at the time of actual relapse (which occurs in up to 25% of the patients). This chemotherapy is called "salvage" therapy.

There are no known prognostic factors that can be used to determine the likelihood of complete response or of maintaining a response in patients with stage I or II disease other than bulky mediastinal and/or hilar disease, a negative factor. A significant percentage of such patients have pulmonary disease at initial examination and relapse relatively soon after radiotherapy. These patients therefore should be considered for initial combined modality treatment. The usual histologic subtype in such situations is nodular sclerosis. Combination chemotherapy used alone as a single modality approach without radiotherapy has not been evaluated in these patients or in patients with stage IIB disease.

Therapy for patients with stage IIIA disease is a controversial subject. A recent study in England compared TNI with combination chemotherapy and demonstrated a higher number of complete responses and a longer disease-free survival with TNI. A second approach uses both radiotherapy and chemotherapy, with initial treatment with TNI followed by 6 months of treatment with Mustargen, Oncovin, prednisone, and procarbazine (MOPP therapy; Table 77-1). As with stage IIB disease, 90% of the patients respond and maintain a complete response for years following this combined approach, whereas only 67% of the patients with stage IIIA disease receiving TNI alone achieve and maintain a prolonged disease-free status. However, of the patients with relapse following TNI, nearly half will have a second remission with salvage chemotherapy or radiotherapy. Thus the salvage approach gives a prolonged, relatively disease-free state in more than 80% of stage IIIA patients.

Recently patients with stage IIIA disease have been substaged into those with upper abdominal (splenic, celiac, hepatic, and/or portal) nodes (stage III_1A) and those with lower abdominal (para-aortic, iliac, and/or mesenteric) nodes (stage III_2A). With the salvage therapy approach, more than 60% of the patients with stage III_1A disease have prolonged disease-free survival following TNI treatment. A significant percentage of those who respond and then relapse following TNI have a durable second response to combination chemotherapy. Patients with stage III_2A disease, however, have a poor chance of prolonged disease-free survival following TNI alone and therefore warrant combined modality therapy initially. This approach produces a prolonged disease-free survival in 75% of the patients.

Thus patients with either stage IIB or III_2A disease warrant combined modality treatment with TNI initially, followed immediately by combination chemotherapy. Long-term complications in the form of second malignancies (primarily acute leukemia) may occur after combined modality treatment, and this accounts for the hesitancy to recommend such treatment to all who may initially benefit. This is a significant risk and must be considered in the design of any treatment program.

Patients with stage IIIB, IVA, or IVB disease are currently treated with combination chemotherapy. In 1965 the National Cancer Institute introduced the cytotoxic chemotherapy combination known as MOPP (Table 77-1), which established combination chemotherapy as a successful form of treatment in patients with malignancy and induced the first cures in what had been a uniformly fatal disease. This combination, now the most widely used chemotherapy regimen, has stood the test of 15 years. Seventy percent of patients with stage IIIB, IVA, or IVB disease attain a complete response during a 6-month course of MOPP, and 75% of those have a sustained response of at least several years and apparent cure of their disease. Two other combination chemotherapy approaches (Table 77-1), one comprised of BCNU, cyclophosphamide, vinblastine, procarbazine, and prednisone (BCVPP), and the other comprised of Adriamycin, bleomycin, vinblastine, and DTIC (ABVD), give results comparable to MOPP in appropriate circumstances. ABVD is not cross-resistant with MOPP and thus may be used in patients who have relapses after MOPP therapy.

Toxic effects associated with combination chemotherapy include nausea and vomiting in 50% of the patients and alopecia in 25% to 33%. Late or long-term complications following cytotoxic chemotherapy are pulmonary fibrosis from long-term administration of BCNU, congestive heart failure in patients with long-term administration of doxorubicin, secondary malignancies such as acute myelogenous leukemia and an undifferentiated non-Hodgkin's lymphoma, and sterility. All of these are seen more commonly in patients receiving combined modality therapy. There is thought to be a 2% to 4% risk of secondary malignancies following TNI and combination chemotherapy.

Relatively few prognostic criteria are available to aid in determining which patients may have a complete response or a prolonged disease-free survival. Age is a factor noted in many studies. Patients under 40 years of age are more likely than older patients to respond and remain free of disease. Other, minor favorable factors are white race, female gender, and high lymphocyte count (>1300 cells/mm^3). A lesser stage and the absence of symptoms have also been noted to be beneficial. The histologic subtype, when corrected for stage, appears to have no influence on the prognosis.

Patients with advanced Hodgkin's disease (stage IIB or IV) who had a relapse after radiotherapy and are receiving salvage chemotherapy have a 75% or better chance of attaining a complete response. However, the likelihood of maintaining a disease-free state for a significant period is less in these patients than in those initially treated with chemotherapy. Only about a third maintain their disease-free state for up to 5 years following salvage chemotherapy. Nevertheless, since the use of salvage therapy provides significant benefit to a large group of patients, it may be preferable to an initial combined modality approach in patients who would be subjected to the considerable risk of secondary malignancies, some of them unnecessarily.

NON-HODGKIN'S LYMPHOMA

Non-Hodgkin's lymphoma (NHL) is a heterogeneous group of malignant disorders of lymphoid derivation that range in biologic behavior from relatively indolent to very aggressive. This behavior can in general be predicted by and correlated with the histologic subclassification. NHL accounts for over 60% of all lymphomas. Approximately 23,000 new cases and 12,400 deaths occurred in 1980, according to American Cancer Society estimates. Men predominate (1.7:1), and there is a peak incidence between 50 and 70 years of age. Radiation and immune deficiencies have been implicated as possible etiologic factors. An increased incidence of NHL has been noted in Hiroshima survivors, kidney transplant patients undergoing immunosuppressive therapy, and patients with immune deficiency syndromes such as ataxia-telangiectasia and Wiskott-Aldrich syndrome. The overall 5-year survival of 30% to 40% is lower than that of patients with Hodgkin's disease, but survival is higher in certain histologic subclassifications. Common causes of death in patients with NHL are infection, organ failure, hemorrhage, and disseminated tumor.

CLINICAL MANIFESTATIONS. The clinical presentation is similar to that of Hodgkin's disease, although NHL is more commonly extensive; that is, patients most often have stage III or IV disease on initial examination. However, the original extent of disease varies depending on the histologic classification. Nearly 80% of the patients with nodular lymphocytic lymphomas have stage IV disease, whereas less than 10% have stage I or II disease. Slightly less than a third of patients with diffuse histiocytic lymphoma (DHL) have generalized (stage IV) disease at initial examination. Nodular lymphocytic lymphoma and DHL are the most common histologic variants of NHL. In general, nodular lymphocytic lymphomas occur in older patients, whereas 35% of the patients with DHL are less than 40 years of age. Increased age and advanced clinical stage are negative prognostic factors, but histologic subtype is the single most influential prognostic factor. Although the majority of patients are asymptomatic initially, 10% to 20% have weight loss, fever, or night sweats. The presence of symptoms may also have an adverse prognostic significance. Roughly one fourth of the patients have extralymphatic disease, which will be discussed later in this chapter. Unlike Hodgkin's disease, the cellular immunologic system of patients with NHL generally remains intact until the late stages of the disease, but hypogammaglobulinemia may occur early.

HISTOLOGIC CLASSIFICATIONS. A number of new classifications of NHL are being developed as more sophisticated immunotyping procedures are ultrastructural information become available, but their reproducibility and general applicability have not been established. The classification originally defined by Rappaport is currently the most widely accepted. This system is based on (1) lymph node architecture, (2) cell type, and (3) degree of differentiation. Histologically, these tumors develop in either a nodular fashion (the tumor cells form nodules separated by reticulin and fibrous tissue) or a diffuse fashion (the tumor cells are diffusely distributed throughout the lymph node, effacing its normal architecture). There is roughly an equal distribution of each. It is generally believed that the tumor cell in nearly all patients with NHL is a malignant lymphocyte, in the majority of cases a B lymphocyte. Although the Rappaport classification, devised before the availability of current immunologic typing methods, refers to "lymphocytic," "histiocytic," and "mixed cell" lymphomas, all nodular lymphomas are B-lymphocyte lymphomas. Diffuse lymphomas may have a B-lymphocyte, T-lymphocyte, null cell, or, rarely, truly histiocytic origin. In addition, the lymphocytic lymphomas may be well or poorly differentiated morphologically. Although this morphologic classification may be replaced within the next decade by a more reproducible classification based on functional criteria, it is currently the basis for nearly all therapeutic decisions.

Nodular lymphomas are characterized histologically by nodules of relatively uniform size without a well-defined lymphoid cuff. The malignant cells in these nodules are morphologically either small atypical lymphocytes with scanty cytoplasm and an irregular cleaved nucleus or cells two to three times larger with vesicular nuclei and two or three nucleoli. Although these large cells resemble histiocytes morphologically, it has been determined using immunologic markers that both the small cell with a cleaved nucleus and the large cell with a vesicular nucleus are B lymphocytes. Nodules containing 75% to 80% small atypical lymphocytes are classified as nodular poorly differentiated lymphocytic lymphomas (NPDLL) or nodular well-differentiated lymphocytic lymphomas (NWDLL). Nodules consisting of 30% to 50% large cells are classified as nodular mixed histiocytic-lymphocytic lymphomas (NML). Those with more than 50% large cells are classified as nodular histiocytic lymphomas. Nodular lymphomas tend to progress histologically over the years to a more diffuse pattern and a "histiocytic" cell type.

The diffuse lymphomas histologically are a heterogeneous group of diseases. Diffuse well-differentiated lymphocytic lymphoma (DWDLL), a variant of chronic lymphatic leukemia, is characterized by normal-appearing lymphocytes. Diffuse poorly differentiated lymphocytic lymphoma (DPDLL) is characterized by a diffuse infiltration of small atypical lymphocytes with cleaved nuclei and B-lymphocyte characteristics. It is likely that in most patients with DPDLL an asymptomatic NPDLL stage precedes clinical manifestation. Diffuse mixed lymphoma (DML), a rare disorder characterized by a mixture of small and large cells, probably represents a histologic extension of NML.

Diffuse histiocytic lymphoma (DHL) and diffuse undifferentiated lymphoma (DUL) are characterized by a diffuse proliferation of large cells with vesicular nuclei and prominent nucleoli that may differ morphologically from each other and from those seen in nodular lymphomas. These tumors are heterogeneous and probably morphologically represent the undifferentiated state of a number of cell lines. Biochemical, enzymatic, and surface marker studies reveal that slightly more than half of these tumors are of B-lymphocyte origin, a small number are of T-lymphocyte origin, an even smaller number are of histiocytic origin, and about a third are unclassifiable or of null cell origin. These are the lymphomas that frequently develop in extranodal sites. Three distinctive recognizable variants of DUL are Burkitt's lymphoma, lymphoblastic lymphoma (histologically akin to T-cell acute lymphatic leukemia), and immunoblastic sarcoma. These variants are characterized by a proliferation of an undifferentiated large cell with relatively distinctive morphologic and clinical features.

STAGING. The reasons for staging a tumor in any patient are (1) to obtain prognostic information, (2) to aid in therapeutic decision making, (3) to standardize a system for comparison of results, and (4) to provide an accepted descriptive system to facilitate communication. Although the Ann Arbor staging classification fulfills all four needs for patients with Hodgkin's disease, it is less useful for patients with NHL. When compared with histologic subclassification, clinical staging plays a relatively minor role in influencing therapeutic decisions and almost no role in determining prognosis.

Current staging procedures include a complete history and physical examination, chest roentgenogram, lymphangiography, technetium liver-spleen scintigraphy, gallium scintigraphy, ultrasonographic examination of the abdomen, and bone marrow biopsy. Occasionally a computed tomographic scan of the abdomen and a bone scan are also indicated. A standard chest roentgenogram is usually adequate to assess the mediastinal and hilar areas, and there is generally little added benefit from whole lung tomography. As in patients with Hodgkin's disease, an adequate assessment of the abdominal lymph nodes usually requires ultrasonography, gallium scintigraphy, and/or lymphangiography. Liver function studies (alkaline phosphatase, SGOT, LDH) and technetium liver scintigraphy (occasionally with confirmation from ultrasonography) are generally adequate to document liver involvement. Bone marrow aspiration or biopsy reveals marrow involvement in 30% to 60% of the patients, most commonly those with nodular lymphomas.

It is the rare patient who requires a staging laparotomy. The treatment is generally determined by histologic subtyping and rarely by clinical staging. Only in patients with stage I (and perhaps symptomatic stage II) mixed cell or "histiocytic" histologic findings might pathologic staging influence treatment. Patients with pathologic stage I and perhaps stage II DHL respond to appropriate radiotherapy with a prolonged disease-free interval. Some patients with stage II and all with stage III or IV disease require combination chemotherapy.

MANAGEMENT. The treatment of patients with non-Hodgkin's lymphoma is currently dictated primarily by their histologic subclassification. Patients with well-differentiated lymphocytic lymphomas (NWDLL and DWDLL) and NPDLL should be managed with relatively nonaggressive treatment. There are indications that asymptomatic patients with these subtypes require no treatment at all, since they may remain asymptomatic for 2 to 3 years following diagnosis. With or without immediate treatment, such patients may anticipate a relatively long survival, with the majority surviving more than 10 years after diagnosis. A variety of treatments, including total nodal irradiation; a chemotherapeutic combination of cyclophosphamide, vincristine (Oncovin), and prednisone (COP; Table 77-2); or single-agent chemotherapy with cyclophosphamide, may induce complete responses in three fourths of these patients. Despite this high complete response rate, survival is not significantly improved because all patients subsequently have relapse (15% to 20% annually) and require additional therapy. Treatment for this group of patients therefore is palliative and directed toward symptom and disease control.

Patients with NML, DPDLL, or nodular histiocytic

Table 77-2. Cytotoxic combinations useful in treating non-Hodgkin's lymphoma

COP *(cycle repeated every 21 days)*	
Cyclophosphamide (Cytoxan)	400 mg/m^2 PO days 1-5
Vincristine (Oncovin)	1.4 mg/m^2 IV day 1 (max—2 mg)
Prednisone	100 mg/m^2 PO days 1-5
CHOP *(cycle repeated every 21 days)*	
Cyclophosphamide	750 mg/m^2 IV day 1
Hydroxydaunomycin (Adriamycin)	50 mg/m^2 IV day 1
Vincristine (Oncovin)	1.4 mg/m^2 IV day 1 (max—2 mg)
Prednisone	100 mg/m^2 PO days 1-5
C-MOPP *(cycle repeated every 28 days)*	
Cyclophosphamide	650 mg/m^2 IV days 1, 8
Vincristine (Oncovin)	1.4 mg/m^2 IV days 1, 8 (max—2 mg)
Procarbazine (Matulane)	100 mg/m^2 PO days 1-14
Prednisone	40 mg/m^2 PO days 1-14

lymphoma generally require a more aggressive therapeutic approach and usually have a poorer prognosis. A cytotoxic combination of cyclophosphamide, hydroxydaunomycin, Oncovin, and prednisone (CHOP; Table 77-2) produces a complete response in nearly three fourths of these patients, but the median duration of survival generally does not exceed 2 to 3 years. Patients with DPDLL (like patients with NPDLL) are subject to relatively early and continuous relapse without any indication to date of a significant percentage of patients achieving long-term disease-free survival. However, patients with NML or nodular histiocytic lymphoma may have a prolonged disease-free survival with CHOP or C-MOPP therapy (Table 77-2), and some may be cured of their disease, although longer follow-up is required to verify this.

Patients with DHL are generally considered to have the poorest prognosis, but a substantial number of patients stand a chance of cure with CHOP therapy. Although a number of relapses occur during the first 12 to 24 months following cessation of treatment (usually given for 6 to 9 months), relapses rarely occur in patients who remain disease free for 24 months following treatment. Since patients with DHL are a heterogeneous group, studies are currently under way to define better the population of patients who may be expected to respond and survive following combination chemotherapy.

Thus, although patients with "histiocytic" histologic involvement of either the mixed or pure type generally have an unfavorable prognosis, it is probable that a substantial number of these patients may be cured with chemotherapeutic combinations. However, patients with lymphocytic subtypes tend to have early and continuous relapse and intermittent recurrences of disease for a 5- to 10-year period. The median survival of patients with lymphocytic lymphomas may therefore be relatively long, but disease activity predominates through many of these years and cure is not feasible. Other than histology, there are essentially no clinical variables associated with either disease-free or absolute survival. Age, sex, and clinical stage generally play an insignificant role in predicting survival. Patients who do not have a complete remission with the initial course of treatment generally may expect a short survival.

A substantial number (20% to 25%) of patients have localized (stage I or II) disease when initially examined. A number of centers have adequately staged such patients, including laparotomy, and have then evaluated treatment with radiotherapy or chemotherapy. As in patients with stage III or IV disease, the histologic subtype plays a significant prognostic role. Nearly all patients with pathologically proven stage I DHL may expect to maintain a disease-free state following radiotherapy (4000 rad in 20 daily treatments over a 4-week period). About 50% of the patients with stage II DHL have relapses following radiotherapy, and those with more than three sites of nodal involvement are at substantial risk for relapse. Preliminary results indicate that chemotherapy using either COP or CHOP following irradiation improves the disease-free survival in patients with stage II diffuse lymphoma. Patients with stage I or II nodular lymphocytic disease have a better prognosis than patients with stage III or IV, but chemotherapy with radiotherapy has not been shown to provide substantial improvement or improve the disease-free survival. Approximately half of such patients, however, can expect to be alive and disease free 5 years after radiotherapy.

Extranodal disease

Extranodal disease occurs in 25% of patients with NHL. The two most common sites are the stomach and the head and neck. Less commonly the disease may involve bone, skin, or the central nervous system. Of cases with apparent localized extranodal involvement of the head and neck, nearly three fourths involve Waldeyer's ring and one fourth involve the paranasal sinuses. The symptomatology varies depending on the site of the primary lesion. It is unclear whether the biologic behavior of extranodal lymphomatous disease differs from or is similar to that of nodal disease, but correlations between survival and histology resemble those in patients with nodal presentations. Lymphoma in the gastrointestinal tract most commonly involves the stomach, is more frequently of the diffuse histiocytic subtype, and if localized has a relatively good prognosis. The treatment is frequently surgical and, provided there is no serosal penetration or lymph node involvement, induces a disease-free 5-year survival in 50% of the patients. Radiotherapy is also effective.

BIBLIOGRAPHY

Aisenberg, A.C.: The staging and treatment of Hodgkin's disease, N. Engl. J. Med. **299**:1228, 1978.

Brugère, J., and others: Non-Hodgkin's malignant lymphomata of upper digestive and respiratory tract: natural history and results of radiotherapy, Br. J. Cancer **31** (Suppl. II):435, 1975.

Desforges, J.F., Rutherford, C.J., and Piro, A.: Hodgkin's disease, N. Engl. J. Med. **301**:1212, 1979.

Hellman, S., and others: The place of radiation therapy in the treatment of Hodgkin's disease, Cancer **42**:971, 1978.

Jones, S.E., and others: Non-Hodgkin's lymphomas. IV. Clinicopathologic correlation in 405 cases, Cancer **31**:806, 1973.

Mann, R.B., Jaffe, E.S., and Berard, C.W.: Malignant lymphomas—a conceptual understanding of morphologic diversity, Am. J. Pathol. **94**:105, 1979.

Portlock, C.S., and Rosenberg, S.A.: No initial therapy for stage III and IV non-Hodgkin's lymphomas of favorable histologic types, Ann. Intern. Med. **90**:10, 1979.

Rosenberg, S.A.: Non-Hodgkin's lymphoma—selection of treatment on the basis of histologic type, N. Engl. J. Med. **301**:924, 1979.

Rosenberg, S.A., and Kaplan, H.S.: Evidence for an orderly progression in the spread of Hodgkin's disease, Cancer Res. **26**:1225, 1966.

Rudders, R.A., Ross, M.E., and DeLellis, R.A.: Primary extranodal lymphoma, Cancer **42**:406, 1978.

Schein, P.S., and others: Potential for prolonged disease-free survival following combination chemotherapy for non-Hodgkin's lymphoma, Blood **43**:181, 1974.

Sweet, D.L., Kinnealey, A., and Ultmann, J.E.: Hodgkin's disease: problems of staging, Cancer **42**:957, 1978.

78 • DISEASES OF THE SPLEEN AND RETICULOENDOTHELIAL SYSTEM

Sally D. Lane

The spleen is an organ that operates directly or indirectly in a number of critical body functions. It is the chief organ of the reticuloendothelial system (RES). Along with the liver, lymph nodes, bone marrow, and specialized reticuloendothelial (RE) cells throughout the body (circulating monocytes and fixed tissue macrophages), it participates in the phagocytic and immunologic activities that form one of the body's chief defenses against infection. Destruction of various intravascular particles (including senescent or deformed red blood cells, infectious organisms, and cellular breakdown products) and metabolic processing of their components are additional functions of the RES. Finally, the RES includes multipotential stem cells capable of differentiation along a number of cell lines: hematopoietic, histiocytic (phagocytic and nonphagocytic), and fibroblastic.

Because of its highly vascular nature, the spleen may also be implicated in disorders of the circulatory system, particularly the portal circulation. As such, it may be indirectly affected by portal hypertension (particularly in association with liver disease) and by vascular events such as splenic vein thrombosis.

EVALUATION OF THE PATIENT WITH SPLENOMEGALY

Determination of the cause of splenomegaly presents a diagnostic challenge to the physician. Although it is often difficult to isolate a specific cause for splenomegaly via noninvasive procedures, a number of clinical guidelines exist.

A finding of a palpable or roentgenographically enlarged spleen generally connotes a pathologic condition, but this is not always the case. The spleen, along with the other lymphoid tissues of the body, enlarges promptly in response to any infectious insult in children, and occasionally lymphatic hyperplasia occurs in healthy adults as well. One series demonstrated the finding of palpable spleens in 3% of healthy college freshmen. Of these, a large number can probably be related to prior infection with delayed or incomplete resolution. Furthermore, the presence of emphysema or a low diaphragm may make a normal-sized spleen palpable.

Nonetheless, a definitely enlarged spleen should prompt an evaluation for the more likely benign and malignant causes of splenomegaly. The chief malignant causes of splenomegaly, lymphomas and leukemias (particularly chronic granulocytic and chronic lymphocytic leukemia), are discussed in Chapters 73 and 77. Among nonmalignant causes of splenomegaly, hemolysis, infections, collagen-vascular disorders, hypersensitivity states, vascular congestion, and proliferative and infiltrative diseases of the RES are perhaps most common. The last two of these are discussed in this section. The reader is referred to the appropriate sections of this text for consideration of splenomegaly in association with other disease states.

A finding of massive splenomegaly should suggest portal hypertension, myeloproliferative disorders, the sphingolipidoses (especially Gaucher's disease), malaria, or occasionally splenic cysts. Among patients in whom no cause for splenomegaly can be identified clinically ("idiopathic splenomegaly"), lymphoma will be ultimately identified in a small percentage.

FUNCTIONAL DISORDERS

Hyposplenism

DEFINITION AND PATHOGENESIS. The functional capacity of the spleen is defined primarily by its activity in clearing microorganisms (especially poorly opsonized bacteria), in filtering and processing blood cells, and in synthesizing both IgM immunoglobulin and opsonizing proteins. Thus hyposplenism can be thought of as a state in which any or all of these functions are disrupted. However, it is usually defined by its specific origin. Clearly, absence of the spleen, either congenital or following splenectomy, produces the extreme manifestations of this state. A severe degree of hyposplenism occurs in sickle cell anemia, in which repeated infarctions lead to atrophy and autosplenectomy. The organ may be enlarged in young children and does not function normally. It shrinks with repeated infarctions and is rarely palpable in older children. Other disorders that are frequently associated with hyposplenism include ulcerative colitis (in which splenic function can wax and wane with the activity of the colitis), celiac sprue, and dermatitis herpetiformis.

CLINICAL MANIFESTATIONS AND LABORATORY FINDINGS. Hyposplenism is frequently recognized by the findings of abnormal red blood cell forms in the peripheral blood. Howell-Jolly bodies (nuclear remnants) and target cells are the hallmarks of a hypofunctional or absent spleen; acanthocytes and siderocytes may also be seen. Granulocytosis occurs immediately after splenectomy but is replaced within several weeks by sustained lymphocytosis and monocytosis. Transient thrombocytosis (usually less than 2 weeks in duration) also occurs after splenectomy; it is of little clinical significance unless there is an underlying myeloproliferative disorder, in which sustained platelet counts in excess of 1 million/mm^3 may predispose the patient to bleeding or thrombosis or both.

The most devastating clinical manifestation of hyposplenism is vulnerability to overwhelming infection, particularly pneumococcemia. This most frequently occurs in sickle cell anemia and in young children who have undergone splenectomy, especially within the first 2 years following surgery. The risk of postsplenectomy sepsis may be as high as 20% in patients with underlying RES disorders such as thalassemia major, histiocytosis, and Wiskott-Aldrich syndrome. However, even normal adults undergoing incidental splenectomy appear to have a small but significant risk of fulminant sepsis. The reported fatality rate is as high as 50%. *Streptococcus pneumoniae* is responsible for most cases, but the meningococcus or *Haemophilus influenzae* may be the infectious agent. Extraordinarily high numbers of microorganisms are found in the blood; shock and disseminated intravascular coagulation are frequent accompaniments. The disorder is believed to be related to loss of phagocytic activity of the spleen, decreased IgM levels, changes in the alternative pathway of complement activation, decreased levels of opsonizing proteins, and possibly alteration of lymphocytic function.

MANAGEMENT. The functional capacity of an absent or atrophied spleen clearly cannot be replaced. The most significant therapeutic interventions that can be made include avoidance of unnecessary splenectomy, bacterial (particularly pneumococcal) vaccines for patients with hyposplenism or absent spleens, and in selected situations prophylactic penicillin. The treatment of undiagnosed fevers or documented sepsis in hyposplenic patients is an emergency and requires prompt institution of antibiotics and supportive measures.

Hypersplenism

DEFINITION. Hyperfunction of the spleen is characterized by splenomegaly, reduction in any or all of the formed blood elements (red cells, white cells, and platelets), compensatory bone marrow hyperplasia, and response to splenectomy. An enlarged spleen does not necessarily lead to hypersplenism and may be asymptomatic or produce mechanical disturbances without functional alteration.

PATHOGENESIS. Increased sequestration of blood cells appears to be the primary mechanism for hypersplenism. Normally about 20 to 30 ml of erythrocytes, roughly 30% of the peripheral pool of platelets, and a small fraction of the granulocytes are located in the spleen. In states of splenic enlargement, increased pooling of these cells causes a reduction in peripheral blood counts. Effects on the various elements may vary. Red cell survival is usually shortened in proportion to the size of the spleen. The degree of anemia, if any, that results depends on the compensatory response of the bone marrow. When increased platelet pooling in the spleen occurs, the bone marrow appears to respond more to the total body platelet mass than to the circulating platelet pool. Leukopenia associated with simple sequestration is frequently "balanced," with a normal differential count. Disorders associated with increased RES activity, such as Gaucher's disease, renal transplantation, and Felty's syndrome (rheumatoid arthritis, neutropenia, and splenomegaly), may produce a more severe degree of leukopenia.

CLINICAL MANIFESTATIONS. Hypersplenism may be entirely asymptomatic, or it may produce symptoms resulting from the depression of blood elements. Hemolysis may produce symptomatic anemia. The degree of anemia depends on bone marrow response (often suboptimal in patients with systemic illnesses associated with splenomegaly) and on the presence of other diseases, such as coronary artery disease or pulmonary insufficiency, that alter the patient's tolerance to anemia. When splenic enlargement occurs as a result of work hypertrophy from hemolytic anemia (for example, hereditary spherocytosis, thalassemia), a vicious circle often occurs in which increasing hemolysis produces increasing splenomegaly and vice versa. Platelets sequestered in an enlarged spleen can be mobilized in response to hemorrhage and appear to function normally; thus significant bleeding is infrequently associated with hypersplenic thrombocytopenia. This may not be the case, however, when a qualitative platelet defect exists, as in some myeloproliferative disorders. Furthermore, in Banti's syndrome (chronic congestive splenomegaly with pancytopenia and portal hypertension), significant bleeding can occur, particularly from esophageal varices. In general the mild granulocytopenia seen with splenomegaly is of little clinical concern; however, the leukopenia seen in Felty's syndrome is associated with a significant risk of infection. Immune destruction of granulocytes appears to play a role in this disorder.

LABORATORY FINDINGS AND DIAGNOSIS. The salient laboratory feature of hypersplenism is the reduction of the affected blood element(s). Reticulocytosis is routinely seen unless severe bone marrow dysfunction exists. Examination of the bone marrow in hypersplenism shows compensatory hyperplasia, particularly in the erythroid series. Quantitation of splenic hyperfunction can be made by measuring the survival of transfused ^{51}Cr-labeled red cells with scanning over the spleen. Radioisotope labeling has also been used to study platelet survival.

COURSE AND MANAGEMENT. The clinical course of hypersplenic states may be benign or progressive, depending in large part on the underlying disease. Certain acute infectious causes such as miliary tuberculosis, viral hepatitis, infectious mononucleosis, and subacute bacterial endocarditis may be self-limited or responsive to antimicrobial therapy. When hypersplenism is progressive or severe, splenectomy or splenic irradiation may be indicated.

Extramedullary hematopoiesis

All organs of the RES retain an inherent capacity for hematopoietic function. This function is normally active in the fetus. The liver is the primary hematopoietic organ from the second through sixth months of gestation and remains active until shortly before birth. Lesser contributions are made during the middle third of fetal life by the spleen, lymph nodes, and thymus. From birth onward, the bone marrow is the sole organ of normal hematopoiesis. However, under circumstances of increased stress and particularly in disease states characterized by bone marrow replacement or fibrosis, the organs of the RES (chiefly the liver and spleen) can again become active in blood formation. This syndrome is characterized by splenomegaly, hepatomegaly, and the finding of immature red and white cell precursors in the peripheral blood. A more detailed discussion of this entity is presented in Chapter 75.

THE LIPIDOSES

A number of inherited disorders are characterized by abnormal accumulation of materials in phagocytic cells with resultant enlargement of RE organs. Most often the defect is related to the absence of a critical enzyme. Two of these disorders will be considered here: Gaucher's disease and Niemann-Pick disease (see Chapter 195).

Gaucher's disease

Gaucher's disease is the most common of the lysosomal storage diseases. The metabolic defect is a deficiency of the enzyme glucocerebrosidase, resulting in the accumulation of glucocerebroside (ceramide glucose). This material, one of the sphingolipids, is a metabolic breakdown product of neutrophils and erythrocytes. The enzyme deficiency is inherited as an autosomal recessive trait and in the most common forms shows a predilection for Ashkenazic Jews.

Three clinical forms of Gaucher's disease exist. The most severe is the infantile (acute neuronopathic) form, characterized by rapid progression and commonly death before age 2. The hallmark of the disorder is severe neurologic dysfunction consisting of cranial nerve abnormalities, extrapyramidal signs, hypertonicity, hyperreflexia, and hyperextension of the neck. Splenomegaly and hepatomegaly are usually present, as is pancytopenia. Death frequently results from pulmonary infection.

In the juvenile (subacute neuronopathic) form onset usually occurs between 1 and 8 years of age. Neurologic defects are often present but are more variable. Hepatosplenomegaly is usually rapidly progressive, and thrombocytopenia may produce symptomatic bruising. Bone destruction is common and may be painful. The disease is often fatal but always at a later age than in the infantile form.

The adult (chronic nonneuronopathic) form is the most common. As the name suggests, neurologic findings are absent. The diagnosis may be made at any age from adolescence to late middle age (and rarely in the elderly). Splenomegaly is usually the presenting manifestation; occasionally abnormal bleeding from thrombocytopenia heralds the diagnosis. Often the disease is asymptomatic, but usually some degree of pancytopenia is present. The major difficulties result from splenomegaly and bone lesions.

The sine qua non of Gaucher's disease is the finding of Gaucher's cells in the spleen, liver, bone marrow, and sometimes lymph nodes. These are large cells (20 to 80 μm in diameter) with small eccentric nuclei and coarsely clumped cytoplasm having the appearance of wrinkled tissue paper. They are phagocytic cells filled with glucocerebroside. The other laboratory hallmark is elevated levels of serum acid phosphatase (tartrate resistant, in contrast to prostatic acid phosphatase).

As noted previously, anemia, leukopenia, and thrombocytopenia are present to some degree (usually greater in the more severe forms). The anemia is hypochromic and normocytic. Hypersplenism is believed to contribute to leukopenia and thrombocytopenia in the juvenile and adult forms, but decreased red cell survival is not prominent.

Bone lesions are characteristic of all but the infantile form. They result mainly from replacement of the marrow by Gaucher's cells. The typical roentgenographic finding is expansion of the cortex of the distal long bones, especially the femur. Pathologic fractures may occur.

The combination of the clinical findings with identification of Gaucher's cells in the RES establishes the diagnosis. "Gaucher-like" cells may be seen in leukemia, especially chronic granulocytic leukemia, in which increased breakdown of granulocytes probably results in accumulation of a glucocerebroside precursor.

Niemann-Pick disease

Niemann-Pick disease is a somewhat more heterogeneous group of disorders, all distinguished by hepatosplenomegaly and the finding of characteristic foamy RE cells. Like Gaucher's disease, it is most common in Jews. The metabolic defect in most if not all forms appears to be a deficiency of sphingomyelinase, with accumulation of sphingomyelin. However, abnormal accumulation of cholesterol also occurs and may predominate. Mental impairment and death within the first 3 years of life are characteristic but not universal. At least four clinical subtypes have been identified, based on rapidity of progression and relative importance of hepatosplenomegaly versus central nervous system involvement.

Anemia and thrombocytopenia are much less common than in Gaucher's disease, and the serum acid phosphatase level is normal. The pathognomonic storage cell is as large as the Gaucher's cell but contains a foamy rather than wrinkled-appearing, blue-green cytoplasm when stained with Wright-Giemsa stain.

CHÉDIAK-HIGASHI SYNDROME

The Chédiak-Higashi syndrome is an uncommon inherited lysosomal storage disease characterized by striking inclusion bodies in many cells. These are most commonly seen in neutrophils and lymphocytes of the peripheral blood but are also identified in tissues such as the skin, hair, and nervous system. The abnormal inclusions are most readily identified in mature neutrophils as large reddish purple bodies. They appear to represent abnormal fusion of lysosomal precursors. They are acid phosphatase positive, but other cytochemical stains vary with the specific cell. Some have classified this syndrome as a lipidosis.

Clinically, Chédiak-Higashi syndrome is characterized by increased susceptibility to infection (particularly caused by *S. aureus*) and by death in childhood. The chemotaxis of neutrophils is abnormal, and the large granules do not degranulate normally, leading to poor intracellular killing of some bacteria. Hepatosplenomegaly, anemia, and thrombocytopenia are common. An association with partial albinism and decreased retinal pigmentation is often found.

PROLIFERATIVE DISORDERS
Idiopathic histiocytosis

DEFINITION. The term "idiopathic histiocytosis" (or "histiocytosis X") includes a spectrum of disease processes ranging from focal to widely disseminated proliferation of lipid-laden histiocytes. These disorders were originally described as three separate entities: eosinophilic granuloma of bone (localized histiocytosis), Hand-Schüller-Christian disease (disseminated chronic histiocytosis), and Letterer-Siwe disease (disseminated acute histiocytosis). In 1953 Lichtenstein proposed the concept of a single category, histiocytosis X, to encompass all three, based on similarities in histologic features and on the possible identification of intermediate forms and transition between the subtypes. This concept has been widely debated in the subsequent literature, however, and many authors prefer to maintain the distinction between localized and disseminated forms.

ETIOLOGY AND PATHOGENESIS. The cause of idiopathic histiocytosis remains unknown. Occasional reports suggesting either infectious or genetic factors have appeared, but there are no consistent data to support a particular origin. In its most aggressive forms the disease may take on the features of a neoplastic process. The clinical features are an expression of the location and extent of proliferation of abnormal histiocytes.

CLINICAL MANIFESTATIONS. The most localized and benign form of histiocytosis, eosinophilic granuloma, is characterized by solitary or multifocal lesions of bone, usually in children or young adults. The lesions most often appear osteolytic on roentgenogram, may stimulate periosteal reaction, and occur most commonly in the skull, ribs, pelvis, and scapulae. Pathologically, they are composed of histiocytes with abundant eosinophilic cytoplasm and many polymorphonuclear cells, largely eosinophils. Localized pain is the usual presenting symptom, and systemic manifestations are rare. The disease generally has a benign course and responds well to local excision or radiotherapy.

The chronic disseminated form of histiocytosis is a rare condition of childhood, in which bone lesions similar to those just described are found in association with other manifestations such as diabetes insipidus, exophthalmos, chronic otitis media or externa, or skin infiltration. Involvement of visceral organs such as lymph nodes, liver, spleen, or lung may occur but is not usually prominent. The course is more variable than in the localized form but usually has a good prognosis. In about half the patients the disease eventually burns out, leaving fibrotic lesions at the sites of involvement but no clinical residual. It may be fatal in up to 15% of the cases.

Of the three subtypes, the acute disseminated form is most readily differentiated from the other two. This is an acute, fulminant disease of infants that generally leads to death within the first few years of life. Bone tumors, hepatosplenomegaly, lymphadenopathy, fever, anemia, and bleeding are prominent features. The prognosis is poorer at an earlier age of onset.

MANAGEMENT. Localized tumors are readily treated by surgery or radiotherapy. In the disseminated forms a number of systemic agents have been used with some reports of success. The most experience has been with corticosteroids and vinca alkaloids (especially vinblastine), although a variety of alkylating agents, antimetabolites, and cytotoxic antibiotics have been used as well.

Histiocytic medullary reticulosis (malignant histiocytosis)

Histiocytic medullary reticulosis is a malignant disorder of RE tissues that is believed by some to be a variant of the "histiocytic" lymphomas. It affects all ages and is not uncommon in the first decade of life. The principal clinical features are fever, wasting, purpura, generalized adenopathy, hepatosplenomegaly, severe pancytopenia, and a rapid downhill course. Infiltration of other organs, including the skin, bone, and gastrointestinal tract, may occur. Histologically it is characterized by the proliferation of large, atypical histiocytes in the bone marrow, medullary portions of lymph nodes, and other involved organs. Phagocytosis of blood elements, especially erythrocytes, is a hallmark of the disease and is believed to be largely responsible for the pancytopenia. Although the anemia shows many features of a hemolytic process, there is usually inadequate reticulocytosis, and Coombs' test is typically negative. Histiocytes are infrequently found in the peripheral blood. When the disease occurs in early childhood, the distinction from Letterer-Siwe disease can be difficult but is usually possible on histologic grounds. Malignant histiocytosis is generally unresponsive to radiotherapy or chemotherapy, but occasional long-term responses to combination chemotherapy have been described.

MISCELLANEOUS DISORDERS

Splenic infarction may result from hemoglobinopathies, leukocytic infiltration (as in the chronic leukemias), or large vessel thrombosis. Rupture of the spleen may occur as a result of blunt trauma to the abdomen or "spontaneously" in disorders in which the spleen is abnormal, such as leukemia, infectious mononucleosis, malaria, or typhoid fever.

Space-occupying lesions of the spleen include abscesses, cysts, and tumors. Abscesses may result from bacteremia, extension from a perforated or diseased neighboring abdominal organ, or secondary infection of a sterile infarct. The characteristic signs are fever, chills, abdominal pain, and irritation of either the pleural or peritoneal surface, depending on the location.

Splenic cysts are rare. They may result from parasitic infestation (especially echinococcosis) or from benign neoplasms such as dermoid cysts, cystic lymphangiomas, or cavernous hemangiomas. Primary malignant tumor of the spleen is a debatable entity; rarely a lymphoma can be localized to the spleen, but in almost all cases there is evidence of widespread involvement. On the other hand, metastatic neoplasms involve the spleen with a significant frequency. The most common primary sites are the lung, breast, prostate, colon, and stomach. The involvement may vary from large nodular deposits to diffuse infiltration, and extensively involved spleens may attain enormous sizes.

BIBLIOGRAPHY

Eichner, E.R.: Splenic function: normal, too much and too little, Am. J. Med. **66**:311, 1979.

Frederickson, D.S., and Sloan, H.R.: Glucosyl ceramide lipidoses:

Gaucher's disease. Sphingomyelin lipidoses: Niemann-Pick disease. In Stanberry, J.B., and others, editors: The metabolic bases of inherited diseases, ed. 4, New York, 1978, McGraw-Hill Book Co.

Jacob, H.S.: Hypersplenism: mechanisms and management, Br. J. Haematol. **27:**1, 1974.

Krivit, W.: Overwhelming post-splenectomy infection, Am. J. Hematol. **2:**193, 1977.

Miale, J.B.: Laboratory medicine: hematology, ed. 6, St. Louis, 1982, The C.V. Mosby Co.

Vogel, J.M., and Vogel, P.: Idiopathic histiocytosis: a discussion of eosinophilic granuloma, the Hand-Schüller-Christian syndrome, and the Letterer-Siwe syndrome, Semin. Hematol. **9:**349, 1972.

Warnke, R.A., Kim, H., and Dorfman, R.F.: Malignant histiocytosis (histiocytic medullary reticulosis), Cancer **35:**215, 1975.

Unit C • HEMOSTATIC DISORDERS

79 • INTRODUCTION TO HEMOSTASIS

Patricia M. Catalano

Evaluation of the patient with a history of bruising and bleeding is a common clinical problem. The accurate diagnosis and appropriate management of such patients depend on a thorough understanding of the normal hemostatic mechanisms and the tests of these mechanisms.

It is convenient to consider the normal sequence of events that leads to hemostasis as occurring in two phases. The first phase involves the immediate control mechanisms related to the vasculature and the formation of a platelet plug at the site of vessel injury. The long-term control mechanisms constitute the second phase and consist of a biochemical chain of events that involve the humoral coagulation factors, platelet factors, and calcium, resulting in the formation of a fibrin clot. As understanding of the hemostatic mechanism increases, so does the realization of the complexity of the interactions among the vascular, platelet, and humoral components of the system. Nonetheless, an astute clinician usually is able to determine from the history and initial physical and laboratory findings approximately where the abnormality in an individual patient is most likely to be found and to direct the subsequent evaluation accordingly.

Several aspects of the history of a patient with a suspected bleeding disorder should be emphasized. The nature and severity of the bleeding episodes should be determined. A defect of the immediate control mechanisms is usually manifested by mucous membrane bleeding, with epistaxis, menorrhagia, and gingival bleeding prominent features. Disorders of coagulation factors, on the other hand, are more often associated with massive bleeding following trauma or surgery. Spontaneous hemarthroses are a prominent feature of severe hemophilia, a disorder of coagulation factors.

It is important to ascertain if the disorder is congenital or acquired, and the family history may be extremely valuable. Family members may have a known disorder; when the bleeding tendency is familial but the diagnosis is unknown, its mode of inheritance may be helpful.

Often the most difficult patients to assess are those who are to undergo a surgical procedure and who have only a history of increased bruising but no previous major surgery or family history of bleeding. The significance of the bleeding tendency can often be elucidated in such patients by a careful dental history. The extraction of a permanent tooth is a significant stress to the hemostatic mechanisms and one that the patient seldom thinks to mention if not questioned directly. Any excessive bleeding after dental procedures deserves evaluation, even in an otherwise asymptomatic patient. This history may provide the only clue to a serious bleeding disorder, and the diagnosis of such a disorder before surgery is, of course, extremely important.

A careful drug history is always important in evaluating a patient for a bleeding disorder. This history may uncover the origin of the bleeding, and it is also important to determine if the patient has taken any drugs that may interfere with the evaluation tests, such as aspirin, which will prolong the bleeding time.

The physical examination may provide further clues as to where the defect may be found. For example, petechiae are almost exclusively seen as a manifestation of thrombocytopenia. Arthropathy of the large joints is a common complication of the repeated hemarthroses of severe hemophilia.

The ultimate diagnosis of a bleeding disorder must of course be made in the laboratory. A routine coagulation survey consisting of a platelet count, partial thromboplastin time, prothrombin time, and bleeding time serves as the first screen of the platelet, intrinsic, and extrinsic coagulation pathways. More elaborate tests of platelet function or specific factor assays may, however, be important even when such a screen is normal.

80 • PLATELET AND VASCULAR DISORDERS

Patricia M. Catalano

Platelets are disk-shaped blood cells 3 to 4 μm in diameter, normally present in whole blood in a concentration of 200,000 to 400,000/mm^3. Structurally they consist of a bilipid membrane and cytoplasm that contains a variety of granules, a few mitochondria, and no nucleus. Within the granules are stored calcium, adenosine diphosphate (ADP), serotonin, and platelet factor 4 (platelet coagulant factor). Platelets are formed in the bone marrow from precursor cells called megakaryocytes and circulate with an average life span of 7 to 9 days.

Platelets adhere to a variety of substances, most notably collagen, which is exposed when a blood vessel is interrupted. The adherence of platelets at the site of vessel injury is rapidly followed by the aggregation of large numbers of platelets to form a platelet plug. Interaction of these activated platelets with the coagulation system then leads to the sequence of events that results in fibrin clot formation.

The ability of platelets to adhere normally has proved to be a difficult function to quantitate. The most readily available test of adherence in vitro is the retention of platelets in a glass bead column. In spite of the relatively crude nature of this test, it has been useful in documenting that this function in some way depends on the presence of the "von Willebrand factor" activity of the coagulation protein factor VIII.

Platelet aggregation, on the other hand, has been extensively studied in vitro. The addition of a variety of stimulating agents, such as ADP or epinephrine, to a stirred solution of platelet-rich plasma results in a characteristic response for the particular agent used. Aggregation stimulated by these agents usually proceeds in two phases, a primary reversible aggregation and a second wave of aggregation that is irreversible. The development of a second wave of aggregation is, at least in part, mediated by the platelet prostaglandin pathway. Arachidonic acid is released from the platelet membrane during aggregation and is metabolized by the enzyme cyclo-oxygenase to a variety of prostaglandins, cyclic endoperoxides, and thromboxanes. Thromboxane A$_2$ produced by this pathway is a potent stimulus to aggregation. When thromboxane production is blocked by aspirin, which inhibits cyclo-oxygenase, secondary aggregation does not occur. An alternative pathway for aggregation must also exist, however, since the inhibition of aggregation by aspirin can be overcome by potent aggregating agents such as thrombin. The second phase of aggregation is also accompanied by the phenomenon known as the release reaction, during which the contents of the platelet granules are secreted, further enhancing the aggregation. A special form of aggregation stimulated by the antibiotic ristocetin is also dependent on factor VIII.

Although these methods of studying adherence and aggregation have been invaluable in the development of the understanding of platelet physiology, it is often difficult to interpret subtle abnormalities and the techniques are subject to numerous artifacts. It is therefore extremely important that they be performed by someone experienced in their interpretation.

A bleeding tendency can be the result of an abnormality at any stage of the events just described. Abnormalities of the vasculature, platelet number, and platelet function have all been well documented, and the evaluation of a patient with a bleeding tendency must consider all these aspects of the initial coagulation mechanism.

THROMBOCYTOPENIA

DEFINITION. Thrombocytopenia of clinical significance exists when the whole blood platelet count is below 150,000/mm^3, although the precise limits for normal vary slightly among laboratories. Because of the potential for laboratory error or artifact, the finding of a low platelet count should always be confirmed by examination of the peripheral blood smear.

ETIOLOGY AND PATHOGENESIS. The origins of the thrombocytopenic disorders are many and varied and are often poorly understood. Thrombocytopenia is probably most commonly drug induced (see outline below), but primary bone marrow disorders, infections, and immunologic and inherited disorders have all been associated with thrombocytopenia.

Drugs commonly implicated in thrombocytopenia

I. Marrow suppressive agents
   A. Chemotherapeutic agents
      1. Doxorubicin
      2. Cytosine arabinoside
      3. Cyclophosphamide
      4. Nitrogen mustard
      5. Nitrosoureas
      6. Busulfan
      7. Methotrexate
   B. Other marrow suppressive agents
      1. Chloramphenicol
      2. Phenylbutazone
      3. Thiazide diuretics
      4. Alcohol
      5. Estrogens
II. Immunologic (proven and suspected)
   A. Quinidine
   B. Quinine
   C. Aspirin
   D. Sulfonamides
   E. Rifampin
   F. Aminosalicylic acid
   G. Thiazides

H. Methyldopa
I. Gold salts
III. Unknown mechanism
A. Heparin

Studies using isotopically labeled platelets for the determination of platelet life span have greatly enhanced the understanding of platelet kinetics. Such studies support the intuitive concept that thrombocytopenia results from either decreased production or increased destruction, although thrombocytopenia as a result of abnormal distribution has also been described. Because the mechanism by which the thrombocytopenia occurs has important clinical and therapeutic implications, it is useful to consider the specific disorders that result in thrombocytopenia grouped on the basis of their platelet kinetics.

Thrombocytopenias caused by decreased platelet production

The disorders that cause decreased platelet production have varied origins. The clinical manifestations of the thrombocytopenia that results from these disorders are similar, regardless of the cause. Consequently, these aspects will be discussed after a review of the individual disorders.

Iatrogenic bone marrow suppression. With the advent of successful chemotherapy and radiotherapy for a variety of malignancies, bone marrow suppression has become an accepted consequence of such therapy. Both ionizing radiation and a wide variety of myelosuppressive chemotherapeutic agents cause a fairly predictable decrease in platelet count, with granulocytopenia often the major manifestation. The severity and duration of the suppression are drug and dose related.

Increasingly, chemotherapeutic regimens are being designed as pulses of multiple agents that result in a transient, often severe marrow suppression with its nadir 10 to 14 days after treatment. Rapid recovery usually occurs thereafter. However, long-term continuous treatment or even repeated aggressive pulse therapies may result in a prolonged suppression. Prolonged platelet suppression is commonly seen after aggressive or prolonged treatment with busulfan and has also been noted with nitrosoureas.

Drug-related bone marrow suppression. Other drugs that inadvertently or idiosyncratically suppress the bone marrow have been described. Chloramphenicol, sulfonamides, and phenylbutazone (Butazolidin) are well known for their aplastic effect, with thrombocytopenia a part of this aplasia. Alcohol is a frequent bone marrow suppressant. Thiazide diuretics are among the most common causes of drug-induced thrombocytopenia. Decreased megakaryocytes have been noted in the bone marrow of some of these patients, making marrow suppression one possible mechanism. In other cases, however, an immunologic mechanism seems likely. Estrogens have been described to lower platelets, and variations in platelet count during the menstrual cycle have been noted in some women. It is postulated that this phenomenon is the result of marrow suppression, but the mechanism is uncertain.

Bone marrow infiltration. Bone marrow infiltration is frequently associated with cytopenias. When the disease is diffuse, such as that seen with the leukemias or myelofibrosis, the mechanism for the cytopenias appears to be marrow replacement. However, spotty infiltration with nests of tumor cells has also been associated with cytopenias and occasionally isolated thrombocytopenia. In these instances it appears that the presence of the foreign cells is toxic or suppressive to normal marrow elements in a manner that is poorly understood. This phenomenon has also been noted in nonmalignant invasive disorders such as granulomatous diseases and in Gaucher's disease.

Congenital disorders. Congenital disorders that result in decreased marrow production are rare but well documented. In addition to the congenital aplastic anemia known as Fanconi's syndrome, a form of congenital aplastic anemia specifically associated with the megakaryocyte is sometimes seen. This may occur with other somatic anomalies, most often in the form of a syndrome of thrombocytopenia with absence of the radii.

Other. Viral infections, rubella vaccination, and megaloblastic anemia are all variably associated with thrombocytopenia resulting from decreased production.

CLINICAL MANIFESTATIONS. The clinical manifestations of this group of disorders will, of course, vary with the underlying disease. The manifestation of the thrombocytopenia per se, however, largely depends on its severity. Between the limits of 20,000 and 100,000 cells/mm^3, an inverse correlation has been observed between platelet count and bleeding time. Clinically, platelet counts of 50,000 to 100,000/mm^3 are seldom symptomatic unless the patient is subjected to surgical or traumatic stress. Platelet counts of 20,000 to 50,000/mm^3 may be manifested by an increased bruising tendency, and platelet counts of fewer than 20,000/mm^3 are often associated with petechiae, bruises, and bleeding from the mucous membranes. In spite of these observations, it should be remembered that even a mildly thrombocytopenic patient can have significant bleeding. Such bleeding can be life threatening when it involves intracranial or visceral organs. In addition, the tendency for a thrombocytopenic patient to bleed is aggravated by a variety of conditions. Medications that interfere with platelet function, for example, may greatly increase this tendency and should be studiously avoided. The presence of concomitant infection (a common problem in leukemic patients) is another condition that predisposes to bleeding seemingly out of proportion to the degree of thrombocytopenia.

LABORATORY FINDINGS. The laboratory findings common to all these disorders are a decreased platelet count and decreased numbers of megakaryocytes in the bone marrow. This may be apparent on the bone marrow smear, but often a marrow biopsy gives a better estimate of cellularity and megakaryocyte number. If an isotopic study of platelet life span can be performed, it will be normal. Associated findings depend entirely on the origin of the marrow suppression. For example, the presence of nucleated red blood cells and immature myeloid elements may suggest bone marrow invasion by tumor or fibrosis; hypersegmented neutrophils may be a manifestation of vitamin B_{12} or folate deficiency or an effect of chemotherapy with antimetabolites.

DIAGNOSIS. The diagnosis of decreased platelet production depends on the finding of thrombocytopenia with decreased numbers of megakaryocytes in the bone marrow. The history of the circumstances surrounding the development of thrombocytopenia is critical in the assessment of such patients. A specific drug history or associated illness may in a few circumstances obviate the need for further investigation. The history may raise the suspicion of tumor, in which case a bone marrow biopsy and aspiration are extremely important.

Differentiating marrow suppression from platelet destruction is occasionally a difficult clinical problem. Unfortunately, current techniques for evaluating platelet survival are cumbersome and not widely available. It is therefore occasionally useful diagnostically to determine if a patient is responsive to platelet transfusions as evidence that there is not a large element of platelet destruction contributing to the thrombocytopenia.

COURSE. The course of the illness also depends on the cause. Drug-induced thrombocytopenias, particularly chemotherapeutically induced, usually respond to withdrawal of the drug over a period of 7 to 14 days. Occasionally there is prolonged or even irreversible damage, especially in the idiosyncratically induced aplasias. The resolution of thrombocytopenia associated with marrow replacement or invasion depends on the success of the treatment of the underlying disorder. Congenital disorders generally persist without improvement.

MANAGEMENT. Management of the patient who is thrombocytopenic because of marrow failure is entirely supportive. In conditions in which the underlying disease can be treated (leukemias and lymphomas) and a finite period of thrombocytopenia is anticipated, it has become increasingly common to use prophylactic platelet transfusion to maintain the platelet count over $20,000/mm^3$. When there is no effective treatment for the underlying disorder, the decision to use platelet transfusions is more complex because the patient may become sensitized to the transfusions with the result that their efficacy will decrease with time. In these circumstances it is often necessary to give transfusions only for bleeding episodes. Many clinicians also prescribe low doses of corticosteroids for their effect of stabilization of the vascular endothelium. Rare reports of responses to androgenic steroids, especially in aplastic states, make a trial of their administration (if not precluded by the underlying disorder) useful in some cases of prolonged hypoplasia (see Chapter 62).

Thrombocytopenias caused by increased platelet destruction

IDIOPATHIC THROMBOCYTOPENIC PURPURA

Definition. Idiopathic thrombocytopenic purpura (ITP) is a relatively common disorder in which isolated thrombocytopenia occurs in otherwise healthy individuals. Two clinical forms of the disease are recognized—acute and chronic. Acute ITP is seen most frequently in children but may occur at any age. The onset is usually sudden, with thrombocytopenia manifested by bruising, bleeding, and petechiae a few days to several weeks after an otherwise uneventful viral illness. Acute ITP is a self-limited disease that generally remits permanently without sequelae.

Chronic ITP is usually a disease of adults and can be sudden or insidious in onset. It is three times more frequent in women than in men, and the course is characterized by remissions and exacerbations. In both acute and chronic ITP, thrombocytopenia and its manifestations are the only physical or laboratory abnormalities.

Etiology and pathogenesis. Although the cause of ITP is unknown, the pathophysiologic mechanism is well documented to be the peripheral destruction of platelets. It has long been believed that this destruction has an immunologic basis, and there is now a large body of evidence to support this. The presence of a humoral factor that can cross the placenta is shown by the fact that infants born to mothers with ITP are also thrombocytopenic but recover over a period of 1 to 3 months. Also, infusion of plasma from patients with ITP into normal individuals has been documented to induce thrombocytopenia in the recipients. In vitro antiplatelet activity has been found in the 7S globulin fraction of plasma, and ITP platelets have increased surface IgG. Further circumstantial evidence is the occurrence of ITP-like syndromes in association with other immunologically mediated diseases such as systemic lupus erythematosus and autoimmune hemolytic anemia.

Clinical manifestations. Patients with ITP often manifest severe thrombocytopenia and may have significant bruising and bleeding as a result. Surprisingly, however, they often have less bleeding than would be anticipated for the degree of thrombocytopenia. A patient with fewer than 10,000 platelets/mm^3 may have only a few dependent petechiae and be otherwise asymptomatic. At the other end of the spectrum, some patients have a remarkably acute and devastating course, and 1% of the patients have intracranial bleeding.

It must be emphasized that ITP is a disorder of platelets only, and the presence of any other abnormality should put the diagnosis in question. Occasionally, patients have a concomitant iron deficiency anemia owing to blood loss, but any other hematologic abnormality is inconsistent with straightforward ITP. There are no abnormal physical findings in ITP other than petechiae and ecchymoses. The presence of splenomegaly or lymphadenopathy should raise the possibility that an underlying lymphoproliferative or auto-immune disorder is the cause of the thrombocytopenia.

Diagnosis and laboratory findings. In spite of the volume of circumstantial evidence for the presence of the antiplatelet antibodies in ITP, efforts to develop tests specifically for the antibody have met with only variable success, and consequently the diagnosis of ITP must still be made on clinical grounds. The presence of isolated thrombocytopenia accompanied by plentiful bone marrow megakaryocytes is the significant finding. It must be emphasized that these findings constitute evidence of increased platelet destruction. The diagnosis of ITP remains one of exclusion. Lack of historical, physical, or laboratory evidence of associated disorders or drugs that could result in platelet destruction is confirmatory. An accurate diagnosis is critical. Other disorders that result in platelet destruction, such as disseminated intravascular coagulation or thrombotic thrombocytopenic purpura, require specific management, and misdiagnosis could have devastating consequences.

Some authors have emphasized that the platelets in ITP may be larger than normal, primarily because these platelets are very young. The usefulness of assessment of platelet size on peripheral smear varies with the experience of the examiner. The application of the isotopic platelet survival test in this disorder is limited by its availability. In most instances the destructive mechanism of the thrombocytopenia is apparent, but in occasional therapeutic dilemmas it is appropriate to refer patients to a center where a study to document the decreased platelet life span can be performed.

Course and management. Corticosteroids and splenectomy are the mainstays of therapy for ITP. Steroids apparently diminish antibody production and inhibit phagocytosis of platelets. Splenectomy also results in diminished antibody production as well as removal of the major site of platelet destruction. Childhood ITP usually remits spontaneously, and many clinicians choose not to treat these patients. Most treat all adult patients, and some choose to treat children with severe manifestations. The initiation of prednisone, 1 mg/kg, induces a response in the majority of patients, often with a gratifyingly rapid increase in platelet count and resolution of symptoms. Once a response has occurred, management must be individualized. The ideal goal of therapy is to achieve normalization of the platelet count without medication. In a small percentage of adult patients the steroids can be tapered and the platelet count will remain normal. More frequently, however, the platelets decrease with decreasing steroid dosages, or a relapse occurs after prednisone has been discontinued. In such patients splenectomy usually results in a permanent remission.

If a remission does not occur or cannot be maintained with less than 10 mg/day of prednisone after a trial of 3 months, a splenectomy should be considered. Patients usually have at least a partial response to splenectomy, and in approximately 50%, splenectomy induces a permanent remission. Some patients with no apparent response to splenectomy become responsive to steroid therapy after the procedure.

There remains a small percentage of patients who do not respond to steroids or splenectomy, and it is in this population that immunosuppressive agents such as cyclophosphamide, azathioprine, or vincristine may be useful.

ITP-like syndromes. A number of disorders can be accompanied by ITP-like syndromes. The lymphoproliferative disorders, chronic lymphocytic leukemia, Hodgkin's disease, and non-Hodgkin's lymphomas all have a small but significant incidence of peripheral platelet destruction. Systemic lupus erythematosus is surprisingly frequently accompanied by an apparently immunologically mediated thrombocytopenia. Autoimmune hemolytic anemia is also occasionally associated with ITP (Evans' syndrome). An ITP-like picture may be the presenting symptom in any of these disorders. It is therefore important in the process of diagnostic exclusion to ascertain that the ITP is not simply the presenting symptom of another disorder, since the treatment of an underlying lymphoproliferative disorder, for instance, may be critical to the patient. The management of thrombocytopenia in these disorders is similar to that for straightforward ITP, with steroids and splenectomy.

Drug-related platelet destruction. Among the drugs reported to cause thrombocytopenia, many are suspected to do so via immunologically mediated peripheral platelet destruction. Quinine, quinidine, and their derivatives are the classic examples of drugs that are documented to cause immunologic thrombocytopenia. In susceptible individuals the responsible drug apparently induces an antibody that, in the presence of the drug, has antiplatelet activity. This effect can be demonstrated in vitro. The patient's plasma, in combination with the drug, lyses platelets in an isotopic release assay, whereas the plasma or drug alone does not. The analogous in vivo counterpart is the observation that the platelet destruction ceases as soon after the drug is stopped as it takes for the drug to be cleared from the plasma. These patients are therefore managed simply by discontinuance of the responsible drug, which should result in a prompt rise in the platelet count.

A number of the drugs that have been reported to cause thrombocytopenia by this mechanism are listed on p. 400. It is an important point in the management of patients susceptible to quinine-induced thrombocytopenia that this susceptibility does not extend to quinidine and vice versa. A patient sensitive to one may be treated with the other without adverse effect.

Gold-induced thrombocytopenia is an interesting example of drug-related platelet destruction. Because gold salts are excreted slowly, the duration of the thrombocytopenia is prolonged. Steroid treatment is frequently required in these patients to maintain an acceptable platelet count until the drug is cleared—often a matter of months.

Thrombotic thrombocytopenic purpura. Thrombotic thrombocytopenic purpura (TTP) is a clinical syndrome in which thrombocytopenia, microangiopathic hemolytic anemia, and neurologic abnormalities occur. There are also often fever and renal failure. The origin is unknown, but the pathogenesis is related to the presence of deposits of hyaline material and platelet thrombi in the capillaries and arterioles. Which of these lesions is causative remains obscure. The disorder usually runs a fulminant course, with mortality ranging in different series from 50% to 90%. A chronic form is now also recognized. The clinical picture varies with renal, neurologic, or hematologic manifestations; the most prominent feature depends on the site of the vascular occlusions. It is likely that TTP in adults and the so-called hemolytic-uremic syndrome in children are the same disorder, although the vascular lesions in the latter are confined to the kidneys.

The therapies that have been proposed are difficult to assess because the disease is infrequent and published series are small. Steroids, splenectomy, and antiplatelet agents such as aspirin or dipyridamole have been tried and reported to have some effect. More recently, encouraging reports of responses to plasma exchange, either alone or in combination with antiplatelet agents, have generated enthusiasm for this approach.

Posttransfusion purpura. In a small number of patients severe thrombocytopenia has been found to develop approximately 1 week after blood transfusion. Patients in whom this occurs almost always lack the platelet-associated antigen PL^{A1}, which is present in 98% of the population. Apparently the transfusion induces the development of anti-PL^{A1} antibodies, and the patient's platelets are destroyed as innocent bystanders. Exchange transfusion and plasmapheresis have been reported to result in successful resolution. The same antibody is responsible for isoimmune neonatal purpura.

Disseminated intravascular coagulation. Disseminated intravascular coagulation (DIC) is a disorder in which coagulation factors and platelets are consumed by the formation of fibrin clots. The process is discussed in detail in Chapter 81. DIC is most frequently seen in association with overwhelming infections and with obstetric complications such as abruptio placentae and toxemia. It must always be considered in a patient with unexplained platelet destruction, particularly if bleeding is out of proportion to the degree of thrombocytopenia.

Disorders of distribution

Splenomegaly, which is usually associated with some degree of increased platelet turnover, has been reported to be associated with thrombocytopenia and a normal platelet survival. In these instances the thrombocytopenia probably results from altered distribution, with pooling in the large vascular bed of the spleen.

THROMBOCYTOSIS

Thrombocytosis exists when the whole blood platelet count is above 400,000/mm^3. It may be either primary (the result of a myeloproliferative disorder) or secondary (reactive to a variety of nonhematologic disorders).

Primary thrombocytosis

Primary thrombocytosis occurs as part of the spectrum of myeloproliferative diseases. It may be the only manifestation of myeloproliferation (essential thrombocythemia) or be part of one of the other myeloproliferative disorders, most frequently polycythemia vera. Occasionally, myelofibrosis or chronic granulocytic leukemia has an associated thrombocytosis. The origin is unknown. Presumably thrombocytosis results from overproduction by an abnormal clone of stem cells or megakaryocytes.

The clinical manifestations of primary thrombocytosis are extremely variable, ranging from the asymptomatic to the life threatening. Thrombotic complications may develop, or in patients with abnormal platelet function, bleeding may occur.

The laboratory findings include an increased number of platelets, which are often morphologically abnormal. There may be spurious hyperkalemia. For the most part laboratory findings are related to the underlying myeloproliferative disorder. For example, there may be an elevated serum vitamin B_{12} or leukocyte alkaline phosphatase level. On physical examination some degree of splenomegaly is usually found. Isolated essential thrombocythemia may be difficult to differentiate from reactive thrombocytosis; in these cases the diagnosis is made when evidence of an associated myeloproliferation can be demonstrated. The presence of platelet function abnormalities is strongly suggestive of a myeloproliferative disorder. Functionally normal platelets are the rule in secondary thrombocytosis.

The course and treatment of the disease vary with symptomatology and with the underlying myeloproliferative disorder, but generally busulfan, radioactive phosphorus (^{32}P), or more recently hydroxyurea and uracil mustard have been used to decrease the platelet count. In acutely symptomatic patients, plateletpheresis may be necessary. In patients with thrombotic manifestations, drugs that inhibit platelet function such as aspirin or dipyridamole may be useful.

Secondary thrombocytosis

For unknown reasons platelet counts over 400,000/mm^3 may be associated with a wide variety of disorders. A transient thrombocytosis almost invariably occurs after splenectomy. Patients with severe iron deficiency occasionally have significant thrombocytosis, and in chronic hemolytic states the platelet count may be elevated. A variety of inflammatory and stressful situations have been described as predisposing factors in reactive thrombocytosis. Among the most common causes are tumors of any origin. Clinically, patients are almost invariably asymptomatic, and platelet function is normal. The occurrence of abnormal platelet function is strongly suggestive of a myeloproliferative disorder rather than a reactive thrombocytosis. Thrombotic events, although rare, occur, especially if the thrombocytosis persists for a prolonged period of time and apparently more frequently in patients with hemolytic disease who have persistent hemolysis after splenectomy. The laboratory findings are usually thrombocytosis and those of the underlying disorder. Spurious hyperkalemia may be noted. The platelets are morphologically normal.

The diagnosis is one of exclusion of a myeloproliferative disorder. The documentation of an underlying disorder associated with reactive thrombocytosis is important. The course and treatment are those of the primary disorder, and the thrombocytosis resolves with the underlying cause. In cases of prolonged or extraordinary thrombocytosis (>1 million cells/mm^3) many clinicians choose to employ drugs that inhibit platelet function, such as aspirin or dipyridamole, and most avoid the use of cytotoxic agents. The merits of heparin or warfarin are uncertain, but they may be indicated for other reasons, as in a bedridden patient who is at high risk for thromboembolic disease.

QUALITATIVE PLATELET ABNORMALITIES

Platelet function defects can be congenital or acquired. In either case disorders of any facet of platelet function are possible, and it is useful to categorize these disorders according to the specific physiologic defect. Congenital defects are rare, but acquired defects are surprisingly common, especially when drug-induced platelet function defects are included.

Congenital disorders of platelet function

BERNARD-SOULIER SYNDROME. The Bernard-Soulier syndrome is an autosomal recessive disorder of platelet adhesion. It is characterized by giant platelets that do not aggregate when stimulated with the antibiotic ristocetin. Unlike the similar phenomenon in von Willebrand's disease, this inability to aggregate is not corrected by factor VIII replacement. In fact, all the factor VIII activities are normal in the plasma of these patients. The defect is an intrinsic abnormality of the platelet membrane, which has been shown to have decreased amounts of glycoprotein I. Glycoprotein I is probably the normal receptor for factor VIII–related ristocetin cofactor activity.

In addition to this functional defect, which results in a prolonged bleeding time, patients may have a mild thrombocytopenia. The bleeding may be severe, with epistaxis, menorrhagia, and bruising, and may require treatment with platelet transfusions.

THROMBASTHENIA. Thrombasthenia is also an autosomal recessive disease characterized by a prolonged bleeding time, but unlike the Bernard-Soulier syndrome, platelet adhesion is normal and there is diminished or absent aggregation to almost all stimuli. The platelet count is normal. A glycoprotein membrane abnormality is the apparent cause. The patients have symptoms similar to those of the Bernard-Soulier syndrome, and platelet transfusions are the therapy for bleeding episodes.

STORAGE-POOL DISEASE. Storage-pool disease is an inherited disorder of variable transmission sometimes associated with albinism. It is caused by a deficiency of the dense platelet granules containing the "storage pool" of the adenine nucleotides adenosine diphosphate (ADP) and adenosine triphosphate (ATP), which are normally secreted during the release reaction. This deficiency results in a selective absence of second-wave aggregation. Platelet transfusion may be necessary to treat bleeding episodes in these patients, but treatment with corticosteroids has also been reported to be of benefit.

Acquired disorders of platelet function

DRUG-INDUCED DISORDERS. By far the most frequent platelet function abnormalities seen today are drug induced. The importance of recognizing this effect of many commonly used drugs cannot be overemphasized. Drugs have been found to inhibit all phases of platelet function. Coating of the cell membrane is reported to be the mechanism by which dextran interferes with platelet adhesion. Phosphodiesterase inhibitors such as dipyridamole increase platelet cyclic adenosine monophosphate (cyclic AMP) and consequently inhibit aggregation. The agents that most commonly inhibit platelet function are the nonsteroidal anti-inflammatory agents, which inhibit the platelet prostaglandin pathway and therefore second-wave aggregation. The most extensively studied of these agents is aspirin, which irreversibly acetylates the enzyme cyclo-oxygenase, inhibiting the production of thromboxane A_2 for the duration of the life of the platelet. This means that platelet function is still abnormal several days after even a single dose of aspirin. Other nonsteroidal anti-inflammatory agents such as indomethacin also act by inhibition of cyclo-oxygenase but do so in a manner that is not as well understood and is of a shorter duration. The following is a list of commonly used agents that have been documented to inhibit platelet function:

Nonsteroidal anti-inflammatory agents (cyclo-oxygenase inhibitors)
   Aspirin
   Indomethacin
   Sulfinpyrazone
   Naproxen (Naprosyn)
Phosphodiesterase inhibitors

Dipyridamole
Theophylline
Unknown mechanism
  Penicillins
  Clofibrate
  Dextran

Many other drugs have been described to inhibit platelet function in vitro, but the clinical significance of an isolated in vitro effect is uncertain.

Laboratory findings in patients taking these drugs vary but can include a prolonged bleeding time, abnormal platelet aggregation, and, in laboratories where it can be measured, decreased thromboxane production.

The clinical result is not a severe bleeding disorder but one that can exaggerate bleeding after surgery, particularly if the drugs are continued. Most normal individuals can tolerate a minor surgical procedure after aspirin, but it is especially important to avoid such medications in patients with underlying bleeding disorders. In these patients significant bleeding may occur.

Aspirin is ubiquitous in commercially available remedies, and the current interest in the role of platelet inhibition in the prevention of arteriosclerotic vascular disease further encourages the use of drugs that inhibit platelet function. These drugs are often useful, and the physician need not be afraid to administer them appropriately. Patient and physician awareness is the most important aspect of management. Should bleeding occur, a decision regarding discontinuance of the drug must be made.

MYELOPROLIFERATIVE DISORDERS. All of the myeloproliferative disorders can be complicated by the development of a platelet function abnormality. These are most likely intrinsic defects resulting from the production of abnormal cells by the diseased clone. Thrombocytosis has been associated with prolonged bleeding time, aggregation abnormalities, and even abnormalities of arachidonic acid metabolism. Similarly, patients with myeloid metaplasia often have large, functionally abnormal platelets. Patients with acute myelogenous leukemia or preleukemia may have functionally abnormal platelets, although this is less conspicuous because the patients are often dramatically thrombocytopenic. Support with platelet transfusions is the treatment for bleeding episodes.

UREMIA. Bruising and bleeding are frequent complications of uncontrolled uremia, and the fact that the bleeding time is often prolonged in these patients suggests a platelet function abnormality. The exact nature of the abnormality is uncertain, but it appears to be an extrinsic defect, since it improves when the patients are dialyzed.

VASCULAR PURPURAS

A variety of disorders of the vasculature can result in clinically significant bruising and bleeding in the presence of an otherwise normal coagulation system. Although most are relatively uncommon, they are important to recognize and differentiate from disorders of the coagulation system per se, since management will be entirely different.

Cushing's syndrome

Purpura associated with Cushing's syndrome or more frequently with exogenously administered corticosteroids is a common finding. Petechiae are uncommon. The cause of this purpura is unknown, but it appears to be related to decreased vascular support in the skin with spontaneous or minimally induced bruising.

Amyloidosis

Amyloidosis is a relatively uncommon disorder that can result in vascular infiltration with fibrous amyloid protein. This may or may not be associated with increased vascular fragility. An associated defect in coagulation factor function may, however, complicate this picture.

Vitamin C deficiency

Scurvy is fortunately now a rare disease but may be seen in indigent and alcoholic populations. Unless it is recognized and treated, a syndrome of petechiae and perifollicular hemorrhages may occur in the advanced state and present a diagnostic dilemma. Connective tissue and endothelial abnormalities as a result of the vitamin deficiency appear to be the cause. Bleeding gums are common, and subperiosteal hemorrhages occur in children. The vascular abnormality reverses with the administration of vitamin C.

Autoerythrocyte sensitization

Autoerythrocyte sensitization is a disorder predominantly of young women in whom spontaneous, inflammatory ecchymoses occur. The lesions usually appear at times of stress and can masquerade as a bleeding or thrombotic event. There is no apparent underlying coagulation abnormality. When the patients are tested by the intradermal injection of their own red cells, red cell membrane, or hemoglobin, the lesions can be reproduced. An important differentiating point is the inflammatory nature of the lesions. Steroids and antihistamines, however, have little effect. There is a strong psychologic element, and the therapy is treatment of the underlying depression or hysteria.

Schönlein-Henoch purpura

Schönlein-Henoch purpura is an allergic vasculitis that occurs most often in children 1 to 3 weeks after an upper respiratory infection. It has been postulated to represent a hypersensitivity to streptococci, but evidence for this is controversial.

The skin lesions, which occur predominantly over the extensor surfaces of the lower extremities, are the result of an aseptic vasculitis. They commence as urticarial lesions and then evolve into hemorrhagic lesions. Complement, IgA, and IgG have all been reported to be deposited in the skin capillary bed. Polyarthralgias and abdominal pain may occur, and there is an associated glomerulonephritis. Steroids and immunosuppressive therapy have been tried but are of uncertain benefit. Relapse occurs in 50% of the patients, and some progress to chronic renal failure.

Osler-Weber-Rendu syndrome

Osler-Weber-Rendu syndrome is an inherited disorder in which telangiectasias occur on the mucous membranes. The lesions become more numerous with time, and hemorrhage from these vessels frequently occurs. The size of the lesions and their hemorrhagic tendencies vary. Occasionally lesions are large and result in significant arteriovenous shunting. The bleeding that occurs can be life threatening. Nosebleeds are frequent and often difficult to control. Bleeding from the gastrointestinal tract can be the greatest management problem, often requiring repeated resections to remove the vascular lesions. About 20% of the patients have pulmonary arteriovenous fistulas. There is no specific treatment. Estrogens have been suggested, but they are of questionable benefit.

Various connective tissue disorders

Several congenital connective tissue disorders, including the Ehlers-Danlos syndrome, pseudoxanthoma elasticum, and osteogenesis imperfecta, can result in increased bruising and bleeding.

Other purpuric disorders

Purpura simplex is a syndrome of easy bruisability unassociated with a specific pathologic condition. It may represent a mixture of underdiagnosed mild platelet and coagulation abnormalities. Cryoglobulinemia and a variety of other γ-globulin abnormalities may be associated with purpura. Many vasculitides are manifested by a mild increased bruising tendency.

VON WILLEBRAND'S DISEASE

DEFINITION. Von Willebrand's disease is a common inherited bleeding disorder in which a prolonged bleeding time is associated with abnormalities of factor VIII. It is a disease of great interest, both because of its frequency and because it illustrates the complex relationship between the platelet and the intrinsic coagulation system.

ETIOLOGY AND PATHOGENESIS. Von Willebrand's disease is almost exclusively a congenital disorder, but rare cases of acquired disease have been reported. It has an autosomal dominant pattern of inheritance with variable expression. The basic abnormality in the disease is the diminution of the factor VIII–related "von Willebrand's" activity. Because this "von Willebrand's factor" (VIII_{vonW}) is required for certain normal platelet functions, the disease is manifested as a platelet function abnormality. The bleeding time is prolonged, and there is diminished platelet adherence to subendothelium and glass beads and diminished aggregation of platelets by the antibiotic ristocetin.

Unlike an intrinsic platelet defect, all these abnormalities are corrected by replenishment of the von Willebrand's factor in vivo or in vitro. Factor VIII is a high-molecular-weight glycoprotein with three activities that are readily measured in the laboratory: VIII_c, the clotting activity, which is missing in classic hemophilia A; VIII_{ag}, the antigenic activity, which can be measured by a variety of immunologic techniques; and VIII_{rcof}, the ristocetin cofactor, which is necessary to support ristocetin-induced platelet aggregation. Any or all of these factor VIII–related activities may be abnormal in von Willebrand's disease. The VIII_{ag} and VIII_{rcof} are of particular interest because they are normal in hemophilia A and low in classic von Willebrand's disease. Both have been shown to be produced by endothelial cells and to be present in platelets. They are both associated with the high-molecular-weight fraction of factor VIII, as is "von Willebrand factor" activity. It seems very likely that VIII_{rcof} in combination with VIII_{ag} represents the laboratory equivalent of the functional concept of a "von Willebrand's factor," and it is the diminution of this activity with or without an associated diminution of VIII_c that is the abnormality in von Willebrand's disease.

CLINICAL MANIFESTATIONS. There is great variability in the clinical severity of von Willebrand's disease. Patients with the classic severe form usually have a history of lifelong spontaneous bruising and episodes of bleeding from mucous membranes, especially epistaxis. Menorrhagia is frequent in women with von Willebrand's disease and can be a management problem, sometimes requiring hormonal manipulation for relief of excessive blood loss.

For unknown reasons factor VIII–related activities usually increase during pregnancy and with the use of birth control pills. Although postpartum hemorrhages do occur, they often do not, possibly because of this phenomenon. Hemarthroses, such as occur in hemophilia, are rare, and consequently no arthropathy is usually seen.

Patients with milder disease may have only easy bruisability or a history of excessive blood loss after a dental extraction. It is in this group of patients that a high index of suspicion is invaluable to the clinician, who might otherwise overlook mild symptoms or a suggestive family history in the preoperative evaluation of a generally well patient.

LABORATORY FINDINGS AND DIAGNOSIS. In severe von Willebrand's disease the diagnosis is straightforward, with a prolonged bleeding time in the presence of a normal platelet count and decreased VIII_c, VIII_{ag}, and VIII_{rcof}. Studies of ristocetin platelet aggregation and glass bead retention are abnormal. It is in the wide spectrum of milder disease and its variants that the diagnosis may be difficult, because only one or some combination of these tests may be abnormal. Especially in patients with so-called variant disease, there may be variability in the laboratory tests as well as in the manifestations of the disease at different times. The ristocetin cofactor, alone or in combination, is the most frequent abnormality, but it must be stressed that no single test currently in use can exclude the diagnosis of von Willebrand's disease. Sometimes repeated testing is necessary because of the fluctuations in test results that have been noted in some patients.

Not all laboratories have the capability of performing all the specialized studies that are necessary to exclude von Willebrand's disease. It is therefore often necessary to refer a patient with suspected von Willebrand's disease to a center where such testing can reliably be performed.

COURSE AND MANAGEMENT. Because of the variability of clinical manifestations, the treatment must be individualized. Cryoprecipitate has been shown to contain more von Willebrand factor activity than the more purified factor VIII concentrates and is therefore the treatment of choice when therapy becomes necessary. It is an intriguing observation that, when patients with von Willebrand's disease are transfused with plasma, cryoprecipitate, or purified factor VIII, there is a prolonged rise in VIII_c at a time when VIII_{ag} and VIII_{rcof} are declining (up to 24 hours after transfusion). Most remarkably, a similar rise in VIII_c occurs after the infusion of hemophilic plasma into a patient with von Willebrand's disease. Some clinicians have tried to use this phenomenon when planning treatment regimens, but its effect on the control of bleeding is unknown. Most clinicians treat patients immediately before a surgical procedure for the added benefit of normalization of VIII_{ag} and VIII_{rcof}, although which if any of these parameters determines the normalization of bleeding is still uncertain. The paradoxical rise in VIII_c after transfusion can sometimes be useful as a diagnostic test.

As with any disorder in which blood products are used, the benefits of cryoprecipitate infusion must be weighed in each situation against the small but significant risk of hepatitis. Conservative local measures, especially in a patient with mild disease, may be all that is necessary in many instances.

BIBLIOGRAPHY
Thrombocytopenia
Aster, R.N.: Thrombocytopenia due to enhanced platelet destruction. In Williams, W.J., and others, editors: Hematology, ed. 2, New York, 1977, McGraw-Hill Book Co.
Bolton, F.G., and Young, R.V.: Observations on cases of thrombocytopenic purpura due to quinine, sulphamezathine and quinidine, J. Clin. Pathol. **6**:320, 1953.
Harker, L.A., and Slichter, S.J.: The bleeding time as a screening test for evaluation of platelet function, N. Engl. J. Med. **238**:155, 1972.
Murphy, S.: Hereditary thrombocytopenia, Clin. Haematol. **1**:359, 1972.
Thompson, R.L., and others: Idiopathic thrombocytopenic purpura: long-term results of treatment and the prognostic significance of response to corticosteroids, Arch. Intern. Med. **130**:730, 1972.

Thrombocytosis
Hirsh, J., and Dacie, J.V.: Persistent post-splenectomy thrombocytosis and thrombo-embolism: a consequence of continuing anaemia, Br. J. Haematol. **12**:44, 1966.

Walsh, P.N., Murphy, S., and Barry, W.E.: The role of platelets in the pathogenesis of thrombosis and hemorrhage in patients with thrombocytosis, Thrombosis and Haemostasis **38**:105, 1977.

Qualitative platelet abnormalities
Packham, M.A., and Mustard, J.F.: Critical review—clinical pharmacology of platelets, Blood **50**:555, 1977.

Vascular purpuras
Gottlieb, A.J.: Nonthrombocytopenic purpuras. In Williams, W.J., and others, editors: Hematology, ed. 2, New York, 1977, McGraw-Hill Book Co.
McKusick, V.A.: Heritable disorders of connective tissue, ed. 4, St. Louis, 1972, The C.V. Mosby Co.

von Willebrand's disease
Firkin, B.G., and Howard, M.A.: Annotation: von Willebrand's disease (vWd), Br. J. Haematol. **32**:151, 1976.
Koutts, T., Howard, M.A., and Firkin, B.G.: Factor VIII physiology and pathology in man, Prog. Hematol. **11**:113, 1979.

81 • DISORDERS OF THE COAGULATION MECHANISM
Marc Rosenshein

Abnormalities involving the coagulation factors can lead to a variety of hemostatic disorders. These may be either congenital or acquired and may present a variety of clinical manifestations ranging from severe spontaneous bleeding to disseminated thrombosis.

Essential to understanding these disorders is a basic knowledge of the physiology of the coagulation cascade (Fig. 81-1). In this cascade two separate systems, the intrinsic and the extrinsic, converge in a final common pathway in the formation of fibrin. In the intrinsic pathway, plasma procoagulants are activated in a series of steps initiated by vessel damage. The extrinsic pathway, a more rapid mechanism, involves the interaction of a tissue factor with factor VII. This series of enzymatic reactions and its interactions with the fibrinolytic system, platelets, and blood vessels are designed both to ensure hemostasis when vascular integrity is breached and to prevent or remove clots within the intact vascular system. Congenital abnormalities most often involve either an absolute deficiency or a functional deficiency of a single coagulation factor. Acquired disorders, on the other hand, frequently involve multiple factors, as well as the other components of the hemostatic system mentioned.

A good history is the most important screening test for coagulation disorders, with particular attention directed toward family history and previous abnormal bleeding, especially that associated with dental extractions, surgery, or trauma. A history of abnormal bruising or epistaxis is less specific. Laboratory screening should be directed toward each of the various components of the coagulation cascade

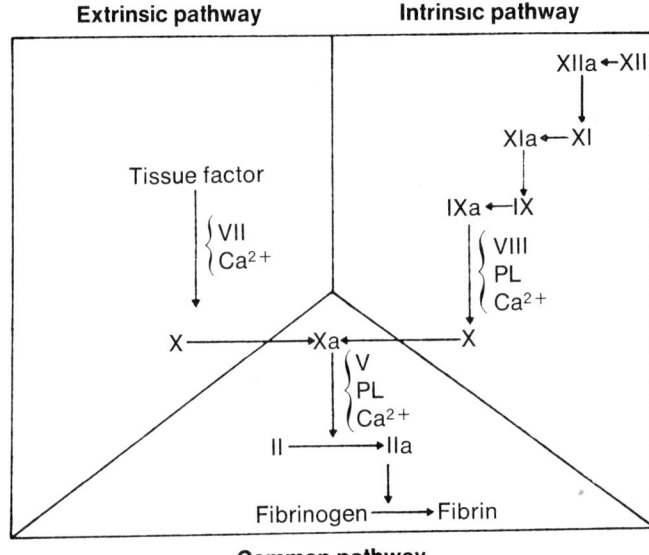

Fig. 81-1. Extrinsic and intrinsic pathways to factor X activation and fibrin formation. In presence of calcium, inactive plasma procoagulants are activated in cascade mechanism to convert inactive factor X to activated Xa. This is intrinsic mechanism. Tissue factor and factor VII in presence of calcium also act on X, converting ti to Xa. After this, Xa in presence of factor V, platelets, and calcium converts factor II (prothrombin) to IIa (thrombin), which in turn converts fibrinogen to fibrin. *a*, Activated; Ca^{2+} calcium; *PL*, platelets. (From Esneuf, M.P.: Br. Med. Bull. 33:213, 1977.)

(Fig. 81-1). The prothrombin time (PT) detects abnormalities of the extrinsic and common pathway factors. The partial thromboplastin time (PTT) screens for abnormalities of the intrinsic and common pathway factors. Both PT and PTT are affected by abnormalities of the common pathway. The thrombin time (TT) and the fibrinogen level can be used to assess the quantitative and qualitative aspects of fibrinogen to fibrin conversion. These four tests (PT, PTT, TT, and fibrinogen level) combined with a platelet count and template bleeding time constitute a complete screen of the hemostatic mechanism. Other more specific tests such as factor assays can be selected using the results of the initial screen.

INHERITED DISORDERS OF COAGULATION

The inherited disorders of coagulation are characterized by a lifelong history of abnormal bleeding. The milder forms, however, may escape early detection and are manifested later in life at a time of stress to the hemostatic mechanism, such as surgery or dental extraction. Of the more common inherited disorders, factor VIII and IX deficiency (hemophilia A and B) are inherited as sex-linked recessive traits, with affected males and carrier females, and von Willebrand's disease is an autosomal dominant trait with variable penetrance.

Hemophilia A

DEFINITION. Hemophilia A is an inherited deficiency of functional factor VIII with an associated bleeding tendency proportional to the severity of the deficiency. It is the most common inherited disorder of coagulation. Severe hemophilia with factor VIII levels less than 1% of the normal value is associated with serious and often apparently spontaneous bleeding. Individuals with mild hemophilia (5% to 25% the normal level of factor VIII) may have little or no increase in bleeding and escape detection for years, whereas those with hemophilia of intermediate severity (factor VIII levels 1% to 4% of normal) usually have no spontaneous bleeding but may have bleeding with surgery or trauma.

ETIOLOGY AND PATHOGENESIS. Although the level of factor VIII as measured by a functional assay of in vitro clotting is depressed in hemophilia A, the antigenic measurement of factor VIII protein reveals normal values. Thus hemophilia A is caused by the presence of a functionally deficient factor VIII molecule rather than by the absence of production of factor VIII. Factor VIII is a very large molecule or perhaps a complex of molecules whose fine structure–function relationships are not well known. For these reasons the molecular defect in hemophilia A is not yet clearly understood. Nearly all cases of hemophilia are inherited, and carrier detection or family history reveals the presence of the trait. In some rare cases, however, it appears that a new spontaneous mutation may be responsible.

Hemophilia is carried on the X chromosome of the female carrier. Although her factor VIII antigen/activity ratio is abnormal, she is unlikely to manifest any bleeding tendency because of the production of normal factor VIII via her other X chromosome. However, 50% of her offspring will inherit the abnormal chromosome, with the daughters being carriers and the sons having the clinical disease. Conceivably, the daughter of a hemophiliac male and a carrier female could be severely affected with two abnormal X chromosomes, but this is obviously a rare occurrence.

CLINICAL MANIFESTATIONS. The clinical manifestations of hemophilia A are directly related to the factor VIII level. Although mild hemophilia is often not detected until later in life, severe hemophilia usually can be diagnosed in infancy or early childhood. Often, postcircumcision bleeding is the initial manifestation. Because of the limited activity of the infant, spontaneous bleeding is frequently not a problem during the first year. With increasing activity come hematomas, oral bleeding, and hemarthroses. Hemarthroses are common clinical problems. In decreasing order of frequency, they involve the knee, ankle, hip, elbow, wrist, and shoulder. There is often a history of preceding trauma or stress, but this may be relatively minor. The affected joints become painful and then swollen, warm, and exquisitely tender. With repeated hemarthroses, extensive destructive changes within the joint may occur, leading eventually to loss of cartilage, osteoporosis, contractures, and functionally useless joints. Hematomas and other soft tissue bleeding may occur into subcutaneous tissues or muscles, most commonly in the calves, thighs, buttocks, or forearms. Pseudotumors, which are recurrent encapsulated hematomas, can mimic malignant tumors and be very destructive locally. Bleeding may also occur in more critical areas such as the tongue, floor of the mouth, or pharynx and may compromise the airway. Retroperitoneal bleeding or intra-abdominal bleeding may occur, mimicking other acute abdominal problems or causing nerve compression. Hematuria is also common. Bleeding from dental extractions, often after apparent initial hemostasis, occurs frequently and can be profuse and prolonged. Intracranial hemorrhage is one of the most feared bleeding manifestations and is a leading cause of death among hemophiliacs. In contrast to platelet disorders, mucosal and cutaneous bleeding are rare in hemophilia.

LABORATORY FINDINGS. Although clinical manifestations may be suggestive, the specific diagnosis of hemophilia is made in the laboratory. The whole blood clotting time is usually abnormal in severe hemophilia but can be normal in milder cases. The PTT, which assesses the intrinsic coagulation pathway, is prolonged, and the PT, TT, and bleeding time are normal. Specific diagnosis requires a functional assay for factor VIII activity demonstrating decreased or absent activity. Antigenic assays for factor VIII reveal normal or elevated values, demonstrating the presence of a functionally deficient factor VIII molecule.

Carrier detection can usually be accomplished by measuring both factor VIII activity and antigen levels in female relatives of hemophiliacs. Carriers generally demonstrate a relative excess of antigen compared to functional activity. However, some carriers cannot be reliably detected with these methods, a situation that can make genetic counseling difficult.

MANAGEMENT. The first principle of therapy should be caution and the avoidance of trauma. This should not exclude the hemophiliac from most normal recreational and vocational activities.

The major therapy for acute bleeding episodes consists of using plasma or factor VIII concentrates to raise the factor VIII to adequate levels for sufficient periods of time for hemostasis to occur. For most major bleeding, this requires factor VIII levels of 30% to 40% of normal, with frequent administration (every 12 to 24 hours) necessary owing to the short half-life of factor VIII in the circulation. Minor hemarthroses or hematomas can be managed with lower factor VIII levels, and major surgery or severe trauma may necessitate higher levels. Dental extractions require meticulous attention to local hemostasis, as well as factor VIII supplements and the use of systemic ϵ-aminocaproic acid to prevent lysis of the clot formed. Circulating antibodies to factor VIII develop in approximately 6% of hemophiliacs. This can be a major therapeutic problem, requiring transfusion with massive amounts of factor VIII concentrate and immunosuppressive therapy to treat bleeding episodes.

Probably the most important advance in hemophilia therapy has been the comprehensive care approach, in which many health professionals assess and treat all aspects of the disorder. These include hematologists, orthopedists, dentists, physical therapists, and vocational and psychosocial counselors. The comprehensive approach combined with early, at-home, patient- or parent-administered factor VIII concentrate therapy for minor bleeding has allowed a more normal life-style and the avoidance of chronic complications for many hemophiliacs.

Hemophilia B

DEFINITION. Hemophilia B or Christmas disease is the functional deficiency of factor IX and is associated with a bleeding tendency.

ETIOLOGY AND PATHOGENESIS. Patients with hemophilia B can be divided into two groups: those with no detectable factor IX antigenic material and those who have antigenic factor IX but a functionally deficient factor IX molecule, similar to the defect in hemophilia A. Hemophilia B is an X-linked recessive trait with genetic considerations identical to those of hemophilia A.

CLINICAL MANIFESTATIONS. The clinical picture of factor IX deficiency is indistinguishable from that of factor VIII deficiency, with the clinical severity directly related to the severity of the deficiency.

LABORATORY FINDINGS. The same coagulation screening tests as those for hemophilia A are used. The assay of factor IV function reveals markedly decreased values. Antigenic factor IX levels are either normal or decreased, which makes carrier detection less reliable.

MANAGEMENT. The overall principles of comprehensive care discussed for hemophilia A also apply to hemophilia B. Treatment of most minor to moderate bleeding episodes can be accomplished with plasma transfusions. Commercial concentrates of the vitamin K–dependent factors (II, VII, IX, X) are available but should be reserved for more severe bleeding episodes because of the increased hepatitis risk and thrombogenicity associated with these concentrates. Clinically significant antibodies to factor IX are rare.

Von Willebrand's disease

Von Willebrand's disease, a hereditary disorder of coagulation characterized by a combination of factor VIII deficiency and a unique platelet function abnormality related to this deficiency, is discussed in Chapter 80, since the clinical manifestations are those of platelet dysfunction.

Other hereditary coagulation disorders

Factor XI deficiency. Factor XI deficiency is an autosomal recessive disorder most common in Jews. The coagulation disorder is usually mild and is manifested by bleeding following surgical procedures.

Factor XII deficiency. Factor XII deficiency and deficiencies of *Fletcher, Fitzgerald,* and *Passovoy* factors are associated with a prolonged PTT but no hemorrhagic manifestations.

Factor V, VII, X, and prothrombin deficiency. Deficiencies of factors, V, VII, X, and prothrombin are rare autosomal recessive traits that may be manifested by mild to severe bleeding episodes requiring plasma transfusion on occasion.

Fibrinogen deficiency and dysfibrinogenemias. Fibrinogen deficiency and dysfibrinogenemias are rare disorders that can be manifested by bleeding, requiring transfusion with plasma or cryoprecipitate. Surprisingly, some dysfibrinogenemias can cause a thrombotic tendency.

Factor XIII deficiency. Factor XIII deficiency is a rare disorder in which there is a deficiency of fibrin stabilization. Clinically, it is manifested by delayed bleeding after initial hemostasis and by poor wound healing. It is the only disorder in which all routine coagulation screening tests are normal. The diagnosis is made by demonstrating the solubility of the patient's fibrin clot in 5M urea. The therapy is plasma transfusion.

ACQUIRED DISORDERS OF COAGULATION
Vitamin K deficiency

Deficiency of vitamin K, which is necessary for the synthesis of prothrombin (factor II) and factors VII, IX, and X, can lead to a hemorrhagic disorder. Vitamin K is responsible for the final activation of the already formed coagulation proteins produced by the liver. This activation of preformed factors accounts for the relatively rapid onset of action of administered vitamin K. The normal diet has a great excess of vitamin K, so dietary lack is not a usual cause of deficiency. Vitamin K, however, is fat soluble, and the malabsorption syndromes, particularly with *steatorrhea,* can be associated with vitamin K deficiency, as well as with deficiencies of the other fat-soluble vitamins A, D, and E. Vitamin K deficiency at birth may lead to *hemorrhagic disease of the newborn,* which can result in serious or even fatal gastrointestinal or intracranial bleeding.

A variety of drugs can interact with vitamin K. *Antibiotics* may interfere with vitamin K production by intestinal bacteria, an important source of the vitamin. *Salicylates* in large amounts and *propylthiouracil* may have vitamin K antagonist properties. *Coumarin*-class anticoagulants are vitamin K antagonists and will be discussed later in the chapter.

The clinical picture of vitamin K deficiency is similar to that of other coagulation factor deficiencies and includes hematomas and gastrointestinal, intracranial, and postoperative hemorrhage. The diagnosis may be confirmed by the rapid reversal of both the clinical and laboratory evidence of the deficiency within several hours after vitamin K administration. In cases of life-threatening hemorrhage, transfusion of plasma can provide more rapid correction of the factor deficiencies. Hemorrhagic disease of the newborn should be prevented with prophylactic vitamin K administration to the infant at birth.

Liver disease

A variety of hepatic diseases can cause a number of different coagulation abnormalities. Obstructive jaundice results in malabsorption of vitamin K and can produce the clinical picture just described, which is easily reversible with parenteral vitamin K administration. Hepatocellular liver disease, on the other hand, can cause a variety of hemostatic abnormalities, including a deficiency of the vitamin K–dependent factors. However, because the basic defect is in the synthesis of the proteins by the hepatocyte and not in the final vitamin K–dependent steps, the deficiencies are not corrected by vitamin K therapy. In addition to the vitamin K–dependent factors, factor V and fibrinogen are frequently depressed in severe parenchymal liver disease, both because of decreased synthesis by the liver and because of increased consumption associated with intravascular coagulation. Fibrinolysis is frequently increased, and fibrinogen degradation products are cleared less effectively than normal. An abnormal fibrinogen is sometimes produced in association with chronic liver disease or hepatocellular carcinoma and can produce a prolonged TT. Thrombocytopenia is frequently present with severe liver disease, particularly in association with portal hypertension and splenomegaly or with disseminated intravascular coagulation. Therapy for the hemostatic abnormalities associated with liver disease is difficult. Plasma in large amounts may temporarily improve the bleeding disorders associated with factor deficiency. Platelet transfusion can be used if severe thrombocytopenia is a problem. Concentrates of vitamin K–dependent factors or ϵ-aminocaproic acid should be used only with great caution.

Acquired anticoagulants

Antibodies to factor VIII are the most common acquired anticoagulants. Those associated with hemophilia were discussed earlier. They may also occur in previously normal patients or in association with drug reactions, lupus erythematosus, or inflammatory bowel disease. Therapy for bleeding associated with these inhibitors can be difficult, requiring large doses of factor VIII concentrates, immunosuppression with steroids or cytotoxic drugs, or even exchange plasmapheresis. Inhibitors of other individual factors are rare. A large percentage of patients with lupus erythematosus have abnormal coagulation tests (PT, PTT,

TT). This so-called lupus anticoagulant is not usually associated with a significant bleeding tendency.

Disseminated intravascular coagulation

DEFINITION. Disseminated intravascular coagulation (DIC), also known as consumption coagulopathy or defibrination syndrome, is an entity characterized by (1) the consumption of platelets and coagulation factors during abnormal intravascular clotting; (2) the deposition of fibrin in the small vessels of various organs and tissues; and (3) the appearance of fibrinogen-fibrin degradation products (FDP) in the circulation as a result of this activation and the lysis of intravascular fibrin. Some degree of activation of the coagulation system occurs in a wide variety of clinical circumstances, but the term "DIC" should be reserved for instances in which significant clinical sequelae result from this activation, such as bleeding or organ dysfunction owing to intravascular clotting.

ETIOLOGY. A wide variety of stimuli can initiate DIC. Among these are bacterial, fungal, viral, and protozoal infections, complications of pregnancy, metastatic carcinoma, leukemia, various liver diseases, surgery, and trauma. A more detailed list is outlined below, but this should not be considered complete. Basically, any condition causing exposure of the circulation to activators of coagulation can result in DIC.

Disorders associated with defibrination*

I. Infections
   A. Gram-negative endotoxinemia with hypotension or shock
      1. Fulminant meningococcemia
      2. Septicemia owing to *Escherichia coli, Pseudomonas, Klebsiella-Enterobacter, Haemophilus influenzae, Proteus,* and so on
   B. Severe gram-positive septicemia
      1. Overwhelming pneumococcal septicemia (often in an asplenic patient)
      2. β-Hemolytic streptococcal septicemia (rare)
      3. Staphylococcal septicemia (rare)
   C. Rocky Mountain spotted fever
   D. Viral infections
      1. Influenza A
      2. Disseminated herpes infection
      3. Hemorrhagic fevers (Korean, Thai)
      4. *Plasmodium falciparum* malaria (overwhelming parasitemia)
II. Complications of pregnancy and delivery
   A. Gram-negative endotoxinemia after septic abortion or amnionitis
   B. Abruptio placentae
   C. Amniotic fluid embolism
   D. Retained dead fetus
   E. Hypertonic saline abortion
   F. Toxemia of pregnancy
   G. Hydatidiform mole
   H. Obstetric hemolytic-uremic syndromes
III. Pediatric disorders
   A. Disorders of the newborn
      1. Defibrination in the infant following abruptio placentae
      2. Multiple pregnancy with retained dead twin fetus
      3. Intrauterine or newborn infection
   B. Purpura fulminans
IV. Malignant diseases
   A. Metastatic carcinoma: prostate, pancreas, lung, stomach, colon, breast
   B. Leukemia: acute promyelocytic (frequent), acute and chronic granulocytic (rare)
V. Liver diseases
   A. Cirrhosis with portal hypertension
   B. Acute severe hepatic necrosis
VI. Complications of surgery
   A. Procedures involving extracorporeal circulation
   B. Prostatic surgery
VII. Disorders producing critical tissue damage
   A. Brain tissue destruction
   B. Massive trauma causing irreversible shock and acidosis
   C. Heatstroke
   D. Extensive burns (with infection)
VIII. Miscellaneous
   A. Hemolytic transfusion reactions
   B. Acute systemic vasculitis
   C. Arterial aneurysms
   D. Massive venous thrombosis
   E. Giant hemangioma
   F. Cardiac arrest
   G. Venomous snakebite

PATHOGENESIS. DIC produces clinical disease either through abnormal bleeding or by tissue damage owing to intravascular fibrin deposition (Fig. 81-2). Consumption of coagulation factors, particularly factors V, VIII, and XIII and fibrinogen itself, contributes to the bleeding tendency, as does thrombocytopenia from the consumption of platelets. Fibrinolysis is accelerated, causing the release of FDPs into the circulation. The FDPs potentiate the bleeding tendency both by interfering with the normal fibrinogen-fibrin conversion and by inhibiting platelet function. Intravascular fibrin deposition can damage a variety of organs, most notably the kidney. Other sensitive organs include the lung, adrenal glands, pituitary gland, liver, bone marrow, brain, and skin. Ischemic tissue damage tends to produce more activation of intravascular coagulation, potentiating and worsening the DIC in a type of "vicious circle." Mechanical damage to red blood cells caused by fibrin strands is responsible for the microangiopathic hemolytic anemia frequently seen.

CLINICAL MANIFESTATIONS. The clinical presentation of DIC is closely linked to its precipitating cause. The sudden appearance of generalized bleeding, such as prolonged

---

*From Rappaport, S.I.: Defibrination syndromes. In Williams, W.J., and others, editors: Hematology, ed. 2, New York, 1972, McGraw-Hill Book Co.

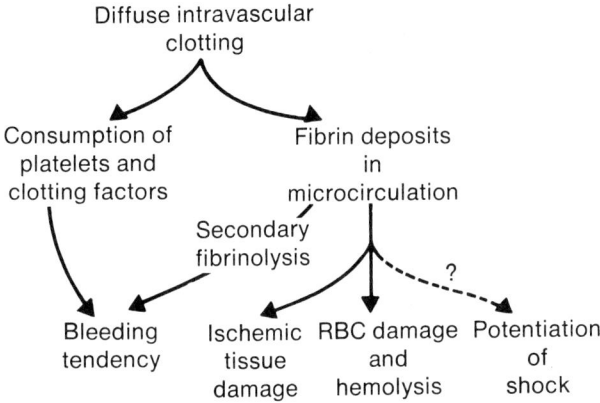

Fig. 81-2. Mechanisms by which diffuse intravascular coagulation produces clinical disease. (From Rappaport, S.I.: Defibrination syndromes. In Williams, W.J., and others, editors: Hematology, ed. 2, New York, 1972, McGraw-Hill Book Co.)

oozing from needle punctures or cutdown sites, is the classic presentation of acute, severe DIC. Often shock, renal failure, and respiratory failure (adult respiratory distress syndrome) accompany the bleeding tendency. More slowly developing or chronic DIC is more often manifested by thrombotic manifestations and organ damage, since there is time for the body to respond to the consumption of factors and platelets with increased production and thus to avoid a severe bleeding tendency.

LABORATORY FINDINGS. The only completely reliable way to make the laboratory diagnosis of DIC is by radioactive-labeled survival studies demonstrating the accelerated consumption of platelets and fibrinogen. These studies are generally not practical or available. When the depletion of coagulation factors in DIC exceeds the body's synthetic abilities, a prolongation of the PT, PTT, and TT and a low fibrinogen level result. FDPs also tend to prolong the TT by acting as inhibitors of fibrin formation. Specific factor assays reveal depletion of a number of factors, particularly factors V, VIII, and XIII and fibrinogen.

Moderate to severe thrombocytopenia can occur. The bleeding time is usually prolonged disproportionately to the platelet count owing to the antiplatelet activity of FDPs.

There are a variety of tests to detect the result of the increased fibrinolysis, the FDPs. These include immunodiffusion, immunoelectrophoresis, tanned red cell agglutination inhibition, and agglutination of coated latex particles. They are all designed to detect fibrinogen- or fibrin-related antigens in serum, which normally has none. These tests effectively detect the larger FDPs but may not detect the smaller fragments, which are also clinically important. They are also not specific for DIC, since levels may be elevated in patients with localized thrombosis such as thrombophlebitis or pulmonary embolism. Tests for serum fibrin monomers, such as the ethanol gelation and prot-

amine sulfate precipitation tests for "paracoagulation," are less specific and less useful.

MANAGEMENT. The most important aspect of the therapy for DIC is treatment or elimination of the underlying cause. If this is accomplished, the DIC will be self-limited and may require no other specific therapy. If bleeding is severe, replacement of volume deficits with whole blood, factors with plasma, platelets with platelet concentrates, and factor VIII and fibrinogen with cryoprecipitate may be lifesaving. The theoretic objection to "adding fuel to the fire" by replacing depleted factors in DIC has not been shown to apply clinically. The use of heparin therapy to arrest the intravascular coagulation is hazardous and can be disastrous, leading to increased severe bleeding. Possible exceptions to this may be prophylactic heparinization before chemotherapy for acute progranulocytic leukemia and in the treatment of purpura fulminans, in which thrombotic manifestations cause much of the clinical problem. Purpura fulminans is a disease with acute necrosis of parts of the body owing to vasculitis and thrombosis; it is associated with DIC.

The use of an inhibitor of fibrinolysis (ϵ-aminocaproic acid) is also not recommended. Fibrinolysis is a secondary phenomenon, and inhibiting it can cause increased organ damage owing to intravascular thrombosis.

Fibrinolytic states

Occasionally a patient manifests an acquired bleeding disorder without either clinical or laboratory evidence of DIC but with evidence of isolated accelerated fibrinolysis. The fibrinogen concentration is usually low, since fibrinogen is also destroyed by plasmin. The platelet count and other coagulation screens are generally normal. The euglobulin lysis time is extremely short, reflecting the increased fibrinolysis. This syndrome may appear as primary fibrinolysis without any obvious precipitating cause or may result from some of the same causes as DIC, such as prostatic carcinoma, amniotic fluid embolism, or heatstroke. There is some disagreement as to whether this fibrinolysis is the primary process or whether it follows a self-limited episode of DIC. For this reason the diagnosis should be certain and DIC should be thoroughly ruled out before ϵ-aminocaproic acid, the treatment of choice, is administered.

ANTICOAGULANT THERAPY
Heparin

Heparin is a powerful anticoagulant that acts at several points in the coagulation cascade. It serves as a cofactor to antithrombin III, a naturally occurring inhibitor of coagulation. Heparin binds to antithrombin III and increases its efficiency as an inhibitor by several thousand times. This complex (heparin plus antithrombin III) inhibits thrombin and the active forms of factors IX, X, and XI.

Heparin can be administered in a number of ways, depending on the indication for anticoagulation. For the treatment of established thrombosis, heparin should be administered intravenously, either by continuous infusion or by intermittent injection. Continuous infusion is just as effective as intermittent injection and has been shown to be associated with fewer serious bleeding complications. Continuous infusion heparin should be administered at a rate that keeps the activated PTT in the range of 1½ to 2 times the control value. Heparin can also be administered in lower subcutaneous doses when used as prophylaxis against thrombosis in bedridden or postoperative patients. It is usually given two or three times daily. The prophylactic dose of heparin should not prolong the PTT but may prolong the TT, which is the most sensitive test for heparin effect.

Should bleeding complications occur during heparin therapy, simply discontinuing treatment may be adequate, since therapeutic levels of heparin are cleared from the circulation quickly. For life-threatening bleeding, protamine sulfate injected intravenously will immediately reverse the anticoagulant effect of heparin on a milligram for milligram basis.

Coumarin anticoagulants

The coumarin-class anticoagulants are vitamin K antagonists. They lower the levels of prothrombin (factor II) and factors VII, IX, and X by interfering with the final steps of synthesis of these molecules. The effect of these drugs on the various factor levels depends on the half-life of the factor. Factor VII levels fall most quickly and recover most quickly owing to its short half-life, and factor IX levels change most slowly owing to its longer half-life. Factors II and X have intermediate levels and half-lives.

The coumarin anticoagulants are administered orally in daily doses. The best laboratory test for monitoring coumarin therapy is the PT, which should be prolonged to 2 to 2½ times control values for adequate and safe anticoagulation.

An important aspect of therapy with coumarin anticoagulants is their interaction with a large number of drugs that may potentiate or lessen their anticoagulant activity through a variety of mechanisms. Barbiturates tend to accelerate coumarin metabolism and lessen its effect. Salicylates can interfere with vitamin K metabolism and potentiate its effect. Phenylbutazone and indomethacin tend to displace coumarin from its protein binding sites and potentiate its effect. A more complete list of coumarin interactions can be found in the article by Koch and Sellers listed in the bibliography.

When excessive bleeding results from coumarin anticoagulants, stopping the drug leads to a gradual return of factor levels to normal over several days. Vitamin K administration can correct the defects in 12 to 24 hours, and plasma transfusion can rapidly correct the coagulation abnormalities if life-threatening bleeding is a problem.

BIBLIOGRAPHY
Inherited disorders of coagulation

Gralnick, I., and others: Factor VIII, Ann. Intern. Med. **86:**598, 1977.
Harker, L.A.: The hemostasis manual, ed. 2, Philadelphia, 1974, F.A. Davis Co.
Hougie, C.: Disorders of hemostasis—congenital disorders of blood coagulation factors. In Williams, W.J., and others, editors: Hematology, ed. 2, New York, 1977, McGraw-Hill Book Co.
Spaet, T.H.: Progress in hemostasis and thrombosis, vol. 1, New York, 1972, Grune & Stratton, Inc.

Acquired disorders of coagulation

Harker, L.A.: The hemostasis manual, ed. 2, Philadelphia, 1974, F.A. Davis Co.
Shapiro, S.: Disorders of hemostasis—acquired disorders of blood coagulation. In Williams, W.J., and others, editors: Hematology, ed. 2, New York, 1977, McGraw-Hill Book Co.

Disseminated intravascular coagulation

Deyken, D.: The clinical challenge of disseminated intravascular coagulation, N. Engl. J. Med. **283:**636, 1970.
Rappaport, S.I.: Defibrination syndromes. In Williams, W.J., and others, editors: Hematology, ed. 2, New York, 1977, McGraw-Hill Book Co.

Anticoagulant therapy

Koch, W.J., and Sellers, E.M.: Drug interactions with Coumarin anticoagulants, N. Engl. J. Med. **285:**487, 1971.
Williams, W.J.: Disorders of hemostasis-thrombosis. In Williams, W.J., and others, editors: Hematology, ed. 2, New York, 1977, McGraw-Hill Book Co.

DENTAL CORRELATIONS

ANEMIAS AND DEFICIENCY STATES
Pernicious anemia
S. Gary Cohen

The onset of pernicious anemia (PA) is usually insidious and progressive. The diverse clinical presentation results in an average period of almost 1½ years between onset of symptoms and the correct diagnosis.

ORAL MANIFESTATIONS. The mucosa may appear pale or icteric. Erythematous macules with irregular borders involving any of the mucosal surfaces may be an early sign of pernicious anemia. The tongue undergoes atrophic or fissural changes in 50% to 60% of these patients. Atrophy of the filiform and later fungiform papillae imparts the classic "beefy red" appearance to the tongue while the fissures may change to lobules as the disease progresses. The progression from fissures to lobules may be secondary to decreased salivary production. Lingual paresthesia, burning, or itching may develop that resolves with therapy. Distortions in taste may accompany the thinned epithelium. Increased susceptibility to irritation and trauma results from the oral epithelium becoming parakeratinized or nonkeratinized.

In long-standing, undiagnosed cases ulcers appear in areas of severe atrophy. These lesions cause significant discomfort, particularly when a patient wears a dental prosthesis. The dentist may be the first clinician to examine the patient and should remember to rule out pernicious anemia in cases of nonspecific stomatitis. If lesions appear in a patient with known pernicious anemia, the practitioner should suspect relapse secondary to cessation of vitamin B_{12} therapy.

DENTAL MANAGEMENT. The oral lesions will heal rapidly when vitamin B_{12} therapy is initiated. There are no contraindications to dental treatment in a patient taking vitamin B_{12} for pernicious anemia.

Folic acid deficiency
S. Gary Cohen

The clinical presentation of a folic acid deficiency is similar to vitamin B_{12} deficiency except that central nervous system symptoms are rare. Individuals with an increased incidence of folic acid deficiency anemia include alcoholics, hemodialysis patients (folic acid is dialyzable), patients taking phenytoin (Dilatin) or oral contraceptives, and those being treated with folic acid inhibitors such as methotrexate.

ORAL MANIFESTATIONS. The most common presentation is a red, sore tongue with varying degrees of papillary atrophy, which progresses until the tongue is smooth and shiny. Angular cheilitis is seen and often becomes secondarily infected with bacteria and fungi. Candidal infections of the mouth and at times the entire gastrointestinal tracts can be found. In some cases ulcerative stomatitis may be present.

Histologically, the epithelium shows an increased nuclear size similar to that seen in vitamin B_{12} deficiency. The cells of the prickle and granular layers of the oral epithelium are found to be enlarged and ballooning. The cytoplasm is lightly stained and nuclear chromatin is clumped in a manner similar to the megaloblastic changes noted in pernicious anemia. Decreased keratinization and extensive shallow ulcerations are also described.

Aplastic anemia
S. Gary Cohen

The clinical picture of aplastic anemia combines the signs and symptoms of severe anemia with those of neutropenia and thrombocytopenia. These patients may present with the mucosal pallor of anemia, but glossitis, glossopyrosis, and papillary atrophy are rare.

One cause of aplastic anemia is the injudicious use of chloromycetin. This antibiotic should only be prescribed when other antibiotics are ineffective.

ORAL MANIFESTATIONS. The purpura and spontaneous gingival bleeding of thrombocytopenia may be seen. These patients are often advised by the dentist to discontinue oral hygiene measures to prevent gingival bleeding, but the accumulation of plaque can intensify gingival ulceration and bleeding. Some oral hygiene measures should be taken to prevent this additional problem.

A severe ulcerative stomatitis and/or pharyngitis is common in all neutropenic patients. These ulcers are necrotic and foul-smelling and may reach several centimeters in diameter. Because of the lack of neutrophils, purulence is absent. Another manifestation is cervical and submandibular lymphadenopathy.

DENTAL MANAGEMENT. A thorough dental evaluation will reveal any source of chronic or potential infection. The elimination of the source will improve the long-term prognosis by decreasing the incidence of septicemia during the neutropenic state (less than $500/mm^3$). In chronic or recurrent cases proper patient management should include an oral hygiene program. Patients should use a soft toothbrush, further softened by hot water and dental tape, which causes less gingival trauma than floss. This technique has been effective in treating patients even with platelet counts of less than $10,000/mm^3$. Gingival ulceration and bleeding may be reduced by decreasing plaque accumulation. This will result in fewer transfusions and a decreased potential for septicemia.

If emergency dental treatment is necessary during periods of severe bone marrow suppression, use of platelet and neutrophil transfusions should be discussed with the hematologist.

The associated ulcerative stomatitis can be severe enough to prevent eating, drinking, and swallowing medication. The management is usually palliative. Good oral hygiene must be maintained, and saline and sodium bicarbonate mouth rinses are recommended to cleanse the surfaces of the ulcers. Use of topical anesthetics will improve comfort during eating. Diphenhydramine (Benadryl) and 0.5% dyclonine (Dyclone) mixed with kaolin/pectin or milk of magnesia has been effective for this purpose.

Antibacterial agents can be used on the ulcers to reduce secondary infection. Use of a vacuformed splint to hold topical medications is recommended. The splint is lined with a 10% neomycin and 1% bacitracin ointment. After the patient wears the splint for 2 hours it is removed and rinsed, and a nystatin (Mycostatin) ointment (10,000 U/g) is applied for the next 2 hours. These alternating medications are used until improvement is noticed. Aqueous chlorhexidine (0.2%) solution has also been used with good results. This potent antibacterial oral rinse is used extensively in Europe and the Middle East, but it has not been approved for use in the United States.

Partial or full dentures should be removed to reduce the chance of ulcers caused by friction. When not in use, dentures are soaked in a nystatin solution (10 ml of a 500,000 U/ml solution in 6 oz water). Orthodontic appliances should be removed because they prevent optimal oral hygiene and can act as a source of irritation.

The most serious complication of dental treatment for neutropenic patients is severe life-threatening infection.

Only necessary dental procedures are performed. If the neutrophil count is less than 2500/mm^3, the patient should receive prophylactic broad spectrum antibiotic coverage. If oral infection develops, specimens of the infection should be submitted for culture and sensitivity testing. While awaiting the results the patient should be started on a broad-spectrum antibiotic or combination of antibiotics.

Another consideration is bleeding secondary to a decreased platelet count. In order to ensure adequate clotting a bleeding profile, including a platelet count, should be obtained before any dental treatment. If the platelet count is less than 50,000/mm^3, posterosuperior and inferoalveolar block injections are dangerous because of the potential for hematoma formation and therefore should be avoided (see section on dental management in thrombocytopenia).

Medical management often includes transfusions and steroids and must be considered during dental treatment. Viral hepatitis is a potential hazard with blood transfusions. Therefore sterilization precautions should be taken (see section on hepatitis). Corticosteroid therapy at adrenosuppressive levels increases susceptibility to shock (see section on adrenals).

Specific dental treatment is limited to infection control and palliation until the patient's blood counts improve. If an acute infection develops and extraction is necessary, a bleeding profile should be obtained. In addition a culture and sensitivity of the areas to be treated are necessary to determine whether unusual oral organisms are present. If the patient is thrombocytopenic, platelet transfusions may be indicated.

Iron deficiency anemia
S. Gary Cohen

The clinical manifestations of iron deficiency anemia generally appear in relatively severe disease and may be discovered during a routine history and examination by a dentist. The signs and symptoms include pallor of the skin and nail beds, progressive fingernail concavity resulting in a spooning effect (koilonychia), a tendency of the nails to crack and split, fatigue, anorexia, headache, and neurologic disturbances. The patient may crave unusual or toxic substances such as paint, starches, or ice.

ORAL MANIFESTATIONS. Gingival and mucosal pallor may be evident along with atrophy of the lingual papillae. Atrophy of the filiform and fungiform papillae continues until the dorsal surface of the tongue becomes totally smooth and its color changes from pale pink to red. The tip and lateral borders are usually affected first, resulting in a patchy effect that may be confused with geographic tongue. However, unlike geographic tongue, these atrophic areas lack a white keratotic border and undergo a progressive increase in size rather than an alteration in distribution. All of these changes cause an increased susceptibility to irritation and traumatic ulceration. Symptoms of soreness and burning may result. Angular cheilitis or leukoplakia gradually develops in some cases. It has been suggested that the oral lesions are caused by a concurrent pyridoxine deficiency rather than the anemia.

DENTAL MANAGEMENT. Wound healing may be prolonged, leading to delayed healing after tooth extraction or other oral surgical procedures. Elective dental procedures should not be done until the hemoglobin level is above 10 g/dl.

Treatment of iron deficiency anemia may include the use of liquid ferrous sulfate, which causes black stains of the teeth and tongue. This can be minimized by drinking the solution through a straw and rinsing the mouth after each dose.

Plummer-Vinson syndrome
S. Gary Cohen

Plummer-Vinson syndrome (sideropenic dysphagia) is associated with stomatitis, pharyngoesophogeal ulcerations, and dysphagia in addition to symptoms of a severe anemia. It occurs almost exclusively in middle-aged females. Nail abnormalities seen in chronic cases include spooning, atrophy of the entire nail bed, or complete loss of the nail. The patient's facial expression and contraction of the lips often create an appearance of "primness" or displeasure.

ORAL MANIFESTATIONS. Oral manifestations are similar to those of an iron deficiency anemia, atrophic glossitis, angular cheilitis, and dysphagia. Xerostomia may also be present. Leukoplakia of the tongue is common and biopsy shows dysplastic changes. Since there is also an increased incidence of pharyngeal and oral squamous cell carcinoma, all suspicious lesions must be biopsied.

DENTAL MANAGEMENT. Patients being treated for Plummer-Vinson syndrome may undergo routine dental treatment as long as the hemoglobin levels are above 10 g/dl. There has been a reported increased risk of infection associated with profound disturbances of iron metabolism. Also, as with all iron deficiency anemias, there may be delayed healing or poor tissue response following surgical procedures. Therefore, these patients should be monitored closely following surgical procedures and maintained on a regular recall basis.

Sickle cell anemia
S. Gary Cohen

The oral manifestations of sickle cell anemia are nonspecific. The most common signs are mucosal pallor due to chronic anemia and jaundice due to hemolysis.

Radiographic changes in the jaw occur in 79% to 100% of patients, in all age groups, and in both the mandible and maxillae. It has been suggested that dental radiographs show bony changes more dramatically than other bone surveys because of the direct juxtaposition of the film to the bone, which results in finer detail and sharpness.

The bony abnormalities are seen on radiographs as decreased radiodensity with a coarse trabecular pattern. These findings are attributed to erythroblastic hyperplasia and medullary hypertrophy with resultant loss of fine trabeculae and increased marrow spaces. This is most commonly seen as radiolucent areas between the apices of the teeth and the inferior border of the mandible. Another presentation, described as "stepladder" because of the characteristic horizontal trabecular arrangement, is most obvious when it occurs in the mandible between the root apices and the alveolar ridge. Some other changes attributed to bone marrow hyperplasia include thinning of the inferior border of the mandible, loss of the cortical layer along the alveolar ridge, interdental cuffing of interproximal bone, loss of alveolar bone height (especially in children under 10), and pronounced lamina dura.

The bony changes are classified into four groups: (1) bone marrow hyperplasia causing osteoporosis, loss of trabeculation, and cortical thinning; (2) thrombosis and infarction producing osteosclerosis, (3) changes subsequent to an infectious process where the bone shows areas of osteoporosis and erosion followed by osteosclerosis, and (4) generalized decreased bone growth caused by hypoxic effects on the growth centers.

These changes should not be considered as definitive diagnostic criteria for sickle cell anemia. Similar changes may be seen in normal individuals as well as in patients with other systemic disorders such as thalassemia, estrogen imbalance, hyperparathyroidism, Paget's disease, and metabolic bone disease. The diagnosis is made with a sickle cell preparation and hemoglobin electrophoresis.

Osteomyelitis of the jaws occurs with increased frequency in patients with sickle cell disease. The inherent vascular abnormalities cause vascular thrombosis and infarction, predisposing the patient to infection. Five cases of osteomyelitis occurring in the mandible of sickle cell patients have been reported in the literature in the past 10 years. In four of the five cases, carious teeth or periodontal disease was considered to be the causative agent. Since the initial manifestations of both vascular infarction and osteomyelitis are similar, only clinical, laboratory, and histologic data can distinguish between the two.

Another significant oral manifestation of sickle cell disease is mental nerve neuropathy. Onset of this symptom is usually preceded by severe pain in the mandible. There have been several reports in which pain in the mandible and lip paresthesia were associated with a sickle cell crisis. Mental nerve paresthesia is thought to be secondary to a vaso-occlusive episode involving the inferior alveolar nerve at or near the mental foramen. Recovery of sensation may be slow, with the paresthesia lasting as long as 18 months.

The results of a cephalometric study noted that sickle cell patients had an increased angulation of the lower border of the mandible with a tendency toward mandibular retrusion. This may be attributed to the generalized bone growth retardation found in these patients.

Hypomineralization of the dentin and enamel and enamel staining occasionally are seen. Thrombus formation resulting in an inadequate supply to the developing enamel organ is thought to be responsible for these changes.

Other head findings include spontaneous hematomas of unknown etiology, headaches, and cranial nerve palsies secondary to cerebral thrombosis.

DENTAL MANAGEMENT. Preventive dental care is important since oral infection may precipitate a sickle cell or aplastic crisis. Dental counseling should begin at an early age and should be maintained throughout life. Preventive therapy should include fluoride application and frequent prophylaxis to prevent caries and periodontal disease.

Once detected, infections must be vigorously treated to prevent an extensive facial cellulitis. The infected area should be carefully debrided, culture and sensitivity tests performed, and the patient placed on appropriate antibiotic therapy. Attentive postinfective monitoring is required. Cellulitis may warrant hospitalization in order to administer high levels of intravenous antibiotics and provide close observation. Endodontics or extraction of the offending teeth should be accomplished. A dental evaluation to rule out a possible dental etiology is recommended in sickle cell patients with fevers of unknown origin.

Routine dental treatment in a noncrisis period may be readily performed, while therapy during a crisis should be directed to palliation. Antibiotic coverage is needed only when active infection is present. Elective oral surgical procedures should not be considered in these patients. However, extensive oral surgical procedures, including orthognathic surgery, can be performed on patients with sickle cell trait. For treatment under general anesthesia, hemoglobin levels should be above 10 mg/dl. Packed erythrocyte transfusions may be administered to obtain an acceptable hemoglobin level. Prophylactic broad-spectrum antibiotic coverage is suggested to minimize the incidence of postoperative wound infection.

If ataractic premedication is required, a non–respiratory depressant drug is recommended to minimize the possibility of potentiating a crisis.

Local anesthesia with vasoconstrictors is a controversial issue. Some clinicians claim that vasoconstrictors may impair circulation locally to cause infarction, while others maintain that vasoconstriction has no effect on the local circulation despite the underlying hypovascularization.

The use of nitrous oxide–oxygen analgesia is another controversial issue. Hypoxia should be avoided with nitrous oxide–oxygen analgesia. A 50% oxygen concentration, high flow rate, and adequate ventilation should allow an adequate safety margin.

General anesthetic techniques for sickle cell patients have been evaluated by many. The technical ability of the anesthesiologist is more important than the choice of anesthetic. Anesthesia for sickle cell patients should only be done in a hospital by a fully trained anesthesiologist.

The oral manifestations and dental management of the other hemoglobinopathies are similar to those described for sickle cell anemia.

Hemolytic disease of the newborn (erythroblastosis fetalis)
S. Gary Cohen

The patient with hemolytic disease of the newborn (HDN) will show discoloration of the crowns of all deciduous teeth that were developing during the period of severe hemolysis. The discoloration may appear yellow, green, blue-green, tan, deep gray, and even blue. This is caused by the bile pigments that are deposited in the enamel and dentin of the developing teeth. The color will usually fade with increasing years. Enamel hypoplasia has also been reported in association with HDN. When kernicterus follows hemolytic disease, enamel hypoplasia was present in 58% to 100% of cases reported. The most common lesion was observed in the enamel and corresponded to the 4½- to 7-month intrauterine period. The hypoplasia can be seen on radiographic examination before tooth eruption.

Since only the deciduous teeth are affected and these will exfoliate, no modifications in dental treatment are needed.

Cold agglutinin disease
S. Gary Cohen

Cold agglutinin disease is an autoimmune hemolytic anemia with no specific oral manifestations. The dentist treating a patient with cold agglutinin disease should be sure that the office is warm (above 65° C). If intravenous fluids are to be used for sedation, they should be warmed before they are administered.

Enzyme deficiency anemias
S. Gary Cohen

The only reported oral manifestations of the Embden-Meyerhof pathway were reported in a case of hexokinase deficiency anemia. The teeth were narrow in the buccolingual dimension and had an abnormally large number of grooves and fissures. The central incisors were screwdriver shaped, with the incisal width narrower than the gingival width. This is similar to patients with thalassemia. Both disorders are caused by the hemolytic process occurring during enamel formation. Other oral signs that may be evident are pallor and jaundice of the mucosa.

Glucose-6-phosphate dehydrogenase deficiency
S. Gary Cohen

Patients with glucose-6-phosphate dehydrogenase (G-6-PD) deficiency have no reported oral manifestations except for the pallor and jaundiced mucosa that occurs during a hemolytic episode. Such episodes can be triggered by dental infection, therefore prevention should be given a high priority. If infection does occur, vigorous treatment is indicated.

Drug sensitivity can also lead to hemolytic episodes. Drugs such as sulfonamides and phenacetin have been implicated and therefore should be avoided.

Thalassemia
S. Gary Cohen

The clinical manifestations of all thalassemias are associated with the reactive extramedullary hemopoietic nature of the disease and are more pronounced than in the hemolytic anemia of sickle cell disease. Painful crises do not occur, as in sickle cell anemia, but bone pain has been reported at low hemoglobin concentrations secondary to marrow hyperplasia. These patients are usually small for their age and often have typical facies (facies Cooley), including separation of the eyes, depression of the bridge of the nose, high bulging cheeks, prominent frontal and parietal bones, and puffy eyes. The degree of cephalofacial deformities is closely related to the severity of the disease and the timing of therapy.

ORAL MANIFESTATIONS. Hypertrophy and remodeling of the maxilla often result in malocclusion. A severe overbite with either protruded and spaced or prominent but crowded maxillary anterior teeth may develop. The posterior segment may be buccally displaced with a concomitant expansion of the alveolar process.

The teeth occasionally show morphologic changes including reduced buccolingual diameters, diminutive premolars and second molars, and increased numbers of grooves, pits, and fissures. The enamel and dentin contain a higher iron concentration, which is related to the number of blood transfusions each year.

The dental radiographic findings are similar to those in sickle cell disease. Osteoporosis, a widening of the trabecular spaces, or generalized rarefactions with a "honeycombed" trabecular appearance may be seen. Occasionally, circular radiolucencies at the root apex can be mistaken for a pathologic lesion. Remaining trabeculae in rarefied areas appear prominent and have been referred to as compensatory lamellar striations. Also, the lamina dura may appear thin. These radiographic changes are caused by the persistent overgrowth of erythrocyte-forming marrow, which results in enlargements of the medullary cavities and thinning of the overlying cortex. Periosteal reactions and focal areas of ischemic necrosis do not occur with any frequency in thalassemia. The skull may show a notable cortical thickening and an unusual sunburst or "hair-on-end" appearance of the trabeculae at the cortex. Obliteration of the paranasal sinuses may occur as a result of the marrow hyperplasia, with only the ethmoid sinuses being spared.

DENTAL MANAGEMENT. Patients with β-thalassemia major require a recent complete blood count, including hemoglobin and hematocrit determinations, before any dental treatment. Only palliative care should be attempted with a hemoglobin level below 8 to 10 mg/dl. All routine dental treatment should be accomplished soon after regularly scheduled transfusions while observing all hepatitis precautions. These patients are more susceptible to infection, and some clinicians advise prophylactic antibiotic coverage before dental treatment. This issue is controversial and should be discussed with the hematologist. A thorough dental evaluation is necessary to rule out an oral source of infection in any fever of unknown origin.

Care should be exercised during surgical procedures to prevent pathologic fractures caused by the large marrow spaces. Orthodontic treatment can be undertaken to correct dental and cosmetic defects, particularly those of the maxillary anterior region.

Patients with thalassemia minor are usually asymptomatic and dental treatment can usually be accomplished without special precautions.

Polycythemia vera
S. Gary Cohen

Patients with polycythemia vera frequently display hypertension, clubbing of the fingernails, and neurologic manifestations such as headache, vertigo, visual disturbances, and paresthesias. These signs and symptoms resolve with therapy. The face may have a ruddy complexion particularly around the ears, nose, and lips. The oral mucosa appears purplish red to crystal violet. The gingivae are congested and edematous and bleed spontaneously from increased intravascular pressure and congestion of the vascular beds. Epistaxis is also seen with this disease. Excessive bleeding may follow oral surgical procedures or slight trauma. Petechiae, ecchymosis, and hematomas are occasionally noted as well as ulcerations of the oral mucosa, gingiva, and tongue.

Hemorrhage and thrombosis are major considerations in dental management. Before treatment a bleeding profile including complete blood count, platelet count, and bleeding time should be obtained. Most bleeding can be controlled with local measures such as pressure, topical thrombin, or microfibrillar collagen. ϵ-Aminocaproic acid (EACA) is contraindicated in these patients because of the possible risk of thrombosis.

BIBLIOGRAPHY

Adelman, A.B.: Cooley's anemia from an orthodontist viewpoint, N.Y. State Dent. J. **31**:405, 1965.

Alexander, W.N., and Bechtold, W.A.: Alpha thalassemia minor trait accompanied by clinical oral signs, Oral Surg. **43**:892, 1977.

Alexander, W.N., and Ferguson, R.L.: Beta thalassemia minor and cleidocranial dysplasia: a rare combination of genetic abnormalities in one family, Oral Surg. **49**:413, 1980.

Biderman, P.D.: The orofacial manifestations of children with sickle cell anemia, Buffalo, 1973, Children's Hospital of Buffalo Press.

Boesen, E., and others: Cytotoxic drugs in the treatment of cancer, London, 1969, Edward Arnold Publisher.

Calandra, J.C.: Oral manifestations of blood disease, Ann. Dent. **16**:109, 1957.

Daramola, J.O.: Massive osteomyelitis of the mandible complicating sickle cell disease, J. Oral Surg. **39**:144, 1981.

Dayal, P.K., and Mani, N.J.: Clinical aspects of the tongue in anemia, Ann. Dent. **38**:21, 1979.

Diner, H.: Therapeutic considerations in handicaps of special interest, Dent. Clin. North Am. **18**:683, 1974.

Friedlander, A.H., Genswer, L., and Swerdloff, M.: Mental nerve neuropathy: a complication of sickle-cell crisis, Oral Surg. **79**:15, 1980.

Garfunkel, A., and others: Iron concentration in teeth of patients with and without beta-thalassaemia major, Arch. Oral Biol. **24**:829, 1979.

Garfunkel, A.A., and others: Local therapeutic approach to agranulocytic oral ulcers, Pharm. Ther. Dent. **4**:21, 1979.

Gillen, G.H., and Trieger, N.: Bilateral mandibular swellings in sickle cell anemia, N.Y.J. Dent. **46**:196, 1976.

Girrasole, R.V., and Lyons, E.D.: Sickle cell osteomyelitis of the mandible: report of three cases, J. Oral Surg. **35**:231, 1977.

Greenberg, M.S.: Clinical and histologic changes of the oral mucosa in pernicious anemia, Oral Surg. **39**:320, 1981.

Halstead, C.L.: Oral manifestations of hemoglobinopathies, Oral Surg. **30**:615, 1970.

Herschfus, L.: Oral manifestations of blood disorders, J. Oral Med. **25**:56, 1970.

Hjorting-Hensen, E., and Bertram, V.: Oral aspects of pernicious anemia, Br. Dent. J. **125**:266, 1968.

Holzman, L., and others: Anesthesia in patients with sickle cell disease, Anesth. Analg. **48**:566, 1965.

Jacobs, A., and Cavill, I.: The oral lesions of iron deficiency anemia; pyridoxin and riboflavin status, Br. J. Haematol. **14**:291, 1968.

Kinsey, R.W., Ballard, J.B., and Matukas, V.J.: Sickle cell hemoglobinopathies: a protocol for management, J. Oral Surg. **37**:441, 1979.

Kirson, L.E., and Tomaro A.J.: Mental nerve paresthesia to sickle-cell crisis, Oral Surg. **48**:509, 1979.

Konutey-Ahulu, F.I.: Mental-nerve neuropathy: a complication of sickle-cell crisis, Lancet **2**:388, 1972.

Lasser, S.D., Camitta, B.M., and Needleman, H.G.: Dental management of patients undergoing bone marrow transplantation for aplastic anemia, Oral Surg. **43**:181, 1977.

Menius, J.W., and Webster, W.P.: Dental management of mild hemophilia with polycythemia vera, Oral Surg. **45**:714, 1978.

Millard, H.D., and Gobetti, J.P.: Non specific stomatitis—a presenting sign in pernicious anemia, Oral Surg. **39**:562, 1975.

Miller, J., and Forrester, R.M.: Neonatal enamel hypoplasia associated with hemolytic disease and with prematurity, Br. Dent. J. **106**:93, 1959.

Mourshed, F., and Tuckson, C.R.: A study of the radiographic features of the jaws in sickle cell anemia, Oral Surg. **37**:812, 1975.

Parkin, S.F.: Dental treatment for children with thalassemia, Oral Surg. **25**:12, 1968.

Peterson, D.E., and Overholser, C.D.: Increased morbidity associated with oral infection in patients with acute nonlymphocytic leukemia, Oral Surg. **51**:390, 1981.

Poyton, H.G., and Davey, K.W.: Thalassemia: changes visible in radiographs used in dentistry, Oral Surg. **25**:561, 1968.

Richard, P.A.: Pathophysiology of dental changes in sickle cell disease, J. Conn. St. Dent. Assoc. **51**:20, 1977.

Robinson, T.B., and Sarnat, B.G.: Roentgen studies of the maxillae and the mandible in sickle cell anemia, Radiology **58**:51, 1952.

Ryan, M.D.: Osteomyelitis associated with sickle cell anemia, Oral Surg. **31**:754, 1971.

Sanger, R.G., and Bystrom, E.B.: Radiographic bone changes in sickle cell anemia, J. Oral Med. **32**:32, 1977.

Sanger, R.G., Greer, R.O., and Averbach, R.E.: Differential diagnosis of some simple osseous lesions associated with sickle-cell anemia, Oral Surg. **43**:538, 1977.

Sanger, R.G., and McTigue, D.J.: Sickle cell anemia—its pathology and management, J. Dent. Handicapped **3**:9, 1978.

Savide, N.L., and Duperon, D.F.: Hexokinase deficiency anemia with dental and other anomalies: report of case, J. Dent. Child. **46**:493, 1979.

Schofield, I.D.F., and Abbot, W.G.: Review of aplastic anemia and report of a rare case (Fanconi type), J. Can. Dent. Assoc. **44**:106, 1978.

Shepherd, N.J., and Samaras, N.G.: Chloramphenicol-induced aplastic anemia, Oral Surg. **29**:689, 1970.

Silling, G., and Moss, S.J.: Cooley's anemia—orthodontic and surgical treatment, Am. J. Orthod. **74**:444, 1978.

Stamps, J.T.: The role of oral hygiene in a patient with idiopathic aplastic anemia, J. Am. Dent. Assoc. **88**:1025, 1974.

Tas, I., Smith, P., and Cohen, T.: Metric and morphologic characteristics of the dentition in beta thalassaemia major in man, Arch. Oral Biol. **21**:583, 1976.

Walker, J.E.G.: Apthous ulceration and vitamin B12 deficiency, Br. J. Oral Surg. **11**:165, 1973.

Winer, H.J., McMahon, R.E., and Olson, R.E.: Palatal necrosis secondary to cytoxin therapy, J. Am. Dent. Assoc. **84**:862, 1972.

NEUTROPHIL DYSFUNCTION SYNDROMES
Martin S. Greenberg

ORAL MANIFESTATIONS. Oral lesions are common and often severe in patients with neutrophil dysfunction syndromes. Three findings repeatedly reported are severe gingivitis, rapidly advancing periodontal disease, and oral ulcers. These oral findings are similar whether they are caused by Chédiak-Higashi syndrome, benign chronic neutropenia, or lazy leukocyte syndrome.

Since periodontal disease is caused by a chronic bacterial infection, it is not surprising that disorders of neutrophils would be accompanied by an increased level of periodontal breakdown. This is a finding generally seen in patients with neutrophil dysfunction. Some investigators have suggested that juvenile periodontitis (periodontosis) may be caused by a neutrophil abnormality. There is evidence to support the fact that individuals with juvenile periodontitis have neutrophils with reduced chemotactic function, decreasing their ability to phagocytize bacteria.

The lazy leukocyte syndrome is characterized by leukocytes that cannot be mobilized due to a defect in chemotactic function. Gingivitis and stomatitis have been noted as prominent manifestations in this disorder. Patients with Chediak-Higashi syndrome have an inherited neutrophil disorder characterized by neutropenia, decreased chemotactic function of neutrophils, and decreased ability of neutrophils to destroy bacteria. This syndrome has prominent periodontal signs that have been described by several workers. In a study of four patients with Chediak-Higashi syndrome, all four had a history of severe periodontal disease. Two patients had their teeth removed during childhood because of severe periodontal breakdown, and the other two patients had gingivitis, mobile teeth, deep periodontal pockets, and severe alveolar bone loss. Oral manifestations of benign neutropenia were reported as well as severe gingivitis and rapidly advancing periodontal disease. It is apparent that the dentist should rule out neutropenia or neutrophil dysfunction syndrome in patients with severe oral ulcers or rapidly advancing periodontal disease that cannot be explained by local factors alone.

DENTAL MANAGEMENT. Patients with abnormal neutrophil function should be under the close supervision of a dentist to minimize local inflammatory factors causing periodontal disease, dental caries, and oral ulcers. Patients should be placed on a strict oral hygiene regimen and periodic dental examinations scheduled. When extensive dental treatment is performed in susceptible patients, broad-spectrum antibiotic coverage should be considered. If surgical procedures are necessary or if oral bacterial infection develop, granulocyte transfusions may be necessary.

BIBLIOGRAPHY

Cianciola, L.J., and others: Defective polymorphonuclear leukocyte function in a human periodontal disease, Nature **265**:445, 1977.

Cohen, D.W., and Morris A.C.: A periodontal manifestation of cycle neutropenia, J. Periodont. **32**:159, 1961.

Deasy, M.J., and others: Familial benign chronic neutropenia associated with periodontal disease: a case report, J. Periodont. **51**:206, 1980.

Kostman, R.: Infantile genetic agranulocytosis, Acta Paed. Scand. **64**:362, 1975.

Kyle, R.A.: Gingivitis and chronic idiopathic neutropenia; report of two cases, Mayo Clin. Proc. **45**:494, 1970.

Lampert, F., and Fesseler A.: Periodontal changes during chronic benign granulocytopenia in childhood: a case report, J. Clin. Periodont. **2**:105, 1975.

Levine, S.: Chronic familial neutropenia with marked periodontal lesions: report of a case, Oral Surg. **12**:310, 1959.

Reichart, P.A., and Dornon H.: Gingivo-periodontal manifestations in chronic benign neutropenia, J. Clin. Periodont. **5**:74, 1978.

Tempel, T.R., and others: Host factors in periodontal disease: periodontal manifestations of Chediak Higashi syndrome, J. Periodont. Res. **7**:Suppl. 1026, 1972.

Weary, P.E., and Bender A.S.: Chediak-Higashi syndrome with severe cutaneous involvement, Arch. Intern. Med. **119**:381, 1967.

LEUKEMIA
Martin S. Greenberg

ORAL MANIFESTATIONS. The most common sign of leukemia observed in a region routinely examined by a dentist is cervical lymphadenopathy due to the infiltration of leukemic cells into the lymph nodes. Intraoral signs and symptoms of leukemia are related to the severity of the deficiency of the mature normal white blood cells, red blood cells, and platelets. Other oral signs may be caused by infiltration of leukemic cells into the oral tissues and side effects of the chemotherapeutic drugs used to treat the disease.

Leukemia may cause a dramatic decrease in the number of normal red blood cells in the peripheral blood. Signs and symptoms noted in these patients are the same as for any other anemic patient, including complaints of dyspnea and dizziness. The oral mucosa will show a generalized pallor.

Thrombocytopenia also results from the replacement of normal marrow elements by the leukemic cells. When the platelet count falls below 25,000 cells/mm^3 spontaneous bleeding will occur that frequently includes petechiae and ecchymosis of the oral mucosa as well as gingival bleeding. The extent of the gingival bleeding depends on a combination of factors including the severity of the platelet deficiency and the amount of local irritants causing gingival inflammation. Oral bleeding may also occur as a result of disseminated intravascular coagulation (DIC). This generalized pathologic coagulation of blood in the vessels causes hypofibrinoginemia, resulting in severe bleeding.

The most common cause of morbidity and fatality in patients with leukemia is infection. This increased susceptibility to infection may be the result of a decrease in normal white blood cells from the disease process itself or of the effects of the chemotherapeutic drugs used to treat the disease. In neutropenic leukemic patients, routine oral infections may lead to septicemia and death. Proper management of these infections may make the difference between the patient dying of a generalized infection or successful remission induced by chemotherapy.

Diagnosis of periodontal abscesses or pericoronal infections may be difficult in patients with leukemia. Normal signs of infection are masked because of the dramatic decrease of normally functioning white blood cells. The usual degree of swelling and redness is often absent, leading clinicians inexperienced in examining oral disease in patients with neutropenia to overlook potentially fatal infections. The dentist must carefully evaluate any clinical complaint in the oral cavity, remembering that a severe bacterial or fungal infection may be present with minimal clinical signs. It is also vital for the dentist to remember that oral infections in hospitalized leukemic patients are often caused by bacteria that are not considered common oral pathogens. It has been shown by several investigators that the oral flora of hospitalized leukemic patients has a greater number of aerobic gram-negative enteric bacilli. Organisms repeatedly reported as causing infection in patients with leukemia include species of *Pseudomonas, Klebsiella, Proteus, Enterobacter,* and *E. coli*. These organisms rarely cause infection in normal individuals but frequently cause infections in hospitalized immunosuppressed patients.

Oral mucosal ulcers are a common finding in patients with leukemia. These lesions may result from bacterial invasion due to severe leukopenia or mucosal atrophy caused by the direct effect of the chemotherapeutic drugs on the epithelial cells. Minor trauma from dental prosthesis or teeth may result in large secondarily infected ulcers progressing to facial cellulitis or occasionally cancrum oris–like lesions causing severe, grotesque tissue destruction. In other instances, oral ulcers may result in septicemia.

Candidiasis is almost universally seen in hospitalized leukemic patients undergoing chemotherapy, but it is important to remember that infections with unusual organisms are common in this group of patients. Several cases of mucosal ulceration from gram-negative enteric bacilli such as *Pseudomonas* and *Klebsiella* have been reported. *Pseudomonas* infection of the oral mucosa appears as a raised, dry, nonpurulent, painless lesion that is sharply demarcated from the surrounding mucosa. Because of the frequency of unusual infections, these ulcers must be cultured to be certain that the patient is treated with the correct antibiotic. Routine treatment with penicillin is often inadequate. Fungal infections with *Aspergillus* or Phycomycetes may also occur. When these lesions are suspected, a biopsy must be taken in addition to a culture.

Oral signs may result from the presence of leukemic infiltrates. These are most frequently reported as gingival infiltrates in patients with acute myelomonoblastic leukemia or acute promyelocytic leukemia. Leukemic infiltrates involving the palate, alveolar bone, dental pulp, and fifth and sixth cranial nerves have also been noted. Disorders of the fifth and seventh cranial nerves in leukemic patients may be caused by vincristine, a commonly used chemotherapeutic drug.

DENTAL MANAGEMENT. The management of oral disease in patients with leukemia is a challenging aspect of dental care. Severe gingival bleeding resulting from thrombocytopenia may often be managed successfully with localized treatment. The use of absorbable gelatin sponge with topical thrombin or placement of microfibrillar collagen will often be sufficient. Some authors have reported successful management of gingival bleeding with oral rinses of antifibrinolytic agents. If these measures are not successful in stopping blood flow from an oral site, platelet transfusions will be necessary. It is important, however, for the dentist to attempt local hemostasis before recommending platelet transfusions, which may lead to transfusion reactions or formation of antiplatelet antibodies. These antibodies will reduce the usefulness of platelet transfusions during severe bleeding episodes that may follow.

Management of oral ulcers in leukemic patients should be directed toward preventing the spread of localized infection and bacteremia, promoting healing of the lesions, and decreasing pain.

Oral ulcers serve as a source of septicemia in patients with leukemia; therefore, ulcers must be cultured to determine the predominant microorganism. Topical antibacterial and antifungal medications should be used on these patients. (Chlorhexidine, which is used extensively in Europe and to date has not been approved for use in the United States is a very successful topical antibacterial agent.) Povidone-iodine solution is a topical drug that can be placed directly over the lesion. Some have reported success in using chlortetracycline compresses over the ulcers. However, the use of topical antibiotics has the potential for increasing the incidence of *Candida* infection as well as risking allergic reactions. Severe ulcers showing clinical signs of infections should be treated with a combination of topical medication and systemic antibiotics. The administration of multiple antibiotics is usually necessary to cover all the organisms commonly found in a group of leukemic patients. The combination of carbenicillin and gentamicin is commonly used for broad coverage of bacterial infections before the results of the culture are known. Candidiasis may be treated with topical nystatin, as a solution or in the form of troches. In severe cases of infiltrating lesions of candidiasis or when the oral lesions are associated with esophageal lesions, systemic use of amphotericin B is recommended.

Dental treatment to eliminate sources of infection before achieving the myelosuppressed effects of chemotherapy is controversial. Most authors recommend postponing all but emergency care until the patient is in remission. Data are now available that indicate that every leukemic patient should have a dental evaluation to remove sources of infection before chemotherapy is begun. This should be done with adequate antibiotic coverage, preparation of the area for surgery with povidone-iodine solution, and, when necessary, preoperative use of platelet and white blood cell transfusions. When dental treatment is performed before chemotherapy, the rate of septicemia is significantly reduced.

BIBLIOGRAPHY

Carey, J.A., and Chuote, R.R.: Dental treatment for the child with acute lymphocytes, J. Dent. Child. **42**:191, 1975.

Dreizen, S., Bodey, G.P., and Brown, L.R.: Opportunistic gram-negative bacillary infections in leukemia, Postgrad. Med. **55**:135, 1974.

Dreizen, S., Bodey, G.P., and Rodriquez, V.: Oral complications of cancer chemotherapy, Postgrad. Med. **58**:75, 1975.

Ferguson, M.M., and others: The presentation and management of oral lesions in leukemia, J. Dent. **6**:201, 1978.

Goepferd, S.J.: Leukemia and its dental implications, J. Dent. Handicapped **4**:44, 1979.

Goodstein, D.B., and Himmelfarb, R.: Allopurinol-induced mandibular neuropathy, Oral Surg. **39**:51, 1975.

Greenberg, M.S., and others: Oral flora as a source of septicemia in leukemia, Oral Surg. In press.

Guggenheimer, J., and others: Clinicopathologic effects of cancer chemotherapeutic agents on human buccal mucosa, Oral Surg. **44**:58, 1977.

Lemongelli, W.A., Clark, M.S., and Williams, A.C.: Nomalike lesion in a patient with chronic lymphocytic leukemia, Oral Surg. **41**:40, 1976.

Lynch, M.A., and Ship, I.I.: Initial oral manifestations of leukemia, J. Am. Dent. Assoc. **75**:932, 1967.

McGowan, D.A., Gorman, J.M., and Otredji, B.W.: Intensive dental care in adult leukemia, Dent. Pract. **20**:239, 1970.

Segelman, A.E., and Doku, H.C.: Treatment of the oral complications of leukemia, J. Oral Surg. **35**:469, 1977.

Sinrod, H.S.: Leukemia as a dental problem, J. Am. Dent. Assoc. **55**:809, 1957.

Smithe, A.C., and Cowman, S.C.: Pulp and periapical involvement in leukemia, N.Z. Dent. J. **65**:32, 1969.

Weinstein, R.A., Choukas, N.C., and Wood, W.S.: Cancrum oris-like lesion associated with acute myelogenous leukemia, Oral Surg. **38**:10, 1974.

Worth, H.M.: Some significant abnormal radiologic appearances in young jaws, Oral Surg. **21**:609, 1966.

MULTIPLE MYELOMA
Martin S. Greenberg

ORAL MANIFESTATIONS. Lesions of the jaws are common in patients with multiple myeloma and may be the first clinical sign of disease. They may present as generalized osteoporosis or as discrete, well-circumscribed, punched-out, radiolucent areas without surrounding bone reaction. Jaw lesions occur more frequently in the mandible than in the maxilla with most lesions detected in the posterior portion of the mandible beneath the premolars or molars and in the ramus of the mandible. A recent report described the initial manifestation of multiple myeloma occurring in the mandibular condyle, affecting function of the temporomandibular joint. Extensive bony involvement has led to pathologic fracture of the mandible.

Some of the lesions of multiple myeloma are detected through symptoms of intraosseous expansion and compression such as paresthesia, pain, and swelling while others are asymptomatic and are identified as a result of routine dental radiographs, particularly panoramic films. Lesions may involve the oral soft tissues and present as a tumor of the gingiva, maxillary tuberosity, or alveolar mucosa. Appearance of these lesions is nonspecific, and they are often not suspected until after the examination has been performed.

Occasionally an isolated plasma cell tumor may be detected in the mouth or jaws without other radiographic or hematologic manifestations of multiple myeloma. A majority of these patients will eventually develop other signs of multiple myeloma and should be evaluated for a number of years with radiographs and blood studies.

Amyloidosis secondary to myeloma may cause generalized infiltration of the muscles of the tongue leading to macroglossia. In other cases, accumulations of amyloid result in the formation of discrete yellow nodules on the tongue, palate, or buccal and labial mucosa. In all patients with amyloidosis detected by oral biopsy the practitioner should rule out multiple myeloma as a cause.

DENTAL MANAGEMENT. The major concerns of a dentist treating a patient with multiple myeloma are bleeding and infection. The increased susceptibility to infection is caused by the effect of the disease on the bone marrow and the decreased levels of normal immunoglobulins. Bleeding tendencies result from thrombocytopenia as well as the high levels of abnormal proteins, which interfere with normal coagulation.

The dentist must carefully evaluate each patient with multiple myeloma before dental therapy to determine whether the patient has chronic renal failure or is receiving chemotherapy, radiotherapy, or adrenal steroids, which may affect the bone marrow or adrenal function. The results of a recent total and differential white blood cell count as well as levels of normal immunoglobulin should be known to decide if the patient requires antibiotic coverage to prevent infection. Elective dental procedures should be performed only for patients in remission who are not taking chemotherapy.

If surgery is necessary in a patient with multiple myeloma, the possibility of hemorrhage is a consideration. A careful history including the symptoms of epistaxis, gingival bleeding, gastrointestinal bleeding, petechiae, or ecchymoses should be obtained by the dentist. If there is suspicion of a bleeding problem, the results of a recent platelet count, prothrombin time, and partial thromboplastin time should be evaluated.

When hyperviscosity syndrome is present, patients may occasionally have a bleeding problem although routine tests are normal. A hematology consultation is indicated in these cases, before oral surgery.

BIBLIOGRAPHY

Bruce, K.W., and Royer, R.Q.: Multiple myeloma occurring in the jaws: a study of seventeen cases, Oral Surg. **6:**729, 1953.

Cataldo, E., and Meyer, I.: Solitary and multiple plasma-cell tumors of the jaws and oral cavity, Oral Surg. **22:**628, 1966.

Jagger, R.G., Helkimo, M., and Carlsson, G.E.: Multiple myeloma involving the temporomandibular joints, J. Oral Surg. **36:**557, 1978.

Shawkat, A.H., and Phillips, J.D.: Muliple myeloma: report of a case, Oral Surg. **37:**969, 1974.

Tabachnick, T.T., and Levine, B.: Multiple myeloma involving the jaws and oral soft tissues, J. Oral Surg. **34:**931, 1976.

MACROGLOBULINEMIA
Martin S. Greenberg

ORAL MANIFESTATIONS. The major oral manifestations of Waldenström's macroglobulinemia are gingival and mucosal bleeding. It is not unusual for the initial complaint to be related to severe, spontaneous gingival bleeding or bleeding after dental extraction. A combination of factors contributed to the bleeding problem. The patient may have thrombocytopenia secondary to bone marrow infiltration with plasma cells and lymphocytes. In other cases the patient will hemorrhage although the platelet count is normal. This is caused by hyperviscosity syndrome, wherein the abnormal serum proteins interfere with the normal function of platelets and coagulation factors.

Bone lesions are uncommon in patients with Waldenström's macroglobulinemia, although radiolucent lesions of the jaw have occasionally been noted. Oral mucosal ulcers related to the disease have been reported by some authors. Infiltration and enlargement of the salivary glands have also been described. This may be confused with Sjögren's syndrome.

DENTAL MANAGEMENT. Bleeding is the most common oral sign and also the most frequent complication of dental treatment. Before initiating dental care, the dentist should order a platelet count, prothrombin time, and partial thromboplastin time. If the patient has hyperviscosity syndrome, a bleeding time should also be performed to evaluate normal platelet function.

If the patient has been recently treated with cancer chemotherapy, the dentist should determine the status of the immune and hematologic systems before proceeding with treatment. A complete blood count, including a total and differential white blood cell count, would be helpful but will not reveal the level of immunoglobulins or lymphocyte function. A medical consultation is required in these cases.

BIBLIOGRAPHY

Gamble, J.W., and Driscoll, E.J.: Oral manifestations of macroglobulinemia of Waldenstrom, Oral Surg. **13:**104, 1960.

Gorden, R.J., and Pindborg, J.J.: Macroglobulinemia of Waldenstrom. In Syndromes of the head and neck, New York, 1976, McGraw-Hill Book Co.

Shteyer, A., and Markitziun, A.: Lymphosarcoma of the mandible associated with macroglobulinemia of Waldenstrom, Int. J. Oral Surg. **7:**585, 1978.

AMYLOIDOSIS
Martin S. Greenberg

The most frequently described oral finding in patients with either primary or secondary amyloidosis is macroglossia. The tongue may have generalized, firm enlargement, often with indurations on the lateral border from the pressure of the teeth or with discrete yellow nodules. In a study of 236 cases of amyloidosis, 12% of the patients with primary amyloidosis and 26% of the patients with amyloidosis related to multiple myeloma had macroglossia. Nodular lesions underlying the palate or buccal and labial mucosa may also be seen. In patients with multiple myeloma amyloidosis may cause tongue or mucosal nodules. Primary amyloidosis has been noted in the temporomandibular joint which significantly limited mandibular movements. Xerostomia may also result from amyloidosis from involvement of the salivary glands.

The relative merit of gingival biopsy in the diagnosis of suspected cases of amyloidosis has been controversial. Gingival biopsy was the desired technique of diagnosis until 1962, when investigators demonstrated positive findings in 75% of rectal biopsies taken from patients with amyloidosis but in only 19% of gingival biopsies. Recent evidence, however, has caused a reevaluation of the efficacy of the oral biopsy in the diagnosis of amyloidosis. The oral biopsy taken from the mucobuccal fold region will show a high percentage of positive results in patients with amyloidosis. These results compare favorably to the rectal biopsy site. Using the mucobuccal fold is sensible since amyloid is found most frequently around blood vessels and muscle tissue, which is found in the mucobuccal fold region and not in the region of the attached gingiva where most of the previous biopsies were taken.

The following plan is recommended when a dentist is consulted regarding "gingival" biopsy to detect amyloidosis. The patient should first be carefully examined for nodules that may be consistent with amyloid deposits. If nodules are noted, they should be biopsied. If nodular areas are not present a biopsy should be taken in the mucobuccal fold. This biopsy site will avoid some of the painful complications associated with rectal surgery, particularly in patients with cardiovascular disease.

BIBLIOGRAPHY

Blum, A., and Sohar, E.: The diagnosis of amyloidosis, Lancet **1:**721, 1962.

Flick, W.G., and Lawrence, F.R.: Oral amyloidosis as initial symptom of multiple myeloma, Oral Surg. **49:**18, 1980.

Kraut, N., and others: Amyloidosis associated with multiple myeloma, Oral Surg. **43:**63, 1977.

Kyle, R.A., and Bayrd, E.D.: Amyloidosis: review of 236 cases, Medicine **54:**271, 1973.

Lehner, T.: Oral biopsy in the diagnosis of amyloidosis, Israel J. Med. Sci. **4:**1000, 1968.

Meyer, I., and others: Amyloidosis of the tongue secondary to multiple myeloma, J. Oral Surg. **36:**459, 1978.

Schwartz, H.C., and Olson, D.J.: Amyloidosis: a rational approach to diagnosis by intraoral biopsy, Oral Surg. **39:**837, 1975.

Schwartz, Y., and others: An unusual case of temporomandibular joint arthropathy in systemic primary amyloidosis, J. Oral Med. **34:**40, 1979.

Timosca, G., and Gavritila, L.: Primary localized amyloidosis of the palate, Oral Surg. **44:**76, 1977.

LYMPHOMA
Martin S. Greenberg

ORAL MANIFESTATIONS. Dentists who examine the neck as part of their routine examination play a significant role in the early detection of lymphoma. The practitioner must be able to distinguish lymph node enlargement suspicious of lymphoma from old fibrotic nodes resulting from resolved infection. Suspicion of lymphoma should be increased when (1) the patient has a recent history of enlarged cervical nodes without localizing signs or symptoms of infection, (2) recently enlarged nodes are nontender and rubbery, (3) there is enlargement of nodes in more than one lymph node chain, and (4) enlargement of a lymph node 1 cm or more in diameter persists for more than 1 month. A patient whose history and examination suggest the possibility of lymphoma should be referred to an oncologist or surgeon for a thorough examination and lymph node biopsy.

Primary lesions of Hodgkin's disease rarely start in an extranodal site, but there are occasional reports of jaw lesions as the initial manifestion. Primary non-Hodgkin's lymphoma occurs wherever lymphoid tissue exists and is therefore much more frequently observed in extranodal sites. Approximately 50% of extranodal lymphomas in the head and neck region occur in the lymphoid tissue of Waldeyer's ring. Therefore all nontender enlargements of pharyngeal or lingual tonsillar tissue occurring in adults should be biopsied to rule out lymphoma.

Several authors have reported non-Hodgkin's lymphoma of the palate. These lesions have been described as slow growing, painless, bluish, soft masses occurring in patients over 50. Due to their presence on the palate they have been often confused with minor salivary glands neoplasms.

Extranodal non-Hodgkin's lymphoma of the mouth mimics other lesions, such as localized gingival enlargements, radiolucent intraosseous lesions, or masses of the tongue. Lesions of the gingiva have been treated for months as infections such as periodontal abscesses or pericoronitis before a biopsy was taken and the proper diagnosis made. To avoid inappropriate dental treatment one should suspect lymphoma in patients over 50 years of age in the following circumstances: slow growing palatal masses, isolated loose teeth, or paresthesia of the lip. Tissue from these sites should always be submitted for pathologic diagnosis, which can include cytologic study by use of a touch preparation.

Biopsy is the only proper method to diagnose lymphoma. Lymphomas have been confused histologically with benign lymphoepithelial lesions or other benign lymphoproliferative disorders. When considering lymphoma one must be sure to take a representative tissue sample from the center of the lesion.

A patient with advanced Hodgkin's disease has decreased cellular immunity and an increased incidence of viral and fungal infection. Particularly significant in the oral region is the incidence of candidiasis and herpes zoster. Herpes zoster may affect the second and third divisions of the fifth cranial nerve, causing pain and unilateral facial and oral lesions along the course of the affected nerve.

DENTAL MANAGEMENT. Radiation and chemotherapy are used to treat the lymphomas. The dose of radiation is much lower in lymphoma than in squamous cell carcinoma, significantly reducing the risk of osteoradionecrosis. The combination of radiation and chemotherapy, however, will depress the bone marrow. Therefore, before providing dental care to the patient who has been recently treated for lymphoma, the dentist should order a complete blood count and evaluate the levels of leukocytes and platelets. Patients about to undergo chemotherapy for lymphoma should have a dental examination before treatment so oral sources of infection can be eliminated.

BIBLIOGRAPHY

Bathard-Smith, P.J., Coonar, H.S., and Maskus, A.F.: Hodgkin's disease presenting intra-orally, Br. J. Oral Surg. **16:**64, 1978.

Blok, P., Van Delden, L., and Van der Waal, I.: Non-Hodgkin's lymphoma of the hard palate, Oral Surg. **47:**445, 1979.

Cline, R.E., and Stenger, T.G.: Histiocytic lymphoma (reticulum-cell sarcoma), Oral Surg. **43:**422, 1977.

Lehrer, S., Roswit, B., and Federman, Q.: The presentation of malignant lymphoma in the oral cavity and pharynx, Oral Surg. **41:**441, 1976.

Mittelman, D., and Kaban, L.B.: Recurrent "non-Hodgkin's lymphoma" presenting with gingival enlargement, Oral Surg. **42:**792, 1976.

Smith, D.B., and others: Soft swelling of the hard palate, J. Am. Dent. Assoc. **102:**199, 1981.

Steg, R.F., and others: Malignant lymphoma of the mandible and maxillary region, Oral Surg. **12:**128, 1959.

Tomish, C.E., and Shafer, W.G.: Lymphoprobferatures disease of the hard palate: a clinico-pathology entity. A study of twenty-one cases, Oral Surg. **39:**754, 1975.

Vickery, L.M., and Midda, M.: Dental complications of cytotoxic therapy in Hodgkin's disease—a case report, Br. J. Oral Surg. **13:**282, 1976.

HISTIOCYTOSIS X
Martin S. Greenberg

ORAL MANIFESTATIONS. Oral findings are present in all three subtypes of histiocytosis X. The review of 13 patients with Hand-Schüller-Christian disease demonstrated that approximately three quarters of the patients had oral findings at some point during the course of the disease.

Rapid alveolar bone loss is a common oral manifestation of histiocytosis X and may be seen as an isolated loose tooth, early exfoliation of deciduous teeth, or multiple permanent teeth loosely retained in soft tissue. Dental radiographs of patients with extensive jaw involvement will demonstrate bone destruction extending beyond the alveolus. The dentist must submit tissue for histopathologic examination when areas of apparent alveolar bone loss cannot be explained by local factors alone.

Although it is common for jaw lesions of histiocytosis X to appear as alveolar bone loss, nonspecific radiolucent lesions may occur. Histiocytosis X mimics many other intrabony lesions, and diagnosis of these cases cannot be made without biopsy.

DENTAL MANAGEMENT. See section on cancer chemotherapy.

BIBLIOGRAPHY
Blevins, C., and others: Oral and dental manifestations of histiocytosis X, Oral Surg. **12**:473, 1959.
Jones, J.C., Lilly, G., and Martlette R.H.: Histiocytosis X, J. Oral Surg. **28**:461, 1970.
Sedano, H.O., and others: Histiocytosis X: clinical radiographic and histologic findings with special attention to oral manifestations, Oral Surg. **27**:760, 1969.
Sleeper, E.L.: Eosinophilic granuloma of bone: its relationship to Hand-Schüller-Christian and Letterer-Siwe's disease with emphasis upon oral symptoms and findings, Oral Surg. **4**:896, 1951.

GAUCHER'S DISEASE
Martin S. Greenberg

ORAL MANIFESTATIONS. Intraosseous lesions of the jaw bone are common in patients with Gaucher's disease. The abnormal Gaucher cells infiltrate bone, causing generalized osteoporosis, unilocular vacuoles, or pseudocysts.

In addition to generalized osteoporosis and specific radiolucencies, thinning of the mandibular cortex and resorption of root apicies have been observed. Cases have been reported where routine dental films with radiolucent areas in the mandible, generalized osteoporosis of the jaws, or widened marrow spaces led to the diagnosis of Gaucher's disease.

DENTAL MANAGEMENT. Infiltration of the marrow by abnormal cells may cause leukopenia, anemia, or thrombocytopenia. Bleeding secondary to thrombocytopenia is the most frequent problem with dental treatment of patients with Gaucher's disease. A platelet count should be obtained in all cases before dental care, and if there is evidence of liver involvement a prothrombin time and a partial thromboplastin time should be obtained as well. The dentist should know total and differential white blood cell count before dental treatment to determine whether the patient has an increased risk for postoperative infection.

BIBLIOGRAPHY
Bender, I.B.: Dental observations in Gaucher's disease, Oral Surg. **12**:546, 1959.
Bildman, B., and others: Gaucher's disease discovered by mandibular biopsy: report of a case, J. Oral Surg. **30**:510, 1972.
Michanowicz, A.E., Michanowicz, J.P., and Stein, G.M.: Gaucher's disease: report of a case, Oral Surg. **23**:36, 1967.
Moch, W.S.: Gaucher's disease with mandibular bone lesions, Oral Surg. **6**:1250, 1946.
Sela, J., and others: Involvement of the mandible in Gaucher's disease, Br. J. Oral Surg. **9**:246, 1972.
Spiegel, L.H.: Gaucher's disease, Oral Surg. **10**:158, 1950.
Weigler, J.M., and others: Gaucher's disease involving the mandible: report of a case, J. Oral Surg. **25**:158, 1967.

PLATELET DISORDERS
Thrombocytopenia
S. Gary Cohen

ORAL MANIFESTATIONS. The oral manifestations of thrombocytopenia may represent its initial signs. Purpura, the most common oral sign, is defined as any escape of blood into subcutaneous tissues and includes petechia, ecchymoses, hemorrhagic vesicles, and hematomas. These may appear on any mucosal surface and are often first seen on the tongue, lips, and occlusal line of the buccal mucosa secondary to minor trauma. Initially, the color may be bright red, resembling vascular dilation. Purpura may be differentiated from vascular lesions by applying pressure directly to the area (diascopy). Purpuric lesions will not blanch and may be induced on the palate from the suction created by a full denture. Other oral signs include spontaneous gingival hemorrhage and prolonged bleeding following trauma, toothbrushing, extractions, or periodontal therapy. Similar purpuric findings are often seen on the skin. The patient may give a positive history of epistaxis, hematuria, melena, and increased menstrual bleeding.

Gingival biopsy is helpful in the diagnosis of thrombotic thrombocytopenic purpura (TTP), since the gingiva is readily accessible, highly vascular, and amenable to hemostasis.

DENTAL MANAGEMENT. Spontaneous gingival bleeding can usually be managed with oxidizing mouthwashes but platelet transfusions may be required to stop the bleeding. Good oral hygiene and conservative periodontal therapy will help to remove plaque and calculus which potentiates the bleeding. Accidental trauma can be avoided by replacing ill-fitting prostheses and removing all orthodontic appliances. These patients should be cautioned not to sleep with any removable prosthesis in place.

Emergency care during severe thrombocytopenic episodes consists of endodontic therapy, antibiotics, and non-salicylate analgesics. A stab incision and drainage may be performed but blunt dissection of an abscessed area is to be avoided. Definitive dental treatment should be delayed until normal platelet function returns. Platelet levels greater than 50,000/mm^3 are desired before dental treatment and further transfusions are given as needed postoperatively to maintain hemostasis. Hepatitis and antiplatelet antibody formation are potential serious side effects of continued platelet transfusions.

An alternative method, developed empirically by some clinicians, utilizes a single preoperative platelet transfusion given ½ hour before dental treatment. Postoperative hemorrhage is minimized by packing all bleeding sites with microfibrillar collagen. Clot integrity is ensured by giving ϵ-aminocaproic acid (EACA) in a 100 mg/kg loading dose, orally or intravenously, just prior to dental treatment followed by 50 mg/kg every 6 hours for 8 days. EACA inhibits fibrinolysis after clot formation. Side effects may be bothersome but are usually not severe enough to warrant discontinuation of the EACA. These include dizziness, diarrhea, nausea, and abdominal pain. EACA in the liquid form may make the required dosages more tolerable, particularly for children.

EACA, 100 mg/kg every 6 hours for 8 days, and local measures may suffice with a platelet count of 20,000 to 50,000/mm^3. Platelet transfusions are used only when local measures fail.

Block injections are to be avoided with a platelet count below 30,000/mm^3 because of the possibility of hematoma formation and airway obstruction. Infiltration or pericemental anesthesia is used instead. Intraligamentary anesthesia using a pressure syringe (Peri-Press syringe, Universal Dental Instruments, Inc.) may be helpful.

Aspirin-containing analgesics are contraindicated since they may potentiate bleeding. Any drug that has previously induced a thrombocytopenic episode is to be avoided. These patients are frequently treated with steroids, which may further complicate dental treatment (see section on adrenal insufficiency).

Thrombocytosis
S. Gary Cohen

A high platelet count can be paradoxically associated with oral bleeding and therefore thrombocytosis should be included in the differential diagnosis of oral bleeding. The oral signs of thrombocytosis include gingival bleeding and mucosal ecchymosis. Petechia rarely occur with this disorder.

The major dental concern is posttreatment bleeding. Dental treatment should be delayed only with rapidly rising platelet levels or counts greater than 800,000/mm^3. Medical intervention may be required to return normal platelet function. The use of a local hemostatic agent, such as microfibrillar collagen, can significantly reduce post-surgical bleeding. Aspirin-containing analgesics should be avoided.

Thrombasthenia

The oral manifestations in Glanzmann's thrombasthenia, as well as in the other functional platelet disorders, are similar to those of thrombocytopenia. Bleeding is the main concern in providing dental care. Dental management is similar to that for patients with thrombocytopenia. The need for fewer platelet transfusions may occur with the use of EACA.

Bleeding secondary to aspirin

A thorough patient history should include the frequency with which aspirin products are used. Aspirin can potentiate prolonged bleeding in patients who (1) have bleeding and clotting disorders, (2) are taking anticoagulants, or (3) have had recent surgery or trauma.

Aspirin use has been implicated in continued oral bleeding following dental extractions, periodontal surgery, and ultrasonic scaling. Bleeding may continue for 24 to 48 hours after discontinuation of aspirin. During this period local hemostatic agents are helpful but occasionally platelet transfusions are required.

BIBLIOGRAPHY

Fox, P.C., Gordon, R.E., and Williams, A.C.: Thrombotic thrombocytopenia purpura: report of case, J. Oral Surg. **35**:921, 1977.

Lemkin, S.A., and others: Aspirin induced oral bleeding: correction with platelet transfusion, Oral Surg. **37**:498, 1974.

McGaul, T.: Postoperative bleeding caused by aspirin, J. Dent. **6**:207, 1979.

Nixon, K.C., Keys, D.W., and Brown, G.: Oral management of Glanzmann's thrombasthenia, J. Periodont. **46**:364, 1973.

Perkin, R.F., White, G.C., and Webster, W.P.: Glanzmann's thrombasthenia: report of two oral surgical cases using a new microfibrillar collagen preparation and EACA for hemostasis, Oral Surg. **47**:36, 1979.

Pogrel, M.A.: Thrombocythemia as a cause of oral hemorrhage, Oral Surg. **44**:535, 1977.

Sugar, A.W.: The management of dental extractions in cases of thrombasthenia complicated by the development of iso-antibodies to donor platelets, Oral Surg. **48**:116, 1979.

Sugimura, M., and others: Tooth extraction in a patient with Glanzmann's thrombasthenia, Int. J. Oral Surg. **4**:130, 1975.

Weiss, J.: Thrombocytopenic purpura: the dentist's responsibility, J. Am. Dent. Assoc. **87**:165, 1973.

Wood, N.: Management of extractions in a case of Glanzmann's disease, Br. J. Oral Surg. **11**:152, 1973.

VON WILLEBRAND'S DISEASE

The oral manifestations of von Willebrand's disease include spontaneous gingival bleeding and prolonged bleeding after dental extractions. Ecchymosis and petechia rarely occur. There is a significant variation in severity among patients with this disorder, and treatment plans must be individualized to account for the degree of bleeding in each patient.

Block anesthesia should be avoided to prevent possible hematoma formation. The use of the rubber dam to protect the soft tissues is recommended in routine restorative procedures. Mild oozing is to be expected at the injection site and around the teeth where the rubber dam clamp or matrix had been placed. This will usually stop within 5 minutes with local application of pressure. Surgical hemostasis can be obtained with microfibrillar collagen and suturing. EACA alone or in combination with either fresh frozen plasma or cryoprecipitate can also be used. EACA reduces the amount of plasma products that must be given and thereby decreases the possibility of antibody formation and the transmission of hepatitis.

BIBLIOGRAPHY

Campbell, H.D., and Payne, R.W.: Dental extractions in a family with von Willebrand's disease, Br. Dent. J. **142**:402, 1977.

Cohen, M.P.: Oral surgical complications with von Willebrand's disease: a case report, J. Oral Med. **30**:115, 1975.

Livingston, R.J., and others: Diagnosis and treatment of von Willebrand's disease, J.Oral Surg. **32**:65, 1974.

Lorson, E.L., and others: Von Willebrand's disease: current concepts and report of case, J. Oral Surg. **34**:655, 1976.

McIvor, E.G.: Von Willebrand's disease, N.Z. Dent. J. **66**:252, 1970.

Pecoraro, F.J., Kelner, A.M., and Deasy, M.J.: Periodontal therapy in von Willebrand's disease: a case report, J. Oral Med. **33**:59, 1978.

Quast, G.L., and Schoetlger, J.D.: Von Willebrand's disease, J. Oral Surg. **32**:840, 1974.

Sydney, S.B., and Ross, R.: Periodontal surgery in a patient with von Willebrand's disease, J. Am. Dent. Assoc. **102**:660, 1981.

Wallack, M.: Periodontal therapy for a patient with von Willebrand's disease: a case report, J. Periodont. **43**:495, 1972.

Westwood, R.M., and others: A new approach to the surgical management of patients with von Willebrand's disease, J. Oral Surg. **31**:483, 1973.

HEMOPHILIA
S. Gary Cohen

The high incidence of dental problems among hemophiliacs is the result of neglect and the fear of bleeding during treatment. These patients will benefit from a comprehensive multidisciplinary treatment plan. An adequate history should include type and severity of the disorder, presence of inhibitors, medications used for pain, replacement therapy, and previous dental treatment. The dentist should be aware of a factoring period so that required dental treatment can be accomplished at that time.

ORAL MANIFESTATIONS. Episodic prolonged bleeding, either spontaneous or traumatic, is the most common oral presentation. Bleeding from the nose, mouth, and lips may be severe. Hemarthroses, which may lead to ankylosis and erosion of the joint surface, are incapacitating and painful. Temporomandibular joint hemarthrosis, although rare, does occur.

Pseudotumors of hemophilia are an uncommon oral manifestation. The hemophilic pseudotumor is a progressive cystic swelling produced by recurrent hemorrhage and may be accompanied by roentgenographic evidence of bone involvement. Pain may be the only presenting symptom. Early diagnosis can often be made with computed tomographic (CT) scanning. Management involves curettage of the lesion after adequate factor replacement therapy.

DENTAL MANAGEMENT. Dental management should be directed toward prevention. Good oral hygiene will aid in the reduction of gingival bleeding. There has never been a reported case of significant bleeding from proper brushing or flossing.

Oral prophylaxis can generally be accomplished without factor replacement. Bleeding caused by supragingival ultrasonic scaling or rubber cup prophylaxis is controlled by the platelets. However deep scaling can cause serious hemorrhage in patients who have not had factor replacement.

Hematomas can be prevented by taking care during x-ray film placement, when utilizing high-speed vacuum and saliva ejectors, and in all oral tissue management. Foam rubber–tipped or gauze-padded instruments can minimize hematoma formation.

The administration of local anesthetics is a major concern in dental treatment. Dissecting hematomas, airway obstruction, and death are known complications of block anesthesia in the hemophiliac patient. The injections should not be given unless the patient has a plasma factor level of 50% or greater. Additional plasma factors are required if blood is aspirated, a hematoma develops, or other symptoms of bleeding such as pain in the area of injection occur. In severe hemophilia (2%) replacement therapy should precede any anesthetic technique. Local anesthesia may be accomplished by infiltration or pericemental injections with an interligamentary injection syringe (see section on thrombocytopenia). Intramuscular injections are also contraindicated because of the potential for hematoma formation.

Most restorative treatment can be performed without factor replacement. A rubber dam should be used to protect the oral tissues against accidental lacerations. Wedges should be placed before any interproximal preparations to both protect and retract the papilla.

Endodontics is preferable to extraction. Pulpal bleeding is readily controlled in any conventional manner. Overinstrumentation and overfilling are to be avoided.

Periodontal therapy, including surgery, is not contraindicated. Periodontal surgery should be performed only if the anticipated therapeutic benefits outweigh the possibility of severe postoperative complications. No factor replacement is needed for probing and careful supragingival scaling. Replacement is recommended preceding deep scaling, currettage, and surgery.

Orthodontic treatment can be performed in the well-motivated patient. Care should be exercised in the placement of bands. Minor intraoral bleeding caused by orthodontics will respond to pressure within 5 minutes.

Primary teeth are to be removed soon after they become loose. When radiographs reveal only soft tissue attachment, a vigorous oral hygiene program is instituted for at least 2 days followed by tooth extraction. Initial bleeding can be controlled by pressure or with local hemostatic measures such as thrombin or microfibrillar collagen (Avitene). Antihemophilic factor (AHF) as a topical agent to prevent postextraction bleeding has been reported to stop the bleeding within 12 hours. The extraction site need not be covered or protected. No replacement therapy is needed when using this technique.

Surgical treatment has often been avoided because of the potential for continued bleeding. Before any surgery complete coagulation studies, factor levels, and red cell type should be obtained. The patient should be tested for inhibitors and replacement therapy should be available. One time-honored management protocol utilizes replacement therapy to achieve a plasma level of 100% 1 hour before the procedure. This is followed by maintaining a 60% level for 4 days and a 20% level for the next 4 days.

A newer protocol consists of a single infusion to raise the plasma levels to 100% 1 hour before the procedure. In addition, a loading dose of EACA (100 mg/kg) is administered. All extraction sockets are packed with microfibrillar collagen and postoperatively the patient receives EACA (50 mg/kg) every 6 hours for 7 days. Because of the amounts required the liquid preparation is more acceptable, especially for children. Additional factor infusion should be instituted only when bleeding continues for longer than 24 hours. Levels should then be increased to 50%.

Inhibitors or circulating antibodies to the deficient factors further complicate dental management. Prevention of bleeding becomes paramount. Systemic replacement is not a reliable alternative for the patient. Topical measures along with the systemic use of EACA must be employed to minimize bleeding.

All elective surgery should be avoided since adequate hemostasis cannot be assured. Should surgery be necessary, the following regimes can be employed.
1. Infusion of sufficient amounts of factor may neutralize the antibody by saturating the mass of antibody and maintaining an antigen excess. The volume of preparation containing factor VIII is the major limiting factor in the saturation process. Therefore this technique is used only when inhibitor levels are low.
2. Infusions of activated factor IX can be used in an attempt to avoid factor VIII antibodies. This activates the "cascade" at a point after the action of factor VIII. This method uses prothrombin complex concentrate (PCC) in doses of 50 to 100 units/kg every 12 hours until the bleeding is controlled. Prothrombin time (PT) and partial thromboplastin time (PTT) are obtained pre- and postoperatively to measure the effectiveness of the PCC. EACA is also given at a dose of 100 mg/kg every 6 hours for 7 days. If bleeding is a problem, EACA can be given as a continuous intravenous drip.

Research on the clinical use of 1-deamino-8-D-arginine vasopressive (DDAVP) may provide an alternative to infusions of plasma derivatives. Its use is primarily indicated in the treatment of central diabetes insipidus but a transient and reliable increase in the factor VIII coagulant activity immediately following DDAVP administration has been shown in patients with hemophilia and von Willebrand's disease.

Chemical cautery or electrosurgery should be avoided because of the possibility of tissue necrosis and secondary bleeding. Aspirin-containing analgesics should not be prescribed. All hemophiliacs should be tested for hepatitis because of the quantity of blood products and transfusions they have received (see section on hepatitis). Dental treatments should be maximized while the patient is receiving replacement therapy.

BIBLIOGRAPHY

Berlocer, W.C., and King, D.L.: Considerations in the dental management of the factor VIII-deficient child with inhibitors, Pediatr. Dent. **1**:188, 1979.

Bjorlin, G., and Nilsson, I.M.: Tooth extractions in hemophiliacs after administration of a single dose of factor VIII or Factor IX concentrate supplemented with AMCA, Oral Surg. **36**:482, 1973.

Chiono, O.: Pulpal therapy for the hemophiliac patient, J. Acad. Dent. Handicapped. **1**:23, 1975.

Cudziwowski, L.: Circulating antibodies in factor VIII deficiency hemophilia: report of case, J. Dent. Child. **46**:54, 1979.

Currier, G.F., Pabisco, T., and McWilliams, N.B.: Restorative dentistry in hemophiliac children, J. Dent. Handicapped **2**:3, 1976.

Evans, B.E.: Dental treatment for hemophiliacs: evaluation of dental program (1975-1976) at the Mt. Sinai Hospital International Hemophilia Training Center, Mt. Sinai J. Med. **44**:409, 1977.

Evans, B.E., and Aledort, L.M.: Hemophilia and dental treatment, J. Am. Dent. Assoc. **96**:827, 1978.

Larson, C.E., and others: Anesthetic considerations for the oral surgery patient with hemophilia, J. Oral Surg. **38**:516, 1980.

Mannucci, P.M., and others: 1-Deamino-8-D-Arginine vasopressive: a new pharmacological approach to the management of hemophilia and von Willebrand's disease, Lancet **1**:869, 1977.

Moss, S.J.: Newer approaches to dental therapy, Ann N.Y. Acad. Sci. **240**:259, 1975.

Mulkey, T.F.: Hemophilic pseudotumors of the mandible, J. Oral Surg. **35**:561, 1977.

Nakajima, T., and others: Topical application of antihemophilia factor after dental extractions in hemophilic patients, J. Oral Surg. **36**:873, 1978.

Ramstrom, G., and Blomback, M.: Tooth extractions in hemophiliacs, Int. J. Oral Surg. **4**:1, 1975.

Sachs, S.A., Lipton, R., and Frank, F.: Management of ambulatory oral surgical patients with hemophilia, J. Oral Surg. **36**:25, 1978.

Storeman, D.W., and Beierl, C.D.: Pseudotumor of hemophilia in the mandible, Oral Surg. **40**:811, 1975.

Walsh, P.N., and others: The therapeutic role of epsilon-aminocaproic acid (EACA) for dental extractions in hemophiliacs, Ann N.Y. Acad. Sci. **240**:267, 1975.

FACTOR DEFICIENCIES
S. Gary Cohen

Hemophilia B—factor IX deficiency

Patients with factor IX deficiencies can be treated similarly to those patients with hemophilia A. Replacement therapy with concentrated factor IX is given before treatment. Bleeding should be minimal if factor IX levels can be kept above 30%.

Factor XI deficiency

Patients can be effectively managed utilizing preoperative infusions of 10 to 20 ml/kg of fresh frozen plasma or cryoprecipitate. This is followed by 5 ml/kg daily or 10 ml/kg every other day for 7 days postoperatively.

ϵ-Aminocaproic acid instead of postoperative infusions or in addition to a lesser volume of fresh frozen plasma and cryoprecipitate has also been used. An alternative method involves the use of prothrombin complex concentrate, a factor XI–containing concentrate. PCC concentrate has been associated with a high risk of transmitting hepatitis.

Factor V, VII, and X deficiency

Patients with deficiencies of factors V, VII, or X can be managed by any of the following methods: (1) no replacement therapy before dental treatment with only local hemostatic measures at the time of treatment and postoperatively, (2) pretreatment infusion of fresh frozen plasma, and (3) utilization of local measures at the time of treatment along with the administration of ϵ-aminocaproic acid alone or in conjunction with preoperative factor infusions.

Afibrinogenemia

The oral manifestations of afibrinogenemia are similar to those seen in mild hemophilia. These patients are unlikely to exhibit spontaneous bleeding but may experience severe hemorrhage after injury or surgery.

DENTAL MANAGEMENT. Dental treatment is preceded by replacement therapy. Cryoprecipitate infusion 1 hour before treatment is the method of choice. Volume considerations usually preclude the use of plasma or whole blood as a source for fibrinogen replacement. The prothrombin time (PT) and partial thromboplastin time (PTT) are used to follow the postinfusion hematologic profile. Once treatment is completed, the patient should receive daily cryoprecipitate infusions for 3 to 5 days. Most minor bleeding episodes will respond to topical fibrinogen. The two major complications related to fibrinogen replacement therapy are hepatitis and antibody development. If antibodies are present, hemostasis may be achieved by saturating the antibodies with large volumes of cryoprecipitate.

BIBLIOGRAPHY

Bhoweer, A.L., Shirwatkar, L.G., and Desai, A.J.: Possible congenital deficiency of factor X (Stuart-Prower): a case report, Ann. Dent. **3**:1, 1977.
Bick, R.L., Adams, T., and Radlack, K.: Surgical hemostasis with a factor XI-containing concentrate, J.A.M.A. **229**:163, 1974.
Blecker, S.M., and Williams, A.C.: Post-extraction bleeding in a patient with an acquired circulating anticoagulant against Factor V, Oral Surg. **32**:538, 1971.
Evian, C.T., and others: Complications of severe bleeding in a patient with undiagnosed Factor XI deficiency, Oral Surg. **52**:12, 1981.
Helpin, M.L., and Morrison, F.S.: Dental treatment of a patient with congenital afibrinogenemia—complications of supportive care, Pediatr. Dent. **3**:42, 1981.
Murphy, J.B., Robinson, K., and Segelman, A.: PTA deficiency (factor XI deficiency), Oral Surg. **42**:26, 1976.
Perhavec, J.C., and Goldberg, J.S.: Management of a patient with factor VII deficiency, Oral Surg. **50**:17, 1980.
Schwartz, H.C., and Stowe, J.D.: Hereditary factor XI deficiency, J. Oral Surg. **34**:453, 1976.
Williams, J.L.: Plasma thromboplastin antecedent deficiency, Br. J. Oral Surg. **10**:126, 1970.

DISSEMINATED INTRAVASCULAR COAGULOPATHY (DIC)
S. Gary Cohen

ORAL MANIFESTATIONS. The oral manifestations of DIC are similar to that seen in the hereditary coagulopathies. Bleeding is usually acute but may present insidiously with petechia, hematomas, or gingival bleeding. It is important to include DIC in the differential diagnosis of thromboses and/or hemorrhage in patients with a negative history of bleeding, especially patients with neoplastic tumors, leukemia, infections, systemic lupus erythematosus, splenectomy, or certain obstetric complications. Interestingly, there have been two reported cases of DIC following simple oral surgical procedures.

DENTAL MANAGEMENT. In the patient with DIC all but palliative emergency care should be deferred until the condition is resolved because, like most disorders in which destruction of coagulation factors occurs, DIC may not be responsive to replacement therapy.

BIBLIOGRAPHY

Falace, D.A., and Kelly, D.E.: Disseminated intravascular coagulation and fibrinolysis as a cause of post-extraction hemorrhage, Oral Surg. **41**:718, 1976.
Kamel, K., and Hoerman, K.C.: Disseminated intravascular coagulation, J. Oral Surg. **31**:95, 1973.
Rawson, D.W., and others: Clinical-pathological conference: disseminated intravascular coagulation, J. Oral Surg. **34**:62, 173, 1976.

ANTICOAGULANT THERAPY
S. Gary Cohen

Heparin

Patients undergoing heparin therapy should receive only emergency care. They can be managed while on continuous anticoagulant therapy by treating postoperative hemorrhage with local hemostatic methods. The effects of heparin will be reversed 6 hours after administration. An alternative method involves discontinuing the heparin 6 hours before treatment and then reinstituting therapy 6 to 12 hours postoperatively. In this way interruption of anticoagulant therapy is minimized. In each case the dentist should consult with the physician prescribing heparin to determine the risk of discontinuing anticoagulant therapy for a short period.

Coumarin

Dental treatment of patients on continuous anticoagulant therapy has been the subject of conflicting reports in both the dental and the medical literature. Many investigators have reported severe hemorrhage following extraction of single teeth. Others have indicated the danger of thrombosis when anticoagulant therapy was suddenly interrupted before dental treatment.

One method used to treat patients while continuing their therapy involves monitoring the patients' prothrombin time (PT) and partial thromboplastin time (PTT) before treatment. If the PT is in the range of 2 to 2½ times the control value and the PTT is in a normal range, treatment can proceed with minimal postsurgical bleeding if adequate local hemostatic methods are obtained. If the levels are above the proposed treatment range, the doses of anticoagulants can be reduced until this range is reached. Another method involves the utilization of a topical preparation of a coagulation-active substance consisting of fibrin, thrombin, and the patient's venous blood for hemostasis.

These methods have been effective for all restorative treatment and simple surgical procedures. If extensive surgery is considered (or the patient is at great risk of thromboembolism) an alternative method should be considered. This involves stopping the patient's coumarin for one dose before admission to the hospital and then initiating heparin therapy on admission. As soon as the prothrombin time has returned to normal, the patient is scheduled for the surgical procedure. Heparin therapy is discontinued 6 hours preoperatively. The PT and PTT are measured preoperatively and if they are found to be in the normal range, the procedure is carried out. Heparin therapy is not resumed for 6 to 24 hours postoperatively, depending on the extent of the surgical procedure. Coumarin is reinstituted at that time and a therapeutic level may be anticipated in 48 to 96 hours. Heparin therapy is then discontinued and the patient is discharged. In this way the patient remains without anticoagulants for 12 to 24 hours as opposed to 3 to 4 days with the traditional method of discontinuing and reinstituting coumarin.

BIBLIOGRAPHY

Christiansen, G.W.: Oral surgery problems for general practitioner, III, Dent. J. **28:**703, 1959.

Cosgriff, S.W.: Prophylaxis of recurrent embolism of intracardiac origin in protracted anticoagulant therapy on ambulatory basis, J.A.M.A. **143:**870, 1950.

Greenberg, M.S., Miller, M.F., and Lynch, M.A.: Partial thromboplastin time as a predictor of blood loss in oral surgery patients receiving coumarin anticoagulants, J. Am. Dent. Assoc. **84:**583, 1972.

Kovacs, K.T., and Kerenyi, G.: Post extraction hemostasis during coumarin anticoagulant therapy with locally applied coagulation-active substance, Int. J. Oral Surg. **5:**3, 1976.

Marshall, J.: Rebound phenomena after anticoagulant therapy in cerebrovascular disease, Circulation **28:**329, 1963.

Poller, L., and Thomson, J.: Evidence for "rebound" hypercoagulability after stopping anticoagulants, Lancet **2:**62, 1964.

Roser, S.M., and Rosenbloom, B.: Continued anticoagulation in oral surgery procedures, Oral Surg. **40:**4, 1975.

Scopp, I.W., and Fredrics, H.: Dental extractions in patients undergoing anticoagulant therapy, Oral Surg. **11:**420, 1958.

Ziffer, A.M., and others: Profound bleeding after dental extractions during Dicumoral therapy, N. Engl. J. Med. **256:**351, 1957.

Section Six
NEOPLASTIC DISEASES

edited by **Rosaline R. Joseph**

82 • INTRODUCTION TO MEDICAL ONCOLOGY

Rosaline R. Joseph

In perhaps no other field of medicine has there been such a rapid evolution of new attitudes, diagnostic tools, and therapeutic strategies as in the area of malignant neoplastic diseases. In contrast to the hopeless and despairing attitude with which physicians previously approached cancer patients, patients are now treated by a team of interested, hopeful medical professionals, who are concerned not only with specific therapy for the primary malignant disease but also with adequate control of symptoms, psychosocial support, and long-term rehabilitative efforts. Proper medical management of patients with cancer demands a multidisciplinary approach, with the treatment plan for each patient representing the optimal combination of surgery, radiotherapy, chemotherapy, experimental modalities, and support services. Advances in all these fields have resulted in potential curability of one of three cancer patients diagnosed in 1980. In many of the remaining cases significant, long-term palliation can be achieved. Innovations in radiotherapeutic techniques, the discovery of new chemotherapeutic agents, and the introduction of new modalities such as hyperthermia and immunotherapy occur with sufficient regularity to render oncology textbooks almost obsolete before they are published. As we constantly learn more about the existing modalities, improvements are made in therapeutic regimens. For this reason details such as dosages and schedules of chemotherapy and radiation have been selectively omitted in this section. The reader is referred to the most current oncologic literature for this information.

83 • AN OVERVIEW OF NEOPLASIA

Rosaline R. Joseph

Cancer, the second leading cause of death in the United States, may be defined as an abnormal proliferation of cells resulting in invasion of adjacent normal tissues, dissemination to distant organs (metastasis), or both. Cancer is not a single disease, since over 100 different forms of malignant neoplasia are recognized, each with different clinical and biologic characteristics. In 1980 over 400,000 Americans died of cancer and 785,000 new cases were diagnosed. It is estimated that one of four Americans will have cancer in his or her lifetime.

The magnitude and complexity of the cancer problem present a challenge to the entire medical community, from the laboratory researcher attempting to unravel the enigma of malignant change, to the physician who first suspects the diagnosis, to the multidisciplinary oncology team who assume responsibility for directing definitive therapy. Since malignant neoplasia occurs in every organ system, specific cancers will be discussed in detail in the sections devoted to the respective systems. This section will present an overview of the current concepts of carcinogenesis; approaches to detection, diagnosis, and staging of malignant tumors; general aspects of their clinical behavior; and principles of treatment.

CARCINOGENESIS

The cause of human cancer remains unknown. Undoubtedly, multiple factors play a role in carcinogenesis, and it appears probable that most cancers are the result of more than one carcinogenic event. Among the most important considerations in human carcinogenesis are environmental factors, genetic predisposition, viruses, and immunologic dysfunction.

Environmental carcinogenesis

Epidemiologic studies suggest that approximately 80% of all cancers are caused by environmental factors. Exposure to carcinogens may be occupational or may result from substances widely distributed in our environment, such as food additives or dyes. Smoking, alcohol consumption, and other social or dietary customs account at least in part for a significant proportion of human cancers.

OCCUPATIONAL CARCINOGENESIS. The first causal relationship between an occupational exposure and the development of cancer was demonstrated in 1775 by Potts, who observed a high incidence of cancer of the skin and scrotum in chimney sweepers exposed to soot. We now know that the carcinogenic agents in soot are benzpyrene and polycyclic aromatic hydrocarbons.

The following are currently recognized occupational carcinogens and their associated neoplasms:

Substance	Site of neoplasm
Asbestos	Pleura, lungs, gastrointestinal tract
Chromium	Lung
Cadmium	Kidney, prostate
Nickel	Lungs, nasal sinuses
Arsenicals	Lungs, skin, liver
Benzene	Acute myelogenous leukemia
Uranium	Lung
Vinyl chloride	Liver
Isopropyl oil	Nasal sinuses
Chloromethyl ethers	Lung

Many other industrial chemicals are suspected of being carcinogens, and the list is constantly growing. The magnitude of the problem of occupational cancer is illustrated by the fact that approximately 20% of all deaths in asbestos workers are caused by carcinoma of the lung; an additional 7% of the deaths are caused by pleural mesotheliomas, rare neoplasms in the general population. Gastrointestinal carcinoma has also been shown to be increased in these workers. The incidence of these neoplasms rises dramatically in exposed individuals who also smoke. Over 30 cases of pleural mesothelioma have been reported in household members whose contact with asbestos was limited to the worker's clothing. The malignancies usually occur after at least a 20-year latent period. This prolonged period between exposure and development of malignancy is characteristic of many environmental carcinogens and necessitates careful history taking in all patients with carcinoma. Important associations may be missed if a complete occupational history is omitted.

GEOGRAPHIC AND SOCIAL FACTORS IN CARCINOGENESIS. Tobacco contains at least 15 identified carcinogens, and smokers have a marked increase in lung cancer. Cancers of the head, neck, esophagus, and bladder also occur more frequently in smokers. Chewing tobacco is associated with a high incidence of oral cancer, as is the chewing of betel nuts, a practice common in Central and Southeast Asia. Aflatoxin, a product of the fungus *Aspergillus flavus,* is a contaminant of certain foods such as peanuts. It is a potent carcinogen, resulting in liver cancer. Nitrates, widely used as food preservatives, have been implicated as a cause of stomach cancer. Carcinoma of the bladder occurs with increased frequency in patients infested with the parasite *Schistosoma haematobium.*

Epidemiologic studies that have not yet identifed specific carcinogens nevertheless point to environmental factors as important in the etiology of some of the most common forms of cancer. These data show a wide geographic variance in the incidence of such cancers. Carcinomas of the lung, colon, breast, and prostate have a high incidence in the United States and western Europe, whereas carcinomas of the stomach and liver occur less frequently in these areas. In contrast, in Japan carcinomas of the stomach and liver are common, whereas carcinoma of the breast is relatively rare. Esophageal carcinoma is frequent in northeast Iran, and nasopharyngeal carcinoma is prevalent in southern China. Both of these cancers are rare in the Western countries. Evidence that these geographic concentrations of cancer are environmentally rather than genetically determined has come from studies of population migration. Daughters of Japanese immigrants to California have an incidence of breast carcinoma similar to that in California rather than the low incidence found in Japan. The change to a high-fat Western diet has been implicated in this phenomenon. On the other hand, the incidence of carcinoma of the stomach and liver in children of Japanese immigrants decreases toward that of the United States, suggesting the removal of an environmental factor, possibly a food preservative. Recently a multination study of the relative incidences of colon cancer revealed a higher incidence in countries whose diets contained a high percentage of meat and refined foods and lacked high-fiber foods.

DRUGS AS CARCINOGENIC AGENTS. Alkylating agents, which are themselves useful in the treatment of a wide variety of neoplasms, have been associated with an increased incidence of acute myelogenous leukemia. Immunosuppressive drugs, usually given to inhibit renal transplant rejection, have been linked to an extraordinary increase (200 times) in lymphoreticular malignancies in transplant patients.

Although synthetic estrogenic hormone administration has been suspected of contributing to the development of breast cancer, no statistically significant correlation has been established. However, administration of the synthetic estrogen diethylstilbestrol to pregnant women has definitely been associated with vaginal adenosis and clear-cell vaginal carcinoma in their daughters. An apparent increased risk for endometrial cancer in adults has been linked to the use of estrogen therapy.

Radiation has been implicated in the induction of many types of malignant neoplasia, including acute and chronic granulocytic leukemia in atomic bomb victims and acute leukemia in patients treated with radiation for ankylosing spondylitis. Thyroid cancer has been detected in large numbers of young people who had radiation therapy during childhood for thymic enlargement or acne. Lymphocytic lymphomas have been noted in patients exposed to radiation, and osteogenic sarcoma is frequent in radium dial painters.

SCREENING FOR CARCINOGENICITY. Since such a wide variety of environmental agents have been incriminated as causal factors in cancer, it becomes imperative to be able to detect potential carcinogens before they result in widespread damage. Traditionally, the standard methods for determining carcinogenicity have been animal bioassays.

So far, all the organic chemicals known to cause cancer in humans have done so in laboratory animals. Besides being very expensive, this method has the disadvantage that doses of the suspected carcinogens used to induce animal tumors are much higher than those to which humans would ordinarily be exposed. Thus animal results might not be applicable in humans. A valuable new screening system, the Ames' assay, rapidly determines potential carcinogenesis by observing the mutagenic effect of a suspect substance on an in vitro bacterial culture system. This test is rapid and has a 90% accuracy in predicting carcinogenicity in rodents.

Genetic factors in carcinogenesis

Only the following few, relatively rare neoplasms have been clearly shown to follow an autosomal dominant pattern of inheritance:

Retinoblastoma
Nevoid basal cell carcinoma
Multiple endocrine adenomatosis (Wermer's syndrome)
Pheochromocytoma and medullary thyroid carcinoma
Polyposis coli
Gardner's syndrome (multiple colon polyps with extra-alimentary tumors)
Tylosis (palmar hyperkeratosis) with esophageal cancer
Trichoepithelioma

A larger group of disorders with a variable inheritance pattern is associated with an increased risk of development of malignancy. This group, known as the preneoplastic or precancerous disorders, follows:

Hamartomas
   Neurofibromatosis
   Tuberous sclerosis
   Von Hippel-Lindau disease
   Multiple exostoses
   Peutz-Jeghers syndrome
Genodermatoses
   Xeroderma pigmentosum
   Albinism
   Polydysplastic epidermolysis bullosa
Chromosomal breakage syndromes
   Bloom's syndrome
   Fanconi's syndrome
Immunodeficiencies
   Ataxia-telangiectasia
   Wiskott-Aldrich syndrome
   Late-onset immunologic deficiencies
   X-linked agammaglobulinemia

Of particular interest within this latter group are the so-called chromosome breakage disorders, Bloom's syndrome and Fanconi's anemia, in which inherited chromosome abnormalities are associated with a high risk of leukemia, lymphoma, and other cancers. Patients with Down's syndrome, or trisomy 21, are subject to a 20- to 50-fold increase in the risk of acute leukemia.

Xeroderma pigmentosum is a rare disorder of special interest because of the clues it may give to the basic mechanism of carcinogenesis. It is an inherited skin disease in which the DNA repair mechanism is ineffective, resulting in a high percentage of multiple skin cancers.

Genetic factors probably play a much greater role in the cause of neoplasia than is evident in the rare malignancies just discussed. Genetic variation in susceptibility to cancer is suggested by the observation that cancer develops in only a small percentage of all people exposed to the same dose of a carcinogen in the same environment. This difference in susceptibility may be due to hereditary variation in the enzymes necessary to process potential carcinogens. It has been suggested that elevated levels of arylhydrocarbon hydroxylase increase the risk of lung cancer in smokers.

Viral oncogenesis

Although viruses are known to cause neoplasms in almost every mammalian species, there is no human cancer that has been definitely proved to be of viral origin. The strongest association thus far has been between African Burkitt's lymphoma and nasopharyngeal carcinoma and the herpes-type Epstein-Barr virus. Viral DNA sequences detected in the tumor cells in both of these neoplasms are the same as those in patients with infectious mononucleosis.

Other strong candidates for viral-induced neoplasia in humans are cancer of the cervix and leukemia. Genetic information and virus-specific antigen of the herpes simplex virus HSV-2 have been found in tumor cells of cervical carcinoma. The finding of a DNA polymerizing enzyme, RNA reverse transcriptase, in human acute leukemia cells may be evidence of viral activity, since this enzyme may be necessary for malignant transformation by oncogenic RNA viruses. Detection of viral components resembling the mouse mammary tumor virus in human breast cancer and detection of type C RNA viruses and viral proteins in tissue culture specimens from patients with lymphoma are further examples of the indirect or "circumstantial" evidence for a viral origin of human cancer.

Immune factors in carcinogenesis

In the 1950s Burnet and Thomas introduced the immune surveillance theory, which states that cancer arises as a result of a breakdown in the patient's natural immune mechanisms. The theory holds that neoplastic cells arise in everyone but do not become evident because they are destroyed by a normal immune system. When a breakdown occurs and the tumor cells are not recognized as "nonself," malignant proliferation takes place. Evidence supporting this theory includes the increased occurrence of lymphoreticular malignancies in the congenital immune deficiency syndromes and the very high incidence of such malignancies in patients who have had long-term administration of immunosuppressive agents. The theory has been weakened by the inability to detect consistent signs of immunodepression in the vast majority of cancer patients, who do not fall into the special and limited categories previously mentioned. The role of immunity in carcinogenesis continues to be explored as new complexities in the human immune mechanism are uncovered.

DETECTION, DIAGNOSIS, AND STAGING OF CANCER
Detection

Early detection and diagnosis remain the most important factors in obtaining optimal cure rates in most cancers. A careful initial history of every new patient, regardless of complaint, with special attention to risk factors such as family history of cancer, occupational exposure, or smoking, will keep the physician's index of suspicion high and direct patients at risk to appropriate screening programs. For example, although annual mammography is not recommended for women under 50 years old, it should be performed regardless of age in women who have a family history of breast cancer. This procedure may detect small cancers before they are palpable. Detailed questioning as to recent changes in appetite, weight, digestion, bowel or bladder habits, voice, or appearance of a mole is of utmost importance in the early detection of cancer.

During the physical examination the clinician should pay particular attention to clues of possible occult malignancy. Inspection of the skin often provides the first such clue. Certain skin conditions, although not in themselves malignant, are so often associated with neoplasia as to arouse a high index of suspicion whenever they are found. Among these are herpes zoster, dermatomyositis, and acanthosis nigricans, a symmetric brownish black pigmentation in body folds. About 20% of cases of dermatomyositis co-exist with a malignant tumor. Intradermal or subcutaneous nodules may be metastases from an occult tumor. Unfortunately, these lesions usually indicate advanced disease. Lymphadenopathy must always be explained. An elarged, hard supraclavicular node on the left side (Virchow's or sentinel node) often points to an intraabdominal malignancy. Femoral (as opposed to inguinal) adenopathy is always significant and is highly suggestive of malignancy, as is the presence of a palpable mass in the umbilicus. Any mass, lump, or unexplained edema should be evaluated for malignancy.

Some parts of the physical examination most valuable in the early detection of cancer are frequently omitted. Careful examination of the oropharynx can identify premalignant or early malignant lesions. Digital rectal examination is invaluable for the detection of both rectal and prostatic carcinoma. Determination of occult blood in the stool is an important screening device for colon carcinoma. Early, asymptomatic gynecologic tumors can often be detected by pelvic examination. The use of Papanicolaou smears to identify abnormalities in cervical cytology has been an important factor in reducing deaths from cervical cancer.

Diagnosis

HISTOLOGIC CONFIRMATION AND CLASSIFICATION. The sine qua non for the diagnosis of cancer is histologic proof of malignancy. Tissue should be obtained by whatever means possible before any therapy is instituted. This rule is relaxed only in the case of suspected gliomas in critical areas of the brain. Besides confirming the presence of malignancy, histologic classification provides prognostic information and guidelines for therapy. The degree of differentiation of the tumor and the presence or absence of vascular invasion are important prognostic factors within each histologic type.

Accuracy in histologic classification is of utmost importance in bronchogenic carcinoma, lymphomas, acute leukemia, and testicular tumors. In all of these situations responses to therapy differ significantly according to cellular type. A most dramatic example of this phenomenon is small or oat cell carcinoma of the lung. Tumors of this cell type are highly sensitive to chemotherapy, whereas other types of bronchogenic carcinoma are much less responsive to available cytotoxic agents.

Malignancy is frequently diagnosed from a biopsy of an accessible metastatic site, such as liver or peripheral lymph node. Occasionally even the most careful search fails to reveal the primary lesion. In these situations procedures such as histochemical analysis or electron microscopy may be helpful in narrowing the list of possible primary sites. Determination of the primary tumor is of utmost importance in planning optimal therapy, since "metastatic" adenocarcinoma can arise from a lesion as resistant to therapy as pancreatic cancer or from one as sensitive as breast cancer.

TUMOR MARKERS. Despite emphasis on early detection, many cancer patients already have advanced disease at the time of diagnosis. Extensive research has been focused on attempts to identify a measurable substance or substances in body fluids that would signify the presence of cancer. This research has led to the discovery of a series of such tumor markers. Besides providing an early detection device, these markers can also be used as a chemical assay of tumor burden. Changes in their levels can serve as a measure of response to therapy or an indication of relapse. Unfortunately, the available markers are not specific for any particular tumor type and in many cases are present in normal individuals or in those with nonmalignant diseases, as well as in cancer patients. Nevertheless, in certain situations such as testicular carcinoma, initial measurement and constant monitoring of tumor markers have made a significant difference in the management of the disease.

Oncofetal antigens are products of gene expression

during fetal life, which normally become repressed when tissue specialization and organization are completed. Malignant transformation of a cell is accompanied by derepression of these genes and reappearance of the fetal antigens.

Carcinoembryonic antigen (CEA), first described in 1965, is a glycoprotein that acts as a specific antigen for adenocarcinoma of the colon and digestive organs of human fetuses in the second to sixth months of gestation. It is also detectable in the feces of normal adults and in the secretion of the pancreatobiliary system and colon. Plasma levels of up to 2.5 ng/ml are detectable in healthy, nonsmoking individuals. Elevated levels have been found in 60% to 90% of patients with carcinoma of the gastrointestinal tract and lung and 50% of patients with advanced breast cancer. The frequency and degree of positivity increase with more extensive disease and more differentiated histology. The development of hepatic metastases is often accompanied by a rapid rise in the CEA level. Elevated CEA levels have also been found in alcoholic hepatitis, alcoholic pancreatitis, and biliary obstruction. There does not appear to be a specific level that separates benign from malignant disorders. Since CEA levels are so nonspecific, they cannot be used for detection or diagnosis of any cancer. The major usefulness of this determination is in monitoring the response to therapy or predicting relapse. Successful therapy should bring elevated CEA levels to normal within 1 month after treatment. A persistent elevation usually means residual disease. A return to normal CEA levels followed by recurrent elevation signifies recurrence of the disease.

α-Fetoprotein (AFP) has a molecular weight of 70,000 and is synthesized by the yolk sac, gastrointestinal tract, and liver of the human fetus. The normal adult level of 40 ng/ml is reached 6 to 12 months after birth. Elevated plasma levels of this protein occur in 70% to 90% of patients with hepatoma and about 70% of patients with nonseminomatous testicular carcinoma. Abnormally high levels also occur in a smaller percentage of patients with cancer of the pancreas, ovary, stomach, and lung, as well as in such benign conditions as viral and alcoholic hepatitis, ataxia-telangiectasia, and hereditary tyrosinemia. AFP determination is useful primarily as a monitor of therapeutic response.

Pancreatic oncofetal antigen (POA) is a glycoprotein found in fetal and malignant pancreatic tissue. Although it is not found in the normal adult pancreas, it is present in the serum of normal adults. Elevated levels have been found in some cases of lung, gastric, colon, and breast cancer, but the highest concentrations and greatest frequency of elevation occur in patients with pancreatic cancer.

Placental proteins may be increased in certain tumors. Human chorionic gonadotropin (HCG) is a glycoprotein normally secreted by the trophoblastic epithelium of the placental villi. It is composed of dissimilar α- and β-subunits. Radioimmunoassay can distinguish between the β-subunit of placental HCG and that of luteinizing hormone. Detectable levels of the β-subunit of HCG in a nonpregnant female or a male signal the presence of a tumor. Ectopic HCG has been found in 40% to 60% of patients with gonadal or extragonadal germ cell tumors and in a lesser percentage of patients with hepatoma and adenocarcinomas of the stomach, pancreas, and ovary. More than 50% of malignant insulinomas secrete HCG, whereas benign islet cell tumors do not. Measurement of HCG levels has been of particular importance in monitoring response to therapy and relapse in germ cell tumors.

Placental alkaline phosphatase (Regan isoenzyme) is synthesized in the trophoblast and can be distinguished from other alkaline phosphatases by heat stability, immunochemical specificity, and electrophoretic mobility. It is elevated in 5% to 15% of patients with cancer of the breast, lung, or female reproductive organs.

Ectopic polypeptides not usually produced by the cell of origin can be secreted by malignant tumors. This phenomenon of ectopic secretion has been explained by the hypothesis that all somatic cells contain a complete genetic complement and that with malignant transformation selective derepression for specific polypeptide production occurs. Elevated concentrations of these substances in body fluids can thus serve as tumor markers. Examples of such markers are adrenocorticotropic hormone (ACTH), antidiuretic hormone (ADH), and calcitonin secreted by small or oat cell carcinoma of the lung; ACTH and serotonin by medullary thyroid cancer; and ACTH or serotonin by islet and germ cell tumors. The finding of increased levels of "big" or pro-ACTH in the serum of most patients with lung cancer has led to the suggestion that ectopic protein secretion may be a universal feature of cancer (see Chapter 192).

Other tumor markers are increased amounts of substances normally secreted by the cells of origin. Detection of this increased secretion may provide a diagnostic clue to the existence of tumors, and monitoring of secretion levels during the course of the disease and its treatment has prognostic and therapeutic significance. Among these substances are the paraproteins produced in the plasma cell dyscrasias, insulin in islet cell tumors, and tartrate-inhibitable acid phosphatase produced by prostatic acinar epithelium. In the last case a recently developed radioimmunoassay can detect approximately one third of patients with occult neoplasms and three fourths of those with palpable but localized prostatic carcinomas.

Staging of tumors

Determining the extent of involvement, or stage, of a tumor at the time of diagnosis is essential to the development of an optimal treatment program for patients with cancer. After a carefully planned series of studies, the patient's disease is classified according to one of several staging systems described later in this section.

Although the specific studies necessary for adequate staging vary with the type of tumor, certain techniques are widely applicable. Radionuclide scanning is useful in determining primary or metastatic tumor involvement of the bones, liver, and spleen. Bone scans generally detect metastatic lesions before they are evident roentgenographically, and they are particularly useful before definitive treatment of large (over 5 cm) breast cancers, since 25% of the patients with such cancers have been shown to have metastatic bone disease at the time of diagnosis. In breast tumors under 2 cm, the positive yield of preoperative bone scans is minimal. In cases of purely lytic lesions, such as those seen in multiple myeloma, the bone scan is usually negative and roentgenographic examination will demonstrate the lesions. Liver scans reveal defects consistent with metastatic disease before either hepatomegaly or abnormal liver function tests are evident.

Computed tomography (CT) is invaluable in the diagnosis of primary and metastatic tumors of the brain. Abdominal CT scans are helpful in detecting mesenteric lymph nodes, liver metastases, retroperitoneal disease, and pelvic masses. Abnormalities in the pancreas, a notoriously difficult area in which to detect early disease, can also be revealed on the CT scan.

Ultrasonography is helpful in the detection of cardiac, pericardial, hepatic, pancreatic, renal, pelvic, and retroperitoneal lymph node abnormalities. It also serves an important function in guiding biopsies of tumor masses.

In certain well-defined situations it is necessary to go beyond the noninvasive studies just discussed to arrive at an adequate staging classification. This is the case when histologic evidence of involvement in a particular area would change the treatment plan for a patient. For example, involvement of mediastinal nodes renders a patient with lung carcinoma inoperable. Mediastinoscopy or exploratory thoracotomy may be required to prove such involvement. In Hodgkin's disease exploratory laparotomy with splenectomy and multiple liver and lymph node biopsies should be performed after clinical staging in cases when the surgical findings might lead to a change in therapeutic approach.

Staging classifications help the physician to estimate the prognosis, plan treatment, and evaluate results. Although a single system applicable to all tumors would seem to be ideal, attempts to establish one have not met with general acceptance. Differences in pathophysiology and natural history among malignant tumors make a single, universal staging classification unwieldy and impractical.

All classifications should be based on anatomic and histologic considerations. The following is a basic system useful for staging the anatomic extent of many solid tumors:

Stage I. Mass limited to organ of origin
Stage II. Local spread into surrounding tissue and first station lymph nodes
Stage III. Extensive primary lesions with fixation to deeper structures, bone invasion, and spread to lymph nodes
Stage IV. Evidence of distant metastases

Recently the tumor-node-metastases (TNM) anatomic classification based on assessment of the primary tumor, lymph nodes, and distant metastases has been advocated by the American Joint Committee for Cancer Staging and Results Reporting. This system, which has been particularly valuable in classifying head and neck tumors, is as follows:

Tumor
  TX. Tumor cannot be assessed
  T0. No evidence of primary tumor
  TIS. Carcinoma in situ
  T1, T2, T3, T4. Progressive increase in tumor size and involvement
Nodes
  NX. Regional lymph nodes cannot be assessed clinically
  N0. Regional lymph nodes not demonstrably abnormal
  N1, N2, N3, N4. Increasing degrees of demonstrable abnormality of regional lymph nodes
Metastases
  MX. Not assessed
  M0. No (known) distant metastasis
  M1. Distant metastasis present; specify sites of metastasis

Histologic staging is based on the degree of differentiation, with G1 being a well-differentiated tumor, G2 moderately well-differentiated, G3 poorly differentiated, and G4 very poorly differentiated.

CLINICAL MANIFESTATIONS

The myriad clinical problems that may be encountered in patients with cancer are the result of the presence of a mass, of invasion or replacement of normal tissue, or of secretory products of the tumor. The specific symptoms depend on the sites of involvement or the particular substances produced.

Obstruction and compression

Obstructive and compressive symptoms caused by the presence of a mass are common in patients with gastrointestinal tract tumors. Dysphagia is the most frequent complaint of patients with carcinoma of the esophagus, pyloric obstruction occurs with carcinoma of the stomach, and intestinal obstruction is a common complication of carcinoma of the left side of the colon. Obstructive jaundice usually results from carcinoma of the pancreas or hepatobiliary tree or less often from pressure by malignant lymph nodes. External compression by such nodes also causes ureteral obstruction in carcinoma of the prostate or ovary and in lymphomas. Bronchogenic carcinomas obstruct bronchi and result in atelectasis. Compression of the spinal cord by epidural tumor produces radicular pain, bladder and bowel dysfunction, and sensory deficits. Progression to complete motor and sensory loss can occur if the compression is unrelieved. Lymphedema and effusions may result from the obstruction of lymphatic flow. Compression or invasion of the superior vena cava by bronchogenic carcinomas, lymphomas, or more rarely other tumors leads to facial swelling, distention of the cervical and upper chest wall veins, conjunctival injection, headache, and convulsions.

Loss or alteration of organ function

Invasion by cancer tissue often results in a loss or alteration of normal organ function. Bone marrow involvement with tumor leads to myelophthisic anemia characterized by the appearance of immature red and white cells in the peripheral blood. Thrombocytopenia is also occasionally seen. Diabetes insipidus, myxedema, or addisonism may arise with tumors involving the posterior pituitary gland, thyroid gland, or adrenal cortex, respectively. Steatorrhea may result from exocrine deficiency of the pancreas. Cardiac arrhythmias occur with invasion of the conduction system by tumor. Hypercalcemia is produced when metastatic tumors, most often carcinoma of the breast and multiple myeloma, directly invade bone.

Tumor secretion

(See Chapter 192.)

Some tumors are characterized by the production of an increased amount of a substance or substances that are normally produced by the cell of origin. In multiple myeloma many of the clinical manifestations result from the excessive secretion of a single or monoclonal immunoglobulin by the malignant plasma cells. Hyperviscosity syndrome, coagulation abnormalities, and renal damage in this disease are directly related to the presence of the malignant paraprotein. The β-cell tumor of the pancreas or insulinoma usually is manifested by hypoglycemia and tumors of the adrenal cortex with hypercortisolism. Carcinoid tumors may produce diarrhea, colic, and malabsorption related to serotonin secretion of attacks of flushing from kallikrein release.

Other tumors are associated with the secretion of substances that are not normally produced by the cells of origin. Bronchogenic carcinomas are the tumors most frequently associated with ectopic hormonal secretion. Clinically apparent hypercortisolism occurs with many carcinomas, particularly small or oat cell carcinoma of the lung. Tumors of the thyroid gland, ovary, prostate, parotid gland, liver, and islet cells and pheochromocytomas also may produce this syndrome. Hypokalemia, weakness, and edema are more common in patients with ectopic ACTH production than in those with other types of Cushing's syndrome. Conversely, truncal obesity, cutaneous striae, and osteoporosis are uncommon in this situation.

Inappropriate secretion of ADH, usually by small or oat cell carcinoma of the lung, results in hyponatremia and excessive urinary sodium excretion. Usually the syndrome is suspected only because of abnormal laboratory values. Occasionally, however, confusion, convulsions, or coma results from profound hyponatremia. The diagnosis may be made by the finding of urine hypertonicity in relation to plasma, normal glomerular filtration rate, and normal adrenocortical function. ADH-like secretion indistinguishable from human pituitary ADH has been isolated from tumors of patients with this syndrome.

Some tumors produce a parathyroid hormone (PTH)–like substance resulting in hypercalcemia, lethargy, weakness, anorexia, nausea, and vomiting. The renal stones or bone disease associated with primary hyperparathyroidism is rarely seen in the ectopic syndrome. Squamous cell carcinomas of the lung and carcinomas of the ovary, kidney, uterus, pancreas, and colon have been associated with ectopic PTH secretion. Prostaglandins produced by tumors also cause nonmetastatic hypercalcemia in cancer patients.

Other hormonal syndromes include hypoglycemia associated with large retroperitoneal or intrathoracic tumors, which may secrete an insulin-like substance, and gynecomastia resulting from gonadotropin secretion by lung, liver, or adrenal tumors.

Miscellaneous paraneoplastic syndromes

Besides the syndromes in which tumor secretion has been demonstrated, there is a heterogeneous group of disorders associated with malignancy for which no explanation has been found. It is presumed that they are effects of secretion of tumor substances, but no such substances have yet been isolated. These syndromes affect many systems and may provide the first clue to the presence of a neoplasm. The symptoms often abate or disappear with successful treatment of the primary tumor.

NEUROLOGIC SYNDROMES. Cerebellar degeneration and many types of peripheral neuropathy including pure sensory, lower motor neuron, and mixed varieties have been described in patients with malignant tumors in the absence of direct involvement of the nervous system. Necrotizing myelopathy, progressive multifocal leukoencephalopathy (probably a papovavirus disease), subacute myelitis, and a myasthenic syndrome (Eaton-Lambert syndrome) have also been observed. Carcinoma of the lung, breast, and ovaries and lymphomas are the tumors most commonly found with these syndromes (see Chapter 153).

RHEUMATIC SYNDROMES. Disorders of connective tissue, such as polymyositis, hypertrophic pulmonary osteoarthropathy, and rheumatoid-like arthropathies, are seen in patients with lung cancer, lymphoid malignancies, and less commonly other tumors. A malignancy is found in 20% of patients with dermatomyositis (see Chapter 19).

HEMATOLOGIC SYNDROMES. A variety of hematologic

abnormalities unrelated to local tumor involvement are recognized in patients with cancer. Autoimmune hemolytic anemia not only occurs in leukemias or lymphomas, where it may be associated with an antibody produced by the tumor cells, but also is seen in certain cystic ovarian tumors in the absence of any detectable anti-red cell antibody. Pure red cell aplasia is often seen with thymomas. Conversely, erythrocytosis occurs with hypernephromas, carcinoma of the lung, prostate, and liver, and cerebellar hemangioblastoma. Erythropoietic activity has been detected in these tumors. Many types of cancer are associated with thrombocytosis and some with thrombocytopenia in the face of normal marrow megakaryocytic activity, pointing to an autoimmune phenomenon. Disseminated intravascular coagulation, particularly of the chronic type, is seen in a wide variety of neoplasms. It is postulated that intravascular coagulation may be initiated by thromboplastins derived from tumor cells, especially of the mucin-secreting types. Migratory thrombophlebitis is common in carcinoma of the lung and pancreas (see Chapter 164).

NEPHROTIC SYNDROME. The nephrotic syndrome has been reported in patients with malignant lymphomas and less frequently with other neoplasms. The mechanism is poorly understood but appears to be immunologic.

DERMATOLOGIC SYNDROMES. A wide variety of nonspecific dermatologic syndromes often herald or coexist with an internal malignancy. The most striking of these is acanthosis nigricans, which is most often seen with carcinoma of the stomach.

TUMOR CACHEXIA SYNDROME. A most puzzling accompaniment of malignancy is the marked cachexia seen in so many advanced cancers. Although anorexia with distortion of taste sensation and aversion to specific foods undoubtedly plays a role, cachexia is often out of proportion to the reduction in caloric intake. The mechanism responsible for this phenomenon is unknown.

COMPLICATIONS OF THERAPY

The therapy for tumors results in a host of clinical problems, some of which, such as infection, augment a tendency already present in a tumor-bearing host, and some of which are unique to a particular therapeutic modality. These are discussed in Chapter 84.

BIBLIOGRAPHY

American Joint Committee for Cancer Staging and End-Results Reporting: Manual for staging of cancer—1978, vol. 1, Chicago, 1978.
Gewirtz, G., and Yalow, R.S.: Ectopic ACTH production in carcinoma of the lung, J. Clin. Invest. **53**:1022, 1974.
Goepp, C.E.: Cancer genetics: a Gordian knot, Semin. Oncol. **5**:61, 1978.
Kardinal, C.G., editor: Historic milestones, Semin. Oncol. **6**:395, 1979.
Rosen, S.W., and others: Placental proteins and their sub-units as tumor markers, Ann. Intern. Med. **82**:71, 1975.
Wynder, E.L., and Rauscher, F.J., Jr., editors: The etiology of cancer, Semin. Oncol. **3**:1, 1976.
Yarbro, J.E., editor: Oncologic emergencies, Semin. Oncol. **5**:123, 1978.

Zambeck, N.: The present status of carcinoembryonic antigen (CEA) in diagnosis, detection of recurrence, prognosis and evaluation of therapy of colonic and pancreatic cancer, Clin. Gastroenterol. **5**:625, 1976.

84 • PRINCIPLES OF SYSTEMIC CANCER THERAPY

Rosaline R. Joseph

The optimal management of patients with malignant tumors changes in response to continuing advances in both basic and clinical cancer research. Since details of therapeutic regimens may be outmoded by the time of publication, this chapter will concentrate on principles of therapy. At present three major therapeutic modalities are available for the treatment of malignant tumors: surgery, radiation, and chemotherapy. Immunotherapy and hyperthermia, although they show promise, are in an experimental stage. Supportive and symptomatic therapy is all-important in maintaining an optimal quality of life. Central to the construction of a treatment plan for each patient should be a consideration of the possible role of each of these modalities in that patient's case, and multidisciplinary consultation should be sought. Traditional roles for surgery, radiation therapy, and chemotherapy are changing, and it is necessary to have expert input in all of these fields. For example, surgery for metastatic disease is no longer always purely palliative. Removal of solitary pulmonary or intracranial metastatic lesions remaining after chemotherapy has resulted in long-term survival in some cancers. Chemotherapy is no longer a "last resort" but is employed after surgery or radiotherapy to prevent or delay clinical recurrence in certain high-risk situations. Preoperative radiation has been shown to be useful in carcinoma of the rectum. The list of such "combined modality" approaches is long and represents a major advance in cancer therapy that has resulted in prolonged survival for many cancer patients and improved quality of life for others. Examples will be discussed under "Management of specific malignancies."

TREATMENT OF LOCALIZED OR REGIONAL DISEASE

Surgery or radiation therapy is usually the treatment of choice in localized disease when careful pretreatment evaluation has revealed no evidence of metastases. If a tumor is accessible and amenable to complete surgical removal, this has traditionally been the recommended procedure. Radiation has been used as primary therapy in situations when surgery is contraindicated (mediastinal node involvement in lung cancer, poor medical condition of the patient) or will cause unacceptable loss of function (some tumors of the head and neck) or when the tumor is highly radiosensitive (lymphomas). Radiation therapy is currently being evaluated as primary therapy for some early breast cancers following "lumpectomy" and for localized rectal carcinoma. Chemotherapy is indicated as "adjuvant" to primary therapy of localized or regional disease when a patient group at high risk for recurrence can be identified and when an agent or agents exist that have demonstrated at least a 20% level of efficacy in metastatic tumors of the type in question.

TREATMENT OF DISSEMINATED MALIGNANCIES

Effective treatment of disseminated malignant neoplasms is based primarily on the availability of chemotherapeutic agents that act systemically, killing tumor cells throughout the body. The potential for curing disseminated human tumors derives from the cell-kill hypotheses and an understanding of tumor cell kinetics. The cell-kill or Skipper hypotheses were originally based on the L-1210 mouse leukemia model but appear to hold true for malignant tumors in general. The major hypotheses state that (1) a single leukemia cell is capable of "cloning" enough cells to kill the host; (2) the life span of the host is inversely proportional to the numbers of clonogenic cells inoculated; (3) the life span of the host is inversely proportional to the number of clonogenic cells remaining at the end of therapy; and (4) first-order kinetics apply to leukemic cell kill by chemotherapy (a given dose of a given drug kills the same percentage, not the same number, of cells in populations varying widely in size). The chances of killing the last cell are calculable in populations that are homogeneous with respect to drug sensitivity.

Although these hypotheses have been useful in the construction of effective chemotherapeutic regimens, their practical value has been limited by the fact that in most human tumors the cells are not uniformly sensitive to chemotherapy. At any one time in any given tumor, only a portion of cells are undergoing division. This is the "growth fraction" of the tumor. The remaining cells are in a resting phase. In the earliest stages of tumor development, growth is exponential, since there is a very large growth fraction. As the tumor enlarges, the growth fraction decreases, possibly because of decreased vascularization, and there is an increase in doubling time of the tumor. Human tumors vary widely in their growth fractions and doubling times.

Replication of the individual cell depends on the cell cycle, which consists of the G_1 or pre-DNA synthetic phase, which varies from 2 hours to infinity; the S phase of active DNA synthesis, which lasts from 6 to 23 hours; the G_2 or premitotic phase lasting 2 to 8 hours; and the M or mitotic phase lasting 0.5 to 2 hours. In addition to the actively dividing cells in the growth fraction, the tumors have a second population of cells that are not actively dividing but have the ability to do so. These are said to be in a G_0 (quiescent) or an extended G_1 phase. Finally, tumors contain a group of cells that are no longer capable of division and cannot reenter the cell cycle.

Many anticancer drugs exert their cytotoxic effects on the dividing cell and are inactive against the quiescent or permanently nondividing population. As previously mentioned, part of the difficulty in achieving total cell kill in humans is derived from the difference in the growth characteristics of the tumor cells and hence their difference in drug sensitivity.

Accurate measurement of cell cycle times of individual cells or doubling times of individual tumors allows precise scheduling so that drugs can be given when the largest number of tumor cells are in the most vulnerable stage. Techniques permitting such measurement are not widely available at this time. Tumors with large growth fractions are generally sensitive to cytotoxic agents. In tumors with low growth fractions, toxicity to normal rapidly dividing cells, such as bone marrow and gastrointestinal mucosal cells, makes effective antitumor chemotherapy more difficult.

Despite these limitations, major advances in the treatment of disseminated malignancy have resulted from the successful use of the best available chemotherapeutic agents in the most effective manner. Some disseminated malignancies such as acute lymphoblastic leukemia of childhood, advanced Hodgkin's disease, diffuse histiocytic lymphoma, nodular mixed lymphoma, nonseminomatous testicular tumors, ovarian carcinomas, choriocarcinomas of pregnancy, and Burkitt's lymphomas are curable by chemotherapy. Wilms' tumor, Ewing's sarcoma, and embryonal rhabdomyosarcoma are curable by multimodality therapy, of which chemotherapy is an integral part. In many other cancers the use of chemotherapy provides significant improvement in the quality and duration of life.

It must be emphasized that chemotherapy, although usually the mainstay of therapy for disseminated cancer, is not the only modality available for these patients. Judicious use of radiotherapy for such situations as bone pain and bronchial obstruction, as well as surgical relief of gastrointestinal obstruction, is invaluable and will be further discussed in the section "Supportive care."

Chemotherapy

Compounds active in cancer treatment are usually cytotoxic. These agents exercise their effects on cell proliferation by interfering with DNA synthesis or transcription, damaging preformed DNA, blocking mitosis, or inhibiting RNA or protein biosynthesis. The following are the major types of chemotherapeutic agents:

I. Antimetabolites
   A. Folic acid antagonists
      1. Methotrexate
   B. Pyrimidine antagonists
      1. Cytosine arabinoside
      2. 5-Fluorouracil

C. Purine antagonists
1. 6-Mercaptopurine
2. 6-Thioguanine
II. Natural products
A. Antitumor antibiotics
1. Dactinomycin
2. Mithramycin
3. Bleomycin
4. Mitomycin C
5. Doxorubicin
6. Daunorubicin
B. Vinca alkaloids
1. Vinblastine
2. Vincristine
C. Enzymes
1. Asparaginase
III. Alkylating agents
A. Mechlorethamine (nitrogen mustard)
B. Cyclophosphamide
C. Melphalan
D. Chlorambucil
E. Busulfan
F. Nitrosoureas (BCNU, CCNU, methyl CCNU, streptozocin)
G. DTIC (Dacarbazine)
IV. Miscellaneous agents
A. Cisplatin
B. Hydroxyurea
C. Procarbazine

These agents are usually classified as cell cycle–specific and cell cycle–nonspecific agents. Cell cycle–specific agents are those that either are active at a specific point in the cell cycle (cycle-phase specific) or kill proliferating cells more effectively than resting cells. For example, cytosine arabinoside inhibits DNA synthesis in the S phase. Other agents that inhibit DNA synthesis, such as methotrexate and 6-mercaptopurine, also inhibit RNA and protein synthesis. These effects slow down the cell cycle and the number of cells entering the S phase, so that the action of these antimetabolites is somewhat self limited. The vinca alkaloids (vinblastine and vincristine) arrest mitosis in metaphase by interfering with the synthesis of proteins necessary for spindle formation. The cell cycle–nonspecific agents are those that interfere in various ways with the function of preformed DNA and are thus not dependent on the cell cycle for their effect. Among the mechanisms of action of these agents are cross-linkage (alkylating agents), depolymerization (procarbazine, dacarbazine or DTIC, cisplatin, nitrosoureas), intercalation with blockage of RNA synthesis (anthracycline antibiotics, actinomycin D, mitomycin C), and scission of DNA strands (bleomycin).

A brief summary of the important properties, indications, and toxicities of the most frequently used chemotherapeutic agents follows. Dosages will not be given because they vary in different protocols, and these protocols are still evolving.

ANTIMETABOLITES

Folic acid antagonists. Methotrexate, the first antimetabolite used clinically as an antitumor agent, acts by inhibiting the enzyme dihydrofolate reductase, which catalyzes the reaction of dihydrofolate to tetrahydrofolate. The result of this inhibition is a block in the conversion of deoxyuridine to thymidylate and thus in DNA synthesis. RNA and protein synthesis are also inhibited by lack of tetrahydrofolate. Methotrexate is readily absorbed orally and is administered either by mouth or intravenously in various dosage schedules. Its plasma half-life is approximately 2 hours, and about half of it is bound to plasma proteins. It is excreted unchanged primarily through the urine.

These properties of methotrexate must be considered when determining dosage of the drug. Displacement from plasma albumin by simultaneous administration of salicylates, sulfonamide, tetracycline, chloramphenicol, or phenytoin can result in a significant increase in toxicity. Likewise, decreased renal function can result in dangerously prolonged blood levels.

Recently, methotrexate in high doses with leucovorin (folinic acid) rescue has been used in the treatment of some malignant tumors in an effort to increase the inhibition of DNA synthesis. Leucovorin is given after the administration of high doses of methotrexate to rescue normal cells. Malignant cells seem less capable of being rescued.

The major toxic effects of methotrexate are myelosuppression, ulcerative mucositis, and alopecia. Rarer complications include interstitial pneumonitis and hepatic dysfunction that occasionally results in cirrhosis.

Methotrexate in standard doses is useful in the treatment of carcinoma of the breast, head, and neck and in acute lymphocytic leukemia. It is curative in about 75% of pregnancy-related choriocarcinomas. Methotrexate in high doses has been particularly successful in osteogenic sarcoma and head and neck cancers.

Pyrimidine antagonists. Cytosine arabinoside is an S phase inhibitor whose principal mode of action appears to be inhibition of DNA polymerase. It is rapidly deaminated to an inactive metabolite that is excreted in the urine. The drug may be administered intravenously or subcutaneously. Its most important toxic effect is severe bone marrow depression with megaloblastic changes. Stomatitis, gastrointestinal disturbances, hepatic dysfunction, dermatitis, and fever also occur. Currently the major indication for cytosine arabinoside is in the treatment of acute myelogenous leukemia, where its combination with daunorubicin results in initial remission rates of 60% to 80%.

5-Fluorouracil (5-FU) is an inhibitor of thymidylate synthetase and thus of DNA synthesis. It is degraded in the liver and excreted in the urine. 5-FU is usually administered intravenously, although there is significant absorption when administered orally. The compound is myelosuppressive and also causes stomatitis, nausea, vomiting, and diarrhea. Hyperpigmentation of the skin and nails and more rarely cerebellar ataxia may occur. 5-FU is used widely in the treatment of solid tumors. It has been applied topically in the form of a cream to treat actinic keratoses and superficial basal cell carcinomas.

Purine antagonists. 6-Mercaptopurine, a hypoxanthine analog, interferes with de novo purine biosynthesis and interconversions. The drug is well absorbed from the gastrointestinal tract and is administered orally. It is metabolized to 6-thiouric acid and inorganic sulfate, which are excreted in the urine. Allopurinol, a xanthine oxidase inhibitor usually used to block uric acid formation, also blocks the metabolism of 6-mercaptopurine. When the two drugs are given simultaneously, the dose of 6-mercaptopurine must be reduced to avoid serious toxicity. The major toxic effect of 6-mercaptopurine is bone marrow suppression. Reversible cholestatic jaundice may develop in up to one third of adult patients taking the drug. Its major use is in acute lymphoblastic leukemia.

6-Thioguanine acts similarly to 6-mercaptopurine and is also usually given orally. It is currently used primarily in combination with other agents in the treatment of acute myelogenous leukemia.

NATURAL PRODUCTS

Antitumor antibiotics. Dactinomycin forms a complex with DNA, resulting in the inhibition of DNA-dependent RNA synthesis. It is administered intravenously and is caustic if extravasation occurs. It causes myelosuppression and gastrointestinal disturbances. Dactinomycin is most useful in Wilms' tumor, testicular tumors, and gestational trophoblastic tumors.

Mithramycin interferes with RNA synthesis and probably inhibits osteoclastic activity. It is administered intravenously and is more often used for its unique calcium-lowering effect than for its antineoplastic activity. The drug must be administered with great care because of the possibility of the development of a severe hemorrhagic diathesis resulting from a combination of thrombocytopenia, multiple coagulation abnormalities, and capillary damage. Other side effects are bone marrow suppression and gastrointestinal, renal, and hepatic abnormalities.

Bleomycin is a mixture of glycopeptide antibiotics that acts both by inhibition of DNA synthesis and by scission of DNA strands. It can be administered either intravenously or intramuscularly and is excreted by the kidneys. Preferential localization occurs in the lung and skin owing to failure of inactivation by the tissues of these organs. This phenomenon probably accounts for the peculiar toxicity of bleomycin. Serious pulmonary damage may occur, usually after a total dose of over 300 mg (units)/m^2. Pulmonary toxicity begins as pneumonitis and in 15% to 20% of cases progresses to fibrosis, which is fatal in about 1% of patients. Multiple dermatologic abnormalities such as ulceration, hyperkeratosis, and hyperpigmentation are common. Stomatitis, alopecia, and fever also sometimes occur. Because of reports of anaphylactoid reactions in patients with lymphomas receiving bleomycin, a test dose of 1 to 2 units is recommended before starting therapy. Bleomycin is not myelosuppressive and is useful in the treatment of lymphomas and testicular and head and neck cancers.

Mitomycin C appears to form a cross-linkage with DNA after intracellular enzymatic reduction. It is administered intravenously, and extravasation may result in serious local tissue damage. Its toxic effect is primarily myelosuppression, with gastrointestinal, renal, pulmonary, and mucocutaneous effects also reported. At present the drug has its greatest use in carcinoma of the stomach.

Doxorubicin and daunorubicin act by binding to DNA with untwisting of the helix to permit intercalation of the drug skeleton. Both these agents are administered intravenously and cause local tissue necrosis if even a small amount is extravasated. Metabolic degradation occurs in the liver, and severe toxicity can result if standard doses are given to patients with reduced liver function. Excretion of the drugs and their metabolites is primarily through the bile. Myelosuppression, nausea, vomiting, and alopecia are all major side effects of these agents. Patients should be warned that their urine will turn red for 1 to 2 days. The most serious toxic effect of these drugs is the development of cardiomyopathy. Two types of cardiotoxicity are recognized. The first or acute variety is characterized by ST-T wave changes, arrhythmias, and an acute reversible reduction in ejection fraction occurring 24 hours after a single dose. This reaction is usually brief and of no serious consequence. Chronic toxicity, however, is cumulative and dose related. It results in congestive heart failure, which is unresponsive to digitalis and carries a mortality rate of greater than 50%. The mechanism of the cardiomyopathy is unclear, but binding to cardiac DNA and oxidative damage have been implicated. Significant cardiotoxicity develops in 20% of patients taking doxorubicin at a total dose greater than 550 mg/m^2, with reports of toxicity at doses as low as 250 mg/m^2. For daunorubicin the critical dose appears to be 600 mg/m^2. Previous irradiation of the mediastinum, treatment with cyclophosphamide, and advanced age increase the risk of cardiotoxicity. No dependable predictive tests are generally available, and the onset of congestive heart failure is often delayed. Half of the cases occur longer than 6 months from the completion of therapy.

Doxorubicin has a broad spectrum of activity with particular usefulness in carcinoma of the breast, thyroid, and lung and osteogenic sarcoma. Daunorubicin is most useful in the treatment of acute myelogenous leukemia.

Vinca alkaloids. Vinca alkaloids are products of the periwinkle plant that interfere with the metaphase through spindle protein damage. Although there is great structural similarity between vinblastine and vincristine, the two alkaloids in current use, there are significant differences in cytotoxic action and little cross-resistance. The compounds are administered intravenously and cause local tissue damage if extravasated. They are cleared rapidly from the bloodstream and are excreted through the biliary tract.

Vinblastine is a bone marrow depressant, and gastrointestinal disturbances are common. Neurotoxicity and alopecia are only minor problems with vinblastine. Its major use is in the treatment of Hodgkin's disease and testicular tumors. Vincristine, unlike vinblastine, is not myelosuppressive. Its major toxic effect is neurologic, with paresthesias, loss of deep tendon reflexes, paresis, ptosis, and double vision. Severe constipation may occur, and all patients receiving vincristine should be given prophylactic stool softeners. Alopecia and inappropriate antidiuretic hormone secretion are other important side effects. Vincristine's greatest use is inducing remission in acute lymphocytic leukemia. It is also effective in Hodgkin's and non-Hodgkin's lymphomas, breast cancer, and Wilms' tumor.

Asparaginase. Asparaginase, an enzyme prepared from *Escherichia coli*, catalyzes the hydrolysis of plasma asparagine to aspartic acid and ammonia. Although normal cells can synthesize asparagine, certain neoplastic cells lack asparagine synthetase and are dependent on exogenous asparagine. When malignant cells are exposed to asparaginase, they develop a selective nutritional deficiency. Although the drug has resulted in remission in up to 60% of children with acute lymphocytic leukemia, its usefulness is limited by anaphylactic and other allergic reactions. Resistance to the enzyme develops rapidly, and remissions are short lived. Other side effects of the inhibition of protein synthesis are mild decreases in hepatic, renal, pancreatic, and coagulation functions.

ALKYLATING AGENTS. The alkylating agents generate highly reactive electrophilic carbonium ions that alkylate with nucleophilic substances by forming covalent linkages. Cross-linkage of adjacent macromolecules may follow, with inhibition of mitosis resulting from prevention of separation of the DNA strands. Cell death may also occur during interphase when many targets, including RNA and protein, are damaged.

Mechlorethamine (nitrogen mustard) is very quickly bound to proteins or intracellular macromolecules. Almost none is excreted in the urine. Intravenous administration of nitrogen mustard must be very carefully performed, usually into the tubing of a rapidly flowing infusion, since thrombophlebitis may occur when high concentrations are in prolonged direct contact with the intima of the injected vein. The drug also has a local vesicant action. Nitrogen mustard may be instilled in body cavities for the control of malignant effusions. Its major toxic effects are myelosuppression, nausea, and vomiting. The agent is useful primarily in the treatment of Hodgkin's disease.

Cyclophosphamide is activated by hepatic microsomal enzymes, and therefore microsomal stimulators such as barbiturates increase its activity and toxicity. It can be administered either orally or intravenously. Bone marrow suppression and alopecia are important side effects. The accumulation of metabolites in concentrated urine causes a sterile hemorrhagic cystitis in about 5% of the patients. To avoid this complication, ample fluid intake and frequent voiding should be recommended to all patients taking cyclophosphamide. Gonadal suppression sometimes resulting in sterility, particularly in males, is not uncommon. Patients should be informed of this possibility before starting the drug. Occasional cases of pulmonary interstitial fibrosis attributed to cyclophosphamide have been reported. Cyclophosphamide is widely used in the lymphoproliferative disorders and carcinoma of the breast, lung, and ovary.

Melphalan (L-phenylalanine mustard) is an orally administered alkylating agent. It is myelosuppressive and is used in the treatment of multiple myeloma and ovarian carcinoma.

Chlorambucil is the slowest acting and least toxic nitrogen mustard derivative in clinical use. It is well absorbed from the gastrointestinal tract and is useful in chronic lymphocytic leukemia and the lymphomas. Moderate bone marrow toxicity does occur, but it is usually readily reversible.

Busulfan is an oral agent that depresses granulocyte production. It has a lesser effect on platelets. Pulmonary fibrosis has been reported following busulfan administration, as have hyperpigmentation of the skin, glossitis, and anhidrosis. Busulfan's major use is in the treatment of chronic granulocytic leukemia.

The mechanism of action of the nitrosourea compounds is closely related to that of the alkylating agents. Active metabolites are probably responsible for their cytotoxic activity. An important feature of the nitrosoureas is their ability to cross the blood-brain barrier, with levels from 15% to 50% of plasma levels attainable in the cerebrospinal fluid. BCNU (carmustine) is administered intravenously through a running infusion. CCNU (lomustine) and methyl-CCNU (semustine) are well absorbed orally. Nausea, vomiting, and delayed bone marrow suppression are prominent side effects of this group of drugs, and pulmonary fibrosis has been reported. The nitrosoureas are useful in lymphomas, brain tumors, and possibly in lung and gastrointestinal tumors. Streptozocin (streptozotocin), a naturally occurring nitrosourea, has a diabetogenic effect and is useful in islet cell tumors. Side effects include mild myelosuppression, nausea and vomiting, hepatic damage, and severe proximal tubular renal toxicity.

Dacarbazine (dimethyltriazmo-imidazole carboxamide, DTIC) behaves like an alkylating agent. It is administered intravenously and activated in the liver. Myelosuppression and gastrointestinal disturbances are the major toxic effects. Fever, myalgias, malaise, alopecia, facial flushing, and hepatotoxicity have also been reported. This is the current drug of choice in the treatment of malignant melanoma.

MISCELLANEOUS AGENTS. The platinum-coordinating complexes are capable of cross-linking with DNA. More than 90% of cisplatin (cis-diamminedichloroplatinum II) is protein bound and appears to be excreted primarily in the urine. Renal tubular toxicity is a major problem, and the drug should be cautiously administered with meticulous attention to concomitant administration of intravenous fluids. Mannitol with or without furosemide has been recommended as an additional safeguard to ensure adequate diuresis. Platinum is also myelotoxic and ototoxic. It is mandatory to obtain baseline creatinine clearance and audiograms before instituting therapy. Platinum shows great promise in testicular, ovarian, bladder, and head and neck malignancies.

Hydroxyurea is an S phase–specific agent that inhibits DNA synthesis. It is well absorbed orally and is largely excreted in the urine. The toxic effects include myelosuppression, gastrointestinal disturbances, and stomatitis. Occasionally alopecia, dermatitis, or neurologic manifestations occur. Hydroxyurea is most often used in the treatment of chronic granulocytic leukemia.

Procarbazine, a compound whose basic mode of action is poorly understood, is capable of inhibiting DNA, RNA, and protein synthesis. It is absorbed from the gastrointestinal tract and metabolized by the liver. The metabolites are excreted in the urine. Bone marrow suppression and gastrointestinal disturbances are the major side effects. Because the drug is a weak monoamine oxidase inhibitor, sympathomimetics, tricyclic antidepressants, and other medications or foods with high tyramine content should not be taken concomitantly. Augmentation of the mild sedative effects of procarbazine has been seen with simultaneous use of central nervous system depressants, and ingestion of ethyl alcohol has resulted in an acetaldehyde syndrome resembling that produced by disulfiram. The major indication for procarbazine has been in the treatment of Hodgkin's disease.

PRINCIPLES OF COMBINATION CHEMOTHERAPY. In almost all situations, combination chemotherapy has proved more effective than single-agent regimens in the treatment of cancer. The principles of rational combinations are listed in the following:
1. Each drug must be individually active in the specific disease being treated.
2. Agents that produce different biochemical lesions should be combined, so that multiple sites of proliferation or function of cells may be attacked.
3. Agents having different toxicities should be selected, allowing a therapeutic dose of each to be employed with little or no increased risk.
4. Combining drugs whose toxicities occur at different times following administration also allows use of larger doses.
5. Agents in which there is a biochemical basis for suspecting synergism should be combined.

In general, intermittent high-dose therapy with these combinations is preferable to continuous low-dose regimens. If these treatment programs have a selective killing effect on tumor tissue rather than normal bone marrow, a 2-week interval is usually sufficient to allow marrow recovery without equal tumor regrowth. Another advantage of intermittent therapy is that this type of schedule permits recovery and even rebound of the host's immunologic defenses rather than the prolonged immunosuppression associated with continuous treatment.

Hormonal manipulation

HORMONAL RECEPTORS. The growth of some tumors appears to be dependent on their hormonal environment, and many patients with carcinoma of the breast, prostate, and endometrium will respond to endocrine manipulation. The mechanism of action of either additive or ablative procedures in carcinoma of the breast has recently been clarified, making the choice of therapy more rational than previously possible. It is known that the initial step in steroid hormone action is the binding of the hormone to highly specialized receptor proteins in the target cells. Cytoplasmic receptors have now been identified for several steroid hormones. Binding of the hormone to the receptor initiates a series of steps, eventually leading to the characteristic hormonal effect on the target tissue. The presence of receptor protein appears to be necessary for hormonal responsiveness. Receptors for estrogen are present in about two thirds of primary breast cancers, with a somewhat lower rate of positivity in metastatic lesions. Tumors in premenopausal women are estrogen receptor (ER) positive in less than 50% of cases, and those in postmenopausal patients are positive in more than 50%. Objective responses to endocrine manipulation occur in 50% to 70% of patients whose tumors are ER positive, whereas only 5% to 10% of ER-negative patients respond. Progesterone receptors (PR) are found in about two thirds of ER-positive tumors and in about 5% of ER-negative tumors. The highest response rate to endocrine therapy (80%) is in tumors that are both ER positive and PR positive. It is of utmost importance to obtain receptor assays in all patients with breast cancer at the time of histologic diagnosis as a guide to future therapy. When metastatic disease occurs, it may involve a site inaccessible to biopsy, and a valuable tool in therapeutic planning is unavailable. The presence or absence of hormonal receptors also appears to have prognostic value. Estrogen receptor positivity seems to be correlated with a prolonged disease-free interval that is independent of other variables. Data relating ER status to response to chemotherapy are conflicting, and further studies are needed to resolve this issue.

Other steroid hormone receptors such as androgen and glucocorticoid receptors are found in some breast tumors.

Their relevance in predicting therapeutic response has not been ascertained. Steroid receptors also exist in carcinoma of the prostate and endometrium and in malignant melanoma. The clinical significance in these tumors is uncertain.

ABLATIVE PROCEDURES. Oophorectomy should be performed in premenopausal women with metastatic or recurrent breast cancer whose tumors are ER positive, who have had a long disease-free interval, and whose metastatic sites are bone and skin rather than viscera. In any other circumstances oophorectomy should be reserved for well-controlled clinical trials.

Bilateral adrenalectomy results in objective improvement in 50% of women with breast cancer who have a relapse after a good response (6 to 18 disease-free months) to oophorectomy. Other patients in whom adrenalectomy may be of benefit are postmenopausal women who have had a relapse following satisfactory response to estrogens or antiestrogens. Surgical adrenalectomy necessitates lifelong replacement therapy. Aminoglutethimide, an inhibitor of the conversion of cholesterol to pregnenolone in the adrenal gland, may be used to effect a "medical adrenalectomy." Administration of this compound together with hydrocortisone replacement has been associated with beneficial results comparable to those with surgical extirpation of the adrenal glands in women with widespread bony metastases. It is preferable to surgery in severely debilitated patients and has the advantage of reversibility if there is no therapeutic effect. Toxic effects include skin rash and lethargy that usually subside spontaneously if therapy is continued.

Hypophysectomy has the same indications as adrenalectomy, with approximately the same success rate. Recently there has been some evidence that this procedure is associated with pain relief apart from its antitumor effect.

Orchiectomy for stage IV (distant metastases) prostatic carcinoma was first suggested by Huggins in 1941. About 80% of the patients respond with reduction of bone pain and size of tumor mass. Occasionally, skeletal metastases show roentgenographic evidence of healing. Orchiectomy is the treatment of choice in men in whom estrogen administration is contraindicated.

HORMONE ADMINISTRATION. The use of estrogens such as diethylstilbestrol in the management of metastatic breast cancer should currently be limited to postmenopausal women with ER-positive or unknown receptor status and in this group should be tried before ablative surgical procedures. The results are best in patients whose metastases are confined to bone and/or soft tissue. In metastatic prostatic carcinoma, estrogens are as effective as orchiectomy in decreasing bone pain. The side effects of estrogen therapy include hypercalcemia in the presence of lytic bone lesions, nausea, vomiting, and edema. In men, doses of 1 mg of diethylstilbestrol daily appear to give a good therapeutic effect. Higher doses lead to a high incidence of hypertension and cardiac complications without increased therapeutic effect. In patients with preexisting cardiac disease, orchiectomy is the treatment of choice for metastatic prostate carcinoma.

Certain estrogen analogs bind to estrogen receptors, antagonizing estrogenic stimulation of target tissue. Tamoxifen is an antiestrogen agent that has a beneficial effect in 60% of the patients with ER-positive metastatic breast cancer. The response appears to be most dramatic in postmenopausal patients. Although tamoxifen generally has fewer side effects than does diethylstilbestrol, thrombocytopenia, leukopenia, and nausea have been reported. An interesting phenomenon associated with tamoxifen administration is the "tamoxifen flare," with increased pain and hypercalcemia occurring shortly after the drug is instituted. This reaction often precedes and predicts a good antitumor response, and it is not a reason to discontinue therapy if the troublesome symptoms can be controlled.

Androgenic steroids are useful in premenopausal women with metastatic breast carcinoma who have previously had responses to primary and secondary hormonal manipulation, that is, oophorectomy and adrenalectomy-hypophysectomy. The masculinizing effects of these hormones, however, are often intolerable to patients, and their usefulness is severely limited.

Progestins have produced significant responses in about 30% of patients with metastatic endometrial carcinoma. There is evidence that some progestins act as antiestrogens and may prove useful in ER-positive metastatic breast cancer. Occasional improvement in metastatic renal cell carcinoma has been observed with progestational agents.

Prednisone is a cornerstone of therapy of the lymphoproliferative disorders. It causes lymphocyte lysis, presumably by inhibition of cellular protein synthesis. Specific receptors for corticosteroids have been found in acute lymphocytic leukemia. The beneficial effect of prednisone in carcinoma of the breast may be due to suppression of adrenocortical estrogen production. Dexamethasone, which is used primarily to reduce edema surrounding brain tumors, may exert a direct antitumor effect against glioblastomas.

Immunotherapy

Attempts to treat cancer by stimulation of the host's immune defenses date to the 1880s, when Dr. W. Coley treated a large series of patients by injecting a mixture of killed bacterial vaccines (Coley's toxins). Although he reported objective tumor regression in a substantial number of patients, his work remains unconfirmed.

The rebirth of interest in immunotherapy was stimulated by the demonstration of specific tumor-associated antigens in animal systems. If the host could mount an immune reaction against these "foreign" antigens, tumor destruction might result. So far, tumor-specific antigens in humans have been demonstrated only in osteogenic sarcoma, although there is circumstantial evidence for their existence in other tumors. Immunopotentiators such as Bacille Calmette-Guérin (BCG) and *Corynebacterium parvum* have been shown to prevent growth or cause regression of transplanted mouse tumors. These observations, together with the popularity of the theory of immune surveillance, which holds that cancer results from a breakdown of the body's natural immune mechanism, were the stimulus for clinical immunotherapeutic trials.

Immunotherapy may be passive, active, or adoptive. The transfer of immune serum into a tumor-bearing host constitutes passive therapy. In adoptive therapy, immune lymphocytes or a dialyzable lymphocytic extract known as transfer factor is administered. Active immunotherapy may be specific or nonspecific. The administration of nonspecific immunomodulators, such as BCG, *C. parvum,* or the antihelminthic agent levamisole, to stimulate the host's immune response has been the most frequently used immunotherapeutic approach. Specific immunotherapy involves immunization of the host with tumor cells or tumor cell extracts.

To be successful, immunotherapy must be used when the tumor burden is low, and it is generally most effective after maximal cytoreduction has been accomplished by other modalities. At the present time immunotherapy of human cancer is experimental. No conclusions can yet be drawn, and trials should be confined to controlled situations.

Interferon

Interferons are potent antiviral glycoproteins that also inhibit the multiplication of tumor cells in experimental systems. The mechanism of their antitumor activity is as yet unknown. Trials are being conducted using interferon of human leukocyte origin in advanced breast cancer, lymphomas, multiple myeloma, and malignant melanoma.

Supportive care

OBSTRUCTION AND COMPRESSION. The superior vena cava syndrome associated with malignancy is most effectively treated by full-dose radiation therapy. Diuretics and corticosteroids may offer some benefit but should not be relied on as definitive therapy. The degree of emergency of each case must be carefully evaluated. In patients for whom no previous histologic diagnosis is available, radiation therapy may render such a diagnosis difficult or impossible. When symptoms are mild, it is often possible to delay irradiation until tissue can be obtained. When there is evidence of significantly increased venous pressure, however, procedures such as mediastinoscopy or bronchoscopy may be hazardous. If a firm diagnosis of oat cell carcinoma has been established, chemotherapy alone may provide rapid relief of symptoms.

Bronchial airway obstruction resulting from direct tumor invasion or external compression by enlarged nodes and neoplastic obstruction of the esophagus should be treated with radiotherapy. Small bowel obstruction caused by malignancy is usually due to extrinsic compression, whereas obstruction of the large bowel is usually the result of a primary colon tumor. In either case surgical removal of the obstructing lesion is the treatment of choice. When the primary tumor is a lymphoma or ovarian carcinoma, radiation may be effective in relieving the obstruction. Partial or complete obstruction of the biliary tree, usually from an infiltrating carcinoma of the head of the pancreas, is treated by surgical decompression. Ureteral obstruction can result from direct invasion by pelvic tumors or from extrinsic compression by enlarged lymph nodes. Uremia due to ureteral obstruction is the major cause of death from cervical carcinoma. If the site of obstruction is identifiable and localized, radiotherapy may be effective. With more diffuse obstruction, diverting surgery may be necessary.

Epidural spinal cord compression should be treated as soon as it is recognized and the diagnosis is established by myelography. Radiation may be used as initial therapy for patients with slowly progressing neurologic symptoms and signs and for those whose tumors are known to be radiosensitive. Decompressive surgery is indicated for patients with rapidly progressive neurologic defects, especially if the tumor is radioresistant. Peripheral nerve or plexus compression of recent onset may be relieved by radiotherapy, but the effects of long-standing compression are usually irreversible.

METABOLIC DERANGEMENT. *Hypercalcemia* of mild to moderate degree usually responds to ambulation, hydration with saline solutions, and diuresis. Severe or refractory hypercalcemia can be effectively treated with mithramycin, 25 µg/kg. Doses can be repeated at 3- to 7-day intervals. Calcitonin, corticosteroids, and prostaglandin inhibitors such as indomethacin are also useful in lowering serum calcium levels.

Hyponatremia resulting from inappropriate antidiuretic hormone (ADH) secretion can be corrected by water restriction. Demeclocycline, which inhibits the action of ADH on the kidneys, is effective in treating this syndrome. As in all ectopic hormonal syndromes, treatment of the primary tumor is the most effective way to eliminate the endocrine abnormalities.

MALIGNANT EFFUSIONS. Intrapleural instillation of sclerosing agents in an attempt to obliterate the pleural space is the standard therapy of recurrent pleural effusions in patients with cancer. Among the agents used have been chemotherapeutic drugs (nitrogen mustard, thioTEPA, 5-FU, bleomycin), quinacrine, talc, and tetracycline. If the effusion is due to central lymphatic obstruction, irradiation of the mediastinum may be beneficial. Malignant pericardial effusions often require the surgical creation of a pleuropericardial window to avoid tamponade. Intrapericardial instillation of sclerosing agents has also successfully controlled such effusions.

Although intraperitoneal instillation of sclerosing agents has been used for intractable ascites in patients with cancer, it is rarely successful, and repeated paracenteses may be the only way to relieve this troublesome complication.

NUTRITIONAL PROBLEMS. Weight loss can seriously limit the cancer patient's quality of life and ability to tolerate intensive antineoplastic therapy. Since anorexia is often a prominent symptom, maintenance of adequate nutrition often requires the use of dietary supplements. These products supply calories in concentrated form. If it is impossible to achieve adequate nutrition orally, total parenteral nutrition (TPN) should be considered for patients in whom primary therapy for tumor control is possible. The solutions of 50% glucose, mixtures of essential amino acids, and vitamins used in TPN can provide up to 3000 calories a day. Gradual increases of glucose concentration will usually prevent the hyperosmolar, nonketotic coma that has occasionally been associated with TPN.

PAIN. Half of all patients with cancer never experience disease-related pain, 30% have mild to moderate pain, and 20% have severe pain. With proper management, all patients with cancer can be rendered essentially pain free. A major stumbling block to achieving this goal has been the fear of addiction. In a patient with advanced cancer and pain that is unresponsive to local measures such as radiation therapy, adequate analgesics should be prescribed on a regular rather than "when necessary" basis. Attention should be paid to the frequency of medication. Meperidine has a short half-life (2 hours) and therefore is ineffective on an every-4-hour schedule. Morphine, hydromorphone, and levorphanol are better choices if narcotics are required. The addition of alcohol, phenothiazines, and cocaine to the analgesic is often helpful, and the use of such mixtures (for example, Brompton's solution) has been successful in relieving some of the anxiety as well as the pain of advanced cancer. Since all the opiates are constipating, stool softeners should be prescribed routinely to patients receiving narcotics. Pain medication should be given orally, whenever possible, to eliminate the discomfort of injections.

INFECTION. Infection is a frequent complication of malignant tumors and of antineoplastic therapy. Advanced cancer itself is often accompanied by a depressed immune response. Intensive chemotherapy and/or radiation therapy results in temporary immunosuppression and granulocytopenia, further increasing the already compromised patient's susceptibility to infection. Finally, local factors such as bronchial or ureteral obstruction make patients susceptible to infection in areas of poor drainage.

A particularly serious problem is the management of infection in the neutropenic, immunosuppressed host. Gram-negative bacteria are the most common pathogenic organisms in these patients, with *Pseudomonas aeruginosa*, *E. coli*, and *Klebsiella-Enterobacter* responsible for the largest number of infections. In many febrile episodes neither the source of infection nor the offending organism is identified despite aggressive diagnostic procedures. Since sepsis in the neutropenic patient can progress rapidly to a fatal conclusion, the physician should institute empiric combination antibiotic therapy while awaiting results of diagnostic studies. The most frequently recommended initial combination is a cephalosporin, an aminoglycoside, and carbenicillin or ticarcillin. This regimen may be appropriately modified when the pathogen is identified and sensitivity studies are completed. An increasing number of serious fungal infections is being recognized in cancer patients, with disseminated candidiasis, aspergillosis, and mucormycosis seen most often. Cryptococcosis is common in patients with lymphoma. The use of amphotericin B in febrile, neutropenic patients who have not responded to antibiotic therapy has been suggested by some. Neutropenic, immunosuppressed patients are particularly susceptible to infection by *Pneumocystis carinii*. If this diagnosis is suspected, the empiric use of trimethoprim-sulfamethoxazole is recommended. Transfusion of HLA-compatible granulocytes appears to be beneficial in controlling infection in patients with persistent neutropenia.

Prophylaxis of infection in immunosuppressed patients should be vigorously pursued. Invasive procedures such as prolonged infusions, indwelling catheters, and endoscopies should be kept to a minimum. Careful attention should be paid to handwashing technique and frequent changes of intravenous infusion sites. Protective environments, such as laminar flow rooms and life islands, and the use of oral nonabsorbable antibiotics have resulted in decreased numbers of infections but not increased overall survival in immunosuppressed patients.

HEMORRHAGE. The most frequent cause of hemorrhage in patients with cancer is thrombocytopenia, which may be a result of the cancer itself but more commonly is a side effect of cytoreductive therapy. Bleeding rarely occurs with platelet counts over $20,000/mm^3$. For counts below this level, prophylactic platelet transfusions should be administered. If repeated transfusions are anticipated, attempts should be made to obtain HLA-matched platelets to delay the appearance of antibodies and resistance to transfusion.

Disseminated intravascular coagulation (DIC) is occasionally responsible for bleeding in patients with cancer. The best treatment for DIC is treatment of the primary disease. Heparin is rarely indicated but may be lifesaving in the treatment of DIC in promyelocytic granulocytic leukemia.

TUMOR LYSIS SYNDROME. The rapid lysis of sensitive tumors following chemotherapy releases intracellular phosphate, resulting in hypocalcemia. Intracellular potassium is also released by lysing tumor cells. Potentially fatal cardiotoxicity from hypocalcemia and hyperpotassemia can be prevented by adequate hydration before chemotherapy. Hyperuricemia results from excessive uric acid production caused by tumor cell breakdown. Allopurinol should be administered whenever substantial tumor lysis is anticipated.

PSYCHOSOCIAL PROBLEMS. Perhaps the greatest challenge to the physician dealing with cancer patients is the management of the enormous emotional, social, and economic impact of the disease on patients and their families. Empathy, tact, and compassion are necessary from the time of diagnosis. It is generally agreed that it is preferable for patients to be aware of the diagnosis, particularly if aggressive therapy is planned. They should be given an honest explanation of the illness and of the proposed treatment in terms they can understand. Every allowable hope should be offered. If patients are not informed of the true nature of their disease, they will lose trust and confidence in their physicians and families as their condition deteriorates. Clergymen, social workers, and oncology nurses all can contribute their own special skills in supporting the patient and family through the difficult postdiagnosis period. It is essential for the physician to keep the family informed throughout the course of the patient's illness and to be available to answer questions.

Vigorous attempts to keep the patient at home for as long as possible should be made, using all existing community agencies. It is often feasible to keep a patient at home with the help of a hospital bed, bedside commode, and a visiting nurse to give parenteral medication. If pain medication must be given frequently, a family member can be taught to administer it.

The hospice movement, emphasizing home care and comfortable homelike surroundings when inpatient care is necessary, is belatedly gaining momentum in the United States. The hospice concept allows unlimited family visits, including children and pets. Meticulous attention is paid to the control of pain, bowel disturbances, and other distressing symptoms of advanced cancer. A most important function of the hospice team is counseling of and continued contact with the bereaved family after the patient's death.

During the terminal period it is essential that the physician not withdraw from dying patients. Hospitalized patients should be seen daily. They should be given the opportunity to talk, and the physician should take the time to listen. Physical contact and continued attention to symptoms will lessen the fears of abandonment and depersonalization characteristic of the last phases of a lingering, fatal disease.

MANAGEMENT OF SPECIFIC MALIGNANCIES
Carcinoma of the lung

Accurate histologic diagnosis is essential to planning proper management of lung cancers. Small cell or oat cell carcinoma, the most rapidly growing of all lung tumors, is usually disseminated by the time of diagnosis, and therefore surgery has no role in the primary management of this disease. The median survival of untreated persons with oat cell carcinoma is under 4 months. Fortunately, this aggressive tumor is responsive to both radiotherapy and chemotherapy. Current drug combinations give response rates of 60% to 100%, with temporary complete response in 20% to 50% of cases. The agents active in the treatment of small or oat cell carcinoma are cyclophosphamide, the nitrosoureas, doxorubicin, vincristine, procarbazine, methotrexate, and the experimental podophyllotoxin derivative VP 16. Multimodality programs combining irradiation of the primary tumor with chemotherapy have produced somewhat higher response rates, but survival appears to be the same with or without radiation. The median survival for treated metastatic small cell carcinoma is approximately 8 to 10 months, and that for apparently limited disease is 12 to 15 months. Some patients are now surviving in a disease-free state for longer than 2 years. Since 10% of patients have intracerebral metastases at the time of diagnosis and 30% have central nervous system involvement at autopsy, prophylactic cranial irradiation is now included in most treatment programs.

Epidermoid or squamous cell carcinoma, the most frequent lung cancer, is slower growing and has the lowest rate of distant metastases and a high frequency of local complications. Only 20% of patients have surgically resectable disease at diagnosis, since the disease has a long asymptomatic period. Even if no distant spread is obvious, involvement of mediastinal lymph nodes or proximity to the great vessels makes surgical removal inadvisable. Potentially curative radiotherapy should be considered as primary therapy for unresectable lesions confined to the hemithorax. The use of adjuvant chemotherapy following curative surgery or radiotherapy has not resulted in prolongation of the disease-free interval or survival and is not recommended except in an investigational setting. Chemotherapy of recurrent or metastatic epidermoid lung cancer has been only minimally effective, and asymptomatic patients should not receive it unless they are participating in a controlled clinical trial. Cyclophosphamide, doxorubicin, methotrexate, procarbazine, cisplatin, and an experimental vinca alkaloid, vindesine, all have shown some activity in this disease.

Adenocarcinoma of the lung is intermediate between small cell and epidermoid carcinomas in its growth rate, speed of hematogenous spread, and resectability. Combination chemotherapy and multimodality trials are in progress in the management of metastatic disease.

Gastrointestinal cancer

CARCINOMA OF THE ESOPHAGUS. Squamous cell carcinoma of the esophagus is rarely resectable at the time of diagnosis, and radiotherapy is usually the treatment of choice. Chemotherapy has been disappointing.

CARCINOMA OF THE STOMACH. Surgery is the treatment of choice for adenocarcinoma of the stomach. Even if there is extensive disease, resection of the lesion to prevent bleeding or obstruction should be performed. Gastric cancer is the most sensitive to chemotherapy of all alimentary tract carcinomas. Various combinations of 5-fluorouracil, nitrosoureas, mitomycin-C, and doxorubicin have proved beneficial in 40% to 50% of cases of advanced or metastatic gastric cancers. Patients who respond show a modest prolongation of survival. Radiotherapy is generally ineffective in this disease. Trials of adjuvant chemotherapy following surgery with curative intent are currently under way.

COLORECTAL CANCER. Early diagnosis and surgical resection constitute the optimal primary management for colorectal cancers. The extent of surgery depends on the operative findings. If curative resection is impossible, the lesion should still be removed to prevent later bleeding or obstruction. The mainstay of medical therapy of metastatic colorectal cancer is 5-fluorouracil, administered intravenously in a variety of schedules. Despite initial enthusiastic reports of improved results with combinations of 5-FU and nitrosoureas, alkylating agents, vinca alkaloids, and other agents, these regimens appear to give no greater survival than the use of 5-fluorouracil alone. About 25% of treated patients have an objective response to this single agent. Repeated trials of postoperative adjuvant chemotherapy with or without immunotherapy have not resulted in any significant increase in 5-year survival, although all these studies have shown some slight benefit. At this time routine adjuvant chemotherapy for colorectal carcinoma is not recommended.

Local symptoms of unresectable or recurrent rectal cancer, such as pain, tenesmus, and bleeding, can often be alleviated with palliative radiotherapy. Occasionally such radiotherapy may render a patient disease free. Since local recurrences account for 50% of relapses after complete resection of rectal cancer, preoperative or postoperative radiation has been employed in an attempt to prevent such recurrence.

PANCREATIC CANCER. Pancreatic cancer, whose incidence is increasing in the United States, has a negligible overall 5-year survival rate. Since only 5% of patients undergoing pancreatoduodenectomy are alive 5 years after the operation, the role of extensive surgery in the primary treatment of pancreatic carcinoma is controversial. Chemotherapy has been disappointing, although various combinations of 5-FU, mitomycin-C, doxorubicin, and streptozocin produce objective responses in a minority of patients. External beam radiation, interstitial instillation of ^{125}I, and fast neutron radiotherapy are currently being evaluated in the treatment of pancreatic cancer.

Breast cancer

The traditional primary treatment of breast cancer has been radical mastectomy, which removes the entire breast together with all axillary nodes and the pectoralis major muscle. Recently, data have emerged suggesting that survival after radical mastectomy is not superior to that following modified radical mastectomy (preserving the pectoralis major muscle) or simple mastectomy followed by radiotherapy to the axilla. Further confirmation of these results is necessary. The use of routine axillary and chest wall irradiation following radical or modified radical mastectomy has proved valueless in prolonging survival, and it should be used only in special situations after careful consultation among the involved surgeon, pathologist, radiotherapist, and medical oncologist.

The single most important prognostic factor in predicting recurrence in breast cancer is the presence or absence of involvement of axillary lymph nodes at the time of primary therapy. Women with four or more positive nodes have an 80% chance of recurrence within 2 years, whereas those with negative axillary nodes have only a 20% chance of recurrence during the same period. Estrogen-receptor negativity has been demonstrated in a large proportion of women with negative nodes whose cancer does recur. Adjuvant use of systemic chemotherapy following surgery in premenopausal women with positive axillary nodes significantly reduces the rate of recurrence up to 5 years after mastectomy. The most widely used regimen is 12 months of combination therapy with cyclophosphamide, methotrexate, and 5-FU. Other combinations and lengths of therapy are currently under investigation. Early studies failed to show a statistically significant advantage for postmenopausal women who have undergone adjuvant chemotherapy, but newer data challenge these conclusions.

Therapy for advanced or recurrent breast cancer must be individualized depending on the sites of disease, menopausal status, and hormonal receptor status of each patient. Premenopausal women with positive estrogen receptors, a relatively long disease-free interval, and metastases limited to bone or soft tissue should have an oophorectomy. Relapse following a good response to oophorectomy is usually followed by a second response to subsequent adrenalectomy or hypophysectomy. ER-positive postmenopausal women with bone or soft tissue metastases should first be treated with estrogens or antiestrogens. In either of these groups, if there is no response to initial hormonal manipulation, if the disease-free interval is very short, or if there are visceral metastases, the patient should receive cytotoxic chemotherapy. Cytotoxic agents should be used as first-line therapy for all ER-negative tumors, since these patients have less than 5% response rate after hormonal manipulation. Chemotherapeutic agents active against carcinoma of the breast are cyclophosphamide, doxorubicin, 5-FU, methotrexate, vincristine, and prednisone. Doxorubicin appears to be the single most effective agent.

Palliative radiotherapy for intracranial metastases and intractable bone pain is most important in achieving optimal quality of life for patients with advanced breast cancer.

Genitourinary tumors

RENAL CELL CARCINOMAS. Renal cell carcinomas should be surgically resected. Progestational agents or hydroxyurea have occasionally produced an objective decrease in the size of metastatic lesions, but both radiation therapy and chemotherapy have been generally disappointing in the treatment of renal cell tumors. There have been reports of regression of metastatic lesions following nephrectomy, and thus debulking of advanced tumors may be useful.

CARCINOMA OF THE BLADDER. Low-grade transitional cell bladder cancers can be successfully treated by fulguration or transurethral resection followed by local instillation of cytotoxic agents. More aggressive tumors that invade the bladder wall require total cystectomy and radical radiotherapy. Metastatic transitional cell tumors show some response to doxorubicin, 5-FU, and cisplatin.

CARCINOMA OF THE PROSTATE. Locally invasive tumors of the prostate may be treated by either radical prostatectomy or primary radiotherapy. Surgery is associated with a higher incidence of incontinence and impotence than is radiation. Symptomatic metastatic disease, especially painful bone lesions, should be treated with either orchiectomy or diethylstilbestrol. Since cardiovascular complications are frequent with diethylstilbestrol, patients with a history of heart disease should have an orchiectomy. The role of cytotoxic chemotherapy in advanced prostate cancer has not been firmly established, but there have been occasional responses to doxorubicin, cyclophosphamide, and 5-FU.

TESTICULAR CARCINOMA. Seminomas are exquisitely sensitive to both radiation therapy and chemotherapy. Almost all patients can be cured with radiation alone. If metastatic disease is present, single-agent chemotherapy is 90% effective.

Radical orchiectomy cures 75% to 80% of nonseminomatous tumors that are truly confined to the testes. The relative importance of lymphadenectomy and radiotherapy in the primary management of nonseminomatous tumors with nodal involvement is controversial. A major breakthrough resulting in potential curability of metastatic nonseminomatous testicular tumors has been the introduction of combination chemotherapy with vinblastine, bleomycin, and cisplatin. Other effective drugs are actinomycin, vincristine, cyclophosphamide, and doxorubicin. The role of adjuvant chemotherapy in patients with para-aortic lymph node involvement at the time of initial surgery is uncertain. Since most of the patients at risk never have metastases because of adequate primary treatment, and since such an effective regimen for advanced disease is available, it may be a more prudent policy to withhold chemotherapy until the appearance of metastases.

Gynecologic cancers

CARCINOMA OF THE OVARY. Regardless of histologic type, the primary treatment of ovarian cancer is hysterectomy and bilateral salpingo-oophorectomy. Prophylactic partial omentectomy is often carried out because of the frequency of omental recurrence. Both single-drug and combination chemotherapy with alkylating agents, cisplatin, and doxorubicin achieve remission rates of up to 80%, with significant prolongation of survival in patients who respond to chemotherapy. The exact role of radiotherapy in the overall management of ovarian carcinomas is under investigation.

ENDOMETRIAL CANCER. Endometrial tumors are most prevalent in obese, nulliparous women who often are diabetic or hypertensive or have a family history of this tumor. The primary treatment is surgery or radiotherapy, depending on the stage at presentation. Favorable responses are occasionally obtained in metastatic disease treated with progesterone, doxorubicin, and cyclophosphamide.

CARCINOMA OF THE CERVIX. Deaths from cervical carcinoma have dropped sharply following the introduction of Papanicolaou smears for early detection. A combined radiotherapeutic and surgical approach to therapy is recommended to achieve the best possible result for each patient. Chemotherapy has no proven value in the management of this disease.

Head and neck cancer

Ninety percent of head and neck tumors are squamous cell carcinomas. Lymphomas, adenocarcinomas, and salivary gland tumors account for the remaining neoplasms in this region. The most frequent primary sites are the lateral borders of the tongue, the floor of the mouth, gums, buccal mucosa, and lips. The majority of head and neck cancers occur in males, and there is a strong association with smoking and alcohol ingestion. Cancers in the oral cavity are often preceded by ''premalignant'' lesions such as leukoplakia or erythroplasia, so that a thorough physical examination can serve as an extremely effective early detection device. Once they become invasive, these tumors spread locally and into regional lymph node chains. Distant metastases, most often to the lungs, are late and relatively uncommon. Head and neck cancers represent one of the most urgent indications for multimodality management. In early stages these lesions are often curable by appropriate surgical, radiotherapeutic, or combined therapy. Even if the tumor appears inoperable at the time of the initial presentation, it is sometimes possible to convert it to operability by chemotherapy with methotrexate, bleomycin, and cisplatin. These drugs also can give dramatic, if short-lived, palliation in advanced local and metastatic disease.

Sarcomas

Osteogenic sarcoma, Ewing's sarcoma, and embryonal rhabdomyosarcoma are rapidly growing, early metastasizing tumors of young people. Appropriate multimodality treatment has resulted in prolonged survival and apparent cure in an increasing number of patients with these malignancies. In all cases as much of the tumor as possible should be removed, and postoperative irradiation of the tumor site should be administered. Systemic chemotherapy should be administered postoperatively even in the absence of detectable metastatic disease, since there is high risk of recurrence and effective chemotherapeutic agents are available.

Embryonal rhabdomyosarcoma responds to a combination of vincristine, dactinomycin, and cyclophosphamide, with 50% of patients enjoying a prolonged disease-free survival even in the face of metastatic disease. High-dose methotrexate with leukovorin rescue and doxorubicin are effective as both adjuvant therapy and treatment of metastatic or recurrent osteogenic sarcoma. Isolated pulmonary metastases, apparently resistant to chemotherapy, can be resected with resultant long-term, disease-free survival. Ewing's sarcoma is highly radiosensitive but has a tendency to metastasize widely. Local therapy should therefore be followed by adjuvant chemotherapy. Since central nervous system involvement is common, prophylactic cranial irradiation should be used.

In the older adult, sarcomas are a heterogeneous group of diseases. They are slower growing than the sarcomas of young people and in general are not responsive to chemotherapy. Surgery is the treatment of choice and radiotherapy is relatively ineffective. Doxorubicin has some activity in treatment of metastatic adult sarcomas and its role as adjuvant therapy following surgery is being explored.

Malignant melanoma

Early diagnosis and adequate surgical resection remain the optimal therapeutic measures for malignant melanoma. Reports of prevention or delay of recurrence following adjuvant bacille Calmette Guérin (BCG) administration have not been confirmed. Intralesional injection of BCG does result in regression of tumor nodules but has no effect on visceral disease. Chemotherapy has been disappointing, although DTIC has shown some activity.

Endocrine tumors

Islet cell tumors often grow slowly, so that symptoms of hormone overproduction are more prominent than those caused either by the physical presence of a mass or by metastatic disease. Malignant insulinomas cause recurrent attacks of hypoglycemia that, if the tumor cannot be completely resected, may be managed by diet, corticosteroids, diazoxide, or phenytoin. In patients with unresectable gastrin-secreting tumors the use of cimetidine results in healing of ulcers and relief of pain and diarrhea.

The most effective chemotherapeutic agent in the treatment of malignant islet cell tumors is streptozocin, which selectively destroys pancreatic β-cells. Objective antitumor and hormonal responses have been obtained in 40% of treated patients. 5-FU and doxorubicin also show some activity against these tumors.

Malignant carcinoid tumors produce symptoms related to serotonin and/or kallikrein secretion. Serotonin-related diarrhea, colic, and malabsorption usually respond to opiates and belladonna. If these symptoms are severe, serotonin antagonists such as cyproheptadine or methysergide provide effective palliation. Flushing attacks brought about by release of kallikrein are partially controlled with anti-α-adrenergic agents such as phenothiazines. More specific blockers including phentolamine and phenoxybenzamine hydrochloride are also useful. Antitumor responses have been obtained with streptozocin, 5-FU, alkylating agents, and doxorubicin.

BIBLIOGRAPHY

Capizzio, R.L.: The pharmacologic basis of cancer chemotherapy, Semin. Oncol. **4**:131, 1977.

Chabner, B.A., and others: The clinical pharmacology of anti-neoplastic agents, N. Engl. J. Med. **292**:1159, 1975.

DeVita, V.T., Young, R.C., and Canellos, G.P.: Combination versus single agent chemotherapy: a review of the basis for selection of drug treatment of cancer, Cancer **35**:98, 1975.

Goepp, C.E., and Hammond, W.: Supportive care of the cancer patient, Semin. Oncol. **2**:283, 1975.

Legha, S.S., Davis, H.L., and Muggia, F.L.: Hormonal therapy of breast cancers: new approaches and concepts, Ann. Intern. Med. **88**:69, 1978.

Levine, A.S., and others: Hematologic malignancies and other marrow failure states: progress in the management of complicating infections, Semin. Hematol. **11**:1401, 1974.

Morton, D.L., and Goodnight, J.E.: Clinical trials of immunotherapy: present status, Cancer **42**:2224, 1978.

Schabel, F.M., Jr.: Rationale for adjuvant chemotherapy, Cancer **39** (suppl.):2875, 1977.

DENTAL CORRELATIONS

CHEMOTHERAPY
Martin S. Greenberg

CLINICAL MANIFESTATIONS. The most common oral manifestations of cancer chemotherapy are ulcers of the oral mucosa. Drugs used in cancer chemotherapy may cause oral ulcers by a direct toxic effect on the epithelium or by increasing the susceptibility of the patient to infection.

These drugs function by decreasing cell division. The side effects of cancer chemotherapy result in large part from the action of the drugs on normal cells. The oral mucosa is particularly susceptible to these drugs due to the normal level of rapid cellular reproduction. The toxic effects are first seen on the oral mucosa well before the epithelium of the skin is involved. Chemotherapeutic drugs frequently associated with oral mucosal ulcers are methotrexate, bleomycin, actinomycin D, and vincristine.

A second cause of oral ulcers in patients undergoing cancer chemotherapy is the bone marrow–suppressing effects of the medication. In patients with severe neutropenia, the invasion of microorganisms of low pathogenicity into the oral mucosa causes large, foul smelling ulcers.

A third cause of oral ulcers in this group of patients is the increased incidence of viral infections affecting the oral mucosa. Herpes simplex and varicella-zoster virus infections are seen in increased frequency in patients undergoing cancer chemotherapy, as a result of immunosuppression. The viral lesions may be distinguished from the lesions already described by the following characteristics: The viral lesions begin as vesicles and quickly break to ulcers. Chemotherapy ulcers do not have a vesicle stage. Patients with a varicella-zoster infection will have significant complaint of pain before the onset of lesions along the course of the affected nerve. The lesions are usually confined to one peripheral nerve trunk. If the diagnosis cannot be made on clinical grounds, laboratory tests may be used to distinguish viral lesions from ulcers caused by neutropenia or the direct effect of chemotherapy. A quick method of diagnosis is the use of cytology smear, which may demonstrate viral changes in the epithelial cells. Use of viral cultures may also be necessary in some cases. Since these patients are immunosuppressed, the viral infection may become generalized, affecting large portions of skin and internal organs.

Fungal infections involving the oral mucosa are frequently observed in patients during cancer chemotherapy. Most common are *Candida* infections, which manifest as yellow-white colonies on the surface of the mucosa. These can be removed, leaving a red, raw tissue base. These lesions are diagnosed by smears showing mycelia and pseudohyphae. Other fungal infections that occasionally occur are aspergillosis or mucormycosis. These infections are often fatal, unless treatment is started early. Diagnosis should not be made by culture alone; suspected lesions must be biopsied.

Oral mucosal infections may also occur with gram-negative bacilli and are commonly noted in patients taking chemotherapy for acute leukemia. These lesions are described in detail in the section on leukemia.

DENTAL MANAGEMENT. The management of oral ulcers resulting from cancer chemotherapy should include treatment to reduce symptoms, minimize infection, and promote healing. Use of topical anesthetics makes eating more comfortable, increasing the nutritional status of the patient. Dyclonine (Dyclone) or diphenhydramine (Benadryl) mixed with milk of magnesia is particularly effective for this purpose. Infections should be prevented by use of antibacterial mouthwash. One medication used effectively is a 0.5% solution of povidone-iodine applied to the ulcers two to three times daily. In severe cases, topical tetracycline compresses may also be used, but these must be combined with nystatin (Mycostatin) to minimize the problem of overgrowth of *Candida*. The clinician should weigh the risks of allergic reactions when prescribing topical antibiotics.

Mild to moderate cases of oral mucosal candidiasis may be effectively treated with topical nystatin oral suspension. In more severe cases, nystatin troches held in the mouth provide more intense topical therapy. In severe cases, especially when esophageal involvement is suspected, intravenous amphotericin B is recommended.

A dental evaluation is indicated prior to cancer chemotherapy to remove potential sources of infection. Dentists in their community should take the responsibility of fostering this concept among their medical colleagues in oncology, hematology, and internal medicine. Patients should have a prophylaxis, periodontal scaling and curettage, and necessary oral hygiene instruction to minimize the risk of infection occurring during bone marrow–suppressing chemotherapy. If emergency dental treatment is necessary during chemotherapy, two major complications must be prevented: hemorrhage and infection. Since chemotherapy may depress the bone marrow, the platelet count should be evaluated before dental treatment. If the dental treatment will require surgery and the platelet count is below 40,000 cells/mm^3, platelet transfusion should be considered. If the patient is severely neutropenic, broad-spectrum antibiotic coverage is indicated before dental treatment. Unusual infections with gram-negative bacilli occur in patients hospitalized for cancer chemotherapy. All infections should be cultured and the area debrided and disinfected with povidone-iodine solution prior to surgery. In cases of severe neutropenia, granulocyte transfusion is a consideration.

BIBLIOGRAPHY

Bottomley, W.K., Perlin, E., and Ross, G.R.: Antineoplastic agents and their oral manifestations, Oral Surg. **44**:527, 1977.

Dreizen, S., Bodey, G.O., and Rodriquez, V.: Oral complications of cancer chemotherapy, Postgrad. Med. **58**:75, 1975.

Thilagaratnam, C.N., and Main, J.H.P.: Metastatic action of vinblastine sulphate on oral epithelia of hamsters, J. Oral Path. **1**:84, 1972.

Vickery, I.M., and Midda M.: Dental complications of cytotoxic therapy in Hodgkin's disease—a case report, Br. J. Oral Surg. **13**:282, 1976.

Section Seven

CARDIOVASCULAR DISEASES

edited by **Toby R. Engel**

---

85 • INTRODUCTION TO CARDIOVASCULAR DISEASE

Toby R. Engel

Cardiologists deal with heart and vascular disease in terms of a physiologic division of symptoms and their managements. They tend to substitute abnormal physiology for pathogenesis and abnormal anatomy for etiology. For example, the cardinal complaints of patients with cardiac disease are chest pain, dyspnea, and edema. Chest pain is discussed in terms of disordered coronary artery and aortic structure in Chapter 96 and 99. Dyspnea and edema are discussed as expressions of disordered hemodynamic physiology, often tempered by structural alterations, in Chapters 86, 90, 94, 95, and 98. The principal findings of abnormal blood pressure, rales, gallop rhythms, and murmurs are discussed in terms of the physiologic mechanisms of their genesis in Chapters 86, 88, 92, 94, and 95. Emboli are discussed in terms of the anatomic derangement that is their cause in Chapters 94 to 96. The vessels obstructed by the emboli (pulmonary versus peripheral) are discussed in Chapters 90 and 100. Syncope and sudden death are discussed principally in terms of physiologic mechanisms in Chapter 97, and the anatomic basis of arrhythmias as a key to understanding their prevention is discussed in Chapter 96. Special diseases, primarily involving younger patients, are dealt with along anatomic lines (Chapter 93) or physiologic lines (Chapter 90).

Thus most patients suffering cardiovascular disease are lumped into just a few rubrics: hypertensive diseases, congenital diseases, valvular diseases, myocardial or pericardial diseases, coronary and other arterial diseases. Some specific tests are detailed in Chapter 89. Physiologic abnormalities and the approach to therapy apply to each disease in a similar manner. An example is the benefit of vasodilation to reduce peripheral vascular resistance in heart failure, hypertension, certain forms of valvular disease, ischemic heart disease, and aortic dissection. The common denominator is an effort to express clinical difficulties and therapy in simple physiologic measurements (for example, pulmonary capillary pressure or the intervals on the electrocardiogram).

86 • CONGESTIVE HEART FAILURE

Joseph A. Franciosa and W. Bruce Dunkman

Congestive heart failure is a common outcome of many cardiovascular lesions and a major cause of physical disability. It should be regarded as a complex clinical syndrome rather than a distinct disease process, since its causes are multiple and its clinical expression variable. Nevertheless, congestive heart failure results from an interplay of pathogenetic mechanisms that are similar despite their development in response to diverse cardiovascular insults. Therefore a common clinical and pathophysiologic entity develops, which usually can be managed by similar interventions. The purpose of this chapter is to emphasize those common pathophysiologic features of congestive heart failure that facilitate understanding of its clinical presentations and from which a rational basis for its management can be derived.

DEFINITION. Congestive heart failure is a clinical syndrome that results from the inability of the heart to adequately perfuse peripheral tissues because of impaired systolic emptying. Perfusion may be considered inadequate when it is absolutely reduced or when it is maintained at normal levels but is accomplished under abnormal hemodynamic conditions that interfere with local tissue function. An example of the latter is acute hypertensive heart failure, in which pulmonary blood flow may be maintained at normal levels but is accomplished at an elevated pressure that can interfere with alveolar capillary gas exchange.

Congestive heart failure must be distinguished from other causes of inadequate tissue perfusion. These include shock of various noncardiac origins such as hypovolemia or sepsis and other states of vascular congestion such as cirrhosis and uremia. In these other conditions the clinical presentation may simulate heart failure, but a cardiovascular lesion is not present, ventricular emptying is not impaired, and the heart usually functions normally for the kind of loading conditions to which it is subjected.

ETIOLOGY. The lesions responsible for heart failure may directly involve the heart or may be located outside the heart in the vascular system but lead to impairment of cardiac function. Some common causes of congestive heart failure are outlined as follows:

I. Intracardiac
  A. Myocardial
    1. Acute myocarditis
      a. Toxic
      b. Infectious
        (1) Viral
        (2) Bacterial
        (3) Fungal
        (4) Parasitic
    2. Infiltrative diseases
      a. Amyloidosis
      b. Hemochromatosis
      c. Tumors
    3. Chronic inflammation
      a. Sarcoidosis
      b. Rheumatic fever
      c. Collagen-vascular diseases
    4. Cardiomyopathies
      a. Congestive
        (1) Ischemic
        (2) Alcoholic
        (3) Postviral
        (4) Postpartum
        (5) Idiopathic
      b. Restrictive
      c. Hypertrophic
      d. Heredofamilial
  B. Endocardial
    1. Valvulopathies
      a. Rheumatic heart disease
      b. Infective endocarditis
      c. Degenerative valvular disease
    2. Collagen-vascular diseases
    3. Endocardial fibroelastosis
  C. Pericardial
    1. Inflammatory
      a. Acute
      b. Chronic
    2. Neoplastic
II. Extracardiac
  A. Systemic hypertension
  B. Pulmonary hypertension
    1. Parenchymal lung disease
    2. Pulmonary embolism
    3. Idiopathic
  C. High-output states
    1. Anemia
    2. Hyperthyroidism
    3. Beri-beri
    4. Alcoholic liver disease
    5. Arteriovenous fistula

Among the cardiac lesions, the *myocardium, endocardium,* and *pericardium* may be involved alone or in combination. The *myocardium* may be the site of inflammatory lesions such as myocarditis of toxic, viral, or bacterial origin. Infiltrative processes such as amyloidosis, sarcoidosis, and tumor, or chronic inflammatory lesions such as rheumatic carditis and rheumatoid arthritis or other collagen-vascular diseases may also involve the heart. Although these forms of myocarditis often are discovered to involve the heart when it is examined pathologically, they are relatively rare as causes of clinically manifest congestive heart failure, either because the disease entities are uncommon or because their cardiac involvement is not extensive.

By far the most common causes of myocardial disease are ischemic and idiopathic cardiomyopathy. Ischemic cardiomyopathy is due to severe coronary obstructive disease and may or may not be associated with typical ischemic events such as acute myocardial infarction or angina pectoris. Pathologically, large coronary arteries are involved, and the lesions are indistinguishable from those observed in patients with other clinical presentations of ischemic heart disease. Although the existence of "small vessel coronary artery disease" has been postulated as a cause of ischemic cardiomyopathy, this has not been clearly demonstrated. Such "small vessel disease" has been seen in patients with diabetes or collagen-vascular diseases. Idiopathic cardiomyopathy is characterized by diffuse myocardial fibrosis with normal coronary arteries. It is seen in association with chronic alcoholism and following pregnancy and viral infections. Alcohol may produce direct cardiac depression, but the cardiomyopathy associated with excessive alcohol ingestion is not usually resolved by cessation of alcohol intake. Idiopathic cardiomyopathies may involve myocardium diffusely and lead to ventricular dilation and the typical clinical presentation of cardiovascular congestion, or they may lead to diffuse interstitial fibrosis resulting in stiffening of the myocardium with restriction of cardiac filling. Finally, the myocardium may be involved predominantly in specific areas leading to localized hypertrophy (hypertrophic cardiomyopathy). The idiopathic and hypertrophic cardiomyopathies are discussed in detail in Chapter 95.

Clinical congestive heart failure also may result from lesions of the *endocardium* or *heart valves*. These may be congenital or acquired, such as after rheumatic fever or bacterial endocarditis. These lesions are discussed in detail in Chapter 94. They lead to heart failure by causing a pressure overload on the ventricle (valvular obstruction) or a volume overload (valvular regurgitation or an abnormal communication between heart chambers).

The *pericardium* can be the site of inflammatory lesions from infection, myocardial infarction, pericardiotomy, or tumor infiltrates. These lesions usually do not lead to heart failure unless they cause pericardial fibrosis severe enough to produce adhesions or constriction great enough to restrict cardiac diastolic filling. Accumulation of fluid in the pericardial cavity as a result of any of these processes may limit cardiac diastolic filling and lead to pericardial tamponade, a low–cardiac output state requiring emergency treatment. Tamponade is seen most commonly with uremic or malignant pericarditis but may rarely occur with other types of pericarditis.

Cardiac dysfunction severe enough to lead to clinically overt heart failure may result from *extracardiac* lesions. The most important of these is systemic hypertension, which is the most common precursor of all forms of congestive heart failure. An explanation for this relationship is that elevated blood pressure increases resistance to left ventricular outflow and this chronic pressure overload leads to ventricular hypertrophy and dilation. Regression of left ventricular hypertrophy follows normalization of blood pressure with agents that inhibit the sympathetic nervous system. However, it does not follow equivalent blood pressure lowering with vasodilator drugs that reflexly increase sympathetic influences. Hypertension is also important as a cause of heart failure because it is a major risk factor for coronary artery disease.

Among other noncardiac lesions, increased venous return to the heart via abnormal arteriovenous communications may induce a congested state. Such volume overload from congenital or acquired arteriovenous fistulas is unusual, and large flow volumes are required before cardiac function is compromised.

Disease processes involving the *pulmonary vessels* or *lung parenchyma* can lead to congestive heart failure by raising pulmonary arterial pressure, thereby overloading the right ventricle and causing failure. Acute right ventricular failure can be caused by sudden increases in pulmonary pressure from pulmonary embolization or severe pneumonia. More commonly, the cause of pulmonary hypertension is chronic obstructive lung disease associated with severe structural changes of pulmonary vessels. Less frequently, pulmonary hypertension is primary and idiopathic (see Chapter 92). This form is most common in younger age groups and has been thought in some cases to be the result of recurrent microembolization to the pulmonary arterial bed.

In "high-output" heart failure, cardiac output is at normal or above-normal levels. This occurs in anemia, hyperthyroidism, beri-beri, and alcoholic liver disease when cardiac output is inadequate to meet metabolic demands or its distribution is altered so that certain tissues are underperfused.

EPIDEMIOLOGY. Since heart failure results from a variety of cardiovascular lesions, its epidemiology reflects its multifactorial origin. Factors determining the incidence and severity of coronary artery disease, rheumatic fever, and hypertension have a great bearing on the prevalence of congestive heart failure in the population. These include age, sex, cigarette smoking, diet, serum cholesterol, blood glucose, body weight, family history, physical activity, and personality type.

In the Framingham study the annual rate of development of heart failure was 2.3 per 1000 for men and 1.4 per 1000 for women. The incidence rose with age, especially after age 50. Hypertension was the most important precursor of congestive heart failure; 75% of patients with heart failure had a history of hypertension.

Hypertension significantly increases the risk of heart failure when it is associated with other heart disease, such as rheumatic or coronary artery disease. Other diseases commonly associated with heart failure include diabetes, cerebrovascular accident, chronic lung disease, and peripheral vascular disease.

NORMAL CARDIOVASCULAR FUNCTION

Myocardial ultrastructure. The light and electron microscopic structure of the myocardium is illustrated in Fig. 86-1. Individual myocardial cells abut on more than two neighboring cells, resulting from branching of myocardial fibers. Within the myocardial cell are multiple crossbanded, parallel myofibrils. The myofibrils are composed of numerous individual contractile elements called sarcomeres, which are connected in series. Investing the myofibrils is the sarcoplasmic reticulum, comprised of the sarcolemma, its inward tubular invaginations called the transverse tubules or T system, and similar tubules oriented lengthwise called the longitudinal system. These structures provide for the intracellular transport of electrolytes and metabolites required for cellular function.

Within the sarcomeres are two types of myofilaments, a set of thinner ones comprised principally of the protein *actin* and thicker ones comprised primarily of the protein *myosin*. Their spatial arrangement, as indicated in Fig. 86-1, gives rise to light and dark bands. The actin and myosin filaments are believed to remain constant in length, with shortening of the sarcomere accomplished by the thin filaments being actively drawn deeper into the lattice of thick filaments during the contractile process (Fig. 86-2). This is achieved by serially making and breaking the linkages between actin and myosin in a process dependent on Ca^{++}, Mg^{++}, and high-energy adenosine triphosphate (ATP). The maximal contractile force that can be produced by the myocardium is determined by the overlap of actin and myosin filaments that allows the greatest number of force-generating bonds between them. This concept fits nicely with the known length-dependent property of skeletal and cardiac muscle (Frank-Starling principle) illustrated in Fig. 86-2. A variety of ultrastructural abnormalities of the myocardium have been described in hypertrophied and failing hearts, although simple alteration of sarcomere length and filament overlap does not appear to be responsible for heart failure.

Myocardial mechanics. Myocardial function can be described in terms of three fundamental parameters: *preload*, *afterload*, and *contractility*. These terms are most easily understood from the study of the isolated cat papillary muscle (Fig. 86-3). One end is attached to a fixed tension transducer, and the other is attached to a fulcrumed lever, whose position is determined by a stop at one end of the fulcrum and a tray, to which various weights can be

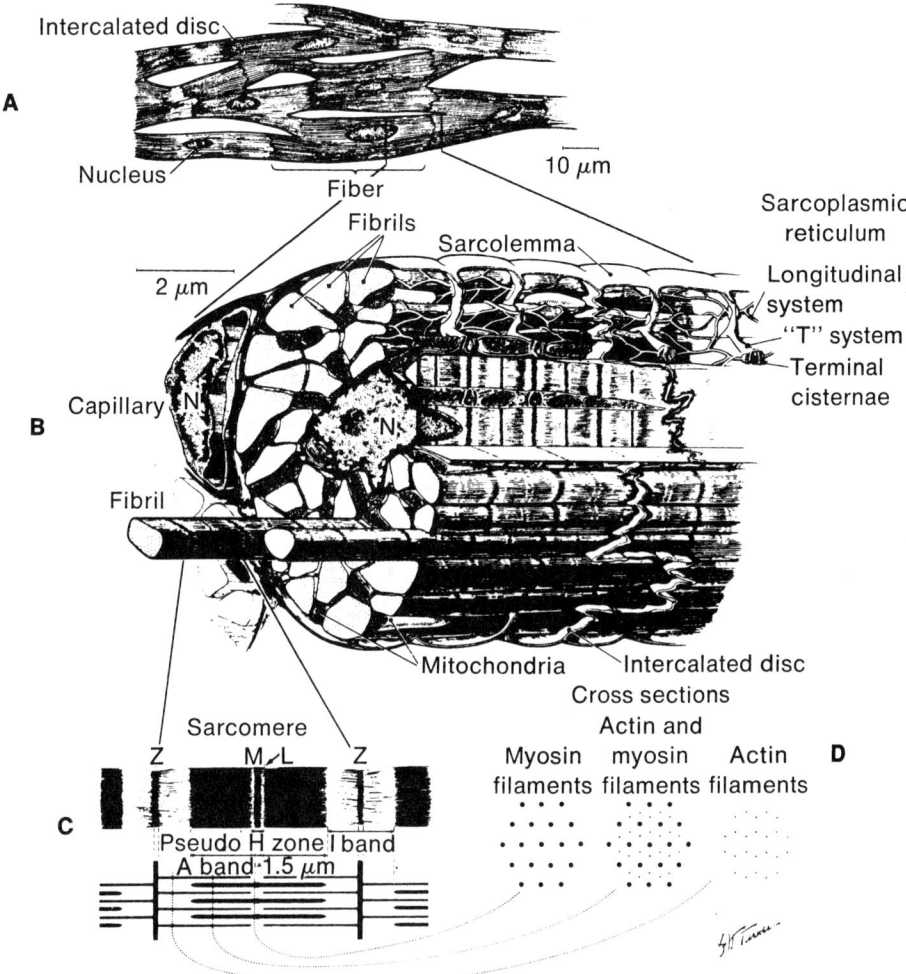

Fig. 86-1. Microscopic structure of heart muscle. **A,** Myocardium as seen under light microscope. Branching of fibers is evident, each fiber containing centrally located nucleus. Fibers or cells are connected by intercalated discs. **B,** Myocardial cell or fiber reconstructed from electron micrographs, showing arrangement of multiple parallel fibrils that compose cell and of serially connected sarcomeres that compose individual fibril (N = nucleus). Sarcotubular system that mediates activation, including sarcolemma and sarcoplasmic reticulum, is also shown. Intercalated disc in center of reconstruction serves to separate two cells. **C,** Individual sarcomere from myofibril, and below it, diagrammatic representation of arrangement of myofilaments that make up sarcomere. Thick filaments, approximately 1.5 μm in length, composed of myosin are localized to the A band, while thin filaments, 1 μm in length and composed primarily of actin, extend from the Z line through the I band into the A band, ending at the edges of the central H zone. The H zone is the central area of the A band where thin filaments are absent. Thick and thin filaments overlap only in the A band. **D,** Diagrammatic cross-section of sarcomere showing specific lattice arrangements of myofilaments. In center of sarcomere *(left)* only thick (myosin) filaments arranged in a hexagonal array are seen. In distal portions of A band *(center)* both thick and thin (actin) filaments are found, with each thick filament surrounded by six thin filaments. In I band *(right)* only thin filaments are present. (From Braunwald, E., Ross, J., Jr., and Sonnenblick, E.H.: Mechanisms of contraction of the normal and failing heart, ed. 2, Boston, 1976, Little, Brown & Co.)

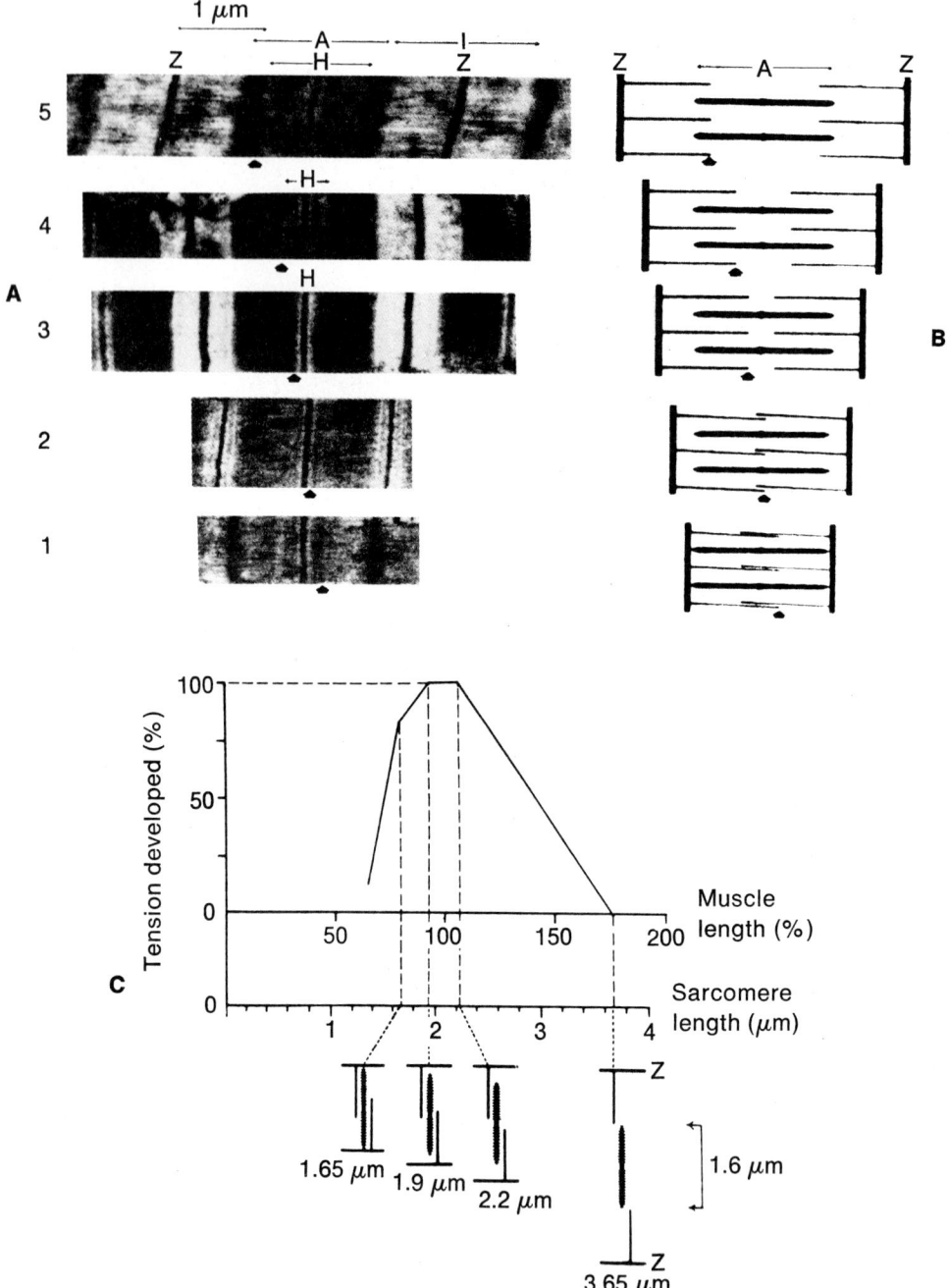

Fig. 86-2. Relationship between electron microscopic band patterns, sarcomere length, and tension development in skeletal muscle (frog sartorius). **A,** Band patterns as seen electron microscopically. **B,** Schematic representation of actin-myosin interaction during contraction of sarcomere. **C,** Maximal tension is developed when actin and myosin filaments are positioned to allow for development of greatest number of sites of interaction. Excessive overlap or separation results in decreased tension development. Similar relationship is probably present in cardiac muscle and may be in part the basis of the Frank-Starling principle. (**A** and **B** from Braunwald, E., and others: Am. J. Cardiol. **20:**705, 1967. Used by permission of the American Heart Association, Inc. **C,** from Hanson, J., and Lowy, J.: Br. Med. Bull. **21:**264, 1965.)

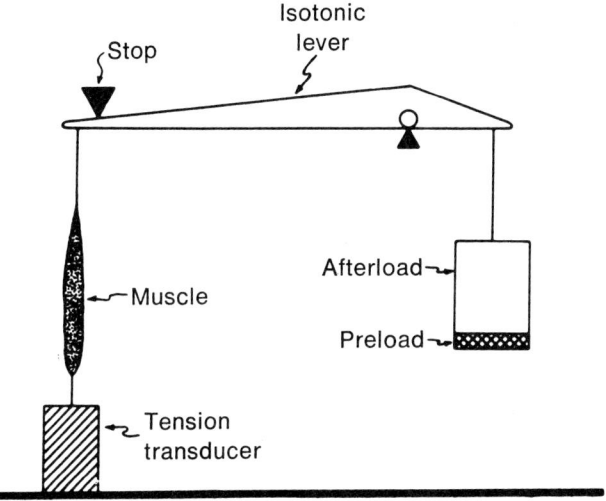

Fig. 86-3. Diagrammatic representation of isotonic lever system. Papillary muscle is stimulated by electrodes along its lateral aspect. Lower end of muscle is attached to extension from tension transducer, while upper free end is attached to end of lever system that is free to move. Fulcrum of lever system is shown at right. Small weight (preload) is placed on opposite end of lever and stretches muscle to length consistent with its resting length-tension relation. Stop is then fixed above tip of lever so that any added weight over and above preload will not be sensed by muscle until it attempts to contract. Additional loads (afterloads) can be added to preload. Total load equals sum of preload and afterloads. (From Braunwald, E., Ross, J., Jr., and Sonnenblick, E.H.: Mechanisms of contraction of the normal and failing heart, ed. 2, Boston, 1976, Little, Brown & Co.)

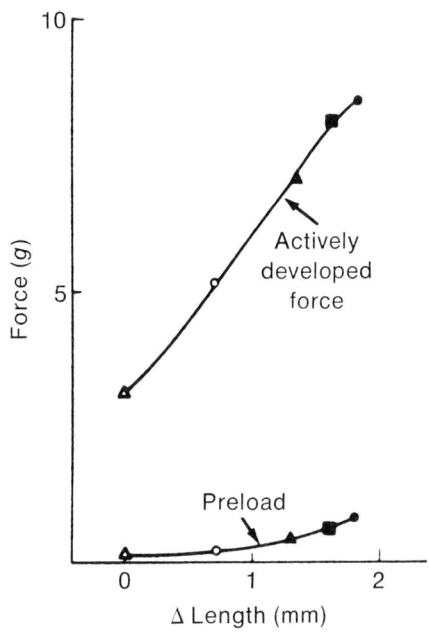

Fig. 86-4. Effects of varying initial muscle length on force-velocity relation of isolated cat papillary muscle. As initial length is increased by increasing preload (lower line), actively developed force increases (upper line), illustrating Frank-Starling principle. (Modified from Sonnenblick, E.H.: Am. J. Physiol. **207**:1330, 1964.)

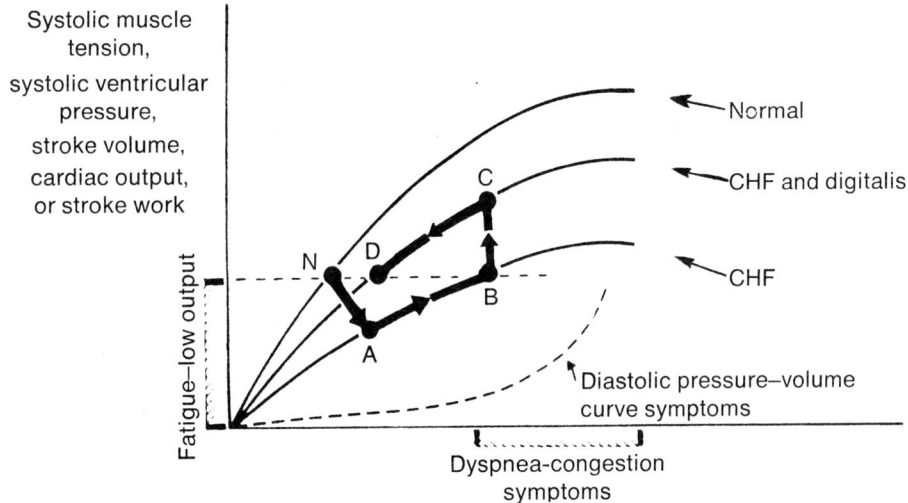

Fig. 86-5. Diagrammatic representation of Frank-Starling principle in congestive heart failure. Three curves represent length-tension or ventricular function curves in normal, congestive heart failure, and heart failure after treatment with digitalis. Points N through D (following the arrows) represent in sequence: depression of contractility, Frank-Starling compensation, increase in contractility with digitalis, and reduction in use of Frank-Starling compensation that digitalis allows. Of note is the fact that points N, B, and D all lie on same line in vertical axis and thus represent same stroke volume, but each is on a different end-diastolic pressure on horizontal axis. Levels at which symptoms of congestion, such as dyspnea, and symptoms of low cardiac output, such as fatigue, occur are represented by crosshatched areas. Dashed curve represents diastolic pressure-volume curve relating end-diastolic pressure on ordinate to end-diastolic volume or muscle length on abscissa. (Modified from Spann, J.F., Mason, D.T., and Zelis, R.F.: Mod. Concepts Cardiovasc. Dis. **39**:79, 1970. Used by permission of the American Heart Association, Inc.)

added, at the other. The length of the muscle before contraction can be determined by the position of the stop, and the force against which the muscle contracts by the weight added to the tray; muscle contraction is initiated by applying an electrical stimulus.

When the weight in the tray is greater than the muscle can lift, an isometric contraction results. The force (tension) that the muscle develops under these circumstances is found to depend on its length. To a certain point of stretch the isometrically contracting muscle develops increasing force with increasing initial length. The weight of the tray and any added weights may also be used as a measure of stretch; thus stretch can be expressed in units of weight or mass as well as length (and in whole heart as pressure, which equals force/area). This length-dependent property of cardiac muscle is the Frank-Starling principle, and the mass (pressure) required to achieve any degree of stretch is termed the *preload*. These relationships are depicted in Fig. 86-4 (force-length curve) and Fig. 86-5 (Frank-Starling curve).

When the weight in the tray is restricted to values that allow the muscle to shorten, it is found that the initial velocity of shortening varies inversely with the weight the muscle is required to lift. The force against which the muscle shortens is termed the *afterload*.

When both preload and afterload are varied, a maximal velocity (V_{max}) of shortening can be extrapolated as if a zero afterload were achieved. Similarly, as the preload and stretch are increased, there is a value beyond which further increases in preload do not result in the development of increased force of contraction. This is the maximal force a given muscle can develop and is termed P_o. Both V_{max} and P_o have been proposed as measures of the third fundamental property of muscle, *contractility*. However, neither measurement is adequate to describe contractility clinically.

Work with the isolated cat papillary muscle appears to confirm the Frank-Starling law of the heart, which states that the force developed by the contracting heart is proportional to its initial length (preload). Changes in contractility are represented as shifts in both the force-length and force-velocity curves, upward in the case of increased contractility and downward in the case of decreased contractility (Fig. 86-5). The Frank-Starling principle fails to describe adequately changes in cardiac function that occur as a result of alterations in afterload. Furthermore, the intact heart operating at pressures in the physiologic range appears to function only on an ascending limb of its force-length relationship (that is, a descending limb of the Frank-Starling curve has not been demonstrated), and the force-length curves for different inotropic states (degrees of contractility) are nonparallel.

Afterload determines the degree of shortening of cardiac muscle, and afterload, as well as the other parameters determining myocardial performance, varies continuously during cardiac contraction. Thus the terms "instantaneous force," "instantaneous length," and "instantaneous shortening" (or "afterload") have been used. These terms serve to emphasize the dynamic nature of the circulatory system. The contracting heart is able to empty until it reaches a point on its maximal force-length curve (contractile state) that is determined by preload and afterload conditions.

Regulation of the circulation. The function of the heart is to provide peripheral tissues with sufficient blood to meet their metabolic requirements. The metabolic requirements of the tissues vary enormously from a basal state to one nearly 20-fold greater as reflected by total oxygen consumption. To account for this required variation, elaborate control mechanisms have evolved.

The mechanisms for regulation of the circulation (determination of the cardiac output and distribution of the cardiac output among the various tissues) may be grouped into two main categories, *neurogenic* and *endocrine*. A third category, *autoregulation*, involves local tissue factors and interplay of the neurogenic and endocrine mechanisms.

The *autonomic nervous system* plays an important role in the regulation of cardiac output. The balance of sympathetic and parasympathetic tone is the prime determinant of heart rate, the former accelerating it and the latter slowing it. Cardiac output is the product of stroke volume and heart rate. Control of heart rate is the principal acute determinant of cardiac output; stroke volume varies less in response to acute changes in physical activity or metabolic status. Changes in stroke volume do occur over time with physical training or in response to regurgitant valvular lesions or arteriovenous shunts. Control of heart rate by the autonomic nervous system is achieved via baroreceptors and other receptors in the blood vessels, heart, and lungs as mediated by various reflex arcs. The autonomic nervous system is critical in the control of regional and total systemic vascular resistance via vasoconstrictor and vasodilatory fibers that are regulated from the medullary vasomotor center, which in turn is influenced by the cerebral cortex, the hypothalamus, and other neural centers.

There are several important endocrine factors regulating the circulatory system. During activity or stress and in certain conditions chronically, the circulating catecholamines epinephrine and norepinephrine influence the heart rate, myocardial contractility, and peripheral vascular resistance. Angiotensin, a peptide produced from activation of angiotensinogen (produced in the liver) by renin (produced in the juxtaglomerular cells of the kidney), is the most potent pressor substance known and exerts its effect directly on arteriolar smooth muscle. Angiotensin, as well as potassium and adrenocorticotropic hormone (ACTH), also stimulates release of the mineralocorticoid aldosterone, which has an important sodium-retaining action, from the adrenal cortex. Antidiuretic hormone (ADH, vasopressin) is synthesized in the hypothalamus and is stored in and released from the posterior pituitary gland. It effects water conservation by the kidney and serves to regulate total body water and circulating blood volume. Other humoral factors such as bradykinin and prostaglandins may also be important in vascular control.

The third major mechanism in the regulation of the circulation is autoregulation, which serves to enhance the blood supply to organs or muscle groups with augmented metabolic needs. Changes in vascular tone are mediated by local changes in pH, Po_2, Pco_2, $[K^+]$, and concentrations of metabolic products. Local tone regulates blood flow in response to varying metabolic needs. The autonomic nervous system and endocrine mechanisms also serve to increase blood flow to regions with increased metabolic demands.

Decreases in total blood volume with change in body posture, venous compression by skeletal muscle during exercise, and changes in intrathoracic and intrapericardial pressures may also have an important influence on cardiac output.

PATHOPHYSIOLOGY. In congestive heart failure of myocardial origin, decreased myocardial contractility is primary. There are changes in preload and afterload that are usually secondary but are of pathophysiologic and therapeutic importance.

Left ventricular failure. Clinically, the most common measure of myocardial contractility is the left ventricular ejection fraction (stroke volume ÷ end-diastolic volume), as determined angiographically or noninvasively by echocardiography or radionuclide blood pool scanning. If the primary defect in left-sided congestive heart failure is impaired contractility evidenced by decreased left ventricular ejection fraction, stroke volume decreases or left ventricular end-diastolic volume increases or both. It follows that generally there is a fall in cardiac output or a rise in left ventricular end-diastolic pressure. The latter tends to augment left ventricular contractility via the Frank-Starling mechanism and thereby to increase stroke volume, compensating for decreased contractility. When the decrease in myocardial contractility is mild or moderate, this compensatory increase in stroke volume may restore cardiac output to normal. However, the consequence of increased left ventricular end-diastolic pressure is increased left atrial pressure and therefore increased pulmonary venous and capillary pressures. These latter increased pressures constitute the hemodynamic criteria for left ventricular failure and are important in symptom production (for example, dyspnea) in so-called backward left-sided congestive heart failure. With failure to maintain a normal cardiac output for the body's metabolic demands, relative peripheral perfusion falls. This results in impaired organ function and the symptoms of so-called forward left ventricular failure.

Right ventricular failure. The most common cause of right ventricular failure is left ventricular failure, although the findings in right ventricular failure are the same regardless of the cause. As indicated previously, the hallmarks of left ventricular myocardial failure are a decreased left ventricular ejection fraction and a rise in the left ventricular end-diastolic pressure, which is transmitted retrograde to the left atrium, pulmonary veins, and pulmonary capillaries. Since the right ventricle provides the active force for delivering blood to the left side of the circulation and the normal pulmonary circulation offers little resistance to forward flow, a rise in the pulmonary capillary pressure dictates a rise in right ventricular systolic pressure. To a degree, the right ventricle is capable of achieving this result without a rise in its filling pressure, but eventually the right ventricular end-diastolic pressure and therefore the mean right atrial pressure rise. These are the hemodynamic and clinical criteria for right ventricular failure.

Physiologic response to cardiac dysfunction. The same factors that regulate the systemic circulation in health have important roles in compensating for cardiac disease; failure of these compensatory mechanisms to return the circulatory system to normal results in symptom production and clinical congestive heart failure. An understanding of these compensatory mechanisms provides an understanding of the pathophysiology of congestive heart failure and its symptoms.

Heart rate. The compensatory response expressed most rapidly is increased heart rate. This may be evident first with modest exercise when increased muscle metabolism calls for increased blood flow (cardiac output). With greater myocardial impairment, tachycardia may be present at rest. Increases in heart rate are mediated by the autonomic nervous system and the endocrine mechanisms discussed previously.

Ventricular dilation and eccentric hypertrophy. Ventricular dilation is a major compensatory mechanism following myocardial injury or in volume overload lesions (regurgitant valvular lesions, atrial or ventricular septal defects, peripheral arteriovenous shunts). The volume of the ventricle increases with the cube of the radius, but thinning of the ventricular wall does not occur. The dilated ventricle may be able to maintain a normal stroke volume despite a decrease in ejection fraction. Ventricular dilation is accompanied by increased muscle mass, even if wall thickness remains normal. This is termed "eccentric hypertrophy."

Concentric hypertrophy. The left ventricular response to systemic hypertension, coarctation of the aorta, aortic valve stenosis, and other lesions, perhaps including ventricular dilation, is an increase in wall thickness ("concentric hypertrophy"). Concentrically hypertrophied myocardium has been demonstrated to have inherently decreased contractility. However, because of an increase in the number of contractile units, even though their individual contractility is less than normal, greater force can be developed by the concentrically hypertrophied myocardium than by normal myocardium, enabling the left ventricle to meet the demand imposed on it.

Thus maintenance of a normal stroke volume, despite decreased left ventricular ejection fraction, and maintenance of normal or higher than normal pressures, despite decreased contractility, are consequences of eccentric and concentric hypertrophy, respectively. Laplace's law indicates that wall stress is directly proportional to the pressure (P) in the chamber and its radius (r) and inversely proportional to the wall thickness (h) (wall stress = Pr/2h). Thus increased pressures and ventricular dilation result in increases in wall stress, but increased thickness of the wall tends to reduce the wall stress. Consideration of the compensatory mechanisms of heart rate, dilation, concentric and eccentric hypertrophy, and their interrelationships affecting wall stress is particularly important when myocardial oxygen delivery is limited owing to obstructive coronary artery disease, since the four major determinants of myocardial oxygen demand are systolic wall stress, myocardial mass, heart rate, and contractile (inotropic) state.

Role of afterload in congestive heart failure. In recent years increased attention has been drawn to the role of afterload in the pathogenesis and treatment of congestive heart failure. Afterload, which is also termed "impedance" or "left ventricular outflow resistance," is the sum of all forces that oppose ejection of blood from the ventricle during systole. As indicated, this value varies with time during the process of ventricular emptying, but instantaneous variation is not easily quantitated. The two major determinants of afterload are the *compliance* of the large arteries that accept the ventricular ejectate and the *peripheral resistance* to blood flow (largely determined at the level of the small arteries and arterioles). These factors determine the systolic pressure rise in the left ventricle and systemic arteries for a given ventricular stroke volume. Other factors affecting the afterload are the viscosity of blood and the inertia of the static blood in the ventricle and proximal aorta, which must be overcome to initiate ventricular ejection.

The normal ventricle adjusts to changes in afterload and maintains a relatively constant stroke volume (homeometric autoregulation). When the ventricle fails, however, its output becomes inversely related to afterload. In congestive heart failure afterload has been found to be increased above normal. The responsible factors appear to be an increase in peripheral vascular resistance owing to enhanced sympathetic tone and an increase in circulating catecholamines and renin. In addition, the compliance of the large arteries is decreased owing either to age (arteriosclerosis) or to vascular smooth muscle congestion. The increased afterload tends to increase the work of the left ventricle at a time when its ability to perform work (inotropic state) is already decreased. In many instances the increased afterload appears to be more an adverse effect of myocardial failure than a beneficial compensatory mechanism; a vicious circle of increasing afterload resulting in further impairment of cardiac performance with resultant further increases in afterload is established.

Production of signs and symptoms in congestive heart failure. The severity of the clinical manifestations of congestive heart failure depends on the degree of myocardial impairment, the demands the individual's activities place on the heart, and the proportion of time spent in activity and at rest. With mild impairment of cardiac function, symptoms may be evident only with strenuous exertion or when the individual is very active for many hours each day. With more severe impairment of cardiac function, symptoms may appear at ordinary levels of activity and subside only slowly with rest. With severe impairment, the patient is symptomatic at rest or with minimal activity. In summary, patients are classified as asymptomatic (I), symptomatic with major exertion (II), symptomatic with mild exertion (III), or symptomatic at rest (IV). Functional capacity does not, however, correlate closely with resting measures of ventricular function.

Consequences of high ventricular filling pressures. The signs and symptoms of "backward" heart failure are the ones most commonly encountered. The cardinal clinical findings in congestive heart failure are *dyspnea* and *edema*. Inability of the failing ventricle to empty completely during systole results in a rise in left ventricular end-diastolic pressure and a subsequent rise in left atrial, pulmonary venous, and pulmonary capillary pressures. The pulmonary venous system becomes engorged with blood, and pulmonary compliance is reduced. This causes an increase in the work of breathing that is perceived by the patient as *dyspnea* (shortness of breath). With milder forms of left ventricular failure, dyspnea may occur only during exertion, whereas it may be present at rest with more severe failure. Dyspnea must be distinguished from *tachypnea,* an appropriate hyperventilatory response that enhances gas exchange but is not perceived as shortness of breath by the patient.

When the elevated pulmonary capillary pressure exceeds the oncotic pressure, transudation of fluid into the alveoli, termed pulmonary edema, occurs. The presence of fluid in alveoli is one cause of pulmonary rales heard on physical examination. The edema results in impaired gas exchange and increases the work of breathing beyond that imposed by pulmonary venous engorgement alone. Pulmonary edema may occur insidiously following prolonged, relatively high levels of physical activity or with the salt and water retention that develops in chronic congestive heart failure. It may also occur abruptly (*acute pulmonary edema*) following acute myocardial infarction, with acute aortic or mitral insufficiency, or without apparent cause in the setting of chronic congestive heart failure.

Orthopnea is dyspnea when the patient is supine, alleviated by elevation of the trunk. Elevation of the thorax above the lower extremities decreases the hydrostatic pressure in the pulmonary capillaries and veins (especially in the upper lobes) and decreases venous return. Both factors contribute to a fall in pulmonary capillary and venous pressure that relieves the dyspnea. With mild orthopnea, sleeping on two or three pillows may provide relief. When orthopnea is more severe, the patient may be able to rest and sleep only bolt upright.

Another symptom of "backward" failure is *paroxysmal nocturnal dyspnea*. Patients with this symptom wake from sleep with shortness of breath that is relieved by sitting up or standing, especially before an open window. The pathophysiology of this symptom is in part similar to that of orthopnea, and sleeping with the thorax and head elevated may prevent it. However, it is possible that depression of the respiratory center during sleep results in hypoxia in the patient with already compromised gas exchange or that decreased adrenergic stimulation of the failing myocardium during sleep is pathophysiologically important.

The consequences of backward failure of the right ventricle are less life threatening than those of left ventricular failure. The sequences of pressure phenomena are identical, but elevation of the filling pressure of the right ventricle (right atrial pressure, jugular venous pressure, systemic venous pressure) does not interfere with as vital a process as respiratory gas exchange. The most common sign of right ventricular failure is *peripheral edema*. This is the result of chronic elevation of systemic venous pressure to a level that exceeds the oncotic pressure. When the patient spends considerable time in the upright position, edema is present at the ankle and pretibially. In the bedridden patient edema is commonly found in the dependent aspect of the trunk ("presacral" edema). Frequently when edema is present, the jugular venous pressure is found to be elevated on physical examination. However, since the right-sided pressures may be elevated only with exertion, this finding may be absent during examination after a period of rest.

A second result of elevation of the systemic venous pressure is *hepatomegaly* and gastrointestinal venous congestion. Hepatic congestion results in parenchymal distention within a less distensible liver capsule, and epigastric or right upper quadrant discomfort is common. Manual compression of the abdomen causes a transient delivery of volume to the right atrium with concomitant elevation of the jugular venous pressure (hepatojugular reflux) visible by inspection. Care must be taken to distinguish this quite specific finding from venous distention produced by a Valsalva maneuver induced by vigorous palpation of the abdomen. Abdominal discomfort may also be due to edema of the gastrointestinal tract with disturbances of digestion and elimination. In severe right-sided heart failure, transudation of edema into the bowel lumen can result in protein-losing enteropathy. In advanced right heart failure ascites may be present.

Pleural effusion is a common finding in congestive heart failure. Since the pleural veins drain into both the pulmonary and systemic venous systems, pleural effusion usually signifies coexisting left and right heart failure. Occasionally pleural effusion may result from marked elevation of pressure in either venous system alone. Modest accumulation of fluid in the pericardium may also occur in heart failure, but pericardial effusions resulting from congestive heart failure are rarely large enough to cause tamponade. Cardiac tamponade may be considered a form of heart failure, but the cause is seldom myocardial. When tamponade is present, a pericardial origin should be sought.

Peripheral edema or accumulation of fluid in the pleural or peritoneal cavities tends to cause an increase in body weight. Anorexia of cardiac or other origin may cause loss of tissue mass concomitant with fluid retention so that no change in body weight occurs or the weight may actually decrease.

Consequences of reduced cardiac output. The "forward" signs and symptoms of heart failure are subtle and more difficult to evaluate than those caused by increased filling pressures. In part, this is because increased filling pressures and other compensatory mechanisms are able to sustain a normal resting cardiac output, as well as increases in the cardiac output sufficient to meet the demands imposed by modest to moderate physical activity.

Normal individuals are able to increase their cardiac output approximately fivefold with exercise and, by increasing peripheral tissue oxygen extraction, can increase oxygen consumption eightfold over resting levels. Trained athletes can raise their cardiac output sevenfold with exercise and their oxygen consumption nearly 20-fold. Neither normal individuals nor trained athletes attain much elevation of ventricular filling pressures to achieve these high levels of performance.

In contrast, the individual with congestive heart failure has a limited capacity to increase cardiac output and oxygen consumption and does so at the expense of elevated ventricular filling pressures, with the consequences previously detailed. Measurement of exercise capacity (work load), cardiac output, oxygen consumption, and the filling pressure required to achieve these maximal values assesses an individual's degree of impaired myocardial performance.

The signs and symptoms of reduced cardiac output in congestive heart failure are related to the changes in distribution of available cardiac output among the organ systems. Although skeletal muscle tends to receive its normal share of the cardiac output at rest, its demands cannot be met during exercise, and *easy fatigability* is a common symptom in congestive heart failure. Because of compensatory vasoconstriction to shift blood to more vital beds, the skin, splanchnic, and renal circulations are subject to the greatest reductions in blood flow when the cardiac output is reduced. Thus *pallor* of the skin and impaired temperature regulation accompany congestive heart failure. Reduced splanchnic circulation adds to the abdominal discomfort and impaired function caused by venous congestion and edema. Hepatic clearance of ADH and aldosterone is reduced.

Renal underperfusion results in reduced glomerular filtration, oliguria, and "prerenal" azotemia (usually without proportionate elevation of the serum creatinine level). Impaired sodium and water excretion contributes importantly to the development of edema. In addition, renal hypoperfusion induces release of renin that results in increased circulating angiotensin and, in turn, increased aldosterone release. Angiotensin contributes to vasoconstriction, and aldosterone further promotes sodium retention and accumulation of fluids.

Cerebral and coronary perfusion is decreased less than that of other organs in congestive heart failure. Perfusion of the hypothalamus is frequently reduced enough to result in the release of increased amounts of ADH. Reduction in cerebral blood flow may result in anxiety or difficulty in concentration and less commonly in confusion (especially if cerebrovascular disease coexists). Marked obtundation and coma rarely result from congestive heart failure. When the coronary arteries are free of atherosclerosis, there is not enough decrease in coronary perfusion in congestive failure to be of clinical importance. However, when the coronary circulation is limited by occlusive atherosclerotic disease, normal autoregulative processes may not be operative and the reduced coronary flow, in combination with the marked increase in myocardial oxygen consumption dictated by ventricular dilation, may cause an increase in angina pectoris or result in myocardial infarction.

LABORATORY FINDINGS. Of the routine laboratory tests, those most commonly affected by heart failure are renal and liver function tests and arterial blood gas studies. Renal function abnormalities result from kidney underperfusion as well as the effect of diuretic agents. Blood urea nitrogen is sensitive to decreases in renal blood flow and tends to rise earlier in congestive failure and to a grater degree than serum creatinine. Diuretic agents may also disproportionately raise blood urea nitrogen via direct renal action or by further decreasing renal blood flow. Serum electrolyte abnormalities occur commonly in heart failure. Hyponatremia may result from water retention or from excess urinary sodium loss in response to diuretics. Hypokalemia occurs commonly as a manifestation of secondary aldosteronism or as a side effect of diuretics. Hypochloremia may also result from diuretic therapy.

Liver function tests are often abnormal in right-sided congestive heart failure because of hepatic venous congestion and hypoxia. Mild to moderate elevations of serum bilirubin, transaminases, and alkaline phosphatase are common. Occasionally these values reach such high levels that distinction from hepatitis is difficult. The prothrombin time is frequently prolonged and may be refractory to correction with vitamin K administration. Since alcoholic or other liver disease may be present in some patients with heart failure, distinction between primary and secondary liver disease is sometimes difficult.

With pulmonary congestion, oxygenation is impaired and arterial hypoxemia occurs. Hypercapnia may occur but only in the most severe cases. In chronic heart failure a low arterial oxygen tension is common, and arterial P_{CO_2} is often low owing to hyperventilation in an attempt to achieve adequate oxygenation. Arterial pH is often alkalotic as a result of both hyperventilation and diuretic-induced metabolic alkalosis. However, in severe low–cardiac output states, arterial pH may be at acidotic levels because of CO_2 retention and anaerobic metabolism.

The *electrocardiogram* may reflect the underlying cardiovascular pathologic condition but does not specifically diagnose congestive heart failure. Common features in heart failure are arrhythmias, left ventricular hypertrophy, conduction defects, and ST-T wave changes that may reflect underlying pathophysiology or the effects of digitalis and diuretics. A completely normal electrocardiogram may occasionally be seen.

The *chest roentgenogram* is a sensitive indicator of the presence of congestive heart failure. It is affected by the duration of heart failure and to some degree by its severity. Acute onset of left ventricular failure usually causes little if any change in heart size or contour, but in its earliest stages it produces pulmonary venous hypertension manifested as dilation and prominence of pulmonary veins. As the severity of pulmonary vascular congestion increases, vascular markings become more prominent, especially in the upper lobes. In the most severe cases transudation of fluid into the alveoli may occur and appears as infiltrates with an alveolar distribution. In chronic heart failure heart size is increased, with the cardiothoracic ratio usually exceeding 50%. Signs of long-standing pulmonary congestion are interstitial edema (Kerley's lines) and pleural effusion. Pericardial effusion may also contribute to increased heart size on roentgenogram. Lateral and oblique views of the heart may be necessary to demonstrate specific chamber enlargement. It should be recognized that neither acute nor chronic roentgenographic changes correlate closely with the hemodynamic findings or symptomatic status of patients.

Echocardiography is discussed in Chapter 89. In left-sided failure the echocardiogram frequently shows left ventricular dilation. Wall motion abnormalities, especially hypokinesis, may also be present. Interpretation of these findings must be cautious, since the single beam view of M-mode echocardiography is subject to errors imposed by the asymmetry of ventricular geometry that frequently accompanies ischemic heart disease. In restrictive and constrictive disease the chamber size may be normal, although valve motion patterns may reflect abnormal hemodynamics. The ability of two-dimensional echocardiography to assess ventricular function appears promising.

Cardiac catheterization is a particular value in diagnosing heart failure and in some instances in determining its cause. Hemodynamic findings indicating heart failure include elevated ventricular filling pressures, decreased cardiac output, and decreased ejection fraction. Depressed contractility is usually evident on ventriculograms.

DIAGNOSIS. The diagnosis of congestive heart failure is usually established from the history and physical findings. In addition to the common symptoms of dyspnea or easy fatigability, presenting features may include weight gain, anorexia, abdominal pain, and coughing with no sputum or production of small amounts of clear sputum. The presence of any of these symptoms in association with a history suggesting a cardiac lesion, such as a murmur from rheumatic disease, angina pectoris, previous myocardial infarction, or hypertension, should lead to a suspicion of congestive heart failure. Physical findings often confirm the diagnosis. The most useful of these are jugular venous distention and a positive hepatojugular venous reflux, which are highly specific. Pulsus alternans is often palpable. More common, but less specific, are an S_3 gallop, pulmonary rales, peripheral edema, and Cheyne-Stokes respirations.

Congestive heart failure must be distinguished from other causes of dyspnea and fatigue. The most common noncardiac causes of shortness of breath are pulmonary disorders, identified by a history of pulmonary disease, abnormal pulmonary function tests, and abnormal blood gas studies. Sometimes the two disorders may coexist, rendering their differentiation more difficult and occasionally requiring hemodynamic measurements to distinguish between heart failure and pulmonary disease as the cause of shortness of breath. Other causes of congested states simulating heart failure include renal failure, cirrhosis, and excess fluid administration. These are usually apparent from the clinical presentation and laboratory tests. However, pulmonary congestion resulting from excess fluid administration should prompt a careful search for the presence of previously unrecognized heart disease, since volume loading is usually well tolerated by patients with normal cardiovascular function. Finally, other causes of low cardiac output must be excluded. These include shock from sepsis, pulmonary embolism, hypoadrenalism, and hypovolemia (see Chapter 88).

COURSE AND PROGNOSIS. Although patients with congestive heart failure frequently have symptomatic improvement following the institution of therapy, the course is usually one of progressive deterioration. According to data collected in the Framingham study, the 5-year survival from the time of diagnosis of congestive heart failure is less than 50%. This ominous prognosis is as bad as or worse than that of all forms of cancer considered together. Patients with moderate to severe heart failure have a mortality as high as 50% to 60% within 12 to 24 months of the time of diagnosis.

This ominous prognosis applies primarily to patients with chronic congestive heart failure of ischemic or idiopathic origin. In other cases congestive heart failure can be "cured." This is most likely when a specific cause such as myocarditis can be found and effectively treated. In patients with acute myocardial infarction, heart failure may be severe during the acute phase but transient and nonrecurrent. Patients with congestive heart failure resulting from valvular heart disease or ventricular aneurysm often improve following surgical therapy. This is more likely in patients whose ventricular function has remained sufficiently unimpaired by valvular disease. Improvement also occurs in cases of ventricular aneurysm when enough functioning myocardium is uninvolved by the aneurysm that correction of the mechanical problem results in good residual function and thus symptomatic relief. The long-term prognosis is very good in such "cured" patients.

Patients with congestive heart failure are subject to other complications of their heart disease. *Arrhythmias* are frequent and range from relatively benign supraventricular to serious ventricular arrhythmias. These occur with ischemic heart disease but are also frequent in other forms of heart disease. The prevalence of arrhythmias appears to be greater in patients with more severe failure, and it is possible that the degree of hemodynamic abnormality, altered cardiac chamber size, and loading conditions are predisposing factors in some cases. *Embolic phenomena* are a common complication of congestive heart failure. Pulmonary embolism usually originates from the peripheral venous bed when there is stasis, particularly in patients with marked peripheral edema and right-sided heart failure. Systemic emboli in the cerebral, renal, and mesenteric beds originate from the left side of the heart (either atrium or ventricle) as a result of clot formation in these chambers. Atrial fibrillation, which is frequently present in patients with congestive failure, facilitates clot formation in the noncontracting atria.

In some patients with stable heart disease, symptoms develop acutely in response to arrhythmias, a new ischemic event, a change in medication, failure to take prescribed medication, or dietary indiscretion. Patients with heart failure are also subject to acute exacerbations of their disease for reasons that are not always apparent. Although it is common when no apparent cause is found to attribute exacerbations to dietary indiscretion or to noncompliance with medical regimens, frequently these factors are not responsible for worsening the patient's clinical status. Excessive salt and fluid ingestion can unquestionably increase the severity of the symptoms of heart failure, but adjustment of diuretic dosage can usually compensate for minor increases in salt and water consumption. It is likely that acute exacerbations of congestive heart failure without apparent cause represent progression of the disease process. The vicious circle of compensatory mechanisms leading to high peripheral resistance, increased afterload, and worsened left ventricular function may account for this steady course punctuated by acute episodes during which therapy must be readjusted.

MANAGEMENT. The major principles in the treatment of heart failure are outlined in Table 86-1. Certain general

Table 86-1. Treatment of congestive heart failure

	Acute heart failure	Chronic heart failure

General measures	Bed rest
	Strict sodium restriction
		Reduced activities
		Moderate sodium restriction
		Control associated disorders:
		  Hypertension
		  Obesity
		  Pulmonary disease
		  Arrhythmias
		Risk factor modification:
		  Smoking
		  Hyperlipidemia

Pharmacologic therapy	Oxygen Morphine Treatment of arrhythmias Correction of pH Diuretics (furosemide) Vasodilators (nitroprusside) Inotropic agents (sympathomimetics)	Inotropic agents (digitalis) Preload reduction (diuretics) Afterload reduction (vasodilators)
Other therapy	Mechanical circulatory assistance Surgery for specific lesions	Surgery for specific lesions

measures are recommended for the majority of patients with congestive heart failure. During periods of marked symptomatology patients are usually advised to *rest* and avoid undue exertion. Such a prescription from the physician is rarely necessary because patients voluntarily curtail activities when their symptoms become more severe with exertion. The prescription of prolonged bed rest (for periods up to 6 months to 1 year) in acute myocarditis or idiopathic cardiomyopathy is no longer enforced in most cases, since it is difficult to achieve and may make patients susceptible to other complications, especially emboli. *Diet* is important, and obesity should be corrected to decrease the metabolic work load on the heart. In addition, patients are advised to curtail sodium intake, but this need not require great patient discomfort because excess sodium accumulation can be controlled by appropriate diuretic administration in all but the most severe cases.

Other factors that may aggravate or impose an increased load on cardiac performance should be controlled. Hypertension should be rigorously controlled by appropriate medications. Caution is advised in the prescription of antihypertensive drugs that may depress cardiac function; these include sympatholytic agents such as methyldopa, β-adrenergic blockers, and reserpine. Other associated disorders such as pulmonary disease must be treated vigorously because they may have significant effects on the circulation by directly imposing a load on the right ventricle, thus limiting systemic oxygen delivery.

The cornerstone of therapy in clinically overt heart failure remains drug treatment. The medications currently used fall into three categories: (1) inotropic agents that enhance contractility and thereby cardiac performance, (2) agents that reduce ventricular filling pressures and thereby decrease pulmonary and systemic venous congestion, and (3) impedance-reducing agents that decrease left ventricular outflow resistance, thereby allowing the failing ventricle to eject a greater portion of its diastolic volume and improve cardiac output.

Oral inotropic agents useful in congestive heart failure currently include only digitalis preparations, of which the most commonly used is digoxin. Although digitalis improves indices of myocardial contractility, several studies in recent years have demonstrated that the effects of digitalis are less than may be desired. Left ventricular filling pressure and cardiac output are not consistently improved by short- or long-term administration of digitalis. Because of the questionable hemodynamic efficacy and relatively high toxicity associated with digitalis administration, its routine use in the long-term management of congestive heart failure has recently been questioned. The use of digitalis (for example, digoxin, 0.125 to 0.375 mg/day) is still recommended in chronic congestive heart failure. In contrast, acute digitalization for hemodynamic improvement does not appear warranted, since the effects of the agent are quite mild and more potent agents are available. The term "digitalization" merely means achievement of effective blood and tissue levels of digitalis, and because of the narrow therapeutic margin with this agent, it is no longer recommended that digoxin be rapidly given or that high doses be used in an attempt to achieve a greater inotropic effect. Other inotropic drugs are currently being developed, but none is now available for long-term oral administration.

The primary preload-reducing agents are diuretics, which decrease intravascular volume, thereby reducing ventricular filling pressures along with pulmonary and systemic venous congestion. Diuretics do not alter cardiac function because they simply shift ventricular performance along the same Frank-Starling curve. The reduction in preload is generally accompanied by no change or a slight fall in cardiac output. These agents should be used with caution in patients operating on a critical volume-dependent portion of the ventricular function curve (the more vertical portions on the left in Fig. 86–5), since a reduction in filling pressure can result in a substantial fall in cardiac output. Hypotension, azotemia, and other signs of low output may ensue. Furthermore, diuretic administration frequently results in electrolyte imbalance, including hyponatremia, hypokalemia, and metabolic alkalosis. Potassium supplementation is usually necessary with diuretic agents, especially when digitalis is used. The most commonly used diuretics are the potent loop diuretics furosemide and ethacrynic acid. In some cases these agents alone produce an insufficient clinical response, but combining them with other diuretics such as thiazides, which act at a different site in the nephron, may lead synergistically to a marked increase in urinary sodium excretion. If hypokalemia becomes prominent, potassium-sparing diuretics such as spironolactone may be beneficial.

Certain vasodilators such as nitrates have a pronounced effect on veins by increasing venous capacitance and thereby reducing preload, filling pressures, and pulmonary congestion. Nitroprusside acts in this manner and also reduces impedance; thus it is useful in pulmonary edema (see below).

The third class of agents used in heart failure are those that decrease resistance to left ventricular ejection. Of these, the most commonly employed are nitroprusside, nitrates, hydralazine, and prazosin. The doses required may be substantially higher than those used to treat angina or hypertension. Captopril, an angiotensin converting enzyme inhibitor, vasodilates and blocks sodium retention caused by excess aldosterone in high renin states. Nifedipine, a calcium antagonist and coronary vasodilator recently made available to treat angina, also works as a systemic vasodilator. Although vasodilators may produce striking hemodynamic and symptomatic improvement in the acute phase of heart failure, their efficacy during long-term management, particularly their effect on morbidity and mortality, is not yet clearly established. Therefore these agents currently are used as adjuncts to conventional therapy with digitalis and diuretics in patients refractory to standard treatment.

Acute pulmonary edema is a medical emergency. The most outstanding abnormality in this condition is marked elevation of the pulmonary venous pressure leading to severe dyspnea. Cardiac output may be normal or occasionally even elevated. The immediate therapeutic goal is to reduce the high filling pressure. Initial therapy includes the administration of oxygen to improve oxygenation and morphine to interrupt disadvantageous cardiopulmonary reflexes and relieve anxiety. Diuretic agents are also useful. If a clinical response is not obtained in 20 to 30 minutes, the addition of impedance-reducing agents should be considered. The agent of choice in this instance is the potent vasodilator sodium nitroprusside.

In patients with symptoms of low output (a shocklike state, oliguria, cerebral underperfusion, and cutaneous vasoconstriction), it may be necessary to add inotropic agents more potent than digitalis for short-term management. These patients usually are already receiving digitalis, and there is no evidence that giving additional digitalis is beneficial. The potent inotropic drugs available are the sympathomimetic agents isoproterenol, dopamine, dobutamine, and norepinephrine. These drugs enhance myocardial contractility and usually raise cardiac output. In high doses their peripheral vasoconstricting effect may limit the rise in cardiac output because of an associated increase in afterload. A useful approach therefore has been the combination of a vasodilating agent such as nitroprusside with a potent inotropic agent such as dopamine or dobutamine (see Chapter 88). This combination raises cardiac output more than either agent alone and is useful in severe low output states. In patients with acute exacerbations of severe chronic congestive heart failure, it is usually necessary to continue these regimens for several days before instituting therapy with oral agents.

BIBLIOGRAPHY

Braunwald, E., Ross, J., Jr., and Sonnenblick, E.H.: Mechanisms of contraction of the normal and failing heart, ed. 2, Boston, 1976, Little, Brown & Co.

Cohn, J.N.: Vasodilator therapy for heart failure: the influence of impedance on left ventricular performance, Circulation **48**:5, 1973.

Cohn, J.N., and Franciosa, J.A.: Vasodilator therapy of cardiac failure, N. Engl. J. Med. **297**:27, 254, 1977.

DelGreco, F.: The kidney in congestive heart failure, Mod. Concepts Cardiovasc. Dis. **44**:47, 1975.

Dodge, H.T., and Baxley, W.A.: Left ventricular volume and mass and their significance in heart disease, Am. J. Cardiol. **23**:528, 1969.

Kannel, W.B., and others: Role of blood pressure in the development of congestive heart failure, N. Engl. J. Med. **287**:781, 1972.

Mason, D.T.: Regulation of cardiac performance in clinical heart disease: interactions between contractile state, mechanical abnormalities and ventricular compensatory mechanisms, Am. J. Cardiol. **32**:437, 1973.

Mason, D.T., and others: Cardiocirculatory responses to muscular exercise in congestive heart failure, Prog. Cardiovasc. Dis. **19**:475, 1977.

McKee, P.A., and others: The natural history of congestive heart failure: the Framingham study, N. Engl. J. Med. **285**:1441, 1971.

Sonnenblick, E.H., and Strobeck, J.E.: Derived indices of ventricular and myocardial function, N. Engl. J. Med. **296**:978, 1977.

Swan, H.J.C., and others: Catheterization of the heart in man with use of a flow-directed balloon-tipped catheter, N. Engl. J. Med. **293**:447, 1970.

Wade, O.L., and Bishop, J.M.: Cardiac output and regional blood flow, Philadelphia, 1962, F.A. Davis Co.

Weber, K.T., and Janicki, J.S.: The heart as a muscle-pump system and the concept of heart failure, Am. Heart J. **98**:371, 1979.

87 • SYSTEMIC HYPERTENSION

Surender Singh

Diseases of the cardiovascular system are the leading causes of death in Western nations. In the United States they account for nearly 1 million deaths each year, 53% of deaths from all causes. There are abundant epidemiologic, clinical, experimental, and pathologic studies indicating that systemic hypertension is one of the most important etiologic factors in cardiovascular disease.

Nearly 35 million Americans have definite hypertension and another 25 million have borderline hypertension. Even with the current campaign for public and professional awareness, only 70% of these people are aware of their high blood pressure. Recent reports suggest that an increasing number of those with hypertension (60% as compared to 40% a few years ago) are currently receiving effective treatment.

Prospective randomized double-blind trials of treated and untreated hypertensive individuals have demonstrated that effective treatment of hypertension can prevent cerebral hemorrhage, cerebrovascular accident, congestive heart failure, renal damage, and dissecting aneurysm and can reduce the risk of heart attack. The major emphasis in the management of hypertension should be placed on the early detection, evaluation, and effective treatment of the vast number of people with untreated or inadequately treated hypertension.

MEASUREMENT OF BLOOD PRESSURE. An annual blood pressure measurement performed by properly trained personnel is recommended for everyone. It is important that the patient be recumbent or seated, resting comfortably for nearly 10 minutes before the pressure is taken, with the arm laid bare to the shoulder to avoid constriction of a rolled-up sleeve. The cuff should be applied evenly to the middle of the upper arm with the middle of the bladder within the cuff on the inner side. The bladder should cover about two thirds of the distance between the shoulder and the elbow. Its length should be sufficient to encircle at least two thirds of the circumference of the arm, but the lower edge of the cuff should not infringe on the antecubital space. If the cuff is too small, falsely high readings are obtained. In obese patients, if a large cuff is unavailable, the approximate blood pressure can be measured by wrapping the standard cuff around the forearm and listening over the radial artery.

The cuff should be inflated 30 mm Hg higher than the level at which radial pulsations disappear and then auscultation should be performed over the brachial artery. On gradual deflation of the cuff (3 to 4 mm Hg per beat), five types of sounds (Korotkoff sounds) are heard. They are defined as follows:

Phase I—Clear tapping sound (Systolic pressure is read at the first regular tapping sound.)
Phase II—Prolonged murmuring sound
Phase III—Reappearance of a loud sharper tone
Phase IV—Appearance of a soft muffled sound
Phase V—Disappearance of all sounds

The Joint National Committee on Detection, Evaluation and Treatment of High Blood Pressure recommends phase V as the diastolic pressure. The World Health Organization recommends that both phase IV and V values be recorded if there is a difference of more than 5 mm Hg. On initial examination blood pressure should be recorded in both arms, for example, right arm 130/82-74 mm Hg, left arm 125/80-74 mm Hg. In subsequent examinations blood pressure should be recorded in the arm found initially to have the higher pressure.

Blood pressure varies from moment to moment, being influenced by several factors such as the following:

1. *Body position.* On passive tilt from recumbent to erect posture, there may be a slight fall in the systolic pressure while the diastolic pressure may rise, thereby decreasing pulse pressure.
2. *Diurnal variation.* Blood pressure is higher in the afternoon and evening than in the morning.
3. *Activity.* Blood pressure is higher in the afternoon and evening than in the morning.
4. *Mentation.* Environmental stimuli can increase blood pressure.

Individual factors determining blood pressure include the following:

1. *Sex.* Blood pressure tends to be higher in males than in females until the age of 55, after which the reverse is true.
2. *Age.* Blood pressure is higher in older individuals. Diastolic blood pressure increases until about age 50 and then levels off. Systolic blood pressure tends to rise more abruptly in later life owing to decreased aortic compliance.
3. *Race.* High blood pressure is more common in blacks.
4. *Family history.* Genetic factors determine both high and low blood pressure patterns. If a family member has hypertension, the chances of a close relative having high blood pressure are increased.
5. *Salt intake.* In some individuals a high salt intake may increase the chances of having high blood pressure.
6. *Weight.* The rise in blood pressure with age is greater in obese individuals.

DEFINITION. There is no precise dividing line between normal and elevated blood pressures. Pressures are normally substantially lower in children and adolescents than in adults. The World Health Organization defines hypertension as a casual blood pressure higher than 160/95 mm Hg. Those with a casual blood pressure less than 140/90 mm Hg in the seated position are considered *normotensive.* Those with blood pressures between 140/90 mm Hg and 160/95 mm Hg are categorized as borderline hypertensives. Currently there is no way of determining in which patients higher pressures will develop. Isolated systolic hypertension is usually defined as systolic pressure greater than 160 mm Hg with a diastolic pressure below 95 mm Hg. This is the more common form of hypertension in the elderly owing to decreased aortic compliance. Labile hypertension is a condition in which blood pressure fluctuates between normal and abnormal levels. However, it should be recognized that the blood pressure in both normotensive and hypertensive individuals also fluctuates widely.

In 90% to 95% of hypertensive patients the cause is unknown and probably represents a heterogeneous group of multifactorial diseases. In only 5% to 10% of hypertensive patients can a cause be discovered. Hypertension is characterized by an abnormal relationship among various homeostatic mechanisms—cardiovascular, renal, neural, hormonal, and others as yet unidentified. Hypertension is easily identified and effectively treated, but if untreated, it can cause abnormalities of "target organs" such as the heart, blood vessels, nervous system, and kidneys with an increase in morbidity and mortality from cardiovascular diseases.

PATHOPHYSIOLOGY. The regulation of arterial blood pressure is complex because several homeostatic mechanisms—cardiovascular, neural, renal, endocrine-metabolic, sodium intake, and genetic—play a role in maintaining blood pressure within a normal range.

Cardiovascular factors. The systolic blood pressure depends mainly on cardiac output (stroke volume × heart rate). Stroke volume in turn depends on left ventricular end-diastolic volume and contractility. Other factors affecting systolic pressure are aortic compliance (distensibility), extracellular fluid volume, and neural and hormonal activity. Diastolic blood pressure depends largely on systemic vascular resistance, which is determined by arteriolar smooth muscle contractions under the influence of the autonomic nervous system and endocrine-metabolic factors. On the basis of hemodynamic determinants (cardiac output and peripheral vascular resistance), hypertension can be divided into the following groups:

1. *Hypertension with high cardiac output.* Young anxious individuals with early labile hypertension frequently have a hyperdynamic circulation and increased cardiac output. Peripheral vascular resistance is usually normal.
2. *Hypertension with increased peripheral vascular resistance.* Elderly individuals with long-standing advanced hypertension frequently have increased peripheral vascular resistance, normal or decreased cardiac output, and vascular changes on pathologic examination.
3. *Hypertension with both high cardiac output and increased peripheral vascular resistance.* Various combinations of the hemodynamic factors, output and resistance, are seen in a large number of patients with hypertension of differing severity. No vascular changes or minimal, usually reversible changes are seen with mild hypertension, whereas patients with severe, long-standing hypertension frequently have irreversible pathologic changes in their arterioles.

Neural factors. Increased arterial pressure in a normal individual causes an increased rate of afferent impulses to the medulla oblongata from stretch receptors (baroreceptors) in the wall of carotid sinuses and the aortic arch via the ninth and tenth cranial nerves, respectively. This results in increased vagal activity (efferent parasympathetic component) and decreased sympathetic activity (efferent sympathetic component). Primarily the latter decreases peripheral vascular resistance, tending to reduce the blood pressure. Decreased sensitivity of baroreceptors was initially thought to be an important etiologic factor in hypertension. It is now believed that resetting of baroreceptors represents an adaptation to the hypertensive state rather than a cause. An increased sympathetic activity and/or reduced vagal tone contributes to *autonomic dysregulation,* which has been demonstrated in some patients with essential hypertension. Although the relationship between the sympathetic nervous system and the pathogenesis of certain forms of clinical hypertension has not been fully delineated, the concept of autonomic dysregulation has been helpful in selecting antihypertensive drugs for some patients.

Renal factors (renin-angiotensin system) (Fig. 87-1). Renin is a proteolytic enzyme secreted by specialized cells, called the juxtaglomerular apparatus, that are found around the afferent arterioles of glomeruli. The stimuli for increased renin production are decreased extracellular fluid volume, low renal perfusion, and decreased sodium content in the macula densa. "Prorenin" (so-called big renin) is an inactive precursor of renin. Renin acts on angiotensinogen to produce angiotensin I, which is converted to angiotensin II by the converting enzyme peptidyldipeptide hydrolase in the lungs. Angiotensin acts in the following ways:

1. *Direct vasoconstriction.* Angiotensin II is a potent pressor agent.
2. *Production of aldosterone.* Angiotensin II stimulates the production of aldosterone by the zona glomerulosa of the adrenal cortex. Aldosterone increases sodium and water retention by distal renal tubules.
3. *Stimulation of sympathetic nervous system.* Stimulation of the sympathetic nervous system (or increasing the effect of sympathetic stimulation) is probably a third route of renin-angiotensin action.

Renin levels in patients with hypertension may be high (20% of patients), normal (60% of patients), or low (20% of patients). Hypertensive patients with intravascular volume expansion (frequently caused by renal disease) have suppressed renin production. This form of hypertension often responds well to diuretics. Patients with renal artery stenosis, malignant hypertension, or renin-producing tumors have high plasma renin activity. They tend to respond favorably to antirenin drugs such as β-adrenergic blockers or to angiotensin inhibitors but poorly to diuretics.

Endocrine-metabolic factors. The endocrine-metabolic

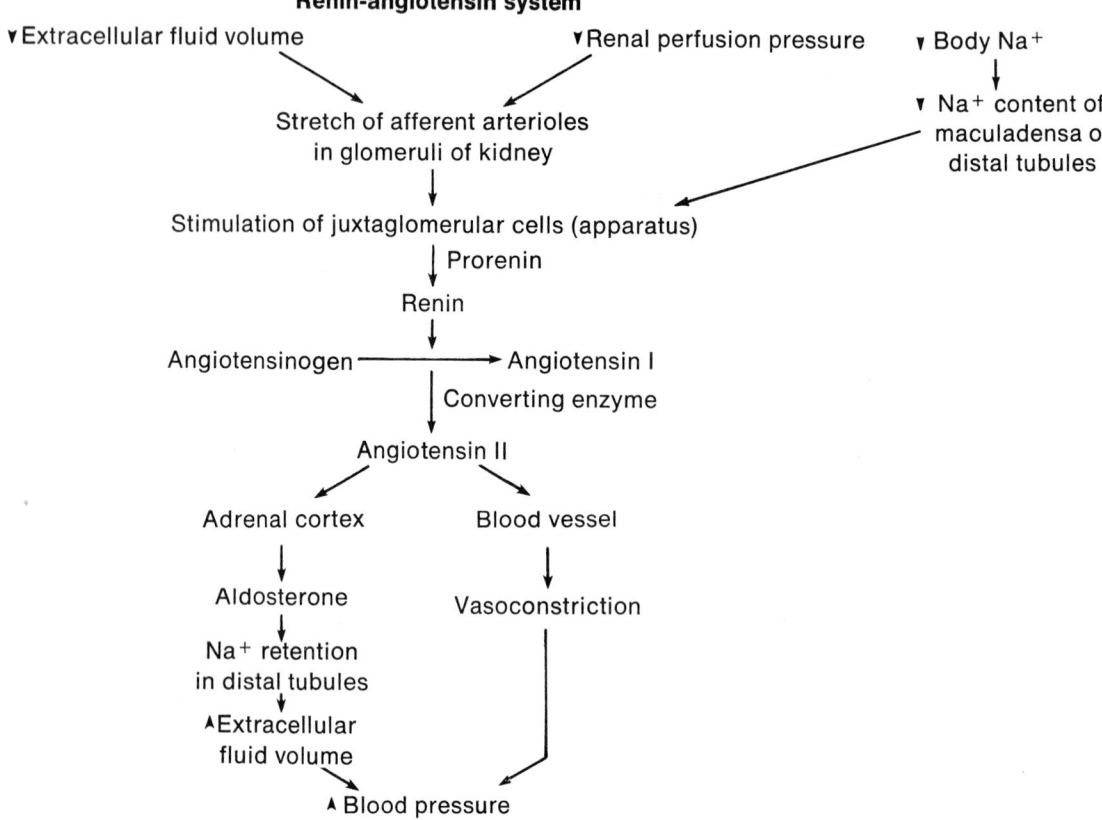

Fig. 87-1. Complex relationship between extracellular fluid volume and pressure as mediated via renal hormonal mechanisms. These involve production of renin and angiotensin. Latter is potent vasoconstrictor and stimulates aldosterone synthesis, resulting in sodium retention and increased volume.

factors include renin-angiotensin, aldosterone and other mineralocorticoids, catecholamines, prostaglandins, kallikrein, bradykinin, and prolactin.

The *renin-angiotensin* system was discussed previously. *Aldosterone* is produced in the zona glomerulosa of the adrenal cortex under the influence of the renin-angiotensin system, potassium intake, and less importantly adrenocorticotropic hormone (ACTH).

Aldosterone has two main physiologic functions: to regulate *extracellular fluid volume* through a direct effect on the renal tubular transport of sodium and to regulate *potassium metabolism*. Aldosterone acts on distal convoluted tubules to increase sodium absorption and potassium excretion. Increased aldosterone production resulting from adrenal adenoma, hyperplasia, or carcinoma (*primary aldosteronism*) is an uncommon but potentially curable cause of hypertension. Secondary hyperaldosteronism develops in patients with accelerated or malignant hypertension. Abnormalities in aldosterone production have not been described in essential hypertension.

Excessive secretion of other mineralocorticoids has been found in some hypertensive individuals. Their role in the cause of essential hypertension is uncertain.

Higher levels of plasma or urinary *catecholamines* and dopamine β-hydroxylase have been demonstrated in certain patients with hypertension. Some hypertensive patients have a reduction in urinary excretion of *kallikrein*, a depressor substance. Renal *prostaglandins* lead to increased sodium excretion. In a recent report of a hypertensive man with normal renin and high *prolactin* levels, both the prolactin level and hypertension responded to the dopaminergic agonist bromocriptine.

Sodium intake. The role of dietary sodium in the genesis of hypertension is unclear. Epidemiologic data have demonstrated a positive correlation between blood pressure and sodium intake. In general, the higher the sodium intake in a given population, the greater the prevalence of hypertension in those with a tendency toward hypertension.

Genetic factors. Essential hypertension is a familial disorder determined by both genetic and environmental factors. A person with essential hypertension inherits an aggregate of multiple genes determining hypertension and is exposed to environmental factors that favor hypertension.

Rare forms of familial and probably genetically determined secondary hypertension are hereditary nephritis, familial multiple endocrine adenomatosis type II (pheochromocytoma, hyperparathyroidism, and medullary carcinoma of the thyroid), and familial fibromuscular hyperplasia of the renal arteries.

CLASSIFICATION

Primary hypertension. Hypertension is called *primary* (essential) if the cause is unknown.

Secondary hypertension. Hypertension may be caused by many defined factors, including the following:

Renal parenchymal disease
    Glomerulonephritis
    Pyelonephritis
    Hydronephrosis
    Polycystic kidney
    Tumors (Wilms', renin-producing)
    Anephric hypervolemia
    After renal transplant
Renal artery disease
    Atherosclerosis
    Fibromuscular hyperplasia
    Aneurysm
    Arteritis
    Embolism
    External compression resulting from mass
Endocrine and metabolic disease
    Pheochromocytoma
    Cushing's syndrome
    Primary aldosteronism
    Adrenogenital syndrome
    Neuroblastoma (in children)
    Acromegaly
    Hypercalcemia
    Acute prophyria
Neurologic, vascular, and other abnormalities
    Coarctation of the aorta
    Increased intracranial pressure
    Neurogenic or psychogenic causes
    Autonomic hyperactivity (for example, mitral valve prolapse)
    Diet and drugs (licorice [causing pseudoaldosteronism], tyramine, alcohol, corticosteroids, oral contraceptives, thyroxine, sympathomimetic agents)

Many etiologic factors are as yet undiscovered.

Accelerated (malignant) hypertension. A patient with very high blood pressure (such as a diastolic pressure greater than 120 mm Hg) is diagnosed as having *accelerated (malignant) hypertension* when the elevated pressure is accompanied by one or more of the following clinical manifestations:

1. *Acute hypertensive retinopathy.* This includes fundal hemorrhages, exudates, or papilledema.
2. *Malignant nephrosclerosis.* This is manifested by unexplained hematuria and proteinuria that clear with the control of blood pressure. In later stages creatinine clearance may be markedly reduced and improvement of renal function with blood pressure control may be only partial. Histologic examination shows intimal hyperplasia and medial hypertrophy of renal arterioles, sometimes with fibrinoid necrosis.
3. *Hypertensive encephalopathy.* This is characterized by diffuse cerebral dysfunction with increasing headache, drowsiness, confusion, convulsions, or coma. Hypertensive encephalopathy must be distinguished from uremic encephalopathy and cerebrovascular accident. The diagnosis is confirmed if there is rapid improvement in the mental state with control of blood pressure.

CLINICAL MANIFESTATIONS

Medical history. Evaluation of the hypertensive patient should include the severity of the hypertension and the presence and extent of target organ damage, a search for curable forms of hypertension, and information concerning other risk factors for cerebrovascular accident and coronary artery disease. The medical history should include a determination of the onset, duration, and progression of high blood pressure and its treatment; symptoms suggesting a secondary cause; symptoms suggesting cardiac, renal, central nervous system, and eye complications; the use of oral contraceptives or other drugs such as corticosteroids or amphetamines; cardiovascular risk factors (smoking, hyperlipidemia, diabetes); a dietary history (salt intake); and a family history of hypertension and its complications, polycystic kidney and familial multiple endocrine adenomatosis type II (pheochromocytoma, medullary carcinoma of the thyroid, and hyperparathyroidism).

Initially most patients with mild to moderate hypertension are asymptomatic. Once high blood pressure is detected, vague symptoms of headache, dizziness, easy fatigability, vertigo, and palpitations develop in a large number of patients. These symptoms may be functional in origin. With severe hypertension, a throbbing suboccipital headache may be present when the patient awakens in the morning, but it disappears spontaneously after several hours. Epistaxis is common in severe hypertension.

A severe and abrupt onset of hypertension before the age of 35 or after the age of 50 probably has a secondary cause. A history of repeated urinary tract infections or proteinuria suggests *renal parenchymal* disease. Hematuria, previous renal trauma, acute flank pain, or abrupt onset of hypertension resistant to medical therapy suggests *renovascular* hypertension. A recent weight loss and intermittent or continuous hypertension associated with paroxysms of head pain, pallor, palpitations, perspiration, anxiety, or tremors precipitated by a change in posture, an intravenous pyelogram, or anesthesia suggest *pheochromocytoma.* Muscle weakness, polyuria, nocturia, polydipsia, tetany, and paresthesias suggest *aldosteronism.*

Cardiac failure is manifested by progressive or paroxysmal dyspnea and can occur after years of mild or moderate hypertension and sooner or even abruptly with severe hypertension. Minor manifestations of central nervous system involvement are headache, dizziness, and vertigo. Patients with major manifestations (hypertensive encephalopathy or cerebrovascular accident) may have severe headache, nausea, vomiting, somnolence, coma, confusion, convulsions, transient paresis, paresthesia, blurred vision, slurred speech, or permanent neurologic deficits. Progressive or sudden loss of vision and field defects occur frequently. Renal involvement occurs late in mild to moderate hypertension. In accelerated or malignant hypertension, renal manifestations such as hematuria may occur early; renal failure and uremia may follow rapidly. The most common cause of death in malignant hypertension is renal failure. Chest pain may be due to myocardial infarction or aortic dissection. Intermittent claudication may be present owing to peripheral vascular disease.

Physical examination. Aside from the blood pressure, the physical examination may initially be entirely normal. Two or more blood pressure readings should be taken (at least one while the patient is standing). Areas to be examined with special attention are the neck for thyroid enlargement, carotid pulsations, bruits, and jugular venous pressure; extremities for peripheral pulses, pedal edema, and femoral delay as compared to radial pulsation; heart for tachycardia, apical heaves, gallops, murmurs, and arrhythmia; lungs for rales; abdomen for bruits, polycystic kidney, and liver enlargement and tenderness; nervous system for neurologic deficits; and fundus for arteriovenous nicking, hemorrhage, exudates, and papilledema.

Examination of the optic fundi is a more reliable index to the severity and prognosis of hypertension than casual blood pressure readings. Unless contraindicated, pupils should be dilated. Retinal changes are graded as follows: grade I, minimal arteriolar narrowing or irregularity; grade II, more marked arteriolar narrowing and irregularity with focal tortuosity or spasm; grade III, very marked arteriolar narrowing and irregularity, with generalized tortuosity, flame-shaped hemorrhages, and cotton wool exudates; grade IV, changes of grade III plus papilledema. Hemorrhages, exudates, and papilledema (grades III and IV) indicate very severe or accelerated (malignant) hypertension. An increased arteriolar light reflex manifested by silver or copper wire changes and arteriovenous nicking or compression is due to arteriosclerosis and correlates with the duration of hypertension.

Young individuals with labile hypertension may have sinus tachycardia, a normal-sized heart with a rapid tapping apical impulse, and a systolic flow murmur along the left sternal border, all indicating a *hyperdynamic circulation*. With long-standing hypertension, there may be a sustained apical lift (ventricular heave), indicating left ventricular hypertrophy, and a visible, palpable presystolic apical impulse and audible fourth heart sound, suggesting diminished left ventricular compliance. There may be an ejection click and systolic murmur along the left sternal border radiating to the neck. An early diastolic blowing murmur caused by a dilated aortic ring may sometimes be audible at the right second intercostal space and left sternal border (usually disappearing after successful treatment of long-standing severe hypertension). Ultimately, hypertensive heart disease leads to *left ventricular failure* (third heart sound, basal rales, or pulmonary edema), *right-sided heart failure* (tender enlarged liver, raised jugular venous pressure, pedal edema), and arrhythmias (atrial fibrillation, ventricular ectopy).

A systolic-diastolic bruit in the epigastrium or flanks usually reflects atherosclerotic disease and may be associated with *renal artery stenosis* in a hypertensive patient. Large, easily palpable kidneys raise the possibility of *polycystic kidneys*. An abdominal aortic aneurysm may be palpable as an atherosclerotic complication of hypertension. Truncal obesity, moon facies, cervicodorsal hump, striae, cutaneous atrophy, and ecchymosis suggest *Cushing's syndrome*. A thin, anxious young adult with excessive sweating, flushed face, tachycardia, and paroxysmal hypertension may have *pheochromocytoma*.

LABORATORY FINDINGS. Recommended laboratory studies to be performed on *all* hypertensive patients are described in Table 87-1. Special investigations are used to identify curable causes of hypertension when there is clinical suspicion or when suggested by routine investigations. These are discussed in the following paragraphs in terms of the specific causes.

Renal artery stenosis. Other than drugs, renal artery stenosis is probably the most common curable cause of hypertension. One or more of the following investigations are performed in patients with suspected renal artery stenosis: rapid-sequence intravenous pyelogram (IVP); renal flow and scan; peripheral plasma renin determination; differential renal vein plasma renin levels (a > 1.5:1 ratio indicates renal artery stenosis on the high side); and arteriography to display the lesion. Chapter 119 gives a description of the tests and their interpretation.

Primary aldosteronism (Conn's syndrome). The hypertension in primary aldosteronism tends to be mild. It is associated with hyperglycemia, hypokalemia, and alkalosis. Evaluation for this condition should be undertaken only if the patient is hypokalemic before diuretic therapy or if diuretic therapy provokes hypokalemia that is severe or poorly responsive to the cessation of diuretics. The diagnosis is suggested by high aldosterone production in the presence of low plasma renin activity. If screening tests are positive, further studies such as adrenal scintiscan, differential adrenal vein aldosterone levels, and adrenal arteriography should be considered. Aldosteronism is not a common cause of hypertension, and if screening tests are negative, further studies can result in unnecessary morbidity and cost. Chapter 188 gives a detailed description of laboratory tests and their interpretation.

Cushing's syndrome. In Cushing's syndrome 24-hour urinary free cortisol excretion is high. Morning and evening plasma cortisol levels demonstrate a lack of diurnal

Table 87-1. Recommended laboratory investigations for all hypertensive patients

Investigations	Purpose
Urinalysis including microscopic examination	To evaluate for renal parenchymal disease such as polycystic kidney, glomerulonephritis, or chronic pyelonephritis
Hematocrit	Decreased in renal insufficiency
Serum potassium	As a baseline before diuretic therapy; increased in renal failure; decreased in primary aldosteronism and with diuretics
Serum creatinine and/or blood urea nitrogen	Increased in renal parenchymal disease
Serum cholesterol and triglycerides	To evaluate and control hyperlipidemia, one of the major risk factors for atherosclerosis
Serum glucose, fasting and/or postprandial	To evaluate for diabetes mellitus
Serum uric acid	As a baseline before diuretic therapy, which may increase the serum uric acid level and rarely precipitate gout or nephropathy
Serum calcium	As a baseline before diuretic therapy, which may increase serum calcium levels, and to rule out primary hyperparathyroidism, which is more common in hypertensive patients than in the general population
Electrocardiogram	To detect left ventricular hypertrophy and coronary heart disease
Chest roentgenogram	To evaluate for left ventricular failure and aortic atherosclerosis

variation. The low-dose dexamethasone suppression test is the screening test of choice (see Chapter 188).

Pheochromocytoma. Pheochromocytoma is a catecholamine-producing tumor of chromaffin tissue. The majority of these tumors are found in the adrenal medulla. Pheochromocytoma is a rare cause of hypertension and can be suspected from the history and physical examination. The diagnosis is confirmed by the detection of excess catecholamine production. Reliable results can be obtained from urine specimens analyzed for metanephrine and normetanephrine, with the results expressed as micrograms per milligram of creatinine. Drugs such as chlorpromazine can cause false positive results. New procedures for determining plasma norepinephrine levels may supplant urinary tests (see Chapter 189).

Renal parenchymal diseases. Renal parenchymal diseases are detected by 24-hour urinary protein and electrolyte determinations, creatinine clearance, microscopic examination of urinary sediment, and urine culture and sensitivity.

MANAGEMENT. Major emphasis should be placed on early detection and adequate treatment of hypertension rather than on extensive diagnostic workup to rule out secondary causes. The patient should be gradually educated to the serious and lifelong nature of hypertension and made aware of the advantages of continuous treatment in preventing future complications. Attempts should be made to identify potential barriers to compliance.

The efficacy of various "general measures" in reducing arterial blood pressure is a matter of controversy, but some have distinct roles in reducing cardiovascular morbidity and mortality. Severe sodium restriction (less than 500 mg/day) lowers blood pressure, but this is highly impractical. Modest sodium restriction, however, enhances the action of most antihypertensive drugs (diuretics, sympatholytics, and vasodilators), which evoke a compensatory response of sodium and fluid retention and plasma volume expansion. The usual recommendations are (1) to omit table salt or salt in cooking; (2) to avoid salted foods such as peanuts, potato chips, and hot dogs; and (3) to limit the consumption of canned, processed, frozen, or prepared foods.

Obese hypertensive patients have a higher incidence of cardiovascular morbidity and mortality than nonobese hypertensive subjects. Caloric restriction is advised in obese individuals to reduce the risk of diabetes mellitus, hyperlipidemia, and probably coronary artery disease. Weight loss may rarely reduce arterial blood pressure but often improves the general health of patients.

Elimination of stressful events, frequent vacations, psychotherapy, transcendental meditation, yoga, biofeedback, and use of tranquilizers or sedatives are various methods for reducing stress. However, there is no strong evidence that these methods reduce arterial blood pressure or its complications other than by placebo effect. Some studies indicate that individuals who lead a sedentary life have a higher risk of heart attack than those who exercise regularly. Regular moderate isotonic physical activity is encouraged as a good health measure and may decrease peripheral vascular resistance. Irregular excessive exercise (particularly isometrics) is undesirable, especially in the presence of uncontrolled hypertension.

Aim of antihypertensive therapy. The aim of treatment is to achieve a normal (<140/90 mm Hg) or nearly normal blood pressure. Individuals with a diastolic blood pressure of 105 mm Hg or higher on three separate occasions need antihypertensive drug therapy. Patients with a diastolic pressure of 130 mm Hg or more should preferably be hospitalized for initial aggressive parenteral therapy.

There is some difference of opinion regarding the treatment of patients with diastolic pressure from 90 to 104 mm Hg. In this group the risk factors that may favor the decision to start drug therapy are young age, male sex, black race, family history of complications of hypertension, diabetes mellitus, or target organ damage.

Antihypertensive agents. Antihypertensive drugs can be classified into the following groups: diuretics, adrenergic inhibitors (sympatholytics), and vasodilators.

Diuretics. Diuretics (especially thiazides) are the most commonly used agents in the treatment of hypertension and are considered the drugs of first choice by most physicians. These agents can be divided into thiazides and their derivatives, loop diuretics, and potassium-sparing diuretics. Commonly used thiazides are *chlorothiazide, hydrochlorothiazide,* and *bendroflumethiazide.* Derivatives are *chlorthalidone* and *metolazone.* They are taken only once or twice daily.

Thiazides decrease extracellular (plasma and interstitial) fluid volume and cardiac output. These agents promote sodium and water excretion by inhibiting sodium reabsorption at the distal convoluted tubules. With prolonged use, they decrease systemic vascular resistance by changing the ionic composition (decreasing the sodium content) of vascular smooth muscle and thereby alter the responsiveness to naturally occurring neural stimuli. They potentiate the effect of other antihypertensive agents. The major antihypertensive effect of the thiazides is through their diuretic action, which decreases intravascular volume.

Periodic serum potassium determinations should be performed. Dietary supplements can usually prevent hypokalemia; however, if hypokalemia develops, dietary therapy is usually insufficient to correct it. Therefore potassium supplements or potassium-sparing diuretics along with thiazides are usually advised when serum potassium is low or the patient is receiving digitalis therapy. Thiazide-induced hyperuricemia does not require treatment in asymptomatic individuals. With marked hyperuricemia or a history of gout, uricosuric agents (probenecid) or xanthine oxidase inhibitors (allopurinol) can be used. Thiazide-induced hyperglycemia is usually mild. It occurs mainly in individuals susceptible to diabetes mellitus. Weight reduction and dietary control are adequate to control the hyperglycemia in most patients. In those receiving insulin the dose must occasionally be altered. Mild hypercalcemia may result from the increased calcium reabsorption accompanying the sodium reabsorption in the proximal tubule induced by hypovolemia. Hypercalcemia may also be caused by potentiation of the renal action of parathyroid hormone by thiazides.

The loop diuretics *furosemide* and *ethacrynic acid* inhibit sodium chloride reabsorption in the ascending limb of the loop of Henle and impair urinary concentrating ability. These agents have a more abrupt and briefer diuretic effect but a weaker antihypertensive effect than thiazides, and they are not used routinely in the treatment of hypertension. They are usually recommended for hypertensive emergencies such as hypertensive heart failure when immediate effect is needed, for patients allergic to thiazides, and for patients with renal insufficiency.

Potassium-sparing diuretics include *spironolactone, triamterene,* and *amiloride.* Spironolactone is a competitive inhibitor of aldosterone in the distal tubule, whereas triamterene and amiloride independently interfere with sodium-potassium exchange. These are weak diuretics used mainly as adjuncts to thiazide therapy to prevent marked hypokalemia. They are the drugs of choice for primary aldosteronism. They should not be used for patients with compromised renal function or given with potassium supplements.

Adrenergic inhibitors. Table 87-2 lists important adrenergic inhibiting agents with their sites of action, dosages, and side effects.

The antihypertensive action of *propranolol* has several mechanisms including β-adrenergic receptor blockade, decreased cardiac output, inhibition of renin release by the kidney, and elimination of sympathetic nerve outflow from the vasomotor center in the brain. Initially it was suggested that propranolol may be more beneficial in hypertensive patients with a hyperkinetic circulation or with increased plasma renin or pheochromocytoma. However, propranolol has been used successfully in hypertensive patients regardless of the level of plasma renin activity. Propranolol is usually administered in combination with other drugs, particularly a thiazide diuretic. It is not indicated for treatment of hypertensive emergencies.

Metoprolol is a cardioselective β_1-adrenergic receptor blocking drug used in a manner similar to propranolol. It has relatively less β-adrenergic blocking effect on bronchi, which are β_2-adrenergic sites.

Nadolol is a nonselective β-adrenergic blocking agent, and *atenolol* is a cardioselective β-adrenergic blocker. Both of these drugs can be administered once daily.

Methyldopa has a moderate antihypertensive effect that is potentiated when it is used with a diuretic. It acts as a false neurohumoral transmitter both centrally (on the hypothalamus) and peripherally (on nerve endings). It also inhibits renin release and decreases renal vascular resistance. Methyldopa tends to maintain renal blood flow in spite of the fall in blood pressure. The direct Coombs' test is positive in 10% to 20% of the patients taking methyldopa, but hemolytic anemia rarely occurs.

Guanethidine blocks peripheral sympathetic nerve terminals and is effective only when the patient is in an upright position. It is one of the most potent antihypertensive agents available for oral administration and should be employed only for severe hypertension because of its unpleasant side effects. It should always be used in combination with diuretics. Amphetamines, chlorpromazine, and tricyclic antidepressants interfere with the antihypertensive action of guanethidine. The advantages of this agent include high potency and absence of central nervous system symptoms, since it does not cross the blood-brain barrier.

Clonidine is a centrally acting stimulator of α-adren-

Table 87-2. Adrenergic inhibitors

Drug	Site of action	Average dose	Side effects
Propranolol	β-Adrenergic receptor blockade	PO 10-80 mg or higher b.i.d. to q.i.d.	Bradycardia, cardiac failure, aggravation of bronchial asthma or peripheral ischemia, masking of hypoglycemia, hallucinosis, sodium retention, Raynaud's phenomenon, weakness, depression
Metoprolol	β-Adrenergic receptor blockade	PO 50-200 mg daily or b.i.d.	Same as above but perhaps less bronchospasm
Methyldopa	Central; peripheral (nerve endings)	PO up to 2 g/day b.i.d., t.i.d., or q.i.d.; IV 250-500 mg every 4-6 hr	Orthostatic hypotension, drowsiness, depression, dry mouth, nasal congestion, impotence, hepatitis, gynecomastia, lactation, positive Coombs' test in 10%-20% but rarely hemolysis
Guanethidine	Peripheral (nerve endings)	PO 5-200 mg/day	Orthostatic hypotension (especially in morning), weakness, diarrhea, bradycardia, impaired ejaculation
Clonidine	Central	PO 0.1-1.2 mg b.i.d.	Dry mouth, drowsiness, impotence, orthostatic hypotension, rebound hypertension when stopped suddenly, hallucinations
Phentolamine	α-Adrenergic receptor blockade; direct vasodilation	IV 1-5 mg (or more) intermittently	Tachycardia, flushing, dizziness
Phenoxybenzamine	α-Adrenergic receptor blockade	PO 10-50 mg daily or b.i.d.	Orthostatic hypotension, tachycardia, nasal congestion, miosis, difficulty in ejaculation
Reserpine	Central; peripheral (nerve endings)	PO 0.1-0.5 mg daily	Drowsiness, sedation, lassitude, nasal congestion, depression, nightmares, gastric hyperacidity, bradycardia, parkinsonian rigidity
Trimethaphan	Peripheral (sympathetic and parasympathetic ganglia)	IV 1-10 mg/min	Orthostatic hypotension, dry mouth, urinary retention, constipation, impotence, visual symptoms

ergic inhibitory fibers. This agent is similar in potency to methyldopa. It is used with a diuretic.

Reserpine is now infrequently used because of its many side effects. *Phentolamine* and *trimethaphan* are used for rapid lowering of blood pressure in emergency situations.

Vasodilators. Hydralazine reduces the blood pressure by dilating arterioles and thereby reducing outflow resistance. It can be used orally or parenterally in conjunction with diuretics and other antihypertensives, particularly β-adrenergic blockers. The side effects of hydralazine are tachycardia, palpitations, severe headache, and angina pectoris. These can be counteracted by prior treatment with propranolol, methyldopa, or reserpine. Systemic lupus erythematosus–like syndromes may occur with large doses of hydralazine. This side effect is usually temporary, does not affect the kidneys, and disappears on withdrawal of medication.

Prazosin is a postsynaptic α-adrenergic blocking agent that dilates arterioles by its smooth muscle–relaxing effect. It is administered orally. The initial dose should be small and is given at bedtime or with the patient recumbent to prevent dramatic hypotension and syncope. After the first dose prazosin can be slowly increased. Side effects include tachycardia, headache, and postural hypotension.

Minoxidil, a newly approved vasodilator, is the most potent oral antihypertensive available. Side effects include tachycardia, for which a β-adrenergic blocker is given concomitantly; sodium retention, for which large doses of diuretics are prescribed; facial hirsutism; and pericardial effusion. The last is most likely to occur in patients with renal insufficiency.

Diazoxide is a nondiuretic benzothiadiazine derivative indicated for the rapid reduction of blood pressure in hypertensive emergencies. Diazoxide is administered by rapid intravenous injection. The maximal antihypertensive effect occurs within 30 seconds. Side effects include sodium and water retention (so a diuretic is usually also administered), hyperglycemia, hyperuricemia, tachycardia, angina pectoris, decrease in uterine contractions, and pain with extravasation into tissues.

Sodium nitroprusside is also used only intravenously. It directly relaxes arteriolar and venular smooth muscle, with reduction in peripheral vascular resistance and blood pressure. The hemodynamic response to infusion occurs within minutes. Nitroprusside is used in hypertensive emergencies or in hypertension associated with acute left ventricular failure. Side effects include thiocyanate and cyanide poisoning (with prolonged administration or renal failure), intrapulmonic ventilation-perfusion mismatch, and decreased platelet aggregation.

Captopril is an angiotensin converting enzyme inhibitor usually used in combination with a diuretic. Serious adverse effects such as neutropenia, agranulocytosis, renal failure, and marked hypotension limit the use of captopril to hypertensive patients resistant to other drugs. It causes hyperkalemia.

A graduated care program is generally recommended, with each drug added in sequence until control of hypertension is achieved. A new agent is added only after the previous drug or drugs have been given an adequate trial.

Step 1—Start a diuretic (usually a thiazide).

Step 2—Add an adrenergic blocker: propranolol, metoprolol, nadolol, methyldopa, clonidine, prazosin, or reserpine.

Step 3—Add a vasodilator: hydralazine or prazosin if not previously used. Minoxidil is reserved for severely hypertensive patients with inadequate response to other drugs or with renal insufficiency.

Step 4—Add or substitute guanethidine for the step 2 agent.

To obtain good compliance, one or two daily doses are superior to more frequent dosage. Initially the patient should be followed at weekly intervals until the blood pressure is under adequate control. Later the patient can be seen at 3- to 6-month intervals to ensure blood pressure control. A complete physical examination, serum potassium study, BUN (or creatinine) determination, urinalysis, electrocardiogram, and chest roentgenogram should be performed every year to detect the complications of hypertension.

Treatment of hypertensive emergencies. Hypertensive emergencies include the following:
1. Hypertensive encephalopathy caused by essential hypertension, renal disease, renal vascular disease, and toxemia of pregnancy
2. Uncontrolled hypertension resulting from malignant hypertension, pheochromocytoma, head injuries, severe burns, cessation of antihypertensives (rebound hypertension), and ingestion of catecholamine precursors in patients taking monoamine oxidase inhibitors
3. Severe to moderate hypertension associated with acute left ventricular failure, cerebrovascular hemorrhage, or a dissecting aortic aneurysm

Patients with hypertensive emergencies should be hospitalized for immediate and intensive care. Parenteral antihypertensive drugs such as diazoxide or nitroprusside can usually control blood pressure within minutes. When blood pressure is adequately controlled and clinical manifestations such as hypertensive encephalopathy improve, oral agents can be started. Parenterally administered nitroglycerin may be preferable to nitroprusside or diazoxide in a hypertensive patient with acute myocardial infarction and left ventricular failure.

Treatment of secondary hypertension

Renovascular hypertension (see Chapter 119). A young patient with severe hypertension of recent onset, clear evidence of unilateral renal artery stenosis owing to *fibromuscular hyperplasia,* and an abnormal differential renal vein renin ratio comparing blood from one renal vein with blood from the other (>1.5:1) usually should have surgical repair. Nearly 75% of such patients have normal blood pressure after surgery. Surgical repair of *atherosclerotic renovascular disease* is comparatively less successful.

Primary aldosteronism (see Chapter 188). Administration of spironolactone usually controls the blood pressure in *primary aldosteronism*. An adrenocortical adenoma accounts for more than 85% of the cases. Surgical removal of the adenoma and affected gland is performed when possible. Adrenal hyperplasia is a second common cause of this syndrome, but surgical treatment of adrenal hyperplasia is controversial. Carcinoma of the adrenal gland causing pure primary aldosteronism is very rare.

Cushing's syndrome (see Chapter 188). Adrenal hyperplasia owing to a pituitary disorder is the most common cause of *Cushing's syndrome* (nearly 60% of cases). Ectopic corticotropin-producing tumors (such as tumor of the lung, pancreas, or thymus gland) and adrenal neoplasms (benign or malignant) are other important causes. Cushing's syndrome is treated with surgery, irradiation, and/or chemotherapy, depending on the underlying cause.

Pheochromocytoma (see Chapter 189). Hypertensive patients with pheochromocytoma are treated preoperatively with prazosin alone or phentolamine or phenoxybenzamine in combination with propranolol. Surgical removal of the tumor is the treatment of choice. During surgery marked hypertension can develop, so a phentolamine infusion should be available. Immediately after removal of the tumor there may be marked hypotension requiring rapid volume expansion and norepinephrine. Nonoperable tumors can be treated with alpha-methyl-para-tyrosine.

Patients with *coarctation of the aorta* should be identified and have surgery performed early in life. If surgery is delayed until late adult life, persistent hypertension and its complications are frequent.

Vasculitis (see Chapter 20). *Polyarteritis nodosa* and *systemic lupus erythematosus* cause hypertension and are treated with corticosteroids, cytotoxic agents, and antihypertensive agents as necessary.

Hypertension, usually gradual (weeks to months) in onset, develops in some individuals receiving *oral contraceptive agents*. The incidence of a positive family history or of preeclampsia-eclampsia is high in such individuals. They usually have high plasma renin activity. The treatment is discontinuation of the oral contraceptive.

Treatment of complications of established hypertension. Severely elevated blood pressure in a patient with intracerebral hemorrhage should perhaps be only partially controlled during the first several days. The Clinical Management Study Group recommends 20% to 30% lowering of systolic pressure if it is more than 200 mm Hg. If hypertension is less severe, the goal should be 160/100 mm Hg.

Long-standing hypertension can cause left ventricular hypertrophy and left ventricular failure. Reduction of blood pressure will benefit left ventricular pump failure.

The use of thiazides should be avoided in hypertensive patients with renal insufficiency because these agents decrease the glomerular filtration rate and diuretic action is lost at a low filtration rate (<20 ml/min). Loop diuretics are still effective in such situations. Potassium-sparing drugs should be avoided because of the danger of hyperkalemia. Guanethidine and propranolol are contraindicated because they may worsen the azotemia. Methyldopa, clonidine, and vasodilators (hydralazine, prazosin, and minoxidil) maintain renal blood flow and can be used if necessary.

Hypertensive patients with end-stage renal failure are managed with dialysis (to remove salt and water) alone or in combination with vasodilators such as hydralazine or sympathetic blocking drugs such as propranolol, methyldopa, or clonidine.

Until recently the practice has been to stop antihypertensive medications long before elective surgery. In general the benefit of control outweighs the risk of anesthesia in the patient receiving antihypertensives, and they should be continued up to the time of surgery. Abrupt withdrawal of propranolol and clonidine may precipitate myocardial infarction and accelerated hypertension, respectively. Propranolol and clonidine may be given with a sip of water even on the day of surgery.

Compliance. Poor compliance is a major problem in the treatment of most hypertensive patients. On every follow-up visit a physician, nurse-practitioner, or physician's aide should reemphasize the importance of continuous treatment. Drug regimens should be as simple and convenient as possible (for example, one or two daily doses) to achieve good compliance. Trial of different drugs to eliminate side effects may further ensure cooperation. Measurement of blood pressure at home and keeping medication records by the patient may improve compliance. The attitude of physicians and other personnel is an important determinant of the patient's acceptance of long-term therapy.

BIBLIOGRAPHY

Biglieri, E.G., and Lopez, J.M.: Clinical and laboratory diagnosis of adrenocortical hypertension, Cardiovasc. Med. **1**:335, 1976.

Bookstein, J.J., and others: Cooperative study of radiologic aspects of renovascular hypertension: bilateral renovascular disease, J.A.M.A. **237**:1706, 1977.

Bumpus, F.M., and Khosla, M.C.: Pathogenic factors involved in renovascular hypertension, Mayo Clin. Proc. **52**:417, 1977.

Dustan, H.P.: Evaluation and therapy of hypertension—1976, Mod. Concepts Cardiovasc. Dis. **45**:97, 1976.

Foster, J.H., and others: Renovascular occlusive diseases: results of operative treatment, J.A.M.A. **231**:1043, 1975.

Frohlich, E.D.: Newer concepts of antihypertensive drugs, Prog. Cardiovasc. Dis. **20**:385, 1978.

Genest, J., Koiw, E., and Kuchel, O., editors: Hypertension: physiopathology and treatment, New York, 1977, McGraw-Hill Book Co.

Kannel, W.B., McGee, D., and Gordon, T.: A general cardiovascular risk profile: the Framingham study, Am. J. Cardiol. **38**:46, 1976.

Koch-Weser, J.: Correlation of pathophysiology and pharmacotherapy in primary hypertension, Am. J. Cardiol. **32**:499, 1973.

Laragh, J.H.: Vasoconstrictor-volume analysis for understanding and treating hypertension: the use of renin and aldosterone profiles, Am. J. Med. **55**:261, 1973.

Low, J., and Oparil, S.: Oral contraceptive pill hypertension, J. Reprod. Med. **15**:201, 1975.

Messerli, F.H., and others: Mineralocorticoid secretion in essential hypertension with normal and low plasma renin activity, Circulation **53**:406, 1976.

Messerli, F.H., and others: Systemic and regional hemodynamics in low, normal and high cardiac output borderline hypertension, Circulation **58**:441, 1978.

The 1980 report of the Joint National Committee on Detection, Evaluation and Treatment of High Blood Pressure, Arch. Intern. Med. **140**:1280, 1980.

Steptoe, A.: Psychological methods in treatment of hypertension: a review, Br. Heart J. **39**:587, 1977.

Stumpe, K.O., and others: Hyperprolactinemia and antihypertensive effect of bromocriptine in essential hypertension, Lancet **2**:211, 1977.

Tarazi, R.C., Dustan, H.P., and Frohlich, E.E.: Long term thiazide therapy in essential hypertension, Circulation **41**:709, 1970.

Veterans Administration Cooperative Study Group on Antihypertensive Agents: Effects of treatment on morbidity in hypertension. I. Results in patients with diastolic blood pressures averaging 115 through 129 mm Hg, J.A.M.A. **202**:1028, 1967.

Veterans Administration Cooperative Study Group on Antihypertensive Agents: Effects of treatment on morbidity in hypertension. II. Results in patients with diastolic blood pressures averaging 90 through 114 mm Hg, J.A.M.A. **213**:1143, 1970.

88 • SHOCK

Carl V. Leier

Shock is an extreme state of circulatory failure in which inadequate perfusion of tissues by blood is the predominant pathophysiologic feature. Impaired tissue perfusion leads to general cellular dysfunction and cell death. The patient prototype, "a patient in shock," is a lethargic or somnolent individual with profound weakness (inability to stand) and cool, pale skin. The hands are often cold and moist ("clammy"). The pulse is weak (diminished amplitude) and rapid. Indirect (sphygmomanometer) blood pressure measurements are unobtainable or very low. Renal dysfunction with a reduction in urine output develops early. If proper therapy is not initiated or if the therapeutic interventions fail, this circulatory collapse state will deteriorate further and cell death will occur; the loss of tissue and cellular viability heralds a state of "irreversible shock" and death of the individual.

CLASSIFICATION. Extreme circulatory failure and shock can be caused by any or a combination of the three major mechanisms outlined below:

I. Reduction in intravascular volume (hypovolemic or cold shock)
   A. Loss of blood volume—hemorrhage
      1. External loss such as gastrointestinal bleeding, trauma
      2. Internal sequestration such as hemothorax, hemoperitoneum, fractures
   B. Loss of plasma volume
      1. Severe burns, exudative lesions
      2. Dehydration caused by vomiting, diarrhea, diabetic ketoacidosis, insensible water loss without replacement, adrenal insufficiency, diabetes insipidus
II. Increased vascular capacitance (warm shock)
   A. Drugs such as anesthetics and antihypertensive agents; overdosage of tranquilizers or sedatives
   B. Toxins and humoral substances such as endotoxin (gram-negative bacillary bacteremia), immune-mediated substances released during anaphylaxis
   C. Neurogenic disorders such as vasodepressor syncope ("faint"), orthostatic hypotension, acute spinal cord injury
III. Failure of the heart as a pump (congestive shock)
   A. Inadequate filling of cardiac chambers as in pericardial tamponade, tension pneumothorax
   B. Inadequate emptying of the ventricles as in myocardial infarction with failure, ruptured papillary muscle, dysrhythmias
   C. Combined inadequate filling and emptying, as from pulmonary embolus and intracardiac tumors

Shock caused by severe reduction in intravascular volume is generally referred to as "hypovolemic shock" because of the low intravascular volume or "cold shock" because of the marked compensatory vasoconstriction with resultant cold extremities. The causes of this form of circulatory shock are related to either the excessive loss of blood or, less commonly, the excessive loss of plasma volume (rate of loss exceeding rate of replacement). The more common causes of acute and excessive blood loss are trauma with disruption of the wall of an artery or large vein or damage to a heavily vascularized structure such as the spleen, lung, liver, or kidney; gastrointestinal disorders such as peptic ulcer disease with erosion of the ulcer into an artery, ruptured esophageal varices in a patient with cirrhosis of the liver and portal hypertension, or hemorrhage from ulcerative colitis; defective mechanisms of blood clotting as seen in leukemia, hemophilia, and thrombocytopenia; and structural defects of the vascular system, exemplified by hereditary hemorrhagic telangiectasia with uncontrolled bleeding from the telangiectasia (nose, gastrointestinal, or lung), rupture of a saccular aneurysm of the aorta or artery, or dissecting aneurysm of the aorta. The more common causes of excessive loss of plasma volume include severe burns, pancreatitis, and peritonitis, with seepage of extracellular fluid (water, electrolytes, and proteins) from the burn or inflamed site. Situations that may lead to severe dehydration and hypovolemia include excessive vomiting or diarrhea, diabetic ketoacidosis (osmotic diuresis of water and electrolytes), inadequate intake of fluids, and untreated adrenal insufficiency, since lack of aldosterone effects a renal loss of water and electrolytes.

The severity of hypovolemic shock is generally related to the amount and rate of loss of the intravascular volume and the responsiveness of the individual's compensatory mechanisms to the sudden or excessive loss of volume. The acute loss of 25% or more of the intravascular volume is required to put a normal subject into circulatory shock; exsanguination in excess of this amount will usually overwhelm the compensatory mechanisms and result in severe hypotension and inadequate tissue perfusion. Loss of the same volume over several days would generally not produce circulatory shock because the compensatory mechanisms would be capable of maintaining an adequate intravascular volume and perfusion pressure. The compensatory mechanisms of circulatory shock will be discussed in the next section of this chapter.

An increase in total vascular capacitance without a change in intravascular volume will produce hypotension and, if severe, circulatory shock. In contrast to the vasoconstricted cold extremities of hypovolemic shock, the extremities in this form of shock are usually warm as a result of generalized vasodilation; the term "warm shock" has been applied to this type of circulatory collapse. The excessive dilation of the vasculature may be caused by any of several factors: drugs—through a primary effect (such as that of antihypertensive drugs), an overdosage, or an idiosyncratic reaction; toxins such as endotoxin produced in certain bacterial infections and responsible for bacteremic or septic shock; humoral substances, examplified by the immune-mediated substances released during an anaphylactic reaction to a drug such as penicillin or lidocaine, insect stings, or food allergies; and abnormalities in neurologic control of the vascular system such as spinal cord injury.

Shock resulting from failure of the heart as a pump may be referred to as "congestive shock" because an elevated venous pressure (systemic and/or pulmonary) is an accompanying feature. Failure of the heart's pumping mechanism may result from inadequate filling or emptying of the ventricles. The prototype for inadequate ventricular filling is pericardial tamponade, in which the pericardial space is filled by fluid or blood under high pressure, preventing adequate filling of the ventricular and atrial chambers by blood. The resultant stroke volume is small, and hypotension with poor tissue perfusion occurs. Failure of the heart to empty adequately or eject enough blood to maintain tissue perfusion is generally referred to as "cardiogenic shock." The most common cause is myocardial infarction. Cardiogenic shock resulting from myocardial infarction has a mortality rate of greater than 60%. Acute valvular insufficiency, such as that caused by rupture of a left ventricular papillary muscle, may lead to shock on the basis of inadequate ejection of blood into the aorta; most of the blood is diverted into the left atrial chamber because of its lower resistance. Certain cardiac dysrhythmias, such as ventricular tachycardia or rapid supraventricular tachycardia, often lead to inadequate emptying of the ventricles. The ventricle in fibrillation or asystole does not eject any blood; if this condition is not corrected, the sudden onset of shock and death is imminent. A massive pulmonary embolus may lead to circulatory shock by preventing the emptying of the right ventricle and the filling of the left ventricle.

Although most causes of circulatory shock can be categorized into one of the three major types outlined previously, many shock states possess features of two or more types. Septic shock is accompanied by ventricular dysfunction (inadequate filling and/or emptying). Hypovolemic shock is in large part a manifestation of poor venous return and diminished ventricular filling.

PHYSIOLOGIC ADAPTATIONS AND COMPENSATORY MECHANISMS. The reduction in arterial pressure and tissue perfusion initiates vital compensatory mechanisms. The major compensatory mechanisms are baroreceptor reflexes, release of endogenous vasoactive substances, and physiologic responses to increase and maintain an effective vascular volume.

Hypotension results in a decrease in the pressure that is sensed by the baroreceptors in the carotid sinuses and aortic arch; this effects a reduction in vagal tone and an increase in sympathetic tone. The enhanced sympathetic tone increases arteriolar and venous vasoconstriction, heart rate, and inotropy of the myocardium. These effects, in turn, increase and maintain perfusion pressure and blood flow to the brain and heart. The clinical manifestations of the increased sympathetic tone in hypovolemic shock are cool, moist extremities and tachycardia. In warm shock, such as sepsis, vasodilation occurs, and as a consequence the extremities may be normothermic or warm; however, the tachycardia from increased sympathetic tone persists. Patients with shock caused by dehydration states usually have cool, dry extremities and tachycardia.

The major endogenous vasoactive substances released during circulatory shock are the catecholamines, vasopressin, and angiotensin. The increased levels of the circulating catecholamines epinephrine and norepinephrine are part of the augmented sympathetic nervous system activity. Vasopressin, a potent vasoconstrictor, is released from the posterior pituitary gland in hypotensive states. Decreased renal perfusion stimulates the release of renin, which converts angiotensinogen to angiotensin. Angiotensin is a powerful vasoconstrictor and, interestingly, stimulates the brain thirst center. The endogenous release of these vasoactive substances contributes to reduction of vascular capacitance and redistribution of flow to the brain and myocardium. The role of the ubiquitous prostaglandins in shock states is not yet defined.

The reabsorption of extravascular fluid and renal conservation of sodium chloride and water constitute a major compensatory mechanism serving to increase and maintain an adequate intravascular volume. These adaptations result in a decrease in hematocrit and plasma oncotic pressure in most forms of shock. Up to 1 L of extravascular fluid may be reabsorbed or autotransfused within the first hour of hypovolemic shock. In addition to serving as a vasoconstrictor, angiotensin stimulates the release of aldosterone from the adrenal gland. Aldosterone, along with increased levels of adenocorticosteroids and vasopressin (antidiuretic hormone), augments the renal reabsorption of sodium chloride and water.

CLINICAL MANIFESTATIONS. The spectrum of circulatory shock is very wide. The event can be transient and mild, as in vasodepressor syncope ("faint"),* or prolonged with a grave prognosis, as in cardiogenic shock caused by a myocardial infarction.

Prolonged hypotension and poor tissue perfusion lead to general cellular dysfunction, which is manifested by varying degrees of organ failure. Although diminished renal perfusion provides certain compensatory mechanisms, prolonged and severe reduction in renal blood flow may lead to renal failure. Hepatic dysfunction and intestinal ileus with ischemia and infarction may occur in severe shock states. Circulatory shock and prolonged bed rest are often accompanied by a progressive deterioration of pulmonary function resulting from accumulating secretions, atelectasis, pneumonia, ventilation-perfusion abnormalities, and interstitial edema from alveolar damage ("shock lung") or from left-sided cardiac events such as ruptured papillary muscle. Abnormalities of the reticuloendothelial system combined with the accumulation of toxic products and vascular injury may complicate circulatory shock by eliciting diffuse intravascular coagulation, a condition characterized by diffuse hemorrhage and by thrombosis of the microvasculature. Failure of the compensatory mechanisms to maintain adequate cerebral blood flow is manifested as lethargy, somnolence, coma, abnormal patterns of respiration (tachypnea, Cheyne-Stokes respiration, or apnea), and loss of central control of the entire nervous system. A reduction in coronary artery perfusion may produce myocardial ischemia and infarction, particularly in patients with underlying atherosclerotic coronary artery

---

*Not classified as a shock state by some investigators because of its transient, self-limited features.

disease or myocardial hypertrophy. The presence and role of a "myocardial depressant factor" in certain shock states have not been well established.

Untreated or intractable circulatory shock thus evolves into a vicious circle of deterioration. The cycle is perpetuated by the progressive development of the complications of shock just noted. Diffuse cell injury and cell death occur with the release of metabolic products (lactate, enzymes, and so forth). Systematically the metabolic products cause acidosis. Locally they disrupt the neural and humoral regulation of vascular smooth muscle, resulting in dilated, nonresponsive blood vessels (further worsening the shock state) and heralding the onset of "irreversible shock." Irreversible shock" is a term applied to terminal shock states incapable of responding favorably to treatment. Circulatory shock (untreated or intractable) is thus a syndrome involving multiple systems and evolves from extreme cardiovascular failure to failure of most of the body systems and death.

MANAGEMENT. The overall therapeutic approach should be concentrated in four major areas: prevention, treatment directed at the cause of the shock state, cardiovascular support, and management of complications.

Each member of the medical community has the responsibility to avoid and prevent events that may lead to circulatory shock. For example, inquiring about drug allergies before the administration of drugs is mandatory. A patient with easy bleeding and bruisability should be evaluated by a medical specialist before a dental or surgical procedure. Salicylates should not be administered to patients with a history of peptic ulcer disease. Bacterial infections should be treated properly and promptly, especially in immunocompromised patients, to prevent overwhelming bacteremia and sepsis.

The initial efforts in managing a patient in circulatory shock should be directed at providing cardiovascular support and determining the cause of the shock state; most often these activities are performed simultaneously. Except for congestive shock states, increasing intravascular volume is the most important part of therapy; infusion of saline and/or other volume expanders should be rapidly initiated, and large volumes (even 5 to 10 L) may be necessary to restore perfusion. To prevent complications of shock, this should be started while monitoring and diagnostic studies are being initiated. Cardiovascular monitoring should be performed in an intensive or coronary care unit and for most forms of shock should include continuous electrocardiography to determine heart rate and rhythm changes and indwelling catheters to measure central and peripheral blood pressures. The flow-directed triple-lumen pulmonary artery catheter (Swan-Ganz catheter) is currently the optimal hemodynamic monitoring device because it provides direct-pressure recordings of the right atrium and pulmonary artery, indirect measurements of the left ventricular filling pressure (via pulmonary arterial occlusive pressure), and cardiac output determinations, generally by a thermodilution technique. The catheter is particularly useful in the management of cardiogenic or congestive shock.

Urine flow of ≥ 30 ml/hr (which may require an indwelling urinary bladder catheter for measurement) indicates adequate renal perfusion. With diminished urine flow, a low urine sodium concentration (<20 mEq/L) indicates sodium reabsorption to conserve intravascular volume. However, the decreased urine flow causes the serum urea nitrogen to be elevated disproportionately (by >10 times) to serum creatinine. When diminished urine flow reflects acute renal tubular necrosis caused by the shock, the urine sodium is high (>20 mEq/L), reflecting failure of reabsorption, and the serum urea nitrogen is elevated proportionately to creatinine (about 10 times that of creatinine). Gastrointestinal bleeding disproportionately elevates urea nitrogen.

Monitoring of the respiratory, metabolic, and hematologic status is accomplished by the intermittent determination of arterial blood gases, lactate concentrations, serum oncotic pressure, hematocrit, and blood clotting parameters. Intensive monitoring provides specific direction in therapeutics. For example, low central venous and left ventricular filling pressures indicate the need for the administration of additional fluids. With a normal or high central venous pressure (>8 mm Hg) and left ventricular filling pressure (a pulmonary wedge pressure >14 mm Hg), there is a need for inotropic agents. Dopamine should be given to increase cardiac output and systemic blood pressure. This drug also dilates the renal and mesenteric arteries.

The determination of the precise cause of shock may permit direct intervention and reversal of the shock state. The history of a penicillin injection immediately before sudden clinical deterioration and shock strongly suggests an acute anaphylactic reaction; the expeditious administration of epinephrine, corticosteroids, and intravenous fluids usually prevents this form of shock from deteriorating into severe and irreversible shock. Hypovolemic shock in a patient with a history of peptic ulcer disease requires the placement of a nasogastric tube and analysis of gastric contents; if gastrointestinal bleeding is present, volume replacement with blood, saline, or volume expanders and control of the bleeding, possibly by surgery, are indicated. In addition to fluid administration, septic shock is treated immediately with antibiotics directed at all the suspected organisms until culture reports are available. Failure to detect and treat a remediable cause of shock often condemns the patient to irreversible shock regardless of how brilliant and aggressive the initial cardiovascular support may have been.

The primary thrust in the management of circulatory shock should be directed at prevention. However, once circulatory shock has developed, the patient's survival depends on aggressive and meticulous interaction of cardiovascular support, cardiovascular and systemic monitoring, and early detection and management of complicating problems.

BIBLIOGRAPHY

Abel, F.L., and Kessler, D.P.: Myocardial performance in hemorrhagic shock in dog and primate, Circ. Res. **32**:492, 1973.
Ledingham, I.M., and McAllister, T.A., editors: Conference on shock, St. Louis, 1972, The C.V. Mosby Co.
McGovern, V.J., and Tiller, D.J., editors: Shock: a clinicopathologic correlation, New York, 1980, Masson Publishing USA, Inc.
Selkurt, E.E., editor: Symposium on the physiologic basis of circulatory shock, Fed. Proc. **29**:1832, 1970.
Selkurt, E.E.: Current status of renal circulation and related nephron function in hemorrhage and experimental shock, Circ. Shock **1**:3, 1974.
Skjoldborg, H., editor: Scanticon shock seminar, Amsterdam, 1978, Excerpta Medica.
Vatner, S.F.: Effects of hemorrhage on regional blood flow distribution in dogs and primates, J. Clin. Invest. **54**:225, 1974.
Weil, M.H., and others: Treatment of circulatory shock, J.A.M.A. **231**:1280, 1975.
Winslow, E.J., and others: Hemodynamic studies and results of therapy in 30 patients with bacteremic shock, Am. J. Med. **54**:421, 1973.
Zeifach, B.W., and Fronek, A.: The interplay of central and peripheral factors in irreversible hemorrhagic shock, Prog. Cardiovasc. Dis. **18**:147, 1975.

89 • DIAGNOSTIC PROCEDURES IN CARDIOLOGY

James A. Joye, Reginald I. Low, Anthony N. DeMaria, Ezra A. Amsterdam, and **Dean T. Mason**

Although much information about cardiac function can be obtained from the patient's history, the physical examination, and routine laboratory studies, the use of specialized laboratory procedures has greatly improved the accuracy of cardiovascular diagnoses. Cardiac catheterization techniques and echocardiography have been particularly important diagnostic procedures developed over the past 30 years. Current advances include the development of radionuclide techniques, application of noninvasive laboratory methods (that is, those that do not require cardiac catheterization, an "invasive" procedure), and testing during exercise to uncover cardiac dysfunction inapparent at rest.

ELECTROCARDIOGRAPHY
Cardiac electrophysiology

Myocardial contraction is induced by electrical depolarization of the heart, an event that can be recorded graphically using electrodes placed on the body. In the resting state most cardiac cells are polarized at -90 mV relative to the extracellular fluid. The cell will depolarize if a certain threshold potential is achieved. This may occur suddenly, as a result of an outside stimulus such as an adjacent cell's depolarization, or slowly and spontaneously, as is characteristic of pacemaker cells. Unlike normal cells, which maintain a stable resting membrane potential, pacemaker cells undergo slow, spontaneous depolarization throughout diastole (a characteristic known as automaticity), with full depolarization after they reach the threshold potential. The cells with the fastest rate of spontaneous depolarization are in the sinoatrial (SA) node at the junction of the superior vena cava and right atrium. Regions of pacemaker cells that are lower in the heart, for example, in the atrioventricular (AV) node or in the His-Purkinje system of the ventricles, have progressively slower rates of spontaneous depolarization and therefore pace the heart more slowly. The pacemaker cells with the highest depolarization frequency override other pacemaker cells and control the heart rate. Cessation of activity in the SA node shifts the cardiac pacemaker to the cells of the next fastest depolarization rate, generally in the AV node. One important characteristic of cardiac tissue compared to other electrically active tissues is the long delay between depolarization and repolarization, or recovery of excitability, resulting in long refractory periods (the interval during which two successive responses cannot occur), thus preventing cardiac tetany.

The polarity of the cardiac cells is the result of ionic gradients, different concentrations of ions across the cell membrane, especially the concentrations of sodium, potassium, and calcium. The resting membrane potential is normally associated with an intracellular sodium concentration of about 10 mEq/L, compared to 132 to 142 mEq/L in the extracellular fluid; the intracellular potassium concentration is approximately 150 mEq/L versus 3.5 to 5 mEq/L extracellularly. The potassium gradient is primarily responsible for the resting transmembrane potential, but the influx of sodium ion causes rapid depolarization and impulse conduction. Partially depolarized cells conduct the impulse more slowly. At membrane potentials of less than -55 mV, depolarization is carried out primarily by calcium ion fluxes and impulse conduction is even slower. The calcium ion flux occurs across the so-called slow channel. As the serum potassium level decreases, the resting membrane potential becomes more negative, depolarization becomes more rapid, and the heart becomes more excitable. As the serum potassium level rises and the transmembrane gradient becomes less, there is less tendency for the cardiac cells to depolarize and conduction is slower. At high serum levels of potassium, usually greater than 8 mEq/L, the heart contracts poorly or ceases to contract altogether.

Depolarization begins in the SA node and spreads through the atria, but it is prevented from entering the ventricles by the insulating effect of the fibrous anulus of the atrioventricular ring, except at the AV node. From the AV node the depolarization wave is carried through the fibrous ring by the specialized conducting tissue of the His-Purkinje system. This tissue rapidly propagates the impulse to the ventricular muscle, which depolarizes at a somewhat slower rate. The most rapidly conducting tissue is in the His-Purkinje system, the slowest conducting tissue is in the AV node, and intermediate conduction is found in muscle tissue of the atria and ventricles.

The AV node is responsive to the autonomic nervous system. The rate of conduction is increased by sympathetic stimulation and decreased by parasympathetic stimulation. The bundle of His carries the impulse from the AV node to the interventricular septum, where the bundle bifurcates into the right and left bundle branches. The left bundle further divides into two collections of fibers known as the anterosuperior and posteroinferior fascicles, corresponding to the regions of the left ventricle they depolarize. There is considerable variation in the structure of the left bundle, and numerous interconnections between the two divisions occur over the surface of the septum. The right bundle, a smaller collection of fibers than the left, passes down the right ventricular side of the interventricular septum and spreads out over the right ventricular subendocardial surface. The cells of the His bundle, bundle branches, and Purkinje network are specialized for rapid conduction so as to achieve a rapid and synchronous depolarization of the ventricles.

Einthoven popularized the useful, although not strictly true, concept that the body represents a large volume conductor with the heart as the center of its electrical activity. The sum of all electrical events in the body can be thought of in terms of an electrical dipole. That is, the net electrical activity at any moment will have a certain magnitude and direction pointing out toward the body surface from the heart as the electrical center. The changes in this net electrical vector during the cardiac cycle can be shown graphically in the familiar electrocardiogram (ECG). When the heart is monitored from several different locations or leads, information can be obtained about the total electrical activity of the heart as well as about the segments of myocardium closest to each monitoring electrode.

Lead systems and recording

The lead system of the ECG is composed of four limb electrodes and electrodes placed over various sites on the precordium (Fig. 89-1). Each ECG lead records the cardiac cycle as changes in electrical potential between two electrodes or between one electrode and a combination of the others. The electrode on the right leg is a ground electrode for all lead systems.

The standard limb lead system is based on the assumption that the leads are symmetric, the body is a homogenous volume conductor, and the heart is a single equivalent dipole at the center of the body. In this system electrodes are placed on the right arm, left arm, and left leg. Lead I records the difference in electrical potential between the two arms, with the left arm electrode positive and the right arm electrode negative. Lead II compares the difference in potential between the right arm and left leg, with the left leg electrode positive. Lead III compares the left arm and left leg, with the left leg electrode positive. Because the major vector of atrial and ventricular depolarization in most normal individuals is directed leftward and inferiorly, placement of the positive electrodes on the legs and left arm usually results in an electrogram with upward deflections for the P wave and QRS complex.

By connecting the right and left arm and left leg electrodes through a standard resistance, potentials from these three points are canceled out (central terminal of Wilson). This reference terminal theoretically remains inactive during the entire cardiac cycle, allowing an exploring electrode to function as a unipolar lead. The unipolar or augmented limb lead system uses the central terminal as the indifferent electrode and one of the three active limb electrodes, labeled aV_R, aV_L, and aV_F, as the exploring one.

The unipolar chest or precordial leads also combine an exploring electrode with the central terminal of Wilson. The exploring electrode is placed in six standard positions over the precordium: V_1 at the right sternal border in the fourth intercostal space, V_2 at the left sternal border in the same interspace, V_4 in the left midclavicular line and fifth intercostal space, V_3 midway between leads V_2 and V_4, V_5 in the left anterior axillary line at the same level as V_4, and V_6 at the left midaxillary line in the same horizontal plane as leads V_4 and V_5. Under certain circumstances the additional leads V_7 through V_9 and right precordial leads V_{3R} through V_{6R} may be used. The latter are used with congenital heart disease or when the heart is positioned more to the right side of the chest. The precordial leads together reflect the total activity of the heart, but each lead monitors activity only in the tissue closest to it.

Normal electrocardiogram

The ECG is generally recorded on graph paper at a standard speed of 25 mm/sec (Fig. 89-2). In the standard ECG recording, 0.1 mV produces a 1-mm positive (upward) deflection.

Although the SA node normally is the pacemaker of the heart, it does not contain enough mass to produce a voltage detectable by the surface ECG. The P wave, caused by depolarization of the atria, is the first evidence of electrical activity in the cardiac cycle. After the P wave the ECG returns to baseline as the depolarization wave is slowed in the tissue of the AV node. When the ventricular muscle depolarizes, the QRS complex is produced. An initial downward or negative deflection is termed a q wave, whereas an initial upward or positive deflection is termed an R wave. A positive deflection following a q wave is also termed an R wave. By convention, r indicates a small

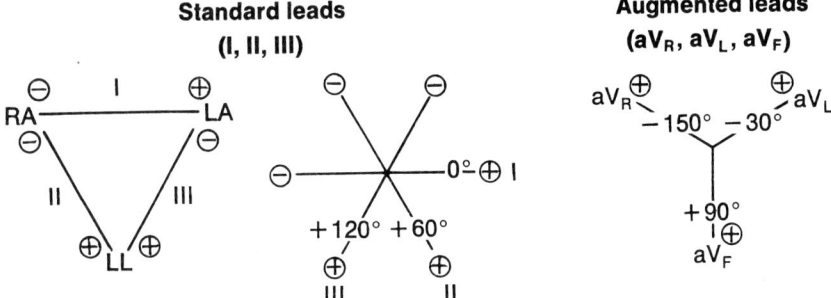

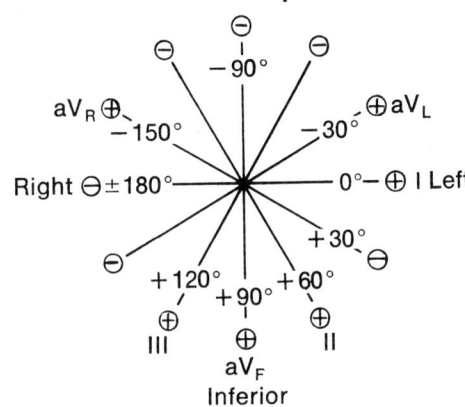

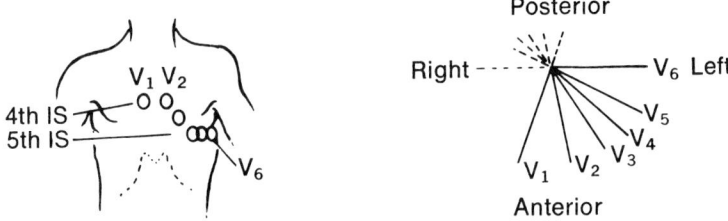

Fig. 89-1. *Standard leads:* electrode position and resultant triaxial reference system of positive and negative polarity along with axes of three leads in frontal plane. *RA*, right arm; *LA*, left arm; *LL*, left leg. *Augmented leads:* unipolar limb leads utilizing indifferent electrode (central terminal of Wilson) for reference with frontal plane axes. *Frontal lead plane:* hexaxial frontal plane reference system with respective axes in degrees. (See text for use of this system to determine axes of cardiac vectors.) *Precordial leads:* unipolar chest leads also use indifferent electrode for reference–V_1 just to right and V_2 just to left of sternum in fourth intercostal space *(4th IS)*, V_4 in left fifth intercostal space *(5th IS)* at midclavicular line, V_3 midway between V_2 and V_4, V_5 in anterior axillary line and V_6 in midaxillary line, both in line with V_4; representation of precordial leads on horizontal plane as axes radiating out of heart and center of chest with 0 degrees being near V_2 and 90 degrees at V_6.

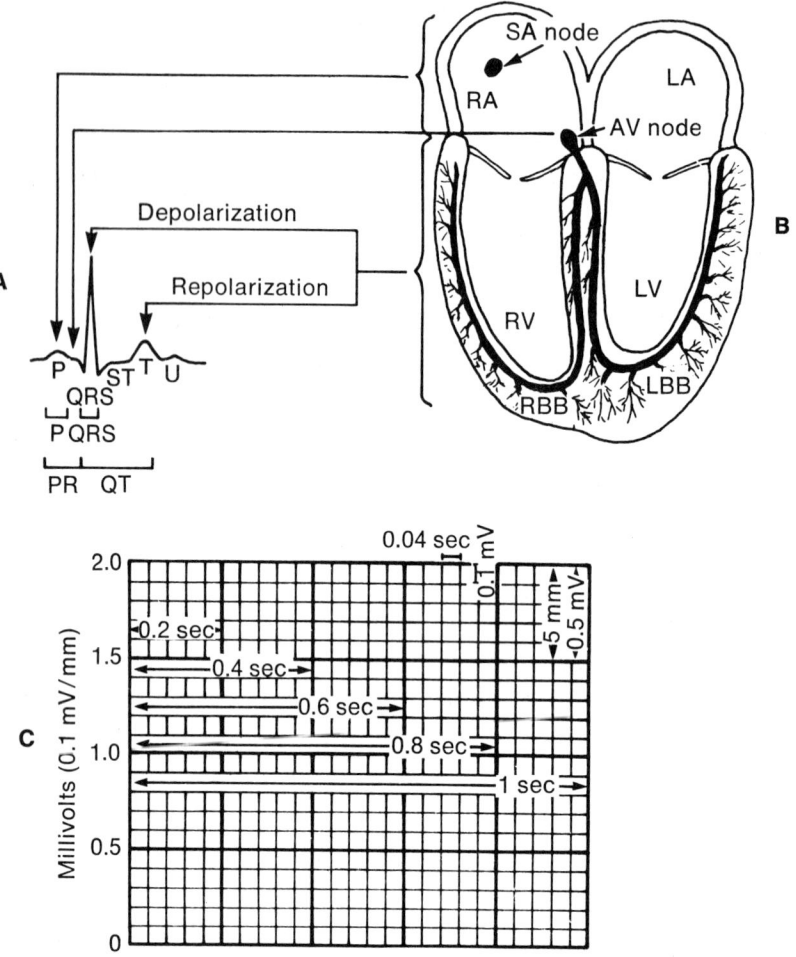

Fig. 89-2. A, Schematic representation of ECG and **B,** its relationship to cardiac electrical activity. *P,* P wave resulting from atrial depolarization; *QRS,* QRS complex resulting from ventricular depolarization; *T,* T wave resulting from ventricular repolarization; *U,* U wave; *PR,* PR interval represents time from onset of atrial depolarization to onset of ventricular depolarization, generally is most affected by atrioventricular nodal *(AV node)* conduction but may be prolonged by block anywhere between atria and ventricular myocardium; *ST,* ST segment; *QT,* QT interval from onset of QRS to end of T wave and measure of complete depolarization and repolarization cycle of ventricles; *LA,* left atrium; *LBB,* left bundle branch; *LV,* left ventricle; *RA,* right atrium; *RBB,* right bundle branch; *RV,* right ventricle; *SA node,* sinoatrial node. **C,** Measurements on standard ECG graph paper. Voltage is measured on vertical scale–smaller interval is 1 mm or 0.1 mV and the larger is 5 mm or 0.5 mV; time is measured on horizontal scale–1 mm equal to 0.04 second, 5 mm equal to 0.2 second, and 25 mm equal to 1 second. At standard paper speed of 25 mm/sec, repetitive events with an interval of 0.04 second (1 mm) occur at 1500/min, those with an interval of 0.2 second occur at 300/min, an interval of 0.4 second equals 150/min, 0.6 second equals 100/min, 0.8 second equals 75/min, and 1 second equals 60/min.

upward deflection and R a large upward deflection. The S wave is a negative deflection following an R wave. If a QRS complex has only a negative deflection without a positive deflection, it is known as a QS complex. In a QRS complex with more than one R wave, the additional positive deflection is labeled R′. Once the ventricles are completely depolarized, the ECG returns to the baseline (ST segment). The T wave that follows represents ventricular repolarization and may sometimes be followed by a small U wave. Atrial repolarization is generally lost in the PR interval and QRS complex because of the small amount of force produced.

ELECTRICAL AXIS. The axes of the electrical vectors generated during sequential depolarization and repolarization of the heart are especially important for interpretation in the frontal plane. These axes can be determined by scrutinizing the ECG leads (Fig. 89-1). For example, a QRS complex that is mostly positive in lead II or mostly negative in lead aV$_R$ represents an electrical vector of ventricular depolarization moving from right to left, superior to inferior. Both leads I and aV_F are more positive than negative as a result of this same QRS vector, a typical finding when the mean QRS axis is normal (0 to +90 degrees). To define the axis more accurately, the ECG is analyzed for the lead in which the QRS complex is isoelectric, equally positive and negative, since the QRS vector will be perpendicular to that lead. If in the previous example the QRS is isoelectric in lead III and slightly more positive than negative in lead aV_L, the axis is +30 degrees. If lead aV_L is isoelectric and lead III slightly positive, the axis is +60 degrees. Another technique for more accurately determining the axis is to compare adjacent leads. In the same example as before, if lead I is as positive as lead aV_F and lead II is as positive as lead aV_R is negative, the QRS axis is +45 degrees. This technique is used to define the axis of the P wave and T wave as well as that of the QRS complex. The most accurate means of defining the vector in any lead is to compare the magnitude and duration of positive deflections with the magnitude and duration of negative deflections. Thus if the QRS complex is all positive, the electrical vector is directed toward the lead. If the QRS complex is all negative, the electrical vector is directed away from the lead. If the positive deflections are equal to the negative deflections, for example, R wave equal to Q wave plus S wave, the vector of depolarization is perpendicular to the lead. If the positive deflections are larger than the negative deflections, the vector is directed more toward the lead than away from it.

P WAVE. The P wave is the graphic representation of atrial depolarization, which begins at the SA node and spreads inferiorly and leftward (Fig. 89-2). The duration of the P wave is normally less than 0.11 second, 2.75 mm on an ECG made at 25 mm/sec. The P wave axis is normally directed between 0 and +60 degrees in the frontal plane and thus is most positive in leads I and II. It tends to be diphasic in leads V_1 and V_2, although it may also be inverted (negative) in a normal individual.

QRS COMPLEX, ST SEGMENT, AND T WAVE. The QRS complex reflects sequential electrical forces resulting from the depolarization of the large mass of ventricular muscle. The duration of the complex is the time required for ventricular depolarization measured from the beginning of the first deflection at the end of the PR segment to the beginning of the ST segment, usually between 0.04 and 0.10 second. The individual waves that comprise the QRS complex are sharp in contour and reflect the sequential changes in the direction of depolarization of the ventricles. As the wave of depolarization travels down the conduction system from the AV node, the left bundle branch depolarizes the interventricular *septum* from the left ventricular endocardium to the right. This anterior and rightward movement results in a small R wave in lead V_1 and a small initial Q wave in leads I, aV_L, V_5, and V_6; these latter leads are referred to as the *lateral* leads. (With horizontal hearts, small initial Q waves may be seen in leads II, III, and aV_F, the inferior leads, because of superior movement of the initial wave front.) These *septal* Q waves are normally <0.04 second long and are of low amplitude. The initial R wave in lead V_1 is normally ≤0.6 mV, >0.02 but ≤0.04 second in duration. The depolarization wave propagates rapidly through the endocardium of both ventricles. The rapid change from the initial rightward and anterior forces of the septum to the leftward and posterior direction of the remaining left ventricular mass is marked by a prominent R wave in the left precordial leads.

In the frontal lead system the lead with the largest R wave depends on whether the electrical axis of the heart is directed horizontally or vertically. Normally the QRS complex has an axis between 0 and +90 degrees. A QRS complex directed between 0 and −30 degrees is said to have left axis deviation. If the axis is more negative than −30 degrees, it is an abnormal left axis deviation. If the QRS axis is +90 degrees or more, it is referred to as right axis deviation (Fig. 89-3). If the QRS axis is directed between −90 and −180 degrees, it is termed extreme right axis deviation, or in some terminologies an indeterminate axis. In the horizontal plane assessed by the precordial leads, the QRS axis is normally directed posteriorly and leftward, resulting in small R and deep S waves in leads V_1 and V_2 and small Q and tall R waves in leads V_5 and V_6.

The ST segment is typically flat and on the same plane as the PR segment. In the precordial leads it may normally rise slowly, with an upward-directed concavity, into the T wave. The T wave axis is normally in the same general direction as the QRS axis, and it should not differ by more than 45 degrees in the frontal plane or by more than 60 degrees in the horizontal plane.

PR AND QT INTERVALS. The PR and QT intervals are also measured as part of the interpretation of the ECG. The PR interval begins with the onset of the P wave and ends at the onset of the QRS complex. It reflects depolarization of the atria, the delay caused by the slow conduction of the depolarization wave through the AV node, and His-Purkinje conduction. The PR interval is greater than 0.12 second but less than 0.20 second in duration in the adult. A prolonged PR interval generally reflects slow conduction through the AV node.

The QT interval is measured from the onset of the QRS complex to the end of the T wave, and care should be exercised to avoid including a U wave, if present, in the measurement. The QT interval approximates the refractory period of the ventricles, the time required for the ventricles to depolarize and repolarize again. Its duration is inversely proportional to the heart rate. The corrected QT interval (QT_c) is the QT interval divided by the square root of the RR interval (the interval between two consecutive QRS complexes) and normally is 0.35 to 0.42 second.

The QT interval may be prolonged by hypocalcemia, hypokalemia, myocardial infarction, quinidine-like antiar-

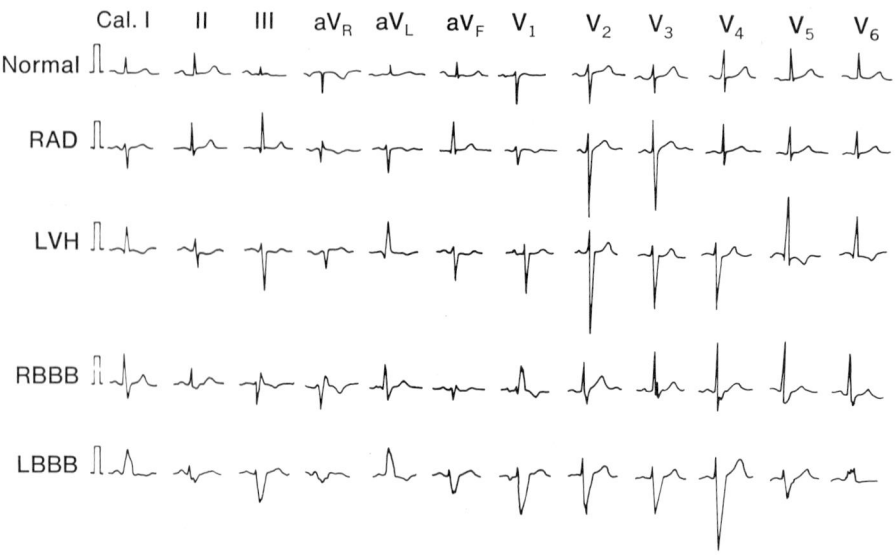

Fig. 89-3. Examples of several ECG patterns as described in text. Normal with QRS axis of +40 degrees and T axis of +35 degrees; *RAD*, right axis deviation with QRS axis of +110 degrees and T axis of +100 degrees; *LVH*, left ventricular hypertrophy demonstrated by limb lead and chest lead voltage criteria and T inversion in lateral leads; *RBBB*, right bundle branch block demonstrating terminal QRS forces directed rightward and anteriorly with rSR′ configuration in lead V_1; *LBBB*, left bundle branch block with slow initial forces and monophasic R complex seen in lateral leads, terminal forces directed to left. *Cal.*, 1 cm or 1 m V ECG calibration.

rhythmic agents, subarachnoid hemorrhage, hypothermia, myocarditis, diffuse myocardial disease, and certain hereditary disorders. The QT interval may be shortened by hypercalcemia or digitalis glycosides. Prolongation of the QT interval is associated with ventricular arrhythmias.

Abnormalities of the electrocardiogram

ACUTE MYOCARDIAL INFARCTION. The ECG changes of acute myocardial infarction represent an evolutionary process characterized by sequential development of ischemia, injury, and infarction (Fig. 89-4). ECG ischemia is defined by T wave changes, injury by ST segment changes, and infarction by QRS abnormalities. The earliest or hyperacute phase is characterized by tall, peaked T waves followed by ST segment elevation as the current of injury develops owing to breakdown of the electrical integrity of the cell membrane. Next, the T waves begin to invert while the ST segment remains elevated. As the infarction progresses, the QRS complex either loses voltage or develops pathologic Q waves. These changes occur in the first few hours of myocardial infarction and are seen in the precordial leads closest to the area of infarction or in the limb leads that best monitor the area of infarction. Leads opposite the region of infarction demonstrate reciprocal changes: depressed ST segment and upright T waves. As the active injury resolves, the ST segments return to baseline. The inverted T waves gradually return to normal over several weeks but may persist for months or possibly years. Pathologic Q waves that appear in leads previously without such waves or that become exaggerated (>0.04 second in duration and >0.2 mV in depth) and the loss of R wave voltage tend to persist. In smaller infarctions some of the voltage may return and the Q waves may become much smaller or disappear, most commonly in the inferior leads.

The area of myocardium infarcted determines the leads involved: II, III, and aV_F if inferior; I, aV_L, V_5, and/or V_6 if lateral; V_2 through V_5 if anterior; and V_1 and V_2 if anteroseptal. If the R waves become more prominent in V_1 and V_2, with R > S and >0.04 second in duration, and with ST segment depression and T wave peaking, this suggests posterior myocardial infarction (these changes in V_1 and V_2 are reciprocal with the usual changes of infarction). Posterior infarction is more likely if there is associated inferior or lateral infarction, since these regions are adjacent to one another. When there are ST depression, T wave changes, and a clinical picture of infarction but Q waves and/or diminution of R waves fails to develop, the diagnosis of nontransmural or subendocardial myocardial infarction is made.

TRANSIENT MYOCARDIAL ISCHEMIA. Asymptomatic individuals with chronic ischemic heart disease may have a normal ECG or minor ST segment depression, flattening or mild inversion of the T waves, or an abnormal shift of the T wave axis. Q waves, a result of an old myocardial infarction, are more specific. The resting ECG of individuals with angina pectoris is the same as for other patients with chronic ischemic heart disease. However, during

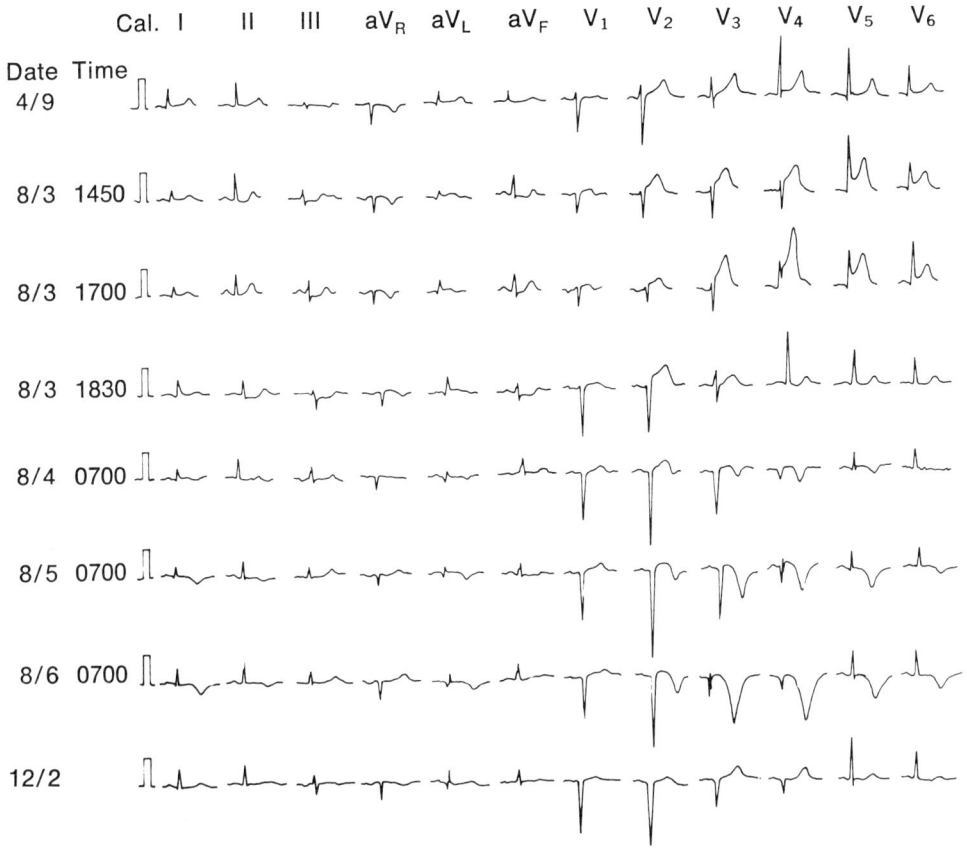

Fig. 89-4. Acute anteroseptal myocardial infarction with evolutionary changes. *4/9*, baseline ECG; *8/3 1450*, ECG after 1 hour of crushing chest pain; *8/3 1700*, 3 hours and 10 minutes after onset of pain (note early ST and T wave elevation with some loss of R wave in chest leads V_1 through V_2); *8/4 0700*, by day following acute event, R waves are diminished, ST segments are decreasing, and T waves have begun to invert; *12/2*, by 4 months following infarction, R waves are gone in leads V_1 through V_4, but ST and T waves have returned to baseline.

spontaneous episodes of angina or during physical or emotional stress, there may be ST segment depression, often horizontal or downsloping, with some flattening or inversion of the T waves. Variant forms of angina pectoris, Prinzmetal's angina resulting from coronary artery spasm, and total occlusion of a coronary artery are associated with epicardial injury and ST segment elevation rather than depression. These changes are the same as those of an acute myocardial infarction but may resolve. Bouts of Prinzmetal's angina may be associated with ventricular arrhythmias and may progress to myocardial infarction.

ECHOCARDIOGRAPHY

In the past 10 years the ability to detect and manage a variety of cardiovascular disorders with echocardiography has been documented. More recently the method has been expanded to provide two-dimensional real-time imaging of the heart and great vessels, permitting evaluation of cardiac structure and function in a manner previously impossible. Accordingly, echocardiography has achieved a primary role in the assessment of patients with cardiac disease.

Clinical echocardiography uses pulsed sonic waves of 2 to 3 million cycles per second (ultrasound), since such waves may be readily directed as a beam that will closely obey the natural laws of reflection and refraction. The sound beam is generated by a piezoelectrode (pressure-electric) crystal that is capable of converting mechanical energy into electrical energy and vice versa. Thus the generator crystal can also convert sound waves reflected from tissue interfaces into electrical signals and can receive returning sound waves during cyclic periods of nonactivation.

The echographic transducer is positioned on the chest wall along the left sternal border and is directed posteriorly. The ultrasound beam emitted travels in a straight line until it encounters an interface between two structures of different acoustic density. The percentage of reflected sound waves (echoes) depends on how nearly perpendicular the transmitted sonic beam is to the interface. Since the velocity at which sound travels through soft tissue is constant, the distance of any interface from the transducer can be calculated from the time required for the transmission and return of a sound wave from a cardiovascular structure. Therefore echographic signals are displayed in terms of their distance from the transducer.

In the most commonly used clinical echo presentation, called motion-mode echocardiography (M-mode echo), the echo from a given structure is represented on an oscilloscope as a dot whose amplitude of reflectance is expressed by intensity and size. This dot first appears on a vertical axis relative to the distance between it and the transducer and then moves along the horizontal axis with time. Thus M-mode echo provides an opportunity not only to record intracardiac anatomy but also to assess the motion of the cardiac structures as they alter their positions relative to the transducer during the phases of the cardiac cycle.

Normal echocardiogram

With the transducer angled inferiorly and to the patient's left, the beam traverses the plane through the cardiac apex, as indicated by sector *1* in Fig. 89-5. When the position of the transducer is progressively angled superiorly and to the patient's right, the echo beam transects the mitral valve, the aorta and aortic leaflets, and the left atrium, as observed in sectors *2* and *3*. The mitral leaflets coapt at the onset of systole (point *C* in Fig. 89-5, *C*), producing echoes that follow a gradual straight-line anterior movement owing to gradual forward motion of the mitral anulus as the left ventricle empties and the left atrium fills. At the onset of diastole (point *D*) the mitral valve opens and the anterior mitral leaflet echo is recorded as a brisk forward motion to point *E*. The anterior leaflet then floats posteriorly toward a closed position in response to rapid ventricular filling and reaches point *F* during the

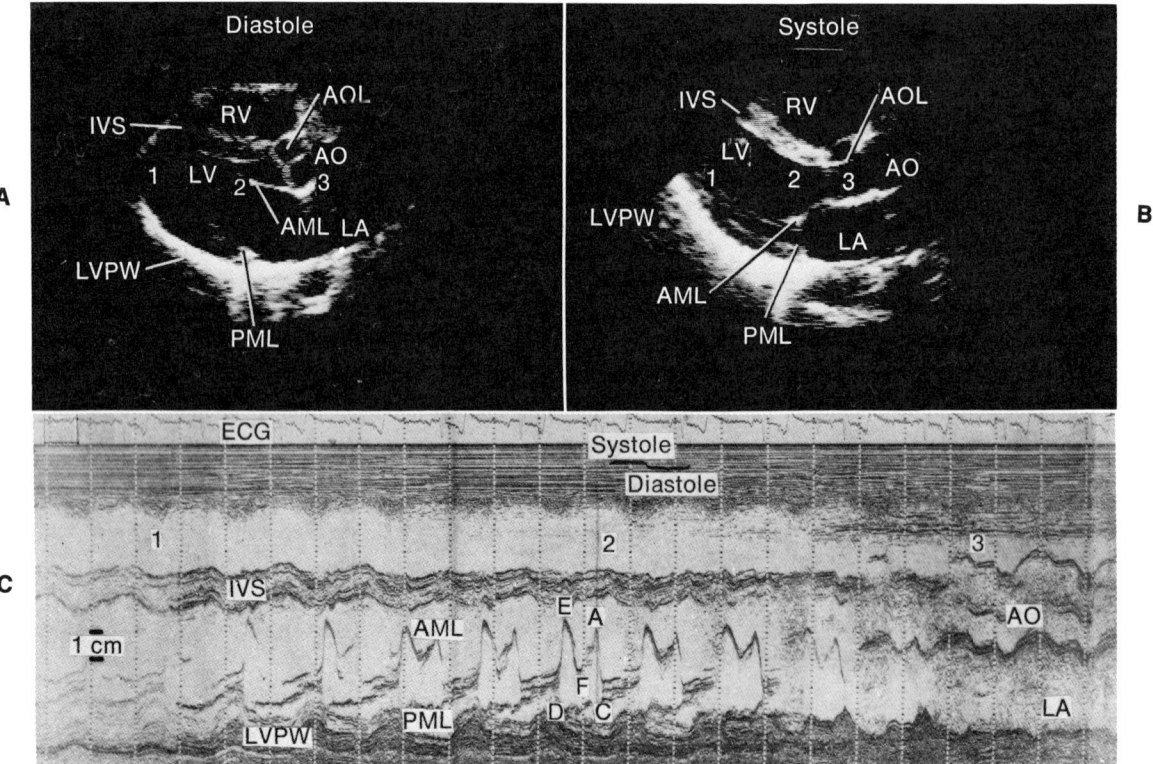

Fig. 89-5. Echocardiogram. **A,** Diastolic and **B,** systolic frames of real-time, 2-D echocardiogram obtained in longitudinal axis as if viewed from left side of heart with anterior at top of pictures, posterior at bottom, base and head to right, and apex and feet to left. **C,** M-mode echocardiogram on sweep from body of left ventricle to base of heart during several cardiac cycles as demonstrated by ECG. Numbers *1*, *2*, and *3* in all three pictures refer to regions of heart: *1*, body of left ventricle; *2*, level of mitral valve leaflets; and *3*, level of aortic valve and left atrium. Letters defining points of mitral valve motion in **C:** *D*, mitral valve opening at beginning of diastole; *E*, point of maximal opening during early diastole caused by rapid flow of blood through valve; *F*, point of low flow in middiastole; *A*, point of maximal opening during atrial systole; *C*, closure point of mitral valve leaflets at beginning of ventricular systole. *AML*, anterior mitral valve leaflet; *AO*, root of aorta; *AOL*, aortic valve leaflets; *ECG*, electrocardiogram; *IVS*, interventricular septum; *LA*, left atrium; *LV*, left ventricle; *LVPW*, left ventricular posterior wall; *PML*, posterior mitral valve leaflet; *RV*, right ventricle; *1 cm*, 1 centimeter. (Slightly retouched for reproduction.)

first third of diastole. In response to atrial contraction during late diastole, the anterior leaflet again moves abruptly forward (point A) and then floats posteriorly to return to a closed position at the onset of systole. The composite diastolic motion of the anterior mitral leaflet therefore describes an **M** configuration, and the posterior mitral leaflet demonstrates a mirror-image **W** contour (sector 2).

In contrast to mitral valve motion, the opening movements of the aortic cusps occur during left ventricular ejection (sector 3). Furthermore, echoes are usually recorded from only two of the three aortic leaflets, believed to be those of the right and noncoronary cusps. Thus the temporal echographic configuration of the aortic valve leaflets consists of single opening and closing motions of two leaflets, which manifest a box-type appearance during systole. Echo signals may also be recorded from the anterior tricuspid and posterior pulmonic valve leaflets and resemble the patterns of the mitral and aortic valves, respectively.

M-mode echocardiography affords only an "ice-pick view" of the heart, and image is restricted to the narrow area within the ultrasonic beam. Two-dimensional (2-D) echo expands the size of the ultrasound beam and provides a second axis. The second dimension offers spatial orientation throughout a large segment of the heart (Figs. 89-5 and 89-6). The increased field of view also allows definition of the perimeter of cardiac structures, thereby affording the capability to determine shape and anatomy. Finally, 2-D echo allows delineation of position or motion in the superoinferior or mediolateral plane as well as the anteroposterior plane recorded by M-mode echo. Accordingly, 2-D echo substantially improves the diagnostic information available.

Traditionally the long axis of the left ventricle, as inscribed by an M-mode scan, remains the cornerstone of 2-D echographic imaging (Fig. 89-5). The ultrasonic beam is directed along an axis from right shoulder to left iliac crest and provides a tomogram of the structures encountered from the plane of the aortic valve leaflets to the apex of the left ventricle. Subsequently the ultrasound transducer is rotated 90 degrees to traverse the heart along an axis from the left shoulder to the right iliac crest (the short axis plane; Fig. 89-6). Short axis views may be obtained at any level; the papillary muscles may be evaluated below the mitral valve leaflets, and the aorta, pulmonary artery, and atria may be imaged from the plane above the mitral valve leaflets.

CARDIAC CATHETERIZATION
Indications

Cardiac catheterization and angiography are indicated to establish definitive diagnoses, to make quantitative anatomic and hemodynamic assessments, to determine whether surgery should be performed, and to assess the results of surgery should signs and symptoms recur. The majority of catheterizations are performed in patients in whom a diagnosis has been made on clinical grounds but whose response to medical therapy is unsatisfactory. In these instances the procedure is pursued to substantiate the diagnosis, determine whether the condition is severe enough to warrant surgical intervention, and detect any associated lesions that may not be apparent clinically. In some circumstances catheterization is performed before the onset of refractory clinical symptoms. Thus in aortic stenosis associated with the onset of left ventricular failure, syncope, or angina, the prognosis can be significantly improved by valve replacement if catheterization demonstrates that the stenosis is severe and that left ventricular function is reasonably well preserved. In severely ill patients, bedside catheterization of the right side of the heart may be used to monitor and optimize pump performance.

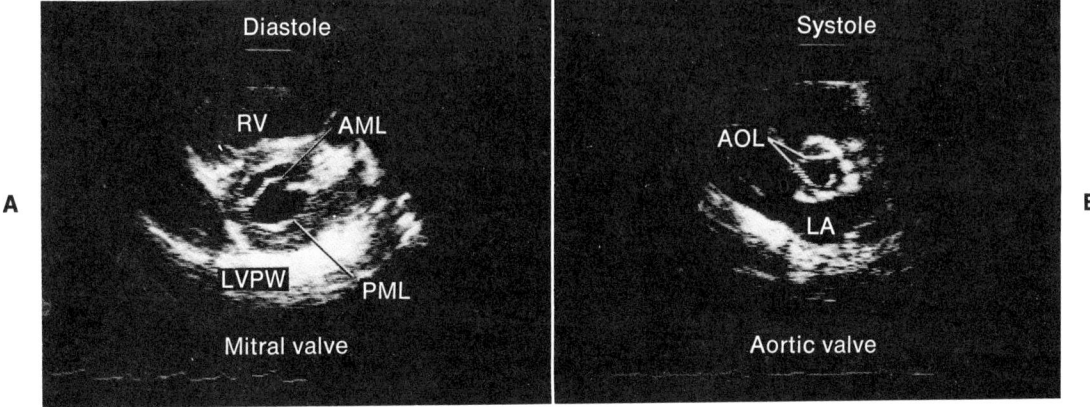

Fig. 89-6. Two-dimensional echocardiogram. Cross section through level of **A,** mitral valve (level 2) during diastole and **B,** aortic valve (level 3) during systole as if looking at heart from feet with anterior at top of the pictures, posterior at bottom, and patient's left to picture's right. All labels as in Fig. 89-5. (Slightly retouched for reproduction.)

Cardiac catheterization provides data concerning intracardiac pressure, cardiac output, vascular resistance, intracardiac shunt detection, valvular stenosis and regurgitation, and ventricular function.

Right-sided heart catheterization

Catheterization of the right side of the heart consists of introducing a radiopaque plastic catheter into a vein of adequate size and under fluoroscopic control passing it to the right-sided heart chambers and pulmonary artery. Pressures are recorded, blood samples are drawn from these sites, and indicator or radiopaque dyes are injected. Catheterization of the coronary sinus via the right atrium allows measurement of coronary blood flow and determination of myocardial metabolites such as lactate. Intracardiac electrocardiography and electrical stimulation are used to diagnose dysrhythmias and to conduct stress studies of the heart by rapid pacing. Recognition of an abnormal catheter course helps the diagnosis of certain congenital anomalies.

Right-sided heart catheterization is frequently indicated in patients with complicated myocardial infarction or in those with cardiac failure of other cause who have not responded to conventional therapy. Such bedside catheterization is facilitated by flow-directed, balloon-tipped catheters that allow performance of the procedure without the need for fluoroscopy. Some catheters can measure cardiac output by the thermodilution method, and the result is rapidly calculated and displayed by a computer. Measurement of cardiac output by the indicator dilution method with automated readout is also available. Multilumen catheter systems can produce, with a single catheter, measurement of right-sided heart pressures, including pulmonary capillary wedge (PCW) pressure, an important indicator of left ventricular performance; cardiac output; and sampling of blood from the chambers of the right side of the heart and pulmonary artery for measurement of gases and pH.

The relationship between PCW pressure and cardiac output, stroke volume, and stroke work defines cardiac function, and these factors are closely related to the prognosis of acute myocardial infarction. The PCW pressure is an important aid in differentiating dyspnea of cardiac origin from that of other causes and in determining whether hypotension is related to hypovolemia or cardiac insufficiency. This information may therefore be important in therapeutic decisions regarding volume expansion or diuresis.

Catheterization of the right side of the heart allows identification of ventricular septal defect and mitral regurgitation in acute myocardial infarction, a distinction that frequently cannot be made on the basis of the physical findings. Mitral regurgitation is recognized by large "v" waves in the PCW pressure pulse, whereas ventricular septal defect produces an increase in blood oxygen saturation between the right atrium and pulmonary artery and a characteristic alteration in the indicator dilution curve, reflecting a left-to-right intracardiac shunt.

The risks of right-sided heart catheterization include infection at the catheter insertion site, sepsis, arrhythmias during passage of the catheter through the right side of the heart, and pulmonary infarction. The complication rate is extremely low when the catheter is left in place 3 days or less.

In summary, right-sided heart catheterization can be readily performed at the bedside in critically ill cardiac patients. It provides important data concerning diagnosis, prognosis, and choice of therapy. The frequency of untoward effects is low.

Left-sided heart catheterization

Although right-sided heart catheterization permits definition of many congenital cardiac malformations, this technique provides only indirect information concerning the left side of the heart, which is primarily affected by most adult types of acquired heart disease. The retrograde arterial approach is the most widely employed in left-sided heart catheterization and can be combined with selective coronary arteriography. Aortography and left ventricular angiocardiography are particularly helpful in defining the size and continuity of the aorta and left ventricle and in assessing the severity of aortic and mitral regurgitation. The transseptal technique consists of right-sided catheterization with atrial septal puncture from the right atrium, with the advantage that both the left atrium and the left ventricle are entered.

Angiocardiography

Angiocardiography is the technique for evaluating the anatomy and function of the chambers of the heart and vascular tree by selective opacification. It requires injection of radiopaque contrast medium through a catheter while recording the event radiographically. Two filming methods, cineangiography and serial angiography, are used. Cineangiography involves motion picture films of fluoroscopic images. Serial angiography uses a rapid film changer and large size roentgenogram films at rates usually of 4 to 12 films/sec. This provides better definition of anatomic detail and a larger field.

Angiographic techniques are an integral part of most cardiac catheterizations to evaluate structure and function. The techniques most commonly employed in cardiology are ventriculography, coronary arteriography, pulmonary angiography, and aortography. Ventriculography and coronary arteriography are usually obtained by cineangiography. Angiography of the pulmonary vasculature and aorta is performed by the serial angiographic method.

Ventriculography of the left or right ventricle is used to demonstrate chamber volume, wall thickness, overall wall motion, segmental abnormalities of contraction (dyssynergy), and regurgitation through the atrioventricular valves. Ventricular ejection fraction (stroke volume divided by end-diastolic volume) is a sensitive, widely used index of ventricular function calculated from the ventriculogram. Coronary arteriography defines structural lesions in the coronary arteries for diagnostic purposes and determines whether myocardial revascularization surgery is indicated and feasible. Pulmonary angiography is used to detect structural abnormalities in the pulmonary circulation, to assess congenital heart disease and pulmonary hypertension, and to diagnose pulmonary embolism. Aortography identifies and measures the severity of structural abnormalities of the aorta and the competence of the aortic valve.

The potential complications of angiography include infection; vascular damage, hemorrhage, and trauma at the catheter insertion site; arrhythmias; and embolism. Serious morbidity (including myocardial infarction, cerebrovascular accident, and limb ischemia) and mortality are rare during cardiac angiography. Mortality is less than 0.5% and serious morbidity is less than 5% when the procedure is performed by skilled, experienced personnel. The incidence is reduced further in laboratories that perform more than 200 procedures per year.

NUCLEAR CARDIOLOGY

Nuclear cardiology is the use of radioisotopes to diagnose cardiac disease. The isotopes used typically emit γ-rays to maximize detection and minimize the radiation dose to the patient. Imaging of the γ-rays is usually accomplished with a scintillation camera. Technologic improvements in scintillation cameras and radiopharmaceuticals and the introduction of computer processing of scintillation data are providing accurate assessment of cardiovascular anatomy and physiology.

Two types of radiopharmaceuticals are currently used: those that label the blood pool and those that label the myocardium. Blood pool labeling requires injection of a radioisotope into the intravascular space, where it remains long enough to image the vascular compartment. First-transit studies, which last less than 30 seconds, can be done with any isotope that does not diffuse out of the intravascular space (especially into the lung parenchyma). Equilibrium blood pool scans require a more stable concentration of isotope in the intravascular space, usually attained by labeling the patient's red cells or human serum albumin with technetium 99m. There are two classes of clinically useful isotopes for labeling the myocardium. Isotopes that are incorporated into normal myocardial cells are used to evaluate myocardial perfusion. The prototype is thallium 201, which has a half-life of 72 hours. These isotopes are also known as "cold spot agents" because an area of decreased perfusion has less scintillation activity than normally perfused myocardium. Radioisotope complexes that are bound only to damaged myocardium, termed "hot spot agents," are used to diagnose myocardial infarction. The prototype is technetium 99m pyrophosphate.

BIBLIOGRAPHY

Berman, D., and Mason, D.T.: Clinical nuclear cardiology, New York, 1981, Grune & Stratton, Inc.
Braunwald, E.: Heart disease, Philadelphia, 1980, W.B. Saunders Co.
Feigenbaum, H.: Echocardiography, Philadelphia, 1976, Lea & Febiger.
Friedman, H.H.: Diagnostic electrocardiography and vector-cardiography, New York, 1977, McGraw-Hill Book Co.
Gensini, G.G.: Coronary arteriography, Mount Kisco, N.Y., 1975, Futura Publications Co.
Grossman, W.: Cardiac catheterization and angiography, Philadelphia, 1980, Lea & Febiger.
Hurst, J.W., and others: The heart, arteries, and veins, New York, 1978, McGraw-Hill Book Co.
Lipman, B.S., Massie, E., and Kleiger, R.E.: Clinical scalar electrocardiography, Chicago, 1972, Year Book Medical Publishers, Inc.
Marriott, H.J.L.: Practical electrocardiography, Baltimore, 1972, The Williams & Wilkins Co.
Mendel, D.: A practice of cardiac catheterisation, London, 1974, Blackwell Scientific Publications.
Strauss, H.W., and Pitt, B.: Cardiovascular nuclear medicine, ed. 2, St. Louis, 1979, The C.V. Mosby Co.

90 • PULMONARY EMBOLISM

Steven G. Meister and Toby R. Engel

PATHOGENESIS. Thrombi and other solid objects that gain access to an arterial system are carried distally until they impact in a branch and cause obstruction. This process is called embolization. Most emboli in the pulmonary arterial tree are thrombi formed in the larger systemic veins (usually in the legs and pelvis) that become detached from the vein wall, float into the right-sided heart chambers, and are expelled into the pulmonary artery. Embolization occurs most commonly to the lower lobes, and more often to the right lung than the left.

Infected thrombi arise in veins that are draining areas of infection, particularly in the pelvis, and become septic emboli, resulting in abscesses when they impact in the pulmonary tree. Less commonly the chambers or valves of the right side of the heart serve as a source of thrombi. Other substances, such as fat, bone marrow, tumor fragments, air, vegetations from infected right-sided heart valves, and even foreign bodies such as shotgun pellets, can embolize to the pulmonary circulation. However, in the following discussion the term "pulmonary embolism" refers to thrombotic material.

Emboli in the pulmonary arterial tree cause complete or partial obstruction of a branch. However, the pulmonary arterial circulation can absorb a remarkable amount of embolic material without an appreciable rise in overall resistance to blood flow. Approximately 50% of the pulmonary tree must be occluded for resistance to rise sufficiently to cause a measurable increase in pressure in the pulmonary artery.

Occasionally a large pulmonary embolus by itself can occude a large portion of the pulmonary vasculature by "saddling" the bifurcation of the main pulmonary artery. More commonly symptomatic emboli are smaller but multiple in number, recurring several times over days and weeks. The effects of multiple emboli are additive and result in a rise in pulmonary arterial pressure when enough of the arterial tree has been occluded. In some patients emboli occur repeatedly and chronically over several weeks and months, creating chronic pulmonary hypertension, right ventricular hypertrophy, and eventual failure. This produces a clinical picture difficult to distinguish from chronic right-sided heart failure of other origins.

Another mechanism whereby pulmonary embolization results in pulmonary hypertension was suggested by infusion of small, fresh, experimentally produced thrombi into dogs, resulting in increased pulmonary vascular resistance and pressure. This effect was observed with emboli much too small to cause pulmonary hypertension from mechanical obstruction, suggesting that a vasoconstrictor substance was released from the thrombus itself. Increased resistance and pressure did not occur in animals pretreated with heparin.

The right ventricle is a thin-walled chamber designed for pumping blood at relatively low pressures. However, when abruptly called on to generate systolic pressures greater than about twice the normal pulmonary pressure of 25 to 30 mm Hg, the right ventricle fails acutely. This in turn results in increased right atrial–systemic venous pressure and reduced cardiac output. On the other hand, a right ventricle that has undergone gradual hypertrophy because of pressure loading, as in mitral stenosis or chronic left-sided heart failure, can frequently sustain substantially higher pressures without failing.

Probably from the moment an embolus arrives in the pulmonary circulation it is subject to thrombolytic mechanisms that work toward its gradual breakdown and eventual absorption. This process can proceed at variable rates and to different stages of completion. Serial angiographic studies in man have emphasized this variability. In some patients massive pulmonary emboli have virtually disappeared in less than 2 weeks. In others, particularly the elderly, the clearing process is much slower and may never be completed.

Unlike most other tissues, the pulmonary parenchyma has a dual blood supply, consisting of the pulmonary arterial system and the bronchial arterial circulation arising from the aorta. This dual supply accounts for the infrequency of parenchymal infarction as a consequence of pulmonary embolization. Nevertheless, infarction and necrosis do occur, particularly in the setting of preexisting left ventricular failure. Necrosis produces a clinical picture similar to lobar or segmental pneumonitis. Infarctions are ultimately converted to relatively avascular scar tissue, causing a permanent loss of pulmonary vasculature.

The consequences of pulmonary embolization are highly variable, depending on whether the embolism is small or massive, whether emboli are single or multiple, whether pulmonary hypertension and right ventricular failure occur, and whether pulmonary infarction results. Therefore the clinical picture is extremely diverse and often confusing.

PREDISPOSING FACTORS. Acute pulmonary embolism is seldom an isolated entity. Its occurrence depends on a source of thrombotic material in either the large systemic veins or the right-sided heart chambers. These in turn seldom occur in the absence of an identifiable predisposing factor, the recognition of which provides important clues to the diagnosis of the pulmonary embolism. Any factor that predisposes to phlebitis of the deep systemic veins predisposes to pulmonary embolism.

Among the most common factors in otherwise healthy individuals are orthopedic injuries, particularly of the lower extremities and pelvis. Leg casts, especially poorly fitting ones that compress the deep veins, are often associated with embolism. Hip fractures are an extremely common antecedent in the elderly. The extent of the orthopedic injury bears no relationship to the magnitude of the embolic syndrome that may be produced: a small cast on the lower leg may initiate a deep venous thrombosis that propagates proximally to the femoral or iliac veins and eventuates in a massive pulmonary embolism.

Major surgery of any type predisposes to deep venous thrombosis and pulmonary embolism so often that many surgeons advocate prophylactic anticoagulation with small doses of heparin before certain major procedures such as hip surgery.

Acute myocardial infarction, cardiogenic shock, and congestive heart failure are also predisposing factors, perhaps because reduction in cardiac output results in sluggish flow and consequent thrombus formation in the larger systemic veins. In congestive cardiomyopathies there is also mural thrombus formation, and thus emboli can arise from the right-sided heart chambers. Myocardial infarction involving the interventricular septum or the free walls of the right ventricle occasionally results in mural thrombosis and subsequent pulmonary embolization.

Pregnancy and oral contraceptives sometimes cause pulmonary embolism in healthy women. Compression of the inferior vena cava by the gravid uterus results in congestion and dilation of the veins of the pelvis and lower extremities, enhancing thrombus formation. The estrogenic component of contraceptives alters platelet adhesiveness and predisposes to thrombus formation.

Malignancies are another predisposing factor for venous thrombosis and pulmonary embolism. Recurrent *migratory* thrombophlebitis sometimes provides the first clue to the presence of a neoplasm. The mechanism whereby neoplasms induce venous thrombosis is not known.

CLINICAL MANIFESTATIONS. The most common symptom of acute pulmonary embolism is dyspnea at rest, typically of abrupt onset. Patients commonly complain of being unable to get enough air. Dyspnea at rest usually subsides after 1 or 2 hours but is often recurrent. Successive episodes are often noted to be of progressive severity and duration. The individual episodes probably correspond to successive embolic events. Subsidence of each episode may correspond to partial breakup and distal migration of the individual embolus. When dyspnea at rest has subsided, patients often describe persistence of dyspnea on slight exertion. Coughing of abrupt onset is also common.

A single massive embolus or many smaller emboli can result in pulmonary arterial obstruction sufficient to cause hypotension, light-headedness, or even syncope, but this is not common. Pain similar to that of acute myocardial infarction is also uncommon; when it occurs, it is probably a manifestation of sudden dilation of the pulmonary artery caused by hypertension.

With pulmonary infarction there is necrosis of a wedge-shaped segment of parenchyma that abuts on the pleura. Inflammation of visceral pleura overlying the infarct causes pain on deep inspiration, coughing, and sneezing. Hemoptysis is a consequence of the hemorrhagic nature of the infarct. Fever may also occur.

Some patients with chronic congestive heart failure complain only of a worsening of their congestive symptoms. Because of this, it is often suggested that acute pulmonary embolism can cause acute pulmonary edema. The dyspnea associated with pulmonary embolism can be acute and severe and suggest pulmonary edema, but it is doubtful that the embolism actually causes pulmonary edema. Cardiac pulmonary edema results from increased pressure within the pulmonary capillary bed because of increased left atrial pressure, and pulmonary arterial obstruction tends to *lower* pulmonary capillary and left atrial pressures. Confusion may result because, as will subsequently be detailed, pulmonary congestion resulting from left-sided heart failure causes false positive results in certain diagnostic tests for pulmonary embolism.

It is important to emphasize that many pulmonary emboli, particularly when small, cause no symptoms. They are often first discovered on the autopsy table. This is partly because physical findings of pulmonary embolism are frequently absent; emboli that cause neither right-sided heart failure nor pulmonary infarction seldom produce physical findings.

Acute right-sided heart failure causes elevated right ventricular diastolic pressure and consequently elevated right atrial and systemic venous pressure. The internal or external jugular veins become distended, with a pulsation at the time of right atrial contraction (timed with an S_4 gallop, preceding the first heart sound). The pulmonic component of the second heart sound may be accentuated. The second sound may be widely split because of resistance to systolic ejection of the right ventricle resulting in delayed closure of the pulmonic valve. Less commonly a right ventricular S_3 gallop can be heard, which is loudest in the third and fourth intercostal space at the left sternal border and increases with inspiration. Occasionally a right ventricular lift is palpable at the lower left sternal border. A very unusual but well-documented finding in acute pulmonary embolism is pulsus paradoxus.

If infarction occurs, the findings are similar to bacterial pneumonia (rales, fever, signs of consolidation, pleural effusion, and/or friction rub).

The local findings of thrombosis of the deep veins of the legs or pelvis provide a clue to the presence of pulmonary embolism. However, deep venous thrombosis can be devoid of physical findings. In fact the loosely attached thrombi that are most likely to detach from the venous endothelium to become emboli are also the least likely to cause the complete venous obstruction and local inflammation responsible for the characteristic signs of thrombophlebitis. Furthermore, the responsible thrombus may well have embolized in its entirety to the lungs by the time the patient is evaluated for acute pulmonary embolism.

LABORATORY FINDINGS. The electrocardiogram shows features of right ventricular overload only when pulmonary embolism is massive. The combination of an S wave in lead I, a Q wave in lead III, and an inverted T wave in lead III occurs with a right ventricular overload. Right precordial T inversion, abnormal rightward deviation of the QRS axis, and right bundle branch block are other signs. Increased right atrial pressure can be accompanied by enlargement of the P wave in leads II, III, and a V_f.

A variety of abnormalities are seen on the chest film. Pulmonary infarction is often associated with an infiltrate, sometimes pyramidal in shape (with the apex pointing toward the hilum), corresponding to the segmental distribution of the occluded vessel. There may be elevation of the diaphragm on the affected side and horizontal streaks at the bases, representing thin irregular bands of atelectasis.

In the absence of pulmonary infarction underperfused areas may appear more radiolucent than adjacent normal areas. In the presence of massive pulmonary embolism the nonembolized segments are overperfused and the resulting vascular engorgement may appear as an infiltrate. In the presence of marked pulmonary hypertension prominence of the main pulmonary arteries is sometimes notable.

It should be emphasized that these findings are inconstant and not specific. In fact a paucity of findings on the chest roentgenogram when the patient complains of severe dyspnea should suggest pulmonary embolism.

Arterial hypoxemia is usually present, regardless of whether there is right-sided heart failure or pulmonary infarction. It was noted in the early 1970s that the partial pressure of oxygen in the blood (Pao_2) was less than 80 mm Hg in most patients and below 90 mm Hg in all patients with pulmonary embolism breathing room air. However there have since been a number of cases of well-documented acute pulmonary embolism with Pao_2 in excess of 90 mm Hg. Thus normal Pao_2 does not exclude acute pulmonary embolism.

It must also be emphasized that an abnormally low Pao_2 is not specific and occurs in a number of conditions that may simulate the clinical picture of acute pulmonary embolus. Among these are congestive heart failure, chronic obstructive lung disease, viral and bacterial pneumonitis, and acute asthmatic attacks.

Other laboratory findings in pulmonary embolism may include decreased arterial $Paco_2$, leukocytosis and elevated erythrocyte sedimentation rate, serum indirect bilirubin, serum lactic dehydrogenase, and fibrin split products. However, these are not constant findings and are therefore of limited diagnostic value.

RADIONUCLIDE STUDIES AND PULMONARY ANGIOGRAPHY. Perfusion scanning of the lungs is a useful screening test for pulmonary embolism. Albumin is treated so that the molecules aggregate to a particle size that will not pass through the pulmonary capillaries and is labeled with a short-lived radioactive isotope of technetium. It is infused intravenously and passes to the pulmonary capillary bed, where the particles are trapped. Scintillation scanning of the thorax creates a series of images corresponding to the distribution of the labeled particles. When embolism is present, the particles are not distributed to lung segments supplied by obstructed arteries, creating filling defects on the scan (Fig. 90-1). The number of particles injected is too small to cause pulmonary vascular obstruction or hemodynamic consequences. (A rare exception is seen with advanced pulmonary vascular disease and extreme pulmonary hypertension, in which the injected particles may aggravate right ventricular failure and induce profound hypotension.)

Perfusion lung scanning is highly sensitive, and for practical purposes a normal scan excludes pulmonary embolism. Unfortunately, like the measurement of Pao_2, perfusion scanning is nonspecific and is abnormal in a variety of conditions, including some that have features resembling acute pulmonary embolism. In congestive heart failure there is reduced flow to the lower lobes that often creates scan defects. Fluid in the lung fissures or at the bases can also cause false positive scans. In obstructive lung disease poorly ventilated segments have reduced perfusion on lung scan. Areas of pneumonitis also result in an abnormal scan.

Improved specificity can be achieved by a variety of strategies. Simple comparison of the lung scan to chest roentgenograms obtained at the same time is helpful in that scan defects corresponding to infiltrates and fluid collections should be disregarded. It is useful to determine whether the filling defects on scan correspond to the known segmental anatomy of the lungs, since the pulmonary artery tree corresponds closely to segmental anatomy.

Combined ventilation-perfusion lung scanning contrasts the images produced on standard perfusion scanning with those made following inhalation of radioactive xenon. Defects in the perfusion scan that are related to reflex under-perfusion of poorly ventilated areas can be identified and disregarded (Fig. 90-1).

Pulmonary angiography is the most specific test for diagnosis of pulmonary embolism. It uses a radiopaque organic iodide-containing contrast material, which is introduced via a catheter passed through the right side of the heart into the main pulmonary artery or its subdivisions. The entire pulmonary arterial tree can be clearly visualized to the level of branches about 2 mm in diameter. Pulmonary embolism is demonstrated by an intravascular thrombus or an occluded ("cutoff") vessel (Fig. 90-2). A variety of normal anatomic features such as overlapping or branching vessels can resemble intravascular clots or cutoff vessels.

MANAGEMENT. The principal therapy for acute pulmonary embolus is anticoagulation. The rationale is prevention of additional thrombus formation at the site of origin to prevent further embolization while natural thrombolytic mechanisms digest the embolized clots. This is effective for the majority of patients. It should be done initially in the hospital with heparin sulfate. It is usually advisable to begin heparin therapy as soon as the diagnosis is strongly suspected while waiting for the diagnostic tests to be performed. Subcutaneous injection, intravenous bolus injection, and constant intravenous infusion are alternative approaches to heparinization. Whichever is used, frequent monitoring of the partial thromboplastin time is useful to select the size and timing of subsequent doses and to avoid inadequate or excessive anticoagulation. A partial thromboplastin time two to two and one half times longer than control values is generally considered optimal. When subcutaneous or intravenous bolus injection is used, the partial thromboplastin time should be drawn 1 hour before the next scheduled dose, when it should be two to two and one half times control values.

There is no evidence that anticoagulation with injected heparin is any more or less effective than with oral warfarin (Coumadin). However, warfarin's effect (against hepatic synthesis of clotting proteins) is not seen for 48 hours. Thus "warfarinization" can be begun after heparinization has been achieved, and heparin should be continued until warfarin has prolonged the prothrombin time (PT) two to three times longer than control values. The doses are adjusted to maintain PT at two to two and one half times control values.

Disadvantages of anticoagulation include bleeding at therapeutic levels in predisposed patients and in others when the therapeutic range is exceeded. Bleeding from heparinization is a common and serious in-hospital cause of drug-induced morbidity. Numerous common prescription and nonprescription drugs accentuate or diminish warfarin's action. Patients receiving long-term warfarin therapy should have PT checked *at least* once monthly. Three to

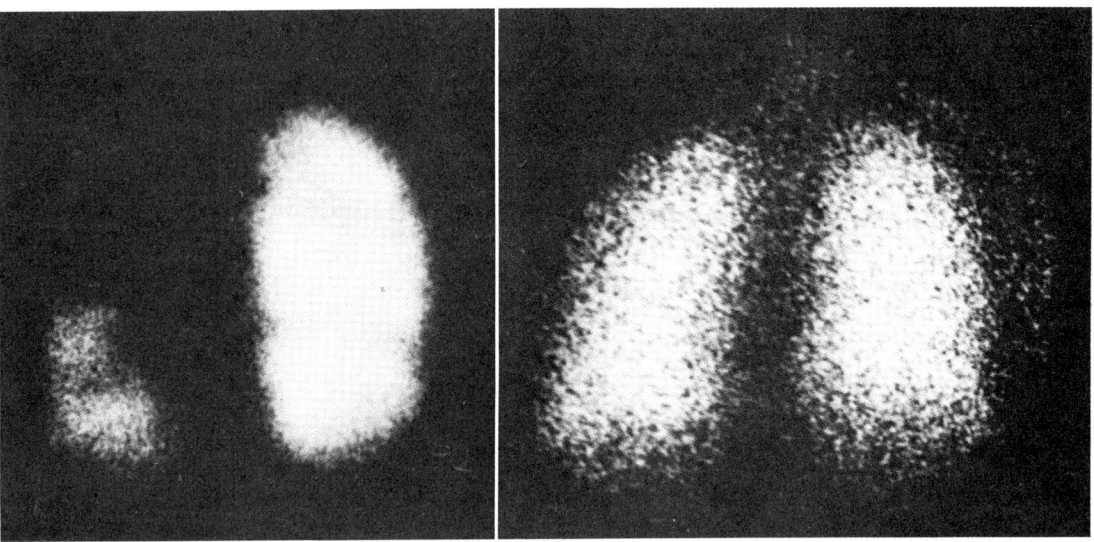

Fig. 90-1. Perfusion *(left)* and ventilation *(right)* scans in patient with massive pulmonary embolism involving lung. Note that one lung is nearly obliterated on perfusion scan and normally represented on ventilation scan.

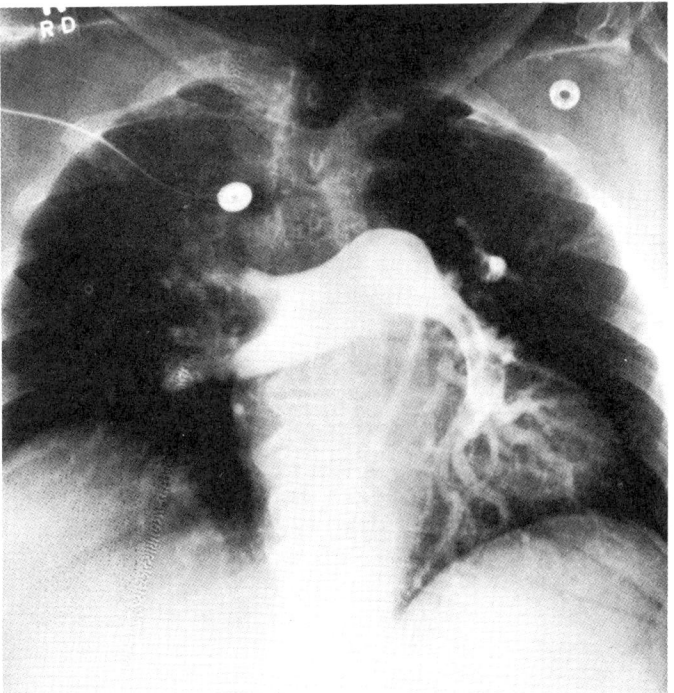

Fig. 90-2. Massive emboli to both lungs seen on pulmonary angiography. Major arteries to entire right lung and left upper lobe are occluded (cutoff). Left lower lobe artery contains several large, serpentine filling defects.

six months of anticoagulation is generally appropriate after embolization. Those with a predisposition to pulmonary embolism who have had documented emboli should be anticoagulated indefinitely.

Patients who cannot be anticoagulated or who have had recurrent pulmonary emboli while on *adequate* anticoagulation can have interruption of their inferior vena cava (IVC). Transverse compartmentalization of the IVC with a series of sutures or a specially designed clip permits continuing blood flow through the vessel without permitting passage of large thrombi. This procedure entails morbidity and potential mortality and should never be done without angiographic documentation of embolization. In the occasional patient who is too ill to undergo an operative procedure, a sievelike device ("umbrella") can be implanted pervenously in the IVC via a specially designed catheter system. Recurrent embolism after IVC interruption has been reported; however, these recurrences generally have not been angiographically documented. Enlarged collateral vessels around the interruption were implicated, but these are less likely when plication is used rather than ligation.

Acute submassive pulmonary emboli can result in asthmatic or shocklike states. This may in part result from release of vasoactive substances from platelets and other components of the emboli that cause bronchial and pulmonary arterial constriction. Initial therapy consists of heparin, oxygen, and agents such as dopamine to increase cardiac output.

In one extensive multicenter trial the thrombolytic agents urokinase and streptokinase were found to induce marginally faster clearing of emboli from the pulmonary vasculature than heparin alone. They may be appropriate in patients in persistent circulatory shock from massive embolization. However, substantial morbidity and mortality from bleeding result, and these agents should be used only when essential. An alternative approach in persistent shock is surgical embolectomy. However, most patients either become normotensive or die in the 1 or 2 hours required to prepare for open heart surgery.

Since the 1960s it has become evident from pathologic studies that pulmonary emboli are often found at autopsy (in some series, in the majority of autopsies following hospital death). The clinical significance of clots found at autopsy has probably been magnified by the association of pulmonary emboli with morbid conditions. For example, dyspnea and hemoptysis in mitral stenosis can be caused by the underlying pulmonary congestion even though mitral stenosis predisposes to pulmonary embolism. Unfortunately, the apparent incidence of pulmonary embolization is magnified by positive diagnostic tests that are quite frequently falsely positive. The chest roentgenogram, serum enzymes, arterial blood gases, electrocardiogram, and lung scan are sensitive but frequently inaccurate.

Anticoagulation carries the risk of morbidity and mortality. The key to proper management is therefore proper diagnosis. At present this still demands pulmonary arteriography whenever possible. In most cases the risk of angiography is less than the risk of anticoagulation. Frequently initiation of therapy, as with heparin, is appropriate before an accurate diagnosis can be established, but continued or chronic anticoagulation can then often be avoided by requiring confirmation with angiography.

BIBLIOGRAPHY

Bell, W.R., and Simon, T.L.: A comparative analysis of pulmonary perfusion scans with pulmonary angiograms (from a national cooperative study), Am. Heart J. **92:**700, 1976.

Burdine, J.A., and Wallace, J.M.: Pulsus paradoxus and Kussmaul's sign in massive pulmonary embolism, Am. J. Cardiol. **15:**413, 1965.

Coon, W.W.: Some recent developments in the pharmacology of heparin, J. Clin. Pharmacol. **21:**337, 1979.

Dalen, J.E., and others: Resolution of acute pulmonary embolism in man, N. Engl. J. Med. **280:**1194, 1969.

Dalen, J.E., and others: Pulmonary embolism, pulmonary hemorrhage and pulmonary infarction, N. Engl. J. Med. **296:**1431, 1977.

Gurewich, V., Cohen, M.L., and Thomas, D.P.: Humoral factors in massive pulmonary embolism: an experimental study, Am. Heart J. **76:**784, 1968.

Gurewich, V., Duncan, P.T., and Rabinov, K.R.: Pulmonary embolism after ligation of the inferior vena cava, N. Engl. J. Med. **274:**1350, 1966.

Hyland, J.W., and others: Effect of selective embolization of various sized pulmonary arteries in dogs, Am. J. Physiol. **204:**619, 1963.

McIntyre, K.M., and Sasahara, A.A.: The hemodynamic response to pulmonary embolism in patients without prior cardiopulmonary disease, Am. J. Cardiol. **28:**288, 1971.

Poulose, K.P., and others: Diagnosis of pulmonary embolism: a correlative study of the clinical, scan, and angiographic findings, Br. Med. J. **3:**67, 1970.

Robin, E.D.: Overdiagnosis and overtreatment of pulmonary embolism: the emperor may have no clothes, Ann. Intern. Med. **87:**775, 1977.

Sagar, S., and others: Efficacy of low-dose heparin in prevention of extensive deep-vein thrombosis in patients undergoing total-hip replacement., Lancet **1:**1151, 1976.

Szucs, M., Jr., and others: Diagnostic sensitivity of laboratory findings in acute pulmonary embolism, Ann. Intern. Med. **74:**161, 1971.

91 • THROMBOPHLEBITIS

Steven G. Meister

PATHOPHYSIOLOGY. Thrombophlebitis is inflammation from thrombus formation within a vein. It is common and results from venous stasis, local injury to venous endothelium, or altered blood coagulability. Factors causing stasis of venous blood include congestive heart failure, myocardial infarction, prolonged bed rest, prolonged maintenance of the legs in a cramped position, pregnancy, tight constricting casts or garments, and obesity. Damage to venous endothelium may result from physical trauma, intravenous lines and needles, infection, and vasculitis. A variety of systemic conditions, including carcinomatosis, the postoperative and postpartum states, polycythemia, and hyperviscosity syndrome, predispose to thrombophlebitis by altering blood coagulability. Thrombophlebitis at multiple sites, simultaneously or in rapid succession, is known as migratory thrombophlebitis. It suggests the presence of polycythemia or occult malignancy.

Thrombophlebitis occurs most commonly in the veins of the lower extremities and pelvis and may involve either the deep or the superficial veins. In the deep veins of the thighs and pelvis portions of thrombi often break loose and are carried proximally to become pulmonary emboli. This rarely occurs with superficial phlebitis or phlebitis of the upper extremities. Deep vein thrombophlebitis can also damage the venous valves, causing them to become incompetent. This causes chronic venous stasis in the lower extremities and predisposes to recurrent phlebitis in the same veins.

CLINICAL MANIFESTATIONS. Superficial thrombophlebitis is an acute inflammation along the course of a superficial vein with redness, induration, and edema. Often the vein itself is visible or, more often, palpable and tender. Symptoms of deep vein thrombophlebitis range from none at all to severe pain. Most patients complain of nothing more than dull aching deep within the involved limb. Fever may be present.

Physical findings, when present, are related to venous inflammation or obstruction. Inflammation can give rise to a palpable, tender cord along the course of the vein. Obstruction produces distal swelling and congestion of the limb. The skin color is dusky, and the skin temperature is appreciably warmer than that of the uninvolved limb. The superficial veins distal to the obstruction also appear distended. Calf tenderness and Homans' sign, midcalf pain elicited by passive dorsiflexion of the foot, are present. Unfortunately, these findings are not always present. In fact, those thrombi most loosely attached to the venous endothelium, and thus *least* likely to be associated with either inflammation or obstruction, are most likely to detach and become emboli. Accordingly, laboratory tests are often needed to establish a diagnosis of acute deep vein thrombophlebitis.

Damage to the venous valves from recurrent deep vein phlebitis results in chronic venous stasis with edema, pigmentation, and skin ulceration (postphlebitic syndrome).

LABORATORY FINDINGS. The most reliable test is injection of roentgenographic contrast medium into the veins of the feet. Serial roentgenograms are made as contrast material progresses through the deep venous system of the legs and pelvis. Thrombi appear as filling defects. This test is definitive; its drawbacks are that it is an invasive procedure involving moderate discomfort and slight risk, as well as considerable expense.

There are several noninvasive but less reliable alternative tests. Radioiodinated fibrinogen is taken up by an actively growing thrombus. Scintillation scanning will reveal a "hot spot" over a thrombus. This is a highly sensitive technique for detecting even small thrombi distal to the midthigh, but it is less reliable for the more important proximal thrombi and is of little value in the pelvis. It is precisely these more proximal leg and pelvic thrombi that have been implicated in pulmonary embolism. Impedance phlebography measures minute fluctuations in electrical impedance of the legs that occur as a consequence of normal respiratory variations in blood volume. Both arterial and venous flow patterns are present and easily distinguishable. Absence of the normal venous fluctuations with inspiration is found when deep veins are obstructed by thrombus. Doppler phlebography uses the phase shift of high-frequency sound waves reflected from moving blood cells to detect blood flow in large veins. It can detect absent flow when there is venous obstruction. Both phlebography tests show 80% to 90% sensitivity to obstructing thrombi in the iliac and femoral veins but are much less sensitive to more distal disease. Both may give negative results when a nonobstructing thrombus is present; this thrombus is less firmly attached and thus is more likely to embolize.

MANAGEMENT AND PREVENTION. Superficial phlebitis is treated with analgesics, moist heat, elevation of the involved extremity, and bed rest. Deep vein phlebitis is treated in the same fashion, and anticoagulation is used as described in Chapter 90. Anticoagulation should be continued for 3 to 6 months. If thrombophlebitis is recurrent, long-term (even lifelong) treatment may be necessary.

Patients at risk for thrombophlebitis because of immobilization (for example, resulting from massive fractures, myocardial infarction, and major surgery) should be considered for prophylactic anticoagulation with heparin.

BIBLIOGRAPHY

Adar, R., and Salgman, W.E.: Treatment of thrombosis of veins of the lower extremities, N. Engl. J. Med. **292:**348, 1975.

Barber, H.M., and others: A comparative study of dextran-70, warfarin and low-dose heparin for the prophylaxis of thrombo-embolism following total hip replacement, Postgrad. Med. J. **53:**130, 1977.

Dmochowski, J.R., Adams, D.F., and Couch, N.P.: Impedance measurement in the diagnosis of deep venous thrombosis, Arch. Surg. **104:**170, 1972.

Nicoliades, A.N., and others: The origin of deep vein thromboses: a venographic study, Br. J. Radiol. **44:**653, 1971.

Provan, J.L., and Thomson, C.: Natural history of thrombophlebitis and its relationship to pulmonary embolism, Can. J. Surg. **16:**284, 1973.

Rabinov, K., and Paulin, S.: Roentgen diagnosis of venous thrombosis in the leg, Arch. Surg. **104:**134, 1972.

Steer, M.L., and others: Limitations of impedance phlebography for diagnosis of venous thrombosis, Arch. Surg. **106:**44, 1973.

Yao, S.T., Gourmos, C., and Hobbs, J.T.: Detection of proximal-vein thromboses by Doppler ultrasound flow-detection method, Lancet **1:**1, 1972.

92 • PRIMARY PULMONARY HYPERTENSION

Nelson M. Wolf

Pulmonary hypertension, as defined by a pulmonary artery pressure of greater than 30/15 mm Hg, may be secondary to cardiac diseases. These include conditions that cause an increase in pulmonary venous pressure, such as left ventricular failure, mitral valve disease, and thrombus or myxoma of the left atrium. In addition, any condition that causes chronic hypoventilation, such as chronic obstructive lung disease, neuromuscular disorders, or severe kyphoscoliosis, may also result in pulmonary hypertension. Disorders that cause a reduction in the pulmonary vascular bed (including pulmonary emboli, arteritis, schistosomiasis, Eisenmenger's syndrome from congenital cardiac defects, and various interstitial parenchymal disorders such as interstitial fibrosis and interstitial granulomatosis) may also cause pulmonary hypertension.

The syndrome of *primary* pulmonary hypertension occurs with a frequency of about 0.2% to 0.17%. It is more common in persons younger than 40, and females outnumber males 3:1. Although no cause has been determined, primary pulmonary hypertension has been associated with collagen vascular disease, Raynaud's syndrome, the use of oral contraceptive agents, and the anorexic agent aminorex.

PATHOLOGY. The histologic changes seen in the pulmonary arteries in primary pulmonary hypertension can be found in severe pulmonary hypertension of other origins. The changes are intimal proliferation, medial hypertrophy, plexiform lesions, fibrinoid necrosis, and arteritis. These pathologic changes involve primarily the pulmonary arterioles and small muscular pulmonary arteries. A grading system has been developed that correlates with altered hemodynamics. Grade 1 shows thickening of the medial and adventitial muscular coat. Grade 2 involves intimal cell proliferation in the smaller pulmonary arteries and arterioles. In grade 3 medial hypertrophy occurs as well as progressive intimal proliferation. In grade 4 dilation of the pulmonary arteries occurs and the plexiform lesion may be seen. In grade 5 chronic dilation occurs with medial and intimal fibrosis. At this point, the intima may be acellular and essentially hyalinized. In grade 6 a necrotizing arteritis occurs. Beyond grade 4 the pulmonary hypertension is thought to be irreversible.

The pathogenesis of the disorder is not understood; however, two mechanisms have been proposed. One involves initial vasoconstriction of the smaller muscular pulmonary arteries and pulmonary arterioles. After prolonged vasoconstriction, the more advanced fixed lesions occur. The second mechanism proposed involves multiple small pulmonary emboli. At the advanced stage of disease the histology cannot be used to support one mechanism over the other.

CLINICAL MANIFESTATIONS. After an asymptomatic period of variable duration, the patient may experience multiple symptoms. As the pulmonary vascular bed becomes destroyed, the cardiac output falls. This results in the heart's inability to increase its cardiac output with exertion. The patient may then suffer from exertional dyspnea, fatigue, effort syncope, or angina. Palpitations may occur as various arrhythmias occur. Eventually right-sided heart failure occurs; sudden death is a common outcome.

The physical findings are a reflection of right ventricular hypertrophy and pulmonary hypertension. The central venous pressure is elevated with prominent a waves (representing atrial contraction). As tricuspid regurgitation develops, this may be replaced by a regurgitant venous wave. The chest is clear to auscultation and percussion. Cardiac examination may reveal a left lower sternal lift; this is a reflection of the right ventricular dilation. The first heart sound is usually well preserved, and the second heart sound is characterized by an accentuated pulmonic valve component (P_2), which may be palpable. The second heart sound is closely split. An ejection sound, which reflects dilation of the main pulmonary artery, is often present. A fourth heart sound, originating from the right ventricle and varying with the respiratory cycle, is often heard. Cardiac murmurs, particularly those of tricuspid regurgitation or pulmonic valvular insufficiency resulting from pulmonary artery hypertension, may be audible in the later phases of the disease. If right-sided heart failure ensues, ascites and peripheral edema may be found. In addition, with tricuspid regurgitation systolic pulsations of the liver may be palpated.

When the cardiac output becomes severely compromised, peripheral cyanosis may develop. In addition, with the elevation of the right atrial pressure, a foramen ovale may be opened and a small right-to-left shunt may occur, resulting in cyanosis.

The electrocardiogram reveals right axis deviation and right ventricular hypertrophy. The chest roentgenogram (Fig. 92-1) shows a prominent right ventricle, right atrium, and main pulmonary arteries. The smaller pulmonary arteries appear attenuated.

The echocardiogram shows an enlarged right ventricle and right atrium. The pulmonic valve motion is characterized by a relatively small a wave, as is noted with any cause of pulmonary hypertension. No evidence for left ventricular enlargement or mitral valvular abnormality is found. The septum may move in an abnormal fashion.

Pulmonary function studies show no appreciable abnormalities. The arterial blood gases reveal normal systemic saturation with some hypocapnia, indicative of hyperventilation.

Cardiac catheterization shows a markedly elevated pulmonary artery pressure with a normal wedge pressure. The calculated pulmonary vascular resistance is high, but no left-to-right shunt, mitral valvular disorder, or left ventricular dysfunction is found. Although the definitive diagno-

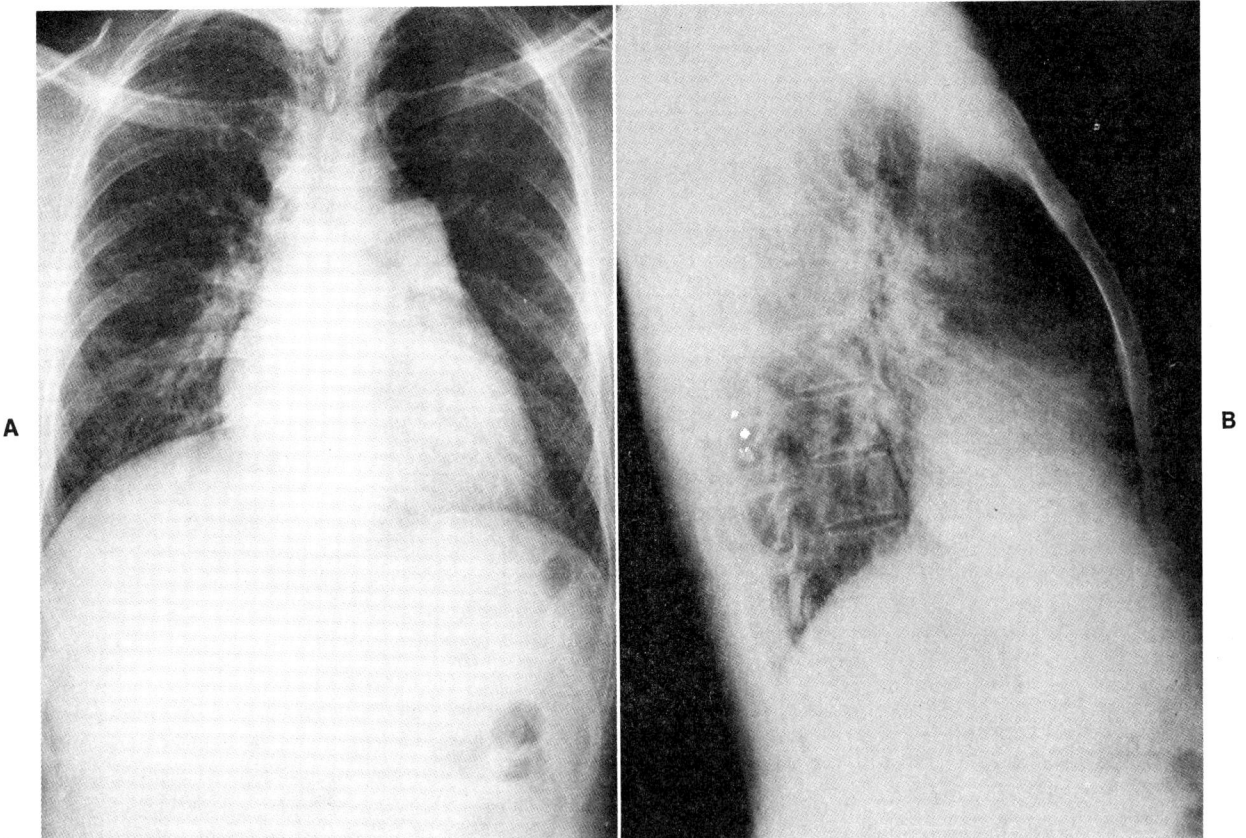

Fig. 92-1. **A,** Posteroanterior and **B,** lateral chest roentgenograms from 26-year-old male with primary pulmonary hypertension, showing cardiac enlargement, particularly of right ventricle, with prominence of main pulmonary arteries and attenuation of peripheral pulmonary arteries.

sis of primary pulmonary hypertension cannot be made before autopsy, a presumptive diagnosis can be made if the secondary causes are excluded.

The course of the disease is variable; however, most patients average a life expectancy of 3 to 7 years once symptoms ensue. A rare patient will survive for longer than 10 years.

Medications have been used to decrease the pulmonary vascular resistance with variable success. These have included oxygen therapy (particularly if hypoxia exists), isoproterenol, hydralazine, and diazoxide. However, systemic vasodilators may increase cardiac output, thereby increasing pulmonary hypertension and worsening symptoms. Since multiple pulmonary emboli cannot be excluded with certainty, anticoagulation has been used. There is no evidence that any of these medicines prolong survival. Patients with primary pulmonary hypertension tolerate pregnancy and procedures such as anesthesia, sedation, surgery, cardiac catheterization, and angiography poorly, often with fatal results.

BIBLIOGRAPHY

Kleiger, R.E., and others: Pulmonary hypertension in patients using oral contraceptives, Chest **69:**143, 1976.

Rubin, L.J., and Peter, R.H.: Oral hydralazine therapy for primary pulmonary hypertension, N. Engl. J. Med. **302:**69, 1980.

Shettigar, U.R., and others: Primary pulmonary hypertension, N. Engl. J. Med. **295:**1414, 1976.

Wagenvoort, C.A., and Wagenvoort, N.: Primary pulmonary hypertension: a pathologic study of the lung vessels in 156 clinically diagnosed cases, Circulation **42:**1163, 1970.

Walcott, G., and others: Primary pulmonary hypertension, Am. J. Med. **49:**70, 1970.

Wang, S.W.S., and others: Diazoxide in treatment of primary pulmonary hypertension, Br. Heart J. **40:**572, 1978.

Whittaker, W., and Heath, D.: Idiopathic pulmonary hypertension: etiology, pathogenesis, diagnosis and treatment, Prog. Cardiovasc. Dis. **1:**380, 1959.

93 • CONGENITAL HEART DISEASE

Iain F.S. Black

Patients with congenital heart disease are referred to the internist, as adults, with increasing frequency and appear in three settings. Many will be asymptomatic after surgical cure or devolution of their defect; for example, a ventricular septal defect may be entirely repaired surgically or may disappear with maturation of the heart. Others will be seen with the evolution of a defect that may become symptomatic after childbirth; for example, atrial septal defect may occur with right-sided heart failure in middle age. Finally, there is an increasing population of patients with the residual effects of anomalies that previously prevented survival past childhood; for example, those patients who have had surgical correction for transposition of the great vessels and no longer have shunts but may develop ventricular muscle dysfunction in adulthood. For these reasons, the principles of pediatric cardiac physiology are directly related to the care of adults.

In 1952 when Dr. John Louis first closed an atrial septal defect using hypothermia and circulatory arrest under inflow occlusion, few people realized that this was to lead to the development of a highly sophisticated specialty for the care of children with congenital heart lesions. Yet despite all the advances that have been made, many children still die in infancy and others have problems for which a surgical solution is not yet available.

The incidence of congenital heart disease is 8:1000 live births. Some anomalies occur as part of chromosomal abnormalities (Table 93-1) and some occur in familial patterns unassociated with any currently detectable chromosomal abnormality. The majority of congenital heart lesions, however, occur in the absence of any known genetic mechanism. Problems occurring in familial patterns without known chromosomal abnormalities include hereditary familial cardiomyopathy, supravalvular aortic stenosis, glycogen storage disease, Holt-Oram syndrome (secundum atrial septal defect, hypoplastic thumb, accessory phalanx), and Laurence-Moon-Bordet-Biedl syndrome (mental retardation, retinitis pigmentosa, hypogonadism). In contrast the occurrence of congenital heart disease resulting from a teratogenic agent is clearly due to an environmental cause. Thus there are many causes of congenital heart disease, and it is likely that many lesions are acquired in utero as a result of interactions between genetic predisposition and subtle factors in the intrauterine environment.

Whereas most examples of congenital heart disease are isolated cases without familial pattern, if a child has congenital heart disease, this warrants some caution in counseling regarding subsequent pregnancy. The risk to a sibling is 2%, or about three times that of the general population.

HEMODYNAMICS OF CONGENITAL HEART DISEASE

All too often the approach to understanding congenital heart disease is to memorize the signs and symptoms of a long list of congenital heart lesions. A simple and more practical approach is to learn the fundamentals of blood flow and structural or vascular resistance as they apply to children with shunts or obstructive lesions. Before dealing with the structural abnormalities, it is necessary first to review normal circulation as it applies to the fetus and the changes that occur after birth.

As the fetus grows, it is essential that the venous return to the right side of the heart be directed away from the lungs and through the patent ductus arteriosus to the mother's placenta. This is accomplished by vasoconstriction of the pulmonary arterioles, a mechanism that develops during the second trimester of pregnancy and persists until birth. The vasoconstriction is maintained by hypertrophy of the medial coat of the pulmonary arterioles in response to the low oxygen tension (19 to 22 mm Hg) of the blood returning to the right side of the heart.

Not all the venous blood returning to the heart enters the right ventricle. The inferior vena cava bloodstream, including the oxygenated blood returning from the placenta, is directed preferentially through a patent foramen ovale into the left atrium and left ventricle. By this method the coronary and cerebral circulations receive blood with a higher oxygen tension (25 to 28 mm Hg). Since a low oxygen tension is necessary to maintain the high pulmonary vascular resistance, the fetus uses a hemoglobin, called fetal hemoglobin, that allows the red blood cells to carry a larger quantity of oxygen for any given oxygen tension.

The placenta itself is an organ with a low vascular resistance, further encouraging the right ventricle to empty through the ductus arteriosus into the descending aorta. As a result the right ventricle functions as a systemic ventricle and maintains this role until birth.

At the time of birth the loss of the placenta establishes the normal systemic vascular resistance, which immediately reduces the right-to-left shunt across the ductus arteriosus. With the first breath the collapsed lungs expand and oxygen enters the alveoli. Sufficient oxygen diffuses across the wall of the alveoli to raise the oxygen tension

Table 93-1. Cardiac anomalies resulting from chromosomal abnormalities

Type	Frequency in live births	Common heart defects
Trisomy 21, Down's syndrome	1:800	Atrioventricular (AV) canal; ventricular septal defect; patent ductus arteriosus
Turner's syndrome	1:5500 females	Coarctation of the aorta
Trisomy 13	1:5000	Ventricular septal defect; patent ductus arteriosus; atrial septal defect; dextropositions
Trisomy 18	1:6000	Ventricular septal defect; patent ductus arteriosus

in the tissues surrounding the arterioles so that the hypoxia is abolished. This causes the vasoconstriction to be relieved and the pulmonary vascular bed to open up. The rate of fall of the pulmonary vascular resistance is determined by the medial coat of the pulmonary arterioles, which, having been markedly hypertrophied, can retain a degree of vasoconstriction for some weeks after birth. Under normal circumstances the pulmonary vascular resistance drops rapidly at first and then more slowly until the normal baseline values are reached. This usually occurs in the first 2 to 4 weeks after birth but may be delayed in some children.

This capacity of the medial coat of the arterioles to retain a degree of vasoconstriction influences the clinical picture and progress of children born with systemic-to-pulmonary shunts. This is best illustrated by the child with a patent ductus arteriosus. It is usual for a patent ductus arteriosus to be closed functionally by 1 day of age and anatomically after approximately 15 days. If the ductus arteriosus remains open after birth, blood will flow through it from the circuit with the higher resistance to the circuit with the lower resistance. In the first hour or so after birth the higher pulmonary resistance will still direct venous blood across the ductus arteriosus into the aorta, but as the pulmonary resistance falls further, the right-to-left shunt will stop and be gradually replaced by one from the aorta into the pulmonary artery. As this shunt increases, excessive pulmonary flow occurs with volume overload of the heart and the clinical picture of congestive heart failure. Since the murmur of a patent ductus arteriosus is caused by the turbulence generated by the left-to-right shunt, if the pulmonary vascular resistance is slow to fall, it is possible for an infant to be discharged home on the third day of life with no abnormal cardiac findings, only to be seen 3 weeks later in the physician's office with an enlarged heart, congestive heart failure, and a loud, continuous murmur as a result of the large shunt. It is often difficult for parents to understand why, if the infant was born with this problem, the murmur was not heard during the hospital stay.

This delay in the appearance of signs and symptoms is common to all children with communications between the pulmonary and systemic circuits. The development of the typical clinical picture for each lesion will depend on the degree and rate of fall of the pulmonary vascular resistance. If the pulmonary vascular resistance remains high at birth, little of the right ventricular output will flow into the pulmonary vascular bed (being shunted instead from the pulmonary artery through the ductus arteriosus into the systemic circuit). This clinical picture is called "persistent fetal circulation," which aptly describes the mechanism involved. Should the high pulmonary vascular resistance persist, the infant will die as a result of hypoxia caused by inadequate pulmonary flow. Occasionally an infant is born in whom the pulmonary vascular resistance does not fall to normal levels. As a result there remains some resistance to pulmonary flow that influences the clinical picture and prevents the development of cardiac failure by limiting the left-to-right shunt. Finally there are cases in which the pulmonary resistance has fallen to normal after birth and then for reasons yet unexplained begins to rise again some months or years later. If the child has congestive heart failure, the gradual reduction in the left-to-right shunt as a result of the increasing pulmonary vascular resistance will bring about an improvement in the clinical picture, which can be misleading if the increasing pulmonary vascular resistance is not appreciated.

The importance of the well-developed medial coat of the arterioles in maintaining vasoconstriction is well illustrated when considering premature infants born toward the end of the second trimester of pregnancy. If the ductus arteriosus remains open, it is essential that the pulmonary arterioles maintain adequate vasoconstriction to protect the lungs from a volume overload. However, since the medial coat of the pulmonary arterioles develops and matures during the last trimester of pregnancy, the premature infant has little muscle in the medial coat to maintain adequate vasoconstriction. It is for this reason that most premature infants with a large ductus arteriosus rapidly develop congestive heart failure and may be extremely difficult to manage medically.

These examples illustrate the important role of the pulmonary vascular bed in determining the clinical picture of children with intracardiac or extracardiac shunts. Although the size of the defect is important, the amount of blood flowing through the defect is in direct proportion to the vascular resistance of both pulmonary and systemic circuits.

THE PEDIATRIC ELECTROCARDIOGRAM

Whereas the pattern of an adult electrocardiogram (ECG) is one of left ventricular dominance, the ECG of the child has a pattern that depends on age. The systemic role of the right ventricle during fetal life requires that it be a hypertrophied chamber; this explains why at birth there is a pattern of right ventricular dominance in the ECG. After birth, as the pulmonary vascular resistance falls, the right ventricle begins to lose its hypertrophy and develops the characteristics of a thinner-walled volume chamber. This development takes months to occur, and it may be a year or more before right ventricular dominance disappears from the ECG and the left ventricle assumes its dominant role. To one unfamiliar with the infant ECG, the prominent right ventricular forces are often incorrectly read as right ventricular hypertrophy.

The criteria listed in Table 93-2 exemplify the changing criteria used for the diagnosis of ventricular hypertrophy. The normal mean frontal QRS axis also reflects changes during the newborn period, moving from 135 degrees to 75 degrees by 3 months. Further progression to

Table 93-2. Criteria for ECG diagnosis of hypertrophy

Type of hypertrophy	Key criteria	Less specific criteria
Right ventricular hypertrophy	R in V_1 > 20 mm 　　　　> 29 mm (< 1 wk of age) S in V_6 > 20 mm (< 1 mo) 　　　　> 10 mm (1-6 mo) 　　　　> 5 mm (> 6 mo) Upright T in V_1, after 4 days	QR in V_1 or V_4 R R/S ratio in V_1 > 2 (> 6 mo) Right axis deviation
Left ventricular hypertrophy	S in V_1 > 25 mm R in V_6 > 20 mm (0-1 yr) 　　　　> 25 mm (1-10 yr) 　　　　> 30 mm (10-20 yr) Q in V_6 > 4 mm	R/S ratio in V_1 < 0.8 (< 1 yr) 　　　　< 0.2 (1-5 yr) 　　　　< 0.1 (> 5 yr)
Combined ventricular hypertrophy	Criteria for right and left ventricular hypertrophy Criteria for right ventricular hypertrophy plus 　R in V_6 > 15 mm or 　Q in V_6 > 3 mm Criteria for left ventricular hypertrophy plus 　R in V_1 > 15 mm	"Normal" ECG in presence of cardiomegaly

the left is gradual after 3 months of age. Right atrial hypertrophy is diagnosed when tall, peaked P waves are present (2.5 mm if less than 1 year of age, 3 mm if older). Broad, notched, or prolonged P waves (0.10 second if more than 1 year of age) suggest left atrial enlargement.

PEDIATRIC ARRHYTHMIAS

Arrhythmias occurring in children are best classified as (1) tachycardias, (2) blocks, (3) extrasystolic rhythms, (4) preexcitation patterns, and (5) sinus node disorders. (See Chapter 97 for a more detailed discussion of these arrhythmias.)

Tachycardias

SUPRAVENTRICULAR TACHYCARDIA. The most common supraventricular tachycardia seen in children is that of the atrioventricular (AV) nodal reentrant type. The next most common is regular tachycardia from an ectopic focus in either atrium. Atrial flutter and fibrillation are relatively rare causes of supraventricular tachycardia.

Treatment is directed either to interrupting the reentrant cycle or suppressing the ectopic focus. In either case digitalis or verapamil is the drug of choice because they act to slow conduction through the AV node, thereby either abolishing the rhythm or slowing the ventricular response. Propranolol (Inderal) is also useful for prolonging AV conduction and suppressing ectopic foci. Quinidine is used to suppress ectopic foci.

VENTRICULAR TACHYCARDIA. Benign ventricular ectopy usually is seen as cycles of ventricular bigeminy or trigeminy. No treatment is indicated. Ventricular tachycardia is most commonly seen in the intensive care unit or cardiac intensive care unit. It is malignant because it frequently produces a lower cardiac output, leading to cardiovascular collapse, and it may be a precursor to ventricular fibrillation. Initial treatment is lidocaine, first as a bolus and then as a continuous infusion. Procainamide and phenytoin are also effective in some cases.

Blocks

Acquired heart block may occur as an isolated finding of rheumatic carditis, myocarditis, or endocardial fibroelastosis. Most cases occur following surgical correction of lesions in which a ventricular septal defect is present. This is because the conducting system lies close to the margin of the defect and may be damaged by a suture as the patch is inserted. Complete congenital heart block is a rare lesion usually found as an isolated problem. Most of the children with this block are active and asymptomatic, but attacks caused by Stokes-Adams disease may occur and are most likely in children whose heart rates fall below 40 to 45 beats per minute. The occurrence of Stokes-Adams attacks is an indication for insertion of a pacemaker.

Preexcitation patterns: Wolff-Parkinson-White (WPW) syndrome

The incidence of WPW syndrome has been estimated to be about 0.1% in infants and children. The pattern results from an accessory conduction pathway that bypasses the AV node, causing early activation of a ventricle. This preexcitation produces a short PR interval and slurring of the upstroke of the QRS (called a delta wave).

The accessory pathway allows retrograde conduction

from the ventricle to the atrium, which sustains an episode of tachycardia. The incidence of tachycardia in children with preexcitation patterns is not known but is thought to be about 50%. Digitalis is the drug of choice for management in children.

Sinus node disorders

Rhythms resulting from blocking of the sinus impulse so that it does not enter the atrium, or sinus node dysfunction, are termed "sick sinus syndrome." Sinus arrest associated with Stokes-Adams attacks is an indication for a pacemaker.

It is becoming apparent that a number of the arrhythmias seen are complicated and require sophisticated diagnostic electrophysiologic study to unravel their origin. The techniques of investigation using His bundle catheters and atrial pacing are similar to those used in adults, with minor modifications to account for the pediatric age.

THE CHEST ROENTGENOGRAM IN CONGENITAL HEART DISEASE

Before the cardiac silhouette is interpreted, the roentgenogram should be evaluated for technique and any extracardiac findings. It is important that the patient be positioned properly with the two clavicles symmetric; this can be difficult in young children and infants and is a frequent cause of a technically poor film. Correct exposure is also important, since over- or underexposure leads to errors in interpretation of the pulmonary vasculature. The degree of inspiration should also be checked, with the crest of the diaphragm being no higher than the sixth anterior rib. Inadequate inspiration makes the heart appear enlarged and the pulmonary vasculature look increased.

Normal growth and individual variation from child to child require that initial roentgenographic evaluation of a heart include a minimum of the frontal, or posteroanterior (PA), and lateral views. Differences in chest configuration could result in errors of interpretation of cardiac size and shape if only a PA film is taken. Oblique views help visualize parts of the heart not readily observed on the standard PA and lateral views. The left anterior oblique view shows the relative size of the two ventricles and allows good visualization of the left bronchus (which becomes elevated in the early stages of left atrial enlargement). The right anterior oblique view is also useful for detecting minimal degrees of left atrial enlargement and gives indirect evidence of right ventricular size by demonstrating how much of the anterior border is in direct contact with the sternum.

In interpreting the chest roentgenogram, it is important to understand the hemodynamics, especially with lesions in which there is enlargement of one or more parts of the heart because of volume overload. Enlargement can be localized to one chamber because of valvular insufficiency or involve a number of chambers and vessels as a result of a left-to-right shunt. One can often deduce the hemodynamics involved by identifying which of the chambers are enlarged. For example, increased pulmonary flow with enlargement of both the left atrium and the left ventricle and dilation of the ascending aorta would be strongly indicative of a patent ductus arteriosus. However, if the increased pulmonary flow were associated with enlargement of the right atrium and right ventricle and the pulmonary artery, the roentgenographic findings would suggest an atrial septal defect (the left atrium would not be enlarged if it were able to empty efficiently across the atrial septal defect as well as through the mitral valve).

The chest roentgenogram is less helpful in the diagnosis of obstructive lesions. In children obstructive lesions are rarely associated with chamber enlargement unless there is associated cardiac failure. Only more subtle changes give a clue to the diagnosis. Dilation of the ascending aorta suggests aortic stenosis; a prominent pulmonary artery segment suggests pulmonary valve stenosis. If the apex of the left ventricle is displaced upward, one has to consider that right ventricular hypertrophy may be the cause. Some of these more subtle changes may be seen only in the oblique views.

The chest roentgenogram is particularly helpful in providing information regarding the pulmonary vascular bed. There is a definite correlation between the volume of blood shunted through the lungs and the size of the pulmonary arteries and veins. The size of any left-to-right shunt is usually expressed as a ratio of the pulmonary/systemic blood flow. In most lesions with a left-to-right shunt at ventricular or ductal level, flow ratios in the range of 1.6:1 to 2:1 correlate with the roentgenographic pattern of a mild increase in vascular markings. Shunts at atrial level rarely show increased pulmonary vascular markings with a flow ratio less than 2:1. Any increase in pulmonary vascular markings requires the presence of a *significant* left-to-right shunt. Conversely, a chest roentgenogram with normal pulmonary vascular markings *does not exclude* lesions with a small left-to-right shunt.

CARDIAC CATHETERIZATION

Cardiac catheterization in infants and children requires a different set of skills and techniques from those used for adults. The majority of studies are done by percutaneous technique from the groin, since not only are the vessels larger than in the arm but approaching the heart from below facilitates passage of the catheter into the left side of the heart if there is a patent foramen ovale; this is useful in small infants when it is not desirable to enter an artery.

The risk to life is less than 1%, although figures as high as 3% or 4% have been quoted for the sick neonate undergoing a diagnostic study. Such risks are justified, since in the absence of definitive treatment survival cannot be expected. Excluding the newborn group, the majority of cardiac catheterizations done in children are for:

1. Diagnosis when the clinical findings are confusing
2. Management when the decision is between the continuation of medical care or surgical intervention
3. Documentation of anatomy when surgery is being considered
4. Electrophysiologic evaluation of complex arrhythmias
5. Postoperative evaluation of reparative surgery
6. Therapeutic purposes such as the creation of an atrial septal defect with a specially designed balloon catheter in infants with transposition of the great arteries, tricuspid atresia, pulmonary atresia, and total anomalous pulmonary venous return

The appearance of cyanosis suggests an unstable cardiac status and the need for early diagnostic intervention. The development of congestive heart failure is another indication for early catheterization unless there is a prompt and satisfactory response to the introduction of digitalis therapy.

The measurement of pulmonary flow and the calculation of pulmonary vascular resistance are an integral part of a pediatric cardiac catheterization. The decision for medical or surgical management frequently depends on the ratio of the pulmonary/systemic flow and on the response of the pulmonary vascular bed to the left-to-right shunt. In the case of an asymptomatic child the decision to recommend surgery is made on the basis of the natural history of the lesion.

Current research is concerned with developing techniques for treatment of congenital heart lesions using cardiac catheters. These techniques include closing atrial septal defects with an umbrella-like fixture that is introduced by the catheter and implanted in the atrial septum. A similar method employing a plug has been used for closing the defect in cases of patent ductus arteriosus. A catheter with a recessed knife at its tip has been developed to cut the atrial septum in children who have had a poor result following the standard balloon septostomy technique.

NONINVASIVE STUDIES

The echocardiogram has become a very useful diagnostic tool for the evaluation of children with heart disease. The elucidation of cardiac anatomy made possible by echocardiography has already eliminated the need for a cardiac catheterization in some children. It is expected that with time echocardiography will assume an even greater responsibility for primary diagnosis.

A major benefit of echocardiography is the addition of sufficient information regarding heart anatomy and function to reduce the necessity for multiple angiocardiographic injections during a cardiac catheterization. This reduces the duration of the study and the incidence of complications.

Echocardiography is being used more frequently as a tool for reevaluation. Repeated echocardiograms have been helpful in monitoring the response to cardiotoxic medications used for treating neoplastic lesions. Echocardiography has also assumed an increasing role in the evaluation of heart function in children with acquired heart disease, including sickle cell anemia, rheumatic heart disease, chronic renal disease, and systemic hypertension.

Exercise tests are also becoming an integral part of the diagnostic evaluation of children with cardiac disorders. The testing is done with either a treadmill or a bicycle ergometer following a strict protocol so that the performance of one child can be compared with others. Most studies report values for work, heart rate, blood pressure, and changes in the ECG at peak voluntary effort.

In children with specific heart lesions such as aortic stenosis a reduction in work performance may be the first sign of a deteriorating cardiac status and an indication for surgery. Testing of a child after major open heart surgery evaluates the capacity to perform work and allows counseling as to how soon the child should return to active sports.

It is likely that more interest will be shown in exercise testing in the next few years. Until recently the only hemodynamic data available were those obtained by cardiac catheterization in children under moderate to heavy sedation. There was no way of knowing how the same heart would perform if the child were active in an upright position. Data now being obtained from exercise testing give a new understanding of cardiac function and assist in determining the child who needs surgical intervention.

SPECIFIC CONGENITAL HEART LESIONS

The malformations discussed in this chapter consist of all the major lesions and occur in over 80% of children with congenital heart disease. For information regarding the less common forms of congenital heart disease, the reader should refer to the bibliography. For convenience, the lesions are separated according to the absence or presence of cyanosis. The acyanotic group is further subdivided into those with left-to-right shunts and those with obstructive lesions.

Acyanotic heart lesions with left-to-right shunts

In this group of lesions the connection between the systemic and pulmonary circulation may either be intracardiac or extracardiac. The left-to-right shunts not only cause murmurs but, if large enough, roentgenographic findings of cardiac enlargement, a prominent pulmonary artery, and increased vascular markings resulting from increased flow. The clinical findings of poor weight gain and congestive heart failure will be present only if the shunt is large. The more common lesions are ostium secundum atrial septal defect, total and partial anomalous pulmonary venous return, endocardial cushion defects (ostium primum atrial septal defect or atrioventricular canal), ventricular septal defects, patent ductus arteriosus, and aorticopulmonary window and truncus arteriosus.

In all these the clinical picture will depend on the magnitude of the left-to-right shunt, which in turn depends on the size of the defect and the level of the pulmonary vascular resistance. Small defects limit the amount of the left-to-right shunt and the increase in pulmonary flow. If the pulmonary vascular resistance is normal, a large septal defect will permit pulmonary flows to be as large as five times normal. In these larger defects the size of the left-to-right shunt is also controlled by the level of the pulmonary vascular resistance. An elevated pulmonary vascular resistance limits total pulmonary flow and reduces the size of the left-to-right shunt. The clinical picture is influenced accordingly.

The clinical picture of congenital heart disease in the premature infant is different from that of the term infant. The earlier the infant is born, the more immature is the pulmonary vascular bed, since the medial coat of the pulmonary arterioles does not develop its full vasoconstrictive capacity until close to term. If a premature infant is born with a shunt lesion, the pulmonary arterioles are ill-equipped to protect the vascular bed from a large blood volume. As a result the clinical picture is that of severe congestive heart failure developing in the first few days after birth.

OSTIUM SECUNDUM ATRIAL SEPTAL DEFECT. Ostium secundum atrial septal defect is the terminology given to an atrial septal defect located in the area of the fossa ovalis. The clinical picture is the direct result of the volume of blood shunting from the left atrium into the right atrium and overloading the right side of the heart. If the shunt is significant, the ECG will show right ventricular enlargement and on the chest roentgenogram there will be cardiac enlargement with increased pulmonary flow.

On auscultation there may be delayed closure of the pulmonic component of the second heart sound because of prolongation of the right ventricular ejection time. A systolic flow murmur is heard across the pulmonary valve and on occasion is soft enough to be mistaken for an innocent murmur. If the pulmonary-to-systemic flow ratio is 2.5:1 or greater, the volume of blood crossing the tricuspid valve generates a diastolic rumble heard best at the third and fourth left interspaces close to the sternum.

The clinical findings of atrial septal defect do not usually appear until at least 3 years of age. For the left-to-right shunt to develop, it is necessary for the right ventricle to lose its systemic characteristics, which are present at birth, and develop the role of a more distensible chamber that is required only to pump blood through the pulmonary circuit. As the right ventricle becomes more distensible, the left-to-right shunt at the atrial level increases. If the pulmonary/systemic flow ratio is 2:1 or greater, the average life expectancy is reduced and congestive heart failure or increased pulmonary vascular resistance is likely to develop after 30 years of age. A pulmonary/systemic flow ratio of 2:1 is therefore an indication for closure of the defect with cardiac bypass. In some centers, because of the low mortality associated with surgery, closure is considered with flow ratios as low as 1.5:1.

ANOMALOUS PULMONARY VENOUS RETURN. The basic malformation is failure of development of the common pulmonary veins from the left atrium. Although the pulmonary venous systems can develop alternative drainage using other venous systems, the return to the heart still has to be via the superior vena cava or inferior vena cava or into the right atrium itself.

For survival it is essential that there be an adequate atrial septal defect with sufficient flow into the left atrium and left ventricle to maintain systemic needs. The rapid fall in pulmonary vascular resistance after birth causes increased pulmonary flow with enlargement of the right side of the heart. The clinical findings are similar to those of atrial septal defect but more pronounced. If murmurs are present, they are flow murmurs and are usually not significant. If the atrial septal defect is of adequate size, many children respond well to digitalization and can be managed medically until corrective surgery with cardiac bypass is done electively at a later age. The clinical findings are different in those children who have a degree of obstruction to their pulmonary veins. Even a moderate degree of obstruction significantly reduces pulmonary flow and the availability of oxygenated blood to the right side of the heart. This in turn reduces systemic saturation, with cyanosis resulting in some cases. Obstruction of the pulmonary veins is an unstable situation frequently requiring open heart surgery, with a high risk of mortality present in the newborn period.

The clinical picture of partial anomalous pulmonary venous return depends on how many of the pulmonary veins are involved. If a small number are affected, the clinical picture is identical to that of the average secundum atrial septal defect, and the correct diagnosis will be established only at the time of cardiac catheterization. Management depends on the number of veins draining anomalously and their hemodynamic effects. A single anomalous pulmonary vein with a normal ECG pattern and chest roentgenogram and a documented small increase in pulmonary flow is compatible with a normal healthy life and does not require surgery.

ENDOCARDIAL CUSHION DEFECTS. In the development of the heart a crucial area is at the site of the endocardial cushions, where the atrial and ventricular septum are in continuity and separate the mitral from the tricuspid valve. Abnormal development in this area causes a spectrum of lesions with various degrees of involvement of the atrial septum, venticular septum, mitral valve, and tricuspid valve. The intracardiac communication is either that of an atrial septal defect, a ventricular septal defect, or a combination of both in which one of the septal defects dominates. The hemodynamic problem resulting from valvular involvement is that of insufficiency, which varies from minimal to severe.

Ostium primum atrial septal defect. This defect is low in the atrial septum and close to the mitral and tricuspid valves. Usually the mitral valve is deformed and often cleft, allowing a varying degree of mitral insufficiency. The clinical picture is that of an atrial septal defect, except the ECG has an axis of -60 degrees as a result of an abnormal pathway of the conducting system, a characteristic of endocardial cushion defects. In most cases the mitral insufficiency is mild and can be detected only by the presence of a systolic murmur at the apex.

Atrioventricular canal. In this situation there is absence of the upper portion of the ventricular septum as well as the lower portion of the atrial septum. This single defect means that there is no septum to which the mitral and tricuspid valves can be attached for support. As a result the mitral and tricuspid valves are in continuity with each other (frequently appearing as one common valve either floating freely or attached to the lower rim of the ventricular portion of the defect). The clinical picture depends on the size of the defect between the two ventricles, the degree of incompetence of the mitral-tricuspid valve, and the level of the pulmonary vascular resistance. Frequently children with this defect are seen with a ventricular septal defect and severe congestive heart failure. The ECG, showing the characteristic axis of -60 degrees, suggests the diagnosis.

Initial management is medicinal with digitalization. The decision for surgery and its timing depend on the nature of the defects present and the status of the pulmonary vascular bed.

VENTRICULAR SEPTAL DEFECTS. Approximately 80% of ventricular septal defects are located in the membranous septum just below the aortic valve; 10% are in the posterior muscular septum behind the septal leaflet of the tricuspid valve, and the rest are situated low in the muscular part of the septum, where they may be multiple.

In defects with a pulmonary/systemic flow ratio of 2:1 or greater, the clinical picture is of cardiac enlargement with increased pulmonary flow. With the left-to-right shunt at ventricular level, the chest roentgenogram shows increased pulmonary flow with enlargement of the left atrium and left ventricle. Similarly the ECG shows left ventricular enlargement unless the shunt is sufficiently large to also increase the size of the right ventricle, in which case combined ventricular hypertrophy will be seen on both ECG and chest roentgenogram.

The turbulence generated at the site of the defect causes a characteristic, harsh pansystolic murmur localized best at the third and fourth left interspaces close to the sternum. It may also be palpated as a thrill. If the pulmonary/systemic flow ratio is 2.5:1 or greater, a flow murmur is generated at the mitral valve and transmitted to the apex as a diastolic rumble.

Small ventricular septal defects (pulmonary/systemic flow ratios less than 2:1) are compatible with a full life. The only risk is of bacterial endocarditis (as high as 8% to 10% in adults). If the pulmonary/systemic flow ratio is greater than 2:1, there is a risk of increasing pulmonary vascular resistance or congestive heart failure in early adult life. In most centers if a child is progressing well but still has a pulmonary/systemic flow ratio greater than 2:1 at 4 or 5 years of age, the defect is closed with cardiac bypass. In infants with severe failure who fail to thrive or have repeated admissions to the hospital for pneumonia, surgery in the first year of life is indicated. The natural history of the lesion indicates that at least 50% of ventricular septal defects undergo a spontaneous reduction in size in the first few years of life; as many as 40% of those decreasing in size undergo spontaneous closure. For this reason conservative management for a 1-year-old child with a large shunt can be justified if the child has a low pulmonary vascular resistance, is making progress, and remains relatively free of serious infections. On the other hand, if the child has systemic pressure in the pulmonary artery with any findings to suggest possible risk for developing increased pulmonary vascular resistance, then surgical intervention would be justified. In some cases a repeat cardiac catheterization may be necessary to determine the correct plan of management.

"Eisenmenger's *complex*" refers to the development of increased pulmonary vascular resistance with cyanosis owing to right-to-left shunting across a ventricular septal defect (the term "Eisenmenger's *syndrome*" is used to describe cyanosis from any left-to-right communication that has resulted in abnormal pulmonary resistance and subsequent right-to-left reversal of the shunt).

PATENT DUCTUS ARTERIOSUS. The ductus that connects the pulmonary artery to the aorta usually closes within the first few hours of birth. If it does not, there is flow from the aorta into the pulmonary artery, which then returns normally to the left side of the heart and the aorta. As the pulmonary vascular resistance falls, the left-to-right shunt occurs in diastole as well as systole. The turbulence in both phases of the cycle generates a continuous machinery-like murmur best heard in the second left intercostal space close to the sternum. The murmur obscures the second heart sound. If the pulmonary/systemic flow ratio is greater than 2.5:1, the increased flow across the mitral valve causes a diastolic rumble heard at the apex. The development of the left-to-right shunt during diastole results in a widened pulse pressure detected as a strong bounding pulse.

Spontaneous closure of a patent ductus arteriosus can occur, particularly if it is associated with prematurity. If spontaneous closure does not occur, surgical ligation is recommended before 2 years of age regardless of the size of the shunt. The justification for closure in an asymptomatic child is the risk of bacterial endocarditis in later life, estimated to be as high as 13%, in comparison to the risk of surgery, which is 1% or less.

AORTICOPULMONARY WINDOW AND TRUNCUS ARTERIOSUS. The aorticopulmonary window is a rare lesion mentioned only because it can be seen with the clinical picture of a patent ductus arteriosus. The defect is a direct communication between the ascending aorta and the main pulmonary artery, with a left-to-right shunt occurring during systole and diastole. The murmur is continuous, and the ECG and chest roentgenogram findings are similar to those of a patent ductus arteriosus. Diagnosis is usually made at cardiac catheterization, and open heart surgery is required for its closure.

Truncus arteriosus is another lesion that must be considered in the differential diagnosis of a patent ductus arteriosus. The intracardiac lesion is a ventricular septal defect with both ventricles emptying into one main arterial trunk arising from the base of the heart. There are varieties of truncus arteriosus, classified according to the method of blood supply to the lungs. The ECG is not diagnostic, showing only the biventricular enlargement of a large left-to-right shunt. The chest roentgenogram shows the same nonspecific findings. However, since some children with a truncus arteriosus have a right aortic arch, if this arch is seen on the chest roentgenogram or if the right pulmonary artery appears to branch higher than normal, the possibility of a truncus arteriosus should be considered. Palliative surgery consists of placing a constriction around the main pulmonary artery or both branches to reduce the flow into both lungs. More definitive surgery, which carries high risk, involves the use of cardiac bypass, at which time the ventricular septal defect is closed and the right ventricle is connected directly to the branches of the pulmonary artery by means of a conduit containing a valve. The left ventricle drains into the arterial trunk and supplies the systemic circuit.

Acyanotic heart disease with obstructive lesions

In discussing the obstructive lesions, it is necessary to separate infants from children more than 1 year of age. Both the clinical picture and the course of management are different. In both age groups congenital mitral stenosis and congenital tricuspid stenosis are rare and will not be discussed.

In children more than 1 year of age the more common lesions are coarctation of the aorta, aortic stenosis, and pulmonary stenosis.

COARCTATION OF THE AORTA. In this lesion there is a localized constriction at or distal to the origin of the left subclavian artery from the aorta. The resulting narrowed pulse pressure distal to the obstruction causes weak or absent pulses in the lower limbs and occasionally in the left arm if the left subclavian artery is compromised by the constriction. There often is hypertension proximal to the coarctation. A systolic murmur is usually heard over the site of the coarctation in the back and transmitted to the left sternal border anteriorly. If the ascending aorta is dilated, there will be an aortic ejection click that is best heard at the apex.

On chest roentgenogram the size of the heart is usually normal. Prominence of the left ventricle may be seen, as well as dilation of the ascending aorta. If the aortic knob and upper descending aorta are well visualized, the break in continuity at the level of the coarctation may be identified. Left ventricular hypertrophy is usually seen on the ECG, although in some cases the finding is that of right ventricular hypertrophy. The reason for this ECG pattern in the absence of an associated right-sided heart lesion is not clear. The most commonly associated cardiac lesion is a bicuspid aortic valve that may occasionally cause aortic valve stenosis.

Turner's syndrome should be considered when a woman has coarctation of the aorta. Patients with Turner's syndrome have short stature, webbing of the neck, widely spaced nipples, a low hairline, and an increased carrying angle of the elbows.

AORTIC STENOSIS. The majority of lesions in aortic stenosis are valvular, although an occasional supravalvular or subvalvular obstruction is seen. Characteristically the aortic valve is thickened, deformed, and often bicuspid. In severe obstructions the left ventricle can generate systolic pressures greater than 200 mm Hg. Despite these high pressures the child may remain asymptomatic. Chest pain or angina is rare and occurs only if there is coronary insufficiency.

The turbulence generated across the obstruction causes a harsh crescendo-decrescendo murmur best heard in the first interspace close to the right sternal border and frequently associated with a thrill. If the ascending aorta is dilated, an apical ejection click will be present. The second heart sound should remain split unless left ventricular emptying delays closure of the aortic valve to the point that it coincides with pulmonic valve closure, making the second heart sound appear single.

The chest roentgenogram may show dilation of the ascending aorta. The heart is usually of a normal size. The ECG may show left ventricular hypertrophy, but it may not reflect the severity of the aortic valve stenosis.

Surgery to relieve the obstruction is helpful, but the valve has an abnormal structure and may re-stenose or become calcified with time. In addition, the deformed nature of the valve may result in aortic valve insufficiency after surgery. Most centers recommend surgery when the gradient across the valve is 50 mm Hg or greater, particularly if there are ST and T wave changes in the ECG. Other centers prefer to wait until the gradient is greater than 75 mm Hg, since the surgery is considered to be palliative and the results are not always satisfactory. In cases where the valve is badly deformed, there may be no choice but to replace it with a prosthetic valve. Although the results from surgery are not optimal, the long-term prognosis without an operation is poor. Fibrosis of the myocardium with the development of left ventricular failure can be expected in adult life. The risk of bacterial endocarditis and, in severe cases, sudden death also has to be considered.

PULMONARY STENOSIS. Pulmonary stenosis with an intact ventricular septum is usually valvular, although it may occur either proximal or distal to the valve. The proximal obstruction is usually at the infundibular level; occasionally it is a result of a muscle band high in the right ventricular cavity. Stenosis of the individual right and left pulmonary arteries is uncommon except following maternal rubella. The obstruction can be bilateral and severe. Regardless of the site of the obstruction, the hemodynamic result is an increase in right ventricular systolic pressure and work.

In valvular pulmonary stenosis the turbulence across the valve generates a harsh systolic murmur heard best at the second left interspace close to the sternum, usually associated with a thrill. In mild to moderate obstruction the pulmonary second heart sound is still split, with both components of normal intensity. An ejection click is heard at the upper left sternal border as a result of the dilation of the main pulmonary artery. The ECG shows right ventricular hypertrophy with right atrial enlargement if the obstruction is severe. The chest roentgenogram is frequently normal except for prominence of the main pulmonary artery because of its dilation.

Unlike aortic stenosis, pulmonary valve stenosis rarely increases in severity. However, in moderate or severe stenosis, fibrosis of the myocardium develops with time, resulting in a gradual loss of right ventricular myocardial function. Congestive heart failure may be a late complication. In most centers a gradient of 50 to 75 mm Hg is considered justification for recommending surgery. As in aortic stenosis, even though the gradient may be abolished, the valve is still abnormal and antibiotic prophylaxis for bacterial endocarditis should be continued for life.

In the first year of life the obstruction to the pulmonary or aortic valve may be so severe that the ventricle dilates and fails. In the case of pulmonary stenosis, if there is a patent foramen ovale, a right-to-left shunt may occur, producing cyanosis. An enlarging right ventricle as a result of pulmonary stenosis is considered an emergency in the newborn period and an indication for immediate surgery.

Cyanotic heart lesions

Most heart lesions produce cyanosis because desaturated venous blood returning to the heart is pumped out into the systemic circuit without having been passed through the lungs for oxygenation. In tetralogy of Fallot, tricuspid atresia, and pulmonary atresia the obstruction to pulmonary flow results in a right-to-left shunt at the ventricular or atrial level. For cyanosis to be visible, it is necessary for at least 5 g/dl of desaturated hemoglobin to be present in the arterial blood. Infants with a mild degree of arterial desaturation may be pink at rest, becoming cyanotic only with crying as the right-to-left shunt increases. If the baby is anemic, cyanosis may still not be appreciated.

The cyanotic lesions discussed are tricuspid atresia, pulmonary atresia, tetralogy of Fallot, Ebstein's anomaly of the tricuspid valve, and transposition of the great arteries.

In the first three lesions there is diminished pulmonary flow as a result of obstruction of flow to the lungs. In the case of tricuspid atresia and pulmonary atresia, venous return to the right atrium cannot advance to the pulmonary artery and therefore crosses the atrial septum into the left atrium to become part of the left ventricular output. For an infant to survive, blood must enter the pulmonary circuit from the aorta through a patent ductus arteriosus. As long as the ductus maintains an adequate size, the child will survive. In tetralogy of Fallot, if there is pulmonary atresia, a patent ductus arteriosus is also necessary for survival. More commonly there is an obstructed but patent pulmonary valve that limits pulmonary flow and causes the remainder of the venous return to the right ventricle to cross the ventricular septal defect and enter the systemic circuit. The degree of cyanosis is proportional to the severity of the pulmonary valve obstruction.

TRICUSPID ATRESIA. Most commonly in this defect there is an atretic tricuspid valve with absence of both the right ventricle and the pulmonic valve. Hemodynamically there is a three-chambered heart, with the left ventricle maintaining not only systemic but pulmonary circulation through a patent ductus arteriosus. Since the usual pattern is for the patent ductus arteriosus to close in the hours or days after birth, the lesion constitutes one of the emergencies of the newborn period.

On examination the second heart sound is single because there is no pulmonary valve, and if a murmur is present, it is nonspecific. Occasionally a continuous murmur from the ductus arteriosus is heard. The chest roentgenogram shows a normal-sized heart with a small or absent pulmonary artery segment and evidence of decreased lung vascularity. The ECG characteristically shows absence of the right ventricular forces with left ventricular dominance and left axis deviation. Although 70% of cases of tricuspid atresia are associated with normally related great arteries, 30% do have transposition of the great arteries. Finally, tricuspid atresia may be associated with a ventricular septal defect, a small right ventricle, and a stenotic pulmonary outflow tract. Because of the ventricular septal defect, children with tricuspid atresia are not dependent for survival on a patent ductus arteriosus, but since many of them have small ventricular septal defects, pulmonary flow is limited and further compromised if the ventricular septal defect becomes smaller.

Even if there is an associated ventricular septal defect, the long-term prognosis is poor without surgery. In the absence of a right ventricle, surgery is palliative and usually consists of an anastomosis between the subclavian artery and the pulmonary artery (Blalock-Taussig operation) or a side-to-side anastomosis of the ascending aorta to the pulmonary artery (Waterston anastomosis). Recently a more physiologic surgical procedure has been introduced called the Fontane procedure. This consists of connecting the right atrium directly to the pulmonary artery either with or without a conduit containing a porcine valve. If care is taken to select patients with low pulmonary artery pressures, the results are encouraging.

PULMONARY ATRESIA. This lesion differs from tricuspid atresia only in that the tricuspid valve is patent and associated with a right ventricular cavity that is usually small or hypoplastic. Hemodynamically the lesion is similar to that of tricuspid atresia, with the venous return shunting from right to left at atrial level. As in the case of tricuspid atresia, there is a single second heart sound and the systolic murmur, if present, is nonspecific. The chest roentgenogram is also similar to that of tricuspid atresia. The ECG has a vertical axis of approximately 90 degrees, and since there is a right ventricular cavity of varying size, right ventricular potentials are also seen. Since survival depends on patency of the ductus arteriosus, management in the newborn period is similar to that of tricuspid atresia.

TETRALOGY OF FALLOT. This lesion consists of a ventricular septal defect, pulmonary stenosis or atresia, and a systemic pressure in the right ventricle with a right-to-left shunt across the septal defect, as well as a 25% incidence of right aortic arch. The pulmonary stenosis is usually valvular or a combination of a valvular and infundibular obstruction. Occasionally pure infundibular stenosis is present.

As a result of the pulmonary obstruction, the pulmonary blood flow is reduced and often inadequate. The reduced venous return from the lungs as well as the right-to-left shunt at the ventricular level cause varying degrees of cyanosis and hypoxia. If cyanosis is not noted at birth, it usually appears in the first 6 months. The cyanosis becomes more noticeable, and as it increases in severity, dyspnea is common. Occasionally the infant or young child develops hypoxic episodes as a result of a sudden reduction in pulmonary blood flow. Irritability is followed by increased cyanosis and the sudden loss of consciousness. Although the majority of these episodes are brief, some may be prolonged and even cause death. One mechanism is thought to be a sudden constriction of the right ventricular outflow tract caused by muscle spasm. The treatment is to administer oxygen, morphine for sedation, and then a β-blocker such as propranolol (Inderal) if there is a poor response to oxygen.

The clinical findings are those of a single second heart sound (pulmonary valve closure not being heard) with a harsh systolic murmur at the upper left sternal border resulting from flow across the stenotic pulmonary valve. The chest roentgenogram shows a normal-sized heart with a small or absent pulmonary artery segment and decreased pulmonary flow. The ECG shows right ventricular hypertrophy.

The long-term prognosis without surgery is poor. In the presence of a severe pulmonary valve obstruction the reduced pulmonary flow leads to fatigue, increasing cyanosis, polycythemia and its complications, and the risk of bacterial endocarditis. The appearance of hypoxic spells is an indication for early surgical intervention in the form of a palliative shunt in small infants. In infants more than 6 months of age consideration is given to more definitive surgery, with closure of the ventricular septal defect and removal of the pulmonary obstruction. The decision to go ahead with a corrective procedure in the first year of life depends on the size of the pulmonary valve and right ventricular outflow tract. If these are of adequate size, corrective surgery is considered. If they are small or hypoplastic, most centers would consider doing a shunt, with corrective surgery being delayed until the child is older. A small right ventricular outflow tract with a hypoplastic pulmonary valve is not a contraindication to surgery, but if it is to handle a normal right ventricular output after closure of the ventricular septal defect, it has to be opened and enlarged with a patch. In such situations, the pulmonary valve ring is often incompetent, and the child may have severe pulmonary valve insufficiency after surgery.

Occasionally a child with a ventricular septal defect develops sufficient right ventricular outflow tract obstruction to cause both diminished pulmonary flow and a right-to-left shunt at the ventricular level. Hemodynamically the combination is behaving as a tetralogy of Fallot, but the anatomy, being that of a ventricular septal defect with infundibular pulmonic stenosis, is different and more favorable for successful corrective surgery. Occasionally the child is seen early with hypoxic spells that are not always recognized as such, since the child is acyanotic and has the clinical picture of a ventricular septal defect. If a child with a ventricular septal defect also had a right aortic arch, the likelihood of infundibular pulmonary stenosis developing is higher than in the child with a ventricular septal defect and a normal left arch.

EBSTEIN'S ANOMALY OF THE TRICUSPID VALVE. The tricuspid valve, instead of being in its usual position, is prolapsed into the right ventricle so that the ventricular cavity is greatly reduced in size. The septal and posterior cusps of the valve are grossly deformed and their attachment tends to separate the right ventricular cavity into two chambers, one at the apex and the other toward the outflow tract. Occasionally there may be a gradient between them. The hemodynamic effect of this anatomy is impairment of right ventricular function with a reduction in pulmonary flow. The right ventricular cardiac output is further compromised by insufficiency of the tricuspid valve. Because of an increase in right atrial pressure, there is frequently a right-to-left shunt at the atrial level with peripheral cyanosis (most noticeable in the early newborn period while the pulmonary vascular resistance is elevated). On auscultation there is frequently a triple rhythm, and a systolic murmur of tricuspid insufficiency is usually heard at the lower left sternal border. Occasionally a diastolic murmur as a result of tricuspid stenosis is present in the same area.

The chest roentgenogram shows a large heart caused primarily by right atrial enlargement. Right atrial enlargement is also a feature of the ECG, which often reveals characteristic conduction patterns of either a right bundle branch block or the Wolff-Parkinson-White syndrome (any supraventricular tachyarrhythmia can occur).

In the asymptomatic child prognosis depends on the ability of the right ventricle to maintain an adequate cardiac output. Of those who survive infancy, 80% die before 30 years of age. Tricuspid insufficiency is a cause of early right-sided congestive heart failure, and serious arrhythmias carry the risk of early death.

TRANSPOSITION OF THE GREAT ARTERIES. This lesion is unusual in that the intracardiac anatomy is normal; the only abnormality is the switching, or transposition, of the great arteries leaving the heart. As a result the venous return to the heart is pumped from the right ventricle into the aorta, and oxygenated blood returning from the lungs is directed from the left ventricle into the pulmonary artery. This situation—return of desaturated blood to the systemic curcuit—is incompatible with life unless there are connections between the two circuits to permit mixing with reasonable oxygenation of the systemic blood. In fetal life adequate communication exists by means of a patent foramen ovale and a patent ductus arteriosus.

The clinical picture develops rapidly after birth as the patent ductus arteriosus begins to close. Cyanosis appears immediately or within a few hours of birth, and if the seriousness of the condition is not recognized quickly, there is rapid deterioration with early death. Management consists of correcting the inadequate mixing between the two circuits by creating an atrial septal defect to allow mixing at that level. Since the mortality is high when this is done by surgery in the newborn period, it is preferable to create one at the time of the cardiac catheterization using a special catheter. The catheter incorporates a balloon at its tip and is passed across the foramen ovale into the left atrium. The balloon is inflated and jerked back hard against the atrial septum. The tear that results is usually large enough to permit adequate mixing.

The diagnosis is difficult to make. On auscultation the second heart sound is normal, although there tends to be accentuation of the aortic component as a result of the anterior position of the aorta. Usually there are no murmurs because the intracardiac anatomy is normal. Frequently the chest roentgenogram is read as normal, although features may be present that would provide a clue to the diagnosis. If there is no thymus present, it may be noted that the mediastinum is narrow because the main pulmonary artery segment is lying more medial than usual. This gives the heart an "egg on a string" appearance, which is characteristic of a transposition of the great arteries.

If a successful balloon septostomy has been done, most infants do well for a number of months. At the age of 6 months or older open heart surgery is performed to restore normal hemodynamics. The current surgical procedure is Mustard's operation, in which the atrial septum is removed and a piece of either the patient's pericardium or prosthetic material is inserted to direct the pulmonary venous return to the right ventricle and the systemic venous return to the left ventricle. It is not yet known what the long-term prognosis for this operation will be, but there is some concern about the ability of the right ventricle to continue to function efficiently as a systemic ventricle for the remainder of a patient's life. Another complication is the moderately high incidence of supraventricular arrhythmias after surgery.

The concern about the role of the right venticle has reawakened interest in the surgical technique of repositioning the transposed great arteries over their appropriate ventricles. A major objection has always been that the coronary arteries would remain with the pulmonary circuit, a contraindication to the operation. Newer surgical techniques have been developed to maintain continuity of the coronary arteries with the repositioned aorta. Unfortunately, the best results with the technique are when the left ventricle has already been functioning in a systemic capacity, which is not the case in a simple, straightforward transposition.

When transposition of the great arteries is associated with a moderately large ventricular septal defect, the presenting clinical picture is usually that of a ventricular septal defect in congestive heart failure. There may be no cyanosis, although intermittent duskiness is often noted. In such patients closure of the ventricular septal defect would not be beneficial unless Mustard's operation was done at the same time. Apart from the congestive heart failure, a major concern of this combination of defects is that increased pulmonary vascular resistance can develop early in life. There are also partial forms of transposition of the great arteries with ventricular septal defects and other associated anomalies such as pulmonary stenosis. The reader should refer to one of the standard pediatric cardiology texts for details of these lesions.

MYOCARDIAL FAILURE IN CONGENITAL HEART DISEASE

Myocardial function can be impaired as a result of a viral infection, rheumatic fever, or a cardiomyopathy. If the ventricle cannot maintain a satisfactory cardiac output, passive congestion will develop with the picture of congestive heart failure. More commonly in infants and children the myocardium is healthy but gradually fatigues as a result of having to cope with prolonged stress. In the presence of a left-to-right shunt the ventricle dilates, increasing the force of contraction by the stretching of each individual myocardial fiber (Starling's law). If the individual muscle fibers stretch to the point that they no longer contract efficiently and the end-diastolic pressure in the ventricle rises, passive congestion occurs and the picture of congestive heart failure becomes more apparent. Digitalis improves contractility and reduces the end-diastolic pressure. Because so many cases of congestive heart failure in children result from fatigue of normal myocardium, the response to digitalis is usually prompt and dramatic. Failure to show any real improvement after an adequate program of digitalization may be considered an indication for surgical intervention in an operable lesion.

SURGICAL MANAGEMENT OF CONGENITAL HEART DISEASE

If surgery is viewed as a method of improving cardiac function to allow a child to live a longer and more active life, the benefits and limitations are more easily understood. The use of the term "corrective surgery" is misleading, since many of the major lesions may have mild residual defects after surgery. For example, the repair of a tetralogy of Fallot involves reconstruction of the right ventricular outflow tract, with the result that there is usually residual mild pulmonary valve insufficiency. The term "definitive surgery" is preferable to "corrective surgery."

Most of the surgery done in the first 6 months of life is palliative in that it does not attempt to correct the causal lesion but compensates for it until such time as definitive repair is feasible. Examples are the Blalock-Taussig and Waterston shunts for infants with tetralogy of Fallot and the balloon septostomy done at the time of catheterization for transposition of the great arteries. Some centers do attempt definitive repair in this age group but only in selected cases. Most surgeons prefer to delay surgery until after 6 months of age, when it is technically easier and the chances for survival are greater.

The aim of definitive surgery is to restore a flow pattern as close to normal as possible. In some lesions, such as ligation of a patent ductus arteriosus or closure of an atrial septal defect, the results are hemodynamically and structurally excellent. In other lesions, such as pulmonary stenosis, tetralogy of Fallot, atrioventricular canal, and aortic stenosis, valvular abnormalities remain even though satisfactory hemodynamic results have been obtained. The family must be made aware that in spite of the obvious immediate benefits, some uncertainty exists regarding the long-term prognosis.

In recent years one of the most important advances in the surgical management of congenital heart disease has been the development of the extracardiac conduit containing a valve. This is used to replace absent or hypoplastic valves and arteries as well as to reroute blood flow patterns in and around the heart. They are being used for many lesions, including transposition of the great arteries with a ventricular septal defect and left ventricular outflow tract obstruction, pulmonary atresia, tetralogy of Fallot with a hypoplastic outflow tract, truncus arteriosus, tricuspid atresia, and single ventricle. Valved conduits are also being used between the left ventricle and the descending aorta when there is severe aortic obstruction that is not suitable for direct repair. Although many children have benefited from the conduit surgery, it now appears that the heterograft pig valve may have a limited life span; some have developed fibrosis and have had to be replaced.

The availability of some form of surgery for even the most complex lesions is prolonging the expected life span for most children with cardiac defects. At this time it is not possible to say what the long-term prognosis will be for most of them. Will the systemic right ventricle of a transposition of the great arteries function efficiently for the rest of a child's life? What is the long-term prognosis for the right ventricle of a child with tetralogy of Fallot in whom the pulmonary valve and right ventricular outflow tract needed to be patched? If complete right bundle branch block develops during the closure of a ventricular septal defect, will it cause problems in the future? Will the scar resulting from a ventriculotomy impair ventricular function at a later date? It is expected that these questions and others will be answered in time.

BIBLIOGRAPHY

James, F.W.: Exercise testing in children and young adults: an overview. In Wenger, N.K., editor: Cardiovascular clinics: exercise and the heart, Philadelphia, 1978, F.A. Davis Co.

Keith, J.D., Rowe, R.D., and Viad, P.: Heart disease in infancy and childhood, New York, 1967, MacMillan, Inc.

Krovetz, L.J., Gessner, I.H., and Schiebler, G.L.: Handbook of pediatric cardiology, New York, 1969, Harper & Row, Publishers, Inc.

Moller, J.H.: Essentials of pediatric cardiology, Philadelphia, 1978, F.A. Davis Co.

Moss, A.J., and Adams, F.H.: Heart disease in infants, children and adolescents, Baltimore, 1977, The Williams & Wilkins Co.

Nadas, A.S., and Fyler, D.C.: Pediatric cardiology, Philadelphia, 1972, W.B. Saunders Co.

Perloff, J.K.: The clinical recognition of congenital heart disease, Philadelphia, 1970, W.B. Saunders Co.

Rudolph, A.M.: The changes in the circulation after birth, Circulation **41:**343, 1970.

Taussig, H.B.: Congenital malformations of the heart, Cambridge, 1960, Harvard University Press.

Vince, D.J.: Essentials of pediatric cardiology, Philadelphia, 1978, F.A. Davis Co.

Watson, D.G.: Pediatric cardiology notes, Jackson, Miss., 1975, University of Mississippi Medical Center Publications.

Watson, H.: Paediatric cardiology, St. Louis, 1968, The C.V. Mosby Co.

Wellens, H.J., Lubbers, W.J., and Losekoot, T.G.: Preexcitation. In Roberts, N.K., and Gelband, H., editors: Cardiac arrhythmias in the neonate, infant and child, New York, 1977, Appleton-Century-Crofts.

94 • VALVULAR HEART DISEASE

Michael J. Barrett

The cause of valvular heart disease has been changing over the last two decades. Rheumatic fever and its valvular sequelae are diagnosed less frequently and are being replaced by congenital valvular disease, such as bicuspid aortic valve and less well-defined disorders such as myxomatous degeneration of the mitral valve. Associated with these changes in the causes is the shifting of the population being treated. For example, with aortic valve disease more and more patients over age 60 undergo successful valvular surgery. With mitral valve disease younger patients continue to predominate, espcially because of mitral valve prolapse. Along with the changing causes and populations, there are new techniques such as two-dimensional (2-D) echocardiography to enable the clinician to identify anatomic valve pathology at a much earlier stage in the patients' disease. Such improvements in diagnostic and therapeutic armamentarium will hopefully result in more optimal timing of valvular surgery and improve survival of patients with valvular heart disease. With all valvular heart disease antibiotic prophylaxis must be considered in association with dental procedures and other types of surgery (see discussion of "Infective endocarditis" in Chapter 40).

MITRAL REGURGITATION

The mitral valve consists of five separate components: the mitral anulus, mitral leaflets, chordae tendineae, papillary muscles, and ventricular myocardium supporting these muscles. All five components must work in synchrony for the mitral valve to remain competent.

Mitral regurgitation results when any one of these five elements is impaired; for example, when the mitral anulus becomes calcified, it loses its sphincterlike action and mild mitral regurgitation results. Rheumatic fever may result in thickening, scarring, and eventual calcification of the leaflets themselves. Commissures become adherent and the chordae shorten and retract the leaflets, thereby preventing adequate apposition of the mitral leaflets and resulting in mitral regurgitation. Another example is myxomatous degeneration of the leaflets, in which the leaflets increase markedly in size so that in systole they prolapse into the left atrium. Papillary muscles may become ischemic or infarcted and fibrotic, resulting in inadequate shortening during systole, which once again results in mitral regurgitation. Finally, the ventricular myocardium may offer inadequate support for the mitral apparatus. This can be a result of myocardial infarction or dilation of left ventricular cavity, causing malposition of the papillary muscles.

CLINICAL MANIFESTATIONS. The most prominent symptom of mitral regurgitation is *dyspnea,* which may progress to orthopnea and paroxysmal nocturnal dyspnea. As mitral regurgitation increases, left atrial pressure rises. This pressure is transmitted into the pulmonary veins, eventually causing exudation of fluid into the capillaries in the lung. The larger the amount of mitral regurgitation, the higher the back pressure in the left atrium and pulmonary veins and the more severe the dyspnea. A second symptom is *fatigue,* which occurs fairly late in the course of the disease. This is due to a diminished cardiac output because a large volume of blood is being regurgitated into the left atrium with each ventricular contraction. Decreased ventricular contractility, a late complication of this disease, may also contribute to a diminished cardiac output.

Mild mitral regurgitation may remain asymptomatic for years. Age at the onset of symptomatology varies with the cause of mitral regurgitation. Rheumatic mitral regurgitation may follow an episode of rheumatic fever by 5 or 10 years and become evident in adolescence. Women experience rheumatic mitral regurgitation almost three times as often as men. In persons over 40 years of age coronary artery disease is often responsible for mitral regurgitation because of either ischemic papillary muscles or ventricular dilation. Men and women are equally affected by this condition. On occasion a chorda tendineae ruptures spontaneously (seen in systemic hypertension or as a consequence of endocarditis) and causes symptoms soon thereafter.

Mitral regurgitation exerts its effect on the left ventricle by increasing the amount of blood required to be pumped to compensate for the regurgitation. When this regurgitant fraction is significant, the left ventricle enlarges, with the apex displaced beyond the midclavicular line. Typically an apical plateau-shaped holosystolic murmur radiating from the apex to the base of the heart or to the axilla is heard. Milder degrees of mitral regurgitation produce only a late systolic murmur, often crescendo in nature. Acute mitral regurgitation resulting from rupture of a chorda tendineae may be found as an early systolic murmur. With the advent of secondary pulmonary hypertension, P_2 (the sound of pulmonic valve closure) will be increased and splitting of the second heart sound will be slightly accentuated. A third heart sound (S_3 gallop) is present in all but the mildest cases. The gallop does not necessarily signify heart failure but may reflect early diastolic filling. Fourth heart sounds (S_4 gallop) are absent until late in the disease.

LABORATORY FINDINGS. The chest roentgenogram shows left ventricular enlargement and cardiomegaly over time. The left atrium also enlarges with time and may be seen as a "double density" under the left mainstem bronchus (see section on "Mitral stenosis" for roentgenographic findings). Late in the course of the disease the pulmonary arteries enlarge, as does the right ventricle. With acute mitral regurgitation there is a normal cardiac silhouette with pulmonary congestion.

The ECG reveals sinus rhythm in the early stages. Left atrial enlargement is reflected by large negative P waves in

V_1. With increasing left atrial dilation, atrial fibrillation is common. Left ventricular hypertrophy causes increased QRS voltage and repolarization abnormalities in the ST segments and the T waves.

The M-mode echocardiogram reveals a dilated left ventricle, dilated left atrium, and perhaps the anatomic disease of the mitral apparatus responsible for the regurgitation, such as vegetations from endocarditis, prolapse, or rheumatic changes on the leaflets. In addition, calcification of the mitral anulus is routinely detected by M-mode echocardiograms. A 2-D echocardiogram permits assessment of left ventricular motion and gives a more precise picture of the valvular deformities, whether they are vegetations, prolapse, or even a flail leaflet.

Cardiac catheterization is required to document the presence and severity of mitral regurgitation. Before marked left atrial dilation, large atrial v waves reflecting the regurgitant blood will be found. Severity of regurgitation into the left atrium is assessed from contrast injection into the left ventricle. As this disease progresses, left ventricular end-diastolic pressure rises when left ventricular contractility falters.

MANAGEMENT. Mild mitral regurgitation is usually asymptomatic and requires no specific therapy. As the mitral regurgitation increases or left ventricular contraction falters, dyspnea, orthopnea, paroxysmal nocturnal dyspnea, and fatigue appear. These symptoms call for dietary sodium restriction and/or diuretic therapy and digitalis (doses determined by symptomatic response and digoxin/digitoxin blood levels). Atrial fibrillation should be converted to sinus rhythm as long as the left atrium is not excessively dilated. Otherwise the rate of the ventricular response to atrial fibrillation is controlled with the digitalis. Patients with dyspnea and fatigue are often benefited by arterial vasodilators such as hydralazine (see Chapter 86).

When patients with mitral regurgitation become dyspneic with mild exertion despite medical therapy, the mitral valve should be replaced. Those whose left ventricular contractility is still normal improve significantly. The risks of surgery rise proportionately to decreased left ventricular function. Mitral valve replacement can be performed using either a prosthetic disk or ball valve or a porcine heterograft. The disk valves function well but require lifelong anticoagulation. Porcine heterografts are preferred in patients with bleeding disorders because they do not require anticoagulation.

MITRAL VALVE PROLAPSE

Mitral valve prolapse is characterized by redundant mitral leaflets that bulge into the left atrium during systole. The clinical hallmarks of this disease are systolic clicks and a late systolic murmur.

Most cases are idiopathic, but a minority are seen with Marfan's syndrome, atrial septal defect, congenital heart disease, or rheumatic valve disease. In some patients microscopic evidence of myxomatous degeneration of the enlarged mitral leaflets has been demonstrated. Prolapse may also occur secondary to bacterial endocarditis of the mitral valve.

CLINICAL MANIFESTATIONS. When isolated systolic clicks appear without a murmur, there is often no mitral regurgitation. Presence of a late systolic murmur indicates mitral regurgitation, usually of a mild degree. In early systole the valve is competent and no murmur is present. However, as the valve prolapses into the atrium, the leaflets separate and regurgitation results. Maneuvers that decrease ventricular volume, such as standing, enhance the prolapse and make the murmur occur earlier and last longer. Maneuvers that increase ventricular volume, such as squatting, move the click later in systole, and the murmur becomes shorter.

The prevalence of mitral valve prolapse is not known, but the disease is common. Estimates vary from 0.3% to 15% and depend on the population studied and criteria used for diagnosis. Most patients are less than 40 years of age, and women far outnumber men. Nonanginal chest pain is common and often causes the patient to seek medical attention. Arrhythmias are frequent, such as atrial or ventricular premature beats and preexcitation syndromes. Sudden death has been reported but is rare. In one report, middle-aged patients with cerebral emboli showed a higher than expected incidence of mitral valve prolapse; the emboli could have emanated from the valve itself or from the left atrium.

Bony abnormalities of the thorax are common, including pectus excavatum, straight back syndrome, and mild thoracic scoliosis. Systolic clicks occur in mid- or late systole. The findings are notoriously variable, even when auscultation is done in the same position. Clicks may come and go, often making the diagnosis difficult.

LABORATORY FINDINGS. Inverted T waves may occur, especially in the inferior leads. Prolonged QT intervals are frequent and are associated with cardiac arrhythmias or sudden death.

The M-mode echocardiogram demonstrates late systolic displacement of one or both leaflets of the mitral valve. Holosystolic prolapse may be seen. With 2-D echocardiography prolapse is diagnosed when any part of the leaflet is seen to protrude into the left atrium during systole. Mild angiographic mitral regurgitation may be present during contrast left ventriculography, which shows the leaflets protruding beyond their closure line into the left atrium.

MANAGEMENT. Many physicians treat patients with mitral valve prolapse with antibiotics during dental and surgical procedures to prevent endocarditis, but such prophylaxis is controversial. Premature contractions are usually not treated. Propranolol may be helpful in treating patients with chest pain, but there is no evidence for its benefit.

MITRAL STENOSIS

Rheumatic fever causes mitral stenosis. The acute episode usually occurs in childhood, but the consequences become evident 10 to 15 years later. Subclinical forms of the disease often occur, and almost half of the patients with rheumatic valvular involvement give no history of prior rheumatic fever.

The rheumatic process results in scarring and thickening of the leaflets, which narrows the valve orifice. In addition shortening and thickening of the chordae tendineae occur and may contribute to associated mitral regurgitation. As the disease progresses, left atrial size increases and there can be thrombus formation as a result of stasis of blood in the left atrium.

CLINICAL MANIFESTATIONS. As the obstruction to flow from the left atrium to ventricle worsens, pressure in the left atrium increases and is transmitted to the pulmonary veins. The patient complains of dyspnea initially and orthopnea eventually. A late complication of mitral stenosis is pulmonary arterial hypertension caused by (1) the transmission of elevated left atrial pressure into the pulmonary veins and (2) a reactive increase in pulmonary arteriolar resistance that occurs as a secondary phenomenon. With the appearance of a dilated atrium, atrial fibrillation is common.

Following an acute episode of rheumatic fever in early childhood, symptoms become evident when persons are in their thirties or forties. Women predominate over men almost 3:1. Patients first complain of dyspnea on exertion, which eventually progresses to dyspnea when lying flat (orthopnea) or paroxysmal nocturnal dyspnea. Symptoms may be heralded by the sudden onset of atrial fibrillation with a rapid ventricular response. Systemic emboli from the left atrium may be the first manifestation of mitral stenosis. With the onset of pulmonary hypertension, right ventricular failure with pedal edema, ascites, and hepatomegaly appears.

The hallmarks of mitral stenosis can be overlooked on physical examination unless specifically sought. The first heart sound is increased and is often palpable at the left sternal border in all but severely calcified valves. Systole is usually quiescent unless there is associated mitral regurgitation. The second heart sound is split with an accentuation of P_2 when there is pulmonary hypertension. An open-

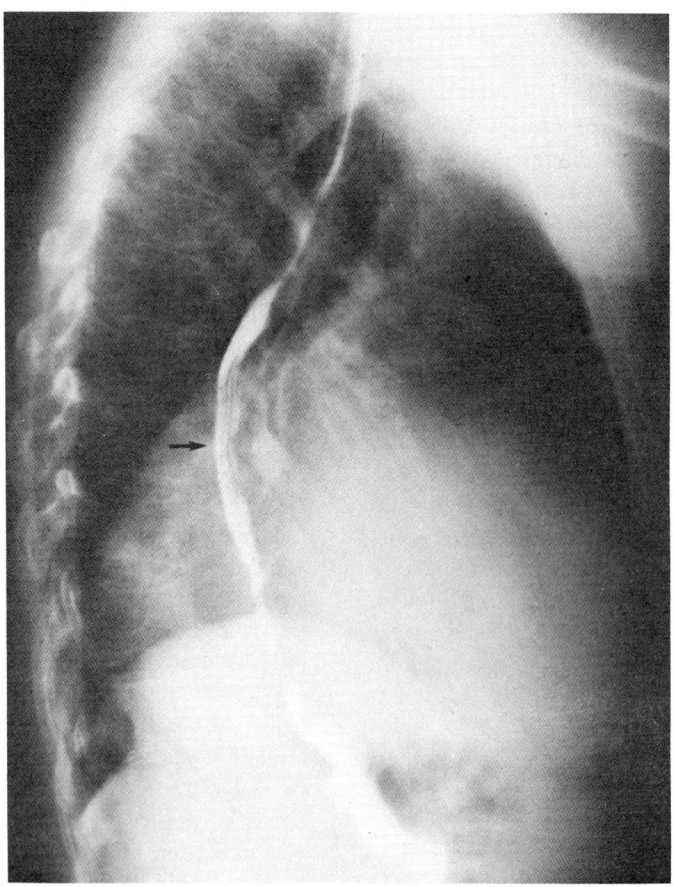

Fig. 94-1. Lateral chest roentgenogram with barium swallow demonstrating left atrial enlargement *(arrow)*. Left atrium enlarges posteriorly, displacing barium-filled esophagus.

ing snap of the mitral valve follows the P_2 by 0.06 to 0.11 second and inaugurates a low-frequency diastolic rumble. This opening snap may soften or even disappear if the valve becomes heavily calcified. The diastolic rumble is heard best with the bell of the stethoscope at the apex of the heart and with the patient in the left lateral decubitus position. In sinus rhythm there is a presystolic accentuation of the rumble timed with atrial contraction. As pulmonary hypertension appears, the right ventricular impulse becomes palpable at the left sternal edge.

LABORATORY FINDINGS. The chest roentgenogram reveals left atrial enlargement, manifested by a double density beneath an elevated left mainstem bronchus. Left atrial size is best demonstrated by a barium swallow in the lateral view (Fig. 94-1). Pulmonary venous congestion may be evident. With pulmonary hypertension there is an increase in pulmonary artery size. A calcified mitral valve may be visible in the lateral chest roentgenogram or on fluoroscopy. Cardiomegaly is rare.

In the early stages of the disease the ECG reveals normal sinus rhythm and left atrial enlargement (manifested by a prominent negative P wave in V_1 and a wide notched P wave in II). As the disease progresses, right axis deviation becomes apparent. The combination of left atrial enlargement and right axis deviation suggests mitral stenosis.

An M-mode echocardiogram will establish the presence of mitral stenosis but cannot quantify the degree of stenosis. A 2-D echocardiogram can measure the mitral valve area (Fig. 94-2) and can detect mitral stenosis (Fig. 94-3). Cardiac catheterization shows a pressure gradient between the left atrium and left ventricle in diastole. Mitral valve area is calculated by taking into account transvalvular blood flow (cardiac output), the pressure gradient, and diastolic filling time.

Atrial myxomas, which may produce the same symptoms as mitral stenosis, may be of right atrial or left atrial origin. The physical findings of atrial myxoma can precisely mimic those of mitral stenosis. Occasionally patients with left atrial myxoma have been followed for years with the mistaken diagnosis of mitral stenosis. Patients in later life are seen with myxoma, often after embolization; true metastases are not seen. At other times patients have unexplained signs of pulmonary hypertension, with syncope or with apparent culture-negative endocarditis. Atrial myxoma can easily be detected by echocardiography.

MANAGEMENT. The symptoms of mild to moderate mitral stenosis are principally those of pulmonary congestion and dyspnea. These usually respond to sodium restriction and/or a diuretic; only atrial fibrillation should be treated with digoxin. Propranolol can be used to control the ventricular rate if there is not regurgitation or diminished ventricular contractility from rheumatic carditis or pulmonary hypertension. Patients in atrial fibrillation should have electrical cardioversion to decrease the risk of emboli. Patients with atrial fibrillation should receive anticoagulation therapy with warfarin (Coumadin) to prevent systemic emboli unless a contraindication is present.

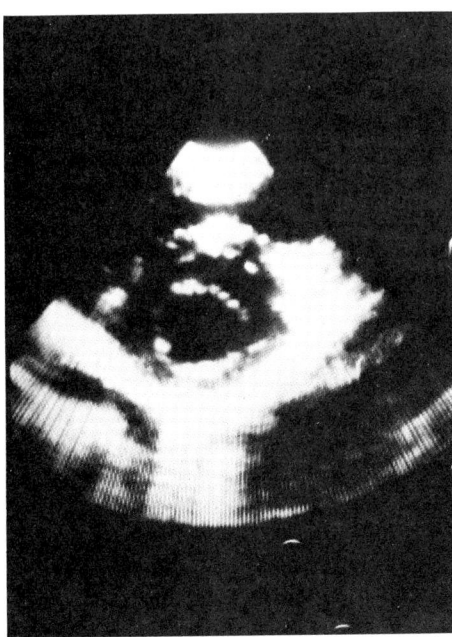
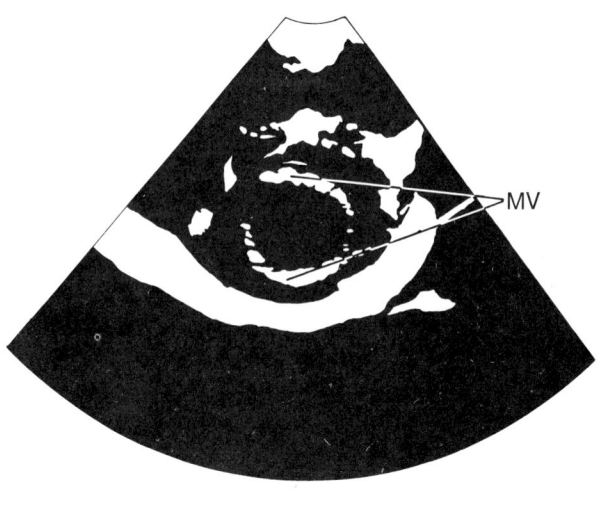

Fig. 94-2. On left is stop frame; on right is idealized drawing from 2-D echocardiogram demonstrating normal mitral valve, *MV,* in short axis view. Anterior leaflet forms top of this valve, and posterior leaflet forms bottom. Left ventricle appears as circle in this view.

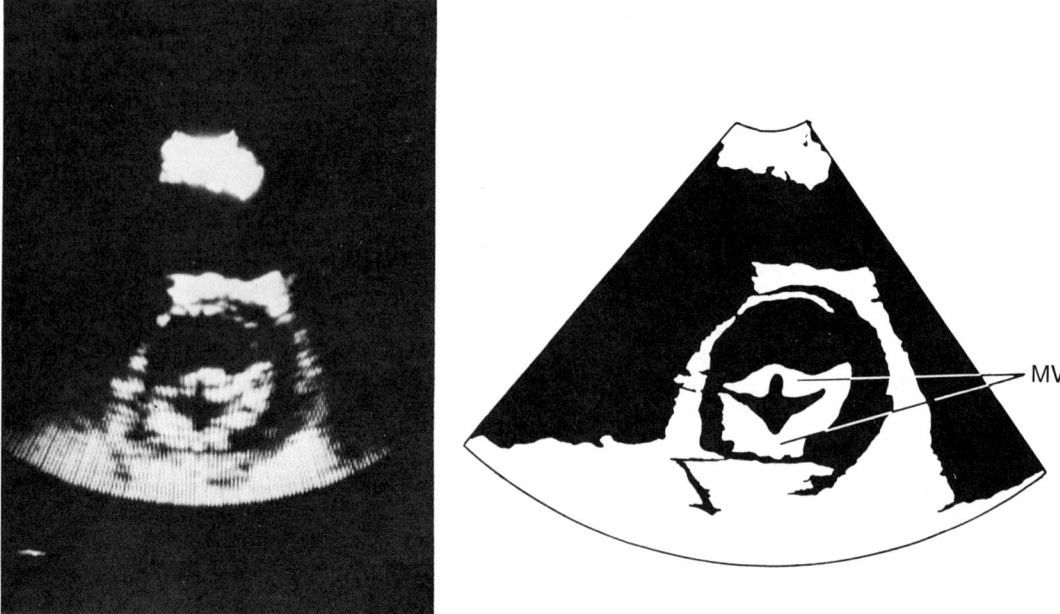

Fig. 94-3. On left is stop frame; on right is idealized drawing from 2-D echocardiograh demonstrating mitral stenosis. Mitral valve, *MV*, is thickened, with a markedly diminished opening compared to normal mitral valve. Mitral valve area can be calculated from this stop frame to quantify degree of mitral stenosis.

When patients become symptomatic with minimal exertion, they should have surgery. Recurrent emboli also are considered by some to be an indication for surgery. Patients with noncalcified valves and without associated regurgitation can have commisurotomy (leaflets directly separated), and this may relieve symptoms for many years. Severely distorted and calcified valves must be replaced with either a prosthesis or a porcine heterograft (if there are contraindications to chronic anticoagulation, procine heterografts are preferred).

AORTIC STENOSIS

The most common cause of aortic stenosis today is congenital bicuspid valves (1% of the general population). Rheumatic disease may also result in stenosis of the aortic valve but is almost always accompanied by mitral disease as well.

CLINICAL MANIFESTATIONS. As the orifice of the aortic valve decreases, the pressure that the left ventricle must generate to eject a normal stroke volume increases. The diminished orifice size causes a pressure gradient across the valve. The turbulence of blood flow generates a murmur. To maintain flow across this narrowed valve, the left ventricle hypertrophies. As the severity increases, flow across the valve becomes fixed and the patient cannot increase cardiac output during exercise. The increased flow to the extremities with exertion causes a decrease in cerebral blood flow and results in dizziness or syncope. Despite severely increased intraventricular pressures, the left ventricle remains compensated as long as its size is normal. Later, myocardial contractility falls and the left ventricle dilates. Diastolic ventricular and left atrial pressures further increase. At this point dyspnea on mild exertion appears. Angina results from the increased oxygen requirements of the massively hypertrophied ventricle, even without coexistent coronary artery disease.

Aortic stenosis occurs in three times as many males as females. The murmur may be present for years before the onset of symptoms. However, from the time of the onset of dyspnea, angina, or syncope, survival is on the average only 5 years. Sudden death may occur when stenosis is severe.

The carotid pulse has a delayed rise with a small pulse volume. A systolic thrill may be felt in the second right intercostal space directly over the aorta. The left ventricular impulse is diffuse, and a palpable fourth heart sound is present. S_1 is normal and S_2 is soft or absent in severe aortic stenosis. The murmur is midsystolic, has a harsh character with a distinct late peaking, and radiates to the carotid arteries with a palpable thrill. With bicuspid valves an ejection sound is often present at the second right intercostal space.

LABORATORY FINDINGS. The chest roentgenogram shows a dilated aorta (poststenotic dilation), but at first the heart size is normal. Cardiomegaly will be present later, as well as pulmonary congestion. A calcified aortic valve is often visible in the lateral chest roentgenogram. The ECG shows left ventricular hypertrophy.

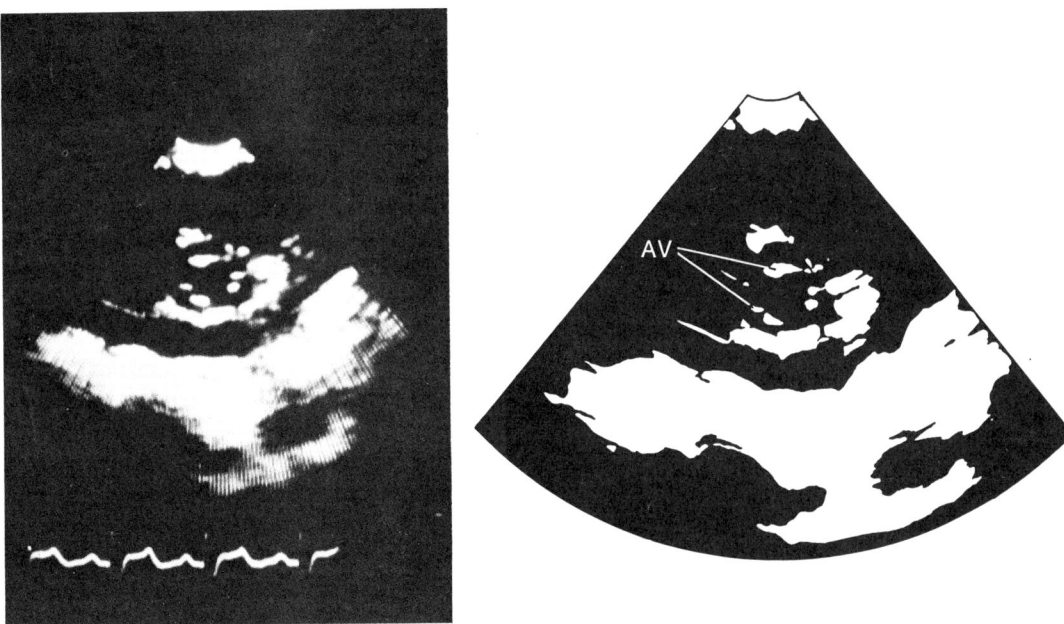

Fig. 94-4. On left is stop frame; on right is idealized drawing from 2-D echocardiogram demonstrating normal aortic valve, *AV*. All three leaflets of this valve are visible, and valve area is space enclosed by these leaflets.

The M-mode echocardiogram can detect thickened aortic leaflets with decreased excursion. A 2-D echocardiogram will allow assessment of the severity of the stenosis (Fig. 94-4). Catheterization reveals a systolic pressure gradient across the aortic valve. The gradient reflects both the severity of the obstruction and the flow (cardiac output). As a rule critical aortic stenosis is present when the pressure gradient across the valve is 50 mm Hg or higher (less with a fall in cardiac output).

MANAGEMENT. Patients with mild aortic stenosis are asymptomatic and require no therapy. When angina, dyspnea, or syncope appears, cardiac catheterization should be done to assess the severity of the stenosis (as well as the coronary anatomy if there is angina). The treatment for severe aortic stenosis is valve replacement. A prosthetic valve requires lifelong anticoagulation. Other complications of prosthetic valves include endocarditis (antibiotic prophylaxis remains indicated), paravalvular leak, and systemic emboli despite anticoagulation. Porcine heterografts do not require anticoagulation and can be used in patients with bleeding abnormalities; these have a resting gradient and may not withstand wear and tear over the years.

AORTIC REGURGITATION

Aortic regurgitation can be secondary to abnormal leaflet structure, such as from endocarditis or rheumatic lesions. Calcific aortic stenosis is often associated with some regurgitation when the leaflets become rigid. Aortic regurgitation may also be due to dilation of the aortic root so that the cusps do not approximate each other normally. Diseases of the aorta such as Marfan's syndrome or cystic medial necrosis, syphilis, ankylosing spondylitis, and dissection cause aortic regurgitation. Cardiac trauma can cause disruption of the leaflets or aortic ring.

CLINICAL MANIFESTATIONS. Blood ejected into the aorta in systole reenters the left ventricle in diastole. To compensate, the left ventricle must increase its stroke volume (by increasing end-diastolic pressure and volume and hence left ventricular size). Unlike mitral regurgitation, left atrial pressure is not elevated because the mitral valve prevents retrograde transmission of the elevated left ventricular pressure. The mitral valve may even close prematurely when diastolic aortic regurgitation quickly causes ventricular pressure to exceed atrial pressure, detracting from ventricular filling. With time the left ventricular enlargement becomes excessive and left ventricular diastolic pressure and hence left atrial pressure become elevated. Mitral regurgitation can then occur as a consequence of malposition of the papillary muscles. The elevated left atrial pressure results in dyspnea. Acute aortic regurgitation from bacterial endocarditis causes a rapid elevation in both left ventricular and left atrial pressures, with prominent symptoms of dyspnea.

Aortic regurgitation is usually well tolerated in its early stages. Exercise tolerance in particular is well maintained, since the vasodilation accompanying exercise serves to enhance forward stroke volume and thereby lessens regurgitation. Patients may become aware of the large stroke volume and note a forceful heartbeat or palpitations. Angina is not typical of aortic regurgitation (as compared to stenosis) and suggests coexistent coronary artery disease. Syncope can occur as a result of an arrhythmia.

The markedly increased stroke volume produces a wide pulse pressure. The carotid, brachial, and femoral artery pulses demonstrate a brisk upstroke with a rapid falloff (water-hammer pulse). In advanced cases the head bobs gently up and down and the nail beds alternately blanch and fill with each cardiac contraction. The left ventricular impulse is displaced beyond the midclavicular line. S_1 is soft. In cases of aortic root dilation there may be an early systolic ejection sound heard in the second right intercostal space. S_2 splits normally, and its aortic component is often increased and may have a tambourlike quality. S_3 and S_4 gallops are common. The murmur of aortic regurgitation is a high-frequency, early diastolic blow often heard best at the third left intercostal space (Erb's point). The duration of the murmur varies with blood pressure and does not necessarily reflect the severity of regurgitation. For instance, mild regurgitation may cause a brief murmur, but acute severe regurgitation may also result in only a very brief murmur that halts when the diastolic pressure equalizes in the aortic root and left ventricle. The majority of patients with aortic regurgitation will have a systolic murmur reflecting the increased flow across the aortic valve. An apical diastolic Austin-Flint murmur caused by the regurgitant jet striking the anterior leaflet of the mitral valve mimics rheumatic mitral stenosis. However, there is no opening snap or presystolic accentuation of the murmur.

LABORATORY FINDINGS. The chest roentgenogram shows dilation of the ascending aortic root. With progressive disease the left ventricle enlarges and cardiomegaly results. Calcium may be seen in the aortic valve on lateral chest roentgenogram. Syphilis results in linear calcifications of the ascending aortic root.

The M-mode echocardiogram reveals the dilated left ventricle and dilated aortic root as well as fluttering of the anterior leaflet of the mitral valve. In acute aortic regurgitation or in severe chronic regurgitation premature closure of the mitral valve may be observed (the mitral valve is considered to close prematurely when its closure precedes the onset of the Q wave). Two-dimensional echocardiography may reveal vegetations on the leaflets or rheumatic involvement of these leaflets. The aortic valve may be seen to prolapse into the left ventricle in diastole.

At cardiac catheterization an elevated left ventricular end-diastolic pressure is usually found because of aortic regurgitation. Severity is estimated from an aortogram.

MANAGEMENT. The first appearance of clear-cut pulmonary edema or other signs of left ventricular failure is an indication for surgical intervention. This is because patients who are allowed to persist for some time in left ventricular failure often have poor surgical results because left ventricular contractility becomes irreversibly impaired. On the other hand, surgery is not recommended for only mild aortic regurgitation because a mild lesion is well tolerated for several years. The usual indications for surgical intervention are increasing heart size on chest roentgenogram or clinical evidence for left ventricular failure. Long-term results of surgery are often good, although there is operative mortality of 10%.

TRICUSPID AND PULMONIC VALVE DISEASE

Tricuspid stenosis is rare as an isolated lesion. Usually it accompanies rheumatic involvement of other heart valves, but it is clinically significant in only 5% of such patients. Other causes of tricuspid stenosis include endocardial fibroelastosis, congenital malformations, and right atrial myxoma.

Tricuspid stenosis should be suspected in patients with multivalve disease who have severe venous congestion in the absence of marked pulmonary hypertension. On physical examination the jugular venous pressure is elevated and, in patients in sinus rhythm, there is a prominent jugular atrial a wave contraction. There is a characteristic slow fall in the jugular v wave caused by obstruction to right atrial emptying. On palpation of the precordium the right ventricle is not enlarged, although a diastolic thrill may be palpated over it. This diastolic rumble of tricuspid stenosis may not be heard unless specifically sought at the lower left sternal border. It resembles mitral stenosis but differs in that it becomes louder with inspiration.

The ECG reveals tall positive P waves in leads II and V_1 when sinus rhythm is present and later reveals atrial fibrillation. There is usually no evidence for right ventricular hypertrophy. Chest roentgenograms may show right atrial enlargement.

Surgical treatment is usually not indicated for mild tricuspid stenosis alone. However, if surgery is to be undertaken for other valvular lesions, the tricuspid valve should first be carefully evaluated, since tricuspid stenosis is sometimes recognized only when unexpected signs of venous congestion develop postoperatively.

Tricuspid regurgitation is usually caused by dilation of the right ventricle, which results from pulmonary hypertension. Tricuspid regurgitation may also result from traumatic injury, congenital defects such as Ebstein's anomaly, or bacterial endocarditis. Regurgitation is reflected by large v waves (regurgitant) in the jugular venous pulse. Systolic hepatic pulsations are often present, and there may be marked hepatomegaly, ascites, and peripheral edema. If pulmonary hypertension is present, a palpable pulmonary artery impulse may be felt in the second left intercostal space and an accentuated P_2 may be evident. With severe tricuspid regurgitation the right ventricle is enlarged and a systolic thrill is palpable at the lower left sternal border. The holosystolic murmur heard over the right ventricle increases with inspiration (Carvallo's sign).

The ECG reveals right ventricular hypertrophy and often atrial fibrillation. Chest roentgenograms show enlargement of the right atrium and ventricle.

Treatment of tricuspid regurgitation consists of sodium restriction, diuretics, and digitalis. If surgery is undertaken for associated mitral or aortic valve disease, functional tricuspid regurgitation improves as pulmonary hypertension is decreased. However, in organic lesions of the tricuspid valve, plication or a prosthetic valve is preferred.

Pulmonic regurgitation in adults is almost exclusively secondary to pulmonary hypertension or bacterial endocarditis. It is difficult to separate from aortic regurgitation. Pulmonic stenosis is almost always congenital, although subpulmonic stenosis may be seen in association with hypertrophic subaortic stenosis.

BIBLIOGRAPHY

Braunwald, E., and others: Aortic stenosis: physiologic, pathological and clinical concepts, Ann. Intern. Med. **58**:494, 1963.
Criley, M.J., and others: Prolapse of the mitral valve: clinical and cineangiographic findings, Br. Heart J. **28**:488, 1966.
Frank, S., Johnson, A., and Ross, J., Jr.: Natural history of valvular aortic stenosis, Br. Heart J. **35**:41, 1975.
Goldschlager, N., and others: The natural history of aortic regurgitation: a clinical and hemodynamic study, Am. J. Med. **54**:577, 1973.
Gorlin, R., and Gorlin, S.G.: Hydraulic formula for calculation of the area of stenotic mitral valve, other cardiac valves and central circulatory shunts, Am. Heart J. **41**:1, 1951.
Jeresaty, R.M.: Mitral valve prolapse click syndrome, Prog. Cardiovasc. Dis. **15**:623, 1973.
Kitchin, A., and Turner, R.: Diagnosis and treatment of tricuspid stenosis, Br. Heart J. **26**:354, 1964.
Korn, E., DeSanctis, R.W., and Sell, S.: Massive calcification of the mitral annulus: a clinico-pathological study of fourteen cases, N. Engl. J. Med. **267**:900, 1962.
Roberts, W.C.: The structure of the aortic valve in clinically isolated aortic stenosis: an autopsy study of 162 patients over 15 years of age, Circulation **42**:91, 1970.
Selzer, A., and Cohn, K.E.: Natural history of mitral stenosis: a review, Circulation **41**:878, 1972.

95 • PRIMARY MUSCLE DISEASES OF THE HEART

Bernadine Healy Bulkley

Cardiomyopathy is a term applied to those diseases characterized by cardiac dysfunction that is caused primarily by an abnormality of the working myocardium. One must exclude valvular disease, coronary disease, and congenital malformations of cardiac structure as the *major* cause of the cardiac dysfunction before diagnosing a cardiomyopathy. Thus primary muscle disease, or cardiomyopathy, is largely a diagnosis of exclusion.

In defining the cardiomyopathies clinically, it is useful to recognize the heterogeneous spectrum and varied pathophysiology that they encompass. Most broadly one can separate the cardiomyopathies into two groups: the primary or idiopathic and the secondary cardiomyopathies (Table 95-1). In both categories there are three functional states: (1) hypertrophic, hyperdynamic; (2) dilated, congestive; and (3) restrictive cardiomyopathies.

Table 95-1. Classification of cardiomyopathies

Functional type	Primary	Secondary
Hypertrophic, hyperdynamic	Idiopathic Familial (ASH) Nonfamilial	Aortic stenosis, systemic hypertension, glycogen storage disease
Dilated, congestive	Idiopathic	Ischemic heart disease, scleroderma, sarcoidosis, hemochromatosis
Restrictive	Idiopathic endocardial fibroelastosis	Amyloidosis, secondary endocardial fibroelastosis, hemochromatosis

The disease classification of primary myocardial disease generally refers to one of the idiopathic cardiomyopathies. Since the secondary cardiomyopathies may mimic the primary ones and require similar therapies, they too must be considered in the definitions of muscle diseases of the heart. Therefore this presentation is divided into idiopathic hypertrophic, congestive, and restrictive cardiomyopathies and secondary cardiomyopathies.

IDIOPATHIC HYPERTROPHIC CARDIOMYOPATHY AND ASYMMETRIC SEPTAL HYPERTROPHY

DEFINITION. Hypertrophic cardiomyopathy has received much attention in recent years. It was first described as a distinct clinical and pathologic entity only a little more than 20 years ago. In this disorder the heart is hypertrophied and hyperdynamic. Systolic ejection is generally in the range of 70% to 90% of left ventricular volume, and heart failure results partly from difficulty in diastolic filling of the hypertrophied, poorly compliant, small-cavity ventricle. A midsystolic subaortic gradient is frequently present, which has led to the subclassification of hypertrophic cardiomyopathy into those with and without "obstruction." Whether the gradient actually measures a true obstruction to flow of blood rather than the "squeeze" of the obliterated cavity around the catheter in systole, however, has never been clear. Furthermore, since patients with gradients do no worse and possibly better than patients without gradients and since the gradient tends to be variable within the same patient, the subclassification by "obstruction" has become less useful.

PATHOGENESIS. Since hypertrophic cardiomyopathy has only recently been defined, it is not surprising that its pathogenesis is as yet unresolved. What has become apparent in recent years, however, is that the clinical spectrum of hypertrophic cardiomyopathy is varied as shown in the outline below:

Clinical spectrum of hypertrophic cardiomyopathy

I. Idiopathic hypertrophic cardiomyopathy with asymmetric hypertrophy and myocardial fiber disarray including familial (Teare type)
II. Idiopathic hypertrophic cardiomyopathy with symmetry and normal histology (non-Teare type)
III. Secondary hypertrophic cardiomyopathy
   A. Systemic hypertension
   B. Aortic stenosis after valve repair
IV. Functional hypertrophic cardiomyopathy
   A. Hyperkinetic heart syndrome
   B. Hypovolemia
   C. Pressor infusion

In some patients hypertrophic cardiomyopathy is a familial disorder associated with *asymmetric hypertrophy* of the heart and abnormal myocardial histology consisting of a disarray of myocardial fibers (Fig. 95-1). This form of hypertrophic cardiomyopathy was originally described in 1958 by Donald Teare, who observed it at autopsy as the cause of sudden death in seven young adults. Teare noted the cardiac structure to be so abnormal that he believed it was most likely caused by some developmental anomaly or congenital lesion in the heart. Familial studies of this form of cardiomyopathy seem to indicate that this condition does reflect an underlying genetic defect that is ultimately manifest in abnormal cardiac structure. The muscle fiber disarray may reflect abnormal wall stress and tension created by the abnormality of cardiac shape, or genetically determined functional abnormalities of left ventricular contraction (as might be seen with some derangement in the sympathetic nervous system), if present early enough in embryonic life, could result in the congenital abnormality of heart structure. The precise interaction of function and structure in this condition remains unknown.

Other forms of hypertrophic cardiomyopathy of the "non-Teare type" exist, in which functional abnormality of the heart is present, with hyperdynamic ejection, abnormal systolic anterior mitral valve motion, and unexplained *symmetric hypertrophy* (without asymmetric hypertrophy or myocardial fiber disarray). Secondary forms of functional symmetric hypertrophic cardiomyopathy may also develop and be difficult to distinguish from the primary varieties. Long-standing systemic hypertension and aortic stenosis can lead to this condition. Even when the aortic valve is replaced, if the hypertrophy is advanced and the left ventricular cavity is normal to small in size, hypertrophic hemodynamics associated with rapid, almost complete systolic ejection and cavity obliteration may occur. Recent studies of HLA typing in hypertrophic cardiomyopathy have pointed out two pathogenetically distinctive forms of this disease—familial, with autosomal dominant inheritance, and sporadic, possibly linked to systemic hypertension.

Patients with normal hearts but hypercontractile states as a result of hypovolemia, pressor administration, or other

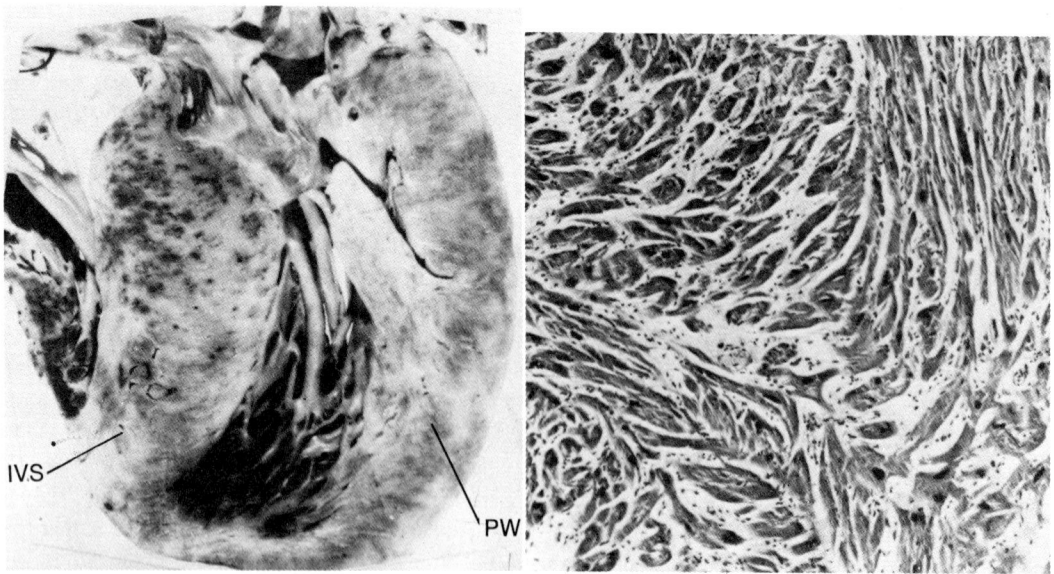

Fig. 95-1. Heart with hypertrophic cardiomyopathy. Interventricular septum, *IVS*, is thicker than posterior wall, *PW*. Histologic section on right shows marked disorganization of myocardium that is especially prominent in septum (hematoxylin and eosin, ×50). (From Bulkley, B.H.: Advances in cardiac pathology. In The heart, update I. by J. Willis Hurst, editor. Copyright © 1979, McGraw-Hill Book Co. Used with the permission of McGraw-Hill Book Co.)

causes may develop a murmur and other clinical features of hypertrophic cardiomyopathy. Thus, in dealing with a patient with clinical features of hypertrophic cardiomyopathy, one must try to identify where they fall in the pathogenetic spectrum of this disorder (see outline on p. 518).

CLINICAL MANIFESTATIONS. Patients with hypertrophic cardiomyopathy may be asymptomatic or may have angina, syncope, congestive heart failure, ventricular arrhythmia, or sudden death. Thus hypertrophic cardiomyopathy may mimic both ischemic heart disease and aortic stenosis. On physical examination, however, the entity reveals itself. Rather than the delayed blunted pulse of aortic stenosis, the carotid pulse in hypertrophic cardiomyopathy has a brisk upstroke, a bifid peak, and a rapid decay. A loud precordial holosystolic murmur is usually present, is most prominent at the left lower sternal border, and increases in intensity with the Valsalva maneuver. The ECG may show a variety of abnormalities, including nonspecific ST and T wave changes, left ventricular hypertrophy, and at times a Wolff-Parkinson-White conduction pattern. Deep septal Q waves are sometimes present in the precordial leads, leading to a "pseudoinfarct" pattern. The chest roentgenogram may be normal or may show cardiomegaly. The echocardiogram, especially useful as a diagnostic tool in the recognition of this disorder, is characterized by increased left ventricular wall thickness and, in those patients who have the familial form of hypertrophic cardiomyopathy, an asymmetric hypertrophy of the septum. Systolic anterior motion of the mitral valve is another useful echocardiographic sign of this condition, as is premature closure of the aortic valve (Fig. 95-2). The left ventricular cavity is usually small, the left atrium may be enlarged, and the ejection fraction is increased. In patients with asymmetric hypertrophy of the septum, the septum usually exhibits poor excursion.

In some patients with hypertrophic cardiomyopathy, arrhythmias may be prevalent. Malignant ventricular dysrhythmias, including ventricular tachycardia and ventricular fibrillation, have been demonstrated in the familial form of this disorder and may account for sudden death in some patients with hypertrophic cardiomyopathy. When present, the malignant ventricular arrhythmias tend also to be present in family members with the disease and may be asymptomatic. Twenty-four-hour ambulatory monitoring would seem indicated in patients with hypertrophic cardiomyopathy and a family history of sudden death. In the differential diagnosis of syncope and sudden death in a young patient with malignant arrhythmias, hypertrophic cardiomyopathy must be considered. Atrial arrhythmias may also occur in patients with this myocardial disease. Atrial fibrillation is especially poorly tolerated because of the hypertrophied ventricle and may lead to development or worsening of heart failure.

DIAGNOSIS. The diagnosis of hypertrophic cardiomyopathy is generally based on the clinical history, symptoms, and laboratory evaluation, particularly the echocardiogram. In the diagnosis of this condition it is useful to determine whether the entity is the familial variety with asymmetric hypertrophy, an idiopathic symmetric form, or the type secondary to long-standing hypertension. Such a diagnostic distinction has implications for prognosis. Studies of the familial form of this condition (when symptom-

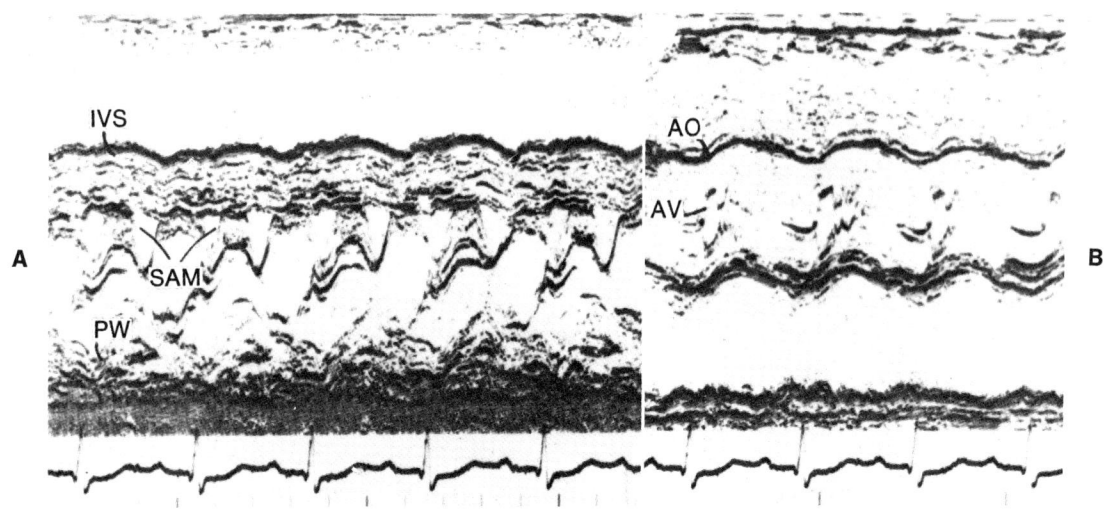

Fig. 95-2. Two echocardiograms from patients with clinical hypertrophic cardiomyopathy. A, Interventricular septum, IVS, is thicker than posterior wall, PW, and systolic anterior motion, SAM, of mitral valve is present. B, Aortic root, AO, area shows premature closure of aortic valve, AV. (From Wei, J.W., Weiss, J.L., and Bulkley, B.H.: The heterogeneity of hypertrophic cardiomyopathy: an autopsy and one dimensional echocardiographic study, Am. J. Cardiol. 45:24, 1980. By permission of the American Heart Association, Inc.)

atic) suggest a 4% annual mortality. For the nonfamilial or asymptomatic form of this condition, however, the prognosis is unknown. Implications for offspring and possible genetic counseling become important if the diagnosis is hypertrophic cardiomyopathy of the Teare type.

MANAGEMENT AND PROGNOSIS. Hypertrophic cardiomyopathy is treated if it is symptomatic. Propranolol has been the mainstay of therapy, and its presumed efficacy is based on its negative inotropic effect on myocardial contractility. Propranolol is usually effective in managing both the congestive heart failure and the angina of this disorder. Additionally, under most circumstances, one should avoid inotropic agents such as digitalis and take care in the use of diuretics, as volume depletion can adversely affect cardiac function in this condition by leading to impaired left ventricular filling. The ventricular arrhythmias of hypertrophic cardiomyopathy may be especially difficult to treat. Propranolol has not been uniformly successful in the management of the ventricular arrhythmias. More recently, the calcium antagonist verapamil has been used in hypertrophic cardiomyopathy with encouraging results. In addition to its value in the management of heart failure and angina, it appears promising for the management of the ventricular dysrhythmias.

For patients who have intractable symptoms despite medical therapy, surgical myectomy and myotomy of portions of the interventricular septum have been performed. Septal myectomy has proved successful in improving symptoms and in diminishing or abolishing the left ventricular outflow tract gradient but does not seem to prolong life. Since patients without outflow tract gradients appear to have the worst prognosis, it is not surprising that surgical abolition of the gradient does not prolong life. Other surgical therapy that has been attempted in this condition is mitral valve replacement, but its value is not widely accepted.

IDIOPATHIC DILATED CONGESTIVE CARDIOMYOPATHIES

DEFINITION. The second major form of cardiomyopathy is the idiopathic dilated congestive cardiomyopathy, which is characterized by hypodynamic function and cardiac dilation with hypertrophy of unknown cause (Fig. 95-3).

The heart in dilated cardiomyopathy is enlarged, with dilation out of proportion to hypertrophy. Although the heart may weigh up to 600 to 700 g (normal is 350 g), the actual wall thickness may be normal or even thinner. The heart is globularly enlarged, the myocardium looks normal grossly, and histologically minor nonspecific changes that include cell hypertrophy and increased interstitial fibrosis are present. Mural thrombi are frequently present in all four cardiac chambers. The coronary arteries and cardiac valves are normal. Ultrastructural changes present in biopsies from patients with dilated cardiomyopathies show nonspecific abnormalities.

PATHOGENESIS. Although the precise cause of these cardiomyopathies has not been proved, they have been lumped into three broad categories with etiologic implications: alcoholic, viral, and drug-induced.

The cause-and-effect relationship of alcohol and cardiomyopathy may be the most widely popularized; for more than a century the link between alcohol and cardiomyopathy has been made and often attributed to a direct toxic effect on the myocardium. Indirect adverse effects of alcohol via its frequent association with nutritional deficiencies have also been suggested. More recently the acute and chronic toxic effects of alcohol on the myocardium have been studied. Although studies have shown temporary depression of myocardial contractility after acute alcohol ingestion, there is little direct evidence that alcohol per se has a direct and irreversible toxic effect on myocardial structure or function. In the animal model prolonged exposure to high doses of alcohol has not been successful in producing cardiomyopathy. In human beings with chronic alcohol ingestion the incidence of cardiomyopathy is low and unpredictable. Thus, although alcohol is in some fashion linked to cardiomyopathy, the strict cause-and-effect relationship is not established. It is likely that alcohol is a contributing factor but not a prime cause of this condition.

Viral infections may affect the heart and lead to a clinical picture of cardiomyopathy. Viruses that have been shown to affect the heart include coxsackieviruses A and B and echoviruses. When viral myocarditis occurs, it is most often asymptomatic with a benign and undetected course. In some patients it may be seen with acute congestive heart failure, cardiac ectopy, or serious conduction disturbances and even sudden death.

The link between acute viral myocarditis and subsequent myocardiopathy is strongly suggested but, as with alcohol, is not well established. The actual role of viral infections, clinical or subclinical, in the subsequent development of chronic congestive cardiomyopathy needs further definition before one can contemplate the feasibility of preventive treatment with vaccines directed against the major cardiotoxic viruses.

Although most recently identified, the relationship between doxorubicin administration and cardiomyopathy is the most firmly established. Cardiotoxicity is the major harmful side effect of this important chemotherapeutic agent. The toxicity may be asymptomatic and manifested only by nonspecific T wave changes, or it may evolve into a full-blown cardiomyopathy with rapidly progressive biventricular heart failure. It is now recognized that the cardiotoxicity is almost always related to the total dose of drug administered, and if that dose is kept below 450 to 550 mg/m^2, the cardiomyopathy is unlikely to occur. Unlike the other cardiomyopathies, doxorubicin cardiomyopathy is associated with distinctive morphologic abnormalities, including focal myocardial cell necrosis, vacuolar

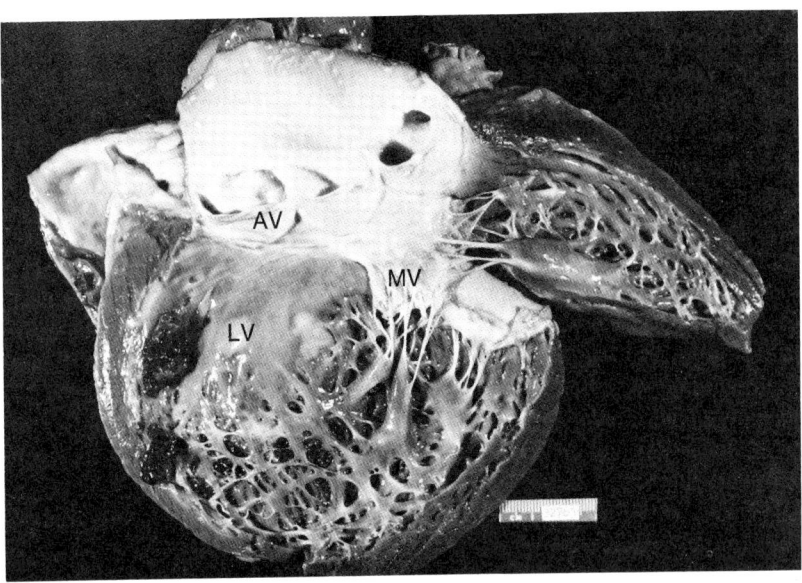

Fig. 95-3. Heart with idiopathic dilated congestive cardiomyopathy. Opened left ventricle, *LV*, has dilated and globular configuration. Aortic, *AV*, and mitral valves, *MV*, are normal. Striking differences between this and hypertrophic cardiomyopathy can be seen by comparing with Fig. 95-1.

degeneration, and myofibrillar dropout. Moreover, these structural abnormalities as detected by right ventricular biopsies have been shown to roughly correlate with functional abnormalities of myocardium.

In addition to these three broad etiologic categories, there are other conditions that on occasion may be linked in some direct or indirect fashion to the development of idiopathic dilated congestive cardiomyopathy. These include the congestive cardiomyopathy of hypothyroidism or that occurring in the postpartum patient; to what extent viral infection or nutritional abnormalities might bear on the latter is not known.

CLINICAL MANIFESTATIONS AND DIAGNOSIS. The clinical picture of patients with congestive cardiomyopathy ranges from unexplained asymptomatic enlargement of the heart and minor abnormalities of ECG to a picture of florid biventricular congestive heart failure with dyspnea and peripheral edema, arrhythmias, and pulmonary and/or systemic embolism.

Chest pain is present in as many as 25% of such patients and may lead to mistaken diagnosis of ischemic heart disease. Physical examination demonstrates an enlarged heart with a right ventricular heave and an outwardly displaced but often poorly palpable apex beat. S_3 and S_4 gallops are usually present, as well as murmurs of mitral regurgitation and at times tricuspid regurgitation. Rales are present in the lungs, and jugular venous distention, hepatomegaly, and peripheral edema may develop. At times patients have acute pulmonary edema or even cardiogenic shock.

The ECG is almost always abnormal, at the very least showing nonspecific ST and T wave changes. Pathologic Q waves may be present in as many as 10% of patients. Conduction disturbances may occur, including bundle branch and complete heart blocks. Atrial arrhythmias and in particular chronic atrial fibrillation may develop in the advanced stages of the disease; recurrent ventricular arrhythmias of all classes of severity may arise and become a major source of morbidity and mortality. Left ventricular hypertrophy may develop over time in some patients with congestive cardiomyopathy and has been viewed as a favorable sign.

Noninvasive techniques have become especially useful in making the diagnosis of congestive cardiomyopathy. The echocardiogram may be useful in sorting out silent valvular or congenital abnormalities that sometimes mimic cardiomyopathy and also in detecting the characteristic dilated diffusely hypodynamic ventricle and enlarged atria of cardiomyopathy. Nuclear myocardial scans using thallium 201 and gated cardiac blood pool scans have also been helpful in some situations in defining congestive cardiomyopathy. On occasion, when the cause of the cardiomyopathy remains unclear and coronary disease is not excluded, a cardiac catheterization may be necessary to precisely define coronary anatomy. This situation infrequently arises with currently available noninvasive techniques.

MANAGEMENT AND PROGNOSIS. Prognosis is usually poor in this condition. The disease tends to run a slowly progressive course with a 5-year mortality in excess of 75% from the time of initial symptoms. There is some evidence that those patients who develop left ventricular hypertrophy (as detected by ECG) have the better prognosis, with some surviving for 10 to 20 years, whereas those without signs of hypertrophy (and possibly without capability of hypertrophy) have a more rapidly progressive downhill course, with some surviving only months.

Treatment of cardiomyopathy is fundamentally treatment of symptoms. The congestive heart failure is treated with digitalis, diuretics, and more recently with vasodilator therapy, including hydralazine and nitrates (see Chapter 86). Arrhythmias are treated with quinidine or procainamide when they cause symptoms (see Chapter 97). There remains no evidence to date that any available therapy for cardiomyopathy interrupts or improves its dismal natural course.

IDIOPATHIC RESTRICTIVE CARDIOMYOPATHIES

DEFINITION. The most infrequent of the muscle diseases of the heart are the restrictive cardiomyopathies. The restrictive cardiomyopathies generally comprise a heterogeneous group of diseases involving endocardium and/or myocardium, including Löffler's endocarditis, endomyocardial fibrosis, and endocardial fibroelastosis. The restrictive cardiomyopathies have in common impaired left ventricular filling but normal systolic function. Clinically and hemodynamically these cardiomyopathies mimic constrictive pericarditis. The restrictive hemodynamics may reflect a diminished left ventricular compliance resulting from infiltration or scarring of myocardium or endocardium.

CLINICAL MANIFESTATIONS AND DIAGNOSIS. Patients with restricitve cardiomyopathy typically have symptoms of biventricular congestive failure with dyspnea and peripheral edema. They may also have atypical chest pain. On physical examination an early and prominent gallop is usually heard, and mitral insufficiency is often present, especially in those with endomyocardial fibrosis. The ECG shows abnormal ST-T wave changes and in some patients evidence of left ventricular hypertrophy. Atrial fibrillation may be present, and as would be expected in a condition associated with restricted diastolic filling, the abrupt onset of atrial fibrillation is often associated with marked deterioration in clinical status. The chest roentgenogram may show cardiac enlargement, but in some patients cardiac size may be entirely normal despite the presence of heart failure.

The diagnosis of restrictive cardiomyopathy ultimately rests on a hemodynamic characterization of the entity. Since the causes of restrictive hemodynamics are so varied, treatable "secondary" causes of restrictive function such as constrictive pericarditis must be considered. The echocardiogram is particularly useful in considering pericardial disease and also in documenting the normal systolic function.

Morphologic features of endomyocardial fibrosis include a small-cavity, thin-walled ventricle and a markedly thickened myocardium. Endocardial thickening is typically more prominent at the apex and the body of both ventricles. The endocardial process may lead to diminished trabeculation and smoothness of the ventricles.

MANAGEMENT AND PROGNOSIS. The cause is unknown, but hypereosinophilia caused by either parasitic infiltration or eosinophilic leukemia may play a role in this disease.

There is no specific treatment for restrictive cardiomyopathy, and the course is generally one of relentless heart failure. In a few cases endocardial resection and valve replacement have been performed with some success. Recent evidence suggests that those patients with restrictive hemodynamics in whom *no* specific cause can be established may have a benign course with resolution of symptoms.

SECONDARY CARDIOMYOPATHIES

Secondary cardiomyopathies comprise a mixed and often unusual assortment of diseases, including glycogen storage disease, hypertension, aortic stenosis, sarcoidosis, scleroderma, ischemic heart disease, amyloidosis, hemochromatosis, and metabolic or nutritional cardiomyopathies.

These secondary cardiomyopathies may behave functionally as a dilated congestive, hypertrophic, or restrictive cardiomyopathy and sometimes as a mixture of these functional states. Diagnosis of the many secondary cardiomyopathies depends first on recognition of the underlying disease process. Therapy includes treatment of the underlying disease, as well as conventional treatment of the heart failure or arrhythmias as they become clinically manifest.

Secondary hypertrophic cardiomyopathies (glycogen storage disease, hypertension, aortic stenosis)

One form of glycogen storage disease, known as Pompe's disease, has been shown to be associated with cardiac dysfunction that is akin to hypertrophic cardiomyopathy clinically. Cardiac catheterization performed in one patient has documented a provokable aortic outflow tract gradient. The secondary hypertrophic state associated with long-standing systemic hypertension or valvular aortic stenosis may be seen as hypertrophic cardiomyopathy, as already discussed, and represents a form of secondary myocardial disease.

Secondary congestive cardiomyopathies (sarcoidosis, scleroderma, ischemic heart disease)

Sarcoidosis may lead to a muscle disorder of the heart by virtue of direct infiltration of myocardium with granulomata (Fig. 95-4). The infiltrative lesions may be so extensive as to replace sizable portions of myocardium and lead to cardiac dilation, arrhythmias, heart failure, and sudden death. As such, the entity may mimic congestive cardiomyopathy.

Similarly scleroderma may involve the heart and lead to extensive necrosis and fibrosis of all four cardiac chambers (likely mediated by a coronary Raynaud's phenome-

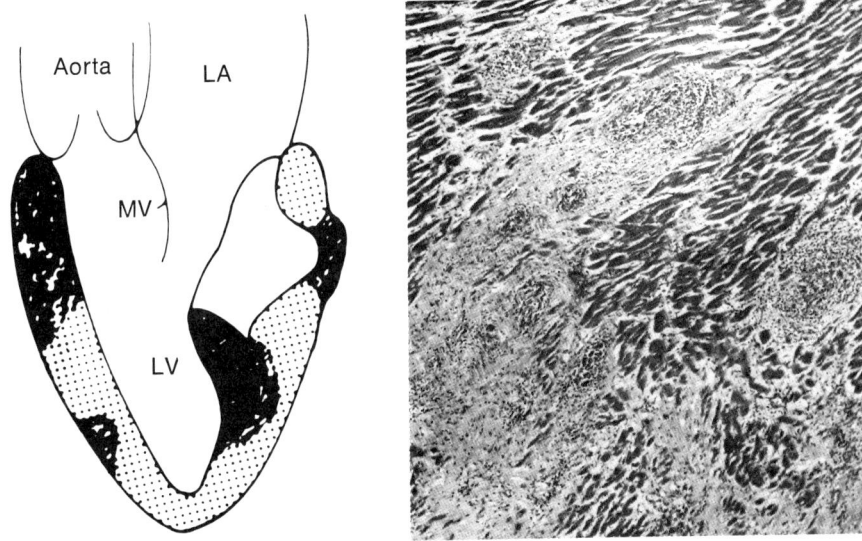

Fig. 95-4. Schematic diagram on left illustrates ways in which sarcoid infiltration (in black) of myocardium can lead to cardiomyopathy. Histologic section on right shows sarcoid granulomata infiltrating and destroying myocardium (hematoxylin and eosin, ×60). (From Bulkley, B.H.: Advances in cardiac pathology. In The heart, update I, by J. Willis Hurst, editor. Copyright © 1979, McGraw-Hill Book Co. Used with the permission of McGraw-Hill Book Co.)

non). Since sclerodermatous myocardial disease involves muscle injury and may lead to cardiac dilation with diffusely impaired function, it also may mimic an idiopathic dilated type of cardiomyopathy.

Perhaps the most common of the secondary cardiomyopathies is that due to ischemic heart disease. Although coronary stenosis may be the underlying disease process, recurrent multivessel myocardial damage as a result of coronary occlusion may lead to a progressive remodeling of heart shape and size such that the heart becomes globular, diffusely dilated, and diffusely hypodynamic. In some patients with ischemic cardiomyopathy the clinical history may be sufficiently vague and the myocardial infarctions clinically silent so that it is not readily apparent that the condition is ischemic. On occasion cardiac catheterization with coronary angiography is necessary to sort out the cause.

Secondary restrictive cardiomyopathies (amyloidosis, hemochromatosis)

Cardiac amyloidosis may lead to a secondary cardiomyopathy by virtue of diffuse infiltration of amyloid in the myocardium. Although cardiac amyloidosis often goes unrecognized in life, when the amyloid deposits around myocardial cells and in small vessels of the heart become extensive enough, abnormalities of cardiac function may become apparent. Cardiac amyloidosis may be seen with a clinical picture of restrictive cardiomyopathy. Increased stiffness of the myocardium leads to impaired diastolic filling of both right and left ventricles, and the typical hemodynamics of cardiac constriction may occur.

Hemochromatosis is another infiltrative disorder that may be seen as a cardiomyopathy of the restrictive or congestive form.

Metabolic or nutritional cardiomyopathies

Another subgroup of secondary cardiomyopathies falls into the broad metabolic or nutritional category and may be related to conditions such as hyperthyroidism, hypothyroidism, beriberi, and chronic anemia. Thyroid abnormalities have received much attention with regard to their effects on myocardium. *Excess thyroid hormone* is associated with an increased cardiac output, coinciding with the overall hypermetabolic state. Thyroid hormone causes enhanced myocardial contractility; it also decreases peripheral resistance. The high-output state of thyrotoxicosis has been cited as a cause of "high-output congestive heart failure." However, that thyroid hormone excess alone can lead to chronic cardiomyopathy in an otherwise normal heart has not been established. Similarly *hypothyroidism* may be associated with decreased cardiac output and depressed myocardial contractility, but the extent to which a chronic cardiomyopathy can be caused by this hormone deficiency is also not clear. Nevertheless, for these nutritional and metabolic "cardiomyopathies," correction of the hormonal, vitamin, or other deficiency leads to correction of the myocardial abnormality in most cases.

BIBLIOGRAPHY

Benotti, J.R., Grossman, W., and Cohn, P.F.: Clinical profile of restrictive cardiomyopathy, Circulation **61**:1206, 1980.

Braunwald, E., and others: Idiopathic hypertrophic subaortic stenosis. 1. A description of the disease based upon an analysis of 64 patients. In Idiopathic hypertrophic subaortic stenosis (American Heart Association monograph 10), Circulation **30** (suppl. IV):IV-3-IV-213, 1964.

Brock, R.C.: Functional obstruction of the left ventricle (acquired aortic subvalvular stenosis), Guy's Hosp. Rep. **106**:221, 1957.

Bulkley, B.H.: IHSS afflicted: idols of the cave and the marketplace, Am. J. Cardiol. **40**:476, 1977.

Bulkley, B.H.: Recent advances in cardiac pathology. In Hurst, J.W., editor: The heart, update I, New York, 1979, McGraw-Hill Book Co.

Bulkley, B.H., and others: Thallium 201 imaging and gated cardiac blood pool scans in patients with ischemic and idiopathic congestive cardiomyopathy: a clinical and pathologic study, Circulation **55**:753, 1977.

Chatterjee, K., and Parmley, W.W.: The role of vasodilator therapy in heart failure, Prog. Cardiovasc. Dis. **19**:301, 1977.

Come, P.C., and others: Hypercontractile cardiac states simulating hypertrophic cardiomyopathy, Circulation **55**:901, 1977.

Epstein, S.E., and others: Asymmetric septal hypertrophy, Ann. Intern. Med. **81**:650, 1974.

James, T.N., and Marshall, T.K.: De subitaneis mortibus. XII. Asymmetric hypertrophy of the heart, Circulation **51**:1149, 1975.

Silverman, K.J., Hutchins, G.M., and Bulkley, B.H.: Cardiac sarcoid: a clinicopathologic study of 84 unselected patients with systemic sarcoidosis, Circulation **58**:1204, 1978.

Teare, R.D.: Asymmetrical hypertrophy of the heart in young adults, Br. Heart J. **20**:1, 1958.

96 • CORONARY HEART DISEASE

James B. Young and Robert J. Luchi

CORONARY ARTERY ANATOMY AND MYOCARDIAL PERFUSION

ANATOMY. The myocardium is perfused by two coronary arteries, the right and the left, arising respectively from the right and left sinuses of Valsalva (Fig. 96-1). It is not uncommon for the *right coronary artery* to arise from two ostia. When this occurs, the upper ostium gives rise to a vessel called the conus artery that supplies the right ventricular outflow tract. When a separate opening for the conus artery is not present, the first major branch from the right coronary artery supplies the right ventricular outflow tract. The major trunk of the right coronary artery descends in the right atrioventricular groove. In this groove it curves around the acute margin of the heart after sending off one or more anterior right ventricular branches. In most patients the right coronary artery continues beyond the acute margin of the heart to extend to or past the crux of the heart, that point where the atrioventricular groove, together with the interatrial and interventricular grooves, forms a cross. Extension of the right coronary artery to or beyond the crux of the heart is termed right coronary artery dominance. As the right coronary artery courses in the posterior atrioventricular groove, it sends branches to the posterior right ventricle, to the interventricular septum, and to the inferior and posterior portions of the left ventricle. In most patients in whom the right coronary artery terminates at or near the acute margin of the heart, the inferior and posterior parts of the left ventricle are supplied by the circumflex artery.

The *left coronary artery* branches after a variable but usually short distance into the *anterior descending* and *circumflex coronary arteries*. The circumflex coronary artery proceeds along the groove between the left atrium and left ventricle, around the obtuse margin of the heart, where it gives off a large vessel called the obtuse marginal artery. The circumflex artery courses a variable distance in the left atrioventricular groove. When left coronary artery dominance is present, that is, when the circumflex artery reaches the crux of the heart, it is the circumflex artery that gives off branches to the inferior and posterior portions of the left ventricle. The left anterior descending coronary artery nourishes a large part of the left ventricle as it descends in the anterior interventricular groove. It sends large perforating branches to the septum and several large diagonal branches that course over the anterior surface of the left ventricle. The anterior descending coronary artery reaches the apex, curves around it, and supplies a variable portion of the inferior wall of the left ventricle. The left coronary artery may trifurcate rather than bifurcate into circumflex and left anterior descending vessels. When a trifurcation exists, the third vessel is termed the *ramus intermedius*. The ramus intermedius generally supplies an area of the lateral left ventricle.

The artery supplying the sinus node arises from the right coronary artery in 55% to 60% of individuals. In the remainder the sinus node artery is a branch of the left circumflex coronary artery. The artery to the atrioventricular node arises at the crux of the heart, from the right coronary artery in approximately 85% of individuals and from the left coronary artery in 15%. The blood supplied to the interventricular septum is provided predominantly from the left anterior descending coronary artery, although a small portion of the posterior and inferior septum is supplied from the right coronary artery. However, in patients in whom the left circumflex artery reaches the crux of the heart, the entire interventricular septum may receive its blood supply from the left coronary artery system.

Occlusions of the left anterior descending coronary artery may result in myocardial infarctions of the left ventricular anterior wall and the septum. Occlusions in the right coronary artery give rise to inferior and posterior wall infarctions of the left ventricle unless the right coronary artery does not reach the crux of the heart. The left circumflex artery supplies the lateral left ventricle; if it extends to the crux of the heart or beyond, occlusions of the

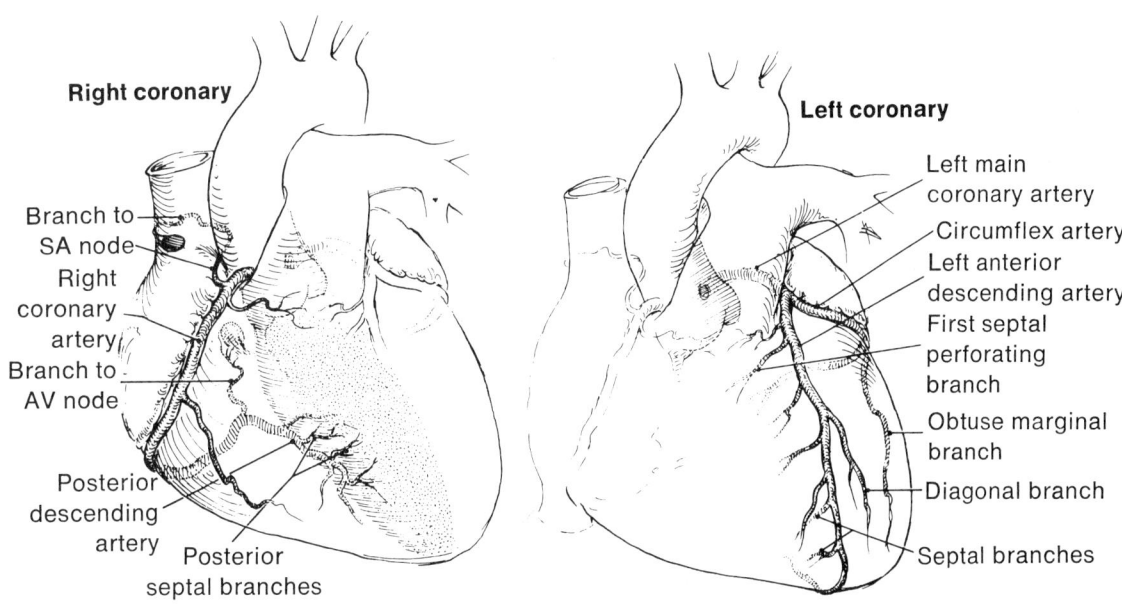

Fig. 96-1. Typical coronary artery anatomy.

circumflex artery give rise to inferior and posterior wall myocardial infarctions.

Occlusions of the right coronary artery may result in infarctions of the right ventricle. Right ventricular infarction usually occurs in conjunction with inferior and posterior wall infarctions of the left ventricle that involve the interventricular septum. Only rarely does right ventricular infarction occur independent of left ventricular infarction.

Anatomically there are only two coronary arteries. Nevertheless, it has become a clinical convention to describe coronary atherosclerosis in terms of one-, two-, or three-vessel disease, the vessels referred to being the *right coronary, left anterior descending,* and *left circumflex coronary arteries.*

The coronary venous system is more variable than the coronary arterial system. In general, veins follow the course of the major coronary arteries, but exceptions are common. The coronary veins draining the left ventricle ultimately empty into the coronary sinus, which lies posteriorly in the atrioventricular groove. The coronary sinus empties into the right atrium. Venous blood draining the right ventricle usually, but not always, also empties directly into the right atrium and right ventricle.

Either the right or the left coronary artery may congenitally be quite small and occasionally absent. The left coronary artery may arise from the pulmonary trunk. Severe symptoms of myocardial ischemia usually are present during infancy in these individuals. There may be a congenital coronary arteriovenous fistula (an abnormal communication between a coronary artery and vein), which, depending on its size, gives rise only to a localized continuous murmur or additionally to signs of ischemia or heart failure.

PHYSIOLOGY. The myocardium consists of cells dependent on oxygen for metabolism. They become injured or die when deprived of oxygen. As just described, the myocardium is supplied by a rich vascular network, although the endocardium is less well supplied than other regions of the myocardial wall. Coronary artery flow depends on the cardiac output and pressure gradient between the aorta and the right atrium, which receives the drainage from the coronary sinus, the major coronary venous channel. Blood flow to the myocardium occurs during both systole and diastole, but diastolic flow is greater because the compressing action of the contracting myocardium on intramyocardial blood vessels raises intramyocardial resistance during systole. Diastolic flow is related to the duration of diastole and is therefore limited during tachycardia when the proportion of the cardiac cycle spent in diastole is shortened.

Resistances along the coronary circuit include (1) a basal viscous resistance defined as the resistance to flow offered by the fully dilated coronary vascular channels during the diastolic phase of the cycle; (2) an autoregulatory resistance determined by tonic contractions of the vascular smooth muscle of the coronary arterioles; and (3) the already mentioned resistance resulting from compression of vascular structures by the contracting myocardium. In the normal, intact, beating heart, overall coronary resistance is predominantly determined by the coronary arteriolar resistance. Resistance in the epicardial coronary arteries is normally small. Commonly, however, resistance in the epicardial coronary vessels is increased by coronary atherosclerosis, a resistance that is either fixed or slowly progressive. Coronary artery spasm produces a reversible and often severe increase in epicardial coronary artery resistance. Occasionally the left anterior descending coronary artery may tunnel through an area of the myocardium capable of active contraction. In this circumstance systolic contraction of the myocardium may sharply increase resistance and may curtail flow in the left anterior descending coronary artery to a clinically significant degree. Elevation of the diastolic pressure in the cavity of the left ventricle may also increase resistance to flow in the endocardial coronary vasculature by exerting a compressive effect on these vessels.

EPIDEMIOLOGY AND PREVENTION OF CORONARY HEART DISEASE

EPIDEMIOLOGY. The prevalence of coronary artery disease (CAD) varies greatly among different populations, and within these cohorts the incidence also varies with age, geographic location, and personal habits. It became clear in the 1930s and 1940s that to study the phenomenon of changing death rates in the world and specifically in the United States, long-range, population-based, prospective epidemiologic studies would be required. Subsequently, the Framingham Heart Study, the National Cooperative Pooling Project, the Tecumseh Study, the Western Collaborative Group Study, the Goteborg Study (Sweden), and the Ni-Hon-Sam Study (Japan) were initiated. To be sure, problems unique to long-term, pooled, epidemiologic studies were evident in these programs. However, they still provide the most accurate data base available to study the natural history of coronary heart disease. The most significant limitation of these surveys is the application of conclusions from data gathered in the 1950s to individuals living in the 1980s.

Important observations in these studies included an assessment of the CAD occurrence rate and discrimination of factors affecting and determining the incidence and natural history of the disease. The studies demonstrated a wide variation in CAD incidence according to individual habits and place of residence. By the 1950s it was realized that CAD was the leading cause of death in North American men and that this disease did not occur randomly. Important variables affecting incidence included age, race, sex, serum cholesterol level, hypertension, hyperglycemia, obesity, cigarette smoking, lack of exercise, high dietary fat intake, genetic factors, and psychosocial influences.

Overall incidence. The United States' crude monthly mortality rate for CAD in 1976 was 301/100,000. However, patterns of geographic variation are evident, with the highest age-adjusted death rate noted in the eastern United States (2310/100,000 along the Atlantic Coast and in the Southern sunbelt, 711/100,000 in the Great Plains region, 925/100,000 in the Western states). Variation in these rates is also noted among industrialized nations. The highest CAD age-adjusted death rate is found in Finland (2399/100,000) and the lowest in Japan (1285/100,000). Poorly kept epidemiologic records in Asia, Africa, and Latin America prevent truly accurate comparison of these areas' CAD death rates with those of the recognized industrialized nations.

Sex. Men have a higher incidence of CAD than do women. In 1976 the male mortality from CAD was 5.2 times greater than the female mortality for the 35- to 44-year-old group and 2.3 times greater for those aged 65 to 74. These differences may be changing as trends and social practices evolve, such as the increased incidence of female smokers and the diminished emphasis on sexual distinction in the workforce.

Time trends. After increasing CAD mortality rates throughout the 1960s for all age, sex, and race groups in the United States, a definite decline in CAD mortality was apparent in the early 1970s. Some have attributed this decline to changes in life-style that altered CAD risk factors. Theoretically, an individual who made such risk factor modifications would have a decreased likelihood of clinically significant CAD.

Age. The incidence of CAD increases with age. When CAD is present in younger individuals, it is usually associated with hyperlipidemia, hypertension, and a strong familial history of CAD.

Lipids. It is useful to precisely characterize the various hyperlipoproteinemias because of their variable implications and treatment. CAD is more closely associated with hypercholesterolemia than with hypertriglyceridemia. Hyperlipidemia may be primary or secondary. The most frequent causes of secondary hyperlipidemia are diabetes, myxedema, alcoholism, cirrhosis, and nephrosis. The ratio of high- to low-density lipoproteins is clearly less in patients with CAD. High-density lipoprotein (HDL) is structurally distinct from the atherogenic lipids and participates in the removal of lipids from cells with subsequent delivery to the liver for metabolism. HDL levels can be increased with fat-controlled diets, exercise, and estrogen use.

Smoking. Smoking is clearly related to death from cardiovascular disease. Male smokers have a fivefold greater risk of cerebrovascular accident and a threefold greater risk of fatal myocardial infarction when compared to nonsmokers. Smoking causes adverse hemodynamic effects (tachycardia and hypertension) that are mediated by adrenergic amines. Nicotine is probably the factor responsible for inciting the adrenergic stimulation. Smoking also causes an increased blood glycerol level and lactate/pyruvate ratio. Carbon monoxide is detrimental because it impairs left ventricular contractility.

Cigarette smoke is also harmful to nonsmokers when they are exposed to the noxious atmosphere created by smokers. Angina is induced at lower workloads in nonsmoking CAD patients exposed to cigarette smoke. It has also been shown that smoke inhalation impairs the diffusion of oxygen into the mitochondria.

Blood pressure. Both systolic and diastolic hypertension are related to the development of CAD, with systolic hypertension better correlated to the prevalence of CAD than either mean or diastolic blood pressure.

There is difficulty in establishing normal values for blood pressure, since both systolic and diastolic pressure have a continuous unimodal association with cardiovascular complications. Prudent points of intervention in any patient would be a systolic blood pressure of 160 mm Hg or greater or a diastolic pressure of 95 mm Hg or higher (see Chapter 87). These levels of hypertension should be aggressively treated, particularly in younger individuals. Despite the fact that systolic hypertension is generally better correlated with cardiovascular catastrophes, it would be unwise to dismiss isolated diastolic hypertension. Indeed, in younger men diastolic hypertension is a more potent risk factor for CAD. Likewise, isolated systolic hypertension should not be regarded as an inevitable concomitant finding of aging. Even in elderly age groups, systolic hypertension carries significant implications for the development of CAD.

Diabetes and obesity. The risk of a cardiovascular event is doubled when diabetes mellitus is present. Obesity may also be a risk factor. The Framingham Study demonstrated an association between obesity and elevated low-density lipoprotein cholesterol. In addition to higher lipid levels, obese patients tend to have systolic hypertension and glucose intolerance.

Physical conditioning. Although reports demonstrate CAD in well-conditioned marathon runners, physical training does seem to be associated with a reduced risk of coronary disease.

Personality. A behavior pattern has been associated with CAD. The "coronary-prone" or "type A" personality describes individuals who have enhanced personality traits of aggressiveness, ambitiousness, and competitiveness, are chronically impatient, and have a passionate sense of time urgency. "Type A" behavior patterns have been associated with increased severity of CAD even when age, sex, blood pressure, smoking, and cholesterol level were comparable.

Coffee. The amount of caffeine intake probably does not affect the risk of CAD. The Boston Collaborative Drug Surveillance Program suggested a relationship between coffee consumption and acute coronary events in a retrospective study. The Framingham Study, a prospective study, failed to corroborate this observation. Also, in reports from the Evans County (Georgia) epidemiologic survey, coronary heart disease mortality was not associated with coffee consumption in several race and sex groups.

Oral contraceptives. It has been suggested that oral hormonal contraception is a CAD risk factor in younger women who smoke. The Lipid Research Clinic Program Prevalence Study demonstrated that patients less than 45 years of age who were taking oral contraceptives had higher serum cholesterol and triglyceride levels. This study also reported that the use of oral contraception in the presence of other major cardiovascular disease risk factors increases the likelihood of death when a myocardial infarction does occur.

Ethanol consumption. Several recent studies have suggested that moderate alcohol consumption plays a *preventive* role in the development of CAD, although others have presented opposing data. The beneficial effects of alcohol may be related to its association with increased serum levels of high-density lipoproteins.

PREVENTION. To avert CAD, prevention and management of adverse risk factors before coronary atherosclerosis becomes clinically apparent seem important. Thus it appears wise to encourage cessation of smoking, control hypertension, modify hypercholesterolemia, and optimize weight and physical conditioning. Oral contraceptives should not be taken by women with other cardiovascular risk factors such as hypertension.

True prevention of CAD might require risk factor intervention in childhood. Reversibility of the atherosclerotic process by dietary manipulation has been demonstrated in animal studies. In humans, however, the process of atherosclerosis resolution may be different. It is difficult to assess the extent of atherosclerosis at the beginning of any study and maintain dietary compliance in human studies. Clearly it is much wiser to prevent the development of CAD than to try to retard its progression or induce regression once it is present.

It would seem that pharmacologic control of glucose intolerance would limit the development and progression of CAD. There is controversy, however, concerning the manner of control of hyperglycemia. The University Group Diabetes Program compared various oral hypoglycemic agents with insulin in amelioration or retardation of the vascular complications of diabetes. This study suggested that diabetic patients controlled with oral agents had a higher incidence of atherosclerotic complications. Therefore it would be prudent to control diabetes with dietary intervention and normalization of weight if possible. Failure to establish reasonable fasting and postprandial glucose levels with this protocol should prompt consideration of insulin administration.

ANGINA PECTORIS

DEFINITION. "Angina pectoris" literally means chest pain. The word "angina," derived from both Greek and Latin, is translated as a choking or strangling sensation. "Pectoris" means of the chest. Although many pathophysiologic events unrelated to the cardiovascular system may cause chest discomfort, convention has decreed that this term be used to refer to chest pains characteristic of ischemic heart disease. The mechanism for production of pain of this nature is always a discrepancy between myocardial oxygen demands and the ability of the coronary arteries to deliver this substrate. Angina pectoris therefore is usually due to atherosclerotic heart disease.

Angina pectoris was first described by William Heberden in 1768. We report his description because of its accuracy and completeness, as well as its historical importance.

But there is a disorder of the breast marked with strong and peculiar symptoms, considerable for the kind of danger belonging to it, and not extremely rare, which deserves to be mentioned more at length. The seat of it, and sense of strangling, and anxiety with which it is attended, may make it not improperly be called angina pectoris.

They who are afflicted with it, are seized while they are walking (more especially if it be up hill, and soon after eating), with a painful and most disagreeable sensation in the breast, which seems as if it would extinguish life, if it were to increase or continue; but the moment they stand still, all this uneasiness vanishes.

In all other respects, the patients are, at the beginning of this disorder, perfectly well, and in particular have no shortness of breath, from which it is totally different. The pain is sometimes situated in the upper part, sometimes in the middle, sometimes at the bottom of the os sterni, and often more inclined to the left than to the right side. It likewise very frequently extends from the breast to the middle of the left arm. Males are most liable to that disease, especially such as have passed their fiftieth year.

ETIOLOGY. Clinically, myocardial ischemia is most commonly associated with coronary atherosclerosis. Atheromas produce clinically significant reduction of coronary blood flow when the internal luminal area is reduced by 50% or more. Myocardial oxygen demands may be met while the patient is at rest, but during exercise, when myocardial oxygen requirements are raised by an increase in heart rate, myocardial contractility, and tension of the ventricular wall, myocardial demands for oxygen exceed the capacity of the coronary arteries to deliver the requisite blood flow. This results in myocardial ischemia.

Myocardial ischemia may also result when there is a primary reduction of blood flow without an increase in myocardial oxygen demands. The most typical example of a primary reduction in blood flow is coronary artery spasm. Coronary artery spasm has been clearly demonstrated to be the major pathogenetic factor in *variant angina* (discussed later in the chapter), and there is evidence that it may be important in classic effort-induced angina, unstable angina, and myocardial infarction. Coronary artery spasm may be caused by mechanical, neural, or chemical factors. Reflex coronary artery spasm on exposure to cold has been demonstrated. Coronary artery spasm has also been documented in association with exercise. Coronary artery spasm appears to be more frequent when atherosclerotic heart disease is present. It is not known whether spasm can occur in a coronary artery completely free from atherosclerosis. A primary reduction in myocardial blood flow may also occur when the left anterior descending coronary artery is compressed during systole by an overlying band of myocardium.

Myocardial ischemia may be produced when there is severe reduction in blood pressure and cardiac output, as in shock, severe aortic stenosis, severe aortic insufficiency, sclerosis of the coronary ostia secondary to syphilitic aortitis, coronary arteritis, coronary embolization, and coronary thrombosis. Anemia and increased diffusion distances from capillary to myocardial cell, as in massive ventricular hypertrophy, worsen the myocardial oxygen deficits caused by any reduction in coronary blood flow. It is not uncommon for many of these factors to act in concert. Thus coronary thrombosis may completely occlude a vessel only partially occluded by atherosclerosis, coronary artery spasm may occur at a point where the vessel is partially obstructed by coronary atherosclerosis and complete the obstruction, or shock in conjunction with coronary atherosclerosis may produce myocardial ischemia more severe than that caused by either alone. Although myocardial ischemia may occur in the absence of coronary atherosclerosis, it is much more common in association with it.

PATHOPHYSIOLOGY. Resting myocardial oxygen consumption is approximately 100 ml of oxygen/100 g of ventricular tissue per minute. Myocardial oxygen extraction averages 70% of the arterial oxygen content. The major determinants of oxygen consumption by the myocardium include the contractile state of the heart, the heart rate, and the tension generated in the myocardium. The tension generated is directly proportional to the pressure developed by the ventricle and the diameter of the ventricular cavity and inversely proportional to ventricular wall thickness. The extent of myocardial shortening, the energy required for activation of myocardial contraction, and "basal" cellular oxygen requirements are other determinants of myocardial oxygen consumption that are of little importance clinically. The so-called double product, that is, the product of the heart rate and the systolic blood pressure, serves as a useful bedside clinical index of myocardial oxygen consumption.

During periods of exercise and stress, myocardial oxygen demands increase. These demands are met primarily by coronary vasodilation, which increases coronary blood flow fourfold or fivefold. Some increase in myocardial oxygen extraction may occur, but only when myocardial oxygen demands are greatly increased. The stimulus to coronary vasodilation is unknown. It is likely that metabolic products (such as adenosine), neural mechanisms, and prostaglandins are involved.

When an imbalance exists between myocardial oxygen demands and coronary blood flow, myocardial ischemia results. There is a rapid release of lactate, phosphate, and potassium from the ischemic myocardial cells. Creatine phosphate and ATP decline in spite of some shift to anaerobic metabolism. If the ischemia is severe or prolonged, anaerobic metabolism may fail to maintain cellular integrity and myocardial infarction results.

Consequences of myocardial ischemia include chest pain, reduced myocardial contractility and diastolic compliance, dyssynergic ventricular contraction, and ECG abnormalities including ST segment elevation or depression, T wave inversion, and arrhythmias. Prolonged or severe myocardial ischemia may result in necrosis of myocardial cells, referred to as myocardial infarction.

Angina pectoris is produced when myocardial ischemia activates visceral efferent pain fibers. The biochemical events and nerve pathways involved are incompletely understood. It is believed that the nerve impulses travel via unmyelinated sympathetic nerve fibers to the upper thoracic and lower cervical cord segments and from there to the thalamus and higher cortical centers. Activation of internuncial neurons in the lower thoracic and upper cervical segments may cause referral of pain to the arm, neck, jaw, and back.

CLINICAL MANIFESTATIONS. The patient's history is the key to the diagnosis of angina pectoris. The hallmark of effort-induced angina pectoris is a history of chest discomfort brought on by exercise or emotion and relieved by rest. Because the chest discomfort arises in a visceral organ, it is often difficult for the patient to characterize and clearly define its location. The discomfort is commonly described as a pain, heaviness, tightness, or squeezing sensation. The location of the discomfort is usually retrosternal, but it may occur in the epigastrium or in the precordial area. When the discomfort is located primarily in the epigastrium or precordial area, careful questioning will often reveal that the retrosternal area is included. When severe, the discomfort commonly radiates to the jaw, neck, back, left shoulder, and/or inner aspect of the left arm down to the ring and little fingers of the left hand. Occasionally the patient may complain of discomfort only in the areas of referral, such as the jaw or left elbow. The duration of the discomfort is variable, usually lasting between 5 and 10 minutes. Attacks lasting less than 5 minutes, however, are not uncommon; an attack persisting beyond 20 minutes suggests a form of unstable angina or myocardial infarction.

Because of the vague nature of the discomfort and the patient's difficulty in describing it precisely, the physician may be misled by the history. The most important characteristic of effort-induced angina pectoris is the relationship between chest discomfort and exertion and emotion and the relief of the chest discomfort by rest.

Severe discomfort may be associated with nausea, salivation, a feeling of generalized weakness, and lightheadedness. The frequency and severity of the anginal discomfort may vary from day to day in spite of similar degrees of exertion. Usually the explanation for this variability can be found in the patient's emotional state (anxiety, for example, increases the metabolic demands of the heart) or in ambient weather conditions. Cold weather, particularly walking into a cold wind, brings on the discomfort sooner and increases its severity. On the other hand, when the amount of exercise and the patient's emotional state can be more or less controlled, as in the exercise laboratory, the amount of exercise that produces chest pain is reasonably constant from test to test.

Examination during an anginal attack may show an increased pulse rate and blood pressure. The patient may have pallor and increased facial sweating. There may be increased salivation. An S_4 gallop may be heard for the first time or may increase in intensity. If there is ischemia of a papillary muscle, a systolic apical murmur resulting from mitral insufficiency may be heard during angina and diminish in intensity or disappear when the attack has passed. Between anginal attacks, examination may be normal or show changes of associated cardiac conditions, such as hypertension or valvular heart disease.

A number of conditions can closely simulate the symptoms of angina periods. One of the more common is pain arising in the precordial chest wall. The nature of this chest pain is poorly understood. It may arise in muscle or in the costochondral or chondrosternal articulations (Tietze's syndrome). The chest wall is often tender to palpation. Pain originating in afferent nerves irritated by arthritis of the cervical and upper thoracic spine may also simulate angina pectoris. The discomfort of esophageal spasm or mucosal inflammation, the pain of peptic ulcer, and the pain of gallbladder disease, particularly chronic calculous cholecystitis, may mimic closely the discomfort of angina pectoris. The physician must consider these conditions in a patient whose symptoms are suggestive of angina. The patient's history and physical signs will help discriminate between angina pectoris and these other conditions. However, the most helpful sign is the relationship of chest discomfort to exercise or emotion and its relief with rest or nitroglycerin in angina pectoris.

LABORATORY ASSESSMENT. The history and physical examination can be complemented by laboratory evaluation when indicated. Conditions such as anemia or thyrotoxicosis, which may exacerbate angina by increasing myocardial oxygen demands, should be excluded. Fasting and 2-hour postprandial blood sugar analyses should be performed to detect carbohydrate intolerance. Measurement of the patient's serum cholesterol and fasting serum triglycerides should be obtained. More sophisticated lipid analyses may be required to define various abnormal lipoprotein states.

DIAGNOSIS. The ECG is an important tool in evaluating patients with angina pectoris. A normal resting ECG does not rule out angina pectoris. A resting ECG showing clear evidence of a previous myocardial infarction supports the clinical impression of angina pectoris. Other changes on the resting ECG such as left bundle branch block and nonspecific ST-T changes cannot be used as evidence to support a diagnosis of angina pectoris. Exercise electrocardiography (exercise stress testing) is important in the diagnosis of angina and in evaluating the response to therapy. The purpose of exercise stress testing is to document the ECG, blood pressure, and symptomatic response. Various exercise protocols are used, but all employ graded increases in exercise with constant ECG and blood pressure monitoring until the patient can exercise no further because of cardiovascular symptoms or fatigue. In a stress test exercise may be stopped at a predetermined heart rate, typically 85% of the maximum predicted on the basis of the patient's age.

One purpose of exercise stress testing is to correlate the patient's symptoms with certain cardiovascular changes suggesting myocardial ischemia. Another is to define the patient's exercise capacity. Although the test is relatively safe, occasionally ventricular tachycardia or ventricular fibrillation may be precipitated, and the physician must be prepared to handle these catastrophes. Exercise stress testing is contraindicated in the first several days after acute myocardial infarction and in patients with unstable angina pectoris with rest pain, severe significant tachycardia or bradycardia, advanced or untreated heart failure, aortic stenosis complicated by effort-induced syncope, and orthopedic or muscular disorders that prevent the patient from exercising adequately.

The normal response is one in which the patient has no episodes of chest discomfort and no horizontal or downsloping ST segment depression of 1 mm or greater after reaching the target heart rate. A normal resting ECG simplifies interpretation of the changes occurring during exercise. A positive test is defined by chest discomfort and a horizontal or downsloping ST segment depression of 1 mm or greater. Greater ST segment depression (for example, 3 to 4 mm) suggests greater degrees of ischemia, as does ST segment depression occurring early in the exercise protocol, failure of the systolic blood pressure to increase with exercise, or a drop in systolic blood pressure after it has risen. ST segment elevation may occur during exercise stress testing. Most often ST elevation appears to be due to abnormal left ventricular patterns of contractions; occasionally it may be due to exercise-induced coronary artery spasm.

If no symptoms or ECG changes occur but the patient cannot reach his assigned heart rate because of poor physical conditioning, the test cannot be used to rule out ischemia. Difficulties in interpretation arise when the resting ECG is abnormal, when the patient has chest discomfort without ST segment change, or when horizontal or downsloping ST segment depression of 1 mm or greater occurs without chest discomfort.

The exercise stress test is often evaluated in terms of its ability to predict occlusive disease in the coronary arteries. Approximately 10% of patients who show a positive test as previously described will have normal coronary arteries of minimal atheromatous change. The reason for false positive tests is unknown; they tend to occur in younger individuals, particularly women. The sensitivity of exercise electrocardiography in predicting critical coronary atheromatous disease is in the range of 60% to 70% of patients with significant obstructive coronary artery disease. Increased specificity can be obtained by using additional endpoints, but when this is done, sensitivity is reduced. Thus exercise stress testing alone is less useful than coronary angiography in predicting cardiovascular mortality or morbidity. The two tests used together are somewhat better than angiography alone in making predictions.

The accuracy of the exercise stress test in predicting critical coronary atheromatous disease can be considerably improved by combining the test with thallium perfusion scintigraphy or blood pool scanning. Thallium uptake by the myocardium is proportional to myocardial blood flow. Areas of ischemia developing during exercise will appear as "cold" areas, that is, areas with reduced thallium uptake. When ischemia is relieved during rest following exercise, former "cold" areas will show normal uptake of thallium. Exercise-induced wall motion abnormalities and reduction in ejection fraction are important indicators of ischemia demonstrable by blood pool scanning. The isotope commonly used in gated blood pool scanning is technetium 99 attached to red blood cells or serum albumin. Images of the blood pool in the right and left ventricles are prepared by computer processing of information derived from precordial counting. Changes in size and configuration of the blood pools can be analyzed separately during systole and diastole. Thus the geometry of ventricular contraction can be recorded, and an ejection fraction (the fraction of the end-diastolic volume ejected during systole) can be calculated.

Coronary angiography determines the anatomy of the coronary circulation, the number and location of critical obstructive lesions, the graftability of the artery distal to a critical obstructive lesion, and coronary artery spasm. Angiography is not indicated in all patients with angina pectoris. There is a definite although small risk of death, myocardial infarction, and cerebrovascular accident. The procedure is expensive. The clearest indication for angiography is to determine coronary anatomy and pathology and the ventricular function of a patient with angina pectoris who requires coronary artery bypass surgery. The procedure may also be used for the evaluation of patients with valvular heart disease in whom both valvular surgery and coronary artery bypass surgery may be required. Another indication is evaluation of patients with atypical chest pain, particularly individuals such as airline pilots on whose cardiovascular health many lives depend. Coronary arteriography and ventriculography also provide the physician with important predictive information concerning patients who suffer from angina or have had a myocardial infarction. Finally, arteriography is the only definitive way of demonstrating coronary artery spasm.

The procedure is performed by inserting a catheter via the brachial artery (Sones' technique) or the femoral artery (Judkins' technique). A 75% reduction in the luminal cross-sectional area (50% luminal diameter reduction seen in two planes) is considered to be "critical" or "significant" obstruction of the coronary artery. It is likely, however, that cross-sectional luminal reductions of less than 75% may be important under stress or exercise when high coronary flow rates are required. The location and extent of intercoronary collateral vessels can be determined. Ventriculography will show areas of reduced and abnormal wall motion, as well as ventricular aneurysms. An ejection fraction can also be calculated.

Despite the availability and importance of these ancillary tests, the diagnosis of angina pectoris still is made mainly by the history.

COURSE. The prognosis of patients with angina pectoris is related both to the extent of critical obstructing coronary artery lesions and to ventricular function. Without intensive medical or surgical treatment, annual mortality is 2% for patients with single-vessel disease, 7% for patients with two-vessel disease, and 11% for patients with three-vessel disease. Critical obstruction of the left main coronary artery increases the annual mortality rate to approximately 30%. These data do not take into account ventricular function. Patients with ejection fractions greater than 55% fare better than those with lesser ejection fractions in a continuum of increasing risk for any combination of coronary vessel involvement.

MANAGEMENT. Attention should be given factors that may precipitate or worsen angina pectoris. Obesity, diabetes mellitus, and hypertension must be controlled. Disorders of cholesterol and triglyceride metabolism should be corrected on the presumption that this may retard the progression of atheromatous disease. Congestive heart failure, anemia, thyrotoxicosis, and tachyarrhythmias, all of which increase myocardial oxygen consumption and worsen angina, should be treated.

A controlled exercise program may be of benefit to some patients with angina pectoris. The exercise prescription should be guided by the results of an exercise stress test. There is no convincing evidence that exercise results in prolongation of life, retardation of atherosclerosis, or an increase in coronary collaterals. Some individuals do show increased serum high-density lipoproteins, which are thought to have a protective effect against the development of atherosclerosis. However, the most important benefit from regular exercise is improved cardiovascular efficiency. Patients who regularly exercise are able to achieve a given level of total body oxygen consumption with less myocardial oxygen consumption because of a lower heart rate and blood pressure. Thus after training any given level of exercise can be sustained by a lower myocardial oxygen requirement.

The nitrates have been used for many years in treatment of and prophylaxis against anginal pain. Beneficial effects of nitrates are thought to be mediated by preload and afterload reduction, by decreased myocardial wall stress and oxygen demand, and possibly by increased blood flow via coronary collateral vessels. Nitrates will also relieve coronary artery spasm, should spasm be important in the genesis of the angina. Nitroglycerin, taken sublingually early in the course of an anginal episode, typically relieves the chest discomfort in 1 to 5 minutes. Sublingual nitroglycerin may also be used prophylactically before climbing stairs or hills—situations likely to precipitate anginal attacks. Longer-acting nitrates are also useful. Isosorbide dinitrate given sublingually exerts a protective effect for a few hours; when isosorbide dinitrate is given by mouth, the protective effect may extend to 4 or more hours. Nitroglycerin preparations applied to the skin are absorbed relatively slowly and may give protection for 6 hours or longer.

Side effects of nitrates include headache and hypotension. A tachyphylaxis to the vasodilation that underlies these effects may occur with time. Nitroglycerin tablets lose their effectiveness after a number of months if not stored in tightly stoppered, colored glass vials.

The β-blocking drugs reduce heart rate, myocardial contractility, and blood pressure, thereby reducing myocardial oxygen consumption and restoring the balance between myocardial blood flow and oxygen consumption. These agents are therefore particularly useful in controlling angina caused by exercise-related tachycardia. They also have a beneficial effect on rest angina. Propranolol and metoprolol are the most commonly used agents. Orally administered propranolol is metabolized by the liver soon after absorption (first-pass effect), but propranolol reduces hepatic blood flow and retards its own metabolism, resulting in a delayed achievement of a steady state after initiation of therapy. One of its metabolites, hydroxypropranolol, retains cardiovascular activity. The drug should be given until the resting pulse rate is between 50 and 60 beats/min. This endpoint is more useful clinically than blood level determinations.

Side effects of propranolol include gastrointestinal upset, diarrhea, insomnia, disturbing dreams, and sometimes loss of sexual desire and performance. Propranolol blocks both β_1-receptors (such as cardiac receptors) and β_2-receptors (such as pulmonary receptors), and therefore it may produce bronchospasm in patients with asthma or chronic obstructive lung disease. It should not be taken by patients who have marked bronchospasm. Metoprolol, a relatively selective β_1-blocker, is preferred for these patients. Because both drugs decrease myocardial contractility, they are contraindicated in congestive heart failure. They are also relatively contraindicated in patients with various forms of bradycardia.

Calcium-blocking agents such as nifedipine have recently been used as alternatives or adjuncts for treating angina pectoris. These agents reduce afterload, increase coronary blood flow by vasodilation, and relieve coronary artery spasm.

Coronary artery bypass grafting. The most direct way to increase myocardial blood flow is by coronary artery bypass surgery. The procedure entails removing a portion of the saphenous vein from the leg and anastomosing one end of it to the aorta and the other end to a suitable coronary artery distal to an obstructing lesion. Occasionally the internal mammary artery is used instead of a saphenous vein. When the internal mammary artery is used, only one anastomosis, to the distal coronary artery, is required. A "suitable" coronary artery is one whose distal ramifications are free from disease and are large enough to receive a graft and nourish a significant amount of myocardium. In appropriately selected patients, coronary artery bypass surgery can be done with an operative mortality of less than 2% or 3%. The left ventricular ejection fraction should be equal to or greater than 30% to reduce risk. The major morbidity is intraoperative myocardial infarction, the incidence of which varies between 10% and 20%.

The major indication for coronary artery bypass surgery is disabling angina pectoris refractory to medical treatment. Approximately 60% of patients have complete relief of angina after surgery, and another 20% or 30% have major or partial relief. Exercise tolerance measured by exercise stress testing also improves in the majority of patients. In patients with critical obstruction of the left main coronary artery, that is, greater than 50% obstruction, coronary artery bypass surgery improves survival. It is uncertain whether coronary artery bypass surgery improves survival in other patients; some studies suggest improved survival in those with good ventricular function and triple-vessel disease, but others do not. There is little evidence that performing this operation in asymptomatic patients is useful in preventing morbidity or mortality. The operation is not indicated as treatment for congestive heart failure.

There are reports of recurrences of anginal pain 5 to 7 years after cure by coronary artery bypass surgery. Continued follow-up examinations, control of risk factors, and medical treatment when indicated are therefore important.

Percutaneous coronary dilation. A new alternative to surgical bypass of atherosclerotic stenoses is to crush the plaques outward via expansion of a balloon placed in the coronary artery by catheter techniques. This investigational procedure seems to restore luminal patency with little risk. It can be done during the coronary angiography, obviating thoracotomy, but its use is limited to incomplete, noncalcific plaques easily reached by the catheter. The long-term results of successful dilation of plaques are unknown.

Unstable angina

Unstable angina pectoris is a syndrome intermediate in severity between classic effort-induced angina and myocardial infarction. The following useful diagnostic formulation encompasses almost all varieties of unstable angina:

Type IA—Twice the number of episodes of exertional angina or twice the severity of anginal attacks as determined by nitroglycerin tablet requirement

Type IB—Rest angina complicating effort-induced angina

Type IC—Recent-onset angina or angina brought on by less than usual exertion

Type II— Severe, prolonged chest pain incompletely or not at all relieved by nitroglycerin, occurring at rest, with either ST segment depression or T wave inversion (Myocardial infarction is excluded by the absence of Q waves and rises in serum cardiac enzyme activity.)

The pathogenesis of unstable angina is unclear. Patients with unstable angina have on the average the same degree of coronary atheromatous changes as patients with effort-induced angina and those with myocardial infarction. It has been postulated that coronary spasm and platelet aggregation may play an important role in the pathogenesis of unstable angina pectoris. Coronary artery spasm was found with significant frequency in one study.

Unstable angina is important because it carries a much more ominous prognosis for myocardial infarction and death than does classic effort-induced angina. Patients judged to have unstable angina by the preceding criteria should be admitted to a coronary care unit. They require monitoring for arrhythmias. Acute myocardial infarction should be excluded by enzyme determinations, ECGs, and perhaps technetium pyrophosphate or thallium scintigraphy. Rapid control of the pain of myocardial ischemia is imperative. Long- and short-acting nitrates and propranolol in doses sufficient to reduce the resting pulse to below 60 beats/min should be given. Oxygen and sedation are also useful. Pain refractory to these measures may respond to intra-aortic balloon pumping. The balloon inflates in diastole, augmenting diastolic coronary blood flow. It deflates just before the next cardiac systole, thereby reducing afterload and hence myocardial oxygen demand. The use of calcium antagonists such as verapamil and nifedipine has not had extensive trial in unstable angina in the United States, but preliminary results are encouraging.

In most patients the acute phase of unstable angina can be controlled by medication alone. Subsequent consideration of a coronary artery bypass procedure should be determined by the patient's frequency of rest and effort-induced angina after discharge from the hospital. In the few cases of unstable angina that cannot be controlled by medication alone, intra-aortic balloon pumping, urgent coronary arteriography, and coronary artery bypass surgery should be considered. However, results of a national prospective randomized trial of medical therapy alone versus surgical therapy plus medical therapy in unstable angina revealed no difference in mortality after 3 years. The incidence of myocardial infarction (comparing perioperative and postoperative infarction in the surgical group with nonoperative myocardial infarction in the medically treated group) was the same. However, pain relief was more complete in patients who underwent a coronary artery bypass procedure, and there was a 35% crossover rate from medical to surgical therapy, the largest portion of which occurred in the first 6 to 12 months.

Prinzmetal's variant angina

Prinzmetal described a variant form of angina pectoris in which the pain occurred only while the patient was at rest. The characteristic ECG change was ST segment elevation rather than ST segment depression, the latter being the hallmark of exercise-induced angina. Prinzmetal postulated that this form of angina was due to coronary artery spasm, and this has been confirmed by coronary angiography done during the course of variant angina. The course of variant angina depends on the nature of the underlying coronary artery pathology. In patients with little or no atheromatous change in the coronary arteries, coronary artery spasm and anginal pain tend to regress with time. This does not mean that Prinzmetal's variant angina is entirely a benign condition; severe hypotension, bradycardia, ventricular tachycardia, ventricular fibrillation, myocardial infarction, and death have occurred in patients with minimal or no atheromatous change but marked coronary artery spasm. In general, however, the prognosis of myocardial infarction and death is more likely in patients with coronary artery atheromatous disease.

Prinzmetal's variant angina is characterized by chest discomfort similar to that of effort-induced angina except that it occurs at rest. It is often cyclic in nature and may occur at the same time of day over a period of days or weeks. ECGs characteristically show ST segment elevation that regresses as the pain regresses. Various atrial and ventricular tachyarrhythmias and bradycardias such as heart block may be seen. Because chest pain occurs at rest with ST segment elevation, myocardial infarction must be excluded in the differential diagnosis.

A rigid separation of Prinzmetal's variant angina from classic effort-induced angina has been challenged. Although spasm is the principal pathogenetic mechanism in variant angina, spasm has also been identified in a few patients as the sole mechanism for classic effort-induced angina. Furthermore, patients with Prinzmetal's angina may show either ST segment elevation or depression.

Treatment of Prinzmetal's variant angina includes the use of nitrates and calcium antagonists (slow channel blocking agents) such as verapamil and nifedipine. Coronary artery bypass surgery should be reserved for those with critical atheromatous narrowing who do not respond to a combination of nitrates and calcium antagonists.

Angina with normal coronary arteries

Chest pain clinically indistinguishable from that of classic angina pectoris has been described in patients who have normal coronary arteries. Some of these patients have an easily identifiable cardiac abnormality that may or may not be related to their chest discomfort, such as hypertrophic cardiomyopathy, the mitral valve prolapse syndrome, aortic stenosis, and (less frequently) aortic insufficiency. The chest pain associated with the mitral valve prolapse syndrome is not understood. In the other conditions, reduced ventricular compliance, increased left ventricular end-diastolic pressure, increased diffusing distances between the capillaries and the center of the hypertrophied myocardial cell, increased myocardial oxygen requirements, and interference with coronary flow because of valvular abnormalities are important in the pathogenesis of the oxygen supply/demand imbalance.

There remains a group of patients with angina pectoris, normal coronary arteries, and no identifiable associated cardiac lesion, among whom women predominate. Their ECGs may show ST segment depression with exercise. Not infrequently, altered carbohydrate metabolism and lipoprotein abnormalities are present. In an appreciable minority of patients, lactate production may be observed when the myocardium is stressed by either pacing or isoproterenol infusion, indicating a shift to anaerobic metabolism. The cause of this condition is unknown. Coronary artery spasm, disease of coronary vessels beyond the resolution of angiography, and an intrinsic disorder of the myocardial cell have all been proposed but with little supporting evidence. The symptomatic response to nitrates and propranolol is poor. Although the condition is generally benign, both myocardial infarction and sudden death have been reported.

ACUTE MYOCARDIAL INFARCTION

DEFINITION. Acute myocardial infarction (MI) results from cardiac muscle ischemia severe and extensive enough to create irreversible necrosis of myocardial cells. Generally MI arises from obstructive coronary atherosclerosis, with limitation of nutrient blood flow producing anoxic, metabolic cellular death.

ETIOLOGY. The majority of MIs occur in patients with ischemic heart disease. Only 2% of all patients with MI and 16% of patients with MI younger than 35 do not have atherosclerotic coronary artery disease. The small subset of infarction patients with normal coronary arteries tends not only to be young but to have few CAD risk factors. In addition, they have none of the usual MI prodromes. Generally they have an acute hospital course no different from that of atherosclerotic patients with infarctions. Postinfarct problems (recurrent MI, heart failure, and sudden death) are fortunately less likely when coronary disease is absent, and these patients usually have no postinfarct angina.

The pathogenesis of MI in patients with no apparent coronary atherosclerosis might be attributed to coronary artery emboli, acute coronary thrombosis with subsequent recanalization, anomalous coronary anatomy, coronary arteriovenous fistulas, trauma, arteritis, or clinically undetected small vessel coronary artery disease. All of these conditions create an oxygen supply/demand disproportion that might predispose a patient to MI.

EPIDEMIOLOGY. Acute MI is an extraordinarily common hospital diagnosis. In the United States alone the diagnosis is made over 1.3 million times yearly. North American men have a 20% likelihood of having an MI or sudden death before they reach 65. Death rates following MI are, unfortunately, four times higher than in the normal population; half of these deaths are sudden.

PATHOGENESIS. Interrelated factors are responsible for the malignant alteration of the normal oxygen supply/demand equation that results in myocardial tissue death. Infarction results whether these changes are acute in situ thrombosis of nutrient vessels previously diseased with atherosclerosis, occlusive spasm of a normal coronary artery, or an embolic episode. Specifically, acute thrombosis may not always be the pathophysiologic event leading to myocardial necrosis, although for many years coronary thrombosis was believed to be synonymous with acute MI. Coronary occlusion has been demonstrated to occur in the absence of tissue necrosis if the collateral circulation is adequate to maintain normal cellular respiration. In addition, infarctions can occur in the absence of coronary occlusion.

Cellular ischemia acutely increases intracellular lactate concentration with the subsequent repression of enzymes in the glycolytic pathway. An increase in cellular acyl CoA occurs (particularly in the mitochondria) when acyl CoA esters inhibit the effective exchange of ADP and ATP between the cytoplasm and the mitochondria. A decline in high-energy phosphate stores occurs, and this, in conjunction with the cellular acidosis and metabolite accumulation, contributes to the rapid development of irreversible ischemic injury that ultimately leads to severe left ventricular dysfunction and death in these individuals.

Grossly visible changes consisting of discoloration and edema occur in the left ventricle 6 to 8 hours after infarction. A serofibrinous exudate develops over the epicardium in transmural infarctions 48 hours later, and in 8 to 10 days there is thinning of the infarct when necrotic muscle is removed by mononuclear cells.

On an ultrastructural level, disruption of sarcomeres, condensation of myofibrillar material, margination of nucleolar chromatin, and granulation in the myocardium occur over a 24-hour period.

CLINICAL MANIFESTATIONS. Chest discomfort is the major complaint of patients with MI. The pain is thought to arise from the nerve endings in injured or ischemic myocardium rather than necrotic muscle. This pain is generally the symptom forcing the patient to consult his physician. The discomfort is usually present at rest, is variable in intensity, and lasts longer than 30 minutes. There is often an eliciting event such as exertional or emotional stress. The discomfort may be characterized many ways by the patient. Frequently it is described not as a "painful" feeling, but rather a constricting, crushing, oppressing, compressing, squeezing, choking, burning, boring, or stabbing sensation. The location of the discomfort is usually retrosternal, with radiation of variable intensity and extent to the neck, jaws, teeth, arms, and back.

Other symptoms may include nausea and vomiting (more frequent in inferior wall MI than in anterior wall MI), diarrhea, weakness, dizziness, perspiration, intractable hiccups, and the symptoms of pulmonary edema (that is, severe dyspnea). Approximately 10% to 15% of MIs are diagnosed retrospectively (particularly in diabetic patients). MI may simulate other diseases such as acute pericarditis, pleurodynia, pulmonary embolism, aortic dissection, costochondritis, pancreatitis, gastritis, cholecystitis, and peptic ulcer disease.

Potentially confounding presentations in which MI must be considered include unexplained congestive heart failure, classic angina pectoris, atypical pain locations (persistent toothache), "bursitis," backache, sudden confusion, mania or psychosis, syncope, overwhelming weakness, acute indigestion, and unexplained peripheral arterial embolization.

Presenting physical findings are trivial unless gross cardiogenic shock or pulmonary edema is present. Usually the patient is anxious and restless and there are findings associated with hypertension, diabetes, or atherosclerosis.

Important signs (by no means specific for MI) include pericardial friction rub, the mitral regurgitation murmur of papillary muscle dysfunction, and gallop rhythms. Signs of abrupt left ventricular failure (pulmonary rales, jugular venous distention, orthopnea, and S_3 gallop) are important. The presence of an S_3 gallop in a patient with an acute MI is an ominous prognostic factor carrying a 30% mortality. There may be signs of shock (hypotension, oliguria, and peripheral cyanosis, in combination with cold, clammy, sweaty skin with an ashen-gray hue). Signs of central nervous system hypoperfusion (transient cerebral ischemic events, overt cerebrovascular accident, confusion) may predominate, particularly in the elderly.

It is important to know that hypotension does not necessarily mean shock in MI patients. Additional causes of low blood pressure in patients with MI include the bradycardia-hypotension syndrome associated with inferior wall myocardial infarction (Bezold-von Jarisch reflex), hypovolemia, occult mitral stenosis, pulmonary emboli, right ventricular infarction, and pericardial effusion.

Additional signs of MI include low-grade fever (most commonly after 24 to 48 hours) and Cheyne-Stokes respiration (secondary to central nervous system hypoperfusion, pulmonary edema, or opiate therapy).

The physical examination can provide prognostic information in the patient with acute MI. Table 96-1 summarizes the Killip classification of acute MI, which categorizes patients according to physical findings. Those with an S_3 gallop and pulmonary rales above the scapula (Killip class III) have at least a 20% hospital mortality and comprise 30% to 50% of patients with MI. Patients with frank cardiogenic shock (Killip class IV) have a 60% to 80% mortality and comprise 10% of MI patients on initial admission.

LABORATORY FINDINGS. Certain enzymes liberated from necrotic myocardial cells are reasonably sensitive and specific indicators of MI. Indeed, the amount of enzyme liberation can grossly quantify the size of an infarction.

Creatine phosphokinase (CPK) may appear in serum as early as 4 hours after the infarction (Fig. 96-2). It is the first enzyme generally measured to become abnormal. Since CPK is liberated in significant amounts from injured brain, liver, thyroid, striated muscle, and smooth muscle cells, CPK elevation might mistakenly be attributed to cardiac muscle when in fact it is due to hepatic, brain, or bowel infarction or more commonly to striated muscle trauma (most often resulting from intramuscular injection of irritating medication). A myocardial band (MB) of CPK can be detected by electrophoresis. If the CPK-MB exceeds 5% of the total CPK, myocardial cell damage can be assumed. The CPK level usually returns to normal within 4 to 6 days. Persistent elevation is an ominous sign, suggesting massive infarction or ongoing necrosis. Serum glutamic-oxaloacetic transaminase (SGOT) rises 6 to 12 hours after MI and returns to normal 5 to 7 days later. SGOT elevation also occurs in patients with liver disease, hepatic congestion, skeletal muscle disease, intramuscular injections, pulmonary emboli, shock, or pericarditis with epicardial involvement.

Lactic dehydrogenase (LDH) is the last enzyme to appear elevated in serum after MI, rising 48 hours after the event and remaining elevated 7 to 9 days. LDH is also liberated in substantial quantities in hemolysis, megaloblastic anemia, leukemia, massive pulmonary emboli, shock, skeletal muscle disease, and myocarditis. Like CPK, LDH has an isoenzyme (hydroxybutyric dehydrogenase, HBDH) that is more specific for myocardial cell necrosis.

Additional abnormal laboratory findings in MI include leukocytosis, myoglobinuria, elevated erythrocyte sedimentation rate, and elevated hematocrit owing to hemoconcentration.

DIAGNOSIS. The diagnosis of acute MI is made by combined assessment of the history, physical examination, serum enzymes, ECG, and, when available, ancillary radionuclide imaging of the heart.

The ECG is generally abnormal in patients with an acute infarction. Indeed, for anterior MIs of reasonable size the ECG will be positive in 95% of the cases. Not only is the ECG important for diagnosing MI, but it also helps to determine extent of injury, age of infarction, and infarction location, as well as the presence of pericarditis or electrolyte disturbances. ECG monitoring is also important for diagnosing rhythm disturbances.

The usual evolutionary pattern of ECG changes is early

Table 96-1. Killip classification of patients with acute MI and their respective mortality

Class	Clinical findings	Mortality (%)
Class I (uncomplicated MI)	No evidence of CHF	5-7
Class II (moderate CHF)	Bibasilar rales and/or S_3 gallop	10-15
Class III (severe CHF/pulmonary edema)	Rales above scapula, S_3 gallop, tachycardia, frank pulmonary edema	20-50
Class IV (cardiogenic shock)	Shock, tachycardia, hypotension	60-80

Adapted from Killip, T., and Kimball, J.T.: Am. J. Cardiol. **20:**457, 1967.

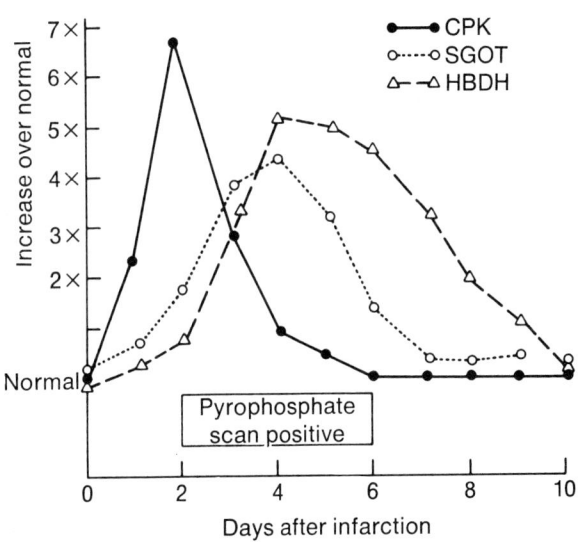

Fig. 96-2. Enzymatic elevation and technetium 99m pyrophosphate scan patterns in patients with acute myocardial infarction. *CPK,* creatine phosphokinase; *SGOT,* serum glutamicoxaloacetic transaminase; *HBDH,* hydroxybutyric dehydrogenase.

ST segment elevation with subsequent T wave inversion and Q wave formation. Q waves localize the region of myocardial necrosis. The usual evolution of ECG changes occurs over several weeks; persistent ST elevation beyond 6 weeks suggests the development of a ventricular aneurysm. Interestingly, 20% to 30% of ECGs normalize entirely after MI, making the retrospective diagnosis particularly difficult at times.

Right ventricular (RV) infarction cannot be diagnosed by ECG. It is important to consider an RV infarct in hypotensive patients with lateral or inferolateral MIs. Generally these patients have jugular venous distention, hypotension, and normal left ventricular filling pressures. The diagnosis must be made by right-sided heart catheterization. A first-pass radionuclide angiocardiogram with an abnormally low RV ejection fraction raises suspicion that there is elevated RV filling (right atrial) pressure despite normal LV filling (pulmonary capillary wedge) pressure. The treatment consists of intravascular expansion with saline, albumin, or crystalloid.

Radionuclide imaging may be useful in other respects. Technetium 99 pyrophosphate is taken up directly by acutely necrosed myocardial cells. This technique of myocardial imaging will allow the recognition, localization (of a "hot spot"), and estimation of size of infarction in most cases of transmural MI, if the study is performed between 2 and 6 days after the acute infarction (pyrophosphate window in Fig. 96-2). In nontransmural MI a pattern of diffuse uptake may occur, which can also be present in non-MI situations.

Thallium 201 imaging, on the other hand, will produce a "cold spot" in regions of diminished myocardial perfusion and therefore would be positive with MIs caused by acute coronary artery occlusion. This study should theoretically diagnose an MI at its earliest inception. However, the filling defect or "cold spot" would remain a persistent finding. Thus imaging with thallium after infarction cannot distinguish hypoperfusion resulting from an old scar from ischemic but viable myocardium. The greatest value of thallium 201 seems to be the imaging of "cold spot" regions with exercise-induced ischemia. (The perfusion scan is abnormal with exercise but normal at rest, suggesting adequate reperfusion.)

Radionuclide angiocardiography can yield serial estimates of left ventricular function by repeated determination of ejection fraction. A left-to-right shunt caused by acute ventricular septal defect (VSD) formation can be diagnosed. Marked mitral regurgitation can also be detected. This procedure can thus differentiate papillary muscle dysfunction or rupture from a VSD. Radionuclide angiocardiography may also prove useful in the differentiation of true and false left ventricular aneurysms.

COURSE AND COMPLICATIONS. It is difficult to determine the actual mortality of acute MI because the majority of patients who die never reach the hospital alive. Some have estimated the prehospital mortality to be as high as 60%. Even patients surviving initial hospitalization have a subsequent high mortality, varying from 4% to 20% per year depending on the amount of left ventricular dyssynergy and number of diseased vessels.

Recently, definite MI has resulted in overall mortality of 16% and unstable angina in mortality of 1% to 2% while both groups were in the coronary care unit. Late hospital death accounted for 5% and 1%, respectively. Hypotension, heart failure, and ventricular arrhythmias are more common in MI patients than in those with unstable angina.

The following observations in the coronary care unit may be risk factors for death in patients with acute MI after discharge from the unit: the development of a new interventricular conduction defect, sinus tachycardia persisting more than 48 hours, ventricular fibrillation, atrial flutter or fibrillation, extensive anterior wall MI, and left ventricular failure.

Hospital mortality depends on the extent of disease and the complications that may occur. Arrhythmias are responsible for most deaths that occur on the first day. Ventricular fibrillation and tachycardia (which may lead to fibrillation) are the most common lethal arrhythmias. Trifascicular heart block may also occur early and is a poor prognostic sign. Shock or pulmonary edema usually occurs on the first or second day and carries a grave prognosis (60% to 80% and 20% to 50% mortality, respectively; Table 96-1). Rupture of the intraventricular septum or papillary muscle may occur after several days and results in a loud systolic murmur and severe heart failure; rupture of the free ventricular wall may result in tamponade. A transient pericarditis (second or third day) from transmural infarction (seen in 15% with transmural MIs) and thromboembolic episodes (usually occurring after several days to weeks) carry a much less ominous prognosis.

Arterial emboli (cerebral, visceral, peripheral, coronary) may be due to dislodgment of an acutely formed left ventricular mural thrombus. Phlebothrombosis, probably related to inactivity, occurs in as many as 10% of patients, and many have subsequent pulmonary emboli. Low doses of subcutaneously injected heparin have routinely been used in many hospitals to ameliorate this problem. Cerebral infarction from episodes of hypotension or tachyarrhythmias may occur in patients with concomitant cerebrovascular and coronary artery disease. It is not uncommon to find an unsuspected MI in patients with cerebral infarction and vice versa. Acute renal failure may be secondary to either frank shock or transient hypotension.

Late complications (weeks to months) include formation of a ventricular aneurysm, delayed heart failure, postmyocardial infarction syndrome (Dressler's syndrome), and shoulder-hand syndrome.

Ventricular aneurysm often leads to heart failure, systemic embolism, or recurrent ventricular tachycardia. Patients often have a palpable double apical impulse, S_3 and S_4 gallops, and persistent elevation of ST segments on ECG. The chest roentgenogram may show a bulge on the heart border, and cineventriculography is diagnostic. If the aneurysm is causing symptoms not responsive to medical therapy, it can be resected.

Dressler's syndrome, thought to be an autoimmune reaction, consists of pericarditis, pleuritis, and pneumonitis. High titers of antimyocardial antibodies are present in the serum. If aspirin does not give symptomatic relief, corticosteroids can be used. Anticoagulants should be avoided in patients with Dressler's syndrome, since life-threatening hemopericardium can result.

The shoulder-hand syndrome is a limitation of mobility in the shoulder and arm (usually on the left side) associated with pain. The treatment is physiotherapy.

MANAGEMENT. Admission to an intensive care unit has become standard practice when a patient's history and clinical findings suggest acute MI. The main benefit of the unit is continuous monitoring that makes possible the early recognition of severe ventricular arrhythmias, ventricular fibrillation, and sudden death. A cardiac care unit is a closely supervised area with well-trained individuals capable of recognizing and treating serious arrhythmias and initiating cardiopulmonary resuscitative efforts and defibrillation when appropriate. In addition, these units provide a place where pacemaker insertion and bedside hemodynamic monitoring with flow-directed pulmonary artery catheters can be accomplished.

Bed rest is important for patients with MI because it places low demand on the myocardium. Depending on the clinical course, the patient should be allowed a bedside commode and reasonable amounts of time for bedside leg dangling and chair rest as early as possible.

Adequate pain relief is important. Since pain is generated in the perinecrotic ischemic zone, its elimination suggests improvement of the oxygen supply/demand ratio in this region, which is at high risk for infarct extension. Morphine sulfate, given slowly intravenously, is the drug of choice. Meperidine may be given intravenously to patients not tolerating morphine. Intramuscular injections should be avoided, especially when heart failure or shock is present, because of the variability of drug absorption in these states and the difficulty with interpretation of cardiac enzyme patterns. Nitrate administration (sublingual, topical, or oral) may also be effective. This maneuver reduces left ventricular filling pressure and intramyocardial wall tension, thus decreasing myocardial oxygen demand and thereby eliminating ischemic chest pain. If pain following MI is particularly severe, prolonged, or intractable, intravenous administration of nitroprusside or nitroglycerin may relieve it.

Sedation to relieve anxiety and continuous psychologic support are usually required. Low-flow oxygen administration should be considered, particularly in patients with hypoxia. The benefits of this maneuver in individuals with normal arterial PO_2 have not been clearly demonstrated, and it should be avoided if the patient reports it to be unpleasant or uncomfortable.

A constipated patient straining at stool produces a Valsalva maneuver that increases peripheral vascular resistance, left ventricular wall stress, and myocardial oxygen demand, therefore potentially furthering ischemic injury. MI patients should receive stool softeners and appropriate laxatives with permission to use a bedside commode as early as possible.

Early mobilization (after 2 to 5 days) of patients following infarction seems reasonable. The decision of when to mobilize an individual is rooted in common sense. However, early ambulation diminishes the likelihood of phlebothrombosis and restores patient self-confidence. With appropriate supervision, early ambulation and exercise after MI are safe.

The routine administration of anticoagulants to patients with acute MI is controversial. Clinically, anticoagulants do not seem to attenuate the complications of ischemia, limit infarction size, or prevent subsequent extension or infarction. Heparin in low doses is beneficial in phlebothrombosis prevention, and its use should always be considered.

Lidocaine should routinely be administered to most patients with acute MI. An intravenous loading dose followed by infusion will generally prevent malignant tachyarrhythmias.

Four special procedures may have to be considered: temporary or permanent pacing, invasive hemodynamic monitoring, balloon counter-pulsation, and immediate surgical intervention.

Temporary transvenous pacemaker placement as prophylactic therapy to prevent sudden asystole or complete heart block and death should be considered in situations of complete heart block with slow idioventricular rhythm; atrioventricular dissociation with symptomatic, slow escape rhythm; symptomatic sinus bradycardia unresponsive to atropine; and new right bundle branch block with left anterior hemoblock, especially with first-degree or Mobitz type II second-degree heart block (see Chapter 97).

Since the physician must attempt aggressively to preserve as much myocardium from necrosis as possible, it is imperative that left ventricular hemodynamics be optimized. It is therefore important to accurately assess cardiac pump function in an individual with MI. Patients can be classified as to whether they have normal hemodynamics, hypovolemic hypotension, left ventricular systolic or diastolic dysfunction, or cardiogenic shock. Since the therapeutic requirements vary for these states, precise diagnosis is mandatory. Frequently this requires invasive hemodynamic monitoring with balloon-tipped, flow-directed, thermistor-equipped catheters passed percutaneously to the pulmonary artery. Invasive monitoring is required because of the frequent disparity between physical findings and actual hemodynamic measurements.

Surgical measures directed toward the heart in MI patients are clearly indicated only when a mechanical lesion such as ventricular septal defect or ruptured papillary muscle is present and clinical deterioration is occurring. Coronary artery bypass surgery in the face of an evolving MI is probably not indicated as a measure to limit infarct size, prevent cardiogenic shock and arrhythmias, or change ultimate mortality. Patients with acute infarctions do not clearly benefit from emergency revascularization and may actually be harmed by the procedure.

SUDDEN DEATH

DEFINITION. A uniformly precise definition of sudden death is unavailable because of the wide-ranging interpretation of this phenomenon by epidemiologists, pathologists, clinicians, coroners, and the public. Three basic components seem interchangeable: (1) that a natural (atraumatic) process is present; (2) that the event was unexpected; and (3) that a short time frame surrounds the event. Thus the unanticipated occurrence of "sudden death" generally refers to an abrupt and unexpected change in continuity of a process (either health or disease) from the state immediately preceding death to the fatal episode itself.

The "suddenness" of the event has varied by definition but generally refers to death less than 6 hours after onset of symptoms when the death is observed, or death occurring within 24 hours of the time the subject is last seen and known to be well.

ETIOLOGY. Sudden death does not always denote cardiovascular pathology, but it is a very strong indicator of it. Heart disease can be inferred from the event of sudden death in 90% of the cases, with cardiovascular disease being present in virtually all cases in which death occurs less than 1 hour after symptoms appear. When confronted with an individual with clinical manifestations of sudden death, it becomes important to determine the most likely cause, since the type of emergency therapy required may be radically different depending on the mechanism. For example, a patient with sudden death owing to ventricular fibrillation is profoundly different from a patient with vasodepressor syncope ("vasovagal reaction" and common "faint"). Indeed, in sudden death, an immediate decision is required as to whether the symptoms are due to a self-terminating derangement, are the result of a cardiac condition, or are noncardiac in origin.

The most common noncardiac causes of sudden death originate in the central nervous system, although death ultimately results from an arrhythmia. Profound metabolic aberrations (sudden hypoxia, hypoglycemia, acidosis, hypercalcemia, and hyperkalemia) may also cause sudden death. Other important causes of sudden death, not primarily cardiogenic, include sepsis, anaphylaxis, electrical shock, and inadvertent drug toxicity (as seen with tricyclic antidepressants, phenothiazines, diuretics, digitalis, quinidine, and procainamide).

Cardiovascular abnormalities precipitating sudden death can be divided into extracardiac problems (aortic dissection, cardiac tamponade, exsanguination, and hypovolemia) and intrinsic cardiac problems (by far the most significant of which are arrhythmias related to ischemic heart disease). Cardiac lesions other than coronary artery disease account for sudden death no more than 10% of the time. These lesions include mitral valve prolapse syndrome, bacterial endocarditis, obstructive cardiomyopathy, myocarditis, rheumatic heart disease, metastatic malignancies, congenital defects, and valvular abnormalities.

EPIDEMIOLOGY. The incidence of sudden death cannot be determined exactly. It appears, however, that 15% to 30% of all natural deaths should be categorized in this fashion. Sudden death seems to have a bimodal population distribution, with highest rates occurring at 1 to 6 months of age (sudden infant death syndrome seen in 3 of 1000 liveborn infants) and 35 to 70 years. Males account for more deaths than females in all age groups. Ninety percent of adults with sudden death occurring within 1 hour of the first symptoms have cardiovascular disease; 80% to 90% of this group have atherosclerotic cardiovascular disease. Significantly, 60% to 70% of atherosclerotic related sudden death occurs out of the hospital, with 30% of patients with CAD having sudden death as their initial disease manifestation.

PATHOGENESIS. The final common pathway in sudden death is always an arrhythmia. Focal cardiac necrosis (acute or old MI) causes ventricular tachycardia and fibrillation. Global ischemic events with chronic heart disease create a setting conducive to asystole and heart block. One study noted that 66% of patients with sudden death had critical CAD (greater than 75% cross-sectional stenosis). This study demonstrated critical left anterior descending lesions in 96% of cases, right coronary lesions in 79%, circumflex disease in 66%, and left main lesions in 34%.

One of the most important, potentially controllable associations with sudden death is the premature ventricular contraction (PVC). Several epidemiologic studies have shown that frequent PVCs indicate an increased risk for sudden death, presumably by inducing unstable ventricular arrhythmias such as ventricular tachycardia and fibrillation. The Framingham data demonstrated, however, that PVCs were a sudden death risk factor only when there was ECG evidence of atherosclerotic cardiovascular disease.

Three basic mechanisms could account for the development of ventricular arrhythmias following ischemic events: (1) unbalanced automaticity in multiple myocardial foci; (2) peri-infarction or ischemic zone reentrant arrhythmias; and (3) depolarization after potentials. In the early period following myocardial necrosis, the important mechanism seems to be reentrant pathways created in the ven-

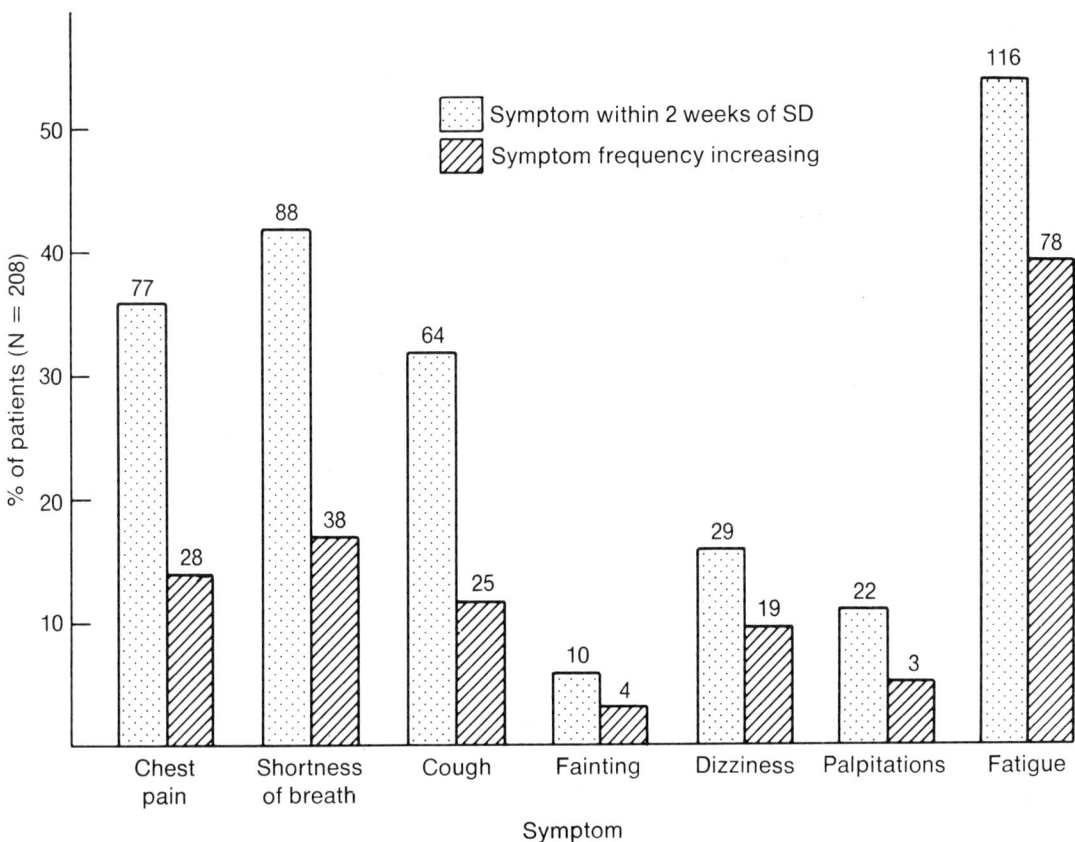

Fig. 96-3. Percentage of patients with atherosclerotic cardiovascular disease and sudden death, *SD*, who exhibited prodromes before their event. (Abstracted from Kuller, L., Cooper, M., and Perper, J.: Arch. Intern. Med. **129:**714, 1972.)

tricular muscle as a result of slow conduction through ischemic or infarcted tissue. Later arrhythmias seem to arise in subendocardial Purkinje fibers, which develop spontaneous diastolic depolarization (and consequently slowed conduction), as well as prolonged action potential duration. A modifying element is parasympathetic/sympathetic imbalance, probably owing to modulating central nervous system factors.

In any event the ultimate consequence of the dysrhythmia (whether it be ventricular tachycardia, ventricular fibrillation, or asystole) is disruption of the cardiac pump function. Ineffectual pump output results in immediate tissue hypoperfusion with lactic acidosis and subsequent cellular death. Unless adequate tissue oxygenation can be maintained with effective cardiopulmonary resuscitation, cellular death with organism demise will ensue. A vicious cycle persists as perpetuation of arrhythmias is encouraged by cellular acidosis and hypoxia.

CLINICAL MANIFESTATIONS. Sudden death may be truly unexpected, or it may follow a short period of prodromal warning. Prodromes are retrospectively recognized in 20% of cases. Fig. 96-3 demonstrates the incidence of different prodromal symptoms in a group of 208 patients with atherosclerosis and sudden death. These symptoms were ignored or minimized by the majority of patients. Table 96-2 compares patients with sudden death and acute MIs to those without documented MIs. The patients with MIs have prodromes, with heralding symptoms present minutes to hours before the event. In addition, patients without associated acute MI are more likely to have recurrence of sudden death and usually have advanced forms of ventricular ectopia.

Table 96-2. Comparison between sudden death patients with MI and those without MI

	Sudden death with acute MI	Sudden death without MI
Prodomes	Yes	No
Duration of symptoms before sudden death	Minutes to hours	Seconds
Presence of PVCs	Yes	Yes (advanced grades)
Recurrence rate of sudden death	<5%	30%

Fortunately, many individuals with sudden death can be saved. Cobb and others have reported on 400 patients who were resuscitated following sudden death owing to ventricular fibrillation. Of this group, 35% had cardiopulmonary resuscitation (CPR) initiated by bystanders.

MANAGEMENT. Sudden death is potentially reversible. The prerequisites for reversibility are appropriate recognition of the event and immediate institution of basic life support measures. The value of CPR has been demonstrated in community-wide studies in which the 1-year survival rate of those successfully resuscitated was 70%.

CPR with effective maintenance of artificial ventilation and circulation must be instituted immediately. This should be followed by advanced life support measures that might include endotracheal intubation, cardiac monitoring for arrhythmias, defibrillation if indicated, maintenance of an intravenous infusion line, and pharmacotherapy to correct metabolic acidosis and aid in establishing an effective cardiac rhythm and circulation.

PREVENTION. Sudden death occurs mainly among patients with CAD. The identification of individuals at risk of sudden death is the subject of active investigation. Certain subsets with recent MI who are predisposed to sudden death can be identified; for example, a patient with anterior infarction and bundle branch block would benefit from prolonged ECG monitoring to predict ventricular tachyarrhythmias, as well as from evaluation for a pacemaker.

Rapid delivery of advanced CPR systems and wide-spectrum community training in CPR are also critical. Initiation of CPR by trained laymen lessens neurologic sequelae in survivors.

Identification of patients at risk for sudden death has been linked to complex forms of PVCs. A large survey demonstrated that the prevalence of ventricular ectopia was 0.6% on resting ECGs of 67,375 asymptomatic military men. Only 6 of 122,043 individuals clinically free from ischemic heart disease had complex ectopia such as multifocal PVCs or ventricular tachycardia. The mere presence of PVCs does not mean cardiovascular disease. Indeed, 24-hour ECG monitoring of asymptomatic medical student volunteers revealed that 50% had one or more PVCs (occasionally multiform). Also, the incidence of PVCs in any given population increases with age.

Several systems of PVC grading have been proposed to identify PVCs predicting sudden death. The PVC grading criteria developed by Lown is summarized in Table 96-3. "Complex" PVCs are those falling into grades 3, 4A, 4B, and 5. These predict sudden death, perhaps because the more malignant forms of PVCs are associated with more severe heart disease, manifested by abnormal systolic left ventricular function (ejection fraction). Furthermore, the distribution of PVCs using Lown's grading is related to the extent of coronary artery involvement. Of patients with multivessel CAD, 41% had grade 4 or 5 PVCs, compared to only 15% of patients with single-vessel disease. Of patients with single-vessel coronary disease, 48% had grade 1A PVCs or none. In addition, only 18% of patients who had no PVCs or grade 1A PVCs had multivessel disease. Among patients with LV end-diastolic pressure greater than 10 mm Hg and LV dyssynergy, 4B PVCs were noted in 40% and 4A in 67%, compared to 6% and 12% in 34 patients without these hemodynamic abnormalities.

Table 96-3. Lown grading criteria for PVCs

Grade	PVC description
0	No PVCs
1A	Occasional isolated PVCs (<30/hr; <1/min)
1B	Occasional isolated PVCs (<30/hr; >1/min)
2	Frequent unifocal PVCs (>30/hr)
3	Multiform PVCs
4A	Repetitive PVCs (couplets)
4B	Repetitive PVCs (salvos)
5	"R-on-T" (early cycle) PVCs

Adapted from Calvert, A., Lown, B., and Gorlin, R.: Am. J. Cardiol. **39**:627,1977.

Identification of those at risk for life-threatening arrhythmias using pacemaker stimulation techniques to induce arrhythmias and catheterization techniques for the selection of drug and surgical therapy is the subject of active and thus far fruitful investigation. The indicators for, and measures of, successful therapy may soon shift away from monitoring PVCs to inducing tachyarrhythmias.

Available data demonstrate the effectiveness of prophylactic medical therapy in patients at risk for sudden death. It has been shown that titration of drug dose with blood levels can reduce sudden death from 30% to 10% in the subset of individuals who have once been resuscitated, although not all the monitored ventricular arrhythmias are abolished.

Finally, since many potentially fatal arrhythmias are linked to foci in the left ventricle and many of these foci are the borderline points of an aneurysm or scar, excision of these regions would seem beneficial. However, left ventricular aneurysmectomy alone has not always been effective in abolishing the dangerous arrhythmias. Endocardial and epicardial mapping techniques during induced ventricular tachycardia identify sites of a tachycardia origination that can be surgically resected. Surgical therapy for recurrent ventricular tachycardia thus can be substantially improved by identification of the endocardial origin of the arrhythmia followed by appropriately guided surgical resection.

BIBLIOGRAPHY

Brodsky, M., and others: Arrhythmias documented by 24 hour continuous electrocardiographic monitoring in 50 male medical students without apparent heart disease, Am. J. Cardiol. **39**:390, 1977.

Brushek, A.V.G., Proudfit, W.S., and Sones, F.M., Jr.: Progress study of 590 consecutive non-surgical cases of coronary disease followed 5-9 years. I. Arteriographic correlations, Circulation **47**:1147, 1973.

Calvert, A., Lown, B., and Gorlin, R.: Ventricular premature beats and anatomically defined coronary heart disease, Am. J. Cardiol. **39**:627, 1977.

Cobb, L.A., and others: Resuscitation from out-of-hospital ventricular fibrillation: 4 years follow-up, Circulation **52**(suppl.):223, 1975.

Dollery, C.T., and George, C.: Propranolol–ten years from introduction, Cardiovasc. Clin. **6**:255, 1974.

Ehrich, D.A., and others: The hemodynamic response to intra-aortic balloon counterpulsation in patients with cardiogenic shock complicating acute myocardial infarction, Am. Heart J. **93**:274, 1977.

Ellestad, M.H., Cooke, B.M., Jr., and Greenbert, P.S.: Stress testing: clinical applications and predictive capacity, Prog. Cardiovasc. Dis. **21**:431, 1979.

Eslami, B., and others: Acute myocardial infarction in the absence of coronary arterial obstruction, Ala. J. Med. Sci. **12**:322, 1975.

Forrester, J.S., and others: Medical therapy of acute myocardial infarction by application of hemodynamic subsets (in two parts), N. Engl. J. Med. **295**:1356, 1404, 1976.

Hinkle, L.E., Jr., Carver, S.T., and Stevens, M.: The frequency of asymptomatic disturbances of cardiac rhythm and conduction in middle-aged men, Am. J. Cardiol. **24**:629, 1969.

Hiss, R.G., Averill, K.N., and Lamb, L.E.: Electrocardiographic findings of 67,375 asymptomatic subjects, Am. J. Cardiol. **6**:96, 1960.

Kannel, W.B., and Feinleib, H.: Natural history of angina pectoris in the Framingham Study: prognosis and survival, Am. J. Cardiol. **29**:154, 1972.

Killip, T., III, and Kimball, J.T.: Treatment of myocardial infarction in a coronary care unit: a two year experience with 250 patients, Am. J. Cardiol. **20**:457, 1967.

Krauss, K.R., Hutter, A.M., Jr., and DeSanctis, R.W.: Acute coronary insufficiency: course and follow-up, Arch. Intern. Med. **129**:808, 1972.

Kuller, L., Cooper, J., and Perper, J.: Epidemiology of sudden death, Arch. Intern. Med. **129**:714, 1972.

Lie, K.I., and others: Lidocaine in the prevention of primary ventricular fibrillation: a double-blind randomized study in 212 consecutive patients, N. Engl. J. Med. **291**:1324, 1974.

McIntosh, H.D., and Garcia, J.A.: The first decade of aortocoronary bypass grafting, 1967-1977: a review, Circulation **57**:405, 1978.

Rubermann, W., and others: Ventricular premature beats and mortality after myocardial infarction, N. Engl. J. Med. **297**:750, 1977.

Russell, R.O., Jr., and others: Unstable angina pectoris: national cooperative study group to compare surgical and medical therapy. II. In-hospital experience and initial follow-up results in patients with one, two, and three vessel disease, Am. J. Cardiol. **42**:839, 1978.

Schultze, R.A., Strauss, H.W., and Pitt, B.: Sudden death in the year following myocardial infarction, Am. J. Med. **62**:192, 1977.

Spain, D.M., Bradess, V.A., and Mohr, C.: Coronary atherosclerosis as a cause of unexpected and unexplained death, J.A.M.A. **174**:384, 1960.

97 • CARDIAC ARRHYTHMIAS

Jerry C. Luck and Toby R. Engel

Cardiac arrhythmia refers to a disturbance of heart rhythm, rate, or conduction. Recognition of arrhythmia is facilitated by specialized monitoring. Cardiac care units with continuous on-line ECG monitoring and ambulatory tape-recorded monitoring enable detection of arrhythmias that were once only recognized during a symptomatic period when the physician was in attendance. Thus many arrhythmias that go undetected by the patient can be recorded. In contrast patients may complain of palpitations or dizziness but have a normal cardiac rate and rhythm at the time, indicating that the symptoms are not related to an arrhythmia.

Characterization of arrhythmia is made more complex by marked spontaneous variation in the frequency of arrhythmia, as with ventricular ectopic beats (VEBs). As exemplified by acute myocardial infarction, the substrate of arrhythmia varies as well. Almost half the heart attack victims die before hospitalization, presumably from ventricular fibrillation. On hospitalization arrhythmias are initially ubiquitous and dangerous for 24 to 48 hours, but then the risk dramatically abates, although severe ventricular ectopy still indicates a isk of sudden death.

This discussion centers on the clinical relevance of arrhythmias, including those incidentally recorded. Mechanisms will be considered with respect to therapy. Classification of arrhythmias is very important in terms of both establishing relevance and selecting therapy. Finally controversial topics of therapeutic importance are discussed separately in detail, including the treatment of ectopic beats and bradycardia.

NORMAL CONDUCTION AND RHYTHM

The primary pacemaker is the sinus node, located at the border of the superior vena cava and the high lateral right atrium. The sinus node is primarily supplied by a single artery that arises from either the proximal right or the circumflex coronary artery. Sympathetic fibers from the right stellate ganglion and parasympathetic fibers from the vagus nerve richly innervate the sinus node and surrounding atrium. A normal beat depends on conduction of the impulse from the node to the atrium (sinoatrial conduction).

The heart has a hierarchy of subsidiary pacemakers that arise from the specialized conduction system. Atrial, atrioventricular (AV) junctional, and ventricular escape pacemakers are slower but become manifest when the sinus node falters.

The AV node lies in the floor of the interatrial septum near the fibrous skeleton that supports the mitral and aortic valves. It is supplied by the AV nodal artery, which arises from the distal right coronary artery 90% of the time. The AV node is richly supplied by both parasympathetic and sympathetic fibers. It mainly serves to modulate the conduction of impulses from the atrium to the common bundle and ventricle. The AV node thus serves as a gate, preventing too many atrial impulses from entering the ventricle. It also can function as a pacemaker when the sinus node or subsidiary atrial pacemakers fail.

Infranodal conduction is through the common bundle (His bundle), which traverses the fibrous body and muscular septum to trifurcate into a right bundle branch and an anterior and posterior fascicle of a left bundle branch. The bundle branches terminate in a complex network of Purkinje fibers throughout the ventricle. Blood flow to the His bundle and proximal bundle branches is mainly from the proximal branches of the left anterior descending coronary artery.

Conduction defects occur at any level. The most prevalent affect the sinus node, AV node, and proximal infranodal structures. The ECG can diagnose conduction disturbances at these levels. Sinus node depolarization is not appreciated on the ECG, and sinoatrial conduction therefore is not discernible. Slow or absent P waves, however, indicate sinus dysfunction. A prolonged PR interval suggests an AV node defect. Bundle branch and fascicular blocks are infranodal defects with characteristic ECG patterns.

Based on anatomic origin, arrhythmias are either supraventricular or ventricular. Further subdivision is based on rate. Normally rhythm is of sinus origin and is 60 to 100 beats/min. Tachycardia refers to rates greater than 100 beats/min, and bradycardia to rates less than 60 beats/min. Other cardiac pacemakers have different ranges of normal; for example, the AV junction has subsidiary pacemakers with rates of 40 to 60 beats/min. Thus AV junctional tachycardia is a junctional rate faster than 60 beats/min., and AV junctional bradycardia is less than 40 beats/min.

Criteria for *normal sinus rhythm* are a P wave of sinus origin (normal axis, upright in lead II); a constant P morphology; and a rate 60 to 100 beats/min, with a fairly constant P-P interval, varying by at most 0.16 second.

Sinus rhythm is influenced by autonomic tone. For example, emotion, position, temperature, drugs, and noncardiac illness alter rate. Heart failure accelerates rate to increase cardiac output.

TACHYCARDIAS
Sinus tachycardia

Sinus tachycardia denotes rates greater than 100 beats/min. Generally, sinus tachycardia does not exceed about 150 beats/min in adults unless there is cardiovascular collapse, hyperthyroidism, or respiratory failure. Adults can increase the rate to 180 to 200 beats/min with maximal exercise. Infants and young children can sometimes increase the rate to 230 beats/min.

Sinus tachycardia always occurs because of a stress, such as emotion, exercise, or fever. Several drugs accelerate the sinus rate by virtue of sympathomimetic action or parasympatholytic action. Pulmonary causes are obstructive lung disease, embolism, asthma, and pneumonia. Any pathologic state that requires increased cardiac output could result in sinus tachycardia. In general sinus tachycardia by itself does not produce symptoms, and therapy is aimed at correcting the underlying cause.

Mechanisms of ectopic tachycardias

Three mechanisms for *tachycardia not of sinus origin* are frequently invoked: *automaticity, reentry,* and *triggered automaticity.* Automaticity occurs when a cell exhibits repetitive spontaneous depolarization to a threshold voltage that causes it to fire itself and also electrically discharge neighboring cells as their pacemaker. *Parasystole* is an automatic ectopic rhythm that is not disturbed by the normal rhythm. Parasystole is characterized by interectopic intervals at fixed multiples, varied coupling of the interval of the ectopic beat to the prior normal beat, and fusion of ectopic and normal beats. Reentry occurs when an impulse enters an abnormal circuit with slowly conducting tissue that leads back to its site of origin (a circus movement). The pathway is small in mass and generates insufficient electrical activity to be recorded on the surface ECG. If there is such slow conduction that the site of origin of the impulse and the surrounding myocardium are again excitable when the impulse returns (if the impulse returns after the refractory period of the original site has terminated), then the heart is again discharged. This is called an ectopic beat. The coupling interval of the ectopic beat to the prior normal beat is fixed, depending on the length of the circuit. Reentry is believed to be the most common cause of ectopy. Tachycardias are generally initiated by premature beats critically timed to be so slowly conducted that they return after the refractory period is over. Most serious tachycardias are treated as reentrant types. But triggered automaticity is a newly described in vitro observation of rapid automatic firing initiated by the same sort of critically timed premature beats that start reentry. Triggering may explain many clinical arrhythmias and therapeutic responses otherwise poorly categorized.

Atrial tachycardia

Atrial tachycardia may be paroxysmal, nonparoxysmal (persistent), or chaotic. Atrial tachycardia is a run of atrial ectopic depolarizations faster than sinus rhythm, with P waves of nonsinus origin, usually at regular intervals. The QRS is usually narrow but can be wide and bizarre when there is a rapid ventricular response. This "aberrant" ventricular conduction occurs because of differences in refractoriness in the bundle branch system, independent of the mechanism of the tachycardia.

Nonparoxysmal atrial tachycardia is frequently caused by digitalis excess or severe heart disease. Often there is AV block, as from the digitalis.

Chaotic (multifocal) atrial tachycardia is different from other atrial tachycardias in that there seem to be several competing ectopic atrial foci. Criteria for chaotic atrial tachycardia (Fig. 97-1) are P waves of at least three different forms seen in the same lead, irregular P-P intervals, and varying PR intervals. Chaotic atrial tachycardia is common with severe obstructive pulmonary disease.

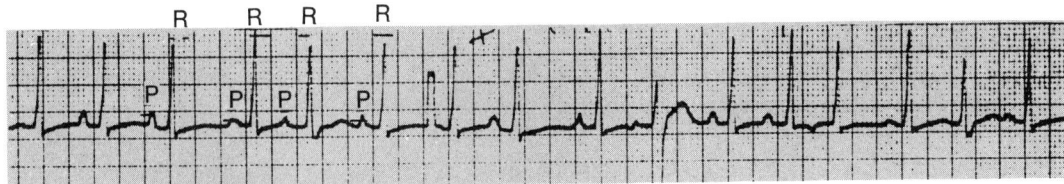

Fig. 97-1. Chaotic multifocal atrial tachycardia. In one lead there are P waves of at least three forms, with varying PR intervals. P-P intervals are also irregular. Aberrant ventricular conduction is best seen in tenth beat (short coupling interval after long interval) but is seen to a lesser degree in fifth and fifteenth beats. This arrhythmia is most frequently seen with pulmonary disease.

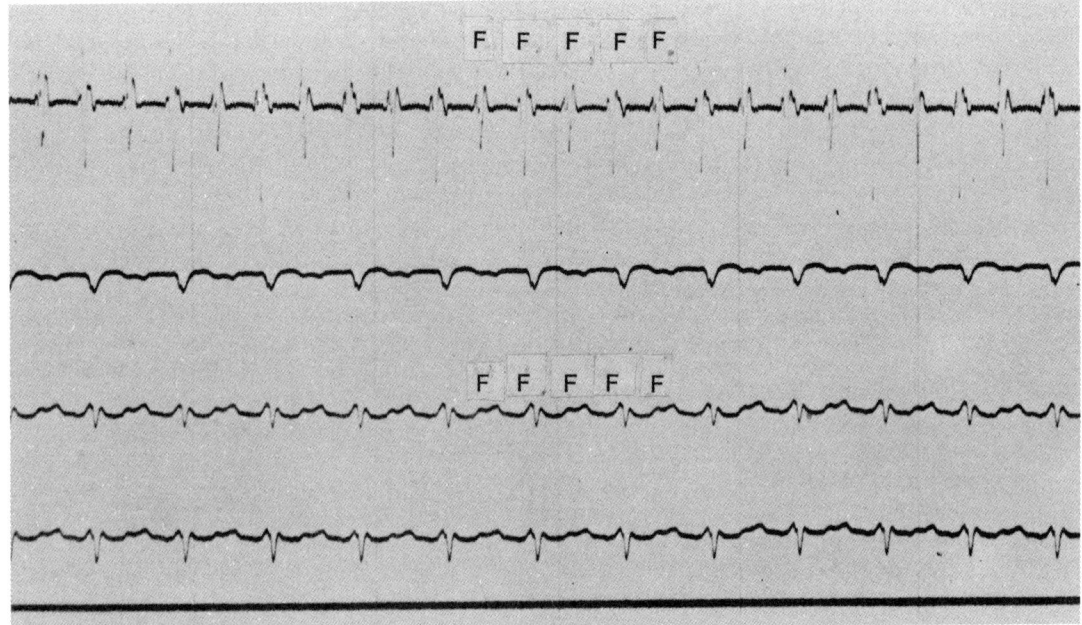

Fig. 97-2. Atrial flutter (250 beats/min). Top trace is intracardiac atrial ECG pattern, and other three are surface leads. There are 1-second time lines. Regular atrial pattern is best seen in middle surface lead when aligned with the atrial recording. There is 2:1 AV block. *F*, flutter waves.

Rarely it can be seen after surgery (with general anesthesia and hypoxia) and with electrolyte imbalance (particularly hypokalemia), pulmonary embolism, septicemia, and ketoacidosis. The patients are mostly elderly and seriously ill. Chaotic atrial tachycardia is commonly mistaken for atrial fibrillation (see "Atrial flutter and fibrillation") because of the irregular rhythm.

Atrial flutter and fibrillation

In atrial flutter the atrial rate is generally about 300 beats/min (Fig. 97-2). Atrial flutter typically occurs with organic heart disease, especially rheumatic mitral valve disease. Type I (classic flutter) is characterized by rates of 240 to 340 beats/min. Type II (so-called impure flutter) is characterized by rates of 340 to 440 beats/min. The ECG pattern of classic atrial flutter is a saw-toothed atrial pattern (best seen in leads II or V_1) and AV block (the ventricular rate is usually half the atrial rate in untreated flutter).

The ventricular response is critical to patient management. Occasionally 1:1 AV conduction is seen. It should suggest superimposed Wolff-Parkinson-White syndrome (discussed later in this chapter). On the other hand high degrees of AV block in the absence of drug therapy suggest concomitant AV junctional disease.

Atrial flutter may be paroxysmal or chronic. The paroxysmal form may degenerate into atrial fibrillation and is frequently seen in the transition from atrial fibrillation to sinus rhythm. Paroxysmal atrial flutter may be seen in apparently healthy individuals, in those recovering from open heart surgery, and in those with hyperthyroidism, Wolff-Parkinson-White syndrome, pulmonary embolism, pericarditis, cardiomyopathy, diphtheria, chest trauma, sick sinus syndrome (tachycardia-bradycardia syndrome), and digitalis intoxication.

Therapy with digitalis, propranolol, or verapamil causes AV block, controlling the ventricular response. Quinidine can terminate the flutter but first slows the atrial rate, which could allow a lesser degree of AV block and thereby a faster ventricular rate. Sinus rhythm can also be achieved by atrial pacing or electrical cardioversion.

Atrial fibrillation (Fig. 97-3) is most frequently seen in patients with organic heart disease. The ECG pattern for atrial fibrillation is replacement of P waves by fibrillatory waves, which resemble irregular oscillations (about 500/min), and a ventricular response that is irregular.

As with atrial flutter the ventricular response determines hemodynamic status, symptoms, and management. In the absence of superimposed AV junctional disease or drugs that slow junctional conduction, the ventricular response to atrial fibrillation is chaotic and rapid (120 to 180 beats/min). When the ventricular response is very rapid (greater than 220 beats/min), Wolff-Parkinson-White syndrome should be considered. Conversely, unusually slow ventricular rates may be seen in the elderly or in patients controlled with drugs (digitalis, propranolol, verapamil). A slow ventricular response in an untreated patient suggests superimposed AV junction disease (block).

Atrial fibrillation is the most common tachyarrhythmia. It is seen in rheumatic heart disease (particularly of the mitral valve), hyperthyroidism, acute myocardial infarction, congestive heart failure, Wolff-Parkinson-White syndrome, and sick sinus syndrome. It is unusual in children. About 6% of patients with paroxysmal atrial fibrillation have no discernible heart disease.

Treatment of atrial fibrillation depends on the cause, the duration of the arrhythmia, and the hemodynamic status of the patient. The ventricular response can be controlled by blocking at the AV junction (as with digitalis, propranolol, or verapamil), or the fibrillation can be converted to sinus rhythm (as with quinidine, treatment of underlying heart disease, or electrical conversion).

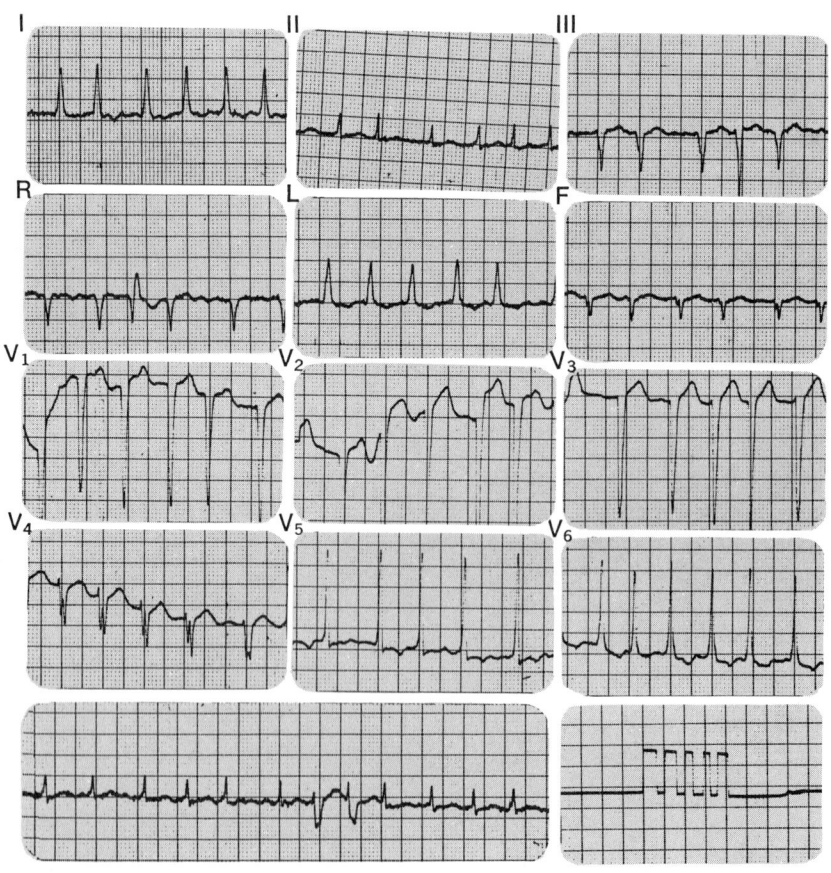

Fig. 97-3. Atrial fibrillation. Atrial activity is represented by irregular oscillations, and there is irregular rapid ventricular response. Some ventricular responses are aberrantly conducted, such as fourth beat in lead III, third beat in aV_R, and two beats in rhythm strip at bottom.

AV junctional tachycardia

AV junctional tachycardia (nodal tachycardia) is paroxysmal or nonparoxysmal (Table 97-1). Junctional pacemakers normally have rates of 40 to 60 beats/min. *Nonparoxysmal AV junctional tachycardia* occurs in a setting of digitalis intoxication, acute inferior myocardial infarction, acute rheumatic fever, myocarditis, and open heart surgery. Thus patients with nonparoxysmal junctional tachycardia almost always have underlying heart disease. *Paroxysmal AV junctional tachycardia* is seen at all ages and in healthy hearts. The mechanism of the paroxysmal form is always reentrant, and dual nodal pathways can be demonstrated physiologically (but not anatomically) in 75% of cases. Most individuals without apparent heart disease tolerate paroxysms well. Paroxysms terminate spontaneously or with AV nodal blocking agents (digitalis, propranolol, verapamil).

Ventricular tachycardia

Ventricular tachycardia is a run of ventricular ectopic beats (VEBs) (Fig. 97-4). The QRS form is wide and bizarre because the ventricular origin results in an abnormal pattern of ventricular depolarization. Ventricular tachycardia may be nonsustained, sustained for minutes to hours, or degenerate into ventricular fibrillation. ECG patterns of ventricular tachycardia are a wide QRS; initiation by a wide complex beat; and AV dissociation, with ventricular capture (supraventricular beats) or partial capture (fusion beats).

Nonparoxysmal ventricular tachycardia is usually only an accelerated idioventricular rhythm (60 to 100 beats/min) and can be from an automatic focus. Since the sinus is about as fast, there is competition with the automatic focus resulting in fusion beats (''parasystole''). Paroxysmal ventricular tachycardia is usually very rapid (often 140 to 240

Table 97-1. Comparison of two types of AV junctional tachycardias

	Paroxysmal	Nonparoxysmal
Rate	150-250 beats/min	65-130 beats/min
Rhythm	Regular	Regular
Mechanism	Reentry	Automatic focus
QRS morphology	Narrow or wide	Narrow
P waves	Present (before, during, or after QRS)	Absent (or dissociated)
Prognosis	Good	Poor

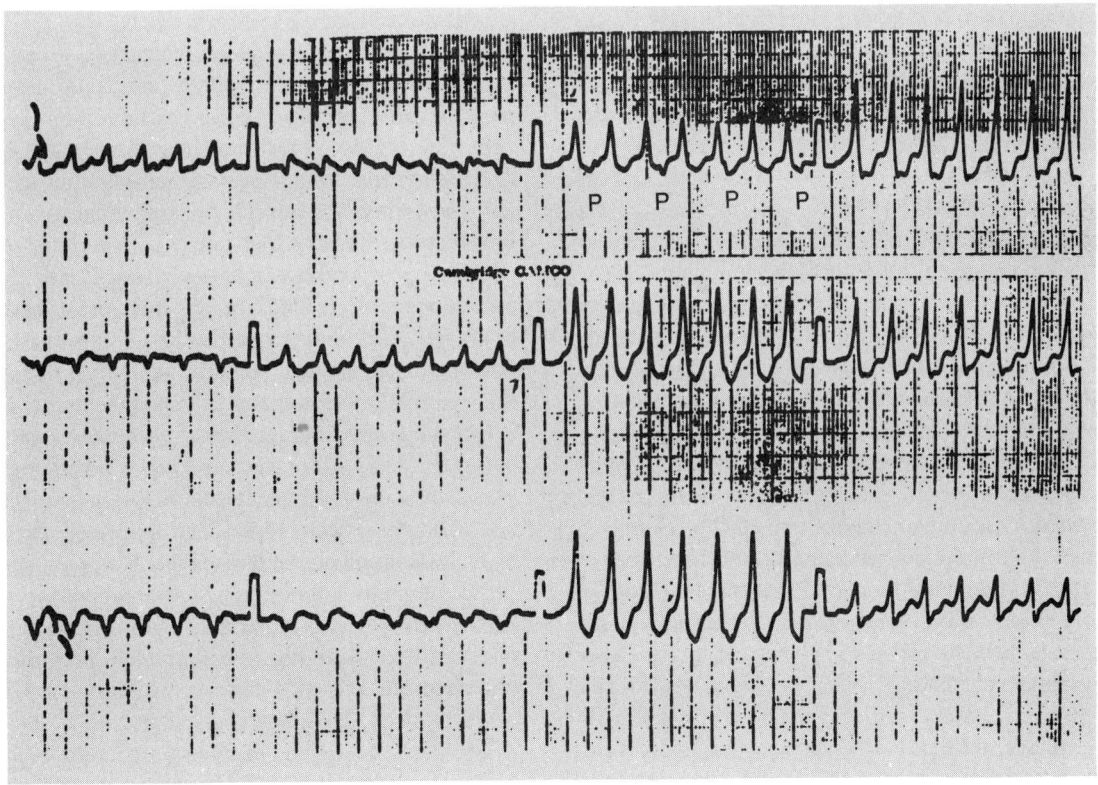

Fig. 97-4. Ventricular tachycardia. There is wide complex tachycardia and AV dissociation because P waves beat independently of tachycardia.

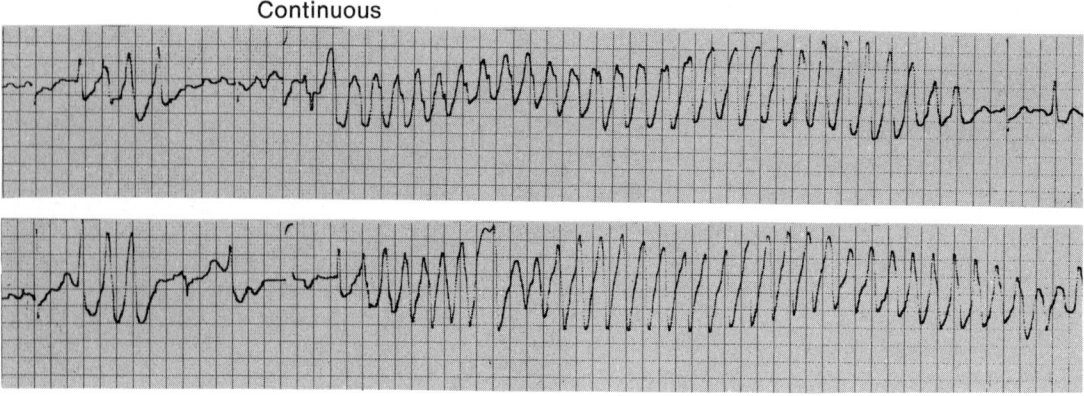

Fig. 97-5. "Torsades de pointes," in this case from quinidine used to treat atrial arrhythmia. There are bursts of rapid ventricular ectopy. Axis of ectopic beats appears to turn about a point, that is, to revolve in a cyclic fashion. The bottom trace is a continuation of the top trace.

beats/min) and reentrant. Ventricular tachycardia usually occurs because of organic heart disease, most commonly coronary heart disease. Ventricular aneurysm consequent to myocardial infarction is frequently a source of recurrent ventricular tachycardia. Digitalis intoxication may also produce ventricular tachycardia. Ventricular tachycardia is also seen in other forms of heart disease, including hypertension, mitral valve prolapse syndrome, cardiomyopathy, and cardiac tumors. Bidirectional tachycardia suggests digitalis excess, whereas a revolving direction or axis ("torsades de pointes") (Fig. 97-5) suggests a prolonged QT interval syndrome, acquired congenitally or from drugs such as quinidine (usually used to prevent reentrant ventricular tachycardia).

Ventricular flutter and fibrillation

Ventricular flutter and fibrillation are not compatible with survival, since they cause rapid hemodynamic deterioration and death. Ventricular flutter has rates of 250 to 350 beats/min and a QRS form resembling a sine wave. With fibrillation there is a chaotic pattern, making QRS complexes difficult to discern.

The most common form of heart disease predisposing to these lethal arrhythmias is coronary heart disease. Other forms of heart disease predisposing to ventricular fibrillation or flutter are cardiomyopathy of any origin, rheumatic heart disease, blunt cardiac trauma, mitral valve prolapse syndrome, and prolonged QT interval syndromes. Digitalis or quinidine intoxication, procainamide or disopyramide excess, and cardiac surgery or catheterization can also cause ventricular fibrillation. Finally, electrolyte imbalance, electrocution, and terminal noncardiac disease will end in ventricular fibrillation. Flutter and fibrillation generally will not abate spontaneously. Rapid, direct current cardioversion is usually the therapy necessary. The underlying cause is the factor determining whether or not electrical cardioversion will be effective.

BRADYCARDIAS AND HEART BLOCK

The hemodynamic consequences of bradycardia depend on age, underlying heart disease, and the rate and focus of the escape pacemaker. Patients with very slow heart rates have fatigue, dizziness, or frank syncope. Slow rates can aggravate congestive heart failure. However, sometimes the patients are asymptomatic.

Sinus bradycardia and sick sinus syndrome

Sinus bradycardia refers to rates less than 50 to 60 beats/min but is often asymptomatic unless the bradycardia is less than 35 beats/min or accompanies heart disease, such as acute inferior myocardial infarction or congestive heart failure. In contrast bradycardia may also be found in healthy athletes. Heart rate decreases with age, and it is not uncommon for an elderly individual to have marked bradycardia. Twenty-four-hour tape-recorded ambulatory monitoring of healthy male medical students revealed that all had periods of sinus bradycardia (25% had rates less than 40 beats/min episodically). Thus periodic sinus bradycardia in an asymptomatic individual is not necessarily abnormal, and therapy is not indicated. Persistent or severe sinus bradycardia should alert one to the possibility of sinus node dysfunction, and those with symptoms such as dizziness or syncope should be further evaluated.

Sinoatrial block represents a defect in conduction at the sinoatrial border and not a defect in automaticity. Since the sinus impulse is not appreciated on the surface ECG, first-degree sinoatrial block (prolonged sinoatrial interval) and third-degree (complete) sinoatrial block go unrecognized. Only second-degree sinoatrial block can be recognized, by analyzing the pattern of the P waves. A Mobitz type I (Wenckebach) sinoatrial block is diagnosed when the P-P intervals progressively shorten until there is a dropped P wave. Mobitz type II sinoatrial block is diagnosed by pauses that are multiples of the basic P-P interval.

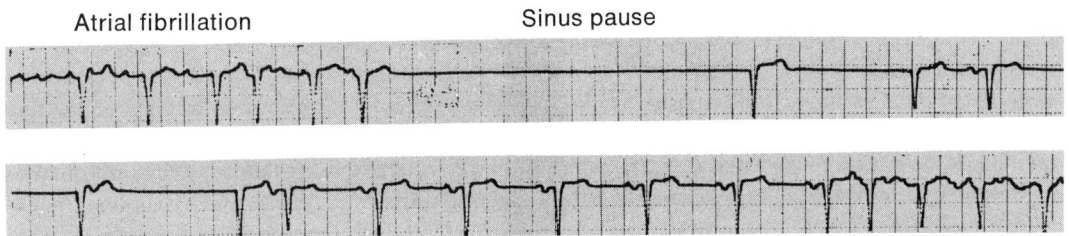

Fig. 97-6. Sinus pauses or arrest. This continuous strip illustrates sinus rhythm punctuated by paroxysms of atrial fibrillation. These paroxysms cause overdrive suppression of sinus node, so that with termination of fibrillation episodes there is sinus pause terminated by escape junctional rhythm. This variety of sick sinus syndrome is called tachycardia-bradycardia syndrome.

With sinus arrest there is no impulse formed, and a pause occurs that is not a multiple of the basic P-P interval (Fig. 97-6). Pauses as long as 2 seconds have been recorded in normal persons during sleep. Pauses longer than 2 seconds are certainly abnormal, since before then subsidiary pacemakers (usually atrial or AV nodal) should provide an escape rhythm. The mechanism of a pause may be (1) complete electrical silence; (2) formation of a subthreshold impulse, producing intrapacemaker block within the node; or (3) sinoatrial exit block.

Symptomatic patients with dizziness, light-headedness, syncope, or fatigue who have evidence of sinus node dysfunction have the sick sinus syndrome. There may be subtle personality changes, convulsions, focal transient neurologic signs, or congestive heart failure. Sick sinus syndrome is most common in the elderly but has been reported in all age groups. Many patients give no clinical evidence of heart disease. The diagnosis of sick sinus syndrome should also be considered if there are tachycardia-bradycardia episodes or there is sinus arrest after cardioversion. Some patients have only persistent, severe, or inappropriate sinus bradycardia. If definitive evidence of sinus node dysfunction (sinus arrest or block) is absent on monitoring, provocative testing should be employed to unmask sinus node dysfunction.

Carotid sinus stimulation may produce pauses or sinoatrial block. Likewise, exercise testing of these patients may show a blunted heart rate response. Atropine, 0.04 mg/kg of body weight intravenously, normally increases heart rate to greater than 90 beats/min (20% to 50% increase over basal rate). Most patients with sick sinus syndrome characteristically fall short of these values. Isoproterenol, 1 to 3 µg/min intravenously, accelerates heart rate by 25% in normal persons. Patients with sick sinus syndrome may have a blunted response, but a normal or even hypersensitive reaction is frequently seen. (A blunted response to isoproterenol correlates with a blunted heart rate response to exercise.) Combining atropine and propranolol denervates the heart, and intrinsic heart rate can be evaluated.

Finally sinus function can be evaluated using atrial overdrive pacing and the atrial extrastimulus technique. The postpacing interval (sinus node recovery time) is a measure of sinus node automaticity. This test of sinus node function is about 90% specific and 75% sensitive. Sinoatrial conduction time is the measure of conduction into and out of the sinus node, estimated by using programmed atrial extrastimulation. Abnormal sinoatrial conduction is associated with sinoatrial exit block but is found in only half of patients with sinus node dysfunction.

Asymptomatic sinus bradycardia at rates of 40 to 55 beats/min should be observed, and pacing is not indicated. The patient with symptomatic sinus bradycardia should be evaluated. A symptomatic patient with a prolonged sinus node recovery time should receive a permanent pacemaker. The patient who has symptoms that monitoring shows are *caused* by bradycardia should also receive a pacemaker. Patients often escape from bradycardia or pauses with supraventricular tachyarrhythmias and vice versa. Tachycardia-bradycardia patients are best treated by pacing to safely allow antiarrhythmic therapy for suppressing the supraventricular tachyarrhythmias. Some investigators have advocated atrial or AV sequential pacing in patients with sick sinus syndrome. But many patients with sick sinus syndrome eventually develop atrial fibrillation. About half of these patients also have associated AV conduction disease. Atrial pacing could increase the vulnerability to supraventricular tachyarrhythmias as well, and thus ventricular pacing is used by many clinicians.

AV block

AV block can occur at the level of the atrium, AV node, common (His) bundle, or bundle branches. Prognosis depends in part on the anatomic site of AV block. The surface ECG does not allow for precise identification of the site of block, but the catheter-recorded His bundle ECG pattern identifies whether conduction abnormalities are above or below the common bundle.

AV block can be first degree (prolonged AV conduction), second degree (intermittent AV block), and third degree (complete AV block). These can occur at any site. The AV node is designed to modulate conduction such that with increasing heart rate there are limits to conduction. With increments in heart rate, the AV node conduction interval progressively lengthens.

Management of patients with chronic AV block depends on the site of the block. First-degree AV block never requires therapy. Permanent pacemaker therapy is recommended for all symptomatic patients with intermittent or chronic third-degree AV block. Asymptomatic patients with second- or third-degree block should undergo evaluation. If the block is above the His bundle or the escape time after ventricular pacing is less than 2 seconds, an asymptomatic patient can be followed without a pacemaker.

VENTRICULAR ECTOPIC BEATS (VEBs)

Normal individuals have VEBs. Fully 0.6% of 67,375 ECGs from asymptomatic healthy individuals, average age 32 years, showed VEBs. When 811 men were monitored for 6 hours, VEBs increased with age; 20% of men aged 35 to 45 years had VEBs, whereas 80% older than 65 had VEBs. Half of healthy medical students showed VEBs on tape-recorded monitoring, although the frequency was low and complex forms were rare. Thus the presence of VEBs does not imply cardiac disease, but frequent and complex VEBs are rare among the healthy.

In one report those with more than 10 VEBs/1000 beats had a tenfold greater risk of sudden death, *but only in the presence of coronary heart disease,* or at least major risk factors. In an 18-year follow-up of 604 individuals free of coronary heart disease, VEBs were not associated with increased mortality. A third study failed to find an increased risk of sudden death in healthy male factory workers with VEBs. Thus, in the absence of associated coronary heart disease, VEBs represent an unimportant risk for sudden death.

Most patients (90%) with coronary heart disease have VEBs. But frequent VEBs imply an increased risk for sudden death. Obviously, the sudden death is not a direct result of frequent or complex VEBs. Rather, it results from ventricular fibrillation, more often in the setting of acute myocardial infarction or in the early months after infarction. For example, in acute infarction frequent VEBs and complex ventricular arrhythmias often, but not necessarily, precede ventricular fibrillation. Lidocaine prevents ventricular fibrillation in acute myocardial infarction but does not suppress all VEBs—a dissociation between VEBs and ventricular fibrillation suppression in acute infarction. Thus VEBs are harbingers of, but are not necessary for, the production of ventricular fibrillation.

After myocardial infarction there is an increased risk of dying suddenly, especially within the first 6 months. Ventricular ectopy is found before death in patients who die suddenly subsequent to their recovery from myocardial infarction. Complex forms (multiformed; very premature; with R-on-T, bigeminy, or couplets; and so on) and especially frequent VEBs are associated with an increased risk, but more than one half of patients have frequent VEBs after hospital discharge following myocardial infarction, and complex VEBs are found in about one third. Although complex VEBs are found in those who die after infarction, most patients with complex VEBs are not victims of sudden death. The highest-risk VEBs are repetitive (couplets and ventricular tachycardia).

The group with complex arrhythmias at risk for sudden death after myocardial infarction will be further defined with new technology. Until then therapy for ectopy must be determined by its clinical setting. Prophylactic treatment with lidocaine to prevent ventricular fibrillation is indicated in acute myocardial infarction for 24 to 48 hours. Ventricular arrhythmias (such as VEBs) after 48 hours are prognostic of sudden death and should be further evaluated or treated. However, therapy may worsen the arrhythmia or increase the risk for sudden death. Treatment is empiric, and subsequent observation with intensive monitoring seems important in high-risk patients.

Asymptomatic patients with VEBs but without associated cardiac disease do not appear at increased risk for sudden death. Antiarrhythmic therapy is thus unwarranted. Even if the treatment of VEBs is felt to be justified, there is evidence that suppression of VEBs may not prevent ventricular fibrillation. Alternatively antiarrhythmic therapy may suppress recurrent cardiac arrest but not significantly reduce asymptomatic arrhythmias.

WOLFF-PARKINSON-WHITE (WPW) SYNDROME

WPW syndrome is a characteristic ECG pattern associated with paroxysmal supraventricular tachyarrhythmias. Recent observations made at the time of surgery for correction of the syndrome have provided an anatomic/physiologic explanation for the ECG and the arrhythmias. There is an accessory AV conduction pathway present at birth, functioning as if a maturational arrest. This pathway provides an alternate route from atrium to ventricle, which has different properties than the AV node: (1) rapid conduction, which responds differently to medications such as digitalis, and (2) short refractoriness, so that the gating function of the AV node is lost and many messages can pass from atrium to ventricle rapidly. Since there are two connections between atrium and ventricle, circus movements are possible between those two chambers, such as down the normal AV node and back up the accessory pathway, allowing for reentrant tachyarrhythmias.

The ECG pattern of WPW syndrome is illustrated in Fig. 97-7. There is a short PR interval, and the His bundle recording illustrates that this is caused by a rapidly conducting pathway that bypasses the AV node and His bundle. The pathway passes from the right or left atrium to the base of the corresponding ventricle, so that depolari-

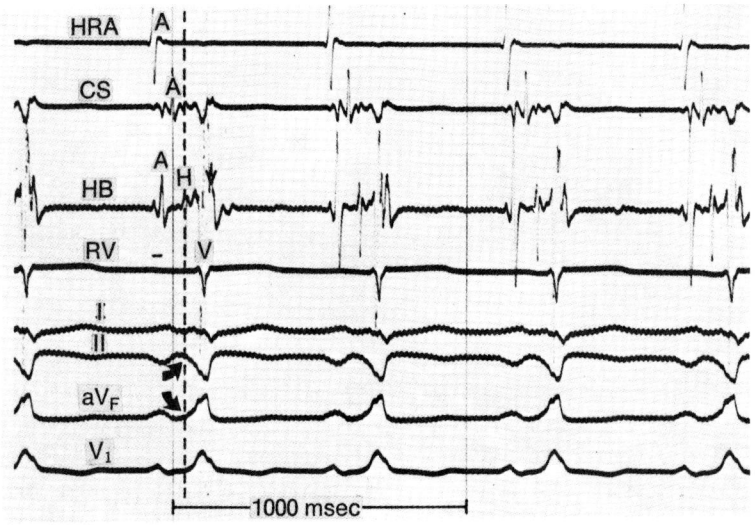

Fig. 97-7. Wolff-Parkinson-White (WPW) syndrome. Top four traces are intracardiac traces from high right atrium, *HRA*, coronary sinus near left atrium, *CS*, His bundle, *HB*, and right ventricle, *RV*. His bundle trace shows sequence of AV conduction from atrium to His bundle to ventricle (see Fig. 97-7). Dotted line indicates that by the time impulse travels from atrium via AV node to His bundle, it has already excited a portion of ventricle. Initial slurred portion of QRS *(dark arrows)* that is inscribed at same time as His bundle (that is, before V or ventricular depolarization via normal pathway) is called "delta" wave. Delta wave and simultaneous excitation of His bundle and ventricle (HV = O) diagnose an accessory pathway from atrium to ventricle.

zation begins in an abnormal pattern, explaining a wide QRS with a slurred upstroke or "delta" wave. There are also associated ST segment and T wave abnormalities because of the abnormal ventricular depolarization sequence. In summary there is a short PR interval and wide QRS complex.

The pattern becomes a syndrome when the patient becomes symptomatic from paroxysmal supraventricular tachycardia. The tachycardias are usually precipitated by atrial ectopic beats, which take the following circus pathway: atrium, anterograde via AV node to ventricle, retrograde via accessory pathway back to the atrium, anterograde via the AV node, and so on. The tachycardias are often much faster than is typical for paroxysmal supraventricular tachycardias and often cause more symptoms. They often are more difficult to prevent with medication.

In addition paroxysmal atrial fibrillation and flutter can occur. Because there is an accessory pathway with rapid conducting properties and curtailed refractoriness, the rapid beating of the atrium with flutter or fibrillation can conduct efficiently to the ventricle, causing such rapid ventricular beating that ventricular fibrillation and sudden death can result. Sudden death is often precipitated by digitalis therapy. Digitalis is one of the drugs of choice for AV nodal reentrant paroxysmal supraventricular tachycardia. With an accessory pathway digitalis often further curtails refractoriness or accelerates conduction velocity. When there is atrial fibrillation or flutter, even more rapid ventricular excitation causes the sudden death. Thus digitalis is contraindicated with paroxysmal supraventricular tachycardia until (1) an ECG in sinus rhythm excludes WPW syndrome (during tachycardia anterograde conduction and the ECG pattern are usually normal) and/or (2) the ability to rapidly conduct to the ventricle or to cause very shortened R-R intervals is assessed, such as by electrophysiologic techniques. Digitalis can be used in children with WPW syndrome, since atrial fibrillation and flutter are unusual.

CARDIOVERSION

Tachyarrhythmias producing hemodynamic collapse, prolonged angina pectoris, or pulmonary edema are treated promptly with direct current cardioversion. Countershock simultaneously depolarizes the entire myocardium, allowing for synchronous repolarization and resumption of sinus rhythm. The energy levels used are determined by the type of arrhythmia. Organized tachycardias (paroxysmal supraventricular tachycardia, atrial flutter, and ventricular tachycardia) generally require low energy levels (10 to 50 joules). Fibrillatory patterns need higher energy outputs. Multifocal atrial tachycardia and drug-induced tachyarrhythmias are resistant to cardioversion. Cardioversion synchronized to the QRS is the recommended mode for all tachycardias except ventricular fibrillation (which is without a QRS). The shock is delivered in the safe period in the cardiac cycle, about 10 msec after the peak of the QRS complex. Nonsynchronized shock may produce ventricular fibrillation when delivered during the T wave.

Digitalis is discontinued before elective countershock of atrial flutter or fibrillation to avoid ventricular fibrillation, anticoagulants are given to avoid thromboembolism on return of atrial systole, and type I agents are started to maintain sinus rhythm after successful cardioversion.

BIBLIOGRAPHY

Akhtar, M., and others: Clinical use of His bundle electrocardiography, Am. Heart J. **91**:520, 660, 805, 1976.

Bigger, J.T., and others: Ventricular arrhythmias in ischemic heart disease: mechanism, prevalence, significance and management, Prog. Cardiovasc. Dis. **14**:255, 1977.

Engel, T.R., Bond, R.C., and Schaal, S.F.: First-degree sinoatrial heart block: sinoatrial block in the sick sinus syndrome, Am. Heart J. **91**:303, 1976.

Ferrer, I.: The sick sinus syndrome, Circulation **47**:635, 1973.

Gallagher, J.J., and others: The Wolff-Parkinson-White syndrome and pre-excitation dysrhythmias: medical and surgical management, Med. Clin. North Am. **60**:101, 1976.

Harrison, D., Fitzgerald, J., and Winkle, R.: Ambulatory electrocardiography for diagnosis and treatment of cardiac arrhythmias, N. Engl. J. Med. **294**:373, 1976.

Lie, K.I., and others: Lidocaine in the prevention of primary ventricular fibrillation: a double-blind randomized study of 212 consecutive patients, N. Engl. J. Med. **291**:1324, 1974.

Moss, A.J., and others: Ventricular ectopic beats and their relation to sudden and nonsudden cardiac death after myocardial infarction, Circulation **60**:998, 1979.

Narula, O.S., editor: Cardiac arrhythmias: electrophysiology, diagnosis and management, Baltimore, 1979, The Williams & Wilkins Co.

Smith, W.M., and Gallagher, J.J.: "Les torsade des pointes": an unusual ventricular arrhythmia, Ann. Intern. Med. In press.

Strauss, H.C., and others: Electrophysiologic evaluation of sinus node function in patients with sinus node dysfunction, Circulation **53**:763, 1976.

Sung, R.J., and others: Mechanisms of spontaneous alternation between reciprocating tachycardia and atrial flutter-fibrillation in the Wolff-Parkinson-White syndrome, Circulation **56**:409, 1977.

Wellens, H.J.J., Lie, K.I., and Janse, M.J., editors: The conduction system of the heart, Philadelphia, 1976, Lea & Febiger.

Winkle, R.A.: Measuring antiarrhythmic drug efficacy by suppression of asymptomatic ventricular arrhythmias, Ann. Intern. Med. **91**:480, 1979.

Wit, A.L., Rosen, M.R., and Hoffman, B.F.: Cardiac antiarrhythmic and toxic effects of digitalis, Am. Heart J. **89**:391, 1975.

98 • PERICARDITIS

Charles A. Bush and John M. Stang

The pericardium is a two-layered membranous structure surrounding the heart and great vessels. In its normal function the pericardium serves mainly as a protective structure, and the absence of or surgical removal of the pericardium does not interfere with normal cardiac function. Like all other organic structures, the pericardium is subject to pathologic disorders resulting in various types of pericardial diseases. Unlike most valvular and congenital cardiac diseases, chronic pericardial disease does not require antibiotic prophylaxis for dental or surgical procedures to prevent endocarditis. Chronic pericardial disease does not contraindicate general anesthesia, but the disease must be accurately distinguished from myocardial ischemic problems.

ACUTE PERICARDITIS

DEFINITION. Acute pericarditis may be defined as active inflammatory disease of the pericardium that develops rapidly and is associated with the sudden onset of symptoms.

ETIOLOGY AND PATHOGENESIS. There are a variety of causes of acute pericarditis. The common infectious causes include both viral and bacterial infections. The most common of the viral causes of acute pericarditis is coxsackievirus. Bacterial causes of acute pericarditis, although less common now with the availability of antibiotics, include suppurative bacterial infections of which pneumococcal, staphylococcal, and streptococcal infections are most prevalent. Prior surgical procedures and uremia are predisposing conditions to bacterial pericarditis. Tuberculosis as a cause of acute pericarditis is still common. Other infectious causes of acute pericarditis include fungal and parasitic infestations. Acute pericarditis is a frequent manifestation of connective tissue disease; common examples are systemic lupus erythematosus, rheumatoid arthritis, scleroderma, and mixed connective tissue disease. Acute pericarditis may also be a manifestation of an immunologic response or a hypersensitivity state. Causes for pericarditis in this subgroup include drug reactions, serum sickness, postmyocardial infarction syndrome, and postcardiotomy syndrome. The last two disorders are apparent immunologic responses to damaged myocardial tissue from infarction or surgery, resulting in pericardial inflammation. A variety of drugs, including procainamide and hydralazine, also cause acute pericarditis. Acute pericarditis frequently occurs with transmural myocardial infarction and is related to direct irritation of the pericardium by the infarcted myocardium. Acute pericarditis may also result from both penetrating and nonpenetrating wounds of the pericardium. Other causes are uremia, bacterial endocarditis, and acute rheumatic fever. However, the most common cause of acute pericarditis may be idiopathic or nonspecific pericarditis. This is usually a benign form of pericarditis for which no specific cause can be determined.

The pathogenesis of acute pericarditis depends on the underlying cause. Some type of infectious, immunologic, toxic, or mechanical insult to the pericardium appears necessary to start the process. The resultant pericarditis may be focal or diffuse. Focal pericarditis may be highly localized or spotty; diffuse pericarditis involves the entire pericardium. Acute pericarditis almost always involves at least the epicardial layer of the myocardium, and some of the manifestations of acute pericarditis are in fact related to myocardial involvement.

CLINICAL MANIFESTATIONS. The most common complaint of the patient with acute pericarditis is chest pain.

The pain is frequently rather sudden in onset and persistent. It is often made worse by inspiration and lying supine; some relief may be obtained with sitting up and leaning forward. Dyspnea or shortness of breath is much less likely to occur in the setting of acute pericarditis. Fever is common in both infectious and noninfectious types of acute pericarditis. The pathognomonic physical finding of acute pericarditis is that of a pericardial friction rub. There are frequently three components to the pericardial friction rub that are synchronous with atrial systole, ventricular systole, and ventricular diastole. Occasionally the pericardial friction rub may be a two-component rub or a one-component rub. In the latter situation it may be difficult to distinguish a pericardial friction rub from a heart murmur.

It is important to point out that any or all of these findings may be absent in the presence of acute pericarditis.

LABORATORY FINDINGS. The specific laboratory findings of the underlying disease causing the acute pericarditis may suggest an examination for pericardial involvement. The white blood count may help indicate the presence of either viral or bacterial infection. Bacterial and viral cultures or viral titers of both acute and convalescent sera may be important in establishing the cause of acute pericarditis. The chest roentgenogram is usually not helpful in making a diagnosis of acute pericarditis, since the cardiac silhouette is often normal. The echocardiogram may be of benefit in identifying a small pericardial effusion. Occasionally a thickened pericardium may also be noted echocardiographically. The ECG is the most useful laboratory study for the diagnosis of acute pericarditis. However, it is important to recognize that the abnormalities in the ECG are not necessarily specific for acute pericarditis, and frequently the ECG may be normal or show only nonspecific changes. In acute pericarditis affecting the pericardium diffusely, the ECG may demonstrate ST segment elevation or deep inverted T waves in all leads. In localized pericarditis the ST segment elevation and T wave inversion may be localized to specific leads. In this latter situation it is vitally important to exclude myocardial injury or infarction as a cause of these ECG changes. The patient with acute pericarditis does not develop Q waves as does the patient with acute myocardial infarction. Another characteristic ECG change of acute pericarditis is depression of the PR segment. Atrial flutter or atrial fibrillation is often present.

DIAGNOSIS. The diagnosis of acute pericarditis is based on the history and physical findings and their correlation with laboratory studies, particularly the ECG. Acute pericarditis may be confused with acute myocardial infarction, dissecting aneurysm of the aorta, pleurisy, pneumonia, pneumothorax, and chest wall pain. It is important to recognize that acute pericarditis may coexist with all of these disease processes but may be particularly difficult to diagnose.

COURSE. Acute idiopathic and acute viral pericarditis are self-limited diseases that usually resolve gradually over days to weeks. Occasionally, acute pericarditis may be recurrent, and it is not unusual to have recurrent acute pericarditis on multiple occasions separated by several months. Acute pericarditis may become a chronic disease of the pericardium and may either result in chronic inflammation of the pericardium or evolve to chronic constrictive pericarditis. The course of acute pericarditis is very dependent on the underlying disease. If the underlying disease is progressive, the course of acute pericarditis is likely to be chronic and progressive as well. Occasionally, acute pericarditis may be rapidly progressive, with either the rapid development of pericardial constriction or rapid fluid accumulation.

MANAGEMENT. The treatment of acute pericarditis necessitates a knowledge of the specific cause. Treatment of the underlying disease causing the acute pericarditis may be necessary for resolution of pericarditis. Management of acute pericarditis in many situations involves supportive care and symptomatic treatment for pain relief. Antiinflammatory agents, including aspirin, indomethacin, and corticosteroids, may be of benefit. Occasionally pericardiectomy (surgical removal of the pericardium) is necessary for total relief of symptoms of pericarditis. This usually is necessary in the setting of chronic inflammatory disease or in recurrent acute pericarditis.

CONSTRICTIVE PERICARDITIS

DEFINITION. Constrictive pericarditis is a chronic disease of the pericardium resulting from fibrosis and scarring of the pericardium that interferes with atrial and ventricular diastolic filling of the heart.

ETIOLOGY. Constrictive pericarditis occurs most commonly as a sequela of inflammatory disease of the pericardium. It is most likely to occur secondary to bacterial infection, tuberculosis, radiation, or trauma. Constrictive pericarditis following open heart surgery is becoming increasingly common.

PATHOGENESIS. Chronic inflammation or irritation of the pericardium leads to increasing fibrosis. This may eventually result in scarring of the pericardium, adhesions of the pericardium to the epicardium, and ultimately dense calcification of the pericardium. This pathologic process results in loss of the normal pericardial viscoelastic properties, with formation of a rigid, nonelastic structure surrounding the heart. Depending on the degree of pericardial involvement and the intravascular volume, the physiology of constrictive pericarditis may be either occult or overt. Eventually the inability to fill the heart appropriately in diastole results in a diminution of cardiac output and an increase in venous pressure.

CLINICAL MANIFESTATIONS. The presentation of a patient with constrictive pericarditis depends on the degree of pericardial involvement and also the intravascular volume. Symptomatology may include vague nonspecific chest pain, dyspnea, and fatigue. In most severe cases the patient may have symptoms of right-sided heart failure, fluid retention, and symptoms of a markedly decreased cardiac output. The physical findings of the patient with constrictive pericarditis are also dependent on the intravascular volume. Frequently the patient demonstrates marked elevation of the jugular venous pressure, with prominent x and y collapses in the jugular venous pressure pulse. There is usually an inspiratory rise in the jugular venous pressure, as opposed to the normal inspiratory fall in pressure. The liver is frequently enlarged, and there may be significant peripheral edema. The heart may be enlarged or normal in size. Examination of the left ventricle is generally normal, and there are no signs of pulmonary congestion. On auscultation an early diastolic sound sometimes referred to as a pericardial knock is frequently heard.

LABORATORY FINDINGS. The ECG in constrictive pericarditis may be normal. Atrial fibrillation may be present, and the only other likely ECG abnormality is nonspecific ST-T wave changes. The chest roentgenogram and cardiac fluoroscopy can reveal a normal or enlarged cardiovascular silhouette. If pericardial calcification is present, it is a striking pathognomonic finding and appears as a dense, white shell around the heart (Fig. 98-1). The echocardiogram may demonstrate dense echoes of a thickened pericardium. Diagnosis of constrictive pericarditis is established best by cardiac catheterization. Classic findings of constrictive pericarditis at catheterization include characteristic pressure pulse configurations in both the right atrium and the right ventricle. The most specific finding of constrictive pericarditis found at the time of catheterization is exact pressure equilibration in all cardiac chambers during ventricular diastole; specifically equilibration of the left ventricular diastolic pressure with left atrial pressure, with pulmonary artery diastolic pressure, with right ventricular diastolic pressure, and with right atrial pressure. This pressure equilibration results from the heart being limited in its filling by the extrinsic shell of the diseased pericardium rather than by the usual limiting factor of individual chamber stiffness. Thus filling the heart results in rapidly attaining a high diastolic pressure that is transmitted equally through all chambers, much as putting air into a basketball results in a rapid rise in pressure within that chamber. When the pressure of filling equals the pressure within the chamber, flow stops and that pressure is maintained until contraction occurs.

DIAGNOSIS. The differential diagnosis of constrictive pericarditis includes valvular heart disease with congestive heart failure, congestive cardiomyopathy, restrictive myocardial disease, and cirrhosis. In each of these entities there are subtle findings that enable the careful observer to differentiate constrictive pericarditis. However, in some cases restrictive myocardial disease may exactly mimic the findings of constrictive pericarditis, and the ultimate diagnosis may rest on a surgical and pathologic examination of the pericardium. It is important to realize that constrictive

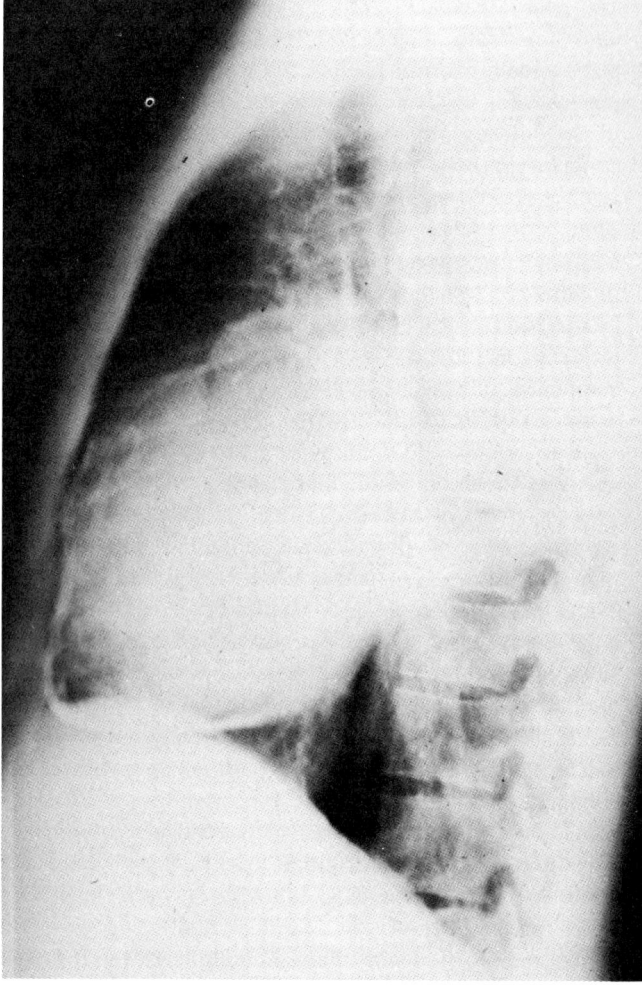

Fig. 98-1. Lateral chest roentgenogram of patient with constrictive pericarditis. Left atrium is enlarged because it is not enclosed within constricted pericardium. Roentgenogram shows dense, white, calcified pericardium surrounding cardiac silhouette.

pericarditis may occur in association with other forms of heart disease. Diagnosis of constrictive pericarditis occurring coincidentally with other types of cardiac disease is difficult.

COURSE. Patients with occult constrictive pericardial disease may have a stable course or only a slowly progressive disease process. Many of these patients have a minor degree of disability from a disease that appears to be anatomically and physiologically stable. Patients with more overt constrictive pericarditis tend to have a progressive course. However, the disease may have a particularly long course, and some patients with calcific constrictive pericarditis appear to be fairly stable with no major sequelae. The most common course of the patient with chronic constrictive pericarditis is one of progressive deterioration of cardiac output and progressive elevation of right-sided heart pressures with peripheral edema and hepatic congestion. The patient may eventually develop end-stage heart failure, with a markedly diminished cardiac output, or develop signs of cardiac cirrhosis with hepatic failure.

MANAGEMENT. Pericardiectomy is the treatment of choice for constrictive pericarditis if the patient is symptomatically disabled from that process. Likewise, pericardiectomy is recommended if there are signs of overt right-sided heart failure, hepatic congestion, or cardiac cirrhosis.

PREVENTION. Some clinicians believe that aggressive use of anti-inflammatory agents early in the course of acute pericarditis prevents the later occurrence of constrictive pericarditis. The use of antibiotic therapy has reduced the incidence of constrictive pericarditis following bacterial pericarditis. Others think that concomitant corticosteroids prevent the development of constrictive pericarditis from tuberculous pericarditis.

EFFUSIVE PERICARDITIS

DEFINITION. When an abnormal amount of fluid accumulates in the pericardial space, this condition is known as effusive pericarditis. Fluid may develop in the pericardial space under little or no pressure, resulting in what is termed a lax pericardial effusion. If fluid develops under pressure and there is cardiac compression, the resulting condition is pericardial tamponade.

ETIOLOGY. Inflammatory disease of the pericardium is frequently associated with pericardial effusion. With bacterial pericariditis the pericardial effusion may be pus. Fluid accumulation can occur in the pericardial space in connective tissue disorders and immunologic disorders; rheumatoid arthritis and systemic lupus erythematosus particularly may have significant pericardial effusions. A frequent cause of pericardial effusive disease is hypothyroidism. Bleeding into the pericardial space may result in a bloody pericardial effusion known as hemopericardium. This is likely to occur in relation to anticoagulant therapy, myocardial infarction, myocardial rupture following myocardial infarction, dissecting aneurysm of the aorta, and penetrating cardiac trauma. The patient with biventricular heart failure from any cause, including valvular heart disease, hypertensive heart disease, and ischemic heart disease, frequently will have a pericardial effusion. Neoplastic disease metastatic to the pericardium is a common cause of large pericardial effusions. Metastatic adenocarcinoma of the lung is the most common primary source for pericardial metastatic disease.

PATHOGENESIS. Fluid accumulation in the pericardium may be related to either excessive production of pericardial fluid or inadequate drainage of the pericardial space. Excessive production of fluid is most likely to occur in inflammatory processes, connective tissue disorders, and metastatic neoplastic processes. Inadequate drainage of the pericardial space frequently results from alterations in lymphatic flow and may be the primary mechanism of fluid accumulation in patients with congestive heart failure. Blood accumulation in the pericardial space results almost exclusively from hemorrhage from a cardiac structure that lies within the pericardial space. The major determining factor as to whether a pericardial effusion is lax or under high pressure resulting in tamponade is the rate of fluid accumulation. The volume of pericardial effusion also plays a role in the intrapericardial pressure but is probably not as important as the rate of fluid accumulation. As little as 100 ml of pericardial effusion developing rapidly may result in a high pressure within the pericardial space, restricting cardiac filling and resulting in tamponade physiology. On the other hand, a pericardial effusion developing slowly over weeks or months may accumulate in excess of 1 L of pericardial fluid but may result in no elevation of intrapericardial pressure and therefore no cardiac compression.

CLINICAL MANIFESTATIONS. The patient with a *lax pericardial effusion* may be symptom free. If symptoms are present, they are likely only those of the underlying disease. The lax pericardial effusion is frequently diagnosed only by noting an abnormal cardiovascular silhouette on the chest roentgenogram. Some patients with a lax pericardial effusion may have vague, nondescript chest discomfort and some associated mild dyspnea or fatigue. The physical findings of a lax pericardial effusion may include an enlarged area of cardiac dullness on percussion, an apex impulse that is difficult or impossible to palpate, and diminished intensity of heart sounds. The patient with *pericardial tamponade* will have symptoms of dyspnea, fatigue, and low cardiac output. Frequently the patient will be acutely ill, demonstrating signs of marked respiratory distress and decreased tissue perfusion. Signs of a severely low cardiac output or shock may be present. Physical findings include hypotension with a narrowed pulse pressure. There is usually a dramatic inspiratory fall in systolic blood pressure (over that normally observed), sometimes associated with a completely absent palpable pulse during inspiration. This finding, with a decrease of more than 10 mm Hg, is known as a "paradoxical pulse"; this is in fact an exaggeration of the normal decrease in blood pressure with inspiration (Fig. 98-2). The jugular venous pressure is markedly elevated. Tachycardia in the range of 100 to 160 beats/min is present.

LABORATORY FINDINGS. The laboratory diagnosis of a pericardial effusion is suggested by the chest roentgenogram, which demonstrates a markedly enlarged cardiac silhouette with a globular configuration. Cardiac fluoroscopy demonstrates diminished pulsation of the cardiac borders. The ECG is likely to demonstrate nonspecific ST and T wave changes. The most common ECG finding is one of diminished voltage in all leads. Alternating voltage (electrical alternans) of the QRS complex is a fairly specific finding for a large pericardial effusion. The echocardio-

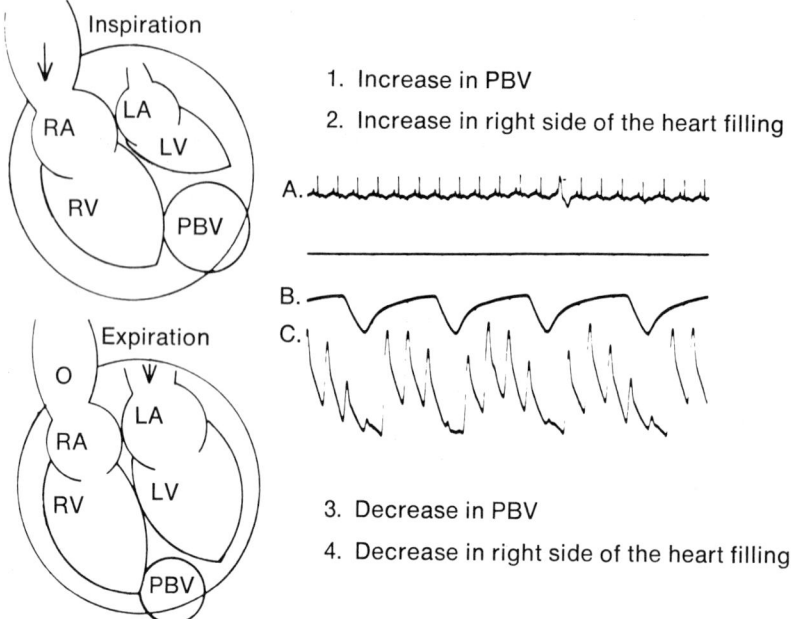

Fig. 98-2. Schematic representation of heart in pericardial tamponade demonstrating mechanism of paradoxical pulse. Arterial pressure tracing demonstrates dramatic fall in pressure with inspiration (marked by downward deflection of line just above pressure pulse). Relative volumes of right atrium, *RA*, right ventricle, *RV*, left atrium, *LA*, left ventricle, *LV*, and pulmonary blood volume, *PBV*, are shown in inspiration and expiration, with corresponding flow (↓) or no or decreased flow *(O)* into right and left atria. Systemic blood pressure falls during inspiration because of decrease in left-sided heart volume, caused by both larger right-sided heart volume in limited pericardial space and pooling of blood in lungs. *A*, ECG; *B*, respirations where downward deflection is inspiration; *C*, arterial pressure tracing.

gram is particularly helpful in establishing the presence of fluid in the pericardial space. Some estimate of the volume of fluid may be obtained by means of the echocardiogram. A nuclear cardiac scan may also demonstrate a large space between the inferior border of the heart and the liver, indicative of a pericardial effusion. Right atrial angiography can demonstrate a discrepancy between the cardiac silhouette and the right atrial wall, which indicates the presence of pericardial fluid. Cardiac catheterization can delineate the physiology of the pericardial effusion.

DIAGNOSIS. The diagnosis of pericardial effusive disease is established by the echocardiographic or scan findings. Differential diagnosis of the enlarged globular cardiac silhouette must include congestive cardiomyopathy with primary myocardial disease and the rather rare entity of Ebstein's anomaly. Documentation of a significant pericardial effusion by echocardiogram and scan with normal-sized cardiac chambers helps to establish the diagnosis of pericardial effusion. It is important to recognize that a pericardial effusion can occur with other cardiovascular disorders and other underlying cardiac conditions, in which case there may be enlargement of the cardiac chambers. The etiologic diagnosis of a pericardial effusion is vital. This can be established by obtaining pericardial fluid for analysis, culture, and cytology. Pericardial biopsy may also be necessary to help establish the etiologic diagnosis.

COURSE. The course of pericardial effusive disease is totally dependent on its cause. If the pericardial effusion is bloody, the course of the hemopericardium may be acute and result in death very quickly. This is particularly true if the cause is cardiac rupture or dissecting aneurysm of the aorta. Occasionally a patient will survive the immediate cause of bleeding into the pericardial space and spontaneously heal the process that resulted in the hemopericardium. However, surgical intervention frequently is necessary to correct the underlying defect. In patients who have had hemopericardium, delayed development of constrictive pericarditis is not uncommon. The patient with pericardial tamponade may develop rapid deterioration related to a suppressed cardiac output, resulting in shock and death. If tamponade physiology gradually resolves, the patient may eventually develop signs of chronic constrictive pericardial disease. Patients with lax pericardial effusions may have them on a chronic basis. The presence of pericardial effusive disease for several years has been well documented and frequently results in little or no symptomatology. Occasionally, such pericardial effusions may spontaneously resolve. Recurrent pericardial effusions are most common in neoplastic metastatic disease, with the recurrence of repeated tamponade physiology not at all uncommon.

MANAGEMENT. Treatment of pericardial effusive disease necessitates exact etiologic diagnosis, and management of the underlying disease is mandatory. Treatment of a pericardial effusion from hypothyroidism consists essentially of treating hypothyroidism. With resumption of the euthyroid state, the pericardial effusion will disappear. Patients with a lax pericardial effusion may respond to drainage of the pericardial space and therapy with anti-inflammatory agents or pericardial sclerosing agents to prevent reaccumulation of the effusion. Occasionally, pericardiectomy is appropriate for management of a recurrent lax pericardial effusion. The management of acute pericardial tamponade is both medical and surgical. The immediate emergency therapy requires the rapid administration of large volumes of intravenous fluids to raise cardiac filling pressures and overcome the compressive effects of the pericardial fluid. Use of potent myocardial inotropic agents such as isoproterenol and dopamine may also be beneficial in aiding cardiac filling by increasing the contractility of the ventricle, thus assisting cardiac filling during the atrial x descent. A drainage procedure either by needle pericardiocentesis or by pericardial window technique is ultimately necessary to relieve cardiac compression and drain the pericardial space. The pericardial window technique involves a subxiphoid incision and placement of a drainage tube in the pericardial space. This procedure is not associated with many of the hazards of needle pericardiocentesis and is preferable for obtaining both fluid and tissue specimens for diagnostic studies.

OTHER PERICARDIAL DISEASES

The entity of *effusive-constrictive pericarditis* is commonly associated with mediastinal irradiation. This form of pericardial disease has a thickened edematous pericardium with fluid in the pericardial space and is characterized by the hemodynamic findings of both pericardial constriction and pericardial effusion. This entity may respond to therapy with corticosteroids or anti-inflammatory agents but most frequently necessitates pericardiectomy for symptomatic relief. *Mediastinal fibrosis* may involve all mediastinal structures, including the pericardium, and has findings not unlike those of constrictive pericarditis. Some *congenital defects* of the pericardium may be associated with near total or partial absence of the pericardium. Occasionally, cardiac structures will evaginate through partial pericardial defects, resulting in strangulation of some cardiac chambers. *Pericardial cysts* are not uncommon and are frequently benign; they may on occasion give rise to acute pericarditis. *Primary tumors* of the pericardium do occur but are rare.

BIBLIOGRAPHY

Agner, R.C., and Gallis, H.A.: Pericarditis: differential diagnostic considerations, Arch. Intern. Med. **139**:407, 1979.

Bush, C.A., and others: Occult constrictive pericardial disease: diagnosis by rapid volume expansion and correction by pericardiectomy, Circulation **56**:924, 1977.

Cohen, M.V., and Greenberg, M.A.: Constrictive pericarditis: early and late complication of cardiac surgery, Am. J. Cardiol. **43**:657, 1979.

Fowler, N.O.: The electrocardiogram in pericarditis, Cardiovasc. Clin. **5**:256, 1974.

Fowler, N.O., and Holmes, J.C: Hemodynamic effects of isoproterenol and norepinephrine in acute cardiac tamponade, J. Clin. Invest. **43**:502, 1969.

Lorell, B., and others: Right ventricular infarction: clinical diagnosis and differentiation from cardiac tamponade and pericardial constriction, Am. J. Cardiol. **43**:465, 1979.

Reddy, P.S., and others: Cardiac tamponade: hemodynamic observations in man, Circulation **58**:265, 1978.

Robertson, R., and Arnold, C.R.: Acute constrictive pericarditis, J. Thorac. Cardiovasc. Surg. **49**:91, 1965.

Rubin, R.H., and Moellering, R.C.: Clinical, microbiologic and therapeutic aspects of purulent pericarditis, Am. J. Med. **59**:68, 1975.

Wood, P.: Chronic constrictive pericarditis, Am. J. Cardiol. **7**:48, 1961.

99 • DISEASES OF THE THORACIC AORTA

James O. Finnegan

The aorta is the largest and most important blood vessel in the human body (Fig. 99-1). It originates from the left ventricle at the level of the anulus fibrosis, rises anteriorly and slightly to the right in the midmediastinum, courses transversely and posteriorly, and then descends via the left posterior chest through the diaphragm to the level of the lumbar vertebrae, where it divides into the common iliac arteries. In its course it gives off branches to the heart, brain, extremities, and gut, carrying more blood than any other vascular channel. The thoracic aorta may be conveniently divided into the ascending, transverse (arch), and descending portions. Although the vessel is a continuum, many aortic diseases involve a specific anatomic section, and these arbitrary anatomic divisions may have important clinical implications in planning the surgical approach for a particular disease entity.

ANATOMY OF THE AORTA
Ascending aorta

The heart, which is roughly the size of a large lemon, is contiguous with the diaphragmatic pericardium as it rests tangentially in the midmediastinum. The heart "ends" and the ascending aorta begins at the level of the anulus fibrosis, the supporting structure for the aortic valve, which sits in the midmediastinum at the level of the third left costal cartilage, just behind the sternum. The lumen of the aorta is widest at its origin and tapers until it finally bifurcates into the iliac vessels. It rises from the

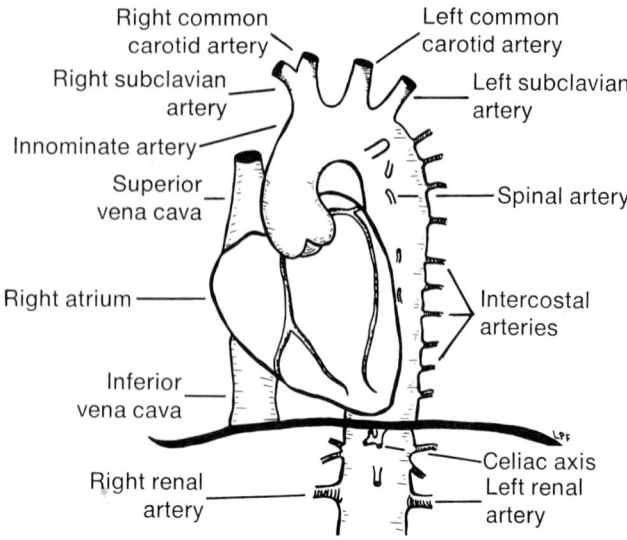

Fig. 99-1. Heart and entire thoracic aorta and its branches. (Illustration by Loretta P. Finnegan, M.D.)

heart vertically and slightly to the right for approximately 5 to 7 cm. The transition from the ascending aorta to the transverse aorta is marked by the branching off of the innominate artery. The ascending aorta is further distinguished from its remainder by pericardial envelopment, which is important to keep in mind in the diagnosis and treatment of pericardial tamponade.

The bulbus aortae is the anatomic designation for the very slight dilation of the aorta at its origin just above the anulus of the aortic valve. The three cusps of the semilunar aortic valve divide this slightly dilated proximal aorta into three sinuses of Valsalva, designated the anterior, left posterior, and right posterior sinuses. The ostium of the right coronary artery is located in the anterior sinus, and the left coronary ostium is found in the left posterior sinus. The right posterior sinus does not contain a coronary ostium; this fact is of some importance in planning surgical procedures in patients with abnormally small aortic anuli, in whom the aortic root is widened by dividing through the noncoronary cusp and inserting a prosthetic patch.

Arch of the aorta

The arch of the aorta may be thought of as beginning at the termination of the pericardial envelopment of the ascending aorta. Frequently referred to as the transverse arch, this portion of the aorta is protected by the upper sternum as it curves upward to the left and posteriorly at the level of the fourth vertebral body. The first major branch of the aortic arch is the innominate artery or brachiocephalic trunk, which subsequently divides into the right subclavian and right common carotid vessels. Most commonly the left common carotid artery arises as a separate vascular branch of the arch 1 to 2 cm lateral to the origin of the innominate vessel. However, in a small percentage of individuals the left carotid artery arises from a common brachiocephalic trunk with the right carotid and right subclavian arteries. The left subclavian artery is normally the last branch of the aortic arch.

A patent ductus arteriosus, when present, arises from the concavity of the thoracic aorta at the junction of the arch and the descending thoracic aorta, connecting the aorta with the left main pulmonary artery. This channel is usually obliterated shortly after birth and exists thereafter as the ligamentum arteriosum.

Within the concavity of the arch can be found the bifurcation of the main pulmonary artery and the left main bronchus. The left vagus nerve crosses the anterolateral portion of the arch, giving rise to the recurrent laryngeal nerve, which curves under the arch and ascends back into the neck, supplying the vocal cords. All operative procedures involving the distal arch of the aorta, patent ductus arteriosus, or coarctation syndromes require careful surgical identification and preservation of the recurrent laryngeal nerve.

Descending aorta

The descending thoracic aorta occupies the left posterior mediastinum from the fourth to the twelfth thoracic vertebrae, moving gradually anteriorly as it descends from a position to the left of the vertebral column to one just in front of it at the level of the diaphragm. The branches of the descending thoracic aorta include the bronchial, esophageal, intercostal, pericardial, superior phrenic, and spinal arteries. As a general rule, all of these branches, with the exception of those supplying the spinal cord, may be ligated with impunity. The blood supply of the spinal cord is of particular concern to thoracic surgeons who perform procedures that require temporary cross-clamping or removal of sections of the thoracic aorta, since these actions cause temporary or permanent spinal chord ischemia that may result in serious neurologic deficits. The important branches of the descending thoracic aorta that supply the spinal cord are seldom identified specifically during a surgical procedure. However, the principles of gentle handling of the aorta, minimal cross-clamping time, and the use of cardiopulmonary bypass or heparinized shunts for maintaining spinal artery blood flow have been the key to avoiding spinal cord ischemia.

CONGENITAL ANOMALIES OF THE THORACIC AORTA
Patent ductus arteriosus

Many patients with patent ductus arteriosus (see Chapter 93) appear to be growing normally and are able to participate in normal activities. This often leads to the false assumption that the condition is compatible with normal longevity. However, it has been found that the subsequent life expectancy of patients with a patent ductus arteriosus who are alive at 17 years of age is approximately half that of the normal population.

Recently, medical treatment aimed at nonoperative closure of patent ductus arteriosus, especially in premature and newborn infants, has been successful. Indomethacin causes closure of the patent ductus in a small percentage of infants, thus avoiding the need for thoracotomy and ligation. However, if symptoms of congestive heart failure persist, surgical intervention is mandatory.

Surgical correction is usually recommended in young children with a persistent patent ductus arteriosus, even in the absence of symptoms. There is minimal operative risk.

Coarctation of the aorta

Coarctation (see Chapter 93) is congenital narrowing of the thoracic aorta, most commonly occurring at the level of the patent ductus arteriosus or ligamentum arteriosum (Fig. 99-2). More unusually the narrowing may occur proximal to the patent ductus; in its most severe form, this variety represents interruption of the aortic arch. The more common so-called postductal coarctation is associated with a bicuspid aortic valve in 25% to 40% of cases, but other cardiac defects are uncommon. Most patients with this defect survive into adult life. Those who have hemodynamic difficulties in the neonatal or infant stages usually have associated intracardiac anomalies.

In patients who survive beyond infancy, the physical and roentgenographic signs of persistent coarctation of the aorta are (1) upper extremity hypertension associated with lower extremity hypotension or absent pulses and (2) collateral arterial beds in the thoracic area. The internal mammary, intercostal, and subscapular vessels may become enlarged to three or four times normal size, are subject to dangerous aneurysm formation, and, in the case of the intercostal vessels, may produce notching of the ribs. Loud bruits may be heard over the posterolateral chest wall.

Most children are asymptomatic. The diagnosis usually results from the discovery of a bruit or upper extremity hypertension. When symptoms do exist, headache, dyspnea, general weakness, palpitations, and intermittent claudication may be present.

The diagnosis is established by comparing upper and lower extremity pulsations and blood pressures. It is essential to evaluate the blood pressure in both upper extremities, since variations may suggest involvement of the left subclavian artery in the coarctation. Systolic murmurs may be audible over the base of the heart or in the midback at the level of the sixth or seventh interspace. A diastolic murmur may represent flow through dilated intercostal arteries. Enlarged collateral chest wall vessels may produce palpable bruits over the chest wall. Evidence of left ventricular enlargement may be present and can be confirmed by an ECG. The definitive study is an aortogram, which

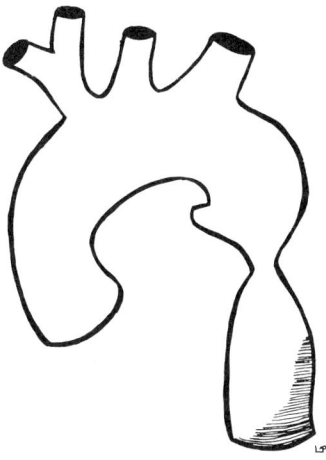

Fig. 99-2. Adult or postductal type of coarctation of thoracic aorta. (Illustration by Loretta P. Finnegan, M.D.)

will demonstrate the site and severity of the coarctation and the most prominent collateral channels.

Surgical therapy is indicated. Several studies have suggested that the life expectancy of an individual with untreated coarctation is approximately 30 to 40 years. Surgery between 7 and 14 years of age is generally recommended. The coarctated segment of aorta is excised. Usually an end-to-end anastomosis is possible. Occasionally it is necessary to insert a tubular Dacron graft. Because Dacron will not grow and because the incidence of recoarctation has been reported to be as high as 35%, alternate methods of handling coarctation of the aorta have been suggested. One is an aortic plastic technique, involving longitudinal opening of the coarctated segment with insertion of a diamond-shaped graft. Another is a procedure in which the subclavian artery is divided distally within the left side of the chest, opened longitudinally in continuity with the coarctation, and folded down as an onlay graft. The advantage of these techniques is, of course, that no prosthetic material is used and the coarctation is repaired with the patient's own tissue. This should allow normal growth of the segment. Follow-up studies have indicated excellent anatomic and hemodynamic results with these techniques.

THORACIC ANEURYSMS

An aneurysm of the thoracic aorta may be defined as a localized outpouching usually secondary to a weakness in the medial layer of the aorta. Aneurysms may occur on a congenital or an acquired basis and may be found anywhere in the thoracic aorta from the sinuses of Valsalva to the iliac bifurcation. The following are the known causes of thoracic aneurysms:

True aneurysms
    Congenital—sinus of Valsalva
    Arteriosclerotic

Cystic medial necrosis
Luetic
False aneurysms
Penetrating injury
Blunt injury
Iatrogenic—infected prosthetic graft or suture line

Dissection of the thoracic aorta secondary to intimal tear or trauma has frequently been associated with the word "aneurysm," hence the term "dissecting thoracic aneurysms." It must be understood that a dissecting hematoma within the wall of the aorta, either spontaneous or traumatic, is a different pathogic process from the formation of an aneurysm and will be discussed separately. Likewise, false aneurysms of the thoracic aorta represent organized hematomas secondary to tears in the thoracic aorta as a result of injury or surgery.

Aneurysms of the sinuses of Valsalva

Aneurysmal dilation of the sinuses of Valsalva may occur in association with Marfan's syndrome and rarely from syphilitic aortitis, and false aneurysms of this area may occur secondary to bacterial endocarditis. However, the most commonly recognized aneurysms of the sinuses of Valsalva are congenital in origin and probably result from defective attachment of the aortic media to the fibrous base of the heart. The resulting localized weakness at the base of the aorta causes aneurysmal development and is most commonly found in the right coronary sinus, occasionally in the noncoronary sinus, and rarely in the left coronary sinus. The male/female occurrence ratio is 5:1.

Congenital aneurysms of the sinuses of Valsalva are extremely unusual except in Japan. Patients are usually asymptomatic until the fourth decade of life when the aneurysm forms a fistula protruding into a cardiac chamber (most frequently the right ventricle or right atrium but sometimes the pulmonary artery or pericardium). Unruptured aneurysms of the aortic sinuses may also produce clinical manifestations, including (1) obstruction of right ventricular outflow by a right coronary sinus aneurysm; (2) tricuspid regurgitation resulting from protrusion of an aneurysm of a noncoronary sinus into the right side of the heart in the area of the tricuspid valve; (3) heart block resulting from compression of the superior portion of the interventricular septum; (4) coronary insufficiency from compression of the left coronary artery; and (5) embolus.

Rupture of an aortic sinus aneurysm typically results in a left-to-right shunt into either the right ventricle or the right atrium. Fistulous communications with the left-sided cardiac chambers are distinctly rare. Although rupture of a sinus aneurysm may cause sudden death from congestive heart failure, most patients live approximately a year after fistula formation. Bacterial endocarditis within the sinus or the fistulous tract is a common cause of death after fistula formation. Sudden rupture of an aneurysm of the sinus of Valsalva into a cardiac chamber may produce severe chest pain, usually precordial in nature and occasionally simulating angina pectoris. Such a rupture may cause distortion of the aortic valve anulus with resultant aortic insufficiency.

Chest roentgenograms and ECGs usually are not diagnostic. The diagnosis can be established by cardiac catheterization and aortography. If rupture has not occurred, the aneurysm will be visualized only as an outpouching of the sinus of Valsalva. If rupture has occurred, aortic root injection will demonstrate flow of dye into the right atrium or ventricle. Chamber oxygen analysis also aids in locating the fistula.

The treatment of a congenital aneurysm of the sinus of Valsalva is surgical. If the aneurysm is unruptured, repair can usually be accomplished through the aorta using cardiopulmonary bypass. Although the aneurysmal sinus can occasionally be repaired by local direct suture methods, it is not uncommon to require replacement of the ascending aorta with a woven Dacron graft. Replacement of the distorted and malfunctioning aortic valve with a prosthetic device may also be necessary. Mortality and morbidity associated with surgical correction of aneurysms of the sinus of Valsalva have steadily decreased, and all such aneurysms, with or without fistula formation and with or without symptoms, should be repaired surgically on discovery.

Aneurysms of the ascending aorta

Aneurysms that involve the entire ascending aorta from the valvular anulus to the branching off of the innominate artery are usually due to cystic medial necrosis. Histologic examination of specimens obtained at surgery or autopsy generally shows thinning of the medial layer of the aortic wall with severe fragmentation or disappearance of the elastic fibers. As a result the ascending aorta becomes very thin and quite dilated. Associated distortion of the aortic valve may produce aortic regurgitation.

If the aortic valve is competent and not involved in the disease process, simple tubular graft replacement of the ascending aorta from a distance approximately 2 cm above the aortic valve to the level of the innominate vessels will suffice. Mild aortic regurgitation may be corrected in some instances by suture fixation of the commissural areas of the valve in such a way as to resuspend the leaflets and restore competence, thus avoiding aortic valve replacement. In cases in which aneurysms of the ascending aorta are associated with severe aortic insufficiency, replacement of the aortic valve and the ascending aorta with a commercially available valved conduit is the procedure of choice. This requires reimplantation of the coronary ostia into the side of the graft.

The advent of open heart surgery has resulted in several new problems in the ascending aorta and surgical methods for their correction. Aortic dissection or rupture at the site of cannulation for bypass surgery or placement of a proximal saphenous vein anastomosis has been reported. Dissection originating in the distal ascending aorta at the site of cannulation can be treated by removal of the cannula, temporary cessation of cardiopulmonary bypass, rapid cannulation of the femoral artery, and reinstitution of bypass in retrograde fashion. The cannulation site is then repaired.

Cracking or rupture of the aorta at the site of aortosaphenous anastomosis can be controlled by excision of that portion of the aorta, replacement with a Dacron patch, and subsequent anastomosis of the vein graft either to the Dacron patch or to other portions of the ascending aorta.

Aneurysms of the aortic arch

Before 1950 most reports indicated that aneurysms involving the arch of the aorta were nearly always luetic in origin and were usually extensions of aneurysms involving the ascending aorta. Now syphilis has nearly disappeared as a cause of major vascular disease and arch aneurysms have become rare. Nearly all aneurysms of the transverse aortic arch reported today are arteriosclerotic in origin. An occasional posttraumatic false aneurysm has been reported in the arch.

A large aneurysm may produce symptoms by compression of branch arteries or adjacent structures including the tracheobronchial tree, esophagus, pulmonary artery, and recurrent laryngeal nerve (producing hoarseness). Compression of the superior vena cava with resultant full-blown superior vena cava syndrome has been reported. Pain associated with rub or vertebral body erosion is not uncommon. Rupture of an arch aneurysm into the mediastinum, pleural space, esophagus, or tracheobronchial tree invariably results in immediate exsanguination.

The presence of aneurysms in the transverse arch may be suspected from simple roentgenograms, but aortography is usually required to define the true nature and extent of the lesion. Aneurysms of the transverse arch commonly involve the origins of the innominate, left carotid, and left subclavian arteries, and therefore surgical procedures designed to correct such aneurysms usually involve not only excision of the arch aneurysm but intraoperative preservation of areas supplied by the branches of the arch, particularly the brain.

Total prosthetic replacement of the aortic arch can be accomplished in a number of ways. Some perform resection and replacement of the ascending thoracic aorta using deep hypothermia, cardiopulmonary bypass, circulatory arrest, and myocardial cooling. Others have described an interesting method of approaching aneurysms of the aortic arch using surgically constructed bypass grafts and ultimately resecting the arch without the use of cardiopulmonary bypass.

Aneurysms of the descending aorta

Most aneurysms of the descending thoracic aorta discovered today have an arteriosclerotic origin. The apparent increasing incidence of this disease may be related to the increased longevity of the population. These aneurysms are usually fusiform and arise just distal to the branching off of the left subclavian artery. Prior studies divided these aneurysms into fusiform and saccular types. However, most of these aneurysms have a common cause (arteriosclerosis), and they run the full spectrum from perfectly saccular to perfectly fusiform, all representing variations of the same disease process. Aneurysms may be reasonably well localized or extend the full length of the thoracic aorta and on into the abdominal area. They are frequently associated with aneurysms in other areas, most commonly the abdominal aorta. As would be expected, many patients with these aneurysms have associated cerebral and coronary vascular disease.

Although patients with descending thoracic aortic aneurysms can be asymptomatic, chest pain is frequent and is usually due to local erosion or compression. Pressure on the origin of the intercostal nerves or spine may produce extreme pain. Although these aneurysms have been reported to rupture into the tracheobronchial tree, esophagus, or pulmonary arterial tree, they most frequently rupture into the left pleural space causing death by exsanguination. The suspicion of the presence of such aneurysms is usually provided by routine chest roentgenograms, although they may often be difficult to differentiate from other mediastinal masses. Aortography will usually resolve the problem and is indicated when surgery is contemplated.

Effective surgical management involves the use of one of several techniques, including (1) cross-clamping of the aorta above and below the aneurysm with excision and rapid replacement with a prosthetic graft; (2) femoral cardiopulmonary bypass to protect the kidneys and spinal cord while the aorta is cross-clamped and the aneurysm is

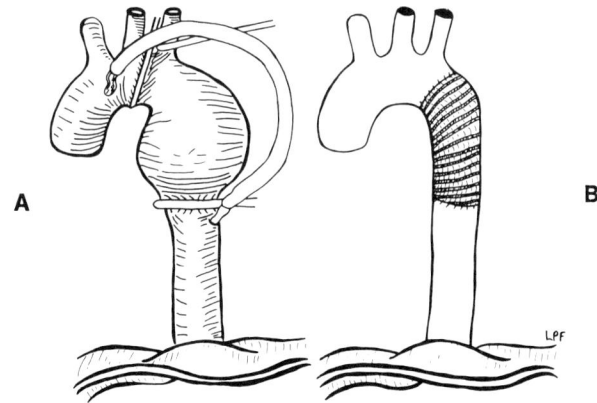

Fig. 99-3. **A,** Aneurysm of proximal descending thoracic aorta. Aorta is clamped above and below aneurysm. Additional clamp is on subclavian artery. Shunt is placed from ascending aorta to descending thoracic aorta, providing for continuous distal flow while aneurysm is repaired. **B,** Replacement of aneurysm with woven Dacron graft. Shunt has been removed. (Illustration by Loretta P. Finnegan, M.D.)

repaired; (3) left atriofemoral bypass providing the same form of renal and spinal protection and ideally decompressing the left heart simultaneously, thereby reducing left ventricular work; and (4) internally heparin-coated shunts from the proximal aorta to the distal aorta, allowing cross-clamping and repair of the aneurysm without heparinization or the use of bypass techniques. The surgery is illustrated by Fig. 99-3.

• • •

Much of the data concerning the natural history of aneurysms of the aorta is derived from patients with luetic disease. Because syphilis has largely disappeared as a cause of vascular disease in this country, these older reports may no longer be applicable. In a more recent series in which most patients had arteriosclerotic aneurysms, none were operated on. Careful follow-up study revealed a 50% 5-year and a 70% 10-year mortality rate. Only a third of these deaths were due to rupture. Half were due to associated cardiovascular disease. Significant risk factors included advanced age, an aneurysm greater than 6 cm in size, hypertension, and the association of other vascular disease, especially cardiac and cerebral disease. The location of the aneurysm did not appear to influence the mortality rate, but the presence of symptoms clearly reduced survival.

AORTIC DISSECTION

The unfortunate term "dissecting aneurysm" is attributed to Laennac. Although this term is well entrenched in the literature, it is incorrect and should be discarded. Aneurysm formation is not part of the pathogenesis of aortic dissection. The terms "aortic dissection" and "dissecting hematoma of the aorta" are more correct. Dissection extends into the media of the aorta.

Acute aortic dissection is the most common acute catastrophe involving the aorta, occurring in about 5 per million population per year and found in about 1 in 500 autopsies. Ruptured abdominal aneurysms occur at a rate of 3.6 per million population per year and ruptured thoracic aneurysms in only about 1 per million population per year.

Dissection of the thoracic aorta occurs most frequently in the 50- to 70-year age group. The male/female incidence ratio is 2:1. It is unusual to see the lesion in patients under 40 years of age unless it is associated with full-blown Marfan's syndrome. Approximately 50% of cases of aortic dissection occurring in women under the age of 40 are associated with pregnancy. Dissection seems to be more common among blacks, possibly owing to the higher incidence of hypertension in that group.

PATHOGENESIS. There is no agreement concerning the cause of aortic dissection. Most agree that intimal tearing is the event that triggers dissection. The cause of the intimal tear is probably a combination of diseases within the aortic wall including cystic medial necrosis, rupture of the vasa vasorum, and loss of elasticity, plus hemodynamic factors. Autopsy studies of patients who died from medial dissection have demonstrated clearly abnormal findings including loss of elastic tissue, pooling of mucoid material, fibrosis, and apparent loss of cellular nuclei. The most common of these changes, cystic medial necrosis, has for decades been thought of as the primary pathologic lesion. However, it is clear that the media of normally aging aortas exhibit the same histopathologic features widely claimed to represent the specific medial defect underlying aortic dissection and that only quantitative differences exist between the pathology of aortic dissection and that of a normally aging aorta. The histologic features of the media, previously implicated as a specific underlying defect, appear to represent the morphologic substrata of a traumatizing and reparative process within the aortic wall consequent to hemodynamic forces. This process may gradually lead to dilation of the aorta. Hemodynamic tensions increase as the aneurysm enlarges. Local circumstances determine whether a dilated aorta will rupture or whether a dissection will occur.

The aorta in patients with Marfan's syndrome shows basically the same structural alterations. The underlying connective tissue disorder in these patients leads to complications at an earlier age.

In addition to the disease process or degenerative changes that must be present within the aortic wall for dissection to occur, the hemodynamic forces acting on the aortic wall are also of major importance. It has been shown experimentally that nonpulsatile flow at pressures up to 400 mm Hg produces no propagation of an aortic dissection. However, pulsatile pressure does cause propagation. Although an intimal tear is found in the majority of aortic dissections, at either surgery or autopsy, there is some controversy as to whether this tear is the primary initiating force in the creation of an aortic dissection or whether it is secondary to hemorrhage within the aortic wall as a result of rupture of the vasa vasorum.

CLINICAL MANIFESTATIONS. Extraordinarily severe chest pain is the most impressive chief complaint in nearly 90% of patients with aortic dissection. Patients usually report abrupt onset of the pain, which can be most severe in the anterior retrosternal area but may also be felt in or radiate to the intrascapular area, the epigastrium, or the back. Arm pain is unusual. It is the simultaneous occurrence of the pain in multiple areas that helps to differentiate aortic dissection from acute myocardial infarction, although this distinction is frequently unclear; indeed, confusion with acute myocardial infarction is the most common diagnostic error made in patients with dissection. Pain may be minimal or absent in patients with spontaneous intimal lacerations, limited dissections, or even extensive classic dissections. It should be recognized that abrupt onset of neurologic symptoms may dull the patient's perception of pain and reduce or eliminate his ability to complain. The presence of neurologic signs in a patient with aortic dissection generally suggests involvement of the aortic arch and partial or complete occlusion of the innominate or left carotid arteries.

Most patients with thoracic aortic dissection appear acutely distressed and have measurable systolic and diastolic hypertension. Renal ischemia secondary to compromise of the renal artery flow by the dissecting channel may aggravate this hypertension. Low blood pressure is found almost exclusively with involvement of the ascending aorta, suggesting rupture into the pericardial sac and tamponade. Since the false channel created by the dissection can compromise the lumen of any branch of the aorta, evaluation of the pulse and blood pressure should be carried out in all four extremities. Occlusion of an arterial branch of the aorta produces definite loss or diminution of a pulse. The baseline pulse examination is especially important because of the possibility of subsequent propagation of the dissection, which is indicated by the loss of a pulse that was originally palpable.

The murmur of aortic regurgitation suggests retrograde dissection of the ascending thoracic aorta. This murmur is audible in approximately one third of all patients with aortic dissection but in less than 10% of those with a dissection distal to the left subclavian artery. Jugular venous distention may suggest cardiac tamponade but can also be caused by mediastinal hemorrhage and compression of the superior vena cava.

Any patient with a widened mediastinum on chest roentgenogram associated with free blood in the left pleural cavity as demonstrated by a limited thoracentesis should be considered to have a ruptured thoracic aorta until proved otherwise. It may occasionally be necessary to carry out emergency surgery without the performance of angiography. The presence of a pericardial friction rub is ominous, usually indicating retrograde dissection into the pericardial cavity. However, there have been survivors, especially when the finding was noted immediately and surgery was undertaken without delay.

The presence of a new murmur of aortic insufficiency should suggest the possibility of the extension of the ascending dissection to involve the aortic anulus and valve. Severe aortic insufficiency may also appear at a later date in patients with healed ascending aortic dissections.

Neurologic complications of thoracic aortic dissection are of various types. One type represents altered states of consciousness in patients who have had profound episodes of hypotension and cerebral hypoperfusion. More focal neurologic disturbances occur when specific branches of the arch are compressed or totally occluded by the dissection. Ischemic paralysis of an extremity results from occlusion of the major vessel to that limb. It is more common in the lower extremities. Central nervous system symptoms including hemiplegia are secondary to carotid artery occlusion and are next in frequency. Paraplegia attributable to spinal cord ischemia occurs secondary to occlusion of intercostal or lumbar vessels. It is important to establish the patient's baseline neurologic status before undertaking surgical correction of the lesion, inasmuch as neurologic deficits as a result of the surgical procedure itself are not uncommon.

Retrograde aortic dissection resulting in coronary occlusion and myocardial infarction occurs in less than 5% of patients. It is usually a fatal event or at least precludes the possibility of major surgery. Two less commonly seen complications of aortic dissection are renal or splenic arterial occlusion and rupture of the dissection at the aortic root. The latter may produce complete heart block resulting from hematoma of the interatrial septum; left-to-right shunts created by rupture into the right atrium, right ventricle, or pulmonary artery; rupture into the left atrium resulting in a continuous murmur; or obstruction of the pulmonary artery.

The following are common findings encountered in plain roentgenograms of patients with suspected or proven aortic dissection:

Mediastinal widening
Aortic root enlargement
Tracheal deviation
Depression of the left mainstem bronchus
An aortic shadow outside a calcified aortic knob
Left pleural effusion

It should be noted that a normal chest roentgenogram does not rule out the possibility of dissection. Possibly one third to one half of patients may initially have a normal chest roentgenogram. Conversely it should be remembered that a supine anteroposterior chest roentgenogram will frequently suggest widening of the mediastinum when actually that is the normal roentgenographic appearance of the mediastinum in that position. Even when the clinical diagnosis of dissection seems well established, ECGs and enzyme determinations should be obtained to rule out the possibility of myocardial infarction.

Angiography is considered essential both to demonstrate the presence and extent of the dissection and if possible to localize the intimal tear, the focal point of the surgeon's subsequent efforts. DeBakey classified dissections on the basis of their origin and extent (Fig. 99-4).

MANAGEMENT. The natural history of acute aortic dissection in patients managed before the introduction of modern pharmacologic and surgical treatment was poor. Of all patients with aortic dissection, 30% died within the first 24 hours, 50% within 48 hours, 70% by the end of 1 week, and 80% by the end of 2 weeks. The prognosis was clearly worst in patients with proximal (ascending aortic) tears and associated hypotension and was best in normotensive or hypertensive patients with distal (descending aortic) dissections.

All patients with any form of aortic dissection should initially be treated medically. A selection process then be-

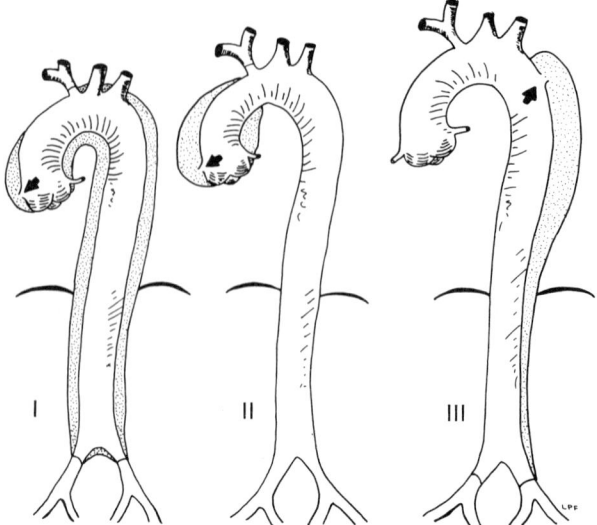

Fig. 99-4. DeBakey's classic categorization of dissection of thoracic aorta. In type *I,* dissection originates in *ascending* aorta *(arrow)* and extends throughout length of aorta. In type *II,* dissection originates in *ascending* aorta *(arrow)* but is limited to ascending aorta or proximal portion of arch. In type *III,* dissection originates in proximal *descending* thoracic aorta *(arrow)* and extends distally. (Illustration by Loretta P. Finnegan, M.D.)

gins in an attempt to identify the patients most likely to benefit from surgical intervention.

The immediate goals of treatment are the reduction of pain, the control of systolic and diastolic blood pressure, and the decrease of tension in the aortic wall. Small intravenous doses of morphine sulfate will reduce the patient's pain and allay anxiety. The intravenous administration of sodium nitroprusside usually results in a dramatic reduction of blood pressure with minimal side effects (see Chapter 87 for dosage); concomitant diuretic therapy (for example, furosemide) may be needed. Nitroprusside can result in transient increases in myocardial contractility that could conceivably contribute to extension of the dissection. For this reason, small intravenous doses of propranolol (1 mg every 3 minutes to a total of 10 mg) are used to decrease contractility and aortic wall tension. Patients who cannot tolerate sodium nitroprusside or whose blood pressure is not controlled with sodium nitroprusside can be treated with trimethaphan camphorsulfonate (Arfonad).

As soon as the patient is stable, normotension has been achieved, and pain has been relieved, angiography can be accomplished. A percutaneous technique using the femoral approach is recommended. The purposes of the angiographic examination are (1) to confirm the diagnosis of aortic dissection, (2) to identify the site of origin (intimal tear) of the dissection, (3) to define the extent of the dissection, (4) to rule in or rule out involvement of the major branches of the aorta, and (5) to quantitate blood flow within the false lumen. The identification of the origin of the dissection is essential to the proper planning of surgery. In an otherwise stable patient, surgery is relatively contraindicated if the intimal origin of the dissection cannot be identified.

Failure to opacify the false lumen roentgenographically, suggesting that the false lumen is clotted, indicates a more favorable prognosis for the patient. In one series long-term survival without surgery in patients without false lumen opacification was 89%, as compared to 43% of patients in whom the false channel could be filled with contrast media.

There is general agreement that surgery is the treatment of choice for proximal dissection (type A or DeBakey types I and II) involving the ascending aorta or the arch because progression of the hematoma in the direction of the aortic valve or branches of the aortic arch may have the devastating consequences of aortic insufficiency, pericardial tamponade, or neurologic compromise. It should be noted that a small group of patients with proximal dissection, who refused surgery or in whom surgery was contraindicated because of age or associated medical illness, were treated successfully with long-term medical therapy. As mentioned, some authorities believe that failure to identify the intimal tear within the proximal aorta is a relative contraindication to surgery in an otherwise stable patient.

Patients with a distal (type B or DeBakey type III) dissection should be treated medically as long as the dissection remains stable and uncomplicated. The slight advantage of medical therapy in this group probably results from the fact that patients with distal dissection tend to be somewhat older and have an increased incidence of associated atherosclerotic and cardiopulmonary disease. However, surgical therapy must be undertaken in patients with distal disease if there is evidence of rupture, impending rupture, pericardial tamponade, vital organ compromise, aortic insufficiency, or inability to control hypertension.

AORTIC ARCH SYNDROME

The term "aortic arch syndrome" refers to a variety of acquired conditions that produce partial or total occlusion of one or all of the branches of the aortic arch. Although there are many known causes of aortic arch syndromes, in the United States over 90% of these lesions are secondary to atherosclerotic occlusive disease. Other causes to consider are trauma, neoplasm, luetic aortitis, Takayasu's arteritis or pulseless disease, and emboli. Also, many other diseases mimic aortic arch syndrome or produce brachiocephalic arterial obstruction. These include collagen vascular disease, thoracic outlet syndrome, and superior sulcus tumor.

When atherosclerosis is the cause of aortic arch syndrome, the left subclavian artery is the most commonly affected vessel, followed by the innominate and left common carotid arteries. In nearly half of the patients, multiple branches are involved.

CLINICAL MANIFESTATIONS. Although aortic arch syndrome is most common between the ages of 50 and 70, it is not rare in younger patients. The majority of patients show cerebral ischemia, which can be divided into four types: (1) a fixed neurologic deficit secondary to frank cerebrovascular accident, (2) transient ischemic attacks (TIAs), (3) reversible ischemic neurologic deficits somewhere between a cerebrovascular accident and a TIA, and (4) chronic deficits from hypoperfusion.

Physical examination should emphasize the evaluation of all peripheral pulses with particular attention to the carotid, temporal, brachial, and radial pulses. The detection of bruits along the course of any vessel demands additional evaluation by ultrasound. The definitive study is the angiogram. The aortic arch can be approached through either the brachial or the femoral artery, although most angiographers prefer the femoral approach.

Subclavian steal syndrome

Perhaps the best known of all the aortic arch syndromes is the subclavian steal syndrome. Ordinarily the pressure head is somewhat higher in the subclavian artery than in the basilar cerebral system, allowing antegrade flow in the vertebral vessel. However, with significant stenosis of the *proximal subclavian artery,* the pressure in that vessel may fall below that of the basilar system, causing a reversal of flow in the vertebral artery system and subsequent diversion of blood from the brain. Exercise of the involved upper extremity may increase flow beyond the subclavian lesion and pull even more blood from the cerebral circulation, which will intensify the cerebral symptoms associated with the flow reversal. The same syndrome has been described for the *innominate artery.* Significant stenosis at the base of this latter vessel can result in cerebral flood flow reversal. The possible greater danger is reversal of flow in the right carotid artery as well as the right vertebral artery, intensifying the blood flow deficit in the brain.

In both steal syndromes, surgical correction is easily accomplished by attaching a bypass graft of Dacron or bovine heterograft from the aorta to the involved vessel beyond the obstruction.

Takayasu's arteritis

Takayasu's arteritis or pulseless disease is an inflammatory panarteritis that may involve all the branches of the thoracic and the abdominal aorta. It has been reported worldwide but is rare in the United States. It is most commonly seen among young women of Oriental extraction.

Three major varieties of Takayasu's occlusive arteritis have been described, depending on the area of the vascular tree involved. In one variety, affecting approximately 50% of the patients, the aortic arch is the primary site of involvement. The second group, approximately one third of the patients, demonstrate involvement of all of the aorta. The third group, about 10% to 15% of the patients, have involvement of the distal thoracic and abdominal aorta.

Most patients with Takayasu's arteritis or pulseless disease are under 40 years of age and women predominate. Patients generally have systemic symptoms such as malaise, fever, anorexia, and weight loss. Many have cardiopulmonary complaints including tachycardia, shortness of breath, and peripheral edema. The laboratory evaluation is not diagnostic, although many patients have anemia and leukocytosis.

Although the arteritis per se becomes inactive in many patients, the vascular obstructive lesions persist. If the inflammatory process continues unabated, early death owing to cardiac or cerebral complications is the rule. Corticosteroids have produced clinical remission in some patients. The value of anticoagulation therapy is unproved. Surgical correction may be indicated in the later fibrotic phase of the disease. However, because of the small size of the vessels involved, the revascularization effort is frequently less than ideal.

Syphilitic aortitis

Before the introduction of penicillin, syphilis was the most common cause of proximal aortitis and was responsible for most branch occlusions of the aortic arch. The occurrence of syphilitic aortitis today is rare. The diagnosis may be suggested if serologic tests for syphilis are positive and an angiogram confirms aortic arch involvement. Proper treatment consists of appropriate antibiotic therapy and prosthetic replacement grafts as indicated.

BIBLIOGRAPHY

Adams, H.D., and Van Geertruyden, H.H.: Neurologic complications of aortic surgery, Ann. Surg. **144:**547, 1956.

Bergen, J.J., and Yao, J.S.T.: Surgery of the aorta and its branches, New York, 1979, Grune & Stratton, Inc.

Borrie, J.: Management of thoracic emergencies, New York, 1980, Appleton-Century-Crofts.

Hirst, A.E., Jr., Johns, V.J., Jr., and Kime, S.W., Jr.: Dissecting aneurysm of the aorta: a review of 505 cases, Medicine **37:**217, 1958.

Lam, R., Robinson, M.J., and Morales, A.R.: Aortic dissection complicating aortocoronary saphenous vein bypass, Chest **68:**729, 1976.

Nasu, T.: Pathology of pulseless disease: a systematic study and critical review of twenty-one autopsy cases reported in Japan, Angiology **14:**255, 1963.

Reivich, M., and others: Reversal of blood flow through the vertebral artery and its effect on cerebral circulation, N. Engl. J. Med. **265:**878, 1961.

Rob, C.G.: The surgical treatment of occlusive disease of the extracranial cerebral arteries. In Dale, W.A., editor: Management of arterial occlusive disease, Chicago, 1971, Year Book Medical Publishers, Inc.

Ross, R.S., and McKusick, V.A.: Aortic arch syndromes, Arch. Intern. Med. **92:**701, 1953.

Schlatmann, T.J.M., and Becker, A.E.: Histologic changes in the normal aging aorta: implications for dissecting aortic aneurysm, Am. J. Cardiol. **39:**13, 1977.

Schlatmann, T.J.M., and Becker, A.E.: Pathogenesis of dissecting aneurysm of aorta, Am. J. Cardiol. **39:**21, 1977.

Taguchi, K., and others: Surgical correction of aneurysm of the sinus of Valsalva, Am. J. Cardiol. **23:**180, 1969.

Wheat, M.W., Jr., and others: Treatment of dissecting aneurysms of the aorta without surgery, J. Thorac. Cardiovasc. Surg. **50:**364, 1965.

100 • DISEASES OF THE DISTAL AORTA AND BRANCHES OF THE AORTA

Marian F. McNamara

Mortality and morbidity from atherosclerotic arterial disease have reached epidemic levels in the United States. As the average age of the population increases, a further rise in atherosclerotic disease can be expected. Multiple risk factors including hyperlipidemia, hypertension, cigarette smoking, and diabetes mellitus are linked to the development of atherosclerotic plaque. Once symptoms are present, manipulation of these risk factors rarely results in palliation. Furthermore, early lesions are commonly asymptomatic, and the initial signs and symptoms are catastrophic events such as cerebrovascular accident, myocardial infarction, or severe limb ischemia resulting from arterial occlusion.

During the past three decades the natural history, pathophysiology, and response to therapy of arterial lesions in the aorta and its branches have been defined. Noninvasive diagnostic techniques and arteriography now allow objective quantification of arterial insufficiency and accurate localization of arterial lesions. Successful palliation is obtained in many patients by surgical treatment of segmental atherosclerotic lesions such as carotid stenosis, abdominal aortic aneurysms, and occlusive plaques in the aorta and limb vessels. The long-term success of these operations, however, depends on the progression of the atherosclerotic process, as well as the surgical techniques employed.

CEREBROVASCULAR DISEASE

Cerebrovascular accident (CVA, stroke) is the third leading cause of death in the United States, with an annual incidence of 1.7 per 1000 population. Morbidity results from paralysis, sensory loss, and speech impairment. In 1951 Fisher drew attention to the importance of the *extracranial* arteries in CVA. Later the Joint Study of Extracranial Arterial Occlusion confirmed his initial opinion, demonstrating by arteriography that 75% of patients with CVA had lesions in surgically accessible sites.

PATHOPHYSIOLOGY. The most common sites of extracranial cerebrovascular disease are the common carotid artery at its bifurcation and the adjacent proximal internal carotid artery. Atherosclerotic plaques at these sites produce symptoms by ulceration with embolization and by stenosis. Ulcerated plaque is a focus for deposition of platelets and cholesterol debris. Embolization of this debris into the cerebral circulation results in transient ischemic attacks, amaurosis fugax, or CVA. Further deposition or growth of the plaque narrows the lumen of the artery. Stenosis of 50% or greater may result in decreased cerebral blood flow.

CLINICAL MANIFESTATIONS. Symptoms of cerebrovascular disease include completed CVA, transient ischemic attacks, and amaurosis fugax. Many lesions remain asymptomatic until CVA occurs. However, when transient deficits precede CVA, these events draw attention to the possibility of extracranial cerebrovascular disease and allow treatment before irreversible neurologic deficits arise. It is estimated that 30% of patients with transient ischemic attacks have a CVA within 5 years. By definition, transient ischemic attacks last less than 24 hours and resolve without residual neurologic deficit. These transient neurologic attacks may be related to the carotid system, vertebrobasilar system, or both. Unilateral motor or sensory loss, dysarthria, aphasia, and amaurosis fugax are indicators of disease in the carotid system. Dizziness, ataxia, vertigo, diplopia, and bilateral motor and sensory symptoms suggest lesions in the vertebrobasilar system. Occasionally bilateral carotid stenosis may cause vertebrobasilar symptoms by reducing total cerebral blood flow.

Physical examination of the patient with cerebrovascular disease should include palpation of the common carotid and upper extremity pulses. The internal carotid pulse is not palpable in the neck. Pulse evaluation may therefore be misleading, since the internal carotid artery is frequently occluded in the presence of a normal common carotid pulse. Bruits audible over the carotid bifurcation indicate stenosis. However, the absence of a bruit does not rule out hemodynamically significant stenosis, since bruits are absent in severe stenosis. In addition, many bruits heard in the neck radiate from the thorax or base of the neck and may be confused with intrinsic carotid bruits.

DIAGNOSTIC TESTS. Arteriography remains the definitive diagnostic test for cerebrovascular disease. Bilateral carotid injections are usually performed via the axillary or femoral route. An arch aortogram is desirable before selective catheterization of the cerebral vessels. If clinical findings suggest vertebrobasilar insufficiency, vertebral artery injections are added. Despite improvement in arteriographic techniques, the complication rate for this study remains 1%.

Recently many noninvasive tests have been introduced for the detection of atherosclerotic disease producing stenosis in the carotid artery. Most of these tests are based on monitoring the ophthalmic artery (the first branch of the internal carotid artery) as an indicator of internal carotid disease. The earliest of these tests was ophthalmodynamometry to measure ophthalmic artery pressure. This test was inaccurate and technically difficult. Ocular pneumoplethysmography allows accurate determination of ophthalmic artery pressure and significant carotid artery stenosis. Fluid-filled oculoplethysmography (OPG) detects changes in ocular volume with retinal artery pulsation. Delay in pulse arrival time between the two eyes indicates hemodynamically significant stenosis in the carotid artery. This test is usually combined with analysis of a carotid bruit by carotid phonoangiography (CPA). Qualitative analysis of bruits by this method differentiates intrinsic carotid bruits from transmitted bruits. Systolic bruits are present with low-grade stenosis and systolic-diastolic bruits are caused by high-grade obstruction. The combination of OPG and CPA correlates with angiographic findings in 90% of cases. Supraorbital Doppler flow testing is yet another method for detection of stenosis in the carotid artery. Flow in the supraorbital artery, a terminal branch of the internal carotid artery, is reversed if there is 60% to 70% stenosis of the proximal carotid artery. Doppler imaging is also used to detect carotid bifurcation lesions. However, calcified plaques may produce false positive results with this method. Unfortunately, none of these noninvasive tests is able to detect an ulcerating plaque in the absence of hemodynamically significant stenosis. For this reason they should not replace arteriography in the symptomatic patient.

MANAGEMENT. The localized nature of atherosclerotic plaque at the carotid bifurcation makes this an ideal lesion for treatment by endarterectomy. Excision of the diseased intima restores luminal diameter and removes ulcerating plaques that may be a source of distal emboli. Indications for carotid endarterectomy include transient ischemic attacks, stable CVA, asymptomatic bruits, and (rarely) chronic cerebral ischemia. During the past 20 years, cerebral protective techniques including surgery under local anesthesia, electroencephalographic monitoring, use of an intraluminal shunt, and monitoring of carotid stump pressure and ophthalmic artery pressure have been suggested to further decrease operative mortality and morbidity. Operative mortality from carotid endarterectomy is now 1% to 2%, with neurologic deficits related to the operation in the range of 2% to 4%. The long-term patency of carotid arteries reconstructed by endarterectomy is high, and the majority of patients undergoing surgery for transient ischemic episodes are asymptomatic in the postoperative period.

Patients with minimal neurologic deficit following CVA are also good candidates for carotid endarterectomy, since the incidence of recurrent CVA is great in this group.

The treatment of the asymptomatic bruit is controversial. It has been demonstrated that asymptomatic stenosis at the carotid bifurcation progresses in 60% of patients and that these patients have a 9% incidence of CVA without antecedent symptoms. A rational approach to the management of the patient with an asymptomatic bruit includes evaluation of its hemodynamic significance with noninvasive testing. In patients with hemodynamically significant lesions, arteriography and endarterectomy or close followup with testing at intervals is indicated to decrease the risk of CVA.

Symptoms caused by inaccessible carotid disease or complete occlusion of the internal carotid artery can now be treated in some patients by extracranial-intracranial bypass using the superficial temporal artery. Although this procedure is more complex than carotid endarterectomy, initial morbidity and mortality rates are acceptable.

Symptoms produced by lesions in the great vessels within the thorax are less common. Extrathoracic bypass procedures are effective in treating these lesions and are associated with lower mortality than direct surgical reconstruction. Innominate endarterectomy may be indicated for ulcerative lesions producing embolic phenomena.

The indications for vertebral artery reconstruction are rare. Many patients with vertebrobasilar insufficiency combined with carotid stenosis are relieved of symptoms of vertebrobasilar insufficiency by carotid endarterectomy.

ANEURYSMS

An aneurysm is a localized dilation of an artery caused by structural weakness in the wall. True aneurysms contain all anatomic layers present in the arterial wall: intima, media, and adventitia. In contrast, false aneurysms begin from a rupture of the arterial wall, surrounded by a fibrous sac or adventitia. Aneurysms are fusiform or saccular in configuration.

ETIOLOGY AND PATHOGENESIS. True aneurysms may be atherosclerotic, mycotic, or syphilitic. These processes weaken the media of the arterial wall and allow the artery to dilate. Increased vessel diameter causes increased lateral wall tension as predicted by the law of Laplace. Increased lateral wall pressure causes further dilation, predisposing the thin vessel wall to rupture. Slow arterial flow through the dilated segment allows layered thrombus to be deposited along the wall. This thrombus does not protect against rupture and may give rise to emboli or complete thrombosis of the artery.

Atherosclerosis is the most common cause of true aneurysms in the United States. Over 95% of true aneurysms are located in the abdominal aorta below the renal arteries. Theories proposed to explain this segmental distribution include degeneration of elastic fibers from aging, turbulent flow, and anoxia caused by the occlusion of sparse vasa vasorum. Many patients with abdominal aortic aneurysms have generalized ectasia of the arterial tree or coexistent aneurysms in the popliteal, iliac, femoral, and renal arteries.

Mycotic aneurysms are rare. Infection of the arterial wall is caused by bacteremia, direct spread from adjacent structures such as osteomyelitis of the vertebral body, or contamination through an aortoduodenal fistula. Frequently, there is an underlying atherosclerotic plaque or aneurysm. Infection results in destruction of the media and subsequent vessel dilation.

False aneurysms are commonly caused by trauma or disruption of vascular anastomoses. The trauma may be blunt or penetrating, acute or chronic. False aneurysms after vascular reconstruction result from disruption of the anastomosis. Degeneration of the arterial wall, fracture of suture material, infection, and degeneration of graft material are underlying causes.

EPIDEMIOLOGY. Atherosclerotic aneurysms are a disease of aging, diagnosed most frequently in the sixth, seventh, and eighth decades. A necropsy study of 4000 male veterans showed an increase in frequency of aortic aneurysms from 6% in the sixth decade to 14% in the ninth decade.

CLINICAL MANIFESTATIONS. Most abdominal aortic aneurysms are asymptomatic and are diagnosed at the time of physical examination or from roentgenograms of the abdomen or urinary tract. Symptoms are caused by compression, rupture, or emboli that pass to peripheral vessels. Vague abdominal pain, back pain, or tenderness over the aneurysm may result from rapid enlargement or be an early sign of rupture. Rupture produces blood in the retroperitoneal space, causing back pain and abdominal pain radiating into the groin. Shock and death follow the initial symptoms of rupture at a time interval dependent on the location and size of the rupture and the cardiovascular stability of the patient. Rarely, abdominal aortic aneurysms are first manifested by emboli to the extremities. These emboli may be small, causing skin discoloration suggestive of petechial lesions, or large, causing major vessel occlusion. Thrombosis of the aneurysm mimicking aortic bifurcation embolus or acute aortic occlusion is rare.

DIAGNOSTIC TESTS. Plain roentgenograms reveal calcification in the aortic wall in 55% to 85% of abdominal aortic aneurysms (Fig. 100-1). However, the right wall of the aorta frequently overlies the vertebral column, obscuring calcification, and variation of the roentgenographic tube-to-patient distance can cause magnification of the lesion.

Ultrasound provides an accurate measurement of the aortic diameter to within several millimeters. This study can detect thrombus in the lumen of the aorta and can differentiate retroperitoneal lesions overlying the aorta from abdominal aortic aneurysms. However, it cannot give exact localization of the aneurysm in reference to the renal arteries or iliac vessels.

Computed tomography detects abdominal aortic aneurysms, assesses the diameter of the aorta, and differentiates residual lumen from overall diameter. Currently it is reserved for paralytic ileus in which ultrasound is ineffective and for detection of suspected retroperitoneal hematoma or infection.

Arteriography is a preoperative study. Since thrombus lining the aneurysm preserves normal luminal diameter in many patients, arteriography may not diagnose an abdominal aortic aneurysm. Current indications for preoperative arteriography include impaired renal function, renovascular hypertension, aneurysms extending above the renal arteries, renal anomalies such as horseshoe kidney, and the presence of lower extremity ischemia.

Elective aneurysm resection

Untreated aneurysms may rupture. Size is the factor correlating best with the risk of rupture; the 5-year risk of rupture of a 4-cm aneurysm is less than 15%, whereas it is over 75% for an 8-cm aneurysm. It is generally agreed that the risk of rupture for an aneurysm of 6 cm exceeds the risk of operative intervention.

Abdominal aortic aneurysms occur in patients with other manifestations of atherosclerosis, including coronary and cerebrovascular disease. In a series of 108 patients with abdominal aortic aneurysms, 43% had cardiac disease, 43% had hypertension, 19% had chronic obstructive pulmonary disease, and 19% had renal disease. Despite the coexistence of other disease processes, an aneurysm greater than 6 cm requires surgical intervention because of the risk of rupture. A survey of representative series published from 1959 through 1978 placed operative mortality in the range of none to 18%. Recent series report operative mortality rates ranging from 3% to 7%. Identification of unusual associated conditions including multiple renal arteries, retroaortic renal veins, double vena cava, horseshoe kidney, and mycotic aneurysms, allowing the most appropriate surgical management, further decreases morbidity.

Complications of aortic aneurysm resection include renal failure, distal arterial insufficiency, colonic ischemia, infection of the prosthesis, and paraplegia. Proper fluid ad-

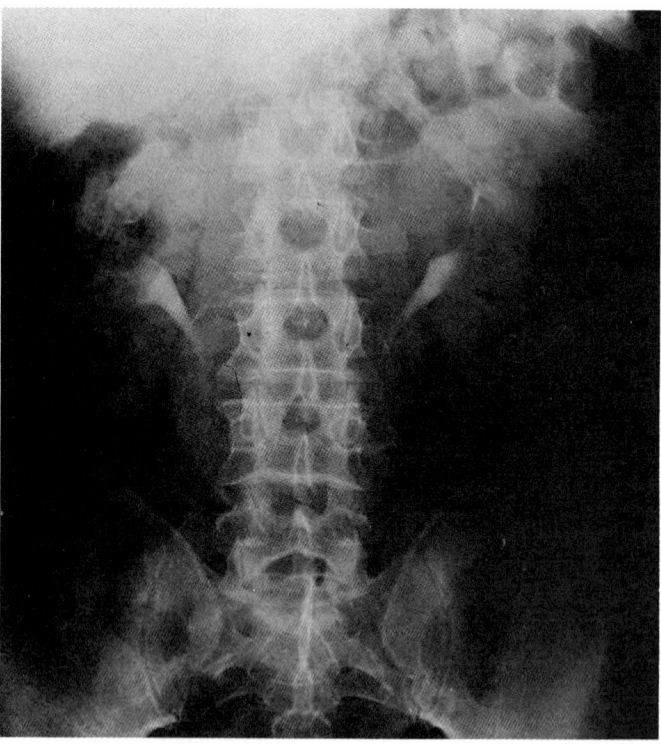

Fig. 100-1. Roentgenogram of abdomen showing calcification in wall of 8.5-cm aortic aneurysm. There is dye in renal collecting system from a urogram.

ministration during and after aortic procedures is critical in preventing hypotension and subsequent renal complications. Early clamping of the iliac arteries and decreased manipulation of the aneurysm reduce distal arterial insufficiency from intraoperative embolization. Bowel ischemia rarely occurs in the absence of superior mesenteric artery stenosis. Evaluation of the colonic blood supply before abdominal closure allows intraoperative correction of this rare problem by reimplantation of the inferior mesenteric artery. Infection of the aortic prosthesis occurs during implantation or from bacteremia after insertion. To decrease the risk of graft infection, patients with aortic implants receive prophylactic antibiotics before and after surgery and during any subsequent procedure that could result in bacteremia. The likelihood of graft infection decreases as the pseudointimal covering develops. Spinal cord ischemia is a rare complication that occurs in patients with severe atheroscleoris and anomalous blood suppy to the cord.

Ruptured abdominal aortic aneurysms

Abdominal aortic aneurysms most commonly rupture into the retroperitoneal space. This results in back pain and hypotension. The initial episode of hemorrhage generally causes transient symptoms followed by an asymptomatic period and then terminal cardiovascular collapse.

Despite improvements in surgical technique, the operative mortality associated with ruptured abdominal aortic aneurysms averages 50%. Factors that adversely influence survival are hypotension (systolic pressure less than 100 mm Hg), age, and severe blood loss. Symptomatic aneurysms require immediate surgery. Despite the high mortality of patients with ruptured abdominal aortic aneurysms, surgery is indicated even with marked hypotension, since the mortality of patients with unoperated ruptured aneuryms is 100%. Complications of resection of ruptured abdominal aneurysms include coagulopathy, bowel ischemia, renal failure, adult respiratory distress syndrome, arterial insufficiency of the extremities, and spinal cord ischemia. Myocardial infarction is a common cause of death despite successful resection. A decrease in mortality can be obtained by elective resection of aneurysms, thereby reducing the risk of rupture.

Popliteal artery aneurysms

Popliteal artery aneurysms are the most common extremity aneurysms, and atherosclerosis is the most common cause. Trauma induced by repeated flexion and extension of the knee joint combined with poststenotic turbulence produced by constriction at the adductor canal is thought to predispose patients to aneurysm formation at this level. Most patients with popliteal artery aneurysms are men in the 40- to 60-year age group.

Aneurysms at other sites are common. Bilateral popliteal aneurysms were found in 59% of patients in one series. In contrast to abdominal aortic aneurysms that result in rupture, popliteal aneurysms produce symptoms of limb ischemia from thrombosis of the aneurysm or distal embolization. Large popliteal aneurysms may compress the adjacent popliteal vein and nerves.

A thrombosed aneurysm may be confused with an abscess, tumor, or Baker's cyst in the popliteal fossa. Likewise, a cyst overlying the popliteal artery may transmit its pulsation and be incorrectly diagnosed as a popliteal aneurysm. Ultrasound of the popliteal fossa allows differentiation between overlying structures and a widened popliteal artery. Most reported symptomatic popliteal aneurysms are 2.5 to 5 cm in diameter. However, isolated reports of larger lesions have appeared in the literature. Arteriography to evaluate the outflow tract is required in the preoperative evaluation of the patient with popliteal aneurysm. Emboli from the aneurysm commonly cause occlusive disease in vessels below the knee.

Treatment of a popliteal aneurysm eliminates the risk of ischemic complications and restores adequate blood flow to the limb. Occasionally, excision of the aneurysm with end-to-end anastomosis of the artery or interposition graft is possible. In most cases ligation of the aneurysm with vein bypass graft is the procedure of choice.

Elective treatment of patients with asymptomatic popliteal aneurysms is associated with low morbidity and mortality. Asymptomatic lesions usually have an intact outflow tract, making reconstruction feasible. In contrast, popliteal aneurysms that are symptomatic as a result of embolization, rupture, or thrombosis are associated with a high amputation rate. Long-term follow-up observation of this patient population is required because of the frequent occurrence of other aneurysms, especially in the opposite popliteal artery and aorta.

ACUTE ARTERIAL INSUFFICIENCY

Acute arterial insufficiency is a sudden and marked decrease in arterial supply to an extremity. Sudden obstruction of a major artery not protected by adequate collateral circulation precipitates symptoms. The clinical manifestations are easily remembered by the mnemonic of five Ps: pain, paralysis, paresthesia, pallor, and pulselessness. Paralysis and paresthesia have important prognostic significance, since they result from ischemia of peripheral nerves and skeletal muscle. If paralysis or paresthesia is present, immediate intervention is required to save the limb.

The most common causes of acute arterial insufficiency are embolic and thrombotic occlusions. In young patients with known rheumatic heart disease, atrial fibrillation, or prosthetic valves, the diagnosis is straightforward. Patients in the atherosclerotic age range who have both significant cardiac disease and peripheral arterial disease present a diagnostic challenge. Less common causes of acute arterial insufficiency are dissecting aortic aneurysms with branch occlusion, intra-arterial drug injection, and vasospasm induced by ergot abuse. Occasionally, extensive venous thrombosis may mimic acute arterial occlusion.

Emboli

The source of the embolus is the heart in 94% of cases. Mitral stenosis, atrial fibrillation, acute myocardial infarction, ventricular aneurysm, left atrial myxoma, bacterial endocarditis, and prosthetic heart valves are predisposing conditions. In a series of 338 patients with emboli, 231 had atrial fibrillation, 50 had acute myocardial infarction, and 7 had atherosclerotic plaques. The source of emboli in the remaining patients was undetermined.

Emboli lodge at branch points or areas of arterial tapering such as the adductor canal. Following impaction of the embolus, stagnant flow in the distal circulation allows distal clotting or formation of a tail thrombus. If collateral circulation is poorly developed, signs and symptoms of acute arterial insufficiency occur. Most emboli lodge in arteries supplying the lower extremities: 46% in the femoral arteries, 18% in the iliac arteries, and 11% in the popliteal tibial tree. Emboli in the upper extremities and the cerebral, renal, and mesenteric arteries are less frequent.

Clinical symptoms occur rapidly. There is pain with decreased sensation and temperature of the limb. Examination of the pulses localizes the arterial occlusion. Neurologic evaluation determines the degree of ischemia. Decreased ability to differentiate light touch occurs before complete anesthesia. Paralysis and impaired motor function are late signs of severe arterial insufficiency. Loss of pliability of muscle mass indicates early tissue necrosis. Acidosis, hyperkalemia, and myoglobinuria result if treatment of acute arterial insufficiency is delayed, especially when large muscle masses are ischemic. Cardiac evaluation should exclude acute myocardial infarction, mural thrombosis, arrhythmia, and valvular disease. Abdominal examination is important at the time of initial evaluation, since there may be emboli in the mesenteric arteries. Abdominal distention or tenderness may indicate early bowel ischemia.

In patients in the atherosclerotic age group, it is difficult to differentiate between embolic and thrombotic occlusion. Arteriography may be helpful in these patients to determine the cause and the extent of the operative procedure required.

MANAGEMENT. Operative removal of the embolus is indicated in all patients except those with terminal disease. During the initial 6 to 12 hours, emboli can be removed with a minor surgical procedure using the Fogarty catheter. This restores arterial blood supply to the limb. Failure to remove emboli in the acute phase frequently results in amputation or major vascular reconstruction with higher morbidity and mortality.

Recently, intra-arterial infusion of large doses of urokinase or streptokinase has successfully restored perfusion in some patients if given early.

Anticoagulant therapy should be initiated as soon as diagnosis of distal embolus is established. Anticoagulation before operative intervention prevents the propagation of distal thrombus and obstruction of collateral flow to the limb. Long-term anticoagulation is important to prevent recurrence. In one study of hospitalized patients, emboli recurred in 9% of those who had received anticoagulant therapy and in 31% of those who had not. Sympathectomy and vasodilating drugs are not indicated.

CHRONIC ARTERIAL DISEASES OF THE AORTA AND ITS BRANCHES

Atherosclerosis is the major cause of chronic arterial insufficiency. Less common causes include Buerger's disease (thromboangiitis obliterans), cystic disease of the popliteal artery, trauma, vasculitis, popliteal entrapment, and Takayasu's arteritis (see Chapter 99). Progressive narrowing of the arterial lumen by atherosclerotic plaque produces symptoms when peripheral demands exceed flow across the narrowed segment. Collateral vessels supplement arterial flow distal to the stenosed or occluded segment. However, arterial flow through collateral arteries is limited by their small size and high resistance.

Branch points, areas of posterior fixation, and areas of compression are preferentially involved in atherosclerosis because of turbulent flow at these points. The terminal aorta below the inferior mesenteric artery, the posterior wall of the common femoral artery, the superficial femoral artery at the level of the adductor hiatus, and the popliteal trifurcation are frequent sites of extensive atherosclerotic plaque. Segmental involvement is treated surgically by the bypass technique.

CLINICAL MANIFESTATIONS. Symptoms of chronic arterial insufficiency include claudication, rest pain, and skin lesions. Claudication is pain in the calf resulting from decreased arterial supply to the gastrocnemius muscle. The pain occurs with exercise because the impaired arterial system cannot meet the metabolic demands of the exercising muscle. Aortoiliac or superficial femoral occlusions may cause claudication. Similar exercise-induced pain in the hip or buttock results from iliac disease. Intermittent claudication varies in intensity and is not a sign of impending limb loss. In a study of 1440 patients with intermittent claudication, survival was 73% at 5 years and 38% at 10 years. Most deaths resulted from coronary or cerebrovascular disease. The amputation rate was 7.2% at 5 years and 12% at 10 years. Conservative treatment of claudication includes abstinence from nicotine, control of hyperlipidemia and hypertension, and exercise. Vasodilating drugs are of questionable benefit. Indications for surgical treatment depend on the degree of disability, site of occlusion, and medical status of the patient.

Rest pain, or pain in the distal portion of the foot and toes, indicates severe arterial insufficiency and impending tissue loss. This pain arises from ischemia of the skin and nerves of the foot. Symptoms initially occur at night because of loss of gravity-induced arterial inflow. Aggressive investigation and treatment by surgical reconstruction are indicated for limb salvage in this group of patients.

Ulcerations may occur spontaneously because of poor nutritional supply to the skin, but minor trauma is more commonly identified as the initiating event. Small traumatic lesions may progress to gangrene in a limb with arterial insufficiency. Signs of arterial insufficiency that precede ulceration or gangrene are atrophic nails and skin and hair loss.

DIAGNOSTIC TESTS. During the past 10 years, development of techniques for noninvasive testing of arteries has introduced objectivity into the evaluation of occlusive disease. Doppler ultrasound (ankle blood pressure determinations and waveform analysis) and various plethysmographic techniques are now used to quantitate the degree of ischemia and define the level of hemodynamically significant arterial lesions. Blood pressure measurement obtained at the brachial, thigh, and ankle levels using the Doppler instrument as a sensor is the simplest of noninvasive testing methods. Blood pressure in the lower extremity should be equal to or greater than the brachial pressure in the absence of arterial obstructive lesions. Expression of the ankle pressure as a ratio over the brachial pressure may be used to quantitate ischemia. An index of 0.5 is compatible with claudication. An index of 0.3 indicates severe arterial insufficiency. Treadmill exercise testing is important to document the degree of disability from claudication and to differentiate neurogenic pain syndromes from arterial claudication.

Noninvasive testing has provided information on the natural history of arterial lesions. Pressure measurements have been used to predict the healing of traumatic ulcers of the foot, the success of revascularization procedures, and the level of amputation. Recently the measurement of penile arterial pressure has aided in the diagnosis of occlusion in patients whose impotence results from decreased arterial blood flow to the pelvis.

Although noninvasive testing gives the most accurate assessment of the effect of arterial occlusion on function of the extremity, arteriography provides a roadmap for the surgeon at the time of operation. High-quality fluoroscopic imaging, rapid sequence filming, and advancements in catheter techniques have provided clear visualization of the arterial tree. Films taken in multiple projections identify lesions in the iliac and femoral arteries previously undiagnosed by isolated anteroposterior projections. These advancements in arteriography allow optimal surgical treatment of arterial lesions by exact localization of the pathologic process. Arteriography is associated with low morbidity and mortality. The mortality rate of 0.5% results predominantly from hypersensitivity reactions to iodine contrast material. Serious complications, which have been reported in 0.3% to 2.3% of patients undergoing arteriography, include acute arterial occlusion caused by thrombus or subintimal dissection, hematoma, renal failure, and distal embolization.

SPECIAL TREATMENT CONSIDERATIONS. Patients with severe arterial insufficiency frequently have occlusion at more than one level. Proximal aortoiliac lesions are corrected first, and usually this results in limb salvage. Bypass procedures to the posterior tibial, anterior tibial, or peroneal artery are now possible. Visualization of the leg vessels and plantar arch on arteriography is critical for the diagnosis of all lesions and may require delayed filming.

If the infrapopliteal arteries communicate with a patent planter arch, patency rates are good. Limb salvage may result even in the presence of graft occlusion if the graft remains patent long enough to heal ischemic lesions. Sequential grafting from the popliteal to the distal tibial vessels has been suggested to improve outflow and patency rates.

The role of sympathectomy in the treatment of atherosclerotic occlusive disease is controversial, but direct arterial reconstruction, when possible, produces superior results. Sympathectomy is not indicated for claudication, since no increase in blood flow to the muscle results. Sympathectomy does increase blood flow to the skin to some extent and may be useful in healing small ischemic skin lesions. Complications include neuralgia and ejaculatory dysfunction or impotence in the male when bilateral sympathectomies at the first lumbar ganglion are performed.

Diabetic patients are at increased risk for lesions at all levels in the arterial tree. Classically, lesions are most likely to occur in the infrapopliteal area. Patients with diabetes mellitus more often require amputation with peripheral arterial disease. This increased risk to the limb results from the preferential distal location of the arterial occlusion, presence of neuropathy, and decreased resistance to infection.

Noninvasive laboratory evaluation is used to localize lesions and distinguish pain caused by peripheral neuropathy from ischemic rest pain. Some diabetic patients have extensive calcification in the arterial wall that invalidates ankle pressure readings. Arteriography is associated with increased risk in patients with diabetic arterial disease. Dye excretion through a kidney with diabetic nephropathy is associated with an increased risk of acute tubular necrosis. Patients should be well hydrated before the evaluation.

Arterial reconstruction is possible in many patients with diabetic arterial disease. Segmental distribution of arterial occlusions and the state of the runoff vessels predict the success of the procedure, as in all patients with atherosclerotic disease. Sympathectomy should *not* be performed in patients with diabetic neuropathy that has resulted in autosympathectomy.

Leriche's syndrome (aortoiliac disease)

In 1940 Leriche described symptoms and signs associated with thrombotic obliteration of the aortic bifurcation in relatively young patients. These symptoms include (1) weariness of the lower extremities with exercise; (2) symmetric atrophy of both lower extremities without trophic skin or nail changes; (3) pallor of the legs and feet; and (4) inability to maintain an erection owing to decreased internal iliac arterial supply. Aortoiliac disease is progressive and may result in limb loss when sequential arterial occlusions develop. Because these patients are predominantly middle-aged (35 to 55 years), symptoms of claudication are more disabling than in the geriatric age group. Operative intervention includes endarterectomy or bypass grafting. Today, aortofemoral bypass grafting is the preferred method of treatment in most hospitals. Mortality rates are in the range of 1% to 5%, with good 5- and 10-year patency rates. Complications include graft thrombosis, intraoperative embolization, false aneurysms at anastomosis, and graft infection. Retrograde ejaculation may result if dissection is performed at the aortic bifurcation.

Extra-anatomic bypass (axillofemoral and femorofemoral grafts) are used for patients with aortoiliac involvement who cannot tolerate the aortoiliac or aortofemoral approach. Femorofemoral grafts are also employed as primary procedures for occlusive disease localized to one iliac artery. Five-year patency rates of 70% to 90% have been reported.

Superficial femoral occlusion

Occlusion of the superficial femoral artery is common in patients over 65 years of age. Symptoms are most severe at onset, and a small percentage of patients require immediate operative reconstruction because of severe arterial insufficiency. Most patients have a gradual improvement in exercise tolerance over a 6- to 12-month period. In this group mild residual claudication often does not require operative intervention. Patients with more severe claudication and poor collateral flow around the lesion are treated by femoropopliteal bypass. A saphenous vein of adequate luminal diameter is the prosthesis resulting in the best long-term patency rate. When a saphenous vein is not available, other materials such as expanded polytetrafluoroethylene and umbilical vein are used. Complications include hematomas, thrombosis of the graft, saphenous nerve injury, edema of the lower extremity, and lymphocele. Patency rates are dependent on the status of the outflow system (runoff).

Buerger's disease (thromboangiitis obliterans)

In 1908 Buerger drew attention to a clinical syndrome caused by inflammation and occlusion of distal arteries by a specific pathologic process distinct from atherosclerosis. He named this syndrome thromboangiitis obliterans (TAO). Despite this precise description, the terms "Buerger's disease" and "thromboangiitis obliterans" have been used by some to characterize distal arterial insufficiency and gangrene from any cause. Others have questioned the existence of the specific pathologic process originally described. These terms should be limited to the pathologic lesion characterized by transmural inflammation of distal arteries accompanied by thrombosis. Histologic evidence of inflammation in adjacent veins and nerves is common.

In contrast to atherosclerosis, Buerger's disease is a rare entity estimated to cause 1% of arterial insufficiency. The disease occurs most commonly in young men of Middle Eastern origin. The cause is unknown, although cigarette smoking has been closely linked to the onset and progression of the disease. Other etiologic factors that have been suggested include infection, genetic predisposition, trauma, and cold injury.

Clinical manifestations of Buerger's disease include rest pain, gangrene, claudication, Raynaud's phenomenon, thrombophlebitis, and hyperhidrosis. Arterial insufficiency caused by the disease usually had a sudden onset. Because of the distal location of the arterial occlusion, rest pain and gangrene are common initial symptoms. Calf or foot claudication is the first symptom in 20% of patients. Both upper and lower extremity involvement occurs in over 10% of the patients. A clinical diagnosis of Buerger's disease is usually made by identifying the following criteria: (1) upper and lower limb involvement, (2) distal site of lesion, (3) history of heavy cigarette smoking, (4) sparing of proximal arteries, and (5) phlebitis. Histologic examination of distal vessels is valuable in establishing the diagnosis and excluding atherosclerosis. Determination of the erythrocyte sedimentation rate, antinuclear antibodies, and rheumatoid factor is helpful in excluding other forms of vasculitis.

Treatment begins with prohibition of cigarette smoking. Smoking is the most important factor in predicting the progression of Buerger's disease. The distal site of arterial occlusion excludes arterial reconstruction in most patients. Rest pain and localized gangrene are therefore treated by sympathectomy and conservative amputation.

BIBLIOGRAPHY

Bernstein, E.F., Harris, R.D., and Leopold, G.R.: Ultrasound and CT scanning in the noninvasive evaluation of abdominal aortic aneurysms. In Bergan, J.J., and Yao, J.S.T., editors: Surgery of the aorta and its body branches, New York, 1979, Grune & Stratton, Inc.

Fogarty, T.J., and Bush, W.S.: The management of embolic and thrombotic arterial occlusion. In Rutherford, R.B., editor: Vascular surgery, Philadelphia, 1977, W.B. Saunders Co.

Greenhalgh, R.M., and Mills, S.P.: On Buerger's "disease": a recognizable syndrome. In Bergan, J.J., and Yao, J.S.T., editors: Gangrene and severe ischemia of the lower extremities, New York, 1978, Grune & Stratton, Inc.

Gross, W.S., and others: Comparison of noninvasive techniques in carotid artery occlusive disease, Surgery **82:**271, 1977.

Hight, D.W., Tilney, R.L., and Couch, N.P.: Changing clinical trends in patients with peripheral arterial emboli, Surgery **79:**172, 1976.

Kartchner, M.M., and McRae, L.P.: Clinical application of oculoplethysmography and carotid phonoangiography. In Bernstein, E.F., editor: Noninvasive diagnostic techniques in vascular disease, St. Louis, 1978, The C.V. Mosby Co.

Lawrie, G.M., and others: Improved results of operation for ruptured abdominal aortic aneurysms, Surgery **85:**483, 1979.

Malone, J.M., Moore, W.S., and Goldstone, J.: The natural history of bilateral aortofemoral bypass grafts for ischemia of the lower extremities, Arch. Surg. **110**:1300, 1975.

Thompson, J.E., and Garrett, W.V.: Peripheral-arterial surgery, N. Engl. J. Med. **302**:491, 1980.

Thomson, J.E., and Talkington, C.M.: Carotid endarterectomy, Ann. Surg. **184**:1, 1976.

Thompson, J.E., and others: Surgical management of abdominal aortic aneurysms, Ann. Surg. **181**:654, 1975.

DENTAL CORRELATIONS

Louis F. Rose, Philip Godfrey, and Barbara J. Steinberg

CONGESTIVE HEART FAILURE

Heart failure may be the outcome of virtually any aberrant cardiac process; therefore the syndrome must be considered a possibility in all patients of advanced age or indicative cardiac history. Following an evaluation designed to discover a history of specific cardiac lesions, individuals should be questioned about those symptoms classically associated with cardiac decompensation: fatigue, dyspnea on exertion, orthopnea, paroxysmal nocturnal dyspnea, and dependent edema. In patients known to have a history of previous cardiac failure, the answers to these same questions can provide important clues to the current state of compensation and the adequacy of therapy. Any change in such a patient's pattern of symptoms should prompt the dentist to postpone treatment and consult the individual's physician.

As has already been noted, the patient with early heart failure typically presents few signs when unstressed. The anxiety that many patients experience in the dental office can make a dental visit a substantial test of cardiac stamina, requiring the dentist's diligence in seeking out both frank and more subtle evidence of decompensation.

CLINICAL MANIFESTATIONS. Significant hypertension in a patient displaying symptoms of congestive heart failure is reason enough for immediate referral (see section on hypertension). Tachycardia, however, is not uncommon in dental surroundings and need not imply autonomic compensation for declining stroke volume. However, suspicions should be aroused when tachycardia is sustained or associated with other hard evidence of heart failure. An irregularity in the pulse may suggest arrhythmia as the basis of a patient's heart failure, but more often the disordered rhythm will prove to be secondary to the underlying process actually producing the decompensation (such as valvular disease and cardiomyopathy). Since even short episodes of tachypnea are less common in the dental operatory than is tachycardia, respiratory rate may sometimes prove a more accurate barometer of cardiac reserve than heart rate. The reclining dental chair provides the practitioner with the means to observe any respiratory changes associated with recumbency, but one should not assume that all discomforts of the supine patient are attributable to orthopnea.

Mucocutaneous color changes can accompany cardiac decompensation. Peripheral cyanosis (for example, as seen in the nail beds) results from exaggerated local extraction of oxygen from blood sluggishly pumped through reflexly constricted vessels. When mucous membranes become blue (central cyanosis), a more serious condition occurs in which one may surmise the existence of significant intrapulmonary shunt. This latter situation will only be seen when left ventricular filling pressures have risen to levels great enough to produce distressingly obvious pulmonary symptoms, such as pulmonary edema.

Patients suffering limited but chronic impairment of gas exchange may develop polycythemia in response to chronic hypoxia. Alone, absolute increases in hemoglobin level may be expected to produce a ruddiness in the complexion. However, when desaturation persists to the extent that 5 g/dl of hemoglobin remains reduced (the amount necessary for clinical cyanosis), the outcome is a curiously purple coloration of the skin. On occasion, hypoxic stimulation of erythroid marrow elements is so pronounced that myeloid and megakaryocytic activity are depressed. Where significant neutropenia is the result, particularly vigorous treatment of odontogenic infection is indicated. Oral purpuras may develop as a result of associated thrombocytopenia, but the dentist is obligated to exclude other causes of disordered primary hemostasis before settling on such a diagnosis.

Neck vein distention is important to evaluate, but may be easily misinterpreted. Tight collars must be loosened and the patient's position taken into account before tenable conclusions may be drawn. For the dentist's purpose it is sufficient to observe the patient in the upright position, where the jugular veins may be considered as erect water manometers. Visible distention of these vessels will occur only when central venous pressure is sufficient to hold a column of blood above the level of the clavicles (approximately 12 cm H_2O). Such a pressure should be considered abnormal. Questionably abnormal observations may be tentatively corroborated by observation of peripheral veins. *In the absence of any peripheral obstruction to flow,* the veins on the dorsum of the hand should empty when elevated above the level of the heart. Continued distention of these vessels is further evidence for an elevation of central venous pressure.

DENTAL MANAGEMENT. First among the management responsibilities of the dentist is the limitation of stress. Short visits, simple explanation of treatments, and adequate pain control are by far the most important measures to be undertaken. For patients with a long history of anxiety in the dental office, sedation may be appropriate. However, the dentist must be alert for interaction between sedative agents and medicine employed in the treatment of heart failure. (For example, barbiturates and opiates may exaggerate the orthostatic hypotensive responses created by thiazides and loop diuretics.) Patients who have once experienced orthopnea may only begrudgingly shed their fear of recumbency even when treatment has restored them sufficiently to allow supination. The understanding practitioner will accommodate these individuals by treating them in the same semierect position used for those truly orthopneic patients.

The dentist also serves his patients through his diligent search for toxic side reactions to anti–heart failure medicines. The elderly edentulous patient with a complaint of xerostomia may also suffer from lethargy and muscle fatigue that he had assumed to be unrelated. It would indeed be unfortunate if the practitioner did not at least suspect that such complaints might reflect electrolyte imbalance from diuretic therapy. The disturbingly low therapeutic index of digitalis preparations obligates the dentist to seek evidence of their intoxicity as well. The potential gravity of digitalis-toxic arrhythmias makes it possible for the dentist to save a life by simply palpating a pulse or heeding a half-hearted complaint of palpitation.

Acute dyspnea, anxiety, frothy productive cough, and cyanosis herald the onset of acute pulmonary edema. Should such signs occur in the dental office, the following list of actions is recommended:

1. Keep patient erect.
2. Administer oxygen.
3. Administer meperidine hydrochloride (Demerol), 50 mg intramuscularly, or morphine sulfate, 4 mg intramuscularly. (Be prepared to manage airway and support respirations.)
4. Apply tourniquets to extremities to maintain blood pressure above venous pressures and below systolic arterial pressure. (This measure should only be used in extreme situations when patient does not respond to first three measures and hospital transportation is slow in coming.)
5. Arrange for patients' immediate transportation to hospital.

HYPERTENSION

So ubiquitous is hypertension that the practicing dentist is involved in the care of many individuals affected with this disease and its sequelae. Current consensus suggests that the practitioner has a dual role to play in interaction with the hypertensive individual; first, as a clinician who works to ferret out undiagnosed disease, and second, as a member of the medical/dental partnership that is created to ensure that such disease neither prevents access to needed dental therapy nor precipitates cardiovascular crisis in those treated.

A personal and family history of hypertensive cardiovascular disease should be sought from each new patient. Similarly, a systems review designed to discover symptoms of hypertensive sequelae should be standard procedure. One should not be surprised to learn how often a patient with no hypertensive history will admit to symptoms of a disease that ultimately proves to have occurred on a hypertensive basis, for example, orthopnea in a patient with hypertensive left ventricular failure without previous history of high blood pressure. Of course, the depth to which the practitioner questions the patient must depend on the clinical situation; the elderly or those with a positive family history or currently high sphygmomanometric findings deserve the closest scrutiny. Having been acquainted with the major causes of secondary hypertensive disorders, the dentist should search for symptoms of these disorders (Table 1).

CLINICAL MANIFESTATIONS. Essential hypertension presents no standard set of orofacial manifestations on which the dentist can rely for its detection. Sphygmomanometric examination of every new patient should be performed, both as a screening tool and as a method of securing baseline information of potential use in any future cardiovascular crisis. Head and neck examination may reveal evidence of hypertensive sequelae, such as the jugular venous distention of heart failure, or of underlying conditions known to produce secondary hypertension, such as the periorbital edema of nephrotic renal disease. A list of physical findings of particular interest in secondary hypertension is noted in Table 1.

DENTAL MANAGEMENT. Except in those instances when examination reveals blood pressure values that are abnormal in malignant proportion, hypertension is never diagnosed based on a single, isolated reading. Fig. 1 presents a flow chart that may be of some aid to the practitioner in those cases where an abnormal blood pressure is detected. As evidenced by this chart, the dental office should serve not only as a place from which initial referral may originate but also as a site for the appraisal of patient compliance and the relative effectiveness of the antihypertensive regimen.

Although an acute exacerbation of hypertension is always to be avoided, the need to prevent episodes of relative hypotension must be strongly underscored. An individual with significant hypertensive vascular disease may depend on a chronic elevation of pressure to provide adequate perfusion of vital organs, hence the oft-noted circumstance of persistent hypertension in the controlled individual. Therefore interventions that produce significant depression of arterial pressure can be potentially devastating to the end organs, even in situations in which the measured values remain within the normal realm. The dentist should always be aware of the measured values that constitute good control in each individual case.

After detection and the institution of appropriate therapy, the ultimate concern of the dentist is the safe delivery of needed services to the hypertensive community. Because hypertensive patients are known to overreact to both

Table 1. Clinical findings of secondary hypertension

	Signs	Symptoms
Renovascular disease	Hypertension beginning before age 30, after age 50	Symptoms of other vascular disease (peripheral vascular disease, ischemic heart disease, etc.)
Renal parenchymal disease	Uremic syndrome (uriniferous breath, pallor, periorbital edema, purpura, uremic frost, etc.)	Fatigue lassitude, nausea, vomiting, hematuria, polyuria, nocturia, easy bruising, weight loss
Coarctation of the aorta	Decreased pulse and blood pressure in lower extremities, infected dental canal increases in size radiographically	Headache, epistaxis, cold extremities, claudication
Pheochromocytoma	Tremor, mydriasis, signs of multiple endocrine neoplasia syndrome III (marfanoid, prominent lips; neuromas of tongue, lips, conjunctiva) Orthostatic hypotension, jugulotympanic ganglionic tumors with VII-XII palsies	Headache, palpitations, diaphoresis, postural dizziness, anxiety, tremor, weight loss
Cushing's syndrome	Moon facies, acne, hirsutism, truncal obesity, ecchymosis, edema	Weight gain, emotional lability, fatigue, polyuria, polydipsia, amenorrhea
Conn's syndrome	Signs of renal parenchymal disease excluding edema (renal disease on basis of hypokalemia)	Headache, polyuria, polydipsia, muscle weakness
Hyperthyroidism (systolic elevation only)	Tremor, tachycardia, proptosis, lid lag, poor convergence, periorbital edema, onycholysis	Anxiety, palpitations, heat intolerance

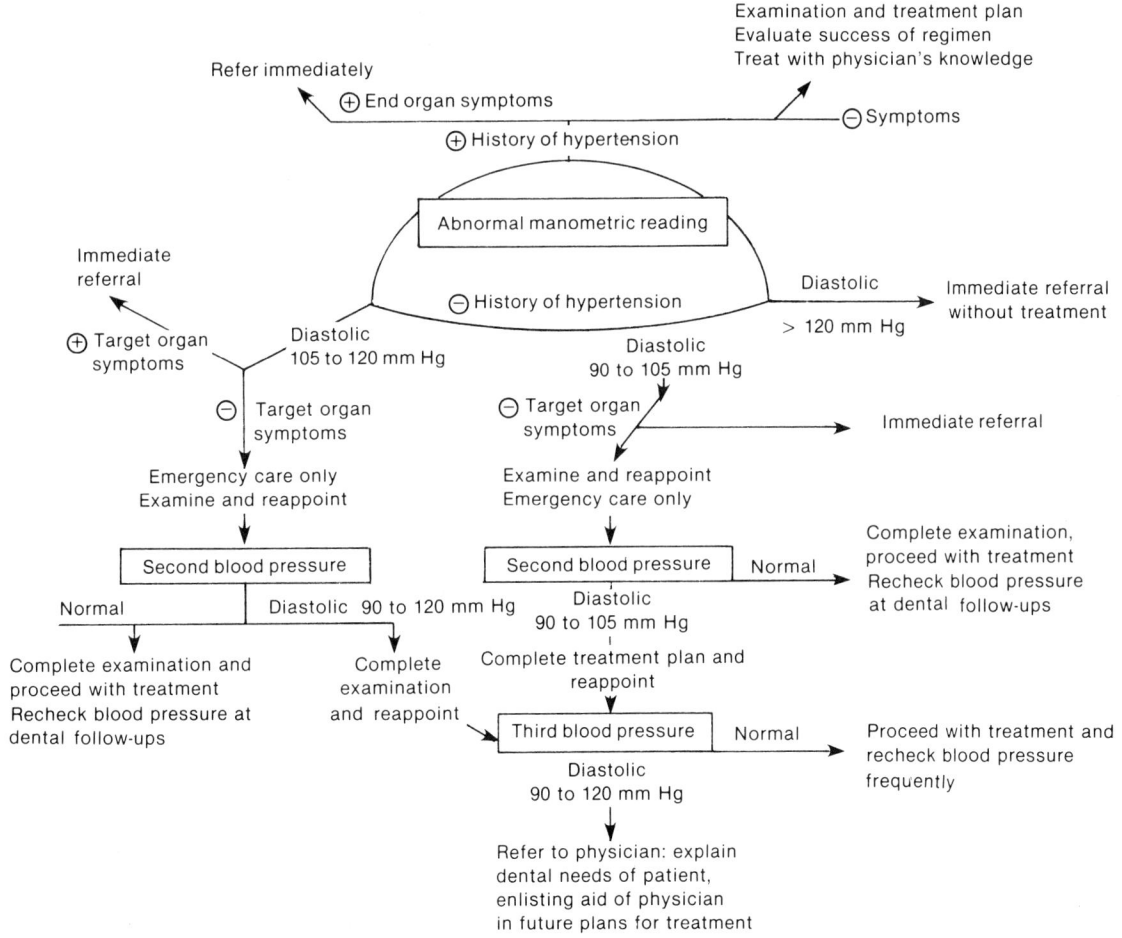

Fig. 1. Evaluation and management of the hypertensive dental patient.

pressor and depressor stimuli, the practitioner should structure every aspect of treatment to optimize the control of anxiety and pain. Significant psychic upheaval during dental treatment, or even in anticipation of such treatment, may precipitate an acute elevation of blood pressure and subsequent emergency, such as heart failure, myocardial infarction, or stroke. Among the dentist's most effective weapons against such a situation are forthrightness and demeanor. No sedative or tranquilizer can equal in importance the influence of good dentist/patient rapport on the well-being of the hypertensive patient. It is therefore of particular importance that the dentist approach all such individuals calmly and confidently, explaining the treatment plan and the design of the team approach used by dentist and physician.

The successful management of the hypertensive patient will also depend on the adequacy of pain control. Both pain and its subsequent relief may produce exaggerated vasomotor responses. It is thus best to provide adequate, long-lasting anesthesia so that the patient need not deal with either the stress or its precipitous removal. The long-expressed notion that pressors should not be used in the local anesthetic management of hypertensive patients has proved to be largely unfounded. It is now generally accepted that situations characterized by anesthesia of insufficient depth or longevity entail the release of endogenous catecholamines in amounts that far exceed those found in anesthetic preparations. This should not be interpreted to mean that these agents may be used with abandon but rather that the dentist should use the smallest quantity of medication consistent with patient comfort. The New York Heart Association has stated that under no circumstances should the total epinephrine dose exceed 0.2 mg in the patient with cardiovascular disease (the equivalent of approximately 18 to 20 ml of solution with 1:100,000 epinephrine or 10 carpules). For the rare patient treated with the monoamine oxidase inhibitor, vasoconstrictor substances are contraindicated.

In those instances where dental manipulations are too involved to be performed effectively under local anesthesia, general anesthetics must, of course, be used. Because of the risks associated with these measures (and particularly the risk for hypotension), it is not recommended that general anesthetics be used on an outpatient basis in patients with significant hypertensive cardiovascular disease. Medical consultation and hospitalization will frequently be in the patient's best interest. For similar reasons, caution must also be exercised in the use of inhalation agents, such as nitrous oxide, for outpatient conscious sedation. Hypoxia may produce startling increases in arterial blood pressure, with calamitous results.

Dentists should be familiar with the actions and side

Table 2. Potential side effects and interactions of commonly used antihypertensive drugs

Antihypertensive drug	Side effects	Interactions
Thiazides	Gastrointestinal upset, weakness, photosensitivity, azotemia, hypokalemia, hyperglycemia	Enhance responsiveness to D-tubocurarine
Propranolol	Bradycardia, congestive heart failure, increased bronchial asthma, hallucinosis, Raynaud's phenomenon, weakness, depression	Epinephrine may produce bradycardia
Loop diuretics (furosemide)	Azotemia, hyperuricemia, hypokalemia, photosensitivity	Enhance D-tubocurarine
Potassium-sparing		
Spironolactone (Aldactone)	Hyperkalemia, gynecomastia, hirsutism	Aspirin may inhibit natriuresis
Triamterene	Hyperkalemia, diarrhea, nausea	
α-Methyldopa (Aldomet)	Orthostatic hypotension, drowsiness, depression, xerostomia, impotence, positive Coombs test, gynecomastia	
Clonidine	Xerostomia, drowsiness, impotence, orthostatic hypotension, rebound hypertension with sudden cessation	
Reserpine	Drowsiness, sedation, weakness, nasal congestion, depression, bradycardia	Hypotension with general anesthesia
Hydralazine	Headache, tachycardia, palpitations, increased angina and congestive heart failure, "lupus" syndrome	
Guanethidine	Orthostatic hypotension	Alcohol increases orthostatic hypotension (hypotension with general anesthesia)
Prazosin	Orthostatic hypotension with syncope, dizziness, weakness, blurred vision, nausea, diarrhea, headache, palpitations	

effects of the commonly used antihypertensive agents. Although less commonly employed today than in the past, reserpine preparations should evoke particular concern in the practitioner, being at times responsible for depression of affect, syncope, and profound hypotension. Because of the drug's mechanism of action (catecholamine depletion), hypotension will be refractory to so-called indirect pressors (such as ephedrine) and should be treated with direct agents (such as norepinephrine or phenylephrine). Table 2 provides information on the side effects of the commonly used antihypertensive medicines.

Also of general interest to the dentist is the frequent occurrence of orthostatic hypotension in individuals taking antihypertensive medication. Routine attention to the need for slow resumption of the erect posture after treatment sessions will help eliminate postoperative dizziness and syncope.

There has long been a question as to the existence of increased bleeding in hypertensive surgical patients. Although the question remains unresolved among those concerned with essential hypertension, there is general agreement that aortic coarctation does contribute to increased bleeding from the inferior alveolar and individual dental arteries. The combination of high blood pressure and dilation of vessels proximal to the coarctation will often produce excessive bleeding after intraoral surgery, and particularly after the extraction of teeth.

If the dentist is alert to the signs and symptoms of target organ insult and employs the management techniques herein described, the likelihood of serious hypertensive crisis occurring in the dental office is small. If and when such crises do occur, one may at least be consoled to know that they are likely a coincidental result of the patient's disease, not the direct result of the dentist's intervention. These crises may take many forms, the most common being acute heart failure, myocardial infarction, cerebrovascular accident, acute renal failure, and hypertensive encephalopathy.

Naturally, the risk for other acute sequelae of hypertension is present as long as the blood pressure remains out of control. Should a crisis occur in the dental office, it is the responsibility of the dentist to provide basic care as in any situation of coma or major seizure (for example, airway management and protection of the patient from convulsive injury). Arrangements for prompt removal of the patient to an appropriate medical facility must be coordinated with these efforts.

The following is a summary of those measures most appropriately used in the management of all hypertensive patients:

1. Obtain a comprehensive medical history.
2. Provide for close coordination of detection and management efforts with the physician.
3. Be aware of the patient's medications, their side effects, and interactions.
4. Arrange short appointments to limit stress.
5. Reduce stress through the establishment of good rapport and the use of sedative agents where indicated.
6. Provide for adequate pain control, with the use of epinephrine kept to the essential minimum.
7. Provide for slow resumption of the erect posture after treatments.

BIBLIOGRAPHY

Abbey, I.M.: Screening for hypertension in the dental office, J. Am. Dent. Assoc. **88**:563, 1974.
Berman, C.L., and others: High blood pressure detection by dentists, J. Am. Dent. Assoc. **87**:359, 1973.
Burch, G.E., and DePasquale, N.P.: Arterial hypertension and the dental patient, J. Am. Dent. Assoc. **73**:102, 1966.
Chue, P.W.Y.: Hypertension: implications for dentistry, J. Dent. Pract. **51**:25, 1975.
Freedman, G.L., and Hooley, J.R.: Medical contraindications to the extraction of teeth, Dent. Clin. North Am. **13**:939, 1969.
Jastak, J.T., and Cowan, F.F.: Patients at risk, Dent. Clin. North Am. **17**:363, 1973.
Little, J.W., and Jakobsen, J.: Management of the hypertensive patient in dental practice, J. Oral Med. **29**:13, 1974.
Stout, F.W.: What about therapy for your hypertensive patients? Fla. Dent. J. **49**:14, 1978.
Vernale, C.A.: Cardiovascular response to local dental anesthesia with epinephrine in normotensive and hypertensive subjects, Oral Surg. **13**:942, 1960.
Wessberg, G.: Role of screening for hypertension in patient management, J. Am. Dent. Assoc. **96**:1040, 1978.

SHOCK

True circulatory shock in the dental office is a rare occurrence. However, the dentist's indiscretion with surgical procedures or in prescribing drugs may make him or her culpable should the patient subsequently arrive at the hospital emergency ward in extremis. Only by eliciting a complete medical history can the practitioner hope to avoid those treatments likely to precipitate crisis in the compromised individual.

Septic and hypovolemic shock

Treatment modifications whose purpose is the prevention of shock are few and easily implemented. When special risk for sepsis exists (for example, in a patient undergoing chemotherapy with steroids), aggressive management of dentoalveolar infection can do much to decrease the incidence of warm shock. The earliest evidence that infection is no longer localized and is spreading is indication enough for hospitalization of such individuals. Analgesic compounds containing aspirin must be prescribed with care so that the anticoagulated individual or ulcer patient is not threatened by serious hemorrhagic complications. Similarly, the patient with bleeding diathesis must command the use of unusual surgical precautions if a normally benign procedure is not to end in exsanguination.

Anaphylactic shock

The medical history may also enable one to avoid anaphylactic shock, a situation more common in the dental office than septic or hypovolemic shock. Devastating anaphylactic reactions can and do occur in dental facilities, and many might be prevented by giving more attention to the allergic history. Specific past reactions to medicines should be sought during all initial evaluations, with particular emphasis given to reports of untoward results from penicillin use. Because patients will commonly ascribe any unpleasant experience with a drug to allergy (for example, upset stomach), the dentist must be prepared to interpret the significance of reported symptoms. The anaphylactoid symptoms that should be sought include antic, urticarial rash (hives), angioedema (swelling of lips, tongue, or larynx), and bronchospastic wheezing with dyspnea. A history of atopy (hayfever, asthma, or eczema) also confers a greater risk for anaphylaxis, even when history of specific drug reactions is wanting.

Although orally administered medications can produce calamitous reactions including shock, parenteral injections are more often the cause. Also, the extent of a reaction can often be foretold on the basis of its rapidity of onset, the response usually occurring within minutes. For these reasons it should be policy to ask that all patients remain in the office for a minimum of ½ hour after any parenteral administration of penicillin. Should symptoms subsequently develop, the dentist will be available to intervene immediately.

Anaphylactoid reactions exist along a continuum stretching from simple hives to circulatory collapse. The dentist must be prepared to provide acute care for any of the phenomena in this continuum. Table 3 describes the signs and symptoms of mild and severe allergic reactions, as well as the preferred course of action in each.

Cardiogenic shock

The dentist will not likely see cardiogenic shock except in the guise of arrhythmic death. The reader is referred to the section on coronary heart disease for a consideration of cardiopulmonary arrest.

Vasovagal syncope

The preceding comments concerning the rarity of shock in the dental office do not, of course, apply if one is to include vasovagal syncope within the definition of circulatory collapse. Syncope refers to an abrupt loss of consciousness, the causes of which are manifold. The common faint is a maladaptive cardiovascular response to stress, not infrequently associated with the sight of blood or hypodermic needles. A prodromal or presyncopal stage may include giddiness, confusion, visual disturbances, pallor, diaphoresis, or nausea and vomiting. If these symptoms are quickly addressed by placing the patient in a Trendelenburg position, loss of consciousness may be prevented. When such is not the case, true syncope will follow, characterized by hypotension, bradycardia, and occasionally limited clonic activity. Treatment includes supination of the patient with elevation of the legs, airway protection, and administration of oxygen. Aromatic spirits of ammonia may be used to stimulate respiration, but only rarely will other forms of medical intervention be required. When consciousness is not restored by these techniques and hypotension and bradycardia persist, slow intravenous administration of 0.5 to 1.0 mg atropine is indicated. The administration of atropine in doses of less than 0.5 mg is to be avoided, as this may produce idiosyncratic exacerbation of bradycardia.

Whenever fainting has occurred, the patient should be allowed to rest comfortably and encouraged to arise slowly. The patient with a history of atherosclerotic dis-

Table 3. Allergic reactions (may be drug induced)

	Signs and symptoms	Treatment
Mild allergic reaction	1. Nasal obstruction with rhinorrhea and sneezing 2. Tearing of eyes 3. Skin—rash with itching 4. Edema of hands, face, eyelids, larynx	1. Diphenhydramine (Benadryl) 50 mg intramuscularly *or* 2. Epinephrine 1:1000, 0.2-0.5 ml subcutaneously
Severe allergic reaction (anaphylactic shock)	1. Pulse—rapid, thready 2. Blood pressure—profound decrease 3. Respiration—dyspnea, bronchial constriction, laryngeal edema 4. Skin—hives, urticaria, petechiae 5. Pain—abdominal	1. Establish airway 2. Oxygen therapy 3. Establish intravenous route 4. Epinephrine 1:1000, 0.5-1.0 ml intravenously 5. Diphenhydramine (Benadryl) 50 mg intramuscularly 6. Hydrocortisone ½-1 g intramuscularly or intravenously

From Rose, L. F.: Continuing dental education, vol. 1, no. 3, Philadelphia, Dec. 1977, The University of Pennsylvania.

ease, who has responded to conservative treatment of syncope, should undergo at least cursory examination for evidence of end-organ damage. Whenever hypotension and bradycardia have been sustained enough to require the use of atropine, it is appropriate to arrange for examination of the patient by the physician. In either case, the patient should be reappointed for dental treatment on a future date, before which time appropriate measures can be taken to deal with the anxiety that precipitated the syncope (for example, a plan for sedation).

PULMONARY EMBOLISM

CLINICAL MANIFESTATIONS. Pulmonary embolism may occur in any setting, including the private dental office, although it is particularly common in the hospital, where patients are predisposed by both infirmity and incapacity. The dentist should be acquainted with those measures most commonly used to help prevent pulmonary embolism and should routinely include these in orders for the hospitalized patient.

It is good to remember that any of three conditions may predispose the patient to venous thrombosis; vascular stasis, vessel wall disease, or disruption and hypercoagulability of blood. Statistically, stasis is the most important of these conditions and is minimized by early postoperative ambulation or the use of support hose and daily leg exercise when extended bed rest is necessary. These measures are of particular importance in patients with a history of phlebitic disease. The hospital dental practitioner should examine all patients at bed rest for signs of thrombophlebitis and should be alert to complaints of leg pain or swelling. Thrombophlebitis is also an important consideration in the differential diagnosis of postoperative fever, especially when such fever occurs several days after surgery and cannot be traced to wound infection or infection of the urinary tract. Although hypercoagulability of blood is an uncommon problem, the abrupt withdrawal of anticoagulants produces rebound hypercoagulation on occasion. For this and other reasons, the dentist should never act apart from the physician in discontinuing or pharmacologically reversing anticoagulant medicines.

DENTAL MANAGEMENT. When medical illness constitutes predisposition to pulmonary embolism, the dentist may consult the physician without hesitation. However, the dental practitioner should have the clinical and pharmacologic knowledge sufficient to allow for the circumspect implementation of the physician's recommendations. It is also critical for the dentist to thoroughly explain the dental therapeutic needs of the patient to the physician, so that the consultant may formulate a plan that reflects a complete understanding of the procedures to be performed.

Anticoagulation. Although chronic anticoagulation is not without its own intrinsic morbidity, the risk for unfortunate sequelae increases when surgery must be performed. The dental surgeon must be versed in the management of the anticoagulated patient in order to avoid numerous and unnecessary referrals. An understanding of hemostatic surgical principles and basic anticoagulant pharmacology is the only requisite to competent management of these patients.

Coumarin. Coumarin preparations (for example, warfarin [Coumadin]) are the only agents currently used for outpatient anticoagulation. They exert their effect through the competitive inhibition of vitamin K, with subsequent depletion of those coagulation factors dependent on that substance for their synthesis (that is, factors II, VII, IX, and X). The half-life of these drugs requires that they be discontinued at least 2 days prior to the time at which normal coagulation studies might be desired. Only rarely, however, will the dentist's need for cessation of therapy be compelling enough to justify the risk for thrombosis pursuant on such action. When contemplating procedures likely to cause bleeding, it is appropriate to ask that the physician make those dosage adjustments necessary to keep the prothrombin time between 1½ and 2 times the control. When this is accomplished, the hypoprothrombinemia is effectively countered with vigorous local hemostatic measures that, depending on the procedure performed, might include tension sutures over foam gelatin or the insertion of stents. Constant local pressure and soft diet are frequently beneficial.

Heparin. Anticoagulation is accomplished on an acute basis through the parenteral administration of heparin. Only infrequently will the dentist be called on to care for individuals so treated. Because effective hemostasis after extraction or mucogingival surgery is extremely difficult, only the most acute dental emergencies can be treated in the heparinized patient. When blood loss is anticipated, heparin must be discontinued for 4 to 6 hours before the procedure and should be reinstituted as soon as effective primary hemostatis has been observed. Definitive dental management is never appropriate in the heparinized patient.

• • •

When local hemostatic measures fail in the anticoagulated patient, pharmacologic manipulation becomes necessary. If the coumadinized patient can tolerate a wait of several hours, vitamin K administration will enhance his hemostatic ability. More urgent situations demand the transfusion of fresh frozen plasma. Where prompt reversal of heparin is in order, protamine sulfate is the drug of choice. (The dentist should seek medical assistance in any situations requiring measures such as these.)

Rules useful in the treatment of the anticoagulated patient are as follows:
1. For treatments likely to cause bleeding (deep scaling, curettage, mucogingival surgery, or extraction)

see that the coumadinized patient has a prothrombin time no greater than 2 times the control.
2. Use strict hemostatic surgical technique.
3. Employ vigorous local hemostatic measures, including primary closure where possible, foamed gelatin, soft tissue packs, and/or stents.
4. Remember that direct pressure is the most effective antihemorrhage measure even in the anticoagulated patient.
5. Whenever possible use the Cavitron for gross scaling, rather than curets, as the latter will more commonly lacerate the gingiva and aggravate bleeding.
6. Acute dental conditions should not be prolonged but rather be given immediate attention.
7. Communicate to the physician the nature of your treatment and enlist the physician's aid in management when medical intervention is required.

PRIMARY PULMONARY HYPERTENSION

Primary pulmonary hypertension is an uncommon disorder that presents no specific clinical findings in the head and neck region. Although evidence of central venous pressure elevation in a patient with "butterfly" rash or Raynaud's phenomenon might suggest the possibility of primary pulmonary hypertension to an astute clinician, such combinations will more often prove to be the result of other processes, such as lupoid pericardial disease, high output heart failure from the anemia of Felty's syndrome, and cardiomyopathy of systemic sclerosis, etc.

It is appropriate to discuss dental manifestations in this case as a platform for the reemphasis of those diagnostic principles most critical to the entire cardiovascular section.

The dentist who would provide competent, complete care to all who might request it should learn to seek syndromes and not diagnose when evaluating the general health of patients. Only by this means can historical questions and examination procedures finally transcend rote to become truly useful and complementary; only by this method may the practitioner develop a true clinical sense of a patient's status, regardless of underlying disorders. Although it is not our intention to minimize the importance of knowledge concerning specific processes and their signs (indeed, these are detailed throughout the text), it is our belief that recognition of the common patterns of physiologic derangement is crucial to any plan for the detection of disease and the management of its victims.

Thus primary pulmonary hypertension will not betray its specific nature to the examining dentist but may well yield historical or physical evidence for the syndromes of heart failure, myocardial ischemia, or disordered cardiac rhythm. These clinical syndromes will then become the center of the dentist's concern in managing the patient (see sections specific to these processes).

DENTAL MANAGEMENT. The limited ability of individuals with primary pulmonary hypertension to tolerate stress has already been emphasized. Counseling and oral hygiene instruction are of obvious value in limiting the need for extensive and stressful dental treatment. Those individuals requiring restorative and/or surgical therapy will benefit from the dentist's efforts to limit anxiety and pain.

Patients taking hydralazide (Hydralazine) may be more prone to syncope in the dental situation; those anticoagulated against pulmonary embolus will require measures commonly employed in the anticoagulated state (see chapter on pulmonary embolus). Although medical management of dental pain or infection is in no way contraindicated, the timing of definitive treatment and the location chosen for its delivery (that is, office or hospital) must depend on the patient's previous dental experience and current state of compensation. Consultation with the physician is always appropriate.

CONGENITAL HEART DISEASE

CLINICAL MANIFESTATIONS. Rarely does the dental patient with congenital heart disease betray his condition during the orofacial examination. Although it is the responsibility of the dentist to be aware of those external physical characteristics that may suggest underlying cardiac abnormality, such as Down's facies or elfin facies, the dentist must also realize that the typical ambulatory patient with congenital cardiac impairment will display little physical evidence of such derangement. The blue mucosa and integument of central cyanosis, so characteristic of right-to-left shunting lesions, is most often observed in those too young and infirm to have come under the dentist's care. When some clinically detectable hypoxemia does persist on a chronic basis, a change in the depth of cyanosis should always be sought by the dentist as evidence of hypoxic decompensation. This may occur in patients who have previously undergone only palliative treatment or in an individual whose formerly marginal shunt has been increased by a second process (such as increasing pulmonary hypertension).

Anomalies of the dentition may bring children with cyanotic disease under the dentist's care, requiring each consultant to be aware of the frequent association between hypoplasia of the primary dentition and cyanotic heart disease. Delay in the formation of the permanent teeth has also been demonstrated in this group. Other reported oral findings, such as furrowed tongue in tetralogy of Fallot and enlargement of maxillary incisor pulp chambers in coarctation of the aorta, are too variable and nonspecific to be of great use in the clinical detection of disease.

Because the upper extremities are easily accessible to the dentist, they should always be examined for clubbing of the fingers. Although this condition is uncommon and may be mimicked by benign disorder, such as familial pachydermoperiostitis, its presence could indicate underlying congenital heart disease.

DENTAL MANAGEMENT. The preceding comments indicate the need for complete history taking, for it is by this method that the patient's congenital disease will most often come to the dentist's attention. Once having elicited a history of congenital disease, the dentist may appropriately seek medical consultation. However, regardless of the specific nature of the patient's lesion, the management must always entail concern for infection, heart failure, and arrhythmia. Exacerbation of heart failure or arrhythmia by the stress of the dental situation or by dental pharmaceuticals is dealt with elsewhere in this section.

INFECTION. Dentoalveolar infection is more common and potentially more devastating in individuals with congenital heart disease. In 1946 Kaner and others demonstrated that dentin is poorly calcified in those with congenital heart disease and that this may predispose such individuals to caries. Such vulnerability is particularly troublesome when it is coupled with the overindulgence of a parent concerned about the child's long-term prognosis. Indeed, studies have shown that oral hygiene and dietary habits are worse among individuals with congenital heart disease than among the general population. Although it is clear that more consistent professional intervention is necessary to improve the oral health of those afflicted with congenital heart disease the high DMF (decayed, missing, and filled teeth) scores found among these patients indicates a poor future prognosis for the general health of the group. As is true for persons with endocardial disease of any variety, those marked by congenital cardiovascular anomaly are at increased risk for infective endocarditis, a risk that increases whenever surgical treatment of the disease requires the insertion of a prosthesis. Given the present recognition of the oral cavity as the most common origin of transient bacteremia, it is clear that the patient risks grave disease from both self-neglect and improper dental treatment. Optimal oral health is necessary to minimize the incidence of significant spontaneous *or* iatrogenic bacteremia. To further decrease risk in the treatment situation, antibiotic chemoprophylaxis is usually indicated. The reader is referred to pp. 581 and 582 concerning accepted antibiotic regimens and the relative risk for endocarditis in each of the disease states. Because those prophylactic schedules presently in favor were derived largely on an empiric basis, the reader is cautioned to remain current with the literature in anticipation of future modifications.

Systemic septic embolization, a form of so-called paradoxic embolization, is common among those with focal infection and congenital heart disease. Brain abscess is a dire consequence of such a process and should be suspected in any child with congenital heart disease who complains of headache. Because cultures of brain abscesses usually grow a mixed spectrum of anaerobic organisms, and because the floral spectrum is so similar to that known to exist within the gingival crevice, oral infection and dental manipulations must be considered as important instigators of brain abscess in the child with congenital heart disease. Valachovic and Hargreaves believe pulpectomy to be contraindicated in the primary dentition of those with congenital heart disease, since root resorption can expose untreated accessory canals that might seed the blood with organisms. Citing a case of brain abscess traced to an endodontically treated primary tooth, they recommend extraction of any tooth with "clinical or radiographic evidence of apical or furcational periodontitis."

In summary, the treatment plan for those with congenital heart disease must include the following:

1. Medical consultation to learn the specific nature of the defect, specific past history, and risk for decompensation or arrhythmia.
2. Antibiotic prophylaxis for all dental procedures in an effort to avoid endocarditis and brain abscess.
3. Prompt and vigorous treatment of all oral infection, with extraction to be considered the preferred treatment for endodontically involved primary teeth.
4. A frank and open discussion with the parents and patient, detailing the importance of strict oral hygiene and regular dental care to both the oral and the general health of the patient.

BIBLIOGRAPHY

Berger, E.: Attitudes and preventive dental health behavior in children with congenital cardiac disease, Aust. Dent. J. **23**(1):87, 1978.

Hakala, P.E., and Haavikko, K.: Permanent tooth formation of children with congenital heart disease, Proc. Finn. Dent. Soc. **70**:63, 1974.

Heineman, H.S., and Braude, A.I.: Anaerobic infection of the brain, Am. J. Med. **35**:682, 1963.

Kaner, A., Losch, P.K., and Green, H.: Oral manifestations of congenital heart disease, J. Pediatr. **29**(3):77, 1946.

Raimondi, A.J., Matsumoto, S., and Miller, R.A.: Brain abscess in children with congenital heart disease, Int. J. Neurosurg. **23**:588, 1965.

Socransky, S.S., and Manganiello, A.D.: The oral microbiota of man from birth to senility, J. Periodontol. **42**:485, 1977.

Sorenson, H.: The pedodontic patient with heart disease, Dent. Clin. North Am. **17**(1):177, 1973.

Valachovic, R., and Hargreaves, J.A.: Dental implications of brain abscess in children with congenital heart disease, Oral Surg. **48**(6):500, 1979.

VALVULAR HEART DISEASE

CLINICAL MANIFESTATIONS. In the modern practice of dentistry an accurate medical history is as essential to proper patient evaluation as the radiograph. Of great importance in this inquiry are those questions designed to discover structural endocardial disease. Although the dentist must remain vigilant for signs of heart failure or arrhythmia in patients with such disorders, the foremost concern remains the entity of endocarditis.

During each patient evaluation a history of congenital or rheumatic heart disease must be sought, as well as a history of heart murmur and rheumatic fever. When rheumatic fever is denied, it is wise to inquire specifically about childhood episodes of polyarthritis, "growing pains," chorea, or prolonged febrile infirmity. It is not uncommon for patients to be unaware that such illnesses

Table 4. Revised Jones criteria for the diagnosis of rheumatic fever

Major manifestations	Minor manifestations
Carditis	Fever
Polyarthritis	Arthralgia
Chorea	Previous rheumatic fever or rheumatic heart disease
Erythema marginatum	Elevated erythrocyte sedimentation rate or positive C-reactive protein
Subcutaneous nodules	Prolonged pressoreceptor interval on electrocardiograph

Plus evidence of antecedent streptococcal infection; positive throat culture, rise in antistreptolysin O or other streptococcal antibodies.

Although the diagnosis of rheumatic fever is made on the basis of clinical judgment, the presence of two major manifestations, or one major and two minor manifestations, is considered highly suggestive if supported by evidence of previous streptococcal infection.

---

may have been episodes of rheumatic fever. (See Table 4 for Jones criteria for the diagnosis of rheumatic fever.)

Because so-called benign or functional cardiac murmurs are relatively common and require no modification of dental management, it is important that the practitioner make some effort to distinguish these from murmurs whose presence indicates organic disease. This can often be done with the help of the patient alone, since most people reporting a murmur will have been concerned enough about its significance to have queried their physicians. Whenever doubt remains, direct consultation with the physician is recommended. Also, since heart failure is the final common pathway in chronic heart disease, specific questions concerning this syndrome are appropriately included in the interrogation (dyspnea on exertion, paroxysmal nocturnal dyspnea, orthopnea, etc.). Although such questions will only occasionally lead to the discovery of new disease, they will always provide valuable information concerning the patient's cardiac reserve and his ability to meet the stress of treatment.

Hard physical findings within the realm of the dentist are not the rule with valvular heart disease, but important information may sometimes be gleaned through careful evaluation of the vital signs and examination of the head, neck, and extremities. The physical findings herein described are variable and should not be considered pathognomonic of valvular disease. They may, however, prove important warning signs when discovered in those individuals with questionable history of rheumatic fever or murmur or known murmur previously assumed to be benign.

Systemic arterial blood pressure is usually normal in the ambulatory patient with mitral valve disease, but the patient with aortic insufficiency will often show systolic hypertension and a widened pulse pressure. In contrast, significant systolic hypertension is uncommon in the stenotic form of aortic valve disease.

Attention should be directed to the carotid pulse, where rate and regularity are noted. An irregular tachyarrhythmia is likely atrial fibrillation, a rhythmic disturbance commonly associated with the dilated left atrium found in rheumatic mitral disease. Frequent extrasystole in a young woman may be the result of the ventricular automaticity seen in mitral valve prolapse.

Considering the pulse's character provides more data, a sharp, regular upstroke being common in mitral regurgitation (where normal sinus rhythm exists) and a slow, weak upstroke with delayed and sustained peak the characteristic of aortic stenosis. Aortic insufficiency classically yields the bounding Corrigan or "water-hammer" pulse mentioned above, and this may have a double or bisferiens character (this latter quality also being seen in hypertrophic cardiomyopathy). Of lesser clinical use but of no small interest are several other pulses associated with aortic insufficiency, two of which were already noted. The head bobbing of Musset's sign and throbbing nail beds of Quincke's disease are equaled in curiosity by a rhythmic pulsation of the uvula named for Müller.

Tachypnea should never be ignored unless it is short lived and obviously related to anxiety. When observed in a patient complaining of dyspnea it should always prompt a search for other signs of decompensation. It is important to remember that some individuals with mitral disease are subject to chronic pulmonary transudation and are at increased risk for respiratory infection. Tachypnea may result from either the underlying problem or its sequelae. Similarly, the persistently febrile patient with known valvular disease may suffer if his fever is too quickly attributed to oral pathosis. Despite its relatively low incidence, infective endocarditis is responsible for morbidity and mortality sufficient in magnitude to justify a septic workup when fever has persisted for more than a week.

Just as symptoms of heart failure may be uncovered in the history, so must physical evidence of decompensation be sought during the examination. Jugular venous distention, ankle edema, and cyanosis are important signs that the dentist should not overlook (see congestive heart failure). The much-touted relationship between a malar-flush and mitral stenosis is, to say the least, controversial, and many believe that this facial ruddiness is more related to the ethnic background of the original study group than to their underlying disease.

Finally, a search for physical evidence of certain predisposing illnesses should be undertaken. The spinal stiffness of ankylosing spondylitis or saddle nose of syphilis may prompt concern for aortic insufficiency. Similarly, a

Marfan's habitus should alert the practitioner to the possibility of mitral valve prolapse, aortic insufficiency, or aortic dissection.

Endocarditis

Risks for the dental patient with valvular heart disease are basically three; heart failure, hemodynamically significant arrhythmia, and infective endocarditis. The first two are compelling problems and are discussed elsewhere in this section. The dental considerations of endocarditis and its prevention are of great concern and will be discussed here.

The medical aspects of endocarditis are treated in detail in the section on microbial disease. Therefore it is sufficient to say that infection of the endocardium is a grave disorder, the incidence of which is largely dependent on the occurrence of transient bacteremia in those with existing valvular heart disease. Particularly distressing is the fact that these heart diseases may render their victims vulnerable to infection with endogenous organisms not ordinarily virulent in the human host.

Studies begun nearly five decades ago have shown the oral cavity to be the single most important area of regular bacterial ingress. Although the early works concerned themselves largely with postextraction bacteremia, more recent papers have established that virtually every dental procedure can seed organisms into the blood. In fact, simple mastication alone with no associated invasive tissue manipulation can produce bacteremia in many individuals. Logically, the risk for such bacterial entry has been found to be related to the level of oral health, and particularly that of the periodontium.

Since the first work of Okell and Elliott in 1935 the significance of *Streptococcus viridans* bacteremia has been widely known. This group of organisms, whose ravages are ordinarily limited to the oral cavity, is one of the most common culprits in subacute bacterial endocarditis. Modern anaerobic culture techniques have also proved that anaerobes commonly found in the gingival sulcus are culpable in increasing numbers of cases.

Based on this knowledge, one might understandably surmise that today's predisposed dental patient is in little peril. Unfortunately, surveys continue to show that such is not the case. Many at risk remain uneducated concerning the need for optimal oral health and special drug prophylaxis before dental surgery. Because these same patients continue to seek and secure regular dental care, it is imperative that dental practitioners be aware of their responsibility to these individuals.

DENTAL MANAGEMENT. It is not at all uncommon to find considerable variability among medical practitioners concerning the approach to chemoprophylaxis. The most recent American Heart Association standards are as follows:

Regimen A—penicillin

1. Parenteral-oral combined:

Adults: Aqueous crystalline penicillin G (1,000,000 units intramuscularly) mixed with procaine penicillin G (600,000 units intramuscularly). Give 30 minutes to 1 hour prior to procedure and then give penicillin V (formerly called phenoxymethyl penicillin) 500 mg orally every 6 hours for 8 doses.†

*Children:** Aqueous crystalline penicillin G (30,000 units/kg intramuscularly) mixed with procaine penicillin G (600,000 units intramuscularly). Timing of doses for children is the same as for adults. For children less than 60 lbs, the dose of penicillin V is 250 mg orally every 6 hours for 8 doses.†

2. Oral:

Adults: Penicillin V (2.0 gm orally 30 minutes to 1 hour prior to the procedure and then 500 mg orally every 6 hours for 8 doses.)†

*Children:** Penicillin V (2.0 gm orally 30 minutes to 1 hour prior to procedure and then 500 mg orally every 6 hours for 8 doses.° For children less than 60 lbs, use 1.0 gm orally 30 minutes to one hour prior to the procedure and then 250 mg orally every 6 hours for 8 doses.)†

For patients allergic to penicillin:

Use either vancomycin (see Regimen B) *or* use:

Adults: Erythromycin (1.0 gm orally 1½-2 hours prior to the procedure and then 500 mg orally every 6 hours for 8 doses.)†

Children: Erythromycin (20 mg/kg orally 1½-2 hours prior to the procedure and then 10 mg/kg every 6 hours for 8 doses.)†

Regimen B—penicillin plus streptomycin

Adults: Aqueous crystalline penicillin G (1,000,000 units intramuscularly) mixed with procaine penicillin G (600,000 units intramuscularly) plus streptomycin (1 gm intramuscularly). Give 30 minutes to 1 hour prior to the procedure; then penicillin V 500 mg orally every 6 hours for 8 doses.†

*Children:** Aqueous crystalline penicillin G (30,000 units/kg intramuscularly) mixed with procaine penicillin G (600,000 units intramuscularly) plus streptomycin (20 mg/kg intramuscularly). Timing of doses for children is the same as for adults. For children less than 60 lbs the recommended oral dose of penicillin V is 250 mg every 6 hours for 8 doses.†

For patients allergic to penicillin:

Adults: Vancomycin (1 gm intravenously over 30 minutes to 1 hour). Start initial vancomycin infusion ½ to 1 hour prior to procedure; then erythromycin 500 mg orally every 6 hours for 8 doses.†

*Children:** Vancomycin (20 mg/kg intravenously over 30 minutes to 1 hour).** Timing of doses for children is the same as for adults. Erythromycin dose is 10 mg/kg every 6 hours for 8 doses.†

Footnotes to Regimens:

*Doses for children should not exceed recommendations for adults for a single dose or for a 24-hour period.

**For vancomycin the total dose for children should not exceed 44 mg/kg/24 hours.

†In unusual circumstances or in the case of delayed healing, it may be prudent to provide additional doses of antibiotics even though available data suggest that bacteremia rarely persists longer than 15 minutes after the procedure. The physician or dentist may also choose to use the parenteral route of administration for all of the doses in selected situations.

> **Categories of risk for subacute bacterial endocarditis**
>
> 1. Greatly increased risk: regimen B
>   a. Prosthetic valve
>   b. Indwelling vascular catheter
> 2. Increased risk: regimen A or B
>   a. Valvular heart disease
>   b. Intracardiac shunts including patent ductus arteriosus, ventricular septal defect, and atrial septal defect of the primary type
>   c. Hypertrophic cardiomyopathy (idiopathic hypertrophic subaortic stenosis, hypermetropic astigmatism)
>   d. Hydrocephalus with ventricular-atrial shunt
> 3. Minimally increased risk: regimen A
>   a. Mitral valve prolapse
>   b. Transvenous cardiac pacemaker
>   c. Artificial atrioventricular fistula for renal dialysis
>   d. Synthetic arterial grafts
> 4. No increase in risk: no antibiotics
>   a. Recent angiography or cardiac catheterization
>   b. Uncomplicated atrial septal defect of secondary type
>   c. Coronary artery surgery
>   d. Shedding primary teeth

A commonly used list of disorders for which prophylaxis is believed to be required, and the relative risk for endocarditis in each, is given in the box above. Although the standards may be considered a near-consensus, they are empirically derived, and hence subject to change.

It is important to note that despite the declining incidence of rheumatic fever, the dentist can still expect to encounter patients with a history of rheumatic heart disease who receive regular chemoprophylaxis against the recurrence of group A β-hemolytic *Streptococcus* infection and rheumatic fever (that is, monthly injections of benzathine penicillin, or daily oral doses). Such treatment should in no way be construed as adequate prophylaxis against subacute bacterial endocarditis. Because oral organisms resistant to the chronically administered medication are known to appear soon after the inception of such therapy, the dentist is advised to consult with the patient's physician to arrange for a substantial increase in the penicillin dose or for the substitution of another drug (usually erythromycin) during dental treatment.

As important as appropriate antibiotic prophylaxis is to the patient's continued health, it must be stated in summation that the dentist's efforts to foster optimal oral health are perhaps even more significant. As has been shown, dental manipulation is in no way essential to the genesis of bacteremia, and it must be assumed that frequent showers of organisms are the rule in individuals with neglected mouths. Perhaps the dentist performs the greatest service for this group when he or she succeeds in significantly modifying their oral hygiene behavior so that septic "suicide" can no longer be inadvertently accomplished.

BIBLIOGRAPHY

Benter, I.B., and others: Comparative effects of local and systemic antibiotic therapy in the prevention of post-extraction bacteremia, J. Am. Dent. Assoc. **57**:54, 1958.

Benter, I.B., and Pressman, R.S.: Antibiotic treatment of the gingival sulcus in prevention of postextraction bacteremia, J. Oral Surg. **14**:20, 1956.

Burket, L.W., and Burn, C.G.: Bacteremia following dental extraction: demonstration of source of bacteria by means of a nonpathogen, J. Dent. Res. **10**:521, 1937.

Eisenbud, L.: Subacute bacterial endocarditis precipitated by non-surgical dental procedures, Oral Surg. **15**:624, 1962.

Feinstein, A.R., and others: Prophylaxis of recurrent rheumatic fever, J.A.M.A. **206**:565, 1968.

Hobson, F.G., and Juel-Jensen, B.E.: Teeth, *Streptococcus viridans*, and subacute bacterial endocarditis, Br. Med. J. **2**:1510, 1956.

Kaplan, E.L., and others: Prevention of bacterial endocarditis, Circulation **56**(1):139A, 1977.

McGowan, D.A., and Tuohy, O.: Dental treatment of patients with valvular heart disease, Dent. J., p. 519, 1968.

Okell, C.C., and Elliott, S.D.: Bacteremia and oral sepsis with special reference to the etiology of subacute endocarditis, Lancet **2**:869, 1935.

Spencer, W.H., and others: Rheumatic fever, chemoprophylaxis, and penicillin-resistance gingival organisms, Ann. Intern. Med. **73**:683, 1970.

CARDIOMYOPATHY

CLINICAL MANIFESTATIONS. Cardiomyopathy does not in general have clinical findings in the cervicofacial structures. Lipoidoses may reveal coarse facies, macrocephaly, or numerous angiomas.

DENTAL MANAGEMENT. Management is the same as that of heart failure and arrhythmia. The reader is referred to the appropriate sections for discussion of these topics.

CORONARY HEART DISEASE

CLINICAL MANIFESTATIONS. Pain is the most perplexing of the chief complaints; no other symptom is at once as demanding of solution and defiant of the doctor's analytic efforts. The discussion of the ischemic heart may provide the most appropriate framework within which to reiterate those clinical principles useful in the general interpretation of pain. Some of these principles may help to distinguish between like discomforts originating from systems as distinct and different as those devoted to circulatory and stomatognathic function.

The dentist should employ a standard protocol in the characterization of pain, in each instance seeking answers to the following questions:

What is the location of the pain?

What is its character? Is it constant or intermittent, sharp or aching?

How long has it been present and what was the nature of its onset?

Is there a pattern of referral?

Are there any initiating or exacerbating factors?

What, if anything, alleviates the pain?

Has the patient experienced similar pain in the past, and if so, how has this episode been different?

Are there any associated symptoms?

Although the location of a pain is often of great help in the elucidation of its nature, too great reliance on this one characteristic has led many practitioners to unfortunate and inaccurate conclusions. A discomfort localized to the jaw, whose other characteristics are atypical of gnathic affliction, demands that related systems be evaluated. That 18% of all cardiac pain is localized solely in the teeth and jaws is ample evidence of the need for full evaluation in each case.

Admittedly, most who suffer with coronary artery disease are aware of the diagnosis before any evaluation is accomplished by the dentist. However, a knowledge of the character of pain is no less important when the history has revealed significant pathophysiology. The determination of a patient's ability to withstand stress must be largely based on the stability of the coronary occlusive process. This is most reliably determined by an evaluation of the ischemic pain pattern, and any change in the frequency or character of painful episodes necessitates postponement of dental treatment and cardiologic reevaluation.

DENTAL MANAGEMENT. Angina sufferers whose pattern of pain is established and unchanging are good risks in the dental office. For those who typically experience frequent bouts of angina after minor exertion, preoperative use of nitroglycerine is indicated. Although sedation can also be of great help in specific instances, it should, of course, be used judiciously. When the hypotension of deep sedation is superimposed on a critical coronary lesion, myocardial infarction may result. Indeed, the dentist must structure treatment to ensure the maintenance of that critical balance between myocardial oxygen demand and the ability of the coronary arteries to supply this substrate. Short morning appointments, adequate anesthesia, and sedation are among the measures that may help to limit stress and therefore myocardial oxygen needs. The avoidance of even small drug-related depressions in blood pressure will protect the coronary perfusion that is so dependent on the maintenance of the gradient between diastolic arterial and left ventricular end-diastolic pressures.

Studies support the view that vasoconstrictors may be used in combination with local anesthetics. Although the New York Heart Association proposes a limit of 0.2 mg epinephrine for those with cardiovascular disease, one is rarely justified in using more than 0.036 mg in patients with symptomatic coronary artery disease (2 carpules of local anesthetic with 1:100,000 epinephrine). The chronotropic, inotropic, and arrhythmogenic potential of catecholamines only amplify the importance of deliberate aspiration before anesthetic deposition. The use of local hemostatic agents such as epinephrine impregnated gingival cord cannot be condoned, since sizable doses of the drug may be absorbed through gingival vessels. Particular care should be exercised when epinephrine is administered to those receiving propranalol. The increased vagal tone resulting from epinephrine-related elevation of blood pressure normally has no bradycardic consequences, owing to the offsetting chronotropy of the drug. When this B-stimulatory effect is blocked by propranalol, however, unopposed vagal stimulation can produce bradycardia and hypotension.

The dentist may also have an impact on the patient's well-being through ongoing concern for the control of atherosclerotic risk factors. Regular sphygmomanometric examinations are important factors in effective antiohypertensive program and may uncover changes in arterial impedance of critical significance to cardiac workload. Surprisingly, the detailing of oral damage attributable to tobacco use and dietary indiscretion may occasionally prove effective in modifying patient behavior.

When angina occurs during dental treatment, the procedure should be halted, nitroglycerine administered, and the patient allowed to rest. If such pain does not represent significant departure from the patient's anginal pattern, dental treatment may be completed. When pain has a new character, such as requiring 2 nitroglycerine tablets for relief rather than the usual single dose, treatment should await reevaluation by the physician. Any pain that remains unrelieved after three doses of nitroglycerine given every 5 minutes, that lasts more than 15 to 20 minutes, or that is associated with diaphoresis, nausea, vomiting, syncope, or hypotension should prompt concern for myocardial infarction. The patient should be given oxygen and 5 to 10 mg of morphine sulfate intravenously for pain and anxiety. Vital signs must be closely monitored while arrangements are made for immediate transportation to hospital facilities.

Should cardiopulmonary arrest occur while aid is still forthcoming, it is the responsibility of the dentist to make the diagnosis and institute treatment. The office staff should be trained in basic life support and the dentist should be knowledgable in advanced life support so that he or she may perform any advanced resuscitative measures that may be required (such as endotracheal intubation or central venous cannulation).

Following myocardial infarction, elective dental treatment is contraindicated for a minimum of 6 months. After complete evolution of the myocardial scar, management will depend on the clinical course, including postinfarction angina and arrhythmias. The physician should always be consulted to determine whether any specific contraindications to elective office therapy exist. If no problems are noted, the dentist may proceed with treatment, employing those principles used when caring for the patient. However, it is good to temper one's treatment, since the reinfarction rate remains disproportionately high for approximately 2 years in the postinfarction group.

ARRHYTHMIA

The dentist's detection of arrhythmia, whether through inquiry or examination, often justifies medical consultation before the initiation of therapy. Not every patient admitting to palpitation requires medical evaluation. Such an evaluation should be reserved for those who report frequent and distressing paroxsyms; associated symptoms such as dizziness, angina, dyspnea, and syncope; or past history of significant heart disease.

CLINICAL MANIFESTATIONS. The dentist's examination may occasionally provide clues to the nature of the arrhythmia, but it should not be expected to substitute for communication with the physician. Regular waxing and waning of heart rate in concert with respiration is characteristic of sinus arrhythmia, a normal phenomenon in children and adults but a common harbinger of sinus node disease in the elderly. Irregular rhythms may have cyclical patterns, as in atrial or ventricular bigeminy, or may be characterized only by chaos (such as atrial fibrillation or multifocal atrial tachycardia).

Indeed, it is in general less crucial to identify an arrhythmia than to observe its circulatory impact. A short-lived paroxysm of supraventricular tachycardia that brings with it angina or syncope commands more of the dentist's concern than a chronic dysrhythmia lacking perfusion compromise. There are then but two major concerns in the evaluation of arrhythmia. The dentist must learn (1) the hemodynamic significance of the rhythm; and (2) the propensity of that rhythm to degenerate into forms of even greater hemodynamic consequence. Both will depend in large measure on the underlying process responsible for the observed alterations.

DENTAL MANAGEMENT. Before considering the dysrhythmias common to each of the major cardiopathologic processes, we should first describe those treatment principles essential to the management of any rhythmic disturbance occurring in the dental office. Cessation of therapy and the administration of oxygen are among those measures appropriate in all situations of new or sustained arrhythmia, as are an immediate hemodynamic evaluation and the summoning of medical help. An appraisal of the patient's mental alertness, blood pressure, heart rate, and skin temperature will provide important clues to the adequacy of perfusion and in no way depends on the presence of sophisticated monitoring equipment.

Hypotension demands the use of the Trendelenburg position but does not in itself justify pharmacologic intervention except when accompanied by persisting symptoms of end-organ oligemia (such as angina, confusion, or coma). In the setting of brady-arrhythmia, symptomatic hypotension is appropriately addressed with the intravenous administration of 0.5 to 1.0 mg atropine sulfate. Similarly, life-threatening hypotension with tachyarrhythmia should be treated with vagal maneuvers. However, the risks of carotid massage require that the dentist use this technique only when it is truly necessary. The practitioner must be prepared to support the patient should syncope, cerebrovascular accident, or vagal arrest ensue.

Because medical treatment directed specifically at the arrhythmia is often impossible without electrocardiographic monitoring, definitive management must usually await the patient's transportation to the hospital. For those practitioners who possess the necessary skill and equipment, interventions beyond those already described may be appropriate. Fortunately, the supportive actions discussed will usually suffice until such time as medical help is available.

Patients with no underlying cardiac disease seldom suffer more than psychic disturbance from arrhythmia. Both atrial and ventricular ectopic beats are common in an otherwise healthy heart. In fact, it has long been held that stress and compulsive activity are the progenitors of much functional heart disease. The practitioner should employ those measures commonly used to reduce stress in the office, so that the patient will not come to expect the precipitation of symptoms with each dental visit.

Valvular heart disease commonly underlies arrhythmia; the atrial dysrhythmias of rheumatic mitral disorders are an example. When atrial fibrillation is chronic and ventricular rate is adequately controlled through digitalization, little need be done by the dentist save the implementation of standard endocarditis precautions. Should new atrial fibrillation develop in the dental office, the measures already described will frequently provide the time required for transportation of the patient to an emergency facility. In those rare instances when fulminant cardiac failure supervenes, rapid digitalization (that is, 0.25 mg digoxin by slow intravenous push) or syncronous electrocardioversion should be considered. (WARNING: Digitalis must be used with caution for the treatment of atrial fibrillation in the setting of acute myocardial infarction.)

The premature ventricular contractions of mitral valve prolapse are rarely of consequence, but paroxysms of supraventricular tachycardia may distress both dentist and patient alike. If the patient is unable to terminate his attack through accustomed vagal maneuvers, sedation and reassurance will often prove effective. Most patients with supraventricular tachycardia do quite well and may be easily transported to hospital facilities if the rhythm persists.

Patients with cardiomyopathy are subject to a host of rhythmic disturbances, with atrial fibrillation, ventricular extrasystoles, and paroxysmal ventricular tachycardia being of particular note. The appearance of frequent multiformed premature ventricular contractions or bursts of ventricular tachycardia require treatment with intravenous lidocaine (50 to 100 mg intravenous push as bolus to be followed by a 2 to 4 mg/min drip when the rescue squad arrives). Ventricular tachycardia with hypotension and obturation demands early asynchronous electric cardioversion.

Although premature ventricular contractions and ventricular tachycardia should also prompt the practitioner to suspect ischemic heart disease, the patient with coronary artery disease may occasionally suffer spontaneous ventricular fibrillation. Immediate 400 watt-second defibrillation will help to avoid the intractable arrhythmias so common with the acidosis of prolonged circulatory arrest. Basic life support measures are called for should defibrillation fail.

Although the dentist's role in the treatment of arrhythmic emergency may be a critical one, his or her part in the prevention of such catastrophies is of more far-reaching import. Combining knowledge of both the individual patient and the disease entities of concern, the dentist must modify the treatment plan in ways that will accurately reflect the risks involved. Both impulsiveness and undue caution may precipitate a medical emergency. The young individual with functional disease or paroxysms of supraventricular arrhythmia should require little more than effective anxiety control. However, the elderly patient with ischemic disease is far more labile and may unexpectedly undergo cardiac arrest if ectopic warning signs are ignored.

Inasmuch as any increase in sympathetic tone may contribute to the frequency of arrhythmia, it behooves the dentist to control the patient's anxiety. Because the group at greatest risk for serious arrhythmia is largely comprised of those with coronary artery disease or heart failure, the dentist will coincidentally ensure against arrhythmic sequelae by attempting to prevent acute exacerbations of these underlying diseases.

Local anesthesia is to be preferred over general agents, since the hypoxia, hypercapnia, and sympathetic outbursts of induction may incite disordered rhythms. If general anesthesia is necessary in those at risk for ventricular arrhythmia, hospitalization and controlled ventilation anesthesia are indicated. The use of narcotics and local anesthetic agents during inhalation general anesthesia can help prevent the instigation of arrhythmias by peripheral stimuli. The fact that halothane is known to sensitize the myocardium to catecholamines is usually reason enough to employ alternative agents. Balanced anesthesia using opiates, nitrous oxide, and high concentrations of oxygen is favored by many anesthesiologists for individuals at cardiac risk.

Table 5. Commonly used antiarrhythmic agents

Agent	Side effects
Procainamide	Muscosal ulcers (secondary to agranulocytosis), lupus-like syndrome
Quinidine	Cinchonism, tinnitus, headache, nausea, vomiting, and visual disturbances
Disopyramide	Xerostomia, dry nose, dry eyes and throat, urinary hesitancy, etc. (anticholinergic)
Propranolol	Light headedness, lassitude, bradycardia, heart failure, hypotension, ulcers (secondary to agranulocytosis), purpuras (thrombocytopenic and nonthrombocytopenic)

As is true in the treatment of any cardiac disease, the need to achieve adequate local anesthesia far outweighs the need to avoid vasoconstrictive agents such as epinephrine. The serial administration of short lived anesthetics can do more to worsen an unstable cardiac rhythm than a single dose of anesthetic with epinephrine.

Pulp testors, motorized dental chairs, belt-driven handpieces, and cavitrons have all at one time been thought capable of producing pacemaker malfunction. Recent evidence suggests that electrosurgery units present the greatest risk to the paced heart. The demand type of pacemaker is the most common variety and the most sensitive to external electromagnetic sources. For these reasons, it is appropriate for the dentist to confirm that all such office equipment is inoperative before the patient with the Demand pacemaker arrives for an appointment.

A basic knowledge of antiarrhythmic pharmacology is essential to the competent treatment of these individuals. Mucosal ulceration may be the earliest evidence of agranulocytosis secondary to procainamide or propranolol toxicity. Xerostomia may be an anticholinergic consequence of disopyramide use. Since antiarrhythmic drugs in toxic amounts may precipitate arrhythmias, the dentist should heed signs of toxic syndromes such as cinchonism and lupus-like syndrome. Table 5 shows some side effects of the commonly used antiarrhythmic agents.

PERICARDITIS

CLINICAL MANIFESTATIONS. Pericarditis produces no cervicofacial manifestations of specific nature. Kussmaul's sign and a paradoxic pulse may uncover an effusive or constructive pericardial lesion in an individual otherwise thought to have right-sided heart failure.

Certain vital organisms known to produce acute pericarditis are commonly to blame for oral vesicular lesions (such as herpes simplex and coxsackie virus)

DENTAL MANAGEMENT. Asymptomatic patients with a history of pericardial disease require no special management save the dentist's regular search for clinical signs of cardiac decompensation. It should be noted that *Streptococcus viridans* pericarditis has been recorded as a sequela of dental extractions in individuals diagnosed as having myeloid metaplasia (myelofibrosis). These patients should therefore receive antibiotic chemoprophylaxis when dental care is provided.

BIBLIOGRAPHY

Ashman, S.G., Kahn S., and Williams, A.C.: Pericarditis secondary to tooth extraction in a patient with myeloid metaplasia: report of a case, J. Oral Surg. **31**:881, 1973.

DISEASE OF THE AORTA AND ITS BRANCHES

Of the disorders discussed previously, cerebrovascular disease is the entity of particular interest to the dentist. Involvements of other portions of the arterial tree are of less dental significance, except when their therapy involves anticoagulation. This latter topic is considered in the chapter devoted to pulmonary embolism.

CLINICAL MANIFESTATIONS. All middle-aged and elderly patients should be queried about neurologic symptoms of vascular character. Those admitting to symptoms consistent with transient cerebral ischemia deserve medical referral. Needless to say, a history of completed stroke is always of note in that it identifies individuals whose cerebra may even yet be tenuously vascularized.

Beyond the carotid findings already mentioned, the head and neck examination usually reveals little in the patient with asymptomatic cerebrovascular disease. Opthalmoscopy may disclose asymmetric retinal deposition of cholesterol crystals in patients with unilateral carotid stenosis, but this is not an observation that the dentist would be expected to make. Thus in the elderly it is perhaps best to assume the existence of some cerebrovascular impairment, even when physical evidence is lacking.

Transient ischemia during the dental visit and fixed deficit from a previously completed stroke will usually reveal themselves during the dentist's examination. Hemiparetic gait or aphasia may betray the history even as the dentist first greets a new patient. Crucial to any examination is an evaluation of the cranial nerves, and the dentist should closely scrutinize the elderly for evidence of cranial nerve palsy. Jaw jerk and zygomatic reflexes may reveal subtle supranuclear fifth nerve involvement; a mild and barely discernible seventh nerve deficit may be the sole physical evidence of an old central nervous system insult. A careful search for infantile reflexes (such as sucking, snouting, and grasping) takes only a moment but can alert the practitioner to the presence of frontal lobe disease that may materially affect the dentist's treatment, especially when there is associated apathy, impaired concentration, lability of affect, or inability to carry out planned tasks. Although these deficits are most commonly found in conjunction with idiopathic dementia, they may also result from ischemic deprivation of prefrontal areas.

The proposed relationship between oral erythrodiapedesis and cerebrovascular accident is noteworthy. It has been observed that the cytologic character of the oral washings may be related to the nature of a cerebrovascular accident. Large numbers of red cells are commonly found in the sediment of individuals with hemorrhagic intracerebral accidents. Subarachnoid bleeding and bland infarctions have low oral erythrodiapedesis, and the former are distinguished by the characteristic bloody or xanthochromic cerebrospinal fluid. These findings could prove useful in instances where a question as to the nature of the stroke creates difficulty in treatment planning (for example, whether or not to anticoagulate the patient).

Despite the fact that the atherosclerotic process is known to affect the facial vessels, it is uncommon for such involvement to be of measurable clinical import. The interpretation of studies designed to investigate the relationship between atherosclerosis and periodontal disease must await the development of reliable indices for rating the severity of these two processes. Fortunately, the collateralization of blood supply in the face all but prevents the occurrence of significant infarction of atheromatous origin. Although studies have shown atherosclerotic disease of the lingual arteries to be common, there exist only a few reports of gangrene traceable to atheromas of these vessels.

DENTAL MANAGEMENT. There are two major concerns in the dental management of those with cerebrovascular disease. The practitioner must (1) attempt to minimize the risk of additional neurologic insult during treatment and (2) contribute to the rehabilitation of the stroke victim.

Essential to the safety of these patients is the avoidance of any substantial variation in cerebral blood flow. Good hypertensive control will limit the incidence of vasospastic or hemorrhagic infarction, and the avoidance of sedative-related hypotension can diminish the risk of bland stroke. For no other patient group are deliberate explanation and calm reassurance more important. The age-related and coincident increase in atherosclerosis and dementia should serve to remind us that the elderly individual is often poorly equipped to deal with the circulatory stress that confusion may provoke. Because disorientation commonly breeds paranoia, the dentist should spare no effort to keep an elderly patient informed. Sedatives may prove to be double-edged swords in these individuals, since small doses can increase disorientation and stress and larger doses may lead to hypnosis and cerebral oligemia. The practitioner should substitute experience and reassurance for sedative pharmaceuticals whenever possible.

There is a greater incidence of carotid sinus sensitivity among those with atherosclerotic cerebrovascular disease;

the dentist will do well to remember this when positioning and examining a patient. All three forms of carotid sinus syncope (vagal, depressor, and central) are potentially devastating for patients whose circulation is already compromised. Gentle palpation of the carotid pulses is essential to avoid such syncope as well as the inadvertent dislodgement and embolization of atheromatous material.

The individual who has sustained permanent cerebral injury presents several technical problems to the dentist, particularly concerning removable prosthetic procedures. The supportive tissues may undergo regressive change because of denture disuse around the time of the cerebrovascular accident. This is sometimes further complicated by the muscular flaccidity of the seventh nerve lesions. For these reasons, denture relining and ultimate rebasing or refabrication are usually needed after a stroke. Other cranial nerve lesions may complicate the treatment process; fifth nerve disease with intraoral hypesthesia may lead to overextension of the denture bases, and ninth nerve palsy increases the chances of impression material aspiration. Frequent postinsertion adjustments and proper patient positioning for impressions are among the measures that may be taken to minimize these problems. Acrylic obliteration of the buccal vestibule on the affected side can be helpful to patients whose mimetic tonus is insufficient to keep the vestibule free of food debris. If and when such tonus returns, the added acrylic may be ground away.

Because stroke often brings dependency and depression to its victims, the dentist should do everything possible to help each patient remain orally self-sufficient. Designing partial dentures with extra clasps on the unaffected side will simplify their removal and eliminate a personal task for which the patient must otherwise enlist another's aid. Suction-mounted denture brushes are also helpful in the hemiplegic's hygiene efforts. Since the central goal is always the maintenance of oral health, however, the dentist must be prepared to encourage a patient to accept assistance, should that assistance prove essential to the success of the rehabilitative program (such as an apraxic individual who may remain unable to insert and remove a prosthesis).

Should a patient develop ischemic symptoms in the dental office, the practitioner must be prepared to support that individual until transportation to hospital facilities is available. The conscious patient will require oxygen and reassurance and should be allowed to rest comfortably in recumbency. When loss of consciousness occurs, airway maintenance, including the removal of prostheses, becomes the cornerstone of treatment. In all instances, the dentist should keep an accurate time record of the patient's level of consciousness, pupillary character, and vital signs. This information may prove invaluable to the medical team that assumes the care of the individual after transfer.

BIBLIOGRAPHY

Bradley, J.C.: A radiological investigation into the age changes of the inferior dental artery, Br. J. Oral Surg. **13**:82, 1975.

Dreizen, S., and others: Human lingual atherosclerosis, Arch. Oral Biol. **19**:813, 1974.

Reed, C., and Ingles, M.J.: Acute massive gangrene of the tongue, Br. Med. J. **2**:575, 1965.

Sakurai, E.H., and Richardson, J.A.: Vascular neck pain: a source of odontalgia, Oral Surg. **25**:553, 1968.

Selbey, W.G.: Dental help for stroke patients, Br. Dent. J., p. 409, 1977.

Stoica, E., and others: Oral erythrodiapedesis at the onset of cerebrovascular accidents, Confin. Neurol. **33**:277, 1971.

Zafran, J.N., and Zayon, G.M.: Prosthodontics and the stroke patient, J. Am. Dent. Assoc. **74**:1250, 1967.

Section Eight

DISEASES OF THE KIDNEY AND DISTURBANCES IN ELECTROLYTE AND ACID-BASE METABOLISM

edited by **Sandra P. Levison**

101 • INTRODUCTION

Sandra P. Levison

Patients with renal, electrolyte, or acid-base disorders may manifest any one of many symptoms or findings on physical or laboratory examination. These include hematuria, dysuria, oliguria, anuria, polyuria, hypertension, edema, stigmata of uremia, proteinuria, pyuria, crystalluria, azotemia, and alterations in the serum concentration of the sodium, potassium, hydrogen, bicarbonate, phosphate, calcium, or magnesium ions.

DETERMINING THE SITE OF INJURY

There may be considerable overlap in the signs, symptoms, and laboratory findings in various renal diseases. Some patients may tolerate well the uremic symptoms of chronic renal failure, whereas similar decreases in renal function may cause severe illness in patients with acute renal failure. Hypertension is usually present in vascular or glomerular disease and variably present in tubular or interstitial disease. Edema may be a feature of tubular or glomerular disease, but it more commonly occurs early in glomerular disease characterized by the nephrotic syndrome or late in interstitial or glomerular disease when sodium excretion is decreased. The nephrotic syndrome rarely occurs with tubular, interstitial, or ureteral disease but is seen in glomerular disease or renal vein thrombosis. Gross hematuria may herald a tumor in the urinary tract, infection, or renal vascular disease, but it is very uncommon in tubulointerstitial disease. Microscopic hematuria is a nonspecific but potentially serious abnormality. Red blood cell (RBC) casts, however, suggest glomerular damage. White blood cells (WBCs) are a nonspecific inflammatory response seen in injury to the glomerulus, tubules, interstitium, or lower urinary tract.

HEMATURIA

Normally fewer than 1.5 million RBCs are excreted in the urine daily. When hematuria increases threefold, it can be detected microscopically. Fresh urine (15 ml collected by clean catch) is centrifuged for 5 minutes at 1500 rpm. After the supernatant is discarded, 0.25 to 0.5 ml of residual urine is used to resuspend the sediment. A drop of this suspension is examined using the high-dry objective ($\times 43$). An abnormal microscopic finding is more than 3 to 5 RBCs in each high-power field when many different fields are examined. Gross hematuria occurs when there is sufficient blood in the urine to make it obvious to the unassisted eye.

The presence of RBC casts or other casts that may accompany RBCs indicates that the kidney is the site of bleeding. Hypotonic urine may produce osmotic lysis of RBCs, and alkaline urine leads to the dissolution of casts. In the presence of gross hematuria, RBC casts are difficult to detect.

The dipstick test is used to detect hematuria. The test results may be negative when the number of RBCs is small and the cells are intact. Since the dipstick test is also positive for hemoglobin and myoglobin, conditions other than those associated with the hematuria should be considered when the test is positive and microscopic hematuria is absent. Myoglobinuria is associated with rhabdomyolysis, the most common causes of which are crushing or thermal injuries. The latter may follow prolonged exposure to extreme cold, heat stroke, or malignant hyperthermia caused by general anesthesia. Muscle injury also may follow vigorous exercise, particularly in unconditioned individuals, in alcoholic persons, and in association with defects such as McArdle's syndrome.

Urine may falsely appear to contain blood in patients who have consumed considerable quantities of foods such as beets or berries or containing red food dyes. A variety of drugs and their metabolites may cause a urine color resembling blood. Red-pink urine may follow the ingestion of phenacetin, sulfanilamide, quinine, phenytoin, methyldopa, doxorubicin, daunorubicin, the laxative phenolphthalein, and phenothiazines. Red-brown urine is seen following the administration of sulfanilamide, quinine, chloroquine, primaquine, metronidazole, phenytoin, the laxatives emodin and cascara, and phenothiazines. Orange-red urine may be seen following the use of phenazopyridine, rifampin, and phenindione.

Hematuria requires thorough investigation to uncover the cause (see following outline). Hematuria usually does not require transfusion except after trauma and postoperatively.

Causes of hematuria

I. Urethral
  A. Foreign body
  B. Local trauma
II. Prostatic
  A. Benign hypertrophy
  B. Acute prostatitis
  C. Carcinoma
III. Bladder
  A. Infection
    1. Bacterial
    2. Viral
    3. Schistosomiasis
  B. Neoplasm
  C. Stones
  D. Foreign body
  E. Trauma
  F. Cyclophosphamide
IV. Ureteral
  A. Malignancy
  B. Stones
  C. Abdominal lesions causing ureteral inflammation
    1. Diverticulitis
    2. Appendicitis
    3. Salpingitis
    4. Gastrointestinal neoplasms
V. Renal
  A. Glomerulonephritis
    1. Not associated with systemic disease
      a. Poststreptococcal glomerulonephritis
      b. Acute nonstreptococcal glomerulonephritis
      c. Berger's disease (IgA nephropathy)
      d. Mesangiocapillary glomerulonephritis
      e. Rapidly progressive glomerulonephritis
      f. Chronic glomerulonephritis
    2. Associated with systemic disease
      a. Lupus erythematosus
      b. Polyarteritis nodosa
      c. Scleroderma
      d. Wegener's granulomatosis
      e. Vasculitis
      f. Goodpasture's syndrome
      g. Thrombotic thrombocytopenic purpura
      h. Preeclampsia, "toxemia" of pregnancy
      i. Hemolytic-uremic syndrome
      j. Infective endocarditis
  B. Infections
    1. Pyelonephritis
    2. Papillary necrosis
    3. Tuberculosis
  C. Neoplasms
  D. Hereditary diseases
    1. Adult polycystic kidney disease
    2. Alport's syndrome
    3. Hemoglobinopathies
      a. Sickle cell anemia
      b. Sickle cell trait
      c. Sickle thalassemia
      d. Sickle cell hemoglobin C
      e. Homozygous hemoglobin C
      f. Homozygous hemoglobin D
    4. Osler-Weber-Rendu disease
  E. Trauma
  F. Malignant hypertension
  G. Acute tubular necrosis
  H. Renal infarct
  I. Renal vein thrombosis
  J. Coagulation defects—hereitary, acquired, or associated with blood dycrasias

PROTEINURIA

The normal urinary protein excretion is less than 150 mg each day. Proteins with molecular weights of less than 10,000 are filtered by the glomerulus and reabsorbed by the tubules. With increasing molecular weight there is a progressive decrease in filtered protein. Most proteins with molecular weights greater than 50,000 are not filtered. In glomerular disease increased amounts of protein appear in the urine, at times reaching as much as 25 g per day. When the proteinuria is "selective," the proteins are of a molecular weight slightly greater than 50,000 with almost undetectable amounts of large-molecular-weight proteins. Selective proteinuria is usually associated with a more favorable prognosis than unselective proteinuria. Large amounts of proteins with high molecular weights appear in the urine of patients with unselective proteinuria. Tubular proteinuria is characterized by incomplete tubular reabsorption of normally filtered proteins, with 1 to 4 g of protein excreted each day.

In patients with increased proteinuria whose protein excretion does not exceed 1 g each day, the problem is distinguishing insignificant proteinuria from that associated with organic disease. With *febrile illnesses* as much as 500 mg to 1 g of protein a day may be excreted. Febrile proteinuria ceases within days of defervescence. Up to 1 g of protein a day may be excreted by an unconditioned person after *strenuous exercise*. Hypertension, edema, azotemia, and abnormal urinary sediment are absent, and the proteinuria disappears within a few days of the exercise. *Orthostatic proteinuria* occurs when the individual is in the lordotic posture and disappears with recumbency. It is usually seen in young adults or children with no other associated symptoms.

The presence of increased urinary protein may be determined by several means. The dipstick is a convenient, simple method that is not specific for albumin nor accurate quantitatively. If the specimen is not dilute (the first morning specimen is optimal), a negative result of a dipstick test precludes albuminuria. It does not rule out the presence of other proteins. Because strongly alkaline urine may give false positive results, dipstick-positive urine should be confirmed by measuring protein excretion in several urine samples before an evaluation for renal disease is undertaken. An aliquot of a 24-hour urine collection is tested with sulfosalicyclic acid and its turbidity is compared wtih standards. The completeness of collection should be determined by measuring the urinary creatinine excretion. False positive results have been reported in the presence of roentgenographic contrast media, chlorpromazine, and tolbutamide metabolites, following high doses of sulfonamides and various penicillins, and occasionally when the urine is extremely alkaline. Paper electrophoresis of the urine proteins separates the proteins according to charge and is helpful in detecting the type of protein present. It distinguishes Bence Jones protein, albumin, and the various immunoglobulins. Techniques of separation based on molecular weight are also available.

PYURIA

Pyuria has been defined as the urinary excretion of more than 3 million WBCs each day. Normal urine has fewer than 5 WBCs in each high-power field. The most common cause of pyuria is the contamination of normal urine by improper collection techniques. Pyuria is rarely an isolated presenting symptom. Bacterial infection of the urinary tract (urethritis, cystitis, pyelonephritis, and prostatitis) is the most common pathologic cause of pyuria. Pyuria is also seen in the following circumstances: (1) granulomatous infections of the urinary tract (for example, tuberculosis); (2) neoplasms of the urinary tract; (3) foreign bodies in the urinary tract (stones or exogenously derived foreign bodies); (4) in association with inflammatory diseases in organs contiguous to the urinary tract (diverticulitis, appendicitis, colitis, ileitis, and pelvic inflammatory disease); (5) as a result of ingestion of large quantities of phenacetin with production of chronic interstitial nephritis (see Chapter 107); (6) as a result of acute interstitial nephritis produced by penicillin analogs and furosemide (see Chapter 1); and (7) in association with other systemic events (fever, congestive heart failure, and exercise).

102 • STRUCTURE AND FUNCTION OF THE KIDNEY

Pedro C. Fernandez

Each human kidney is composed of approximately 1 million anatomic and functional units called nephrons. Each nephron includes a glomerulus, which is continuous with a tubule. The glomerulus consists of a tuft of interconnected capillary vessels that branch off the afferent glomerular arteriole and reunite in an efferent glomerular arteriole. The glomerular capillary wall is comprised of three layers: the fenestrated capillary endothelium, the basement membrane, and the epithelial cells (podocytes). The last exhibit a large number of cytoplasmic extensions (foot processes) that interdigitate with each other, leaving only a narrow slit between them. The glomerular capillary tuft is contained inside a balloonlike structure, Bowman's capsule, that opens into and is continuous with the proximal tubule. The glomerulus is the filtering component of the nephron. Approximately 180 L of plasma is filtered daily by the glomerulus and is subsequently markedly reduced in volume and modified in composition during passage along the tubule.

The tubule is divided into several segments: the proximal tubule, the hairpinlike Henle's loop, the distal tubule, and the collecting duct. The last segment collects urine from several terminal distal tubules and opens directly in the renal papillae. The tubule is lined by a single layer of cuboid epithelial cells resting on a basement membrane. Marked morphologic differences exist among the epithelial cells lining the diverse tubular segments. From a functional point of view the proximal tubule exhibits characteristics quite different from those found in the remaining nephron segments. Whereas the proximal tubule reabsorbs approximately 70% of the glomerular filtrate, only minor or no changes in filtrate composition take place in this nephron segment. It can thus be functionally classified as a high-capacity, low-gradient system. As the filtrate moves distally along the nephron, the amount of filtrate reabsorbed by the remaining tubular segments decreases progressively. However, simultaneously, the ability of the tubule to create and maintain steep ionic concentration differences between tubular urine and blood increases greatly (low-capacity, high-gradient system). Teleologically, the kidney's anatomic distribution of epithelia with different transport characteristics favors formation of urine that may differ markedly in composition from plasma.

In the human kidney there are two main populations of nephrons, with some variations between the two types. The cortical nephrons, located in the outer cortex, have short Henle's loops and are more numerous than the juxtamedullary nephrons. The latter nephrons are more deeply situated near the corticomedullary boundary and have long loops with well-developed descending and ascending limbs. There seems to be a direct relationship between maximal urine-concentrating ability and the relative length of the Henle's loop.

RENAL BLOOD FLOW AND GLOMERULAR FILTRATION

Normally the renal blood flow is approximately 25% of the cardiac output. The corresponding renal plasma flow is 600 ml/min, of which 120 ml/min is filtered at the glomerulus. The relationship between the glomerular filtration rate and the renal plasma flow is described by the filtration fraction, which is the ratio of the glomerular filtration rate to the plasma flow rate and which normally averages 20%.

It is characteristic of the renal circulation that both the renal blood flow and the glomerular filtration rate tend to remain quite constant in the face of changes in mean arterial pressure ranging from 80 to 180 mm Hg. This circulatory autoregulation is mainly a result of changes in the renal vascular resistance at the level of the afferent glomerular arterioles. The mechanisms of circulatory autoregulation are intrinsic to the kidney, and they may be modified by neurogenic and humoral factors (catecholamines, angiotensin, and prostaglandins). The bulk of the renal blood flow (90%) is distributed to the cortical area of the kidneys. Within the cortex itself, the outer part seems to have a larger blood flow than those areas closer to the renal medulla.

Glomerular filtration is a physical process determined by the interplay between the forces favoring filtration (glomerular capillary hydraulic pressure) and those opposing it (glomerular capillary oncotic pressure and hydraulic pressure in Bowman's capsule). The mean net filtration (that is, the difference between the capillary hydraulic pressure and both the hydraulic pressure in Bowman's capsule and the glomerular capillary oncotic pressure) is probably less than 10 mm Hg. Given the magnitude of glomerular filtration (180 L/day in adults), the low mean net ultrafiltration pressure suggests a high hydraulic conductivity of the glomerular capillary wall. This may be in part related to the large surface area displayed by the glomerular capillary bed.

The glomerular filtrate is a virtually protein-free ultrafiltrate of the plasma. Apart from the restriction to the passage of macromolecules, which is purely dependent on the pore size of the glomerular capillary wall, electrical charge also seems to be an important factor in limiting the filtration of plasma proteins. Fixed negative charges that are present in the glomerular capillary wall probably significantly restrict the passage of negatively charged plasma proteins. In pathologic states proteinuria may be at least partly caused by a decrease in the normal electronegativity of the glomerular capillary wall.

As a consequence of the formation of a protein-free ultrafiltrate, the plasma protein concentration and consequently the plasma oncotic pressure increase at the efferent end of the glomerular capillary bed. Since the blood supply to the proximal tubule is derived from the efferent arteriole, the oncotic pressure at the level of the peritubular capillaries is normally higher than that of the systemic blood. This high oncotic pressure represents a driving force for the net reabsorption of salt and water by the proximal tubule. Changes in the filtration fraction may thus influence proximal tubular reabsorption through concomitant changes in the oncotic pressure of peritubular capillaries.

RENAL HANDLING OF SODIUM AND WATER

The renal regulation and maintenance, within a narrow range of variation, of the osmolality and volume of the extracellular fluid are accomplished through changes in the urinary excretion of water and sodium, respectively.

The osmolality of the extracellular fluid is normally maintained between 280 and 290 mOsm/kg water, in spite of highly variable fluid intake, the continuous addition of solute to the body by the diet and its metabolic products, and the continued loss of hypotonic fluids through the skin and respiration. The kidney can excrete a urine ranging in osmolality from one-fifth to four times the plasma osmolality. Thus the osmolality of the intake (taking into account the extrarenal losses of water) is closely matched by the osmolality of the urine, and a constant extracellular fluid osmolality is maintained. A feedback control system normally links the extracellular fluid osmolality to the renal concentrating and diluting mechanisms. This is the osmoreceptor-antidiuretic hormone secretory apparatus, located in the hypothalamus and posterior pituitary gland. Antidiuretic hormone (ADH), which is released in response to increases in plasma osmolality, is required by the kidney for the production of a concentrated urine. In the absence of circulating ADH (decreased plasma osmolality) the renal concentrating mechanisms are interrupted and a dilute urine is excreted.

The intrarenal mechanisms of urine concentration and dilution are located in the tubular segments distal to the proximal tubule. Isotonic fluid escaping reabsorption by the proximal tubule is rendered hypotonic as it emerges at the end of the ascending limb of Henle's loop. This results from the ability of the thick ascending limb to reabsorb sodium chloride (chloride being the actively transported ion in this nephron segment) without water. The reabsorbed sodium chloride renders the medullary interstitium hypertonic to the plasma. The countercurrent disposition of both limbs of Henle's loop accounts for the increase in tonicity observed in the innermost region of the renal medulla (countercurrent multiplication). In addition, the hairpinlike medullary blood vessels act as a countercurrent exchanger, which prevents dissipation of the medullary hypertonicity. The process just described is instrumental in both urine concentration and urine dilution. In the absence of ADH, the tubular segments beyond the loop are impermeable to water, and as they continue to reabsorb sodium chloride, a maximally dilute urine is produced. In the presence of ADH the water permeability of the most distal nephron segments is markedly increased, allowing osmotic equilibration to take place between the tubular fluid and the surrounding interstitium. A maximally concentrated urine is thus produced as the tubular urine osmotically equilibrates with the maximally hypertonic medullary interstitium at the level of the terminal collecting tubule.

Sodium is actively extruded from all cells in the body

and is distributed primarily in the extracellular fluid, where sodium salts account for more than 90% of the osmolality. Changes in sodium excretion by the kidneys are accompanied by parallel changes in the renal excretion of water, as dictated by the ADH-renal mechanisms that control extracellular fluid osmolality. Therefore changes in the body content of sodium result in parallel changes in the volume of the extracellular fluid. The renal regulation of extracellular fluid volume is accomplished through the control of urinary sodium excretion. Normally a neutral sodium balance is maintained, in which the urinary output of sodium equals the intake minus the extrarenal losses of sodium. However, as the volume of the extracellular fluid decreases or increases, appropriate changes in the urinary excretion of sodium rapidly take place to restore the altered volume of that fluid compartment. The feedback control system, which monitors changes in extracellular fluid volume and secondarily dictates the pattern of urinary sodium excretion, has not been completely elucidated. For example, the exact nature and location of the volume receptors are not known, although they are probably related to cardiovascular baroreceptors.

In the kidney, changes in the urinary excretion of sodium seem to be mediated mainly by changes in the tubular reabsorption of sodium rather than by modification of the filtered sodium load (glomerular filtration rate times plasma sodium concentration). About 22,000 mEq of sodium is filtered each day. Normally two thirds of the filtered sodium load is reabsorbed isotonically in the proximal tubule, 20% to 25% in the thick ascending limb of Henle's loop as a result of active chloride transport, and another 10% to 15% in the distal tubule and collecting duct. The amount of sodium finally excreted in the urine is usually 1% or less of the filtered sodium load. Proximal tubular sodium reabsorption is greatly influenced by peritubular physical factors such as colloid osmotic and hydrostatic pressures, whereas in the most distal nephron segments, sodium reabsorption is partly dependent on the levels of aldosterone. Other humoral factors (prostaglandins and kinins) and neurogenic factors also seem to have an influence on sodium reabsorption, although their effect is less clear.

Changes in the tubular sodium reabsorption in response to changes in the extracellular fluid volume occur in different nephron segments. Although changes in the proximal tubular reabsorption are classically associated with changes in the extracellular fluid volume, emphasis has been more recently placed on the crucial role of the collecting duct as the main determinant of the final urinary excretion of sodium. The mechanisms responsible for the volume-induced changes in sodium reabsorption by those most distal nephron segments are not completely understood. They may occur independently of changes in aldosterone levels and possibly may be mediated by poorly identified humoral factors independent of aldosterone ("natriuretic hormone").

ROLE OF THE KIDNEY IN ACID-BASE HOMEOSTASIS

The pH of the blood is normally maintained between 7.36 and 7.44, despite wide variations in the dietary intake of acid or alkali, fecal loss of alkali, and metabolic production of nonvolatile acids, mainly as a result of precise renal regulation of the plasma bicarbonate concentration. At the normal plasma bicarbonate concentration of 24 mEq/L, approximately 4000 mEq of bicarbonate is filtered at the glomerulus in each 24 hours. This amount greatly exceeds the body stores of bicarbonate. From a quantitative point of view the main role of the kidney in acid-base homeostasis is the reabsorption of the filtered bicarbonate. In humans, the renal tubular reabsorption of bicarbonate is practically complete at plasma bicarbonate concentrations below 28 mEq/L. Above this level bicarbonate reabsorption is incomplete and significant bicarbonaturia occurs, preventing the plasma bicarbonate concentration from exceeding the threshold level of 28 mEq/L under physiologic conditions.

The proximal tubule reabsorbs 80% to 90% of the filtered bicarbonate. The remainder is reabsorbed in more distal nephron segments. The tubular reabsorption of bicarbonate is at least partly mediated by the enzyme carbonic anhydrase, which is present in high concentrations in the kidney. Other factors influencing bicarbonate reabsorption are:

1. *The effective volume of the extracellular fluid.* Volume depletion enhances the bicarbonate reabsorptive capacity of the renal tubule, while volume expansion has the opposite effect.
2. *The body stores of potassium.* Potassium depletion increases renal tubular bicarbonate reabsorption, and hyperkalemia decreases it.
3. *The arterial* P_{CO_2}. Changes in the bicarbonate reabsorptive capacity parallel changes in the arterial P_{CO_2}.

One or more of these factors may raise the plasma bicarbonate threshold well above 28 mEq/L.

The metabolism of different foods produces 50 to 100 mEq of hydrogen ion in 24 hours in the form of sulfuric, phosphoric, and several strong organic acids. These nonvolatile acids are instantaneously buffered by intracellular and extracellular buffers; the titrated bicarbonate is converted to water and carbon dioxide, which is eliminated by the lungs. Although these mechanisms provide an immediate defense against wide pH fluctuations, ultimately exhaustion of body buffers and overwhelming acidosis would occur if the kidney were not able to excrete in the urine an amount of H^+ equivalent to that provided by the nonvolatile acids.

Most of the H^+ excreted in the urine is bound to buffers, since only a negligible amount of free H^+ can exist at even the lowest urine pH (4.5 to 5.2). About one third of the daily H^+ load is excreted bound to filtered buffers (phosphate and creatinine); the amount of H^+ excreted in this form (titratable acid) is equivalent to the amount of buffer required to titrate the urine to the pH of the blood. The remainder of the H^+ is excreted in the urine as NH_4^+ (from the titration of NH_3 by H^+). The renal tubular cells produce NH_3 from glutamine. In acidosis NH_3 production may increase tenfold, thus allowing the excretion of increasingly large acid loads. It should be emphasized that H^+ excretion as titratable acid and NH_4^+ is highly dependent on the acidification of the urine to a pH considerably lower than that of the blood.

The cellular mechanisms of urinary acidification seem to involve the secretion of H^+ in exchange for reabsorbed Na^+. The secreted H^+ probably originates from the dissociation of H_2CO_3 into H^+ and HCO_3^-; the reabsorbed Na^+ together with HCO_3^- is then transferred to the blood. Thus for each milliequivalent of H^+ secreted into the urine, 1 mEq of HCO_3^- is added to the blood.

RENAL HANDLING OF POTASSIUM

Of the 3500 to 4000 mEq of potassium present in the normal adult, less than 100 mEq is distributed in the extracellular fluid; potassium is the main intracellular cation. However, the concentration of potassium in the extracellular fluid is closely maintained between 3.5 and 5.5 mEq/L. Fluctuations outside this range may have deleterious effects on the function of excitable tissues, since the ratio of intracellular to extracellular potassium concentration is the main determinant of the cell membrane resting potential.

A normal diet provides 60 to 120 mEq of potassium daily. Normally, less than 10 mEq is excreted in sweat and stools, and the remainder is excreted in the urine. Although the kidney maintains day-to-day potassium balance, the immediate disposition of large potassium loads is largely effected via transfer of potassium into the cells. The factors controlling cellular uptake of potassium are not well understood, but they may involve insulin and aldosterone and are significantly influenced by the acid-base status.

The renal handling of potassium is complex. Potassium is freely filtered at the glomerulus and is reabsorbed in the proximal tubule and Henle's loop. Studies in experimental animals have shown that regardless of the amount of potassium excreted in the final urine, the amount of potassium present in the early distal tubule remains quite constant, normally less than 10% of the filtered potassium. This suggests that neither the proximal tubule nor the loop contributes significantly to the renal maintenance of potassium homeostasis. Changes in the urinary excretion of potassium are mediated primarily through changes in potassium secretion by the distal tubule and by the collecting duct.

The mechanisms underlying distal tubular potassium secretion represent a complex interplay between the potassium content of the distal tubular cells, the chemical concentration gradients, and the electrical potential differences existing across the different cell membrane barriers of the distal tubular epithelium. The large intraluminal electrical negativity normally present in the distal tubule results in a passive mechanism of potassium secretion. However, potassium secretion depends mainly on cellular rather than transcellular events. Thus the tubular cell content of potassium, which is influenced by the total body potassium stores, by the acid-base status, and probably by aldosterone, seems to be a major determinant of distal tubular potassium secretion.

Factors influencing distal tubular potassium secretion are:

1. Aldosterone, which increases potassium secretion
2. The rate of delivery of sodium and fluid to the distal tubule, since potassium secretion increases with increasing delivery rates
3. The body stores of potassium
4. The acid-base status, since alkalosis enhances and acidosis impairs potassium secretion
5. The type of anions accompanying sodium in the distal tubular fluid (Poorly reabsorbable anions increase potassium secretion, probably by increasing the intraluminal electrical negativity.)

BIBLIOGRAPHY

Andreolli, T.E., and others: Questions and replies: renal mechanisms for urinary concentrating and diluting processes, Am. J. Physiol. **235F**:1, 1978.

Brenner, B.M., and Humes, H.D.: Mechanics of glomerular ultrafiltration, N. Engl. J. Med. **297**:148, 1977.

De Wardener, H.E.: The control of sodium excretion, Am. J. Physiol. **235F.**:163, 1978.

Rector, F.C., Jr.: Renal acidification and ammonia production. In Brenner, B.M., and Rector, F.C., Jr., editors: The kidney, Philadelphia, 1976, W.B. Saunders Co.

Tisher, C.C.: Anatomy of the kidney. In Brenner, B.M., and Rector, F.C., Jr., editors: The kidney, Philadelphia, 1976, W.B. Saunders Co.

Wright, F.S.: Sites and mechanisms of potassium transport along the renal tubule, Kidney Int. **11**:415, 1977.

103 • DISTURBANCES IN FLUID, ELECTROLYTE, AND ACID-BASE METABOLISM

Hugh J. Carroll and Man S. Oh

SODIUM AND WATER METABOLISM

Preservation of the proper biochemical milieu requires the maintenance of normal ionic strength. The osmolality of cellular and extracellular fluid (ECF) is about 280 mOsm/L. The osmolality of the body fluids is defended by the combined action of the thirst mechanism and antidiuretic hormone (ADH). When the patient is dehydrated, the serum sodium concentration rises and the total body fluid osmolality rises. This has the effect of stimulating the release of ADH from the posterior pituitary gland and simultaneously stimulating the thirst mechanism. In states of overhydration, when the osmolality and serum sodium concentration are low, ADH allows the kidney to excrete dilute urine, and osmolality returns toward normal. When the control mechanisms are operating normally, hyponatremia is prevented by the appropriate excretion of water, and hypernatremia is prevented by the retention of water. Thus hyponatremia and hypernatremia are observed clinically when there is an abnormality of the control mechanisms.

Hyponatremia

Hyponatremia is found in conditions in which the natural tendency to excrete a dilute urine is prevented, although the failure to excrete water allows a low serum sodium concentration to persist. The mechanisms capable of overriding hypo-osmolality and causing the retention of water in the body incude (1) hypovolemia and hypotension; (2) hormonal disturbances such as hypopituitarism, hypoadrenalism, and hypothyroidism; (3) physical and psychologic stress such as that caused by surgery; and (4) drugs such as chlorpropamide, vincristine, acetaminophen, and a number of medications used in psychiatry. Pseudohyponatremia occurs in states of hyperlipidemia and hyperproteinemia because a given volume of plasma contains less water and therefore less sodium than normal. Under these circumstances the measurement of plasma Na^+ gives an erroneously low estimate of the extracellular Na^+ concentration even if the serum osmolality is normal or elevated.

PATHOGENESIS. There are four mechanisms by which the extracellular Na^+ concentration may be reduced: (1) retention of water, (2) loss of sodium, (3) shift of sodium into the cell, and (4) shift of water from the cell to the ECF.

Primary water retention may occur either because of a greatly increased water intake, such as may occur in psychogenic polydipsia, or because of reduced water excretion. Reduced water excretion may be caused by renal failure, increased levels of ADH, or reduced urine flow through the distal nephron, as is seen in conditions with a low effective arterial volume. Reduced urine flow results from reduced glomerular filtration and enhanced reabsorption of water and sodium in the proximal nephron. Increased ADH activity may be caused by the low effective arterial volume in states in which edema develops, such as congestive heart failure, the nephrotic syndrome, and ascites, or in the syndrome of inappropriate ADH secretion (SIADH). In SIADH the hormone is released from a tumor or from the posterior pituitary gland in response to the following stimuli:

Causes of SIADH
I. Tumors
  A. Oat cell carcinoma of the lung
  B. Adenocarcinoma of the duodenum or pancreas
  C. Lymphosarcoma
  D. Hodgkins's disease
  E. Thymoma
  F. Carcinoma of the ureter
II. Central nervous system
  A. Head injury
  B. Brain tumor
  C. Brain abscess
  D. Cerebrovascular accident
  E. Guillain-Barré syndrome
  F. Encephalitis
  G. Meningitis
  H. Schizophrenia
  I. Lupus cerebritis
  J. Acute intermittent prophyria
  K. Seizure disorders
III. Intrathoracic diseases
  A. Pulmonary tuberculosis
  B. Pneumonia
  C. Lung abscess
  D. Positive-pressure respirator
IV. Drugs
  A. Chlorpropamide
  B. Barbiturates
  C. Vincristine
  D. Vinblastine
  E. Morphine
  F. Indomethacin
  G. Carbamazepine
  H. Amitriptyline
  I. Oxytocin
V. Surgical and emotional stress
VI. Addison's disease and myxedema
VII. Idiopathic disorders

Hyponatremia may be primarily a result of sodium loss caused by sweating, diarrhea, vomiting, diuretic therapy, adrenal insufficiency, or certain types of renal disease. It may be caused in part by the shift of sodium into the cell in exchange for cell potassium in potassium-depleted states. Any osmotically effective nonsodium solute in the ECF, such as mannitol or an excess of glucose, can shift water from the cell and produce hyponatremia. In the condition referred to as reset osmostat syndrome, mild asymptomatic hyponatremia is observed in patients with chronic, debilitating disease. The body regulates water balance around a serum Na^+ level that is fixed at a lower than normal level.

DIAGNOSIS AND MANAGEMENT. Hyponatremia is usually associated with hypo-osmolality. However, hyponatremia may be associated with increased osmolality when it is caused by hyperglycemia or mannitol infusion; in this case the patient can have the same signs and symptoms of cellular dehydration as in hypernatremia. The patient with hypo-osmolality and hyponatremia can be assigned to one of three categories depending on the ECF volume. The ECF volume is estimated by the physical examination of the patient and is described as low, expanded (edema), or apparently normal. Patients who have hyponatremia in the presence of volume depletion have lost salt from the body, either from the kidney or by an extrarenal route. In extrarenal salt loss the kidney attempts to conserve sodium and the urinary Na^+ in the urine exceeds 25 mEq/L. The exception to this rule is hyponatremia caused by diuretic therapy. The urinary sodium excretion is high until the diuretic is discontinued, at which time values usually fall to less than 10 mEq/L. The patient with hyponatremia and a diminished extracellular volume is treated by the administration of isotonic sodium chloride. The kidney excretes whatever water is not needed and retains the salt. In some types of renal salt loss it is impossible to diminish the renal excretion of sodium, and the patient must be given sufficient salt replacement to prevent the recurrence of hyponatremia.

Patients with severe edema have an expanded extracellular space and increased total body sodium but a low effective arterial volume. The low arterial volume impairs urinary dilution and produces hyponatremia. These patients should be treated with the careful use of diuretics combined with inhibition of excessive water intake.

Hyponatremic patients with an apparently normal ECF volume usually have SIADH. They may also have the reset osmostat syndrome or certain of the hormonal disorders just described. Patients with SIADH can be treated with water restriction, but their sodium intake should not be lowered. When the excess body water has been lost and the arterial volume is reduced to a normal level, the stimulus to excessive salt excretion is eliminated and the serum Na^+ returns to normal.

When acute hyponatremia develops or there is chronic severe hyponatremia (serum Na^+ less than 115 mEq/L) and the patient manifests symptoms of cerebral water intoxication (seizures or decreased consciousness), treatment with the administration of hypertonic sodium chloride must be initiated. When administering hypertonic saline, it is advantageous to give intravenous furosemide concomitantly because furosemide produces relatively greater water loss than sodium loss by preventing urinary concentration.

Hypernatremia

PATHOGENESIS. Hypernatremia is usually caused by excessive water loss (see the following outline). It also can be caused by the addition of salt to the body along with the loss of water or in some instances by the retention of salt alone. An example of the latter is the iatrogenic entry of hypertonic salt into the maternal circulation when it is used as an abortifacient.

Causes of excessive water loss
I. Renal
  A. Diabetes insipidus
    1. Hypothalamic or posterior pituitary (central diabetes insipidus)
      a. Primary and metastatic brain tumors
      b. Sarcoidosis
      c. Tuberculosis
      d. Surgery
      e. Trauma
      f. Encephalitis
      g. Guillain-Barré syndrome
      h. Alcohol
      i. Phenytoin
    2. Nephrogenic diabetes insipidus
      a. Congenital
      b. Drug-induced (lithium, demeclocycline, methoxyflurane)
  B. Osmotic diuresis
    1. Glucose
    2. Urea
    3. Mannitol
II. Extrarenal
  A. Cutaneous
    1. Sweating
    2. Burns
  B. Pulmonary
    1. Hyperventilation with fever
  C. Gastrointestinal
    1. Osmotic diarrhea
    2. Loss of gastric fluid

Hypernatremia of clinical importance occurs in persons who lack a normal thirst mechanism, since hyperosmolality provokes severe thirst and drinking water corrects the hypernatremia. However, in patients who are confused, comatose, physically unable to drink, or without access to water, hypernatremia is also common.

DIAGNOSIS. Examination of the urine osmolality can help determine the cause of hypernatremia. If the urine osmolality is greater than 800 mOsm/L, the patient is simply water depleted and his kidneys are responding normally. If the dehydrated patient with severe hypernatremia is unable to raise the urine osmolality even to the level of the plasma osmolality, he is suffering from severe central diabetes insipidus or severe nephrogenic diabetes insipidus (inability to respond to ADH because of acquired or congenital renal disease). If the urine osmolality is greater than plasma osmolality and less than 800 mOsm/L, the patient has either severe osmotic diuresis or moderately severe central diabetes insipidus. Osmotic diuresis is obvious when the patient is excreting large amounts of solute. Central diabetes insipidus can be distinguished from nephrogenic diabetes insipidus because patients with the latter do not respond to the infusion of ADH with a significant increase in urine osmolality; patients who lack ADH show a marked rise in urine osmolality when ADH is administered.

MANAGEMENT. Hypernatremia is treated by the administration of water in the form of isotonic or hypotonic glucose solution. The quantity of water required to treat a given degree of hypernatremia in a patient with water loss alone can be estimated from the following formula:

Water requirement = Estimated total body water (L) × $\left(\dfrac{\text{Observed serum sodium}}{\text{Normal serum sodium}} - 1\right)$

For patients whose hypernatremia is also caused in part by salt accumulation, it may become necessary to use diuretics such as furosemide if urinary excretion of the extra salt does not promptly follow the administration of water. When hypernatremia complicates renal failure, the excess salt can be removed by dialysis.

Volume depletion states

EFFECTIVE OSMOLALITY AND TONICITY. The terms "effective osmolality" and "tonicity" both refer to the solute concentration that determines osmotic water movement across the cell membrane. Thus, if the body fluid is hypertonic or effective osmolality is increased, water is pulled from the cell; if the body fluid is hypotonic or effective osmolality is decreased, water enters the cell. In contrast, if the body fluid osmolality is increased by increased levels of urea or alcohol (which can enter the cell freely), the effective osmolality remains normal, as does tonicity. An increase in extracellular osmolality by hypernatremia or by glucose or mannitol causes a shift of water from the cell, since sodium, glucose, and mannitol are virtually or completely restricted to the ECF; thus effective osmolality is increased.

Hypernatremia is always associated with increased effective osmolality, but hyponatremia is not always associated with decreased effective osmolality. Hyponatremia caused by hyperglycemia or by mannitol is associated with increased effective osmolality.

The total serum osmolality can be measured by an osmometer or can be estimated by using the following equation:

Serum osmolality = Sodium × 2 + $\dfrac{\text{Glucose (mg/dl)}}{18} + \dfrac{\text{Urea (mg/dl)}}{2.8}$

However, because the osmometer does not distinguish between the solutes that can diffuse into the cell freely and those that cannot, the effective osmolality can only be estimated:

Effective osmolality = Serum osmolality (measured or calculated) − Osmolalities of freely diffusible solutes (urea, alcohol, and so on)

ROUTES OF FLUID LOSS. About 200 to 300 ml of pure water is lost daily via the lungs. This volume increases with fever and hyperventilation. About 300 ml of pure water is lost through the skin in the absence of sweat. This amount is increased with fever and sweating, since sweat contains about 50 mEq/L of sodium and 5 mEq/L of potassium. The renal excretion of water and salt varies with intake, but the minimum water loss without renal failure is about 500 ml daily. An abnormal fluid loss through the kidney can occur with diuretic therapy, osmotic diuresis, metabolic acidosis, aldosterone deficiency, salt-losing renal disease, and the diuretic phase of acute tubular necrosis. Normally about 100 ml of water and 7 to 10 mEq of potassium are lost daily in the stool. An abnormal fluid loss can occur with vomiting or gastric lavage, diarrhea, drainage through a fistula, or enterostomy. When there is evidence of volume depletion without an obvious loss, fluid may be sequestered in the intestinal lumen because of mechanical obstruction or adynamic ileus, in the pleural cavity and peritoneal cavity, in the skin with burns, or in the extremities with thrombophlebitis.

TYPES OF DEHYDRATION. Dehydration can be divided into three types—isotonic, hypertonic, and hypotonic—depending on the effective osmolality (tonicity) of the ECF.

Isotonic dehydration. Isotonic fluid loss may occur through the kidney or the gastrointestinal tract or directly from the ECF by drainage of pleural effusions, ascites, and so on. Since water moves across cell membranes only in response to a change in the effective osmolality of the ECF, the intracellular volume remains normal and the fluid loss is only from the ECF space. The treatment consists of isotonic salt solution in the amount of the estimated ECF deficit.

Hypertonic dehydration. The primary aberration in hypertonic dehydration is loss of water because of either inadequate water intake or excessive water loss. Inadequacy or cessation of water intake may be caused by a defective thirst mechanism, as occurs with central nervous system lesions; impaired consciousness; lack of access to water because the patient is neglected, restrained, or paralyzed; or inability to drink water because of continuous vomiting or esophageal or pharyngeal tumors. Excessive water loss results from osmotic diuresis, diabetes insipidus, and sweating.

Dehydration caused by reduced water intake is usually slower to develop than that caused by abnormal water loss. Even when excessive water loss is the cause of hypertonic volume depletion, one of the conditions necessary for the limitation of water intake must be present to maintain hypertonicity. Otherwise, the stimulation of thirst by increased osmolality leads to increased drinking of water and the correction of hypernatremia.

In hypertonic dehydration the salt content of the body may be normal, increased, or decreased. It is decreased if salt loss accompanied the water loss, as in osmotic diuresis or vomiting, but the salt loss must always be less than the water loss. In pure desiccation the salt content is normal because the renal excretion of salt promptly stops as dehydration develops. If salt is administered to or ingested by a water-deficient person, it will be largely retained because of volume depletion and the salt content of the body will increase. In this case hypernatremia is the result not only of water loss but also of sodium retention.

In pure water loss without a gain or loss of salt the serum sodium concentration may be used as a fairly accurate index of the degree of desiccation. The estimated water deficit can be replaced with 2.5% or 5% glucose solution. (See "Management" in the discussion of "Hypernatremia" for calculation of water deficit.)

If salt retention is a cause of the hypernatremia, administration of the total amount of water lost calculated on the basis of altered serum sodium leads to an overexpansion of the ECF volume. If the kidney is functioning normally, the excess salt and water are excreted. If renal function is impaired, the correction of hypernatremia in patients with sodium excess may require the removal of sodium from the body by diuretics or dialysis in addition to the administration of water.

Hypotonic dehydration. If renal function is adequate, a loss of salt alone does not occur because the resultant hyponatremia suppresses ADH and the kidney excretes water. A loss of salt in excess of water loss is more commonly encountered.

Patients with hypotonic dehydration may present more evidence of compromised circulation for a given degree of fluid loss than patients with isotonic or hypertonic dehydration because acute hypotonicity may itself significantly diminish vascular tone and cardiac output. In addition, the reduction in the ECF for a given amount of total body water loss is greater because water is lost from the body as well as into the cells.

Hypotonic dehydration may be treated by administering hypertonic saline to restore the serum sodium concentration to normal and adding normal saline to complete the restoration of the ECF volume. The amount of sodium necessary to normalize serum sodium is calculated as:

$$140 - \text{Serum sodium (mEq/L)} \times \text{Total body water (L)}$$

The total body water is used instead of the ECF volume for this calculation because an increase in extracellular sodium and hence osmolality would cause a shift of water from the cell. Hypotonic dehydration can also be treated by administering isotonic saline. As the ECF volume increases, ADH is suppressed, free water is excreted, and both the ECF volume and the serum sodium concentration return to normal. Isotonic saline should be given when symptoms of hypovolemia are the major concern.

Edema

An inappropriate collection of interstitial fluid may be caused by a rise in capillary pressure (as a consequence of increased hydrostatic pressure), low plasma oncotic pressure (hypoalbuminemia), increase in capillary permeability (often idiopathic), or obstructed lymphatics. In all instances of generalized edema there is a reduced effective arterial volume that produces renal salt and water retention. The treatment of edema involves restriction of salt intake and, if renal function is adequate, the use of diuretics. Various diuretics work at different parts of the nephron. The diuretics that operate in the proximal tubule include acetazolamide and osmotic diuretics. The diuretics that operate in the ascending limb of Henle's loop include furosemide and ethacrynic acid. The thiazide-like group— hydrochlorothiazide, chlorthalidone, and metolazone—operate in the early distal tubule. These diuretics have different degrees of potency and durations of action; metolazone is particularly potent. Diuretics that act on the area proximal to the distal tubule cause potassium depletion, since excess amounts of salt are delivered to the distal sodium-potassium exchange site. The diuretics that act in the distal tubule and the collecting duct and that cause potassium retention include spironolactone, triamterene, and amiloride. Combinations of diuretics can be used for their synergistic effect or to allow the side effects of one (such as potassium loss) to offset the side effects of the other (such as potassium retention).

POTASSIUM METABOLISM

Most of the potassium in the body is contained in the cells where the concentration is about 160 mEq/L of cell water; the plasma potassium concentration in normally 4 to 5 mEq/L. Clinical problems in potassium metabolism are caused by hypokalemia, a result of potassium loss or a shift of potassium into the cells, or by hyperkalemia in which potassium is retained in excess or shifted from the cells to the ECF. The mechanism of urinary potassium excretion involves the secretion of potassium into the urine in the distal tubule and the collecting duct. A number of factors modify the rate at which potassium secretion takes place (see Chapter 102).

Hypokalemia

PATHOGENESIS. Hypokalemia is defined as a reduction in the extracellular potassium concentration. Potassium may be lost through the kidney or by extrarenal routes, the most important of which is the gastrointestinal tract. Gastrointestinal losses may be caused by diarrhea, laxative abuse, villous adenomas of the rectum, vomiting, or surgical drainage of the gastrointestinal tract. A shifting of potassium into the cells can be caused by metabolic or respiratory alkalosis, ingestion of barium salts, glucose or insulin infusion, and hypokalemic periodic paralysis.

Excessive renal potassium loss may occur when there is (1) increased aldosterone production, as in primary or secondary hyperaldosteronism (loss may not occur in these conditions if delivery of sodium to the distal nephron is markedly reduced); (2) excessive production of deoxycorticosterone (as in adrenal cancer, ectopic ACTH-secreting tumor, 11- or 17-hydroxylase deficiency); (3) excessive ingestion of mineralocorticoid-like substances such as natural licorice or of exogenous mineralocorticoids; (4) increased delivery of bicarbonate to the distal tubule as in proximal renal tubular acidosis; (5) excessive delivery of sodium to the distal nephron with normal or increased plasma concentrations of aldosterone as in diuretic therapy, metabolic acidosis, or Bartter's syndrome; (6) increased delivery of poorly reabsorbable anions such as sulfate, penicillin, or ketone to the distal nephron; or (7) unclear mechanisms such as magnesium deficiency, leukemia, or Liddle's syndrome.

It can be concluded that the kidney is the route of potassium loss if the daily potassium excretion in the urine exceeds 40 mEq while the patient has a low serum potassium concentration. If a hypokalemic patient excretes less than 20 mEq of potassium in the urine daily, the route of potassium loss is extrarenal. It is often useful to measure the plasma renin activity and the plasma aldosterone concentration for the differential diagnosis of hypokalemia caused by renal potassium loss. Some of the important patterns are as follows:

1. Low plasma renin activity with high aldosterone concentration—primary hyperaldosteronism caused by adrenal adenoma or bilateral adrenal hyperplasia
2. Increased plasma renin acitivity and increased aldosterone concentration—"secondary hyperaldosteronism," such as malignant hypertension, renal artery stenosis, and Bartter's syndrome
3. Decreased plasma renin activity and decreased aldosterone concentration—increased mineralocorticoid concentration other than that of aldosterone; ingestion of natural licorice; exaggerated salt reabsorption by the nephron without excess mineralocorticoid concentration (Liddle's syndrome)

CLINICAL MANIFESTATIONS. The important effects of hypokalemia are on the neuromuscular system. The involvement of skeletal muscle is manifested by muscle weakness or paralysis. The involvement of visceral muscle may be represented by adynamic ileus. The effects on the heart include various types of heart block and arrhythmias.

MANAGEMENT. The treatment of hypokalemia involves correction of the underlying cause when possible, administration of potassium by the oral or intravenous route, and when it is required and feasible, a reduction in the urinary potassium loss. The last can often by accomplished by the use of potassium-sparing diuretics such as spironolactone and by a reduction in sodium intake.

Hyperkalemia

PATHOGENESIS. Hyperkalemia is defined as an increase in the extracellular potassium concentration. True hyperkalemia must be distinguished from pseudohyperkalemia, which is an elevated concentration of potassium only in vitro or in the local blood vessel from which blood is being drawn. Pseudohyperkalemia may be caused by the release of potassium in vitro from platelets or from leukocytes in thrombocytosis or severe leukocytosis. Since the potassium is released during blood clotting in these situations, only the serum potassium concentration is high and the plasma concentration is not elevated. In vitro hemolysis—as occurs with the use of a tourniquet with fist exercise or the use of tybes containing fluoride or potassium-EDTA—may also lead to in vitro "hyperkalemia." Hyperkalemia can be caused by reduced renal excretion, a shift of potassium from the cell to the ECF, and increased potassium intake. Increased potassium intake can only be a contributing factor; if potassium is excreted normally, increased intake alone is almost never responsible for an elevation in the serum potassium level. Potassium may be caused to shift out of the cell by acute acidosis, rhabdomyolysis, hemolysis, increased catabolism, hyperosmolar states, and hyperkalemic periodic paralysis.

Causes of reduced renal potassium excretion

I. Aldosterone deficiency
   A. Addison's disease
   B. Selective deficiency of aldosterone
      1. Chronic heparin therapy
      2. Hyporeninemic hypoaldosteronism
II. Tubular unresponsiveness to aldosterone (pseudohypoaldosteronism)
   A. Congenital
   B. Acquired
III. Use of potassium-sparing diuretics
   A. Spironolactone
   B. Triamterene
   C. Amiloride
IV. Reduced delivery of sodium to the distal nephron—marked reduction in effective arterial volume such as hepatorenal syndrome, severe heart failure
V. Advanced renal failure

Diagnosing renal causes of hyperkalemia. When it has been established that hyperkalemia is due to deficient excretion of potassium by the kidney, the pattern of plasma renin activity (PRA) and plasma aldosterone concentration may be useful in establishing the cause:

1. High PRA and low plasma aldosterone concentration—selective aldosterone deficiency caused by adrenal disease, Addison's disease; chronic heparin therapy (heparin interferes with aldosterone synthesis)
2. High PRA and high aldosterone concentration—reduced delivery of sodium to the distal nephron; tubular unresponsiveness to aldosterone; potassium-sparing diuretics
3. Low PRA and low aldosterone concentration—hyporeninemic hypoaldosternism syndrome, in which patients usually have diabetes or interstitial renal disease and aldosterone secretion is suppressed because of suppressed renin secretion

CLINICAL MANIFESTATIONS. Isolated in vitro hyperkalemia is clinically unimportant. True hyperkalemia causes changes in myocardial excitability, which vary from electrocardiographic abnormalities of tall T waves and decreased P waves to eventual atrial asystole, intraventricular block, and ultimately ventricular standstill. Neuromuscular symptoms occur only with severe hyperkalemia.

MANAGEMENT. Hyperkalemia is treated by combinations of three basic modalities:

I. Reduction in body potassium content
  A. Reduced potassium intake
  B. Increased intestinal loss by use of sodium-potassium exchange resin (sodium polystyrene sulfonate [Kayexalate])
  C. Increased renal potassium excretion by increased sodium intake, diuretics, and mineralocorticoid therapy (fludrocortisone acetate [Florinef])
  D. Peritoneal dialysis or hemodialysis
II. Shift of potassium into the cell
  A. Administration of alkali
  B. Intravenous insulin and glucose
III. Antagonism of potassium in the heart
  A. Intravenous administration of calcium salts (chloride, lactate, or gluconate)
  B. Administration of hypertonic sodium salts, usually as bicarbonate

ACID-BASE BALANCE

The concentration of hydrogen ion (H^+) in the body fluid must be maintained within a very narrow range for cellular biochemical reactions to perform properly. The H^+ concentration of body fluids is 40 nEq/L. Current convention expresses this concentration as the pH, which is the negative of the logarithm of the H^+ concentration. In the normal state, the blood pH is 7.4. The body is constantly threatened by an excess of H^+, or alkalosis. To prevent gross deviation from the normal pH, the body is equipped with a set of buffering mechanisms that prevent an excessive rise or fall in the H^+ concentration. These buffers include the bicarbonate–carbonic acid system, which is the predominant buffering system of the ECF, and a variety of intracellular buffers, most of which are phosphates and proteins. The bicarbonate–carbonic acid system is not only the most important buffer system of the body but is also one that is readily available for study in the form of the arterial blood gases. Since extracellular buffers are in equilibrium with cell buffers, evaluation of the arterial blood gases gives a clue to the state of all the buffers in the body. Bicarbonate is produced by metabolic processes, and primary disturbances in bicarbonate concentration cause metabolic disturbances in acid-base regulation. Carbonic acid is produced by the reaction of CO_2 with water, and inappropriate retention or loss of CO_2 causes respiratory disturbances in acid-base regulation. There are four types of primary acid-base disturbances:

1. Metabolic acidosis, a primary decrease in bicarbonate
2. Metabolic alkalosis, a primary increase in bicarbonate
3. Respiratory acidosis, a primary increase in P_{CO_2}
4. Respiratory alkalosis, a primary decrease in P_{CO_2}

Metabolic acidosis

Each day the body produces about 70 to 100 mEq of acid from the metabolism of foods. This acid is buffered by the various body buffers and is subsequently excreted by the kidney. In the process of the renal excretion of acid, bicarbonate is formed by the kidney and returned to the circulation to restore the body buffers to the normal state.

PATHOGENESIS. Metabolic acidosis may be caused by one of two general mechanisms: extrarenal acidosis and renal acidosis. In extrarenal acidosis the kidney is unable to maintain the body buffers in a normal state. The serum bicarbonate concentration falls because acid production or ingestion is so great that it exceeds the renal excretory ability. Examples of extrarenal acidosis include the generation of organic acids in diabetic ketoacidosis and lactic acidosis, the intestinal loss of bicarbonate, and ingestion of acid or precursors of acid. Renal acidosis occurs because the kidney is unable to excrete the normal amounts of metabolic acid needed to regenerate the normal quantities of bicarbonate. In this instance there may be specific tubular defects, as in distal renal tubular acidosis or aldosterone deficiency, or there may be a reduction in the number of functioning nephrons as a result of renal disease, as in uremic acidosis.

COMPENSATORY MECHANISMS. The mechanisms by which the body protects itself from the effects of metabolic acidosis and restores itself to normal may be summarized as follows:

1. Buffering by bicarbonate and cellular buffers, proteins, and phosphates
2. Respiratory compensation in which the low pH of the blood stimulates ventilation. The P_{CO_2} appropriate for a given fall in bicarbonate can be calculated by the following equation:

$$\Delta P_{CO_2} = \Delta HCO_3^- \times 1.2 \pm 2$$

Thus a patient whose serum bicarbonate level fell from 24 to 12 mEq/L (ΔHCO_3^- 12 mEq/L) should respond with a decrease in arterial P_{CO_2} by $12 \times 1.2 = 14.4$ mm Hg.

3. Excretion of acid by the kidney with simultaneous regeneration of bicarbonate. Phospate and ammonia serve as urinary buffers for the process.
4. Conversion of organic anions (lactate and keto acid) to bicarbonate

MANAGEMENT. Most diabetic patients with ketoacidosis have prompt reversal of the acidotic state following the administration of insulin; they convert the sodium salts of keto acids present in their tissues to bicarbonate and rely on the kidney to generate whatever additional bicarbonate is needed. Lactic acidosis can be reversed only if the cause is corrected, but intravenous bicarbonate may be used to ameliorate acidosis while the basic problem is being managed. Severe acidosis requires the administration of bicarbonate to restore the pH to approximately 7.2, particularly in older subjects or those with compromised myocardial reserve. A good initial dosage is 1 mEq of bicarbonate per pound of body weight. Subsequent repetition of this dosage can be ordered as determined through arterial blood gas studies.

Patients with renal acidosis have no bicarbonate precursors circulating in the blood, and their kidneys are unable to regenerate sufficient bicarbonate to reverse the acidosis. Such patients must be treated by the administration of bicarbonate or by a bicarbonate precursor such as sodium citrate (Shohl's solution).

Metabolic alkalosis

PATHOGENESIS. There are two pathogenetic mechanisms required for the maintenance of a high serum bicarbonate concentration (see the following outline). One mechanism establishes the high serum bicarbonate level, and the other prevents the excretion of bicarbonate in the urine by raising the renal threshold for bicarbonate.

Mechanisms producing and maintaining high serum bicarbonate

I. Mechanisms that produce a high serum bicarbonate concentration
   A. Gastrointestinal or renal H^+ loss
   B. Intracellular shift of H^+ in potassium depletion states
   C. Ingestion of alkali or precursors of alkali
   D. Conversion of organic anions to bicarbonate
   E. Loss of extracellular volume without loss of bicarbonate (contraction alkalosis)
II. Mechanisms that increase the renal threshold for bicarbonate excretion
   A. Low effective arterial volume
   B. Potassium depletion
   C. Hypercalcemia; hyperphosphatemia; hypoparathyroidism
   D. Chloride depletion (associated with volume depletion)
   E. Renal failure

CLINICAL MANIFESTATIONS. The major clinical categories of metabolic alkalosis are those with reduced ECF and those with expanded ECF (see the following outline). The disorders associated with low effective arterial volume are described as "chloride responsive" and are characterized by low urine chloride concentrations (less than 10 mEq/L). Exceptions are Bartter's syndrome and diuretic therapy. The disorders associated with increased effective arterial volume are called "chloride resistant" metabolic alkalosis and are characterized by normal urinary chloride concentrations.

Categories of metabolic alkalosis

I. Causes of metabolic alkalosis with reduced effective arterial volume
   A. Gastrointestinal H^+ loss caused by vomiting, gastric suction, congenital chloridorrhea (rare)
   B. Renal H^+ loss: diuretic abuse
   C. Bartter's syndrome
II. Causes of metabolic alkalosis with increased effective arterial volume
   A. Primary aldosteronism, renin-secreting tumor, renal artery stenosis
   B. Cushing's syndrome (pituitary-adrenal and ectopic ACTH)
   C. Liddle's syndrome (resembles mineralocorticoid hyperresponsiveness)
   D. Excess licorice or carbenoxolone (resembles mineralocorticoid effect)

COMPENSATORY MECHANISMS. There are three ways in which the body compensates for metabolic alkalosis: (1) tissue buffering by intracellular buffers; (2) renal loss of bicarbonate when the cause is extrarenal; and (3) respiratory compensation. Hypoventilation with an increase in carbon dioxide can help to ameliorate the rise in pH caused by increase in bicarbonate. However, this is the least satisfactory of all acid-base compensatory mechanisms because it may be limited by the hypoxemia that results from hypoventilation. Total absence of compensation in mild to moderate metabolic alkalosis is common. The compensatory rise in P_{CO_2} rarely exceeds 60 mm Hg, regardless of the extent of rise in bicarbonate, except in azotemic patients with metabolic alkalosis. The following equation predicts the normal compensation of metabolic alkalosis:

$$\Delta P_{CO_2} = \Delta HCO_3^- \times 0.9 \pm 5$$

MANAGEMENT. If possible, attempts should be made to remove factors that raise the serum bicarbonate concentration or prevent renal bicarbonate excretion. In volume-depleted states administration of chloride accomplishes this, and in potassium-depleted states replacement of potassium or administration of potassium-sparing diuretics is necessary. Alternatively, direct titration of bicarbonate can be provided with ammonium chloride, dilute (0.1N) hydrochloric acid, lysine, or arginine hydrochloride. The enhancement of renal excretion of bicarbonate by acetazolamide may be effective in the presence of heart failure. Hemodialysis is useful in metabolic alkalosis with severe renal failure.

Respiratory acidosis

PATHOGENESIS. Since carbon dioxide can be readily expelled by the body through ventilation, elevated levels of carbon dioxide in the body are traceable to disturbances of ventilation rather than to overproduction of carbon dioxide. Hypoventilation may be caused by a variety of mechanisms that involve the lung itself, the thoracic respiratory muscles and nerves, and the respiratory center in the brain (see the following list).

Causes of respiratory acidosis

I. Central nervous system disease or pharmacologic suppression
II. Neuromuscular disorder—Guillain-Barré syndrome, myasthenia gravis, potassium depletion
III. Airway obstruction—aspiration, laryngeal edema, bronchospasm
IV. Acute lung disease—pneumonia, massive embolism, pulmonary edema
V. Chronic lung disease—emphysema, bronchitis, interstitial lung disease
VI. Alveolar hypoventilation—primary or caused by obesity
VII. Thoracic disease or trauma, kyphoscoliosis, flail chest, pneumothorax

COMPENSATORY MECHANISMS. Compensation for the retention of carbon dioxide is accomplished through the generation and retention of bicarbonate. Bicarbonate is produced by two mechanisms: (1) tissue buffering, which is rapid but increases the serum bicarbonate by at most 3 to 4 mEq/L, and (2) renal excretion of H^+ with the simultaneous generation of bicarbonate. This renal process requires 3 to 5 days for its maximal effect, and the increase in bicarbonate appropriate for a given rise in P_{CO_2} is calculated by the following equation:

$$\Delta HCO_3^- = \Delta P_{CO_2} \times 0.4 \pm 3$$

MANAGEMENT. Obvious causes of hypoventilation such as obstruction of the airway must be removed and mechanical ventilation should be applied as necessary. In patients who have pulmonary failure, efforts must be made to reestablish adequate ventilation so that oxygen can be administered at an appropriate rate. Care must be taken to avoid carbon dioxide narcosis in patients with protracted hypercapnia who are treated with oxygen. Dehydration and infection must be appropriately treated. Deficits of potassium and chloride, if present, must be restored. The arterial pH must be monitored to avoid posthypercapnic alkalosis. When ventilation is restored and carbon dioxide levels decline, the alkaline pH allows renal excretion of bicarbonate and restoration of serum bicarbonate to a normal level. The factors that may prevent the excretion of bicarbonate have been previously listed in the section on "Metabolic alkalosis"; in posthypercapnic states the most common reasons for persistent alkalosis are low effective arterial volume and potassium deficiency.

Respiratory alkalosis

PATHOGENESIS. Respiratory alkalosis is caused by the excessive loss of carbon dioxide as a result of hyperventilation (see the following list).

Causes of respiratory alkalosis

I. Hypoxia resulting from high altitude, ventilation perfusion abnormalities, alveolar capillary block
II. Drugs and toxins such as salicylate, progesterone, and epinephrine
III. Central nervous system disorders such as meningitis, brain tumor, cerebrovascular accident, and trauma
IV. Psychogenic hyperventilation
V. Reflex stimulation caused by pneumothorax, pulmonary congestion, or embolism
VI. Sudden recovery from metabolic acidosis
VII. Miscellaneous causes such as hepatic failure, severe anemia, gram-negative sepsis, and assisted ventilation

COMPENSATORY MECHANISMS. Compensation of respiratory alkalosis is accomplished by a reduction in the serum bicarbonate concentration. The bicarbonate concentration falls 3 to 4 mEq/L because of rapid tissue buffering. Renal compensation requires 2 to 3 days for maximal effect and consists of excretion of bicarbonate and reduced net acid excretion. The generation of lactic acid is increased, and the lactic acid may titrate some of the body buffers. The appropriate degree of compensation is calculated using the equation:

$$\Delta HCO_3^- = \Delta P_{CO_2} \times 0.5 \pm 2.5$$

The excellent compensation predicted by this equation often results in the return of blood pH to normal.

MANAGEMENT. The treatment of respiratory alkalosis is very difficult. Whenever possible the underlying disorder should be corrected. For hyperventilation caused by anxiety, rebreathing of carbon dioxide into a bag may help, along with reassurance that calms the patient sufficiently to terminate the hyperventilation. Sedation with agents that suppress the respiratory center, such as chlordiazepoxide (Librium) and phenobarbital, may sometimes be indicated. In extreme cases pharmacologic paralysis and mechanical ventilation must be employed.

Mixed acid-base disorders

The arterial blood gases serve to confirm the diagnostic impression of an acid-base disturbance, to determine the severity of a disturbance, and to permit an assessment of the appropriateness of the degree of compensation for the primary acid-base disturbance. Fig. 103-1 shows the primary and compensatory changes noted in uncomplicated acid-base disturbance. For each of the disorders in this scheme the factor used to determine if an appropriate degree of compensation is present has been supplied. If the patient seems to be undercompensated or overcompensated, he has an additional, unrelated primary acid-base disturbance. There are five types of mixed acid-base disorders:

1. Respiratory acidosis with metabolic acidosis
2. Respiratory alkalosis with metabolic alkalosis
3. Respiratory alkalosis with metabolic acidosis

Disorder	pH	HCO$_3^-$	P$_{CO_2}$
Metabolic acidosis	↓	↓ 1°	↓ 2°
Respiratory acidosis	↓	↑ 2°	↑ 1°
Metabolic alkalosis	↑	↑ 1°	↑ 2°
Respiratory alkalosis	↑	↓ 2°	↓ 1°

Fig. 103-1. Primary and secondary events in acid-base disturbances. (From Carroll, H.J., and Oh, M.S.: Water, electrolyte and acid-base metabolism, Philadelphia, 1978, J.B. Lippincott Co.)

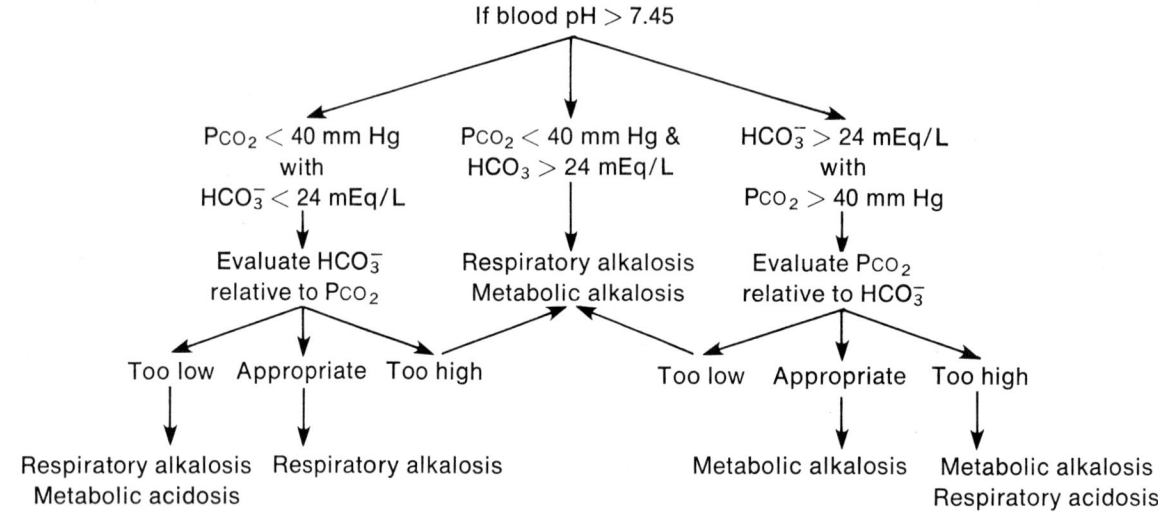

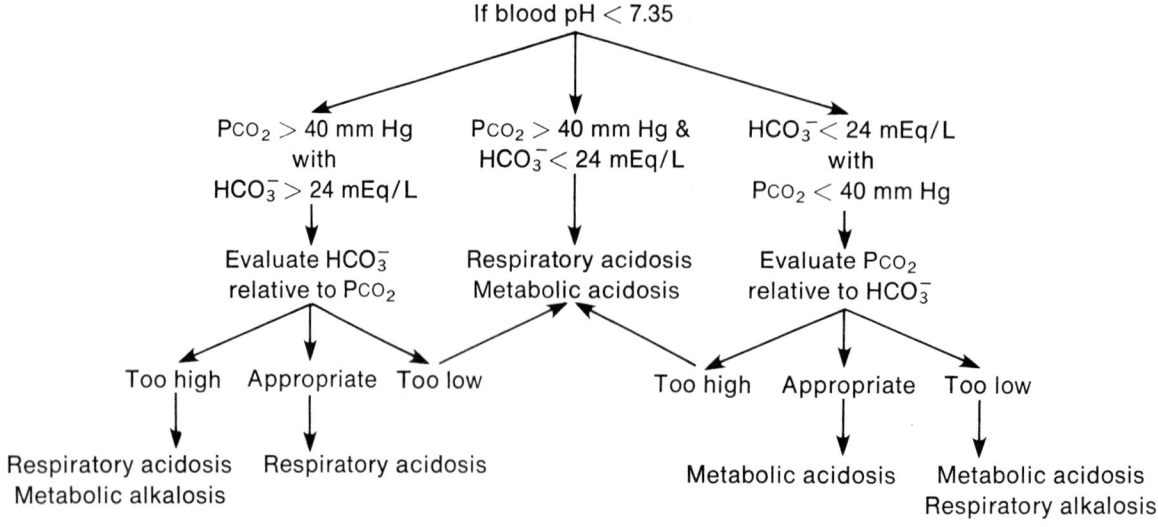

Fig. 103-2. Diagnosis of mixed acid-base disorder. (From Carroll, H.J., and Oh, M.S.: Water, electrolyte and acid-base metabolism, Philadelphia, 1978, J.B. Lippincott Co.)

Table 103-1. Normal compensation of acid-base disorders

Type of disorder	Degree of compensation	Duration required for compensation
Metabolic acidosis	$\Delta P_{CO_2} = \Delta HCO_3^- \times 1.2 \pm 2$*	12-24 hours
Metabolic alkalosis	$\Delta P_{CO_2} = \Delta HCO_3^- \times 0.9 \pm 5$†	12-24 hours
Acute respiratory acidosis	$\Delta HCO_3^- = \Delta P_{CO_2} \times 0.07 \pm 1.5$	Within minutes
Chronic respiratory acidosis	$\Delta HCO_3^- = \Delta P_{CO_2} \times 0.4 \pm 3$	3-5 days
Acute respiratory alkalosis	$\Delta HCO_3^- = \Delta P_{CO_2} \times 0.2 \pm 2.5$	Within minutes
Chronic respiratory alkalosis	$\Delta HCO_3^- = \Delta P_{CO_2} \times 0.5 \pm 2.5$	2-3 days

From Carroll, H.J., and Oh, M.S.: Water, electrolyte and acid-base metabolism, Philadelphia, 1978, J.B. Lippincott Co.
*In severe metabolic acidosis, the P_{CO_2} should be less than 18 mm Hg for a pH less than 7.1, and the P_{CO_2} less than 15 mm Hg for a pH less than 7.
†The P_{CO_2} should not exceed 60 mm Hg, and a total absence of compensation is not considered abnormal if the HCO_3^- is less than 37 mEq/L.

4. Respiratory acidosis with metabolic alkalosis
5. Metabolic acidosis with metabolic alkalosis

DIAGNOSIS. The clinical findings are often sufficient to allow the strong suspicion of a mixed acid-base disturbance. For example, metabolic acidosis develops in a patient who has acute renal failure following an operation because his kidney is not able to excrete metabolic acid. If that patient undergoes gastric suction, the removal of acid from the stomach is accompanied by the retention of bicarbonate in the blood. This patient therefore has a mixture of metabolic acidosis and metabolic alkalosis. A patient with diabetic ketoacidosis who had a massive pulmonary embolism could have a mixture of metabolic acidosis and respiratory alkalosis. The diagnosis of a mixed acid-base disturbance is made when the blood gases show ΔP_{CO_2} or ΔHCO_3^- outside the range predicted for the primary disturbance. Thus, for a given ΔP_{CO_2}, ΔCO_3^- will be too high or too low; for a given ΔHCO_3^-, ΔP_{CO_2} will be too high or too low. In some instances an apparently inadequate degree of compensation may be explained by an insufficient time interval for complete compensation to occur. A summary of the factors used for the calculation of appropriate degrees of compensation is shown in Fig. 103-2 and Table 103-1.

BIBLIOGRAPHY

Bartter, F.O.: The syndrome of inappropriate secretion of antidiuretic hormone, D.M., November 1973, p. 1.
Brenner, B.M., and Stein, J.H., editors: Acid-base and potassium homeostasis, vol. 2, New York, 1978, Churchill Livingstone Inc.
Carroll, H.J., and Oh, M.S.: Water, electrolyte and acid-base metabolism, Philadelphia, 1978, J.B. Lippincott Co.
Lindeman, R.D., and Dapper, S.: Therapy of fluid and electrolyte disorders, Ann. Intern. Med. **82:**64, 1975.
Maxwell, M.H., and Kleeman, C.R., editors: Clinical disorders of fluid and electrolyte metabolism, ed. 3, New York, 1979, McGraw-Hill Book Co.
Shrier, R.W., editor; Renal and electrolyte disorders, ed. 2, Boston, 1980, Little, Brown & Co.
Shrier, R.W., and Berl, T.: Non-osmolar factors affecting renal water excretion, N. Engl. J. Med. **292:**81, 1975.
Winters, R.W., editor: The fluids in pediatrics, Boston, 1973, Little, Brown & Co.

104 • INVESTIGATION OF RENAL FUNCTION AND STRUCTURE

Pedro C. Fernandez

CLINICAL ASSESSMENT OF RENAL FUNCTION
Clearance measurements

The urinary excretion of any substance can be expressed in terms of its plasma clearance, which is equal to the urine/plasma concentration ratio for that substance times the urine volume ($C = U/P \times V$). The clearance of substances that are freely ultrafiltrable and not subjected to either tubular reabsorption or secretion equals the glomerular filtration rate (GFR). If a substance were completely extracted from the plasma and excreted in the urine in each single pass through the kidneys, its clearance would equal the renal plasma flow. Substances that undergo net tubular reabsorption have clearances lower than the GFR. When the clearance of a substance exceeds its GFR, that substance is subjected to net tubular secretion by the kidney.

The overall renal excretory function is best assessed clinically by determination of the GFR. The determination of the clearance of inulin or polyfructosan represents the most reliable method of measuring the GFR. However, since these clearance determinations are cumbersome to perform, measurement of the clearance of endogenous creatinine can be substituted in most clinical situations. Practically all the creatinine excreted in the urine is formed in the muscles at a relatively constant rate for a given individual. In humans, creatinine is not only filtered at the glomerulus but also undergoes tubular secretion. The latter probably accounts for a larger fraction of the urinary creatinine when renal function is decreased. Thus in normal persons the clearances of creatinine and inulin are almost equal, but when the GFR is decreased, the creatinine clearance exceeds the inulin clearance. In spite of these reservations the clearance of creatinine is a useful parameter for determining the progression of renal disease. For clinical purposes, the creatinine clearance is best determined using a 24-hour urine collection, which reduces the error caused by inaccurate timing and defective emptying of the bladder. The creatinine concentration in the plasma should be determined in the morning of the urine collection period. Although various analytic methods may be used to measure the urine creatinine, the method employed for the plasma creatinine determination should measure the true creatinine and not the so-called noncreatinine chromogens. Automated laboratory methods provide an adequate measurement of the plasma creatinine concentration. The determination of the creatinine clearance is valid only if the patient's renal function is in a steady state, that is, not changing while the clearance is being determined. The clearance of creatinine normally averages 120 ± 20 ml/min in men and 110 ± 15 ml/min in women.

The GFR may be estimated from the plasma concentration of creatinine. This is based on the fact that, if creatinine production remains constant, the plasma creatinine concentration varies with changes in the GFR. The inverse relationship between the plasma creatinine concentration and the GFR is given by a rectangular hyperbola, so that a doubling of the plasma creatinine concentration would mean that the GFR has been halved. Although this relationship is grossly correct, it should be mentioned that normal plasma creatinine concentrations range from 0.7 to 1.4 mg/dl, depending mainly on the body muscle mass. Consequently, the plasma creatinine concentration changes reliably reflect changes in the GFR only when the plasma creatinine concentration and creatinine clearance were previously known. In advanced renal failure this relationship does not hold true because of the decreased creatinine production and the increased contribution of tubular secretion to the urinary excretion of creatinine.

There is also an inverse relationship between the blood urea nitrogen (BUN) concentration and the GFR. Although the BUN increases with deteriorating renal function, this parameter is a less reliable indicator of renal function than the plasma creatinine concentration, mainly because urea production is very variable and markedly influenced by factors such as protein intake and degree of protein catabolism.

The determination of the renal blood flow is rarely carried out for clinical purposes. The renal clearance of para-aminohippurate (PAH), a substance that in humans has a 90% index of extraction in a single pass through the kidney, closely approaches the value of the renal plasma flow. However, the adequacy of the blood supply to the kidney more often is clinically assessed by means of radioisotope studies, as discussed later in this chapter.

Measurements of renal concentrating ability

Although the ability to maximally concentrate the urine is lost by the diseased kidney, the direct investigation of the renal concentrating ability is indicated mainly in the diagnosis of nonglucosuric polyuria. The test requires complete fluid deprivation for 12 hours or until the patient's body weight is reduced by 3% to 5%, whichever comes first. A patient with marked polyuria should be carefully observed to prevent the development of severe intravascular volume depletion. The patient empties the bladder at the end of the fluid deprivation period, and the osmolality of the urine voided in the next half hour is determined. Five units of aqueous vasopressin is then injected subcutaneously, and the osmolality of the subsequent urine sample is determined. Normal individuals excrete a urine with an osmolality of at least 800 mOsm/kg H_2O following 12 hours of fluid deprivation. Moreover, the osmolality of their urine is not increased further by the exogenous administration of vasopressin.

Urinalysis

The urinalysis is the simplest, most economical, and most reliable screening test for the detection of renal disease. It should be performed on a freshly voided, midstream, clean-catch urine specimen. Samples collected in the morning after an overnight fast allow estimation of the concentrating ability of the kidney. A specific gravity greater than 1.020 in the absence of glucosuria is a strong argument against the presence of significant renal failure.

The urine should be routinely tested for the presence of protein, sugar, and blood. The widely available dipsticks impregnated with several reagents provide a simple and reliable method for the qualitative chemical testing of urine samples.

The bromphenol-impregnated protein indicator reacts more strongly in the presence of albumin than of globulins and does not detect Bence Jones protein. False positive results may be seen with very alkaline urines. The detection of persistent proteinuria by routine urinalysis should be followed by its quantification on a 24-hour urine sample, by means of the sulfosalicylic acid, biuret, or Kjeldahl methods. The amount and type of proteins being excreted may also be determined by electrophoretic and immunologic techniques.

Glucose, but not other sugars, is specifically detected by the glucose oxidase–impregnated dipstick. The ortho-tolidine reagent of the dipstick detects both heme pigments and myoglobin; microscopic examination of the urinary sediment should be used to confirm the presence of red blood cells in patients with hematuria.

The pH indicator of the dipstick is of little clinical value, although the presence of a highly alkaline urine (pH of 8 or higher) suggests a urinary tract infection caused by urea-splitting organisms, usually *Proteus*.

An essential part of the urinalysis is the careful microscopic examination of the urinary sediment. Ten to 15 ml of urine should be centrifuged, the supernatant decanted, and the sediment resuspended in 0.5 ml of urine. A thin film of the sediment, as obtained by depositing a coverslide over a droplet of the sediment, should then be examined with a subdued light under the low-power objective (×10) and the high-dry-power objective (×40), screening 15 to 20 different fields. Attention should be paid to the presence and type of cells, urinary casts, and crystals. Cell and cast quantification is expressed as the number of formed elements per high-dry-power field.

The normal urinary sediment contains one or no red blood cells and not more than three to five white blood cells in each high-power field in men and three or fewer red blood cells and six to eight white blood cells in women. Although hyaline casts may be seen in small numbers in normal persons, other types of casts (granular, waxy, red cell, white cell, and renal tubular cell casts) are abnormal. Since urinary casts are formed exclusively inside the renal tubules, the presence of cellular casts suggests a pathologic condition in the kidney itself, rather than or in addition to disease elsewhere in the urinary tract. The presence of red blood cell casts in patients with hematuria is strong evidence for the presence of glomerulitis. Other types of casts, specifically granular casts, are not useful for localizing disease.

In the presence of 3+ or 4+ proteinuria the sediment should be examined under polarized light for double-refractile bodies ("Maltese crosses"), which may be free in the sediment, encased in casts (fatty casts), or inside degenerated renal tubular cells (oval fat bodies). These double refractile bodies are fat globules seen most often in patients with the nephrotic syndrome.

Assessment of proteinuria

Normal individuals excrete less than 150 mg of protein in the urine in each 24 hours. The most abundant protein in normal urine is the Tamm-Horsfall protein or uromucoid, a glycoprotein not present in the plasma. This protein is secreted by the distal nephron segments and tends to precipitate inside the tubules in pathologic states. It is the main constituent of the matrix of urinary casts. Most of the other urinary proteins, including albumin and various globulins, are normal plasma proteins. Some urinary proteins are derived from prostatic and urethral secretions or are enzymes released from renal tubular cells.

Pathologic proteinuria is usually persistent and may range in severity from less than 500 mg protein to more than 30 in each 24 hours. Animal experiments indicate that the normal glomerular filtrate contains less than 30 mg protein/L urine, mainly albumin. Since this protein does not appear in the excreted urine, most of it must be reabsorbed by the tubules. Tubular reabsorption of protein occurs, at least in part, by a process of endocytosis and seems to be a saturable process.

Three main mechanisms account for the development of pathologic proteinuria:

1. *The presence in the plasma of abnormal proteins, which can easily cross the glomerular wall owing to their low molecular weight (≤40,000).* This type of proteinuria is exemplified by the urinary excretion of light chains of immunoglobulins (Bence Jones protein) in patients with multiple myeloma and sometimes those with amyloidosis.
2. *Abnormal tubular reabsorption of normally filtered plasma proteins, seen mainly in the tubulointerstitial type of renal disease.* This "tubular" proteinuria is usually mild (less than 1.5 g daily), and most of the proteins appearing in the urine are low-molecular-weight globulins, especially β_2-microglobulin.
3. *Abnormal permeability of the glomerular capillary wall to normal plasma protein constituents, mainly albumin.* This is the most common cause of pathologic proteinuria. The proteinuria of glomerular disease may be of any degree of severity. Practically all patients with urinary protein in excess of 3 g a day ("nephrotic range" proteinuria) have some form of glomerular disease, as do a majority of patients with 24-hour urinary protein ranging from 1.5 to 3 g.

Mild abnormal proteinuria (usually less than 1.5 g protein/24 hours) is occasionally seen in the absence of renal disease, such as in patients with congestive heart failure, in febrile illnesses, following heavy exercise, and in so-called orthostatic proteinuria. This last condition is characterized by the presence of proteinuria when the patient is erect, but not when he is recumbent. It is most commonly seen in young adults, and if associated with normal renal function and the absence of abnormalities in the urinary sediment, it has an excellent prognosis, often disappearing spontaneously.

ROENTGENOGRAPHIC AND ULTRASONOGRAPHIC EXAMINATION OF THE KIDNEYS

Roentgenographic examination of the kidneys provides the physician with detailed anatomic information about the kidneys and the collecting system. Plain roentgenography of the abdomen may yield valuable information concerning the size and contour of the kidneys and the presence of opacities (renal calcifications or calculi) in the region of the kidney or the collecting system. This noninvasive examination represents the preliminary step to the more accurate renal roentgenographic examinations in which radiopaque contrast material is administered to the patient. Triiodinated sodium or meglumine diatrizoate, iothalamate, and metrizoate are radiopaque contrast agents excreted only be glomerular filtration and concentrated in the urine by the tubular reabsorption of salt and water. The contrast agent is injected into a peripheral vein, and the renal concentration and excretion of the agent are then followed by means of an intravenous pyelogram or excretory urogram. Another technique is to insert a thin catheter percutaneously into a large peripheral artery or vein (usually the femoral vessels at the groin) and subsequently to move it into the renal arteries or veins. This allows the direct injection of the radiopaque dye into the renal arteries (renal arteriography) or veins (renal venography) to assess the renal vasculature in detail. In certain cases the contrast material is injected directly into the collecting system. This may be done in two ways: (1) via a catheter passed percutaneously into the renal pelvis (antegrade pyelography), or (2) through a catheter inserted during cystoscopy into the ureter via the ureteral bladder orifices (retrograde pyelography).

The administration of iodinated roentgenographic contrast material may be followed by allergic reactions ranging in severity from an urticarial rash to bronchospasm and anaphylactic shock. Unless studies requiring the administration of these dyes are absolutely necessary, they should not be performed in individuals with a history of allergy to contrast agents. If they must be performed, pre-treatment of the patient with corticosteroids under expert guidance and availability of an emergency resuscitation team at the time of the procedure are mandatory.

Acute renal failure following the intravascular injection of roentgenographic contrast agents has been reported relatively frequently in recent years. Predisposing factors to the development of acute renal failure are (1) preexisting renal insufficiency (serum creatinine concentration greater than 2 mg/dl; (2) diabetes mellitus, especially if long standing and associated with renal insufficiency; (3) multiple myeloma; (4) dehydration, which probably increases the inherent risk in otherwise predisposed patients, particularly those with multiple myeloma; and (5) advanced age, hypertension, and hyperuricemia, which are thought to constitute additional risk factors. Although the condition is usually transient and full recovery is the rule, diabetic patients with severe renal insufficiency (serum creatinine concentration greater than 5 mg/dl) may not regain renal function.

Intravenous urography

In intravenous urography the intravenous administration of a bolus of a radiopaque contrast agent is normally followed by progressive opacification of the renal parenchyma within the first minute of the injection (the nephrogram). This is followed in the next 1 to 3 minutes by the successive opacification of the calices, renal pelvis, and ureters (urogram). Disappearance of the dye normally occurs between 30 and 60 minutes after the injection.

Visualization of the renal parenchyma and perirenal structures is improved by tomographic sections, which eliminate overlying bowel gas from the renal image. Nephrotomography combined with the continuous intravenous infusion of contrast material is particularly valuable in the evaluation of renal masses. The detailed visualization of the collecting system is facilitated by external compression of the distal ureters by means of a pneumatic device applied over the lower abdominal wall. This prevents the rapid flow of contrast material into the bladder.

Intravenous urography remains the best initial study in the roentgenographic evaluation of renal disease. The nephrogram shows the size and contour of the kidneys. Visualization of renal masses is best accomplished by nephrotomography. If the mass is cystic, a thin, regular wall suggests a benign cyst. The nephrogram may also provide useful functional information. In cronic renal failure the nephrogram is delayed and faint, whereas acute renal failure may present a rapidly appearing and abnormally persistent nephrogram. In urinary tract obstruction the nephrogram appears late and increases progressively in intensity.

The urogram makes it possible to study the anatomy of the collecting system. Distortion of the calices may be due to renal mass lesions or to previous inflammatory disease of the kidneys. The calices and renal pelvis are dilated in urinary tract obstruction. Ulcerations and excavations of the renal papillae may be seen in renal tuberculosis and papillary necrosis. Stones or primary tumors of the collecting system appear as filling defects on the urogram. The urogram also provides diagnostically valuable functional information. In hypertension caused by stenosis of one renal artery, the urogram is delayed in the affected side in films taken at 1 or 2 minutes (rapid-sequence intravenous urogram). The urogram is also delayed in obstruction, and films taken at 6, 12, and 24 hours may show a dilated collecting system.

Retrograde pyelography

Retrograde pyelography is indicated mainly in two clinical situations. In the presence of renal failure the patient's history and other diagnostic procedures (ultrasonography, intravenous urography, radionuclide scanning) may lead the physician to suspect that urinary tract obstruction is the cause. In these cases the procedure is usually done on one side only (preferably the one on which the kidney is larger), since bilateral obstruction is implied when obstruction is the cause of renal failure. If obstruction is found and the catheter can be passed beyond the point of obstruction, it may be left in place to ensure urine drainage until a more definitive procedure is performed. Retrograde pyelography is also useful in the differential diagnosis of unexplained unilateral hematuria or filling defects in the collecting system that have not been sufficiently visualized with the intravenous urogram.

The main complication of retrograde pyelography is the introduction of infection. For this reason, as well as the frequent need for general or spinal anesthesia with retrograde pyelography, antegrade pyelography is favored in the diagnosis and immediate management of urinary tract obstruction.

Antegrade pyelography

The major indication for diagnostic antegrade pyelography is suspected obstruction, as just discussed. In addition, the antegrade insertion of draining catheters may be the temporary procedure of choice in the relief of confirmed urinary tract obstruction. This is chiefly because antegrade pyelography is a more sterile procedure than retrograde pyelography and it is performed with local anesthesia.

Renal angiography

The main renal arteries can be visualized by injecting the contrast material into the aorta (aortography). Digital subtraction angiography is a new technique for visualization of the renal vasculature following intravenous injection of contrast material. However, detailed visualization of the intrarenal vasculature requires direct injection of the dye into the main renal artery or one of its branches (selective renal arteriography). The renal veins are faintly visible on the arteriogram within a few seconds of the injection. For more precise definition the contrast agent must be injected directly into the renal veins (renal venography).

The main indications for renal arteriography are (1) for evaluation of renal masses that have not been clearly defined by other examinations, (2) for confirmation of the diagnosis of hypertension associated with stenosis of the renal arteries, (3) in cases of renal trauma and posttransplant renal failure, and (4) therapeutically for the obliteration, by means of local embolization, of the vascular supply to tumors, arteriovenous fistulas, and lacerated blood vessels.

Renal venography is performed to determine if renal call carcinoma has spread beyond the parenchyma into the renal veins. The procedure is also needed to confirm the presence of renal vein thrombosis, which may complicate the nephrotic syndrome. Finally, renal vein catheterization is often performed to obtain blood samples in cases of hypertension associated with renal artery stenosis. Renal vein renin concentration ratios of 1.5 or greater between the affected and the unaffected sides are the best criterion for surgical treatment of the hypertension.

Computed tomography

Computed tomographic scanning provides high-resolution transverse images of the kidneys, adrenal glands, and perirenal areas. The investigation is noninvasive and safe, except for the potential hazard of complications induced by iodinated contrast material, which is generally used in renal computed tomography.

Computed tomography is indicated in the further evaluation of mass lesions identified by intravenous urography of renal ultrasonography. The computed tomographic scan allows differentiation between cystic and solid lesions. The benign or malignant nature of arteriographically avascular masses can at times be ascertained by computed tomography. The technique is also valuable in the assessment of the regional spread of proven renal malignancies. In addition, it is useful in the evaluation of suspected cases of hydronephrosis, adrenal tumors, and other perirenal and retroperitoneal disease processes.

Renal ultrasonography

Ultrasonic waves from 1 to 10 MHz in frequency travel at a characteristic uniform velocity through a homogeneous medium, but they become refracted or reflected at the interface of two media with different acoustic properties. The combination of this basic principle with amplification and computer analysis of the reflected ultrasound beam ("echo"), as exemplified by gray-scale ultrasonography, allows the demonstration of the contour, size, and morphologic details of the renal parenchyma.

Longitudinal and transverse ultrasonographic sections of the kidney are usually obtained. The normal renal cortex is echogenic, whereas the renal medulla and intrarenal collecting system are relatively echo free. Fluid-filled areas such as renal cysts or a dilated collecting system appear as sonolucent areas with occasional internal echoes owing to tissue debris from infection or tumor necrosis. Solid masses within the kidney may produce increased echoes, but they are frequently difficult to differentiate from normal parenchyma.

Renal ultrasonography is a benign, noninvasive procedure that is rapidly gaining popularity as the screening test for the study of the renal anatomy. In this respect it is particularly useful when there are absolute or relative contraindications to the intravenous urogram. Moreover, renal ultrasonography is mandatory in the evaluation of renal masses. With lesions 1.5 cm in diameter or greater, ultrasonography allows differentiation between solid masses (usually tumors) and fluid-filled structures. In the latter a smooth and sharply defined wall and the absence of internal echoes are highly characteristic of a benign cyst. If ultrasonographic findings are equivocal, the cystic lesion may be punctured under ultrasonographic guidance and the fluid processed for cytologic and chemical analysis.

Ultrasonography is also useful in the detection of urinary tract obstruction and the diagnosis of polycystic kidney disease. The performance of a percutaneous renal biopsy or antegrade pyelography is greatly facilitated by determining the exact location of the kidney with ultrasonography.

Radioisotope imaging

A large number of radiopharmaceuticals that are excreted by the kidney are currently available. The renal handling of different radiopharmaceuticals varies. Among the most commonly used agents are (1) technetium-labeled diethylenetriamine penta-acetic acid (Tc 99m DTPA), which is excreted almost exclusively by glomerular filtration; (2) radioactive iodine–labeled orthoiodohippuric acid

(Hippuran I 131), which is excreted primarily by tubular secretion; (3) technetium-labeled dimercaptosuccinic acid (Tc 99m DMSA), which is bound by cortical tubular cells; and (4) technetium-labeled glucoheptonate (Tc 99m GHA), which combines the properties of DTPA and DMSA.

Current gamma camera external scanning techniques can produce roentgenographic images of the kidneys and collecting system (renal scan). In addition, curves plotting the accumulation of the radioactive compound in the renal areas versus time can be constructed (isotopic renogram). Finally, since the early accumulation of radioactive tracers in the kidneys depends mainly on the blood supply, the magnitude of the renal blood flow can be estimated by isotopic techniques. The choice of agent depends on the problem to be investigated; consequently the physician performing the test should be provided with the pertinent clinical information.

The imaging procedure is safe, since the radiation exposure risk of isotopic studies is generally less than that of standard urography. Its indications are quite broad and include (1) the screening evaluation of patients suspected of having hypertension caused by renal artery stenosis; (2) the evaluation of solid renal masses to distinguish between tumor and pseudotumor; (3) the diagnostic evaluation of patients with acute and chronic renal failure, particularly to assess renal blood supply and the presence or absence of obstruction; and (4) the postoperative follow-up monitoring of renal function in renal transplant recipients.

RENAL BIOPSY

Although renal biopsy specimens may be obtained surgically, percutaneous renal biopsy is usually the procedure of choice in the morphologic evaluation of medical ailments of the kidney. The procedure is relatively simple and safe in experienced hands. The lower pole of the right kidney is usually chosen, its exact position being determined roentgenographically or by renal ultrasonography. With the patient under local anethesia, the kidney is first located by means of a thin-bore spinal needle, and subsequently renal tissue is obtained using the Franklin modification of the Vim-Silverman biopsy needle or with a specially designed disposable needle (Travenol needle). Complete bed rest is prescribed, and the patient is carefully observed for the following 24 hours. The obtained tissue should be processed for light microscopy (and stained with hematoxylin-eosin, periodic acid—Schiff [PAS], PAS—silver methenamine, Masson trichrome, and if indicated other special stains), electron microscopy, and immunofluorescence studies. Light microscopy sections should not exceed 3 μm in thickness. For a biopsy specimen to be diagnostically adequate, it should contain at least 5 to 10 glomeruli.

The absolute or relative contraindications to percutaneous renal biopsy are patient uncooperativeness, the presence of a single kidney, bleeding and/or coagulation abnormalities, uncontrolled hypertension, and small, contracted kidneys. In the case of active or suspected renal infection or neoplasm, needle biopsy should not be performed owing to the risk of dissemination.

Renal biopsy is particularly useful in the diagnosis of glomerular diseases, which are currently classified mainly on the basis of clinicopathologic correlations. Thus biopsies are commonly performed in patients with the nephrotic syndrome, acute nephritic syndrome, and persistent urinary abnormalities to diagnose the underlying disease, establish a prognosis, and select therapy. Renal biopsy is also frequently indicated to determine the degree and type of renal involvement in certain systemic diseases. Acute renal failure of obscure cause or protracted course is another indication for renal biopsy.

The immediate complications of percutaneous renal biopsy are laceration of the kidney or other intra-abdominal organs and severe bleeding. Infection and perirenal hematomas are uncommon. The formation of an arteriovenous fistula manifested by hematuria and/or severe hypertension is a rare late complication.

BIBLIOGRAPHY

Heinemann, H.O., Maack, T.M., and Sherman, R.L.: Combined clinical and basic science seminar: proteinuria, Am. J. Med. **56**:71, 1974.

Kassirer, J.P., and Gennari, J.F.: Laboratory evaluation of renal function. In Earley, L.E., and Gottschalk, C.W., editors: Strauss and Welt's diseases of the kidney, ed. 3, Boston, 1979, Little, Brown & Co.

Muehrcke, R.C., and Pirani, C.L: Renal biopsy: an adjunct in the study of kidney disease. In Black, D., editor: Renal disease, ed. 3, Oxford, England, 1972, Blackwell Scientific Publications.

Morrison, R.B.I.: Urinanalysis and assessment of renal function. In Black, D., editor: Renal disease, ed. 3, Oxford, England, 1972, Blackwell Scientific Publications.

Rosenfield, A.T., Glickman, M.G., and Hodson, J.: Diagnostic imaging in renal disease, New York, 1979, Appleton-Century-Crofts.

105 • PRIMARY GLOMERULAR DISEASE

Pasha Agarwal and **Brajesh Agarwal**

Glomerular disease includes all renal conditions in which structural and functional abnormalities of the glomeruli are the primary features. The kidneys may be affected in multisystem diseases of known cause, but in the majority of cases of glomerulonephritis the cause remains unknown. Basically, two immunologic mechanisms have been implicated in the pathogenesis of glomerulonephritis. Anti–glomerular basement membrane antibodies play a role in a few cases, but the more common pathogenetic mechanism involves the deposition of circulating antigen-antibody complexes in the glomeruli, which initiates an inflammatory reaction leading to glomerular damage. Recent studies suggest that free circulating antibodies may react with antigens already present in the glomerulus, resulting in in situ immune complex formation. The activation of the complement system plays a major role in the resultant inflammatory process.

The clinical manifestations of the glomerular diseases may be in three different forms: asymptomatic urinary abnormalities, nephritic syndrome, or nephrotic syndrome.

ASYMPTOMATIC URINARY ABNORMALITIES

Asymptomatic proteinuria or hematuria may be associated with a benign course; mild to moderate proteinuria is present, sometimes only with lordotic posture. Gross or microscopic hematuria may be persistent or recurrent. Hypoproteinemia, hypertension, edema, and renal failure are absent.

NEPHRITIC SYNDROME

The nephritic syndrome is characterized by evidence of inflammation of the glomeruli and is manifested by the abrupt onset of macroscopic or microscopic hematuria, erythrocyte casts, and proteinuria. Usually it is associated with edema and circulatory congestion, hypertension, and some degree of renal failure, and occasionally it is seen with oliguria. The course may be acute, subacute, or chronic. Most patients with acute glomerulonephritis have a short clinical course and recover spontaneously. Subacute or rapidly progressive glomerulonephritis is more insidious in onset and progressive in course. Patients usually are markedly oliguric, and severe renal failure rapidly develops. In patients with chronic glomerulonephritis caused by various inherited and acquired glomerular diseases, progressive renal functional impairment gradually develops, accompanied by varying degrees of proteinuria, hematuria, and hypertension.

Acute poststreptococcal glomerulonephritis

Acute poststreptococcal glomerulonephritis is a prototype of the acute nephritic syndrome that can be seen in a variety of conditions including some nonstreptococcal infections (pneumococcal pneumonia, bacterial endocarditis, infected ventriculoatrial shunt, sepsis, leptospirosis, infectious hepatitis, infectious mononucleosis, coxsackievirus type B infection, mumps, varicella, echovirus infection, toxoplasmosis, malaria), collagen-vascular disorders, other systemic diseases, and some primary glomerular diseases (membranoproliferative glomerulonephritis, benign focal glomerulonephritis, and IgA nephropathy).

Only a few strains of group A β-hemolytic streptococci are nephritogenic. These strains are typed according to the M protein antigen present on the cell wall of the organism. The strains most frequently associated with nephritis include 1, 2, 4, 12, 18, 25, 49 (Red Lake), 55, 57, and 60. Poststreptococcal glomerulonephritis is an immune complex disease, but the nature of the antigen is not well defined. However, it appears to be derived from the streptococcal organism.

PATHOLOGY. Acute poststreptococcal glomerulonephritis is characterized histologically by diffuse cellular proliferation involving all glomeruli. There is an increase in endothelial and mesangial cells along with an infiltration of neutrophils. The capillary lumen may be narrowed and sometimes obliterated. In severe cases there may be necrotizing changes, extravasation of debris, fibrin, and neutrophils in Bowman's space, and formation of crescents because of proliferation of epithelial cells of Bowman's capsule. The tubules may be dilated and filled with red blood cells and casts. Edema and infiltration of inflammatory cells in the interstitium may also be noted. In the healing phase, sclerotic changes in the glomeruli may occur. In some series a persistent increase in the cellularity in the mesangial stalk region has been described. This is a nonspecific finding and can occur in patients without a history of acute infection. Electron microscopy characteristically shows scattered subepithelial deposits of electron-dense material in the form of humps. Immunofluorescence reveals diffuse granular deposits of IgG, complement (C3), properdin, and fibrinogen.

CLINICAL MANIFESTATIONS. Poststreptococcal glomerulonephritis occurs in all age groups but most commonly in children. The peak incidence is between the ages of 3 and 7 years, and the disease is more frequent in males. Characteristically there is a latent period of a few days between the onset of acute streptococcal infection (in the throat or skin) and clinical findings suggestive of acute glomerulonephritis. The clinical features in the elderly may be very atypical.

The onset may be heralded by vague constitutional symptoms. Usually the patient has a history of gross hematuria. Sometimes the urine is described as smoky or cola colored. Hematuria may be microscopic, and the disease may remain undetected if urinalysis is not performed carefully. Oliguria and anuria are uncommon and, when present, indicate a poor prognosis. Dull, aching pain in the abdomen or loins may also be present. In most symptomatic patients some degree of edema develops, most prominently in the face and eyelids in the morning. Later in the disease course, dependent edema and anasarca may develop. The patient may also have mild to moderate hypertension, circulatory congestion, and in some cases pulmonary edema caused by volume expansion. During the acute phase, one possible development is severe hypertension resulting in hypertensive encephalopathy. In the majority of cases in adults the course is that of slow healing with clinical improvement and return of the blood pressure to normal. Abnormal urinary findings such as mild proteinuria and microscopic hematuria may persist as long as 2 years after clinical resolution with a normal glomerular filtration rate. In the acute stage up to 5% of patients die of complications despite dialysis. A rapidly progressive decline in renal function leading to end-stage renal failure within a few weeks occurs in a few patients. In most of these cases extensive crescent formation is seen in renal biopsy specimens. Chronic glomerulonephritis can also develop occasionally after apparent clinical healing of acute poststreptococcal glomerulonephritis.

LABORATORY FINDINGS. Urinalysis is the most important test in diagnosing glomerulonephritis. The urine appears red or brownish, and red blood cells and some degree of proteinuria are almost always present. Red blood cell casts are commonly seen. Occasionally, leukocytes, other casts, or proteinuria in the nephrotic range may be found.

The glomerular filtration rate varies from normal in asymptomatic patients to markedly decreased in symptomatic patients. The renal plasma flow and tubular functions are less affected, and the filtration fraction is decreased. The urine-concentrating ability is preserved until advanced renal failure supervenes. Some degree of normocytic normochromic anemia and hypoalbuminemia resulting from excessive fluid retention may be present. Intrinsic myocardial function remains normal, and pulmonary congestion with or without cardiac enlargement reflects an expanded vascular volume caused by sodium retention. The throat culture may be positive for group A β-hemolytic streptococci during the acute phase when the pharynx is the site of infection. Measurements of changing antibody titers to streptococcal antigens (antistreptolysin O [ASO], anti-hyaluronidase, anti-NADase, or streptozyme) help confirm the diagnosis. There seems to be no correlation between the degree of titer increase and the severity of disease. Titers may remain elevated for 6 months. Both the classic and alternate pathways of the complement system are activated in poststreptococcal nephritis. The total serum hemolytic complement (CH_{50}) and C3 components are decreased during the first 3 to 8 weeks.

MANAGEMENT. Streptococcal infection should be treated with antimicrobial drugs. Whether antibiotic treatment prevents the development of acute glomerulonephritis in patients who are already infected with nephritogenic streptococci is controversial. Once glomerulonephritis develops, no treatment modality changes the clinical course. There is no evidence that steroids, cytotoxic agents, or anticoagulants are of benefit, and their use is not recommended. Complications such as circulatory congestion, hypertension, and metabolic abnormalities should be prevented or treated promptly with appropriate diet, fluid and sodium restriction, diuretics, antihypertensives, and dialysis as indicated.

Rapidly progressive glomerulonephritis

Rapidly progressive glomerulonephritis is a clinicopathologic syndrome characterized by a rapid deterioration of renal function leading quickly to uremia and by proliferation of extracapillary cells of Bowman's capsule (crescents). It may be of unknown cause (idiopathic) or associated with other diseases, for example, poststreptococcal glomerulonephritis, hypersensitivity angiitis, Goodpasture's syndrome, Wegener's granulomatosis, systemic lupus erythematosus, Schönlein-Henoch purpura, hemolytic-uremic syndrome, thrombotic thrombocytopenic purpura, mixed cryoglobulinemia, and membranoproliferative glomerulonephritis.

PATHOGENESIS AND PATHOLOGY. The most striking findings are the proliferation of extracapillary cells and the formation of crescents in more than 60% of the glomeruli. Necrosis, neutrophilic infiltration, and fibrin deposition are present to a variable degree. Gross examination reveals a large, pale kidney with petechiae on the surface. In most cases of idiopathic, rapidly progressive glomerulonephritis, linear deposits of immunoglobulins in an uninterrupted continuous pattern along the glomerular basement membrane (GBM) are found. This finding, along with the presence of circulating anti-GBM antibodies in the serum of many of these patients, indicates that the pathogenesis of glomerular injury is immunologically mediated through anti-GBM antibodies. However, anti-GBM anti-bodies and their linear deposition along the GBM are not seen in all cases, and in some of these patients the pathogenesis of the disease may be the deposition of immune complexes.

CLINICAL MANIFESTATIONS. The onset may be abrupt or insidious. A patient may have nonspecific constitutional complaints. At the time of the initial examination, oliguria or anuria is commonly present. Proteinuria, hematuria, and red blood cell casts, indicating glomerular damage, are almost always found. The blood urea nitrogen and creatinine values are elevated. Hypertension and edema may sometimes be present. In many cases there is no obvious predisposing cause.

MANAGEMENT. In 90% of patients with rapidly progressive glomerulonephritis, end-stage renal failure develops within a short time. No treatment has been proved to be consistently effective. Steroids, immunosuppressive drugs, anticoagulants, and antiplatelet drugs alone and in various combinations have been tried. Recently, large doses of steroids (prednisone, 30 mg/kg) given intravenously as a pulse therapy in varying regimens have been shown to be beneficial in some cases, especially those in which the glomerulonephritis is not induced by anti-GBM antibodies. Plasmapheresis to reduce the circulating levels of anti-GBM antibodies, in combination with steroids and immunosuppressive drugs, has been found effective in reducing mortality and long-term mobility. Even though recurrence of glomerulonephritis induced by anti-GBM antibodies is common in transplanted kidneys, patients do well for extended periods. Therefore transplantation of the kidney is not contraindicated.

Goodpasture's syndrome

The syndrome of pulmonary hemorrhage associated with glomerulonephritis is called Goodpasture's syndrome. This clinical picture is nonspecific and can be seen in other diseases (Wegener's granulomatosis, systemic lupus erythematosus, mixed cryoglobulinemia, and necrotizing vasculitis).

Renal biopsy reveals focal glomerulonephritis early in the disease, but with progression of lesions, crescent formation is seen in the majority of the glomeruli. Linear deposits of immunoglobulin along the GBM are characteristically found on immunofluorescence studies.

Goodpasture's syndrome is usually seen in young men. Associations with influenza and with exposure to volatile hydrocarbons have been reported in a few cases. Hemoptysis usually precedes the apparent onset of glomerulonephritis. Iron deficiency anemia develops, and the sputum contains hemosiderin-laden macrophages. Urinalysis reveals erythrocytes, casts, and proteinuria. Renal failure develops rapidly. Anti-GBM antibodies are present in the circulation. The most common course is that of waxing and waning pulmonary hemorrhages and the development of progressive, often irreversible, renal failure. Treatment is similar to that of rapidly progressive glomerulonephritis (discussed in preceding section). Bilateral nephrectomy and maintenance dialysis have been recommended to prevent possibly fatal pulmonary hemorrhage. Success with plasmapheresis appears to make this obsolete.

Focal glomerulonephritis

Focal glomerulonephritis includes several conditions in which some of the glomeruli are affected while others remain normal. Various syndromes in which focal glomerulonephritis is seen are recurrent or persistent hematuria, benign hematuria with focal glomerulonephritis, IgA nephropathy (Berger's disease), and hereditary nephritis. This lesion also occurs in some systemic diseases such as subacute bacterial endocarditis, Schönlein-Henoch purpura, systemic lupus erythematosus, and hypersensitivity angiitis.

The clinical features of the various syndromes of undetermined cause are similar, and it is possible that they may have the same pathogenesis. Patients usually have recurrent or persistent hematuria and mild proteinuria. Hypertension, the nephrotic syndrome, and renal failure are uncommon, and the prognosis is generally good.

IgA NEPHROPATHY (BERGER'S DISEASE). The most clearly defined syndrome associated with focal nephritis is IgA nephropathy, or Berger's disease, which is characterized by deposits of IgA in the mesangial area of the glomeruli. IgG and complement are also present but stain less intensely on immunofluorescence. Light microscopy shows a variable histologic picture, but segmental or diffuse proliferative changes may be seen.

This disease is more common in boys and young men. Most patients have either episodes of gross hematuria, frequently preceded by an acute respiratory illness, or persistent microscopic hematuria. Heavy proteinuria has occasionally been noted, and renal failure may develop in as many as 20% of the cases. The response to corticosteroid treatment is variable. In patients requiring renal transplantation, the recurrence of IgA nephropathy is common.

Glomerulonephritis associated with bacterial endocarditis and ventriculoatrial shunt infection

Glomerulonephritis may develop in patients with bacterial endocarditis and ventriculoatrial shunt infection. Usually this follows chronic indolent infection with organisms such as streptococci or *Staphylococcus albus*. However, development of the acute nephritic syndrome has also been seen in association with fulminant infections such as those caused by *S. aureus*.

Kidney biopsy specimens show focal or diffuse proliferative changes in the glomeruli. In severe cases the proliferation of epithelial cells (crescents) can also be seen. The development of the renal lesion appears to be related to the deposition of immune complexes rather than to bacterial embolization, since granular deposits of IgG and complement can be detected in the peripheral capillaries. Electron microscopy shows electron-dense material in the basement membrane in the subendothelial area of the capillary loops. During the acute phase rheumatoid factor, circulating immune complexes, and cryoglobulins can be detected in the serum, and serum levels of C1q, C3, and C4 are diminished. The symptoms and clinical course vary from asymptomatic hematuria and proteinuria to oliguria and advanced renal failure. The prognosis is good if the infection is promptly and successfully treated.

Hereditary nephritis (Alport's syndrome)

Hereditary nephritis, or Alport's syndrome, consists of nephritis and nerve deafness. The mode of inheritance seems to be autosomally dominant with variable penetrance. Males are more severely affected, and the disease is more often transmitted through an afflicted female.

Histologic findings of mixed glomerular and tubulo-interstitial diseases are usually present. The glomeruli may show segmental hypercellularity, sclerosis, and at times crescent formation. Foam cells in the interstitium and tubular dilation and atrophy are commonly found. The electron microscopic finding of splitting and lamellation of the glomerular capillary basement membrane is characteristic of hereditary nephritis.

The disease may be clinically latent for many years, although laboratory abnormalities are present. A defect in hearing, which may be unilateral nerve deafness, is present in one third of the patients. Ocular abnormalities such as cataracts, keratoconus, myopia, and nystagmus may also be present in some cases.

Hematuria is the most common renal manifestation of the disease. Proteinuria is mild or absent in the early stages, but in the advanced stage heavy proteinuria may be present. Renal failure, often accompanied by hypertension, develops in the late second or third decade of life. The patients are treated with dialysis or transplantation or both.

NEPHROTIC SYNDROME

The nephrotic syndrome is characterized by heavy proteinuria (more than 3.5 g protein/1.73 m^2 body surface area/day) and is usually associated with hypoalbuminemia, hyperlipidemia, and edema. Lipiduria is a constant finding and can be demonstrated by light microscopy as oval fat bodies and fatty casts or as "Maltese crosses" under polarizing light. Abnormal tubular functions such as aminoaciduria and glycosuria are also noted in some patients. The following outline includes some of the conditions associated with the nephrotic syndrome:

Causes and conditions associated with the nephrotic syndrome

I. Primary glomerular diseases (idiopathic)
   A. Lipoid nephrosis
   B. Membranous nephropathy
   C. Membranoproliferative glomerulonephritis
   D. Proliferative glomerulonephritis
   E. Focal glomerular sclerosis
II. Allergens
   A. Bee sting
   B. Pollen
   C. Poison oak
   D. Poison ivy
   E. Insect repellent
III. Drugs
   A. Penicillamine
   B. Bismuth
   C. Gold
   D. Probenecid
   E. Trimethadione
IV. Collagen-vascular diseases
   A. Systemic lupus erythematosus
   B. Polyarteritis nodosa
V. Metabolic diseases
   A. Diabetes mellitus
   B. Amyloidosis
   C. Multiple myeloma
VI. Infectious diseases
   A. Quartan malaria (*Plasmodium malariae*)
   B. Bacterial endocarditis
   C. Schistosomiasis
   D. Secondary syphilis
VII. Neoplastic diseases
   A. Bronchogenic carcinoma
   B. Hodgkin's disease
   C. Colonic carcinoma
VIII. Vascular diseases
   A. Constrictive pericarditis
   B. Renal vein thrombosis
   C. Inferior vena cava obstruction
IX. Congenital nephrotic syndrome
X. Heredofamilial nephrotic syndrome
XI. Pregnancy

More than 70% of cases of nephrotic syndrome in Western countries are related to primary glomerular diseases. In the remaining cases the most common causes of the nephrotic syndrome are diabetes, amyloidosis, multiple myeloma, and collagen-vascular diseases. The clinical course, prognosis, and response to treatment in patients with the nephrotic syndrome correlate with the underlying disease.

PATHOGENESIS OF PROTEINURIA AND EDEMA. Increased glomerular basement membrane permeability caused by an immunologic, inflammatory, or metabolic abnormality results in proteinuria. Usually proteins of low molecular weight, such as albumin and α-globulin, are excreted in excessive amounts, while the higher molecular weight proteins are retained in the blood. When albumin synthesis cannot keep pace with the excretion and catabolic process, hypoalbuminemia develops. The plasma oncotic pressure falls, and in accordance with Starling's law, fluid shifts to the interstitial space from the intravascular compartment. A decrease in intravascular volume causes a reduction of the effective renal blood flow, a decrease in the glomerular filtration rate, and stimulation of the production of aldosterone (secondary to renin-angiotensin) and antidiuretic hormone. All these hemodynamic and endocrine changes result in excessive sodium and water retention and edema formation.

CLINICAL MANIFESTATIONS. Except for cases in which heavy proteinuria is detected during routine urinalysis, most patients with the nephrotic syndrome initially show edema in the lower extremities, followed by anasarca. Later, fluid accumulates in the serosal (peritoneal, pleural, and pericardial) cavities.

When the protein loss is massive, patients may show manifestations of malnutrition. Transverse white bands appear on the nails as the result of hypoalbuminemia. Unless accompanied by severe renal failure, anemia is uncommon. However, the patient appears pale. Hypertension develops in some patients. The incidence of myocardial infarction and atherosclerotic heart disease is high. A transient deterioration of renal function as evidenced by elevation of blood urea nitrogen and creatinine values and orthostatic hypotension may occur as a result of overtreatment with diuretics and strict sodium restriction.

LABORATORY FINDINGS. Examination of the urine shows heavy proteinuria and lipiduria. In the blood the typical findings are hypoalbuminemia and hyperlipidemia. The pathogenesis of hyperlipidemia is unclear but may be related to increased synthesis of lipoproteins. Characteristically, patients with the nephrotic syndrome also have decreased α_1-globulin levels and increased α_1- and β-globulin levels. Increased concentrations of fibrinogen, fibrinolytic inhibitors, and factors V, VII, VIII, and X have been observed. The serum T_4 level may be low, but the patients are clinically euthyroid. Hypomagnesemia has also been reported.

MANAGEMENT. All attempts should be made to diagnose the cause of the nephrotic syndrome, and therapy should be guided accordingly (see the following and Chapter 106). A diet rich in protein (2 to 3 g protein/kg body weight/day) is recommended, since edema is a direct consequence of hypoalbuminemia. Supplementary vitamins are also suggested because vitamins may be lost with the proteinuria. Some restrictions on salt intake should be made, but with the availability of modern diuretics a severe restriction of salt intake is not needed. Mild edema does not necessitate diuretic therapy, but patients with marked fluid retention are treated with the thiazide group of diuretics, and in resistant cases loop diuretics may be used. Because some bacterial infections in these patients may be caused by a loss of immunoglobulins in the urine, appropriate antibiotics should be promptly started to prevent overwhelming infection. The beneficial effects of pneumococcal polysaccharide vaccination in patients with the nephrotic syndrome are being investigated. Attempts to decrease massive proteinuria with iatrogenic embolization through the renal arteries, surgical nephrectomy, and administration of indomethacin should be discouraged because they may be harmful.

Primary glomerular diseases resulting in the nephrotic syndrome

LIPOID NEPHROSIS. Lipoid nephrosis, also called minimal lesion disease or nil disease, is characterized by the absence of significant glomerular abnormalities on light microscopy. Glomerular abnormalities can be seen only with the electron microscope. Fusion of the foot processes of the epithelial cells is consistently present. The basement membrane itself shows no abnormality. No immunologic abnormality in the blood or renal tissue has been demonstrated. The cause is unknown, but some patients have a history of exposure to an allergen. There is an increased incidence of this lesion in patients with Hodgkin's disease.

In the age group of 1 to 5 years 95% of patients with nephrotic syndrome have lipoid nephrosis, whereas only 20% of nephrotic adults have it. The disease is characterized by an insidious onset of edema. The renal function remains stable for several years. Persistent hematuria and hypertension are absent. The prognosis is good; spontaneous remission occurs in 60% of the cases, and 90% show remission with corticosteroids. Initially prednisone, 1 mg/kg body weight/day, is recommended. The daily dosage is reduced to 15 to 20 mg after remission is obtained. The complications associated with steroids may be minimized by alternate-day prednisone therapy. Cylophosphamide is used for patients with frequent relapses or those requiring high doses of prednisone.

MEMBRANOUS NEPHROPATHY. Membranous nephropathy is characterized by diffuse thickening of the basement membrane of the glomerular capillary walls without cellular proliferation. Early in the disease the basement membrane may not show much change on routine light microscopy. However, spikelike projections of the epithelial surface of the basement membrane may be demonstrated with silver methenamine staining, and electron microscopy reveals subepithelial deposits of electron-dense material. In the advanced stages, diffuse thickening of the basement membrane becomes apparent on light microscopy. Immunofluorescence studies reveal deposits of immune complexes containing IgG and complement in a granular pattern in capillary walls. These morphologic lesions have also been seen in patients with systemic lupus erythematosus, carcinoma, sarcoidosis, renal vein thrombosis, diabetes mellitus, hepatitis B antigenemia, secondary syphilis, and schistosomiasis. Certain toxic drugs such as mercury (organic and inorganic), gold, penicillamine, and trimethadione can also cause the nephrotic syndrome with similar histologic findings. However, in idiopathic membranous nephropathy no specific antigen has been demonstrated.

Idiopathic membranous nephropathy is a disease of adults and is rare in children. The mode of onset is insidious, and the clinical course varies. About 20% to 25% of the patients show spontaneous remission. Of the remaining patients, some have very rapid deterioration of renal function leading to end-stage renal disease within 3 to 5 years. In others the course is indolent, and the rate of decline in renal function is slow. Hypertension may be present, and in some cases microscopic hematuria has also been noted. Interestingly, renal vein thrombosis frequently occurs in these patients and seems to be the result rather than the cause of the disease.

Steroid therapy has been tried, but no consistent beneficial effect has been seen. In a recent study the early initiation of steroid treatment prevented a decrease in glomerular filtration in patients with membranous nephropathy and a normal glomerular filtration rate. Alkylating agents are not effective.

MEMBRANOPROLIFERATIVE GLOMERULONEPHRITIS. At least two and perhaps three subgroups comprise the disorder called membranoproliferative glomerulonephritis or mesangiocapillary glomerulonephritis. The glomeruli are usually enlarged, and marked accentuation of the lobular pattern is usually visible. The characteristic findings are hypercellularity of the mesangial or centrilobular area with subendothelial extension of mesangial cells and matrix into the periphery of capillary walls, giving an appearance of duplicated basement membranes. In type I a close relationship between membranoproliferative glomerulonephritis and classic lobular glomerulonephritis is found. Finely granular subendothelial and mesangial deposits are commonly demonstrable on electron microscopy. Immunofluorescence staining shows C3 and IgG along capillary walls. Complement is activated through the classic pathway. In type II, dense intramembranous deposits giving an appearance of ribbonlike thickening of the basement membrane are found. On immunofluorescence, these deposits stain only for complement. This disease usually occurs in adolescents or young adults. There may be an acute onset of hematuria associated with proteinuria, but more commonly the onset is insidious. The disease may also be manifested by asymptomatic proteinuria and mild or no edema. In many cases hypertension develops. Partial lipodystrophy in women is sometimes associated with the type II lesion. The characteristic feature of this disease is persistent hypocomplementemia, which is more commonly seen with the type II lesion. The serum of these patients contains a factor (C3 NeF) that is capable of activating the alternate pathway of complement at the C3 step Complement factors preceding C3 in the complement activation cascade may be normal while the level of C3 is low. There is a high incidence of recurrence of the disease in transplanted kidneys. Corticosteroid and alkylating agents do not seem to have any beneficial effect.

PROLIFERATIVE GLOMERULONEPHRITIS. Proliferative glomerulonephritis is a heterogeneous group of diseases causing the nephrotic syndrome in 30% of nephrotic patients. There is a definite increase in glomerular cellularity. The classic picture is seen in poststreptococcal acute glomerulonephritis (described previously). In some of these patients the nephrotic syndrome follows an acute attack of glomerulonephritis. Generally the prognosis is good, and renal function returns to normal. Remission of the nephrotic syndrome can occur as long as 12 to 18 months after onset. Proliferative glomerulonephritis with marked glomerular damage is usually associated with a poor prognosis. A good prognosis has been documented in patients with mild mesangial proliferative glomerulonephritis. These patients also show improvement with steroid treatment.

FOCAL GLOMERULOSCLEROSIS. The characteristic lesion in focal glomerulosclerosis is segmental sclerosis and hyalinization of some glomeruli, especially those in the deeper cortex. Usually only part of the capillary tuft is involved, but occasionally the affected glomeruli may be totally hyalinized. The capillary lumina are obliterated, and the involved capillary tuft shows adhesion to the adjacent Bowman's capsule. Tubular atrophy and interstitial fibrosis are often present. Electron microscopic examination may reveal various combinations of paramesangial, subendothelial, and intramembranous electron-dense deposits. No specific findings are consistently reported on immunofluorescence. The presence of fibrin or fibrinogen has been described in one third of the cases. Focal and segmental hyalinosis is not a specific disease entity. Similar histopathologic changes are seen in Alport's syndrome, hypertension, pyelonephritis, and persistent idiopathic proteinuria. However, when seen in nephrotic patients, hyalinosis is a significant finding. Focal and segmental hyalinosis should not be confused with focal and segmental glomerulonephritis in which proliferation of the cells and not hyalinization of the capillary tuft is the diagnostic finding.

Focal glomerulosclerosis most commonly affects children, but such lesions can also be seen in adults. The mode of onset is insidious. The disease is characterized by edema and heavy proteinuria. Microscopic hematuria is common. Hypertension and decreased renal function may be found at the time of detection of focal glomerulosclerosis. In drug addicts with the nephrotic syndrome, focal glomerulosclerosis is usually the main histologic finding.

The prognosis is poor, and renal function deteriorates rapidly. Patients with total hyalinization of the glomeruli have a better prognosis than those with segmental sclerosis. The response to corticosteroids is poor.

CHRONIC GLOMERULONEPHRITIS. Chronic glomerulonephritis is the final outcome of several different types of renal disease. Histologically, the most striking feature is hyalinization of most of the glomeruli. Undamaged glomeruli show a proliferation of cells. The capillary walls are usually thickened. In moderate chronic proliferative glomerulonephritis, tubular atrophy and interstitial scarring may not be extensive. There is often no history of renal disease, infection, or any systemic disease. Frequently the disease is manifested by the nephrotic syndrome and symptoms and signs of renal failure. The prognosis and response to treatment are poor.

BIBLIOGRAPHY

Bacani, R.A., and others: Rapidly progressive (nonstreptococcal) glomerulonephritis, Ann. Intern. Med. **69:**463, 1968.

Baldwin, D.S., and Schacht, R.G.: Late sequelae of poststreptococcal glomerulonephritis, Annu. Rev. Med. **27:**49, 1976.

Cameron, J.S., and others: The nephrotic syndrome in adults with "minimal change" glomerular lesions, Q. J. Med. **43:**461, 1974.

Coggins, C.H.: An interhospital study of the adult idiopathic nephrotic syndrome and its response to treatment, Kidney Int. **8:**408, 1975.

Donado, J.V., Jr., and others: Idiopathic membranoproliferative (mesangiocapillary) glomerulonephritis: a clinicopathologic study, Mayo Clin. Proc. **54:**141, 1979.

Glassock, R.J.: Clinical aspects of acute, rapidly progressive and chronic glomerulonephritis. In Earley, L.E., and Gottschalk, C.W., editors: Strauss and Welt's diseases of the kidney, ed. 3, Boston, 1979, Little, Brown & Co.

Gluck, M.C., and others: Membranous glomerulonephritis: evolution of clinical and pathologic features, Ann. Intern. Med. **78:**1, 1973.

Gutman, R.A., and others: The immune complex glomerulonephritis of bacterial endocarditis, Medicine **51:**1, 1972.

Habib, R.: Focal glomerular sclerosis (editorial), Kidney Int. **4:**355, 1973.

Hayslett, J.P., and others: Clinicopathological correlations in the nephrotic syndrome due to primary renal disease, Medicine **52:**93, 1973.

McKenzie, P.E., and others: Plasmapheresis in glomerulonephritis, Clin. Nephrol. **12**:97, 1979.
Merrill, J.P: Glomerulonephritis, N. Engl. J. Med. **290**:257, 1974.
Nissenson, A.R., and others: Poststreptococcal acute glomerulonephritis: fact and controversy, Ann. Intern. Med. **91**:76, 1979.
Pierides, A.M., and others: Idiopathic membranous nephropathy, Q. J. Med. **182**:163, 1977.
Sherman, R.L., Churg, J., and Yudis, M.: Hereditary nephritis with a characteristic renal lesion, Am. J. Med. **56**:44, 1974.
Wilson, C.B., and Dixon, F.J.: Antiglomerular basement membrane antibody induced glomerulonephritis, Kidney Int. **3**:74, 1973.
Wilson, C.B., and Dixon, F.J.: Immunopathology and glomerulonephritis, Annu. Rev. Med. **25**:83, 1974.
Zimmerman, S.W., and Burkholder, P.M.: Immunoglobulin A nephropathy, Arch. Intern. Med. **135**:1217, 1974.

106 • RENAL LESIONS IN SYSTEMIC DISEASE

Brajesh Agarwal and **Pasha Agarwal**

COLLAGEN-VASCULAR DISEASES
Systemic lupus erythematosus

(See Chapter 16.)

Renal involvement is seen clinically in two thirds of the cases of systemic lupus erythematosus. In many patients the kidney is the initial organ involved. Although lupus nephritis is commonly accompanied by other systemic findings, it may be the sole manifestation during the entire course of the disease.

PATHOLOGY. Although the pathologic changes are present primarily in the glomeruli, very occasionally only interstitial nephritis is present. Renal involvement may occur in the absence of abnormalities in urinalysis or renal function. The renal lesion in lupus may be (1) minimal, with some increase in mesangial structure, (2) focal proliferative glomerulonephritis, (3) diffuse proliferative glomerulonephritis, or (4) membranous glomerulonephritis. Typical "wire looping" (a rigid-appearing eosinophilic glomerular capillary) wall is seen in association with proliferative lesions. Lupus nephritis is a classic example of immune-complex disease. The complexes are initially deposited in the mesangium and later extend to the subendothelial areas of the glomerular capillary walls. In the membranous form, immune complexes are deposited in the subepithelial aspect of the basement membrane. The clinical course of the disease seems to correlate with the histologic findings and with the amount and site of immune-complex deposition.

CLINICAL MANIFESTATIONS. The clinical presentation and course of the disease vary from mild asymptomatic urinary abnormalities to the nephritic syndrome and rapidly progressive glomerulonephritis. The nephrotic syndrome or renal failure rarely develops in patients with minimal histologic changes, and therefore these patients have a better prognosis. Patients with diffuse proliferative changes and subendothelial deposits have a worse prognosis. They usually have proteinuria and hematuria, and renal failure develops rapidly. Patients with membranous lupus nephritis often show the clinical symptoms of the nephrotic syndrome. The rate of deterioration of renal function is slow. Various immunologic abnormalities such as a low serum complement concentration and the presence of antinuclear antibodies, anti-DNA antibodies, circulating immune complexes, cryoglobulins, and rheumatoid factors can be detected in the serum.

MANAGEMENT. Treatment regimens for lupus nephritis are varied, and results are controversial. Extrarenal manifestations of the disease must be considered in planning reasonable treatment. Since there is no accurate way of correlating renal histology with urinary sediment and protein excretion and serologic abnormalities, a renal biopsy is often performed.

Patients with minimal histologic lesions can be treated with small oral doses of steroids (prednisone, 0.5 mg/kg/day). The serious morbidity and increased mortality associated with high doses of prednisone or cytotoxic drugs must be weighed against the inherent risk of the lesion. If there is no improvement or if toxicity develops, the steroid dosage should be tapered. The patient should be observed for signs of progression of the lesion to the diffuse form.

Suggestions for the management of membranous lupus nephritis with the nephrotic syndrome vary from no therapy to a 6-week trial of prednisone (1 mg/kg/day), followed by a lower dose or alternate-day therapy if a remission is induced. There is uniform agreement that diffuse proliferative glomerular lesions with proteinuria or azotemia should be treated aggressively, but therapeutic approaches vary. Regimens consisting of oral cyclophosphamide (2 to 2.5 mg/kg/day) and high doses of prednisone (1 mg/kg/day) alone or in combination have been advocated. Comparison studies of the treatment of diffuse proliferative glomerulonephritis with high doses of oral prednisone (1 mg/kg/day) versus short-term intravenous steroid regimens (1 g methylprednisolone daily for 3 days) followed by low doses of steroids are in progress. Recently, uncontrolled studies using plasmapheresis followed by cytotoxic drugs have reported improvement of rapidly deteriorating renal function in patients with diffuse proliferative glomerulonephritis and circulating immune complexes.

Scleroderma

(See Chapter 17.)

PATHOLOGY. Renal involvement in scleroderma (progressive systemic sclerosis) is not uncommon and adversely affects the prognosis. Pathologic changes such as concentric intimal proliferation and the deposition of mucoid material are seen mainly in the arcuate and interlobular arteries. The vessel lumen may be partly or totally occluded. The arterioles show fibrinoid necrosis, and the glomeruli are often ischemic. Patchy bilateral renal cortical necrosis is found in patients with oliguric renal failure. Immunofluorescence studies show fibrinogen in the damaged vessels and glomeruli.

CLINICAL MANIFESTATIONS. Mild proteinuria, often intermittent, is the most common renal manifestation. Patients may have an abrupt onset of malignant hypertension, and renal failure rapidly develops. Some patients have normotensive oliguric renal failure. Azotemia with or without hypertension indicates a poor prognosis.

MANAGEMENT. No definite improvement in scleroderma has been seen with any specific therapy. Patients with hypertension and renal failure should be vigorously treated with antihypertensive medications and dialysis. With the use of antirenin drugs (propranolol and captopril) and vasodilators (minoxidil) in patients with severe hypertension, an improvement in renal function has been documented. Bilateral nephrectomy and maintenance dialysis are recommended for patients with uncontrolled hypertension and irreversible renal failure. Transplantation has been performed successfully in a few patients.

Polyarteritis nodosa

(See Chapter 20.)

PATHOLOGY. Renal pathologic changes are very common in polyarteritis nodosa. Arteritis and obliteration of the vessel lumen with aneurysm formation may occur. In classic polyarteritis the medium-sized vessels are involved and renal cortical infarcts are common. Small vessels are diseased in the microscopic form of hypersensitivity angiitis. Diffuse or focal glomerulitis may be seen, with fibrinoid necrosis and microthrombus formation in glomerular capillaries. Crescent formation may occur, especially when small vessels are involved. There may be interstitial infiltrates of inflammatory cells and tubular atrophy.

CLINICAL MANIFESTATIONS. Renal manifestations of polyarteritis are usually seen in association with symptoms and signs of other systemic involvement. The patients may have gross hematuria, and the clinical picture may resemble that of acute glomerulonephritis. There is a urine sediment containing erythrocytes, erythrocytic casts, fat cells, fatty casts, broad casts, granular casts, and waxy casts; this is referred to as a "telescoped" sediment. Hypertension, the nephrotic syndrome, and a rapid deterioration of renal function are common.

MANAGEMENT. In most cases renal lesions contribute in some way to the death of the patient. High doses of corticosteroids (prednisone, 1 mg/kg/day) are recommended. Azathioprine or cyclophosphamide may be used if there is an inadequate response to the initial corticosteroid treatment.

Wegener's granulomatosis

(See Chapter 22.)

Wegener's granulomatosis is characterized by a necrotizing granulomatous vasculitis that may involve the nasopharynx, paranasal sinuses, lungs, ears, eyes, heart, nervous system, skin, and joints. In the generalized form, renal involvement is common and can be fatal.

PATHOLOGY. The classic renal lesion is a focal and segmental glomerulonephritis with proliferative changes and fibrinoid necrosis. In severe cases diffuse changes and crescent formation occur. In some cases localized subepithelial deposits of dense material are seen on electron microscopy. Immunofluorescence studies show staining for IgG and complement along the basement membrane.

CLINICAL MANIFESTATIONS. The presentation and urinary findings (proteinuria, erythrocytes, and erythrocyte casts) are typical of acute glomerulonephritis. Sinusitis, hemoptysis, and pulmonary infiltrates are often present. The renal function can deteriorate rapidly.

MANAGEMENT. Early diagnosis, frequently by biopsy, is important because Wegener's granulomatosis is a fatal disease if not treated promptly. Long-lasting remissions have been induced with cyclophosphamide (1 to 2 mg/kg/day).

Schönlein-Henoch purpura

(See Chapter 21.)

With Schönlein-Henoch purpura (anaphylactoid purpura), renal damage is more common in children than in adults. Other manifestations of this syndrome (arthritis, rash, and gastrointestinal hemorrhage) are also present in most cases.

PATHOLOGY. Focal and segmental proliferation occurs with fibrinoid necrosis of the glomerular capillary tuft and intracapillary deposition of fibrin. In severe cases crescent formation may occur. Immunofluorescence studies commonly show granular staining of the mesangium for fibrinogen, IgA, IgG, and C3, suggesting that the pathogenesis of renal damage is associated with the deposition of immune complexes in the glomeruli. Serum complement and immunoglobulin levels are usually normal, however.

CLINICAL MANIFESTATIONS. Patients may remain asymptomatic or have hematuria, proteinuria, or renal failure. The clinical course is usually benign with spontaneous remission. However, in some patients with crescentic glomerular changes, advanced renal failure necessitating dialysis may develop.

MANAGEMENT. Besides symptomatic treatment, corticosteroids may be given to treat the extrarenal manifestations of Schönlein-Henoch purpura (see Chapter 21). In patients with progressive renal failure a trial of azathioprine or mercaptopurine may be used.

Hemolytic-uremic syndrome and thrombotic thrombocytopenic purpura

The hemolytic-uremic syndrome occurs most frequently in children, whereas thrombotic thrombocytopenic purpura is more common in adults. Both disorders are characterized by microangiopathic hemolytic anemia and thrombocytopenia. Platelet thrombi are seen in small arteries and capillaries throughout the body. In thrombotic thrombocytopenic purpura, pulmonary and cerebral manifestations may be significant and more marked than the renal involvement. In the hemolytic-uremic syndrome, disseminated intravascular coagulation occurs, and renal involvement is severe. The local deposition of fibrin and platelets in the subendothelial space may result in focal or generalized renal cortical necrosis. The syndrome is characterized by oliguria or anuria, proteinuria, hematuria, and impaired renal function. The prognosis is poor, and the patients usually die of renal failure. The response to treatment with steroids and immunosuppressive drugs is inconsistent. Recently, good results have been reported with exchange transfusion and plasmapheresis.

METABOLIC AND OTHER SYSTEMIC DISEASES
Diabetes mellitus

PATHOLOGY. The common renal lesions in diabetes mellitus are diffuse and nodular intracapillary glomerulosclerosis. Vascular lesions in the form of arteriosclerosis involving vessels of all sizes and hyaline thickening of arterioles, especially the efferent arterioles, are frequent findings. Interstitial fibrosis, glycogen deposition in renal tubules, pyelonephritis, and papillary necrosis are also seen.

CLINICAL MANIFESTATIONS. Proteinuria is usually the first manifestation of diabetic nephropathy. The nephrotic syndrome may occur. Initially, the kidney size and glomerular filtration rate may be above normal. With progression of the disease, hypertension and edema develop and the glomerular filtration rate drops. Hematuria is uncommon. In the majority of cases other evidence of diabetic microangiopathy, particularly diabetic retinopathy, is also present.

Patients with acute papillary necrosis and pyelonephritis may have chills, fever, flank pain, oliguria or anuria, and rapid deterioration of renal function. Acute renal failure may also develop in diabetic patients following the use of radiopaque contrast media.

MANAGEMENT. Diabetic nephropathy may be delayed by good control in insulin-dependent diabetic patients. Diabetic patients maintained with hemodialysis have a much poorer prognosis than nondiabetic patients. They have frequent problems with vascular access and have higher morbidity and mortality because of vascular complications. Blindness and loss of extremities commonly occur. Encouraging results with renal transplantation, especially if performed at an early stage, have been demonstrated in some centers. Long-term peritoneal dialysis may be the therapy of choice, particularly if vascular access is a problem.

Renal amyloidosis

(See Chapter 76.)

Accumulation of amyloid in the kidney occurs frequently in primary or secondary amyloidosis. This is most marked in the glomeruli but may also occur in the peritubular basement membrane, interstitium, and blood vessels. Characteristic amyloid fibrils can be seen by electron microscopy, or affected tissues can be stained with Congo red to demonstrate green birefringence under polarized light.

Proteinuria is the main manifestation of renal amyloidosis. Clinically, the patient may have the nephrotic syndrome or renal insufficiency. Renal tubular disorders such as Fanconi's syndrome or distal renal tubular acidosis may also be present and be associated with Bence Jones proteinuria. Hypertension, although uncommon, may occur. The kidney size may remain normal in spite of advanced renal failure. Death from renal causes is uncommon. There is no effective therapy directed specifically at preventing or reducing amyloidosis. Cases associated with multiple myeloma show remission with alkylating agents, and those following chronic infection may resolve with cure of the infection. Patients with advanced renal failure are treated with dialysis or transplantation or both. However, recurrence of the disease in transplanted kidneys is common.

Multiple myeloma

(See Chapter 76.)

The kidneys are frequently affected in multiple myeloma. Many factors may contribute to renal injury, including hyperuricemia, hypercalcemia, plasma hyperviscosity, interstitial infiltration of plasma cells, pyelonephritis, urinary tract obstruction, and amyloidosis. Renal insufficiency is slowly progressive over several months. Bence Jones proteins (light chains) may have a direct toxic effect on the renal tubules and may result in tubular atrophy and dysfunction. Large eosinophilic casts are commonly seen in tubular lumina. Glomerular changes are minimal. Isolated tubular defects without a reduction of glomerular filtration, such as Fanconi's syndrome, distal renal tubular acidosis, and urine-concentrating defects, are seen in association with the excretion of light chains. Dehydration, use of roentgenographic contrast materials, use of nephrotoxic antibiotics, and hypercalcemia are some of the factors that may precipitate acute renal failure in patients with myeloma who have not previously had renal impairment.

Symptomatic treatment (correction of volume depletion, hypercalcemia, and hyperuricemia) and avoidance of use of nephrotoxic antibiotics and roentgenographic contrast materials are recommended. An improvement in renal function has been noted with the use of alkylating agents. Acute renal failure is treated with forced alkaline diuresis, dialysis, and chemotherapy. In patients with acute renal failure associated with an increased excretion of urinary light chains, plasmapheresis has been successful in restoring renal function. Patients with end-stage renal failure and multiple myeloma can be considered for dialysis and transplantation.

Waldenström's macroglobulinemia

(See Chaper 76.)

In contrast to multiple myeloma, in which glomerular disease is rare, Waldenström's macroglobulinemia may be manifested by large eosinophilic thrombi, nonspecific glomerulitis, or the deposition of amyloid material in the glomeruli. Immunofluorescence studies and electron microscopic examination show intraluminal deposits of IgM between the endothelium and the inner aspect of the glomerular basement membrane. The tubules are rarely affected, but the interstitium may have infiltrates of lymphoid cells. Proteinuria is the most common clinical finding and may be nonselective or may have only light chains. Therapy includes the use of alkylating agents and plasmapheresis.

Essential cryoglobulinemia

Essential mixed cryoglobulinemia, usually of an IgG-IgM combination, may result in renal damage. There is glomerular proliferation with deposition of IgG and IgM. In some cases only one immunoglobulin is present. Occasionally, crescent and intracapillary thrombus formation occurs. The clinical picture is that of acute glomerulonephritis, at times leading to acute renal failure. In some cases both renal lesions and symptoms disappear completely when the exacerbating condition is alleviated. In others, renal failure may persist. In almost all cases, renal lesions are associated with purpura. Extrarenal manifestations of mixed essential cryoglobulinemia include arthralgia, Raynaud's syndrome, extrarenal necrotizing angiitis, and peripheral neuropathy. In rapidly progressive renal failure, plasmapheresis is recommended. Adrenal corticosteroids and immunosuppressive drugs have not been found to be very effective.

Sickle cell disease

(See Chapter 67.)

Although a variety of functional abnormalities are noted in patients with sickle cell disease or uncomplicated sickle cell trait, morphologic defects are seen mainly in sickle cell disease.

PATHOLOGY. The kidneys show enlarged glomeruli, with engorged capillaries filled with sickled red blood cells. In a few cases thickening of glomerular basement membrane, membranoproliferative glomerulonephritis, and segmental glomerular sclerosis have also been described. Patchy interstitial fibrosis, especially in the medulla, and papillary necrosis are common.

CLINICAL MANIFESTATIONS. Microscopic hematuria is the most common renal manifestation of both sicle cell disease and sickle cell trait. There may be recurrent bouts or a single episode of gross hematuria leading to severe anemia. Some patients have the nephrotic syndrome. Papillary necrosis, seen in sickle cell disease, is usually insidious. Advanced renal failure is uncommon. Early in the disease the glomerular filtration rate may be supernormal. Maximal urine-concentrating ability is defective in both the disease and the trait. Initially this defect can be reversed by the transfusion of normal hemoglobin A, but eventually it is irreversible. The pathogenesis of the defect seems to be related to the loss of normal medullary and papillary architecture, as well as to changes in the pattern of vasa recta caused by sickling of the cells. Impaired renal acidification of the urine has also been described.

MANAGEMENT. The treatment of patients with massive hematuria has been frustrating, and no consistently successful regimen is available. A combined regimen of intravenous mannitol to promote osmotic diuresis, potent loop diuretics (furosemide or ethacrynic acid), and sodium bicarbonate to alkalinize the urine, along with infusion of hypotonic fluid, is recommended but often is unsuccessful. ϵ-Aminocaproic acid has been found to be effective. In some patients the massive hematuria is caused by the association of von Willebrand's disease and sickle hemoglobin. Such patients respond to factor VIII infusion. Nephrectomy should be discouraged. For terminal renal failure, hemo-dialysis and transplantation have been used.

Sarcoidosis

(See Chapter 24.)

The kidneys are frequently affected in diffuse sarcoidosis. Although sarcoid granuloma formation is common, it rarely leads to severe renal failure. Impairment of renal function is correlated with the associated hypercalcemia, nephrocalcinosis, and hyperuricemia, and the therapy is directed specifically at those problems. Glomerular changes in the form of membranous glomerulopathy, focal glomerulosclerosis, and proliferative glomerulonephritis have also been reported. Patients with glomerular changes may have the nephrotic syndrome; otherwise, proteinuria usually is mild.

BIBLIOGRAPHY

Alleyne, S.A.O., and others: The kidney in sickle cell anemia, Kidney Int. **7**:371, 1975.

Aster, R.H.: Thrombotic thrombocytopenic purpura: new clues to the etiology of an enigmatic disease, N. Engl. J. Med. **297**:1400, 1977.

Baldwin, D.S., and others: The clinical course of the proliferative and membranous forms of lupus nephritis, Ann. Intern. Med. **73**:929, 1970.

Baldwin, D.S., and others: Lupus nephritis: clinical course as related to morphologic forms and their transitions, Am. J. Med. **62**:12, 1977.

Brouet, J.-C., and others: Biologic and clinical significance of cryoglobulins: a report of 86 cases, Am. J. Med. **57:**775, 1974.
Cannon, P.J.: Medical management of renal scleroderma, N. Engl. J. Med. **299:**886, 1978.
DeFronzo, R.A., and others: Renal function in patients with multiple myeloma, Medicine **57:**151, 1978.
Falls, W.F., and others: Nonhypercalcemic sarcoid nephropathy, Arch. Intern. Med. **130:**285, 1972.
Fauci, A.S., Haynes, B.F., and Katz, P.: The spectrum of vasculitis: clinical, pathologic, immunologic, and therapeutic considerations, Ann. Intern. Med. **89:**660, 1978.
Gundersen, H.J., and others: Early and late changes in the diabetic kidney, Adv. Nephrol. **8:**43, 1979.
Hecht, B., and others: Prognostic indices in lupus nephritis, Medicine **55:**163, 1976.
Jacobs, C., and others: Treatment of end-stage renal failure in the insulin-dependent diabetic patient, Adv. Nephrol. **8:**101, 1979.
Kaplan, B.S., and Drummond, K.N.: The hemolytic-uremic syndrome is a syndrome (editorial), N. Engl. J. Med. **298:**964, 1978.
Kyle, R.A., and Bayrd, E.D.: Amyloidosis: review of 236 cases, Medicine **54:**29, 1975.
McCoy, R.C., and Tisher, C.C.: Glomerulonephritis associated with sarcoidosis, Am. J. Pathol. **68:**339, 1972.
Morel-Maroger, L., and Verroust, P.: Glomerular lesions in dysproteinemias, Kidney Int. **5:**249, 1974.
Sebastian, A., and others: Renal amyloidosis, nephrotic syndrome, and impaired renal tubular absorption of bicarbonate, Ann. Intern. Med. **69:**541, 1968.
Wolff, S.M., and others: Wegener's granulomatosis, Ann. Intern. Med. **81:**513, 1974.
Zlotnick, A., and Rosenmann, E.: Renal pathologic findings associated with monoclonal gammopathies, Arch. Intern. Med. **135:**40, 1975.

107 • INTERSTITIAL NEPHRITIS
Paul J. Kovnat

DEFINITION AND ETIOLOGY. "Interstitial nephritis" refers to a group of renal disorders characterized by functional and morphologic alterations in the renal tubules and interstitium. In this category of nephropathies the tubular and interstitial findings are increased out of proportion to the glomerular changes. Other terms for this disorder include "tubulointerstitial disorder," "interstitial nephropathy," "interstitial renal inflammation," and "tubulointerstitial disease." Many of the renal findings are nonspecific responses to noxious substances and systemic disease.

Until a few years ago chronic interstitial nephritis was known as chronic pyelonephritis and was thought to be caused by infection. Studies of patients with urinary tract infections, however, have led to the generally held view that urinary infections rarely if ever cause significant renal damage in adults in the absence of underlying kidney disease or urinary tract obstruction. Furthermore, the majority of patients with interstitial nephritis and infection have the infection as a complication of their underlying disease rather than as the primary process. The infection may be the factor that causes symptoms and therefore triggers the investigation and identification of interstitial nephritis. It is estimated that at least 90% of cases of chronic interstitial nephritis are preventable or reversible with identification and removal or treatment of the underlying causes, which are listed in the following outline:

Causes of interstitial nephritis
I. Obstruction of urinary collecting system
II. Physical factors and environment
   A. Radiation nephritis
   B. Balkan nephritis—limited to Danube Valley (obscure environmental cause)
III. Metabolic causes
   A. Hypercalcemia or hypercalciuria
   B. Hypokalemia
   C. Hyperuricemia or hyperuricosuria
   D. Oxalosis or hyperoxaluria
IV. Hereditary causes
   A. Medullary cystic disease (nephronophthisis)
   B. Sponge kidney
V. Vascular causes
   A. Sickle cell disease
   B. Atheroembolic disease
   C. Nephrosclerosis
VI. Infiltrative causes
   A. Lymphoma
   B. Leukemia
   C. Myeloma
   D. Amyloidosis
VII. Immunologic and granulomatous causes
   A. Transplant rejection
   B. Systemic lupus erythematosus
   C. Sarcoidosis
   D. Sjögren's syndrome
VIII. Hypersensitivity
   A. Antibiotics—sulfonamides, penicillins (especially methicillin), rifampin
   B. Nonsteroidal anti-inflammatory agents
   C. Anticonvulsants
   D. Diuretics
IX. Toxicity
   A. Heavy metals
      1. Cadmium
      2. Copper
      3. Uranium
      4. Lead
   B. Analgesic abuse
   C. Aminoglycosides (gentamicin and tobramycin)
X. Infection
   A. Tuberculosis
   B. Fungus
   C. Bacterial pyelonephritis (?)
XI. No known cause

PATHOLOGY. Interstitial nephritis is characterized by cellular infiltration, edema, and fibrosis of the potential space between nephrons, tubular dilation, and tubular cell atrophy. If edema and infiltration with polymorphonuclear cells are the major findings, the descriptive term "acute interstitial nephritis" is preferred. If tubular atrophy and fibrosis are the major findings, the disease is called "chronic interstitial nephritis." When eosinophils predominate in the interstitium, "allergic interstitial nephritis" is the preferred term. Papillary necrosis may occur, with sloughing of the renal papillae. Fibrosis around Bowman's capsule with secondary glomerular changes may be an attendant finding. In the patient with end-stage renal disease, the histologic findings of chronic interstitial nephritis may be similar to those of the end-stage kidney of chronic glomerular disease.

CLINICAL MANIFESTATIONS. Interstitial nephritis may come to the attention of the physician in one of several ways:

1. Patients may have known systemic disease or known exposure to a toxin, and investigation may show the findings of interstitial nephritis.
2. Patients may have urinary tract infections, and investigation may show evidence of underlying chronic interstitial nephritis as the predisposing factor.
3. Acute flank pain with fever and hematuria may signal papillary necrosis or urinary calculi as the first sign of interstitial nephritis.
4. After seeking treatment for other problems, patients may be found to have abnormal urinary findings, azotemia, or stigmata of chronic interstitial nephritis.
5. Patients may complain of polyuria or nocturia because of early loss of urine-concentrating ability.
6. Evidence for chronic interstitial nephritis may be found during investigation of family members or associates of patients with hereditary or environmental causes of kidney disease.

Interstitial nephritis should be considered in a patient with renal disease (elevated blood urea nitrogen and creatinine levels or abnormal findings on urinalysis) in whom characteristics of primary glomerular disease are absent. Because of its potential reversibility, interstitial nephritis must be differentiated from glomerulonephritis (Table 107-1). Tubular dysfunction may be seen as a specific defect such as salt wasting, loss of urine-concentrating ability (polyuria), or tubular acidosis.

Although tubular and interstitial abnormalities predominate, secondary changes occur in the microcirculation and glomeruli, with a resultant decline in the glomerular filtration rate.

DIAGNOSIS. Evaluation of a patient with interstitial nephritis should include a historical view for (1) exposure to radiation or heavy metal such as lead or cadmium; (2) symptoms of partial urinary obstruction or of gross hematuria, suggestive of stone disease or papillary necrosis; (3) family history of renal disease or sickle cell disease; (4) therapy with drugs such as penicillins, sulfonamides, rifampin, anticonvulsants, aminoglycosides, or methoxyflurane anesthetics; or (5) chronic diarrheal states.

Table 107-1. Comparison of glomerulonephritis and interstitial nephritis

Factor	Glomerulonephritis	Interstitial nephritis
Urinary sediment	Many cells and casts	Few cells and casts
Sodium excretion	Normal until late	Sodium wasting common
Hyperkalemia	Mild until oliguria	May occur early
Proteinuria	>3 g/day	<1 g/day
Type of protein	Primarily albumin	Nonselective with β-microglobulins and lysozyme
Hypertension	Usual	<50% of cases and usually mild
Acidosis	Normochloremic with increased anion gap	Hyperchloremic
Uric acid level	Mildly elevated	Frequently markedly elevated
Anemia	Moderate until renal failure	Disproportionately severe for degree of renal failure
Kidney biopsy	Often diagnostic	Usually nonspecific
Urine volume	Unremarkable	Frequently increased with poor concentrating ability

The physical examination and laboratory screening of patients with interstitial nephritis should search for evidence of systemic disease; elevated urine or serum levels of calcium, uric acid, or oxalate; hypokalemia; or bacteriuria. Intravenous urography may be helpful in papillary necrosis or sponge kidney, but results are not often specific. Renal biopsy is usually not diagnostic, but eosinophils may suggest acute interstitial nephritis.

MANAGEMENT. The cornerstone of therapy is identification and removal or reversal of the underlying cause. A short course of corticosteroid therapy is indicated in some patients with allergic interstitial nephritis. Complicating factors, such as infection, obstruction, volume depletion, congestive heart failure, hypertension, electrolyte disturbances, and administration of nephrotoxins, must be prevented or, if present, appropriately treated. Hemodialysis, peritoneal dialysis, and transplantation may be used for patients with interstitial nephritis in whom renal failure develops despite therapy.

HYPEROXALURIA

Excessive urinary excretion of oxalic acid is caused by excessive production or excessive colonic absorption of oxalic acid. The hyperoxaluria leads to calcium oxalate nephrolithiasis or interstitial nephritis or both.

Causes of hyperoxaluria include (1) primary hyperoxaluria, an autosomal recessive disorder of glyoxalate metabolism; (2) toxicity from drinking antifreeze (ethylene glycol); (3) methoxyflurane-induced anesthesia; and (4) (more recently described) steatorrhea.

Steatorrhea commonly develops in people with chronic inflammatory bowel disease or jejunoileal bypass. In the presence of steatorrhea the calcium in the small-bowel lumen, which normally combines with oxalate to make a nonabsorbable compound, is bound by unabsorbed fatty acids. This leaves oxalate as sodium oxalate rather than as insoluble calcium oxalate, making it abnormally available for absorption. The treatment is aimed at reversing the steatorrhea.

ANALGESIC ABUSE NEPHROPATHY

Analgesic abuse nephropathy, or analgesic nephropathy, is a form of interstitial nephritis usually characterized by papillary necrosis, which is attributable to excessive consumption of analgesics (for example, over 1 kg of phenacetin—six tablets a day for 3 years). This disorder was originally called "phenacetin nephropathy," but in recent years as many as one third of patients with analgesic nephropathy have had no history of significant phenacetin intake. Usually patients have consumed a mixture of analgesics, especially aspririn, phenacetin, and caffeine.

Many analgesic and nonsteroidal anti-inflammatory agents, including phenylbutazone, mefenamic acid (Ponstel), indomethacin (Indocin), sulindac (Clinoril), and propoxyphene (Darvon), have produced papillary necrosis in laboratory animals. More recently, clinical reports have implicated these and other nonsteroidal anti-inflammatory agents as causes for nephropathy.

Analgesics and their metabolites are concentrated in the medulla of the kidney where they inhibit local prostaglandin synthesis, which in turn reduces medullary blood flow. Papillary ischemia, fibrosis, and necrosis result. Salicylate, by uncoupling oxidative phosphorylation and thus inhibiting normal repair of the damaged renal medulla, further contributes to this process.

Analgesic abuse nephropathy may be manifested by symptoms of papillary necrosis such as flank pain, colic, and hematuria. However, patients may also have symptoms of chronic interstitial nephritis, such as nocturia, anemia, salt wasting, and metabolic acidosis, as well as evidence of chronic renal failure. Patients usually have a history of headaches and backaches and may have gastrointestinal symptoms of analgesic excess, such as gastritis or gastrointestinal bleeding. Some patients may not report analgesic use because of embarrassment or failure to recognize the importance of mentioning these nonprescription drugs.

Discontinuance of the use of all analgesics is an essential objective in the care of patients with analgesic abuse nephropathy. The prognosis is good if renal failure is not severe and marked proteinuria has not developed. Even patients with elevated serum creatinine concentrations may display some improvement. Recent evidence suggests an increased risk for the development of transitional cell carcinoma of the bladder in patients with a history of analgesic abuse nephropathy.

BIBLIOGRAPHY

Alfrey, A.: Chronic renal failure: manifestations and pathogenesis. In Schrier, R., editor: Renal and electrolyte disorders, ed. 2, Boston, 1980, Little, Brown & Co.

Cotran, R.S.: Tubulo-interstitial diseases. In Brenner, B.M., and Rector, F.C., Jr., editors: The kidney, ed. 2, Philadelphia, 1981, W.B. Saunders Co.

Freedman, L.: Interstitial renal inflammation, including pyelonephritis and urinary tract infection. In Earley, L.E., and Gottschalk, C.W., editors: Strauss and Welt's diseases of the kidney, Boston, 1979, Little, Brown & Co.

Gower, P.E.: Analgesic nephropathy. In Black, D., and Jones, N., editors: Renal disease, Oxford, England, 1979, Blackwell Scientific Publications.

Heptinstall, R.H.: Pathology of the kidney, Boston, 1974, Little, Brown & Co.

Kincaid-Smith, P.: Analgesic abuse and the kidney, Kidney Int. **17**:250, 1980.

Murray, T., and Goldberg, M.: Etiologies of chronic interstitial nephritis, Ann. Intern. Med. **82**:453, 1975.

108 • OTHER RENAL DISEASES

Steven J. Peitzman

NEPHROGENIC DIABETES INSIPIDUS

Polyuria occasionally results from a tubular inability to generate concentrated urine, even in the presence of antidiuretic hormone (ADH). The polyuria is usually less abundant than that seen in classic central diabetes insipidus, which is characterized by a lack of ADH. An otherwise healthy and alert person with nephrogenic diabetes insipidus therefore usually has little difficulty ingesting enough water to replace the amount voided. On the other hand, impaired access to water for any reason favors dehydration and hypernatremia. A rare congenital nephrogenic diabetes insipidus occurs, but most cases reflect toxic, inschemic, or mechanical damage to the distal tubule and collecting duct. Drugs capable of inducing this disorder include lithium, demeclocycline, and methoxyflurane. They probably interfere with the activation of ADH of adenyl cyclase—mediated cyclic AMP and its effects on increasing the water permeability of the collecting duct. The polyuria caused by methoxyflurane appears to be attributable to a toxic effect of the fluoride ion released metabolically; fortunately, it rarely persists beyond several days. Other causes of nephrogenic diabetes insipidus include hypokalemia, hypercalcemia, obstructive nephropathy, sickle cell trait or disease, pyelonephritis, medullary cystic disease, Sjögren's syndrome, and amyloidosis.

The definitive diagnosis is established when the concentrating defect fails to respond to exogenous ADH (5 mU/min of aqueous vasopressin given intravenously slowly for 1 hour or 5 units vasopressin tannate in oil given intramuscularly).

HYPOKALEMIC NEPHROPATHY

When available for examination, renal tissue from persons with marked potassium depletion reveals a distinct vacuolation of proximal tubular cells. The vacuoles have a striking foamy appearance in advanced cases, but several follow-up biopsies have shown reversal of the histologic derangement with replenishment of body potassium. Although this visible disturbance appears in the proximal tubules, a functional distal effect—loss of concentrating ability—is associated with hypokalemic nephropathy. Hence polyuria (nephrogenic diabetes insipidus) may exacerbate the volume contraction commonly occurring in patients with protracted vomiting, prolonged nasogastric suctioning, or diarrhea, all of which can lead to a cumulative potassium loss. In the absence of volume contraction, hypokalemia itself does not impair the glomerular filtration rate (GFR), and if the potassium loss is through the gastrointestinal tract, little potassium appears in the urine. Profound hypokalemia may rarely produce rhabdomyolysis and myoglobinuric acute renal failure.

HYPERCALCEMIC NEPHROPATHY

"Hypercalcemic nephropathy" is a regrettably indistinct term that comprises several adverse effects of calcium on the kidney. Acute renal failure is said to occasionally follow a rapid and severe rise of the plasma calcium level; the association has been documented most commonly in the hypercalcemia of multiple myeloma. Chronic hypercalcemia of any cause (see Chapter 193) more predictably leads to several phenomena. It may blunt concentrating ability and, much like hypokalemia, may bring on reversible nephrogenic diabetes insipidus. Ample evidence supports hypercalcemia as a cause of moderate hypertension, which may vanish on correction of the calcium elevation. Whether this effect is mediated by a renal disturbance is uncertain.

Nephrocalcinosis is the roentgenographic or pathologic finding of diffuse calcium deposition, which usually is most intense in the renal interstitium. Although it may be wholly asymptomatic, nephrocalcinosis (at least when caused by primary hyperparathyroidism) may correlate with a gradual reduction in the GFR. If associated with hypercalciuria, hypercalcemia predisposes the patient to renal calculi. The treatment of any renal disorder resulting from hypercalcemia would obviously include attention to the underlying cause, as well as specific measures to lower the plasma calcium content (see Chapter 193).

URIC ACID NEPHROPATHY

Throughout the later nineteenth century and most of the twentieth, physicians concerned with renal disease confidently held gout to be a common source of renal failure with chronic interstitial nephritis. Over the last decade, however, a remarkable revision of this understanding has occurred. Careful and prolonged prospective studies of patients with gout indicate that gout in itself rarely induces renal failure. Hence the relationship between the histologic picture (interstitial sodium urate deposits with surrounding inflammation) and the clinical event (decrease in the GFR) now seems uncertain. Many gouty persons undeniably suffer renal insufficiency but usually as a consequence of other disorders known to often accompany gout, such as uric acid stones with infection or obstruction, hypertension, and renal atherosclerotic vascular disease. One relatively distinct entity, lead poisoning, also produces the association of gout and renal failure. Chronic plumbism causes interstitial nephritis, hypertension, and, at least under some circumstances, hyperuricemia and saturnine gout. This confluence of findings occurs in some parts of the United States in those who drink "moonshine" alcohol, which is often distilled in improvised devices rich in lead.

Although gouty nephropathy has declined as an important disease concept—either in actuality or in the eyes of physicians—a new and important recognition of *acute* uric acid nephropathy has emerged. In this acute form a massive bulk of uric acid suddenly appears, is filtered or secreted into the tubular lumina, and precipitates. The crystalline material forms an effective intrarenal obstruction to urinary flow; the patient clinically seems to have oliguric acute renal failure. Most patients reported to have this complication had been recently treated with chemotherapeutic agents for leukemia or lymphoma. With the lysis of a large number of abnormal cells, abundant nuclear purines become available for metabolism to their end product, uric acid. The administration of allopurinol reduces the conversion of purines to uric acid and may be used to prevent renal failure in this setting. Rarely, acute intrarenal uric acid obstruction also occurs following the use of uricosuric drugs.

RENAL TUBULAR ACIDOSIS

In a sense all renal acidosis is tubular; the kidneys excrete the body's metabolic acid load by tubular secretion, not by filtration of hydrogen ion, which exists free in plasma only in negligible amounts. In addition, the tubules, especially the proximal tubules, reabsorb from the luminal fluid all of the existing plasma bicarbonate that had been filtered. The retention of this bicarbonate, along with distal generation of new bicarbonate equivalent to metabolic acid generation, maintains normal pH and buffering capacity. The term "renal tubular acidosis" (RTA), however, is conventionally reserved to describe certain diseases marked not by an overall loss of renal function (filtration and tubular transport) but rather by a specific tubular decline in acid excretory capacity.

The patient with *proximal* (type 2) RTA possesses only partial ability to proximally reabsorb bicarbonate from luminal filtrate. A stable metabolic acidosis occurs, and administered sodium bicarbonate is excreted through the urine without raising the plasma bicarbonate concentration or correcting the acidosis. Although distal acidification is normal in proximal RTA, the large quantities of sodium bicarbonate unclaimed by the proximal tubule exceed the bicarbonate reclaiming ability of the distal tubule, resulting in bicarbonaturia. Proximal RTA occasionally appears as an isolated defect, but more often it is associated with other proximal defects, such as those seen in Fanconi's syndrome, cystinosis, Wilson's disease, hereditary fructose intolerance, multiple myeloma, medullary cystic disease, and some forms of heavy metal toxicity.

With severe acidosis bicarbonaturia stops and the urinary pH falls to normal, since with lowered plasma bicarbonate concentration the small filtered load of bicarbonate can be reabsorbed in the proximal tubule.

The underlying disorder associated with the RTA should be treated. If this is not feasible, large quantities of sodium bicarbonate (5 to 10 mEq/kg/day) are necessary to correct the acidosis. Potassium supplementation in increasing quantities is required with bicarbonate therapy.

Patients with the more common *distal* (type 1) RTA can reabsorb all filtered bicarbonate proximally but are unable to maximally acidify the distal tubular fluid; the quantitative excretion of acid as fully saturated buffer requires a low luminal pH. Some patients with distal RTA have a defect in the hydrogen ion secretory pump and do not achieve the maximal hydrogen ion gradient, which produces a maximally acid urinary pH. Other patients exhibit a backleak of bicarbonate. Like patients with proximal RTA, those with the distal form show hyperchloremic metabolic acidosis, which may be associated with hypokalemia. The hypokalemia is sometimes severe and can cause distressing muscle weakness, a symptom that may call attention to the disease. Part of the daily metabolic acid load not excreted is buffered by the skeleton; bone pain, osteomalacia, and rickets (in children) may result. The consequent dissolution of bone releases excess calcium into the plasma and hence into the urine. The hypercalciuria, along with a relatively high urinary pH and other less well-understood factors, contributes to the high incidence of calcium renal stones and renal parenchymal calcification (nephrocalcinosis) seen in distal RTA. Distal RTA may be an independent disorder or accompany other diseases, as shown in the following outline:

Disorders associated with distal RTA

    I. Primary distal RTA
       A. Infantile
       B. Adult sporadic
       C. Genetic defect in carbonic anhydrase
   II. Nephrocalcinosis
  III. Hypergammaglobulinemic states (for example, Sjögren's syndrome, lupus erythematosus)
  IV. Cirrhosis
   V. Renal transplantation
  VI. Drug-induced distal RTA
       A. Amphotericin B
       B Toluene
       C. Lithium
       D. Spironolactone
 VII. Medullary sponge kidney
VIII. Obstructive nephropathy

The diagnosis of distal RTA is confirmed by infusing ammonium chloride, 0.1 g/kg body weight, and demonstrating that the urine pH does not drop below 5.4 within 6 to 8 hours.

When an underlying cause of distal RTA cannot be identified or cannot be specifically corrected, the acidosis should be treated with alkali replacement. Usually only modest quantities of sodium bicarbonate (1 to 3 mEq/kg/day) are required, and with this supplementation renal potassium loss may stop. Children require more bicarbonate to ensure growth.

HYPORENINEMIC HYPOALDOSTERONISM

A newly recognized but common disease entity, categorized by some as a form of RTA, is variably called isolated hypoaldosteronism, selective hypoaldosteronism, and hyporeninemic hypoaldosteronism. Patients with this defect usually have chronic mild renal insufficiency, often caused by diabetes mellitus or some type of interstitial nephritis. Hyperkalemia and hyperchloremic metabolic acidosis, seemingly out of proportion to the GFR loss, occur in these patients because their ability to generate renin and aldosterone is blunted or absent. Why relatively few persons with early chronic renal disease show this disorder, whereas most maintain activity of the renin-aldosterone axis, remains controversial. Some may have lost renin-producing cells; others seem to be chronically but subclinically volume expanded with a secondary suppression of renin and hence of aldosterone responsiveness. These patients are treated with diuretics. At least in some cases mineralocorticoid replacement must be given to prevent life-threatening hyperkalemia. When this is unsuccessful, sodium polystyrene sulfonate resins may be used regularly to prevent severe hyperkalemia.

BIBLIOGRAPHY

Berger, L., and Yu, T.: Renal function in gout, Am. J. Med. **59**:605, 1975.

DeFronzo, R.A., and others: Acute renal failure in multiple myeloma, Medicine **54**:209, 1975.

DeFronzo, R.A.: Hyperkalemia and hyporeninemic hypoaldosteronism, Kidney Int. **17**:118, 1980.

Gonick, H.C., editor: Current nephrology, vol. 3, Boston, 1979, Houghton-Mifflin Co.

Heptinstall, R.H.: Pathology of the kidney, ed 2, vol. 2, Boston, 1974, Little, Brown & Co.

Mallette, L.E., and others: Primary hyperparathyroidism; clinical and biochemical features, Medicine **53**:127, 1974.

Massry, S.: Effects of electrolyte disorders on the kidney. In Earley, L.E., and Gottschalk, C.W.: Strauss and Welt's diseases of the kidney, ed. 3, Boston, 1979, Little, Brown & Co.

Morris, R.C., and Sebastian, A.: Renal acidosis, Kidney Int. **1**:322, 1972.

Narins, R.G., and Goldberg, M.: Renal tubular acidosis, D.M. **23**:1, 1977.

Perez, G.O., and others: Hyporeninemia and hypoaldosteronism in diabetes mellitus, Arch. Intern. Med. **137**:852, 1977.

Priest, J.N., Ahmed, M., and Nuttall, F.Q.: Pathologic hypofunction of the renin-angiotensin-aldosterone system, Postgrad. Med. **59**:86, 1976.

Robinson, R.R., and Yarger, W.E.: Acute uric acid nephropathy, Arch. Intern. Med. **137**:839, 1977.

Schambelan, M., Sebastian, A., and Biglieri, E.G.: Prevalence, pathogenesis, and functional significance of aldosterone deficiency in hyperkalemic patients with chronic renal insufficiency. Kidney Int. **17**:89, 1980.

109 • TOXIC NEPHROPATHY

Michael R. Rudnick, Christine P. Bastl, and Robert G. Narins

Acute tubular necrosis (ATN) develops most often in the settings of hypotension and sepsis and in the presence of potentially nephropathic drugs and toxins. An ever-lengthening list of common medications and poisons capable of injuring the kidneys has greatly increased the incidence of toxic nephropathy.

PATHOGENESIS

Several intrinsic properties of the kidney sensitize them to drug- and toxin-induced damage. Although the kidneys make up less than 1% of the body weight, they receive 25% of the cardiac output, thereby greatly enhancing their exposure to circulating toxins. Nephrotoxins are concentrated in tubular fluid by the reabsorption of more than 98% of toxin-free glomerular filtrate and by their direct secretion into the lumen. Some toxins are reabsorbed from the glomerular filtrate and accumulate within tubular cells, thereby directly compromising renal epithelium. Thus the kidneys' unique functional and anatomic properties render them susceptible to toxic damage from various agents at blood concentrations not injurious to other organs.

Toxic nephropathy may be mediated by various processes, including immunologic mechanisms, direct epithelial damage, or obstruction.

Necrotizing vasculitis, polyarteritis, the nephrotic syndrome, and acute glomerulonephritis may all be caused by drug-induced *hypersensitivity* reactions. The administered agent, a metabolic product, or an associated contaminant may act as the antigen in sensitized individuals, evoking an antibody response and acute serum sickness. When immune complexes are deposited with the kidney, acute vasculitis or a variety of glomerular and tubular nephritides may result. The enormous endothelial surface provided by the renal blood vessels ensures a fertile ground for the development of allergic vasculitis. The potential for immune complex formation is present with almost any exogenously derived material, such as foreign sera, toxoids, or drugs. Common offending drugs include the penicillins and sulfonamides. The hypersensitivity reactions usually give evidence of diffuse systemic involvement, manifested by some combination of fever, urticaria, arthralgias, and arthritis.

Toxins may also produce a chronic glomerulonephritis with the nephrotic syndrome or slowly progressive renal insufficiency or both. The deposition of antigen-antibody complexes mediates this lesion. The membranous nephritis associated with gold or penicillamine is a clear example of toxin-induced, chronic glomerulonephritis (see the discussion of "Glomerulopathies" later in this chapter). Evidence suggests that these drugs complex with tissue proteins, forming an antigen to which antibodies are produced. The deposited complex evokes an inflammatory reaction in the glomerulus.

Tubular and interstitial damage may also occur through immunologic mechanisms. Acute interstitial nephritis is a well-recognized reaction to therapy with the penicillins, especially methicillin. Patients usually have fever, eosinophilia, eosinophiluria, and rash, suggesting that their nephritis has an allergic basis. The penicilloyl haptenic group complexes with the tubular basement membrane, forming an antigen that incites an antibody response. Other drugs that may cause immune complex–mediated interstitial nephritis are rifampin, sulfonamides, furosemide, cephalothin, phenindione, and allopurinol.

Nephrotoxins also produce acute renal failure by direct damage to proximal renal tubular cells. ATN is probably the most common clinically recognized syndrome produced by nephrotoxins; however, the pathophysiologic events producing cell death remain unclear. The agents most commonly associated with ATN are listed in Table 109-1. Toxic epithelial cell damage may occur with minimal or no impairment of glomerular function. A diffuse defect of proximal tubular transport, *Fanconi's syndrome*, is caused by a variety of drugs and toxins. Outdated tetracyclines caused this syndrome in the past, but it has also resulted from exposure to heavy metals such as lead and mercury. Although gentamicin commonly causes acute renal failure, it can also cause renal tubular wasting of magnesium and potassium. Distal renal tubular acidosis is caused when amphotericin B disrupts luminal membrane integrity, thereby allowing secreted protons to diffuse back to blood. Hypokalemic renal alkalosis may result from the ability of high doses of penicillin, ticarcillin, or carbenicillin to cause distal tubular potassium and hydrogen ion wasting. Impaired distal tubular potassium secretion has been found with indomethacin and propranolol. Nephrogenic diabetes insipidus resulting from blockade of the tubular effects of antidiuretic hormone (ADH) is caused by lithium and demethylchlortetracycline.

Various agents can also produce acute uremia by obstructing urine flow. Ureteral obstruction may be caused by retroperitoneal fibrosis related to methysergide use. Most obstructive uropathies related to toxins are intrarenal in nature. The obstruction may be caused by crystallization and precipitation of the agent within the renal tubule, as occurs with large doses of methotrexate. Obstruction may also occur as a result of drug-induced generation of relatively insoluble substances such as uric acid, as seen with cancer chemotherapy. The acute renal failure associated with roentgenographic contrast material is thought to be at least partially caused by tubular obstruction. Although not well defined, the obstructing agent may be contrast dye, uric acid, Tamm-Horsfall proteins, or a combination of these. Endogenously released substances that cause obstructive uropathy by precipitation in distal tubules include myeloma proteins, myoglobin, and hemoglobin.

Chronic renal failure caused by chronic tubulointerstitial nephritis is most commonly seen with the combination analgesic drugs containing aspirin and phenacetin or acetaminophen. The cumulative consumption of large quantities of these drugs and their concentration in the papilla and medulla produces oxidative tissue damage.

The remainder of this chapter deals with a general review of the drug and toxin-induced glomerular, tubular, interstitial, renal vascular, and obstructive syndromes; this review is in turn followed by a more detailed outline of the effects of specific disorders caused by selected drugs and toxins.

CLINICAL SYNDROMES ASSOCIATED WITH NEPHROTOXICITY

The clinical presentations of the toxic nephropathies are dictated largely by which renal structures are involved (Table 109-1). Certain toxic nephropathies lead to renal failure that may evolve over a period of days or more insidiously progress over many months. Differentiation of toxin-induced renal failure into acute and chronic forms carries important diagnostic and therapeutic implications.

Acute renal failure

Rapidly occurring renal insufficiency may be caused by acute injury to any of the aforementioned anatomic areas.

Table 109-1. Localization of the toxic nephropathies

Anatomic site	Urinary sediment	Proteinuria	Hypertension	Miscellaneous	Commonly associated drugs and toxins
Glomeruli	Red blood cells (RBCs); lipid; oval fat bodies; casts: RBC, pigmented, white blood cell (WBC)	2-4+	Unusual in rapidly progressive glomerulonephritis, common in other forms of acute glomerulonephritis	Look for signs of nephrotic syndrome	Penicillamine, gold, sulfonamides, penicillin, heroin, antiepileptics, nonsteroidal anti-inflammatory drugs, mercury, probenecid
Tubules (ATN)	Renal tubular epithelial cells (RTE); casts: RTE, finely granular, coarsely granular, pigmented	1-2+	Variable	Sepsis, hypotension, renal tubular acidosis, diabetes insipidus, Fanconi's syndrome	Aminoglycosides, cephalosporins, lead (acute), glycols, hydrocarbons, roentgenographic dyes, lithium, methoxyflurane, amphotericin B, trichlorethylene, cisplatin, methotrexate, demeclocycline
Interstitium	RTEs, WBCs, eosinophiluria, RBCs; casts: RTE, WBC, RBC (rare)	1-2+	Variable	Fever, rash, eosinophilia, drug allergy	Penicillin homologues, thiazides, furosemide, cimetidine, phenacetin, anesthetics, lithium (?), phenytoin
Blood vessels	RBCs are scant if preglomerular; RBCs with RBC casts if glomerular	2-4+	Variable but may be severe	Signs of multisystem disease, drug allergy, hepatitis-associated antigen positive, renal aneurysms	Sulfonamides, amphetamines, penicillin homologues, allopurinol, potassium iodide
Ureter	Bland sediment	0-1+	Reversible hypertension with unilateral or bilateral hydronephrosis	Insidious renal failure, back pain in migrainous patients	Methysergide, ergots (rarely), methicillin

A carefully taken history, physical examination, and laboratory evaluation permit rapid differentiation of acute intrinsic renal insufficiency into discrete glomerular, tubular, interstitial, vascular, and obstructive syndromes (Table 109-1). Drug- or toxin-induced ATN may occur as oliguric (less than 400 ml of urine excreted daily) or nonoliguric renal failure.

Chronic renal failure

Several drugs and toxins are capable of slowly destroying the kidneys, leading to the insidious onset of progressive renal failure. Prolonged exposure to certain analgesic compounds and heavy metals is the most common cause of this form of toxic nephropathy. In advanced cases the presence of small, shrunken kidneys, chronic anemia, or osteopenia allows these disorders to be differentiated from the acute syndromes of acute renal failure.

Glomerulopathies

Acute glomerulonephritis may develop as part of a systemic hypersensitivity reaction to drugs such as penicillin or sulfonamides (Table 109-1). The patients show deteriorating renal function, hypertension, proteinuria, and edema. Red blood cells (RBCs) and white blood cells (WBCs), both free and trapped within casts, are found in the urinary sediment, reflecting the acute glomerular inflammation. The deposition of immune complexes within the glomerulus or the presence of glomerular microvasculitis results in an aggressive proliferation of mesangial, endothelial, and occasionally epithelial cells. An influx of WBCs and their penetration, along with RBCs, of the disrupted glomerular barrier account for the sedimentary changes observed.

Other nephrotoxins, also acting through immune mechanisms, produce a somewhat less dramatic and more indolent glomerulopathy characterized by varying degrees of proteinuria. Such patients often show a recent onset of edema or the serendipitous finding of albuminuria on routine urinalysis. Gold, penicillamine, and nonsteroidal antiinflammatory agents are only a few of the drugs capable of this more selective alteration of glomerular permeability. A renal biopsy usually reveals either minimal changes or thickening of the basement membrane and capillary wall. Portions of some glomeruli may reveal mild proliferative changes. These "bland" glomerular alterations are usually mirrored by an equally bland urinary sediment. Occasional RBCs, finely granular and hyalin casts, and oval fat bodies are typically found in the urine.

Tubular disorders

A variety of drugs and toxins (Table 109-1) may impair proximal or distal tubular function and thereby cause dramatic clinical syndromes. Agents damaging the proximal tubule may appear as isolated defects in the transport of phosphorus, glucose, uric acid, amino acids, or bicarbonate. Fanconi's syndrome is characterized by the impaired transport of several of these substances normally processed by the proximal nephron. Bone pain, osteomalacia, and fractures reflect the phosphaturia, whereas muscle weakness, paresthesias, and cardiac arrhythmias are the consequences of bicarbonate and potassium wasting. Blood chemistries reveal hypobicarbonatemia and hyperchloremia, reflecting the presence of bicarbonaturia. Certain heavy metals, hydrocarbons, and antibiotics have been shown to cause these syndromes.

The ability of the distal nephron to reabsorb sodium, to secrete potassium and protons properly, and to process water effectively may be impaired by several drugs and toxins. Ingesting amphotericin B or lithium or sniffing glue (trichloroethylene) impairs distal hydrogen ion secretion and urinary acidification, thereby initiating a series of events that lead to potassium and calcium wasting. Lithium and demeclocycline inhibit the hydro-osmotic effect of ADH and thereby cause polyuria and nephrogenic diabetes insipidus. Tubular reabsorptive defects are induced by some drugs as part of a more diffuse picture of renal damage. Magnesium wasting, for example, may complicate the acute renal failure occurring with gentamicin or cisplatin nephrotoxicity.

Interstitial disorders

The list of drugs causing acute diffuse interstitial nephritis is increasing rapidly (Table 109-1). The clinical picture usually includes some manifestation of hypersensitivity such as fever, rash, or peripheral or urinary eosinophilia. WBCs, including eosinophils, renal epithelial cells, and finely and coarsely granular and cellular casts, characterize the urinary sediment. Salt wasting and potassium retention may be seen in some patients. The rising blood urea nitrogen and creatinine levels may be associated with oliguria or nonoliguria. A biopsy of these swollen, edematous kidneys reveals diffuse round cell infiltration often accompanied by eosinophils, whereas the glomeruli and tubules are usually well preserved.

Penicillins (especially methicillin), thiazides, furosemide, phenytoin, and many other drugs have been incriminated as causing this form of reversible renal failure.

Vascular disorders

Large and small vessel vasculitides can be caused by various drugs. The intravenous use of amphetamines may cause a polyarteritis nodosa–like syndrome that commonly attacks the kidney. Inflammation of medium-sized to small renal cortical arteries leads to the formation of vascular aneurysms that occasionally rupture. Progressive azotemia, hypertension, and a bland urinary sediment occur in many patients. The microvasculitides are characterized by proliferative glomerulitis (see previous discussion of "Glomerulopathies").

Obstruction

Methysergide (Sansert) therapy may lead to progressive retroperitoneal fibrosis with entrapment of one or both ureters, causing the insidious onset of progressive renal failure. Hypersensitivity reactions to drugs such as methicillin may occasionally lead to obstructive ureteral urticaria. Crystalluria, as occurs with hyperuricosuria and oxaluria, may cause intrarenal obstruction.

SPECIFIC NEPHROTOXINS

Specific toxins causing nephropathies are listed in Table 109-2.

Heavy metals

(See Chapter 138.)

Inorganic *mercurial salts* avidly bind to sulfhydryl groups on key cellular proteins. Poisoning, industrial exposure, or more rarely mercurial diuretic therapy may result in ATN or the nephrotic syndrome. The clinical picture is characterized by a metallic taste, various signs and symptoms in the upper and lower gastrointestinal tract, and shock. The therapy includes an emetic, gastric lavage with charcoal, and the intravenous use of the chelating agent dimercaprol (BAL) in doses of 3 mg/kg every 4 hours. If renal failure is present, hemodialysis must be initiated to remove the dimercaprol-mercury complex.

Gold salts as therapy for rheumatoid arthritis may cause membranous nephropathy with the nephrotic syndrome. Although glomerular deposition of gold-induced immune complexes is the putative cause, there is no unequivocal proof for this mechanism. Neither the cumulative dose nor the serum or urinary gold levels are well correlated with the proteinuria that occurs in a small number of treated patients. Dermatitis and bone marrow depression may be associated findings. The proteinuria remits within weeks of the discontinuance of therapy. Steroids are of unproven benefit in proteinuria, and their use should be avoided.

Acute *lead* intoxication, as seen with a pica syndrome or the inhalation of tetraethyl lead fumes, causes reversible acute renal failure with proximal tubular damage and Fanconi's syndrome. Chronic exposure causes interstitial nephritis and irreversible chronic renal failure.

The acute lead syndrome occurs primarily in children 1 to 5 years of age who have repeatedly swallowed chips of lead-based paint. Industrial exposure, as with lead storage batteries or leaded gasoline products, causes intoxication in adults. Phosphaturia, glycosuria, aminoaciduria, and less often uricosuria and bicarbonate wasting are part of the acute renal failure caused by a brief, high-dose lead exposure. Motor neuropathy, abdominal colic, and anemia with basophilic stippling of RBCs are often associated signs. Varying degrees of epithelial cell damage and acid-fast intranuclear inclusions in normal or damaged proximal tubular cells characterize this disorder.

Sustained exposure to lead insidiously leads to chronic renal failure resulting from interstitial nephritis. Industrial exposure or protracted use of illicit ("moonshine") alcohol produced in leaded stills causes most cases in adults. Gout occurs in more than 50% of patients and is a strong clue to the presence of chronic lead nephropathy. Extrarenal signs of lead toxicity are not usually found in the chronic syndrome. Interstitial scarring, round cell infiltration, and an occasional intranuclear inclusion are histologic findings.

The chelation of lead with parenteral EDTA is effective treatment for acute renal and extrarenal manifestations of toxicity. Chronic lead nephropathy is best treated by simply avoiding further exposure. Chelation therapy is of unproven benefit for this irreversible renal disease.

Acute *cadmium* toxicity may lead to the abrupt onset of reversible renal failure but more frequently causes Fanconi's syndrome. The proximal reclamation of low-molecular-weight (15,000 to 40,000 daltons) proteins normally filtered, reabsorbed, and metabolized in the early nephron is impaired, causing lysozymuria and light-chain protein-

Table 109-2. Specific nephrotoxins

Group	Agents
Heavy metals	
Common	Mercury, gold, lead, cadmium, cisplatin, beryllium
Rare	Bismuth, arsenic, copper, silver, thallium, uranium
Antibiotics	
Aminoglycosides	Streptomycin, neomycin, gentamicin, kanamycin, tobramycin
Cephalosporins	Cephaloridine, cephalothin
Sulfonamides	Sulfathiazole, sulfadiazine, sulfapyridine, sulfamethoxazole
Penicillins	Penicillin G, methicillin, ampicillin
Antituberculous drugs	Rifampin, aminosalicylate sodium, capreomycin
Others	Tetracyclines, amphotericin B, bacitracin, polymyxin, colistin
Analgesics and nonsteroidal anti-inflammatory drugs	Phenacetin, aspirin, phenylbutazone, indomethacin, fenoprofen, naproxen
Hydrocarbons and glycols	Carbon tetrachloride, trichloroethylene, tetrachloroethylene, ethylene glycol
Anesthetics	Methoxyflurane, enflurane, fluroxene
Diuretics	Thiazides, furosemide
Pigments	Hemoglobin, myoglobin
Antiepileptics	Trimethadione, paramethadione, phenytoin
Miscellaneous	Lithium, streptozotocin, vitamin D, heroin, probenecid

uria. Toxic exposure occurs primarily in the alkaline storage battery and metallurgic industries. Bone disease and acidosis resulting from renal tubular damage are the major clinical manifestations. Advanced renal failure has not been well documented, and therapy is limited to the avoidance of further exposure.

Beryllium may cause a chronic granulomatous interstitial kidney and lung disease when it is inhaled in the manufacture of fluorescent lights. Hyperuricemia and small urinary calculi containing beryllium or calcium oxalate may occur, but the major clinical manifestation is chronic pulmonary disease.

Silver is a rare cause of ATN that occurs in film developers.

Both *copper* and *ferrous sulfate* intoxication have resulted in acute renal failure, although part of the renal damage may be explained by shock and, in the case of copper, the development of hemolysis and sulfhemoglobinemia.

Antimony therapy for kala-azar and *cisplatin* therapy for various genitourinary tract malignancies have resulted in acute renal failure. Cisplatin causes acute interstitial nephritis characterized by magnesuria, hypomagnesemia, and tetany. Chronic renal insufficiency may ensue.

Thallium, used in rat poison and ectoparasiticide, has been reported to cause renal proteinuria.

Arsenic intoxication, in addition to causing well-recognized neurologic and gastrointestinal symptoms, may also cause ATN. The exposure may be intentional or may occur accidentally with certain fertilizers, agricultural sprays, or arsine gas (used in the petroleum industry).

Roentgenographic dyes

Absorbed or parenteral iodinated contrast dyes cause ATN in some patients. The risk of nephrotoxicity appears to be greatest in patients with dehydration, azotemia, or diabetes mellitus, and in the elderly. The pathogenesis of dye-induced renal failure is uncertain. Dehydration, dye-induced uricosuria, precipitation of Tamm-Horsfall or light-chain proteins, direct cellular toxicity, reduction in renal blood flow, and idiosyncratic reactions are possible but unproven mechanisms.

Cholecystographic, angiographic, and pyelographic dyes have all been injurious to the kidney. No clear relationship exists between the total dose of dye and the development of nephrotoxicity. Renal failure usually occurs within 24 to 72 hours of exposure to dye. Acute renal failure is typically mild and nonoliguric with peak serum creatinine levels of 5 to 6 mg/dl. Most patients show improved renal function within 5 to 7 days. Dialysis is usually not required, and severe hyperkalemia is unusual. Azotemic diabetic patients whose preexposure serum creatinine concentration exceeds 5 mg/dl tend to have more severe and often permanent renal failure. Appropriate substitution of ultrasonography and avoidance of dehydration may limit this complication.

Antibiotics

All *aminoglycosides* are potential nephrotoxins, but the more widespread use of gentamicin and tobramycin makes them by far the most common offenders. Restriction of the poorly absorbable neomycin to oral and topical therapy and further purification of streptomycin have markedly limited their renal toxicity. As with gentamicin and tobramycin, kanamycin causes ATN, but its use has greatly diminished over the years.

The pathogenesis of aminoglycoside-induced ATN is imperfectly understood, although decreased glomerular permeability and lysosomal and mitochondrial damage of proximal tubular epithelium have been demonstrated experimentally. Factors predisposing patients to aminoglycoside-induced ATN include excessive dosage, advanced age, dehydration, low salt intake, hypokalemia, and concomitant exposure to furosemide, cephalosporins, or methoxyflurane.

Although exceptions are common, aminoglycoside-induced renal failure is typically mild and nonoliguric with serum creatinine concentrations frequently peaking at 6 to 10 mg/dl before returning to baseline levels. Magnesium and potassium wasting may accompany the disorder. The concomitance of this otherwise mild renal failure with sepsis and other medical and surgical disorders makes the prognosis for survival guarded.

Cephaloridine unequivocally causes a dose-dependent acute renal failure. High doses of other *cephalosporins*, especially when associated with the same factors that sensitize patients to aminoglycoside nephrotoxicity, may also cause acute renal failure.

Sulfonamide antibiotics may cause acute renal failure by such mechanisms as precipitation in and obstruction of renal tubules and induction of hypersensitivity vasculitis or acute interstitial nephritis. Newer sulfonamides are far more soluble than older preparations, making drug precipitation and intrarenal obstruction an extremely rare event. Nevertheless, in the presence of dehydration, high dosage can still lead to sulfonamide crystalluria and obstruction. Vasculitis and interstitial nephritis are usually associated with fever, rash, ad eosinophilia. Trimethoprim-sulfamethoxazole is mildly nephrotoxic but may also cause a functional decrease in the creatinine clearance by impairing the renal tubular secretion of creatinine, with true glomerular filtration being unimpaired.

Amphotericin B commonly causes a dose-dependent, nonoliguric ATN that is frequently associated with hypercalciuria, hypokalemia, and a distal renal tubular acidosis. Avoidance of excessive dosage and maintenance of brisk urine flows may limit toxicity.

The severe nephrotoxicity of *bacitracin, polymyxin,* and *colistin* limits their use mainly to topical therapy. *Capreomycin* and *rifampin,* antituberculous drugs, may cause acute renal failure. Rifampin nephrotoxicity, which is often associated with light-chain proteinuria, develops most commonly when patients resume therapy following discontinuance. Extrarenal metabolic effects of *tetracyclines* cause azotemia by impairing the anabolism of protein. Changes in the preservatives used in the manufacture of tetracyclines have eliminated the drug-induced Fanconi's syndrome. Demethylchlortetracycline causes a dose-dependent nephrogenic diabetes insipidus that may lead to hypernatremia and azotemia.

Acute interstitial nephritis may be caused by the *penicillins,* especially methicillin, less commonly ampicillin, and least commonly penicillin G. Hypersensitivity-induced vasculitis is a reported but infrequent complication of these drugs.

Analgesics, nonsteroidal anti-inflammatory agents, and drug abuse

The cumulative ingestion of 2 to 7 kg of *phenacetin,* usually in association with aspirin, causes chronic renal failure as a result of interstitial nephritis. Papillary necrosis and an increased incidence of transitional cell carcinoma have been noted. Acetyl-*p*-aminophenol, phenacetin's major metabolite, concentrates in the renal medulla, causing oxidative tissue damage. Discontinuance of the drug often halts progressive azotemia and may result in improvement.

Methysergide, used to treat migraine headaches, not uncommonly causes retroperitoneal fibrosis. The resulting hydronephrosis may lead to insidious renal failure.

Nonsteriodal anti-inflammatory drugs (NSAID) such as indomethacin, fenoprofen, and naproxen have been associated with reversible lipoid nephrosis and acute interstitial nephritis. Renal prostaglandins, the synthesis of which is inhibited by NSAID, are regulators of renin secretion. The hyperkalemia sometimes associated with NSAID is caused by induced hyporeninemic hypoaldosteronism. Loss of the vasodilating prostaglandins may severely compromise renal blood flow and lead to acute renal failure in patients with preexisting dehydration, the nephrotic syndrome, liver disease, or congestive heart failure or in those undergoing surgery. Patients with systemic lupus erythematosus appear particularly sensitive to the inhibitory effects of NSAID on the glomerular filtration rate and renal blood flow.

Heroin abuse causes the nephrotic syndrome and renal failure by mechanisms that are unclear. Focal glomerular sclerosis is the most commonly associated lesion. Intravenously administered *amphetamines* are known to induce a polyarteritis nodosa–like syndrome with renal insufficiency and aneurysms of intrarenal vessels.

Hydrocarbons and glycols

Inhalation or ingestion of *carbon tetrachloride,* a household cleaner, industrial solvent, and fire extinguisher, leads to severe hepatitis and oliguric renal failure. *Tetrachloroethylene,* a dry-cleaning and degreasing agent, causes a similar syndrome. Sniffing spot remover or glue containing *trichloroethylene* also leads to liver and renal failure. Fanconi's syndrome and distal renal tubular acidosis are often associated findings.

Ethylene glycol (antifreeze) is metabolized to oxalic and glycolic acids and impairs central nervous system activity, leading to renal and cardiopulmonary failure. An elevated anion gap metabolic acidosis caused by glycolic acid accumulation and calcium oxalate crystalluria are typical findings. The therapy entails the use of hemodialysis and parenteral ethanol to block metabolic conversion of ethylene glycol to its more toxic metabolites.

Pigments

Transfusion reactions or drug-induced hemolysis may lead to acute renal failure. *Alcohol,* hypokalemia, or hypophosphatemia may induce rhabdomyolysis, myoglobinuria, and acute renal failure. Obstructing pigment casts or direct epithelial or glomerular damage may cause the nephrotoxicity. The early use of sodium bicarbonate and furosemide or mannitol diuresis may prevent failure in these cases.

Miscellaneous toxins

The metabolism of the general anesthetic *methoxyflurane* (Penthrane) forms oxalic acid and releases fluoride. Nephrogenic diabetes insipidus and acute renal failure develop in some patients. Interstitial fibrosis and calcium oxalate crystallization are the hallmarks of this disorder. Other related anesthetics, *fluroxene* (Fluoromar) and *enflurane* (Ethrane), have also caused acute renal failure.

Lithium salts, used in treating certain psychiatric conditions, may cause a dose-dependent, slowly reversible, nephrogenic diabetes insipidus. Lithium has been associated with chronic interstitial nephritis, but the causality has not been firmly established.

Hypersensitivity reactions to *thiazides, furosemide,* and the anticoagulant *phenindione* have all been reported to cause acute renal failure. Biopsy has shown acute interstitial nephritis.

Penicillamine, used in treating cystinuria, Wilson's disease, and a variety of collagen-vascular disorders, causes an immune-complex, membranous glomerulonephritis and the nephrotic syndrome. Continued use of the drug may lead to a rapidly progressive, crescentic glomerulonephritis. The membranous lesion is usually reversible with the discontinuance of therapy.

BIBLIOGRAPHY

Agarwal, B.N., Cabebe, F.G., and Hoffman, B.I.: Diphenylhydantoin-induced acute renal failure, Nephron **18**:249, 1977.

Appel, G.B., and Neu, H.C.: The nephrotoxicity of antimicrobial agents (in three parts), N. Engl. J. Med. **296**:663, 722, 784, 1977.

Bastl, C.P., Rudnick, M.R., and Narins, R.G.: Diagnostic approaches to acute renal failure. In Brenner, B.M., and Stein, J.H., editors: Contemporary issues in nephrology, vol. 6, New York, 1980, Churchill-Livingstone.

Border, W.A., and others: Antitubular basement-membrane antibodies in methicillin associated interstitial nephritis, N. Engl. J. Med. **291**:381, 1974.

Byrd, L., and Sherman, R.L.: Radiocontrast-induced acute renal failure: a clinical and pathological review, Medicine **58**:270, 1979.

Carling, P.C., and others: Nephrotoxicity associated with cephalothin administration, Arch. Intern. Med. **135**:797, 1975.

Citron, B.P., and others: Necrotizing angiitis with drug abuse, N. Engl. J. Med. **283**:1003, 1970.

Cogan, M.C., and Arieff, A.I.: Sodium wasting, acidosis and hyperkalemia induced by methicillin interstitial nephritis, Am. J. Med. **64**:500, 1978.

Gault, M.H., and others: Syndrome associated with the abuse of analgesics, Ann. Intern. Med. **68**:906, 1968.

Graham, J.R., and others: Fibrotic disorders associated with methysergide therapy for headache, N. Engl. J. Med. **274**:359, 1966.

Hestbech, J., and others: Chronic renal lesions following long-term treatment with lithium, Kidney Int. **12**:205, 1977.

Johansson, S., and Wahlqvist, L.: Tumors of urinary bladder and ureter associated with abuse of phenacetin-containing analgesics, Acta Pathol. Microbiol. Scand. **85**:768, 1977.

McCurdy, D.K., Frederic, M., and Elkinton, J.R.: Renal tubular acidosis due to amphotericin B, N. Engl. J. Med. **278**:124, 1968.

Porter, G.A., and Bennett, W.M.: Toxic nephropathies. In Brenner, B.M., and Rector, F.C., Jr., editors: The kidney, ed. 2, Philadelphia, 1981, W.B. Saunders Co.

Rao, T.K., Nicastri, A.D., and Friedman, E.A.: Natural history of heroin associated nephropathy, N. Engl. J. Med. **290**:19, 1974.

Schilsky, R.L., and Anderson, T.: Hypomagnesemia and renal magnesium wasting in patients receiving cisplatin, Ann. Intern. Med. **90**:929, 1979.

Singer, J., and Rotenberg, D.: Demeclocycline-induced nephrogenic diabetes insipidus, in vivo and in vitro studies, Ann. Intern. Med. **79**:679, 1973.

110 • ACUTE RENAL FAILURE

T.K.S. Rao

DEFINITION. Acute renal failure (ARF) may be defined as an abrupt reduction in glomerular and renal tubular function resulting in azotemia. Oliguria (daily urine output less than 400 ml) and anuria (daily urine output less than 50 ml) with azotemia have long been considered hallmarks of this syndrome, yet a nonoliguric form is commonly encountered in clinical practice. ARF may be dramatic, at times a life-threatening syndrome, or alternatively subtle in severity and gradual in onset. Reduced renal function from any cause is associated with retention of blood urea nitrogen (BUN), creatinine, phosphorus, uric acid, and several other substances not usually measured in clinical practice. During ARF the serum creatinine concentration usually increases by 1 to 2 mg a day and the BUN level by 10 to 20 mg a day. In disease states associated with hypercatabolism such as follows trauma or rhabdomyolysis, the increase in BUN and creatinine levels may be three to five times this rate. The major emphasis in this chapter is on the variety of ARF known as acute tubular necrosis (ATN). Synonyms for ATN include shock kidney, lower nephron nephrosis, nephrotoxic nephropathy, and vasomotor nephropathy.

ETIOLOGY AND PATHOGENESIS. In a recent review of 2200 cases of ARF collected from around the world, 43% were related to surgery, 26% occurred in a medical setting, 13% were related to complications of pregnancy, 9% were related to trauma, and 9% were a result of nephrotoxins. A rational approach to the patient with ARF requires differentiation of the causes of azotemia into prerenal, renal, and postrenal, as in the following outline:

Causes of ARF

I. Prerenal
 A. Gastrointestinal losses (vomiting, diarrhea, nasogastric suction, colostomy, ileus)
 B. Excessive sweating
 C. Hemorrhage
 D. Burns with sequestration of fluids
 E. Renal losses (diuretics, renal salt wasting)
 F. Cardiovascular failure
  1. Congestive heart failure
  2. Myocardial infarction with shock
  3. Cardiac tamponade
 G. Hepatic failure
  1. Cirrhosis with ascites
  2. Hepatorenal syndrome
 H. Vascular obstruction
  1. Renal artery thrombosis, embolism, dissecting aneurysm
  2. Bilateral renal vein thrombosis (rare in adults)
  3. Vena caval occlusion

II. Intrinsic renal
 A. Acute tubular necrosis (vasomotor nephropathy)
  1. Hypovolemia
  2. Septic shock
  3. Drug-induced (aminoglycosides, sulfonamides, amphotericin B)
  4. Roentgenographic contrast media
  5. Anesthetics (methoxyflurane)
  6. Nephrotoxins
   a. Carbon tetrachloride
   b. Methyl alcohol
   c. Heavy metals (bismuth, lead, uranium, inorganic mercurials)
  7. Posttraumatic and postoperative
  8. Rhabdomyolysis with myoglobinuria (trauma, fever, heat stroke, overdosage with methadone or heroin, hypokalemia, viral infections)
  9. Hemolysis with hemoglobinuria
  10. Obstetric (septic abortion, uterine hemorrhage)
 B. Bilateral cortical necrosis
 C. Glomerular
  1. Poststreptococcal glomerulonephritis
  2. Anti–glomerular basement membrane antibody disease
  3. Systemic lupus erythematosus
  4. Hemolytic-uremic syndrome
  5. Thrombotic thrombocytopenic purpura
  6. Schönlein-Henoch purpura
  7. Rapidly progressive glomerulonephritis
 D. Vasculitis

1. Polyarteritis
2. Wegener's granulomatosis
E. Malignant hypertension
F. Accelerated scleroderma
G. Allergic interstitial nephritis (antibiotics, anticonvulsants)
H. Miscellaneous—hypercalcemia, hyperuricemia, multiple myeloma, homograft rejection

III. Postrenal
A. Bilateral ureteric obstruction or ureteric obstruction in a solitary kidney
1. Retroperitoneal fibrosis
2. Tumor
3. Stones
4. Surgical ligation
5. Papillary necrosis
B. Bladder obstruction (prostatic hypertrophy, stones, neurogenic)
C. Disruption of bladder with intraperitoneal extravasation of urine
D. Urethral obstruction (stones, strictures)

Prerenal failure. Hypovolemia from any cause, including excessive blood loss resulting from hemorrhage, sequestration of fluids following severe burns, intestinal obstruction, or cardiac failure, can lead to a fall in effective arterial volume and a reduction in renal perfusion and renal function. The common pathophysiologic factor in these states is a reduction in renal blood flow without intrinsic injury to glomeruli and tubules. The renal response to hypovolemia is an attempt to maintain the extracellular fluid volume by retaining salt and water. Initially this is associated with the excretion of concentrated urine. The other changes seen in prerenal azotemia include oliguria and a benign urinary sediment. Prompt restoration of vascular volume and improvement in cardiac function result in increased urine output and correction of azotemia.

Intrinsic renal failure. Of the various causes of intrinsic renal failure listed in the preceding outline, this chapter is limited to the discussion of the syndrome of ATN. This term is a misnomer because renal tubular necrosis is not always present, and little correlation exists between histologic lesions in the kidney and the severity of renal failure (that is, histologic findings may be normal despite uremia). Renal ischemia and nephrotoxic agents are the two major factors involved in the pathogenesis of ATN. In both, significant intrarenal hemodynamic alterations account for the development of renal failure. Consequently, many have proposed the term "acute vasomotor nephropathy" to better describe this variety of ARF.

Renal ischemia. Excessive blood loss from trauma, surgery, or obstetric cause, and hypotension resulting from anesthesia or septicemia are some of the principal causes of renal hypoperfusion and renal ischemia. The renal ischemia rapidly reduces renal function and eventually leads to ATN. Many believe there usually is an initial prerenal phase of ATN that is of variable duration and during which restoration of blood volume and mannitol infusion (which relieves vasoconstriction and redistributes renal blood flow) can reverse the renal insufficiency. In clinical situations there is a great variation among patients in the duration and severity of renal hypoperfusion necessary to produce ATN. In some patients transient periods of hypotension may result in ATN, whereas others successfully tolerate prolonged periods of renal ischemia. At the present time it is unclear what other factors in addition to renal ischemia are needed to induce the development of ATN. Excess renin-angiotensin production, intrarenal (vascular) coagulation with fibrin deposition, and other unknown factors, although unsubstantiated, are implicated in the pathogenesis of ATN.

Nephrotoxins. Industrial chemicals (carbon tetrachloride and ethylene glycol), heavy metals (mercury and lead), nephrotoxic drugs (aminoglycoside antibiotics), anesthetic agents, and roentgenographic contrast media (intravenous pyelography, oral cholecystography, and angiography dyes) are some of the commonly encountered agents implicated in the production of ATN in humans. The release of large amounts of hemoglobin (intravascular hemolysis) or myoglobin (in rhabdomyolysis) into the circulation in patients who are dyhydrated and acidotic may also result in ATN. These agents produce renal tubular injury, probably by a direct toxic mechanism.

In both ischemic and nephrotoxic ATN, once the initiating events result in an acute reduction of renal function, numerous factors including persistence of profound renal vasoconstriction, renal tubular obstruction by inspissated debris, and back leakage of tubular fluid through disruptions in the tubular wall are responsible for the maintenance of renal failure.

Postrenal failure. In the postrenal group of disorders renal failure is caused by obstruction to urine flow in various segments of the urinary tract. Surgical correction of obstructions generally results in an improvement in renal function.

CLINICAL MANIFESTATIONS

Oliguric phase. In most patients with ATN the endogenous creatinine clearance falls to values of 1 ml/min or less. Within a day of the precipitating event oliguria with azotemia is usually seen, but at times it may be delayed for 1 or 2 weeks. The average duration of oliguria is 7 to 14 days, but it may be as short as a few hours or persist for several weeks. The daily urine output averages 200 to 300 ml, and anuria is rare. In the nonoliguric form of ATN, the glomerular filtration rate (GFR) is still markedly reduced, but the creatinine clearance is not less than 3 to 5 ml/min and the daily urine output is generally more than 500 ml. Regardless of urine volume there is a progressive increase in the concentration of BUN, creatinine, uric acid, phosphorus, and other products of nitrogen metabolism. The retention of 50 to 100 mEq of fixed acids daily results in metabolic acidosis, which is reflected biochemically as a decrease in plasma bicarbonate concentration, an increase in the anion gap, and a reduction in arterial pH. Hyperkalemia generally develops, the severity of which depends on potassium intake, release of potassium from the tissues, and arterial pH. The effects of hyperkalemia on the electrocardiogram (ECG) include (in sequence) tall, peaked T waves in the precordial leads, prolongation of the P-R interval, complete heart block, absent P waves, prolongation of the QRS complexes, ventricular fibrillation, and cardiac arrest. The electrophysiologic effects of hyperkalemia on the myocardium are potentiated by hyponatremia and hypocalcemia.

Salt and water retention with the development of peripheral edema and pulmonary congestion is a frequent complication in ATN. With persistent renal failure, the uremic syndrome develops and includes many of the following abnormalities. Neurologic manifestations may include stupor, mental confusion, asterixis, convulsions, and coma. Gastrointestinal bleeding resulting from uremic gastritis or colitis may at times be severe enough to require blood transfusion. Anemia, hypocalcemia, poor wound healing, and an increased tendency to develop infections are some of the other findings that may be present. Pericardial effusion and tamponade may rarely occur.

Diuretic phase. After 1 to 2 weeks of oliguria, if there is to be recovery, there is a progressive increase in urine output, generally 2 to 3 L a day but at times exceeding 5 to 10 L daily. The onset of diuresis signals the beginning of recovery from ATN. Since diuresis precedes the decline in BUN and creatinine levels by a few days, uremic symptoms may progress, requiring dialysis. The magnitude of the diuresis depends on three factors: (1) the degree to which urea and other endogenous solutes accumulate during oliguria, (2) the degree of extracellular volume expansion caused by salt and water retention, and (3) the rate of recovery of tubular reabsorptive capacity. Significant fluid and electrolyte losses occasionally occur because the inability of the recovering tubules to concentrate the urine causes severe hypovolemia. Following the onset of diuresis, the GFR improves gradually as reflected by a fall in BUN and creatinine levels. Normal values are usually achieved in 2 to 3 weeks. The recovery of renal function following more than 3 weeks of oliguria is uncommon but does occur. Infection is the major complication during the diuretic phase. Urinary tract infection from indwelling bladder catheters and septicemia from intravenous infusions and operative and trauma sites are common during the diuretic phase.

Recovery phase. During the recovery phase, renal function continues to improve and achieves a level compatible with normal life. After a few months testing reveals a minor reduction in the GFR and a diminution in the ability of the kidneys to concentrate and acidify the urine. These functional derangements are of no practical clinical significance except when ARF is superimposed on chronic renal failure. Rarely, patients with ATN fail to recover, and irreversible renal failure requiring maintenance hemodialysis develops.

DIAGNOSIS. The approach to the patient with an acute onset of oliguria and azotemia should be as follows.

Tests for prerenal azotemia. A careful history is taken and a physical examination is performed to uncover underlying predisposing factors such as evidence of a toxin, dehydration, hypovolemia, and cardiac failure. Laboratory studies (Table 110-1) can also help distinguish prerenal azotemia from ARF. In prerenal azotemia, oliguria is associated with a concentrated urine (specific gravity greater than or equal to 1.020), a urine/plasma osmolality ratio greater than 1.4:1, a low urinary sodium concentration (less than 20 mEq/L), and a fractional sodium excretion of less than 1. The BUN/creatinine ratio is abnormally increased (greater than 10:1) because urea clearance is more sensitive to urine flow than creatinine clearance. However, in the oliguric patient with ARF the urine sediment shows broad granular casts, the urine is isosmolar to blood, the urine sodium concentration and fractional excretion of sodium are high, and BUN and creatinine levels rise proportionately. If the diagnosis of prerenal azotemia is made, rapid and appropriate expansion of the plasma volume should be initiated with saline, albumin, plasmanate, or blood while the patient's cardiovascular status is monitored by auscultation of the lungs for rales and central venous or pulmonary wedge pressure measurements. Patients with prerenal azotemia resulting from hypovolemia generally respond to expansion of their intravascular volume. The heart rate falls, the blood pressure rises, and urine output increases. If oliguria persists, 25 g of mannitol should be administered as an intravenous bolus. A satisfactory response consists of an increase in urine volume to greater than 50 ml/hour. Additional mannitol should not be given if there is no response. Despite the absence of controlled

Table 110-1. Differential characteristics of prerenal azotemia and acute renal failure

Laboratory study	Prerenal azotemia	ARF
BUN/serum creatinine concentrations	>10:1	10:1
Urine/plasma osmolality	>1.4:1	1
Urinary sodium concentration	<20 mEq/L	>20 mEq/L
Fractional excretion of sodium*	<1	>4
Urine output	500-600 ml/day	<400 ml/day
Urine sediment	None	Renal failure, broad granular casts

*Fractional excretion of sodium = $\dfrac{\text{Urine Na}^+ \times \text{Plasma creatinine}}{\text{Urine creatinine} \times \text{Plasma Na}^+} \times 100$

studies, some suggest the administration of 200 to 400 mg of furosemide intravenously if mannitol is ineffective. If the urine output improves, diuresis is maintained by the parenteral infusion of fluids, 10% mannitol solution (not to exceed 100 g a day), or repeated doses of furosemide. If all these measures fail to induce diuresis, a diagnosis of ATN is made and the treatment outlined in the next section should be followed. Diuresis may occasionally be produced with these measures, but follow-up laboratory studies show persistent elevations in creatinine and BUN levels, suggesting the development of nonoliguric renal failure.

Tests for urinary tract obstruction. The extent of the search for obstruction is variable and depends on the clinical situation. Prostate hypertrophy causing outlet obstruction can be determined after rectal examination and measurement of the residual urine volume by percussion of the bladder, bladder sonography, and bladder catheterization. Plain films of the abdomen can detect radiopaque calculi. A renal sonogram and an intravenous pyelogram can detect the presence of enlarged kidneys and dilation of the urinary collecting system. Computed tomographic scans of the abdomen can be obtained to uncover extrinsic mass lesions that may be compressing the ureters. If ureteral obstruction is likely, retrograde ureteral catheterization is performed. The risks are infection and edema of the ureter.

Tests for intrinsic renal diseases. Since ARF can be caused by systemic diseases, as well as bilateral primary renal diseases other than ATN, a careful search via the history and physical and laboratory examination is made. ATN is suggested by the findings listed in the preceding outline of "Causes of ARF."

MANAGEMENT

Oliguric phase. ATN usually follows its own self-limited course, and currently there is no specific therapy to hasten the recovery of renal function. Consequently the treatment is aimed at careful management of the primary surgical, traumatic, or obstetric problem while avoiding additional nephrotoxic injury and minimizing the complications of uremia.

The principles of management during the oliguric phase of ATN consist of fluid restriction while maintaining nutrition, potassium restriction, treatment of septicemia, and early dialysis before the development of complications.

Fluids and nutrition. The daily fluid intake in oliguric patients should be restricted to an amount equal to the sum of urinary output and extrarenal losses (from insensible sweating, nasogastric suction, colostomy drainage, and diarrhea). The fluid balance is determined by weighing the patient daily and accurately recording all intake and output volumes, as well as measuring electrolyte excretion. Nutrition is maintained by prescribing a diet consisting of 40 g of high-biologic-value protein and a high carbohydrate content to provide at least 30 calories/kg/day. If the patient is unable to tolerate oral feeding, aseptic hyperalimentation techniques must be instituted to provide adequate caloric intake. A hypertonic glucose solution containing 50 to 75 mEq/L of sodium and no added potassium is used. In severely hypercatabolic patients the use of essential amino acids and hypertonic glucose has been shown to reduce mortality and slow the rise in BUN and creatinine levels. Further evaluation is required before the routine use of hyperalimentation in uncomplicated ATN can be recommended. Appropriate fluid and nutritional intake is associated with no weight gain (for example, from edema fluid) and in fact loss of ½ to 1 pound each day, which results from tissue catabolism.

Multivitamins are prescribed to prevent a vitamin deficiency. If significant metabolic acidosis (pH less than 7.3) is present, sodium bicarbonate should be administered (see Chapter 103). The use of sodium bicarbonate in oliguric-phase patients is limited by the high sodium content of each ampule (which has equal quantities of sodium and bicarbonate) and can precipitate volume overload and pulmonary edema. Severe acidosis generally requires intervention with dialysis. Other measures include the use of antacids containing aluminum to prevent absorption of phosphate from the gut and the avoidance of products containing magnesium.

If significant pulmonary congestion develops in spite of the preceding measures, dialysis should be instituted as early as possible. During dialysis ultrafiltration and the removal of excess fluid can be accomplished. In an emergency situation, if dialysis or ultrafiltration cannot be immediately instituted, phlebotomy with the removal of 250 to 500 ml of blood (if the hematocrit level is greater than 30%) may be indicated for the treatment of severe fluid overload.

Hyperkalemia. The myocardial effects of hyperkalemia can provoke the most rapid lethal complications of ATN. Efforts to prevent hyperkalemia include avoiding the use of potassium supplements, potassium-rich foods, and potassium-sparing diuretics (spironolactone and triamterene). Since hyponatremia and acidosis accompany renal failure and aggravate myocardial sensitivity to potassium, it is difficult to label any specific potassium concentration as safe. During the oliguric phase of ATN, frequent determinations of sodium, potassium, and bicarbonate concentrations and ECG monitoring are essential for the early detection of hyperkalemia. Despite severe potassium restriction, hyperkalemia commonly occurs in the course of ATN, particularly in hypercatabolic patients.

The method for the treatment of hyperkalemia depends on the speed required to lower the serum potassium. In the presence of arrhythmias or ominous ECG changes hyperkalemia can be treated by methods that rapidly transport potassium into the cell (for example, intravenous sodium bicarbonate or calcium gluconate or lactate have an almost immediate onset of action). Sodium bicarbonate (88 to 132 mEq) can be infused intravenously when there is no evidence of fluid overload. The infusion can be repeated as indicated by the deterioration in ECG. Bicarbonate has the additional advantage of correcting the metabolic acidosis of renal failure. Calcium gluconate or lactate, 10 to 30 ml, can be given intravenously at a rate of 2 ml/min, with ECG monitoring if the patient is not receiving a digitalis preparation.

The infusion of 50 to 100 ml of 50% glucose solution along with 5 to 10 units of regular insulin lowers the potassium level after a short delay. Hypoglycemia may develop if the glucose infusion is terminated abruptly while the insulin effect remains. It is preferable to avoid this form of therapy for an unconscious patient. Therapy aimed at removing potassium from the body should always be instituted, since bicarbonate, calcium, and glucose infusions have only a temporary effect. A cation exchange resin such as sodium polystyrene sulfonate (Kayexalate) can be given orally (15 to 20 g three to four times a day together with 20 to 30 ml of 70% sorbitol solution) or by retention enema (50 g in a mixture of 50 ml of 70% sorbitol and 100 ml of tap water). The enema can be repeated every 2 hours. Each gram of the resin extracts 1 mEq of potassium, and sorbitol prevents fecal impaction by inducing diarrhea. Since the sodium in the resin is exchanged for potassium, repeated use can result in sodium retention. Dialysis is the most efficient way to remove excess potassium from the body and should be instituted early. Hemodialysis, because of its high efficiency, is preferable to peritoneal dialysis in the management of hyperkalemia.

Infection. Every attempt should be made to prevent the development of sepsis in patients with ATN, including the avoidance of indwelling catheters in the bladder, proper surgical management of trauma, adequate pulmonary toilet, and antiseptic care of infusion sites. The physician must be vigilant to recognize early infection because there may be a blunted response to infection in uremia and because infection is a common cause of morbidity and mortality in ATN. If infection does develop, a careful search for the source and identification of the organism and its antibiotic sensitivity should be undertaken. Aggressive therapy should be initiated promptly to prevent overwhelming sepsis. When nephrotoxic antibiotics (aminoglycosides) are needed, the dosage should be modified according to the residual renal function and dialyzability of the drug. As soon as the organism is identified and sensitivities are available, regimens can be established that avoid nephrotoxic antibiotics whenever possible.

Dialysis. When the conservative regimen just outlined fails to maintain an optimal clinical status, dialysis therapy

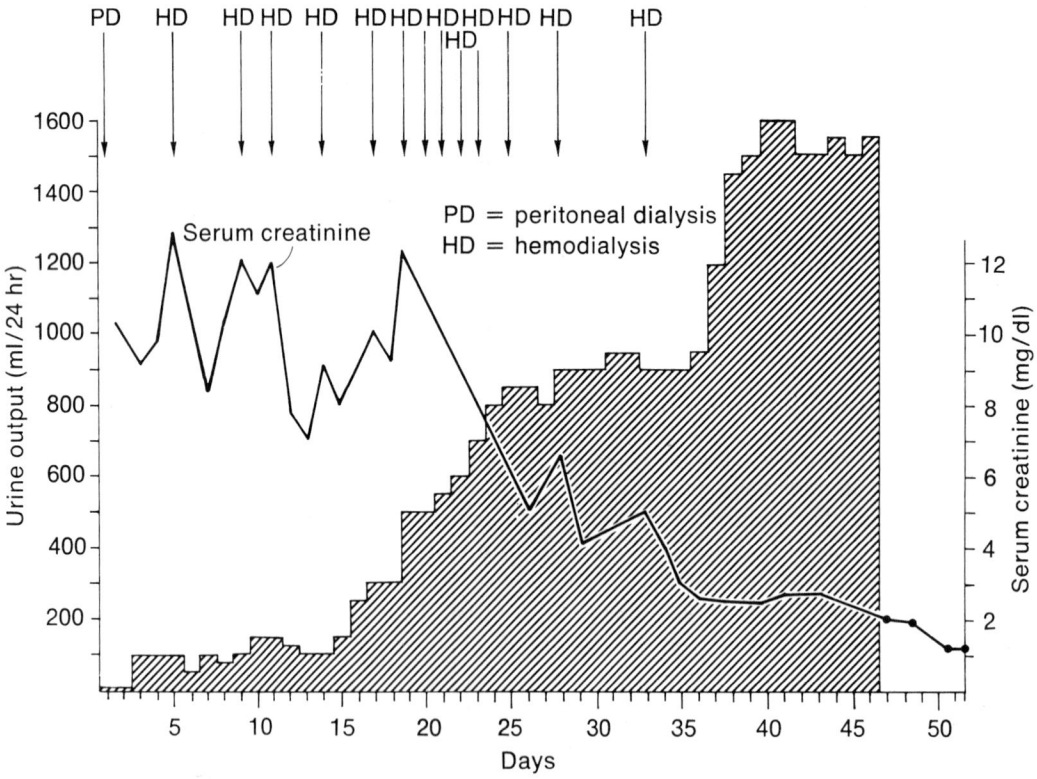

Fig. 110-1. Protracted oliguria in rhabdomyolysis-induced acute renal failure. Note prolonged oliguria, hypercatabolic state requiring intensive hemodialysis, diuretic phase, and excellent recovery.

should be instituted. Indications for dialysis include hyperkalemia, acidosis, fluid overload, septicemia, bleeding diathesis or pericarditis resulting from uremia, asterixis, and uremic coma. Early dialysis is currently recommended to avoid these serious complications. Both peritoneal dialysis and hemodialysis are acceptable modes of treatment in ATN; the mode selected depends on the clinical state of the patient and the hospital resources. Generally patients are dialyzed every other day, but if there is a deterioration of the clinical status or existence of a hypercatabolic state, daily dialysis may be needed. Aggressive dialysis with maintenance of the serum creatinine concentration below 5 mg/dl and the BUN below 70 mg/dl has been reported to reduce mortality in ATN.

Diuretic phase. During the diuretic phase the goal of management is to maintain a normal fluid balance. At this time most patients excrete the excess fluid retained during the oliguric phase. Occasionally, however, dehydration may occur because of excessive diuresis, and provisions should be made for the replacement of fluid and electrolytes to maintain a normal vascular volume. Body weight, urinary output, tissue turgor and edema, and serum and urinary electrolyte levels serve as guides in proper replacement therapy. Infection and uremic complications are still a problem during the diuretic phase, and the principles previously outlined should be followed. Hyperkalemia is rare during diuresis.

PROGNOSIS. Death in ATN is usually a result of the underlying disease. The highest mortality occurs when renal failure is precipitated by trauma, surgery, or infection. Reported fatality rates in such patients range from 50% to 75% and are largely attributable to respiratory insufficiency, sepsis, and gastrointestinal bleeding. The mortality in obstetric-related or nephrotoxin-induced ATN is generally less than 10%. The prognosis is good for patients who recover from ARF because the residual renal damage is minimal. The course of a patient with ARF resulting from rhabdomyolysis is depicted in Fig. 110-1.

BIBLIOGRAPHY

Anderson, R.J., and others: Nonoliguric acute renal failure, N. Engl. J. Med. **296:**1134, 1977.

Friedman, E.A., and Eliahou, H.E., editors: Proceedings, Acute Renal Failure Conference, HEW Pub. No. (NIH) 74-608, Washington, D.C., 1973, U.S. Government Printing Office.

Kleinknecht, D., and others: Uremic and non uremic complications in acute renal failure, evaluation of early and frequent dialysis on prognosis, Kidney Int. **1:**190, 1972.

Levinsky, N.G., Alexander, E.A., and Venkatachalam, M.A.: Acute renal failure. In Brenner, B.M., and Rector, F.C., Jr., editors: The kidney, ed. 2, Philadelphia, 1981, W.B. Saunders Co.

Lewers, D.T., and others: Long term follow up of renal function and histology after acute tubular necrosis, Ann. Intern. Med. **73:**523, 1970.

Patak, R.V., Lifschitz, M.D., and Stein, J.H.: Acute renal failure: clinical aspects and pathophysiology, Cardiovasc. Med. **4:**19, 1979.

111 • CHRONIC RENAL FAILURE
T.K.S. Rao

DEFINITION. Chronic renal failure (CRF) can be defined as a progressive loss of renal function that is often irreversible. Regardless of the causes and pathophysiology of this disorder, uremia generally develops. The term "uremia," derived from Greek and meaning urine in the blood, implies the retention of constituents normally excreted in the urine, for example, urea, creatinine, uric acid, phosphorus, and several other substances. However, clinical experiences have shown that the manifestations of uremia result not only from the retention of nitrogenous end products but also from a wide variety of other metabolic and hormonal alterations influencing many organ systems. The development of CRF may be very rapid, as in some forms of glomerulonephritis, or gradual over years, as in polycystic kidney disease. In general, the signs and symptoms of uremia develop when renal impairment is advanced and the creatinine clearance is less than 20 ml/min. In most patients the loss of renal function progresses to end-stage renal failure and death unless treated by dialysis or renal transplantation.

ETIOLOGY AND INCIDENCE. The number of new patients with uremia treated by dialysis or renal transplantation in the United States is estimated to be between 50 and 81 per 1 million population per year. These numbers translate to approximately 10,000 to 15,000 new patients with uremia every year. About two thirds of these patients are males, and blacks are more commonly afflicted than whites. The incidence of CRF is quite low below the age of 12 (5:1 million yearly).

Establishing an accurate tissue diagnosis in newly diagnosed end-stage renal failure is often difficult. Frequently the primary diagnosis is made on clinical grounds. The leading cause of uremia is chronic glomerulonephritis, comprising a group of disorders of varying renal histology (see Chapter 105), which accounts for 40% to 50% of cases. Interstitial nephritis, another group of poorly defined disorders that includes pyelonephritis, Balkan nephropathy, and analgesic and other drug-related diseases, accounts for about 20% of CRF in Europe. Diabetic nodular and diffuse glomerulosclerosis is responsible for about 20% to 25% of new cases of uremia in the United States. The low prevalence of diabetes as a cause of end-stage renal failure in Europe is probably a result of the selective exclusion of diabetic uremic patients from European dialysis facilities. Hypertensive renal vascular disease, which is more common in blacks than in whites, is another common cause of severe renal failure. Other categories of irreversible uremia include hereditary renal diseases (polycystic and medullary cystic kidneys and hereditary interstitial nephritis), collagen vascular diseases (systemic lupus erythematosus and scleroderma), and other miscellaneous disorders such as obstructive uropathy.

PATHOPHYSIOLOGY. Uremia is a complex clinical and biochemical syndrome in which clinical manifestations can be found in every organ system in the body. At one extreme uremic coma resembles systemic intoxication in which there are seizures, hypothermia, shallow respirations, a bleeding diathesis, cardiac arrhythmias, and coma, whereas at the other end there may be few symptoms in spite of advanced renal insufficiency. Since the symptoms of CRF are reversible by dialysis, the cause of uremic toxicity is presumed to be a dialyzable toxin or toxins. The quest for the so-called uremic toxin still continues, and no specific single toxin has yet been identified. Several substances, including methylguanidine, guanidinosuccinic acid, indoles, phenols, hydrogen ion, urea, and parathyroid hormone (PTH), have been partially incriminated.

Because no single toxin can sufficiently account for the various manifestations of renal failure, the complexity of the uremic syndrome can be looked on as a combination of (1) excretory failure (retention of nitrogenous products, salt, and water), (2) regulatory failure (inappropriate loss of salt, water, and minerals), (3) biosynthetic failure (diminished synthesis of ammonia leading to acidosis and decreased erythropoietin resulting in anemia), (4) excessive production (PTH excess causing bone disease and renin excess causing hypertension), and (5) decreased renal clearance (hyperinsulinemia resulting in hypoglycemia and hypergastrinemia resulting in peptic ulcer disease).

Excretory failure. With progressive renal impairment and diminution in the glomerular filtration rate (GFR), fewer and fewer remaining nephrons are called on to handle the daily excretory load. Consequently, although the concentration of urea and creatinine in the blood does not rise above normal until more than 50% of renal function is lost, any subsequent reduction is associated with a steep increase. Renal failure also leads to the retention of other nitrogenous substances, uric acid, phosphorus, sulfates, and many products not usually measured in clinical practice (as described previously). Initially there are polyuria and nocturia, which result from the combination of increased solute clearance by the few remaining nephrons, and then diminution in the ability of the renal tubules to conserve salt and water. In late stages the decreased sodium and water excretory ability results in oliguria and the retention of sodium and water, leading to hypertension, edema, and congestive heart failure. A diminished excretion of potassium may result in hyperkalemia with its attendant effects on the myocardium (see Chapter 110).

Regulation of volume. In many diseases that lead to CRF the kidney loses the ability to regulate the extracellular fluid volume by modulating the excretion of sodium and water. Accordingly, if adequate intake is not maintained to replace the obligatory loss of salt and water in the urine, hypovolemia and further deterioration in renal function may occur. Diseases that usually exhibit the renal salt-losing state include medullary cystic kidneys, polycystic kidneys, pyelonephritis, and some types of interstitial nephritis.

Biosynthetic failure

Acidosis. Reduced renal function is initially associated with a normal anion gap, hyperchloremic acidosis caused by volume expansion, and inhibition of proximal bicarbonate resorption.

A normal man consuming 70 g of protein daily produces 40 to 60 mEq of acid (H^+), primarily sulfuric and phosphoric acids. About half the load of H^+ appears in the urine as NH_4^+, and the rest is excreted buffered with phosphates. With a reduction in renal mass the capacity to produce NH_3 and hence NH_4^+ is diminished, leading to the retention of H^+ and metabolic acidosis.

Biochemical findings seen in the acidosis of advanced uremia typically include an increase in the anion gap, a lowering of the plasma bicarbonate concentration, a normal serum chloride concentration, and a reduction in arterial pH with compensatory hyperventilation (low Pco_2).

Anemia. The anemia associated with CRF is primarily a result of decreased renal erythropoietin secretion and suppression of red blood cell production by the bone marrow along with decreased red blood cell survival. The morphology of red blood cells in renal failure is usually normocytic and normochromic. In advanced stages of uremia, poor dietary intake, bleeding problems, and iatrogenic blood sampling contribute to deficiencies of folic acid, vitamin B_{12}, and iron, which aggravate the severity of anemia.

Excessive hormone production

Renal osteodystrophy. The term "renal osteodystrophy" is used to describe the complex bone changes that develop as a result of renal failure. The pathogenesis of bone disease in uremia is multifactorial in origin, and at least two basic mechanisms can be identified. Osteitis fibrosa is related to the presence of excess PTH, and osteomalacia to a deficiency of the active form of vitamin D. Two other bony lesions, osteoporosis and osteosclerosis, are also found in renal failure, but the pathogenesis is poorly understood.

A progressive loss of renal function results in the retention of dietary phosphate. To maintain a normal calcium and phosphorus product, the serum calcium is reciprocally depressed. The resulting hypocalcemia stimulates the secretion of PTH. The serum calcium concentration rises as a result of PTH action on the bone, and the level of phosphate is reduced by enhanced renal tubular excretion of phosphorus. The concentration of calcium and phosphorus in the blood is restored to normal at this lower level of renal function, but it is associated with higher PTH levels. This process is repeated with each decrement in renal function, resulting in increasingly higher levels of PTH. When the GRF falls below 20 ml/min, normal serum phosphorus levels cannot be maintained even with maximal stimulation of the parathyroid glands. Along with the development of secondary hyperparathyroidism, the kidneys also cannot hydroxylate 25-hydroxycholecalciferol (25-OHD) to 1,25-dihydroxycholecalciferol (1,25-[OH]$_2$D), the biologically most active form of vitamin D. The absence or deficiency of 1,25-(OH)$_2$D produces hypocalcemia as a result of diminished calcium absorption from the gut and osteomalacia as a result of defective bone formation.

The roentgenographic findings of secondary hyperparathyroidism can best be demonstrated in the skull (salt-and-pepper appearance), hands (subperiosteal resorption of the middle phalanx), clavicles (resorption of the distal third), and spine (alternate areas of rarefaction and osteosclerosis, so-called rugger-jersey spine). Rarely, cystic lesions or giant-cell tumors may develop in the mandible and in long bones. The roetgenographic changes appear late in the course of renal osteodystrophy, whereas histologic changes in bone can occur quite early.

Hypertension. Hypertension can cause kidney failure, but hypertension and kidney disease are so closely related that on many occasions it is impossible to identify the primary event. Eight-five percent of patients with uremia are hypertensive. In uremic patients hypertension contributes significantly to the mortality and morbidity from cardiac and cerebrovascular disease. The mechanism of hypertension in uremia is twofold: an expanded extracellular fluid volume resulting from increased salt and water retention and excessive vasoconstriction mediated by renin and angiotensin. Volume-related hypertension, present in about 40% of patients with CRF, is generally mild (diastolic blood pressure less than 100 mm Hg) and responds to salt restriction, diuretics, and ultrafiltration during dialysis. Renin-mediated hypertension is usually severe (diastolic blood pressure greater than 120 mm Hg), is present in about 15% of patients, and is difficult to control with conventional antihypertensive drugs. In the remaining 30% of hypertensive patients with chronic renal failure, the hypertension is of moderate degree (diastolic blood pressure 100 to 120 mm Hg) and is caused by a combination of increased volume and excess renin production.

Other endocrine abnormalities. The endocrine abnormalities in uremia are complex. Some are caused by a combination of regulatory and biosynthetic failure, and excessive production and decreased renal clearance of various hormones account for others. Apart from the previously discussed PTH excess, deficient 1,25-(OH)$_2$D synthesis, and decreased erythropoietin production, functional abnormalities in the pituitary, thyroid, and adrenal glands and the testes and ovaries are reported but are less clearly understood. A derangement of sexual functions with decreased fertility is frequently present in patients with renal failure. In women menstrual irregularities and anovulatory cycles are common, and in advanced uremia successful full-term pregnancies are extremely rare. Uremic men have oligospermia, decreased sperm motility, impotence, and reduced libido. Although decreased plasma testosterone and increased luteinizing hormone levels have been reported, these findings do not sufficiently explain the various sexual dysfunctions occurring in renal failure. Normal kidneys clear about 30% of the circulating insulin; in renal failure this clearance is decreased and much less insulin is catabolized. Consequently, in diabetic patients with CRF there is a marked diminution in the insulin requirement, and if the dose is not reduced, hypoglycemia is a common occurrence. In nondiabetic patients with renal insufficiency, there is carbohydrate intolerance because of poor peripheral utilization and delayed insulin release. Similarly, elevated levels of gastrin resulting from diminished renal clearance may be responsible for the increased incidence of peptic ulcer disease in uremia.

CLINICAL MANIFESTATIONS (Table 111-1). The clinical onset of uremia may be abrupt, as in some forms of rapidly progressive glomerulonephritis, or gradual over several years, as in polycystic kidney disease. Patients are generally sicker and more symptomatic when the renal loss is rapid, whereas in slowly progressive disease there may be few symptoms. The presence of coexisting systemic diseases may worsen the severity of symptoms, and therefore

Table 111-1. Clinical manifestations of uremia

System	Manifestations
Cardiovascular	Hypertension, edema, congestive heart failure, pericarditis, cardiomyopathy, accelerated atherosclerosis, vascular calcifications
Dermatologic	Pruritus, pallor, urochrome pigmentation, excoriation, ecchymosis, purpura, calcium deposits, uremic frost
Endocrine	Hyperparathyroidism; decreased erythropoietin; insulin resistance and insulin sensitivity; excessive secretion of renin, gastrin, glucagon, and growth hormone; sexual dysfunction; thyroid function abnormalities
Gastrointestinal	Anorexia, nausea, vomiting, diarrhea, gastrointestinal bleeding owing to uremic gastritis and colitis, pancreatitis, peptic ulcer
Hematologic	Anemia, bleeding diathesis
Neurologic	Inability to concentrate, poor memory, headache, irritability, insomnia, reversed sleep pattern, drowsiness, muscle twitching, restless legs, asterixis, neuropathy, coma, seizures
Oral	Uremic fetor, bleeding from gums
Psychologic	Depression, agitation, anxiety, suicidal tendencies, denial, psychosis
Pulmonary	Edema, calcifications, hemorrhage

the signs and symptoms of uremia vary from person to person. Although in CRF the correlation between the degree of loss of renal function and the appearance of clinical symptoms is not accurate, several stages can be distinguished. In the initial stage with modest decreases in the GFR (creatinine clearance 50 to 90 ml/min), patients are generally asymptomatic with an elevation of the PTH level in the blood. The concentrations of BUN and creatinine do not rise until more than one half of the renal function is lost, a result of compensatory adaptation by the remaining nephrons. With greater reductions in filtration (creatinine clearance 20 to 50 ml/min) patients may have azotemia, anemia, hypertension, hyperlipidemia, carbohydrate intolerance, inability to concentrate the urine, nocturia, and polyuria. They may report weakness, fatigue, diminished work tolerance, and a decreased ability for mental concentration. When the creatinine clearance falls to between 5 to 20 ml/min, patients may have advanced azotemia with severe anemia, acidosis, hypocalcemia, hyperphosphatemia, hypertension, anorexia, weight loss, restless leg syndrome, sleep disturbances, weakness, and urochrome pigmentation of the skin. There may be polyuria, and hypovolemia may develop because of the obligatory loss of salt and water in the urine. Edema may develop if sodium intake exceeds renal excretory power. When the creatinine clearance is between 1 and 5 ml/min, patients are obviously sick, with the manifestations of nausea, vomiting, diarrhea, weight loss, uremic fetor, asterixis, bleeding disorders, pericarditis with or without cardiac tamponade, neuropathy, seizures, hyperkalemia with cardiac arrythmia, and finally coma and death.

DIAGNOSIS AND MANAGEMENT. The treatment of end-stage renal failure involves either lifelong maintenance dialysis or kidney transplantation; both forms of therapy are associated with significant morbidity and mortality. In addition, the cost of treating chronic uremia is prohibitively expensive, exceeding 1 billion dollars in the United States in 1980. Consequently, a principal concern in the evaluation of patients with CRF is to identify and correct reversible and remediable causes of uremia, as described in the following outline:

Steps in the diagnosis and management of patients with CRF

I. Establishing the diagnosis
   A. Exclude prerenal, postrenal and reversible causes
   B. Look for hereditary and systemic diseases
   C. Perform renal biopsy when indicated
II. Quantitating renal and other organ functional status
   A. Perform tests for endogenous creatinine clearance, urine culture, and protein and salt excretion
   B. Check for anemia, hypertension, and diabetes
III. Initiating conservative management
   A. Initiate appropriate diet
   B. Treat urinary tract infection, systemic disease, hypertension, congestive heart failure, and secondary hyperparathyroidism
   C. Educate patient and family; liaison consultation when needed
   D. Establish vascular access
   E. Avoid dehydration and nephrotoxic agents
IV. Individualizing long-term management
   A. Prepare for and initiate hemodialysis—home, center, self-care, or satellite unit
   B. Prepare for and initiate peritoneal dialysis—center, home, or continuous ambulatory
   C. Consider and prepare for renal transplantation—living or cadaver donor

Establishing the diagnosis. As outlined in Chapter 110, prerenal azotemia and reversible acute tubular necrosis are identified by the appropriate clinical signs and symptoms, urinary sodium, and osmolality measurements, urinary microscopic findings, therapeutic trials with fluids, mannitol, or furosemide, and the self-limiting natural history of the disease. The kidney size is normal in both these forms of renal failure. When uremia is caused by obstruction, there is dilation of the urinary collecting system (hydronephrosis) and hydroureters, which can be identified by renal sonography, by intravenous, retrograde, or antegrade pyelography, or by computed tomography.

A proper medical history, a physical examination, and appropriate clinical and biochemical tests may establish the cause of intrinsic renal disease in systemic lupus erythematosus, diabetes mellitus, scleroderma, polycystic kidneys, and hereditary nephritis. Identifying genetically transmitted renal disease is important to screen relatives for early detection of the disease and provide family counseling to prevent further transmission. A renal biopsy may be necessary to clarify the diagnosis when the cause of renal failure is unknown or when clinical evidence of the nephrotic syndrome is present. A renal biopsy can identify diseases that respond to appropriate therapy with an improvement in renal function (for example, Wegener's granulomatosis, anti–glomerular basement membrane antibody glomerulo-nephritis, urate nephropathy, and analgesic nephropathy). If only one kidney is functioning or if sonography or roentgenography indicates that both kidneys are small, a kidney biopsy is generally contraindicated and an accurate diagnosis of the cause of renal failure may not be possible.

Quantitating renal function. Once the diagnosis of CRF is established, the GFR should be determined. Although the endogenous creatinine clearance is only a crude indicator of the GFR at low filtration rates, it is useful in clinical practice. Serial creatinine clearance measurements may be necessary to monitor changes (both improvement and deterioration) in renal function and to time the initiation of appropriate therapy.

A urine culture should be obtained for bacterial studies because persistent infection can accelerate the loss of renal function. Quantitative determinations of protein, sodium, and potassium excretion in the urine are helpful in formulating a suitable diet for the uremic patient. Appropriate investigations should be performed to identify iron loss from bleeding as well as folic acid and vitamin B_{12} deficiency. An assessment of the status of coexisting problems such as congestive heart failure, hypertension, diabetes mellitus, or systemic lupus erythematosus determines the need for concomitant therapy.

Initiating conservative management. Conservative management of renal failure is generally feasible until the creatinine clearance has fallen to about 5 ml/min. The principles of management include the following.

Dietary prescription. The rationale of diet therapy in patients with a creatinine clearance of less than 20 ml/min is to limit protein intake and minimize the retention of nitrogenous products while preventing tissue catabolism. Studies have indicated that a daily diet containing 40 g of high-biologic-value protein (0.5 g/kg body weight) along with an adequate amount of calories (30 calories/kg) promotes anabolism and prevents negative nitrogen balance. In patients with significant proteinuria the protein content in the diet should be increased to match the protein loss. Protein restriction also limits the intake of phosphorus and helps prevent the development of renal osteodystrophy. The intake of dietary sodium is adjusted according to daily measurements of body weight, urinary sodium excretion, and blood pressure and the presence or absence of peripheral edema and pulmonary congestion. Although some patients may require 10 to 20 g of salt in the daily diet to keep up with obligatory urinary losses, severe sodium restriction (1 to 2 g) is necessary in others with limited urinary excretion. Most patients with CRF (creatinine clearance 5 to 15 ml/min) excrete about 2 to 6 g of salt (34 to 102 mEq of Na^+) a day in the urine. Initially a salt restriction to 4 g (68 mEq Na^+) a day can be prescribed for the patient with recently detected uremia. The dietary sodium can subsequently be increased (for weight loss and hypotension) or decreased (for weight gain and hypertension). In some patients gradual and incremental dietary sodium increases are accompanied by increases in filtration. If the patient has metabolic acidosis (pH less than 7.25), sodium bicarbonate tablets are prescribed, taking into account the sodium content of the preparation and its effects on the cardiovascular and volume status. Limiting potassium intake to 2 g daily, especially in patients with a creatinine clearance of less than 10 ml/min, is another integral part of a proper dietary prescription. Patients are advised to eliminate from the diet foods rich in potassium, potassium supplements, and potassium-sparing diuretics (spironolactone and triamterene). It is seldom necessary to use potassium-binding resins such as sodium polystyrene sulfonate (Kayexalate) until the urine output is less than 1 L a day.

Hypertension. Hypertension should be vigorously treated because of its contribution to further renal loss. A stepwise approach should be implemented. Initially sodium and fluid restriction and diuretics should be prescribed. Diuretics such as furosemide, ethacrynic acid, and metolazone are safe and effective, but their use should be carefully monitored to prevent excessive diuresis with contraction of the extracellular fluid volume. If hypertension does not respond to diuretic therapy, antihypertensives such as methyldopa, hydralazine, clonidine, prazosin, and propranolol can be effectively employed in renal failure. However, if the hypertension is severe, more potent drugs such as guanethidine and minoxidil may be necessary. Use of the new drug captopril, an inhibitor of angiotensin-converting enzyme, has been reported to be successful in the hypertension complicating scleroderma. All therapy and dosages must be individualized according to patient needs.

Anemia. Anemia, which is almost universally found in patients with a creatinine clearance of less than 10 ml/min, is difficult to treat. The use of anabolic steroids (testosterone and nandrolone), which stimulate renal and extrarenal erythropoietin production, is associated at times with an improvement in hemoglobin levels. Associated deficiencies of iron, folic acid, and vitamin B_{12} should be corrected by adequate supplementation, and blood loss by iatrogenic means should be minimized.

Bone disease. In all patients with CRF attempts should be made to prevent the development of renal osteodystrophy, which contributes to morbidity and limits rehabilitation. Serum calcium, phosphate, alkaline phosphatase, and PTH levels should be monitored. The primary aim of therapy is to maintain a normal phosphorus level. This is achieved by restricting phosphate in the diet (low protein intake) and by the use of phosphate-binding agents (aluminum hydroxide or aluminum carbonate). If hypocalcemia persists even after normalization of the serum phosphorus level, calcium supplementation (1 g of elemental calcium daily) and one of the commercially available vitamin D preparations should be prescribed. Serial calcium determinations are necessary to monitor vitamin D therapy and to prevent hypercalcemia and metastatic calcifications. In severe cases of hyperparathyroidism, subtotal or total parathyroidectomy may be necessary.

Other coexisting systemic diseases. Although asymptomatic bacteriuria is not treated except when there is coexistent obstruction, symptomatic urinary tract infection is treated. The antibiotic selected depends on the sensitivity of the organism; nephrotoxic drugs should be avoided whenever possible. Coexisting systemic diseases should be treated appropriately. Management of diabetes with careful monitoring of blood glucose levels, reduction of insulin dosage to avoid hypoglycemia, surveillance of the retinopathy, and control of hypertension prolong the survival of the diabetic patient.

Individualizing long-term management

Preparing and initiating hemodialysis and transplantation. Since CRF usually pursues a relentless course, it is essential to educate the patient and the family about the various options available for the treatment of end-stage renal failure. The principles, techniques, and complications of peritoneal dialysis or hemodialysis (performed in a hospital, at home, or in a satellite clinic) and renal transplantation (using a cadaver or a living related donor) should be discussed. A lifetime plan is formulated for each patient, and the treatment is individualized according to medical indications and personal preference.

Preparation for hemodialysis involves the early establishment of an adequate vascular access. The proper time to establish a suitable vascular access is when the creatinine clearance is about 15 ml/min. However, if rapid deterioration is anticipated, vascular surgery should be performed when the creatinine clearance is 25 ml/min or more. Creating a 3-mm fistulous communication between the radial artery and an adjacent vein at the wrist in the nondominant arm enables arterial blood to flow into the veins. The forearm veins, which are numerous and superficial, become engorged and thick walled in 2 to 6 weeks. Subsequently needles can be inserted easily into these arterialized superficial veins, and adequate blood flow (200 to 300 ml/min) can be obtained to perform effective hemodialysis.

Peritoneal dialysis catheters can be used as soon as they are inserted. Education for self-care such as chronic ambulatory peritoneal dialysis takes several weeks.

The preparation for renal transplantation includes an inventory of suitable and willing living relatives (such as siblings or parents), tissue typing of the donors and the patient, and medical evaluation of acceptable live donors. If a living donor is not available, arrangements are made for the patient to await transplantation from a cadaver, and maintenance dialysis may be required during this interval.

It is preferable to institute dialysis therapy before the development of severe complications of uremia such as pericarditis, neuropathy, convulsions, and coma. The indications for dialysis include gastrointestinal symptoms (anorexia, nausea, and vomiting) resulting in weight loss, pericarditis with or without cardiac tamponade, heart failure unresponsive to diuretics, neuropathy, asterixis, convulsions, and unexplained deterioration of the patient's condition. In general, maintenance dialysis should begin when the creatinine clearance falls below 5 ml/min. In patients with multisystem diseases, including diabetes mellitus, scleroderma, systemic lupus erythematosus, and cardiac failure, dialysis may have to be initiated at higher filtration rates.

The timing of renal transplantation varies from patient to patient. Whereas live donor transplantations can be carried out electively at a time convenient to both the recipient and the donor, most cadaver donor transplants are performed as an emergency procedure.

PROGNOSIS. Up until the early 1960s all patients with end-stage renal failure died. The annual mortality in treated uremic patients is currently under 15% because of advances in the technical aspects of dialysis and renal transplantation.

BIBLIOGRAPHY

DeLuca, H.F.: The kidney as an endocrine organ involved in the function of vitamin D, Am. J. Med. **58**:39, 1975.

Eastwood, J.B., Bordier, P.H.J., and DeWardener, H.E.: Some biochemical histological, radiological and clinical features of renal osteodystrophy, Kidney Int. **4**:128, 1973.

Friedman, E.A., editor: Strategy in renal failure, New York, 1978, John Wiley & Sons, Inc.

Friedman, E.A., Delano, B.G., and Butt, K.M.H.: Pragmatic realities in uremia therapy, N. Engl. J. Med. **298**:368, 1978.

Knochel, J.P., and Seldin, D.W.: The pathophysiology of uremia. In Brenner, B.M., and Rector, F.C., Jr., editors: The kidney, ed. 2, Philadelphia, 1981, W.B. Saunders Co.

Manis, T., and Friedman, E.A.: Dialytic therapy for irreversible uremia, N. Engl. J. Med. **301**:1260, 1979.

112 · TREATMENT OF IRREVERSIBLE RENAL FAILURE BY DIALYSIS

Lois Anne Katz

Patients with uremia caused by acute or chronic renal failure are treated with peritoneal dialysis or hemodialysis. These techniques may also be used to remove poisons or to correct severe fluid or electrolyte abnormalities. During dialysis, solutes diffuse down a concentration gradient and across a semipermeable membrane that separates blood from a balanced salt solution (dialysate). This protein-free solution approximates the composition of normal plasma water, although the sodium concentration is slightly lower than the normal physiologic level and the potassium concentration varies depending on the patient's serum potassium level. The dialysate does not contain those substances (urea, creatinine, and uric acid) that are to be removed from the patient but does have relatively high concentrations of buffer (usually acetate) and calcium so that these solutes can diffuse into the patient's plasma. Metabolism of the acetate to bicarbonate corrects acidosis. How quickly solutes are removed from the blood depends on their size, the area and permeability of the membrane, and blood flow.

PERITONEAL DIALYSIS

In peritoneal dialysis a plastic catheter is inserted percutaneously into the abdominal cavity and dialysate is infused. The peritoneum, which has a functional surface area of about 1 m^2, acts as the semipermeable membrane. It is permeable to small- and middle-molecular-weight (500 to 6000 daltons) solutes; some proteins also cross this membrane. In adults 1 to 2 L of sterile dialysate warmed to body temperature is infused rapidly, allowed to remain in the abdomen for a variable period (up to 30 minutes), and then drained by gravity. Each complete exchange takes 30 to 60 minutes. Small amounts of heparin may be added to the dialysate to maintain catheter patency. Fluid removal depends on the osmolality of the dialysate, which is determined by its glucose concentration. Commercially available dialysate containing 1.5 g/dl dextrose is slightly hypertonic to plasma and leads to some water loss. To remove more fluid from overhydrated patients, solutions containing 4.25 g/dl of dextrose are available. In acute dialysis, exchanges are continued for 36 to 48 hours or until the desired correction of plasma abnormalities is obtained.

Because peritoneal dialysis is a relatively simple technique requiring no complicated equipment, it is widely available. There are few contraindications, although it may be difficult to perform in a patient with previous abdominal surgery and adhesions. Technical problems include abdominal discomfort or pain, intra-abdominal bleeding, inadequate drainage, and leakage around the catheter site. When 4.25% dextrose solutions are used, hyperglycemia may develop, especially in diabetic patients. Removal of too much water may result in hypernatremia. Perforation of a viscus (such as the colon or bladder) or blood vessel may complicate catheter placement. The most common problem is peritonitis, subclinical (cloudy fluid and positive cultures) or clinical (with fever and abdominal pain). Intraperitoneal and systemic antibiotics are used to treat peritonitis when it occurs.

Chronic peritoneal dialysis may be used in the treatment of end-stage renal failure. A permanent Silastic catheter with Dacron cuffs is inserted sugically. Patients are dialyzed intermittently for 8 to 12 hours three or four times a week in a hospital unit or at home, or continuously using a newly developed technique, chronic ambulatory peritoneal dialysis (CAPD). Patients undergoing CAPD use dialysate in plastic bags that are connected by tubing to the permanent catheter. After the dialysate is instilled into the abdomen, the empty bag is rolled up and worn for several hours. Then the bag is unrolled, used to drain the dialysate, and discarded. Four or five exchanges are done daily. Patients receiving CAPD are independent and ambulatory even while being dialyzed. Because the dialysis is continuous, they have fewer dietary and fluid restrictions than those receiving intermittent dialysis, and their blood pressure is usually normal without medications. Since protein losses are significant with CAPD, high-protein diets are prescribed. The main disadvantage of CAPD is frequent peritonitis, which usually responds to antibiotics but sometimes requires removal of the catheter. It is hoped that refinements in technique will reduce the incidence of infection. The long-term effects of CAPD remain to be determined.

HEMODIALYSIS

When hemodialysis is performed, dialysate and anticoagulated blood flow on opposite sides of a synthetic semipermeable membrane contained in a disposable dialyzer or artificial kidney. Types of dialyzers include coil, hollowfiber, and plate dialyzers; most have membranes made of Cuprophan with surface areas of 1 to 2.5 m^2. Most patients with no residual kidney function are dialyzed three times a week for 4 to 6 hours at each treatment.

Vascular access is necessary. Surgically constructed internal arteriovenous (AV) fistulas are commonly used; in patients whose own vessels are poor, synthetic vascular prostheses may be used to create a fistula. Once the veins near the fistula dilate, one or two needles can be inserted to provide flow of blood to and from the dialyzer. An alternative method of access is the cannulation of vessels to form an external AV shunt. Shunts obviate the need for venipunctures but are easily infected or thrombosed. Catheters can be inserted into the femoral or subclavian veins for blood access; this method is usually reserved for acute dialyses. Blood flows of 200 to 300 ml/min are used.

Dialysate is mixed, heated, monitored, and pumped at flow rates of about 500 ml/min to the dialysate compartment of the artificial kidney. Urea and creatinine are easily cleared; the removal of toxins of middle molecular weight is dependent on the dialyzer size and the length of treatment. Hydrostatic pressure across the membrane, not dialysate osmolality, determines fluid removal or ultrafiltration. Positive pressure can be created on the blood side or negative pressure in the dialysate compartment with the transmembrane pressure gradient adjusted to remove an appropriate amount of fluid.

To prevent blood from clotting when it is exposed to the tubing or membrane, heparin is infused systemically. In patients who are actively bleeding or likely to bleed, it is possible to use low doses of heparin or regional heparinization (heparin infused into blood going to the dialyzer and protamine infused into blood returning to the patient). However, significant bleeding and hypotension or cardiovascular instability are contraindications to hemodialysis.

The technical complications of hemodialysis include blood leaks, air emboli, and hemolysis caused by contaminated or improperly prepared dialysate. Hypotension, bleeding, muscle cramps, cardiac arrhythmias, fever, infection, pruritus, and disequilibrium (headaches, nausea and vomiting, and seizures) may occur during dialysis.

Patients undergoing hemodialysis are commonly infected by the hepatitis B virus, and many become chronic carriers, with the virus found in blood, saliva, and other body secretions. Most dialysis units routinely test for hepatitis B surface antigen (HBsAg) and isolate patients who are carriers.

Because of the risk of septicemia and endocarditis in patients with AV fistulas, such patients should probably receive prophylactic antibiotics for dental or surgical procedures. Well-dialyzed patients have normal coagulation profiles between dialyses; however, patients with AV shunts are anticoagulated with warfarin (Coumadin). Patients receiving dialysis often have occult or overt gastrointestinal bleeding resulting from duodenal ulcer disease or gastritis; therefore, for routine analgesia acetaminophen is prescribed instead of aspirin. Drugs containing magnesium should not be given. Many other drugs such as antibiotics, which are normally excreted by the kidneys, must be given in reduced dosage to dialyzed patients.

Patients receiving dialysis must follow certain dietary limitations; protein, salt, and potassium are moderately restricted and fluid intake is severely reduced to avoid excessive weight gain between treatments.

Hemodialysis may be done in a hospital, in a satellite clinic, or at home. Most patients feel well following dialysis; their urea and creatinine levels are significantly lowered, and their fluid and electrolyte metabolism is normalized. Dialysis substitutes for the excretory functions of the kidney but not for its endocrine functions.

Dialysis treatments are usually begun when a patient's creatinine clearance is less than or equal to 5 ml/min or when uremic signs or symptoms supervene. Advanced age and systemic illnesses are no longer contraindications to maintenance dialysis. Currently, most patients are hemodialyzed, although children and elderly and diabetic patients may do better with peritoneal dialysis. Peritoneal dialysis does not require vascular access or anticoagulation; because it is less efficient than hemodialysis, changes occur slowly, and hypotension and disequilibrium are seen less frequently. For these reasons peritoneal dialysis may be the preferred mode of therapy in patients who have small or fragile veins, bleeding, severe angina, or neurologic problems likely to be complicated by disequilibrium.

NEW DEVELOPMENTS

In addition to CAPD, several new developments in the treatment of uremia are being investigated. These include hemoperfusion, hemofiltration (convectional dialysis technique in which clearance of large and small molecules is equal), sequential dialysis (ultrafiltration without dialysis followed by dialysis without fluid removal), and oral sorbents. Work is under way to construct a wearable, continuously working hemodialyzer. More efficient dialyzers and new types of membranes are also being tested.

COMPLICATIONS

Even if patients tolerate the dialysis treatments without serious problems, patients undergoing hemodialysis or peritoneal dialysis are subject to numerous long-term complications. Many dialyzed patients have hypertension, usually related to volume overload but occasionally renin dependent. Hypertension and lipid abnormalities may predispose patients to accelerated atherosclerosis. There is a high incidence of fatal and nonfatal cardiovascular complications, especially atherosclerotic heart disease.

Most patients have chronic anemia, which may be treated with iron or androgens. Neurologic abnormalities include peripheral neuropathy, autonomic neuropathy (which may be manifested as orthostatic hypotension), and dialysis dementia, a progressive dementia of unknown cause but possibly related to accumulation of aluminum in the brain. Another problem is disordered calcium-phosphorus metabolism leading to secondary hyperparathyroidism and bone lesions known as renal osteodystrophy. High serum phosphorus concentrations, hypocalcemia caused by decreased production of the active metabolite of vitamin D (an endocrine function of the kidney not corrected by dialysis), and acidosis contribute to the hyperparathyroidism. An early sign may be loss of the lamina dura of the teeth. The use of phosphate-binding antacids, active vitamin D metabolites, dialysate with a high calcium content, and calcium supplements may prevent the development of parathyroid hyperplasia. Dialyzed patients are susceptible to all kinds of infections; pneumonias, tuberculosis, and skin infections commonly occur. Most dialysis-related deaths are a result of cardiovascular disease or infection. Mortality is highest in the first year of treatment; the overall mortality is about 8% to 15% a year. Despite the medical and psychosocial problems associated with the treatment of uremia, dialysis does restore many individuals to happy and productive lives.

BIBLIOGRAPHY

Alfrey, A.C., LeGendre, G.R., and Kaehny, W.D.: The dialysis encephalopathy syndrome: possible aluminum intoxication, N. Engl. J. Med. **294**:184, 1976.

Bennett, W.M., and others: Drug therapy in renal failure: dosing guidelines for adults (in two parts), Ann. Intern. Med. **93**:62, 286, 1980.

Goldsmith, R.S.: The effects of calcium and phosphorus in hemodialysis, Annu. Rev. Med. **27**:181, 1976.

Manis, T., and Friedman, E.A.: Dialytic therapy for irreversible uremia (in two parts), N. Engl. J. Med. **301**:1260, 1321, 1979.

Merrill, J.P.: Dialysis versus transplantation in the treatment of end-stage renal disease, Annu. Rev. Med. **29**:343, 1978.

Popovich, R.P., and others: Continuous ambulatory peritoneal dialysis, Ann. Intern. Med. **88**:449, 1978.

Vaamonde, C.A.: Peritoneal dialysis: current status, Postgrad. Med. **62**:148, 1977.

113 • RENAL TRANSPLANTATION

Robert A. Grossman

Dialysis and transplantation must be considered complementary forms of therapy for chronic renal failure. Although dialysis can exist without transplantation, the reverse is not true. Virtually all patients receiving a renal transplant require a period of dialysis before surgery. In addition, dialysis may be required during the immediate postsurgical period to assist the patient through the initial acute tubular necrosis, for maintenance therapy during periods of severe rejection, and if irreversible rejection should occur. About 4000 renal transplantations are performed each year in the United States at about 150 renal transplantation centers.

PATIENT SELECTION AND PREPARATION

Since the indications for renal transplantation have become so broad, it is simpler to list the contraindications: extremes of age, metastatic cancer, active infection, and active destructive psychosis. In addition, severe vascular disease affecting the heart, the extremities, or the brain and severe chronic lung disease enjoin strongly against transplantation. Systemic diseases such as diabetes mellitus, systemic lupus erythematosus, Wegener's granulomatosis, scleroderma, and amyloidosis are no longer contraindications to renal transplantation.

The patient should be in optimal condition at the time of transplantation to have the best chance of surviving the stresses of surgery and immunosuppression. Hypertension should be controlled, calcium and phosphate problems rectified, and anemia corrected as much as possible. Active infection must be cured and potential infectious sources must be eliminated before transplantation and concomitant immunosuppression can proceed. The most common potential source of infection is the urinary tract. Infected hydronephrotic, calcareous, or pyelonephritic kidneys must be removed. The lower urinary tract must function normally; if not, it must be repaired or a bowel conduit created before transplantation.

Bilateral nephrectomy is not a routine procedure and is reserved for patients with active renal infection or severe unremitting hypertension. Splenectomy is not routinely performed except for correction of leukopenia and thrombocytopenia unresponsive to other forms of therapy.

Histocompatibility determination

An absolute prerequisite for transplantation is donor-recipient compatibility for the major ABO (red cell) antigens. The major human histocompatibility complex, HLA, is located on the short arm of chromosome 6. There are at present four known loci on each chromosome 6: HLA-A, -B, -C, and -D. The loci are each paired. The A, B, and C loci are found on virtually all cells of the body and are detectable by serologic means. The HLA-D antigens are expressed on a limited number of cells, mainly B lymphocytes, monocytes, and endothelial cells. The A and B loci can be determined within a few hours and serve as the basis for cadaveric transplantation. The C locus is a "weaker" system; the availability of good antisera for determination of the C loci is rare. Furthermore, the C locus seems to have little importance in clinical transplantation. It is probable that the most important antigens for which to match are at the D locus. These are the first foreign antigens recognized by the recipient's immune system. At the present time D locus antigens can be accurately determined only by the mixed lymphocyte culture reaction, in which lymphocytes of the potential donor and recipient are mixed in tissue culture and the intensity of blast cell transformations is graded. The time required to identify D locus antigens in a cadaver kidney, 4 to 6 days, exceeds the "shelf-life" of the kidney. However, the test is useful for selecting the best donor from several potential living related donors. There has recently been considerable interest in the serologically determined D-related (DR) antigens found on B lymphocytes because they can be rapidly determined.

The importance of the HLA-A and -B loci is threefold. First, foreign A and B antigens serve as targets against which the recipient makes antibody. Second, the A and B loci exist in some degree of linkage disequilibrium with the D locus; matching for the A and B loci occasionally results in matching for the D locus. Third, presensitization to A and B loci can occur, usually from pregnancies, blood transfusions, or previous transplants. The presence of preformed circulating cytotoxic antibodies against certain A and B loci precludes the use of a kidney containing those antigens. This is determined by a pretransplantation cross-match, in which donor lymphocytes are incubated with recipient serum in the presence of rabbit complement. A positive cross-match is determined by lympholysis. Transplantation between a donor and recipient with a positive cross-match almost uniformly results in hyperacute rejection.

The meaning of the HLA system in family donor transplantation is quite clear. There are two number 6 chromosomes, one from each parent. Therefore, in parent-child transplants one chromosome (haplotype) is shared, indicating sharing of at least one A, B, and D locus. Among siblings, 25% share both chromosomes (a two-haplotype or HLA-identical match), 50% share one chromosome as with a parent donor, and 25% have both chromosomes (two haplotypes) mismatched. There is a clear increment in transplant success going from a two-haplotype mismatch in which success is scarcely better than with a kidney from an unrelated donor, through a one-haplotype match, to a two-haplotype (HLA-identical) match with success exceeding 95%. In cadaver organ transplantation the situation is much more complex; matching at the A and B loci does not necessarily imply identity of the D locus. In the United States identity at the A and B loci gives about a 10% increment in success over transplantation with kidneys completely mismatched at these loci. Statistically there has been no difference between matching for one, two, three, or no antigens. The chances of any individual being A and B locus identical with any other unrelated individual vary between 1:100 and 1:1 million. Because of this it is difficult to find an unrelated donor who is A and B locus identical with any specific recipient.

In Europe the situation is somewhat different. It is possible to draw survival curves for cadaver grafts showing a gradual but statistically significant decrement in graft survival going from four antigen matches to none. The reason postulated is related to the greater genetic homogeneity of the native European population. Matching for A and B loci has a far greater chance of matching for the D locus in a country such as the Netherlands than it would in the genetic melting pot of the United States.

Cadaver donors

Although a kidney from a family donor with one or two matching haplotypes has a better chance of survival than does a kidney from an unrelated source, the trend in the United States and around the world is toward cadaver donation rather than family donors, for ethical rather than medical reasons.

CADAVER DONOR PROCUREMENT. Even though surveys have suggested that an adequate supply of potential cadaver kidney donors exists, the kidneys are actually obtained from only about 20% of suitable potential donors. The reason for this low rate is public and physician ignorance of the need for these organs.

Any patient under the age of 60 years with actual or possible brain death and normal renal function is a suitable potential donor. The presence of malignancy (except for nonmetastasizing cerebral tumors), infection, renal disease, prolonged diabetes, or severe hypertension makes a donor unacceptable. The majority of donors who meet the medical criteria for brain death are patients with severe head trauma or spontaneous cerebral hemorrhage. Organ procurement is simpler in states where uniform anatomic gift statutes have been enacted.

The pretreatment of cadaver donors with large doses of cytotoxic drugs before kidney removal has been advocated to reduce the presence of ''passenger leukocytes,'' a postulated source of immunization. At present controlled studies showing the efficacy of this technique are lacking.

ORGAN PRESERVATION. There are two methods of cadaver organ preservation. Once removed, the kidneys can be flushed with a hyperosmolar solution such as Collins' solution and stored in iced slush for up to 24 hours before transplantation. Alternatively, a pulsatile perfusion apparatus can perfuse the kidney with an oxygenated plasma or albumin solution at 40° F (4° C). With pulsatile perfusion, kidneys can be maintained for up to 48 hours and occasionally up to 72 hours before transplantation. This technique also allows examination of pressure-flow relationships of the prefusate through the kidney, occasionally making it possible to predict severe ischemic damage to the organ.

SURGICAL PROCEDURE

Cadaveric and living donor kidney transplantations are performed with identical surgical techniques. The kidney is placed in a heterotopic position retroperitoneally in the iliac fossa. An end-to-end arterial anastomosis is usually performed with the divided internal iliac (hypogastric) artery of the host and the renal artery. If the host internal iliac artery is unsuitable, the renal artery can be placed end to side into the external iliac artery. The renal veins are usually placed end to side into the host external iliac or common iliac veins. Ureteral continuity is obtained by one of three techniques. Most commonly the donor ureter is tunneled into the bladder by a technique similar to that used for ureteral reimplantation for reflux (ureteroneocystostomy). Alternatively, the donor ureter can be sutured to the recipient ureter (ureteroureterostomy) or the recipient ureter can be fixed to the pelvis of the donor kidney (ureteropyelostomy). The last two techniques require nephrectomy of the recipient's ipsilateral kidney.

IMMUNOSUPPRESSIVE THERAPY

Azathioprine and prednisone are the backbone of immunosuppressive therapy in renal transplantation. Therapy with azathioprine is usually started a few hours before surgery in cadaveric transplantation and 1 to several days in advance with living donor transplants. Most medical centers consider an adequate dosage of azathioprine to be 2 to 3 mg/kg body weight/day. The dosage is regulated according to the white blood cell count; every effort is made to avoid leukopenia. Cyclophosphamide can be substituted if azathioprine cannot be used.

Prednisone is usually started on the day of transplantation at a dosage of 1.5 mg/kg/day, usually about 100 mg. The dosage is gradually tapered to 0.5 mg/kg/day 1 month after the transplantation unless rejection supervenes.

Antilymphocyte globulin (ALG), a heterologous serum directed against human lymphocytes, has been widely used over the past decade. There is yet no evidence that ALG prolongs graft survival, although it can ameliorate rejection reactions while it is being administered.

A new, potent immunosuppressive drug of fungal origin, cyclosporin A, has been developed. This drug appears to have a substantially greater effect in enhancing graft survival than present immunosuppressives. However, its use has been associated with an approximate 10% incidence of malignant lymphomas in animal studies and a small number of human studies.

It has been noted that patients who have received blood transfusions before transplantation do significantly better than those who have never received transfusions. The mechanism is unclear. This may be a preselection phenomenon; patients who are immunologically ''reactive'' form cytotoxic HLA antibodies with transfusion and may never receive a transplant because of difficulties in matching with a suitable donor. Alternatively, the transfusions may result in immunologic enhancement or the formation of blocking antibodies. At present it is unclear what blood preparation and how much blood to use and when it should be given.

COMPLICATIONS
Rejection reactions

Rejection can be divided into three types: hyperacute, acute, and chronic.

Hyperacute rejection, the most dramatic type, occurs when the recipient has preformed circulating antibodies against the HLA loci of the donor kidney. It takes place within minutes to hours after the arterial anastomosis and always results in loss of the graft. Cytotoxic antibodies against the kidney are presumably involved in an antigen-antibody reaction at the vascular endothelium. There is subsequent activation of the clotting, complement, and kinin cascade with thrombosis of small and large vessels and more distal necrosis. Hyperacute rejection can be avoided by careful pretransplantation cross-matching of donor and recipient. However, an occasional patient with a level of cytotoxic antibodies too low to be detected suffers a hyperacute rejection. This type of rejection is usually recognized during surgery; the kidney never "pinks up" but stays soft and blue even though the arterial anastomosis is clearly patent.

Acute rejection generally occurs between the first and fourth weeks after transplantation. It is recognized by a decrement in graft function usually associated with fever, weight gain, hypertension, graft enlargement and tenderness, and a decrease in urine output with a fall in the urinary sodium concentration. Despite a multitude of reports there is no test specific for the diagnosis of acute rejection. Acute rejection is characterized by an interstitial infiltration of mononuclear cells, lymphocytes, and plasma cells and extensive edema. The appearance is one of pure cellular immunity, with the absence of vasculitis, fibrin deposition, or polymorphonuclear infiltration. Most rejection episodes are a mixture of cellular and humoral immune responses.

The treatment of acute rejection is limited, and there are no controlled studies showing the effectiveness of therapy. Most centers increase steroid dosage during acute rejection (intravenous methylprednisolone, 0.5 to 1 g daily for 3 to 7 days). Alternatively, oral prednisone can be increased to 3 to 5 mg/kg/day for several days, or both forms of therapy can be used. When the rejection has abated, the steroid dosage is tapered to pretreatment levels. Some centers treat acute rejection with external irradiation of the graft at a dose of 150 rad daily for 3 to 5 days, but there is no proof of the efficacy of this therapy.

Chronic rejection is an insidious process causing a gradual loss of renal function over months to years. It is characterized pathologically by interstitial fibrosis and endarteritis obliterans caused by endothelial proliferation. Chronic rejection usually occurs following one or more episodes of acute rejection but can occur in its absence. Treatment with increased doses of steroids has not been shown to be effective and increases the risk of intercurrent infection.

Graft nonfunction

A majority of grafts from living donors and about 50% of cadaver grafts function immediately. Most kidneys that do not function immediately have acute tubular necrosis (ATN). This condition does not affect the eventual outcome; the only treatment is watchful waiting. ATN may persist for up to 6 weeks, and the graft may still recover and develop adequate function. Other conditions causing immediate nonfunction are arterial or venous thrombosis and ureteral obstruction. The diagnosis of these conditions can be determined easily by a combination of radionuclide imaging and ultrasonographic examination of the kidney. Late graft failure usually results from rejection but can be caused by vascular or ureteral obstruction. Noninvasive imaging techniques, sometimes along with renal biopsy, allow diagnoses to be made.

Infection

Infection is the major complication and cause of death in renal transplantation. Infections range from cystitis in about 50% of patients to life-threatening pulmonary and systemic infections. With more able management of immunosuppressive drugs, routine bacterial infections have become less common. At present many of the infections are opportunistic or viral. Cytomegalovirus, herpes simplex or zoster, and *Listeria, Nocardia,* and *Pneumocystis* infections may develop because of T-cell suppression. If suspected, infection must be rapidly and fully evaluated, often with special microbiologic techniques, since overwhelming infections can occur in a matter of hours.

Hypertension

Hypertension occurs in a majority of renal transplant recipients. Its evaluation and treatment do not differ substantially from those in a normal patient.

Recurrent disease

The incidence of recurrence of the original disease in the transplanted organ is remarkably small, perhaps because of the immunosuppressive therapy. Focal segmental glomerulosclerosis, type II membranoproliferative glomerulonephritis, Goodpasture's disease, and IgA nephropathy (Berger's disease) have all been reported to recur in a small number of patients.

Malignancy

There is a 5% to 6% incidence of a new malignancy developing in the first few years after transplantation. About three fourths of these are skin, lip, or uterocervical carcinomas that can be adequately treated by local excision. Of the remaining one fourth a majority are reticulum cell sarcomas, which often involve the central nervous system and are almost uniformly fatal.

Other complications

Urinary leakage and fistula formation or lymphocele may result from surgical technical difficulties. Any of the recognized complications of steroid therapy (aseptic necrosis of bone, peptic ulcer, diabetes, and posterior subcapsular cataract formation) may occur in the recipient. Vesicoureteral reflux occurs in the absence of infection and may be associated with reduced graft survival.

Table 113-1. Graft and patient survival following renal transplantation

	1-year survival (%)		10-year survival (%)	
	Graft	Patient	Graft	Patient
HLA-identical sibling (four-antigen match)	>95	≅100	85-90	≅100
One haplotype (two-antigen match)	70-75*	90	50-55	70-75
Cadaver	50†	75-80‡	20-25	25§

*Falls to 60% graft survival at 5 years.
†Falls to 35% graft survival at 5 years.
‡Selected centers have improved patient survival to 90% to 95%.
§Same range as survival with hemodialysis.

OUTCOME

The results of renal transplantation can be expressed in two ways, graft survival and patient survival (Table 113-1).

In living donor transplantation a graft from an HLA-identical sibling (four-antigen match) has by far the best chance of success. Patient survival 10 years after cadaver renal transplantation is in the same range as survival with hemodialysis. Therefore living donor transplantation offers advantages in success rate and life span as compared with cadaveric transplantation or dialysis. With cadaveric transplantation the advantage over hemodialysis lies only in lifestyle; no statement can be made about life span.

BIBLIOGRAPHY

Advisory Committee to the Renal Transplant Registry: The 13th Report of the Human Renal Transplant Registry, Transplant. Proc. **9:**9, 1977.
Calne, R.Y., and others: Cyclosporin A as the only immunosuppressant in 34 recipients of cadaveric organs: 32 kidneys, 2 pancreases, and 2 livers, Lancet **2:**1033, 1979.
Guttmann, R.D.: Renal transplantation (in two parts), N. Engl. J. Med. **301:**975, 1038, 1979.
Monaco, A.P.: Transplantation. In Earley, L.E., and Gottschalk, C.W., editors: Strauss and Welt's diseases of the kidney, ed. 3, Boston, 1979, Little, Brown & Co.
Opelz, G., and Terasaki, P.I.: Dominant effects of transfusions on kidney graft survival, Transplantation **29:**153, 1980.
Porter, K.A.: Renal transplantation. In Heptinstall, R.H.: Pathology of the kidney, ed. 2, Boston, 1974, Little, Brown & Co.

114 • NEPHROLITHIASIS

Mary Catherine Stom and Elizabeth D. Labovitz

Kidney stones predominate in industrialized areas, whereas bladder stones are more common in underdeveloped and nonurban areas. Kidney stones occur in 1% to 5% of the U.S. population and are responsible for 1 of every 1000 hospitalizations. If infectious stones are eliminated, men have four times as many stones as do women. The prevalence is higher in whites than in blacks and in white-collar workers than in laborers. The peak incidence of initial stone formation is in the third decade of life. Most patients average more than 3.5 stones in their lifetime, with 50% of patients having a second stone within 5 years and 60% within 9 years. There appear to be "stone belts"; in the southeastern United States, stones are responsible for 2 in 1000 hospitalizations.

Calcium stones predominate. Of all analyzed stones, calcium oxalate and calcium phosphate account for more than 80%, struvite for 10% to 15%, uric acid for 5% to 10%, and cystine for 1% to 3%.

The presentation of kidney stones ranges from asymptomatic hematuria and minimal proteinuria to dysuria, colic, costovertebral angle tenderness, and the passing of clots, sludge, or stones. The initial syndrome may result from the complications of stones, including obstruction, renal failure, infection, and hematuria.

Normal urine is commonly supersaturated with calcium, oxalate, and phosphate. Stone formation, however, is multifactorial and is affected by the saturation and solubility of salts, promoters and inhibitors of crystal growth and aggregation, and local physical factors (obstruction, infection, and urine pH). The crystal nidus may be homogeneous or heterogeneous. Crystals of similar lattice size may grow on one another; thus calcium oxalate, calcium phosphate, and monosodium urate crystals, all of similar dimensions, augment the precipitation of one another. The existence of inhibitors has been known for more than 20 years. The main inhibitors in vivo seem to be inorganic phosphate, citrate, and magnesium; however, in vitro studies have identified other inhibitors such as urine, zinc, polyelectrolytes, and proteins. Inhibitors delay nidus formation, growth, and aggregation. One theory of the mechanism of inhibition is based on the fact that less than 1% of the crystal surface need be bound by an inhibitor to prevent crystal growth. It is not known if patients with stones overall have less inhibitors.

The physical chemistry involved in stone formation has clinical and therapeutic relevance. The therapy should be directed at increasing solubility, decreasing saturation, increasing inhibitors, and impairing crystal nidus formation. Therapeutic maneuvers include hydration, drugs, and alteration in the urine pH.

CALCIUM STONES

Nephrocalcinosis, in distinction to kidney stones, is the deposition of calcium within *renal* tissue. It may be demonstrable roentgenographically or histologically. Hypercalciuria and/or hypercalcemic states, infection, and renal degenerative changes predispose patients to nephrocalcinosis. Nephrocalcinosis is an asymptomatic phenomenon and may or may not be associated with calcium stones.

Table 114-1. Metabolic and clinical disorders in 460 consecutive calcium stone formers

Disorder	No. of patients	%
Idiopathic hypercalciuria	95	20.7
Marginal hypercalciuria*	53	11.5
Hyperuricosuria†	67	14.6
Hypercalciuria and hyperuricosuria‡	54	11.7
Hyperuricemia	26	5.7
Primary hyperparathyroidism	24	5.2
Renal tubular acidosis§	17	3.7
Inflammatory bowel disease‖	21	4.6
Medullary sponge kidney	7	1.5
Sarcoidosis	3	0.7
No disorder found	93	20.2
TOTAL	460	

Reproduced with permission from Coe, F.L.: Nephrolithiasis—Pathogenesis and Treatment. Copyright © 1978 by Year Book Medical Publishers, Inc., Chicago.
*Urine calcium > 140 mg/g creatinine.
†Urine uric acid above 800 mg (men) and 750 mg (women) in at least one of two 24-hour urine collections.
‡Marginal hypercalciuria not included.
§Distal hereditary form.
‖Regional enteritis, ulcerative colitis, granulomatous ileocolitis.

The following discussion is limited to kidney stones.

Although there are two types of calcium stones (oxalate and phosphate), there are diverse metabolic causes that must be delineated to devise appropriate therapy. In one study that evaluated 460 consecutive calcium stone–forming patients, it was found that 80% had known causes of stone disease (Table 114-1).

Hypercalciuria

The most widely accepted normal levels of daily calcium excretion are 250 mg for women and 300 mg for men, or 4 mg/kg body weight. These values are based on studies showing that 95% of non-stone-forming patients excreted less than 250 to 300 mg of calcium a day and that over 30% of stone-forming patients excreted more than this. Marginal hypercalciuria is defined as excretion of more than 150 mg calcium/1 g creatinine/day.

If hypercalciuria occurs with hypercalcemia, the approach to the patient is directed toward diagnosis of the hypercalcemia, for example, hyperparathyroidism, tumor, Paget's disease of bone, vitamin D excess, sarcoidosis, immobilization, milk-alkali syndrome, hyperthyroidism, adrenocortical insufficiency, infantile hypercalcemia, renal transplantation, and the recovery phase of acute renal failure. If the patient is normocalcemic, several causes of hypercalciuria must be excluded, for example, hyperparathyroidism, renal tubular acidosis, sarcoidosis, Cushing's disease, hyperthyroidism, Paget's disease, immobilization, medullary sponge kidney, and drugs such as vitamins A and D, furosemide, ethacrynic acid, and perhaps spironolactone. Therapy for the hypercalciuria is then directed at the underlying cause.

Hyperparathyroidism is the most common cause of hypercalcemic hypercalciuric stone formation. An inappropriately high serum parathyroid hormone (PTH) level is the prime indicator of the diagnosis. Hypercalcemia of neoplasm is common, but stones are rare. Sarcoid patients have normal or high serum calcium concentrations, low serum PTH levels, and hypercalciuria from both increased levels of and increased gut sensitivity to hydroxylated vitamin D_3, or 1,25-dihydroxycholecalciferol (1,25$[OH]_2D_3$). In sarcoidosis the hypercalciuria is reversed in 5 to 14 days with 15 mg of prednisone daily.

Distal renal tubular acidosis is a disease associated with metabolic acidosis caused by renal inability to secrete H^+ and acidify the urine to a pH less than 5.8 (see Chapter 108). It is a cause of normocalcemic, hypercalciuric stone formation. Patients with this disease have hypercalciuria, phosphaturia, and lowered urinary citrate levels. The hypercalciuria, phosphaturia, alkaline urine (a result of the basic metabolic defect), and low urine levels of citrate (a necessary inhibitor), are associated with the common occurrence of calcium phosphate stones. Specific therapy for the hypercalciuria is directed toward resolution of the acidosis with 0.5 to 2 mEq base/kg body weight/day in four equally divided doses.

In medullary sponge kidney 50% of patients have calcareous deposits in the cysts and 40% have hypercalciuria (see Chapter 116). Hypercalciuria should be treated with thiazide diuretics.

Idiopathic hypercalciuria is the syndrome of normocalcemia, recurrent calcium stones, and hypercalciuria of undetermined cause. Controversy exists concerning the definition and pathogenesis of idiopathic hypercalciuria. Two pathogenetic mechanisms—renal hypercalciuria and absorptive hypercalciuria—have been described. In renal hypercalciuria the primary defect is an impairment of renal tubular calcium reabsorption, perhaps as a result of renal phosphate leak and phosphate depletion. Regardless of the cause, the calcium loss stimulates PTH release and further phosphate depletion, both of which lead to increased 1,25$(OH)_2D_3$ formation. This enhances the intestinal absorption of calcium.

Absorptive hypercalciuria has as its primary defect an increased intestinal absorption of calcium. This presents an increased calcium load to the kidney, suppresses PTH, and results in hypercalciuria. One third to one half of these patients have elevated levels of 1,25$(OH)_2D_3$. Some suggest that the primary defect is again renal tubular phosphate wasting, with phosphate depletion stimulating formation of the active vitamin D. It is believed that phosphate depletion and 1,25$(OH)_2D_3$ decrease PTH release.

In both renal and absorptive hypercalciuria the urine calcium, $1,25(OH)_2D_3$, and intestinal calcium absorption is high and serum phosphate concentrations are normal or low. The higher PTH concentration in renal hypercalciuria helps distinguish the two conditions. In renal hypercalciuria a high urinary calcium level persists after both a low-calcium diet (400 mg/day for 5 to 7 days) and a high-calcium diet (1000 mg/day for 5 to 7 days), whereas in absorptive hypercalciuria increased urine calcium results only after the high-calcium diet. In addition, after overnight fasting a 2-hour urine sample shows a calcium/creatinine excretion ratio of less than 0.11 in absorptive hypercalciuria and greater than 0.12 in renal hypercalciuria.

The therapy for idiopathic hypercalciuria is directed toward lessening the urine calcium concentration. Thiazide diuretics accomplish this (1) by stimulating calcium resorption via PTH, (2) by producing volume depletion, which increases proximal tubular calcium resorption, and (3) perhaps by potentiating the action of PTH by inhibiting the degradation of renal cyclic AMP. Impairment of the effectiveness of thiazides may be a result of volume repletion and hypoparathyroidism. Decreased stone formation is found in as many as 90% of treated patients. Suggested mechanisms for this include hypocalciuria, increased urine volume, reduced oxalate excretion, or increased urine phosphate and magnesium. In some patients treated with thiazides there may be a slight rise in the total serum calcium concentration. The serum PTH level should not rise and in fact may decrease if the renal phosphate ''leak'' of renal hypercalciuria is resolved with thiazides. If the serum calcium concentration remains at 11 mg/dl for more than 4 to 6 weeks, despite discontinuing the thiazides, other causes of hypercalcemia, especially hyperparathyroidism, should be pursued. Agents that bind calcium in the intestinal tract are also used in the therapy for idiopathic hypercalciuria. Orthophosphates (1.5 to 2 g/day in divided doses) decreased stone activity in 90% of study patients. Stone prevention may result from decreased gatrointestinal calcium absorption, increased urine phosphate levels, or decreased urine calcium levels. Neutral phosphate preparations are preferable to acid preparations because acidosis decreases renal calcium resorption. Diarrhea, the most common side effect, may be obviated by prescribing the phosphates for postprandial use. An increased urine oxalate level may occur, which in theory may increase calcium oxalate stone formation. Phosphates should be avoided in patients with renal failure or phosphate stones (for example, patients with renal tubular acidosis and those with struvite stones). Cellulose phosphate is a nonabsorbable cation-binding resin that binds calcium and magnesium in the intestine, thus decreasing absorption. A negative calcium-magnesium balance may ensue. For these reasons the drug should be reserved for patients with absorptive hypercalciuria who do not respond to other therapies. Although diphosphonates are potent inhibitors of stone formation, the required doses cause bone disease and these drugs should not be used.

Hyperuricosuric, calcium oxalate nephrolithiasis

Both hyperuricosuria (urinary uric acid excretion greater than 750 mg/day in females and greater than 800 mg/day in males) and hyperuricemia have been recognized as risk factors for calcium stones. With allopurinol treatment, stone formation is reduced to 6% of predicted cases. These patients have a different clinical syndrome than other stone-forming patients; the onset is later, the formation rates are higher, the interval times are shorter, and surgical manipulation is more common.

Hyperoxaluria

Hyperoxaluria (oxalate excreted in urine greater than 40 mg/day) results from increased intestinal absorption or overproduction of oxalate. Increased absorption occurs with overingestion (rare), small bowel bypass surgery (because of fatty acid malabsorption), and ingestion of cellulose phosphate. Fatty acids and cellulose phosphate bind intestinal calcium, leaving oxalate free to be absorbed. The overproduction of oxalate may be primary (hereditary) or secondary. Ascorbic acid, ethylene glycol, and methoxyflurane are converted to substrate for oxalate formation, causing hyperoxaluria. Cholestyramine, a low-fat diet, calcium tablets, and oxalate restriction should be therapeutic in hyperabsorption states. Pyridoxine may be used in overproduction states.

Idiopathic calcium stones

In patients with idiopathic calcium stones, treatment with low-calcium diets and hydration produces modest success. Thiazides, allopurinol, and orthophosphates have caused decreased stone activity in some studies.

STRUVITE STONES

Struvite stones are associated with infection. Urease-forming bacteria (most often *Proteus*) form an alkaline urine, resulting in magnesium–ammonium phosphate (struvite) stones. This begins a vicious circle, since the stone harbors the infection, which in turn increases growth of the stone. Struvite stones can grow rapidly in this infectious environment and are often staghorn calculi when the patients (usually young women, elderly men, and patients with indwelling Foley catheters and ileostomies) are discovered. The diagnosis involves metabolic evaluation (any stone may have been the nidus), definition of the bacteria, and roentgenographic evaluation for an anatomic defect. The therapy is then directed at eradication or long-term suppression of the infection, surgical removal of all stones, repair of the anatomy, and treatment of any metabolic disorder. The recurrence rate after surgical removal is high. Urease inhibitors have recently been found effective in patients refractory to treatment.

URIC ACID STONES

Uric acid stones account for 10% of all cases of renal stones in the United States, but this varies in other parts of the world. Pure uric acid stones are radiolucent, but often calcium oxalate or phosphate crystals are part of the stone, which is then radiopaque.

Hyperuricosuria may result from hyperuricemia or an abnormality in renal proximal tubular transport. Because of the low pK of uric acid (5.75), it is almost completely dissociated at blood pH into its ionized soluble form, monosodium urate. In the tubules, as the pH falls, ionized urate is transformed into free undissociated uric acid, whose solubility is much less. The precipitation of uric acid crystals depends on the quantity excreted and a urinary pH of less than 6. Decreased ammonia excretion rates in patients with uric acid stones, leading to increased urinary acidity, may be important in the pathogenesis. Other clinical techniques and syndromes (ileostomies, diarrhea, and volume depletion states) that dispose patients to aciduria may be manifested by normal serum uric acid levels but uric acid stones as well.

Uric acid stone formation is correlated with hyperuricemia and hyperuricosuria. The disorders of uric acid overproduction include gout, myeloproliferative diseases, Lesch-Nyhan syndrome and other enzyme deficiency states, and glycogen storage diseases. The therapy is directed at alkalinizing urine (pH 6 to 7), increasing urine volume (3 L/day), and decreasing serum and urine uric acid levels (as with allopurinol).

CYSTINE STONES

Cystine stones, a familial disease, occur in males and females with equal frequency and at any age. They are moderately radiopaque because of their sulfur bonds. Of stones passed by cystinuric patients, 50% are pure, 40% are mixed, and almost 10% have no cystine; thus stone analysis alone is insufficient, and the diagnosis is based on the urinary excretion of cystine. Hexagonal flat crystals on urinalysis are strong evidence. The excretion of increased amount of cystine is determined with nitroprusside screening test of the urine, which detects greater than 75 mg cystine/1000 mg creatinine. False positive results occur in patients with cystinosis, homocystinuria, or acetonuria. The normal excretion of cystine is less than or equal to 30 mg/day. Decreased solubility occurs in an acid pH. The therapy includes hydration, urinary alkalinization (pH greater than 7), and possibly penicillamine, which complexes with and solubilizes cystine. Penicillamine side effects may be significant.

MANAGEMENT OF ACUTE UROLITHIASIS

The initial therapy for acute symptomatic urolithiasis involves administering adequate analgesics and ensuring a fluid intake of more than 3 L/day. Infection should be treated, and if gram-negative bacillary bacteremia with shock occurs, emergency surgery may be required to remove an obstructing stone.

Most ureteral and bladder stones are passed spontaneously over a period of days; however, urologic intervention either surgically or through a cystoscope may be required. Calculus chemolysis has recently been undertaken to lyse renal stones via a nephrostomy tube. However, this therapy may cause systemic toxicity or renal damage.

Eradication of bacteriuria or long-term suppression may help prevent the formation of new stones or the propagation of stones already present.

BIBLIOGRAPHY

Broadus, A.E., and Thier, S.: Metabolic basis of renal-stone disease, N. Engl. J. Med. **300**:839, 1979.

Coe, F.L., editor: Nephrolithiasis—pathogenesis and treatment, Chicago, 1978, Year Book Medical Publishers, Inc.

Labovitz, E.D.: Hyperuricemia and the kidney. In Jepson, J.H., editor: Hematologic problems in renal disease, Reading, Mass., 1979, Addison-Wesley Publishing Co., Inc.

Pak, C.Y., editor: Symposium on urolithiasis, Kidney Int. **13**:341, 1978.

Pak, C.Y.: Physiological basis for absorptive and renal hypercalciurias, Am. J. Physiol. **237**:415, 1979.

115 • MALFORMATIONS OF THE URINARY TRACT

Linda B. Hiner

RENAL ANOMALIES
Renal agenesis

Bilateral renal agenesis occurs in about 1 in 4000 births and is incompatible with life. The absence of intrauterine micturition leads to oligohydramnios with ensuing lung hypoplasia and facial (Potter facies) and limb anomalies.

Unilateral renal agenesis is sporadic, occurring in about 1 in 1000 births. It is commonly associated with ipsilateral agenesis of the ureter and bladder hemitrigone and is occasionally associated with abnormalities of the genital tract such as absence of a gonad, the uterine horn, or the adrenal gland. The contralateral kidney is usually large from birth; it may be more susceptible to infection, stone formation, and tumor.

Renal hypoplasia

Renal hypoplasia describes a kidney whose histology is normal but whose total size or number of ureteral divisions is reduced (there may simply be too thin a cortex). Unilateral renal hypoplasia occurs in about 1 in 500 live births. Hypoplasia can result from abnormal intrauterine or postnatal growth. The diagnosis of renal hypoplasia requires histologic evaluation. Because these kidneys are prone to develop infection, stones, and vascular disease, the diagnosis is usually discovered incidentally during evaluation for one of these complications.

The Ask-Upmark kidney is a form of segmental renal hypoplasia or perhaps atrophy characterized by bands of aglomerular or hypoglomerular tissue that cut deep clefts into the cortex and medulla of the involved kidney. The cause of the malformation is unknown. It may be associated with severe childhood hypertension, which is usually corrected by nephrectomy or segmental nephrectomy.

Oligomeganephronia is a nonfamilial form of bilateral renal hypoplasia associated with a reduced number of calyceal divisions. The few nephrons present are very large and hypertrophied. Affected individuals tend to "outgrow" their fixed, reduced renal functional capacity within the first decade of life. There may be associated progressive interstitial fibrosis and glomerulosclerosis.

True bilateral renal hypoplasia is rare. Both kidneys appear as miniatures with a normal number of calyceal divisions. This defect may occur together with other congenital anomalies, especially those of the central nervous system.

Renal dysplasia

Gross disorganization of tissue differentiation results in dysplasia of the kidney. Dysplastic kidneys may also be hypoplastic, but the term "hypoplasia" is reserved for kidneys with normal tissue differentiation. The disorganized renal tissue may contain areas of squamous epithelium, fibrous tissue, and even cartilage and bone. Renal cysts are common.

Renal dysplasia is usually sporadic. However, there may be concurrence within families for mechanically or functionally obstructive lesions that may lead to renal dysplasia. It is generally believed that abnormal differentiation results from in utero obstruction to urine flow. Such obstruction may be of varying degrees as a result of such causes as ureteral atresia, functional or mechanical obstruction to bladder emptying, or obstruction at the ureteropelvic junction.

Multicystic kidneys that occur with bilateral ureteral atresia are large, grossly cystic, and have a completely disorganized structure. This condition is not compatible with life. Affected children are oliguric in utero and have oligohydramnios, Potter facies, and pulmonary hypoplasia.

Unilateral multicystic renal dysplasia is associated with severe in utero urinary obstruction on the involved side and is usually discovered in the newborn. The treatment is nephrectomy. The remaining kidney may not be entirely normal and may have associated bladder or ureteral abnormalities. Usually, however, the prognosis is good.

Anomalies of renal position

Abnormal renal migration or rotation may lead to such anomalies as horseshoe kidney, ectopic placement, and even pancake or "crossed" ectopic kidneys. There may be areas of dysplasia within abnormally placed kidneys. There is an increased susceptibility to infection and nephrolithiasis. There may also be an increased incidence of progressive interstitial fibrosis with a loss of renal function.

URETERAL ANOMALIES

A complete duplication of the collection system, "double kidney," refers to a double pelvis within the substance of one kidney. Either there is a single, terminal ureter or the ureters reach the bladder separately. The occurrence of a true supernumerary kidney is rare. The ureter that drains the upper pole of a completely duplicated system usually opens ectopically into the bladder, urethra, vagina, rectum, or some other place in the urogenital tract.

Although a variety of anomalies of the bladder and ureters are described, often with associated abnormal renal morphogenesis, clincally the most significant are those leading to vesicoureteral reflux. Reflux of bladder urine into the ureter results from incompetent flap-valve function of the bladder wall and the intravesical ureter.

Anatomic situations associated with vesicoureteral reflux include a shortened intramural ureteral tunnel, a large-diameter intramural ureter, abnormal placement of the ureteral orifice with a loss of integrity of normal detrusor function, and decreased pliability of the bladder wall.

Urine that has refluxed into the ureter and kidney serves as a reservoir and increases the risk of urinary infection (see discussion of "Urinary tract infection and perirenal abscess" in Chapter 40). There may be mechanical damage to the kidney, especially if there is an associated obstruction. Although it is commonly thought that refluxed urine exposes the upper tract to bacteria, bacteria may ascend the ureters in the absence of vesicoureteral reflux. Severely involved individuals with massive hydroureteronephrosis often have dysplastic kidneys, the function of which cannot be much improved by ureteral reimplantation.

Although vesicoureteral reflux is uncommon in adults with urinary tract infection, it is found in 30% of young girls evaluated for cystitis. Such reflux is more common in girls than in boys and in whites than in blacks. It probably results from a shortened intramural ureter and decreased pliability of the inflamed edematous bladder wall.

Reflux can be evaluated by its appearance during voiding, a cystourethrogram, and the cystoscopic appearance of the ureteral orifice, which can be calibrated according to the diameter and length of the intramural ureter as follows:

1. Normal—little cone, slit on top
2. Stadium orifice—flatter cone, stretched slit
3. Horseshoe orifice—no cone, slit stretched with one side flat
4. Golf-hole orifice—gaping hole, often abnormally placed

The roentgenographic appearance of vesicoureteral reflux can be categorized as follows:

1. Grade I—lower ureter only
2. Grade IIa—ureter and kidney; no calyceal dilation
3. Grade IIb—ureter and kidney; mild calyceal dilation
4. Grade III—ureter and kidney; ureteral dilation and calyceal clubbing
5. Grade IV—massive hydroureteronephrosis

Since ureteral orifices that are slightly abnormally placed may develop competent valve function as a result of growth and freedom from infection, a conservative approach is acceptable for some children with reflux. However, ureters with severe reflux or markedly abnormal ("golf-hole") orifices should be treated surgically. Correction of the reflux may not stop loss of renal function; such kidneys may be congenitally dysplastic.

Reflux may produce a nephropathy associated with hypertension, proteinuria, glomerular sclerosis, interstitial nephritis, and progressive renal insufficiency over a period of years.

BLADDER ANOMALIES

Congenital bladder anomalies are rare. The more severe ones require urinary diversion in childhood. Agenesis of the bladder, hypoplasia, duplications, and diverticula have been described. Failure of closure involving the rectum (cloacal exstrophy) can occur. Children with sacral agenesis or meningomyelocele may have an accompanying neurogenic bladder.

URETHRAL ANOMALIES

Minor urethral anomalies include urethral stenosis, which may require surgical correction to prevent urinary obstruction or infection. *Hypospadias* (presence of a proximal ventral meatus) is the most common urethral abnormality in males and often requires surgical correction. *Epispadias* (abnormal dorsal opening of the urethra) occurs in both sexes and is either entirely asymptomatic or produces incontinence. Two other rare anomalies include megalourethra, which is associated with lack of development of the erectile bodies of the penis, and urethral diverticula.

BIBLIOGRAPHY

Bernstein, J.: Congenital malformations of the kidney. In Earley, L.E., and Gottschalk, C.W., editors: Strauss and Welt's diseases of the kidney, ed. 3, Boston, 1979, Little, Brown & Co.

King, L.R.: Vesicoureteral reflux: history, etiology, and conservative management. In Kelalis, P.P., and King, L.R., editors: Clinical pediatric urology, Philadelphia, 1976, W.B. Saunders Co.

Stephens, F.D.: The ureteric orifice: the embryologic key to radiologic status of the ureter, J. Pediatr. Surg. **10**:473, 1975.

Stickler, G.B., and others: Primary interstitial nephritis with reflux: a cause of hypertension, Am. J. Dis. Child. **122**:144, 1971.

Torres, V.E., and others: The progression of vesicoureteral reflux nephropathy, Ann. Intern. Med. **92**:776, 1980.

116 • RENAL CYSTS AND CYSTIC DISEASES OF THE KIDNEY

Linda B. Hiner

Renal cysts may be "simple" or may occur within a renal tumor. Cysts may appear in congenital dysmorphic syndromes, may be the primary manifestation of hereditary disease, or may occur in malformed, dysplastic kidneys. The cysts may arise from the renal parenchymal epithelium, from the renal capsule, or within the peripelvic renal lymphatics.

SIMPLE CYSTS

By definition simple renal cysts do not arise in nephrocarcinoma. Unless they are very large, renal cysts are usually asymptomatic and are discovered fortuitously during uroroentgenographic or ultrasonographic studies performed for other purposes. Renal cysts are common and occur in more than 50% of individuals over 50 years old. Since they are uncommon in childhood, they are probably an acquired anomaly.

Simple renal cysts may vary in size from a few milliliters to liters in volume. Their walls are translucent and parchmentlike. The fluid within them is usually straw colored and resembles an ultrafiltrate of plasma. The lining cells are flattened epithelium with occasional papillary projections. The cyst capsule contains some collagen, some mononuclear cells, and occasionally focal deposits of hemosiderin or calcium salts.

Renal cortical cysts may be solitary, multiple, or bilateral. With excretory urography they appear as smooth, radiolucent defects. Cortical cysts may occasionally distort the calyces. If large enough, renal cysts may be palpable through the abdominal wall. The appearance of calcium in a renal cyst should suggest nephrocarcinoma.

Ultrasonography of the simple cyst reveals a space without internal echoes and with good sound transmission. Angiography demonstrates the presence of a smooth-walled structure without neovascularization. The evaluation of a renal cyst involves the use of ultrasonography, cyst puncture with fluid analysis, cytology, and angiography (see Chapter 118). If the cysts rupture, hemorrhage, or become infected, they may cause pain and bleeding. Hemorrhage into a renal cyst suggests nephrocarcinoma.

POLYCYSTIC DISEASE

Polycystic disease of the kidneys is a special designation for the two heritable forms of cystic renal disease associated with progressive renal failure. It should not be applied to cystic renal dysplasia, renal involvement with many simple cortical cysts, or renal cysts associated with the phakomatoses or dysmorphic syndromes.

Adult polycystic disease

Adult polycystic disease of the kidney is an autosomal dominant inherited disorder. Penetrance approaches 100% if individuals at risk are followed into their eighth or ninth decade of life. Polycystic disease can occur in the absence of a family history as a spontaneous mutation. Adult polycystic disease tends to become clinically apparent within any one family at approximately the same age, usually in the fourth or fifth decade of life. Adult-type polycystic disease has also been seen in the newborn. Since polycystic disease is not usually apparent until an individual has reached reproductive age, some individuals at risk may want sonographic or urographic evaluation for purposes of genetic counseling. Because the onset may be very late, however, negative evaluation in the third decade of life does not necessarily mean that the individual is unaffected.

The cause of polycystic disease is unknown. A similar entity may be induced by chemical means in genetically predisposed mice. When raised in a germ-free environment, these mice do not manifest the disease.

The involved kidneys may be huge. The cysts are distributed throughout the parenchyma and may vary in size from a few millimeters to several centimeters. The walls of most cysts are transparent, and in most cysts the contents are clear but can be muddy or cloudy when there has been hemorrhage or infection. The cysts are derived from tubular segments, and analysis of their contents may indicate their tubular sites of origin. Some glomerular cysts simply dead-end. Most cysts are lined with a single layer of cuboidal or columnar epithelium. They may be continuous with the glomerular tuft. There is interstitial fibrosis of varying amounts but no dysplasia.

Electron microscopy reveals splitting and lamination of the basement membrane of the renal tubules. There is no suggestion of the presence of immune complexes. Cysts may be found in organs other than the kidney, including the liver, spleen, lung, ovary, endometrium, epididymis, and seminal vesicles.

The primary symptom is commonly pain, usually described as dull, aching heaviness. Severe pain may occur with nephrolithiasis, cyst rupture, or hemorrhage into a cyst. Hypertension is common. There may be intracranial hemorrhage from aneurysms of cerebral vessels, which are present in more than 20% of affected individuals. Cerebral hemorrhage accounts for as many as 10% of the deaths among patients with polycystic disease. The kidneys are commonly large enough to be easily palpated. The enlargement may be asymmetric.

Hematuria is common in polycystic disease, but casts are uncommon. Bleeding may result from pressure, cyst rupture, or nephrolithiasis. Although proteinuria is common, it is usually not of sufficient quantity to cause the nephrotic syndrome. Hyperuricemia is the rule, but it is too nonspecific to be used as a marker within families. Polycythemia may be present as a result of increased erythropoietin production; these patients may not become anemic when uremia develops.

In early polycystic disease the collecting system may not appear distorted by intravenous urography, but sonographic evidence for the cysts may be present. Radioisotope renal scanning does not define the cysts well. In some cases a renal angiogram is required to demonstrate the characteristic features. The diagnosis is confirmed by a positive family history. The therapy involves control of hypertension and urinary tract infection, maintenance of acid-base and electrolyte equilibrium, and treatment of renal osteodystrophy. It is best to avoid the use of potent diuretics, which may increase cyst size. Patients with polycystic disease and end-stage renal disease are excellent candidates for renal transplantation and dialysis.

Infantile polycystic disease

Infantile polycystic disease is a genetic recessive disorder that is always associated with hepatic fibrosis and intercommunicating bile duct ectasia. The clinical expression is variable. In some children the renal involvement is so severe that renal failure ensues in infancy or early childhood. In others the renal involvement is less severe, but portal hypertension and gastrointestinal bleeding occur. Oligohydramnios develops when there is oliguria in utero. This is associated with Potter facies, pulmonary hypoplasia, and limb deformities. Large flank masses may be palpable at birth. If not discovered in the newborn, infantile polycystic disease is usually diagnosed during infancy. Hepatomegaly occurs early or late in infancy. Renal infection, lithiasis, and hemorrhage do not occur as often as in adult polycystic disease.

With severe involvement, the kidneys are large, spongy-looking organs with dilated cortical collecting ducts seen as radial stripes on the renal surface. The kidneys are not hypoplastic, the numbers of nephrons and amount of ureteral and ductular branching are normal, and progressive cyst formation does not occur. There is some glomerular obsolescence, interstitial fibrosis, and tubular atrophy. The renal size may appear to diminish with somatic growth.

High-dose excretory urography may show a prolonged "nephrogram" effect, demonstrating either radial streaking like a sunburst or diffuse cortical mottling, but the function is sufficiently diminished that good visualization of the renal collecting system is rare. In these cases ultrasonography may be of great benefit to establish the absence of a dilated bladder or collecting system.

Extrarenal cysts occur less commonly in infantile polycystic disease than in the adult form and may be functionally insignificant. Cerebral artery aneurysm formation is rare.

For children who do not die shortly after birth, renal transplantation may offer hope for a normal childhood.

MEDULLARY CYSTIC DISEASE (NEPHRONOPHTHISIS)

The terms "medullary cystic disease" and "nephronophthisis" refer to the same type of kidney disease, characterized by a variation in age of expression, inheritance, and associated clinical findings.

On gross examination involved kidneys show cysts within the medulla or the cortex, most commonly at the corticomedullary junction. The cysts are diverticula from dilated distal tubules and collecting ducts. These findings may not be evident on gross examination of the kidneys from individuals who die very young. There is interstitial fibrosis with an accumulation of periodic acid-Schiff (PAS)–positive hyaline-like material around the tubules. The tubular basement membranes are thickened. The glomeruli are either normal or hyalinized but are not hypercellular.

The disease can be divided into three clinical subgroups. In the first group are patients with genetically recessive disease that becomes apparent within the first decade of life without apparent retinal disease. The second group is similar to the first, but the disease is associated with a pigmentary retinopathy; blindness may precede renal failure by several years. In the third group renal disease becomes apparent in early adulthood, and autosomal dominant inheritance is likely. The renal pathologic and functional manifestations are the same for the three subgroups. The disease is usually discovered within the first decade of life and leads to end-stage renal disease sometime within the second decade. Occasionally families have individuals who maintain normal renal function into early childhood. The first manifestations of the disease are often the consequences of renal insufficiency such as renal osteodystrophy, growth failure, and anemia. Hypertension is uncommon. Proteinuria is minimal and the urinary sediment often normal; thus renal disease may not be diagnosed until growth failure or azotemia intervenes. Defective urine-concentrating ability is the rule. Occasionally children have associated central nervous system problems such as progressive ataxia, poor coordination, and even learning disabilities.

The diagnosis is usually suspected clinically by the presence of a predisposing family history, renal concentrating defects, and retinopathy. The confirmation is made by deep renal biopsy. Roentgenographic studies are not very helpful. Ultrasonography assists in detecting the absence of obstructive urinary tract lesions.

The treatment is similar to that of other progressive renal diseases of uncertain etiology.

MEDULLARY SPONGE KIDNEY

Medullary sponge kidney is usually an asymptomatic entity detected incidentally by roentgenography. It is characterized by the pooling of contrast material in the papillary collecting ducts, which appears as a cortical "blush" or as contrast-filled papillary lakes and puddles. This finding occurs in about 0.5% of excretory urograms. Papillary nephrocalcinosis can sometimes be demonstrated on plain films because of the precipitation of calcium in the stagnant urine of the dilated terminal ductules. Clinical symptoms of renal infection, calculi, and obstruction may occasionally occur. The glomerular filtration rate is usually normal, but more than two thirds of these patients show some loss of urine-concentrating ability. There is no sex or genetic predisposition.

BIBLIOGRAPHY

Bernstein, J.: Polycystic disease. In Edelmann, C.M., Jr., editor: Pediatric kidney disease, ed. 1, Boston, 1978, Little, Brown & Co.

Bernstein, J.: Congenital malformations of the kidney. In Earley, L.E., and Gottschalk, C.W., editors: Strauss and Welt's diseases of the kidney, ed. 3, Boston, 1979, Little, Brown & Co.

Gardner, K.D., Jr.: The medullary cystic diseases: the nephronophthisiscystic renal medulla complex and medullary sponge kidney. In Earley, L.E., and Gottschalk, C.W., editors: Strauss and Welt's diseases of the kidney, ed. 3, Boston, 1979, Little, Brown & Co.

Grantham, J.J.: Polycystic renal disease. In Earley, L. E., and Gottschalk, C.W., editors: Strauss and Welt's diseases of the kidney, ed. 3, Boston, 1979, Little, Brown & Co.

Kissane, J.M.: Congenital malformations. In Heptinstall, R.H., editor: Pathology of the kidney, ed. 2, Boston, 1974, Little, Brown & Co.

Kuiper, J.J.: Medullary sponge kidney. In Gardner, K.D., Jr., editor: Cystic diseases of the kidney, New York, 1976, John Wiley & Sons, Inc.

Lieberman, E., and others: Infantile polycystic disease of the kidneys and liver: clinical, pathological and radiological correlations and comparison with congenital hepatic fibrosis, Medicine **50**:277, 1971.

Steele, B.T., Lirenman, D.S., and Beattie, C.W.: Nephronophthisis, Am. J. Med. **68**:531, 1980.

Werder, A.A., Cuppage, F.E., and Nielson, A.H.: Naturally occurring polycystic renal disease in CFW_w mice, Kidney Int. **8**:464, 1975.

117 • OBSTRUCTIVE UROPATHY

Clarence Martin and **Sandra P. Levison**

DEFINITION AND ETIOLOGY. Obstruction to urine flow is referred to as obstructive uropathy and can cause back pressure on ureters and the calyceal system (hydronephrosis).

Obstructive uropathy can result from functional defects or from intrinsic or extrinsic mechanical blockage of urine anywhere along the genitourinary tract. The obstruction can be unilateral or bilateral, partial or complete, or acute or chronic and can cause temporary or permanent damage to the kidney. The normal physiologic points of narrowing along the genitourinary tract are more susceptible to obstruction; these points include the ureteropelvic junction, ureterovesical junction, bladder neck, and urethral meatus.

Urinary tract obstruction may be caused by various disease states that can be grouped in terms of location and type, as shown in the following outline:

Causes of urinary tract obstruction

I. Any location
   A. Calculi
   B. Papillary tissue
   C. Tumor
   D. Trauma
   E. Blood clot
   F. Fungus ball

II. Tubule
   A. Uric acid
   B. Multiple myeloma
   C. Acute tubular necrosis

III. Renal pelvis
   A. Tumor
   B. Ectopic kidney
   C. Fibrous bands at ureteropelvic junction
   D. Strictures
   E. Aberrant vessels
   F. Tuberculosis
   G. Cyst
   H. Neoplasm

IV. Ureter
   A. Congenital malformations
     1. Strictures
     2. Ectopic kidney
     3. Vesicoureteral reflux
     4. Ureteral valves
     5. Adynamic ureteral segment
   B. Retroperitoneal disease
     1. Lymphoma
     2. Primary or metastatic cancer
     3. Retroperitoneal fibrosis
     4. Retroperitoneal hemorrhage
     5. Retroperitoneal abscess
     6. Inflammation or metastatic cancer of nodes
   C. Primary genitourinary disease
     1. Cancer of the ureter
     2. Cancer of the bladder
     3. Ureteral polyp
     4. Tuberculosis
     5. *Schistosoma haematobium* infection
   D. Others
     1. Abdominal and pelvic neoplasms
     2. Granulomatous bowel disease
     3. Congenital absence of the abdominal musculature (prune belly)
     4. Endometriosis
     5. Pregnancy
     6. Trauma
     7. Radiation
     8. Iatrogenic (surgical)

V. Bladder and prostate
   A. Benign prostatic hypertrophy
   B. Foreign bodies
   C. Congenital disease
   D. Carcinoma of prostate
   E. Neurogenic bladder
   F. Prostatic abscess
   G. Inflammatory diseases of the prostate
   H. Carcinoma of the bladder
   I. Contraction of the bladder

VI. Urethra
   A. Congenital valves or diverticula
   B. Meatal stenosis
   C. Strictures
   D. Foreign bodies
   E. Phimosis
   F. Carcinoma of the urethra
   G. Carcinoma of the penis
   H. Hypospadias and epispadias
   I. Polyps

Although calculi, sloughed papillary tissue, tumor, trauma, blood clot, or fungus ball can cause obstruction at any level, most processes causing obstruction are confined to a specific level. Uric acid, myeloma protein, or acute tubular necrosis can obstruct tubules. Tuberculosis (and other granulomatous diseases), polycystic kidney disease (and other cystic diseases), aberrant vessels, and renal tumors obstruct from within the renal pelvis. The ureteropelvic junction, an area of normal narrowing, is especially susceptible to strictures (acquired or congenital), fibrous bands, and aberrant vessels. The ureter may be obstructed by retroperitoneal disease (fibrosis, lymphoma, primary or metastic tumor, tumor invasion of nodes, hemorrhage, or inflammatory nodes), congenital malformations, primary carcinoma of the ureter, abdominal or pelvic neoplasms, strictures, prune-belly syndrome, endometriosis, pregnancy, and surgical trauma. The most common cause of obstruction to urine flow from the bladder is benign prostatic hypertrophy, but other causes include presence of foreign bodies, cancer, and inflammatory disease of the prostate. The urethra can be blocked by valves, diverticula, strictures (congenital or acquired), infection, foreign bodies, polyps, congenital malformations such as hypospadias, and carcinoma. Functional causes of obstructive uropathy include neurogenic bladder, vesicoureteral reflux, and adynamic ureteral segment.

PATHOLOGY AND PATHOPHYSIOLOGY. In obstructive uropathy urine distends the ureters and the renal pelvis and backs into the tubules and then into the lymphatic and venous channels. In advanced cases the kidney may be transformed into a thin-walled cystic structure. Initially the total size of the kidney and pelvis is increased, but eventually only a thin rim of atrophic renal parenchymal tissue remains. In unilateral obstruction there is compensatory hypertrophy of the remaining contralateral kidney; an as yet unidentified humoral factor is probably responsible. Obstruction leads to urinary stasis and increased susceptibility to ascending or hematogenous infection that hastens renal damage.

Obstruction to urine flow causes alteration of renal function that may be permanent. The longer and more severe the obstruction, the greater the functional changes. However, well-documented cases of some return of renal function have been reported in patients completely obstructed for more than 90 days.

Renal function in hydronephrosis is characterized by three disturbances: loss of concentrating ability, inability to excrete an acid load, and decreased glomerular filtration rate (GFR).

Changes in the GFR depend on the duration, degree, and location of the obstruction. Partial obstruction may result in only minimal changes in the GFR, whereas acute complete obstruction causes a more rapid and severe decrease. Lower tract obstruction produces a smaller decrease in the GFR than upper ureteral obstruction, since the ureter is less abruptly dilated when pressure is transmitted over a greater length of ureter. The net filtration pressure is decreased because of the increased hydrostatic pressure in the obstructed ureters. This increased pressure in the renal pelvis and calyces may compress the arcuate arteries directly over them, decreasing blood flow. Chronic obstruction also decreases the GFR by an effect on arteriolar resistance. It appears from experimental data that there is a decrease in the GFR in the juxtamedullary nephrons that is greater than that in superficial nephrons.

Changes in renal blood flow following unilateral ureteral obstruction are also variable and depend on the degree and duration of obstruction. For the first 24 hours there is an increase in renal blood flow, probably caused by renal vasodilation. Thereafter renal blood flow falls and remains low, returning to normal with relief of the obstruction. Twenty-four hours after total bilateral obstruction there is no change in renal blood flow, perhaps as a result of vasodilation in the nephrons with residual function. The renal blood flow is redistributed, with greater flow to the inner cortex. Marked differences between the filtration fraction of superficial and juxtamedullary nephrons occur and may be responsible for the defects in sodium handling and concentrating ability.

The inability to concentrate urine is the earliest and most consistent finding in both unilateral and bilateral obstructive uropathy. The concentrating defect is unresponsive to vasopressin and is thought to be caused by impaired solute transport or disturbances in medullary blood flow. In the presence of partial ureteral obstruction there is increased water and electrolyte resorption.

Impaired urinary acidification (ammonia excretion, titratable acidity, and bicarbonate absorption) can be demonstrated in the obstructed kidney. With unilateral obstruction significant metabolic acidosis is absent because of the normal contralateral kidney. Persistent obstruction for more than 90 to 120 days results in irreversible renal damage; however, it is not unusual for patients with obstructive uropathy to be well until azotemia is far advanced.

With relief of obstruction most patients have either no significant natriuresis or a physiologic diuresis that releases the excess amounts of retained sodium, urea, and water, reducing total body sodium and volume to normal. The term "postobstructive diuresis" has been used to describe the period (hours or a few days) of negative fluid and sodium balance that follows the release of lower urinary tract obstruction. Several different functional states may be responsible: (1) sodium and fluid retention during obstruction, (2) administration of diuretics, (3) presence of acute tubular necrosis, or (4) less commonly, inappropriately large sodium and water losses. When the last condition occurs, it is caused by relatively acute and severe obstruction with advanced but reversible renal failure. During diuresis the renal tubular sodium reabsorption is diminished. Occasionally phosphaturia, uricosuria, or aminoaciduria accompanies the relief of obstruction.

CLINICAL MANIFESTATIONS, LABORATORY FINDINGS, AND DIAGNOSIS. Clues to the type of obstruction are age and sex. The most common cause of obstruction in children is congenital malformation. Women commonly have obstruction caused by pregnancy, stones, or a tumor, whereas in men the cause is often prostatic disease, stones, spinal cord injuries, or strictures.

Obstruction should be sought in any patient with unexplained renal failure, sudden worsening of renal function, or decreased urine output. Although these patients are usually asymptomatic, the history may imply the cause, such as gout, diabetes, sickle cell anemia, and multiple myeloma.

Symptoms of lower urinary tract obstruction include hesitancy in urination, poor stream, overflow incontinence, inability to empty the bladder completely, stop-and-start urination, and postmicturition dribbling. Upper tract symptoms include colicky pain radiating into the groin, associated with nausea and weakness. Nocturia and polyuria can develop as results of a loss of concentrating ability, especially with partial obstruction; with complete obstruction oliguria develops. When significant renal failure is present, the symptoms of uremia are evident.

The physical examination may show signs of the uremic syndrome if renal failure has developed. Physical examination may uncover an abdominal or rectal mass, an enlarged prostate in the male, or a pelvic mass in the female, but is often unrewarding. Hypertension commonly develops either as a result of salt retention and volume expansion or with unilateral obstruction caused by increased renin secretion.

Urinalysis can be helpful if there are sediment changes, as seen with debris from calculi, sloughed papillae, or uric acid crystals. The urinalysis may otherwise be completely normal in the presence of obstruction. An abnormal blood urea nitrogen/creatinine ratio (greater than 10:1) occurs in obstruction but must be distinguished from prerenal azotemia, which causes similar ratios. This abnormal ratio results from increased urine backflow caused by obstruction and the reabsorption of urea in the presence of decreased tubular flow; creatinine is not reabsorbed.

An estimation of residual bladder urine can be made at the bedside by catheterizing the bladder after the patient voids or by performing bladder ultrasonography. The retention of more than 50 to 100 ml of urine after voiding suggests bladder obstruction. Evaluation of the urethra, bladder, ureters, and kidneys should be undertaken.

The first step in this evaluation should be a plain roentgenogram of the abdomen (kidneys, ureters, and bladder [KUB]) to look for stones, distortion, and abnormal kidney size. A small kidney implies chronic disease.

The time-honored test for the localization of obstructive uropathy is the intravenous pyelogram. Unfortunately, with significantly decreased function and destruction in the kidney there may be poor visualization. However, the typical findings of obstruction, such as delayed and intense opacification, may be seen if subsequent films are taken hours or even days later.

Ultrasonography has been used very successfully; it not only documents hydronephrosis but also can localize the site of obstruction. A negative ultrasonographic study does not completely rule out acute obstruction, and a repeat study should be scheduled several days later. If clinically indicated, more definitive studies should be obtained.

Either antegrade or retrograde pyelography can demonstrate and relieve obstruction. The risk of introducing infection, however, is a complication of retrograde pyelography, especially when the catheters remain in place for the relief of obstruction. Antegrade pyelography with the placement of percutaneous nephrostomy drainage tubes can be performed with sonogram localization under local anesthesia.

MANAGEMENT. The treatment is aimed at relieving obstruction to preserve renal function. Infection and sepsis require immediate surgical relief in addition to appropriate antibiotic therapy. The patient may rarely require dialysis to withstand surgical correction.

If there is obvious congenital malformation, primary repair is indicated. Calculi can often be managed conservatively with observation, hydration, and analgesics, since they are frequently passed spontaneously, particularly those less than 1 cm in diameter. Lower tract calculi may be removed transurethrally with the basket apparatus or surgically. Calculi obstructing the ureters near the kidneys often require surgical repair. In some instances primary surgical repair is not feasible, and secondary diversion (nephrostomy, cystostomy, ureteroileostomy, and so on) of the stream is needed; however, recurrent pyelonephritis, urolithiasis, and metabolic acidosis may occur. Nephrectomy is occasionally the best mode of therapy; however, renal tissue should be preserved whenever possible.

Functional obstruction can at times be treated nonsurgically, such as with frequent voiding, repeated daily catheterization of the bladder, cholinergic drugs, and bladder training maneuvers. Surgery is required when there is progressive renal damage, recurrent pyelonephritis with sepsis, or massive vesicoureteral reflux.

Indwelling catheters or tubes may be placed for permanent diversion and drainage, especially in poor surgical candidates, but they may lead to chronic infection.

BIBLIOGRAPHY

Beck, L.H., Stein, J.H., and Earley, L.E.: Obstructive uropathy. In Earley, L.E., and Gottschalk, C.W., editors: Strauss and Welt's diseases of the kidney, ed. 3, Boston, 1979, Little, Brown & Co.

Gillenwater, J.Y.: Hydronephrosis-induced changes in renal hemodynamics and function, Cardiovasc. Med. 4:701, 1979.

Gillenwater, J.Y. and others: Renal function after release of chronic unilateral hydronephrosis in man, Kidney Int. 7:179, 1975.

Klahr, S.R.: Obstructive uropathy, Semin. Nephrol. 2:1, 1982.

Wright, F.S., and Howards, S.S.: Obstructive injury. In Brenner, B.M., and Rector, F.C., Jr., editors: The kidney, ed. 2, Philadelphia, 1981, W.B. Saunders Co.

118 • NEOPLASMS OF THE URINARY TRACT

Linda B. Hiner

RENAL NEOPLASMS

Renal neoplasms can be derived from any of the tissue types of the kidney, its vasculature, or its capsule. Benign renal tumors are usually discovered incidentally or at autopsy. Among the more common benign renal tumors are angiolipomas, renal adenomas, fetal renal hamartomas, and leiomyomas. Rare tumors such as hemangiopericytomas may be benign or malignant but are often dramatic because of secondary effects such as hypertension.

Renal cell carcinoma and nephroblastoma (Wilms' tumor) account for the majority of renal malignancies.

Renal cell carcinoma

The most prevalent malignant renal neoplasm among adults is renal cell carcinoma (hypernephroma). It is more common in men than in women and occurs rarely in children. The incidence of the adult form is increasing. Exposure to certain viruses, estrogens, some nitrosamines, aromatic hydrocarbons, aflatoxins, and heavy metals may be associated with its development.

PATHOLOGY. There are three major cell types of renal tumor: clear cells that resemble renal tubular epithelial cells, granular eosinophilic cells, and spindle cells. The cells may arrange themselves as tubular structures, acini, or papillae. They may form cystic or solid masses.

Tumors are graded according to their most anaplastic segments. Although the clear cells may appear reasonably differentiated, grading is done by degree of *nuclear* anaplasia: grade I—normal, grade II—some pyknotic nuclei and some irregular nuclei, grade III—enlarged irregular pleomorphic prominent nucleoli, and grade IV—enlarged irregular nuclei. The tumor stage (I to IV) is related to the extent of the spread of these cells at the time of diagnosis and surgery: stage I—the tumor is confined within the renal capsule; stage II—the tumor does not extend beyond Gerota's fascia; stage III—the tumor has invaded the renal vein and/or regional lymph nodes or the inferior vena cava or has extended into the perirenal fat; and stage IV—the tumor has invaded adjacent viscera or distant metastases are evident.

The patient outcome has been examined in relation to cell type, nuclear morphology, and stage at presentation. Survival at 1, 5, and 10 years after presentation falls with increasing nuclear anaplasia. Patients with clear cell tumors have a somewhat better prognosis than those with granular cell types. Both groups do better than those whose tumors are composed of spindle cells. Patients with stage I tumors have about a 65% survival after 5 years and nearly 60% at 10 years. Approximately 50% of patients with stage II and III tumors are living after 5 years, but fewer than 10% with stage IV tumor are living at 5 years.

Renal cell carcinoma spreads by lymphatic or hematogenous extension. Between 25% and 50% of the patients have distant metastases (for example, to lung and bone) at the time of diagnosis.

CLINICAL MANIFESTATIONS. Renal cell carcinomas are among the "great imitators" of medicine. Painless hematuria is the initial symptom in 60% of the patients. Fever is another common presenting complaint. Varicoceles and leg edema occur uncommonly and suggest extension of tumor into the inferior vena cava or gonadal vein.

The systemic effects of renal cell carcinoma include fever caused by tumor pyrogen, a high erythrocyte sedimentation rate, and anemia. Amyloidosis and neuropathy may occur as a result of immune responses to the tumor. A variety of syndromes have been seen, including erythrocytosis caused by tumor production of erythropoietin-like hormones, syndromes secondary to corticotropin (ACTH) or ACTH-like substance production, ectopic alkaline phosphatase isoenzyme production, masculinizing effects resulting from tumor production of gonadotropin, and systemic and portal hypertension resulting from tumor renin production or vascular compression, respectively.

Hypercalcemia may result from the destruction of bone because of metastasis, tumor production of parathyroid hormone (PTH), or "humoral nonparathyroid hypercalcemia," in which hypercalcemia and hypophosphatemia occur in the absence of detectable levels of PTH. It is thought that prostaglandin E secretion from the tumor or metastasis stimulates bone resorption; the hypercalcemia may respond to the administration of a prostaglandin inhibitor such as indomethacin.

Hepatosplenomegaly and hepatic dysfunction, hypoprothrombinemia, increased haptoglobin, increased alkaline phosphatase, and increased indirect bilirubin may be present in patients with hypernephroma but *without* hepatic metastases. Liver biopsies demonstrate proliferation of Kupffer's cells with hepatocellular degeneration and portal triaditis. The abnormalities in liver function are reversible following nephrectomy. Many of these patients have undifferentiated clear cell tumors with extrarenal extension. They have constitutional symptoms, but hematuria is uncommon.

DIAGNOSIS. The diagnostic approach to the patient with an asymptomatic renal mass attempts to identify the mass as benign or malignant. Cytologic examination of the urinary sediment is an unreliable means of determining the diagnosis. Urinary activity of lactic dehydrogenase (LDH) is increased in 90% of patients with tumors but is not increased in patients with cysts.

Invasive or metastatic hypernephromas may be associated with significant elevations of serum haptoglobin, whereas normal levels are found in patients with localized hypernephromas. The increase in serum α_2-globulins that may be seen in patients with renal cell carcinoma is caused by increased haptoglobin. The carcinoembryonic antigen (CEA) level in serum is normal or slightly increased in patients with localized hypernephromas. Elevated titers may be associated with advanced and metastatic tumors.

If the renal mass is discovered on physical examination or is an incidental finding on an intravenous urogram, an ultrasonographic study or computed tomography of the kidneys may be performed. A calcified mass or cyst on intravenous urography is highly suggestive of malignancy, and sonography may be omitted. Renal angiography provides a definitive diagnosis, as well as demonstrating vascular anatomy that is important for surgery. If the mass is solid or shows complex internal echoes by sonography, angiography is used to further delineate it. If the mass is cystic, cyst puncture is performed. Simple cysts can occur in association with renal cell carcinoma, but occasionally the malignancy may not involve the cyst cavity.

The fluid is analyzed for cell block cytology, LDH levels, lipid levels, and the presence or absence of blood. If the fluid is bloody or the fluid and cytologic findings suggest malignancy, angiography is performed to delineate the tumor before surgery. If the fluid is not suggestive of tumor or the sonogram shows what appears to be a normal kidney, no further study is necessary. Injection of contrast material into the cyst may be confusing and is no longer recommended.

MANAGEMENT. Radical nephrectomy offers hope of cure if the tumor is removed intact. A spread to regional nodes or the invasion of neighboring organs worsens the prognosis. Ex vivo segmental nephrectomy and autotransplantation have been performed when nephrocarcinoma occurs in a solitary kidney. Removal of a solitary metastasis along with nephrectomy is occasionally recommended because of evidence for improved survival.

Although irradiation may not increase survival after 5 years, it may provide a longer tumor-free interval within that time. Progestational or androgenic agents in combination with various chemotherapeutic agents may have palliative effects in some patients with extensive metastases. Immunotherapy is experimental.

Nephroblastoma (Wilms' tumor)

Nephroblastoma, or embryonal carcinosarcoma, is the most common renal neoplasm of childhood, accounting for 20% of all childhood cancer. Although this tumor is occasionally seen in adults and adolescents, it most often appears before 8 years of age; the mean age at diagnosis is 3.6 years. There seems to be no racial or sex predilection for this tumor, but there have been reports of concurrence within families. There is an increased incidence in individuals with congenital aniridia, hemihypertrophy of the face or extremities, urogenital anomalies, and certain chromosomal abnormalities.

PATHOLOGY. Nephroblastomas contain both epithelial and mesenchymal elements, which may be well or poorly differentiated. The outcome for patients with Wilms' tumor can be related to the degree of tissue differentiation, the extension of tumor to lymph nodes and blood vessels, the age at diagnosis, and the primary tumor size. Staging and grading of these tumors are somewhat complicated. The National Wilms' Tumor Study (NWTS) has divided the patients into five groups according to the extent of the tumor's spread and the success of surgical resection. Patients in group I have the tumor limited to the kidney, and resection is complete. In group II the tumor has spread locally beyond the capsule or into para-aortic lymph nodes of blood vessels outside the kidney, but no residual tumor remains beyond the resection. In group III a residual tumor confined to the abdomen remains postoperatively because of tumor rupture during surgery, presence of peritoneal implants, node involvement beyond the abdomen, or inability to completely resect the tumor. In group IV hematogenous metastases to distant organs occur. In group V there is bilateral renal involvement.

CLINICAL MANIFESTATIONS. The child with nephroblastoma is usually discovered because of a palpable abdominal mass. The child may occasionally complain of abdominal pain or have hematuria. Hypertension and fever are common. Patients with these tumors occasionally have signs of tumor spread or rupture, such as varicocele, enlarged testes, congestive heart failure, hydrocephalus, pleural effusion, abdominal emergency, or acute anemia.

DIAGNOSIS. The initial laboratory investigation of the child with an abdominal mass likely to be a neoplasm includes a urinalysis and tests to assess renal function. Erythropoietin and α_2-H-fetoprotein levels may serve as markers for tumor recurrence. The initial roentgenographic investigation includes studies of the chest and intravenous urography. Abdominal ultrasonography can help define the tumor and even inferior vena cava involvement in some cases. Echocardiography may show tumor extension if it has occurred. Venography in children can be performed during intravenous urography if a lower extremity vein is used for the injection. If hematogenous metastases are evident initially, bone and liver scans and a bone marrow aspiration should be done. Abdominal arteriography delineates the tumor, its vasculature, and its presence or absence in the other kidney.

MANAGEMENT. The treatment includes surgical removal (even in the presence of metastases) with abdominal exploration, postoperative irradiation (since the tumor is radiosensitive), and chemotherapy. These tumors are often massive but are usually well encapsulated. Removal of the tumor permits more effective irradiation and chemotherapy. The approach to patients with bilateral Wilms' tumor must be individualized. Patients with pulmonary metastases may be treated with whole lung irradiation and chemotherapy.

Nephroblastoma occurs at an early age, and the long-term survival now being achieved for many patients has revealed the complications of treatment that become apparent in later childhood, adolescence, and early adulthood. These complications include scoliosis of the spine, vascular abnormalities caused by irradiation, and secondary tumors in the field of irradiation (1% annual incidence). Follow-up monitoring into adulthood is necessary for such long-term survivors.

UROTHELIAL TUMORS OF THE KIDNEY

Tumors of the renal pelvis and upper ureters are uncommon. Transitional cell tumors of both the upper and lower urinary tract are associated with certain industrial exposures. Men with transitional cell tumor outnumber women, which may reflect greater exposure to potential carcinogens. Two groups of individuals have an increased incidence of urothelial tumor of the renal pelvis without an associated increased risk of bladder tumor. These are individuals with so-called Balkan nephropathy and those with interstitial nephritis caused by the chronic use of analgesics, usually those containing aspirin and a phenacetin-like compound. In both groups of patients the usual male preponderance for these tumors is absent.

PATHOLOGY. Urothelial tumors are graded by the degree of cellular differentiation. The transitional cell carcinomas can occur in situ or can invade locally, as well as metastasizing to distant organs. Urothelial tumors tend to spread first to regional lymph nodes and adjacent organs. The stage is determined by the extent of the tumor's spread. Transitional cell tumors are commonly multiple, and in these cases the classification of the patient is determined by the tumor with the worst grade and stage.

CLINICAL MANIFESTATIONS. Urothelial tumor of the renal pelvis and upper ureter may have an insidious onset. Since the muscular wall of these structures is thin, the tumor may extend quite easily. About 75% of the patients with these tumors have hematuria at the time of diagnosis; about 50% complain of pain, either a vague ache or ureteral colic from the passage of a blood clot.

Unless there is massive hydronephrosis, there is rarely a palpable mass. In some individuals a varicocele develops from local interference with blood flow or a psoas sign appears from retroperitoneal tumor extension. Such patients commonly have associated bladder tumors and symptoms of bladder irritability.

DIAGNOSIS. Tools available for the diagnosis and evaluation of the patient who may have a urothelial tumor of the upper urinary tract include intravenous urography, cystoscopy with retrograde pyelography, and cytologic study of ureteral washings obtained with or without brush biopsy. Angiography and operative nephroscopy are also used in some cases. A lucent defect in the renal pelvis or upper ureter seen on excretory urography may be confused with a blood clot, radiolucent stone, pyelitis cystica, an area of leukoplakia with squamous metaplasia, or even an indentation from a parapelvic renal cyst or a branch of the renal artery. Chest roentgenograms and bone and liver scans assist in determining the presence of distant metastases.

MANAGEMENT. Until fairly recently the treatment has been nephroureterectomy with removal of a cuff of bladder adjacent to the site of ureteral entry. In certain instances when the tumor is bilateral or of an apparently low grade and stage, segmental nephrectomy has been used. Segmental nephrectomy may be tried for a tumor in a solitary kidney. Operative nephroscopy at the time of segmental nephrectomy determines if the remainder of the kidney appears free of tumor. Neither radiation nor chemotherapy has been helpful.

The outcome of management seems related more to the grade and extent of tumor than to the procedure performed. Forty percent of these patients already have or will have a urothelial bladder tumor (most within 2 years).

BLADDER NEOPLASMS

Carcinoma of the bladder is the second most prevalent genitourinary tract tumor (carcinoma of the prostate is the primary cause of death from genitourinary tract malignancy). Bladder carcinoma occurs more commonly in men than in women and in whites than in nonwhites. It may occur in any age group but is more prevalent after age 50, with a peak occurrence between ages 75 and 84. A predisposition to carcinoma of the bladder occurs in those with chronic infestation with *Schistosoma haematobium*, in some habitual cigarette smokers after many years, and in individuals exposed to products used in the manufacture of aniline dyes. Ribonucleic acid (RNA) virus has been present in some of these bladder tumors, possibly suggesting a causal relationship. Patients with nephropathies associated with analgesic abuse or Balkan nephropathy are predisposed to bladder cancer. Papillary and solid tumors are the two forms of bladder carcinoma.

Papillary tumors

Papillary tumors may be single but tend to be multiple. Painless hematuria is the most common manifestation. In the absence of bladder wall invasion, endoscopic resection and fulguration or the instillation of triethylenethiophosphoramide may be effective. Cystoscopy and similar repetitive treatment are used to follow and control recurrence. The tumors may become invasive.

Solid carcinomas

Solid carcinomas may be sessile or ulcerating, and painless hematuria is the most common symptom. Dysuria and frequency of urination in the absence of infection are also common. The lesion is evaluated with cystoscopy, biopsy, and bimanual examination under anesthesia. Intravenous pyelography to detect ureteral obstruction (seen with bladder wall invasion) is required. The prognosis depends on the degree of anaplasia and the depth of tumor invasion. Poorly differentiated tumors that invade the perivesicular tissues are rarely curable. Preoperative irradiation, total cystectomy, and urinary diversion are the modes of treating bladder tumors that involve the lateral walls of the bladder base. If the tumor is confined to the dome of the bladder, a partial cystectomy is performed. Supervoltage irradiation alone is used when the patient is a poor surgical candidate or for palliation; the results approach those of surgery. Radiation cystitis and proctitis may complicate therapy and cause significant morbidity.

PROSTATIC CARCINOMA

Carcinoma of the prostate is the second most common cause of cancer in men, accounting for 17% of cancers in American men (lung cancer is the most common cancer). Prostate cancer is rare before age 45 and the incidence of carcinoma in situ exceeds 40% by the eighth decade. It is more common in blacks. Adenocarcinoma accounts for 95% of prostatic cancers, with primary transitional cell carcinoma accounting for the rest. Although the cause is unknown, suggested predisposing factors have included environmental pollution, viruses, hormones, changes in steroidogenesis, tobacco smoking, alcohol consumption, circumcision, and certain blood groups.

PATHOLOGY. Two thirds of prostatic carcinomas arise in the peripheral or juxtarectal prostate glands. By contrast, benign prostatic hyperplasia involves the submucosal prostate glands. The degree of malignancy based on histologic grading has been correlated with survival; poorly differentiated carcinomas have a less favorable prognosis. Carcinoma spreads from the prostate by direct extension to the seminal vesicles, bladder, urethra, and pelvic sidewalls. It rarely invades the rectum. Lymphatic spread is via the obturator, iliac, presacral, and periaortic lymph nodes. Mediastinal, supraclavicular, inguinal, and axillary nodes are occasionally involved.

CLINICAL MANIFESTATIONS. Localized symptoms are usually those of bladder irritation or outlet obstruction. Bladder or ureteral obstruction may be manifested by decreased renal function or evidence of uremia. Symptoms from metastases depend on the location and degree of involvement. Lymph node involvement is usually asymptomatic unless leg edema or ureteral obstruction occurs. Small, bony lesions are usually painless, but large lesions of the vertebral column, hips, or ribs may be painful. Bony metastases are usually osteoblastic, may be mixed, and less commonly are purely osteolytic.

DIAGNOSIS. The diagnosis of prostatic carcinoma is suspected on the basis of the rectal examination and confirmed by needle biopsy. Staging must be done to determine the appropriate therapy. In addition to a digital rectal examination to determine local spreading of the tumor, the extent of spread is determined by cystoscopy to discover bladder or urethral invasion, by excretory urography to define ureteral obstruction, by bone roentgenograms and scans to detect metastases, and by measurements of acid phosphatase and serum calcium levels. A normal prostatic acid phosphatase concentration does not completely exclude metastasis. Elevated levels can be seen with prostatic infarction, recent prostate manipulation, catheterization, and surgery, as well as metastatic prostatic carcinoma.

MANAGEMENT. Attempts at cure of localized tumor involve surgery or irradiation or both. Chemotherapy, hormonal therapy, or orchiectomy is used once the tumor has spread; these measures improve symptoms but do not prolong life (see Chapter 84).

BIBLIOGRAPHY

Clayman, R.V., Williams, R.D., and Fraley, E.E.: The pursuit of the renal mass, N. Engl. J. Med. **300:**72, 1979.

D'Angio, G.J., and others: Childhood cancer: the National Wilms' Tumor Study: a progress report, Urology **3:**798, 1974.

Deming, E.L., and Harvard, B.M.: Tumors of the kidney. In Campbell, M.F., and others, editors: Urology, ed. 3, Philadelphia, 1970, W.B. Saunders Co.

Friedell, F.H., and others: Histopathology and classification of urinary bladder cancer, Urol. Clin. North Am. **3:**53, 1976.

Gittes, R.F.: Urothelial tumors of the kidney. In Campbell, M.F., and others, editors: Urology, ed. 3, Philadelphia, 1979, W.B. Saunders Co.

Green, D.M., and Jaffe, N.: Wilms' tumor—a model of a curable pediatric malignant solid tumor, Cancer Treat. Rev. **5:**143, 1978.

McLaughlin, A.P., III: Tumors of the kidney. In Earley, L.E., and Gottschalk, C.W., editors: Strauss and Welt's diseases of the kidney, ed. 3, Boston, 1979, Little, Brown & Co.

119 • VASCULAR DISORDERS OF THE KIDNEY

Sal A. Lofaro and Sandra P. Levison

RENAL ARTERY STENOSIS

DEFINITION. Renovascular hypertension refers to the hypertension caused by renal ischemia. The incidence varies between 1% and 15% of all hypertensive patients, depending on whether the patients are unselected or referred for diagnostic evaluation. Severe malignant and accelerated forms of hypertension are seen in about one third of patients with renovascular disease. Although potentially curable, not all renal artery stenosis may be severe enough to produce sufficient ischemia to cause hypertension. Varying degrees of renal artery stenosis have been demonstrated in normotensive patients and in autopsy series of otherwise normal persons. It is important to prove the functional significance of this lesion to prevent surgery (nephrectomy or vascular repair) that would not normalize blood pressure.

ETIOLOGY. Atherosclerotic disease is responsible for most renal artery stenosis. Fibromuscular and atherosclerotic lesions together cause 95% of renovascular hypertension. There are several ways of classifying renovascular lesions. In the simplest classification the lesions are divided into atherosclerotic, fibromuscular, and other lesions.

The atherosclerotic lesions occur primarily in the fifth through the seventh decades of life and more often in men than in women. The lesions are progressive and often bilateral. They generally involve the aortic orifice and the proximal one third of the renal arteries. There is usually atherosclerotic involvement of medium-sized vessels throughout the body.

Fibromuscular lesions generally occur in women in the third or fourth decade of life. The fibrous lesions are usually located in the distal two thirds of the main renal arteries and also involve portions of the primary and secondary renal arteries. Cylindric fibromuscular disease may involve the entire renal artery and its primary and secondary branches. Other lesions that occasionally cause renal artery occlusion include thrombosis, embolus, arteriovenous fistula, aneurysm, arteritis, radiation injury, surgical ligation of the renal artery, tumor, neurofibromatosis, renal transplant, congenital unilateral renal hypoplasia (Ask-Upmark kidney), and extrinsic lesions (pheochromocytoma, congenital fibrous bands, retroperitoneal fibrosis, metastatic tumors, and perirenal hematomas).

The location of the lesion in the vessel wall is the basis of another classification of renovascular disease: (1) *intimal* lesions occur as a result of atherosclerosis or intimal fibroplasia; (2) *medial* lesions are caused by fibromuscular dysplasia, which can be further divided into medial fibroplasia, perimedial fibroplasia, medial hyperplasia, and medial dissection; and (3) *adventitial* and *periarterial* lesions result from periarterial fibroplasia, among other causes.

PATHOPHYSIOLOGY. With significant renovascular occlusion (greater than 60% reduction in lumen diameter or 84% reduction in cross-sectional area) there is a reduction in renal perfusion and a decreased pulse pressure against the juxtaglomerular cells. This increases renin secretion by the affected kidney. The level of angiotensin II is increased (see Chapter 87), causing a rise in peripheral resistance, which results in systemic hypertension and the suppression of renin from the contralateral normal kidney. The increased renin also results in increased aldosterone production (secondary aldosteronism), which produces renal sodium retention, systemic volume expansion, and renal potassium wasting.

Bilateral renal arterial involvement is not uncommon and may be severe enough to produce renal insufficiency. Even though the disease may show predominantly unilateral involvement, the detection of bilateral renovascular disease is important to ensure the selection of the appropriate therapeutic approach. The diagnosis of bilateral renal vascular disease should be considered in young patients with severe hypertension and in older patients with diffuse atherosclerotic disease if sudden and significant worsening of hypertension or renal function occurs.

DIAGNOSIS AND LABORATORY FINDINGS. The diagnosis of renal artery stenosis should be considered whenever hypertension is severe. Physical findings such as the presence of abdominal bruits can be misleading because they can be produced by celiac or splenic artery disease as well as by renal artery stenosis. A high-pitched, systolic-diastolic abdominal bruit that radiates to the flank or a flank bruit is more specific than an epigastric bruit. Unfortunately, flank bruits are often absent despite significant stenosis. The diagnosis of renovascular disease depends on laboratory and roentgenographic studies, which are not ideal because they may give false positive and negative results, many are expensive, and some are hazardous.

An evaluation for renovascular hypertension should not be undertaken in every hypertensive patient but should be reserved for those who have an increased likelihood of having the disease, who are not at undue risk from the hazards of the diagnostic or surgical procedures, and who have an excellent likelihood of being cured by the surgery. Patients under the age of 25, patients whose blood pressure is difficult to control medically, or patients in whom antihypertensive drug therapy substantially decreases the quality of life should be evaluated for renovascular hypertension.

A variety of screening studies can suggest the diagnosis but do not predict the blood pressure response to surgical correction. High peripheral vein plasma renin activity may occur with renovascular hypertension, but low or normal peripheral values may also be found. Peripheral plasma renin concentrations are more accurately expressed as a function of urinary sodium excretion. Renal ultrasonography may detect a disparity in renal size. Radioisotope renography is a noninvasive technique that can lateralize difference in renal function. In one series 88% of patients with renal artery stenosis and hypertension had renographic abnormalities. The renogram, however, is not specific for renovascular hypertension and indicates evidence of reduced renal function from other renal diseases. Early rapid sequence urography suggests renal artery stenosis when the affected kidney displays (1) a pole-to-pole diameter 1.5 cm smaller than that of the opposite kidney, (2) delayed appearance of the contrast material in the collecting system, (3) delayed excretion and hyperconcentration of the contrast material, (4) decreased volume of the collecting system, (5) ureteral notching caused by collateral vessels to the ischemic kidney, and (6) cortical thinning caused by renal infarction. Rapid sequence urography is an excellent screening test for severe renal artery stenosis, with one of the six positive findings occurring in 80% of cases of severe unilateral disease. A normal study, however, does not exclude renovascular hypertension.

The infusion of saralasin, the specific competitive blocker of angiotensin II, produces a greater depression in the blood pressure of patients with high renin hypertension than of those with other causes of high blood pressure. This research tool has been successfully applied to detect patients with renovascular hypertension.

Renal vein renin determination and renal arteriography are invasive studies performed to make a definitive diagnosis of renovascular hypertension; the decision to perform them should be made on an individual basis. The studies are indicated in the case of a young woman with significant hypertension who has neither a bruit nor an abnormal urogram. Renal vein renin determination should also be ordered for all patients with an abnormal urogram suggestive of renal ischemia. Selective renal vein renin sampling should be performed in the moderately sodium-depleted patient after renin-suppressing antihypertensive therapy has been discontinued. The results can be expressed as a function of urinary sodium excretion. The ratio of affected kidney renin to contralateral kidney renin is also determined; a ratio greater than 1.5:1 with evidence of contralateral renin suppression (contralateral renal effluent/plasma level ratio no more than 1.3:1) indicates a favorable surgical response. The infusion of an angiotensin-converting enzyme inhibitor increases sampling differences in plasma renin activity between the involved and noninvolved kidney in unilateral renovascular hypertension. At present this is a research tool. In the past, urine obtained from bilateral occlusive ureteral catheters was compared according to volume and sodium and creatinine excretion. These split function tests are no longer performed because of the morbidity (pyelonephritis, sepsis, and renal failure) associated with the studies. More reliable functional data can be obtained from other studies, particularly renal vein renin determinations.

Selective renal angiography including oblique views is required to locate and delineate a renovascular lesion. The demonstration of renal artery stenosis on an angiogram, however, does not predict that correction of the stenosis will cure hypertension.

MANAGEMENT. Antihypertensive drugs used to lower blood pressure in renovascular hypertension are the same as those used in essential hypertension. The use of the angiotensin-converting enzyme inhibitors already mentioned is specific and effective therapy when clinically available. Medical therapy should be proposed for patients more than 50 years old or those with coexisting disease (such as coronary or cerebrovascular disease, pulmonary insufficiency, or renal insufficiency) that increases surgical morbidity and mortality.

Surgery should be considered (1) in the young patient who faces a life of taking medications, (2) when hypertension is severe and poorly controlled, or (3) when poor compliance or the side effects of medication significantly interfere with the patient's life-style. Renal artery reconstruction rather than nephrectomy is preferred. In patients with bilateral renal artery stenosis, vascular repair on the side with the greatest involvement should be undertaken. Thereafter, if hypertension persists, the patient should be reassessed for the need to operate on the other side. Patients with atherosclerotic disease have a poorer response to surgery and a greater operative mortality than patients with fibromuscular disease. Recently, percutaneous transluminal angioplasty has been used for patients with renal arterial disease. The risks of angioplasty are similar to those of arteriography and include perforation, aneurysm, thrombosis, peripheral embolization, and restenosis. In experienced hands the technique appears to have a significantly lower morbidity and mortality than surgery. The short- and long-term morbidity in patients previously considered at high risk for the development of operative complications awaits study.

PROGNOSIS. The definitive therapy for renovascular hypertension is surgical. With careful preoperative assessment, blood pressure control is substantially better with surgical than with medical management. The 10-year mortality is also lower in the surgical group than in the medical group. The most common cause of death in both groups is myocardial infarction followed by cerebrovascular disease and renal failure.

RENAL VEIN THROMBOSIS

The precise prevalence of renal vein thrombosis is unknown because of variability in presentation. In very young children it produces renal failure and therefore is detectable, whereas in adults it may cause only a slight reduction in the filtration rate along with hematuria and proteinuria. The thrombosis may be unilateral but more commonly is bilateral. The rapidity, extent, and location of venous occlusion are the main factors determining the clinical presentation. The ability to develop collateral circulation also helps determine the presentation. Acute bilateral renal vein obstruction is characterized by flank or abdominal pain, enlargement of the kidneys, subsequent development of proteinuria, and deterioration of renal function. After several months the kidneys are bilaterally small. In contrast, chronic (insidious) obstruction is often manifested only by proteinuria, with preservation of renal function. A collateral venous blood supply can develop via the lumbar, adrenal, renal capsular, ureteral, and gonadal veins.

ETIOLOGY. Although the exact mechanism producing renal vein thrombosis is unclear, there is evidence that a hypercoagulable state, hypovolemia (especially in children), and renal disease are predisposing conditions (see the following outline). The nephrotic syndrome is often but not invariably associated with renal vein thrombosis. Renal vein thrombosis appears to be a complication rather than a cause of the nephrotic syndrome.

Causes of renal vein thrombosis

I. Intrinsic factors
   A. Primary renal disease
      1. Glomerulonephritis (mainly membranous and membranoproliferative)
      2. Pyelonephritis
      3. Amyloidosis
      4. Sickle cell anemia
      5. Polyarteritis nodosa
      6. Systemic lupus erythematosus
   B. Hypercoagulable states, including the nephrotic syndrome
   C. Neoplasm (hypernephroma, Wilms' tumor)
   D. Hypovolemia (mainly in children) caused by severe dehydration, hemorrhage, or gastrointestinal losses
   E. Blunt or surgical trauma
II. Extrinsic factors
   A. Retroperitoneal tumors
   B. Lymphomas
   C. Pregnancy
III. Functional factors (causing increases in venous pressure)
   A. Tricuspid insufficiency
   B. Constrictive pericarditis
   C. Congestive heart failure (treated with mercurial diuretics)

The renal lesions most commonly associated with the nephrotic syndrome and renal vein thrombosis are membranous glomerulonephritis and membranoproliferative glomerulonephritis. Lipoid nephrosis is rarely associated with renal vein thrombosis.

PATHOPHYSIOLOGY. Histologic findings include (1) diffuse thickening of the glomerular basement membrane, (2) tubulointerstitial changes (edema and/or fibrosis) out of proportion to the glomerular changes, (3) glomerular basement membrane deposits (mainly subepithelial, coarsely granular deposits of immunoglobulins IgA and IgM and β_1

C-globulin), (4) granulocyte margination in the glomerular capillaries, and (5) glomerular capillary lumen narrowing.

DIAGNOSIS AND LABORATORY FINDINGS. Two thirds of adult patients lack symptoms or laboratory findings suggestive of renal vein thrombosis. The diagnosis is often suspected if symptoms of pulmonary embolism or infarction develop. Children, however, more frequently than adults have acute symptoms of severe loin pain, hematuria, and renal failure. The classic findings of flank pain, swollen kidney, gross hematuria, massive proteinuria, and severe oliguric renal failure are acute manifestations and are uncommon. The most common clinical findings are:

1. Extreme variability of proteinuria and glomerular filtration rate
2. Microscopic hematuria
3. Sterile pyuria
4. Hyperchloremic acidosis
5. Decreased tubular threshold for glucose
6. Pulmonary embolization and other thromboembolic phenomena
7. Increased fibrin degradation products
8. Hypertension
9. Left testicular swelling (rare)

The diagnosis of renal vein thrombosis is suggested by an abnormal intravenous urogram that shows enlarged kidneys, a poor concentration of the dye because of the decreased renal function, and the notching of the upper ureters by collateral veins, occurring in 25% of patients. Kidney enlargement is an inconstant finding, and progressive shrinkage and atrophy may occur over months when there is extensive obstruction. Other roentgenographic findings include a shortened nephrographic phase, compression of the collecting system by interstitial edema, and poor opacification of the collecting system. The intravenous urogram is occasionally normal despite renal vein thrombosis. Selective renal vein phlebography is the most reliable technique for making the diagnosis. There is, however, a risk of dislodging clots with subsequent pulmonary embolization. In addition to a filling defect caused by the clot, involvement of collateral vessels may be demonstrated. Tumor invasion of the renal vein can also appear as a filling defect. Renal arteriography avoids the risk of pulmonary embolism and can demonstrate involved collateral vessels in the venous phase, but it is a somewhat unsatisfactory method of diagnosis because of inconsistency of opacification and lack of detail.

MANAGEMENT. Thrombectomy for renal vein thrombosis, even in acute cases, is *not* recommended. Surgery has failed in some cases to reestablish patency and has extended the thrombi distally. Severe proteinuria usually persists, and renal function is unimproved. Long-term anticoagulation should be instituted whenever possible to preserve renal function and prevent embolization. Neither steroid nor cytotoxic therapy is useful. Steroids may actually exacerbate the existing thromboembolic tendency.

There is no evidence to justify the prophylactic administration of anticoagulants to patients with the nephrotic syndrome, particularly membranous glomerulonephritis, to prevent renal vein thrombosis.

BIBLIOGRAPHY

Baum, N.H., Moriel, E., and Carlton, C.E.: Renal vein thrombosis, J. Urol. **119**:443, 1978.

Cade, R., and others: Chronic renal vein thrombosis, Am. J. Med. **63**:387, 1977.

Davis, B.A., and others: Prevalence of renovascular hypertension in patients with grade III or IV hypertensive retinopathy, N. Engl. J. Med. **301**:1273, 1979.

Foster, J.H., and others: Renovascular occlusive disease: results of operative treatment, J.A.M.A. **231**:1043, 1975.

Harrison, E.G., and McCormack, L.J.: Pathologic classification of renal arterial disease in renovascular hypertension, Mayo Clin. Proc. **46**:161, 1971.

Juncos, L.I., Strong, C.G., and Hunt, J.C.: Prediction of results of surgery for renal and renovascular hypertension, Arch. Intern. Med. **134**:655, 1974.

Kees, C.J., and Harrell, R.S.: Radiographic manifestations of renal vein thrombosis, J. Urol. **108**:830, 1972.

Kuhlmann, U., and others: Renovascular hypertension: treatment by percutaneous transluminal dilatation, Ann. Intern. Med. **92**:1, 1980.

Llach, R., Arieff, A.I., and Massry, S.G.: Renal vein thrombosis and nephrotic syndrome—a prospective study of 36 adult patients, Ann. Intern. Med. **83**:8, 1975.

Rosemann, E., Pollak, V.E., and Pirani, C.L.: Renal vein thrombosis in the adult—clinical and pathologic study based on renal biopsies, Medicine **47**:269, 1968.

Stewart, B.H.: Correlation of angiography and natural history in evaluation of patients with renovascular hypertension, J. Urol. **104**:231, 1970.

Trew, P.A., and others: Renal vein thrombosis in membranous glomerulonephropathy—incidence and association, Medicine **57**:69, 1978.

Vaughan, E.D., and others: Renovascular hypertension: renin measurements to indicate hypersecretion and contralateral suppression, estimate renal plasma flow, and score for surgical curability, Am. J. Med. **55**:402, 1973.

120 • RENAL DISEASE IN PREGNANCY

Sal A. Lofaro and **Sandra P. Levison**

CHANGES IN RENAL PHYSIOLOGY ASSOCIATED WITH NORMAL PREGNANCY

During normal pregnancy and for up to 4 months after delivery, the kidney increases approximately 1 cm in length and the collecting system dilates. The latter is thought to be caused by hormonal factors and mechanical obstruction at the pelvic brim. This is associated with urinary stasis and an increased likelihood of urinary tract infection. Changes in the glomerular filtration rate (GFR) and renal plasma flow occur during pregnancy, but there is some controversy as to the exact findings. It has been thought that the GFR increases much more than renal plasma flow (RPF), so that the filtration fraction $\left(FF = \dfrac{GFR}{RPF}\right)$ increases during pregnancy; placental lactogen has been suggested as a mediator. Recent studies suggest that the filtration fraction decreases, especially in early pregnancy, but again increases in the third trimester. Both blood urea nitrogen and creatinine levels decrease, so that values greater than 13 mg/dl and 0.8 mg/dl, respectively, suggest renal insufficiency and merit further investigation.

The usual weight gain of about 12.5 kg (28 pounds) can be attributed mainly to the retention of water and 500 to 900 mEq of sodium that does not appear to be mediated by aldosterone. Serum sodium and albumin concentrations decrease because of water retention. There is an increase in plasma volume mainly in the second trimester, whereas interstitial volume rises the most in the third trimester. Diastolic blood pressure falls, reaching a nadir in the second trimester, and rises again in the third trimester.

The glycosuria occurring in pregnancy is believed to result mainly from an increased GFR, but there may also be defective tubular reabsorption of glucose. Increases in urinary excretion of most amino acids, some soluble vitamins, and protein (up to 300 mg a day) may occur. The plasma uric acid concentration also decreases, presumably as a result of increased uric acid clearance or increased extracellular fluid volume.

ACUTE RENAL FAILURE

Acute renal failure occurring during pregnancy has a bimodal distribution, with an early peak caused mainly by septic abortion along with associated sepsis, hemolysis, hypovolemia, hypotension, and subsequent acute tubular necrosis. The increase in late pregnancy is predominantly a result of preeclampsia but may also be caused by bilateral cortical necrosis associated with abruptio placentae. Bilateral cortical necrosis usually occurs before the thirtieth week and usually follows prolonged oligoanuria. Recovery from bilateral cortical necrosis can occur; however, it commonly results in end-stage renal disease.

GLOMERULONEPHRITIS

Glomerulonephritis may occur during pregnancy (1:40,000 pregnancies) and generally results in fetal death. In early pregnancy it is relatively easy to diagnose and may resolve. Glomerulonephritis occurring in late pregnancy may be confused with preeclampsia because of its similar clinical course and urine sediment. The serum complement may be depressed in glomerulonephritis.

There seems to be no increased risk to mother or neonate if a pregnancy occurs more than 3 years following an episode of acute glomerulonephritis; however, these neonates seem to have lower birth weights than those born of unaffected mothers. Women with chronic glomerulonephritis appear to have an increased risk of early preeclampsia, preterm deliveries, low-birth-weight infants, and fetal and neonatal deaths, especially if hypertension of azotemia is present. The early occurrence of toxemia is suggestive of preexisting renal disease. Although preexisting renal disease usually does not worsen with pregnancy, exacerbations of focal sclerosing glomerulonephritis have been reported. Deterioration in renal function has developed in pregnant patients with preexisting asymptomatic proteinuria. It is prudent, therefore, to consider renal biopsy in women of childbearing age who have significant asymptomatic proteinuria. These women may need counseling about the effects of pregnancy on maternal and fetal survival.

Maternal and fetal survival appears to correlate best with excellent control of hypertension (if present) and close monitoring of renal function. If renal failure develops, the patient should be dialyzed vigorously as soon as possible.

POSTPARTUM RENAL FAILURE

Postpartum renal failure occurs 3 to 6 weeks after delivery with an otherwise uncomplicated pregnancy. The cause is unknown. The renal failure is usually associated with severe hypertension and often with microangiopathic hemolytic anemia and diffuse intravascular coagulation, with arteriolar and intraglomerular thrombosis, and with malignant nephrosclerosis. Unfortunately, most of the women die. There is controversy concerning the success of anticoagulant therapy or plasmapheresis. Dialysis is generally helpful when indicated.

NEPHROTIC SYNDROME

Nephrotic syndrome of pregnancy is very uncommon, occurring in only 1 in 4000 pregnancies. It is usually caused by preeclampsia, which generally is manifested by only moderate proteinuria. The proteinuria resolves completely after delivery and may recur during a subsequent pregnancy. The degree of proteinuria correlates with the severity of glomerular damage. Reports of abnormal histologic findings are sparse. Subendothelial deposits of IgG and β_1C-globulin have been described.

In women with nephrosis that antedates the pregnancy, proteinuria may increase during pregnancy, presumably as a result of the increased GFR. Renal function in these patients does not appear to worsen during pregnancy; however, as with chronic glomerulonephritis, if there is concurrent azotemia or hypertension, the risk of preeclampsia and fetal loss is greater.

Birth weight correlates with serum albumin levels, and severe hypoproteinemia frequently results in premature births. Pregnant women with the nephrotic syndrome are more prone to thromboembolic disease and renal vein thrombosis. Premature births are more common in women with nephrosis and hypertension. There may also be increased infection caused by the loss of v-globulin. The diagnosis of nephrotic syndrome of pregnancy is more easily made in early pregnancy, since later it is difficult to differentiate from preeclampsia.

TOXEMIA

PATHOGENESIS. The term "toxemia" includes eclampsia and preeclampsia and describes hypertensive disorders of pregnancy that improve with delivery and are associated with edema and proteinuria. With eclampsia, convulsions and/or coma develops as well. Toxemia occurs in 5% to 10% of all pregnancies; the recurrence rate is 25% after a primiparous toxemia. Although the pathogenesis is unknown, possible causes include (1) uterine ischemia with subsequent premature placental aging (ischemic chorionic villi are thought to induce vasospasm and hypertension); (2) diminished production of the vasodilators, prostaglandins E and A, with subsequent unopposed vasoconstrictor action of angiotensin; (3) increased estrogen-, progesterone-, or metabolite-induced arteriolar sensitivity to vasoconstriction; (4) nutritional deficiencies; and (5) abnormal protein metabolism. Despite increases in aldosterone, plasma renin activity, and angiotensin II in normal pregnancy, there is a decrease in blood pressure. This may represent a decreased sensitivity to angiotensin II. However, with pregnancy-induced hypertension this refractoriness to angiotensin II is lost and may be mediated by decreases in local prostaglandin synthesis or increased prostaglandin catabolism. An increased predisposition to toxemia occurs when there is associated or preexisting hypertension, diabetes mellitus, multiple fetuses, primigravidity (65% of all cases), polyhydramnios, hydatidiform mole, a very young (under age 17) or older (over age 35) mother, malnutrition, or familial predisposition.

DIAGNOSIS. True toxemia generally occurs after the twenty-fourth week and most commonly after the thirty-second week, although it may occur as early as the twentieth week with hydatidiform mole. In toxemia the systolic blood pressure rises 30 mm Hg or more and the diastolic pressure 15 mm Hg or more on two readings taken 6 or more hours apart. In some women whose usual blood pressures are low, convulsions have been documented at a blood pressure as low as 140/90 mm Hg. In addition to increasing blood pressure, other associated findings include weight gain greater than 2 pounds a week even before edema is detected, more than 300 mg of protein excreted in the urine each day, and hyperuricemia. Headache may be mild initially but becomes more severe as the disease progresses. Visual blurring is a late symptom. Epigastric pain, hemoglobinemia/hemoglobinuria, thrombocytopenia, hyperbilirubinemia, and pulmonary edema are rare but ominous signs. Convulsions occur in eclampsia. Retinal hemorrhages and exudates are rare with preeclampsia, although a "retinal sheen" or glistening retina is seen. Spinal reflexes may be accentuated and are a good monitor of central nervous system activity.

Despite these criteria, toxemia is often confused with chronic hypertension. Chronic hypertension is more likely than toxemia (1) when hypertension is noted before the twentieth week, (2) if there is a history of hypertension but not toxemia in a previous pregnancy, (3) with an absence of toxemia during the first pregnancy but its appearance in subsequent ones, (4) if there is absence of proteinuria and edema, and (5) with evidence of sustained and severe hypertension with target organ involvement.

MANAGEMENT. Women with hypertension who become pregnant should be maintained with antihypertensive therapy to prevent maternal and fetal complications. However, sodium restriction and diuretics are not used. There has been considerable safe experience with oral methyldopa and hydralazine. The safe use of clonidine, prazosin, β-adrenergic blockers, and minoxidil in pregnancy is yet to be demonstrated. Once the diagnosis of preeclampsia is made, immediate hospitalization and delivery are urged. Toxemia is associated with fetal intrauterine growth retardation. When delivery is delayed to allow the fetus to mature, there are associated stillbirths in utero and an increased risk of maternal morbidity and mortality. Attempts to lower the maternal blood pressure and prolong pregnancy have been associated with fetal death in utero.

In addition to fetal monitoring, the mother is carefully and rapidly prepared for delivery. Fluid and electrolyte balance is restored, and the patient's neurologic and cardiovascular system should be stabilized. Sedation may be needed to control agitation and hyperreflexia; phenobarbital, 250 mg intramuscularly every 6 hours; diazepam, 5 to 10 mg parenterally every 2 hours; or thiopental, 250 mg intravenously, is used for short-term control of neuroirritability. The anticonvulsant of choice is magnesium sulfate; the goal is to attain therapeutic blood levels of 6 to 8 mEq/L but avoid toxicity. Magnesium sulfate is not an antihypertensive. The lowering of maternal blood pressure may be initiated, particularly when the blood pressure is very high or when anesthesia induction may be required. The use of intravenous antihypertensives, particularly those with action that can be carefully regulated, would seem desirable. However, nitroprusside is now thought to be contraindicated because data from animal studies indicate accumulation of cyanide in the fetus. Diazoxide can precipitously lower blood pressure and depress labor, but small boluses (30 to 60 mg intravenously) are safest. Intravenous hydralazine or methyldopa has been used successfully. Neither diuretics nor sodium restriction is used despite the presence of edema, since there is already a contracted intravascular volume.

PROGNOSIS. Maternal mortality associated with eclampsia is 2% to 5%. Fetal mortality is increased, but the precise mortality is difficult to assess because values may vary greatly among medical facilities. The maternal blood pressure generally returns to normal within 2 weeks of delivery, whereas proteinuria may persist longer. Sequelae rarely occur. The incidence of recurrent toxemia is 25% after a primiparous toxemia.

PYELONEPHRITIS

(See Chapter 40.)

Significant bacteriuria develops in about 5% of pregnant women during pregnancy, whereas the incidence of acute pyelonephritis is about 1%. About 75% of those with bacteriuria during pregnancy have it at the first prenatal visit. Twenty percent of these patients (as well as 20% of those whose bacteriuria develops later) will have acute pyelonephritis later in the pregnancy.

Susceptibility to bacteriuria during pregnancy has been attributed to the changes in hormones, collecting system dilation, urinary stasis, and glycosuria. The clinical presentation varies from asymptomatic bacteriuria to cystitis with dysuria to acute pyelonephritis with fever, flank pain, and sepsis. With acute pyelonephritis, cortical abscesses may develop.

Pregnancies complicated by acute pyelonephritis are associated with high neonatal mortality and more frequent preterm deliveries. These are caused mainly by the commonly associated hydramnios, amniotic fluid bacterial infections, and abruptio placentae. Asymptomatic bacteriuria may also increase the complication rate. Urinary calculi generally cause minimal problems during pregnancy.

The complications of pyelonephritis during pregnancy can be significantly decreased by routine prenatal urine cultures followed by the appropriate antibacterial treatment of bacteriuria.

SYSTEMIC LUPUS ERYTHEMATOSUS AND OTHER COLLAGEN-VASCULAR DISEASES

There is controversy about the effect of pregnancy on systemic lupus erythematosus (SLE) and vice versa. Pregnant women with SLE generally show no change and in some cases have improvement in symptoms. There is an increased incidence of spontaneous abortions. Controversy exists as to whether there is a tendency toward relapse of SLE during puerperium. Patients with SLE and normal renal function generally have no added risks during pregnancy; however, in those with SLE nephropathy the pattern is similar to patients with chronic glomerulonephritis, with an increased incidence of preeclampsia and fetal loss, especially if there are associated hypertension and azotemia. The transmission of a variety of antibodies and possibly viral particles via the placenta appears to occur. Pregnant patients with active SLE should continue drug therapy. There are reports of deliveries of normal infants despite therapy with cytotoxic drugs.

Patients with scleroderma or periarteritis nodosa generally have difficult pregnancies, possibly because of associated severe hypertension.

BIBLIOGRAPHY

Davison, J.M., and Lindheimer, M.D.: Renal disease in pregnant women, Clin. Obstet. Gynecol. **21**:411, 1978.
DeAlvarez, R.R.: Preeclampsia—eclampsia and renal diseases in pregnancy, Clin. Obstet. Gynecol. **21**:881, 1978.
Ferris, T.f.: Postpartum renal insufficiency, Kidney Int. **14**:383, 1978.
First, M.R., and others; Preeclampsia with the nephrotic syndrome, Kidney Int. **13**:166, 1978.
Leppert, P., and others: Antecedent renal disease and the outcome of pregnancy, Ann. Intern. Med. **90**:747, 1979.
Lindheimer, M.D., and Katz, A.I., editors: The kidney in pregnancy (symposium), Kidney Int. **18**:147, 1980.
Naeye, R.L.: Causes of the excessive rates of perinatal mortality and prematurity in pregnancies complicated by maternal urinary-tract infections, N. Engl. J. Med. **300**:819, 1979.
Peyser, M.R., and others: Late follow-up in women with nephrosclerosis diagnosed at pregnancy, Am. J. Obstet. Gynecol. **132**:480, 1978.
Rosen, S.: Pathology of renal disease during pregnancy, Clin. Obstet. Gynecol. **21**:875, 1978.
Taylor, J., and others: Focal sclerosing glomerulonephropathy with adverse effect during pregnancy, Arch. Intern. Med. **138**:1695, 1973.

DENTAL CORRELATIONS

Burton H. Goldstein
edited by **James T. Amsterdam**

It is appropriate to discuss the dental aspects and management of renal disease as a single systemic problem rather than to discuss the oral and dental problems related to specific kidney disorders. Patients with renal disease generally have clinical manifestations related to the functional status of their kidneys regardless of the cause of the disease. Their problems are frequently associated with the various life-saving treatment modalities such as dialysis and transplantation.

ORAL MANIFESTATIONS. Oral lesions related to renal disease are generally nonspecific. However, many of the metabolic and physiologic body alterations that accompany renal disease have oral manifestations. Clinicians should be aware that some of the signs and symptoms manifested in the oral cavity may suggest the presence of renal disease, especially in the more advanced stages. Due to more reliable, sophisticated laboratory techniques, renal and electrolyte disorders are frequently discovered before the patient is symptomatic.

Elevation of blood urea nitrogen in renal failure results in a high concentration of urea in the saliva; a breakdown product, ammonia, results. The increased concentrations of ammonia result in some distinguishing oral manifestations. Dysgeusia, often described as a salty or metallic bad taste and frequently perceived as halitosis, is a common occurrence. Uremic stomatitis may occur in severe untreated renal failure. This is most often noted in patients with a blood urea level exceeding 30 mmol/L. Baries' classification of uremic stomatitis consists of two types. *Type I, erythemopulaceous,* initially manifests a red thickening of the buccal mucosa, which later includes a gray, thick, pasty, gluey exudate and pseudomembrane covering the gingiva, fauces, and oral mucosa. When the pseudomembrane is removed with a tongue blade, a swollen, dry, red but not ulcerated mucosa is found. Associated manifestations for type I include fetor oris, dry burning sensation, excessive saliva, and perversion of taste. *Type II, ulcerative form,* is similar to type I but includes loss of integrity of the mucosa with frank ulceration. The ulcers may be superficial or deep and frequently involve the gingiva. Purpura may also be visualized on the mucosa as a result of thrombocytopenia due to bone marrow depression. Excessive salivation is again noted. Parotid and submandibular gland swelling may be seen in patients with chronic renal failure without accompanying uremic stomatitis.

The cause of uremic stomatitis is partially related to the high salivary urea level with consequent breakdown into ammonia and to the presence of other harmful metabolites, which are not being executed by the kidneys. Histologic uremic stomatitis appears as an intense polymorphonuclear inflammation and extensive necrosis of mucosa; the friable mucosa is highly susceptible to secondary infection. The most common bacteria involved are Vincent's organisms, fusobacterium. As in the treatment of acute necrotizing ulcerative gingivitis (ANUG), local debridement and systemic antibiotics (e.g., penicillin or erythromycin) are useful therapy.

Patients with uremic stomatitis are severely ill, and the oral lesions may take 2 to 3 weeks to resolve after the onset of dialysis. During this period dental management is generally palliative (e.g., hydrogen peroxide, mouth rinses, or topical anesthetics).

Bleeding disorders are associated with uremia and have nonspecific oral manifestations such as ecchymoses, petechiae, and spontaneous gingival bleeding. The same bleeding disorders also contribute to the crusting seen in uremic stomatitis. The mechanisms of these hemostatic defects is complex, and although thrombocytopenia may occur in as many as 50% of uremic patients, the major cause of the clinical bleeding problem is considered to be platelet dysfunction. This abnormality is caused by a dialyzable substance, and the control of the bleeding and associated oral manifestations is related to systemic improvement by dialysis.

Chronic renal failure is frequently accompanied by anemia. The anemia may be severe with hemoglobin levels of 5 g/dl or less. Oral mucosal and gingival pallor may be present in such situations. This anemia is often well tolerated by the patient and does not usually respond to treatment of renal failure. If other factors compound the anemia of chronic renal failure, such as pernicious anemia, a glossitis may be seen.

Several other factors also cause oral signs in uremic patients. Hyperuricemia secondary to renal failure may cause deposition of urate crystals in the temporomandibular joint or oral soft tissues. Edema, secondary to decrease in osmotic pressure from loss of plasma protein (as in nephrotic syndrome), manifests itself orally in the tissues of low resistance. Therefore the uvula is apt to show signs of congestion with edema. Passive venous congestion secondary to cardiac insufficiency may be evident by swelling on the base and lower surface of the tongue.

Neuropathy occurring with severe renal failure may be manifested as dysesthesia of the lingual nerve. The patient may complain of tingling or numbness of the tongue.

Severe orofacial and odontogenic infections sometimes associated with unusual oral flora may also occur in the debilitated or immunosuppressed renal failure patient. In a series of immunosuppressed and control patients dental infection occurred as frequently as pneumonia or urinary tract infections in the transplant patients. Patients who developed acute alveolar abscesses tended to be immunosuppressed for more than 5 years and had lymphocyte counts less than 400 ml^3. The importance of good dental health before transplantation and maintenance of dental health was emphasized, although none of the patients in the study died as a result of dental infection–related sepsis. (See dental management section.)

Renal osteodystrophy—first described in 1937 by Albright, Drake, and Sulkowitch and also known as renal osteitis fibrosa cystica—is the adult counterpart of renal rickets in children. The apparent cause is renal insufficiency leading to decreased excretion of phosphate, acidosis, and impaired absorption of calcium from the gut. This in turn stimulates hyperplasia of the parathyroid glands (secondary hyperparathyroidism). The degree of renal osteodystrophy has been shown to be secondary to the duration of the disease. The histologic picture is that of replacement of spongy bone with an immature coarse fibrillar type and fibrosis of the bone marrow–infected areas. There is evidence of osteoclastic resorption and the fibrous marrow was found to contain giant cells and small cysts.

The most commonly seen changes on dental radiographs of patients with chronic renal failure are altered trabeculation, altered radiodensity, subperiosteal cortical bone resorption, and partial loss of the lamina dura. Periapical and panoramic radiography may reveal both osteoporotic and osteosclerotic appearances, often termed "chalky," "ground glass," or "granular" due to the delicate, finely meshed trabecular pattern. The much discussed loss of lamina dura associated with chronic renal failure, while present in some patients, should not be considered diagnostic or specific for renal disease since it may occur in localized inflammatory disorders as well as in many systemic diseases. The associated "triad" of loss of lamina dura, altered trabecular pattern, and density changes is suggestive of renal osteodystrophy. Temporomandibular joint involvement has been documented to include decreased bone density, subcortical cysts of the condyle, irregularity of the condyle and/or glenoid fossa, and in the most severe cases, complete resorption of the condylar head and process with resultant acquired dentofacial deformity.

If the process of renal osteodystrophy begins at an early age, during the development of the teeth, the teeth may appear highly calcified, because teeth are depositories of calcium but they do not release calcium. Cystic lesions of the jaws (osteoclastomas) may also be evident. These giant cell lesions can cause a thinning of the cortex and may be palpable as surface swellings. Such lesions may be seen in the calvarium, mandible, and maxilla as well as the long bones, pelvis, and phalanges.

The oral manifestations of hyperparathyroidism secondary to renal failure during childhood are important since they affect growth and development of the dentoalveolar complex. Young patients, especially those undergoing dialysis, must be provided with sufficient calcium for proper development of teeth. These patients generally have a low caries incidence. Although excessive calculus deposits are detected on the teeth secondary to an increased calcium-phosphate solubility product.

Vitamin D-resistant rickets caused by renal tubular defects cause unique oral manifestations involving the structure of the tooth. Such defects cause the formation of globular dentin with clefts and defects in the dentinal tubules. Pulp horns become elongated and extend to the dentinoenamel junction. The abnormality in dentin formation is a direct cause for frequent bacterial invasion of the pulp without evidence of tubular destruction of the dentin normally seen in the cariously involved tooth. Periapical involvement is seen without apparent tooth involvement. Dental radiographs reveal the presence of lamina dura and an abnormal alveolar bone pattern.

Dental alterations observed in patients with renal disease include both intrinsic staining from previous tetracycline administration and extrinsic staining from iron medications. Enamel hypoplasia, retarded growth, and tooth eruption may be seen, and an increased tendency toward heavy dental calculus formation has been reported.

Malignant renal tumors may metastasize to the jaws and/or the oral structures. Renal cell carcinoma has been reported to represent 15% of the primary cancers with jaw metastases. The mandible was more frequently involved than the maxilla. These tumors may be accompanied by soft tissue swelling and mobility of the teeth in the area of the lesion. Such rare lesions may be suspected if an extraction socket fails to heal. Direct soft tissue involvement is also rare, in which case the carcinoma may be found in the gingiva, lips, tongue, or salivary glands. The lesions have been described as red-brown in appearance, friable, and cystlike.

Orofacial abnormalities are seen in a number of syndromes that involve renal abnormalities. Patients with chromosomal syndromes, especially trisomy 18 or Turner (XO) syndrome, may have associated renal anomalies, including horseshoe kidney. Cleft palate patients have a higher incidence of renal anomalies than the general population and warrant investigation. Any family history of an infant death related to renal disease should be investigated for the possible presence of renal agenesis or renal dysplasia, which can be associated with Potter syndrome (oligohydramnios syndrome) and bilateral renal agenesis, also associated with micrognathia and cleft lip/palate. Patients with Reiter's syndrome may have oral lesions and occasionally their involvement of the urinary tract may include nephritis. Multiple oral fibromas are seen in tuberous sclerosis (Bourneville-Pringle syndrome), and 40% of these patients have renal hamartomas. Oral and facial angiokeratomas (multiple red-purple pinpoint lesions especially on the lips) are seen in Fabry's syndrome (angiokeratoma corporis diffusum). These patients suffer progressive renal failure from the accumulation of a glycosphingolipid. Further specific discussion of these and the many other syndromes that may be associated with both oral and renal involvement is available.

DENTAL MANAGEMENT. It is estimated that by 1984 more than 55,000 patients in the United States will be undergoing dialysis for end-stage renal disease and over 5200 patients will have renal transplants. Dental treatment for these people is increasingly recognized as an essential health service. Dental management is complicated because of the oral disease and the medical problems seen in this population. These patients survive under narrowly controlled conditions of intake and activity as well as under great physiologic and psychologic stress with medications, diet, invasive treatments, limited life-style, and dependency on others. Dental treatment, even minor dental procedures, may present major problems and should be considered particularly stressful when superimposed on such situations.

Hemodialysis is by far the most prevalent therapy for end-stage renal disease. In a survey of 100 hemodialysis patients, more than 60% were in need of dental treatment and 88% had natural teeth present in one or both arches. All renal dialysis patients should be informed of the importance of oral health in preventing complications due to infection or dietary difficulties. Comprehensive oral evaluation and dental treatment are part of the basic health care of the end-stage renal disease patient. Many hospitals provide dental services, although most medically controlled renal failure patients may be safely and adequately treated in the private dental office.

A healthy dentition and oral cavity should be considered a basic precondition to renal transplantation. The consequences of oral infection may be life-threatening in the immunosuppressed patient. Dental management of the transplant patient is complicated by the potent medications often used to prevent or treat graft rejection. In 21 patients with fever of unknown origin after renal transplantation, 16 had oral pathology including infected nonvital teeth, impacted teeth with the possiblity of oral communication, advanced periodontitis with furcation involvement and pockets over 5 mm in depth, and osteomyelitis. Six of these patients' fevers resolved within 12 hours of dental treatment.

The following considerations are important when evaluating and treating the dental patient with renal disease.

Timing. The best time for dental treatment is the day after dialysis. This will avoid bleeding problems related to systemic anticoagulation as well as provide an optimal metabolic condition for the patient. Individual dental or medical considerations may be coordinated with regional anticoagulation techniques, in-hospital dental treatment, and other treatment modifications as suited to individual patient needs.

Asepsis. All patients with end-stage renal disease including renal transplant recipients are potential carriers of hepatitis B. Laboratory testing to determine the status of hepatitis B antigenicity should be routinely obtained for these patients before dental treatment and updated frequently. HBsAg-negative or HBsAb-positive patients may be treated routinely, and HBsAg-positive patients should be treated with currently recommended procedures to minimize the potential transmission of hepatitis B. The presence of hepatitis B antigen is not a contraindication to dental office treatment but rather is an indication of the need for special care and meticulous techniques. It is recommended that appropriate aseptic techniques be used for all dental patients.

Hematologic and physiologic status. The multiple hematologic abnormalities that accompany renal disease and the treatment of renal failure must be considered for each patient as potential modifying factors for dental treatment. Clinical and laboratory evaluation for anemia, bleeding disorders, and white cell abnormalities may be indicated, depending on the status of renal disease or therapeutic modality and the type of dental treatment anticipated. Fluid and electrolyte balance may also be subject to wide ranges of alterations in patients undergoing dialysis and with varying stages of renal failure. Evaluation and stabilization of these alterations should be accomplished before dental treatment.

Maintenance of the vascular access device of the hemodialysis patient is important. The location of the shunt or fistula should be noted and care taken to avoid renipuncture, blood pressure cuff compression, or any trauma to the area.

Immunosuppression and corticosteroid medications. Many renal transplant patients are on a regimen of antiinflammatory and immunosuppressive medications. These medications may mask the early signs and symptoms of infection and inflammation, making timely diagnosis difficult as well as producing a tendency toward more severe problems when first recognized. The prophylactic use of antibiotics for dental treatment must be considered for each patient and each procedure. At present, there is no documented evidence of the efficacy of antimicrobial prophylaxis in the renal transplant patient; however, many dentists and physicians believe the benefits of potential protection far outweigh the risks of potential infection. The nature of each dental procedure as well as the individual patient's physical and psychologic status must also be considered. Chronic systemic steroid administration suppresses the patient's ability to respond to stress by causing adrenal atrophy. Supplemental steroids should be considered before stressful dental procedures.

Medications and drug therapy for dental purposes. The practitioner prescribing or administering medications to patients with compromised renal function must be familiar with the metabolism and excretion of each of the agents involved and the functional status of the individual patient's kidneys. To provide safe, yet effective drug therapy, modification of the usual dosage regimen may be necessary. Distinction regarding the amount of kidney function for purposes of drug administration may be made; mild to moderate renal failure or renal insufficiency and severe renal failure or a functionally anephric patient are satisfactory for dental purposes. Guidelines are presented in tabular form and discussed according to the therapeutic use. (See Table 1.)

Local anesthesia. Renal failure, renal dialysis, renal transplantation, and other medically controlled conditions related to end-stage renal disease, such as hypertension, do not contraindicate the use of local anesthetics or vasoconstrictors in dentistry. Provision of adequate pain relief for dental procedures sometimes necessitates the use of vasoconstrictor-containing local anesthetic solutions. The kidney is the main excretory organ for all the local anesthetics commonly used in dentistry and their metabolites. The amide-type local anesthetic agents are excreted approximately 15% or less unchanged, and the ester-type agents are excreted unchanged in even smaller amounts. Significant impairment of renal function may, therefore, result in increased blood levels of the local anesthetic or its metabolites (which are generally less toxic than the parent compounds), which may cause adverse systemic effects. The use of cocaine is specifically contraindicated since it is excreted entirely unchanged in the urine. On the basis of clinical experience, it is recommended that the slow administration of not more than 25% of the maximum total recommended dosage for the "normal" patient is a practical and safe guideline for local anesthetic injections for dental purposes in the medically controlled patient with absent renal function and not more than 50% of the maximum "normal dose" in the patient with renal insufficiency. Specific information regarding a safe local anesthetic dosage in the patient with end-stage renal disease is not available.

Inhalation sedation. The administration of nitrous oxide and oxygen to produce conscious sedation and analgesia should be carefully performed in the patient with impaired renal function. The degree of anemia and oxygen-carrying capacity of the blood must be considered. However, it appears to be clinically safe and well tolerated to administer up to 50% nitrous oxide and 50% oxygen to the monitored and medically controlled patient with end-stage renal disease. A knowledge of the patient's hemoglobin level and serum potassium is helpful before the use of inhalation sedation agents.

Parenteral sedation. Anxiety control in dentistry sometimes requires the use of sedative drugs. In patients with end-stage renal disease, diazepam is the safest and most commonly used agent. Whether given orally, intramuscularly, or intravenously, careful administration and especially titration of the intravenous dose should be employed. Diazepam is removed by hemodialysis, and modification of the dosage for single episodic sedative purposes is usually unnecessary. Diazepam and its metabolite oxazepam may linger. All sedated patients should be monitored closely after the procedure and should have someone accompany them home when discharged.

General anesthesia. The administration of general anesthesia to the patient with impaired renal function should be performed by a specialist with knowledge, training, and ability to manage the complex potential problems associated with an anemic hypertensive and metabolically unstable patient. Efficient use of general anesthetic time to accomplish maximal services should be considered and hospitalization is indicated. The clinician should know that inhalation or parenteral sedation is on a continuum with general anesthesia. Therefore the dentist should be able to manage and support the unconscious patient if the administration of any of these agents is considered.

Analgesics. Doses of the nonnarcotic analgesics commonly used in dentistry must be modified for patients with renal failure (Table 1). Both aspirin and acetaminophen are removed by hemodialysis. The use of acetaminophen should be avoided in severe renal failure, as should phenacetin, due to nephrotoxic side effects. Doses of the narcotic analgesics are usually not modified since they are detoxified primarily by the liver.

Antibiotics. Penicillin is the drug of choice for the treatment of most oral and odontogenic infections. It may be prescribed in usual doses (less than 3 million units/day) for periods up to 5 days. However, high-dose or long-term therapy requires regimen modification, with special cau-

Table 1. Guidelines for drug therapy in dental treatment of patients with renal disease

Drug	Normal dosage regimen	Dosage adjustment in Renal insufficiency	Dosage adjustment in Anephric patient
Analgesics			
Acetaminophen	q3-4h	Unchanged	Avoid
ASA	q3-4h	q4-6h	q8-12h
Phenacetin	q3-4h	Avoid	Avoid
Codeine	q4h	Unchanged	Unchanged
Meperidine	q4h	Unchanged	Unchanged
Morphine	q4h	Unchanged	Unchanged
Pentazocine	q4-6h	Unchanged	Unchanged
Sedatives			
Diazepam	q8h	Unchanged	Unchanged
Antimicrobial agents			
Clindamycin	q6h	Unchanged	Unchanged
Erythromycin	q6h	Unchanged	Unchanged
Tetracycline	q6h	Avoid	Avoid
Doxycycline	q24h	Unchanged	Unchanged
Penicillin G	q8h	Unchanged	q12-16h*
Penicillin V	q8h	Unchanged	q12-16h*
Amoxillin	q8h	q8-12h	q12-16h
Ampicillin	q6h	q8h	q12h
Cloxicillin	q6h	Unchanged	Unchanged
Dicloxicillin	q6h	Unchanged	Unchanged
Oxacillin	q6h	Unchanged	Unchanged
Methicillin	q6h	Unchanged	Unchanged

These guidelines are suggested estimates aimed at providing optimal therapeutic effects with minimal side effects. Individual patient variation in serum levels may be significant, and this table in no way implies that these regimens are "safe" or rigid requirements. Modified and adapted from Bennett, Singer, and Coggins: J.A.M.A. **230**:1544, 1974; Heard, Staples, and Czerwinski: J. Am. Dent. Assoc. **96**:792, 1978; Kelly and others: Oral Surg. **50**:372, 1980.
*The potassium salt has 1.7 mEg K^+ per 1 million units.

tion in using the potassium salt of penicillin G or penicillin V (Table 1). Amoxillin, ampicillin, and carbenicillin are removed by hemodialysis while the other commonly used penicillins are not. Tetracyclines are usually avoided with renal functional impairment due to their catabolic effects, but if they must be prescribed doxycycline is recommended for uremic patients. Erythromycin and clindamycin may be given in usual doses.

SUMMARY

Oral manifestations of renal and electrolyte disorders are generally nonspecific, with few exceptions. The entity of uremic stomatitis was rare when dialysis was unavailable and is rarer now with the advent of adequate treatment of uremia. Mild forms of stomatitis are evident and are a frequent complaint in many patients. Clinicians should be aware of the frequency of secondary infection. Renal osteodystrophy is still seen and is a serious manifestation of renal disease. Jaw findings occur late and indicate more serious skeletal involvement. This complication can be monitored via dental radiographs and is preventable to an extent with proper calcium and phosphate balance. Dental management of the renal patient is complicated due to the physiologic and psychologic problems in these patients.

Dental appointments must be timed with regard to dialysis therapy. Treatment modalities and the medications used must be altered depending on the physical status of the patient. Although most patients with renal failure can be managed in the office setting, hospital dental care may be required in order to provide the appropriate treatment.

BIBLIOGRAPHY

Alexander, R.E.: Hepatitis risk: a clinical perspective, J. Am. Dent. Assoc. **101**:182, 1981.

Bennett, W.M., Singer, I., and Coggins, J.: A guide to drug therapy in renal failure, J.A.M.A. **230**:1544, 1974.

Cappellini, G., and others: Temporomandibular joint changes in renal osteodystrophy, Radiol. Clin. **47**:330, 1978.

The choice of antimicrobial drugs, Med. Letter **549**(22):9, 1980.

Chow, M., and Peterson, D.: Dental management for children with chronic renal failure undergoing hemodialysis therapy, Oral Surg. **48**(1):34, 1979.

Clausen, F., and Poulsen, H.: Metastatic carcinoma to the jaws, Acta Pathol. Microbiol. Scand. **57**:361, 1963.

Comore, B., Collins, L., and Crane, M.: Internal medicine in dental practice, Philadelphia, 1943, Lea & Febiger.

Covino, B.G., and Vassallo, H.G.: Local anesthetics: mechanisms of action and clinical use: the scientific basis of clinical anesthesia series, New York, 1976, Grune & Stratton, Inc.

Epstein, S.R., Mandel, I., and Scopp, I.W.: Salivary composition and calculus formation in patients undergoing hemodialysis, J. Periodontol. **51**:336, 1980.

Fletcher, P., Scopp, I., and Hersh, R.: Oral manifestations of secondary hyperparathyroidism related to long term hemodialysis, Oral Surg. **43**(2):1218, 1977.

Gorlin, R.J., Pindborg, J.J., and Cohen, M.M., Jr.: Syndromes of the head and neck, ed.2, New York, 1976, McGraw-Hill Book Co.

Greenberg, M., and Cohen, G.: Oral infection in immunosuppressed renal transplant patients, Oral Surg. **43**(6):874, 1977.

Guttman, R.D.: Renal transplantation, N. Engl. J. Med. **301**:975, 1979.

Heard, E., Jr., Staples, A.F., and Czerwinski, A.W.: The dental patient with renal disease: precautions and guidelines, J. Am. Dent. Assoc. **96**:792, 1978.

Hovinga, J., Roudvoets, A.P., and Gaillard, J.: Some findings in patients uraemic stomatitis, Dent. Health **17**:15, 1978.

Kelly, W.H., and others: Radiographic changes of the jawbones in end stage renal disease, Oral. Surg. **50**:372, 1980.

Krekeler, G., Wilms, H., and Akuamoa-Boateng, E.: Inflammatory pathology in the dental system in renal transplantation, Int. J. Oral Surg. **9**:383, 1980.

Payne, W., and others: Reconstruction of the temporomandibular joints in a patient with renal osteodystrophy, J. Oral Surg. **35**:394, 1977.

Potter, J.L., and Wilson, N.H.F.: A dental survey of renal dialysis patients, Public Health, **93**:153, 1979.

Shafer, W., Hine, M., and Levy, B.: Oral pathology, Philadelphia, 1974, W.B. Saunders Co.

Sowell, S.B.: Dental care for patients with renal failure and renal transplants, J. Am. Dent. Assoc. **104**:171, 1982.

Spolnick, K.J., and others: Dental radiographic manifestations of end-stage renal disease, Dent. Rad. Photog. **54**:21, 1981.

Thoma, K.H.: Oral Pathology, St. Louis, 1950, The C.V. Mosby Co.

Van Scoy, R.E., and Wilson, W.R.: Antimicrobial agents in patients with renal insufficiency, Mayo Clin. Proc. **52**:704, 1977.

Westbrook, S.D.: Dental management of patients receiving hemodialysis and kidney transplants, J. Am. Dent. Assoc. **96**:464, 1978.

Wintrobe, M.M., and others: Clinical hematology, ed. 7, Philadelphia, 1974, Lea & Febiger.

Section Nine
RESPIRATORY DISEASES
edited by **William L. Morrissey**

121 • INTRODUCTION TO THE RESPIRATORY SYSTEM
Sanford Levine and **Samuel T. Kuna**

DEFINITIONS

"Respiration" can be defined as those processes concerned with gas exchange between an organism and its environment. The term "respiratory system" is used to describe the organs and tissues involved in the process of respiration: the nose, mouth, oropharynx, extrapulmonary airways, thoracic cage, respiratory muscles, pleura, lungs, nerves, spinal cord, brain, and cardiovascular system. In this chapter, discussion of pathologic conditions of the respiratory system is restricted to the extrapulmonary and intrapulmonary airways, lungs, pleura, chest wall, and muscles of respiration.

OVERVIEW OF RESPIRATION

The major function of the lung is to add oxygen to and remove carbon dioxide from venous blood. To accomplish this task, the lung is composed of two different conducting systems: a gas-conducting system and a blood-conducting system. The gas-conducting system terminates in blind pouches, or alveoli; the major function of the gas-conducting system is to maintain gas tensions in these alveoli in the direction of ambient gas. The blood-conducting system transports venous blood to alveolar walls; this venous blood in alveolar walls is contained in thin-walled exchange vessels, or pulmonary capillaries. The surface area of the pulmonary capillary-alveolar interface constitutes the major area of gas exchange. In adults the surface area of this interface is about 70 m^2, or approximately 40 times the surface area of the body. To further facilitate gas transfer between alveoli and pulmonary capillary blood, the membrane separating these structures is only 1 or 2 μm thick.

The gas-conducting system begins at the two nasal passages (sometimes a third passage, the mouth, is also used), which subsequently merge into one tube, the trachea. The trachea subdivides into two main branches, the left and right mainstem bronchi. Each mainstem bronchus passes to its corresponding lung (for example, the left mainstem bronchus to the left lung) and then has 20 to 33 further subdivisions (or bifurcations). These subdivisions have about 1 million terminal conducting tubes, and the 300 million alveoli (the number in the two lungs of adults) arise from these terminal conducting tubes. The diameters of the alveoli range from 75 to 300 μm.

During quiet breathing the diaphragm is the principal muscle of inspiration and accounts for the movement of more than two thirds of the air that enters the lung. Contraction of the diaphragm causes its domes to descend and the chest to expand longitudinally. At the same time, because of the vertically oriented attachment of the diaphragm to the costal margins, its contractions also elevate the lower ribs.

Contraction of the intercostal muscles (external intercostal and parasternal intercartilaginous muscles) also raises the ribs during inspiration. As the ribs are elevated, the anteroposterior and transverse dimensions of the thorax enlarge because of the pattern of movement of the ribs around the axes of their necks. Upward displacement of the upper ribs is accompanied by an increase in the anteroposterior dimension, whereas elevation of the lower ribs is associated with an increase in the transverse dimension of the chest.

In addition to the diaphragm and intercostal muscles, other inspiratory mucles may also play a role in enlarging the thorax in certain circumstances. The scalene muscles make their major contribution during high levels of ventilation when the upper parts of the thorax must be enlarged. These muscles arise from the transverse processes of the lower five cervical vertebrae and insert into the upper aspect of the first and second ribs. Contraction of these muscles elevates and fixes the uppermost part of the rib cage.

Another accessory muscle, the sternocleidomastoid, normally becomes active only at high levels of ventilation. Contraction of the sternocleidomastoid muscle is frequently apparent during severe asthmatic or bronchitic episodes. The sternocleidomastoid muscle elevates the sternum and slightly enlarges the anteroposterior and longitudinal dimensions of the chest.

In contrast to inspiration, expiration during quiet breathing occurs passively as a result of lung recoil. However, expiration does not become active at higher levels of ventilation and when movement of air out of the lungs is impeded. The muscles involved in active expiration include the internal intercostal muscles and the transversus and rectus abdominis muscles, which compress the abdominal contents, depress the lower ribs, and pull down the anterior part of the lower chest.

TOTAL VENTILATION VERSUS ALVEOLAR VENTILATION

Total ventilation is the volume of air entering or leaving the respiratory system during each breath (tidal volume) or each minute (minute ventilation or minute volume).

Alveolar ventilation is the volume of gas entering the alveoli during each breath or each minute. This gas entering the alveoli arises from two sources. In early inspiration the alveoli are filled with gas remaining in the conducting airways after the last expiration, whereas during the latter portion of inspiration, freshly inspired gas enters the alveoli. Alveolar ventilation is always less than total ventilation; the difference between the two depends on the anatomic dead space (the internal volume of the conducting airways), tidal volume, and respiratory frequency.

ALVEOLAR VENTILATION AND ARTERIAL CARBON DIOXIDE TENSION

The following relationship exists between alveolar ventilation, arterial carbon dioxide tension ($PaCO_2$), and CO_2 production:

$$PaCO_2 \propto \frac{CO_2 \text{ production}}{\text{Alveolar ventilation}}$$

This indicates that $PaCO_2$ represents a quantitative statement of the ratio between tissue CO_2 production and alveolar ventilation. Strictly speaking,

$$PaCO_2 \text{ in mm Hg} = \frac{CO_2 \text{ production} \times 0.863}{\text{Alveolar ventilation}}$$

where CO_2 production is stated in milliliters per minute at standard temperature and pressure of dry gas (STPD), and alveolar ventilation is stated in milliliters of gas per minute at body temperature and pressure saturated with water vapor (BTPS). In normal humans at sea level, a $PaCO_2$ of 36 to 42 mm Hg represents an appropriate value. The terms "hypoventilation" and "hyperventilation" are used to describe abnormal relationships between alveolar ventilation and tissue CO_2 production. Hypoventilation is characterized by an increase in $PaCO_2$ (that is, greater than 42 mm Hg); this disorder indicates a decrease in alveolar ventilation per unit of CO_2 production. In contrast, hyperventilation is characterized by a decrease in $PaCO_2$ (that is, less than 36 mm Hg); this latter disorder exhibits an increase in alveolar ventilation per unit of CO_2 production.

Some clinicians erroneously use $PaCO_2$ as a quantitative measure of alveolar ventilation, believing that a constant $PaCO_2$ implies no change in alveolar ventilation. This generalization is true only for circumstances in which tissue CO_2 production remains constant. However, during moderate muscular exercise an unchanged $PaCO_2$ accompanies twofold to sixfold increases in both alveolar ventilation and tissue CO_2 production.

COMPOSITION OF ALVEOLAR GAS AND ARTERIAL OXYGEN TENSION

Alveolar gas can be thought of as a compartment of gas lying between atmospheric air and alveolar capillary blood. O_2 is continuously added to it by blood flowing through alveolar capillaries. Alveolar gas tensions (PAO_2, $PACO_2$) exhibit three important phenomena: (1) in each alveolus the gas tensions vary throughout every breath; PO_2 is highest and PCO_2 is lowest at end-inspiration; (2) in the same alveolus gas tensions vary from breath to breath; and (3) considerable differences exist in gas tensions between different alveoli.

Despite these statements about the heterogeneity of alveolar gas, calculation of the *mean* PAO_2 is useful. Even in normal subjects, mean PAO_2 is always greater than PaO_2. The difference between alveolar and arterial PO_2 is termed the "alveolar-arterial (A-a) O_2 tension difference," or $P(A-a)O_2$; it is a measure of the lung's efficiency in tranferring O_2 between the alveolus and blood. In normal young subjects breathing room air the $P(A-a)O_2$ is usually less than 12 mm Hg, whereas in patients with lung disease this difference is greater than 15 mm Hg. When patients with lung disease hyperventilate, their PaO_2 is sometimes raised to normal values; however, their $P(A-a)O_2$ remains abnormally high (greater than 15 mm Hg).

Calculation of mean PAO_2

An approximate clinical method of calculating mean PAO_2 is as follows:

$$PAO_2 = PIO_2 - \frac{PaCO_2}{R}$$

where

PAO_2 = Mean alveolar PO_2
PIO_2 = Moist inspired PO_2, that is, $FIO_2 \times$ (barometric pressure − water vapor pressure)
$PaCO_2$ = Mean arterial PCO_2
R = Respiratory exchange ratio, that is, milliliters of CO_2 excreted/milliliters of O_2 uptake
FIO_2 = Fractional concentration of O_2 in inspired gas

For normal humans in steady-state conditions at sea level, the PIO_2 of moist inspired air (that is, tracheal gas) is approximately 150 mm Hg. $PaCO_2$ approximates 40 mm Hg, and R varies between 1.0 and 0.7. For an R of 1.0, PAO_2 = 110 mm Hg, whereas an R of 0.7 results in a PAO_2 of 93 mm Hg. For clinical purposes an R of 0.8 is usually assumed.

PULMONARY PERFUSION

The lung has a dual blood supply: the pulmonary circulation and bronchial circulation. Bronchial arteries arise from the thoracic aorta and hence have systematic pressures. They perfuse the tracheobronchial tree and anastomose with the pulmonary circulation. Most hemoptysis is caused by abnormalities of the tracheobronchial tree and represents bleeding from the bronchial circulation. Some of the blood in the bronchial circulation does not come into contact with the alveoli and is desaturated when it enters the left atrium. Blood from the bronchial circulation and the thebesian veins of the left ventricle accounts for the normal right-to-left anatomic shunt that is about 6% of the resting cardiac output.

The pulmonary circulation arises from the right ventricle. It is a low-pressure system. The normal pulmonary artery pressure (PAP) is 20/10 mm Hg with a mean of 14 mm Hg. Although the pulmonary circulation has almost the same blood flow as the systemic circulation, the pressures are lower in the former because of the low pulmonary vascular resistance (PVR). The normal PVR is less than 1 mm Hg/L/sec and is less than 10% of systemic vascular resistance. With increases in pulmonary blood flow, as during exercise, there is a decrease in PVR and only a slight increase in mean PAP. This decrease in PVR results from an increase in the total cross-sectional area of the vascular bed from distention of vessels that already contain circulating blood and recruitment of previously collapsed vessels. The ability of the pulmonary circulation to adapt to changes in blood flow is dramatically demonstrated after a pneumonectomy. Despite doubling of blood flow to the remaining normal lung, PAP remains normal. Greater than a 50% obliteration of the pulmonary vascular tree must occur to be the sole cause of increased PAP. Other factors that can cause an increase in PAP are (1) increased left atrial pressure, (2) alveolar hypoxia, (3) acidemia, and (4) humoral substances such as histamine, catecholamines, and angiotensin. Release of these humoral substances is the proposed mechanism for the rise in PAP after major pulmonary emboli that occlude less than 50% of the pulmonary vascular bed.

RELATIONSHIP BETWEEN ALVEOLAR VENTILATION AND PULMONARY CAPILLARY BLOOD FLOW
Distribution of pulmonary capillary blood flow

Gravity plays a major role in the distribution of pulmonary capillary blood flow. In the upright human lung, capillary blood flow decreases almost linearly from bottom to top. When the subject lies supine, the apical zone blood flow increases significantly, and the blood flow distribution from the apex to base becomes fairly uniform. However, in this posture, blood flow in the posterior (dependent) regions of the lung exceeds flow in the anterior parts. Measurements on human subjects suspended upside down show that apical blood flow exceeds basal blood flow in this position.

The role of gravity in accounting for the vertical distribution of pulmonary capillary blood flow in upright humans can be explained by hydrostatic pressure differences in the pulmonary blood vessels. Viewing the pulmonary arterial system as a continuous column of blood, the difference in pressure between the top and bottom of a vertically suspended lung 30 cm high is about 30 cm of water, or 23 mm Hg. This is a large pressure difference for the low-pressure pulmonary circulation (normal pressure = 20/10), and its effects account for the distribution of pulmonary capillary blood flow in the upright position.

Distribution of alveolar ventilation

Not all alveoli are uniformly ventilated in the lungs of humans. Some alveoli are hyperventilated, whereas others are hypoventilated. The presence of nonuniform alveolar ventilation can be demonstrated by many tests, such as nitrogen washout, closing volume, and radionuclide techniques.

Matching of alveolar ventilation and pulmonary capillary blood flow

For the entire respiratory system, the matching of alveolar ventilation to pulmonary capillary blood flow is usually quantitated by the ventilation-perfusion ratio ($\dot{V}_A/\dot{Q}_C$). In healthy humans under basal conditions (that is, 4 L/min of alveolar ventilation and 5 L/min of pulmonary blood flow), the $\dot{V}_A/\dot{Q}_C$ for the entire respiratory system is 0.8.

Just as there is a $\dot{V}_A/\dot{Q}_C$ ratio for the entire respiratory system, each of the 300 million alveoli in the two lungs has its own $\dot{V}_A/\dot{Q}_C$ ratio. The $\dot{V}_A/\dot{Q}_C$ of each alveolus is determined by the ratio of ventilation to blood flow for that alveolus. Fig. 121-1 presents a schematic diagram of three representative alveoli. Alveolus B has a normal $\dot{V}_A/\dot{Q}_C$ ratio, approximately 0.8. In Fig. 121-1 this alveolus has a P_{O_2} of 100 mm Hg and a P_{CO_2} of 40 mm Hg. Alveolus A is distal to an obstructed bronchus; since this alveolus is not ventilated, it has a $\dot{V}_A/\dot{Q}_C$ ratio of 0. The gas tensions in this alveolus are in equilibrium with mixed venous blood; the P_{O_2} is 40 mm Hg and the P_{CO_2} is 45 mm Hg. Perfusion has been eliminated in alveolus C; since this alveolus is not perfused, its $\dot{V}_A/\dot{Q}_C$ ratio is infinite. The gas tensions in this alveolus are identical to those in moist ambient gas; the P_{O_2} is 150 mm Hg and the P_{CO_2} is 0 mm Hg. Even in the normal individuals there may be a few alveoli with a ratio of 0 or infinity, but the majority are close to four fifths, or 0.8. Patients with pulmonary disease have more alveoli with a ratio of 0 or infinity and many more that deviate significantly from 0.8.

Effects of $\dot{V}_A/\dot{Q}_C$ abnormalities on Pa_{CO_2}

Fig. 121-2, A, indicates that over the physiologic range, a linear relationship exists in blood between P_{CO_2} and CO_2 content. Alveoli with infinite $\dot{V}_A/\dot{Q}_C$ ratios have no blood flow and therefore play no role in determining Pa_{CO_2}. However, alveoli with high $\dot{V}_A/\dot{Q}_C$ ratios are extremely effective. Alveoli with high $\dot{V}_A/\dot{Q}_C$ ratios can

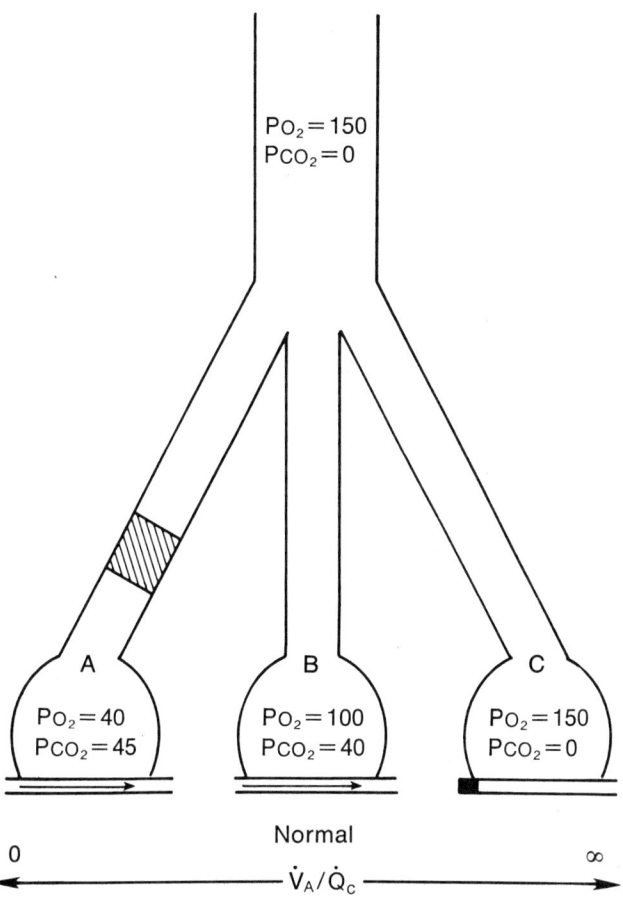

Fig. 121-1. Relationships of alveolar ventilation to pulmonary capillary blood flow ($\dot{V}_A/\dot{Q}_C$).

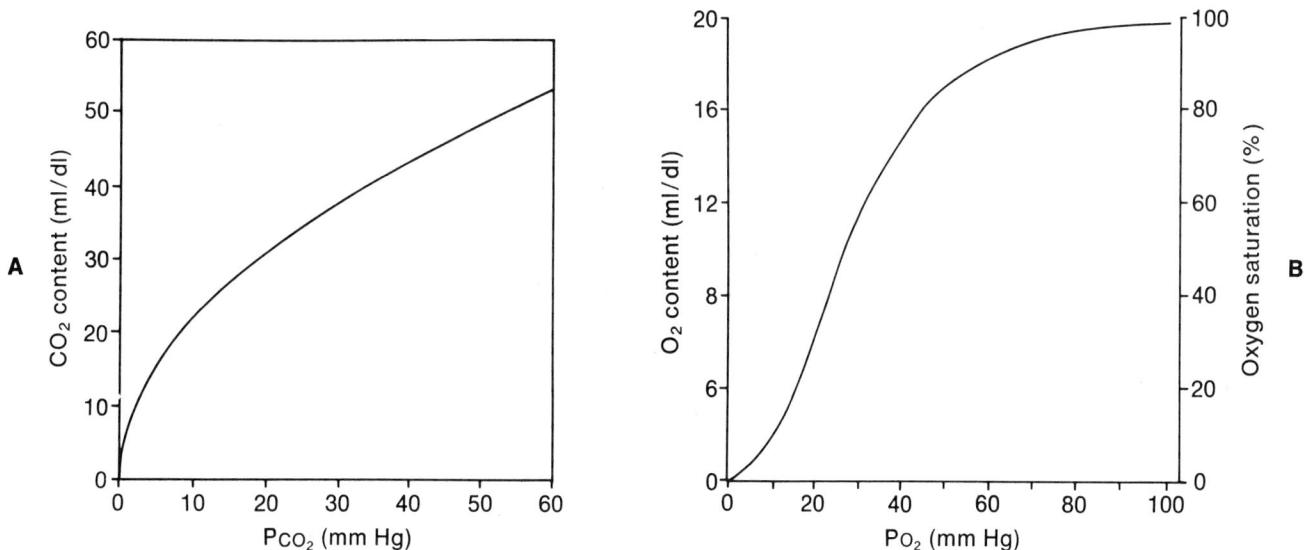

Fig. 121-2. Relationship between gas contents and partial pressure. **A,** Relationship between P_{CO_2} (abscissa) and CO_2 content (ordinate). **B,** Relationship between P_{O_2} (abscissa) and O_2 content and percent of saturation (ordinate). O_2 content data assume 15 g hemoglobin/dl blood.

compensate for alveoli with low $\dot{V}_A/\dot{Q}_C$ ratios with respect to pulmonary CO_2 elimination and thereby maintain a normal $Paco_2$.

Effects of ventilation-perfusion abnormalities on Pao_2

Alveoli with low $\dot{V}_A/\dot{Q}_C$ ratios cause arteria hypoxemia regardless of the presence of alveoli with high $\dot{V}_A/\dot{Q}_C$ ratios. Fig. 121-2, B, shows the oxyhemoglobin dissociation curve. Because of the nonlinear shape of this curve, the decrement in arterial blood O_2 content caused by alveoli with low Po_2 cannot be compensated for by alveoli with relatively high Po_2.

ROLE OF DIFFUSION IN ALVEOLAR-CAPILLARY GAS TRANSFER

Diffusion is the process by which gas transfer occurs between the alveolus and the capillary; it is determined by the following variables: surface area of the alveolar-capillary membrane, thickness of the alveolar-capillary membrane, and difference in partial pressure between the two sides of the membrane (that is, the alveolar-capillary gradient). Decreases in tissue surface area of the alveolar-capillary membrane, increases in thickness of this membrane, and decreases in the alveolar-capillary gradient all decrease the rate of gas transfer between the alveolus and pulmonary capillary. This rate of gas trnasfer is also proportional to a diffision constant that depends on the properties of the tissue and the particular gas.

Under resting conditions the red blood cell (RBC) spends about 0.75 second in its passage through the pulmonary capillary. The Po_2 in an RBC entering the pulmonary capillar is about 40 mm Hg. Since the alveolar Po_2 is 100 mm Hg, this large pressure difference causes the Po_2 in the RBC to rise rapidly; RBC Po_2 very nearly reaches Pao_2 by the time the RBC is one third of its way along the capillary. Under normal circumststances there is no measurable Po_2 difference between alveolar gas and end-capillary pulmonary blood; therefore diffusion is not a rate-limiting factor in alveolar-capillary O_2 exchange in resting humans.

During severe exercise the time spent by the RBC in the pulmonary capillary may diminish to 0.25 second. Therefore the time available for oxygenation is less, but in normal subjects breathing ambient air there is still no alveolar—end pulmonary capillary Po_2 gradient. However, if the alveolar-capillary membrane is abnormal (thickened), the rate of transfer of O_2 across the alveolar-capillary membrane occurs at a slower rate and the end-capillary RBC Po_2 may be less than the Pao_2, in this case, diffision constitutes a rate-limiting process in oxygenating pulmonary capillary blood.

Another method of demonstrating diffusion limitation of O_2 transfer to reduce Pao_2 (for example, to 50 mm Hg). In this case the Po_2 of RBCs entering the pulmonary capillaries may be only about 20 mm Hg; however, the alveolar-capillary O_2 gradient has been reduced from a normal of 60 mm Hg to 30 mm Hg. Therefore the rate of transfer of O_2 occurs at a slower rate. In the normal individual an alveolar–end capillary Po_2 gradient may not occur under these circumstances: however, in cases in which the alveolar-capillary membrane is abnormal, end-capillary Po_2 is less than Pao_2. Thus once again in the abnormal lung, diffusion constitutes a rate-limiting process in oxgyenating pulmonary capillary blood.

The role of diffusion as a rate-limiting factor in the oxygenation of pulmonary capillary blood in normal subjects remains controversial. However, some authorities believe that exhausting exercise at high altitudes (that is, hypoxic conditions) constitutes a situation in which diffusion impairment of O_2 transfer can be demonstrated in normal humans. Therefore it follows that an individual with an abnormal blood gas barrier would probably show diffusion impairment of oxygenation in the laboratory while breathing hypoxic gas mixtures during exercise.

Measurements of diffusing capacity

Carbon monoxide (CO) is generally used in diffusion capacity measurements because it provides certain technical advantages; in addition, this gas is transported and absorbed in the same manner as O_2. The CO diffusing capacity (D_{LCO}) is equal to CO uptake per minute divided by the mean pressure gradient for CO between alveolar gas (P_{ACO}) and pulmonary capillary blood.

Clinical relevance of D_{LCO}

The major clinical problem with D_{LCO} is that it is not a specific test of abnormality of the alveolar-capillary membrane: for example, a patient who has undergone a pneumonectomy with no obvious pathologic condition in the remaining lung has a significant decrease in D_{LCO}. After many years of use, most experts now agree that D_{LCO} is affected by the following variables: lung volume, pulmonary capillary blood volume, blood hemoglobin concentration, and $\dot{V}_A/\dot{Q}_C$ mismatch. Decreases in lung volumes, pulmonary capillary blood volume, and hemoglobin concentration all decrease D_{LCO}; increases in $\dot{V}_A/\dot{Q}_C$ mismatch also decrease D_{LCO}. Because so many pathologic processes other than diffusion can cause decreases in D_{LCO}, the British literature uses the less specific term ''CO transfer factor'' rather than ''diffusing capacity.''

The precise relationship between decreases in D_{LCO} and resting arterial hypoxemia remains somewhat controversial. However, most authorities believe that patients with interstitial lung disease without obvious $\dot{V}_A/\dot{Q}_C$ abnormalities can show decreases in D_{LCO} in the absence of resting arterial hypoxemia.

CONTROL OF VENTILATION

The respiratory center in the medulla oblongata regulates the neural drive to the muscles of ventilation; the output from this center is modulated by multiple inputs. Afferents from the cerebral cortex can bring ventilation under conscious control. Other afferents relay information about the effectiveness of gas exchange by monitoring the tensions of O_2 and CO_2 in arterial blood. The input from these chemoreceptors is referred to as the chemical drive to ventilation. The PO_2 of arterial blood is monitored by the carotid and aortic bodies. This information is transmitted to the brain via the glossopharyngeal and vagus nerves. Removal of the carotid bodies in humans ablates the ventilatory response to arterial hypoxia. However, although both the carotid and aortic bodies respond to increases in arterial PCO_2, removal of these structures does not ablate the ventilatory response to hypercapnia; the reason for this is that an important CO_2 or H^+ receptor is located on the surface of the medulla oblogata.

Receptors in the trachea and lungs transmit information about the mechanical state of the lung to the respiratory center via the vagus nerves and spinal cord. Receptors innervated by the vagus nerves include irritant receptors, stretch receptors, and J receptors; inputs from these receptors constitute the mechanical drive to ventilation. In the absence of an increased chemical drive to ventilation, an increased mechanical drive may explain the tachypnea seen in lung disorders such as pulmonary edema and asthma.

EVALUATION OF PULMONARY PERFORMANCE
Measurement of lung volumes and capacities

Fig. 121-3 presents a schematic diagram of the lung volumes and capacities. When the lungs are fully expanded the amount of gas they contain is called the total lung capacity (TLC), TLC is determined by the point at which the pressure developed by the inspiratory muscles is equal and opposite to the combined recoil pressures of the lungs and chest wall (principally the lungs, which become very stiff at high lung volumes). Loss of lung recoil in conditions such as emphysema allows the inspiratory muscles to shorten further, resulting in increased TLC.

Vital capacity (VC) is defined as the amount of gas that a person can exhale from TLC. The VC is always decreased in restrictive ventilatory disorders (such as pulmonary fibrosis), and it may or may not be decreased in obstructive pulmonary disease.

Residual volume (RV) is the amount of gas remaining in the lung at the end of a maximal expiration. In young individuals the RV is determined by the point at which the inward pressure developed by the expiratory muscles and the lung is equal and opposite to the outward recoil of the chest wall. (Actually at RV the inward recoil pressure of the lung is quite small; on the other hand, the outward recoil of the chest wall is large.) In older persons the RV is governed mainly by factors that regulate the caliber and patency of peripheral airways: thus even though the expiratory muscles are capable of greater thoracic compres-

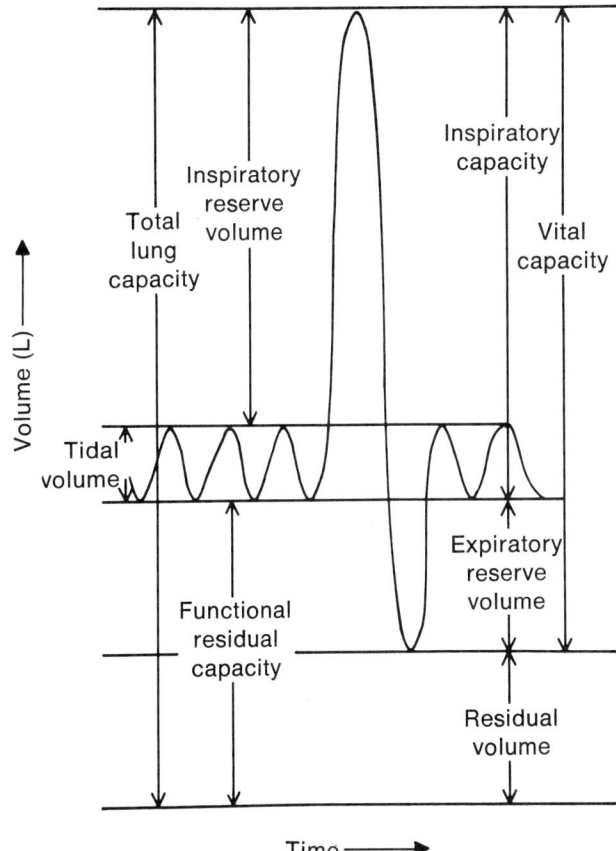

Fig. 121-3. Lung volumes and capacities.

sion, further exhalation of gas is prevented by airway closure.

Lung volumes and capacities vary among healthy persons according to their age, sex, and physical characteristics (especially height). Because body build varies slightly from one ethnic group to another, it is important to have normal data that pertain to the population being studied. Measured lung volumes and capacities are usually expressed as both the observed value and the percentage of the predicted value for a normal subject of the same age, sex, and height:

$$\text{Percent predicted} = \frac{\text{Observed value}}{\text{Predicted value}} \times 100$$

Measured values for lung volumes and capacities should not be considered abnormal unless they are clearly outside the range of values likely to be found in normal persons (100% ± 20% for VC, TLC, and RV).

Measurement of the forced expiratory vital capacity

Measurement of the forced expiratory vital capacity (FVC) is probably the most commonly used test of pulmonary performance. In this test the subject (wearing

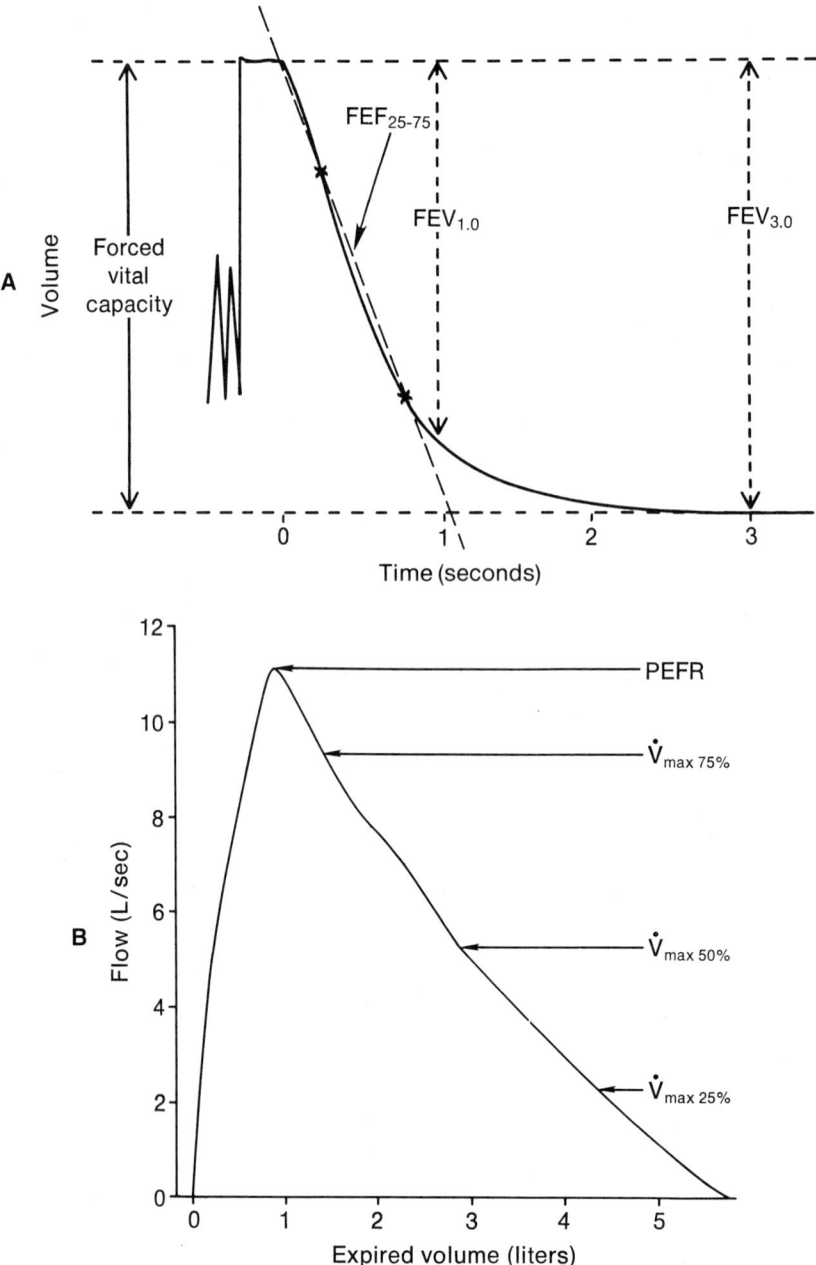

Fig. 121-4. Forced expiratory vital capacities. **A,** Volume-time representation, FEF_{22-75} mean flow rate between 25% and 75% of vital capacity; $FEV_{1.0}$ forced expired volume in 1 second; $FEV_{3.0}$ forced expired volume in 3 seconds. **B,** Flow-volume representation of forced expiratory vital capacity. *PEFR,* peak expiratory flow rate; other markings on flow-volume loop indicate maximal flow rates at 75% of FVC($V_{max75\%}$). 50% of FVC ($V_{max50\%}$). and 25% of FVC ($V_{max25\%}$).

noseclips) inspires maximally to TLC and then forcefully expires into a spirometer until RV is reached. The most commonly used spirometer, the water-filled spirometer, presents a record of volume on the ordinary versus time on the abscissa; Fig. 121-4, *A,* presents a representative volume-time record of an FVC of a normal subject. In normal persons the FVC equals the VC from a slow or nonexpulsive maneuver. However, in patients with obstructive airways disease, vigorous expiration may cause airways to narrow or close so that the FVC may be less than the slow VC.

Additional information about airway function can be obtained from the forced expiratory volume in 1 second ($FEV_{1.0}$), the forced expiratory volume in 3 seconds ($FEV_{3.0}$), and the flow rate between 25% and 75% of the VC (FEF_{25-75}). The volume-time plot in Fig. 121-4, *A,* shows all of these measurements. In normal individuals the ratio between $FEV_{1.0}$ and FVC ($FEV_{1.0}$/FVC) is greater than 75% and the ratio between $FEV_{3.0}$ and FVC ($FEV_{3.0}$/FVC) is greater than 97%. In patients with obstructive pulmonary disorders, $FEV_{1.0}$/FVC is less than 75%, $FEV_{3.0}$/FVC is less than 97%, and FEF_{25-75} is appreciably less than the predicted normal measurement.

Other types of spirometers (such as a rolling seal) present a recording of flow on the ordinate versus volume on the abscissa: Fig. 121-4, *B*, presents a representative flow-volume record of an FVC of a normal subject. The markings on this diagram indicate peak expiratory flow rate (PEFR) and maximal flow rates at 75% of FVC ($V_{max\ 75\%}$), 50% of FVC ($V_{max\ 50\%}$), and 25% of FVC ($V_{max\ 25\%}$). From the flow-volume loop, all of the maximal flow rates at any fraction of the VC can be determined and reported as percentages of the predicted values for a subject of the same age, sex, and body size.

The early portion of the maximal expiratory flow-volume curve, which includes peak flow and probably $V_{max\ 75\%}$, is determined largely by the effort exerted by the subject and is called the effort-dependent segment. Below 75% of the VC, increasing expiratory effort fails to augment the velocity of airflow; therefore this latter portion is called the effort-independent segment. Effort independence of expiratory flow (at intermediate and low lung volumes) is explained by a combination of circumstances through which increasing expiratory effort narrows airways by the phenomenon of dynamic compression and increases airway resistance by the amount necessary to offset the effect of the increased driving pressure.

Measurement of functional residual capacity

Functional residual capacity (FRC) is the volume of gas remaining in the lungs at the end of a normal expiration. At present, two techniques are used to measure FRC: inert gas dilution and body plethysmography.

The closed-circuit helium dilution method is the most commonly employed inert gas dilution method. In this method a spirometer is initially filled with a mixture of approximately 10% helium in air. Starting precisely at FRC, the patient begins to breath from the closed spirometer system. The spirometer contains a CO_2 scrubber to absorb all the CO_2 produced by the patient. This scrubbing of CO_2 would decrease the total volume of gas in the spirometer; however, O_2 is added by the operator to maintain a constant volume. As the helium in the spirometer mixes with the gas in the patient's lungs, the concentration of helium continuously falls until a constant level is achieved. Since helium does not cross the alveolar-capillary membrane, the total volume of helium in the patient's lungs plus the spirometer system does not change during the rebreathing period. Therefore the initial concentration of helium multiplied by the initial volume of the spirometer system must equal the final concentration of helium multiplied by the total volume of the spirometer-patient system at the end of the test (that is, the sum of the patient's FRC and the final volume of gas in the spirometer system). The patient's FRC can be easily computed from the relationship previously noted. However, FRC measurements by all of the inert gas dilution techniques measure only the volume of gas that freely communicates with the airways during the breathing maneuver; dilution techniques do not detect gas trapped beyond closed (or narrowed) airways and in poorly communicating regions such as those with bullae.

Body plethysmography involves placing the patient in the plethysmograph, a large, airtight box resembling a telephone booth. The patient initially breathes through a mouthpiece, which is then occluded by a shutter at the end of a normal expiration (that is, FRC). The subject then pants against the occluded mouthpiece. During panting, with its associated thoracic volume changes, pressure is measured at the mouth and in the plethysmograph; changes in the plethysmograph pressure reflect changes in thoracic volume. From application of Boyle's law, which states that the pressure times the volume of gas is constant if the temperature remains the same, the volume of gas in the thorax can be calculated. The body plethysmograph measures all of the gas present during breathing, including that in feely communicating airspaces and any that may be trapped behind poorly communicating airways or in closed spaces (pneumothorax).

At FRC the inward recoil pressure of the lungs is equal but opposite to the outward recoil pressure of the chest wall. Therefore the FRC is reduced by conditions characterized by an increased recoil pressure of the lungs (such as pulmonary fibrosis); similarly, the FRC is increased in conditions characterized by a decreased recoil pressure of the lungs (such as emphysema).

Exercise testing

Muscle O_2 consumption and CO_2 production increase greatly during exercise. Coincident with these alterations in muscle metabolism, mixed venous blood shows decreases in Po_2 and increases in Pco_2. In addition, the time that a given volume of blood spends in the pulmonary capillary is significantly decreased. Nonetheless, the normal respiratory system maintains Pao_2 at resting levels and $Paco_2$ at or below resting levels. Exercise-induced hypoxemia is commonly the first abnormality noted in early interstitial lung disease; this abnormality is a good indicator for evaluating therapy in interstitial lung disease. Many patients with obstructive lung disease also manifest exercise-induced arterial hypoxemia. Last, in all types of lung disease, exercise testing provides the physician with objective measurements of work tolerance (such as maximal O_2 consumption); these measurements should enable the physician to provide better occupational guidance to the patient.

Airway resistance

The driving pressure producing airflow along the tracheobronchial tree is the difference between alveolar pressure and pressure at the airway opening. Airway resistance (R_{aw}) is defined as the quotient of driving pressure divided by the rate of airflow. Resistance to airflow is affected chiefly by the caliber of the airways. R_{aw} is measured in a plethysmograph similar to that used for FRC determinations.

The diameter of individual members of each successive generation of airways decreases from the trachea to the peripheral airways. However, the total cross-sectional area of the tracheobronchial tree progressively increases from the trachea to the peripheral airways. These anatomic observations indicate that most of the resistance of the human tracheobronchial tree resides in large airways; direct measurements reveal that about 80% of total R_{aw} originates in airways greater than 2 mm in diameter. A corollary of this observation is that decreases can occur in the caliber of the small peripheral airways (that is, less than 2 mm), without having much effect on total R_{aw}. Therefore small peripheral airways are sometimes referred to as the lung's "quiet zone."

Changes in the cross-sectional area of the airways can be effected by the following mechanisms (1) changes in lung volume, (2) diseases of the lung parenchyma, and (3) diseases of the airways. First, the caliber of individual airways progressively increases as the subject approaches TLC; conversely, airway caliber decreases as the subject approaches RV. The reason underlying this association between airway caliber and lung volume is that lung parenchyma normally serves as radial supports to maintain the patency of airways: at high lung volumes these tethers are taut, increasing the elastic recoil of the lung and maintaining the airways in a fully patent state. However, at low lung volumes the tethers are lax, decreasing the elastic recoil of the lung and allowing the airways to be partially collapsed. In diseases such as emphysema the airways are not maintained in a fully patent state because of a decrease in elastic recoil of the lung at any given lung volume. Airway narrowing can also result from bronchospasm, edema of the mucosal lining, and secretions within the lumen.

CATEGORIZATION OF LUNG DISEASE

Lung diseases that cause abnormalities of ventilation are usually divided into two categories: restrictive and obstructive ventilatory disorders. It has been pointed out that this classification is somewhat unsatisfactory, since it ignores the fact that disturbances of the distribution of ventilation are the earliest and probably the most common abnormality of ventilation. Moreover, abnormalities in the distribution of ventilation can occur in the absence of manifestations of either obstructive or restrictive disorders. Table 121-1 presents characteristic changes in both lung volumes and flow rates in patients with restrictive and obstructive ventilatory disorders.

Table 121-1. Characteristic changes in lung capacities, volumes, and forced expiratory spirograms in patients with restrictive and obstructive ventilatory disorders

Test	Restrictive	Obstructive
FVC	Decreased	Decreased or normal
RV	Decreased	Increased
TLC	Decreased	Normal or increased
RV/TLC	Normal or increased	Significantly increased
$FEV_{1.0}$/FVC	Normal or increased	Decreased
$FEV_{3.0}$/FVC	Normal or increased	Decreased
FEF_{25-75}	Normal or decreased	Decreased

Restrictive ventilatory disorders

Restrictive ventilatory disorders are characterized by reductions in lung volumes. The hallmark of restriction is a decreased VC and TLC. A decrease in VC also sometimes occurs in obstructive ventilatory disorders; therefore if only the VC is measured, the presence of airway obstruction must be ruled out by the ratios $FEV_{1.0}$/FVC and $FEV_{3.0}$/FVC.

Restrictive ventilatory disorders can develop in conditions that (1) affect the chest wall or respiratory muscles (myasthenia gravis), (2) cause infiltrates in the lung parenchyma or airspaces (diffuse interstitial fibrosis and pulmonary edema), (3) involve the pleura (pleural thickening), (4) occupy space within the thorax (tumors, effusions, and cardiac enlargement), and (5) occur after lung resection.

Obstructive ventilatory disorders

Obstructive ventilatory disorders are characterized by abnormalities in the FVC; an $FEV_{1.0}$/FVC ratio less than 75% is a widely used criterion for diagnosis of these disorders. However, maximal flow-volume relationships (particularly flow rates obtained at low lung volumes) are being increasingly used in the diagnosis of obstructive pulmonary disorders, and these relationships appear to be more sensitive for the early diagnosis of peripheral airway obstruction.

Obstructive ventilatory disorders are found in patients with asthma, bronchitis, emphysema, advanced bronchiectasis, and other diseases that cause narrowing of the tracheobronchial system. When the term "obstructive disorders" was originally coined, it was not possible to differentiate among these various entities; therefore they were lumped together in the nonspecific category of chronic obstructive pulmonary disease (COPD). However, specialized tests can now sort out these various diseases even when they coexist.

INITIAL EVALUATION OF ARTERIAL BLOOD GAS MEASUREMENTS

Blood gas measurements are subject to technical error, and therefore the physician must determine whether a given set of blood gas values is theoretically possible for the F_{IO_2} being delivered to the patient. As an example of this principle, we analyze the measurements of PaO_2 and $PaCO_2$ in a patient with severe COPD who was spontaneously breathing room air; in a measured blood sample PaO_2 = 80 mm Hg and $PaCO_2$ = 65 mm Hg. Assuming a respiratory exchange ratio (R) of 0.8 and substituting in the simplified alveolar air equation:

$$P_{AO_2} = 150 - 65/0.8 = 69 \text{ mm Hg}$$

The $P(A\text{-}a)O_2$ is determined as follows:

$$P(A\text{-}a)O_2 = 69 - 80 = -11 \text{ mm Hg}$$

Since the $P(A\text{-}a)O_2$ can never be negative, it is assumed that an error exists in the reported blood gas measurements. Although clinicians often blame the laboratory for such errors in blood gas determinations, faulty technique in drawing arterial blood gas specimens (such as allowing room air into the syringe) may be responsible for these erroneous measurements.

ARTERIAL HYPERCAPNIA

In determining a therapeutic approach to the patient with arterial hypercapnia, the physician must first determine if the arterial hypercapnia is acute or chronic and what deleterious effects (if any) the hypercapnia is causing.

Acute versus chronic arterial hypercapnia

Acute increases in $PaCO_2$ cause significant decreases in arterial pH levels. On the other hand, in response to chronic increases in $PaCO_2$, renal mechanisms increase the blood bicarbonate concentration; therefore chronic hypercapnia is accompanied by only a small decrease (if any) in arterial pH levels. Another excellent clue is provided by the patient's past record; did the patient have arterial hypercapnia when last discharged from the hospital or seen as an outpatient at the physician's office?

Patients with COPD commonly have acute hypercapnia superimposed on chronic hypercapnia. In these situations the patient's history, previous records, and nomograms (graphs showing the relationship between arterial pH levels and $PaCO_2$ for both acute and chronic hypercapnia) allow the physician to estimate the magnitude of the acute increase in $PaCO_2$.

Physical signs of hypercapnia

The clinical signs of hypercapnia are nonspecific, and these effects are often difficult to distinguish from those of hypoxemia in ventilatory failure. Minor degrees of hypercapnia usually produce an increase in systemic blood pressure, drowsiness, irritability, and headache. Significant elevations of $PaCO_2$ result in muscle twitching a further deterioration of mental function that can progress to coma. However, the cerebral effects of hypercapnia depend to a large extent on the acuteness of the change, so that in some instances a patient with chronic CO_2 retention at a level of 80 mm Hg may be fully conscious, whereas another patient with acute elevation of $PaCO_2$ to 80 mm Hg may be stuporous.

Therapy for acute symptomatic hypercapnia

If acute hypercapnia and coma are due to a drug overdose, specific pharmacologic antagonists to the offending drug should be immediately administered if available. If the acute hypercapnia and associated coma are not caused by a drug overdose, the patient should be intubated and receive mechanical ventilation.

Relationship of arterial hypercapnia to lung disease

Patients with restrictive ventilatory disorders rarely manifest arterial hypercapnia throughout the course of the disease. However, hypercapnia sometimes develops in these patients as a terminal event.

In contrast, hypercapnia commonly develops in patients with COPD. The development of arterial hypercapnia is poorly correlated with most tests of pulmonary function. However, in patients with COPD hypercapnia rarely develops until the $FEV_{1.0}$ decreases to below 1.25 L. If arterial hypercapnia develops in a patient with COPD and $FEV_{1.0}$ greater than 1.25 L, he should be evaluated for the following clinical entities: (1) administration of drugs capable of depressing ventilatin, (2) metabolic alkalosis, or (3) a disorder of respiratory regulation.

ARTERIAL HYPOXEMIA

Five physiologic mechanisms are known to cause arterial hypoxemia: (1) inspiring air (or a gas mixture) with low PO_2, (2) hypoventilation, (3) decreased diffusion, (4) ventilation-perfusion mismatching, and (5) right-to-left shunting of blood.

Inspiring air (or a gas mixture) with a low PO_2

At sea level individuals trapped in a fire inspire air with a low PO_2, since the ambient PO_2 has been reduced by the consumption of O_2. Obviously, the therapy for this condition is to remove the individual from the environment of the fire.

The most common cause of arterial hypoxemia is a sojourn at a high altitude. The decreased barometric pressure at high altitudes quantitatively accounts for the hypoxemia seen in mountain dwellers; in these individuals the $P(A\text{-}a)O_2$ is normal. The magnitude of altitude-induced hypoxemia can be quite severe. For example, normal individuals living at 10,000 feet (3050 m) above sea level exhibit an arterial PO_2 of 53 mm Hg. In most of the United

States, altitude-induced hypoxemia is of little practical importance. However, in Denver (altitude 5200 feet [1560 m]) the normal Pa_{O_2} is approximately 70 mm Hg. Therefore patients with lung disease may require supplemental O_2 earlier in the course of their disease when living at high altitudes.

Alveolar hypoventilation

Alveolar hypoventilation is manifested by an increase in both arterial and alveolar P_{CO_2}. Since the sum of the partial pressures of the alveolar gases must equal barometric pressure, increases in Pa_{CO_2} must be accompanied by decreases in Pa_{O_2} because of the alveolar pressures of nitrogen and water vapor remain virtually constant. At sea level "pure alveolar hypoventilation" is the only disease causing arterial hypoxemia with a normal $P_{(A-a)O_2}$.

Since the $P_{(A-a)O_2}$ is normal in pure alveolar hypoventilation, this entity cannot result from intrinsic lung disease in itself. Rather, pure alevolar hypoventilation is usually caused by depression of the central nervous system resulting from anesthetic agents or sedatives. It can also be a result of neuromuscular disease such as myasthenia gravis or Guillain-Barré syndrome.

The principal point in the management of pure alveolar hypoventilation is the realization that the patient is rarely if ever in a steady state; he will continue to hypoventilate, and Pa_{CO_2} will continue to increase progressively. Therefore this medical emergency must be treated promptly. A patient suffering from a drug overdose should be given a specific antidote for the offending agent (such as naloxone for opiate intoxication). If the patient does not show a notable improvement following the administration of the pharmacologic antagonist or if no history of drug ingestion is obtained, the patient must be intubated and undergo mechanical ventilation.

Diffusion

Diffusion abnormality in the absence of ventilation-perfusion mismatch does not cause resting arterial hypoxemia.

Ventilation-perfusion mismatch

The most common cause of arterial hypoxemia at sea level is $\dot{V}_A/\dot{Q}_C$ mismatch, and this mechanism accounts for the hypoxemia of both obstructive and restrictive ventilatory disorders. The fact that alveoli with low $\dot{V}_A/\dot{Q}_C$ ratios can result in hypoxemia has been previously noted.

The patient with acute hypoxemia caused largely by $\dot{V}_A/\dot{Q}_C$ mismatch, who also manifests severe signs of acute hypercapnia (such as coma and depressed breathing), should be intubated and undergo mechanical ventilation.

If acute hypoxemia resulting from $\dot{V}_A/\dot{Q}_C$ mismatch is associated with hypercapnia in the absence of clinical manifestations of hypercapnia, controlled O_2 therapy (that is, small increases in FI_{O_2}) is begun. The goal of this therapy is to raise the Pa_{O_2} to approximately 60 mm Hg; the oxyhemoglobin dissociation curve indicates that the arterial O_2 saturation is approximately 90% at this point.

If the Pa_{O_2} is raised above 60 mm Hg (or even in some patients to 60 mm Hg), the hypoxemia-induced chemical drive to ventilation is eliminated, and the patient may hypoventilate further. If after the administration of O_2 therapy the patient shows severe clinical manifestations of acute hypercapnia, he should be intubated and receive mechanical ventilation.

Right-to-left shunt

A right-to-left shunt is characterized by the failure of some mixed venous blood to come into contact with ventilated alveoli; rather, this fraction of mixed venous blood passes directly into the left side of the heart. The thebesian and bronchial veins account for the normal anatomic right-to-left shunt. Many types of congenital heart disease are characterized by pathologic right-to-left shunts (such as tetralogy of Fallot, tricuspid atresia, and pulmonary atresia). Other types of congenital heart disease initially appear as a left-to-right shunt and then develop pulmonary hypertension. Once pulmonary hypertension has become established, these conditions become transformed into right-to-left shunts; examples of this type of condition include atrial septal defect, ventricular septal defect, and patent ductus arteriosus. Pulmonary arteriovenous fistulas and blood flow to a collapsed lung are examples of intrapulmonary right-to-left shunts.

Arterial hypoxemia from a right-to-left shunt can be distinguished from that caused by $\dot{V}_A/\dot{Q}_C$ mismatch by having the patient inspire 100% O_2. The breathing of 100% O_2 flushes nitrogen out of the lungs and creates a high gradient for O_2 across the alveolar-capillary membrane; this gradient for O_2 across the alveolar-capillary membrane; this gradient is sufficiently large to fully oxygenate even pulmonary capillary blood passing through low $\dot{V}_A/\dot{Q}_C$ regions. Thus when arterial hypoxemia is caused by a ventilation-perfusion imbalance, the $P_{(A-a)O_2}$ difference becomes normal (about 80 mm Hg) when the patient is breathing 100% O_2. In contrast, in a right-to-left shunt the shunted desaturated blood never comes in contact with the O_2-enriched alveoli, and the $P_{(A-a)O_2}$ difference remains elevated.

The presence of a major right-to-left shunt in such a common pulmonary disease as adult respiratory distress syndrome (ARDS) has important implications. As noted, breathing 100% O_2 does not appreciably correct the arterial hypoxemia. On the other hand, inspiration of 100% O_2 for a prolonged time results in pulmonary O_2 toxicity (whether arterial hypoxemia is present or not). Therefore when faced with hypoxemia resulting from a right-to-left shunt caused by ARDS, the physician must resort to such therapeutic modalities as positive end-expiratory pressure (PEEP).

BIBLIOGRAPHY

Bates, D.V., Macklem, P.T., and Christie, R.V.: Respiratory function in disease: an introduction to the integrated study of the lung, ed. 2, Philadelphia, 1971, W.B. Saunders Co.

Campbell, E.J.M., Agostoni, E., and Davis, J.N.: The respiratory muscles: mechanics and neural control, ed. 2, Philadelphia, 1970, W.B. Saunders Co.

Comroe, J.H., Jr.: Physiology of respiration: an introductory text, ed. 2, Chicago, 1974, Year Book Medical Publishers, Inc.

Comroe, J.H., Jr., and others: The lung: clinical physiology and pulmonary function tests, ed. 2, Chicago, 1962, Year Book Medical Publishers, Inc.

Fenn, W.O., and Rahn, H., editors: Handbook of physiology: respiration, vols. 1 and 2, Washington, D.C., 1965, American Physiological Society.

Fishman, A.P.: Pulmonary diseases and disorders, New York, 1980, McGraw-Hill Book Co.

Jones, N.L., and others: Clinical exercise testing, Philadelphia, 1975, W.B. Saunders Co.

Murray, J.F.: The normal lung: the basis for diagnosis and treatment of pulmonary disease, Philadelphia, 1976, W.B. Saunders Co.

Nunn, J.F.: Applied pulmonary physiology, London, 1977, Butterworth & Co., Ltd.

West, J.B.: Respiratory physiology: the essentials, ed. 2, Baltimore, 1979, The Williams & Wilkins Co.

122 • RESPIRATORY DIAGNOSTIC PROCEDURES

Samuel T. Kuna and **Sanford Levine**

A patient is evaluated for pulmonary disease because of respiratory symptoms or because of an abnormality fortuitously noted in the general physical examination. When examining a patient for respiratory diseases or disorders, the physician commonly uses specialized diagnostic procedures. These diagnostic techniques range from a specialized physical examination of the respiratory system that is not associated with morbidity to complex invasive procedures that may produce morbidity (and in rare cases mortality). Deciding which of the more invasive diagnostic procedures to perform depends not only on the medical indications but also on the expertise available at each medical facility. This chapter presents the following respiratory diagnostic techniques: specialized physical examination, chest roentgenographic examination, sputum examination, radionuclide scans, ultrasonography, thoracentesis, bronchoscopy, bronchography, percutaneous needle aspiration, open lung biopsy, mediastinoscopy and mediastinotomy, and pulmonary angiography. Arterial blood gas studies and other tests of pulmonary performance are discussed in Chapter 121.

SPECIALIZED ASPECTS OF THE PHYSICAL EXAMINATION OF THE RESPIRATORY SYSTEM
Examination of nonthoracic areas

CYANOSIS. The physician should note the color of the nailbeds and lips. A bluish discoloration of these areas is termed cyanosis. The relationship between cyanosis and arterial hypoxemia requires amplification. The physician usually perceives cyanosis when the concentration of reduced hemoglobin in the skin capillaries reaches 5 g/dl of blood. Alternatively, cyanosis usually accompanies a capillary methemoglobin concentration of 1.5 g/dl of blood or a sulfhemoglobin concentration of 0.5 g/dl of blood.

The distribution of cyanosis frequently provides a clue to the cause. Generalized systemic arteriolar vasoconstriction, as occurs in congestive cardiac failure, and localized systemic arteriolar vasoconstriction involving the fingers such as in Raynaud's disease are associated with cyanosis of the nailbeds; however, systemic arteriolar vasoconstriction does not usually cause perioral cyanosis. Another peculiar distribution of cyanosis is observed in patients with patent ductus arteriosus associated with pulmonary hypertension and a predominant right-to-left shunt; in this complicated condition a pink right upper extremity is accompanied by cyanosis of the left upper and both lower extremities. Thus patients with cardiovascular lesions may show various patterns of cyanosis; these patterns strongly suggest that arterial hypoxemia caused by intrinsic lung disease cannot account for the observed cyanosis.

The relationship between an abnormal red blood cell count, such as in anemia and polycythemia, and cyanosis is important. Patients with severe anemia (hemoglobin concentration less than 5 g/dl of blood) never exhibit cyanosis regardless of the severity of the arterial hypoxemia. Conversely, patients with significant degrees of polycythemia may manifest cyanosis coincident with moderate arterial hypoxemia.

Occasionally, significant "global" cyanosis is observed in patients whose measured arterial O_2 tension (PaO_2) is perfectly normal (100 mm Hg). This combination of findings suggests that the blood of the patient contains an abnormal hemoglobin such as methemoglobin or sulfhemoglobin. The physician can confirm this by drawing another blood specimen from the patient (venous blood is adequate) and demonstrating that the blood fails to become red when it is aerated in a syringe with room air or a hyperoxic gas mixture. Although exact definition of the abnormal hemoglobin must await specialized hematologic tests, this simple test allows the astute physician to conclude that the perceived cyanosis is unrelated to arterial hypoxemia.

CLUBBING. "Clubbing" is the term used to refer to changes in the distal segment of a digit that result from an increase in soft tissue. This selective increase in soft tissue is accompanied by sponginess at the nail base, widening of the angle formed at the junction of the nail base and periungual skin, and increased curvature of the nails in both the coronal and longitudinal planes.

Clubbing occurs with primary or metastatic carcinoma of the lung and with diseases of chronic pulmonary suppuration, including bronchiectasis, empyema, and lung abscess. It also occurs with pulmonary fibrosis and cystic fibrosis. However, clubbing is not a specific sign of pulmonary disease; it can also be associated with hepatic cirrhosis, regional enteritis, ulcerative colitis, subacute bacterial endocarditis, and congenital cyanotic heart disease. Clubbing also occurs on a genetic basis as an isolated abnormality (hereditary clubbing). In addition, clubbing can occur coincident with subperiosteal new bone formation in the rare disease pachydermoperiostosis.

Clubbing is an unusual finding in chronic obstructive lung disease in the absence of chronic infection and is also unusual in tuberculosis unless there is significant pulmonary fibrosis or empyema.

Examination of the thorax

Examination of the thorax includes inspection, palpation, percussion, and auscultation.

INSPECTION. Mouth breathing, as opposed to nasal breathing, decreases the work of breathing. Therefore most if not all severely dyspneic patients use mouth breathing to diminish the work of breathing. Patients with obstructive pulmonary disease and dyspnea invariably use the accessory muscles of respiration such as the sternocleidomastoids.

Most patients with obstructive pulmonary disease exhale through pursed lips. This pursed lip breathing (PLB) relieves dyspnea both at rest and during exercise. PLB presumably maintains the patency of bronchi during expiration. Two possible mechanisms account for the subjective benefit elicited by PLB: (1) a change in the length-tension relationship of the respiratory muscles or (2) relief from any discomfort incurred because of narrowing or collapse of larger bronchi.

INSPIRATORY MUSCLE FATIGUE. Within the past several years many authors have pointed out that fatigue of the inspiratory muscles may account for exercise intolerance in patients with chronic obstructive pulmonary disease (COPD), as well as inability to wean these patients from a ventilator. Both in patients with COPD and in normal subjects breathing through inspiratory flow-resistive loads, recent investigations have demonstrated that inspiratory muscle fatigue is manifested by a triad of physical signs: (1) the development of rapid shallow breathing; (2) inward movement of the abdomen during inspiration, indicating that the diaphragm is failing to contract on some inspirations; and (3) an alternation between predominantly abdominal and predominantly rib cage displacements during inspiration. At present it is believed that these physical findings constitute the most sensitive signs of inspiratory muscle failure (or fatigue) during attempts to wean patients from mechanical ventilation.

PALPATION. Palpation should include a meticulous search for axillary and supraclavicular lymph nodes. The trachea is palpated in the suprasternal notch to check for mediastinal shifts.

Palpation is also used to perceive vocal fremitus. To produced fremitus, the patient should slowly repeat some phrase such as "ninety-nine" loudly and in as low a pitch as possible; the physician should be able to palpate vibrations induced by these sounds over all areas of the chest wall covering the lung. Fremitus normally is decreased or absent if the patient's voice is not sufficiently forceful and resonant. It is also diminished by a thick layer of fat in the thoracic wall and especially by large breasts.

Fremitus is pathologically increased whenever the ratio of lung tissue or solid matter to air in a particular lung region is increased, provided that the bronchus to that area is patent. An example is the increased fremitus palpable over a pneumonic infiltrate with a patent bronchus. However, fremitus is decreased or absent if the bronchus supplying that region is occluded by extrinsic compression, endobronchial tumor, foreign body, or retained secretions.

Air in the pleural cavity (pneumothorax) or any type of pleural effusion tends to block the transmission of vibrations from the lung to the chest wall; in these situations fremitus is diminished or abolished.

PERCUSSION. The percussion note over the thorax is determined by the ratio of air to solid tissue. A relative increase in the amount of air gives a more booming note; a relative decrease results in a duller or flatter sound. The term "resonant" describes the percussion note over healthy lung tissue.

Dullness represents the composite sound produced by resonance from the lung, plus a more pronounced element from solid, airless tissue. It is normally present over the heart, mediastinum, upper portion of the liver, and spleen—organs that are solid but also adjacent to the air-containing lung.

The finding of dullness over normally resonant areas of the chest indicates a pathologic change in the underlying tissues. Among the abnormal conditions causing dullness are pleural effusion, atelectasis, pneumonia, and primary or metastatic tumor.

AUSCULTATION. Auscultation of the respiratory system can be subdivided into breath sounds at the mouth and breath sounds transmitted to the chest wall; a stethoscope is required only for the latter category.

Breath sounds at the mouth. The breath sounds of healthy individuals are inaudible at a distance of a few centimeters from the mouth unless the patient is panting, gasping, or sighing. In contrast, the resting ventilation of many patients with obstructive airways disease is accompanied by noise that can be heard across the room. In chronic bronchitis and asthma the intensity of the *inspiratory* noise correlates well with the forced expiratory volume in 1 second ($FEV_{1.0}$), peak expiratory flow rate, and other indices of obstruction to airflow. However, in emphysema the sound of inspiration at the mouth is faint, even in the presence of severe airflow obstruction. Therefore the amplitude of the inspiratory sound can be used to distinguish emphysema from chronic bronchitis and asthma.

Breath sounds transmitted to the chest wall. Breath sounds vary according to the location of the stethoscope. The breath sounds heard over the trachea have a short inspiratory phase and a long expiratory phase; these breath sounds remain audible to the end of expiration. They have been called bronchial breath sounds. Normal breath sounds heard over the chest (formerly termed "vesicular" breath sounds) have a long inspiratory phase and a short expiratory phase, becoming inaudible throughout the major portion of expiratory airflow. Normal breath sounds over the chest are believed to originate in the lobar, segmental, and perhaps even more peripheral branches of the bronchial tree. The aerated lung and chest wall act as a low-pass filter that attenuates this sound. Fluid or air in the pleural space establishes a complete acoustic barrier. Consolidated lung tissue transmits breath sounds almost without attenuation. The breath sounds over such areas of consolidation are similar to those over the trachea. Over areas of lung consolidation there is also increased transmission of voice resulting in the clinical sign of bronchophony.

Adventitious lung sounds include crackles and wheezes. Crackles are discontinuous popping sounds that are believed to be caused by the reequilibration of pressure with sudden reinflation of collapsed alveoli and peripheral airways. Crackles can occur during inspiration and expiration. They can be scanty or profuse, loud or faint, and high pitched or low pitched. Crackles are a characteristic physical finding in pneumonia, pulmonary edema, atelectasis, and interstitial diseases.

Wheezes are continuous musical sounds. They are believed to be generated by the oscillation of the walls of airways between the closed and barely open positions. Wheezing can be elicited in normal individuals during the dynamic airway compression of a maximal forced expiration. Nonetheless, wheezing should be thought of as a clinical sign of partial airway obstruction. Wheezing may consist of constant musical notes that start and stop at different times during inspiration and expiration. Such a pattern is characteristic of asthma. Alternatively, wheezes can be variable musical sounds occurring throughout expiration. These wheezes occur in many chronic pulmonary diseases.

CHEST ROENTGENOGRAPHIC EXAMINATION
Posteroanterior and lateral chest views

The chest roentgenographic examination is an invaluable diagnostic tool in the evaluation of diseases of the thorax. Although different pulmonary diseases may have similar clinical presentations, they can often be distinguished on the basis of their characteristic roentgenographic appearance in conjunction with the history and physical examination. These criteria usually determine the diagnostic and therapeutic approach to a particular clinical problem. The importance of past films cannot be overemphasized. An abnormality that is roentgenographically stable over a 2-year period may not warrant further evaluation. Conversely, a changing roentgenographic appearance identifies an active process that requires further investigation. In the workup of any pulmonary disorder, every effort should be made to obtain results of previous studies.

The standard posteroanterior and lateral views reveal whether a disorder is intraparenchymal or extraparenchymal or both. If the abnormality is not apparent on both of these films, oblique views can help make this distinction. An intraparenchymal infiltrate may be alveolar or interstitial. An alveolar infiltrate is fluffy and irregular. As these shadows become confluent, the infiltrate assumes a more homogeneous pattern. Airways surrounded by fluid-filled alveoli produce air bronchograms. Common respiratory disorders that produce an alveolar pattern include pneumonias and pulmonary edema. The location of the infiltrate is helpful in establishing a differential diagnosis. For example, whereas a bilateral perihilar alveolar infiltrate is typical for pulmonary edema, a unilateral alveolar infiltrate is much more likely to result from an infectious process.

An interstitial infiltrate is more discrete and sharp. Air bronchograms are not characteristic. Interstitial patterns can be micronodular, reticular, or linear. The type of interstitial pattern as well as its location can help determine its cause. For example, a micronodular pattern with predominance in the apices would be a typical roentgenographic presentation for sarcoidosis. A micronodular interstitial infiltrate uniformly distributed throughout the lung fields would be a representative presentation for miliary tuberculosis.

Usually the roentgenographic examination gives the first indication of a solitary pulmonary nodule. This often initiates an extensive diagnostic evaluation. Of the many possible causes of a solitary pulmonary nodule, bronchogenic carcinoma, tuberculosis, and fungal infections are the most common. The roentgenographic appearance of the nodule may help determine its cause. The presence of "popcorn calcifications" on tomography is suggestive of a hamartoma. In general, well-circumscribed lesions are more likely to be benign. As previously noted, past films are important to determine if the nodule is changing in size or is roentgenographically stable. Pneumonitis can also appear as a nodule. If previous films are not available, it is important to document that the lesion is not evanescent by repeating the roentgenographic examination after an interval of at least a week.

An increased density on the film may represent atelectasis. Obstruction of airways leads to resorption of air distally and collapse of these lung units. When involving peripheral airways, this collapse can appear as discoid or platelike opacities on the film. Atelectasis is particularly common after upper abdominal surgery and is manifested clinically by fever. Obstruction of a central bronchus can result in the collapse of a lobe or even an entire lung. Collapse of each individual lobe has a characteristic roentgenographic appearance. The central obstructing lesion is usually the result of a mucous plug, endobronchial tumor, or foreign body.

The film can also show areas of decreased density in the lung. Localized hyperlucent airspaces may represent bullae, blebs, or cysts. Bullae are airspaces within the lung that occur in association with emphysema. Blebs are collections of air adjoining the visceral pleura, usually in the apices. Cysts are airspaces that have an epithelial lining. Some are congenital malformations of the bronchial tree; others result from persistent postinfectious cavities that reepithelialize. Hyperlucent areas can also be caused by a decrease in vascular perfusion, for example, from pulmonary embolus. Diffuse hyperlucency is typical in emphysema, a disease of lung destruction. In contrast, a unilateral hyperlucent lung suggests the following possibilities: (1) a technical error resulting when one side of the chest is not flush with the film cassette, (2) a difference in soft tissue mass overlying each hemithorax, for example, after mastectomy, (3) a unilateral pleural effusion in a film taken with the patient in a supine position, and (4) decreased perfusion to one lung caused by postinfection ventilation abnormalities (Swyer-James or Macleod's syndrome).

The film may reveal an extrapulmonary abnormality involving the heart, mediastinum, pleura, and so on. Pleural disease frequently escapes detection during physical examination. The most common pleural abnormality is a pleural effusion. Accumulation of fluid between the visceral and parietal pleura appears in the dependent portion of the thorax and initially causes blunting of the costophrenic angle. Blunting on a posteroanterior film occurs only after 300 to 500 ml of fluid has formed.

Special views

Small pleural effusions can be seen on the lateral projection, but a lateral decubitus view is the most sensitive roentgenographic technique to document pleural fluid. The lateral decubitus view also differentiates blunting caused by pleural fluid from other causes of blunting such as pleural fibrosis. A subpulmonic effusion, which follows the contour of the diaphragm on an upright film with relative preservation of the costophrenic angles, also layers out on the decubitus view. A loculated pleural effusion, however, does not change position but can be diagnosed as fluid with ultrasonography (see later section).

In the standard posteroanterior view of the chest, parenchymal abnormalities in the lung apex may be obscured by the overlying clavicles and first rib. In an apical lordotic view these structures are no longer superimposed, enabling better interpretation of the apical infiltrate.

Abnormalities in other areas of the film that are difficult to interpret can be better defined by oblique views and tomography. Lung tomograms provide roentgenographic slices of lung tissue. They are indicated to outline cavitation that is only suggested on standard films, look for calcification in a solitary pulmonary nodule, and show blood vessels leading into and out of a lesion, identifying it as an arteriovenous malformation. Whole lung tomograms may reveal evidence of multiple pulmonary metastases. Tomograms also give a good outline of the trachea and bronchi and are useful in evaluating a possible central obstructing lesion.

The potential applications of computed tomography to diseases of the thorax are still being evaluated. Initial studies indicate that this technique is more sensitive than linear tomography for detecting calcification in a solitary pulmonary nodule and in screening the lung for multiple metastatic nodules. Computed tomography can also be useful in delineating pleural and mediastinal abnormalities that are confusing on the more conventional roentgenograms. The indications for computed tomography will undoubtedly evolve as more experience is gained.

SPUTUM EXAMINATION

A cough can produce sputum that is mucoid or purulent. Diagnostically, the presence of mucoid sputum is not helpful. Copious frothy sputum suggests bronchoalveolar carcinoma, whereas pink frothy sputum can result from pulmonary edema. Sputum that appears purulent can indicate either an infectious or an allergic disorder. Purulent sputum with a foul odor suggests an infection caused by anaerobic organisms. Sputum from bronchiectasis forms three distinct layers when collected and allowed to stand. However, these findings should be confirmed with additional diagnostic studies.

Microscopic examination of the sputum can yield important information. A useful routine is to examine a wet mount of the sputum specimen before staining it. A drop of sputum is spread under a coverslip and screened for the presence of squamous cells and alveolar macrophages. The presence of many squamous cells indicates that the specimen must have originated above the level of the larynx. In contrast, the presence of alveolar macrophages indicates that the specimen originated from the tracheobronchial tree and is an appropriate sample for staining. The number of eosinophils on the wet mount can also be determined and could suggest an allergic disorder reponsive to steroids. After the coverslip is removed, the slide dries and is stained for bacteria or acid-fast mycobacteria. The presence of many leukocytes, as well as bacteria, on a sputum Gram stain is indicative of infection. Appropriate antibiotic coverage is determined by the morphologic structure of the organisms and the appearance of the roentgenographic film. A sputum culture is used to help verify this therapeutic decision.

Cytologic examination of the sputum is useful in daignosing neoplasms located in endobronchial sites. The diagnostic yield of this procedure increases with up to five separate sputum collections. Since sputum is also composed of extrapulmonary secretions, malignant cells on sputum cytologic examination may originate from the extrathoracic airway or an esophageal tumor.

RADIONUCLIDE SCANS
Perfusion scan

One type of radionuclide scan assesses the distribution of perfusion in the lungs. The perfusion scan is performed by intravenous injection of technetium Tc 99m human albumin microspheres. These particles have a diameter larger than that of the capillary lumen and are retained in the pulmonary capillary bed. This microembolization is transient and of no clinical consequence. The distribution of pulmonary blood flow is determined by quantifying the relative distribution of the radioactive-labeled albumin with scintillation scanning over the thorax.

Ventilation scan

Another type of radionuclide scan assesses the distribution of ventilation in the lungs. The ventilation scan is performed by having the patient breathe a radioactive gas, usually xenon 133, from a spirometer. Scintillation scanning that monitors the distribution of xenon is used as a marker for the distribution of ventilation. The distribution of ventilation is evaluated under the following circumstances: (1) initially, on inspiration to TLC, (2) during equilibration of the labeled xenon in the lungs with normal tidal breathing (wash-in), and (3) during elimination of the labeled xenon from the lungs when breathing room air (washout). Areas of decreased ventilation are characterized by delayed appearance of the radionuclide during wash-in and prolonged retention of the radionuclide on washout.

Use of radionuclide scans in the diagnosis of pulmonary emboli

In most institutions perfusion scans are routinely used in the diagnostic workup for pulmonary emboli. Embolic occlusion of branches of the pulmonary arterial tree results in segmental areas of decreased or absent perfusion. Therefore an entirely normal perfusion or absent perfusion. Therefore an entirely normal perfusion scan constitutes strong evidence against the diagnosis of pulmonary emboli.

An abnormal perfusion scan, however, is somewhat difficult to interpret. First, disorders such as pneumonia that cause decreases in ventilation to specific areas of the lung can elicit secondary decreases in perfusion to the same area of the lung. Therefore it is important to correlate the results of the perfusion scan with a concurrent chest roentgenographic examination. For example, an alveolar infiltrate on the film can explain decreased perfusion of the same area on the perfusion scan.

Second, in patients with obstructive pulmonary disease, regions characterized by low V_A/Q_C ratios may show up as areas of decreased perfusion on the perfusion scan. However, a ventilation scan can demonstrate that the perfusion defects are occurring in areas of low V_A/Q_C ratios.

Use of perfusion lung scans in the preoperative assessment of patients undergoing lung resection

Perfusion lung scans are used in the preoperative assessment of patients with marginal respiratory reserve who are scheduled for lung resection. If the area of the lung to be removed has poor perfusion, resection will probably not significantly impair respiratory function. In evaluating a patient for pneumonectomy, the perfusion lung scan can quantify the percentage of pulmonary blood flow to each lung. On this basis it is possible to estimate from routine tests of pulmonary performance (see Chapter 121) the pulmonary function that will remain following removal of the involved lung and to predict whether the patient can tolerate a pneumonectomy.

ULTRASONOGRAPHY

Ultrasonography is often helpful in determining the presence and location of fluid in the pleural space. When the high-frequency sound waves are directed into the normal thoracic cavity, the sound is almost completely reflected by the air-containing lung at the surface. However, when pleural fluid is present, an echo-free space is demonstrated between the chest wall and the aerated lung. The fluid transmits the sound so that echoes are produced only when the sound waves are reflected from the underlying lung.

THORACENTESIS

There are both diagnostic and therapeutic indications for thoracentesis. The diagnostic indication is to elucidate the cause of the pleural effusion, whereas the therapeutic indication is symptomatic relief from dyspnea.

Methodology and complications

To perform a thoracentesis in a free-flowing effusion, the best site for introduction of the needle in a sitting subject is the posterior eighth intercostal space at the midscapular line. A helpful landmark is the scapular tip that overlies the seventh rib when the arms are flush with the body. A loculated pleural effusion should be localized by ultrasonography before a decision is made concerning the site for introducing the needle.

The complications of thoracentesis include pneumothorax, hemothorax, reexpansion pulmonary edema, and rarely air embolism. Leakage of air into the pleural space through the thoracentesis needle is the most common cause of pneumothorax associated with thoracentesis. However, in a few instances pneumothorax follows laceration of the visceral pleura; the leak usually seals itself quickly. If the pneumothorax is large or causes dyspnea, aspiration of the air or even placement of a chest tube is indicated. Hemothorax usually follows trauma to an intercostal vessel.

Reexpansion pulmonary edema is believed to result from the more negative intrathoracic pressure following removal of a large amount of fluid. The balance of forces across the alveolar-capillary membrane, described in Starling's law, is disrupted, resulting in transudation of fluid into the alveoli. The incidence of this complication can be decreased by limiting fluid aspiration during each thoracentesis to 1 L or less.

In rare instances lacerations of lung tissue by the thoracentesis needle allows air from alveoli to enter adjacent pulmonary veins, producing air embolism. When this complication is suspected, the patient is placed on his left side with the head lower than the trunk to trap gas in the right atrium, thereby minimizing pulmonary and systemic air embolism.

Pleural fluid analysis

If pus is aspirated from the pleural space or organisms are present on stains of the pleural fluid, an infection is the cause of the pleural effusion and should be treated appropriately. Even if there is no initial evidence to suggest bacterial infection, a specimen of fluid is still sent for culture. In addition, chemical studies of the fluid are made to determine whether it is a transudate or an exudate. Table 122-1 presents simple chemical criteria for distinguishing between transudative and exudative pleural effusions.

The cellular profile of pleural fluid may provide some suggestions regarding cause. Bloody pleural effusions with red blood cell counts greater than 100,000/ml result most commonly from trauma, malignancy, and pulmonary thromboembolism. A lymphocytic pleural effusion with greater than 50% lymphocytes suggests a tuberculous or malignant origin. Eosinophilia in pleural fluid is a nonspecific finding.

Transudative effusions

Pleural fluid formed through normal capillary membranes is termed a transudate; transudates contain little protein or other large molecules (Table 122-1). Transudates occur when normal relationships between capillary hydrostatic pressure and colloid osmotic pressure are disturbed so that fluid formation at one pleural surface exceeds reabsorptive capacity at the other. The following physiologic disturbances favor the accumulation of a transudate in the pleural space: increases in systemic capillary pressure, increases in pulmonary capillary pressure, decreases in the colloid osmotic pressure of plasma, and significant decreases in intrapleural pressure. Common causes of transudates are left ventricular failure, the nephrotic syndrome, and cirrhosis with ascites. The finding of a transudative pleural effusion in the appropriate clinical setting should focus attention on treating the underlying clinical disorder.

Exudative effusions

Pleural fluid formed through abnormally permeable capillary membranes is termed an exudate; exudates contain higher concentrations of protein than transudates (Table 122-1). The altered membrane permeability is usually produced by inflammatory changes in the pleura caused by infection, pulmonary infarction, or neoplasm. Because it can have many causes, an exudative pleural effusion usually requires further diagnostic studies that are dictated by the clinical findings. The pleural fluid amylase concentration is elevated when the effusion is caused by pancreatitis or esophageal rupture. The complement concentration is decreased in pleural fluid resulting from systemic lupus erythematosus. The rheumatoid factor level is elevated and the glucose concentration is characteristically less than 10 mg/dl in pleural fluid associated with rheumatoid arthritis.

Frequently, after empyema is ruled out, the chemical profile of the exudative fluid does not establish its cause. It then becomes important to exclude two diagnoses: tuberculous pleural effusion and malignant pleural effusion. For this purpose another thoracentesis is performed in conjunction with biopsies of the parietal pleura. Several biopsies are submitted for histopathologic examination to look for tumors or granulomata. Another biopsy is sent for mycobacterial culture. The addition of this low-risk procedure greatly increases the diagnostic yield of the thoracentesis. Repeating the pleural biopsies and thoracentesis, if the first attempt does not establish the diagnosis, also increases the likelihood of identifying a tuberculous or malignant pleural effusion. Continued failure to establish a diagnosis may necessitate an open pleural biopsy.

BRONCHOSCOPY

The fiberoptic bronchoscope is an invaluable diagnostic tool in the evaluation of pulmonary diseases, providing diagnoses that previously could be made only by thoracotomy. Bronchoscopy is a low-risk procedure. In one large series the mortality was 0.01% and the morbidity 0.08%. With direct vision for guidance, the flexible bronchoscope can reach the first generations of subsegmental bronchi.

Table 122-1. Criteria for distinguishing pleural transudates from exudates

	Transudate	Exudate
Pleural fluid specific gravity	<1.016	>1.016
Pleural fluid total protein	<3 g/dl	>3 g/dl
Pleural fluid total protein / Serum total protein	<0.5	>0.5
Lactic dehydrogenase	<200 IU	>200 IU
Pleural fluid LDH / Serum LDH	<0.6	>0.6

More distally the airways become too narrow to allow further passage of the bronchoscope. When an abnormality is identified using direct vision, endobronchial biopsies and brushings are performed. Many abnormalities, however, are more peripheral in location and are beyond the field of bronchoscopic vision. In these situations forceps and brushes are advanced through the bronchoscope and guided into the lesion with the aid of fluoroscopy. A biopsy using fluoroscopy should include alveoli, as well as bronchiolar tissue, and is called a transbronchial biopsy. Thus, regardless of location, specimens can be obtained directly from the abnormal area and sent for culture, as well as cytologic and histologic examination.

Bronchoscopy is of particular value in the evaluation of hemoptysis, atelectasis, and mass or cavitary lesions found on roentgenographic examination. With transbronchial biopsy the diagnostic yield in sarcoidosis is said to be greater than 80%. Bronchoscopy is generally of limited use in establishing the infectious cause of bacterial pneumonias, but newer techniques such as the use of sterile catheter-sheathed brushes are currently being evaluated. In contrast, bronchoscopy with biopsy is an excellent means of detecting pulmonary infection in the immunocompromised host by unusual pathogens such as *Pneumocystis* and *Aspergillus* organisms.

Because of its versatility the flexible bronchoscope has virtually replaced the rigid bronchoscope. However, the rigid bronchoscope is still preferable to obtain large endobronchial biopsy specimens, to remove foreign bodies, to evaluate tracheal lesions, and to allow bronchoscopy in the presence of profuse bleeding.

BRONCHOGRAPHY

Bronchography visualizes the tracheobronchial tree with a roentgenographic dye. With the patient under local or general anesthesia, a catheter is advanced into the area of interest. The contrast material, propyliodone oil suspension, is injected to coat the airways. In general, bronchography is valuable in obtaining better definition of the tracheobronchial tree before surgery when the usual diagnostic evaluation does not provide sufficient information. Bronchoscopy has greatly decreased the indications for bronchography and should always precede bronchography. Although bronchography is an excellent technique for diagnosing bronchiectasis and determining whether there is localized involvement, it is rarely indicated unless surgical removal is planned. Bronchography should not be performed for 6 weeks following a pneumonia, since reversible postpneumonic dilation of the bronchial tree can be interpreted as bronchiectasis. Bronchography is also used in the evaluation of tracheal stenosis, hemoptysis of undetermined cause, and congenital malformations of the tracheobronchial tree. The procedure may be dangerous in patients with an iodine sensitivity and in the presence of severe airway narrowing or respiratory distress. The propyliodone oil suspension may cause an inflammatory reaction. A newer contrast material, aerosolized tantalum powder, has been approved only for experimental use but holds promise of being a safer agent.

PERCUTANEOUS NEEDLE ASPIRATION

Percutaneous needle aspirations are playing an increasingly important role in the diagnostic evaluation of nodules and masses in the chest. Use of a narrow-gauge needle has decreased the incidence of bleeding and pneumothorax, but the risk of complications appears to be greater than with bronchoscopy. Percutaneous needle aspiration provides a cytologic, rather than a histologic, diagnosis. Seeding of the needle tract with tumor is very rare but appears to occur more commonly with mesothelioma.

OPEN LUNG BIOPSY

Failure to establish the cause of a parenchymal abnormality with any of these techniques may lead to an open lung biopsy. This surgical procedure requires general anesthesia. Open lung biopsy provides a larger specimen of lung tissue, permitting an analysis of lung architecture. This is of particular importance in reaching a diagnosis in the diffuse nonnodular interstitial infiltrates. Open lung biopsy is also useful in diagnosing opportunistic pulmonary infections in the immunocompromised host.

MEDIASTINOSCOPY AND MEDIASTINOTOMY

Mediastinoscopy is an operative procedure performed by blunt dissection along the thoracic trachea and paratracheal structures through a transverse incision across the suprasternal notch. Lymph nodes visualized through a mediastinoscope can be biopsied. It is technically difficult to reach left-sided structures by this approach. The left side of the mediastinum can be evaluated by mediastinotomy, dissecting down into the mediastinum through a transverse incision over the left, second, anterior costal cartilage. These procedures are used to stage a bronchogenic carcinoma for local spread to hilar and paratracheal nodes. There are few false negative results, and the mortality should be no greater than that from general anesthesia. Finding carcinomatous mediastinal lymph nodes usually obviates the need for thoracotomy. In addition, when the roentgenographic examination shows lymphadenopathy consistent with such diagnoses as sarcoidosis, Hodgkin's disease, and tuberculosis, mediastinoscopy or mediastinotomy can be used to obtain lymph node tissue for pathologic examination. The superior vena cava syndrome and prior mediastinoscopy are considered to be contraindications to mediastinoscopy.

PULMONARY ANGIOGRAPHY

Pulmonary angiography provides a visualization of the pulmonary vascular tree. This invasive procedure is the most sensitive technique available for diagnosing pulmonary thromboembolism. It is indicated (1) when findings on the lung scan are equivocal; (2) in the presence of an underlying pulmonary disease such as emphysema, which would make the interpretation of the lung scans difficult; and (3) for firmly establishing the diagnosis of pulmonary thromboembolism in a patient who is at high risk of complications from anticoagulant therapy.

Other indications for pulmonary angiography are as follows: (1) to differentiate whether the hilar prominence on the chest film represents a vascular shadow or lymphadenopathy, (2) to determine if a unilateral hyperlucent lung on roentgenographic examination is caused by proximal vascular obstruction such as from tumor impingement, (3) to diagnose an arteriovenous malformation, and (4) to preoperatively assess the amount of collapsed lung adjacent to a giant bulla. Complications of pulmonary angiography include arrhythmias, hematoma formation, and vasovagal reactions.

Angiography of the bronchial circulation, although not of diagnostic usefulness, is currently performed in some medical centers in the treatment of significant hemoptysis. Angiography is used to guide therapeutic embolization of the bronchial circulation in an effort to stop bleeding from the tracheobronchial tree. Angiography also identifies whether a spinal artery arises from the bronchial artery, which is a contraindication to embolization.

BIBLIOGRAPHY

Epstein, R.L.: Constituents of sputum: a simple method, Ann. Intern. Med. **77**:259, 1972.

Fishman, A.P.: Pulmonary diseases and disorders, New York, 1980, McGraw-Hill Book Co.

Forgacs, P.: The functional basis of pulmonary sounds, Chest **73**:399, 1978.

Fraser, R.G., and Pare, J.A.P.: Diagnosis of diseases of the chest, Philadelphia, 1978, W.B. Saunders Co.

Hinshaw, H.C., and Murray, J.F.: Diseases of the chest, Philadelphia, 1980, W.B. Saunders Co.

Light, R.W., and others: Pleural effusions: the diagnostic separation of transudates and exudates, Ann. Intern. Med. **77**:507, 1972.

Roethe, R.A., and others: Transbronchoscopic lung biopsy in sarcoidosis, Chest **77**:400, 1980.

Sackner, M.A.: Bronchofiberscopy, Am. Rev. Respir. Dis. **111**:62, 1975.

Zavala, D.C., and Schoell, J.E.: Ultrathin needle aspiration of the lung in infectious and malignant disease, Am. Rev. Respir. Dis. **123**:125, 1981.

123 • CHRONIC BRONCHITIS AND EMPHYSEMA

Paul D. Siegel and Frank Barch

Chronic obstructive pulmonary disease (COPD) may be the consequence either of primary airway disease, typified by chronic bronchitis, or of parenchymal disease, represented by emphysema. These two diseases have many overlapping characteristics such as a reduction in expiratory flow rates and a relationship to smoking. These similarities allow them to be considered jointly. In addition, the two diseases frequently coexist, and it is often impossible to separate out the various facets of each disease as they occur in a particular patient. If a patient has significant chronic bronchitis with obstruction that is resistant to bronchodilators, associated emphysema is a likely pathologic finding. In addition, the patient with predominantly emphysematous lung disease may exhibit features of chronic bronchitis.

Airway obstruction is usually defined in terms of a diminished flow of air during forced expiration, and a variety of tests have evolved to measure this. The volume of air exhaled in the first second of forced expiration ($FEV_{1.0}$) is one of the most commonly used measures; predictive equations based on sex, height, and age have been devised. Values less than 75% of the patient's predicted $FEV_{1.0}$ levels are likely to be abnormal, values less than 65% of those predicted strongly suggest abnormality, and values less than 1 L for the $FEV_{1.0}$ indicate severe disease and are often associated with CO_2 retention.

The airway obstruction found in COPD can be compared to flow obstruction in a water pipe. If deposits on the pipe wall reduce the size of the lumen or if the walls have been squeezed together in some areas, the resistance to flow will increase, turbulence may develop and further increase resistance, and transport of fluid through the pipe takes longer. Although this conception describes an airway partially occluded by mucus or narrowed by bronchospasm in chronic bronchitis, it does not explain the airway obstruction that occurs in emphysema. In this form of COPD the forces that must be overcome to exhale during a forced expiratory effort must be considered. Chest wall and lung inertia and tissue viscous resistance are minimal, and therefore airway resistance is the major component. Airway pressure must be greater than atmospheric pressure to allow flow to occur. This pressure is produced by a combination of pressures generated by the expiratory muscles of the chest cage and by the elastic recoil of the lung itself. The bronchioles lack cartilage and are surrounded by lung tissue that is under compressive force generated by the chest wall during expiration. The driving pressure for flow through the bronchioles is equal to the static recoil pressure of the lung plus the pressure generated by the expiratory muscles of the chest wall. Along the airway from alveolus to mouth, the pressure decreases as a consequence of flow resistance. At some point (the equal pressure point) this pressure within the lumen equals the pressure in the surrounding lung. Because the pressure closer to the mouth along this airway is less than the surrounding lung pressure, "dynamic compression" of the airway tends to occur. However, at this point in the normal lung there is sufficient rigidity of the bronchioles to prevent collapse.

If lung elastic recoil is diminished, as in emphysema, the alveolar driving pressure and the retractile force of the lung, acting to increase airway pressure and keep the bronchiole lumen patent, are diminished. The point of dynamic compression then occurs more distally in less rigid bronchioles, decreasing expiratory flow. If a stronger expiratory effort is applied, driving pressure is increased along with dynamic compression, and little change in flow occurs.

CHRONIC BRONCHITIS

DEFINITION. Chronic bronchitis is a pulmonary response to chronic irritant exposure. It is defined as the presence of a productive cough on most days for at least 3 months of at least 2 consecutive years. Some patients with chronic bronchitis manifest a reduction in forced expiratory flow rates, wheezing, shortness of breath, or dyspnea on exertion. Patients with "simple" chronic bronchitis have been said to lack evidence of airway obstruction, but sensitive tests of small airway function show abnormal lung function in many of these patients. In this discussion the term "chronic bronchitis" implies significant associated airway obstruction.

EPIDEMIOLOGY. COPD is a major cause of chronic disability in the United States. Valid statistics concerning COPD are difficult to accumulate. Much disease probably goes undiagnosed, and data collected from sources such as death certificates underrepresent its prevalence. An associated disease such as pneumonia or lung cancer is commonly the terminal event for patients with COPD.

Epidemiologic studies using questionnaires suggest that 10% to 25% of the adult American population have chronic bronchitis; however, the National Health Survey in 1970 reported a more conservative prevalence rate of 29.5:1000 adults. According to the Social Security Administration, COPD ranks second only to coronary artery disease as a cause of disability. A male/female ratio of 9:1 has been reported, but this number may be changing to reflect the increasing use of cigarettes by women. More recent data suggest a 7:1 ratio.

ETIOLOGY. Chronic airway irritation from cigarette smoking is the primary cause of chronic bronchitis and emphysema. Nonsmoking Seventh-Day Adventists show reduced mortality from COPD, suggesting that smoking is important in its development.

Air pollution can play a significant role in COPD, especially in smokers, since the mortality from COPD correlates with worsening of air quality. Chronic bronchitis is twice as common in London as in rural England. In normal children ventilatory function after exercise is impaired by air pollutants. Exposure to a dusty atmosphere is associated with chronic bronchitis, including evidence of airflow obstruction. Hereditary factors also play a role in COPD, as demonstrated in *Kartagener's syndrome,* which consists of chronic bronchitis with bronchiectasis, sinusitis, and situs inversus.

Impaired airway clearance increased by alterations in the phagocytic activity of macrophages and polymorphonuclear leukocytes in COPD allows deposited bacteria to proliferate for prolonged periods before removal; however, a causative role of infection in COPD is not clear. Antibiotic treatment of acute exacerbations of symptoms in chronic bronchitis appears to decrease morbidity. Although the use of these drugs prophylactically seems to decrease the duration of exacerbations, the total number of episodes does not change, implying that viral infections may initiate or exacerbate symptoms and that bacteria contribute to the persistence of the worsened symptomatology. The role of antibiotics is widely accepted clinically, although its scientific foundation is unproved. *Diplococcus pneumoniae* and *Haemophilus influenzae* are commonly cultured from the sputum of patients with chronic bronchitis; *Mycoplasma* and L-forms have also been implicated in exacerbations, but their ubiquity in bronchitic patients and the lack of host-antibody response to their presence make assessment of their role difficult. Recurrent exacerbations seem to be related to the gradual progressive decline in pulmonary function exhibited by patients with chronic bronchitis.

PATHOGENESIS AND PATHOLOGY. Chronic bronchitis is a clinical diagnosis with variable pathologic findings. Characteristic findings include hypertrophy of mucous glands and hyperplasia of goblet cells. The Reid index is an attempt to quantify these and is defined as the ratio of mucous gland depth to bronchial wall thickness with the upper limit of normal being 0.4. A correlation between the Reid index and the volume of sputum produced exists; however, this correlation is a bell-shaped curve skewed toward patients with chronic bronchitis rather than a bimodal distribution of both normal persons and bronchitic patients. An associated inflammatory infiltrate is frequently found in and around the bronchial walls but is of highly variable severity. There may also be associated mucous plugging or even obliteration of smaller airways.

Airway irritants, especially cigarette smoke, impair pulmonary defense mechanisms, decrease ciliary activity, interfere with normal scavenger cell activity, cause bronchospasm, increase scavenger cell populations, and increase mucus viscosity and volume. Mucus stasis and impaired phagocytic cell function promote colonization of the airways by bacteria. Retained secretions plus inflammation may account for the reduction in small airway function.

CLINICAL MANIFESTATIONS. COPD is usually a combination of chronic bronchitis and emphysema. In most cases a chronic productive cough that was insidious in onset has been present for many years. The patient may even deny having this symptom initially and later admit to having a "smoker's cough." Episodes of tracheobronchitis with mucopurulent secretions occur later. These episodes tend to resolve spontaneously, although slowly.

Accounts of repeated "colds" characterized by cough

and sputum production and lasting for a protracted period can commonly be elicited. Dyspnea on exertion, wheezes, rhonchi, and diminished expiratory flow rates are found. Posttussive wheezing and cough provoked by forced expiratory effort underscore the irritable airways found in chronic bronchitis with associated obstructive airways disease.

The patient with chronic bronchitis may have less dyspnea than the patient with relatively pure emphysema who demonstrates comparable ventilatory insufficiency, but hypoxemia and CO_2 retention are usually more severe in bronchitis. Hypoxemia and hypercarbia induce pulmonary vasospasm, which can lead to right-sided heart strain and eventual right ventricular failure. The disorder may occasionally be erroneously diagnosed as biventricular heart failure, since the patient complains of orthopnea (caused by worsening ventilation-perfusion matching when the patient is supine), paroxysmal nocturnal dyspnea (from retained pulmonary secretions), dyspnea on exertion, shortness of breath even at rest, and dependent edema. Lethargy and somnolence may also be present.

The physical examination may demonstrate wheezing (as in cardiac asthma), rhonchi, and rales. In addition, the patient may show signs of right ventricular failure with neck vein distention, hepatojugular reflux, and bipedal edema. If the absence of a left ventricular gallop is not appreciated, the presence of a right ventricular gallop, an increased P_2, and a right ventricular heave may lead to an erroneous diagnosis of biventricular heart failure.

To differentiate chronic bronchitis with cor pulmonale from biventricular failure sometimes requires an exhaustive history and a careful physical examination. The physical examination of patients with chronic bronchitis should reveal evidence of airway obstruction with a decrease in forced expiratory flow rates. A simple test showing fair correlation with spirometric testing results requires the patient to make a forced expiratory effort from full inspiration with his mouth wide open while the physician listens over the trachea with a stethoscope. If air movement can still be heard after 4 seconds of expiration, significant airway obstruction is suggested. Hyperinflation, decreased respiratory excursion, use of the accessory muscles of respiration, and depression of the diaphragmatic position are less marked than in advanced emphysema.

Digital clubbing is rare in chronic obstructive bronchitis and should raise the suspicion of complicating bronchiectasis or lung tumor. Cyanosis may be noted but is an unreliable sign of arterial hypoxemia.

LABORATORY FINDINGS. Although chest roentgenography cannot establish the diagnosis of chronic bronchitis, it plays an important role in the evaluation of chronic cough by helping to rule out other causes of the symptom such as neoplasia, inflammatory lesions, and left ventricular failure. The chest roentgenogram is abnormal in up to 80% of patients with chronic bronchitis, with common findings including hyperinflation (best detected by finding a flattened diaphragm on the lateral film), ring shadows and parallel lines (representing thickened bronchial walls), and increased peripheral markings.

The electrocardiogram (ECG) is frequently abnormal in COPD. Atrial and ventricular arrhythmias are common in the presence of pulmonary hypertension, hypoxia, or respiratory acidosis. About one half of hospitalized patients demonstrate arrhythmias, with atrial tachycardia and multifocal atrial tachycardia (MAT) being the most common. With 72-hour monitoring the incidence of arrhythmias approaches 90%, often occurring together with severe hypoxemia, which may be found in patients with chronic bronchitis during REM sleep. Other ECG abnormalities generally reflect pulmonary hypertension: tall, peaked P waves, a shift to the right of the P wave axis, and evidence of right ventricular hypertrophy.

In patients with COPD the leukocyte count is usually normal unless a bacterial infection has supervened. Hematocrit values and hemoglobin levels may be elevated, reflecting secondary polycythemia resulting from hypoxemia, "stress," or diuretic therapy. These changes may be obscured by the increased plasma volume of right ventricular failure.

Sputum examination in the patient with chronic bronchitis is usually of minor help, since leukocytes are often found in the patient's sputum regardless of the clinical status; colonization of the lower respiratory tract with a variety of organisms is the common finding. Nevertheless, gross and microscopic sputum examination should be performed, since the finding of pus or the predominance of a single organism may influence therapy.

Early in the course of chronic bronchitis, routine pulmonary function tests often reveal normal findings. In contrast, the more sensitive tests, which reflect small airway function such as frequency dependence of compliance, closing volume, maximal midexpiratory flow rate, and change in flow rates at lower lung volumes when the patient breathes helium-oxygen mixtures instead of air (volume of isoflow), are often abnormal. These tests are not in general clinical use because of their poor standardization, technical difficulty, and expense. Furthermore, they are often abnormal in young, healthy smokers. As the obstructive defect worsens, there is evidence of a decrease in maximal expiratory flow rates, such as the $FEV_{1.0}$ and peak expiratory flow, as well as a decrement in the maximal voluntary ventilation. Such flow reduction may or may not respond to bronchodilators. The residual volume may be elevated with a relatively unchanged total lung capacity. The diffusing capacity is frequently unimpaired, although this test can be affected by a severe ventilation-perfusion mismatch.

Compliance measurements are occasionally used in the evaluation of COPD, although they tend to be time consuming and uncomfortable for the patient. Compliance is a means of expressing the volume-pressure relationship of the lung and thorax. The tidal volume generated by a measured change in transpulmonary pressure is divided by that pressure change. Static compliance is calculated at a time when air flow has ceased, whereas dynamic compliance is measured during an uninterrupted respiratory cycle. Static compliance is normal or reduced in bronchitis, clearly distinguishing it from emphysema, in which the static compliance is increased. Dynamic compliance, however, is diminished in both diseases and decreases more with increasing respiratory frequency (frequency dependence of compliance).

MANAGEMENT. The avoidance of bronchoirritants, especially cigarettes, should be the mainstay of patient management, especially during exacerbations of respiratory symptoms. Smoking contributes to bronchospasm, mucus production, and decreased ciliary motion and raises the carboxyhemoglobin levels.

Therapy should also be directed toward relieving airway obstruction, reducing cough and sputum production, treating infections, preventing complications, and managing acute respiratory insufficiency. Airway obstruction is usually managed with oral bronchodilators. specifically theophylline or other xanthines.

Adrenergic agonists, especially selective β_2-agents (such as terbutaline) are of potential benefit, not only for their bronchodilator activity but also for their capacity to increase the speed of mucus transport. Unfortunately, their systemic use is frequently limited because of side effects such as tremor occurring at therapeutic dosages. Aerosolized β_2-adrenergic agonists are often administered by intermittent positive-pressure breathing (IPPB) machines, hand-bulb nebulizers, or propellant-driven nebulizers (for example, metaproterenol, two to three inhalations no more frequently than every 4 hours). IPPB therapy with saline, detergents, or mucolytic agents is of little if any benefit; these agents may induce rather than relieve bronchospasm. If O_2 is used to power the IPPB machine, the resulting high inspired O_2 concentration can aggravate CO_2 retention in the O_2-sensitive, severely compromised patient with COPD. Physical therapy involving the chest and postural drainage may help to loosen and raise thick, viscous secretions, especially in the presence of decreased cough or severe debility.

Oral expectorants have less than convincing benefit. Atropine-like agents, including antihistamines, have been thought to be contraindicated because of their adverse effect on sputum viscosity, but recent work using inhalable anticholinergic agents for the treatment of bronchospasm suggests that a reevaluation is indicated.

The role of corticosteroids is not clearly defined. Methylprednisolone has been shown to improve $FEV_{1.0}$ when used with bronchodilators in hospitalized patients with chronic bronchitis. Some stable outpatients may demonstrate an improvement in expiratory flow rates with steroids (such as prednisone) administered in association with their usual bronchodilators. Long-term metabolic side effects may seriously impair the usefulness of steroids in this group of chronically ill patients.

Antibiotics have been widely used to treat exacerbations of symptoms. Ampicillin, tetracycline, erythromycin, and trimethoprim-sulfonamide combinations have been shown to be effective in decreasing morbidity. A common indication for therapy is a change in sputum consistency, amount, or color associated with a worsening of dyspnea. A sputum Gram stain usually confirms an increased number of leukocytes. Frequent exacerbations may be managed with prophylactic antibiotics. Regimens have included daily therapy during the winter, 4 days a week during the winter, or a 5- to 7-day course at the first sign of exacerbation. Unfortunately, although such prophylactic therapy has reduced the severity and duration of exacerbations, their frequency has been generally unaffected.

The use of O_2 in the treatment of advanced chronic bronchitis is currently under investigation. Improvement in performance of mental tasks and a reduction of pulmonary hypertension have been reported. O_2 therapy may be warranted when a patient demonstrates severe hypoxemia on mild exercise or when O_2 improves exercise tolerance. Cough suppressants, sedatives, and hypnotic agents pose a serious threat to patients with severe chronic bronchitis. Patients with hypercapnia are particularly susceptible to respiratory depression. The suppression of cough may lead to retention of pulmonary secretions with resultant worsening of hypoxia and hypercapnia; this in turn causes central nervous system depression.

Cor pulmonale. Except for reducing pulmonary hypertension, little can be done to treat cor pulmonale. If polycythemia is significant, a decrease in resistance to blood flow may occur with a decrease in the hematocrit. This is best accomplished by reducing hypoxia with supplemental O_2; however, phlebotomy is occasionally indicated. The use of diuretics may control peripheral edema but further compromise cardiac output and contribute to electrolyte abnormalities. Abnormalities of left ventricular function in patients with cor pulmonale are usually minor. Digoxin has been used to improve right ventricular function but usually is without significant benefit, and these patients may be particularly susceptible to drug-induced side effects.

EMPHYSEMA

DEFINITION. Emphysema is an abnormal morphologic finding consisting of alveolar enlargement with destruction of alveolar walls. It is usually subdivided into centrilobular, panlobular, and localized forms. Centrilobular emphysema is commonly ascribed to chronic bronchitis and is associated with disease of the conducting airways. Panlobular emphysema is a parenchymal abnormality, typically represented by the patient with α-1-antitrypsin deficiency.

EPIDEMIOLOGY. Emphysema has been estimated by the National Health Survey to have a prevalence of 9.8:1000 adults, or about one third that of chronic bronchitis. In the patients surveyed, activity limitation from emphysema was present in about 35%, whereas such limitation affected only 5% of the bronchitis group. Although much attention has been given to patients deficient in α-1-antitrypsin because of implications regarding pathogenesis, this autosomal recessive gene appears in its homozygous form in only about 0.1% of the U.S. population.

PATHOGENESIS AND PATHOLOGY. A clear distinction between centrilobular and panlobular emphysema frequently cannot be made. Such differentiation is clinically of little consequence. The hypotheses of pathogenesis receiving the greatest attention at present are those involving lung damage from proteolytic enzymes in the presence of abnormal controlling factors. This reasoning grew out of the discovery that some nonsmoking patients with pure emphysema of early onset lacked certain serum proteins originally termed α-1-antitrypsin but more accurately described as α-1-antiproteases. Various degradative enzymes inhibited by these proteins have been shown to cause emphysema when administered to experimental animals. The effect of smoking on the balance between proteolytic enzymes and inhibitor proteins is under investigation.

ETIOLOGY. Genetic predisposition is more clearly present in emphysema than in chronic bronchitis. The homozygous antitrypsin-deficient patient is rare and very susceptible to panlobular emphysema. The heterozygous antitrypsin-deficient patient may be at increased risk for COPD especially if subjected to stress such as cigarette smoke. Cigarette smoking remains the greatest risk factor for the development of emphysema, although air pollution and infection may contribute by provoking chronic bronchitis.

CLINICAL MANIFESTATIONS. In relatively pure emphysema there is a gradual onset of dyspnea on exertion without a productive cough. Over the ensuing years shortness of breath at rest, fatigue, and weight loss develop. The physical examination demonstrates the findings of the classic "pink puffer"; a thin and sometimes wasted acyanotic patient with a hyperinflated (barrel) chest and low-lying diaphragms. There is increased use of the accessory muscles of respiration. The chest wall appears to move more vertically and on inspiration lacks the normal increase in the antero-posterior diameter and widening of the intercostal spaces. Intercostal and supraclavicular retractions may be noted. The lungs are hyperresonant to percussion with diminished breath sounds. Dry, crackling rales are occasionally heard.

The cardiac examination is frequently difficult because of the air-filled lung interposed between chest wall and heart. The heart frequently assumes a rather vertical position behind the sternum. The apical impulse and cardiac sounds may be best noted in the subxyphoid area. A loud pulmonary closure sound suggests pulmonary hypertension, and a right-sided gallop indicates right ventricular failure.

Abdominal examination may demonstrate a palpable liver edge; however, percussion of the superior border usually reveals a low-lying rather than an enlarged liver. Clubbing of the extremities is not present unless complicating disease such as lung cancer has developed.

LABORATORY FINDINGS. Moderate or advanced emphysema can often be diagnosed from a routine chest roentgenogram, although a normal chest film does not exclude significant disease. The roentgenographic findings reflect two major physiologic changes: lung hyperinflation and damage to lung parenchyma. The more reliable signs of hyperinflation are an increased retrosternal airspace and flat or scalloped diaphragms. Less specific findings are low-lying diaphragms, hyperlucency of the lung fields, increased intercostal spaces, and an increased anteroposterior diameter (Fig. 123-1). Vascular changes include prominent hila with diminished peripheral vessels and a "pruned" appearance (loss of visible distal divisions) of the vascular tree. The cardiac silhouette may appear narrow with a vertical axis. Irregular patches of lucency suggest emphysema. The diagnosis of a bulla is usually reserved for a radiolucent area clearly surrounded by a visible ring of lung tissue.

The ECG changes in emphysema are comparable to those in chronic bronchitis but tend to occur later in the disease process. Diffuse low voltage may also be seen.

Infectious airway disease is not a typical feature of pure emphysema; when it occurs, it is usually associated with tracheobronchitis or pneumonia. Sputum is usually minimal in the patient with stable emphysema, and hematologic abnormalities are likewise absent. A serum protein electrophoresis may show near absence of the α-1 region in the α-1-antitrypsin-deficient homozygote. A normal α-1 region on serum protein electrophoresis does not rule out the heterozygous state or an abnormal α-1-antiprotease. Further studies are indicated if a low α-1 level is noted.

Tests for airway obstruction show similar results in both chronic bronchitis and emphysema with the exception of the static lung compliance, which is increased in emphysema, and the diffusion capacity, which is generally more severely impaired in emphysema. Pure emphysema demonstrates bronchodilator-resistant airway obstruction, but so may chronic bronchitis. Flow rates in emphysema may show a disproportionate reduction in comparison with lung volumes, which may be increased. Arterial O_2 levels are commonly depressed, but CO_2 retention is less common and occurs later in the course of emphysema.

MANAGEMENT. Little can be done at present for the patient with pure emphysema. Avoidance of smoking, of carbon monoxide exposure, and of the stress of other ill-

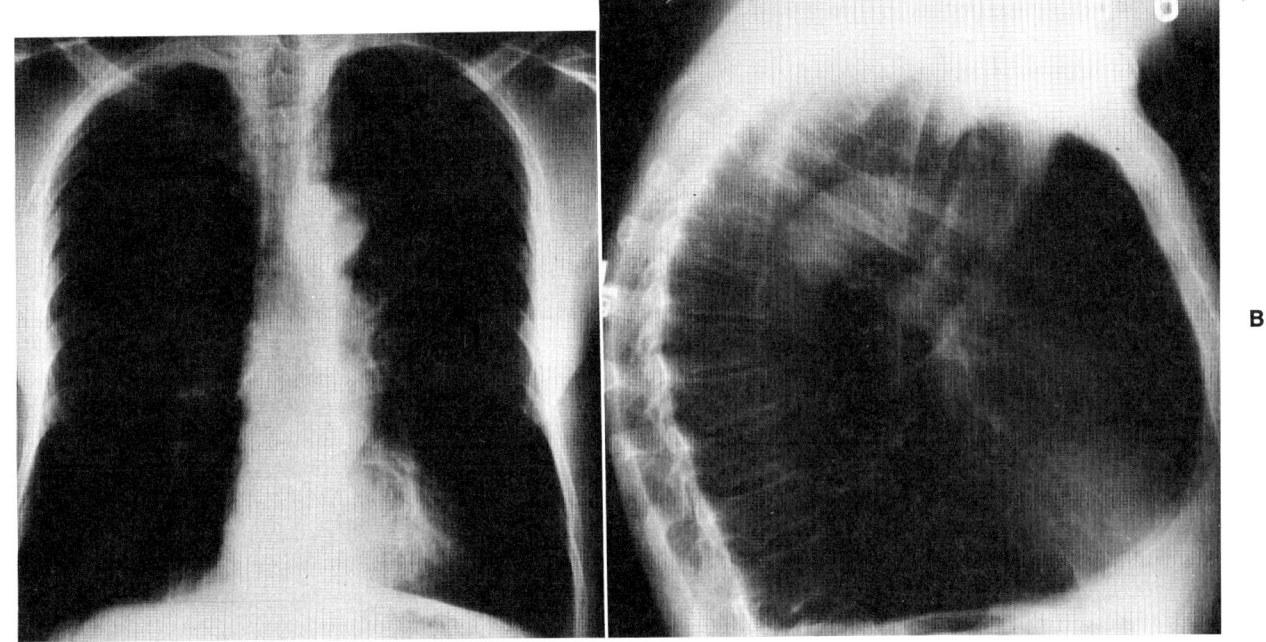

Fig. 123-1. A, Posteroanterior and, **B,** lateral chest roentgenograms of 67-year-old man with emphysema. Note increased retrosternal air space, flat diaphragms, and increased anteroposterior diameter. (Courtesy of George Popky, M.D.)

nesses is important. When hypoxia-related polycythemia, central nervous system dysfunction, or pulmonary hypertension occurs, O_2 therapy may be of help. Cor pulmonale, however, is not usually the result of pulmonary vasospasm but often reflects the decreased pulmonary vascular bed. O_2 usually fails to significantly improve the cor pulmonale associated with emphysema. The decision to intubate and artificially ventilate a patient with emphysema-related ventilatory failure is always difficult. This reflects the recognition that the respiratory failure resulting from emphysema, in the absence of acute correctable complications such as pneumonia, is not associated with a reversible condition, and artificially ventilated patients with emphysema may be dependent on the ventilator for the remainder of their lives.

BIBLIOGRAPHY

Ayers, S.: Cigarette smoking and lung diseases, Basics of Respiratory Disease, vol. 3, no. 5, 1975.

Boushay, H., and others: Bronchial hyper-reactivity, Am. Rev. Respir. Dis. **121:**389, 1980.

Brashear, R., and Rhodes, M.: Chronic obstructive lung disease, clinical treatment and management, St. Louis, 1978, The C.V. Mosby Co.

Burrows, B., and Earle, R.: Course and prognosis of chronic obstructive lung disease, N. Engl. J. Med. **280:**397, 1969.

Fishman, A.: Chronic cor pulmonale, Am. Rev. Respir. Dis. **114:**775, 1976.

Fletcher, C., and Peto, R.: The natural history of chronic airflow obstruction, Br. Med. J. **1:**1645, 1977.

Goldsmith, J.: Health effects of air pollution, Basics of Respiratory Disease, vol. 4, no. 2, 1975.

Gump, D., and others: Role of infection in chronic bronchitis, Am. Rev. Respir. Dis. **113:**465, 1976.

Hogg, J., and others: Site and nature of airway obstruction in chronic obstructive lung disease, N. Engl. J. Med. **278:**1355, 1968.

Hugh-Jones, P., and Whimster, W.: The etiology and management of disabling emphysema, Am. Rev. Respir. Dis. **117:**337, 1978.

Jeanne, J.: The clinical pharmacology of bronchodilators, Basics of Respiratory Disease, vol. 6, no. 1, 1977.

Kueppers, F., and Black, L., Alpha-1-antitrypsin and its deficiency, Am. Rev. Respir. Dis. **110:**176, 1974.

Lertzman, M., and Cherniack, R.: Rehabilitation of patients with chronic obstructive pulmonary disease. Am. Rev. Respir. Dis. **114:**1145, 1976.

Macklem, P.: Disease in small airways, Basics of Respiratory Disease, vol. 4, no. 5, 1976.

Rodman, T., and Sterling, F.: Pulmonary emphysema and related lung disease, St. Louis, 1969, The C.V. Mosby Co.

Thurlbeck, W.: Chronic obstructive lung disease—a comparison between clinical, roentgenologic, functional and morphologic criteria in chronic bronchitis, emphysema, asthma and bronchiectasis, Medicine **49:**81, 1970.

Thurlbeck, W.: Chronic bronchitis and emphysema—the pathophysiology of chronic obstructive lung disease, Basics of Respiratory Disease, vol. 3, no. 1, 1974.

U.S. Department of Health and Human Services: Smoking and health, a report of the Surgeon General, Pub. No. 79-50066, Washington, D.C., 1979, U.S. Government Printing Office.

124 • PULMONARY HYPERTENSION AND COR PULMONALE

William L. Morrissey

When the right ventricle faces increased pressures in the pulmonary vascular system, right ventricular enlargement and dilation ensue. These changes of right ventricular overload are manifested clinically by the signs and symptoms of right-sided heart failure, including right ventricular prominence, right ventricular gallop rhythm, jugular venous distention, and peripheral edema. The electrocardiogram shows evidence of right atrial hypertrophy (peaked P waves, or P pulmonale) and right ventricular strain.

Most commonly the increased pulmonary vascular pressures merely reflect the elevated left-sided heart pressures caused by left ventricular failure or mitral valve disease. However, pulmonary hypertension may develop in spite of normal left-sided pressures. The resultant right ventricular failure is then termed "cor pulmonale," or heart disease resulting from lung disease. This form of pulmonary hypertension is the result of either pulmonary parenchymal disease or airways hypoxia, or it may be primary, as in primary pulmonary hypertension.

Pulmonary parenchymal disease may involve loss of alveoli with concurrent loss of associated capillaries, as in emphysema, or isolated loss of the capillary bed, as in pulmonary vasculitis resulting from collagen vascular disease or illicit intravenous drug use. Other causes of a diminished vascular bed include recurrent pulmonary emboli, primary pulmonary hypertension, and pulmonary veno-occlusive disease. Primary pulmonary hypertension is a disease of unknown cause occurring predominantly in young women and confirmed histologically by finding pulmonary arterial hypertrophy and hyperplasia. Pulmonary veno-occlusive disease begins with fibrous narrowing of pulmonary venules and progresses to occlusion and subsequent pulmonary arterial changes. Therapy for pulmonary vascular diseases is generally unsatisfactory, although prevention of pulmonary emboli is a worthwhile goal.

Hypoxia, usually caused by chronic obstructive pulmonary disease, results in pulmonary hypertension by inducing vasoconstriction. This apparently inappropriate reaction to hypoxia is the unfortunate extension of the body's normal and appropriate attempt to divert blood from areas in which it is being poorly oxygenated. The therapy is directed at the underlying lung disease, but relief of hypoxia is crucial to improvement. The administration of supplemental oxygen to raise the arterial oxygen level to 50 to 60 mm Hg is usually required. Diuretic therapy may improve peripheral edema, but digitalis is not particularly helpful.

BIBLIOGRAPHY

Fishman, A.P.: Chronic cor pulmonale: state of the art, Am. Rev. Respir. Dis. **114**:775, 1976.

125 • BRONCHIECTASIS

Paul D. Siegel and **Frank Barch**

DEFINITION. Bronchiectasis is a morphologic change consisting of persistent abnormal dilation of bronchi. It may occur diffusely throughout the tracheobronchial tree, usually in a patchy distribution, or it may be localized to a segment or lobe. It may be associated with recurrent cough, fever, pneumonia, or sporadic hemoptysis, or it may be of no clinical importance and unaccompanied by symptoms.

ETIOLOGY AND EPIDEMIOLOGY. Bronchiectasis has a number of causes and predisposing factors. It can also occur without any discernible cause, in which case it is often presumed to have followed an unrecognized bronchopulmonary infection.

Bronchiectasis is associated with several congenital anomalies. Pulmonary sequestration is a localized abnormality usually accompanied by bronchiectasis. The yellow nail syndrome is a condition in which bronchiectasis coexists with lymphedema and yellow nails. Bronchiectasis is a common complication of cystic fibrosis (mucoviscidosis).

The association of bronchiectasis, sinusitis, and situs inversus has been referred to as Kartagener's syndrome or triad. Bronchiectasis occurs in 15% to 25% of patients with situs inversus, strongly suggesting a congenital origin. In Kartagener's syndrome structural abnormalities of the bronchial cilia have been described, with subsequent impaired motility of the cilia. Spermatozoa of these patients are also immotile and have the same microtubular deficiency.

Bronchiectasis commonly occurs as a complication of congenital or acquired disorders of humoral immunity. A defect in humoral immunity renders a patient susceptible to pyogenic bacterial infections. Recurrent pneumonia with *Streptococcus pneumoniae* is common, and *S. pyogenes*, *Pseudomonas aeruginosa*, and *Haemophilus influenzae* are also commonly found pathogens. Presumably, bronchiectasis is the result of repeated injury to the tracheobronchial tree as a consequence of infection with these organisms.

Bronchiectasis may occur following childhood pneumonia, especially that subsequent to measles or pertussis. Bronchial obstruction by a tumor, foreign body, or stenosis is also commonly followed by bronchiectasis. Tuberculosis may be associated with bronchiectasis that persists after the organism is eradicated. A localized, proximal form of bronchiectasis can be seen in asthmatic patients whose bronchi are colonized by *Aspergillus* species.

Exposure to the oxides of sulfur or nitrogen most commonly results in obliterative bronchiolitis as a late sequela, but occasionally bronchiectasis may occur. This was seen more often in the past after exposure to mustard gas.

PATHOLOGY AND PATHOPHYSIOLOGY. Bronchiectasis can be divided into a cylindric type, a saccular form, and an intermediate irregular ectasia known as varicose. Cylindric bronchiectasis may occur following pneumonia and is reversible, whereas saccular bronchiectasis is usually considered irreversible.

In addition to luminal dilation, there are substantial inflammatory changes in the bronchial walls. All layers of the wall may be infiltrated with inflammatory cells, and smaller branches may be plugged by mucus or fibrous tissue. Large anastomotic channels develop between the bronchial and pulmonary circulations, with an increase in bronchial artery blood flow. These changes result in a ventilatory pattern resembling that of chronic bronchitis. The vital capacity is decreased, with more severe decreases found in the expiratory flow rates. The maximal voluntary ventilation is decreased, and the ratio of residual volume to total lung capacity is increased. The venous admixture is increased because of abnormal ventilation-perfusion ratios and a decrease in diffusing capacity.

CLINICAL MANIFESTATIONS. Although patients with bronchiectasis may be asymptomatic, the symptoms are characteristically those of recurrent bronchopulmonary infections. Cough, producing copious three-layered sputum containing pus on the bottom, saliva in the center, and mucus on the top, is a classic symptom. This type of presentation is currently less common because of widespread antibiotic therapy. Recurrent fevers are frequently present, and chronic fatigue is common. Hemoptysis is not uncommon and may be massive. Hemoptysis may be the initial symptom in cases of upper lobe bronchiectasis, since excessive sputum production is uncommon. These cases are often referred to as dry bronchiectasis or bronchiectasis sicca. The most characteristic finding in bronchiectasis is the detection of crackles over the affected lung lobe or segment. These may be accompanied by wheezes and usually persist even when the patient is asymptomatic. Clubbing of the fingers is also a common occurrence in bronchiectasis.

LABORATORY FINDINGS. Routine chest roentgenograms are rarely normal in bronchiectasis but can seldom establish the diagnosis. Bronchography, in which a radiopaque contrast medium is instilled into the tracheobronchial tree, provides a morphologic diagnosis of bronchiectasis and also delineates the extent of involvement. Patients with impaired pulmonary function should be evaluated with caution, since bilateral bronchography produces a temporary 30% to 50% decrease in lung function. Care must be taken not to diagnose irreversible bronchiectasis when cylindric changes are found in a lobe or segment for up to 4 months following an episode of pneumonia; these changes may be reversible.

DIAGNOSIS. The diagnosis of bronchiectasis is based on the clinical history and the findings of persistent crackles and wheezes during the physical examination. If clubbing of the fingers is present, this diagnosis is even more likely. Asthma is often confused with bronchiectasis, but in asthma the physical examination should not reveal persistent crackles and the airway obstruction should be largely reversible. Chronic bronchitis closely resembles milder forms of bronchiectasis, and bronchography may be required to differentiate the two disorders. If the disease is localized, bronchoscopy should be performed to rule out an obstructing lesion. The only definitive way to establish the diagnosis is through bronchography.

COURSE AND PROGNOSIS. The course and prognosis of bronchiectasis depend largely on the extent and severity of the disorder. Bronchiectasis localized to a lobe or segment often causes little or no difficulty and is amenable to surgical correction. Generalized bronchiectasis with recurrent infections and sepsis formerly resulted in death within several years after the diagnosis. The introduction of antibiotics has enabled most patients to live more than 15 years after the diagnosis is first established. Those with cystic fibrosis or immunologic deficiencies continue to have a much poorer prognosis. Pulmonary function tends to decline rather slowly, so that respiratory insufficiency and cor pulmonale develop rather late in the course of the disease, if at all.

MANAGEMENT. The mainstay of medical therapy for bronchiectasis is the maintenance of a clear airway, which prevents pooling of secretions and subsequent infection. This can be accomplished by postural drainage, in which the bronchi draining the involved segments or lobes are placed in a dependent position for 10 to 20 minutes at least twice daily. Chest percussion or vibration over the involved area may further facilitate drainage. If nebulized acetylcysteine is used to loosen viscid secretions, it should be combined with a bronchodilator aerosol. The use of bronchodilator and decongestant aerosols before postural drainage may make the latter more productive. Oral antibiotics are usually reserved for the treatment of exacerbations of bronchopulmonary infection. Selected patients with persistently purulent sputum or frequently recurring attacks of bronchopulmonary infection have been reported to benefit from the intermittent administration of tetracycline or ampicillin. Acute infections should be treated with an appropriate antibiotic chosen on the basis of a sputum Gram stain and culture results.

Ampicillin or tetracycline is usually effective except in cystic fibrosis, in which the frequent occurrence of staphylococcal and *Pseudomonas* infections often requires use of a penicillinase-resistant penicillin or an aminoglycoside, respectively.

Hemoptysis is usually managed adequately with rest, cough suppressants, and treatment of infection. Blood replacement is rarely necessary. Emergency resection of a segment or lobe to stop life-threatening bleeding is even less commonly needed. Elective surgical resection is reserved for cases in which the disease is localized to a segment or lobe. In these individuals failure to control recurrent infection, hemoptysis, or chronic debilitating cough might be considered an indication for surgery. Before any surgery, bronchography should be performed to outline the extent of the disease. Pulmonary function studies are useful to indicate the patient's ability to tolerate the surgery.

PREVENTION. The prevention of bronchiectasis requires an understanding of the role of bronchial obstruction and infection. Aspirated foreign bodies should be promptly removed, and the prevention or prompt reexpansion of postoperative atelectasis is also important. Vigorous treatment of bronchopneumonia is mandatory, and slowly resolving pneumonias must be followed to full resolution. If this does not occur spontaneously within an appropriate time (generally 6 weeks), measures such as bronchoscopy, physiotherapy, and respiratory therapy should be taken to encourage resolution. If there is no response to initial therapy or if there is evidence of an obstructing lesion, bronchoscopy should be considered much sooner. Prompt treatment of primary tuberculosis may prevent bronchial compression and atelectasis with the subsequent development of bronchiectasis.

BIBLIOGRAPHY

Guenter, C.A., and Welch, M.A.: Pulmonary medicine, Philadelphia, 1978, J.B. Lippincott Co.

Rosenberg, M., and others: Clinical immunologic criteria for the diagnosis of allergic bronchopulmonary aspergillosis, Ann. Intern. Med. **86:**405, 1977.

Sturgess, J.M., and others: Cilia with defective radial spokes, N. Engl. J. Med. **300:**53, 1979.

126 • LUNG ABSCESS

Donald Kaye

ETIOLOGY AND PATHOGENESIS. Lung abscess occurs when lung parenchyma in an area of infection undergoes necrosis. Many of these areas communicate with bronchi and therefore undergo cavitation with formation of an air-fluid level. Cavitation may occur as a part of acute bacterial pneumonia; it is common in staphylococcal, *Klebsiella, Pseudomonas,* and other pneumonias, except for those caused by pneumococci, *Mycoplasma pneumoniae,* and *Haemophilus influenzae.* However, the term "lung abscess" is often reserved to describe a more chronic process in which the most common cause is a combination of anaerobic and microaerophilic bacteria, often in association with aerobes.

The most common pathogenetic mechanism of lung abscess is identical with that of mixed flora pneumonia—aspiration of the contents of the mouth. The material aspirated plugs off a bronchus or bronchiole, providing an anaerobic environment and allowing the anaerobic bacteria that are always present to grow. An acute aspiration or necrotizing mixed flora pneumonia that is cavitary may result, or a lung abscess may be discovered after days or weeks of fever.

Aspiration most often occurs during an episode of unconsciousness (for example, from alcohol, drug overdose, head trauma, anesthesia, seizure, or coma from any cause), in association with neuromuscular disease of the oropharynx or esophagus, or following operative procedures in the mouth. The patient's oral hygiene is often poor, and a gag reflex may be absent.

Lung abscess also tends to occur beyond obstructive disease of the bronchus such as beyond a tumor. Lung abscess in an edentulous person who has few anaerobes in the mouth suggests tumor. Bronchiectasis is another predisposing factor. Lung abscess occasionally results from secondary infection of a bronchogenic cyst, uninfected cavity or bulla, or from infection of a bland infarct. Lung abscess may also occur from a subdiaphragmatic process extending to the lung, such as amebic abscess of the liver causing right lower lobe infection.

Solitary or multiple lung abscesses may occur as the result of metastasis from suppurative pelvic or jugular thrombophlebitis, usually caused by anaerobes; from right-sided endocarditis, usually caused by *Staphylococcus aureus* (particularly in intravenous drug abusers); and occasionally from bacteremia from other sites.

CLINICAL MANIFESTATIONS. The patient with aspiration pneumonia has an acute onset of fever and cough productive of purulent sputum with or without blood. Pleuritic chest pain may be present if empyema develops. The physical examination reveals evidence of dullness to percussion and rales.

Patients with lung abscess often give a history of fever, anorexia, weight loss, malaise, and cough for days, weeks, or even months, with or without an initial acute onset. The sputum is commonly blood tinged and in most patients has a foul odor. Physical examination of the chest may reveal dullness, amphoric breathing, and rales but is often negative. Clubbing of the fingers may occur.

LABORATORY FINDINGS. The microscopic examination of sputum in both aspiration pneumonia and anaerobic organism lung abscess reveals many polymorphonuclear leukocytes and a mixed flora of gram-positive cocci in chains, mixed gram-negative bacilli, gram-negative cocci, and/or gram-positive bacilli. Cultures usually reveal "normal flora." In fact, sputum cultures are of no value because the organisms that cause lung abscess are present in the mouth in huge numbers. The diagnosis is usually apparent clinically and from the roentgenographic examination. Although percutaneous transtracheal aspiration is not usually indicated clinically, proper culturing of the aspirate reveals a mixed flora of anaerobes with or without aerobes. The

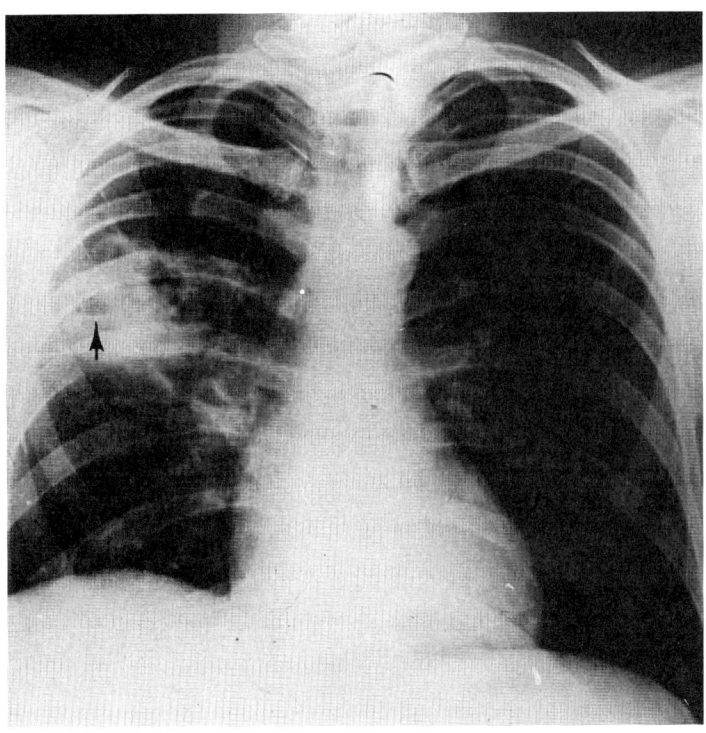

Fig. 126-1. Lung abscess demonstrating air-fluid level *(arrow)*.

organisms most commonly isolated are *Fusobacterium, Peptostreptococcus, Peptococcus,* microaerophilic streptococci, and *Bacteroides melaninogenicus.*

Chest roentgenography reveals the infiltrate of pneumonia, often with multiple cavities in aspiration pneumonia. In lung abscess there is usually a well-defined cavity surrounded by a rim of infiltrate. Air-fluid levels are common and strongly suggest abscess rather than tuberculosis (Fig. 126-1). The infiltrate is usually in the midlung fields, since most patients aspirate while lying on their backs or sides and aspirate into the dependent areas of the lungs, most commonly the posterior segment of the right upper lobe, the posteroapical segment of the left upper lobe, or the superior segments of the lower lobes.

If empyema occurs, the roentgenographic examination reveals pleural effusion, and an aspirate yields pus containing one or more of the etiologic agents. The fluid may have a foul odor. Blood cultures are positive in patients with metastatic lung abscesses. Cavitating carcinoma, tuberculosis, fungal infection, and Wegener's granulomatosis may simulate lung abscess.

MANAGEMENT. In contrast to abscesses elsewhere, surgical drainage is rarely indicated in lung abscess. Postural drainage is important, and drainage usually occurs through the bronchi provided they are unobstructed. In the presence of apparent obstruction, such as with atelectasis, bronchoscopy should be performed promptly to determine the patency of the airways.

The primary approach to the treatment of mixed flora lung abscess and aspiration pneumonia is antibiotic therapy directed toward the mouth flora (mainly anaerobic microorganisms) that cause most of these infections. Many of the anaerobes isolated from the mouth are sensitive to penicillin G; therefore penicillin is considered the drug of choice by many. Because some of the anaerobic gram-positive cocci are relatively resistant to penicillin, high doses (for example, 10 to 20 million units intravenously each day) should be used. After response the doses can be decreased to 600,000 units of procaine penicillin every 12 hours intramuscularly. For the nonseriously ill, ambulatory patient, oral penicillin V may be effective. Ampicillin, amoxicillin, and penicillin V are all equivalent in activity against anaerobes. Cephalosporins such as cephalothin, cefazolin, and cephalexin are also active against many of the anaerobes isolated from the mouth and have been used successfully.

B. melaninogenicus is commonly isolated in lung abscesses and aspiration pneumonias and often produces β-lactamase. Furthermore, lung abscesses and aspiration pneumonias occasionally (10% to 15%) contain *B. fragilis.* Many of these bacteria are sensitive to high concentrations of penicillin G, ampicillin, and carbenicillin and to cofoxitin. However, clindamycin and chloramphenicol are more reliably active.

Aspiration pneumonia usually requires 2 weeks of therapy. There is no established duration of therapy required to prevent relapse after the treatment of anaerobic organism lung abscess. Although some lung abscesses have been cured with 2 or 3 weeks of therapy, those acquired by the bacteremic route usually require 4 to 6 weeks of therapy, and some acquired following aspiration may require 6 or even more weeks of therapy.

The lung abscesses that occur as a result of infection by single organism such as *S. aureus* or *Klebsiella* are treated with antimicrobial agents directed specifically at the causative organism, for example, nafcillin for *S. aureus*.

Empyema should be drained. Abscesses at distant sites, such as a pelvic abscess in a patient with metastatic lung abscesses, should also be drained. Heparin therapy and vein ligation may be required in patients with septic phlebitis who continue to have pulmonary emboli.

PROGNOSIS. The prognosis in appropriately treated aspiration pneumonia depends partially on the underlying disease, but the overall mortality is about 20%. With multiple cavities the course is more severe. Anaerobic organism lung abscess has a mortality of about 10%. Pneumonias caused by *S. aureus, Klebsiella,* and other gram-negative bacilli have a mortality of 25% or higher even with appropriate therapy.

BIBLIOGRAPHY

Bartlett, J.G., and Finegold, S.M.: Anaerobic pleuropulmonary infections, Medicine **51**:413, 1972.
Bartlett, J.G., and Finegold, S.M.: Anaerobic infections of the lung and pleural space, Am. Rev. Respir. Dis. **110**:56, 1974.
Bartlett, J.G., and others: Bacteriology and treatment of primary lung abscess, Am. Rev. Respir. Dis. **109**:510, 1974.

127 • CYSTIC FIBROSIS

Paul D. Siegel and **Frank Barch**

Cystic fibrosis (mucoviscidosis) is caused by an autosomal recessive gene. It is one of the most common inherited disorders of whites in the United States. The heterozygous carrier state is present in about 5% of the population, and the disease occurs in about 1 in 2000 live births. The basic abnormality appears to be an elevation of viscosity of the mucous secretions of the body. In the pancreas this results in the obstruction of secretory ducts with subsequent exocrine insufficiency and malabsorption. In the bronchi, extensive plugging occurs with obstruction, infection, and consequent destruction of bronchial walls. The inadequate clearance of secretions and resultant bronchiectasis commonly involve the upper lobes, whereas the usual idiopathic bronchiectasis preferentially affects the lower lobes.

The secretory abnormality that provides confirmation of the diagnosis of cystic fibrosis is elevation of the concentration in sweat of both sodium and chloride to greater than 70 mEq/L.

Infection with *Staphylococcus aureus* and *Pseudomonas* species is common, and death before the age of 20 was formerly the rule. Recently, however, with better bronchial hygiene and more appropriate antibiotic treatment, more than 30% of patients with cystic fibrosis survive past the age of 18. The treatment includes aggressive respiratory and physical therapy in addition to antibiotics.

BIBLIOGRAPHY

Stern, R.C, and others: The course of cystic fibrosis in 95 patients, J. Pediatr. **89**:406, 1976.
Tomashefski, J.F., Christoforidis, A.J., and Abdullah, A.K.: Cystic fibrosis in young adults, Chest **57**:28, 1970.

128 • BULLOUS EMPHYSEMA AND LUNG CYSTS

Paul D. Siegel and **Frank Barch**

BULLOUS EMPHYSEMA

DEFINITION. A bulla is an emphysematous space exceeding 1 cm in diameter. In contrast, blebs are collections of air within the visceral pleura, and cysts are airspaces lined completely by epithelium. Bullous emphysema is said to exist when one or more bullae are present.

ETIOLOGY AND PATHOGENESIS. Bullae can be associated with chronic bronchitis or panacinar (panlobular) emphysema. They also complicate the late stages of both pneumoconiosis and pulmonary sarcoidosis. In addition, bullae can appear without accompanying disease of the airways or interstitium. This latter type comprises true bullous disease of the lung or bullous emphysema, whereas the others are more properly referred to as emphysema with bullae, sarcoidosis with bullae, and so on.

Bullae are formed by the same processes responsible for emphysema, including atrophy and overinflation and destruction of lung tissue. Progressive trapping of air causes bullae to enlarge and in some cases to eventually reach remarkable size.

CLINICAL MANIFESTATIONS. Bullae that occur in a relatively normal lung are usually detected at the time of routine chest roentgenography as areas of hyperlucency bordered by curvilinear densities. Occasionally they may become large enough to interfere with the function of the remaining normal lung and can then cause shortness of breath. A sudden enlargement of a bulla or the development of spontaneous pneumothorax from rupture of a bulla can result in acute dyspnea or severe pleuritic chest pain. Bullae may become infected, leading to cough, fever, chills, and sputum production. The physical findings are those of decreased or absent breath sounds with a hyperresonant percussion note over the bulla, in addition to the signs of any underlying lung disease.

LABORATORY FINDINGS. The roentgenographic findings consist of areas of increased radiolucency that are sharply defined and bordered, at least to some extent, by fine opaque lines representing fused connective tissue septa. Perfusion lung scans show an absence of perfusion in the bullae. However, ventilation scans may show normal, diminished, or absent ventilation depending on the patency of the bronchus leading to the bulla.

The results of pulmonary function studies in patients with bullae and normal intervening lungs are normal except for an increase in functional residual capacity when measured by body plethysmography. If the bullae communicate very poorly with the airway, this increase may not be reflected in the functional residual capacity measured by dilutional techniques.

In patients with underlying emphysema or chronic bronchitis the pulmonary function studies are abnormal and consistent with the severity of the underlying disease.

MANAGEMENT. Bullae in an asymptomatic patient with normal lung function require no therapy other than cessation of smoking and periodic evaluation for enlargement of the bullae. Infected bullae should be treated with appropriate antibiotics as determined by a sputum smear and culture. The major decision to be made in the management of bullae is whether surgical removal or obliteration of the bullae should be performed. Each case must be considered on an individual basis, but generally the indications for surgery include dyspnea, recurrent pneumothorax, infection, and hemoptysis. The best results from surgery are obtained in patients with giant bullae (especially if confined largely to one lung), with evidence of compression of adjacent tissue, with lesser degrees of chronic obstructive pulmonary disease, and in whom simple plication or excision of bullae rather than lobectomy is possible.

LUNG CYSTS

DEFINITION. A lung cyst is defined as an abnormal space lined with bronchial epithelium. This space may be either fluid- or air-filled.

BRONCHOGENIC CYSTS. Bronchogenic cysts are rare developmental abnormalities resulting from abnormal budding of the developing foregut; they may lie within either the mediastinum or the lung. They are usually first discovered in the patient's third decade of life as an incidental finding on the chest roentgenogram. Pathologically a cyst is usually thin walled and lined with either ciliated or nonciliated epithelium. If it is centrally located, it may contain mucous glands, cartilage, muscle tissue, and elastic fibers. Central cysts are usually solitary and do not communicate with the major bronchi. In contrast, peripheral cysts, usually located within the parenchyma, are more often multiple and may retain communication with normal bronchi. The presence of ciliated or nonciliated respiratory epithelium is noted in the absence of infection; however, infection may destroy the epithelium. Mucous glands and cartilage are usually absent in peripheral bronchogenic cysts; muscle is nearly always absent, whereas elastic fibers are more common. Calcium deposits in either central or peripheral bronchogenic cysts are rare.

ACQUIRED CYSTS. Acquired lung cysts are more common than the congenital variety. The term implies that the abnormal space is air filled. The terms, "bulla," "bleb," and "cyst" are somewhat variable, in part reflecting the fact that pathologic examination is often necessary to distinguish among them. A postinfection cavity is one of the most common precursors of such cysts.

CLINICAL MANIFESTATIONS. Most cysts are asymptomatic. If a cyst is intrapulmonary, hemoptysis is the most common symptom. Although pneumothorax is rare, air embolism has been noted following decompression in tunnel workers with pulmonary bronchogenic cysts. In contrast, mediastinal cysts give rise to symptoms produced by local pressure, especially when present in confined areas such as near the carina. Cough, dyspnea on exertion, stridor, and dysphagia may also be reported.

Roentgenographic discovery of these lesions unfortunately does not often allow a definitive diagnosis. The cysts are usually sharply marginated, round, dense tissue masses that are commonly stable in size but may occasionally change. Intrapulmonary cysts favor the lower lobes of both lungs.

Mediastinal cysts often occur as sharply defined masses below the carina. Esophageal displacement or tracheobronchial compression may be reported. Infection eventually occurs in a high proportion of lung cysts. In the presence of infection it may be difficult to differentiate, even pathologically, between a bronchogenic cyst and an acquired lung cyst resulting from an abscess that has already healed. A definitive diagnosis may require thoracotomy. If symptoms occur, surgical resection may be necessary.

BIBLIOGRAPHY

Fraser, R., and Paré, J.: Diagnosis of diseases of the chest, vol. 1, Philadelphia, 1977, W.B. Saunders Co.

Landing, B.: Congenital malformations and genetic disorders of the respiratory tract, Am. Rev. Respir. Dis. **120**:151, 1979.

Murphy, D.M.F., and Fishman, A.P.: Bullous emphysema. In Fishman, A.P.: Pulmonary diseases and disorders, New York, 1980, McGraw-Hill Book Co.

Poe, R.H., and others: Perfusion-ventilation scintiphotography in bullous disease of the lung, Am. Rev. Respir. Dis. **107**:946, 1973.

Wesley, J.R., Macleod, W.M., and Mullard, K.S.: Evaluation and surgery of bullous emphysema, J. Thorac. Cardiovasc. Surg. **63**:945, 1972.

129 • ATELECTASIS

Paul D. Seigel and **Frank Barch**

DEFINITION. Atelectasis is the collapse of lung tissue that has been previously expanded. Since the alveoli in the affected portion of the lung are no longer filled with air, blood flowing past this area is not oxygenated and the area functions as a venoarterial or right-to-left shunt.

ETIOLOGY. Any lesion obstructing a bronchus to a lung, lobe, or bronchopulmonary segment can cause atelectasis of that portion of lung. These lesions can include foreign bodies, such as dental bridges or portions of teeth, aspirated mucus or food, and endobronchial tumors. Extrabronchial compression by lymph nodes or tumors may be of sufficient magnitude to cause bronchial obstruction. Broncholiths caused by the erosion of calcified lymph nodes into a bronchus can also cause bronchial obstruction.

Atelectasis may develop without bronchial obstruction following radiotherapy. Small areas of collapse, termed "microatelectasis," may develop whenever respiration is impaired and pulmonary surfactant is diminished, as in the postanesthetic state or in the adult respiratory distress syndrome. Linear or platelike atelectasis may also develop as a result of pulmonary infarction, pleural effusion, or other conditions that restrict or limit chest wall or diaphragm motion. These include obesity, ascites, pleuritic pain, paralytic or obstructive ileus, and subdiaphragmatic masses or abscesses. Basilar atelectasis may develop in the postoperative period, especially after upper abdominal or thoracic surgery.

PATHOGENESIS. When a bronchus is occluded, the air distal to the obstruction is quickly absorbed into the blood. This occurs because the sum of the partial pressures of the gases in venous blood is less than that in alveolar air, since the fall in Po_2 in tissue greatly exceeds the rise in Pco_2 in the same tissue. If room air is being breathed, the area distal to an obstruction will collapse in several hours. If O_2 is being breathed, the pressure gradient is greater and collapse may occur in a few minutes. With occlusion of a smaller bronchus, collapse may be prevented by openings in the alveolar wall that allow passage of air from one lobule to another. However, it is known that collapse can occur even under these circumstances, probably because of blockage of the collateral channels or local loss of surfactant.

A sharp reduction in vital capacity occurs following upper abdominal and thoracic surgery. Small areas of atelectasis subsequently develop, presumably because of impaired expansion of the lung or because of deactivation of surfactant. As the vital capacity becomes smaller, more alveolar units approach their closing volume and thus become atelectatic, requiring greater than normal pressures to reexpand. In many critically ill patients, persistent collapse of lung tissue results from retained secretions in the airway, impaired regional ventilation, and altered compliance of lung tissue.

CLINICAL MANIFESTATIONS. If a main bronchus to the right or left lung is occluded, respiratory distress with tachypnea, tachycardia, and eventual fever (probably from pneumonia) follows. Arterial O_2 saturation drops initially, and cyanosis may become evident. If atelectasis involves only one lobe or part of a lobe, the only symptoms may be fever or dyspnea. Tachypnea and tachycardia may also occur but may be less pronounced.

LABORATORY FINDINGS. The findings on physical examination depend on the location and extent of the atelectasis. Uninflated portions of the lung generally show dullness to percussion, decreased or absent breath sounds, and sometimes rales and egophony. With a major loss of volume there is a shift of the trachea and mediastinum toward the involved side or an elevation of the diaphragm. The only significant laboratory findings are usually the abnormalities in arterial blood gases. The Pao_2 is decreased as a result of the shunt effect from blood perfusing the unventilated lung. The $Paco_2$ may drop significantly as the result of the compensatory hyperventilation of the remaining lung. The white blood cell count is often elevated.

DIAGNOSIS. The diagnosis is suspected by recognizing the patient at risk and heeding the clinical findings described previously. For major areas of atelectasis the chest film is the most important diagnostic tool, showing collapsed lobes and an abnormal location of interlobar fissures (Fig. 129-1).

Air bronchograms produced by the contrast between

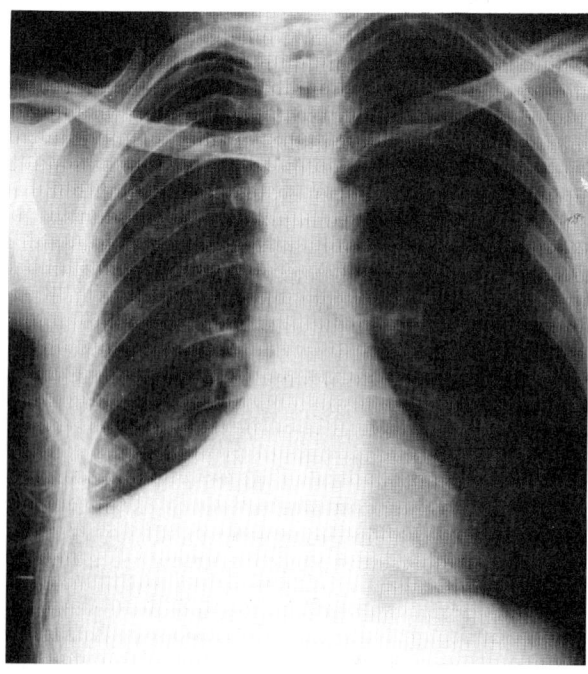

Fig. 129-1. Right lower lobe atelectasis with obliteration of shadow of diaphragm. There is no bronchogram. (Courtesy of George Popky, M.D.)

endobronchial gas and collapsed tissue on the chest roentgenogram may have therapeutic significance, since they correlate with patency of major airways. In atelectasis caused by proximal airway obstruction, usually there is no air remaining in the bronchus, and an air bronchogram is not found; this suggests that bronchoscopy may be helpful in relieving the obstruction.

COURSE, MANAGEMENT, AND PREVENTION. If untreated, atelectasis, particularly if caused by an obstructed bronchus, can lead to secondary infection and bacterial pneumonia. The secretions retained in the obstructed or unventilated portion of the lung serve as a medium for bacterial growth and eventual pneumonia. If the bronchus to the atelectatic area is obstructed, infection is likely to be caused by anaerobic bacteria and to result in lung abscess. Whether pneumonia develops or not, atelectasis can progress to eventual fibrosis and permanent volume loss if the affected pulmonary tissue is not reexpanded. As with almost any pathologic process, prevention is preferable to treatment.

Since atelectasis is a rather common complication of upper abdominal and chest surgery, this situation has been intensely studied. Although there remains considerable controversy as to the best technique, the major factor in the prevention of postoperative atelectasis appears to be periodic expansion of the lungs with large volumes of air. Formerly intermittent positive-pressure breathing (IPPB) therapy was used to achieve this result, but more recently incentive spirometry and other techniques have been used. At present it would appear that none of these methods offers any advantages over the others in most cases.

The patient's own bronchoalveolar clearing mechanisms should also be used. This requires training in cough techniques, encouragement to cough, early postoperative mobility, and avoidance of suppression of the cough reflex with sedation or pain medication. Chest percussion to loosen secretions and adequate airway hydration to prevent excessive drying and inspissation of mucus are also important in the prevention of atelectasis. Once atelectasis has occurred, the treatment depends to some extent on the cause. If there is proximal airway obstruction by a foreign body, this should be promptly removed by rigid bronchoscopy. If there is no proximal obstruction or obstruction only by mucus plugs, vigorous respiratory therapy, including airway humidification, aerosolized bronchodilators, mucolytic agents, chest percussion, and postural drainage techniques, should be employed. If these measures are unsuccessful, fiberoptic bronchoscopy is recommended for aspiration of mucus plugs and saline lavage of occluded areas. In addition, bronchodilators, decongestants, and mucolytic agents may be instilled locally to aid in the removal of mucus plugs.

MIDDLE LOBE SYNDROME

Middle lobe syndrome is atelectasis of the right middle lobe, with the cause generally attributed to compression of the lobe's orifice by enlarged peribronchial nodes. Recently, however, this concept of cause has been challenged, since numerous cases have been reported in which no bronchial obstruction could be documented by bronchoscopy and bronchography. The right middle lobe has been singled out for special consideration because chronic atelectasis, with no readily discernible cause, appears to occur most commonly in this lobe. Theories advanced for the predilection of this lobe to volume loss now include (1) the prominent collection of lymph nodes surrounding the right middle lobe bronchus, (2) the drainage of much of the right lung and some of the left lung into these nodes, (3) the acute angulation of the right middle lobe bronchus, (4) the relatively narrow caliber of the right middle lobe bronchus compared to other bronchi subserving similar lung volumes, (5) the relatively long length and easy compressibility of the right middle lobe bronchus, and (6) the relatively poor collateral ventilation of the right middle lobe, attributed to the greater ratio of pleural surface to nonpleural surface of this lobe when compared to other lobes.

The symptoms of right middle lobe syndrome are variable and include a history suggestive of bronchial asthma or episodes of recurrent respiratory infections. Chronic cough, fever, anterior chest pain, and hemoptysis may also be complaints.

The roentgenographic findings are those of volume loss in the right middle lobe. This may be difficult to detect unless a lateral film of the chest is carefully scrutinized. When right middle lobe atelectasis is discovered, bronchoscopy and possibly bronchography are required to evaluate the lesion, since in the adult population about 40% of such lesions are caused by malignant tumors. Treatment of the right middle lobe syndrome is the same as that for any other lobar atelectasis, except that the tendency toward chronicity may necessitate long-term respiratory therapy on an outpatient basis. Because of the chronicity and recurrent nature of right middle lobe atelectasis, surgical removal of the lobe is required more frequently than in other forms or areas of atelectasis, but this is still rarely necessary.

BIBLIOGRAPHY

Culiner, M.M.: The right middle lobe syndrome, a non-obstructive complex, Dis. Chest **50:**57, 1966.

Fraser, R.G., and Paré, J.A.: Diagnosis of diseases of the chest, Philadelphia, 1977, W.B. Saunders Co.

Inner, C.R., and others: Collateral ventilation and the middle lobe syndrome, Am. Rev. Respir. Dis. **118:**305, 1978.

Iverson, L., and others: A comparative study of IPPB, the incentive spirometer and blow bottles: the prevention of atelectasis following cardiac surgery, Ann. Thorac. Surg. **24:**197, 1978.

Latimer, R.G., and others: Pulmonary complications after upper abdominal surgery by pre-operative and post-operative computerized spirometer and blood gas analysis. Am. J. Surg. **122:**622, 1971.

Mahajan, V.K., Catron, P.W., and Huber, G.L.: The value of fiberoptic bronchoscopy in the management of pulmonary collapse. Chest **73:**817, 1978.

Marini, J.J., Pierson, D.J., and Hudson, L.D.: Acute lobar atelectasis: a prospective comparison of fiberoptic bronchoscopy and respiratory therapy, Am. Rev. Respir. Dis. **119:**971, 1979.

Schlenker, J.D., and Hubay, C.A.: The pathogenesis of post-operative atelectasis, Arch. Surg. **107:**846, 1973.

130 • ASTHMA
Gregory S. Lenchner

(See Chapter 4.)

DEFINITION. Asthma is a syndrome characterized by intermittent shortness of breath and wheezing. It is associated with increased responsiveness of the trachea and bronchi to various stimuli, producing bronchospasm. There is widespread narrowing of the airways that changes in severity either spontaneously or as a result of treatment. Asthma differs from chronic bronchitis and emphysema in that it is an episodic disease with airflow obstruction that is at least partially reversible.

Asthma can be divided into extrinsic (or atopic or allergic), intrinsic (or nonallergic), and combined intrinsic and extrinsic forms and some miscellaneous types. Although patients often do not strictly fit one category, categorization is useful for historical reasons and to help in understanding asthma.

EXTRINSIC ASTHMA. Extrinsic asthma is caused by exposure to an allergen. Asthmatic patients with this condition often have a strong history of allergies and a family history of asthma. Skin tests often give evidence of multiple allergens. The attacks tend to be seasonal. Patients commonly have a history of hay fever and eczema, and their asthma usually begins before age 35. Asthma with onset in childhood usually stops before adulthood but may recur in later years. Patients with a strong history of atopy, such as eczema and hay-fever, may have high levels of IgE antibodies in their blood. This IgE or reagin antibody is produced in allergic individuals in response to a particular antigen or allergen. IgE antibodies are bound to mast cells in the submucosa of bronchial epithelium. On exposure to the appropriate antigen, an antigen-antibody reaction occurs, causing release of substances from the mast cell (see "Pathogenesis and pathophysiology" later in this chapter). These substances cause various reactions resulting in the acute syndrome known as asthma. Substances that increase cyclic adenosine monophosphate (AMP) inhibit mast cell release of the asthma-provoking agents, and substances that increase cyclic guanidine monophosphate (GMP) facilitate their release. In some patients who have extrinsic asthma as children, intrinsic asthma develops in adulthood.

INTRINSIC ASTHMA. In certain asthmatic patients no extrinsic substance can be demonstrated to cause the asthma. Attacks are often preceded by an upper respiratory infection. These patients tend to be older than 35 years of age and to have more persistent, less successfully treatable bronchial obstruction. Like patients with extrinsic asthma, they may have high eosinophil counts in both blood and sputum. Their IgE levels, however, tend to be normal. Results of skin tests for allergies are usually negative, and family and personal histories tend to be lacking for atopy. These patients often become reliant on long-term steroid therapy for adequate control.

MISCELLANEOUS FORMS OF ASTHMA

Drug-induced asthma. Certain drugs and chemicals may provoke a potentially severe asthmatic attack by causing the release of substances from mast cells without using the IgE pathway. Such substances include aspirin, various nonsteroidal anti-inflammatory drugs such as indomethacin and mefenamic acid, and tartrazine, a yellow dye used in foods. Some patients also have nasal polyps and sinusitis. It is believed that the mechanism involved is not allergic but is related to prostaglandin inhibition. Curiously, sodium salicylate ingestion by these patients does not precipitate an asthmatic attack.

Exercise-induced asthma. Many asthmatic patients tend to have worsening of bronchospasm with exercise, but there is a subgroup whose bronchospasm is brought on only with exercise. This condition, called exercise-induced asthma, may be related to heat and moisture loss in the upper airways. Certain exercises, such as jogging in cold weather, are more asthmogenic than others, such as swimming in warm water. Cromolyn sodium and/or a β-adrenergic agonist used before asthma-provoking exercise may prevent attacks.

Occupational asthma. (See Chapter 133.) Various occupational exposures may also provoke an asthmatic attack. These occupational asthmatic syndromes may be related to allergic or nonallergic factors; some are mediated by IgE antibody and others are not. The incidence varies with the occupation. For example, some form of asthma develops in 10% of bakers, 50% of those exposed to toluene-di-isocyanate (TDI), and a majority of those who work with platinum. A detailed occupational history should be elicited from all asthmatic patients to search for provocative agents. Occupational asthma may be confirmed by skin testing, but the best technique for confirming the diagnosis is bronchial provocation testing. Serial pulmonary function tests are obtained before and after exposure to the suspected offending agent to determine if a deterioration in pulmonary function occurs after exposure. If such testing is not possible, the physician may get indirect evidence that the patient has occupational asthma by having him avoid the suspected agent (for example, by taking a vacation) to see if the asthma then improves only to recur on the patient's return to work. Occupationally induced asthma should also be suspected if bronchospasm is worse during the week and improves over weekends or holidays.

Allergic bronchopulmonary aspergillosis. Allergic bronchopulmonary aspergillosis is a form of asthma associated with recurrent pulmonary infiltrates and peripheral eosinophilia. The roentgenographic findings are associated with the expectoration of brownish plugs that, when cultured and stained, show the presence of the fungus *Aspergillus*. Criteria for the diagnosis are (1) underlying asthma, (2) blood eosinophilia, (3) immediate skin reaction to *Aspergillus* antigen, (4) precipitating antibodies to *Aspergillus* antigen, (5) increased IgE levels, (6) a history of transient or fixed pulmonary infiltrates, and (7) central bronchiectasis. Less specific criteria include *A. fumigatus* in the sputum, a history of expectoration of brown plugs or flecks, and Arthus reactivity (delayed skin reaction) to the *Aspergillus* antigen.

It is important to recognize allergic bronchopulmonary aspergillosis because of its long-term complications. If left untreated, the patient will have repeated episodes of bronchospasm and worsening obstruction, and central bronchiectasis will eventually develop. When a diagnosis of allergic bronchopulmonary aspergillosis is made, steroid therapy of relatively long duration is necessary to prevent sequelae.

Bronchopulmonary aspergillosis must be distinguished from other forms of *Aspergillus* disease such as invasive aspergillosis in the immunocompromised host, hypersensitivity pneumonitis caused by *Aspergillus,* and fungus ball formation resulting from *Aspergillus* infection (aspergilloma).

Cough as the only manifestation of asthma. It has been shown recently that some people may have persistent cough without evidence of bronchospasm. This cough may be the only manifestation of asthma. These people can have normal results of routine pulmonary function studies; only when they are challenged with methacholine does a greater than expected increase in airway obstruction develop. The diagnosis of cough caused by asthma is most appropriately based on the methacholine challenge test. However, if this test is unavailable, a trial with antiasthmatic medications may be indicated for a patient with unexplained chronic cough. If the patient responds to the medications with alleviation of the cough, a diagnosis of cough asthma is presumed.

PATHOLOGY AND PATHOPHYSIOLOGY. Early in the acute asthmatic attack there is smooth muscle contraction. As the attack becomes prolonged, more bronchoconstriction caused by mucosal edema, mucosal gland hypertrophy caused by increased inflammatory cells, and mucous plugging of the bronchial tree occur.

In the allergic type of asthma there are numerous mast cells (and possibly basophils) with attached IgE antibodies in the submucosa of the bronchi. When the antibodies combine with specific antigens, various preformed and newly synthesized substances are released from the mast cells. These substances include histamine, eosinophilic chemotactic factor of anaphylaxis (ECF-A), slow-reacting substance of anaphylaxis (SRS-A), platelet activating factor, lipid chemotactic factors, and prostaglandins. Some of these substances cause a contraction of bronchial smooth muscle and an increase in vascular permeability.

The release of these mediators is affected by various cholinergic and adrenergic drugs that alter the cellular levels of cyclic AMP and cyclic GMP. Drugs that increase cyclic AMP prevent the release of the chemical mediators from the mast cell. Drugs that increase cyclic GMP facilitate the release of the chemical asthmatic mediators. β-Adrenergic agonists and certain prostaglandins (such as E_1 and E_2) tend to increase cyclic AMP by activating the enzyme adenyl cyclase, which converts adenosine triphosphate (ATP) to cyclic AMP. Other drugs increase cyclic AMP levels by acting on the enzyme phosphodiesterase, which is responsible for the breakdown of cyclic AMP. Methylxanthines inhibit phosphodiesterase and thus result in increased levels of cyclic AMP. Acetylcholine, methacholine, and other parasympathomimetic drugs tend to increase cyclic GMP by activating guanyl cyclase and converting guanidine triphosphate (GTP) to cyclic GMP. The ratio between cyclic AMP and cyclic GMP is very important. With an increased ratio fewer mediators are released; with a decreased ratio more mediators are released.

The parasympathetic nervous system, acting through the vagus nerve, may be important in causing asthma. In the lung there exists a vagally mediated, cholinergic, broncho-constriction-irritant reflex that, when activated (possibly by histamine), causes bronchoconstriction. When the vagus nerve is either cooled or cut in experimental animals, experimentally induced asthma is considerably diminished. Some believe there are decreased numbers of β-adrenergic receptors in the asthmatic patient, resulting in an increased tendency for bronchoconstriction.

CLINICAL MANIFESTATIONS. Asthma may be manifested by various symptoms and signs depending on the degree of bronchoconstriction. Classically asthma is characterized by cough, shortness of breath, and wheezing; the asthmatic attacks may be episodic. In some asthmatic patients the symptoms are worse in the early morning, probably because levels of epinephrine are decreased at that time. Cough may be the only manifestation of asthma. Status asthmaticus is usually defined as persistence of severe bronchospasm despite bronchodilator therapy. After several hours muscle fatigue may result in hypoventilation and hypercapnia.

Physical examination of an asthmatic patient may be unremarkable. Routine spirometric testing may show normal results between attacks. With increased severity the physician may observe an increase in the anteroposterior diameter of the chest because of air trapping, wheezing, increased shortness of breath, an exaggerated decrease in systolic blood pressure on inspiration (pulsus paradoxus), and increased use of the accessory muscles of respiration.

When pulsus paradoxus is present, the patient is using his accessory muscles to breathe. This indicates that the attack is very severe and that the patient's expiratory airflow is significantly diminished. Generally at this point the patient should be hospitalized for intensive therapy.

In some cases airflow obstruction is so pronounced that the physician hears nothing on chest examination ("silent chest") and may be lulled into thinking that the patient is not having a serious attack. Only with therapy and improvement in the patient's condition is audible wheezing appreciated. Since it can be difficult to assess the severity of an asthmatic attack, various laboratory studies should be employed to assess and follow the clinical course of the attack.

LABORATORY FINDINGS. Laboratory studies for an asthmatic patient may be normal between attacks. During an attack the 1-second forced expiratory volume ($FEV_{1.0}$) is decreased with a normal forced vital capacity (FVC), and the ratio of $FEV_{1.0}$ to FVC is reduced. The expiratory flows at low lung volumes are also markedly diminished. Peak flow and $FEV_{1.0}$ are reliable, easily reproducible tests and good indicators of airway obstruction and are thus excellent for following and assessing the asthmatic patient. In all patients with asthma who are thought to be seriously ill, arterial blood gases should be measured. It is difficult to estimate the amount of hypoxemia by clinical examination. The asthmatic patient classically has a reduced Pa_{O_2} and a reduced Pa_{CO_2}. With extremely severe asthma the Pa_{CO_2} may rise to normal or higher. At the point when the Pa_{CO_2} reaches normal, bronchial obstruction is extremely severe, the $FEV_{1.0}$ is probably less than 25% of the predicted value, and the patient may require mechanical assistance for ventilation. With therapy including bronchodilating agents, the bronchi may not only dilate, but there may also be increased perfusion, caused by pulmonary vasculature dilation, to areas of reduced ventilation. Because of this effect there tends to be a decrease in the Pa_{O_2} in the asthmatic patient with the onset of treatment, making it all the more necessary to check levels of arterial blood gases. Even when both the patient and the physician believe that the asthma has receded, the spirometric values ($FEV_{1.0}$ and forced expiratory flow between 25% and 75% of vital capacity) remain abnormal. The test result that remains abnormal for the longest period, perhaps even 3 weeks after the acute attack, is the residual volume, which may be much greater than normal. This abnormality stresses the importance of continued treatment even after the clinical symptoms of the attack have disappeared.

In following the asthmatic patient, the physician may use daily $FEV_{1.0}$ and peak expiratory flow rate measurements. Other expiratory flow rates and Pa_{CO_2} may also help in judging the severity of an attack.

MANAGEMENT. Prevention is the primary goal of asthma therapy. Precipitating factors (as with aspirin-induced asthma) should be avoided when possible. The patient should stop smoking and should avoid other irritants. The patient who has hypertension should not be given β-adrenergic blockers such as propranolol. If the patient has occupational asthma, exposure to the occupational allergen should be eliminated. Food allergens rarely cause asthmatic attacks in adults, but when they do, the attacks are often accompanied by urticaria or gastrointestinal symptoms. Desensitization, although useful in some patients, has not been shown to be beneficial for the majority of adult asthmatic patients. In some individuals emotional stress may precipitate an attack, and minor tranquilizers may be useful.

For the acute attack requiring immediate therapy in the physician's office or hospital emergency department, the traditional initial management is the administration of serial injections of adrenergic agents (epinephrine, terbutaline) subcutaneously. Persistent bronchospasm requires the use of parenteral methylxanthines (aminophylline). The therapy may have to be altered for the individual with hypertension, coronary artery disease, or arrhythmias. O_2 supplementation, hydration, and aerosolized bronchodilators may also be useful. The roles of intermittent positive-pressure breathing (IPPB) and tranquilizers in treating acute attacks are controversial. When bronchospasm does not improve, parenteral steroid therapy and hospitalization are required.

Theophyllines. The methylxanthine compounds have been used for many years and remain the primary agents in the treatment of asthma. They act by inhibiting phosphodiesterase, which results in an increase in cyclic AMP and bronchodilation.

β-Adrenergic agonists. The β-agonists reduce obstruction by activating adenyl cyclase, thereby increasing cyclic AMP. The original β-agonist is epinephrine, which is still a commonly used and reliable drug for the acute asthmatic attack. $β_2$-Agonists are newer agents that more selectively affect β-receptors in the lung ($β_2$-receptors), causing bronchodilation, and less significantly activate cardiac receptors ($β_1$-receptors). The $β_2$-agonists theoretically cause less cardiac toxicity and are more specific for the bronchial smooth muscle receptors. The recently approved $β_2$-agonists that are used in the United States include metaproterenol, terbutaline, and albuterol. These substances may be given orally, subcutaneously, or by inhalation. It has been shown recently that $β_2$-agonists administered by the inhalation route may give more prompt relief of an asthmatic attack than does a full dose of intravenous aminophylline.

Cromolyn sodium. Cromolyn sodium is of greatest benefit in the childhood or extrinsic form of asthma. This agent is of no value in treating an acute attack but is used for prophylaxis. It stabilizes the mast cell, thereby preventing the release of the various mediators that can result in bronchospasm. It is very useful in preventing exercise-induced asthma and may decrease the steroid dosage that is required to control some asthmatic patients. It is administered by inhalation via a "spinhaler."

Steroid therapy. When to use steroids, how much to use, how effective steroids are, and how long it takes steroids to act are still controversial matters. Most physicians specializing in the treatment of pulmonary disease agree that steroids should be used for the severely asthmatic patient who requires hospitalization and the patient who has had an unsatisfactory response to therapeutic β-agonists and theophylline. Vigorous attempts should be made to quickly wean patients from steroids. Occasionally, particularly in the adult asthmatic patient, a maintenance regimen of steroids is required. If possible, an alternate-day regimen should be used to minimize side effects. When the patient's condition is stable, the use of a topically inhaled steroid such as beclomethasone may make it possible to decrease the maintenance dosage of oral steroids. The steroids administered by inhalation exert their action locally and when used properly are not significantly absorbed systemically. As a result they are preferred over orally administered steroids in maintenance therapy. The use of inhaled topical steroids should probably be preceded by an inhaled β-adrenergic agonist to produce bronchodilation and ensure that the steroid is delivered to the deepest parts of the lung. Converting from oral to inhalation steroids may worsen the patient's nasal symptoms. On a long-term basis the use of inhalation steroids may result in oral candidiasis; to avoid this, the patient should rinse his mouth after each use of the inhalation steroid.

Oxygen and hydration. Asthmatic patients should be given O_2 liberally, since the initial effect of bronchodilators may cause a decrease in the arterial Po_2. In addition, these patients should be well hydrated to mobilize secretions and prevent their inspissation.

PROGNOSIS. The long-term prognosis for patients with asthma is excellent. In the absence of recurrent infections there is little evidence for a progressive deterioration of pulmonary function.

BIBLIOGRAPHY

Barnes, P., and others: Nocturnal asthma and changes in circulating epinephrine, histamine and cortisol, N. Engl. J. Med. **303**:263, 1980.

Corrao, W.M., Braman, S.S., and Irwin, R.J.: Chronic cough as the sole presenting manifestation of bronchial asthma, N. Engl. J. Med. **300**:633, 1979.

McFadden, S.R., Jr., and Ingram, R.H., Jr.: Exercise-induced asthma, N. Engl. J. Med. **301**:763, 1979.

Rosenberg, M., and others: Clinical and immunologic criteria for the diagnosis of allergic bronchopulmonary aspergillosis, Ann. Intern. Med. **86**:405, 1977.

Rossing, T.H., and others: Emergency therapy of asthma: comparison of the acute effects of parenteral and inhaled sympathomimetics and infused aminophylline, Am. Rev. Respir. Dis. **122**:365, 1980.

Weiss, E.B., and Segal, M.S.: Bronchial asthma, mechanisms and therapeutics, Boston, 1976, Little, Brown & Co.

131 • RESPIRATORY FAILURE

Sandeep Dhand

Since the primary function of the lungs is gas exchange, that is, O_2 uptake and CO_2 elimination, a failure of the respiratory system implies a reduction in O_2 and CO_2 exchange. Normal pulmonary physiologic mechanisms (see also Chapter 121) must be discussed briefly before embarking on a discussion of respiratory failure.

OXYGEN TRANSPORT

O_2 transport to tissues depends on O_2 content and cardiac output. The former is a function of hemoglobin (Hb), O_2 saturation of Hb (So_2), and arterial O_2 tension (or partial pressure) (Pao_2), as shown in the equation:

$$O_2 \text{ content} = O_2 \text{ carried by Hb} + O_2 \text{ dissolved in plasma}$$
$$= (1.34 \times g\,Hb \times So_2) + (0.003 \times Pao_2)$$

For a normal Hb concentration (15 g%), Pao_2 (100 mm Hg), and So_2 (100%) the value of O_2 content carried by Hb is 20.1 vol%. The Hb is the major determinant of the total amount of O_2 carried by blood under normal conditions.

The normal oxyhemoglobin dissociation curve is shown in Fig. 131-1. A Pao_2 of 60 mm Hg is usually acceptable. A shift of the curve to the right or to the left indicates a change in the Hb affinity for O_2 and is measured as the Pao_2 at which 50% of the Hb is saturated with O_2. This pressure of O_2 is called P_{50}, with the normal value being approximately 27 mm Hg. A shift of the curve to the right (increased P_{50}) occurs with acidemia, high

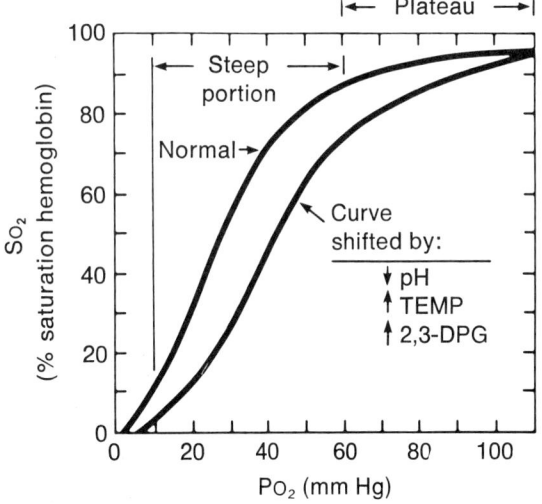

Fig. 131-1. Normal oxyhemoglobin dissociation curve, with pH 7.4 and temperature 98.6° F (37°C). Shifted curve depicts rightward shift caused by decrease in pH, increase in temperature, and increase in red blood cell 2,3-diphosphoglycerate.

Paco₂, high temperature, and increased red blood cell 2,3-diphosphoglycerate; it results in reduced O_2 content but aids in the transfer of O_2 from blood to tissue.

The Fick equation ($\dot{V}_{O_2} = \dot{Q}[Ca_{O_2} - C\bar{v}_{O_2}]$), in which $\dot{V}_{O_2}$ is O_2 consumption, $\dot{Q}$ equals cardiac output, Ca_{O_2} is arterial O_2 content, and $C\bar{v}_{O_2}$ equals mixed venous O_2 content, indicates that if $\dot{V}_{O_2}$ is constant, cardiac output is inversely related to the arterial-to-venous O_2 content difference ($C[a-\bar{v}]_{O_2}$). A reduction in $C\bar{v}_{O_2}$ or increase in $C(a-\bar{v})_{O_2}$ signifies decreased cardiac output. The $C\bar{v}_{O_2}$ can be measured in pulmonary artery blood via a Swan-Ganz catheter, or cardiac output can be estimated directly by a thermodilution technique.

In summary, the O_2 transport equation shows that a normal Pa_{O_2} does not necessarily guarantee normal O_2 transport if either hemoglobin or cardiac output is reduced.

CARBON DIOXIDE TRANSPORT

The Henderson-Hasselbalch equation indicates the relationship of pH, HCO_3^- and P_{CO_2}:

$$pH = pK' + \log \frac{[HCO_3^-]}{0.03 \times P_{CO_2}}$$

where pK' is the dissociation constant in plasma at 98.6° F (37° C). In the normal situation this equation becomes

$$7.4 = 6.1 + \log \frac{(24)}{0.03 \times 40}$$

In chronic respiratory acidosis the rise in the Paco₂ is chronic, thus allowing time for the renal compensatory response, which results in an increase in HCO_3^-. Hence the fall in pH is not significant. In acute respiratory acidosis, however, an acute increase in Paco₂ results in a significant drop in pH because of the lack of time for a compensatory rise in HCO_3^-.

HYPOXEMIA AND ITS MECHANISMS

Hypoxia is the state in which there is inadequate delivery of O_2 to meet the oxidative requirements of tissues. Hypoxemia, on the other hand, indicates a reduced level of oxygen in the blood (low Pao₂). The four basic causes of hypoxemia are ventilation-perfusion ($\dot{V}_A/\dot{Q}_C$) mismatch, right-to-left shunting of blood (venous admixture), diffusion defects, and alveolar hypoventilation. Of these, $\dot{V}_A/\dot{Q}_C$ mismatch is the most common.

The alveolar-arterial (A-a) oxygen gradient is the difference between the P_{O_2} in alveolar air and that in arterial blood; it is normally less than 12 mm Hg in a subject breathing room air. This difference is related to some normal intrapulmonary right-to-left shunting of blood and some $\dot{V}_A/\dot{Q}_C$ match. $P(A-a)_{O_2}$ is increased with most causes of hypoxemia, except pure alveolar hypoventilation.

Normal values of arterial blood gases measured during room air breathing are 80 to 90 mm Hg Pao₂ (decreasing with increasing age), 36 to 42 mm Hg Paco₂, 7.38 to 7.42 pH, and 95% to 100% So₂. The mixed venous O_2 ($P\bar{v}_{O_2}$) is normally about 40 mm Hg. A reduction in Pao₂ below 50 mm Hg with or without an elevation of the Paco₂ above 50 mm Hg indicates respiratory failure.

CLASSIFICATION OF RESPIRATORY FAILURE

Respiratory failure may be acute or chronic and hypoxemic alone or hypoxemic and hypercarbic. Acute respiratory failure is characterized by a rapid change in the Pao₂ or Paco₂ either in individuals with previously normal lungs or in those with underlying chronic respiratory failure. It is a medical emergency. Chronic respiratory failure is suggested by the presence of chronically elevated Paco₂ and a reduction in the Pao₂. The increase in the Paco₂ is compensated by an increase in bicarbonate. The causes of respiratory failure include:

I. Failure to oxygenate arterial blood (hypoxemic respiratory failure)
   A. Adult respiratory distress syndrome (ARDS)
   B. Cardiac pulmonary edema
   C. Neurogenic pulmonary edema (includes elements of ARDS)
II. Failure of CO_2 excretion (hypoxic and hypercarbic respiratory failure)
   A. Chronic obstructive pulmonary disease (COPD)
   B. Severe bronchial asthma
III. Failure with normal lungs (predominantly hypercarbic respiratory failure)
   A. Brain—sedative overdose, central and obstructive sleep apneas, primary alveolar hypoventilation
   B. Spinal cord and chest wall (chest bellows)—obesity-hypoventilation syndrome, kyphoscoliosis, thoracoplasty, flail chest, cervical cord injury, other neuromuscular diseases
   C. Upper airways—severe laryngospasm, foreign body, tumor, stenosis

ADULT RESPIRATORY DISTRESS SYNDROME (ARDS)

ARDS is one of the most common causes of acute hypoxemic respiratory failure. Other synonyms for this disorder are shock lung, traumatic wet lung, and Da Nang lung. The causes of ARDS include viral pneumonia, hypotension, fat emboli, aspiration, drug overdose, trauma, multiple transfusions, and pancreatitis.

The patient usually has no underlying cardiac or pulmonary disease. Symptoms and signs develop after a latent period of up to 48 hours following an insult. The earliest features are tachypnea and apprehension. These gradually worsen and then are accompanied by grunting respirations and the use of the accessory muscles of respiration. Rales and rhonchi may be audible during auscultation of the chest. Hypoxemia minimally responsive to oxygen therapy (indicating intrapulmonary right-to-left shunting of blood) is evident. The chest roentgenogram shows bilateral patchy, fluffy infiltrates that gradually progress to a "lung whiteout." Air bronchograms are commonly prominent.

The increase in extravascular lung water in ARDS may occur from a number of mechanisms (based on Starling's law). The permeability of the alveolar-capillary membrane is increased in ARDS with a resultant increase in fluid flux. This increase may be related to direct damage, as from aspiration of gastric contents with a low pH, or to release of proteolytic enzymes and complement activation, as from microthrombi in the pulmonary capillaries, particularly in pancreatitis and sepsis. Low protein osmotic pressure and increased hydrostatic pressure may play a small role in some cases of ARDS. The pulmonary capillary wedge pressure (PCWP), as measured by a Swan-Ganz catheter, is normal (less than or equal to 12 mm Hg), thus differentiating ARDS from cardiogenic pulmonary edema, in which the PCWP is elevated.

In ARDS there is alteration of lung mechanics, lung volumes, and gas exchange. The lung compliance is decreased as a result of increased lung water and decreased surfactant. The functional residual capacity (FRC) is consistently reduced as a result of atelectasis and reduced compliance. There is hypoxemia indicated by widening of the $P_{(A-a)}O_2$. An intrapulmonary right-to-left shunt is suggested by the lack of response of the hypoxemia to inhalation of 100% O_2. This shunt occurs when lung units become filled with edema fluid and are not ventilated. Perfusion continues so that the $\dot{V}_A/\dot{Q}_C$ ratio in these involved lung units approaches 0. Hypercarbia in patients with ARDS is a late and ominous sign. The diagnosis of ARDS is made by finding appropriate clinical circumstances, diffuse alveolar shadows on the chest roentgenogram with a normal heart size (Fig. 131-2), hypoxemia resistant to O_2 therapy, decreased lung compliance and FRC, and normal PCWP.

MANAGEMENT. The aim of treatment in ARDS is to maintain adequate O_2 transport and thus good tissue oxygenation. Swan-Ganz catheters help in the measurement of $P\bar{v}O_2$, cardiac output, and PCWP. The last is a better indicator of left ventricular function and overall fluid status than is the central venous pressure.

Adequate oxygenation in patients with ARDS can be obtained by proper fluid management guided by PCWP (keeping it between 10 and 12 mm Hg to reduce the lung water), diuretics as necessary, supplemental high concentrations of oxygen, and early mechanical ventilation. The value of positive end-expiratory pressure (PEEP) in ARDS has been well documented. Recruiting collapsed alveoli and hence increasing FRC reduces the areas of low $\dot{V}_A/\dot{Q}_c$ or shunt. This increases the PaO_2 obtained with a given inspired O_2 concentration (FIO_2) and helps prevent O_2 toxicity by allowing reduction of the FIO_2.

The hazards of PEEP include barotrauma and hemo-

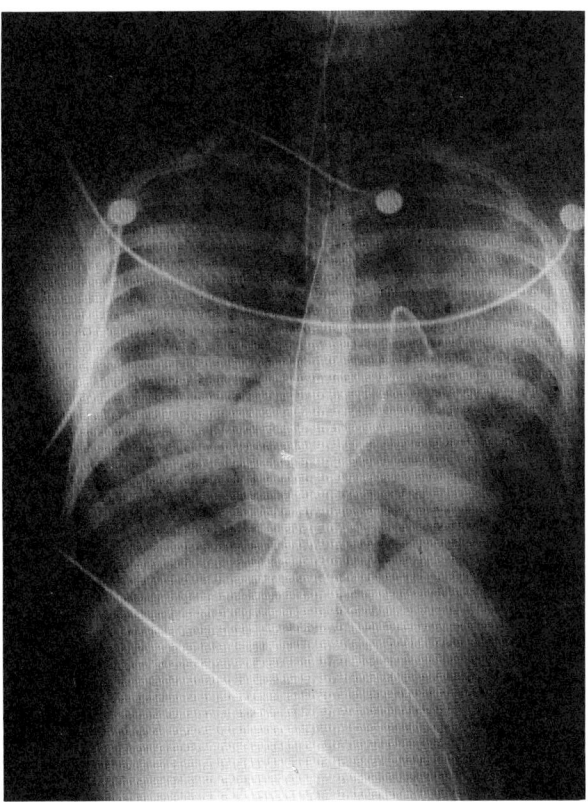

Fig. 131-2. Acute respiratory distress syndrome in 17-year-old girl with overwhelming bacteremia. There are bilateral alveolar infiltrates with normal heart size.

dynamic impairment. The former consists of subcutaneous emphysema, pneumothorax, and pneumomediastinum. Hemodynamically, with increasing levels of PEEP there is a reduction in venous return to the heart, and hence cardiac output falls. The decrease in cardiac output may offset any advantage gained by an increase in PaO_2, since systemic O_2 transport is dependent on both of these factors. The $P\bar{v}O_2$ and effective compliance can be used as guides for the level of PEEP that leads to the most favorable combination of PaO_2 and cardiac output. Ideally, the PaO_2 is kept between 60 and 80 mm Hg, the $P\bar{v}O_2$ above 30 mm Hg, the FIO_2 at 0.5 or lower, and the PCWP between 10 and 12 mm Hg.

The use of corticosteroids and heparin in ARDS remains controversial. No controlled clinical traits are available regarding the use of either of these agents. Steroids may be indicated in fat embolism, aspiration, and septic shock. Antibiotics should be used when there is evidence of infection. The role of the extracorporeal membrane oxygenator (ECMO) is limited, since it fails to increase survival. The prognosis for patients with fully developed ARDS is poor, and the mortality ranges from 50% to 70%. Death usually results from decreased cardiac output, gastrointestinal bleeding, or sepsis.

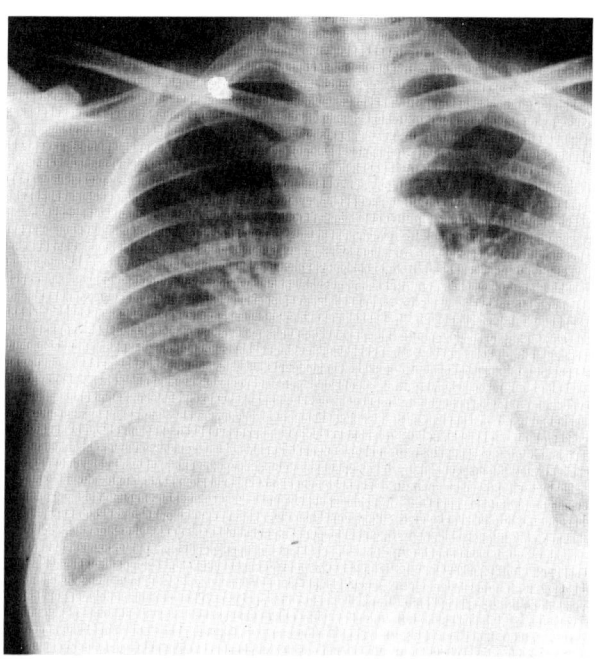

Fig. 131-3. Heart failure in 42-year-old man demonstrating enlarged heart with marked venous congestion and pulmonary edema. (Courtesy of George Popky, M.D.)

PULMONARY EDEMA

Cardiac pulmonary edema is characterized by increased lung water, bilateral infiltrates, cardiomegaly, and increased PCWP, as measured by means of the Swan-Ganz catheter (Fig. 131-3). In accordance with Starling's law, the increase in pulmonary capillary hydrostatic pressure related to left ventricular failure or mitral stenosis leads to increased fluid flux into the lung interstitium and then into the alveoli.

Patients with pulmonary edema have tachypnea, cardiac enlargement, and an S_3 gallop. They usually have an underlying cardiac condition and respond quickly to diuretics, digitalis, and fluid restriction. Hypoxemia and respiratory alkalosis are common in the early phases, but with severe pulmonary edema, respiratory acidosis supervenes and assisted ventilation may be necessary. Usually, however, supplemental O_2 administered by nasal prongs or a mask is sufficient.

Neurogenic pulmonary edema (usually following head injury) is also related in part to high hydrostatic pressure. The mechanism is thought to be hypothalamic stimulation leading to pulmonary venoconstriction and shifting of blood from the systemic to the pulmonary circulation. Adrenergic blocking agents may be helpful in this form of edema.

CHRONIC OBSTRUCTIVE PULMONARY DISEASE AND ASTHMA

The majority of patients with COPD who have respiratory failure also have severe chronic bronchitis (giving the characteristic "blue bloater" appearance). Severe bronchial asthma (status asthmaticus) and cystic fibrosis are uncommon causes of respiratory failure. Patients with these disorders usually have a long history of disease. The chronic bronchitis group may have chronic well-compensated respiratory failure, and acute respiratory failure may be superimposed on chronically abnormal blood gas levels. Acute exacerbations of COPD are the cause in one third of cases of acute respiratory failure in intensive care units.

The mechanisms of airway obstruction in patients with COPD or asthma are intraluminal obstructions (mucous plugs), intramural narrowing (edema and smooth muscle contraction), and loss of extramural support (decreased elasticity in emphysema). Airway obstruction leads to non-homogeneous distribution of ventilation and hence to areas with abnormal $\dot{V}_A/\dot{Q}_C$ ratios. Low $\dot{V}_A/\dot{Q}_C$ ratios lead to hypoxemia, and increased $\dot{V}_A/\dot{Q}_C$ ratios result in increased alveolar dead space and ultimately hypercapnia. Increased work of breathing caused by the abnormal airway resistance may also worsen gas exchange abnormalities.

The sudden deterioration of already abnormal blood gas levels can lead to acute respiratory failure and is caused by infection, bronchospasm, congestive heart failure, injudicious use of sedatives, or high concentrations of O_2.

The clinical manifestations of the acute phase are those of hypoxemia and hypercapnia. The former results in confusion, restlessness, tachycardia, supraventricular tachyarrhythmias, and peripheral vasoconstriction, whereas hypercapnia leads to headache, drowsiness, coma, papilledema, hypertension, and tachycardia. Semicoma or coma is generally observed only when the $PaCO_2$ exceeds 75 mm Hg or the PaO_2 is less than 35 mm Hg. The patient with chronic respiratory failure has similar symptoms of hypoxemia, but the increased $PaCO_2$ is well compensated for and the symptoms of CO_2 narcosis are less prominent. Features of chronic hypoxemia are evident in the form of pulmonary hypertension, cor pulmonale, and polycythemia.

MANAGEMENT. Since hypoxemia provides a more immediate danger to life than hypercapnia, correction of the low PO_2 is of utmost importance. The goal is to increase the PaO_2 to 50 to 60 mm Hg, that is, above the steep portion of the oxyhemoglobin dissociation curve. Patients with COPD and acute respiratory failure are very O_2 sensitive. Since their ventilatory drive is dependent on hypoxemia, removing this hypoxic stimulus with excessive O_2 may cause them to hypoventilate and retain CO_2. Controlling O_2 at a fixed FIO_2 is very important in these patients. Venturi masks or nasal prongs administering O_2 at 1 to 2 L/min can be used. Nasal prongs allow for better patient comfort and expectoration, which should be encouraged. Arterial blood gas measurements must be repeated at frequent intervals to ensure a safe PaO_2 and to avoid significant CO_2 retention. However, the fear of CO_2 retention should not be a contraindication to O_2 therapy, since hypoxemia poses a more immediate threat to life.

Bronchodilators help by reducing the airway narrowing and thus improving the $\dot{V}_A/\dot{Q}_C$ abnormality and the work of breathing. The drugs available include theophyllines (intravenous and oral), adrenergic agonists (oral, inhaled, and subcutaneous), and anticholinergics.

Inhaled bronchodilators can be delivered by an intermittent positive-pressure breathing (IPPB) device, a handheld nebulizer, a freon-propelled metered-dose inhaler, or a compressor-powered nebulizer. In the dyspneic patient an IPPB device may be more easily tolerated because it allows slow, deep inspirations that maximize bronchodilator deposition. Hydration and chest physical therapy help in clearance of secretions and may improve gas exchange.

Antibiotics such as tetracycline or ampicillin may be indicated, especially if the sputum is purulent and the Gram stain reveals pus cells. The most common organisms found are *Streptococcus pneumoniae* and *Haemophilus influenzae*. Pneumonia, if present, must be aggressively treated because it may be the precipitating cause of the respiratory failure. Viral infections are also important in exacerbations.

The role of corticosteroids is controversial, and no controlled studies are available demonstrating their benefit in COPD patients with acute respiratory failure. They may help by reducing inflammation and by sensitizing adrenergic receptor sites to adrenergic agonists. Significant wheezing, unresponsiveness to bronchodilators, and sputum or blood eosinophilia are considered by some to be indications for using steroids.

Approximately 15% to 25% of patients with COPD who are undergoing acute respiratory failure require therapy with an artificial airway and mechanical ventilation. Indications for this therapy include apnea, marked respiratory acidosis with a pH of less than 7.2, and an associated metabolic acidosis related to hypotension or hypoxemia.

In patients with acute respiratory failure, cor pulmonale, and right ventricular failure, the use of digitalis is controversial and may be associated with an increased incidence of arrhythmias. Respiratory stimulants have no proven benefit.

Roughly 70% of patients with COPD survive a given episode of acute respiratory failure. However, the long-term prognosis is poor, with 1-year survival rates of 50% and 2-year survival rates of 30% reported following episodes of acute respiratory failure in COPD patients.

RESPIRATORY FAILURE WITH NORMAL LUNGS

Breathing is under the control of two centers in the central nervous system: voluntary ventilation is controlled by the cerebral cortex and involuntary ventilation is controlled by centers in the brainstem.

Chemoreceptors and neuroreceptors send signals to the centers in the brainstem. Chemoreceptors in the carotid and aortic bodies are sensitive to changes in the O_2 level in the blood. Chemoreceptors in the brainstem respond to changes in the hydrogen ion level. A reduction in blood O_2 tension or an elevation of hydrogen ion content is detected by these chemoreceptors and results in increased levels of ventilation.

Neuroreceptors in the lung include stretch, irritant, and juxtapulmonary capillary receptors. Neuroreceptors detect changes in the mechanical status of the lung and send impulses to the medullary brain centers.

Abnormal respiratory control

Alveolar hypoventilation is most commonly caused by changes in the lung parenchyma or airways, but it can also occur in patients with normal lungs. Abnormal respiratory mechanics can be the result of severe obesity, one of the sleep apnea syndromes, or primary alveolar hypoventilation. A number of disease entities fall into this category of respiratory failure with normal lungs (see previous outline).

Hypoventilation related to sedative overdose is manifested as coma, with the patient having slow, shallow respirations. At times ventilation has to be immediately supported mechanically without waiting for arterial blood gas results.

The sleep apnea syndromes (central and obstructive) are recently described entities. Central sleep apnea is the occurrence of frequent episodes of cessation of respiration caused by failure of the normal neurologic impulses to reach the respiratory muscles. These episodes must occur during non-REM sleep, last longer than 10 seconds, and recur more than 30 times in a night to be considered significant. Obstructive sleep apnea differs from the central type only in that neurologic impulses and respiratory muscle activity persist throughout the apneic episode, and transient upper airway obstruction temporarily interrupts airflow. Chronic disease is characterized by cyanosis, somnolence, polycythemia, pulmonary hypertension, and cor pulmonale. Most of the clinical abnormalities are explicable on the basis of chronic hypoxemia and hypercapnia. Snoring is an obvious finding in obstructive sleep apnea, particularly when it is associated with obesity. Sedation or a lower respiratory tract infection exacerbates the gas exchange abnormality and can lead to acute respiratory failure. The treatment includes controlled O_2 therapy, especially at night when the O_2 desaturation is more likely to occur. Respiratory stimulants such as progesterone or theophylline are often used. Tracheostomy may be required in obstructive sleep apnea. In the acute respiratory failure phase, mechanical ventilation may be necessary.

Alveolar hypoventilation resulting from defective brainstem regulation (primary alveolar hypoventilation) is uncommon but not rare. Some cases are associated with neurologic disorders such as encephalitis, whereas others are not associated with central nervous system disease other than loss of respiratory control. In this disorder the respiratory centers do not respond to CO_2 or acid stimuli and depend on hypoxic drive to maintain respiration. The suppression of hypoxic drive by the use of excessive O_2 or the administration of sedative or tranquilizing drugs results in CO_2 narcosis. Such patients can voluntarily ventilate to normal levels.

The treatment is directed at maintaining safe but not excessive levels of oxygenation. Assisted ventilation with mechanical devices, rocking beds, and electrophrenic pacemakers may be required, particularly at night.

Chest bellows disease

Chest bellows disease can be divided into mechanical and neuromuscular categories. The former includes obesity-hypoventilation syndrome (pickwickian syndrome), kyphoscoliosis, and thoracoplasty; the latter includes amyotrophic lateral sclerosis, poliomyelitis, myasthenia gravis, multiple sclerosis, spinal cord injury, and Guillain-Barré syndrome. Respiratory failure is fairly common with these diseases, and in most it is slowly progressive.

In chest bellows disease, lung function is impaired because of reduced ability to cough, leading to retained secretions, infections, and atelectasis. These can result in a severe degree of $\dot{V}_A/\dot{Q}_C$ mismatch. The reduction of vital capacity (VC) is progressive, and its measurement is a better prognostic indicator than are arterial blood gases. A VC greater than 1 L, exceeding three times the tidal volume, or above 10 to 15 ml/kg body weight is usually adequate. Any reduction below these levels leads to significant hypoventilation, $\dot{V}_A/\dot{Q}_C$ abnormalities, and respiratory failure. The chest wall compliance in this group of diseases is low, and the work of breathing is high. This coupled with the reduction in FRC below the level of closing capacity causes further impairment of gas exchange. With increasingly severe disease patients cannot maintain the high level of respiratory work required and alveolar hypoventilation ensues. Lower respiratory infections, sedatives, or underlying obstructive lung disease may precipitate acute respiratory failure.

Although many obese patients maintain normal levels of oxygen tension and alveolar ventilation, some have hypoxemia while others have both hypoxemia and hypoventilation. The obesity hypoventilation syndrome is characterized by alveolar hypoventilation with $Paco_2$ elevation, hypersomnia, cyanosis, and polycythemia; cor pulmonale is common (such patients have been called "pickwickian" because of their resemblance to a character in Charles Dickens' *Pickwick Papers*). The pulmonary tissue remains normal and there are no obstructive airway changes. Inspiratory capacity, tidal volume, and total lung capacity are preserved, but the FRC and expiratory reserve volume are reduced. Hypoxemia can be an early development because of inadequate ventilation to perfused units at the bases of the lungs.

A complete understanding of the cause of the pickwickian syndrome is not yet available, but some factors appear related if not causative. The work of breathing is increased and the chest wall compliance is reduced in obese patients with this syndrome, but both remain at normal levels in obese patients who do not have the syndrome. In addition, decreased responsiveness of the respiratory center to CO_2 has been demonstrated. Intermittent obstruction of the upper airways, such as at the glottis, is another feature of this disorder. Treatment of this syndrome includes drastic weight reduction, which is sometimes successful in reversing the syndrome. Relief of nocturnal airway obstruction and correction of hypoxemia are also important in management. Correction of acid-base status, appropriate use of diuretics, and pharmacologic agents such as theophylline and medroxyprogesterone to stimulate ventilation are useful in some patients.

In kyphoscoliosis the angle of scoliosis determines the degree of functional impairment. The risk of respiratory failure increases with an angle of scoliosis exceeding 70 degrees, and at more than 120 degrees alveolar hypoventilation commonly results. In patients with scoliosis or thoracoplasty the use of periodic hyperinflation with an IPPB device or an incentive spirometer has been shown to improve lung compliance and hypoxemia for several hours. Chronic hypoxemia should also be treated with controlled O_2 therapy. The use of orthopedic procedures for correcting kyphoscoliosis and thereby attempting to prevent progression of ventilatory impairment shows little long-term benefit.

Hypercapnia is rare in flail chest, and hypoxemia occurring in this condition is related to lung contusion, which causes decreased FRC and $\dot{V}_A/\dot{Q}_C$ mismatching.

Patients with injury to the cervical spinal cord cephalad to the third cervical vertebra have no diaphragmatic function; with injury at the third to fifth cervical vertebrae diaphragmatic function is partially lost. Either situation can cause the neuromuscular type of respiratory failure. Guillain-Barré syndrome at times may develop rapidly accompanied by respiratory failure. Patients with myasthenia gravis may have intermittent episodes of respiratory failure.

Respiratory infections must be vigorously treated. The use of tracheostomy in obstructive sleep apnea or in the obesity-hypoventilation syndrome and of diaphragmatic pacing in cervical cord paralysis should be considered. Prophylactic intubation or tracheostomy may be required, especially in the neuromuscular group, if the VC shows a progressive decrease.

If these measures do not suffice and chronic respiratory failure persists, measures such as a cuirass respirator, a rocking bed, or frog breathing can be used.

In the acute phase of respiratory failure assisted mechanical ventilation may be necessary. It may also be needed during respiratory infection in a patient with kyphoscoliosis, during the acute phase of cervical cord injury, in the obesity-hypoventilation syndrome with severe congestive heart failure, or during periods of marked neuromuscular weakness in the Guillain-Barré syndrome or myasthenia gravis.

Upper airway obstruction

Upper airway obstruction is frequently overlooked in the initial evaluation of dyspnea and wheezing. It is often not considered among the classic causes of airway obstruction, since these involve peripheral airways. However, upper or large airway obstruction can be more acute in onset than asthma or more subtle in presentation than emphysema. It may also produce acute or chronic respiratory failure.

Obstruction of the trachea may occur precipitously, as in the "café coronary" with foreign body obstruction. The individual will be in acute respiratory distress but silent, since the obstruction prevents airflow. Wheezing will not be heard. The therapy consists of attempts to relieve the obstruction by abdominal thrusts (Heimlich maneuver), back pounding, or as a last resort manual removal with the fingers. Failure to relieve the obstruction obviously results in death. Less than complete obstruction should be evident by noisy respiration and is best handled by transferring the victim to an emergency care facility. More aggressive intervention may only convert partial into complete obstruction.

Tracheal obstruction can also result from tracheal or vocal cord tumor and from stenosis caused by prior tracheal intubation or injury, in which case signs and symptoms develop more slowly. Although inspiratory stridor is usually obvious when listened for over the trachea, the condition is often initially diagnosed as asthma. These patients have even occasionally been admitted to an intensive care unit for treatment of status asthmaticus before the correct diagnosis was made. The findings, in addition to inspiratory stridor, may be limited to an abnormal laryngoscopic or bronchoscopic examination. The therapy includes maintenance of the upper airway by careful intubation or tracheostomy. The definitive therapy is usually surgical.

Obstruction of a major bronchus by a tumor or foreign body also usually develops insidiously. Occasionally a history that suggests foreign body aspiration can be elicited. The presentation more commonly is one of recurrent or persistent wheezing localized to one lung area, with eventual development of postobstructive pneumonia resistant to or recurrent after antibiotic therapy. The definitive therapy is again usually surgical removal.

Respiratory failure related to upper airway obstruction responds rapidly to removal of the obstruction or tracheostomy. Prolonged ventilatory support and oxygen therapy are rarely indicated.

BIBLIOGRAPHY

Bergofsky, E.H., and others: Cardiorespiratory failure in kyphoscoliosis, Medicine, **38**:263, 1959.

Campbell, E.T.M.: The J. Burns Amberson Lecture: the management of acute respiratory failure in chronic bronchitis and emphysema, Am. Rev. Respir. Dis. **96**:626, 1967.

Feldman, N.T., and McFadden, E.R.: Asthma therapy, old and new, Med. Clin. North Am. **61**:1239, 1977.

Guillerinault, C., and Dervent, W., editors: Sleep apnea syndromes; Kroc Foundation Series, vol. 2, New York, 1978, Alan R. Liss, Inc.

Murray, J.F., and the staff of the Division of Lung Diseases, National Heart Lung and Blood Institute: Mechanisms of acute respiratory failure, Am. Rev. Respir. Dis. **165**:1071, 1977.

Pontoppidan, H., and others: Acute respiratory failure in the adult, N. Engl. J. Med. **287**:743, 760, 799, 1972.

Staub, N.L.: Pulmonary edema, Physiol. Rev. **54**:678, 1974.

Wilson, R.S., and Pontoppidan, N.: Acute respiratory failure: diagnostic and therapeutic criteria, Crit. Care Med. **2**:293, 1974.

Zwillich, C.W., and others: Complications of arrested ventilation: a prospective study of 354 consecutive episodes, Am. J. Med. **57**:161, 1974.

132 • DIFFUSE LUNG DISEASES
Morton Rubenstein

PULMONARY FIBROSIS
Idiopathic pulmonary fibrosis

Idiopathic pulmonary fibrosis (IPF) typifies many of the clinical, roentgenographic, and physiologic features of the diffuse or interstitial lung diseases. It is characterized by dyspnea, interstitial infiltrates on the chest film, inflammation and fibrosis of the alveolar walls, and a relatively poor response to therapy. After the known causes are excluded, IPF accounts for about 40% to 60% of interstitial disease. It most commonly occurs in the fourth and fifth decades of life, but there is no clear-cut sexual, racial, or geographic predilection.

ETIOLOGY. Although no single pathogenetic mechanism has been described that accounts for all features of IPF, recent evidence suggests the participation of the immune system, perhaps in response to alveolar injury. Autoantibodies such as rheumatoid factor and antinuclear antibody, circulating immune complexes, alveolar deposition of IgG and complement, increased amounts of immunoglobulins and inflammatory cells in lavage fluid, and the occasional improvement following treatment with steroids or immunosuppressive agents support the concept of an immune mechanism. The presence of circulating immune complexes and the alveolar deposition of immunoglobulin and complement most commonly occur in the more cellular types of IPF.

CLINICAL MANIFESTATIONS. The cardinal symptom of IPF is dyspnea, which often develops insidiously. A dry cough may also be present. On auscultation, bilateral basilar crackling rales may be heard. As the disease advances, there may be tachypnea, tachycardia, and cyanosis. When pulmonary hypertension develops, jugular venous distention, a right ventricular "tap," pulmonic flow murmur, S_3 and S_4 heart sounds, hepatomegaly, and peripheral edema may be found. Digital clubbing is common in advanced cases. IPF and the collagen-vascular diseases have certain features in common, including digital vasculitis, Ray-

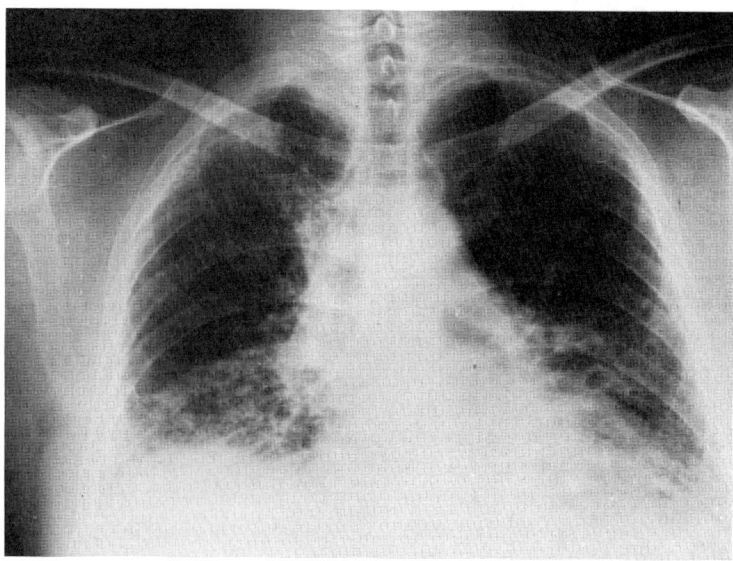

Fig. 132-1. Idiopathic pulmonary fibrosis (IPF) in 39-year-old man. There is bilateral interstitial infiltration, most pronounced at bases and obliterating diaphragms and cardiac borders.

naud's phenomenon, arthralgias, and discoid lupus erythematosus.

DIAGNOSIS. The chest film typically shows bilateral reticular or reticulonodular densities, predominantly in the lower lung zones, and loss of volume (Fig. 132-1). In advanced cases, "honeycomb" changes and evidence of pulmonary hypertension develop. Small cystic spaces may occasionally rupture, resulting in the development of a pneumothorax.

Routine laboratory studies usually contribute little additional diagnostic information. An elevated sedimentation rate is often found. The presence of rheumatoid factor, antinuclear antibody. Coombs' -positive hemolytic anemia, and idiopathic thrombocytopenic purpura has been reported. Pulmonary function tests typically reveal arterial hypoxemia and decreased lung volumes and diffusing capacity. Early in the course of the disease the chest film, resting arterial blood gas values, and pulmonary function tests may be normal, but an exercise study usually reveals evidence of impaired oxygenation.

Although the diagnosis of IPF requires the exclusion of the known causes of interstitial pneumonitis, the clinical picture usually suggests the diagnosis. Because a number of other disorders closely resemble IPF, because the course, prognosis, and therapy of some of these may differ, and because the course of IPF is often defined by the histologic features, a lung biopsy is often needed for diagnosis. In some medical centers transbronchial biopsy is performed first, and this is followed by open biopsy if the nature of the disease process is still unclear.

MANAGEMENT AND PROGNOSIS. Corticosteroids are the mainstay of therapy. They presumably decrease inflammation and subsequent fibrosis. The exact role of these drugs is difficult to define because of the variability of the natural history of IPF and because of the paucity of prospective controlled trials of steroid therapy. The finding of cellular infiltration and tissue immunoglobulin deposition in lung biopsy specimens and the presence of circulating immune complexes imply continued active inflammation and a good chance for a favorable response to corticosteroids, whereas extensive fibrosis suggests that a response to corticosteroids is unlikely. Controlled studies to evaluate the role of immunosuppressive agents and other types of drugs in the treatment of IPF are currently in progress.

The best methods for evaluating efficacy of treatment in IPF have not been clearly established. Symptoms, physical findings, and chest films are generally considered inadequate criteria. Measurement of lung volumes, diffusing capacity, and Pa_{O_2} during exercise may be useful. Recently the gallium scan has been used to assess the degree of inflammation, but its adequacy in following patients remains to be proved. The evaluation of lavage fluid obtained by fiberoptic bronchoscopy has also been described and may eventually prove to be a useful means of monitoring these patients.

Patients with IPF are susceptible to infection and may need antibiotic therapy and chest physical therapy. Supplemental oxygen may improve cor pulmonale and right-sided heart failure, decrease an elevated red cell mass, and improve exercise tolerance. Nutritional supplementation may also be useful.

The course and prognosis of IPF are variable. A fulminant course leading to death within 1 year, called the Hamman-Rich syndrome, is unusual; the mean survival in IPF is about 4 years, and many patients survive 10 years or longer. The duration of survival seems to correlate with the severity of functional impairment at the time of recognition; the appearance of the chest film correlates poorly with survival. The most common cause of death is respiratory failure, often accompanied by pulmonary infection.

Lymphocytic interstitial pneumonitis

Lymphocytic interstitial pneumonitis (LIP) is characterized by a histologic pattern of pulmonary interstitial infiltration with a uniform population of lymphocytes, associated with little fibrosis. The mode of onset, physical findings, appearance of the chest film, and pulmonary function data are indistinguishable from those of IPF, except that digital clubbing is relatively uncommon, chest infection is possibly more common, and the pattern of infiltration on the chest film may be more coarsely nodular at the lung bases. A number of patients with LIP have been reported to have dysproteinemias, defects in delayed hypersensitivity, and a variety of other presumably autoimmune disorders. Lymphocytic infiltrates may also involve the salivary glands, thyroid, kidney, and liver. Patients may have a Sjögren's-like syndrome, Hashimoto's thyroiditis, renal tubular acidosis, or chronic active hepatitis.

The clinical course of LIP seems to be variable, although only a limited number of cases have been observed. Respiratory failure does not appear to be a common cause of death in LIP. The disorder has been treated with corticosteroids, but response has been infrequent.

Systemic lupus erythematosus

(See Chapter 16.)

The pulmonary manifestations of systemic lupus erythematosus (SLE) may take the form of pleural disease, atelectasis, acute pneumonitis, and chronic interstitial disease. Pleural involvement may occur in as many as 50% of patients. Pleuritic pain is a frequent symptom, and pleural effusion is often present. Transient atelectasis, commonly consisting of linear or patchy involvement of the lung bases, is often found. Acute lupus pneumonitis is relatively uncommon; it is characterized by fever, dyspnea, cough, and patchy infiltrates. Since patients with SLE are susceptible to infectious pneumonitis because of their underlying disease and treatment with corticosteroids or immunosuppressive agents, a diagnosis of acute lupus pneumonitis should be considered only after infection has been carefully excluded.

The chronic interstitial abnormalities seen in SLE include an interstitial pneumonitis and fibrosis, a lymphocytic interstitial reaction, hemosiderosis, and a small-vessel vasculitis. Clinically apparent interstitial disease, most commonly fibrosis, occurs in about 10% of SLE cases.

Scleroderma (progressive systemic sclerosis)

(See Chapter 17.)

Scleroderma or progressive systemic sclerosis (PSS) is the collagen-vascular disease most frequently associated with interstitial disease. Dyspnea develops in approximately 40% of patients with PSS, and a similar percentage have chest film evidence of increased interstitial density. At autopsy as many as 90% of patients have evidence of lung involvement that commonly resembles IPF, but occasionally a hypersensitivity angiitis picture is found. Pleural disease is unusual.

The interstitial fibrosis seen in PSS seems to progress more rapidly than that associated with the other collagen-vascular diseases, yet less rapidly than with IPF. The 5-year survival in patients with PSS-related interstitial fibrosis is about 50%, and death from PSS is more commonly related to renal or cardiac failure.

The high incidence of disorders of esophageal motility and swallowing associated with PSS may lead to aspiration and recurrent pulmonary inflammation, infection, and scarring. PSS has also been reported to be associated with an increased incidence of bronchoalveolar cell carcinoma.

Rheumatoid arthritis

(See Chapter 10.)

Interstitial fibrosis of the IPF type appears to be the most common pulmonary manifestation of rheumatoid arthritis (RA), although it is usually milder and less progressive than IPF, and death resulting from respiratory failure is uncommon. Interstitial fibrosis is more common in males. There is no clear-cut correlation of fibrosis with the duration and extent of articular disease nor with the titer of rheumatoid factor. Pulmonary function abnormalities are present in about 40% of patients with RA, but only half of these have detectable chest film abnormalities.

The diagnosis is based on the presence of clinical features of RA in a patient with concomitant interstitial fibrosis. The diagnosis is complicated by the facts that about 20% of IPF patients may have either arthralgias or a positive test for rheumatoid factor and that in RA interstitial disease can occasionally precede the development of joint symptoms.

Other pulmonary manifestations of RA include pleural disease, pulmonary nodules, and pulmonary vasculitis. Pleural effusion is more common in males, is associated with high titers of rheumatoid factor and with extra-articular disease, tends to follow the development of joint symptoms, and is seldom massive. The fluid is an exudate that commonly has a markedly reduced glucose content (often less than 20 mg/dl). Lung nodules may be single or multiple, solid or cavitary, and variable in size. They usually occur in patients who also have subcutaneous nodules that are identical histologically to the pulmonary lesions. The treatment of nodules is unnecessary unless hemoptysis or rupture into the pleural space occurs. In Caplan's syndrome there is formation of pulmonary nodules in patients with coexisting RA and pneumoconiosis.

Polymyositis-dermatomyositis

(See Chapter 19.)

Pulmonary fibrosis resembling IPF is an uncommon complication of polymyositis, occurring in less than 5% of patients. Bronchogenic carcinoma may be associated with adult polymyositis.

Mixed connective tissue disease (overlap syndrome)

(See Chapter 17.)

In mixed connective tissue disease, also called the overlap syndrome, the features of two or more of the collagenvascular diseases coexist. In a substantial number of patients with overlap syndrome, pulmonary abnormalities develop that are similar in histopathology to IPF.

Sjögren's syndrome

(See Chapter 10.)

Recent data suggest a 3% incidence of interstitial pulmonary disease in Sjögren's syndrome. An IPF-like disorder may occur with or without an associated collagenvascular disease. There may be LIP-like infiltrates that follow a benign course and cause minimal dysfunction but occasionally progress rapidly to end-stage fibrosis. Malignant lymphoma has also been reported to follow the LIP of Sjögren's syndrome.

Ankylosing spondylitis

(See Chapter 12.)

Patients with ankylosing spondylitis occasionally have upper lobe fibrosis. This is usually bilateral and on a chest film may resemble tuberculosis. In its early stages the fibrosis may appear as linear fibrotic stranding, later becoming coarser to form large, dense infiltrates. Cavitation is common and may be the site of mycetoma formation. As fibrosis advances, lung distortion and bronchiectasis can lead to the development of cough, sputum production, and recurrent chest infection.

INTERSTITIAL DISEASES OF UNKNOWN CAUSE
Sarcoidosis

(See Chapter 24.)

Sarcoidosis is a systemic granulomatous disease of unknown cause. It most often affects young adults and is commonly manifested by bilateral hilar adenopathy, lung infiltrates, ocular disease, or cutaneous lesions. Other commonly occurring features include abnormalities of the immune system and hypercalciuria, occasionally associa50d with hypercalcemia. The diagnosis is based on clinical and roentgenographic evidence coupled with histologic evidence of noncaseating epithelioid-cell granulomata.

EPIDEMIOLOGY. The worldwide distribution and prevalence of sarcoidosis have proved difficult to determine because of variability in both diagnostic criteria and availability of diagnostic modalities. In the United States the disease occurs over a wide range but the highest incidence is in young adults. There is a slight female preponderance. American blacks are affected about 10 times more frequently than whites. About 50% have respiratory symptoms, about 25% have systemic symptoms such as fever, anorexia, and weight loss, less than 10% manifest symptoms of localized extrathoracic disease, and 20% are asymptomatic and are discovered by chest roentgenography.

CLINICAL MANIFESTATIONS. Pulmonary involvement is the leading cause of disability and death in sarcoidosis, and about one third of the patients with this disorder have dyspnea at some time. Even in patients with only hilar adenopathy and roentgenographically clear lung parenchyma, abnormalities may be present on pulmonary function testing, and granulomata may be demonstrated by lung biopsy. Cought develops in about one third of patients and may be due to endobronchial granulomata. If parenchymal fibrosis and secondary bronciectasis occur, purulent secretions and chronic pulmonary infection can develop. Chest pain occurs in less than 20% of cases and hemoptysis in less than 5%.

The physical examination may reveal no abnormality referable to the lungs. With advanced disease there may be tachypnea, harsh breath sounds, or bibasilar roles. Wheezes suggest the presence of endobronchial disease. Diminished breath sounds may signify the development of bullae or compensatory emphysema as pulmonary fibrosis occurs. Pleural effusion develops in only a small percentage of cases, generally as a small, unilateral, asymptomatic exudate. The fluid contains predominantly lymphocytes, and the pleural biopsy may reveal noncaseating granulomata. End-stage pulmonary fibrosis, which occurs in less than 5% of cases, resembles end-stage fibrotic lung disease of other causes.

A host of extrathoracic manifestations are known to occur. Palpable adenopathy is usually nontender. Splenomegaly, which occurs in 10% to 20% of cases, rarely leads to clinical complications. Erythema nodosum, a nonspecific cutaneous vasculitis of the lower extremities, occurs in less than 5% of patients. Erythema nodosum and bilateral hilar adenopathy *Löfgren's syndrome)* are said to portend a favorable outcome.

Skin lesions, which are seen in 30% of cases, often consist of small papules that on biopsy reveal typical granulomata. *Lupus pernio* is a severe destructive cutaneous infiltration occurring over the nose, cheeks, lips, and ears.

Ocular involvement (in 20% of cases) is most commonly manifested as acute anterior uveitis. Chronic uveitis, glaucoma, corneal and lenticular opacities, retinitis, papillitis, and blindness may occur. The association of uveitis with granulomatous involvement of the salivary glands has been designated *Heerfordt's syndrome*. Central nervous system involvement (in 5% of cases) may take the form of cranial nerve palsies, basilar meningitis, or intracerebral granulomatous disease.

Granulomatous disease of the myocardium is found at autopsy in 20% of patients. Clinical disease occurs less often and is most commonly manifested by conduction disturbances, ventricular arrhythmias, or left ventricular failure. In end-stage lung disease there may be cor pulmonale. Although percutaneous biopsy shows granulomatous disease of the liver in 50% to 80% of the patients, hepatomegaly occurs in only 10% to 20% and clinically significant liver disease is rare. Less than 5% of patients have detectable renal involvement, with nephrocalcinosis and nephrolithiasis being most frequent.

Almost all patients with sarcoidosis have decreased plasma levels of parathyroid hormone, 10% to 30% have hypercalciuria, and 2% to 3% have hypercalcemia. Increased absorption of calcium from the gastrointestinal tract, suggesting a heightened sensitivity to vitamin D, seems to underlie the abnormalities of calcium metabolism. Musculoskeletal complaints may include transient polyarthralgias and polyarthritis, usually involving the knees and ankles. Muscle biopsy (especially of the gastrocnemius muscle) may demonstrate granuloma formation, but overt myopathy is rare.

LABORATORY FINDINGS AND DIAGNOSIS. A variety of largely nonspecific laboratory findings have been associated with sarcoidosis. Hematologic studies may demonstrate mild anemia or lymphocytopenia. Thrombocytopenia, hemolytic anemia, eosinophilia, and pancytopenia resulting from hypersplenism are rare. Urinalysis may demonstrate an impaired concentrating ability owing to diabetes insipidus (from pituitary involvement) or to hypercalcemic nephropathy. About 10% to 20% of patients have hyperuricemia. Elevated levels of hepatic enzymes such as alkaline phosphatase may also be found. About 50% of patients have abnormalities of the resting electrocardiogram, mostly of a nonspecific nature.

There has been recent interest in the angiotensin-converting enzyme as a serologic marker of this disease. The blood level of this enzyme has been reported to be elevated in 30% to 80% of patients but may also be elevated in other granulomatous diseases and Gaucher's disease. Its role in diagnosis is not yet clearly defined, but it may correlate with activity of the disease process.

Often the chest film provides the initial clue to the correct diagnosis. The roentgenographic findings have been divided into four categories:

1. *Stage 0.* Patients in this category (10%) have a normal chest film.
2. *Stage I.* In these patients (50%) bilateral hilar adenopathy is present, but the parenchyma is clear. The enlarged lymph nodes are smooth and lobulated. A clear space is usually present between the nodes and the remainder of the hilus (Fig. 132-2). Right paratracheal adenopathy is present in about half.
3. *Stage II.* These patients (25% to 30%) have parenchymal infiltrates in addition to bilateral hilar adenopathy. The pattern is usually nonspecific and can be quite variable with diffuse small nodules, linear densities, reticulonodular changes, larger confluent shadows, and/or atelectasis.
4. *Stage III.* These patients (10% to 15%) have infiltrates without evidence of hilar adenopathy. Linear fibrotic strands, cystic changes, and bullous disease may occur.

Other roentgenographic changes include nephrolithiasis and lytic bone lesions of the phalanges. The latter are most likely to be found when there are pain and swelling in the overlying soft tissues.

Pulmonary function tests are generally more sensitive than the chest film in detecting parenchymal lung involvement. Serial measurements of pulmonary function serve as important guides to therapy, but the initial severity of impairment is not an accurate predictor of the future clinical course. The diffusing capacity is perhaps the most useful test with which to follow the patient with sarcoidosis, and it is diminished in more than half of the patients with stage I disease.

In more advanced parenchymal disease the lung volumes and diffusing capacity are diminished in a manner

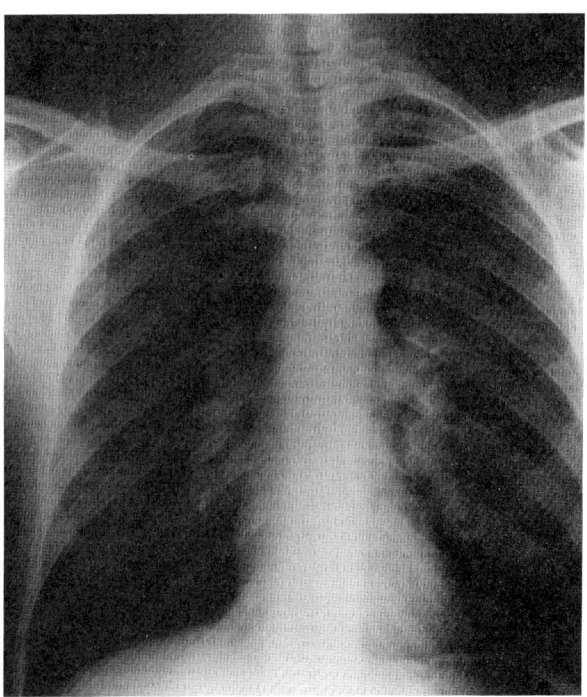

Fig. 132-2. Bilateral hilar adenopathy in patient with sarcoidosis. No parenchymal involvement can be seen (stage I). (Courtesy of George Popky, M.D.)

typical for restrictive disease. There may be arterial hypoxemia, and exercise testing may reveal significant exertional limitation and widening of the alveolar-arterial oxygen difference. Airway obstruction can be attributed to endobronchial or peribronchial involvement or to airway distortion owing to parenchymal fibrosis.

Sarcoidosis is associated with a variety of abnormal findings related to the immune system. However, it has proved difficult either to identify a causative antigen or to fit the known immunologic abnormalities into a clearly defined pathogenetic mechanism. Among the features that suggest involvement of the immune system are polyarthralgias and erythema nodosum, evidence of increased B-cell activity (such as increased serum immunoglobulin concentrations, circulating immune complexes, and the presence of autoantibodies), and evidence of depressed cellular immunity (such as lymphopenia, decreased numbers of circulating T cells, impaired T-cell proliferative response to mitogens, and cutaneous anergy to skin test antigens and synthetic skin sensitizers). In patients with inactive or resolved disease many of the abnormalities disappear. The defect in cellular immunity is relatively mild, and sarcoidosis is not associated with an increased incidence of opportunistic infection. Cells obtained from patients with sarcoidosis by lung lavage reveal an increased number of T lymphocytes, a finding that seems to support the belief that the lung is the site of an immune response.

Since there are no pathognomonic features, the diagnosis must be based on a compatible clinical picture, biopsy evidence of noncaseating granulomata, and exclusion of other granulomatous disorders. The biopsy procedures that most often yield noncaseating granulomata are mediastinoscopy, open lung biopsy, and multiple transbronchial biopsies. These are positive in over 90% of patients with roentgenographic evidence of disease. Percutaneous liver biopsy has a high yield (60% to 90% positive), but hepatic noncaseating granulomata may be seen in a variety of other illnesses. Skin lesions and palpably enlarged lymph nodes frequently yield granulomata. Other sites used to obtain material for histologic study include the lacrimal glands, salivary glands, labial salivary glands, and gastrocnemius muscle.

The Kveim test, performed by injecting intracutaneously a suspension of human sarcoid tissue and performing a biopsy of the resulting papular lesion 4 to 6 weeks later, yields typical noncaseating granulomata in 60% to 80% of cases. The test results are usually positive in patients with adenopathy but often negative in patients who have stage III disease or who are in remission or receiving steroid therapy. The false positive rate is less than 2% to 3% with properly prepared material. Because of difficulties in obtaining material with which to make the Kveim antigen and problems in standardizing and validating the reagent, this test is seldom used.

MANAGEMENT. Steroids appear to diminish the granulomatous inflammation, but whether the final degree of fibrosis is modified is unknown. As a rule, patients with minimal or no pulmonary function impairment are not treated. Patients with symptomatic lung disease, marked function changes, or evidence of progressive lung disease on serial chest films and pulmonary function tests generally receive steroid therapy. Treatment is also indicated for disfiguring skin lesions, myocardial or central nervous system disease, severe constitutional symptoms, and ocular disease. Mild anterior uveitis may be controlled with topical steroid therapy, but this should be carried out under the supervision of an ophthalmologist. Hypercalcemia also responds to steroid therapy, which may minimize or prevent nephropathy. In patients whose lung disease progresses to fibrosis and bronchiectasis, bronchial infection may occur and require antibiotic therapy. Massive hemoptysis may require surgical resection of the source of bleeding. Mycetoma formation is generally asymptomatic, but surgery may be needed if hemoptysis results.

Elevated levels of angiotensin-converting enzyme in blood, a gallium scan with lung parenchymal uptake, and pulmonary lavage demonstrating increased numbers of activated T lymphocytes correlate with the activity of the disease and may be helpful guides to the need for therapy.

PROGNOSIS. The prognosis is variable. The mortality resulting from sarcoidosis is less than 5%. The causes of death most commonly include respiratory insufficiency, massive hemoptysis, and severe disease of the heart, brain, kidneys, or liver. Of patients with stage 1 disease, 75% achieve remission within 2 years of diagnosis and 25% develop pulmonary infiltrates. Of those with infiltrates at the time of diagnosis, 50% are improved within 2 years; in the rest the infiltrates either do not change or worsen. Roughly 10% of all sarcoid patients show roentgenographic evidence of fibrosis. Chronic uveitis, skin lesions, bone cysts, and upper respiratory granulomata are said to portend the development of major pulmonary impairment.

Histiocytosis X

(See Chapter 78.)

Histiocytosis refers to three rare diseases: eosinophilic granuloma, Hand-Schüller-Christian disease, and Letterer-Siwe disease. However, about half the patients do not fit unequivocally into any one of these three disease categories. The common histologic feature in an infiltration containing large, irregularly shaped histiocytes with pale, eosinophilic, "foamy" cytoplasm. Other cells, including eosinophils, may also be seen, but the number of eosinophils present is variable. Their absence on histologic examination may occasionally lead to diagnostic confusion.

Eosinophilic granuloma is the form most often associated with pulmonary disease in adults. In about 25% of cases the disorder is generalized, but in most adults the disease is confined to the lungs. Eosinophilic granuloma may be detected in an asymptomatic patient on routine chest film, may be characterized by dyspnea and cough, or occasionally may be associated with acute spontaneous pneumothorax. The disease may have systemic manifestations such as fever, weakness, and cachexia. Early in the disease the chest film reveals a widespread symmetric interstitial infiltrate, usually distributed uniformly from base to apex but occasionally more prominent in the upper lobes. The diagnosis requires identification of the characteristic histiocytes in a tissue biopsy specimen. Rodlike structures (X bodies) may also be identified by means of electron microscopy in the cytoplasm of the histiocytes and in cells obtained by bronchial lavage. The course and prognosis are variable, ranging from a single stable bone lesion to a multisystem progressive disease with a rapidly fatal course. Similarly, lung involvement may be functionally mild or may evolve into a progressive fibrotic process resulting in extensive cystic change and respiratory insufficiency. Most adult cases that are confined largely to the lungs have a benign course. The disease has been treated with steroids, but although apparent benefit has occasionally been noted, the rarity of eosinophilic granuloma and the variability of its natural history have made it difficult to assess the usefulness of this therapy.

Hand-Schüller-Christian disease, occurring most often in childhood, is a widespread disease whose manifestations include skin lesions, bone lesions, otitis media, mastoiditis, adenopathy, splenic enlargement, and interstitial lung disease. Exophthalmos, diabetes insipidus, and bony lesions of the skull are a characteristic triad. The course is variable. Recovery may occur, although occasionally with persistence of the diabetes insipidus.

Letterer-Siwe disease affects children under 3 years of age and is regarded as a lymphomatous proliferation of histiocytes. The manifestations include adenopathy, hepatosplenomegaly, skin and bone lesions, and marrow involvement with pancytopenia, bleeding, and infection. The illness usually is rapidly fatal.

Amyloid

(See Chapter 76.)

Amyloid may involve the lung parenchyma as one or more nodular deposits (usually asymptomatic) or in the form of widespread interstitial infiltrates. The latter usually accompanies generalized amyloidosis and may produce significant lung restriction. Tracheobronchial amyloid deposits occasionally produce signs and symptoms of localized obstruction.

PULMONARY VASCULITIDES
Polyarteritis nodosa and related vasculitides

(See Chapter 20.)

At one time medical textbooks described asthma, eosinophilia, and pulmonary infiltrates as manifestations of polyarteritis nodosa. However, it is now recognized that polyarteritis nodosa is largely a necrotizing disorder of me-

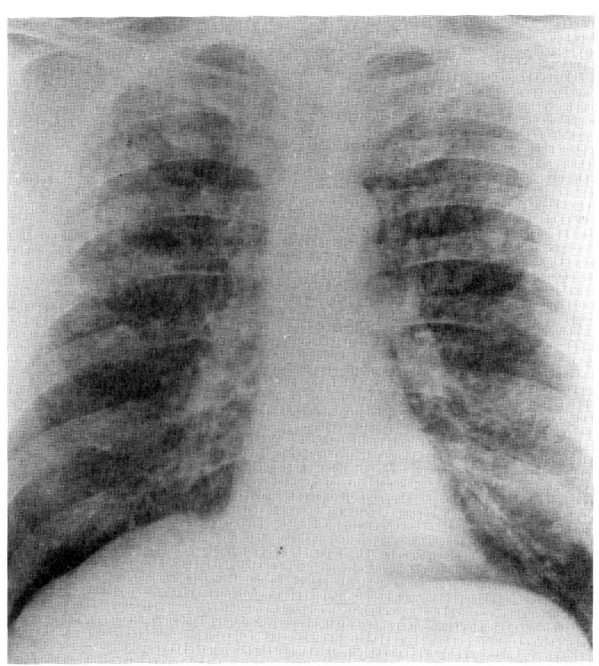

Fig. 132-3. Diffuse pulmonary disease (Churg-Strauss syndrome). (Courtesy of George Popky, M.D.)

dium-sized muscular arteries that is unlikely to affect pulmonary vessels and rarely is associated with lung disease. Patients with the constellation of wheezing, fever, eosinophilia, and vasculitis are more likely to have *Churg-Strauss syndrome,* a disorder essentially confined to asthmatic individuals and most commonly involving the lung (diffuse alveolitis with granulomata and fibrosis), skin, gastrointestinal tract, and peripheral nerves (Fig. 132-3).

Hypersensitivity (allergic) angiitis is a systemic small-vessel vasculitis that may be associated with both alveolitis and interstitial fibrosis. About half the cases are of unknown cause; drugs or infection appears to precipitate some cases. The disorder is thought to result from the deposition of immune complexes in the walls of small blood vessels, activation of complement, and subsequent inflammation.

Some patients with necrotizing vasculitis cannot be easily classified as having one of the well-defined vasculitides such as polyarteritis nodosa, Churg-Strauss syndrome, or hypersensitivity angiitis. The term "overlap vasculitis" has been employed to describe such patients, who often have pulmonary involvement characterized by interstitial fibrosis and necrotizing vasculitis.

Wegener's granulomatosis

(See Chapter 22.)

Wegener's granulomatosis is a multisystem disorder characterized by necrotizing vasculitis of the upper and lower respiratory tract, glomerulonephritis, and disseminated vasculitis involving small vessels. Respiratory tract involvement is usually clinically evident, whereas the renal disease may be subclinical. A renal biopsy may show focal glomerulonephritis. Upper respiratory tract involvement may include paranasal sinusitis, otitis media, scleroiritis, and nasopharyngeal ulceration. With nasal involvement there may be bacterial infection, septal perforation, and saddle nose deformity. Involvement of the lung may take the form of transient infiltrates associated with few or no symptoms. Commonly, however, there are nodular lesions that may cavitate and may be associated with fever, cough, chest pain, or hemoptysis. Pleural effusion and adenopathy are uncommon.

The major recent therapeutic advance in this once rapidly fatal disorder was the discovery that cyclophosphamide may induce long-term remission.

DIFFUSE HEMORRHAGIC LUNG DISEASE AND PULMONARY HEMOSIDEROSIS

Among the disorders associated with lung hemorrhage or the widespread deposition of iron in lung tissue are mitral stenosis, long-standing left ventricular failure, repeated blood transfusions or excessive administration of parenteral iron preparations, Goodpasture's syndrome (lung hemorrhage with nephritis), and idiopathic pulmonary hemosiderosis. In all these entities the parenchymal iron deposition may lead to pulmonary fibrosis and restriction.

Goodpasture's syndrome

Goodpasture's syndrome is an immune-complex disease manifested by interstitial and intra-alveolar hemorrhage (with or without gross hemoptysis), iron deficiency anemia, and acute glomerulonephritis. It is a disease of young adults (usual age range 18 to 25 years), with more than 75% of the cases occurring in males. About 20% of the cases follow viral respiratory illnesses.

The pathogenesis is believed to be related to the antigenic similarity of alveolar and glomerular basement membranes. Injury to one of these membranes may result in the release of membrane antigen that triggers the production of anti-basement membrane anti-body. This antibody attaches to the alveolar and glomerular basement membrane, binds complement, and causes a cytotoxic reaction that damages the involved structures. In the lung there is bleeding from the damaged pulmonary capillaries into the interstitial spaces and alveoli.

Hemosiderin remains in the lung parenchyma as a result of the breakdown of blood; this eventually leads to fibrosis and may contribute to iron deficiency anemia (because iron from the lung hemorrhage apparently remains sequestered in the lung, unavailable for hemoglobin synthesis). The finding of linear deposits of IgG along the glomerular basement membrane with immunofluorescent staining, the discovery of acute glomerulonephritis by means of kidney biopsy, and the demonstration of bound immunoglobulin and complement in the lung support this hypothetical immune mechanism.

Hemoptysis is often the initial symptom. Although massive hemorrhage may occur, repeated small hemorrhages resulting in pulmonary fibrosis are more common. Macrophages take up the breakdown products of blood in the lung parenchyma, and hemosiderin-laden macrophages may be recovered in the sputum or on bronchoscopy, which is otherwise usually normal. Other manifestations include rales and rhonchi as the result of lung hemorrhage and pallor as the result of anemia. Systemic symptoms such as weight loss, malaise, and extertional dyspnea may also occur. The chest film may show patchy densities that vary in appearance from day to day, reflecting the recurrence or resolution of hemorrhage. Eventually an interstitial pattern develops, and there may be fibrosis that appears indistinguishable from fibrosis caused by other diffuse parenchymal diseases.

Progressive renal disease causes the appearance of albuminuria, microscopic hematuria, and cellular and granular casts. Uremia may develop rapidly and was formerly the most common cause of death. Because this complication has been postponed in some cases by dialysis and renal transplantation (glomerulonephritis may also develop in the transplanted kidney), death now more often results from lung hemorrhage and respiratory insufficiency. Bilateral nephrectomy may lead to a cessation of lung hemorrhage, presumably by removing the source of antigen. The therapy also includes the use of steroids and immunosuppressive agents. Plasmapheresis to remove circulating anti–basement membrane antibody may occasionally lead to sustained remissions. It may prove useful to follow such patients with serial measurements of the diffusing capacity, since a sudden increase in diffusing capacity, presumed to result from carbon monoxide uptake by the red blood cells in areas of lung hemorrhage, may serve as an indication for repeated plasmapheresis.

Idiopathic pulmonary hemosiderosis

Idiopathic pulmonary hemosiderosis most often affects children and is rare in individuals over age 20. The sex distribution in affected children is about equal, although males seem to be more commonly affected in the young adult age group. The clinical and roentgenographic manifestations are indistinguishable from those of Goodpasture's syndrome, except for the absence of renal involvement. The histologic findings in the lung are also indentical, except that in idiopathic pulmonary hemosiderosis, anti-IgG antibody is not demonstrated by immunofluorescent staining.

The diagnosis is based on the clinical picture of hemoptysis, iron deficiency anemia, chest film abnormalities (as previously described for Goodpasture's syndrome), the finding of hemosiderin-laden macrophages in the sputum, and the absence of renal involvement. The disorder is usually fatal with a course of several weeks to several years. Death may result from large hemorrhages with hypoxemia or from recurrent smaller hemorrhages leading to the development of interstitial fibrosis and cor pulmonale.

EOSINOPHILIC DISEASES
Pulmonary infiltrates with eosinophilia (PIE syndrome)

The PIE syndrome (infiltrative lung disease with blood eosinophilia) may follow either a brief, self-limited course or a more severe and protracted one. Cases occur that are not easily classified as one of the two major idiopathic varieties of the PIE syndrome, Löffler's syndrome and chronic eosinophilic pneumonia. In addition, there are now recognized a large number of disorders (principally neoplasms, infections, and drug-induced diseases) that may also cause eosinophilia and pulmonary infiltrates. The following outline lists the types of the PIE syndrome:

Classification of the PIE syndrome
I. Löffler's syndrome
II. Chronic eosinophilic pneumonia
III. Known causes
  A. Tumor
    1. Leukemia, lymphoma (especially Hodgkin's disease)
    2. Metastatic carcinoma
    3. Bronchogenic carcinoma
  B. Parasitic disease
    1. Infection with *Ascaris, Strongyloides, Ancylostoma,* and so on
    2. Visceral larva migrans *(Toxocara canis)*
    3. Tropical eosinophilia (microfilaria)
  C. Other infections, especially viral pneumonitis
  D. Sarcoidosis
  E. Drug reactions such as those caused by nitrofurantoin, para-aminosalicylic acid, penicillin, sulfonamides, chlorpropamide, isoniazid, aspirin, methotrexate, disodium cromoglycate
  F. Bronchopulmonary aspergillosis
  G. Vasculitis such as Churg-Strauss syndrome

LÖFFLER'S SYNDROME. Löffler's syndrome is a self-limited disorder that usually runs its course in several weeks. There are transient migratory infiltrates and blood eosinophilia. Patients may be asymptomatic or may manifest symptoms such as cough, fever, headache, and malaise. Wheezing may be present. The histologic picture is not well defined; patients have such mild symptoms and the illness is of such short duration that a lung biopsy is usually not performed.

CHRONIC EOSINOPHILIC PNEUMONIA. Chronic eosinophilic pneumonia is clinically a more severe disorder than Löffler's syndrome. It is characterized by cough, dyspnea, and occasionally hemoptysis. There may be systemic symptoms such as weight loss, fever, chills, and diaphoresis. The blood eosinophil count may be normal in one third of the patients. The chest film characteristically shows peripherally located infiltrates that spare the perihilar areas. A biopsy shows increased numbers of eosinophils in the tissues. The disorder may persist for months or years, but both the symptoms and roentgenographic densities clear rapidly with corticosteroid therapy.

FAMILIAL DISEASES
Gaucher's disease

(See Chapter 195.)

Gaucher's disease, a lipid storage disease caused by a deficiency of the enzyme glucocerebrosidase, is associated with the accumulation of lipid material in reticuloendothelial cells. The resulting "Gaucher's cells" may infiltrate a number of organs. Involvement of the pulmonary interstitium and pulmonary fibrosis may occur.

Niemann-Pick disease

(See Chapter 195.)

Niemann-Pick disease, another lipid storage disease, is caused by a deficiency of the enzyme sphingomyelinase. It is associated with the accumulation of sphingomyelin in histiocytes, giving them a foamy appearance. These foam cells, in addition to infiltrating the liver, spleen, lymph nodes, and central nervous system, may cause interstitial pulmonary fibrosis.

Familial interstitial pneumonitis

An interstitial pneumonitis indistinguishable from idiopathic pulmonary fibrosis may occur on a familial basis. The mechanism of inheritance has not been clarified but may be autosomal dominant with incomplete penetrance.

Neurofibromatosis

(See Chapter 156.)

Neurofibromatosis, also known as von Recklinghausen's disease, is an autosomal dominant disorder characterized by neurofibromas in the skin and peripheral and central nervous system and by cutaneous café au lait spots. About 10% of 20% of the cases in adults are associated with interstitial fibrosis that is histologically indistinguishable from the idiopathic variety.

Tuberous sclerosis

(See Chapter 156.)

Tuberous sclerosis is a rare disorder characterized by mental deficiency, seizures, adenoma sebaceum, and hamartomatous involvement of multiple organs. Interstitial pulmonary fibrosis occurs in about 10% to 20% of the cases.

DRUG-INDUCED DISEASE

The wide variety of drugs in clinical use today and the large quantities administered have significantly increased the risk of adverse drug reactions. The problem is heightened by the almost routine use of multiple drug therapy, which increases the opportunities for adverse drug interactions, by the ready availability and widespread use of nonprescription drugs, and by the surreptitious use of narcotic and mood-altering drugs. The lung parenchyma may be affected by drugs through a variety of mechanisms. The most common types of drug-induced disease and some of the agents that cause them are outlined below.

Common agents causing drug-induced lung disease

I. Acute pulmonary infiltrates
   A. Amitriptyline
   B. Azathioprine
   C. Chlorpropamide
   D. Imipramine
   E. Isoniazid
   F. Mephenesin
   G. Methotrexate
   H. Nitrofurantoin
   I. Para-aminosalicylic acid
   J. Penicillin
   K. Procarbazine
   L. Sulfonamides

II. Chronic interstitial fibrosis
   A. BCNU
   B. Bleomycin
   C. Busulfan
   D. Cyclophosphamide
   E. Hexamethonium
   F. Mecamylamine
   G. Melphalan
   H. Methotrexate
   I. Oxygen

III. Increased permeability of alveolar-capillary membrane
   A. Chlordiazepoxide
   B. Ethchlorvynol
   C. Heroin
   D. Methadone
   E. Propoxyphene
   F. Salicylates
   G. Thiazides

IV. SLE syndrome
   A. Hydralazine
   B. Isoniazid
   C. Mephenytoin
   D. Methyldopa
   E. Methylthiouracil
   F. Phenytoin
   G. Procainamide
   H. Propylthiouracil
   I. Reserpine

RADIATION PNEUMONITIS AND FIBROSIS

(See Chapter 138.)

Radiation damage to the lung results most commonly from the therapeutic use of radiation in a variable percentage of patients treated for malignancies of the breast, mediastinal structures, and lung. Such damage is usually divided into an early stage (radiation pneumonitis) and a late reaction (radiation fibrosis). Although radiation pneumonitis may occasionally resolve completely and without sequelae, it is more often followed by at least some degree of fibrosis.

Radiation pneumonitis develops insidiously, usually 2 to 6 months after radiation therapy but occasionally as early as 4 weeks. Earlier reactions are associated with more severe damage. The degree of lung involvement is related to the volume of lung irradiated, the total dose of radiation and its rate of delivery, the concomitant use of chemotherapeutic agents, the withdrawal of steroid therapy during or after radiation therapy, and the administration of radiation to an area previously irradiated. Radiation damage is likely to be tolerated poorly by individuals with previously impaired pulmonary function.

An early symptom of radiation pneumonitis is cough, usually hacking and nonproductive (although scant amounts of pink-tinged sputum may be produced). The major symptom of radiation pneumonitis is dyspnea, present only on exertion in most cases but progressing to severe respiratory distress at rest in some. Fever and other constitutional symptoms may accompany severe cases as well. There may be rales, signs of consolidation, a pleural friction rub, and skin changes overlying the port of radiation.

Histologic findings include engorged and thrombosed pulmonary capillaries, hyperplasia and desquamation of alveolar lining cells, hyaline membranes, and edema and mononuclear cell infiltrates of the interstitial space. Roentgenographic changes initially consist of diffuse haziness in the area of involvement, and the normal lung markings become indistinct. As the process progresses, alveolar infiltrates may develop, and in advanced cases consolidation accompanied by air bronchograms may be seen. Pleural and pericardial effusions may develop, and the mediastinum may become widened and blurred. Lung cavitation is unusual; its occurrence should suggest the development of infection or necrosis of the underlying tumor. Classically, the roentgenographic density has relatively sharp margins that correspond to those of the radiation port, but diffuse and poorly marginated pneumonitis may also occur. Corticosteroid therapy may be of benefit, but data concerning efficacy in controlled trials are lacking.

Radiation fibrosis, which in some degree usually follows symptomatic radiation pneumonitis by 6 months or more, may occasionally result in severe dyspnea and even chronic respiratory failure. With unilateral irradiation there may be volume loss with a shift of the mediastinal structures toward the affected side. The involved area becomes progressively contracted, the diaphragms may become tented, and pleural thickening may develop. Finally a densely fibrotic and contracted portion of lung may be left, and bronchiectatic changes may develop in the area. There is no known effective therapy for the fibrotic stage.

BIBLIOGRAPHY

Baum, G.L., editor: Textbook of pulmonary diseases, ed. 2, Boston, 1974, Little, Brown & Co.
Carrington, C.B., Addington, W.W., and Goff, A.M.: Chronic eosinophilic pneumonia, N. Engl. J. Med. **280**:787, 1969.
Carrington, C.B., and others: Natural history and treated course of usual and desquamative interstitial pneumonia, N. Engl. J. Med. **298**:801, 1978.
Colp, C.: Sarcoidosis: course and treatment, Med. Clin. North Am. **61**:1267, 1977.
Daniele, R.P., Dauber, J.H., and Rossman, M.D.: Immunologic abnormalities in sarcoidosis, Ann. Intern. Med. **92**:406, 1980.
Dreisin, R.B., and others: Circulating immune complexes in the idiopathic interstitial pneumonias, N. Engl. J. Med. **298**:353, 1978.
Fulmer, J.D., and Crystal, R.G.: Interstitial lung disease. In Simmons, D.H., editor: Current pulmonology, Boston, 1979, Houghton Mifflin Co.
Hinshaw, H.D., and Murray, J.F.: Diseases of the chest, ed. 4, Philadelphia, 1980, W.B. Saunders Co.
Liebow, A.A., and Carrington, C.B.: The eosinophilic pneumonias, Medicine **48**:251, 1969.
Mitchell, D., and Scadding, J.G.: Sarcoidosis, Am. Rev. Respir. Dis. **110**:774, 1974.
Morrissey, W.L., and others: Chronic eosinophilic pneumonia, Respiration **32**:453, 1975.
Schwartz, M.I.: Idiopathic interstitial lung disease, Semin. Respir. Med. **1**:47, 1979.
Sostman, H.D., Matthay, R.A., and Putman, C.E.: Cytotoxic drug-induced lung disease, Am. J. Med. **62**:608, 1977.
Strimlan, C.V., and others: Lymphocytic interstitial pneumonitis, Ann. Intern. Med. **88**:616, 1978.
Weinberger, S.E., and others: Bronchoalveolar lavage in interstitial lung disease, Ann. Intern. Med. **89**:459, 1978.
Zeck, R.T., and Cugell, D.S.: Diffuse infiltrative lung diseases, Med. Clin. North Am. **61**:1251, 1977.

133 • ENVIRONMENTAL (OCCUPATIONAL) LUNG DISEASE

David M.F. Murphy

Lung diseases that result from exposure to organic or inorganic dusts or gases form an important subgroup of environmental diseases. Knowledge of environmentally related disease has been increasing remarkably, and with the accelerating progress in industrial technology, new forms of these diseases are constantly being recognized.

Awareness of the common environmental lung disorders is necessary in order that the potential for disease may be recognized when a patient describes his occupation. If an occupational lung disease is suspected, it is essential to take a detailed occupational history. Previous exposure to injurious agents may be closeted in the patient's memory, their significance apparent only to the enlightened questioner. Although most environmental lung disease is occupationally related, in some cases neighborhood or leisure time exposure can be implicated. In most cases a diagnosis can be made on the basis of the occupational history, physical examination, and roentgenographic interpretation. It is only in exceptional circumstances that invasive procedures such as open lung biopsy are required. Determination of the impairment attributable to these conditions requires objective tests of lung function.

Lung disease may develop in workers who are exposed to organic or inorganic dusts, chemical fumes, radiation, or infectious agents. Inorganic dusts can cause industrial bronchitis, pulmonary neoplasms, occupational asthma, and the pneumoconioses. Pneumoconiosis is defined as the accumulation of dust in the lungs and the reaction of lung tissue to its presence. In susceptible subjects organic dusts may produce a syndrome characterized by an allergic inflammation of the alveolar walls known as hypersensitivity pneumonitis. Farmer's lung and mushroom worker's lung are examples of this syndrome. Toxic gases may cause an outpouring of fluid from the alveoli, producing pulmonary edema or lesser degrees of immediate irritation and injury.

For a dust particle to penetrate the gas-exchanging part of the lung, that is, beyond the terminal bronchioles, it must be sufficiently small to bypass the filtering mechanism of the upper airways and nasal passages. In general only partiles less than 7 μm in diameter can penetrate beyond the distal airways; particles of this size represent the respirable fraction. These particles are deposited on the walls of the airways by inertial impaction, sedimentation, or diffusion and are subsequently removed by scavenging macrophages that then enter the lymphatic system. Inorganic dusts tend to accumulate around the respiratory bronchioles, whereas organic dusts give rise to immunologic reactions at the alveolar level or, in the case of occupational asthma, cause smooth muscle contraction in the bronchioles.

SILICOSIS

ETIOLOGY AND EPIDEMIOLOGY. Silicosis, probably the most common occupational lung disease in the United States, is defined as a fibrotic lung disease resulting from the inhalation of dust containing silicon dioxide, or silica. More than 1 million workers in the United States are believed to be exposed to free silica. Industries associated with a silica hazard include metal mining, coal mining, and foundry work, as well as stone, clay, and glass production. The sandblasting of stone and metal is regarded as particularly hazardous.

Simple silicosis is rarely seen in workers with less than 10 years of exposure to free silica, but an accelerated form of silicosis occurring after 10 to 15 months of exposure has been described in sandblasters.

PATHOGENESIS. When deposited in the alveoli, silica particles are ingested by alveolar macrophages and enclosed within their phagosomes. A reaction between the phagosomal wall and the inhaled silica particle subsequently takes place, leading to the release of phagosomal proteolytic enzymes within the macrophage; this results in destruction of the macrophage and ultimately in release of the silica particle. The released silica particle is then ingested by another macrophage and the process repeats itself. Destruction of the macrophage also leads to release of at least two factors: a chemotactic factor for other macrophages and a factor involved in the production of collagen. The continual formation of fibrous tissue leads to the production of the characteristic "silicotic nodule," which has a whorled appearance caused by concentric layers of connective tissue. Silicotic nodules are usually seen adjacent to respiratory bronchioles or pulmonary arterioles. In certain people, for reasons unclear at present, large numbers of nodules tend to conglomerate in the upper lobes with increased fibrosis. This advanced stage of the disease is known as "conglomerate silicosis."

Silicosis is sometimes associated with infection with *Mycobacterium tuberculosis;* in these cases the pathologic findings of pulmonary tuberculosis may also be found in the lungs. Cavitation of the conglomerate masses may result from either ischemia or tuberculous infection. An abnormal immunologic reaction may be important in the pathogenesis of silicosis, since there is an increased prevalence of autoimmune disease in patients with this disorder.

CLINICAL MANIFESTATIONS. Silicosis can be classified into three main types: simple silicosis, conglomerate silicosis, and acute silicosis. The simple type is characterized by few symptoms other than shortness of breath and cough, which occur only in its later stages. Conglomerate silicosis, on the other hand, is associated with more severe dyspnea and paroxysmal coughing and in the later stages of the disease with tachypnea and use of the accessory muscles of respiration. Acute silicosis is associated with rapidly progressive dyspnea, cough, and a fulminant course.

The physical signs include some degree of dullness to percussion over areas of conglomeration, which are usually in one or both upper lobes. Bullous emphysema, which often complicates conglomerate silicosis, may mask this decreased resonance. Distortion of the airways by the large masses can cause signs of airflow obstruction. Pulmonary hypertension may develop as a result of hypoxemia and reduction in the pulmonary vascular bed and may lead to cor pulmonale and ultimate death.

LABORATORY FINDINGS. Simple silicosis is characterized on the chest roentgenogram by multiple small nodules, predominantly in the upper lobes. These nodules are usually fairly uniform in size and vary from 1.5 to 10 mm in diameter. They occasionally calcify; more commonly, calcification of hilar lymph node capsules gives rise to "eggshell" calcification (Fig. 133-1).

Conglomerate silicosis is characterized rotengenographically by fibrotic masses greater than 1 cm in diameter. These develop in the upper lobes in patients with

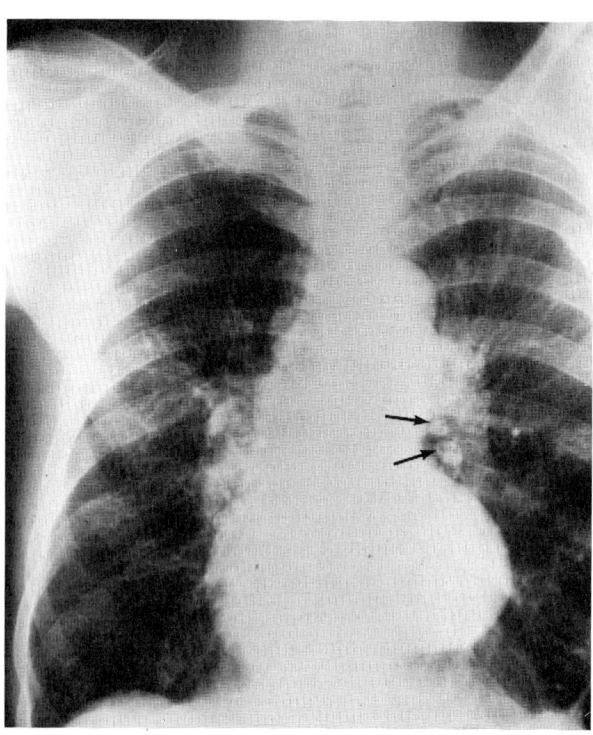

Fig. 133-1. Silcosis showing "eggshell" calcifications of hilar lymph nodes *(arrows)*. There is mild fibrosis in midlung regions. (Courtesy of George Popky, M.D.)

simple silicosis and migrate toward the hilum, causing upward retraction of the hilum. A peripheral zone of bullous emphysema often develops beyond the mass. Bullae may also develop at the lung bases. It is usually impossible to distinguish the presence of concomitant tuberculosis using roentgenography alone.

Acute silicosis is sometimes seen in subjects exposed to high levels of respirable free silica over relatively short periods. Roentgenograms of the chest show a bilateral alveolar filling pattern spreading out from the hila.

Simple silicosis has little effect on lung function, whereas conglomerate disease may give rise to an obstructive pattern and/or a restrictive pattern accompanied by a reduction in diffusing capacity.

PREVENTION AND MANAGEMENT. Prevention is the best form of treatment. If a dust hazard is recognized, the concentration of silica dust must be maintained below levels believed to be associated with an acceptable incidence of disease. Because even simple silicosis may progress, workers with the disease should avoid further exposure to free silica.

Patients with conglomerate silicosis may require supplemental oxygen, cardiac glycosides, and antibiotics to counter respiratory infections. Concomitant tuberculosis should be treated with appropriate antimicrobials. A positive skin test for tuberculosis (in the absence of active tuberculosis) is an indication for prophylactic chemotherapy, such as isoniazid. Acute respiratory failure may require temporary mechanical ventilation.

COAL WORKERS' PNEUMOCONIOSIS

ETIOLOGY AND EPIDEMIOLOGY. Coal workers' pneumoconiosis (CWP) results from the prolonged inhalation of coal dust of respirable size. In most cases at least 10 years' exposure is required before roentgenographic disease is evident. The condition is defined as the accumulation of coal dust in the lungs and reaction of tissue to its presence. The disease takes two forms: simple and complicated. Although originally believed to have little effect on life expectancy, CWP was recognized in the 1930s as an important cause of excessive mortality in the coal miners of south Wales in the United Kingdom.

Coal dust of respirable particle size accumulates in the lungs. It is first deposited in the alveoli and ingested by alveolar macrophages, which migrate to the region of the respiratory bronchiole. Coal dust is not toxic to the macrophages if it does not contain free silica. Accumulation of coal dust around the respiratory bronchiole produces a pathologically distinct lesion, the "coal macule." In addition to the coal dust, a few fibers of reticulin are also laid down. In some cases atrophy of the smooth muscle of the respiratory brochiole, along with traction on the wall of the bronchiole by the macule, leads to "focal emphysema." Collections of coal dust may also be found in the hilar lymph nodes and in the lymphatics leading to the nodes.

Complicated CWP, or progressive massive fibrosis (PMF), usually develops in the presence of advanced simple CWP. The precise factors responsible for the development of the complicated form remain a mystery, but the condition is characterized by the development of large, unilateral or bilateral, black fibrotic masses, greater than 1 cm in diameter, in the upper lobes of the lungs. The fibrotic masses tend to increase progressively in size, resulting in distortion of the airways and destruction of the pulmonary vasculature. The condition may be complicated by pulmonary tuberculosis, but this occurs less commonly than in silicosis. The massive lesions may cavitate because of ischemic central necrosis or coincident mycobacterial infection.

CLINICAL MANIFESTATIONS AND LABORATORY FINDINGS. Simple CWP gives rise to few symptoms and signs. Chronic cough and sputum production are most likely to result from coincident chronic bronchitis caused by cigarette smoking. PMF is associated with shortness of breath, as well as a local decrease in tone of the percussion note. If cor pulmonale develops, signs of right-sided heart failure are present. Clubbing of the fingers is not seen in CWP or silicosis.

Simple CWP appears roentgenographically as uniform nodules, usually more profuse in the upper lung zones and varying in size from 1.5 to 10 mm. Bilateral masses can cause an "angel wings" appearance in complicated CWP. Since this form is associated with simple CWP, which is usually obvious roentgenographically, these large masses are usually not confused with others such as carcinoma of the lung or pulmonary tuberculosis.

Simple CWP is not associated with clinically significant decreases in ventilatory capacity. Complicated CWP, on the other hand, may be associated with airflow obstruction. The large masses may cause a reduction in lung volume, and the diffusing capacity is decreased in proportion to this reduction in lung volume. Exercise is often accompanied by a reduction in arterial oxygen tension.

MANAGEMENT AND PREVENTION. Prevention is the only effective treatment. The reduction of dust levels in the coal mines will eventually reduce the prevalence of the disease. Symptomatic management as described previously in the discussion of silicosis may be of value in some cases.

ASBESTOS-RELATED DISORDERS

Asbestos is a naturally occurring fibrous silicate that has two main forms: serpentine or curly fibers and amphibole or needlelike fibers. Chrysolite, or white asbestos, is of the serpentine form and is mined particularly in Canada and Russia. The amphibole group includes crocidolite, or blue asbestos, found especially in South Africa, amosite, or brown asbestos, from the Transvaal in South Africa, and anthophyllite, a white asbestos mined in Finland. Tremolite and actinolite are less common forms of asbestos.

The use of asbestos in industry has increased remarkably over the last century; at present, more than 1 million tons of asbestos is used annually in the United States. Because of its great resistance to heat and chemical destruction, asbestos is used mainly for insulation and fireproofing. The lagging (covering) of pipes and electrical lines with asbestos produces a significant hazard when the dry lagging is removed. Asbestos was sprayed on the inside of the holds of ships and is still used as grouting material in furnaces. It is also used in cement products, tiles, gutters, roofing materials, and brake lining, as well as in paper, plastic, and paint manufacturing.

Exposure to asbestos may occur in occupations that do not involve the direct use of asbestos, since workers in the vicinity of asbestos use are also frequently exposed. Environmental exposure can occur in residents living near asbestos dumps, mines, or mills. Other forms of exposure occur in family members who may be exposed to the dusty overalls of asbestos workers and even in barbers of these workers.

Asbestos particles are of a fibrous nature, that is, their length/diameter ratio is greater than 3:1. Those fibers able to penetrate to the small airways are less than 3 μm in diameter. The amphibole fiber is needlelike and can travel farther into the peripheral airways with the axial airstream than can the serpentine form, which is curly and tends to impact higher in the airways, particularly at the bifurcation sites.

Smaller fibers are ingested by alveolar macrophages and taken up into the phagosome where endogenous iron (ferritin) is deposited, giving the fibers a yellow or brown color. They may subsequently be released and lie free in tissue. The fiber coat consists of an iron-containing protein and is segmented along the length of the fiber and bulbous at the ends. These coated fibers or ferruginous bodies are not peculiar to asbestos but may occur with other types of fibers as well. When the central fiber is asbestos, they may accurately be called asbestos bodies. Ferruginous bodies have been found in 40% to 60% of urban dwellers with no known exposure to asbestos. The finding of asbestos bodies in the sputum is evidence only of asbestos exposure and not of asbestos-related disease. Uncoated asbestos fibers can be detected by electron microscopy.

Lung conditions associated with asbestos exposure include pleural plaques, asbestosis, malignant mesothelioma of the pleura, and bronchogenic carcinoma.

Pleural plaques

Pleural plaques are evidence of asbestos exposure. They may occur over the diaphragm or on the parietal surface of the costal pleura and may be hyaline or calcified. When uncalcified, they appear as linear or protuberant densities along the walls of the chest, commonly in the middle or lower zones. When calcified, they are often visible as thin, linear calcifications over the surface of the diaphragm or along the costal margins. Oblique views are often helpful in detecting pleural plaques, which may be bilateral. At present there is no evidence that they precede the development of malignant mesothelioma of the pleura.

Asbestosis

Asbestosis is defined as fibrosis of the lungs caused by inhaled asbestos dust. Up to a certain level, the greater the amount of asbestos dust inhaled, the greater the fibrosis that results. Progression from moderate to severe fibrosis, however, seems to be related to other factors. Progressive fibrosis is associated with a progressive decrease in total lymphocyte count. Antinuclear antibody occurs more commonly in exposed subjects in whom clinical disease develops than in those in whom it does not.

Fibrosis develops first in subpleural areas and then extends farther into the lobe. Lower lobes tend to be affected first, with the disease then spreading to middle and upper lobes. Honeycomb cysts and emphysema may be seen later. Lesions similar to the massive fibrosis of complicated CWP are very uncommon. The earliest stage identified microscopically is a peribronchiolar fibrosis with subsequent fibrosis of the alveolar walls. Ferruginous bodies or uncoated asbestos fibers may also be seen. The initial symptom is usually inappropriate breathlessness following exertion. Nonproductive cough and chest pain also occur.

Cellophane-like late inspiratory crackles are audible on auscultation at the lung bases. Clubbing of the fingers also occurs in some cases.

Irregular or round opacities are seen roentgenographically, particularly in the lower zones. A ground-glass appearance may also occur, and cystic changes or "honeycomb lung" may be seen. Pleural plaques are often associated with asbestosis and may be calcified. When a mixed dust exposure occurs (for example, with silica), the opacities tend to be more rounded. The opacities seen roentgenographically in asbestosis may be classified using the International Labor Organization/University of Cincinnati (ILO/UC) classification.

Usually, asbestosis results in a restrictive pattern of functional abnormality with a reduction in the vital capacity (VC) and a reduction in total lung capacity (TLC). The diffusing capacity is frequently decreased, and arterial oxygen desaturation may be demonstrated on exercise. About 20% of cases demonstrate an obstructive pattern with reduction in the ratio of the 1-second forced expired volume to the forced vital capacity ($FEV_{1.0}/FVC\%$), and a further 20% reveal a mixed obstructive and restrictive pattern.

The diagnosis is established when an appropriate exposure history is obtained in association with roentgenographic changes of parenchymal disease, lung function impairment, and appropriate clinical findings. There is no evidence that removal from the source of exposure will affect the outcome of the disease. Treatment of infections may be important, since it has been suggested that nonspecific inflammation may contribute to progression of the fibrosis. Corticosteroid therapy is not advocated. Supplemental oxygen may provide symptomatic relief of dyspnea.

Malignant mesothelioma

There is a clear association between pleural or peritoneal mesothelioma and inhalation of crocidolite asbestos, mined in the northwest Cape Province of South Africa. The tumor is not related to the amount of inhaled asbestos fiber, and there is a latent period of about 40 years from exposure to development of the tumor. There have been cases of mesothelioma reported in association with other types of asbestos.

A definite diagnosis can be made only by histologic examination of the tumor tissue. Since these tumors contain a variety of cell types and arrangements, the diagnosis is often difficult. If a mesothelioma is suspected, tissue should be obtained by open pleural biopsy rather than needle biopsy, since the latter technique usually provides an insufficient specimen and the tumor may grow down the needle track. Cytologic examination of the pleural fluid is usually not helpful.

Although various treatment modalities, including surgical resection, chemotherapy, and radiotherapy have been tried, there is no curative therapy. The average survival time is about 6 months from the onset of symptoms. Surgery has been the most effective treatment in the past but does not affect the median survival rate. Installation of radioactive colloidal gold into the pleura has occasionally prolonged survival.

Bronchogenic carcinoma

It has been clearly established that significant exposure to asbestos is associated with an increased risk for the development of lung cancer. About 20% of men with asbestosis die of lung cancer. When asbestos exposure is combined with cigarette smoking, the risk is multiplied; a heavily exposed smoker has 90 times as great a risk of developing lung cancer as a nonexposed nonsmoker. Most are adenocarcinomas or squamous cell type, whereas oat cell carcinomas are uncommon.

Other cancers shown to be associated with asbestos exposure include carcinoma of the larynx and gastrointestinal carcinomas.

HYPERSENSITIVITY PNEUMONITIS

The hypersensitivity pneumonitis conditions are defined as a group of pulmonary disorders in which inhalation of organic dust results in hypersensitivity reactions at the alveolar level, usually associated with the production of serum precipitins. Many of these disorders are occupationally related. Table 133-1 lists the more common conditions.

In the majority of cases hypersensitivity pneumonitis results from the inhalation of organic dust containing proteinaceous material that acts as an allergen. Although precipitating antibodies against the allergens have been detected in exposed workers, not all subjects with precipitating antibodies develop disease and not all cases of disease demonstrate precipitating antibodies. It is not known why the disease, which occurs in both acute and chronic forms, develops only in some workers. Many of the allergens identified have been bacterial or fungal spores. These spores are less than 5 μm in diameter and so can penetrate to the alveolar level. Spores from thermophilic bacteria have been particularly associated with the condition. These bacteria grow in the high temperatures generated in moldy hay, bagasse, or mushroom compost. It is believed that large number of spores are liberated when moldy hay is turned, and in exposed workers up to 750,000 spores can be deposited in the lung each minute.

In affected subjects a cellular reaction occurs at the alveolar level. In the early stages this consists of infiltration of the alveolar walls with lymphocytes, plasma cells, and foamy histiocytes. Alveolar macrophages are found in the alveolar spaces. Loosely formed granulomata are an important histologic characteristic of this disorder. In some cases bronchiolitis obliterans also occurs. In the late stages irreversible interstitial fibrosis and honeycombing are the predominant findings. It has been suggested that the immunologic mechanism involved in initiating the cellular reaction is a hypersensitivity response. It is characterized by the onset of systemic symptoms, including fever, malaise, or myalgia, 4 to 6 hours after exposure to the organic

Table 133-1. Common types of hypersensitivity pneumonitis

Clinical condition	Source of offending agent	Agent
Farmer's lung	Moldy hay	*Micropolyspora faeni*
		Thermoactinomyces vulgaris
Bagassosis	Moldy bagasse	*Thermoactinomyces vulgaris*
Mushroom worker's lung	Mushroom compost	*Micropolyspora faeni*
		Thermoactinomyces vulgaris
Suberosis	Cork dust	Cork dust
Maple bark disease	Maple bark	*Cryptostroma corticale*
Sequoiosis	Redwood sawdust	*Aureobasidium pullulans*
Wood pulp worker's disease	Wood pulp	*Alternaria* species
Malt worker's lung	Moldy barley	*Aspergillus clavatus*
		Aspergillus fumigatus
Wheat weevil disease	Wheat flour	*Sitophilus granarius*
Furrier's lung	Animal hairs	None shown
Coffee worker's lung	Coffee bean	Coffee bean dust
Paprika splitter's lung	Paprika	*Mucor stolonifer*
Cheese washer's lung	Moldy cheese	*Penicillium caseii*
Bird fancier's lung (pigeon breeder's lung)	Pigeon, parrot, and other bird droppings	Serum and droppings
Pituitary snuff taker's lung	Bovine and porcine pituitary snuff	Pituitary antigens
Turkey raiser's disease	Turkey protein	Turkey serum
Chicken raiser's disease	Chicken protein	Chicken feathers, serum, and droppings

dust, associated with rales on auscultation of the chest and a mixed reticular-nodular pattern on the chest roentgenogram. Lung function tests reveal a restrictive pattern with an associated defect in gas transfer. Precipitating antibodies of the IgG class may be demonstrated against the allergen. Bronchial inhalation challenge with the appropriate allergen is valuable in establishing the diagnosis.

The treatment involves avoidance of the allergen, which may entail a change of occupation. Acute hypersensitivity pneumonitis may be rapidly fatal and should be treated with steroids, supplemental oxygen, and mechanical ventilation if respiratory failure ensues.

OCCUPATIONAL ASTHMA

Occupational asthma is a respiratory disorder related to an occupational inhalant and characterized clinically by shortness of breath, wheezing, chest tightness, and cough. The prevalence of the disorder ranges from 5% to 9% in certain industries in the United States. Both organic and inorganic substances may give rise to the condition. Inorganic sources of exposure include fumes, chemicals, and drugs; organic sources include dusts, danders, and enzymes. Sources commonly encountered in industry are listed in the following outline:

Materials associated with occupational asthma

I. Fumes
   A. Ammonia
   B. Sulfur dioxide
   C. Chlorine
   D. Ozone
II. Chemicals
   A. Phthalic anhydride
   B. Trimellitic anhydride
   C. Ethylene diamine
   D. Toluene di-isocyanate
   E. Polyvinylchloride products
   F. Formalin
   G. Formaldehyde
   H. Platinum salts
   I. Nickel salts
   J. Soldering fluxes
III. Drugs
   A. Ampicillin
   B. Spiramycin
   C. Piperazine
   D. Amprolium
IV. Dusts
   A. Cotton
   B. Flax
   C. Hemp
   D. Castor bean
   E. Coffee bean
   F. Grain
   G. Flour
   H. Wood
V. Danders
   A. Rat
   B. Guinea pig
   C. Cat
   D. Dog
   E. Horse
   F. Bird
VI. Enzymes
   A. *Bacillus subtilis*
   B. Hog trypsin
VII. Insecticides—organic phosphorus

Three mechanisms have been proposed as being important in the pathogenesis. These are the allergic, pharmacologic, and toxic factors. Allergic mechanisms are important in occupational asthma caused by coffee and castor beans (and other agents just listed), enzymes, platinum salts, and the epoxy resin—curing agents, phthalic anhydride and trimellitic anhydride. Specific IgE has been described in the serum of subjects with asthma caused by these agents. On the surface of mast cells it can combine with the allergen or hapten, resulting in the release of chemical mediators. These mediators are believed to be responsible for the smooth muscle contraction, mucosal edema, and subsequent mucous plugging that occurs in the condition. Positive immediate skin tests, characterized by a wheal and flare reaction occurring in about 1 hour, have been demonstrated in occupational asthma resulting from organic materials and metal salts.

The condition is characterized by wheezing, chest tightness, and shortness of breath. Cough, particularly nocturnal cough, is also a common symptom. Symptoms may occur within 1 hour of exposure, but a delayed reaction occurring after 4 hours is also seen.

The diagnosis is based on the physical examination and history of exposure. Pulmonary function tests show an obstructive pattern when the subject is symptomatic. Confirmation can be obtained with a positive bronchial inhalation challenge with the appropriate agent.

The treatment consists of avoidance of the offending agent and the use of bronchodilators, antihistamines, and aminophylline. Steroid therapy may be required in severe cases. Disodium chromoglycate may also be useful in preventing attacks.

LUNG DISEASE CAUSED BY INHALED GASES AND VAPORS

Most toxic gases exert a direct effect on the respiratory mucous membrane. The site of injury and extent of damage are determined to a large degree by such factors as the amount of the exposure, the solubility of the agent, and the individual's ability to recognize and minimize exposure. For example, certain substances may rapidly produce highly irritating symptoms in the upper airway such as sneezing and coughing, as well as ocular discomfort; an individual with such symptoms is likely to avoid prolonged exposure. On the other hand, individuals trapped in an enclosed space with a pulmonary irritant who do not imme-

Table 133-2. Inhaled gases and vapors commonly involved in direct respiratory tract injury

Substance	Source
Ammonia	Fertilizer production
	Commercial refrigerant
Cadmium	Heating or smelting of ores and metals
	Welding
Chlorine	Manufacture of alkalies and bleaches
	Water purification
Nitrogen oxides	Silage (silo filler's disease)
	Arc welding in enclosed spaces
	Burning of nitrogen-containing substances
	Manufacturing processes
Ozone	Inside high-altitude, high-performance aircraft
	Photochemical smog
	Arc welding
Sulfur dioxide	Multiple industrial processes (especially manufacturing of paper and chemicals)
	Smog

diately recognize the exposure or who cannot escape because of physical incapacity such as loss of consciousness are more likely to sustain a severe exposure. A variety of potentially damaging pulmonary irritants are in widespread industrial use or are commonly encountered as by-products of industrial or occupational processes (see Table 133-2); a full listing is beyond the scope of this chapter. The diagnosis of inhalational lung disease is facilitated when there is a well-defined history of exposure and a rapid development of symptoms. However, insidious exposure and a latent period of up to 12 hours before the development of symptoms and roentgenographic changes may lead to diagnostic confusion. Serial measurements of arterial blood gases over the first few hours after the inhalational injury may demonstrate hypoxemia and precede the development of clinical and roentgenographic changes.

The therapy for inhalational injuries includes attention to airway maintenance (intubation or tracheostomy are occasionally required for upper airway edema or spasm), humidification of inspired gases, treatment of atelectasis by respiratory therapy measures, removal of desquamated debris by suctioning or bronchoscopy, and supportive treatment for chemically induced pulmonary edema (oxygen administration, positive end-expiratory pressure, and mechanical ventilatory support).

Smoke inhalation

Exposure to the products of combustion generated by fire may result in any or all of four distinct insults to the individual. The fire may consume all available oxygen with resultant asphyxiation of the victim. Incomplete combustion may produce carbon monoxide with its consequent cardiac and neurologic effects of angina, arrhythmia production, myocardial infarction, confusion, coma, seizures, and death. Thermal injury to the upper airway, although uncommon, can result in edema, mucosal sloughing, and airway obstruction. Severe thermal injury carries a poor prognosis.

True smoke inhalation damage is a chemical injury resulting from the inhalation of multiple toxic agents such as acrolein and phosgene absorbed onto carbon particles. The extent of injury depends on the material burned, the amount of smoke particles, and the humidity of the inspired gas. Injury is greater in the burn victim who has been exposed to open flames, been unconscious, suffered facial burns, or been injured in a closed-space fire.

Smoke injury can consist of any or all of three phases. Initially there may be acute respiratory distress with edema and bronchospasm that may require bronchodilator or steroid therapy. Alveolar-capillary injury may subsequently be manifested as the adult respiratory distress syndrome, requiring assisted ventilation, O_2, and the use of positive end expiratory pressure. During the recovery phase and possibly for up to 2 weeks following the initial injury there is a significant risk of bacterial pneumonia, usually as a result of *Staphylococcus aureus* or *Pseudomonas* species.

With improved techniques for caring for the burn injury itself, concomitant respiratory injury is becoming responsible for a progressively increasing proportion of death caused by burns. The therapy remains unsatisfactory.

Oxygen toxicity

Although humans need oxygen to exist, human tolerance for this gas is limited. In a classic example of too much of a good thing, exposure to greater than normal partial pressures of O_2 can result in lung injury. This generally occurs because of therapeutic intervention during disease states causing hypoxia, but divers, aviators, and workers in hyperbaric chambers may also be exposed to increased pressures of O_2, and it is the pressure of inspired O_2 rather than the concentration that appears to be the major determinant of toxicity.

Some studies have shown impairment of mucociliary transport mechanisms and alveolar macrophage activity at relatively low levels of O_2 supplementation, but at normal atmospheric pressure up to 40% O_2 is considered safe. Most agree that concentrations greater than 60% are generally toxic, but there is disagreement about the safety of intermediate concentrations. However, the consensus is that (1) O_2 supplementation is indicated only for the treatment of hypoxia, (2) other means of improving oxygenation should also be used, (3) the minimal concentration necessary to relieve hypoxia should be employed, and (4) O_2 supplementation should be decreased and discontinued as soon as feasible.

The initial manifestations of O_2 toxicity are increasing discomfort on inspiration and dry cough. Lung volumes are reduced, and diffusion is impaired. Arterial O_2 pressure begin to fall as the alveolar-arterial O_2 difference increases. If hypoxia is present, O_2 supplementation may have to be further increased even though this can exacerbate the degree of toxicity. Pathologically, interstitial edema, cellular infiltration, patchy atelectasis, and hemorrhagic pneumonitis develop. Often the pathologic picture is complicated by the presence of the initial disease entity that necessitated O_2 supplementation. Therapy other than that directed at the initial underlying disease process and other than continued efforts to decrease the pressures of O_2 being employed is unsatisfactory.

BIBLIOGRAPHY

Bailey, W.C., and others: Silico-mycobacterial disease in sandblasters, Am. Rev. Respir. Dis. **110**:115, 1974.

Becklake, M.R.: Asbestos related diseases of the lung and other organs: their epidemiology and implications for clinical practice, Am. Rev. Respir. Dis. **114**:187, 1976.

Criteria document—recommendations for an occupational exposure standard for crystalline silica, U.S. Department of Health, Education and Welfare, Washington, D.C., 1974. U.S. Government Printing Office.

Elmes, P.C., and Simpson, M.J.C.: The clinical aspects of mesothelioma, Q. J. Med. **45**:427, 1976.

Jacobson, G., and Lanihart, W.S.: ILO/UC 1971 international classification of radiographs of the pneumoconioses, Med. Radiogr. Photogr. **48**:67, 1972.

Legha, S.S., and Muggic, F.M.: Therapeutic approaches in malignant mesothelioma, Cancer Treat. Rev. **4**:13, 1977.

Morgan, W.K.C.: Byssinosis and related conditions. In Morgan, W.K.C., and Seaton, A., editors: Occupational lung diseases, Philadelphia, 1975, W.B. Saunders Co.

Morgan, W.K.C., and Lapp, N.L.: Respiratory disease in coal miners, Am. Rev. Respir. Dis. **113**:531, 1976.

Schlueter, D.P.: Response of the lung to inhaled antigens, Am. J. Med. **57**:476, 1974.

Slavin, R.G.: Asthma in adults. III. Occupational asthma, Hosp. Pract. **13**:133, 1978.

Wagner, J.C., Sleggs, C.A., and Marchand, P.: Diffuse pleural mesothelioma and asbestos exposure in the north-west Cape Province, Br. J. Ind. Med. **17**:260, 1960.

Weil, H., and Ziskind, M.M.: Occupational pulmonary diseases. In Fishman, A.P., editor: Pulmonary diseases and disorders, New York, 1980, McGraw-Hill Book Co.

134 • DISEASES OF THE PLEURA

Maurice Sones

The pleura is the very thin covering or lining of the lung and is composed of connective tissue. It contains lymphatics, blood vessels, smooth muscle fibers, and pain fibers.

The parietal pleura lines the inner surface of the chest wall and becomes the visceral pleura at the hilum; thus pleura encases the entire lung. It creates a saclike structure, the pleural cavity, that has no air within it but does contain a thin layer of fluid that serves to decrease the friction between the two layers of pleura. This lymph fluid within the pleural space is not static but is constantly being formed and removed. The presence of this fluid can be demonstrated by roentgenographic techniques in 10% of normal individuals and up to 40% of postpartum women. The turnover of pleural fluid may amount to several hundred milliliters daily. The physiologic mechanisms by which this fluid enters and leaves the pleural space are the result of several pressures. The parietal capillary hydrostatic pressure (30 cm water) plus the negative pleural space pressure (5 cm water) plus the pleural fluid osmotic pressure (6 cm water) totals 41 cm of water pressure. The colloid osmotic pressure of the blood within the capillaries is 32 cm of water. The resulting difference of 9 cm of water pressure produces a flow of fluid from the parietal pleura into the pleural space. In the visceral pleura, however, the capillary hydrostatic pressure is only 11 cm of water as opposed to 30 cm in the parietal pleura. This reduced pressure allows a constant movement of fluid from the pleural space into the visceral pleura, that is, from the area of higher pressure to one of lower pressure. Any interruption of this balance of pressures can interfere with normal fluid transport or result in increased friction between pleural layers.

PLEURITIS

Pleuritis is an inflammation of the pleura. Most commonly it is caused by tuberculosis, bacterial pneumonia, lung abscess, malignancy, or pulmonary embolism. One type of tumor affecting the pleura is mesothelioma, usually related to asbestos exposure. By interfering with the normal fluid transport, all of these conditions result in increased friction between the layers of pleura.

The most prominent symptom associated with pleurisy is pain, which is usually sharp and lancinating and is accentuated by inspiration. (The most severe pain is noted in Bornholm disease, frequently called the "devil's grip"; it is more likely a result of involvement of the intercostal muscle or nerve than of the pleura and is caused by coxsackievirus type B.) Cough is common and aggravates the pain. Other symptoms may be present and are usually related to the underlying disease process. The cardinal physical finding is a pleural friction rub, which may be absent if marked splinting of the affected side occurs. Chest wall tenderness may be present. Breathing can become very distressing and consequently can be quite shallow. Fever may also be present, especially with infections. An insidious onset of pleuritis with gradual progression of poor health in patients over 40 years of age suggests malignancy. Laboratory studies should be directed at the suspected underlying cause. Chest films generally reveal poor expansion and/or the presence of underlying parenchymal disease or pleural fluid. An examination of pleural effusion, if present, is critical (see following discussion of "Pleural effusion"). The progression of pleuritis can result in the formation of a pleural effusion either by increasing fluid production or by inhibiting its uptake by the visceral pleura. The therapy is symptomatic once the underlying cause has been identified and removed.

PLEURAL EFFUSION

The systematic approach to abnormal fluid accumulation in the pleural space, or pleural effusion, begins with a complete history and physical examinaiton, followed by appropriate chest films that include posteroanterior and lateral decubitus views. Skin tests for tuberculosis, as well as examination of the pleural fluid for bacteria, tubercle bacilli, fungi, malignant cells, and *Entamoeba histolytica,* are mandatory. A chemical analysis of pleural fluid can also be helpful. In effusion of unclear cause the examination of the pleura itself by needle biopsy can often be revealing. Ultrasonography, lymph node biopsy, mediastinoscopy, sputum examination, and exploratory thoracotomy are other modalities that may have to be considered in the evaluation of pleural effusions.

An area of dullness to percussion found posteriorly above the diaphragm, which becomes resonant when the patient bends forward, suggests the presence of shifting or mobile pleural fluid. Breath sounds are absent in the area. Clubbing of the fingers can be seen with effusions caused by chronic infections such as bronchiectasis or empyema and also with malignancies. The chest roentgenogram shows a homogeneously increased density above the diaphragm and adjacent to the chest wall (Fig. 134-1). A decubitus view allows detection of lesser amounts of fluid.

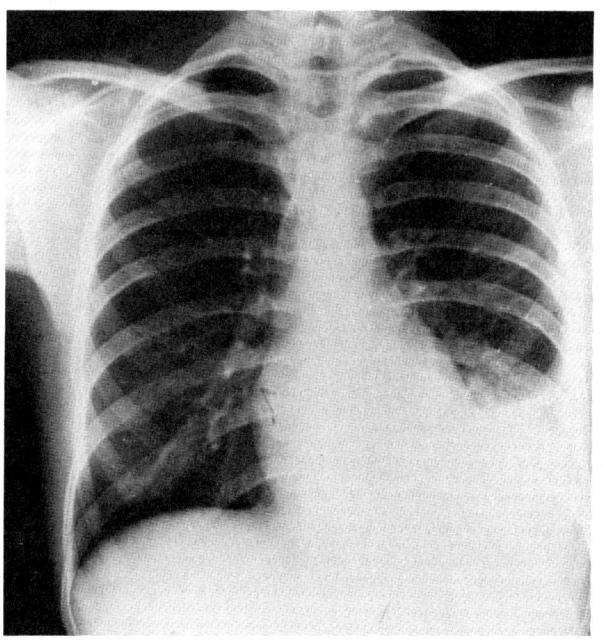

Fig. 134-1. Left pleural effusion in 21-year-old woman who has tuberculosis without parenchymal involvement. (Courtesy of George Popky, M.D.)

Pleural effusions may be a prominent finding in patients with congestive heart failure, tuberculosis, pneumonia, and pulmonary embolism. Rheumatoid arthritis may also result in the formation of a pleural effusion. Pleural effusion with pelvic tumors in females is called *Meigs' syndrome*. The nephrotic syndrome may be associated with pleural effusions, as well as marked peripheral edema and ascites.

Pleural effusions have also been reported in pancreatitis, chylothorax resulting from traumatic or surgical injury to the thoracic duct, ankylosing spondylitis, cirrhosis of the liver with ascites, amebiasis, sarcoidosis, disseminated lupus erythematosus, insertion of central venous cannulas, and uremia. There is about a 50% incidence of small pleural effusions after abdominal surgery.

Pleural effusions can be divided into transudates and exudates. A transudate is a filtrate of plasma containing little protein that has passed through a membrane as a result of an alteration in the mechanics of fluid homeostasis. An exudate is the result of the passage of fluid, protein, and white blood cells through vessel walls that have been made permeable because of localized disease and interference with lymphatic drainage. Transudates occur in congestive heart failure, cirrhosis, and the nephrotic syndrome, whereas exudates are found in pneumonia, tuberculosis, malignancy, and embolism.

Transudates are usually clear with a specific gravity of 1.015 or less, a protein content of less than 3 g/dl, and a serum lactic acid dehydrogenase (LDH) concentration of less than 200 IU. The ratio of pleural fluid to serum protein is generally less than 0.5 and that for pleural fluid to serum LDH less than 0.6.

With exudates these parameters are increased: protein content is greater than 3 g/dl, the pleural fluid to serum protein ratio is more than 0.5, and the pleural fluid to serum LDH ratio greater than 0.6.

Milky fluid (chylothorax) is most often seen following trauma or with disease involving the thoracic duct. Long-standing effusions containing excessive amounts of cholesterol and exhibiting a satinlike sheen are called pseudochylous effusions.

A pH less than 6 suggests gastric contents from esophageal rupture, and a pH between 6 and 7 implies empyema. Samples for pH determination must be collected anaerobically.

If the pleural fluid is bloody or turbid, with the red cell count exceeding 100,000/mm^3, malignancy is found in more than 50% of cases. Bloody fluid may also be found in trauma or pulmonary embolism and rarely in congestive heart failure, infections, and cirrhosis of the liver.

A white blood cell count of more than 1000/mm^3 in the absence of red cells suggests that the fluid is related to infection, such as bacterial or tuberculous infection. If at least 50% of the white blood cells are polymorphonuclear, bacterial infection is usually the cause of the effusion. A preponderance of lymphocytes is seen in effusions caused by tuberculosis. Neoplasm or cirrhosis with ascites may also occasionally cause pleural fluid leukocytosis. Congestive heart failure rarely results in pleural white cell counts greater than 1000/mm^3.

Eosinophil counts of 5% to 50% can be seen in Löffler's syndrome, polyarteritis nodosa, tropical eosinophilia, and Hodgkin's disease. When blood eosinophilia coexists, the hypersensitivity diseases are suggested. Pleural fluid eosinophilia in the absence of blood eosinophilia is often of occult origin but has been related to pulmonary infection, trauma, malignant tumor, pulmonary infarction, or cirrhosis of the liver with ascites. The presence of pleural fluid eosinophilia argues strongly against tuberculosis or fungal infections.

Glucose should be measured during the fasting state, and if it exceeds 85 mg/dl in pleural fluid, the fluid is probably not due to infection in the pleural space. In the absence of acute bacterial infection, levels of glucose less than 60 mg/dl suggest tuberculosis or malignancy, and a glucose concentration under 30 mg/dl is most commonly seen in patients with rheumatoid arthritis.

When abdominal pain accompanies pleural effusion, pancreatitis should be suspected, and in that case the pleural fluid amylase level will be higher than the serum amylase concentration. Pleural fluid that is gelatinous and bloody and contains elevated levels of hyaluronic acid suggests an underlying malignant mesothelioma.

In pleural effusions caused by malignancy there is a 50% chance of finding tumor cells by cytologic examination of a single specimen. If three or more specimens are obtained and a pleural biopsy is performed, the majority of malignant effusions can be correctly diagnosed.

Cultures of pleural fluid are often positive in empyema but are not diagnostically helpful in the patient with pneumonia and a sterile sympathetic effusion. If the fluid is foul smelling, anaerobes are the cause, but they may be difficult to isolate. Tuberculosis can be diagnosed by direct smear and culture in less than 30% of cases, possibly because pleural effusions resulting from tuberculosis are often caused by a hypersensitivity reaction to the tubercle bacillus, and thus few bacilli may be present. If possible, large amounts of fluid should be examined to improve the chances of obtaining a positive culture.

Biopsy techniques may be important in the evaluation of pleural effusions. A pleural biopsy should be performed in the case of an exudative effusion if the diagnosis has not been made by other means. Complications are uncommon but may include pneumothorax and bleeding. Implantation of carcinoma in the needle tract is also reported rarely. The contraindications to pleural biopsy are an uncooperative patient, severe coagulation defects, and limited respiratory reserve. A tissue diagnosis can be made in 75% of cases of tuberculous fluid accumulation and in more than 50% of cases of effusion caused by malignancy or rheumatoid disease. Biopsy of the internal mammary nodes via the second intercostal space gives positive findings in up to 50% of cases of effusions resulting from tuberculosis or malignancy. The diagnosis can be established by thoracoscopy or pleuroscopy (procedures that allow direct visualization of the pleura) in 90% of cases caused by tuberculosis or malignancy. Ultrasonography and computed tomography may prove helpful in the diagnosis of pleural disease. Thoracotomy as a diagnostic procedure should be considered only when all other procedures have failed.

The causes of pleural effusions are numerous and are listed as follows:

Causes of pleural effusion

Common
Malignancy
Congestive heart failure
Pulmonary infarction
Infection (bacterial, fungal, parasitic, tuberculous, viral)
Pancreatitis
Cirrhosis with ascites
Collagen diseases
Renal diseases
Subphrenic abscess
Trauma to lung, mediastinum, or spine
Postmyocardial infarction (Dressler's syndrome)
Idiopathic

Rare
Amebiasis
Catamenial pneumothorax
Central venous cannula insertion
Coagulation defects
Emphysema
Hepatitis B infection
Hydrocarbon ingestion
Hypoproteinemia
Iatrogenic (surgery, instillation of drugs)
Infectious mononucleosis
Löffler's syndrome
Malignant mesothelioma
Familial Mediterranean fever
Meigs' syndrome
Methysergide therapy
Myxedema
Niemann-Pick disease
Pneumoconioses
Obstructed superior vena cava or azygos vein
Radiation therapy
Respiratory distress syndrome
Ruptured aneurysm
Ruptured dermoid cyst
Ruptured esophagus
Sarcoidosis
Spontaneous chylothorax
Trapped lung syndrome
Waldenström's macroglobulinemia
Wegener's granulomatosis
Whipple's disease
Yellow nail syndrome

The most common causes of pleural effusions are cancer, congestive heart failure, infection, and pulmonary embolism. If there is evidence of congestive heart failure, the fluid should resolve with drug treatment and nothing more need be done. If it does not resolve, however, or if there is no evidence of congestive heart failure, thoracentesis should be performed. A protein measurement, cell count, and differential and cytologic examinations should be routinely ordered. If the primary diagnosis being considered is cancer or lymphoma, depending on the characteristics of the pleural fluid, only protein measurement and cytologic studies need ordinarily be obtained. If the effusion is chylous in nature, a determination of fat content (triglyceride and cholesterol) is also in order. If the fluid is purulent, routine culture and Gram stain should be added. However, other studies that have a high correlation with the specific diagnosis being considered should be included, such as the glucose concentration in rheumatoid disease, the amylase level in pancreatitis, and appropriate stains and cultures in tuberculosis and fungal infections. If the diagnosis has still not been established, pleural biopsy and other studies are indicated. This approach to the diagnosis of pleural effusion is more reasonable and cost effective than ordering all studies at the initial examination without taking the time to evaluate and proceed in an orderly fashion.

The therapy depends on the underlying cause and nature of the fluid, but repeated thoracentesis or instillation of sclerosing agents such as tetracycline may be necessary for recurring effusions.

PNEUMOTHORAX

Spontaneous pneumothorax most commonly occurs in young men; a bleb ruptures allowing air to escape into the pleural space and resulting in partial or total collapse of a lung. Occasionally the tension of the air may increase from the trapping of more air, which results in the collapse of a large part of the lung with a shift of the heart and mediastinum to the opposite side; this is a tension pneumothorax, an extremely dangerous situation because it compromises the opposite lung (Fig. 134-2). The patient may note pain initially, followed by increasing dyspnea. Inadequate blood supply to the lungs and heart may result in a pale, sweaty, dyspneic patient.

The physical examination reveals hyperresonance with absent breath sounds over the pneumothorax. The chest film exhibits an area of hyperlucency with an absence of lung markings. The collapsed lung may be evident as an area of increased density. With tension pneumothoras the diaphragm is pushed down and mediastinal structures are displaced to the contralateral side.

Chronic obstructive pulmonary disease, pneumonia and other infections, malignancies, the pneumoconioses, and sarcoidosis are other conditions in which spontaneous pneumothorax may occur. If done incorrectly, cannulation of a subclavian vein may also result in this complication.

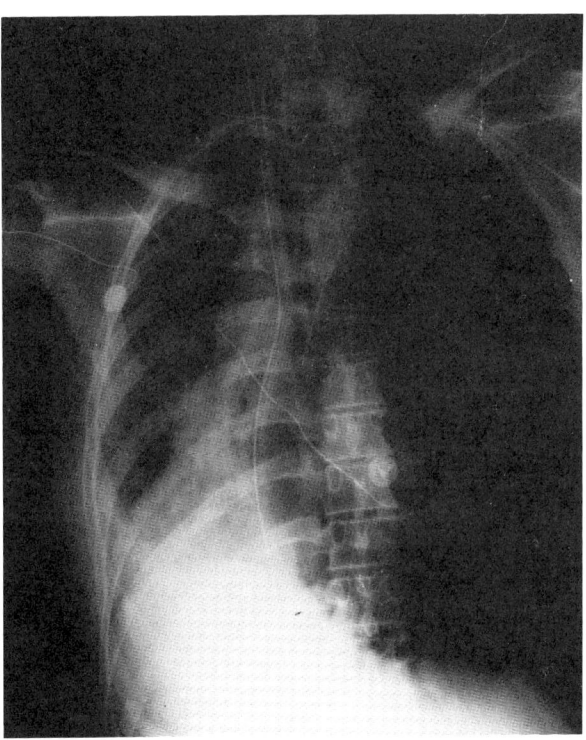

Fig. 134-2. Tension pneumothorax on left side resulting from introduction of central venous pressure catheter. Left lung is collapsed and mediastinum is shifted to right side. (Courtesy of George Popky, M.D.)

Pneumothorax is a common finding in infants with respiratory distress syndrome, the incidence varying with severity of the syndrome, intensity of respiratory assistance, and use of continuous positive airway pressure (CPAP) or positive end-expiratory pressure (PEEP).

Recurring spontaneous pneumothorax may be associated with menses. This entity, catamenial pneumothorax, is found predominantly on the right side and is usually associated with endometriosis. The management of patients who have received respiratory therapy is also occasionally complicated by subcutaneous emphysema, pneumomediastinum, and pneumothorax.

Pneumothorax can be relieved by inserting a large-bore needle or catheter under a water seal to allow the air to escape, thus permitting the lung to reexpand and the dyspnea and pain to be relieved. In the case of a tension pneumothorax a medical emergency exists until the air is released. A conservative approach should be used in clamping or removing a tube thoracostomy. Before removal there should be no air leak and full lung expansion. Removal should be preceded by a trial of tube clamping for 24 to 48 hours with no recurrence of the pneumothorax.

The rent in the lung frequently closes over and the lung completely reexpands; however, recurrence is common, and if three or more episodes occur, surgical intervention is usually necessary. Poudrage can be accomplished with talc or tetracycline instillation; if this does not correct the situation, pleurectomy may be required.

PLEURAL TUMORS

Primary pleural tumors are of two varieties: a localized fibrous mesothelioma that is often pedunculated, benign, and treated by localized excision, and a highly malignant, diffuse mesothelioma related to asbestos exposure in up to 40% of cases (see Chapter 133).

The benign mesotheliomas are often associated with hypoglycemia and rheumatoid-like symptoms, both of which are curved with removal of the tumor. The chest film, often the first evidence of abnormality, reveals a localized, encapsulated lesion commonly along pleural planes. The therapy is surgical removal, and the prognosis is good.

Malignant mesothelioma is often characterized chiefly by the signs and symptoms of a pleural effusion. It may be manifested by pleuritic pain, dull, aching chest pain, or shortness of breath. Chest roentgenograms reveal a pattern similar to that of a rapidly progressing pleural effusion. Instillation of tetracycline, quinacrine, or radioactive phosphorus may obliterate the pleural space and temporarily prevent the further formation of fluid, but the treatment of malignant mesothelioma is often unsatisfactory. A patient will occasionally respond to total pleurectomy and chemotherapy using a variety of drugs. The overall outlook is generally grave, with most patients dying within the year following diagnosis.

Metastatic tumors arising from the lung, breast, pancreas, ovary, and colon may involve the pleura. Thymoma and lymphoma can also spread to the pleura. The therapy includes local irradiation for pain relief and management appropriate for the primary lesion.

BIBLIOGRAPHY

Arai, H., and others: Significance of the quantification and demonstration of hyaluronic acid in tissue specimens for the diagnosis of pleural mesothelioma, Am. Rev. Respir. Dis. **120**:529, 1979.

Ayvazian, L.: Diagnostic aspects of pleural effusion, Bull. N.Y. Acad. Med. **53**:532, 1977.

Barrocar, A.: Catamenial PNX: case report and review of the literature, Am. Surg. **45**:340, 1979.

Ellis, K., and Wolff, M.: Mesotheliomas and secondary tumors of the pleura, Semin. Roentgenol. **12**:303, 1977.

Felson, B., editor: Causes of pleural fluid, Semin. Roentgenol. **12**:327, 1977.

Herman, M.A.: Recurring spontaneous pneumothorax associated with menses, South. Med. J. **69**:488, 1976.

Light, R.W., and George, R.B.: Incidence of pleural effusion after abdominal surgery, Chest **69**:621, 1976.

Light, R.W., and others: The diagnostic separation of transudates and exudates, Ann. Intern. Med. **77**:507, 1972.

Ogata, E.S., and others: Pneumothorax in the respiratory distress syndrome: incidence and effect on vital signs, blood gases and pH, Pediatrics **58**:177, 1976.

Sahebjami, H., and Loudon, R.G.: Pleural effusion: pathophysiology and clinical features, Semin. Roentgenol. **12**:269, 1977.

Storey, D.D., Dines, D.E., and Coles, D.T.: Pleural effusion, a diagnostic dilemma, J.A.M.A. **236**:2183, 1976.

Zimmerman, J.E., Dunbar, B.S., and Klingenmaier, C.H.: Management of subcutaneous emphysema, pneumomediastinum and pneumothorax during respirator therapy, Crit. Care Med. **3**:69, 1975.

135 • DISEASES OF THE MEDIASTINUM, DIAPHRAGM, AND CHEST WALL

Stanley L. Altschuler

MEDIASTINAL DISEASE

The mediastinum is located in the midthorax and separates the two pleural cavities. From the thoracic inlet to the diaphragm the mediastinum is divided into three major compartments: anterior, middle, and posterior. The anterior mediastinum is situated in front of the heart and contains the thymus gland, the anterior mediastinal lymph nodes, and the internal mammary arteries and veins. The middle mediastinal compartment contains the pericardium and heart, the great vessels, the phrenic and part of the vagus nerves, the trachea and main bronchi, and lymph nodes. The posterior mediastinum contains the descending thoracic aorta, esophagus, thoracic duct, azygos and hemiazygos veins, the sympathetic nerves and portions of the vagus nerve, and posterior mediastinal lymph nodes. Diseases of the mediastinum are predominantly infectious, tumor related, or the result of abnormalities of the contained structures. Chest roentgenograms are often crucial to the diagnosis.

Mediastinitis

Acute infections of the mediastinum usually result from esophageal perforation. The esophagus may be perforated from carcinoma, from an impacted foreign body, as a complication of esophagoscopy, or spontaneously after vomiting. Infection from adjacent tissues can also spread into the mediastinum. The clinical manifestations include severe retrosternal pain associated with chills and high fever. Subcutaneous emphysema may be present in the soft tissues of the neck. The diagnosis is suggested by the clinical presentation and substantiated by roentgenographic findings, including widening of the mediastinum, the presence of air in the mediastinum or soft tissues of the neck, and the presence of pneumothorax or hydropneumothorax. Untreated mediastinitis can result in abscess formation, with perforation of the abscess into the pleural cavity, esophagus, or bronchus. The treatment involves the use of appropriate antibiotics, maintenance of fluid balance, and identification and treatment of the originating insult.

Chronic mediastinitis usually develops slowly and

asymptomatically. The diagnosis is often first suspected on the basis of a routine chest roentgenogram or occasionally because of symptoms related to pressure on one of the mediastinal structures. Chronic mediastinitis can be granulomatous or sclerosing.

The cause of granulomatous mediastinitis is seldom established, but histoplasmosis or tuberculosis is sometimes implicated. Sarcoidosis, silicosis, and other fungal infections can also be responsible. Most patients are asymptomatic, but obstruction of the superior vena cava and the esophagus may be the initial manifestation. The *superior vena caval syndrome* is characterized by puffiness of the face and neck, cyanosis, headaches, epistaxis, and lightheadedness.

The cause of sclerosing mediastinitis is only rarely established; it is sometimes associated with retroperitoneal fibrosis or other sclerosing conditions, leading to the concept of a multifocal fibrosclerosis. This association has been reported in cases of systemic lupus erythematosus, rheumatoid disease, and during treatment with methysergide maleate. The diagnosis is suspected by finding a widening of the upper half of the mediastinum on chest film, but a biopsy is required for confirmation. The clinical manifestations include superior vena caval obstruction and obstruction of the tracheobronchial tree and esophagus. The treatment is directed at correcting the underlying cause and relieving obstruction.

Pneumomediastinum

The presence of gas in the mediastinum, or pneumomediastinum, is relatively rare. It usually occurs spontaneously but may result from trauma or follow rupture of the esophagus or tracheobronchial tree during bronchoscopy. Spontaneous pneumomediastinum usually results from severe coughing or vomiting, deep inspiratory efforts, or Valsalva's maneuver and may occur in the mother during the time of delivery, particularly when labor is prolonged. Gas accumulates in the mediastinum and hilar areas and can also result in pneumothorax. These findings are evident on the chest roentgenogram as abornmal hyperlucent areas. The air usually passes into the neck, resulting in gas in the tissues or subcutaneous emphysema. If the gas is unable to leave the mediastinal compartment, pressure may develop, causing compression of vascular or respiratory structures. Air may also enter the mediastinum as a result of dental extractions or following trauma to the neck.

The clinical manifestations include the sudden onset of retrosternal pain radiating to the shoulders and arms. Swallowing and respiratory efforts may increase the pain, and dyspnea may be severe. Subcutaneous emphysema is sometimes noted in the neck or over the thoracic wall. Pneumomediastinum usually resolves spontaneously or after correction of the underlying cause. Chest tube drainage of air for reexpansion of the lung may be required if a pneumothorax also develops.

Anterior mediastinal masses

Thymomas, germinal tumors, thyroid lesions, and lipomas comprise the majority of abnormal masses in the anterior mediastinum.

Thymomas are the most commonly occurring neoplasms in the anterior mediastinum and may be benign or malignant. Thymomas are often associated with myasthenia gravis, and most of the symptoms related to thymomas are the result of this condition.

Germinal tumors include dermoid cysts, teratomas, seminomas, choriocarinomas, and embryonal carcinomas. These tumors arise from primitive germ cell nests and are present from birth although they are manifest only later in life. Dermoid cysts contain only epidermis and its appendages, whereas teratomas contain all three embryonic derivatives. The majority of these lesions are benign and asymptomatic and are discovered on routine chest roentgenograms. Thoracic seminomas are histologically similar to testicular seminomas and ovarian tumors. Most choriocarcinomas of the mediastinum occur in males; they grow rapidly and produce symptoms such as dyspnea, hemoptysis, Horner's syndrome, and gynecomastia. The possibility of metastasis from the testes must be eliminated in both seminoma and choriocarcinoma.

Thyroid goiters are usually asymptomatic and also are discovered on routine chest roentgenograms. Clinical manifestations include respiratory distress caused by tracheal compression, as well as stridor and hoarseness resulting from involvement of the recurrent laryngeal nerve. Usually an enlarged gland can be palpated in the neck region when a thyroid-related mediastinal mass is present.

Lipomas can occur in any of the mediastinal compartments but are usually found anteriorly. They are often visualized on chest roentgenograms and appear to have a density lower than surrounding tissues. Occasionally fatty deposition in the anterior mediastinum can be the result of corticosteroid administration. Fibromas, hemangiomas, and lymphangiomas are other mesenchymal tumors that may rarely appear in the anterior mediastinum.

Middle mediastinal masses

Lymph node enlargement in Hodgkin's disease and non-Hodgkin's lymphoma usually occurs in the middle mediastinum. Metastasis from cancer in lungs, gastrointestinal tract, prostate, or kidneys can also result in lymph node enlargement; other causes include tuberculosis, histoplasmosis, and sarcoidosis.

Bronchogenic cysts are congenital abnormalities usually located near the carina. They often have a cavitary appearance on chest films. These cysts are mostly asymptomatic but occasionally cause tracheal compression. Pericardial cysts are usually located in the cardiophrenic angles and remain asymptomatic but sometimes cause dyspnea.

Dilations or aneurysms of major vessels in the mediastinum can also occur as mediastinal masses. Dilation of the main pulmonary artery is usually the result of pulmonary hypertension or a left-to-right shunt. Aortic aneurysms may result from arteriosclerosis, syphilis, trauma, dissection, stenosis, or infection. Patients with aortic aneurysms are commonly asymptomatic, but symptoms related to compression of the superior vena cava, recurrent laryngeal nerve, or tracheobronchial tree may develop. Dissecting aneurysms usually result in severe retrosternal pain radiating to the back.

Posterior mediastinal masses

Neurogenic neoplasms can arise from nerve sheaths, nerve cells, or all nerve elements and usually occur in the posterior mediastinum. Nerve sheath tumors are usually benign, whereas tumors arising from other nerve elements are often malignant. Mediastinal neurofibromas and neurilemomas arise from peripheral nerves. Sympathetic ganglia may give rise to neuroblastomas and pheochromocytomas. Chemodectomas arise from paraganglionic cells.

Esophageal lesions, including neoplasm, diverticulum, hiatus hernia, and megaesophagus, are located in the posterior mediastinum. Esophageal neoplasms are frequently malignant, although benign lesions also occur. Esophageal diverticula are of three types and can be differentiated on the chest film on the basis of location. Zenker's diverticula are located in the pharyngeal region. Traction diverticula are commonly the result of granulomatous processes such as histoplasmosis or tuberculosis and are located in the middle portion of the esophagus. Pulsion diverticula are located in the lower esophagus and are the result of mucosal outpouchings. Dilation of the esophagus may be caused by scleroderma, carcinoma, achalasia, or gastric regurgitation.

All of the various mediastinal masses can appear as localized lesions on chest roentgenograms. Surgical exploration is often required for both diagnosis and therapy.

DIAPHRAGMATIC DISEASE

The diaphragm is a musculotendinous structure that separates the thoracic and abdominal cavities. Muscle fibers arise from the thoracic ribs, lumbar vertebrae, and the xiphoid process and insert into a central tendon. Contraction of the muscles results in a downward movement of the diaphragm and expansion of the thoracic cage. In the normal individual diaphragmatic contraction is responsible for most of the air that is inspired during ventilation. Diaphragmatic excursion can be measured by roentgenographic techniques as well as by physical examination and is usually approximately 3.5 cm.

Abnormalities of motion

Although paralysis of the diaphragm may have any of several casues, the most common is phrenic nerve invasion by carcinoma. Other causes of diaphragmatic paralysis include disc degeneration in the cervical area, abnormalities of nerve roots from the third to the fifth cervical vertebrae, and viral neuritis. Other disorders of diaphragmatic motion include tonic contractions, diaphragmatic flutter, and persistent hiccups. Pain and dyspnea may result from these abnormal contractions. Elevation of a hemidiaphragm, abnormal motion during respiration, mediastinal swing during respiration, or paradoxic motion with sniffing can be demonstrated fluoroscopically in patients with abnormal diaphragmatic acitivity. The therapy is directed at the underlying cause.

Eventration

Eventration is a rare congenital anomaly with abnormal muscular development of a hemidiaphragm. A portion of the diaphragm consists of a thing, membranous sheath rather than the normal muscle fibers. The abnormality is usually found on a routine roentgenographic study, and the diagnosis can be confirmed if necessary by the induction of a pneumoperitoneum. This abnormality is usually asymptomatic but occasionally results in respiratory or cardiac distress. Generally no therapy is required.

Herniation

Herniation of abdominal contents into the thoracic cavity can occur as a result of trauma or disruption through congenitally weak areas of the diaphragm. Herniation through the esophageal hiatus (hiatus hernia) is the most common form of diaphragmatic hernia. Most patients with esophageal hiatus hernia are asymptomatic; however, retrostrenal pain, particularly when the patient lies flat, is the most frequent clinical manifestation. On occasion the entire stomach may herniate through the esophageal hiatus and become incarcerated or strangulated. Hiatus hernia may result in an air-fluid level in the stomach, seen behind the heart on a chest roentgenogram. The treatment includes the avoidance of recumbent positions and the use of antacids.

Herniation through the posterior hiatus, or the foramen of Bochdalek, occurs in infants but rarely in adults. Herniation through the anteriorly situated Morgagni's foramen is also rare. These two unusual forms of hiatus hernia are relatively asymptomatic in adults.

Miscellaneous conditions

Other abnormalities of the diaphragm include intradiaphragmatic cysts, known as extralobar sequestration, and tumors of the diaphragm. Extralobar sequestration of lung tissue results when a lung bud develops within the diaphragm during embryonic development. The sequestrated lung is aerated via the tracheobronchial tree. Blood is supplied by the abdominal aorta, and drainage occurs via systemic veins. Tumors of the diaphragm can be benign or malignant, but both types are quite rare. The diagnosis is suspected when an abnormal diaphragmatic mass is noted on the chest film, but a definitive diagnosis often requires open biopsy. The therapy depends on the tumor type, but surgical removal at the time of diagnostic thoracotomy is the common procedure.

CHEST WALL DISEASE
Rib lesions

Accessory ribs arising from the seventh cervical vertebra are known as cervical ribs and are often asymptomatic; they are roentgenographically evident as simply a smaller set of ribs. These accessory ribs can compress subclavian vessels or the brachial plexus. The symptoms include arm pain, reduction of the peripheral pulse, and weakness of the upper extremities. If the symptoms are disabling, surgical removal of the cervical rib is required.

Notching of the ribs seen on the chest film is most commonly caused by the dilation of intercostal arteries, which usually results from coarctation of the aorta. Rib notching may be associated with various other congenital cardiovascular defects.

Costochondral osteochondritis, or Tietze's syndrome, involves inflammation of the costochondral or costosternal joints. The disorder usually occurs in patients 20 to 40 years old and is a self-limited disease characterized by anterior chest wall pain. Acute myocardial infarction may have to be ruled out in patients with this syndrome. In addition to chest pain with movement and respiratory effort, there is localized tenderness over the costosternal junction or cartilaginous aspect of the anterior rib cage. Roentgenographic studies are unrewarding. This condition is treated with aspirin or other anit-inflammatory agents.

Neoplasms of the rib cage are almost always metastatic, with the primary source usually the lung or breast. Multiple myeloma and Hodgkin's disease less commonly involve the rib cage. Paget's disease may also be observed on roentgenographic examination of the ribs.

Sternal abnormalities

Pectus excavatum, or "funnel chest," is a depression of the sternum with the ribs protruding anteriorly. It is often associated with connective tissue disorders such as Marfan's syndrome or with multiple congenital defects. Most patients with pectus excavatum have normal pulmonary function studies and little or no respiratory disability. Surgery is required to correct the defects, but it is only rarely indicated and usually performed primarily for cosmetic purposes.

Pectus carinatum, or "pigeon breast," is a deformity in which the sternum protrudes anteriorly more than normal. This disorder is frequently associated with atrial or ventricular septal defects of the heart and occasionally associated with severe asthma of early childhood. Surgical correction is rarely if ever indicated.

Thoracic spinal abnormalities

Kyphosis is an abnormal posterior curvature of the thoracic spine, and *scoliosis* is an abnormal lateral curvature.

Kyphoscoliosis can be classified as congenital, paralytic, or idiopathic. Congenital kyphoscoliosis may be associated with neurofibromatosis, Marfan's syndrome, or other hereditary disorders. Poliomyelitis is the most common cause of paralytic kyphoscoliosis. The cause of kyphoscoliosis may remain unknown, and in this case there is a female sex predominance.

Kyphoscoliosis can alter the mechanical properties of the respiratory system. Chest wall compliance is reduced, and the work of breathing is increased. Lung volumes, including tidal volumes, are smaller than normal. Eventually alveolar hypoventilation ensues, and complications associated with respiratory failure develop. These include pulmonary artery hypertension and right-sided heart failure, hypoxemia and hypercapnia, acid-base disturbances, and recurrent respiratory infections.

Corrective surgery and orthopedic devices may be helpful in the adolescent patient with kyphoscoliosis. Straightening of the curvature followed by fixation of the spine results in increased lung volumes and diminished mechanical abnormalities of the thoracic cage. The treatment of kyphoscoliosis in the advanced stage is directed at correction of hypoxemia and heart failure, as well as prevention of respiratory infections. Assisted ventilation by means of positive-pressure machines, negative-pressure devices such as cuirass respirators, or rocking beds can improve alveolar ventilation. Surgery is not usually recommended for advanced disease.

Ankylosing spondylitis

(See Chapter 12.)

Ankylosing spondylitis is a rheumatologic condition in which bony ankylosis of zygapophyseal joints and ossification of paravertebral structures result in fixation of the chest cage in inspiration. The male-to-female ratio is approximately 8:1. The association of ankylosing spondylitis with the histocompatibility antigen HLA-B27 supports a genetic relationship.

Low back pain and stiffness, sometimes associated with fever, fatigue, and weight loss, herald the onset of ankylosing spondylitis. Symptoms progress cephalad, eventually involving the thorax. Respiratory mechanics are altered, and alveolar hypoventilation with carbon dioxide retention develops. Pulmonary function testing reveals an increased residual volume and reduced vital capacity without evidence for airway obstruction.

Some patients with ankylosing spondylitis also develop pulmonary interstitial fibrosis. Other extra-articular manifestations include iridocyclitis, aortic insufficiency, and cardiac conduction abnormalities. The diagnosis is confirmed by the classic roentgenographic features, which include a "bamboo spine."

Treatment involves the use of exercise, physical therapy, and suppression of pain and inflammation. Indomethacin and phenylbutazone are the most effective anti-inflammatory agents, but an initial trial of salicylates is recommended.

BIBLIOGRAPHY

Bergofsky, E.H.: Respiratory failure in disorders of the thoracic cage, Am. Rev. Respir. Dis. **119**:643, 1979.

Caillet, R.: Scoliosis diagnosis and management, Philadelphia, 1975. F.A. Davis Co.

Dines, D.E., and others: Mediastinal granuloma and fibrosing mediastinitis, Chest **75**:320, 1979.

Gacad, G., and Hamosh, P.: The lung in ankylosing spondylitis, Am. Rev. Respir. Dis. **107**:286, 1973.

Gale, A., and others: Neurogenic tumors of the mediastinum, Ann. Thorac. Surg. **17**:434, 1974.

Gibson, G.J., and others: Pulmonary mechanics in patients with respiratory muscle weakness, Am. Rev. Respir. Dis. **115**:389, 1977.

McCredie, M., Lovejoy, F.W., and Kaltreider, N.L.: Pulmonary function in diaphragmatic paralysis, Thorax **17**:213, 1962.

Proceedings of the International Symposium on the Diaphragm, Am. Rev. Respir. Dis. **119**:1, 1979.

Salyer, D., Salyer, W., and Eggleston, J.: Benign developmental cysts of the mediastinum, Arch. Pathol. Lab. Med. **101**:136, 1977.

136 • PRIMARY MALIGNANCIES OF THE LUNG

William Weiss

Pulmonary tumors may be benign or malignant. They have been classified by the World Health Organization into 13 types, with the distribution varying somewhat with geographic location and population subgroup. Almost 50% of the cases occurrinv in the general U.S. male population are squamous cell carcinomas, 15% to 20% are small cell carcinomas, 15% to 20% are adenocarcinomas, 10% are large cell carcinomas, and the remainder includes mixtures of squamous cell carcinoma and adenocarcinoma, carcinoids, bronchial gland tumors, and a few rarer types. In females squamous cell and small cell carcinomas are less common, and adenocarcinomas account for a larger proportion of the cases.

ETIOLOGY AND EPIDEMIOLOGY. Lung cancer is a disease of increasing importance, not only because of its frequency but also because current knowledge about its chain of causation makes prevention a possibility. Primary lung cancer has increased strikingly in incidence during this century, from a rare disease to the most common cause of cancer mortality in men and the second most common cause in women. More than 100,000 deaths result from lung cancer each year in the United States. It is almost entirely a disease of people 45 years of age and over, with an age-specific peak in the seventh decade of life. The drop in incidence after the seventh decade is primarily because of a cohort effect, that is, the oldest people today were born into cohorts whose lifelong risks of lung cancer were lower than those of later birth cohorts, probably as a result of lower exposure to carcinogens. Individual birth cohorts show a steadily increasing risk with increasing age. In recent years the risks have become higher in blacks than in whites. The reason for this is unclear. There has also recently been some slowing in the increase of the rates among men but an exponential increase in the rates among women. As a result, the male-to-female ratio has been falling from about 7:1 two decades ago to about 3:1 at present.

The explanation for these age, sex, and temporal characteristics lies in a strong association between the incidence of lung cancer and the prevalence of cigarette smoking in a given population, allowing for a lag of 20 to 40 years. The judgment that this association is one of cause and effect is based on a great deal of corroborated evidence that includes the following: (1) the incidence is negligible in people who have never smoked; (2) there is a strong dose-response relationship between the number of cigarettes smoked daily and the incidence of the disease; (3) this relationship holds for all histologic types of lung cancer, although it is not as strong for adenocarcinoma as for the other major types; (4) the association is consistent with what is known about lung cancer, such as its predilection for men, who in the past have been smokers more commonly than have women; (5) the incidence decreases among people who stop smoking until at 10 to 15 years after cessation it reaches a level almost as low as the incidence in nonsmokers; and (6) lung cancer has been produced in animals exposed to cigarette smoke.

The relationship of lung cancer to cigar and pipe smoke is much weaker, probably because most smokers of these forms of tobacco inhale relatively little smoke. At present smoking can account for 95% to 99% of lung cancer in men and 60% in women. Since women contribute only about 16% of the cases, it can be calculated that smoking can account for more than 90% of all cases. Therefore smoking must be taken into account when evaluating other causes of this disease.

A small proportion of lung cancer cases is caused by occupational exposure such as to asbestos, ionizing irradiation, coke oven fumes, arsenic, nickel, chromates, chloromethyl ethers, and mustard gas. When it has been studied, the interaction of these agents with cigarette smoke varies. It is one of synergism in asbestos workers and uranium miners but one of antagonism in chloromethyl ether and arsenic workers.

It is not clear whether ambient air pollution plays any significant role in causing lung cancer. The association is weak, inconsistent, and possibly spurious when positive because people in lower socioeconomic levels tend to live in more polluted areas and also are more commonly smokers than those in higher socioeconomic levels.

Lung cancer does not develop in everyone exposed to a pulmonary carcinogen. The lifetime risk of a heavy cigarette smoker is probably about 15%. Host factors must also be important in determining susceptibility, but much of the explanation for lung cancer not developing in most smokers lies with the induction-latent period, which may range from 30 to 60 years; thus competing causes of death remove many people from risk before the malignant process reaches clinical proportions.

The histologic type is important when considering etiologic factors. Recent data show that small cell carcinomas are commonly found in uranium miners and chloromethyl ether workers.

PATHOGENESIS. The evolution of changes in the bronchial epithelium in relation to the most common carcinogenic exposure, cigarette smoke, has been carefully studied. There is a loss of epithelial cilia, an increase in the number of cell rows, and the development of squamous metaplasia and cellular atypia. These abnormalities show a dose-response relationship to cigarette consumption and are less common in pipe and cigar smokers, presumably because they inhale less smoke. Eventually foci of carcinoma in situ develop in multiple areas, and sooner or later one or more of these become invasive. This observation accounts for the 10% of patients who have multiple cancers. People who stop smoking show regression of the epithelial abnormalities.

Lung cancer is predominantly a tumor of the medium-sized and small bronchi; thus it most often originates as a peripheral lesion. Tumors occur most commonly in the upper lobes. The lobar distribution is consistent with the pattern of particulate deposition in hollow casts of the human bronchial tree. Cancers that develop in the larger bronchi tend to produce enlargement of the hilar structures and bronchial obstruction. If the obstruction is partial, it may cause localized obstructive emphysema through a check-valve mechanism, but more commonly it progresses to produce atelectasis, distal pneumonitis, or suppuration. Occasionally the tumor itself cavitates and may be mistaken for an abscess. Sometimes there is direct invasion of surrounding organs. Characteristically lung cancer metastasizes early to regional nodes, mediastinal nodes, the liver, bone, adrenal glands, and the brain and less often to many other organs.

CLINICAL MANIFESTATIONS. The symptoms and signs of lung cancer are related to the primary tumor, extension to neighboring structures, metastases, and systemic effects. Some patients are asymptomatic at the time of tumor detection, usually by routine chest roentgenograms, but a majority have clinical manifestations.

Symptoms related to the primary lesion most commonly include dyspnea and a chronic cough productive of small amounts of nonpurulent sputum. However, since most patients with this disease are cigarette smokers, chronic bronchitis and emphysema are common and often account for the cough and dyspnea. Less common symptoms include hemoptysis, usually limited to blood-streaked sputum, and rarely unilateral wheezing caused by partial obstruction of a major bronchus by the neoplasm. Distal infection may produce manifestations of pneumonia or suppuration, including chills, fever, and purulent sputum. Obstruction can also lead to signs of atelectasis of a lobe or an entire lung. When ths tumor extends beyond the lung, many other symptoms and signs may develop. Pleural extension causes pleuritic pain and pleural effusion. Chest wall involvement often produces chest pain of a dull, boring, and persistent nature. Extension to the esophagus may cause dysphagia. Involvement of the recurrent laryngeal nerve paralyzes a vocal cord with resultant hoarseness. Superior vena caval obstruction is followed by edema of the face, neck, and upper extremities and dilated veins in these areas, sometimes with headache, dizziness, and vertigo *(superior vena caval syndrome)*. Invasion of the brachial plexus by a neoplasm at the apex of the lung causes pain along the nerve distribution, muscle weakness, sensory disturbances of the upper extremity, and other abnormalities caused by neural involvement such as *Pancoast's syndrome* (Fig. 136-1).

Distant metastases may produce visible or palpable superficial tumors, bone pain, headache, and paralyses or other neurologic manifestations. Lymph node enlargement, especially in the neck, is common. Hepatic involvement may cause epigastric distress and jaundice.

Systemic effects include anorexia, weight loss, fatigue, and weakness. In a small percentage of patients, endocrine

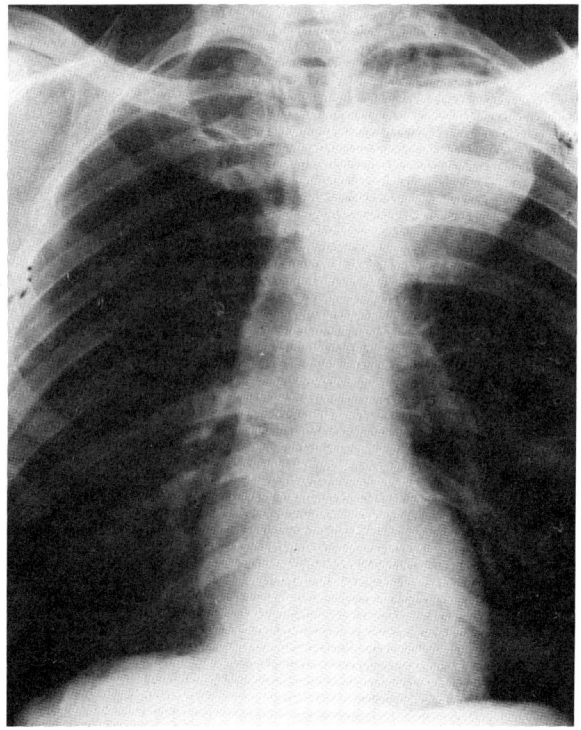

Fig. 136-1. Bronchogenic carcinoma at apex of left lung and invading brachial plexus (Pancoast's tumor). (Courtesy of George Popky, M.D.)

syndromes develop because of the secretion of hormone-like substances by the tumor; these syndromes include the syndrome of inappropriate antidiuretic hormone secretion (SIADH), Cushing's syndrome, gynecomastia, and hypercalcemia (see Chapter 192). Hypertrophic pulmonary osteoarthropathy, usually of the long bones, may cause pain, limitation of motion, and tenderness and is often associated with clubbing of the digits. Clubbing also often occurs alone. These manifestations tend to disappear after successful complete resection of the tumor.

Some neurologic and neuromuscular syndromes not caused by metastases may occur, such as cerebellar degeneration, neuropathy, and myopathy. These usually do not regress after resection of the tumor. Thrombophlebitis is fairly common, and nonbacterial thrombotic endocarditis with embolic phenomena may develop.

LABORATORY FINDINGS. Useful laboratory studies in lung cancer are limited mainly to the chest roentgenogram and cytologic examination of the sputum. Other laboratory studies depend on the clinical evidence of disease beyond the lung or of systemic syndromes. A chest film should be obtained when pulmonary disease is suspected. Its use as a periodic screening device has been disappointing in improving the cure rate because metastases have usually occurred by the time a tumor is large enough to be seen on the chest film. Most lung cancers can be seen on a posteroanterior film, but other views and tupes of examination may be useful. Early in the course of the disease the majority of cancers are manifested as peripheral lesions; of these approximately one half are round nodules or masses and the other half are ill-defined nonhomogeneous infiltrates that are sometimes mistaken for inflammatory disease (Fig. 136-2). Most of the remaining cancers, especially small cell carcinomas, arise in the central bronchi and are manifested as enlarged hilar shadows or mediastinal widening. Occasionally a pleural effusion or localized obstructive emphysema may be the first sign. Rarely, but particularly when the tumor is entirely endobronchial, the chest film may be normal.

With time atelectasis and pleural effusion become more commonly noted on the roentgenogram. These are most frequently found when the diagnosis is made after serious symptoms have led the patient to seek medical care. Lung cancers sometimes develop gross necrosis and excavate, producing cavities whose walls are characteristically irregular and nodular; these are usually best demonstrated by tomographic techniques.

Cytologic examinations of sputum are simple to perform, but good, deep cough specimens are essential in these studies and at least three should be examined. The inhalation of hypertonic saline vapor may be used to induce sputum. Cytologic studies of sputum occasionally show the presence of tumor cells even though the chest film is normal. The diagnosis can often be confirmed by this method, but frequently it is not possible to determine the histologic type of cancer. A tissue specimen is preferred for this purpose.

DIAGNOSIS. The steps in making a diagnosis of lung cancer, in order of increasing complexity, cost, and hazard, are as follows: history, physical examination, chest roentgenogram, cytologic examination of sputum, bronchoscopy with cytologic examination of secretions and brushings, biopsy of easily accessible lesions, mediastinoscopy, and thoracotomy. A diagnosis can be only presumptive until cytologic or histologic evidence is obtained. Such evidence is highly desirable because, although surgery is the treatment of choice for other types, it is essentially worthless for small cell carcinoma.

Bronchoscopy is a minor, essentially risk-free procedure and, since the advent of the fiberoptic instrument a decade ago, offers little discomfort. Its efficacy in confirming the diagnosis is high as a result of cytologic examination of bronchial secretions and brush specimens and transbronchial biopsy. With these techniques it is possible to establish the presence of lung cancer in 80% to 90% of cases. In addition, bronchoscopy can help to determine the extent of the disease within the lung.

Biopsy of these lesions may be accomplished in other ways. In cases of peripheral lesions in the lung that cannot be reached with the bronchoscope, a needle biopsy under fluoroscopic control sometimes can provide a diagnostic specimen. If the cancer is large and adjacent to the chest wall, this technique offers no particular difficulty, but if it is small and deep in the lung, the procedure should be

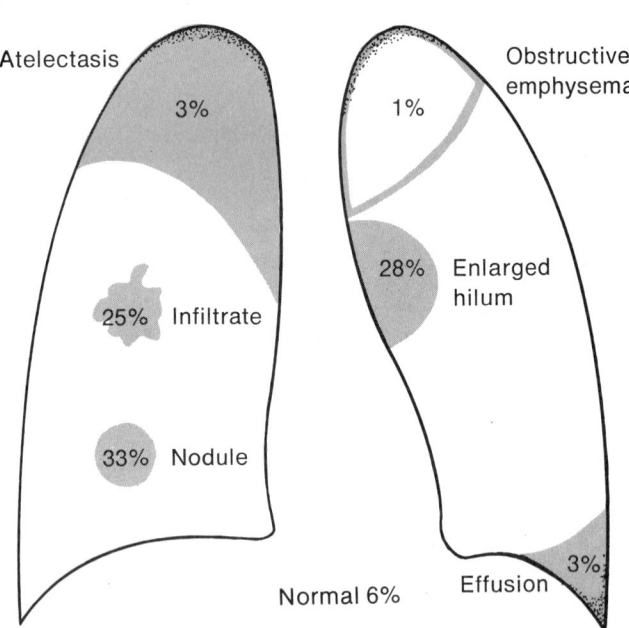

Fig. 136-2. Early roentgenographic appearance of lung cancer found as result of semiannual chest x-ray screening of older men in Philadelphia Pulmonary Neoplasm Research Project (From Weiss, W.: J. Respir. Dis. 1[3]:41, 1980.)

performed by an experienced physician with the recognition that pneumothorax and hemoptysis may result. Some metastases are readily sampled by biopsy, and thus the diagnosis may be easily made.

In a small percentage of cases an important step in establishing a diagnosis is mediastinoscopy. This is a minor procedure taking only ½ hour. It can be performed with the patient under local anesthesia; the associated morbidity is about 1.5%, and the mortality is negligible. The procedure consists of making a small incision in the suprasternal notch, entering the superior mediastinum anterior to the trachea, and employing blunt dissection and an instrument similar to a laryngoscope. A biopsy of a lymph node may be made through the mediastinoscope. Mediastinoscopy can also be used in the staging of lung cancer.

Thoracotomy, the ultimate step in the diagnostic evaluation, is seldom necessary today. It should not be undertaken lightly because the type of patient (aged and often with cardiac problems or chronic obstructive lung disease) who has lung cancer has a significant operative mortality of 2% to 10%, depending on how carefully patients are selected for surgery.

COURSE. Much of the natural history of lung cancer has been learned piecemeal and some from prospective periodic screening studies. Although many pieces of the puzzle are still missing, a fairly clear picture is emerging, as diagrammed in Fig. 136-3.

The growth rate of cancer cells is probably close to exponential, since one cell divides to form two, two make four, and so on. This growth rate can be seen as a straight line by plotting the number of volume doublings on an arithmetic scale along the horizontal axis and the tumor size or diameter (which in a sphere bears a constant relationship to the volume or number of cells) on a logarithmic scale along the vertical axis. To simplify calculations, this model assumes that the average diameter of a cancer cell is 0.001 cm (10 μm); changing the cellular diameter would make little difference in the details.

A tumor diameter of 1 cm is at the threshold of detectability by chest film, and some tumors are missed even at diameters of 2 or 3 cm. About 30 doublings are required for the tumor to reach a diameter of 1 cm, and symptoms rarely appear before this point. However, by 40 doublings the tumor reaches a diameter of 10 cm, at which point only a few patients survive. Metastases probably begin very early, arbitrarily designated in Fig. 136-3 at the tenth doubling. They are discernible in 85% of patients by the fortieth doubling. This model suggests that the diagnosis of lung cancer is usually made in the last quarter of a tumor's life cycle. Early diagnosis, allowing time for cure by resection, is possible only in the few patients whose cancers spread very late or not at all. This happens sometimes in squamous cell carcinoma but seldom in small cell carcinoma or adenocarcinoma. It is difficult to relate the number of volume doublings to units of time because doubling time varies in individual tumors by an order of magnitude.

MANAGEMENT. The treatment of choice for lung cancer is resection whenever feasible, except in patients with small cell carcinoma, which has almost always metastasized by the time of diagnosis and thus is rarely amenable

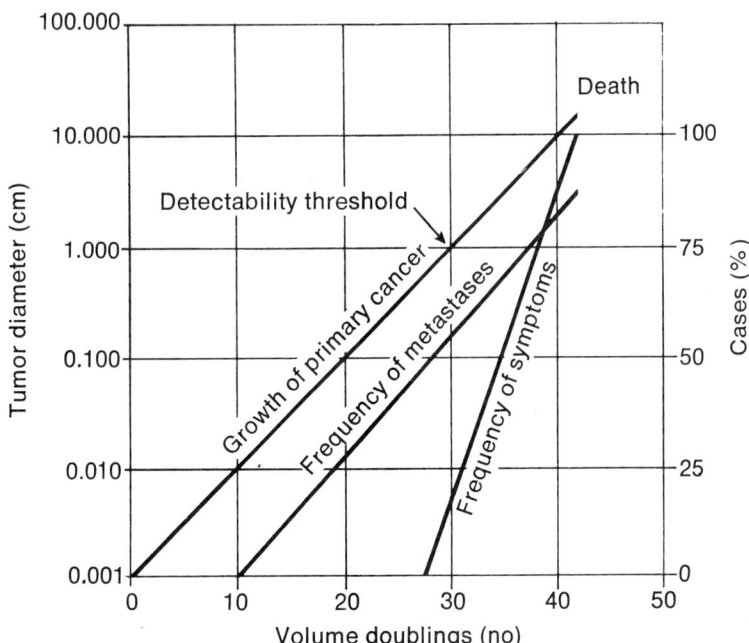

Fig. 136-3. Diagram of hypothetical natural history of lung cancer (see text for explanation). (From Weiss, W.: J. Respir. Dis. **1**:41, 1980.)

to removal. The decision for resection depends on the stage of the disease and the patient's ability to tolerate major chest surgery.

A lung cancer may be staged after clinical evaluation, which includes all the steps taken to arrive at a diagnosis except thoracotomy. An elaborate classification of the extent of disease has been devised, but the final criteria for the decision against surgical treatment include: (1) the presence of distant metastases, (2) evidence of spread beyond the confines of the lung, or (3) a distance of less than 2 cm from the neoplasm to the carina of the trachea. If there is no evidence of such involvement by history, physical examination, chest film, or bronchoscopy, the logical next step is mediastinoscopy. In preoperative evaluation the results of this simple procedure distinguish the resectable from the unresectable cases with considerable accuracy. Even small peripheral cancers may involve mediastinal nodes in up to 30% of the cases. Such an extension is considered a contraindication to surgery by most physicians. The low morbidity and negligible mortality of mediastinoscopy make it an excellent method for avoiding the hazards of thoracotomy.

There is some question as to how far the search for distant metastases should go if the clinical evaluation up to and including mediastinoscopy shows no evidence of spread. Liver and brain scans are warranted only if chemical tests of liver function show abnormalities or there are abnormal neurologic manifestations. In the absence of such abnormalities, scans seldom add information and are sometimes falsely positive. Roentgenographic bone surveys and scans in asymptomatic patients are similarly unjustified. Gallium nitrate Ga 67 scans are currently under investigation.

Since lung cancer is a disease of middle to old age, the patients often have other health problems, some of which make chest surgery unfeasible. Most common among these problems are cardiac disease and chronic obstructive pulmonary disease. A patient with severe coronary disease or any other condition that suggests survival of less than 1 year is not generally considered a candidate for resectional surgery.

Because lung cancer patients are usually smokers, chronic bronchitis and emphysema are common complications that require an evaluation of pulmonary function. In some cases the clinical assessment suffices to determine the very good and the very bad risk cases. For cases between these extremes, pulmonary function tests should be performed. Unfortunately, there are no hard and fast rules or reliable critical values that allow more than a reasonable estimation of who is at low risk for surgery. It is also unfortunate that surgery may make the patient a respiratory cripple even though it cures his cancer. The judgment of operability is further complicated by the question of how much of the patient's dysfunction is caused by the cancer and how much is the result of other pulmonary diseases.

Given 100 patients, with a conservative approach to surgery, a clinical evaluation including bronchoscopy is likely to eliminate 75 cases as surgical candidates; mediastinoscopy may remove another 10, so that only 15 are candidates for thoracotomy. Of these, only 13 are likely to have a completely resectable lesion. If the approach is more radical, a larger proportion of patients will undergo surgery, but the result will be essentially the same, with only a 5% to 10% 5-year survival rate.

Rarely does any other form of treatment have a significant curative impact. Radiotherapy often shrinks the primary tumor and may even kill all the malignant cells in it, but the distant metastases are unaffected. It may, however, provide palliation for superior vena caval syndrome, brain metastases, and bone pain. Early results of trials with multiple drug regimens in patients with small cell carcinoma suggest some prolongation of life. Since this type of cancer is almost never detected before metastases occur, radiotherapy and chemotherapy are the treatments of choice. These therapies may also be of some value in patients unsuitable for surgery for other reasons.

PREVENTION. Because of the overall poor results in the management of lung cancer, prevention deserves more attention. Campaigns against cigarette smoking and exposure to carcinogens in the workplace are important. It is likely that the elimination of tobacco and industrial carcinogens would result in the almost complete disappearance of this dread disease and return its incidence to the rarity it had early in this century—a far cry from the approximately 100,000 deaths it now causes annually in the United States.

BIBLIOGRAPHY

Archer, V.E., Gillam, J.D., and Wagoner, J.K.: Respiratory disease mortality among uranium miners, Ann. N.Y. Acad. Sci. **271**:280, 1976.

Ashbaugh, D.G.: Mediastinoscopy, Arch. Surg. **100**:568, 1970.

Auerbach, O., and others: Changes in bronchial epithelium in relation to sex, age, residence, smoking, and pneumonia, N. Engl. J. Med. **267**:111, 1962.

Benfield, J.R., and others: Current and future concepts of lung cancer (UCLA Conference), Ann. Intern. Med. **83**:93, 1975.

Doll, R., and Peto, R.: Mortality in relation to smoking: 20 years' observations on male British doctors, Br. Med. J. **2**:1525, 1976.

Fox, W., and Scadding, J.G.: Medical Research Council comparative trial of surgery and radiotherapy for primary treatment of small-celled or oat-celled carcinoma of bronchus, Lancet **2**:63, 1973.

Geddes, D.M.: The natural history of lung cancer: a review based on rates of tumor growth. Br. J. Dis. Chest **73**:1, 1979.

Hammond, E.C., Selikoff, I.J., and Seidman, H.: Asbestos exposure, cigarette smoking, and death rates, Ann. N.Y. Acad. Sci. **330**:473, 1979.

Tisi, G.M.: Preoperative evaluation of pulmonary function, Am. Rev. Respir. Dis. **119**:293, 1979.

Weiss, W.: Lung cancer due to chemicals, Comp. Ther. **5**:18, 1979.

Weiss, W.: The Philadelphia Pulmonary Neoplasm Research Project, Appl. Radiol. **8**:50, 138, 1979.

Weiss, W.: Lung cancer: diagnosis and preoperative evaluation, J. Respir. Dis. **1**:41, 1980.

Weiss, W., and others: Risk of lung cancer according to histologic type and cigarette dosage, J.A.M.A. **222**:799, 1972.

137 • TUMORS OF THE LUNG OTHER THAN BRONCHOGENIC CARCINOMA

William L. Morrissey

Although primary malignant lung tumors comprise the most common and most serious form of pulmonary tumors, other lung tumors are not uncommon. Included in the latter category are bronchial adenomas, lymphomas, fibromas, chondromas, papillomas, lipomas, hamartomas, and metastatic tumors. Benign neoplasms comprise less than 10% of primary pulmonary neoplasms.

BRONCHIAL ADENOMA

Bronchial adenoma accounts for somewhat less than 5% of all tumors of the lung but may represent 50% of benign lesions. Recently there has been a tendency to classify it as malignant because of its aggressive local invasion and rare distant metastases. Bronchial adenoma originates from cells in the bronchial wall, usually in proximal airways. It generally is only locally invasive and histologically is either of the carcinoid or cylindromatous (cystadenoma) type; 90% are carcinoid. Bronchial adenoma is associated with hemoptysis or the sequelae of obstruction such as pneumonia in patients over 30 years of age. Rarely the carcinoid form may produce the carcinoid syndrome with wheezing, episodic flushing, cyanosis, diarrhea, right-sided valvular heart disease, increased serum levels of 5-hydroxytryptamine (serotonin), and increased urine levels of 5-hydroxyindoleacetic acid (5-HIAA). This syndrome may also occur with carcinoid tumors of the intestinal tract, invariably after hepatic metastasis, and with oat cell or undifferentiated bronchogenic carcinoma.

The carcinoid syndrome is treated symptomatically if local resection for the adenoma is not curative. Although endoscopic removal has been attempted in the past, this has proved unsatisfactory and should be reserved for patients unable to tolerate thoracotomy. The prognosis for long-term survival is good, although extensive local spread or (rarely) distant metastasis may be fatal.

LYMPHOMA AND LYMPHOPROLIFERATIVE DISORDERS

Primary pulmonary lymphoma without extrathoracic or mediastinal involvement is rare, but lymphomatous involvement of the lung, including both parenchymal and pleural manifestations, may occur in up to 40% of patients with disseminated lymphoma. Hilar adenopathy, nodular or infiltrative parenchymal lesions, and, less commonly, pleural effusions may all occur. The symptoms include dyspnea, pain, cough, localized wheezing, hemoptysis, and systemic manifestations.

Other lymphoproliferative disorders affecting the lungs include lymphocytic interstitial pneumonia, Sjögren's syndrome, pseudolymphoma, Waldenström's macroglobulinemia, leukemia, amyloidosis, and multiple myeloma.

BENIGN TUMORS

Benign endobronchial tumors include fibroma, chondroma, papilloma, and lipoma, with the first two accounting for 80% of these lesions. They are usually manifested by obstructive related symptoms, may be confused with bronchial adenoma, and require local or endoscopic removal.

Hamartomas are benign but disorganized collections of normal tissue. In the lung they usually contain primarily muscle, collagen, or cartilage. Most are discovered in asymptomatic individuals in whom the chest roentgenogram was obtained for other reasons. The lesion usually is round, less than 5 cm in diameter, and may be flecked with calcium (popcorn calcification) (Fig. 137-1). Resection may be necessary to confirm the diagnosis and to rule out malignancy.

METASTATIC TUMORS

Metastatic tumors may involve the lung in several ways. Multiple nodular densities, particularly from kidney, breast, thyroid, or testicular primary sites, may be seen on the chest roentgenogram. Diffuse spread of tumor cells throughout pulmonary lymphatics (lymphangitic carcinomatosis) results in rapidly progressive lung disease termi-

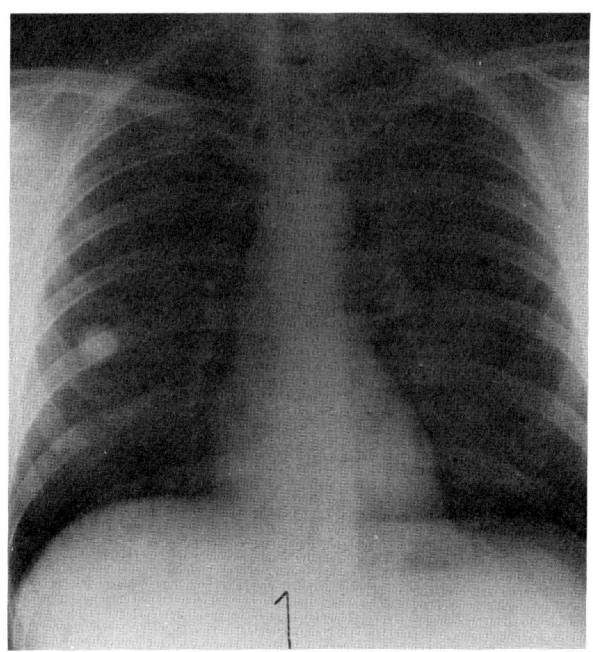

Fig. 137-1. Hamartoma manifested as solitary pulmonary nodule containing calcium. (Courtesy of George Popky, M.D.)

nating in respiratory failure; the most common primary sites for this type of tumor spread include the stomach, colon, bronchus, larynx, breast, prostate, and pancreas. Progressively severe dyspnea is common, but pleuritic chest pain, cyanosis, tachypnea, shallow respirations, and signs and symptoms of cor pulmonale may develop. The chest film usually shows bilateral diffuse linear shadows or fine nodular shadows. Less commonly, hilar enlargement or a parenchymal mass lesion may also be seen. The syndrome may be difficult to distinguish from other causes of diffuse lung disease without resorting to lung biopsy. In patients receiving chemotherapy or irradiation of the thorax, lymphangitic tumor spread may have to be differentiated from radiation-induced or drug-induced changes as well as from opportunistic infections, such as those caused by *Pneumocystis carinii*. The therapy available is generally unsatisfactory, although steroids may provide some symptomatic relief.

SOLITARY PULMONARY NODULE

The solitary pulmonary nodule discovered on routine roentgenographic examination of the chest in the asymptomatic individual may have one of many origins. Because of this, it represents a difficult diagnostic and therapeutic problem.

Referred to as a coin lesion, this nodule appears as a rounded abnormal shadow on the chest film. It is well circumscribed, round or oval, surrounded by normal lung, smooth bordered, homogeneous, noncavitated, and with no associated satellite lesions. Overall it appears that about 5% are malignant, although some surgical series report up to a 50% rate of malignancy. The risk of malignancy is increased in males, smokers, and those over 40 years of age. The differential diagnosis includes granulomata (the most common benign cause), hamartomas, and other benign lung tumors. Pulmonary infarcts and interlobar effusions (vanishing tumor) are other possibilities. Additional causes include primary lung malignancies and metastatic lesions. If metastatic, the primary site is most often the kidney, colon, or nasopharyngeal area.

Although age, smoking history, previous granulomatous infections, and positive skin and serologic tests for fungi or tuberculosis may be helpful, they rarely allow a definitive diagnosis. The availability of previous chest films may diminish the need for further evaluation, since the doubling time for carcinomatous lesions varies from about 6 weeks to 18 months. More rapid growth suggests an inflammatory process, whereas roentgenographic stability longer than 2 years makes malignancy unlikely. The presence of laminated or stippled calcification also suggests a benign lesion. The introduction of computed tomography has recently been reported to increase the ability to detect calcium.

Bronchoscopy or percutaneous transthoracic needle biopsy can sometimes establish the diagnosis, but generally thoracotomy is required. Extensive workup for a primary tumor elsewhere before thoracotomy is unwarranted unless there are specific symptoms or laboratory abnormalities referable to another organ system. Mediastinoscopy is rarely helpful in the diagnosis.

Resection has therapeutic as well as diagnostic value. Surgical removal of a primary lung tumor occurring as a solitary nodule may result in a 50% 5-year survival rate. Resection of a solitary metastasis from a known primary tumor may be indicated if the primary tumor has been completely eradicated and there are no other known metastases; the best results have been obtained in cases of sarcoma and colonic cancer.

BIBLIOGRAPHY

Filly, R., Blank, N., and Castellins, R.A.: Radiologic distribution of intrathoracic disease in previously untreated patients with Hodgkin's disease and non-Hodgkin's lymphoma, Radiology **120**:277, 1976.

Goodwin, J.D.: Carcinoid tumors: an analysis of 2837 cases, Cancer **36**:560, 1975.

Heitzman, E.R., Markarian, B., and DeLise, C.T.: Lymphoproliferative disorders of the thorax, Semin. Roentgenol. **10**:73, 1975

Lillington, G.A.: The solitary pulmonary nodule—1974, Am. Rev. Respir. Dis. **110**:699, 1974.

Okike, N., Bernatz, P.E., and Woolner, L.B.: Carcinoid tumors of the lung, Ann. Thorac. Surg. **22**:270, 1976.

Yang, S., and Lin, C.: Lymphangitic carcinomatosis of the lungs, Chest **62**:179, 1972.

DENTAL CORRELATIONS

B. Kyle DeMartino and Stuart L. Fischman

Respiratory disease is frequently an insidious complication revealed in a patient's medical history. Because of the subtle aspects of serious respiratory compromise and its ubiquitous presence in our society, there is a tendency to ignore the danger signs of respiratory disease states, especially if the patient is capable of getting to the dental office without assistance. Therefore, this is a potential danger area for the dentist conducting a traditional outpatient dental practice. The anecdotal comment often heard years ago, when guidelines for treating medically compromised patients were initially introduced to the profession, was that if the patient could climb one or two flights of stairs to reach the dental office he was probably in good enough health to undergo dental treatment. That attitude was deplorable in the past and inexcusable in the present. Each dentist must be prepared *not* to perform dental treatment if that is what is dictated by a patient's physical condition.

There are numerous entities associated with respiratory disease, each with its own diagnosis, primary, secondary, and tertiary areas of affliction, symptoms, and functional impact. Developing a rational treatment methodology when faced with this myriad of potential complications would appear to be difficult. Even more confusing is making the decision as to whether the patient's respiratory status requires special considerations at all—and if it does, is the existing disease state of such magnitude that treatment should be denied?

There are three major factors that must be considered when approaching the decision of whether the patient with respiratory disease is well enough to be managed as an ambulatory patient.

1. Patient status. *Is the patient's ability to exchange oxygen and carbon dioxide so severely impaired that he has experienced or is experiencing difficulty during his normal activities?* The implication is that if the patient is unstable without the added insult of dental treatment, the prudent dentist will devote the time and effort to avoid treating the patient until ability to safely withstand the therapy has been established. This determination should involve discussions with the physician responsible for the patient's medical condition.

2. Planned procedure. *Is the dental treatment contemplated likely to contribute to ths patient's difficulties?* If it is thought that the treatment could compound the respiratory problem, then the risk-benefit ratio must be very carefully analyzed. In the case of inhalation or intravenous sedatives and anesthesias (whether "conscious" or unconscious), a patient with moderate to severe respiratory disease may be at extreme risk. Should the dentist fail to fully appreciate the effects that sedative agents have on the respiratory system, however benign those effects are thought to be, serious morbidity or mortality may ensue.

3. Style of delivery of dental care. *Will the mechanical aspects of the dental delivery method contribute to the patient's difficulties?* The presently popular supine operating position could seriously jeopardize the safety of a patient with a full stomach should he receive sedative or analgesic agents. Subsequently, the patient may regurgitate and aspirate the low pH gastric contents. Without any other contributing factors, placing an obese individual in the supine position can compromise the individual's mechanical ability to ventilate. Adding a prolonged dental procedure such as periodontal surgery or prosthetic reconstruction using intravenous sedation may set the stage for a life-threatening emergency.

Many of the respiratory diseases previously discussed may be so serious that the entire question of dental care is moot and patients suffering from them are already hospitalized. By contrast, the ambulatory patient with moderate to severe disease can appear to be in sufficiently good health to encourage ill-advised dental treatment that results in exacerbating the patient's disease or precipitating a crisis of major proportions. It seems apparent that a format for evaluating respiratory status and overall candidacy for dental treatment would be of prime importance. Relating the degree of pathology present and its functional impact to the planned procedure would provide the dentist with a guide to how dental therapy could be accomplished with minimum danger to the patient.

Chronic bronchitis

PROMINENT SYMPTOMS. Chronic productive cough, often referred to by the patient as "smoker's cough," has often been present for many years. The patient usually has a history of repeated colds or upper respiratory tract infections characterized by cough with mucopurulent sputum production and lasting for a protracted period of time. He may demonstrate shortness of breath on exertion. Wheezes, rhonchi, and diminished expiratory flow rates are common, and post-tussive wheezing may be provoked by forced expiratory effort.

PHYSIOLOGIC FEATURES. There is a reduction in expiratory flow rates as a consequence of airway obstruction by mucus and/or bronchospasm resulting as a response to chronic irritant exposure. Characteristically, there may be hypertrophy of mucous glands; there may also be decreased ciliary activity, increased mucous viscosity and volume, mucous plugging of smaller airways, inflammatory infiltrates, and colonization of the airways by bacteria. Hypoxemia and hypercapnia may also be present.

Orthopnea (the feeling that one is short of breath when supine) may be caused by ventilation-perfusion mismatching as the hemodynamics of the lung change in the reclining position.

RISK FACTORS. Whenever a patient's respiratory system is compromised to the extent that he experiences shortness of breath, a chronic productive mucopurulent cough, or wheezing, dental treatment may trigger complications that could culminate in a serious disease encounter. For example, a patient such as the one described would be an extremely poor risk for general anesthetic requiring the administration of anticholinergic drugs such as atropine or scopolamine, since these agents and their related compounds tend to reduce ciliary activity in the tracheobronchial tree, leading to mucous plugging of the smaller airways, reduction in the efficiency of an already compromised system, and possibly postanesthetic pneumonitis. Additionally, since these patients may suffer from hypercapnia and hypoxia, they are particularly sensitive to circumstances that depress the ventilatory mechanism further. In the traditional system for delivery of dental care the patient is seen, treated, and sent away; thus the postoperative respiratory status in these marginal patients is not monitored and the connection may not be made between the dental treatment experience and subsequent respiratory difficulties.

DENTAL MANAGEMENT. The dentist must refrain from using techniques or agents that may affect the respiratory system. These patients are not good candidates for sedation or general anesthetic procedures. Drying agents and respiratory depressants are to be avoided.

If the patient has orthopnea, he should not recline in the chair. It may be necessary to proceed with the patient in a sitting or upright position rather than supine.

Supplemental oxygen may be beneficial.

Pulmonary emphysema

PROMINENT SYMPTOMS. Symptoms are related to the degree of damage; typically, emphysema appears in combination with chronic bronchitis. Persistent dyspnea on exertion is the most significant clinical symptom. There may also be enlarged chest fixed in the hyperinflated position.

PHYSIOLOGIC FEATURES. Because of the alterations in alveolar morphology, increased airway resistance, and degeneration of elastic tissue, these patients suffer from mild oxygen arterial unsaturation that progresses to hypoxemia with carbon dioxide retention and respiratory acidosis. There may be a secondary polycythemia, and the work of the right side of the heart is increased, leading to cor pulmonale.

RISK FACTORS. Patients with chronic obstructive pulmonary disease including emphysema may present for dental treatment at virtually any point in the disease process. The decision to provide dental treatment is made on the basis of the severity of the dental problem when weighed against the possible injury to the patient's respiratory status posed by the planned treatment. As with the patient with chronic bronchitis, the emphysema patient may be a generally poor risk and should be protected from procedures that will further compromise the respiratory status, including sedation techniques involving respiratory depressants, general anesthesia, drying (anticholinergic agents), and use of the supine position.

DENTAL MANAGEMENT. Treatment should be managed in a fashion consistent with the degree of disease.

1. Respiratory depressants should not be used. This includes both narcotics and barbiturates.
2. Atropine, scopolamine, and similar anticholinergics as well as antihistamines should be avoided because of their adverse effects on the viscosity of secretions.
3. "Physiologic shunting" associated with posture may dictate that these patients be managed in an upright position rather than supine or semirecumbent.
4. Because acute respiratory failure may occur without an obvious trigger event, it is essential that the dentist be prepared to administer oxygen and support ventilation.

Modifications to treatment deemed prudent by the presence of existing disease are entirely up to the individual dental practitioner; however, there are philosophic guidelines that help in designing safe and effective treatment.

Patients with chronic respiratory and cardiovascular disease are seen in increasing numbers for dental treatment. Any patient who is under medical care for any condition should be thoroughly examined and should give a detailed history of the disease before a specific dental procedure is undertaken.

No dental procedure is so sacred that it takes precedence over a patient's life. Treatment and technique must always bow to the demands of a patient's overall medical condition. Most particularly in the case of respiratory problems that may not appear particularly serious, the dentist has a responsibility to become acquainted with the details of the patient's disease and make an effort to alter dental treatment to reduce risk to a minimum.

Bronchiectasis

Bronchiectasis represents a morphologic change that may be unaccompanied by symptoms. When symptoms do occur they resemble those associated with recurrent bronchopulmonary infections.

PROMINENT SYMPTOMS. Symptoms include productive cough, chronic fatigue, and hemoptysis.

PHYSIOLOGIC FEATURES. Decreased vital capacity with decreased expiratory flow rates and an increased venous admixture may be found.

RISK FACTORS. The risk factors for bronchiectasis are essentially the same as for chronic bronchitis.

Lung abscess

PROMINENT SYMPTOMS. Symptoms of lung abscess include fever, cough, anorexia, and malaise of varying duration.

PHYSIOLOGIC FEATURES. Necrotic areas of lung parenchyma that communicate with bronchi are found. Bronchiectasis predisposes toward lung abscess, but abscess is most frequently associated with aspiration of the contents of the mouth.

RISK FACTORS. Unless there is a dental emergency, these patients should be sent to a hospital for immediate aggressive treatment of the lung abscess.

DENTAL MANAGEMENT. Lung abscess is one of the few respiratory disease entities that the dentist actually has the opportunity of creating. As stated earlier, the pathogenesis of lung abscess is frequently associated with aspiration of the oral contents. This can occur when a patient in a supine position receiving sedation or general anesthesia regurgitates and aspirates into the tracheobronchial tree. The original study of postpartum aspiration pneumonia by Mendelsohn in 1946 implicated "the full stomach" in combination with nitrous oxide–oxygen analgesia as a cause. Changes in dental operating position (supine rather than upright) may have set the stage for an increase of this disease unless dentists, like their physician counterparts, start insisting that patients remain fasting prior to the use of sedative or analgesic agents.

Cystic fibrosis

Because of the complexity of this disease and its treatment, it would not serve the best interests of either the patient or the dentist to provide a formula for dealing with the dental requirements of those suffering from this problem. The patients are predominantly young and from the respiratory standpoint "fragile." Medical consultation is imperative prior to treatment. Anhydrous gases (such as nitrous oxide and oxygen) tend to dry the lung by lowering the humidity and are relatively contraindicated unless humidified prior to inhalation (a difficult task in the dental office).

In the past most patients suffering from cystic fibrosis died before reaching school age, but now expert medical attention has increased the expected life span to age 21.

According to the Cystic Fibrosis Foundation aggressive therapy and early diagnosis are the keys to survival. The disease itself is one that may masquerade as bronchitis, asthma, whooping cough, pneumonia, or other respiratory problems. Although there is involvement of other systems the principal concern of the dentist should be oriented toward protection of the patient's respiratory system. For example, the use of a rubber dam is highly advisable to prevent aspiration of infectious particles. By contrast the use of sedative agents is not indicated because of the possible contribution of respiratory depression, however slight.

Bullous emphysema and lung cysts

PROMINENT SYMPTOMS. There is an alteration in the parenchymal architecture represented by large emphysematous spaces. They represent an acute danger because of the possibility of rupture with subsequent tension pneumothorax.

RISK FACTORS. Although no treatment may be required if the patient is asymptomatic, there is relative risk if general anesthesia with supported or controlled ventilation is required, because a "blow out" of the bulla is possible when the respiratory system is pressurized during the inspiratory phase of the ventilatory cycle.

DENTAL MANAGEMENT. Circumstances, treatments, or techniques that could require ventilating the patient under pressure must be avoided. Simply stated, this means that general anesthesia is to be avoided.

Asthma

PROMINENT SYMPTOMS. Symptoms include wheezing and shortness of breath.

PHYSIOLOGIC FEATURES. There may be airway narrowing secondary to bronchiolar smooth muscle spasm.

RISK FACTORS. Probably no other respiratory disease has the same potential for catastrophe as asthma in regard to dental care. With the more serious debilitating respiratory disease syndromes, the patient is usually chronically ill between exacerbations of the disease. In asthma, however, the patient enjoys periods of remission between attacks only to be subject to the full fury of an attack once the particular criteria for his "disease trigger" have been met. It is for this reason that an asthmatic individual must be very thoroughly evaluated prior to dental treatment and possibly denied ambulatory care if the asthma history is such that frequent hospitalization has been necessary.

Risk evaluation must be based on the following criteria:

1. Frequency of attacks
2. Severity of attacks (is hospitalization necessary)
3. Precipitating factors
    a. Stress or anxiety
    b. Allergy
    c. Drugs (β-adrenergic blockers)

DENTAL MANAGEMENT. The extent of the treatment and the stress it may provoke must be evaluated, since stress has been implicated as a precipitating factor for asthmatic attacks. Techniques that may have direct bearing on the disease must be modified or eliminated. This includes a prescription against the use of narcotics and barbiturates, which have both been implicated in precipitating asthmatic attacks. Medications and emergency treatment protocol should be readily available and well rehearsed in the event that a patient has an attack in the dental office.

The temptation to evaluate a patient's physical condition solely on the basis of appearance and affect is strong in dentistry, and the dentist should be mindful that respiratory disease states often coexist with the look and demeanor of health.

Diffuse lung disease

PROMINENT FEATURES. Symptoms of this disease include dyspnea, coughing, tachypnea, cyanosis, digital "clubbing," and rales.

DENTAL MANAGEMENT. The patients in this general category may present in varying stages of disease, since this group of maladies is chronic and debilitating. Additionally, the dentist may have to deduce the presence of the disease from the patient's medical history and/or from an examination of the respiratory system.

When disease is suspected or confirmed, medical consultation is demanded to determine the degree of impairment. Whereas the dentist may feel inadequate in *some* areas of physical medicine, physicians *are* inadequate in *all* areas of dentistry and may have to be educated by the dentist in such information as the fact that turbine handpieces generate aerosols of bacteria and debris that may create complications if inhaled by the respiratorily compromised patient.

Environmental diseases

PROMINENT FEATURES. Symptoms include bullous emphysema, pulmonary hypertension/cor pulmonale, chronic cough and sputum production, malignancy, fibrosis, and occupational asthma.

DENTAL CONSIDERATIONS. In mining towns it is quite common to deal with large populations of patients suffering from occupationally linked respiratory disease. The same is true for the asbestos worker. The dentist who practices in an area with such facilities should be prepared to evaluate levels of impairment.

The dentist should guard against:
1. Drying or dehumidification of the respiratory system
2. Respiratory depression secondary to reductions in ventilatory rate, volume, or both
3. Shunting (increases in arteriovenous admixture related to hemodynamic changes in the lung tissue secondary to position in the chair)
4. Drugs or chemicals that might trigger bronchoconstriction (asthma), including β-adrenergic blockers (two that come to mind are propranolol and amyl nitrite)

BIBLIOGRAPHY

Bendixen, H.H., and others, Respiratory care, St. Louis, 1965, The C.V. Mosby Co.

Goodman, L.S., and Gilman, A.: The pharmacological basis of therapeutics, ed. 6, New York, 1980, Macmillan Inc.

Harrison, T.R., and Adams, R.D.: Principles of internal medicine, ed. 9, New York, 1980, McGraw-Hill Book Co.

Selkurt, E.E.: Physiology, Boston, 1978, Little Brown & Co.

Section Ten
ENVIRONMENTAL INJURIES
edited by **Donald Kaye**

138 • CHEMICAL AND ENVIRONMENTAL INJURIES
Geoffrey Lefferts and David T. Lush

RADIATION INJURY

DEFINITION. Common types of ionizing radiation are particulate (α- and β-rays) and electromagnetic (γ-rays and x-rays). α-Rays are composed of two protons and two neutrons; they are positively charged and are converted to helium atoms by the acquisition of two electrons. β-Rays are electrons ejected from the nucleus of an atom undergoing radioactive decay. γ-Rays have great penetrating power and are electromagnetic radiation emitted by the nucleus of a radioactive substance. X-rays are similar waves of even shorter wavelength and greater penetrating power; they are produced by the bombardment of a substance by a stream of electrons at very high velocity, as in a vacuum tube.

Several terms and concepts are required to understand the expressions of amounts of radiation. The roentgen (abbreviated R) is a measure of the amount of radiation passing through air. However, for medical use and for damage to tissue to occur, the radiation must be absorbed by tissue and not just pass through air. The rad is a unit defined as the amount of radiation energy equal to the absorption of 100 ergs of energy per gram of material. The type and thickness of tissue absorbing the rad are important; the greatest absorption is on ths surface, which decreases absorption by the deeper tissues. The length of time during which a certain amount of radiation is absorbed is also important; the greater the time, ths less tissue damage resulting from the exposure. This is of great use in radiation oncology because of tumoricidal dose can be given with less damage to normal tissues.

PATHOPHYSIOLOGY. At the molecular level the penetrating radiation starts a cascade reaction that culminates in cellular death or injury. First, penetrating particles or waves react with nuclei or intracellular atoms to produce ion pairs; these then react with water molecules to produce the toxic products H_2O_2 and HO_2. Finally, these products react with essential intracellular regulators such as deoxyribonucleic acid (DNA) and enzymes, leading to altered function or death of the irradiated cells. At the cellular level the type of damage done depends on the dosage factors mentioned previously. Very low doses may produce chromosomal mutations such as breaks or deletions; somewhat higher doses can cause a transient abnormal chromosomal function such as slowed mitosis. A few hundred rad can cause permanent cessation of mitotic activity without altering the other cell functions. Higher doses directly kill cells by preventing normal metabolic functions.

On the tissue level, rapidly reproducing areas are affected earliest and by the lowest radiation dosages; for instance, bone marrow and skin are affected by much smaller doses than are needed to affect bone, muscle, or the central nervous system, which are very slowly proliferating or nonproliferating tissues.

There is currently considerable debate concerning the amount of radiation needed to produce an effect on cell components, especially on DNA. One school of thought advocates a "threshold effect," with no damage of any kind occurring until a variable and unknown threshold dosage level is reached and with a linear relationship between dosage and damage above this threshold. The other school believes that current evidence suggests there is no safe lower limit and that the linear dose-damage relationship starts at dose0 and increases from there; this group argues that the time from exposure to noticeable effect can be so long for some minor chromosomal aberrations that the ultimate damage is easy to overlook.

CLINICAL MANIFESTATIONS. As can be seen in Table 138-1, the part of the body affected by a particular amount of radiation is hard to predict, especially since the dosage received is not usually known in the individual case. Most exposures are accidental and thus specific details on dose or distribution are unknown; only by observation of the clinical course can a retrospective conclusion be reached. The side effects of radiation are commonly divided into acute and delayed effects. Diffuse or local exposure is another useful way to categorize the syndromes.

Acute diffuse exposure results in three syndromes. One is the cerebral syndrome, a usually fatal result of massive exposure. The course is progressive loss of consciousness followed by irreversible cardiovascular collapse, developing over 1 to 2 days. The second is the hematopoietic syndrome. This has many variations, as noted in Table 138-1, depending on which bone marrow cell line is the most

Table 138-1. Effects of radiation on body systems

Organ or effect	Time to onset	Time to maximal effect	Total time from first dose to recovery	Dose required to cause injury (rad)	Major consequences
Cerebral syndrome	Few hours	1-2 days	Usually fatal	300	Irreversible coma and cardiovascular collapse
Hematologic syndrome					
Granulocyte depletion	1-2 weeks	4 weeks	6-8 weeks	200-400	Bacterial infection
Lymphocyte depletion	Few hours	1-2 days	4-8 weeks	200-400	Nonbacterial infection (virus, tuberculosis)
Platelet depletion	1-2 weeks	4 weeks	6-8 weeks	200-400	Bleeding
Gastrointestinal syndrome	3-4 days	6-7 days	2 weeks	600-2000	Fluid and electrolyte loss from mucosal sloughing
Skin lesions					
First-degree burn	Few hours	2-3 weeks	6-8 weeks	200	—
Second- or third-degree burn	Few days	1-2 weeks	8-12 weeks	1000	May need skin grafts
Hair loss	—	3 weeks	3-4 months	300	Permanent if greater than 700-800 rad
Sterility	—	Few days to few weeks	—	600-700	Permanent infertility
Hypothyroidism	—	Several years	—	Variable	Myxedema
Cataract	—	Several years	—	300-600	Visual loss
Leukemia	—	5-7 years	—	Unknown	Fatal
Solid tumors (thyroid, bone, breast, lung)	—	Many years	—	Unknown	Usually fatal, except thyroid tumors

affected. In terms of rapidly fatal effect, the loss of neutrophils is most threatening, since fatal bacterial infection commonly occurs rapidly once cell counts fall below a few hundred cells per cubic millimeter. The third syndrome, the gastrointestinal syndrome, results when radiation damage prevents the normal rapid turnover of gastrointestinal epithelial cells. This leads to the rapid loss of fluid and electrolytes and severe dehydration. Regeneration can occur if the patient receives supportive therapy through the first few weeks.

Acute local exposure can cause severe damage to the skin and its appendages (hair) even if no internal organs or systems are damaged. Depending on the dosage and duration of exposure, changes may range from mild redness and itching, resembling a sunburn, to very painful, full-thickness necrosis. Hair loss can occur with doses that do not cause much obvious skin damage, and it may or may not be permanent, depending again on dosage and duration of exposure.

Delayed effects are arbitrarily defined as those that take years to become noticeable. Sterility, hypothyroidism, lenticular cataracts, and neoplasia are the most common late effects. Leukemias ars the most publicized cancers, but various solid tumors such as those of the thyroid, bone, lung, and breast are also noteworthy.

MANAGEMENT. For the treatment of the acute cerebral syndrome only supportive measures are available, such as intravenous fluids, respiratory support, and anticonvulsant therapy. For the more common hematologic syndrome the object is to support the patient through the stage of absence of the various cell lines until recovery can occur. If bacterial infection can be prevented or successfully treated until granulopoiesis is reestablished, the patient should recover. For example, selective transfusion of the various blood components is lifesaving; there is no indication for whole blood transfusion, but red blood cells, granulocytes, or platelets are administered as needed. The prevention of infection is also important; avoidance of instrumentation or invasive procedures (if possible), administration of prophylactic antibiotics, and reverse isolation can be used, depending on the individual situation and severity. The gastrointestinal syndrome, as mentioned previously, is best managed by vigorous support with fluids and electrolytes; intravenous hyperalimentation is useful because this syndrome is theoretically reversible.

Local injury to skin and appendages is managed in much the same way as a burn. Mild lesions need no specific treatment, whereas third-degree, full-thickness lesions may require debridement and grafting. Permanent hyperpigmentation may result from even mild lesions. Neither prophylactic nor therapeutic treatment is available for hair loss.

Treatment of the delayed effects is the same as when these conditions arise for any other reason and is beyond the scope of this chapter. These conditions may appear even many years after the exposure; periodic examination for them is important so that they can be diagnosed in the earliest and, ideally, most treatable stage.

Dental radiation dosage
Robert Beiderman

Dental radiation doses are generally well below those delivered by medical colleagues. Nevertheless, low, repeated x-radiation doses delivered to limited body sites over a period of days, weeks, or years should be considered. In 1959 the National Council on Radiation Protection and Measurement (NCRP) established that available evidence was not sufficient to establish the dose-response relationship at low doses and so proposed that the direct proportional relationship be assumed to exist until proved otherwise. In effect this statement requires that all dentists realize that *any* exposure to themselves or their patients may carry some potential somatic and/or genetic effect. On June 29, 1981, before the National Center for Health Care Technology Assessment Forum: Dental Radiology, Dr. Lauriston S. Taylor, Honorary President of the NCRP, commented that;

1. The public tends to believe that it is at much greater risk of harm from radiation than actually exists.
2. The doses of radiation normally used in dental radiology are so low as to pose little, if any, risk. Nevertheless, because any exposure to radiation might possibly cause harm, x-rays should be used only when the patient is expected to benefit. . . .

Total oral radiation doses to the head and neck region for a complete mouth series range from 4 to 6 rads. Although this seems small, it is possible for the lenses of the eyes and the thyroid gland to receive a total dose of somewhat less than 2 rads. To date it is not known if this is significant, especially if dental needs dictate repeating this dose serially over several years. For this reason, available thyroid shields may be indicated.

Genetic doses from head and neck irradiation are extremely small. About $1/10,000$ rad reaches the unshielded reproductive cells per rad of head and neck exposure. Again, the dose is low, but perhaps significant, and body shielding of dental patients is recommended.

Elective oral radiology is generally delayed until the last two trimesters of pregnancy. The reason for this is usually patient apprehension or physician recommendation to pregnant patients. According to available indications, a pregnant patient who is properly shielded could receive dental x-ray doses at any time. However, the procedure of exposing first-trimester pregnant females is usually confined to emergency dental situations. These patients, of course, should be shielded.

The specific effects of dental radiation doses are not well known. The effects of usually larger medical doses cannot be extrapolated down in direct proportion. The result is the recommendation that dentists get a clinical history and perform clinical examinations of patients in order to minimize patient exposure yet maximize necessary diagnostic information. The practitioner should consider dose rate, age, sex, individual variations, and relative tissue radiosensitivity variations before prescribing oral radiographs.

ELECTRICAL INJURY

EPIDEMIOLOGY. Including accidents caused by lightning, over 1200 deaths each year result from electrical injury. Most occur in people below the age of 40, and the great majority of the victims are males. Presumably this is because most electrical accidents are job related.

PATHOPHYSIOLOGY. Two main types of severe electrical injury occur. The first is cardiorespiratory arrest, usually caused either by massive amounts of electricity or by small amounts of current transmitted more directly to or through the myocardium. Ventricular fibrillation is induced by the current, and this may persist even if the current is transient; immediate resuscitation is needed to prevent death.

The second type of severe injury is similar in many ways to a crush injury. The devitalization of large amounts of muscle can result from the heat generated by the passage of large currents, or blood vessels can be damaged as the current travels along them. The damaged vessels may then cause thrombosis, leading to necrosis of muscle or damage to almost any organ whose blood supply is affected. Muscle and skin are more severely damaged when the victim comes in contact with alternating current than with direct current because alternating current causes tetanic muscle contractions that keep him from releasing his contact with the source. The location of the entrance and exit points of the current is important because a short path may cause less damage than a path through the entire length of the body. The amount of current passing through the body is crucial; the flow of the current is directly proportional to the difference in voltage between its source and destination and inversely proportional to the electrical resistance between these points (Ohm's law). Because water is an excellent conductor with very low resistance, its presence in contact with the body can increase the severity of the injury. Furthermore, the conductivity of the various body tissues is directly proportional to their water content, blood (and therefore blood vessels) and muscle being the best conductors and thus the tissues most sensitive to injury.

CLINICAL MANIFESTATIONS. The severity, nature, and time course of clinical signs of electrical injury can vary widely for the reasons previously indicated. The most immediate and severe symptom is coma caused by apnea and cardiac standstill. This is usually fatal unless the accident is witnessed, the victim is removed from electrical contact, and resuscitation is begun within 2 to 4 minutes. Fractures, especially of the spine or proximal long bones owing to tetanic contracture of axial or proximal muscles, require early diagnosis and immobilization. Within the next 4 to 24 hours hypotension or shock may result from the loss of plasma volume into a large area of necrotic muscle or other tissue. Oliguria may follow, caused by shock or by the release of myoglobin from damaged muscle. The presence of hyperkalemia and metabolic acidosis must be sought, since they are potential causes of death during this stage.

In the 2 to 3 days following the injury, several problems may arise. Stress ulcers with secondary gastric bleeding may occur. Delayed hemorrhage from damaged arterial vessels or thrombosis in these vessels can also occur, even in areas removed from the area of necrosis.

Late damage, which may not be apparent for several days to weeks, is mostly neurologic or psychologic. The common neurologic sequelae are peripheral neuropathy or spinal cord injury manifested mainly by motor signs; psychologic sequelae as a result of the severity or nature of the injury vary widely depending on the patient's personality, but some reaction needing at least supportive therapy is almost certain to occur.

MANAGEMENT. The first priority in treatment is removal of the victim from contact with the source of current. Either turning off the current, if possible rapidly, or pulling the victim away is essential; if the source cannot be turned off, the rescuer must use a nonconductive (wood, leather, or rubber) shield or guard when touching the victim to avoid becoming part of the electrical circuit. After this, if the victim is not breathing or has no pulse, cardiopulmonary resuscitation must be started at once and continued until breathing or circulation has returned or until an hour has passed with no response, indicating that response is unlikely.

Treatment in the next few hours centers on wound care, fracture diagnosis and management, and fluid and electrolyte therapy. As mentioned previously, fractures may have resulted from tetany; careful physical and roentgenographic examination of deformed or tender bony areas is important. The vertebrae are especially susceptible to fracture. The wound management is standard, with debridement, irrigation, and review of tetanus immunization status most important. Fluid management can be crucial because a large portion of plasma volume can escape into the muscle compartments. Close monitoring of the pulse rate, blood pressure, urine volume and specific gravity, and serum electrolytes is necessary. Intravenous fluids are needed if any of these parameters indicate the presence of hypovolemia.

After these initial stabilization steps, taken during the first few hours of hospital care, several more definitive steps are needed over the next several days.

1. Devitalized tissue, usually skin or muscle, may require removal and eventual grafting. If the current has caused the death of an area of muscle, it must be surgically removed to prevent infection and sloughing.

2. Late vascular damage in the form of thrombosis or hemorrhage may occur at sites distant from the entrance or exit wounds, and close observation for several days is needed to detect and treat these problems. Bowel, extremity, or renal tissue and arterial or venous vessels may be involved.

3. Renal sequelae related to large tissue injury may occur; myoglobin released from damaged muscle may precipitate in the renal tubules and cause acute renal failure. This is manifested by oliguria, rising BUN and creatinine concentrations, and a positive result of urine test for myoglobin. Standard treatment for acute renal failure is needed. Recovery may take several weeks, and the mortality is high (25% to 50%).

4. There is a high incidence of gastritis and stress gastric ulcers in patients with severe injuries of any type, and electrical injury is no exception. Monitoring of hematocrit and stool for occult blood loss is important. Prophylaxis with frequent (every 2 to 3 hours) administration of antacid and/or cimetidine is always indicated.

5. Neurologic sequelae may result from damage to the peripheral nerves, spinal cord, or brain; discovery of this may be delayed by the other complications and may take several weeks. The nature of the deficit depends on the particular nerve or cord level involved; the treatment is supportive and rehabilitative, and no preventive measures are known.

POISONINGS
Heavy metal toxicity

Heavy metal poisoning is noteworthy for two reasons. First, although not an everyday occurrence, these diseases are common enough to warrant a basic knowledge of them by all practitioners. Second, most are treatable if the diagnosis is made early enough.

The treatment is described here rather than with the individual metals because it is similar for most of the metals. The most important and most obvious step is to locate and remove the source of the offending substance. The next step is to remove accumulated metal ions from the body. This is crucial because the metals do their damage by combining with various intracellular molecules: sulfhydryl groups in enzymes in the case of mercury and arsenic and other enzyme components in the case of lead. These attachments can be reversed by the intense attraction between the metal ions and the following three drugs.

Dimercaprol (BAL) binds to arsenic, mercury, and antimony; the complex is then at least partly removed from the body by renal filtration. BAL is given intramuscularly in a gradually tapered 10-day course, starting as soon after the poisoning as possible. The dosage is 5 mg/kg body weight given every 4 hours on the first day, every 6 hours on the second day, then every 8 hours for the next 8 days.

Edetate (Versenate) also forms stable complexes with most metallic ions. Since it binds the essential ion calcium as well as it binds most metal ions, it must be given as a calcium salt to avoid serious hypocalcemia. It is administered intravenously, 2 g a day in adults in two divided doses for a 5-day course.

Penicillamine also chelates lead and mercury, as well as copper. It can be given orally, making it more advantageous than the other agents for ease of administration. It is generally less toxic than BAL but is less effective than edetate for the chelation of lead. The dosage is 1 to 2 g each day in four divided doses for 10 days.

LEAD POISONING

Etiology. Ingestion and inhalation are the ways lead enters the body. Ingestion is much more common, occurring mostly from eating paint made with various lead compounds. Children less than 5 years of age are the usual victims; inhabitants of older housing that has not been repainted for years are commonly affected, since paints made in recent years contain no or much less lead. The ingestion of lead also occurs in minor epidemic form among users of homemade whiskey distilled in auto radiators containing lead. Inhalation usually occurs in an industrial setting, especially in the production of leaded gasoline and in the production or the burning for reuse of storage batteries.

Once lead is ingested, about 10% is absorbed from the gastrointestinal tract; it is then transported to the liver, released into the circulation, and deposited in bone marrow and red cell precursors and in bone. The lead stored in bone is inert and does not contribute to toxicity unless mobilized. Lead is cleared rapidly from the blood by these storage sites. Inhaled lead is absorbed directly into the blood through the respiratory mucosa.

Clinical manifestations. The signs of lead poisoning usually develop slowly because prolonged exposure is needed for enough lead to accumulate to cause symptoms and signs. A high index of suspicion is needed because the early symptoms are vague and may be intermittent.

The symptoms fall into three main groups. The first is abdominal pain or "lead colic." Bouts of severe pain occur in varying locations with or without nausea and vomiting. An examination while pain is present does not show abdominal tenderness or other signs of intraperitoneal inflammation. The cause of the pain is spasm of the bowel wall musculature. Fever and leukocytosis do not occur. A useful diagnostic (and therapeutic) maneuver is the intravenous administration of 1 g of calcium gluconate; this at least temporarily relieves the pain if lead colic is the cause.

Peripheral neuropathy is the second symptom complex; paralysis without sensory loss is the key finding. The upper extremities are affected more severely than the lower. Recovery after treatment is common if the condition has not resulted in severe atrophy by the time of diagnosis.

Encephalopathy is the third and most life-threatening symptom complex. The mortality is approximately 25%, and many nonfatal cases result in permanent brain damage. The encephalopathy is seen mostly in children and does not seem to occur with inhalation of lead. The early symptoms are behavioral changes, irritability, restlessness, and confusion. Memory loss may follow. A rapid progression to ataxia, convulsions, stupor, and coma occurs if the diagnosis is not made early in the course. Although the accumulation of lead is slow and chronic and the earlier encephalopathic symptoms are usually present, the patient may initially require emergency treatment because seizures or coma is the first manifestation that brings the patient to medical attention.

In patients with poor oral hygiene, lead sulfide may be deposited in a black line along the gingival margin of the teeth (lead line).

Laboratory findings and diagnosis. Anemia occurs in most patients with lead poisoning. It is microcytic in appearance, and the cells often have basophilic stippling. The anemia is usually not severe and is reversible with treatment.

Two urine tests are useful in the diagnosis. Coproporphyrin III excretion is increased because lead interferes with enzymes in the heme synthesis pathway. Measurement of urinary porphyrin is a good screening test. Urinary lead levels should also be determined; levels greater than 0.1 mg/L are probably significant. Measurement of urinary lead after the administration of edetate can be a useful test; if the excretion is greater than 0.5 mg/24 hours after three doses, the diagnosis is almost certain.

The determination of blood lead levels is not especially useful for two reasons. First, as mentioned previously, lead is rapidly cleared from the blood by storage sties and the blood level may be normal in spite of a large accumulated load. Second, the collection of specimens without contamination by needle or container is difficult.

Management. The permanent elimination of the source of lead is essential. Encephalopathy requires emergency treatment by lowering the intracranial pressure with osmotic agents or steroids. Next, edetate is used as a chelating agent, followed by penicillamine, in the dosages mentioned previously.

MERCURY POISONING.

Mercury can cause three quite different syndomres—acute inorganic poisoning, chronic inorganic poisoning, and organic mercurial toxicity—that are dissimilar in presentation. Acute inorganic poisoning can result from the ingestion of mercuric chloride. This industrial corrosive does extensive damage to any gastrointestinal mucosa with which it has contact; after absorption it denatures enzymes by combining with their sulfhydryl groups, especially in the renal tubular cells where the substance is concentrated for potential excretion. Severe diffuse enteritis and uremia result. There is an early need for massive replacement of the fluid loss of enteritis and a later need for fluid restriction and a program for the treatment of renal failure. The prognosis is poor.

Chronic intoxication is usually the result of industrial exposure. Photoengraving, the manufacture of scientific and electrical instruments, scientific research laboratories, mining, and the production of industrial and marine paints are all enterprises using large amounts of mercury, and workers in these industries can come in long-term contact with the substance. The symptoms and signs are diffuse and can appear unrelated if they wax and wane over months or even years. Painful bleeding gums, often with a blue, metallic-appearing line along the margin, loosening of teeth, and a generally painful stomatitis are common. Neuropsychiatric manifestations of facial or distal extremity tremors, irritability, and bizarre behavior or frank psychosis constitute a second large group of symptoms. The nephrotic syndrome with its massive proteinuria may appear early or late in the course. Treatment with BAL or penicillamine as a chelating agent is effective is used early in the therapy, but residual damage is not unusual.

The organic mercurials ethyl and methyl compounds seem to concentrate in the nervous system, causing ataxia, peripheral neuropathy, loss of vision, and a dementia or retardation syndrome. As with the chronic inorganic syndrome, once high tissue levels have been present for a prolonged period, treatment with chelating agents is often not helpful.

POISONING WITH OTHER METALS. Arsenic is a main ingredient of many insecticides and pesticides used in homes and commercial agriculture. Poisoning usually occurs by accidental or intentional ingestion of one of these products; in rare cases agricultural workers have enough exposure to cause symptoms.

Acute arsenic poisoning can cause death in just a few hours from cardiovascular collapse and shock, following a period of severe vomiting, diarrhea, and abdominal pain. Chronic poisoning depends on the frequency and amount of exposure. Since several weeks are required for the excretion of just one dose, very small doses at even weekly intervals can gradually accumulate to cause a problem. Arsenic is stored in nervous tissue, liver, and keratin-containing tissue such as hair and nails. Neurologic signs of severe mixed peripheral neuropathy, headache, depressive symptoms, fatigue, and even convulsions are common. Skin signs are also important, especially hyperpigmentation, hyperkeratosis, scaly dry rash, and transverse white lines in the fingernails.

The diagnosis is confirmed by the analysis of urine, hair, or nails for arsenic. Since arsenic exists in very low levels in food and water, some arsenic is normally present in the body. A ruine excretion greater than 0.2 mg/L or hair levels greater than 0.1 mg/100 g of hair strongly indicate arsenic poisoning. The treatment is removal of the source of toxicity, plus BAL for the acute syndrome; BAL is not very effective for chronic poisoning.

Even though the use of thallium in household products was banned by the U.S. government in 1965, it is still found in insecticides and pesticides that are left over. Accumulation in nervous tissue and hair loss dominate the clinical picture of thallium poisoning. The treatment is purely supportive because the chelating agents do not have much effect on thallium.

Other common poisons

In addition to the heavy metals and carbon monoxide, there are a number of other substances that can cause actue poisoning. Those commonly found in the home are discussed here in terms of the types of damage they cause and the intial therapeutic measures required.

ACIDS, ALKALIES, AND BLEACHES. Lye (sodium hydroxide), washing soda (sodium carbonate), and other strong alkalies and acids are commonly used as cleansing agents and drain solvents. Ingestion of these substances causes severe and almost immediate irritant burns of all mucosal surfaces contacted; the esophagus and stomach may be perforated from the lesion. Death usually results from peritonitis or mediastinitis caused by perforation. The initial treatment is dilution of the poison with large amounts of water or milk. Neither induced vomiting nor gastric tube drainage should be used, since both increase the risk of perforation. Beyond this, the treatment is that of shock or intestinal perforation.

INSECTICIDES. Chlorinated insecticides such as DDT are seen much less often since they were banned by the U.S. government. However, they are still found in many households and can cause diffuse central nervous system and muscle hyperexcitability if ingested in large doses. The treatment is induced emesis followed by supportive measures for seizures and ventilatory failure.

Cholinesterase inhibitor–type insecticides are quite common; they can be inhaled, ingested, or absorbed through the skin. Their damage is done by allowing acetylcholine to accumulate at the nerve endings and cause diffuse autonomic and central nervous system effects. Central depression occurs, leading to coma; peripheral muscle weakness or fasciculation, vomiting or diarrhea, blurred vision, excess salivation, and sweating also occur. The combination of signs makes the diagnosis likely. The initial treatment is induced emesis to remove the poison, followed by atropine injections to block the central and parasympathetic acetylcholine effects.

Fluorinated insecticides are also common. Their damage is caused by enzyme inhibition, which blocks cellular chemical reactions. Fluoride can also precipitate with calcium and thus deplete serum calcium, leading to neuromuscular hyperirritability. Ingestion is treated by the administration of oral calcium to precipitate the fluoride before it is absorbed. This is followed by general supportive measures.

PETROLEUM PRODUCTS. The accidental or intentional ingestion of gasoline or kerosene can lead to aspiration of the material into the lungs, where pulmonary edema and chemical pneumonitis may result. Induced emesis and gastric lavage are not indicated as emergency measures unless a cuffed endotracheal tube is in place to reduce the danger of aspiration of these products. Otherwise, the treatment is symptomatic.

ABNORMALITIES OF TEMPERATURE REGULATION

Body temperature is closely controlled by neural, vascular, and metabolic mechanisms that permit only a few degrees of variation despite wide fluctuations in ambient temperature. The temperature of circulating blood is sensed by regulatory cells in the hypothalamus, which initiates compensatory changes if the blood is too warm or too cool. The range of normal is 96.5° F (35.8° C) to 99° F (37.2° C); a diurnal rhythm occurs with the lowest values in the early morning and a peak of 1° to 2° F higher in the early evening.

Excess body heat is lost through four different mechanisms. *Conduction* is direct transfer by contact from one surface to another and is a minor consideration, except during water immersion, in humans. *Convection* is transfer from the body surface to the ambient air; wind accelerates this considerably. *Radiation* is transfer of heat energy by nonparticulate means; this can be responsible for the loss of half of the body's heat production at temperatures near freezing. *Evaporation* of water cools the body surface and is the main object of sweating. Heat is produced by metabolic reaction (breakdown of glucose) by body tissues, the largest component of which is muscle tissue. Shivering is a reflex response to cool circulating blood that increases head production in muscle tissue. The main regulating device of these mechanisms of heat production or loss is blood flow to skin vessels, which contract or dilate depending on the need to conserve or lose heat; the amount of sweat produced can also vary because sweat glands of the skin respond to sympathetic nerve stimulation.

Abnormalities of local tissue damage such as burns or frostbite are beyond the scope of this chapter, as are the temperature abnormalities caused by infectious diseases. The systemic effects of high ambient temperature are discussed first, followed by the effects of low temperature.

Heat syndromes

Two major mechanisms cause heat syndromes. The first is prolonged sweating without adequate replacement of water and sodium chloride; the second is cessation of sweating and failure of the evaporation mechanism of heat loss. Heat cramps, heat syncope, and heat exhaustion are related to the first mechanism, and heat stroke is caused by the second.

HEAT CRAMPS. Heat cramps are painful spasms of the voluntary muscles, usually following sudden or strenuous use of the involved muscle during hot weather and after excess sweating. The replacement of sodium chloride and water is therapeutic, and the use of sodium chloride tablets before such activity may be prophylactic.

HEAT SYNCOPE. Heat syncope occurs when a person working in a hot, humid environment becomes light headed or weak and then faints without other discoverable cause. Cutaneous vasodilation, loss of circulating volume resulting from excess sweating with inadequate water intake, lack of salt replacement, and lack of acclimatization to the hot surroundings contribute to the event. The physical findings are tachycardia, hypotension, and cool sweaty skin. The treamtent is usually quick and easy and consists of rest, a supine position, and replacement of water and salt.

HEAT EXHAUSTION. Heat exhaustion is a general term used to describe a more prolonged and generalized syndrome than either heat cramps or syncope, although both are usually part of the picture. Prolonged sweating for several days leads to a symptom complex of weakness, nausea, unsteadiness, thirst, loss of concentration, muscle cramps, and eventual collapse or delirium. Again, the cause is thought to be prolonged underreplacement of salt and water. Treatment is replacement of salt and water by the oral or intravenous route, whichever is needed to replace 6 to 8 L of fluid each day. This syndrome is common and can occur with little physical work in people with chronic diseases such as heart failure or arteriosclerosis or those in the geriatric age group. Nursing home patients are especially susceptible during prolonged periods of high heat and humidity.

HEAT STROKE. Heat stroke, or heat pyrexia, results from the cessation of sweating despite a high ambient temperature and humidity. The cause is unknown. As with heat syncope, the incidence is higher in older people and those with chronic circulatory ailments. Symptoms similar to those of heat exhaustion may or may not precede the onset. Cessation of sweating and rapid rise of the body temperature to 105° or 106° F (41.1° C) signal the onset. The skin is very hot and dry, and the patient is tachycardic and disoriented or delirious. Complications can follow quickly if the treatment is not immediate; shock, coagulopathy with diffuse bleeding, heart failure, or renal failure can occur within 1 to 2 days. Treatment should begin as soon as the diagnosis is made and consists of immersion in cold water; drastic as this seems, it is the quickest and most effective way to lower the central body temperature. If the very high temperature is not reduced, it will cause permanent damage to intracellular enzymes in neural, renal, and other tissues. Once the temperature falls to about 101° F (38.3° C), immersion can be stopped and general supportive measures are continued. The intravenous administration of fluids and electrolytes is guided by laboratory measurements and hemodynamic parameters. The prognosis is guarded, especially for older and chronically ill persons.

Hypothermia

Hypothermia occurs when heat loss exceeds heat production for long periods, at least hours. The numerical definition is a central (rectal or esophageal) temperature less than 95° F (35° C). Since standard medical thermometers are not calibrated lower than this, incubator thermometers or other wider-range instruments must be used to confirm the diagnosis. The treatment and prognosis correlate to some extent with how low the temperature falls, and thus it is important to measure it exactly. Rectal probe thermocouples can give a continuous reading and are useful during treatment.

The physiologic effects of sustained low temperature are mainly neurologic and cardiac. Early in the course a period of confusion, irrationality, and even mania can occur, followed by a gradual lapse into stupor and coma. Cardiac irritability is the cause of death in fatal cases; this can occur during rewarming as well. Hypotension, diversion of blood from skin and peripheral tissues, and nonfatal cardiac arrhythmias may also occur.

Mild hypothermia can be caused by various disease states. Hypothyroidism is probably the most common, and hypoadrenalism, hypopituitarism, advanced cirrhosis, stroke, and ingestion of phenothiazines or alcohol are also occasional causes. However, these conditions do not cause fatal hypothermia, and the low temperature is almost an incidental finding among a host of more obvious symptoms and physical signs.

Environmental exposure causes most cases of severe or fatal hypothermia. Several groups are especially susceptible. Elderly people of low income in colder climates are the largest group; a combination of inadequate heating, other chronic diseases, and borderline caloric intake can cause the syndrome even if the ambient temperatures are not strikingly low. Alcoholics and derelicts are also susceptible; falling asleep outside, especially after alcohol has dilated the skin vasculature, is probably the most common cause of cases seen in city hospitals. The third group at risk is hikers and campers in mountainous areas; a hike that starts in 70° F weather at the bottom of the mountain can end at 40° F with 30 mph winds at the top. Those who do not dress for the colder climate are subject to a rapid loss of body heat accelerated by the muscular effort of hiking. Significant and even fatal hypothermia can develop over just a few hours under these conditions even though the temperature is above freezing.

Unfortunately, the diagnosis is easy to overlook in an emergency room setting. In a stuporous patient with cold skin, traumatic, vascular, or infectious causes are often sought first. If a special thermometer is not used to find how far below 95° F (35° C) the temperature is, treatment can be delayed. Bradycardia, hypotension, slow shallow respirations, and stiffness of muscles and joints accompany the neurologic signs. In extreme cases the patient may actually appear dead with no palpable pulse and imperceptible respirations; however, electrocardiographic recording or penetration of a central vessel proves that circulation is present. Death should not be declared prematurely in a potentially hypothermic patient.

The treatment obviously is rewarming the patient, but the best way to do this is not obvious. The options are passive versus active rewarming and, if active rewarming is used, external versus invasive means. Passive rewarming is simply removing the patient from the exposed environment and wrapping him in blankets. This is all that can be done in the mountainous or hiking setting, and it should be done at once. Active external rewarming includes immersion in warm water or the use of electric blankets or heating pads. The trouble with this method is that studies have shown that it may worsen hypotension and hypovolemia by dilating skin and superficial muscle vessels before affecting brain or heart function; this may worsen the prognosis.

The other alternative is active invasive rewarming with techniques such as peritoneal dialysis with warmed dialysate, hemodialysis with a warming device in the circuit, lavage of an intragastric balloon with warm fluid, and inhalation warming. All of these require a hospital environment; they are recommended for patients with temperatures below 85° F and for those with coma.

BIBLIOGRAPHY

Baxter, C.R.: Present concepts in the management of major electrical injuries, Surg. Clin. North Am. **5**:1401, 1970.

Chisolm, J.J., Jr.: Poisoning due to heavy metals, Pediatr. Clin. North Am. **17**:591, 1970.

Clowes, G.H.A., and O'Donnel, I.F., Jr.: Current concepts: heat stroke, N. Engl. J. Med. **291**:564, 1974.

Dalrymple, G.V., and others: Medical radiation biology, Philadelphia, 1973, W.B. Saunders Co.

Ennis, L., Berry, H., and Phillips, J.: *Dental roentgenology*, Philadelphia, 1967, Lea & Febriger, p. 57.

Guinee, V.F.: Lead poisoning, Am. J. Med. **52**:283, 1972.

Jablon, S., and Kato, H.: Studies of the mortality of A-bomb survivors. V. Radiation dose and mortality, 1950-1970, Radiat. Res. **50**:649, 1972.

Joselow, M.M., Louria, D.B. and Browder, A.: Mercurialism: environmental and occupational aspects, Ann. Intern. Med. **76**:119, 1972.

Kay, N.R.M., and others: The management of electrical injuries of the extremities, Surg. Clin. North Am. **53**:1459, 1973.

Reuler, J.B.: Hypothermia: pathophysiology, clinical settings and management, Ann. Intern. Med. **89**:519, 1978.

Review of the current state of radiation protection philosophy, NCRP Report no. 43, January 15, 1975.

Rouse, R.G., and Dimick, A.R.: The treatment of electrical injury compared to burn injury: a review of pathophysiology and comparison of treatment protocols, J. Trauma **18**:43, 1978.

Stannard, J.N.: Toxicology of radionuclides, Annu. Rev. Pharmacol. **13**:325, 1973.

Section Eleven
NEUROLOGIC DISEASES
edited by **Rosalie A. Burns**

139 • INTRODUCTION TO NEUROLOGY
Rosalie A. Burns

The subject of neurology deals with diseases of the brain, spinal cord, nerve roots, peripheral nerves, neuromuscular junctions, and muscles. These are often referred to using the Greek or Latin derivative as encephalopathies, myelopathies, radiculopathies, neuropathies, myoneural junction disturbances, and myopathies. Encephalopathies can be further broken down into encephalopathies mainly affecting gray matter, or polioencephalopathies, and encephalopathies affecting white matter, or leukoencephalopathies. For the most part, neurologic disorders are destructive, with symptoms reflecting loss of function or deficits. Irritative phenomena occur with lesions in the cerebral cortex, however, resulting in seizure activity. Neurologic disorders may be focal, as in a cerebral infarction or hemorrhage; may be diffuse, as in a metabolic encephalopathy; or may follow an anatomic pattern in which specific combinations of anatomic pathways or systems are affected, as in motor neuron disease or combined system disease (so-called system disorders).

Whereas the neurologic examination points to lesion localization, the case history suggests the cause and the differential diagnosis. To be effective, the case history must indicate the nature of the problem, the type of onset, and whether progression or improvement has occurred. Specific information of importance in a neurologic history includes detail regarding headaches, vertigo, hearing loss, disturbed vision, speech disturbance, dysphagia, sensory or motor disturbance, seizures, syncope, sphincter disturbances, sexual dysfunction, and disorders of cerebration. The patient's medical history may disclose underlying relevant medical illnesses such as pernicious anemia in combined system disease or a previous myocardial infarction in an embolic cerebrovascular accident. A previous head injury may be the cause of a seizure disorder, or meningitis may be the cause of eventual normal pressure hydrocephalus. The patient's educational history is important as background for evaluating dementia. The family history is relevant, for example, in diagnosing many degenerative disorders. An occupational history and a history of exposure to toxins and the use of medications, drugs, or alcohol are also important for diagnosing a variety of central and peripheral disorders (see Chapter 143). The emotional impact of neurologic disorders must always be assessed.

Because the deficits discovered during the neurologic examination correlate with the localization of lesions, a basic knowledge of neuroanatomy is a prerequisite for analyzing a neurologic problem. Any case analysis should begin with anatomic localization. The cerebral hemispheres are well visualized using computed tomography (Fig. 139-1). In appropriate horizontal sections, for example, it is possible to see the frontal, parietal, temporal, and occipital lobes, the cortical sulci, the sylvian fissures, the basal ganglia, the ventricular system with the lateral and third ventricles, the fourth ventricle, the cerebellum, and the brainstem.

NEUROLOGIC LESIONS
Lesions of the frontal lobe

Lesions of the frontal lobe affecting the motor cortex result in a contralateral hemiplegia or paresis affecting fine and skilled movements to a greater extent than gross movements. Weakness is classified as paresis when the paralysis is partial and as plegia when the paralysis is complete. The paralysis may be initially flaccid (hypotonic), but ultimately spasticity develops (an increased tone of the limbs, noted maximally during initial passive movement). Spasticity is generally greater in the adductors and flexors of the arm and the extensors of the leg. Associated with this tone change are increased deep tendon reflexes, pathologic reflexes such as the Babinski sign, and absent superficial abdominal reflexes. Whereas the lower face and the limbs are affected by unilateral corticobulbar and corticospinal tract involvement, various midline structures are uninvolved because their innervation derives from both cerebral hemispheres (upper face, pharynx, larynx, neck muscles, diaphragm, and trunk). There may be minor degrees of motor deficit such as a minimal flattening of the nasolabial fold, decreased arm swing during walking, a slight downward drift of an outstretched arm, or an eversion of the leg while the patient is reclining. The frontal eye field, lying anterior to the motor cortex, is thought to be the source of a saccadic (rapid voluntary) polysynaptic eye movement pathway (frontomesencephalic) from the cerebral hemisphere to the opposite pontine paramedian re-

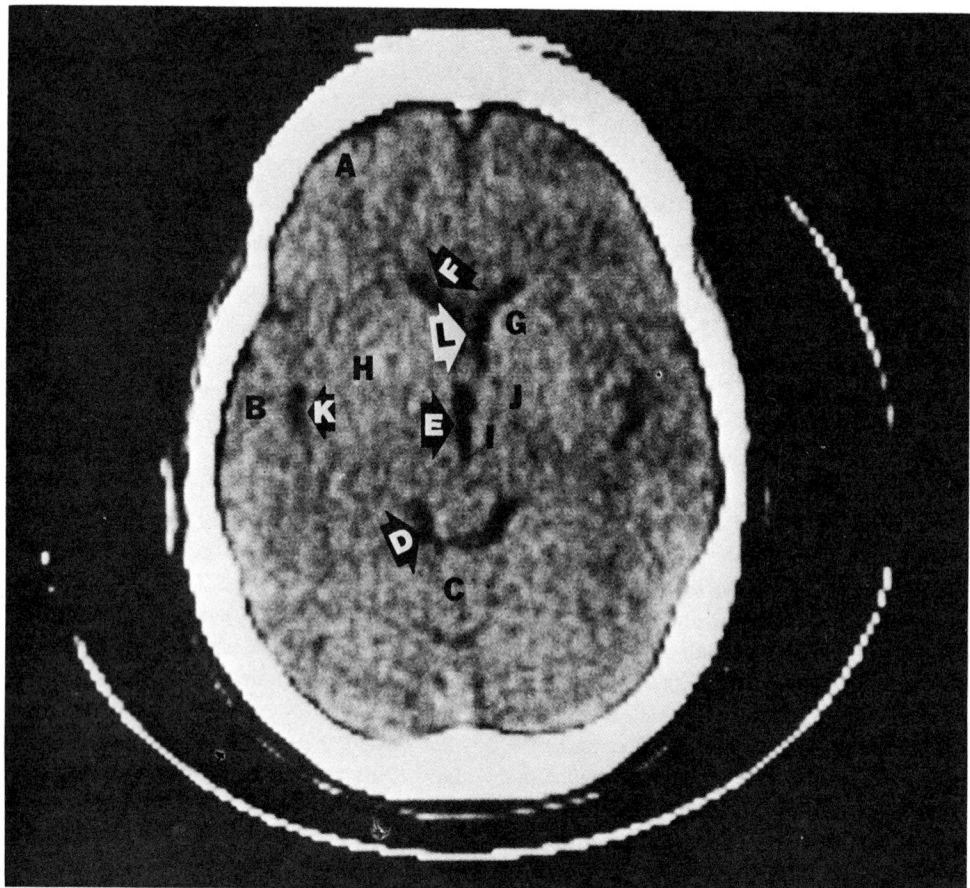

Fig. 139-1. Anatomic designations of computed tomogram. *A,* frontal lobe; *B,* temporal lobe; *C,* superior vermis of cerebellum; *D,* quadrigeminal cistern; *E,* third ventricle; *F,* frontal horn of lateral ventricle; *G,* caudate nucleus; *H,* lenticular nucleus; *I,* thalamus; *J,* internal capsule; *K,* sylvian cistern; *L,* septum pellucidum.

ticular formation (PPRF). Patients with lesions in this cerebral region tend to look toward the side of the lesion. This is commonly transient and can be overcome by using ice-water labyrinthine stimulation or the doll's head maneuver. Seizure discharges in this region cause the head and eyes to turn toward the opposite side.

Focal lesions affecting the dominant frontal lobe are likely to cause an expressive language disturbance known as nonfluent aphasia, or Broca's aphasia, and may cause some forms of apraxia. Apraxia, the inability to perform a motor act when the necessary motor, sensory, and cerebellar skills are intact, occurs with disconnection lesions of white matter pathways coursing between the dominant parietal and frontal areas, the corpus callosum, and the nondominant frontal area. An example of apraxia would be the inability of a patient to mimic eating on command, although the patient understands the command and has no difficulty handling his own meals (see Chapter 142). A patient who has difficulty in walking, with small steps, a narrow base, shuffling, and the feet seemingly stuck to the floor, is said to suffer from apraxia of gait. It has been attributed to bilateral frontal lobe disease.

A variety of pathologic reflexes known as primitive reflexes or frontal release signs are common with frontal lobe lesions and resemble the reflexes seen in an infant. These include the suck, snout, rooting, and grasp reflexes. The suck reflex is a pouting movement in response to tactile stimulation of the lips; the snout reflex is a pursing of the mouth in response to pressure on the upper lip; the rooting reflex involves a movement of the angle of the mouth toward a stimulus on the corner of the lips or cheek; and the grasping reflex involves a flexion of the patient's fingers over the examiner's fingers with moving palmar stimulation. Paratonia, or gegenhalten, is also seen with frontal lobe lesions; it is a seeming inability of the limbs to relax for testing of passive movements.

Lesions of the parietal lobe

Manifestations of parietal lobe lesions may include cortical sensory loss, agnosias, apraxia, seizures, visual field defects, and disruption of optokinetic nystagmus.

Cortical sensory loss resulting from the involvement of the postcentral gyrus may include deficits in pain, touch, and temperature. This loss is generally considered to affect discriminative sensations, so that deficits may involve position sense, touch localization (atopognosia), tow-point discrimination, the ability to identify an object by modalities such as texture, size, and weight (astereognosis), the identification of numbers outlined on the palm (agraphesthesia), and the appreciation of double simultaneous stimuli (extinction). Vibration sense is thought by many to be a thalamic function.

The term "agnosia" is used when the patient has impaired recognition or awareness of something through otherwise intact sensory modalities—visual, auditory, or tactile (see Chapter 142). Some patients with lesions of the nondominant parietal lobe may be unaware of their deficit or illness (anosognosia). They may neglect one half of the body or space (amorphosynthesis) and may have spatial disorientation. They may also have constructional apraxia, which is a difficulty with drawing and copying.

Patients with lesions of the dominant parietal lobe may have difficulty in carrying out acts because of apraxia. They may have Gerstmann's syndrome, in which they cannot distinguish right from left (right-left disorientation), have difficulty handling figures (acalculia), are unable to identify or name body parts, particularly digits (finger agnosia), and are unable to write spontaneously (agraphia).

Seizure disorders manifested by sensory phenomena may occur with irritative lesions of the parietal lobe. Lesions involving the optic radiations produce inferior quadrantanopsias. Optokinetic nystagmus (OKN) is a normal phenomenon that may be disrupted with parietal lobe disease. A series of stripes or bars moved across the patient's field of vision produces OKN. This visually induced nystagmus consists of two phases, a slow (pursuit) phase in the direction of the moving objects and a fast (saccadic) phase in the opposite direction. Although the precise pathways have defied elucidation and abnormalities are not dependent on visual field defects, two clinicoanatomic correlations deserve mention. First, because vision is a prerequisite, OKN is absent if the patient is blind (for example, cortical blindness) but is present if the patient is feigning blindness (that is, functional blindness). Thus the presence of OKN proves that there must be *some* residual vision. Second, if the moving objects are directed toward a damaged parietal lobe, OKN may be abnormal in rate, rhythm, or amplitude. Thus unilateral disruption of OKN is a clinical sign of parietal lobe damage.

Lesions of the temporal lobe

Manifestations of temporal lobe lesions include Wernicke's aphasia, complex partial (psychomotor) seizures, and memory disorders (see Chapters 142, 144, and 145). Cortical deafness is uncommon; it requires bilateral lesions of the primary auditory cortex located in the superior temporal gyri. Involvement of the optic radiations may produce superior quadrantanopsias. The anterior 5 cm of one temporal lobe can be removed without causing a significant deficit.

Lesions of the occipital lobe

Manifestations of occipital lobs lesions involve mainly disorders related to vision. There may be homonymous hemianopsias caused by involvement of the geniculocalcarine system. Central vision, or macular vision, is often preserved; this is called "macular sparing." Homonymous scotomas in the macular or paramacular visual fields may occur. Cortical blindness with preservation of pupillary light reflexes may develop with bilateral occipital lobe infarction (see Chapter 152). Occipital lobe seizures are manifested by the patient perceiving abstract forms and colors. A polysynaptic occipitomesencephalic pathway is involved with horizontal slow pursuit or following movements of the eyes.

Lesions of basal ganglia

Evaluating lesions of the basal ganglia (extrapyramidal lesions) involves assessing muscular tone, looking for rigidity (increased resistance throughout a range of passive movement), and observing for abnormal involuntary movements such as chorea, athetosis, hemiballismus, or dystonia (see Chapter 150).

Lesions of corticospinal pathways

Lesions of the corticospinal pathways anywhere in their course produce the upper motor neuron signs of increased deep tendon reflexes, spasticity, and weakness. A unilateral corticospinal lesion at the level of the internal capsule results in hemiparesis or hemiplegia.

Lesions of the thalamus

Lesions of the thalamus may produce nondiscriminative sensory deficits (for example, with pain, touch, temperature, and vibration) resulting from involvement of the ventral posterior nucleus. Thalamic pain may develop (see Chapter 152). Lesions of the dorsal medial nucleus of the thalamus have been associated with the amnestic syndrome (Korsakoff's psychosis) in Wernicke's disease (see Chapter 154).

Lesions of the cerebellum

Lesions of the cerebellum in general may affect equilibrium (involvement of midline cerebellum or vermis) or limb coordination (involvement of cerebellar hemispheres). Patients with midline cerebellar lesions have gait ataxia and truncal ataxia. The gait is often described as wide based. These patients perform tandem gait poorly and may be unable to stand with their feet together and eyes open. With lesions of the cerebellar hemispheres, patients display dysmetria and intention tremor on a variety of coordination tests such as the finger-to-nose and heel-to-shin maneuvers and the performance of rapid rhythmic alternating movements. Diffuse cerebellar lesions may produce an intermittent explosiveness of speech known as "scanning." Patients may have hypotonia on passive movement and may be unable to check movement, resulting in a rebound phenomenon when resistance to muscle contraction is suddenly removed.

Lesions of the brainstem

Lesions of the brainstem produce cranial nerve, motor, sensory, and cerebellar system deficits. Involvement of the reticular system results in a loss of consciousness. A review of the vascular disorders of the brainstem (see Chapter 152) gives an overview of the anatomy of this region. The cranial nerve deficits are ipsilateral to the site of the lesion, and the sensory and motor deficits are usually contralateral. A major portion of the brainstem can be assessed by evaluating pupillary responses to light, voluntary extraocular movements, and reflex extraocular movements such as the oculocephalic or doll's head response and the oculovestibular or caloric response (see Chapter 140). Ophthalmoplegias may be internal (pupillary paralysis) or external, involving eye movements. Involvement of the extraocular muscles supplied by cranial nuclei three, four, and six or their nerves (nuclear or infranuclear) results in dysconjugate gaze (unequal limitation of eye movement) and diplopia. Internuclear ophthalmoplegia or the syndrome of the medial longitudinal fasciculus is a supranuclear dysconjugate gaze abnormality (see discussion of multiple sclerosis in Chapter 148). The paralysis of horizontal conjugate gaze that occurs with lesions of the pontine gaze center (PPRF) is usually persistent and involves both saccadic and pursuit movements. It is not overcome by icewater labyrinthine stimulation.

Nystagmus is an oscillation of the eyes that occurs with brainstem disease. It also may be normally induced, as in OKN, may be congenital (pendular), may be associated with a severe reduction in visual acuity, may be related to ingesting drugs such as phenytoin, may reflect labyrinthine disease, or may result from a supranuclear gaze paresis (to the side of the paresis). The oscillatory eye movements in nystagmus may be pendular (of equal amplitude in both directions) or have a jerklike quality with slow and fast components. Jerk nystagmus is usually named by the direction of the more easily visualized fast component (for example, horizontal to the right); it occurs in brainstem disease and may be horizontal, rotatory, or vertical. Conjugate horizontal nystagmus on lateral gaze may be gaze evoked ipsilaterally as a result of either a conjugate gaze paresis or a cerebellar pathway involvement with a pontine lesion. It may also be caused by involvement of the vestibular nuclei, occurring either in the primary position or as a gaze-evoked nystagmus to the side opposite the lesion. Rotatory nystagmus suggests involvement of the vestibular nuclei. Vertical nystagmus always indicates brainstem disease if drug intoxication is excluded. Upbeat nystagmus can be more specifically localized to the medullary area when it is present in the primary position but increases in intensity on downward gaze. A large-amplitude upbeat nystagmus in the primary position that increases during upward gaze suggests a lesion in the anterior vermis of the cerebellum. Downbeat vertical nystagmus suggests a medullary lesion, commonly associated with Arnold-Chiari malformations or other abnormalities of the craniovertebral junction. A horizontal nystagmus in the primary position that changes direction periodically is known as periodic alternating nystagmus and requires careful observation to be noted. It suggests a lesion in the caudal medullary region. Seesaw nystagmus (one eye up and one down) suggests a diencephalic lesion. Retraction nystagmus and convergence nystagmus are associated with paralysis of upward gaze (Parinaud's syndrome) and suggest a pretectal lesion.

Although evaluating the trigeminal nerve assesses pontine function, lesions of the spinal tract of the trigeminal nerve, which descends as low as the upper cervical cord, may decrease peripheral facial pain sensation. Whereas involvement of supranuclear or corticobulbar fibers to the seventh cranial nerve nucleus results only in weakness of the contralateral lower face, a lesion of the seventh nerve nucleus in the pons or in the nerve itself involves both the upper and the lower halves of the face on the same side. A peripheral seventh cranial nerve palsy may decrease lacrimation and possibly salivation and taste on the same side and may produce hyperacusis by involving respectively branches to the greater superficial petrosal nerve, the chorda tympani, and the nerve to the stapedius muscle.

Nerve deafness and vestibular disturbances are discussed in Chapter 147. Bulbar palsy, with the patient having difficulty in speaking and swallowing (dysarthria and dysphagia), occurs with lesions involving the ninth, tenth, and twelfth cranial nuclei or cranial nerves. With twelfth cranial nerve lesions, atrophy and fasciculations of the tongue are present, with deviation of the protruded tongue toward the side of the lesion.

Lesions of the spinal cord

Lesions of the spinal cord may be localized at a transverse level, involving segmental structures such as the secondary sensory neurons for pain and temperature that cross in the anterior commissure, or long tract functions below the level of the lesion such as ipsilateral proprioception in the posterior columns, contralateral pain and temperature sensations in the lateral spinothalamic tracts, and ipsilateral motor function in the corticospinal pathways. The perception of touch is commonly spared as compared to the perception of pain (dissociated sensory loss) with spinal cord disease, since touch sensation traverses the anterior spinothalamic tracts and posterior columns bilaterally, providing alternate pathways. Involvement of corticospinal tracts results in weakness below the level of the lesion with increased deep tendon reflexes and increased tone (in acute spinal shock, flaccidity and decreased deep tendon relexes are noted). The Babinski sign may be present, and incontinence may occur. Preservation of sacral sensation, or "sacral sparing," may occur with intramedullary mass lesions. Pain is commonly associated with extramedullary mass lesions. Localized spinal cord disorders may include transverse myelitis as from multiple sclerosis, intramedullary syrinx or tumor, or extramedullary compression by mass lesions. Other lesions of the spinal cord may involve combinations of particular tracts or systems, as in the posterior column and corticospinal tract involvement of combined system disease.

Diffuse involvement of anterior horn cells, as in amyotrophic lateral sclerosis, results in widespread atrophy, weakness, fasciculations (contraction of muscle fibers of a single motor unit), and a decrease in deep tendon reflexes.

Lesions of nerve roots, peripheral nerves, neuromuscular junction, and muscle

Lesions of nerve roots and peripheral nerves result in atrophy, weakness, fasciculations, a decrease in deep tendon relexes, and sensory deficit, all appropriate to their myotomal oc dermatomal origin. Deep tendon relexes are mediated by specific spinal cord segmental levels as follows: biceps—fifth and sixth cervical; radial—fifth and sixth cervical; triceps—sixth, seventh, and eight cervical; patellar—third and fourth lumbar; and Achilles—first sacral.

Lesions of the neuromuscular junction, such as myasthenia gravis, are characterized by a weakness of muscle that varies with activity. The muscle mass is usually retained, and deep tendon reflexes may be decreased during muscle fatigue.

In muscle disease, weakness is often proximally distributed. Deep tendon reflexes are lost only with significant muscle atrophy, which may occur with time (see Chapter 155).

DIAGNOSTIC TESTS

To correctly use the variety of diagnostic tests available for neurologic disorders, it is essential to base the study selection on a careful assessment of the history and physical examination. Details regarding diagnostic tools are specifically discussed in appropriate sections of this book. Some generalizations are mentioned here regarding selected procedures.

Computed tomography (CT) is a roentgenographic technique using computer analysis of digitized fine beam roentgen ray transmission data. It produces a cross-sectional anatomic image with extremely high tissue density discrimination and represents a major advance in detecting destructive, hemorrhagic, neoplastic, atrophic, and demyelinative brain lesions. There are pitfalls in using CT scanning of the head. Studies both with and without contrast medium should be obtained when the patient does not have an allergy to iodinated material. This increases the likelihood of demonstrating one of the many lesions associated with a breakdown in the blood-brain barrier. Some subdural hematomas may be difficult to define because they may be isodense with the surrounding brain and may be bilateral without a shift of intracranial structures. Arteriovenous malformations and aneurysms may not be demonstrated by a CT scan. Current scanners do not always define brainstem infarction. Because of its high density discrimination, however, the CT scan may detect faint calcification and small hemorrhages and may distinguish intracerebral brain abscesses, tumors, and infarctions. Using echoencephalography for determining a shift of the midline structures is rarely warranted when a CT scan can be obtained.

The skull roentgenogram remains useful in detecting skull fractures and abnormalities in the region of the sella turcica and at the base of the skull, as in foraminal erosions. The isotope brain scan with dynamic and static studies is used as a screening test for occlusive vascular disease in the carotid system. It may also detect lesions sometimes missed with a CT scan, such as arteriovenous malformations, chronic subdural hematomas, small meningiomas, and blood-brain barrier abnormalities as in herpes encephalitis. It takes second place to the CT scan in diagnosing the specific pathologic conditions in most intracranial lesions.

Cerebral angiography, accomplished most often today by catheterization via the femoral artery, is performed to diagnose lesions not outlined by other techniques, when management will be influenced by the findings. Examples are the demonstration of a potentially surgically accessible arteriovenous malformation not visualized on a CT scan or a radionuclide scan or documentation of a venous sinus thrombosis when anticoagulation is being considered. Another purpose of cerebral angiography is to visualize stenosed or occluded extracranial or intracranial cerebral vessels, with the goal of endarterectomy or bypass surgery, or to visualize aneurysms when surgery is comtemplated after a subarachnoid hemorrhage.

Computed digital angiography and dynamic CT scanning are techniques using the rapid injection of an intravenous bolus of contrast media. They appear to be promising methods that may replace some arterial vascular studies.

Pneumoencephalography has been almost entirely replaced by CT scanning. Introducing air into the subarachnoid space and the ventricular system is no longer necessary to outline the anatomic structures. At times, however, introducing metrizamide (Amipaque) into the subarachnoid space may help to outline a mass poorly defined on a CT scan, as for example, with suprasellar craniopharyngioma.

Positron emission tomography (PET) is a research technique using appropriately labeled positron-emitting isotopes, which can be imaged in a manner similar to roentgenographic CT scanning, to study metabolism and physiologic alterations in the brain.

Spine films are important in demonstrating subluxations, dislocations, compression fractures, erosions, and intervertebral disc space abnormalities. Myelography, the introduction of nonsoluble (isophendylate [Pantopaque]) or water-soluble (metrizamide) contrast agents into the spinal subarachnoid space, is still necessary for diagnosing the majority of spinal canal disorders for which surgery or radiotherapy would be advised. This would include intramedullary mass lesions and extramedullary mass lesions (for example, tumors, syrinx, and arteriovenous malformations) of the spinal cord, foramen magnum, and cauda equina. Spinal CT scanning, with and without metrizamide, is becoming more important, since with appropriate equipment it can demonstrate extramedullary spinal lesions and some intramedullary spinal cord lesions. Spinal CT scanning may sharply delineate lumbar disc protrusions. With the use of intrathecal water-soluble contrast media (metrizamide), many intradural lesions can be better defined than they are with routine myelography.

Spinal angiography is important in diagnosing spinal arteriovenous malformations, but because of the danger of spinal cord injury is should be reserved for patients in whom the index of suspicion is very high and for whom surgery is justified.

Lumbar puncture, with the assessment of intracranial pressure and the evaluation of cerebrospinal fluid for cells, protein, sugar, serology, and organisms, is essential in the diagnosis and differentiation of meningitis and encephalitis. It remains important in the diagnosis of subarachnoid hemorrhage if blood in the subarachnoid space is not defined on a CT scan. Whereas lumbar puncture presents the real danger of cerebral herniation when increased intracranial pressure is present, it is not contraindicated and must be performed if a CT scan fails to define a mass and a central nervous system infection remains possible (for example, pseudotumor cerebri). Patterns of altered cerebrospinal fluid are described under specific disorders in this text.

Audiograms, caloric testing, and electronystagmography are discussed in Chapter 147.

Noninvasive extracranial vascular diagnostic tests are discussed in Chapter 100.

Electromyography (EMG) may be used to differentiate nerve and muscle disease and to evaluate neuromuscular disorders. Measurement of nerve conduction velocity is particularly helpful in detecting the demyelinative neuropathies and compression peripheral neuropathies. Details regarding these procedures and muscle biopsy are discussed in Chapter 155.

Electroencephalography, recording the electrical activity of the most superficial layers of the cerebral cortex, is important in the diagnosis of seizure disorders, metabolic encephalopathies, dementia, focal versus diffuse pathologic conditions, and cerebral death. The normal background activity consists of α-waves at 8 to 12 Hz, most prominent posteriorly, and low-voltage fast β-waves at 13 to 30 Hz anteriorly. Significant degrees of slower activity such as δ-waves at 0.5 to 3 Hz and θ-waves at 4 to 7 Hz, either diffusely or focally distributed, can be correlated with destructive lesions. Metabolic encephalopathies should be associated with diffuse slow-wave activity. Destructive focal lesions, such as tumor or infarction, may cause focal slow-wave activity. Cerebral dysrhythmias are associated with seizure disorders (see Chapter 144 and 145). Provocative techniques that may be used to bring out seizure activity include sleep tracings, photic stimulation, hyperventilation, and in special instances pentylenetetrazol (Metrazol) activation. Special sleep tracings may be useful in diagnosing sleep disorders such as narcolepsy and sleep apnea.

Within the last decade the scope and usefulness of electrophysiologic methods employed in neurologic diagnosis have expanded. Whereas standard electroencephalography (EEG) and EMG techniques are still the main methods, using a minicomputer with them has increased their usefulness. By using computer averaging, the evoked potentials for a series of visual, auditory, or somatosensory stimuli can be calculated and compared to normal levels for stimulus latency, interwave latency, and amplitude. The visual evoked response (VER) is very useful in diagnosing dysfunction in the optic nerve and optic chiasm, as is seen with multiple sclerosis and chiasmatic tumors. The brainstem auditory evoked response (BAER) can localize dysfunction in the auditory system from the cochlea to the medial geniculate body. Lesions that impair the auditory pathways include multiple sclerosis, tumors, and vascular disease. The somatosensory evoked response (SER) is increasingly useful in defining peripheral nerve plexus dysfunction and spinal cord dysfunction, but the clinical applicability of this technique is less well defined than with the VER and BAER. Nonetheless, these new clinical neurophysiologic techniques often show abnormalities earlier than other studies.

BIBLIOGRAPHY

Baker, A.B., and Baker, L.H., editors: Clinical neurology, New York, 1980, Harper & Row Publishers, Inc.

Critchley, M., O'Leary, J.L., and Jennett, B., editors: Scientific foundations of neurology, Philadelphia, 1972, F.A. Davis Co.

Haymaker, W.: Bing's local diagnosis in neurological diseases, St. Louis, 1969, The C.V. Mosby Co.

140 • ALTERATIONS IN CONSCIOUSNESS

Leopold Canales

The behavior of the human central nervous system alternates between wakefulness and sleep in periods closely tied to circadian rhythms. During wakefulness, objective interaction with the environment is always accompanied by the awareness of private brain events intimately related to behavior, called thoughts, occurring in an uninterrupted stream called *mentation*.

Introspectively we can distinguish two components of human mentation. *Cognition* produces a coherent view of the environment by identifying, computing, classifying, and storing data collected by the senses; *affect,* or *emotion,* identifies innate sensations that occur spontaneously or by learned association with cognitive functions. Awake behavior is then the result of the integration of cognitive patterns of response, learned and perfected through experience (learned behavior), and built-in patterns of emotional nature (instinctive behavior).

Anatomically and physiologically, at least three parts of the brain are involved in producing awake behavior. One, phylogenetically ancient, located in the reticular core of the upper brainstem and diencephalic region, activates and coordinates the most general patterns of reactivity to the environment, giving the animal the appearance of alertness and vigilance. When these structures are destroyed or when their physiology is disturbed, the waking behavior decreases or ceases completely, resulting in the pathologic states known as stupor and coma.

The second anatomic part consists of phylogenetically recent structures, such as the cortical mantle and its connections, that have developed simultaneously with an increasing variety and complexity of the cognitive aspects of vertebrate behavior. The great development of these structures in the human is the anatomic feature that most distinctively separates us from other animals, allowing us to be in contact with a large and complex environment and simultaneously to draw the detailed distinctions between the environment and ourselves that we call self-awareness. Damage to ths neocortex or its connections results in pathologic states characterized by a decrease in the capacity to analyze data and a decrease in the versatility of responses to the environment (learned behavior). Localized damage may result in isolated deficits of cognition in one sensory modality (agnosia) or in the impairment of language (aphasia), memory (amnesia), or motility (apraxia). Diffuse damage may result in a general impoverishment of all cognitive functions and learned behavior, called dementia.

The third part is the anatomic substrate of emotional or instinctive behavior. It is located in the phylogenetically ancient part of the brain called the limbic lobe and mediates some patterns of behavior that determine the survival of the individual or the species, such as mating, aggression, fear, and affection. Damage to the limbic system or interference with its physiology results in distortions of perception or inappropriate responses of behavior that constitute the psychopathologic syndromes primarily dealt with in psychiatry.

STUPOR AND COMA

In clinical neurology the term "consciousness" has been used to imply not only the appearance of wakefulness but also the expression of some form of mental function.

Table 140-1. Classification of stupor and coma

Level of consciousness	Response to stimuli*		Comments
	Verbal	Pain	
Awake	+	+	Alert and fully oriented
Sleep	+	+	Returns to alertness and orientation when stimulated
Delirium	+	+	Confused, disoriented, agitated, combative; hallucinations may occur
Obtundation	+	+	Remains drowsy, confused, and disoriented when awakened; wakefulness maintained only by continuous stimulation
Light stupor	−	+	Withdraws quickly and forcefully from moderately intense pain, localizing the stimulus
Deep stupor	−	+	Responds only to a strong stimulus but is unable to localize it; decerebration or other stereotyped responses may be present
Coma	−	−	Although unresponsive to stimuli, vital signs may be stable without assistance; some brainstem and spinal cord reflexes may still be present; EEG shows electrical activity
Cerebral death	−	−	Vital signs artificially maintained- no reflexes; electrical silence on EEG

*+, Responds to stimulus; −, no response to stimulus.

(Progressive loss of consciousness ↓)

The general reactivity of the nervous system to stimuli that we call wakefulness or alertness depends on the interaction of the reticular activating system located in the upper brainstem and diencephalic region with the cerebral hemispheres. Structural or metabolic damage to these structures produces states of decreased alertness or unconsciousness that range from mild drowsiness to stupor to the complete unresponsiveness of coma (Table 140-1).

A practical way to classify the level of consciousness of a patient is to observe responses to two types of stimuli: verbal and pain. A normal person during wakefulness responds readily and appropriately to verbal and painful stimuli. At the end of a period of wakefulness, which for most people is around 16 hours, or in the presence of a nonstimulating environment, the nervous system drifts into sleep, but when aroused it rapidly regains an alert and fully oriented mental state.

The earliest stages of a pathologic decrease of alertness that are clearly distinguishable are *delirium* and *obtundation*. In delirium the impairment of consciousness is not severe enough to completely abolish voluntary behavior but impairs mentation sufficiently to produce confusion, disorientation, distortions of perception, dysphoria, and psychomotor agitation. This is seen commonly in metabolic encephalopathies and transiently in patients who are going slowly into coma or recovering from coma. In obtundation the impairment of consciousness has progressed to what looks like deep sleep, but when aroused the patient is unable to regain a normal state of alertness, remains confused and disoriented, and can be kept awake only through constant stimulation.

In the further deteriorated state of consciousness called stupor, the patient no longer responds to verbal stimuli but still responds to pain. In lighter states of stupor the response to pain is quick and well coordinated, sometimes including verbal manifestations of anger and defensive movements. When a deeper state of stupor is present, a stronger stimulus is needed to elicit a response; at this point the patient is unable to localize the stimulus and the response is slower and usually stereotyped. In the deeper state of unconsciousness called coma, the patient no longer responds to painful stimuli but still is able to maintain stable vital signs and to manifest some brainstem and spinal cord reflexes. This is often seen in severe barbiturate intoxication and transiently in postictal states.

Unfortunately, no unanimity in the medical literature exists concerning ths nomenclature used to define different states of unconsciousness. Some authors call any degree of unresponsiveness stupor or use terms such as ''semicoma'' or ''semistupor'' without precisely describing the degree of patient responsiveness. Because of this lack of agreement, the physician should always add a brief description of the behavior of the patient and the type of stimulus employed to clarify the meaning of the terms.

Some states of consciousness exist in which the degree of interaction between a patient and the environment is greatly reduced, giving the appearance of unresponsiveness. On closer inspection, however, there is sometimes evidence of preserved alertness or at least some degree of mental function.

The locked-in syndrome or de-efferented state is a condition in which a lesion in the ventral portion of the brainstem severely damages the corticospinal and corticobulbar tracts, producing extensive paralysis and in some cases sparing only vertical eye movements. Some patients with this condition have learned to translate their remaining movement into Morse code, revealing an intact mind.

The apallic state refers to the state of severely decreased responsiveness resulting from extensive bilateral lesions in the cerebral hemispheres. The combination of cortical lesions and deeper white matter and gray matter lesions produced by trauma, prolonged anoxia, hypoglycemia, carbon monoxide exposure, or the end state of a degenerative disease damages motor, cognitive, and affective mechanisms, sparing only arousal centers and homeostatic centers.

Akinetic mutism is a state in which the patient gives the appearance of vigilance by following objects with his eyes and occasionally chewing and swallowing food but remains otherwise relatively immobile and mute. This condition, also called coma vigil, has been associated with a variety of brain lesions, such as communicating hydrocephalus, septal and hypothalamic lesions, craniopharyngiomas destroying the walls of the third ventricle, and paramedian infarctions in the mesencephalic region.

Catatonic stupor is seen most commonly in young people affected by catatonic schizophrenia. The patient lies with eyes open or tightly closed, resisting passive eye opening; he has no spontaneous movements, but optokinetic stimulation and caloric testing produce nystagmus. Sometimes the phenomenon of catalepsy is found in which passive postures of the limbs are maintained for a prolonged time. This state of unresponsiveness may be interrupted by catatonic excitement in which the patient is wildly agitated and combative. The electroencephalogram (EEG) during catatonic stupor usually shows low-voltage fast activity instead of the slow frequencies found in unconscious patients.

Although in hysterical unresponsiveness the patient may appear to have no response to verbal and painful stimuli, neurologic examination reveals normal pupillary reflexes, nystagmus in response to caloric stimulation, and an EEG pattern indicating an awake state.

PATHOPHYSIOLOGY OF UNCONSCIOUSNESS

Early pathologic accounts of patients with encephalitis suggested that lesions in the tegmental region of the upper midbrain were responsible for the decrease in consciousness. The classic animal experiments of Bremer in 1935 demonstrated that transections through the lower part of the brainstem (encephale isolé) show the behavior and EEG characteristics of cycles of wakefulness and sleep, whereas transections through the upper midbrain (cerveau isolé) put the animal into a state resembling perpetual sleep. The initial interpretation of these experiments followed pavlovian doctrines indicating that sensory inflow was responsible for maintaining wakefulness, until in 1949 Magoun and Moruzzi discovered the ascending reticular activating system (ARAS). This system, within the reticular formation of the midbrain and the diencephalic regions, produced awakening of the animal with electrical stimulation. Destruction of the ARAS produced the behavior and EEG patterns of coma that were irreversible to stimulation via intact sensory pathways. Further experience with pathologic specimens and experimental preparations indicates that, to produce unconsciousness, lesions in the brainstem reticular formation must be bilateral and rostral to the lower third of the pons. Patients with pontine lesions that cause unconsciousness may show awake EEG patterns.

Lesions of the cerebral hemispheres also can produce a decrease in consciousness, but whereas in the brainstem a discrete well-localized lesion can devastate wakefulness, hemispheric lesions must be bilateral, extensive, and acute.

Experimental evidence in animals shows that local cooling of the hypothalamus induces sleep and that destruction of the posterior nuclei produces coma. The medical literature shows instances of somnolence and inversion of the sleep-wake cycle as a symptom of hypothalamic dysfunction, and it is known that progressively destructive lesions in this area eventually produce coma, Because of the closeness of the mesencephalic reticular formation, however, it has been hard to determine whether the mesencephalic reticular formation is also affected by the pathologic process.

INITIAL PHYSICAL AND NEUROLOGIC EXAMINATION OF THE PATIENT IN COMA

When the cause of a decreased level of consciousness is unknown, immediate steps should be taken to rule out causes that, if neglected, could produce irreversible damage to the nervous system. Checking vital signs and administering 50% glucose intravenously, after a blood sample has been drawn to document the serum glucose level, should indicate whether the problem is caused by inadequate blood supply, ventilatory problems, or hypoglycemia. Hypothermia is an often neglected sign. It may be a primary cause of coma in cases of accidental exposure to cold, or a sign of hypothyroidism, hypoglycemia, or barbiturate coma.

A general physical examination should precede the neurologic evaluation. Evidence of trauma should be sought carefully by palpating the scalp and looking for an accumulation of blood in the subcutaneous orbital and mastoid regions and behind the tympanic membranes. Blood in these locations or leakage of cerebrospinal fluid (CSF) through the nose or ear canal is evidence of a basilar skull fracture. Obvious signs of head trauma should alert the physician to the possibility of an accompanying cervical spine injury, and passive neck movements should be avoided until adequate roentgenograms are taken. Inspection of the mouth may show evidence of tongue biting and hypertrophic gums (a side effect of the anticonvulsant phenytoin) that point to seizures as the cause of the loss of consciousness. The general physical examination also may show evidence of bleeding diathesis, cirrhosis, respiratory disease, or ohter systemic illness that could be the primary cause of or a contributing factor to the loss of consciousness.

The neurologic examination of an unconscious patient is a challenge to a clinical neurologist. Since the patient is unable to cooperate, the examination is limited to reflex responses and is directed toward establishing the degree of responsiveness to specific stimuli (level of consciousness) and the anatomic localization of the lesion.

The parameters that are most informative in unconscious patients ars the ocular fundi, pupillary reflexes, spontaneous and reflex motor behavior, spontaneous and reflex eye movements, and respiration.

OCULAR FUNDI. Careful observation of the ocular fundi, without using mydriatics that interfere with pupillary reflexes, may produce information about chronic arterial hypertension, diabetes, subhyaloid hemorrhages (the result of sudden severe intracranial hypertension, as in subarachnoid hemorrhage), and the presence or absence of papilledema.

PUPILLARY REFLEXES. Pupillary reflexes depend on the correct functioning of centers situated in the diencephalon, the midbrain, and the pons and therefore provide important clues to the localization of lesions in the brainstem. Damage to the anterior hypothalamic region affects the sympathetic outflow, causing Horner's syndrome (ptosis, miosis, and anhidrosis). The sympathetic fibers continue from the hypothalamus along the brainstem and the cervical spinal cord toward the second neuron in the upper thoracic region, returning to the cranium to dilate the pupil via peripheral sympathetic nerves accompanying ths carotid artery. Any lesion along this circuitous route could produce Horner's syndrome, but in the presence of stupor or coma a diencephalic lesion or a brainstem lesion is likely Pupils that are midposition in range and unreactive to light suggest a midbrain lesion in the tectal or pretectal region, but the additional presence of bilateral external oculomotor paralysis points to a more tegmental location involving third nerve nuclei or fibers. Bilateral pinpoint pupils indicate a pontine lesion. The light reflex is still present, although a magnifying lens may be required to observe it.

A unilaterally dilated pupil suggests a peripheral lesion in the third nerve. The pupillary fibers are located in the periphery of the nerve and are the first to be affected in the process of transtentorial herniation when the uncus of the temporal lobe presses on the nerve, stretching its fibers.

Systemic metabolic processes leading to unconsciousness do not affect pupillary reflexes except for intoxication with atropine-like drugs, glutethimide, and opiates. Atropine-like drugs produce fully dilated unresponsive pupils in addition to dry skin, dry mucous membranes, and hyperthermia. Glutethimide is a hypnotic; an overdose produces midposition pupils or moderately dilated pupils. Opiates such as heroin or morphine constrict the pupils to pinpoint size but preserve the light reflex.

SPONTANEOUS AND REFLEX MOTOR BEHAVIOR. In cases

in which unconsciousness progresses from obtundation into coma, a concomitant deterioration of spontaneous and reflex motor behavior occurs. In obtundation it is common to see the patient spontaneously changing posture in bed, drawing up the bed sheets, and trying to pull out intravenous needles and indwelling catheters. When painful stimuli are used (touching the cornea, rubbing the sternum, pinching the Achilles tendon, pressing on a nail bed, or caloric stimulation), the patient accurately localizes the stimulus and fights forcefully, sometimes accompanying the response with vocalization and grimacing. Asymmetry of spontaneous movement, confirmed by a similar pattern of response to pain, may indicate a hemiparesis or monoparesis. As unconsciousness deepens, the resting posture becomes less natural and spontaneous movements no longer occur. Motor asymmetries become less apparent as the response to pain becomes less elaborate and forceful; they may be replaced by stereotyped responses having specific anatomic or pathologic connotations. These responses include the following:

1. *Decorticate posture.* The arms and wrists are flexed and the legs are extended with internal rotation and plantar flexion. This posture is seen in cases of extensive hemispheric lesions involving the corticospinal pathways.
2. *Decerebrate posture.* In this posture there is extension and pronation of the arms and extension of the legs with plantar flexion (sometimes accompanied by trismus and opisthotonos), occurring spontaneously or as a response to pain. A lesion between the red nuclei and the vestibular nuclei of the brainstem is implicated.
3. *External rotation of one leg.* In the absence of hip fracture this indicates leg weakness, most probably caused by hemiparesis.
4. *Focal seizures.* This may be manifested by deviation of gaze, usually with a clonic quality, head rotation, and twitching of the face or fingers.
5. *Myoclonus.* Manifested by generalized myoclonic contractions (sudden, generalized asynchronous muscle contractions), this is commonly seen in uremia or anoxia. Coarse and irregular tremor and asterixis (palmar flapping) are often seen in metabolic encephalopathies.

SPONTANEOUS AND REFLEX EYE MOVEMENTS. Unconscious patients in whom the centers that mediate eye movements are intact commonly have a slightly divergent straightforward gaze and slow, horizontal conjugate movements (roving eye movements). In these patients turning the head briskly from side to side elicits conjugate eye movements directed opposite to the head rotation. This is the oculocephalic or doll's head reflex, which is absent in the alert normal individual. Stimulation of the semicircular canals by irrigating the external ear canal with cold water (caloric stimulation) produces tonic eye deviation toward the stimulated side. In a normal awake individual this type of stimulation causes nystagmus with the rapid component away from the stimulated side.

Full horizontal excursion of the eyes to both sides is possible only when the nuclei and the internuclear connections between the third and the sixth nerves are preserved. Because these structures are located in the tegmentum of the pons and the midbrain, the presence of horizontal eye movements suggests that the immediately adjacent reticular activating system is also intact and that the cause of unconsciousness is not a structural brainstem lesion.

Unilateral lesions in the pontine gaze center (region of the abducens nucleus) produce a paralysis of ipsilateral conjugate gaze and a contralateral conjugate deviation of the eyes. Caloric stimulation fails to move the eyes beyond the midline.

The pathway connecting the pontine gaze center to the midbrain oculomotor nuclei is called the medial longitudinal fasciculus (MLF). When its fibers are damaged, the ipsilateral medial rectus muscle fails to contract when required for voluntary or reflex conjugate horizontal gaze. This is called internuclear ophthalmoplegia and can be demonstrated by oculocephalic or caloric testing in the unconscious patient.

Skew deviation of the eyes (one up or down) is an indication of brainstem lesions. Forced downward deviation of the eyes (looking at the tip of the nose) has been described in cases of thalamic hemorrhage and is usually accompanied by nonreactive pinpoint pupils.

RESPIRATION. The abnormal respiratory patterns most commonly identified in unconscious patients are Cheyne-Stokes respiration, central neurogenic hyperventilation, and apneustic and ataxic breathing.

Cheyne-Stokes respiration is the respiratory rhythm that alternates between periods of hyperpnea (increased rate and depth of ventilation) and apnea (absence of respiratory movements). After the apnea the hyperpnea starts in a crescendo fashion until a peak is reached, after which a decrescendo period starts, ending in apnea again. It is commonly caused by deep, bilateral hemispheric lesions, either structural or metabolic.

Central neurogenic hyperventilation is a pattern of rapid, regular respiration described with tegmental lesions of the upper brainstem, but probably pulmonary in origin.

Apneustic breathing is the result of a lesion in the pontine respiratory center. The inspiratory and expiratory phases of the respiratory cycle are separated by pauses of 2 or 3 seconds.

Ataxic respiration is a disorganized pattern of inspiratory and expiratory movements seen in association with lesions of the medullary respiratory center.

From these descriptions it can be concluded that if the respiratory cycle (an inspiratory movement followed by an expiratory one) is disturbed, there is a lesion in the pontomedullary respiratory center. Lesions above this level affect only the respiratory rhythm.

LESIONS PRODUCING UNCONSCIOUSNESS

Lesions producing unconsciousness can be divided into three groups: supratentorial mass lesions, infratentorial lesions, and metabolic encephalopathies.

Supratentorial mass lesions

The intracranial cavity is divided into two compartments by a portion of ths dura called the tentorium cerebelli. The supratentorial compartment harbors the cerebral hemispheres and the diencephalon, whereas the infratentorial compartment or posterior fossa contains the cerebellum and the brainstem. The anterior attachment of the tentorium is to the edges of the petrous bone and the clinoid processes of the sella turcica. Between the clinoid attachments ths edge of the tentorium recedes to form an opening called the incisura, through which the midbrain, the CSF contained in the mesencephalic subarachnoid cisterns, and the posterior cerebral arteries enter the supratentorial space. This incisura is the only space connecting the supratentorial and infratentorial spaces.

Because of the nondistensible properties of the skull after its sutures close, a continuously expanding mass in the supratentorial space produces progressive displacement of brain parenchyma and increased intracranial pressure that will eventually push the tissues through the only possible exit, the incisura. The passage of the supratentorial structures through the incisura is called transtentorial herniation and causes a number of clinical signs that can be grouped into two syndromes: central and uncal herniations.

Central transtentorial herniation occurs when the displacement of tissues is symmetric enough that the resultant vector of forces converges in the midline region to push the diencephalon through the incisura. Acute hydrocephalus and vertex, frontal, and occipital mass lesions are the most common causes of central transtentorial herniation. The impairment of diencephalic function and the downward displacement of the brainstem initially produce obtundation or light stupor accompanied by Cheyne-Stokes respirations and small pupils. Roving eye movements may be present, and the eyes move conjugately toward the side of caloric stimulation, implying the structural integrity of the brainstem. Preexisting hemiparesis may worsen, whereas paratonia (active resistance to passive movements) develops in contralateral limbs accompanied by bilateral Babinski signs and decorticate posture. As the herniation progresses, signs of hypothalamic distress (diabetes insipidus, hyperthermia, or hypothermia) may occur, and signs of midbrain involvement begin to characterize the clinical picture. Cheyne-Stokes respiration is replaced by central hyperventilation, the pupils enlarge to midpoint, caloric testing produces dysconjugate movements, and decorticate posture is replaced by spontaneous, or pain-elicited, decerebrate rigidity.

Further progression shows signs of lower brainstem involvement with the development of generalized flaccidity and an absent response to caloric stimulation. At this point the combination of pressure and downward displacement of the brainstem produces ischemia and herniation of the medulla and the cerebellar tonsils through the foramen magnum, resulting in respiratory depression and hypotension. Respiratory arrest and dilated pupils signal the end of the process. If vital signs are artificially maintained with ventilators and pressor agents, the intracranial pressure may continue to rise, becoming equal to the arterial systolic pressure, at which point no brain perfusion is possible.

The inferior surface of the temporal lobe rests on the tentorium, and the most medial portion, the uncus, slightly overhangs the edge. Expanding temporal or parietal lesions produce a medial displacement of the hemisphere, which, in addition to the increased intracranial pressure, pushes the ipsilateral uncus through the incisura. This is called uncal herniation. The third cranial nerve runs parallel to the incisural edge in such a way that the herniated uncus descends on the nerve, stretching its fibers and producing ipsilateral pupillary dilatation. At this point consciousness may be normal or impaired, depending on how much the supratentorial displacement of the tissues is affecting the diencephalic region. Further herniation of the uncus compresses the midbrain against the opposite edge of the tentorium. Signs of progressive deterioration of brainstem function include further depression of consciousness, abnormal respiratory pattern, sluggish or absent caloric response, decerebrate posture, dilatation of the pupil opposite to the one originally dilated, and hemiparesis ipsilateral to the mass lesion. Such hemiparesis has been explained as the result of the pressure of the cerebral peduncle contralateral to the herniating temporal lobe against the tentorial edge (Kernohan's notch). The time between the initial pupillary dilatation and the signs of midbrain distress can be quite short if the expanding lesion is rapidly enlarging (for example, in epidural hematoma). After this point the clinical picture is identical to central transtentorial herniation. Postmortem specimens from patients who have sustained prolonged herniation have shown that the compression and displacement of the brainstem result in tegmental hemorrhagic lesions.

Infratentorial lesions

Two types of posterior fossa lesion (infratentorial lesions) cause unconsciousness: destructive lesions that directly destroy the reticular activating system in the brainstem tegmentum and expanding lesions that compress the brainstem or CSF pathways.

In destructive lesions there is a rapid loss of consciousness occurring simultaneously with signs of midbrain or pontine dysfunction. Brainstem infarction caused by basilar artery thrombosis and pontine hemorrhage are the most common pathologic conditions destroying the brainstem tegmentum.

Expansive lesions, or mass lesions, produce a disturbance of consciousness either by directly compressing the brainstem or by blocking CSF flow through the fourth ventricle and thereby producing acute hydrocephalus. Cerebellar hemorrhage, infarction, tumor, and abscess account for the majority of these cases.

Metabolic encephalopathies

Metabolic encephalopathies, diffuse disturbances of neuronal function, occur when the substrates required for neuronal energy metabolism are in short supply, when the internal environment of the cell is disturbed by external agents such as drugs or environmental poisons, or as a complication of the failure of another organ system such as the kidneys, the liver, or the endocrine, cardiovascular, or respiratory system.

Metabolic encephalopathy is the most common cause of decreased consciousness and accounts in any large hospital for more than half of the patients with coma of unknown origin. The metabolic causes of unconsciousness are listed in Table 140-2.

When the metabolic impairment is mild, the onset of symptoms can be insidious and nonspecific. Subtle changes in mentation such as decreased attention span, mild drowsiness, dullness of affect, and decreased motor coordination precede for variable periods of time the more overt pathologic picture of an advanced metabolic impairment. As neuronal dysfunction progresses, confusion, disorientation, and perceptual distortions such as illusions, delusions, or hallucinations, accompanied by combativeness and agitation, may dominate the clinical picture for a prolonged time or may be a short prelude to a more severe impairment of consciousness.

Motor phenomena such as coarse irregular tremor, asterixis, myoclonus, or seizures are usually seen during the course of the disease. There are often fluctuations of the level of consciousness, so that a patient who is at one moment confused and agitated may quiet down to a stuporous state for a variable period and then return spontaneously to psychomotor agitation.

Metabolic encephalopathy is generally characterized by an impairment of consciousness without signs of focal neurologic deficit. Nevertheless, exceptions exist. Focal signs suggestive of a structural lesion such as hemiparesis, aphasia, and focal seizures may occur in hypoglycemia. Hemiparesis, gaze palsies, and bilateral Babinski signs may be present transiently in hepatic failure. Signs of meningeal irritation, with CSF pleocytosis and focal seizures, can be seen in uremic encephalopathy. The opposite situation, in which focal or multifocal pathologic conditions behave clinically as diffuse brain disorders, is also important to remember in the differential diagnosis. Chronic subdural hematoma, frontal and temporal lobe tumors, fat embolism, systemic lupus erythematosus, cerebral malaria, and thrombotic thrombocytopenic purpura are examples of such a situation.

Elderly demented patients seem to be more susceptible to metabolic encephalopathies than younger patients with healthy brains and take longer to recover from them. In this respect the prolonged use of drugs, especially sedatives and analgesics, is of particular concern because it is one of the most common causes of such problems in these patients.

LABORATORY DATA IN THE DIAGNOSIS OF UNCONSCIOUSNESS

The basic battery of tests supplementing the clinical analysis of the history and physical examination consists of computed tomography (CT scans), EEG, and serum chemistry tests. The CT scan produces information about structural lesions in the supratentorial and infratentorial spaces and is the ideal test for diagnosing tumors, hematomas, hydrocephalus, cerebrovascular accidents, and brain swelling. Intrinsic brainstem lesions are still difficult to visualize with current techniques.

The EEG tests neuronal physiology and is therefore important in the diagnosis and follow-up of metabolic encephalopathies. Serum chemistry tests should cover the spectrum of biochemical abnormalities that may result from an organ system failure or fluid and electrolyte imbalance capable of impairing brain function.

Table 140-2. Metabolic causes of unconsciousness

General causes	Specific manifestations and drugs
Lack of energy substrate	Anoxia, hypoglycemia, decreased brain blood flow, deficient thiamine and niacin
Endogenous causes	
Organ system failure	Liver, kidney, lung, endocrine system
Fluid and electrolyte imbalance	Dehydration/water intoxication, hyponatremia/hypernatremia, hypomagnesemia/hypermagnesemia, hypocalcemia/hypercalcemia, acidosis/alkalosis
Toxic products or direct effect of infection	Sepsis, meningitis
Disturbance of temperature regulation	Hypothermia/hyperthermia
Exogenous causes	Sedative drugs, ethanol, anticholinergics, opiates, heavy metals, cyanide, methyl alcohol, ethylene glycol, organic phosphates

CSF examination is important when the differential diagnosis includes a central nervous system infection or a subarachnoid hemorrhage. Screening serum and urine for toxic agents becomes necessary in metabolic encephalopathies when suggested by the patient's history or when endogenous causes have been excluded.

Skull roentgenograms, isotope brain scans, or cerebral angiograms may become important in the diagnosis of coma if a CT scan is not available. Skull roentgenograms should be obtained in every case of craniofacial trauma.

BIBLIOGRAPHY

Fisher, C.M.: The neurological examination of the comatose patient, Acta Neurol. Scand. **45**(suppl. 36):1, 1969.

Plum, F., and Posner, J.: The diagnosis of stupor and coma, ed. 2, Philadelphia, 1972, F.A. Davis Co.

141 • SLEEP DISORDERS

Leopold Canales

The physiology of the human nervous system demands a period of sleep lasting 5 to 8 hours every 24 hours. Roughly speaking, we spend one third of our lives asleep. Until about 50 years ago sleep was assumed to be a period of cerebral rest, simple and homogeneous. The development of the electroencephalogram (EEG) as a clinical tool gave the first indication that cerebral function during sleep was active and multivariable.

From the EEG point of view there are basically two types of sleep: rapid eye movement (REM) and non-REM. In REM sleep, in addition to low-voltage fast cerebral activity, there are extremely low muscle tone, variations in the heart and respiratory rates, penile erection, dreaming, and of course rapid eye movements. REM sleep occurs in periods lasting 5 minutes to 1 hour. The first period is usually the shortest and does not occur until 70 to 90 minutes after the onset of sleep.

Non-REM sleep is characterized by three stages of the progressive slowing of cerebral frequencies, with low-voltage fast activity in light sleep or stage 1, the presence of bursts of 12 to 14 cps (Hz) activity (sleep spindles) and slow negative deflections followed by positive deflections (K complexes) in stage 2, and slow high-amplitude waves in stages 3 and 4, also called delta sleep.

Current concepts about the neurologic basis of sleep indicate that it is the result of the interaction between the wake system (reticular activating system) and the sleep circuitry. The anatomic and biochemical basis of sleep circuitry has not been completely elucidated, but structures such as the serotonergic nuclei of the pontine raphe, the medial forebrain area, and the nucleus ceruleus and gigantocellular tegmental field in the pons seem certain to be components.

A recent diagnostic classification formulated by the Association of Sleep Disorders Centers lists more than 60 separate disorders of sleep and arousal. In general, sleep disorders can be divided into the disorders of excessive daytime sleepiness (DOES) and the disorders of initiating and maintaining sleep (DIMS) or the insomnias.

The physician may have difficulty distinguishing DOES from the transient sleepiness that a patient may experience following a sleepless night. Excessive daytime sleepiness does, however, differ from the transient states in its duration, intensity, and inappropriateness. DOES may seriously affect the patient's ability to work and function normally in society. These disorders can be assessed by the patient's history and by polysomnography (all-night and occasional daytime monitoring of various physiologic parameters such as EEG, eye movement, and respiration). The two most common disorders of excessive daytime sleepiness are narcolepsy and the hypersomnia–sleep apnea syndrome.

Classic narcolepsy includes the following tetrad:

1. *Sleep attacks.* Along with chronic drowsiness, frequent attacks of sleep lasting from 10 minutes to 2 hours occur during the daytime.
2. *Cataplexy.* Episodic paralysis of voluntary muscle activity of sudden onset is triggered by emotional states (laughing, crying, or excitement) and lasts a few seconds to a few minutes.
3. *Hypnagogic hallucinations.* Vivid dreams occur when the patient is falling asleep but while he is still aware.
4. *Sleep paralysis.* With the exception of the eye and respiratory muscles, the patient feels paralyzed when falling asleep or on awakening; this lasts from a few seconds to several minutes.

Unlike normal subjects, narcoleptic patients may enter a REM period immediately at sleep onset, and despite their chronic drowsiness, their nocturnal sleep is often fragmented and poor. Symptoms usually appear in the second decade of life. Relatives of narcoleptics have a significantly greater risk of having the disease than individuals in the general population.

The treatment available is not completely satisfactory. Stimulants are used to control drowsiness. Pemoline is the preferred medication and may be administered in a dosage of 18.75 to 112.5 mg a day. Methylphenidate (5 to 60 mg a day) and less often dextroamphetamine (5 to 60 mg a day) may be tried. Cataplexy may be treated with imipramine (25 to 100 mg a day or in individual doses as needed).

Sleep apneas are episodes in which the patient stops breathing during sleep. The apnea may last up to 3 minutes and is terminated by an arousal that the patient may or may not remember. This pattern may recur during the entire night, or episodes may recur for only minutes to hours and alternate with normal sleep. In severe cases, in addition to chronic daytime drowsiness, essential hypertension and cardiac arrhythmias may develop. Most cases of sleep apnea syndrome are caused by upper airway obstruction in men who tend to be obese and heavy snorers. Weight reduction has helped some patients, but when it fails and the problem is severe, tracheostomy may be necessary. Less often sleep apnea may be caused by lesions in the central nervous system (for example, in the cervical spinal cord). In this case upper airway obstruction is not present.

In Kleine-Levin syndrome a periodic excessive sleepiness is accompanied by increased sexual and food appetites in young men. This rare syndrome tends to disappear with age.

There are many causes of insomnia (DIMS), which is a symptom rather than a disease. Among the common causes are drug dependence, poor sleep habits and scheduling problems, and emotional problems. Iatrogenic sleep disorders, such as the severe insomnia caused by the habitual use of hypnotics, may occur. The typical situation is a temporary disturbance of sleep treated with hypnotics that continue to be carelessly prescribed for months or years until natural sleep becomes impossible. Individuals who keep irregular hours, work on varying shifts, or travel across time zones may find it difficult to sleep during their desired bedtime.

Poor sleep is a well-known sign of depression. Early morning awakening and difficulty falling asleep are the common patterns. Early REM periods have been described in primary depression. Patients with nocturnal myoclonus often have difficulty initiating sleep.

An additional category of sleep disorder is the parasomnias. These include phenomena such as sleepwalking, sleep-talking, bedwetting, nightmares, and nocturnal seizures.

BIBLIOGRAPHY

Kales, A., and Kales, J.A.: Sleep disorders: recent findings in the diagnosis and treatment of disturbed sleep, N. Engl. J. Med. **290**:487, 1974.

Roffwaig, H.P., Chairman, Sleep Disorders Classification Committee, Association of Sleep Disorders Centers: Diagnostic classification of sleep and arousal disorders, Sleep **2**:1, 1979.

Zarcone, V.: Narcolepsy, N. Engl. J. Med. **288**:1156, 1973.

142 • DISORDERS OF COGNITION

Leopold Canales

The study of cognitive disorders has been historically based on clinical descriptions of abnormal behavior associated with brain lesions. In general, when the predominant feature is a failure to identify or recognize a stimulus, the syndrome is called *agnosia,* and when there is a failure to execute a response (in the absence of paralysis), it is called *apraxia.* Disorders of language production and comprehension are called *aphasias,* and disorders of memory are known as *amnesias.*

A sizable body of literature has accumulated over the years producing conflict and controversy in the classification, anatomic correlation, and inferred pathophysiology of the cognitive dysfunctions. At the core of the problem is our ignorance of the pertinent normal anatomic structures and physiologic mechanisms involved. Without such knowledge, the various definitions, classifications, and anatomic inferences are made in a vacuum and often turn out to be incomplete and inaccurate. The problem is compounded because some forms of human behavior such as language are highly complex, and when they disintegrate, the remnants left are so intricate that they easily conform to almost any form of classification.

In searching for a useful conceptual tool to help understand the clinical literature, it is best to look for the most basic common denominator of brain function and to evaluate it in both the normal state and the clinical syndrome. The nervous system is clearly concerned with processing information. Anatomically, the great development of the cerebral hemispheres is the most striking phylogenetic feature differentiating the human brain from the brains of other mammals. This development is based primarily on the increase in the area occupied by the association cortex and its connections. The human brain therefore possesses additional machinery that enables it to process information quantitatively and qualitatively better than any other comparable nervous system. We can also assume that damage to the hemispheres would result in syndromes that in one way or another would be failures of information processing.

To use information processing as a conceptual tool requires a correlation between our knowledge of anatomy and physiology and a general model of human information processing. This correlation is unavoidably tentative because of the need to generalize about complex mechanisms that at present cannot be defined more precisely and because of our modest knowledge of the anatomy and physiology of the different sensory channels. In recent years knowledge about information processing by the visual cortex has become available, and there are indications that the same type of processing occurs in other sensory modalities.

The basic premises of the model can be summarized as follows: each sensory modality undergoes some degree of processing before entering the pool of multimodal information; this pool is integrated in different ways by special areas of the association cortex, leading to unique forms of behavior (Fig. 142-1).

INFORMATION PROCESSING AND FOCAL HEMISPHERIC LESIONS

Different types of environmental energy are constantly stimulating our peripheral receptors. The transduction of

INFORMATION PROCESSING OPERATIONS

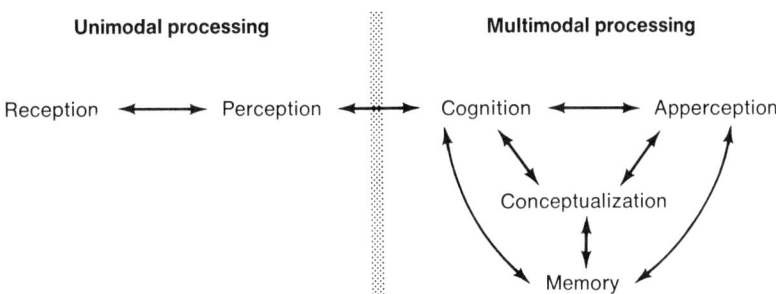

Fig. 142-1. Model for information processing. Each sensory modality undergoes some degree of unimodal processing before entering the pool of multimodal information, which is integrated by special areas of the association cortex.

energy taking place at the receptor area (for example, in the retina and cochlea) generates a signal that contains all the information of the modality at a given moment. This operation, called *reception,* constitutes the first step of the information processing model. Lesions at this point produce unimodal and primary deficits. The lesion affects only one sensory modality, destroying raw information (for example, a complete lesion destroys all information, producing blindness or deafness).

From the receptor area the information is transported to the primary receptive cortex of each modality via thalamic nuclei that are also modality specific. This anatomic arrangement is common to most sensory channels. Once the information reaches the primary receptive cortex, it travels to the immediately adjacent cortical regions, called the association cortex. In the primary and association cortices the raw information begins to be analyzed and organized into familiar patterns by feature detection mechanisms. This constitutes the second operation of sensory processing, called *perception.* Lesions limited to these cortical regions are very rare; the few cases reported have been caused by carbon monoxide poisoning or anoxia. These cases are forms of visual agnosia in which, in the presence of good visual acuity and intact visual fields, the patient is unable to identify or copy objects.

In the association cortex the information travels via subcortical fibers to the nonspecific thalamic nuclei, to other association cortical regions and limbic structures ipsilaterally, and via commissural fibers to the homotopic cortex in the contralateral hemisphere. In the association cortex and its connections the unimodal information coming from the primary receptive cortices is integrated and further elaborated into multimodal levels. In this process, called *gnosis* or *cognition,* perceptions are identified and classified on the basis of past experience (recognition) or by association with other simultaneous perceptions along other sensory modalities (cross-modality reference).

Discrete lesions of the association cortex or its connecting fibers result in disconnection syndromes. Many types of agnosias and apraxias are easily explained by this mechanism. Alexia without agraphia and color anomia results from a combined lesion of the left occipital cortex and the splenium of the corpus callosum. Surgical section of the corpus callosum results in an "aphasic right hemisphere" (alexia and anomia in the left visual field and apraxia and tactile anomia in the left hand). In visual association agnosia the patient can copy drawings without difficulty but is unable to identify them. In visual object agnosia the patient has an inability to name objects that can be described in detail and can be identified when touched. Both visual association agnosia and visual object agnosia suggest a disconnection between the visual and language centers.

The extraction of information from the multimodal pool progresses in the human brain through the operations performed by three special areas of multimodal convergence: the parietal, language-processing, and prefrontal cortices.

Based on visual and somesthetic information, the parietal cortex is able to abstract the *concepts* of self-image (somatognosia) and external space. Arithmetical calculation, the sensing of volume and shape (stereognosis), the sensing of weight (barognosis), and the ability to read and write are also made possible by the capacity of the parietal cortex to codify, abstract, and integrate information into conceptual levels.

Lesions of the parietal cortex produce syndromes that represent the conceptual loss of self-image, external space, and their relationship. Neglect of the contralateral space or of the limbs, spatial disorientation, right versus left confusion, dressing apraxias, constructional apraxias, and astereognosis are the predominant features of right-sided lesions. Alexia, agraphia, acalculia, and finger agnosia are more commonly seen with left-sided lesions.

The language-processing cortex is located at the convergence of the temporal, parietal, and frontal regions and is in the left hemisphere in most people. This area of the association cortex with its connections is able to encode cognitive and affective information into a system of symbols called verbal language and is also able to produce the reverse process of decoding verbal language into cognitions and emotions. This process of codifying information provides the brain with an extraordinary capacity to receive, extract, store, and transmit vast amounts of information that would be otherwise inaccessible. The operations possible with the use of this code (including abstraction, association, synthesis, induction, and deduction) result in what is called the *verbal conceptual* level of information processing. It occupies the major portion of mentation and has become the most important mental instrument to interpret the environment.

Damage to the language-processing cortex results in syndromes called aphasias. If the lesion affects the posterior aspect of this area, the patient's difficulty is primarily with the decoding process (an inability to understand spoken and written language). It includes the patient's inability to repeat when the lesion includes the posterior region of the superior temporal gyrus or Wernicke's area (Wernicke's aphasia). Lesions situated in the anterior aspect, toward the posterior and inferior portions of the frontal lobe, result in difficulty or inability to encode language (Braca's aphasia) with a difficulty in verbal expression. Subcortical lesions between the temporal and frontal lobes can produce difficulty in repeating on command even when the patient has good comprehension and fluent production of language (conduction aphasia).

Another special area of multimodal convergence is the prefrontal cortex. It is extensively connected with the rest of the cortex and the limbic system, which suggests that its function deals with the interface between cognition and emotion. In general the prefrontal cortex seems to be concerned with integrating cognitive information and emotional needs, resulting in forms of behavior that produce the most adequate emotional response to a given environmental situation. From the clinical description of patients with bilateral lesions, it seems clear that these patients, suffer changes in their emotional reactions. The terms "witzelsucht" and "moria" have been used to describe the facetiousness and silly joking these patients often display. Changes in goal-oriented behavior are commonly prominent and are manifested as a lack of insight and foresight, a loss of the sense of what is socially appropriate, and a loss of ethical and esthetic values.

The next operation in information processing is *apperception*. This involves the choice of material to be brought from cognition and emotion into the stream of thought (mentation). Apperception also determines what information is to be incorporated as memories. Its anatomic and physiologic substrates represent the collective effort of cortical and limbic structures in addition to the diencephalic mechanisms that deal with arousal and attention. Damage to any of these structures impairs mentation in many different ways.

The last operation in information processing is *memory*. The ability to store and retrieve information is one of the most important features of human information processing. It is the basis of learned behavior because without it the nervous system would depend entirely on a limited repertoire of built-in responses (reflex behavior).

The anatomic structures that have so far been implicated in memory function are located mainly in the limbic system, suggesting a link between emotions and memory. Assuming a nervous system model in which emotions are the primary impulse for action, the learning process is directed to retaining data that produce emotional experiences intense enough to induce a motor response (pursuit or avoidance depending on the nature of the emotional experience). The learning process is demonstrated when the same response is repeated sooner in the same circumstances or with only a fraction of the original stimulus. Our conscious experience with memory processes clearly shows the vestiges of such a model. Data related to intense emotional situations enter our memory without difficulty and are not only easy to remember but often impossible to forget, whereas daily events with a minimum of emotional association escape our memory completely or are retained for only short periods. The purposeful use of memory, unrelated to emotional experience, requires laborious recruitment of attention, tedious repetition, and periodic rehearsal to prevent decay. Lesions of the hippocampi, fornices, mammillary bodies, dorsomedial nuclei of the thalamus, and temporal cortex have been associated in different degrees with amnestic syndromes. The most consistent evidence so far concerns lesions of the hippocampi; their bilateral excision produces the most severe and discrete amnestic syndrome sparing all other cognitive functions.

Memory can be clinically categorized and selectively affected in the following ways.

Immediate memory is the ability to retain data long enough to maintain a coherent thread of thought, to execute sequential tasks, or to perform mental calculation and digit span (repeating a series of digits after hearing them). Immediate memory can be maintained for several minutes if there is no distraction, even in some patients with bilateral hippocampal lesions or Korsakoff's syndrome. It is impaired in processes that decrease the attention span, such as metabolic encephalopathies and dementia.

Short-term memory is the ability to retain and retrieve data for more than a few minutes. Its loss represents the amnestic syndrome and can be produced by thiamine deficiency (Korsakoff's syndrome) or by bilateral hippocampal lesions; old memories and skills are retained, but new learning is impossible (anterograde amnesia). Transient forms of short-term memory defect have been described in cases of temporal lobe epilepsy or idiopathic transient global amnesia. Patients with the latter usually have difficulty recalling recent events before the attack (retrograde amnesia) in addition to having the memory defect during the attack. A unilateral hippocampal lesion on the left side may impair verbal recent memory, whereas a lesion on the right side may impair nonverbal memory.

Long-term memory is the ability to retain and retrieve data extending from events of a few months back to events of childhood. It is affected in the form of retrograde amnesia most commonly seen in cases of severe head injury; the defect rarely persists beyond a few months and tends to lessen with time.

In summary, focal lesions to the hemispheres produce clinical syndromes through the following deficits of information processing:

1. Deterioration of the signal through damage to the thalamocortical projections, producing deficits of primary sensation such as visual field defects or hypoesthesia
2. Perceptual disorders resulting from failure to complete the processing of unimodal information because of damage to the cortical extraction mechanisms
3. Disconnection syndromes resulting from failure of cross-modality referencing and multimodal processing because of lesions affecting connecting fibers (commissural or subcortical) or their neurons of origin
4. Inability to integrate multimodal information to a conceptual level because of damage to the special areas of multimodal convergence such as the parietal, language-processing, and prefrontal cortices
5. Inability to store or retrieve information because of damage to limbic structures or thalamic nuclei

These syndromes are seldom found in pure form because hemispheric lesions rarely remain limited to the cortex or to discrete connecting fibers. The most common syndrome is a mixture of these mechanisms, the result depending on the type and location of the lesion.

INFORMATION PROCESSING DEFICIT AND DIFFUSE HEMISPHERIC PATHOLOGY (DEMENTIA)

DEFINITION AND DIAGNOSIS. The impairment of all cognitive functions and learned behavior is called dementia. It can be caused by diffuse damage to the cortex or its connections or by one or several focal lesions large enough that the resulting cognitive loss severely impairs general behavior and cannot be compensated for by the remaining healthy tissue. Dementia is a common and nonspecific clinical syndrome that can result from any of the pathologic processes known to affect the central nervous system.

It is estimated that dementia is severe enough in about 5% of the population over 65 years of age to render them unable to cope with the activities of daily living. It is the most common reason for needing nursing home care. Alzheimer's disease, its most common cause, currently has no specific treatment. Dementia is expected to increase in prevalence as the older segment of the population increases. For many years the classification of dementia has included a division between senile and presenile types. This is unjustified because no specific clinical or pathologic characteristics exist to differentiate dementias starting before or after 65 years of age.

Because many different causes of dementia exist, there may be variations in the chronology of the evolution and in the neurologic signs accompanying the cognitive impairment. Clinically, generalized cognitive and behavior deterioration is manifest in the neurologic examination as an impairment of data processing (a decrease in memory, abstraction, and attention span) and as an inappropriate response to the environment (impaired judgment and affect). The physician tests these parameters first while taking the history. The patient's ability to maintain a coherent thread of thought, his attention span, and the information content of his language give the physician a general idea of his intellectual capacity. In direct mental testing every parameter should be tested in progressive degrees of complexity; it is always important to test attention span and language function first because they are the main factors limiting the degree of complexity possible in the rest of the neurologic examination. The physician should test attention using well-memorized series repeated forward and backward in escalating degrees of difficulty (counting from 1 to 10, naming the days of the week and months of the year, and then subtracting serial sevens). Memory can be tested by asking the patient to repeat three items several minutes later or to retell immediately a simple but detailed story. Abstraction is tested by asking the patient to interpret the similarities between proverbs and their meaning. The evaluation of judgment and affect is best obtained from relatives and co-workers. The remainder of the neurologic examination may show severe deficits of cortical function involving visuospatial tasks, body scheme, apraxias, and agnosias of different kinds.

Motor testing is of great interest because the findings point to a process of disintegration of function that reverses ontogenic development. Infants react to the environment reflexly. Stimulating the lips or circumoral region causes the infant to pursue the stimulus and to begin sucking. Stimulating the palmar surfaces of the hands and feet causes grasping, dorsiflexion of the foot elicits a stepping reaction, and stroking the thenar eminence produces contraction of the mentalis muscle. In infancy myelination of the hemispheres has not yet taken place, and therefore the command of motor behavior occurs mainly at the diencephalic, limbic, and brainstem levels. With the progressive maturation of the nervous system, learned behavior replaces reflex behavior, culminating years later in mature individuals who have at their disposal an immense repertoire of responses. This process of learning has been preceded by the progressive myelination of the hemispheres that become incorporated in processing information and commanding motor behavior (cortication).

In a degenerative process such as Alzheimer's disease, which is characterized by progressive cortical neuronal loss, the cerebral hemispheres begin to lose their role in behavior (decortication), sending the command back to the diencephalic and brainstem reflex levels. The reappearance of infantile reflexes and findings of motor impersistence, perseveration, and generalized hyperreflexia are classic in advanced dementia. In the end state of motor deterioration the patient returns to the fetal position (pelvicrural contraction).

ALZHEIMER'S DISEASE. Alzheimer's disease, characterized pathologically by neuronal loss, senile plaques, and neurofibrillary tangles, affects primarily the association cortex and hippocampi and in some series accounts for up to 55% of cases of dementia. The early manifestations of Alzheimer's disease can be quite insidious and more obvious to relatives and co-workers than to the physician examining the patient for the first time or to the patient himself. The account by an observant relative, familiar with the patient's emotional and intellectual characteristics, will point to a subtle but progressive personality change. Negative personality traits, which in an unaffected person are kept in bounds because of good judgment, begin to express themselves more overtly at the same time that positive aspects of the personality begin to diminish. Suspiciousness may turn into paranoia, assertiveness into belligerence, and tenaciousness into stubbornness, and intellectual drive, a sense of humor, and subtlety of observation begin to be lost. At this point the patient may be aware of his inability to cope with the environment as effectively as before; consequently, in up to 25% of these patients a mild reactive depression develops.

As the disease progresses, the abnormalities of behavior become more obvious. Relatives become increasingly aware of the patient's unreliability in handling money, conveying messages, and making decisions. Accidents resulting from carelessness begin to occur at home or at work, and the patient's social life and outside interests are greatly reduced or become nonexistent. Disorientation in space progresses so that the patient is easily lost when away from home, and the conversation is reduced to clichés and formula courtesies. At this point the diagnosis of dementia is obvious with mental testing, and other signs of dysfunction are usually present during the neurologic examination.

A more advanced state of Alzheimer's disease renders the patient unable to perform activities of daily living. The patient has to be dressed, bathed, and fed. Sphincter control disappears, and apathy and mutism ensue. The patient may spend the whole day sitting in a chair staring at the walls, and motor behavior is reduced to occasional clumsy attempts to stand up.

OTHER CAUSES OF DEMENTIA. Among other disorders that cause dementia are mass lesions such as tumors or chronic subdural hematomas, the spongiform encephalopathies such as Creutzfeldt-Jakob disease, Pick's disease, Huntington's chorea, parkinsonism (see Chapter 150), progressive supranuclear palsy, Hallervorden-Spatz disease, normal pressure hydrocephalus, dementia paralytica caused by syphilis or other chronic central nervous system infections (see Chapter 51), subacute sclerosing panencephalitis (see Chapter 151), and a variety of storage diseases and leukodystrophies in childhood (see Chapters 148 and 195). A variety of toxic and metabolic derangements such as those induced by drug ingestion, hypothyroidism, hypercalcemia, and vitamin B_{12} deficiency may result in impaired mentation. Vascular disease may cause dementia when multifocal infarcts or lacunes are present. Other diseases with multifocal lesions such as multiple sclerosis and progressive multifocal leukoencephalopathy can produce a decline in intellect. The following are selected causes of dementia.

Creutzfeldt-Jakob disease. Although the spongiform encephalopathy Creutzfeldt-Jakob disease accounts for a very small number of cases of dementia, it has become the subject of much attention recently since its infectious origin as a slow virus was demonstrated in 1969. It is characterized by dementia, myoclonic jerks, rigidity, cerebellar incoordination, and occasionally motor neuron disease. The course of the illness is relatively rapid; the average duration is 15 months, although some patients have survived up to 6 years. It is characterized by diffuse neuronal loss in the cortex, basal ganglia, and cerebellum. The treatment is symptomatic. Because of the possibility of contagion, caution is advised in handling tissues and cerebrospinal fluid (CSF) from both patients and contaminated instruments.

Pick's disease. Pick's disease is a rare cause of dementia. Its course is progressive and lasts from 2 to 15 years. Pathologically, atrophy of the frontal and temporal cortices is prominent, the parietal cortex is less involved, and the occipital lobes are usually spared. Pick's disease is clinically indistinguishable from Alzheimer's disease. The treatment is symptomatic.

Huntington's chorea. Huntington's chorea is a degenerative hereditary disorder characterized by choreic movements and progressive dementia. Symptoms begin around the fourth decade of life, although there is a range from 15 to 65 years of age. Sporadic cases have been found, but its transmission is almost exclusively in a dominant hereditary pattern. Pathologically there is atrophy of the caudate nucleus and the cerebral cortex. Less prominent degenerative changes are also found in other subcortical gray structures. No specific treatment for this condition exists, but choreic movements have been lessened by using reserpine, phenothiazines, or haloperidol.

Progressive supranuclear palsy. Progressive supranuclear palsy is a degenerative disorder that begins late in life and is characterized clinically by supranuclear ophthalmoplegia, pseudobulbar palsy, and axial dystonia. Mild dementia may also be present. L-Dopa may produce some improvement.

Hallervorden-Spatz disease. Hallervorden-Spatz disease is a recessively inherited disorder characterized by deposits of iron in the basal ganglia. It produces neuronal degeneration affecting primarily the red nucleus, globus pallidus, and substantia nigra. Rigidity, dystonia, choreoathetosis, spasticity, and progressive dementia are all present. The onset is in late childhood, and the treatment is symptomatic.

Normal pressure hydrocephalus. Normal pressure hydrocephalus (NPH) is a rare but treatable cause of dementia. Besides its idiopathic origin, known causes include head trauma, subarachnoid hemorrhage, and meningitis. Progressive dementia, urinary incontinence, and gait apraxia accompany the dilatation of the ventricles, which probably results from the impairment of CSF flow through the subarachnoid space. The progressive dilatation of the ventricles accounts for the CSF pressure being maintained within normal limits. The most important diagnostic test is the computed tomographic (CT) scan, which shows severe dilatation of the entire ventricular system in the absence of cortical atrophy. Another important test is isotope cisternography, which studies the flow of radioactive-labeled substances in the subarachnoid space. In cases of NPH the radioactive material injected into the lumbar sac enters the ventricular system instead of flowing toward the cerebral convexities and concentrating along the sagittal sinus. Isotope retention in the ventricular system for more than 48 hours has been associated with a good prognosis for improvement with CSF shunting procedures.

MANAGEMENT. Because of the large number of diseases included in the differential diagnosis of dementia, it has been considered practical to direct clinical efforts to ruling out the treatable causes of dementia. Chronic central nervous system infections (lues and fungi), mass lesions (tumors and chronic subdural hematoma), chronic intoxication (sedatives), deficiency states (pellagra and vitamin B_{12} deficiency), hormonal dysfunction (of thyroid, parathyroid, and adrenal glands), and NPH should be investigated before assuming that an untreatable degenerative disorder is the cause.

LABORATORY FINDINGS. A CT scan of the head is imperative in the diagnosis of dementia. Hydrocephalus, brain atrophy, and mass lesions are easily demonstrated with this test. A lumbar puncture is essential to rule out infection, and serum chemistry tests can detect the other possible causes.

Depression in the elderly can produce manifestations of behavior that resemble dementia. In most cases the patient has a history of psychiatric care, and in some patients crying spells, sadness, and self-deprecatory statements may betray the underlying depression. In cases in which the diagnosis remains in doubt, a therapeutic trial with antidepressants is warranted.

BIBLIOGRAPHY

Brown, J.: Aphasia, apraxia, and agnosia, Springfield, Ill., 1974, Charles C Thomas, Publisher.

Hecaen, H., and Albert, M.: Human neuropsychology, New York, 1978, John Wiley & Sons, Inc.

Heilman, K., and Valanstein, E.: Clinical neuropsychology, New York, 1979, Oxford University Press.

143 • CENTRAL NERVOUS SYSTEM INTOXICATIONS

Paul L. Schraeder

The clinical practitioner is often confronted with patients having varying degrees of central nervous system (CNS) intoxication, ranging from mild isolated exposure to intoxicants to full-blown chronic drug abuse. Persons of all ages and social and educational levels are affected. The patient may also be taking more than one type of drug with combined toxicity, producing a more complicated problem such as when the toxicity of alcohol is enhanced with use of a sedative drug of the barbiturate or benzodiazepine group. Although self-inflicted CNS intoxications are common, all too often the patient's problems are a result of the physician's overreliance on the prescription pad as a substitute for empathic listening.

CNS DEPRESSANTS

The most commonly encountered CNS depressant is ethyl alcohol, although laymen widely believe that it is a CNS stimulant. Up to 7% of the adult population of the United States is estimated to have major alcohol-related problems. Symptoms of alcohol intoxication result in about 50% of those persons who achieve a blood alcohol level of 50 mg/dl or greater, although habitual imbibers have fewer signs of intoxication at this blood level. (A blood alcohol level above 400 mg/dl produces stupor or coma.) The widespread potential for alcohol abuse can be appreciated when one realizes that two thirds of the adult population in the United States use alcohol at least intermittently and that an increasingly higher percentage of alcoholics are in their teens. The common symptoms of adult alcohol intoxication are well known and include dysarthria, ataxia, and changes in behavior. With increasing blood alcohol levels, the generalized CNS depressant effect becomes increasingly manifested by impaired sensory, motor, and judgmental functions.

An uncommon but dramatic manifestation of alcohol ingestion is pathologic alcoholic intoxication. This violent and at times self-destructive state can be associated with hallucinations or delusional thinking and may be more likely to occur in persons with underlying psychopathologic conditions. In a susceptible person pathologic intoxication may result from ingesting a relatively modest amount of alcohol.

The withdrawal states that occur as the depressant effect of alcohol wears off are a major problem encountered among alcohol abusers. The most benign set of symptoms is the self-limited, morning-after hangover that includes irritability, malaise, slight tremulousness, and headache. If the person has been drinking heavily for several days or longer, a more severe state of tremulousness may occur. The patient has tremors that are often quite severe, with mental irritability, mild disorientation, insomnia, and autonomic symptoms including tachycardia, nausea, and vomiting. The symptoms usually subside after a few days but can take as long as 2 weeks to disappear.

Withdrawal seizures or "rum fits" occur 6 to 48 hours after the patient has had the last drink. One or more seizures can occur and are usually generalized; if any focal component is present, cerebral pathologic conditions are highly suspect. Anticonvulsants have no place in treating these seizures. Alcoholics are unreliable, take anticonvulsants irregularly, and commonly withdraw from alcohol and anticonvulsants simultaneously when treated with anticonvulsants, almost guaranteeing that they will have severe withdrawal seizures. It should be remembered, however, that alcohol withdrawal, even of a minimal degree, can aggravate an independent seizure disorder. A thoughtfully obtained, nonjudgmental medical history should easily clarify which patients also have seizures occurring independently of the withdrawal state. This important information can usually be obtained by asking the patient or the friends and family whether the patient has ever had seizures while abstaining from alcohol for extended periods. Likewise, a history of childhood seizures is very suggestive of an independent seizure disorder. To make a diagnosis of alcohol withdrawal seizure alone, it must be determined that the seizures occur only when the patient is withdrawing. Status epilepticus (continuous seizure activity) or two or more seizures occurring without a return of consciousness should be treated in the manner discussed in Chapter 145.

Delerium tremens, or the "DTs," is the most severe form of alcohol withdrawal. Delirium tremens may be mild or severe, with onset 1 to 4 days after the beginning of abstinence. Although not the usual case, this state may be preceded by one or more seizures. In the milder syndrome the patient is diaphoretic, confused, tremulous, fearful, and often has hallucinations. In the majority of cases the symptoms are more severe, manifested by frighteningly vivid auditory and visual hallucinations with prominent autonomic overactivity (including diaphoresis, tremulousness, and tachycardia). Without treatment the mortality is usually 5% to 15% but has been reported to be as high as 50%. A rare but dramatic withdrawal syndrome is alcoholic hallucinosis, in which auditory hallucinations are the major symptom, without tremulousness or clouding of consciousness. Repeated bouts of this syndrome may indicate an underlying schizophrenic state.

The treatment of the alcohol withdrawal state starts with the presumption that underlying intracranial disease is present. Cerebral trauma often precedes or accompanies the withdrawal state, and a subdural hematoma should be suspected. Likewise, CNS infection should be considered in the debilitated chronic alcoholic patient who has fever with confusion or seizures. The initial evaluation should include a computed tomographic (CT) scan. A lumbar puncture is indicated if there are symptoms of meningitis such as unexplained fever or nuchal stiffness. The parenteral administration of fluids is very important but must include vitamins, especially thiamine, from the very beginning, particularly if glucose solutions are given initially. The specific drug treatment of alcohol withdrawal is often the subject of heated discussion among knowledgeable professionals, but as a general rule drugs cross-tolerant (that is, producing a similar clinical response) with alcohol are best; these include benzodiazepines and paraldehyde. Phenothiazines should not be used in treating withdrawal because they are not cross-tolerant with alcohol and can aggravate a seizure diathesis. Barbiturates may cause excessive sedation and respiratory depression. As can be guessed, many drug regimens are used, but several studies have shown that modern drugs have minimal or no advantage over paraldehyde, which may be given in doses of 7.5 to 10 ml, either orally or as oil retention enemas every 4 hours. Parenteral administration of this drug is potentially hazardous because sterile abscesses can result from an intramuscular injection, and the presence in old vials of the breakdown product acetaldehyde, a metabolic poison, makes intravenous injection risky. In severe delirium tremens the successful treatment of withdrawal symptoms requires frequent doses of drugs, with such totals as 40 to 80 ml of paraldehyde or 400 to 500 mg of chlordiazepoxide being administered over the course of treatment. The most important aspect of drug treatment, however, is to choose a drug that works and to learn to use it safely and effectively.

The outpatient management of patients with suspected delirium tremens is to be discouraged because there is no way of determining the prognosis based on a cursory evaluation of early symptoms. Likewise, the physician should keep in mind that delirium tremens develops in one third of patients with withdrawal seizures, and these patients should be observed for at least 72 hours. Status epilepticus should be treated in the manner discussed in Chapter 145.

Because *methyl alcohol* is found occasionally in illegally produced alcoholic beverages, methyl alcohol poisoning deserves mention. This compound is oxidized to formic acid and formaldehyde, which produce delayed toxic manifestations. Severe acidosis and blindness may result, the blindness caused by retinal ganglion cell damage. The treatment consists primarily of giving bicarbonate intravenously, with hemodialysis reserved for severe poisoning.

Intoxication with depressant drugs other than ethanol is a major problem, in part brought on by the public expectation that medication can effect cures for all human ills, whether physical or emotional. Barbiturates are ubiquitous and consequently are responsible for a major proportion of intoxications. Acute intoxication with the shorter-acting barbiturates is more hazardous; the patient rapidly becomes comatose with relatively low blood levels (as low as 10 μg/ml). Long-acting drugs such as phenobarbital require higher blood levels (60 μg/ml) to produce coma, and consequently they take more time to achieve the same degree of CNS depression than with the shorter-acting barbiturates. The varying signs of acute barbiturate intoxication are similar to alcohol intoxication, ranging from minimal mental dysfunction, dysarthria, ataxia, and nystagmus to more severe depression and apnea. In the early differential diagnosis of drug intoxication, serum blood levels are very important. Likewise, the electroencephalogram (EEG) is sometimes useful as a diagnostic tool because mild degrees of intoxication result in very prominent fast (greater than 13 cps) beta activity, whereas more severe degrees of intoxication result in slower (1 to 3 cps) delta activity intermixed with the beta rhythm. Bilateral burst suppression patterns, that is, periodic complexes (repetitive waveforms) mixed with the absence of EEG waves, are often present on the EEG in severely intoxicated persons.

The treatment of acute barbiturate intoxication consists of maintaining respiration, using endotracheal intubation and artificial respiratory support if needed. Diuresis aided by alkalinization of the urine is the major means of ridding the body of barbiturates. Although hemodialysis is also effective, it is usually reserved for patients who have renal failure.

In persons withdrawing from chronic barbiturate abuse, prominent symptoms include tremulousness, insomnia, seizures, and a hallucinatory delirium similar to that in alcohol withdrawal. To suppress the symptoms, pentobarbital substitution is often used in doses to cause mild intoxication. Usually, 200 to 400 mg every 6 hours is sufficient to achieve stabilization; 1 to 2 days thereafter the pentobarbital is gradually withdrawn at a rate of 100 mg daily. Temporary increases in dosage may be needed to suppress symptoms during withdrawal.

Other depressants besides barbiturates are often the cause of CNS intoxication. Although once commonly used, bromides are now infrequently prescribed. Nonetheless, occasional intoxication cases appear as a result of abusing over-the-counter agents containing bromides. Chronic bromism can be manifested by confusion, memory problems, delirium, and, in severe cases, coma. Skin lesions, conjunctivitis, and gastritis are common. Blood bromide levels above 75 mg/dl are in the toxic range. A high sodium intake and diuretic treatment cause bromide excretion diuresis; hemodialysis is effective in severe cases of intoxication.

Benzodiazepines, including chlordiazepoxide, diazepam, and flurazepam, are among the most commonly abused CNS depressants. The symptoms of intoxication are nonspecific and include gait ataxia, drowsiness, slurred speech, and confusion. Other types of nonbenzodiazepine depressant drugs, including glutethimide and methaqualone, have similar clinical properties. Chronic abuse of most of the depressant drugs can result in the same symptoms on withdrawal as described with alcohol and the barbiturates; these symptoms require the same type of treatment. As in the withdrawal from alcohol, phenytoin is of little use in preventing the seizures that are often the early part of the abstinence syndrome. Phenothiazines should be avoided in any form of abstinence syndrome.

CNS STIMULANTS

The most commonly used CNS stimulant is caffeine. The average cup of coffee or tea contains 80 to 150 mg of the drug, and a 12-oz bottle of cola contains 35 to 50 mg. Caffeine counteracts fatigue and promotes wakefulness while producing clearer thinking and a better appreciation of sensory stimuli. Overdosage leads to insomnia, diuresis, tachycardia, and cardiac arrhythmias.

Amphetamines are commonly abused drugs. Although their mechanism of action is unclear, it appears that they may cause the release of norepinephrine from the brain. The CNS effects include stimulated alertness, diminished appetite, mood elevation, and increased motor and speech activity. Prolonged use results in a debt of wakefulness that must be paid off by a significant degree of fatigue and depression. The acute CNS toxic effects of amphetamines are exaggerations of the therapeutic effects and include arrhythmia, irritability, insomnia, and weakness. Confusion, anxiety, delirium, and even suicidal or homicidal tendencies can occur, particularly in persons predisposed to mental illness. The treatment of acute intoxication includes increasing urinary secretion by acidifying the urine with ammonium chloride in conjunction with chlorpromazine and antihypertensives. Chronic amphetamine intoxication results in many of the same symptoms found in acute intoxication. Profound weight loss and a paranoid psychosis, however, are also usually present. The intravenous use of amphetamines has been associated with the occurrence of autoimmune vasculitis and endocarditis.

Methylphenidate is structurally related to the amphetamines, having similar therapeutic and toxic properties. As with the amphetamines, the only valid clinical indications for its use are for the childhood hyperactivity syndrome and narcolepsy.

OTHER COMMONLY ABUSED DRUGS

The opiates and other analgesic drugs, cocaine, and various illegal compounds constitute other commonly abused drugs that have had a profound socioeconomic impact. Both compulsive drug use and physical dependence are widespread problems with which all groups of medical practitioners must deal. It is important that all prescriptions for potentially addicting drugs be written only after the physician thinks carefully about the specific needs of the patient. Opium derivatives must be used only when no other category of drug provides relief. A balance must be maintained between the need to relieve unnecessary suffering and the concern for prescribing a potentially addicting drug (for example, for a patient with a terminal malignancy).

The most common cause of drug-related deaths in the United States is acute opiate intoxication (for example, from heroin, morphine, or meperidine). The symptoms of opiate intoxication include respiratory depression, pinpoint pupils, hypothermia, hypotension, and bradycardia. Death results from acute respiratory failure. Pulmonary edema is commonly seen. A patient with the combination of coma, pinpoint pupils, and depressed respirations should prompt suspicion of acute opiate intoxication; another important and easily apparent clue is needle marks on the arm.

If the drug has been taken orally, the treatment starts with gastric intubation and aspiration, since opiates cause gastric retention. Because of the high risk of respiratory arrest, an endotracheal tube is needed along with respiratory support. The opiate antagonist naloxone (Narcan) should be given in a dose of 0.5 to 0.7 mg intravenously to improve spontaneous respirations. Subsequent intramuscular doses can be used as needed to maintain the response. Since many persons suffering from acute opiate intoxication are also habitual users of opiates, the patient must be observed for the precipitation of acute withdrawal symptoms.

Opiate addiction is a major public health problem. Various studies estimate that more than 500,000 heroin addicts live in the United States, with two thirds of these having used these drugs before 21 years of age. With repeated use increasingly larger doses are needed to produce the desired euphoria, so that in many cases massive doses are eventually tolerated. The severity of the abstinence symptoms is proportional to the daily dosage of the drug and the length of time the patient has been addicted. The abstinence symptoms are both purposive, that is, related to the environment and oriented toward obtaining more drugs, and nonpurposive, which includes uncontrolled symptoms and signs such as mydriasis, muscle twitching, gooseflesh, extreme restlessness, vomiting, diarrhea, and alternating feelings of hot and cold. The symptoms start at 8 to 16 hours after the last dose, peak at 2 to 3 days, and are usually gone within 1 to 1½ weeks. Although complete abstinence as a treatment is usually not life threatening as long as a sufficient fluid and electrolyte balance is maintained, modern withdrawal management includes an initial dose of methadone of 15 to 20 mg orally. Further maintenance doses are given at a ratio of 1 mg methadone for 4 mg of morphine, 2 mg of heroin, or 20 mg of meperidine, followed by a reduction of 20% of the total dose each day. After 10 days the withdrawal is usually complete. Avoiding further addiction at this time involves using daily methadone doses that block the euphoria of intravenously injected heroin. Neurologic complications of opiate addiction include transverse myelopathy, various types of neuropathies, acute myopathies, and CNS infections (meningitis and abscess). Some of these complications may be the result of contaminating agents mixed with the opiates.

After many years of being a relatively minor source of drug abuse, cocaine again is becoming much more widely used. The drug produces a euphoria often indistinguishable from that caused by amphetamines. With high doses increased CNS irritability, including seizures, appears. High body temperatures are a common symptom of cocaine intoxication, and signs of increased sympathetic activity are evident. Thus the symptoms of cocaine intoxication include restlessness, tachycardia, fever, mydriasis, delirium, convulsions, and finally respiratory arrest. The treatment involves intravenous administration of sedatives such as barbiturates or benzodiazepines.

Although a wide variety of other drugs show varying degrees of popularity with drug users, cannabis (marijuana) and lysergic acid diethylamide (LSD or "acid") are the best known. The active agent in cannabis is tetrahydrocannabinol. The desired effect is a feeling of euphoria, relaxation, and sleepiness. A sense of unreality about self is also reported, along with more vivid sensory perceptions and altered time perception. High doses produce a toxic psychosis. The so-called hard drug effect of hallucinogenic agents such as LSD is typically described as a feeling of being a passive spectator to one's own experiences, which also acquire a unique meaning to that person. Visual illusions and hallucinations are common, and complex sensory and affective interactions frequently occur. Auditory hallucinations, however, are rare. A common adverse reaction is the so-called bad trip or panic response. Flashbacks, or recurrences of drug effects previously experienced, are common. The treatment for these phenomena is sedation, using agents such as diazepam, and talking down the patient. Habitual use of LSD can result in a permanent psychosis.

In recent years phencyclidine (PCP, or "angel dust") has become a major illegal drug. It is used as a veterinary anesthetic and is related to the commonly used human anesthetic ketamine. Its psychotomimetic effects preclude its legal use in humans. Phencyclidine can be taken orally or smoked. The symptoms and signs of phencyclidine intoxication include nystagmus, hypertension, tachycardia, flushing, sweating, ataxia, and CNS depression. Abnormal meiosis is a variable finding. Patients exhibit a dramatic variation between hyperactivity resembling mania and hypoactivity resembling catatonia. Complex bizarre behavior is also commonly seen. Laryngeal stridor, seizures, and renal failure may occur with overdosage. In contrast to LSD, hallucinations are uncommon. Phencyclidine intoxication must be suspected in any young person with an acute psychosis and hypertension. The treatment includes gastric lavage and increasing urinary excretion by acidifying the urine with ascorbic acid or ammonium chloride. Treatment with phenothiazines tends to lower the blood pressure too precipitously, but diazepam or haloperidol therapy may be useful. In mild intoxication a dark, quiet environment is sufficient treatment. As with any illegal drug use, patients often take mixtures of several drugs, making a diagnosis of any particular drug as the cause of the patient's symptoms a difficult task.

NEUROLOGIC EFFECTS OF COMMONLY PRESCRIBED DRUGS

This section describes the various CNS and peripheral nervous system complications that may be seen with drugs in the phenothiazine, antidepressant, antibiotic, antituberculous, steroid, and antimetabolite groups.

Phenothiazines are indicated for various psychoses, but they are commonly and inappropriately used in treating less severe symptoms such as anxiety. The major neurologic side effects are extrapyramidal. Typical symptoms of parkinsonism may be seen, including rigidity, tremor, masked faces, and bradykinesia. Various types of extrapyramidal symptoms and dyskinetic symptoms are common in sensitive persons after only one dose of a phenothiazine, but they usually respond quickly to intravenous administration of 25 to 50 mg of diphenhydramine (Benadryl). Unfortunately, the most chronic movement disorder, tardive dyskinesia (continuous facial, lip, and chewing movements as a result of long-term phenothiazine use), is not responsive to therapy. It must also be remembered that phenothiazines tend to lower the seizure threshold. Anticholinergic drugs diminish the parkinsonian symptoms but may increase the tardive dyskinesia.

The antidepressant drugs most commonly used today are in ths tricyclic group (for example, imipramine, amitriptyline, and desipramine). The neurologic side effects of these drugs are of a wide variety. A fine tremor is common in 1 out of 10 patient. As with phenothiazines, elements of parkinsonian symptoms can also be found. Likewise, generalized major motor seizures have been reported to follow high doses of these drugs. In severe poisoning, hyperpyrexia, elevated blood pressure, choreoathetosis, delirium, and seizures can ocur. The treatment for overdosage is intravenous physostigmine to reverse these CNS anticholinergic symptoms. Propranolol and lidocaine may be needed to control cardiac arrhythmias.

Another commonly used drug is lithium carbonate, which is very important in treating manic depressive illness. At therapeutic levels of 0.9 to 1.4 mEq/L neurologic symptoms such as ataxia, slurred speech, and fine tremor appear. Higher levels result in more severe manifestations such as impairment of consciousness or even coma, severe tremor, hyperreflexia, fasciculations, and convulsions. The treatment involves diuresis, intravenous administration of sodium bicarbonate, and in severe cases dialysis.

The atropine group of drugs can produce delirium, as can any agent with major anticholinergic effects (for example, phenothiazines, antidepressants, and antiparkinsonian agents). With increasing dosages they can also produce memory loss and visual hallucinations. Older patients seem to be more susceptible to these symptoms, and for such patients any of these drugs should be used cautiously. Physostigmine is used to treat anticholinergic overdose.

Peripheral polyneuropathies can be caused by many different drugs. In the past, before the concurrent use of pyridoxine (vitamin B_6), using isoniazid to treat tuberculosis commonly resulted in the appearance of a neuropathy after several months. This neuropathy was thought to result from interference with the production of pyridoxal phosphate. Nitrofurantoin, a drug commonly used to treat urinary tract infections, also can produce peripheral neuropathy after several weeks of use. In both instances the earliest symptoms are paresthesias of the feet, followed by an increasing diffuse sensory loss, primarily in the lower extremities, along with increasing weakness and loss of deep tendon reflexes. Other common drug-related polyneuropathies are produced by disulfiram and vincristine.

Corticosteroids are implicated as the cause of several types of neurologic symptoms. Pseudotumor cerebri (increased intracranial pressure not caused by structural disease) is an uncommon but well-established reaction to withdrawal from these compounds. A myopathy, with the usual emphasis on proximal limb weakness, can be seen in patients undergoing long-term, high-dose corticosteroid therapy. Even with withdrawal, this weakness resulting from muscle dysfunction may persist. In addition, these compounds commonly produce psychiatric symptoms such as depression or psychosis of a schizophrenic type.

BIBLIOGRAPHY

Adams, R.D., and Victor, M.: Principles of neurology, New York, 1977, McGraw-Hill Book Co.

Goodman, L.S., and Gilman, A., editors: The pharmacological basis of therapeutics, ed. 5, New York, 1975, MacMillan, Inc.

Kissin, B., and Bigleitto, H.: The biology of alcoholism. Vol. 2, Physiology and behavior, New York, 1972, Plenum Publishing Corp.

Kissin, B., and Bigleitto, H.: The biology of alcoholism. Vol. 3, Clinical pathology, New York, 1972, Plenum Publishing Corp.

Kissin, B., Lowinson, J.H., and Millman, R.B., editors: Recent developments in chemotherapy of narcotic addiction, Ann. N.Y. Acad. Sci. **311:**1, 1978.

144 • SYNCOPE

Paul L. Schraeder

Syncope, or fainting, refers to an impairment of consciousness with an associated loss of postural tone. Although syncope is one of the most common symptoms encountered by the physician, patients often considerably confuse terms when attempting to describe their symptoms. Patients often describe dizziness, light-headedness, unsteadiness, and other ill-defined feelings of weakness as fainting spells. One of the common yet difficult differentiations to make is between fainting and seizures. In making this differentiation, no series of laboratory tests is as important as a carefully taken history. Because the patient may poorly recall what happened, the sequence of events as related by friends or family usually is very important in helping the physician to determine the cause of the patient's symptoms.

Syncope of whatever cause usually is preceded by symptoms of varying duration. Commonly, feelings of light-headedness are accompanied by sweating, pallor nausea, impaired vision, and an inability to think. The patient with a seizure often receives no warning, or if there is a warning or an aura, the symptoms are more specific and quite stereotyped before each event. The patient with syncope often complains of palpitations before losing consciousness. Likewise, at the time of the event the patient may have an occasional convulsive jerk. These so-called syncopal seizures are not to be confused with a seizure disorder. Usually, as the patient assumes a recumbent posture, the symptoms rapidly abate because of an improvement of blood flow to ths brain. In contrast to the patient with a seizure who is often confused for varying periods after regaining consciousness, the patient with syncope rapidly resumes a fully alert state with no hint of confusion, lethargy, or headache.

The causes of fainting are divided into two broad categories. The cardiovascular category includes events that cause diffusely impaired cerebral blood flow because of changes in vascular resistance or a drop in cardiac output. The metabolic category encompasses causes such as hypoglycemia and hypoxia. The following are the most common etiologic factors in each category.

In the cardiovascular category the most common cause of fainting is vasovagal syncope, which usually occurs in healthy persons. Almost every physician can recall classmates who fainted when first confronted with venipuncture, illustrating that sudden, severe, emotional stress or pain can cause peripheral vasodilatation with a resulting drop in brain perfusion. Likewise, most people at one time or another have felt close to fainting in closed, hot, unventilated quarters. The patient with vasovagal syncope often is pale, sweaty, nauseated, and mildly short of breath before losing consciousness. Because of excessive vagal stimulation, the cardiac rate does not increase in compensation for the drop in blood pressure. Placing the patient in a recumbent position usually restores consciousness with no sequelae.

Micturition syncope is probably also related to excessive vagal reflex activity, occurring in males emptying an overfull bladder. This nonpathologic state, often unwitnessed, is commonly confused with a nocturnal seizure. The patient, however, may be able to relate a sequence of symptoms that are compatible with a rapidly progressive onset of faintness and with a rapid return of alertness after lying on the floor. In these circumstances head injury and some urinary incontinence may give the erroneous impression of a seizure.

Some patients have episodes of decreased cerebral perfusion because of postural hypotension. Often such persons are taking diuretics or antihypertensive medications and typically experience the rapid progression of symptoms associated with syncope when standing up quickly from a recumbent position. Also susceptible to postural hypotension are persons taking phenothiazine drugs or L-dopa. Diabetic patients commonly have an autonomic component as part of a peripheral polyneuropathy, with vasomotor instability on arising. It should be kept in mind, however, that many otherwise normal persons may suffer syncope if they arise too quickly from a prolonged state of recumbency. The diagnosis of postural hypotension usually can be suspected from the patient's history. The diagnosis is confirmed by having the patient lie supine for several minutes, taking a baseline blood pressure reading, and then having the patient stand up suddenly; the blood pressure determination is repeated several times. Any more than a minor transient drop in blood pressure is considered suspect, especially if the patient complains of appropriate symptoms in conjunction with a significant drop in pressure. The treatment consists of readjusting dosages of any offending medication, advising the patient to arise from a recumbent position gradually, and recommending that the patient wear supportive hose. In nonhypertensive patients, extra salt in the diet may raise intravascular volume.

Cardiac syncope most commonly results from an arrhythmia. Whether it is a form of bradycardia or tachycardia, the net result is impaired cerebral circulation. The best-known cause of cardiogenic syncope is Stokes-Adams syndrome resulting from a cardiac conduction block. In these patients ventricular standstill may last for several seconds with a very rapid onset of unconsciousness. Often there are a few clonic jerks, which are not to be confused with seizures. The episodes of syncope can occur several times daily and are unrelated to posture. It is important to obtain continuous 24-hour electrocardiographic monitoring for patients suspected of having Stokes-Adams syndrome.

Carotid sinus syncope is the result of an exaggerated normal response to stimulation, although in some instances no history suggestive of a sensitivity to carotid sinus stimulation can be obtained. In susceptible persons a very minor stimulus such as shaving over the sinus and tilting back or turning the head can result in an attack with a sudden loss of consciousness, falling, and some clonic motor activity. The unconsciousness lasts no more than a few minutes, with a complete return of alertness when consciousness returns. Three mechanisms are used to explain the syncope: (1) the vagal type of response, resulting in cardiac slowing of varying degrees; (2) the depressor type of response, resulting in a fall of arterial pressure without a change in heart rate; and (3) the central type of response, with an impairment of cerebral perfusion caused by carotid artery stenosis. The treatment is preventive, with efforts to remove offending stimuli such as tight collars. Atropine may occasionally be needed to prevent bradycardia, whereas sympathomimetic drugs such as ephedrine may be useful for persons susceptible to hypotensive episodes. Neither cardiac pacemakers nor carotid sinus denervation is usually needed, but they may produce dramatic results in severely affected persons. Finally, it should be kept in mind that frequently a carotid artery arteriosclerotic plaque may predispose a patient to hypersensitivity; in such instances too much pressure on the sinus may actually impair the blood supply to the brain.

Hypoglycemia is a common noncardiovascular cause of syncope or near-syncope. Usually, reactive hypoglycemia occurs 2 to 4 or more hours after eating a high-carbohydrate meal. The history is of a gradual onset of sweating, tremor, confusion, and often an urge to eat. Coma and seizures occur only when blood sugar levels are below 20 mg/dl. In such severe cases islet-cell pancreatic tumors, endocrinopathies of the pituitary-adrenal axis, or excessive doses of exogenous insulin in diabetic patients should be considered as possible causes. The diagnosis, as always, hinges on a good history, especially in the patient with reactive hypoglycemia. The relationship of the syncope to meals is the most important point to seek, and the diagnosis can be confirmed with a glucose tolerance test. Treatment focuses on avoiding unusual glucose loads.

Hyperventilation syndrome can cause a faint feeling but uncommonly results in a complete loss of consciousness. Along with the causative anxiety, the patient complains of having a pounding in the chest. Patients may admit feeling short of breath when asked, but many times patients are unaware of any such feeling even when the question is emphasized. Associated symptoms include paresthesias of the fingers and the perioral area. Hyperventilation results in hypocapnia, with concomitant cerebral vasoconstriction and decreased cerebral blood flow. Transient systemic alkalosis may contribute to protein binding of calcium, with resultant peripheral nerve symptoms in the form of paresthesias and muscle spasms. The treatment consists of telling the patient to breathe into a paper bag or voluntarily inhibiting the respiratory rate to rapidly elevate the carbon dioxide pressure. Explaining the cause and mechanism of these often frightening symptoms to the patient usually is sufficient to provide relief. In cases of severe recurrent anxiety and hyperventilation, however, psychotherapy is indicated.

BIBLIOGRAPHY

Adams, R.P., and Victor, M.: Principles of neurology, New York, 1977, McGraw-Hill Book Co.

145 • EPILEPSY (SEIZURE DISORDERS)

Paul L. Schraeder

DEFINITION. A seizure is an uncontrolled paroxysmal discharge of the central nervous system that interferes with normal function; epilepsy is a term used to denote the repeated occurrence of any of the various forms of seizures. A prodrome refers to the mood or behavior change that often precedes a seizure by hours or even days. An aura is the localized symptom that may be the first part of a seizure originating from a localized region of the cerebral cortex, but often it can occur without a clinical seizure following. Neither seizure nor epilepsy defines a disease state but rather is only a symptom of some underlying disease of the brain, whether structural, biochemical, or genetic. In many, if not the majority, of patients a concise mechanism cannot be defined. This uncertainty and lack of understanding contribute to the difficulty in management of these patients and to the negative attitudes toward epileptic persons that are frequently encountered.

Despite the relative ease of defining prodrome and aura on paper, it should be remembered that patients often cannot clearly describe what they have experienced. A reliable patient may only be able to say, "I just knew that I was going to have a seizure." Likewise, the amnesia commonly associated with the seizure often precludes an accurate description of the prelude to the seizure. Auras may be considered as minor, recurrent symptoms that stand alone, making them psychologically debilitating occurrences, since the patient can never be certain when the aura will proceed to a severe seizure. The aura acts as a pointer, indicating from which part of the brain the seizure originated.

CLASSIFICATION AND PATHOPHYSIOLOGY. The classification of epileptic seizures is of much more than academic importance. Until a decade ago seizures were listed as focal motor (jacksonian), psychomotor (temporal lobe), grand mal, and petit mal. As knowledge of the electroencephalographic (EEG) and clinical manifestations accumulated, it became evident that many observed phenomena did not fit into these categories. Seizures originating in the temporal lobe also can be so complex as to escape recog-

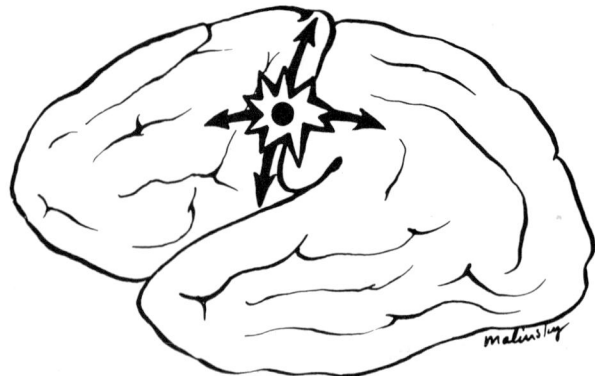

Fig. 145-1. Focal seizure involves spread of discharge over limited area of cerebral cortex.

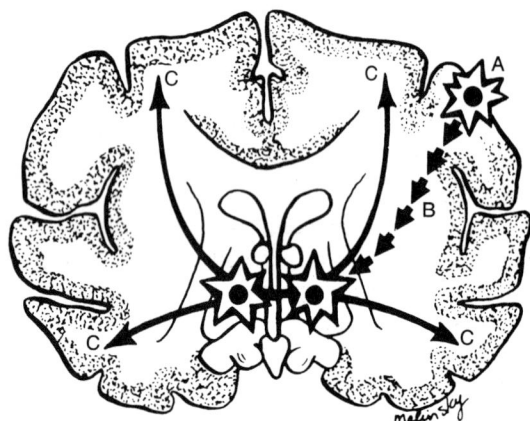

Fig. 145-2. *A* is cortical focus of epileptogenic discharge. *B* indicates spread of discharge to thalamus and reticular activating formation. *C* is secondary spread to both hemispheres, causing generalized seizure. *C* without *A* and *B* is what occurs in idiopathic epilepsy.

nition as a seizure by all but the most experienced observer. In the 1960s, a major effort was made by the International League Against Epilepsy to formulate a more rational and useful classification, based on both clinical and EEG observation of seizures of all types.

Before describing this classification further, it is important to consider the possible pathophysiologic nature of epilepsy, keeping in mind that the actual mechanisms of seizures are still unknown. Seizures may be focal or generalized or both. If a population of cortical neurons loses inhibitory control, it can start firing in a synchronized fashion. One of the results can be a localized seizure that involves only the cortex contiguous to the focus. At most this activity will involve only one hemisphere (Fig. 145-1). If this focal seizure activity involves the reticular activating formation and the diencephalic structures, however, a secondarily generalized seizure can occur with a loss of consciousness. Although the mechanism is not entirely understood, these deep midline structures are thought to play an important primary role in causing primarily generalized (idiopathic) seizures (Fig. 145-2). The International Classification of Epileptic Seizures (see following outline) is a categorization of seizures that can be easily understood, keeping in mind the concepts just described.

International Classification of Epileptic Seizures

I. Partial seizures (seizures beginning locally)
   A. Partial seizures with elementary symptomatology (generally without impairment of consciousness)
      1. With motor symptoms (includes jacksonian seizures)
      2. With special sensory or somatosensory symptoms
      3. With autonomic symptoms
      4. Compund forms
   B. Partial seizures with complex symptomatology (generally with impairment of consciousness; temporal lobe or psychomotor seizures)
      1. With impairment of consciousness only
      2. With cognitive symptomatology
      3. With affective symptomatology
      4. With ''psychosensory'' symptomatology
      5. With ''psychomotor'' symptomatology (automatisms)
      6. Compound forms
   C. Partial seizures secondarily generalized
II. Generalized seizures (bilaterally symmetric and without local onset)
   A. Absences (petit mal)
   B. Bilateral massive epileptic myoclonus
   C. Infantile spasms
   D. Clonic seizures
   E. Tonic seizures
   F. Tonic-clonic seizures (grand mal)
   G. Atonic seizures
   H. Akinetic seizures
III. Unilateral seizures (or predominantly unilateral)
IV. Unclassified epileptic seizures (because of incomplete data)

Partial seizures. Partial seizures are so named because they originate from a localized area of the brain and usually do not involve the whole brain as do generalized seizures. A partial seizure with elemental symptomatology produces symptoms of which the patient is conscious, whether they are focal motor, sensory, or autonomic. When elemental or simple partial seizures are of the focal motor type, they usually originate in the contralateral precentral gyrus, with the first symptoms occurring in the body part controlled by that brain region (for example, the hand or face and less commonly the foot). This motor activity can spread (as seen in the classic jacksonian seizures) to involve the whole limb and often the entire half of the body. Continuous, well-localized, clonic seizure activity usually occurring in the face or hand is known as epilepsia partialis continua. Elemental sensory seizures are uncommon, originate from the postcentral gyrus, and are manifested by various degrees of paresthesias or numbness. Simple focal seizures commonly have mixed motor and sensory symptoms.

Partial seizures with complex symptoms (also known as psychomotor seizures or temporal lobe seizures), in contrast to partial seizures with elemental symptoms, are often associated with an impairment of consciousness. Indeed, as seen in the classification, an impairment of consciousness may be the only manifestation and may be difficult to differentiate from the petit mal absence described in the following section. Three of the main differentiating features are the older age of onset, the presence of an aura, and varying periods of postictal confusion in the partial seizure. Commonly occurring auras include a visceral rising sensation from the epigastrium to the throat, olfactory sensations, and overwhelming feelings of familiarity (déjà vu). The most common observable manifestation of complex partial epilepsy is the ictal automatism. These uncontrolled motor activities are stereotyped and include lip smacking, chewing movements, fumbling movements of the fingers, inappropriate verbalizations, and even complex acts. These seizures can also consist of impairment or distortions of perceptions, including complex delusions and hallucinations. In many cases varying combinations of symptoms occur at different times. Common interictal symptoms experienced by patients with complex partial seizures include feelings of dissociation from the body or the environment and a distortion of visual perceptions, such as objects appearing to become smaller (micropsia) or closer and larger (macropsia). Unexplained fearfulness is another common affective symptom. These subjective symptoms are probably the result of minor degrees of epileptogenic discharge without observable seizure activity. As a rule, purposeful, directed, violent behavior is not an epileptic phenomenon; however, often the patient reacts defensively if efforts are made at restraint during complex partial seizures or periods of postictal confusion.

Generalized seizures. Generalized seizures without onset from a focal cortical discharge are usually either absences (petit mal) or tonic-clonic (grand mal). Since there is no focal component, prodromes, auras, and focal motor or sensory symptoms are not expected. No brain disease is diagnosable, and the seizures are thought to be the result of a diathesis involving corticoreticular interaction. Except in the case of psychogenic pseudoseizures, the diagnosis of tonic-clonic activity is obvious. Petit mal absences, however, often have very subtle manifestations. The onset of absence seizures is usually between 4 and 10 years of age, with the frequency of episodes tending to wane after puberty. Children with this disorder are often diagnosed as having behavior or learning problems, when in reality their functioning may be altered by repetitive periods of impairment of consciousness occurring each day. In recent years automatisms have been observed as part of petit mal seizures, making differentiation from complex partial seizures difficult without the use of the EEG. It should also be remembered that generalized tonic-clonic seizures develop in up to 50% of persons with a petit mal seizure disorder, usually at puberty.

Generalized seizures also can be the result of the secondary generalization of focal cortical discharges and clinically are often difficult to differentiate from primarily generalized tonic-clonic seizures. Tonic-clonic seizures resulting from a focus of cortical irritability tend to have an onset after adolescence. The older the patient when the first seizure occurs, the more probable that it results from a cortical pathologic condition. In secondarily generalized tonic-clonic seizures an aura may occur or the patient may also have a focal (simple partial or complex partial) seizure just before the tonic-clonic activity. One of the most common clinical problems in neurology is making the differentiation between primarily and secondarily generalized tonic-clonic seizures.

Finally, generalized seizures such as infantile spasms (massive myoclonic seizures), clonic seizures, tonic seizures, and atonic seizures (sudden loss of muscle tone with falling) require brief mention. These seizure types are usually found in childhood and are often associated with the presence of various types of perinatal, metabolic, and genetic brain disease. The prognosis for normal development in these young patients is, unfortunately, often poor, and the treatment is less successful than with other seizure types.

ETIOLOGY

Genetic factors. In general, epilepsy is not a predictable, inherited entity except in rare autosomal dominant diseases such as tuberous sclerosis, Sturge-Weber syndrome, and neurofibromatosis. For the more common types of primarily generalized seizures, the patterns of inheritance are not fully understood. The only well-defined inherited pattern is that of the classic 2.5 to 3/sec spike-and-wave pattern on the EEG. More than 40% of siblings of patients with petit mal seizures have this EEG trait, yet less than 8% of siblings have seizures. The EEG trait has its highest prevalence before 15 years of age, then diminishes rapidly; it is a marker of a dominantly inherited seizure diathesis with incomplete penetrance of the trait. In a broader population of epileptic patients with diverse seizure types, 3.2% of near relatives also have epilepsy. This incidence increases to 7.6% of relatives of infants with seizures. If the seizure onset is after 30 years of age, the incidence in relatives is much lower, less than 2%. Although inheritance is thought to be a major risk factor in ths development of seizures, environmental risk factors play a significant role. For example, certain circumstances such as head trauma, brain tumor, and stroke are known to result in the development of seizures. Persons with a family history of epilepsy are in a higher risk category of developing epilepsy as a result of such environmental risk factors than persons without such a family history.

Acquired factors. Although many disorders of brain

structure and metabolism cause seizures, the following are the most common etiologic factors. Head injury is one of the major causes of epilepsy and is the most commonly acquired cause of seizures in the young adult. The more severe the head trauma, the greater the chance of seizures, with the risk approaching 50% in persons with open head injuries. Over 90% of seizures resulting from head trauma occur within 2 years. Paradoxically, if seizures occur within 1 week after head trauma, the risk of subsequent seizures developing is small. In persons whose onset of seizures occurs after age 21 and who have no known history of trauma or alcohol abuse, the next most likely cause is a tumor, with a probability of 10%. After age 50 the chance of a tumor as a cause of adult-onset seizures approaches 15%; if the seizure is focal, the risk of neoplasm is even greater. Cerebrovascular disease, nonetheless, is the most common cause of seizure onset after age 50, with more than 7% of persons with brain infarction ultimately having seizures. The risk is higher if hemorrhage is present. As in the case of head trauma, the patients whose seizures develop early in the postinfarction period have less risk of subsequent seizures than those with later (after 2 weeks) onset of seizures.

Alcohol withdrawal seizures are common in urban emergency rooms and are usually generalized without focal features. These seizures typically occur 7 to 48 hours after the cessation of drinking. Unfortunately, it is often difficult to differentiate so-called rum fits from an underlying seizure disorder that is precipitated by alcohol withdrawal. If focal seizures occur during withdrawal states, other causes must be considered, including subdural hematoma and brain contusion.

As a generalization, an adult onset of seizures implies serious structural disorders until proved otherwise. The physician must avoid the pitfall of categorizing the cause of a seizure (for example, alcohol withdrawal) on the basis of a superficial evaluation and must remember that a seizure is a symptom, not a diagnosis.

CLINICAL EVALUATION AND MANIFESTATIONS

History. A thorough history is the most important factor in establishing the probable nature of the patient's problem. Every effort must be made to obtain information from observers and family members, as well as from the patient. Specific points that must be covered include the presence of a prodrome or an aura, whether the seizure onset was focal, a clear description of the seizure, and the number and length of seizures. The physician should also inquire about acute precipitating causes such as noncompliance with anticonvulsant medication, alcohol or drug withdrawal, and the relation of the seizure to menses. The previous seizure history (that is, types and frequency of seizures), anticonvulsant medication used, and family history are very important. Additional information concerning specific medical and neurologic causes of seizures should include inquiries about head trauma, headaches, fever, focal neurologic symptoms, visual symptoms, personality change, prior neurologic disorders (for example, encephalitis or stroke), diabetes, heart disease, renal disease, liver disease, and hypertension.

Examination. The general physical examination should include some emphasis on observation. For example, tremulousness might indicate alcohol withdrawal or other drug withdrawal, fetid breath might indicate metabolic derangement (for example, hepatic failure), cyanosis might indicate hypoxia, and skin lesions such as café au lait spots or adenoma sebaceum (collections of raised lesions resembling pimples, primarily around the nasolabial fold on the face) could indicate neurofibromatosis or tuberous sclerosis, respectively, as probable causes of the seizure. Evidence of trauma such as scalp ecchymosis or other injuries to the head should be sought. The tympanic membranes should be visualized for evidence of blood in the middle ear, as is seen in basilar skull fractures. A cardiovascular examination should be performed, since cardiac arrhythmias may cause cerebral emboli accompanied by seizures.

In examining the patient neurologically, one should note the state of consciousness, for subsequent comparison, to see if the patient is becoming more alert or less so. If the patient is having a seizure while being examined, the seizure should be described and its duration noted. Any focal signs during the seizure (for example, focal motor activity or tonic deviation of the eyes) should be noted, as should any focal signs postictally (for example, transient focal paralysis). The presence of nuchal rigidity raises the question of a subarachnoid hemorrhage or a CNS infection. The extraocular movements should be evaluated, and if the patient is unresponsive, the oculocephalic or doll's head eye response should be observed. Pupillary responses are important to note because asymmetries could be the result of eary brain herniation with pressure on the third nerve. The funduscopic examination is necessary, with emphasis on looking for signs of elevated intracranial pressure such as loss of venous pulsation, early disc elevation, or hemorrhage. The patient should be examined for any focal motor weakness, but if he is unconscious, the examiner may have to depend on looking for asymmetries of withdrawal to painful stimuli or for any differences in muscle tone. A unilateral Babinski sign is important in localization, as is an asymmetry of the deep tendon reflexes. Testing cerebellar function usually includes evaluating the patient's equilibrium or gait, as well as evaluating coordination by finger-to-nose movements and the performance of rapid alternating hand movements; however, in a confused or stuporous patient it is often impossible to perform this aspect of the examination. The same is true for the sensory examination, which, if it is to be performed adequately, requires the patient's full alertness and cooperation. In a postictal patient the response to superficial pain or deep pain may often be the only sensory information available to the examiner.

In short, the examination of the patient with a recent or ongoing seizure should focus on observations of possible acute causes, such as trauma, CNS hemorrhage, metabolic disease, infection, or cardiovascular disorders. Emphasis during the neurologic examination should be directed toward seeking evidence of deterioration of the state of consciousness and any focal signs indicating recent localized brain disease (for example, a subdural hematoma with early brainstem herniation) or long-standing localized brain disease (for example, an old perinatal injury).

Diagnostic procedures. The diagnostic procedures used to evaluate an initial seizure in an adult in the acute phase should, at a minimum, include a complete blood count, urinalysis, and tests for blood glucose, serum calcium, phosphorus, electrolytes, blood urea nitrogen, blood alcohol level, and urine screening for various medications. If there is evidence of trauma or of increased intracranial pressure, a computed tomographic (CT) scan should be obtained immediately to look for the structural causes of seizures that might warrant early treatment. If emergency CT scans are unavailable, a skull roentgenogram should be obtained to look for fractures or for evidence of a shift of a calcified pineal gland, and if the pineal gland is not visualized, an echoencephalogram might give additional information about a possible midline shift of brain structures. A lumbar puncture should not be performed routinely unless there is a strong suspicion of a CNS infection or a subarachnoid hemorrhage; lumbar puncture is contraindicated in patients who have signs of increased intracranial pressure (for example, papilledema, third nerve palsy, space-occupying mass on a CT scan, shift of the pineal gland on a skull roentgenogram, or abnormalities of the echoencephalogram). When performing a lumbar puncture, the physician should use a small (20-gauge) needle and examine the cerebrospinal fluid immediately. In young children who have a febrile seizure, a lumbar puncture is absolutely necessary to rule out a CNS infection, provided that there is no evidence of increased intracranial pressure.

After the initial studies are completed, more definitive procedures should be considered. Today the CT scan has virtually replaced the radionuclide brain scan except in selected instances, as in evaluating abnormal flow patterns (such as arteriovenous malformations) and isodense subdural hematomas. CT scanning has been revolutionary in allowing definitive evaluation for most structural causes of seizures, with little or no attendant discomfort or risk to the patient. A CT scan is a required study for all adults with recent onset of seizures or person with a change in established seizure patterns. Pneumoencephalography is no longer a common procedure. Cerebral angiography has continued to be useful, particularly in looking for various types of vascular abnormalities and for evaluating a subdural hematoma.

The EEG is very important in evaluating persons with seizures. An epileptogenic discharge on an EEG often clarifies an otherwise equivocal seizure history. Although up to 50% or more of persons with epilepsy will eventually have abnormal discharges on the EEG, a negative EEG does not exclude epilepsy. The probability of finding a positive EEG is a function of the severity of the seizure disorder, the number and duration of EEGs, and the use of procedures that activate epileptogenic activity, such as sleep, photic stimulation, and hyperventilation. Photic stimulation and hyperventilation are useful in certain patients with petit mal seizures, whereas sleep and hyperventilation are useful in complex partial seizures. Sleep is a benign activating procedure that, when used in combination with noninvasive nasopharyngeal electrodes, increases the yield of epileptogenic activity by 25% or more over a routine awake study. It should be remembered that the differentiation between petit mal absences or automatisms and complex partial absences or automatisms may hinge on finding classic 3/sec bilateral symmetric spike-and-wave discharges as opposed to temporal lobe discharges. This differentiation is very important because the therapeutic regimen for these two seizure types is quite different. Nonetheless, despite all of our sophisticated technology, the most useful diagnostic procedure is a thorough history, a careful neurologic examination, and consistent and careful follow-up of the patient.

MANAGEMENT. The immediate treatment of the patient with a seizure is less involved than the long-term management of the epileptic patient. A soft object should be placed under the head of the patient having a seizure to protect him from hurting himself. Positioning the patient on his side with his head extended also minimizes the danger of aspiration; there is no need to use the traditional padded tongue blade. Intravenous medication is not needed for the patient with a single, short, self-limited seizure. In prescribing long-term maintenance anticonvulsant drugs, every physician should adhere to the following basic principles:

1. Use the correct drug for the type of seizure.
2. Use one drug until enough is given to achieve seizure control or until the appearance of toxicity.
3. Monitor blood drug levels in patients with poor seizure control or with signs of toxicity.
4. If the first drug inadequately controls seizures at therapeutic levels, add a second drug to achieve therapeutic levels, without discontinuing the first drug.
5. Do not abruptly withdraw any drug because status epilepticus may ensue.

Table 145-1 lists the major anticonvulsants useful for the common types of seizures, along with the usual dosage schedule and the therapeutic blood levels.

In an adult, phenytoin can be given safely at an initial oral loading dose of 900 to 1000 mg, which achieves therapeutic blood levels quite rapidly. Intravenous use of this

Table 145-1. Commonly used initial antiepileptic agents

Seizure type	Drugs	Usual adult dose	Therapeutic level	Common side effects	Monitoring
Grand mal, simple partial, and complex partial seizures	Phenobarbital	90-180 mg/day	20-40 μg/ml	Dose related—nystagmus, ataxia, drowsiness Idiosyncratic—megaloblastic anemia, rash, paradoxical hyperkinesis	Annual complete blood count (CBC)
	Phenytoin (Dilantin)	300-400 mg/day	10-20 μg/ml	Dose related—nystagmus, ataxia, lethargy, diplopia Idiosyncratic—rash, adenopathy of pseudolymphoma, lupus erythematosus, blood dyscrasias Other—gum hyperplasia, hypertrichosis, hyperglycemia, hypocalcemia, megaloblastic anemia	Annual CBC
	Primidone (Mysoline)	750-1500 mg/day	8-12 μg/ml	Essentially similar to phenobarbital	Annual CBC
	Carbamazepine (Tegretol)	900-1600 mg/day	6-10 μg/ml	Dose related—ataxia, nystagmus, dizziness, diplopia Idiosyncratic—agranulocytosis and thrombocytopenia, rash, hepatic dysfunction	CBC with platelet count, urinalysis, liver function studies monthly for 1 year, then quarterly
Petit mal	Ethosuximide (Zarontin)	Up to 2 g/day	40-80 μg/ml	Dose related—nausea, vomiting, fatigue, vertigo, lethargy Idiosyncratic—rash, leukopenia, lupus erythematosus	CBC every 3 months for 1 year, then annually

drug is reserved only for status epilepticus, and intramuscular use is not recommended under any circumstances because of the marked unpredictability of absorption by this route of administration. Within 12 hours of the loading dose, the patient should receive another 300 to 400 mg to maintain the therapeutic blood level. Thereafter, the patient can take phenytoin once every 24 hours to maintain seizure control, but in some individuals who are rapid metabolizers the anticonvulsant half-life may be sufficiently short (for example, 12 hours) to require divided dosage.

Phenobarbital is a long-respected and effective drug that is forgiving of occasional missed doses because of its long half-life. It can be administered routinely as a single oral daily dose. In using primidone, carbamazepine, and ethosuximide, divided doses are needed to achieve a relatively stable therapeutic level of anticonvulsant medication. No matter which drug is used, however, unless a consistent therapeutic blood level is maintained, effective seizure control is unlikely. Nonetheless, if the patient is seizure free with less than therapeutic levels in the blood, raising the dosage is usually not helpful. In contrast, if a patient necessarily maintains higher than therapeutic serum levels of medication to achieve seizure control yet shows no signs of toxicity, no diminution of dosage is indicated. In summary, the physician should treat the patient, not the levels, and should rely on levels only when poor seizure control or drug toxicity is present.

Drug interactions should be kept in mind. For example, valproic acid inhibits phenobarbital metabolism and results in an elevation of the phenobarbital blood level. Likewise, valproic acid lowers total serum phenytoin levels yet increases the amount of active unbound phenytoin. Isoniazid is metabolized by the same pathways as phenytoin; thus when it is used in combination with standard doses of phenytoin, toxic levels of phenytoin often result. Warfarin (Coumadin), in contrast, tends to lower the phenytoin level.

Several other important points are relative to an adequate therapeutic approach in managing the patient with a seizure disorder. Consideration must be given to dietary and personal habits, other drug use, and emotional factors, since these may significantly influence the patient's seizure control. For example, an unusually high intake of caffeine in the form of coffee, tea, or cola drinks may impair seizure control. Likewise, some persons with a seizure disorder may find that seizures occur after they imbibe even moderate amounts of alcohol. Insufficient rest is another factor that increases seizure frequency, and every patient with a seizure disorder should have regular sleeping habits. Some college students with a seizure disorder have seizures after staying up all night studying for an examination. Many times patients receive medications from more than one physician so that inadvertent incompatibilities may occur. Some persons with seizure disorders are subject to increased frequency of seizures as the result of taking antihistamines, phenothiazines, and tricyclic antidepressants. The local anesthetic lidocaine (Xylocaine) also can induce seizures in susceptible persons, although this is an uncommon occurrence. Finally, the importance of emotional factors in increased seizure frequency should be mentioned. Emotional stresses of various types may precipitate seizures, but often this factor remains unknown unless the patient is asked about any adverse circumstances that may be occurring at home or at work.

The treatment of the patient who has a history of alcohol or drug withdrawal seizures is follow-up, abstinence, and multivitamin therapy. If the patient had a recent seizure that is thought to be the result of withdrawal, however, that person has a 30% risk of fulminating delirium tremens. Consequently, despite the reluctance of many physicians to deal with alcoholic patients, it is important that all patients with so-called rum fits be admitted for at least 48 to 72 hours of observation, since the withdrawal seizure can precede the full abstinence syndrome by that much time. The specific therapy for the withdrawal or abstinence state is discussed in Chapter 143. Except for the rare patient who has status epilepticus, the use of anticonvulsants is not indicated. One of the consequences of prescribing antiepileptic medication for a known alcoholic patient without specific indication is introducing the opportunity for subsequent withdrawal from both alcohol and the antiepileptic agent. Unfortunately, some alcoholic patients also have an independent seizure disorder, often the result of the many head traumas they have sustained. The history may be difficult to obtain, and the patient may be noncompliant; he may need long-term anticonvulsant therapy and often presents a therapeutic dilemma that can be resolved only if he can resolve his drinking problem.

STATUS EPILEPTICUS

Pathogenesis. Status epilepticus is defined as two or more seizures occurring without the patient regaining alertness, or a state of continuous seizure activity. This clinical state may be most dramatically manifested by tonic-clonic seizure activity but is also demonstrated by continuous focal motor seizures without an impairment of consciousness. In addition, petit mal status epilepticus and psychomotor status epilepticus (although usually not recognized as seizure activity) are manifested by a confusional state or inappropriate behavior. The greatest risk of complications such as anoxia or aspiration pneumonia occurs as a result of generalized grand mal or tonic-clonic status epilepticus. The risk of cardiac arrhythmias also increases. Common causes of status epilepticus include abrupt anticonvulsant withdrawal, various metabolic derangements such as electrolyte imbalance, hypoglycemia, renal failure, or hypoxic encephalopathy, CNS infections, and hemorrhage. Blood samples for a complete blood count and for determination of levels of calcium, phosphorus, magnesium, blood urea nitrogen, glucose, and electrolytes should be drawn. Arterial blood gas values should also be obtained if circumstances permit.

Management. The most important early steps in treating status epilepticus are to establish an airway, provide oxygen, properly position the patient on his side with the head slightly extended and cushioned, and start administering drugs intravenously. A discussion of the drug therapy for status epilepticus among a group of neurologists usually results in as many opinions on the correct approach as there are members of the group. The fundamental principle, however, is to give enough medication intravenously as is necessary to stop the seizure. More important than discussing which drug is best is the principle of having a plan before being faced with the emergency. The following plan is one approach to treating status epilepticus:

1. Initially, after drawing blood glucose, give 50% dextrose intravenously.
2. If this is unsuccessful, give diazepam (Valium) intravenously at a rate of 2.5 mg/min until the seizure stops or to a maximum of 20 to 25 mg. The diazepam is infused through a separate vein or through intravenous tubing containing a 0.9% saline solution (diazepam and phenytoin are poorly soluble in glucose solution).
3. Next, 900 to 1000 mg of phenytoin should be given to an adult at a rate no faster than 50 mg/min intravenously, through a separate vein or through intravenous tubing containing saline. An ECG monitor should be used. Phenytoin should be given as soon as the diazepam stops the seizure because of the very short time (15 to 20 minutes) that intravenous diazepam is effective.

In the uncommon event that this dosage schedule does not work, phenobarbital should be given intramuscularly at a dose of 200 to 400 mg. The concurrent use of diazepam and phenobarbital intravenously may produce severe respiratory depression. If the patient is adequately intubated and has adequate respiratory assistance, however, 200 to 400 mg of phenobarbital can be given intravenously if the seizures continue unabated. As an alternative 5 to 10 ml of paraldehyde as an oil retention enema may be tried. If all else fails, general anesthesia with a short-acting barbiturate is needed.

BIBLIOGRAPHY

Adams, R.D., and Victor, M.: Principles of neurology, New York, 1977, McGraw-Hill Book Co.

Aird, R.B., and Woodbury, D.M.: The management of epilepsy, Springfield, Ill., 1974, Charles C Thomas, Publisher.

Goodman, L.S., and Gilman, A., editors: The pharmacological basis of therapeutics, ed. 5, New York, 1975, MacMillan, Inc.

Schmidt, R.P., and Wilder, B.J.: Contemporary neurology series: epilepsy, Philadelphia, 1968, F.A. Davis Co.

Soloman, G.E., and Plum, F.: Clinical management of seizures: a guide to the physician, Philadelphia, 1976, W.B. Saunders Co.

146 • HEADACHE AND FACE PAIN

Vasant Dhopesh

Headache is an exceedingly common symptom. Fortunately, most causes of head pain are benign and self-limited. In understanding the pathophysiology of head and face pain, it is important to realize that the brain parenchyma itself is insensitive to pain. Additional structures that are insensitive to pain include the ependymal lining of the ventricles, the choroid plexuses, the pia arachnoid membrane, parts of the dura mater, and the skull itself. The intracranial pain-sensitive structures include the venous sinuses and their tributaries, parts of the dura at the base, the dural arteries, and the arteries at the base of the brain. Extracranial structures sensitive to pain include the skin, scalp, and mucosa. The fifth cranial nerve contains the pain fibers above the tentorium cerebelli, with pain referred to the frontal and temporal areas as far back as a line drawn coronally above the ears. Below the tentorium cerebelli, pain is mediated by the ninth and tenth cranial nerves and the first two or three cervical nerve roots, with pain usually located in the occipital areas or in the upper cervical areas.

As indicated anatomically, headaches may arise from intracranial or extracranial locations and may be classified this way clinically. Trigeminal neuralgia and other more atypical facial pain syndromes also must be considered in the differential diagnosis of head and face pain.

VASCULAR HEADACHE

Extracranial causes of headache most commonly include vascular and muscle contraction mechanisms. In vascular headache, pain is caused by extracranial vasodilatation involving branches of the external carotid artery.

Migraine

Migraine, a major category of vascular headache, is characterized by recurrent unilateral throbbing headache often associated with autonomic symptoms. It is often familial and has some predilection for young women. In classic migraine, which occurs in the minority of cases, an aura or prodrome occurs, consisting most often of visual phenomena in which scintillating scotomata appear in half of the visual field. This is thought to be caused by an ischemia of the occipital cortex resulting from vasoconstriction of the cerebral arteries. Severe throbbing unilateral headache follows most commonly in the temporal and frontal regions but also in the retro-orbital, parietal, or occipital areas. Almost always there are anorexia and nausea. Other regularly accompanying features are photophobia and sonophobia, and most patients prefer to lie down in a darkened and quiet room. Variations include common migraine, the most common variety of vascular headache, in which the aura is absent, and rare varieties such as hemiplegic and ophthalmoplegic migraine in which transient neurologic signs and symptoms occur.

Many factors have been known to precipitate a migraine attack. Migraine sufferers are said to be perfectionists and at times to have a compulsive personality structure. Any undue stress or fatigue may provoke a headache. In dietary migraine, certain tyramine-rich foods (aged cheese, chicken liver, broad beans, and certain red wines) bring on an attack. There is some association with hormonal changes, although the exact relationship is unknown. Migraine is not uncommonly associated with menstruation and often disappears during pregnancy. Oral contraceptives increase the frequency and severity of migraine attacks.

The exact pathogenesis of migraine is unclear. Recent studies have shown that serotonin levels rise during the prodromal phase and drop during the headache phase and that the urinary excretion of 5-hydroxyindoleacetic acid (5-HIAA), a metabolite of serotonin, is increased during the attack. Platelet aggregability, which increases just before a migraine episode, is presumably responsible for the release of serotonin. Migraine is not thought to be an allergic phenomenon.

The treatment of migraine can be divided into two parts, symptomatic and prophylactic. Because the headache is caused by extracranial vasodilatation, the therapy for an acute attack is vasoconstrictor agents such as the ergot alkaloids. The most commonly used drug is ergotamine tartrate, which can be given orally or rectally, 1 to 2 mg hourly until relief to a maximum of 6 mg/day or 10 mg/week. Various commercial preparations are available in which ergotamine tartrate is combined with antiemetic, anticholinergic, or sedative agents. Toxic doses may cause intense vasoconstriction and gangrene in the limbs and rarely in the tongue. The prophylactic treatment consists of avoiding known precipitating factors such as foods containing high levels of tyramine. Methysergide, a lysergic acid derivative, is effective prophylactically. Resembling serotonin in its structure, methysergide is thought to be a competitive serotonin inhibitor that simulates the vasoconstrictor-potentiating effects of serotonin on catecholamines. The dosage is 2 mg three times daily. Retroperitoneal fibrosis is a serious side effect. A β-adrenergic blocker, propranolol, has also been found prophylactically effective; the dosage is 40 to 80 mg three times a day. In recent years either electromyographic or thermal biofeedback is increasingly being used because the results have been somewhat encouraging.

Many other conditions are known to produce vascular headache, including febrile states, bacteremia, carbon monoxide inhalation, nitrite ingestion, hypoxia, the postictal state following seizures, and caffeine withdrawal. Because the knowledge of these conditions is obtained readily by eliciting a thorough history, the diagnosis is relatively straightforward, and an elaborate differential diagnosis is unnecessary. The treatment is directed toward the primary offending agent.

Cluster headache

Cluster headaches (Horton's, or histamine, headache) are unilateral and vascular and belong to the migraine family; however, the characteristic features are distinct enough for them to be classified as a separate entity. Cluster headache can mimic face pain. It is more common in males, usually occurring in the third and fourth decades of life. The outstanding clinical feature is the periodicity of the headache, occurring in small groups or clusters separated by brief intervals (chronic, nonremitting forms, however, have been described). The pain is commonly nocturnal, recurring at the same time, and is usually located in and behind the eyeball, temple, and forehead. It is throbbing and so severe that patients cannot sit still and may walk around in the hope of getting some relief. There is no prodrome or appreciable nausea. Other autonomic symptoms, however, such as eye tearing and nasal congestion on the same side, are prominent. A Horner's syndrome manifested by partial lid ptosis and pupillary miosis may be seen, and this occasionally can be permanent. Although the recurrent brief attacks of headache continue for hours or weeks, they abruptly disappear sometimes for months or even years, only to recur again in another cluster. Cluster headaches must be differentiated from atypical facial neuralgia and may mimic Raeder's syndrome, both of which are discussed later in this section. The exact mechanism of the production of cluster headache is unknown, although increased histamine with resultant vasodilatation has been incriminated. Although cluster headaches are vascular, the response to ergot preparations is less impressive than in migraine, and other approaches have been tried. Prednisone (40 mg/day for 5 days and then tapered over 3 weeks) has been used to abort attacks. Recently, lithium in doses up to 900 mg/day has shown encouraging results as a prophylactic agent. Methysergide is also helpful as a prophylactic agent but has a potential risk.

A variation of the cluster headache, chronic paroxysmal hemicrania, has recently been recognized. These headaches occur daily without remission and respond dramatically to indomethacin in doses of between 25 and 50 mg three times a day.

MUSCLE CONTRACTION (TENSION) HEADACHE

Muscle contraction headache, also known as tension headache, is the most common type of head pain encountered clinically. Most series report a preponderance of this condition in women and a higher incidence in adults ranging from 20 to 40 years of age, but symptoms may persist in later years. The headache pain characteristically is slow in onset and develops into a steady ache of mild to severe intensity. It may be confined to the frontal, temporal, or parietal regions or be diffuse, and although most often bilateral, it may have a unilateral component. Some patients describe it as a tightness, pressure, or bandlike sensation around the head. Other associated symptoms such as nausea, vomiting, and photophobia are absent unless the headaches are very severe or there is a vascular component. Muscle contraction headache may also be caused by local diseases of the spine, eyes, teeth, or paranasal sinuses.

The role of emotional factors such as anxiety, repressed hostility, and unresolved dependency in the causation of muscle contraction headache is well established. The observation that many patients with muscle contraction headache are depressed and have other somatic complaints such as anorexia and insomnia has led some authorities to believe that the headache is a symptom of depression.

The aim of treatment is to reduce both muscle tension and emotional tension. Mild headaches respond to simple analgesics. Minor tranquilizers such as diazepam are of considerable value. Amitriptyline in doses of 50 to 150 mg daily is useful, especially in depressed patients. Massage, warm baths, and manipulation are important adjunct treatments. In severe and more resistant cases psychotherapeutic intervention may be necessary. Various other modalities such as biofeedback, hypnosis, and acupuncture are being used in some centers to treat resistant cases.

OTHER FORMS OF HEADACHE
Posttraumatic headache

Posttraumatic, or postconcussion, headache may develop as a sequela to head injury along with other symptoms such as dizziness, light-headedness, and lack of concentration. These headaches are thought to be caused by muscle contraction, vascular dilatation, or direct injury to the scalp. They are notoriously resistant to any form of treatment but eventually subside.

Hypertensive headache

Hypertensive headache occurs in about 10% to 15% of hypertensive patients. These headaches are more common after awakening, are predominantly occipital, and are throbbing in type. They are thought to have both vascular and muscle contraction components and may be relieved with effective antihypertensive treatment.

Headache in temporal arteritis

Temporal arteritis is also called cranial arteritis and giant-cell arteritis. A biopsy of the superficial temporal artery and other cranial and noncranial arteries may reveal the presence of giant cells and perivascular inflammatory exudate. Intracranial arteries, especially the ophthalmic arteries, may be involved. Temporal arteritis is included in the group of so-called collagen-vascular diseases because the pathogenesis of this condition is thought to be caused by an autoimmune mechanism. It typically affects patients over 60 years of age. The headache is commonly located in the temporal area and may be accompanied by visual loss caused by ophthalmic artery involvement. Temporal arteries may be seen as enlarged, tortuous vessels or may be felt as firm, tender cords on palpation. The most useful laboratory test is determination of the erythrocyte sedimentation rate (ESR), which usually is markedly elevated. The diagnosis may be confirmed by a temporal artery biopsy. The condition dramatically responds to corticosteroids such as oral prednisone in a dosage of 60 mg daily, which should be instituted early to prevent visual loss. The prednisone should be tapered to 40 mg daily after 1 week, and after 4 to 6 weeks it should be reduced further to a maintenance dosage of 5 to 10 mg daily, which should be continued for about 2 years.

Headache from sinus or eye disease

Headache in sinusitis results from an inflammation of the ostia and the turbinates. The pain is characteristically dull and aching and is present in the morning with improvement as the day progresses. Tenderness may be present over the affected sinus. Pain in frontal sinusitis is felt over the forehead, in ethmoid sinusitis between the orbits, and in maxillary sinusitis over the cheek and upper jaw. The treatment consists of decongestants, antibiotics, and surgical drainage if a fluid level is present on roentgenograms of the sinuses. Errors of refraction, glaucoma, or inflammatory conditions of the eye produce headache, with pain usually localized to the eye. Careful ophthalmologic evaluation can determine pathologic conditions of the eye.

Traction headache

The brain is not sensitive to pain but is surrounded, especially at the base, by pain-sensitive structures (arteries, veins, and cranial nerves) that produce referred head pain when stretched or displaced by a mass lesion. Although a mass lesion classically suggests a tumor, other conditions such as an abscess, hematoma, or brain edema can produce headache through a similar traction mechanism. These traction headaches are usually deep and dull, with a steady ache that is usually worse in the morning and is aggravated by the coughing and straining that result in transiently increased intracranial pressure. The location of the pain may serve as a rough guide to the location of the mass, corresponding in position in 70% to 80% of the cases in the absence of diffusely raised intracranial pressure. For example, in posterior fossa tumors, the headache is almost always occipital. Focal neurologic signs suggestive of a structural lesion may be found, and papilledema, when present, supports the impression of increased intracranial pressure caused by a mass lesion.

Appropriate laboratory tests pinpoint the location and nature of the tumor. Computed tomographic (CT) scanning has essentially eliminated the need for more complex roentgenographic procedures. Electroencephalography may be useful. The therapy usually consists of surgically removing the mass, although in specific instances such as metastatic disease to the brain, radiation therapy may be advisable.

Lumbar puncture headache

Lumbar puncture headache also is classified as traction headache because the mechanism is presumed to be a leakage of cerebrospinal fluid (CSF) following puncture of the dural sac, with a subsequent minimal displacement of pain-sensitive structures. These headaches are occipital, are precipitated or worsened by assuming an erect posture, and are relieved by recumbency. Simple analgesics and bed rest usually bring relief. Rarely, in incapacitating cases, intravenous fluids and small doses of codeine may be necessary for 24 hours.

Headache in pseudotumor cerebri

Pseudotumor cerebri, also called benign intracranial hypertension, is a syndrome seen mainly in young, obese women. The patient has diffuse headaches caused by increased intracranial pressure without any other associated symptoms. On examination, the only sign elicited is papilledema. The CSF is normal expect for increased pressure. The pathogenesis of this increased pressure is unknown, but various factors have been associated with it, such as venous sinus thrombosis, vitamin A excess, and taking birth control pills. As the name implies, the prognosis is often good.

Headache in subarachnoid hemorrhage

Subarachnoid hemorrhage may be caused by the rupture of a cerebral artery aneurysm with the onset of sudden severe and generalized headache. Patients may or may not lose consciousness and may or may not have focal neurologic signs. As a result of chemical meningitis caused by the presence of blood, nuchal rigidity frequently develops, and a spinal tap reveals red blood cells and xanthochromia of the supernatant fluid. If an aneurysm is suspected, angiography is indicated to confirm its presence and suitability for surgical treatment.

Headache in meningitis

Headaches that occur with various forms of meningitis have a variable onset, are very severe, and are aggravated by any movement of the head. Patients with these headaches are febrile and have signs of meningeal irritation. The pain is thought to be caused by a chemical irritation of the nerve endings in the meninges. A spinal tap with careful CSF examination is essential to establish the diagnosis.

TRIGEMINAL NEURALGIA

Trigeminal neuralgia (tic douloureux) is characterized by brief paroxysmal attacks of severe pain in the distribution of one of the three divisions of the trigeminal nerve. The pain is so excruciating that it often causes the patient to wince with obvious facial contraction; hence the name tic douloureux. Similar paroxysmal attacks of pain in the throat are known as glossopharyngeal neuralgia.

The pathogenesis of trigeminal neuralgia is unknown. There is no structural lesion demonstrable along the course of the nerve. The term "neuralgia" is therefore used. A similar secondary syndrome can offer in cases of multiple sclerosis, gasserian ganglion or cerebellopontine tumor, or brainstem infarction. These cases have an obvious neurologic deficit. In recent years compression of the root entry zone of the trigeminal nerve by anomalous loops of basilar artery branches has been shown to be responsible for a number of cases of trigeminal neuralgia.

The idiopathic form of this disorder occurs in midlife or late life and is slightly more common in females. The second and third divisions of the fifth nerve are most commonly involved. The pain is described variously as like lightning jabs or electrical shocks and lasts only a few seconds. The attacks are recurrent over weeks or months, although there may be spontaneous remissions. Frequently there are tender areas or trigger zones, and any mechanical activity such as smiling, talking, chewing, or touching the face sets off an attack. A neurologic deficit in the distribution of the fifth cranial nerve demands an urgent search for structural causes. The diagnosis is based on the characteristic history. Differentiation from atypical facial neuralgia is discussed later in this chapter.

Because it is believed that the pain of trigeminal neuralgia is caused by the temporal summation of afferent impulses in the spinal nucleus of the fifth cranial nerve, anticonvulsants have been tried; these agents have been found to be effective. The drug of choice is carbamazepine (Tegretol) in doses of 400 to 1000 mg/day, starting with a smaller dose to avoid the side effect of drowsiness. Rarely, severe bone marrow depression can occur as an idiosyncratic reaction; therefore frequent blood counts are advisable. Another anticonvulsant, phenytoin (Dilantin), in doses of 300 to 600 mg/day also has been useful. If medical treatment fails and pain renders the patient incapacitated, surgical treatment may be undertaken. In the past a popular procedure consisted of cutting the appropriate root proximal to the gasserian ganglion or destroying a selective portion of the gasserian ganglion by alcohol injection or thermal coagulation. Currently, in patients less than 60 years of age and in otherwise good health, the preferred surgical method is the microvascular decompression procedure developed by Jannetta, in which, through a posterior fossa approach, pressure by a branch of the superior cerebellar artery on the root entry zone of the fifth nerve is relieved by separating the vessel from the nerve with a prosthetic implant.

ATYPICAL FACIAL NEURALGIA

There are as many syndromes as there are structures of the head and face that are characterized by forms of antypical facial neuralgia, or "lower half headache." Sluder's sphenopalatine ganglion neuralgia and Vail's vidian neuralgia are included in this category, and the profusion of eponyms compounds the confusion. It is often impossible to pinpoint the exact source of the pathologic condition. Frequently patients with this condition are diagnosed as having trigeminal neuralgia. They are differentiated from those with trigeminal neuralgia, however, by the absence of trigger zones, by the occurrence in a younger age group, and by the character of the pain, which may be dull, throbbing, boring, and either constant or episodic. There may be some autonomic symptoms such as eye tearing, nasal congestion, and nausea. The pain is located at the base of the nose or in the orbit, upper cheek, jaws, and teeth and may radiate to the temple or forehead. Sluder believed that the cause was in the sphenopalatine ganglion and termed the disorder "sphenopalatine ganglion neuralgia." Vail ascribed the same condition to an irritation of the vidian nerve caused by sphenoid sinusitis and coined the term "vidian neuralgia." Destroying either the sphenopalatine ganglion or the vidian nerve does not abolish the pain in all cases. It is therefore believed that atypical facial neuralgia is caused by multiple factors, including vascular phenomena. It may resemble vascular headache of the migraine type, especially cluster headache, from which it may be difficult for the physician to differentiate. Unfortunately, the therapeutic response to various treatments, including ergot alkaloids, is poor.

Raeder described patients with orbital pain and supraorbital pain associated with oculosympathetic paralysis. Raeder's syndrome is also referred to as paratrigeminal neuralgia, since a lesion in the paratrigeminal location could involve the ophthalmic division of the trigeminal nerve and the oculosympathetic fibers traveling with the internal carotid artery. Most often no definitive cause is found. Men are affected more commonly than women. The oculosympathetic paralysis is believed to be caused by pressure from dilatation of the internal carotid artery in the cavernous sinus. The resultant partial Horner's syndrome is manifested by miosis and partial ptosis. Usually there is normal facial sweating or loss of sweating only in a localized supraorbital area, since the lesion involves sympathetic fibers along the internal carotid artery and sudomotor fibers to the face travel along the branches of the external carotid artery. If studies exclude a parasellar lesion, the treatment of Raeder's syndrome is the same as that for cluster headaches.

Atypical facial pain is a term that is used when pain does not have the characteristics of any of the conditions described previously. The pain usually persists for months or years and in some cases attains the status of a delusion. It is presumed to be psychogenic and therefore may be resistant to any kind of therapy.

CAROTIDYNIA

Carotidynia is pain that occurs on one side of the neck in the area of the bifurcation of the common carotid artery.

It may radiate to the face, jaw, and temple and characteristically occurs in young or middle-aged adults. Swelling and tenderness in the carotid artery at the carotid sinus may be present. The treatment is symptomatic.

• • •

From the foregoing discussion, it is clear that for a patient with the complaint of headache or face pain, a detailed history is essential. One should ask pertinent questions about onset, location, quality, intensity, relationship to the time of day, and associated symptoms. Although in the majority of instances pain involving the head and face falls into well-defined syndromes, it may be difficult to determine whether the pain results from diseased teeth, temporomandibular joint disease, a sinus disorder, vascular headache, or neuralgia. In such cases a multidisciplinary evaluation is required so that patients are spared unnecessary treatments such as extraction of teeth. Conversely, patients with dental dysfunction or temporomandibular joint disease should not be subjected to neurosurgery or other inappropriate procedures.

BIBLIOGRAPHY

Adams, R. D., and Victor, M.: Principles of neurology, New York, 1977, McGraw-Hill Book Co.

Dalessio, D. J.: Wolff's headache and other head pain, ed. 3, New York, 1972, Oxford University Press.

147 • VERTIGO, DIZZINESS, AND HEARING LOSS

Joseph U. Toglia

VERTIGO

The term "vertigo" implies a sensation of rotation in space of either the patient or his environment, caused by altered physiology of the labyrinth or the central vestibular pathways of the ear. Vertigo may be physiologic, as experienced after sudden rotatory acceleration or deceleration (Bárány's test), or pathologic, as experienced with disorders of the labyrinth such as Meniere's disease or with lesions of the central vestibular pathways, as in multiple sclerosis.

The differential diagnosis between peripheral or labyrinthine vertigo and central or neurogenic vertigo is based on clinical observations and a laboratory evaluation.

CLINICAL MANIFESTATIONS. In labyrinthine vertigo the onset is sudden and the intensity is influenced by the position of the head in space. The duration varies from hours to days and in some patients may last for a few weeks. The patient loses his balance and has a tendency to fall always to one side. A jerky, horizontal-rotatory unidirectional nystagmus is associated with the vertigo and is usually inhibited by visual fixation. Past pointing and falling occur toward the slow phase of the nystagmus. Autonomic symptoms such as sweating, pallor, nausea, and vomiting occur almost constantly. Tinnitus and hearing loss are often present, and other neurologic symptoms are characteristically absent. If the patient has a severe vertiginous attack, he may black out momentarily.

In neurogenic vertigo the onset is sudden. The intensity is not influenced by the position of the head in space but in some cases may be influenced by rotating and extending the neck. Autonomic symptoms are variable in their occurrence, and audiologic symptoms are usually absent. Other neurologic symptoms such as diplopia, dysarthria, dysphagia, ataxia, paralysis, and loss of consciousness suggest a neurogenic origin. Nystagmus may be elicited on neurologic examination, beating in any direction or in multiple directions. It may be of any degree and form and usually is not abolished by visual fixation. Past pointing and falling occur toward the fast phase of the nystagmus.

LABORATORY FINDINGS. Labyrinthine function is examined by means of caloric tests, and the results of these tests may be recorded with an electronystagmograph. The tests are performed by irrigating the ear canal with cold and warm water while the patient's head is positioned in the midsagittal plane, so that a line between the external ear orifice and the lateral canthus of the eye is perpendicular to the floor. About 30 seconds after the irrigation stops, the eyes of the patient develop a jerky, horizontal-rotatory nystagmus, with the fast phase beating away from the ear irrigated by cold water or toward the ear irrigated by warm water. The nystagmus lasts about 1 minute, and nausea and other autonomic symptoms may develop. The caloric responses are evaluated with relation to latency, duration, amplitude, and frequency. Electronystagmography records the velocity of eye movements and is based on the existence of a biologic corneoretinal potential; it allows recording of the parameters of the caloric response.

Additional tests of value in specific instances include audiograms, brainstem auditory evoked potentials (see discussion of "Hearing loss" in this chapter), skull and mastoid roentgenograms, complex motion tomography of the temporal bone, computed tomography of the brain, high-resolution computed tomographic (CT) scans of the inner ear, CT cisternography with air or metrizamide, Pantopaque encephalography, electroencephalography, cervical spine roentgenograms, cerebrospinal fluid (CSF) examination, and occasionally cerebral angiography. The selection of these additional tests depends on the clinical history and the physical examination.

Diseases causing vertigo

DISEASES OF THE LABYRINTH. The function of the labyrinth may be disrupted by a variety of pathologic processes, including infectious labyrinthitis, drugs (gentamicin, streptomycin, kanamycin, and neomycin), metabolic disorders (diabetes, dysproteinemia, and uremia), vascular diseases, and head trauma. The most common diseases of the labyrinth are labyrinthitis, traumatic labyrinthopathy, Meniere's syndrome, and benign positional vertigo.

Labyrinthitis usually occurs with chronic middle ear infection, especially associated with cholesteatoma. Vertigo, ataxia, nausea, and vomiting are always present, and there may be a loss of hearing. Nystagmus beats to the opposite side, and the caloric responses are diminished on the side of the pathologic condition. Usually there is no fever. Bacterial labyrinthitis or suppurative labyrinthitis, in which there are abnormaities in hearing, should be distinguished from a viral form or from vestibular neuronitis, in which cochlear signs and symptoms are conspicuously absent. The prognosis in labyrinthitis is usually benign, and recovery takes place within several days to a few weeks. Occasionally bacterial infection spreads to the central nervous system, produces a middle ear cholesteatoma, or causes a fistula of the labyrinth. The therapy is with antibiotics, myringotomy, and/or symptomatic medication for vertigo and nausea. Mastoidectomy is indicated in cases of chronic osteitis and fistula of the labyrinth.

Head trauma is a common cause of labyrinth dysfunction, or traumatic labyrinthopathy. The trauma may cause extravasation of blood into the labyrinth, producing permanent damage, or may result only in a transient loss of labyrinthine function (labyrinthine concussion). An acute flexion-extension injury of the neck also causes labyrinthine dysfunction, through concussion of the labyrinth, through ischemia in the distribution of branches of the vertebral artery, or through disruption of proprioceptive cervical impulses. Vertigo occurs in the immediate posttraumatic period. Several days later the vertigo is usually present only after the assumption of certain postures, and the patient may complain only of postural disequilibrium. Nystagmus and abnormal results of caloric tests recorded by electronystagmography occur in about 40% of these patients. The degree of tinnitus and hearing loss varies according to the severity and type of head trauma and is particularly severe with fractures of the petrous bone.

The prognosis varies according to the severity of the trauma. Even minor injuries may cause protracted symptoms, especially when a medicolegal settlement is pending or if the patient has a psychiatric disorder. The therapy is symptomatic. These patients often require mild tranquilizers and psychotherapy.

Meniere's syndrome usually is attributed to hydrops of the membranous labyrinth caused by a defective reabsorption of the endolymph. Its cause is unknown, although it has been associated with allergies, metabolic and endocrine disturbances, and dysfunction of the autonomic nervous system.

Symptoms and signs include a fluctuating fullness and hearing loss in one ear associated with episodes of vertigo, tinnitus, unsteadiness, nausea, and vomiting. Most symptoms abate within several hours. These attacks occur periodically and at varying intervals. Nystagmus is very active during the acute attack and may persist for weeks after the vertigo has subsided. Caloric test results are always abnormal. Audiologic tests show specific abnormalities (see discussion of "Hearing loss" in this chapter).

The attacks become less frequent after several years, but the hearing loss gets progressively worse. In about 10% of these patients the other ear also will eventually become involved. When possible, therapy should be addressed to a specific cause. Nevertheless, medications such as antihistaminics are needed for acute symptoms. A variety of regimens, including diuretics, anticonvulsants, and desensitization, have been used prophylactically. When medical therapy has failed and the attacks continue to be incapacitating, and particularly if the hearing loss is already severe, various surgical procedures should be considered. These include labyrinthotomy, labyrinthectomy, and vestibular nerve section.

DISEASES OF THE CENTRAL NERVOUS SYSTEM. Vertigo occurs in many diseases of the central nervous system (CNS), including intracranial infections (cerebellar or temporal lobe abscess), vascular disease (vertebrobasilar artery insufficiency, brainstem and cerebellar infarction, and cerebellar hemorrhage), multiple sclerosis, migraine, epilepsy, encephalitis, CNS trauma, degenerative diseases, and CNS neoplasms. Only a few of these conditions are discussed here in detail.

Vascular diseases

Vertebrobasilar artery insufficiency. Patients with vertebrobasilar artery insufficiency have transient neurologic symptoms and deficits that may result from combinations of intrinsic vascular disease and from mechanical causes of decreased perfusion pressure. A not uncommon example of the latter is obstruction of the vertebral arteries by arthitic osteophytes.

Patients with vertebrobasilar artery insufficiency may experience vertigo, transitory visual disturbances, syncope dysarthria, drop attacks, or numbness. The symptoms may be induced by postural changes of the neck, by sudden arising from a sitting or supine position, or by exercise of the upper extremities (subclavian steal syndrome). Special test include cervical spine roentgenograms, electronystagmography, and in some cases angiography.

Infarctions and hemorrhages. Infarctions and hemorrhages cause vertigo when they are localized in the posterolateral area of the medulla or in the cerebellum.

The symptoms include many of those seen in cases of vertebrobasilar artery insufficiency, but the deficits are not transient. They often can be grouped in specific syndromes according to the anatomic blood supply (for example, Wallenberg's syndrome). Electronystagmography and brainstem auditory evoked potentials are particularly useful tests for diagnosing brainstem lesions.

The prognosis varies with the severity of the vascular disease and the localization of the lesion in the brainstem.

Multiple sclerosis. Although vertigo is a common complaint of patients with multiple sclerosis, the latter disorder begins with vertigo in only about 5% of the cases.

Paroxysmal vertigo with or without autonomic symptoms or loss of balance may suggest multiple sclerosis in a young patient, particularly if it is associated with other oculomotor abnormalities or with visual abnormalities. Vertigo in this instance is seldom associated with tinnitus or loss of hearing. The diagnosis depends on the course of the illness and the elevation of CSF v-globulins. Nystagmus occurs in a variety of forms, especially monocular and vertical. Vestibular test results are almost always abnormal. Visual and auditory evoked potentials are very useful tests. The prognosis and therapy are discussed further in Chapter 148.

Epilepsy. An epileptogenic lesion in the temporal lobe may cause vertiginous seizures, in which case the vertigo usually occurs as the aura of a generalized attack. It is frequently associated with an epigastric sensation but not with hearing loss or nystagmus. The diagnosis is established by electroencephalography.

Migraine. Vertigo may occur in place of a migraine attack (migraine equivalent) or as one of the multiple manifestations of basilar artery migraine. Vertigo typical of Meniere's syndrome may replace the attacks of migraine in later life. At times migraine and vertigo may occur separately in the same patient.

POSITIONAL VERTIGO. Positional vertigo may be seen with disorders of the labyrinth, such as vestibular neuroniti and head trauma, or with central lesions involving the cerebellum or brainstem. The vertigo occurs when the patient is suddenly placed in a supine position from an initial sitting position, with his head hanging off the examining table. In the peripheral type there is a rotatory nystagmus beating toward the undermost (pathologic) ear, and this nystagmus reverses direction when the patient returns to the sitting position. The nystagmus appears after 3 to 5 seconds of latency and lasts for 10 to 15 seconds. Neither the nystagmus nor the vertigo recurs if several positional tests are performed consecutively. In the central type there is no latency period, no specific directionality, and no fatigability. The caloric tests show abnormalities in both the peripheral and central types. The treatment is directed at specific pathologic conditions when evident.

In many instances patients with positional vertigo have no evidence of peripheral or central vestibular dysfunction, and the caloric test results are normal. In this type, called benign paroxysmal positional vertigo, the condition is self-limited and no specific therapy is indicated.

DIZZINESS

The term "dizziness" implies a sensation of disequilibrium, as may occur when patients wear glasses with the wrong refractive correction, have cataracts, or have lost their proprioceptive sensations, such as with peripheral neuropathy or cervical spondylosis. In addition to such ophthalmogenic and somatosensory dizziness, anxiety can cause a psychogenic dizziness as a result of hyperventilation. The overbreathing and resultant hypocapnia produce cerebral vasoconstriction and a diminished cerebral blood flow. The patient with hyperventilation syndrom also complains of paresthesias of the extremities and lips. Nystagmus is absent, and caloric test results are normal. The treatment consists of mild sedatives, reassurance, and having the patient rebreathe into a paper bag.

Odontogenic dizziness has been associated with abnormal dental occlusion and temporomandibular joint disease. Other symptoms include tinnitus, hearing loss, facial pain, and nausea.

If more than one of these situations occur, with various combinations of opthalmogenic, somatosensory, or odontogenic types, the dizziness may become incapacitating. Such combinations often happen in elderly patients with multisystem disorders such as diabetes, cataracts, and cervical spondylosis.

The term "vertigo" should be restricted to the rotatory hallucination caused by acute vestibular dysfunction. All other sensations of disequilibrium or physical disorientation in space should be identified as dizziness. Labyrinthine dysfunction may itself cause a nonrotational hallucination of disequilibrium or dizziness.

HEARING LOSS

The human ear detects tones ranging in frequency between 16 cycles per second (cps) and 16,000 cps (Hz). The greater the frequency, the higher will be the pitch. Persons who clearly detect frequencies between 500 and 2000 cps can hear adequately, but may not appreciate the many qualities of sound. The loudness of sound depends on the amplitude of the sound wave. The greater the amplitude, the louder is the sound.

Normal hearing levels are defined by an international standard. The intensity of sound is defined in decibels (db), with 0 being barely audible. A patient's hearing level is the difference in decibels between the faintest pure tone that he can hear and the normal reference level given by the standard. Normal conversation has a level of about 60 db. Mild hearing loss often starts at 4000 cps and is rather common after 65 years of age, but it is noted also among younger people, especially those exposed continuously to intense noise. A hearing loss of 15 db at the frequencies of 500, 1000, or 2000 cps is considered a minor impairment, and a loss of 80 db at the same frequencies may be considered deafness, at least in a social context. Hearing loss may be caused by diseases of the middle ear (conductive hearing loss), the cochlea and cochlear nerve (sensorineural hearing loss), and the central auditory pathways (central hearing loss).

Hearing loss may be evaluated as a screening procedure (Weber's and Rinne tests) with a tuning fork at either

256 or 512 cps or more thoroughly in special environments with audiometry. In Weber's test the tuning fork is struck and placed on the forehead. If hearing is equal in both ears, the patient does not lateralize the vibratory sound to either ear. If the sound is lateralized to the right ear, for example, this means that either the left ear has sensorineural hearing loss or that the right ear has conductive hearing loss. In the Rinne test the tuning fork is struck and placed alternately near the ear and against the homolateral mastoid bone. If the hearing is normal, the sound is heard about twice as long by air conduction as by bone conduction. If bone conduction is equal to or greater than air conduction, the hearing loss is conductive and not sensorineural.

Conventional pure tone audiometric testing reveals the patient's level and configuration of hearing loss by both air and bone conduction. Speech audiometry tests measure the patient's threshold for speech and his ability to discriminate its finer qualities. Special auditory tests (impedance audiometry, Békésy audiometry, and loudness balance and tone decay tests) are useful clinically in differentiating conductive hearing disorders, cochlear and retrocochlear lesions, and pathologic conditions of the CNS.

The three basic types of hearing loss are conductive, sensorineural, and central.

Conductive hearing loss

Conductive hearing loss is caused by pathologic conditions of the external or middle ear; common causes are otitis media and otosclerosis. Otitis media may be infectious (suppurative) or noninfectious (serous). Suppurative otitis may spread to the inner ear, mastoid, and CNS. Chronic otitis may produce a cholesteatoma; this tumor may invade the inner ear, resulting in mixed conductive and sensorineural hearing loss. In otosclerosis, which is commonly familial, there is decreased mobility of the middle ear ossicles, the hearing loss begins in late adolescence, and the deficit is conductive. Audiometric tests in middle ear disease reveal an essentially normal level of hearing for pure tones by bone conduction and a substantial loss of air conduction.

Sensorineural hearing loss

Sensorineural hearing loss, typical of Meniere's disease and acoustic neuroma, is caused by lesions of the cochlea or the cochlear nerve. Patients note difficulty in understanding conversation in a noisy place and cannot tolerate loud speech.

In sensorineural hearing loss, air conduction is greater than bone conduction on the Rinne test, although both are diminished; on Weber's test the sound is lateralized to the normal ear. Audiometric tests reveal that pure tone air and bone conduction thresholds are both impaired, mostly in the higher frequencies. The presence of recruitment (a disproportionate increase in loudness perceived relative to intensity delivered) suggests a lesion of the cochlea, as in Meniere's disease, and early impairment of speech discrimination suggests a nerve lesion, as in a tumor of the eighth cranial nerve (acoustic neuroma).

In Meniere's disease the hearing loss is almost always unilateral and of moderate degree for all frequencies, and hearing sensitivity fluctuates in the early stage of the disease. Tinnitus and vertigo are the other two complaints in this syndrome.

In the past, acoustic neuroma was rarely seen until the involved ear was essentially deaf. Today, however, thanks to specific roentgenographic tests, the tumor may be diagnosed when the hearing loss is as little as 15 db. Tinnitus is the earliest symptom, and vertigo is either absent or seen in the later stage of the disease. Other neurologic signs of later stages are paralysis of lower cranial nerves, cerebellar ataxia, and signs of increased intracranial pressure. Diagnostic tests include complex motion tomography of the temporal bone, computed tomography of the posterior fossa, high-resolution CT scans of the inner ear, CT cisternography with air or metrizamide, Pantopaque encephalography, brainstem auditory evoked responses, and electronystagmography. The surgical prognosis is good, especially in cases that are diagnosed early.

Sudden hearing loss may be caused by acute ischemia in the distribution of the internal auditory and anterior inferior cerebellar arteries, which supply the labyrinth and brainstem cochlear nuclei. Other causes of sensorineural hearing loss include trauma, presbycusis, and ototoxicity.

Central hearing loss

Central hearing loss is caused by pathologic conditions of the central auditory pathways (cochlear and dorsal olivary nuclei, inferior colliculi, medial geniculate bodies, and temporal lobe cortex). This is rather uncommon, although it may be seen in multiple sclerosis, encephalitis, and brainstem infarction. The hearing loss is evident most often against a background of multiple sensory stimuli.

Audiometry tests reveal normal pure tone audiometry and conventional speech audiometry. Localization audiometry and brainstem auditory evoked potentials are the most useful tests for diagnosing central hearing loss.

The technique of brainstem auditory evoked potentials is relatively simple: the responses to auditory stimuli are averaged in an evoked response recording device via scalp electrodes. A normal response is characterized by a series of seven electrical potentials that are generated in the auditory nerve, the cochlear nuclei, and the interconnecting pathways. Lesions of the central auditory pathways alter the latencies and amplitude of these evoked responses.

BIBLIOGRAPHY

Paparella, M.M., and Shumrick, D.A., editors: Otolaryngology, Philadelphia, 1973, W.B. Saunders Co.

Spector, M., editor: Dizziness and vertigo, New York, 1967, Grune & Stratton, Inc.

Toglia, J.: Electronystagmography: technical aspects, Springfield, Ill., 1976, Charles C Thomas, Publisher.

148 • DEMYELINATING, DEGENERATIVE, AND HEREDOFAMILIAL DISEASES OF THE CENTRAL NERVOUS SYSTEM

Michael J. Walsh and Wallace W. Tourtellotte

DISEASES OF WHITE MATTER

Diseases of white matter constitute a very heterogeneous group of disorders, with damage confined predominantly to the white matter, loss of the oligodendrocytes and their myelin sheaths, and relative sparing of the neurons and the axons. It is useful to divide these disorders into *demyelinating* and *dysmyelinating* types. Demyelinating refers to disorders in which myelin is apparently formed normally but because of various insults is broken down; dysmyelinating refers to disorders in which it is presumed that the myelin membrane is abnormal qualitatively or quantitatively at the time of formation. Most demyelinating disorders are of unknown origin, but some are thought to be virally and immunologically mediated, whereas dysmyelinating disorders are caused by known or presumed genetically determined disturbances of myelin formation and breakdown. These two categories of white matter disease differ epidemiologically, clinically, and prognostically. Multiple sclerosis and its variants are the prototypes of the demyelinating diseases, and metachromatic leukodystrophy and its relatives are the best characterized of the dysmyelinating diseases. Also included with the dysmyelinating diseases are adrenoleukodystrophy, globoid cell leukodystrophy, sudanophilic leukodystrophy, spongy sclerosis, fibrinoid leukodystrophy, and some of the aminoacidurias (phenylketonuria) and lipidoses. Phenylketonuria is potentially treatable if the diagnosis is made at birth, but no therapy is yet available for the other disorders. The metabolic disturbance that is presumed to underlie most of these disorders is known in only a few instances, and diagnosis is sometimes impossible during life. The advent of computed tomography (CT) of the brain has made possible a noninvasive differentiation of gray matter from white matter and may reveal changes in white matter such as decreased density focally or diffusely that may be very helpful in the differential diagnosis. This roentgenographic study may also confirm the presence of bilateral disease when the patient has focal symptoms suggesting a mass lesion. Enhancement of the lesion may be demonstrable when there is considerable inflammation and disruption of the blood-brain barrier.

Demyelinating diseases

MULTIPLE SCLEROSIS. Multiple sclerosis (MS) is the most common of the human demyelinating diseases. The disease has been known as a clinical and pathologic entity for the past century, but its cause is still not established and there is no known therapy that will reverse the demyelination or prevent the progression of this disease. There is no diagnostic test for this disease, although a constellation of clinical and laboratory findings is suggestive when a restricted number of other disorders have been excluded. The disease derives its name from the autopsy picture of the brain, where grossly apparent and microscopic plaques are scattered throughout the white matter of the central nervous system (CNS). The clinical picture also reflects the presence of multiple disseminated lesions of the brain. Another remarkable feature of this disease is the tendency for serious symptoms such as blindness and hemiplegia to remit. These aspects—dissemination over time and evidence of multiple lesions in the CNS—are prerequisites for a clinical diagnosis of MS. Not all patients, however, meet the stringent clinical criteria for diagnosis, and laboratory investigations may be equivocal. In these instances the physician may have to perform exhaustive studies to exclude other diseases and may have to postpone making a definitive diagnosis. However, it is usually possible to make the diagnosis with assurance, and recently developed techniques for noninvasive investigation of the CNS sometimes provide strong support for the clinical diagnosis.

Etiology. No single hypothesis with experimental validation has emerged that explains adequately all the features of MS. Morphologic, genetic, virologic, epidemiologic, immunologic, and clinical peculiarities abound in this disease more than any other disorder of the CNS. Because MS affects so many young people and seems potentially treatable if the inciting events and the factors that induce its exacerbation and progression are identified, an enormous research effort has been under way for almost a century to establish the cause and therapy for this disorder. The following are the most reliable observations on which an etiologic hypothesis might be established.

Morphology. The lesions of MS, particularly perivascular lymphocyte cuffing and periplaque and white matter infiltration by plasma cells and lymphocytes, are characteristic of lesions seen in viral and postvaccinal disorders of the CNS, leading some to consider a viral cause. The morphologic conditions are also reminiscent of those seen in experimental allergic encephalomyelitis, a disorder induced by immunization with brain homogenate combined with adjuvant.

Genetic aspects. An individual who has an identical twin affected with MS has a 20% risk of the disease. This is 300 times the risk for the general population. The risk of a nonidentical twin is less than 15%, and for siblings the risk is 1%. First-degree relatives are also at increased risk. Immunogenetic data have accumulated over the past few years that tend to implicate certain histocompatibility antigens in the genesis of MS. It appears that certain HLA antigens are significantly overrepresented in patients with MS.

Virology. Patients with MS tend to have higher titers of antibody in both serum and cerebrospinal fluid (CSF) to a large number of viruses, most notably measles, rubella, mumps, parainfluenza, Epstein-Barr virus, and herpes simplex type 1 virus. The observed differences, although significant, are relatively small in most studies, generally on the order of a twofold or smaller titer elevation. Morphologic studies using electron microscopy sometimes demonstrate filamentous structures resembling paramyxovirus nucleocapsid in mononuclear cell nuclei in MS brain lesions, but no immunologic evidence points to this material as being a virus. Efforts to culture virus from the brain have been unsuccessful except in a few instances. Clustering of MS in families and communities may suggest a common agent such as virus, but other environmental and genetic hypotheses are also plausible explanations.

Epidemiology. Numerous studies have confirmed the well-known association between disease prevalence and distance from the equator. Geographically, MS is most common in western Europe, southern Canada, southern Australia, and New Zealand. Clusters of the disease have occurred in such places as the Faroe Islands. Although these islands had not experienced a high incidence of MS, there was a virtual epidemic of disease attributed to the presence of British forces on the islands during World War II. The epidemiologic studies in the Faroe Islands seem compatible with a transmissible viral infection of the CNS introduced at that time. Other studies have evaluated the impact of migrations of populations on the prevalence of MS. It appears that individuals who move from areas of higher prevalence to areas of lower prevalence after 15 years of age retain the risk of MS of their previous environment. Those who move before 15 years of age acquire the risk prevalence of their new environment. Various hypotheses may account for these differences. Children from areas of high prevalence may have an infection in the early years of life that predisposes them to subsequently having MS. Alternatively, infection may be common in areas of low risk for MS and may provide protection later against the disease. Virus infection may also affect age groups differently. For example, when poliomyelitis occurs at an early age, it may be asymptomatic, whereas in later life it tends to produce paralytic disease. Lifelong immunity occurs in both instances. Epidemiologic investigations have also raised the question of a dietary factor (deficiency of unsaturated fats) being associated with the increased incidence of MS in certain regions of the world.

Immunologic aspects. The CSF shows abnormalities in 90% of patients with MS, most notably increased IgG and oligoclonal bands revealed by electrophoresis. Evidence exists that some of the immunoglobulin is synthesized in situ within the CNS independent of the systemic immune system. It has long been speculated that this immunoglobulin is directed against MS antigen(s), but studies to determine the specificity of this IgG have been inconclusive.

It seems that suppressor lymphocyte function is altered in MS and that acute deteriorations in this disease are accompanied or perhaps preceded by defective immunoregulation that allows unimpeded damage to oligodendrocytes and the myelin membrane. Remission, however, is accompanied by a rebound elevation in suppressor function. Whether the suppressor abnormality is of pathogenetic significance or is merely a secondary manifestation of a more complex immune perturbation is unknown.

It is obvious that both virally and immunologically mediated injury may give rise to human demyelination with features identical to those seen in MS. Genetic factors play a role in MS, but there is no haplotype or genetic characteristic yet known that is obligatory for disease expression. Some evidence exists that a disturbance of fatty acid and prostaglandin metabolism may play some part in the disease's pathogenesis. Such a disturbance may render myelin more susceptible to an immune attack and permit injury to the oligodendrocytes and the myelin membranes by cytotoxic cells and serum factors that gain access to them. It is also possible that MS is not one disorder but a consequence of various insults to the CNS acting alone or in unison.

Neuropathology. The external surface of the brain is normal. Sometimes the brain weight is diminished and the ventricles are enlarged. Staining of the myelin sheath in sections of the cerebral hemispheres, brainstem, cerebellum, and spinal cord may reveal multifocal discrete plaques of demyelination. In the cerebral hemispheres there is a predilection for plaques to be present in the periventricular areas, particularly around the third and fourth ventricles. The optic nerves are often shrunken because of demyelination. A mild lymphocytic meningitis may accompany the parenchymal changes, predominantly a perivenulitis that is most apparent in the deep sulcal recesses. Although MS is primarily a disorder of myelin, some axonal damage may occur, and gliosis develops with time. The peripheral nerves are not involved.

Pathophysiology. Demyelination leads to four important central disturbances that are relevant to the clinical appearance of MS: decreased nerve conduction velocity, differential rate of transmission of impulses resulting from slowing in the fibers of particular nerves or tracts, frequency-related conduction block, and complete failure of impulse transmission.

It has been known for a long time that minor fluctuations in temperature may produce major changes in the severity of signs and symptoms of MS. Increases of $0.2°$ F may produce decreased visual acuity, additional weakness, and pathologic reflexes. The disease's tendency to be aggravated by increasing temperature is the basis for the hot bath test still used diagnostically by some physicians. It has also been observed that hyperventilation may produce transitory amelioration of some manifestations such as scotomas; sodium bicarbonate infusions may have similar effects. This is believed to result from an effect on ionized calcium, since hypocalcemia increases the excitability of damaged fibers and may facilitate conduction in demyelinated nerves and tracts.

Clinical manifestations. The clinical manifestations of MS reflect the effect of the widespread and multifocal demyelination of the CNS both in place and time (that is, multiple sites and episodes). The disease process tends to affect some systems preferentially, so that certain manifestations commonly occur whereas other signs and symptoms occur only rarely. Furthermore, not all lesions of the CNS are manifested clinically, and the lesions at autopsy may be extensive although the known manifestations in life were trivial. As electrophysiologic and roentgenographic techniques continue to develop, it is likely that more clinically inapparent lesions will be identified; for example, evoked potential recordings of the brainstem and visual system are often abnormal even though clinical testing shows no abnormality.

The cardinal manifestations of MS are caused by injury to the visual, motor, and sensory fiber systems and are easily categorized.

Visual manifestations are of great importance because 60% or more of patients have significant temporary or permanent visual complaints. Moreover, some eye signs elicited by the physician, causing little or no symptoms, are extremely helpful in supporting a diagnosis in difficult cases. The interrogation of the patient is very important in establishing past evidence for disease dissemination with time. Some patients initially deny all visual complaints, but when queried repeatedly and by different examiners, they may recall long-forgotten episodes of temporary visual disturbances.

Optic neuritis is the most serious of the visual manifestations. It may be the first symptom of MS, preceding other manifestations by many years, or may appear at the onset or at any time during the course of the disease. It may be unilateral or bilateral and the eyes may be affected together or separately. Patients may complain of the sensation of having a patch or a fog over one eye, or they may complain of visual blurring. When a central scotoma is the main feature, the patient may appreciate that the peripheral field of vision is unaffected. Paracentral scotomas, quadrantanopsia, altitudinal field defects, and less commonly homonymous field defects may occur. Optic neuritis is usually subacute at onset, with gradual and maximal visual impairment developing over several days; this is in contrast to ischemic optic neuropathy, in which visual loss is usually acute and total. Sudden visual loss, however, does occur. Frontal headache or pain on moving or touching the eye is common, as is photophobia. Visual acuity in most patients falls to 20/100 or worse. Gradual recovery occurs over 2 to 4 weeks in most patients, but many are left with subjective residua of the primary attack. Some notice that colors appear desaturated, and defects in color perception may be elicited. Vision may be **transiently** reduced with vigorous exercise or increased **temperature** (Uhthoff's sign).

During the episode of optic neuritis, disc edema resembling papilledema may occur; however, in papilledema the visual acuity if normal. The edema is now considered to be caused by a disturbance of axoplasm flow at the optic nerve head. The term "retrobulbar neuritis" is used when funduscopy is normal. An important physical sign to be sought in every patient is an afferent pupillary defect (Marcus Gunn's pupillary sign, or the swinging flashlight sign). This test is positive in most patients who have had unilateral optic neuritis and also may be elicited in patients in whom there is no clear history to suggest previous eye disease. To elicit this sign, the physician shines the light in each eye separately. When the light is swiftly shifted from the normal to the affected eye, the pupil is seen to dilate rather than to constrict to direct light stimulation. The optic disc becomes pale in patients with previous optic neuritis, chiefly temporally at first. Optic pallor, however, is not a useful sign because it depends on a subjective evaluation. A more reliable assessment is possible by counting the small vessels intervening on the disc between the major grouping of superior and inferior retinal vessels; normally there are six to eight small vessels, but in optic neuritis there may be only two to four.

MS eventually develops in 40% or more of all patients with optic neuritis. Predictive tests, however, are of no value at this time in attempting to predict which patients will have multifocal demyelinating disease.

Another category of visual system abnormality reflects disease of the oculomotor system. Whereas palsies of individual muscles and nerves occur infrequently, internuclear ophthalmoplegia is a common sign and should be carefully sought. The cardinal manifestations of internuclear ophthalmoplegia are unilateral nystagmus in the abducting eye and contralateral impaired adduction. The signs are indicative of a lesion of the medial longitudinal fasciculus on the side contralateral to the nystagmus.

Motor manifestations are common and occur in almost all patients at some stage of the illness; they are responsible for most of the chronic disability seen in MS. Excessive fatigue may herald disease onset and may be prominent at a time when there is no easily identifiable objective motor finding. A sense of stiffness or heaviness, especially in the lower extremities, is a common patient complaint. Dragging of an extremity or stumbling may occur. Involvement of the upper extremities is usually preceded by or is simultaneous with involvement of the lower extremities. Unilateral upper extremity monoparesis is manifested by "the useless hand," a clumsiness or diminished facility for tasks requiring skilled motor function, such as handwriting or typing. A feature of the motor signs and symptoms is their tendency to fluctuate from day to day or hour to hour at disease onset. This is especially true for signs such as the Babinski sign, which may alternate from flexor to extensor with repeated testing. Exercise or an increase in body temperature may render an equivocal plantar response plainly extensor. The important accompaniments of motor involvement are increased tone, spasticity, increased reflexes, and alteration in cutaneous reflexes. The Babinski sign is found in most patients with established disease, and clonus at the ankle and knee is elicited. The superficial abdominal and cremasteric reflexes are altered and lost, but abdominal reflexes are often difficult to assess when the patient is obese or has abdominal scarring. A downward drift of the outstretched arms is a useful indication of disease. The motor disability may remit or progress to paraparesis or paraplegia, sometimes with equal severity in the upper extremities. Cerebellar signs commonly accompany the corticospinal disturbance, but not invariably. At times chronic spastic paraparesis, as either a stable or a slowly progressive deficit, is the only manifestation, and the diagnosis is then difficult to make because the criteria of the dissemination of the disease in place and time cannot be confirmed.

The prominence of cerebellar abnormalities has been known since the time of Charcot, and the triad of scanning speech, nystagmus, and intention tremor is sometimes known by his name. Along with corticospinal tract involvement, this is the most disabling of the major manifestations of MS. Incoordination, disequilibrium, falling, and stumbling are distressing. Skilled use of the hands for writing and work may be impossible. Sometimes only mild tremor is present; this is predominantly a proximal tremor and is accentuated greatly with the initiation and persistence of movement. The tremor may be predominantly truncal, in which case the patient has difficulty with gait and has titubation of the head. Marked dysarthria may make speech unintelligible. The tremor may be so manifest and powerful that the patient's bed or wheelchair may shake in synchrony.

Sensory manifestations are common, and patient complaints related to sensory disturbance may greatly exceed what might be demonstrable on physical examination. Paresthesias are the most common complaint, but the patient may describe a very complex pattern of sensory alteration. The impairment may be so great that the patient is unaware of the position of a limb in space and needs to visually identify its location. Patients complain of both lower extremities feeling dead, heavy, or like wood. They may note sensations like a constricting bandage, for example, around all or part of the circumference of the abdomen. Disturbance of temperature, with an entire limb or the lower half of the body unable to appreciate the degree of heat or cold, such as while swimming and bathing, is a feature in some cases. Lhermitte's sign refers to a sensation of electricity or shock that may extend down the arms and back in association with sudden neck flexion. Although this is described by some patients with MS, it also occurs after trauma and with cervical spondylosis or cord tumor. Testing of sensory function usually discloses that the most prominent disturbance is in posterior column modalities, including vibration sense and position sense.

Bladder complaints are found in most instances of established disease. Urgency, precipitancy, poor urinary stream, frequency of urination, and urinary incontinence are found in various degrees. It is common for the examiner to be able to identify some disturbance of corticospinal disease when urinary complaints are prominent. Abnormalities in the bladder muscle (detrusor) reflex function in MS arise from either an interruption of the corticoregulatory tracts or a demyelination in the conus medullaris; the former leads to detrusor hyperreflexia and the latter to detrusor areflexia. Almost all patients have abnormalities, hyperreflexia being twice as common as hyporeflexia. Diminished facility and frequency of penile erection and actual impotence may result from the disease in some cases. Psychologic factors may be at fault and should be assessed fully in any evaluation. Cystometrography and anal sphincter electromyography are useful to categorize the urinary and sexual complaints.

Other manifestations such as aphasia and myoclonus occur uncommonly. Some authors report an increased frequency of epilepsy. Cranial nerve palsies are rare; facial palsy is usually of the central type but peripheral seventh nerve palsy can occur. It is rare for the acoustic division of the eighth nerve to be affected, but vestibular symptoms occur occasionally and a severe episode with vertigo, nausea, and vomiting may herald the onset of MS. An important paroxysmal syndrome seen in 2% to 5% of patients is trigeminal neuralgia. Other painful syndromes include glossopharyngeal neuralgia, atypical facial pain, and shooting pains akin to the pain of tabes dorsalis. Some patients have facial myokymia, a movement disorder affecting the facial muscles and manifested by undulant, poorly synchronized movements that may occur bilaterally or unilaterally. Paroxysmal syndromes, including tonic spasms, facial myokymia, and trigeminal neuralgia, may arise from cross-communication between nude axons. Intellectual impairment is not a prominent feature of MS but may result from the cumulative effects of long-standing disease and extensive demyelination.

Diagnosis. Because multiple lesions in the CNS are expected in MS, any patient with neurologic signs pointing to a single lesion should be investigated for a localized disorder such as a spinal cord or foramen magnum tumor, a cervical disc, or a spinal malformation. In spinal cord or foramen magnum tumors, cervical discs, or spinal malformations pain may occur, and the course is more likely to be one of progression rather than of remission and exacerbation. Spinocerebellar degenerations have characteristic patterns of inheritance and involve particular pathways in the CNS. Subacute combined degeneration gives signs characteristic of symmetric involvement of posterior and lateral columns of the spinal cord, generally in a patient with a low serum vitamin B_{12} level. Syringomyelia commonly includes a segmental sensory involvement not typical of MS. Collagen disorders, particularly lupus erythematosus, may mimic MS, since vasculitis can cause multifocal CNS disease. A diagnosis of hysteria is sometimes considered early in MS, when nuerologic signs may be transient or not prominent. Such a psychiatric diagnosis should be suggested by a history of psychiatric disturbances and not by the absence of neurologic signs. Multiple sclerosis generally does not produce signs of peripheral neuropathy or anterior horn cell disturbance, and its onset is uncommon beyond 50 years of age.

Laboratory findings. No definitive laboratory tests exist for MS. The physician should perform a CSF analysis for every patient suspected of having this disorder. This analysis should include a cell count with differential count, estimation of total protein and IgG concentration, and electrophoresis to check for the presence of oligoclonal IgG bands. The CSF leukocyte count is greater than five cells (lymphocytes)/mm^3 in about 30% of cases. A count that exceeds 50 cells/mm^3 or the presence of polymorphonuclear leukocytes should cast doubt on the diagnosis or suggest a complication. The total protein level in the CSF is usually normal. A protein value greater than 100 mg/dl warrants a reevaluation of the diagnosis. An increase in the γ-globulin fraction of the CSF total protein, however, is found in two thirds of patients with MS. De novo synthesis of IgG in the CNS in MS is demonstrated by a relative increase in the ratio of CSF IgG (produced in the CNS) to CSF albumin (derived from serum). This abnormal quantitative index and a qualitative demonstration of oligoclonal IgG bands on electrophoresis are found in approximately 90% of patients with definite MS. This profile may be mimicked in part by neurosyphilis, subacute sclerosing panencephalitis, and certain other diseases, including chronic infections. The serum IgG concentration should be normal in MS. In addition, myelin basic protein can be measured in the CSF by radioimmunoassay and may be increased in the CSF during an acute exacerbation, reflecting the myelin breakdown process. Concentrations of measles antibodies and other common viral antibodies are increased, more in CSF than in blood.

CT of the brain may show areas of low attenuation surrounding the ventricles, and ventricular enlargement and cerebral atrophy are seen with long-standing disease. A large plaque of demyelination may be difficult to differentiate from a tumor if no other lesions are demonstrable.

Electrophysiologic studies of sensory function have been useful in evaluating the patient with suspected MS. This has involved using auditory, visual, and somatosensory evoked potentials. The visual evoked response is abnormal in acute optic neuritis. Delayed latency of the response, an altered waveform, and an altered amplitude of the response occur. The amplitude of the response recovers with improving visual acuity, but the delayed latency, once established, persists indefinitely. Visual evoked responses are impaired in more than 85% of patients with definite MS regardless of the findings on ophthalmologic examination. Similarly, spinal cord, subcortical, and rolandic somatosensory responses may show abnormalities in MS, and brainstem evoked responses are often abnormal. These recordings may be made before, during, and after artificially raising the body temperature and may yield additional information on disease dissemination. Thus a combination of electrophysiologic recordings can facilitate assessing the major fiber tracts in the CNS for clinically inapparent disease, can provide evidence for disease dissemination in the presence of isolated signs and symptoms, and may be useful in following the course of the illness and the response to various putative therapies.

Course. Remissions, which may be complete or partial, are common, particularly in cases beginning in young adult life. The course is more likely to be progressive, without remissions occurring, in cases of MS beginning at a later age. The mechanism of relapse and remission has long been a perplexing problem in MS. Pathologic studies suggest that remyelination may take place; however, this is usually very limited in extent and may not contribute much to restoring lost function. An alternative mechanism of recovery involves structural and cytochemical alterations in the internodal axon that permit a continuous conduction of impulses along the nerve fiber. This may involve the development of new sodium channels along the entire extent of the axon. Recovery from some acute deficits may simply result from resolution of the edema that is known to accompany acute lesions. Steroids may be of some benefit in accelerating this resolution.

Remissions tend to become less complete with time. Despite varying degrees of disability, longevity is better than generally believed; more than 70% of patients with MS are alive 25 years after the onset.

Management. The treatment of MS is symptomatic and is aimed at alleviating the neurologic and psychologic consequences of demyelination and its complications. The uncertainty of diagnosis in some instances and the tendency of the disease to go into remission and then to relapse have made quantifying responses to various interventions difficult.

Incoordination, spasticity, and bladder difficulties constitute the three symptoms that are most disabling for patients with MS. At this time no drug is reliably hopeful for tremor and incoordination. Propranolol in low doses (40 to 240 mg daily) is sometimes helpful for short periods in reducing the intensity of the tremor. When tremors are severe and disabling for long periods, contralateral thalamotomy may give relief for some years. Spasticity and flexor spasm can be both painful and disabling. Baclofen (Lioresal) has proved to be a significant development in the symptomatic management of such patients. The dose is 5 mg three times a day, increasing until an optimal effect is achieved (usually 15 to 25 mg three times a day). Diazepam may be useful in moderating the intensity of spasticity, but the required doses often lead to sedation.

In bladder disorders anticholinergic agents such as propantheline and methantheline reduce detrusor reflex activity and diminish urgency and precipitancy in some cases. Baclofen is also helpful. Bethanechol may help patients with decreased detrusor reflex contraction and bladder tone. Various surgical procedures have been devised, such as intermittent urinary catheterization, which prevents excessive bladder distention. When neurologic impotence is present, a penile prosthesis may be inserted. Dorsal column stimulation has not been useful in treating any of these complications of MS.

Every attempt should be made to maintain patient mobility and to prevent deformities and contractures. Because premature fatigue may be an overwhelming symptom in MS, physiotherapy should be modified in accordance with the stamina of the patient. Hydrotherapy is of great value to patients with MS because buoyancy permits more vigorous and precise movement and dissipates the heat that so frequently aggravates MS symptoms.

Steroids do not appear to alter the progression of neurologic injury or to reverse preexisting injury to the CNS. Clearly there are potentially serious complications from their use over long periods in immobilized patients with bladder dysfunction and increased liability to infection and osteoporosis. Steroids should be reserved for instances of acute neurologic deterioration, such as optic neuritis with severe visual impairment, bilateral optic neuritis, acute transverse myelitis, and the uncommon instances when the lesion ascends with quadriparesis and bulbar paresis. In these situations, adrenocorticotropic hormone (ACTH) or prednisone (40 to 60 mg daily) is used for 8 to 10 days. Nonspecific immunosuppressive therapy (for example, azathioprine and cyclophosphamide) should be considered highly experimental in treating MS.

ACUTE DISSEMINATED ENCEPHALOMYELITIS AND ACUTE NECROTIZING ENCEPHALOMYELITIS. Acute disseminated encephalomyelitis (ADE) and acute necrotizing encephalomyelitis (ANE) constitute a spectrum of pathologic injury to the CNS characterized chiefly by a white matter injury, often with a predilection for the white matter of the cerebrum, brainstem, and spinal cord. The peripheral nervous system may also be affected. The relationship of ADE to ANE is controversial, but present evidence suggests that both are responses to an immune-mediated injury to the CNS. In both disorders perivenous inflammation with myeloclasis is common, but the destruction of white matter may be more extensive in ANE.

ADE is most common in childhood but also occurs in adult life. A history of preceding viral infection may be obtained, or both may occur concurrently. Sometimes the disorder is consequent to immunization, in which case the term "postvaccinal encephalomyelitis" is appropriate. Postvaccinal encephalomyelitis has been seen after rabies and smallpox vaccination. The clinical picture in ADE is characterized by the acute onset of headache, high fever, stiff neck, and alteration in mental status with delirium and obtundation. Seizures may occur. Focal signs depend on the predominant site of injury. In cases of predominant spinal cord injury, areflexic flaccid paraplegia or quadriplegia with sensory disturbance and sphincter failure may occur as a manifestation of transverse myelitis. Guillain-Barré syndrome with neuropathic features may be the major manifestation. A brainstem syndrome may predominate, in which nystagmus, ophthalmoplegia, facial paresis, and various motor and sensory findings are combined. The CSF demonstrates pleocytosis with increased protein concentration but is occasionally normal.

ANE may be similar clinically to ADE but is more fulminating and more frequently characterized by focal symptoms and signs. The disease tends to occur in children and young adults and often is preceded by an upper respiratory tract infection.

Both disorders may be fatal in hours or days, but patients with ADE commonly recover partially or fully. In occasional instances both disorders may recur after full recovery, sometimes in association with some new antigenic stimulus such as drug ingestion or vaccination. Most clinicians believe that steroids are useful if given in time.

Dysmyelinating diseases

METACHROMATIC LEUKODYSTROPHY. Metachromatic leukodystrophy is the most common of the leukodystrophies. The disease is inherited as an autosomal recessive trait; late infantile, juvenile, and adult forms occur. In the late infantile form development seems normal until the end of the first year of life. At this time incoordination and gait disturbance appear. The patient has flaccid paraparesis or quadriparesis with absent or diminished reflexes. Rarely, spastic diplegia without increased stretch reflexes occurs. Speech deteriorates because of dysarthria and dysphasia. Optic atrophy may be seen. Eventually the patient has quadriplegia with decorticate or decerebrate posturing. Dysphagia caused by bulbar and pseudobulbar palsy occurs. Dementia ensues, and the patient usually dies 2 to 4 years after the onset of symptoms.

The progression of the juvenile form is similar to the infantile variety, except deterioration is not as rapid.

The adult form of metachromatic leukodystrophy may be difficult to diagnose because for many years the patient may appear to suffer from a functional disorder. Later, seizures, movement disorders with extrapyramidal signs, and intellectual impairment confirm the organic nature of the disease.

In this disease galactosyl ceramide esterified with sulfuric acid accumulates in nervous tissue, the kidney, and the biliary system. The defect in this disease results from a lack of arylsulfatase A, which hydrolyzes the sulfuric acid ester from galactose. Patients excrete large quantities of this material, and it also accumulates in the nervous tissue. The material is stained with the dye cresyl violet, and the orange-brown color produced is known as metachromasia.

Pathologically, there is extensive involvement of the white matter, usually symmetrically. The ventricles may be enlarged because of shrinkage of the white matter. Myelin is principally affected, but axons and neurons also undergo degeneration. Macrophages filled with debris are evident in areas of myelin breakdown. Nerve cells are ballooned and swollen, containing cerebroside sulfatide. Metachromatic material is seen also in oligodendrocytes, some neurons, and Schwann cells.

The diagnosis is made by measuring urinary arylsulfatase A activity or by demonstrating metachromatic material in tissue from the kidney or peripheral nerve. The diagnosis of the heterozygote state can be made by assaying enzyme levels in cultured fibroblasts. The CSF almost always shows an increase in total protein. CT scans may show decreased density surrounding the lateral ventricles, which is consistent with a diffuse demyelinating process. Nerve conduction velocities are slowed, and a sural nerve biopsy stained with acidified cresyl violet may show the metachromatic staining of stored sulfatide. Prenatal diagnosis is possible by amniocentesis.

ADRENOLEUKODYSTROPHY. The typical age at onset of adrenoleukodystrophy is between 5 and 10 years. The initial symptoms are behavior disturbance and intellectual failure. Visual loss (cortical) and motor deficits occur, and later seizures may develop. Unilateral symptoms may initially predominate. In children signs of adrenal insufficiency are not prominent, although their skin may show a bronze pigmentation. When familial, the disease shows an X-linked recessive pattern of inheritance. An enzyme defect is presumed in this disorder, but its nature is unknown. A brain biopsy shows the key feature of demyelination. Subcortical arcuate fibers are usually not involved. On light microscopy adrenoleukodystrophy may look identical to multiple sclerosis. An ultrastructural study may reveal characteristic trilaminar cytoplasmic inclusions within the macrophages. Similar changes are found in the peripheral tissues, and a biopsy of one of these peripheral sites may allow a diagnosis to be made in life. CT scanning is useful in excluding tumor and shows extensive, usually symmetric low-density lesions in the white matter. Some lesions may be enhanced with injection of contrast media. ACTH stimulation reveals an impaired adrenal reserve. The CSF total protein is often increased. Many cases of adrenoleukodystrophy were described in the past under the eponym "Schilder's disease."

GLOBOID CELL LEUKODYSTROPHY (KRABBE'S DISEASE). Globoid cell leukodystrophy, or Krabbe's disease, is a rare dysmyelinating disease in which symptoms begin within the first 3 to 6 months of life with irritability, stiffness of the extremities, and febrile episodes. The infant becomes sensitive to external stimulation and cries constantly for no apparent reason. Progressive intellectual deterioration, decorticate posturing, and death within months to several years ensue. The disorder is associated with a deficiency of a β-galactosidase (cerebrosidase) and is transmitted as an autosomal recessive trait. There is extensive demyelination of the brain and spinal cord. The gray matter is usually spared. Large multinucleated globoid cells with abundant cytoplasm and containing para-aminosalicylic acid (PAS) positive staining material are found in the CNS. Peripheral nerve involvement is present. The urine sediment shows galactosyl ceramide. Reduced levels of β-galactosidase (cerebrosidase) are found in leukocytes and fibroblasts. Nerve conduction velocities are slowed. A CT scan may show the white matter loss. The CSF protein is increased. Prenatal diagnosis is possible by amniocentesis.

SUDANOPHILIC LEUKODYSTROPHY (PELIZAEUS-MERZBACHER DISEASE). Sudanophilic leukodystrophy, or Pelizaeus-Merzbacher disease, is a rare dysmyelinating disorder affecting principally the white matter. It is most commonly a sex-linked recessive disorder. The clinical picture is variable; it may begin in the first few months of life or later in childhood. The earliest and most characteristic signs are pendular and rotary nystagmus, chaotic eye movement, and intermittent shaking movements of the arms and the head. The disease may progress slowly over many decades. In cases occurring later in life, spasticity, dysarthria, ataxia, and choreoathetosis occur. In all cases intellectual deterioration occurs and seizures are common. Optic atrophy and blindness eventually appear. The characteristic pathologic condition is a symmetric, diffuse hypomyelination with areas of gliosis interspersed with islands of normal myelination. The white matter disturbance, interpreted as an arrest of myelination, is most prominent in the cerebrum and cerebellum. The subcortical U fibers and the axons are spared. Diagnostic tests and treatment are not available for this disease.

SPONGY DEGENERATION OF THE WHITE MATTER (CANAVAN'S DISEASE). Spongy degeneration of the white matter, or Canavan's disease, is an autosomal recessive disorder usually classified with the dysmyelinating diseases. More than 30% of reported cases have occurred in Ashkenazi Jews (of eastern European descent), but cases have been reported in all races. Most cases begin in infancy with hypotonia of the head and neck noticeable at 3 or 4 months of age. Megalencephaly and psychomotor retardation are apparent by 6 months of age. Decerebrate and decorticate posturing in response to sensory stimuli is superimposed on generalized hypotonia. Myoclonic seizures and choreoathetosis are added to the evolving clinical picture. Autonomic crises (for example, blood pressure fluctuations and diaphoresis) may occur. Optic atrophy, nystagmus, and rolling eye movements are noted. Most patients die in the first 2 years of the disease. The first signs of Canavan's disease may be noted later in the first decade, in which case a cerebellar syndrome with optic atrophy, spasticity, and intellectual deterioration occurs, but megalencephaly is usually not present. Pathologically, the brain is enlarged. There is little stainable myelin, along with marked vacuolation of the myelin sheaths and secondary degeneration of the myelin membrane. The water content of the brain is increased, and both edema and a spongy state have been described on microscopic examination. There is a generalized enlargement of the protoplasmic astrocytes, which contain bizarre and enormously elongated mitochondria with a crystalline substructure. Alzheimer's type 2 cells are also present in great numbers. Diagnostic tests and therapy are not available for this disorder.

FIBRINOID LEUKODYSTROPHY (ALEXANDER'S DISEASE). Fibrinoid leukodystrophy, or Alexander's disease, is the rarest of the hereditary disorders of myelin. Its mode of transmission is unknown, but the disease affects males much more frequently than females. Neurologic deterioration with a rapidly enlarging head begins early in infancy. The head enlargement usually results from megalencephaly, but hydrocephalus may occur. Seizures and spasticity are characteristic symptoms. If hydrocephalus results from stenosis of the aqueduct of Sylvius, there may be a temporary response to shunting. Most affected children die before 5 years of age. At autopsy the brain is heavier and larger than normal. There is a pronounced lack of myelin staining of the cerebral and cerebellar white matter. Multiple hypertrophic astrocytes with eosinophilic inclusions within their cytoplasm are seen; these inclusions are known as Rosenthal fibers and are thought to represent glial degradation products. The axis cylinders are preserved. No inflammatory cells are present. No degenerating sudanophilic material exists to indicate myelin breakdown. There is no diagnostic test for this disease, and its cause is unknown.

OTHER DYSMYELINATING DISEASES. Other dysmyelinating diseases include phenylketonuria, an autosomal recessive disorder classified in the aminoacidopathies, and the lipidoses (for example, Tay-Sachs disease) (see Chapter 195).

DEGENERATIVE DISORDERS
Motor neuron disease

The term "motor neuron disease" refers to a group of disorders characterized pathologically by injury and a loss of motor neurons in the cerebral cortex, brainstem, and spinal cord and clinically by muscular atrophy, spasticity, and weakness. Significant sensory symptoms are absent in all instances. The nomenclature established for these diseases is reasonably descriptive of the clinical and pathologic findings. Amyotrophic lateral sclerosis (ALS) refers to cases in which upper motor neuron findings are prominent, in addition to atrophy and fasciculations as manifestations of lower motor neuron involvement. Involvement of the bulbar muscles usually occurs at some point during the course of the disease. Progressive bulbar palsy is a variant of ALS; its chief features are paresis and wasting of muscles innervated by the lower cranial nerves, and it is characterized clinically by dysphonia, dysphagia, dysarthria, and difficulty with respiration and clearing of secretions. Progressive muscular atrophy is characterized by findings chiefly reflecting an injury to anterior horn cells. It is not a single entity and includes a number of disorders with differences in age of onset, severity, genetics, and prognosis, such as Werdnig-Hoffman syndrome of infancy and Kugelberg-Welander disease of late childhood or early adulthood. The neuronal form of Charcot-Marie-Tooth disease may be included in this category.

AMYOTROPHIC LATERAL SCLEROSIS. ALS is the most common variant of motor neuron disease, with an estimated prevalence of 2 to 7:100,000 persons in the United States. A clustering of cases occurs in the western Pacific region, where the disease is perhaps 50 times more common than in other regions. The mean age of onset is between 50 and 60 years of age, but the disease also may occur in the very aged. ALS has a slight male preponderance, and familial cases occasionally occur.

Etiology. The cause of ALS is not established. The clustering of cases found in the western Pacific, especially in Guam, and the occasional occurrence of an ALS syndrome many years after a poliovirus infection have raised the question of the disease being a slow virus infection. Efforts to transmit this disease have not been successful, virologic studies have not disclosed any disease-specific abnormality, and the majority of ultrastructural studies for virus material have been negative or inconclusive. Immunologic factors involved in its pathogenesis are suggested by the finding of immune complex deposition in the glomeruli of some patients with ALS and the cytotoxicity of ALS serum to anterior horn cells in tissue culture. Histocompatibility typing in some studies has shown a preponderance of some HLA types.

Pathology. In the cerebrum, atrophy of the cortex, particularly of the precentral gyrus, may be grossly apparent. Microscopic changes are confined to the upper motor neurons and to the lower motor neurons and their tracts. The Betz cells of the motor cortex are reduced in number and size. There is loss of the motor neurons of the brainstem except for those subserving the extraocular muscles. In the spinal cord a loss of large motor neurons is found and corticospinal tract degeneration is noted. In the Guamanian form neurofibrillary degeneration is prominent. In some familial cases of ALS, degeneration of the posterior columns and spinocerebellar tracts occurs, linking this subtype to other degenerations of the nervous system.

Clinical manifestations. Signs of anterior horn cell disease may predominate initially, or the patient may have pyramidal tract signs alone. Eventually, combinations of findings develop in which, despite atrophy and fasciculations of anterior horn cell disease, reflexes may be increased pathologically and there may be reflex spread. The principal symptom is weakness that begins in the upper extremities and is often unilateral at onset. Atrophy, cramps, and fasciculations develop. The weakness and wasting often are first apparent in the small muscles of the hand and result in loss of dexterity for fine hand movements and in clumsiness. In a minority of patients the weakness and atrophy are first apparent proximally in the shoulder girdle muscles. At a time when the hands and upper extremity muscles have been greatly damaged by disease, the lower extremities may be unimpaired, although examination may disclose fasciculations and brisk reflexes. Conversely, spastic paraparesis may occur. Unilateral involvement may be present for a long time, sometimes masquerading as a localized lesion. In such cases, however, careful examination for fasciculations throughout the body, using reflected light and muscle percussion, commonly discloses multifocal twitching. Sometimes the first evidence of ALS is in the lower extremity, manifested by footdrop and mimicking a mononeuropathy of the peroneal nerve for some time. The time of onset and rate of progression of bulbar palsy are variable; the first signs usually include fasciculations and atrophy of the tongue. The patient complains of dysphagia, and dysphonia and dysarthria appear. Significant sensory findings do not occur; if present, they are caused by some complicating process such as metabolic disease, entrapment neuropathy, radiculopathy, or spondylosis. Sphincter involvement does not usually occur except in the later stages of the illness.

Differential diagnosis. The neurologic examination usually is adequate to establish the differential diagnosis. Nevertheless, some conditions may mimic ALS. Foremost among these disorders are spinal cord disease such as cervical spondylosis with myelopathy and radiculopathy. Tumors of the spinocranial junction, especially foramen magnum meningiomas, may be missed if this region is not carefully examined by myelography. Demyelinating disease must be considered when the patient is young and complains of such symptoms as a useless hand. Syringomyelia may be considered when there are atrophy in the arms and spasticity in the legs, but prominent and characteristic sensory signs establish the diagnosis of syringomyelia.

Laboratory findings. No specific laboratory abnormality occurs in ALS. Creatine phosphokinase may be elevated to twice its normal values. Circulating immune complexes may be found, but the antigen has not been identified. The CSF may show a mild elevation of total protein with a normal IgG concentration and a normal cell count. The myelography may be normal or may show a shrunken spinal cord. CT scanning of the brain is normal or shows cerebral atrophy. The electromyogram may show remarkable abnormalities and is useful in confirming a diffuse process in patients who have monoparetic or unilateral forms of disease; it typically shows widespread fibrillations associated with giant polyphasic potentials and fasciculations. Motor and sensory nerve conduction velocities are typically normal. A muscle biopsy usually shows the abnormalities and changes of denervation.

Course. The course of ALS is usually unremittingly progressive. Patients survive for 3 to 5 years or less, although the survival rate may range from 1 to 10 years. Variations in the initial symptoms and in the course of ALS occur, and since the prognosis depends to a large extent on the degree of the involvement of the bulbar musculature, the early development of bulbar paralysis is associated with a shorter course compared to that found with its late onset. One familial variant of ALS is characterized by an illness of long duration.

Management. No specific treatment for ALS is known. Immunosuppressive therapy and snake venom are not useful. Patients should maintain their mobility, and their morale may be helped by an active hydrotherapy exercise program. When spasticity and clonus are painful or cause gait difficulty, either diazepam (5 mg three times a day) or baclofen (5 mg three times a day, increasing to its optimal effect, usually 15 to 25 mg three times a day) may be used. Drug therapy may help to reduce secretions in bulbar paresis, and a cricopharyngeal myotomy may alleviate dysphagia.

PROGRESSIVE SPINAL MUSCULAR ATROPHIES

Werdnig-Hoffman disease (infantile muscular atrophy) and Fazio-Londe atrophy. Werdnig-Hoffmann disease (infantile muscular atrophy) is an anterior horn cell disease of infancy that runs a rapid course; it begins in the first year of life with death resulting in several months to years. Sometimes the clinical picture is more slowly progressive. The disorder is autosomal recessive. The infant's mother may have noted diminished fetal movements in the last trimester. At birth the child is limp and flaccid and cries feebly. The child's reflexes are unobtainable, and feeding is difficult because of the child's weakness. Tongue fasciculations may be found. Eye movements are intact, giving the child an alert appearance despite the widespread weakness. The laboratory and pathologic findings resemble those found in ALS.

A progressive bulbar palsy of childhood is known as Fazio-Londe atrophy. There is no known treatment for these disorders.

Kugelberg-Welander disease (juvenile progressive spinal muscular atrophy). Kugelberg-Welander disease, or juvenile progressive spinal muscular atrophy, is an anterior horn cell disease of childhood or adolescence. It is slowly progressive and, although usually beginning in the first or second decade of life, may not be diagnosed until the patient is 30 or more years of age. The disorder is being recognized more frequently in recent years. Some of these cases may represent infantile muscular atrophy with a long survival. A male preponderance is noted in the juvenile group. Weakness begins in the lower extremities, with the hip flexors affected first. Patients may have atrophy at this stage or only much later. The proximal weakness may lead to difficulty in rising from a low chair or walking up stairs. When the disease is established in the lower extremities, the patient may also have proximal upper extremity weakness, and there may be some bulbar involvement. The distribution of the weakness may easily lead the physician to diagnose myopathy or dystrophy, especially facioscapulohumeral and limb-girdle muscular dystrophy. Most patients have fasciculations. An electromyography and a muscle biopsy also support the diagnosis of a neuropathic process and exclude primary muscle disease. Muscle enzymes are sometimes elevated.

Other chronic spinal muscular atrophies. A variety of other chronic spinal muscular atrophies of adult onset occur either sporadically or with varied patterns of inheritance and different distributions of muscle wasting and weakness. Those with proximal involvement, such as facioscapulohumeral and scapulohumeral muscular atrophy, may be confused with muscular dystrophy. Scapuloperoneal spinal muscular atrophy involves the face, neck, and shoulder girdle, as well as footdrop. A neuronal rather than a neuropathic form of Charcot-Marie-Tooth disease can be categorized with the spinal muscular atrophies. Unlike other forms of Charcot-Marie-Tooth disease, the nerve conduction velocity is normal to borderline, and hypertrophic neuropathy is not found on sural nerve biopsy.

SYNDROMES OF PROGRESSIVE HEREDITARY ATAXIA

The progressive hereditary ataxias constitute a significant proportion of the chronic disorders seen by neurologists. A scientifically based classification is not possible at this time because the cause of these disorders is not known in most instances. The clinical symptoms are diverse, and the pathologic findings can vary from a discrete degeneration of one neuronal system and tract to multifocal and multisystem degeneration. Eponyms are still used to describe a few of these disorders in spite of some clinical and pathologic heterogeneity. Although the site of disease in the hereditary ataxias is basically the cerebellum and its pathways, classifications often include disorders that involve other neural systems because they can be found in the same kinships. The various syndromes demonstrate clinical or pathologic evidence of involvement of the following systems: spinocerebellar tracts, cerebellum, retinal ganglion cells or optic nerve, basal ganglia, midbrain, pons, olives, cochlea, dorsal columns, corticospinal tracts, ventral horn cells, and peripheral nerves. The cerebral hemispheres, especially the cortical neurons, are involved in some instances. There is often an array of associated musculoskeletal abnormalities, including kyphoscoliosis and pes cavus, and cardiac lesions, including myocarditis and cardiac rhythm disturbances. Epilepsy, mental retardation, and dementia may occur. Endocrine abnormalities are seen in some cases. The following are the better known syndromes.

FRIEDREICH'S ATAXIA. Friedreich's ataxia is the best characterized of all the hereditary ataxias, with degeneration involving posterior and lateral columns of the spinal cord and the cerebellum. The common form of inheritance is autosomal recessive, and the symptoms begin soon after the first decade. Another atypical pattern, in which the pattern of inheritance is dominant, has been described with the onset at about 20 years of age. Cases of Roussy-Lévy syndrome and Charcot-Marie-Tooth disease have been reported in families with Friedreich's ataxia.

Pathology. The conspicuous pathologic conditions are in the spinal cord, which is visibly shrunken. The fiber loss in the fasciculus gracilis is complete, and the fasciculus cuneatus is affected less intensely. The pyramidal tracts show progressive attenuation as they descend caudally in the spinal cord. Degeneration is constant in the posterior spinocerebellar tracts and common in the anterior spinocerebellar tracts. The cerebellar cortex is normal or shows some loss of Purkinje cells, but the white matter is gliotic and the dentate nuclei show severe cell loss. The vestibular nuclei are also shrunken and gliotic. Nerve fiber loss may be noted in the optic tract and when severe is accompanied by corresponding abnormalities in the lateral geniculate body. The cerebral cortex is usually normal. Myocardial muscle may show degeneration and replacement by macrophages and fibroblasts.

Clinical manifestations. Ataxia of the lower extremities is almost always the first symptom; the trunk and upper extremities are affected later. Antecedent injury and infection may sometimes be noted. The incoordination that occurs is caused by lesions in both the cerebellum and its pathways. Lesions in the posterior columns result in a Romberg's sign with a profound loss of position and vibratory senses. Later there may be some impairment of spinothalamic sensory modalities. The hands usually become clumsy after the gait disturbance is well developed. Dysarthric speech usually follows the development of appendicular and truncal ataxia. Sometimes the patient has prominent head titubation and side-to-side movements, called choreiform by some, which are probably caused by combined sensory and motor disturbances. The mentation is usually normal. Muscle atrophy is uncommon unless there is associated neuropathy of the peroneal muscular atrophy type. The stretch reflexes are lost early, but flexor spasms and extensor plantar responses occur as manifestations of corticospinal (pyramidal) tract involvement. The superficial abdominal reflexes usually are maintained. Ocular abnormalities are found when the disease is established. Horizontal, rotary, vertical, and periodic alternating nystagmus may occur. Optic atrophy, pigmentary degeneration of the retina, and extraocular nerve palsies may develop. A syndrome of progressive external ophthalmoplegia has been described with Friedreich's ataxia. Deglutition may be impaired later in the disease. Cardiac rhythm disturbances and respiratory disease are important causes of morbidity and mortality.

Laboratory findings. The diagnosis is apparent from the characteristic clinical picture. No laboratory abnormality is diagnostic. A disturbance of pyruvate metabolism occurs, but it is not known how this may be related to the nervous manifestations. Overt diabetes or chemical diabetes mellitus may be found. Electrocardiograms may be abnormal; echocardiography may demonstrate evidence of asymmetric septal hypertrophy. Sensory action potentials are absent or markedly reduced in amplitude at an early stage of the disease. In contrast, motor nerve conduction velocities remain normal or decrease only slightly with disease progression. The prominent alteration of sensory action potentials reflects involvement of large myelinated nerve fibers and neurons in dorsal root ganglia.

Differential diagnosis. In the differential diagnosis various other hereditary and sporadic disorders may be considered, including congenital spastic paraplegia, muscular dystrophies, tabes dorsalis, multiple sclerosis, and the olivopontocerebellar degenerations. Bassen-Kornzweig syndrome (abetalipoproteinemia), a familial disorder with posterior and lateral column degeneration, pes cavus, and cardiac abnormalities, may mimic Friedreich's ataxia but is associated with abnormalities in the peripheral blood smear (acanthocytosis) and in blood lipids.

Management. No specific treatment for Freidreich's ataxia exists. An exercise program, especially hydrotherapy, is important. Orthopedic correction of the symptomatic skeletal disorders should be carried out. Infection, arrhythmia, heart failure, and diabetes are treated in the usual way. Acetazolamide, physostigmine, and ketogenic diets are undergoing evaluation for treatment of the ataxic components of this disease, but the benefits appear questionable or short lived.

ROUSSY-LÉVY SYNDROME. Roussy-Lévy syndrome is an autosomal dominant disorder that usually begins in childhood, but there are instances in which the disorder begins later in life. Features of this neuropathy include skeletal disorders such as clubfood and kyphoscoliosis, wasting of the muscles of the lower extremity and the small hand muscles, generalized areflexia, unsteady gait, and tremor of the hands resembling intention tremor. Other cerebellar signs are absent. Cataracts and deafness may occur. Sensory disturbance is generally absent, although in some instances posterior column modalities are greatly impaired, thus linking this disorder with the spinocerebellar ataxias. Roussy-Lévy syndrome has been viewed by some as intermediate between Friedreich's ataxia and Charcot-Marie-Tooth disease (see Chapter 155). Demyelination and onion bulb formation (layering secondary to proliferation of Schwann cells and fibroblasts) are seen pathologically. Nerve conduction velocities are prolonged. The disease runs a very slowly progressive ourse.

REFSUM'S DISEASE. Refsum's disease is a rare disorder with an autosomal recessive pattern of inheritance, which may resemble Charcot-Marie-Tooth disease (see Chapter 155). The cardinal disturbances are retinitis pigmentosa with night blindness, chronic sensorimotor polyneuropathy, and cerebellar ataxia. In most instances deafness and cardiomyopathy occur. Other reported occurrences include pupillary abnormalities, cataracts, anosmia, skeletal abnormalities, ichthyosis, and palpably enlarged nerves. The age of onset varies from early childhood to the second and third decades of life. The disorder is slowly progressive, and in some instances striking exacerbations and then remissions without obvious cause have occurred. Sometimes the deficits are static. Findings of laboratory studies are normal, but the serum phytanic acid level is markedly elevated. The CSF protein concentration may be significantly elevated. Pathologically, peripheral nerves are hypertrophied and onion bulb formation is seen. Loss of myelin and some axonal loss are demonstrable. Administered early in the course of the disease, vitamin A may reverse or delay some of the retinal manifestations of this disease. Similarly, dietary exclusion of phytol and phytanic acid may be beneficial, but information is not adequate at this time.

OTHER HEREDITARY ATAXIAS. Soon after Friedreich's studies of hereditary ataxis, a number of reports appeared describing individuals and families with features of Friedreich's ataxia but with more extensive pathologic changes in the cerebellar cortex, inferior olivary nuclei, brainstem, and in some cases the basal ganglia and cerebral cortex. These patients with olivopontocerebellar atrophy have a predominance of spasticity and hyperreflexia over sensory findings in the lower extremities.

Another type of predominantly spinal ataxia but also with spasticity, in contrast to Friedreich's ataxia, is Sanger Brown spinal ataxia. Menzel described a patient with many of the pathologic features typical of Friedreich's ataxia but also with conspicuous atrophy involving mainly the middle cerebellar peduncle, the pontine nuclei, and the olivary nuclei. A sporadically occurring disorder was described by Dejerine and Andre-Thomas, differing from the Menzel form pathologically in that the spinal cord was spared. Late cortical cerebellar atrophy was described by Marie, Foix, and Alajounine. The Ramsay Hunt syndrome, in which dentatorubral atrophy occurs, is characterized clinically by myoclonus and cerebellar ataxia. Many of these syndromes may be accompanied by manifestations of disease above the brainstem, including mental retardation, dementia, seizures, movement disorders, optic atrophy, and pigmentary retinal degeneration. The diagnosis of these disorders is based on the clinical features, and no consistent diagnostic test is available, although visual and brainstem evoked potentials, electromyography, and CT scanning may be helpful.

SYRINGOMYELIA

Syringomyelia (from *syrinx,* meaning tube) refers to a tubular dilatation of the spinal cord extending over many segments. Syringobulbia sometimes occurs in association with syringomyelia and refers to a cavitation extending above the foramen magnum but usually not extending above the medulla. This disease has a serious morbidity, its cause is still in dispute, and a consensus does not exist on management.

PATHOPHYSIOLOGY. Syringomyelia may be divided into the following several different categories:

1. *A form communicating with the fourth ventricle.* This is seen most commonly in association with developmental abnormalities of the craniospinal junction such as Arnold-Chiari malformation. It may occur with acquired disease such as arachnoiditis, tumors, and cysts. It has been suggested that syringomyelia develops as a result of blockage of the outlet of the fourth ventricle, combined with downward pulsations of CSF into the central canal over time.
2. *An accompaniment of spinal cord tumors, especially those that are intramedullary in location, such as ependymoma and hemangioblastoma.* Some studies report intramedullary tumors in 25% of all cases of syringomyelia. Cavitation also may occur in association with an extramedullary tumor.
3. *As a sequel to spinal cord trauma, including traumatic paraplegia and quadriplegia.* The injury is usually serious, but it has been reported to follow minor trauma.
4. *Not associated with any of these circumstances*

PATHOLOGY. Externally at surgery or autopsy the spinal cord may appear swollen and tense. The syrinx is mot apparent at the cervical region but may extend infrequently to involve the lumbosacral enlargement. When the lesion is large, it may appear to occupy the entire cross section of the spinal cord, sparing only the peripheral islands of nervous tissue. Typically the gray matter is most damaged. The cavity fluid is commonly a clear, slightly yellowish liquid. If the cavity is lined by ependyma, the term "hydromyelia" may be used.

CLINICAL MANIFESTATIONS. Syringomyelia in its classic form is a progressive disorder of young people, especially those in their second and third decades of life. It is characterized by muscle atrophy, dissociated anesthesia, and paraparesis with neurotrophic changes, including neurogenic arthropathy and kyphoscoliosis. The age of onset varies between 10 and 60 years, but cases have also been seen at the extremes of life. The precise clinical manifestations depend on the location of the cavity. Since the cavity is usually most obvious initially in the cervical enlargement, the initial signs reflect disease there. The disease may be unilateral and monosymptomatic at the outset but usually becomes characteristic with time.

Involvement of the ventral horns of the spinal cord leads to weakness of the hand and the forearm muscles and striking atrophy, scoliosis, and a characteristic loss of lumbrical and interosseous function with resulting claw-hand and main en griffe deformities. Deep reflexes in the upper extremity are lost early in the course of the disease. Interruption of the spinothalamic fibers (which decussate just anterior to the central canal) before cavitation extends into the dorsal columns induces dissociated anesthesia, with impairment of temperature and pain sensations but retention of light touch and proprioceptive sensibilities. Spastic paraparesis results from the lateral extension of the cavitation to affect the corticospinal tracts. The paraparesis starts asymmetrically but ultimately becomes symmetric with the development of clonus, extensor plantar responses, and a loss of superficial abdominal reflexes. Sphincter involvement is late. Cavitation at the first dorsal (thoracic) segment leads to ipsilateral Horner's syndrome. Extension of the disease into the medulla leads to weakness and wasting of the tongue, dissociated fifth nerve sensory loss, palatal weakness, and nystagmus. Pain in the neck and shoulders occurs, mimicking radicular pain. In advanced cases the disease is very recognizable, but in the early stages it must be differentiated from other disorders such as intramedullary cord tumors and the central cord syndrome that may result from trauma and hematomyelia. If the onset is asymmetric with sensory complaints, root compression must be excluded. Demyelinating disease, tumors of the spinocranial junction, and arachnoid cysts may be considered in some instances. Muscle wasting and fasciculations require that motor neuron disease be considered.

LABORATORY FINDINGS. The confirmation of the diagnosis of syringomyelia requires roentgenographic studies. Myelography demonstrates an enlargement of the spinal cord and narrowing of the subarachnoid space. Air myelography accurately demonstrates the diameter of the spinal cord and may identify tonsillar herniation if present. By manipulation of the air and fluid at myelography, changes in the collapsibility of a syrinx may be demonstrated and thus the syrinx can be differentiated from a tumor. CT scanning of the spinal canal combined with a contrast study of the subarachnoid space also permits a good visualization of syrinx anatomy.

MANAGEMENT. The optimal treatment for syringomyelia has not been established. A number of procedures have been advocated. These include posterior fossa decompression with or without plugging of the obex, myelotomy, and sectioning the filum terminale. A shunt also may be placed between the cavity and the spinal subarachnoid space. The variety of procedures suggests that none is optimal for every patient, and repeat surgery may be necessary.

COMBINED SYSTEM DISEASE (VITAMIN B_{12} DEFICIENCY)

(See also Chapter 61.)

Combined system disease primarily affects the lateral and dorsal columns of the spinal cord and is related to vitamin B_{12} deficiency. Vitamin B_{12} is a coenzyme not synthesized by man but derived from foodstuffs, the best sources being liver, kidney, meat, and milk. Plants contain no vitamin B_{12}. In the United States the average daily diet contains 15 to 39 μg of vitamin B_{12} of which perhaps 5 μg is absorbed in the ileum with the aid of intrinsic factor, a glycoprotein from gastric secretions. The most important cause of vitamin B_{12} deficiency in humans is pernicious anemia, a presumed autoimmune disease associated with atrophic gastritis and the absence of intrinsic factor necessary for vitamin B_{12} absorption. Inadequate dietary intake and malabsorption syndromes also rarely may lead to neurologic involvement.

PATHOLOGY. The pathologic condition is confined to the white matter of the spinal cord and occasionally involves the cerebrum and optic nerve. Disturbances in L-methylmalonyl coenzyme A may lead to abnormalities of myelin. The earliest lesion is a separation of the myelin lamellae and the formation of intramyelin vacuoles, leading eventually to complete destruction of myelin. As in wallerian degeneration, numerous lipophages appear and come to lie within the perivascular spaces of blood vessels. Axonal degeneration occurs later. The result is a severe depletion of myelin and damage to axons. Tese changes give the tissue a spongy, vacuolated appearance. Marked gliosis ensues with time. The lesions, which are spotty initially and later become confluent, begin in the posterior columns and move forward into the lateral columns. Scattered lesions, however, are seen in the other tracts of the spinal cord, including the spinothalamic tracts. Lesions are sometimes found in the optic nerve and cerebral white matter.

CLINICAL MANIFESTATIONS. Paresthesias of all four extremities are usually the first manifestation. The lower extremities are sometimes the first to become symptomatic. Motor manifestations, predominantly increased fatigue, weakness, and stiffness, then occur in the lower extremities. The motor signs, combined with the prominent defect in postural sensation resulting from dorsal column disease, lead to an unsteadiness of gait and falling episodes. Behavior change and intellectual alterations may be prominent. Rarely, visual impairment with centrocecal scotomas and later optic atrophy may occur, apparently sometimes in isolation, as a manifestation of vitamin B_{12} deficiency.

The clinical findings demonstrate a loss of vibration and position senses. The muscle tone of the lower extremities is increased, with extensor plantar responses and clonus. If treatment has been delayed, spastic paraplegia may be noted. In most instances the stretch reflexes are exaggerated, but occasionally they are diminished or absent, returning with treatment. Distal impairment of pain, light touch, and temperature may be found, suggesting a peripheral neuropathic process. In infants born to vegetarian mothers, florid encephalopathy, anemia, hyperpigmentation, and methylmalonic aciduria may develop in the first year of life.

LABORATORY FINDINGS. The neurologic picture may mimic other metabolic, inflammatory, and degenerative diseases of the spinal cord. The hematologic picture may be normal. A consistent finding is methylmalonic aciduria. The serum vitamin B_{12} level is reduced. The Schilling test establishes the diagnosis of intrinsic factor deficit; since it involves a flushing dose of vitamin B_{12}, treatment begins at the time of the test. The disease should be considered for an infant who was born to a vegetarian mother and has an obscure and unexplained encephalopathy. Visual evoked responses may be abnormal in amplitude and velocity in patients without obvious damage to the optic system.

MANAGEMENT. Treatment involves administering one of the various preparations of vitamin B_{12} intramuscularly and continuing for life, usually monthly (see Chapter 61). Generally all the manifestations respond, but the extent of the response depends on the duration of symptoms. Patients who have had gait disturbance for less than 6 months show the best response. Improvement may continue for months and sometimes years.

NEUROCUTANEOUS SYNDROMES

The neurocutaneous syndromes, or phakomatoses, are congenital conditions, usually dominantly inherited and characterized by various cutaneous, ocular, neurologic, and mesenchymal abnormalities. The term "phakomatoses" is descriptive and has no causal or pathogenetic basis. The syndromes are remarkable for the wide spectrum of individual variation in clinical expression among members of the same affected family; for example, neurofibromatosis may be represented by a few café au lait spots in one family member and by generalized neurofibromatosis with cutaneous, neuroectodermal, and mesenchymal abnormalities in another.

Neurofibromatosis (von Recklinghausen's disease)

Neurofibromatosis is the most common of the phakomatoses. The disorder has autosomal dominant transmission with variable penetrance. The cutaneous hallmark of this disease is café au lait spots; these are brownish, pigmented macules that may be found on any part of the skin surface. Some suggest that any person with more than six café au lait spots, each greater than 1 cm in broadest diameter, may be presumed to have the disease. Freckles in the axillae are particularly significant. Cutaneous and subcutaneous hard and soft fibromas and lipomas also occur. A variety of associated abnormalities are involved, including bony abnormalities such as spinal fusion defects, posterior orbital roof defects, basilar impression (see Chapter 149), syringomyelia, and pheochromocytoma. Schwannomas and neurofibromas are common. Parencymal brain tumors occur, of which astrocytoma is the most common. There is a high incidence of optic nerve glioma, acoustic neuroma (which may be bilateral), and meningiomas (which may be multiple). The clinical abnormalities reflect these diverse lesions. Mental retardation occurs in 10% of patients, and seizures occur with the same frequency. Optic nerve glioma may lead to papilledema, visual field disturbance, proptosis, optic atrophy, and blindness. Tumors of the eighth cranial nerve are manifested by mild vestibular symptoms and progressive hearing loss. Brainstem and cerebellar symptoms and signs may result, as well as obstructive hydrocephalus. Tumors of other cranial nerves are less common.

Neurofibromas may involve the entire extent of multiple roots and peripheral nerves, causing pain, disfigurement, paresis, and sometimes spinal cord compression. The diagnosis is suggested by the skin lesions. Every patient with such lesions and neurologic symptoms should be screened for intracranial mass lesions. This is now aided by CT scanning. Tumors of the eighth nerve cause widening of the internal auditory meatus demonstrated by petrous ridge conventional tomography; a posterior fossa contrast reontgenographic study using air, metrizamide, or Pantopaque will define the extent of the lesion. Myelography is required for investigating spinal cord tumors. The CSF protein concentration is almost always elevated with spinal neurofibroma and with acoustic tumors.

Von Hippel-Lindau disease

Von Hippel-Lindau disease is an autosomal dominant disorder, but the expression of the disease varies greatly between and among families. The range of onset of ocular and neurologic signs extends from the first to the fifth decade of life. The syndrome includes retinal, neurovascular, and visceral components. The first manifestations are usually referable to retinal hemangiomas, which are sometimes multiple and are bilateral in one third of these cases. Examination of the fundus reveals dilated, tortuous arteries entering the lesion and enlarged draining veins. Bleeding from the lesion may lead to retinal detachment, glaucoma, cataract, uveitis, and blindness. Enucleation is sometimes necessary because of pain. Photocoagulation is useful in controlling the vascular lesion. Cerebellar hemangioblastoma occurs in 10% to 20% of the affected patients and may appear in the absence of retinal lesions. The first symptom of this tumor is often headache, followed by manifestations of obstructive hydrocephalus (vomiting and papilledema) and cerebellar symptoms, usually gait and speech disturbance. These tumors are readily operable. They are usually benign but may recur and may be multiple. Abnormalities associated with cerebellar hemangioblastoma include syringomyelia, hemangioma of the brainstem, spinal cord angioblastic tumors, polycythemia, and pheochromocytoma. The visceral manifestations of von Hippel-Lindau disease include angiomas and cysts of various organs. A serious associated lesion is renal cell carcinoma, which may be bilateral.

Ataxia-telangiectasia

Ataxia-telangiectasia is a relatively rare autosomal recessive disorder, the cardinal manifestations of which are progressive cerebellar ataxia, oculocutaneous telangiectasia with oculomotor apraxia, a tendency to frequent sinopulmonary infection, lymphoreticular malignancy, and other malignancies. The ataxia begins early, but the bulbar telangiectases are not evident until the third to eighth years of life; they first appear on the bulbar conjunctivae as horizontal symmetric streaks and give the eyeball a bloodshot appearance; later they may spread to include the eyelid, face, and neck. Unlike Sturge-Weber syndrome and other neurocutaneous syndromes, the telangiectases do not involve the CNS. The finding of choreoathetosis may be so striking as to overshadow the cerebellar disturbance. Patients surviving until adolescence may develop features of spinocerebellar disease and clinical and electromyographic features of peripheral neuropathy. With time, intellectual impairment occurs in more than one third of patients. Endocrine disorders, especially female hypogonadism, and signs of premature aging of hair and skin are found. Immunologic disturbance is prominent, manifested by frequent infection, especially sinopulmonary infection, a profound deficiency or absence of IgA and sometimes IgE, thymic hypoplasia or aplasia, and depressed cellular and humoral immunity. Lymphopenia is found in 30% of patients. The incidence of all types of tumors, especially lymphoid tumors, is at least 10%; there is also an increased incidence of all tumor types in relatives. The α-fetoprotein serum concentration is elevated and serves as a marker for this disease. The increased levels of this protein may reflect a defect of hepatic maturation.

Two remarkable features of ataxia-telangiectasia are exquisite radiosensitivity and a tendency toward violent transfusion reactions (related to infusion of IgA, to which the patient can make antibodies). Chromosome anomalies may be one factor predisposing the patient to oncogenesis. The most striking pathologic findings are in the cerebellum, where there is almost selective cortical cerebellar degeneration, especially affecting Purkinje cells and to a lesser extent granular cells and basket cells. Neuronal degeneration is also common in the vermis and in the dentate and olivary nuclei. Demyelination with variable axonal loss is common in the dorsal columns. Minor changes, including gliosis and gliovascular malformations, may be found in the cerebral hemispheres.

Sturge-Weber syndrome

The hallmark of Sturge-Weber syndrome is a unilateral facial nevus that predominantly involves the upper face, especially the upper eyelid, and is associated with a thin-walled vascular nevus on the surface of the ipsilateral cerebral cortex. The nevus is flat or only very slightly elevated, unlike the common cutaneous, cavernous strawberry hemangioma. Involvement of the face by the nevus in the absence of involvement of the upper eyelid may be confidently used to exclude a diagnosis of Sturge-Weber syndrome. Other features of this disorder include buphthalmos, epilepsy, hemiparesis, hemianopsia, and progressive intellectual disturbance. The diagnosis of Sturge-Weber syndrome should be suspected in all children with the typical facial nevus and neurologic symptoms, especially focal motor seizures and hemiparesis. Skull roentgenograms may show "tram-track" calcification in the cerebral cortex. Calcification is rarely demonstrated on roentgenograms before patients are 2 years of age but is apparent earlier with CT scanning. Histologic examination shows excessive vascularization of the pia, usually in the parietal and occipital regions. Fliosis and calcium concretions are found in the underlying cortex. Management should involve early commencement of anticonvulsant therapy because intellectual decline seems to result partly from intractable seizures. Consideration should be given to early ablative surgery (for example, lobectomy) to control intractable seizures and halt intellectual decline.

Tuberous sclerosis (Bourneville's disease)

Seizures and mental retardation are the most common neurologic manifestations of tuberous sclerosis (Bourneville's disease). The earliest cutaneous lesions are multiple, dull white depigmented macules, leaf shaped and increasing in size with age. Ultraviolet light helps in recognizing them in fair-skinned persons. The other common skin manifestations are adenoma sebaceum, a nodular facial eruption resembling acne but without pustules; shagreen patches, which are indurated excrescences usually over the sacrum; and café au lait spots. Seizures and mental retardation become apparent in the first decade of life. The seizures may precede the characteristic skin lesions by many years. A funduscopic examination may disclose nodules that histologically are formed from retinal ganglion cells, fibroblasts, and glial cells. Nodules also occur in the parenchyma of the brain or on the surface; they may also line the surface of the ventricles to create the "candle guttering" commonly mentioned in descriptions of this disease. Other tumors, including vascular malformations, meningiomas, gliomas, and hamartomas, are also recognized.

Incontinentia pigmenti (Bloch-Sulzberger syndrome)

Incontinentia pigmenti, or Bloch-Sulzberger syndrome, an uncommon disorder in which epilepsy and mental and motor retardation are prominent, is occasionally familial. The majority of reported cases have been in females, and it has been suggested that the condition in males is fatal in utero. In the early days of life widespread erythematous and bullous lesions appear, becoming crusted and indurated; this is followed by persistent secondary pigmentation with linear streaks over the trunk, arms, and legs. These disappear by the end of the second decade of life. Eye lesions, suggesting dysplasia or glioma, may occur and may be mistaken for retrolental hyperplasia. Local application of steroids is helpful in treating the skin lesions.

BIBLIOGRAPHY

Barnett, H.J.M., Foster, J.B., and Hudgson, P.: Syringomyelia, Philadelphia, 1974, W.B. Saunders Co.
Cuzner, M.L., and Davison, A.N.: The scientific basis of multiple sclerosis. In Baum, H., and Gergely, J., editors: Molecular aspects of medicine, vol. 2, no. 3, New York, 1979, Pergamon Press Inc.
Davison, A.N., and others, editors: Multiple sclerosis research, London, 1975, Her Majesty's Stationery Office.
Jacob, E., and Herbert, V.: Vitamin B_{12} and the nervous system. In Kumar, S., editor: Biochemistry of brain, New York, 1980, Pergamon Press Inc.
Kark, R.A., Rosenberg, R., and Schut, L.:Advances in neurology, vol. 21, The inherited ataxias, New York, 1978, Raven Press.
Konigsmark, B.W., and Weiner, L.P.: The olivopontocerebellar atrophies: a review, Medicine **49:**227, 1970.
Rubinstein, L.J., and others: Disseminated necrotizing leukoencephalopathy: a complication of treated central nervous system leukemia and lymphoma, Cancer **35:**291, 1975.
Vinken, P.J., and Bruyn, G.W.: Handbook of clinical neurology—vol. 10, Leukodystrophies and poliodystrophies, 1970; vol. 14, The phakomatoses, 1972; vol. 22, part II, System disorders and atrophies, 1975, Amsterdam, North Holland Publishing Co.
Wright, D.G., Laureon, R., and Victor, M.: Pontine and extrapontine myelinolysis, Brain **102:**361, 1979.

149 • ABNORMALITIES OF THE CRANIOVERTEBRAL JUNCTION

Paul L. Schraeder

Disorders of the craniovertebral junction, including platybasia and basilar impression or basilar invagination, Arnold-Chiari malformations, and Klippel-Feil syndrome, occur in varying degrees of severity. They may be clinically asymptomatic but can have associated signs and symptoms that range from subtle to severe as a result of the involvement of the brainstem, cerebellum, cranial nerves, spinal cord, or nerve roots. Although each can occur singly, various combinations of these abnormalities are commonly found in the same patient.

PLATYBASIA AND BASILAR IMPRESSION

Platybasia is a flattening of the base of the skull in which, on a lateral skull roentgenogram, the angle created by lines connecting the nasion, tuberculum sellae, and the anterior margin of the foramen magnum is greater than 143 degrees. The term is often incorrectly used synonymously with basilar impression, since these anomalies commonly coexist. In basilar impression one half or more of the odontoid process of the axis protrudes above Chamberlain's line (a line drawn from the back of the hard palate to the posterior margin of the foramen magnum). These deformities are usually congenital and can be associated with varying degrees of atlanto-occipital assimilation, Klippel-Feil syndrome, and Arnold-Chiari malformations. Basilar invagination, also defined by Chamberlain's line, is acquired in diseases in which the bones of the skull are softened, such as rickets, osteomalacia, Paget's disease, and osteogenesis imperfecta.

The clinical findings are variable and more likely to be associated with the congenital anomalies. Often the patient has only a short neck with limited motion. In more severe cases abnormalities of the lower cranial nerves, cerebellum, and motor and sensory long tracts are found. A syrinx of the cervical spinal cord and medulla or an Arnold-Chiari malformation may be present. The importance of considering craniovertebral junction anomalies in the differential diagnosis of multiple sclerosis and foramen magnum tumors cannot be overemphasized, since the diagnosis can usually be based on a technically adequate plain skull roentgenogram. Surgical decompression is indicated if symptoms are progressive.

ARNOLD-CHIARI MALFORMATIONS

Arnold-Chiari malformations include several congenital hindbrain anomalies, the most important of which are the displacement of the cerebellum and an elongated medulla through the foramen magnum into the cervical spinal canal (type 2) and the displacement of the cerebellar tonsils into the cervical canal (type 1). Basilar impression is often present. Hydrocephalus, aqueductal stenosis, and anomalies of the cerebral hemispheres, such as the absence of the septum pellucidum and heterotopias, may occur.

The patient with the type 2, or infantile, form usually has communicating hydrocephalus early in life; the downward displacement of posterior fossa structures probably interferes with cerebrospinal fluid (CSF) flow. It is most commonly associated with a spinal midline defect such as spina bifida, meningocele, or myelomeningocele in the lumbosacral region. Myelomeningocele is a saccular, soft mass covered with friable skin, weeping CSF, and containing elements of the spinal cord and cauda equina. The patient usually is paraplegic and subject to recurrent bacterial meningitis originating from the lumbosacral defect. The treatment involves shunting procedures for the hydrocephalus and repair of the myelomeningocele. The latter procedure is performed only to prevent infection, however, because the paraplegia almost invariably persists after surgery. Diagnosis of this disorder in utero is possible via ultrasound, roentgenograms of the fetus, and amniocentesis to determine whether the α-fetoprotein concentration is increased.

The type 1, or adult, form is often asymptomatic until adulthood. The symptoms and signs include varying degrees of dysfunction of the cerebellum, motor and sensory long tracts, and cranial nerves. If present, a particularly helpful sign of medullary dysfunction is downbeat nystagmus (a nystagmus in the primary position of gaze, with the fast phase beating downward). Syringomyelia of the cervical cord and medulla is often present, as are associated bony abnormalities such as fusion of cervical vertebrae. Hydrocephalus is less common than in type 2. Foramen magnum tumors must be considered in the differential diagnosis. The diagnosis depends on a high index of suspicion. The common finding of basilar impression on the plain skull roentgenogram and the characteristic findings of a herniated cerebellum and brainstem on cervical myelography confirm the diagnosis. Treatment in the form of decompression by an upper cervical laminectomy and by a suboccipital craniectomy may be helpful for patients with progressive symptoms.

KLIPPEL-FEIL SYNDROME

In Klippel-Feil syndrome an asymptomatic congenital fusion of two or more cervical vertebrae is not uncommon. In the more extreme situation a congenital fusion of the second to sixth cervical vertebrae in association with a narrow spinal canal may be found. The patient has a very short, squat neck, with the head appearing to rest on the shoulders and significant limitation of movement of the head and neck. This deformity is commonly associated with basilar impression, Arnold-Chiari malformations, and an undescended scapula (Sprengel's deformity). Evidence of spinal cord compression (that is, hyperreflexia, an extensor plantar response, and loss of position and vibration senses) is an indication for obtaining a myelogram and performing cervical cord decompression.

BIBLIOGRAPHY

Adams, R.D., and Victor, M.: Principles of neurology, New York, 1977, McGraw-Hill Book Co.
Blackwood, W., and others: Greenfield's neuropathology, Baltimore, 1976, The Williams & Wilkins Co.
Taveras, J.M., and Wood, E.H.: Diagnostic neuroradiology, Baltimore, 1976, The Williams & Wilkins Co.

150 · BASAL GANGLIA DISORDERS AND RELATED CONDITIONS

Roger Duvoisin

PARKINSONISM

DEFINITION. Parkinsonism is a distinctive symptom complex comprised of tremor, muscular rigidity, bradykinesia, and characteristic alterations of posture and attitudes of the limbs. The tremor is usually a resting tremor, that is, most marked when the affected part is at rest. Muscular rigidity refers to a hypertonicity of the musculature that can be noticed during passive manipulation of the limbs, as a uniform resistance to movement. It differs from spasticity, which is more marked in the antigravity muscles (for example, the flexor muscles of the arm and the extensor muscles of the leg), and gives way, often suddenly, in the "clasp-knife" phenomenon during sustained stretching of the muscles. Bradykinesia comprises a slowness of all bodily movement, a loss of automatic motor activity such as eye-blinking and swallowing, a loss of associated movements such as the swing of the arms on walking, hesitation on initiating a motor act, and rapid fatigue during continuing or repetitive motor actions.

ETIOLOGY. The most common cause of parkinsonism the physician encounters today is Parkinson's disease, also referred to as idiopathic parkinsonism or paralysis agitans. Most authorities believe that Parkinson's disease represents a specific morbid entity with no known cause. Iatrogenic parkinsonism closely resembling Parkinson's disease may be induced by various drugs, principally the major tranquilizers or, rarely, methyldopa, α-methyl-para-tyrosine, reserpine, and other agents that interfere with the synthesis or the storage of dopamine or that block the striatal dopamine receptors. Drug-induced chemical parkinsonism is always reversible, usually within 1 or 2 weeks after the offending agent is discontinued. A form of parkinsonism occurring as a sequela of *encephalitis lethargica (von Economo's encephalitis)*, termed "postencephalitic parkinsonism," was common in the years 1920 to 1940 but has subsequently declined in incidence and is now quite rare. There are still a few survivors of the epidemics of encephalitis lethargica; strangely, the epidemics ran their course from 1916 to 1926, then subsided, and the disease has not occurred since. Parkinsonism may also occur as part of the clinical manifestation of several distinct degenerative disorders of the nervous system such as olivopontocerebellar atrophy, striatonigral degeneration, and progressive supranuclear palsy. Juvenile parkinsonism may on rare occasions represent an unusually early onset of Parkinson's disease but more often represents Wilson's disease.

EPIDEMIOLOGY. Parkinson's disease occurs throughout the world in all racial and ethnic groups. Differences in prevalence in different groups are difficult to assess because of the differences in medical practice. Population surveys have shown a prevalence of about 130:100,000 standard population. Parkinson's disease is uncommon in people under 40 years of age; the mean age at onset is about 60 years and the prevalence increases with age. Approximately 1% of the population over 60 years of age has Parkinson's disease. Although genetic factors have long been suspected of playing a significant role in causing Parkinson's disease, little evidence exists proving familial concentrations of the disease. Family studies have shown that only about 2% of the adult siblings of patients with Parkinson's disease also have the disease. Reports of families with multiple cases usually represent another disorder, most commonly olivopontocerebellar atrophy, which can often mimic Parkinson's disease and occurs in both recessive inheritance and dominant inheritance patterns.

PATHOGENESIS. Parkinsonism is presently regarded as a pathophysiologic state reflecting primarily a dysfunction of the brain dopamine neuronal systems. The most consistent pathologic feature found at autopsy is a degeneration of the pigmented neurons of the substantia nigra. These neurons contain a melanin pigment that can be seen during a gross inspection of sections cut through the midbrain of normal human specimens. This pigment is lost in Parkinson's disease because of a neuronal degeneration of the substantia nigra. Any morbid process that produces a degeneration of these neurons will be associated with a parkinsonian state.

The substantia nigra projects its axons principally to the striatum (the caudate nucleus and the putamen), which normally contains dopamine. The concentration of dopamine in the striatum is significantly reduced in Parkinson's disease and in experimental animals with lesions of the substantia nigra. The hypothalamus has important dopamine neurons. The degeneration of these neurons in Parkinson's disease may be correlated with autonomic dysfunctions such as seborrhea, excessive sweating, orthostatic hypotension, and anorexia. The dopaminergic neurons of the substantia nigra also extend to the limbic lobe, especially to the medial temporal lobe. The involvement of these neurons may account for the behavior changes typical of the disease. The sympathetic neurons of the spinal cord and the peripheral autonomic ganglia may also degenerate in Parkinson's disease, contributing to the orthostatic hypotension and other autonomic dysfunctions.

The cause of the neuron degeneration of Parkinson's disease is unknown. Because of the high degree of the selective involvement of widely dispersed neuron groups including the substantia nigra, the locus ceruleus, the peripheral autonomic ganglia, and the dopaminergic neurons of the hypothalamus, the disorder has been classified as a system degeneration, and many physicians believe it may have a metabolic or viral cause.

CLINICAL MANIFESTATIONS. The most common initial symptoms are a slight weakness and a tendency to tremble, usually appearing in one hand or less often in one foot. Often the patient has some slowness or awkwardness in using the affected limb, a tendency to posture the arm flexed at the elbow, some loss of facial expression, and a deliberate quality of speech even though complaining only of the tremor. The symptoms at first are mild and may persist with little change for 1 to 2 years. Gradually, however, they become more marked and similar manifestations appear on the opposite side of the body. Subsequently, the posture becomes less erect and the patient stands gently stooped and walks with a shuffling gait without swinging the arms. With further progression of the disease, all movement becomes gradually very slow, walking becomes difficult, and the tremor and rigidity become generalized. The patient may have tremors in the lips, tongue, jaw, and facial muscles, as well as in the limb muscles and axial muscles. In general, the rigidity is most marked in the spinal musculature.

As bradykinesia becomes gradually more severe, all movement is marked by abrupt interruptions. Thus the patient's feet suddenly seem to stick to the floor on walking, and there is inability to move them for a moment. The patient may also suddenly walk with short shuffling steps that become progressively shorter and faster, a phenomenon termed "festination." During festination the patient's trunk may lean farther and farther with each step, and falling may occur. The patient seems to be pushed forward by an unseen force or to be chasing after his center of gravity. This phenomenon is termed "propulsion." Similar backward stepping is termed "retropulsion" and similar sidewise stepping is termed "lateropulsion." These phenomena are usually associated with the loss of the normal "righting" of the body to sudden displacement and with an impairment of equilibrium. The patient may fall, resulting in injury. Because these patients lack not only normal postural responses to an impending fall but also protective movements, they fail to raise their hands to protect themselves and may suffer blows to the head and face.

In advanced stages of the disease the patients are largely immobile, are confined to a bed or wheelchair, and require assistance in the acts of daily living. Impaired deglutition results in the pooling of saliva in the fauces, drooling, weight loss because of the difficulty in ingesting adequate amounts of food, and the risk of aspiration and secondary bronchopneumonia. The failure of the cricopharyngeal muscles to relax appears to delay swallowing. The patient may point to the larynx and explain that the food remains stuck at that point.

In approximately one half of patients with Parkinson's disease the later course of the illness is complicated by gradual dementia. Initially the patient may be forgetful and have a tendency to develop minor confusional episodes that may be ascribed to medication. Reducing the dosage of anticholinergic drugs or discontinuing them entirely may result in a clearing of these symptoms, but gradually the sumptoms reappear. The patient may be confused and irritable and have paranoid ideas. Many patients have a typical pattern of complex visual hallucinations. The patient may see strange people wandering about or may claim to have seen a deceased relative. Initially the patient may be aware that the hallucinations are unreal. With the advent of dementia, however, the patient reacts to the hallucinations, often with paranoia. The patient may have frank delirium. Drugs with anticholinergic properties, including not only the antiparkinsonian drugs but also antihistamines, tricyclic antidepressants, and many tranquilizers, may induce the patient's hallucinations and increase confusion. The drug-induced exacerbation of dementia usually clears in several days after the offending agent is withdrawn.

Typically, the parkinsonian patient's speech is soft, monotone, and rapid. The patient loses the normal rhythm of speech and runs syllables together without pause or inflection. The first few words may be spoken clearly but then the voice becomes softer, articulation becomes slurred, and the patient utters words with increasing speed (tachyphemia). Voice amplitude may dwindle rapidly to a whisper and speech may cease altogether. The patient's handwriting shows analogous changes; the letters become progressively smaller (micrographia) and tremulous until the patient ceases writing, the hand apparently frozen in immobility for a moment before resuming the task.

The stooped posture characteristic of Parkinson's disease may be quite marked in some patients, yet it disappears when the patient sits back in a reclining chair or lies down. Many patients also have a mild scoliosis with the thoracic spine gently curving in most cases away from the side of the initial symptoms. In some cases the patient leans to one side, with a lateral tilt of the trunk of as much as 10 to 15 degrees from the vertical while standing. Usually the tilt is more pronounced in the sitting position and the patient tends to slump to one side. Patients are often unaware of these postural aberrations.

Characteristic changes in the attitude of the hands occur in parkinsonism, even in the drug-induced form. The patient holds the fingers extended with the metacarpophalangeal joints flexed about 30 degrees. The abnormal attitude of the fingers abruptly disappears when the patient grasps an object with the hand but reappears when the hand is at rest. Patients often have flexion of the toes with dorsiflexion of the proximal phalanges. Sometimes the first toe assumes a constant dorsiflexed position simulating the position of the first toe in Babinski's sign.

Symptoms of autonomic dysfunction are very common in Parkinson's disease. Increased secretion of sebum (seborrhea) is evident in an oiliness of the skin, especially of the face. When seborrhea is marked, the patient has a scaly erythematous eruption of the skin, especially along the nasolabial folds, behind the ears, at the eyebrows, and in the scalp. Some patients have intermittent, sometimes profuse, bouts of diaphoresis. Chronic constipation with reduced bowel motility is a ubiquitous feature of Parkinson's disease. Mild impairment of micturition with urgency and hesitation is common, especially in elderly male patients. A small percentage of patients have orthostatic hypotension. These patients complain of dizziness on standing up or on suddenly arising from a sitting position. Such patients may have *Shy-Drager syndrome,* in which peripheral autonomic failure is coupled with extrapyramidal manifestations.

LABORATORY FINDINGS. Laboratory findings may include a mild microcytic anemia in some cases, presumably representing a nonspecific feature of chronic illness. Chest roentgenograms may show a slight scoliosis. Skull roentgenograms and computed tomographic (CT) brain scans should be normal. Patients with dementia, however, may have some cortical atrophy and ventricular enlargement. The electroencephalogram (EEG) is either normal or shows minimal slowing and disorganization. Such changes, however, may be the result of drug therapy, especially therapy involving anticholinergic agents. The EEG of patients with marked bradykinesia and those with dementia may show moderate to marked slowing and diffuse disorganization.

Cineradiographic studies of swallowing often reveal an abnormal pattern caused by a delayed relaxation of the cricopharyngeal muscles. Contrast radiography of the gastrointestinal tract commonly reveals some hypomotility of the intestines, delayed stomach emptying, and varying degrees of distention of the large bowel. A frank megacolon may rarely be found in patients with severe constipation.

DIAGNOSIS. The diagnosis of parkinsonism is based primarily on the clinical manifestations. The presence of the triad of tremor, rigidity, and bradykinesia, plus the characteristic postural changes, the seborrhea, and the monotone tachyphemic speech, forms a distinctive clinical picture. In early cases with minimal physical findings a diagnosis may be difficult to make, and one may need to do a reevaluation after a period of time. The differential diagnosis comprises a wide variety of disorders. The clinical setting helps make the diagnosis easier. Thus parkinsonism in a young patient should suggest Wilson's disease. One should consider the possibility of arteriosclerotic cerebrovascular disease in an elderly patient. The patient who has suffered several minor strokes and has mild bilateral hemipareses may have what is termed "arteriosclerotic parkinsonism." Dementia is more common in such cases. The patient's speech is slurred rather than monotone and tachyphemic. The lower extremities are more involved than the upper extremities. There should be a mild spasticity rather than a rigidity. The plantar reflexes may be extensor. No seborrhea is present. Despite all of these distinctive features, however, differentiation in individual cases may be difficult. The CT scan may be helpful in showing evidence of multiple previous cerebral infarcts.

Rarely, patients with brain tumors may have symptoms resembling Parkinson's disease. More commonly, patients with Parkinson's disease may also coincidentally have brain tumors. The appropriate thyroid function tests can exclude hypothyroidism. Hypoparathyroidism may on rare occasions mimic parkinsonism. Thus one should check serum calcium levels, especially in patients with a history of a thyroidectomy in the past.

Differentiating among the various parkinsonian syndromes may be difficult in early cases. A patient with a history of encephalitis lethargica (in lay terms, "sleeping sickness") and of oculogyric crises (uncontrollable uprolling of the eyes) may have postencephalitic parkinsonism. Signs of cerebellar dysfunction in addition to parkinsonian features should suggest an olivopontocerebellar atrophy. A history of treatment with tranquilizers or of psychiatric care should arouse a suspicion of drug-induced parkinsonism. Patients having a primarily bradykinetic syndrome with little or no tremor may have striatonigral degeneration, which may be difficult to distinguish from Parkinson's disease. Additional clues that the patient has striatonigral degeneration may be a failure to respond to levodopa therapy and evidence on the CT scan of a striatal atrophy affecting particularly the putamen. The diagnosis of striatonigral degeneration can be established with reasonable certainty only on postmortem examination.

COURSE. The course of Parkinson's disease is one of slow gradual progression over many years. There is great variability from one patient to another; some have unilateral symptoms for 10 years or more, whereas others may reach a stage of significant disability within 10 years. Before the introduction of levodopa therapy the life expectancy of patients with Parkinson's disease was significantly reduced. With present treatment, life expectancy has approached the norm. Patients with advanced disease may succumb to intercurrent infections, but Parkinson's disease is not generally fatal.

MANAGEMENT. The most effective treatment available today is levodopa (L-dopa), which is the immediate metabolic precursor of dopamine. The rationale for this treatment is to replenish the cerebral stores of dopamine. Levodopa may be given alone but is most conveniently given in combination with an inhibitor of dopa decarboxylase to protect the levodopa from decarboxylation to dopamine in the kidney, bowel, and other extracerebral tissues and to permit a larger proportion of the levodopa taken by mouth to reach the brain. The decarboxylase inhibitor alphamethyldopa hydrazine (carbidopa) is generally employed in a combination tablet (Sinemet) containing levodopa and carbidopa in a 10:1 ratio. The inhibitor does not cross the blood-brain barrier and so does not prevent the conversion of levodopa to dopamine in the brain. One must carefully adjust the dosage and the dosing schedules to the individual patient to obtain optimal results. The average dose is 25 mg of alphamethyldopa hydrazine in combination with 250 mg of levodopa three times daily. The major dose-limiting side effect of this treatment is the induction of choreiform involuntary movements. If these are excessive, the dosage should be reduced. Orthostatic hypotension and sinus tachycardia may occur and may require special measures. The patient may have agitation, insomnia, nightmares, and rarely hallucinations and even frank delirium.

A variety of drugs possessing central anticholinergic properties are useful secondary agents that one may use as an initial treatment in mild cases or as an adjunct to levodopa therapy. These include trihexyphenidyl (Artane), benztropine (Cogentin), and amantadine (Symmetrel). The tricyclic antidepressant drugs imipramine (Tofranil) and amitryptyline (Elavil) are useful for patients with depression complicating the parkinsonism. The phenothiazines and haloperidol should be avoided because they block the desired actions of levodopa therapy.

Stereotactic surgery to produce a small lesion in the ventrolateral nucleus of the thalamus can effectively alleviate tremor and rigidity on the opposite side of the body. To alleviate symptoms on both sides, bilateral operations are required. The risk of the second operation is considerably greater than that of a single unilateral procedure. About 15% of patients who have had a bilateral thalamotomy have suffered a significant pseudobulbar palsy. Bradykinesia, speech impairment, disturbances of gait and equilibrium, and other features have not been altered by surgery, nor has the progression of the disease been modified. Levodopa therapy has largely supplanted the surgical treatment of parkinsonism. Surgery may still be useful, however, in carefully selected patients who have a unilateral tremor as their major problem and who have failed to respond to drug treatment.

Recently a new class of drugs that act directly at dopamine receptor sites has been under investigation for the treatment of parkinsonism. These dopamine receptor agonists have been shown to have substantial therapeutic efficacy, comparable in some instances to that of levodopa. One of the agents, bromocriptine (Parlodel), has recently been approved for this use.

Physical therapy and a sensible program of exercise are useful in maintaining patient mobility and general well-being. Attention to maintaining good bowel habits is needed to counter the chronic constipation so common among parkinsonian patients.

ESSENTIAL TREMOR

DEFINITION. Essential tremor is a benign hereditary condition characterized by a postural tremor usually affecting the hands, the head, and often the voice. Other terms for this condition are "benign essential tremor," "familial tremor," and "senile tremor."

ETIOLOGY. Essential tremor is a genetic trait transmitted in an autosomal dominant pattern with considerable variation in its severity. Curiously, families harboring this trait appear to enjoy unusual longevity. There are no observable pathologic lesions, and the nature of the underlying neural dysfunction is a subject of speculation.

CLINICAL MANIFESTATIONS. The patient has a tremor of the hands, perhaps best described as a trembling, with a frequency of about 8 to 10 Hz symmetrically in both upper extremities. The patient is usually an adult, but rarely the disorder may appear in childhood or adolescence. In some members of affected families the tremor may not appear until the patient reaches advanced age and it may then be termed "senile tremor." At first the tremor may only appear during periods of stress, and the patient feels it as a transient "nervousness." Unlike the tremor of parkinsonism, it tends to disappear at rest and is most noticeable when the hands are held up with the arms outstretched or when the patient attempts to hold a fixed posture for a moment; hence its description as a postural tremor. The tremor diminishes during movement and consequently in most cases causes relatively little disability. There is no rigidity or bradykinesia as in parkinsonism and no loss of coordination as in the intention tremor of multiple sclerosis or of cerebellar disease.

Patients commonly have a rhythmic bobbing of the head. The tremor may also involve the thorax, diaphragm, and abdomen resulting in a vocal tremor. Rarely, the tremor may involve the lower extremities.

The tremor is more marked during stressful moments and may be absent when the patient is relaxed. It is often most prominent when the patient arises in the morning and diminishes somewhat during the day. When the tremor is severe, it may interfere with tasks requiring dexterity and steadiness. Patients with this tremor tend to write rapidly and in large letters to minimize the trembling.

Aside from the tremor there are no abnormalities of nervous function. A slight hypotonia of the musculature and a slight hyperextensibility of the joints may occur in many cases.

DIAGNOSIS. The diagnosis rests on observing the tremor, noting its distribution in the body and the lack of any other neurologic abnormality. Also helpful is the family history. The condition is often mistaken for parkinsonism, especially in elderly patients. Differentiation may be made readily by noting the absence of the bradykinesia, rigidity, and postural aberrations of parkinsonism. The micrographic handwriting of the parkinsonian patient is conspicuously absent. In contrast to the parkinsonian patient, the patient with essential tremor has a lively facial expression, a normal speed and spontaneity of body movement, and normal associated movements.

The characteristic head tremor of essential tremor is rarely, if ever, seen in parkinsonism. Rather there may be a tremor of the lips, jaw, tongue, and facial muscles but not a rhythmic tremor of the entire head.

The evolution of the disease also helps in making the diagnosis. The patient who has had a symmetric tremor of the hands for many years, with no other stigmata of parkinsonism, almost certainly has essential tremor. The tremor of Parkinson's disease, moreover, usually has a unilateral onset and spreads first to the lower extremity of the same side before appearing on the opposite side, whereas essential tremor develops in both upper extremities simultaneously and more or less symmetrically, rarely spreading to involve the lower extremities.

The differential diagnosis of essential tremor includes considering the tremor of hyperthyroidism, chronic alcoholism, anxiety, and cerebellar degeneration. The absence of associated features should exclude these conditions.

COURSE. The tremor increases very slowly in severity and bodily distribution over many years. Most patients with essential tremor live a normal life with little or no disability.

MANAGEMENT. Patients with essential tremor are frequently aware that an alcoholic beverage temporarily suppresses the tremor. Alcohol often induces a rebound effect, however, with increased tremor a few hours later or the following day. Various sedatives and minor tranquilizers such as the benzodiazepines are commonly employed in attempts to control the tremor. Although the tremor may be significantly reduced, it is never completely abolished. Propranolol (Inderal) may be more effective in some persons, but it has significant side effects and should be employed cautiously. It may lower the blood pressure, slow the pulse, and provoke congestive heart failure. Propranolol may induce bronchospasm and should not be given to patients with a history of asthma.

Stereotactic thalamotomy can effectively abolish essential tremor in the contralateral limbs, but the condition is rarely sufficiently disabling to warrant brain surgery.

CHOREA

The term "chorea," derived from the Greek word for "dance," is applied to a state of motor hyperactivity in which the speed, amplitude, and frequency of body movement are abnormally increased. Given that there is a broad range of normality, it is understandable that minor degrees of chorea may pass unnoticed or be taken simply as representing nervousness or fidgetiness. Careful observation, however, may reveal brief twitches of the hands, fleeting facial grimaces, and a slight irregularity of movement. In overt chorea, brief irregular jerky movements of the limbs, head, trunk, face, and tongue are observed. The patient has a sudden flexion and extension of a limb, inappropriate gestures, exaggerated blinking, involuntary protrusions of the tongue, and abrupt contractions of major muscle groups. When these phenomena are mild, the patient may be unaware of them or regard them as normal voluntary movements. The automatic movements that are normally outside awareness are particularly affected. Thus the patient may walk with an excessive armswing. Normal gestures become flamboyant. Stepping is exaggerated. The patient appears "loose jointed" and moves excessively rapidly. In severe cases all movement is distorted and impaired by violent involuntary jerks and twitches. High stepping, flinging movements of the arms, sudden starts and stops, bowing, and turning abruptly reduce walking to a caricature of the norm. Respiration may be irregular, with hyperventilation, deep sighs, and panting breaths occurring in a random sequence. Speech becomes slurred with an explosive quality. Choreic patients may also be emotionally labile, impulsive, and aggressive. The common underlying feature of chorea appears to be a disinhibition of all motor activity.

The patient with chorea has difficulty maintaining a fixed posture for more than a fleeting moment. For example, a handgrip cannot be maintained; the grip is relaxed intermittently, producing an effect picturesquely termed "milkmaid's grasp." The patient cannot keep his mouth open steadily. Instead, the mouth opens and closes at irregular intervals, and the tongue relaxes and protrudes in rapid darting movements while the patient is constantly changing position, apparently squirming in his seat. When attempting to stand still, the patient constantly shifts his weight from one foot to the other, and a continuous motion of the legs and feet causes him to sway and rock back and forth.

Chorea is a pathophysiologic state reflecting a dysfunction of the basal ganglia that may be regarded as the opposite of parkinsonism. Chorea occurs in association with a variety of disorders; the motor disturbances are similar, although the clinical settings may differ. All choreas show similar pharmacologic responses. Postulations include increased sensitivity of striatal dopamine receptors or hyperactivity of striatal dopaminergic systems. The major tranquilizing drugs, which interfere with dopaminergic function, induce parkinsonism but reduce chorea. In contrast, drugs useful in treating parkinsonism, notably levodopa, induce or exacerbate chorea. The major side effect of levodopa in the treatment of parkinsonism is the induction of choreiform involuntary movements.

Huntington's chorea

DEFINITION. Huntington's chorea, or Huntington's disease, is a chronic progressive hereditary disorder of adult life characterized by choreic involuntary movements, behavioral changes, and dementia.

ETIOLOGY AND PATHOGENESIS. Huntington's chorea is transmitted in an autosomal dominant pattern with virtually complete penetrance. There are no formes frustes nor does the condition skip generations. The disease may be expected to develop in half of the offspring of an affected parent. Unfortunately, the initial symptoms usually do not appear until after the patient is 40 years of age, which has ensured the continued prevalence of the disease.

The abnormality is confined to the brain, which in advanced cases shows an extensive atrophy of the cerebral cortex, basal ganglia, and cerebellum. The caudate nucleus and putamen are particularly affected and may be reduced to thin layers of gliotic tissue. There is severe and widespread loss of neurons and nerve fibers. The cause of the neuron degeneration is unknown. Recent studies have indicated that there may be a generalized defect of cell membranes.

Postmortem biochemical investigations have shown a selective loss of γ-aminobutyric acid (GABA) in the caudate nucleus and putamen. GABA is a prominent and widespread neurotransmitter in the brain, and its loss appears to result from the degeneration of the striatal neurons that normally synthesize and store it. A decrease in angiotensin also has been noted in the striatum.

EPIDEMIOLOGY. Huntington's chorea occurs throughout the world in all ethnic and racial groups. The prevalence varies from 4 to 7:100,000 standard population. In certain communities the prevalence is much higher.

CLINICAL MANIFESTATIONS. The main clinical manifestations are a gradual development of choreic phenomena and mental deterioration, usually after the patient is 40 years of age. Considerable variations in symptoms, age of onset, and rate of progression may be noted. Mental disturbances may precede the chorea by a number of years. Behavior changes marked by impulsive or antisocial acts, depression, or withdrawal suggestive of schizophrenia may be the initial manifestations. Conversely, some patients may exhibit chorea for a number of years before mental changes become apparent. In such cases severe involuntary movements of the face, tongue, and head may profoundly limit speech and render a clinical evaluation of the mental state difficult. Rarely, the disease may become symptomatic in childhood or adolescence. Juveniles tend to have a rigid bradykinetic syndrome instead of the more usual chorea. The rigid form of Huntington's chorea may resemble Parkinson's disease.

Mild at first and sometimes dismissed as mannerisms, the chorea gradually becomes more severe. Violent flinging movements, rapid darting movements of the tongue, sudden jerking of the head, irregular respiration, contortions of the trunk, and thrashing and kicking of the limbs combine to create a dramatic clinical picture. Falls and injuries may result from the violent involuntary motor activity; physical exhaustion from the constant and excessive activity contributes to the death of patients with advanced disease.

The mental changes are usually those characteristic of organic brain disease. Impairment of memory, a gradual decline in intellectual capacity, apathy, and a disregard for personal hygiene are seen as in other organic dementias. Patients may also be irritable or have sudden bursts of aggressive behavior, fits of depression, and impulsive behavior. Because of the prominence of mental changes, many patients need to be committed to a psychiatric facility. Some patients may be hospitalized for psychotic reactions, and only much later, when the chorea appears, is the correct diagnosis established.

LABORATORY FINDINGS. Laboratory findings include an EEG that is most often diffusely abnormal. A CT scan may show enlargement of the lateral cerebral ventricles with a "butterfly" appearance on coronal sections, especially in advanced cases. Plasma growth hormone levels are elevated, and an exaggerated response to insulin-induced hypoglycemia is usually found. GABA levels in the spinal fluid have been reported to be reduced.

DIFFERENTIAL DIAGNOSIS. The diagnosis rests primarily on clinical findings. With the combination of mental disturbance, the choreic involuntary movements, and a positive family history, it is usually quite easy to make the diagnosis. In the absence of one of these elements, diagnosis may be difficult. In the absence of a family history, the diagnosis must remain presumptive and alternatives must be considered. Patients with Alzheimer's disease have similar mental changes and occasionally may have involuntary movements. The involuntary movements are never a prominent feature, however, and other neurologic deficits may be found. Cerebrovascular disease may lead to chorea, but usually the involvement is unilateral, acute or subacute in onset, and associated with other neurologic abnormalities. Lupus erythematosus can be a cause of chorea and may result in behavior changes and psychotic reactions. Usually the nervous system is involved late in the course of the lupus after the diagnosis has been established. Rarely, thyrotoxicosis and hyperparathyroidism may induce choreic manifestations and behavior changes. Sydenham's chorea differs because it affects mainly children and adolescents and is not associated with dementia. Occasionally, psychiatric patients who have undergone long-term neuroleptic therapy and have tardive dyskinesia may have abnormal movements that strikingly resemble those of Huntington's chorea. With these patients the predominance of oral dyskinesia and the lack of progression with time should help distinguish this disorder from Huntington's chorea.

COURSE. The severity of the chorea and dementia gradually increases over 10 to 20 years or more. Patients with advanced disease are disabled, are largely confined to a bed and chair, and may need to be placed in a chronic care facility. In terminal stages the chorea may subside to be replaced by widespread muscular rigidity.

MANAGEMENT. Only symptomatic therapy is available. Haloperidol and the phenothiazines may reduce the chorea, but it is rarely possible to suppress the involuntary movements completely. The tranquilizers may help control the psychotic behavior. Cholinergic treatment has been attempted with physostigmine and more recently with choline chloride or lecithin, but the results have been disappointing. Experimental treatment with isoniazid to retard the catabolism of GABA has been reported, but the reports of results are conflicting. Minor tranquilizers such as the benzodiazepines may sometimes help control mild agitation or hyperactivity.

PREVENTION. The main hope of preventing Huntington's chorea lies at this time in genetic counseling. All offspring of patients with this disease should be advised of its genetic character.

Hemichorea

DEFINITION. Unilateral chorea, usually termed "hemichorea" or "hemiballism," is an uncommon disorder of acute or subacute onset, commonly occurring in association with cerebrovascular disease.

ETIOLOGY AND PATHOGENESIS. Postmortem studies in patients with hemichorea have usually shown a vascular lesion, either an infarct or a hemorrhage in the internal capsule damaging the subthalamic nucleus or its connections to the globus pallidus. Unilateral chorea also may occur as a consequence of an infarction of the head of the caudate nucleus resulting from atherosclerotic vascular disease.

CLINICAL MANIFESTATIONS. Hemichorea usually develops subacutely over weeks and sometimes over several months following recovery from a cerebrovascular accident (posthemiplegic chorea). It begins insidiously with mild adventitious involuntary movements of the hand, slowly progressing to involve the entire upper extremity, the face, and to a lesser extent the lower extremity of the same side. In the most severe cases the patient's movements are violent and flinging; the resemblance to throwing movements has led some neurologists to prefer the term "hemiballism" for severe hemichorea. In these cases the movements are disabling, and the exhaustion resulting from the continuous motor activity may hasten the patient's death.

Some cases of hemichorea develop in the absence of a previous cerebrovascular accident, although the manifestations are otherwise similar. Hemichorea also has occurred as a complication of stereotactic brain surgery used to treat parkinsonism.

COURSE. In patients surviving the cerebrovascular accident responsible for the hemichorea, the activity usually stabilizes and in most cases gradually subsides spontaneously. The patient may then be left with a residual deficit in the form of a hemiparesis.

MANAGEMENT. The major tranquilizing drugs can suppress or greatly reduce the movements, although often only at dosages producing some degree of parkinsonism on the opposite side. Stereotactic thalamotomy has been successfully employed in a number of cases.

Sydenham's chorea

(See the discussion of "Streptococcal infections and rheumatic fever" in Chapter 45.)

DEFINITION. Sydenham's chorea, the most important form of chorea in childhood and adolescence, is associated with rheumatic fever. Sydenham's chorea, carditis, migratory polyarthritis, subcutaneous nodules, and erythema marginatum comprise the major clinical manifestations of rheumatic fever.

ETIOLOGY AND PATHOGENESIS. The association of Sydenham's chorea with rheumatic fever is clear, but the nature of the underlying cerebral disorder is uncertain. The chorea is not fatal, and opportunities for studying the neuropathology of rheumatic chorea are few. A mild diffuse vasculitis has been found, presumably reflecting the widespread involvement of connective tissue characteristic of rheumatic fever. Some degenerative changes in the neurons in the cerebral cortex, basal ganglia, and cerebellum also have been described. Evidence exists indicating that patients with rheumatic chorea have antibodies to streptococcal antigens that react with neurons of the subthalamic nuclei and the caudate nuclei. Thus the chorea, as in other manifestations of rheumatic fever, may be related to immune mechanisms triggered by streptococcal infections.

EPIDEMIOLOGY. Sydenham's chorea has become quite rare with the significant decline of rheumatic fever since the advent of antibiotics. It is almost exclusively confined to patients 7 to 14 years of age, the peak incidence being at 8 years of age. It is rare after puberty. Girls are affected more frequently than boys. It sometimes occurs in association with pregnancy in the patient's late teens or early twenties. Seasonal variation paralleling that of rheumatic fever has been noted; cases of chorea are uncommon in the summer.

CLINICAL MANIFESTATIONS. The onset is usually insidious; "nervousness" develops in a child who was previously well. Some stressful incident may be thought responsible for the change in behavior, but as the condition worsens, emotional lability, aimless involuntary movements, impaired coordination, and muscular weakness appear. The weakness may be so marked that the child is unable to get up out of bed, walk unassisted, or even sit up unsupported. The child drops things, fumbles, and has difficulty speaking. Involuntary movements of the tongue, mouth, and palate give the child's speech a slurred, explosive quality. Facial grimacing, sudden jerks of the head, and flinging movements of the limbs complete the picture of generalized chorea. In some cases the chorea may be more pronounced on one side of the body, but bilateral involvement is usual. There is great variability in the severity of the involuntary movements, which usually become much more pronounced when the affected child is disturbed and under stress.

Muscle tone is reduced, and the reflexes are sometimes pendular. At times delayed relaxation results in a "hung-up" reflex. Mental changes are commonly present. The child usually is irritable and is sometimes listless and apathetic.

The child may have other signs of rheumatic fever such as a cardiac murmur. Concurrent arthritis is unusual, but arthritis may precede or follow an attack of the chorea.

DIFFERENTIAL DIAGNOSIS. The acute onset of choreiform involuntary movements in a child or an adolescent should immediately bring to mind the possibility of Sydenham's chorea. Acute chorea also may be a manifestation of various drug intoxications, jimsonweed poisoning, or a complication of anticonvulsant therapy with phenobarbital, phenytoin, or ethosuximide. Acute chorea has been associated with pertussis, encephalitis, lupus erythematosus, and Schönlein-Henoch purpura. The presence of tics and habit spasms occasionally may make the differential diagnosis difficult. They should be distinguished by a more chronic course and by their stereotyped character.

LABORATORY FINDINGS. Laboratory findings may include a mild anemia and a slight eosinophilia. Leukocytosis and an elevated erythrocyte sedimentation rate usually indicate cardiac involvement. Studies of the cerebrospinal fluid (CSF) are within normal limits in most cases. A mild pleocytosis has been reported. Serum titers of streptococcal antibodies may be elevated.

The EEG usually shows some diffuse slowing and disorganization. In the rare case of unilateral chorea the EEG abnormalities may be greater over the opposite cerebral hemisphere. Radionuclide brain scans and CT brain scans show no abnormalities.

COURSE. Sydenham's chorea is a benign condition that usually subsides within 1 to 2 months. Minor choreic phenomena may persist up to 6 months, but complete recovery is the norm. Recurrences are common and have been observed in about one third of cases after several months and even after several years. Long-term follow-up studies have suggested that neurotic personality traits may persist indefinitely.

MANAGEMENT. The traditional treatment of having the patient rest in a darkened room may suffice in mild cases. Involuntary movements may be reduced to some extent by sedating the patient with barbiturates, chloral hydrate, or mild tranquilizers. The phenothiazines or haloperidol can effectively control the chorea and are recommended when the involuntary movements are severe.

Sydenham's chorea is considered a major diagnostic sign of rheumatic fever and an indication to initiate prophylactic antibiotic therapy to prevent the subsequent development of other manifestations of rheumatic fever.

TORSION DYSTONIAS

The torsion dystonias are a heterogeneous group of disorders characterized by slow, involuntary turning and twisting movements of the neck, trunk, and limbs produced by forceful muscle contractions and culminating in sustained abnormal postures. Their cause is unknown. The manifestations may be confined to one body part (for example, the neck in torticollis) or the process may be generalized. Several clinical types of the disorder are distinguished by the body distribution of the movements and postures, the clinical manifestations, the pattern of the disorder's progression, the familial history, and other clinical features. Some of these clearly represent distinct entities, but the nosologic identity of most of these disorders remains uncertain, and the classification of individual cases may often be speculative. The most important syndromes are spasmodic torticollis, dystonia musculorum deformans, and dystonic writer's cramp. Additional rare entities are oromandibular dystonia and spasmodic dysphonia.

Spasmodic torticollis

DEFINITION. Spasmodic torticollis is the most familiar type of torsion dystonia, characterized by a deviation of the head to one side. The spasm begins with a slow, usually tremulous or jerky movement producing a turning of the head to one side and elevation of the shoulder. Contractions of the sternocleidomastoid muscle and the trapezius muscle bring the ear close to the shoulder of the same side. The deviation of the head is maintained for 1 to 2 minutes and then a period of relaxation follows, with the head returning toward the normal midline position but not reaching it.

CLINICAL MANIFESTATIONS. The torticollis comprises both a slow, involuntary movement and a sustained abnormal posture. The movement can often momentarily be overcome by an effort of will or by sensory contact. The patient may temporarily arrest the spasm simply by stroking the cheek with a finger. Many patients also have a rhythmic nodding head tremor and a postural tremor of the hands very similar to essential tremor. Inspection and palpation reveal hypertrophy of the sternocleidomastoid muscle.

ETIOLOGY. In most cases the cause is completely unknown. In some cases spasmodic torticollis may represent the initial manifestation or an oligosymptomatic expression of dystonia musculorum deformans. In many cases the patient may have a history of trauma to the head or neck that appears to have precipitated the symptoms. The significance of such trauma is unclear.

PATHOGENESIS. Little is known of the pathogenesis of spasmodic torticollis. An analysis of the lesions producing similar posture abnormalities of the head in animals suggests that the involvement of various structures in the brainstem can cause spasmodic torticollis. An abnormal response to vestibular stimuli has been postulated as one explanation. Thus far, no consistent pathologic lesions have been found.

LABORATORY FINDINGS. Electromyography of the involved muscles shows rhythmic discharges and increased activity on the abnormal side.

COURSE. Spasmodic torticollis may begin in childhood but more commonly makes its appearance in adult life. It increases in severity very gradually over many years and may remain stable and essentially unchanged throughout a normal life span. A mild scoliosis and later some tortipelvis may be noted in many cases. As the spasms become more severe, they may be quite painful. Secondary osteoarthritic changes may occur in the cervical spine. During periods of emotional stress the intensity of the spasms often increases.

MANAGEMENT. No satisfactory treatment is available at present. Various tranquilizing drugs are commonly employed and often yield some relief for painful spasms. Diazepam and related drugs have been most frequently used for this purpose. Major tranquilizers, including haloperidol and the phenothiazines, also may benefit some patients. Amantadine, alone or in combination with haloperidol, has been recommended by some clinicians. Anticholinergic agents such as trihexyphenidyl (Artane) may help, especially in younger patients. Psychotherapy may help alleviate secondary neurotic reactions, especially during periods of stress.

Surgical denervation of the cervical musculature may reduce the torticollis. The diffuse and variable involvement of the neck muscles generally limits the benefits of limited denervation, however, whereas more extensive denervation produced by sectioning all the upper cervical motor nerve roots is disfiguring. Stereotactic lesions of the thalamus have been made as a last resort, but the results often have been transitory and bilateral procedures are required to yield a significant benefit. Dramatic initial benefits have been reported, but because of the common recurrence of the spasms and the significant incidence of complications of the bilateral operation, thalamotomy is now rarely performed for spasmodic torticollis.

Physical therapy emphasizing range-of-motion exercises and training the patient to become more aware of the head position has been useful in some cases. Supplemented with biofeedback monitoring techniques, such exercises have helped many patients.

Dystonia musculorum deformans

DEFINITION. Dystonia musculorum deformans is a chronic, slowly progressive disorder beginning in childhood or adolescence and characterized by slow, involuntary twisting movements of the limbs, neck, and trunk culminating in fixed abnormal postures.

ETIOLOGY. The disorder is inherited; two genetic patterns have been recognized. One is transmitted in an autosomal recessive pattern and occurs almost exclusively in patients of Ashkenazi Jewish descent. It appears to be associated with high intelligence. The other major form is an autosomal dominant disorder with an extremely variable expression. A rare sex-linked form occurring only in females in which dystonic spasms are induced or exacerbated by exercise recently has been recognized.

PATHOGENESIS. Despite the inexorable progression of dystonia musculorum deformans over years resulting in severe disability, there is at present no known morbid anatomic alteration of the nervous system. Postmortem studies have revealed no consistent abnormality. The pathogenesis of this disorder is also unknown. From the evidence of cases of torsion spasms associated with brain tumors and in hepatolenticular degeneration (Wilson's disease), a basal ganglia dysfunction is suspected.

CLINICAL MANIFESTATIONS. A tendency to invert the foot while walking is the most common initial symptom, especially in children. Minimal at first and perhaps regarded as a mannerism, the phenomenon gradually becomes more pronounced with exaggerated stepping movements lending the gait a bizarre quality. The child may step squarely on the lateral border of the foot. Abnormal posturing of the arm in internal rotation and extension may then appear. Within a few years the process becomes generalized with torticollis, retrocollis, tortipelvis, kyphoscoliosis, and athetoid posturing of the hands. The wrists become hyperflexed and the fingers become extended. Although at the outset the abnormal movements occur only as adventitious muscle contractions superimposed on and altering the pattern of normal voluntary movement, the torsion spasms in time become sustained and result in abnormalities of posture that become fixed and constant. Patients with long-standing cases have extraordinary contortions and skeletal deformities. All voluntary movement becomes slow, awkward, and laborious. Dysphagia and dysarthria may occur at an advanced stage of the disease. Many patients also have a postural tremor similar in appearance to essential tremor.

LABORATORY FINDINGS. Concentrations of serum dopamine β-hydroxylase (DBH) have been reported to be elevated in the autosomal recessive form of dystonia musculorum deformans, but this finding has not been confirmed.

DIAGNOSIS. Torsion spasms may be symptomatic of Wilson's disease, cerebral birth injury, encephalitis, and rarely brain tumor. The development of the torsion spasms and abnormal postures in childhood, in the absence of evidence for another cause, leads to the diagnosis of dystonia musculorum deformans. Evidence of a similar disorder in other members of the family may help establish the diagnosis. Some individuals in a given family may have only a very mild scoliosis of which they may be unaware. Thus an examination of the parents and siblings, even if they deny having symptoms, may be useful. The bizarre nature of the initial symptoms and their marked fluctuation in intensity has often led physicians to suspect that they are psychogenic or "hysterical." This may delay the establishment of the correct diagnosis and result in inappropriate therapy. Differentiation from focal forms of dystonia may be difficult early in the course of the disease until the generalized nature of the affliction becomes evident.

MANAGEMENT. No satisfactory treatment is available. Diazepam and related drugs may diminish the intensity of the spasms and the consequent pain. Major tranquilizers such as haloperidol and anticholinergic drugs such as trihexyphenidyl (Artane) and benztropine (Cogentin) may also provide slight benefits. Treatment with levodopa in small doses has been reported to help in some cases. Levodopa appears especially to help in the exercise-induced form of dystonia. Carbamazepine (Tegretol) also has been effective in certain cases.

A stereotactic thalamotomy may induce a partial alleviation of distressing symptoms for a few years. Bilateral surgery is usually necessary, and the subsequent progression of the disease may require another operation to maintain the initial benefit. Surgery does not alter the course of the disease.

Writer's cramp

The term "writer's cramp" refers to spasms of the muscles of the forearm and hand provoked by attempts to perform fine movements such as writing, buttoning, or working with small tools. It has been regarded as an occupational neurosis, and many varieties have been described in different occupational settings, such as instrumentalist's cramp and violin player's cramp. Psychologic factors have often been implicated. Some cases represent a highly localized dystonic process that very slowly increases to involve the entire upper extremity after many years. Its cause and pathogenesis are entirely unknown. There is no known effective treatment. Training the patient to use the opposite unaffected hand may help.

Oromandibular dystonia

Oromandibular dystonia is a rare condition characterized by spasms of the jaw muscles and has been described as a form of focal dystonia. Patients with this disorder suffer from a slow, involuntary forceful opening of the mouth and a deviation of the jaw with a protrusion of the tongue. The phenomenon is somewhat similar to the acute dystonic reactions that may be provoked by the phenothiazines. Several features typical of other dystonias may be observed. For example, the patient may be able to abort a spasm by stroking his chin with his hand. The spasm may be sufficiently forceful to dislocate the jaw and fracture the teeth.

The cause and pathogenesis of this remarkable disorder are unknown. There is no satisfactory treatment. As in other dystonias, haloperidol, the phenothiazines, and anticholinergic agents may yield partial relief.

GILLES DE LA TOURETTE'S SYNDROME

DEFINITION. Gilles de la Tourette's syndrome (Tourette's syndrome) is the syndrome of multiple tics including corprolalia (uttering frequent obscenities) and impulsive behavior, named after the neurologist who gave the first full description of this remarkable disorder.

ETIOLOGY. The cause of Tourette's syndrome is unknown, but genetic factors are suspected. A biochemical defect in purine metabolism, presumably genetically determined, has been suggested as the cause at least in some cases. Psychologic factors were formerly considered causally significant.

PATHOGENESIS. The underlying pathogenesis is unknown. The effectiveness of major tranquilizers in controlling many of the symptoms, however, has suggested an abnormal predominance of brain dopaminergic neural systems. A dysfunction of other transmitter systems, notably serotonin and γ-aminobutyric acid, has been suggested, but a clear model of neurotransmitter imbalance comparable to that available for parkinsonism has not yet been established.

CLINICAL MANIFESTATIONS. Tourette's syndrome usually commences in childhood with minor involuntary movements, chiefly frequent eye-blinking, facial twitches, and grunting, or "clearing the throat" noises. These may be disregarded as mannerisms or ascribed to an irritation of the eyes or the throat by allergies or other factors for some time before they are recognized as tics. Hyperactive behavior is commonly noted and may be the initial manifestation in some children. Later in the course of the disease, shrugs of the shoulders, sudden jerks of the head, and sudden inappropriate vocalizations appear. After several years the abrupt jerking movements spread from the muscles of the neck and shoulders to the arms and legs. Subsequently, the patient may constantly make repetitive vocalizations, grunts, barks, and cooing noises and ultimately may utter frequent obscenities. The impulsive behavior, vocalizations, and coprolalia understandably interfere with the patient's social adjustment and frequently prevent regular attendance at school. The involuntary nature of the tics and vocalizations is often unrecognized, and disciplinary measures are applied inappropriately. Self-mutilation such as lip biting and gnawing the tips of the fingers has been noted in some cases.

COURSE. Tourette's syndrome has a variable course. Usually the progression is gradual, from one or two tics in childhood to the full-blown syndrome in adolescence or young adulthood. Some patients have spontaneous remissions that may rarely be of long duration, but in general the disorder persists essentially unchanged through adult life.

DIFFERENTIAL DIAGNOSIS. The syndrome is so remarkable and distinctive that, when all the elements are present, the correct diagnosis is usually not difficult to make. Some individuals may suffer only one or two tics throughout life, never having coprolalia or other features. Although these cases may represent fragments of the disorder, there is general agreement that in the absence of verbal tics they should not be designated as Tourette's syndrome. The major difficulty in diagnosis has been the tendency to consider the motor and behavior abnormalities as expressions of a psychologic disorder. Many such patients have been thought to be psychotic or hysterical. The motor disturbances are sometimes similar to those of chorea but differ in their stereotyped character. Characteristically, the patient experiences a sense of inner pressure and frustration when attempting to control the tic by an effort of will and a sense of relief when allowing the tic to occur. This sense of release does not accompany choreic movements. The vocalizations and coprolalia clearly distinguish Tourette's syndrome from the choreas.

MANAGEMENT. The major tranquilizing drugs are remarkably effective in suppressing the tics, impulsive behavior, vocalizations, and coprolalia. In contrast, amphetamines and levodopa may exacerbate the tics. The potent tranquilizer haloperidol is most commonly used today. The dosage and the therapeutic response may be limited by sedation and drug-induced parkinsonism to a level yielding only a partial control of the tics. Recently the noradrenalin receptor-blocker clonidine (Catapres) has been reported to be effective; its place in the tratment of Tourette's syndrome awaits further study.

WILSON'S DISEASE

DEFINITION. Wilson's disease is a genetic disorder characterized by the signs and the symptoms of basal ganglia dysfunction and hepatic cirrhosis described in 1912 by Wilson, who named it hepatolenticular degeneration.

ETIOLOGY AND PATHOGENESIS. Wilson's disease is a familial disorder occurring in an autosomal recessive pattern. The pathogenesis involves an abnormality of copper metabolism. There is a failure of synthesis of the serum copper-binding protein ceruloplasmin. As a result, copper accumulates gradually in the tissues, ultimately producing pathologic changes in the brain, liver, kidney, and other organs. In a sense the disease is a form of copper poisoning caused by a defect in the transport of copper that renders the patients unable to handle the trace amounts of copper normally present in the diet. The accumulation of copper in the liver in abnormal amounts can be detected in infancy. Ultimately the concentration of copper in the liver reaches levels hundreds of times greater than normal and induces a form of cirrhosis. The accumulation of copper in the brain results in degenerative changes involving mainly the basal ganglia but also the cerebral cortex, cerebellum, and other parts of the nervous system. In severe cases necrosis and cavitation of the globus pallidus and putamen may occur. Copper deposits in the cornea result in a golden-brown ring of pigment visible at the outer margin of the cornea.

EPIDEMIOLOGY. Wilson's disease is relatively rare. Little data are available on its prevalence, but it has been estimated that in some areas as many as 1% of the inmates of chronic mental hospitals may have this disorder. Neurologic manifestations develop in most cases in adolescence or early adulthood. Its onset as early as 4 years of age and as late as the fifth decade of life has been reported.

CLINICAL MANIFESTATIONS. Many cases are diagnosed in children when they have the signs and symptoms of hepatic disease. If proper treatment is instituted at this time, neurologic manifestations may never appear. With improved diagnosis in recent years, some cases have been identified in the neonatal period or in early childhood before the appearance of clinical manifestations.

The first manifestation of nervous system involvement is usually a decline in intellectual function. Deterioration in schoolwork is a frequent early sign. The patient may then become depressed and withdrawn and exhibit some slowness of movement, loss of facial expression, and slurring of speech. A tendency to keep the mouth open constantly is often noted. Voluntary movement becomes abnormal, with athetoid posturing of the arms and hands. Involuntary movements may develop such as slow, writhing movement of the limbs, a tremor similar to that of Parkinson's disease, and wing-beating movements of the arms. Patients becoming symptomatic in childhood tend to have dystonic and athetoid features, whereas those who become symptomatic later have dysarthria and a tremor of the hands. Muscular rigidity and bradykinesia may then develop, leading to a clinical picture resembling that of Parkinson's disease; Wilson's disease is probably the most common cause of juvenile parkinsonism. There is considerable variability, and many cases show features of both the childhood and adult forms.

The Kayser-Fleischer ring, a golden-brown ring of pigmentation at the outer margin of the cornea, is almost always present in patients with neurologic manifestations. This ring may easily be seen when the iris is lightly pigmented; in dark-eyed patients it can be seen with slit-lamp examination. Convulsions, unexplained periods of coma, and mental changes simulating psychosis or affective disorders may occur in rare cases.

LABORATORY FINDINGS. If the cirrhosis is sufficiently severe, the results of liver function tests may be abnormal. The serum uric acid level is often decreased and may be a useful clue to the correct diagnosis. Urinary amino acid excretion may have an abnormal pattern, and urinary copper excretion is increased. A 24-hour urine sample must be obtained in a copper-free container for the assay or urinary copper. Measurement of the concentration of copper in hepatic tissue obtained by needle aspiration shows a significant elevation. Copper-free needles must be used for this purpose. The major diagnostic laboratory abnormality is finding a low serum ceruloplasmin concentration.

DIAGNOSIS. The childhood cases of Wilson's disease are apt to be confused with cerebral palsy and rarely with dystonia musculorum deformans. Cases with a later onset are often erroneously classified as juvenile parkinsonism. Patients with prominent mental changes may be thought to have schizophrenia. The possibility of Wilson's disease should always be kept in mind when a young patient shows chronic progressive mental changes and extrapyramidal features. A history of a previous hepatic disorder, possibly diagnosed at the time as a form of hepatitis, may be a helpful clue. Finding a low serum uric acid level in the routine chemistry profile may be another helpful clue. The diagnosis can be established with considerable confidence by finding the Kayser-Fleischer ring in the cornea. If it cannot be seen by direct visual inspection, the patient should be referred to an ophthalmologist for a slit-lamp examination of the cornea. Determining the serum ceruloplasmin level is the definitive diagnostic test.

COURSE. In the absence of treatment the clinical course of the disease is one of gradual decline culminating in advanced cases in severe rigidity, ataxia, and dementia. Ultimately the patient dies of inanition and intercurrent infection. Some patients die of the hepatic disease or of the complications of cirrhosis such as a hemorrhage from ruptured esophageal varices.

MANAGEMENT. Specific treatment should begin as soon as the diagnosis has been established, even in asymptomatic cases. The goal of therapy is to remove the copper from the tissues and to prevent its reaccumulation. Copper removal is achieved with chelating agents such as penicillamine (usually 1 g daily), and the reaccumulation of copper is prevented by maintaining the patient on a copper-poor diet and administering potassium sulfide to reduce copper absorption. Chelating agents must be given in dosages adequate to produce a copper diuresis. The 24-hour urinary excretion of copper is measured during the treatment to ensure that an adequate diuresis is achieved. The potassium sulfide is given by mouth (20 mg three times daily as sulfurated potash) following meals to precipitate copper in the bowel in the form of the highly insoluble copper disulfide. Penicillamine may cause a pyridoxine deficiency; to prevent this, a pyridoxine supplement (50 mg daily) is usually given in conjunction with the chelating agent. Improvement of the neurologic manifestations, fading of the Kayser-Fleischer rings, and improvement of the hepatic dysfunction can be expected. Even very severe manifestations may be markedly or completely reversed. Treatment must, however, be continued indefinitely.

IDIOPATHIC ORTHOSTATIC HYPOTENSION

DEFINITION. Orthostatic hypotension reflecting an insufficiency of the autonomic nervous system occurs in diabetes mellitus, polyneuritis, Parkinson's disease, the hereditary ataxias, and other disorders of the nervous system. It may also occur following the administration of tranquilizers, antidepressants, antihypertensives, and other drugs. In a small group of patients orthostatic hypotension develops (usually in middle age) without other clinical manifestations of a nervous system dysfunction. These have been designated idiopathic orthostatic hypotension or primary orthostatic hypotension. Nearly all patients with this disorder, however, subsequently have impotence, anhidrosis, and an atonic bladder; many also have parkinsonism and ataxia. Patients exhibiting such evidence of diffuse involvement of the nervous system have been designated as having Shy-Drager syndrome following the description by Shy and Drager of the postmortem findings in a typical patient. It remains uncertain whether idiopathic orthostatic hypotension with or without manifestations of the additional involvement of the nervous system represents a distinct morbid entity.

ETIOLOGY. Idiopathic orthostatic hypotension is a degenerative disorder of the nervous system of unknown cause. It may be grouped among the multiple system atrophies of the central nervous system, including striatonigral degeneration and Parkinson's disease.

PATHOLOGY. The most common feature found during postmortem examination is a degeneration of the intermediolateral cells of the spinal cord. Intracytoplasmic inclusion bodies (Lewy bodies) may be found in these cells and also in the paravertebral sympathetic ganglia. Neuron degeneration and Lewy bodies may also be found in the substantia nigra, the locus ceruleus, various cranial nerve motor nuclei, and the olivary nuclei. In some cases the cerebral cortex may show atrophic change.

CLINICAL MANIFESTATIONS. Light-headedness, faintness, or even a loss of consciousness on assuming the erect posture is the major clinical symptom of this disorder. Initially the patient may have only weakness, dizziness, and faintness when suddenly standing up from a seated or supine position, as in arising from bed in the morning. If questioned, the patient may report more subtle symptoms including impaired sexual performance in men (with an inability to maintain penile erection and delayed ejaculation), loss of sweating, urinary urgency, and urinary frequency. The orthostatic hypotension may become so severe after several years that the patient cannot assume the upright position and remains confined to a bed and chair. When the patient stands up, the blood pressure drops precipitously, and syncope usually occurs when the blood pressure falls below 80/50 mm Hg. Such a drop can be appreciated by palpating the radial pulse. The heart rate fails to increase in response to the fall in pressure. The pallor and sweating that normally occur in response to hypotension fail to occur in these patients because of the dysfunction of the peripheral autonomic nerves. The autonomic deficiency can be demonstrated by studying the response to Valsalva's maneuver. Hypotension is readily produced, but tachycardia during the maneuver, hypertension on conclusion of the maneuver, and subsequent bradycardia (all observed in normal subjects) do not occur.

In patients with the Shy-Drager syndrome the signs and symptoms of central nervous system involvement also develop. Usually these include a parkinsonian state with bradykinesia, mild rigidity, tremor, monotone speech, ataxia, and dysarthria. Distal wasting of the limb muscles may also be found. Shy and Drager noted atrophy of the iris in their cases.

COURSE. The course of the disease is one of gradual

progression. Patients with advanced disease are usually confined to bed by the severe hypotension. Ultimately the patients may succumb to myocardial infarction, cerebral infarction, inanition, or intercurrent infections. Sleep apnea complicating the late course of the illness has been implicated as a cause of death in some cases.

MANAGEMENT. Orthostatic hypotension may be treated symptomatically with sodium chloride supplements or with fludrocortisone, 0.1 to 1 mg daily titrated gradually, to increase blood volume. Wearing elastic hose and abdominal binders may help prevent the pooling of large volumes of blood in the legs and in the splanchnic circulation in the erect position. Ephedrine (25 mg three times a day) and phenylephrine administered orally may also be helpful. The combined use of a monoamine oxidase inhibitor and tyramine or levodopa has been described by some investigators. The levodopa may help relieve the parkinsonian symptoms seen in many cases, but when used alone usually aggravates the orthostatic hypotension.

BIBLIOGRAPHY

Aaron, A.M., Freeman, J.M., and Carter, S.: The natural history of Sydenham's chora, Am. J. Med. **38**:83, 1965.

Bird, M.T., Palkes, H., and Prensky, A.L.: A follow up study of Sydenham's chorea, Neurology **26**:601, 1976.

Calne, D.B.: Parkinsonism, London, 1969, Butterworth, Inc.

Chase, T., Wexler, N.J., and Barbeau, A., editors: Huntington's disease, New York, 1979, Raven Press.

Costero, I.: Cerebral lesions responsible for death of patients with active rheumatic fever, Arch. Neurol. Psychiatry **62**:48, 1949.

Critchley, M.: Observations on essential (heredofamilial) tremor, Brain **72**:113, 1949.

Diess, A., and others: Long-term therapy of Wilson's disease, Ann. Intern. Med. **75**:57, 1971.

Duvoisin, R.C.: Clinical diagnosis of the dyskinesias, Med. Clin. North Am. **56**:1321, 1972.

Duvoisin, R.C.: Parkinsonism: a guide for patient and family, New York, 1978, Raven Press.

Eldridge, R.: The torsion dystonias: literature review and genetic and clinical studies, Neurology **20**(suppl.):1, 1970.

Herz, E., and Glaser, G.H.: Spasmodic torticollis: clinical evaluation, Arch. Neurol. Psychiatry **61**:227, 1949.

Hughes, R.O., Cartlidge, N.E.F., and Millac, P.: Primary neurogenic orthostatic hypotension, J. Neurol. Neurosurg. Psychiatry **33**:363, 1970.

Marsden, C.D.: Dystonia: the spectrum of the disease, Res. Publ. Assoc. Res. Nerv. Ment. Dis **55**:351, 1976.

Marsden, C.D., and Harrison, M.J.G.: Idiopathic torsion dystonia (dystonia musculorum deformans), Brain **97**:703, 1974.

Martin, J.P., and Alcock, N.S.: Hemichorea associated with a lesion of the corpus luysii, Brain **57**:504, 1934.

Shapiro, A.K., and others: The Gilles de la Tourette syndrome, New York, 1977, Raven Press.

Shy, G.M., and Drager, G.A.: A neurological syndrome associated with orthostatic hypotension: a clinical-pathologic study, Arch. Neurol. **2**:511, 1960.

Sternlieb, I., and Scheinberg, I.H.: Penicillamine therapy for hepatolenticular degeneration, J.A.M.A. **189**:146, 1964.

Sternlieb, I., and Scheinberg, I.H.: Prevention of Wilson's disease in asymptomatic patients, N. Engl. J. Med. **278**:352, 1968.

Strickland, G.T., and Leu, M.-L.: Wilson's disease, Medicine **54**:113, 1975.

Wilson, S.A.K.: Progressive lenticular degeneration: familial nervous disease associated with cirrhosis of the liver, Brain **34**:295, 1912.

Yahr, M.D., and Duvoisin, R.C.: The drug treatment of parkinsonism, N. Engl. J. Med. **287**:20, 1972.

151 • VIRAL AND SLOW VIRAL INFECTIONS OF THE CENTRAL NERVOUS SYSTEM

David P. Dunn

(See also Chapter 37.)

Many viruses can cause infections of the central nervous system. Most of them are complications of systemic infections by common viruses that normally do not involve the nervous system. Some viruses have an affinity for the nervous system and are known as neurotropic viruses. Most infections involve the meninges instead of the neural parenchyma and produce the syndrome of aseptic meningitis. When the brain is involved, the patient has encephalitis. Meningoencephalitis refers to the involvement of the brain and the meninges. Myelitis is an infection of the spinal cord. The sensory ganglia are involved in herpes zoster. Clinically apparent viral infections of the nervous system have an acute onset, a period of illness for the patient, and either eventual recovery or permanent neurologic sequelae or death. Some encephalopathies develop after systemic viral infections and are not caused by direct viral invasion of the nervous system. Certain viruses can enter a cell and remain latent, reactivating in later years to produce a disease. A few progressive neurologic diseases previously thought to be degenerative and of unknown cause are known now to be caused by slow viruses. Some viruses cause a specific disorder, but in the overwhelming majority of cases specific identification is possible only through serologic tests or through the recovery and growth in culture of the virus. Other diseases of the nervous system may resemble viral infections, but clinical suspicion and various laboratory tests often can indicate the nonviral cause.

ASEPTIC MENINGITIS

DEFINITION. Aseptic meningitis is a relatively benign, nonpurulent infection of the meninges of the nervous system. It is probably more common than is recognized.

ETIOLOGY AND PATHOGENESIS. A myriad of viruses are responsible for causing aseptic meningitis, and new ones are discovered each year. Often the specific virus involved is not identified. The enteric viruses that are temporary occupants of the alimentary tract are common offenders. Viruses that are neurotropic such as poliovirus and arbovirus may cause only meningitis. Mumps virus, herpes virus, varicella virus, Epstein-Barr virus (infectious mononucleosis), measles virus, and other viruses have been implicated. Lymphocytic choriomeningitis is a less common cause of meningitis than the other viruses, and it rarely produces a severe infection.

CLINICAL MANIFESTATIONS AND COURSE. The symptoms and signs are similar to those of bacterial meningitis except they are less fulminant and devastating. The patient has an acute onset of headache, stiff neck, fever, photophobia, nausea, and vomiting. The patient may be irritable but retains consciousness. The course is self-limited over 1 or 2 weeks, and recovery is complete. The main clinical concern is not to mistake aseptic meningitis for a more serious problem.

LABORATORY FINDINGS. Laboratory findings include a cell count in the cerebrospinal fluid (CSF) that is elevated and predominantly lymphocytic. Polymorphonuclear leukocytes may predominate early in the course of the disease, but lymphocytes rapidly increase to become the dominant type of cell. The glucose level in the CSF, with few exceptions, is not reduced as it is in bacterial infections. The protein level is normal or slightly elevated. Serologic tests and cultures are necessary to identify the specific virus causing the infection.

DIAGNOSIS AND MANAGEMENT. The clinical manifestations and the laboratory findings in the CSF suggest the diagnosis of aseptic meningitis. It should be realized that the predominantly lymphocytic cellular reaction in the CSF may be found in partially treated bacterial infections, tuberculous and fungal infections, tumors, sarcoidosis, vasculitis, and brain abscesses. The evaluation of the protein and glucose levels and staining and culturing the fluid are essential for making the correct diagnosis. Other laboratory tests may be necessary to identify lesions that produce a lymphocytic reaction in the CSF. Once the diagnosis is confirmed, treatment is supportive.

ENCEPHALITIS

Encephalitis is a diffuse, nonpurulent inflammatory disease of the brain. The invading virus attacks and may destroy the brain cells, and inflammatory cells accumulate in the parenchyma. The meninges are usually involved to some degree, and a variable increase in lymphocytes is found in the CSF. The protein concentration is often increased, and with few exceptions the glucose concentration is not lowered. Besides the manifestations of aseptic meningitis, encephalitis produces neurologic deficits that range from lethargy to a deep coma. Convulsions are common, and patients may have muscular weakness, sensory disturbances, and alterations in behavior. With some infections the mortality is high. The clinical manifestations and the epidemiologic pattern are occasionally suggestive of a particular viral infection but serologic tests and cultures are usually necessary to incriminate a specific virus.

Arbovirus encephalitis

DEFINITION. Arbovirus (arthropod-borne) encephalitis is an epidemic encephalitis transmitted by arthropod vectors, most commonly by mosquitoes.

ETIOLOGY AND PATHOGENESIS. Vertebrate wildlife are the reservoirs for arbovirus. The mosquito acquires the virus from the blood of infected wildlife. When the mosquito bites a human it introduces the virus into the bloodstream. Encephalitis develops in a minority of infected people. When the right combination of weather, mosquitoes, and reservoir hosts exists, humans become accidental victims and a localized epidemic occurs. California, St. Louis, western equine, and eastern equine are the most common arthropod-borne encephalitides in the United States. The severity of the cell destruction and the inflammatory reaction in the brain varies, depending on which arbovirus is involved.

CLINICAL MANIFESTATIONS AND COURSE. Headache or other minor symptoms may be the only clinical manifestations, or the disease may progress to convulsions, focal neurologic deficits, coma, and death. California encephalitis usually causes only a mild meningoencephalitis. St Louis encephalitis is widespread and causes severe neurologic deficits and death in the elderly; the mortality is about 10%. Eastern equine encephalitis is the least common, but it has a mortality of 70%. Young children are particularly susceptible to it. Western equine encephalitis has a mortality of only 2%, and serious neurologic sequelae are less common than with the eastern form.

LABORATORY FINDINGS. The CSF protein concentration is often moderately increased, and cells, most of which are mononuclear, can be found in the fluid. Polymorphonuclear leukocytes may be found in the CSF in the earliest phase of the disease. Serologic tests can identify the specific arbovirus.

DIAGNOSIS AND MANAGEMENT. The diagnosis depends on the clinical manifestations, the laboratory tests, and the epidemiologic pattern. The treatment is supportive.

Herpes simplex encephalitis

DEFINITION. Herpes simplex encephalitis is the most common sporadic, or nonepidemic, type of severe encephalitis.

ETIOLOGY AND PATHOGENESIS. Most brain infections are caused by type 1 herpes simplex virus, which is a common quiescent inhabitant of the trigeminal ganglion. When it reactivates and moves down the nerve, it causes herpes labialis, or fever blisters. Encephalitis is produced when the reactivated virus travels to the brain and attacks and damages the brain cells. The virus has a proclivity for the temporal lobes, where it causes edema and hemorrhagic necrosis. Type 2 herpes simplex virus in infants usually causes a disseminated infection in which the brain is not always involved.

CLINICAL MANIFESTATIONS AND COURSE. The first manifestations are headache, fever, and symptoms of meningeal irritation. Changes in behavior, memory defects, and peculiar sensations of taste and smell occur next. Focal neurologic signs, seizures, and increasing lethargy progress to coma. The usual outcome is death or severe neurologic sequelae in the survivors.

LABORATORY FINDINGS. The CSF pressure is increased, as is the cell count, which is predominantly mononuclear. The CSF may be bloody or xanthochromic, and the glucose level may be reduced, which is an unusual finding in viral infections. Various roentgenographic tests can demonstrate the predominant temporal lobe involvement.

DIAGNOSIS AND MANAGEMENT. The clinical manifestations of encephalitis with temporal lobe involvement are suggestive of herpes simplex virus. The specific diagnosis rests on the identification of the herpes simplex virus or the herpes simplex antigen in the brain tissue. Adenine arabinoside, an antiviral drug, may be of value if given early in the course of the disease.

Cytomegalovirus

Cytomegalovirus is a member of the herpesvirus family and is a widespread, clinically inapparent inhabitant of healthy humans. Serologic studies indicate that most adults have had contact with cytomegalovirus. Infants can be infected in utero or in early postnatal life and either remain symptomless or have cytomegalic inclusion body disease. This generalized disease is characterized by enlarged cells with intranuclear inclusion bodies. It varies in severity from a mild illness to a fatal one. Many organs, including the brain, can be infected, especially the spleen, salivary glands, lungs, liver, and kidneys. The involvement of the brain can vary from a fatal encephalitis to mild mental retardation. The cerebral cortex may show maldevelopment. Calcifications and hydrocephalus are found in mentally retarded survivors. Infants are more vulnerable because of their immature immunologic defenses. The disease occurs in adults who have altered immunologic responses, and some of these patients have encephalitis. The virus is identified by culture and serologic tests. No specific treatment is available.

Rabies

From 1960 to 1978 the annual rate of reported human rabies cases in the United States has varied from none to four. With very few exceptions rabies is a fatal disease. Although it is usually transmitted to humans by the infected saliva of a rabid animal, a few cases of aerosol transmission in laboratories and bat-infested caves have occurred. It has also been transmitted by a corneal transplant. Rabies exists in plentiful supply in wildlife, which is a reservoir for the virus. In recent years infections of skunks, bats, and raccoons have far outnumbered those of dogs and cats. The incubation period varies from weeks to months while the virus multiplies at the site of the bite and travels up the nerve to the central nervous system. It attacks the neurons and spreads via the nerves to the salivary glands and to other organs. Usually the clinical disease lasts less than 1 week. The patient feels peculiar sensations at the site of the initial infection and becomes apprehensive. Salivation and lacrimation increase, and agitation, delirium, or frank mania develops. The patient has painful spasms when trying to swallow; this is followed by terminal seizures and a lapse into a coma. If rabies exposure is suspected, the wound should be thoroughly washed and the victim should consult a physician. Nonprovoked wild animal bites are particularly suspect (see Chapter 38 for a discussion of prophylaxis of rabies).

POLIOMYELITIS

Poliovirus is an enteric virus that has three antigenic types. It spreads from person to person via the alimentary tract. The virus enters through the mouth, multiples in the alimentary tract, and is excreted in the feces for a period of time. Clinical disease develops in only a small number of infected people. Aseptic meningitis and mild disturbances of the upper respiratory tract and the gastrointestinal system can occur. The severe infection poliomyelitis usually follows one of these illness. The virus spreads to the gray matter of the spinal cord and the cranial nerves, where it attacks the large motor neurons. The involvement of these cells produces a flaccid paralysis of the muscles. The weakness is usually most severe at onset and varies from muscle to muscle. A small minority of cases are fatal, most often because of respiratory paralysis. Usually a partial or complete recovery takes place, depending on the extent of the damage to the neurons. The virus can be cultured from the throat and rectum, and a rise in the antibody titer can be found in the serum. An infection produces type-specific immunity. Vaccination has dramatically reduced the incidence of poliomyelitis. Today it is a rare disease in the United States. Some of the other enteric viruses can cause a more benign but clinically similar disease.

HERPES ZOSTER (SHINGLES)

DEFINITION. Herpes zoster (shingles) is a sporadic painful eruption of the skin in an area supplied by one or two adjacent sensory nerve roots.

ETIOLOGY AND PATHOGENESIS. Varicella, or chickenpox, is a common childhood disease caused by the varicella-zoster virus. In the adult the same virus causes a different clinical entity, herpes zoster (shingles). The virus is a member of the herpesvirus family and can remain quiescent in the sensory ganglia of the spinal and cranial nerve roots. Some stimulus in later years reactivates the virus. It attacks the neurons of the ganglion, presumably travels down the nerve, and appears as a vesicular eruption in the area of skin innervated by the damaged ganglion.

CLINICAL MANIFESTATIONS AND COURSE. A severe, burning, lancinating pain develops in the area of skin supplied by the sensory nerve of the infected ganglion. After a few days a vesicular eruption appears in the same area. The eruption eventually clears, but persistent postherpetic pain is a common complication, especially in debilitated patients. The spinal ganglia of the thoracic region are the most commonly affected. Of the cranial nerves, the fifth is usually involved with the first or ophthalmic division most often affected. Herpetic lesions of this division may develop on the cornea, resulting in scars that can seriously impair vision. The geniculate ganglion of the seventh nerve occasionally is involved. The virus can disseminate and produce a chickenpox-like illness; this is likely when a patient takes immunosuppressive drugs or has a disease that compromises the immunologic response.

LABORATORY FINDINGS. The virus can be isolated from the skin lesions, and a rise in antibody titers can be found in the serum.

DIAGNOSIS AND MANAGEMENT. The diagnosis can be made clinically. The treatment is symptomatic. Postherpetic pain or neuralgia can be intractable; surgical procedures on the nerve root or the ganglion seldom relieve it. The medical management of persistent postherpetic neuralgia is similar to that of trigeminal neuralgia (see Chapter 146).

REYE'S SYNDROME

DEFINITION. Reye's syndrome is a rare sequela to a variety of viral illnesses of childhood. Swelling of the brain and fatty degeneration of the liver develop rapidly a few days after the onset of an antecedent illness.

ETIOLOGY AND PATHOGENESIS. Influenza, particularly B type influenza, and chickenpox have been incriminated in many cases of Reye's syndrome. Often the antecedent illness is a mild and ill-defined upper respiratory tract infection. How the viral infections produce the syndrome is unknown. Damaged mitochondria and fat droplets are found in the hepatocytes of the liver. There may be a fatty infiltration of the heart and kidneys. The brain swelling or edema is severe, and damaged mitochondria may be seen in the brain cells. Mitochondrial enzyme deficiency, circulating fatty acids, increased ammonia levels in the blood, and hypoglycemia have all been implicated as causes of the edema.

CLINICAL MANIFESTATIONS AND COURSE. Severe and repetitive vomiting ushers in the syndrome. Fever and hyperexcitability followed by lethargy, seizures, stupor, and coma develop in the course of a few days. Death or serious neurologic sequelae usually can be prevented in patients who receive early treatment.

LABORATORY FINDINGS. Laboratory findings vary according to the severity and course of the syndrome. Abnormal tests of hepatic function, electrolyte derangements, hypoglycemia caused by the liver involvement, increased blood ammonia levels, increased CSF ammonia levels resulting from the breakdown of the urea cycle, and increased CSF pressure can be found.

DIAGNOSIS AND MANAGEMENT. The diagnosis is based on the history, the clinical manifestations, and appropriate laboratory tests. The intracranial pressure is monitored and reduced enough to ensure an adequate blood circulation in the brain. Exchange transfusions may be performed if the prothrombin time is prolonged. A normal blood glucose level should be maintained and other metabolic derangements corrected.

POSTINFECTIOUS ENCEPHALOMYELITIS AND POSTVACCINAL ENCEPHALOMYELITIS (ACUTE DISSEMINATED ENCEPHALOMYELITIS)

DEFINITION. Postinfectious encephalomyelitis and postvaccinal encephalomyelitis are acute demyelinating diseases that follow a viral infection or a vaccination. Occasionally the encephalomyelitis may be parainfectious when it develops concurrently with the viral infection.

ETIOLOGY AND PATHOGENESIS. The antecedent viral diseases are usually those that produce a rash, but influenza, mumps, and other respiratory infections have been implicated as causes of these disorders. Smallpox vaccine and rabies nerve tissue vaccine, both of which are no longer used in the United States, were the main source of postvaccinal encephalomyelitis. All of these agents produce the same lesion. An acute inflammatory reaction with destruction of the myelin develops around the blood vessels in the white matter of the brain and the spinal cord. Some cases in which early neurologic manifestations appear may be caused by a direct viral invasion of the nervous system. Most authorities believe delayed manifestations are allergic reactions in white matter set off by viral illness.

CLINICAL MANIFESTATIONS AND COURSE. The clinical manifestations vary depending on the affected region of the brain or spinal cord. Neurologic deficits usually appear a few days after the onset of the rash. Lethargy, convulsions, muscle weakness, visual problems, and coma may progress to death. Measles, probably the most common provoking condition, produces encephalomyelitis in only about 1 in 1000 cases.

LABORATORY FINDINGS. The CSF may be normal or have an increased total protein level and lymphocyte count. Cultures and serologic tests for viruses are necessary.

DIAGNOSIS AND MANAGEMENT. The history and clinical manifestations should suggest the diagnosis. A search for viruses should be undertaken so that the diagnosis is not mistaken for an encephalitis in which the nervous system is directly invaded. No specific treatment is known.

SLOW VIRAL INFECTIONS OF THE CENTRAL NERVOUS SYSTEM

The discovery that slow viruses can cause progressive neurologic diseases in humans has altered many previously held conceptions about infections of the central nervous system. Some diseases thought to be degenerative are actually slow virus infections. The term "slow" does not refer to a specific virus but rather indicates the timespan from infection to death. In humans and animals a long incubation period precedes the onset of clinical disease, but after the onset the disease progresses inexorably to death.

Kuru

Kuru is a progressively disabling, fatal disease of a linguistically related group of natives in the highlands of New Guinea. Thought to be transmitted by the various rituals of cannibalism, it was very prevalent at the time of the first report in 1957. Since the cessation of cannibalism it is disappearing. New cases do occur, probably from exposure to the causative agent many years earlier. When the brains of kuru victims were examined microscopically, an extensive vacuolation was found in the cells. This change was similar to that found in scrapie, a disease of sheep that was known already to be a transmissible disease. The brain tissue of kuru victims was inoculated into chimpanzees, and after 1 to 2 years they developed a disease marked by vacuoles in the brain cells. A specific virus has not yet been isolated, but the transmissible quality indicates the presence of an infectious agent.

Creutzfeldt-Jakob disease

Creutzfeldt-Jakob disease is a rare and fatal disorder that occurs throughout the world, mostly in middle-aged people. Dementia that progresses to death in usually less than 2 years is accompanied by other neurologic deficits, especially rapid jerks of the trunk and limbs (myoclonus). The electroencephalogram usually shows a typical pattern. Brain tissue from patients has produced the disease months to years later in inoculated chimpanzees. A corneal transplant from a demented donor transmitted the disease to the recipient, and instruments implanted in the cerebrum of a patient and later used again were responsible for two other cases. Vacuoles similar to those in scrapie and kuru are present in the brain cells. Because the cell vacuolation has a spongy appearance microscopically, these diseases are called subacute spongiform encephalopathies. The slow virus is probably similar to that of kuru and is resistant to many of the usual viral inactivators. Dental and medical personnel do not face an unusual risk from contact with this disease, but they should take precautions similar to those used with carriers of chronic hepatitis if procedures are to be performed on a patient with an undiagnosed type of dementia. Instruments should be autoclaved. Known virus inactivators include povidone-iodine (Betadine), hexachlorophene, Dakin's fluid (antiseptic solution), and household bleach. They should be used on inadvertent skin wounds.

Subacute sclerosing panencephalitis

Subacute sclerosing panencephalitis, a rare and fatal disease of children and young adults, is caused by a measles virus that lacks the envelope of a mature virus. School-aged males are most commonly affected, and they usually have a history of measles during the first 2 years of life. The patient usually has an insidious deterioration of mental function followed by myoclonic jerks, muscle weakness, seizures, and severe dementia. Most patients die within 1 year. High levels of antibodies to measles virus are found in the serum and CSF. Measles virus has been recovered from infected brains. It is thought that an abnormal immunologic response has allowed the virus to remain in the cells after the patient has recovered from the initial attack of measles. At a later date the virus reactivates, and the disease ensues.

Progressive multifocal leukoencephalopathy

Progressive multifocal leukoencephalopathy is a rare disease that usually arises in patients who already have severe systemic disorders such as lymphomas, leukemias, and other disorders that reduce the immunologic defense mechanisms. The progress is rapid, the average course from onset to death being 6 months. Multiple foci of demyelination appear, enlarge, and often coalesce in the brain. The clinical manifestations are diverse because they depend on the regions of the brain that are affected. Mental deterioration is common. No specific laboratory tests are available, although computed tomographic scans can show the multifocal white matter lesions. Papovaviruses are present in the nuclei of diseased oligodendroglia cells, the cells necessary for the maintenance of myelin. The papovavirus most often present is the JC virus, which is a common, usually nonpathogenic, virus. The altered immunologic response allows it to opportunistically invade and destroy these cells. Demyelination follows.

BIBLIOGRAPHY

Davis, L.E., and Johnson, R.T.: An explanation for localization of herpes simplex encephalitis? Ann. Neurol. **5:**2, 1979.

Gajdusek, D.C., and others: Precautions in medical care of, and in handling materials from, patients with transmissable virus dementia (Creutzfeldt-Jakob disease), N. Engl. J. Med. **297:**1253, 1977.

Houff, S.A., and others: Human-to-human transmission of rabies virus by corneal transplant, N. Engl. J. Med. **300:**603, 1979.

Johnson, R.T., and Mims, C.A.: Pathogenesis of viral infections of the nervous system, N. Engl. J. Med. **278:**23, 1968.

Narayan, O., and others: Etiology of progressive multifocal leukoencephalopathy: identification of papovavirus, N. Engl. J. Med. **289:**1278, 1973.

Trauner, D.A.: Treatment of Reye syndrome, Ann. Neurol. **7:**2, 1980.

Venes, J.L., Shaywitz, B.A., and Spencer, D.D.: Management of severe cerebral edema in the metabolic encephalopathy of Reye-Johnson syndrome, J. Neurosurg. **48:**903, 1978.

152 • VASCULAR DISEASES OF THE CENTRAL NERVOUS SYSTEM

Rosalie A. Burns

Various diseases of the cerebral vessels set the stage for what is commonly known as a stroke or a cerebrovascular accident (CVA). CVA is the third leading cause of death in the United States and a major cause of disability. The general term "cerebrovascular accident" is so broad, however, that it is insufficient as a diagnosis. More specific and meaningful diagnostic categories to which therapy can be related include cerebral infarction caused by either an arterial thrombosis or an embolus; transient cerebral ischemia or transient ischemic attacks (TIAs); cerebral hemorrhage, either subarachnoid or parenchymal; and infarction and hemorrhage caused by a venous thrombosis.

The diagnosis for a patient who has sustained a CVA cannot rest with a description of the presumed pathophysiologic conditions alone. An attempt to localize the lesion in the central nervous system, thereby suggesting which cerebral vessel is involved, is important for both therapy and prognosis. An example is the situation in which prophylactic surgery on extracranial cerebral vessels is contemplated. The cause of the vascular wall abnormality must be considered. For example, a cerebral thrombosis can be superimposed on a vessel showing atherosclerotic change, or it may be associated with a vasculitis. In an older patient, vascular disease frequently occurs in conjunction with diabetes or hypertension. Hypertension is a frequent cause of underlying cerebrovascular disease, producing hyalinization, a fibrinoid change of the arterioles, and Charcot-Bouchard microaneurysms. A history of hypertension is frequently obtained in patients with a cerebral thrombosis, is commonly present in patients with an intracerebral (parenchymal) hemorrhage, and is usual for patients with the lacunar state (état lacunaire). Severe hypertension may lead to hypertensive encephalopathy. For the older patient, temporal arteritis should be considered as a cause of CVA. For a younger patient, less common but pertinent causes of CVA that must be considered include collagen-vascular disease, infections such as meningovascular syphilis, drug ingestion (for example, amphetamines or LSD), hyperlipidemia, migraine headache, fibromuscular dysplasia, mitral valve prolapse, atrial myxoma with emboli, homocystinuria, polycythemia vera, sickle cell disease, hyperviscosity syndromes, various coagulopathies, pregnancy, the use of oral contraception, and moyamoya disease.

Finally, hemodynamic causes of ischemia, which may be superimposed on a compromised cerebral circulation, should be considered. These would include, for example, various causes of hypotension. The clinical manifestations of cerebrovascular disease are characterized by a sudden onset, in contrast to the gradual downhill progression of a cerebral tumor, an abscess, or a subdural hematoma. In most instances a clinical diagnosis can be made on the basis of a thorough history and physical examination, but 5% to 20% of seemingly straightforward CVAs turn out on further study to warrant an alternative diagnosis. Thus is is important that all patients with a presumed CVA undergo a basic diagnostic workup.

ANATOMY AND PHYSIOLOGY OF THE CEREBRAL CIRCULATION

The flow of blood to the brain, approximately 50 ml/100 g of brain each minute, is normally regulated by a process called autoregulation. This mechanism operates through alterations in the caliber of the cerebral arterioles and the small arteries. This intrinsic myotonic blood vessel reactivity maintains the cerebral blood flow at a relatively constant level between the mean arterial blood pressures of approximately 60 mm Hg and 150 mm Hg in the normal individual. In the hypertensive patient with arteriolar wall thickening, normal blood flows are maintained at higher mean pressures. Autoregulation is transiently disturbed by an acute cerebral insult such as a seizure, head trauma, or a CVA. Without autoregulation the cerebral blood flow passively follows the blood pressure.

The cerebral circulation is commonly divided into the extracranial circulation, referring to the major vessels originating from the aortic arch and traversing the neck to the base of the skull, and the intracranial circulation, referring to the intracranial portions of the internal carotid and the vertebral arteries and their branches (Fig. 152-1). The extracranial arteries arising from the aortic arch are the innominate artery, giving rise to the right common carotid artery and the right subclavian artery, and the separate left common carotid and subclavian arteries. The vertebral arteries are the first branches of each subclavian artery. As they ascend, the vertebral arteries pass through the foramina in the transverse processes of the upper six cervical vertebrae and then turn around the atlas to enter the skull through the foramen magnum. Intracranially the vertebral arteries unite to form the basilar artery. The basilar artery divides into the two posterior cerebral arteries that join the circle of Willis.

The common carotid arteries bifurcate in the neck into the external carotid artery and the internal carotid artery, the internal carotid artery continuing intracranially through the base of the skull. The portion of the internal carotid artery just distal to the bifurcation of the common carotid artery is the carotid sinus. The ophthalmic artery arises from the internal carotid artery intracranially and proximal to the origin of the anterior cerebral artery, the middle cerebral artery, and the posterior communicating artery. The posterior communicating branch of the internal carotid artery forms a major connection through the circle of Willis

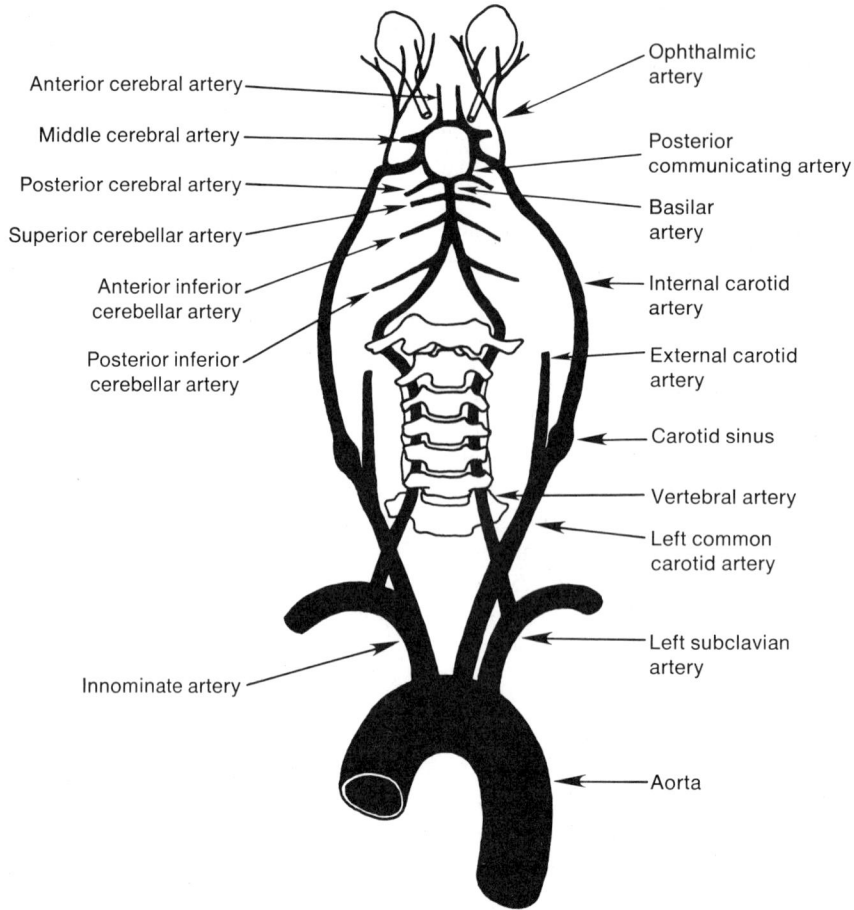

Fig. 152-1. Cerebral circulation.

with the posterior basilar-vertebral circulation. The intracranial arteries may receive collateral blood flow, bypassing occluded vessels, by means of communication with the extracranial vessels or with other intracranial vessels. An example of the communication with the extracranial vessels is the retrograde blood flow that may occur through the ophthalmic branch of the internal carotid artery by way of external carotid vessel anastomoses. Intracranially, distal anastomoses occur between the subarachnoid arterial branches of the various cerebral arteries. The circle of Willis also provides a means of collateral blood flow; for example, it unites the carotid arterial system with the basilar-vertebral arterial system through the posterior communicating artery. Frequent anomalies of the circle of Willis make the adequacy of this source of collateral circulation unpredictable.

INFARCTION OF THE BRAIN

PATHOGENESIS. In an infarction of the brain a localized drop in cerebral blood flow results in permanent structural change to a focal area of the brain. Vessel occlusion may be caused by a thrombosis with an underlying vessel wall disease or by an embolus. Sites of predilection for underlying atherosclerosis include the carotid sinus in the neck, the intracranial internal carotid artery at the siphon (near the origin of the ophthalmic artery), the middle cerebral artery at its first major bifurcation, the vertebral arteries at their entrance to the cranial cavity and at their junction forming the basilar artery, the basilar artery itself, the posterior cerebral arteries at their origin, and the anterior cerebral arteries as they bend around the genu of the corpus callosum. In hypertensive patients, arteriosclerosis and thrombosis occur in the smaller cerebral arteries.

Infarctions may be pale or hemorrhagic. Pale infarctions involve tissue softening, liquefaction, and eventual glial scarring and cavity formation. Hemorrhagic infarctions are usually caused by an embolus and show abundant petechial hemorrhages.

In an infarction caused by an embolus, the embolic material may arise from an intracardiac mural thrombus following a myocardial infarction, from the diseased valves of rheumatic heart disease, from prosthetic valves, from mitral valve prolapse, from the heart in atrial fibrillation, as a complication of cardiac surgery, or from plaques in the extracranial cerebral arterial system. Infrequently, an embolus from a peripheral vein may reach the brain by way of an atrial septal defect, a so-called paradoxical embolus. Septic emboli can arise from vegetations of acute and subacute bacterial endocarditis. Emboli may arise from an atrial myxoma or from the nonbacterial valvular vegetations of Libman-Sacks endocarditis in lupus erythematosus.

The neurologic deficits that occur with a brain infarction are directly related to the functional anatomy of the disturbed region. The acute symptoms of a cerebral infarction may be magnified by local cerebral edema, and improvement may occur with time as the edema subsides and collateral circulation develops. An area of remaining encephalomalacia persists, and clinically the patient has a residual deficit of varying degree that warrants efforts at physical rehabilitation.

CLINICAL MANIFESTATIONS. In an infarction caused by a thrombosis the onset is sudden and the neurologic deficit commonly appears abruptly; the patient may simply awaken with the deficit. In some instances the progression may be over a matter of hours, in which case the term "thrombosis in evolution" is appropriate, or there may be a stuttering onset with small increments of increasing deficit that may occur over a matter of days to weeks. The patient may have had previous TIAs. Symptoms associated with a cerebral thrombosis at its onset may include headache or, for a small percentage of patients, seizures.

The onset of an infarction caused by an embolus is sudden, commonly even more abrupt than with an infarction caused by a thrombosis. Because small branches may become occluded, neurologic deficits may be confined to the distribution of single branches, and monoparesis, for example, would not be unusual. A cortical localization in the cerebrum is common. A higher incidence of seizures at onset has been noted than with a thrombosis or with a hemorrhage. Because the emboli may dissolve or move further downstream, blood may gain access to a previously occluded vessel, resulting in a hemorrhagic infarction. Identifying a site of origin is one of the more useful criteria for differentiating features are the presence of multiple occlusions in the peripheral arteries and the arteries supplying the brain, as in the showering of multiple emboli, and an absence of cerebral atherosclerosis.

In contrast to the progressive course expected with a tumor, an abscess, a subdural hematoma, or a massive intracerebral hemorrhage, the patient with an accomplished cerebral infarction caused by a thrombosis or by an embolus commonly reaches a plateau period of stabilization, followed by improvement. Mortality early in the disease is approximately 15%. There is a substantial recurrence rate for cerebral infarction in the first several years, ranging from approximately 20% to 40%.

LABORATORY FINDINGS. Laboratory studies for patients with an accomplished cerebral infarction are aimed at de-

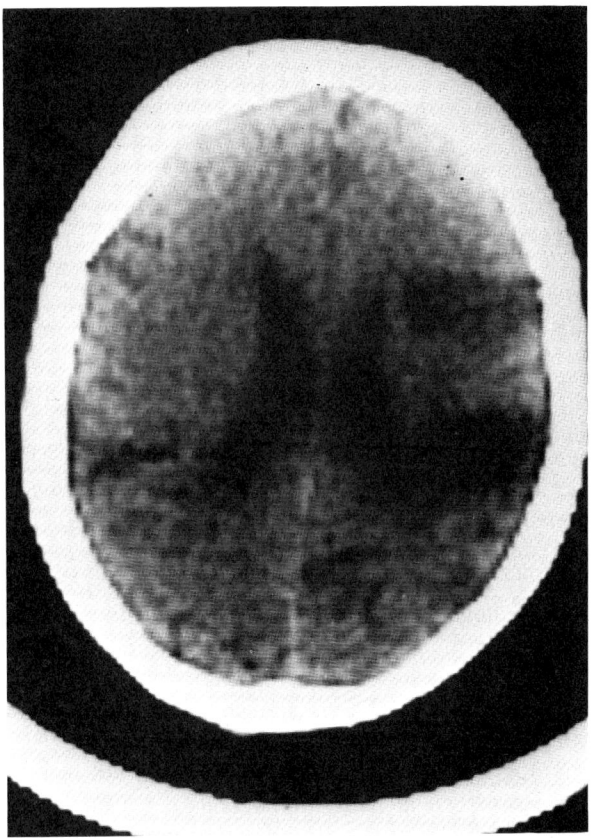

Fig. 152-2. Computed tomogram demonstrating decreased attenuation of infarction (right side of photograph).

tecting the small but significant percentage of nonvascular central nervous system disorders that may masquerade as an infarction (mainly a brain tumor or a subdural hematoma). For the most part this can be accomplished with screening studies such as computed tomographic (CT) scanning with and without injecting contrast material, the isotope brain scan, and serial electroencephalograms (EEGs).

The CT scan of a cerebral infarction (Fig. 152-2) may show an area of decreased density (decreased attenuation) as early as 8 hours after the onset, but it is more often positive approximately 72 hours after the onset. The detection of lesions depends on the timing of the study in relation to the onset of the illness and on the resolution of the equipment used. After approximately 7 days the injection of contrast material may show an enhancement suggesting a tumor. Interpreting such a finding may require coordinating clinical and laboratory data with repeated observations of the clinical course and the performance of serial roentgenographic studies. In an embolic infarction the CT scan may show single or multiple areas of decreased attenuation, earlier contrast enhancement than with a thrombotic infarction, and evidence of a hemorrhage after 3 to 5 days if the lesion evolves from a pale infarction to a red infarction. The isotope brain scan is usually normal for the first 48 to 72 hours. In approximately 75% of cases it may then show a wedge-shaped area of isotope density corresponding to a region of presumed breakdown in the blood-brain barrier. The isotope brain scan may also demonstrate the occasional subdural hematoma that is isodense on the CT scan.

Cerebral infarctions may produce focal slow wave activity on the EEG. Serial testing may be required to differentiate them from mass lesions because it is common for the EEG abnormality to improve with infarctions but not with tumors. Infarctions of the brainstem or cerebellum are unlikely to produce EEG changes. Other diagnostic tests that aid in determining the cause of a CVA include blood and cerebrospinal fluid (CSF) serologic tests for syphilis, blood lipid tests for hyperlipidemia, and antinuclear antibody tests for vasculitis. The possibility of a silent myocardial infarction should be investigated by performing electrocardiography and cardiac enzyme tests early and then later in the course of the disease. In infarction, the CSF obtained by lumbar puncture may reveal a small increase in white blood cells and protein. A total protein level greater than 100 mg/dl suggests a cerebral neoplasm. Hemorrhagic fluid may be found after 24 or 48 hours in instances of a hemorrhagic infarction seen with an embolus.

MANAGEMENT AND PREVENTION. The treatment of a patient with an accomplished infarction caused by a thrombosis is generally supportive. Any associated cardiac disease must be treated to improve and maintain the cerebral blood flow, but no attempt should be made to lower hypertensive blood pressure levels to less than 110 mm Hg diastolic pressure in the first several weeks. Because the baseline range of autoregulation is elevated in hypertensive patients, and because autoregulation is impaired following a CVA, the cerebral blood flow is very vulnerable to the lowering of the systemic blood pressure. An adequate fluid balance should be maintained, but the treatment of cerebral edema with steroids or hyperosmolar agents has not been routinely beneficial. Although the infarction resulting from a cerebral embolus is treated similarly, consideration should be given to using anticoagulants to prevent the production of further emboli if no evidence exists to suggest a hemorrhagic infarction and if no other major medical contraindication such as blood dyscrasia, severe hypertension, severe liver disease, or gastrointestinal bleeding is present. In this situation a continuous intravenous infusion of heparin (5000 units initially followed by approximately 1000 units an hour, extending the partial thromboplastin time to two to two and one half times the control level) may be used after a 24-hour period of observation, with the use of the CT scan and a lumbar puncture to exclude hemorrhage. Warfarin (Coumadin) should be initiated and maintained so that the prothrombin time is approximately one and one half to two times the control level. Heparin may then be discontinued. Surgery may be a possible option for removing the source of the embolic material, as in valvular disease. To treat a patient with thrombosis in evolution, after excluding hemorrhage, the physician should consider the urgent use of heparin to prevent the presumed propagation of a thrombus or an embolization from a thrombus. If heparin cannot be given, an alternative is the use of the antiplatelet agents, aspirin, 300 to 600 mg twice a day, and/or dipyridamole (Persantine), 50 mg three times a day.

Syndromes of the cerebral arteries

The neurologic deficits in cerebral occlusive vascular disease are generally related to the functional anatomy of the disturbed region. An infarction in the distribution of the middle cerebral artery, supplying the motor and sensory regions of the cerebral convexity, may result in hemiparesis and hemisensory disturbance (the arm more involved than the leg) with various forms of aphasia when the dominant cerebral hemisphere speech centers are involved. An occlusion of the middle cerebral artery may be indistinguishable from a thrombosis of the internal carotid artery and commonly results from an embolus from this extracranial vascular source. An occlusive vascular retinopathy may occur with occlusion of the internal carotid artery or with emboli from the internal carotid artery to the retinal arteries. With an infarction of the medial surface of the cerebral hemisphere, supplied by the anterior cerebral artery, the motor weakness and sensory deficit are more apparent in the leg than in the arm, in contrast to the situation with a middle cerebral artery disturbance. The patient may have gait apraxia. The involvement of the paracentral lobule on the medial surface of the hemisphere may produce urinary incontinence.

Decreased blood flow through the posterior cerebral artery, which supplies the occipital lobe, results in homonymous hemianopsia, and the involvement of its thalamic branches can produce hemisensory deficits. These deficits are associated at times with a persistent and disagreeable sensation known as thalamic pain. The syndrome of Dejerine-Roussy consists of a transient motor deficit, a hemisensory impairment, spontaneous pain, and abnormal involuntary movements of a choreoathetoid type, all developing contralateral to the lesion. An infarction of the left calcarine cortex and the splenium of the corpus callosum results in a right homonymous hemianopia, a difficulty in identifying colors, and alexia (difficulty in reading) without agraphia (difficulty in writing). When both posterior cerebral arteries are involved, cortical blindness may result, and if the patient is unaware of this blindness, he is said to have Anton's syndrome. A persistent amnesia may result from a bilateral infarction of the hippocampal gyri with an occlusion of both posterior cerebral arteries.

The involvement of a perforating thalamic branch of

the posterior cerebral artery to the subthalamic nucleus may result in contralateral hemiballismus. The involvement of the branches to the paramedian midbrain (also supplied by small rostral paramedian branches of the basilar artery) may result in Weber's syndrome, in which a third nerve palsy is present on the side of the infarction with contralateral upper motor neuron signs. When the third nerve nucleus is involved, because of its midline configuration, a contralateral superior rectus palsy also appears. Both internal ophthalmoplegia (dilated and fixed pupil) and ptosis, when present because of the involvement of the third nerve nucleus, are bilateral. In Benedikt's syndrome, in addition to the features of Weber's syndrome, the involvement of the regions of the red nucleus and the medial lemniscus results in chorea and hemisensory deficits on the opposite side.

Upward gaze paralysis may occur from unilateral infarctions involving the posterior commissure in the midbrain or from the bilateral involvement of the pretectum, the posterior commissure, or the dorsal midbrain tegmentum. Downward gaze paralysis may result from bilateral involvement dorsal and medial to the red nuclei. Bilateral lesions of the rostral pontine tegmentum and the midpontine tegmentum may also cause a paralysis of either upward or downward gaze in some cases. The involvement of branches of the posterior cerebral artery may produce isolated manifestations of these various syndromes.

Syndromes of the basilar artery and its branches

In the basilar arterial system there may be an occlusion of the small paramedian vessels supplying the medial pontine structures, involvement of the short circumferential branches involving the lateral pons and the long circumferential branches producing involvement of the cranial nuclei and the nerves as in the superior cerebellar artery syndrome and the anterior inferior cerebellar artery syndrome, or involvement of the basilar artery itself, commonly with a loss of consciousness caused by lesions of the reticular formation. These brainstem syndromes are commonly partial or incomplete because of the overlapping distribution of the arterial supply. It is common for a patient to have bilateral brainstem signs when a drop in the blood flow through the basilar arterial system affects branches on both sides of the brainstem.

The descriptive term "locked-in syndrome" has been applied to the situation occurring with a lesion in the caudal basis pontis in which the patient is quadriplegic or quadriparetic, with a retention of consciousness and vertical eye movements. In this de-efferented state the patient is mute and uncommunicative unless communication can be achieved by response with the retained eye movements to appropriate questioning.

A jerky conjugate movement of the eyes in the vertical plane, occurring spontaneously in a patient with a pontine infarction or a hemorrhage, is known as ocular bobbing.

The involvement of the paramedian branches of the basilar artery to the medial and superior pons can produce an internuclear ophthalmoplegia (the syndrome of the medial longitudinal fasciculus with paralysis of adduction on the side of the lesion and nystagmus in the abducting eye), an ipsilateral ataxia, and a contralateral hemiparesis. The involvement of the dentato-rubro-thalamo-olivary pathway in the brainstem may be followed after a period of time by the development of continuous rhythmic movements of the palate, called palatal myoclonus. The patient may also have an associated rhythmic titubation of the head and nystagmus.

When the paramedian branches of the basilar artery to the medial inferior pons are affected, there may be a combination of an involvement of the abducens nucleus, the seventh nerve as it curves around this nucleus, and the corticospinal pathways, producing Millard-Gubler syndrome. Patients with this syndrome have a paralysis of the lateral rectus muscle, a peripheral facial palsy on the side of the infarction, and a contralateral hemiparesis.

Pontine lesions involving the pontine paramedian reticular formation (PPRF) are characterized by a paralysis of conjugate horizontal gaze to the side of the lesion (Foville's syndrome). If the medial longitudinal fasciculus should also be involved on the same side, the so-called 1½ syndrome may result from the additional paralysis of adduction on the side of the lesion. The resulting condition is a paralysis of abduction and adduction in the eye on the side of the lesion, and a paralysis of adduction in the opposite eye. Ipsilateral ataxia and contralateral paresis of the arm and leg may also be noted in the medial pontine syndromes at the midpons and the inferior pons.

In an occlusion of the short circumferential branches of the basilar artery, an infarction occurs in the lateral midpons and is manifested by ipsilateral incoordination or ataxia. The patient may have impaired facial sensation and a paralysis of the muscles of mastication on the side of the lesion. Contralateral hemianesthesia may occur.

Involvement of the long circumferential branches of the basilar artery produces the syndromes of the superior cerebellar artery and the anterior inferior cerebellar artery. The superior cerebellar artery supplies the lateral area of the caudal midbrain and the rostral pons in its course to the cerebellum. An infarction in this distribution produces a syndrome involving ipsilateral involuntary movements and ataxia. A sensory deficit for pain and temperature may involve the entire contralateral body. Horizontal nystagmus may be associated with an ipsilateral paresis of conjugate gaze. The patient may have partial deafness, Horner's syndrome, bulbar myoclonus, and dysarthria. Horner's syndrome consists of miosis, ptosis, and decreased sweating on the ipsilateral face and may be partial. It is caused by an interruption of the sympathetic nervous system pathways in the brainstem.

In the syndrome of the anterior inferior cerebellar ar-

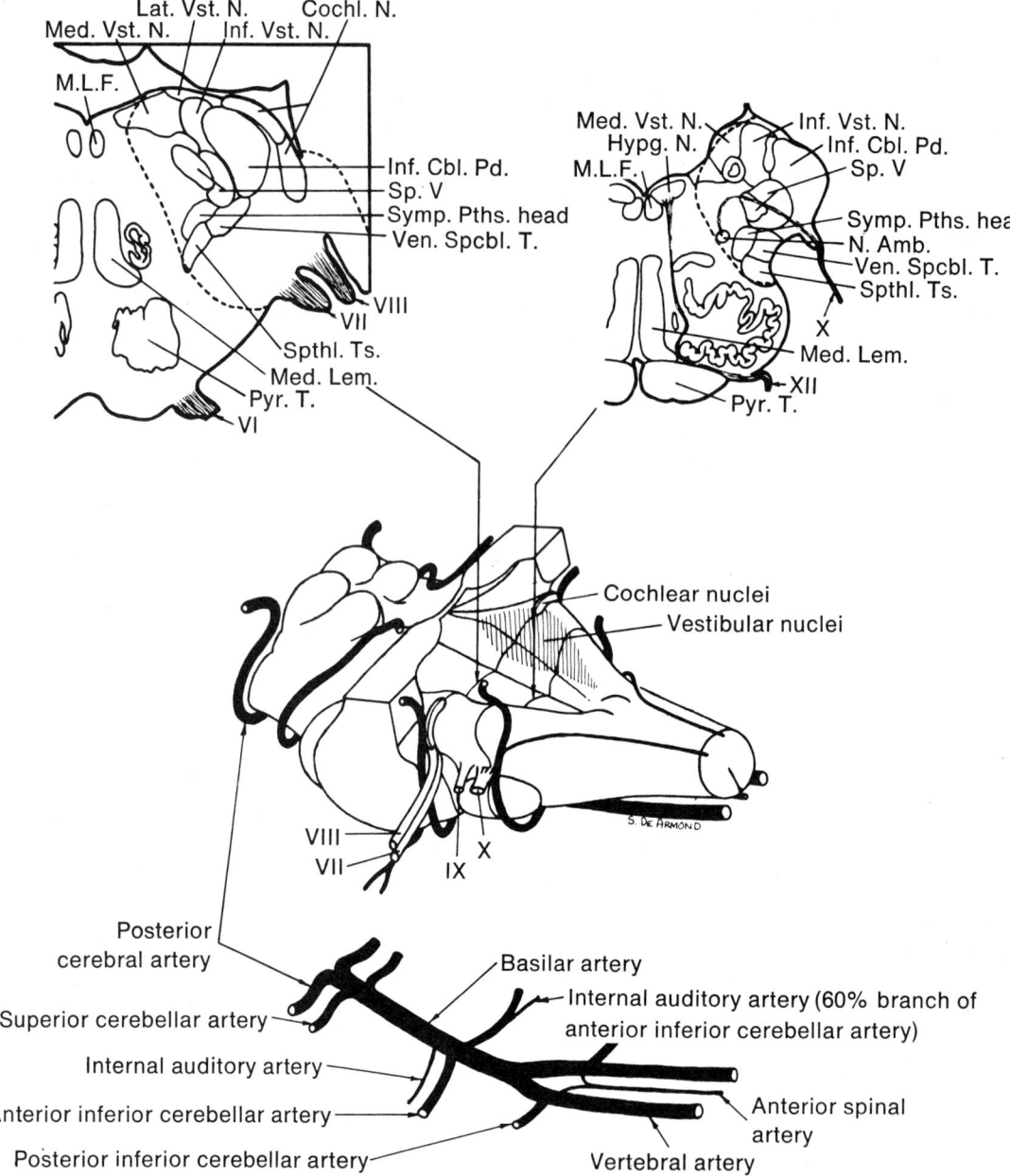

Fig. 152-3. Anatomy of brainstem showing cross sections at level of blood supply by anterior cerebellar artery (upper left) and posterior inferior cerebellar artery (upper right); longitudinal view od extent of cochlear and vestibular nuclei and relation of blood vessels to brainstem (middle); and a view of long circumferential branches of basilar-vertebral artery system (below). Regions of cochlear and vestibular nuclei are crosshatched. Dotted lines in cross sections (at top) outline sites of ischemia in syndrome of anterior inferior cerebellar artery (upper left) and posterior inferior cerebellar artery (upper right). *Cochl. N.*, dorsal and ventral cochlear nuclei; *Hypg. N.*, hypoglossal nucleus; *Inf. Cbl. Pd.*, inferior cerebellar peduncle; *Inf. Vst. N.*, inferior vestibular nucleus; *Lat. Vst. N.*, lateral vestibular nucleus; *M.L.F.*, medial longitudinal fasciculus; *Med. Lem.*, medial lemniscus; *Med. Vst. N.*, medial vestibular nucleus; *N. Amb.*, nucleus ambiguus; *Pyr. T.*, pyramidal tract; *Sp. V*, Spinal tract and nucleus of the fifth cranial nerve; *Spthl. Ts.*, lateral and ventral spinothalamic tracts; *Symp. Pths. head*, pathways controlling sympathetic outflow to head; *Ven. Spcbl. T.*, ventral spinocerebellar tract. (From Burns, R.A.: Otolaryngol. Clin. North Am. 6:287, 1973.)

tery (Fig. 152-3), vertigo occurs, as well as sudden ipsilateral deafness, facial paralysis, Horner's syndrome, ipsilateral cerebellar ataxia, nystagmus, nausea, vomiting, paresis of conjugate lateral gaze, ipsilateral loss of touch sensation on the face, possible contralateral hemisensory impairment of pain and temperature perception, and hemiplegia. With an occlusion of the internal auditory artery, which supplies the structures of the inner ear, ipsilateral sudden deafness also may occur, along with tinnitus and vertigo. A syndrome of an occlusion of the labyrinthine branch of the internal auditory artery may be recognized clinically, producing only vertigo and a diminished ipsilateral labyrinthine response to caloric stimulation.

Syndromes of the vertebral arteries

An occlusion of the vertebral artery can result in the syndrome of the posterior inferior cerebellar artery or can produce the medial medullary syndrome. The syndrome of the posterior inferior cerebellar artery (Fig. 152-3) is also known as Wallenberg's syndrome or the lateral medullary syndrome. The pathologic condition involves the inferior portion of the vestibular nuclei, and vertigo is a significant symptom. Other signs include ipsilateral facial hypoesthesia for pain and temperature, paralysis of the palate, pharynx, and larynx with dysphagia and dysarthria, cerebellar ataxia, Horner's syndrome, and contralateral hypoesthesia for pain and temperature.

In the medial medullary syndrome the hypoglossal nerve is involved in the medulla with weakness and atrophy of the tongue on the same side. The patient has a paresis of the arm and leg on the contralateral side, but the face is spared. Because of the involvement of the medial lemniscus, the patient has a loss of position and vibratory perception on the contralateral side.

An infarction of the cerebellum is often not suspected while the patient is alive. It is caused most often by a vertebral artery occlusion. Its signs may be overshadowed by those brainstem deficits that occur with a decreased blood flow in the long circumferential branches supplying both the brainstem and the cerebellum. An acute onset is associated with vomiting, dizziness or vertigo, gait ataxia, dysmetria, dysarthria, and nystagmus. Progressive neurologic deterioration may occur after a latent interval of 24 to 96 hours. A cerebellar hemorrhage or an expanding mass lesion in the posterior fossa must be considered in the differential diagnosis; a CT scan can help in this differentiation. If accompanied by significant edema, infarctions of the cerebellum may become life threatening through compression of the brainstem. If signs of progressive brainstem dysfunction develop, there should be an immediate decompression of the infarcted cerebellar hemisphere or shunting of the CSF.

Lacunar syndromes

The lacunar syndromes occur mostly in hypertensive patients and are the result of small infarctions (0.5 to 15 mm) called lacunes (état lacunaire). Lacunes characteristically occur in the corona radiata, basal ganglia, internal capsule, or pons and result in several discrete syndromes. In the pure motor stroke the lacune may be located in the internal capsule or the pons. Sensory, speech, or visual deficits are not noted. In the pure sensory syndrome the thalamus is implicated, and the deficit, as the descriptive name implies, is confined to the sensory system. In the syndrome of homolateral ataxia with crural paresis the lesion is thought to involve corticopontine pathways in the corona radiata. Contralateral ataxia and weakness are found (both on the same side of the body), with the leg more involved than the arm. The dysarthria–clumsy hand syndrome suggests a pontine lacune and is manifested mainly by a marked dysarthria and difficulty with fine movements of the hand contralateral to the lesion. Contralateral central facial weakness and finger-to-nose wavering are also present, along with a deviation of the protruded tongue away from the side of the lesion and some dysphagia. In the lacunar syndromes each episode tends to have a good prognosis, but multiple episodes may develop in time, resulting in a pseudobulbar palsy. In a pseudobulbar palsy the involvement of the bilateral corticobulbar fibers results in dysarthria and dysphagia. The patient may also lose control over emotional outbursts such as laughing and crying (emotional incontinence), and may have a gait with small steps (marche à petits pas). Multiple lacunes or multiple infarcts may result in dementia (multi-infarct dementia).

Because the lacunar syndromes are commonly caused by the hyalinization of intracerebral arterioles, evaluating for large vessel disease with arteriography is not usually necessary.

INFARCTION OF THE SPINAL CORD

The blood supply to the spinal cord consists of one anterior spinal artery, which supplies the anterior two thirds of the cord, and two posterior spinal arteries, which supply the dorsal root entry zones and the posterior columns. These vessels originate superiorly from the branches of the vertebral arteries, but they receive major contributions in their course along the length of the spinal cord from the radicular arteries, which derive from branches of the vertebral arteries and subclavian arteries, the aorta (intercostal and lumbar branches), and the iliac arteries. A major contributing branch is the great anterior medullary artery of Adamkiewicz, which is a branch of the aorta supplying the spinal cord at approximately its first or second lumbar levels.

The spinal cord is particularly vulnerable to an infarction at the watershed area in the midthoracic cord, where ascending and descending branches meet and where a decrease in the blood flow in one of the major contributing branches would be most likely to produce symptoms.

The syndrome of the anterior spinal artery is most commonly the result of a proximal vascular occlusion such as occurs with a dissecting aneurysm of the aorta, or an occlusion of the artery of Adamkiewicz (iatrogenic at surgery or with catheterization in aortography). Atherosclerosis of the anterior spinal artery is uncommon. In the spontaneous disorders, back pain is common initially. The sudden onset of quadriplegia (with cervical cord lesions) or paraplegia (with the more common thoracic or lumbar lesions) may be associated in the early stages with spinal shock (flaccidity and decreased reflexes). Ultimately, spasticity and increased deep tendon reflexes (corticospinal tract signs or pyramidal tract signs) prevail. Sensory signs reflect the bilateral involvement of the spinothalamic tracts with a decrease in pain and temperature sensations. Position sense, vibration sense, and variable degrees of touch sense remain intact because of the preservation of the posterior columns. The patient becomes incontinent. The prognosis for the recovery of function is poor, and myelography may be necessary to determine that there is no spinal cord compression.

The syndrome of the posterior spinal artery is uncommon. Because the findings reflect the relatively small area of the spinal cord involved (the posterior horns and the posterior columns), deficits are not striking. Ipsilateral proprioceptive deficits may be present, and some physicians have noted hemiparesis.

TRANSIENT ISCHEMIC ATTACKS

DEFINITION. Transient ischemic attacks (TIAs) are syndromes in which focal neurologic deficits develop abruptly and last for either a period of minutes or up to an arbitrary maximal duration of 24 hours. They are a common forerunner of a CVA. The transient symptoms or signs reflect focal areas where the decreased cerebral blood flow temporarily has been unable to satisfy the metabolic requirements but where an accomplished infarction has not occurred. Although most TIAs last only minutes and are completely reversible, there can be borderline situations with a more prolonged or persistent residual deficit of a minimal degree such as a reversible ischemic neurologic deficit (RIND) or transient ischemic attacks with incomplete recovery (TIA-IR). The focal ischemic symptoms generally occur in either the distribution of the carotid arterial system or the basilar-vertebral arterial system. Symptoms of involvement in the carotid arterial system include ipsilateral monocular blindness (amaurosis fugax), contralateral motor deficits or sensory deficits, aphasia when the dominant hemisphere is involved, and headache. These symptoms reflect an ischemia in the distribution of the branches of the internal carotid artery: the ophthalmic artery, the anterior cerebral artery, and the middle cerebral artery. Patients may describe amaurosis fugax, or fleeting blindness, either as a curtain ascending or descending in front of one eye or as merely monocular blurring. Funduscopic examination in some patients will show cholesterol emboli, platelet-fibrin emboli, or calcific retinal emboli such as Hollenhorst plaques (refractile cholesterol deposits) seen at the retinal arterial bifurcations. Unilateral visual blurring in combination with contralateral motor signs or sensory signs is highly suggestive of carotid artery disease. Symptoms of disease in the basilar-vertebral arterial system reflect its supply to the brainstem, the inferior temporal lobe, the occipital lobe, and the cerebellum. Because of the compact nature of the structures in the brainstem, isolated symptoms are unusual. Symptoms of TIAs in the basilar-vertebral arterial system include vertigo, visual disturbances, dysarthria, facial paresthesias, headache, disorders of equilibrium, vomiting, dysphagia, alternating weakness of the opposite sides of the body, loss of consciousness, drop attacks, and transient global amnesia. A drop attack is a sudden fall without a loss of consciousness. Transient global amnesia describes a brief episode of difficulty with short-term memory that may result from a bilateral hippocampal ischemia in the distribution of the posterior cerebral arteries. Vertigo is the most common symptom of an insufficiency of the basilar-vertebral arterial system, although vascular disease accounts infrequently for the complaint of dizziness, and isolated vertigo without other brain-stem symptoms is more often labyrinthine in origin. The physician should also consider other diagnoses, such as myasthenia gravis and drug toxicity, in the presence of isolated and recurrent dysarthria or diplopia.

ETIOLOGY AND PATHOGENESIS. Approximately 70% of patients with TIAs have atherosclerotic lesions of the extracranial cerebral vessels, with the region of the carotid sinus being a major site. These vessels can be stenotic, occluded, or patent but containing an ulcerating atheroma. Stenotic lesions must narrow the vessel lumen by 90% to decrease the flow significantly. Platelet-fibrin aggregates or cholesterol emboli from these atheromatous lesions are probably a major factor in producing attacks. Microembolic material may produce only a temporary occlusion, with symptoms resolving as the microemboli disintegrate or disappear or as the collateral channels open. Emboli derived from the heart are more likely to result in an infarction. Decreased cardiac output resulting in a decreased cerebral perfusion pressure does not result in focal neurologic symptoms (TIAs) unless this hemodynamic change is superimposed on significantly narrowed cerebral vessels. For example, syncope caused by a decreased cardiac output is not a TIA. In the basilar-vertebral arterial system emboli are less easily demonstrated and hemodynamic causes may be more significant. Mechanical compression by skeletal or muscular structures may be responsible for the blood flow changes in some cases. Occasionally, no apparent basis for TIAs can be found.

CLINICAL MANIFESTATIONS. In the face of a negative neurologic examination or one with minimal residual signs, the general physical examination, particularly the cardiac evaluation, becomes particularly important. Cardiac murmurs and arrhythmias should be sought. The blood pressure should be measured for evidence of hypertension, orthostasis, or a difference in systolic pressure of 20 mm Hg or more in the two arms. The difference in systolic pressure, although uncommon, suggests an occlusion of a proximal subclavian artery resulting in a reversal of the blood flow down the vertebral artery and producing brainstem symptoms (subclavian steal syndrome). The neurovascular examination includes palpating the carotid, superficial temporal, and radial artery pulses. Auscultation for bruits is performed with the bell of the stethoscope over the carotid bifurcations, the supraclavicular areas, and the orbits. A bruit caused by stenosis at the carotid bifurcation, heard best at the angle of the mandible, is generally not prominent over the more proximal common carotid artery, where murmurs that are transmitted from the heart may be heard.

LABORATORY FINDINGS. Laboratory studies include those described for an accomplished infarction, but other tests are aimed at guiding a course for CVA prevention. Studies to determine a cardiac source of embolism include performing a 24-hour Holter monitor and echocardiography. Noninvasive screening tests for extracranial cerebrovascular disease such as Doppler scanning of the carotid arteries, supraorbital directional Doppler scanning, ophthalmodynamometry, and oculoplethysmography can provide gross information about the presence of a carotid artery stenosis or occlusion (see Chapter 100). These techniques do not identify the patient with an ulcerated plaque or a small plaque, do not reveal intracranial disease, and are not useful in evaluating the basilar-vertebral arterial circulation. They are a safe means of confirming a suspicion of extracranial carotid vascular disease, but they do not establish the pathogenesis because atherosclerosis is common. On occasion, when the noninvasive diagnostic screening tests are not sufficiently helpful to satisfy clinical suspicion or when they point to the need for further study, cerebral angiography may be warranted. Because this procedure carries a mortality of approximately 0.1% and can result in a 0.6% incidence of permanent severe focal neurologic deficit, it should not be undertaken lightly and is not needed to confirm the diagnosis of TIA.

Cerebral angiography is the only definitive method of localizing a vascular lesion, although it does not prove the vascular nature of the symptoms. Aortic arch studies do not show the intracranial vessels satisfactorily, and selective filling of nondiseased carotid arteries may be indicated for a more complete evaluation. These procedures should be performed only when the diagnosis is in doubt and the determination would significantly alter patient management or when prophylactic surgery for a remediable lesion is contemplated. Digital intravenous angiography will make the visualization of these vessels safer and more practicable as this technique is improved in the future.

COURSE. Because somewhere between 25% and 40% of patients who have TIAs will have a CVA within 3 to 5 years, the goal in identifying them is prophylactic and is intended to prevent the development of an accomplished infarction. These patients most often die of cardiac disease.

MANAGEMENT. No unanimity exists about the best treatment. The methods of treatment can be directed toward correcting the hemodynamic and cardiac irregularities, regulating the blood clotting mechanisms, or repairing the arterial vessel wall. There is statistical support for the effect of aspirin in decreasing platelet aggregability. Doses of between 300 and 600 mg twice a day are recommended. Other antiplatelet agents that are used but lack the same statistical validation clinically include sulfinpyrazone (Anturane), 100 to 200 mg twice a day, and dipyridamole (Persantine), 50 mg three times a day. Frequent recent TIAs warrant a brief course of intravenous heparin if there are no contraindications such as a diastolic blood pressure of 110 mm Hg or greater, blood in the CSF or apparent on the CT scan, blood dyscrasia, gastrointestinal bleeding, or severe liver disease.

The acute period is not the time for vigorous antihypertensive management, which may decrease the cerebral blood flow. The diastolic blood pressure, however, should be gradually lowered to 110 mm Hg. For patients who are good surgical candidates and who are willing to have surgery, a carotid endarterectomy should be considered for eroded plaques or for stenoses of 50% or more. The best surgical response with occlusive disease is in unilateral carotid stenosis. Investigation with cerebral angiography, including the aortic arch, is necessary. When performed by an experienced surgeon, carotid surgery has a mortality of 1% and a morbidity for transient or permanent neurologic deficits of approximately 1% to 2%. Vertebral stenoses are rarely treated surgically. The proximal subclavian artery is surgically accessible for treating the subclavian steal syndrome. Some physicians perform surgery on major carotid artery stenoses to increase the blood flow to an insufficient basilar-vertebral circulation if the posterior communicating artery is adequate, but the benefits have not been consistently demonstrated.

For patients in whom standard extracranial surgical techniques are ruled out by completely occluded lesions or by inaccessible lesions, microsurgical cerebral revascularization to bypass the occluded vessel may be considered. These procedures, such as the superficial temporal artery to middle cerebral artery (STA-MCA) bypass, involve an anastomosis of the small extracranial arteries to the cortical arteries. An alternative course of treatment is a 3- to 6-month maintenance course of warfarin (Coumadin) if no contraindications are present. Warfarin has been shown to decrease TIAs, at least in the first several months of use, although no consensus exists regarding its role in preventing thrombosis and an accomplished infarction. The prothrombin time should be maintained between one and one half and two times the control levels, and there should be no contraindications such as blood dyscrasia, evidence of blood on a CT scan or in the CSF, severe hypertension, liver disease, or patient noncompliance.

CEREBRAL HEMORRHAGE

PATHOGENESIS. Intracerebral hemorrhage or parenchymal hemorrhage occurs with increased frequency in hypertensive patients. The bleeding into the substance of the brain is caused by a rupture of microaneurysms of the arteriolar vessels (Charcot-Bouchard aneurysms), the result of hypertensive vascular disease. The most common site for these hemorrhages, accounting for about 60% of cases, is in the area of the putamen. Other common locations, with an incidence of about 10% each, are the thalamus, the tegmentum of the pons, the cerebellum, and the cerebral white matter.

When an intracerebral hemorrhage occurs in the absence of hypertension, it is appropriate to consider other sources of bleeding: a cerebral aneurysm, an arteriovenous malformation (AVM), a hemorrhage into a tumor, arteritis, an obscure angiopathy, a blood dyscrasia, anticoagulation, or the rupture of a mycotic aneurysm in bacterial endocarditis.

Bleeding may occur into the substance of certain brain tumors, either as the patient's initial problem or during the course of the tumor. Tumors with a predilection for hemorrhage include glioblastoma multiforme, hemangioblastoma, pituitary tumors (pituitary apoplexy), renal cell carcinoma, melanocarcinoma, and choriocarcinoma. The physician may suspect a tumor as an underlying cause of an intracerebral hemorrhage from a history of progressive symptoms preceding the hemorrhagic event, from findings on a CT scan, or if the hemorrhagic CSF reveals an elevation in total protein concentration exceeding the 1 mg/dl for each 1000/mm^3 red blood cells normally occurring from blood alone.

Arteritides that may result in a hemorrhage include tuberculous arteritis and lupus erythematosus. An infrequently described amyloid angiopathy occurs in the cortex of nonhypertensive older patients and may result in a lobar hemorrhage.

CLINICAL MANIFESTATIONS. The clinical manifestations of an intracerebral hemorrhage are characterized by an abrupt onset, often said to develop during a period of activity rather than during rest. Headache is common at the onset. Seizures are infrequent, occurring in about 10% of patients. With a massive intracerebral hemorrhage, a loss of consciousness in the ictal period is common and the course is rapidly downhill, the intracerebral hematoma acting as a mass lesion and causing cerebral herniation. The neurologic deficit at onset depends on the location and amount of bleeding. Smaller hemorrhages in the cerebral hemisphere may mimic a cerebral infarction. Bleeding into the basal ganglia is associated with varying degrees of hemiparesis, hemisensory deficit, and homonymous hemianopsia. Conjugate deviation of the eyes toward the side of the lesion can be overcome by ice-water labyrinthine stimulation. If the hemorrhage is massive, bilateral pyramidal tract signs develop early, with respiratory irregularities and pupillary changes reflecting brainstem compression from herniation. Thalamic hemorrhages are commonly associated with medial and downward deviation of the eyes. Pontine hemorrhages are associated with a rapid loss of consciousness, flaccid quadriplegia, miotic but still reactive pupils, ocular bobbing, abnormalities of conjugate lateral gaze that persist during a doll's head eye maneuver and ice-water caloric testing, and at times hyperpyrexia. The patient with a cerebellar hemorrhage may have an occipital headache, gait ataxia, a paralysis of lateral gaze, seventh nerve palsy, and lateralized incoordination on the side of the hemorrhage. The patient's condition often progresses rapidly to coma and death as pressure causes further brainstem compromise.

The prognosis for a patient with a massive intracerebral hemorrhage is exceedingly grave. The mortality is 90%. Since the advent of CT scanning, smaller intracerebral and brainstem hemorrhages can be differentiated from infarctions, and the overall prognosis for patients with a cerebral hemorrhage is more optimistic than previously realized.

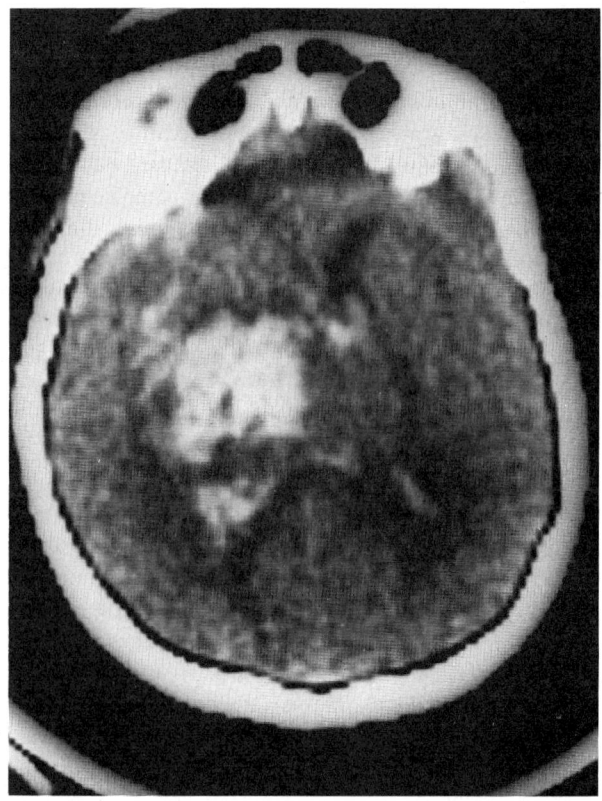

Fig. 152-4. Computed tomogram demonstrating increased attenuation of hemorrhage (left side of photograph).

LABORATORY FINDINGS. The most important laboratory study is the CT scan, which clearly shows the increased attenuation of intracerebral blood (Fig. 152-4). A lumbar puncture is unnecessary to document the bleeding, may introduce a danger of cerebral herniation, and in deep noncommunicating bleeding may be negative in 15% of the cases.

MANAGEMENT. The treatment is mainly supportive. Dehydrating agents such as mannitol (0.25 to 1.5 g/kg body weight in a 20% solution given rapidly intravenously) may be tried for the prevention of herniation. Corticosteroids are commonly used (10 mg dexamethasone intravenously followed by 4 mg every 6 hours, tapering the dosage after 7 days) but are of questionable value for this disorder unless vasogenic edema is present. Surgical evacuation of large intracerebral hematomas has not proved generally beneficial with the exception of a hemorrhage in the cerebellum. The cerebellar hematoma is more readily accessible, and early surgical intervention, either the evacuation of the hematoma or the placement of an intraventricular shunt, is essential. The intraventricular shunt also has been of use when a cerebellar infarction has been associated with local edema and increased intracranial pressure.

SUBARACHNOID HEMORRHAGE AND OTHER MANIFESTATIONS OF VASCULAR ANOMALIES

The most common cause of a subarachnoid hemorrhage is probably trauma. A spontaneous subarachnoid hemorrhage, however, which accounts for 5% of cerebrovascular accidents, is caused by a rupture of a berry aneurysm or an arteriovenous malformation directly into the subarachnoid space.

Aneurysms

BERRY ANEURYSMS. Berry aneurysms are believed to arise from areas of congenital weakness in the vessel wall at bifurcations of the major branches of the circle of Willis in the subarachnoid space. They usually do not appear in childhood, and only rarely do they produce neurologic signs by a local nonhemorrhagic compression of the adjacent structures (paralytic aneurysms). The occurrence of a spontaneous subarachnoid hemorrhage from a ruptured berry aneurysm correlates best with aneurysmal size, being most likely with aneurysms 1 cm or greater in diameter.

The majority of berry aneurysms are found on the anterior circle of Willis. They occur, for example, at the first major bifurcation of the middle cerebral artery, at the origin of the anterior cerebral artery, adjacent to the anterior communicating artery, and at the junction of the posterior communicating artery and the internal carotid artery. These posterior communicating aneurysms are commonly associated with signs of a third nerve palsy, including pupillary dilatation, ptosis, and extraocular palsies, because the third nerve is in close anatomic proximity.

FUSIFORM ANEURYSMS. Fusiform aneurysms appear to be dilatations of the entire circumference of a vessel for several centimeters, returning at each end to the vessel's normal caliber. These rarely rupture, although they may compress nearby structures. Most often patients with them are asymptomatic. Although they are commonly attributed to atherosclerosis and are more common in hypertensive patients, their presence in some younger patients has suggested a congenital abnormality.

CLINICAL MANIFESTATIONS. The initial clinical manifestation of a subarachnoid hemorrhage from a ruptured aneurysm is of sudden onset with a severe and commonly generalized headache that the patient may describe as feeling "like the top of my head is coming off." The initial bleeding is associated with sudden collapse and death in many instances. However, a patient coming to an emergency room with a severe headache from a subarachnoid hemorrhage may have no focal neurologic deficits during the clinical examination. Focal signs are present if the arterial bleeding also produces an intracerebral hemorrhage. Blood in the subarachnoid space also may be associated with cerebral vasospasm, which may produce ischemia with focal signs. The pressure of arterial bleeding directly into the subarachnoid space may produce preretinal subhyaloid hemorrhages (that appear as large, boat-shaped hemorrhages). Subhyaloid hemorrhages seen on the funduscopic examination suggest the diagnosis. Nuchal rigidity and Kernig's sign (restriction of straight leg raising as a result of meningeal irritation) are common.

LABORATORY FINDINGS. A diagnosis of a spontaneous subarachnoid hemorrhage can be suspected clinically and confirmed with either a CT scan, which may show subarachnoid blood in the first several days, or a lumbar puncture, which shows bloody CSF with a xanthochromic supernatant fluid in essentially all instances. A reliable method of distinguishing a subarachnoid hemorrhage from blood introduced into the CSF by a traumatic lumbar puncture is to compare an accurate count of red blood cells in the first and last tubes of fluid collected. The number should not decrease in the pathologic situations. The opening pressure is also likely to be elevated in a subarachnoid hemorrhage. Calcification in the wall of an aneurysm may allow it to be seen on plain skull roentgenograms or CT scans even before a subarachnoid hemorrhage. Cerebral angiography is required to demonstrate the loction of a cerebral aneurysm. Because berry aneurysms may be multiple, a complete angiographic study of the intracranial circulation usually is required before surgical intervention. At that time one should obtain appropriate roentgenograms of the kidney to look for commonly associated polycystic kidneys. Coarctation of the aorta may also be associated.

PROGNOSIS AND MANAGEMENT. A significant percentage of initial subarachnoid hemorrhages result in sudden death. Of those patients who survive, approximately 30% will rehemorrhage within a 2-week period and again have a significant mortality. The preferred treatment for a patient who is a good surgical candidate is one of a variety of techniques that attempt to clip the aneurysm or to decrease the blood flow through it. Experience has shown that, despite the urgency, these procedures are best deferred for a period of stabilization, usually from 10 days to 2 weeks, because cerebral vasospasm is common during this early period.

A medication that is commonly used during the stabilization period, but still a subject of some controversy, is ϵ-aminocaproic acid (Amicar), an antifibrinolytic agent that may decrease the incidence of rehemorrhaging. This is administered by continuous intravenous drip at 24 to 36 g each 24 hours for several days following the hemorrhage. It has been associated, however, with some reports of cerebral thrombosis, multiple pulmonary emboli, and other complications of hypercoagulability.

Another complication of a subarachnoid hemorrhage is the development of a communicating hydrocephalus with ventricular enlargement, because the subarachnoid blood may obstruct the absorption of CSF. Normal pressure hydrocephalus may result, and shunt procedures may be required.

Arteriovenous malformations

Arteriovenous malformations (AVMs) are abnormal direct communications between the arterial and venous systems, occurring both within and on the surface of any portion of the central nervous system. These are congenital abnormalities in which venous channels contain blood under arterial pressure, so that a rupture is a common problem. They account, however, for only 0.1% of cases of subarachnoid hemorrhage. The hemorrhage may occur at any time in life and may be associated with signs of a subarachnoid hemorrhage or with all the clinical manifestations of an intracerebral hemorrhage. Since a seizure disorder may be the initial symptom and may begin at any age, AVMs should be considered in the diagnostic evaluation of seizure problems. The patient may have a history of headaches. The abnormal shunting of blood has been said to steal blood from other cerebral regions, producing ischemic symptoms on rare occasions.

AVMs may be associated with a cranial bruit, audible with the bell of the stethoscope applied to the skull. Calcification may be noted on skull roentgenograms or a CT scan. The dynamic isotope brain scan and the CT scan with injection of contrast material may indicate the presence of an abnormal blood flow or a pooling of blood. Angiography is, however, often required for delineation. Small, ruptured AVMs may be so disrupted by a hemorrhage that they may not be detected even by an angiogram. At times delayed or repeat studies, when the hemorrhage has resolved, will show a malformation not previously seen.

Treatment of AVMs is primarily surgical when they are accessible and is aimed at preventing a further hemorrhage after the initial episode of bleeding. Interventional roentgenographic techniques, with embolization or acrylic injections of the malformation, may be tried for nonresectable lesions.

Arteriovenous fistulas

Arteriovenous fistulas, which can occur between the internal carotid artery and the cavernous sinus (through which the artery passes), are most often caused by cranial trauma and basilar skull fracture, although they can occur spontaneously or develop from rupture of aneurysms. Blood enters the venous system under high pressure, resulting in proptosis, chemosis, blindness, extraocular muscle palsies, and a local cranial bruit.

SPINAL CORD HEMORRHAGE

A spinal cord hemorrhage may be subarachnoid or intramedullary. A primary spinal cord subarachnoid hemorrhage is an infrequent occurrence and is caused most often by a ruptured spinal AVM. Back pain is common and headache, mimicking that of a ruptured intracranial berry aneurysm, may occur as blood circulates in the subarachnoid space. Intramedullary hemorrhage (hematomyelia) may also occur as a result of an AVM, trauma, or blood dyscrasia, with the patient having severe back pain and sudden paraplegia.

The diagnosis of spinal AVM is difficult to make, and these lesions are often mistaken for herniated discs or spinal tumors. There is nothing absolutely characteristic about their natural history, which is often that of progressive spinal cord disease, thought possibly to be caused by compression. Less often there is a sudden onset caused by a subarachnoid or intramedullary hemorrhage. Progression followed by regression and repeated subsequent events is common. Pain, weakness (with combined upper and lower motor neuron signs), sensory deficits, and early micturition difficulties are frequent. Males are affected more often than females. Symptoms may occasionally vary with posture, exercise, and the menstrual cycle.

The majority of lesions occur in the midthoracic and lower thoracic and thoracolumbar cord, and their length can be extensive. Occasionally cutaneous angiomas are present on the back, making it possible to localize the spinal AVM to the same segment. Less often an audible bruit may be heard over the spine, defining an otherwise undiagnosed myelopathy. The CSF is commonly but nonspecifically abnormal. Laboratory investigation requires performing roentgenographic contrast studies such as myelography (with a visualization of the posterior surface of the cord) or arteriography for a definitive diagnosis. The surgical excision of some localized AVMs is possible.

VENOUS THROMBOSIS

A thrombosis may occur in the cortical veins or in any of the dural venous channels draining blood into the internal jugular veins, such as the superior sagittal, transverse, or cavernous sinuses. Infection is a common predisposing cause, as with underlying chronic otitis media, mastoiditis, or cellulitis of the face or neck, and it has been associated with dehydration, cachexia, congestive heart failure, shock, and sepsis. Other associations include the postpartum or postoperative period, debilitation, thrombocytopenia, cryofibrinogenemia, disseminated intravascular coagulation, hemolytic anemia, paroxysmal nocturnal hemoglobinuria, leukemia, diabetic ketoacidosis, ulcerative colitis, polycythemia, or sickle cell disease. The use of oral contraceptives may be a predisposing factor. A tumor may also invade the venous sinuses.

The patient's initial symptoms vary with the site of the thrombosis, but headache, increased intracranial pressure, and seizures are not uncommon. Papilledema may be present. With a thrombosis of the sagittal sinus the patient has intracranial hypertension resulting from an obstruction of CSF reabsorption and may have jacksonian seizures. Motor weakness may be greater in the legs than in the arms, and either a lower extremity monoparesis or a paraparesis may develop. With a thrombosis of the cavernous sinus and an obstruction of the ophthalmic veins the patient has proptosis, chemosis, and frequent involvement of the third, fourth, and sixth cranial nerves (resulting in ophthalmoplegia) and the sympathetic nerves that also traverse this sinus. Focal features including seizures are characteristic of a primary cortical vein thrombosis.

Pathologically, there may be various combinations of infarction, hemorrhage, and associated cerebral edema. Diagnostic studies include performing a prolonged serial cerebral angiogram, particularly studying the late venous phase. A CT scan without the injection of contrast material may show a dense sinus early and with the injection of contrast material may demonstrate the so-called delta sign, in which a triangular filling defect is visible in the sagittal sinus. The treatment of a venous thrombosis is directed at any known infection, and anticoagulation is often considered when a hemorrhage is not demonstrated by a CT scan or lumbar puncture. Fever and peripheral leukocytosis are indications for a lumbar puncture to exclude meningitis if the CT scan does not show an intracranial mass effect.

HYPERTENSIVE ENCEPHALOPATHY

(See Chapter 87.)

Infrequently, the systemic blood pressure may rise to an extent that overcomes the ability of the cerebral arterioles to maintain the cerebral blood flow within a normal range. With this breakdown in autoregulation, cerebral edema develops and multiple small infarctions and petechial hemorrhages occur. This situation is seen in patients with severe malignant hypertension, acute glomerulonephritis, and eclampsia.

Clinically, the patient with hypertensive encephalopathy has severe hypertension, headache, vomiting, confusion, obtundation, and commonly seizures. The course is subacute and can be reversed dramatically by appropriate antihypertensive therapy. Hypertensive retinopathy is usually present, and papilledema is common. The CSF pressure is elevated, and the protein levels may be high. Focal signs may be found, in which case care must be taken to determine if a cerebral infarction has occurred. This differentiation is particularly important because a marked lowering of the blood pressure is contraindicated in an infarction with its associated disturbance of autoregulation.

UNCOMMON VASCULAR DISEASES OF THE CENTRAL NERVOUS SYSTEM

Arteritis caused by collagen-vascular disease can result in infarction and less frequently in hemorrhage. The collagen disorder most commonly implicated is lupus erythematosus, in which the central nervous system signs may be the patient's initial problem. Polyarteritis nodosa also, but less frequently, involves the cerebral vessels. Determination of the erythrocyte sedimentation rate (ESR) is a valuable screening test for collagen disorders. Cerebral angiography may show evidence of arteritic changes in the cerebral vessels.

In the older patient, temporal arteritis, a giant cell arteritis affecting the cranial vessels and associated with polymyalgia rheumatica, may result in headache, occlusion of retinal arteries, and occasionally cerebral infarction. The ESR is significantly elevated in temporal arteritis. Cerebral angiography may show evidence of arteritic changes in the superficial temporal artery and scattered areas of involvement in other branches of the external carotid artery. The intracranial cerebral arteries are rarely involved by the pathologic process, although the vertebral arteries and the cavernous portion of the internal carotid arteries may be affected. If temporal arteritis is suspected, a biopsy of a lengthy portion of the superficial temporal artery may establish the diagnosis, and corticosteroid therapy is urgently warranted, particularly to prevent blindness.

A giant cell arteritis described originally in young Oriental women is known as Takayasu's disease or pulseless disease. This disorder affects major branches of the aortic arch with, for example, carotid and subclavian artery stenosis, and may produce cerebral infarction. The sedimentation rate is increased in this disorder. Patients may have cataracts and retinal atrophy.

Granulomatous arteritis involves the small and medium-sized cerebral vessels, may have an autoimmune basis, and at least in some instances may be related to infection with herpes zoster ophthalmicus. The CSF in granulomatous arteritis shows a moderate mononuclear pleocytosis and an elevation of the total protein concentration, frequently exceeding 100 mg/dl. Women are affected somewhat more commonly than men, and the disorder may occur at any age with the majority of patients being affected in the fifth to eighth decades of life. A leptomeningeal biopsy should be considered before therapy, with prednisone if the diagnosis is obscure.

Inflammatory changes in the cerebral blood vessel walls may occur with a variety of meningeal infections. In meningovascular lues, a secondary form of syphilis, the cerebral blood vessels in the subarachnoid space are affected by meningitis. This is reflected by the meningeal response noted in the CSF, with pleocytosis and an elevated total protein concentration.

Mucormycosis is an opportunistic fungal disease. The fungus gains access to the central nervous system through the nose and sinuses in debilitated diabetic patients and those with blood dyscrasias, causing cerebral thromboses. Pyogenic and tuberculous arteritides occur infrequently, and other rare causes of infarction are typhus, schistosomiasis, falciparum malaria, and trichinosis.

The term "vasospasm" should be avoided except in very specific situations. Vasospasm does occur in the presence of a subarachnoid hemorrhage. It is *not* a cause of transient cerebral ischemia, with the exception of the vasoconstrictive phase of migraine headaches. During this vasoconstrictive phase the patient may have a variety of focal signs, including visual field defects and unilateral motor and sensory deficits, the so-called hemiplegic migraine. On a rare occasion such deficits may not reverse and may result in an infarction. Platelet hyperaggregability may contribute to a thrombosis in patients with migraine headaches.

Fibromuscular dysplasia is an infrequent nonatheromatous vascular disorder involving an intimal and medial fibroplasia of the extracranial internal carotid and vertebral arteries, as well as other large systemic vessels such as the renal arteries. Cerebral angiography shows a beaded appearance of the vessel caused by segmental sections of narrowing alternating with areas of dilatation. The intracranial arteries are usually not involved. This disorder is far more common in women than in men, and its cause is poorly understood. It is most often discovered as an incidental angiographic abnormality, and occasional symptoms of progressive cerebral ischemia may warrant the use of anticoagulants, vascular bypass surgery, endarterectomy, or intra-arterial dilatation.

Mitral valve prolapse (see Chapter 94) caused by a myxomatous degeneration is a common cardiac disorder that may account at times for the development of cerebral platelet-fibrin emboli.

Atrial myxomas are tumors of endothelial or subendothelial origin with myxoid degenerative changes. These tumors arise most often from the left side of the heart's atrial septum, but they also may be present on the right side or in the ventricles. They most commonly occur in the middle years of life, with cardiac, systemic, and embolic effects. The patient may have a recent history of the rapid development of heart failure, weight loss, fatigue, and fever. An embolus from an atrial myxoma should be suspected in any patient with a cerebral embolus who has a normal sinus rhythm and no evidence of bacterial endocarditis. On auscultation of the heart the findings of rheumatic mitral valve disease may be suggested, or a characteristic tumor plop may be detected. There may be a variability in the auscultatory findings with position change on different examinations. The histology of the embolus can be useful in making the diagnosis.

The more definitive diagnostic tests include two-dimensional ultrasonic cardiac imaging and angiocardiography. A long-term neurologic follow-up is warranted after myxoma removal because there may be a delayed invasion of a previously embolized vessel wall leading to aneurysm formation or metastatic tumor growth.

Homocystinuria (see Chapter 195) is an inborn error of metabolism in which there is an increased incidence of arterial and venous thrombosis. Other stigmata such as Marfan's-like appearance and dislocated ocular lenses should suggest this diagnosis. Other features include generalized osteoporosis, mental retardation, and bony abnormalities such as scoliosis and chest deformity. The diagnosis can be substantiated by urinary testing for homocystine and by measuring a low level of cystathionine synthetase in a skin tissue culture or a liver biopsy specimen.

Various hematologic disorders have been associated with cerebrovascular disease. Hyperviscosity syndromes associated with other systemic diseases may result in small vessel occlusion and multiple areas of infarction or hemorrhage. Various neoplasms may be associated with disseminated intravascular coagulation and cerebral infarction. In polycythemia the increased blood viscosity may predispose the patient to cerebral arterial thrombosis, venous thrombosis, and small hemorrhages. A venous sinus thrombosis may occur, and the retinal veins may become occluded. Sickle cell disease should be suspected in young black patients who have had multiple episodes of neurologic disturbance. In sickle cell disease, dural sinus thrombosis and cerebral arterial or venous occlusion may occur. There may be an associated hemorrhage. A vasculopathy occurs in sickle cell disease, involving arterial vessels in the anterior part of the circle of Willis. Repeated transfusions aimed at keeping hemoglobin S levels below 30% can decrease the incidence of recurrent CVA.

Patients with thrombotic thrombocytopenic purpura have a characteristic triad of thrombocytopenic purpura, hemolytic anemia, and neurologic symptoms; the neurologic symptoms may be the first manifestation or the main manifestation. Patients may have alterations in mentation, seizures, and focal neurologic deficits. The small cerebral vessels show hyperplasia and platelet thrombi. The treatment of this disorder has been generally unsatisfactory.

An association with pregnancy or the postpartum period has been noted in approximately 35% of young women with a CVA in the carotid system. It has been speculated that known alterations of clotting factors in pregnancy such as a decrease in fibrinolysins and an increase in fibrinogen, as well as other clotting factors, may be significant. Venous sinus thrombosis and cortical vein thrombosis have been associated with both the postpartum period and the use of oral contraceptives. Consumptive coagulopathies resulting in a CVA have been reported with abruptio placentae, septic abortion, intrauterine fetal death, amniotic fluid embolism, uterine rupture, saline abortion, hydatidiform mole, placenta accreta, transfusion reaction, eclampsia, and severe preeclampsia. The low platelet count is the single most important finding in the diagnosis of a consumptive coagulopathy complicating one of these gynecologic situations. Thrombotic thrombocytopenic purpura occurs with increased frequency during pregnancy, and the renal dysfunction with hematuria and proteinuria may suggest the diagnosis of eclampsia.

The association of oral contraceptives with an increased risk of CVA appears well established. Several multi-institutional controlled studies have noted that women who use oral contraceptives have a significantly increased relative risk of a thrombotic CVA and a lesser risk of a hemorrhagic CVA. The risks are increased with age and hypertension. Smoking is a risk factor for hemorrhage; preparations higher in estrogen and probably progestin content are associated with a greater risk of thrombosis.

Moyamoya disease is a condition in which there are occlusions of one or more cerebral vessels in and around the circle of Willis with the development of a telangiectatic network in the lenticulostriate and thalamo-perforating arteries. This telangiectatic network acts as a source of collateral circulation to circumvent the occluded vessels and has the angiographic appearance of a haze or a puff of smoke. The Japanese name "moyamoya" is derived from this description. A rete mirabile is also commonly seen, which is a transdural anastomotic network of small vessels between the external and internal carotid arterial branches. This was originally described as a syndrome in young Orientals, but a similar syndrome may occur in children and in some adults with a slowly progressive occlusive disease of the circle of Willis from any cause. Both cerebral infarction and hemorrhage may occur. Cerebral angiography is necessary to establish this diagnosis.

BIBLIOGRAPHY

Buonanno, F., and Toole, J.F.: Management of patients with established ("completed") cerebral infarction, Stroke **12**:7, 1981.
Committee on Cerebro-Vascular Disease: A classification and outline of cerebrovascular diseases II, Stroke **6**:565, 1975.
Easton, J.D., and Sherman, D.G.: Management of cerebral embolism of cardiac origin, Stroke **11**:433, 1980.
Millikan, C., and McDowell, F.: Treatment of transient ischemic attacks, Stroke **9**:299, 1978.
Oral contraception and increased risk of cerebral ischemia or thrombosis, N. Engl. J. Med. **288**:871, 1973.
Sundt, T.M., Jr., and Whisnant, J.: Subarachnoid hemorrhage from intracranial aneurysms, surgical management and natural history of disease, N. Engl. J. Med. **299**:116, 1978.
Toole, J.F., and Patel, A.N.: Cerebrovascular disorders, New York, 1974, McGraw-Hill Book Co.

153 • EFFECTS OF PRIMARY AND METASTATIC TUMORS ON THE CENTRAL NERVOUS SYSTEM, AND PSEUDOTUMOR CEREBRI

George Paulson

BRAIN TUMORS

Brain tumors include both malignant and benign space-occupying lesions. These tumors produce symptoms by local destruction, by irritating the surrounding areas, and by producing increased intracranial pressure. The term "benign" generally refers to the tissue type, but unfortunately many tumors called benign are ultimately lethal because of their location and the limited possibility of their total removal. All age groups may be affected by brain tumors, and all structures and areas of the brain are vulnerable. Growth rates vary, ranging from the explosive growth of glioblastomas to the desultory and almost imperceptible changes of some meningiomas. In contrast to some types of tumors, environmental factors seem insignificant in the development of brain tumors, although in some varieties genetic factors are relevant.

CLASSIFICATION AND PATHOLOGY. Tumor taxonomy for the primary neoplasms has been traditionally based on the presumed cell of origin, often with specific comments or titles reflecting regional and anatomic factors. The taxonomy often seems confused, and there may be uncertainty regarding the cell of origin or only an indefinite linkage of the cell type with the prognosis for an individual case. The location of the tumor may be as relevant as the cell type. Some neoplasms originate from specific areas or cells, such as in the pituitary gland or the pineal gland, and therefore classifications reflect this; for example, a chromophobe adenoma or a pinealoma.

An oligodendroglioma is assumed to originate from the oligodendroglia cells, but the clinical response of an individual patient who harbors the oligodendroglioma is unpredictable. It may vary over a period of decades, and the clinical manifestations may reflect the varying locations. This tumor is one of several that evolve slowly and might be detected on a routine skull roentgenogram because intracranial calcification may occur. Microscopically it is composed of small, round cells with spherical nuclei. The clinical pattern of an oligodendroglioma is indistinguishable from that of a benign astrocytoma.

Astrocytic tumors originate from the astrocytes and can be partially defined by location (for example, a cerebellar astrocytoma). Astrocytic neoplasms are the most common primary tumors, and the group includes several types of tumors representing a transformation of the normal stellate astrocytes into a more fibroblastic appearance. Cavities or pseudocysts may form, and some astrocytomas may become more malignant with time. One common type of astrocytic neoplasm is the fibrillary astrocytoma, which comprises 90% of all astrocytic tumors. The graded terms are from I to IV; grade I suggests that this form of astrocytoma is the most benign neoplasm within the fibrillary group of tumors.

The astrocytoma grade IV, also called glioblastoma multiforme, is the most anaplastic form, and the tissue reveals evidence of marked dedifferentiation. In glioblastoma multiforme the nuclear-cytoplasmic ratio is increased and mitoses are common, with prominent cellular necrosis and changes in the surrounding blood supply. Angiograms may show a network of abnormal vessels. Frequently more than one lobe of the brain is involved. Glioblastomas unfortunately are among the more common gliomas, with a peak incidence in the productive fifth and sixth decades of life. They are not completely resectable, and death usually occurs within 18 months. There are numerous astrocytic variants, as well as the very benign or very malignant ones, and differences in the clinical state noted in the astrocytic tumor largely depend on the tumor's location in the brain.

As an example of the importance of the location of tumors, the astrocytic neoplasms of the cerebellum deserve particular note. Patients may have classic cerebellar symptoms, morning vomiting, and cranial nerve signs (particularly involving the sixth cranial nerve). The tumor may be a solitary mass in the cerebellum, but it may also be a nodule with a slow accumulation of fluid leading to a cystic area within the cerebellum. Surgery is feasible for several types of cerebellar astrocytomas with elective drainage or removal of the tumor. With, and even without, concomitant roentgenographic therapy, prolonged survival and even total remission have been reported for patients with cerebellar astrocytomas. Much more alarming is the pontine astrocytoma, which is widespread and diffuse with a wildly spongiform and degenerative appearance. Like the cerebellar tumors, this variety is more common in childhood. Polymorphism, necrosis, and glial proliferation are characteristic of this type of astrocytoma, a variety that responds poorly to both roentgenographic therapy and chemotherapy and is in a location where total surgical removal is impossible.

If the histologic pattern of the cerebellar tumor is that of a medulloblastoma, it is considered to have developed from a primitive cell in the cerebellum. In a child the midline signs of truncal ataxia and vomiting may be the initial symptoms of medulloblastoma, and later the nerve roots may also be involved because these tumors often seed along the spinal canal.

Ependymomas are primary tumors that originate from the walls of the ventricular system and may invade tissue or obstruct the ventricles, leading to death within 5 years.

Other subtypes of tumors besides the primary brain tumors each have a distinctive clinical pattern and merit mention, including adnexal tumors such as primary tumors of the choroid plexus and tumors of the various cranial nerves. A patient with a colloid cyst of the third ventricle, arising from the choroid plexus region, can have hydrocephalus, variable confusion, and intermittent headache. An acoustic neuroma can cause not only tinnitus and hearing loss but also signs of pressure on the seventh or fifth cranial nerves or even cerebellar symptoms resulting from pressure on nearby pathways.

Some tumors seem congenital and by their natural history invoke the concept of "cell rests." Examples are the giant cell astrocytoma or gemistocytic astrocytoma of tuberous sclerosis and the colloid cyst in the area of the foramen of Monro. In these conditions abnormal cells have presumably been present since birth but begin to grow in early adolescence. The tumors linked with von Recklinghausen's disease include acoustic neuroma and fibromas on the nerve roots or on the peripheral nerves. Granulomata, chromaffin-cell tumors, or tumors of vascular origin are rare enough to be only an infrequent consideration. Occasionally tumors are seen that are even more obviously congenital than the astrocytomas of tuberous sclerosis. Dermoid tumors and teratomas, for example, can be found in the midline posteriorly or at the base of the skull and may include evidence of very primitive cell types.

Tumors that arise from the meninges assume an importance beyond their incidence because of their insidious onset and their potential for total removal. These meningiomas grow slowly but can be exceedingly vascular, and removal is not always possible when the tumor has invaded critical structures. They include several cell types, and differences in prognosis may be postulated on the basis of the cellular variety. The cells are often uniform and may form characteristic whorls. The meningiomas, along with cholesteatoma and metastatic disease, often affect the skull.

Metastatic disease is one of the most frequent sources of brain tumor in adult life, with the most common sources being lung tumors in men and breast tumors in women. The metastatic tumors may be multiple or solitary, and in favorable locations some transient benefit may follow removal of the solitary lesions. Patients with tumors at the base of the skull may have face pain or numbness. Nasopharyngeal growths, which include carcinoma, can be difficult to diagnose, but roentgenograms of the base of the skull or computed tomographic (CT) scans can be helpful. Some patients require a nasopharyngeal biopsy.

Other intracranial masses occur in addition to the brain tumors just reviewed. An abscess may have the same symptoms as a tumor. Abscesses can be characterized both by the systemic symptoms such as fever and by increased pressure, but they may be indistinguishable from neoplasia until surgery is performed. Young patients with subdural hematomas may have focal weakness and headache, but an aged patient may only remain in bed with no local signs apparent.

In meningeal carcinomatosis a diffuse infiltration of the meninges by tumor cells takes place. Pleocytosis, a low value for cerebrospinal fluid (CSF) sugar, and an elevated value for protein in CSF are common in these patients. The syndrome may be overlooked when the presence of generalized cancer is unknown. Patients may have cranial nerve signs such as facial numbness or diplopia, complaints of back pain or neck ache, or the infiltrating sheets of cancer cells can produce generalized weakness with areflexia in the legs.

PATHOPHYSIOLOGY. The skull is filled with incompressible substances, and a tumor may produce effects by an increase in pressure, by regional edema, or by destroying tissue. Regardless of the pathologic type, the location of the tumor is of great importance. Supratentorial tumors often involve the motor or sensory systems, and many patients have seizures. A substantial percentage of patients have an adult onset of seizures as the initial manifestation of an infiltrative tumor. The traditional triad of papilledema, projectile vomiting, and headache occurs late in the course of the disease and results from the increased intracranial pressure. The diagnosis is usually possible before this stage, and in modern medicine few patients are seen with this triad as the initial clinical manifestation of a supratentorial tumor. Instead, focal seizures in an adult, changes in mental function, dull, inexplicable headaches, and a slowly progressive weakness may be among the first recognizable features. It is not recognized sufficiently that tumors may fluctuate in their manifestations through partial and abortive seizures, small hemorrhages, shifts in intracerebral pressure, or vascular involvement. Some patients seem to be having transient ischemic attacks, although a neoplasm is eventually discovered. The memory can be defective, particularly when the frontal or temporal lobes are involved. Extracerebral structures such as the first cranial nerve can be involved when meningiomas are present, and these more slowly growing tumors often have very few initial signs. Glioblastomas, on the other hand, are likely to begin with changes over a matter of weeks or months, and commonly the patient is obviously ill when first seen.

Infratentorial tumors are much more subtle in their effect and are relatively more common in childhood when the history is more difficult to obtain. When the cerebellopontine angle is involved, as in adult acoustic neuroma, the patient shows cerebellar dysfunction, difficulty with hearing and with the vestibular system, or complex disturbances in eye movements. Pressure on the sixth cranial nerve may produce diplopia.

Hydrocephalus, the dilatation of the ventricular system by the obstruction of CSF pathways, can result from tumors. It may occur independent of a neoplasm, for example, with congenital aqueductal stenosis, even during adult life. Hydrocephalus following the obstruction of the subarachnoid space by blood or a previous meningitis can produce a mixed clinical picture, with an initial improvement after the insult and then late deterioration. Signs of hydrocephalus include leg weakness or spasticity, presumably resulting from stretching of the long periventricular fibers arising from the parasagittal region, or symptoms of increased intracranial pressure plus a generalized cerebral dysfunction.

SYMPTOMS THAT SIGNAL THE POSSIBILITY OF TUMOR

Progressive focal neurologic disturbance. Whereas cerebrovascular disease can have a stepwise or stuttering onset, a sudden catastrophic insult, or a transient defect with a complete recovery, the brain tumor commonly has a more insidious onset. Punctuated by gradually increasing weakness, by a subtle sensory less, or by adult-onset seizures that are not always relieved by medications, the progressive nature of the decline from a tumor generally becomes obvious when the history is adequate. Often the findings and the complaints are less obvious for patients with a tumor than for patients with cerebrovascular accidents (CVAs) or degenerative disease.

Mentation. A personality change and an insidious decrease in mentation may occur. Frontal lobe disease in particular is associated with striking behavior changes, including facetiousness or inappropriate comments. Depression, or the appearance of a loss of joy of life, is common with brain tumors, and a few patients with infiltrative tumors may have a striking deficit in their memory or judgment.

Onset of seizures in adult life. The onset of seizures in adult life always raises the specter of a tumor unless alcoholism or another logical explanation is readily apparent. Even when the diagnostic workup does not document a tumor, a follow-up may reveal a more ominous diagnosis later. The patient who most needs an evaluation and a follow-up by a neurologic specialist is the patient who develops unexplained seizures in adult life.

Change in the character of headaches. Many patients with vascular headache have repetitive headaches throughout their life with a diminution in the middle years, whereas patients with brain tumors may have persistent, steady, or intractable dull pain rather than intermittent severe episodes. Consistently unilateral pain, or a pain that changes in character over a few weeks, suggests a need for an additional workup. Intermittent sharp pains in the head or the face as with tic douloureux and dull facial pains are only very rarely associated with tumors, and then more often with growths at the base of the skull than with growths in the brain. Stress-induced headaches (for example, pain resulting from cough, sneeze, or strain, and even repetitive headache that results from routine exercise) may require a more intensive evaluation for a tumor than is necessary for nonspecific headaches. This is particularly true if the headache is severe and persistently triggered by exercise or cough and even more so if the pain is unilateral. A dull headache that occurs in the morning seems to be more common with tumors than a headache that occurs at other times of the day. The headache caused by a brain tumor may respond to aspirin.

Signs and symptoms of increased intracranial pressure. Besides local symptoms produced by tumor, there are signs and symptoms caused solely by the diffuse increase in intracranial pressure. The classic triad suggesting this increase in intracranial pressure includes headache, vomiting, and papilledema. Further symptoms reflect the effects of pressure on vital centers in the diencephalon and the hindbrain and damage to the cranial nerves. With the compression of the third nerve by the herniation of the uncus of the temporal lobe over the tentorial edge, the pupil dilates and may not react reflexly by constriction to light, and eventually the lid droops. In many instances mydriasis is a late sign, and pupillary dilatation resulting from increased intracranial pressure is often an indication that something already should have been done to reduce the pressure. Because 10% of normal people have slightly unequal pupils, a minimal asymmetry in pupil size is often irrelevant. Although not every dilated pupil implies an increase in intracranial pressure, dilatation, especially with an impaired pupillary reflex and decreasing consciousness, remains a time-honored and valuable sign of an impending cerebral herniation. The cerebellar tonsils may herniate through the foramen magnum, and such a herniation may produce a stiff neck or a tilting of the head caused both by the reflex tonic neck responses and by the conscious efforts of the patient to prevent pain whenever the neck is flexed. With these patients a search for papilledema is desirable, but papilledema is not present in every patient with increased intracranial pressure. A loss of venous pulsations at the optic disc is usual with markedly increased pressure, but some unaffected people have retinal venous pulsations that are difficult to see, and a few patients have no visible pulsations even when the CSF pressure is normal. A loss of previously observed pulsations can, however, signify a recent increase in pressure. In the assessment of increased pressure it is often a change from the result of the previous examination that is of the greatest consequence.

Unfortunately, occasional patients, particularly if the changes have developed very slowly, may have almost no signs of increased intracranial pressure until the disease is in a dangerously late stage. Most neurologists have seen patients in whom papilledema was an incidental finding or in whom the only complaint was diplopia caused by third nerve pressure, or patients with repetitive morning vomiting followed by an abrupt herniation. The clinician must remain alert to detect this kind of case, which is often potentially very treatable. There is no substitute for informed clinical suspicion to detect a cerebral herniation.

In some instances, such as benign intracranial hypertension (pseudotumor cerebri) or lead encephalopathy, there is increased pressure in the absence of a tumor.

DIFFERENTIAL DIAGNOSIS. CVAs are likely to have a different temporal pattern than a brain tumor, although either can sometimes have a stepwise or episodic onset. Patients with brain tumors occasionally can have a sudden deterioration in function of the central nervous system, particularly if there is a change in pressure, a seizure, or a hemorrhage into the tumor, but sudden changes are more typical of vascular disease. Patients with subdural hematomas can have moderate hemiparesis and headache, but they can also have only apathy and an apparently depressed state with few other symptoms. Fortunately, the current techniques of CT and radioisotope scans can distinguish subdural hematomas from brain tumors. Multiple sclerosis, particularly when its course lacks classic remissions and exacerbations, can be confused with a brain tumor, and a brain tumor at the base of the skull or in the area of the foramen magnum can be falsely labeled as a case of multiple sclerosis. When in doubt the physician should perform ancillary diagnostic techniques. Dementia of the type seen in Alzheimer's disease often leads to an evaluation to rule out a tumor of the frontal or temporal lobe. The severe cortical dementia with intact motor and sensory systems that is so characteristic of Alzheimer's disease is in fact uncommon with brain tumors. Brain tumors often affect mentation but rarely lead to severe dementia in early stages. Patients with Alzheimer's disease may have profound memory deficits with intact social graces and no motor or sensory deficits. As mentioned earlier, for the diagnosis of a brain tumor, lesser and more subtle signs can be particularly significant. Extreme dementia is more common in patients with Alzheimer's disease than in patients with a brain tumor; complete hemiparesis is more common in CVAs than in brain tumors; and severe ataxia is more commonly seen with a degeneration of the cerebellum than with brain tumors. Epilepsy can be an initial complaint of patients with brain tumors and deserves a detailed evaluation and a close follow-up. In some cases only time may clarify the diagnosis. With abscesses the clinical manifestations can resemble those of a subacute tumor, and the diagnosis may be apparent only during surgery. In fact an abscess is a "tumor" in the sense of swelling, and it may manifest any of the clinical features of neoplastic disease.

LABORATORY FINDINGS. Skull roentgenograms are usually performed when increased pressure is suspected, seeking an erosion of the posterior clinoid processes. An erosion of the posterior clinoid processes or the presence of intracranial calcifications may confirm the need for further laboratory studies. As a rule, however, plain roentgenograms are of little benefit in detecting a brain tumor, and in fact a chest roentgenogram to look for a primary lung tumor or metastatic disease is more valuable. CT has, however, revolutionized the management of patients in whom a brain tumor is suspected. This test is especially useful with contrast enhancement to identify the presence of the more vascular tumors. Changes in ventricle size and shifts of the midline structures also are readily apparent with CT. CT has greatly reduced the need for pneumoencephalography, with the exception of tumors near the chiasm and a few other specialized purposes. The rapidly developing techniques of radioisotope scanning have been overlooked in the glamorous surge of CT scanning, but for the detection of infections such as herpes simplex encephalitis, and even for abscess, radionuclide scans are of great ancillary benefit. Both isotope and CT scans can often detect the tumor when the patient is first seen. The appearance of a lesion with an infarction may be anatomically more consistent with the distribution of a major vessel and, although possibly normal immediately after a major CVA, within a week is usually positive. Electroencephalography is still a desirable test, particularly because it is a harmless screening technique. Slow-growing tumors may produce no change in the electroencephalogram (EEG) or may result in focal epileptic discharges. Rapidly developing tumors and abscesses generate marked focal slowing in the EEG. With increased intracranial pressure, rhythmic, periodic, and high-voltage slowing may be noted, particularly frontally. Examination of CSF for protein and cytologic analysis is of value in selected cases, but a lumbar puncture is not usually necessary and may be harmful to patients with rapidly growing tumors. In the presence of a mass, downward herniation may occur when pressure is suddenly reduced from below. If increased pressure is discovered inadvertently during a lumbar puncture, the immediate use of antiedema agents such as steroids or mannitol should be considered and the patient must be monitored carefully. The fluid available in the manometer should be studied even though the additional amount removed must be limited. The purposes of performing the lumbar puncture should be met and cultures should be obtained as needed, since the problems after a lumbar puncture in this situation appear to be related to the further flow of CSF from the sustained subarachnoid puncture site and not to the CSF removed for study.

NEUROLOGIC COMPLICATIONS OF CANCER THERAPY

It has become increasingly apparent that necrosis resulting from radiation occurs in the brain tissue and its supportive tissues and that the late effects of radiation can be extremely insidious in onset. Vulnerability to the effects of radiation varies from person to person, and the precise limits of therapy are uncertain, but any patient whose brain receives over 4000 rad may have secondary effects. It seems likely that chemotherapy has an additive effect. Radiation-induced spinal cord lesions are particularly common following therapy for pulmonary or breast lesions. Brown-Séquard syndrome, spasticity, and a moderate elevation in CSF protein concentration are among the clinical observations in these cases. No useful therapy exists for radiation-induced changes in the central nervous system, but steroids may slow the progressive course of what seems to represent not only a deterioration of neural tissue but also scarring and a breakdown in the local blood supply to the nerve tissue. At times radiation effects may even appear as a tumorous swelling and may require surgery for adequate diagnosis. Whenever there is a recurrence of symptoms in an area of previous radiation therapy, the possibility of radiation-induced symptoms must be considered.

Almost all chemotherapeutic agents are potentially neurotoxic when used in large doses. The most common toxic effect from these chemicals is a peripheral neuropathy with paresthesias, weakness, and sensory loss. The paresthesias reflect the type and amount of drug used, as well as the duration of the therapy. The use of vincristine in particular is almost universally associated with some degree of neuropathy. Intrathecal injections of methotrexate may cause catastrophic generalized weakness, paresthesias, or severe cerebral irritation. Periventricular gliosis also can result from using intrathecal injections of methotrexate, which is nevertheless often the best available agent to treat meningeal carcinomatosis.

EFFECTS OF REMOTE TUMORS ON THE NERVOUS SYSTEM

The nervous system can react to the presence of a tumor in numerous ways, and immunologic or toxic factors associated with a tumor are difficult to separate from the direct effects of local metastases. Nevertheless, in some patients who have no local metastasis a cerebellar syndrome develops, with a slowly progressive deterioration in balance and coordination. A few patients without a focal spread of the cancer have combined muscle and nerve disease (neuropathy and myopathy) that appears as paresthesias, sensory loss, and a weakness in the proximal musculature. Classic polymyositis can also be linked to a tumor, again without any obvious metastatic nodules in the muscle. These entities may be mixed in complex clinical patterns and can be confused at times with the overlapping and direct effects from metastatic foci. For example, in rare cases a mild dementia may be linked to the presence of a tumor outside the brain, although an unrecognized depression or a local metastatis is a more common explanation for the mental change with neoplasia. The syndrome of a remote effect of cancer, particularly the sensory neuropathies, is most often seen with carcinoma of the lung, but cancer of the breast, ovary, or stomach also has been associated with remote effects on the central nervous system. The syndrome of inappropriate antidiuretic hormone (ADH) secretion also has been reported secondary to carcinoma and appears in the usual fashion with usually only a mild hyponatremia.

Another paraneoplastic syndrome is the tendency in the late stage of carcinoma, particularly after treatment with radiation therapy or chemotherapy, for a patient to have superimposed infections. These infections may consist of an easily recognized bacterial meningitis, but in addition, subtle fungal infections such as with *Cryptococcus* often are noted in patients with neoplasia. The involvement of the brain tissue by the papovavirus in the syndrome of progressive multifocal leukoencephalopathy (occurring primarily in patients with leukemia, lymphoma, or immunosuppression) produces mental deterioration, motor deterioration, and death within weeks.

MANAGEMENT. Surgical therapy for brain tumors depends on the type of lesion and its location, and ranges from decompression for the palliation of headaches to total extirpation. Cases must be considered individually, and even in the therapy for metastatic tumors each patient deserves careful evaluation to avoid fruitless surgery or nihilistic neglect. For solitary primary tumors, palliative surgery may be very helpful.

Radiotherapy and sometimes chemotherapy, which remains somewhat experimental, can prolong useful life in selected patients. Medical therapy can offer support with anticonvulsants, antiedema agents, and general supportive care for the patient and his family.

The management of tumors or of a new growth of the skull is similar to that of any other bony structure, and in fact the skull often is surgically more accessible than other bony areas. With the exception of a massive thickening such as with Paget's disease, the intracranial contents usually are not affected by an overgrowth of bone. The cranial nerves are impinged on in some cases, and if the outflow tracts for the CSF are compromised in the foramen magnum area by thickened bone or meninges, hydrocephalus can result.

Patients with tumors of the pituitary gland often have a hormone imbalance and disturbances in their visual fields. These tumors may require a combination of surgical, radiation, and endocrinologic management. Pituitary microadenomas can be detected with high-resolution CT scans. These small tumors produce endocrinologic symptoms without neurologic signs. They may be treated medically (for example, with bromocriptine) or surgically.

PSEUDOTUMOR CEREBRI, OR BENIGN INTRACRANIAL HYPERTENSION

Pseudotumor cerebri, or benign intracranial hypertension, involves increased intracranial pressure in the absence of an intracranial mass lesion, obstructive hydrocephalus, meningitis, hypertensive encephalopathy, or any other demonstrable structural lesion. The patient has an intractable headache and papilledema associated with a measurable increase in intracranial pressure but is alert and nonsomnolent and has no focal neurologic signs, in contrast to the patient with a lesion. The patient may have a sixth nerve palsy. The major physical threat posed by pseudotumor cerebri is a potential decrease in visual acuity or a defect in the visual fields, so these clinical signs must be carefully monitored. Pseudotumor cerebri may occasionally appear without papilledema. The syndrome is more common in women than in men, and although it can occur at any age, it has a peak age incidence in the third decade of life.

Although the pathogenesis of pseudotumor cerebri is not well formulated, this disease has been found in association with a number of other disorders, including Addison's disease, steroid treatment or withdrawal, pregnancy, the use of oral contraceptives, hypoparathyroidism, hypervitaminosis A, hypovitaminosis A, the administration of drugs (tetracycline, nalidixic acid, or the phenothiazines), the time of the menarche or the menopause, and commonly in young obese women with menstrual irregularities. The increased intracranial pressure associated with a thrombosis of the venous sinuses is often included as a cause of benign intracranial hypertension. This form is known as otitic hydrocephalus because of an association with otitis media in some cases, although hydrocephalus is not present.

The differential diagnosis of pseudotumor cerebri includes considering midline ventricular tumors, tumors of the nondominant, silent frontal lobe, malignant hypertension with retinopathy, and variations of the optic fundi (pseudopapilledema).

The definitive diagnostic tests for pseudotumor cerebri include a CT scan to exclude a mass lesion and a lumbar puncture to record the pressure and also to eliminate the possibility of a chronic meningeal process such as sarcoid or fungal meningitis by an analysis of the CSF. The CT reveals small- or normal-sized ventricles without a shift in their location, and without any focal abnormality. The CSF itself should be normal.

The treatment of an uncomplicated pseudotumor cerebri includes using diuretics (for example, furosemide, 40 mg four times a day, or acetazolamide, 500 mg twice a day) and weight reduction when appropriate. Repeated lumbar puncture with the removal of CSF is often recommended. Steroids (dexamethasone, 16 mg daily in a divided dosage, or prednisone, 60 to 80 mg a day for short courses) have been used. Immediate and aggressive surgical treatment such as a lumboperitoneal shunting of CSF, and rarely a subtemporal decompression, should be considered when the patient's vision is threatened. Although pseudotumor cerebri is considered a relatively self-limited condition, chronic elevations of CSF pressure have been described and patients may have acute recurrences.

BIBLIOGRAPHY

Armstrong, R.M.: Effects upon the nervous system from remote tumors. In Goldensohn, E.S., and Appel, S.H., editors: Scientific approaches to clinical neurology, vol. I, Philadelphia, 1977, Lea & Febiger.

Burger, P.C., and Vogel, F.S.: Surgical pathology of the nervous system and its coverings, New York, 1976, John Wiley & Sons, Inc.

154 • NUTRITIONAL DISORDERS OF THE NERVOUS SYSTEM

David P. Dunn

Many dietary factors, particularly vitamins, are essential to the nervous system. Vitamins are used in various enzymatic reactions required for the normal metabolism of nerve tissue. The most common nutritional disorders of the nervous system are caused by vitamin deficiencies, usually deficiencies of the B complex vitamins. The clinical manifestations of vitamin deficiencies can be variable because many patients have multiple deficiencies of varying degrees and even the lack of one vitamin may adversely affect the use of others. The vitamin deficits produce an abnormal metabolism and eventual structural defects in various levels of the nervous system. The ensuing signs and symptoms reflect the regions most involved. Deficiencies are apt to arise as the result of many situations such as fad diets, starvation, malabsorption problems, neoplasia, and other debilitating disease. In North America the most common situation in which a nutritional disorder of the nervous system occurs is when the chronic alcoholic forsakes a normal diet.

PERIPHERAL NEUROPATHY

DEFINITION. The peripheral neuropathy produced by a vitamin deficit is a subacutely evolving polyneuropathy, a symmetric disorder of the distal peripheral nerves.

ETIOLOGY AND PATHOGENESIS. Thiamine deficiency has been implicated as the cause of the nutritional neuropathies, the classic example being beriberi. Beriberi is usually associated with a subsistence diet of thiamine-deficient rice, but it also has occurred in Western populations during periods of famine. Although emphasis has been placed on the lack of thiamine in alcoholic polyneuropathy, and many patients have responded to the administration of thiamine, most alcoholic nutritional neuropathies are found in patients who have a mixed deficiency state. The cell bodies of the motor and sensory neurons are affected metabolically, resulting in an axonal degeneration that involves the distal parts of the neurons.

CLINICAL MANIFESTATIONS AND COURSE. Clinical manifestations include sensory deficits, muscle weakness, and atrophy that are more prominent in the legs than in the arms, start in the distal regions of the legs, and progress proximally and symmetrically. Diverse sensory symptoms begin insidiously in the feet and calves. Patients complain of numbness, coldness, pain, aches, burning sensations, a "dead" sensation in the feet, and just not feeling right. One patient complained of a sensation that felt like a thousand ants with cold and hot feet marching around his legs. As the disease progresses, the hands may become similarly affected. The involved areas are often extremely tender, and even the pressure of bedsheets can cause pain. Stroking the sole of the foot can feel like a hot knife to the patient, almost causing him to leap from the bed. Eventually a complete sensory loss may develop in a stocking and glove distribution. Weakness is variable from very slight to so severe that the patient cannot stand or walk. As the disease progresses, the muscle weakness ascends. The deep tendon reflexes, especially the ankle jerks, disappear early in the course of the disease.

LABORATORY FINDINGS. Underlying causes of malnutrition such as malabsorption need to be evaluated with the appropriate laboratory tests. Nerve conduction velocities may be preserved in nutritional neuropathies, as opposed to other common neuropathies in which the myelin sheath around the axon is primarily involved.

DIAGNOSIS AND MANAGEMENT. The diagnosis of neuropathy may be suggested by the patient's history, but it is confirmed by the neurologic findings during a clinical examination. An accurate history is essential to identify the cause more specifically as a nutritional deficit related to alcoholism. The possibility of toxins found in illegally distilled liquor causing or contributing to a neuropathy should be kept in mind. Treatment consists of abstinence from alcohol, vitamin therapy (especially with B complex vitamins), and a nutritious diet. The use of other drugs that interfere with the metabolism of vitamins should be carefully evaluated. The carbohydrate load found in some intravenous solutions can precipitate further problems in a patient who is thiamine deficient.

WERNICKE'S ENCEPHALOPATHY AND KORSAKOFF'S PSYCHOSIS

DEFINITION. Wernicke's encephalopathy is an acutely evolving disease manifested by confusion, a wide-based stumbling walk (gait ataxia), and disturbances of eye movement, among which involuntary oscillations (nystagmus) are the most common. Korsakoff's psychosis usually occurs as a chronic sequela to Wernicke's encephalopathy. The patient has a loss of recent memory with the rest of the cognitive functions left intact. The overwhelming majority of patients with this combination are chronic alcoholics.

ETIOLOGY AND PATHOGENESIS. Vitamin B_1 deficiency is central to the production of this syndrome. Ingested thiamine is phosphorylated to form the coenzyme cocarboxylase, which is essential in energy-producing pathways of carbohydrate metabolism. Cocarboxylase is necessary to the activity of the enzyme pyruvate decarboxylase in the initial reaction of the tricarboxylic acid cycle and to the function of the enzyme transketolase in the hexose monophosphate shunt. Exactly how the metabolic abnormalities produce the various lesions in this disorder is unknown. Presumably those regions of the brain that have the most enzyme activity at risk are the most involved. Some patients have a genetic abnormality of transketolase. With a normal diet such a patient has no problems, but when the diet is thiamine deficient, the disease develops. Tissue necrosis and blood vessel changes are produced in the hypothalamus, especially the mammillary bodies, the central gray matter of the brainstem, and the thalamus. Atrophy occurs in the cerebellum. The abnormalities of the eye movements are caused by the brainstem lesions, the gait ataxia is caused by the cerebellar atrophy, and the memory defects have been linked to the involvement of the thalamus.

CLINICAL MANIFESTATIONS AND COURSE. Although nystagmus is the most common ocular manifestation, the eye muscles that cause each eye to move laterally, the lateral recti, are often partially or completely paralyzed. The patient may be unable to move the eyes conjugately up and down and horizontally. When thiamine is administered, the eye abnormalities may start to improve in a matter of hours. Nystagmus may be a permanent sequela. The gait ataxia does not improve as quickly as do the ocular manifestations, and often the improvement is incomplete. The disorder of mentation initially consists of a quiet state of disorientation, memory loss, apathy, decreased concentration, and misperceptions of people and objects, described as the global confusional state. Some patients have delirium tremens in which agitation, hallucinations, and tremors are prominent.

Treatment may reverse all the mental changes. The persistence of a memory loss as the other signs return to normal indicates the presence of Korsakoff's psychosis. The patient cannot remember recent events but retains older pieces of information. When a patient cannot remember an object or a number after 5 minutes, he will have difficulty learning new information. Confabulation is often used to fill in the gaps of information. One patient, when asked where he was in the morning, although actually in the hospital, responded with a detailed description of the boarding house where he had lived for several years. The response of the memory loss to thiamine is poor. Most patients do not recover completely, and the intellectual deficits persist to a varying degree.

The majority of patients have an associated nutritional polyneuropathy and a plethora of other diseases. Death can occur after treatment has started and is probably related to the severity of the lesions in the brainstem.

LABORATORY FINDINGS. Laboratory findings include increased levels of blood pyruvate, but the increase is not specific for this disorder. The blood transketolase assay is the preferred test. The activity of transketolase is markedly decreased when thiamine is deficient.

DIAGNOSIS AND MANAGEMENT. The clinical manifestations in a malnourished alcoholic patient should lead to a correct diagnosis. Laboratory tests and the response to thiamine can confirm the diagnosis. Initially 100 mg of thiamine should be administered parenterally. This dose should be continued daily in the acute phase of the disease. In Korsakoff's psychosis the response to thiamine is much less evident. Other associated diseases must be sought and treated. Because of the general nutritional depletion, these patients require more than just thiamine replacement, and both a good diet and multivitamin therapy must be instituted.

NUTRITIONAL AMBLYOPIA

Nutritional amblyopia, a characteristic type of amblyopia (decreased vision) is found in undernourished individuals. The patient complains of a slowly progressive, usually bilateral, visual loss for close work or reading. An examination of the central visual fields reveals decreased vision corresponding to the point of fixation or extending from it to the blind spot (central scotoma or centrocecal scotoma). The peripheral vision is intact, and unless the disease is far advanced, the optic nerve appears normal. The amblyopia is caused by the involvement of the papillomacular bundle, which carries the nerve fibers for central vision. In the past tobacco and alcohol have been suggested as causal agents, but a good diet and vitamin B therapy have resulted in the return of vision even with the continuance of smoking and drinking. Amblyopia has been found in association with other vitamin deficiency syndromes and has been present in undernourished patients who did not use alcohol and tobacco.

PELLAGRA

Niacin deficiency, pellagra, can cause a wide spectrum of neurologic deficits in the central nervous system. Mental change is an early symptom; the patient may appear anxious, confused, and even frankly psychotic. Without treatment the brain damage may result in a permanent dementia. A weakness of the legs and a loss of position sense in the feet with resulting unsteadiness in walking are indicative of the spinal cord involvement, which clinically mimics vitamin B_{12} deficiency. Peripheral nerve abnormalities are less common and may be caused by associated vitamin deficits and protein deficits. Niacin deficiency first causes the neurons to swell, but if it is persistent, they eventually disintegrate. Niacin therapy reverses the neurologic defects, but because other concurrent deficiencies are common, B complex vitamins also should be given.

CEREBELLAR CORTICAL DEGENERATION

Although cerebellar cortical degeneration is usually found in chronic alcoholic patients, it has occurred in nonalcoholic patients with severe malnutrition. The anterior superior cortex of the cerebellar vermis, the central region of the cerebellum, becomes atrophic with a selective loss of Purkinje cells. This regional atrophy causes gait ataxia. The anterior lobes of the lateral hemispheres may be involved, but not as much as the vermis. Thiamine is essential to some of the nerve cell transmitters in the cerebellum. The role of the other nutritional factors and their relation to thiamine are unknown.

VITAMIN B₁₂ DEFICIENCY (PERNICIOUS ANEMIA)

(See Chapter 148.)

The most commonly recognized neurologic defect in vitamin B_{12} deficiency is a demyelination of the posterior and lateral columns of the spinal cord, known as subacute combined degeneration (SCD). Less commonly recognized is the cerebral involvement producing a progressive dementia. The peripheral and optic nerves can be demyelinated. Usually the neurologic manifestations are concurrent with pernicious anemia. It must be strongly emphasized, however, that the neurologic manifestations can be present in the absence of anemia. Besides a lack of gastric intrinsic factor, surgery and diseases of the gastric tract can result in a failure of vitamin absorption.

SCD starts with numbness and tingling in the toes and fingers. Position sense is lost in the feet. The deep tendon reflexes are lost when the fibers of the reflex arc are damaged in the cord. Babinski's sign (upgoing great toe on stroking the sole of the foot) reflects the lateral column involvement that eventually causes muscle weakness. Dementia can be mild or severe depending on the tissue damage in the cerebrum. Some loss of pain distally in the extremities indicates a neuropathy. Cyanocobalamin therapy may reverse the deficits completely or to a lesser degree depending on the severity of the disease. The dosage is 250 μg by injection twice weekly for several months, then 250 μg twice each month for a year, then 100 μg each month of life.

BIBLIOGRAPHY

Victor, M., Adams, R.D., and Collins, G.H.: The Wernicke-Korsakoff syndrome, Philadelphia, 1971, F.A. Davis Co.

155 • PROBLEMS OF NERVE AND MUSCLE

Hiroshi Mitsumoto and **Theodore L. Munsat**

STRUCTURE AND FUNCTION

Anterior horn cells (α motor neurons) are located in the anterior horn gray matter of the spinal cord (Fig. 155-1). Their motor axons leave the spinal cord via the anterior roots, form large mixed peripheral nerves with other motor and sensory axons, and finally reach the innervated muscle through the independent motor nerves. The anterior horn cell and the totality of muscle fibers innervated by it are called a motor unit. The synaptic region between the nerve and the muscle is the neuromuscular junction. At this synapse acetylcholine is released from the presynaptic motor terminal and initiates the excitation-contraction events.

Muscle contraction is monitored by the muscle spindles (intrafusal fibers) and the Golgi tendon organs through

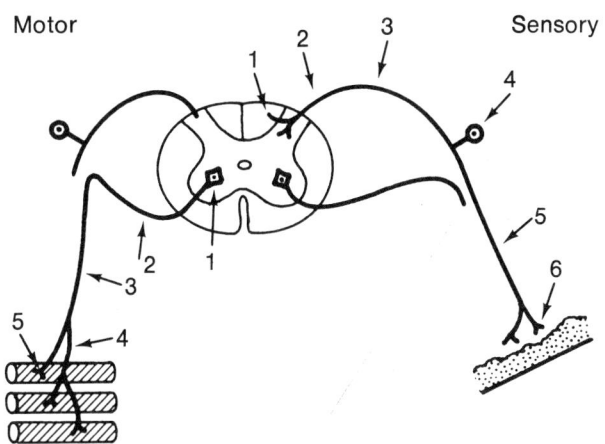

Fig. 155-1. Motor system: *1*, anterior horn cells: *2*, anterior root; *3*, peripheral nerve; *4*, motor nerve terminal; *5*, neuromuscular junction. Sensory system: *1*, posterior horn and posterior column, *2*, root entry zone; *3*, posterior root; *4*, dorsal root ganglion; *5*, peripheral nerve; *6*, sensory nerve terminal (cutaneous). (From Bradley, W.G.: Disorders of peripheral nerves, Oxford, Eng., 1974, Blackwell Scientific Publications.)

larger-sized sensory fibers. These sensory fibers return to the spinal cord through the posterior roots. Their cell bodies are located in the dorsal root ganglion. Cutaneous sensation is transmitted by small-sized sensory fibers. Voluntary and involuntary control of muscle contraction is mediated by pyramidal and extrapyramidal systems in the central nervous system. The muscle fiber is a long, cylindric, syncytial cell connected to a tendon at each end. It contains numerous myofibrils running parallel to the muscle fiber. Myofibrils are composed of regularly oriented repeating units, sarcomeres, which appear histologically as cross-striations and consist of a series of alternating dark (A) and light (I) bands containing the fundamental contractile proteins. The I band consists of thin actin-containing myofilaments, which penetrate into the A band as well. The A band contains the thick myosin-containing filaments in addition to the ends of the thin filaments. When muscle fibers contract isotonically, thin filaments on either side of the A band move toward each other, between thick filaments. Thus the I band, the sarcomeres, and the total length of the muscle shorten by the interdigitation of these contractile elements.

The contraction is triggered by calcium ions released from the sarcoplasmic reticulum, an intracellular cistern, which stores calcium and is adjacent to the myofibrils. At the neuromuscular junction acetylcholine molecules are released from the presynaptic motor terminal and reach the receptor site of the postsynaptic membrane, resulting in a depolarization of the sarcolemma. The depolarization is rapidly transmitted to the entire muscle fiber through a tubular (T) system that is a direct extension of the outer sarcolemma. The T system makes contact with the sarcoplasmic reticulum at the A-I band junction, forming a so-called triad. Calcium ions are then resequestered into the sarcoplasmic reticulum, and the contraction is ended.

There are basically two fiber types in human muscle, present in roughly equal proportions. Each human skeletal muscle is composed of random admixtures of both fiber types. The type I fibers have high oxidative activity and are slow-twitch fibers physiologically. The type II fibers have low oxidative capacity, high adenosine triphosphatase activity, and are fast-twitch fibers physiologically.

SIGNS AND SYMPTOMS

Weakness is the cardinal manisfestation of neuromuscular disorders. It can occur in any muscle group such as the limb, trunk, ocular, swallowing, or respiratory muscles. Weakness involving primarily proximal muscles is seen in myopathies. A characteristic maneuver of using the arms on the thighs while arising from the floor (Gower's sign) is typically seen in Duchenne type muscular dystrophy. Vertebral column alterations are common in advanced neuromuscular disorders that begin in childhood. Increased lumbar lordosis is often seen in the ambulatory child with Duchenne type muscular dystrophy. Specific distributions of muscle weakness and atrophy are seen in certain neuromuscular disorders such as peroneal atrophy, facioscapulohumeral muscular dystrophy, and limb-girdle muscular dystrophy. Increased muscle size in a weak muscle is known as pseudohypertrophy and is particularly characteristic of Duchenne type muscular dystrophy. Fasciculations are visible, discrete, rapid, spontaneous muscle twitches typically seen in motor neuron diseases. Muscle tone is generally decreased in myopathies and neuropathies but is increased in amyotrophic lateral sclerosis (ALS). The deep tendon reflexes are lost early in neuropathies and late in myopathies. Muscle contracture is a common sequela of unused muscle in advanced neuromuscular disorders, especially myopathies. Aches, cramps, and pains may be an early complaint in neuromuscular disorders. Sensory symptoms such as numbness and paresthesias are manifestations of peripheral (sensory) neuropathies. Graded loss of sensation in the distal part of the extremities (stocking and glove distribution) is typical of peripheral neuropathies. Sensory loss in the distribution of a specific single peripheral nerve is seen in a mononeuropathy. Loss of pain, touch, and temperature sense is a result of small sensory fiber involvement, whereas loss of vibration and position sense is a result of large sensory fiber involvement.

PATHOPHYSIOLOGY
Pathology

Investigating morphologic changes is of prime importance for the correct diagnosis of neuromuscular disorders. The tissue must be properly processed and interpreted, however, by an experienced neuromuscular morphologist.

The pathologic changes of muscle basically consist of those resulting from denervation in which muscle fibers undergo atrophy, at times in groups, and myopathies in which muscle fibers undergo random degeneration and often regeneration. Certain myopathies can be diagnosed correctly only with histochemical techniques that involve processing muscle quick-frozen at the time of the biopsy.

Biopsy of a peripheral nerve, particularly the sural nerve, is being performed with increasing frequency. Fascicular biopsies are almost as useful as whole nerve biopsies and have a much lower incidence of postbiopsy discomfort. Two main forms of peripheral nerve damage have been identified: axonal degeneration (axonal neuropathy) and segmental demyelination (demyelinating neuropathy). In axonal degeneration the presumed defect is inherent in the axon or cell body, whereas in segmental demyelination the presumed defect is in the investing Schwann cell and its myelin production or maintenance.

Electrophysiology

The measurement of nerve conduction velocities (NCVs) of individual peripheral nerves and the needle electrode examination of muscle (electromyography, EMG) provide valuable pathophysiologic data on neuromuscular disorders. NCVs are normal in myopathies but are impaired in many neuropathies. When the myelin sheath surrounding the axon is damaged (demyelinating neuropathies), nerve conduction is markedly delayed in contrast to nerve conduction in axonal neuropathies, which is not delayed as regularly or to the same degree. The loss of nerve fibers (axonal neuropathies) results in markedly diminished or even absent evoked potentials in sensory nerve fibers (sensory neuropathies) and motor fibers (motor neuropathies).

In disorders of nerve and muscle the EMG may demonstrate (1) changes in the motor unit potentials, (2) alternations in the recruitment of motor units on increased voluntary contraction, and (3) spontaneous muscle fiber activities at rest (whereas a normal EMG is entirely silent when the tested muscle is at rest). In myopathies, motor unit potentials are decreased in amplitude and are polyphasic because of the scattered loss of muscle fibers. In active denervation, as seen in acute and subacute axonal motor neuropathies, the remaining motor units may be normal. In chronic motor neuropathies, however, they become polyphasic, broadened, and of high amplitude because of reinnervation. Recruitment is prominent and rapid with low-level voluntary muscle contraction in myopathies but is diminished in neuropathies. A normal EMG is entirely silent when the muscle is at rest. Spontaneous fibrillation potentials and positive waves occur at rest in active denervation and in some necrotizing myopathies. Spontaneous fasciculations are most often present in motor neuron disease. Myotonic discharge sounding like a racing car when the audio is amplified represents muscle membrane instability and is characteristic of the myotonic disorders. The function of the neuromuscular junction can be studied by the repetitive stimulation of a motor nerve at various rates and by recording the motor response.

Clinical enzymology

Serum enzymes such as creatine phosphokinase (CPK), lactic dehydrogenase (LDH), serum glutamic-oxaloacetic transaminase (SGOT), and aldolase are increased in necrotizing myopathies, particularly in Duchenne type muscular dystrophy, polymyositis, and muscle necrosis associated with myoglobinuria. These sarcoplasmic enzymes are released from the muscle cells because of necrosis or leakage through the sarcolemma. In denervated muscle CPK is generally normal but may occasionally be mildly elevated. The level of CPK elevation helps differentiate Duchenne type muscular dystrophy, when it is very high, from other myopathies of young children. CPK is a particularly sensitive and specific enzyme for carrier detection in Duchenne type muscular dystrophy. A study of CPK isoenzymes can detect the origin of the enzyme (that is, muscle, heart, or brain).

PERIPHERAL NEUROPATHIES
Nutritional deficiencies

ALCOHOLIC NEUROPATHY. Alcoholic neuropathy is one of the most common neuropathies. Clinically, the patient has a painful and predominantly sensory symmetric polyneuropathy that may have a subacute or chronic course. Paresthesias of the feet are often very disturbing, and in advanced cases motor impairment with footdrop prevents successful ambulation. It is generally believed that alcoholic neuropathy is caused by nutritional deficiency. Recent evidence, however, suggests that alcohol itself may be neurotoxic. Vitamin replacement therapy rarely results in complete recovery.

VITAMIN B_{12} DEFICIENCY (PERNICIOUS ANEMIA). (See Chapters 61, 148, and 154.) Vitamin B_{12} deficiency affects the nervous system at several levels. Cerebral involvement results in dementia, spinal cord damage results in defective motor and sensory pathways (combined system disease), and peripheral nerve damage causes a symmetric motor and sensory neuropathy with prominent paresthesias. There is often a marked loss of vibration and position sense with upper motor neuron signs such as spasticity and increased reflexes. Folic acid therapy may improve the hematologic findings, but the neurologic manifestations continue or may even worsen. Vitamin B_{12} should be given parenterally and often results in a dramatic improvement within a few days.

OTHER NUTRITIONAL POLYNEUROPATHIES. Other nutritional polyneuropathies occur with pyridoxine and niacin deficiency. A peripheral neuropathy may also occur with the malabsorption syndrome.

Toxic and metabolic neuropathies

HEAVY METALS. Acute arsenic poisoning causes a rapidly progressive polyneuropathy and an acute encephalopathy. In more chronic arsenic toxicity a mixed sensory-motor peripheral neuropathy develops. The nails may show white tranverse lines (Mees' lines). Lead poisoning typically results in a pure motor neuropathy in the arms. Radial nerve palsy is common. Lead necephalopathy is common in children and rare in adults. Toxic levels of arsenic are best detected in the hair or nails, and toxic levels of lead are best detected in the serum and urine. These neuropathies are potentially reversible depending on the degree of damage. The source of toxic exposure should of course be eliminated. Dimercaprol treatment is used for both arsenic and lead poisoning. Penicillamine is particularly effective for the treatment of lead neuropathy.

ORGANIC COMPOUNDS. Various organic solvents, insecticides, and herbicides are neurotoxic. Triorthocresylphosphate and acrylamide may produce a mixed sensory-motor polyneuropathy. The pathologic changes are primarily those of axonal damage. These neuropathies are usually associated with industrial or accidental exposures. Glue sniffing (*n*-hexane) can result in a severe axonal neuropathy.

DRUG-INDUCED NEUROPATHIES. Anticonvulsants (phenytoin), chemotherapeutic agents (isoniazid, nitrofurantoin), and antimitotic drugs (vinca alkaloids, nitrogen mustard) may prdouce a chronic mixed sensory-motor neuropathy. Vitamin B_6 (pyridoxine) should always be given with isoniazid therapy because isoniazid interferes with pyridoxine metabolism. A severely painful, predominantly sensory polyneuropathy has been reported with the recreational abuse of nitrous oxide. Cases of nitrous oxide neuropathy have been found among dentists and dental technicians who are exposed to nitrous oxide in this way.

DIABETIC NEUROPATHY. Diabetes mellitus is one of the most common causes of neuropathy. There are three main clinical presentations. (1) The first is a distal, symmetric, predominantly sensory neuropathy that is primarily of the demyelinating type. Schwann cells are damaged by an ill-defined metabolic distrubance. The pathogenesis has not been clarified. Approximately 5% of all diabetic patients have a significant clinical neuropathy. A larger number have electrophysiologic abnormalities. The damage is greater with poorly controlled diabetes of long duration. (2) There may be a proximal acute mononeuropathy characterized by a painful motor deficit, particularly of the femoral or oculomotor nerve. An occlusion of the vasa nervorum is probably the cause of this form of neuropathy. (3) Autonomic neuropathy is the least common type but may be very disturbing to the patient. Impotence in males, diarrhea, and orthostatic hypotension are a result of autonomic dysfunction.

UREMIC NEUROPATHIES. Patients with chronic renal disease often have a predominantly sensory axonal polyneuropathy characterized by burning paresthesias. This neuropathy may develop or worsen in patients undergoing hemodialysis, although hemodialysis usually results in a modest benefit. Renal transplantation is usually beneficial. Objective neurologic improvement is often delayed many months. The pathogenesis remains uncertain.

ACUTE INTERMITTENT PORPHYRIA. Acute intermittent porphyria is a dominantly inherited metabolic disorder that is associated with decreased levels of urobilinogen I synthetase. It results in a proximal sensory-motor polyneuropathy, prominent emotional disturbances, constipation, abdominal pain, nausea, and vomiting. The neuropathy is of an axonal type. Acute attacks may be precipitated by barbiturates, alcohol, and sulfonamides.

OTHER METABOLIC NEUROPATHIES. Chronic mixed sensory-motor neuropathies occur in certain patients with hepatic cirrhosis, serum hepatitis, hypothyroidism, and hypoglycemia. Chronic polyneuropathies associated with paraproteinemias occur in patients with macroglobulinemia, lymphoproliferative disorders, multiple myeloma, and cryoglobulinemia.

Systemic disorders

POLYARTERITIS NODOSA. Of all patients with polyarteritis nodosa, 20% to 30% have peripheral nerve lesions, usually appearing as an acute mononeuritis multiplex. Necrotizing vasculitis involves the nutrient vessels of individual large nerves, resulting in actual nerve infarction. Later in the course of the disease, after many individual nerves have been damaged, the clinical manifestation is a distal symmetric sensory-motor neuropathy. The neuropathy of polyarteritis nodosa responds poorly to corticosteroid therapy.

RHEUMATOID NEUROPATHY. Four types of neuropathy are commonly seen in patients with seropositive rheumatoid arthritis. (1) Acute lesions of the major nerves of the upper and lower extremities comprise about 40% of all rheumatoid neuropathies. These lesions are the result of nerve compression by joint effusion or osteophytes. The lateral popliteal nerve at the fibular head is a common site. Local corticosteroid injection or surgical decompression is the preferred treatment. (2) An occlusion of the small digital arteries results in a digital neuropathy manifested by distal sensory loss in one finger. (3) A distal symmetric sensory polyneuropathy of insidious onset is seen less frequently and is attributed to a poorly defined metabolic process. (4) Distal symmetric mixed sensory-motor neuropathy is the least common type of rheumatoid neuropathies. This type is usually more severe and has a poor prognosis. Vasculitis is usually present on a tissue biopsy in patients with this neuropathy.

SYSTEMIC LUPUS ERYTHEMATOSUS. In systemic lupus erythematosus peripheral nerve lesions are relatively uncommon. A diffuse neuropathy may occur and a vascular occlusion of the vasa nervorum may produce a mononeuritis multiplex.

PRIMARY AMYLOIDOSIS. (See Chapter 76.) Primary amyloidosis may occur as a sporadic disease or as a familial disease. Besides the systemic manifestations of amyloidosis, the peripheral nerves are also frequently involved. Three main types of familial amyloidosis have been described: (1) the Andrade type, which is a peripheral neuropathy characterized by prominent pain with distal ulcer formation and prominent autonomic manifestations; (2) the Rukavina type, which is a progressive, distal, large fiber polyneuropathy; and (3) the Van Allen type, which is a painful, distal symmetric sensory-motor neuropathy. Neuropathy is rarely seen in secondary amyloidosis.

Infectious and parainfectious neuropathies

ACUTE IDIOPATHIC POSTINFECTIOUS POLYRADICULONEUROPATHY (GUILLAIN-BARRÉ SYNDROME)

Definition. This is an acute, monophasic polyneuropathy often following a nonspecific infectious process.

Etiology. More than 50% of patients have had a prior nonspecific infectious event, usually 10 to 14 days before the onset of the neuropathy. It has been suggested that sensitized lymphocytes produce the demyelination that characterizes this neuropathy. It is unclear, however, how these peripheral lymphocytes become sensitized. The participation of a humoral factor cannot be excluded. The basic mechanism is similar to that of a postviral encephalomyelitis.

Clinical manifestations. The neurologic illness usually starts with limb paresthesias. Occasionally patients have severe pain, particularly in the back and limbs. The most characteristic feature is weakness. In 50% of the patients weakness is diffuse from the onset, whereas in the other 50% it spreads upward from the lower limbs to sequentially involve the upper limbs, the respiratory muscles, and then the bulbar muscles in the most severe cases. The neuropathy usually peaks at 3 to 4 weeks. Tracheostomy and mechanical respiratory support are necessary in the most severe cases. The cerebrospinal fluid (CSF) findings are very helpful. The CSF protein level increases within a few weeks after the onset, but CSF cells remain normal. The EMG commonly shows a marked slowing of nerve conduction consistent with the demyelination. A nerve biopsy may reveal active demyelination and perivenular lymphocytic infiltration, but biopsy is rarely necessary to establish the diagnosis. Improvement usually starts within 5 to 6 weeks after the onset and continues slowly. The recovery period may be prolonged, lasting several months or even a few years. The mortality is about 10%. Most patients recover satisfactorily.

Management. During the acute phase the patient should be watched closely for respiratory impairment, which can develop quickly. Respiratory assistance should be instituted early. Proper positioning and passive stretching of the limbs are essential for preventing bedsores and contractures. The benefit of corticosteroid therapy has not been proved. The effect of plasmapheresis is under investigation.

IDIOPATHIC RECURRENT POLYNEUROPATHY. The first attack of idiopathic recurrent polyneuropathy may be similar to that of the Guillain-Barré syndrome. Its course is more subacute in evolution, however, and it reaches its maximal severity months after the onset. It is characterized by recurrent similar attacks spaced many months or even years apart. Patients with this neuropathy often respond well to steroid therapy or plasmapheresis.

DIPHTHERITIC NEUROPATHY. Demyelination caused by the diphtheria neurotoxin is usually delayed for 15 to 40 days after the onset of a pharyngitis. Paralysis often begins in the palate but then rapidly spreads to all the nerves, both motor and sensory. The patient may require a tracheostomy and artificial respiration. Recovery usually occurs rather quickly (within 15 to 30 days). With adequate immunization this neuropathy is rarely seen today.

LEPROSY. (See Chapter 50.) In lepromatous leprosy the skin lesion is the most dominant feature. The nerves, however, are frequently affected. The neuropathy, when it occurs, is distal, symmetric, and predominantly sensory. In the tuberculoid form there is a mononeuritis multiplex with severe anesthesia in the involved distribution.

HERPES ZOSTER (SHINGLES). (See the discussion of "Viral infections of the central nervous system" in Chapter 37.) This is a neurocutaneous manifestation of the varicellazoster virus. The patient usually has a severe girdle-like pain on one side lasting 3 or 4 days. This is followed by a vesicular eruption in the same dermatomal distribution. The virus is thought to remain dormant in the dorsal root ganglia for many years following an episode of varicella (chickenpox). The reactivation of the virus then leads to the clinical symptoms. Herpes zoster often occurs along with an underlying illness such as a tumor or in patients who have been immunosuppressed. The infection may spread to the spinal roots, the leptomeninges, and the spinal cord, producing muscle weakness and spasticity. Postherpetic neuralgia is one of the most difficult types of pain to control. Recent therapies include using membrane stablizers such as phenytoin or carbamazepine, transcutaneous nerve stimulation, and antidepressants.

Hereditary neuropathies

CHARCOT-MARIE-TOOTH DISEASE (PERONEAL MUSCULAR ATROPHY). This is the most commonly encountered hereditary neuropathy. Both autosomal dominant and recessive inheritance occurs, although the latter is infrequent. The disease may start in the first or second decade of life or later, with slowly progressive weakness and wasting in the distal legs. This results in a "reversed champagne bottle" appearance. The sensory involvement is considerably less than the motor deficit, but a decrease in position and vibration senses is usual. In the demyelinating form, enlarged peripheral nerves may become palpable. The EMG is characterized by a marked slowing of NCVs. A nerve biopsy reveals segmental demyelination and an onion-bulb formation that results from recurrent demyelination and remyelination. In the axonal form the NCVs may be relatively normal despite prominent muscular weakness.

HYPERTROPHIC NEUROPATHY (DEJERINE-SOTTAS DISEASE). This autosomal recessive neuropathy usually starts with progressive sensory and motor neuropathy in the first few years of life. There is a marked onion-bulb formation and severe segmental demyelination. The nerves are prominently enlarged.

HEREDITARY SENSORY NEUROPATHY. The hereditary sensory neuropathies are a group of progressive neuropathies that are characterized by the severe loss of various sensory modalities. Both dominant and recessive forms of inheritance are described. The clinical characteristics include distal ulcers and mutilation of the hands and feet.

REFSUM'S DISEASE. Refsum's disease is a metabolic neuropathy with increased serum levels of phytanic acid. Retinitis pigmentosa, ataxia, cutaneous lesions (ichthyosis), and a hypertrophic sensory-motor polyneuropathy develop. Improvement follows use of a special diet excluding phytols. Plasmapheresis has recently been reported to be effective.

Carcinomatous (paraneoplastic) neuropathies

Neoplasms can affect the peripheral nerves in a variety of ways. Neuropathies can result from a direct tumor infiltration or from compression, chemotherapeutic agents, or malnutrition. However, neuropathies unrelated to these definable causes (that is, paraneoplastic neuropathies) also are seen. Carcinomatous (paraneoplastic) neuropathy occurs in 4% to 5% of all cancer patients. Both a mixed sensory-motor axonal neuropathy and a pure sensory axonal neuropathy occur. The pure sensory axonal neuropathy is caused by degeneration of the dorsal root ganglia. Pulmonary, ovarian, breast, and stomach carcinomas are the major tumors found.

NEUROMUSCULAR JUNCTION DISORDERS
Myasthenia gravis

DEFINITION. Myasthenia gravis (MG), first described by Willis in 1792, is characterized by weakness and abnormal fatigability. It most commonly affects the facial, oculomotor, laryngeal, pharyngeal, and respiratory muscles. Partial recovery characteristically follows rest and therapy with anticholinesterase drugs.

ETIOLOGY. The fundamental abnormality in MG is at the neuromuscular junction. There is a reduction of acetylcholine (ACh) receptors on the muscle because of autoimmune damage. Elevated serum antibodies to the ACh receptor are found in most patients. The origin of the autoimmune process is still poorly understood. Of these patients 75% have thymic abnormalities with hyperplastic glands or an actual thymoma. The thymoma is rarely malignant. The role of the thymus in the pathogenesis is unclear, but it has been suggested that primitive myoid cells found in the gland serve as the initiating antigenic stimulus.

CLINICAL MANIFESTATIONS. The incidence of MG is approximately 1:20,000. The female to male ratio is 3:2. The most characteristic clinical features are pathologic fatigability and weakness, worsened by exertion and improved by rest. When first seen, 50% of these patients have ocular palsies, 33% have bulbar weakness, and 20% have limb muscle weakness. Ptosis and diplopia are common symptoms of ocular muscle involvement; in fact, MG may be limited to the ocular muscles. Facial weakness often produces a typical snarl expression when the patient smiles. The voice becomes nasal and indistinct. Severe respiratory distress is seen in the advanced stages. The limb weakness differs from that of other neuromuscular diseases by the abnormal fatigability and the absence of wasting. Fluctuations in the severity of the disease are common and occur unpredictably. The weakness may be intensified by an increasing dosage of anticholinesterase agents, aminoglycoside antibiotics, membrane stablizers (such as quinine, procainamide, and phenytoin), and infections. Intravenous edrophonium (Tensilon) in a test dose of 2 mg followed by 8 mg over 1 minute is used for diagnostic purposes. A rapid but temporary improvement of the weakness should result. A saline control should always be used.

LABORATORY FINDINGS. The repetitive stimulation of a motor nerve provides the most useful diagnostic information. The amplitude of the evoked muscle contraction declines with both slow and fast rates of stimulation. A newer method of single fiber EMG can be of diagnostic help. A roentgenogram and preferably a computed tomographic (CT) scan of the chest may demonstrate the presence of a thymoma. A muscle biopsy generally reveals nonspecific changes and is less useful. The ACh receptor antibody levels provide important evidence of autoimmunity and are helpful in establishing a diagnosis. Only a fair correlation exists between the severity of the illness and the titer of the ACh receptor antibody.

MANAGEMENT. The treatment consists of administering the anticholinesterase agents neostigmine (Prostigmin), 15 mg three times daily initially, or pyridostigmine (Mestinon), 60 mg three times daily initially, for early and mild cases. The dosage should be carefully adjusted to avoid excessive levels that might block the neuromuscular junction. Cortcosteroids suppress the autoimmune process, and their therapeutic benefit has been clearly demonstrated. A single-dose, alternate-day program is preferrred, using the smallest effective dosage. Early thymectomy is indicated for most patients. At least 75% of patients improve after a thymectomy, and many go into remission. Recently it has been demonstrated that plasmapheresis has a significant beneficial effect in controlling acute exacerbations of MG. Plasmapheresis has become an important addition to the therapeutic armamentarium of this disease.

Eaton-Lambert (myasthenic) syndrome

The Eaton-Lambert (myasthenic) syndrome is a unique and uncommon defect of neuromuscular transmission, occurring occasionally in association with small cell carcinoma of the lung and less frequently with other cancers. It also has been reported without any evidence of cancer. Men are affected more than women in a ratio of 5:1. The defect of the neuromuscular transmission is caused by a decreased number of ACh packets released at the presynaptic nerve terminals. Clinically, the weakness differs from that of MG in being particularly prominent soon after the patient arises in the morning. Exercise may help for a brief period. Patients often complain of a dry mouth. Deep tendon reflexes are usually absent. Repetitive nerve stimulation (10 to 50 Hz) produces a marked facilitation of the amplitude of the muscle contraction, which is in contrast to the declining amplitude seen in true MG. Treatment of the underlying cancer may result in improvement. Guanidine, which facilitates ACh release at the neuromuscular junction, is of benefit in some patients; 20 mg/kg of body weight is administered daily in three divided doses.

Botulism

(See the discussion of "Botulism" in Chapter 41.)

Botulism results from the ingestion of the exotoxin of *Clostridium botulinum*. The illness is characterized by progressive descending bulbar and skeletal muscle paralysis. Botulinum toxin is the most powerful poison known. It interferes with the release of ACh by blocking exocytosis at the motor nerve terminal.

The illness often starts with a blurring of vision, diplopia, and difficulty in chewing and swallowing. The weakness rapidly becomes generalized, and respiratory failure often develops quickly. Intensive respiratory care, including a tracheostomy and assisted respiration, is mandatory. The effectiveness of botulinum antitoxin has not yet been proved. Guanidine facilitates ACh release at the neuromuscular junction and is effective in certain patients; the dosage is 20 mg/kg of body weight daily in three divided doses.

DISORDERS OF MUSCLE
Muscular dystrophies

DEFINITION. The diagnosis of muscular dystrophy rests on clinical, genetic, and histologic features. It has been suggested that the term "muscular dystrophy" be reserved for cases of progressive, genetically determined, primary, degenerative myopathy. It has been further suggested that only X-linked types (Duchenne and Becker types) are clinically, genetically, pathologically, and biochemically homogeneous enough to warrant the term "dystrophy."

X-LINKED DYSTROPHIES

Duchenne type muscular dystrophy (DMD). This is the most uniform clinical entity among the muscle disorders. The disease, when inherited, is transmitted by a defective

X chromosome in the asymptomatic female carrier. It is clinically expressed only in males. About one third of cases of DMD, however, appear to be caused by spontaneous mutations and are not inherited. The incidence of DMD has been estimated at from 20 to 30:100,000 liveborn males. The incidence in the general population is approximately 3:100,000.

Pathogenesis. The pathogenesis of DMD has not been elucidated. Recent hypotheses have suggested (1) a decreased intramuscular blood flow leading to muscle necrosis, (2) an altered neural control, and (3) underlying defects in the muscle fiber membrane wherein increased calcium inside the muscle cell leads to poorly regulated muscle contraction and subsequent degeneration.

Clinical manifestations. The patient becomes symptomatic at 2 to 4 years of age with clumsiness, weakness, and occasional falling. He often walks on his toes because of heel cord contractures. He has pseudohypertrophy, particularly of the calves, with accentuated lumbar lordosis. He requires increasing amounts of hand support to arise to an upright posture (Gowers' sign).

The disease progresses inexorably, confining the patient to a wheelchair at 9 to 11 years of age. At this stage scoliosis and multiple contractures ensue, and respiratory difficulty develops. Patients inevitably die by their late twenties.

The ocular muscles are rarely involved. Verbal intelligence is often impaired. Most patients have cardiomyopathy but become symptomatic only in its late stages.

Laboratory findings. The serum CPK determination is one of the most valuable tests for DMD. Before the patient is 10 years of age, the serum CPK level is dramatically elevated, often more than 200-fold. Usually the CPK level falls later in life and may approach normal by the time the patient is 20 years of age. In fact, a significant CPK elevation is a prerequisite for the diagnosis of DMD before the patient is 10 years of age. The electrocardiogram shows a tall R wave in the anterior precordial leads in about 70% of patients. The EMG shows the classic changes of myopathy. A muscle biopsy reveals large hyalinized muscle fibers, groups of regenerating fibers, profound connective and fat tissue proliferation, and other myopathic features.

Carrier detection. All families should receive genetic counseling. The serum CPK level is the most sensitive indicator of the carrier state. It tends to fall, however, after patients are 20 years of age. Carrier detection therefore should be carried out early. Attempts to identify an affected male fetus prenatally have been unsuccessful. Prenatal sex determination, however, can often be of help to a pregnant carrier.

Management. At the present time DMD is an incurable disease. Incurable and untreatable are not synonymous terms, however, and much can be done to make the life of these patients more rewarding and comfortable. Proper management is best carried out by a team consisting of the neurologist, pediatrician, orthopedic surgeon, physiotherapist, occupational therapist, and social worker. Supportive therapy has prolonged a useful life into the third decade in many instances.

Becker type muscular dystrophy. This is milder form of dystrophy that also is inherited as an X-linked recessive trait. The clinical signs and symptoms are much less severe than with DMD, and patients survive well into adult life.

FACIOSCAPULOHUMERAL (FSH) MUSCULAR DYSTROPHY. This is an autosomal dominant disorder of multiple pathologic types. The affected patient becomes symptomatic by the end of the first decade or during the second decade of life. Facial weakness usually appears first. Gradually a weakness of the upper arms and shoulders develops; later the weakness may involve the hip muscles. The neck and shoulder muscles become atrophied, but the trapezius muscle is preserved. Scapular winging is prominent. The muscles of the upper arms are atrophied out of proportion to those of the forearms. Some features are only minimally expressed, and spontaneous arrest occurs in certain patients. The laboratory investigation should include serum enzyme studies, EMG, and a muscle biopsy. The CPK concentration may be slightly elevated but is more often normal. The muscle biopsy may show various types of abnormality, including inflammation, denervation, lipid storage, or necrotizing myopathy, in patients with identical clinical deficits.

LIMB-GIRDLE MUSCULAR DYSTROPHY. In this autosomal recessive condition weakness involves the proximal muscles of all limbs and the muscles of the shoulder and hip girdles. The condition is pathologically heterogeneous. The CPK concentration may be slightly elevated but is more often normal. Identical clinical manifestations occur with anterior horn cell disease (spinal muscular atrophy), storage diseases, metabolic diseases, and mitochondrial myopathies.

OCULAR MYOPATHY AND OCULOPHARYNGEAL DYSTROPHY. In these conditions ptosis is the first symptom and progresses insidiously with or without an external ophthalmoplegia. Later, proximal muscle weakness may occur in the arms or even in the legs. In ocular myopathy the symptoms begin in early adulthood and the inheritance is autosomal dominant.

Oculopharyngeal dystrophy occurs with high frequency in patients of French-Canadian extraction. This condition begins in late adult life with slowly progressive ptosis and dysphagia. It is almost always inherited as an autosomal dominant trait. Yet another group of disorders, termed "ophthalmoplegia plus," is characterized by ophthalmoplegia, myopathy, heart block, retinal pigmentary changes, and central nervous system dysfunction. Many patients with these disorders have mitochondrial abnormalities detected by muscle biopsy. The pathogenesis of these conditions is unclear, and the classification is unsettled. The **CPK** concentration infrequently is slightly elevated in the **ocular** myopathies.

Inflammatory myopathies

POLYMYOSITIS AND RELATED CONDITIONS. Polymyositis is characterized by a noninfectious, nonsuppurative inflammation of the striated muscle (polymyositis) and the skin (dermatomyositis). Progressive muscle weakness is the paramount sign (see Chapter 19 for details).

POLYMYALGIA RHEUMATICA. This condition occurs almost exclusively in patients over 60 years of age. Females are affected twice as often as males. The chief symptoms consist of severe, proximal muscle pains and stiffness without weakness. Approximately 20% of patients with polymyalgia rheumatica also have a temporal arteritis that may result in acute blindness. Almost all patients have a very high erythrocyte sedimentation rate. If there is any hint of temporal arteritis, a temporal artery biopsy may be helpful and corticosteroids should be administered. The EMG and muscle biopsy findings are normal (see Chapter 23 for details).

TRICHINOSIS. Muscle infestation with the larvae of *Trichinella spiralis* produces severe muscle pain and frequently weakness. Early symptoms consist of periorbital edema or a skin rash with petechiae. Pain while attempting to open the jaw or with chewing is common because of the masseter muscle involvement. Eosinophilia is characteristic. The muscle biopsy reveals numerous larvae and inflammation (see Chapter 55 for details).

Metabolic myopathies

HYPOTHYROID MYOPATHY. In adults hypothyroidism is associated with a slowness of movement, cramps, muscle hypertrophy, and weakness. In congenital cretinism the infant may appear robust, but the muscle is actually hypotonic and weak. Myoedema (mounding of the muscle on percussion) and a delayed relaxation of the muscle stretch reflex are commonly present.

MALIGNANT HYPERPYREXIA OR MALIGNANT HYPERTHERMIA. Malignant hyperpyrexia or hyperthermia is a rare but potentially fatal condition triggered by anesthesia. It occurs in 1:14,000 to 75,000 patients who undergo anesthesia. When inherited, it is transmitted as an autosomal dominant trait. Patients may have signs of myopathy such as muscle hypertrophy, lumbar lordosis, mild hip weakness, and percussion myotonia. On exposure to anesthetic agents, particularly halothane and succinylcholine, the patient demonstrates fasciculations and increased muscle tone, particularly of the masseter muscle. Jaw clenching during the induction of anesthesia is a typical early sign. The body muscles become rigid, and excessive body heat is produced. Marked lactic acidosis develops.

The anesthesia should be discontinued, oxygen should be administered, and the patient should be cooled. Intravenous dantrolene sodium has a therapeutic effect. Renal failure can occur as a result of massive myoglobinuria.

PERIODIC PARALYSES

Definition. The periodic paralyses are characterized by episodes of weakness usually associated with alterations of serum potassium levels. These attacks of weakness are classified according to whether the serum potassium level is low or high during an attack. The so-called normokalemic periodic paralysis is most likely a variant of hyperkalemic periodic paralysis.

Hypokalemic periodic paralysis. In this disorder the serum potassium level may be as low as 1.5 mEq/L during an attack. The weakness affects the limb and trunk muscles but not the respiratory, bulbar, or ocular muscles. The inheritance is autosomal dominant. Attacks usually begin in the second decade of life. Rest after exercise or after heavy carbohydrate meals may precipitate an attack. Potassium salts, in doses of 5 to 10 g of oral potassium chloride, and terminate an attack. Acetazolamide, 250 mg or more daily as needed, is the preferred therapy for prevention.

Hyperkalemic periodic paralysis. This is also autosomal dominant in its form of inheritance. Attacks of weakness begin shortly after exercise and are generally brief compared to those in the hypokalemic form. There is often a symptomatic myotonia that is best demonstrated by a slowness of eye opening after tight closure. The serum potassium level may be elevated or normal during an attack. Acute attacks usually require no treatment. Acetazolamide is effective prophylactically in this form of periodic paralysis.

GLYCOGEN STORAGE DISEASE

Acid maltase deficiency (glycogenosis type II). Acid maltase is a lysosomal enzyme that splits the terminal glucose from glycogen. Its absence results in a marked glycogen accumulation in the lysosome and in the sarcoplasm. The infantile form of acid maltase deficiency is the most severe. Generalized glycogen accumulation, cardiopulmonary failure, and severe generalized weakness result in early death. The later infantile and juvenile forms may resemble muscular dystrophy, and their courses are more benign. Adult-onset acid maltase deficiency may mimic limb-girdle muscular dystrophy or polymyositis. Acid maltase deficiency is autosomal recessive in its inheritance.

McArdle's disease (glycogenosis type V). The enzyme myophosphorylase that degrades glycogen in anaerobic glycolysis is defective in this muscle disease. Typical clinical manifestations include postexertional muscle cramps and myoglobinuria. The patient usually becomes symptomatic in the second decade of life. The failure of lactic acid to rise with ischemic exercise is a diagnostic indicator, as is an absence of phosphorylase detected with histochemical studies. Similar clinical manifestations are seen in fructokinase deficiency (glycogenosis type VII).

LIPID STORAGE DISEASES

Carnitine deficiency myopathy. This disorder is caused by a deficiency of carnitine that helps transfer fatty acids into the mitochondria for β-oxidation. Patients have slowly progressive proximal muscle weakness. A biopsy shows increased fat droplets in the muscle fibers. Because of the hepatic involvement there is no ketone production during fasting. A biochemical analysis of muscle carnitine is required to confirm the diagnosis.

Carnitine palmityl transferase (CPT) deficiency. CPT is an enzyme that facilitates oxidative metabolism of fatty acids. In this myopathy, postexertional muscle cramps and myoglobinuria are typical symptoms. A muscle biopsy shows no significant fat accumulation, unlike carnitine deficiency, and often is normal.

ALCOHOLIC MYOPATHIES

Acute alcoholic myopathy is characterized by muscle tenderness, rhabdomyolysis, and myoglobinuria and occurs along with both high blood alcohol levels and acute protein depletion and vitamin depletion. Acute renal tubular necrosis may be a serious complication. Chronic alcoholic myopathy occurs infrequently and is largely related to malnutrition. It is characterized by proximal muscle weakness, particularly in the legs. In acute alcoholic myopathy, muscle enzyme levels may be elevated 300-fold, whereas in the chronic form they may be elevated only threefold to fourfold.

Myotonic disorders

MYOTONIC DYSTROPHY

This is an autosomal dominant disease characterized by myotonia, distal muscle wasting, cataracts, testicular atrophy, and other polysystemic abnormalities. The cause is unknown, but recent evidence suggests a generalized membrane abnormality.

The incidence is estimated at 3 to 5:100,000. Myotonic dystrophy becomes symptomatic in adolescence or early adult life. The patient's face is expressionless, and there are temporal muscle wasting and frontal balding. Myotonia can be elicited with direct percussion or with the voluntary contraction of the muscle. The EMG shows typical myotonic discharges with myopathic changes. Besides the neuromuscular abnormalities the patient has cataracts, testicular atrophy, abnormal glucose tolerance, cardiac conduction blocks, and pulmonary hypoventilation. Myotonic dystrophy may appear in neonates born to affected mothers. Prominent signs are severe hypotonia and facial paralysis. The myotonia is mild.

The muscle histologic findings are characterized by type I (high-oxidative) fiber atrophy and marked central nucleation. The treatment is with membrane stabilizers such as quinine, procainamide, and especially phenytoin. Genetic counseling is very important to prevent unwanted affected offspring.

MYOTONIA CONGENITA (THOMSEN'S DISEASE)

This also is transmitted as an autosomal dominant trait. The muscles are stiff, but with continued exercise they loosen and movement becomes almost normal. Muscle hypertrophy may be present, but weakness does not occur. Exposure to cold makes the symptoms worse. The Becker type of myotonia congenita is autosomal recessive in its inheritance, and muscle wasting and weakness may occur.

Congenital myopathies

The congenital myopathies are characterized clinically by hypotonia and a slowly progressive proximal weakness with or without a family history. They are a pathologically heterogeneous group. Peculiar structural alterations of the muscle have been observed.

CONGENITAL FIBER TYPE DISPROPORTION

The type I muscle fibers are less numerous and smaller than type II (low-oxidative) fibers. This condition is occasionally inherited as an autosomal dominant trait. One third of the patients have congenital hip dislocation. Weakness may improve or worsen with time.

CENTRAL CORE DISEASE

The weakness in this disorder usually progresses slowly throughout life. Mitochondria and oxidative enzyme activity are deficient in the center of the muscle fiber, and the central portion of the muscle fiber is abnormal histologically. Skeletal deformities are a result of the early onset of the muscle disease. Malignant hyperthermia has been reported in some patients with central core disease.

NEMALINE MYOPATHY

This congenital myopathy is characterized by the presence of small, rodlike inclusions in the oxidative (type I) muscle fibers. There may be type I fiber predominance and atrophy. The rods are composed of α-actinin similar to Z-band material. Both inherited and sporadic cases have been described. Adult-onset nemaline myopathy has been reported.

CENTRONUCLEAR (MYOTUBULAR) MYOPATHY

The term "myotubular" refers to the similarity of these fibers to fetal myotubes. The nuclei are central rather than peripheral in location. The inheritance varies. There may be extraocular muscle involvement, cardiopulmonary failure, and EEG abnormalities.

Myoglobinuria

Myoglobin is the reddish brown respiratory pigment that helps transport oxygen from the blood to the muscle fiber. A breakdown of the muscle fiber results in the release of myoglobin into the serum. Excessive myoglobin in the serum may produce renal tubular necrosis and renal failure.

PRIMARY MYOGLOBINURIA

Primary myoglobinuria is a myoglobinuria of unknown cause, often precipitated by sepsis or exercise. Apparently, myoglobinuria may occur in otherwise normal people after unusually exhausting exercise.

SECONDARY MYOGLOBINURIA

Metabolic myopathies such as McArdle's disease, phosphofructokinase deficiency, and carnitine palmityl transferase deficiency often appear with postexertional myoglobinuria. In malignant hyperthermia massive myoglobinuria may occur. Other causes of myoglobinuria include a crush injury, excessive long-term ethanol intake, a lightning injury, and drug reactions.

A striking elevation of serum muscle enzymes almost always accompanies myoglobinuria. In cases of severe myoglobinuria, renal function should be carefully monitored. Diuresis should be maintained with fluid replacement, diuretics, and mannitol, and the urine should be kept alkaline.

DISORDERS OF THE SPINAL ROOTS, BRACHIAL PLEXUS, AND SPINAL CORD
General signs and symptoms

SPINAL ROOTS. Damage to the spinal anterior (ventral) root results in segmental weakness, whereas posterior spinal root damage produces dermatomal sensory loss of all modalities and radicular pain in the same distribution. An examination reveals weakness and wasting only in the muscles belonging to the root in question with a corresponding sensory loss. This specific distribution of the muscle weakness and sensory change can distinguish a root lesion from a plexus or nerve lesion. When multiple roots are involved, however, localization becomes difficult. In such situations the EMG becomes an important ancillary test.

SPINAL CORD. Damage to the spinal cord produces a loss of neuron function at the level of the lesion, resulting in paralysis and atrophy of the muscles in the territory of the damaged motor neurons. Sensory function is also lost in the territory of the dermatome belonging to the segment of the lesion. The lesion also interrupts the ascending and descending spinal cord tracts. Damage to the ascending tracts results in a loss of sensation of all modalities below the level of the lesion. Damage to the descending tracts (corticospinal tracts) produces a paralysis followed by spasticity and pathologic reflexes below the level of the lesion. Sphincter disturbances result from interrupted descending tracts controlling the bladder and bowel. The signs vary depending on the size of lesion, whether it is intrinsic or extrinsic, and the rapidity of damage. For example, a small tumor arising in the center of the cervical spinal cord at the fifth segmental level (C5) produces a loss of cutaneous sensation in the fifth cervical dermatome. If the lesion is larger, the muscles belonging to the nerve roots at this level become weak and atrophied. Fasciculations may appear. When the lesion is even larger, the white matter fiber tracts are affected. The muscles below the level of the fifth cervical spinal segment become spastic with brisk and pathologic reflexes. A sensory examination in the early stages may show only a loss of sensation in the legs because of the topographic arrangement of the nerve fibers. Later sensory loss is complete below the fifth cervical level (C5) of the spinal cord.

Specific disorders

DEGENERATIVE VERTEBRAL OSTEOARTHRITIS (SPONDYLOSIS). Common neurologic sequelae of spondylosis include shoulder and neck pain (cervical spondylosis) and low back pain (lumbosacral spondylosis). There may be no objective neurologic deficit in the early stages. In advanced spondylosis neurologic damage may occur. Compression of the spinal roots at the intervertebral foramen and of the spinal cord because of narrowing of the spinal canal are major complications. Root compression produces radicular pain, muscle weakness, and wasting in the territory of the root. Spinal cord compression occurs most commonly at the cervical level and produces slow progressive spastic paraparesis (spondylitic cervical myelopathy). A narrowing of the spinal canal at the lumbosacral level results in lumbosacral canal stenosis, causing intermittent exercise-induced leg pain. When physical therapy and other conservative measures do not help and neurologic deficits are progressive, surgical decompression is indicated.

DISC DISEASE. When the intervertebral disc undergoes degenerative changes, its soft nucleus pulposus may extrude and compress the nerve root laterally. It also may compress the spinal cord anteriorly at the cervical and thoracic levels. Disc herniation is often a result of sudden or excessive movement in the cervical or lumbar regions. Severe radicular pain develops in the distribution of the compressed root. The nerve roots most commonly compressed are the fifth and sixth cervical roots, the fifth lumbar root, and the first sacral root. Stretching the lumbar and sacral nerve roots by straight leg raising or increasing spinal canal pressure by sneezing may precipitate severe radicular pain. The diagnosis of disc disease can be confirmed by myelography. Conservative treatment consists of prescribing bed rest, analgesics, and traction for cervical radiculopathy. When conservative measures are unsuccessful, surgical treatment is often necessary.

SPINAL CORD TUMOR. Expanding lesions within the spinal canal can compress the nerve roots and spinal cord. The most common intramedullary tumor is a glioma. Intraspinal extramedullary tumors also produce a compression of the spinal roots and the spinal cord. These tumors include schwannomas, neurofibromas, and meningiomas. Epidural masses may be associated with the bony destruction of the adjacent vertebral bone and are commonly caused by metastatic carcinoma. Lymphoma may produce an epidural mass without any bony destruction. A sudden onset of paraplegia, fever, and localized tenderness over the spinal column suggests an epidural abscess. Cauda equina lesions may be caused by tumors or herniated discs. Sphincter disturbances are common with these masses.

BRACHIAL PLEXOPATHY (NEURALGIC AMYOTROPHY). This is an unusual neuropathy involving only the brachial plexus. It may occur in association with infection, trauma, immunization, or surgery. Males are four times more frequently affected than females. Occasionally familial occurrence is seen. The cause is unknown. The disease is characterized by a severe pain in one or both shoulders that may last for 1 day to 3 months. Motor symptoms occur, and the affected muscle rapidly becomes paralyzed and atrophied. One cord of the brachial plexus or a single nerve root may be involved. The patient usually recovers function in 6 months to 2 years.

BIBLIOGRAPHY

Bradley, W.G.: Disorders of peripheral nerves, Oxford, Eng., 1974, Blackwell Scientific Publications.

Brooke, M.H.: A clinician's view of neuromuscular diseases, Baltimore, 1976, The Williams & Wilkins Co.

Drachman, D.B.: Myasthenia gravis, N. Engl. J. Med. **298:**136, 1978.

Dyck, P.J., Thomas, P.K., and Lambert, E.H., editors: Peripheral neuropathy, Philadelphia, 1975, W. B. Saunders Co.

Merritt, H.H.: A textbook of neurology, Philadelphia, 1979, Lea & Febiger.

Munsat, T.L.: The classification of human myopathies. In Vinken, P.J., and Bruyn, G.W., editors: Handbook of clinical neurology, vol. 40, Amsterdam, 1979, Elsevier North-Holland Inc.

Simpson, F.A.: Myasthenia gravis and myasthenic syndromes. In Walton, J.N., editor: Disorders of voluntary muscle, London, 1974, Churchill Livingstone Inc.

DENTAL CORRELATIONS

Vernon J. Brightman

SLEEP DISORDERS
Nocturnal bruxism

Excessive and repeated contraction of the masticatory muscles with nonfunctional grinding and clenching of the teeth is a frequently observed phenomenon that is considered to be an important etiologic factor in periodontal disease, excessive tooth wear, pulpal involvement, fracture of restorations, and temporomandibular joint myofascial dysfunction. It may be observed during waking hours or while sleeping. However, the intensity of the contractions during sleep and their association with a specific phase of the sleep cycle strongly suggest that nocturnal bruxism is a separate entity from that experienced during the waking hours.

Nocturnal bruxism occurs only in association with REM sleep and usually accompanies movements of the limbs and periods of increased heart rate. REM sleep represents a state of partial arousal, as may occur with dreaming. If dreaming occurs, however, the subject's recollection of the dream does not include awareness of jaw movement. Usually, the patient is unaware of nocturnal bruxism and attention is drawn to it by a spouse or parent. Like other phenomena associated with REM sleep, nocturnal bruxism may be instigated by any stimulus that disturbs sleep, whether it be external, internal, physical, or emotional.

Nocturnal bruxism occurs in about 5% of the population with prevalence as high as 15% among students. A familial distribution of affected individuals has been recorded, suggesting a genetic predisposition. It is often a transient and inconsistent phenomenon and may disappear entirely. There is no evidence to associate psychologic abnormality or brain lesions with nocturnal bruxism, and the sleep EMG records of affected individuals are normal.

Alcohol has been implicated as an important stimulus of nocturnal bruxism. Alcohol may act as a stimulant for the reticular activating system rather than as a central nervous system depressant. As few as one or two cocktails in the evening will result in a fourfold increase in the frequency of nocturnal bruxism and an even greater increase in the length of time the patient grinds and clenches. On the average periods of nocturnal bruxism last only 9 seconds, but they recur during periods of REM sleep to occupy on the average 40 seconds/hour of sleep. Characteristically, the intensity of masseter muscle contraction during a period of nocturnal bruxism results in a noise level that cannot be achieved by conscious activity.

There are no specific treatments for this problem, and the majority of recommended treatments have not been tested in a sleep laboratory, which is essential for the study of nocturnal bruxism. A full-arch maxillary occlusal splint (night guard), when tested under these conditions, will reduce the level of nocturnal masseter electromyographic activity in about 50% of patients, and it is an effective treatment modality for some patients with this problem.

Sleep apnea syndrome

In patients with sleep apnea syndrome considered to be secondary to upper airway obstruction, investigation of the possibility that mandibular retrognathism is the cause of the obstruction should be considered. Such obstruction may be secondary to mandibular fractures, ankylosis of the temporomandibular joint, or developmental malposition of the mandible. A number of cases in which surgical correction of mandibular retrognathism with elimination of airway obstruction has led to cure of the sleep apnea syndrome have been described in the dental literature in recent years.

Sleep disturbance associated with depression

Unrecognized and untreated depression not uncommonly complicates the diagnosis and treatment of a number of dental problems and causes otherwise unexplained oral symptoms such as burning tongue, dysgeusia, and atypical facial pain. While not specific for depression, disturbances of sleep pattern are often a major concern to many of these patients and may be the first clue to the dentist to consider psychiatric abnormality in the differential diagnosis of an oral complaint. Disturbances of sleep patterns are often sufficiently distressing, particularly to older patients, that they will accept psychiatric consultation even when they reject this as a causative factor.

BIBLIOGRAPHY

Bear, S.E., and others: Sleep apnea syndrome: correction with surgical advancement of the mandible, Oral Surg. **38**:543, 1980.

Brightman, V.J.: Oral symptoms without apparent physical abnormality. In Lynch, M.A., editor: Burket's oral medicine, ed. 7, Philadelphia, 1977, J.B. Lippincott Co., pp. 343-368.

Robinson, J.E., and others: Nocturnal teeth-grinding: a reassessment for dentistry, J. Am. Dent. Assoc. **78**:1308, 1969.

Suzuki, J.B.: Etiology of parafunction: a brief review of psychological and occlusal genesis, Periodont. Abst. **27**:48,1979.

ALCOHOLISM AND DRUG ABUSE

Habitual use of alcohol, "hard drugs" (heroin and other opiate derivatives, cocaine, amphetamines, tranquilizers, LSD, phencyclidine), and other commonly abused substances (sleeping pills, antidepressants, nitrous oxide, nitrites, and other inhalants) may be associated with persisting behavioral and mood changes, as well as specific oral and systemic pathologic changes. Both the behavioral and the tissue changes can be of considerable significance in the dental treatment of these patients.

A variety of psychotic and unpredictable behaviors are seen in association with drug and other substance abuse, often reflecting underlying behavioral problems that become more prominent with drug use, as well as more direct CNS effects of the drugs themselves. While it is unwise, therefore, to speak of characteristic alcoholic and drug abuse personalities, awareness of the following traditional patterns of behavior can be of help to the dentist who encounters these problems. Abusive, boisterous, and physical behavior is commonly accepted as standard in an intoxicated alcoholic, as is the alcoholic's frequently repeated intention to stop drinking and "do better." The apparently compliant, repentent alcoholic is also common and can lead the unwary dentist into planning lengthy treatment, even when there is clear evidence of consistent dental neglect. Failure to keep appointments; elaborate explanations for not undertaking dental treatment or home care; garrulous, argumentative, or obtunded behavior; and consistent alcoholic odor to the breath can be useful clues to alcohol habituation.

The dentist must also be aware of the narcotic addict who uses dental pain as an excuse for obtaining additional drugs. While it may be difficult to withhold a narcotic prescription when an obviously painful dental infection is present, usually prescribed doses of Percodan or other opiate derivatives may be relatively ineffective for the habituated or addicted patient. Paradoxic responses to opiate derivatives are also common, these medications making some individuals less able to handle dental pain. Addictive behavior should be suspected when a patient persistently defers definitive dental or surgical treatment and repeatedly consults one or several dentists for a prescription for control of dental pain, "just until he has a chance to get the tooth treated." Elaborate and quite convincing ruses are devised by addicts to obtain prescriptions for narcotics and other abused substances, and the dentist should be wary of the patient who is "just moving into the neighborhood but doesn't yet have an address," the patient whose doctor "usually prescribes a narcotic prescription but is unfortunately away," or the patient with atypical, chronic, and unexplicable jaw pain that "requires" continuous narcotics. Drug addiction is seen in all classes of society, and some of the more elaborate ruses are perpetrated by physicians, nurses, and dentists on their colleagues.

Burglary of dental offices for drugs and prescription forms still occurs, and the dentist who maintains prescription blanks with a preprinted narcotic license number or even limited stocks of barbiturates or narcotics is particularly liable in this regard. Theft and employee abuse of nitrous oxide cylinders also occur. Finally, the addict experiencing withdrawal symptoms may select a dental office as a likely place for both drugs and cash and seek to obtain them by means of armed assault.

Numerous publications in recent years have documented the effects of narcotic addiction on the oral cavity. Rampant dental caries, especially involving the gingival third region as an indolent hard brown lesion, is described in heroin addicts and may be related to opiate-induced xerostomia. Poor oral hygiene is characteristic as well and contributes to both rampant caries and gingival and periodontal disease, including acute necrotizing ulcerative gingivitis. Excessive occlusal wear and other evidences of grinding are common and probably relate to central effects of drugs, a similar phenomenon occurring in response to alcohol ingestion (see section on nocturnal bruxism).

Maxillofacial trauma is common in addicts and alcoholics and frequently brings them to the attention of the oral surgeon and hospital dental service. Neurotic behavior regarding oral hygiene and dental treatment may also be seen in the addict, for whom loss of a tooth, an oral infection, or even a carious cavity may produce intolerable pain or inappropriate concern about dental health. Diminished smell and taste sensation often occur, particularly as a result of sniffing cocaine or volatile chemicals or as a result of CNS damage from alcohol and a variety of other abused toxic substances; these symptoms and other oral sensory disturbances may be presenting problems for the dentist.

The dentist must also be aware of numerous systemic disease problems that occur commonly in alcoholics and drug addicts. Toxic damage to the liver from continued alcohol abuse leads to cirrhosis, which if severe may seriously compromise the formation of intrinsic blood coagulation factors and predispose the patient to hemorrhage following dental surgery. These deficiencies may or may not be reversed by administration of vitamin K. Decreased detoxification of estrogens in the compromised liver may result in the formation of spider telangiectases on the skin, which should be distinguished from petechial hemorrhages due to platelet deficiency that also can occur as a result of the toxic effect of alcohol on the red bone marrow. Hypoalbuminemia and anemia due to toxic effects of alcohol on the liver and bone marrow or to an associated nutritional deficiency may occur and complicate hospital management and the administration of general anesthetic agents. Obstructive pulmonary disease occurs with prolonged heroin abuse and may be the basis of dyspnea and wheezing in these individuals, who usually have abnormal pulmonary function tests but often normal auscultatory and radiographic chest examinations. The nephrotic syndrome (with raised BUN, proteinuria, and generalized edema) and cardiac arrhythmias and conduction defects are also described in association with narcotic addition.

Administration of general anesthetic to the narcotic addict and the alcoholic pose special problems relating to premedication and withdrawal of the abused drugs and substitution of a defined purified medication (such as methadone or diazepam) that will serve to control any withdrawal symptoms and also provide adequate preanesthetic sedation. Hypotension and respiratory depression secondary to narcotic abuse also render general anesthesia more hazardous and, along with concerns regarding additional liver toxicity, emphasize the need for careful selection of anesthetic agent and adequate monitoring of blood pressure and respiration. The postoperative period also requires special management to control pain and establish methadone maintenance without significant withdrawal problems.

Intravenous administration of abused substances allows the introduction of a variety of infectious and toxic substances that further complicate management of the addict. Hepatitis B infection, often with chronic active hepatitis and persistently positive hepatitis B_s antigenemia, and bacterial endocarditis are notable problems in this regard that must be considered by the dentist both for personal protection (hepatitis) and for protection of the patient (endocarditis) when extractions and other oral surgical procedures are involved. Transmission of miscellaneous other infectious agents has been traced to use of contaminated "street" drugs, which are often diluted with unknown foreign materials to increase their sales value. This problem is not restricted to "mainlining"; a recent epidemic of salmonellosis, for example, was traced to contaminated marijuana. The peculiar epidemic of hepatitis B, Kaposi's sarcoma, and cytomegalovirus infections documented in a number of male homosexual communities and thought to be associated with an immune deficiency has also been associated with abuse of nitrites and other drugs by members of these communities.

Nitrous oxide, widely used as a gaseous analgesic and anesthetic in dentistry, is probably the most commonly abused anesthetic gas, due partly to its ready availability in dental offices, hospitals, and industrial situations (and at one time in households, as a propellant for whipped cream) and partly to the mistaken belief that it is harmless when inhaled with adequate oxygen. Repeated and heavy abuse of this substance, however, has been associated with the development of a characteristic type of myeloneuropathy, and access to nitrous oxide machines and gas lines by unauthorized personnel should be strictly controlled. Reports of similar problems in dentists and dental personnel who have habitually used nitrous oxide as a relaxant further emphasize the potential for abuse of anesthetic agents.

Of primary concern in recent years has been the recognition that patterns of habituation and addiction often involve more than one abused substance. The importance of taking histories of other drug use in alcoholics cannot be overemphasized, since more than 20% of alcoholics in recent surveys commonly abuse a number of substances in addition to alcohol. Mutual potentiation of the various substances usually occurs, and it has been estimated that alcohol used in combination with other drugs accounts for over 20% of drug-related accidental and suicidal deaths each year. This problem of multiple drug abuse, which has been highlighted by the U.S. Surgeon-General in recent years, also includes unrestricted and incautious prescription of sedatives, hypnotics, narcotics, antidepressants, tranquilizers, and antihistamines to patients who also habitually consume alcohol. It is important that the dentist who prescribes drugs in these categories also take an adequate history of alcohol use, review the package insert for known drug interactions, restrict the quantities of drugs prescribed, and estimate the likelihood patients will comply with warnings regarding potentiation of the drug's effects by alcohol and restrict their consumption while using the prescribed drugs.

Methods for detecting and quantitating the more commonly abused substances present in blood and urine have been developed, and these procedures are readily available at minimal cost from most diagnostic laboratories providing toxicologic assays, usually by means of gas chromatographic and mass spectrophotometric procedures. Confirmation of suspected drug abuse and monitoring of blood levels are therefore possible and often desirable before major surgery and general anesthesia.

BIBLIOGRAPHY

Foltz, R.L., and others: GC/MS assays for abused drugs in body fluids, Natl. Inst. Drug Abuse Res. Monogr. Series **32**:1, 1980.

Gotta, A.W, and others: Anesthetic management of the narcotic addict. I. Pre-operative evaluation, J. Hosp. Dent. Pract. **11**(3); 13,1977.

Gotta, A.W., and others: Anesthetic management of the narcotic addict. II. Intra-operative and post-operative care, J. Hosp. Dent. Pract. **12**(1); 17, 1978.

Gutmann, L., and others: Nitrous oxide-induced myelopathy-neuropathy: potential for chronic misuse by dentists, J. Am. Dent. Assoc. **98**:58, 1979.

Jaffe, L., and Schuckit, M.A.: The importance of drug use histories in a series of alcoholics, J. Clin. Psychiatry **42**:224, 1981.

Layzer, R.B., Fishman, R.A., and Schafer, J.A.: Neuropathy following abuse of nitrous oxide, Neurology **28**:504, 1978.

Novak, A., and others: The deliberate inhalation of volatile substances, J. Psychedelic Drugs **12**:105, 1980.

SYNCOPE

Snycope is a relatively common event in the dental office, most often associated with the administration of local anesthesia or a surgical procedure. The cause of the syncopal episode (or "common faint") may vary from patient to patient (see medical section), but an increased catecholamine level as a result of anxiety and pain or the injection of epinephrine or other vasopressor substances is frequently the common immediate cause.

Syncopal episodes are sometimes mistaken for allergic or toxic reactions to local anesthetic agents when they follow infiltration or regional block anesthesia, particularly if the patient is rigid or subject to isolated convulsive jerks while unconscious. A patient may claim to be "allergic to novocaine and dental anesthetic" as a result of such an experience. It is important that a record of any untoward reaction be entered in the patient's chart to establish the true nature of the episode in the event of future inquiry. For the same reason, an attempt should be made to identify the type of snycopal reaction involved, using the guidelines set out in Chapter 144. Pulse and blood pressure recorded during the episode, a history of the events leading up to the episode, and any unusual sensations that immediately preceded it are useful data in establishing a differential diagnosis. Measurement of blood pressure in the recumbent and standing position and measurement of blood glucose at a subsequent appointment may help identify episodes caused by postural hypotension and hypoglycemia. In the older patient, a review of the patient's medications frequently reveals a cause of postural hypotension (usually an antihypertensive drug), which sometimes occurs when a patient suddenly stands from a recumbent position after a lengthy period of dental treatment.

The management of a syncopal episode is straightforward, and most observers will respond automatically, placing the patient in a supine position with the legs elevated slightly (Trendelenburg position). Manipulation and movement of the extremities frequently will increase the return of blood from the periphery. An upright position in the chair may cause prolonged cerebral anoxia, which can precipitate convulsions, nausea, and the like. The proper positioning is the most important aspect of treatment since the majority of clinical manifestations in this emergency result from inadequate flow of cerebral blood.

The establishment of a patent airway is the next step in treatment. Frequently the head-tilt position will be sufficient to develop a patent airway, stimulating spontaneous respiration. Occasionally it will be necessary to administer oxygen when the head tilt is not successful. The patient should immediately regain consciousness once the appropriate position of the patient is instituted and the airway is patent.

If the patient is not responding rapidly to these measures, a respiratory stimulant, such as aromatic spirits of ammonia, should be crushed and placed under the patient's nose so that he may inhale the spirits. This acts as a chemical stimulant to breathing. In addition, it is helpful to loosen the patient's tight clothing, such as belt or necktie. Placing a cold towel on the patient's forehead may be soothing and may assist the patient in feeling comfortable.

During the episode, vital signs must be monitored, including blood pressure, pulse, and respiration. They must be compared to the patient's baseline values in order to determine the severity and progression of the emergency. A temporary drop in blood pressure will usually occur, and the pulse may be rapid and thready or slow and steady. Dilated pupils, pale skin, excessive perspiration, and nausea and vomiting may occur. When difficulty is experienced in detecting either a peripheral pulse or a heartbeat, cardiac failure should be considered as a possibility and appropriate CPR measures instituted. However, recovery from a syncopal episode is usually prompt and without residual complication, and it occurs once cerebral circulation is regained. On rare occasions, a syncopal patient may remain hypotensive for a more extended period, requiring administration of phenylephrine or other vasopressor substance to counteract peripheral vasodilation.

Once the patient has regained consciousness he should remain seated until vital signs are stable and all discomfort and anxiety have passed. The patient should not be allowed to stand quickly or walk unattended. Dental treatment should be discontinued and the practitioner should attempt to discover the syncopal precipitant so that future therapy may be modified to prevent recurrence.

PATIENT WITH A HISTORY OF EPILEPSY

Epilepsy is a very common disorder that is said to affect 0.5% of the North American population. The two major concerns of the dentist providing dental treatment for a patient with a history of epilepsy are:

1. How to minimize the oral side effects of long-term administration of phenytoin and how to treat these complications once they occur
2. How to prevent the dental visit from becoming an occasion of increased seizure activity, and how to manage the patient should a seizure occur during the dental visit

While it is true that seizures may occur at times with no or only minimal warning and that a generalized convulsive seizure can be a frightening event, especially in the confines of a dental operatory, such drama is not a daily event for the majority of treated, noninstitutionalized epileptic persons. With some few exceptions, discussed here, routine dental procedures do not increase the risk of seizures. Dental care for many epileptic individuals thus can be provided safely by the general practitioner using the following guidelines.

History

Since the term "epilepsy" covers a wide spectrum of disease activity and equally well defines a patient who has had one convulsion of undetermined cause and is maintained on anticonvulsant medications prophylactically, patients with temporary impairment of consciousness without convulsive activity, and also patients with recurrent tonic/clonic, generalized (grand mal) convulsions, an accurate record of the patient's seizure history is essential. This should be obtained from a member of the family as well as from the patient, corroborrated if possible by a physician who has been consulted for diagnosis and management of the patient's seizures. Given the changing classification of convulsive disorders and the likelihood that treatment will have modified the patient's seizure experience, a description of the events associated with recent seizure activity (when, where, and what happened; frequency; prodrome, aura, seizure, and postictal events) and recent medical history (failure to take medication; side effects of additional medications, alcohol, etc.; association of seizures with sleep, menstrual cycle, fever, or other events) will often be more helpful than a diagnosis. Timing and dose of all medications should also be recorded.

Examination

The oral examination of the epileptic patient usually focuses on evidence of side effects of chronic anticonvulsive therapy, but it also provides an opportunity for noting facial and intraoral lacerations and scars indicating damage during convulsive episodes. Close observation of some epileptic patients during dental care will also reveal episodes of decreased consciousness or inattention, eye movements, and muscular spasms, which may give a better idea of the frequency of partial seizures and drug effects than the history revealed. Laboratory evaluations (CBC and liver function tests) are not routinely indicated for epileptic patients before dental treatment unless general anesthesia is being considered but are useful screening procedures for side effects of prolonged anticonvulsive therapy. They may also provide a way of securing medical consultation for the patient who continues on a medication for many years without follow-up. Laboratory measurement of serum and urinary drug levels may also be required following consultation with the patient's physician, when control of seizures is poor, and when additional medication before dental treatment is being considered.

Medical consultation

Communication with the physician is helpful in obtaining a diagnosis of the patient's seizure disorder and corroborating the details of the patient's history. Consultation is also essential if a general anesthetic is considered and if the oral side effects of phenytoin are severe and unacceptable to the patient.

Phenytoin-induced gingival hyperplasia

Phenytoin-induced gingival hyperplasia affects at least 40% to 50% of those who use the drug longer than 3 months. The more severe effects may not develop until after several years of continued use of the drug. Evidence from animal studies, individual case reports, and clinical trials indicates that both the drug and the local irritation from plaque, calculus, restorations, or appliances are causative factors. If gingival irritation can be eliminated, gingival hyperplasia will at the most be only minimal. Continuous and obvious irritation, such as that associated with banded orthodontic appliances, is often associated with very severe hyperplasia. The pathogenesis of the gingival changes caused by this drug is still unsettled; earlier suggestions that the gingival collagen is modified or that reduced serum and salivary IgA associated with continued use of phenytoin are the cause of the hyperplasia have not been confirmed. In fact, the available data indicate that the mature fibrous-type phenytoin-induced gingival lesion represents neither hypertrophy, hyperplasia, nor fibrosis but is an example of uncontrolled growth of a connective tissue of apparently normal cell and fiber composition. The term phenytoin (or DPH)-induced "hyperplasia" is still commonly used, however.

ORAL MANIFESTATIONS. The clinical appearance of phenytoin-induced gingival hyperplasia is usually characteristic, although numerous variants are seen depending on the location of the lesion, the particular irritant involved, and the extent of secondary inflammatory changes. The diagnosis is made from the history of long-term phenytoin use and the clinical appearance of the lesions; biopsy and estimation of the serum levels of phenytoin offer no additional diagnostic information. With very rare exceptions, the hyperplasia is restricted to the gingivae, and following extraction of teeth and excision of the hyperplastic tissue there is no recurrence.

DENTAL MANAGEMENT. Treatment of phenytoin-induced gingival hyperplasia should emphasize elimination of local gingival irritants, scrupulous oral hygiene, and interdental massage. In a number of patients, seizures can be controlled by other nonhydantoin derivatives, and the physician, the patient, and the family may be willing to experiment with supervised alteration of the patient's anticonvulsive medications in order to reduce the hyperplasia. The menarche frequently begins a period of difficult management, partly because of the increased frequency of seizures that may occur at this time, partly because orthodontic treatment is usually begun about this time, and partly because of the patient's increased awareness of any orofacial cosmetic defects as adolescence progresses. Some authors advocate that phenytoin be routinely avoided in treating female adolescents to exclude the possibility of both gingival hyperplasia and hirsutism. The epileptic patient's medication should at least always be reviewed before orthodontic treatment is begun.

Topically applied medications including antiplaque agents such as chlorhexidine have no effect on the gingival changes once hyperplasia is established. Hyperplasia of any degree also will not resolve simply by removing local gingival irritants, and surgical removal of hyperplastic gingivae, root planing, and elimination of rough margins on restorations are usually necessary before adequate gingival hygiene and plaque control can be established. If surgical procedures to eliminate the hyperplastic gingivae are not followed by institution of adequate oral hygiene and use of interdental massage, the hyperplasia will recur.

The brain-damaged and retarded epileptic patient often presents a difficult management problem, particularly if neither parents nor nurses can provide adequate tooth brushing and gingival hygiene. In such cases, the value of surgery must be carefully considered and resorted to only when the overgrowth interferes with closure of the teeth or lips or is a source of severe halitosis or hemorrhage.

Anesthesia

Routine dental local anesthetic procedures with lidocaine, carbocaine, and related agents with or without vasoconstrictors are not associated with any increased risk of seizures and do not interact with the commonly used anticonvulsant medications. Seizures have been reported when Intravenous lidocaine is used for the treatment of cardiac arrhythmias, but the amount contained in dental local anesthesia is unlikely to cause a seizure, particularly if care is taken to aspirate before injection of the solution. General anesthesia including nitrous oxide sedation may induce seizures, and local anesthesia is preferred where practical. General anesthetic agents also may precipitate anticonvulsant drug toxicity, and some anesthetics, such as ketamine, are known to produce high-frequency EEG activity and convulsions. While intravenous diazepam is frequently used to control persistent seizures and is considered a relatively safe drug for this purpose, cardiopulmonary arrest may occur when it is administered with barbiturates.

Since emotional upsets may induce seizures in some patients, medication to control anxiety is often prescribed for epileptic patients before dental treatment. An additional 10 to 20 mg of phenobarbital 1 or 2 hours before the dental visit is usually well tolerated without significantly increased drowsiness by epileptic individuals who are already using this drug routinely. Temporary increase in the dose of other anticonvulsive agents (phenytoin, carbamazepine, primidone, and ethosuximide) for prophylactic control of seizures in the dental office is usually not recommended.

Removable appliances

Poorly retained crowns, bridges, and partial dentures, as well as loose and grossly carious teeth, are generally considered a hazard for the epileptic patient with recurrent generalized seizures, who could conceivably aspirate any of these items while unconscious. Plastic bridges and dentures should be fabricated to include a radiopaque marker in the event an examination of the gastrointestinal and respiratory tracts has to be made following a seizure. The decision of whether to make a removable appliance or not should be conditioned by an estimate of the frequency of convulsive seizures.

Managing a patient having a seizure

The majority of seizures are brief, self-limiting events resulting in no permanent ill effects, provided the patient is prevented from harming himself while unconscious. Patients who are subject to seizures with some regularity should not be left alone during the dental visit, and auxiliaries and other office personnel should be taught to observe the epileptic patient and be acquainted with proper procedures if a seizure occurs. Partial seizures, manifest by some impairment of consciousness, ictal automatism, and inappropriate speech or sounds, usually pass in a few minutes, leaving the patient confused and tired but otherwise unaffected; restraint is not needed in this case and may at times produce a violent defensive response.

In the event that a partial or generalized seizure occurs in the dental chair, the chair should be placed in a supine position; often the floor offers a firm, flat treatment surface. The patient's head is placed sideways in order to allow saliva and vomitus to exit and thereby prevent the possibility of aspiration. Efforts should be directed to maintaining a patent airway by the use of the head tilt position as long as all secretions have been suctioned from the patient's mouth so as not to create a situation where the patient may aspirate. Occasionally during seizure activity there are periods of apnea. At times the use of oxygen may be helpful, via face or nose mask. Patients should be protected from injuring themselves by gently restraining their extremities from uncontrolled movements but still allowing for some freedom of movement.

There is some controversy as to the use of an object such as a tongue depressor covered with gauze to prevent tongue, cheek, and lip biting. Many believe that this is not necessary and that the improper placement of these devices may cause tissue injury and bleeding as well as compromised airway patency.

During the postictal phase the patient must be observed very carefully to be sure that respiratory depression or airway obstruction does not occur. The emergency situation is not over until all vital signs are normal and the patient is alert and oriented. The patient should not be discharged from the dental office unaccompanied. It is recommended that the patient relax for the remainder of the day and not carry on any strenuous activity since the potential for a subsequent seizure exists.

If a patient suffers more than one seizure without regaining consciousness, status epilepticus should be considered and an emergency team summoned. In the interim, and intravenous line should be established and 50% dextrose administered. Where the dentist is experienced in the use of Intravenous diazepam, a dose not exceeding 10 mg may be given over a 2-minute period using a different vein, repeating the dose in 20 to 30 minutes if convulsions continue. Intravenous barbiturates will also usually terminate a convulsion, but when given along with diazepam they may cause respiratory depression and are not advised unless an electrocardiographic monitor if available. An antiepileptic drug such as phenytoin may be given intravenously once diazepam has stopped the seizure, but it is *not* used as the primary drug for treatment of suspected epileptic patients.

BIBLIOGRAPHY

Evans, D.E.N.: Anesthesia and the epileptic patient—a review, Anesthesia **30**:34, 1975.
Hassel, T.M., and others: Summary of an international symposium on phenytoin-induced teratology and gingival pathology, **99**:652, 1979.
Livingstone, S., editor: The medical treatment of epilepsy, Pediatr. Ann. **8**:110, 1979.
Smith, Q.T.: Gingival fibrosis during phenytoin-ingestion, Northwest Dent. **57**:23, 1978.

AURAL SYMPTOMS ASSOCIATED WITH TEMPOROMANDIBULAR JOINT DYSFUNCTION, ODONTOGENIC DIZZINESS, AND THE OTOMANDIBULAR SYNDROME

Otalgia (pain in or around the ear) and other aural complaints are frequently included among the symptoms of temporomandibular joint dysfunction. For the most part, otalgia is the predominant aural symptom mentioned, but some published series also include dizziness, vertigo, tinnitus, and deafness in the syndrome. Dentists are familiar with the patient who returns from an otologic consultation with the statement that no ear problem has been found to account for the patient's aural symptoms and that they must be due to dental or Temporomandibular joint (TMJ) problems. The media have also tended to emphasize a very broad concept of TMJ dysfunction that attributes ear, neck, shoulder, and even more distant musculoskeletal and sensory abnormalities, as well as the more localized orofacial symptoms, to masticatory muscle tension.

Otalgia seems to be convincingly established as a symptom of the TMJ dysfunction, and it occurs in over three fourths of patients in some series. Despite a long history of association between TMJ problems and dizziness, however (commencing with Costen's description in the 1930s), there still are very few data to support this correlation, other than theoretical considerations based on the shared innervation of the masticatory, tensor tympani, and tensor palati muscles. Careful evaluation of patients with both TMJ and aural symptoms in one recent critical study also led to the conclusion that the coexistence of these two sets of symptoms (TMJ dysfunction and aural symptoms excluding otalgia) was entirely coincidental.

As currently stated, the *otomandibular syndrome* includes complaints of pain in and around the ear, fullness in the ear, hearing loss, tinnitus, and a loss of equilibrium. The patient with the otomandibular syndrome may have one or more of these symptoms with no pathologic changes evident on otologic examination and always has one or more of the muscles of mastication in a state of spasm.

The theoretical justification for relating these otologic symptoms to masticatory muscle function lies in the fact that the tensor tympani muscle is innervated by the mandibular branch of the trigeminal nerve, which also innervates the medial pterygoid muscle. It is postulated that early in embryologic development, neural patterns are established within the brainstem where the jaw bone and ear ossicle movements are integrated. The tensor palati muscle is also innervated by the mandibular branch of the trigeminal nerve, being the only muscle of the soft palate so innervated. As such, it could conceivably go into spasm when other masticatory muscles do so, leading to eustachian tube dysfunction and concomitant aural symptoms.

In one sense, the otomandibular syndrome is a restatement of Costen's syndrome, in which spasm within the masticatory muscle system has replaced mechanical infringement of the condyle on the glenoid fossa, ear canal, and related nerves, as the pathogenesis of TMJ disorders. Spasm within the masticatory muscle system is a currently well accepted and to some extent an experimentally established explanation for jaw pain, mandibular deviation, and joint dysfunction. Spasm of the tensor tympani and tensor palati, however, have not been convincingly demonstrated, and conceivably other abnormalities, such as vasomotor swelling of the lining of the eustachian tube and similar changes in the inner ear, could account for the dizziness, tinnitus, and hearing loss in the patient with other signs of TMJ dysfunction. A recent study reviewing 45 patients with TMJ dysfunction, otalgia, and other aural symptoms demonstrates clearly that with thorough otologic evaluation, otolaryngologic pathology will be found in the majority of these patients and that allergic and estrogen-induced vasomotor changes could well account for the others.

DENTAL MANAGEMENT. Treatment is the same whether otherwise unexplained aural symptoms are present or not. Well-maintained daily doses of aspirin, heat to the masticatory muscles, anti-inflammatory agents, muscle relaxants, bite splints, and biofeedback relaxation are all effective in acute TMJ myofascial dysfunction, and also quite helpful in more chronic forms of the disorder. Debate continues over the value of joint surgery when there is evidence of intrinsic disease of the joint. Irrespective of the treatment modality used, however, the major improvement will be in eliminating painful masticatory muscle spasm, trismus, mandibular deviation, pathologic joint sounds, and the characteristic superficial skin tenderness and sensory abnormalities experienced over the joint, ear, and surrounding areas by these patients. Symptoms of fullness in the ear, tinnitus, and dizziness, on the other hand, should not be expected to improve with any certainty, although they may. Rehabilitation of the occlusion with the sole aim of curing otherwise unexplained aural symptoms other than otalgia should not be undertaken until the effect of repositioning the patient's mandible utilizing removal appliances has been evaluated.

BIBLIOGRAPHY

Appelberg, D.B., and others: TMJ disease: results of a 10 year study, Postgrad. Med. **65**:167, 1979.

Appelberg, D.B., and others: Otological manifestations in TMJ dysfunction, J. Oral Rehab. **7**:249, 1980.

Arlen, H.: The otomandibular syndrome. In Gelb, H., editor: Clinical management of head, neck, and TMJ pain and dysfunction, Philadelphia, 1977, W.B. Saunders Co.

Brookes, G.B., and others: "Costen's syndrome"—correlation or coincidence: a review of 45 patients with temporo-mandibular joint dysfunction, otalgia and other aural symptoms, Clin. Otolaryngol. **5**:23, 1980.

Costen, J.B.: Neuralgias and ear symptoms associated with disturbed function of the temporomandibular point, J.A.M.A. **107**:252, 1936.

Jonck, L.M.: Ear symptoms in TMJ disturbance, South Afr. Med. J. **54**:782, 1978.

DEMYELINATING, DEGENERATIVE, AND HEREDOFAMILIAL DISEASES OF THE CENTRAL NERVOUS SYSTEM

Demyelinating and degenerative diseases of the CNS possibly associated with transmissible agents

Amyotrophic lateral sclerosis (ALS, "Lou Gehrig's disease") and multiple sclerosis (MS) are of particular interest because they are possibly caused by infectious agents. These should be contrasted with those that are more certainly associated with slow virus infection, like Kuru (a progressive and fatal neurologic disorder occurring exclusively among highland natives of New Guinea), Creutzfeldt-Jakob disease,* and progressive multifocal leukoencephalopathy. The evidence for an infectious etiology is still obscure as far as multiple sclerosis and amyotrophic lateral sclerosis are concerned, but transmissible infectious agents have been demonstrated in nervous tissue from patients with both kuru and Creutzfeldt-Jakob disease, and the diseases have been transmitted to both humans and experimental animals by means of the viral agents concerned.

While an infectious etiology for both MS and ALS remains a useful working hypothesis, it is no more than that. It is unfortunate that at times the hypothesis has been confused with fact and patients with these diseases have been actively discouraged from seeking dental care for fear of transmission of the disease to the dentist. As far as MS and ALS are concerned, there is no rationale for such prohibitions, and usual standards of hygiene and instrument sterilization that are used in dental practice are recommended.

Because of the hazards associated with the infectious agent of Creutzfeldt-Jakob disease, however, it is currently recommended that dentists should use the same precautions now used for known carriers of chronic hepatitis when they treat confused or demented adults. Because of the great variability of clinical findings in Creutzfeldt-Jakob disease, any adult who acquires rapidly progressive dementia without having a space-occupying intracranial lesion should be handled in this fashion. Exposure to breath, saliva, and nasopharyngeal secretions is not considered hazardous; however, percutaneous exposure to blood and nervous tissue including pulp fragments should be avoided.

MULTIPLE SCLEROSIS. Since multiple sclerosis is the most common of the demyelinating diseases and usually runs a protracted course, dental care is often needed. The problems involved are similar to those encountered with other physically handicapped patients and include inability to maintain adequate oral hygiene, accumulation of food debris with loss of facial and masticatory muscle tonus, inability to support the head, and, in some cases, the development of muscle spasms, involuntary movements of the jaws, and rigidity.

The miscellaneous sensory abnormalities characteristic of multiple sclerosis, including localized paresthesias, numbness, and pain, may affect the oral cavity, jaws, and face. Particular attention has also been paid in the literature to tic douloureux and atypical facial pain in multiple sclerosis patients, the coexistence of two largely unexplained problems in one patient being of especial interest. Sensory impairment over the distribution of the Trigeminal nerve occurs in 1% to 4% of cases of multiple sclerosis. Among selected samples of patients, such as those seen at the Mayo Clinic, as many as 0.9% of the multiple sclerosis patients have trigeminal neuralgia; conversely, 2% of their trigeminal neuralgia patients have multiple sclerosis. Autopsy studies suggest that plaquelike lesions at the point of entry of the roots of the fifth nerve into the pons are the source of the neuralgic pains in these cases, although the disseminated character of the intracerebral lesions of multiple sclerosis leave this somewhat uncertain in some cases. Multiple sclerosis should always be considered in the differential diagnosis of unexplained orofacial pain, especially if the pain is accompanied by symptoms of numbness or other sensory abnormality. On rare occasions, multiple sclerosis has been diagnosed as the result of a

---

*See also Chapter 142.

neurologic consultation for unexplained orofacial pain, but no one set of symptoms consistently characterizes the presenting complaints for this protean disease.

Since the etiology of multiple sclerosis remains obscure, it is not surprising that many different factors have been suspected as the cause of both initial and subsequent episodes of the disease. At one time, injections of novocaine were considered to be hazardous for patients with multiple sclerosis and the exciting cause of recurrent episodes. This phase seems to have passed with the advent of xylocaine as a dental anesthetic, and one now rarely hears of a patient who has been cautioned against having dental local anesthetic injections for this reason. It is well to remember, however, that it may be difficult for the multiple sclerosis patient to distinguish the lingering effects of a local anesthetic from an episode of paresthesia; informing the patient about the sequelae of an anesthetic is always a good practice, but it is particularly important with the multiple sclerosis patient.

AMYOTROPHIC LATERAL SCLEROSIS. To quote a recent text dealing with this disease, "The diagnosis of ALS has traditionally been surrounded by an aura of hopelessness. Such a diagnosis means helplessness, despair and ultimate death." Since ALS is an insidiously progressive disease, with severe effects on respiration and deglutition, patients do not usually seek routine dental care other than in the early stage of the disease. This diagnosis, however, also generates an attitude of denial in some patients, who may continue to seek medical and dental care from numerous consultants even though there is no doubt about the diagnosis. Such patients vainly hope that a new denture or a tooth extraction or medication will cure their symptoms and will at times argue forcefully for treatment. It is important that the dentist, through adequate history taking and communication with the various physicians the patient has consulted, become aware of the patient's diagnosis and participate in this "game" only with full understanding of the reality of the patient's condition.

Syringomyelia

Syringomyelia, a relatively rare disease, appears in the dental literature under two headings: (1) as one of the causes of intractable jaw and face pain of *central* origin (distinct from pain of peripheral or neuropathic origin); and (2) because of the severe lacerations and other injuries that can occur to the face and jaws as well as to other parts of the body, from trauma to areas of permanently anesthetized tissue.

Vitamin B$_{12}$ deficiency

See Chapter 154.

Phakomatoses

Patients with a number of conditions described under this heading, such as neurofibromatosis, tuberous sclerosis, Sturge-Weber syndrome, ataxia telangiectasia, and incontinentia pigmenti, may have oral or facial evidences of the disease. Neurofibromatosis and tuberous sclerosis also are of special interest because of their association with predisposition to malignancy elsewhere in the nervous system even though the local oral lesions are themselves without any precancerous potential.

Approximately 5% of the patients with *neurofibromatosis* have well-developed oral lesions with macroglossia (the tongue being the most common oral location of neurofibroma). The lesions are generally asymptomatic and discovered only on routine oral examination. The lesions of solitary neurofibromas are indistinguishable histologically from those of multiple neurofibromatosis, the diagnosis of neurofibromatosis being made on the basis of multiple macules or nodules, café-au-lait spots, and a positive family history.

The characteristic skin lesions of *tuberous sclerosis,* the so-called adenoma sebaceum, occur usually over the nose in a "butterfly distribution," in the nasolabial folds, and over the chin and forehead, appearing either as telangiectases or small firm, yellow, gray, or red, elevated nodules. Similar lesions may occur intraorally. Fibromas and enlargement of the gingivae have also been described even when the patient had not received any hydantoin to control seizures. A characteristic pitting of the labial and buccal enamel of the permanent dentition has also been reported, as have miscellaneous other oral abnormalities, including hyperkeratosis, jaw cysts, facial asymmetry, high palate, cleft lip and palate, and retarded eruption.

Oral changes occur in about a third of the cases of *Sturge-Weber syndrome* and may include massive growths of the gingiva and asymmetric jaw growth and tooth eruption sequence (due to differential blood flow to the affected area). It is important to differentiate angiomatous lesions of the jaw from the gingival hyperplasia induced by phenytoin, especially if gingivectomy is planned. Classically, the intraoral lesions in this syndrome occur on the same side of the body as the other angiomas the patient exhibits.

The fine, symmetric, bright red streaks that develop in the temporal and nasal areas of the conjunctiva in patients with the *ataxia telangiectasia syndrome* usually extend with age to the "butterfly" area of the face and neck as well to the extremities. Rarely these changes may also be manifest on the hard and soft palate and throughout the nasal mucosa. A small stature, thin sad face, and stooping shoulders are said to be characteristic of the syndrome along with excessive drooling and poor quality of speech.

The oral changes of *incontinentia pigmenti* are limited to the dentition, which exhibits delayed eruption and missing or peg-shaped teeth. These anomalies affect both deciduous and permanent dentitions and occur with a familial distribution.

BIBLIOGRAPHY

Brightman, V.J.: Benign tumors of the oral cavity. In Lynch, M.A.L., editor: Burket's oral medicine, Philadelphia, 1977, J.B. Lippincott Co.

Cohen, L.: Disturbance of taste as a symptom of multiple sclerosis, Br. J. Oral Surg. **2**:184, 1965.

Gajdusek, D.C., and others: Precautions in medical care of, and in handling materials from patients with transmissible virus dementia (Creutzfeldt-Jakob disease), N. Engl. J. Med. **297**:1253, 1977.

Gorlin, R.J., and Pindborg, J.J.: Syndromes of the head and neck, Ed. 2, New York, 1979, McGraw-Hill Book Co.

Mulder, D.W., editor: The diagnosis and treatment of amyotrophic lateral sclerosis, Boston, 1980, Houghton-Mifflin Co.

Pisanti, S.: Burn injuries in a patient with syringomyelia—case report, J. Oral Med. **32**:104, 1977.

Roller, N.W., and others: Amyotrophic lateral sclerosis, J. Oral Surg. **37**:46, 1974.

Rushton, J.G., and Olafson, R.A.: Trigeminal neuralgia associated with multiple sclerosis, Arch. Neurol. **13**:383, 1965.

Scully, C.: Orofacial manifestations in tuberous sclerosis, J. Oral Surg. **44**:706, 1977.

Vinken, P., and Bruyn, G.W.: *Handbook of clinical neurology,* vol. 9: Multiple sclerosis and other demyelinating disorders, Amsterdam, 1970, North-Holland Publishing Co.

TREMORS AND OTHER ABNORMAL INVOLUNTARY JAW MOVEMENTS

A variety of degenerative diseases of the central nervous system (CNS) are associated with abnormal and repetitive movements of the jaws and facial muscles. The majority of these problems appear with advancing age and may seriously interfere with the fitting and wearing of dentures. In younger patients with a natural dentition, pressure generated by these involuntary jaw movements may have a destructive effect on both the dentition and the periodontium. Those most commonly discussed in the dental literature include senile tremor (also referred to as spontaneous bucco-linguo-facial dyskinesia, or BLFD), parkinsonism, the relatively rare dyskinesia induced by levodopa (currently the most effective drug used to treat parkinsonism), the miscellaneous group of conditions often referred to as the tardive dyskinesias, and the destructive ruminatory jaw movement seen in some decerebrate patients. Miscellaneous other conditions are also associated with abnormal jaw movements.

In some patients with these problems, neurologic consultation is effective in specifying medication or other treatment that is helpful in reducing the tremor and allowing the dentist to complete necessary dental care satisfactorily. In others, a means of controlling the abnormal movements is not found or is rejected because of undesirable side effects of an otherwise effective drug. The following comments may prove useful to the dentist called upon to treat a patient who is so affected.

Intention tremors of the jaws and head are often temporarily worsened when a patient is required to perform specific jaw movements (for example, during bite registration for dentures) and may be of less consequence when the patient is in a more relaxed situation. Loss of proprioceptive jaw sensation through extraction of teeth will usually worsen a tremor, the patient in effect not being able to sense where to put his jaw. In like fashion, construction of dentures may entirely eliminate a jaw tremor, just as resting the hands on a table or in pockets may alleviate mild tremors in patients with parkinsonism.

The development of *rigidity* in some affected muscle groups as often occurs in Parkinson's disease may prove a greater problem for dental treatment than the presence of tremor. In particular, when rigidity of one or more facial and masticatory muscle groups is present, accurate muscle trimming of a dental impression and bite registration become impossible. Some authors have claimed success in such cases by use of a Myomonitor, allowing the patient to develop the borders of an impression or a bite pathway at his own rate. Passage of low level electric stimuli through the masticatory muscles using the same device may also assist in relaxing rigid muscles. In some patients, small oral doses of diazepam before the dental visit may achieve greater relaxation during treatment. In severely affected patients, intravenous sedation supplemented with nitrous oxide and oxygen will control all tremors.

Repetitive tongue movements that bring the lingual mucosa into forceful contact with the teeth not uncommonly produce depapillation, abrasion, and ulceration of the tongue. Patients with parkinsonism may also complain of burning sensations in the tongue, which often as not appear to be caused by such repetitive trauma and constant tension in the tongue, forcing it against the teeth. Construction of acrylic night guards or modification of existing appliances can be helpful in controlling such symptoms. Because of the complex interaction of all elements of the masticatory system, correction of major occlusal disharmonies and other occlusal and dental defects can sometimes alleviate both tremors and related sensory complaints by ensuring a more comfortable and smoothly functioning dentition.

A number of medications used in the treatment of Parkinson's disease, either alone or in combination with levodopa, are strongly anticholinergic and produce considerable inhibition of salivary flow. Benztropine (Cogentin), trihexyphenidyl (Artane), cycrimine (Pagitane), biperiden (Akineton), procyclidine (Kemadrin), and amantadine (Symmetral) all possess this property, as do the tricyclic antidepressants (for example, imipramine and amitriptyline) and the antihistamines themselves. While this property can be useful in controlling the sialorrhea exhibited by many of these patients, the anticholinergic effect often predominates and contributes to the symptoms of dryness and soreness of the tongue and oral mucosa, which may bring these patients to the dentist's attention. Development of root surface and recurrent caries should also be a concern in patients maintained on these medications for prolonged periods; suppurative parotitis has also been observed in this situation.

The main side effects of levodopa of dental concern are the possibility of postural hypotension and the development of choreiform and dystonic movements of the head and jaws. Burning sensations of the tongue and bitter taste are also listed as side effects of this medication.

Tardive dyskinesia describes a broad group of extrapyramidal motor disorders that have been observed as long-term side effects of the administration of neuroleptic drugs (for example, phenothiazines such as trifluoperazine [Stelazine], thioridazine [Mellaril], and chlorpromazine [Thorazine]; butyrophenone tranquilizers such as haloperidol [Haldol]; and reserpine derivatives such as Serpasil. The minor benzodiazepine tranquilizers (Librium, Valium, Ativan) are free of this side effect. Both short- and long-term dyskinetic side effects of these medications are believed to result from hypersensitivity of the basal ganglia to dopamine. The effects may be manifest as either symptoms of agitation or jitteriness; dystonic problems such as spasm of the neck muscles, trismus, swallowing difficulties, and protrusion of the tongue; or Parkinson-like symptoms. These symptoms usually subside within 24 to 48 hours after the drug is discontinued; when they appear after long-term therapy with the drug, the term "tardive" dyskinesia is used.

While the manifestations of tardive dyskinesia are not limited to the head, neck, and jaws, a characteristic syndrome has been described in which there are rhythmic involuntary movements of the tongue, face, mouth, and jaws. Involuntary mouthing, lip tremor ("rabbit syndrome"), as well as chewing or puckering of the lips and fasciculation or darting movements of the tongue have all been described as part of this syndrome. The risk of tardive dyskinesia is higher for elderly females taking high drug doses, and symptoms frequently persist after the offending drug is discontinued. Some control of the symptoms is usually possible, however, with the various medications used to treat other basal ganglia abnormalities. Such dyskinetic symptoms usually prevent the wearing of dentures, and attempts at controlling them should be made for this reason, as well as to alleviate the patient's suffering.

The incidence of tardive dyskinesia is not accurately known. The majority of cases are seen in persons in mental institutions, where similar symptoms may often equally well be blamed on psychiatric and neurologic mannerisms and to senile dyskinesias.

In an entirely different category from the standpoint of both cause and management are the *powerful ruminatory* (circular, grinding) *movements of the mandible seen in essentially decerebrate patients* as a result of injuries to the cerebral cortex, trigeminal nuclei, and hypothalamus. These movements represent reinstitution of primitive rhythmic jaw movements during which pressures as high as 270 psi may be exerted on molar teeth. Lack of coordination of tongue, lip, and cheek movements with the jaw movements rapidly leads to severe self-inflicted wounds of the oral cavity with through-and-through lacerations of the soft tissues. The majority of dental appliances cannot withstand these forces and special stents (such as the Minnesota Tongue Stent), which are ligated to the molar teeth to elevate the tongue from the floor of the mouth, are needed to minimize the self-inflicted damage. Spasm of the masseter muscles usually complicates the problem, and an oral examination including Dental impressions can usually be performed on these patients only after the administration of 0.05 mg/kg curare or succinylcholine chloride to relax the spasm.

BIBLIOGRAPHY

Cohen, C.I.: A case report: periodontal surgery in parkinsonism utilizing intravenous sedation, N.Y. State Dent. J. **44**(1):19, 1978.

Delwaide, P.J., and others: Spontaneous bucco-linguo-facial dyskinesia in the elderly, Acta Neurol. Scand. **56**(3):256, 1977.

Fielding, M.L.: Case report: construction of complete dentures for Parkinson patient, Dent. Survey **53**(12):36, 1977.

Hanson, G.E., and others: A tongue stent for prevention of oral trauma in the comatose patient, Crit. Care Med. **3**(5):200, 1975.

Jackson, M.J.: The use of tongue-depressing stents for neuropathologic chewing, J. Prosth. Dent. **40**(3):309, 1978.

Simpson, G.M., and Kline, N.S.: Tardive dyskinesia: manifestations, incidence, etiology and treatment. In Yahn, M.D., editor: The basal ganglia, Res. Publ. Assoc. Res. Nerv. Ment. Dis. **55**:427, 1976.

STROKE

Cerebrovascular accidents remain a leading cause of death and disability in the United States. Detection of blood glucose abnormalities and elevated blood pressure in dental offices contributes to the national effort to control this problem, since the majority of strokes, in the older segment of the population at least, occur in blood vessels that have been previously compromised by preexisting diabetes and hypertension.

In general, the untoward effects of hypertension on the cerebral vasculature are long-term and include degenerative changes and weakening of the walls of cerebral arterioles that predispose to thrombosis, microaneurysms, and hemorrhage, as well as changes in the endocardium, aorta, and carotid tree that contribute emboli to the cerebral vasculature. The peak systolic reading noted at a given dental office visit is thus of less significance in the pathogenesis of stroke than are chronic untreated elevations of the diastolic pressure, which lead to severe atherosclerosis and the variety of arteriosclerotic changes that provide the setting for most cerebrovascular accidents.

However, vascular changes underlying cerebrovascular accidents (transient ischemic attacks, in particular) are not restricted to the cerebral vasculature, and similar changes are often demonstrable in both the intra- and extracranial portions of the entire carotid artery system. Detection of occlusion in an oral or superficial facial branch of the external carotid may therefore have a significance beyond any associated local oral symptomatology and should lead to referral for a decision concerning more detailed examination of the carotid artery system. Excessive calcification of these arteries, detected in radiographs, and swellings and bruits noted over the major carotid vessels in the neck likewise should suggest the possibility of more extensive carotid artery problems that could predispose to a stroke. Recently, Doppler (pulsed ultrasound) screening of the branches of the carotid system has been extended to include the lingual artery, and irregularities of pulse rhythm and periodic reductions of the flow have been noted in the lingual arteries of stroke patients.

ORAL MANIFESTATIONS. Oral symptoms and functional disability of varying degrees may develop as a result of a stroke, the extent and character of the oral problems depending on the location and extent of cerebral damage. Oral sensory dysfunction, ranging from mild dysesthesia, through prickling and burning sensations, to pain of sufficient severity to require analgesics and even tractotomy, may be seen. The more mildly affected patients will usually accept these problems as part of the complex of symptoms that resulted from the stroke, and often are not reported in the face of a more severely handicapping hemiplegia. Alternatively, the dentist may consult with stroke patients about oral sensory dysfunction in hope that dental treatment may assist with a persistent and annoying oral symptom. Thorough evaluation of such patients to rule out other possible causes for these symptoms, such as moniliasis, denture irritation, dental defects, fractured teeth, drug-induced xerostomia, and dysgeusia, is indicated, although in many cases cerebral damage will finally have to be accepted as the diagnosis of the problem.

Patients occasionally will present with taste abnormalities following a stroke. At other times, when cerebral damage results from obstruction of the inferior cerebellar artery, pain control centers may be affected with resultant intractable and usually poorly localized facial pain associated with other neurologic abnormalities (Wallenberg's syndrome).

Some degree of oral motor dysfunction usually accompanies oral dysesthesia secondary to a stroke, and motor dysfunction affecting the muscles of mastication, deglutition, and facial expression contributes heavily to the unfortunate effects of a stroke on the orofacial area. Problems with speech (articulation in particular), dribbling of saliva, difficulties in swallowing, choking episodes, and nasal regurgitation of fluids may all be encountered. Lack of muscle tone and inability to control the muscles of mastication cause problems with retention of dentures and with the clearing of the food bolus from buccal and lingual sulci. Plaque and food debris are retained around the teeth, and weakness or paralysis of the arm and shoulder on one side may significantly reduce the effectiveness of whatever oral hygiene measures are possible.

Malformations of the cerebral vasculature may occur in the various angiomatous syndromes, some of which also involve the face and oral tissues with a visible hemangiomatous birthmark or phakos, such as Sturge-Weber and von Hippel-Lindau syndromes. Neurologic changes secondary to cerebral angiomatosis are common complications of these syndromes. Orofacial hemangiomatosis in patients with evidence of focal neurologic disease should be considered to be possibly part of one of these phakomatoses, until an alternate explanation for the neurologic problem is established. Surgical treatment of an orofacial hemangioma in such a patient should only be attempted after the extent of the vascular malformation and its collaterals have been adequately defined.

Arteritis, a rare cause of cerebral infarction or hemorrhage, may be generalized throughout the carotid system and may manifest as localized tenderness over the temporal or facial arteries or as chronic pain in the areas supplied by those vessels. These problems and migraine are considered in more detail in Chapter 146.

DENTAL MANAGEMENT. The patient who has a hemiplegia or other major physical disability often presents a management problem for the dentist, particularly the dentist working in a small operatory that makes no provision for the physically handicapped. These patients may need to bring their wheelchairs next to the dental chair, in order to lift themselves or to be assisted into the chair. Others may need wider spaces to manipulate poorly functioning limbs and prosthetic aids. Still others may need to be treated in a wheelchair, hospital bed, or litter. The American Society for Dentistry for the Handicapped has developed a number of devices to assist the dentist and the patient in these areas, and most hospital dental centers and some dental offices are equipped to offer these special services.

The practice of deferring elective dental treatment for patients who have persistent blood pressure elevations beyond 160-95 is designed to encourage patients of obtain and follow an antihypertensive therapeutic regimen including medication and appropriate diet if required. In general, the blood pressure (BP) reading itself is a poor predictor of the likelihood of a cerebrovascular accident occurring at a given office visit. Even with elevations as high as 200/120, there is no direct correlation between the BP reading and the likelihood of a stroke. However, most dentists would customarily defer even emergency dental procedures when a pressure is recorded at this level. Spasm of the cerebral arterioles has been detected as a response to peak elevations of systolic blood pressure in patients with malignant hypertension and probably contributes to the cerebral edema, petechial hemorrhages, and small infarctions that underlie the syndrome of hypertensive encephalopathy that characteristically occurs in malignant hypertension. These patients apart, however, the risk that dental procedures will trigger transient cerebral ischemic attacks, cerebral hemorrhage, or any other type of cerebrovascular accident in a patient with a markedly elevated blood pressure is essentially unknown. Efforts are usually made to allay nervousness, to limit the length of a visit, to avoid vasoconstrictors, and to monitor the blood pressure during dental treatment of a patient with markedly elevated readings. The wisdom of such management procedures remains unquestioned, although their contribution to the prevention of strokes may be minimal.

Cerebral venous thrombosis, including cavernous sinus thrombosis, remains a possible and very serious complication of oral surgical procedures, facial and jaw fractures, and dental infection with facial cellulitis, particularly in the anterior maxillary and pterygoid plexus regions. While less common than in the preantibiotic era, this problem is still reported in the oral surgical literature, emphasizing the well-established connections known to exist between the intra- and extracranial venous circulations in these locations. Cerebral venous thrombosis is not a cause of cerebral infarction and stroke, although small emboli may reach the cerebral arterial circulation through arteriovenous anastomoses, confusing the signs and symptoms characteristic of cerebral venous thrombosis.

A number of oral prosthetic devices have been designed to address some of the problems faced by patients after a stroke, and they may be very effective in assisting the stroke patient to overcome his handicap without disastrous oral complications. A partial listing of such appliances is included here, but it should be emphasized that success in this area depends as much on the willingness of both the dentist and the patient to experiment and persist with an appliance as it does on the ingenuity of the dentist and dental laboratory to design and adapt existing prosthetic techniques to this end. Timing of efforts to correct oral functional disability is important. Initially all that may be needed is an attempt to make the patient's mouth more comfortable by prophylaxis, polishing of dentures, institution of a regular program of denture and oral hygiene (even if only daily use of mouthrinses can be achieved), and relining of loose dentures.

Retention of large amounts of food debris, particularly in the buccal sulcus of the affected side, is a fairly common problem in stroke patients and may be of sufficient extent to block the orifice of the parotid duct, if daily oral hygiene is omitted. Processing of an acrylic extension to the buccal flange of an existing lower denture aids considerably in controlling this problem and may also assist in the retention of the denture by lax muscles. Such a flange is fabricated out of the mouth and subsequently adjusted to the patient's comfort. Simple bite splints or night guards will often protect the tongue from irregularities in the dental arch, which aggravate lingual dysesthesias and glossodynia, particularly in patients with hypermobile lingual musculature. A wire or acrylic palatal extension added to the posterior edge of an upper denture is said to aid considerably in the control of nasal regurgitation and certain types of speech defects following a stroke; improved control over swallowing and a number of oropharyngeal muscular problems are also said to result from use of this device. An electronically controlled visual speech aid unit has also been developed in association with the palatal extension to help coordinate palatal movements. In the stroke patient with remaining natural teeth, use of an electric toothbrush and water irrigating units considerably improves oral hygiene. A number of devices have been fabricated to aid the physically handicapped patient with weak or poorly controlled hand and arm movements to use these and other oral hygiene aids.

BIBLIOGRAPHY

Childs, H.G., and Courville, C.B.: Thrombosis of the cavernous sinus secondary to dental infections, Am. J. Ortho. **28**:367, 1942.

Myers, D.E., and others: Evaluation of lingual artery hemodynamics in stroke patients using Doppler ultrasound, J. Oral Surg. **51**:252, 1981.

Selley, W.G.: Dental help for stroke patients, Br. Dent. J. **143**:409, 1977.

Tatoian, J.A., and others: Meningitis and temporal lobe abscess of dental origin: report of a case, J. Oral Surg. **30**:423, 1972.

PROBLEMS OF NERVE AND MUSCLE
Neuromuscular disease

The masticatory and facial muscles may exhibit evidences of neuromuscular disease at the same time that other regional muscle groups are affected, or they may be the location of the presenting complaint in the early stages of some neuromuscular disorders. Patients who complain of difficulties with speaking and swallowing, those who find they can no longer manage full dentures, and those with trismus and TMJ dysfunction should always be carefully evaluated for signs of unequal masticatory muscle strength, facial muscle palsy, unexplained deviation on opening, and tremors and fasciculations. An evaluation of this type is not usually included in the standard dental head and neck examination but should at least be part of the routine for dental evaluation of patients with these particular problems. In the majority of cases, isolated spasms affecting one or more masticatory muscles or a major occlusal disharmony will be the explanation of the abnormal function observed, but on occasions evidence of masseter or pterygoid muscle weakness will be detected. At other times, some evidence of neuromuscular dysfunction will be noticed by the patient in another region of the body, such as the shoulder girdle or hands, before signs and symptoms develop in the muscles of the face and jaws.

The technique for evaluating facial and masticatory muscle function has been fully described by Bosma. It is hoped that his estimate that dentists, by virtue of their day-to-day experience with the ranges of orofacial neuromuscular function, are best equipped to carry out such an evaluation will be matched by an increasing interest and involvement with these techniques on the part of dental consultants.

When evidences of orofacial neuromuscular dysfunction are noted, either as a presenting complaint suggesting a neuromuscular disorder or along with other previously diagnosed problems, consultation with the patient's private physician or appropriate specialist is desirable. In a number of circumstances, treatment of the neuromuscular problem will greatly assist the dentist in managing the patient's dental problems

With the exception of electromyographic recording of the masticatory cycle, little work has been done recording the various parameters that are currently available as clinical measurements on limb muscles, for example. Nerve conduction velocities of the branches of the facial nerve are sometimes measured as part of the management of a facial palsy, but in general data on orofacial neuromuscular function of current clinical usefulness are minimal.

Peripheral neuropathy

ORAL MANIFESTATIONS. Symptoms of burning tongue, unexplained orofacial pain (especially if atypical), and other oral sensory deficits are frequently attributed to peripheral neuropathy affecting the trigeminal nerve. In most cases, there is minimal evidence to support such an impression, and the range of tests available for documenting such a diagnosis for similar symptoms affecting a limb is not customarily applied to this region. The diagnosis of peripheral neuropathy of the trigeminal nerve is usually tacitly accepted in a diabetic individual who has well-documented evidence of peripheral neuropathy elsewhere, and the same reasoning by analogy is usually used in cases of peripheral neuropathy of other types. The dental literature also emphasizes a causative role for diabetes as far as oral dysesthesias are concerned, but there is no direct evidence to implicate diabetic peripheral neuropathy as the pathologic change underlying these symptoms. There is also some question whether the long-stated relationship between burning tongue, atypical facial pain, and other oral dysesthesias is valid. Screening tests for diabetes carried out on dental patients with these symptoms will at times reveal mild glucose intolerance or even undiagnosed frank diabetes and justify medical consultation and treatment of the problem. There are no data available, however, to indicate how often treatment of glucose (and lipid) abnormalities that occur with some frequency in these patients leads to resolution of the orofacial neurologic complaint.

DENTAL MANAGEMENT. While the treatment of orofacial symptoms resulting from a peripheral neuropathy is essentially whatever treatment is available for the particular type of neuropathy involved, acrylic bite splints and night guards also may help in resting the jaw and protecting the tongue from additional local trauma.

Myasthenia gravis

ORAL MANIFESTATIONS. The primary signs and symptoms of myasthenia gravis occur in the orofacial-pharyngeal area and may be quite prominent, even when the patient is not in crisis. A flat expressionless face, drooping corners of the mouth, paresis of the orbicularis oris and oculi muscles, and a general affect of tiredness and depression, accentuated by weakness of the neck muscles (causing drooping of the head) and a flat weak voice, produce a characteristic picture. Not uncommonly, a mistaken diagnosis of depression has been made in some cases. Intraorally, protrusive movements of the tongue appear weak and limited, leading at times to posterior collapse of the organ with airway obstruction. Sterterous breathing and dyspnea may also be apparent even with the patient at rest. The soft palate hangs low, lax, and motionless, and the cheeks hand closely along the buccal surfaces of the teeth. Dysphagia and regurgitation of food into the mouth are common symptoms. Masticatory, facial, and neck muscles are often among those primarily affected, leading to inability to keep the jaws closed without guiding and holding it in place by hand. The anticholinesterase drugs stimulate saliva production as a side effect, and the patient may have difficulty handling the copious saliva if swallowing and masticatory and facial muscle function are weak.

DENTAL MANAGEMENT. Ability to manage full dentures may be compromised in the patient with myasthenia gravis because of inability to maintain a peripheral seal or retain the lower denture by muscular control. Construction of a thin peripheral border to the denture is recommended, and the maximum muscle trimming possible is desirable. The laxity of the buccinator and masseter muscles brings them in close contact with the sides of the upper denture, often blocking the flow of parotid saliva or causing it to accumulate under the upper denture and dislodge it.

Infection, including dental abscesses, and stress may induce a crisis in the myasthenia gravis patient, and this should be kept in mind by a dentist treating a patient with this problem. Ideally, in the patient subject to repeated crises, dental care should be provided in a hospital dental center or other location where facilities for intubation and artificial respiration are available. Excessive saliva will often need to be controlled by working on the upright patient and using an effective aspirator.

Inflammatory myopathies

ORAL MANIFESTATIONS. Myofascial dysfunction affecting the muscles of mastication (usually referred to as TMJ myofascial dysfunction) is assumed to be the result of localized inflammatory changes in one or more of these muscles as a result of trauma, excessive movement under stress, or even minor ruptures in ligaments or muscle fibers. For the most part, there is no clear evidence to establish the nature of the pathologic changes underlying the dysfunction syndrome, and the exact nature or cause of the change remains a mystery.

It is fairly clear, however, that other localized inflammatory changes occurring in these muscles can lead to symptoms indistinguishable from those of TMJ dysfunction syndrome. In particular, dental consultants should keep in mind two conditions, polymyalgia rheumatica and trichinosis, as possible causes of an inflammatory myopathy of the masticatory muscles. Appropriate screening tests (sedimentation rate and eosinophil count, respectively) should be done to rule out these possibilities. On occasion, muscle biopsy is required, but the effects of most inflammatory myopathies are widespread and more appropriate locations for a biopsy than the masticatory muscles should be found.

DENTAL MANAGEMENT. Management of an inflammatory myopathy of the masticatory muscles is the same as that used for control of TMJ myofascial dysfunction. A routine of local application of heat, anti-inflammatory agents, and rest to the joint and associated muscles should be followed.

Malignant hyperthermia

Malignant hyperthermia during general anesthesia continues to be associated with a high mortality despite the availability of intravenous dantrolene sodium, which is used as a direct muscle relaxant and to control the amount of calcium released during a hyperthermic crisis. The problem persists largely because the signs of the disease are often not diagnosed until widespread and irreversible cellular damage has occurred. To a limited extent, a suspicion in this regard should be raised if any of the following are noted in the history: malignant hyperthermia during a prior general anesthesia, a family history of the problem, serum biochemical abnormalities (elevated creatine phosphokinase [CPK] levels), and musculoskeletal disease in a patient or close relative. Unfortunately, only about one third of patients with malignant hyperthermia manifest a musculoskeletal abnormality, so the presence of muscle disease is a useful guide only when one or more of these conditions are also present. Of those who develop malignant hyperthermia, many do display skeletal muscle rigidity as part of their neuromuscular problem. The presence of elevated CPK levels is also nonspecific for this condition, raised levels being found in a number of conditions such as coronary thrombosis, severe neuromyopathies, myxedema, and late pregnancy. Where available, muscle biopsy with evaluation of the in vitro response to halothane remains the most accurate predictor of susceptibility.

BIBLIOGRAPHY

Aldrete, J.A., and Britt, B., editors: Second international symposium on malignant hyperthermia, New York, 1977, Grune & Stratton, Inc.

Bigot, C., and others: Dental and periodontal incidence in two systemic diseases; Friedrich's ataxia and Duchenne de Boulogne's disease, Inform. Dent. **59**:23, 1977.

Bosma, J.F.: Sensorimotor examination of the mouth and pharynx, Frontiers Oral Physiol. **2**:78, 1976.

Bottomley, W.K., and others: Management of patients with myasthenia gravis who require maxillary dentures, J. Prosth. Dent. **38**:609, 1977.

Hawada, T., and others: Masticatory function in the patient with Kugelberg Welander disease, J. Hiroshima Univ. Dent. Soc. **8**:216, 1975.

Hawada, T., and others: Roentgenocephalometric analysis of open bite in patients with progressive muscular dystrophy, J. Hiroshima Dent. Soc. **8**:55, 1976.

Hawada, T., and others: Masticatory performance in patients with progressive muscular dystrophy, J. Hiroshima Dent. Soc. **8**:61, 1976.

Kamiiski, H., and others: Correction of myopathic face associated with myotonic muscular dystrophy, J. Maxillofacial Surg. **5**:48, 1977.

Kent, J.N., and others: Correction of severe dentofacial deformity associated with myotonia congenita, J. Oral Surg. **36**:129, 1978.

Section Twelve

SKIN DISEASES AND THEIR ORAL MANIFESTATIONS

edited by **Bernard A. Kirshbaum** and **Robert N. Arm**

Many dermatologic diseases and systemic diseases with dermatologic manifestations have oral manifestations. The dentist may have a problem in diagnosis and management of the oral lesions or in general dental management. This chapter is intended to acquaint dentists with some dermatologic conditions that may be encountered during routine oral examination.

ORAL MANAGEMENT OVERVIEW

While each disease may present individual management problems, many will have similar precautions. Specific precautions will be covered in each section.

The two major problems encountered in a patient with oral lesions are relieving the symptoms and maintaining dental preventive therapy. Symptomatic relief can generally be obtained by avoiding irritating agents and using topical anesthetics. Spicy or acid food and alcoholic drinks and solutions, including most mouthwashes, may bring added discomfort to a patient with oral ulcers. It is best to recommend a bland diet when symptoms are severe. For mouth rinsing, a baking soda rinse of about 1 tablespoon soda to 8 ounces warm water may be best. New non-alcoholic mouthwashes can be used and can be especially helpful for dental health if they contain fluoride.

Many agents can be applied for topical relief. Some, such as emollient mixtures (Orabase), will provide a topical protective barrier. Others will provide anesthetic relief as well. For single lesions or those in a limited area, 5% lidocaine ointment can be used. For longer action an anesthetic in an emollient base may be helpful. For diffuse mucosal involvement a rinse may be best. Viscous lidocaine, while commonly used, is often disliked because of its viscosity and taste. A solution of 0.5% dyclonine (Dyclone) or 0.5% aqueous diphenhydramine (Benadryl) will provide excellent relief and, if swallowed, slight sedation. Generally 1 teaspoon (5 ml) is used, either alone or on crushed ice, and swished in the mouth. It can be used every hour if needed. The elixir must be avoided since it will cause a severe burning sensation.

In some diseases patients complain of sialorrhea or xerostomia. Increased salivation should be explained to the patient but treatment avoided. A false saliva solution may help the xerostomic patient. Commercially available sprays (Salivart) and solutions (Sal-eze) can be obtained. One can make a 2% methylcellulose solution or a solution of 5% glycerin, 1% methylcellulose, flavoring agent, and sodium bicarbonate to buffer to pH 7. In severe xerostomia fluoride should be included in the mouthrinse.

Once the patient is comfortable, good mouth care will be easier. Comprehensive treatment should be avoided during acute flare-up. Hygiene should always be stressed since good hygiene will avoid secondary infections, allow lesions to heal faster, and avoid dental breakdown. If toothbrushing, even with a small brush, is not possible a 4 × 4 gauze may be used to gently clean the mouth. If tolerated, a sponge with baking soda (Toothette) may be helpful. The lemon glycerine swabs provided in hospitals for oral hygiene may irritate the lesions and, if used for a long period, may cause enamel decalcification because of the acidity. As soon as possible the patient should be restored to normal hygiene aids. Baking soda rinses may be helpful. Peroxide solutions can aid healing and periodontal health, but one should be cautious about fungal overgrowth. A water irrigating device (Water-Pik) at low pressure may allow cleaning of difficult areas.

156 • CONGENITAL DISEASES

Robert N. Arm, Bernard A. Kirshbaum, Anthony V. Benedetto, and Karen Lipinski

ANHIDROTIC ECTODERMAL DYSPLASIA

Anhidrotic ectodermal dysplasia is a rare familial disorder characterized by scanty hair, thin dry skin, and dental abnormalities. The hair is thin, sparse, and dry on the scalp, eyebrows, eyelashes, bearded areas, axillae, and pubic areas. Eccrine and sebaceous glands are almost totally absent, hence there is no sweating, no sebum production, and dry skin. The nails may also be absent or malformed. There have been reports of ophthalmologic abnormalities, sensorineural hearing deficit, and mental deficiencies. There is a characteristic facies suggestive of congenital syphilis, with frontal bossing, saddle nose (depressed nasal bridge), prominent supraorbital ridges, and pointed chin. The lips are often thickened, especially the upper, and there may be furrows, especially at the buccal commissures, often giving a "pouting" expression. The cheek bones are characteristically high and wide with narrowing of the lower half of the face. The eyebrows are scanty with the outer two thirds usually absent; the eyes slant upward producing a somewhat oriental appearance. The cheeks present telangiectasia and small papules simulating milia and adenoma sebaceum. These patients are often short.

This condition is familial, probably transmitted by an X-linked recessive gene; only males fully express the disorder. Female carriers have milder abnormalities of teeth and breasts and have diminished ability to sweat. Autosomal recessive and dominant forms have also been reported. The basic defect causing the disease is unknown.

Since these patients do not sweat, they are uncomfortable in hot weather due to elevation of body temperature. With exertion they experience fatigue and asthenia. Many of these patients tolerate infections poorly and succumb to complications of bacterial and viral illnesses. There is no specific treatment for this disorder; in order to function relatively normally, these patients must modify their living conditions to avoid the dangers of increased temperatures.

Genetic counseling is indicated for those afflicted with this condition, as well as those who are known carriers of the trait.

ORAL MANIFESTATIONS. These patients have oligodontia or anodontia. The remaining teeth are affected by a delayed eruption pattern and developmental abnormalities ranging from cone- or peg-shaped teeth to teeth with hypoplastic hypocalcified enamel. Some reports suggest that these teeth may be more vulnerable to carious lesions. The tongue may also appear enlarged, filling the edentulous areas. Oligodontia and alveolar aplasia give the patient's face an older appearance.

DENTAL MANAGEMENT. The dentist plays a major role in psychologic management of the child by creating a positive self-image by providing a normal appearing mouth. Maintenance of the natural teeth is the key to a successful prosthesis. Edentulous patients may have problems retaining prosthetic devices due to the frequent occurrence of xerostomia, aplastic knifelike alveolar ridge, and alveolar aplasia. Cases of successful complete dentures have been reported. Microbial infection must be avoided since the patient may develop hyperthermia during the fever.

BIBLIOGRAPHY

Bartlett, R.C., Eversole, L.R., and Adkins, R.J.: Autosomal recessive hypohidrotic ectodermal dysplasia: dental manifestations, Oral Surg. 33:736, 1972.

Giansanti, J.S., Long, S.M., and Rankin, J.L. The "tooth and nail" type of autosomal dominant ectodermal dysplasia, Oral Surg. 37:576, 1974.

Gold, R.J.M.: The characterization of hereditary abnormalities of keratin: Clouston's ectodermal dysplasia. Birth Defects 7:91, 1971.

Lowry, R.B., Robinson, G.C., and Miller, J.R.: Hereditary ectodermal dysplasia: symptoms, inheritance patterns, differential diagnosis, management, Clin. Pediatr. 5:395, 1966.

Reed, W.B., Lopez, D.A., and Landing, B.: Clinical spectrum of anhidrotic ectodermal dysplasia, Arch. Dermatol. 102:134, 1970.

Saunder, K.D.: Consideration in dental treatment of children with ectodermal dysplasia, J. Am. Dent. Assoc. 93:1177, 1976.

Tocchini, J.J., West, F.T., and Barlett, R.W.: An unusual development pattern in a case of hypohidrotic ectodermal dysplasia, J. Dent. Child. 37:158, 1970.

Witkop, C.J., Brearley, L.J., and Gentry, W.C.: Hypoplastic enamel, onycholysis, and Hypohidrosis inherited as an autosomal dominant trait: a review of ectodermal dysplasia syndromes, Oral Surg. 39:71, 1975.

EPIDERMOLYSIS BULLOSA DYSTROPHICA

Epidermolysis bullosa dystrophica is a hereditary vesiculobullous disorder that involves both skin and mucosa. There are several diseases included under this name including autosomal dominant and recessive forms. Lesions may occur spontaneously but often arise from trauma.

In the simplex form, lesions generally appear shortly after birth at frictional sites and heal without scarring. One fifth of the patients have affected nails. As the child grows, the condition improves, especially after puberty. Lesions are generally caused by trauma or heat. Transmission is autosomal dominant.

The dominant dystrophic form is also an autosomal dominant trait. Bullae, generally of the ankles, knees, hands, and elbows, heal, leaving scars. Most patients have thick, dystrophic nails. One fifth of the patients have onset of lesions by the age of 1, and there may be improvement with age.

The recessive dystrophic form is unlike the dominant form since it has conjunctival and corneal involvement and is autosomal recessive. The bullae will arise at any pressure or trauma site. The bullae easily rupture, leaving raw lesions, and heal leaving scars and pigment changes. The scarring can lead to clawhand. Nails are absent or dystrophic. A positive Nikolsky sign is present. Scarring of the esophageal mucosa can lead to stenosis and dysphagia.

The letalis form is most severe, causing death during the first few months of life. No scarring or pigment changes are noted. Shortly after birth lesions appear, and nails may be shed. The entire body except the palms and soles can be involved. Vesicular changes can occur in other organ systems.

Therapy for all forms is generally symptomatic. Steroids and vitamin ointments may be of some benefit.

ORAL MANIFESTATIONS. Oral involvement will vary with each form of the disease. In the dominant simplex form only 2% of patients may exhibit oral lesions. A biopsy will show cleavage through the basal layer. The bullae will heal without scars. In the dominant dystrophic form, 2% of patients may have oral involvement with resulting scarring. No odontogenic changes have been noted.

In the recessive dystrophic form 16% of patients have oral involvement. Some lesions appear soon after birth, possibly from the sucking reflex, and leave scars. When the lesion is biopsied, a cleavage may be seen below the basement membrane. Enamel hypoplasia has been reported with "pock-marked" appearance seen. The dentin appears uninvolved. Other reported changes include maxillary atrophy with mandibular prognathism.

All patients with the letalis form have oral lesions. When these lesions are examined microscopically, cleavage may be noted between the cell membranes of the epidermal and dermal layers. The bullae are most commonly present at the junction of the hard and soft palates. Severe alterations of enamel formation have been reported as well as microscopic dentinal changes. Gardner et al. believes the enamel problems arise from ameloblastic dysfunction.

DENTAL MANAGEMENT. Dental management must be aimed at the prevention of oral disease and of trauma to tissues. Atraumatic sponges or soft toothbrushes can be used for daily debridement. Palliative oral treatment of topical anesthetics may aid in the total systemic management.

Care must be taken to protect the entire body when treating patients with generalized involvement. The chair, head rest, operating table, and head ring should be covered with padding. The body should be lightly covered or protected in a burn tent. All cases reported were treated in the operating room. The concern of causing a lesion from the trauma of placing a throat pack has been mentioned. Howden reports two cases using throat packs with no complications.

Patients have tolerated restorations, prophylaxis, and extractions, but prosthodontics are poorly tolerated because the trauma may create new large lesions.

BIBLIOGRAPHY

Endruschat, A.J., and Keenan, D.S.: Anesthetic and dental management of a child with epidermolysis bullosa dystrophica, Oral Surg. **36**:667, 1973.

Gardner, D.G., and Hudson, C.D.: The disturbances in odontogenesis in epidermolysis bullosa hereditaria letalis, Oral Surg. **40**:483, 1975.

Gorlin, R.J.: Epidermolysis bullosa, Oral Surg. **32**:760, 1971.

Howden, E.F., and Oldenburg, T.R.: Epidermolysis bullosa hystrophica: report of two cases, J. Am. Dent. Assoc. **85**:1113, 1972.

NEUROFIBROMATOSIS (VON RECKLINGHAUSEN'S DISEASE)

Neurofibromatosis is a form of hereditary dysplasia with manifestations in the skin, soft tissues, bone, and nervous system. The skin lesions include neurofibromas, café au lait spots, axillary freckling, freckling on the neck and perineal areas (Crowe's Sign), and bronzing (diffuse hyperpigmentation) of the skin. There may also be associated nevus anemicus, pigmented hairy nevi, sacral hypertrichosis, and cutis verticis gyrata (deep furrows and folds of skin and subcutaneous tissues extending vertically over the scalp). The bone findings include spina bifida, dislocations, and fractures but are mainly erosive changes producing kyphosis, lordosis, and pseudarthrosis. Neuromas of the spinal nerves may occasionally cause paralyses. Tumors of the cranial nerves, as well as brain tumors, epilepsy, mental retardation, and dementia, also occur in von Recklinghausen's disease.

The cutaneous neurofibromas (fibroma molluscum) are tumors that vary in size from pinhead to large pendulous flabby masses; the skin over these is usually coarsened and may become deeply pigmented. Many of the soft tumors are pedunculated, and an underlying cutaneous defect can be felt as a ring or buttonhole at the base of the lesion. Plexiform neuromas are subcutaneous neurofibromas that form along the course of peripheral nerves in large, irregular beaded masses. Neurofibromas may be found over any part of the skin surface, although usually not on the palms and soles.

Café au lait spots are brownish macules, often round to ovoid, varying from 0.5 to 15 cm or more in diameter. Some believe the presence of six or more café au lait spots 1.5 cm or more in diameter is sufficient to establish the diagnosis of neurofibromatosis even in the absence of tumors (Fig. 156-1). However, café au lait spots are not pathognomonic of von Recklinghausen's neurofibromatosis. Though they may vary in appearance, they can be seen in the orbital glioma syndrome (which may have neurofi-

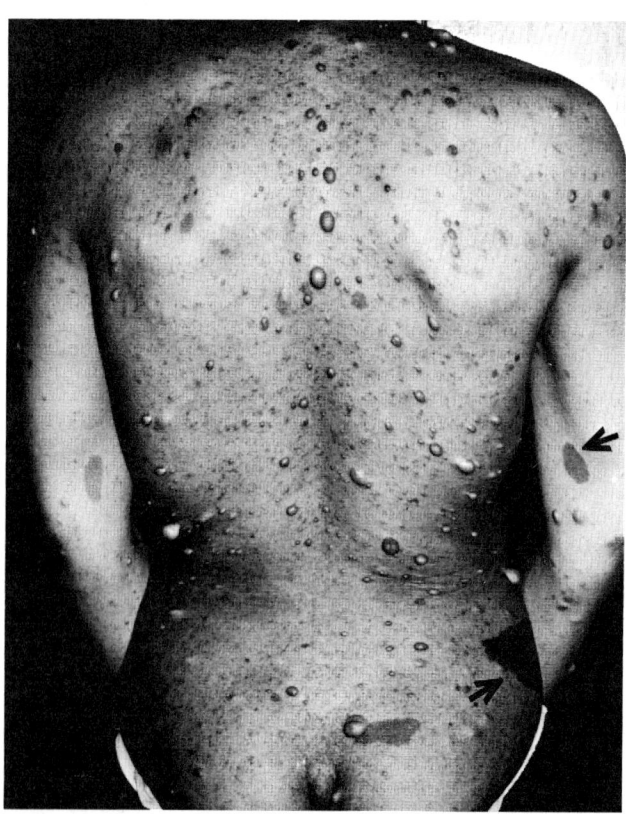

Fig. 156-1. Neurofibromatosis. Note café au lait spots *(arrows)* and multiple neurofibromas.

bromas), Silver syndrome, Albright's syndrome, and tuberous sclerosis. In Albright's syndrome (polyostotic fibrous dysplasia) and precocious puberty, the café au lait spots generally have a more irregular outline, often called "coast of Maine" appearance. Silver syndrome should be recognized by the triangular face caused by a disproportionately large head for a small facial mass (pseudohydrocephaly) tapering to a narrow jaw, short stature, and significant asymmetries. The patient may have syndactylism of the second and third toes and short, incurved fifth finger; about one third will be retarded. "Turned-down" corners of the mouth have also been reported.

Many other organ systems may be involved. Endocrine disorders such as acromegaly, cretinism, hyperparathyroidism, myxedema, precocious puberty, and growth retardation have been described. From 5% to 10% of patients with pheochromocytoma have neurofibromatosis. Retinal tumors (phakomas) may also be found.

Neurofibromatosis is an autosomal dominant inherited disease without sex linkage; skipped generations do not occur. It is found in approximately 1 in 3000 births. About 50% of the cases are sporadic, have no familial history of the disease, and probably represent new mutations. Once established, the disorder is transmitted in a mendelian dominant pattern, but the expression of the defect in successive generations can vary from café au lait spots to extensive neurofibromas. The basic defect explaining the tendency of the neural sheath (Schwann) cells to form tumors is not known.

The diagnosis is based on the clinical findings and is fairly easy when typical lesions and café au lait spots are present. Confusion can occur with other diseases with pigmented spots.

Another syndrome often confused with neurofibromatosis is the multiple endocrine neoplasia syndrome, often called Sipple's syndrome. The affected individual may have neuromas or neurofibromas and pheochromocytomas. The neuromas are generally mucosal and histologically resemble traumatic neuromas. The major characteristics of the syndrome are thyroid nodules, which generally become medullary thyroid carcinoma. The clinician should be alerted that *any* thyroid nodule in this syndrome should be treated with aggressive surgery. Often multiple parathyroid adenoma occur. There have been reports of associated intracranial hemangiomas, Cushing's disease, and diabetes.

While neurofibromatosis is generally a benign, disfiguring disease, deaths have been reported from associated meningiomas and gliomas, as well as sarcomatous degeneration of the lesions. From 5.5% to 16% malignant degeneration has been reported. Excision of the disfiguring superficial lesions remains the only accepted treatment, but when the neurofibromas are numerous, this can become a formidable task.

Genetic counseling is indicated for those afflicted with von Recklinghausen's disease, to make sure all options are understood. Careful periodic examinations are needed to avoid and treat complications.

ORAL MANIFESTATIONS. The patient with neurofibromatosis can often be recognized by the multiple neurofibromas of the face. These nodules may also appear in the mouth. They are generally nonulcerated, mucosal colored masses or pendulous polyps. They are most commonly located on the tongue and lips. While the neurofibromas are generally benign, they can undergo malignant transformation. A biopsy is indicated for lesions that change appearance.

Maxillary and mandibular bone abnormalities with resulting facial asymmetry have been reported. Some of these abnormalities are related to osteoclastic resorption by pressure atrophy from tumor growth. Radiographically, a radiolucent area will be seen. Cases of stimulation of bone growth resulting in hyperplasia with focal hypoplasia due to restructuring have been reported, as has hypoplasia of the ramus. Muller reported radiolucencies of the ascending ramus in the area of the sigmoid notch, as well as increased depth of the notch with exostosis of the zygoma. At surgery, the radiolucencies were proved to be neurofibromas. Some of the lytic lesions have been known to disappear spontaneously.

Macroglossia has been seen in patients without lesions or thyroid problems, though it is more common in patients with cretinism or myxedema.

DENTAL MANAGEMENT. Early recognition and biopsy are important. The asymmetries lead to major occlusal problems and reconstructive difficulties. Orthognathic intervention via surgery may help, as may removal of lesions that interfere with function. It is virtually impossible to remove all lesions, and careful observation must be made to rule out malignant change.

The systemic problems in von Recklinghausen's disease will have a great effect on dental treatment. Many patients may have seizures and may be taking anticonvulsants (for dental management refer to Chapter on epilepsy). Pheochromocytomas may cause intermittent headaches that are often mistaken for "temporomandibular joint problems." Of greater significance is the labile hypertension, which must be closely watched.

BIBLIOGRAPHY

Barone, D.A.: Neurofibromatosis, a clinical review, Postgrad. Med. 66(2):73, 1979.

Bartlett, R.C., and others: A neuropolyendocrine syndrome: mucosal neuromas, pheochromocytomas and medullary thyroid carcinomas, Oral Surg. 31:206, 1971.

Bergsma, D.: Birth defects, atlas and compendium, Baltimore, 1973, The Williams & Wilkins Co.

Brasfield, R.D., and DasGupta, T.K.: VonRecklinghausen's disease: a clinicopathological study, Ann. Surg. 175:86, 1972.

Casino, A.J., and others: Oral facial manifestations of the multiple neoplasia syndrome, Oral Surg. 51:516, 1981.

Feinman, N.L., and Yakovac, B.A.: Neurofibromatosis in childhood, J.Pediatr. 76:339, 1970

Gorlin, R.J., and others: Multiple mucosal neuromas, pheochromocyto-

mas and medullary carcinoma of the thyroid—a syndrome, Cancer **22:**293, 1968.
Johnson, B.L., and Charneco, D.R.: Cafe au lait spots in neurofibromatosis and in normal individuals, Arch. Dermatol. **102:**442, 1970.
Lewin-Epstein, J., and Michmann, J.: Multiple neurofibromatosis with oral lesions: report of a case, J. Oral Surg. **20:**507, 1962.
Muller, H., and Slootweg, P.J.: Maxillofacial deformities in neurofibromatosis, J. Maxillofac. Surg. **9:**89, 1981.
Riccardi, V.M.: VonRecklinghausen neurofibromatosis, N. Engl. J. Med. **305:**1617, 1981.
Rittersma, J., and others: Neurofibromatosis with mandibular deformities, Oral Surg. **33:**718, 1972.

TUBEROUS SCLEROSIS; ADENOMA SEBACEUM; EPILOIA (BOURNEVILLE-PRINGLE SYNDROME)

Epiloia encompasses the triad of adenoma sebaceum, mental deficiency, and epilepsy. The term "tuberous sclerosis" represents central nervous system involvement. The primary cutaneous finding is adenoma sebaceum, characterized by mostly pinhead-sized, yellowish red, translucent waxy papules on the face. They are located mainly in the rostral and paranasal areas, circumorally, and on the nose, cheek, and chin in a symmetric distribution. The forehead is usually less involved, and periorbital lesions are generally minimal. Although the papules remain discrete, they may form large aggregates in the affected areas; they persist indefinitely and may increase in number. They usually appear after early childhood. Other associated findings that may be present include subungual fibromas, "shagreen" patches on the skin, white leaf-shaped macules, poliosis, café au lait spots, and oral fibrous papules. Subungual fibromas are small digitate asymptomatic fibromatous tumors that may be found protruding from beneath the fingernails or toenails. Shagreen patches are irregular areas of "knobby" skin varying from 1 to 8 cm that may occur on the trunk, most often in the lumbosacral area. They are a form of connective tissue nevi. White lanceotate leafshaped macules are present in 50% of the cases of tuberous sclerosis. They may sometimes be the only manifestation of this condition and often are the first sign of epiloia in the newborn. These lesions are not vitiligo but are hypomelanotic macules containing less melanin in the melanocytes. Depigmented eyelashes or eyebrows (poliosis) may occur as the result of leukoderma affecting the hair follicles. Café au lait spots may also be found but not as frequently as in neurofibromatosis.

Mental deficiency is usually observed early in life and varies from slight to profound mental impairment. Epilepsy is likewise variable, ranging from minimal to severe; myoclonic seizures may occur quite early in life. Mental deficiency and epilepsy are frequently associated with a notable tendency to tumor formation and the finding of potato-like nodules in the brain. Roentgenographic examination may reveal intracranial calcification ("brain stones") in the region of the basal ganglia.

Other organ systems may be involved. Cortical thickening may be seen in long bones, sclerotic lesions in the skull and vertebrae, and cystic changes (similar to those of sarcoidosis and hyperparathyroidism) in the phalanges. Renal hamartomas and cardiac tumors, as well as cystic changes in the lungs, have been reported. Retinal tumors (phakomas) are similar to those occurring in von Recklinghausen's disease.

Epiloia is an inherited disease with an autosomal dominant pattern, equal sex distribution, and varied expression in successive generations. Some individuals have only the adenoma sebaceum; others have epilepsy or other manifestations. Although 90% of facial lesions appear by late childhood, there are rare instances of affected individuals without facial lesions. The reproductive capacity of these patients is low, and it is estimated that over 50% of cases probably arise as spontaneous mutations. The defective gene may be present in up to 1 in 50,000 of the population; the mechanism by which it causes its effects is unknown.

The term "adenoma sebaceum" for the skin lesions is a misnomer—they are neither adenomas nor of sebaceous origin. Histologically they are essentially a vascular and connective tissue tumor (angiofibromatous hamartoma), with giant cells, hyperplasia of the hair follicles, and nervelike structures. The retinal tumors (phakomas) are gliomas; renal hamartomas may be angiomyolipomas, and cardiac tumors are rhabdomyomas.

The course varies with the degree of involvement. Relatively unaffected individuals may lead fairly normal lives. The skin lesions do not undergo malignant change. Spontaneous pneumothorax may occur in those with pulmonary involvement, and hematuria and renal failure in those with kidney lesions. Mental deficiency and seizures may be severe, and many patients die in the third and fourth decades of life as a result of progressive neurologic deterioration.

The facial lesions of adenoma sebaceum may be treated by dermabrasion. Management of seizures and other neurologic manifestations is the major therapeutic concern. There is no known gene marker that is useful in prenatal diagnosis. Genetic counseling is important for those who manifest any of the clinical traits, but this probably does not affect the incidence of new cases, since more than half seem to arise as spontaneous mutations.

ORAL MANIFESTATIONS. The most common oral manifestation is a fibrous growth, generally found on the anterior gingiva but also reported on the lips, cheeks, and tongue. While they are generally mucosal colored, they may also be bluish, red, or yellow. Gingival hyperplasia may be caused by phenytoin (Dilantin) therapy used to control the epilepsy. Periodontitis caused by poor hygiene is common in retarded individuals. Stirrups recently reported a patient who exhibited gingival hyperplasia that could not be explained by drug therapy or by poor oral hygiene. He believed it might have been related to the fibrous growth of the syndrome.

Hyperostosis causing alveolar enlargements, high

vaulted palate, and cystic mandible lesions have been found. The teeth have been involved with a delayed eruption pattern. Hoff has reported enamel hypoplasia believed to be caused by defective amelogenesis.

Since descriptive information on the oral lesions varies, biopsy should be taken and all tissue including gingivectomy specimens submitted for histopathology.

DENTAL MANAGEMENT. Patient management is frequently difficult. Seventy-five percent of the patients are retarded and many are epileptic. Pulmonary problems will alter management if general anesthesia is required. Many of the patients have progressive dyspnea from lung involvement and are prone to spontaneous rupture of pulmonary cysts, leading to a pneumothorax.

BIBLIOGRAPHY

Bergsma, D.: Brith defects, atlas and compendium, Baltimore, 1973, The Williams & Wilkins Co.
Choa, D.H.C.: Congenital neurocutaneous syndromes in childhood. II. Tuberous sclerosis, J. Pediatr. **55**:447, 1959.
Hoff, M., and others: Enamel defects with tuberous sclerosis, Oral Surg. **40**:261, 1975.
Lagos, J.C., and Gomez, M.R.: Tuberous sclerosis: reappraisal of a clinical entity, Mayo Clin. Proc. **42**:26, 1967.
Mackler, S.B., and others: Tuberous sclerosis with gingival lesions, Oral Surg. **34**:619, 1972.
Marshall, D., Saul, G.B., and Sachs, E.: Tuberous sclerosis, N. Engl. J. Med. **261**:1102, 1959.
Nickel, W.R., and Reed, W.B.: Tuberous sclerosis, Arch. Dermatol. **85**:209, 1962.
Reed, W.B., Nickel, W.R., and Campion, G.: Internal manifestations of tuberous sclerosis, Arch. Dermatol. **87**:715, 1963.
Rushton, M.A.: Some less common bone lesions affecting the jaws, tuberous sclerosis with jaw lesions, Oral Surg. **9**:289, 1956.
Stirrups, D.R., and Inglis, J.: Tuberous sclerosis with nonhydantoin gingival hyperplasia, Oral Surg. **49**:211, 1980.

STURGE-WEBER SYNDROME (ENCEPHALOTRIGEMINAL ANGIOMATOSIS)

Sturge-Weber syndrome consists of craniofacial angiomatosis and cerebral calcification. The cutaneous vascular nevus ("port wine stain," nevus flammeus) may be large or small and is present at birth, usually located along the course of the superior and middle branches of the trigeminal nerve (Fig. 156-2). There is an associated meningeal hemangioma on the same side, with calcification and cortical atrophy of adjacent brain tissue, often resulting in contralateral jacksonian convulsions, paralysis, sensory deficit, and mental retardation. While the nevus flammeus is usually unilateral with a sharp border, it may be bilateral or midline. The oral mucous membranes may be affected on the same side. Glaucoma may be present in the ipsilateral eye. This is not an inherited disorder, although occasionally more than one member of a family may be affected. The cause of the Sturge-Weber syndrome is unknown.

Characteristic calcification in the outer layers of the cerebral cortex may be seen in roentgenograms of the skull

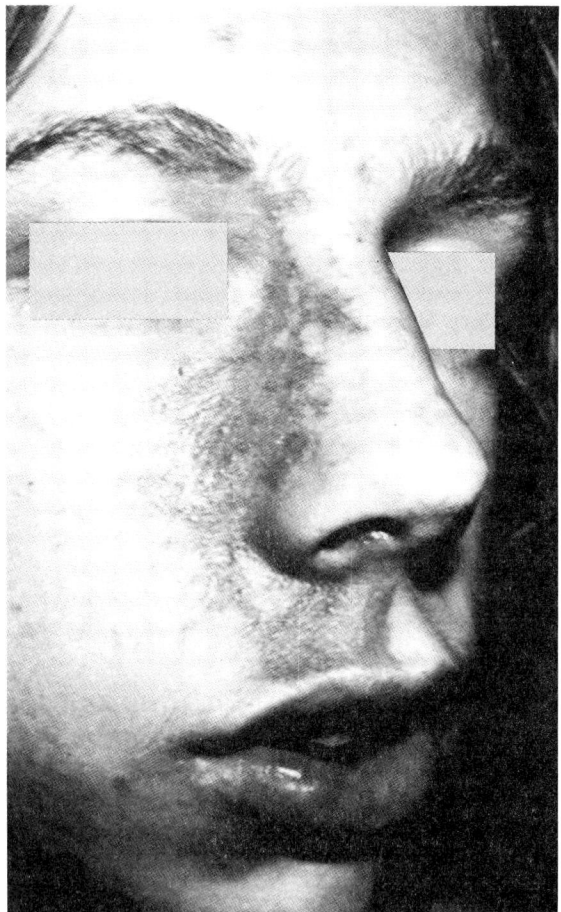

Fig. 156-2. Encephalotrigeminal angiomatosis (Sturge-Weber syndrome) in mentally retarded adolescent. Color of lesion is that of port wine.

as sinuous, double-contoured lines ("tram lines") that follow the convolutions of the cerebral cortex on the affected side. The treatment is directed at the neurologic manifestations and is primarily asymptomatic. Since the occurrence is sporadic and cannot be determined before birth, there are no preventive measures available.

Confusion in texts and literature often occur between Sturge-Weber syndrome and Klippel-Trenaunay syndrome (angio-osteohypertrophy). They will often occur together. Klippel-Trenaunay syndrome consists of hypertrophy of soft tissue and bone secondary to vascular supply with cutaneous and bony hemangiomas and varicose veins in the long bones. The orofacial region may be involved with or without Sturge-Weber syndrome.

ORAL MANIFESTATIONS. Angiomas of the face and mucosa are readily seen. Generally a cutaneous vascular nevus ("port wine" stain) will occur over an area of the trigeminal nerve. Oral involvement, seen in about 40% of patients, consists of a bluish red lesion that blanches on pressure and is found most commonly on the buccal mucosa and lips. Less commonly seen are lesions involving the gingiva of the ipsilateral maxilla and the palate. Rarely the mandibular gingiva, floor of the mouth, and tongue are involved. The lesions resemble a vascular hyperplasia or large tumorlike mass. Microscopy reveals thin wall vessels in a cavernous-type hemangioma. Pyogenic granuloma and possibly early eruption of teeth have been reported from increased vascularity. Gingival problems secondary to phenytoin (Dilantin) and poor hygiene can be seen. Ninety percent of the patients have epilepsy and may be taking phenytoin. Up to 50% are retarded and may be unable to maintain hygiene. Hemiplegia, seen in 30% of the cases, may also lead to oral hygiene problems. One report indicated that the gingival hyperplasia may not be caused by phenytoin, poor hygiene, or angiomas but by a true hyperplasia.

In Klippel-Trenaunay syndrome vascular lesions involving bone, bony hypertrophy, and early eruption have been reported.

DENTAL MANAGEMENT. The major problem is possible hemorrhage from the angiomas. If the involved area is treated, hospitalization with standby pressure splints and blood may be indicated. For general anesthesia, oral intubation may be safer so unseen angiomas may be avoided. All dental treatment must be done with care. Diagnostic angiography may be needed before treatment. Treatment of the vascular areas have included sclerosing solutions, carbon dioxide snow, and electrodissection. Problems from epilepsy and retardation must be dealt with. Special hygiene aids may help the patient, especially if hemiplegia is present.

In the Klippel-Trenaunay syndrome, the bony hypertrophy can lead to occlusal problems or tilting of the teeth. The bony shape may also create problems with prosthesis. The bony angiomas create difficult, possibly life-threatening bleeding problems during surgery. Patients may suffer from thrombocytopenia because of chronic hemorrhage of the vascular lesions. Reports of arterial insufficiency with secondary heart disease due to arteriovenous fistulas may alter the treatment plan.

BIBLIOGRAPHY

Alexander, G.L., and Norman, R.M.: The Sturge-Weber syndrome, Bristol, England, 1960, John Wright & Sons, Inc.

Bergsma, D.: Birth defects, atlas and compendium, Baltimore, 1973, The William & Wilkins Co.

Chao, D.H.: Congenital neurocutaneous syndromes of childhood. III. Sturge-Weber disease, J. Pediatr. **55**:635, 1959.

Crinzi, R.A., and others: Management of a dental infection in a patient with Sturge-Weber disease, J. Am. Dent. Assoc. **101**:798, 1980.

Morgan, G.: Pathology of the Sturge-Weber syndrome, Proc. R. Soc. Med. **56**:422, 1963.

Ykna, R.A., Cassingham, R.J., and Carr, R.F.: Periodontal manifestations and treatment in a case of Sturge-Weber syndrome, Oral Surg. **47**:408, 1979.

BLOOM'S SYNDROME

Bloom's syndrome is a rare hereditary disorder characterized by telangiectatic erythema in the "butterfly area" of the face, sunlight sensitivity, and dwarfism. The skin changes of face and hands consist of telangiectatic erythematous patches resembling lupus erythematosus. There may also be bullous crusted lesions on the lips. These manifestations develop usually in the first months or few years of life and become exacerbated in the summer months by sunlight. Eczematization and vesiculation of the involved areas can result in atrophy, mainly on the face. In addition, there may be café au lait spots, acanthosis nigricans, ichthyosis, prominent ears, hypospadias, cryptorchidism, syndactyly, and hypertrichosis. These individuals are quite small at birth and subsequently show a pituitary type of retarded growth in height and weight in the early years of life. The skeletal frame is small; the body is delicate but well proportioned. Growth may resume later in life, and these dwarfs may eventually appear fairly normal. Intelligence and sexual maturation are normal.

This syndrome is a primary ectodermal dysplasia, with a high frequency of chromosomal breaks and rearrangements. Abnormalities of immunoglobulins have been reported, but no abnormalities in endocrine function or porphyrin metabolism, and the basic defect has not been identified. An autosomal recessive gene is assumed to be responsible. The condition occurs in Jews more often than in other ethnic or racial groups. Aside from deficiencies in the immunoglobulins there are no unusual laboratory findings.

Differential diagnosis includes lupus erythematosus, ataxia-telangiectasia (Louis-Bar syndrome), and Cockayne's syndrome (trisomy 10). Patients with Bloom's syndrome are more prone to repeated infections; some have developed leukemia and other malignancies. This points to the chromosomal structural changes with resultant malignant transformation as well as impaired immunologic defenses.

There is no specific therapy for Bloom's syndrome, only symptomatic treatment and sunlight avoidance to prevent exacerbation of lesions. Genetic counseling is indicated for those who manifest the trait.

ORAL MANIFESTATIONS. Intraoral lesions have not been found but reports of delayed eruption and absence of the maxillary lateral incisors have appeared. The patient may have an erythematous rash on the lips in addition to the "butterfly" facial rash.

Since the patient is sensitive to sunlight, caution should be used with long-term or high-power light sources.

DENTAL MANAGEMENT. The major management problem will center on related systemic disease. This can be linked to the decreased immunoglobulins or development of leukemia. (See chapter on immunodeficient patients and leukemia.)

BIBLIOGRAPHY

Bloom, D.: Congenital telangiectatic erythema resembling lupus erythematosus in dwarfs, Am. J. Dis. Child. **88**:754, 1954.

Bloom, D.: The syndrome of congenital telangiectatic erythema and stunted growth, J. Pediatr. **68**:103, 1966.

German, J., Bloom, D., and Passarge, E.: Bloom's syndrome. VII. Progress report for 1978, Clin. Genet. **15:**361, 1971.
Goodman, R.N., and Gorlin, R.J.: Atlas of the face in genetic disorders, St. Louis, 1977, The C. V. Mosby Co.
McKusick, V.A.: Mendelian inheritance in man, Baltimore, 1974, John Hopkins Press, p. 366.
Rauh, J.L., and Soukoup, S.W.: Bloom's syndrome, Am. J. Dis. Child. **116:**409, 1968.
Smith, D.W.: Recognizable patterns of human malformation, Philadelphia, 1970, W.B. Saunders Co., pp. 68-69.
Warkeny, J.: Congenital malformations, Chicago, 1970, Year book Medical Publishers, pp. 157-158.

BASAL CELL NEVUS SYNDROME (NEVOID BASALIOMA SYNDROME; NEVOID BASAL CELL CARCINOMA SYNDROME)

Basal cell nevus syndrome is a hereditary disorder characterized by multiple basal cell carcinomas, pitted depressions of the palms and soles, bony abnormalities of the ribs and spine, odontogenic keratocysts, and abnormalities of the nervous system and other organs.

The basal cell epitheliomas are usually multiple, can occur in the hundreds, and may appear early in life. They can occur on any part of the body but tend to affect the central facial area (eyelids, periorbital areas, nose, cheeks, and about the lips). In addition to the characteristic presentations, they may be nodular or pigmented or resemble nevi or seborrheic keratoses, but microscopically they have the typical appearance of basal cell carcinomas. From puberty onward, newer lesions that appear grow more rapidly, with the true invasive character of basal cell carcinoma. They may metastasize to the brain and lung.

Pitting of hands and feet is a distinguishing feature, usually developing during the second decade of life or later, becoming more apparent with advancing age. Pitting occurs in at least 70% of patients with this syndrome. The pits are discrete, shallow, 2- to 3-mm depressions found on the palms and soles.

Various bony abnormalities may occur, including spina bifida, scoliosis and kyphosis, shortening of the fourth metacarpal, and rib deformities such as bifid and splayed ribs, synostoses, and partial agenesis.

Calcification of the dura, especially the falx cerebri and cerebelli, may be seen on roentgenograms of the skull. Mental retardation and neurologic abnormalities may be encountered, as well as occasional medulloblastomas and other brain tumors.

The characteristic facial appearance includes hypertelorism, lateral displacement of the medial canthi, frontoparietal bossing, accentuated supraorbital ridges, and a broad nasal root. Mesenteric, ovarian, and mammary cysts, fibromas, and calcifications may occur. Some patients have pseudohypoparathyroidism.

This genetic disorder has an autosomal dominant pattern, with up to 95% penetrance and variable expression. Not all patients exhibit all of the features of this syndrome, and varying formes frustes are often seen. It occurs mainly in whites; males and females are equally affected.

If the basal cell carcinomas are allowed to go untreated, the invasive, aggressive nature of this disorder may result in large, eroding ulcerations and occasional metastases. Curettage and electrofulguration may suffice for most of the lesions; some may require surgical excision. Radiotherapy may be indicated for a few of the lesions, but because of the great number that develop, cumulative dose effects make this modality impractical. Odontogenic cysts of the jaws require surgical intervention. Genetic counseling is indicated.

ORAL MANIFESTATIONS. Usually the first clinical sign is the multiple basal cell carcinomas of the face. The Panorex radiograph will generally show multiple, multilocular, cystlike areas. They often resemble soap bubbles. These cysts are odontogenic keratocysts. They can occur in children as young as 7 years old and may be an initial key finding for this syndrome. The lesions are often painful and may drain into the oral cavity, possibly leading to pathologic fracture. The keratocysts may be associated with unerupted teeth and can displace erupted teeth. Unfortunately, they may be diagnosed simply as a "cyst of the jaw" instead of the clinically significant "keratocyst." Other reported findings include cleft lip and palate, frontal bossing, hypertelorism, and oligodontia.

DENTAL MANAGEMENT. The patient may present with pain, swelling, trismus, and fever secondary to an infected cyst. Complete radiographs are needed to fully delineate the involved area. A CAT scan may help. The cysts should be treated because the keratocyst tends to be more aggressive than other cysts. Surgical removal should be complete to avoid possible recurrence, generally due to a "daughter" cyst. To avoid deformity, reconstruction must be considered as part of the surgical treatment plan. Maintenance of remaining teeth may be important for prosthetic retention. The facial basal cell carcinomas are aggressive and will also lead to deformity and create a possible need for a facial prosthesis.

BIBLIOGRAPHY

Clendenning, W.E., Block, J.B., and Radde, I.C.: Basal cell nevus syndrome, Arch. Dermatol. **90:**38, 1964.
Correl, R.W.: Bilateral cysts of the jaw occurring with multiple skin lesion, J. Am. Dent. Assoc. **101:**978, 1980.
Ellis, D.J., Akin, R.K., and Bernhard, R.: Nevoid basal cell carcinoma syndrome: report of a case, J. Oral Surg. **30:**851, 1972.
Gorlin, R.J., Vickers, R.A., Kellen, E., and Williamson, J.J.: The multiple basal cell nevi syndrome, Cancer **18:**89, 1965.
Howell, J.B., and others: Identification and treatment of jaw cysts in the nevoid basal cell carcinoma syndrome, J. Oral Surg. **25:**129, 1967.
Jackson, R., and Gardere, S.: Nevoid basal cell carcinoma syndrome, Can. Med. Assoc. J. **125:**850, 1971.
Miller, A.S., and others: Nevoid basal cell carcinoma syndrome, Oral Surg. **36:**533, 1973.
VanDijk, E., and Neering, H.: The association of cleft lip and palate with basal cell nevus syndrome, Oral Surg. **50:**214, 1980.
Zackheim, H.S., Howell, J.B., and Loud, A.V.: Nevoid basal cell carcinoma syndrome, Arch. Dermatol. **93:**317, 1966.

PSEUDOXANTHOMA ELASTICUM (GRÖNBLAD-STRANDBERG SYNDROME)

Pseudoxanthoma elasticum is a rare, inherited disorder of elastic tissue, involving the skin, retina, and blood vessels. It is transmitted primarily as an autosomal recessive trait; women are more frequently affected than men.

The skin lesions are small, yellowish papules that initially form parallel to the skin lines and then coalesce. They are usually found in flexural areas—the sides of the neck, axillae, antecubital fossae, abdomen, groin, thighs, and perineum. The lesions have the appearance of plucked chicken skin. They often develop in early childhood but may be overlooked. They generally appear by the second decade. The skin becomes lax and redundant. Gastric, rectal, and vaginal lesions may also occur.

Retinal lesions called angioid streaks are the result of tearing of the elastic tissue in Bruch's membrane and are found radiating along the vessels outward from the optic discs. Retinal hemorrhages and exudates also occur as a result of changes in the elastic tissue of the retinal vessels, leading to varying degrees of blindness.

Arterial involvement can result in epistaxis and hematemesis. Peripheral vascular calcification may produce intermittent claudication. Hypertension, cerebral hemorrhage, and myocardial infarction may occur, contributing to the morbidity and mortality in this disease.

There is no specific treatment; vitamin E (tocopherol) may be helpful. Plastic surgery for cosmetic reasons may be tried.

ORAL MANIFESTATIONS. Yellowish white patches of the mucosa have been reported in about 5% of the cases. They resemble Fordyce granules when seen on the buccal mucosa but are not sebaceous glands. They may also occur on the labial mucosa, soft palate, and lips.

DENTAL MANAGEMENT. Although the lesions present no problem, the systemic involvement due to arterial elastic fiber degeneration may. Arterial breakdown and rupturing may cause gastrointestinal bleeding and occlusion causing myocardial and cerebral infarctions. Arterial calcification has been noted radiographically. Hypertension is also a common problem. Caution should be used in treatment of the patient, especially because of the vascular alterations. (See chapter on cardiovascular disease for management of hypertensive patient.)

BIBLIOGRAPHY

Bergsma, D.: Birth defects, atlas and compendium, Baltimore, 1973, The Williams & Wilkins Co., p. 757.

Ebeling, F.J., Rook, A., and Wilkinson, D.S.: Textbook of dermatology, Oxford, 1979, Blackwell Scientific Publications Ltd, pp. 1642-1644.

Fleischmajer, R., and Matus, N.: Diseases of the corium and subcutaneous tissues. In Moschella, S.L., Pillsbury, D.M., and Hurley, H., editors: Dermatology, Philadelphia, 1975, W.B. Saunders Co., pp. 985-987.

Goette, D.K., and Carpenter, W.: The mucocutaneous Marker of Pseudoxanthoma elasticum, Oral Surg. **51**:68, 1981.

Gorlin, R.J., and Goldman, H.M.: Thoma's oral pathology, St. Louis, 1970, The C. V. Mosby Co. p. 690.

Pope, F.M.: Historical evidence for the genetic heterogeneity of pseudoxanthoma elasticum, Br. J. Dermatol. **92**:493, 1975.

157 • ENDOCRINE AND METABOLIC DISORDERS

Bernard A. Kirshbaum, Anthony V. Benedetto, Karen Lipinski, and Robert N. Arm

DIABETES MELLITUS

The skin changes found in diabetes mellitus can be related to infection, arteriosclerosis, neuropathy, microangiopathy, long-term insulin therapy, and metabolic abnormalities. About 30% of diabetic patients have cutaneous manifestations. The susceptibility to bacterial and fungal

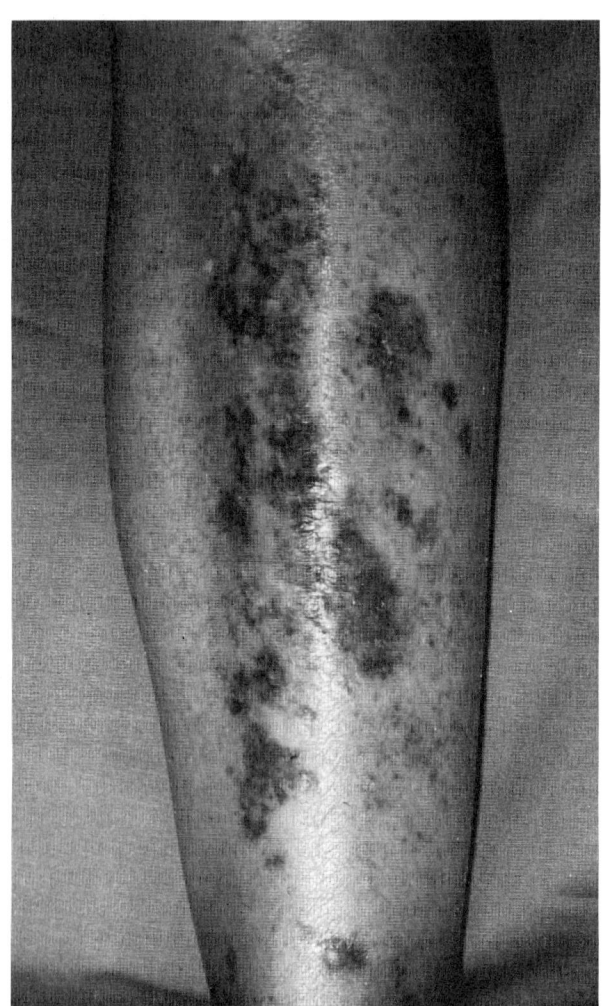

Fig. 157-1. Diabetic dermopathy (shin spots).

infections is influenced by the degree of hyperglycemia. Most of the other skin conditions of diabetic patients are not necessarily related to or dependent on control of the blood glucose.

Pruritus is common in diabetic patients. It is often localized to the lower extremities but may be generalized. Frequently the skin is dry (xerotic). When the anogenital region is involved, a fungal infection may be the cause of the pruritus. The treatment includes less bathing and using mild soaps and topical therapy with moisturizing lotions containing menthol or hydrocortisone or both. Fungal infections are treated with clotrimazole, miconazole, or other topical antifungal agents. For severe infections, systemic antifungal agents are needed.

Diabetic dermopathy, also known as diabetic shin spots, occurs on the lower legs and thighs and resembles traumatic scars. They are small, depressed, pigmented (from hemosiderin) scars that may have a superficial scale (Fig. 157-1). They are a useful skin marker, but they show no relationship to the severity of the diabetes nor to its complications. There is controversy as to whether shin spots are related to diabetic microangiopathy. There is no specific treatment.

Patients with diabetes mellitus are often chronic nasal carriers of *Staphylococcus aureus*. They are more susceptible to styes, pyodermas, furuncles, and carbuncles. The treatment is directed toward control of the infection, which can alter insulin requirements. Recurrent infections may be related to uncontrolled blood glucose levels.

Monilia *(Candida)* infections are associated with diabetes mellitus. Vaginitis, pruritus ani, paronychia, interdigital infections, intertrigo, and balanitis can occur. These entities should arouse the suspicion of diabetes, especially if there are no other reasons for their occurrence.

Superficial fungal infections (dermatophytosis) involving the groin and feet require prompt therapy, since bacterial superinfection may occur.

Papular eruptive xanthomas can occur. They appear as firm, pinkish yellow nodules and papules, symmetrically located on elbows, knees, buttocks, and dorsa of the hands and feet. Less than 1% of diabetic patients have them (usually young men).

Bullosis diabeticorum is most often associated with peripheral neuropathy. It is very rare. Painless blisters develop rapidly on the hands, feet, toes, fingers, and forearms. They are slow to heal and generally leave no scar. The blister fluid is clear and syrupy.

Granuloma annulare has two forms. In both, the color is pale yellow to salmon pink. A localized annular form, found most often on the extremities, is not as closely associated with diabetes mellitus as is the disseminated form, which consists of diffuse, small, confluent annular lesions. This usually occurs on sun-exposed areas of older adults. The localized form is more common in children. Screening for diabetes should be done in both cases.

Necrobiosis lipoidica diabeticorum is similar histologically, but not clinically, to granuloma annulare. It is the best-known cutaneous marker for diabetes, but its relation-

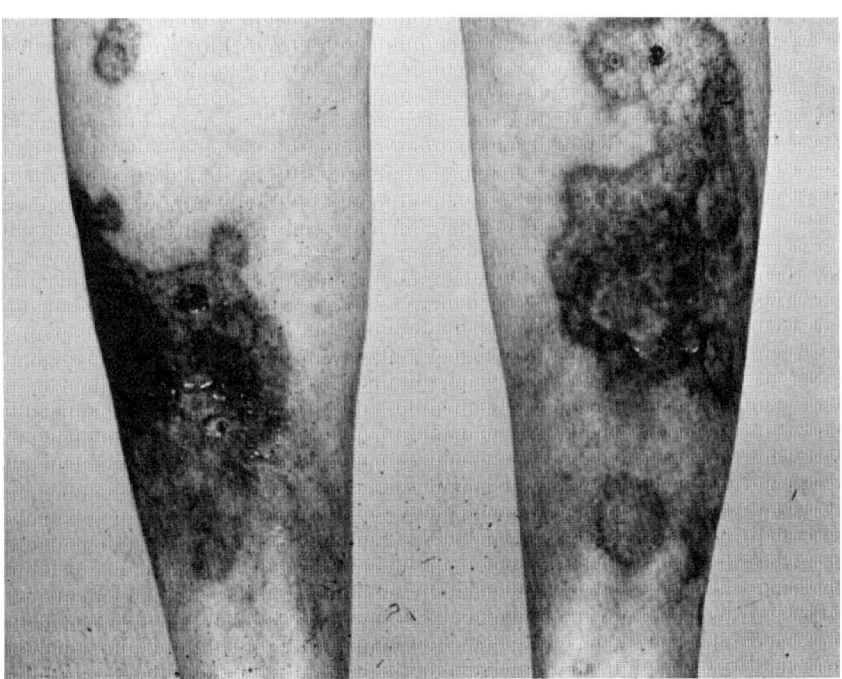

Fig. 157-2. Necrobiosis lipoidica diabeticorum. Lesions are initially paler and atrophic. In advanced stages, as here, there is marked atrophy with hyperpigmentation.

ship to the clinical disease is unclear. It is found in only 3 in 1000 patients with established diabetes. However, the lesions may occur in the absence of diabetes; in these cases there is often a strong family history of diabetes, steroid-induced hyperglycemia, or previously abnormal blood sugar levels in the absence of overt diabetes. Diabetes eventually develops in some of these patients. The majority of patients with necrobiosis lipoidica diabeticorum are women.

The development of necrobiosis lipoidica diabeticorum does not appear to be altered by control of the diabetes. The lesions are characteristic in the fully developed state: oval or irregular indurated plaques with a glazed surface, central atrophy, yellow-orange discoloration, and prominent telangiectases, surrounded by a violaceous border. The lesions usually occur on the lower extremities, but in 15% of patients they are found on the arms, hands, trunk, and scalp. Atypical forms also occur (Fig. 157-2).

The progression of necrobiosis lipoidica diabeticorum is slow. Ulceration and variable scarring occur. Topical or intralesional administration of corticosteroids may help, but these agents should be used carefully because they also induce atrophy.

ORAL MANIFESTATIONS AND DENTAL MANAGEMENT. See pp. 1294-1295.

THYROID DISEASE
Hyperthyroidism

In hyperthyroidism the skin is warm and moist owing to increased cutaneous blood flow and sweating. The skin feels soft and is described as being "fine." This connotes its texture and does not imply thinness, since studies show the skin to have normal thickness. Palmar erythema and onycholysis (separation of the nail distally from the nail bed) may be seen in some patients with hyperthyroidism, but neither sign is specific for this condition. The scalp hair may be fine, friable, and shed diffusely during active hyperthyroidism, but it regrows when the disease is controlled.

An addisonian type of pigmentation is occasionally noted in chronic cases of active hyperthyroidism. This may be caused by increased secretion of melanocyte-stimulating hormone (MSH) by the pituitary. Vitiligo occurs in about 7% of thyrotoxic individuals. Other skin conditions found in association with hyperthyroidism include atopic dermatitis and, infrequently, chronic urticaria and generalized pruritus.

Perhaps the most striking complication of hyperthyroidism is the syndrome of pretibial myxedema, which consists of thickened nodules and plaques on the anterior tibial surfaces of the legs.

The nodules and plaques on the shins have a waxy, translucent appearance and may be flesh colored to pink or violaceous. They are formed by the deposition of acid mucopolysaccharides, which cause dilation of the follicular orifices as the material accumulates, resulting in a peau d'orange appearance. It is accompanied by exophthalmos and usually develops after surgical or radioactive iodine therapy for thyrotoxicosis.

Hypothyroidism

In primary myxedema caused by insufficiency of the thyroid gland, the skin becomes rough and dry, mainly on the extensor surfaces of the extremities, and sometimes appears ichthyotic. The skin of the face becomes puffy, especially around the eyes and on the cheeks. The facial features become coarsened, with a broad thick nose and fat lips, producing a dull expression. The feet and hands may also become swollen, but this is a nonpitting edema owing to the deposition of mucin. The swelling is not to the extent found in pretibial myxedema (see the preceding discussion of "Hyperthyroidism"). The skin may develop a yellowish tint as a result of carotenemia, and the skin temperature falls below normal. The hair becomes universally sparse, dry, and thin and is lost from the outer third of the eyebrows. The nails are brittle, show striations, and break readily at the edges. The tongue is enlarged, and the oral mucous membranes become thickened. The dentition becomes poor, and the teeth may break easily. When hypothyroidism develops as a result of pituitary failure, the skin and hair changes are milder than those found in primary myxedema.

ORAL MANIFESTATIONS AND DENTAL MANAGEMENT. See pp. 1205-1206.

ACROMEGALY

With acromegaly, an increase in dermal collagen causes the skin to become thicker, and ridges (cutis verticis gyrata) may form over the forehead and scalp. The facial features become coarse with a large nose and thickened lips. The tongue may be large and deeply furrowed. The skin becomes coarse and leathery, often with excessive sweating and oiliness. The body hair is coarse and increased in amount. Hyperpigmentation of the skin develops, probably as a result of increased MSH secretion. Hypothyroidism may develop when the normal pituitary tissue is destroyed.

ADRENAL INSUFFICIENCY (ADDISON'S DISEASE)

One of the skin manifestations of Addison's disease is the gradual onset of diffuse hyperpigmentation, which ranges from brown to black and is more pronounced on exposed areas of the body. It is also found on the tongue, gums, buccal mucosa, areolae, genitalia, and areas of friction (such as the knees, elbows, knuckles, and belt line). Scars, pigmented nevi, and hair may become darker, with brunettes showing deeper pigmentation than blonds. The oral pigmentation develops in spots, rather than diffusely, and may be dark brown, blue, or black. Vitiligo develops in 15% of individuals with Addison's disease.

The diffuse hyperpigmentation is induced by an increased secretion of β-MSH from the pituitary, which occurs because adrenal cortisol is not present to function in the feedback system of hypothalamic-pituitary-adrenal control. The differential diagnosis must include other sources of hyperpigmentation such as scleroderma, lupus erythematosus, chronic renal and hepatic diseases, hemochromatosis, melanemia, thyrotoxicosis, and the ingestion of busulfan, actinomycin D, and arsenic. Replacement therapy with corticosteroids can reduce the pigmentation gradually.

ORAL MANIFESTATIONS AND DENTAL MANAGEMENT. See p. 1207.

ADRENAL CORTICAL HYPERPLASIA (CUSHING'S SYNDROME)

Patients with Cushing's syndrome have a characteristic "moon" facies, with telangiectasia over the cheeks and often a dusky plethoric flush. There is an increase of hair on the face, with thinning scalp hair more noticeable in females, as well as hypertrichosis of the body and extremities.

Acneiform lesions of the face, consisting of perifollicular papules and pustules, can occur, but this "steroid acne" does not produce the comedones and deep cystic lesions seen in adolescent acne vulgaris.

Some patients have a brownish pigmentation of the addisonian type because of increased secretion of β-MSH from the pituitary. Acanthosis nigricans may develop in intertriginous areas of the neck, axillae, and groin. Because of the atrophic skin, blood vessels are more prominent, producing cutis marmarata (marble-like mottling of the skin). With loss of dermal collagen and elastin, the skin becomes thin, dry, and fragile. The blood vessels have less support, and purpura and ecchymoses develop. Purple atrophic striae appear on the abdomen and sometimes on the thighs.

Patients with Cushing's syndrome are more susceptible to superficial fungal infections such as *Trichophyton rubrum,* and tinea versicolor (caused by *Pityrosporum orbiculare*). Although *T. rubrum* is an organism commonly found in fungal involvement of the feet, inguinal area, and nails, in Cushing's syndrome the infection becomes disseminated over the trunk and buttocks. These superficial infections often clear spontaneously after adrenalectomy.

ORAL MANIFESTATIONS AND DENTAL MANAGEMENT. See pp. 1206-1207.

ACANTHOSIS NIGRICANS

The lesions of acanthosis nigricans are hyperpigmented, velvety surfaced, or slightly verrucous plaques occurring in the axillae, sides and back of the neck, anogenital region, groin and other flexural surfaces, and submammary, umbilical, and even palmar-plantar regions (Fig. 157-3). The lips and oral mucosae are rarely involved.

Acanthosis nigricans can occur in association with

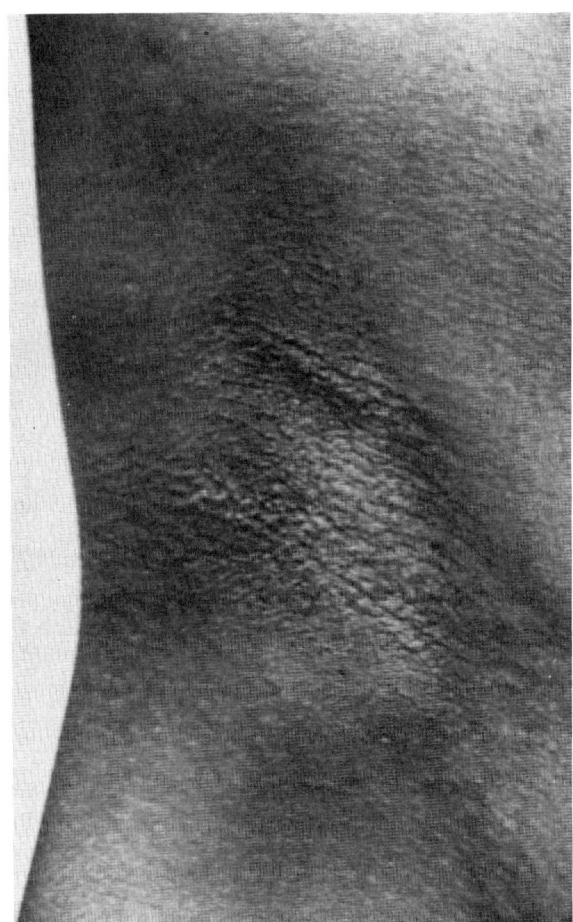

Fig. 157-3. Acanthosis nigricans in axilla. It is hyperpigmented and papular.

a variety of endocrinopathies, such as acromegaly, Cushing's syndrome, polycystic ovaries (Stein-Leventhal syndrome), testicular disorders, adrenal insufficiency, pituitary adenomas, diabetes mellitus, hypothyroidism, hyperthyroidism, hepatolenticular degeneration (Wilson's disease), and lipodystrophy with hyperlipemia. Acanthosis nigricans is often permanent and improves in only a few cases after the endocrine disease is successfully treated.

In addition, acanthosis nigricans may also be found in several non-endocrine-related disorders, including an autosomal dominant hereditary trait that appears during childhood or puberty and persists. Flexural surfaces (axillae and neck) are involved to a limited extent, and there is no association with underlying disease. Drugs such as nicotinic acid and diethylstilbestrol have been reported to induce acanthosis nigricans. In these cases the acanthosis nigricans generally resolves when the drug is discontinued.

Pseudoacanthosis nigricans (idiopathic type) is seen in obese, darker-skinned patients. In these individuals there is no genetic predisposition or endocrine disorder, and weight reduction generally leads to resolution of the lesions.

There is a "malignant" form of acanthosis nigricans

that is not truly malignant but is associated with underlying carcinoma (see Chapter 164).

ORAL MANIFESTATIONS. Oral lesions of acanthosis nigricans have been seen in half the patients. They generally occur on the lips and tongue, appearing as verrucous plaques. The tongue may be hypertrophic and have elongated papillae resembling a fissured tongue. Other mucosal lesions have been reported on the palate and buccal mucosa. All three forms—benign, malignant, and pseudo—can occur in the mouth, though the pseudo form only rarely has oral lesions. All have the same histopathology, consisting of a papillary surface with hyperkeratosis. Widening of the prickle zone with a suggestion of acanthosis with atrophy and occasional hyperpigmentation are also noted.

DENTAL MANAGEMENT. The malignant form is of most concern because the clinician must realize that while the biopsy of the mucosa is benign, there may be an underlying malignancy. The malignancy is often of the gastrointestinal tract, especially the stomach. About one fifth of the lesions occur before the malignancy is diagnosed.

Generally, no treatment of the lesion other than "surgical shaving" is needed. Topical steroids have helped.

Other problems in dental management have been related to the underlying systemic disease, be it endocrine or malignant, and therapy for them. (Refer to chapter on particular disease for treatment.)

BIBLIOGRAPHY

Bang, G.: Acanthosis nigricans maligna, Oral Surg. 29:370, 1970.
Bergsma, D.: Birth defects, atlas and compendium, Baltimore, 1973, The Williams & Wilkins Co., p. 135.
Brown, J., and Winkelmann, R.K.: Acanthosis nigricans, a study of 90 cases, Medicine 47:33, 1968.
Ebeling, F.J., and Rook, A.: Disorders of keratinization. In Rook, A., Wilkinson, D.M., and Ebeling, R.J., editors: Ltd., Textbook in Dermatology, Oxford, 1979, Blackwell Scientific Publications, Ltd., pp. 1307-1310.
Gorlin, R.J., and Goldman, H.M.: Thoma's oral pathology, St. Louis, 1970, The C. V. Mosby Co., p. 688.

PORPHYRIA

The porphyrias are a group of inherited and acquired disorders of porphyrin metabolism. Except for acute intermittent porphyria, all varieties show photosensitivity reactions, which usually present as vesiculobullous eruptions on sun-exposed areas. Subsequent cigarette paper–like scars, milia, hyperpigmentation, and hypertrichosis may develop.

The porphyrins are products of hemoglobin and myoglobin synthesis. These compounds absorb sunlight in the ranges of 400 to 410 nm (Soret band) and 500 to 600 nm. Problems occur as a result of overproduction of porphyrin precursors. Both the liver and the bone marrow red blood cells may be involved.

Erythropoietic porphyrias. In these forms, the blood and bone marrow will fluoresce. They are all inherited.

Congenital erythropoietic porphyria (Gunther's disease). The photosensitivity in this rare autosomal recessive variant is mutilating. Shortly after birth, vesicles and bullae appear on sun-exposed areas. Milia, hypertrichosis, scarring alopecia, ectropion, loss of nasal cartilages, loss of the terminal phalanges, and erythrodontia eventually occur. Frequently, there is an associated hemolytic anemia with splenomegaly. Sunlight avoidance is mandatory; β-carotene has been reported to be of some help. Splenectomy may ameliorate the hemolytic anemia as well as photosensitivity and porphyrin excretion.

Erythropoietic protoporphyria. This variant is inherited as an autosomal dominant disorder. The disease begins in childhood, with burning and tingling on sun exposure. Urticarial plaques and eczematous areas develop and a papular thickening of the skin with a "cobblestone" appearance occurs. Sunlight through window glass can also precipitate symptoms. Micronodular cirrhosis has been reported as part of the complex. Minimal hypertrichosis, scarring, and hyperpigmentation develop. Frequently, the disease improves after the first decade of life. Protection from sunlight via opaque sunscreens and oral administration of β-carotene are useful.

Erythropoietic coproporphyria. This is clinically similar to erythropoietic protoporphyria.

Hepatic porphyrias. These are both inherited and acquired.

Acute intermittent porphyria. This autosomal dominant form often presents as an "acute abdomen." Clinical manifestations also include psychotic episodes and neurologic abnormalities similar to lead poisoning. There are skin changes.

Porphyria variegata. This form has acute attacks that are similar to acute intermittent porphyria, as well as photosensitivity reactions. It is inherited as an autosomal dominant trait. The disease usually begins in young adults. Vesicles develop on the dorsum of the hands, face, and neck on sun exposure. Tissue-paper scars, milia, plaques of lichenified skin, hypertrichosis, and hyperpigmentation occur. These patients have fragile skin and often appear older than their chronologic age. Exposure to sunlight must be minimized, sunscreens are useful, and trauma to the extremities should be avoided.

Porphyria cutanea tarda. This acquired variant has cutaneous manifestations similar to porphyria variegata. Alcohol, hexachlorobenzene, chlorinated hydrocarbons, griseofulvin, and estrogens can all precipitate attacks. The onset is in later adult life. Photosensitivity occurs in late summer and autumn. Vesicles, milia, tissue-paper scars, and sclerodermoid skin changes are found. Treatment includes the use of sunscreens (minimal help), avoidance of alcohol and other substances that might provoke an attack, and very low doses of chloroquine. Currently, phlebotomy, at intervals of 2 to 4 weeks with removal of 500 ml of blood each session, is most helpful. This induces anemia and a low serum iron, which helps prevent symptoms from developing.

Hereditary coproporphyria. This is a rare, autosomal dominant form, clinically similar to porphyria variegata.

ORAL MANIFESTATIONS. The most remarkable manifestation in the oral cavity is the reddish brown tooth discoloration. This erythrodontia will show a red fluorescence in ultraviolet light. Other signs that may be seen in the various forms will include vesiculobullous lesions that heal slowly on the sun-exposed surfaces of the face. The patients also tend to have deformed ears, noses, and eyelids.

DENTAL MANAGEMENT. Dental esthetics presents a problem because of the severe tooth discoloration. Various forms of esthetic coverage may be tried. The new tooth veneering system using composite resins should be attempted, but no results have been published to date. Because of the patient's photosensitivity, night appointments are recommended. The use of facial protection, like a mask, may be beneficial if bright light is used.

The systemic involvement will vary with the type of porphyria, thus consultation is mandatory. Problems reported include hemolytic anemia, neurologic disturbances, behavioral disorders, and fluid imbalance. The neurologic involvement can vary from epileptic-like convulsion to a uniplegia or paraplegia. Behavioral problems include emotional disturbances and frank psychosis. The fluid problems may lead to need for fluid restriction despite signs the patient may need fluid. This fluid problem may lead the physician to request improvement of masticatory capabilities.

Some medications cause a problem by either exacerbating or precipitating the porphyria or affecting involved organs. Barbiturates, sulfonamides, antileptics, and anticonvulsives may exacerbate porphyria. Additional caution must be taken due to liver and hemopoietic problems. (For management see appropriate chapters.)

BIBLIOGRAPHY

Benedetto, A.V., and others: Porphyria cutanea tarda in three generations of a single family, N. Engl. J. Med. **298:**358, 1978.

Brenner, D.A., and Bloomer, J.R.: The enzymatic defect in variegate porphyria, N. Engl. J. Med. **302:**765, 1980.

Brodie, M.J., and others: Hereditary coproporphyria, Q. J. Med. **46:**229, 1977.

Cripps, D.J., Gocman, A., and Peters, H.A.: Porphyria turcica, Arch. Dermatol. **16:**46, 1980.

Dean, G.: The porphyrias, Philadelphia, 1963, J.B. Lippincott Co.

DeLeo, V.A., and others: Erythropoietic protoporphyria, Am. J. Med. **60:**8, 1976.

Goldberg, A.: Acute intermittent porphyria: study of 50 cases, Q. J. Med. **28:**183, 1959.

Harber, L.C., and Bickers, D.R.: The porphyrias: basic science aspects, clinical diagnosis and management. In Malkinson, F., and Pearson, R., editors: Yearbook of dermatology, Chicago, 1975, Year Book Medical Publishers, Inc., pp. 9-47.

Lever, W.F., and Schaumberg-Lever, G.: Histopathology of the skin, ed. 5, Philadelphia, 1975, J.B. Lippincott Co., pp. 396-399.

Levere, R.D., and Kappa, A.: The porphyric disease of man, Hosp. Pract. **5:**61, 1970.

Meyer, U.A., and Schmid, R.: The porphyrias. In Stanbury, J.B., and others, editors: The metabolic basis of inherited disease, ed. 4, New York, 1978, McGraw-Hill Book Co., pp. 1166-1220.

Reed, W.B., and others: Erythropoietic protoporphyria: a chemical and genetic study, J.A.M.A. **214:**1060, 1970.

Taddeini, L., and Watson, C.J.: The clinical porphyrias, Semin. Hematol. **5:**335, 1968.

HYPERLIPIDEMIAS

Xanthomas are papular or nodular yellow-orange lesions that develop as the result of deposition of lipid in cells (xanthoma cells). They generally appear in association with disorders of lipid metabolism but may occasionally occur without any evidence of abnormal lipids or lipproteins. The importance of xanthomatous lesions lies in their indication of possible systemic disease with cardiovascular complications.

The lipoproteinemias (hyperlipidemias) are classified into five major types on the basis of electrophoresis and ultracentrifuge separation of serum. The dermatologic manifestations are type I, eruptive cutaneous xanthomas; type II, tuberous, tendinous, palpebral (xanthelasma), and childhood xanthomas; type III, tuberous and tendinous xanthomas, xanthoma palmaris (xanthoma along the palmar creases), and sometimes palpebral and eruptive xanthomas; type IV, generally no external manifestations but when present, eruptive xanthomas are the characteristic skin finding; and type V, eruptive xanthomas and, rarely, tuberous xanthomas.

Most lesions develop in adulthood, except in type II, in which the disease may start in childhood. Eruptive xanthomas are pinhead- to pea-sized, reddish yellow papules. They occur in crops and may be pruritic. Extensor and pressure surfaces are involved. The lesions may ulcerate and sometimes may be evanescent. They are an indication of elevated triglyceride levels, and may vary as the triglyceride levels fluctuate. They are seen in types I, II, IV, and V.

Tendinous xanthomas occur as nontender nodules on tendons, fascia, and periosteum. The Achilles tendon and extensor tendons of the fingers are most commonly involved.

Tuberous xanthomas are located on the knees, elbows, knuckles, and other extensor surfaces. They are yellowish plaques or patches of papules that do not ulcerate and, once developed, are stable. Tendinous and tuberous xanthomas are usually associated with types II and III.

Xanthelasma or palpebral xanthomas are yellow, slightly raised plaques on the upper eyelids. They are often bilaterally symmetric and are the most common cutaneous xanthomas. In two thirds of patients with xanthelasma no lipid abnormality can be found. When an abnormality is present, it is type II or III.

Obstructive liver disease (xanthomatous biliary cirrhosis) leads to a type of hyperlipidemia in which serum levels of phospholipids and cholesterol increase. The triglyceride levels are elevated, and the plasma is clear, showing no chylomicrons. The xanthomatous lesions are planar xanthomas that occur on the face, flexor surfaces of the extremities, and trunk. Striate palmar and plantar lesions and xanthelasmas are also seen. Hepatomegaly is present, and pruritus is extremely severe.

Xanthomatosis in myxedema is due to an increase of pre-β-lipoproteins. These eruptions respond to treatment with thyroid medication.

Eruptive xanthomas may occur as a result of diabetes mellitus (xanthoma diabeticorum). This is especially true in patients who are unresponsive to insulin. When the diabetes is brought under control, the triglyceride levels are lowered and the lesions involute. Weight reduction and carbohydrate intake restriction are mandatory. Identical phenomena may be seen in von Gierke's disease.

Xanthomatoses may result from a number of hematopoietic diseases, including chronic leukocytosis, histiocytosis, and myelomas. Plane xanthomas are usually the eruptive lesions found in these diseases.

In chronic pancreatitis the lipoprotein concentrations are increased, with elevated triglyceride and cholesterol levels. Xanthoma disseminatum is seen along with a pre-β-lipoprotein increase that responds only when the pancreatitis is controlled. The nephrotic syndrome may also be associated with eruptive xanthomatosis and occasionally with chylomicronemia.

If a patient has isolated xanthelasma, generally no workup beyond determination of the cholesterol level and preprandial and postprandial glucose concentrations is needed. Other forms of xanthomas require evaluation of serum cholesterol and triglyceride levels, examination of serum turbidity, and lipoprotein electrophoresis.

ORAL MANIFESTATIONS AND DENTAL MANAGEMENT. See p. 903.

HEMOCHROMATOSIS

Hemochromatosis (bronze diabetes) is characterized by increased deposition of iron in the skin, liver, heart, pancreas, and endocrine organs, with impairment of their function. Hyperpigmentation is generalized and is more prominent in exposed areas, although it may be noted on the gums, palate, buccal mucosa, and conjunctivae. The spectrum of pigmentation can vary from brown to slate gray, and these colors may be present simultaneously. The increased pigmentation is usually due to melanin rather than iron deposition in the skin.

Patients with hemochromatosis tend to have dry and scaly skin. The disorder occurs in men more frequently than women and usually develops between the ages of 40 and 60 years. In addition to diabetes mellitus and hyperpigmentation, these individuals also have hepatic cirrhosis with the accompanying features of spider angiomas, sparse body hair, ecchymoses, and gynecomastia.

ORAL MANIFESTATIONS AND DENTAL MANAGEMENT. See Chapter 69.

BIBLIOGRAPHY

Benedetto, A.V., and Taylor, J.S.: Porphyria cutanea tarda: update 1978, Cutis **21**:483, 1978.

Benedetto, A.V., and others: Porphyria cutanea tarda in three generations of a single family, N. Engl. J. Med. **298**:358, 1978.

Bernstein, J.E., and others: Bullous eruption of diabetes mellitus, Arch. Dermatol. **115**:324, 1979.

Bleechen, S.S.: Metabolic and nutritional disorders. In Rook, A., Wilkinson, D.S., and Ebling, F.J.G., editors: Textbook of dermatology, ed. 3, Oxford, Eng., 1979, Blackwell Scientific Publications.

Braverman, I.M.: Skin signs of systemic disease, ed. 2, Philadelphia, 1981, W.B. Saunders Co.

Brenner, D.A., and Bloomer, J.R.: The enzymatic defect in variegate porphyria, N. Engl. J. Med. **302**:765, 1980.

Brodie, M.J., and others: Hereditary coproporphyria, Q. J. Med. **46**:229, 1977.

Brown, J., and Winkelmann, R.K.: Acanthosis nigricans: a study of 90 cases, Medicine **47**:33, 1968.

Chevrant-Breton, J., and others: Cutaneous manifestations of idiopathic hemochromatosis, Arch. Dermatol. **113**:161, 1977.

Cripps, D.J., Gocmen, A., and Peters, H.A.: Porphyria turcica, Arch. Dermatol. **16**:46, 1980.

Dean, G.: The prophyrias, Philadelphia, 1963, J.B. Lippincott Co.

DeLeo, V.A., and others: Erythropoietic protoprophyria, Am. J. Med. **60**:8, 1976.

Domonkos, A.N., Arnold, H.L., and Odom, R.B., editors: Andrew's diseases of the skin, ed. 7, Philadelphia, 1982, W.B. Saunders Co.

Ebling, F.J.G., and Rook, A.: Disorders of keratinization. In Rook, A., Wilkinson, D.S., and Ebling, F.J.G., editors: Textbook of dermatology, ed. 3, Oxford, Eng., 1979, Blackwell Scientific Publications.

Fitzpatrick, T.B., and others: Dermatology in general medicine, New York, 1979, McGraw-Hill Book Co.

Frederickson, D.S., and others: The familial hyperlipidemias. In Stanbury, J.B., and others, editors: Metabolic basis of inherited disease, New York, 1978, McGraw-Hill Book Co.

Goldberg, A.: Acute intermittent porphyria: study of 50 cases, Q. J. Med. **28**:183, 1959.

Gordon, D.A., Hill, F.M., and Ezrin, C.: Acromegaly: a review of 100 cases, Can. Med. Assoc. J. **87**:1106, 1962.

Gouterman, I.H., and Sibrach, L.A.: Cutaneous manifestations of diabetes, Cutis **25**:45, 1980.

Gross, M.E., and others: Porphyria cutanea tarda: clinical features and laboratory findings in 40 patients, Am. J. Med. **67**:277, 1979.

Harber, L.C., and Bickers, D.R.: The porphyrias: basic science aspects, clinical diagnosis and management. In Malkinson, F., and Pearson, R., editors: Yearbook of dermatology, Chicago, 1975, Year Book Medical Publishers, Inc.

Harber, L.C., and Bickers, D.R.: Photosensitivity diseases: principles of diagnosis and treatment, Philadelphia, 1981, W.B. Saunders Co.

Johnson, S.A.M.: The skin in internal disease, Postgrad. Med. **41**:438, 1967.

Lerner, A.B., and McGuire, J.S.: Melanocyte-stimulating hormone and adrenocroticotrophic hormone: their relationship to pigmentation, N. Engl. J. Med. **270**:539, 1964.

Lever, W.F., and Schaumberg-Lever, G.: Histopathology of the skin, ed. 5, Philadelphia, 1975, J.B. Lippincott Co.

Malkinson, F.D.: Hyperthyroidism, pretibial myxedema and clubbing, Arch. Dermatol. **88**:303, 1963.

Mason, A.S., and others: Epidemiological and clinical picture of Addison's disease, Lancet **2**:744, 1968.

Meyer, U.A., and Schmid, R.: The porphyrias. In Stanbury, J.B., and others, editors: The metabolic basis of inherited disease, ed. 4, New York, 1978, McGraw-Hill Book Co.

Moschella, S.L.: Cutaneous xanthomatoses: a review and their relationship with the current classification of the hyperlipoproteinemias, Lahey Clin. Found. Bull. **19**:106, 1970.

Muller, S.A.: Dermatologic disorders associated with diabetes mellitus, Mayo Clin. Proc. **41**:689, 1966.

Orth, D.N., and Liddle, G.W.: Results of treatment in 108 patients with Cushing's syndrome, N. Engl. J. Med. **285**:243, 1971.

Perdrup, A., and Poulsen, H.: Hemochromatosis and vitiligo, Arch. Dermatol. **90**:34, 1964.

Reed, W.B., and others: Erythropoietic protoporphyria: a chemical and genetic study, J.A.M.A. **214**:1060, 1970.

Ross, E.J., Marshall-Jones, R., and Friedman, M.: Cushing's syndrome: diagnostic criteria, Q.J. Med. **35**:149, 1966.

Scoggins, R.B., and Harlan, W.R., Jr.: Cutaneous manifestations of hyperlipidemia and uremia, Postgrad. Med. **41**:537, 1967.

Taddeini, L., and Watson, C.J.: The clinical porphyrias, Semin. Hematol. **5**:335, 1968.

Watanakunakorn, C., Hodges, R.E., and Evans, T.C.: Myxedema: a study of 400 cases, Arch. Intern. Med. **116**:183, 1965.

158 • GASTROINTESTINAL DISORDERS WITH CUTANEOUS LESIONS

Bernard A. Kirshbaum, Anthony V. Benedetto, Karen Lipinski, and Robert N. Arm

GARDNER'S SYNDROME

Gardner's syndrome is a hereditary autosomal dominant disorder characterized by polyps of the colon and rectum that commonly undergo malignant degeneration and are associated with cutaneous, osseous, and dental lesions.

The skin manifestations consist of large sebaceous or epidermal cysts located mainly on the face but also occurring on the trunk, scrotum, and extremities. They may be present at birth or appear in early childhood, many years before the intestinal polyps develop. Simple fibromas and other fibrous tissue tumors (desmoids), as well as lipomas, may also be noted.

Osteomas of the skull, maxillae, or mandibles may be palpable in the skin or may be found only on roentgenographic examination. The long bones are seldom involved.

Dental abnormalities include odontomas, dentigerous cysts, and unerupted and supernumerary teeth.

Polyps are uncommon in childhood, but half of the patients with this syndrome have polyps by the age of 20 years, which is often when malignant changes begin. Carcinomatous degeneration of polyps develops in about 50% of these individuals.

The treatment consists of removal of the sebaceous cysts (particularly if they are large or disfiguring), appropriate correction of the dental abnormalities, and extirpation of involved sections of the large bowel and rectum.

ORAL MANIFESTATIONS AND DENTAL MANAGEMENT. See pp. 1093-1095.

PEUTZ-JEGHERS SYNDROME (MELANOSIS-POLYPOSIS)

Peutz-Jeghers syndrome is characterized by pigmentation and intestinal polyps. The pigmentation consists of brown to bluish or black macules on the lips, especially the lower lip, which appear in early childhood or may be present at birth. Macular lesions may also occur elsewhere on the face, perinasally, and periorbitally, but mainly circumorally. Slate gray to brown lesions may be found on the oral mucosa, tongue, palate, and gingivae. Associated macules have been occasionally noted on the hands, feet, and elbows. The macules are irregular and may vary in size from 1 mm to 1 cm; they may be relatively light or dark. In later years the facial pigmentation may fade or even disappear completely, but the mucosal pigmentation persists. The oral pigmentation resembles that normally found in blacks and individuals with adrenal insufficiency.

The polyps occur almost exclusively in the small intestine but may also be found in the stomach, large bowel, and rectum. These polyps are hamartomas, which rarely undergo malignant change in the small bowel. Most of the reported carcinomas occur in the gastric, colonic, or rectal areas.

The syndrome is inherited as an autosomal dominant trait, but sporadic noninherited cases may occur. In some involved families there may be certain individuals who exhibit either the pigmentation or the polyposis alone. Prevention of the disorder requires genetic counseling.

ORAL MANIFESTATIONS AND DENTAL MANAGEMENT. See pp. 1093-1095.

CRONKHITE-CANADA SYNDROME

Cronkhite-Canada syndrome is a rare disorder consisting of generalized gastrointestinal polyposis, alopecia, nail changes, and pigmentation. There may be a sudden onset of abdominal cramps and diarrhea, with loss of albumin and electrolytes, steatorrhea, and sometimes melena. There is resultant hypoproteinemia, anemia, edema, tetany, and weight loss. These are associated with alopecia of the scalp, eyebrows, axillary, pubic, and other body hair, as well as pigmentation of the hands, arms, face, body folds, palmar creases, and occasionally buccal surfaces. The nails become brittle and atrophic and may be shed.

Benign adenomatous polyps of the stomach, small bowel, colon, and rectum, as well as cystic glandular dilation, have been described. Patients with the Cronkhite-Canada syndrome are usually middle aged to elderly. Manifestations may improve after bowel resection of the involved segments, and spontaneous remission has also been reported. The protein-losing enteropathy may improve with the use of corticosteroids; the hair may regrow and pigmentation may disappear.

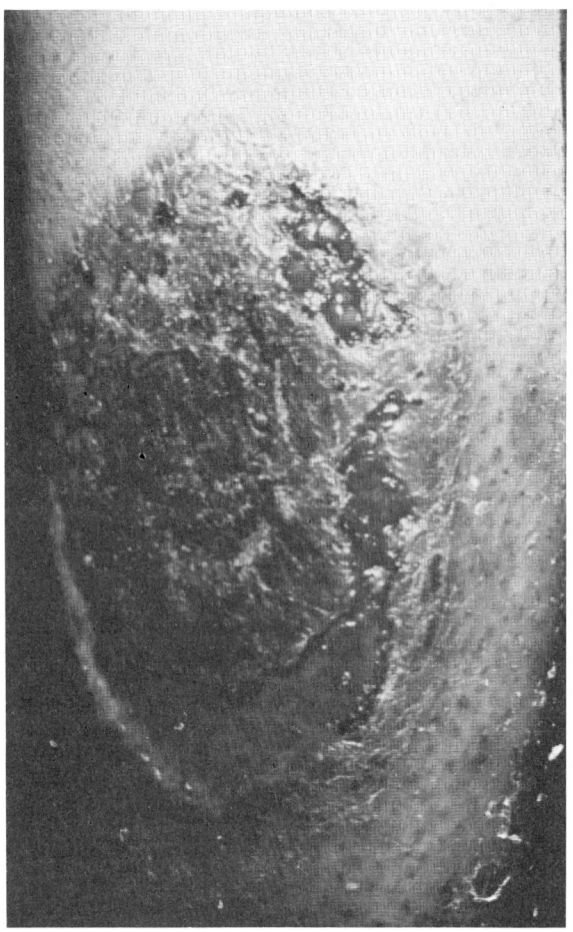

Fig. 158-1. Pyoderma gangrenosum on anterior surface of leg. There is ulceration with rolled, undermined edges and purulent (but sterile) drainage.

ULCERATIVE COLITIS WITH PYODERMA GANGRENOSUM AND PYOSTOMATITIS VEGETANS

Skin and oral lesions occur in approximately one third of patients with ulcerative colitis. Aphthous stomatitis occurs commonly; the minute ulcers, which are indistinguishable from the usual variety, appear with acute exacerbations of the bowel disease. Erythema nodosum also may occasionally develop during the acute phase.

Pyostomatitis vegetans is a rare oral lesion associated with chronic ulcerative colitis. It consists of papillomatous projections with minute ulcerations and pockets of pus at their tips. They may be numerous and form aggregates on the palate, buccal mucosa, gums, and lips. The tongue is not involved. Pyostomatitis follows the course of the underlying ulcerative colitis.

Other dermatologic findings associated with ulcerative colitis include perianal abscesses and fistulas (reported in 10% to 20% of patients), palmar erythema, and clubbing of fingers. Thrombophlebitis (in up to one third of patients) and arterial thromboses also occur; a hypercoagulable state is apparently associated with ulcerative colitis.

Pyoderma gangrenosum appears mainly on the legs but occasionally on the trunk and upper extremities; it occurs in up to 10% of patients with active ulcerative colitis. It is characterized by boggy, bluish black, undermined ulcers that develop rapidly, almost explosively. The lesion begins as an erythematous papulovesicle or pustular nodule that quickly becomes necrotic and ulcerates. The ulcers have rolled edges surrounded by an erythematous halo (Fig. 158-1). Satellite lesions may develop, break down, and fuse to form large, peripherally extending phagedenic ulcerations. When healing occurs, a thin atrophic scar is formed. The histologic findings are nonspecific inflammation in the dermis and around the vessels, with ulceration of the epidermis; there is no evidence of necrotizing angiitis. Despite the term "pyoderma," bacterial cultures from these ulcers are frequently sterile.

ORAL MANIFESTATIONS AND DENTAL MANAGEMENT. See pp. 1095-1096.

REGIONAL ENTERITIS (CROHN'S DISEASE)

The skin findings associated with regional ileitis include multiple perianal fistulas, erythematous nodular (erythema nodosum–like) and ulceronodular skin lesions, pyoderma gangrenosum, local or "metastatic" extension of the granulomatous disease to involve perianal or distant skin, and skin changes owing to resultant malabsorption. Rosacea-like eruptions and digital clubbing have also been reported.

ORAL MANIFESTATIONS AND DENTAL MANAGEMENT. See pp. 1096-1097.

DERMATITIS HERPETIFORMIS

Dermatitis herpetiformis is a chronic, recurrent, intensely pruritic disease usually presenting as grouped, annular, or gyrate erythematous vesicles. The eruption is polymorphous and may also include urticarial, maculopapular, papulovesicular, and (rarely) bullous lesions with a generally symmetric distribution. The lesions most commonly affect the scapulae, extensor surfaces of arms and legs, sacral regions, and buttocks, although any area of the body can be affected. Postinflammatory hyperpigmentation and scarring may remain when the lesions regress. Pruritus, often described as having a concomitant burning sensation, can be severe at times. The onset may be sudden, with no associated constitutional symptoms.

The disease is relatively uncommon. The onset occurs generally between the second and fifth decades of life; children may rarely be affected. The incidence is twice as frequent in men as in women; it is found in all races, but there is no familial incidence or genetic transmission. Often severe emotional stress is seen in persons afflicted by this disease, though it is sometimes difficult to differentiate between cause and effect. The disease has also been related to hormonal changes and vaccination, but the true cause remains unknown. Occasionally, severe bullous forms have been associated with internal malignant disease, usually regressing after the carcinoma has been successfully treated. Conversely, there is no increased risk of malignancy in patients with dermatitis herpetiformis.

There may be an eosinophilia in the blood of 10% or higher; numerous eosinophils are found in the fluid of the vesicles and bullae, at times comprising up to 90% of the cellular elements. No specific abnormalities of circulating immunoglobulins or serum complement levels have been demonstrated. Direct immunofluorescent staining for immunoglobulins is positive at adjacent uninvolved perilesional skin at the dermoepidermal junction; the pattern may be microgranular, fibrillar, and linear continuous along the basement membrane. Although IgA is the predominant demonstrable immunoglobulin, IgG and IgM may be deposited; complement is also deposited in the tips of the dermal papillae. These findings can aid in differentiation from bullous pemphigoid. Similar immunofluorescent patterns in the upper gastrointestinal tract have also been reported.

In more than two thirds of patients with dermatitis herpetiformis there may be atrophy of the villi in the proximal small bowel mucosa indistinguishable from celiac sprue. The enteropathy is less pronounced than that seen in the celiac syndrome, and a gluten-free diet has been reported as helpful to a few patients with dermatitis herpetiformis.

The disease responds dramatically to sulfapyridine and the sulfones (dapsone and others). Systemic corticosteroids may also be required when the disease is severe. The side effects of each of these modalities must be considered when treatment is undertaken with any of them. Topical steroids and oral antipruritic agents are important adjuncts.

ORAL MANIFESTATIONS. The oral cavity is rarely involved. When lesions appear, they are generally reddish brown bulla, which undergo degeneration and ulcerate. The common locations are the buccal mucosa and tongue. In addition, atrophy of filiform and fungiform papillae of the tongue have been reported. This disease has been reported in association with Sjögren's disease.

ORAL MANAGEMENT. The oral lesion will respond to sulfapyridine treatment. (NOTE: Long-term use of sulfapyridine may affect the kidneys.) For oral hygiene, alkaline rinses (bicarbonate) or saline rinses may help.

Sensitivity to halogens has been reported, which may contraindicate the use of fluorides and certain antiseptic rinses and preparations containing iodine.

BIBLIOGRAPHY

Fraser, N.G., and others: Dermatitis herpetiformis and Sjögren's syndrome, Br. J. Dermatol. **100**:213, 1979.
Fry, L., and others: The small intestine in dermatitis herpetiformis, J. Clin. Pathol. **27**:811, 1974.
Katz, S.I.: Dermatitis herpetiformis: Clinical, histologic, laboratory and therapeutic clues, Int. J. Dermatol. **17**:529, 1978.
Marks, J.M., and others: Small bowel changes in dermatitis herpetifomis, Lancet **2**:1280, 1966.
Russotto, S.B., and Ship, I.I.: Oral manifestations of dermatitis herpetiformis, Oral Surg. **311**:42, 1971.

MALIGNANT ATROPHIC PAPULOSIS (DEGOS' DISEASE)

Malignant atrophic papulosis is a fatal cutaneointestinal syndrome of unknown cause, characterized by an endovasculitis of skin, gastrointestinal tract, and sometimes other viscera. It is a rare disorder occurring chiefly in men between 20 and 40 years of age. The average survival is 2 years, but a few patients have lived for 6 years or more after the disease has developed.

Clinically the manifestations consist of discrete asymptomatic pale rose to erythematous rounded edematous papules measuring 2 to 10 mm. The eruption is mainly on the trunk, more often involving the back, with an average of 30 lesions. Sometimes hundreds of lesions may be present. Other areas of the skin may be affected, but the face, palms, and soles are spared. The lesions evolve slowly over a period of weeks to months, becoming umbilicated with a central depression covered by a distinctive porcelain-white crust. The periphery becomes livid red and telangiectatic. When healing occurs, there is an atrophic white scar. There may be successive crops of lesions, with a few new ones appearing at intervals over several years. Urticaria-like ulceropustular and gummatous nodular lesions have been described.

Abdominal complaints, which result from anemic infarcts of the intestines, generally develop a few months after the onset of skin lesions. The gastrointestinal symptoms include nausea, vomiting, hematemesis, epigastric and abdominal pain, colic, diarrhea, malabsorption, ileus, and melena. Occasionally these symptoms may precede the skin lesions. Death generally ensues within a few months from hemorrhage and multiple perforations of the intestine, leading to fulminant peritonitis.

Other viscera that may be involved are the heart, pericardium, kidneys, and bladder. White plaques similar to those in the skin and gastrointestinal tract may involve the cerebral cortex. Neurologic symptoms in this disease include headache, numbness in the extremities, ataxia, and diplopia. There may also be retinal and scleral plaques and microaneurysms of the bulbar conjunctival vessels.

The basic pathogenic mechanism is vascular obliteration from endovasculitis and thrombosis with resultant ischemic infarction of the involved tissues. Histologically, there is small arterial endothelial swelling and proliferation with fibrinoid necrosis of the intima and thrombosis, producing wedge-shaped infarcts brought on by the obliteration of small arteries and arterioles. Abnormal increases of serum IgA and plasma fibrinogen have been found. No effective therapy is known; administration of corticosteroids is usually of no value.

ORAL MANIFESTATIONS. Lesions of the oral cavity are rare. The few that occur resemble the cutaneous lesions. Erythematous papules may change to lesions with a white atrophic center and an erythematous border. The lips are most likely to be involved. A biopsy is indicated.

DENTAL MANAGEMENT. Management must be directed at symptomatic relief of the limited oral involvement in this rare cutaneous disease. No therapy is known, though steroids have been tried. Systemic involvement will be fatal. Consultation is indicated to learn the extent of organ involvement before treatment.

BIBLIOGRAPHY

Gorlin, R.J., and Goldman, H.M.: Thoma's oral pathology, St. Louis, 1970, The C. V. Mosby Co., p. 699.
May, R.E.: Degos' syndrome, Br. Med. J. **1:**161, 1968.
Roenigk, H.H., Jr., and Farmer, R.G.: Degos' disease (malignant papulosis), J.A.M.A. **206:**1508, 1968.
Strole, W.E., Jr., Clark, W., Jr., and Isselbacher, K.J.: Progressive arterial occlusive disease (Kohlmeier-Degos), N. Eng. J. Med. **276:**195, 1967.

HEREDITARY HEMORRHAGIC TELANGIECTASIS (WEBER-OSLER-RENDU DISEASE)

Hereditary hemorrhagic telangiectasia is characterized by telangiectasia of the skin of the face, fingers, and toes, mucous membranes, and gastrointestinal tract, with frequent nosebleeds and gross or occult blood in the bowel. The dilated capillaries are seen mainly in the mouth, nasal mucosa, ears, palms, fingertips, nail beds, and feet. Arteriovenous fistulas of the lungs may develop in later life, leading to pulmonary hemorrhages. Bleeding may also occur in the kidney, bladder, liver, meninges, and brain.

The telangiectasia usually appear at puberty and tend to increase in number in middle age. Epistaxis is the most frequent and persistent sign, especially in childhood. The disease is inherited as an autosomal dominant trait.

Treatment of telangiectasia by surgical resection, local destruction, and sclerosing agents has been tried, as well as control of bleeding tendencies by estrogen and steroid therapy.

ORAL MANIFESTATIONS. The telangiectasia can be seen throughout the oral cavity. They appear as dilated capillaries or spiders that blanch on pressure. The lips and tongue are most commonly involved. The number of lesions increase with age. To avoid rupturing the gingival vascular lesions, the patient may avoid brushing and have poor hygiene, leading to periodontal problems.

DENTAL MANAGEMENT. Dental treatment may be done normally as long as trauma to lesions is avoided. Major complications will arise from the systemic involvement including pulmonary and cerebral hemorrhages. While telangiectasia are easy to recognize, the family history is helpful but not always positive. These patients tend to exhibit hemorrhaging gingiva with both spontaneous bleeding and bleeding secondary to trauma. This often makes home care and periodontal therapy difficult. Splints, pressure packs, and hemostatic agents will be beneficial to control bleeding after periodontal or oral surgical procedures. Telangiectasia are often treated like hemangiomas with sclerosing solutions and cautery. Often a gingival vascular area must be eliminated for the patient to maintain the periodontium. Dental prostheses have caused rupture of the vascular lesions, necessitating their removal or elimination of the vascular anomaly. Multiple lesions may make prosthetic devices difficult for the patient to tolerate.

BIBLIOGRAPHY

Bean, W.B.: Vascular spiders and related lesions of the skin, Springfield, Ill., 1958, Charles C Thomas, Publisher.
Harrison, D.F.N.: Familial haemorrhagic telangiectasia: 20 cases treated with systemic oestrogen, Q.J. Med. **33:**25, 1964.
Hashimoto, K., and Pritzker, M.S.: Hereditary hemorrhagic telangiectasia—an electron microscopic study, Oral Surg. **34:**751, 1972.
Hattler, A.B., and Summers, R.B.: Hereditary hemorrhagic telangiectasia—report of case and clinical consideration, J. Am. Dent. Assoc. **103:**421, 1981.
Hodgson, C.H., and others: Hereditary hemorrhagic telangiectasia and pulmonary arterio-venous fistula, N. Engl. J. Med. **261:**625, 1959.
Weber, F.P.: Some telangiectatic and other anomalous vascular groups, especially those of dysplastic origin, Med. Press **210:**219, 1943.

ACRODERMATITIS ENTEROPATHICA

There are hereditary and acquired forms of acrodermatitis enteropathica. The syndrome, resulting from zinc deficiency, is characterized by a distinctive dermatitis located about the body orifices and extremities, with alopecia, diarrhea, and mental changes. Clinical symptoms are marked by exacerbations and remissions.

The skin eruption consists of symmetric, grouped, vesiculobullous lesions on a bright red erythematous base around the mouth, nose, eyes, ears, genitalia, perineum, buttocks, elbows, knees, hands, feet, and scalp. The vesiculobullous lesions progress to crusted seborrhea-like and psoriasiform patches, with exudates. These lesions become altered by bacterial and candidal infections (Fig. 158-2). Healing occurs without atrophy or scarring.

The fingers and toes may show marked redness and swelling of the paronychial areas, with subungual thickening and transverse grooving of the nails. There often is blepharitis and photophobia. These patients have an increased susceptibility to bacterial and candidal infections.

Alopecia involves not only the scalp but also the eyebrows, eyelashes, and sometimes the rest of the body hair. The alopecia is usually reversible when the disease is controlled by appropriate treatment.

Diarrhea is found in most patients, and at times there may be severe malabsorption. In children body growth is often stunted and there are personality and mental changes. These children are apathetic and depressed and appear mentally dull.

The hereditary disease is inherited as an autosomal recessive trait and begins early in infancy. Cutaneous manifestations usually develop shortly after breast feeding is

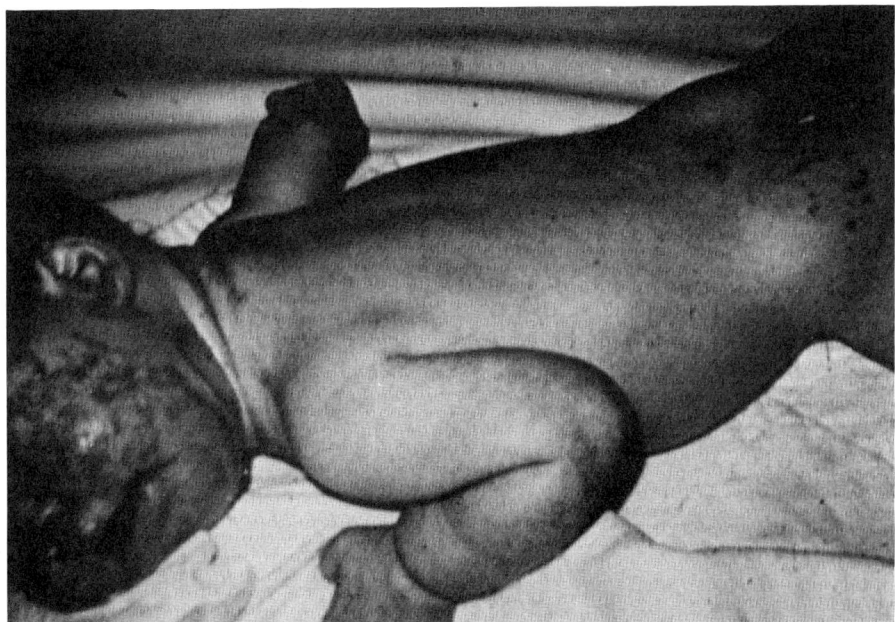

Fig. 158-2. Acrodermatitis enteropathica in infant. Note perioral and perianal lesions appearing as exudates on erythematous base.

stopped or up to 2 years of age (rare cases may occur as late as 10 years). There is usually an insidious onset; the affected child fails to thrive and develops erythematous, scaling, pustular lesions around the body orifices. The zinc deficiency is probably related to malabsorption.

The "acquired" form of acrodermatitis enteropathica is most often seen in patients receiving total parenteral nutrition (intravenous hyperalimentation) when zinc supplements have not been added to the nutritional fluid. Many of these patients have inflammatory bowel disease and have a partial zinc deficiency at the outset. Patients with the acquired form develop seborrhea-like and candidal eruptions in the groin and orbital and circumoral regions. An eczema picture with dry, brittle, fissured skin may appear. Angular stomatitis, alopecia, and chronic paronychia have also been noted. Frequently the eruption is mistaken for *Candida* or other fungal infection, eczema, or seborrheic dermatitis.

Treatment for both the hereditary as well as the "acquired" forms of this disease is zinc replacement, by either oral or intravenous routes. The response is dramatic and rapid. In the inherited form, replacement therapy must be lifelong.

ORAL MANIFESTATIONS. Perioral vesiculobullous lesions surrounded by bright red erythematous zone are common. Perleche, glossitis, and stomatitis have been reported. The tongue and buccal mucosa may have white patches of varying sizes. Secondary infection from *Candida* will alter the appearance, and a coated tongue may be seen. Classic candidal lesions of the mucosa will leave a raw erythematous area after rubbing off the white surface.

DENTAL MANAGEMENT. The major therapy must be aimed at treating the *Candida* by use of antifungal agents. Allowing a nystatin troche to dissolve in the mouth slowly two to four times a day will give better results than the oral suspension. A more recent drug, ketoconazole (Nizoral), appears to provide excellent results. One must remember to treat dental prostheses with nystatin soaks.

The vesiculobullous lesions resolve after zinc therapy.

Elective dental treatment should be delayed when acute lesions are present. The stomatitis and glossitis may be relieved using bland mouthrinses and avoiding alcoholic rinses.

Bright dental lights may affect the patient, who has photophobia. Reported depression in adults may create management problems.

BIBLIOGRAPHY

Bergsma, D.: Birth defects, atlas and compendium, Baltimore, 1973, The Williams & Wilkins Co., p. 142.

Bernstein, B., and Leyden, J.: Zinc deficiency and acrodermatitis after intravenous hyperalimentation, Arch. Dermatol. **114:**1070, 1978.

Brazin, S., and others. The acrodermatitis enteropathica–like syndrome, Arch. Dermatol. **115:**597, 1979.

Danbolt, N.: Acrodermatitis enteropathica, Br. J. Dermatol. **100:**37, 1979.

Gorlin, R.J., and Goldman, H.M.: Thoma's oral pathology, St. Louis, 1970, The C. V. Mosby Co., p. 691.

Graves, K., Kestenbaum, T., and Kalivas, J.: Hereditary acrodermatitis enteropathica in an adult. Arch. Dermatol. **116:**562, 1980.

Hirsh, F.S., Michel, B., and Strain, W.H.: Gluconate zinc in acrodermatitis enteropathica, Arch. Dermatol. **112:**475, 1976.

Moynahan, E.J.: Acrodermatitis enteropathica: a lethal inherited human zinc deficiency disorder, Lancet **2:**399, 1974.

Nelder, K.H., and others: Acrodermatitis enteropathica, Int. J. Dermatol. **17:**380, 1978.

159 · LIVER DISORDERS

Bernard A. Kirshbaum, Anthony V. Benedetto,
and **Karen Lipinski**

The cutaneous signs of liver disease are related to the severity of the underlying condition.

Urticaria, as well as fever and arthralgias, may be part of the prodrome of hepatitis B. A scarlatiniform eruption limited to the trunk and proximal portions of the extremities, with sparing of the face, may be present at the onset; this usually fades within a week.

Pruritus may be present if there is biliary obstruction; the cause of the itching is the high concentration of retained bile acids in the blood. The pruritus caused by retained bile acids can be relieved by agents such as cholestyramine that bind bile acids and their metabolites in the intestinal lumen to prevent their absorption.

Xanthomatous lesions (planar xanthomas) may appear on the face, extremities, and trunk in patients with obstructive biliary disease such as biliary cirrhosis.

Spider angiomas, which consist of a central vascular punctum and radiating telangiectatic "legs," occur commonly in chronic liver disease. They may also appear during the acute stage of viral hepatitis and regress after the illness is over. However, spider angiomas are not pathognomonic signs of liver disease; they are also often seen in pregnant women, patients with other hyperestrogen states, and otherwise normal young adults and children.

Palmar erythema ("liver palms"), a blotchy erythema on the thenar and hypothenar eminences and fingertips, may be found in persons who exhibit spider angiomas. A similar erythema may be noted in pregnancy and is also associated with rheumatoid arthritis, thyrotoxicosis, and malnutrition. In lupus erythematosus the palmar erythema tends to be more violaceous and discrete.

ORAL CONSIDERATIONS AND DENTAL MANAGEMENT. See pp. 1097-1101.

BIBLIOGRAPHY

Braverman, I.M.: Skin signs of systemic disease, Philadelphia, 1981, W.B. Saunders Co.
Sarkany, I.: The skin lesions associated with liver disease, Prog. Dermatol. **4:**1, 1969.

160 · RENAL DISORDERS

Bernard A. Kirshbaum, Anthony V. Benedetto,
and **Karen Lipinski**

There are a number of hereditary syndromes that affect the skin and may also show renal involvement. These include, among others, hereditary hemorrhagic telangiectasia (Osler-Weber-Rendu disease) with vascular anomalies; pseudoxanthoma elasticum (Grönblad-Strandberg syndrome) with vessel changes and calcium renal stones; angiokeratoma corporis diffusum (Fabry's disease) with glomerular and tubular glycolipid storage; tuberous sclerosis (Bourneville's disease) with hamartomas and angiomyolipomas; neurofibromatosis (von Recklinghausen's disease) with tumors in the kidney; von Hippel-Lindau disease with cystic kidneys and hypernephroma; and sickle cell disease with hematuria, isosthenuria, renal infarcts, and the nephrotic syndrome.

Vasculitides (Schönlein-Henoch anaphylactoid purpura and "allergic" vasculitis) may be manifested by both skin and glomerular effects. The connective tissue diseases (systemic lupus erythematosus, progressive systemic sclerosis, polyarteritis nodosa, and Wegener's granulomatosis) may produce profound changes in the skin and the kidneys.

Metabolic diseases can bring about significant alterations in function and structure of the kidneys as well as cutaneous changes, although not always simultaneously in the same patient. Thus, diabetes mellitus produces nodular intercapillary glomerulosclerosis (Kimmelstiel-Wilson syndrome) and necrobiosis lipoidica diabeticorum. Gout results in nephritis caused by tophi in interstitial tissue of the renal pyramids and tophaceous deposits in subcutaneous tissues. Systemic amyloidosis causes amyloid deposition in glomeruli, blood vessels, and interstitial tissue around tubules and also results in cutaneous deposits in the dermis and subcutis. Dysproteinemic states (paraproteinemia and cryoglobulinemia) cause glomerulonephritis and purpura, livedo reticularis, Raynaud's phenomenon, acrocyanosis, and ulceration of the skin. "Metastatic" calcinosis produces deposition of calcium in the tubular epithelium and the cutis.

Some neoplasms that affect the skin can also infiltrate the kidney, including Kaposi's sarcoma, urticaria pigmentosa (mastocytoma), leukemia, lymphoma, and multiple myeloma.

Skin findings occur in advanced renal failure. Uremic frost is due to a greatly increased concentration of urea in the sweat and its subsequent precipitation on the skin. This is rare but is a serious prognostic sign when it occurs. Dry scaly skin (xerosis), itching, and excoriations are more frequent findings. They may be associated with linear purpura and secondary pyoderma. The pruritus may be intractable; ultraviolet therapy has sometimes been successful. Dialysis may be helpful in relieving the intense itching. Secondary hyperparathyroidism has been implicated in renal pruritus. Burning, painful paresthesias of the dorsal or plantar surfaces of the feet is a common early sign of peripheral neuropathy.

Soft tissue calcification in uremia is due mainly to hyperphosphatemia. Calcinosis cutis may be present in the skin and subcutaneous tissues as infiltrated plaques, firm white papules and nodules from which a milky substance can be expressed. It may also occur in the conjunctiva and cornea, periarticular tissue, arteries, and viscera. A hemorrhagic diathesis caused by a platelet defect and increased capillary permeability may be present, resulting in easy bruisability, bleeding from the gums and nasal mucosa, and purpura and ecchymoses. Pallor of the skin, mucous membranes, and nail beds is the result of anemia. The accumulation of urinary pigments gives the skin a sallow complexion. A brownish discoloration of the skin may be due to the deposition of hemosiderin from repeated transfusions and hemodialysis. There may be loss of hair on the extremities. Poor wound healing is attributed to the connective tissue changes, an increase in dermal elastic fibers with decreased collagen turnover.

Uremic onychopathy is of two types: a brown arc spanning the distal part of the nail proximal to the line of its separation from the nail bed and the "half-and-half nail" characterized by a whiteness proximally and a dark brown or reddish discoloration of the distal portion.

A porphyria cutanea tarda—like syndrome has been noted in some patients undergoing long-term hemodialysis. This is manifested as a bullous eruption on the dorsa of the hands, pruritus, skin fragility, and even hemorrhagic bullae that may appear on areas exposed to sunlight. A photosensitizer present in the dialysis fluid or the tubing is believed to be a cause of the reaction.

In patients undergoing immunosuppressive therapy for renal disease, fungal and viral infections are more frequent and more extensive. *Candida,* herpes simplex, molluscum contagiosum, and warts are more persistent in these patients and may respond only when the dosages of the immunosuppressive drugs are reduced for a short period. Steroid-induced acne has also been noted in prolonged therapy.

ORAL MANIFESTATIONS AND DENTAL CONSIDERATIONS. See pp. 666-671.

BIBLIOGRAPHY

Bergfeld, W., and Roenigk, H.H., Jr.: Cutaneous complications of immunosuppressive therapy, Cutis **22:**169, 1978.
Bluefarb, S.M., and Caro, W.A.: Cutaneous manifestations of renal diseases, Mod. Med. **37:**159, 1969.
Gilchrist, B., and others: Relief of uremic pruritus with ultraviolet light therapy, N. Engl. J. Med. **297:**136, 1977.
Gruskin, S.E., and others: Oral manifestations of uremia, Minn. Med. **53:**495, 1970.
Lever, W.F., and Schaumberg-Lever, G.: Histopathology of the skin, Philadelphia, 1975, J.B. Lippincott Co.
Lindsay, P.G.: The half and half nail, Arch. Intern. Med. **119:**583, 1967.
Massey, S.G., and others: Intractable pruritus as a manifestation of secondary hyperparathyroidism, N. Engl. J. Med. **279:**697, 1968.
Parfitt, P.M.: Soft tissue calcification in uremia, Arch. Intern. Med. **124:**544, 1969.
Poh-Fitzpatrick, M., and others: Porphyria cutanea tarda associated with chronic renal disease and hemodialysis, N. Engl. J. Med. **116:**191, 1980.
Scoggins, R.B., and Harlan, W.R., Jr.: Cutaneous manifestations of hyperlipidemia and uremia, Postgrad. Med. **41:**537, 1967.

161 • HEMATOLOGIC DISORDERS

Bernard A. Kirshbaum, Anthony V. Benedetto, and **Karen Lipinski**

POLYCYTHEMIA VERA

The skin changes in polycythemia vera are due primarily to an increase of red blood cells. There is vascular engorgement of the viscera and skin. The overdistended cutaneous vessels ultimately produce an intense red color, mainly on the face, neck, and distal extremities. Because there is facial erythema with superimposed telangiectasia, rosacea may be mistakenly diagnosed. Not all patients with polycythemia vera are deeply erythematous, and the intensity of color can vary from day to day. Sometimes erythema may persist after normal hematocrit values have been achieved.

The vessels of the oral mucous membranes are also dilated in polycythemia vera, and a deep reddish blue color may be present on the tongue, pharynx, and tonsils. The engorgement may cause macroglossia. Bleeding gums and epistaxis are commonly encountered. Petechiae and ecchymoses may be produced in the skin by relatively mild injury, and intramuscular injections may result in hematomas. Cyanosis may be present.

Pruritus may be severe in patients with polycythemia vera. This is especially true after a hot shower or bath, when skin sensations of burning may develop and persist to an extent far greater than that encountered in persons with eczema and ichthyosis. The intense pruritus and burning paresthesias have been correlated with increased histamine levels and with the overdistention of cutaneous vessels that are unable to respond to localized heating by further vasodilation.

Acne urticata is a chronic, severely pruritic eruption consisting of pale red, wheal-like papules, sometimes surmounted by vesicles and appearing in crops on the face and extensor aspects of the extremities. These often result in scarring and hyperpigmentation following excoriations. Although acne urticata is considered a specific sign of polycythemia vera, it has also been found in patients with lymphomas and carcinomas.

Erythromelalgia (erythermalgia) is a peculiar vascular response consisting of sensations of burning accompanying erythematous swelling of the legs. This may develop after exercise or exposure to heat or if the legs have been in a dependent position for a long time. Elevation and cooling of the legs help to alleviate the symptoms. Leg ulcers and cold sensitivity are the result of increased blood viscosity produced by the increased red cell mass.

SICKLE CELL DISEASE

Cutaneous ulcerations are found in 25% to 75% of patients with sickle cell anemia and 2.6% of heterozygotes (patients with sickle cell trait). The sickled red blood cells become trapped in capillaries, leading to further stasis, deoxygenation, decreased pH, and increased sickling. Packing of these cells in the small vessels causes thrombosis and infarction. This results in "punched-out," sharply marginated, painful ulcers that tend to be unilateral and are generally found about the malleoli. The ulcers may be deep or shallow and are out of proportion to the trauma that precedes them. They are chronic and indolent and heal slowly, with atrophic scars that readily break down again. The scars are often hypopigmented with a peripheral zone of hyperpigmentation. Patients with sickle cell disease tend to have long, slender extremities (asthenic habitus). The mucous membranes, nail beds, and palms are pale, the conjunctivae are icteric, and the lower areas of the legs show residual hyperpigmentation, often as the result of hemosiderin deposition.

THROMBOCYTOPENIA AND OTHER PLATELET ABNORMALITIES

Purpura is caused by extravasation of blood into the skin or mucous membranes, usually resulting from rupture of the capillary walls and appearing as distinctive macules that may vary from bright red to brownish, rust colored, or purplish. They may be petechiae—superficial, pinhead-sized (less than 3 mm), round, hemorrhagic macules—or ecchymoses ("black and blue marks"), which form flat, irregularly shaped, bluish-purplish patches that signify deeper and more extensive interstitial hemorrhages. They gradually assume a yellowish hue as they fade.

Purpura caused by thrombocytopenia may be the result of decreased platelet production or increased destruction. Purpura may also be caused by various thrombopathies including hereditary thrombasthenia, by a phospholipid defect, by metabolic states (uremia or liver disease), and by dysproteinemias (cryoglobulinemia, macroglobulinemia, or hyperglobulinemia). In addition, purpura may be caused by an increase in platelets (thrombocythemia) as in myeloproliferative disorders.

LEUKEMIAS
Specific lesions

The lesions of leukemia are the same as those found in the malignant lymphomas and consist of macules, papules, nodules, tumors, and plaquelike infiltrations that range in color from pink to reddish brown to purple (violaceous to plum colored). The solid lesions are firm but not stony hard and are composed of leukemic infiltrates. These lesions may rarely appear before the disease is expressed in the bone marrow or peripheral blood. Leukemic infiltrates may be found at sites of trauma, including intramuscular injections, recent surgical scars, burns, herpes zoster, and herpes simplex. Leukemia cutis may resemble mycosis fungoides by forming arciform lesions and plaques, with massive infiltration producing a leonine facies, especially in patients with chronic lymphocytic leukemia. Sometimes the facial involvement may resemble rosacea or lupus erythematosus; subcutaneous periarticular nodules may simulate juxta-articular nodes; ulcerations in genital areas may mimic venereal disease; infiltration of erectile tissue may produce priapism. Oral lesions are an especially prominent finding in acute leukemia but may also occur in chronic leukemia. Leukemic infiltrates often produce hyperplasia of the gums that sometimes completely covers the teeth. The red and friable gingival tissue bleeds spontaneously or after minimal trauma. The gums and buccal mucosa frequently ulcerate, producing a necrotic appearance.

Lymphocytic leukemia is characterized by leukemic infiltrates consisting of discrete nodules and tumors, with occasional widespread diffuse swellings and infiltration accompanied by erythroderma. Leonine facies is more commonly found in chronic lymphocytic leukemia. Infiltrates may begin as one or more discrete, bluish red or plum-colored, painless, rubbery nodules in the skin, or as nodular subcutaneous infiltrations under otherwise normal skin.

Tumors and plaques may become ulcerated, especially on the genitalia. A diffuse infiltrated erythroderma may develop as a generalized swelling and redness of the skin with intense pruritus. The skin surface may vary from smooth to lichenified, slightly scaly, eczematous, or severely exfoliative.

Granulocytic leukemia may be associated with chloroma. Chloroma, named for its green color, is the only lesion that is pathognomonic in any of the leukemias. It is a granulocytic sarcoma and is the only facial tumor that is green. The green pigment is due to the enzyme myeloperoxidase (verdoperoxidase), which fades in a few hours after the cut tumor is exposed to air. Chloroma is rare and occurs mainly in childhood; it is caused by the infiltration of immature granulocytic cells in the periosteum primarily of the orbital and cranial bones, although the sternum, vertebrae, pelvis, and long bones may be involved. Chloromas can expand epidurally and subdurally, causing compression of the brain, cranial nerves, and spinal cord. Chloroma may develop at the same time as acute granulocytic leukemia or may precede it by as much as 1 year.

The cutaneous nodules seen in leukemia have a predilection for the trunk, but they may also occur on the face and extremities; they may be firm or elastic and livid red to mahogany in color.

Monocytic leukemia may present two types of cutaneous lesions. The macular form may resemble an acute exanthem or secondary syphilis; these lesions subsequently turn from pink to slate blue. The other variety consists of pale discrete papules deep in the skin; these may later soften and undergo necrosis, forming multiple small ulcers. Acute monocytic leukemia tends to have more florid oral lesions than the other forms of leukemia.

Nonspecific lesions

Leukemids are the nonspecific cutaneous eruptions found in leukemia. They are polymorphous and may present urticarial, bullous, and erythema multiforme–like pictures, as well as papulonecrotic and eczematous lesions. Diffuse erythroderma, hemorrhagic exanthems, and ulcerations are common in all types of leukemias.

Pruritus is probably the most common nonspecific manifestation of the leukemias, especially the lymphocytic type. Prurigo-like papules may develop that are pale, edematous, and surmounted by minute vesicles. With exfoliative erythroderma, pruritus may become unbearably severe.

Herpes zoster occurs especially in lymphocytic leukemia and also in Hodgkin's disease and myeloma; it may become hemorrhagic or gangreous and sometimes generalized. Bullae may form in the mouth, simulating pemphigus.

Other nonspecific cutaneous findings commonly found in leukemias include pallor caused by anemia, purpura and hemorrhage in the skin and mucous membranes caused by thrombocytopenia, and the general wasting of malignant disease.

MULTIPLE MYELOMA

The skin lesions of multiple myeloma are usually direct extensions or metastatic from bone lesions. They are reddish blue subcutaneous nodules 1 to 2 cm in diameter, generally occurring on the trunk and consisting of collections of malignant plasma cells. They usually appear after the diagnosis of multiple myeloma has already been established on the basis of other findings. Primary cutaneous plasmacytomas unrelated to bony lesions are rare. There are no characteristic clinical features that enable a diagnosis without a histologic examination. The lesions may sometimes be present for years before there is other evidence of multiple myeloma

Amyloidosis is found in 10% of patients with myeloma. The lesions are usually located on the skin, mucosal surfaces, tongue, gastrointestinal tract, heart, blood vessels, and muscle. When involved, the gingivae appear spongy, thickened, and nodular and bleed readily following minor trauma. Amyloid deposited diffusely in the tongue produces induration, usually painless macroglossia with uniform enlargement, and sometimes protrusion of the tongue. The surface of the tongue may be smooth, pale, and atrophic. If the involvement is spotty, erythematous nodules and papules occur. On the buccal, nasal, conjunctival, vaginal, and anal mucosa there may be yellowish to pale red papules or plaques in which purpura may be noted after minor trauma. A biopsy of these sites will confirm the presence of amyloid.

Amyloid in the skin is evidenced by translucent waxy yellow to pink superficial and slightly elevated lesions varying from 1 mm to several centimeters. The lesions occur on the eyelids, nasolabial folds, and circumorally, as well as on the neck, axillae, chest, periumbilical areas, and perineum, Because of their shiny translucent quality, they may appear vesicular, but they are solid papules that develop purpura when they are rubbed or pinched because amyloid deposited in the vessel walls makes them fragile. When there is diffuse involvement of an area of the skin, it may take on the appearance of scleroderma. Infiltration of the face may resemble myxedema, with coarse facial features and a rigid expression. Alopecia may develop when hairy sites (scalp, eyebrows, axillae, and pubic areas) become infiltrated. There is generally no pruritus with this form of amyloidosis.

Cryoglobulinemia is found in about 5% of patients with multiple myeloma. The clinical findings are blotchy cyanosis following exposure to cold, Raynaud's phenomenon (sometimes causing digital gangrene), purpura, and necrosis. There may be hemorrhagic bullae leading to cutaneous ulcers (which appear especially on the ankles, hands, and ears), bleeding gums, epistaxis, and cold urticaria that becomes hemorrhagic on rewarming.

Severe hyperlipoproteinemia may result from the dysproteinemia of multiple myeloma, with the formation of cutaneous and visceral xanthomatosis. Normolipemic patients may have diffuse flat xanthomas that can appear before the diagnosis of systemic myelomatosis.

Nonspecific skin findings associated with myeloma include pruritus, pallor (caused by anemia), ichthyosiform dermatitis, pemphigoid, dermatomyositis, uremic frost (when severe renal impairment develops), and disappearance of the lunulae of the nails.

Purpura occurs as a result of thrombocytopenia, amyloidosis of cutaneous vessels, and hyperglobulinemia. The incidence of herpes zoster infections is increased.

MALIGNANT LYMPHOMA

Cutaneous manifestations occur at some time during the course of the disease in about 50% of patients with lymphomas. The morphology of specific cutaneous lesions and nonspecific eruptions is similar in leukemia and lymphoma. Malignant lymphoma of the skin is usually metastatic from some internal organ but may occasionally be a primary event in the skin.

The specific lesions in which the characteristic malignant cells may be found include papules, nodules, and tumors, infiltrations and plaques, ulcerated lesions, and erythroderma. The most distinctive specific lesions are violaceous to plum-colored papules or subcutaneous firm nodules of various sizes. A solitary nodule, especially one occurring on the scalp, may be present for years before causing symptoms. These tumors are firm but not stony hard (unlike metastatic carcinoma), have a rubbery consistency, and may vary from dusky red to a dark violet color. The specific lesions can occur anywhere on the body surface or in the oral cavity, the conjunctivae, and the genitalia. They may be distributed in a generalized manner, may form clusters or circinate or arciform patterns, or may coalesce into large plaques. Nodules and ulcerations may occur on the tonsils, palate, tongue, and nasopharynx. There may be symmetric swelling of the lacrimal, orbital, and salivary glands owing to infiltration with malignant cells. The lymph nodes may become necrotic, resulting in the formation of sinus tracts with ulcerations of the overlying skin.

Any of the lymphomas can occasionally begin with skin lesions that may remain localized in the skin for months or years before there is visceral involvement. Generally, however, the reverse is true; by the time specific lesions are found in the skin, the diagnosis of the underlying problem has usually been made. In Hodgkin's disease, skin lesions usually appear in the late stages and indicate widespread involvement with a poor prognosis.

The nonspecific manifestations include pruritus, prurigo-papular eruptions, pigmentation, erythema multiforme, erythema nodosum, and urticaria. Eczematous and psoriasiform dermatitis, exfoliative dermatitis, and bullous lesions may also occur. Pallor may be noted when anemia develops, and purpura may be seen when thrombocytopenia occurs. In addition, infections of the skin may supervene as the patient's immune state becomes compromised. These infections can be bacterial, superficial or deep fungal, or viral (herpes simplex or herpes zoster).

The nonspecific lesions mentioned previously are more commonly associated with Hodgkin's disease, whereas specific lesions are seen more frequently with reticulum cell sarcoma and lymphosarcoma. Generalized pruritus and excoriations may be the only manifestation of Hodgkin's disease for years before other evidence of the disease appears. Exfoliative dermatitis is likewise associated mainly with Hodgkin's disease and infrequently with reticulum cell sarcoma and lymphosarcoma. It may begin as an erythrodermic patch that becomes generalized with pronounced scaling. Pruritus may become intense, and the patient feels chilly owing to the heat loss resulting from vasodilation and increased blood flow in the skin. The nails may become dystrophic and are shed, and the hair may fall out. Exfoliative dermatitis is associated with lymphomas or leukemias in up to 25% of cases. Acquired ichthyosis may be found in association with lymphomatous diseases, more often with Hodgkin's disease than the other lymphomas. It can be manifested by mild dry skin or severe fishlike scales; there may be hyperkeratosis of palms and soles. The ichthyosis may subside when the lymphoma is in remission.

MYCOSIS FUNGOIDES

Mycosis fungoides has many attributes of the malignant lymphomas: it is a neoplastic disorder involving the lymphoreticular system and it has the ability to undergo transition to the other types of malignant lymphoma. It is different from the monomorphous lymphomas such as reticulum cell sarcoma and lymphosarcoma in its natural history and histopathologic features and is more akin to Hodgkin's disease. However, unlike patients with Hodgkin's disease, those with mycosis fungoides have an intact delayed hypersensitivity response.

Mycosis fungoides occurs more commonly in men than in women; it may develop as early as adolescence but is diagnosed most often in patients who are 40 to 60 years of age. Its duration may be 1 year or it may last for several decades, becoming progressively more severe. The average course is about 10 years, but when the tumor stage develops, survival is usually less than 3 years.

Three phases of the disease are recognized: (1) a premycotic phase consisting of erythematous, eczematous, and psoriasiform lesions, usually accompanied by intense pruritus; (2) an infiltrated plaque phase; and (3) a tumor phase. These phases do not always follow in sequence; the disease may begin with any of these forms and one may exist without the others. Generally, however, the onset is insidious, with a premycotic phase lasting from months to many years. Pruritus, at times intense, may be the sole initial manifestation, or it may accompany various clinical presentations resembling seborrheic dermatitis, psoriasis, eczema, neurodermatitis, parapsoriasis, and erythema multiforme, as well as urticarial lesions and scaly patches. The eruptions may be transitory or persistent; they may remit spontaneously and recur later. In many patients with parapsoriasis en plaques (pale, erythematous, fingerlike to palm-sized patches) and poikiloderma (diffuse variegated erythema) of the trunk, mycosis fungoides eventually may develop.

The configuration of lesions may be bizarre; arciform, large ring, crescent, and ribbonlike forms occur. The color is often vivid, predominantly shades of red such as scarlet, salmon, rose, and crimson, sometimes with a bluish or yellowish tinge. Erythroderma and exfoliative dermatitis may develop and become generalized. The universal redness (l'homme rouge) and scaling are accompanied by edematous and thickened skin, with leonine facies, ectropion, scanty hair, and dry ridged nails; enlargement of the spleen and lymph nodes (dermatopathic lymphadenopathy) may be noted.

In the plaque stage (Fig. 161-1) the premycotic lesions become infiltrated, sometimes resulting in a pebbly surface. Induration may initially be present in only a few of the lesions, and infiltrated plaques may arise in previously

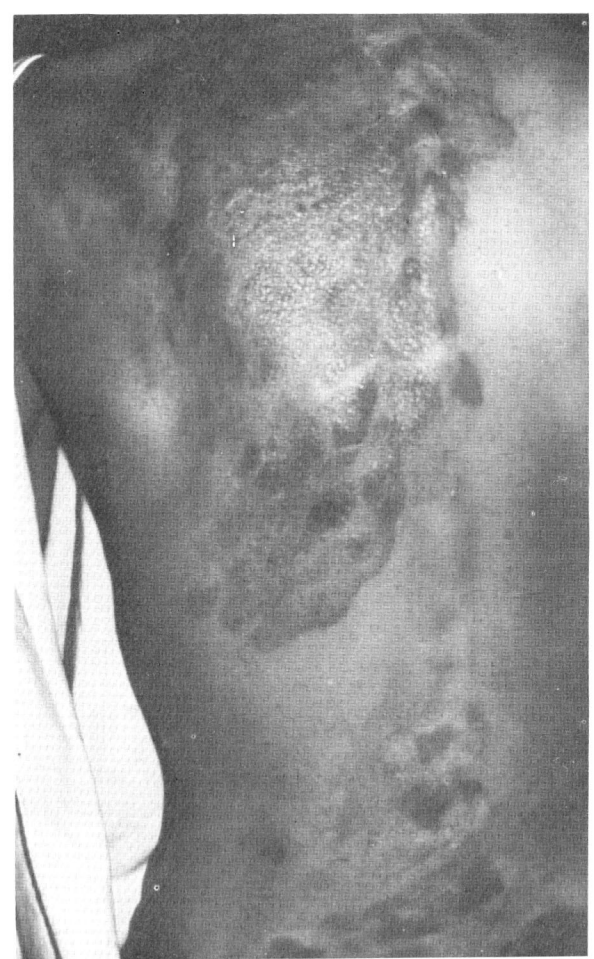

Fig. 161-1. Mycosis fungoides on back. Plaque stage with beginning early tumor formation is shown. Lesions are erythematous and slightly infiltrated.

uninvolved areas. These lesions also assume bizarre shapes and the pruritus continues; the color varies from shades of red to brownish or purple. The infiltration becomes progressively more marked, leading to extensive plaques that coalesce to produce widespread involvement, interspersed with some patches of normal skin. Eventually almost the entire skin surface may become infiltrated, resulting in a universal erythroderma with thickened skin. Exceedingly painful superficial and sometimes large ulcerations may develop.

The tumor stage is characterized by nodules and tumefactions of varying sizes and shapes that develop in the infiltrated plaques, in the erythrodermic areas, or on previously uninvolved surfaces. These tumors most commonly occur on the trunk, but they may occur anywhere on the skin and occasionally in the mouth or upper respiratory tract. The colors are those seen in the plaques, often a dusky bluish red. The tumors tend to break down and form deep necrotic ulcers with rolled edges. Despite this, and even with extensive involvement, the patient at first does not seem gravely ill, and the pruritus tends to diminish somewhat with the onset of the tumor stage. Occasionally tumors spontaneously regress and disappear, as the lesions in the premycotic and infiltrative (plaque) stages sometimes do, but recurrence and progression are inevitable. Lesions in all three stages may be present at the same time.

The d'emblée form of mycosis fungoides is the name applied to the disorder when large tumors appear de novo without the first two stages of the disease being present. This may sometimes be a manifestation of a malignant lymphoma. The Sézary syndrome is simply a variant manifestation of mycosis fungoides. It is an erythrodermic phase of mycosis fungoides in which a percular atypical monocytic cell is found in the circulating blood, as well as in the lymph nodes and the cutaneous infiltrate. The Sézary cell is considered to be a giant abnormal lymphocyte with a large convoluted nucleus and a narrow rim of cytoplasm. The nucleus is cerebriform with lobulations and indentations; the cytoplasm is vacuolated. The Sézary syndrome is characterized by severe pruritus accompanying a generalized erythroderma that is often fiery red; there is a leonine facies, with edema of the eyelids and ectropion, diffuse alopecia, hyperkeratosis of palms and soles, dystrophic nails, splenomegaly, and diffuse superficial lymphadenopathy, in addition to the finding of the aforementioned unusual cell. There is generally a leukocytosis in the range of 20,000 cells/mm^3 with an absolute lymphocytosis, up to 19% eosinophils, and the abnormal Sézary cell. This has led to the belief that the Sézary syndrome may be a leukemic phase of mycosis fungoides.

The therapy for mycosis fungoides is based on the stage of the disease and includes topical, intralesional, and systemic administration of corticosteroids; topical administration of nitrogen mustard and nitrosourea; intralesional administration of nitrogen mustard and bleomycin; immunotherapy with BCG vaccine, levamisole, and other agents; chemotherapy with cytotoxic or immunosuppressive agents including azaribine, methotrexate, procarbazine, and bleomycin; physical agents including ultraviolet light and grenzray therapy in the early stages; and electron beam therapy, teleroentgen therapy, and conventional radiation therapy in the later stages of the disease.

BIBLIOGRAPHY

Amorosi, E.L., and Ultmann, J.E.: Thrombotic thrombocytopenic purpura; report of 16 cases and review of the literature, Medicine **45:**139, 1966.

Baxter, D.L., and Lockwood, J.H.: Acne urticata polycythemia; report of a case, Arch. Dermatol. **78:**325, 1958.

Block, J.B., and others: Mycosis fungoides: natural history and aspects of its relationship to other malignant lymphomas. Am. J. Med. **34:**228, 1963.

Bluefarb, S.M.: Cutaneous manifestations of malignant lymphomas, Springfield, Ill., 1959, Charles C. Thomas, Publisher.

Bluefarb, S.M.: Leukemia cutis, Springfield, Ill., 1969, Charles C. Thomas, Publisher.

Boggs, D.P., and others: The acute leukemias: analysis of 322 cases and review of the literature, Medicine **41**:163, 1962.

Braverman, I.M.: Skin signs of systemic disease, ed. 2, Philadelphia, 1981, W.B. Saunders Co.

Burg, G., and others: Monocytic leukemia: clinically appearing as "malignant reticulosis of the skin," Arch. Dermatol. **114**:418, 1978.

Cyr, C.P., Goekas, M.C., and Worsley, G.H.: Mycosis fungoides, Arch. Dermatol. **94**:558, 1966.

Domonkos, A.N., Arnold, H.L., and Odom, R.B., editors: Andrew's diseases of the skin, ed. 7, Philadelphia. 1982, W.B. Saunders Co.

Edelson, R.L., and others: Preferential cutaneous infiltration by neoplastic thymus-derived lymphocytes, Ann. Intern. Med. **80**:685, 1974.

Fromer, J.L., and Geokas, M.C.: Cutaneous manifestations in lymphomas, N.Y. J. Med. **63**:3222, 1963.

Hegde, U.M., and others: Platelet anitbodies in thrombocytopenic patients, Br. J. Haematol. **35**:113, 1977.

Karayalcin, G., and others: Sickle cell anemia: clinical manifestations in 100 patients and review of the literature, Am. J. Med. Sci. **269**:51, 1975.

Klein, H.: Polycythemia: theory and management, Springfield, Ill., 1973, Charles C. Thomas, Publisher.

Levin, H.A., and others: Multiple extramedullary plasmacytomas, Arch. Dermatol. **96**:456, 1967.

Mikhail, G.R., Spindler, A.C., and Kelly, A.P.: Malignant plasmacytoma cutis, Arch. Dermatol. **101**:59, 1970.

River, G.L., and Schorr, W.F.: Malignant tumors in multiple myeloma, Arch. Dermatol. **93**:432, 1966.

Sergeant, G.R.: Leg ulceration in sickle cell anemia, Arch. Intern. Med. **133**:690, 1974.

Waldenstrom, J.: Diagnosis and treatment of multiple myeloma, New York, 1970, Grune & Stratton, Inc.

Wintrobe, M.M., and others: Clinical hematology, ed. 7, Philadelphia, 1974, Lea & Febiger.

Yoder, F.W., and Schuen, R.L.: Aleukemic leukemia cutis, Arch. Dermatol. **112**:367, 1976.

162 • CONNECTIVE TISSUE DISORDERS

Bernard A. Kirshbaum, Anthony V. Benedetto, Karen Lipinski, and **Robert N. Arm**

LUPUS ERYTHEMATOSUS

Lupus erythematosus (LE) appears in two basic forms: a purely cutaneous form called chronic discoid lupus erythematosus (CDLE) and systemic lupus erythematosus (SLE).

The cutaneous lesions of CDLE are usually discrete, heliotrope-colored plaques with disklike and irregular configurations. They heal centrally with slight scaling and usually a moderate amount of scarring (Fig. 162-1). In active lesions the borders remain edematous and scaly with telangiectasia contributing to the lesion's bright red color. In hairy areas follicular hyperkeratosis and plugging occur. Atrophy usually is accompanied by depigmentation and hyperpigmentation. Darker-skinned patients are more severely affected with leukoderma. Typically the lesions are found on the exposed areas of the face, ears, and scalp, but they can also be found on the neck, shoulders, back, forearms, and legs. Lesions can appear singly or can be localized to a small area of the body (usually the face); some patients manifest a generalized distribution of discoid lesions. SLE is more likely to develop in individuals with widespread lesions.

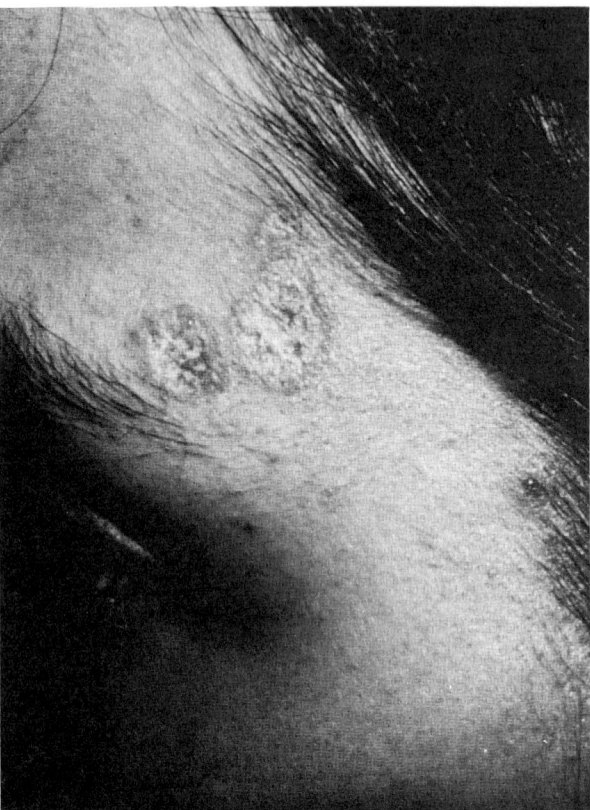

Fig. 162-1. Lesions of chronic discoid lupus erythematosus. Note scarring. Lesions are surrounded by erythema. (Courtesy of Department of Dermatology, The Cleveland Clinics.)

Oral lesions occur in 25% to 50% of patients with CDLE. These lesions often begin with an irregular whitish area that extends peripherally. A centrally depressed red area develops, while the border expands and remains white, elevated, and hyperkeratotic. Surrounding this border there may be a somewhat erythematous hyperemic halo. If healing occurs in the central portion or if the entire area goes into remission, there may be a slightly atrophic scar or no residua.

The cause of LE is unknown, but sunlight and local physical trauma precipitate the lesions. Women are affected more frequently than men in a ratio of 2:1.

The results of laboratory tests are characteristically normal for patients with CDLE, although abnormalities are found in patients with SLE. The treatment of skin lesions of LE consists of avoiding precipitating causes (heat, light, cold, physical trauma, and emotional stress). Intralesional and topical administration of corticosteroids and oral chloroquine, quinacrine, or hydroxychloroquine is usually effective. Therapy with these agents should be undertaken only with due regard to ocular and other potential side effects.

ORAL MANIFESTATIONS AND DENTAL CONSIDERATIONS. See pp. 111-112.

SCLERODERMA

Scleroderma is characterized by progressive fibrotic changes in dermal collagen and the connective tissues of other involved organs. The disease may be localized or systemic and has an insidious course. The cause is unknown, but an autoimmune mechanism may be involved. There is a general increase in sclerotic collagen, a marked increase, thickening, and condensation of the connective tissues, and an increase in collagen-bound hexosamine. Sclerosis is also noted in the subcutaneous tissues.

LABORATORY FINDINGS. Laboratory findings that may be present in scleroderma include an elevated erythrocyte sedimentation rate and mild anemia. Immunologic changes also occur, including the presence of rheumatoid factor and occasionally a false positive serologic reaction for syphilis. Antinuclear antibodies are present in a majority of patients but are usually of low titer as compared to SLE. The LE cell test is seldom positive. Hypergammaglobulinemia with a marked increase of IgG may be found, and antithyroid antibodies have been noted.

MANAGEMENT. The treatment of scleroderma consists mainly of physiotherapy (warmth, massage, exercise, and baths) to prevent ankylosis, contractural deformities, and immobility. Sundry therapeutic modalities have been tried, including para-aminobenzoic acid, chelating agents, D-penicillamine, dimethyl sulfoxide, and azathioprine. Some of these have been highly touted, but all have been found wanting. Vasodilators are helpful, and sympathectomy may improve the cutaneous circulation for a while. Systemic corticosteroids reduce joint symptoms and give patients a feeling of well-being.

Morphea (circumscribed scleroderma)

Morphea is a localized form of scleroderma. It may occur as multiple guttate lesions mainly on the chest and neck or as oval or linear plaques of hard, dry, smooth skin primarily on the chest, face, or scalp. These lesions are often ivory colored or white with a faint violaceous border. Bandlike lesions may form along the course of a rib, on the long axis of an extremity, or vertically on the forehead. Solitary linear lesions that develop on the scalp and forehead are called en coup de sabre ("saber stroke") because of their appearance and are sometimes associated with facial hemiatrophy. Linear scleroderma usually appears in the first decade of life and occurs in females twice as often as males. It rarely leads to the generalized forms of scleroderma. There is no satisfactory treatment, but some lesions reach an end point beyond which the sclerosis does not progress and many undergo spontaneous resolution (especially in children and adolescents).

ORAL MANIFESTATIONS. The lip may be involved in morphea. The elastic qualities will be lost, often causing a stricture. A localized white scar may also be seen on the lip. The alveolar ridges, gingiva, and mucosa underlying the affected area can also be involved. A roentgenogram of an involved bone will show a radiolucency. This absence of bone is caused by fibrosis. Teeth in the area may have enamel defects. In one case, a cleft developed after the shedding of teeth.

In the en coup de sabre form, hemifacial atrophy can lead to esthetic and functional problems.

DENTAL MANAGEMENT. Because the oral cavity may be inaccessible in patients exhibiting perioral involvement, increased caries and periodontal disease may occur. The lip strictures may also make placement of removable prosthesis impossible. A "hinge" may allow for flexibility needed to place the appliance. Widening of the periodontal ligament and bone necrosis have been reported in systemic scleroderma. Some of the deformities may be corrected by surgery.

BIBLIOGRAPHY

Saad, M.N., and Khoo, C.T.K.: Localized scleroderma of the premaxilla and upper lip, Br. J. Plast. Surg. 33:245, 1980.

Progressive systemic sclerosis

Progressive systemic sclerosis appears in two forms: acrosclerosis and diffuse scleroderma.

Acrosclerosis. Acrosclerosis, which accounts for 95% of all cases of scleroderma, is characterized by cutaneous sclerosis of the digits (sclerodactyly) and Raynaud's phenomenon, but there is also visceral involvement. It occurs chiefly in young women, usually in late adolescence or early adult life. It begins with Raynaud's phenomenon and arthralgias or symptoms like rheumatoid arthritis. In the early phases there are transient and recurrent erythema and edema, especially of the hands and fingers; sometimes the onset is insidious, without edema. The sclerodermatous changes and atrophy shortly supervene; the skin becomes yellowish, smooth, shiny, and firm, and retraction occurs so that it is bound to the underlying structures. The face becomes expressionless and appears drawn and taut with a loss of normal lines. The patient's mouth cannot be opened to its full width, and the forehead cannot be wrinkled; the patient may have a fixed stare and the lips form a permanent grimace. The hands become clawlike, with sclerodactyly, tapered fingers, and shiny hidebound skin. Contractures of the fingers occur, not only from the tight skin but also from fibrosis of muscles, sclerosis of the synovia, and disuse atrophy. The fingers become semiflexed and immobile. Gradual resorption of bone occurs in the terminal phalanges, with shortening of the fingers. There is a progressive increase of induration extending from the forearm and hand to the fingertips.

Raynaud's phenomenon, which is almost universally present in acrosclerosis, varies from mild vasospasm to severe attacks of vascular insufficiency resulting in gangrene. Small pitted scars and ulcerations on the fingertips are characteristic. Trophic ulcers of the knuckles, toes, and ankles occur as the result of the combination of trauma and chronic vascular insufficiency. Changes occurring in the feet and toes are similar to those in the hands and fingers but are generally less severe.

Roentgenograms may show small areas of calcification at the base and borders of the ulcers. Calcium is also deposited around major joints and in the fingers; this is called Thibierge-Weisenbach syndrome. The skin over these firm, whitish nodules erodes, and bits of calcium are discharged at the surface; this is often accompanied by cellulitis and secondary bacterial infection. Calcinosis cutis develops relatively late in the course of scleroderma, unlike dermatomyositis in which it appears earlier and is more disabling.

Telangiectatic lesions are commonly noted on the face, lips, buccal mucosa, and hands of patients with scleroderma. The lesions range from dusky to bright red or pink and from 1 to 5 mm. They are oval to square or multiangular with sharp or indistinct borders. Although telangiectasia is also seen in the other collagen diseases, these "telangiectatic mats" with their characteristic shapes occur most commonly in scleroderma. Linear telangiectases are also found on the posterior nail fold in scleroderma and the other connective tissue diseases.

The combination of calcinosis, Raynaud's phenomenon, sclerodactyly, and telangiectasia has been called the CRST syndrome. This is simply a relatively benign form of scleroderma in which visceral involvement is uncommon or minimal.

Conversely, visceral scleroderma without cutaneous sclerosis is known to occur. Patients with this condition usually have Raynaud's phenomenon and some telangiectasia that may be overlooked.

Cutaneous pigmentary changes occurring in scleroderma are of three types:
1. Hyperpigmentation and hypopigmentation are postinflammatory changes appearing in areas of sclerosis.
2. Patches of perifollicular pigmentation develop in sites of complete pigment loss and resemble repigmenting vitiligo.
3. A generalized hyperpigmentation, especially of exposed areas and mucous membranes, mimics the pigmentation of adrenal insufficiency.

Diffuse scleroderma. Diffuse scleroderma is an uncommon form of scleroderma. It begins with edema and subsequent hardening of the skin over the chest and spreads rapidly to the head and extremities. The sclerotic areas appear yellowish brown and waxy. The visceral involvement resembles acrosclerosis, but Raynaud's phenomenon is not encountered and sclerodactyly does not develop because the disease is rapidly fatal. Visceral involvement affects mainly the gastrointestinal tract and the lungs.

ORAL MANIFESTATIONS AND DENTAL MANAGEMENT. See chapter on collagen vascular disorders.

BIBLIOGRAPHY

Braverman, I.M.: Skin signs of systemic disease, Philadelphia, 1970, W.B. Saunders Co.

Christianson, H.B., and others: Localized scleroderma—a clinical study of 235 cases, Arch. Dermatol. **74:**629, 1956.

Curtis, A.C., and Jansen, T.G.: The prognosis of localized scleroderma, Arch. Dermatol. **78:**749, 1958.

Domonkos, A.N.: Andrew's diseases of the skin, Philadelphia, 1971, W.B. Saunders Co.

Rodnan, G.P.: Progressive systemic scleroderma. In Samter, M., editor: Immunologic diseases, Boston, 1965, Little, Brown and Co., pp. 769-783.

Rodnan, G.P., and Fennel, R.H., Jr.: Progressive systemic sclerosis *sine* scleroderma, J.A.M.A. **180:**665, 1962.

Tuffanelli, D.L., and Winkelmann, R.K.: Diffuse systemic scleroderma: a comparison with acrosclerosis, Ann. Intern. Med. **57:**198, 1962.

DERMATOMYOSITIS

Dermatomyositis is a necrotizing inflammatory disease of unknown cause that affects striated muscles, skin, and subcutaneous tissue. Muscle weakness resulting from polymyositis is often the major symptom. Although myositis is sometimes found in association with SLE, scleroderma, rheumatoid arthritis, and rheumatic fever, it is not a prominent finding in these conditions. Dermatomyositis is a relatively rare condition. It may occur as early as 1 year of age or as late as 70 years of age. Although most cases are found in adults, about 15% develop in children and young adolescents; females are twice as frequently affected as males. There is no racial or geographic predilection. Dermatomyositis follows a variable course. It may be acute and intense, ending fatally within a year, or there may be long periods of remission and recurrence, progressing slowly for a decade or more. Permanent remission occurs in a few cases. The disease has been noted following infection, physical trauma, immunization, and drugs. It is not caused by any of these but is probably a hypersensitivity reaction or the result of an autoimmune mechanism. The presence of malignancy has frequently been associated with dermatomyositis, which may appear before the signs and symptoms of carcinoma are manifest. Patients with dermatomyositis should be studied carefully to rule out visceral cancer.

There may be a vague prodrome or a febrile episode, followed by muscle inflammation and degeneration associated with edema and dermatologic changes. Erythema, telangiectasia, and pigmentary changes occur; ultimately interstitial calcinosis may develop. The classic manifestation is a pinkish violet erythema and puffy swelling of the eyelids and face (the characteristic heliotrope eruption), which may also involve the upper part of the trunk, with or without edema. This stage may last for months but is eventually superseded by lupus-like skin changes akin to those in SLE, affecting not only the face but also the neck, shoulders, arms, and chest. This is accompanied by deep tenderness and a firm, slightly pitting brawny edema over the shoulder girdle, arms, and neck. Linear telangiectases are noted on the cuticles and fingernail folds in dermatomyositis as in the other collagen diseases, and there may occasionally be ulceration of the fingertips, although this is not a regular feature as in scleroderma. Gottron's papules are a pathognomonic sign; these are flat-topped, faintly violaceous lesions on the dorsa of the fingers over the interphalangeal joints. They occur relatively late in the disease in about one third of the patients. When they regress, atrophy, telangiectasia, and hypopigmentation remain in these sites.

Sometimes the earliest signs of dermatomyositis may be transient violaceous blotchy lesions on the trunk, extremities, and face, which may be accompanied by a fine scale. In this stage the disease may be diagnosed as seborrheic dermatitis, contact dermatitis, or an allergic reaction. Occasionally urticarial lesions, vesicular and bullous lesions and erythema multiforme-like lesions may be seen; photosensitivity may occur. Sun-exposed areas develop a confluent violaceous, telangiectatic, slightly scaling eruption, which becomes fixed as minute hyperpigmented and hypopigmented macules with telangiectasia and atrophy. This speckled appearance of the skin, called poikoloderma atrophicans vasculare, occurs in the late stages of dermatomyositis, rarely in SLE, and not at all in scleroderma. Poikilodermatomyositis is the name given to this stage of the disease.

Vasomotor disturbances (Raynaud's phenomenon) occur in less than one third of patients; alopecia of the scalp may also be seen. When the disease regresses, a bronze discoloration develops that mimics the hyperpigmentation of adrenal insufficiency, and hypertrichosis may occur in the sites of previous cutaneous involvement. Sclerodactyly, diffuse sclerodermoid changes in the skin, hyperpigmentation, and hypopigmentation develop in about 25% of the patients. The term "sclerodermatomyositis" has been applied to this condition, which may appear in 6 months to 3 years after the onset of the myositis. When the sclerodermatous features become prominent, the myositis is usually less active.

There is no relation between the extent of skin lesions and the degree of muscle involvement in dermatomyositis. The skin lesions may be minimal with pronounced myositis, or conversely there may be extensive cutaneous disease with relatively little muscle involvement.

The earliest symptoms of dermatomyositis are soreness and weakness of muscles, sometimes accompanies by swelling and tenderness. It is symmetric and affects primarily the shoulder girdle and pelvic region as well as the neck and proximal muscles of the arms. Patients have difficulty raising their arms, rising from chairs, and walking up stairs. The muscles initially feel doughy, later firm, and ultimately become atrophic and fibrotic, with calcification noted especially in children. Dysphagia and dysphonia result from involvement of the striated muscles of the pharynx, palate, and esophagus. Esophageal motility changes may be seen on radiographic examination. Cardiac muscle may also become involved, ultimately with cardiac failure.

Calcinosis cutis occurs in dermatomyositis; it tends to be more diffuse and appears earlier than in scleroderma. It is found in the subcutaneous tissue, dermis, and muscle and is demonstrable roentgenographically. Unlike scleroderma, it rarely affects the fingers. Calcification develops in children more frequently than in adults. Laboratory findings include elevation of serum enzymes including glutamic oxaloacetic transaminase (SGOT) and lactic dehydrogenase (LDH), with creatine phosphokinase (CPK) being a more specific marker. Since the enzyme levels reflect the degree of activity of the myopathy, they have prognostic significance and can be used to measure therapeutic efficacy. Creatinuria is relative to the amount of muscle damage and may reflect disease activity more accurately than serum enzymes. Proteinemia also occurs and in severe cases myoglobinuria may be seen.

The erythrocyte sedimentation rate is usually increased in patients with dermatomyositis. Leukocytosis may be present in acute cases, and subsequently leukopenia may be noted. Anemia occurs in chronic cases. Antinuclear antibodies are found in one third of cases; serum γ-globulin levels may be elevated. Rheumatoid factor is present in 10% of the cases. Electromyographic studies are useful to distinguish this disease from other myopathies and neuropathy.

The treatment consists of the administration of corticosteroids and supportive therapy. Corticosteroids help control the inflammatory process and induce remissions but do not appreciably alter the ultimate course of the disease. Prednisone should be used with due regard to all of its potential side effects. Bed rest, warmth, and analgesics are essential in acute cases; physiotherapy is necessary to prevent contractures. The disease tends to be progressive with remissions.

ORAL MANIFESTATIONS. A diffuse stomatitis and pharyngitis are nonspecific clinical findings in dermatomyositis. Facial edema and erythema are generally noted. Twenty percent of the patients may have lesions on the palate, tongue, and buccal mucosa. They present as erythema, papules, shallow ulcers, and white patches. These lesions are often similar to those seen in lupus erythematosus.

The muscle involvement can affect the facial and jaw muscles, making it difficult to speak and eat and preventing normal facial expression. The muscle dysfunction can lead to alteration of the temporomandibular joint, and myofascial pain syndrome may develop. Calcinosis, especially in the tongue, may be seen and the tongue can become large and immobile. Roentgenographs can show the calcified masses in the soft tissue. There have been reports of telangiectatic lesions of the lips and cheeks. Altered tooth morphology has been seen, especially shortened roots, calcified pulp chambers, and pulp stones. An increased incidence of teeth fracturing during extraction indicates dentinal involvement.

DENTAL MANAGEMENT. Because of the poor response to therapy, these patients will be hard to manage. Little can be done to benefit these patients. They have systemic involvement as well as oral lesions. Teeth will fracture. There will be a lack of muscle control. Of major concern is the extent of systemic organ involvement, especially heart and lungs. The drugs the patient is taking must also be evaluated.

BIBLIOGRAPHY

Barnes, B.: Dermatomyositis and malignancy, Ann. Intern. Med. **84:**68, 1976.
Bohan, A., and Peter, J.B.: Polymyositis and dermatomyositis, N. Engl. J. Med. **292:**344, 1975.
Braverman, I.M.: Skin signs of systemic disease, ed. 2, Philadelphia, 1981, W.B. Saunders Co.
Domonkos, A.N.: Andrew's diseases of the skin: clinical dermatology, Philadelphia, 1971, W.B. Saunders Co.
Everett, M.A., and Curtis, A.C.: Dermatomyositis, Arch. Intern. Med. **100:**70, 1957.
Sanger, R.G., and Kirby, J.W.: The oral and facial manifestations of dermatomyositis with calcinosis, Oral Surg. **35:**476, 1973.

MIXED CONNECTIVE TISSUE DISEASE (OVERLAP SYNDROME)

Mixed connective tissue disease, or overlap syndrome, is seen in patients, mostly female, who have features of SLE, dermatomyositis, polymyositis, and scleroderma.

The most common symptom is joint pain. The cutaneous manifestations include nonscarring alopecia, discoid lupus erythematosus, swelling of the hands with sclerodactyly, and pigmentary abnormalities. The pigmentary changes, resembling those seen in scleroderma, are a "salt and pepper" discoloration owing to retention of pigment in the follicles. Raynaud's phenomenon also occurs. Fever, splenomegaly, lymphadenopathy, hypergammaglobulinemia, esophageal motility abnormalities, violaceous suffusion of the eyelids, and proximal muscle weakness are seen in these patients.

RHEUMATOID ARTHRITIS

Rheumatoid nodules occur in 20% of patients with rheumatoid arthritis. They are associated with the more severe forms of the disease, higher levels of rheumatoid factor, more severe joint manifestations, and vasculitis. Nodules are rarely the initial symptom; more often they develop during the course of the disease. They occur over bony prominences, especially the olecranon and its vicinity; they are also found on the heels, ears, knuckles, and ischial tuberosities. Ulceration and breakdown of the nodules are common. The nodules persist and may recur after excision.

Linear subcutaneous bands have been described in patients with nodules. These are fixed, subcutaneous bands, 3 to 5 mm wide and several centimeters long. They are nontender and are located on the trunk.

Pyoderma gangrenosum occurs rarely, manifested by an ulceration surrounded by violaceous discoloration. The lesions may appear as "punched-out" draining areas or as papules with a bluish red rim. The response to systemic corticosteroid therapy is often dramatic.

Rheumatoid vasculitis, which is slightly more common in men, involves the venules and small and medium-sized arteries. There is deposition of IgG, IgM, and the third component of complement (C3). Ulcerations, livedo reticularis, Raynaud's phenomenon, ecchymoses, and gangrene may occur. Painful ulcerations develop on the legs and ankles. They heal slowly and may be preceded by ecchymoses and palpable purpura.

Small infarctions are seen in the paronychial areas. These are asymptomatic, last only 3 to 4 days, and heal leaving a residual brown macule. Necrosis of the digits occurs more frequently in patients with high titers of rheumatoid factor. Painful nodules may develop in the digital pulp, sometimes in crops, healing with scars, hyperkeratosis, and brown discoloration.

Patients undergoing long-term corticosteroid therapy are susceptible to steroid-induced purpura and ecchymoses.

ORAL MANIFESTATIONS AND DENTAL MANAGEMENT. See pp. 105-106.

WEGENER'S AND LYMPHOMATOID GRANULOMATOSIS
Wegener's granulomatosis

Cutaneous lesions are present in about one half of patients with Wegener's granulomatosis. Ulcerated nodular, petechial, papulovesicular, pyoderma gangrenosum-like, and urticarial lesions have been described. The lesions are frequently bilateral and nonspecific. A histologic examination usually shows a necrotizing vasculitis with thrombosis; occasionally a granulomatous reaction is found. A persistent, crusted, hemorrhagic granuloma of the nostrils, nasal septum, pharynx, trachea, or larynx should suggest Wegener's granulomatosis. Painful proliferative granular gingivitis starting in interdental papillae and coalescing rapidly is highly suggestive of this disease.

BEHÇET'S DISEASE

Behçet's disease is a progressive, systemic, multisystem disease of unknown cause. The syndrome was first recorded by Hippocrates as he described patients with aphthous ulcers in the mouth, discharge and sores about the genitalia, and watery inflammation of the eyes with loss of sight in some cases. It is believed related to vasculitis, with 60% of patients having an increased erythrocyte sedimentation rate and about 80% having dysproteinemia. Unlike the female dominance of aphthae, about 5:1 more males have Behçet's disease. It most commonly affects men between 15 and 45 and consists of iritis and oral and genital ulcerations. Pyoderma, erythema nodosum–like lesions, polyarthritis, and central nervous system, cardiac, and pulmonary involvement also occur.

The initial manifestations are oral or genital ulcers. Mucosal lesions resemble recurrent aphthae. Genital ulcers occur on the scrotum and penis in men and the labia in women; they tend to be smaller than ulcers in the mouth and pharynx.

Ocular manifestations include photophobia, conjunctivitis, iritis, uveitis, neuritis, and vitreous opacification. Eye involvement is the major cause of disability.

About 80% of patients with Behçet's disease have skin lesions, which consist of follicular and perifollicular pustules, inflamed dermal nodules, cellulitis, and furunculosis. These develop on the trunk, limbs, and flexural areas. Sterile pustules developing at the sites of venipuncture should alert the physician to the possibility of Behçet's disease.

Systemic symptoms of malaise, fever, and arthralgias are variable. Thrombophlebitis, which may be superficial or deep, develops in 20% of the cases. Central nervous system involvement may be fatal.

The prognosis is variable. The disease can wax and wane, with spontaneous remissions and exacerbations. One organ system involvement may remain active while the others are in remission, but in general the disease activity diminishes and finally ceases after many years.

ORAL MANIFESTATIONS. Oral ulcers are often the initial sign of Behçet's disease and are present in about 95% of the cases. The lesions are often indistinguishable from aphthae. They generally begin as vesicles or pustules and evolve into superficial ulcers. They commonly occur in the buccal vestibule, tongue, floor of mouth, and lips. The extent of the lesions vary, and often there are spontaneous exacerbations or remission after years. They can also erode into the deeper submucosa and take a long time to heal. The patient may have persistent lesions for years, often with a fetid breath, dysphagia, and pain. In severe cases the palate, pharynx, and esophagus are also affected.

The distinguishing feature of Behçet's disease is that about 65% of the patients also have genital ulceration and 80% have iritis. Other common associations are skin lesions (80% of patients) and arthritis (60% of patients). The arthritis may affect the temporamandibular joint. Trauma may make any of the lesions worse. Sepsis and thrombosis have been reported at venipuncture sites.

REITER'S SYNDROME

Reiter's syndrome is a symptom complex consisting of nongonococcal urethritis, conjunctivitis, arthritis, and dermatitis. A predisposition to this complex is strongly associated with the HLA-B27 antigen. Two forms of the syndrome exist: a postinfectious form and a venereal form.

The postinfectious variant occurs after dysenteric infections caused by *Shigella, Salmonella, Campylobacter,* and *Yersinia*. The venereally transmitted form affects men 50 times more commonly than women; no specific etiologic agent has been substantiated, but *Chlamydia* and *Mycoplasma* have been suggested as possible causes.

Reiter's syndrome is variable and recurrent. Often it is chronic with multiple relapse, but it may be self-limiting. The onset is usually abrupt, often with no prodromal symptoms, generally a few weeks after sexual exposure. The subjects are generally 25 to 35 years old. Diarrhea, especially in the enteric form, may be the first sign. Often heel or ankle pain and polyarthritis causes the patient to seek professional care. Initial constitutional symptoms of fever, weakness, anorexia, weight loss, and anemia may be present along with a purulent urethral discharge. The bilateral catarrhal conjunctivitis rarely has a purulent exudate and is generally not painful. Keratitis may occasionally develop with painful ulcerations. The eye symptoms may clear spontaneously in a few days or weeks or may progress to iridocyclitis.

Keratoderma blenorrhagicum refers to the hyperkeratotic, scaling, serpiginous lesions that develop on the palms, soles, legs, and scalp of patients with Reiter's syndrome. Lesions on the abdomen and buttocks tend to be psoriasiform. This eruption develops about 1 month after the onset of urethritis and follows the appearance of the arthritis; it is self-limited and may last weeks to months. Nail and paronychial involvement may be severe and can lead to onycholysis, nail thickening, and dystrophy. Penile lesions occur in 25% of the cases. Balanitis is the most common mucocutaneous manifestation. Painless, shallow erosions with keratotic margins occur near the corona of the glans penis. Dry scaling of the glans penis may be noted, and scaling erosive plaques may appear on the scrotum. Rarely an exfoliative dermatitis may develop; this may be fatal in severely ill patients who have a protracted course. As in psoriasis, the skin lesions are treated with tar and topical corticosteroids.

The arthritis is an inflammatory polyarthritis often resembling rheumatoid arthritis. The lower extremities are more commonly involved, especially knees, heels, and ankles. The arthritis can be disabling. Occasionally only one joint may be involved. Classic treatment for rheumatoid arthritis has been tried but is not successful.

Systemic complications may include urethral stricture, prostate vesiculitis, and less commonly neurologic and cardiac manifestations. A cervical or lumbar radiculopathy and seizure disorder have been reported. In patients with widespread dermatitis a polyneuritis may be present. Aortic insufficiency and first-degree atrioventricular heart blocks can occur years after initial onset of Reiter's syndrome.

ORAL MANIFESTATIONS. While Reiter's syndrome involves eyes, mouth, and genitals, like Behçet's disease, the lesions are different. Oral mucosal lesions are present in 30% to 80% of the cases but are often missed because of the mild symptoms. The oral lesions in this disease last only a few days. They usually are concomitant with the other classic manifestations but may be the initial sign. The generally painless lesions can occur anywhere but more commonly on the tongue, palate, buccal mucosa, and tonsillar pillars. The lesions are psoriasiforme. They initially exhibit a vesicular area with erythematous surrounding and quickly form a shallow ulcer. Confluence of patches of denuded papillae may look similar to geographic tongue (p. 937). Many clinicians suggest that geographic tongue is common in Reiter's syndrome. Some patients have reported a slight burning, loss of taste, and pain.

DENTAL MANAGEMENT. Aimed at symptomatic relief, therapy for each entity is much the same. For pain, topical anesthetic ointment (5% lidocaine) applied to each lesion or a rinse (0.5% aqueous diphenhydramine [Benadryl], 2% viscous lidocaine) for multiple lesions will be beneficial. To avoid pain when eating, a bland diet with no citrus fruit is indicated. A neutral mouthrinse (sodium bicarbonate, calcium bicarbonate for the hypertensive patient) or a peroxide rinse will help keep the mouth clean. The patient should avoid alcohol-containing mouthrinses, elixirs, and beverages.

Multiple therapies have been tried without success, yet many clinicians continue therapeutic measures. None cures the patient. The most favorable records have resulted from use of tetracycline ointment or topical corticosteroids. Other modalities have included administering ether, acidophilus tablets, and zinc. Recent trials of levamisole, a drug affecting the immune system, have shown little promise. While cautery agents, such as phenol or silver nitrate, may initially decrease pain, they enlarge the lesions and prolong healing.

Vitamins have helped in cases where a deficiency was documented. Some researchers suggest obtaining folate, iron, and vitamin B_{12} levels routinely, since one study showed 15% of Reiter's syndrome patients low in all three. When the patients were treated for their deficiency, 60% were cured. Other studies have demonstrated only a 5% to 7% rate of deficiency.

A complete medical history prior to dental treatment is required because of effects on treatment by generalized involvement and drug therapy. Generalized involvement can include cardiac, CNS, vascular (thrombophlebitis in up to 20% of patients with Behçet's disease, probably requiring anticoagulants), and various autoimmune diseases. (For management, see pp.110-111.)

Drug therapy may also alter treatment. Treatment of arthritis with aspirin may alter platelet function. Phenylbutazone, also used in arthritis, may cause aplastic anemia. If long-term steroids are used the increased risk of shock and infection must be evaluated.

BIBLIOGRAPHY

Arnet, G.F.: Reiter's syndrome: report of case, J. Oral Surg. **38**:382, 1980.

Baker, H.: Reiter's disease. In Rook, A., Wilkinson, D.S., and Ebeling, F.J.G., editors: Textbook of dermatology, ed. 3, Oxford, 1979, Blackwell Scientific Publications, pp. 1369-1376.

Berlin, C.: Behçet's disease as a multiple symptom complex, Arch. Dermatol. Syph. **82**:73, 1960.

Callen, J.P.: The spectrum of Reiter's disease, J. Am. Acad. Dermatol. **1**:75, 1979.

Chajek, T., and Fainaru, M.: Behçet's disease: report of 41 cases and review of the literature, Medicine **54**:179, 1975.

Cohen, L.: Etiology, pathogenesis and classification of aphthous stomatitis and Behçet's syndrome, J. Oral Pathol. **7**:347, 1978.

Ersoy, F., and others: HLA antigens associated with Behçet's disease, Arch. Dermatol. **113**:1720, 1977.

Fox, R., and others: The chronicity of symptoms and disability in Reiter's syndrome, Ann. Intern. Med. **910**:190, 1979.

Francis, T.C.: Recurrent aphthous stomatitis and Behçet's disease, Oral Surg. **30**:476, 1970.

Good, A.E.: Reiter's disease, Postgrad. Med. **61**:153, 1977.

Good, A.E.: Reiter's disease: a review with special attention to cardiovascular and neurologic sequellae, Semin. Arthritis Rheum. **3**:253, 1979.

Good, A.E.: Reiter's disease, Cutis **24**:514, 1979.

Graykowski, E.A., and Hooks, J.J.: Summary of workshop on recurrent aphthous ulcers, South. Med. J. **70**:559, 1977.

Lehner, T.: Progress report: oral ulceration and Behcet's syndrome, Gut **18**:491, 1977.

Merchant, H., and others: Zinc sulfate supplementation for treatment of recurrent aphthous ulcers, South. Med. J. **70**:559, 1973.

Meyer, J., and others: Levamisole in aphthous stomatitis, evaluation of three regimes, Br. Med. J. pp. 671-674, 1977.

Miller, M.F., and others: The inheritance of recurrent aphthous stomatitis, Oral Surg. **49**:409, 1980.

Miller, M.F., Ship, I.I., and Ram, C.: A retrospective study of the prevalence and incidence of recurrent aphthous ulcers in a professional population, Oral Surg. **43**:532, 1977.

Moschella, S.L.: Hypersensitivity and miscellaneous inflammatory disorders. In Moschella, S., Pillsbury, D.M., and Hurley, H., editors: Dermatology, Philadelphia, 1975, W.B. Saunders Co., pp. 402-404.

Nally, F.F.: Behçet's syndrome with autoimmune findings, Oral Surg. **25**:357, 1968.

Nicholas, K.D., Bays, R.A., and Lyons, E.D.: Periadenitis mucosa nerotica recurrens, J. Oral. Surg. **33**:65, 1975.

Pindborg, J.J.: Disorders of the oral cavity and lips. In Rook A., Wilkinson, D.M., and Ebeling, F.J.G., editors: Textbook of dermatology, ed. 3, Oxford, 1979, Blackwell Scientific Publications, pp. 1882-1883.

Rosenberg, A.M., and Petty, R.E.: Reiter's disease in children, Am. J. Dis. Child. **133**:394, 1979.

Sharp, J.T.: Reiter's syndrome, Curr. Prob. Dermatol. **5**:157, 1973.

Ship, I.I., Merritt, A.D., and Stanley, H.R.: Recurrent aphthous ulcers, Am. J. Med. **32**:32, 1962.

Silverman, S., and others: Recurrent aphthous stomatitis: current status of etiology and treatment, J. Calif. Dent. Assoc. **5**:38, 1977.

Stanley, H.R.: Management of patients with persistent recurrent aphthous stomatitis and Sutton's disease, Oral Surg. **35**:174, 1973.

Walden, C.A.: Psoriasiform lesions of the oral mucosa, Oral Surg. **37**:872, 1974.

Wray, D., and others: Nutritional deficiencies in recurrent aphthous ulcers, J. Oral Pathol. **7**:418, 1978.

Zizic, T.M., and Stevens, M.B.: The arthropathy of Behçet's disease, Johns Hopkins Med. J. **136**:243, 1975.

163 • MISCELLANEOUS SKIN DISORDERS

Bernard A. Kirshbaum, Anthony V. Benedetto, Karen Lipinski, and Robert N. Arm

MASTOCYTOSIS

Mastocytosis is an uncommon disorder characterized by aggregates of mast cells in the skin and occasionally the internal organs.

Urticaria pigmentosa

Urticaria pigmentosa is the accumulation of mast cells in pigmented lesions of the skin that vary from yellowish brown to reddish brown macules and papules and occasionally nodules. The lesions may be few or numerous, scattered discretely or forming large coalescent areas. Sometimes they are present at birth, but they appear mainly within the first year of life, occasionally later in childhood, and rarely after puberty. The condition clears spontaneously and pigmentation disappears in most cases by the midteens but sometimes may persist into adult life. When lesions appear for the first time in adult life, they are less likely to undergo spontaneous regression. The lesions of urticaria pigmentosa are located mainly on the trunk, but they also occur on the extremities and to a lesser extent on the head and neck. The palms and soles are not involved, and lesions are rarely found on mucous membranes.

Firm stroking or rubbing of the lesions causes them to urticate (Darier's sign). Vesicles and bullae containing clear fluid may develop at sites of mast cell infiltrates in the skin of children. This may persist for a few years but is not found in older people with urticaria pigmentosa.

Mastocytoma

Mastocytoma is a mast cell infiltrate occurring usually as a solitary nodule in infancy. Sometimes there may be a few lesions on the trunk, neck, or forearm. Rubbing the lesion sometimes produces systemic symptoms (flushing and colic) caused by the release of histamine.

Telangiectasia macularis eruptiva perstans

Telangiectasia macularis eruptiva perstans is a rare presentation of mastocytosis that occurs primarily in adults, seldom in children. Numerous hyperpigmented telangiectatic macules appear mainly on the trunk and sometimes on the extremities. Telangiectasia is notable in the lesions, and there is marked erythema. Dermatographism and urtication on rubbing (Darier's sign) are present along with pruritus. There may be bone lesions caused by collections of mast cells, and these patients have an increased incidence of peptic ulcer.

Diffuse mastocytosis

Diffuse mastocytosis is a rare event in which large portions of the skin is infiltrated with mast cells, giving a doughy, boggy, thickened appearance. The skin is leathery and lichenified as a result of enormous aggregates of small papules, with a generalized erythroderma. Mild trauma produces blistering, and there is generalized intense pruritus.

Systemic mastocytosis

Systemic mastocytosis implies infiltrates of mast cells occurring in organs other than the skin. It is most often associated with urticaria pigmentosa and diffuse mastocytosis, but in rare instances it may occur without cutaneous lesions. Bone, liver, spleen, and the gastrointestinal tract are most commonly involved; the brain and central nervous system are not affected. Bone involvement is uncommon in children but occurs in up to 30% of other patients with systemic mastocytosis; it is seen roentgenographically as osteoporosis and osteosclerosis. Mastocytomas account for approximately 25% of bone lesions; there may be associated bone pain. Mast cell infiltrates of the liver generally do not cause symptoms, but there may be hepatomegaly and fibrosis. Splenomegaly may also be caused by collections of mast cells. Infiltration of mast cells in the small bowel is not usually associated with symptoms but occasionally may result in malabsorption.

The majority of patients with mastocytosis are asymptomatic; about one third have pruritus or flushing. The degranulation of mast cells in large quantities with a release of histamine may result in symptoms of headache, flushing, pruritus, diarrhea, cardiac palpitations, hypotension, and syncope. This can be induced in a number of ways, including vigorous rubbing of skin, hot baths, exercise, ingesting spicy foods or alcohol, and ingesting or injecting certain drugs, including codeine, morphine, aspirin, atropine, and polymyxin B. Heparin release from mast cells may account for the purpuric appearance of some of the skin lesions. Rare instances of mast cell leukemia or lymphoma have been reported.

Mastocytosis occurs in all races, but most cases reported have been in whites; males and females are equally affected. Because some cases have appeared in familial patterns, credence has been given to heritable factors, but most instances of mastocytosis are single events and genetic transmission is therefore unlikely.

Since most cases of mastocytosis regress spontaneously, there is little need for intervention. Solitary mastocytomas may be excised if troublesome. Systemic mastocytosis tends to persist. The management is usually symptomatic, with reliance on antihistaminics, antiserotonin agents, and the avoidance of foods, drugs, and activities that may produce pruritus and flushing.

ORAL MANIFESTATIONS. Mucosal lesions are rare and cannot be definitely diagnosed without a biopsy. If the patient has systemic signs (especially skin lesions), one may assume the diagnosis. The lesion would generally appear pigmented, suggesting a hematoma. The clinician will more commonly see lesions on the face.

In systemic mastocytosis, a facial flush may suggest the systemic involvement. The patient may report histamine headache, which he may confuse as being of dental origin. Bone lesions may occur throughout the skeleton, especially in marrow spaces. Radiographically, lesions appear stippled with areas of sclerotic and lytic changes. There have been reports of generalized osteoporosis and osteosclerosis and pathologic fractures. While involvement of the skull has been mentioned, no specific reports on the jaws have been found and a biopsy is indicated. Histopathology of bone lesions shows rapid bone turnover with a mast cell infiltrate (mostly round cells but some spindle and stellate forms), amorphous material, and a woven bone pattern under polarized light. Eosinophilia has also been reported. Lymph node involvement may confuse the diagnosis and can suggest myelofibrosis, myeloproliferative process, or malignancy.

DENTAL MANAGEMENT. Once a diagnosis is made the major problem may be the hypotension and headaches associated with systemic involvement. Antihistamines may help control the headaches. Caution should be used with drugs that may precipitate histamine release, such as codeine (meperidine appears safe) and aspirin. Events such as marked temperature changes should be monitored. Careful radiographic analysis should reveal possible complications to surgical procedures. Though such complications are unlikely, the surgeon and anesthesiologist must be aware of them. Histamine release, even in patients with asymptomatic cutaneous disease, has been reported to give severe reactions including cardiovascular collapse and death. No evidence of inhalation anesthesia causing histamine release has been found, but halothane may increase the hypotension. Prophylactic antihistamine therapy has been suggested for trauma procedures and surgery.

BIBLIOGRAPHY

Caplan, R.M.: Urticaria pigmentosa and systemic mastocytosis, J.A.M.A. **194:**1077, 1965.
Demis, D.J.: The mastocytosis syndrome: clinical and biochemical studies, Ann. Intern. Med. **59:**194, 1963.
Fine, J.D.: Mastocytosis, Int. J. Dermatol. **19:**117, 1980.
Klaus, S.N., and Winkelman, R.K.: Course of urticaria pigmentosa in children, Arch. Dermatol. **86:**68, 1962.
Mills, E., Dunstan, C.R., and Evans, R.A.: Bone metabolism in systemic mastocytosis, J. Bone Joint Surg. **63A:**665, 1981.
Sagher, F., and Evan-Paz, Z.: Mastocytosis and the mast cell, Chicago, 1967, Year Book Medical Publishers, Inc.
Webb, T.A., and others: Systemic mast cell disease: a clinical and hematopathologic study of 26 cases, Cancer **49:**927, 1982.
Yam, L.T., Yam, C., and Li, C.Y.: Eosinophilia in systemic mastocytosis, Am. J. Clin. Pathol. **73:**48, 1980.

SARCOIDOSIS

Sarcoidosis (Boeck's sarcoid) is a granulomatous (reticular) disorder of unknown cause that involves the skin and the internal organs, including the lungs, mediastinal and peripheral lymph nodes, myocardium, liver, spleen, kidneys, central nervous sytem, eyes, lacrimal and parotid glands, and phalangeal bones.

The disease usually has its onset in early adult life, progressing insidiously and generally following a persistent course marked by remissions and relapses. The common patient in the United States is a 20- to 40-year-old black female. The cutaneous manifestations are diverse; papules, nodules, plaques, and tumors may appear virtually anywhere on the skin surface. The lesions are usually multiple, firm but slightly elastic to the touch, and involve the entire dermis. The overlying epidermis is somewhat thinned, with red to purple or brownish discoloration. Alopecia has been associated with scalp lesions.

In generalized sarcoidosis there may be a number of papules or small nodules on the face, eyelids, neck, and shoulders. They may be lichenified and show central pitting. This is known as miliary sarcoid. Over an extended time these papules may gradually involute to faint macular lesions. They must be differentiated from syringoma, trichoepithelioma, xanthelasma, and lichen planus.

Moderately large plaques, called Hutchinson's plaques, may appear symmetrically on the cheeks, nose, and arms. These plaques are slightly elevated with a flat, nodular, or lobulated surface.

Lupus pernio is manifested by smooth, shiny, violaceous plaques that may appear on the forehead and acral areas, including nose, ears, toes, and fingers. Lupus pernio is often found in connection with granulomas of the bones, which are seen roentgenographically as "punched-out" cysts, especially in the distal phalanges.

Erythema nodosum with fever and polyarthralgia may precede the other skin manifestations. These tender, red nodules are generally seen on the face, extensor surfaces of upper and lower extremities, and upper part of the back of young women. Constitutional symptoms of fever, weight loss, fatigue, and malaise may accompany these findings.

Ocular involvement, mainly as granulomatous uveitis, is found in approximately 25% of patients. There may also be nodular lesions of the iris (keratotic "mutton fat" precipitates) and lesions of the sclera, retina, choroid, and optic nerve. The lacrimal gland may show painless, nodular swelling unilaterally or bilaterally. There may be associated involvement of the submaxillary salivary glands or the parotid glands. Uveitis with fever and enlargement of the parotid gland and lacrimal gland is called uveoparotid fever or Heerfordt's syndrome. This may last from 2 to 6 months.

There may be sharply delineated plaques with psoriasiform scaling on the trunk and extremities. Sarcoid lesions resembling keloids may also develop in old scars of various causes (burns, surgical scars, or trauma). Subcutaneous calcium deposits, prurigo, and erythema multiforme have also been described with sarcoidosis.

Deep-seated nodules 1 to 3 cm in diameter may occur on the trunk and extremities. They are subcutaneous but are attached to the overlying skin, which may be slightly violaceous. This form is known as Darier-Roussy sarcoid. Papules may also form on mucous membranes.

The characteristic histologic finding is a "naked tubercle" consisting of large pale-staining epithelioid cells, with histiocytes, lymphocytes, and Langhan's giant cells but without evidence of caseation. Often nonspecific giant cell inclusions are seen, including conchoid bodies (Schaumann bodies) and asteroid bodies.

Immunologic abnormalities include significant elevations of serum IgA, IgM, and IgG levels. Most patients (85%) with sarcoidosis are negative tuberculin reactors. Delayed hypersensitivity reactions are impaired (anergy). Anergy can be seen with *Trichophyton, Candida,* and mumps antigens. Circulating antibody formation is preserved, and immediate-type reactions are not impaired. There is also a delayed granulomatous response to intracutaneous injection of sarcoidosis tissue extracts; this is the basis of the Kveim test.

Treatment of the systemic disease is with judicious use of steroids. The skin lesions will often respond to topical and intralesional corticosteroid administration. Occasionally systemic steroid therapy may be required for extensive or disfiguring skin lesions.

ORAL MANIFESTATIONS. The common findings a clinician may see in the head and neck area are involvement of salivary glands and lymph nodes. While oral lesions have been reported, few have been proved. In one review only 12 documented mucosal lesions and 16 documented intraoral minor salivary gland lesions were found. Mucosal lesions resemble lesions of other granulomatous processes and often mimic cancer. They are often slightly raised maculopapular lesions, varying in color from pale to reddish, often nontender, occasionally coalescing into a plaque, and possibly ulcerated. They are commonly located on the hard palate, uvula, and faucial pillars.

The salivary gland lesions occur more often in the major glands, as mentioned before. Bilateral involvement can occur. Glandular involvement may lead to various degrees of xerostomia. Mucosal dryness, atrophy, and burning may follow in severe cases of xerostomia. Parotid and lacrimal involvement is part of Heefordt's syndrome.

While bone lesions are not common, they do occur. They are generally cystlike lytic areas with intact periosteum and thinning of medullary trabecular areas. They often appear diffuse without obvious cause and with loss of lamina dura. Clinically, they may cause tooth mobility and delayed or abnormal healing at extraction sites. Resolution may occur after the patient is treated systemically.

DENTAL MANAGEMENT. The major concerns during dental treatment are the effect of steroid therapy and the extent of systemic involvement. Supplemental steroids may be needed during treatment and any alterations in the tissue response must be watched for. Topical steroids may help the patient with rare symptomatic lesions. In severe xerostomia, an artificial saliva solution would be helpful, especially where removable prosthetics are indicated. The clinician should avoid endodontics and extractions if the teeth are asymptomatic and vital despite lytic areas since the cystic areas may be of sarcoid origin. Nonspecific oral lesions should be confirmed by a biopsy.

BIBLIOGRAPHY

Betten, B., and Koppany, H.S.: Sarcoidosis with mandibular involvement of the mandibular condyle, J. Oral Surg. **34:**1026, 1976.

Cohen, C., Krutchoff, D., and Eisenberg, E.: Systemic sarcoidosis: report of two cases with oral lesions, J. Oral Surg. **39:**613, 1981.

Hamner, J.E., and Scofield, H.H.: Cervical lymphadenopathy and parotid gland swelling in sarcoidosis: a study of 31 cases, J. Am. Dent. Assoc. **74:**1224, 1967.

James, D.G., and others: A worldwide review of sarcoidosis, Ann. N.Y. Acad. Sci. **278:**321, 1976.

Mayock, R.L., and others: Manifestations of sarcoidosis: analysis of 145 patients with a review of nine series selected from the literature, Am. J. Med. **35:**67, 1963.

Orlian, A.I., and Birnbaum, M.: Intra-oral localized sarcoid lesion, Oral Surg. **49:**341, 1980.

Scadding, J.G.: Sarcoidosis, London, 1967, Eyre & Spottiswoode, pp. 174-194.

Scadding, J.G.: The definition of sarcoidosis, Postgrad. Med. J. **46:**465, 1970.

Siltzbach, L.E.: Sarcoidosis: clinical features and management, Med. Clin. North Am. **51:**483, 1967.

Thomas, R.G., and Merkow, L.: Sarcoidosis with involvement of the mandibular condyle, J. Oral Surg. **34:**1026, 1976.

Tillman, H.H., and others: Sarcoidosis of the tongue: report of a case, Oral Surg. **21:**190, 1966.

ANGIOKERATOMA CORPORIS DIFFUSUM (FABRY'S DISEASE)

Angiokeratoma corporis diffusum (Fabry's disease) is manifested by minute black to bluish black vascular papules varying from pinpoint size to 3 or 4 mm and sometimes surmounted by a fine keratotic scale. They are generally concentrated between the umbilicus and the knees, usually in clusters of various size papules. The angiokeratomas appear in the thousands and tend to aggregate in the lumbosacral region, on the buttocks, scrotum, and penis. Groups of lesions may also be found in the mouth, on the lower extremities, and the elbows, and around the nails. Involvement of the gastrointestinal, respiratory, and genitourinary tracts has also been noted. The face, scalp, and ears are spared.

Fabry's disease is a hereditary sex-linked systemic glycolipid storage disorder caused by deficiency of the enzyme ceramidetrihexosidase. The neutral glycolipid ceramidetrihexoside is stored abnormally in many cells, including neurons; smooth, striated, and cardiac muscle fibers, renal tubules and glomeruli, histiocytes, and vascular endothelial cells.

The disease is familial, and the complete clinical picture occurs only in males. Characteristic lesions begin to develop in late childhood or early adolescence. Other clinical features include pain in the fingers, toes, or an entire extremity that may be precipitated by heat, cold, or exertion; diminished sweating with heat intolerance; cataracts and corneal opacities; tortuous retinal and conjunctival vessels with sausage-link constrictions and dilations; diarrhea and proctocolitis; fever; signs of central nervous system involvement that are sometimes transient, such as tremor, paresis, paresthesias, unconsciousness, and aphasia; occasionally arthritis of the distal interphalangeal joints; and edema of the ankles. Death generally results from renal insufficiency with uremia; other causes are hypertension, cerebrovascular accidents, and cardiac disease with congestive heart failure. Death usually occurs in the patient's thirties or forties. Heterozygous females, as carriers of the disease trait, show only mild or no features of the disease; they sometimes have skin lesions or cataracts and usually have a normal life span.

Laboratory findings include albuminuria. The urinary sediment reveals large "mulberry cells" containing doubly refractile glycolipid granules. Polaroscopy reveals the characteristic birefringent "Maltese cross" material. These findings may also be noted in the bone marrow.

No specific treatment is known. The therapy is usually supportive, aimed at relieving pain and treating associated renal, cardiac, and cerebrovascular problems.

ORAL MANIFESTATIONS. Lesions may occur on the lips, buccal mucosa, and soft palate. They appear as punctate lesions or linear and reticular telangiectasia that are bluish red in color. No oral mucosal involvement has been reported in the female carrier. Individual angiokeratomas unrelated to Fabry's disease have been reported, one being a large spontaneously regressing angiokeratoma of the palate.

DENTAL MANAGEMENT. While the vascular lesions may resemble the telangiectasias seen in hereditary hemorrhagic telangiectasia, they present no major problem if caution is taken to avoid hemorrhage. Treatment is similar to that of hemangiomas with sclerosing solutions and cautery. Hypertension is common as are vascular effects in the kidney and heart leading to uremia and possible heart disease. Central nervous system involvement may cause tremors and paresthesia.

BIBLIOGRAPHY

Arm, R.N., and others: A recurrent intraoral vascular lesion: abstract presentation, Am. Assoc, Oral Pathol. April, 1975.
Bergsma, D.: Birth defects, atlas and compendium, Baltimore, 1973, The Williams & Wilkins Co., p. 400.
Danehower, C.C., and Moyer, D.G.: Angiokeratoma corporis diffusum, Arch. Dermatol. **94**:628, 1966.
DeGroot, W.P.: Angiokeratoma corporis diffusum Fabry, Dermatologica **128**:321, 1964.
Gorlin, R.J., and Goldman, H.M.: Thoma's oral pathology, St. Louis, 1970, The C. V. Mosby Co., p. 694.
Gorlin, R.J., and Sedano, H.O.: Stomatologic aspects of cutaneous diseases: angiokeratoma corporis diffusum (Fabry's syndrome), J. Dermatol. Surg. Oncol. **5**:180, 1979.
Hayen, D.O.: Thrombosed angiokeratoma simulating malignant melanoma, Arch. Dermatol. **93**:358, 1966.
Orpitz, J.M., and others: The genetics of angiokeratoma corporis diffusum (Fabry's disease) and its linkage relations with the X_z Lucus, Am. J. Human Genet. **17**:335, 1965.
Von Gemmingen, G., Kierland, R.R., and Opitz, J.M.: Angiokeratoma corporis diffusum (Fabry's disease), Arch. Dermatol. **91**:206, 1965.
Wise, D., Wallace, H.J., and Jellinek, E.H.: Angiokeratoma corporis diffusum: a clinical study of 8 affected families, Q. J. Med. **31**:177, 1962.

164 • CUTANEOUS SIGNS OF INTERNAL MALIGNANCY

Bernard A. Kirshbaum, Anthony V. Benedetto, and **Karen Lipinski**

Numerous signs occur in the skin that can alert the practitioner to the possibility of internal malignancy. These range from direct cutaneous metastases to remote effects of the tumor or paraneoplastic syndromes. The more common signs are discussed here.

Cutaneous metastases occur with several internal malignancies; lung, gastrointestinal, breast, and ovarian carcinomas and melanoma are the most frequent. The metastatic lesions may be nodular, papular, or plaquelike; they may be single or multiple. Usually they are identified by performing a biopsy when the diagnosis of the skin condition is in question. They may overlie the tumor or be distant. Breast cancer is the most common underlying malignancy, followed by cancer of the stomach, lung, uterus, and kidney.

Acquired ichthyosis is associated with lymphomas and Hodgkin's disease. It can appear as generalized dryness or may resemble the "fish scales" of the inherited ichthyosis vulgaris. It is surmised that liver damage with subsequent impairment of vitamin A metabolism may cause the ichthyosis.

Intense, generalized, recalcitrant pruritus is a well-recognized symptom of Hodgkin's disease. Severe pruritus may indicate a poor prognosis. Intractable itching of the nose has been reported in patients with brain tumors.

Acquired hypertrichosis lanuginosa is linked to internal malignancy such as carcinoma of the bronchus, gallbladder, colon, rectum, uterus, or urinary bladder. It is marked by the sudden appearance of fine, silky, lanugo-like hair on the face and eventually the whole body. The development of the hair may precede the malignancy by several years.

The Leser-Trélat sign is the sudden development of numerous seborrheic keratoses with pruritus. This sign, which occurs with gastrointestinal malignancies, is very rare and requires careful interpretation, since multiple seborrheic keratoses commonly develop in the absence of cancer.

Erythema gyratum repens may resemble a wood grain

or knotty pine. It is associated with carcinoma of the breast and oat cell tumors of the lung. Festooned lesions appear on the trunk and extremities.

Migratory thrombophlebitis is linked to carcinoma of the pancreas and other types of malignancies.

Torre's syndrome (sebaceous adenomas) should suggest an underlying gastrointestinal malignancy, usually of the colon. The lesions are usually multiple, occurring on the trunk as smooth, elevated, pedunculated tumors. These patients have quite a good prognosis, considering that many of them have multiple primary cancers. These cancers are usually of low malignancy and often respond well to radiotherapy. Whenever a sebaceous adenoma is removed, a more complete history and a further search are needed to rule out visceral disease.

The so-called malignant form of acanthosis nigricans is always associated with an underlying malignancy. Adenocarcinomas of the stomach, gastrointestinal tract, lung, ovary, breast, and prostate have been found. It has also been seen in patients with lymphoma and Hodgkin's disease. The lesions occurring in the malignant form are severe and widespread. Palmar thickening may be noted. Mucosal involvement occurs in more than 50% of cases. Lesions may precede the overt malignancy by several years. Treatment of the underlying cause leads to resolution of the acanthosis nigricans.

Subcutaneous nodular fat necrosis occurs in 2% to 3% of patients with pancreatitis and pancreatic carcinoma. Subcutaneous nodules develop in the pretibial regions and rarely on the scalp, arms, and face. The nodules may be asymptomatic. Liquefaction degeneration may occur with resultant discharge of an oily liquid. Synovitis of the small joints, causing polyarthritis, has been reported. The syndrome is probably caused by the release of pancreatic lipases that reach the fat via lymphatics.

In the glucagonoma syndrome, necrolytic migratory erythema is associated with a pancreatic α-islet cell tumor that secretes glucagon. The skin manifestations consist of gyrate and circinate erythemas that involve the trunk, groin, perineum, and limbs and undergo necrosis with scarring. Perioral erythema and crusting and a red tongue are also present. New lesions develop as old lesions heal. Weight loss, diabetes, refractory anemia, diarrhea, and venous thrombosis are other features of the syndrome. Most patients are postmenopausal women. The condition responds to removal of the tumor. It is important to recognize this disease, since the tumor is potentially curable.

BIBLIOGRAPHY

Andree, V.C., and Petkov, I.: Skin manifestations associated with tumors of the brain, Br. J. Dermatol. **92:**675, 1975.
Binnick, A., and others: Glucagonoma syndrome, Arch. Dermatol. **113:**749, 1977.
Brownstein, M.H., and Helwig, E.B.: Metastatic tumors of the skin, Cancer **29:**1298, 1972.
Brownstein, M.H., and Helwig, E.B.: Patterns of cutaneous metastases, Arch. Dermatol. **105:**862, 1972.
Curth, H.O., and others: The site and histology of the cancers associated with malignant acanthosis nigricans, Cancer **15:**364, 1962.
Feiner, A.S., and others: Prognostic importance of pruritus in Hodgkin's disease, J.A.M.A. **240:**2738, 1978.
Holt, P., and Davis, M.: Erythema gyratum repens, Br. J. Dermatol. **96:**343, 1977.
Leonard, D.D., and Deaton, W.R.: Multiple sebaceous gland tumors and visceral carcinomas, Arch. Dermatol. **110:**917, 1974.
Liddel, K., and others: Seborrheic keratoses and carcinoma of the large bowel, Br. J. Dermatol. **92:**449, 1975.
Mallinson, C.N., and others: A glucagonoma syndrome, Lancet **2:**1, 1974.
Rosenberg, F.W.: Cutaneous manifestations of internal malignancy, Cutis **20:**227, 1977.
Roulon, D.B., and Helwig, E.B.: Multiple sebaceous neoplasms of the skin, Am. J. Clin. Pathol. **60:**745, 1973.
Sibrack, L.A., and Gouterman, I.H.: Cutaneous manifestations of pancreatic disease, Cutis **21:**703, 1978.
Swanson, K., and others: The glucagonoma syndrome, Arch. Dermatol. **114:**224, 1978.

165 • NEOPLASMS OF THE SKIN

Robert N. Arm, Bernard A. Kirshbaum, Anthony V. Benedetto, and **Karen Lipinski**

Cutaneous neoplasia can be categorized as benign, premalignant, and malignant.

SEBORRHEIC KERATOSIS

Of the many benign cutaneous tumors, seborrheic keratosis is the most commonly encountered. Devoid of any tendency for malignant degeneration, seborrheic keratosis usually occurs as a hyperpigmented, firm but soft, sessile tumor. It may feel waxy, manifesting numerous furrows and keratin-filled, follicle-like openings scattered over its surface, which contributes to its overall verrucous character (Fig. 165-1). It can also appear to be "stuck onto" the surface of the skin, demonstrating distinct margins and occasionally yielding to the slightest amount of picking or lifting, resulting in moderate bleeding and delayed regrowth.

Seborrheic keratosis is more commonly found in older persons, with equal distribution in males and females. There is little tendency for these tumors to disappear spontaneously. Dermatosis papulosa nigra, a variant of seborrheic keratosis, usually appears as multiple lesions over the face and neck in dark-skinned individuals, generally at a younger age than with seborrheic keratosis. The sign of Leser-Trélat occurs when a profuse number of seborrheic keratoses appear rapidly over a matter of months, heralding the presence of possible occult malignancy, most often in the gastrointestinal tract. Seborrheic keratosis is treated with superficial surgical procedures such as cryosurgery, curettage, and chemical cautery or electrocautery. Unnecessary deep surgery should be avoided to ensure the best cosmetic results.

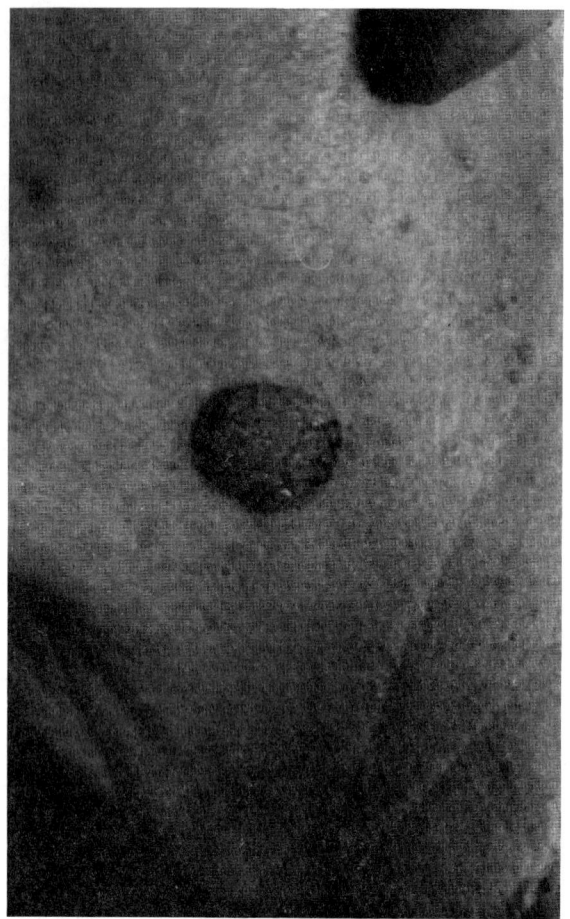

Fig. 165-1. Seborrheic keratosis of neck. Lesion is elevated and nodular with waxy crenated surface.

PREMALIGNANT LESIONS—ACTINIC KERATOSIS AND BOWEN'S DISEASE

Of the premalignant lesions common to the skin, actinic keratoses (solar keratoses) and Bowen's disease are encountered most frequently. Given a sufficient amount of time and the necessary host response, many of these lesions undergo malignant transformation into invasive epidermoid (squamous cell) carcinoma. Actinic keratoses (formerly designated as senile keratoses) are adherent, hyperkeratotic lesions found on exposed, sun-damaged skin, usually on an erythematous base. They are most often seen in multiple numbers in light-skinned individuals who have obvious weather-beaten (solar elastotic) skin. This lesion has a fine, white scale on the surface that is easily detached from the less well-defined erythematous base, producing punctate areas of bleeding. Histologically, the actinic keratosis presents numerous dyskeratotic cells with many mitoses in the epidermis. The presence of actinic keratoses is predicated on how much radiation and physicochemical damage an individual's skin has sustained and the relative susceptibility of the tissues. This includes ultraviolet light exposure as well as exposure to ionizing radiation, radiant heat, and pitch and other coal and petroleum distillate by-products.

Because of their tendency to transform into malignant lesions, actinic keratoses should be treated. If there is no invasion into the dermis, treatment is by superficial destruction. This can be accomplished by cryosurgery, curettage, and chemical cautery or electrocautery. Topical application of 5-fluorouracil has proved to be useful in treating multiple lesions over a large surface area. Prophylaxis can be accomplished by avoidance of the destructive causative radiation, especially excessive and persistent sunbathing, and by the routine use of tropical sunscreening agents.

Bowen's disease is intraepidermal squamous cell carcinoma in situ. It can occur as a single lesion or as multiple lesions. The possibility of prolonged exposure to arsenicals should be suspected when numerous lesions of Bowen's disease are found, especially if they involve the palms and soles. The lesions occur in skin areas not exposed to the sun, including the genitalia and perineum. They are somewhat more well defined, more hyperkeratotic, and often larger than actinic keratoses but much less common. After the keratotic roof is removed, the base of the lesion is usually redder and thicker than in actinic keratosis, appearing plaquelike or verrucous.

When similar changes are found on the male genitalia, especially the glans, they are usually referred to as erythroplasia of Queyrat. These generally appear as a circumscribed, erythematous, velvety, often moist and shiny patch. A tissue biopsy is the only sure way to differentiate Bowen's disease from other papulosquamous lesions, Paget's disease, and invasive carcinoma, especially when the genitalia are involved.

At one time it was thought that systemic malignancies were more common in patients who manifested multiple lesions of Bowen's disease, but this concept has largely been abandoned.

The treatment is surgical; however, a high rate of recurrence can be attributed to the frequent involvement of the epithelium of the follicular apparatus, through which the intraepithelial dysplastic changes are carried deep into the dermis instead of remaining relatively superficial. Therefore deep wedge excisions are recommended rather than cryosurgery and topical chemotherapeutic agents when the lesions are large and especially where hair is present.

MALIGNANT NEOPLASMS

Basal cell and squamous cell carcinomas and malignant melanomas constitute the majority of the malignant neoplasms of the skin. Basal cell carcinoma is the most commonly occurring cutaneous carcinoma, account for 85% of skin malignancies; it rarely metastasizes. Squamous cell carcinomas comprise approximately 10% of all skin malignancies and occasionally become aggressive and metastasize. Malignant melanoma, representing 4% to 5% of skin malignancies, is the most lethal and devastating of all skin tumors.

Squamous cell carcinoma

Squamous cell carcinoma (epidermoid carcinoma) is characterized by invasive keratinizing epithelial anaplasia with a potential for metastasis. Long-term ultraviolet light (sun) exposure, ionizing radiation (repeated small doses of roentgen rays), chemical carcinogens (arsenicals and coal distillate by-products), chronic trauma, and ulcerations (old burns and long-standing granulomatous lesions, as with tuberculosis, lupus erythematosus, and osteomyelitis) are the main causes for squamous cell carcinoma. These are associated with a more favorable prognosis, since all de novo squamous cell carcinomas and those of mucous membranes have a more aggressive behavior that more frequently results in treatment failures and metastasis. Dark-skinned individuals show less tendency for formation of these skin cancers than do lightly pigmented individuals.

Clinically, lesions of squamous cell carcinoma, whether early or late, are diverse in appearance, occurring initially as a nonhealing papular or verrucous lesion. Eventually, as the tumor enlarges in depth and breadth, it becomes fixed to underlying structures and the center usually becomes ulcerated.

Histologically, the more undifferentiated a tumor appears, the more malignant it is, and the higher the grade of malignancy, the less tendency for keratinization and usually the deeper the tumor extends within the dermis.

The therapy includes any of the various techniques of radiation, excision, and electrothermic destruction, provided the tumor is extirpated in its entirety. An adaption of standard excisional surgery is the Mohs technique (called chemosurgery), which entails complete histologic examination of all the excised tissue. This establishes beyond doubt whether the surgical excision was complete. This method is now preferred for more difficult tumors. Topical chemotherapeutic agents have no place in the treatment of invasive squamous cell carcinoma.

Basal cell carcinoma

Basal cell carcinoma is the least malignant but the most common of all the skin cancers. A basal cell carcinoma is an epithelial cutaneous tumor arising from the basal layer of cells of the epidermis and its appendages; it is composed of cells resembling the immature cells of these structures.

Basal cell carcinoma is found in younger adults as well as the elderly, usually in tissue damaged by ultraviolet and ionizing radiation; hence it is less common in darkly pigmented individuals. Increased exposure to chemical carcinogens probably also contributes to the pathogenesis. Clinically, the basal cell carcinoma takes on a characteristic appearance. Initially a small, smooth-surfaced papule appears over an area that might show evidence of actinic damage (Fig. 165-2). Eventually the papule becomes fria-

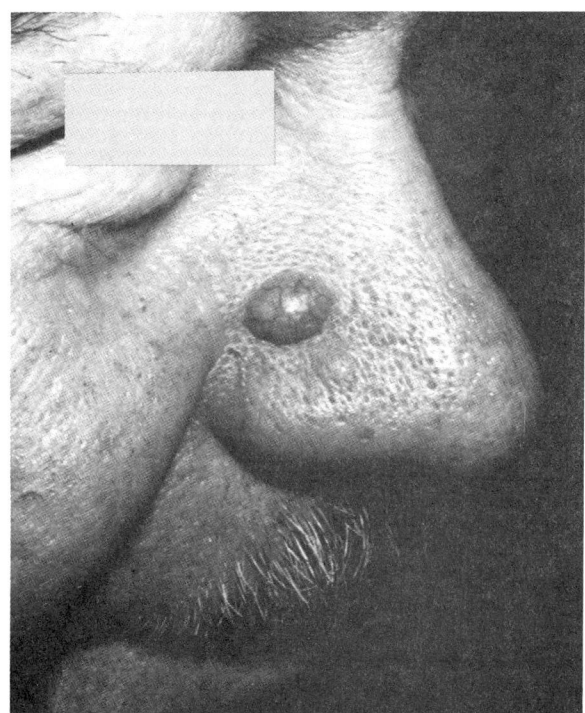

Fig. 165-2. Early basal cell carcinoma. Papulonodular lesion with pearly surface and telangiectasia. (Courtesy of Department of Dermatology, The Cleveland Clinics.)

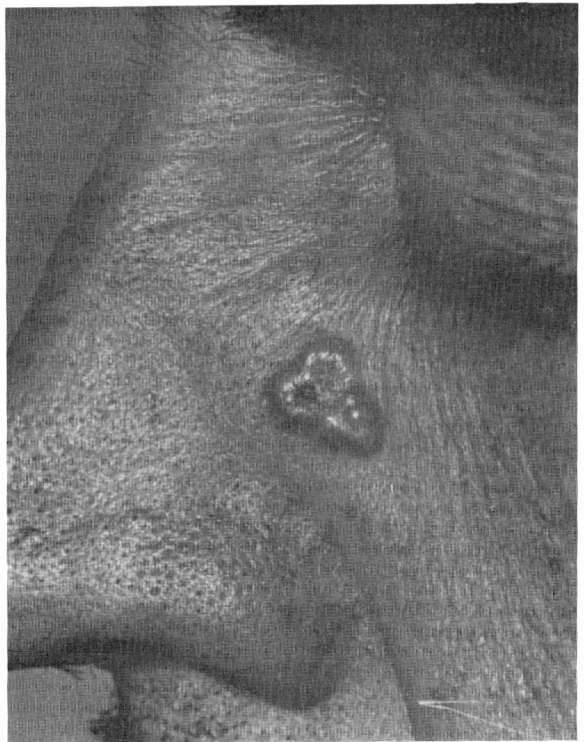

Fig. 165-3. More advanced basal cell carcinoma than in Fig. 165-2 with rolled pearly borders, depressed center, and early ulceration. (Courtesy of Department of Dermatology, The Cleveland Clinics.)

ble and bleeds with slight trauma. The tumor slowly enlarges with a depressed, slightly sclerotic center that subsequently may ulcerate. At this point the edges of the tumor thicken, giving the appearance of being rolled upon themselves (Fig. 165-3). Tumors can also be pigmented, making differentiation from melanoma sometimes difficult.

A basal cell carcinoma can show variations in its clinical presentation. Some of the more troublesome types of basal cell carcinoma, which may be recurrent and sometimes relatively resistant to therapy, include the following. (1) The superficial basal cell carcinoma resembles a papulosquamous lesion (psoriasis) but occurs in multifocal islands, some of which are clinically inapparent. (2) The morpheiform (sclerotic) basal cell carcinoma simulates a superficial cicatrix whose borders may not be distinct. Histologically, small groups of tumor cells are trapped in a fibrous tissue stroma. (3) The metatypical or basosquamous cell carcinoma is characteristically ulcerated, conforming to the old description of the "rodent ulcer" (Fig. 165-4). In this type elements of squamous cell carcinoma are seen interspersed among tumor islands of basal cell carcinoma, and occasionally the biologic behavior is that of an aggressive squamous cell carcinoma rather than that of a basal cell carcinoma.

The treatment is either surgical or with roentgen radiation. Mohs chemosurgery is perferred for the more aggressive types of basal cell carcinoma or those resistant to other forms of therapy. Cryosurgery has been used in the treatment of basal cell carcinoma; however, many believe that it is just a temporary palliative procedure, since it sometimes does not fully obliterate the tumor. For total extirpation, considerable freezing of the deep tissues is necessary. Prophylaxis might be accomplished by consistently using sunscreens and by avoiding any form of direct radiation to the skin.

Patients with the basal cell nervus syndrome (formerly nevoid basal cell carcinoma) present a host of ectodermal defects, as well as myriad basal cell carcinomas over the entire body, which can start to appear as early as the first decade of life (see discussion of "Basal cell nevus syndrome" in Chapter 156).

Malignant melanoma

Malignant melanoma is a potentially grave, aggressive, and metastasizing tumor that originates from anaplastic melanocytes. It is currently thought that there are precursor and premalignant pigmented lesions as well as four types of malignant melanomas.

In the past decade there has been an increased incidence of melanoma in the United States. It is believed that contributing factors are more leisure time spent out in the sun and the increased population in the South and Southwest. In most large study series the sex ratio of occurrence approximates 1:1. The occurrence of melanomas in whites is six to seven times greater than in blacks in the same geographic localities, and the incidence ranges from 4 to 8:100,000 population annually.

Whites may have melanomas anywhere on the body, with the sun-exposed areas affected most frequently, whereas blacks and Orientals tend to have melanomas of the palms, soles, nail beds, and mucous membranes.

Clinically and histopathologically, there are now four identifiable types of melanoma: lentigo maligna melanoma, superficial spreading melanoma, nodular melanoma, and acrolentiginous melanoma.

Lentigo maligna is considered the precursor of lentigo maligna melanoma. It is a pigmented macule usually found on exposed areas (especially the face) in the elderly. Variations in color, size and shape occur with time. When the atypical melanocytic cells become invasive, penetrate the epidermal basement membrane, and enter the dermis, the lesion becomes a lentigo maligna melanoma. It is postulated that one third of all lentigo maligna lesions give rise to melanomas.

The treatment of choice for lentigo maligna is simple excision. Care must be taken with large lesions, since frequently atypical melanocytes can be found deep within the dermis along the basal layer of the external root sheath of hair follicles. For this reason the more precise, microscopically controlled excision of the Mohs chemosurgical technique is preferred. Curettage and electrodesiccation can be counterproductive. Since superficial roentgen ray therapy

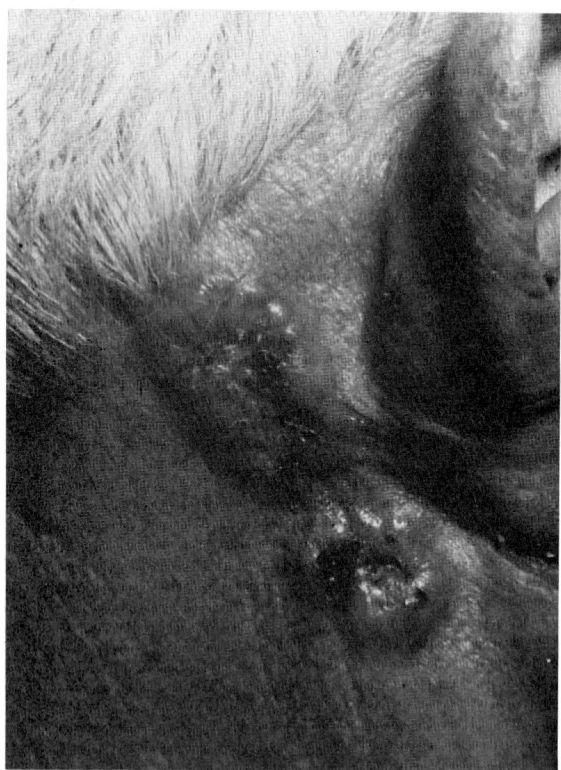

Fig. 165-4. Basal cell carcinoma at slightly more advanced stage than in Fig. 165-3 (rodent ulcer). (Courtesy of Department of Dermatology, The Cleveland Clinics.)

has resulted in recurrences of lentigo maligna and in some cases the development of lentigo maligna melanoma, this form of therapy is not recommended.

Other precursor lesions to melanomas are the congenital nevi and the atypical nevi found in members of families who have familial melanomas. There are two types of congenital nevi: the giant hairy nevus and the smaller congenital melanocytic nevus. Since both tend to transform into a melanoma usually before puberty, extirpation of any congenital melanocytic nevus, however large, is recommended. In families whose members have malignant melanoma, an irregularly shaped and pigmented acquired nevus has been observed. These nevi may have hues of pink to red or blue to gray and are known to transform into melanoma. They have been observed in family members without melanoma and in unrelated normal individuals.

The most common type of melanoma is the superficial spreading melanoma, which constitutes 70% of all melanomas. It usually occurs as a slightly elevated, irregularly shaped, arciform notched lesion with variations in color (brown, blue, black, pink, and gray) (Fig. 165-5). It is thought to undergo a lateral phase for 1 to 7 years before nodular formation and vertical growth.

About 15% of all melanomas appear as nodular, or polypoidal, melanoma. This probably arises as an invasive nodule de novo without any lateral growth phase; histologically, the epidermis is the last layer to be involved in such melanomas. Nodular melanomas are blueberry shaped with variation in color ranging from black to gray (Fig. 165-6). They are the quickest to grow and metastasize.

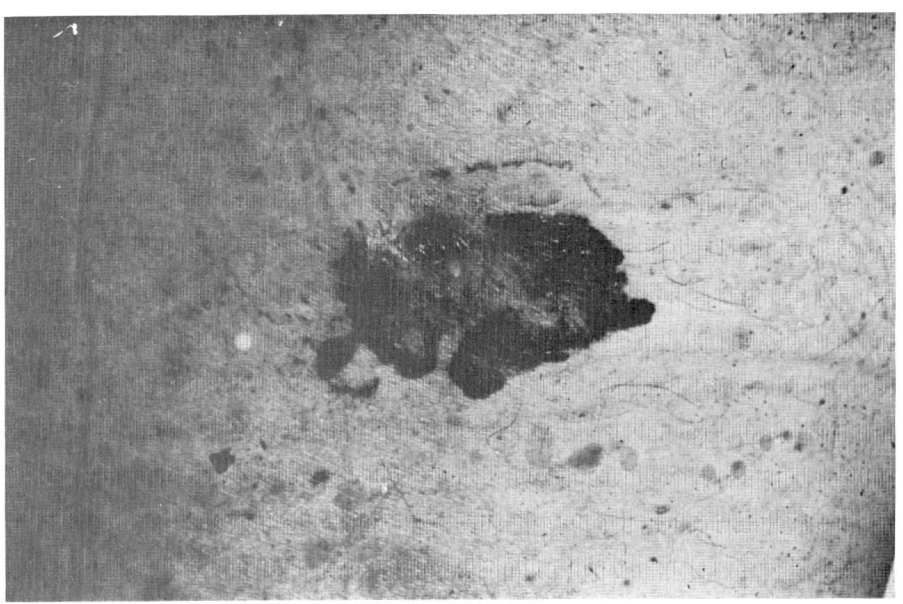

Fig. 165-5. Malignant melanoma, superficial spreading type, with mottled blue-black pigmentation.

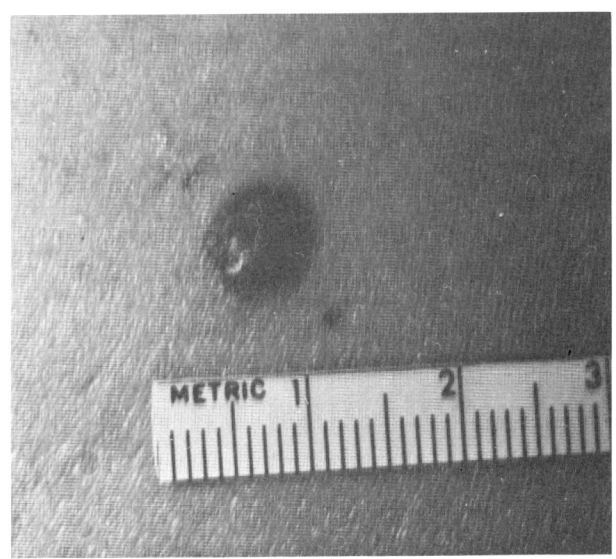

Fig. 165-6. Nodular malignant melanoma. This was an intensely blue-black lesion.

A fourth type of melanoma recently identified in the acrolentiginous, or palmar-plantar subungual-mucosal, melanoma. This type is similar in appearance to a lentigo maligna melanoma (a macule with variegate pigmentation), but it is much more aggressive. It is found most commonly on the hands, feet, oral mucous membranes, and genitalia of blacks and Orientals and rarely in whites.

Two relatively recent developments have helped to classify the biologic behavior, and thus the prognosis, of the various types of melanoma. The prognosis can be estimated from the depth of invasion of the tumor cells within the skin. This classification if referred to as Clark's levels of invasion, and no diagnosis of melanoma should be made without it. Level I indicates that tumor cells still lie within the epidermis; in level II tumor cells are within the papillary dermis but not filling it; in level III the papillary dermis is filled; in level IV tumor cells enter the reticular dermis; and in level V the tumor has penetrated the subcutaneous fat. In the second (Breslow) classification, the thickness of a primary lesion from the granular layer of the epidermis down to the deepest tumor cell in the skin is measured with a calibrated ocular micrometer mounted in the eyepiece of a microscope. Lesions less than 0.75 mm deep are associated with a 5-year survival rate of 100%; those of 1.5 mm in depth have a 75% to 80% survival rate in 5 years; but those deeper than 3 mm have a guarded prognosis.

The controversy of prophylactic lymph node dissection rages on. The overall 5-year survival for disease involving the regional nodes is approximately 30%. It has been found that lesions on the trunk, as opposed to those on acral areas, have a worse prognosis, probably because on the extremities there is a more definite pattern of lymphatic drainage and involved nodes are more accessible. Whether removal of lymph nodes containing microscopic foci of tumor ultimately improves survival is debatable. Of nonpalpable regional nodes, 15% to 20% show tumor involvement. Surgical excision is the treatment of choice. Malignant melanoma has a relatively high spontaneous regression rate (15% total and 13% partial). Moreover, following removal of the primary tumor, there can be a delay in invasion and metastasis of up to 35 years.

Level I lesions require only wide local excision. For level II lesions less than 0.75 mm thick, the Melanoma Clinical Cooperative Group recommends a wide local excision with a 3- to 5-cm border and primary closure using a split thickness skin graft. For lesions of levels III, IV, V, and thicker than 1.5 mm, a wide local excision with graft is followed by lymph node dissection, whether the nodes are palpable or not. For isolated local recurrence, wide local excision is also recommended. Mohs, who developed chemosurgery, advocates using zinc chloride paste fixation along with his microscopically controlled excisions. In his series the 10-year cure rate was at least 30% better in all levels of tumor invasion; however, the concept of measuring tumor thickness with a micrometer was unknown at the time of his study.

Adjuvant chemotherapy is usually reserved for metastatic melanoma. Single-drug therapy has been shown to be as effective as combination chemotherapy. Current drugs of choice are dimethyltriazenoimidazolecarboxamide (DTIC) and the nitrosoureas (CCNU and methyl CCNU). Chemotherapy along with immunotherapy with intralesional injection of bacille Calmette Guérin (BCG) or vaccinia is currently under investigation.

Neoplasms of the mouth

Pigmentation may be seen as normal racial pigmentation or secondary to tumors, syndromes (like Peutz-Jeghers), endocrine problems (such as Addison's disease), drugs (like antimalarials), systemic disease (such as jaundice), foreign bodies (such as amalgam tattoo), and organisms (for example, black hairy tongue).

Benign lesions. The clinician should recognize facial lesions but difficulty arises in ruling out basal cell carcinomas. Thus referral and biopsy are often needed. Seborrheic keratosis and actinic keratosis occur on the face, generally in older people. Actinic keratosis is common on the lips and is usually seen in conjunction with a ruddy "weatherbeaten" complexion resulting from ultraviolet exposure of the sun. The lips appear dry, scaly white, and hyperkeratotic with surrounding erythema. Because of possible malignant transformation, surgical treatment is indicated. This usually consists of a superficial lip "shave." A sun screen (such as zinc oxide or PABA) may prevent further irritation. Careful follow-up is needed.

Nevi inside the oral cavity are not as common as epidermal nevi. Some estimate about 15 skin nevi per white patient, making surgery impossible. This is not the case orally. Rarity can, in part, be explained by a lack of diagnosis. The lesions are generally small, asymptomatic, and easily confused with amalgam tattoos. Oral nevi have been reported in patients from age 10 to 80, though mostly in persons in their third and fourth decades. Unlike skin nevi, where male occurrences equal female, oral nevi are more frequently found in females. Approximately two fifths are found on the hard palate. Less frequently nevi are also seen on the labial mucosa, gingiva, vermilion border of lips, and buccal mucosa. The lesions are small, generally between 0.1 and 3.0 cm, slightly raised, and sessile. About 80% are pigmented, ranging in color from blue, gray, brown, or black. They appear well circumscribed and superficial, often looking like normal racial pigmentation. All nevi types have been reported, but their ratios of occurrence are unlike the skin. Over half are intradermal and over one third are blue nevi. Together, compound and junction nevi account for less than 10%. While the other nevi occur about equally on the hard palate and buccal mucosa (25% each), the blue nevus occurs mostly on the hard palate (60%) and labial mucosa (20%). The blue nevus is generally a light to deep blue color.

It is not clear whether a benign nevi can transform into a malignant one. There is a high ratio of melanoma to nevi in the mouth, and often it may be impossible to distinguish a nevus from melanoma in early stages. Removal of pigmented lesions is suggested even if they are asymptomatic.

A related entity appearing in the oral cavity is the melanotic macule (ephelis, melanosis, lentigo). These generally occur in the sixth decade, though they range from 4 to 82 years old. They are twice as frequent in females. They are generally singular, 0.1 to 2 cm, brownish, blue, black, or gray macules. Commonly, they are well-circumscribed lesions located on the vermilion border of the lower lip (30%), gingiva (23%), and buccal mucosa (16%). Up to 20% are nonpigmented but have the same histology as the pigmented macules.

Amalgam tattoos often look the same as the melanotic macules and nevi and are often confused with them. Radiographically, amalgam fragments are sometimes seen. Because of diagnostic problems pathologists recommend removal of pigmented lesions if no diagnosis is known.

Premalignant lesions. Oral dysplasias occur but often resemble malignancy and need biopsies for definitive diagnosis. Multiple entities have been reported to be "premalignant" but proof is mostly speculative. Generally accepted as premalignant are syphilitic glossitis, radiation changes, and field changes. The most common is syphilitic glossitis, where reports of 20% to 50% malignant transformations have been reported. The "field" change is in the diagnosed cancer patient who often develops a second primary site. Radiation therapy, immunosuppressive drugs, and other agents (tobacco, especially chewing tobacco, snuff, alcohol, etc.) can lead to an increased likelihood of malignant change. Debatable premalignant relations are spoken in conjunction with nicotine stomatitis, epulis fissuratum, and lichen planus. Careful examination should be given at routine dental check-ups.

Malignant lesions. Basal cell carcinomas are rare in the mouth; squamous cell carcinomas are the most common malignancy. Since some believe basal cell carcinomas to be associated with epidermal adnexal structures, they say such carcinomas cannot occur in the mouth. Histologically proven lesions have been reported on the gingiva. In the oral cavity, basal cell nevi have been reported on the lower lip, palate, and gingiva (generally anterior labial). They are slightly raised, grayish or white, with a pebbly surface and hyperemic surrounding. Circumferential induration has been reported. Most patients are over 60 years old and are asymptomatic. Most have had a history of cutaneous basal cell carcinoma. Treatment involves total wide excision.

Squamous cell carcinoma is the most common oral malignancy and generally occurs on the posterior lateral borders of the tongue and the floor of the mouth. It can, however, occur anywhere. Carcinomas have multiple appearances, generally white or red and speckled, and are often indurated and ulcerated. A suspicious, nonhealing, undiagnosed lesion should be biopsied. Treatment will include surgery and/or radiation, possibly in combination with chemotherapy.

Malignant melanomas of the mouth represent less than 1% to 2% of all melanomas. Most are pigmented and may have bleeding but no pain. The prognosis is very poor since most lesions are already metastasizing by the time of diagnosis. The cure rate of oral melanomas is less than that of cutaneous lesions. Oral melanomas have been reported more frequently in males (2:1), unlike the oral nevi, which are more common in females. Reports of metastasis from skin lesions have also appeared. Treatment varies with the staging.

DENTAL MANAGEMENT. All treatment modalities of the malignancy can present difficulties during operative dentistry, making consultation and collaboration a must. Radiation probably presents the most serious problems. All patients should have a thorough dental evaluation before radiation. Radiation may cause xerostomia, radiation caries (severe cervical caries), and slow or no healing. After radiation, extractions can and generally do lead to osteoradionecrosis with possible sloughing of parts of the jaws, especially the mandible because of its decreased vascularity. All teeth in poor or debatable condition or in a poorly motivated patient should be extracted before radiation. Those teeth saved must be treated with daily fluorides. Fluoride gel in a tray is best and easiest. An artificial saliva solution may aid the xerostomia. A topical anesthetic, such as 0.5% aqueous diphenhydramine (benadryl) or 2% viscous lidocaine, will help relieve radiation stomatitis—an erythematous "burn" of the mucosa. Frequent dental visits with close scrutiny of oral hygiene is a must.

The patient undergoing chemotherapy may present a problem due to alterations in bone marrow, the painful oral ulcerations, or secondary infections. The dentist can help avoid problems by limiting oral infection prior to chemotherapy, removing sharp cusps, and maintaining oral hygiene. This will help decrease the incidence of ulcers and help avoid systemic infections.

BIBLIOGRAPHY
Seborrheic keratoses

Domonkos, A.N.: Andrew's diseases of the skin: clinical dermatology, Philadelphia, 1971, W.B. Saunders Co.

Sanderson, K.V.: The structure of seborrheic keratoses, Br. J. Dermatol. **80:**588, 1968.

Bowen's disease

Gorlin, R.J.: Bowen's disease of the mucous membrane of the mouth: a review of the literature and a presentation of six cases, Oral Surg. **3:**35, 1959.

Graham, J.H., Bendl, B.J., and Johnson, W.C.: Solar keratosis with squamous cell carcinoma: a new biologic concept, Am. J. Pathol. **55:**26a, 1969.

Graham, J.H., and Helwig, E.B.: Pre-malignant cutaneous and mucocutaneous diseases. In Graham, J.H., Johnson, W.C., and Helwig,

E.B. editors: Dermal pathology, New York, 1972, Harper & Row Publishers, pp. 561-624.

Olson, R., Nordquist, R., and Everett, M.A.: Dyskeratosis in Bowen's disease, Br. J. Dermatol. **81**:676, 1969.

Basal cell carcinoma and squamous cell carcinoma

Andrade, R., and others, editors: Cancer of the skin, Philadelphia, 1976, W.B. Saunders Co.

Helm, F.: Cancer dermatology, Philadelphia, 1979, Lea & Febiger.

Mobs, F.E.: Chemosurgery: microscopically controlled surgery for skin cancer, Springfield, Ill., 1978, Charles C Thomas, Publishers.

Neoplasms of the skin and malignant melanoma—a collection of papers presented at the 20th Annual Clinical Conference on Cancer, 1975, at the University of Texas Cancer Center, M.D. Anderson Hospital and Tumor Institute, Houston, Texas, Chicago, 1976, Year Book Medical Publishers Inc.

Melanoma

Breslow, A.: Thickness, cross-sectional areas and depth of invasion in the prognosis of cutaneous melanoma, Ann. Surg. **172**:902, 1970.

Clark, W.H., Jr., Goldman, L.I., and Mastrangelo, M.J., editors: Human malignant melanoma, New York, 1979, Grune & Stratton, Inc.

Clark, W.H., Jr., and others: The histogenesis and biologic behavior of primary human malignant melanomas of the skin, Cancer Res. **29**:705, 1969.

Kopf, A.W., and others, editors: Malignant melanoma, New York, 1979, Masson Publishing USA, Inc.

McGovern, V.J.: The classification of melanoma and its relationship with prognosis, Pathology **2**:85, 1970.

Mihm, M.C., Jr., and others: The clinical diagnosis, classification and histogenetic concepts of the early stages of cutaneous malignant melanomas, N. Engl. J. Med. **284**:1078, 1971.

Mihm, M.C., Jr., and others: Early detection of primary cutaneous malignant melanoma: a color atlas, N. Engl. J. Med. **289**:989, 1973.

Reed, R.J.: Acrolentiginous melanoma. In Reed, J.R., editor: New concepts in surgical pathology of skin, New York, 1976, John Wiley & Sons, Inc., pp. 89-90.

Reimer, R.R., and others: Precursor lesions in familial melanoma, J.A.M.A. **239**:744, 1978.

Neoplasm of the mouth

Buchner, A., and Hansen, L.S.: Melanotic macule of the oral mucosa, Oral Surg. **48**:244, 1979.

Buchner, A., and Hansen, L.S.: Pigmented nevi of the oral mucosa: a clinicopathologic study of 32 new cases and review of 75 cases from the literature, Oral Surg. **49**:55, 1980.

Chaudhry, A.P., Hamped, A., and Gorlin, R.J.: Primary malignant melanoma of the oral cavity, Cancer **11**:923, 1958.

Devildos, L.R., and Langlois, C.C.: Intramucosal cellular nevi, Oral Surg. **52**:162, 1981.

Dummett, C.V., and Barens, G.: Oromucosal pigmentation: an updated literary review, J. Periodontol **42**:726, 1971.

Fejerskov, O., and Nybroe, L.: Primary malignant melanoma of the hard palate: report of case, J. Oral Surg. **31**:53, 1973.

Hatziotis, J.C., and Mylona-Hatziotis, A.J.: Blue nevi of the oral cavity: review of the literature and report of two cases, J. Oral Surg. **31**:772, 1973.

Jackson, D., and Simpson, H.E.: Primary malignant melanoma of the oral cavity, Oral Surg. **39**:553, 1975.

Liroff, K.P., and Zeff, S.: Basal cell carcinoma of the palatal mucosa, J. Oral Surg. **30**:730, 1972.

Marlett, R.H.: Generalized melanoses and non-melanotic pigmentations of the head and neck, J. Am. Dent. Assoc. **90**:141, 1975.

Mosby, E.L., Sugg, W.E., and Hiatt, W.R.: Gingival and pharyngeal metastasis from a malignant melanoma, Oral Surg. **36**:6, 1973.

Silverman, S., Greenspan, J.S., and Christie, T.M.: Junction nevus of the oral mucosa, Oral Surg. **39**:259, 1975.

Teles, J.C.B., Corodoso, A.S., and Goncalves, A.R.: Blue nevus of the oral mucosa, Oral Surg. **38**:905, 1974.

Weathers, D.R., and others: The labial melanotic macule, Oral Surg. **42**:196, 1976.

Squamous cell carcinoma/radiation therapy

Beume, J., Curtis, T.A., and Morrish, R.B.: Radiation complications in edentulous patients, J. Prosth. Dent. **26**:193, 1976.

Carl, W., Schaaf, N.G., and Sako, K.: Oral surgery and the patient who has had radiation therapy for head and neck cancer, Oral Surg. **36**:651, 1973.

Cox, F.L.: Endodontics and the irradiated patient, Oral Surg. **42**:679, 1976.

Curtis, T.A., Griffith, M.R., and Firtell, D.N.: Complete denture prosthodontics for the radiation patient, J. Prosth. Dent. **36**:66, 1976.

Daly, T.E., and Drane, J.B.: The management of teeth related to the treatment of oral cancer, Seventh National Cancer Conference Proceedings, Head and Neck Cancer, pp. 147-154, 1973.

Greenberg, M.S., and others: The oral flora as a source of septicemia in patients with acute leukemia, Oral Surg. **53**:32, 1982.

Karmioi, M., and Walsh, R.F.: Dental caries after radiotherapy of the oral regions, J. Am. Dent. Assoc. **91**:838, 1975.

Montgomery, S.: Endodontic complications in an irradiated patient, J. Endodont. **3**:277, 1977.

Nakomoto, R.Y.: Use of a saliva substitute in post-radiation xerostomia, J. Prosth. Dent. **42**:539, 1979.

Pappas, G.L.: Bone changes in osteoradionecrosis, Oral Surg. **27**:622, 1969.

Schofield, I.D.E., Abbott, W., and Popowich, L.: Osteoradionecrosis of maxillae, Oral Surg. **45**:692, 1978.

Shannon, I.L., McCrary, B.R., and Starcke, E.N.: A saliva substitute for use by xerostomic patients undergoing radiotherapy to the head and neck, Oral Surg. **44**:656, 1977.

Kaposi's hemorrhagic sarcoma

Kaposi's multiple idiopathic hemorrhagic sarcoma is a neoplastic disease marked by abnormal proliferation of lymphoreticular and endothelial cells. The disease is found worldwide but predominantly in Europe (especially Central and Eastern European countries and Italy), Equatorial and South Africa (primarily among Bantus), and North America. In the United States it occurs mainly among Jews of Galician, Polish, or Russian extraction and Southern Italians, with some cases in blacks. In Western countries the peak incidence is in the sixth and seventh decades of life, whereas in Africa the disease tends to appear in much younger age groups. It is seen in men 10 to 15 times more frequently than in women. Recent reports have suggested an increased incidence in homosexuals. The average duration of the disease is about 10 years, but death may occur from 3 to 50 years after onset. Death infrequently is the direct result of the disease and is attributed to the disease when it progresses rapidly and acts as a true sarcoma. If the course is more prolonged, death may be from other causes such as hemorrhage, intestinal perforation with peritonitis, septicemia, or bronchopneumonia.

Kaposi's sarcoma develops primarily in the skin, but multicentric visceral involvement usually follows to a variable degree. The initial sites are usually the feet, toes, and legs; dark reddish blue to purplish, sharply demarcated macular, papular, or nodular lesions appear. Sometimes

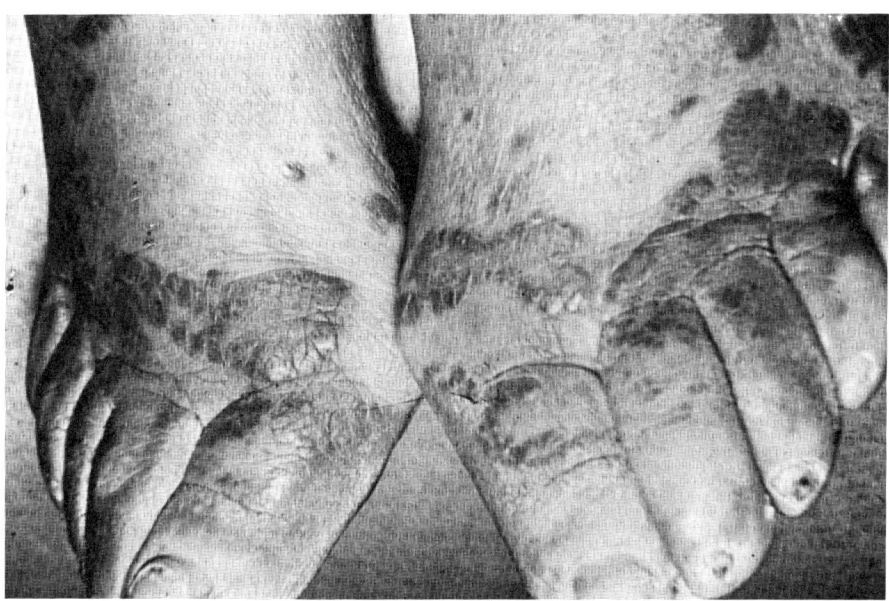

Fig. 165-7. Kaposi's hemorrhagic sarcoma with plaque lesions on dorsa of feet and toes.

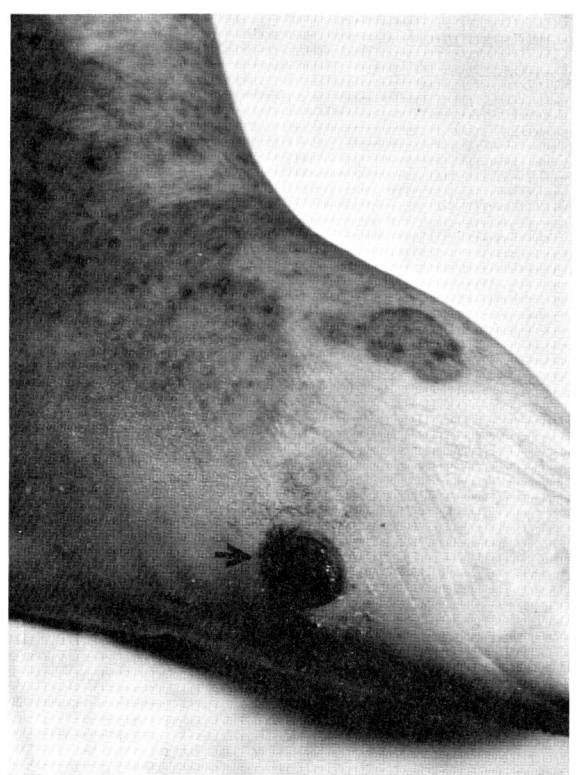

Fig. 165-8. Kaposi's hemorrhagic sarcoma with nodular and plaque lesions. Nodule *(arrow)* is dusky and erythematous. Plaques are infiltrated and reddish brown.

there is a reddish brown component that later becomes bluish. Lesions may sometimes appear first on the hands, forearms, ears, nose, or genitalia but most often are found in these locations after the appearance of lesions on the lower extremities. The macular and papular lesions may coalesce to form infiltrated plaques, from which nodules may develop (Fig. 165-7). Nodules may occasionally be the initial lesion, appearing as dusky violaceous angiomas with a firm rubbery consistency (Fig. 165-8). There is often a brawny edema of the affected extremity, with subsequent development of lymphedema. Elephantiasis of the legs and verrucous, ichthyotic lesions may also develop on the feet, ankles, and lower half of the legs as the result of chronic edema and stasis. Ulcers are uncommon and occur as the result of trauma rather than spontaneous necrosis.

The gastrointestinal tract is the most common extracutaneous site of Kaposi's sarcoma. Characteristic bluish nodules may be noted on the tongue, palate, pharynx, and esophagus and throughout the intestinal tract and may lead to internal hemorrhage as the most serious complication. The respiratory tract is the next most common area of involvement. Lesions may be found in the lungs, pleura, and larynx, but bleeding from these sites is uncommon. Kaposi's sarcoma has been reported to occur in virtually every organ, including the heart, liver, spleen, kidneys, adrenal glands, testes, and lymph nodes, but these lesions are not generally clinically significant.

Occasionally there may be periods of spontaneous remission of the lesions, especially early in the disease. Kaposi's sarcoma has also been associated with other neoplastic diseases (mycosis fungoides, Hodgkin's disease, lymphosarcoma, leukemia, and multiple myeloma). Histologically, Kaposi's sarcoma consists of masses of spindle cells, fibroblasts, and proliferating capillaries. Its behavior is that of a multifocal proliferative and reactive process originating in the reticuloendothelial system.

Treatment with conventional roentgen ray therapy is often very effective; the lesions are quite radiosensitive. Chemotherapy has been used with various cytotoxic agents (nitrogen mustard, chlorambucil, methotrexate, 5-fluorouracil, and vinblastine) administered intravenously and by regional intra-arterial perfusion.

Recently a malignant form of Kaposi's sarcoma has been recognized to occur with high frequency in young male homosexuals and occasionally in debilitated patients. The initial lesions may be anywhere on the body, and dissemination to skin and internal organs occurs rapidly. The pathogenesis seems to be related to impaired cellular immunity, and cytomegalovirus (CMV) infections and *Pneumocystis* pneumonia are associated. This disease has been called *acquired immune deficiency syndrome (AIDS)*.

ORAL MANIFESTATIONS. Oral lesions may occur without skin lesions, but generally skin lesions are present either before or during the oral manifestation. Several cases of primary oral malignancy have been reported. They are most common on the palate but can appear on alveolar ridges, lip, and tongue. They appear as a raised, reddish to mucosal-colored mass similar to a pyogenic granuloma. The patient is generally 50 years or older. Secondary infection and hemorrhage often occur from trauma.

DENTAL MANAGEMENT. Biopsy of the lesion is the key to early diagnosis and success. Often treatment may be needed for secondary infection or hemorrhage. Since Kaposi's sarcoma occurs frequently in patients undergoing immunosuppressive therapy, complications for dental therapy may be related to the drugs as well as the disease. Radiation may be used to treat the sarcoma, which may lead to problems mentioned during discussion of squamous cell carcinoma.

BIBLIOGRAPHY

Ackerman, L.V., and Murray, J.F.: Symposium on Kaposi's sarcoma, New York, 1962, S. Karger.
Bluefarb, S.M.: Kaposi's sarcoma, Springfield, Ill., 1957, Charles C Thomas, Publisher.
Braverman, I.M.: Skin signs of systemic disease, Philadelphia, 1970, W.B. Saunders Co.
Centers for Disease Control: Kaposi's sarcoma and pneumocystis pneumonia among homosexual men—New York and California, M.M.W.R. **30**:305, 1981.
Centers for Disease Control: Update on acquired immune deficiency syndrome (AIDS)—U.S., M.M.W.R. **31**:507, 1982.
Davis, J.: Kaposi's sarcoma: present concept of clinical course and treatment, N.Y.J.Med. **68**:2067, 1968.
Domonkos, A.N.: Andrew's diseases of the skin: clinical dermatology, Philadelphia, 1971, W.B. Saunders Co.
Durack, D.T.: Opportunistic infections and Kaposi's sarcoma in homosexual men, N. Engl. J. Med. **205**:1465, 1981.
Howard, W.R., Roenigk, H.H., and Bergfield, W.F.: Kaposi's hemorrhagic sarcoma, Cutis **21**:503, 1978.
Safai, B., and Good, R.A.: Kaposi's sarcoma: a review and recent developments, Clin. Bull. **10**:62, 1980.

166 • ERYTHEMAS

Robert N. Arm, Bernard A. Kirshbaum, Anthony V. Benedetto, and Karen Lipinski

ERYTHEMA MULTIFORME

Erythema multiforme is an acute inflammatory syndrome that involves the skin and mucous membranes and in the more severe forms, various internal organs. As the name "multiforme" implies, the lesions appear in many varieties, including macular, papular, nodose, vesicular, and bullous. They may be the classic iris shaped (so-called target or bull's-eye lesions). There may also be annular and circinate or purpuric and urticarial lesions (Fig. 166-1). They are not only polymorphous but variable in color as well, sometimes with exudation. Most often the lesions are found on the face, neck, forearms, and legs (especially the extensor surfaces), and the dorsa of hands and feet, frequently with a symmetric distribution. Mucous membranes are also occasionally involved. The onset of the eruption is usually fairly rapid, developing within 12 to 24 hours after a short prodromal period. Recurrent attacks may appear at regular intervals; the lesions usually heal without scarring.

The disease is more commonly seen in the spring and fall and seldom in summer. More cases are noted during viral epidemics. Although erythema multiforme may occur at any age, it is seen mainly between ages 10 and 40. The severe bullous form is more often seen in adolescents and young adults. The disease is rare in children less than 3 years old and adults over 50. When it is found in adults of the older age group, the possibility of an occult carcinoma must be considered.

Although the exact cause of erythema multiforme is unknown, it is generally considered to be a toxic or hypersensitivity syndrome, developing as the result of an antigen-antibody interaction following sensitization of the small cutaneous vessels. Different types of skin lesions may be produced by the same causative agent, and conversely, different causative agents may evoke similar clinical reactions on the skin and mucous membranes. The symptom complex has been associated with a number of viral and chlamydial infections (herpes simplex virus, coxsackievirus B-5, influenza virus type A, and echovirus infection; mumps; psittacosis; and lymphogranuloma venereum), viral immunizations (vaccination and poliovirus), deep fungal infections (histoplasmosis and coccidioidomycosis), bacterial infections (typhoid fever, leprosy, and *Mycoplasma pneumoniae* infection), bacille Calmette Guérin (BCG) vaccination, collagen diseases (dermatomyositis, allergic vasculitis, lupus erythematosus, and polyarteritis nodosa), malignancies (carcinoma and lymphoma), following radiation therapy, spontaneously, and as a result of drug reactions (penicillins, sulfonamides and related compounds, iodides, bromides, phenytoin, phenol-

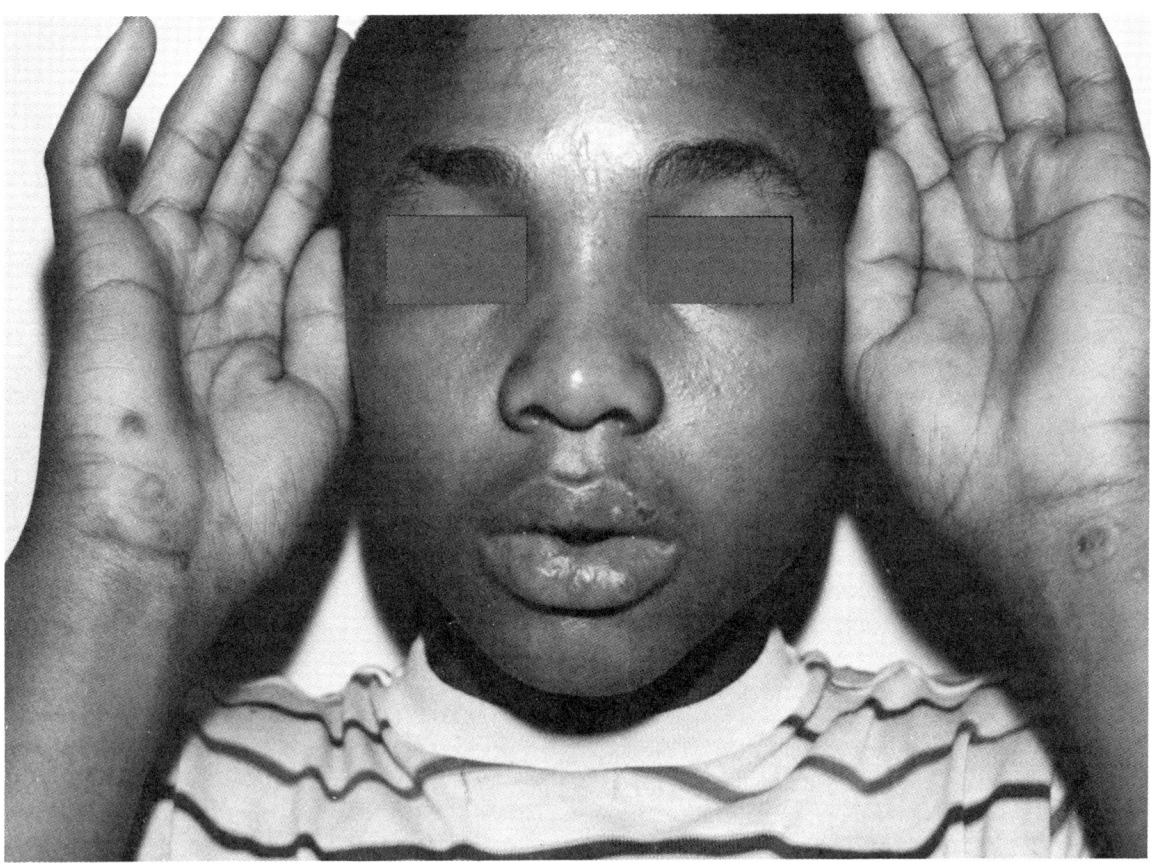

Fig. 166-1. Erythema multiforme. Lesions on lips are ruptured vesicles, and those on hands are vesicles and iris lesions.

phthalein, salicylates, and barbiturates). The eruptions in children and young adults are more often related to infections, whereas in older persons they are associated with drugs and malignancies. No cause is found in many patients.

There is a wide clinical spectrum in this disease, with gradations varying from a relatively localized minor eruption on the skin and mucous membranes to a major multisystem disorder with a potentially fatal outcome. The maculourticarial form usually occurs on the extremities, especially extensor surfaces, and the mucous membranes. The characteristic target (iris) lesion is urticarial with a dusky center that sometimes forms a vesicle, surrounded by the brighter erythematous rings; fine petechiae may be noted. The trunk may become involved, but usually this follows severe involvement of the extremities. Lesions tend to appear in crops for a few weeks, healing in about a week and leaving residual hypopigmentation or hyperpigmentation but no scarring. The vesiculobullous form may develop in preexisting lesions; this form often involves the mucous membranes more than the skin and sometimes affects the mucous membranes alone. Recurrences are more common in the vesiculobullous type than in the maculourticarial form.

The Stevens-Johnson syndrome is considered to be an extreme form of erythema multiforme. There is usually a prodrome of 1 day to 2 weeks that may variably consist of fever, malaise, sore throat, rhinitis, cough, chest pain, arthralgias, myalgias, vomiting, and diarrhea. This is followed by an abrupt eruption of bullae on the skin and mucous membranes, including the conjunctivae, nose, lips, mouth, tongue, genitalia, and rectum. The bullae rupture and become erosions and ulcerations, sometimes with hemorrhagic crusting and pseudomembranous coverings. Eye involvement includes bullae, catarrhal or purulent conjunctivitis, corneal ulcerations, anterior uveitis, and occasionally panophthalmitis, sometimes with resultant corneal opacities and blindness. Vulvovaginitis may end in fibrotic bands or stenosis of the vagina; balanitis may result in adherence of the prepuce to the glans. Shedding of nails may also occur.

The roentgenographic changes in the lung are seen as patchy infiltrates, resembling the pattern of atypical pneumonia. Lymphadenopathy may be present, and proteinuria, hematuria, tubular necrosis, and progressive renal failure have been noted. Mortality in the severe forms of erythema multiforme is 5% to 15%.

Mild cases of erythema multiforme usually clear in a

few weeks and require only local symptomatic treatment to allay symptoms of burning and itching and to drain bullae. Removal of underlying causes, when these are known, is important in both minor and major forms of the disease. Severe cases require systemic administration of corticosteroids, along with supportive therapy that includes mouthwashes and oral hygiene, eye irrigations, mydriatics, lubricants, and local antibiotics to prevent secondary infection. Antihistaminics are sometimes useful, but in general, drugs (laxatives, analgesics, and sedatives) should be avoided because there may be cross-reactivity with drugs responsible for the eruption.

ORAL MANIFESTATIONS. When a clinician hears the name "erythema multiforme," blood-encrusted lips are envisioned; this need not be the case. The variable features of this disease can present a diagnostic challenge. Often skin and oral lesions are independent of each other and vary from mild to severe. The mild lesions, if found only intraorally, will present the hardest problem for diagnosis, with a differential ranging from recurrent aphthous stomatitis and primary herpes to pemphigus in the older age groups. When limited to the oral cavity the disease is often self-limiting and resolves after a period of time, often 2 to 4 weeks. If lesions remain, a biopsy may help rule out other disease. Biopsy features of erythema multiforme are not pathognomonic. The histopathology will generally show a nonspecific inflammatory infiltrate, mild acanthosis, and occasionally a perivascular chronic inflammatory cell infiltrate. A study by Lozada showed 24% of cases with oral lesions only, 38% with oral and lip lesions, and 38% with oral, lip and skin lesions.

The lesions generally develop rapidly, beginning as an erythematous area where vesicles form, break down, and quickly ulcerate. Often the lesions coalesce, forming a grayish white pseudomembrane and leaving a yellowish white exudate. During the lesion formation the patient may complain of sialorrhea and dysphasia. A mild fever and lymphadenitis may accompany the lesions.

In Stevens-Johnson syndrome, the severe form of erythema multiforme, visceral lesions also occur in addition to cutaneous, oral, ocular, and genital mucosal lesions. The oral lesions generally appear more necrotic and the skin rash more maculopapular than the classic "target" lesions of erythema multiforme. It is not uncommon for oral lesions to precede the others, often starting during a prodromal period that may resemble a common respiratory infection.

DENTAL MANAGEMENT. In the mild form, treatment is symptomatic. The severe form requires systemic steroid treatment.

The patient generally is most concerned over the pain and inability to eat and drink. Decreased fluid intake can lead to dehydration, for which the young patient especially may need intravenous therapy. Systemic corticosteroids are the treatment of choice and beginning resolution will be seen within days. Symptomatic therapy will include topical anesthetics, neutral mouthrinses, and a switch to a liquid and then to a soft bland diet.

The patient should be instructed to avoid alcohol-containing mouthrinses and trauma to the mucosa. A soft sponge-type toothbrush or gauze can be used.

BIBLIOGRAPHY

Bianchine, J.R., and others: Drugs as etiologic factors in Stevens-Johnson syndrome, Am. J. Med. **44**:390, 1968.

Fulghum, D.D., and Catalano, P.M.: Stevens-Johnson syndrome from clindamycin, J.A.M.A. **223**:318, 1973.

Helligren, L., and Hersle, K.: Erythema multiforme: statistical evaluation of clinical and laboratory data in 224 patients and matched healthy controls, Acta Allergol. **21**:45, 1965.

Lozado, F., and Silverman, S.: Erythema multiforme, Oral Surg. **46**:628, 1978.

Meyers, W.: Erythema multiforme, Arch. Dermatol. **101**:707, 1970.

Mok, C.H., and Stevens, F.R.T.: Stevens-Johnson syndrome, Med. J. Aust. **2**:591, 1964.

Shklar, G.: Oral lesions of erythema multiforme; histologic and histiochemical observations, Arch. Dermatol. **92**:495, 1965.

Webster, G.M., and Simon, J.F.: Erythema multiforme limited to the oral cavity: report of case, J. Am. Dent. Assoc. **83**:1106, 1971.

ERYTHEMA NODOSUM

Erythema nodosum is a transitory syndrome of acute inflammatory erythematous nodules in the skin that are generally limited to the extensor surfaces of the extremities, especially the legs. It is not a specific entity but represents a hypersensitivity reaction to a number of infectious and other systemic processes; it is seen most often in relation to group A β-hemolytic streptococcal infections (pharyngitis, tonsillitis, and scarlet fever) and tuberculous infections, as well as sarcoidosis. Other infections associated with this syndrome include bacterial infections (*Yersinia*), deep fungal infections (blastomycosis, histoplasmosis, and coccidioidomycosis), superficial fungal infections (tinea capitis in the kerion formation stage), and chlamydial and viral infections (psittacosis, cat-scratch fever, and lymphogranuloma venereum). The eruption appears in relation to deep mycoses and tuberculosis when skin tests for these diseases show conversion to a positive reaction. Other noninfectious conditions in which erythema nodosum may be seen include ulcerative colitis, regional enteritis (occasionally), Behçet's syndrome, leukemia, Hodgkin's disease, and following radiation therapy of some pelvic malignancies. Rarely erythema nodosum may be seen with use of drugs, (especially sulfonamides, iodides, bromides, and contraceptive pills).

Erythema nodosum occurs more often in spring and fall and least often in summer. The greatest incidence is found in patients 20 to 35 years of age; the disease is rare after age 50. It occurs three times more often in women than in men. The incidence has been diminishing as the result of control of many infectious diseases. There may be prodromal symptoms of fever, chills, malaise, and arthralgia. The lesions consist of tender nodules, 1 to 5 cm in diameter, mainly on the anterior tibial surfaces, around the knees and ankles, occasionally on the thighs, forearms, and face, and rarely on the trunk. Episcleral nodules may develop in the palpebral fissures bilaterally. The cutaneous nodules are initially bright red, and the skin is smooth and shiny. Later the color may go through changes similar to those of a bruise (erythema contusiformis). There are usually few nodules, but there may be dozens, sometimes coalescing into large plaques producing induration and edema in the affected areas, resembling erysipelas. The usual duration of erythema nodosum is 3 to 6 weeks, but sometimes it may last for months. During healing a fine scale may evolve, but there is neither suppuration or resultant scarring.

Hilar adenopathy may be seen on chest roentgenograms if the erythema nodosum is caused by sarcoidosis. Löfgren's syndrome, associated with sarcoidosis, consists of fever, erythema nodosum skin lesions, periarticular swelling of the ankles, and a palpable paratracheal node.

The treatment of erythema nodosum is directed mainly at the underlying cause (sarcoidosis, tuberculosis, or drug reaction) of the eruption. Bed rest and intralesional corticosteroids are sometimes beneficial. Systemic corticosteroid therapy gives only temporary symptomatic relief and do not shorten the course of the eruption. There are sometimes recurrences after withdrawal of corticosteroids, and these agents should be used only where there is no evidence of an underlying infectious process.

ORAL MANIFESTATIONS. Erythema nodosum is initially a secondary finding of an underlying systemic disease. While the lesions are generally located on the extremities, intraoral lesions related to underlying disease may be seen. If the patient reports erythematous lesions of the extensor surface of the arms or legs, a careful history must be taken and referral for diagnosis made to determine the underlying cause. Cases of erythema nodosum have been reported before the onset of Behçet's syndrome.

BIBLIOGRAPHY

Fine, R.M., and Meltzer, H.D.: Erythema nodosum: form of allergic cutaneous vasculitis, South. Med. J. 61:680, 1968.
Fine, R.M., and Meltzer, H.D.: Chronic erythema nodosum, Arch. Dermatol. 100:33, 1969.
Frayha, R.A., and Nasr. F.W.: Erythema nodosum—arthropathy complex as an initial presentation of Behçet's disease: report of 5 cases, J. Rheumatol. 5:244, 1978.
Soderstrum, R.M., and Krull, E.A.: Erythema nodosum: a review, Cutis 21:806, 1971.
Weinstein, L.: Erythema nodosum, DM. 6:1, 1969.

ERYTHEMA CHRONICUM MIGRANS

Erythema chronicum migrans (ECM) is an annular, expanding, erythematous lesion caused by a tick bite (family Ixodidae). The lesion begins as a papule and gradually expands peripherally to form a palpable ring with central clearing (Fig. 166–2). There may be regional lymphadenopathy. The lesion can persist for several months. Re-

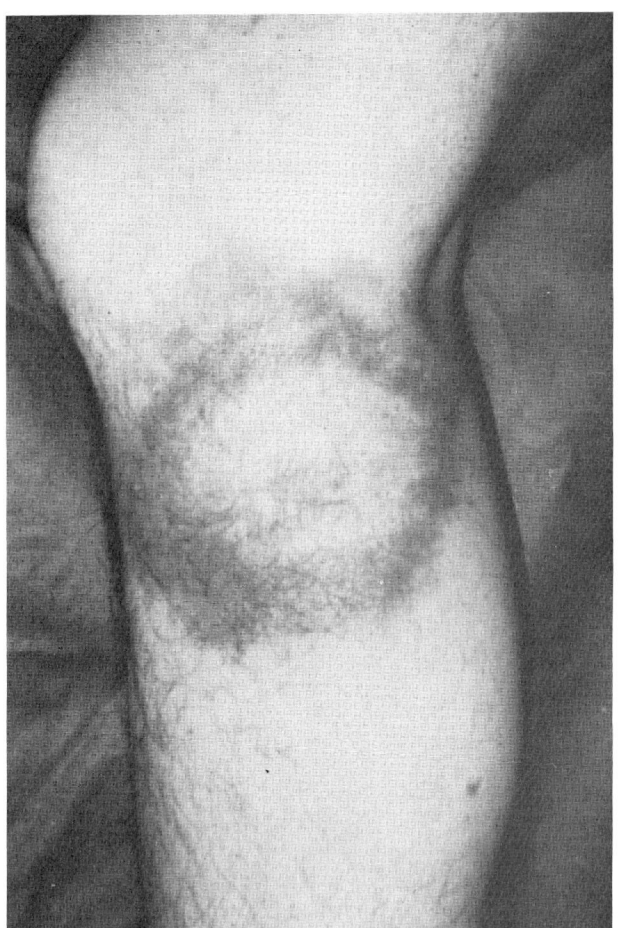

Fig. 166-2. Erythema chronicum migrans. Note central clearing. (Courtesy of Westwood Pharmaceuticals.)

cently, ECM has been associated with a form of arthritis called Lyme arthritis (named after Lyme, Connecticut, where a clustering of the disease occurred). A month or so after the initial lesion develops, an arthritis manifests itself, usually involving the knee, although other joints can be affected. It remains monarticular, lasts about 1 month, and may recur. Synovial biopsy findings are indistinguishable from those of rheumatoid arthritis.

The cause of ECM may be rickettsiae living within the gut of the ticks. The arthritis is probably immune complex mediated.

ORAL MANIFESTATIONS. A review of the literature fails to reveal oral involvement in erythema chronicum migrans. It does not appear to be related to erythema migrans (geographic tongue, migratory glossitis) for which no proven etiology has been found. (See psoriasis.) (See p. 937)

Lyme disease may present head and neck complaints including headaches and stiff necks. The patient may seek dental care because of these headaches. There have been reports of cranial or spinal neuropathies, especially unilateral or bilateral Bell's palsy. Neuropathies and lesions of erythema chronicum migrans would suggest a diagnosis of Lyme disease.

BIBLIOGRAPHY

Centers for Disease Control: Lyme disease—United States, 1980, MMWR **30**:489, 1981.

Gross, G.P., and others: Erythema chronicum migrans with purpura and polymorphonuclear infiltrate, Arch. Dermatol. **115**:873, 1979.

Hardin, J.A., and others: Immune complexes and the evolution of Lyme arthritis, N. Engl. J. Med. **301**:1358, 1979.

Mast, W.E., and Burrows, W.M.: Erythema chronicum migrans in the United States, J.A.M.A. **236**:859, 1976.

Smith, R.L., and others. Erythema chronicum migrans, Cutis **17**:962, 1976.

Steere, A.C., and others: Erythema chronicum migrans and Lyme arthritis, Ann. Intern. Med. **86**:685, 1977.

167 • INFECTIONS

Bernard A. Kirshbaum, Anthony V. Benedetto, and Karen Lipinski

VIRAL INFECTIONS
Herpes simplex

Herpes simplex virus (HSV) infects humans, who are its only natural host. Antibodies to HSV can be detected in 50% of some adult populations and may occur in 100% of certain childhood populations. The virus is spread by direct contact and is very contagious. Most primary infections occur in children, and many are subclinical. Type 1 virus usually causes oral, mucosal, and skin lesions above the waist; type 2 virus usually causes genital and skin lesions below the waist. Conversely, oral mucosal lesions may be caused by type 2 virus and genital lesions may be caused by type 1 virus.

The HSV infections can be divided into primary and recurrent. The incubation period for the primary infection is 4 to 5 days but can be as long as 12 days. There are several forms of primary infection.

PRIMARY HERPES

Gingivostomatitis. Gingivostomatitis is the most common form of primary herpes, occurring usually in children but sometimes in adults. It may be asymptomatic, but generally there is a prodrome of fever, malaise, restlessness, and drooling. The buccal mucosa, tongue, palate, and pharynx become covered with vesicles that eventually ulcerate. There is regional lymphadenopathy and considerable pain in oral tissues. Recovery is complete in about 2 weeks.

Genital herpes. In genital herpes a circumscribed patch of vesicles on an erythematous base appears on the penis, labia, vaginal wall, or cervix. The primary infection may be very painful, with urinary retention caused by dysuria, whereas cervical or vaginal wall infection may go unnoticed. Lesions may also occur on the thighs and perianally. Regional lymphadenopathy is present.

Keratoconjunctivitis. HSV can cause a purulent conjunctivitis and a very painful dendritic keratitis. Autoinoculation of the eye may occur from another site on the body by way of the fingers. An ophthalmologist should be consulted when eye involvement is suspected. Topical antiviral agents that are effective in the eye include idoxuridine and adenosine arabinoside.

Inoculation herpes. Inoculation herpes can occur when an abrasion in the skin comes in contact with HSV. The most common sites are the index and middle fingers. Medical and dental personnel are at higher risk of this "herpetic whitlow," which is extremely painful. Swelling, erythema, and vesiculation of the fingertip or finger pad occur. Inoculation herpes is often confused with a pyogenic infection, but incision, drainage, and antibiotics are of no help in the herpes infection.

RECURRENT HERPES. Recurrent HSV infection occurs in up to 40% of patients. The virus persists in the local nerve ganglia, from which recurrent invasion of the skin occurs. Sunlight, menses, fever, infection, debilitation, stress, trauma, and pregnancy can trigger recurrence. Often no initiating factor can be found. Lesions are often painful.

The most common type of recurrence is the fever blister or cold sore, also known as herpes labialis. The lesions recur at almost the identical site each time. A tingling or burning sensation generally precedes the development of the lesion. This prodrome may last from a few hours to 2 days; then vesicles erupt for a period of 2 to 4 days. These vesicles evolve into crusts lasting 8 to 11 days. Healing follows, without scarring unless secondary bacterial infection supervenes. The lesions remain infectious for varying periods, and thus the patient should be told that the lesions are infectious until the crusts fall off.

Recurrent HSV infections can also occur on the cheeks or other areas such as the buttocks. The same prodome occurs. Circumscribed vesicles on an erythematous base develop and evolve as already described.

Recurrent genital HSV infection is an escalating problem. The recurrent infection is often shorter in duration and less symptomatic than the primary infection, but very contagious. Particularly important are the devastating effects that genital HSV infections have on the neonate and the developing fetus. Cesarean section is needed for delivery of the infant if active vaginal infection is present.

In patients with severe atopic dermatitis, a condition of disseminated cutaneous infection called eczema herpeticum can develop. Severe disseminated infection can occur in patients receiving immunosuppressive agents and those with certain malignancies.

There is no cure for recurrent HSV infections at present. Compresses, medications to relieve pain, a sympathetic physician, and understanding by the patient of the disease process and its implications comprise the therapy.

Herpes zoster

Herpes zoster, also called "shingles" or zoster, is caused by the reactivation of varicella (chickenpox) virus that remains dormant in the sensory ganglia. The disease is characterized by a vesiculopustular eruption in a dermatomal arrangement. Zoster occurs only in someone who has had chickenpox. It is infectious for a person who has not had chickenpox (that is, a person who has not had varicella can get the infection from someone with zoster), but a patient with chickenpox cannot transmit zoster to another person.

The frequency of herpes zoster increases with age. Two thirds of the patients are over 45 years old. It is rare in children, and the incidence is thought to be 2:1000 in the general population. Increased frequencies of zoster are found in association with Hodgkin's disease, other lymphomas, leukemia, and renal transplantation. Antineoplastic agents, corticosteroids, and radiation therapy have also been implicated in the induction of zoster, as well as its dissemination.

The prodrome usually consists of painful burning, tingling, or tenderness along one or more contiguous sensory nerves. The dermatomes affected are along thoracic nerves (50%), cervical nerves (20%), lumbosacral nerves (10%), and trigeminal nerves (10% to 15%). Bilateral involvement is rare. Three to 4 days after the initial symptoms, grouped papulovesicles erupt along the involved nerve. These evolve into pustules. There may be regional lymphadenopathy. Once the eruption appears, the symptoms may decrease, but not in all cases. In young adults the lesions resolve in 2 to 3 weeks, whereas in older patients it may take longer. It is not unusual to see a few scattered vesicles or pustules outside the involved dermatome.

Cutaneous disseminiation, occurring 6 to 10 days after the onset of dermatomal lesions, develops in about 2% of patients. However, cutaneous and systemic dissemination may occur in 25% of patients with Hodgkin's disease, other lymphomas, or leukemia and in those receiving corticosteroids or immunosuppressive agents. Systemic zoster can involve the gastrointestinal tract, myocardium, lungs, and central nervous system. The patients most susceptible to zoster encephalitis are those with ophthalmic zoster. Adenosine arabinoside has recently been used to treat disseminated zoster.

Postherpetic neuralgia is a complication of herpes zoster. An intractable and disabling pain develops in the area of the healed zoster. This occurs in about 30% of patients over the age of 40. These patients frequently have a more aggressive form of dermatomal zoster, with deeper, more necrotic lesions and at times very severe pain during the zoster attack.

The treatment includes analgesics for the pain, drying compresses, and topical corticosteroid sprays. Systemic corticosteroids administered early in the course of the disease suppress the inflammatory response and prevent or considerably reduce the likelihood of postherpetic neuralgia. When there is the possibility of eye involvement, an ophthalmologist should be consulted.

Warts

Warts (verrucae) are viral-induced benign turmors of the epidermis and mucous membranes. They are caused by papovaviruses and occur at some time in 80% of the population; at any given time 10% of children and 5% of adults have warts. There are several varieties of warts: vulgaris (common), plantar (sole of the foot), flat (facial and other body areas), periungual, and condyloma acuminatum (genital or perirectal). It has been shown recently that different types of human papovaviruses induce these various forms.

Antibodies to warts develop, and it is thought that this may cause partial immunity to recurrence. However, patients with active warts often have low titers of IgM antibody. During regression of warts, either spontaneous or induced, wart antibody titers rise, and both IgG and IgM antibodies can be found. Among patients with recurrence, 25% have IgG antibodies. It is uncertain at present what role antibodies may play.

Warts regress spontaneously. One third of warts are usually gone within 6 months, and two thirds disappear within 2 years. However, some lesions may persist for years.

Patients who are pregnant, immunosuppressed, or have immune deficiency states show a higher rate of wart infection, and the warts are often extensive and recalcitrant to treatment. This includes renal transplant patients, patients undergoing immunosuppressive therapy for other diseases, and those with lymphomas, Hodgkin's disease, chronic lymphocytic leukemia, and Wiskott-Aldrich syndrome.

There are many ways to treat warts. It is best to begin conservatively because of the benign nature of the condition. Irritants (salicylic acid compounds), carbolic and trichloroacetic acid, liquid nitrogen freezing, and podophyllin solutions (best for condyloma acuminatum) are established therapies. Surgery is useful for isolated or persistent lesions. Immunotherapy with dinitrochlorobenzene should be avoided because it results in permanent sensitization of the skin.

Molluscum contagiosum

Molluscum contagiosum is caused by a pox virus. It is spread by direct contact and is seen most often in children. However, the lesions can develop in adults, often through sexual contact. Patients with atopic dermatitis may be susceptible to widespread, generalized infection.

The virus infects the skin. The incubation period ranges from 14 to 50 days. The lesions appear as dome-shaped, umbilicated papules that are translucent or whitish. They occur on the face, neck, arms, inner aspect of the thighs, pubic area, and buttocks. Some lesions involute spontaneously, but many persist for months to years. Occasionally a giant molluscum occurs, requiring surgical excision.

The skin lesions are benign and should be treated delicately. A curette can be used to shell out the molluscum body, which is the central core, or the body can be expressed and the central dell cauterized with carbolic acid. Freezing with liquid nitrogen is also effective.

ORAL MANIFESTATIONS AND DENTAL MANAGEMENT. See pp. 298-301.

FUNGAL INFECTIONS

Superficial fungal infections, also known as tineas and dermatophyte infections, are limited to the keratin layer of the skin. There are several forms: tinea corporis (ringworm of the body), tinea pedis (athlete's foot), tinea capitis (ringworm of the scalp), tinea cruris (jock itch), and onychomycosis (fungal infection of the nails). These infections are caused by a number of fungi, the most common being *Trichophyton rubrum, T. mentagrophytes, Microsporum canis,* and *Epidermophyton floccosum.* The topical anti-fungal agents miconazole and clotrimazole and the systemic agent griseofulvin are used for therapy. Ketoconazole is a new systemic agent that shows great promise.

Tinea corporis affects all ages. *T. rubrum, T. mentagrophytes,* and *M. canis* are the fungi most commonly isolated in this infection. The classic "ringworm" of the glabrous skin is an annular, erythematous, scaling patch with a spreading, active border and central clearing (Figs. 167-1 and 167-2). Lesions may be located on the face, trunk, and extremities, as well as intergluteally. The lesion tends to be pruritic. An eczematous form that has vesicles and pustules and is oozing may also be encountered; this is most often caused by *T. mentagrophytes.* These infections respond well to topical antifungal agents. When infection is severe, extensive, or prolonged, griseofulvin or ketoconazole may be required to control the lesions.

Tinea pedis can be a persistent and disabling problem. A chronic, fine, dry scaling in the "moccasin distribution" on the feet is common in both men and women; the infecting agent is *T. rubrum.* An inflammatory, pustular, and vesicular variant occurring on the plantar surfaces is caused by *T. mentagrophytes.* Interdigital infections usually involve the third and fourth interspaces but may also be found in the other toe spaces. These areas commonly become secondarily infected, and antibiotic therapy may be required in addition to topical (or, if needed, systemic) antifungal agents.

Tinea capitis is almost exclusively a disease of children. It may appear as a diffuse, dandrufflike scaling, as an alopecic patch, as black dots on the scalp, or as a boggy, tender, oozing mass with crusts and alopecia. The form described last is called a kerion and is probably a hypersensitivity reaction to the fungal infection. Many

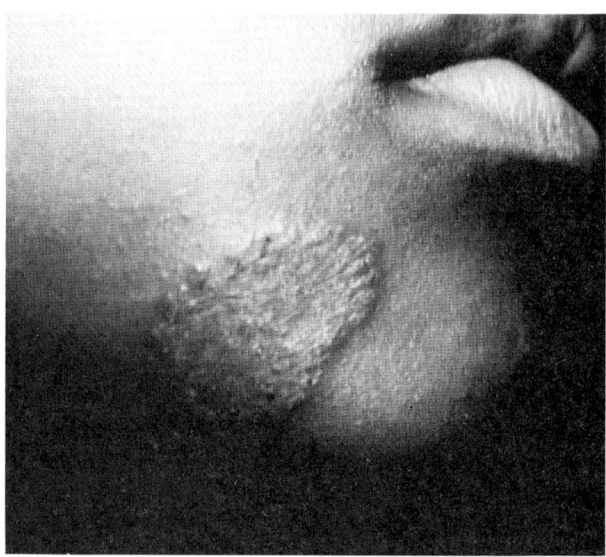

Fig. 167-1. Tinea on face of child. Elevated, sharply demarcated lesion with erythematous border is present.

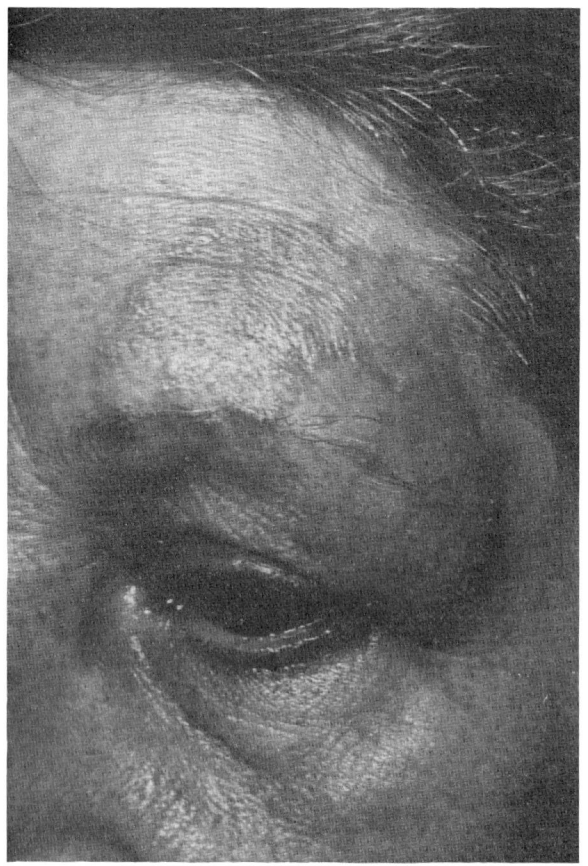

Fig. 167-2. Tinea on face of adult is less elevated and less inflamed than in children. (Courtesy of Department of Dermatology, The Cleveland Clinics.)

species of superficial fungi (mainly in the *Microsporum* and *Trichophyton* groups) can cause tinea capitis. All scalp dermatophyte infections require griseofulvin therapy, since topical antifungal agents do not penetrate the follicles sufficiently.

Tinea cruris is an erythematous, scaling, pruritic eruption involving the groin. It is more common in men and tends to occur in warmer months. *E. floccosum* is the most common causative agent, but *T. rubrum* and *T. mentagrophytes* are frequently responsible. Topical antifungal therapy is indicated, and sometimes systemic agents (griseofulvin or ketoconazole) may be needed. Healing occurs with residual hyperpigmentation that fades slowly. Because of the thinness of scrotal skin and its inability to support an environment for fungal growth, the scrotum is usually not involved. When tinea cruris is found in women, it is usually caused by yeast organisms.

Onychomycosis is dermatophyte infection of the nails. The nails become thickened and discolored with subungual debris. Usually only one or a few nails are involved; infection of all the nails simultaneously rarely occurs. Toenails do not respond as well as fingernails to therapy, which includes griseofulvin (or ketoconazole), sometimes required for months. Surgical avulsion of the nails also may be helpful and is followed by griseofulvin and topical therapy.

ORAL MANIFESTATIONS AND DENTAL MANAGEMENT. See pp. 306-308.

YEAST *(CANDIDA)* INFECTIONS

Infections with the yeast *Candida albicans* are also known as thrush and moniliasis (from the former genus name for *Candida*). They may appear as monilial intertrigo and may be found in chronic paronychia. Factors predisposing patients to *Candida* infection include obesity, diabetes mellitus, pregnancy, use of oral contraceptives, use of broad-spectrum antibiotics, chronic debilitating illness, cancer chemotherapy, and deficiencies in cell-mediated immunity.

Thrush occurs most commonly in patients receiving antibiotics or immunosuppressive drugs. The buccal mucosa, tongue, and gums become red and may have clumps of white material that are easily scraped off. Cultures of these patches reveal *Candida*. The treatment includes local topical anesthetics and nystatin rinses or troches. Zinc is an important adjunct when there is an accompanying deficiency (see discussion of "Acrodermatitis enteropathica" in Chapter 158).

Vaginal moniliasis (candidiasis) can be passed back and forth between sexual partners. Women have a curdy, white discharge, as well as burning and itching. Men may have only a persistent erythematous patch, which may be asymptomatic. Fungal infection involving the penis is almost invariably monilial. The predisposing factors are the same as for other forms of *Candida* infection.

Intertrigo appears as a fiery red, burning, itching, uncomfortable groin rash in adults or as a "diaper" rash in infants. Other areas of involvement are under pendulous breasts and intergluteally. "Satellite" lesions are usually noted at the periphery of the eruption (Fig. 167-3). Topical antiyeast agents (nystatin and amphotericin B) and drying compresses are used in treatment.

Chronic mucocutaneous candidiasis is a spectrum of diseases, all of which are chronic, recurrent, and recalcitrant (Figs. 167-4 and 167-5). Other associated abnormalities include deficiencies in cell-mediated immunity, various endocrine disorders such as diabetes, hypoparathyroidism, hypothyroidism, and hypoadrenalism, iron deficiency anemia, zinc deficiency, and dermatophyte infections. Some forms of the disease are thought to be inherited. Ketoconazole has been very effective in treatment.

ORAL MANIFESTATIONS AND DENTAL MANAGEMENT. See pp. 307-308.

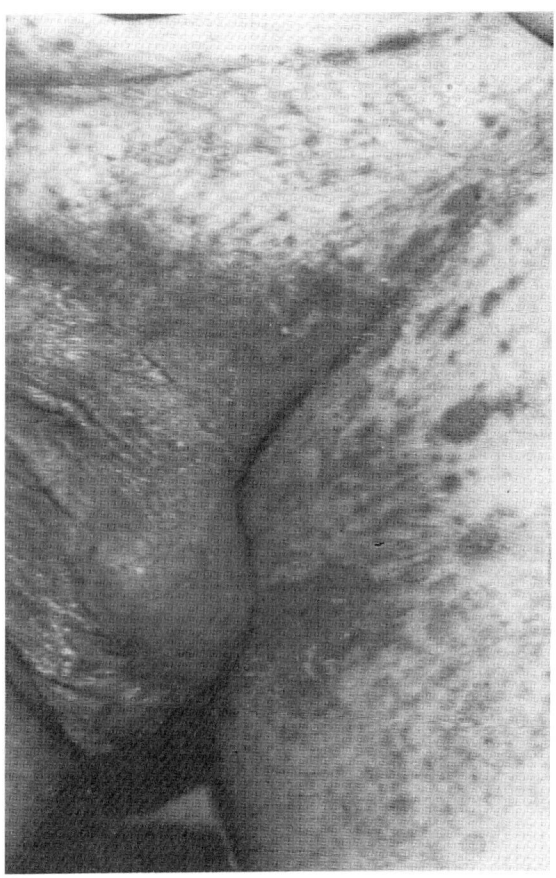

Fig. 167-3. Genital intertrigo in candidiasis. This is a moist and erythematous eruption. Note satellite lesions, highly suggestive of *Candida*. (Courtesy of Department of Dermatology, The Cleveland Clinics.)

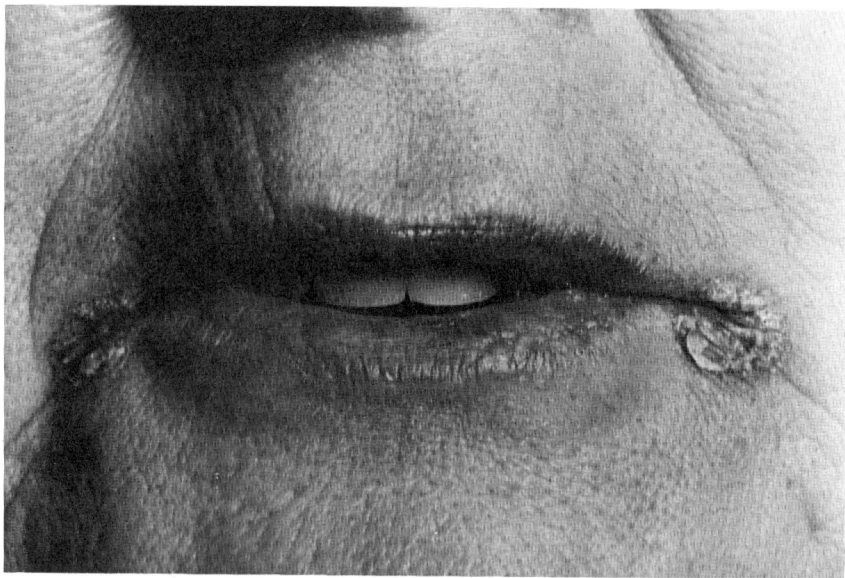

Fig. 167-4. Angular cheilitis in candidiasis. Note white scale on erythematous base. (Courtesy of Department of Dermatology, The Cleveland Clinics.)

BIBLIOGRAPHY

Bader, C., and others: The natural history of recurrent facial-oral infection with herpes simplex virus, J. Infect. Dis. **138:**897, 1978.

Baxter, D.L.: Superficial and deep mycotic infections. In Moschella, S., Pillsbury, D.M., and Hurley, H.J., editors: Dermatology, Philadelphia, 1975, W.B. Saunders Co.

Briggaman, R.A., and Wheeler, C.R.: Immunology of human warts, J. Am. Acad. Dermatol. **1:**297, 1979.

Chang, T.W., Fiumara, N.G., and Weinstein, L.: Genital herpes: some clinical and laboratory observations, J.A.M.A. **229:**544, 1974.

Curry, S.S.: Cutaneous herpes simplex infections and their treatment, Cutis **26:**41, 1980.

Dolin, R., and others: Herpes zoster-varicella infections in the immunosuppressed patient, Ann. Intern. Med. **89:**375, 1978.

Edwards, J., and others: Severe candidal infections, Ann. Intern. Med. **89:**91, 1978.

Gardner, S.D.: The new human papovaviruses: their nature and significance. In Waterson, A.P., editor: Recent advances in clinical virology, Edinburgh, 1977, Livingstone.

Gilbert, G.J.: Herpes zoster ophthalmicus and delayed contralateral hemiparesis, J.A.M.A. **229:**302, 1974.

Hilton, A.L., and others: A trial of adenosine arabinoside in genital herpes. Br. J. Vener. Dis. **54:**50, 1978.

Jacobs, P.H.: Fungal infections in childhood. In Symposium on Pediatric Dermatology, Pediatr. Clin. North Am. **25:**357, 1978.

Juretic, M.: Natural history of herpetic infection, Helv. Paediatr. Acta **21:**356, 1966.

Mazur, M.H., and Dolin, R.: Herpes zoster at the NIH: a 20 year experience, Am. J. Med. **65:**738, 1978.

Morrison, W.: Viral warts, herpes simplex, and herpes zoster in patients with secondary immune deficiencies and neoplasms, Br. J. Dermatol. **92:**625, 1975.

Nagington, J., and Rook, A.: Virus and related infection. In Rook, A., Wilkinson, D.S., and Ebling, F.J.G., editors: Textbook of dermatology, ed. 3, Oxford, Eng., 1979. Blackwell Scientific Publications.

Pass, F.: Warts, biology and current therapy. Minn. Med. **57:**844, 1974.

Plummer, G., and others: Herpes simplex viruses: discrimination of types and correlation between different characteristics, Virology **60:**206, 1974.

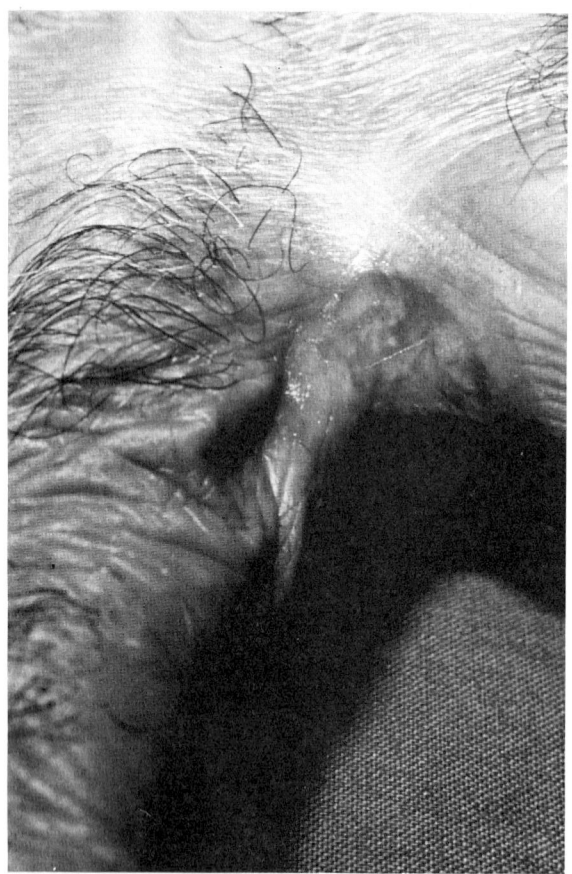

Fig. 167-5. Candidiasis of finger web (erosio interdigitalis blastomycetica). Lesion is moist and erythematous and occurs in patients, such as bartenders, whose hands are continually wet. (Courtesy of Department of Dermatology, The Cleveland Clinics.)

Pravda, D.J., and Pugliese, M.M.: Tinea facei, Arch. Dermatol. **114:**250, 1978.
Rebell, G., and Taplin, D.: Dermatophytes, their recognition and identification, ed. 2, Coral Gables, Fla., 1970, University of Miami Press.
Rifkind, D.: The activation of varicella-zoster virus infections by immunosuppressive therapy. J. Lab. Clin. Med. **68:**463, 1966.
Roberts, S., and MacKenzie, D.W.: Mycology. In Rook, A., Wilkinson, D.S., and Ebling, F.J.G., editors: Textbook of dermatology, ed. 3, Oxford, Eng., 1979, Blackwell Scientific Publications.
Roseman, N.: Chronic mucocutaneous candidiasis, Postgrad. Med. J. **55:**611, 1979.
Rosenberg, E.W., and Yusk, J.W.: Molluscum contagiosum. Arch. Dermatol. **101:**439, 1970.
Rowson, K.E.K., and Mahy, B.W.J.: Human papova (wart) virus, Bacteriol. Rev. **31:**110, 1967.
Ruckdeschel, J.C., and others: Herpes zoster and impaired cell associated immunity to the varicella-zoster virus in patients with Hodgkin's disease, Am. J. Med. **62:**77, 1977.
Spruance, S.L., and others: History of recurrent herpes simplex labialis, N. Engl. J. Med. **297:**69, 1977.
Whitley, R.J., and others: Adenosine arabinoside therapy of herpes zoster in the immunosuppressed, N. Engl. J. Med. **294:**1193, 1976.
Wright, E.T., and Winer, L.H.: Herpes zoster and malignancy, Arch. Dermatol. **84:**242, 1971.

168 • SKIN DISEASES

Robert N. Arm, Bernard A. Kirshbaum,
Anthony V. Benedetto, and Karen Lipinski

TOXIC EPIDERMAL NECROLYSIS (LYELL'S DISEASE)

Toxic epidermal necrolysis (Lyell's disease) is an extensive, but relatively superficial, blistering disease. There is a toxic erythema of the skin with necrosis and peeling, which gives a scalded appearance. The mortality can be high, and there may be associated debilitating secondary adverse reactions, such as infection, dehydration, electrolyte imbalance, and scarring.

In adults the disease is caused by a hypersensitivity reaction to a wide variety of drugs, whereas in children the necrolysis is usually induced by a toxin produced by coagulase-positive staphylococci and thus is called the staphylococcal scalded skin syndrome (SSSS).

Adult disease

In adults onset is abrupt with nonspecific prodromal symptoms including burning, skin tenderness, fever, fatigue, diarrhea and vomiting, malaise, and arthralgias. The condition may become grave within hours. A morbilliform rash or urticarial lesions appear predominantly on the face and extremities and lead to an erythroderma. Vesicles then appear that rapidly become confluent, producing large flaccid bullae and leading to epidermal denudation over large areas of the body. The epidermis may peel off in large sheets, leaving a raw, red, scaled-appearing skin surface (Fig. 168-1). Nikolsky's sign (dislodging of the epidermis adjacent to and surrounding a bullous lesion by sliding pressure applied with a finger) is usually present. Mucous membranes including lips, buccal mucosa, and conjunctivae can be severely affected, and there may be onycholysis of fingernails and toenails. There may also be purpuric and hemorrhagic manifestations in the skin. The extensive sloughing of epidermis allows much plasma loss, resulting in fluid and electrolyte imbalance. Other associated systemic complications are fever, liver damage, renal failure, and shock.

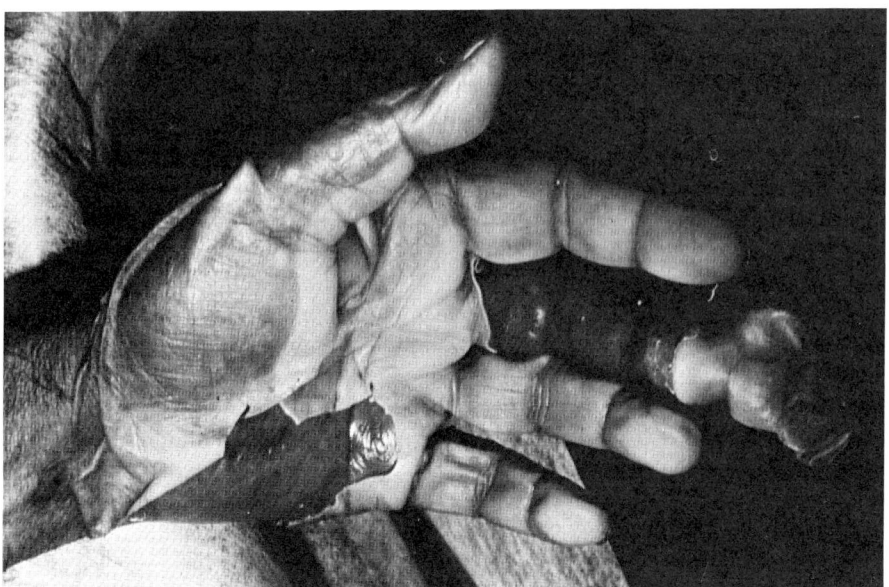

Fig. 168-1. Toxic epidermal necrolysis showing extensive exfoliation. (Courtesy of American Academy of Dermatology.)

Histopathologic examination of early lesions shows vacuolization and bulla formation at the basal cell layer. There is little or no inflammatory infiltrate in the dermis. Later, subepidermal bullae form. Dermal vessels show endothelial swelling, but no necrosis or vasculitis.

The treatment is usually systemic corticosteroids in high doses, adequate replacement of fluids and electrolytes, topical and systemic antibiotics, and skilled nursing care. The mortality is approximately 30%. In patients who recover, symblepharon and ectropion, trichiasis, corneal opacities, alopecia, and anonychia may result from the scarring.

Staphylococcal scalded skin syndrome

The staphylococcal scalded skin syndrome (SSSS) is usually linked to infection with group 2 phage types of *Staphylococcus aureus* (usually type 71). A staphylococcal exotoxin (epidermolysin) is responsible. Children, in particular newborns in their first 3 months, are prime victims of this disease. It rarely develops in adults.

SSSS usually occurs in a child or infant with a severe purulent conjunctivitis, otitis media, or nasopharyngeal infection who develops a faint yellow amber eruption, with circumoral predilection. The child may complain of skin tenderness. Within 24 to 48 hours there is a positive Nikolsky's sign, and large bullae develop over massive areas of the body. Sheets of epidermis separate easily, leading to loss of plasma and body heat. The fluid loss may subside quickly, followed by dry desquamation within the first week. Mucous membrane involvement is rare, and cultures taken from intact bullae are usually sterile.

A histopathologic examination shows epidermal splitting within the middle to upper epidermis just beneath the stratum corneum. Bullae contain acantholytic cells with virtually no dermal reaction. This is unlike the toxic epidermal necrolysis of adults in which the bullae develop at the basal layer or the basement membrane zone.

Treatment with appropriate antibiotics has markedly reduced associated mortality.

ORAL MANIFESTATIONS. The mucosa can be extensively involved with vesicobullous lesions in toxic epidermal necrolysis. The staphylococcal scalded skin syndrome has less frequent oral involvement. The lesions resemble Stevens-Johnson syndrome. When lesions are present, the Nikolsky sign will usually be positive. In a short period of time the mucosal lesion will become erosive.

Increased severity of the disease process will lead to excessive pain, especially when the patient attempts to eat or drink.

DENTAL MANAGEMENT. While the systemic management is indicated for definitive treatment, the patient should be made as comfortable as possible. Topical anesthetic solutions such as 0.5% aqueous diphenhydramine (Benadryl) will be of great assistance for sensitivity. The lesions may be made worse by rough cusps and restorations. All elective dental treatment should be deferred.

With increased use of nonsteroidal anti-inflammatory drugs in dentistry, one should take note that ibuprofen (Motrin) and sulindac hypersensitivities have been related to Stevens-Johnson–like toxic epidermal necrolysis syndrome.

PEMPHIGUS AND PEMPHIGOID

The most important group of bullous dermatoses in terms of morbidity and mortality is the pemphigus/pemphigoid group. In pemphigus, autoantibodies appear within the epidermis. In the diseases of the pemphigoid group autoantibodies are found beneath the epidermis at the basement membrane zone. In both conditions bullae appear de novo with no surrounding erythema.

Pemphigus

PEMPHIGUS VULGARIS. Pemphigus vulgaris is reported to have a higher incidence in Jews but is seen throughout the world. Most commonly the age group 40 to 60 is affected. It may remain localized for some months, often in the mouth, with the bullae being small and flaccid. If bullae persist, erosions and ulcers can occur, and the disease may progress to widespread skin and mucosal distribution, including the nose, pharynx, larynx, esophagus, vulva, penis, and anus. Secondary bacterial infection with crusting can occur and accounts in part for the characteristic mousy odor. Lesions that heal spontaneously or with therapy do not leave scars. Histologically, there is primary acantholysis with intraepidermal splitting and bulla formation. A positive Nikolsky's sign (dislodging of the epidermis adjacent to and surrounding a bullous lesion by a sliding pressure applied with a finger) is present in blistered and adjacent normal-appearing skin. If the condition is left untreated, there is steady deterioration with eventual death, the average time being about 14 months (Fig. 168-2).

The treatment of all forms of pemphigus depends on the severity. Treatment includes hospitalization for intensive local skin care and high doses of corticosteroids. Immunosuppressive agents such as methotrexate, azathioprine, and cyclophosphamide can be used for their adjunct corticosteroid-sparing effects.

Oral manifestations. As noted previously, pemphigus is often localized in the mouth and is frequently the initial site of involvement. The lesions are vesicobullous in nature, often "weeping," and may produce painful ulcers. The rupturing generally occurs immediately after vesicle formation due to trauma, unlike the skin lesions, which can remain intact for days. The ulcerations vary in size, are often covered with yellowish gray pseudomembrane, and may often be confused with other lesions.

Differential diagnosis of pemphigus includes aphthosis, lichen planus, benign mucous membrane pemphigoid (which may resemble early mucosal lesions of pemphigus vulgaris), and Stevens-Johnson's syndrome (which appears clinically similar, but the disease has a more abrupt onset and acute febrile course). Other blistering diseases such as

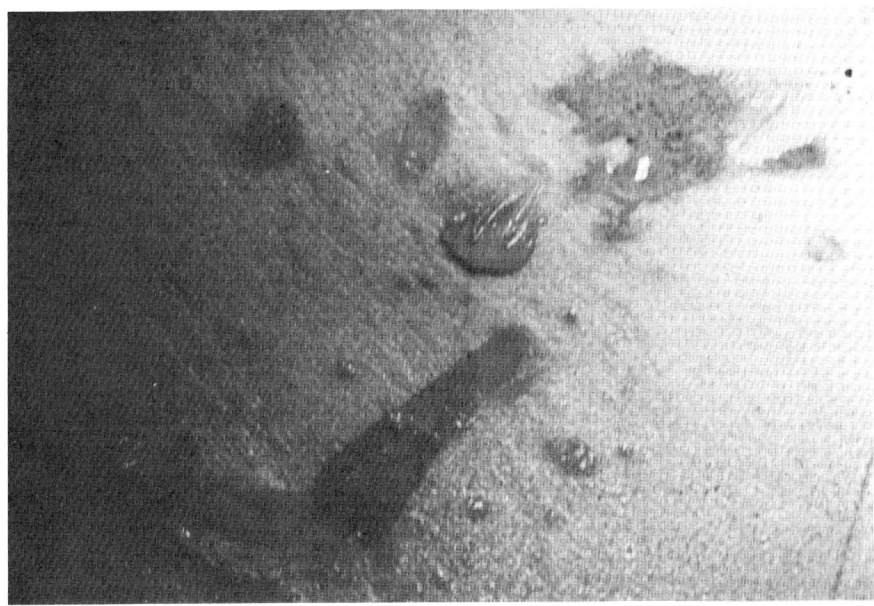

Fig. 168-2. Flaccid bullae in pemphigus vulgaris. There is no erythema around lesions (lesions arise from uninflamed skin).

toxic epidermal necrolysis, dermatitis herpetiformis and bullous erythema multiforme, candidiasis, and desquamative gingivitis should also be considered.

Examination should include testing for Nikolsky's sign; however if Nikolsky's sign is positive it is not pathognomonic since it may also be positive for other disorders. A biopsy is therefore needed. Early lesions that have not undergone degenerative changes should be selected for biopsy, especially if a vesicle is present. If pemphigus is included in the differential diagnosis, arrangements for immunofluorescence should be done before biopsy. Oral cytologic study may suggest a diagnosis but cannot replace the biopsy.

Dental management. The treatment for pemphigus is generally systemic but topical oral corticosteroids can be helpful for severe lesions or if the disease is limited only to the oral cavity. For prolonged gingival contact steroids can be applied beneath a splint or denture. Topical anesthetics, especially a rinse of 0.5% aqueous diphenhydramine (Benadryl), will alleviate the pain. Hygiene can be promoted by use of neutral mouthrinse and/or peroxide rinse. Occasionally antibiotics may be needed for secondary infection.

Of major concern to the dentist is the systemic use of corticosteroids and immunosuppressants, which may lead to increased infection and delayed healing. Supplemental steroids may be needed before treatment.

PEMPHIGUS VEGETANS. Pemphigus vegetans is variant of pemphigus vulgaris that occurs in patients with increased resistance to the disease. There are two types of pemphigus vegetans. The Neumann type begins with flaccid bullae resembling pemphigus vulgaris, most often found in the intertriginous areas. These bullae become eroded, forming fungoid vegetations and papillomatous proliferations. The onset may sometimes be insidious, with lesions found in the nose, mouth, axillae, genitalia, perineum, or umbilicus. After the bullae rupture, they develop verrucous vegetations on their moist bases, covered by crusts and a surrounding inflamed border. These lesions may coalesce into large patches or form irregular patterns. Initially the symptoms are mild, with long periods of spontaneous remission of the disease. Later there may be febrile episodes with other constitutional symptoms. The terminal phases are like pemphigus vulgaris, with intercurrent infection aggravated by the use of corticosteroid therapy.

The Hallopeau type (dermatitis vegetans, pyodermite vegetans) follows a more benign course, and the lesions are pustules rather than bullae. Large areas of exuberant granulation tissue and moist verrucous vegetating plaques form, become crusted, and exude serum and pus with a distinctive foul odor. They may break down and form central ulcerations with vesicles and pustules at the periphery of the plaques. Characteristically there is development of large granulomatous masses in the intertriginous areas of the axillae and groin. Occasionally single lesions may be localized to the ankles, but there may be disseminated lesions that develop as vegetating masses and multiple ulcers on various parts of the body and mucous membranes, including lips, buccal mucosa, and vagina. This form of the disease may be an abnormal tissue reaction to various infectious processes, including a viral-bacterial symbiosis, in persons who are immunologically deficient. Although it tends to follow a chronic, prolonged course, it can behave like pemphigus vulgaris and terminate fatally.

Oral manifestations. Oral lesions of pyodermite vegetans were reported in two of the five first described cases by Hallpeau. While cutaneous involvement is generally present, McCarthy reported several cases of oral involvement only and used the term "pyostomatitis vegetans." One of his patients later developed the skin lesions. Many patients with oral involvement also have gastrointestinal problems. The oral lesions are often asymptomatic and start as small (less than 5 mm.) red, inflamed areas. They have a yellowish gray necrotic surface that can be rubbed off easily, leaving a raw exposed surface. The lesions are generally ovoid, well delineated, and slightly raised, and they often coalesce. Common areas involved are the buccal mucosa, mucobuccal fold, and labial gingiva.

A biopsy is usually needed and will show various patterns. An early lesion will resemble an epithelial abscess, with many eosinophils. Areas of intraepithelial separation are seen, like the acantholysis of pemphigus. Older lesions generally have ulcerated surfaces and fewer eosinophils. In both, an infiltrate of lymphocytes and plasma cells is seen in the connective tissue.

While the oral lesions can resemble pemphigus histopathologically, there are many differences, including the presence of an inflammatory infiltrate and clinical differences such as painless lesions. Clinically, pyostomatis vegetans may be a separate entity. The oral lesion will follow a course similar to the gastrointestinal disease, with periods of spontaneous remissions.

Dental management. Systemic management will be indicated for diffuse disease. Pain of oral lesions may be lessened with topical corticosteroids. A gastrointestinal work-up as part of a complete physical examination may be indicated. Antibiotics seem to be of limited value when pustules are seen.

PEMPHIGUS FOLIACEUS AND PEMPHIGUS ERYTHEMATOSUS. Pemphigus foliaceus and pemphigus erythematosus are considered to be variant forms of pemphigus vulgaris. Epidemiologically, pemphigus foliaceus occurs worldwide without any racial or ethnic prevalence but is endemic in Brazil where it is known as fogo selvagem. It usually occurs in adults 30 to 60 years of age, except in Brazil, where adolescents and young adults in a family, especially women, are affected. It begins locally and insidiously, usually on the scalp and face, advancing to flaccid bullae with prominent scaling and crusting of the scalp, face, and upper areas of the trunk. The mucous membranes are usually not affected. Histologically there are acantholysis and a subcorneal split with bulla formation high within the epidermis. Autoantibodies occur at the site of bulla formation. Pemphigus foliaceus, other than that in Brazil, tends to present a more generalized exfoliative dermatitis, with similar histologic and immunologic findings. The prognosis is relatively good, but the response to corticosteroid therapy is less favorable in the non-Brazilian form.

Pemphigus erythematosus (Senear-Usher syndrome) clinically resembles a mixture of pemphigus vulgaris, seborrheic dermatitis, and lupus erythematosus. Red, greasy, crusted, eroded lesions occur on the malar and sternal areas, on the scalp, and occasionally in the mouth. The course is more chronic than that of pemphigus vulgaris.

The lesions of pemphigus foliaceus and pemphigus erythematosus are caused by an intradermal blister associated with a neutrophilic infiltrate and the presence of many eosinophils. The blisters are small, flaccid, and easily broken. Direct immunoflourescence of involved skin shows the presence of IgG, C1, C4, C3, properdin, and factor B in the intercellular spaces surrounding the cells of the epidermis. Over 90% of patients develop circulating IgG antibodies against the intercellular cement of the epidermis. Increases in the amount of antibody precede clinical flares of the disease; the antibody-antigen combination probably fixes complement by the classic pathway, causing acantholysis and cell separation. Another possibility is that the antibody alone (without complement activation) releases epidermal proteases that cause acantholysis.

The treatment of all forms of pemphigus depends on the severity. Treatment includes hospitalization for intensive local skin care and high doses of corticosteroids. Immunosuppressive agents such as methotrexate, azathioprine, and cyclophosphamide can be used for their adjunct corticosteroid-sparing effects.

HAILEY-HAILEY DISEASE (BENIGN FAMILIAL CHRONIC PEMPHIGUS). Hailey-Hailey disease, or benign familial pemphigus, is a rare hereditary disorder characterized by recurrent vesicular and bullous eruptions most commonly appearing on the neck, axillae, upper part of the trunk, and groin. It is caused by an irregularly dominant gene in 70% of cases. There appears to be an epidermal defect involving a fault in the synthesis or maturation of the tonofilament and desmosome complex or a fault in the synthesis of intercellular substance. External agents such as friction, freezing, and ultra-violet irradiation may precipitate acantholysis. Infection (especially with *Candida albicans* and staphylococci) is another important precipitating factor. Histologically, Hailey-Hailey disease appears very much like pemphigus vulgaris except for the following characteristics: Hailey-Hailey disease has more extensive acantholysis but less damage to acantholytic cells, with a few intercellular bridges remaining so that neighboring cells still adhere loosely to one another, giving the appearance of a dilapidated brick wall. Clinically, groups of small vesicles erupt on normal or erythematous skin with initially clear contents that soon become turbid. The lesions extend peripherally, and the center may heal or show soft, flat, moist vegetations. Sweating and heat usually aggravate this condition, whereas cold may cause regression of the lesions. Diseases to be considered in the differential diagnosis include chronic bacterial intertrigo, mycotic infections, infectious eczematoid dermatitis, and impetigo.

The treatment is accomplished with topical and systemic antibiotics, corticosteroid preparations, and the removal of external precipitating factors when possible. Grenz-ray therapy has been used with some success. Dapsone has also been reported to be effective.

Pemphigoid

BULLOUS PEMPHIGOID. Bullous pemphigoid occurs worldwide with no racial prevalence. It usually affects those over 60 years of age, beginning as a generalized erythema lasting several days or weeks, followed by the development of large, tense, tough bullae that remain intact or, if ruptured, heal rapidly. It predominates on the limbs and trunk and seldom affects mucous membranes. This disease may undergo spontaneous remission, but recurrent attacks occur. Death may occur from complications.

Histologically, there is subepidermal bulla formation without acantholysis. Autoantibodies are evident in the basement membrane zone. The subepidermal bullae contain a neutrophilic infiltrate, often with eosinophils. Direct immunoflourescence of the skin shows linear or tubular IgG (sometimes IgA or IgM) in the basement zone. Often C1q, C4, C3, and C5, properdin, and factor B are present. The specific IgG antibody combines with a basement membrane antigen and fixes complement by the classic pathway, attracting neutrophils to the dermal-epidermal junction, thus initiating release of proteolytic enzymes and tissue destruction. The alternate pathway of complement may also be activated. Electron microscopy shows IgG binding to the stratum lucidum of the basement membrane in the region of the anchoring filaments. Complement components are decreased in the blister fluid of bullous pemphigoid.

Differential diagnosis includes eczematous eruptions and pemphigus vulgaris. Patients with pemphigus vulgaris, however, have severe mucosal lesions and small, flaccid, easily broken bullae rather than the tense, tough, large bullae of pemphigoid. The treatment consists of corticosteroids and immunosuppressive agents.

Benign mucosal pemphigoid (cicatricial pemphigoid, ocular pemphigus). Benign mucosal pemphigoid (cicatricial pemphigoid, ocular pemphigus) is a disabling but nonfatal vesiculobullous eruption of the mucous membranes, especially the conjunctivae. Some patients show skin lesions. The disease is most commonly seen in individuals over 65 years of age; women are affected twice as often as men. The cause is unkown. Histologically, formation of subepidermal bullae without acantholysis is seen. Autoantibodies to basement membrane are found infrequently. Constant care by an ophthalmologist is necessary to relieve eye problems. Combined treatment with corticosteroids and immunosuppressive agents may be helpful, and sulfapyridine may give a temporary response, but therapy is generally ineffective.

The two striking clinical features are the bullae on the mucous membranes (conjunctivae, mouth, nose, larynx, pharynx, esophagus, penis, vulva, vagina, and anus) and the formation of scars. It must be differentiated from pemphigus vulgaris and ulcerative lichen planus. Treatment with corticosteroids, and immunosuppressives may be helpful.

Oral manifestations. This nonfatal, painful, chronic disease may resemble the vesicobullous lesions of pemphigus and other similar diseases. Unlike pemphigus, the bullae appear thicker walled and remain visible for a longer period of time. The sloughed mucous membrane will be raw and bleeding but will heal in about 2 weeks. Gingival lesions are common in benign mucous membrane pemphigoid and resemble a desquamative gingivitis with an erythematous appearance.

Because of local trauma, the gingival lesions may remain for a long time. A biopsy using immunofluorescent studies is necessary for definitive diagnosis.

After the lesion heals, scarring may occur. They may cause decreased vestibular depth leading to later problems with prosthetics.

Dental management. Since the disease is often limited to the oral cavity, diagnosis and local management may fall upon the dentist. The easy sloughing of the mucosa will lead to a nondiagnostic tissue specimen, and care must be taken during the biopsy to avoid this. Once the diagnosis is established, treatment can include systemic steroids or intralesional injections. Use of splints may help topical steroids stay in place. Oral hygiene will be a problem and may be supplemented by topical steroids, peroxide solutions, and other rinses. A topical anesthetic may be helpful for painful lesions. Since prosthetic device may be hard to use because of both the lesions and the scarring, maintenance of the dentition must be stressed. One study has shown successful use of a split-thickness skin graft to gain vestibular depth. The patient successfully used a full denture. It should be noted, however, that grafting has had limited success on the skin and is a difficult procedure.

BIBLIOGRAPHY

Asboe-Hansen, G.: Diagnosis of pemphigus, Brit. J. Dermatol. **83**:81, 1970.

Behlen, C.H., II, and Mackay, D.M.: Benign mucous membrane pemphigus, Arch. Dermatol. **92**:566, 1965.

Cataldo, E., Covino, M.D., and Tesone, P.E.: Pyostomatitis vegetans, Oral Surg. **52**:172, 1981.

Eversole, L.R., Henney, E.B., and Sabes, W.R.: Oral lesions as the initial signs in pemphigus, Oral Surg. **22**:354, 1972.

Hasler, J.F.: The role of immunofluorescence in the diagnosis of oral vesicobullous disorders, Oral Surg. **33**:362, 1972.

Jordan, R.E., Triftshauser, C.T., and Schroeder, A.L.: Direct immunofluorescent studies of pemphigus and bullous pemphigus, Arch. Dermatol. **103**:486, 1971.

Laskaris, G., and Angelopoulos, A.: Cicatrical pemphigoid: direct and indirect immunofluorescent studies, Oral Surg. **51**:48, 1981.

Laskaris, G., Sklavounoy, A., and Bovopoulou, O.: Juvenile pemphigus vulgaris, Oral Surg. **51**:415, 1981.

Lever, W.F.: Pemphigus and bullous pemphigoid. Springfield, Ill., 1965, Charles C. Thomas, Publisher.

Lever, W.F., and Hashimoto, K.: The etiology and treatment of pemphigus and pemphigoid, J. Invest. Dermatol. **53**:373, 1969.

McCarthy, F.P.: Pyostomatitis vegetans: report of 3 cases, Arch. Dermatosyph. **60**:750, 1949.

McCarthy, P., and Shklar, G.: A syndrome of pyostomatitis vegetans and ulcer colitis, Arch. Dermatol. **88**:281, 1963.

McCarthy, P.L.: Benign mucous membrane pemphigoid, Oral Surg. **33**:75, 1972.

Meurer, M., and others: Oral pemphigus vulgaris: a report of 10 cases, Arch. Dermatol. **113**:1520, 1977.

O'Hara, P.B., and others: Split thickness skin graft for treatment of oral benign mucous membrane pemphigoid, Oral. Surg. **49**:487, 1980.

Perry, H.O., and Brunsting, L.A.: Pemphigus foliaceous, Arch. Dermatol. **91**:9, 1965.

Pisanti, S., and others: Pemphigus vulgaris incidence in Jews, Oral Surg. **38**:382, 1974.

Shklar, G., Meyer, I., and Zacarian, S.A.: Oral lesions in bullous pemphigoid, Arch. Dermatol. **99**:663, 1969.

Urbanek, V.E., and Cohen, L.: Benign mucous membrane pemphigoid, Oral Surg. **31**:772, 1971.

Wright, E.T., Epps, R.L., and Newcomer, V.D.: Fluorescent antibody studies in pemphigus vulgaris, Arch. Dermatol. **93**:562, 1966.

Zegarelli, D.: Pemphigus, Oral Surg. **44**:384, 1977.

PSORIASIS

Psoriasis is a chronic, papulosquamous skin disease characterized by systemic lesions of fine, silvery white scales over a thickened erythematous base (Fig. 168-3). It involves all areas of the body, including glabrous skin, scalp, and mucous membrane. The major areas of involvement are the extensor surfaces of the extremties and the scalp.

The age of onset can be from infancy to late adult life, with no predilection to sex. Psoriasis may affect various family members without conformity to the laws of mendelian genetics. With the recent emphasis of HLA typing, B locus antigens HLA-B13 and HLA-BW17 have been observed to be significantly increased in psoriasis. HLA-BW17 portends early onset of the disease, and patients possessing HLA-BW16 and HLA-BW17 probably will demonstrate a more severe form of the disease.

The etiology of psoriasis is unknown. Pathophysiologically, epidermal cell turnover rate is increased, resulting in a more rapid growth rate of the epidermal cells. The usual 28 days required for basal cells to become skin surface cells can be telescoped into 2 to 5 days. This helps to account for the clinical appearance of thickened epidermis with persistent and exuberant scaling and for the elevated serum uric acid levels because of the consequent increased nucleic acid degradation.

When the semiadherent scale is lifted off a plaque of psoriasis, minute punctate bleeding is often found (Auspitz sign). This characteristic feature of psoriasis, although not exclusively associated with this disease, can be supported by the histologic finding of increased capillary vascularization in the dermal papillae just beneath the thickened (acanthotic), rapidly proliferating areas of epidermis.

Another interesting feature of psoriasis (again not exclusive for this disease) is the Koebner or isomorphic phenomenon, the appearance of morphologically identical skin lesions over normal skin areas that have been recently traumatized. This isomorphic response can be elicited by trauma such as scratching or rubbing, sunburning, or undergoing surgery involving the skin.

Many descriptive terms are used to identify the various configurations of the erupting lesions of psoriasis. For instance, guttate (droplike) psoriasis most commonly occurs in children and young adults following an upper respiratory tract infection with group A β-hemolytic streptococci or following acute emotional or physical trauma such as a sunburn. Linear lesions of psoriasis are characteristic of

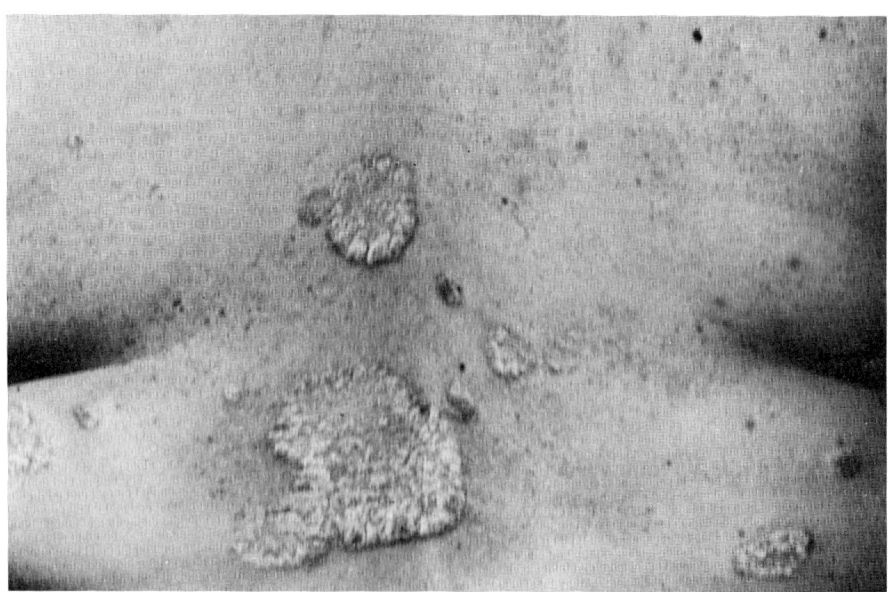

Fig. 168-3. Psoriasis. Note scaly surface of patches. (Courtesy of Department of Dermatology, The Cleveland Clinics.)

the Koebner reactions following scratching. Exfoliative erythroderma (total body involvement with scaling and hyperemia) is an acute uncontrolled flare usually following a severe illness or toxic reaction to medication. Exfoliative erythroderma occurs under comparable circumstances in many other papulosquamous diseases such as various forms of eczema, atopic dermatitis, and pityriasis rubra pilaris. Exfoliative erythroderma is a serious medical emergency resulting in considerable morbidity and occasional mortality because of excessive heat loss and fluid and electrolyte imbalance.

Approximately 50% of patients with psoriasis manifest some form of nail dystrophy, which varies from minor pitting on the surface of the nail plate to onycholysis with partial and incomplete nail growth.

PUSTULAR PSORIASIS. There are two forms of pustular psoriasis, the localized and the generalized. In either case sterile pustules, in groups or singly, appear in psoriatic plaques or in previously uninvolved sites. No pyogenic organisms have been implicated as the causative agents of either the localized or the generalized form of pustular psoriasis. Localized pustular psoriasis can have varying manifestations. There may be groups of pustules localized on the palms, soles, or periungual areas, with or without associated lesions of psoriasis elsewhere on the body; this is known as palmoplantar pustulosis. Pustular lesions may or may not by symmetric and may cover very large areas. Onycholysis may occur because lakes of pus beneath the nail lift it from the nail bed.

Generalized pustular psoriasis of von Zumbusch is an acute generalized eruption of superficial sterile pustules associated with high fever, leukocytosis, lymphopenia, heat and fluid loss, electrolyte imbalance, hypocalcemia, and hypoalbuminemia. Bacteremia and cardiopulmonary decompensation may result. The mortality may be appreciable. Pustules appear episodically over generalized erythroderma. The cause is unknown, but the disorder sometimes occurs during treatment of psoriasis with or after withdrawal of systemic corticosteroids, occasionally in association with extremely potent topical corticosteroids, or after indiscreet use of irritating topical therapy.

PSORIATIC ARTHRITIS. The arthritis associated with psoriasis is usually a sero-negative, polyarticular erosive joint disease, characteristically involving the small joints, especially the distal interphalangeal joints. When psoriatic arthritis is present, some form of nail dystrophy usually exists. With progressive disease, skin and joints may flare simultaneously. In patients with spinal involvement there is a high incidence of HLA-B27 tissue type.

MANAGEMENT. The safest treatment for psoriasis, which is as old as the disease, is ultraviolet light. This may be in the form of natural sunlight or ultraviolet light treatment.

Photochemotherapy, the combined use of ultraviolet light and medication, can be administered topically or systemically. Topical photochemotherapy may include topical tar preparations or topical corticosteroids with ultraviolet light. Recently, systemic photochemotherapy has been developed; this combines oral ingestion of 8-methoxypsoralen and exposure to ultraviolet light. The combination of light and medication works synergistically, whereas individually they would be less effective.

Other effective therapy includes topical corticosteroids (with or without occlusion), topical anthralin and tars, and systemic methotrexate for severe skin and arthritic disease. Systemic corticosteroids are usually contraindicated because they can precipitate pustular psoriasis.

Treatment of localized pustular psoriasis is varied and not very effective. Topical corticosteroids, grenz-ray therapy, Dapsone, tars, or ultraviolet light may result in a remission. The treatment for generalized pustular psoriasis is intravenous methotrexate and supportive measures.

ORAL MANIFESTATIONS. Psoriasis of the face and mouth is rare. Some deny the existence of oral psoriasis and believe it may be another entity, but there have been histologically proven lesions that show the same remission pattern as the skin lesions. These lesions may be seen on the buccal mucosa, lips, palate, tongue, gingiva, and floor of the mouth. They have a variable appearance ranging from sharply demarcated plaques of gray to yellowish white to ring-shaped striae. Raised beefy red lesions and elevated ulcerative masses have been reported. One study of 100 patients reported 11% as having angular cheilosis, 6% having fissured tongue, and 5% exhibiting geographic tongue. Reports of *Candida* infections and desquamative gingivitis have appeared. Poor oral hygiene resulting from hand involvement may also cause gingivitis.

Biopsies of geographic tongue lesions (migratory glossitis, erythema migrans) and lesions of Reiter's syndrome appear similar to those of psoriatic lesions. It is possible all these diseases may be related.

While the arthritis in psoriasis generally affects the fingers, the temporomandibular joint may also be involved.

DENTAL MANAGEMENT. Usually the lesions are asymptomatic and require no therapy, but sore mouths have been reported during mastication. Symptomatic relief can be gained with topical anesthetics. Intralesional steroid injections may eliminate discrete lesions but are impractical for diffuse lesions; topical steroids may help. Neutral rinses and a bland diet will prevent some of the soreness.

While no therapy is contraindicated, there have been reports of problems in obtaining a clear incision line during periodontal surgery. Lesions seem to flare up if traumatized. Patients have tolerated prosthetic appliances. Arthritis in the temporomandibular joint may be a problem and hard to treat, but anti-inflammatory drugs and injections of steroids may help. Special hygiene aids may be needed in a patient with severe hand problems.

Systemic involvement may also present a problem. Diabetes, myopathia, ulcerative colitis, and *Candida* infections may affect oral treatment. The *Candida* infection may be treated with nystatin or ketoconazole. The systemic effects of drug therapy (steroids, methotrexate) will alter working conditions and the patient taking steroids may require supplemental steroids as well as have altered healing. Methotrexate may alter bone marrow function and cause oral ulcerations.

BIBLIOGRAPHY

Baker, H.: Psoriasis: a review, Dermatologica **150**:16, 1975.
Baker, H., and Ryan, T.J.: Generalized pustular psoriasis: a clinical and epidemiological study of 104 cases, Br. J. Dermatol. **80**:771, 1968.
Buchner, A., and others: Oral lesion in psoriatic patients, Oral Surg. **41**:327, 1976.
DeGregori, G., Pippon, R., and Davies, E.: Psoriasis of the gingiva and tongue: report of a case, J. Periodontol. **42**:97, 1971.
Doben, D.I.: Psoriasis of the attached gingiva, J. Periodontol. **47**:38, 1976.
Farber, E.M., and Cox, A.J., editors: Psoriasis: proceedings of the second international symposium, New York, 1977, Yorke Medical Books.
Farber E.M., and Nall, M.L.: The natural history of psoriasis in 5600 patients, Dermatologica **148**:118, 1974.
Fischman, S.L., Barnett, M.L., and Nisengard, R.J.: Histopathologic, ultrastructural and immunologic findings in an oral psoriatic lesions, Oral Surg. **44**:253, 1977.
Jones, L.E., and others: Desquamative gingivitis associated with psoriasis, J. Periodontol. **42**:35, 1972.
Pisanty, S., and Ship, I.I.: Oral psoriasis, Oral Surg. **30**:351, 1970.
Salmon, T.N., and others: Oral psoriasis, Oral Surg. **28**:48, 1974.
Svejgaard, A., and others: HL-A in psoriasis vulgaris and in pustular psoriasis population and family studies, Br. J. Dermatol. **91**:145, 1974.
White, D.K., Lewis, H.J., and Miller, A.S.: Interoral psoriasis associated with widespread dermal psoriasis, Oral Surg. **41**:174, 1976.

ERYTHEMA MIGRANS

Erythema migrans or geographic tongue has the histopathology of a psoriatic lesion. Some authors suggest an infectious agent, nutritional alteration, allergy, or psychosomatic process as a probable cause. While the process is commonly thought of as being limited to the tongue, it has been reported in other areas of the mouth. Clinically, the lesions of stomatitis or glossitis migrans appear to migrate daily, with the margins changing shape. They appear as well-circumscribed areas of red, depapillated, desquamating epithelium with a yellow to white border and slightly raised in comparison to other surrounding areas. The process is self-limited and may remain present in some form for long periods or at times may completely resolve.

DENTAL MANAGEMENT. No treatment is indicated for geographic tongue or stomatitis, except rare palliative treatment for burning, pain, or itching such as a bland diet (avoid citrus fruits) and topical anesthetics in extreme cases.

BIBLIOGRAPHY

Hume, W.J.: Geographic stomatitis: a critical review, J. Dent. **3**:25, 1975.
Marks, M.B.: Recognizing the allergic person, Am. Fam. Phys. **16**:72, 1977.
Rahaminoff, P., and Muhsam, H.V.: Some observations on 1246 cases of geographic tongue Am. J. Dis. Child. **93**:519, 1957.
Redman, R.S., and others: Psychological component in the etiology of geographic tongue, J. Dent. Res. **45**:1403, 1966.
Sapiro, S.M., and Shklar, G.: Stomatitis areata migrans, Oral Surg. **36**:28, 1973.
Weathers, D.R., and others: Psoriasiform lesions of the oral mucosa (with emphasis on "ectopic geographic tongue"), Oral Surg. **37**:872, 1974.

LICHEN PLANUS

Lichen planus is a unique eruption of symmetrically distributed, flat-topped, polyhedral, violaceous papules usually involving flexural surfaces and mucous membranes either as single lesions or in groups. There is no predilection for race or sex. The cause is unknown, but the finding of immunoglobulins at the dermal-epidermal interface has led some to hypothesize an immune pathogenesis for this disease. The appearance of lichen planus is linked to emotional stress and has also been attributed to viral infections and genetic predisposition. Lesions of the oral mucosa are found in two thirds of all cases of lichen planus of the glabrous skin. There are many pattern variations, of which the most important are annualar lesions, most commonly found on the genitalia; hypertrophic lesions, seen over the distal lower extremities; follicular or cicatricial alopecia of lichen planopilaris, occurring in hair-bearing regions; and the typical pterygia of lichen planus found on the nail plate. Histopathologically, there are characteristic changes that distinguish lichen planus from other disease processes. The treatment is usually symptomatic, including topical, intralesional, and systemic corticosteroids depending on the severity of the symptoms. In most cases the lesions resolve spontaneously within 8 to 12 months; however, in some cases years may pass before lesions disappear. Recurrences are common.

ORAL MANIFESTATIONS. As mentioned, oral lesions occur in about two thirds of all patients with skin lesions, but these represent only half of the cases of oral lichen planus. Only about 30% to 50% of patients with oral lichen planus may have skin lesions. The most common location is the buccal mucosa opposite the molars (generally bilaterally), but lesions can occur on the palate, tongue, lips, and gingiva.

The classic lesion is the reticular form. This has been described a slightly raised, radiating, bluish white or gray, lacy, velvety, threadlike papule in a linear, annular, or netlike arrangement. Wickham's striae are commonly seen. Occasionally the lesions coalesce to a large plaque with radiating striae. Another form is the erosive or vesicular form. Here the lesions are vesicles or blisters that promptly rupture, leaving a raw red erosion of irregular shape and size. Occasionally a pseudomembrane may cover the lesion. On the gingiva, it may resemble desquamative gingivitis. A rarer form is the atrophic type. These may be found on the tongue and have a smooth flat atrophic red appearance that is poorly defined and has peripheral striae.

A biopsy may be needed for diagnosis. Like the skin, the histopathology will be diagnostic and shows "saw toothed" rete ridges, a subepithelial bandlike infiltrate of lymphocytes, liquefaction degeneration of the epithelial basement membrane, and hyperparakeratosis.

DENTAL MANAGEMENT. The lesions are generally asymptomatic, but burning has been reported, especially in the erosive form. Symptomatic relief with topical anesthetics and the use of neutral mouthrinses and bland food and avoidance of alcoholic mouth rinses and temperature extremes in food will help. Treatment of the lesions has included intralesional steroids for small areas and topical steroids such as betamethasone. Dentures in contact with the lesions appear to be a problem only when ulcers are present. Topical applications of steroids under the denture may help. Oral hygiene must be stressed and the patient aided, especially when erosive gingival lesions are present.

The most severe problem is found in the patient who is high strung, emotional, and overanxious. "Cancer phobia" is common, and a biopsy may help "treat" the patient's fear. Cancer has been reported in less than 1% of the cases, although some reports indicate a higher precent in erosive lichen planus. There is debate as to whether or not diabetes is related to oral lichen planus. Some research shows no increased incidence, but an earlier report by Howell showed that out of 316 patients with "lichen planus" 13% had diabetes (20% in erosive lichen planus).

BIBLIOGRAPHY

Altman, J., and Perry, H.C.: The variations and course of lichen planus, Arch. Dermatol. **84**:47, 1961.

Al-Ubaidy, S.S., and Nally, F.F.: Oral lichen planus—a clinical evaluation of 120 cases over a 12 year period, J. International Dent. Assoc. **20**:257, 1974.

Andreasen, J.O.: Oral lichen planus, Oral Surg. **25**:31, 1968.

Boozer, C.H.: Benign migratory glossitis associated with lichen planus, J. Oral Med. **29**:58, 1974.

Christensen, E.: Arterial blood pressure in patients with oral lichen planus, J. Oral Pathol. **6**:139, 1977.

Christensen, E.: Glucose tolerance in patients with oral lichen planus, J. Oral Pathol. **6**:143, 1977.

Fellner, M.J.: Lichen planus—a review, Int. J. Dermatol. **19**:71, 1980.

Greenspan, J.S.: Oral lichen planus—a double blind comparison of treatment with betamethasone valerate aerosol and pellets, Br. Dent. J. **144**:83, 1978.

Herschfus, L.: Lichen planus, J. Mich. Dent. Assoc. **57**:170, 1975.

Holmstrup, P.: The frequency of *candida* in oral lichen planus, Scand. J. Dent. Res. **82**:584, 1974.

Howell, F.V., and Rick, G.M.: Oral lichen planus and diabetes: a potential syndrome, J. Calif. Dent. Assoc. **1**:58, 1973.

Jolly, M.: Lichen planus and its association with diabetes mellitus, Med. J. Aust. **1**:990, 1972.

Kay, L.W.: Corticosteroids in disease of oral mucosa, Int. Dent. J. **26**:405, 1976.

Kritchkoff, D.J.: Oral lichen planus: evidence regarding potential malignant transformation, J. Oral. Pathol. **7**:1, 1976.

Lund, W.S.: Treatment of superficial lesions of the mouth and pharynx, J. Laryngol. Otol. **90**:105, 1976.

Randell, S.: Erosive lichen planus, management of oral lesions with intralesional corticosteroid injections, J. Oral Med. **29**:88, 1974.

Reisman, R.J.: The malignant potential of oral lichen planus—diagnostic pitfall, Oral Surg. **38**:227, 1974.

Section Thirteen
DISORDERS OF THE DIGESTIVE SYSTEM
edited by **Walter Rubin**

169 • THE STRUCTURE AND FUNCTION OF THE DIGESTIVE SYSTEM

Walter Rubin

OVERVIEW

The gut is a long, muscular tube that propels ingested food and accumulated secretions caudad from its origin at the bottom of the hypopharynx to the rectum and anus, where its contents are evacuated during defecation. The major role of the gut is to assimilate from the diet the nutrients that are essential for good health: adequate calories, proteins, fats, carbohydrates, vitamins, minerals, and water. The normal assimilation of most ingested proteins, fats, and carbohydrates depends on two processes: (1) the intraluminal digestion or hydrolysis of large, nonabsorbable molecules into smaller ones, a process mediated largely by digestive enzymes secreted into the lumen of the gut, and (2) the transport or absorption of digested substances by the lining epithelial cells from the lumen of the gut into its wall, from which they are transported by the blood and lymphatic vessels to the liver and other organs of the body. Normally almost all dietary calories, proteins, carbohydrates, lipids, and water are assimilated, with the exception of cellulose, some oligosaccharides, and other dietary fiber and roughage that cannot be digested.

The gut is divided into several anatomic divisions—esophagus, stomach, small intestine, and large intestine—each of which performs certain specialized functions. The esophagus serves merely as a conduit to move food from the hypopharynx into the stomach. The stomach serves primarily as a secretory organ and a reservoir. It secretes acid (to kill swallowed bacteria), mucus, and pepsinogen (a proteolytic enzyme that helps digest dietary protein), but the stomach's only essential secretion is intrinsic factor, a glycopeptide that permits adequate absorption of dietary vitamin B_{12}. The reservoir function of the stomach is also important. The stomach collects food that has been hurriedly swallowed and empties it slowly into the duodenum, the proximal small intestine, so that its acidity can be rapidly neutralized, its osmolality quickly made isotonic, and its nutrients comfortably digested and absorbed. This proximal region of the small intestine is the principal site of digestion and absorption and therefore is the most important region of the gut. When chyme enters the duodenum, it stimulates the pancreas to secrete sodium bicarbonate into the duodenum, which neutralizes the gastric acid, and more important, to secrete many digestive enzymes that are essential for the normal digestion of food. Chyme in the duodenum also stimulates the gallbladder to contract and discharge stored bile through the common bile duct and the relaxed distal Oddi's sphincter into the duodenum. Although most nutrients are absorbed in the proximal small bowel, vitamin B_{12} is absorbed predominantly in the distal small intestine (ileum), which contains receptors for the vitamin B_{12}–intrinsic factor complex. The bile acids that promote fat absorption in the proximal small intestine are themselves also reabsorbed primarily in the distal small bowel, returned to the liver, and resecreted into the bile, to be brought once again into the duodenum; this process is called enterohepatic circulation.

A large amount of water and electrolytes is transported across the gut. Each day about 9 L of fluid enters the upper small intestine: about 2 L from the diet, 1.5 L from saliva, 2.5 L from gastric secretion, 1.5 L from the pancreas, 0.5 L from bile, and 1 L from intestinal secretions. Most of this fluid, about 8 L, is absorbed in the small intestine; only about 1 L enters the large intestine, whose major role is to extract most of the remaining water, store the feces in the rectum and sigmoid colon, and evacuate them when desired. About 100 to 200 g of feces is normally defecated daily. Diarrhea is present by definition when more than 300 g or 300 ml of stool is defecated in a day. If more than approximately 2 L of fluid enters the large bowel each day, even a normal colon cannot absorb enough water to reduce the daily fecal weight to less than 300 g. Thus diarrhea may result from a failure of either the small or large intestine to function normally. Net absorption is the net result of influxes into and outfluxes from the gut lumen. Thus diarrhea may result either from a failure of true absorption (outflux) or from excessive secretion (influx). The tremendous diarrhea associated with cholera, for example, results from extraordinary secretion in the small bowel. Cyclic adenosine monophosphate (AMP) in intestinal epithelial cells promotes their secretion, and thus any cause of elevated intestinal cyclic AMP promotes secretory diarrhea.

Although the histology of the gut is fundamentally similar in all its segments, there are variations, especially of the epithelial cells, that reflect the specialized functions of each of the divisions. The basic histologic structure of the gut wall consists of four layers, or tunicae. The innermost layer, the mucosa, consists of a surface epithelium resting on a layer of loose connective tissue (lamina propria) that is delimited below by a narrow layer of smooth muscle (muscularis mucosae). In most regions of the gut the epithelial cells extend from the surface into the lamina propria—and sometimes even below, as in the duodenum—to form a network of glands. Below the muscularis mucosae, the second layer, the submucosa, consists of a denser connective tissue through which numerous larger arteries, veins, and lymphatics traverse. The third layer, the muscularis externa, which is largely responsible for the contractile or motor activity of the gut, is a thick layer of smooth muscle formed in most regions by an inner layer of circumferentially oriented fibers and an outer layer of longitudinally oriented fibers. In the proximal third of the esophagus and distal rectum and anus, the smooth muscle is replaced in part or entirely by skeletal (voluntary) muscle, thus subjecting these areas to diseases that affect skeletal rather than smooth muscle. The fourth or outermost layer of gut, the adventitia, consists of a narrow layer of connective tissue and contains many larger traversing vessels. Along much of its length this layer is covered by a flat epithelium or mesothelium (mesentery) and in such areas is referred to as the serosa.

The epithelial cells that line the gut and form its glands are the most important constituent cells because they largely determine most of the specialized functions characteristic of each segment and play an important protective role in each. These cells are continually turning over; they die, are desquamated into the lumen of the gut, and are replaced through the replication, differentiation, and migration of undifferentiated epithelial cells located within the glands or, in the esophagus, at the base of the epithelium. This process is extremely important for the maintenance of normal populations of epithelial cells and therefore for the structural and functional integrity of the gut. Impairment of this process in the stomach, for example, by some forms of experimental stress can lead to ulceration of the surface. In celiac disease the rapid death of mature epithelial cells and their inadequate replacement through an increased rate of replication and differentiation lead to atrophy of the surface lining and malabsorption. Normally the cells lining the surface of the gut are completely renewed approximately every 3 to 7 days. Many of the cells in the glands, however, have a much longer life span; the parietal cells in the stomach, for example, are thought to live for many weeks.

Most of the gut epithelial secreting cells are exocrine cells; that is, they secrete mucus, digestive enzymes, acid, or other substances directly into the lumen of the gut or into the duct of a gland. The gut is also, however, the largest endocrine organ in the body and contains many different morphologic types of endocrine epithelial cells that secrete in a basal direction, into the lamina propria. These cells produce polypeptide hormones and biogenic amines, such as 5-hydroxytryptamine (serotonin). Some of these polypeptide hormones have been identified, and many of their apparent physiologic functions are understood: for example, secretin, the first hormone discovered, and cholecystokinin-pancreozymin (CCK-PZ), both from the proximal small intestine, and gastrin from the distal stomach and the proximal small intestine. Many other gut hormones and putative hormones have been discovered only recently, however, and their physiologic roles have yet to be defined. This group includes somatostatin, enteroglucagon, gastric inhibitory polypeptide (GIP), vasoactive intestinal polypeptide (VIP), probably located in nerves, bombesin, motilin, and enkephalin, also in nerves. When released, these substances may act locally rather than at distal sites; that is, they may serve "paracrine" rather than endocrine functions. The gut endocrine cells exhibit many morphologic and cytochemical characteristics of neurons, synthesize and secrete many polypeptides and amines also found in the nervous system, and have been considered a possible part of a neuroendocrine system. There are many similarities among different polypeptide and amine-synthesizing endocrine cells in the body. It has been suggested (perhaps erroneously) that these cells arise embryologically from neural ectoderm (neural crest) rather than entoderm. These cells have been named APUD (amine precursor uptake decarboxylation) cells, and tumors derived from them have been called apudomas.

The gut is also an important immunologic organ, active in both cell-mediated and humorally mediated immunologic processes. Lymph follicles are present along its length and are most prominent in the submucosa and mucosa particularly in the distal ileum, where they often form visible aggregates called Peyer's patches, and in the appendix and large intestine. Gut lymphocytes are recirculated: they drain from the gut back into the systemic circulation through the intestinal lymphatics and thoracic duct. Disease processes that block the drainage of lymph and lymphocytes from the gut into the systemic circulation, such as Whipple's disease and lymphangiectasia, characteristically reduce the numbers of lymphocytes observed in peripheral blood counts. The lamina propria of the gut normally contains numerous plasma cells that produce all classes of immunoglobulins but predominantly IgA (see Chapter 3). Much of this IgA, sometimes called secretory IgA, can be found within the gut lumen; much is along the surface of the lining epithelium in the form of a dimer bound to a glycopeptide, which is produced by the epithelial cells and has been called secretory piece and transport piece. How the IgA is secreted into the gut lumen and the possible role of secretory piece in this process have not been clearly defined. The gut may be the site of primary immunizations; secretory IgA and local immunologically competent cells are thought to play important roles in protecting the gut and body from potentially harmful substances, microorganisms, and other agents that enter the body by the intestinal route. It is also thought that immunologic processes occurring in the gut may go awry and cause some poorly understood inflammatory diseases, such as ulcerative colitis and granulomatous ileocolitis.

The gut has millions of intrinsic neurons whose cell bodies are arranged largely within two plexuses: the myenteric (Auerbach's) plexus, located between the circular and transverse muscle layers of the muscularis externa, and the submucous (Meissner's) plexus, located along the submucosa. Much of the motor activity of the gut is intrinsic, regulated in large measure by this intrinsic nervous system. It is also modulated in part, however, by the innervation of extrinsic nerves—the classic postganglionic sympathetic (thoracolumbar) and preganglionic parasympathetic (craniosacral) nerves—and by humoral agents. Parasympathetic stimulation has classically been thought to have excitatory effects on the gut and sympathetic stimulation inhibitory effects, but this view is proving to be much too simplistic. The extrinsic nerves, particularly the vagus, are mixed nerves containing numerous afferent as well as efferent fibers and releasing many neurohumoral mediators, with varying physiologic effects. In general, gut contractility, secretion, and blood flow vary together. Whenever the motor activity of the gut is stimulated, its secretory activity and blood flow are also usually increased. Eating is the usual physiologic stimulus that activates the digestive system.

ESOPHAGUS AND SWALLOWING

The esophagus, the first part of the gut, extends from the hypopharynx, where the cricopharyngeus muscle forms its upper esophageal sphincter, through the posterior aspect of the chest, to join the stomach just below the diaphragm. The lower esophageal sphincter is a nonanatomic, physiologic high-pressure zone that extends along the last few centimeters of the esophagus and normally prevents the regurgitation of the gastric contents, including acid, back into the esophagus. The esophagus is the least sophisticated part of the gut; it serves only as a conduit to bring swallowed food and saliva from the hypopharynx to the stomach. Thus it is lined by a stratified squamous epithelium to protect against "wear and tear."

Swallowing is a complex physiologic process integrated through a swallowing center in the medulla oblongata. After food is chewed into small pieces and lubricated with alkaline mucous saliva, which also contains amylase and some lipase enzymatic activities, the tongue moves a bolus of food back into the pharynx to initiate swallowing. The pharyngeal muscles contract and the soft palate is elevated, occluding the passage between the pharynx and nasopharynx and preventing the regurgitation of food into the nose. The glottis closes and the epiglottis folds over it, preventing the aspiration of food into the respiratory passages. The contraction of the pharyngeal muscles moves the food into the hypopharynx, and the upper esophageal sphincter relaxes, permitting the bolus to enter the esophagus. A primary peristaltic wave is initiated in the upper esophagus, which with the aid of gravity moves the bolus down the esophagus. Finally, the lower esophageal sphincter relaxes, permitting the bolus to enter the stomach, the fundus of which relaxes (receptive relaxation) to receive it. Each of these processes—the blockage of the nasopharynx and respiratory tract, the relaxation of the sphincters, and the initiation of the primary peristalsis—is independently initiated by deglutition and is integrated through the swallowing center. Impairment of any of these processes, for example, by a neurologic or muscular disorder, can result in serious consequences while eating, such as the aspiration of food into the lungs, the regurgitation of food through the nose, or the inability of food to enter the esophagus. If the esophagus is distended, for example, by a piece of food that is stuck or regurgitated from the stomach, a secondary peristaltic wave is initiated at a level just above the distention to move the piece down into the stomach.

STOMACH

The stomach, the short second segment of gut, is a secretory organ and more usefully functions as a reservoir. However, its secretion of the glycoprotein intrinsic factor, which is necessary for the adequate absorption of dietary vitamin B_{12}, is actually its only essential function. Intrinsic factor and essentially isotonic hydrochloric acid are secreted by the parietal (oxyntic) cells, a major constituent of the gastric glands throughout most of the gastric mucosa. Pepsin, a proteolytic enzyme secreted as the proenzyme pepsinogen, which is activated by acid and pepsin itself, is produced by the chief cells, the second major constituent of the same gastric glands, although immunologically identifiable pepsinogens are also produced by gastric mucous cells. The surface of the stomach and the numerous pits (foveolae) that connect the surface with the gastric glands below are lined by mucous cells. These are largely responsible for the neutral mucus or glycoprotein that coats and lubricates the surface of the stomach and is thought to play some protective role as well. The glands in the pyloric antrum, the most distal portion of the stomach, and also in the cardia, a narrow segment of stomach encircling the esophagogastric junction, are lined by a different type of mucous cell (pyloric gland cell) and contain few if any parietal or chief cells. Also present within the gastric glands, although these are usually not apparent in routine hematoxylin- and eosin-stained histologic sections, are at least four morphologic types of endocrine cells. The G cells, located in pyloric glands, produce the hormone gastrin; the D cells produce somatostatin; and the EC cells produce serotonin (5-hydroxytryptamine); the product of the ECL cells has not yet been identified. The replicating undifferentiated cells that maintain the populations of the differentiated epithelial cells are located in the upper regions (necks) of the glands.

The surface of the stomach is quite impermeable to water and ions, a property probably resulting largely from the tightness of the junctions between the adjoining epithelial cells. As a result, hypotonic and hypertonic solutions can be maintained for some time within the gastric lumen. The impermeability of the surface to ions permits an electric potential of about -40 to -60 mV, possibly generated largely by a parietal Cl^- pump, to be maintained between the luminal and serosal surfaces of the mucosa. The impermeability to H^+—the so-called mucosal barrier to acid back-diffusion—plays an important protective role by preventing the acid secreted into the lumen from diffusing back into the mucosa. When this barrier is broken, for example, by agents such as aspirin and ethanol, acid can diffuse back into the mucosa, often causing erosions, ulceration, and even hemorrhage. This is thought to be the mechanism by which alcohol and aspirin cause erosive gastritis. Damage to the mucosal barrier can be detected by a decrease in or loss of the normal transmucosal potential difference. In recent years certain prostaglandins have been discovered to possess cytoprotective properties; by some poorly understood mechanism, these seem to protect the stomach and maintain its structural and functional integrity.

During the interdigestive (fasting) period the stomach is usually inactive; it exhibits little motor activity and secretes little fluid, most of which resembles an ultrafiltrate of plasma and little of which is thought to arise from the parietal cells. In fact, the normal fasting person secretes only about 2 to 5 mEq acid an hour. The act of eating or even hunger, the thought of food, or the desire to eat stimulates gastric motor and secretory activity; a normal meal usually stimulates this activity for about 3 to 4 hours. Although the stimulated secretions contain mucus from mucous cells and pepsinogen from chief cells, most of the volume is probably produced by the parietal cells, which secrete intrinsic factor and approximately isotonic hydrochloric acid. Thus the composition of gastric juice secreted during a meal approaches that of the parietal cells, and its pH may approach 1 (100 mEq H^+/L) or even lower. Many substances stimulate the parietal cells to secrete, including Ca^{++}, caffeine, amino acids, and peptides, but acetylcholine, gastrin, and histamine are probably the most potent and physiologically important stimulants. The parietal cell membrane seems to have receptors for each of these three stimulants, and the effect produced by one seems to be related to the actions of the other two. If the receptor for histamine is blocked by a histamine H_2-receptor blocking agent (for example, cimetidine) or if the muscarinic effects of acetylcholine are reduced with atropine or a vagotomy, the responsiveness of the parietal cells to the other two respective agents is markedly reduced. That is the reason, for example, why acid secretion can be almost abolished with cimetidine even though this agent in essence only eliminates the "histamine tone" on the parietal cell. The role played by possible second messengers, such as cyclic AMP or GMP, remains unclear, but the final secretion of H^+ at the cell membrane seems dependent on a K^+, H^+-ATPase that promotes an exchange of H^+ for K^+. The secreted H^+ comes from carbonic acid formed from the reaction of carbon dioxide and water, which is mediated by the enzyme carbonic anhydrase. Thus for every H^+ molecule secreted, a HCO_3^- molecule is released into the lamina propria, thus accounting for the alkaline venous blood, or alkaline tide, that flows from the stomach during a meal.

Although a meal stimulates gastric secretion for 3 to 4 hours, the maximum rate of acid secretion is reached in about 1 hour. Monitoring the acidity of the gastric contents during a meal often reveals a rather precipitous fall in the pH after about 1 hour. During the first hour the secreted acid is usually well buffered by the ingested food, especially by the protein. After this hour, however, much of the food has left the stomach and much of the buffering capacity of the retained food has been exhausted; the acid that is now being secreted at about its maximal rate can no longer be adequately buffered and the pH usually falls toward 1, where it generally remains for several additional hours. Thus patients with peptic ulcers often have immediate symptomatic relief by eating because the food buffers the gastric acid, but their pain often returns 1 or more hours later because of the presence of unbuffered gastric acid produced by the very food they may have originally ingested to relieve their pain. The dietary protein, the greatest buffer of gastric acid, is also the major stimulus of its secretion.

The stimulation of gastric secretion and motor activity by a meal is traditionally divided into three phases: cephalic, gastric, and intestinal. The cephalic phase is the stimulation before the food even reaches the stomach. Feeling hungry, thinking of eating, smelling food, hearing the dinner bell (as with Pavlov's dogs), chewing, tasting, and swallowing all stimulate gastric secretion. The efferent limb of this stimulation is mediated by the vagus nerves, which stimulate secretion largely by their release of acetylcholine in the wall of the stomach, which in turn stimulates the parietal cells not only directly but possibly indirectly by stimulating a release of gastrin from the antral G cells. The cephalic phase of gastric secretion can be eliminated by a vagotomy or reduced by anticholinergic drugs or by the traditionally bland, unseasoned diets that make eating tasteless and unattractive. The gastric phase of gastric secretion is initiated by the presence of food in the stomach. This stimulation is mediated by gastrin, whose release is stimulated by dietary constituents such as peptide and Ca^{++}; by intrinsic and extrinsic nerves, which are activated at least in part by gastric distention and which lead again to the release of acetylcholine; and by dietary substances such as peptides, amino acids, caffeine, and Ca^{++}, which directly stimulate the parietal cells. The intestinal phase of gastric secretion is stimulated by the entrance of the chyme into the small intestine and is mediated probably again by both neural and humoral factors and at least in part by the release of gastrin from the duodenum. In all three phases the three major stimulants at the site of the parietal cells are probably acetylcholine, gastrin, and histamine, released from cholinergic nerve terminals, endocrine cells, and mast cells, respectively.

The control of acid secretion is very complex; in fact, there are humoral and neural feedback mechanisms that tend to reduce its secretion. For example, when secreted acid bathes the antrum, it suppresses the secretion of gastrin, inhibiting it completely when the pH is reduced to approximately 1. When acid enters the duodenum it also tends to reduce gastric acid secretion, perhaps in part through its stimulation of the release of secretin and possibly other enterogastrones, humoral agents (hormones) released from the small intestine that inhibit gastric activity.

The acid secretory function of a patient's stomach can be assessed clinically. A nasogastric tube is passed into the subject's stomach while he is fasting, and the gastric secretions are continually aspirated and titrated to neutrality with sodium hydroxide. In this way the basal acid output (BAO), the rate of acid secretion during fasting, is determined. The patient then receives a stimulant of gastric secretion—usually histamine, histalog, or more commonly pentagastrin, a synthetic pentapeptide containing the active tetrapeptide of gastrin—in a dose to elicit a maximal secretory response from the patient's stomach. The aspirates are collected during four subsequent 15-minute periods and again are titrated. The largest amount of acid secreted in a period, usually during the second or third period, multiplied by four gives the maximal acid output (MAO) or peak acid output (PAO), that is, the maximal rate at which that patient's stomach can secrete acid. The MAO is actually a measurement of the number of parietal cells in a subject's stomach: the more parietal cells, the more acid the stomach can secrete when maximally stimulated. The values obtained vary somewhat among different laboratories, but the BAO of most normal subjects is about 2 to 5 mEq acid on hour, and the MAO is about 20 to 30 mEq acid an hour. Patients with atrophic changes in their stomachs (atrophic gastritis or gastric atrophy) and therefore with diminished numbers of parietal cells secrete smaller amounts, whereas patients with duodenal ulcer disease as a group secrete more acid than normal subjects in both the basal and stimulated states, findings that indicate these patients have more parietal cells and are less successful in reducing or ceasing acid secretion during the basal (fasting) state. The marked hypersecretory characteristics observed in patients with gastrinomas (Zollinger-Ellison syndrome) are discussed in Chapter 173.

As already noted, in the interdigestive period the stomach exhibits little motor activity as well. Even then the stomach is thought to contain an electrogenic pacemaker, located high on the greater curvature of its body, which emits myoelectric waves at a rate of about 3 waves a minute. These waves are conducted along the outer longitudinal muscle layer. They produce few muscle depolarization spikes and contractions. When motor activity is stimulated by eating or by hunger (hunger pangs probably result from gastric peristalsis, possibly initiated through the vagus by a low or falling blood sugar), peristaltic contractions arise in the mid to distal body of the stomach at the same pacemaker rate and sweep caudad through the antrum toward the muscular pyloric sphincter, which forms the junction between the distal stomach and duodenum. The rate at which the gastric contents are emptied into the duodenum probably depends not only on the physical nature of the contents (liquids and solids of varying size and consistency) but also on the completion of the peristaltic waves, the force of antral contractions, the squeeze and tension in the pyloric sphincter, the pressure generated in the proximal duodenum (bulb), and the interrelationships of these ever-changing factors. This motor activity that regulates the rate of gastric emptying is in turn controlled by the intrinsic and extrinsic nerves, humoral agents, and locally released, active paracrine substances, the same factors that affect gastric secretion.

As noted previously a major physiologic function of the stomach is to act as a reservoir. Although meals may be eaten in only a few minutes and the food passes rapidly through the esophagus, the food is stored in the stomach, is churned in the antrum by its motor activity, and is slowly emptied into the proximal small intestine, the major site of digestion and absorption. The regulation of gastric emptying is extremely important in avoiding impaired absorption and the unpleasant symptoms commonly produced when the gastric contents are rapidly emptied or dumped into the small intestine (dumping syndrome). These symptoms are often observed in patients who have undergone gastric surgery, usually for ulcer disease or tumors.

Many factors affect the rate of gastric emptying: the amount and physical state of the gastric contents and the pH, osmolality, lipid content, and caloric content of the chyme being emptied into the duodenum. These factors presumably affect gastroduodenal motor activity largely through the neural and hormonal mechanisms already mentioned. The greater the gastric content and distention, the more rapid gastric emptying tends to be. Liquids are emptied more rapidly than solids, and small solids more easily than large ones. The greater the acidity, hyperosmolality (and in part hypo-osmolality), fat content, and caloric content of the chyme entering the duodenum, the stronger is the feedback from the duodenum to slow down the rate of gastric emptying. These feedback regulatory processes initiated in the duodenum permit the acid chyme to be rapidly neutralized and made isotonic within the duodenum and the fat and other nutrients to be more leisurely and adequately digested and absorbed in the proximal small intestine, as described more fully in the following section.

SMALL INTESTINE, PANCREAS, AND LIVER

The small intestine, about 20 feet (6 M) in length, is composed of the duodenum, jejunum, and ileum. The duodenum, the short first segment, consists of the bulb, just beyond the stomach, and the descending, transverse, and ascending portions, which are retroperitoneal and partially encircle the head of the pancreas. At the ligament of Treitz, where the duodenum assumes a mesenteric covering and penetrates into the peritoneal cavity at the base of the mesentery, it becomes the jejunum, the proximal half of the remaining small intestine; the distal half is the ileum. The junction between the two halves is arbitrary and involves no structural or functional demarcation. The ileum ends at the ileocecal valve, the muscular sphincter between the small and large intestines.

The surface area of the small intestine is enhanced by the presence of many visible folds (plicae circulares) and numerous finger-shaped projections of the mucosa, the intestinal villi, which can be seen with a magnifying glass or low-power microscope. The villi are lined by tall columnar epithelial cells (differentiate villous epithelial cells) that have numerous tall apical microvilli, seen with a light microscope as a prominent striated (brush) border. These are the most important cells in the gut because they are responsible for the absorption of digested nutrients from the bowel lumen into the lamina propria; many of the important enzymes and carrier systems for this transport are associated with the brush border membrane. At the base of the villi, the epithelium forms glands, or crypts, that extend into the lamina propria to the muscularis mucosae. The crypts are lined predominantly by undifferentiated cells but also contain, especially at their bases, serous cells, the Paneth's cells, that contain prominent apical secretory granules, the nature and function of which have yet to be clearly defined. Goblet cells, mucous cells that secrete an acid mucus and that resemble brandy goblets when distended with mucus, are located along the crypts and villi. Again, several morphologic types of endocrine cells are present, predominantly in the crypts, but these are usually not apparent in routinely stained sections.

The pancreas is a retroperitoneal gland whose head is encircled by the duodenum and whose body and tail extend to the left and upward, behind the stomach and lesser sac, to the hilus of the spleen. The pancreas is actually a dual organ. Its islets of Langerhans, which are more numerous in its body and tail, are aggregates of at least four types of endocrine cells that secrete insulin, glucagon, somatostatin, and pancreatic polypeptide. Most of the organ, however, functions as an exocrine gland whose acinar cells synthesize, store, and secrete many digestive enzymes, which flow through small ducts into the main duct of Wirsung or the accessory duct of Santorini and through the ampulla of Vater and Oddi's sphincter into the descending segment of the duodenum. The secretion from the acinar cells contains relatively little water in volume but is rich in the digestive enzymes, as follows:

1. *The proteolytic enzymes trypsinogen, chymotrypsinogin, procarboxypeptidase, proaminopeptidase, and elastase.* The trypsinogen is activated in the duodenum to trypsin by means of enterokinase, an enzyme in the brush border of the epithelial cells. In turn, trypsin activates trypsinogen and the other proenzymes to change to their active moieties.
2. *Amylase.* Amylase catalyzes the hydrolysis of α-1,4-glucosidic bonds and thereby converts dietary starch and glycogen to glucose, short straight-chain oligosaccharides (maltose and the like), and isomaltose.
3. *Lipolytic enzymes.* These are lipase, which hydrolyzes the 1 and 3 bonds of triglycerides, mechanically assisted by another secreted protein, colipase; phospholipases A_1 and A_2, which hydrolyze phospholipids, including the conversion of lecithin to lysolecithins; and other lipases that hydrolyze cholesterol esters and water-soluble esters of fatty acids.
4. *Ribonuclease and deoxyribonuclease*

In addition to the acinar secretion, the duct cells secrete a large volume of alkaline water that is rich in sodium bicarbonate.

The liver is also an endocrine and exocrine organ. Bile, its exocrine secretion, is secreted by the hepatocytes (liver parenchymal cells) into the canaliculi, the small excretory channels formed by adjacent hepatocytes. Bile drains into the bile ductules and ducts, which like the pancreatic ducts are lined by cells that secrete alkaline water rich in sodium bicarbonate into the bile. The bile flows from the left and right main hepatic ducts into the common hepatic duct and common bile duct. In the interdigestive (fasting) state, when Oddi's sphincter at the distal end of the common bile duct is closed, little bile enters the duodenum; most of it flows back through the cystic duct into the gallbladder, where it is stored and concentrated by the absorption of water and electrolytes by the lining epithelial cells. During a meal, however, the gallbladder is stimulated to contract and Oddi's sphincter to open, thereby permitting both stored and newly formed bile to flow into the duodenum.

Bile contains bile pigment, predominantly bilirubin

diglucuronide, which gives bile its yellow color. Bile also contains bile acids, lecithin, and cholesterol; the detergent bile acids and lecithin serve to solubilize insoluble cholesterol by incorporating it into mixed micelles. The bile acids are synthesized in the liver from cholesterol and are conjugated largely with glycine and taurine to form the principal primary bile acids: glycocholic, taurocholic, glycochenodeoxycholic, and taurochenodeoxycholic acids. These are stored mainly in the gallbladder bile during the fasting state and are released into the duodenum when the gallbladder empties during eating. They aid fat absorption mainly by solubilizing the fatty acids and monoglycerides produced by the digestion of dietary fat, thereby bringing them more rapidly to the surface of the absorbing intestinal epithelial cells. Although this physiologic function is performed predominantly in the proximal small intestine, the bile acids themselves are absorbed primarily in the distal ileum, returned to the liver, resecreted into the bile, and returned to the duodenum or gallbladder. In this way an individual bile acid molecule may be returned two or three times to the proximal small intestine during a single meal to aid in the absorption of the ingested lipid. This enterohepatic circulation helps to maintain the body's bile acid pool of 2 to 4 g. Only about 15% of this pool is lost in the feces each day, and this amount is readily restored by the synthesis of new bile acid in the liver. If the fecal loss of bile acid is increased because of disease, surgical removal, or a bypass of the distal ileum, hepatic synthesis also increases in an effort to maintain a normal pool of bile acid. The enhanced synthesis can compensate satisfactorily for a moderate loss of bile acid, but a greater rate of fecal loss results in a significant reduction in the bile acid pool.

The rate of bile secretion by the liver cells is greatly influenced by the rate at which the hepatocytes secrete bile acid, which in turn is influenced largely by the enterohepatic circulation and the rate at which bile acid is returned to the liver. In the fasting state, when most of the bile acid pool is stored in the gallbladder (or possibly in the intestine if there is no gallbladder), the liver cells usually make little bile. This bile is also often lithogenic; that is, it contains too much cholesterol in relation to its bile acid content, such that the bile is supersaturated in respect to cholesterol. The composition of this hepatic bile is usually corrected, however, when it enters the gallbladder and mixes with the stored bile there or when during a meal the contents of the gallbladder and its stored bile acids are emptied into the intestine, thereby causing the bile acids to move through the enterohepatic circulation and thus increase the rate of hepatic bile formation. Some individuals, however, especially those with diseased or absent terminal ileums and therefore reduced bile acid pools and those who have some metabolic derangement of hepatic function, secrete a more persistent lithogenic bile, making them more susceptible to the formation of cholesterol gallstones in the gallbladder.

DIGESTION, ABSORPTION, AND MOTILITY IN THE SMALL INTESTINE

When chyme enters the small intestine (duodenum), it initiates many rapid physiologic processes functioning principally to promote efficient and rapid digestion and absorption. Although the stomach can retain hyperosmolar and hypo-osmolar solutions, these are rapidly rendered isotonic when introduced into the duodenum. This occurs through active absorption, rapid fluxes of water across the mucosa, and dilution with the isotonic secretions of the pancreas, bile, and intestine. If much hypertonic solution is rapidly dumped into or produced during digestion in the small intestine, as may occur when the reservoir function of the stomach is impaired by gastric surgery, rapid fluxes of water from the blood into the intestinal lumen may quickly deplete the blood volume and lead to the symptoms of dumping syndrome (weakness, light-headedness, faintness, palpitations, sweating, and diarrhea).

When gastric acid enters the duodenum, it stimulates a quantitative release of the hormone secretin from the wall of the duodenum, which in turn stimulates the epithelium of the pancreatic and biliary ducts to secrete a large volume of their alkaline juices into the duodenum. In this way the acidic chyme is neutralized, the feedback slowing of the gastric emptying of acid in the duodenum permitting a more rapid and complete neutralization within the proximal duodenum. The neutralization of acid chyme within the proximal intestine is essential for normal absorption because an acid pH impairs the ability of the bile acids to solubilize the fatty acids and monoglycerides and also impairs the digestive action of the pancreatic enzymes. Lipase may be irreversibly denatured by an acid pH.

When chyme enters the duodenum, it stimulates the release of another hormone. CCK-PZ, largely because of its content of fatty acid. CCK-PZ in turn stimulates the gall-bladder to contract, the pancreatic acinar cells to secrete their enzyme-rich juice, and Oddi's sphincter to open, thereby permitting bile and pancreatic secretions to enter the duodenum easily. CCK-PZ and secretin are synergistic, each augmenting, the physiologic activity of the other. Even before chyme enters the duodenum, the act of eating produces some stimulation, especially of pancreatic secretion, through the cephalic and gastric phases; vagal cholinergic fibers and released gastrin, which structurally resembles CCK-PZ and engages in some of the same activity, stimulate some acinar secretion.

The pancreatic enzymes are essential for normal digestion. Salivary amylase, active at a neutral or alkaline pH, and gastric pepsin, active at an acid pH, play a digestive role but are unnecessary. Within the proximal small intestine the pancreatic enzymes digest dietary protein into amino acids and small peptides; starch and glycogen into glucose, maltose, other short-chain straight oligosaccharides, and isomaltose; and triglycerides (neutral fat) into fatty acids and 2-monoglycerides. These products of digestion together with other dietary substances, such as the disaccharides lactose from milk and milk products and sucrose (table sugar), must then be transported by the lining intestinal epithelial cells from the intestinal lumen into the lamina propria.

As already noted, the fatty acids and monoglycerides, as well as fat-soluble vitamins and cholesterol, are solubilized in mixed micelles by the bile acids so that they can move rapidly through the unstirred water layer to the surface membrane of the lining cells, which they penetrate passively. Within the epithelial cells most of the fatty acids and monoglycerides are resynthesized into triglyceride, which in turn is converted into chylomicron particles with the addition of phospholipid and β-lipoprotein to the surface. The chylomicrons are secreted into the lamina propria and drained by the lacteals (lymphatics) through the thoracic duct into the systemic circulation. Short- and medium- chain triglycerides, containing more soluble fatty acids with fewer than 10 and 10 to 14 carbon atoms, respectively, are more rapidly hydrolyzed within the intestine. They do not require solubilization within micelles, and most of their absorbed fatty acids are drained directly into the vascular capillaries of the portal circulation. The bile acids also aid fat digestion by promoting and stabilizing emulsions of fat particles within the intestinal lumen and by stabilizing and protecting lipase and colipase.

The amino acids are actively transported by the epithelium to the lamina propria. Some small peptides are hydrolyzed by peptidases in the brush border and cytosol of the epithelial cells, and the resultant amino acids are also transported across. A few small peptides cross the epithelial cells intact. All these products derived from dietary protein are absorbed mainly into the portal circulation.

Glucose and galactose are also actively absorbed by the lining epithelium. Several disaccharidase enzymes, located in the brush border of these lining cells, are also essential for the normal absorption of dietary carbohydrate. For example, luminal maltose and isomaltose, produced from the digestion of starch and glycogen, must be split by brush border maltase and isomaltase before their contained glucose can be satisfactorily transported across these cells. Similarly, milk sugar lactose must be split by lactase and sucrose by sucrase (invertase) to ensure normal absorption of their component hexoses, glucose-galactose and glucose-fructose, respectively. A deficiency of intestinal lactase, a common clinical occurrence, may result in the malabsorption of ingested lactose, the fermentation of lactose by intestinal bacteria, especially in the colon, and cramps and osmotic diarrhea if appreciable milk or dairy products are ingested.

The active absorption of glucose, galactose, and amino acids is coupled with the absorption of Na^+. Thus in certain secretory diarrhea states such as cholera, in which large amounts of body water and salt are lost by their voluminous secretion into the gut (because of activation of adenylate cyclase), the absorption of Na^+ and water can be promoted and partially restored by the oral administration of isotonic Na^+-containing fluids that also contain glucose or sucrose (which is split to glucose and fructose). The intestinal epithelial cells also contain a sodium pump that extrudes Na^+ from the cell into the interstitial fluid and thereby provides for the active absorption of Na^+ from the intestinal lumen. The absorption of the products of digestion and of Na^+ also provides for the secondary passive absorption of water from the lumen. The intestine can also absorb Cl^- actively, coupled in the jejunum and ileum with HCO_3^- secretion, and thus the chyme contains a higher concentration of HCO_3^- and becomes more alkaline toward the distal ileum.

The absorption of most vitamins (except B_{12}), iron, and calcium is also maximal in the proximal small intestine; the absorption of some is complex and is still not entirely understood. Calcium absorption is promoted by vitamin D, possibly because of its effects on binding protein, whereas iron absorption is enhanced by the presence of anemia.

The motor activity of the small intestine, quiescent during the interdigestive state, is aroused by eating, an effect also mediated by intrinsic and extrinsic nerves and hormones. The small intestine exhibits little peristaltic activity but rather has prominent multiple segmental contractions that squirt the chyme forward and backward, thereby mixing it with the digestive enzymes and other secretions and promoting digestion and absorption. Because these contractions are more frequent in the proximal than in the distal small bowel, the net effect is to propel the chyme forward toward the large intestine. When the distal ileum contracts, the ileocecal sphincter is stimulated to relax, permitting the chyme to be squirted into the cecum of the large intestine. An increased pressure in the cecum, produced by distention or contractions of the cecum, for example, in turn stimulates the ileocecal sphincter to contract to prevent the contaminated cecal contents from regurgitating back into the ileum. The normal small intestine is practically sterile, largely because its motor activity effectively propels the chyme forward, but the large intestine, which is essentially a large, stagnant loop, contains high titers of bacteria. Whenever the contents of the small intestine are in stasis because of either impaired motor activity or a mechanical blockage, abnormal numbers of bacteria proliferate in the stagnant small intestine and may lead to malabsorption of fat and vitamin B_{12} (bacterial overgrowth or stagnant loop syndrome).

LARGE INTESTINE

The colon, or large bowel, is divided into several segments: (1) the cecum, the blind pouch into which the ileum empties and from which the small rudimentary appendix extends, (2) the ascending colon, (3) the hepatic flexure, (4) the transverse colon, (5) the splenic flexure, (6) the descending colon, (7) the sigmoid colon, (8) the rectum, and (9) the anus. The ascending colon, descending colon, rectum, and anus are extraperitoneal and relatively fixed.

In contrast the cecum (usually), transverse colon, and sigmoid colon are invested with a mesentery, are located within the abdominal cavity, and are much more movable. The rectum begins where the sigmoid colon exists from the abdominal cavity, a point about 16 cm from the anal orifice. The anus, or anal canal, comprises the distal 2 to 3 cm of the large bowel, from the point where the columnar epithelium of the rectum becomes stratified squamous epithelium to the anal orifice where the anus joins the skin. The outer longitudinal muscle of the colon does not form a complete layer but rather is organized into three longitudinal bands, the taeniae coli. The final muscular sphincter at the end of the large bowel, which is ultimately responsible for fecal continence, is actually a dual sphincter: the internal anal sphincter, prominent smooth muscle that is continuous with the muscularis externa, and the external anal sphincter, a surrounding sheath of skeletal or voluntary muscle (the levator ani) that is innervated by neurons emanating from sacral segments of the spinal cord and allows for voluntary control of defecation. The parasympathetic innervation of the proximal two thirds of large bowel is received through the vagus nerves from the "cranial outflow," whereas the parasympathetic innervation of the distal third including the internal anal sphincter is derived from the "sacral outflow" and sacral nerves.

The mucosal surface of the large intestine is relatively flat because there are no villi and the folds are relatively inconspicuous, with the exception of three semicircular folds in the rectum, the so-called rectal valves, which can serve as landmarks during proctoscopy, and several short longitudinal folds at the rectum-anus junction, the so-called rectal columns of Morgagni. The surface of the colon is lined by tall columnar epithelial cells with a narrow brush border. Long, straight crypts of Lieberkühn extend from the surface to a prominent muscularis mucosae. The undifferentiated cells are located predominantly in the lower halves of the crypts, which also contain numerous goblet cells, differentiated columnar cells along the upper portions, and endocrine cells. Paneth's cells are usually not present in the normal large bowel. The lamina propria usually contains more connective tissue cells than other parts of the gut, and lymph nodules are relatively abundant in the mucosa and submucosa. The mucosal and submucosal veins in the distal rectum and anus—the internal and external hemorrhoidal plexus—are especially prominent and subject to becoming distended, varicose, and thrombosed.

The small appendix, the blind-ending evagination of the cecum, is lined by columnar epithelium. Its crypts are less regular in shape and length and contain a relatively large number of endocrine cells, which probably give rise to the relatively common carcinoid tumors (argentaffinomas) that develop in the appendix. The muscularis mucosae is poorly developed, and numerous lymph nodules and lymphocytes fill much of the mucosa and submucosa.

The major role of the large intestine is to receive the ileal effluent, about 1 L a day, to absorb most of its water and salt to produce about 100 g of solid feces, and to store and evacuate the feces. The colon actively absorbs Na^+ and Cl^- and along with them passively absorbs water. The colon also secretes HCO_3^- and K^+, some of the K^+ in exchange for Na^+ under the control of aldosterone. Because of the small amount of stool normally evacuated, relatively little K^+ is lost, but with diarrhea appreciable quantities of body K^+ can be lost.

The motility of the colon is extremely slow and sluggish. It exhibits multiple short segmental contractions, some contractions of larger segments, and occasional peristaltic activity. In the interdigestive state the colonic contents are thought to be forwarded at a net rate of only about 5 cm an hour, but when colonic motility is stimulated by eating, this net rate is approximately tripled. This enhanced motility often moves feces into the rectum and initiates a defecation reflex. Whenever the rectum is distended, usually by the addition of new feces, the rectal muscle is stimulated to contract and the internal sphincter to relax, and the subject experiences an urge to defecate. The tension in the external sphincter, however, is reflexly increased by tension in its muscle spindles, thereby preventing the evacuation of feces. A person who does not wish to defecate can voluntarily maintain the tension in the external sphincter, and in this case the contraction and tension in the rectal muscles are reflexly decreased, the tension in the internal sphincter is increased, and the urge to defecate is abated until additional feces distend the rectum even further. If the person wishes to defecate, the defecation reflex can be voluntarily facilitated by sending neural impulses from the cerebral cortex to the defecation center in the medulla. Impulses from the center largely to sacral segments of the spinal cord result in the relaxation of the external sphincter and other perineal muscles, the continued relaxation of the internal sphincter, further contraction of the rectal and sigmoid muscles, and finally the evacuation of the feces. Defecation is assisted by increasing intraabdominal pressure through Valsalva's maneuver and the contraction of abdominal muscles.

SPLANCHNIC BLOOD FLOW

The motor activity, secretory activity, and blood flow of the digestive system generally vary together. Thus eating also increases the splanchnic blood flow such that it constitutes a larger percentage of an enhanced cardiac output. The enhanced perfusion of the digestive organs is essential to provide the water and electrolytes necessary for secretion, to provide the nutrients and oxygen to support the increased metabolic activity and work of the cells involved, and to transport the aborbed nutrients from the intestine into the portal and systemic circulation. The control of the splanchnic circulation and local perfusion is not clearly defined but is influenced by intrinsic neural, hormonal, and metabolic factors as well as by the extrinsic autonomic nervous system and humoral agents. The increased cardiac output associated with eating results sometimes is postprandial angina pectoris in patients with coronary artery disease. The increased oxygen required by the activated gut during and following a meal has been considered responsible for the postprandial abdominal pain (intestinal angina) occasionally experienced by patients with intestinal vascular disease and thought to be caused by intestinal ischemia.

BIBLIOGRAPHY

Davenport, H.W.: Physiology of the digestive tract, ed. 4, Chicago, 1977, Year Book Medical Publishers, Inc.

Rubin, W.: The epithelial "membrane" of the small intestine, Am. J. Clin. Nutr. 24:45, 1971.

Rubin, W., and others: The normal human gastric epithelia: a fine structural study, Lab. Invest. 19:598, 1968.

Weiss, L., and Greep, R.O.:Histology, New York, 1977, McGraw-Hill Book Co.

170 • MANIFESTATIONS OF DISORDERS OF THE DIGESTIVE SYSTEM

Walter Rubin

NATURE AND SYMPTOMS OF DIGESTIVE DISORDERS AND APPROACH TO EVALUATING PATIENTS

Disorders of the digestive system are among those most commonly encountered in clinical medicine. They produce a multitude of symptoms, including pain and discomfort, alterations in bowel habit as with diarrhea and constipation, nausea, vomiting, abdominal distention, dysphagia, hemorrhage, anemia, gaseousness, edema, jaundice, alterations in mental status, arthritis and arthralgias, rashes, visual disturbances, and constitutional symptoms such as fever, malaise, weakness, anorexia, and weight loss. Digestive system disorders are associated with a variety of etiologic agents and pathologic alterations: infections with viruses, bacteria, and parasites; toxins such as alcohol and lead; many drugs (most prescribed drugs may produce gastrointestinal symptoms); benign and malignant neoplasms; acute, chronic, and granulomatous inflammatory processes; acute and chronic ulcerations; primary neurologic, muscular, or vascular disorders; connective tissue diseases; congenital and acquired enzyme deficiencies; and allergic and immunologic disorders.

In many patients—probably more than half of those with chronic or recurrent symptoms—the symptoms are not, however, associated with any identifiable cause, pathology, or overt pathophysiologic process. The disorders of such patients have been labeled "functional bowel disease," "irritable bowel syndrome," "functional dyspepsia," and other similar names; that is, these have been considered psychosomatic disorders whose symptoms are the somatic results of life's stresses. Such disorders are better considered, however, as having an unknown cause or probably many causes, some of which may be related at least in part to emotional factors. For example, many patients with chronic cramps and diarrhea whose conditions were diagnosed a few years ago as the irritable bowel syndrome are today recognized as having a lactase deficiency and lactose intolerance. This condition has been appreciated for only about 15 years and is easily treated if correctly diagnosed. In addition to common gastrointestinal symptoms without recognizable causes, symptoms associated with recognized pathologic processes are often not clearly understood, for example, the pain or discomfort produced by peptic ulcers and gastroesophageal reflux. Finally, the causes of many pathologic processes involving the digestive system are still unknown or not well understood, for example, the causes of peptic ulcer disease, ulcerative colitis, and granulomatous ileocolitis.

In the evaluation of patients with gastrointestinal disorders, as with many other diseases, a careful history and physical examination are essential. Many digestive disorders can be tentatively diagnosed, or at least the diagnostic possibilities can be greatly narrowed, by means of a good history in itself. The physician must have a clear picture of the patient's symptoms: their nature, characteristics, location, onset, duration, and temporal relationships; their relationships to body postures, movements, functions, and stresses; and their associated symptoms and systemic manifestations such as fever, malaise, anorexia, and weight loss. Are the symptoms acute or chronic, persistent or intermittent, progressive or remittent? How are they elicited and how are they relieved? When do they occur? Do they wake the patient at night? How are they affected by eating, belching, defecating, and passing flatus and by body postures, movements, and respirations? Because eating stimulates the digestive system into action—the gut to increase its motor activity, the gallbladder to contract, the stomach and pancreas to secrete, and the splanchnic circulation to increase—symptoms resulting from gastrointestinal disorders are often precipitated or enhanced by eating. Are the symptoms affected by particular foods? What drugs is the patient receiving? Is there a family history of the same or similar symptoms or related diseases? The complete physical examination should include careful abdominal, rectal, and, with most females, pelvic examinations. A careful search should be made for direct and rebound abdominal tenderness, spasm, masses, organomegaly, hernias, distention, ascites, abnormal bowel sounds, and bruits, and any findings should be carefully characterized.

The symptoms and physical signs associated with specific diseases are discussed at length in the following chapters describing specific disorders of the digestive system.

This chapter, however, briefly discusses a few of the common manifestations of digestive disorders, such as pain, diarrhea, constipation, nausea and vomiting, gastrointestinal bleeding, protein-losing enteropathy, gaseousness, dysphagia, and distention, and some of the common systemic manifestations, such as fever, anorexia, satiety, weight loss, rash, and arthralgia.

PAIN

Pain and various kinds of discomfort are common symptoms of disorders of the digestive system. The sensory fibers to the abdominal viscera are carried with the sympathetic (first thoracic to second lumbar) and parasympathetic nerves. The mechanisms by which the abdominal viscera generate pain are not fully understood. Stretching of the hepatic or splenic capsules, distention or tension of the gut wall smooth muscle, and traction on the mesenteric attachment each stimulate sensory fibers and produce pain. The discomfort produced by peptic ulcers and peptic esophagitis, however, is not well understood, because the mucosa of most of the gut is anesthetic. Such tissue can be removed in a biopsy, for example, without causing discomfort to the patient. Perhaps the pain generated by mucosal ulcerations or inflammations is produced by associated muscle tensions or spasms, its threshold having been lowered by the inflammation. The quality of pain produced by esophageal spasm (often a severe, angina-like pain) is, however, usually distinctly different from that produced by reflux esophagitis (often a burning or gnawing pain). Visceral pain tends to be deep, not clearly localized, central or bilateral, and aching, dull, burning, or vague in quality, often producing more suffering or discomfort than actual sharp pain. In contrast, somatic (parietal) pain such as that produced by inflammation or irritation of the parietal peritoneum is usually well localized, lateral, sharp, and discrete. Visceral pain is usually referred to the somatic dermatomes corresponding to the spinal levels from which its sensory fibers emanate. As mentioned, however, it may not be clearly localized and often includes a few spinal segments above and/or below the level from which its major innervation originates. Thus pain arising from the esophagus is usually referred to the chest; stomach, duodenal, biliary, and pancreatic pain to the upper abdomen above the umbilicus; pain in the small intestine to the periumbilical area; and colonic pain to the lower abdomen. Pain arising from the central portions of the diaphragm is usually referred to the ipsilateral shoulder. Severe pain, especially when associated with acute inflammation of the parietal peritoneum, commonly leads to a reflex spasm of the musculature innervated by the same spinal segments; this is the involuntary abdominal spasm or guarding that should be carefully sought in the physical examination.

As discussed previously, a careful history often reveals the probable cause of a discomfort or at least restricts the likely causes. The following descriptions of classic symptoms associated with some common gastrointestinal disorders demonstrate the value of the history in establishing or suggesting the nature of these disorders.

Heartburn (pyrosis) resulting from gastroesophageal reflux is usually perceived as a recurrent retrosternal or high epigastric burning, gnawing, or heaviness and is usually brought on by eating or recumbency, is accompanied by the regurgitation of sour juice (gastric acid) or a sour taste, and is relieved by antacids. Odynophagia, or retrosternal discomfort occurring when food is swallowed, usually suggests inflammation (esophagitis) or occasionally neoplasia of the esophagus. The diagnosis of esophageal spasm is suggested by severe persistent retrosternal pain that often recurs and frequently mimics the pain of myocardial infarction, sometimes even radiating to the neck and arms and often relieved by nitroglycerin; esophageal spasm is also associated with dysphagia with both liquids and solids. The more serious disorders, such as myocardial infarction, coronary insufficiency, dissecting aneurysm, and perhaps pulmonary embolus, should be excluded from the diagnosis.

Peptic ulcer disease classically produces an epigastric burning, aching, or gnawing discomfort recurring 1 or more hours after eating or during sleep and relieved immediately by eating or ingesting an antacid; the pain occurs in the presence of unbuffered gastric acid and is relieved by its neutralization.

Gallbladder disease, usually cholelithiasis in which a gallstone obstructs the cystic duct, is suggested by recurrent attacks of persistent epigastric or right upper quadrant pain that sometimes radiates to the tip of the right scapula, is often promoted by eating, commonly lasts ½ to 2 hours, and is frequently associated with nausea and belching. Choledocholithiasis, the presence of a stone in the common duct, may cause similar symptoms although it may also cause left upper quadrant or left chest pain. If the pain persists, especially if it is associated with fever and tenderness in the right upper quadrant, the probable diagnosis is acute cholecystitis.

Persistent upper abdominal or periumbilical pain that is usually severe and lasts many hours, that often radiates straight through to the back and is commonly relieved by bending forward (jackknifing or assuming a fetal position), and that commonly is accompanied by nausea and vomiting is suggestive of acute pancreatitis, especially in an alcoholic patient. Similar symptoms can be produced by a posterior penetrating ulcer. If this type of pain arises and persists in an otherwise healthy middle-aged or older person, especially if it is associated with weight loss, a diagnosis of pancreatic carcinoma is likely.

Pain associated with biliary tract disease as described previously has been called biliary colic. The terms "colic" and "colicky pain" have generally been used in two senses. When used to describe pain associated with biliary tract disease or with the passage of a kidney-ureteral stone (renal colic), these terms generally refer to a severe persistent discomfort during which the patient can find no comfortable position or relief and usually keeps moving around attempting to escape the pain. Renal colic is usually a severe persistent pain in the lumbar area or flank that often radiates into the groin, testis, or penis and is commonly accompanied by nausea and vomiting. The second and more accurate usage of the term refers to a rhythmic recurring pain, each recurrence usually starting mildly and increasing in severity to be followed by an interval of absent or reduced discomfort. Such pain, like that occurring during labor, is characteristic of a hollow muscular viscus contracting recurrently against an obstruction. This colicky abdominal pain is characteristic of an intestinal obstruction, especially an early obstruction before any strangulation or embarrassment of the intestinal circulation has occurred. It is usually associated with abdominal distention, audible borborygmi, nausea and vomiting, and the inability to pass feces or gas. Milder and more common forms of this type of colicky pain are commonly called cramps.

In contrast to the restlessness of the patient with renal colic, when the parietal peritoneum is inflamed or irritated in acute peritonitis, the patient lies perfectly still because any movement of the peritoneum results in extreme aggravation of the pain. The physician need only tap the side of the bed lightly or percuss or palpate the abdomen gently to elicit marked superficial or rebound tenderness. The acute, catastrophic onset of abdominal pain followed by peritonitis suggests the perforation of a viscus, such as a peptic ulcer; a similar but somewhat less acute pain in an older patient with vascular disease might suggest a vascular catastrophe such as an embolus or acute occlusion of the superior mesenteric artery.

Upper abdominal discomfort that is subsequently localized in the right lower quadrant and is accompanied by focal superficial and rebound tenderness (focal peritoneal signs) and fever is of course classically symptomatic of acute appendicitis. Similar symptoms and signs in the left lower quadrant in an older person suggest diverticulitis, but similar symptoms and signs can be produced by other disorders such as a twisted ovarian cyst or mittelschmerz in a younger woman. Therefore a careful rectal and pelvic examination is needed in addition to a full history and routine physical examination.

An acutely swollen liver, such as may be produced by congestive failure, hepatitis, alcoholic hepatitis, metastatic cancer, and fatty infiltration, commonly produces persistent upper abdominal pain that is often more pronounced on the right side and is sometimes worsened by body movements and even respirations; the detection of a large, tender liver during the physical examination reveals the origin of the pain.

Abnormalities of the abdominal wall, such as hernias, may cause recurrent or persistent (as with an incarcerated or strangulated hernia, abdominal wall hematoma, or myositis) abdominal pain that is often intensified by movement and straining and by contracting the abdominal musculature. The cause of this pain is confirmed by eliciting focal tenderness in the abdominal wall that is increased when the supine patient lifts his head and thereby contracts his rectus sheath and, when applicable, by demonstrating a hernia at the site of tenderness.

Abdominal pains of primary *neural* origins sometimes pose diagnostic problems. Pain of *radicular* origin is often sharp and shooting, is usually worsened by movements of the spine or by coughing, sneezing, and straining, and is often accompanied by tenderness over the spine. Tabes dorsalis and diabetic neuropathy can lead to severe, recurrent, puzzling pains. Pain resulting from herpes zoster is usually diagnosed by its dermatomic distribution and classic skin lesions, but when it occurs without a rash or after a rash has been forgotten, it can be puzzling. The recurrent pains of porphyria are usually severe, persistent, deep, visceral-like pains that mimic acute visceral disease such as gallbladder disease.

Acute severe abdominal pain accompanied by minimal physical findings suggests an ischemic episode to the gut resulting from a vascular catastrophe or strangulation of a portion of the gut caused by an internal hernia or twisting of a loop of gut or vascular pedicle. Puzzling recurrent postprandial periumbilical pain that is sometimes associated with diarrhea, especially in an older person with vascular disease, is suggestive of a more insidious chronic vascular insufficiency, the rare intestinal angina.

Chronic recurrent abdominal pain, commonly in a young or middle-aged woman who has previously consulted many physicians and has undergone many studies with negative results and who may have undergone an operation such as cholecystectomy or the lysis of adhesions, is suggestive of functional bowel disease. This pain is often associated with other gastrointestinal symptoms such as constipation or less commonly diarrhea; sometimes alternating constipation and diarrhea; gaseousness with eructations, borborygmi, or flatulence; nausea; and abdominal distention. The pain is usually worsened by eating and is relieved somewhat by a bowel movement, belching, or the passing of flatus. Rarely do these symptoms interrupt a sound sleep. The symptoms are often promoted or aggravated by periods of emotional stress, and the patient often exhibits other neurotic symptoms. Evidence of depression should be carefully sought in the history of patients suspected of having functional symptoms; constipation is often associated with depression. If the history suggests that abdominal cramps often accompanied by diarrhea, flatulence, and distention are produced by the ingestion of milk, ice cream, and other dairy products, a diagnosis of lactase deficiency and lactose intolerance is suggested.

The onset of abdominal pain in previously healthy middle-aged and elderly patients should be treated with great respect. The onset of functional symptoms in these patients is not common in the absence of depression. An organic cause of the pain should be suspected and sought, with due concern for the high incidence of malignancy in these circumstances. The physician should elicit a complete drug history from all patients because drugs are common causes of gastrointestinal disturbances including pain.

Finally, it should be remembered that referred abdominal pain may be produced by disease affecting other organ systems: the lungs, heart, and genitourinary tract. Thus pneumonia, pulmonary infarction, and myocardial infarction occasionally produce pain in the upper abdomen and sometimes, surprisingly, even tenderness. The careful history, physical examination, and laboratory tests usually reveal the correct cause of the pain. Pain arising in the pelvis, such as that produced by pelvic inflammatory disease, or in the bladder, such as that produced by acute urinary retention, is commonly perceived in the lower abdomen. Pain of kidney origin, such as with acute pyelonephritis, is commonly felt in the lumbar and flank region but may also be perceived more anteriorly in the abdomen.

DIARRHEA

Acute diarrhea and chronic diarrhea are common manifestations of gastrointestinal disorders. When a patient complains of diarrhea, the physician should elicit a careful history to determine exactly what the patient means, including the number of bowel movements each day; whether they wake the patient at night; the patient's usual bowel habits; whether the symptoms are acute, recurrent, or chronic; the presence of associated symptoms; and a clear description of the character of the stools including their approximate volume and consistency and whether they contain blood, mucus, pus, or fat. An estimate of the daily volume of stool may be helpful; an accurate weight should be obtained in cases of chronic diarrhea of puzzling cause. Diarrhea to one patient may mean passing a single somewhat soft or mushy stool each day, whereas to another it may mean the "runs," sitting on the toilet often and passing numerous large volumes of water.

The normal bowel habit varies tremendously among individuals. Most people comfortably pass about one formed stool each day, whereas others may pass two or three, and still others may defecate only every 2, 3, or 4 days. As discussed in Chapter 120, the average person puts out approximately 100 to 200 g of stool each day, about 70% of which is water. Diarrhea, defined as the passage of more than 300 g of stool each day, may result from a disorder of either the small or large bowel, owing to an impairment of absorption or secretion in either.

The normal ileal effluent introduced into the colon is approximately 1 to 1.5 L each day. If it exceeds approximately 2 to 3 L, diarrhea ensues. Excessive ileal effluent may result from a disease of malabsorption, an inflammatory disease of the small intestine, or excessive secretion in the small intestine, which is commonly produced by a number of toxins, hormones, and other humoral substances, some of which seem to act by stimulating adenylate cyclase and elevating epithelial cyclic AMP levels. Among such agents are numerous bacterial toxins, such as cholera toxin and those of toxigenic *Escherichia coli;* certain prostaglandins as may be produced by medullary carcinomas of the thyroid; and vasoactive intestinal polypeptide and possibly gastrin, hormones produced in excessive amounts of some non-β islet cell tumors of the pancreas.

Several factors can impair the colon's net absorption of water and its ability to form solid stool: a reduced colonic mucosa from previous surgery, a diseased mucosa from inflammatory disease, and a rapid transit through the colon caused by enhanced motor activity, especially peristaltic activity. In addition, increased fatty acids in the colon, particularly the hydroxylated acids resulting from a malabsorption syndrome, or excessive bile salts in the colon resulting from ileal resection or disease reduce the net absorption of salt and water and cause diarrhea. Osmotic diarrhea may be produced by the presence in colonic chyme of increased amounts of nonabsorbable, soluble, osmotically active substances, such as salt cathartics or the bacterial metabolites of the unabsorbed lactose ingested by patients with lactase deficiency. An occasional cause of diarrhea, especially in older patients, is a villous adenoma, a tumor that often secretes much water, mucus, and potassium. The presence of increased nondigestible and nonabsorbable hydrophilic roughage and fiber in the diet (as is found in the normal diets of many nonwesternized societies such as rural Africa) results in the passage of more stool and water each day. Thus a fecal output normal in many parts of the world would be considered diarrhea in Americans.

Diarrhea caused by dietary factors, as is the case with diseases of malabsorption and with the osmotic diarrhea produced by lactose in patients with lactase deficiency, may be eliminated or markedly reduced by fasting. In contrast, a secretory diarrhea caused by a bacterial enterotoxin or hormone is usually affected little by fasting. A choleretic diarrhea produced by excessive bile salts in the colon also tends to improve with fasting because most of the bile salts are then retained in the unstimulated gallbladder.

Acute diarrhea is extremely common. When it occurs in otherwise healthy people who are not under stress or taking some recently initiated medication, it is most often produced by infectious agents, usually thought to be viruses because routine stool cultures are generally negative. Several types of bacteria may also cause acute diarrhea, either by producing enterotoxins that cause secretory diarrhea or by directly invading the mucosa, predominantly in the distal ileum and colon, or by both mechanisms. Organisms that predominantly invade and ulcerate the mucosa, such as *Shigella,* often produce a dysentery-like symptomatology, including fever, constitutional symptoms, and blood and pus (leukocytes) in the stools. In contrast, the enterotoxin forms of diarrhea such as those produced by cholera and staphylococcal enterotoxin are usually associated with little fever and few constitutional symptoms. *Clostridium perfringens* and *Bacillus cereus* are predominantly enterotoxin producers, whereas *Yersinia enterocolitica, Vibrio parahaemolyticus,* and *Campylobacter* are predominantly invaders. Many bacteria can both invade and produce toxins, their relative abilities varying among strains. Most instances of *E. coli* diarrhea in the United States and contracted by American tourists in Mexico are produced by predominantly toxigenic strains, but some cases are caused by strains that mainly invade. Even some strains of *Shigella,* the classic invader, produce toxins. Although *Salmonella* strains may produce toxins, they predominantly invade; these usually affect the distal small bowel, rarely ulcerating the mucosa, and thus they do not usually produce the ulcerative dysenteric picture commonly produced by *Shigella* (see discussion of ''Shigellosis'' in Chapter 41).

Acute diarrheas may also be produced by protozoan parasites, especially by *Giardia lamblia* and *Entamoeba histolytica.* The incidence of parasitic diarrheas varies, of course, among populations and geographic areas.

A careful history should be elicited from the patient with acute diarrhea, not only for clues to possible noninfectious causes but also to determine whether other close associates are similarly affected and thus whether a common food or water source can be implicated as the cause. Acute diarrheas, especially in children, are often seen at times when an intestinal disease, presumably caused by a virus, is known to be prevalent.

Most cases of acute diarrhea are self-limited, usually last from 1 to a few days, and are often accompanied by variable other symptoms such as abdominal cramps, nausea, vomiting, anorexia, fever, myalgia, and headache. These cases are usually viral. The physician should probably perform few diagnostic tests, especially if the case is mild, there is no blood in the stool, and the patient looks well. If the patient does not look well, however, and has profound diarrhea, dehydration, prominent constitutional symptoms, bloody stools, or the symptoms of dysentery, proctoscopy should be performed and the stools should be examined for blood, leukocytes, and parasites and should be cultured. Most patients should be treated supportively with fluids, electrolytes, restricted activity, and probably an antidiarrheal agent such as an opiate or diphenoxylate. Some recent studies have suggested, however, that infectious diarrheas resulting from bacterial agents such as *Shigella* may be worsened by antiperistaltic agents, presumably because they retard the intestinal elimination of the organisms. Fluids and electrolytes can usually be replaced orally, possibly with the addition of glucose or sucrose to salt solutions for secretory diarrheas. This replacement should be performed parenterally if patients are markedly depleted or cannot take oral medications.

Whereas acute diarrhea is usually self-limited and requires little diagnostic effort, chronic diarrhea must be evaluated more aggressively to establish an accurate diagnosis and to institute proper therapy. Again a complete, careful history, physical examination, and routine laboratory tests are essential to discover evidence of inflammatory bowel disease, a malabsorption syndrome, an endocrine disturbance, and previous illnesses or surgical procedures that might be relevant. The history should include any travel by the patient, fever, abdominal pain, tenesmus, rectal urgency, distention, blood or fat in the stools, nausea, vomiting, anorexia, weight loss, anemia, rashes, allergies, arthralgias, arthritis, and eye symptoms. All medications should be stopped, if possible. The workup of such patients should usually include examination of the stool for blood, leukocytes, eosinophils, mucus, fat, and ova and parasites, especially *Giardia* and *E. histolytica* but also others such as *Strongyloides* and *Schistosoma.* The stool could be cultured, although bacteria are not expected to be the cause of chronic diarrhea. The patient should usually undergo proctosigmoidoscopy, a rectal biopsy in most cases, a barium enema examination, and a gastrointestinal and small bowel series.

If the diagnosis is still unclear, the presence of steatorrhea indicating a disease of malabsorption should be sought by a quantitative determination of fecal fat. If a malabsorption syndrome is present, the specific disease should be diagnosed as outlined in Chapter 174. Lactase deficiency as possible cause of the patient's diarrhea can be determined by performing a lactose tolerance test and/ or by assessing the response to a lactose-free diet. The presence of a functioning carcinoid tumor as the cause of the diarrhea can usually be detected by means of a urinary 5-OH-indole acetic acid (5-HIAA) determination. The possible existence of other endocrine abnormalities, such as hyperthyroidism and adrenal insufficiency, should be determined by additional appropriate tests.

The history, physical examination, routine laboratory tests, elimination of medications, and other diagnostic tests and procedures suggested should usually detect or strongly suggest the cause of the patient's chronic diarrhea. They should reveal or suggest the presence of most cases of ulcerative colitis; granulomatous ileocolitis; diverticulitis; other, rarer intestinal inflammatory diseases such as tuberculosis, fungal infections, some cases of eosinophilic gastroenteritis, and amyloidosis; villous adenomas, lymphomas, carcinoid tumors, and other intestinal tumors; diseases causing the malabsorption syndrome; choleretic diarrhea; partial intestinal obstruction; fecal impaction with overflow diarrhea; parasitic diseases; lactase deficiency; drug-induced diarrhea, including pseudomembranous enterocolitis (usually acute); endocrinopathies such as hyperthyroidism, adrenal insufficiency, and hypoparathyroidism; uremic colitis; and pellagra. A diagnosis of ischemic bowel disease or ischemic colitis is usually suggested by the presence of "thumbprinting" or other roentgenographic intestinal changes and often by fecal blood, usually in an older person with vascular disease, congestive failure, and often abdominal bruits. The diabetic patient with diarrhea resulting from a visceral neuropathy also usually exhibits peripheral neuropathic signs and other evidence of a visceral neuropathy, such as postural hypotension. Diabetic patients also have malabsorption resulting from bacterial overgrowth or celiac disease, the incidence of which is increased in diabetes. A diagnosis of functional bowel disease is suggested by a history of chronic diarrhea in an otherwise healthy young or middle-aged patient (usually a woman) when tests are negative, there are other neurotic manifestations, and stress frequently aggravates the symptoms.

If the diagnosis is still uncertain, especially in patients who do not seem to have a functional disorder, the search should be continued and additional tests should be performed. The daily fecal weight should be measured to determine whether the diarrhea is of large or small volume; large volumes suggest a secretory diarrhea. The fecal Na^+, K^+, and osmolality concentrations should be determined to detect the presence of a significant quantity of unidentified osmotically active substances indicating an osmotic diarrhea. The normal stool is usually moderately hyperosmolar, averaging 375 mOsm, because of the presence of organic substances produced by colonic bacteria. The effects of fasting on the fecal output can be assessed as noted previously, to help determine the nature of the diarrhea. Surreptitious diarrhea resulting from the ingestion of laxatives should be suspected in puzzling cases, especially in patients exhibiting neurotic or psychotic symptoms. Alkalinization of the stool can reveal the presence of phenolphthalein by its red color, and the presence of melanosis coli on proctosigmoidoscopy suggests the use of anthraquinone laxatives. Melanosis coli is a benign, brown-black discoloration of the colonic mucosa that results from the presence of pigmentladen macrophages in the lamina propria. The pigmentation is associated with constipation and the habitual use of anthraquinone laxatives and may disappear when the laxatives are discontinued.

If the cause is still not evident, more unusual types of endocrine abnormalities that cause secretory diarrhea should be considered. The watery diarrhea syndrome (pancreatic cholera), often caused by a tumor that secretes vasoactive intestinal polypeptide (VIP) (vipoma) in the pancreas and occasionally in neural or other organs, is suggested by secretory diarrhea usually associated with hypokalemia and gastric hypochlorhydria (hyposecretion). Serum VIP levels can be determined by an immunoassay at certain medical centers. Serum gastrin levels should be determined to detect a *gastrinoma* because about 10% of such tumors are initially associated with diarrhea rather than with the more classic manifestations of the Zollinger-Ellison syndrome. Serum calcitonin levels should also be determined to detect the presence of a medullary carcinoma of the thyroid. Abnormal prostaglandin secretion has been implicated as the cause of diarrhea in cases of medullary thyroid carcinoma and in other cases of obscure, puzzling secretory diarrhea. Immynoassays of serum prostaglandins should become increasingly available in the future. If prostaglandins are suspected of being the cause of a puzzling case of secretory diarrhea, the effects of inhibiting prostaglandin synthesis with indomethacin or some other agent can be determined.

Food allergies may be the cause of puzzling diarrhea, commonly in children but also occasionally in adults. This diarrhea is often accompanied by abdominal pain and other gastrointestinal symptoms. These patients often have a family history of allergy, exhibit eosinophilia and elevated IgE levels, and also have allergic reactions of other organs, such as hives, eczema, rhinitis, and asthma, that may be initiated by the same dietary antigen. About 20% of patients with eosinophilic gastroenteritis are found to have an allergy to a dietary antigen and improve after it is eliminated. This poorly defined syndrome, which often produces diarrhea, is characterized by the inflammation of portions of the gut, predominantly with eosinophils, and is usually accompanied by peripheral eosinophilia and often fever. When the mucosa is predominantly involved, diarrhea and varying degrees of malabsorption, protein-losing enteropathy, and occult or gross blood loss are the usual manifestations. Predominant involvement of the tunica muscularis, especially of the stomach and upper intestine, often results in obstructive symptoms. Involvement of the serosa and peritoneum can lead to ascites. The gastrointestinal series may reveal no apparent abnormality or may show changes suggestive of Crohn's disease, a malabsorption syndrome, or a focal tumor or nodules. When a food allergy is suspected as the cause of diarrhea, skin testing may be of some help, but usually the elimination of milk and other dietary proteins must be empirically assessed.

The proper treatment of patients with diarrhea depends on establishing an accurate diagnosis of the specific disorder. The following chapters describe in greater detail the diseases that cause diarrhea and their pathology, clinical manifestations, physical and laboratory abnormalities, method of diagnosis, and specific therapy. General supportive therapy of these patients should include the assessment of water, electrolyte, and nutritional losses and deficiencies and their repletion. General supportive therapy for mild diarrheas that are not controlled by a specific therapy has also included agents such as opiates and anticholinergics that inhibit gut motility and sometimes also hydrophilic bulk agents such as psyllium seed preparations that absorb water and harden the stools.

CONSTIPATION

Constipation, both actual and perceived, is a common gastrointestinal complaint. It is a cause of chronic discomfort and concern and a major focus of attention of thousands of people, especially those in middle and old age. As discussed previously, the normal bowel habit varies tremendously among individuals; some apparently normal, asymptomatic people evacuate only once every 2 or 3 days or even less frequently without any appreciable difficulty. True constipation should therefore be judged not solely by the frequency of evacuation but by the character of the feces and evacuation. If the stools are so dehydrated and hard that evacuation is difficult or painful or cannot be attained without mechanical or therapeutic assistance, the person can be said to be constipated. Constipation may cause abdominal pain and cramps and even intestinal obstruction as a result of fecal impaction. Many constipated individuals complain of sluggishness, dullness, weakness, malaise, fatigue, anorexia, and headaches. The extent to which such symptoms are functional in nature or are caused, perhaps in part, by the constipation is unclear. By metabolizing feces, colonic bacteria produce "toxins" such as ammonia and short-chain fatty acids that can dull the sensorium and impair the intellect. These toxins are normally drained, however, into the portal circulation and to the liver where they are metabolized. Only in the presence of liver disease, when this metabolism is impaired or when the toxins are shunted from the portal circulation to the systemic circulation, are sufficient quantities of these substances thought to reach the systemic circulation and central nervous system to produce appreciable effects such as hepatic encephalopathy, which is clearly promoted or aggravated by constipation, presumably because of the increased toxin production. Whether constipation can affect the brain of an otherwise normal person has not been established.

Because of the marked variability of the normal stooling habit and the uncertainty of symptoms attributed to constipation, it is often difficult for a physician to decide whether an individual is truly constipated and should be treated. One asymptomatic young woman, for example, always defecated with firm but not hard or voluminous stools, once every 2 weeks without difficulty. Her workup, including a rectal examination, proctosigmoidoscopy, barium enema, and thyroid studies, was normal. It was not clear if she was constipated or if she should have been treated to promote more frequent evacuations. In contrast, many patients, often middle-aged or older women, feel sluggish, weak, and dull or have headaches unless they have at least one complete movement each day. These patients often believe they cannot completely evacuate their stool. Regardless of whether these individuals have ever been truly constipated, they often have become so habituated to the use of laxatives, suppositories, or enemas that it has become almost impossible for them to defecate satisfactorily without assistance.

Most cases of chronic constipation are thought to be functional in nature and thus have been given names such as spastic colon, spastic colitis, functional constipation, and functional bowel syndrome. The pathogenesis of functional constipation is unclear. Perhaps some of these patients had so successfully learned to suppress their defecation reflex at the time of rigorous toilet training that at times of rectal distention they no longer recognize the urge to defecate and unconsciously inhibit the reflex. Some of these patients have alternating periods of constipation and diarrhea. Patients with functional constipation often pass small, hard fecal pellets similar to those produced by rabbits. Many of these patients are bothered most by abdominal cramps and pain. Studies in recent years have demonstrated that patients with chronic constipation and pain often exhibit abnormal, severe contractions or spasms of their sigmoid colons that cause the pain. Some of these patients have learned to control these spastic contractions through operative conditioning and have thereby been relieved of their pain. The abnormal sigmoid contractions observed in these patients are similar to those associated with colonic diverticulosis, and it is now thought that these patients, because of the abnormal colonic pressures, are prone to diverticulosis.

Almost everyone has become acutely constipated at some time, an experience often promoted by travel and being away from familiar bathrooms, diet, and habits, by an intercurrent illness, by hospitalization, by a period of unaccustomed inactivity, by some unusual emotional stress, by a medication, by the development of perianal condition that makes defecation painful, or by an injury or illness that impedes Valsalva's maneuver and the ability to increase intra-abdominal pressure and thereby defecate. Most of these experiences are of short duration, and the cause of the constipation is usually evident; the individual usually requires little more than a mild laxative to prevent fecal impaction. Some cases of acute constipation or obstipation are of course more serious, such as an intestinal obstruction or an ileus resulting from a severe acute illness, but the primary underlying disorders in these instances are usually readily recognizable.

If constipation of recent onset persists, however, or if a patient with chronic constipation has never been fully evaluated, a more thorough investigation is warranted to determine the cause of constipation. Most patients should receive a complete history and physical examination, including careful neurologic, rectal, and pelvic examinations; the usual laboratory tests; and proctoscopy, a barium enema, and usually a gastrointestinal and small bowel series. What cause is considered most likely for the altered bowel habit depends largely on the age of the patient and clinical setting. Causes that should be considered include medications; inactivity; an emotional disorder, especially in inapparent depression; a metabolic disorder such as hypothyroidism, hypercalcemia, or rarely porphyria or lead poisoning; a mechanical obstruction, especially a rectal or colonic carcinoma in a middle-aged or older person; diverticulitis; an ileus or an intestinal pseudo-obstruction such as motor abnormality of the gut, usually resulting from a disease involving the nerves or muscle, such as scleroderma; megacolon; a neurologic or muscular disorder that impairs the ability to perform Valsalva's maneuver successfully and to defecate; and laxative abuse that may impair a person's ability to defecate normally, perhaps by damaging the enteric nerves of the bowel and its motility. The habitual use of irritant laxatives may in fact also alter the roentgenographic appearance of the colon, producing the so-called cathartic colon in which there are a loss of haustra and an effacement of the mucosal pattern, especially on the right side, and occasionally even a megacolon. These roentgenographic features may erroneously suggest the presence of ulcerative or granulomatous colitis or other diseases.

In most cases of chronic constipation, no correctable underlying cause can be identified. In the management of these patients the physician's goal is to promote a regular, comfortable bowel habit with minimal concern, effort, and laxative assistance, to divert the patient's attention and energies to more important and enjoyable matters, and to promote the patient's emotional and psychologic well-being. A caring, devoted physician should lend sympathetic support. Serious emotional or psychologic problems such as depression should be identified and treated, with the aid of a psychiatrist if necessary. The patient should be encouraged to exercise regularly, to maintain good hydration with a liberal fluid intake, and to increase the fiber and roughage of his diet. He should be encouraged to eat vegetables and fruits, including prunes, figs, and prune juice. Bran and/or a hydrophilic bulk laxative such as a psyllium seed preparation should be added to the diet. The patient should be taught about the defecation reflex in terms he can understand. He should be encouraged to sit relaxed in a comfortable familiar bathroom with pleasant reading material one to three times each day at the same time and after the same meal(s). If additional therapy is necessary, the smallest necessary amount of the mildest laxatives should be used.

NAUSEA AND VOMITING

Nausea and vomiting often are manifestations of gastrointestinal disorders but also commonly result from diseases of other organs. A vomiting center located in the medulla oblongata is responsible for the integrated act of vomiting. Outflow from this center causes a sensation of nausea, a spasm of the duodenum and gastric antrum, the relaxation of the body and fundus of the stomach and the lower esophageal sphincter, and forceful contractions of the abdominal muscles and diaphragm that force the gastric contents into the esophagus. Slow deep inspirations with a partially closed glottis reduce intrathoracic pressure and promote the reflux of the gastric contents into the esophagus, which are then swept back into the stomach by secondary peristalsis. Repetition of this process constitutes retching. Vomiting ensues when strong contractions of the abdominal muscles force the diaphragm up, the intrathoracic pressure increases, the upper esophageal sphincter opens, and the esophageal contents are propelled out of the mouth. Vomiting is commonly accompanied by autonomic manifestations such as salivation, sweating, pallor, and tachypnea. The vomiting center receives afferent impulses from many areas including the cortex, the eighth nerve (labyrinth mechanism), abdominal and other viscera, and a chemoreceptor trigger zone nearby in the medulla that may be stimulated by substances in the circulation, such as drugs like apomorphine. Thus nausea and vomiting may be initiated by stimuli from all over the body, including the cortex (with willful vomiting), the labyrinth (as in motion sickness, labyrinthitis, and Meniere's disease), and a host of chemical and metabolic irritants. Nausea and vomiting may accompany many acute illnesses of many organ systems, such as myocardial infarction, pyelonephritis, and meningitis. Nausea and vomiting also commonly accompany many acute illnesses of the digestive system, such as gastroenteritis, appendicitis, pancreatitis, cholecystitis, peritonitis, and viral and alcoholic hepatitis.

A number of patients have acute, subacute, recurrent, or chronic nausea and vomiting without such obvious associated acute illnesses. The possibility of pregnancy, a common cause of nausea and vomiting in susceptible patients, should be excluded before any roentgenographic studies are performed. Drug toxicity, metabolic disorders such as uremia or hypercalcemia, and increased intracranial pressure must also be considered and eliminated as possible causes.

Abnormalities of the digestive system, especially obstructing lesions, are in such patients common causes of nausea and vomiting and also regurgitation, which may be mistaken for vomiting but which is usually unaccompanied by nausea, abdominal contractions, and associated autonomic symptoms. A careful description of the vomitus or regurgitated material may reveal something about the nature and location of the disorder. If the vomitus contains bile—if it is yellow and tastes bitter—then it is unlikely that there is an obstructing lesion of the esophagus, stomach, or duodenal bulb. If the material contains acid—tastes sour—then it is unlikely that there is an obstructing lesion of the esophagus. Identifiable food that is regurgitated probably comes from either the esophagus or stomach; if it is expelled many hours after it was ingested, obviously the esophagus or stomach is not emptying normally. Thus if the patient's problem is in the esophagus (an obstructing lesion such as a tumor or stricture, a motor disorder such as achalasia, or a diverticulum that catches and retains the food), the regurgitated material often contains food but usually not acid or bile. If the stomach fails to empty because of an obstructing peptic ulcer or cancer or because of a motor disorder such as a diabetic gastric atony, the vomitus usually contains acid (if the patient's stomach can secrete it) and food but no bile. A distended stomach can usually be suspected by the finding of a succussion splash in the physical examination (the splash heard with a stethoscope over the stomach when the patient is shaken from side to side). Active ulcers may cause vomiting without obstructing the stomach, but an obstruction should be suspected in known ulcer patients. The regurgitation commonly associated with an incompetent lower esophageal sphincter and gastroesophageal reflux (often with heartburn) usually contains acid and therefore tastes sour, but it may also contain bile. If an obstruction exists high in the intestine but below the ampulla of Vater, bile is usually prominent in the vomitus, and the patient may exhibit little distention. If an obstruction exists lower in the small intestine or in the large intestine, distention is usually prominent and the vomitus is more apt to be feculent or putrid, the result of bacterial metabolism of intestinal contents. Intestinal obstructions, especially mechanical obstructions, are usually associated with prominent abdominal cramps and pain as well. With obstructions, especially those that are high in the gut, the vomiting is often marked after eating. In metabolic abnormalities such as pregnancy. early uremia, and alcoholic toxicity, the vomiting is often prominent in the morning.

The evaluation of patients with persistent or recurrent nausea and vomiting usually includes a flat plate roentgenogram of the abdomen (after excluding the possibility of a pregnancy), the passage of a nasogastric tube and the aspiration of gastric contents (if an obstruction is suspected), and barium studies of the esophagus, stomach, and intestines. A functional cause of chronic vomiting is not unusual, but possible gastrointestinal, metabolic, drug-related, and other organic causes should first be excluded from the diagnosis of these patients. Vomiting may be the sole symptom in patients with a functional disorder or may be associated with other manifestations of a functional bowel syndrome. As discussed previously, the physician should attempt to make a positive diagnosis, rather than a diagnosis based solely on exclusion, by correlating the symptoms with periods of stress and identifying other abnormal emotional and psychologic symptoms. A severe emotional disorder must be identified and treated with psychiatric assistance. Vomiting, especially in young women, may be a manifestation of unrecognized anorexia nervosa.

The management of nausea and vomiting depends on the cause being identified. Significant dehydration and electrolyte and metabolic derangements must be recognized and corrected as rapidly as necessary. Severe acute hypokalemic metabolic alkalosis can result from losses of potassium and gastric acid. Vomiting, especially by intoxicated patients, may also lead to aspiration pneumonia. Severe retching may lead to a mucosal tear, usually near the esophagogastric junction (Mallory-Weiss syndrome) with resultant bleeding, or even to an esophageal rupture (Boerhaave's syndrome) with mediastinitis and serious consequences.

GASTROINTESTINAL BLEEDING

Bleeding from the gastrointestinal tract revealed as either an acute hemorrhage or occult blood in the stool is a common manifestation of gastrointestinal disease. A gastrointestinal hemorrhage is a serious, potentially lethal medical emergency. The patient usually has hematemesis, the vomiting of red blood or a dark material resembling coffee grounds, and/or the passage through the rectum of red blood (hematochezia) or black, tarry, sticky stools (melena). The coffee-ground material results from the conversion of hemoglobin to hematin by the acid in the stomach, whereas a melenic stool results from the alteration of at least 50 ml of blood in the gut, usually requiring several hours and probably bacterial action. Hematemesis usually means the bleeding is at a site proximal to the ligament of Treitz; continual vomiting or nasogastric aspiration of large amounts of red blood from the stomach usually suggests that the stomach or esophagus is the site of the hemorrhage, the duodenum being a less likely possibility. Melena also suggests the upper gastrointestinal tract as the site of bleeding, although bleeding from the jejunum, ileum, or even the right side of the colon can produce melena if the transit is slow. The passage of red blood through the rectum suggests that the bleeding site is distal to the ligament of Treitz, usually in the colon or rectum, but brisk bleeding from the upper gut with rapid intestinal transit also produces red rectal blood.

Even before a hemorrhage is apparent, bleeding patients often have symptoms of acute blood loss, the severity of which depends on the rate and magnitude of loss. Such symptoms include weakness, malaise, dyspnea, palpitations, faintness, sweating, and even syncope.

The physician's first concern with bleeding patients should be for the vital signs and the perfusion of the vital organs: the heart, brain, and kidneys. An acute blood loss of less than 500 ml or 10% of the blood volume rarely affects the vital signs significantly. A loss of more than 2 L or 35% to 40% usually produces frank hypovolemic shock. A loss of 1 to 2 L or 15% to 35% usually produces tachycardia and decreased blood pressure (pulse greater than 100 and systolic blood pressure less than 110 mm Hg) and "tilting" (when the patient rises from the prone position, the systolic blood pressure falls more than 10 mm Hg, the pulse increases more than 20 beats, and the patient often feels faint or light headed). Blood should be drawn immediately for a hemoglobin and hematocrit determination and type and cross-match; a large-bore intravenous needle should be inserted immediately and an infusion begun; and if the patient shows signs of shock, he should immediately receive saline or preferably a colloidal volume expander (plasma or dextran), to be replaced with blood as soon as it can be obtained. The patient should receive only enough blood to maintain satisfactory blood pressure, pulse, and perfusion of the brain, heart, and kidneys. His mind should be clear, he should not feel faint, he should be free of angina and ischemic electrocardiographic changes, and he should be excreting good volumes of urine.

In addition to treating shock and observing and maintaining the patient's vital signs, circulation, and vital functions, the physician's goal is to diagnose the cause of bleeding, to control it, and to treat the underlying lesion. A surgeon and gastroenterologist, if available, should be consulted to help in the workup and management and to perform endoscopy or surgery if necessary. A history, physical examination, and laboratory tests should be performed as quickly and thoroughly as the patient's condition permits. All pertinent historical data should be elicited, including previous known diseases and bleeding and any use of drugs or toxins that can cause gastrointestinal bleeding (such as aspirin, alcohol, and anti-inflammatory agents) or impair clotting (such as anticoagulants). The nose and throat should be examined as possible sites of the bleeding. If there is any question of actual bleeding having occurred, the presence of blood in the stool, vomitus, or gastric aspirate should be confirmed by a guaiac or benzidene test. The ingestion of iron, bismuth, or licorice can turn the stools dark (although not sticky), and beets can make them red. The hemoglobin and hematocrit determinations obtained soon after a hemorrhage do not reflect the severity of blood loss but continue to decline over many hours as the plasma volume is reexpanded by the addition of interstitial fluid. The finding of hypochromic, microcytic red cells suggests that the blood loss is chronic as well as acute. The finding of marked anemia in a patient with a good blood pressure and pulse also suggests a chronic slow loss of blood or antecedent anemia. Soon after bleeding the patient usually exhibits moderate leukocytosis and thrombocytosis and, if the bleeding site is in the upper gut, usually an elevation of blood urea nitrogen, even when renal function is normal.

The site of bleeding should be determined. A nasogastric tube should be passed, and the gastric contents aspitated. The presence of blood in the gastric contents (or a history of hematemesis) indicates that the site of bleeding is proximal to the ligament of Treitz; the absence of blood means either that the bleeding has stopped or that the site is not in the esophagus or stomach. If bile but no blood is recovered with continuous aspiration, there is no active bleeding in the proximal duodenum. If blood is recovered from the stomach, the stomach should be washed with ice-cold saline or water in an effort to stop or slow the bleeding. If lower gastrointestinal bleeding is suspected because of the rectal passage of red blood and the absence of hematemesis and blood in the stomach, usually anoscopy and proctoscopy should be performed to determine if the rectum or anus is the site of bleeding or if the blood is coming from above these areas.

Common causes of acute severe upper gastrointestinal hemorrhage include peptic ulcers, erosive gastritis, esophageal and gastric varices, esophagitis, Mallory-Weiss tears, and less commonly polyps, benign and malignant tumors, vascular malformations, ruptured aneurysms, hematobilia, inflammatory bowel disease, and diverticula. Stress erosions or ulcerations are common causes of hemorrhage in patients susceptible to them because of severe trauma, severe illness, burns, central nervous system trauma or operations, and sepsis and other severe infections. Common causes of acute lower gastrointestinal hemorrhage include hemorrhoids and, in patients over 50 years of age, colonic diverticulosis and angiodysplasia. Less common causes include inflammatory bowel disease, colonic polyps, other benign and malignant tumors, gut ischemia, and radiation enteritis. Inflammatory bowel disease, including proctitis, is a relatively common cause of hematochezia or bloody diarrhea but an uncommon cause of severe hemorrhage. A Meckel's diverticulum is a relatively common site of gastrointestinal bleeding in young patients. Patients with impaired clotting resulting from anticoagulants or thrombocytopenia may have gastrointestinal bleeding; the less impaired the clotting, the more likely is an underlying lesion such as an ulcer whose bleeding was promoted by the anticoagulation.

The initial diagnostic procedures and therapy depend on the likely diagnosis derived from the history, the physical examination, the routine laboratory results, and the probable site of bleeding. A patient who has ingested aspirin or alcohol may very well be bleeding from erosive gastritis. If the patient has a history of ulcer disease and has ulcer symptoms, a peptic ulcer is most likely the cause of upper gastrointestinal bleeding. If the patient has cirrhosis as established by the history or physical examination, varices may be the cause; alcoholics, however, even with established cirrhosis and varices, commonly bleed because of other causes such as erosive gastritis, a peptic ulcer, esophagitis, and Mallory-Weiss tears. A patient, especially an alcoholic, who has hematemesis after much retching and initial vomiting of nonbloody material is likely to be bleeding from a Mallory-Weiss tear. A patient who is taking anticoagulant drugs or who is found to have petechiae, ecchymoses, or blood in the urine probably has a bleeding diathesis causing or contributing to the gastrointestinal hemorrhage. The physical finding of abnormal pigmentation or vascular lesions of the hands, face, lips, or mouth may reveal the presence of a Peutz-Jeghers syndrome or Osler-Weber-Rendu disease, respectively, as the cause of the bleeding.

In general, if the bleeding is from the upper gut, an emergency or early endoscopy (esophagogastroduodenoscopy) should be performed if the technique is available and the patient's condition permits. Although studies have not yet clearly demonstrated that emergency endoscopy alters the outcome of patients with gastrointestinal bleeding, the procedure usually establishes a rapid diagnosis for bleeding in the esophagus, stomach, or duodenum and permits proper therapy to be initiated immediately. Even if the bleeding is too brisk to permit complete visualization, the site of bleeding can usually be determined, and some diagnostic possibilities such as varices and diffuse erosive gastritis can be excluded. Endoscopy is especially helpful in patients such as alcoholics who are likely to have many possible causes for their bleeding. Their varices may be demonstrable by an esophagogram, but endoscopy is usually required to determine these as the source of the bleeding rather than gastritis or some other lesion. Endoscopy is usually required to identify many lesions, such as erosive gastritis, esophagitis, duodenitis, a Mallory-Weiss tear, or small vascular lesions such as occur in patients with Osler-Weber-Rendu disease. Therapeutic procedures such as the use of laser beams and electrocautery will in the future be used with endoscopes to control some types of bleeding. Angiography is helpful in some cases of upper gastrointestinal bleeding, especially if the bleeding site cannot be successfully demonstrated by endoscopy or if a vascular anomaly is the cause of bleeding. Angiography can demonstrate the bleeding site usually when the bleeding is arterial and occurs at a rate of 0.5 ml/min or more. The dye can be seen collecting in the gut lumen. Esophagography and gastrointestinal series are performed in many cases, but once barium has been introduced into the stomach in an emergency study, it impedes subsequent endoscopic and especially angiographic examinations for some time. A patient who has a classic history suggesting peptic ulcer disease and who has apparently stopped bleeding requires only a gastrointestinal series.

If brisk lower gastrointestinal bleeding continues and arises at a level above the reach of the proctoscope, angiography is usually the procedure of choice. If the bleeding site cannot be found in the colon, it should be sought in the small intestine and even in the stomach. Emergency barium enemas and small bowel series are usually less determinative in patients with severe lower gastrointestinal bleeding, especially older patients in whom diverticulosis and angiodysplasia, a vascular lesion of the right side of the colon, are common causes of such bleeding. In at least 50% of the cases of brisk diverticular bleeding the bleeding site is on the right side of the colon even though diverticula are much more common on the left. If the bleeding is not brisk, especially in a patient below the age of 45 and especially if polyps, a neoplasm, or inflammatory bowel disease is suspected, a barium enema and small bowel series should be performed before angiography is considered. Colonoscopy usually cannot be successfully performed when the bleeding is appreciable but may be used after the bleeding has ceased, ideally after a period of bowel preparation (see Chapter 171).

Therapy for gastrointestinal bleeding, in addition to general supportive measures, depends on the specific cause and must often be individualized according to the condition and associated medical problems of the patient. If the bleeding is so brisk that an adequate blood volume and adequate perfusion of vital organs cannot be maintained, usually emergency surgery must be performed to control it. Even if vital signs and functions can be maintained by means of transfusions, the physician should try to avoid the need for massive transfusions of 15 units or more, to avoid the attendant complications and increased possibility of death. Acid-peptic related disorders such as ulcers, gastritis, and esophagitis are usually treated by controlling gastric acidity with antacids, cimetidine, or constant gastric suction, although it is usually advisable not to leave nasogastric tubes in patients with gastric or esophageal lesions. Patients with bleeding varices should receive intravenous vasopressin (Pitressin) in an effort to reduce the splanchnic blood flow and portal pressure and perhaps tamponade with the Sengstaken-Blakemore tube. Some physicians do not use the tamponade because of the attendant risks, and still others advocate early surgery, especially in low-risk patients. The local arterial perfusion of vasopressin has been used in many medical centers to reduce local blood flow and persistent bleeding. It is perfused into a branch of the superior mesenteric artery or inferior mesenteric artery to control colonic diverticular bleeding or into the left gastric artery to control bleeding from erosive gastritis, a gastric ulcer, or a Mallory-Weiss tear. Some angiographers occlude local arterial branches to a persistently bleeding site by injecting an autologous clot or gelatin sponge (Gelfoam). Some angiographers have even been able to introduce catheters into the portal circulation and inject bleeding varices with sclerosing agents. These latter procedures are available in relatively few medical centers and should still be viewed as experimental. With the remarkable capabilities of angiographers to introduce catheters into increasingly more vessels, however, new angiographic as well as therapeutic endoscopic techniques will become available for rapidly controlling gastrointestinal bleeding and thereby avoiding surgery.

The slow, inapparent loss of blood from the gastrointestinal tract is another common manifestation of gastrointestinal disorders. These patients often have iron deficiency anemia or an occult fecal blood loss detected by routine testing of the stool with guaiac or benzidine. These tests are usually positive if the daily blood loss is at least 5 ml. The benzidine test is more sensitive but less specific, and thus in some weakly positive cases dietary meat may have to be restricted to be certain the test is positive. Many gastrointestinal lesions have been alleged to produce occult blood loss and hypochromic microcytic anemia, the more common of which are cancers of the colon, stomach, ampulla of Vater or pancreas, and esophagus; colonic and gastric polyps; peptic ulcers; and gastritis, usually produced by drugs such as aspirin. Colon cancer in particular tends to produce occult blood loss, and thus the examination of three stool specimens for occult blood with the Hemoccult test has been advocated as a regular screening test for the detection of early colon cancer. Other lesions thought to produce occult blood in the stools and iron deficiency anemia include almost all other known gastrointestinal lesions, including hiatus hernia and diverticulosis. These two conditions are very common and may certainly be associated with acute hemorrhage. Their presence should not be accepted, however, as a cause of occult blood loss. Patients found to have occult fecal blood or unexplained iron deficiency anemia should usually undergo proctoscopy, an air-contrast barium enema, esophagography, and a gastrointestinal and small bowel series. If the cause has still not been satisfactorily determined, colonoscopy and esophagogastroduodenoscopy should be performed as well.

GASEOUSNESS

Gaseousness is a common gastrointestinal complaint resulting in excessive belching, abdominal bloating or distention associated with cramps and pain, or excessive flatulence.

Gas can usually be observed in the stomach and large intestine of the normal person, about 50 ml in the stomach and 100 ml in the intestine. The gas in the gut is derived from swallowed air, nitrogen therefore usually forming a large percentage of the gas, from the rapid fluxes of gases between the bowel lumen and blood, and from gas produced in the lumen. Carbon dioxide is formed in the duodenum from the neutralization of gastric acid and fatty acids by the secreted sodium bicarbonate, 22.4 ml of carbon dioxide resulting from each mEq of acid neutralized. In the colon hydrogen and carbon dioxide are produced largely from the bacterial fermentation of nonabsorbed food or, in the case of carbon dioxide, in part from the reaction of secreted HCO_3^- with fatty acids produced by the bacteria. About one third of adults also have bacteria that produce methane, but its production is independent of food ingestion and persists even when fasting. The hydrogen and methane formed in the colon are absorbed in part into the circulation and cleared effectively in the lungs, and thus the rates of colonic formation of these gases can be estimated by analyzing expired breath. Trace amounts of malodorous gases are also formed in the colon and account for the repugnant odors of flatus.

The gas in the stomach is largely swallowed air with the addition of some carbon dioxide. When a person is erect, the gastric air bubble accumulates in the upper part of the stomach near the esophagogastric junction, and much of it can be readily eructated. When a person is supine, however, most of the air accumulates in the antrum, and the esophagogastic junction is covered with gastric fluid; thus little of the swallowed air is eructated, and most of it passes into the duodenum. Because of its low viscosity, gas moves rapidly through the small intestine. The large volume of carbon dioxide produced in the duodenum, about half or more of the duodenal gas after a meal, is rapidly absorbed in the small intestine. The hydrogen, carbon dioxide, and methane formed in the colon occasionally account for over half of the colonic gas and flatus in some patients, although in most patients nitrogen usually accounts for 50% to 90%. Little oxygen is found in the colon or flatus because of its rapid utilization by bacteria. The amount of flatus and its content of hydrogen and carbon dioxide are appreciably increased when the amounts of fermentable substrates entering the colon are increased, for example, by increasing undigestible dietary substances such as the oligosaccharides found in beans and other roughage and fiber, in the presence of a malabsorption syndrome, or by the ingestion of lactose by a person with lactase deficiency.

About 2 to 3 ml of air is thought to enter the stomach with each swallow; the occasional eructation following a meal or the drinking of a carbonated beverage emanates from the gastric air bubble. On the other hand, patients who have frequent recurrent belching have usually been observed to swallow or aspirate air before each belch. Most of this air moves only partway down the esophagus before being expelled (esophageal eructations). Thus chronic excessive belching is usually a functional habit that is often promoted or aggravated by emotional stress rather than the result of excessive gas formation in the stomach or intestine. The mechanism and functional nature of the eructations should be explained to these patients, whose symptoms often improve with the reassurance that no significant disease exists.

Many patients complain of chronic abdominal bloating and cramps or pain attributed to the presence of excessive intestinal gas. These patients have in the past been thought to have excessive aerophagia—the swallowing of too much air with meals or when swallowing saliva—which leads to excessive gas. Recent studies have shown, however, that such patients have normal amounts of intestinal gas and that when their intestines are perfused with volumes of gas tolerated by normal subjects, the abdominal pain is reproduced. Thus it appears that these patients have some sort of motor disorder or that they are abnormally sensitive to the usual distentions of the gut. These patients also benefit from the reassurance that they do not have a serious disease. Because they react even to normal quantities of intestinal gas, it should be reduced if possible. They should be warned against repetitive belching, because some of the swallowed or aspirated air may reach the stomach. They should remain erect after meals to promote eructation of gastric gas and to minimize the amount passing into the intestine. The amount of carbon dioxide produced in the duodenum can theoretically be reduced by neutralizing or inhibiting gastric acid secretion (with antacids or inhibitors) and by reducing dietary fat. The amount of gas produced in the colon can be decreased by reducing the intake of nondigestible foods such as beans, roughage, fiber, and lactose, especially with patients with lactase deficiency. Finally, anticholinergics and antispasmodics may be tried, although their efficacy in reducing this pain has not been established.

An effort can also be made to reduce the intestinal gas of patients complaining of excessive flatus. In some medical centers the amount of flatus can be measured, or a sample of colonic gas can be more easily collected for analysis with a syringe and rectal tube. If the gas is predominantly nitrogen, the problem is excessive aerophagia and the patient can be advised accordingly. On the other hand, if hydrogen and carbon dioxide are major constituents (hydrogen can also be detected in expired breath), the major problem is the colonic presence of excessive nonabsorbed fermentable substrates; the major therapeutic thrust then should be to reduce dietary beans, other roughage and fiber, and lactose (especially with patients with lactase deficiency) and to exclude the possibility of a malabsorption syndrome.

OTHER MANIFESTATIONS OF GASTROINTESTINAL DISORDERS

Many other symptoms, which are discussed in greater detail in subsequent chapters, may be the initial or associated manifestations of disorders of the digestive system. Jaundice is a common manifestation of hepatic or biliary disease and pancreatic cancer. Abdominal distention may result from gaseous intestinal distention (such as that resulting from an intestinal obstruction or ileus), ascites, an abdominal mass, a hernia, or organomegaly such as a large liver, spleen, or uterus. Dysphagia, the sensation of food or drink sticking when swallowed, is a common manifestation of disorders of the esophagus. The presence of fever in a patient with a gastrointestinal disorder suggests an inflammatory or, less commonly, a neoplastic process. Anorexia commonly accompanies obstructive, neoplastic, and inflammatory processes, especially of the liver, and must be differentiated from early satiety, the loss of appetite and the feeling of fullness after eating little. Satiety may occur with a milder form of anorexia but is also often experienced with obstructing, infiltrating, or exophytic lesions of the stomach, usually neoplasms, that prevent its normal filling. An appreciable weight loss commonly accompanies inflammatory and neoplastic processes of the digestive system as well as diseases of malabsorption. Rashes, arthralgias, or arthritis may accompany digestive diseases, especially acute and chronic hepatitis and inflammatory bowel disease.

BIBLIOGRAPHY

Brooks, F.B.: Gastrointestinal pathophysiology, New York, 1974, Oxford University Press.

Greenberger, N.J., and Winship, D.H.: Gastrointestinal disorders: a pathophysiologic approach, Chicago, 1976, Year Book Medical Publishers, Inc.

Sleisenger, M.H., and Fordtran, J.S.: Gastrointestinal disease, ed. 2, Philadelphia, 1978, W.B. Saunders Co.

171 • SPECIAL TECHNIQUES FOR DIAGNOSING DISORDERS OF THE DIGESTIVE SYSTEM

William O. Frank

The purpose of this chapter is to discuss the various specialized diagnostic tests available to detect pathologic conditions in various segments of the gastrointestinal tract. For the sake of clarity, the gastrointestinal tract is considered in the following segments: esophagus, stomach, small bowel, colon (large bowel), liver, hepatobiliary tree, and pancreas. For each of these segments the appropriate specialized diagnostic tests are discussed. The indications for their use are emphasized, their technical aspects are briefly discussed, and when applicable, modifications being made to permit therapeutic intervention are described. New tests and instruments for the diagnosis and treatment of digestive disorders are being developed almost daily; a few of the more promising new ones are included, even though they may not yet be routinely available or their value clearly established. Finally, abdominal sonography, computed tomography, and angiography are discussed.

ESOPHAGUS

A battery of tests is available for evaluating the competence of the lower esophageal sphincter, esophageal peristaltic activity, and esophageal mucosal inflammation or masses. Esophageal mucosal inflammation and masses are diagnosed directly by esophagoscopy, biopsy, and cytologic specimens. (Endoscopy is discussed under "Stomach.") Other diagnostic tests include the Bernstein test, esophageal manometry, pH probe test, and esophageal scintigram. As mentioned in other chapters, these tests are used in a select group of patients with reflux esophagitis or in whom an esophageal motility disorder is suspected.

Bernstein test

The Bernstein test endeavors to reproduce the patient's symptoms by perfusing the esophageal mucosa with acid to determine whether the symptoms originate from the esophagus, presumably from reflux esophagitis.

In this test a tube is positioned in the upper one third of the esophagus with its opening 30 cm (12 inches) from the teeth. A Y-tube is connected to the other end of this tube, which in turn is connected to reservoirs of 0.1N HCl and saline. After an initial drip of saline, the acid solution is permitted to flow until symptoms appear or until 30 minutes has elapsed. If the patient's usual symptoms are reproduced, the drip is switched back to saline. If the symptoms vanish within 3 to 4 minutes, redripping the acid reproduces them rapidly if they result from an esophageal lesion.

Superficially, this test appears to be easy to interpret. In some patients, however, the acid perfusion of the esophagus elicits discomfort or pain different from the patient's original pain. It has not been clearly determined whether these patients should be considered to have a positive Bernstein test result. In addition, the test results may be negative in patients with an esophageal stricture caused by reflux esophagitis. Despite these limitations, this test is an invaluable clinical tool for diagnosing reflux esophagitis.

Esophageal manometry

Esophageal manometry is a technique used to assess the functioning of the upper and lower esophageal sphincters and the motor activity of the body of the esophagus. A bundle of catheters is passed into the esophagus. The open tips of the catheters are separated from one another by a known distance. By means of pumps, water is infused through each catheter at a constant rate. Another arm of each catheter is connected to a low-volume displacement transducer to record pressures on a calibrated recorder. When the outflow of water from a catheter is impeded by the contraction of esophageal muscle or by the tightening of a sphincter, the event is recorded as an increase in pressure occurring at the tip of that catheter. In this way the resting pressures of the sphincters and the degree of their relaxation after swallowing can be determined, as well as the amplitude, velocity, and coordination of the peristaltic waves in the body of the esophagus. The test is performed on patients suspected of having esophageal motor disorders. In achalasia, for example, the test reveals a hypertonic lower esophageal sphincter that fails to relax normally on swallowing and the absence of peristaltic waves in the body of the esophagus. Diffuse esophageal spasm is detected by the simultaneous recording of high-pressure contractions in several catheters at the same time.

pH probe test for reflux

In the pH probe test a pH electrode attached to a manometric catheter is positioned 2 cm above the lower esophageal sphincter, which is located by its high pressure recorded by the catheter. The pH in the esophagus is normally about 6, but if acid is refluxed from the stomach, it falls to about 2. The patient is asked to perform certain maneuvers that tend to promote reflux (Valsalva's maneuver, vigorous sniffing, and elevation of the legs). If no reflux is demonstrated, the catheter is passed into the stomach, 300 ml of 0.1N HCl is infused into the stomach, the catheter assembly is withdrawn to the same location in the esophagus, and the maneuvers are repeated. Because the stomach clearly now contains acid, reflux should readily be detected by observing an acid pH of about 2 in the esophagus. Occasionally pH probes may be left in the esophagus for several hours, for example, during sleep, to record the frequency of reflux and the rate at which refluxed acid is cleared from the esophagus.

Gastroesophageal scintigram

Of all the tests discussed in the preceding paragraphs, none actually demonstrates reflux of gastric juice into the esophagus. The demonstration of the reflux of a radioactive isotope, technetium, into the esophagus during scanning of the esophagogastric area documents reflux of gastric contents. This test is a recent development, but clinical trials suggests that it will prove to be a simple, reliable test for reflux.

Esophagoscopy

Esophagoscopy is discussed in the following section on endoscopy.

STOMACH

Several tests are available for evaluating pathologic lesions in the stomach, for measuring gastric emptying of solids and liquids, and for evaluating the physiology of a stomach altered by surgery. Upper endoscopy permits the gastroenterologist to directly inspect superficial mucosal disease, masses, and ulcers in all areas of the stomach. The measurement of gastric emptying of solids or liquids provides an indirect measure of gastric motility. A scintigraphic technique to assess enterogastric reflux also detects altered gallbladder emptying and simultaneously measures gastric emptying. Each of these tests is discussed in the following sections.

Endoscopy

UPPER ENDOSCOPY. The flexible fiberoptic endoscope is a diagnostic tool used to detect pathologic conditions in the esophagus, stomach, and duodenum. These instruments are forward viewing, have a flexible tip that can be deflected 180 degrees in any direction, and have channels to permit the passage of biopsy forceps, cytology brushes, irrigating or injecting cannulas, and snares or cautery equipment for operative procedures. The examination of the upper gastrointestinal tract with an endoscope permits the physician with direct vision to inspect and perform a biopsy in all portions of the esophagus, stomach, and duodenum. The procedure can be easily performed with little risk and discomfort to the patient, although serious complications such as perforation have been known to occur.

Because upper endoscopy is a common procedure, the

indications for its use are important. Most gastroenterologists agree that upper endoscopy should be performed in patients with (1) upper gastrointestinal hemorrhage, (2) an abnormal roentgenographic appearance of the upper gastro-intestinal tract, (3) unexplained chest or abdominal pain and negative upper gastrointestinal roentgenographic studies, and (4) unexplained symptoms and a history of previous upper gastrointestinal surgery.

An endoscopic examination of a patient with upper gastrointestinal hemorrhage is a rapid and accurate way to determine directly the site of bleeding. Upper endoscopy should probably by the first diagnostic test for evaluating most patients with upper gastrointestinal hemorrhage, for reasons based on several important observations. It is now recognized that upper gastrointestinal roentgenographic studies commonly do not reveal superficial mucosal lesions such as erosions or inflammation. Furthermore, several potential sites of gastrointestinal bleeding sometimes coexist in the same patient, and roentgenograms cannot determine which site is bleeding. Upper endoscopy circumvents these problems. Upper endoscopy should be performed within the first 24 to 48 hours after the episode of bleeding, however, because superficial mucosal lesions may heal within 48 hours. Thus the advantages of upper endoscopy over upper gastrointestinal roentgenograms are (1) superficial mucosal lesions are routinely detected, (2) the clinician is able to determine the site of hemorrhage rapidly and accurately in virtually all patients, including patients with multiple potential sites of bleeding, and (3) a rapid, accurate diagnosis enables the clinician to render appropriate medical or surgical therapy.

When upper gastrointestinal series have detected filling defects, masses, ulcers, and strictures in the esophagus, stomach, and duodenum, upper gastrointestinal endoscopy, should be performed (except for duodenal ulcers). A major advantage of an endoscopic study in these patients is that biopsy and cytology specimens can also be obtained from lesions or suspicious areas of the gut for pathologic study, which enables the clinician to differentiate malignant from benign disease. If the mass is intramural or extrinsic to the gut and no mucosal break is present, however, an appropriate biopsy sample cannot be obtained using conventional endoscopic biopsy techniques.

An upper gastrointestinal series may not reveal ulcers in the upper gastrointestinal tract and, as mentioned previously, commonly does not detect superficial mucosal lesions. Because these lesions may produce symptoms referable to either the thorax or abdomen, upper endoscopy should probably be performed in patients with unexplained chest or abdominal pain and negative gastrointestinal roentgenograms.

Contrast studies of the upper gastrointestinal tract are often difficult to interpret after operations. The gastric emptying time and gastrointestinal transit time are commonly dramatically altered. Therefore good air-contrast studies may be unobtainable, and it may be difficult to differentiate postoperative changes from intrinsic disease. For these reasons the upper gastrointestinal series may not be satisfactory, and careful endoscopic evaluation may be necessary in such postoperative cases.

THERAPEUTIC ENDOSCOPY. The use of upper endoscopy in diagnosing upper gastrointestinal pathologic conditions is well accepted. In addition to its diagnostic capabilities, a therapeutic and operative role for upper endoscopy is now being rapidly developed. Because upper gastrointestinal lesions are commonly associated with bleeding, it would seem appropriate to combine the diagnostic and therapeutic roles of upper endoscopy. Specialized equipment and double-channel upper endoscopes are currently being developed to control gastrointestinal hemorrhage by topical spraying of clotting factors, laser cautery, heater probe, electrocautery, and tissue adhesives. Other therapeutic roles for endoscopy include the removal of foreign bodies and the insertion of prosthetic tubes to relieve an obstruction.

Gastric motility studies

Research into the electromechanical events of gastric motility has shown that the stomach can be divided into two distinct physiologic segments, the proximal and distal portions. The proximal stomach serves as a reservoir. This portion relaxes to receive food boluses from the esophagus—a phenomenon called *receptive relaxation*—and adapts to increasing volumes with little change in pressure, a phenomenon called *accommodation to distention*. These two phenomena maintain a low intragastric pressure as the stomach fills. The distal stomach acts as the gastric mixer and grinder. Peristaltic waves, progressive circular rings of contraction, begin in the corpus and sweep down the stomach to the pylorus. The terminal antrum contracts forcefully and the pylorus closes tightly. This electromechanical activity causes propulsion, squeezing, and retropulsion of the gastric contents and thoroughly mixes, grinds, and triturates gastric solids. It also permits a slow passage of chyme into the small bowel.

Because disturbances of gastric motility alter gastric emptying, tests to measure the gastric emptying of solids and liquids can detect disturbances of gastric motor function. Several techniques have been devised to measure gastric emptying. The classic clinical test is to use a nasogastric or Ewald tube to measure the volume of food and secretions retained in the stomach at a given time after a meal. Newer, more sophisticated tests of gastric emptying include monitoring the emptying of roentgenographic contrast agents, of a saline load, of labeled nonabsorbable markers, or of plastic spheres. A promising new method monitors the rate of disappearance of radioactive-labeled food from the stomach using a gamma camera or scintillation deflector.

Abnormal gastric motility and therefore abnormal gastric emptying are found in at least two groups of patients: those with diabetes mellitus and those who have had gastric surgery. With the advent of new drugs such as metoclopramide, which may prove of value in treating gastric motor disorders, it is especially important to differentiate such disorders from mechanical obstructions and other disorders that may require surgery. Although many of the tests of gastric motility and emptying are not now routinely available, they are being improved and are becoming more widely available.

Scintigraphic technique to measure enterogastric reflux

The reflux of bile and digestive enzymes from the small bowel into the stomach has been described in patients with postsurgical alkaline gastritis (Billroth II surgery), gastric ulcers, reflux esophagitis, and functional dyspepsia; it is unclear what role enterogastric reflux plays in the pathogenesis and symptomatology of these patients. Recently a new scintigraphic technique has been developed to measure enterogastric reflux.

The test is performed in the following manner. ^{99m}Tc-HIDA (N,N'-[2,6-dimethylphenylcarbamoylmethyl]iminodiacetic acid) is administered intravenously. This agent is excreted by the hepatobiliary tree, and when counts are maximal over the gallbladder, the patient drinks a liquid test meal mixed with indium 111 and DTPA (diethylenetriamine penta-acetic acid). Windows are set for each of these radioactive-labeled agents, which are counted over a specified time interval. In essence the small bowel contents become labeled with ^{99m}Tc-HIDA and the gastric contents with ^{111}In-DTPA. Reflux of ^{99m}Tc-HIDA and into the stomach therefore reflects enterogastric reflux. This test is still experimental but may prove to be an important clinical test for the groups of patients listed previously. The test also measures rates of gallbladder and gastric emptying.

SMALL BOWEL

Diseases of the small bowel, apart from peptic ulcer disease of the duodenum and some acute infectious disorders, are relatively uncommon. Abdominal pain, diarrhea, and intestinal obstruction are common symptoms produced by disorders of the small intestine. Barium-contrast roentgenograms (small bowel series) are generally the most useful tests for diagnosing diseases of the small bowel, especially neoplasms and inflammatory disorders such as regional enteritis. Endoscopy will undoubtedly play a larger role in the future. At the present time the distal ileum can be directly viewed with the colonoscope and at least the duodenal bulb and descending duodenum with the duodenoscope. Undoubtedly new endoscopes that are introduced orally or rectally will be in the future permit the direct viewing of and the biopsy of more portions of the small bowel. In certain patients suspected of having a parasitic infection such as giardiasis or an abnormal growth of bacteria in the small bowel, a thin tube can be passed into the small intestine to obtain intestinal aspirates for microscopic examination and appropriate culture studies. In many patients with a malabsorption syndrome diagnosed by the detection of excessive fat in the stool (steatorrhea), a peroral biopsy of small intestine mucosa is necessary for diagnosing the specific cause of the malabsorption.

Small bowel biopsy

The available instruments for a relatively safe peroral biopsy of the small intestine include (1) the *multipurpose biopsy tube* (also called the Rubin or Quinton tube;, which obtains one to four mucosal samples with one passage; (2) the *Crosby capsule,* which obtains one large mucosal sample; and (3) the *hydraulic suction biopsy tube,* which obtains several samples during a single passage. These tubes are passed under floroscopic control through the mouth and the stomach to the ligament of Trietz, the duodenojejunal junction. Obtaining biopsy tissue samples from this site permits histologic comparisons of the mucosa among patients and in the same patient at different times.

To be definitive and free of artifacts, peroral biopsy samples must be obtained, processed, and interpreted correctly. For a small bowel biopsy to have maximal diagnostic value, (1) the biopsy site must be precisely radiologically localized, (2) the biopsy samples must be properly oriented and promptly fixed, (3) the gross specimen should be examined with a dissecting microscope or a low-power microscope, mainly to determine the presence or absence of normal villi, and (4) serial sections cut perpendicular to the lumen and extending to the muscularis mucosae to include the full width of the mucosa should be examined microscopically.

This procedure has a relatively low morbidity and mortality. Complications include perforation and hemorrhage at the biopsy site. The diseases that may be diagnosed by means of an intestinal biopsy include adult and childhood celiac disease, tropical sprue, giardiasis, Whipple's disease, congenital β-lipoprotein deficiency, hypogammaglobulinemic enteritis, and occasionally lymphangiectasia, eosinophilic gastroenteritis, amyloidosis, and intestinal lymphoma.

COLON

The colon (large bowel) is the most common site for cancer. In addition other diseases of the colon such as polyps, diverticulosis and diverticulitis, inflammatory bowel disease (ulcerative colitis and Crohn's disease), and bacterial and parasitic infections are common. Because colonic disease is prevalent, there has been a strong impetus to improve diagnostic techniques. The double-contrast roentgenographic method (introduction of barium followed by air insufflation) is superior to the former single-contrast method and postevacuation roentgenograms for detecting colonic lesions. Colonoscopes now permit direct inspection of the entire colon from the anus to the cecum.

Colonoscopy

Colonoscopes are flexible fiberoptic instruments 160 to 180 cm (64 to 72 inches) long. They have one or two channels for the passage of biopsy forceps, cytology brushes, snares, and electrocautery equipment. In addition there are channels for suction and air insufflation.

Colonoscopes can be passed to the cecum either blindly or with fluoroscopic guidance. Considerable skill is required, but an experienced colonoscopist can reach the cecum in approximately 90% of patients. The colon can be inspected thoroughly as the colonoscope is slowly withdrawn from the cecum. Biopsy samples are taken from suspicious areas of mucosa, and polyps are removed by the snare and electrocautery equipment. Successful colonoscopy usually requires several days of colon preparation (involving a residue-free diet and use of laxatives and enemas) to eliminate fecal residue. Emergency endoscopy is rarely successful because the suction capacity of present colonoscopes is inadequate to remove the usual fecal contents satisfactorily.

Colonoscopy should be performed in (1) patients in whom barium enemas reveal abnormalities, (2) patients who have iron deficiency anemia and Hemoccult-positive stools but whose gastrointestinal tract has a normal roentgenographic appearance, (3) selected patients with inflammatory bowel disease or diverticulosis, and (4) patients with colonic polyps. The indications for colonoscopy are obvious in the first group of patients. Patients in the second group commonly have colonic lesions such as polyps despite a normal barium enema examination. Patients with inflammatory bowel disease often have abnormalities revealed by barium enemas. Patients with chronic idiopathic ulcerative colitis have an increased risk of colon cancer; these patients should routinely undergo colonoscopy. Colonoscopy should usually be deferred, however, in patients with severe, acute inflammation because of the increased risk of perforation. Colonic polyps are considered premalignant lesions, and the larger the polyp the greater the likelihood of malignant transformation. If colonic polyps removed by colonoscopic polypectomy are found to have carcinoma that does not extend into the stalk, their removal can be considered a cure. This important technical advance underlies the significance of this diagnostic tool.

Colonoscopy is not a benign procedure, but it is associated with a low morbidity and mortality. The complications include perforation and bleeding, especially after polypectomy, that may require surgical intervention. A barium enema study should not be performed for at least 7 to 10 days in patients who have had biopsies, especially after a polypectomy, because the high intraluminal pressures generated during a barium enema may theoretically cause perforation at the site of a mucosal biopsy or polypectomy.

Fiberoptic sigmoidoscopy

Fiberoptic sigmoidoscopy is currently being used in place of rigid sigmoidoscopy. A fiberoptic sigmoidoscope is a flexible endoscope with channels similar to those of the colonscope but is only 60 cm (24 inches) long. The advantages of this flexible sigmoidoscope over the rigid sigmoidoscope are currently being studied.

LIVER

A liver biopsy is often necessary for diagnosing liver disease because the symptoms, signs, and results of liver function tests often do not allow for reliable discrimination among various liver diseases. A definitive diagnosis of liver disease is therefore commonly based on characteristic histologic findings. For example, a liver biopsy is required to distinguish chronic active hepatitis from chronic persistent hepatitis and may be necessary to detect hepatic tuberculosis, sarcoidosis, or metastases. A liver biopsy may be performed blindly or under direct vision during laparoscopy (peritoneoscopy); either procedure is acceptable. A major advantage of peritoneoscopy, however, is that the liver, peritoneal cavity, and other organs (spleen, stomach, and gallbladder) can also be inspected. In the following sections the transthoracic (blind) liver biopsy and laparoscopy are discussed separately.

Transthoracic liver biopsy

In a transthoracic liver biopsy, liver dullness is first localized through percussion at the anterior axillary line in the right ninth, tenth, or eleventh intercostal space during inspiration and expiration. The site is marked and anesthetized, and a small incision is made. During expiration, a biopsy needle (such as the Vim-Silverman, Menghini, or Jamshuti needle) is directed toward the liver. As the needle approaches the liver capsule, suction is applied to the glass syringe, and the needle is passed into the liver and rapidly withdrawn.

The procedure has a low morbidity and mortality. Associated complications are intrahepatic or peritoneal hemorrhage, bile leakage and bile peritonitis, the creation of traumatic arteriovenous shunts, and vasovagal shock. Before the liver biopsy is performed, the patient's platelet count and prothrombin time should be checked. A liver biopsy can be performed if the platelet count is greater than 50,000/mm^3 and the prothrombin time is less than 3 seconds more than is normal. Contraindications to a liver biopsy are an uncooperative patient, an extrahepatic biliary tract obstruction existing longer than 2 months, a low platelet count, prolonged prothrombin time, significant ascites, and the suspected presence of ascending cholangitis.

Laparoscopy

Laparoscopy permits direct inspection of the peritoneal cavity and intra-abdominal organs and thus is a valuable and safe technique for diagnosing intra-abdominal pathologic conditions. A state of pneumoperitoneum is produced with carbon dioxide or nitrous oxide using a Verres needle inserted through the anterior abdominal wall into the peritoneal cavity, usually in a lower abdominal wall into the peritoneal cavity, usually in a lower abdominal quadrant. A small incision is then made in the skin, usually at the inferior margin of the umbilicus. The laparoscope trocar and cannula are introduced through this incision into the peritoneal cavity; the trocar is then withdrawn and replaced by the laparoscope.

Many manipulating and operating instruments can be safely introduced into the peritoneal cavity through a second smaller trocar under direct visual guidance. These are used for palpation, manipulation, and exposure of intraabdominal organs. Insulated instruments capable of applying a high-frequency cutting or coagulating current are used for hemostasis, lysis of adhesions, and procedures such as tubal sterilization. Biopsy forceps and combined suction-coagulation instruments can be used for safe and accurate tissue sampling as indicated.

Laparoscopy is indicated (1) to evaluate liver disease, (2) to solve abdominal diagnostic problems, and (3) to determine the stage of a malignant disease. Liver biopsies performed under direct vision using the laparoscope are superior to blind liver biopsies in diagnosing and ascertaining the stage of chronic liver disease, primary and metastatic hepatic cancer, and lymphomas. In addition, laparoscopy is a valuable technique for performing certain invasive roentgenographic procedures.

Hepatic radionuclide imaging

Disease within or adjacent to the liver is often difficult to detect and is even more difficult to localize accurately. Hepatic radionuclide imaging is a fairly sensitive noninvasive technique for detecting and localizing a pathologic condition within or adjacent to the liver. Several available radioactive-labeled colloids are taken up by the liver after being injected intravenously. Rose bengal sodium I 131 is concentrated in hepatocytes and is excreted through the biliary tract. In contrast, gold Au 198, iodinated I 131 human serum albumin aggregated, and technetium Tc 99m sulfur colloid are sequestered by the reticuloendothelial cells (Kupffer's cells). Hepatic lesions that replace or displace normal liver tissue usually appear as an area of di-

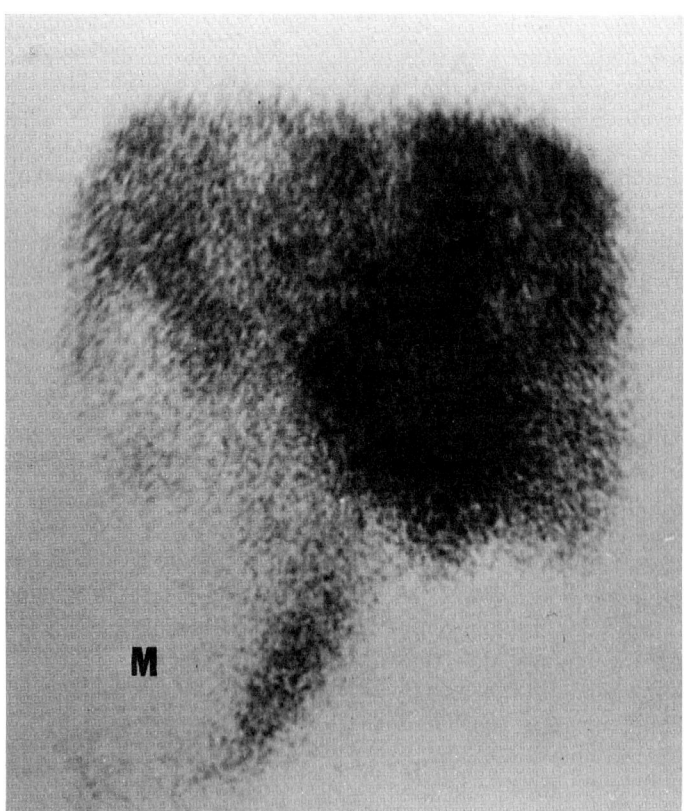

Fig. 171-1. Liver scan with technetium Tc 99m sulfur colloid reveals multiple defects owing to metastatic colon carcinoma. Large metastatic mass *(M)* has replaced much of right lobe. (Courtesy of George Popky, M.D.)

minished activity (Fig. 171-1). A lesion must be at least 2 cm before it can be detected and larger if it is located deep within the hepatic parenchyma.

Hepatic scans are useful for detecting a hepatic tumor (primary or secondary) (Fig. 171-1), abscess, or traumatic injury to the liver. In addition, with hepatic scans the clinician can follow such lesions at various intervals to evaluate the response to appropriate therapy. The liver scan is a poor test for detecting hepatic involvement in systemic disease, however; commonly it is falsely positive or negative. The scan is of little value in patients with cirrhosis because it often exhibits many small filling defects; it may be useful, however, in demonstrating a change in the liver or the presence of splenomegaly. Hepatic scans are probably indicated in patients suspected of having hepatomegally or splenomegaly.

A filling defect noted on a liver scan does not indicate whether the lesion is solid or cystic or whether it is an abscess, tumor, or area of trauma. Liver scanning and gallium citrate Ga 67 can distinguish a primary tumor from a secondary tumor because it is taken up by viable hepatoma cells but not by metastatic tumor cells. In addition, a pyogenic hepatic abscess concentrates ^{67}Ga, but an amebic abscess does not.

HEPATOBILIARY TREE

Obstruction of the hepatobiliary tree (biliary tract) by either malignant or benign disease commonly requires surgical intervention. The aim of the clinician is to determine the presence, location, and cause of an extrahepatic biliary obstruction, which often cannot easily be differentiated from cholestatic (medical) jaundice by its symptoms, signs, or liver function tests. Roentgenographic studies such as the oral cholecystogram or intravenous cholangiogram cannot achieve a complete view of the biliary tree when the serum bilirubin exceeds a certain level, even if no obstruction is present. The ideal diagnostic test should therefore differentiate patients with cholestatic jaundice from those with extrahepatic biliary tract obstruction, should accurately detect the site of the obstruction, and should achieve a complete view of the biliary tree even in the presence of high serum bilirubin levels. Ultrasonography and computed tomography, discussed in later sections, may demonstrate the presence of dilated intrahepatic and extrahepatic ducts, a dilated gallbladder, gallstones, and enlargement of the head of the pancreas, but the usefulness of these techniques is often limited.

Diagnostic tests that fulfill the above criteria have re-

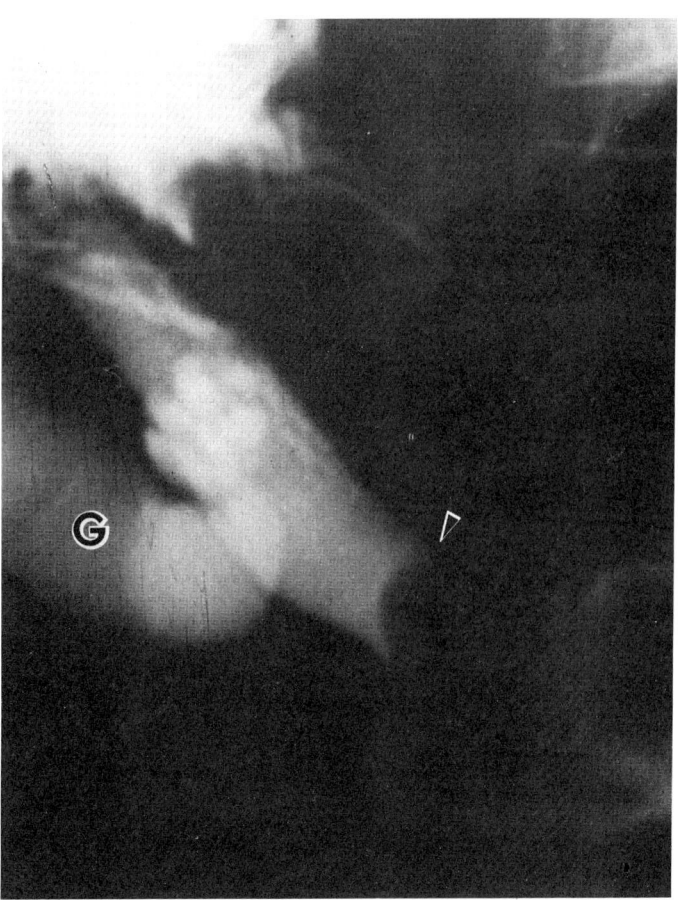

Fig. 171-2. Chiba needle percutaneous cholangiography in patient with deep jaundice reveals large gallstone *(arrow)* completely obstructing dilated common duct. Part of gallbladder *(G)* is visualized on left. (Courtesy of George Popky, M.D.)

cently become available. The transhepatic cholangiogram using the very fine Chiba needle and endoscopic retrograde cannulation of the pancreaticobiliary tree (ERCP) are especially useful. In addition, the recently introduced HIDA and PIPIDA, which permit noninvasive radionuclide imaging of the hepatobiliary tree, are helpful in many cases.

Transhepatic cholangiography with the Chiba needle

Transhepatic cholangiography using the Chiba needle is performed as follows. With fluoroscopic guidance the needle is passed into the liver and is slowly withdrawn while contrast dye is slowly injected through it. When a biliary duct is visualized, the rest of the contrast dye is injected rapidly until the entire biliary tree is opacified, and then the needle is rapidly withdrawn.

This procedure allows visualization of the biliary tract even in the presence of deep jaundice (Fig. 171-2). Other advantages are that it does not require specialized equipment or extensive clinical experience, it is readily available in most hopsitals, and it commonly identifies the site and type of obstruction. Before the procedure is performed, the patient's coagulation profile should be satisfactory (as is required for a liver biopsy). The procedure's complication rate (of bleeding, bile peritonitis, and perforation of the gallbladder) is at least 10%. Most gastroenterologists consider this test a preoperative procedure and before performing it consult with a surgeon and prepare an operating room.

In addition to its diagnostic value, several innovative therapeutic applications of the procedure have been recently developed. These include the decompression of the biliary tree in patients who have a malignant obstruction, the insertion of endoprostheses for internal biliary tract drainage, and dislodgment of stones from the common duct.

Endoscopic retrograde cannulation of the pancreaticobiliary tree

Endoscopic retrograde cannulation of the pancreaticobiliary tree is performed as follows. A side-viewing endoscope is passed into the distal duodenum and is slowly withdrawn until the ampulla of Vater is localized. When the ampulla is visualized, a cannula is passed via the endoscope through the ampulla into the common duct, and contrast dye is injected through the annula while fluoroscopy detects and monitors the opacification of the biliary and pancreatic ducts (Fig. 171-3). When the ductal systems of the pancreas and biliary tract have been amply opacified, the cannula is withdrawn, the endoscope is removed, and roentgenograms are obtained.

This technique demands considerable expertise and sophisticated equipment and is not routinely available in most hospitals. Like transhepatic cholangiography with the Chiba needle, this test should be a preoperative procedure because of the appreciable incidence of associated complications (cholangitis, pancreatitis, and rupture of a pancreatic pseudocyst).

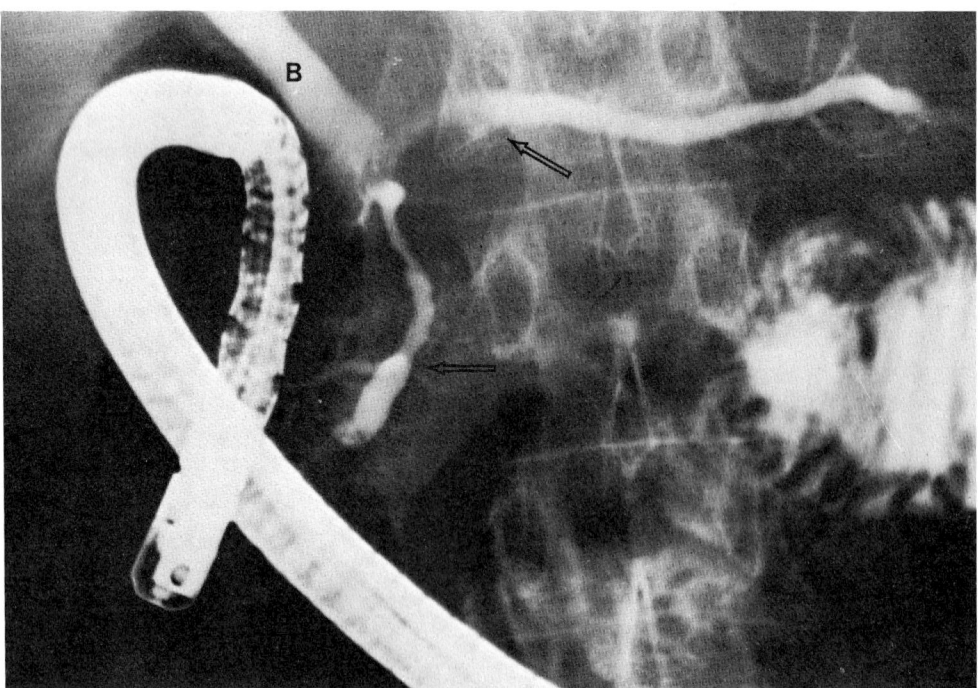

Fig. 171-3. ERCP reveals infiltration and displacement of main pancreatic duct *(between arrows)* by carcinoma of pancreas. *B* denotes partially emptied common bile duct. (Courtesy of Harvey Lefton, M.D.)

A therapeutic role for the procedure has recently been developed. Side-viewing endoscopes have now been refined to permit the endoscopist to remove stones from the common duct and to perform sphincteroplasties. These two adaptations are available, however, at only a few major medical centers.

HIDA and PIPIDA imaging

^{99m}Tc-HIDA (N,N'-[2,6-dimethylphenylcarbamoylmethyl]imminodiacetic acid) and ^{99m}Tc-PIPIDA (paraisopropyl iminodiacetic acid) have recently been used for imaging of the hepatobiliary tree. These agents are taken up by the hepatocytes and excreted into the biliary tree where they are concentrated and thus can detect a site of obstruction. This test enables the clinician to distinguish between intrahepatic and extrahepatic jaundice by noninvasive techniques and is an excellent means of diagnosing cystic duct obstruction in patients suspected of having acute cholecystitis.

PANCREAS

Until recently it has been difficult to study the pancreas without resorting to invasive tests such as angiography. Ultrasonographic examination and computed tomography are noninvasive tests currently available for assessing pancreatic disease, as discussed in following sections. The pancreatic ducts can also be studied directly with the endoscopic retrograde cannulation technique outlined previously, and the very fine Chiba needle can be passed transabdominally under fluoroscopic control into the pancreas to obtain tissue for cytologic analysis.

Endoscopic retrograde cannulation of the pancreaticobiliary tree

Endoscopic retrograde cannulation can be performed with the main pancreatic duct in the same manner as with the common bile duct (Fig. 171-3). In addition, some endoscopists have advocated flushing the pancreatic ductal system with saline to obtain secretions for cytologic analysis and to determine carcinoembryonic antigen levels, but the results have been disappointing.

Pancreatic biopsy

In the literature pancreatic biopsy is said to be dangerous and unreliable even though morbidity and mortality figures have not been cited. Some surgeons recommend resecting an apparent pancreatic malignancy after surgical inspection and palpation alone, even though 3% to 25% of such lesions turn out to be benign. Because the mortality for pancreatic resection is approximately 22% and the 5-year survival rate after surgery for pancreatic carcinoma is less than 1%, the operative risk does not seem justified if there is no histologic proof of malignancy.

The diagnosis of and choice of appropriate therapy for pancreatic cancer require histologic confirmation. Noninvasive diagnostic tests such as computed tomography and ultrasonography and invasive diagnostic tests such as angiography and endoscopic retrograde cholangiopancreatography can locate disease and masses in the pancreas and may suggest their malignant nature, but these tests do not provide histologic proof. Despite the prevailing opinion about the danger and unreliability of pancreatic biopsy, several safe approaches may be used to obtain tissue from the pancreas preoperatively and intraoperatively.

The focus here is on preoperative techniques available for biopsy of the pancreas. Preoperative pancreatic biopsy tissue can be obtained during endoscopic retrograde cholangiopancreatography or by percutaneous fine needle aspiration using an imaging technique. In the former technique, material can be aspirated from the pancreatic duct through the cannula, or a brush can be inserted into the pancreatic duct to obtain cytologic specimens. The yield with this technique appears to be good, and the technique is free from major complications. In the fine needle aspiration technique, the mass is located by an imaging technique such as endoscopic retrograde cholangiopancreatography, angiography, ultrasonography, or computed tomography. A point on the skin perpendicular to the lesion is identified, and a thin needle (20 to 23 gauge) 10 to 15 cm (4 to 6 inches) long is introduced through this site after appropriate local preparation. This needle is then passed transabdominally into the mass. Cytologic specimens are aspirated by applying suction to the attached syringe while moving the needle up and down in the mass. The yield from this technique is good, and the procedure is virtually free from complications. Several authors suggest that endoscopic retrograde cholangiopancreatography and fine needle aspiration should be used in patients with suspected cancer in the tail or body of the pancreas because these patients do not require a bypass operation. For patients with suspected cancer in the head of the pancreas, however, the intraoperative biopsy technique is more applicable because these require a bypass procedure.

OTHER DIAGNOSTIC METHODS

The use of ultrasonography, computed tomography, and angiography in the past decade has greatly improved the roentgenographic diagnosis of digestive disorders; such diagnosis is far superior to that achieved with conventional barium studies alone.

Abdominal ultrasonography

Ultrasound is a mechanical vibration of a frequency in the range above human hearing (greater than 20,000 cycles per second) produced by applying an electrical pulse to a transducer. When a pulse of ultrasonic energy is reflected from an interface in the abdomen to the transducer, a minute voltage change is produced that is amplified, processed, and converted into an image on the screen of an ultrasonic scanner. A tissue interface occurs between tissues of different composition. Ultrasonic imaging does not involve organ function, and thus a nonfunctioning organ can be visualized as adequately as a functioning one. Because gas and barium sulfate strongly reflect sound, an ultrasonogram cannot be made of a gas- or barium-filled bowel.

ULTRASONIC DIAGNOSIS OF PANCREATIC DISEASE. A normal pancreas often cannot be visualized by ultrasonography. The area of the pancreas, however, can be defined precisely because of its close relationship to the splenic and portal veins, which are visible with ultrasonography in most patients. In acute pancreatitis an enlarged and edematous pancreas is visible ultrasonically as an almost echo-free band running across the abdomen 2 cm anterior to the aorta and inferior vena cava. A pancreatic pseudocyst may be shown as a single or multilocular echo-free area. Serial ultrasonograms are a noninvasive means of detecting the rupture, migration, or resolution of the pseudocyst. An ultrasonogram showing chronic pancreatitis is similar to that showing acute pancreatitis except when fibrosis or calcification is present and obscures the ultrasonic outline of the pancreas. Pancreatic carcinoma appears as a localized enlargement with few internal echoes, a ragged margin, and attenuation or obliteration of retropancreatic organs such as the aorta. Ultrasonography reveals only carcinomas at least 2 to 3 cm in size. An ultrasonogram can usually differentiate pancreatitis from pancreatic carcinoma.

ULTRASONIC DIAGNOSIS IN THE LIVER AND BILIARY TREE. Ultrasonography of the gallbladder is performed after an overnight fast because the gallbladder is then at its maximal size. Once the gallbladder has been ultrasonographically identified, its long axis is scanned. Gallstones, detected in over 90% of patients with cholelithiasis, are characterized by strong linear echoes near the posterior wall and a marked attenuation of the sound beam posterior to them (Fig. 171-4). Dilated intrahepatic and extrahepatic biliary tracts, including the common bile duct, are visualized as enlarged echo-free areas on ultrasonograms. Intrahepatic mass lesions such as cysts, primary or metastatic malignancy, and cirrhosis can be demonstrated by ultrasonograms, but ultrasonography is probably not the best diagnostic tool for this purpose.

ULTRASONIC DIAGNOSIS OR INTRA-ABDOMINAL ABSCESSES. Ultrasonic examination of the abdomen is an excellent method for diagnosing intra-abdominal abscesses; ultrasonography demonstrates abscesses directly and has a level of accuracy over 95%. The abscess appears as an echo-free zone with sharply defined walls. In addition its relationship to other organs and the skin surface can be plotted, and its size can be measured in three dimensions. Abscesses must be distinguished, however, from normal fluid-filled structures, especially the gallbladder.

ULTRASONIC DETECTION OF ASCITES AND OTHER INTRAPERITONEAL FLUIDS. Ascites, except when it is loculated by intraperitoneal adhesions, collects in dependent portions of the peritoneal cavity, especially in the hepatorenal space. The depth of the fluid layer in the most dependent part of the abdomen can be measured by an ultrasonogram;

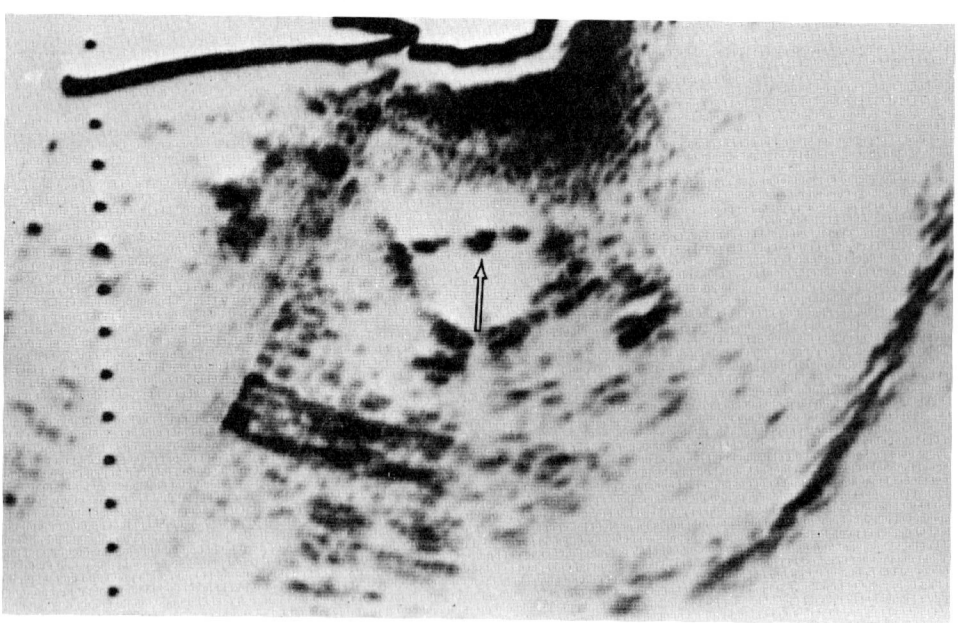

Fig. 171-4. Ultrasonography of gallbladder reveals presence of three "floating" gallstones *(arrow)*. (Courtesy of George Popky, M.D.)

layers of fluid as little as 1 cm deep can be detected by this method. Other free intraperitoneal fluids, however, such as peritoneal dialysates and blood, cannot be distinguished from ascites by their ultrasonic properties.

OTHER INDICATIONS FOR ULTRASONOGRAPHY. Ultrasonography can be used to localize lesions accurately for needle aspiration and radiotherapy planning and to estimate an organ's volume.

Computed tomography

Computed tomography (CT scanning) is a roentgenographic technique that records minor differences in roentgen ray absorption and records an image by computer processing of roentgen rays transmitted through the body. Anatomic definition by CT scanning is more precise than that achieved by ultrasonography, but the equipment is extremely expensive and the radiation dose is substantial. Intestinal gas does not interfere with abdominal CT scanning, but the absence of fat impairs the quality of the scan. CT scans are used in detection of (1) liver metastases, cysts, and abscesses, (2) pancreatitis and pancreatic carcinoma (Fig. 171-5), and (3) biliary tract obstruction. Parenchymatous disease of the liver cannot be defined clearly by CT scanning. In many cases CT scanning and ultrasonography are complementary diagnostic examinations.

Visceral angiography

The ability to perform selective catheterization and the subsequent magnification of intra-abdominal blood vessels has dramatically improved the diagnostic capability of visceral angiography (Fig. 171-6). Therapeutic capabilities have been developed for visceral angiography as well. The selective occlusion of vessels can be accomplished through an arterial catheter for the control of gastrointestinal bleeding, preoperative devascularization of tumors, and treatment of arteriovenous malformations. Techniques of pharmacoangiography, the injection of drugs through an arterial catheter, can be used to enhance opacification, differentiate between normal and tumor vessels, control gastrointestinal bleeding, and treat hepatic metastases.

With the introduction of ultrasonography and CT scanning it has been necessary to reevaluate the role of visceral angiography in the diagnosis of tumors of the pancreas and liver. Visceral angiography of the pancreas cannot readily differentiate pancreatic carcinoma from chronic pancreatitis or detect pancreatic carcinoma in a curable stage. Ultrasonography and CT scanning are superior to pancreatic visceral angiography in these respects. On the other hand, hepatic visceral angiography is superior to ultrasonography and CT scanning in the diagnosis of vascular tumors of the liver such as angiomas, hemangioendotheliomas, benign hepatic adenomas, and most primary hepatomas. Metastatic disease involving the liver, however, is better diagnosed by radionuclide scanning, ultrasonography, or CT scanning. In such instances angiography should be reserved for special situations in which the results from the other tests cannot determine the diagnosis. Although visceral angiography is an excellent method for diagnosing splenic and hepatic ruptures, peritoneal lavage should be performed to detect intraperitoneal bleeding before visceral angiography; peritoneal lavage often eliminates the need for angiography. Visceral angiography, like endoscopy of

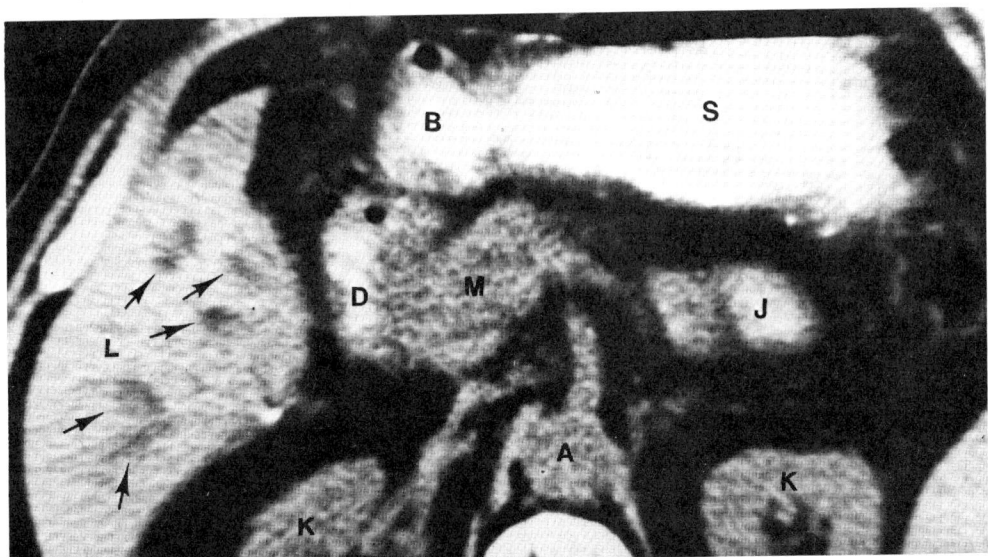

Fig. 171-5. CT scan of abdomen in jaundiced patient reveals large mass *(M)* in head of pancreas and probably dilated ducts *(arrows)* within liver *(L)*. Also identifiable are contrast-filled stomach *(S)*, duodenal bulb *(B)*, descending duodenum *(D)*, loop of jejunum *(J)*, aorta *(A)*, and kidneys *(K)*. (Courtesy of George Popky, M.D.)

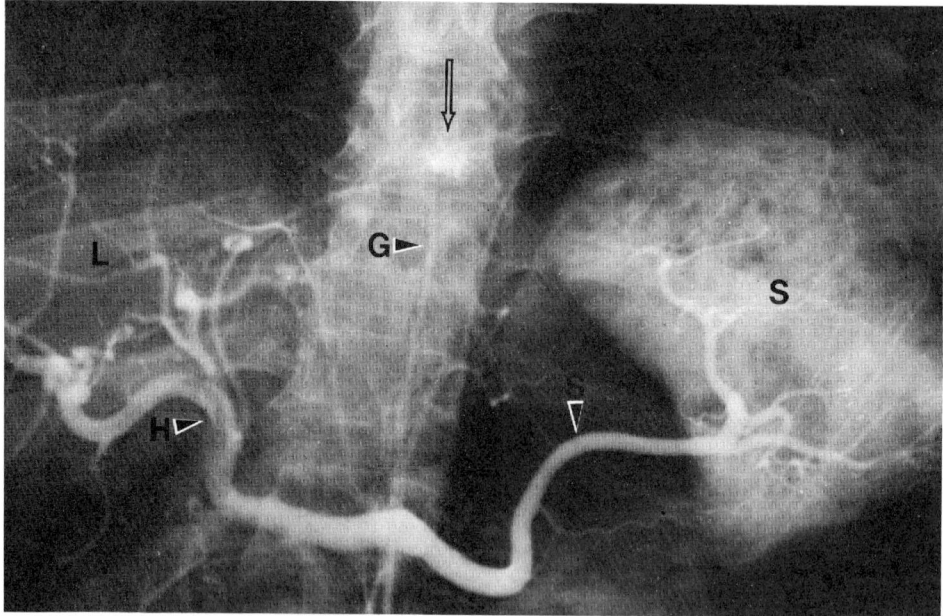

Fig. 171-6. Angiography performed through celiac axis of patient with gastrointestinal bleeding reveals intraluminal collection of contrast material *(upper arrow)* that arises from left gastric artery *(arrow at G)* and accumulates at esophagogastric junction. Hemorrhage at this site was due to Mallory-Weiss tear. Splenic artery is denoted by arrow at S, hepatic artery by arrow at H, spleen by S, and liver by L. (Courtesy of Linda Griska, M.D.)

the gastrointestinal tract, is indicated for both localization and therapy in the management of patients with acute gastrointestinal bleeding. The intra-arterial infusion of vasopressin is effective in controlling gastric mucosal bleeding, bleeding esophageal varices, and colonic diverticular bleeding.

BIBLIOGRAPHY

Bruguera, M., Bordas, J.M., and Rodes, J.: Atlas of laparoscopy and biopsy in the liver, Philadelphia, 1979, W.B. Saunders Co.

Burcharth, F., Jensen, L.I., and Olesen, K.: Endoprosthesis for internal drainage of the biliary tract: technique and results in 48 cases, Gastroenterology **77**:133, 1979.

Demling, L.: Recent advances in gastrointestinal edoscopy, Am. J. Gastroenterol. **69**:533, 1978.

Gudjonsson, B., and Spiro. H.M.: Biopsy techniques in the diagnosis of pancreatic cancer, Gastroenterology **75**:726, 1978.

Kreek, J.M.J., and Balint, J.A.: "Skinny needle" cholangiography: results of a pilot study of a voluntary prospective method for gathering risk data on new procedures, Gastroenterology **78**:598, 1980.

Ogoshi, K., and others: Endoscopic pancreaticocholangiography in the evaluation of pancreatic and biliary disease. Gastroenterology **64**:210, 1973.

Perrault, J., and others: Liver biopsy; complications in 1000 patients and outpatients, Gastroenterology **74**:103, 1978.

Sleisenger, M.H., and Fordtran, J.S.: Gastrointestinal disease, ed. 2, Philadelphia, 1978, W.B. Saunders Co.

Tolin, R.D., and others: Enterogastric reflux in normal subjects and patients with Billroth II gastroenterostomy: measurement of enterogastric reflux, Gastroenterology **77**:1027, 1979.

Wolff, W.I., and others: Colonofiberoscopy: a new and valuable diagnostic modality, Am. J. Surg. **123**:130, 1972.

172 · DISORDERS OF THE ESOPHAGUS

Steven Nussbaum

The esophagus is a muscular tube approximately 25 cm in length that lies in the posterior mediastinum and connects the pharynx with the stomach. It functions to convey food from the oropharynx to the stomach and to prevent reflux of gastrointestinal contents into the body of the esophagus and subsequently into the tracheobronchial tree. At both ends of the esophagus is a sphincter that is tonically closed by muscular contraction. Although its function appears simple and straightforward, its physiologic processes are far from completely understood.

ANATOMY AND PHYSIOLOGY OF THE ESOPHAGUS

The esophagus begins 15 to 18 cm from the incisor teeth and ends at the lower esophageal sphincter, an average 40 cm from the incisor teeth in men and 37 cm in women. The length of the esophagus varies directly with the height of the individual. Its lateral diameter is approximately 30 mm and its anteroposterior diameter approximately 19 mm.

In its course through the mediastinum the esophagus lies in proximity to the thyroid gland, vertebral bodies (sixth cervical to fourth thoracic), the aortic arch, the tracheal bifurcation, and the left atrium. Diseases of these structures may impinge on or involve the esophagus and vice versa.

The upper esophageal sphincter is a transverse slitlike opening formed by the fibers of the cricopharyngeus muscle. The fibers of this muscle, which is the lowermost portion of the inferior pharyngeal constrictor, arise on the posterolateral margin of the cricoid cartilage and pass laterally around the pharyngoesophageal junction to join posteriorly. The superior margin of the muscle is attenuated, creating a zone between it and the inferior constrictor where diverticula may form. The upper esophageal sphincter at rest is tonically closed, separating the oropharynx, which is at atmospheric pressure, from the body of the esophagus, which is at the lower pressure of the thorax, and preventing the entrance of air into the esophagus. It relaxes during deglutition, allowing the bolus of food to enter the esophagus.

The body of the esophagus is lined by stratified squamous epithelium that is separated from the columnar gastric mucosa below by a jagged line, the ora serrata or Z line. The normal epithelium is divided into two layers: the superficial layer, composed of stratified, flat epithelial cells, and the basal layer, composed of several layers of basophilic cells with dark nuclei. Below the mucosa is the lamina propria, composed of loose connective tissue. Characteristic of this zone are papillae, or dermal pegs, that extended into the epithelium normally less than half the distance to the luminal border. A thin band of smooth muscle, the musclaris mucosae, separates the lamina propria from the underlying submucosa. The submucosa consists of both elastic and collagen fibers as well as the deep esophageal glands, the busmucosal venous plexus, and Meissner's neurogenic plexus. Below the submucosa are the outer muscular coats of the esophagus. The inner coat has a circular orientation, whereas the outer coat is longitudinal. Between the two muscular coats lie the ganglion cells of Auerbach's nerve plexus.

The upper one fourth to one third of the muscular coats of the esophagus consists of striated muscle, and the lower two thirds consists of smooth muscle. There is a gradual transition of these two types in the middle one third. Unlike other areas in the gastrointestinal tract, the esophagus has no serosa except in its lower one quarter, where it is surrounded by the phrenicoesophageal ligament in its passage through the diaphragmatic hiatus.

Unlike the upper esophageal sphincter, the lower esophageal sphincter in humans is not anatomically distinct. There is a zone 3 to 4 cm wide, beginning about 40 cm from the incisors, that tonically maintains a resting pressure, thus separating the negative intrathoracic pressure of the body of the esophagus from the positive intraabdominal pressure of the gastric cardia. This high-pressure zone prevents the reflux of gastric material into the esophagus but relaxes after deglutition, allowing the bolus to enter the stomach. Despite years of controversy among anatomists, physiologists, and radiologists, the anatomic components of this sphincter still have not been precisely determined. It would appear, however, that the lower 3 to 4 cm of the esophageal musculature behaves differently from the remainder of the esophagus in response to various neurohumoral stimuli.

Our understanding of the motor physiologic functions of the esophagus has been greatly facilitated in recent years by the development of cineradiography and esophageal motility catheters. The control of esophageal function, however, especially that of the lower esophageal sphincter, remains poorly understood.

After the food bolus is prepared in the oral cavity under voluntary control, the remainder of deglutition proceeds automatically. On entering the pharynx the bolus stimulates afferent nerve endings, resulting in a series of reflex arcs that rapidly complete the swallowing act. Respiration is inhibited, and the suprahyoid muscle contracts, displacing the larynx forward and upward to lie under the base of the tongue, effectively sealing off the respiratory tract. Beginning with the superior pharyngeal constrictor, perstaltic wave moves the bolus downward. The upper esophageal sphincter simultaneously relaxes, and as the peristaltic wave sweeps into the upper esophagus, the bolus enters the cervical esophagus. These events can be clearly shown in esophageal motility studies. The upper esophageal sphincter maintains a zone of tonically increased pressure, as shown by manometry. This zone is 2 to 3 cm wide, and the pressure varies from 40 to 100 mm Hg depending on the orientation of the recording catheter; the zone is asymmetric. With this recording system the upper esophageal sphincter can be shown to relax to the baseline pressure of the esophagus simultaneously with the arrival of the pharyngeal pressure wave. This sphincter appears to be tonically stimulated by excitatory neural activity that is inhibited coincident with the sphincter's relaxation. The control of the pharyngeal phase of deglutition and upper esophageal sphincter motility appears to reside in the medulla and is carried by the vagus nerve.

The continuation of the pharyngeal pressure wave into the esophagus initiates the primary peristaltic wave. Sequential contraction of the esophagus produces a shearing wave that pushes the bolus to the distal esophagus. The control of peristalsis in the striated portion of the esophagus appears to reside in the medulla, whereas in the smooth muscle portion it lies predominately in the peripheral, intramural nerve plexus.

With manometric catheters placed several centimeters apart in the body of the esophagus, the sequential progress of the peristaltic wave can be traced. The waves have a characteristic pattern and often reach 100 mm Hg pressure. A balloon distended in the body of the esophagus, an arrested food bolus, or a reflux of material from the stomach initiates an organized peristaltic wave that originates locally in the esophagus and progresses downward to the lower esophageal sphincter. This secondary peristaltic wave is identical to the primary wave except that it arises locally. It is important in completing the movement of food that has been pushed into the stomach by the primary wave and in ridding the esophagus of refluxed material.

In many individuals, particularly the elderly, tertiary esophageal contractions are often observed. These nonperistaltic contractions arise locally in the esophagus, especially the lower portion, and often occur simultaneously in several locations. They may produce a corkscrew or curling pattern on barium esophagograms.

Coincident with the onset of the primary peristaltic wave the lower esophageal sphincter relaxes to the level of intragastric pressure. Manometric catheters demonstrate that the high-pressure zone at the lower esophagus is 3 to 4 cm wide with a normal resting pressure of 15 to 20 mm Hg. This pressure is not static, and its level may vary according to the recording system used. In contrast to the upper esophageal sphincter, the lower esophageal sphincter remains tonically closed because of the intrinsic property of the muscle in this region. The strength of closure is affected by a great variety of neurohumoral substances and drugs. The control of the opening of the sphincter is poorly understood but seems to reside in an intramural myenteric plexus in this region. The neural transmitter of these inhibitory neurons is neither acetylcholine nor catecholamine but is thought by some to be vasoactive intestinal polypeptide or cyclic adenosine monophosphate (AMP).

SYMPTOMS OF ESOPHAGEAL DISEASE

As with many diseases, the diagnosis of esophageal disorders can often be made from the history. Symptoms of esophageal disease arise from the malfunction of one or both of its primary functions: transporting food to the stomach and preventing reflux of gastric contents.

Dysphagia

Dysphagia, or difficulty with swallowing, is a serious symptom of esophageal disease. Its presence almost always implies a serious disorder, and thus it should never be attributed to neurosis. Dysphagia should be distinguished from globus hystericus, the sensation of a lump in the throat, which is a continual sensation and is independent of swallowing. Although globus hystericus may have a physiologic basis, more commonly no pathologic condition is found.

Dysphagia is perceived by the patient as food sticking or being held up after swallowing. The patient can often precisely localize the point of obstruction but commonly refers the obstruction to the suprasternal notch even when it lies in the lower esophagus. Dysphagia may develop suddenly or gradually and may be so insidious that the patient ignores it until nothing at all can be eaten. It is occasionally helpful to question the patient's family, who might have noted, for example, that the patient was still eating long after everyone else in the family had finished.

Dysphagia may be caused by disorders of the oropharynx or the esophagus. Oropharyngeal dysphagia can usually be differentiated from esophageal dysphagia by means of careful history alone.

Oropharyngeal dysphagia is characterized by difficulty in initiating the act of swallowing. Liquid as well as solids cannot be propelled from the parynx into the upper esophagus. The patient may be unable to move food out of the mouth, or food may seem to stick in the upper neck. Oropharyngeal dysphagia may be associated with aspiration immediately after swallowing. It is occasionally associated with pain. The most common causes include a mechanical obstruction secondary to a tumor or extrinsic mass, central nervous system diseases, and primary muscular diseases. In cases of primary muscular diseases dysphagia may be associated with a nasal quality of the voice and the regurgitations of liquids into the nose.

Esophageal dysphagia may be clinically subclassified as disorders caused by mechanical narrowing or obstruction. The mode of onset and symptoms help to differentiate these disorders. Mechanical narrowing of the lumen can result from mucosal lesions such as carcinoma, strictures (peptic or corrosive), and webs or from extrinsic lesions such as mediastinal tumors, aortic aneurysms, and so on. Motor disorders associated with dysphagia include achalasia, diffuse esophageal spasm, and reflux esophagitis.

Patients with mechanical narrowing of the lumen often have progressive dysphagia. Typically they first have difficulty swallowing solid foods with an elastic or spongy quality, such as breads and meat. Over time, usually weeks to months, the dysphagia progresses until the lumen is totally obstructed and even liquids cannot be swallowed. Occasionally a patient has a sudden, complete obstruction resulting from the impaction of a food bolus above the area of narrowing.

In dysphagia resulting from motility disorders the patient has difficulty initially with both liquids and solids; there is no progression. The symptoms often occur intermittently at first and may have a gradual onset. Extremes in food temperatures and anxiety-producing situations may exacerbate the dysphagia of patients with motility disorders.

The impaction of food bolus above a mechanical obstruction may cause the patient extreme distress that can be relieved only by regurgitation of the bolus. Patients with motility disorders, on the other hand, may cause the bolus to pass by repeatedly swallowing a liquid or by performing Valsalva's maneuver.

Heartburn

Heartburn, or pyrosis, has been experienced at one time or another by nearly everyone. It is described as a hot or burning sensation that moves upward from the epigastrium, beneath the sternum, and often into the neck. It is frequently accompanied by belching and a sour or bitter taste in the mouth resulting from the reflux of gastric contents into the esophagus. It commonly follows a meal and may be precipitated by maneuvers that increase intra-abdominal pressure, such as bending or lifting. The patient often has heartburn on lying down, particularly after a large meal or at bedtime. Pyrosis is usually relieved by the ingestion of antacids, although this relief may be temporary. The failure of antacids to relive heartburn suggests that the symptom might be caused by a disorder other than reflux. Heartburn may be exacerbated by acidic liquids such as citrus juices or precipitated by smoking or drinking coffee or alcohol.

Pyrosis may be associated with regurgitation, the backflow of gastric contents into the patient's mouth without preceding nausea. Occasionally the patient may note the appearance of a clear, salty fluid in the mouth accompanying heartburn. This unusual symptom, water brash, probably results from the release of salivary secretions. Patients with heartburn may regurgitate in their sleep, resulting in nocturnal coughing, wheezing, and morning hoarseness caused by aspiration, and may find the pillow is wet in the morning because of this nocturnal regurgitation.

Odynophagia

Odynophagia, or pain on swallowing, usually results from inflammatory disorders of the esophageal mucosa. It is seen when the mucosa is invaded by organisms such as *Candida* or herpesvirus. Mucosal inflammation caused by ingestion of a corrosive chemical may give rise to odynophagia. Patients with reflux esophagitis commonly have odynophagia in varying degrees and occasionally may have bolus awareness, a sensation of the bolus moving down the esophagus.

Esophageal spasm

Esophageal spasm may cause severe pain that may mimic precisely the symptoms of angina or a myocardial infarction. The patient has substernal pain that may radiate to the neck or arm or straight through to the back. The spasm is caused by a motility disorder and therefore may also be associated with dysphagia. Attacks of pain may occur spontaneously, even during sleep, or may be triggered by the ingestion of cold liquids or by emotional upset.

Hematemesis

Inflammatory and neoplastic disorders of the esophagus may give rise to gastrointestinal bleeding. Chronic blood loss is common in patients with reflux esophagitis and paradiaphragmatic hernias. Massive bleeding with hematemesis occasionally occurs as a result of reflux esophagitis, esophageal carcinoma, or esophageal varices.

DISORDERS OF ESOPHAGEAL MOTILITY

Primary disorders of the musculature of the esophagus or its innervation result in defects in esophageal motility. Symptoms vary according to the location and type of musculature involved.

Disorders of striated muscle

OROPHARYNGEAL DYSPHAGIA

Definition. Grouped under the term "oropharyngeal dysphagia" are a variety of disorders that primarily affect the striated muscle of the oropharynx and upper esophagus. They share in common the symptom of difficulty in the initiation of swallowing.

Etiology. Primary degenerative and inflammatory disorders of striated musculature may produce the syndrome of oropharyngeal dysphagia. Inflammatory disorders such as dermatomyositis or polymyositis may involve the striated musculature of the esophagus. Two types of familiar muscular dystrophy, oculopharyngeal myopathy and myotonia dystrophica, may produce the syndrome. Metabolic myopathies such as are produced by hyperthyroidism or hypothyroidism may rarely cause the syndrome. Myasthenia gravis, a disorder of the motor end-plate affects all striated muscle including the esophagus.

Diseases of the central and peripheral nervous system may result in defects in the coordination of the pharyngeal musculature. Cerebrovascular accidents (especially those involving the brainstem), Parkinson's disease, Huntington's chorea, amyotrophic lateral sclerosis, multiple sclerosis, tabes dorsalis, brainstem tumors, and other congenital and degenerative disorders of the central nervous system may produce oropharyngeal dysphagia. Bulbar poliomyelitis, peripheral neuropathies (diabetic mononeuritis multiplex), and even sectioning of the last four cranial nerves (Vernet's syndrome) may similarly produce the syndrome.

In a third group of patients with oropharyngeal dysphagia no primary disorder can be found. These patients are said to have cricopharyngeal spasm or cricopharyngeal achalasia. This syndrome is commonly associated with Zenker's diverticulum, an outpouching of the esophagus above the cricopharyngeal muscle.

Clinical manifestations. The primary symptom is difficulty in the initiation of swallowing. Patients with this syndrome either are unable to move the bolus of food out of the mouth or complain of its sticking in the region of the Adam's apple. They may have pain or odynophagia in the region of the upper neck and may lose weight because they are afraid of eating. Nasal or oral regurgitation of food or liquid may occur immediately after swallowing. Misdirection of the bolus into the tracheobronchial tree may result in an immediate postdeglutitive cough, acute pulmonary infection, or even chronic lung disease. In addition to the symptoms of the underlying disease, there patients may manifest a nasal quality of speech or even dysarthria.

Laboratory findings. The laboratory findings are those of the underlying disease. Polymyositis or dermatomyositis is manifested by elevations of muscle enzymes such as creatine phosphokinase and aldolase. Hypothyroidism and hyperthroidism are diagnosed by appropriate thyroid studies. There are no specific laboratory studies for the syndrome of cricopharyngeal achalasia.

Diagnosis. Roentgenographic studies are helpful in the diagnosis of oropharyngeal dysphagia. A barium esophagogram may demonstrate the pooling of contrast material in the valleculae and pyriform sinuses, areas that normally are rapidly cleared. A posterior indentation or bar may be seen in the barium column; this is caused by a spasm of the cricopharyngeal muscle. Occasionally barium may not pass this area at all, a situation that has given to the term "cricopharyngeal achalasia." Aspiration of barium into the lungs may be seen after swallowing.

Cineradiography is perhaps the most useful diagnostic tool, permitting detailed examination of the coordination of swallowing.

Manometric recordings of the pharynx and upper esophagus have produced conflicting results in these disorders, perhaps because of the difficulty in studying this area. Defects in the strength and coordination of the pharynx and upper esophageal sphincter have been found but are not universally accepted.

Course. The course is that of the underlying disorder. Occasionally a patient who suffers oropharyngeal dysphagia after a cerebrovascular accident gradually regains the ability to swallow. If untreated, however, patients with oropharyngeal dysphagia may die of the results of inanition or pulmonary aspiration.

Management. Medical treatment consists of treating the underlying disorder. Patients with Parkinson's disease may benefit from L-dopa therapy. Anticholinesterases may improve swallowing in patients with myasthenia gravis. Corticosteroids may occasionally produce remissions in patients suffering from dermatomyositis or polymyositis. Quinine and procainamid have been used in the therapy of myotonic dystrophy. Appropriate treatment can improve the myopathy responsible for oropharyngeal dysphagia in thyroid disorders.

Bougienage and mechanical dilation have been advocated by some as treatments for oropharyngeal dysphagia, but there have been no large series with follow-up studies to support this therapy.

Cricopharyngeal myotomy, in which the circular muscles of the cricopharyngeal muscle are sectioned, has produced perhaps the best results. In one series good results were obtained in 64% of cases. The most consistently good results have been produced in patients with the idiopathic disorder called cricopharyngeal achalasia. There have been scattered case reports of success in patients with neuromuscular disorders such as amyotrophic lateral sclerosis. The poorest results are obtained in patients with a central nervous system disorder such as occurs after a cerebrovascular accident. Cricopharyngeal myotomy is indicated in patients with significant dysphagia, weight loss, or aspiration. In patients with a large Zenker's diverticulum, resection of the diverticulum in addition to myotomy is indicated. The resolution of small diverticula has been noted after cricopharyngeal myotomy, an observation that suggests that cricopharyngeal incoordination or spasm plays a role in the development of diverticula.

A gastrostomy or jejunostomy for feeding is occasionally necessary in a refractory patient who is unable to eat.

Disorders of smooth muscle

Included as disorders of the smooth muscle are those that primarily affect the smooth muscle of the lower esophagus and lower esophageal sphincter.

ACHALASIA

Definition. Achalasia is a disorder of the esophageal smooth muscle characterized by an absence of peristalsis and a defect in the normal relaxation of the lower esophageal sphincter. The failure of the sphincter to relax to the resting gastric pressure results in a functional obstruction to the emptying of the esophagus. Measurements of the resting pressure of the sphincter led to achalasia originally being designated cardiospasm. As a result of its failure to empty, the esophagus dilates progressively over time.

Etiology and pathogenesis. Although achalasia was the first motility disorder of the esophagus to be described, its cause remains unknown. Most observers agree that the defect lies in the neural control of esophageal motility and lower esophageal sphincter relaxation. Autopsy and operative specimens seem to support this theory because in almost all cases the ganglion cells in Auerbach's plexus are reduced in number. Most observers agree that these changes can be found in the body of esophagus, but there is controversy about the finding in the sphincter. Defects in the esophageal motor nerves found in the vagal nerve trunk and the degeneration of neurons in the dorsal motor nucleus of the vagus nerve have also been described and likened to wallerian degeneration. Research into these defects has been hampered by the lack of a true animal model for achalasia.

The response of the esophagus to cholinergic drugs supports the theory of denervation. When patients with achalasia are given synthetic acetylcholine-like drugs such as methacholine, both the esophageal body and sphincter react more vigorously than is normal. This reaction has been interpreted by some as a sign of denervation hypersensitivity (Cannon's law).

Another interesting finding in these patients is that the esophageal sphincter is hypersensitive to gastrin, which causes increased contraction. The lower esophageal sphincter has a lower threshold and responds submaximally at lower doses of gastrin than is the case normally. There is little correlation, however, between lower esophageal sphincter pressure and gastrin levels, and the role of gastrin in the production of achalasia is unknown.

The closest analogy to achalasia is Chagas' disease, an infection with *Trypanosoma cruzi,* whose symptoms and clinical findings may mimic achalasia. Unlike achalasia, however, Chagas' disease is often associated with megaureter, megaduodenum, and megacolon. Examination of the esophagus and other involved organs reveals destruction of Auerbach's ganglion cells, a finding that has led some to suggest that an infective organism, perhaps a neurotropic virus, is responsible for the lesions in achalasia. The lack of a pattern in the cases and serologic data, however, do not support this theory.

Epidemiology. Achalasia is a rare syndrome affecting perhaps 1 in 100,000 people. It affects both sexes equally and is found in all races.

Clinical manifestations. The onset of symptoms occurs usually in those from 20 to 40 years of age; however, cases have been described at both extremes of age and even in infancy. The classic symptom is dysphagia with both solids and liquids that is gradual in onset and may be precipitated or made worse during times of stress. Dysphagia is usually painless, but an occasional patient may experience odynophagia or esophageal colic early in the disease. The patient may learn to promote emptying of the esophagus with a variety of maneuvers such as throwing the head back and performing Valsalva's maneuver.

The regurgitation of undigested food retained in the esophagus is a common symptom that may lead to severe complications. Regurgitation is especially noted at night. The aspiration of retained food may result in pulmonary complications. The patient may complain of wheezing, coughing, and choking, especially at night. Frequent episodes of bronchopneumonia or lung abscess may result from soiling of the pulmonary tree.

Weight loss is uncommon in the early stages of the disease but may become marked later in its course. Some patients complain of halitosis, which results from the fermentation of retained material. Occasionally a patient has hematemesis caused by esophageal erosion or, rarely, esophageal varices. Heartburn is an unusual symptom in patients with achalasia and thus makes the diagnosis of achalasia questionable.

The physical findings are generally unremarkable. Weight loss and cachexia are seen in advanced cases. Signs of pulmonary consolidation are present in patients with bronchopulmonary aspiration. Rarely a widened area of mediastinal dullness may be noted.

Diagnosis. The esophagus dilates progressively over time and in its final stage may have sigmoid appearance. Occasionally on chest roentgenograms the dilated esophagus appears as a mediastinal mass and may even contain an air-fluid level resulting from retained food and fluid. A common findings is the absence of a stomach bubble on chest roentgenograms.

A barium esophagogram often produces helpful diagnostic information (Fig. 172-1). The classic appearance is a dilated esophagus with an air-fluid level and a smooth, symmetric, beaklike narrowing of the distal esophagus. Early in the disease the esophagus may not be dilated, but the fluoroscopist may note an absence of peristalsis in the distal two thirds of the esophagus and its failure to empty when the patient is in the supine position. Purposeless movements of the distal esophagus may occasionally be noted. A hiatus hernia is very unusual in achalasia, and its presence makes this diagnosis doubtful. Occasionally, however, an epiphrenic diverticulum is noted just above and to the right of the lower esophagus.

Esophagoscopy and biopsy of the esophagus are indicated in every patient with achalasia. In addition to ruling out other causes of esophageal obstruction, such as benign stricture or carcinoma, with these tests the endoscopist may note characteristic findings. The lumen of the esophagus may be dilated, and prevously ingested material may be present. Peristalsis is of course absent, and the lower esophageal sphincter does not open despite the continued insufflation of air. The esophageal mucosa may be inflamed. With gentle pressure at the lower esophageal sphincter the instrument easily passes the obstruction. Although these findings are characteristic of achalasia, they cannot determine the diagnosis.

The definitive diagnosis of achalasia should always be established with manometry. The upper portion of the esophagus has normal motility. Examination of the remainder of the esophagus reveals four characteristic abnormalities: (1) elevated resting pressure in the body of the esophagus, (2) absence of peristalsis following a swallow, although nonperistaltic waves occasionally may be seen, (3) a high resting pressure at the lower esophageal sphincter (usually about twice normal, or 40 to 50 mm Hg above gastric pressure), and (4) failure of the resting sphincter pressure to fall to the gastric baseline pressure following a swallow. Although the sphincter does relax after a swallow, it rarely falls more than 10 to 20 mm Hg. As a result a high-pressure zone is maintained, preventing food and fluid from entering the stomach.

When patients with achalasia are given methacholine (Mecholyl) by injection, intraluminal catheters may measure a dramatic, sustained rise in pressure, usually in excess of 25 mm Hg. Although the methacholine test is characteristic of achalasia, it may have a positive result with other disorders. Because it is uncomfortable for the patient and because the diagnosis can be established by manometric abnormalities, the methacholine test should not be used for the diagnosis of achalasia.

Achalasia must be differentiated from other causes of esophageal obstruction, most importantly from carcinomas and benign strictures. Carcinomas rarely produce a dilated esophagus and can usually be diagnosed by endoscopic biopsies. A benign stricture should be suspected in a pa-

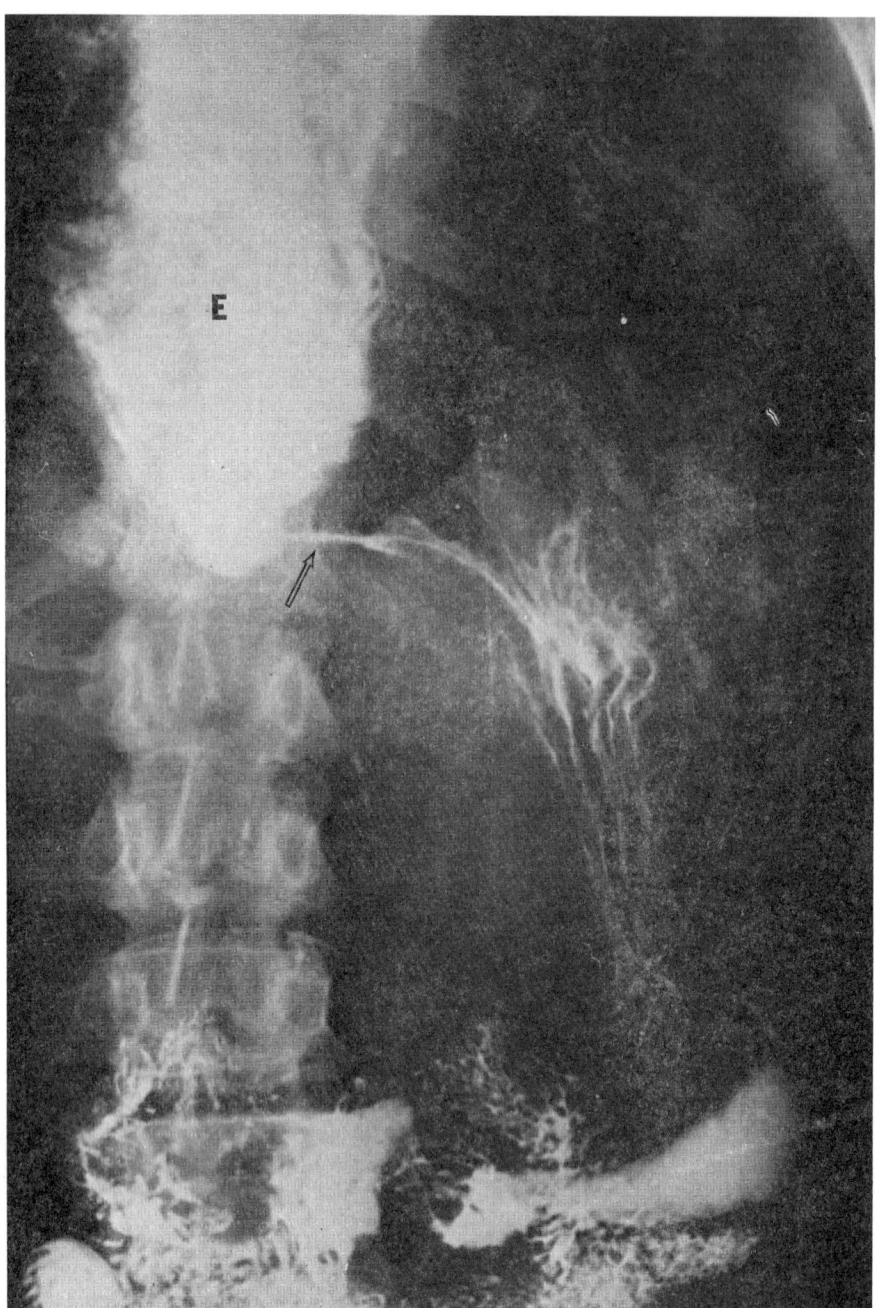

Fig. 172-1. Gastrointestinal series from 72-year-old man with achalasia. Note markedly dilated esophagus *(E)* with retained barium, food, and secretions and symmetrically narrowed distal esophagus *(arrow)*. (Courtesy of George Popky, M.D.)

tient with a long history of heartburn or a hiatus hernia revealed by a barium esophagogram. With benign strictures and carcinomas, the esophagoscope commonly cannot pass the obstruction. Achalasia can of course be diagnosed by manometry.

Occasionally a carcinoma that involves the distal esophagus and arises in the gastric cardia or is metastatic from another primary carcinoma may produce a syndrome that mimics achalsia clinically, reoentgenographically, and manometrically. This syndrome is thought to arise from carcinomatous destruction of Auerbach's ganglia. Diagnosis can be made in most cases endoscopically.

Course. Untreated, the esophagus progressively dilates. The patient may be asymptomatic for years but in time begins to suffer weight loss and inanition. Death may result from pulmonary aspiration and infection.

An increased incidence of squamous carcinoma in cases of achalasia has been noted. The carcinoma arises usually in the midesophagus and in patients younger that those with carcinoma but without achalasia. In patients in whom it is found, achalasia commonly has been present for years. The early diagnosis of carcinoma in patients with achalasia is complicated by these patients already being symptomatic and esophagograms only occasionally detecting the carcinoma because of the dilation and retained material. The incidence of carcinoma has been reported to be 2% to 7% in those with achalasia. The reason for this increased incidence is unknown, although chronic stasis and bacterial overgrowth have been implicated. Because of this increased tendency toward carcinoma, it has been advocated that patients with achalasia undergo yearly endoscopy and cytologic biopsy. Unfortunately, there is no evidence that the early treatment of achalasia lessens the incidence of carcinoma.

A rare complication of achalasia is the production of "downhill" varices from the obstruction of periesophageal, azygos, and hemiazygos venous channels by the pressure of the dilated esophagus. These may give rise to massive bleeding.

Management. The medical treatment of achalasia has been disappointing. Although anticholinergic agents, glucagon, and β-adrenergic drugs may reduce the pressure of the lower esophageal sphincter, they must not been shown to be clinically effective. Two modes of therapy are currently employed in the treatment of achalasia: pneumatic dilation and esophageal myotomy. Both these forms of therapy have the goal of weakening the musculature of the lower esophageal sphincter so that food may pass into the stomach.

Bougienage, even with the largest avaiable dilators, achieves only a temporary relief of symptoms. Several mechanical devices are now available that forcefully and rapidly disrupt the muscle of the lower esophageal sphincter. The most commonly used device employs a balloon that is placed across the gastroesophageal junction, rapidly inflated to a pressure of 300 to 500 mm Hg, and held for 15 to 60 seconds. The procedure is often painful but provides symptomatic and often long-lasting relief in 60% to 75% of patients. Occasionally a patient may even regain peristaltic activity after dilation, an as yet unexplained phenomenon. If it is unsuccessful, the dilation may be repeated, but more than two dilations are not recommended. The most serious complication of the procedure is esophageal perforation or rupture, which occurs in 5% of patients. Pneumatic dilation is not indicated in a patient with a massively dilated, sigmoid esophagus.

The surgical procedure of choice is Heller's myotomy or a variation of this operation, which consists of a limited incision of the circular smooth muscle of the lower esophageal sphincter. About 80% of patients obtain symptomatic relief after a Heller's myotomy. The chief complication is reflux esophagitis, which occurs because the chief barrier to reflux, the lower esophageal sphincter, has been destroyed and because the esophagus is unable to clear the refluxed material owing to its peristaltic defect. Although this complication occurs in a minority of patients, many surgeons have recommended the inclusion of an antireflux procedure in the surgical treatment of achalasia.

There is controversy about whether pneumatic dilation or surgery should be initially attempted. Both appear to be efficacious, and the difficulty of the decision is a compounded by the lack of controlled trials comparing them. The decision must be based on the experience of the treating physician.

SYMPTOMATIC IDIOPATHIC DIFFUSE ESOPHAGEAL SPASM

Definition. Symptomatic idiopathic diffuse esophageal spasm is a rare disorder of esophageal motility in which chest pain or dysphagia is produced by repetitive, high-pressure, simultaneous contractions of the smooth muscle of the esophagus.

Etiology and pathophysiology. The cause and pathophysiologic nature of symptomatic idiopathic diffuse esophageal spasm are essentially unknown. The most common pathologic change reported has been marked thickening of the smooth musculature of the lower esophagus. Abnormalities in the innervation of the esophagus have been reported but are not universally accepted.

Epidemiology. Diffuse spasm is a rare disorder. Patients are usually over 50 years of age, although this disorder has been reported in younger age groups.

Clinical manifestations. The most common symptom of diffuse spasm is esophageal colic. The patient experiences a crushing substernal chest pain that may radiate through to the back and may be associated with diaphoresis. Esophageal colic may closely simulate the pain of myocardial infarction or angina pectoris. Pain may be precipitated by emotional upset or by the ingestion of hot or cold foods. Reflux of gastric contents has been reported as a precipitating factor. The pain may also occur spontaneously and often awakens the patient from sleep.

The patient may have dysphagia that is usually not associated with pain; dysphagia occurs with both solids and liquids and is intermittent and not progressive. Forceful regurgitation occasionally occurs.

The physical examination is unremarkable.

Diagnosis. In addition to the patient's history, barium esophagography and manometry are required to make the diagnosis.

The barium swallow examination reveals spontaneous, uncoordinated, nonperistaltic movements of the lower two thirds of the esophagus. Occasionally the smooth muscular portion of the esophagus can be seen to contract as a unit simultaneously with the onset of pain. These tertiary contractions may produce a picture of pseudodiverticula or sacculations, a condition that has been called a corkscrew esophagus (Fig. 172-2).

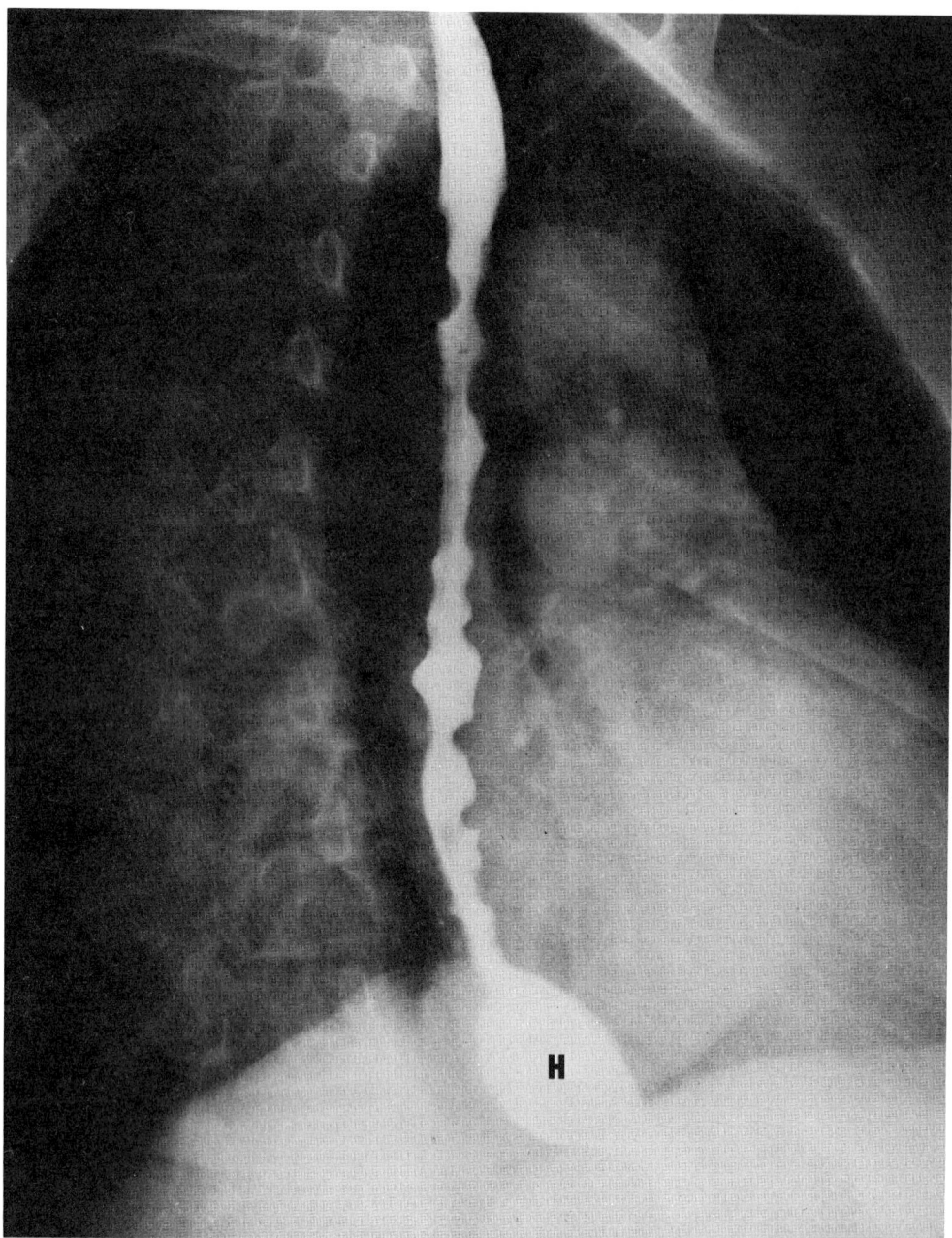

Fig. 172-2. Patient with recurrent episodes of chest pain and dysphagia exhibits "corkscrew" appearance, sacculations, and pseudodiverticula of esophagus, findings indicative of esophageal spasm. He also has hiatus hernia *(H)*. (Courtesy of George Popky, M.D.)

Manometry of the upper esophageal sphincter and upper esophagus reveals normal motility. In the esophageal body most swallows, especially of cold liquid, are followed by nonperistaltic, high-amplitude repetitive waves that may be prolonged. In addition, spontaneous, nonperistaltic high-pressure waves may occur without swallowing. Occasionally a swallow is followed by normal peristalsis. The pressure and relaxation of the lower esophageal sphincter are normal in most of these patients, but abnormal relaxation or a high resting pressure occurs in about 30%.

As in achalasia, most patients with symptomatic idiopathic diffuse esophageal spasm are hypersensitive to cholinergic stimulants such as subcutaneous methacholine. These patients have also been found to be supersensitive to intravenous gastrin, responding with an increased amplitude and duration of esophageal body contractions.

Course. The course of diffuse spasm is unknown. In 3% to 5% of patients the disorder may progress from classic diffuse spasm to achalasia, an observation that has led some to suggest that diffuse spasm may represent an early stage of achalasia or that there is a spectrum of neurologic damage with spasm on one end and achalasia on the other.

Management. Some patients obtain relief with nitrites such as nitroglycerin, an observation that further compounds the confusion of diffuse spasm and angina pectoris. A few patients obtain relief from pain with anticholinergic drugs.

Pneumatic dilation of the lower esophageal sphincter has provided relief from symptoms in a small number of patients. This technique is currently under evaluation.

When dysphagia becomes so severe that it causes weight loss or pain becomes intractable, surgery must be considered. Good results with a long myotomy of the lower esophagus have been reported.

OTHER PRIMARY ESOPHAGEAL MOTILITY DISORDERS. A number of patients have motility disorders that cannot be classified as either classic achalasia or diffuse spasm. These disorders are variants of the two syndromes and may exhibit a mixture of motility disturbances seen in the classic disorders. In one type of disturbance chest pain and high-pressure spontaneous contractions are associated with an elevated pressure and abnormal relaxation of the lower esophageal sphincter; this variant has been labeled vigorous achalasia. Other patients have been described with aperistalsis but normal function of the lower sphincter or normal peristalsis and elevated sphincter pressures. The progression of some of these disorders to achalasia has also been documented. Several of these patients have achieved relief of dysphagia and/or pain by pneumatic dilation. The existence of these ''intermediate'' syndromes has led some observers to suggest that achalasia and diffuse esophageal spasm are part of a spectrum of related motor disorders.

CHRONIC IDIOPATHIC INTESTINAL PSEUDO-OBSTRUCTION. Chronic idiopathic intestinal pseudo-obstruction is a motility disorder of the entire gastrointestinal tract that is characterized by recurrent episodes of intestinal obstruction. Esophageal involvement results in mild symptoms, and the motility disorder resembles achalasia. Manometric recordings have demonstrated aperistalsis and an impaired relaxation but a normal pressure of the lower esophageal sphincter. Two variants have been described, one resulting from a degeneration of the innervation of the intestinal tract and the other from a degeneration of gut smooth muscle.

Motility disorders of the esophagus in systemic diseases

COLLAGEN VASCULAR DISEASES. Esophageal motor dysfunction has been described in a number of patients with collagen vascular diseases but occurs most commonly in association with scleroderma (systemic sclerosis). Involvement is manifested by aperistalsis and the incompetence of the lower esophageal sphincter.

Etiology and pathophysiology. Both the cause of the systemic disease and its esophageal involvement remain unknown in all of these disorders. Almost without exception Raynaud's phenomenon is present when esophageal motility disorders can be demonstrated, leading to the suggestion that disturbances in motility in these disorders result from a defect in the neurologic control of the esophagus or from the effects of ischemia. In the case of scleroderma, this hypothesis is supported by the autopsy finding that portions of the esophagus with abnormal peristaltic activity may still contain histologically normal muscle. Late findings in the disease are patchy atrophy and replacement of smooth muscle with fibrous tissue. Supporting the hypothesis of a neurologic defect is the fact that the lower esophageal sphincter is responsive to cholinergic drugs acting directly on smooth muscle but not to cholinesterase inhibitors such as edrophonium.

Epidemiology. The esophagus is involved in about 75% of patients with scleroderma and mixed connective tissue disease. The incidence of esophageal involvement in systemic lupus erythematosus, dermatomyositis, rheumatoid arthritis, and Raynaud's disease is unknown but probably is much lower than in scleroderma except when these diseases are associated with Raynaud's phenomenon.

Clinical manifestations. The chief symptoms of esophageal involvement are reflux esophagitis and dysphagia. Reflux arises from an impaired lower esophageal sphincter function and impaired ability of the esophagus to clear itself of refluxed material.

Reflux results in heartburn, regurgitation, and a sour or bitter taste in the mouth. Dysphagia initially may occur with both solids and liquids and may be most severe when the patient is in the supine position and gravity cannot assist in emptying the esophagus. Esophagitis is often progressive and leads to stricture formation in about 40% of patients; as a stricture forms in the esophageal lumen, dysphagia becomes progressively more severe, especially with solids. Interestingly, esophageal dysfunction and Raynaud's phenomenon may precede skin involvement in scleroderma by years.

Diagnosis. In chest roentgenograms air may be seen in the esophagus. Barium esophagography reveals an absence of peristalsis and the presence of free esophageal reflux, retention of barium in the supine position, dilation of the lumen, and often a smoothly tapered stricture.

Motility studies reveal a diminution of peristaltic force early in the disease that progresses to a total lack of peristaltic activity in the distal two thirds (smooth muscle portion) of the esophagus. The lower esophageal sphincter is incompetent and has a pressure usually below 5 mm Hg.

Management. As is the case with collagen vascular diseases, no completely effective treatment is available for esophageal motility disorders. Antireflux measures such as elevating the head of the bed and administering antacids should be taken and are often helpful. Cimetidine has been reported to provide symptomatic relief and heal involved mucosa. Metoclopramide, a drug that directly stimulates smooth muscle, may increase the strength of peristalsis and the pressure of the lower esophageal sphincter early in the disease; it is currently under evaluation.

Antireflux operations, especially fundoplication, have been reported to lead to symptomatic improvement but must be performed with extreme caution when peristalsis is absent. Occasionally colonic interposition or esophagogastrostomy may be necessary because of a stricture formation.

MISCELLANEOUS SYSTEMIC DISEASES. A number of motor defects have been demonstrated by manometry in diabetic patients with neuropathic disorders. These motility disorders rarely lead to clinical symptoms. Long-term alcoholics, usually with peripheral neuropathic disorders, have been shown to have a loss of peristalsis in the distal esophagus, but this rarely is clinically evident. Degenerative defects in primary peristalsis have been reported to occur with aging, a condition referred to as presbyesophagus. Recent studies have not found such abnormalities, and the existence of presbyesophagus is now questioned.

GASTROESOPHAGEAL REFLUX DISEASE AND HIATUS HERNIA

The reflux of gastric contents into the esophagus may lead to mucosal damage. Reflux is manifested clinically by the symptom of heartburn and by the sequelae of mucosal injury, esophagitis, esophageal ulceration, stricture, and metaplasia.

ETIOLOGY AND PATHOGENESIS. Incompetence of the lower esophageal sphincter is now thought to be the primary defect in the reflux of acid-pepsin, bile, and pancreatic and intestinal secretions from the stomach. Although acid-pepsin is probably responsible for most mucosal damage, bile salts may enhance their detrimental effects.

In the majority of patients the failure of the lower esophageal sphincter results from a primary disorder of the sphincteric muscle. The cause of this disorder is unclear. In some individuals failure of the sphincter is caused by the effects of another disorder, medications, or a congenital defect, including scleroderma, surgical myotomy for achalasia, certain drugs (anticholinergics, coronary vasodilators, nicotine from smoking, and progesterone and estrogens), and pregnancy. In pregnancy or the use of oral contraceptives, estrogen-progesterone combinations have been shown to directly lower esophageal sphincter pressures.

The cause of lower esophageal sphincter incompetence is unknown, but it does not appear to be mechanical. The presence of a hiatus hernia was once thought to be responsible for reflux symptoms, but it has been found that the presence of a hiatus hernia does not alter the sphincter's pressure and that there is no strong correlation between reflux symptoms and the presence of a hernia. In addition, in animal studies the displacement of the lower esophageal sphincter above the diaphragm does not alter its pressure.

The majority of patients with reflux symptoms are found to have sphincter pressures below 10 mm Hg. In 20% of patients, however, the pressure is normal, and the cause of symptoms in these patients remains unexplained. Symptomatic patients also commonly exhibit diminished responsiveness of the lower esophageal sphincter to increases in intra-abdominal pressures and decreased sphincter pressure changes after a meal.

Esophageal mucosal damage may itself lead to a further lowering of the sphincter pressure and a secondary decrease in motility with an impaired ability of the esophagus to clear itself of refluxed material. This process may lead to a vicious circle of reflux, esophagitis, and further reflux.

Gastrin is thought to promote normal pressures in the lower esophageal sphincter. There is some evidence to suggest that the sphincter in patients with reflux may be less responsive to this effect of gastrin and that following a protein meal, the serum gastrin in these patients fails to rise to normal levels. The importance of these unconfirmed observations, however, is not yet clear.

CLINICAL MANIFESTATIONS. The most characteristic symptom of reflux disease is heartburn, the sensation of heat or burning that spreads upward from the epigastrium to the neck. It is uncomfortable but not painful. Heartburn most commonly occurs about 1 hour after a meal, especially if the patient is in a supine position. It commonly occurs at night when the patient first lies down in bed and is also induced by lifting heavy objects or straining. Certain foods such as coffee or citrus juices may produce heartburn.

Heartburn is often associated with belching and a sour or bitter taste in the mouth. The regurgitation of sour-tasting fluid into the mouth is common and probably indicates rather severe reflux. The patient may complain in particular of coughing and wheezing at night and hoarseness in the morning. These severe symptoms indicate bronchopulmonary aspiration and require immediate attention. Recurrent episodes of pulmonary infection with an unknown cause should always provoke a search for reflux disease.

Dysphagia, usually with solid foods, and odynophagia are occasionally experienced by patients with reflux esophagitis. Dysphagia that becomes progressively worse suggests the development of an esophageal stricture.

Bleeding may result from mucosal inflammation caused by reflux. Although this bleeding most commonly is occult, massive bleeding and hematemesis may develop.

The physical examination is usually unremarkable in reflux disease unless pulmonary complications have occurred. Laboratory tests usually are not helpful although occasionally a patient may have iron deficiency anemia.

DIAGNOSIS. No one test is diagnostic of reflux disease, but various clinical and physiologic tests are available for assessing different aspects of the disease. These tests can be classified according to which of three questions they answer: (1) Is esophagitis or its complications present? (2)

Is reflux present? and (3) Do the patient's symptoms result from reflux?

The barium swallow examination is not a sensitive method by which to diagnose the presence of esophagitis. Occasionally, particularly with double-contrast studies, minute ulcerations may be seen, and this method may show the presence of a stricture or large ulcer. Esophagoscopy performed with a fiberoptic endoscope is the method of choice for diagnosing esophagitis. The early signs of esophagitis include erythema and a blurring of the ora serrata. The manifestations of more advanced esophagitis include friability, superficial and often linear ulcerations, and exudate. Deep ulcers and strictures may be seen. Up to 50% of patients with heartburn, however, have no visible signs of esophagitis. A biopsy specimen of esophageal mucosa removed through the endoscope or with a suction biopsy tube often demonstrates changes consistent with reflux esophagitis. Acute inflammation and ulceration of the mucosa are characteristic. The thickening of the basal layer to over 15% of the entire thickness of the mucosa and the elongation of the papilla are chronic changes that may be seen. It is unfortunate, however, that normal biopsy results may be obtained in patients with visible evidence of esophagitis and that, conversely, evidence of esophagitis may be found by a biopsy of areas that appear normal.

The presence of reflux can be documented by the barium swallow examination, esophageal manometry, and radionuclide scanning. The barium swallow examination may demonstrate the reflux of barium from the stomach into the esophagus but is insensitive in that only 15% to 20% of patients with heartburn can be shown to have reflux. Esophageal manometry may demonstrate that the sphincter has a low resting pressure. The placement of a pH-sensing catheter above the lower esophageal sphincter with manometric guidance is an extremely sensitive test of the presence of reflux. Normally the esophageal pH is 6. If the intraesophageal pH falls to 2 spontaneously or after maneuvers to increase intra-abdominal pressure are performed, reflux is indicated. If these maneuvers do not demonstrate a fall in pH, 0.1N HCl can be infused into the stomach and the test repeated. In addition to demonstrating the reflux of acidic material from the stomach, this test assesses the ability of the esophagus to clear itself of acid and return the lumen to a normal pH. The monitoring of esophageal pH over 24 hours is perhaps the most sensitive test for reflux. Bouts of reflux can be demonstrated in most individuals, particularly at night, but are more frequent and prolonged in patients with symptoms. Scanning of the stomach and esophagus after the instillation of normal saline containing the radioisotope technetium Tc 99m sulfur colloid has successfully demonstrated reflux in over 90% of subjects with reflux demonstrated by a pH probe.

The most reliable available test for assessing whether the patient's symptoms result from reflux is the Bernstein or acid-perfusion test. A tube is positioned in the lower esophagus 30 cm from the incisor teeth through which normal saline is infused. After a baseline period of 5 minutes, the infusion solution is changed to 0.1N HCl without the patient knowing of this change. The acid infusion is continued for 30 minutes or until symptoms develop. If symptoms develop, the infusion is changed to normal saline, again without the patient's knowledge. Symptoms should disappear in several minutes, and acid perfusion is then performed again to confirm the findings. This reproduction of the patient's symptom complex confirms that the pain is of esophageal origin. It is unfortunate, however, that this test can be inconclusive or even have a negative result in a patient with esophagitis demonstrated by biopsy or endoscopy.

In the majority of patients a diagnosis can be made on the basis of the history and the response to medical therapy. In patients in whom the history is atypical or in whom therapy is unsuccessful, the clinician must use a combination of the available tests to determine whether reflux is present, whether it is responsible for the symptoms, and whether it has produced complications.

COURSE. Almost everyone has had heartburn from time to time, but the majority of individuals never require medical management. The incidence of individuals requiring medical treatment is unknown. Of those who do require therapy, very few develop the complications of reflux: esophageal stricture, esophageal ulceration, hemorrhage, pulmonary aspiration, and Barrett's esophagus (the replacement of squamous esophageal epithelium by columnar epithelium).

Severe inflammation caused by reflux esophagitis can incite the development of fibrosis, the result of which is a stricture. This is accompanied by progressive dysphagia. The stricture is usually located in the distal esophagus but occasionally may extend to the midesophagus. On a barium esophagogram the lumen may be seen to taper smoothly (Fig. 172-3). The stricture, however, may not always be circumferential. Endoscopy should be performed to rule out the possibility of a carcinoma.

Another complication of severe reflux esophagitis is deep ulceration. Severe reflux commonly causes superficial ulceration of the mucosa, but deep ulceration into the muscular layer is unusual. These patients usually complain of severe intractable pain. The diagnosis should be made by barium esophagography or endoscopy. Complications include esophageal perforation and massive bleeding.

Although occult bleeding is common in reflux esophagitis, massive hemorrhage is rare. Severe esophagitis may occasionally result in life-threatening hemorrhage requiring emergency surgery.

The aspiration of gastric contents into the tracheobronchial tree may result in recurrent pulmonary infections. The presence of recurrent pulmonary infections in an adult or child, even when symptoms are not present, should stimulate a search for reflux.

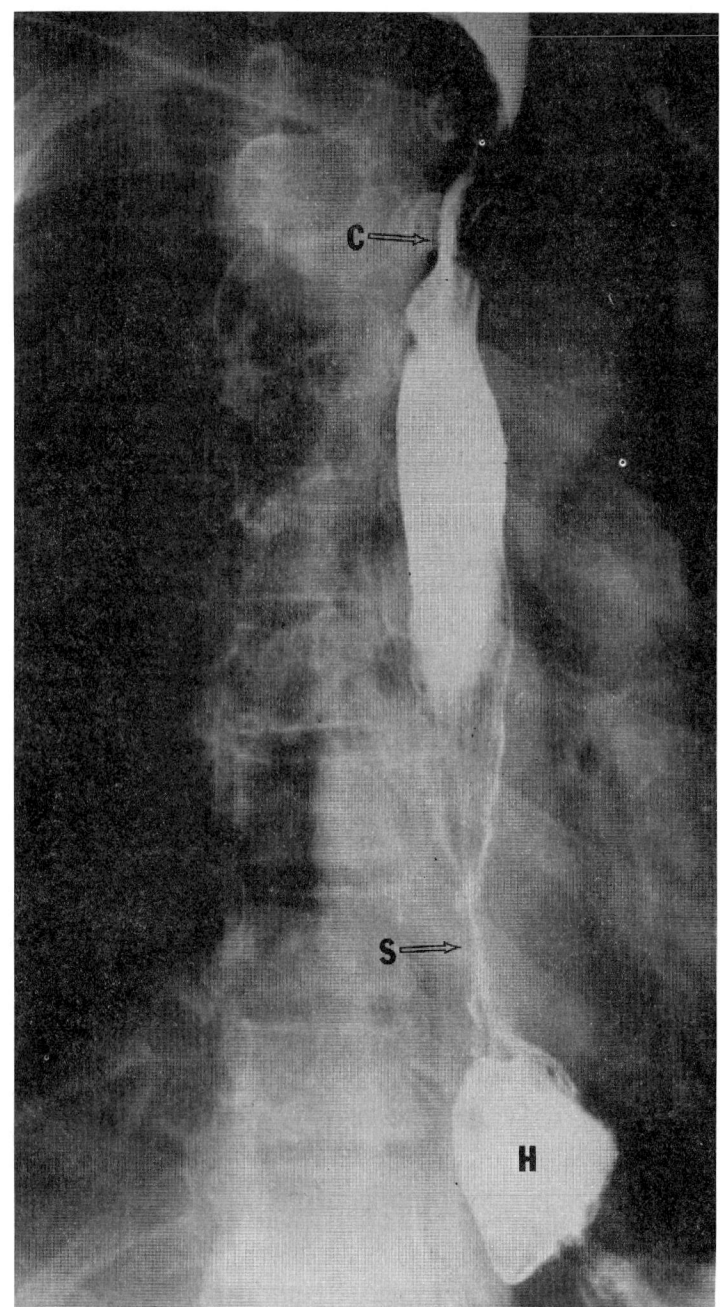

Fig. 172-3. Patient with dysphagia has peptic stricture *(arrow at S)* located above hiatus hernia *(H)*. Of graver consequence, he is also found to have constricting carcinoma in upper esophagus *(arrow at C)*. (Courtesy of George Popky, M.D.)

Chronic gastroesophageal reflux may lead to the replacement of normal squamous epithelium by columnar epithelium. Barrett, who first described this condition, thought that the columnar-lined segment was a congenital anomaly, but serial biopsies have demonstrated the development of Barrett's epithelium in patients with reflux esophagitis. Three types of mucosal changes have been described: (1) a true metaplastic epithelium consisting of villiform folds without foveolae and containing goblet and mucous cells but no parietal or chief cells, (2) a junctional type of mucosa similar to that found in the gastric cardia, and (3) a gastric fundus–like mucosa containing chief and parietal cells. Patients with Barrett's esophagus may have a high esophageal stricture, deep peptic ulceration in the esophagus, and severe reflux symptoms. The incidence of adenocarcinoma of the esophagus is increased to perhaps 10% in this condition. Barrett's esophagus may be a premalignant condition, and these patients should have repeated endoscopy and cytology. Regression of Barrett's epithelium following antireflux surgery has been reported.

MANAGEMENT. Medical therapy for gastroesophageal reflux symptoms is successful in most patients. Patients should avoid tight-fitting garments that increase intra-abdominal pressure. If nocturnal symptoms are bothersome, the force of gravity should be used to strengthen the barrier against reflux by elevating the head of the bed by 20 to 30 cm (8 to 12 inches); wood or cinder blocks can be used for this elevation. The patient should avoid nighttime snacks, which stimulate nocturnal acid production, and should avoid foods and medications that lower the pressure of the lower esophageal sphincter, including alcohol, cigarettes, and chocolate.

Antacids are usually effective in ameliorating symptoms, and thus any failure of antacids to lessen the symptoms at least temporarily should raise doubts about the diagnosis of reflux. For severe symptoms hourly antacids are indicated. A liquid mixture of aluminum hydroxide antacid and alginic acid (Gaviscon) has been claimed to coat the esophagus and form a barrier against reflux and is often effective in controlling symptoms. Cimetidine, an H_2-receptor antagonist, markedly decreases acid production and has been demonstrated by double-blind trials to be beneficial, but its use for reflux esophagitis is still awaiting the approval of the Food and Drug Administration.

Drugs that increase the pressure of the lower esophageal sphincter have been shown in some clinical trials to be effective. Bethanechol, a cholinergic agent, may be beneficial in patients refractory to antacids or cimetidine. Metoclopramide, a direct stimulant of smooth muscle, can increase sphincter pressure and esophageal emptying and is currently undergoing clinical trials.

Esophageal strictures can usually be managed by a combination of bougienage and medical therapy. Various dilators are available for this purpose.

Surgery is never indicated for a hiatus hernia. The major indications for surgery are the severe complications of gastroesophageal reflux: stricture, hemorrhage, and pulmonary aspiration. Surgery is indicated rarely for severe symptoms resistant to medical management. The object of surgery is not to replace the lower esophageal sphincter below the diaphragm but to produce an effective barrier against reflux, as can be accomplished by a variety of procedures such as Belsey's, Hill's, and Nissen's procedures. Surgical opinion is divided concerning which procedure is most effective.

TUMORS OF THE ESOPHAGUS

See Chapter 180.

ESOPHAGITIS RESULTING FROM INFECTIOUS AND PHYSICAL AGENTS
Infectious diseases

Esophagitis caused by a *Candida albicans* infection has become an important clinical disorder. It is often found in diabetic patients or those with abnormalities in cellular immunity but is most commonly found in patients with a malignancy, particularly those under treatment with chemotherapeutic, antibiotic, and steroidal agents. It can occur in normal individuals as well. The symptoms usually are dysphagia and odynophagia, and the diagnosis is accomplished by barium esophagography and endoscopy. The barium swallow examination may reveal multiple small ulcerations and nodular filling defects; in about 50% of patients, particularly those with mild disease, the study is normal. Endoscopy reveals hyperemia, friability, ulceration, and exudate. Direct smear tests of the exudate demonstrate the presence of organisms more often than biopsy. These findings may be present in the esophagus even when the oral cavity is not involved. Taking a nystatin suspension orally or sucking on vaginal systatin tablets may be an effective treatment. In severe cases the intravenous administration of amphotericin B may be necessary.

Infections of the esophagus with herpes simplex have also been reported. As with *Candida* esophagitis, herpes esophagitis occurs most commonly in patients with a malignancy, particularly lymphomas and leukemias, but may occur also in normal individuals. Clinical and endoscopic findings are similar to those with candidiasis. The presence of herpetic cutaneous lesions or stomatitis is helpful in establishing the diagnosis, but esophagitis may occur in the absence of mucocutaneous lesions. Brushings and an exfoliative cytologic examination are most helpful in determining the diagnosis because they reveal intranuclear inclusion bodies. No specific treatment is available. The infection is usually resolved with improvement in the underlying condition.

Physical agents

INGESTION OF CAUSTIC AGENTS. The ingestion of strong alkaline or acidic corrosive agents such as lye results in severe esophagitis; such ingestion usually results from an attempted suicide or an accident, usually with children. The patient experiences prostration and severe pain in the mouth and chest. Odynophagia is severe, and the patient may be unable to swallow. Burns are usually noted in the oropharynx but may be absent even when severe esophagitis is present. If the patient survives the acute episode, extensive strictures may form in the esophagus (Fig. 172-4). Endoscopy should be performed within 24 hours to determine whether caustic ingestion has resulted in an esophageal burn. If esophagitis is present, therapy aimed at preventing stenosis is initiated. Various forms of therapy have been used, but there have been no double-blind trials to prove their effectiveness. Emergency esophagogastrectomy has been recommended for severe extensive burns. For the average case, however, analgesics, supportive care, and antibiotics are indicated. Large doses of corticosteroids, early bougienage, and the use of a large nasogastric tube have been advocated for preventing strictures, but definitive evidence of their effectiveness is lacking.

If stricture formation occurs, the patient is treated with repeated dilations to maintain the esophageal lumen. Co-

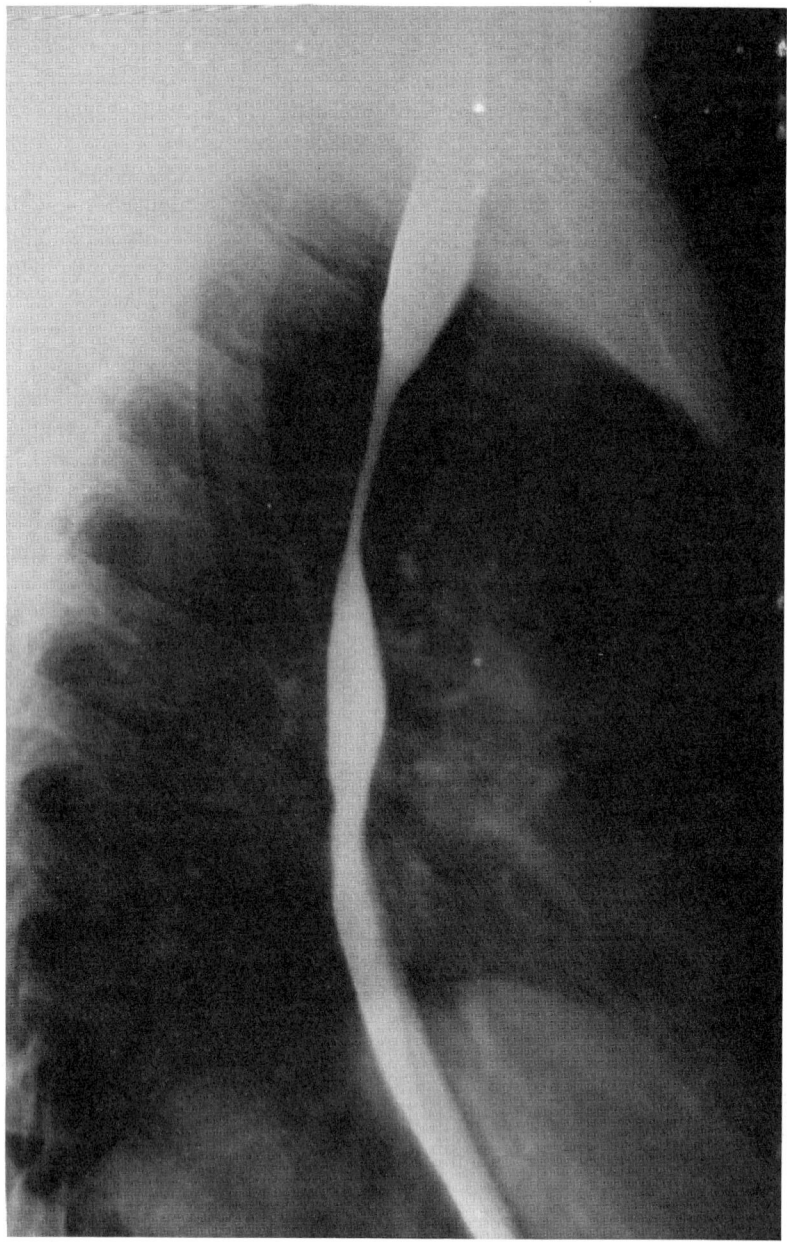

Fig. 172-4. Lye ingestion was cause of this esophageal stricturing. (Courtesy of George Popky, M.D.)

lonic interposition is occasionally necessary. An increased incidence of esophageal carcinoma has been reported in these patients.

RADIATION. Esophagitis may result from the irradiation of the esophagus during the treatment of mediastinal and lung tumors or esophageal carcinomas. Patients have odynophagia and dysphagia. *Candida* esophagitis should always be excluded from the diagnostic possibilities by endoscopy in these patients. The esophagitis resolves with time.

LACERATION AND PERFORATION OF THE ESOPHAGUS

Laceration of the esophageal mucosa or perforation of the entire esophageal wall most commonly results from trauma. Vomiting, external trauma to the body, and instrumentation by a physician are the most common causes.

Mallory-Weiss syndrome

Mucosal laceration, or Mallory-Weiss syndrome, most commonly results from emetic trauma, particularly after excessive ingestion of alcohol. The typical history includes repeated episodes of vomiting followed by hematemesis. Hematemesis occurs initially, however, in 25% of these patients. The laceration usually is on the posterolateral aspect of the esophagus and is longitudinal. Bleeding in the majority of cases is short lived but may be massive. The diagnosis should be made with endoscopy. Massive bleeding may respond to intra-arterial vasopressin (Pitressin), but surgery is occasionally required.

BIBLIOGRAPHY

Behar, J., and others: Evaluation of esophageal tests in the diagnosis of reflux esophagitis, Gastroenterology **71**:9, 1976.
Bennett, J.R., and Henrix, T.R.: Diffuse esophageal spasm: a disorder with more than one cause, Gastroenterology **59**:273, 1970.
Castell, D.O.: Achalasia and diffuse esophageal spasm, Arch. Intern. Med. **136**:571, 1976.
Cohen, S.: Motor disorders of the esophagus, N. Engl. J. Med. **301**:184, 1979.
Goyal, R.K., and others: Lower esophageal ring, N. Engl. J. Med. **282**:1298, 1970.
Kilman, W.J., and Goyal, R.K.: Disorders of pharyngeal and upper esophageal motor function, Arch. Intern. Med. **136**:592, 1976.
Kodsi, B.E., and others: *Candida* esophagitis: a prospective study of 27 cases, Gastroenterology **71**:715, 1976.
Pope, C.E., II: Pathophysiology and diagnosis of reflux esophagitis, Gastroenterology **70**:445, 1976.

173 • ACID-PEPTIC DISEASES

Walter Rubin

This chapter focuses on several disorders whose pathogenesis is not well understood but is dependent at least in part on the secretion of acid by the stomach. These conditions include peptic ulcer disease, the Zollinger-Ellison syndrome, stress erosions, and some varieties of gastritis. Gastroesophageal reflux disease, another common acid-related disorder, is discussed in Chapter 172. Additional types of gastritis and other disorders of the stomach unrelated to acid secretion are included at the end of this chapter.

PEPTIC ULCER DISEASE

A peptic ulcer is a benign (nonmalignant) ulceration in the mucosal surface of the gut. Most peptic ulcers are located in the stomach (gastric ulcer) or duodenal bulb (duodenal ulcer), the first part of the small intestine just beyond the stomach. Duodenal ulcers are three times as common as gastric ulcers. On occasion ulcers develop just beyond the bulb in the duodenum (postbulbar ulcer) or rarely even more distally in the duodenum or jejunum (jejunal ulcer). Peptic ulcers occasionally occur in the esophagus of patients with esophagitis from gastroesophageal reflux. When patients or physicians refer to ulcers or ulcer disease, they are usually referring to a duodenal or gastric ulcer. Ulcers usually occur singly, but occasionally two or even more may be present at the same time.

The incidence of peptic ulcer disease seems to be declining in the United States, but it is still a common disorder, developing at some time in approximately 10% of the population. Because ulcers may cause no symptoms and their presence therefore may not be apparent, their incidence may be even greater. Most victims of ulcer disease, however, have recurrent pain and consult their physicians time and again for relief of the symptoms and with the hope of preventing the recurrences that most of these patients inevitably have. About 10% to 20% of these patients at some time have a life-threatening complication: a hemorrhage, perforation, or obstruction. Failure to assess and manage these patients properly on these occasions can be tragic.

New techniques, drugs, and knowledge have in the past few years modified the methods of diagnosing and treating ulcer disease. The development of better and more tolerable flexible fiberoptic endoscopes has enlarged the role of endoscopy in diagnosing and sometimes treating disease in communities where this technique is available. The development of an immunoassay test for serum gastrin has made the diagnosis of the Zollinger-Ellison syndrome much easier. The use of dietary and anticholinergic therapy has been losing favor, whereas a better understanding of the proper use of antacids has been developed. Finally, a new class of drugs, the histamine H_2-receptor blockers, has become the most effective practical means for controlling gastric acidity and treating ulcer disease.

ETIOLOGY AND PATHOGENESIS. Despite much research, the causes and pathogenesis of peptic ulcers and their associated symptoms are still poorly understood. Genetic and psychosomatic factors and a failure of the mucous membrane to maintain its integrity and normal resistance have been thought to play possible roles in causing peptic ulcers, but the acid secreted by the stomach is still believed to play a major role and still receives the most attention. Patients who secrete no acid, such as those with pernicious anemia, rarely if ever have benign peptic ulcers, whereas patients who secrete huge amounts of acid, such as those with the Zollinger-Ellison syndrome, have a marked tendency to develop ulcers and associated complications. Patients with ulcers often have pain when there is unbuffered acid in their stomachs, and characteristically this pain is often rapidly relieved when that acid is neutralized or diluted with antacid, food, or even water. Acid secretion seems to play an especially large role in the pathogenesis of duodenal ulcers, which are statistically associated with the production of large amounts of acid; however, many individual patients with duodenal ulcers secrete normal quantities. In contrast, patients with benign gastric ulcers commonly exhibit atrophic changes of the stomach and secrete normal or even decreased amounts of acid.

The role that diet, such as a diet of spicy foods, and drugs play in producing peptic ulcers remains unclear. Although many still believe that anti-inflammatory agents such as aspirin, steroids, indomethacin, and phenylbutazone promote peptic ulceration, especially of the stomach, this belief has not been substantiated with good objective studies. An increased incidence of ulcer disease is associated with cigarette smoking, but its association with alcohol ingestion, which clearly causes gastritis, has not yet been established.

Emotional stress has also been thought to play a possible role in the development of ulcers. Strong emotional reactions such as anxiety, anger, or frustration seem to activate ulcers or produce symptoms in many patients with ulcer disease. Obviously emotional stress cannot be a sole cause of ulcers, because most people under stress do not have them.

CLINICAL MANIFESTATIONS. Peptic ulcers may be asymptomatic. The most common symptom of an uncomplicated ulcer is pain, most often in the epigastrium but sometimes in one or both upper quadrants, and less commonly in the back, lower abdomen, or chest. The pain is often perceived as a burning or gnawing sensation but may also be described as a hunger pain, a heaviness, an ache, a cramp, or even a sharp pain. The pain characteristically occurs when the stomach is empty or when not enough of a meal remains in the stomach to buffer adequately the secreted acid stimulated by the meal. Therefore it often begins 1 or more hours after eating and at night when the patient is asleep. The pain is characteristically relieved, usually within a few minutes, by buffering or diluting the gastric acid with the ingestion of an antacid, milk, food, or even water; the pain returns some time later, presumably when the gastric acidity has again increased. Most duodenal ulcers produce classic symptoms, whereas the pain of gastric ulcers tends to be somewhat atypical; pyloric channel ulcers classically produce pain when the patient eats.

Because peptic ulcers recur in the majority of patients, many patients have a history of similar recurrent pains lasting a few days or weeks. Some patients, especially those with duodenal ulcers, experience seasonal attacks of pain, in the spring or autumn. Sometimes patients can correlate episodes of pain with precipitating factors such as emotional stress, an alcoholic binge, or some dietary indiscretion such as the ingestion of particularly spicy foods.

Nausea and vomiting may be associated with uncomplicated ulcer disease, but these symptoms in a patient with an ulcer suggest the presence of an obstruction, in which case the vomitus is usually nonbilious. When an ulcer perforates, the patient usually has sudden, severe abdominal pain, becomes acutely ill, may even go into shock, and develops signs of peritonitis. When an ulcer hemorrhages, the patient often vomits gross blood or material with the appearance of coffee grounds (hematemesis) and usually notes that his stools have become black (melena) or sometimes grossly bloody if the bleeding is brisk and intestinal transit rapid. Because of a rapid loss of blood he may feel weak, light headed especially on standing, and short of breath; he may have palpitations and may even faint or go into shock. A slower chronic rate of bleeding may produce iron deficiency anemia and symptoms of chronic anemia.

The physical examination of ulcer patients is usually not very helpful in reaching a diagnosis. It commonly reveals some nonspecific abdominal tenderness, usually in the epigastrium. Especially in patients with duodenal ulcer, the tenderness is often localized. Occasionally a patient with an obstruction may exhibit a succession splash produced by the retained food and secretions in the stomach. A specimen of feces should be obtained in the rectal examination and examined for the presence of gross or occult blood.

DIAGNOSIS. The diagnosis of a peptic ulcer is not difficult in most patients. A careful history alone suggests the correct diagnosis with the majority of patients, especially those with duodenal ulcer disease. Many patients with ulcers have atypical symptoms, however, and many patients with typical ulcer symptoms (epigastric pain that begins 1 or more hours after eating and is relieved by antacids) have no demonstrable abnormality or less commonly have some other disease. Thus a diagnosis of a peptic ulcer must be confirmed in every new patient by appropriate laboratory tests, particularly a gastrointestinal series or endoscopy if it is available. Patients who have well-established duodenal ulcer disease with typical recurrent symptoms may be treated and followed to be certain that the expected response is obtained without repeating the roentgenographic and endoscopic studies each time.

Many disorders can cause upper abdominal pain possibly suggestive of ulcer disease. Gallbladder disease may cause recurrent pain in the epigastrium rather than in the right upper quadrant or over the right scapula, but this pain is commonly brought on by eating and is not usually relieved by the ingestion of food or antacid; however, the use of an antacid and the concomitant belching occasionally produce some relief. Biliary colic is more often accompanied by nausea and vomiting than is pain resulting from a peptic ulcer. When the gallbladder is acutely inflamed (acute cholecystitis), there are usually right upper quadrant tenderness, fever, and leukocytosis.

Heartburn (reflux esophagitis), caused by the reflux of gastric acid into the esophagus, is usually perceived by the patient as a burning, gnawing, or heaviness behind the sternum or sometimes high in the epigastrium. Although the discomfort may wake the patient at night or may be relieved by antacids, the symptoms commonly are felt while eating or soon after eating, are often worse when the patient is lying down, and are frequently accompanied by the regurgitation of food or acid (marked by its sour taste) into the throat (pyrosis). It should be noted, however, that a significant number of patients with ulcer disease also have reflux and heartburn.

The pain of acute pancreatitis occurs usually in the upper abdomen but characteristically lasts many hours and is a persistent, severe pain usually accompanied by nausea and vomiting and unrelieved by food or antacid. The pain commonly radiates directly through to the back, and patients often seek relief by assuming a flexed fetal position. A posterior peptic ulcer penetrating into the pancreas may produce identical symptoms and may even be associated with elevated serum amylase levels, presumably a result of the pancreatitis it has caused.

Diseases above the diaphragm such as myocardial infarction, pulmonary embolus, and pneumonia sometimes produce abdominal pain, but a careful history, physical examination, and appropriate laboratory tests should readily differentiate these conditions from ulcer disease.

The first symptom of acute appendicitis is often an epigastric pain that might suggest ulcer disease, but the more classic symptoms and abdominal findings of appendicitis usually develop within a few hours, and the temperature and white blood cell count are usually elevated.

Vascular disease sometimes produces acute or even recurrent upper abdominal pain (intestinal angina), but this pain is not relieved by antacids and may characteristically be produced or intensified by eating.

Functional bowel disease (functional dyspepsia) is the most common imitator of ulcer disease. Its symptoms, however, are often produced or worsened by eating, are often associated with much belching resulting from aerophagia, and tend to be more persistent.

An acutely swollen liver associated with congestive failure, metastatic cancer, fatty infiltration, hepatitis, or alcoholic hepatitis can produce upper abdominal pain, but eating usually has little effect on this symptom. The liver is usually found to be tender by palpation, and a careful history and physical examination usually reveal a probable cause for the acutely enlarged liver.

Cancers of the digestive system, especially of the stomach and pancreas, may produce upper abdominal pain, but this pain is usually more persistent and is usually unaffected or increased by eating.

Many drugs commonly cause dyspepsia-like symptoms. Any drugs suspected of causing such symptoms should be discontinued in symptomatic patients.

When abnormalities of the abdominal wall such as hernias cause upper abdominal pain, the pain is usually unaffected or is occasionally worsened by eating and is usually intensified by straining (increasing intra-abdominal pressure) or by contracting the abdominal musculature, and the focal tenderness is usually increased when the reclining patient lifts his head (flexes his neck) and contracts his rectus muscles.

LABORATORY FINDINGS. The usual laboratory tests should include a complete blood count for detecting anemia and leukocytosis, an examination of the stool for occult blood, and a serum calcium test for detecting an occasional elevation resulting from an associated hyperparathyroidism or more likely from multiple endocrine tumors with the Zollinger-Ellison syndrome. The serum gastrin level should also be determined if the test is available, especially if the patient also has chronic diarrhea, atypical or multiple ulcers, or severe ulcer disease—manifestations suggestive of the Zollinger-Ellison syndrome.

The diagnosis of a peptic ulcer is usually confirmed by a gastrointestinal series, which demonstrates the presence of the ulcer crater in 80% to 90% of patients with a peptic ulcer (Fig. 173-1). In some cases of duodenal ulcer the roentgenogram may fail to demonstrate the crater's presence but may show some deformity or spasm of the duodenal bulb and thus suggest the presence of an ulcer or at least scarring from previous ulcer disease. If the gastrointestinal series fails to reveal an ulcer despite a suggestive history, a gastroenterologist (if available) should be consulted, and endoscopy should be performed (esophagogastroduodenoscopy) to examine the mucosal surfaces directly. This procedure identifies some ulcers and even other lesions sometimes not apparent on the gastrointestinal roentgenograms and occasionally reveals duodenitis, an inflammation of the duodenal bulb without frank ulceration, a condition that may produce symptoms similar to those of an ulcer. If both the gastrointestinal series and endoscopy fail to reveal an ulcer or other cause for the patient's symptoms, other appropriate tests such as cholecystography should be performed to detect the cause.

If the gastrointestinal series demonstrates the presence of a duodenal ulcer, endoscopy is unnecessary and proper therapy can be instituted or continued. If, however, a gastric ulcer is revealed, further tests must be performed to eliminate the possibility that the lesion is one of the 3% to 8% of gastric ulcers that are actually ulcerated cancers. A gastric secretory study should be performed to confirm that the patient can secrete acid, and a gastroenterologist should be consulted to perform a gastroscopy to observe the lesion, take multiple biopsy samples along its circumference for pathologic examination, and obtain brush specimens of its surface for cytologic examination. If the patient can secrete acid and all the other tests suggest a benign disease, vigorous medical therapy should be instituted, and a gastrointestinal series (an endoscopy in some cases) should be repeated at later dates to confirm normal healing of the ulcer.

If an obstruction of gastric outflow is suspected, a nasogastric or Ewald tube should be passed into the stomach to detect, measure, and evacuate any retained food and secretions. A gastrointestinal series and endoscopy should be performed after evacuation, but often these procedures,

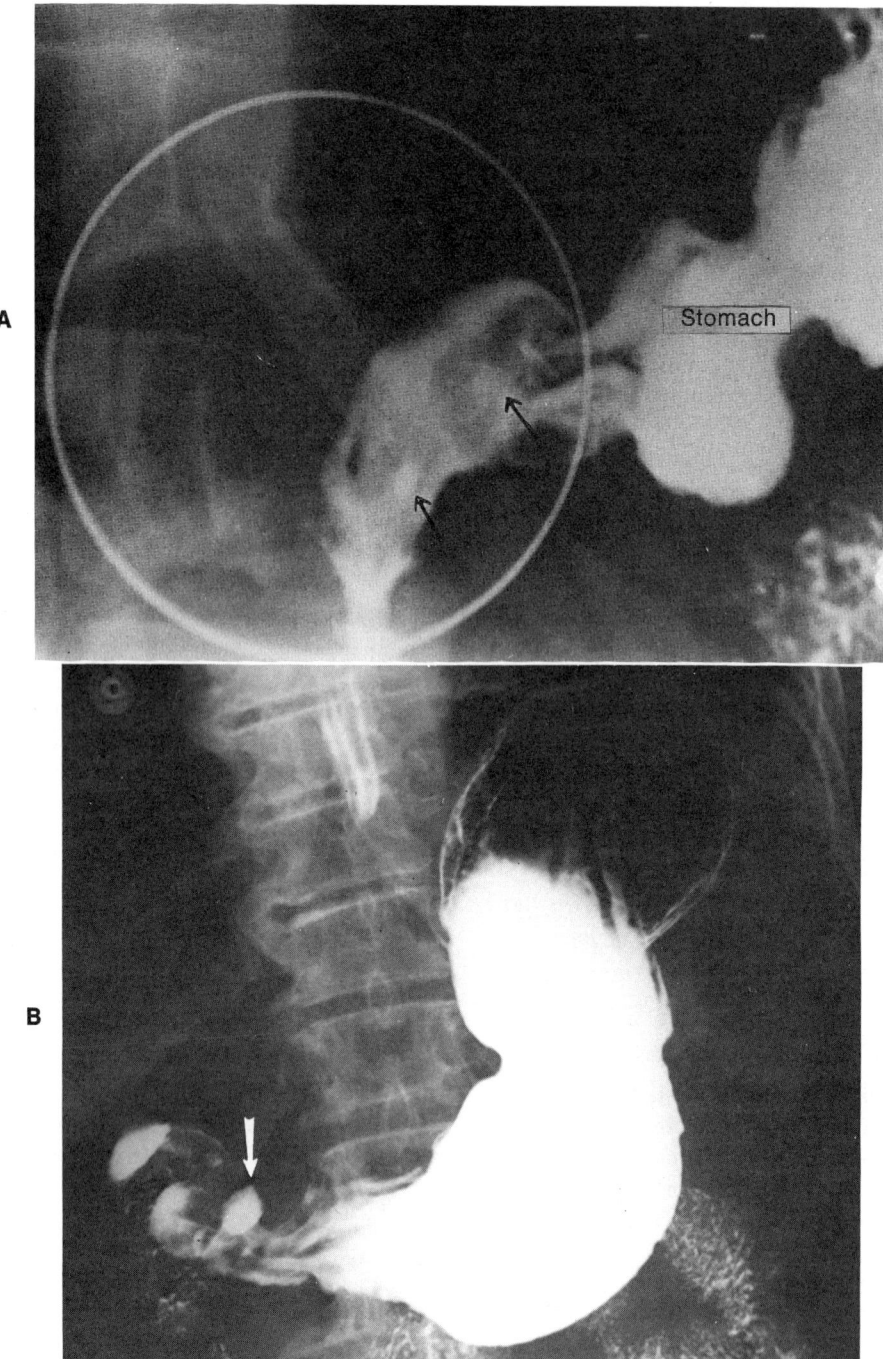

Fig. 173-1. Gastrointestinal series demonstrates **A**, duodenal and **B**, gastric ulcers. Barium is collected in ulcer craters or niches *(arrows)*. (Courtesy of George Popky, M.D.)

especially roentgenography, reveal only an obstruction to the outflow of the stomach but not the cause. In this instance these procedures have to be repeated after a period of treatment with nasogastric suction. In patients with an obstruction the degree of dehydration should be immediately assessed, and the levels of serum electrolytes, blood urea nitrogen, and creatinine should be determined.

Bleeding ulcers must be differentiated from other causes of upper gastrointestinal hemorrhage while the patient's vital signs are monitored and while he is being given blood necessary for maintaining satisfactory blood pressure and adequate perfusion of the heart, brain, and kidneys. If the patient has blood in the stools but not hematemesis, the stomach should be aspirated with a nasogastric tube to determine whether blood is present and thereby to confirm the upper gastrointestinal tract as the site of bleeding. If the patient's condition is reasonably stable and the bleeding indeed seems to be arising from the upper gastrointestinal tract, a gastroenterologist (if available) should be consulted, and emergency endoscopy should be performed to establish a diagnosis and institute proper therapy as soon as possible. Endoscopy is especially helpful in patients who are likely to have many possible causes for their bleeding. Alcoholics, for example, especially those with liver disease, have bleeding commonly caused not only by ulcers but also by esophageal or gastric varices, gastritis, esophagitis, and Mallory-Weiss tears of the esophagus or stomach. Endoscopy often makes possible a rapid specific diagnosis. If the bleeding is very brisk and thus prevents complete visualization, at least the site of the bleeding can usually be determined and some causes such as varices and diffuse erosive gastritis can usually be excluded from diagnostic possibilities.

If a perforation is suspected, a plain roentgenogram of the abdomen should be obtained for the detection of free air in the peritoneal cavity.

Other laboratory tests such as routine chest roentgenograms and electrocardiograms are usually helpful with most patients, especially if a disease of the chest or heart is suspected. If other diseases are strongly suspected or if the diagnosis of an ulcer cannot be made, other pertinent laboratory tests should be performed such as a serum amylase test if acute pancreatitis is suspected, liver function tests if liver disease is suspected, or cholecystography if gallbladder disease is suspected.

COURSE. Peptic ulcer disease must be viewed as a chronic illness. Most ulcers heal by themselves and become asymptomatic but then recur at a later time. Indeed, approximately 50% to 75% of patients whose duodenal ulcers heal have a reactivation of their ulcers within 1 year of healing. About 10% to 20% of ulcer patients at some time have a life-threatening complication such as a hemorrhage, perforation, or obstruction.

MANAGEMENT

Uncomplicated ulcers. There are four goals in the treatment of the patient with uncomplicated ulcer disease: (1) to alleviate symptoms, (2) to promote healing, (3) to prevent recurrences, and (4) to prevent complications. Achieving the first two goals is not difficult in most cases, especially because ulcers usually heal by themselves although they recur later. Good medical therapy, however, is designed primarily to reduce gastric acidity by inhibiting acid secretion or by neutralizing secreted acid and thus alleviating symptoms more rapidly and hastening healing. The prevention of recurrences and complications has been a more difficult problem, and physicians have generally been unable to resolve this problem with medical therapy. The long-term use of the histamine H_2-receptor blockers such as cimetidine, however, promises perhaps to be a practical and effective way of reducing ulcer recurrences and complications.

Patients are traditionally encouraged to get adequate rest, relaxation, and sleep. Anxiety and anger should be reduced as much as possible by whatever practical means seem effective, such as instructing the patient, encouraging him to let out his feelings, manipulating his environment, encouraging participation in sports, the use of tranquilizers, and so on. Drugs thought to be ulcerogenic, such as aspirin, should be avoided or replaced with alternatives. Smoking and alcohol ingestion should be minimized or completely eliminated if possible.

The role of diet in the treatment of peptic ulcers has been extensively debated in recent years. An increasing number of gastroenterologists think that the traditional restrictive bland diets eaten in frequent small meals are unnecessary or possibly even harmful. They advocate just three regular meals a day and the avoidance of highly seasoned and spicy foods or any foods noted to cause symptoms. Caffeine-containing beverages such as regular coffee, tea, and colas may also be restricted. The frequent meals traditionally advocated are not only inconvenient but also continually stimulate the secretion of acid they are intended to reduce. The traditional bedtime snack is especially harmful because it stimulates acid secretion for about 4 hours while the patient is asleep and unable to take an antacid. The traditional bland diets are not only unattractive to patients but generally contain much milk sugar lactose, which causes abdominal cramps, gas, and even diarrhea in many patients who have lactose intolerance (lactase deficiency). The bland diet also tends to be high in calories and, because of its high fat content, possibly atherogenic.

Anticholinergic drugs have long been used to reduce gastric acid secretion in ulcer patients, but because of their limited effectiveness and disturbing side effects they are losing favor. When taken in the optimal dosage, four times a day (½ hour before each meal and at bedtime), they reduce meal-stimulated acid secretion by only about 30% to 50%. They do not significantly reduce acid secretion without producing at least some dryness of the mouth and commonly other more disturbing side effects such as urinary retention, constipation, heartburn, tachycardia, drying of bronchial secretions, visual disturbances, and precipitation or aggravation of glaucoma.

The agents recommended for the control of gastric acidity in ulcer patients are the long-used antacids, which neutralize secreted acid, or the new drug cimetidine (Tagamet), which effectively inhibits acid secretion. Because these drugs work differently, they may be used together if desired.

The antacids are effective, relatively safe drugs when used properly, but the physician should be aware of the problems they may cause. Absorbable antacids such as sodium bicarbonate can produce an appreciable alkalosis, especially in patients with renal disease, and if appreciable amounts are taken along with much calcium (from calcium carbonate or a large quantity of milk products), occasionally the very rare but serious milk-alkali syndrome (hypercalcemia and alkalosis) may develop. The antacids containing calcium have been losing favor not only because they can cause hypercalcemia and renal impairment but also because they are thought to stimulate acid secretion. The aluminum antacids, when used in large amounts, can occasionally cause phosphate depletion (by forming insoluble precipitate in the gut) and thereby anorexia, weakness, and bone pain. Antacids must be used especially carefully in patients with renal failure because the cations (calcium, magnesium, or aluminum) can cause toxicity. The aluminum antacids tend to cause constipation whereas the magnesium antacids tend to produce diarrhea; thus the physician may have to change preparations or use more than one type in accordance with the effects on the individual patient. Some antacids, especially the aluminum antacids, may bind various drugs such as tetracyclines within the gut and thereby affect their absorption. The physician must be aware of this phenomenon and check the effects that antacids have on the absorption of the other medications required by the patient. If a patient requires a salt-restricted diet, a low-sodium antacid must be used.

Antacids must be used in adequate amounts and at proper times to ensure satisfactory acid neutralization. Different preparations vary in terms of potency, the rate of neutralizing acid, and the length of time they remain effective in the stomach. If taken when the stomach is empty, most antacids rapidly leave the stomach and therefore are effective for only 10 to 20 minutes. When taken an hour after a meal, however, when the acid secreted in response to the meal is no longer adequately buffered by the food remaining in the stomach, the antacid is usually effective for 2 to 3 hours. The amount of antacid required depends not only on the potency of the preparation used but also on the amount of acid the individual patient secretes; this of course is usually difficult for the physician to know without performing secretory tests, which are neither always available nor usually desirable. The physician should be aware, however, that if a patient's symptoms are not responding satisfactorily, that patient might require more antacid. The solid chewable antacid preparations are much less effective than their liquid counterparts and should not be used.

If antacid therapy is the choice, the physician should usually prescribe about 100 mEq of a liquid aluminum and magnesium antacid (usually about 1 ounce [30 ml] of the more potent antacids or 2 or 3 ounces [60 or 90 ml] of the weaker ones) to be taken 1 hour and 3 hours after each of the three meals and every 2 hours thereafter. If symptoms are not well controlled by this regimen, the antacid can be taken more frequently, even every hour. The physician must consider whether a low-salt antacid should be used and whether the chosen antacid might interfere with the absorption of other drugs the patient requires. It may be necessary to change or alternate preparations if diarrhea or constipation develops.

Cimetidine is a histamine H_2-receptor antagonist that effectively inhibits the gastric acid secretion stimulated by histamine. Histamine has long been known to be a powerful stimulant of acid secretion, but the conventional antihistamines used to treat allergic patients block only the histamine H_1-receptors and have essentially no effect on gastric acid secretion. When 300 mg of cimetidine in tablet form is taken four times a day (with meals and at bedtime), or if necessary every 6 hours intravenously, the drug effectively controls gastric acidity in almost all patients by inhibiting about 70% or more of the acid normally secreted. Of particular importance, the dose taken at bedtime inhibits most nocturnal acid secretion during the period when the patient is asleep and unable to take antacids. Because the drug is eliminated mainly through the kidneys, the dosage should be reduced in patients with renal disease; it is usually taken only two or three times a day by these patients. The Food and Drug Administration has approved the use of cimetidine in the United States for the treatment of active duodenal and gastric ulcer disease for no longer than 8 weeks.

To date cimetidine seems to be very safe. Slight inconsequential reversible elevations of serum creatinine and serum glutamic-oxaloacetic transaminase are commonly observed. Mild and transient diarrhea, rashes, muscle aches, and dizziness occur in about 1% of patients. Neutropenia has been reported rarely, and mild gynecomastia has developed in about 4% of patients with the Zollinger-Ellison syndrome who have been on long-term therapy and in about 0.3% of other patients. Occasional mental confusion has been reported, especially in elderly patients taking the drug. A slightly increased incidence of benign testicular tumors has been reported in rats when the drug was administered over a long period in high dosages to a susceptible strain.

Thus cimetidine offers a simple alternative method of medical therapy with which patients can easily comply. Patients may also take an antacid for relief of ulcer pain, as is usually necessary during the first few days of cimetidine therapy while the symptoms are being brought under control. The patient can continue to use antacid during treatment with cimetidine, but this is probably unnecessary. Antacid should probably not be ingested within 1 hour of oral cimetidine therapy because it may reduce the absorption of the cimetidine. Many new effective drugs will become available for the treatment of ulcers. Some, like the newer histamine H_2-receptor antagonists, will also inhibit acid secretion, but others, like sucralfate, will have other mechanisms of action.

Treatment with either antacids or cimetidine should be continued for 6 weeks. The pain in most patients is usually controlled within the first week of therapy, and most ulcers heal by the sixth week.

Special aspects of gastric ulcers. If gastrointestinal roentgenograms or endoscopy suggests a malignancy, if the stomach cannot secrete acid even after maximal stimulation with histamine, betazole (Histalog), or pentagastrin, or if the pathologic or cytologic specimens reveal malignancy, a surgeon should be consulted and an appropriate resection performed if possible. If all these tests suggest a benign disease, the vigorous medical therapy outlined previously should be instituted. The gastrointestinal series (and endoscopy in some cases) should be repeated in 3 weeks to confirm that the ulcer is healing and again at 6 weeks (if it is not healed at 3 weeks), at which time the ulcer should be healed or at least reduced by 90% in size. Another gastrointestinal series should be performed at 12 weeks to confirm complete healing. If the series at any time reveals a possibility of malignancy or if the ulcer is not healing by 3 weeks, not almost healed by 6 weeks, or not completely healed by 12 weeks, surgery should probably be recommended if the patient is a reasonable candidate. Some large benign ulcers with craters wider than 2.5 cm may require more than 12 weeks to heal. If such an ulcer appears benign and seems to be healing well, medical therapy can be continued beyond 12 weeks and a follow-up gastrointestinal series and/or endoscopy can be performed in a few weeks to confirm complete healing.

Surgery. Surgery for peptic ulcer disease should be reserved mainly for patients with the complications of perforation, recurrent significant hemorrhage or an acute severe or persistent hemorrhage, or an obstruction that fails to open satisfactorily despite good medical therapy. Gastric ulcers that are suspected of being carcinomas or that fail to heal satisfactorily with medical therapy should also be treated surgically. The poorest indication for surgery is apparent intractability, that is, persistent or very frequent recurrent symptoms despite good medical therapy. Such patients should be carefully evaluated, even with endoscopy if necessary, to make sure that their symptoms result from active ulcers, that they are following their prescribed therapy, and that they do not have the Zollinger-Ellison syndrome.

The results of surgery vary with the talent of the individual surgeon, the hospital where it is performed, and the selection of patients; the overall mortality is about 1% to 2% (lower in some medical centers), and the recurrence rate probably well below 10%. The two most widely used procedures in the United States are truncal vagotomy with a drainage procedure (usually a pyloroplasty) and truncal vagotomy with a gastric resection and gastrojejunostomy (Billroth II procedure). The former procedure probably has a somewhat lower mortality and morbidity, whereas the latter procedure probably results in a somewhat lower incidence of recurrent disease.

Although surgery seems to prevent recurrent disease in most cases, it unfortunately also causes postoperative symptoms (postgastrectomy syndrome) in up to 50% of patients. Patients selected for surgery should be warned that they may be exchanging their ulcer symptoms for other discomforts. Although these symptoms are usually most prominent during the months immediately after the operation, many patients suffer chronic symptoms for years. Common postoperative complaints include diarrhea, weight loss, weakness, early satiety, and postprandial distress.

Some patients have a postprandial syndrome consisting of light-headedness, weakness, sweating, palpitations, nausea, and diarrhea. When these symptoms occur an hour or later after eating, they are usually the result of reactive hypoglycemia. More often they occur during the meal or soon afterward; this is known as the dumping syndrome. The syndrome probably results from a rapid emptying of the stomach, causing the accumulation of hypertonic chyme in the small intestine, and the rapid flux of water from the blood into the intestinal lumen, causing a rapid reduction of blood volume.

Complications. When a patient with ulcer disease has a perforation, hemorrhage, or obstruction, he should be hospitalized and a surgeon and ideally a gastroenterologist should be consulted immediately. A patient with a perforation usually requires immediate surgery. A patient with an obstruction should be treated with continuous nasogastric suction, intravenous fluids and electrolytes, and intravenous cimetidine (300 mg every 6 hours if renal function is normal). After 3 days of suction the nasogastric tube should be withdrawn and the patient put on a liquid diet and antacids. If intravenous cimetidine cannot be continued, a full antacid regimen should be employed, as outlined previously. The stomach should be aspirated at least once a day, about 1 hour after a meal. If the outlet obstruction seems to be improving, that is, if the retention is less than 500 ml and progressively improves, the medical therapy can be continued and the diet advanced to include soft food. If the obstruction does not improve, if a low-grade chronic obstruction persists, or if the patient has a history of recurrent obstruction, surgery is recommended. If the diagnosis of a mechanical outlet obstruction could not be confirmed by the gastrointestinal series or endoscopy when the patient was first seen, these procedures should be repeated after the period of nasogastric suction, especially if surgery is contemplated. A mechanical outlet obstruction must be differentiated from gastric atony, a motility disturbance that may result from diabetic gastroparesis, other severe diseases, drugs, or unknown causes.

Patients with bleeding ulcers should receive blood, usually whole blood, to maintain a satisfactory blood pressure and the adequate perfusion of the heart, brain, and kidneys and should be treated with antacids and/or cimetidine (intravenously if necessary). Most patients with bleeding ulcers require no blood or only a few units. If the bleeding is so brisk and persistent that vital signs cannot be easily maintained, or if 6 or more units of blood is required during the first 24 hours, surgery should probably be performed if the bleeding still continues. If brisk bleeding is permitted to continue such that the patient requires massive transfusions (10 or more units over a 24- or 48-hour period), the mortality risk increases considerably. Such patients should therefore be identified as soon as possible so that surgery can be performed and the arterial bleeder ligated before the patient needs massive amounts of blood and serious complications develop. If a patient continues to bleed for more than 3 days, even if his blood requirements are not great, surgery should probably be recommended as well. The decision must be made individually for patients, however, and the decision of whether to operate is often affected by their clinical condition and the presence or absence of associated diseases.

PREVENTION. Recurrent ulcer disease and its complications are difficult if not impossible to prevent. The patient who has only occasional short attacks of active disease is unlikely to follow any prescribed prophylactic regimen even if a practical effective one could be devised. The patient who suffers more frequent attacks, especially if they are precipitated by recognizable factors, can be educated to avoid the precipitating circumstances or to institute a medical program prophylactically whenever such circumstances arise or as soon as the first symptoms appear. Thus if the patient finds himself under undue stress, if he ingests an excessive amount of alcohol or too much spicy food, or if he must take some drug thought to be ulcerogenic, he can begin taking antacids frequently or cimetidine and a tranquilizer if necessary in the hope of preventing or aborting a recurrence of symptoms. The patient with frequent or continual ulcer symptoms should be encouraged to follow an intensive long-term medical program to determine whether the symptoms can be controlled and prevented. Patients who have disease apparently uncontrollable with good medical treatment should be carefully evaluated to determine whether their symptoms indeed result from active ulceration (with endoscopy if the gastrointestinal series does not definitely reveal an ulcer) and to make sure they understand and are following the prescribed medical program. If they are found to have active ulcer disease, they should be carefully tested for the Zollinger-Ellison syndrome by determining their serum gastrin level. Many truly intractable ulcers are found to be penetrating ulcers (extending beyond the wall of the stomach) and may require surgery.

It is difficult to maintain patients on long-term antacid therapy, especially in quantities adequate to control gastric acidity most of the time. A dosage of 400 mg of cimetidine taken each day at bedtime, however, has been shown to be an effective prophylactic treatment for patients who suffer frequent recurrent duodenal ulcer disease, and the Food and Drug Administration has approved this use of cimetidine for a period up to 1 year. In controlled clinical studies, duodenal ulcers were found to recur in about 50% to 75% of patients within 1 year after healing, whereas the prophylactic use of cimetidine reduced the recurrence rate to about 15%. It should be noted, however, that cimetidine is still a relatively new drug, and although it seems safe, its long-term safety has not been established.

ZOLLINGER-ELLISON SYNDROME

DEFINITION AND ETIOLOGY. The Zollinger-Ellison syndrome, thought to be present in fewer than 1% of ulcer patients, is usually caused by a non-β islet cell tumor of the pancreas, a gastrinoma, that continually secretes the hormone gastrin and produces high blood levels. Gastrin causes hyperplasia of the acid-secreting parietal (oxyntic) cells in the stomach and continually stimulates them to secrete, and thus the patient produces large amounts of acid even when fasting. As a result, almost all of these patients eventually have ulcer disease that is usually severe.

The tumors of the pancreas tend to be small and difficult to find. About 50% of these patients have multiple tumors in the pancreas, and about 10% to 20% of patients have multiple endocrine adenomatosis type I syndrome with additional adenomas, hyperplasia, or carcinomas in the parathyroid, pituitary, or adrenal glands. In about 5% of patients with Zollinger-Ellison syndrome the gastrinoma is located in the proximal duodenum, and in another 5% the tumor is in the stomach, hilus of the spleen, or some other organ. About two thirds of gastrinomas are malignant, usually low-grade malignancies that metastasize slowly to the duodenum, local lymph nodes, and eventually the liver and other organs. In the past, however, when the diagnosis and treatment of the syndrome were often unsatisfactory, the patients usually died of the complications of ulcer disease rather than the malignancy. Gastrinomas are apudomas, tumors arising from a group of endocrine cells, the amine precursor uptake decarboxylation (APUD) cells, that synthesize polypeptide hormones and biogenic amines. Some gastrinomas also produce other polypeptides and amines, such as corticotropin (ACTH), glucagon, insulin, vasoactive intestinal polypeptide, and serotonin. Zollinger-Ellison syndrome may rarely result from a hyperplasia of the gastrin-producing cells (G cells) in the antrum of the stomach rather than from a gastrinoma.

CLINICAL MANIFESTATIONS. In about 75% of patients with Zollinger-Ellison syndrome, ulcers develop in the duodenal bulb or occasionally in the stomach, whereas in the rest ulcers develop more distally in the duodenum or in the jejunum. The ulcers are usually single but may be multiple. Patients usually have a virulent form of ulcer disease. They commonly have intractable ulcers causing pain that is unusually resistant to traditional medical therapy. These patients have a high incidence of ulcer complications, especially perforations and hemorrhages, and they commonly require surgery because of these complications or the intractability. If the syndrome is not recognized and a conventional ulcer operation is performed, ulcers and their complications usually continue to develop even after surgery. Because of the virulence of the disease, if it is not diagnosed and managed properly, many patients will die, primarily from a complication.

About 40% of Zollinger-Ellison patients have diarrhea, and in about 10% the diarrhea precedes the ulcer disease. Several causes of the diarrhea have been proposed: (1) the large volumes of water and acid secreted by the stomach, (2) malabsorption resulting from an acid pH in the proximal small intestine and the consequent inhibition of the pancreatic digestive enzymes, especially lipase, and of the ability of the bile acids to form micelles, (3) acid damage to the proximal small intestinal mucosa, (4) impaired salt and water absorption in the small intestine, and (5) altered intestinal motility. Regardless of the precise cause, if the voluminous secretion of the stomach is stopped or prevented from entering the small intestine by nasogastric suction, surgery, or the use of cimetidine, the diarrhea usually ceases.

DIAGNOSIS. The Zollinger-Ellison syndrome should be suspected in any patient with severe or intractable disease, postbulbar or jejunal ulcers, multiple ulcers, recurrent ulcers after surgery, ulcers associated with chronic diarrhea, hypercalcemia (possible type I syndrome), or prominent gastric or small intestinal folds incidentally discovered by roentgenography or endoscopy. If the syndrome is suspected, the diagnosis is not difficult to establish. Gastric secretory studies usually reveal markedly elevated fasting and stimulated acid outputs. The basal acid output is usually at least 10 mEq/hour, and in about half the cases it is at least 60% of the maximal acid output, the maximal rate the stomach can secrete when stimulated with histamine, betazole (Histalog), or pentagastrin. The diagnosis is confirmed by demonstrating a very high serum gastrin level by immunoassay. In questionable cases the serum gastrin level can be induced to rise even higher (by 50% or 400 pg/ml) by infusing calcium or injecting secretin. The secretin injection test is especially helpful because in patients who do not have Zollinger-Ellison syndrome secretin usually depresses serum gastrin levels or has little effect. The rare cases of antral G-cell hyperplasia can be differentiated from the syndrome by the secretin injection test (with a normal response) or by feeding the patient a standard meal. Postprandial serum gastrin levels usually rise more than 50% above fasting levels in normal individuals and in those with G-cell hyperplasia but not in patients with gastrinomas, which are usually little affected by eating. Zollinger-Ellison syndrome can also be differentiated from other conditions that may be associated with high serum gastrin levels, such as pernicious anemia, atrophic gastric mucosa, or a retained gastric antrum following a Billroth II operation. The patients with pernicious anemia and atrophic gastritis secrete no gastric acid or reduced amounts, and patients with a retained antrum can probably be differentiated by their normal response to secretin. About 20% to 40% of gastrinomas can be demonstrated by arteriography, and some by computed tomography.

Because the ulcers associated with the Zollinger-Ellison syndrome can be very mild, and because the immunoassay for serum gastrin is now simple and readily available, some physicians suggest that a routine serum gastrin determination should be obtained for all patients with peptic ulcer disease.

MANAGEMENT. Because most of the tumors and their local metastases cannot be found or satisfactorily removed by surgery, and because conventional ulcer surgery is usually not adequate in controlling the disease, total gastrectomy has become the conventional therapy. In perhaps 10% to 20% of patients a discrete solitary pancreatic tumor can be identified, often in the duodenum, and can be entirely removed, making gastric resection unnecessary. Such patients should be followed postoperatively with serum gastrin and gastric secretory studies. In the past few years long-term cimetidine therapy has been shown to be an effective alternative to total gastrectomy for patients with Zollinger-Ellison syndrome, and the drug has been approved for this use. Patients with this treatment, however, should be carefully followed and their gastric secretion monitored, since they often require higher dosages of cimetidine for the control of their gastric acidity and symptoms. The addition of an anticholinergic drug often permits satisfactory control in patients whose symptoms cannot be controlled with a reasonable dosage of cimetidine alone.

STRESS EROSIONS

Acute erosions or superficial ulcerations commonly develop in the stomach and/or duodenum of patients under conditions of severe stress such as are associated with shock, severe trauma, burns, sepsis, surgery, and renal, respiratory, or hepatic failure. The lesions are characteristically superficial, limited to the mucosa, and often multiple. The so-called Cushing's ulcer, associated with trauma to the head, brain surgery, or increased intracranial pressure resulting from a brain tumor or other cause, is commonly located high on the lesser curvature of the stomach, whereas the so-called Curling's ulcer, associated with burns, is characteristically located in the duodenum. The lesions develop rapidly, often within 24 to 48 hours of the stressful episode, and if clinically apparent, usually cause gastrointestinal bleeding resulting in either hematemesis or melena. Less commonly lesions cause significant epigastric pain, nausea, or vomiting. Since they are superficial, they are usually not detectable by a routine gastrointestinal series, but they are more often demonstrable by double-contrast techniques. They are best diagnosed by endoscopy, which also reveals their numbers and the extent of gastric involvement with erosive changes.

The pathogenesis of stress erosions remains unclear. Although the presence of gastric acid seems necessary, only in the case of Cushing's ulcer has gastric hypersecretion been demonstrated. In some types of stress ulceration a breakage of the gastric mucosal barrier to acid back-diffusion seems to occur, thereby permitting luminal acid to gain access to and perhaps damage the mucosa. This postulated mechanism, however, does not account for duodenal erosions or for cases apparently associated with intact mucosal barriers. In some experimental animal models the applied stress seems to interfere with the normal process of epithelial replication, which maintains normal populations of surface cells. Evidence in recent years, however, suggests that stress erosions may be caused by mocosal ischemia, a result of altered mucosal blood flow.

The best therapy for stress erosions is prevention. The continual maintenance of the gastric pH level above 3.5 or preferably 5 by means of antacids and/or cimetidine markedly reduces the incidence of these erosions in identified high-risk patients. This preventice therapy is increasinly being adopted in intensive care units. If erosions and bleeding develop, the patient should undergo diagnostic endoscopy and his stomach should be lavaged with ice-cold saline or water in an effort to control the bleeding. The patient should receive blood as needed (see Chapter 170) and antacids and/or cimetidine to control gastric acidity. If the stomach is the site of persistent bleeding, infusion of vasopressin (Pitressin) into the left gastric artery may be considered in institutions where this technique is available. If these measures fail, however, surgery may be necessary, even though these patients are usually in poor condition and thus have a high surgical risk and often develop additional ulcers after surgery. The patient with a single pumping erosion, who may require only ligation or local resection, is usually a better surgical candidate than one with many diffuse erosions involving much of the stomach and occasionally requiring a total gastrectomy.

GASTRITIS

Acute and chronic inflammations of the gastric mucosa are common pathologic processes.

Acute erosive gastritis, if symptomatic, usually causes hematemesis and/or melena but may also cause abdominal pain, nausea, and vomiting. The acute erythema, friability, and erosions may be limited to a small area of the gastric mucosa or may be more diffuse, sometimes involving the entire stomach. The cause of the gastritis may be inapparent but commonly is alcohol, which is thought to act by breaking the mucosal barrier to acid back-diffusion, or anti-inflammatory agents, which also break the barrier or inhibit prostaglandin synthesis. Aspirin is the most prominent of these agents, but phenylbutazone, indomethacin, corticosteroids, and others have also been incriminated as causes. These same anti-inflammatory agents have also been thought by some to promote ulcer formation.

The management of acute erosive gastritis is similar to that of stress erosions discussed previously. The general measures for gastrointestinal bleeding should be instituted (see Chapter 170). The stomach should be lavaged with ice-cold saline or water in an effort to stop or retard bleeding. Endoscopy should be performed to establish the diagnosis and to ascertain the extent of gastric involvement. Gastric acidity should be controlled with antacids and/or cimetidine. If significant bleeding continues, the infusion of vasopressin into the left gastric artery may be considered if this technique is available. If significant bleeding continues despite these measures, surgery must be considered. Surgery for acute gastritis, however, especially a diffuse gastritis, is not very satisfactory, and the procedure of choice is unclear. Most surgeons first attempt to control the bleeding with a vagotomy and pyloroplasty or a vagotomy and antrectomy and resort to a total gastrectomy only if these more conservative procedures fail. Some surgeons, however, advocate early total gastrectomy for diffuse involvement that cannot be successfully managed with vigorous medical therapy.

Acute necrosis and inflammation of the stomach that are often severe can be caused by corrosive agents (corrosive gastritis) or rarely by an acute pyogenic infection of the wall of the stomach (phlegmonous gastritis). The ingestion of a strong alkali or acid, usually in an attempted suicide, can cause necrosis of the stomach wall as well as burns of the mouth and esophagus. The necrosis may lead to perforation and peritonitis, hemorrhage, or a later stricture formation. (See Chapter 172 for the management of such patients.)

Chronic gastritis, the chronic inflammation of the gastric mucosa, occurs commonly, especially in older people. Because this condition is usually asymptomatic, its presence is often discovered when an associated gastric lesion such as an ulcer, polyp, or cancer leads to a biopsy or resection of the stomach. The classification of types of chronic gastritis has been somewhat arbitrary and controversial. Superficial gastritis is an inflammation in which acute and chronic inflammatory cells are largely limited to the upper portions of the mucosa between the gastric pits. In atrophic gastritis the inflammation extends deeper to involve the glands, and there is a concomitant loss of normal glandular cells and their variable replacement with intestinal types of cells (intestinal metaplasia) and pyloric gland cells (pseudopyloric metaplasia). The progressive loss of parietal cells is accompanied by a comparable reduction in their ability to secrete acid and intrinsic factor. The loss of most of the parietal cells is associated with achlorhydria, inadequate absorption of dietary vitamin B_{12} (measured by the Schilling test), and the possible eventual development of pernicious anemia. When such severe atrophy is associated with little or no inflammation, the lesion is called gastric atrophy.

Chronic gastritis is often limited solely or largely either to the area of the stomach that contains the fundic or gastric glands (chronic fundal gland gastritis) or to the area of the pyloric glands (antral gastritis). The causes of these forms of chronic gastritis are unknown, but the frequent association between atrophic fundal gastritis and certain immunologic phenomena suggests a possible role of immunologic processes in its pathogenesis. About 60% of patients with atrophic fundal gastritis and 90% of those with pernicious anemia have antibodies to parietal cells in their circulation. Most patients with pernicious anemia also have antibodies to intrinsic factor and, along with many others who also have severe atrophic fundal gastritis, have high serum gastrin levels, a result of increased numbers of pyloric G cells and the absence or reduction of acid secretion to inhibit G-cell secretion.

In contrast, predominant antral gastritis is not usually associated with parietal cell antibodies, an appreciable reduction in acid secretion, or elevated serum gastrin levels. Antral gastritis is commonly observed in patients with peptic ulcer disease and has been thought by some to result from the reflux of bile and bile acids from the duodenum into the stomach. Indeed, in patients who have undergone a gastrojejunostomy and thereby have regular reflux of bile through the anastomosis into the stomach, gastritis regularly develops around the stoma (stomal gastritis). Stomal gastritis is usually asymptomatic but it has occasionally been considered the possible cause of epigastric pain, nausea, and vomiting and is sometimes the source of gastrointestinal bleeding. After a partial gastric resection and especially after a Billroth II procedure, atrophic gastritis with a loss of parietal and chief cells often develops in the gastric remnant. The pathogenesis of this alteration is unclear, but the reflux of bile and the elimination of the antral G cells and the trophic effects to their gastrin have been suggested as playing a role. These gastric remnants appear to have an increased risk of developing carcinoma 15 years or more after the operation, and some physicians thus have advocated following these patients with regular endoscopic examinations.

A biopsy or resection performed because of the presence of gastric ulcers, polyps, or cancer usually reveals atrophic gastritis, and stomachs known to have atrophic gastritis seem to have an increased risk of developing these lesions. It remains unclear whether the presence of gastritis predisposes or leads to the development of ulcer, polyps, and cancer or whether the gastritis is an unrelated result of pathologic gastric processes that independently lead to the development of these lesions.

The term "hypertrophic gastritis" or gastropathy usually refers to the presence of thickened gastric mucosa and enlarged gastric folds, which are often difficult to differentiate roentgenographically and endoscopically from lymphomas and infiltrating carcinomas. Menetrier's disease is characterized by giant gastric folds and/or nodules, especially in the body of the stomach, marked hyperplasia of the surface and pit mucous cells, atrophy of the normal glandular cells, the hypersecretion of mucus, and the hyposecretion of acid. It is one of the causes of protein-losing enteropathy, and patients sometimes have edema resulting from a low serum albumin level (see Chapter 170) but more commonly have epigastric pain. The diagnosis may be determined by endoscopy and biopsy, but sometimes a laparotomy and full-thickness mucosal biopsy are required. Patients with the Zollinger-Ellison syndrome often have large gastric folds, an increased thickness of the mucosa, and hyperplasia of the fundic glands, especially of the parietal cells. These changes result from the trophic effects of the elevated levels of circulating gastrin, and these patients of course exhibit marked hypersecretion of gastric acid rather than the hypochlorhydria usually found in patients with Menetrier's disease. Hypersecretory hypertrophic gastropathy involves changes that resemble the gastric changes associated with the Zollinger-Ellison syndrome, with large gastric folds and thickened fundic mucosa, mainly because of an increased number of parietal and chief cells. These patients, however, do not have gastrinomas, elevated serum gastrin levels, or the markedly elevated acid secretions associated with that syndrome. Their acid secretions are often elevated, however, and the condition seems to be associated with an increased incidence of duodenal ulcer disease. These patients may sometimes exhibit an abnormal enteric loss of plasma proteins and, as in patients with Menetrier's disease, hypoalbuminemia may develop.

OTHER GASTRIC DISORDERS

Several other disorders of the stomach are discussed in other chapters, such as the common benign and malignant neoplasms (Chapter 180), the rare Crohn's disease (Chapter 175), eosinophilic gastroenteritis (Chapter 174), and motor disturbances such as pseudo-obstruction and diabetic gastroparesis (Chapter 177).

Acute gastric dilation

Acute gastric dilation is an acute motor disturbance in which the stomach fails to empty and therefore accumulates food and secretions in an enlarging "third space." It may be produced by drugs, such as anticholinergics, but is more commonly associated with many, often severe illnesses such as trauma, surgery, pneumonia, myocardial infarction, and sepsis. The condition can be recognized by the presence of a succussion splash and by means of an abdominal roentgenogram or nasogastric aspiration and must be differentiated from a mechanical obstruction. The patient must be placed on constant nasogastric suction while the resultant fluid and electrolyte disturbances are corrected.

Adult hypertrophic pyloric stenosis

Adult hypertrophic pyloric stenosis, an unusual hypertrophy of the pyloric muscle, causes symptoms of pyloric obstruction in adults: nausea, vomiting, and gastric retention. The gastrointestinal series and endoscopy reveal a symmetric narrowing of the pylorus and an "umbrella defect" in the base of the duodenal bulb. The lesion must be differentiated from an infiltrating carcinoma, from the scarring or inflammation of peptic ulcer disease, and from inflammatory processes such as Crohn's disease, eosinophilic gastroenteritis, and tuberculosis or tertiary syphilis, which rarely affect the stomach. Surgery may be required to relieve the symptoms or occasionally to determine the definitive diagnosis.

Gastric volvulus

Gastric volvulus (torsion), a rare acute or chronic twisting of the stomach, may cause severe upper abdominal pain and the regurgitation of saliva rather than gastric contents. The abdominal roentgenogram usually demonstrates the diagnosis. Surgery may be required if an acute volvulus does not subside but progresses to strangulation or if a chronic volvulus produces repeated symptoms.

Gastric diverticula

Gastric diverticula are rare lesions that occur most commonly just below the cardia on the posterior wall near the lesser curvature. They can usually be diagnosed by a gastrointestinal series, but occasionally endoscopy is required to differentiate them from an ulcer. They are usually asymptomatic and require no treatment except in the rare cases of bleeding, perforation, or severe pain that therefore may require surgery.

Bezoars

Bezoars, aggregates of organic and/or inorganic matter, occasionally develop in the stomach, especially in a gastric remnant after a partial gastrectomy. They often cause anorexia, satiety, nausea, and vomiting. These usually large masses can be differentiated from tumors by gastrointestinal roentgenograms and endoscopy. Often bezoars can be fragmented at the time of the endoscopy and removed by repeated lavage. Some phytobezoars (composed of vegetable matter) may be partially digested with the aid of cellulase and/or papain and then successfully removed with lavage. Trichobezoars (composed of hair) are more resistant to digestion. Rarely aggregates of inorganic substances are found. If the bezoars cannot be successfully removed by lavage after mechanical or enzymatic fragmentation, surgery may be necessary. Other swallowed foreign bodies occasionally lodged in the stomach may also be gripped and removed at the time of endoscopy.

BIBLIOGRAPHY

Sleisenger, M.H., and Fordtran, J.S.: Gastrointestinal disease, ed. 2, Philadelphia, 1978, W.B. Saunders Co.

174 • DISORDERS OF ABSORPTION—THE MALABSORPTION SYNDROME

Gerald H. Escovitz

The malabsorption syndrome is caused by many disorders that impair the body's ability to assimilate dietary fats and often other dietary substances such as proteins, carbohydrates, vitamins, minerals, and water.

NORMAL PHYSIOLOGY

Most people in the United States and other developed countries ingest 50 to 100 g of fat in their daily diet. Normally less than 5 g of fat can be recovered from the stool daily, and the excretion of more than 6 g is considered abnormal. The lipids in the normal diet are primarily triglycerides that contain long-chain fatty acids usually 16 and 18 carbon atoms in length. After ingestion, the first important action occurs when triglyceride, a large water-insoluble molecule, is hydrolyzed into free fatty acids (FFA) and a β-monoglyceride (β-MG) by the action of the pancreatic enzyme lipase (Fig. 174-1). The FFA and β-MG are also water insoluble but are reaily solubilized by the detergent properties of bile salts, which are brought to the intestine in the bile.

Bile salts, detergents with special physicochemical properties, are amphipaths; that is, they have both hydrophilic and hydrophobic regions. The bile salts aggregate into water-soluble particles called micelles by aligning themselves so that their hydrophilic regions align at the aqueous surface and their hydrophobic regions cluster away from the aqueous solution. The bile salts solubilize the FFA and β-MG by incorporating them within their hydrophobic regions to form mixed micelles. This formation occurs when the concentration of bile salts is greater than the critical micellar concentration (CMC) of 2 to 5 mM, when the medium is at a proper pH, and when the bile salts are conjugated to taurine or glycine.

This solubilization of fat is apparently essential for its absorption at normal rates, possibly by making the fat more accessible to the epithelial cells lining the small intestine. At this stage the large, water-insoluble fat particles have been transformed into smaller water-soluble particles. The fat-soluble vitamins (A, D, E, and K) are also incorporated in the interior part of the micelles.

FFA and β-MG dissociate from the bile salts at the intestinal surface and diffuse passively into the epithelial cells of the upper small intestine. There are four stages in the passage of lipids from the intestinal lumen to the circulation: (1) their uptake into the mucosal cells, (2) the reesterification of FFA and β-MG into triglycerides, (3) the formation of chylomicrons, and (4) the secretion of chylomicrons into the lymphatic circulation.

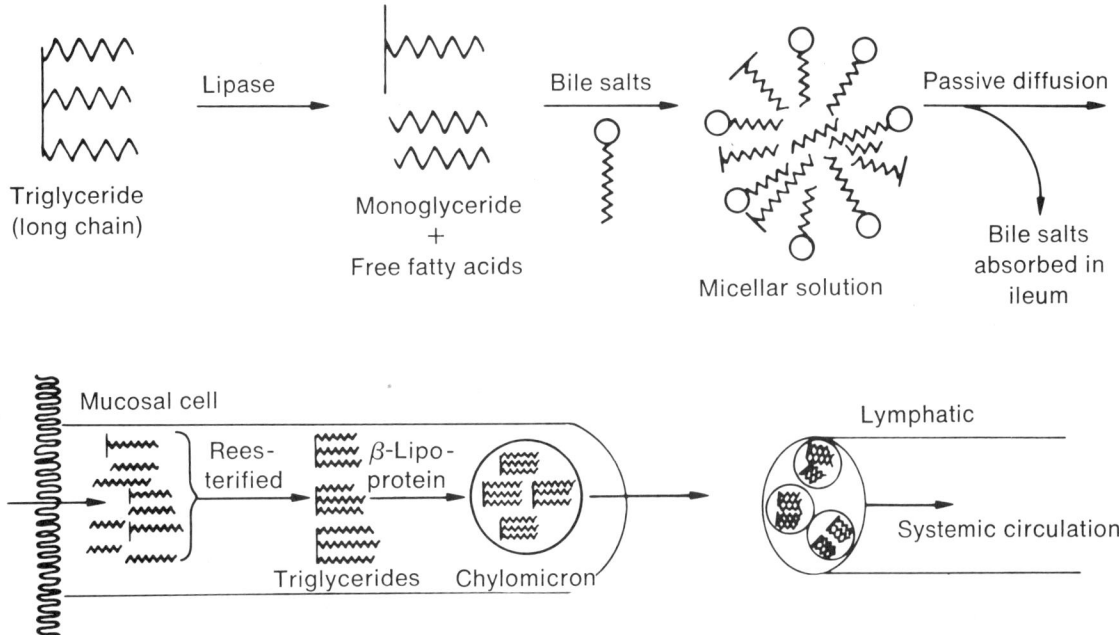

Fig. 174-1. Sequence of steps in normal absorption of dietary lipids. Malabsorption may result when any of these essential steps is disturbed by disease processes. See text for details.

The first stage of the passage is the passive, non-energy-dependent transport of FFA and β-MG through the lipophilic membrane of the brush border. Intracellular passage is facilitated in the aqueous medium of the cell by a small protein that binds the FFA and the β-MG. In the smooth endoplasmic reticulum FFA and β-MG are resynthesized into triglycerides, with each step requiring a different activating enzyme. The resulting triglyceride molecules coalesce into larger particles that are coated with a lipoprotein. These large particles, chylomicrons, exit from the base of the cell and enter the lymphatic circulation. The lipoprotein coating is necessary for the normal departure of the triglyceride from the intestinal cell.

The bile salts themselves are not absorbed with the lipids they solubilize but pass on to the distal ileum where they are actively absorbed. They are then returned to the liver via the portal circulation, are resecreted into the bile, and are used again in the formation of micelles. This enterohepatic circulation preserves the total body pool of bile salts at approximately 4 g. Only about 15% of the bile salt pool, or about 600 mg, is lost in the stool each day, and the loss is readily replaced by hepatic synthesis of new bile salts.

Triglycerides whose FFA is of shorter length (from 6 to 10 carbon atoms) are called medium-chain triglycerides (MCT) and are able to bypass steps in absorption that are necessary for triglycerides with longer FFA. MCT may be absorbed intact, requires lower concentrations of lipase for hydrolysis, forms micelles at concentrations of bile salts below the CMC, and may avoid the process of intracellular reesterification by being absorbed directly into the portal venous system. These properties of MCT make it an effective therapeutic agent in a variety of conditions that cause malabsorption.

PATHOPHYSIOLOGY

Disorders that interfere with any of the steps necessary for normal fat absorption may produce steatorrhea. The several clinical entities that cause pancreatic insufficiency also cause steatorrhea consisting mainly of undigested triglycerides. Impaired micelle formation caused by bile salt deficiency, altered pH, or deconjugation of bile salts also leads to impaired fat absorption. Many disorders directly affect the small bowel mucosa and thereby inhibit fat absorption. These clinical entities include intestinal resection, which simply eliminates part of the bowel; a wide variety of mucosal diseases such as celiac sprue that inhibit the transport of FFA and β-MG across the mucosal cell; disease processes that selectively impair the normal metabolism within the mucosal cell, such as congenital β-lipoprotein deficiency; specific defects of the transport of chylomicrons into the lymphatics, such as lymphangiectasia; and disease processes that involve several steps, such as the malabsorption that occurs after a Billroth II gastric resection, in which there may be bacterial overgrowth in a stagnant loop and/or relative pancreatic insufficiency because of an inadequate mixing of ingested lipids with pancreatic secretions.

In addition, a wide variety of metabolic defects may accompany fat malabsorption. Hypoproteinemia, usually caused by an abnormal protein loss through diseased mucosa, commonly occurs in patients with celiac sprue, eosinophilic gastroenteritis, radiation enteritis, diffuse ileojejunitis, and Crohn's disease. Severe malabsorption may produce both hyponatremia and hypokalemia. Hypocalcemia and hypomagnesemia, both of which may contribute to muscle irritability and even tetany, may occur in patients with chronic diseases of the mucosa such as celiac sprue, after intestinal resection, and in other conditions causing significant malabsorption such as pancreatic insufficiency. Hypocalcemia may be made more severe by vitamin D malabsorption. Anemia is often present. Mucosal diseases such as celiac sprue may lead to several types of anemia with deficiencies of iron, folate, and vitamin B_{12}. Vitamin B_{12} absorption may also be decreased in diseases that cause bacterial overgrowth because it may be bound to the bacteria and thus not be absorbed. Vitamin B_{12} absorption may also be decreased as a result of diseases or surgical procedures involving the terminal ileum, the site of vitamin B_{12} absorption. A tendency toward bleeding in cases of vitamin K deficiency is seen both in diffuse mucosal disease and in conditions that affect micelle formation.

In general, disorders that involve minimal fat malabsorption have fewer metabolic side effects than those with more severe malabsorption. Mucosal diseases usually have the most severe accompanying metabolic disorders; the steatorrhea of pancreatic insufficiency is next in severity.

CLINICAL PRESENTATION

Patients with the malabsorption syndrome may have symptoms of general malabsorption or symptoms caused by the deficiency of a specific substance such as vitamin A, D, or K, calcium, magnesium, iron, or folate. The patient with malabsorption syndrome classically has bulky, oily, malodorous stools associated with significant weight loss, muscle wasting, weakness, edema, anemia, ecchymoses, abnormal bleeding, a smooth tongue, hyperkeratosis of the skin, skeletal pain, and even tetany. The oral cavity manifestations of malabsorption occur when vitamin deficiencies are part of the clinical presentation. These may include reddening and ulceration of the mucosa and tongue, swelling and burning of the tongue, and fissuring of the corner of the mouth (cheilosis), all of which are associated with vitamin B deficiencies. If vitamin B_{12} deficiency is prominent, atrophy of the tongue may be present.

In the United States dramatic symptoms of malabsorption syndrome are rare, and the physician must be alert to more subtle symptoms. Stools may be watery, and occasionally a patient may be constipated. Weight loss may be slight. There may be abdominal pain. Symptoms of deficiencies of vitamins A, K, and D may occur as isolated phenomena. Edema caused by hypoalbuminemia and the glossitis, stomatitis, or neuropathy related to vitamin B deficiencies may also occur as isolated phenomena.

An unexplained laboratory finding may also be the first clue to the presence of malabsorption syndrome, such as an unexplained anemia, hypocalcemia, hypocholesterolemia, hypoalbuminemia, hypoprothrombinemia, or a flat glucose tolerance curve.

In many patients the diagnosis of the clinical condition causing malabsorption is readily apparent from the history, such as with patients who have had a massive small bowel resection, abdominal irradiation, or a pancreatic resection. The symptoms of malabsorption are also not difficult to interpret in patients with a history of alcoholism and recurrent pancreatitis, in patients from a geographic area where tropical sprue is endemic, in patients taking one of the medications associated with malabsorption, in patients with the obvious skin findings of scleroderma or dermatitis herpetiformis, and in patients with diabetes mellitus and severe peripheral neuropathy.

In many cases, however, the history is not helpful in diagnosing the cause of malabsorption, either because there is no significant history or because the symptoms are nonspecific. Abdominal pain and distention, often associated with conditions causing malabsorption, also occur in a multitude of conditions not associated with malabsorption. The causes of diarrhea, weight loss, anorexia, anemia, and so on are many, and these symptoms are only as clues to be evaluated in the context of other findings.

The results of the physical examination of patients with malabsorption vary greatly. Some patients appear essentially normal or even overweight. There may, however, be signs of weight loss, muscle wasting, or the specific nutritional deficiencies just described. Hypotension and tachycardia may be present. Pallor, skin atrophy, hyperkeratosis, ecchymoses, clubbing, cheilosis, glossitis, and peripheral edema may all be present. The abdomen may be protuberant, with loops of small intestine visibly distended. Peripheral neuropathy or findings of combined system disease are occasionally observed.

CLINICAL APPROACH

Several steps must be taken when approaching the evaluation of a patient suspected of having the malabsorption syndrome:

1. Objective confirmation of malabsorption
2. Diagnosis of the specific disorder responsible for the syndrome
3. Institution of specific and supportive therapy
4. Evaluation of the patient's responses to the therapy, since in many conditions that cause malabsorption the therapeutic trial is also a diagnostic step

OBJECTIVE CONFIRMATION OF STEATORRHEA. A quantitative analysis of fecal fat is the best single test for confirming the presence of steatorrhea. Stools should be collected for at least 3 consecutive days while the patient is ingesting at least 70 g (ideally, 100 g) of fat daily. The excretion of more than 6 g daily confirms the diagnosis of fat malabsorption.

Other tests, such as the serum carotene test, the radioactive triolein excretion test, the vitamin A absorption test, and the urinary indican test, are not sufficiently specific or reliable and should not be used. The qualitative evaluation of fat in the stool, by means of microscopic examination using Sudan stain, is of some value as a screening procedure when the quantitive method is unavailable. This test is, however, subject to both false positive and false negative results, and the result should generally be regarded as an additional clue rather than a confirmation of the diagnosis.

SPECIFIC DISORDERS CAUSING MALABSORPTION
Pancreatic insufficiency

In the United States chronic pancreatitis (usually caused by alcoholism) is the most common cause of pancreatic insufficiency. In such cases the patient usually has a lengthy history of recurrent episodes of pancreatitis with progressive, persistent, debilitating pain. The malabsorption in these patients is generally severe (measured fecal fat greater than 30 g daily) and is accompanied by weight loss, vitamin and mineral deficiencies, and often diabetes mellitus. The secretin test is rarely necessary in these patients. The response of the patient with malabsorption to commercial preparations of pancreatic digestive enzymes (often given with supplementary antacids) is usually excellent, including a resultant weight gain and the correction of metabolic abnormalities.

Other, less common causes of pancreatic insufficiency are a pancreatic resection for either chronic pancreatitis or pancreatic cancer, a pancreatic carcinoma that blocks the main pancreatic duct at the head of the pancreas, cystic fibrosis occurring in children or young adults, and rarely insufficiency caused by the gastric hypersecretion occurring in patients with the Zollinger-Ellison syndrome or by a massive small bowel resection, which inactivates pancreatic enzymes by lowering the duodenal pH.

Patients with these less common causes of pancreatic insufficiency show a malabsorption pattern similar to that of chronic pancreatitis. Patients with cystic fibrosis, however, may have milder symptoms. The secretin test is often helpful in confirming the diagnosis in these cases. The D-xylose test, bile acid–breath test, and small bowel roentgenogram, all of which are normal in these patients, are useful in ruling out other possible causes. In some patients the diagnosis of pancreatic insufficiency can be made only after a successful response to a therapeutic trial of pancreatic enzymes. This approach to diagnosing pancreatic insufficiency is valid when the more specific measures already described are not helpful or when they are unavailable to the physician.

Mucosal disease

CELIAC DISEASE. Celiac disease (celiac sprue, or gluten enteropathy) is a prototype of the malabsorption syndrome. Its cause is unknown, but the therapeutic response to the elimination of gluten from the diet indicates that this protein, through either a direct toxic effect or an immunologic reaction, is the major contributing factor. The importance of genetic factors is demonstrated by the high incidence of histologic abnormalities of the intestinal mucosa in asymptomatic relatives of patients with celiac disease and the high incidence of HLA-8 or DW3 tissue antigens in these patients. Many patients also have a history compatible with childhood celiac disease.

Steatorrhea in these patients is often moderate to severe (25 to 40 g daily) and is often accompanied by hypoproteinemia, hypocalcemia, hypomagnesemia, hypokalemia, and anemia. In some patients an occult anemia, ecchymoses, osteomalacia, or tetany may be symptoms. In patients with celiac sprue the D-xylose test results are abnormal, and small bowel roentgenograms usually show nonspecific findings of dilation, coarsening of the folds, flocculation, and clumping of barium. Because the disease is most severe in the upper small bowel and relatively spares the terminal ileum, the vitamin B_{12} absorption test results may be normal. These patients often have a secondary lactose intolerance.

The abnormal D-xylose results and roentgenograms only indicate an intestinal mucosal disease, for which there are many possible causes. A small bowel biopsy must be performed; the typical findings with celiac disease are flattened villi and an increase in the infiltration of inflammatory cells. Even then, because celiac sprue is not the only condition that causes this histologic picture, a therapeutic response to a gluten-free diet is necessary for an absolute confirmation of the diagnosis. Most patients with gluten enteropathy respond to a gluten-free diet with both clinical and histologic improvement, although rarely a very ill patient may require supplemental therapy with corticosteroids. The response to the gluten-free diet is usually observed within 1 or 2 weeks but occasionally only after many weeks of therapy. A lack of response to a gluten-free diet should cause the physician to reconsider the diagnosis, since this therapeutic trial is an important part of the diagnostic evaluation. However, the diet should be reviewed carefully, since inadvertent gluten ingestion is a common cause of apparent therapeutic failure.

DISEASES THAT MAY BE CONFUSED WITH CELIAC DISEASE
Tropical sprue. Tropical sprue causes histologic findings similar to those of gluten enteropathy, but these as well as the malabsorption and metabolic abnormalities are often less severe. Macrocytic anemia is usually present. This condition is endemic in certain tropical and subtropical regions such as Southeast Asia, the Indian subcontinent, and the Caribbean. When this condition appears in a temperate climate, the patient has usually previously resided in an endemic area.

The cause of this condition is unknown, but patients usually respond to broad-spectrum antibiotics, folate, and parenteral vitamin B_{12}. Some patients may require up to 6 months of therapy before a significant clinical response is seen. Antibiotic and folic acid administration should be continued as long as the clinical and laboratory improvement continues.

Collagenous sprue. Collagenous sprue is similar to celiac sprue in many ways, but biopsy reveals a dense band of collagen in the lamina propria. These patients do not respond to a gluten-free diet. The prognosis for these patients is grim and death is almost certain.

Intestinal lymphoma. An intestinal lymphoma may be either a secondary development in patients with longstanding gluten enteropathy or a primary condition that may be confused with celiac sprue. Patients with malabsorption caused by intestinal lymphoma usually have severe, persistent abdominal pain, fever, and severe malabsorption; their small bowel biopsy results are similar to those of celiac sprue, and the patients fail to respond to a gluten-free diet. Whereas celiac sprue is most severe in the upper small intestine, lymphoma affects the entire small bowel. Diffuse intestinal lymphoma is common in patients from the Mideast and is most often seen in young adults and teenagers.

The treatment of patients with diffuse intestinal lymphoma associated with malabsorption syndrome is generally ineffective. In one series of nine patients, none survived beyond 4 years.

Dermatitis herpetiformis. Two thirds of the patients with dermatitis herpetiformis have histologic changes that are revealed by small bowel biopsy. Some of these changes are identical to the findings with classic celiac sprue, whereas in other patients the changes may be less severe and less specific. In patients with dermatitis herpetiformis, steatorrhea, and histologic abnormalities of the small intestine, the malabsorption responds to a gluten-free diet with no effect on the skin disease. On the other hand, the skin disease responds to dapsone or sulfapyridine with no effect on the malabsorption. Thus these appear to be two separate diseases that may often coexist. The patient with dermatitis herpetiformis should be evaluated for malabsorption in the manner previously described.

IATROGENIC CAUSES. Malabsorption of mucosal origin is often caused by therapy applied for other conditions. Such therapies include an intestinal resection or bypass, radiation therapy, and medications.

Surgical resection. Resection of 50% or more of the small intestine usually results in significant malabsorption. Resection of a smaller portion of small bowel in the distal ileum may also lead to significant steatorrhea. Patients who have had a significant resection of small bowel should be carefully evaluated for steatorrhea, which is often severe, and for all of the other metabolic abnormalities associated with a severe malabsorption syndrome.

In these patients hypoproteinemia and vitamin and mineral deficiencies and their sequelae are the rule and must be evaluated and treated vigorously.

Radiation enteritis. Patients with a known history of radiation therapy to the abdomen who have any of the symptoms of malabsorption should be evaluated for malabsorption syndrome. The symptoms may occur soon after the therapy or after months or even years have elapsed. The mechanism for malabsorption in these patients may be direct and generalized damage to the small bowel mucosa. If this damage includes the distal ileum, a quantitative deficiency of bile salts may result and contribute to the malabsorption, whereas if there is a stricture, the resulting stasis may lead to bacterial overgrowth and the deconjugation of bile salts.

The malabsorption may be severe, especially when severe mucosal damage occurs. The therapy should be directed to the specific cause: surgery for a stricture, MCT for a damaged terminal ileum, and so on. A diet free of gluten, lactose, and milk protein may be of value.

Medications. Colchicine therapy may result in mild steatorrhea and abnormal results on the D-xylose test. The mechanism of action appears to be an inactivation of mucosal intracellular enzymes that resynthesize triglycerides from FFA and β-MG. Neomycin also causes mild malabsorption by a direct toxic effect on mucosal enzymes, by inhibiting lipase action, by precipitating bile salts, or by some combination of these. Cathartic agents may cause mild malabsorption, perhaps because of an increase in motility and intestinal transit time. Malabsorption occurs only in habitual users of relatively large amounts of cathartic agents. Podophyllin, bisacodyl, colocynth, and jalap have been found to cause malabsorption under these conditions. Cholestyramine is often used to decrease the diarrhea associated with bile salt malabsorption, that is, choleretic enteropathy. Although the cholestyramine mitigates diarrhea in these cases, it further diminishes the bile salt pool and may exacerbate the malabsorption. The extent of malabsorption in these patients is generally related to the dosage of cholestyramine. Para-aminosalicylic acid may also cause malabsorption if given in a high dosage.

In all of these conditions malabsorption is generally mild and stops when the medication is discontinued.

MISCELLANEOUS CAUSES OF MALABSORPTION OF MUCOSAL ORIGIN

Whipple's disease. Whipple's disease is an uncommon disease that causes moderate to severe malabsorption and is associated with a wide spectrum of systemic manifestations that may include arthritis, arthralgia, fever, an increase in skin pigmentation, pleuritis, pericarditis, central nervous system symptoms, and anemia. The classic histologic finding for this disease is an infiltration of the lamina propria with macrophages that stain red with periodic acid–Schiff stain. Over the years many observers have described small rodlike structures detected in biopsies, and electron microscopy clearly shows the presence of small bacilli (0.25 μ wide and 2 μ long). These, however, have not yet been cultured successfully.

Patients with Whipple's disease are generally ill from both the malabsorption and the systemic involvement and in the past have almost invariably died. Treatment with antibiotics, however, has completely altered this grim prognosis, and most patients become asymptomatic within several weeks. Penicillin and tetracycline are both effective agents.

Small intestinal ischemia. Although malabsorption associated with small bowel ischemia is rare, the increase in life expectancy in the United States and the resultant increase in visceral ischemia will undoubtedly lead to an increased incidence of this disorder. Malabsorption that is usually mild may be seen with diffuse arteriosclerosis, vasculitis, polycythemia vera, and Kohlmeier-Degos disease (necrotic skin lesions and vasculitis of the small bowel). Therapy is directed at the underlying disorder.

Eosinophilic gastroenteritis. Eosinophilic gastroenteritis, which has been considered an allergy to foods, is characterized by an increase in eosinophils both in the lamina propria and in the peripheral blood and may be accompanied by malabsorption of fat and protein-losing enteropathy. Patients with this condition usually have an increased incidence of allergic disorders and often a dramatic increase in symptoms when certain foods are ingested. The objective of therapy is to eliminate foods from the diet in a sequential manner, but usually the long-term use of corticosteroids is also required.

Amyloidosis. Both primary and secondary amyloidosis may be associated with malabsorption, which is usually moderate but may be associated with protein-losing enteropathy. The infiltration of amyloid protein may cause a motility disorder, and a bacterial overgrowth may also occur. Encroachment on the vascular supply may cause ischemia with resultant pain and diarrhea.

The small bowel biopsy may or may not reveal the amyloid deposits. For that reason, a rectal biopsy is often performed to confirm the presence of amyloidosis in patients with suspected amyloidosis and malabsorption.

There is no treatment for amyloidosis; the disease is usually relentless and fatal.

Disorders of lymphatic transport

INTESTINAL LYMPHANGIECTASIA. Intestinal lymphangiectasia is a rare disorder characterized by abnormally dilated lacteals that may distort the villous architecture. The cause of this disorder is unknown, but it leads to the accumulation of chylomicrons between the intestinal cells and the lamina propria as a result of an inability to transport the chylomicrons into the lacteals. Malabsorption is moderate and is associated with protein-losing enteropathy, hypoproteinemia, lymphocytopenia, and peripheral edema. The disease usually affects children and young adults.

The diagnosis can usually be made with a small bowel biopsy. The specific therapy uses MCT, which not only corrects the fat malabsorption but also corrects the intestinal protein loss and its sequelae. The prognosis with early diagnosis and treatment is good.

A clinical picture similar to that of lymphangiectasia may be seen in patients whose abdominal lymphatics are blocked by disseminated carcinoma or lymphoma.

Miscellaneous causes of malabsorption

PARASITIC DISEASES. (See also Chapters 54 and 55.) A variety of parasitic diseases may be associated with malabsorption, including giardiasis *(G. lamblia)*, strongyloidiasis *(S. stercoralis)*, hookworm disease, coccidiosis *(Isospora belli)*, and capillariasis *(Capillaria philippinensis)*. In the United States the last three diseases are extremely rare and strongyloidiais is also rare, but giardiasis is increasingly common. Giardiasis may cause malabsorption, often in patients with IgA deficiency but also in patients with normal immunoglobulins. A severe *Strongyloides* infestation is usually seen in patients whose immune system has been compromised either by chemotherapy for cancer or by corticosteroids. In these instances malabsorption may be more severe, and the patient may be very ill.

When a parasitic origin is suspected for a patient's malabsorption, the stool examination may reveal the parasite. Duodenal aspiration and a small bowel biopsy may be necessary, however, to confirm the diagnosis. Because the ingestion of barium may "wash out" the parasite, it should be delayed in patients suspected of having a parasitic infestation until the aspiration and biopsy have been performed.

Parasitic conditions generally respond well to specific therapy (metronidazole for *Giardia* and thiabendazole for *Strongyloides*), leading to the remission of malabsorption and other symptoms of the infestation.

DIFFUSE ILEOJEJUNITIS. Diffuse ileojejunitis is a rare, poorly defined inflammatory disease of the small bowel. Patients often have fever, malaise, abdominal cramps, diarrhea, and malabsorption. The diagnosis usually requires an exploratory laparotomy and biopsies of the inflamed bowel. The intestinal mucosa may exhibit patchy areas of villous atrophy resembling that of celiac disease. Some patients respond to steroid therapy, but for most the prognosis is poor. The mortality is high.

VIRAL AND BACTERIAL GASTROENTERITIS. Mild to moderate fat malabsorption may be found in patients with acute viral gastroenteritis. The malabsorption is generally self-limited. Metabolic complications other than transient electrolyte changes do not occur. Gastroenteritis caused by *Shigella, Escherichia coli,* cholera, *Clostridium,* staphylococci, and *Yersinia* may also have an associated self-limited malabsorption.

DIABETES MELLITUS. Malabsorption associated with diabetes mellitus usually occurs in patients who have peripheral and autonomic neuropathy. Malabsorption is usually mild to moderate, but a persistent, frequent, watery diarrhea that causes patients considerable annoyance is common. It is assumed that the diarrhea and malabsorption are caused by an enteric neuropathy. Bacterial overgrowth is occasionally present, and some patients have been found by the small bowel biopsy to have flattened villi. Most patients, however, have neither bacterial overgrowth nor histologic changes in the small bowel.

The treatment is symptomatic and directed at reducing the frequency of stools. The malabsorption may make the control of the diabetic patient's blood sugar difficult and may lead to episodes of both hyperglycemia and hypoglycemia. In these patients a complete reversal of diarrhea and malabsorption is rare.

MALABSORPTION ASSOCIATED WITH ENDOCRINE DISEASE. Malabsorption that is usually mild has been reported in cases of hyperthyroidism, adrenal insufficiency, hypoparathyroidism, carcinoid, and systemic mast cell disease. In all of these conditions the endocrinopathy is usually obvious and severe, and the malabsorption is a rather unimportant aspect of the patient's problem. The malabsorption responds to the treatment of the primary disease.

Somewhat more common is the malabsorption occurring in patients with the Zollinger-Ellison syndrome. In these patients the disorder probably results from the excessive gastric secretion and consequent acid pH in the proximal small bowel, which impairs fat digestion and micelle formation. Malabsorption in these patients always responds to treatment of the primary problem.

SCLERODERMA. The smooth muscle fibrosis of scleroderma may also involve the small bowel with a resultant dilation of bowel, decreased motility, and stasis. Although originally reported in patients with obvious skin manifestations, small bowel involvement with scleroderma may occur in patients with minimal skin changes or none at all. The malabsorption is usually mild to moderate and often is the result of bacterial overgrowth caused by intestinal stasis. The malabsorption usually responds to antibiotic therapy with a total or partial remission.

POSTGASTRECTOMY SYNDROME. Postgastrectomy malabsorption may be seen in patients who have had a gastric resection such as the Billroth II operation. The malabsorption is usually mild to moderate, but it can be severe. Because of the relatively rapid gastric emptying the patient may also have bloating and symptoms referable to dumping or reactive hypoglycemia. Symptoms related to decreased vitamin D and calcium absorption are common, as is iron deficiency anemia.

The principal cause of the malabsorption seems related to the rapid gastric emptying, which results in inadequate mixing of ingested food with bile salts and pancreatic enzymes. Rarely, there may also be bacterial overgrowth in a stagnant afferent loop.

Patients with a stagnant afferent loop and bacterial overgrowth usually require corrective surgery. For others, a trial of multiple small feedings with supplemental pancreatic enzymes may mitigate all or most of the malabsorption. Patients whose malabsorption is serious and fails to respond to these measures may need surgical revision. Many patients with gastric resection, even those without malabsorption, may require supplemental vitamins and minerals, especially vitamin D, calcium, and iron. These needs are even more intense when malabsorption is present.

DISORDERS OF CARBOHYDRATE ABSORPTION
Normal physiology

Most carbohydrates are ingested as starch and glycogen and to a lesser extent as the disaccharides lactose and sucrose. In the intestinal lumen the starch and glycogen are digested by α-amylase secreted by the salivary glands and pancreas, to form oligosaccharides of 2 to 10 glucose molecules. These molecules are further broken down at the brush border–lumen interface by oligosaccharidases, which are located on the outer surface of the intestinal brush border. These enzymes hydrolyze the glucose α-dextrins to glucose. Specific brush border enzymes act on lactose to form glucose and galactose (lactase) and on sucrose to form glucose and fructose (sucrase). The monosaccharides are then transported across the intestinal epithelium by specific active transport systems that are energy dependent.

As is the case with fat malabsorption, conditions that inhibit any of these steps can lead to malabsorption of sugars. The intraluminal phase is rarely a clinical problem in carbohydrate malabsorption because amylase is rarely so reduced in quantity that it becomes a clinical problem. Thus disorders of carbohydrate absorption result either from a deficiency or absence of oligosaccharidases located at the brush border or from a defect in one or more specific transport systems.

When any of these disorders exist, unabsorbed disaccharides or monosaccharides remain in the intestinal lumen where they have an osmotic effect. The net flow of water into the intestinal lumen results in bloating, increased intestinal transit, and crampy abdominal pains. The unabsorbed sugars are fermented by colonic bacteria and create an acid pH that appears to inhibit the absorption of water and electrolytes in the colon. In addition, the bacterial fermentation produces gas, which adds to the abdominal cramping. The net result, depending on the severity of the problem, is diarrhea, crampy abdominal pain, flatulence, and bloating.

There are several specific disorders of carbohydrate malabsorption, but lactase deficiency (lactose intolerance) is by far the most common and is clinically the most important.

Lactose intolerance (lactase deficiency)

Although a premature infant may have transient lactase deficiency, lactase activity is usually very high in the neonatal period. This activity declines in childhood, however, and much of the world's population over 10 years of age has a lactase deficiency. This is called acquired lactase deficiency. Whites of Northern European ancestry are an exception to this acquired deficiency, but even in this group up to 20% may have this deficiency. An acquired deficiency therefore may be considered normal. Certain racial groups, notably blacks, Asians, and Eskimos, have an incidence as high as 70% to 95%. The deficiency of lactase is minimal in some persons and more severe in others of the same race, and thus there is wide individual variation in the ability to absorb lactose even within a "pure" racial group. In the United States there is clearly a major difference in incidence between whites of Northern European origin and all others.

It has been demonstrated that lactase deficiency is inherited as an autosomal recessive condition. It has been postulated that the decrease in intestinal lactase seen in adults (the acquired form) is secondary to the decrease in milk ingestion after childhood and the subsequent lack of enzyme stimulation by ingested lactose. This hypothesis however, is not supported by evidence. There has also been controversy about the extent to which milk proteins or other constituents contribute to the symptoms. Recent evidence supports the theory that lactose—and lactose alone—is responsible for symptoms in lactase-deficient persons.

In the congenital form of lactose intolerance there is virtually no lactase present at birth, and the reaction to ingested lactose is immediate and severe. Whereas the acquired form of lactase deficiency has been viewed as a genetic (autosomal recessive) defect in enzyme regulation, the congenital form has been regarded as a structural change in the gene itself. More recent studies of patients with the congenital form, however, reveal minute quantities of lactase that is qualitatively indistinguishable from normal lactase. Thus the congenital form of this disorder may just be one end of a spectrum of the defect in enzyme regulation.

The third form of lactase deficiency is secondary lactase deficiency, that is, a deficiency that occurs in association with other diseases and is resolved when the primary disease is treated. Secondary lactase deficiency is most common in conditions that affect large areas of small bowel mucosa, such as sprue, acute gastroenteritis, and bowel ischemia. Postgastrectomy diarrhea is often caused by rapid gastric emptying in which ingested lactose does not have adequate time to make contact with intestinal lactase. Lactose intolerance has also been found to be the cause of some cases of so-called spastic colon; patients thus diagnosed may in fact have occult lactose intolerance. In these patients a lactose-free diet eliminates the symptoms of the irritable colon syndrome.

DIAGNOSIS. In most instances a history of the symptoms described occurring 1 to 4 hours after the ingestion of milk or milk products suggests the diagnosis of lactase deficiency. Many patients are aware of this association and inform the physician of it, but many others are not and with these the burden of diagnosis rests with the physician. The usual diagnostic test is the lactose tolerance test, in which 50 g of lactose is given orally and the clinical response noted. In more than 90% of patients with lactase deficiency who are given this test, abdominal cramps and diarrhea develop. It is also possible to measure the blood glucose in these patients, as with a glucose tolerance test, because those with lactase deficiency have a flat curve. Patients with a normal lactase content, however, may also have a flat curve. A more accurate confirmation of the diagnosis can be obtained with a biopsy of the small bowel and an assay of lactase content. This test, however, is not readily available and involves added discomfort, cost, and risk (although minimal) to the patient. It should be used only with carefully selected patients when other tests are equivocal and when it is important to confirm the diagnosis.

It is also possible to test for lactose intolerance by administering ^{14}C-labeled lactose and measuring the amount of radioactive carbon dioxide in the patient's breath within 4 hours. Lactase-deficient patients discharge measurably less ^{14}C than is normal.

MANAGEMENT. The treatment consists of removing lactose from the diet, a regimen that may not be as simple as it seems because many foods, such as all milk products, bakery goods made with milk, and canned and frozen fruits and vegetables, contain lactose. In time both the physician and the patient will learn just how much lactose the patient can tolerate and in what form. Because the degree of lactase deficiency varies from patient to patient, the extent to which each patient can tolerate lactose also varies. For this reason the dietary restrictions should be individualized.

BIBLIOGRAPHY

Benson, G.D., Kowlessar, O.D., and Sleisenger, M.H.: Adult celiac disease with emphasis upon response to the gluten free diet, Medicine **43**:1, 1964.

Finlay, J.M., Hogarth, J., and Wightman, K.J.R.: A clinical evaluation of the D-xylose tolerance test. Ann. Intern. Med. **61**:411, 1964.

Fromm, H., and Hofmann, A.F.: Breath test for altered bile-acid metabolism, Lancet **2**:621, 1971.

Gray, G.M.: Congenital and adult intestinal lactase deficiency, N.Engl. J. Med. **294**:1057, 1976.

Ochner, R.K., and Isselbacher, K.J.: Recent concepts of intestinal fat absorption. Rev. Physiol. Biochem. Pharmacol. **71**:107, 1974.

Rubin, C.E., and Dobbins, W.O., III: Peroral biopsy of the small intestine: a review of its diagnostic usefulness, Gastroenterology **49**:676, 1965.

Sleisenger, M.H., and Fordtran, J.S.: Gastrointestinal disease, ed. 2, Philadelphia, 1978, W.B. Saunders Co.

Spiro, H.: Clinical gastroenterology, New York, 1977, Macmillan, Inc.

175 • INFLAMMATORY DISEASES OF THE INTESTINES

Harvey B. Lefton

INFLAMMATORY BOWEL DISEASE

DEFINITION. Inflammatory bowel disease is a general classification of inflammatory processes affecting the large and small intestines. Ulcerative colitis is one such inflammatory condition involving the mucosa and submucosa of the colon. The disease may inflame part or all of the large intestine. Occasionally when the entire colon is involved, 5 to 10 cm of the most distal terminal ileum is inflamed; this is referred to as backwash ileitis. A milder form of ulcerative colitis may affect only the rectum and sigmoid; this is called proctosigmoiditis. This inflammatory process is also limited to the mucosa and submucosa.

Crohn's disease is an inflammatory condition involving all layers of the gut. The disease may inflame segments of the colon or small intestine. Although ulcerative colitis is usually contiguous, beginning in the rectum and extending retrograde to involve various portions of the colon, Crohn's disease is usually segmental, and there is normal intestine between areas of inflammation. Most commonly, the terminal ileum and right colon are involved. The colon may be affected and the rectum not affected. Lesions also have been reported in the esophagus, stomach, and duodenum.

In the last 20 years a greater effort has been made to differentiate the histologic and clinical course of patients with ulcerative colitis and Crohn's disease. The approach to treatment is based on this differentiation. Despite an improved understanding of these diseases, the inflammation in about 10% of patients is still indeterminate because it shares features of both processes.

ETIOLOGY. Possible causes of inflammatory bowel disease have been investigated since these conditions were first recognized. Infectious agents have been considered as causes. Bacillary dysentery was not distinguished from idiopathic ulcerative colitis until about 100 years ago.

Sophisticated techniques have been used in the search for infectious agents. Speculation has centered around L-forms of *Pseudomonas,* viruses, and atypical bacteria. Using homogenates of diseased colon, investigators have produced granulomata in the foot pads of mice and inflammatory lesions in the small intestine of rabbits. These lesions are nonspecific and have not been uniformly reproduced in different laboratories. The evaluation of gut flora has shown increased numbers of anaerobes in patients with regional enteritis. Advocates of a "slow virus" hypothesis have isolated an agent with the physical characteristics of an RNA-like picornavirus, and animal transmission studies have been conducted with varying results. The question of whether this virus is the pathogen of inflammatory bowel disease or is an innocent passenger has not been resolved. No one has been able to fulfill the requirements of Koch's postulates.

Immunologic factors have been cited as a possible cause of inflammatory bowel disease. Hypersensitivity reactions characterized by increased mast cell degranulation have been studied. An increased incidence of allergic reactions in colitis patients with asthma, hay fever, and eczema has also been noted. The presence of extraintestinal lesions in patients with inflammatory bowel disease has also been cited as evidence of immunologic changes in patients with inflammatory bowel disease. Colon antibodies have been found in the sera of patients with inflammatory bowel disease, but these have not been demonstrated on the colonic epithelium, suggesting that the antibodies are caused by the inflammatory process rather than initiating agents. These antibodies have also been found in the sera of patients with pernicious anemia, collagenopathies, and colon cancer.

Prostaglandins have been implicated in the pathogenesis of inflammatory bowel disease. These agents are the principal mediators of the inflammatory process throughout the body. Elevated prostaglandin levels have been found in rectal biopsy tissues from patients with ulcerative colitis and infectious diarrhea. Although no evidence as yet suggests this is the cause of inflammatory bowel disease, prostaglandins appear to play a role in propagating the inflammatory response. Drugs that have been found to inhibit prostaglandins play a major role in the treatment of inflammatory bowel disease.

Inflammatory bowel disease can occur in several members of the same family. Although no genetic mode of inheritance has been determined, there is a familial history of inflammatory bowel disease in one fifth of the patients with the disease. No evidence exists that a single dominant gene is involved. An increased incidence of inflammatory bowel disease in monozygous twins has been shown; when one twin has the disease, the sibling has an increased risk. Several studies have shown that high numbers of Ashkenazi Jews have the disease in the United States and South Africa. Similar studies in Tel Aviv, however, indicate a much lower than predicted incidence in the same group in Israel, an observation that emphasizes the difficulty in separating hereditary from environmental factors. The lack of a higher than normal incidence of the disease in spouses of patients with inflammatory bowel disease is evidence against environmental factors. The association between ankylosing spondylitis, a classic genetically determined disease, and inflammatory bowel disease further supports a genetic role in its cause. It has been reported that in some families that share histocompatibility antigens, several members have inflammatory bowel disease. A major concern in these family studies is whether true genetic forces have a role or whether the common environment plays a role.

Much has been written about psychologic factors associated with inflammatory bowel disease. The "colitis personality" distinguished by feelings of helplessness, dependency, anxiety, and despair is not unique to patients with inflammatory bowel disease but characterizes a common response to any chronic debilitating disease. That many people have these personality traits without having the disease is further evidence against this association. In fact, one study of the emotional profile of patients with inflammatory bowel disease showed that they had less life stress than patients with irritable bowel syndrome. Although the onset of symptoms may be associated with a major life crisis, the emotional stress itself is not a causative factor.

Whatever the cause of Crohn's disease may be, the disease seems to be relatively new, to be increasing in its incidence, and to be three to five times more common in whites and two to three times more common in Ashkenazi Jews.

Chronic ulcerative colitis

PATHOLOGY. The hallmark of chronic ulcerative colitis is an inflammatory reaction of the mucosa and submucosa. The disease begins in the rectum and involves the bowel contiguously.

Macroscopically, the mucosa may have a granular appearance if the disease is mild. Ulcers and hemorrhage occur in the active phase. The disease when fulminant may include the stripping of the mucosa with actual areas of sloughing; normal mucosa may remain between these areas. When the healing phase is completed, these islands of normal mucosa may be pushed up by surrounding fibrous tissue, giving a polypoid appearance to this normal tissue that is referred to as pseudopolyps. Marked hyperemia is present in ulcerative colitis, accounting in part for the bleeding that occurs when the mucosa is swabbed or stool passes over it. As healing occurs, submucosal scarring may develop and give rise to residual pitting of the mucosa. This may be the only sign remaining after a mild attack. The submucosal fibrosis may also cause the rectal valves to lose their contours and have a blunted or rounded appearance. Perianal disease is uncommon but may cause a hyperpigmentation of the perianal skin that remains after an attack. Shallow rectal fissures are occasionally present.

Microscopically, changes related to the activity of disease can be observed. In severe disease there is loss of goblet cells and marked vascular congestion. The submucosa and lamina propria may contain mononuclear cell infiltrates. Collections of neutrophils may occur in the epithelial crypts and give rise to crypt abscesses that usually penetrate the mucosa and drain into the bowel lumen. Burrowing ulcers do not occur unless there is necrosis of the myenteric plexus, such as occurs with toxic megacolon. With healing the epithelial lining of the bowel is restored, and the inflammatory infiltrate is diminished. Complete healing observed macroscopically is usually reflected microscopically in the diminished numbers of crypts and in the presence of some degree of submucosal fibrosis. Pseudopolyps appear in areas of normal mucosa, and the numbers of goblet cells are diminished. Vascular congestion appears to be an early finding in the inflammatory picture. Rectal biopsies of patients with quiescent disease may reveal vascular congestion as a harbinger of recurrent inflammation. The rectal biopsy is also important in detecting precancerous changes in the colon. The loss of goblet cells, severe dysplasia in the absence of an inflammatory process, and glandular elements in the submucosa may serve as the first signs of malignant degeneration. The recognition of such changes is important because colonic cancers are often multifocal, flat, infiltrative lesions that are metastatic by the time they have been recognized.

CLINICAL MANIFESTATIONS. The hallmark of ulcerative colitis is rectal bleeding and diarrhea. The frequency of bowel movements and the amount of blood present reflect the activity of the disease. Scant bleeding and a minimal change of consistency of stools may occur in patients with mild disease or inflammation limited to the rectosigmoid. Moderate to severe disease is characterized by more frequent bleeding. The patient may experience tenesmus with rectal pressure, the urge to have repeated bowel movements, and the passage of scant amounts of bloody mucoid material. Abdominal cramps may precede each episode and may be only partially relieved by defecation. Along with the change in the pattern of bowel movements, the patient may have nocturnal diarrhea. Although patients may not recognize a minor change in daytime stool habits, nocturnal symptoms are quite troublesome. Abdominal bloating and gas may accompany bloody diarrhea. Fatigue and malaise may result from anemia caused by rectal bleeding. In patients with severe disease a decrease in serum albumin levels can occur and lead to edema. Profuse mucoid diarrhea can also cause an electrolyte imbalance. Fever and tachycardia may accompany severe exacerbations and are especially prominent when toxic dilation of the colon (toxic megacolon) occurs. In patients with toxic megacolon the abdominal wall is tender. Large, dilated loops of bowel are palpable, and tympany is noted with percussion.

Extraintestinal manifestations may be prominent. Skin manifestations may include erythema nodosum, characterized by red, swollen nodules usually on the thighs and legs. A severe form of ulcerating skin disease with a purulent discharge (pyoderma gangrenosum) may occur on the arms or legs. Cultures from these lesions reveal only normal skin flora. Healing usually occurs when the colon inflammation comes under control.

Pyoderma gangrenosum may also occur in the mouth in the form of deep ulcers that sometimes ulcerate through the tonsillar pillar. Pyostomatitis vegetans, a purulent inflammation of the mouth, may also occur; inflammatory vegetations are usually sterile lesions like those in pyoderma gangrenosum and respond not to local therapy but rather to control of the disease. Aphthous stomatitis, gingivitis, and oral *Candida* infections may also occur.

Eye changes, such as episcleritis, uveitis, corneal ulcers, and retinitis, may cause eye pain or photophobia.

Joint symptoms occur in up to 20% of patients with the disease. "Colitic arthritis" usually affects the ankles, knees, and wrists. Ankylosing spondylitis and sacroiliitis are common findings in patients with colitis. Conversely, there is an increased incidence of colitis in patients with these arthritic disorders. Ankylosing spondylitis occurs 20 times more commonly in patients with colitis than in the general population. Patients with colitis who have backache should have a careful roentgenographic search for narrowing of the sacroiliac joints, osteophytes, and calcification of paraspinal ligaments. The arthritic disease may not improve with control of the colitis. Patients with spondylitis and colitis are HLA-B27 positive, whereas those with only peripheral arthritis do not have this histocompatibility antigen.

Perhaps the most pernicious complication of ulcerative colitis is liver disease. Pericholangitis may occur with an intense inflammation of portal areas. Fatty infiltration of the liver, bile duct carcinomas, sclerosing cholangitis, chronic active liver disease, granulomatous hepatitis, and primary biliary cirrhosis have occasionally been noted in these patients. Although the other extraintestinal manifestations usually undergo remission with medical or surgical control of the colon inflammation, liver disease may continue and progress to cirrhosis and liver failure.

Thrombophlebitis is a serious complication in patients with colitis. Hypercoagulable states occur in patients with severe disease and may promote thrombosis of major veins throughout the body.

LABORATORY FINDINGS. Anemia is commonly associated with inflammatory bowel disease. It may be caused by iron deficiency, chronic disease, or severe bleeding. Leukocytosis occurs in active disease, but a white blood cell count greater than 15,000/mm^3 is rare and is usually a sign of intra-abdominal abscess or toxic megacolon. Hypoalbuminemia may occur along with an electrolyte imbalance. Low serum magnesium and potassium levels are often found along with profuse diarrhea. Smears of stool specimens show many red blood cells, neutrophils, and eosinophils. The sedimentation rate also is elevated.

DIAGNOSIS. A careful history and physical examination are important in establishing the presence of inflammatory bowel disease and may help to exclude gonorrheal proctitis, ischemic colitis, and irritable bowel syndrome. A full evaluation is necessary to exclude Crohn's colitis (Table 175-1). The presence of abdominal tenderness and a dilated colon may indicate toxic dilation. The rectal examination reveals bleeding. Pseudopolyps may also be palpable in the digital examination.

Sigmoidoscopy should precede roentgenographic studies. The presence of diffusely inflamed rectal mucosa along with discrete ulcers and mucus indicates active disease. During the healing phase or with quiescent disease the mucosa may have a granular appearance, and friability can be confirmed by swabbing the mucosa. The rectal valves are usually blunted in this stage, indicating submucosal edema. A rectal biopsy may be helpful in distinguishing between ulcerative colitis and Crohn's disease.

Stool cultures should be obtained to rule out the possibility of shigellosis and *Campylobacter* infection. A stool examination should also be performed to exclude the possibility of amebiasis.

Table 175-1. Comparision of inflammatory bowel diseases

Site and symptoms	Ulcerative colitis	Crohn's colitis
Usual location	Rectosigmoid and left colon	Right colon
Small bowel involvement	Rare "backwash ileitis"	Common
Area of spread	Contiguous	Noncontiguous segments
Fistulas	Uncommon	Common
Abscesses	Uncommon	Common in fistulas
Rectal bleeding	In most patients	In 50% of patients
Ulcers	Small mucosal ulcers	Large deep ulcers
Strictures	Rare	Common
Pseudopolyps	Common	Never occurs
Carcinoma	Risk increases 10% with each decade	Increased risk

A barium enema examination can help to determine the extent of the disease and to rule out a carcinoma (Fig. 175-1). It is imperative that patients with inflammatory bowel disease are gently prepared for roentgenography. Harsh cathartics aggravate an electrolyte imbalance and may cause shock. Saline enemas help to cleanse the colon and allow for suitable roentgenograms. A severely ill patient should not undergo any contrast study, however, until the condition is stabilized and improved. The barium enema may show the disease limited to the rectosigmoid, as in proctosigmoiditis, in which there is a widening (greater than 2 cm) of the space between the sacrum and the barium-filled rectum, as shown on lateral films. The amount of the colon involved can also be gauged with the barium study. A granular appearance along with small ulcerations is characteristic. With severe disease a loss of haustra occurs. As healing proceeds, marked narrowing and shortening of the colon develop, giving the colon a tubular appearance. Intense spasm may occur, and areas may mimic strictures. Residual pseudopolyps may be present from previous attacks. Care must be taken to evaluate these areas closely, and any area of narrowing must be considered a carcinoma until proven otherwise. Often agents that relax the colon open up these areas. Barium studies should not be performed on patients who are severely ill, but a plain film of the abdomen may reveal air in the bowel outlining irregular mucosa. A plain film of the abdomen should be made with patients who have abdominal pain and distention to confirm a diagnosis of megacolon. A transverse colon greater than 6.5 cm in diameter indicates such a process, which should be watched closely because surgical intervention may be necessary.

Persistently narrowed areas should be evaluated with

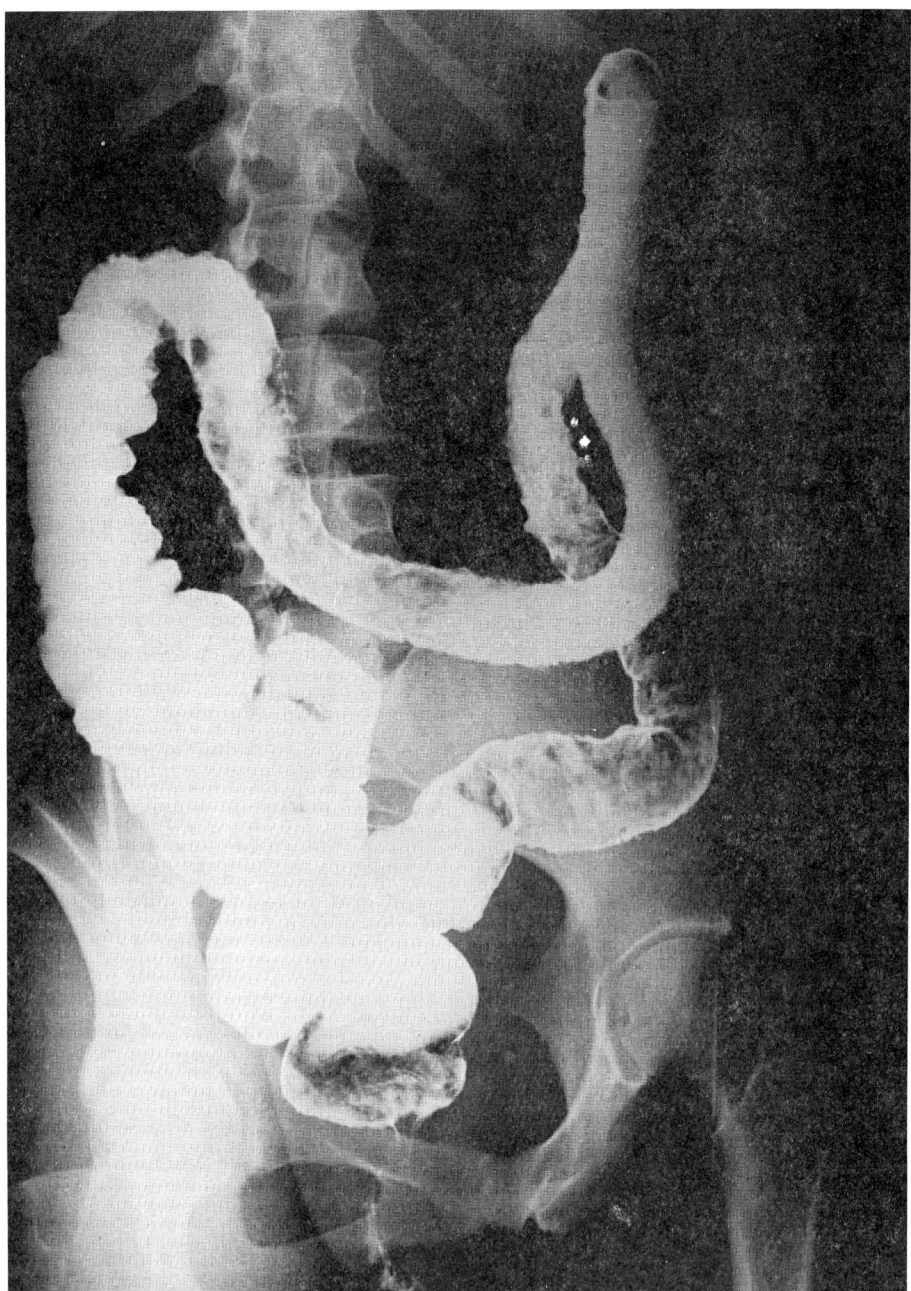

Fig. 175-1. Barium enema in 34-year-old woman with bloody diarrhea reveals classic changes of diffuse ulcerative colitis. Note loss of normal mucosal pattern, loss of haustra, and diffuse ulcerations along surfaces.

colonoscopy and biopsy. A colonoscopy should also be performed on patients with normal roentgenograms and persistent symptoms. These patients usually are found to have proctosigmoiditis or mild inflammatory bowel disease. Colonoscopy can make a more accurate determination of the extent of colon involvement. Colonoscopy should be performed reluctantly and then only with great care in patients with colitis, especially in ill patients with acutely inflamed colons, because the risk of perforation is significantly increased.

COURSE. Ulcerative colitis is a chronic disease that may be characterized by acute attacks and remissions, a continual lower degree of activity, or an initial episode followed by quiescent disease. Those who have the disease during childhood are a major concern because they often fail to grow and develop normally and because they have a risk of developing carcinoma increasing by 10% each decade after the first 10 years of disease. Up to 75% of patients have only one or two attacks that can be quickly controlled by medical therapy; the remainder have recurrent exacerbations and require further treatment. Patients may have increased flare-ups during the first trimester of pregnancy or after delivery, but during the second and third trimester the disease is usually quiescent. Patients with frequent active disease have a higher incidence of massive hemorrhage, perforations, and colon cancer and have an increased risk of dying of a disease complication or developing amyloidosis. Statistical analysis of patients with inflammatory bowel disease reveals that those with severe disease have an annual mortality of 14%, whereas quiescent disease is associated with a 2% to 4% mortality. The mortality of the first attack is much higher for patients over 60 years of age.

Patients with proctosigmoiditis have the best outlook; in 90% of these patients the disease is limited to this area of the bowel. Usually inflammation subsides over 3 to 5 years, and residual scarring is minimal. These patients do not appear to have an increased risk of cancer.

The incidence of colon carcinomas is increased in patients with a long history of colitis. The major problem is that a carcinoma is often metastatic by the time it is symptomatic. There is also an increased incidence of multifocal neoplasms that are not revealed by roentgenography. The monitoring of these patients should be strict and should consist of yearly roentgenography and semiannual sigmoidoscopy. Colonoscopy is also a valuable tool of surveillance. Although more precise recommendations will no doubt evolve in the next decade, any suspicious area revealed on a roentgenogram should be evaluated colonoscopically. Some authors have advocated alternating barium enemas with colonoscopy and biopsy at 6-month intervals for the better detection of early cancers. Measurements of the carcinoembryonic antigen (CEA) may be helpful in spotting the early development of cancers. A rising CEA titer in a patient should trigger a search for neoplastic disease.

MANAGEMENT. The therapy for ulcerative colitis is aimed at reducing the inflammation and correcting the effects of the disease. Patients with weight loss and dehydration may require intravenous electrolyte replacement. Transfusion is required if the patient has severe anemia. The dietary treatment may include low-residue, high-nitrogen prepared supplements. A bland diet may be most easily tolerated during exacerbations. Dietary restrictions have occasionally been imposed automatically rather than with good logic, but this approach should be avoided because the aim is to provide calories and amino acids in the most palatable form. High-residue foods, caffeinated beverages, and spices stimulate peristalsis and should be avoided. Milk products may contribute to diarrhea because of either a long-standing lactose intolerance or a newly acquired lactase deficiency.

The medical treatment is directed to reducing inflammation. Sulfasalazine is used to initiate and maintain a remission in ulcerative colitis. Its active moiety, 5-aminosalicylate, has a direct anti-inflammatory effect in dosages of 2 to 8 g a day. Although the colon flora are not altered by sulfasalazine, colon bacteria are required to split the drug. Patients can be maintained in remission by doses of 1 to 2 g a day. The drug is not without side effects. Nausea and abdominal distress may result but can be ameliorated by the use of enteric-coated tablets that dissolve in the small bowel. Severe skin reactions may also occur including exfoliative dermatitis and photosensitive reactions. Because hemolytic anemia, agranulocytosis, pancytopenia, and thrombocytopenia may also occur, frequent blood counts are mandatory. Although most side effects of the drug develop within the first month of therapy, delayed skin and hematologic reactions have been reported in patients who had taken the medication for 1 to 2 years. Sulfasalazine interferes with folate metabolism, and supplemental folic acid may be needed in the treatment.

Corticosteroids and corticotropin (ACTH) should be used in patients with severe disease or in those who have not responded satisfactorily to sulfasalazine. These steroids have an anti-inflammatory effect on the bowel. They are administered in high dosages that are adjusted as the patient improves. Therapy is initiated with 40 to 80 units of ACTH by intramuscular or intravenous injection or with 40 to 60 mg of oral prednisone each day. Maintenance therapy consists of 20 to 40 units of ACTH or 10 to 20 mg of prednisone daily. Alternate-day therapy with eventual discontinuance of the medication is indicated when the patient goes into remission. Often steroids can be discontinued and remission maintained by sulfasalazine. Anemia, electrolyte imbalance, and negative protein states should be treated because patients may not respond to the steroid treatment until these problems are corrected. Several studies have suggested that patients receiving steroids have a higher risk of complications requiring surgery. Analysis of these reports, however, indicates that it is the patient with severe disease who receives steroids and that the complications are related to the severity of disease rather than to the treatment. Patients with proctosigmoiditis may benefit from the instillation of steroids in specially prepared enemas. These preparations may induce a remission by themselves or in conjunction with oral steroids. Because at least 25% of rectally administered steroids are absorbed, systemic effects may occur. The use of steroid suppositories and steroid rectal foams should be avoided in patients with active disease. These agents contain small amounts of steroids and have a minimal area of penetration.

Many side effects are associated with the use of ACTH and steroids. The development of cushingoid facies, fluid retention, hypokalemia, and muscle cramps may be troublesome. Emotional instability and severe depression or hypermania may also develop but usually subside promptly when the drug is discontinued. Hypertension and diabetes are serious side effects that may require treatment or discontinuance of the steroid therapy. Long-term therapy may cause osteoporosis and vertebral compression fractures as well as cataracts. Steroid-induced myopathy characterized by quadriceps wasting may be debilitating and may impair the patient's ability to climb stairs. Steroids increase the patient's susceptibility to many infections, including oral candidiasis. Young patients undergoing steroid treatment may have growth failure or alterations in the menstrual cycle. Patients undergoing surgery require increased doses of steroids before and after the operation because their own adrenal response to stress is blunted. Patients treated with ACTH should have their therapy maintained and react to the stress of surgery without difficulty. Patients requiring long-term steroid treatment should be closely evaluated for a possible colectomy because the risks of steroid side effects and carcinoma associated with active long-term disease are greater than those of surgery.

Immunosuppressive medications such as azathioprine have been used as treatment for ulcerative colitis with varying results. Some authors have reported that lower steroid dosages are effective when azathioprine is given concomitantly. To date there has been no good study to support the efficacy of immunosuppressive agents. The risk of hematologic suppression and superinfection is increased in patients taking these medications, and therefore they should be reserved for patients who have not responded to more traditional medical therapy.

Surgery for ulcerative colitis is indicated in patients with intractable disease. Patients with severe recurrent diarrhea and bleeding that have not responded to medical therapy require surgery. The presence of a perforation, intra-abdominal abscess, stricture, or premalignant biopsy changes is an indication for surgery. Patients with toxic megacolon must be followed closely; if there is evidence of further colonic dilation or if the patient does not improve in 24 to 72 hours, surgery is required.

Proctocolectomy along with the construction of a permanent ileostomy is the usual operative procedure. The timing of surgery is important because the mortality of elective surgery is less than 5% but rises to 15% to 20% if emergency surgery becomes necessary. If the patient is very ill, the surgeon may elect to perform a subtotal colectomy and ileostomy initially and to remove the rectal stump at a later time. If the rectum is in good condition, an ileorectal anastomosis may rarely be performed, but the rectal segment still has a risk of developing recurrent disease and carcinoma. The English experience with this procedure has been better than the American. Proctectomy may impair the sexual function in men if the parasympathetic nerves are not carefully removed from the rectal serosa. A patient with toxic megacolon may undergo a decompression cecostomy initially and a proctocolectomy later after the patient's condition improves. There has been much concern about the psychologic implications for patients after an ileostomy. With the new disposable ileostomy equipment available today, however, patients find they can enjoy athletics, perform strenuous work, and have normal sexual activity despite the operation. Women can have normal pregnancies. Patients who are relieved of much suffering and disability find ileostomy acceptable. Proctocolectomy combined with ileostomy is a curative procedure for ulcerative colitis; most patients can look forward to a normal life expectancy after successful surgery.

Crohn's disease

PATHOLOGY. Crohn's disease is an inflammatory disease of the small or large intestine. The inflammation involves all the layers of the gut, and thus the term "transmural colitis" has been used to describe this disease in the colon. Gross examination may reveal mucosal ulceration: aphthous ulcers within mucosa that appears normal, deep ulcers within areas of swollen mucosa, and long linear serpiginous ulcers. Punctate areas of mucosal hemorrhage may alternate with areas of gross hemorrhage. If edema is pronounced in the submucosa, ballooning of the mucosa may give rise to a cobblestone-like appearance of the intestinal surface. Perianal fistulas may occur with either colonic or small bowel disease and produce copious drainage of purulent and fecal material. The perianal region may have scarring and darkening of the surrounding skin as a result of severe inflammation.

With the involvement of either the colon or small intestine in Crohn's disease, microscopic examination reveals inflammatory infiltrate in all layers of affected bowel, with plasma cells and lymphocytes predominating in the lamina propria. The serosa may be congested. Deep ulcers may extend into the muscularis, and fistulous tracts may extend from the ulcers, through the bowel wall, and into adjoining segments of intestine. Granulomata composed of epithelioid multinuclear cells are observed in almost 60% of cases. They may be present in areas of severe inflammation or in relatively normal-appearing intestine far removed from other areas of inflammation; they often occur near the lymph channels in the intestine. Granulomata have also been found in bone marrow and muscle tissue. The intestinal muscularis is often hypertrophied and may remain thickened even after the inflammation subsides. Fibrosis may occur in the submucosa and serosa, but the degree of bowel shortening that occurs in ulcerative colitis is not present in Crohn's disease. Dense areas of fibrosis may produce a narrowing or stricturing of the intestinal lumen. Regional lymph nodes often are enlarged in cases of intense inflammation and may contain granulomata. The mesentery may be edematous, and mesenteric nodes may be matted together.

CLINICAL MANIFESTATIONS. Although bleeding is a prominent feature of ulcerative colitis, it is present in only 50% of patients with transmural colitis. Bleeding is rare in cases of small bowel Crohn's disease. Diarrhea is the most common feature in both large and small bowel disease. Patients with disease limited to the terminal ileum may have a tender right lower quadrant mass and obstructive symptoms of pain, nausea, vomiting, and distention. Weakness, fatigue, anorexia, and fever are common symptoms of active disease. An intra-abdominal abscess or enterocutaneous fistula may be the initial manifestation of the disease or may develop during its course.

The disease is solely perianal in 5% of cases. More often, however, perianal disease accompanies ileocolitis or colonic disease. Severe perianal disease, sometimes occurring with numerous fistulous tracts, may lead to an undermining and sloughing of the entire perineum. Enterovesical fistulas may occur and produce stool in the urine and pneumaturia. Compression of the right ureter by an inflamed terminal ileum may lead to hydronephrosis and pyelonephritis.

Other manifestations depend on the location of the disease. Inflammation of the small intestine may impair its absorption of vital nutrients. Calcium, iron, and folate are absorbed in the duodenum, and disease in this region may lead to malabsorption and deficiencies of these substances. Disease in the terminal ileum may interfere with the absorption of bile salts and vitamin B_{12}, although marked malabsorption of these substances more commonly follows surgical resection of the distal ileum. The malabsorption of bile salts may result in their introduction in increased amounts into the colon and the production of choleretic diarrhea. More severe malabsorption, as occurs usually after the resection of at least 100 cm of terminal ileum, can lead to a critical reduction of the bile salt pool and the malabsorption of dietary fat and fat-soluble vitamins. An impaired ileal absorption of bile salts may also cause the bile to become lithogenic (containing too much cholesterol in respect to bile salts), thereby increasing the incidence of gallstones. Ileal disease or resection has also been associated with hyperoxaluria and an increased incidence of oxalate kidney stones. It is not clear whether this association results from an enhanced intestinal absorption of oxalic acid caused by the intraluminal binding of calcium by malabsorbed fatty acids or from the ileal malabsorption of glycine-conjugated bile salts, their conversion into glyoxalate by colonic bacteria, and the subsequent conversion of absorbed glyoxalate into oxalate. Inflammation of the small or large intestine may impair the intestinal absorption of salt and water and may also cause excessive intestinal protein loss, hypoalbuminemia, and possibly pedal edema.

Extraintestinal manifestations also develop in Crohn's disease, usually in association with colonic involvement. Arthritis, pyoderma gangrenosum, erythema nodosum, uveitis, and liver disease have all been reported. In patients with long-standing disease, amyloidosis may develop, often first indicated by the presence of proteinuria or hepatosplenomegaly.

Many patients initially have the symptoms and signs of acute appendicitis, and the diagnosis of Crohn's disease is made at the time of laparotomy. An incidental appendectomy should not be performed at this time because there is an increased risk of postoperative fistula formation.

The physical findings reflect the involvements just described, including the presence of an abdominal tenderness, mass, and distention. The rectal examination may reveal perianal complications, rectal tenderness, blood, or narrowing and induration.

LABORATORY FINDINGS. The absorptive function of the small bowel is more likely to be altered in patients with Crohn's disease than in those with ulcerative colitis. Electrolyte abnormalities and low albumin levels commonly occur in cases of severe disease. Anemia, usually resulting from an iron or sometimes a folate deficiency, may also be present. Leukocytosis may be present, but white blood cell counts greater than $15,000/mm^3$ suggest an abscess or perforation. Stool specimens may show red blood cells and eosinophils. Cultures are negative for enteric pathogens. Fresh stool specimens should also be examined for ova and parasites.

DIAGNOSIS. The diagnosis of Crohn's disease depends on effective barium studies. As with ulcerative colitis, caution must be exercised to avoid the use of cathartics. A barium enema administered with filling of the terminal ileum and a small bowel series (Fig. 175-2) help determine the extent of the disease. In ileitis there is classically a narrowing of the terminal ileum with ulcerations and cobblestoning of the mucosa. The classic string sign indicates a luminal narrowing of the distal ileum produced either by the inflammation and edema of active disease or by fibrosis from an old inflammation. The presence of ulcers helps identify this as active disease. The barium study may reveal an abnormality of the terminal ileum in cases of tuberculosis, lymphoma, actinomycosis, periappendiceal abscess, and cecal cancer. The history should help to distinguish the disease from these entities, but a lymphoma may be difficult to differentiate from inflammatory bowel disease. Long intestinal segments are usually involved in lymphomas, and regional adenopathy may be present. Lymphomas are more common in middle-aged men and may be associated with symptoms of malabsorption. Because Crohn's disease can occur in any part of the bowel, there may be fibrosis, ulcers, and cobblestoning in the duodenum, jejunum, or colon as well as the ileum. Fistulas between segments of bowel are common, as are sinus tracts, especially extending from the large bowel to the perineum. In older patients diverticulitis and ischemic bowel disease must also be differentiated from Crohn's disease. Associated arteriosclerotic cardiovascular disease and atrial fibrillation make a diagnosis of ischemic disease of the large or small bowel more likely. Diverticulitis may be suspected if there is the appearance of local disease in the sigmoid colon on roentgenograms.

Sigmoidoscopy may be helpful in determining the presence of proctitis and sigmoiditis but usually cannot differentiate granulomatous colitis from ulcerative colitis.

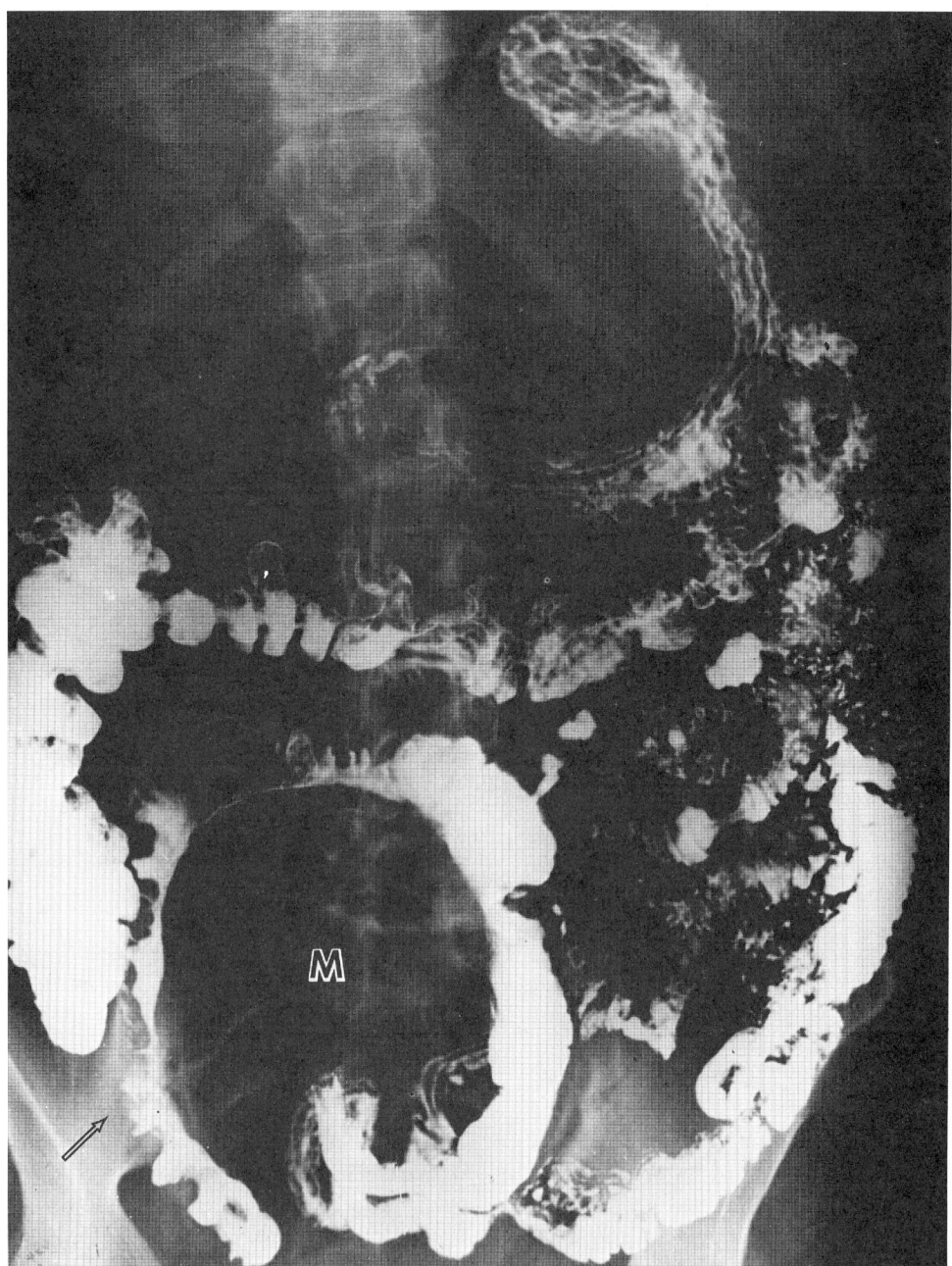

Fig. 175-2. Small bowel series reveals irregularity and nodularity of diseased distal ileum *(arrow)* and extrinsic pressure and displacement of distal small bowel by large inflammatory mass *(M)*. These changes are due to regional ileitis.

A rectal biopsy may be helpful in diagnosing Crohn's disease, especially if it reveals granulomata. Occasionally colonoscopy may be helpful in a patient who has diarrhea, weight loss, or bleeding but no roentgenographic signs, by demonstrating typical aphthous ulcerations in the upper colon.

COURSE. Crohn's disease is a protean illness characterized by exacerbations and remissions. It is estimated that 5% to 10% of affected patients die of the illness. The initial location of the disease may provide some clue as to its probable course. Life tables indicate that up to 80% of patients require surgery within 20 years. Patients who undergo surgery appear to have a 60% chance of requiring additional surgery. Patients whose initial disease is ileocolic have a 73% surgical rate; if the initial site is the colon or small intestine, the rate is 50%. Ileocolic disease in at least 50% of patients eventually "burns out," causing minimal symptoms.

The incidence of carcinomas of the small bowel is increased in patients with Crohn's disease. Whereas most small bowel tumors occur within 20 cm of the ligament of Treitz, in Crohn's disease most cancers develop in involved segments of small intestine. There is also an increased risk of colon cancer in patients with transmural colitis, but the incidence is much less than with ulcerative colitis. Although there are good statistical data indicating rates of carcinomas in patients with ulcerative colitis, none is available for patients with Crohn's disease of the colon.

About 25% of patients who have Crohn's disease before the age of 21 experience growth failure. The risk of severe disease requiring multiple operations is also greater in this younger group.

The assessment of recurrent disease after surgery is problematic. Because the surgeon cannot be sure he has removed all of the diseased area, and because the pathologist often finds microscopic disease in normal-appearing portions of gross specimens, much of what has been called recurrent disease is probably residual disease not appreciated during the operation. Although some maintain that the disease does not extend along the intestine unless surgery is performed, an accurate natural history of the disease cannot be ascertained until more sensitive methods are developed for the detection of all areas of affected bowel.

MANAGEMENT. Crohn's disease may recur and remit without the patient receiving any treatment. Certainly some patients in later life have been incidentally found with a barium enema to have the classic narrowed terminal ileum. If carefully interviewed, such patients may indicate that they have had episodes of diarrhea and cramps during their life but that the symptoms were never severe enough for them to seek medical attention. Indeed, many patients may reveal that they have seen their doctor over the years for cyclic bouts of what was considered intestinal flu. It is therefore easy to understand that most reports of treatment have been anecdotal. It was not until the National Cooperative Crohn's Disease Study (NCCDS) was completed recently that some firm facts about the modalities of treatment emerged. The goal of this multicenter study was to establish quantitative estimates about the disease's activity and to measure the responses of patients to various treatments. The study showed that prednisone was effective in inducing remission in 78% of patients during the 4 months of study. Prednisone was most effective in patients with disease of the small intestine and in the reduction of arthritic symptoms. Ileocolic and colonic disease responded well to sulfasalazine, but small intestinal disease did not, probably because colonic bacteria are needed to break sulfasalazine into its active component 5-aminosalicylate and the inactive sulfapyridine moiety. The study showed that the antimetabolite azathioprine was no more effective than a placebo but that it was the most toxic of the drugs used in the treatment of Crohn's disease. The drug had to be discontinued in 12% of the patients receiving it; pancreatitis developed in half of these patients. Of the patients taking a placebo, 30% achieved remission during the study.

Thus there are effective drugs for the treatment of Crohn's disease. Sulfasalazine in a daily dosage of 4 to 8 g is used to treat ileocolic and colonic disease, and there is evidence that perianal disease and fistulas respond well to this medication. Sulfasalazine therapy can be tapered off when remission occurs and eventually discontinued. Unlike the situation with ulcerative colitis, the remission of transmural colitis does not appear to be sustained by sulfasalazine; the NCCDS report seems to indicate that no drug is effective in maintaining remission. Prednisone and ACTH have a role in suppressing the symptoms of the disease. Prednisone is initially given in oral dosages of 40 to 80 mg daily. ACTH may be given intravenously in a soluble form or intramuscularly in a gel in a daily dosage of 40 to 80 units. An observable response to this therapy may appear only after 2 to 4 weeks. The patient's sense of well-being and appetite are often restored before the diarrhea and abdominal cramps are controlled. Once remission is achieved, this drug therapy should be tapered off. Giving the drug only every other day can reduce the side effects. As already noted, the NCCDS report indicates that steroids do not maintain remissions of Crohn's disease. Some patients have recurrent symptoms when the drug is discontinued and respond again when it is reinstituted in small dosage. It seems unwise to discontinue the drug in these patients. This observation underscores the need to individualize the therapy. Recent studies have suggested that metronidazole in dosages of 3 g daily may help heal perineal fistulas.

Symptomatic and supportive treatment is important in Crohn's disease in the large and small intestines. Diarrhea and cramping may be controlled by loperamide in a dosage of 2 mg four times daily or diphenoxylate in a dosage of 2.5 to 5 mg up to four times a day. Atropine analogs may also be helpful in reducing abdominal spasm when used alone or in conjunction with these other drugs. Patients with severe disease involving the terminal ileum and those who have had surgical removal of the distal ileum may have diarrhea resulting from bile salt malabsorption rather than from inflammation. In these patients the bile salts pass unabsorbed into the colon, where they exert a cathartic effect. With the administration of the bile salt resin cholestyramine in dosages of 4 to 12 g daily, bile salts are bound and the diarrhea is diminished. Because Crohn's disease often affects the small intestine, malnutrition is often a major problem, as may be reflected by a moderate weight loss or cachexia with hypoalbuminemia. In patients with symptoms of partial obstruction a low-residue elemental diet supplying 1500 to 2400 calories daily helps maintain a positive nitrogen balance. Dietary supplements have the advantage of being absorbed in the upper bowel and thereby reducing the flow of material through diseased distal segments of the intestine. Reducing the residue in the diet and thereby the solid material flowing through the ileum may prove helpful even for patients with less severe disease. Some patients with ileal disease develop a lactase deficiency and become intolerant of dietary lactose. If such patients avoid milk and dairy products, their cramps and diarrhea may be reduced.

Some patients do not respond well to dietary changes or are too ill to take in adequate oral nutrition. These patients benefit from a therapy of total parenteral nutrition, which involves the continuous infusion of fluid rich in elemental amino acids and hypertonic glucose through a catheter in the subclavian vein. Fat solutions also are available for this therapy. This technique has the advantage of removing all absorptive requirements from the bowel and putting it at rest. Reports have indicated that a positive nitrogen balance is achieved, that patients gain weight, and that the drainage through fistulas decreases. This technique may allow patients who are resistant to steroids to correct their negative nitrogen and caloric balance and to respond to therapy. Parenteral alimentation has also been used to improve patients' nutritional status before major surgery. In patients who have had an extensive resection of bowel, the absorptive surface of the small intestine may be so reduced that adequate oral nutrition will never be possible. In these individuals total parenteral nutrition administered on an outpatient basis has been successful. Parenteral alimentation is not without risk, however. Infection at the intravenous site, sepsis, and the development of fatty liver and a phosphorus deficiency are some of the more common complications.

As in ulcerative colitis, anemia in Crohn's disease should be corrected with oral administration of iron and folate and if necessary with blood transfusions. Because vitamin B_{12} is absorbed in the terminal ileum, a deficiency may occur if severe disease occurs in the terminal ileum or if there has been a resection of more than about 60 cm of this region. Monthly injections of 1000 μg of cyanocobalamin are indicated in such patients. Electrolyte abnormalities should be corrected by intravenous replacements. Serum magnesium levels may fall in severe disease, causing secondary hypocalcemia that should be corrected by intravenous replacement. If a loss of bile salts leads to a malabsorption and deficiency of the fat-soluble vitamins (K, D, A, and E), causing clotting disturbances, bone resorption, and possibly even visual problems, these vitamins must be replenished, preferably with water-soluble analogs.

Surgery is not curative in Crohn's disease as it is in ulcerative colitis. Therefore surgery is reserved for patients who have not responded to medical treatment or who have disorders such as an abscess, free perforation, or unremitting obstruction that do not respond to medical management. Several series have shown that patients do better postoperatively if their disease had been brought under control by medical treatment before surgery. The most common procedure for ileocolic disease is the segmental removal of the distal ileum and right colon. In the past a simple bypass procedure creating an anastomosis between the ileum and the transverse colon was commonly performed, but its common failure to control the disease activity has put this procedure in disrepute. A small area of intestinal disease may be treated by resection of as much diseased area as is feasible, but the removal of large areas of small intestine may lead to serious malabsorption problems and cause serious nutritional problems for patients. Such patients may require long-term parenteral nutrition, as already discussed. Patients with enteroenteric fistulas may benefit from resections that eliminate the short circuit of nutrients from the upper to lower small intestine. Enterocutaneous fistulas that occur from the small bowel to the abdominal wall or from the rectum to the perineum are best treated medically along with surgical drainage of any local abscesses that form. The disease occasionally involves the duodenum, and a gastric outlet obstruction may occur; these patients often do well with a simple gastrojejunostomy, leaving the diseased segment in place. Patients with colonic disease pose a different problem. Strictures may cause obstruction in the large bowel; occasionally these can be resected. Severe colonic disease may be treated with a colectomy. If the rectum is not diseased, a subtotal colectomy along with the creation of an ileorectal anastomosis may be performed, but at least one third of these patients then require proctectomy within 3 years for subsequent rectal disease that cannot be adequately managed medically. If the total colon is diseased, the patient requires proctocolectomy and ileostomy. Unlike patients with ulcerative colitis, however, about one third to one half of these patients experience recurrent disease in the remaining ileum. A significant number of patients have inflammation of the ileostomy stoma, which can often be treated with topical steroids. Patients who have inactive disease and those in whom ileal disease does not develop are able to live normal productive lives despite the ileostomy.

APPENDICITIS AND APPENDICEAL ABSCESS

DEFINITION. The appendix is an anatomic remnant of the base of the cecum. Inflammation and perforation of this structure can occur, causing an abscess, generalized peritonitis, and death. Although appendicitis is a disease of decreasing incidence, it is still the most common cause for abdominal surgery in patients 10 to 20 years of age.

EPIDEMIOLOGY. Like diverticular disease, appendicitis is most prevalent in industrialized urban communities. Whether the diet is a precipitating factor is still conjectural. This disease occurs most commonly in communities where low-fiber diets are the standard and a high meat intake is common. The incidence of disease is markedly lower in vegetarians and in rural cultures that have high-fiber diets.

PATHOGENESIS. Most commonly the symptoms arise from the occlusion of the appendiceal lumen by stool. Occasionally food particles or barium sulfate may obstruct the lumen. An obstruction of the lumen does not always cause inflammation; asymptomatic calcified concretions (fecaliths) are often seen in abdominal roentgenograms. In children the appendiceal lumen may be obstructed by hyperplasia of lymphatic follicles, a mechanism possibly accounting for the increased association of appendicitis with viral respiratory and enteric infections in children. The appendix may occasionally be occluded by pinworms, ascarides, or other parasites. In older patients a carcinoma of the cecum may obstruct the appendiceal orifice. Patients with collagen vascular disease occasionally have arteritis of the appendix leading to necrosis and perforation. Occlusion of the appendiceal lumen leads to edema and congestion of the wall, pain, and ulceration and necrosis of the mucosa. The appendix fills with pus, swells, and ruptures, leading to a localized abscess, peritonitis, or septicemia.

CLINICAL MANIFESTATIONS. The patient usually notes the onset of generalized mild abdominal pain or cramping, symptoms often confused with the presence of a mild intestinal flu. Anorexia and nausea with emesis may occur. The patient may or may not have a low-grade fever. As the inflammation increases in the appendix, especially when it extends to the adjoining parietal peritoneum, the generalized pain subsides and localized right lower quadrant pain and tenderness develop, classically at McBurney's point (2 to 5 cm from the iliac crest on the line between the iliac crest and umbilicus). If the appendix is retrocecal, back pain may occur. If the cecum is low-lying and the appendix is in the pelvis, tenderness may be elicited only by a digital examination of the rectum or a pelvic examination. Patients with malrotation of the cecum may have pain in the right upper quadrant or periumbilically, and the examining physician may note tenderness and guarding in the right upper quadrant. Tenderness may occur when the patient flexes the right hip if the inflamed appendix is resting on the psoas muscle; pain is also elicited when the examiner forcibly extends the right hip (the psoas sign). As the inflammation progresses, or if perforation occurs, the patient's fever rises and tachycardia and lethargy may become prominent. In elderly patients the symptoms often are minimal up to the time of perforation. Diffuse abdominal pain, diffuse peritoneal signs, and the absence of bowel sounds suggest that perforation has occurred.

LABORATORY FINDINGS. The leukocyte count is mildly elevated early in the disease. A leukocytosis of more than 15,000/mm^3 along with a marked shift to the left signals severe inflammation. In elderly or debilitated patients leukopenia may occur. The sedimentation rate is elevated but is not a basis for the diagnosis.

DIAGNOSIS. The clinical history and physical examination are the most important factors in making the diagnosis of appendicitis. A plain film of the abdomen may reveal an ileus, but usually roentgenograms are not helpful. The use of a barium enema can be carefully considered for undiagnosed patients who are stable. Appendicitis may cause perforation and peritoneal soilage, but more commonly edema occurs at the tip of the cecum without filling of the appendix. Regional enteritis may be discovered by the barium enema; occasionally a small bowel roentgenogram is needed to fill the terminal ileum and show disease in this region. A careful history may reveal that the symptoms of a patient in the middle of her menstrual cycle are the result of ovulation (mittelschmerz symptoms). Other causes of pelvic disease in women should be considered, such as salpingitis, an ectopic pregnancy, or a twisted ovarian cyst. In older patients the possibility of a perforating cecal cancer should be considered. Diabetic ketoacidosis in children may cause abdominal pain, but proper urine and blood tests should reveal its presence. Hematuria or pyuria with bacilluria should alert the physician to the possibility of a renal calculus or infection as the cause of the pain. Right-sided diverticulitis in an adult may appear clinically identical to acute appendicitis.

COURSE. The mortality of surgery for nonperforative appendicitis is less than 3%. Most deaths result from pneumonia, embolism, or myocardial infarction. Patients with an abscess formation have a much greater risk of death. Generalized peritonitis and miliary liver abscesses are serious complications with a mortality up to 50%. Pylephlebitis (pus in the portal vein) may lead to portal thrombosis and liver abscesses. Anaerobic bacteria and Enterobacteriaceae have a major role in these infections. These patients have chills, fever, and jaundice. Broad-spectrum antibiotics can help control the infection, but surgical drainage of liver abscesses may be needed. An intestinal obstruction caused by adhesions may be a late complication of surgery in patients with acute appendicitis or an appendiceal abscess.

MANAGEMENT. The preferred treatment is the surgical removal of the appendix, which should be carried out as soon as the diagnosis seems certain and the patient is stabilized. Dehydration should be corrected preoperatively. Gastric or intestinal intubation should be initiated preoperatively in patients with obstructive symptoms. The removal of the appendix and drainage of an abscess, if present, help to decrease postoperative complications. If a perforation has occurred, it may be impossible to identify the appendix; surgical drainage of the abdomen is then indicated. In this situation there is an increased incidence of colocutaneous fistulas, which require later surgical resection. Appendicitis may complicate a pregnancy, but most surgeons agree that appendectomy is indicated regardless of the risk to the fetus. Nonoperative therapy has occasionally been advocated in cases of acute nonperforative appendicitis. The patient fasts and is treated with large dosages of antibiotics and intravenous fluids to allow the inflammatory process to subside. This therapy should be considered only when surgical treatment is not available or when the general condition of the patient is so poor that surgery is contraindicated.

DIVERTICULAR DISEASE OF THE COLON

DEFINITION. Diverticulosis is a disease in which small saclike outpouches of mucosa and submucosa are present in any or all regions of the colon, most often in the sigmoid colon. Patients may be asymptomatic, have recurrent episodes of pain, have bleeding, or develop inflammation from an intramural, pericolic, or intra-abdominal perforation.

EPIDEMIOLOGY. Diverticulosis is a disease of urban society; studies have shown a lower incidence among rural populations. The incidence increases as well in those people who have moved from the country to industrialized centers. Decreased fiber in the diet is strongly correlated with the incidence of diverticulosis. Indeed, studies have shown diverticular disease to be one fourth as common in vegetarians as in age-matched controls on standard diets. There is a low incidence of colonic disease in Africans on high-fiber diets and an increased incidence of diverticular disease in those Africans on Western diets. The consumption of refined sugar, wheat, and much meat is correlated with a tendency to diverticulosis. Colonic diverticula are rare in patients below the age of 40, but thereafter the incidence in the United States increases to include about 50% of patients at age 80.

PATHOGENESIS. The motor activity of the colon—the contractions of colonic muscle—gives rise to segments of high pressure. If the stool lacks residue and bulk, higher colonic pressures are generated, especially in the sigmoid colon, as a result of the decreased caliber of the lumen (Laplace's law). The colonic wall is weakened in areas where the nutrient vessels penetrate the wall along the mesenteric border, and the increased pressure causes ballooning of the mucosa through these areas to form saccular outpouches. Marked hypertrophy of the colonic muscle also occurs and further increases these pressures.

CLINICAL MANIFESTATIONS. Most patients with diverticulosis remain asymptomatic. As a result of the abnormal spasm or pressure of the sigmoid colon, however, some patients have recurrent left lower quadrant pain and during the physical examination may be found to have a tender loop of sigmoid colon. The diverticula may perforate the wall of the bowel, producing inflammation or diverticulitis. Perforation beyond the wall may lead to a pericolic or more distant abscess or even to frank peritonitis. The abdominal wall may be rigid and marked guarding may be present if there is severe inflammation or abscess formation. Fever may occur, and a high fever with shaking chills signals the perforation of a diverticulum along with an abscess or peritonitis. The inflammation may cause an intestinal obstruction or diarrhea. An extended inflammation in the bladder or left ureter may cause a urinary tract infection, hydronephrosis, or even fistula between the colon and bladder. Diverticula are a common cause of lower gastrointestinal bleeding in patients over the age of 50, usually unaccompanied by active inflammation, pain, or fever. The bleeding is usually self-limited, but massive blood loss and shock may occur, in which case the site of bleeding is often in the right side of the colon.

LABORATORY FINDINGS. Patients with mild disease may have an elevated leukocyte count. A high leukocyte count with a marked shift to the left is associated with severe inflammation and abscess. Anemia may be present if bleeding has occurred. If anemia is present in the absence of overt bleeding, a search should be made for a neoplasm or another inflammatory process, although diverticula too have been alleged to be a source of occult blood loss.

DIAGNOSIS. The diagnosis of diverticular disease depends on a good history, physical examination, and barium study. If active inflammation is present, the barium enema may be deferred to avoid the risk of perforating the bowel or soiling the peritoneal cavity through a perforation already present. Sigmoidoscopy usually has negative results in these patients. The barium enema may not resolve the possibility of a neoplasm being present. Indeed, a carcinoma may occur in areas of diverticular narrowing. In addition, the muscular hypertrophy that occurs in patients with diverticulosis may appear as luminal narrowing. Colonoscopy and biopsy may be helpful in making the diagnosis of cancer in these areas. Great care must be exercised during colonoscopy because an overdistention with air may cause diverticular perforation. If an abscess formation is suspected, colonoscopy should be deferred. Colonoscopy may be helpful in differentiating Crohn's disease and ischemic bowel disease from diverticular disease.

MANAGEMENT. Recurrent attacks of left lower quadrant pain may be treated with bed rest and a bland diet. Severe pain requires hospitalization and the administration of meperidine or pentazocine. These agents decrease colon spasms and do not increase intraluminal pressure. The use of anticholinergics is controversial, although many physicians use them to decrease spasms. Intravenous glucagon has also been used for this purpose with some success.

Bulk agents such as psyllium seed preparations have also been used to reduce spasms and prevent attacks. These agents cause water retention in the feces and increase their size, thus reducing colonic pressure so that less force is exerted during defecation. Studies have shown that a higher contraction pressure is required for the expulsion of small stools and a lower pressure for bulky bowel movements. Patients who find bran unpalatable may use psyllium or methylcellulose preparations in a glass of water at bedtime. These patients may note some abdominal distention and increased flatus initially with these bulk agents because they are partially digested by colonic bacteria. The addition of fruit and vegetables to the diet also helps to increase the dietary fiber. The long-term preventive effects of bran and fiber are still conjectural.

Patients who have bleeding should be monitored closely because transfusion may be necessary, but bleeding is often self-limited. If a patient's bleeding is vigorous or unremitting, angiography may be helpful in identifying the bleeding site and allows the selective infusion of vasopressin (Pitressin), which may be helpful in controlling the bleeding. If bleeding recurs, surgical resection is indicated.

Patients suspected of having a perforated diverticulum should receive intravenous antibiotics. If the patient's condition does not improve in 24 to 48 hours, surgical intervention is probably necessary. The draining of abscess material and a diverting colostomy are indicated. When the infection has been controlled, the patient may undergo a resection of the involved area along with anastomosis of the bowel and closure of the colostomy.

For patients with severe pain, an elective sigmoid resection can be helpful. Rarely, a subtotal colectomy along with an ileorectal anastomosis is needed for extensive colonic diverticular disease.

PSEUDOMEMBRANOUS ENTEROCOLITIS AND ANTIBIOTIC-INDUCED DIARRHEA

DEFINITION. Diarrhea may occur in patients receiving antibiotic therapy as a result of an alteration of the fecal flora. Often this condition is mild and subsides when the antibiotic therapy is discontinued. Occasionally a severe disease results with the development of thick mucosal exudate that has the appearance of a membrane. This condition is extremely serious and demands aggressive treatment.

ETIOLOGY. When diarrhea develops while an individual is receiving antibiotics, the cause of the altered bowel habit is usually evident. Because this symptom may also occur several days or even weeks after the antibiotic is discontinued, however, a careful history must be obtained. Pseudomembranous enterocolitis has commonly been associated with the use of clindamycin but also occurs in association with amoxicillin, cephalosporins, ampicillin, and other agents. Patients who are debilitated or have renal failure or low-output syndromes seem to have a higher risk of contracting the disease. Pseudomembranous enterocolitis has been reported as a complication of major abdominal surgery, but most of these patients had been receiving antibiotics, which can be implicated as a cause of superinfection. Many early reports of pseudomembranous enterocolitis, especially of postoperative cases of the disease, stressed the finding of *Staphylococcus aureus* in the stool, but the role played by this organism remains unclear at present. Recent studies have shown a major role for *Clostridium difficile* in the pathogenesis of antibiotic-produced pseudomembranous enterocolitis. This bacterium has been found in the stool of many patients with the disease, and an identified cytopathic toxin of the *Clostridium* has also been found in the stool of patients with pseudomembranous enterocolitis. This toxin has also been found in up to 25% of patients with milder forms of antibiotic-related diarrhea. When antibiotics are administered, presumably the normal colonic flora are inhibited, allowing *C. difficile* to proliferate (especially if it is resistant to the antibiotic) and produce toxin.

PATHOLOGY. The gross appearance of the bowel affected by antibiotic-related diarrhea can vary greatly. Mild hyperemia and granularity may occur. In fully developed cases of pseudomembranous enterocolitis raised yellow plaques of exudate can be seen coalescing to form a membrane. This can occur throughout the gut and may be patchy. The underlying mucosa may be edematous and hyperemic and sometimes necrotic and ulcerated. The microscopic examination shows that the membrane contains leukocytes, mucus, and fibrin, and the mucosa exhibits edema, congestion, inflammation, and occasionally ulceration and necrosis.

CLINICAL MANIFESTATIONS AND DIAGNOSIS. A careful history of patients with diarrhea is needed to determine whether they have received antibiotics. Bowel movements may occur every 15 to 20 minutes, but the severely ill patient may be unaware of them. The patient may describe his stool as mucoid, usually without blood, and a greenish brown liquid mucoid material may be detected in the rectum in the absence of solid stool. The patient may be febrile and may have lost considerable fluid, electrolytes, and protein. Sigmoidoscopy may reveal mild or severe inflammation along with yellow raised membranous plaques of exudate. Carefully performed colonoscopy may be helpful in demonstrating these lesions if sigmoidoscopy does not. A barium enema examination may reveal nodular filling defects in the colon, but often the patient is too ill to undergo this study. Stool cultures may demonstrate the presence of *C. difficile* if appropriate anaerobic cultures are made.

MANAGEMENT. Pseudomembranous enterocolitis is a life-threatening disease with a 50% mortality. Patients must be placed in isolation to avoid danger of the infection spreading to others. Infected individuals must be treated aggressively with massive fluid and electrolyte replacement. Potassium supplements may be needed, and intravenous sodium bicarbonate may be required to correct acidosis. Intravenous albumin may be necessary to improve the patient's plasma protein levels and to prevent shock. Vancomycin given orally is effective in a dosage of 250 to 500 mg four times daily for 10 to 14 days. Shorter courses of therapy are associated with a high relapse rate. Cholestyramine, a bile acid–binding resin, may also be given to bind the toxin of *C. difficile* and to help reduce the diarrhea. Antispasmodics have been used cautiously.

RADIATION ENTERITIS

DEFINITION. Radiation injury to the bowel occurs after pelvic or abdominal radiation therapy for a malignant disease. The disease appears more commonly in patients who have also had prior pelvic surgery or an abdominal inflammation that gives rise to adhesions that cause the fixation of loops of bowel. Radiation injury rarely results with radiation doses of less than 3000 rad but is very common when more than 4500 rad is given. Symptoms may occur immediately or be delayed for several years after treatment.

PATHOGENESIS. Radiation damage is greatest in tissues that have a rapid cell turnover because cells undergoing differentiation and growth are more sensitive than cells that have matured. Because cell renewal is constant in the gut, this area is very sensitive to radiation effects. Mucosal cells are most susceptible to radiation effects, and severe sloughing of the mucosa may result if the radiation is intense. The small arterioles of the gut are also very sensitive to radiation and may become inflamed and degenerate; this process may occur soon after treatment or be a late effect. Fibrosis of the arterioles occurs along with resultant ischemia, which may lead to intestinal necrosis and ulceration. Patients with an underlying arteriolar disease are most susceptible to these effects. Severe fibrosis of the gut along with stricture formation is a late effect of radiation injury. The histologic findings are marked inflammation, arteriolar narrowing or thrombosis, and foam cells in the submucosa. If present, ulcers may be deep, giving rise to the formation of abscesses or fistulas.

CLINICAL MANIFESTATIONS. Nausea is a common symptom of a radiation injury in the gut, probably resulting from a central nervous system effect of radiation because nausea can occur in patients undergoing radiotherapy in other parts of the body. A change in bowel habits, abdominal cramping, and diarrhea may occur. If the damage is severe, a bloody mucoid diarrhea may develop. Abdominal distention along with diarrhea may result from the late effects of stricture formation. Malabsorption may occur if a severe small bowel disease, stasis (with bacterial overgrowth), or significant enteroenteric fistulas are present. Malabsorption is manifested by severe diarrhea and weight loss. Obstipation occurs if strictures develop in the rectosigmoid.

LABORATORY FINDINGS. If bleeding or malabsorption occurs, anemia and hypoalbuminemia may result. Pyuria or stool in the urine develops if the fistulization extends into the bladder.

DIAGNOSIS. Sigmoidoscopy should be performed in all patients suspected of having radiation colitis. Erythema, friability, and cyanosis of the mucosa may be present. Occasionally ulcers occur. If sigmoidoscopy has a negative result, a barium enema should be performed and may demonstrate ulceration, stricture formation, internal fistulas, or areas of abscess. Colonoscopy is helpful in delineating ulceration, but care must be exercised to avoid the perforation of inflamed segments. Small bowel roentgenograms are necessary to demonstrate the disease in the small intestine.

MANAGEMENT. Patients with inflammatory radiation disease may respond to steroid enemas. No studies have demonstrated the efficacy of oral steroids for the treatment of this disease. If stagnant loops of bowel are present and give rise to bacterial overgrowth, antibiotics may reverse the associated diarrhea and malabsorption. If the patient has abdominal cramping, antispasmodics and bulk agents should be given. Low rectal strictures can be dilated with rubber dilators. Strictures elsewhere often are asymptomatic or cause occasional abdominal cramps and diarrhea. Long, symptomatic strictures require surgical resection. A diverting colostomy may be needed for low colonic strictures.

INTESTINAL ULCER

Isolated intestinal ulcers, although unusual, have been found in the cecum, sigmoid colon, and rectum. The presenting symptoms are related to the ulcer's location. Cecal ulcers have been found incidentally in autopsies or in patients with right lower quadrant pain that mimics that of appendicitis. Sigmoid ulcers may cause no abdominal pain and may develop into a perforation. Unlike solitary ulcers elsewhere, rectal ulcers are usually asymptomatic and have been discovered incidentally by sigmoidoscopy, but they occasionally cause rectal bleeding. The cause of these lesions is unknown. They usually range in diameter from 5 mm to 5 cm, and occasionally the ulcers are multiple. The histologic findings are necrosis, inflammatory exudate, and an increased number of fibroblasts in the submucosa. These findings are nonspecific and give no clues about the cause of the lesions. Barium roentgenograms may reveal a solitary ulcer with surrounding edema. Rectal lesions may be followed by sigmoidoscopy, and some have been reported to remain static for years. The advent of colonoscopy allows the examination, removal of biopsy samples, and following of sigmoid and cecal ulcers under direct vision; previously when these ulcers were detected on roentgenograms, they were often surgically resected because carcinoma was suspected. The methods of treatment that have been used for rectal ulcers include steroid enemas, electrocoagulation, topical sclerosing agents, and antibiotics. None of these therapies has been successful, leaving surgery as the only consistently successful measure for treating symptomatic intestinal ulcers.

BIBLIOGRAPHY

Banks, B., Zetzel, L., and Richter, H.: Morbidity and mortality in regional enteritis: report of 168 cases, Am. J. Dig. Dis. **14:**369, 1969.

Bartlett, J.G., and others: Antibiotic-associated pseudomembranous colitis due to toxin-producing clostridia, N. Engl. J. Med. **298:**531, 1978.

Block, G.E.: Surgical management of Crohn's colitis, N. Engl. J. Med. **302:**1068, 1980.

DeCosse, J.J., and others: The natural history and management of radiation induced injury of the gastrointestinal tract, Ann. Surg. **170:**369, 1969.

Devrode, G.J., and others: Cancer risk and life expectancy of children with ulcerative colitis, N. Engl. J. Med. **285:**17, 1971.

Fawaz, K.A., and others: Ulcerative colitis and Crohn's disease of the colon: a comparison of the longterm postoperative course, Gastroenterology **71:**372, 1976.

Gennaro, A.R., and Rosemond, G.P.: Diverticulitis of the colon, Dis. Colon Rectum **17:**74, 1974.

Gitnick, G.L.: Etiology of inflammatory bowel diseases: are we making progress? Gastroenterology **78:**1090, 1980.

Glotzer, D.J., and others: Comparative features and course of ulcerative and granulomatous colitis, N. Engl. J. Med. **282:**582, 1970.

Kirsner, J.B., and Shorter, R.G., editors: Inflammatory bowel disease, Philadelphia, 1975, Lea & Febiger.

National cooperative Crohn's disease study, Gastroenterology **77:**825, 1979.

Painter, N.S., and Burkitt, D.P.: Diverticular disease of the colon: a disease of Western civilization, Chicago, 1970, Year Book Medical Publishers, Inc.

176 • VASCULAR DISEASES OF THE GUT

Ralph M. Myerson

Although a variety of localized or systemic disorders may involve the vasculature of the gut, the most important are those that produce the ischemic syndromes of the bowel. The intra-abdominal portions of the gastrointestinal tract are nourished almost entirely by three major unpaired arterial trunks arising from the ventral surface of the aorta: the celiac axis, the superior mesenteric artery, and the inferior mesenteric artery. Any or all of these may be involved in a process producing an ischemic syndrome of the bowel.

It has relatively recently been recognized that vascular disease of the intestine in the ischemic syndromes may be either occlusive or nonocclusive. Either type may be acute or chronic and segmental or extensive. In occlusive disease there is an actual occlusive process of either a major arterial vessel or a minor branch. Nonocclusive vascular disease of the gut, comprising about 80% of all cases of ischemic bowel disease, results from decreased perfusion without an actual occlusion although some component of occlusive vascular disease is usually also present.

OCCLUSIVE VASCULAR DISEASE OF THE GUT

The nature of the occlusive process is usually atherosclerotic, but other causes include embolus, aneurysm, and rare disorders such as vasculitides.

CELIAC AXIS. Occlusive disease of the celiac axis is rare. A controversial syndrome of celiac axis compression has been described in which a vascular insufficiency allegedly results from the compression of the celiac axis by the median arcuate ligament. The clinical symptoms are usually vague. The diagnosis is made with angiography. The surgical relief of symptoms has been described.

SUPERIOR MESENTERIC ARTERY. Occlusion of the superior mesenteric artery may be acute or chronic. Acute occlusion is an abdominal catastrophe; some series have reported a mortality of 90%. Acute occlusion usually involves the main arterial trunk, resulting in extensive infarction of the gut. The degree of collateral circulation has an important bearing on the extent of the damage. Abdominal pain is invariably present periumbilically or in the epigastrium and is severe, sudden in onset, and constant. About 80% of patients have vomiting, and diarrhea that is often bloody is present in about 30%. In most cases this occlusion results from a thrombus; an embolus is a less common cause. Cardiac arrhythmia suggests the latter.

The first 6 hours after occlusion of the superior mesenteric artery are critical. A delay in the diagnosis beyond this point leads to increasing difficulty in management and a rapidly rising mortality. The clinical picture in a patient over 60 years of age should suggest the diagnosis. There are no ancillary aids in making the diagnosis other than arteriography.

The treatment is surgical. Whether thrombectomy, a bypass graft, or an intestinal resection is performed depends on the findings during surgery.

Chronic vascular insufficiency of the superior mesenteric artery is usually not a clinical problem. Some degree of atherosclerotic change is invariably present in older patients, but the gut does not seem to suffer as a consequence, perhaps because of the rich collateral supply of vessels. Rarely, chronic vascular insufficiency gives rise to a syndrome known as abdominal angina. Typically the patient has dull or cramping pain 15 to 30 minutes after a meal; the pain lasts up to a few hours. The mechanism of this pain is inadequate vascular perfusion during digestion and absorption. Weight loss and steatorrhea may result. Abdominal angiography is helpful in making the diagnosis, and the treatment of choice is the appropriate surgical procedure.

INFERIOR MESENTERIC ARTERY. Colonic ischemia resulting from thrombosis or embolism of the inferior mesenteric artery, resulting in a similar clinical picture, is distinctly rare. This artery can be sacrificed during surgery, with ischemic colitis occurring as a consequence in only about 1% of these cases.

NONOCCLUSIVE VASCULAR DISEASE OF THE GUT

The pathogenesis of nonocclusive ischemic syndromes is poor perfusion. In the presence of an inadequate cardiac output and generally poor tissue perfusion, the blood flow distribution favors the brain and other vital organs and the splanchnic blood flow falls disproportionately. The use of vasoconstrictors may compound the problem. Nonocclusive intestinal ischemia may be manifested by widespread, patchy, or segmental infarction involving a varying depth of the bowel wall from the mucosa through the muscularis to the serosa.

CLINICAL MANIFESTATIONS. This syndrome occurs in the elderly. In a report of 227 patients, the average age was

71 years, and 77% had a serious organic heart disease. All types of heart disease were associated with the syndrome, and there was no sex predilection. Symptoms are often precipitated by a sudden drop in cardiac output resulting from myocardial infarction, the onset of an arrhythmia, or the additional stress of another illness. Many patients are already in the hospital for treatment of cardiac or other diseases when their abdominal symptoms begin. Abdominal pain is usually present and may be localized or diffuse and constant or colicky. Vomiting and diarrhea are present in one third of these cases, and about 25% of the patients with diarrhea have gross blood in the stool. Tenderness and distention are the most common objective findings, but the findings may be unimpressive until peritonitis develops. The laboratory findings are nonspecific; leukocytosis is common.

DIAGNOSIS. Plain roentgenograms of the abdomen may reveal nonspecific findings related to an abnormal distribution of intestinal gas or fluid or both. The changes include a small bowel obstruction pattern, splenic flexure cutoff sign (gas present up to but not beyond the splenic flexure), or an absence of gas in the abdomen. Findings considered more specific include an altered mucosal contour involving regular or irregular indentations ("thumbprinting") and outpouchings, obliterated valvulae conniventes, a thickened bowel wall, a narrowed lumen, a stiff appearance of the bowel along with abrupt bends, and the presence of gas in the bowel wall or portal vein.

Arteriography is valuable in ruling out an actual occlusion. The smooth, tapered narrowing of arterioles has been interpreted as an indication of vasoconstriction. Most observers agree that the information obtained by this examination is not sufficiently precise to influence the decision of whether surgery is required.

MANAGEMENT. Although various measures have been used in an attempt to increase the splanchnic blood flow, such as ganglionic blockade and the intra-arterial infusion of vasodilator substances, none has convincingly demonstrated its effectiveness. Treatment is therefore best directed toward the correction of the underlying responsible condition.

The decision of whether a patient with bowel infarction and an underlying severe cardiac disease should undergo surgery is a dilemma. Inasmuch as the mortality in patients without treatment approaches 100%, the presumption is that despite the risk entailed, surgery is indicated so that frankly necrotic areas of bowel may be resected.

ISCHEMIC COLITIS

It has become apparent recently that a number of less catastrophic variants of ischemic disease involving the colon may occur. These are usually associated with a more localized ischemia, although this is not necessarily the case. Particularly vulnerable are the areas of the colon that lie in the "watershed" between two major arterial sources: the splenic flexure (between the superior and inferior mesenteric arteries) and the rectosigmoid (between the inferior mesenteric and the internal iliac arteries).

CLINICAL MANIFESTATIONS. Most patients with ischemic colitis are over 50 years of age and have evidence of atherosclerotic disease elsewhere. They characteristically have an abrupt onset of lower abdominal pain, rectal bleeding, and variable amounts of vomiting and fever. The findings are suggestive of acute diverticulitis.

MANAGEMENT. The initial therapy is supportive and usually includes antibiotics. Depending on the situation, clinical judgment may dictate early surgical exploration. Some patients require resection of the ischemic bowel with a reanastomosis or a colostomy.

A substantial number of patients with ischemic colitis do well without surgery, but close monitoring is indicated. Barium enemas and even plain films of the abdomen in these cases commonly reveal "thumb-printing," narrowing of the lumen, and an irregularity and sacculation of the bowel (Fig. 176-1). About one third of these patients go on to complete healing, about one third have the formation of a permanent stricture, and about one third require surgery or have an acute process terminating in death.

DIFFERENTIAL DIAGNOSIS. The possibility of acute diverticulitis and the risk of performing a barium enema must be weighed against the benefits of an accurate diagnosis. Most experts agree that the risk of producing a perforation with a barium enema is small in an acutely ischemic colon.

In cases of rectal involvement sigmoidoscopy reveals submucosal hemorrhage, ulcerations, and mucosal slough. A biopsy may be helpful in determining the diagnosis, but usually it is difficult to differentiate the condition from ulcerative colitis.

In cases progressing to stricture formation it appears likely that there is transmural involvement leading to fibrotic constriction (Fig. 176-2). Continued bleeding and the presence of obstructive signs may suggest this process. The patient should be followed with serial barium enema examinations; some strictures may improve with time. Some patients with ischemic strictures have obstructive symptoms without having had any apparent prior symptoms. In these cases the physician must differentiate ischemic colitis from carcinoma of the colon and inflammatory bowel disease. Colonoscopy may be useful in these cases, but surgery may be necessary if carcinoma cannot be ruled out with certainty.

VENOUS THROMBOSIS

Mesenteric venous thrombosis is much less common than arterial ischemia. It occurs in hypercoagulable states, in myeloproliferative disorders, with vascular congestion, in disseminated intravascular coagulopathy, in association with oral contraceptives, or spontaneously without an apparent cause. The clinical picture may be insidious or catastrophic and is characterized by abdominal pain, a change

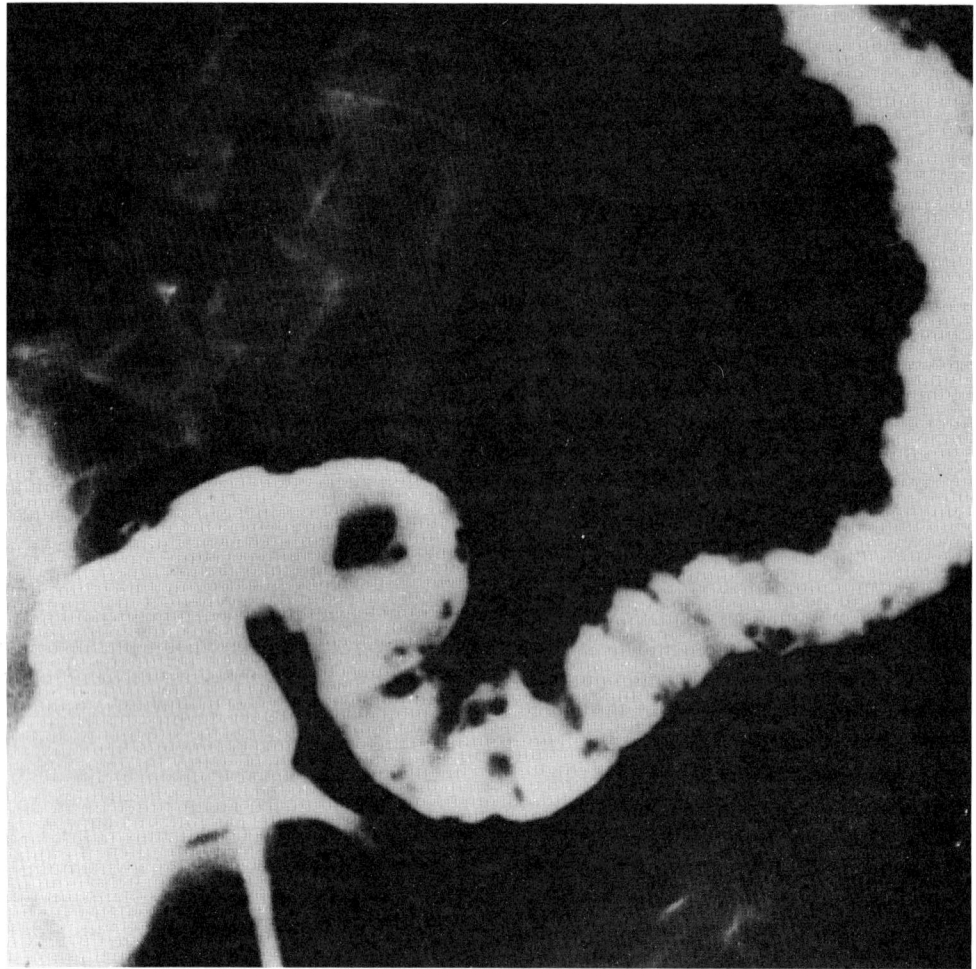

Fig. 176-1. Barium enema in ischemic colitis showing mucosal ulcerations and filling defects suggestive of pseudopolyposis. Same changes are seen in ulcerative colitis.

in bowel habits, gastrointestinal bleeding, and serosanguineous ascites. The diagnosis of venous thrombosis is difficult to establish but should be suspected in the presence of a precipitating factor and the described clinical picture. A prolonged arterial phase in an angiogram of the superior mesenteric artery suggests the diagnosis. The treatment if supportive and surgical. A bowel resection is favored over a vascular reconstruction procedure. The prognosis is considerably more favorable than that following an arterial ischemic episode.

OTHER VASCULAR DISORDERS
Vasculitis

The gastrointestinal tract is involved in systemic vascular diseases such as systemic lupus erythematosus, polyarteritis, and acute vasculitides of the hypersensitivity type. These disorders may be manifested in prominent gastrointestinal findings. Patients with systemic lupus erythematosus show acute peritoneal signs as a result of serositis of the peritoneal lining. Polyarteritis nodosa, a disorder of medium-size arterioles, commonly exhibits striking abdominal findings secondary to involvement of intra-abdominal arterioles. Cystic artery involvement may produce the signs and symptoms of acute cholecystitis.

Schönlein-Henoch purpura is a type of small vessel vasculitis. Gastrointestinal involvement is present in over 50% of these patients, manifested most commonly by abdominal pain and gastrointestinal bleeding. The underlying pathologic condition is localized upper or lower bowel ischemia and ulceration.

Rarer forms of vasculitis such as rheumatoid vasculitis, Takayasu's disease, and essential mixed cryoglobulinemia may involve the mesenteric arteries. Enteric-coated potassium chloride tablets have been incriminated as a cause of vasculitis.

Arteriovenous malformations

Arteriovenous malformations may involve the circulation of the gastrointestinal tract. These not only may give rise to hemodynamic complications but may be a cause of

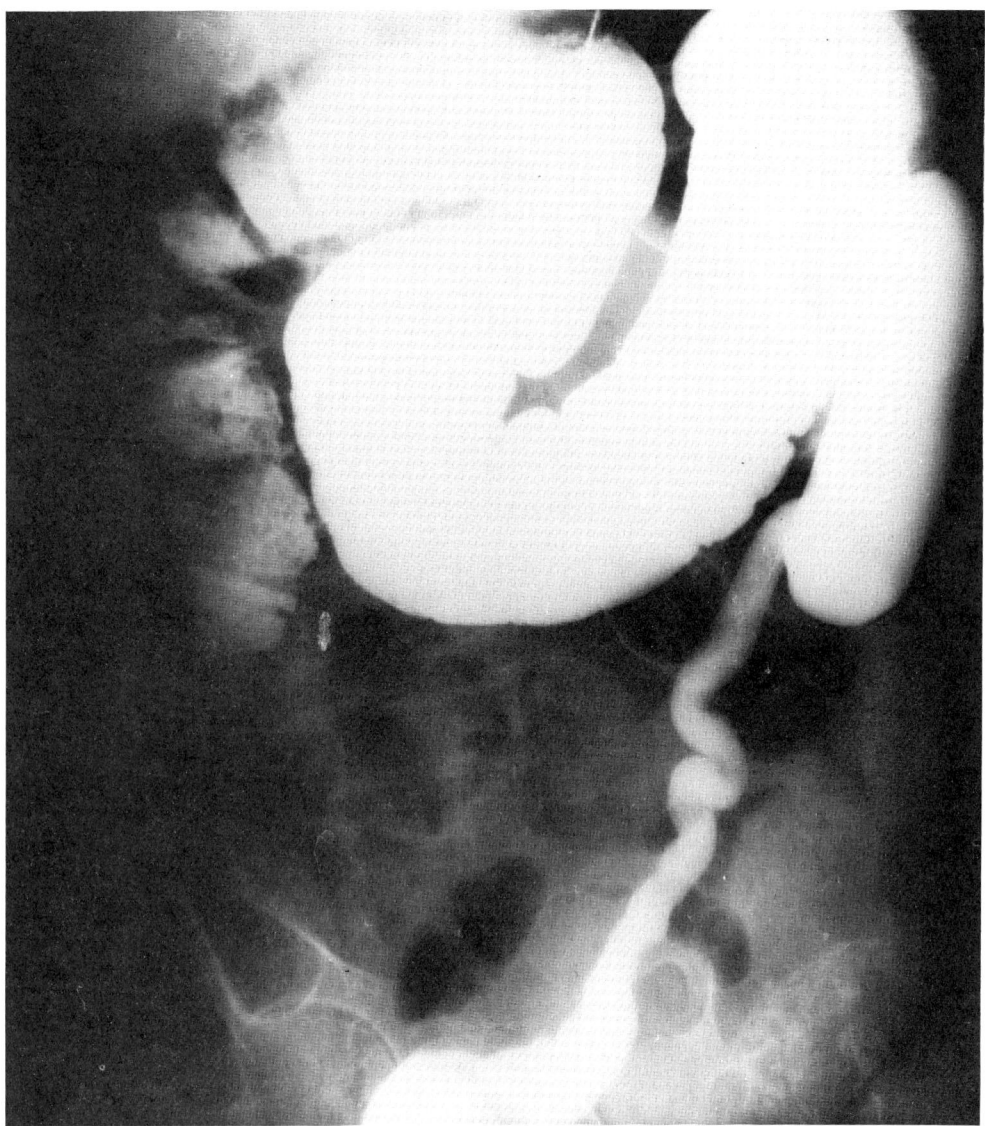

Fig. 176-2. Stricture of rectosigmoid following ischemic colitis.

bleeding. The diagnosis is established with selective angiography. Of particular interest are mesenteric-portal fistulas, the sequelae of penetrating wounds, or surgical trauma. These patients have crampy abdominal pain, diarrhea, and an abdominal bruit. The major complication is portal hypertension.

Hereditary hemorrhagic telangiectasia

Hereditary hemorrhagic telangiectasia (Osler-Weber-Rendu disease) is a vascular anomaly transmitted as a simple dominant trait by both sexes. It is characterized by multiple dilations of capillaries and venules in the skin and mucous membranes. Although lesions may be found in children, they increase in number as the individual grows older, and bleeding may not occur until the individual reaches adult life.

The lesions range from the size of a pinpoint to 3 mm in diameter, are bright red or violaceous, and blanch when pressure is applied. Bleeding may occur in any location and may be provoked by minimal trauma. Lesions on the skin are less likely to bleed than those on mucous membranes.

Lesions of the gastrointestinal tract are found from the mouth to the anus. The diagnosis should be suspected in every case of gastrointestinal bleeding whose origin is inapparent. Bleeding is usually chronic and low grade but may also be acute and massive. Telangiectasias of the skin and oral cavity, particularly sublingually, should alert the physician to the diagnosis of hereditary hemorrhagic telangiectasia. The diagnosis is confirmed by the demonstration of typical lesions with endoscopy, particularly gastroscopy.

The treatment of hereditary hemorrhagic telangiectasia has been unsatisfactory. Many prophylactic procedures and medications have been employed without success, including androgens and estrogens. Hemostatic agents are useful in controlling bleeding from the skin and nasal and oral mucosa but are of little value with bleeding in the stomach and intestine. Cauterization with electrocoagulation and more recently with a laser beam has been employed with limited success.

BIBLIOGRAPHY

Byrne, J.J., and others: Ischemic diseases of the bowel. II. Ischemic colitis, Dis. Colon Rectum **13**:283, 1970.
Fagin, R.R., and Kirsner, J.B.: Ischemic diseases of the colon, Adv. Intern. Med. **17**:343, 1971.
Price, W.E., Rohrer, G.V., and Jacobson, E.D.: Mesenteric vascular diseases, Gastroenterology **57**:599, 1969.
Williams, L.F., Jr.: Vascular insufficiency of the intestine, Gastroenterology **61**:757, 1971.
Williams, L.F., Jr., and others: Ischemic diseases of the bowel. I. Ischemia of the small bowel, Dis. Colon Rectum **13**:275, 1970.

177 • INTESTINAL OBSTRUCTION

Steven Nussbaum

MECHANICAL OBSTRUCTION AND ILEUS

DEFINITION. An intestinal obstruction exists when the normal flow of intestinal contents is prevented either by an obstruction of the bowel lumen or by a defect in peristalsis.

ETIOLOGY. An obstruction may be caused by mechanical or nonmechanical disturbances. Mechanical occlusion of the bowel lumen results from three types of abnormalities: (1) an obturation obstruction, (2) an intrinsic bowel lesion, and (3) an extrinsic bowel lesion. The causes of an obturation obstruction include gallstones, foreign bodies, intussusception, fecal impaction, meconium, bezoars, and polypoid tumors. Intrinsic bowel lesions include congenital and acquired atresia and stenosis. Acquired strictures may result from inflammatory disorders such as regional enteritis, diverticulitis, or radiation enteritis or from neoplastic disorders. Occasionally a stricture may follow chronic ischemia of the bowel wall or result from a failed surgical anastomosis. An extrinsic obstruction may result from occlusion by adhesions, internal and external hernias, extrinsic masses, and volvulus.

A nonmechanical obstruction, or paralytic ileus, results from a failure of peristalsis caused by one of several neurohumoral defects. Adynamic ileus is commonly found after abdominal surgery and may follow any peritoneal insult. Ileus may be associated with spinal and pelvic fractures, retroperitoneal hemorrhage, trauma, pyelonephritis, and ureteral calculi. Thoracic diseases associated with ileus include pneumonia, rib fractures, and myocardial infarction. Ileus commonly occurs with sepsis. Metabolic abnormalities, particularly hypokalemia, may cause paralytic ileus, as does intestinal ischemia.

For purposes of diagnosis and treatment, an intestinal obstruction can be classified as a small bowel obstruction or a large bowel obstruction. Small bowel obstructions are caused most commonly by adhesions (70%), internal and external hernias (8%), and cancer (9%). Obstructions of the large intestine are rarely caused by adhesions; carcinoma (67%), volvulus (9%), and diverticulitis (7%) are the most common causes.

PATHOPHYSIOLOGY. An obstruction in the normal flow of intestinal contents results in distention of the bowel with gas and fluid. Most of the retained gas is swallowed air and thus is predominantly nitrogen, which is poorly absorbed by the intestines. The accumulation of ingested matter and the daily 7 to 10 L of gastrointestinal secretions adds to the distention. As a result of vomiting and the inhibition of absorption caused by the obstruction, large amounts of fluid are lost from the intravascular space. After 24 hours of obstruction there is a net secretion of water and electrolytes into the lumen, further compounding the distention and fluid loss. In addition to hypovolemia and a loss of electrolytes, an obstruction results in dramatic rises in intraluminal pressure, especially in closed-loop obstruction, the obstruction of a loop of intestine at both ends such as is caused by a hernia or adhesive band. A form of closed-loop obstruction may result from a colonic obstruction when the ileocecal valve is competent. An impairment of mucosal blood flow results from the effects of distention, torsion, or extrinsic pressure, resulting in ischemia, necrosis, bacterial invasion, and eventually peritonitis.

CLINICAL MANIFESTATIONS. A mechanical obstruction of the small bowel is manifested by midabdominal paroxysmal colicky pain and vomiting. The higher the obstruction, the more frequent and severe are the paroxysms of pain. Between episodes of pain the patient may be relatively comfortable. In cases of high intestinal obstruction vomiting has an early onset, and the vomitus may be profuse and may contain bile. In cases of distal small bowel obstruction vomiting is delayed, and the vomitus may contain feculent material resulting from the action of bacteria on retained intestinal contents. With continued distention the pain may gradually diminish, probably because of an impairment of motility. The development of a continuous, localized pain may signal the onset of strangulation, but it is usually not possible to differentiate the symptoms of strangulation from those of a simple obstruction. Early in the course of an obstruction some loose stools or flatus may be passed, but complete obstipation and a failure to pass gas ensue.

The physical examination begins with a search for scars of previous surgery. Early in the course of a small bowel obstruction the distention may be minimal. With prolonged obstruction, particularly of the distal small bowel, the abdomen becomes distended and tympanic. Bowel sounds characteristically are heard coincident with the onset of pain, are hyperactive and high pitched, and often have a muscial or tinkling quality. Late in the course of an obstruction or strangulation these findings may be absent. Tenderness and rigidity are usually minimal, as is fever. Unless a sausagelike abdominal mass can be palpated, the physical findings of strangulation may be no different from those of a nonstrangulating obstruction. Shock, fever, rigidity, and rebound are late findings and usually indicate peritoneal soilage.

In cases of adynamic ileus the patient's most prominent complaints are distention and obstipation. Colicky pain is not present, and vomiting, although frequent, is usually not profuse. Distention and tympany may be prominent in the physical examination, but tenderness and rigidity are absent. Bowel sounds are usually absent.

Mechanical obstruction of the colon is manifested by a more prominent distention than occurs with a small bowel obstruction. Pain may be colicky and tends to localize in the hypogastric area in cases of left colonic lesions or in the epigastrium and right upper quadrant in cases of right-sided lesions. In cases of colonic obstruction pain tends to have a more delayed onset and is less severe than with a small bowel obstruction. Vomiting occurs late and, surprising, is rarely feculent. A history of blood in the stool or of a recent change in bowel habits is common, resulting from the underlying cause of the obstruction. Although the patient may pass small amounts of stool and gas early in the course of colonic obstruction, obstipation and a failure to pass gas follow rapidly. In the physical examination the abdomen is found to be distended and tympanic. Bowel sounds are less frequent and lower pitched than in cases of small bowel obstruction. The rectal examination may reveal a fecal impaction, mass, or blood; if the obstruction is above the rectum, the rectum may be essentially empty.

In all forms of obstruction, dehydration and hypovole-

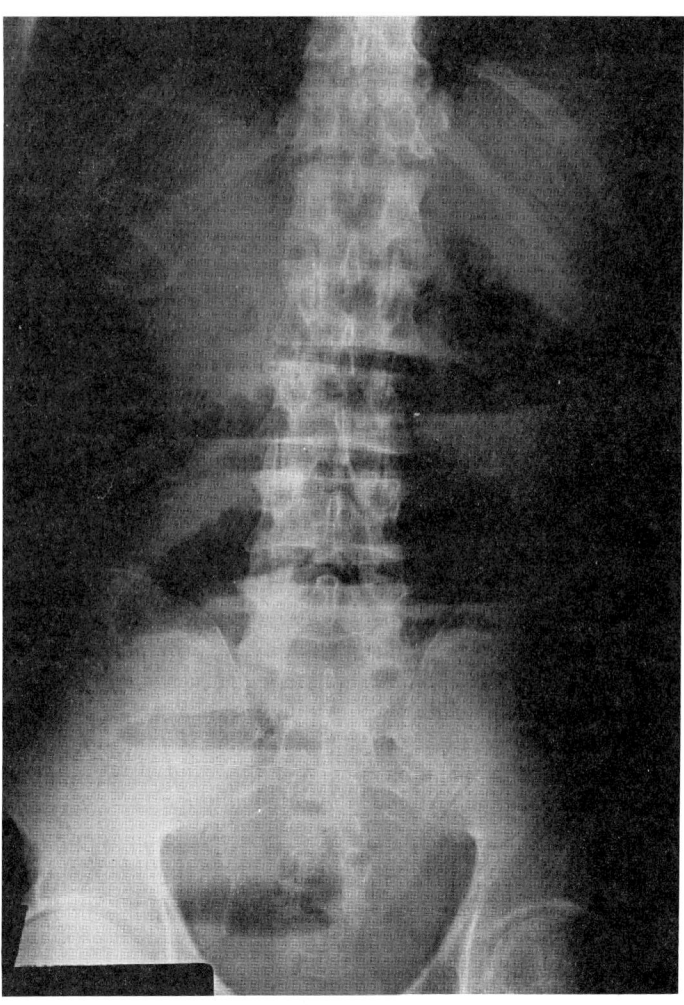

Fig. 177-1. Erect film of abdomen reveals multiple distended loops of small bowel with air-fluid levels in patient with small intestinal obstruction owing to incarcerated inguinal hernia. (Courtesy of George Popky, M.D.)

mia ensue and are manifested by a fall in urine output and eventually by shock.

LABORATORY FINDINGS. The loss of fluids and electrolytes leads to hemoconcentration and is reflected by a fall in the levels of serum chloride and potassium and a rise in the level of blood urea nitrogen. Although the hemoglobin level may rise initially with hemoconcentration, prolonged obstruction leads to severe congestion of the intestine and a loss of blood into the lumen. A significant loss of blood may result in a fall in the level of hemoglobin. The leukocyte count may be normal early in the course of obstruction but may rise appreciably with a shift to the left, particularly if strangulation ensues. The level of serum amylase occasionally rises as it diffuses from the obstructed lumen into the circulation.

Roentgenograms of the abdomen are extremely helpful in confirming the clinical diagnosis and determining the point of obstruction (Fig. 177-1). Repeated roentgenograms are necessary to assess the progress of the patient. In cases of a mechanical small bowel obstruction loops of distended small bowel arranged in a stepladder pattern may occur in a central location. Air-fluid levels can be seen on roentgenograms made with the patient erect. Little or no gas is seen in the colon. In cases of strangulating obstruction a single distended loop may occur, but in at least 50% of these cases roentgenograms are not helpful.

In cases of a bowel obstruction with a competent ileocecal valve, distended loops of colon can be seen arrayed along the lateral aspects of the abdomen. The colon is distinguished from the small bowel by the haustral markings, which do not traverse the entire diameter of the bowel. In a distended small bowel the valvulae conniventes can be seen encircling the entire lumen. In cases of a colonic obstruction with an incompetent ileocecal valve, the roentgenographic appearance may resemble that of a partial small bowel obstruction with dilated loops of small and large bowel. When the obstruction results from fecal impaction, masses of feces can usually be seen in the rectum and extending proximally.

Adynamic ileus is manifested by the dilation of all levels of the intestinal tract, commonly including the stomach. Air-fluid levels may be seen on lateral and upright films.

Barium should never be given by mouth to determine the point of obstruction until the possibility of a colonic obstruction has been ruled out. Barium may become inspissated above a colonic obstruction and make the situation worse. A colonic obstruction can be excluded from diagnostic possibilities by performing a barium enema. Once colonic obstruction has been ruled out, barium can safely be given orally because it is not inspissated above a small bowel obstruction.

MANAGEMENT. With a few exceptions, a mechanical intestinal obstruction is treated surgically. Before surgery, electrolyte and fluid balances should be restored, and decompression by means of nasogastric suction or a long intestinal tube should be attempted. Decompression may lessen the symptoms but should not give the physician a false sense of success. Surgery should not be delayed unless there is unequivocal evidence that the obstruction has resolved. During the period before surgery broad-spectrum antibiotics are given. The choice of surgical procedure is dictated by the site of the obstruction and the experience of the surgeon.

Certain situations can be managed nonsurgically, including the following. (1) Adynamic ileus, particularly following an abdominal operation, is treated by decompression using a long intestinal tube. (2) Sigmoid volvulus may be treated by decompression with a colonoscope or sigmoidoscope. (3) Children with intussusception may be managed with hydrostatic reduction. Adults with intussusception should be treated surgically. (4) An obstruction caused by Crohn's disease may abate with supportive and decompressive therapy. (5) When the obstruction results from fecal impaction, disimpaction may be accomplished by gently breaking up and removing feces digitally or with a proctoscope or by means of water, saline, or oil retention enemas.

MEGACOLON

Megacolon is characterized by the massive enlargement of the diameter of all or a portion of the colon. Megacolon is usually accompanied by severe constipation or obstipation. It may result from acquired or congenital abnormalities.

Congenital megacolon, or Hirschsprung's disease, is a disorder of intestinal motility usually manifested in infancy by intractable constipation. The disease is familial, is more common in males, and results from a congenital absence of myenteric ganglion cells in the colonic wall. The defect is usually confined to the distal colon but occasionally may involve long segments of colon. The aganglionic segment is unable to relax; that is, it is tonically contracted. This segment acts as a functional obstruction, and the portion of colon proximal to it becomes massively dilated. Roentgenographic examination with a barium enema reveals colonic dilation proximal to a narrowed segment. The diagnosis is made by detecting an absence of ganglion cells in a surgical biopsy specimen of the involved segment. Surgical excision of the abnormal segment with a "pull-through" and anastomosis of normal colon to the rectal stump is the procedure of choice.

Psychogenic megacolon, a common disorder of childhood, results from chronic stool holding. Its onset occurs later in childhood than Hirschsprung's disease, but it must be differentiated from that disease by means of a barium enema and rectal biopsy. The treatment involves changing the toilet habits and giving large doses of mineral oil and enemas. A similar condition may occur in adults, particularly in psychotic patients being treated with phenothiazines.

Acquired megacolon may result from a number of infectious, metabolic, and neuromuscular disorders. Chagas' disease, commonly found in South America, results from an infection with *Trypanosoma cruzi* and is manifested by megacolon, megaesophagus, megaduodenum, and/or megaureter. It is caused by the destruction of Auerbach's plexus by a tissue reaction to the parasite. Chronic megacolon may also occur in association with scleroderma, amyloidosis, lead poisoning, and myxedema. Neurologic disorders associated with megacolon include parkinsonism, multiple sclerosis, spinal cord lesions, and diabetic visceral neuropathy. Narcotic, anticholinergic, and phenothiazine drugs may cause severe constipation and dilation. Habitual laxative abuse has been associated with megacolon. Any chronic partial obstruction of the distal colon may cause megacolon. The treatment is that for the underlying disorder.

Acute toxic megacolon may result from any inflammatory disorder of the colon but most commonly is associated with chronic ulcerative colitis or Crohn's disease of the colon (see Chapter 175).

BIBLIOGRAPHY

Cohn, I., and Atik, M.: Strangulation obstruction: closed loop studies, Ann. Surg. **153**:94, 1961.

Cope, Z.: The early diagnosis of the acute abdomen, ed. 14, London, 1972, Oxford University Press.

Ehrenpreis, T.: Hirschsprung's disease, Chicago, 1970, Year Book Medical Publishers, Inc.

Miller, L.D., and others: The pathophysiology and management of intestional obstruction, Surg. Clin. North Am. **42**:1285, 1962.

Silen, W., and others: Strangulation obstruction of the small intestine, Arch. Surg. **85**:121, 1962.

178 • FUNCTIONAL BOWEL DISEASE

Julian Katz

DEFINITION. Functional bowel disease is a group of clinical features probably best viewed as a syndrome rather than a disease. There are no demonstrable anatomic abnormalities, and there are a variety of causes. The recognition in recent years of lactase deficiency in some patients previously thought to have functional symptoms suggests that additional "organic" abnormalities will in the future be identified in some of these patients, leading to the development of more specific therapies.

Functional bowel disorders are heterogeneous, but the symptoms include abdominal pain, excessive borborygmi, abdominal bloating, and alterations in stool frequency. A morphologically demonstrated organic disease such as a peptic ulcer, celiac disease, ulcerative colitis, or a bowel tumor may produce the same symptoms. Distention, relief of pain with a bowel movement, and more frequent and looser stools along with the onset of pain are significantly more common with functional bowel disease than with organic disease. Other symptoms of functional bowel syndrome are notable mucus in the stool and a sensation of incomplete evacuation. Most patients have abdominal discomfort, but painless runny stools are another symptom of functional bowel disease. Different terms have been used to describe the syndrome. *Spastic colitis* emphasizes the disturbed bowel motility that may be present, but in functional disorders there is no mucosal inflammation. *Psychophysiologic gastrointestinal reaction* emphasizes that certain patients have an altered physiologic response to stress, often with lower pain thresholds. *Irritable bowel or colon* is another commonly used term.

ETIOLOGY. Intestinal motility studies suggest that there may be abnormal motor patterns in patients who have the irritable bowel syndrome of pain and problems with bowel movements. These differences are evident in the basal state and in response to physiologic and pharmacologic stimuli. On the right side of the colon segmental contractions normally result in retrograde and forward mixing and churning movements, with a periodic mass movement of the stool into the left colon. In the left colon normal segmental contractions retard the passage of the stool into the rectum. Manometric studies demonstrate that the segmental contractions of the sigmoid colon are increased in frequency and amplitude in patients with irritable bowel syndrome, particularly during periods of symptoms. Abdominal cramps are correlated with increased intraluminal pressures and with the contraction of the circular layer of smooth muscle. Patients with painless diarrhea have a decrease in the activity of sigmoid segmental contractions.

The control and coordination of the contractile patterns of the colon are related to intrinsic myoelectric activity. Pacemakers are located in the circular muscle of the colon, and a basic electrical rhythm can be recorded. Patients with the irritable bowel syndrome have abnormal myoelectric patterns demonstrable by intraluminal mucosal electrodes. An increased percentage of slower frequency waves is found in these patients.

Bowel contractions are affected by many factors, including food intake, the autonomic nervous system, physical activity, and psychologic states. Altered responses to meals, cholinergic and anticholinergic drugs, humoral agents, and emotional stresses occur in patients who have an irritable bowel syndrome. In patients with notable postprandial symptoms there is an exaggeration of the normally occurring increase in segmental contractions following eating. Cholecystokinin and gastrin, which are released in the gut in response to eating, also cause an exaggerated increase in colonic muscular activity. Patients with abdominal pain and constipation often respond to stress by showing an increased amplitude and frequency of sigmoid segmental contractions, and those with diarrhea have a decreased contractile activity.

The syndrome includes clinical symptoms that patients

attribute to intestinal gas. These include belching, bloating, and excessive flatus. Bowel gas is 99% composed of odorless gases: nitrogen, oxygen, hydrogen, carbon dioxide, and in about 30% of adults, methane. Intestinal gas derives from swallowed air, gases produced within the colon, and gases that diffuse from the blood into the gut lumen. Air is swallowed as part of food, in association with eating and drinking, and by the habit of aspirating air into the esophagus. Eructation occurs in some people as an annoying but benign response to air swallowing. Further gas is produced in the intestine as acid reacts with bicarbonate to form carbon dioxide. An additional important source of gas production is the fermentation by colonic bacteria of carbohydrates that are not entirely absorbed in the small intestine. Lactose intolerance is a common cause of bloating and flatulence. The milk sugar lactose is a disaccharide composed of glucose and galactose; if there is insufficient lactase in the small intestine to digest the carbohydrate into its two component sugars, the lactose is utilized by colonic bacteria, resulting in the release of hydrogen, carbon dioxide, and organic acids that react with bicarbonate to produce additional carbon dioxide. Lactase insufficiency is genetically determined and is very common in certain ethnic groups such as Orientals and American blacks. Other carbohydrates not digested by enzymes in the intestine, such as the oligosaccharides in beans, are fermented by colonic bacteria.

Abdominal discomfort and bloating, particularly after meals, have been attributed to excessive gas. Yet the total volume of intestinal gas in patients with these clinical gas syndromes is not increased over the normal volume, either in the fasting state or following a large meal. Rather, these patients show a retarded passage of gas through the intestine and a retrograde movement of gas in the gut. The introduction of gas into the intestine in an amount tolerated by normal subjects provokes pain in these patients. Thus these problems are related to a motility disturbance in the small intestine and an increased perception of distention of the bowel.

EPIDEMIOLOGY. Of all patients seen by gastroenterologists, 20% to 40% have functional bowel symptoms. A survey of apparently healthy people showed that 30% had recurrent abdominal pain and alterations in bowel habits. Epidemiologic studies have suggested that the fiber content of the diet may play a role in the pathogenesis of functional bowel disease, but other factors as well as the type of fiber may cause patients to complain of bowel problems. East Europeans and rural Africans both consume large amounts of fiber, but Europeans are more troubled by functional bowel distress.

No environmental or emotional stress pattern, personality type, sex, age group, or psychiatric disturbance is correlated with the functional bowel syndrome. The alterations in colonic motility and myoelectric activity that occur in patients with irritable bowel syndrome can be found in many patients who are not bothered by gastrointestinal symptoms. The response of patients to the motility disturbance is determined by their attitude, conditioning, and cultural background. Some patients have a definite lower pain threshold to distention of the gut.

CLINICAL MANIFESTATIONS AND COURSE. Different functional syndromes have been described that may have disparate mechanisms and that would therefore respond to different treatment programs. Usually the symptoms can be expected to return, provoked often by changes in the patient's life pattern or psychologic stress. In 20% of an otherwise well population, abdominal pain occurs more than six times a year. Pain below the navel that is relieved by defecation or the passage of flatus is a characteristic of the irritable bowel syndrome. Some patients may have painless diarrhea, whereas others have staining at stool and obstipation, culminating in ill-formed stools. There may be another pattern of upper abdominal distress with features suggesting acid-peptic disease but without readily demonstrable mucosal inflammation.

DIAGNOSIS. The diagnosis should not merely be made by excluding other disorders. A history compatible with a bowel motility disorder is necessary for the diagnosis of an irritable bowel syndrome. Roentgenographic studies show no specific abnormalities. Diverticulosis of the colon may be present, however; it has been associated with similar increased sigmoid pressures and abdominal pains such as occur in irritable bowel syndrome. Endoscopic examination of the gastrointestinal tract is unrevealing in the evaluation of dyspeptic symptoms. Perhaps most important, the circumstances that contribute to an enhanced physiologic bowel response to varied stresses should be identified. The recent onset of seemingly functional symptoms without obvious precipitating causes or a nocturnal prominence of these symptoms should mandate a more vigorous search for an organic origin, such as pancreatic carcinoma. Often the best test, after the preliminary evaluation, is a therapeutic trial, as discussed in the following section.

MANAGEMENT. The scientific basis of most dietary regimens for the treatment of functional bowel syndrome is questionable. Vigorous dietary restriction of the composition and consistency of the diet is not helpful. Regular balanced meals that are moderate in nonabsorbed spices and food temperatures are a sufficient recommendation. The elimination of specific dietary carbohydrates is helpful in treating distention, cramps, and flatulence in some patients; a decrease in foods that contain large amounts of nonabsorbable carbohydrates such as beans and cabbage reduces gas production in the gut. Lactose is not completely absorbed even by patients without an obvious lactase deficiency, and a diet limited in milk, ice cream, and soft cheeses might be tried. A low-fat diet may reduce carbon dioxide production in the upper small intestine.

The role of added dietary fiber in the treatment of functional bowel symptoms is controversial. In a high-fiber diet there is an increase in stool weight and probably a decrease in the transit time of the stool, and a reduction in intraluminal pressures in the sigmoid colon has been described. Symptomatic relief has not been clearly demonstrated with such a diet, however, and large amounts of fiber must be ingested for alterations in bowel function to occur. Supplementary mucilloid bulk agents should probably be tried as a means of adding measured amounts of fiber.

Convincing studies of the efficacy of anticholinergic agents are lacking. Some such drugs do cause the myoelectric patterns of the irritable bowel to become more normal. A trial of one of these drugs for a few weeks is justified. Antidiarrhea agents such as diphenoxylate, loperamide, or even codeine may give confidence to the patient who suffers from diarrhea. Recent work with the operant conditioning (biofeedback) of colonic motility shows some positive results. The use of psychotherapeutic modalities of therapy may often be necessary, but reassurance, education, and careful and compassionate follow-up are most important.

BIBLIOGRAPHY

Almy, T.P.: Irritable bowel syndrome. In Sleisinger, M.H., and Fordtran, J.S., editors: Gastrointestinal disease, ed. 2, 1978, Philadelphia, W.B. Saunders Co.
Burns, T.W.: Colonic motility in the irritable bowel syndrome, Arch. Intern. Med. **140:**247, 1980.
Drossman, D.A.: Diagnosis of the irritable bowel syndrome, Ann. Inter. Med. **90:**431, 1979.
Levitt, M.D., and Bond, J.H.: Flatulence, Annu. Rev. Med. **31:**127, 1980.
Thompson, W.G., and Heaton, K.W.: Functional bowel disorders in apparently healthy people. Gastroenterology **79:**283, 1980.

179 • ANORECTAL DISORDERS

Harvey B. Lefton

DEFINITION. Disease in the anorectal region may result from infectious, inflammatory, or neoplastic processes. Pain is a common feature of disease of the lower anus, whereas bleeding, difficulty with defecation, and rectal fullness characterize disease in the upper canal and rectum.

ANATOMY. The location of the pathologic process determines they symptoms. The perianal region and lower anal canal are lined with squamous epithelium and are innervated by somatic nerves with pain receptors. The venous drainage is to the inferior vena cava, and lymphatics drain to the inguinal nodes. The pectinate line is the beginning of the portion of the upper anus lined with mucous membrane. The upper anal canal is innervated by sympathetic nerve fibers that do not carry pain impulses. Lesions in this area produce discomfort by triggering spasms of the rectum or by putting pressure on the surrounding musculature. Venous drainage in the upper anus is to the portal system, and the lymphatics drain to the lumbar nodes. At the pectinate line are epithelial bulges called papillae (Fig. 179-1). Proximal to this line are the rectal columns of Morgagni, consisting of mucosal folds separated by crypts.

The anal canal has an internal sphincter consisting of rectal smooth muscle and an external sphincter that joins with the puborectal muscles, the levator ani coccyx. The internal sphincter is under autonomic control and relaxes as stool is propelled against it. The external sphincter is controlled voluntarily once toilet training is completed. Although cutting the internal sphincter does not produce

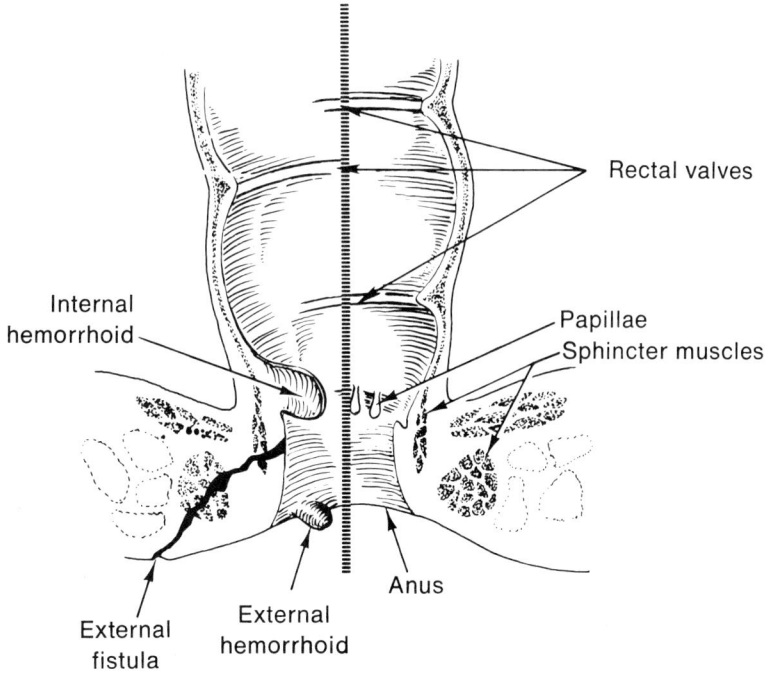

Fig. 179-1. Normal and abnormal findings of anorectal region.

symptoms, chronic inflammation or surgical injury of the external sphincter results in soilage and incontinence.

The ischiorectal and perirectal spaces contain large deposits of fatty tissue. When an infection invades this region from the anus or rectum, large, painful abscesses can develop.

SKIN DISORDERS

The most common symptom of anal disease is pruritus, which may result from psoriasis, atopic dermatitis, seborrhea, or lichen planus of the anal canal. Infection with *Trichophyton* or *Candida albicans* may also produce anal pruritus. Surgical injury to the anal canal, hemorrhoids, and recurrent anal infection can cause incontinence resulting in chronic soilage with alkaline rectal contents and eventually producing intense pruritus and hyperpigmentation of the perianal skin. *Enterobius vermicularis* (pinworm) infestation may cause nocturnal anal pruritus, especially in children.

Commonly no identifiable dermatologic or inflammatory process is present. In some patients a severe emotional upset may precede the onset of pruritus; these patients benefit from treatment with mild tranquilizers. Improvement in anal hygiene alleviates the discomfort related to soilage. If the patient has anal incontinence and incomplete rectal emptying, the administration of a tap water enema after defecation can remove the alkaline rectal fluid; this should be followed by drying the perineum. The use of medicated pads rather than toilet paper also reduces perianal irritation. Mild tranquilizers or sleeping aids should be given if anxiety accompanies incontinence.

Rarely, pruritus may be associated with anal condylomata caused by a papovavirus infection, a condition common in homosexual patients. Treatment with a podophyllin solution may eradicate these anal warts. Occasionally surgery or cautery is necessary.

HEMORRHOIDS

Hemorrhoids are varicose veins occurring in the anus. Precipitating factors include pregnancy, prolonged sitting, straining at stool because of constipation, recurrent diarrhea, and portal hypertension. The incidence of hemorrhoids increases with advancing age, and 70% of people over age 50 have hemorrhoids.

External hemorrhoids are covered by skin. They become symptomatic when the vessels become thrombosed, causing the surrounding tissues to swell and become painful. Initially the patient notes a palpable anal mass and marked rectal throbbing. Anoscopy reveals soft bluish masses covered by skin. Often these lesions remit with a treatment of sitz baths, emollients, and stool softeners; complete resorption of the clot usually occurs in 2 to 4 weeks. Severe pain may necessitate the surgical removal of the clot, however, leaving an open wound that is subject to a secondary infection. Occasionally spontaneous healing produces a prolapsed skin tag. These markers of healed hemorrhoids are usually asymptomatic and do not require surgical excision.

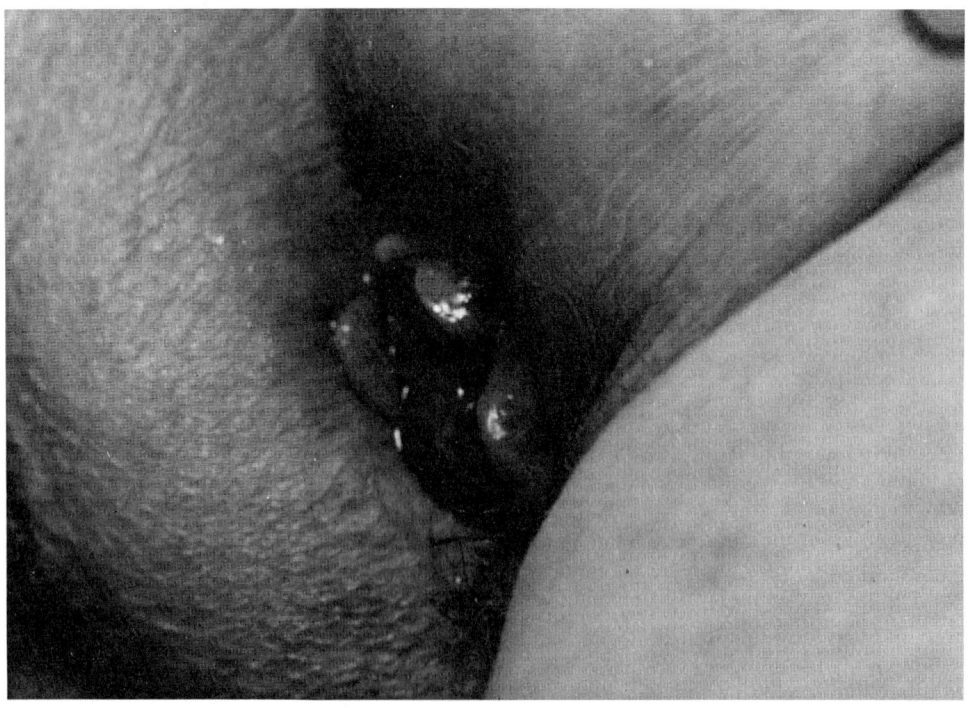

Fig. 179-2. Prolapsed thrombosed internal hemorrhoids.

Internal hemorrhoids are varicosities covered by mucous membrane that cause rectal bleeding. Because this region lacks sensory innervation, pain is not a common feature. Patients may have the sensation of rectal fullness if hemorrhoids are large. The prolapse of swollen internal hemorrhoids may cause anal pruritus and soilage. Prolapsed internal hemorrhoids also may become strangulated by the anal sphincter, producing pain (Fig. 179-2). The most important aspect of the treatment of uncomplicated internal hemorrhoids usually involves reassuring the patient that a rectal cancer is not present. Local anesthetics, cortisone suppositories, and sitz baths help promote healing. Sclerosing agents can be injected into the hemorrhoid to promote fibrosis. More recently the ligation of internal hemorrhoids with rubber bands has been performed to cause a sloughing of the lesion; this procedure is associated with few problems. Surgical excision is indicated when significant bleeding develops or hemorrhoids remain prolapsed.

FISSURES

A break in the lining of the anal canal causes a painful ulceration. Such a break develops in the posterior midline of the anal canal as a result of a paucity of muscular support fibers in this region and the high pressure of defecation. The pain from an anal fissure is often so severe that the administration of opiates is required. Topical anesthetics must be used before digital examination or anoscopy. The examiner may seen a sentinel skin tag resulting from anal thickening. Because of the repeated trauma of defecation, untreated fissures do not heal. Surgical treatment is necessary to resolve this lesion. Anal stenosis is a late feature of an untreated fissure or an improper surgical resection.

FISTULAS

Burrowing infections of the anal crypts and altered anal immunologic mechanisms are thought to play a role in the development of anal fistulas. Infections may drain to the perianal region or burrow internally to adjacent areas in the bowel, bladder, or vagina. Patients may have a history of recent anal abscesses or may note pus or fecal soilage on their underclothing. Fistulas may also occur in patients with Crohn's disease, tuberculosis, carcinoma, or lymphogranuloma venereum. Fistulas not associated with inflammatory bowel disease should be surgically probed and resected. In patients with Crohn's disease, surgical resection often leads to indolent ulcers. Such patients should have abscesses drained and should be treated with oral sulfasalazine or metronidazole. A recurrent anal abscess leads to anal stenosis.

TUMORS

Malignant tumors are rare in the anus. An epidermoid carcinoma may originate as a small mass that goes on to ulcerate and cause pain. This is a slow-growing tumor that is locally invasive and spreads through the lymphatics. The treatment consists of abdominoperineal resection. When the inguinal nodes are involved, the prognosis is poor, but radiation therapy may have palliative value for these patients.

Several other tumors may occur in the anus. A basal cell carcinoma of the anus may develop as an anal nodule in elderly patients. This is a superficial cancer that responds well to excisional therapy. Bowen's disease (intraepithelial squamous cell carcinoma) of the anus first appears as a draining reddish anal plaque; this also responds to excisional therapy. Malignant melanoma is a vary aggressive lesion of the anus that appears as a tender bluish nodule. The lesion may have the appearance of a hemorrhoid but on palpation is very hard. The mortality with malignant melanoma is high even with the most radical surgical procedures. A cloacogenic carcinoma may occur in the transitional epithelium of the proximal anus; this extensive carcinoma requires abdominoperineal resection and is associated with a high mortality.

BIBLIOGRAPHY

Alexander-Williams, J., editor: Disease of the anus and rectum. Clinics in gastroenterology, vol. 7, Philadelphia, 1975, W.B. Saunders Co.

180 • TUMORS OF THE GUT
Paul B. Weisberg

Gastrointestinal neoplasms are a common cause of morbidity and mortality throughout the world. The relative incidence of some types of tumors varies widely, however, among different populations according to geographic location and dietary habits. Both benign and malignant lesions may arise in any level of the gastrointestinal tract, and any of the cell types found there can be the source of tumor formation. The vast majority, however, originate in the mucosa. With the exception of certain colonic polyps, benign neoplasms do not pose clinical problems as commonly as malignant tumors. With the current advances in diagnostic and therapeutic technology, particularly endoscopy, there should be increasing success in the diagnosis and management of this group of disorders.

ESOPHAGEAL NEOPLASMS
Benign tumors

LEIOMYOMAS. Leiomyoma, a smooth muscle tumor, is the most common of the benign esophageal neoplasms, but its incidence is less than 10% of that of malignant tumors. Leiomyomas are usually clinically silent; about half of the reported cases are found in autopsy studies. When large, they may produce dysphagia by causing a partial obstruction, but only rarely do they ulcerate and bleed as gastric leiomyomas do. The diagnosis is usually made with a barium roentgenogram, in which the lesion appears as a smooth, constant filling defect. Endoscopy reveals a mass with normal overlying mucosa, and for this reason an endoscopic biopsy is usually not helpful in determining the diagnosis. The only treatment is surgical enucleation of the tumor.

OTHER BENIGN TUMORS. Other benign tumors are extremely rare in the esophagus and usually are present as polyps. A long pedicle is characteristic of the fibrovascular polyp. Other lesions that have been reported include lipomas, fibromas, squamous papillomas, neurofibromas, lymphangiomas, and cysts.

Malignant tumors

EPIDERMOID CARCINOMA. Carcinoma arising in the squamous epithelium is the most common of the esophageal tumors. Epidemiologic data show that the incidence of such carcinomas is much higher in some populations than in others. Men in certain regions of the Soviet Union, Iran, and China have an incidence 10 to 30 times that of American white males. American black males have an incidence almost 4 times that of American white males—15.6 compared to 4:100,000—and males in general have a higher incidence than females. A number of causative associations have been identified. The incidence of carcinoma is increased among patients with a history of alcohol abuse, cigarette smoking, lye stricture, exposure to ionizing radiation, achalasia, and Plummer-Vinson syndrome.

Clinical manifestations. Epidermoid carcinomas usually occur in middle-aged or older people. The most common initial symptom is progressive dysphagia (first with solids, then with soft foods, and finally with liquids), which results from gradual narrowing of the esophageal lumen. Odynophagia also occurs but is less common. As the obstruction becomes marked, there may be retention of food and secretions resulting in symptoms of tracheal aspiration. A constant substernal or back pain is a poor prognostic sign because it usually signifies a local extension of the tumor outside the esophagus. Gross hemorrhage is unusual, but occult bleeding is common, and these patients commonly become anemic as a result of an iron deficiency. Anorexia and weight loss also accompany the illness. If advanced, the tumor may erode into adjacent organs, leading to the development of a tracheoesophageal fistula or rarely an aortoesophageal fistula. The physical examination may reveal nonspecific findings such as evidence of weight loss, anemia, supraclavicular adenopathy or hepatomegaly resulting from metastases, and signs of aspiration pneumonitis.

Diagnosis. When a carcinoma of the esophagus is suspected, the diagnostic procedure of choice is the barium swallow examination with an upper gastrointestinal series (Fig. 180-1). The usual finding is of a localized, often circumferential luminal narrowing with irregular or shelflike boundaries and mucosal destruction. Occasionally the tumor may appear to involve only one side of the lumen or may appear as a smooth tapered lesion, in which case it is difficult to differentiate a carcinoma from a benign stricture. When feasible, fiberoptic endoscopy should be performed after roentgenography in an effort to determine the extent of the lesion and to confirm the diagnosis with biopsy and brush cytology. When both biopsy and brush cytology are performed, the diagnostic accuracy approaches 96%. When endoscopy cannot be performed, an exfoliative cytologic examination may be made of gastric aspirates and washings taken from the region of the tumor through a nasogastric tube; this method has a diagnostic accuracy only slightly less than that of endoscopic studies. Computed tomography of the mediastinum can also be of value in selected cases to determine the extent of the lesion. Newer techniques of radioisotope scanning with materials that are preferentially picked up by squamous cell carcinomas are under investigation.

Management. The two major therapeutic modalities available are radiation therapy and surgical extirpation, performed either alone or in combination. The choice of therapy for a given patient depends on many factors, the most important of which is the location of the lesion in the esophagus. Lower-third lesions (50%) are most accessible to surgical removal, middle-third lesions (30%) are somewhat more difficult, and upper-third lesions (20%) are technically very difficult to remove surgically. For this reason, high-dose radiation therapy has traditionally been used for most upper- and middle-third tumors and less commonly for lower-third lesions. Any patient with evidence that the tumor has spread should probably be treated with radiation rather than resection, regardless of the location. The symptoms can be palliated with either modality, and the overall 5-year survival rate, approximately 5%, is the same with both therapies. Recent studies using a combination of preoperative radiation and surgical excision, however, have shown that this approach may significantly increase the survival rate for selected patients. For symptomatic palliation at any stage of the disease, esophageal dilation or insertion of a prosthetic tube can be performed.

ADENOCARCINOMA. The true incidence of primary adenocarcinomas of the esophagus is difficult to determine because many of these lesions originate in the columnar epithelium of the stomach and grow upward in the esophageal wall. An adenocarcinoma in an otherwise normal esophagus accounts for less than 1% of all esophageal malignancies. If patients with Barrett's esophagus are included, the rate increases to 3% to 7%. The columnar epithelium in Barrett's esophagus is considered by many to be a premalignant lesion because of its strong association with esophageal adenocarcinoma.

This disease is most common in the same age group as epidermoid carcinomas and usually appears in a similar

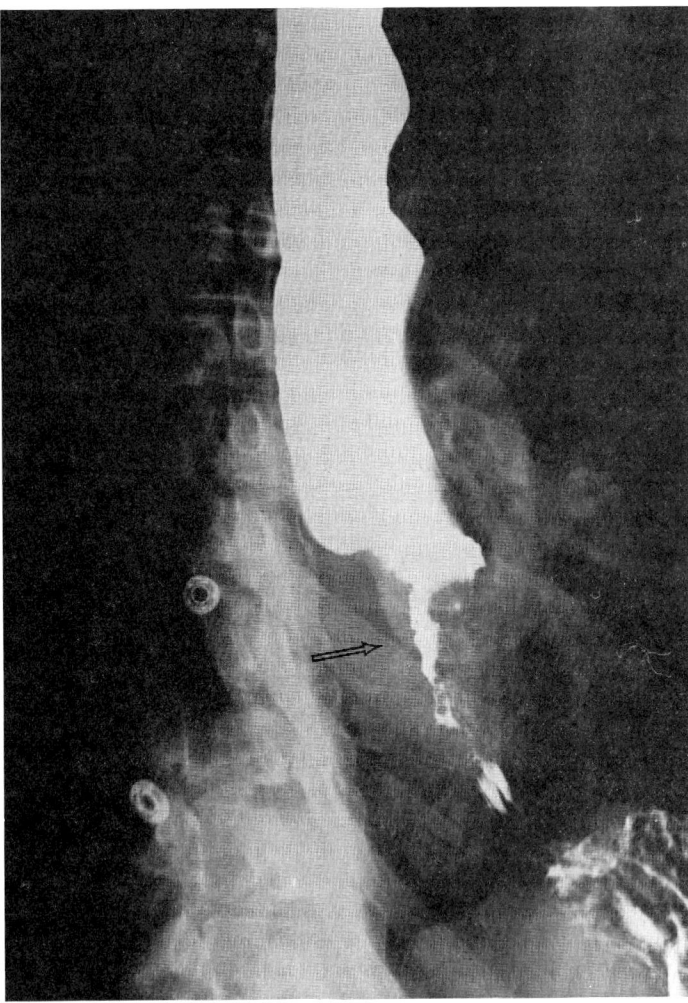

Fig. 180-1. Esophagogram reveals obstructing carcinoma *(arrow)* in lower esophagus of patient with progressive dysphagia and weight loss. (Courtesy of George Popky, M.D.)

fashion, with dysphagia as one of the earliest and most prominent symptoms. Other clinical manifestations are likewise very similar. The diagnosis can be established with the same approach, using roentgenographic and endoscopic techniques.

Because conventional radiation therapy is relatively ineffective in treating patients with an adenocarcinoma, surgery for the palliation of obstructive symptoms or a curative resection should be performed on those who are operative candidates. The routine resection of the lesion results in a 9% 5-year survival rate.

OTHER MALIGNANT TUMORS. Malignant tumors of the esophagus other than squamous cell carcinomas and adenocarcinomas are extremely rare. Other types that have been reported include carcinosarcomas, pseudosarcomas, verrucous carcinomas, melanomas, and argyrophil cell carcinomas. Metastatic lesions of the esophagus are also distinctly uncommon, but the contiguous spread of tumors from adjacent organs does occur, particularly from the lungs and the thyroid gland.

GASTRIC NEOPLASMS
Benign tumors

GASTRIC POLYPS. Benign gastric polyps are relatively rare lesions; their incidence revealed by autopsies is about 0.5%. Histologically they are either hyperplastic (80%) or adenomatous (20%), but the two types may coexist. Villous adenomas occur rarely. Achlorhydria occurs in 95% of patients with benign gastric polyps and in virtually all patients with multiple polyps, although no causal relationship has been proved. Only 2% of all achlorhydric patients develop polyps. Polyps are present in 5% of patients with pernicious anemia. Gastric polyps are important primarily because of their association with malignancy; 25% to 35% of patients with polyps also have a gastric carcinoma. True hyperplastic polyps never contain malignancy, but 20% to 40% of adenomatous polyps are cancerous. In addition, 30% to 60% of patients with adenomatous polyps have a coexisting cancer. The rate is much lower for patients with hyperplastic lesions. Polyps that are sessile and greater than 2 cm in diameter are much more likely to be malignant than lesions that are stalked and less than 1 cm in diameter. Multiple polyposis is rarely associated with cancer, probably because these lesions are almost always the hyperplastic type.

Clinical manifestations. Most patients with gastric polyps are over 50 years of age, and the disease shows no sex predilection. Many patients are asymptomatic, but others describe a vague upper abdominal discomfort that is usually not related to eating. Gross bleeding is rare, but occult blood loss producing iron deficiency anemia and the attendant symptoms is common. Occasionally a large antral polyp may prolapse into the pylorus and produce a transient gastric outlet obstruction. The physical examination usually reveals little except for the signs of iron deficiency anemia or pernicious anemia. Likewise the laboratory evaluation if nonspecific, showing some form of anemia and, if gastric analysis is performed, total achlorhydria in 95% of these patients.

Diagnosis. The upper gastrointestinal series, particularly an air contrast study, reveals most lesions as round, translucent filling defects (Fig. 180-2). Gastroscopy is somewhat more sensitive than roentgenography in detecting small lesions and has the added advantage of allowing the direct removal of biopsy and brush cytology tissue samples Exfoliative cytology may also be useful.

Management. If a polyp is thought to be the cause of symptoms or complications, or if it is sessile or greater than 2 cm in diameter, it should be removed. Removal can be performed through the gastroscope with a snare-cautery if the polyp has a stalk. Otherwise, surgical excision is indicated. If an associated malignancy can be excluded from the diagnosis, patients with small or even multiple polyps can be observed instead.

LEIOMYOMAS. Leiomyomas are the most common benign tumors of the stomach. Leiomyomas are usually found incidentally during surgery or an autopsy; they rarely produce clinical symptoms unless they are larger than 3 cm in diameter. When large, they have a tendency to ulcerate and may cause gross hemorrhage. On roentgenograms they appear as large, smooth, filling defects that may have a central ulceration. Gastroscopy shows a mass with normal overlying mucosa and the ulcer if one is present. Because the lesion is intramural, an endoscopic biopsy and brush or exfoliative cytology usually cannot establish the diagnosis preoperatively. Symptomatic lesions as well as those found during surgery should be excised.

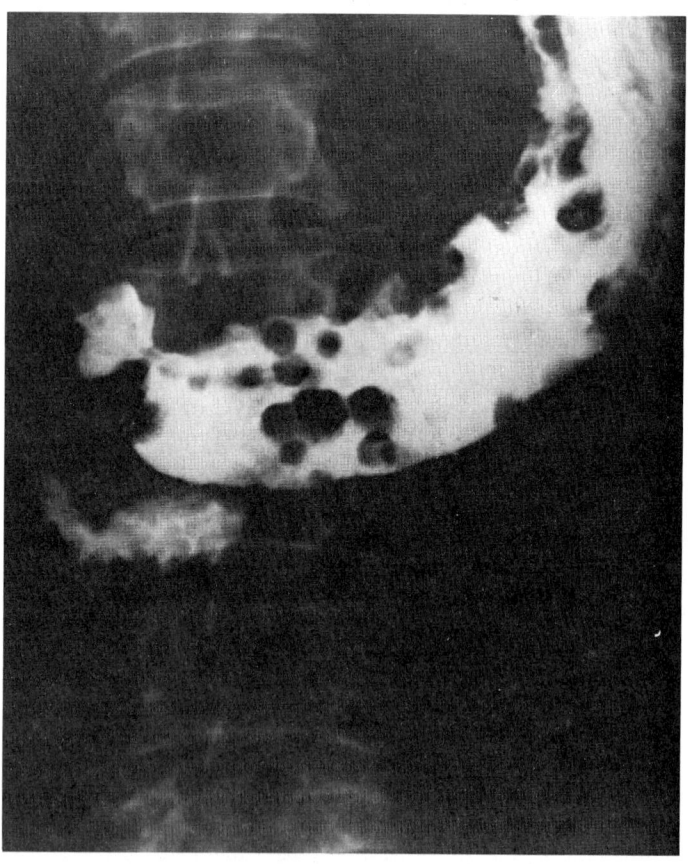

Fig. 180-2. Translucent filling defects in this barium-filled stomach represent multiple polyps (gastric polyposis). (Courtesy of George Popky, M.D.)

OTHER BENIGN TUMORS. Very few other benign tumors of the stomach occur. About 25% of ectopic pancreatic tissue occurs in the stomach, usually on the greater curvature of the distal antrum. Rarely more than 2 cm in diameter, about half of these lesions produce vague abdominal symptoms. Roentgenographically and endoscopically they appear as smooth submucosal masses with a central umbilication that represents the duct. Symptomatic lesions are treated by a distal gastrectomy.

Malignant tumors

ADENOCARCINOMA. Gastric carcinoma is one of the most insidious and lethal of all malignancies and accounts for the majority of gastric malignancies. Fortunately, its incidence in the United States has been declining over the last several decades, and the 5-year survival rate has increased to 9%. A comparison of the relative incidences of gastric carcinoma among various populations around the world reveals that there are marked differences. The reason for this is unknown, but it is probably related to genetic or, more likely, environmental factors. In all populations mostly older individuals are affected, males are affected more often than females, and nonwhites are affected more often than whites.

Gastric carcinomas have been associated with a number of factors that are thought to be predisposing influences. Genetic factors undoubtedly operate in certain situations, such as in kindreds in which the incidence of gastric malignancy is unusually high. People with blood group A have a 10% higher risk than others, and there is a vague relationship of gastric carcinoma with the secretion of the Lewis substance in the saliva. In addition to genetic factors, several disease states are associated with a higher incidence of gastric cancer, such as acanthosis nigricans, in which the associated malignancy commonly develops in the stomach. Certain pathologic and physiologic changes in the gastric mucosa are also known to be related to malignancy; these abnormalities are hypochlorhydria, achlorhydria, atrophic gastritis, and chronic gastritis. A causative role for these disorders, however, has not been established. Gastric polyps, pernicious anemia, hypertrophic gastropathy (Menetrier's disease), and gastric resection with gastroenterostomy are also associated with higher rates of cancer; the incidence of cancer in the last of these usually does not begin to rise until many years after surgery. In the past a chronic benign gastric ulcer was thought to be a predisposition to cancer, but it is extremely doubtful that such a relationship exists. A malignant degeneration of benign gastric ulcers probably does not occur.

Clinical manifestations. The gross morphologic form of a gastric adenocarcinoma can be of several different types: a sessile or pedunculated polypoid mass; a superficial spreading plaque that may be elevated, flat, or depressed; and ulcerated lesion with or without a mass effect; or an infiltrating intramural tumor (linitis plastica). Regardless of the growth pattern of the tumor, the early stages of the disease when it is limited to the mucosa and submucosa are generally symptom free. The lesion eventually grows out of the confines of the stomach, extends locally into adjacent organs, and metastasizes via the lymphatic and hematogenous routes to distant organs such as the liver, lungs, bones, and central nervous system. By the time symptoms appear, the tumor is usually in an advanced stage, but distant metastases are not necessarily present.

The symptoms of gastric carcinoma are nonspecific, but some are encountered regularly. Weight loss occurs in 96% of these patients, pain in 70%, and nausea and vomiting in 50%. The pain is generally vague and may or may not be affected by meals or medications such as antacids. Anorexia and early satiety are also common. Other symptoms include weakness, easy fatigability, abdominal bloating, fever, and changes in bowel habits. Although gross hemorrhage is unusual, occult bleeding is common and leads to iron deficiency anemia.

The physical findings in patients with an advanced gastric carcinoma are related to the local spread and metastases of the tumor and to its systemic effects. About half have a palpable abdominal mass, but only 20% have tenderness. The liver may be enlarged, but unless it is nodular, the presence of metastases cannot be assumed. Metastatic lesions may occur as Virchow's node (left supraclavicular node), as pelvic metastases revealed as Blumer's shelf in the rectal examination, and as Krukenberg's tumor in the ovary. Physical signs of anemia are common, but severe cachexia occurs in only about 20% of these patients.

The laboratory findings are nonspecific and usually show an anemia of the iron deficiency type, macrocytic type (if the patient has pernicious anemia of folate deficiency), combined type, or normochromic and normocytic type. There is usually occult blood in the stool, and many patients are hypoproteinemic. In patients with hepatic metastases, the bilirubin and alkaline phosphatase levels may be elevated. A gastric analysis may be performed, and if no acid is secreted with maximal stimulation and there is an ulcerating lesion of the stomach, a malignancy is almost certainly present; no conclusions can be drawn, however, if any acid at all is present. In 25% of patients with gastric cancers achlorhydria is present. Varying amounts of acid are secreted in the remaining 75%.

Diagnosis. The diagnostic procedure of choice when gastric carcinoma is suspected is a barium roentgenographic study (Fig. 180-3). The double-contrast study is preferred to the traditional study because the latter is not as sensitive in detecting small lesions; this is especially true for small superficial spreading tumors and small polypoid masses. Large intraluminal tumors and ulcerating masses can generally be detected with either study. A tumor infiltrating the wall of the stomach (linitis plastica) usually appears only as a nondistensible, poorly motile or-

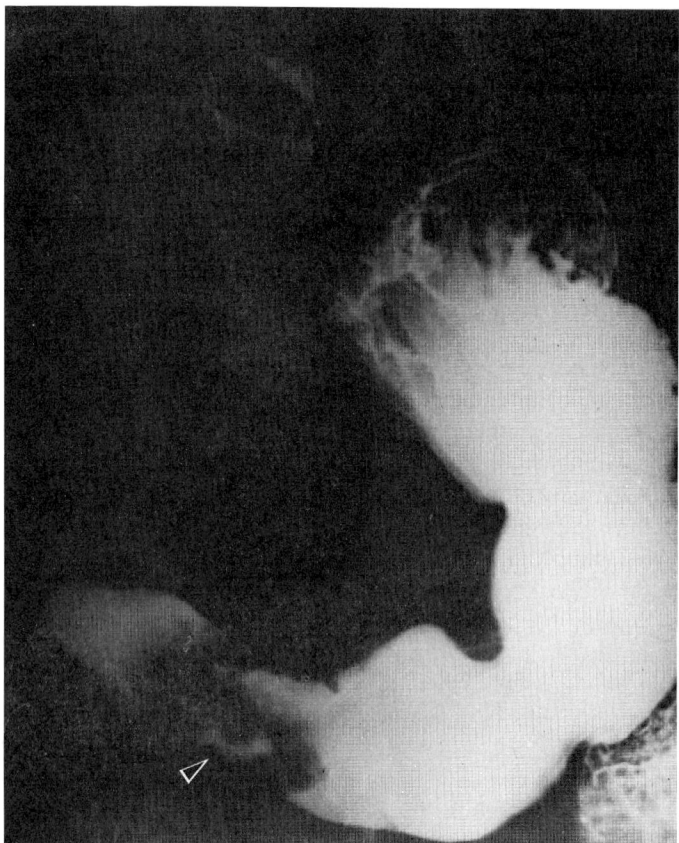

Fig. 180-3. Ulcerating mass *(arrow)* in antrum of this barium-filled stomach is adenocarcinoma. Patient also has hiatus hernia. (Courtesy of George Popky, M.D.)

gan with no apparent mass. Although roentgenographic criteria alone can correctly identify a gastric lesion as benign or malignant in 80% of cases, there are many false positive and false negative results. For this reason endoscopy is of great value in the differential diagnosis of gastric lesions. With the questionable exception of very small gastric ulcers that appear benign on roentgenograms, most lesions in the stomach should be examined endoscopically, and tissue samples should be obtained for biopsy and cytologic examination. The diagnostic accuracy for carcinomas when this approach is applied is 96% to 98%. An exfoliative cytologic examination can also be used to confirm the diagnosis of malignancy. This technique has a 90% accuracy rate and a false positive rate of 1% to 2%. The time-honored approach of obtaining serial roentgenograms to document the healing of gastric ulcerating lesions as an indication of benignity is inappropriate because malignant ulcerations also may seem on roentgenograms to heal. Computed tomography may be helpful in selected cases.

Management. Patients with an untreated gastric carcinoma have a 5-year survival rate of about 1% or less. The surgical removal of the entire tumor mass offers the only hope for a cure, but this is possible in only a small number of patients. Any patient in whom a spread of the tumor outside the stomach cannot be shown, however, should undergo surgery. A partial or subtotal gastrectomy is usually performed, except for lesions high in the cardia, in which case a total gastrectomy is almost always performed. Attempts at more extensive resections commonly result in a higher operative mortality. Occasionally palliative surgery alone must be performed for a complication such as an obstruction, hemorrhage, or perforation.

Metastatic disease is managed with a combination of chemotherapy, radiation therapy, and immunotherapy, all of which result in only a small lengthening of the patient's life span.

MALIGNANT LYMPHOMA. Malignant lymphomas account for about 5% of all gastric malignancies in the United States. Lymphomas of all cell types have been reported, and the gastric involvement may be the primary tumor or a manifestation of more diffuse disease, as is seen in 40% of patients with a disseminated lymphoma. A gastric lymphoma may occur in patients at a younger age than does gastric carcinoma, but the clinical manifestations are otherwise very similar. Most patients have abdominal pain, and many have weight loss, nausea, vomiting, and constitutional symptoms. When the lymphoma is confined to the stomach, the physical examination is usually unremarkable. In cases of disseminated disease hepatosplenomegaly and peripheral adenopathy may occur. Occasionally signs of iron deficiency anemia are found. A gastric analysis usually shows an acid-secreting capability.

The roentgenographic findings in patients with gastric lymphoma commonly mimic the appearance of other benign and malignant gastric lesions. A marked enlargement of the rugal folds may be more indicative of a lymphoma. It is also impossible to differentiate a lymphoma from a carcinoma endoscopically by its gross appearance. An endoscopic biopsy and brush cytologic examination may be of some value in making the diagnosis. An exfoliative cytologic examination is considered by some to be the best way to establish the diagnosis preoperatively.

The treatment of a localized gastric lymphoma consists of the surgical excision of the tumor followed by postoperative radiation therapy. With this regimen the 5-year survival rate is more than 50%. Chemotherapy is indicated for patients with a disseminated lymphoma or diffuse intraabdominal disease.

LEIOMYOSARCOMA. Leiomyosarcomas comprise 1% of all gastric cancers. They tend to occur in patients at a younger age than carcinomas but result in the same kinds of symptoms. Ulceration and gross hemorrhage are more common than with other gastric malignancies. Of these patients, 75% have a palpable epigastric mass that may be tender. Roentegenograms show a round, intramural mass that may have a central ulceration. The endoscopic findings are similar, but with these studies it is usually not possible to differentiate a leiomyosarcoma from a benign leiomyoma, although the larger it is, the more likely it is that the tumor if a sarcoma. Exfoliative cytology has reportedly been helpful in making a preoperative diagnosis. The only treatment is surgical resection, which is curative in more than 50% of these cases.

SMALL BOWEL NEOPLASMS
Benign tumors

Small bowel tumors account for fewer than 5% of all gastrointestinal neoplasms; about 40% of small bowel tumors are malignant. Of the benign tumors, the most commonly occurring type is the adenoma, which may consist of ectopic islet cell tissue or Brunner's gland hyperplasia or may be a true neoplasm similar to adenomatous polyps that occur elsewhere in the gastrointestinal tract. Juvenile polyps also occur but usually are part of an inherited polyposis syndrome. Leiomyomas occur less commonly than adenomas but are more likely to cause symptoms. Lipomas are still less common and occur most often in the distal ileum and ileocecal valve area. Hemangiomas are very rare but are important in that 70% of these patients have gross hemorrhage from the lesion.

Most patients with benign small bowel tumors are over 50 years of age, and the symptoms are usually related to obstructive phenomena, intussusception, or gross or occult bleeding. The physical examination rarely reveals a palpable mass. The diagnosis generally must be made with roentgenographic studies such as small bowel barium contrast roentgenography, arteriography, or computed tomography. Fiberoptic enteroscopy may be available in some medical centers. The treatment of symptomatic benign small bowel tumors is surgical removal.

Malignant tumors

In order of decreasing incidence, adenocarcinomas, lymphomas, and leiomyosarcomas are the most common small bowel malignancies. Adenocarcinomas occur in the older age groups and are almost always found within 20 cm on either side of the ligament of Treitz, usually in the duodenum. Several disease states have been associated with an increased incidence of enteric carcinoma: celiac sprue, dermatitis herpetiformis, chronic regional enteritis, and the Peutz-Jeghers syndrome. Abdominal pain, bleeding, constitutional symptoms, and occasionally acute small bowel obstructions are the usual presenting symptoms. An ulcerating lesion may sometimes be confused on roentgenograms with atypical peptic ulcer disease. The therapeutic approach is surgical.

A lymphoma of the small bowel may be a primary lesion or secondary to disseminated disease. The involvement of the bowel may also be localized or diffuse. Patients with a lymphoma are generally younger than those with other gastrointestinal malignancies. Abdominal pain and bleeding are common symptoms, and when the involvement is focal, a tender abdominal mass commonly can be palpated. Hepatosplenomegaly and peripheral adenopathy occur in disseminated disease. In some cases of diffuse primary intestinal lymphomas, malabsorption is significant and the disease may closely resemble celiac sprue. The disease can be suspected on the basis of small bowel roentgenograms and confirmed by the examination of tissue obtained by biopsy or surgery. Focal lesions are treated with surgery and radiation and/or chemotherapy. Surgery is of no value if the involvement is diffuse except to treat complications such as an obstruction, perforation, or hemorrhage.

Leiomyosarcomas are usually large tumors and tend to occur in the jejunum and ileum. Pain and bleeding are common symptoms, and perforation may occur but is not as common as with lymphosarcomatous lesions. A palpable abdominal mass is common. Surgical removal is the only effective therapy.

Carcinoid tumors are lesions arising from the enterochromaffin cells of the gastrointestinal tract. Although these tumors may occur anywhere, they are usually found between the duodenum and the transverse colon, and the highest incidence is in the appendix. Metastases may occur, but the tumor is considered a very low-grade malignancy. Most lesions are asymptomatic except when hepatic metastases have occurred, in which case the carcinoid syndrome results. This complex of symptoms includes abdominal cramps and diarrhea, cutaneous flushing, cyanosis, bronchospasm, telangiectasia, pellagra-like skin lesions, and valvular lesions of the heart. These manifestations result from the secretion by the tumor tissue of a number of biogenic amines and other substances, the most characteristic of which is serotonin. When a carcinoid tumor is suspected on clinical grounds, the diagnosis may be established by the finding of elevated levels of 5-hydroxyindoleacetic acid (5-HIAA) in the urine. Barium contrast studies of the gastrointestinal tract may show filling defects, and arteriography has also been used to determine the diagnosis. Radionuclide scanning, ultrasonography, and computed tomography may document hepatic lesions that are accessible for a needle biopsy. Symptomatic and incidentally discovered lesions may be removed surgically if the patient does not have the carcinoid syndrome. If the disease is metastatic, the therapy is symptomatic and includes the special use of serotonin antagonists. Chemotherapy has also been successful in alleviating symptoms, but survival data are inconclusive because few patients actually die as a direct consequence of their disease.

COLONIC AND RECTAL NEOPLASMS
Benign tumors

EPITHELIAL POLYPS. Benign polyps of the large bowel are a common medical problem occurring in up to 8% of the population. Their clinical significance lies not only in the symptoms they may produce but also in their relationship to colorectal cancer. This association of epithelial polyps with malignancy has been reported in terms of several descriptive categories, including size, location, number, presence or absence of a stalk, and histologic characteristics. The histologic classification seems the most important. Four major types have been described. (1) Hyperplastic polyps, which are simply overgrowths of normal colonic cellular elements, account for 25% of all polyps but constitute the majority of smaller polyps, especially those under 5 mm in size. They are not associated with malignancy. (2) Adenomatous polyps are neoplasms that consist of abnormal glandular tissue that may show varying degrees of dysplasia from a mild atypia to a carcinoma in situ. They may undergo malignant degeneration or may be found concurrently with or in proximity to a frank carcinoma (sentinel polyp). (3) Villous adenomas, characterized by multiple frondlike projections, arise from cells at the base of the crypts of Lieberkühn; 25% to 50% of these lesions undergo malignant change. (4) Mixed villoglandular polyps, also described as adenovillous or tubulovillous polyps, contain components that are both adenomatous and villous and therefore are considered likely to be premalignant lesions.

A polypoid lesion has an increased probability of containing carcinoma if it is large, especially over 2 cm in size, if it is present in a greater number, if it lacks a pedicle, and perhaps if it is located in the left side of the colon, because most polyps and most carcinomas occur there. These relationships do not preclude the likelihood that a carcinoma may develop de novo without going through an adenomatous stage.

Clinical manifestations. Most polyps occur in middle-aged and older patients, and most are asymptomatic. The most common symptom is gross or occult bleeding. A change in bowel habits or pain may also occasionally be reported, the pain usually resulting from intussusception or an obstruction caused by a large lesion. Villous adenomas have been associated with the passage of large amounts of protein-rich mucus, which rarely may lead to hypoproteinemia and hypokalemia.

Diagnosis and management. A diagnosis of polyps in most patients being evaluated either because they have symptoms or for screening purposes can be made with routine sigmoidoscopy and/or a barium enema (Fig. 180-4). Flexible fiberoptic sigmoidoscopy and an air-contrast barium enema can detect more and smaller lesions, however, Fiberoptic colonoscopy has also come to play an extremely important role in the diagnosis and management of polypoid colonic lesions. A colonoscopic examination of the whole colon commonly detects lesions not detectable with other techniques. In addition, most polyps can be removed endoscopically by means of snare cautery, even if they are large or sessile. Laparotomy is indicated for only those lesions that cannot be removed endoscopically or, in the case of malignant polyps, if the possibility of residual cancer exists. As a rule, most colonic polyps should be removed, regardless of their size and even if they are asymptomatic, because of their association with cancer. Lesions less than 1 cm, however, have an incidence of malignancy of only about 1%.

After polypectomy, periodic follow-up examinations are mandatory. The stool guaiac test, flexible sigmoidoscopy, an air-contrast barium enema, and colonoscopy should all be part of the program. Though there is no generally accepted protocol for these studies, stool guaiac tests and sigmoidoscopy should probably be performed yearly, whereas the air-contrast barium enema and colonoscopy can be alternated every 2 to 3 years. Patients who have had multiple polyps or polyps with foci of carcinoma and who otherwise have a high risk of carcinoma should have full evaluations annually.

OTHER BENIGN TUMORS. Benign lesions of the colon other than epithelial polyps are rare. Juvenile polyps are large, pedunculated hamartomas that usually occur in childhood, most commonly in the rectum. They may bleed, may cause a rectal prolapse or intussusception, and commonly autoamputate. They also occur as a part of several inherited multiple polyposis syndromes. Pseudopolyps consist of inflammatory and normal elements and usually occur in conjunction with ulcerative colitis, but they may

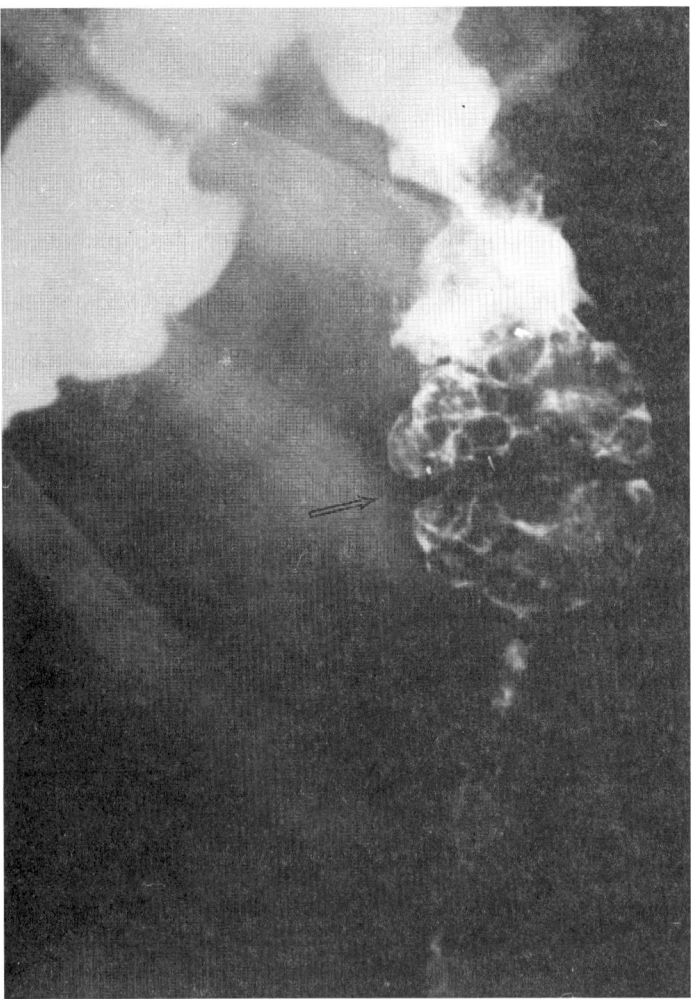

Fig. 180-4. Large villous adenoma *(arrow)* is revealed by barium enema in proximal portion of descending colon. (Courtesy of George Popky, M.D.)

occur in any inflammatory disease of the colon. Lipomas are sometimes found in the cecum near the ileocecal valve. Leiomyomas rarely occur in the colon but when present may ulcerate and cause hemorrhage much as they do in the stomach and small bowel.

Malignant tumors

ADENOCARCINOMA. Colorectal cancer is one of the most common causes of death resulting from a malignancy; it comprises almost half of the gastrointestinal cancers in the United States. Adenocarcinomas account for over 95% of all colorectal malignancies. As is the case with many other tumors, there is wide variation in the incidence of colon cancer among different populations around the world. As a rule, the more industrialized nations have a significantly higher incidence than less industrialized societies. Many explanations have been proposed to account for this difference. In industrialized societies the relatively high-fat, low-residue diet, food additives, ingested carcinogens, and less frequent bowel movements have all been postulated as possible causative factors. A high-fiber diet, frequent stools, and lack of exposure to industrial carcinogens and additives are thought by some to explain the lower incidence in less industrialized cultures. Because none of these relationships has been proved, they remain interesting but speculative factors.

A number of medical conditions, however, have a definite association with the development of colon cancer, including the presence of adenomatous, villous, or mixed polyps, familial multiple polyposis and Gardner's syndrome, and chronic ulcerative colitis, especially universal colitis beginning before adulthood or of more than 10 years' duration. Genetic factors are probably associated in many cases as well, as is apparent both in cases of multiple polyposis, in which the development of carcinoma is virtually certain, and in data showing that the chances of having colon cancer are increased for family members of patients with the disease. In addition there is evidence that a "cancer family" syndrome exists in which many members are affected.

Adenocarcinomas may occur anywhere in the colon, but approximately 75% occur in the sigmoid colon or rectum. Fewer than 15% occur proximal to the hepatic flexure, and the rest are in the transverse or descending colon. Four types of growth patterns have been described: ulcerating, polypoid, colloid, and scirrhous. Except for possible difference in the presenting symptoms, there is no practical importance in this classification.

Clinical manifestations. The symptoms of adenocarcinomas vary depending on their gross morphologic form and location in the colon. Abdominal pain is a common complaint in a majority of patients with lesions proximal to the peritoneal reflection but occurs in only about 25% of those with rectal tumors. The majority of colon cancers bleed, but gross blood in the stool is more common with left-sided lesions. Iron deficiency anemia, sometimes profound, is more common in cecal and ascending colon tumors. Changes in bowel habits commonly occur, especially with left-sided lesions. Patients may complain of recent constipation, diarrhea, or a change in the timing, frequency, consistency, or caliber of the stools. Weight loss occurs in 25% to 50% of patients. Other nonspecific symptoms such as anorexia and malaise may also occur. Colloid tumors commonly cause large amounts of mucus to appear in the stool. The more common ulcerating and scirrhous types may occasionally appear more catastrophically, causing an intestinal obstruction or confined or free perforation, particularly with left-sided tumors.

The physical examination may reveal signs of anemia, evidence of recent weight loss, an enlarged and nodular liver or jaundice if there are hepatic metastases, or, less commonly, ascites if peritoneal seeding has occurred. An abdominal mass can be palpated in many patients, particularly those with right-sided lesions. A mass can be palpated directly or through the bowel wall in the rectal examination of many patients with tumors of the rectum or rectosigmoid. A Blumer's or rectal shelf resulting from a pelvic spread may also be detected. Fecal masses proximal to partially obstructing lesions are sometimes present, but with a more acute obstruction there are abdominal distention, tympany, abnormal or absent bowel sounds, and other accompanying signs. Localized or diffuse peritonitis is found if perforation has occurred.

The laboratory findings in patients with colonic cancer are nonspecific. The majority of these patients show evidence of anemia, usually of the iron deficiency type. Most also have positive results on the stool guaiac test, although some lesions may bleed intermittently, occasionally causing negative results. In patients with liver metastases the serum alkaline phosphatase level may rise, but some tumors can themselves produce an alkaline phosphatase isoenzyme. When the hepatic involvement is extensive, the level of serum bilirubin is usually elevated. The peripheral leukocyte count may be elevated in the presence of inflammatory complications such as tumor necrosis and perforation. Carcinoembryonic antigen is present in most patients with a colorectal carcinoma, but the diagnostic value of this determination is unproved because it is also found in patients with other gastrointestinal malignancies and in some benign disorders of the alimentary tract, liver, and lung. The presence of carcinoembryonic antigen may be of prognostic value, however, in proven cases of colon and rectal cancer.

Diagnosis. Any patient whose clinical presentation even remotely suggests the possibility of colorectal cancer should be evaluated for this disease. The initial studies should include a stool guaiac test, a digital rectal examination, sigmoidoscopy, and a barium enema (Fig. 180-5). About 50% to 60% of all colon cancers can be visualized with the conventional 25-cm (10-inch) sigmoidoscope. With flexible fiberoptic sigmoidoscopy about 75% can be seen. With endoscopy the lesions appear as friable, stalked, or sessile polypoid intraluminal masses; as circumferential, constricting lesions that partially or completely occlude the lumen; or as localized areas of inflamed, ulcerated tissue. On roentgenograms colon cancer can appear as an intraluminal, polypoid filling defect; as an abrupt localized stenosis, sometimes with overhanging edges giving it an apple core appearance; or just as an area of focal mucosal irregularity and stiffness. It is very difficult to differentiate benign from malignant polyps on roentgenograms except to ascertain probabilities. In general, almost half of all lesions over 2 cm in diameter contain malignancy, about 10% of lesions between 1 and 2 cm in diameter are malignant, and only 1% of polyps under 1 cm in size contain cancer. As is true with upper gastrointestinal barium contrast studies, an air-contrast barium enema detects more and smaller lesions than the conventional procedure.

Fiberoptic colonoscopy should also be employed as a complement to the barium enema in the workup of most patients. Because about 3% of colon cancers occur with a second synchronous malignancy and also because the incidence of other simultaneous benign neoplasms is increased, colonoscopy is appropriate even in cases in which a lesion has already been detected by sigmoidoscopy or a barium enema. It is certainly indicated when there is a strong clinical suspicion and other studies are negative or inconclusive. Colonoscopy is most productively used to determine the nature of roentgenographically or clinically suspected lesions by direct visualization, by snare-cautery removal of polypoid masses when possible, and by biopsy and cytologic studies of nonremovable lesions. Several benign diseases may mimic carcinoma of the colon very closely. The diagnosis must differentiate an adenocarcinoma from other diseases such as a colonic stricture resulting from inflammatory disease such as ulcerative colitis or granulomatous colitis, lymphogranuloma venereum, an ischemic stricture, and diverticulitis. Cecal involvement with an appendiceal abscess, tuberculosis, an amebic granuloma, or actinomycosis may also be difficult to distinguish roentgenographically from carcinoma. Colonic sar-

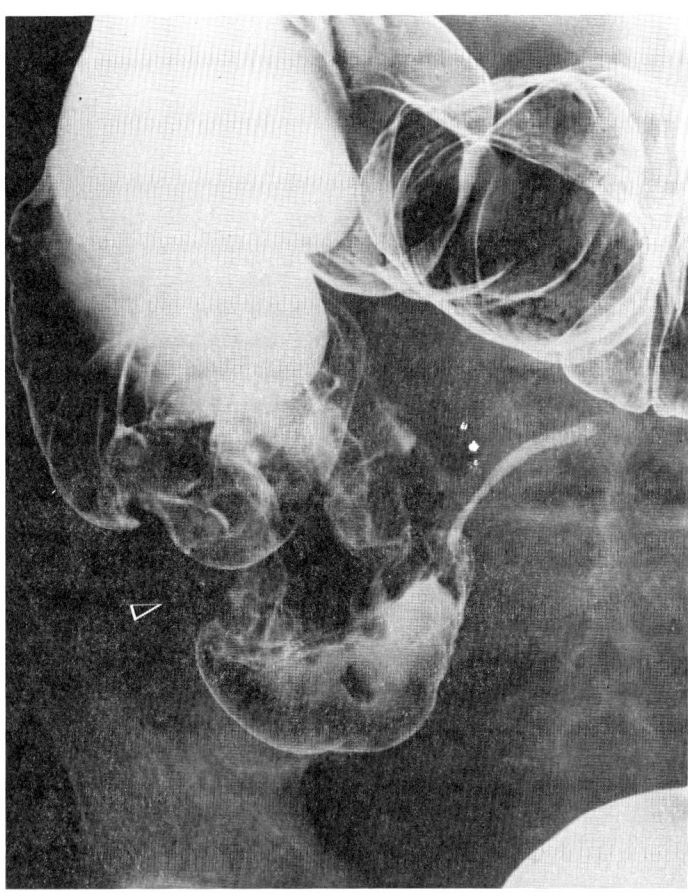

Fig. 180-5. Air-contrast study of colon reveals constricting carcinoma *(arrow)* in ascending colon, just above cecum. (Courtesy of George Popky, M.D.)

comas, although rare, must also be differentiated.

Management. The only potentially curative therapy for colorectal cancer is surgical extirpation of the tumor. Colonoscopic snare-cautery removal of polypoid lesions is probably curative if the malignancy does not extend to the line of resection. In all other circumstances laparotomy is advised. Lesions above the peritoneal reflection can usually be handled by a wide resection and end-to-end anastomosis. Lesions below this level may require an abdominoperineal resection that necessitates performing a permanent colostomy. The patient's level of carcinoembryonic antigen should be obtained before surgery for reference in the follow-up period. A preoperative evaluation to detect local and distant spread should be performed with an intravenous urogram and a radionuclide scan of the liver, perhaps supplemented by a liver needle biopsy if it is indicated. If these studies have positive results, attempts at curative surgery should not be made, but palliative procedures should not be avoided to correct or even prevent complications such as an obstruction, hemorrhage, or perforation. Rectal lesions in patients who are not surgical candidates can be managed with fulguration or local excision. Radiation therapy and chemotherapy have been tried in combination with and without surgery, resulting in an increased length of survival.

Prognosis. Although the overall 5-year survival rate for patients with colorectal carcinoma treated with surgery is about 37%, the prognosis in individual cases depends on several factors. In general, the survival rate is negatively correlated with an increasing degree of penetration by the tumor through the bowel wall, increasing numbers of positive regional lymph nodes, and the degree of histologic dedifferentiation. In 3% of these patients a second primary colon cancer develops, and in the majority there is a recurrence of the primary tumor within 5 years after surgery. For this reason a program of follow-up care should be instituted that includes periodic physical examination, stool guaiac tests, liver function tests, sigmoidoscopy, and an air-contrast barium enema or colonoscopy. If a high preoperative level of carcinoembryonic antigen decreases significantly after surgery, periodic determinations of its level have prognostic value because a tumor recurrence may be signaled by a rise toward the preoperative level.

Other malignancies

Lymphomas rarely occur as a primary colorectal lesion. When present, a lymphoma commonly causes abdominal pain and gross bleeding or may result in intussusception. A lymphoma usually appears similar to an adenocarcinoma on roentgenograms but may mimic ulcerative colitis. The treatment is a combination of radiation therapy and surgery. Leiomyosarcomas are also rare but almost always involve the rectum or sigmoid colon, producing pain, bleeding, and constipation. Carcinoid tumors of the colon are most common in the rectum and rarely produce the carcinoid syndrome. Epidermoid carcinomas of the anus account for about 2% of large bowel cancers and usually cause local pain and a bleeding mass. The rare mucinous adenocarcinoma of the anal glands may appear as recurrent anorectal fistulas. Malignant melanoma has also been reported to arise in the anal skin.

GASTROINTESTINAL POLYPOSIS SYNDROMES

The gastrointestinal polyposis syndromes are a group of interesting but exceedingly rare disorders that have in common the presence of large numbers of polyps in the alimentary tract and that are with one exception of genetic origin. They are differentiated from one another on the basis of histopathologic findings, the distribution of lesions, patterns of inheritance, and extraintestinal manifestations. At least six different syndromes have been described.

Familial polyposis coli

Familial polyposis coli is the most common of the polyposis syndromes. It is characterized by the appearance in childhood or early adulthood of adenomatous polyps that are usually confined to the colon but have also been reported in several patients in the stomach and small intestine. The lesions may be pedunculated or sessile, and they generally remain small. With time, however, they increase in number until there may be literally hundreds of polyps carpeting the colon from the rectum to the cecum. The disease is transmitted as an autosomal dominant trait.

The symptoms, when they occur, consist of abdominal pain, diarrhea with or without blood, and occasionally weight loss. Some patients remain asymptomatic, and their disease is diagnosed only because they are known to be members of an affected kindred. The early diagnosis of this disease is extremely important because the incidence of adenocarcinoma of the colon approaches 100%, usually developing between the ages of 20 and 40 years.

The diagnosis can usually be made with a barium enema, sigmoidoscopy, or colonoscopy and biopsy. Because of the almost universal tendency of familial polyposis coli to develop into carcinoma, the preferred management is early total proctocolectomy.

Gardner's syndrome

Gardner's syndrome is characterized by multiple polyposis of the colon in association with bony and soft tissue tumors. The colonic lesions are adenomatous polyps similar to those occurring in familial polyposis coli but may not be as numerous. They may also occasionally be found in the small intestine, particularly the ileum. The disease is inherited as an autosomal dominant trait, and the clinical features related to the colon are the same as in familial polyposis coli.

The extraintestinal manifestations of Gardner's syndrome usually precede the appearance of the colonic lesions by many years. The most common bony lesions are osteomas, which have a tendency to affect the mandible and facial bones leading to a noticeable deformity. There may also be multiple exostoses and a thickening of the cortices of the long bones. The soft tissue lesions affect mostly cutaneous and subcutaneous tissues but may also affect other areas of the body. The most common abnormalities are epidermoid cysts, lipomas, fibromas, and connective tissue tumors. In addition there is a tendency for masses of fibrous tissue hyperplasia to form, leading to keloids in scars, adhesions after surgery in the abdomen, and fibrous tumors of the retroperitoneum and peritoneal space.

The potential of these intestinal lesions to become malignant is the same as in familial polyposis coli. The preferred management is an early total colectomy.

Peutz-Jeghers syndrome

The Peutz-Jeghers syndrome is defined by the association of generalized gastrointestinal polyposis with mucocutaneous pigmentation. It is transmitted as a single pleiotropic gene that has a high degree of penetrance. The histologic examination reveals that these polyps are hamartomas or juvenile polyps with a prominent smooth muscle component. They occur most often in the small intestine, particularly in the jejunum and ileum, but may affect the stomach and colon as well. Polyps have also been reported in the respiratory and urinary tracts. The lesions appear in childhood and may produce symptoms related to the polyps, such as hemorrhage, intestinal obstruction, intestinal infarction resulting from torsion, or intussusception.

Mucocutaneous pigmentation occurs in Peutz-Jeghers syndrome as hairless melanin spots usually found on the lips, buccal mucosa, face, forearms, hands, soles, digits, and the perianal region. Other associated findings include ovarian cysts and tumors, exostoses, and digital clubbing. Not all features of the syndrome are present in every patient.

The incidence of gastrointestinal carcinomas in this syndrome is about 2% to 3%, an incidence greater than that in the general population. The only treatment for the disorder, however, is aimed at management of the complications; preventive surgery is not indicated.

Juvenile polyposis

Two forms of juvenile polyposis, a heritable disorder, have been recognized: juvenile polyposis coli and generalized juvenile polyposis. The histologic examination reveals that the lesions are hamartomas that differ from the Peutz-Jegher polyp in lacking smooth muscle components but that are histologically the same as those found in the

Cronkhite-Canada syndrome. The disease typically develops in childhood, but the polyps may also be found in adults in the same families. It is thought to be transmitted as an autosomal dominant trait.

Regardless of whether the polyps are limited to the colon or are distributed throughout the gastrointestinal tract, the symptoms are usually the result of a complication such as hemorrhage or intussusception. It is not unusual with sigmoidoscopy or colonoscopy to find stalks without tumors as a result of autoamputation. Juvenile polyps are not considered to be premalignant, but various carcinomas have occurred in nonaffected members of some kindreds. Some patients have had congenital anomalies, but the ectodermal abnormalities seen in the Cronkhite-Canada syndrome do not occur. There is no treatment except for the management of complications.

BIBLIOGRAPHY

Hancock, R.J.: An 11-year review of primary tumors of the small bowel including the duodenum. Can. Med. Assoc. J. **103**:1177, 1970.

McNeer, G., and Pack, G.T.: Neoplasms of the stomach, Philadelphia, 1967, J.B. Lippincott Co.

Nagayo, T., and Yokoyama, H.: Cancer of the gastrointestinal tract: early phases and diagnostic features, J.A.M.A. **228**:888, 1974.

Nakayama, K., and Kinoshita, Y.: Surgical treatment combined with preoperative concentrated irradiation, J.A.M.A. **227**:178, 1974.

Sherlock, P., and others: Malignant lymphoma of the gastrointestinal tract. In Glass, G.B.J., editor: Progress in gastroenterology, vol. 2, New York, 1970, Grune & Stratton, Inc.

Welch, C.E., and Hedberg, S.E.: Polypoid lesions of the gastrointestinal tract, vol. 2, Major problems in clinical surgery, ed. 2, Philadelphia, 1975, W.B. Saunders Co.

Wennstrom, J., Pierce, E.R., and McKusick, V.A.: Hereditary benign and malignant lesions of the large bowel, Cancer **34**(suppl.):850, 1974.

Winawer, S.J., Sherlock, P., and Miller, D.C.: Screening for colon cancer, Gastroenterology **70**:783, 1976.

Witzel, L., and others: Evaluation of specific value of endoscopic biopsies and brush cytology for malignancies of the esophagus and stomach. Gut **17**:375, 1976.

Wolf, W.I., and Shinya, H.: Comparison of colonoscopy and the contrast enema in five hundred patients with colorectal disease. Am. J. Surg. **129**:181, 1975.

181 • DISEASES OF THE PERITONEUM AND MESENTERY

William O. Frank

ANATOMY AND PHYSIOLOGY

ANATOMY. The peritoneal cavity and the organs it contains are lined by a serous membrane, the peritoneum. The visceral peritoneum encases the abdominal organs and forms the mesenteries from which they are suspended. The parietal peritoneum lines the anterior, lateral, and posterior walls of the abdominal cavity. Retroperitoneal organs such as the duodenum, ascending and descending colon, and portions of the pancreas, kidneys, and adrenal glands are lined anteriorly by the parietal peritoneum.

BLOOD SUPPLY. The majority of the peritoneal surface and mesentery is supplied by the splanchnic arteries and drained by the splanchnic and portal venous system. A much smaller portion of the peritoneal surface is supplied by the intercostal, subcostal, lumber, and iliac arteries and drained by the lumbar and iliac veins that enter the inferior vena cava.

INNERVATION. The innervation of the parietal peritoneum differs from that of the visceral peritoneum. Twigs from the spinal nerves that supply the abdominal wall innervate the respective areas of the parietal peritoneum. An irritation of the parietal peritoneum thus gives rise to afferent stimuli transmitted via the intercostal nerves and perceived as *somatic pain*. In contrast, an irritation of the visceral peritoneum gives rise to afferent stimuli transmitted via the distribution of the respective visceral sympathetic nervous system. The diaphragmatic peritoneum has a double innervation: the phrenic nerves innervate its central portion and the intercostal nerves its peripheral portion. A pathologic condition involving the parietal peritoneum has a more precise pain localization and more definite physical signs than a pathologic condition involving the visceral pertoneum because the parietal peritoneum is innervated by somatic afferent nerves. An irritation of the diaphragmatic peritoneum may refer pain to the shoulder (phrenic innervation) or to the thoracic and abdominal wall (intercostal innervation).

PHYSIOLOGY. The movement of fluid and both high- and low-molecular-weight solutes across the peritoneal membrane occurs by means of simple passive diffusion. Peritoneal lymphatics remove the solid and liquid material from the peritoneal cavity. The intercellular gaps between the mesothelial cells that line the peritoneal cavity and the endothelial cells of the terminal lymphatics permit this passive passage of fluid and solutes.

The clearance of peritoneal fluid from the abdominal cavity is biphasic; a rapid initial clearance is followed by a slower constant clearance phase. Studies in humans using intraperitoneal saline and radioactive-labeled albumin indicate that an equilibration of saline between the serum and peritoneal fluid occurs within 2 hours, after which fluid is absorbed at a relatively constant rate of 33 ml an hour. In the initial 2 hours the rate of absorption varies with the osmolar gradient and becomes constant after equilibration.

DIAGNOSIS OF PERITONEAL DISEASES

HISTORY AND PHYSICAL EXAMINATION. The cardinal manifestations of peritoneal disease are abdominal pain and ascites. Direct tenderness, rebound tenderness, and involuntary spasm of the anterior abdominal musculature are the major signs of peritoneal irritation.

ROENTGENOGRAPHY. Ascites may reflect the presence of peritoneal disease. Large amounts of fluid are detected on plain abdominal roentgenograms as abdominal haziness, an increased density shifting to the pelvis on upright films, a separation of bowel loops, and the obliteration of the psoas muscle shadows. Smaller amounts of fluid (800 to 1000 ml) are detected by an obliteration of the hepatic angle, an increased thickness between the air-filled bowel lumen and extraperitoneal fat layer, and a widening of the flank strip (the line formed by the lateral colonic wall and peritoneum). A sonographic examination of the abdominal cavity can also detect ascites.

Other specialized roentgenographic techniques are available for detecting peritoneal disease, such as the introduction of pneumoperitoneum for demonstrating nodules on the parietal peritoneum. Barium contrast studies of the gastrointestinal tract may demonstrate bizarre angular patterns of the intestinal loops, rigidity of the bowel along with diminished peristalsis, or altered mucosal patterns along with filling defects or flattened folds and indirectly reflect the visceral peritoneal involvement of the small bowel.

ABDOMINAL PARACENTESIS. Diagnostic paracentesis for the detection of obvious or suspected ascites can be easily performed at the bedside with the patient sitting or supine after having emptied his bladder. The midline area located midway between the umbilicus and pubis is anesthetized, and a needle or catheter is inserted using a sterile technique. The aspirated fluid is evaluated by gross inspection and the following examinations: the determination of specific gravity, a cell count and differential cell count, a Gram stain, a bacterial culture and cultures of tuberculosis and fungi, a cytologic examination, a Sudan stain evaluation, and determinations of protein, glucose, amylase, lactic dehydrogenase, and lipid concentrations.

PERITONEAL BIOPSY. Cope's needle or the Vim-Silverman needle can be used to perform a biopsy of the peritoneum. With this technique hemorrhage is the major complication, usually from enlarged intra-abdominal veins, but a perforation or infections may also occurr. Adequate tissue for histologic study can usually be obtained with either needle, but the diagnostic yield with the blunt-ended Cope's needle is probably higher.

PERITONEOSCOPY. With peritoneoscopy the clinician can directly inspect the peritoneum or abdominal organs and perform a biopsy of a suspected pathologic lesion under direct vision. The technique is described under fully in Chapter 171.

ASCITES

PATHOPHYSIOLOGY. Ascites is the accumulation of fluid within the peritoneal cavity. The mechanisms of this accumulation have not been exactly defined, but the development of ascites is associated with several abnormal physiologic factors. Alterations in the protal venous pressure, colloidal osmotic pressure, hepatic lymph formation, splanchnic lymphatic drainage, sodium metabolism, and subperitoneal capillary permeability have been thought to contribute to ascitic fluid accumulation.

An elevated portal venous pressure increases the hydrostatic pressure in the splanchnic capillary bed and increases the filtration pressure. The elevated filtration pressure is balanced by the plasma collodial osmotic pressure, which primarily reflects the albumin concentration. According to the Frank-Starling law, a rise in the portal venous pressure or a fall in the plasma albumin concentration leads to ascites formation. In addition, an increased hepatic lymph formation and decreased splanchnic lymphatic reabsorption may cause an ascitic fluid accumulation, especially in patients with cirrhosis. Renal sodium retention leads to an expansion of plasma volume and secondarily to ascites because of an overflow phenomenon. Renal sodium retention may occur in patients with cirrhosis for a number of reasons, including an impaired hepatic inactivation of aldosterone or renin, a hepatic production of the humoral stimulator of aldosterone secretion, or a deficiency of an unknown natriuretic hormone. Alterations in renal hemodynamics in cases of cirrhosis, particularly an intrarenal vasoconstriction that reduces cortical perfusion, may also cause renal sodium retention. Excessive sodium reabsorption and impaired water diuresis at the proximal or distal tubules may possibly also account for the increased sodium retention in cases of cirrhosis. Finally, an increased permeability of the subperitoneal capillaries in patients with inflammatory and neoplastic diseases of the peritoneum may cause ascites formation. The relative importance of these possible mechanisms, however, undoubtedly varies according to the underlying disorder and the individual patient, and the mechanism remains uncertain in most cases.

CLINICAL AND LABORATORY FINDINGS. Abdominal distention is the major symptom of ascites, and when a large amount of fluid is present, the patient may also complain of dyspnea and abdominal discomfort. In the physical examination the flanks can be seen to bulge, and a fluid wave may be elicited. If 1.5 to 2 L of fluid is present, a shifting dullness can usually be detected. Placing the patient on his hands and knees and percussing the flatness over the dependent abdomen (puddle sign) may detect as little as 300 to 400 ml of fluid.

A laboratory evaluation of the peritoneal fluid is essential. Exudative and transudative ascitic fluid are differentiated by their protein concentrations and specific gravity. Peritoneal fluid with protein concentrations greater than 3 g/100 ml or a specific gravity greater than 1.016 is classified as an exudate; peritoneal fluid with values below these is designated as a transudate. *Transudative ascites* is usually associated with congestive heart failure, an inferior vena cava obstruction, the Budd-Chiari syndrome, hypoalbuminemia, cirrhosis, Meigs' syndrome, and vasculitis. *Exudative ascites* is usually found in cases of a peritoneal malignancy, tuberculous peritonitis, myxedema, pancreatic ascites, and bacterial peritonitis, although exudative ascites may also occur in cases of uncomplicated congestive heart failure or cirrhosis. Glucose concentrations less than 60 mg/dl suggest a neoplastic effusion. Amylase or lipase levels are increased in patients with pancreatic ascites. Triglyceride levels are higher in the peritoneal fluid than in the plasma in patients with chylous ascites. Bloody ascites usually indicates a neoplasm, particularly a hepatoma or ovarian carcinoma. A leukocyte count of 250 cells/mm^3 or more in the ascitic fluid is an indication of a peritoneal irritation caused by an infection, inflammation, or tumor infiltration. The white blood cell differential count is important. Polymorphonuclear leukocytes reflect an acute bacterial infection, whereas mononuclear cells characterize a chronic inflammatory disease. A cytologic examination to detect a malignancy is valuable; it has positive results in 60% to 90% of these cases.

DIFFERENTIAL DIAGNOSIS. Ascites may be found in patients with or without direct involvement of the peritoneum. Portal hypertension and hypoalbuminemia are common causes of ascites in patients without direct involvement.

PORTAL HYPERTENSION

Cirrhosis. Cirrhosis is the most common cause of ascites in North America. The causes of cirrhotic ascites involve many factors including portal hypertension, hypoalbuminemia, alterations in lymph flow, and the renal retention of sodium and water. Ascites in patients with cirrhosis is discussed in Chapter 183.

Cardiac causes of portal hypertension. A mechanical or functional impedance to hepatic venous flow is often associated with ascites. Cases of congestive heart failure, particularly right-sided and constrictive pericarditis; are included in this chapter. Constrictive pericarditis should be considered in cases of ascites of obscure origin, and appropriate diagnostic tests should be performed, including cardiac catheterization if necessary.

Inferior vena cava and hepatic vein obstruction. Inferior vena cava and hepatic vein obstructions characteristically cause acites and hepatomegaly (the Budd-Chiari syndrome). This syndrome occurs when thrombi, venous fibrosis, anomalous venous valves, or a tumor occludes the hepatic venous outflow. Thrombosis may result from polycythemia vera (and other causes of hyperviscosity or thrombocytosis) or from hemoglobinopathies such as sickle cell disease or may be associated with the use of oral contraceptives. An idiopathic membranous obstruction of the inferior vena cava, a surgically correctable condition, has been reported in Japan.

The clinical presentation and course of this disorder may be acute, subacute, or chronic. The signs and symptoms include abdominal pain with ascites and tender hepatomegaly. Splenomegaly and jaundice are much less common, and the results of liver function tests are often not dramatically abnormal. The diagnostic workup commonly shows an elevated femoral venous pressure along with normal pressures in the superior vena cava, and a liver biopsy reveals centrilobular necrosis and congestion and/or centrilobular fibrosis and occasionally cirrhosis. Hepatic venography may show a vena cava obstruction or a narrow, occluded main hepatic vein with a network pattern of neighboring veins.

HYPOALBUMINEMIA. Approximately 12% of patients with the nephrotic syndrome have ascites. These patients almost invariably have a level of serum albumin lower than 2.5 g/dl and usually lower than 1.5 g/dl. Protein-losing enteropathy and malnutrition are rare causes of hypoalbuminemic ascites in North America.

OTHER ASCITES. Ascites may occur in patients with myxedema or ovarian disease or in the form of pancreatic ascites, bile ascites, or chylous ascites.

Myxedema. Patients with myxedema often have significant exudative ascites that responds poorly to diuretics. The peritoneal fluid is yellow and gelatinous and has a protein concentration greater than 4 g/dl; the protein electrophoresis of ascitic fluid is similar to that of the serum. This ascites is thought to result from an increased capillary permeability and an escape of protein-rich fluid. The ascites is rapidly cleared after the start of thyroid therapy.

Ovarian disease. Ovarian carcinoma, Meigs' syndrome, and the ovarian overstimulation syndrome are causes of ascites in female patients. Meigs' syndrome consists of ascites and hydrothorax associated with ovarian fibromas or cystadenomas. *Struma ovarii* is a rare, unilateral ovarian teratoma that contains thyroid tissue. Patients may have the symptoms of hyperthyroidism, ascites, or an ovarian mass. The diagnosis should be suspected if abdominal roentgenograms demonstrate ovarian calcification and if iodine 131 uptake is localized in the abdomen. After treatment with clomiphene citrate and human menopausal gonadotropin, the ovarian overstimulation syndrome may occur, leading to massive ascites, pleural effusions, and hypovolemia with enlarged ovaries.

Pancreatic ascites. Ascites may develop in patients with acute pancreatitis, chronic pancreatitis, or a pancreatic carcinoma. Occasionally a massive, intractable, exudative ascites develops in patients with chronic pancreatitis. This pancreatic ascites usually results from a leaking pseudocyst or a break in the pancreatic duct. The leaking pancreatic juice in either case causes a chemical peritonitis with elevated levels of protein, amylase, and lipase in the ascitic fluid. These patients rarely respond to conventional medical management and often require surgical intervention to correct the pancreatic pathologic condition before the ascites resolves.

Bile ascites. Bile ascites, which results from the leakage of bile from the hepatobiliary tree, usually occurs in patients who have had bile duct surgery. Its onset may be delayed until 2 months postoperatively. The magnitude and severity of the ascites usually reflect the magnitude of the leakage. A peritoneal tape reveals bile in the fluid, and the diagnosis can virtually be made on this basis. Occasionally the bile ascites resolves after the paracentesis, but the majority of patients require surgical correction of the leaking biliary tree.

The acute leakage of bile into the peritoneal cavity, as is sometimes observed after a percutaneous liver biopsy, may result in acute severe peritonitis (bile peritonitis) and the rapid progression of the patient into shock; such cases may require immediate surgical intervention to drain the peritoneal cavity and repair the hepatic or biliary tear.

Chylous ascites. Acute or chronic chylous ascites occurs when there is assumulation of lipid-rich lymph in the peritoneal cavity. Malignant or benign neoplasms are the cause in 80% of the chronic cases. These patients usually have weight loss, hypoproteinemia, and inanition but not abdominal pain. The cause of acute chylous ascites may be an obstruction, trauma, or rupture of chyle-containing cysts, but in the majority of patients no cause is found. These patients have an abrupt onset of crampy abdominal pain, usually after a heavy meal and usually localized in the right lower quadrant.

The peritoneal fluid in patients with chylous ascites is turbid, separates into lipid and aqueous layers on standing, and stains positively for fat. The fluid is sterile and has an elevated lymphocyte count and a high lipid content (the triglyceride levels exceed those of plasma). *Pseudochylous ascites* is also opalescent but contains phospholipid-protein material from degenerating cells rather than large amounts of triglycerides.

The cause of chylous ascites is often discovered only with laparotomy. Intravenous hyperalimentation or the administration of medium-chain triglycerides may be helpful. Acute or idiopathic cases usually clear spontaneously, but chronic cases usually lead to progressive debilitation and death, depending on the underlying neoplasm.

TREATMENT OF ASCITES. The successful treatment of ascites often depends on the treatment of underlying disease. In patients with cirrhotic ascites the mainstays of medical therapy are sodium restriction (250 to 500 mg/day) and diuretics. Judicious use of this medical regimen should not cause complications. Some patients with a refractory ascites that does not respond to conventional medical therapy may be candidates for the LeVeen shunt, which continuously infuses the ascitic fluid into the patient's systemic venous circulation. (See Chapter 183 for further discussion of the therapy of ascites.)

INFECTIONS OF THE PERITONEUM
Tuberculous peritonitis

Tuberculous peritonitis, one of the most important diseases involving the peritoneum, is an unusual form of tuberculosis. The incidence is approximately 0.5%. Tuberculous peritonitis may commonly be mistaken for a neoplastic disease or for ascites caused by cirrhosis. Cirrhosis in fact predisposes the patient to tuberculous peritonitis.

PATHOGENESIS. A tubercle bacillus infection of the peritoneum may occur as the result of (1) an activation of a long-latent tuberculous focus in the peritoneum, (2) a primary focus in the lung or elsewhere, (3) infected mesenteric lymph nodes, (4) a contamination from tuberculous enteritis, and (5) tuberculous salpingitis. Although an extraperitoneal site of infection is present in the majority of patients, it is often not clinically apparent. The extraperitoneal site of infection may be active or inactive. In fact, many patients with tuberculous peritonitis appear to have a reactivation of a latent peritoneal focus established at the time of earlier hematogenous spread from a primary focus, usually in the lung. A hematogenous spread from active pulmonary tuberculosis or diffuse miliary tuberculosis can, however, also cause active tuberculous peritonitis.

EPIDEMIOLOGY. Tuberculous peritonitis is most commonly found in an inner-city population in which cirrhosis is common and many patients are poorly nourished and debilitated. There is no sex or age predilection, but 80% to 90% of the patients in previously reported clinical series were black.

CLINICAL MANIFESTATIONS. Tuberculous peritonitis should be suspected in patients with ascites, fever, and unexplained constitutional symptoms with or without diffuse abdominal pain or tenderness. Symptoms are usually constitutional and nonspecific. The majority of patients have an insidious onset and have constitutional symptoms for several months before the diagnosis; fever, anorexia, weakness, malaise, and weight loss are present in 80% of these patients. Abdominal pain is usually described as being vague, dull, and diffuse but is present in only one half of the patients. Rarely, tuberculous peritonitis may appear as an acute condition of the abdomen. Vomiting, diarrhea, and constipation are variable symptoms. The physical examination reveals the presence of ascites along with diffuse abdominal tenderness in approximately 70% of these patients. Hepatomegaly or a palpable mass caused by loculated fluid or inflamed mesentery is present in one fourth of these patients. A lymphadenopathy may be present, but the classic doughy abdomen is rare. The "dry" form of tuberculous peritonitis involves little or no ascites, but extensive peritoneal adhesions are present.

LABORATORY FINDINGS. Routine blood studies are usually normal, including the white blood cell and differential counts, level of hemoglobin, and hematocrit. The tuberculin skin test is positive in most patients. If the disease is generalized, other studies may prove useful. A chest roentgenogram shows pulmonary infiltrates in about 15% of these patients and pleural effusions in 40%. Contrast studies of the gastrointestinal tract, pyelograms, and salpingograms are rarely useful. A transthoracic liver biopsy or lymph node biopsy may show caseating granulomata but does not prove that there is also peritoneal involvement.

Less than one half of these patients have evidence of disease outside the peritoneum.

The most important initial diagnostic test is an examination of the peritoneal fluid. In patients with tuberculous peritonitis the protein concentration is greater than 2.5 g/dl and the count of leukocytes, predominantly monuclear, is greater than 250 cells/mm^3. Acid-fast stains of the peritoneal fluid have positive results in less than 5% of patients and cultures in only 40%; however, if 1 L of ascitic fluid is removed and centrifugally concentrated before being cultured, the yield is increased to 80%. A peritoneal biopsy shows granulomata in 70% of these patients, but the culture yield from peritoneal biopsies is not well known. Peritoneoscopy or laparotomy is probably the best method for diagnosing tuberculous peritonitis. Peritoneoscopy should be performed first, however, and laparotomy then only if the results of peritoneoscopy are inconclusive and the diagnosis is still suspected.

PROGNOSIS AND MANAGEMENT. Before appropriate chemotherapy was available, the mortality of tuberculous peritonitis was approximately 60%. With the introduction of antituberculous chemotherapy, the disease is now curable. After chemotherapy begins, the constitutional symptoms should resolve within 1 to 2 weeks, and fever should disappear by the fourth week. The role of steroids in the treatment of tuberculous peritonitis to reduce the incidence of late fibrotic complications is unclear.

Intra-abdominal abscess

Abscesses in the abdomen are usually caused by anaerobic bacteria (particularly *Bacteroides fragilis* and gram-positive cocci) mixed with enteric gram-negative bacilli. The most common locations are in and around the liver, around the appendix, and in the area of the distal colon. Abscesses usually follow a spontaneous perforation of the bowel (such as from a diverticulum or the appendix), surgery on the large bowel, or infection in the biliary tract. From an abscess in the abdomen the infection may spread to the liver via the lymphatics, the venous channels, or the arterial system or by direct extension. Certain anaerobic bacteria are likely to cause septic phlebitis along with resultant septic emboli carried to the liver through the portal system or to the lungs through veins draining the lower rectum or pelvis. (See discussion of "Infections caused by nonsporeforming anaerobes" in Chapter 49.)

Patients with intra-abdominal abscesses have fever with or without symptoms or signs related to the abdomen. Although the patient may have pain, tenderness, or a mass, there may be no physical findings or complaints referable to the abdomen. Leukocytosis is usually present along with a shift to the left in the white cell series. Blood cultures may have a positive result. The abscess may be deomonstrable with ultrasonography, a liver-spleen scan, computed tomography, or a gallium scan (gallium is concentrated in pus).

The therapy consists of surgical drainage and treatment with antibiotics directed against the likely bacteria. Clindamycin (600 mg intravenously every 6 hours in adults), chloramphenicol (12.5 mg/kg intravenously every 6 hours), or metronidazole (7.5 mg/kg intravenously every 6 hours) is administered for anaerobes. In addition, an aminoglycoside (such as gentamicin, 1.7 mg/kg intravenously or intramuscularly every 8 hours when renal function is normal) is administered for Enterobacteriaceae. Therapy is continued for at least 2 weeks. If metronidazole is used, a penicillin or cephalosporin should be added to the regimen because of metronidazole's poor activity against gram-positive anaerobes.

NEOPLASMS OF THE PERITONEUM
Primary mesothelioma

Primary mesotheliomas, which are rare, arise from the epithelial and mesenchymal components of the mesothelium. The majority of patients with primary mesotheliomas have a history of asbestos exposure and pathologic evidence of pulmonary asbestosis. Although asbestos appears to play a role in the pathogenesis of mesothelioma, the exact pathophysiologic mechanism is unknown. The tumors usually involve the visceral and parietal peritoneum extensively, but the histologic characteristics are quite variable. Patients with mesotheliomas have abdominal pain, nausea, vomiting, weight loss, abdominal distention, and commonly ascites. A peritoneal biopsy or cytologic examination of the peritoneal fluid may suggest the diagnosis, but an exploratory laparotomy is usually required, often to rule out some other primary neoplasm. Systemic and intraperitoneal chemotherapy and radiation have been tried as therapeutic methods but have not proved helpful. The prognosis is poor, and most patients survive less than 2 years after the diagnosis is made.

Secondary carcinomatosis

Metastatic cancer or the extension of a neighboring primary tumor is a common cause of peritoneal disease. Approximately 80% of these cases are metastatic adenocarcinomas; other metastatic tumors are extremely rare. One third of the patients with leukemia or a lymphoma, however, have an infiltration into the peritoneum. Patients with peritoneal carcinomatosis have diffuse abdominal pain, weight loss, nausea, and vomiting and commonly have ascites. The pathophysiologic mechanism by which peritoneal metastases induce ascites is unknown. The ascitic fluid may be either a transudate or an exudate and often contains red cells or gross blood. Peritoneal carcinomatosis is diagnosed by a cytologic examination of ascitic fluid, a peritoneal biopsy, or peritoneoscopy. The long-term prognosis is poor; however, cytotoxic agents, radioactive implants, or quinacrine instillation leads to a good response in about 50% of these patients.

FAMILIAL PAROXYSMAL POLYSEROSITIS

ETIOLOGY AND PATHOLOGY. Familial paroxysmal polyserositis, or familial Mediterranean fever, is an inherited disease characterized by recurrent, acute, self-limited attacks of fever associated with signs of peritonitis, pleuritis, and arthritis. The cause of familial Mediterranean fever is unknown, but it appears to be inherited as a single autosomal recessive trait and is found predominantly in patients of Mediterranean or Middle Eastern origin. During an acute attack inflammatory changes occur in the serosa that are reversible; however, repeated attacks may lead to secondary inflammatory adhesions. The major complication in these patients is an increased susceptibility to amyloidosis; amyloid is deposited in the intima and media of arterioles and the subendothelial area of venules. There are a characteristic pattern of parenchymal distribution of amyloid and an extensive involvement in the renal glomeruli, adrenal glands, spleen, and pulmonary alveolar septa but usually a sparing of the liver sinusoids and heart muscle (see also Chapter 15).

CLINICAL MANIFESTATIONS. The first attack usually begins when patients are in their first or second decade. The acute attacks are of relatively short duration, 24 to 48 hours, and are unpredictable. Between attacks these patients are completely asymptomatic. An interesting, recently recognized phenomenon is that attacks do not occur during pregnancy. An acute attack is associated with a high fever and the classic signs of peritonitis, pleuritis, and arthritis. The symptoms and signs of peritonitis are virtually universally present in all patients. The disease sometimes cannot easily be differentiated from an acute abdominal catastrophe, and therefore laparotomy occasionally must be performed. An injudicious use of narcotics by these patients may result in drug addiction. Laboratory findings are nonspecific.

DIAGNOSIS. When the characteristic clinical pattern of recurrent self-limited attacks is present in a person of the appropriate ethnic background, the diagnosis is not difficult. Occasionally, however, there is a failure to consider the possibility of this disease, and as a result the patient is subjected to one or more unnecessary laparotomies before the diagnosis is made. Abdominal attacks must be differentiated from acute abdominal disorders such as appendicitis, pancreatitis, cholecystitis, perforations, and intestinal obstructions. In addition, porphyria and hyperlipidemia with acute abdominal symptoms must be excluded from diagnostic possibilities.

MANAGEMENT. The treatment of choice is colchicine therapy. Controlled trials have shown that the prophylactic use of colchicine reduces the frequency of attacks in most patients with familial Mediterranean fever. Furthermore, if colchicine is administered at the onset of the prodrome, attacks may be aborted. The mechanism by which colchicine affects this disease is uncertain, but it is postulated to interfere with the cellular phase of the inflammatory response. Because long-term colchicine therapy may cause azoospermia and chromosomal abnormalities, a course of intermittent therapy should be tried.

PROGNOSIS. If amyloidosis or drug addiction does not develop, the prognosis is excellent and normal longevity can be expected.

OTHER DISEASES OF THE PERITONEUM
Peritoneal vasculitis

The autoimmune vascular diseases such as systemic lupus erythematosus and periarteritis nodosa, as well as the allergic vasculitis associated with Schönlein-Henoch purpura, are rare causes of isolated peritonitis. Both categories of these vasculitis syndromes, however, more commonly involve the arteries of the gut and thereby may cause a hemorrhage, ulceration, perforation, obstruction, or infarction of the gastrointestinal tract. Laparotomy may be the only way to distinguish isolated peritonitits from a gastrointestinal complication in these groups of patients. Cases of isolated peritonitis usually resolve with steroid therapy.

Granulomatous peritonitis

Sarcoidosis, Crohn's disease, and foreign bodies may cause noncaseating granulomata in the peritoneum, which may be associated with ascites. Tuberculous peritonitis must be excluded from the diagnostic possibilities in these patients by means of appropriate cultures and tests.

DISEASES OF THE MESENTERY AND OMENTUM
Mesenteric inflammatory disease

Mesenteric inflammatory disease is a poorly defined pathologic condition ranging from inflammatory to fibrotic lesions of the mesentery. It is commonly called mesenteric panniculitis or retractile mesenteritis, depending on its predominant pathologic features.

ETIOLOGY AND PATHOGENESIS. Trauma, infection, or ischemia is the causative agent that initiates the pathologic sequence. It is postulated that the underlying pathogenetic defect involves an excessive growth of normal fat tissue that undergoes degeneration, necrosis, and xanthogranulomatous inflammation. Abnormal lipid material is released from the degenerating lipocytes and causes granulomatous inflammation that progresses to fibrotic scarring.

CLINICAL MANIFESTATIONS. Patients with mesenteric panniculitis have recurrent episodes of localized or generalized crampy abdominal pain, weight loss, nausea, vomiting, and low-grade fever. In certain patients mesenteric panniculitis progresses to retractile mesenteritis. These patients have the same symptoms but in addition may have a bowel obstruction, mesenteric thrombosis, and an intestinal obstruction. Roentgenographic evaluation of the gastrointestinal tract may reveal displacement, extrinsic pressure deformities, separation, and a distortion of mucosal patterns of intestinal segments.

PATHOLOGY. Laparotomy in patients with mesenteric panniculitis reveals a thickened mesenteric root, usually limited to the small bowel mesentery. In patients with retractile mesenteritis the mesentery is thickened, fibrotic, retracted, and studded with pale gray plaques. The histologic examination reveals varying degrees of mesenteric fat, inflammation, and fibrosis.

PROGNOSIS AND MANAGEMENT. Because mesenteric panniculitis is a rare disease, its prognosis and the most appropriate therapy have not been established.

Mesenteric cysts

Mesenteric cysts are usually chylous lymphatic cysts. These cysts are sequestrations of lymph vessels that may or may not communicate with the lymphatic system. The cause of these mesenteric cysts is unknown. They are usually asymptomatic but may produce symptoms that are usually related to their site and size. When they are symptomatic, surgical excision or enucleation is required.

Mesenteric tumors

Mesenteric tumors are rare but may arise from any of the cellular elements of the mesentery.

Mesenteric hernias

Various forms of herniation of the mesentery result from an anomalous intestinal rotation along with fusion of the mesentery and parietal peritoneum during embryonic development.

Omental torsion and infarction

Torsion of the omentum is an acute surgical condition that may mimic acute appendicitis or acute cholecystitis. Cases of omental infarction have a similar clinical picture.

BIBLIOGRAPHY

Berkowitz, H.D., and others: Improved renal function and inhibition of renin and aldosterone secretion following peritoneovenous (LeVeen) shunt. Surgery **84**:120, 1978.

Dinarello, C.A., and others: Colchicine therapy for familial Mediterranean fever; a double-blind trial, N. Engl. J. Med. **291**:934, 1974.

Dineen, P., Homan, N.P., and Grafe, W.R.: Tuberculous peritonitis: 43 years experience in diagnosis and treatment, Ann. Surg. **184**:717, 1976.

Donowitz, M., Kerstein, M.D., and Spiro, H.M.: Pancreatic ascites, Medicine **53**:183, 1974.

Gregory, P.B., and others: Complications of diuresis in the alcoholic patient with ascites: a controlled trial, Gastroenterology **73**:534, 1977.

Sleisenger, M.H., and Fordtran, J.S.: Gastrointestinal disease, ed. 2, Philadelphia, 1978, W.B. Saunders Co.

Tavill, A.S., and others: The Budd-Chiari syndrome: correlation between hepatic scintigraphy and the clinical, radiological and pathological findings in nineteen cases of hepatic venous outflow obstruction, Gastroenterology **68**:509, 1975.

182 • DISORDERS OF THE PANCREAS

Ralph M. Myerson

The pancreas has both endocrine and exocrine components. Although this chapter deals primarily with the exocrine pancreas, the endocrine pancreas also has important gastroenterologic implications.

ENDOCRINE PANCREAS. The specialized cells of the endocrine component of the pancreas, the islets of Langerhans, secrete at least five hormonal substances. The β-cells secrete insulin, and the α-cells secrete glucagon. The effects of these hormones on glucose metabolism and their role in the pathophysiology of diabetes mellitus are discussed in Chapter 198. Glucagon also appears to inhibit pancreatic secretion in man. Other specialized islet cells, the δ-cells, secrete somatostatin, a polypeptide whose exact physiologic role is as yet undetermined. It is believed to have an inhibiting effect on the release of pituitary growth hormone, which has a pancreaticotrophic influence. Other polypeptide hormones believed to be produced in the islets include vasoactive intestinal polypeptide (VIP), pancreatic polypeptide, and possibly gastrin. Normally none of these hormones is secreted in any substantial quantity. The pancreatic islets are, however, the most common site for a gastrinoma, a gastrin-producing tumor responsible for the gastric hypersecretory condition known as the Zollinger-Ellison syndrome. VIP-secreting tumors arising from the islets have been related to a severe diarrheal state commonly referred to as pancreatic cholera.

EXOCRINE PANCREAS. The exocrine component of the pancreas is composed of small groups of acini separated into lobules by connective tissue stroma. Each acinus drains into a small pancreatic duct. These ducts unite to form a herringbone pattern eventually draining into the major excretory ducts of Wirsung and Santorini.

The general function of the exocrine pancreas is twofold: (1) the secretion of enzymes important for the digestion of dietary fat, carbohydrates, and protein, and (2) the secretion of water and bicarbonate to create an alkaline medium within the pancreatic ducts and the duodenum. Pancreatic enzymes are inactivated in the presence of acid.

The pancreatic enzymes are synthesized by the acinar cells and play an important role in intraluminal digestion by hydrolyzing food substances into a form that can be absorbed. Four classes of pancreatic digestive enzymes have been identified. *Amylase* acts to hydrolyze starch into maltose and has properties similar to those of salivary amylase. Pancreatic juice contains at least three *lipolytic enzymes:* lipase to hydrolyze triglycerides into monoglycerides and fatty acids, and phospholipase to hydrolyze phospholipids, and a carboxylesterase. The pancreas also synthesizes a number of *proteolytic enzymes* in the form of inactive zymogens that are rapidly activated on their entrance into the duodenum. The major proteolytic enzymes thus formed are trypsin, chymotrypsin, elastase, and carboxypeptidase A and B. In essence these enzymes act by cleaving the peptide bonds of ingested dietary proteins, thus forming smaller protein factions. The nucleolytic enzymes comprise the fourth group of pancreatic enzymes. These are ribonuclease and deoxyribonuclease, which act to hydrolyze the phosphodiesterase bonds that unite mononucleotides in nucleic acids.

The bicarbonate present in pancreatic juice is secreted by the cells of the pancreatic ducts by a complex process not yet completely understood. The origin of the bicarbonate excretion appears to be extracellular, and its pH, its bicarbonate concentration, and the partial pressure of carbon dioxide seem to be important variables. Carbonic anhydrase is present in ductular epithelium.

PHYSIOLOGY OF PANCREATIC SECRETION. Pancreatic secretion is controlled by a complex interaction of neural and hormonal influences. Stimulation of the vagus nerve results in the secretion of pancreatic enzymes from the acini, but the vagus nerve does not stimulate the ducts to secrete bicarbonate. The hormones gastrin, secreted by the antrum of the stomach, and especially cholecystokinin-pancreozymin (CCK-PZ), secreted by the small intestine, similarly stimulate the secretion of enzymes but are only weak stimulants of pancreatic bicarbonate secretion. On the other hand, secretin, another hormone secreted by the small intestine, plays little or no role by itself in the secretion of pancreatic enzymes but is a very strong stimulant of bicarbonate secretion by the pancreatic ducts.

The so-called *cephalic phase* of pancreatic secretion occurs when a person sees, smells, or chews food. It is medicated by the vagus nerve, which stimulates pancreatic secretion directly, and also indirectly by causing the secretion of gastrin and acid in the stomach.

Once food reaches the stomach, the *gastric phase* of gastric and pancreatic secretion takes place. The distention of the stomach stimulates gastrin release, probably by vagal reflexes. The release of gastrin is also stimulated by products of protein digestion and by certain substances such as calcium. The released gastrin and neural reflexes stimulate the gastric parietal cells to secrete acid and the pancreas to secrete its enzymes.

The *intestinal phase* of pancreatic stimulation, which accounts for most of the pancreatic secretion, is initiated when acid enters the duodenum. Secretin is released when the pH of the duodenal contents falls to 4.5 or lower. Its action in stimulating the pancreatic ducts to secrete bicarbonate is essential in maintaining the alkaline pH of the duodenum. Another component of the intestinal phase of pancreatic secretion is the stimulation of the secretion of CCK-PZ by certain food substances. Fatty acids, especially those with long chains (16 to 18 carbon atoms), are particularly potent stimulants of CCK-PZ. Certain amino acids and some polypeptides also stimulate the secretion of CCK-PZ. There is evidence that CCK-PZ and secretion protentiate the actions of each other.

DISORDERS OF THE PANCREAS

The disorders of the exocrine pancreas may be classified in the following categories: congenital abnormalities, acute pancreatitis, chronic pancreatitis, and tumors.

Congenital abnormalities

Primary congenital abnormalities of the pancreas may be of an anatomic or a functional nature.

Numerous *anatomic anomalies* of the pancreas exist, but with the exception of the annular pancreas and ectopic pancreas they are rarely of clinical significance. In cases of annular pancreas a ring of pancreatic tissue arising from the head of the pancreas encircles the descending part of the duodenum. This tissue ring is one of the causes of obstructive vomiting in the neonate, and surgical correction is required. Most cases are accompanied by other congenital anomalies such as Down's syndrome and congenital heart disease.

An ectopic pancreas results from the dislocation of pancreatic tissue from the primitive endodermal buds and its migration to another site during embryologic development. The most common sites for an ectopic pancreas are the distal stomach, duodenum, and jejunum. The roentgenographic and endoscopic findings are those of an intramural lesion with a central umbilication. In most instances the lesion is asymptomatic and is discovered serendipitously. Rarely, bleeding may occur from superficial ulceration.

Congenital cysts are usually asymptomatic. They may occur as part of a polycystic disease in many organs including the liver and kidney. They are clinically insignificant, in contrast to acquired cysts that occur as the result of a carcinoma or parasitic infection. Pseudocysts, an important complication of pancreatitis, are discussed in a later section.

Functional anomalies include congenital deficiencies in any or all of the pancreatic secretions; these are quite rare. Cystic fibrosis, or more properly, mucoviscidosis, is an autosomal recessive disorder that affects the function of many exocrine glands including the exocrine pancreas, the mucous glands of the bronchi, the salivary and sweat glands, and others. The disease is characterized by an increased viscosity of the mucus in these glands. As a result the pancreatic ducts become obstructed by inspissated material, producing dilation of the ducts, retention cyst formation, and atrophy and fibrosis of the pancreas. Pancreatic insufficiency along with a resultant weight loss and poor growth and maturation follow. The involvement of the respiratory tract in cystic fibrosis leads to recurrent infections, pansinusitis, and pulmonary insufficiency. The involvement of the sweat glands results in an inability to conserve sodium, potassium, and chloride. The measurement of the sodium or chloride content in sweat is the basis of a diagnostic test for cystic fibrosis. The treatment consists of replacement therapy with pancreatic enzymes and the prophylaxis and therapy of respiratory infections.

Acute pancreatitis

ETIOLOGY AND PATHOGENESIS. Acute pancreatitis is characterized by enzymatic autodigestion of the pancreas. The disorder may be produced by a variety of causative mechanisms. Alcoholism and biliary tract disease account for the majority of cases. The predominant cause depends on the life-style of the patient, especially the consumption of alcohol. The following are causative mechanisms:

Alcohol
Biliary tract disease
Trauma
Contiguous spread of an infection or a penetrating duodenal ulcer
Hyperlipidemia
Hyperparathyroidism and hypercalcemia
Viral causes such as mumps
Familial disorders
Drugs
Idiopathic and miscellaneous causes

The mechanisms whereby alcohol produces pancreatitis are not clearly understood. Alcohol is known to stimulate the secretion of pancreatic juice and at the same time may produce an obstruction to the flow within pancreatic ducts. Presumably alcohol also has a direct deleterious effect on the acinar cell, perhaps disrupting its integrity and allowing the escape of pancreatic enzymes into pancreatic tissue.

In patients with biliary tract disease pancreatitis is most often associated with the passage of a gallstone from the common duct through the ampulla of Vater into the duodenum. A common distal channel for both the bile and pancreatic ducts, as occurs in many cases, presumably causes a predisposition for the reflux of bile into the pancreatic duct, resulting in pancreatitis. In addition, refluxed bile may contain altered components that are especially harmful, such as biliary lecithin, which may be converted to lysolecithin by pancreatic phospholipase, and deconjugated bile, which may occur in the presence of bacteria in the common bile duct and duodenum. Both lysolecithin and deconjugated bile produce pancreatitis in experimental animals when refluxed into the pancreatic duct.

The mechanisms by which hypercalcemia, hyperparathyroidism, and hyperlipidemia produce pancreatitis are unclear. In hyperparathyroidism, pancreatic calcification may occur, but its presence is not essential for the development of pancreatitis. Types I, IV, and V hyperlipidemia may predispose a patient to pancreatitis, and its appears that chylomicronemia may be the responsible factor by a mechanism not yet understood (see Chapter 202).

Contiguous infections occurring postoperatively or as a consequence of an abdominal catastrophe such as a perforated viscus may produce pancreatitis by direct spread of the inflammatory process to the pancreas. A penetrating duodenal ulcer may also produce pancreatitis. Mumps virus has a predilection for the pancreas, a phenomenon related to the histologic and functional similarities between the salivary glands and the pancreas.

A number of drugs have been implicated in the development of pancreatitis. A causal relationship has been most convincingly demonstrated for azathioprine, thiazides, sulfonamides, furosemide, estrogens, and tetracycline. There is suggestive evidence as well for a causative role played by L-asparaginase, chlorthalidone, corticosteroids, ethacrynic acid, phenformin, and procainamide. Little is known about the pathogenesis of drug-induced pancreatitis.

CLINICAL MANIFESTATIONS. There are no specific or pathognomonic features that distinguish pancreatitis with certainty from other diseases. Pancreatitis involves a wide spectrum of clinical patterns ranging from clinically inapparent involvement to fulminant cases that rapidly lead to death.

The clinical picture is correlated with the pathophysiologic process. Milder cases are usually associated with edema of the pancreas, more severe cases are associated with hemorrhage and suppuration, and the most severe cases are associated with pancreatic necrosis and the necrosis of adjacent and occasionally distant adipose tissue.

Abdominal pain is by far the most common symptom of acute pancreatitis and is present in almost all of these cases. The pain is usually epigastric and commonly radiates through to the back. The pain is steady and is made worse by eating and helped somewhat by sitting upright or leaning forward. As inflammation spreads throughout the pancreas and is accompanied by exudation and peritonitis, the pain spreads and becomes generalized throughout the abdomen. Nausea and vomiting are symptoms in the majority of patients.

In milder cases abdominal tenderness is confined to the epigastrium and is usually not accompanied by fever or tachycardia. In severe cases the abdominal findings are more impressive and include marked tenderness, abdominal wall spasm, and the absence of peristaltic sounds. There may be abdominal distention, and the findings may mimic those of peritonitis resulting from a perforated viscus. If there has been hemorrhage into the peritoneal cavity, ecchymoses may be present in the flanks (Turner's sign) or periumbilically (Cullen's sign). Tachycardia is present, and a temperature of 100° to 102° F (37.8° to 38.9° C) is common. The patient may be restless or lie motionless and may be confused or semiconscious. If the cause is alcohol, the clinical picture may be complicated by the findings of acute alcoholic intoxication or an alcoholic withdrawal syndrome such as delirium tremens.

The patient may have accompanying shock and hypotension if there has been significant pancreatic exudation and loss of fluid into the peritoneal space. The extremities may be cold and clammy, and signs of dehydration may be present. Renal insufficiency and a left pleural effusion may accompany acute pancreatitis. Some of the pathophysiologic events occurring in cases of pancreatitis are thought to be initiated and medicated by vasoactive substances released into the peritoneal cavity and subsequently absorbed into the bloodstream or passing directly into the blood from their pancreatic origin.

The examiner may get a clue as to the cause of the pancreatitis from the associated physical findings, such as biliary tract disease, an alcoholic syndrome, parotid swelling, band keratopathy, eruptive santhoma, and so on.

LABORATORY FINDINGS. The most reliable laboratory test for the diagnosis of acute pancreatitis is the serum amylase test. An elevated level of serum amylase, although it is not pathognomonic for acute pancreatitis, is very strong supportive evidence of the diagnosis when the clinical presentation is compatible. This elevation occurs rapidly as a result of a disruption of the integrity of the acinar cell wall and an escape of amylase into the blood. The increased serum amylase level is reflected in the urine as well as in the ascitic or pleural fluid that may accompany acute pancreatitis. Amylase originating from the pancreas is filtered by the kidney at a faster rate than amylase from other sources. A reliable method of documenting an increased urinary amylase is to simultaneously determine the renal clearances of amylase and creatinine. The ratio of the clearance of amylase to the clearance of creatinine is normally 1% to 5%; in cases of acute pancreatitis it is over 5%.

Although the amylase level may become elevated within hours of an attack, elevation of the serum lipase level occurs later in the course of the disease and persists for a longer period of time. Serum lipase elevations occur much less commonly than hyperamylasemia. Leukocytosis is common, and the hemoglobin may be elevated because of a loss of fluid into the abdomen. Subsequent drops in the hemoglobin and hematocrit may be associated with a hemorrhage into the pancreas or the peritoneal cavity. Hyperglycemia and glycosuria commonly accompany acute pancreatitis, even in nondiabetic patients. The impairment in glucose metabolism is related to the involvement of the contiguous islets of Langerhans. Renal failure caused by acute tubular necrosis resulting from shock may accompany acute pancreatitis.

Signs of an extrahepatic biliary obstruction in pancreatitis are common because of inflammatory changes in the head of the pancreas in the region of the papilla of Vater. Serum alkaline phosphatase and bilirubin elevations commonly occur. Alcoholic liver disease may contribute to these abnormalities.

Lactescent serum resulting from hyperlipidemia involving triglycerides and/or chylomicrons may accompany acute pancreatitis. Inasmuch as hyperlipidemia may produce acute pancreatitis, it is important that the levels of serum lipids are followed through the patient's recovery and convalescent period so that the cause can be differentiated from its effects.

Hypocalcemia is a fairly common laboratory finding in cases of acute pancreatitis. It has been attributed to the precipitation of ionized calcium in areas of fat necrosis. Hypercalcemia or a normal serum calcium level in the presence of acute pancreatitis raises the distinct possibility of underlying hyperparathyroidism. Hypomagnesemia has also been observed in cases of acute pancreatitis, and it too has been attributed to the deposition of magnesium in areas of fat necrosis, although alcoholism may contribute to its presence.

Abdominal roentgenograms may be helpful in establishing a diagnosis of acute pancreatitis. Opaque biliary calculi may appear, suggesting the possibility that the pancreatitis may have occurred in association with biliary tract disease. Calcifications within the pancreas indicate that the patient has previously had damage to the pancreas.

Several roentgenographic findings are considered suggestive of acute pancreatitis although they are by no means pathognomonic. Most commonly observed is the so-called sentinel loop, a localized segment of small bowel ileus usually involving the jejunum. The transverse colon may be spastic as a consequence of irritation caused by pancreatic exudation. The ascending colon and hepatic flexure proximal to the area of spasm may become distended, suggesting the presence of an obstructing lesion. This finding is referred to as the colon cutoff sign. Widening of the duodenal loop caused by the pressure of an edematous head of the pancreas may be seen on a plain film of the abdomen or with a barium meal examination. The stomach may be anteriorly displaced. Ultrasonography and computed tomography may be helpful in demonstrating an enlargement of the pancreas. Ultrasonography in particular may be helpful also in demonstrating the presence of pseudocysts or gallstones, especially because for several weeks following an attack of acute pancreatitis the successful visualization of the gallbladder by cholecystography or intravenous cholangiography may be prevented. Endoscopic retrograde cholangiopancreatography, if its use is considered, should be deferred until the acute pancreatitis has subsided because this procedure may cause flare-ups of existing pancreatitis. Superior mesenteric angiography probably has no place in the diagnosis of acute pancreatitis.

DIFFERENTIAL DIAGNOSIS. It may be difficult to differentiate acute pancreatitis from other acute abdominal disorders. The emphasis should be on excluding from the diagnostic possibilities an acute surgical emergency, especially a perforated peptic ulcer. The patient with a perforated peptic ulcer usually assumes an immobile supine position with knees tightly flexed. Signs of generalized peritonitis commonly develop more quickly when there is a perforation. The presence of free air in the abdomen, of course, a valuable aid in differentiating the two conditions. In patients with acute biliary tract disease the localization of the discomfort in the right upper quadrant is a helpful finding. The serum amylase level usually is normal or only slightly elevated. The use of radionuclide imaging (HIDA and PIPIDA scans) may be helpful in the differential diagnosis.

Other conditions to be differentiated from acute pancreatitis include an expanding or dissecting aortic aneurysm, mesenteric vascular occlusion, and volvulus of the bowel. Rarer conditions to be excluded from the diagnostic possibilities include a sickle cell crisis, tabetic crisis, porphyria, Schönlein-Henoch purpura, and lead poisoning.

The presence of an elevated level of serum amylase caused by acute pancreatitis must be differentiated from macroamylasemia, in which abdominal discomfort may occur. The diagnosis of macroamylasemia is confirmed by the presence of a low or normal rather than elevated urinary amylase.

MANAGEMENT. Because of the complexities involved and the monitoring required, patients with severe pancreatitis may require treatment in an intensive care unit. There is no specific or definitive therapeutic modality for acute pancreatitis. Every effort should be made to put the pancreas at rest, presumably because continuing pancreatic secretion may perpetuate the process. Because of the stimulating effect of gastric acid on the pancreas, efforts have been made to control acidity. Gastric suction and the administration of the H_2-receptor antagonist cimetidine and antacids have been employed therapeutically for this purpose. In addition, the patient is given nothing orally, so that the gastric phase of acid secretion is slowed. The results of these measures to combat gastric acidity are equivocal in terms of altering the course of acute pancreatitis. There is little doubt that nasogastric suction is beneficial, but its benefit may be derived from its decompressing effects rather than from its removal of gastric acid. There is as yet no convincing evidence about the benefits of antacids or cimetidine and especially of any benefit of anticholinergics, which have been used in the past.

The profound hemodynamic and electrolyte disturbances that accompany pancreatitis make it mandatory that the patient's fluid and electrolyte balances and urinary output be closely monitored. The central venous pressure should be employed for this purpose in a severely compromised patient. Colloid infusions may be necessary, as well as occasionally blood transfusions, if there has been significant hemorrhage.

The alleviation of pain is an important component of this therapy. The decompression of the stomach with a nasogastric tube helps ease the pain of distention. Morphine should be avoided because of its tendency to constrict Oddi's sphincter. Small doses of meperidine may be administered as needed. The tendency for patients with pancreatitis, particularly chronic pancreatitis, to become dependent on narcotics is noteworthy, and the physician should be on guard for addicted patients who may be adept at feigning the signs and symptoms of acute pancreatitis.

Acute pancreatitis in itself does not require the use of antibiotics, but when this condition is accompanied by acute cholecystitis, an infection contiguous with the pancreas, or a pancreatic abscess, antibiotics are indicated. Ampicillin and/or one of the cephalosporins, along with an aminoglycoside such as gentamicin, is most commonly employed.

Pulmonary and cardiac complications should be treated appropriately. Respiratory aid may be required in the form of oxygen and intermittent positive pressure. Complicating pulmonary infections should be treated promptly. Patients with cardiac disease may require the administration of digitalis and diuretics.

Various agents have been tried empirically as treatments for acute pancreatitis without noteworthy success. Steroids have not proved helpful, nor has the use of aprotinin (Trasylol), a polypeptide that inhibits trypsin and kallikrein.

Surgery may be necessary for acute pancreatitis in certain circumstances. Surgical intervention in the case of gangrene or empyema of the gallbladder may abort the occurrence of secondary pancreatitis. Surgery is also recommended for the drainage of a pancreatic abscess, but differentiating an abscess with certainty from a phlegmonous infiltration of the pancreas or from a pseudocyst of the pancreas is extremely difficult. These conditions may mimic one another even in their appearance with ultrasonography and computed tomography. A meticulous individualization of each patient that correlates clinical findings with the results of special studies is required.

Peritoneal lavage in the treatment of acute pancreatitis has received favorable reports but is not yet generally accepted as a therapeutic modality.

Once the acute pancreatitis has subsided, surgery has an important role in cases in which biliary tract disease or hyperparathyroidism has been demonstrated as the underlying causative mechanism.

PROGNOSIS AND COMPLICATIONS. The prognosis of patients with acute pancreatitis depends largely on the severity of the inflammatory response. In mild edematous pancreatitis the mortality is less than 5%, but the mortality rises to above 50% in cases in which there is hemorrhage and/or necrosis. Shock, renal failure, infection, bleeding, and respiratory failure increase the mortality.

The complications of an acute episode of pancreatitis were discussed previously. The potential late complications include pseudocyst formation, abscess, pancreatic ascites, recurrence, and chronicity. Chronic pancreatitis may be accompanied by endocrine insufficiency (diabetes mellitus) and/or exocrine insufficiency.

LATE COMPLICATIONS

Pseudocyst. A pseudocyst of the pancreas is a nonepithelialized cavity containing blood, serum, pancreatic secretions, and inflammatory exudate. Pseudocysts that develop as a complication of acute pancreatitis are almost invariably of alcoholic origin. With the continuing secretion of pancreatic juice into the pseudocyst, a pseudocyst may expand to a considerable size, producing pain, a palpable and sometimes tender mass, and evidence of impingement on the stomach, duodenum, or other abdominal organs (Fig. 182-1). A pseudocyst may cause nausea and vomiting and occasionally obstructive jaundice. Leakage or an overt rupture into the peritoneal cavity may occur, often with dire consequences. A rupture into the stomach or intestine sometimes occurs, often causing gastrointestinal bleeding. Pseudocysts are usually present singly but may be multiple; their size is variable. They may occur within the pancreatic tissue or may be located within the lesser peritoneal sac, within the mesentery, behind the peritoneum, or as far distant as the mediastinum.

Evidence is accumulating that many pseudocysts regress spontaneously, but symptomatic ones should be approached surgically. The procedure of choice is a cystenterostomy into an adjacent portion of the stomach or intestine. Results of surgery are generally quite satisfactory.

Pancreatic abscess. A pancreatic abscess is a rare complication of acute pancreatitis. It usually occurs within a few weeks of an acute episode and is characterized by a high fever and a tender abdominal mass. Leukocytosis is common. Enteric organisms and probably anaerobes such as *Bacteroides fragilis* are usually responsible for the inflammatory reaction, but occasionally *Staphylococcus aureus* or a species of *Streptococcus* is involved. If surgical drainage is not performed, the mortality is high.

Pancreatic ascites. Persistent ascites may develop after a bout of acute pancreatitis, especially in cases of a poorly walled-off pseudocyst. Abdominal paracentesis reveals ascitic fluid with a high amylase content, which differentiates pancreatic ascites from ascites caused by cirrhosis of the liver. Drainage of the fluid may result in a lasting remission, but many cases are resistant to conservative therapy and may require surgery.

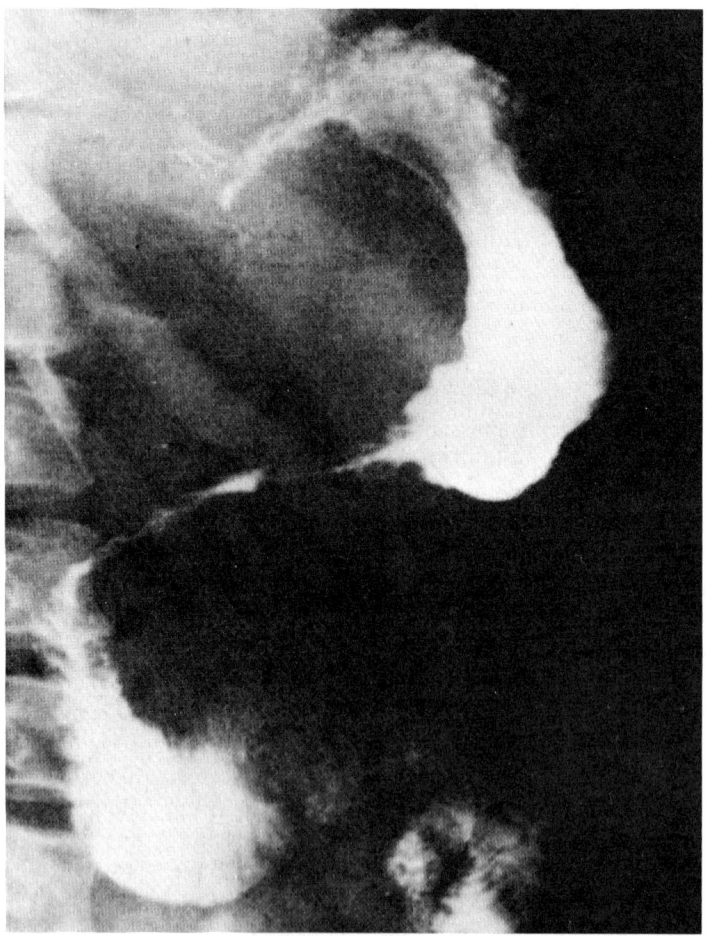

Fig. 182-1. Barium meal examination reveals large pancreatic mass (pseudocyst) causing pressure on lesser curvature of stomach, narrowing of distal stomach and proximal duodenum, and widening of duodenal loop.

Relapsing acute pancreatitis

In some cases when the underlying cause of pancreatitis remains, as in patients with alcoholism or cholelithiasis, attacks of acute pancreatitis may recur. Recurrences may result in chronic pancreatitis, especially if the underlying causative mechanism is not remedied.

Chronic pancreatitis

When the pancreas is subjected to repeated bouts of pancreatitis, regardless of the cause, it may undergo irreversible inflammatory changes, fibrosis, and eventual calcification. Alcohol is the most common cause of chronic pancreatitis, either because of a specific toxic effect of alcohol or because pancreatitis associated with biliary tract disease is more amenable to corrective therapy.

The clinical course is characterized by recurrent attacks of pain and disability, although in some patients chronic pancreatitis may occur without preceding pain. In fully developed cases of chronic pancreatitis, especially when there is pancreatic calcification, pain may be steady and unrelenting, suggesting a mechanical cause, or it may be intermittent. The pain is boring and poorly localized and tends to radiate to the midback. Characteristically it is relieved when the patient sits upright and bends forward. Other symptoms are caused by the endocrine and exocrine pancreatic insufficiency that develops in these patients.

Glucose intolerance is common in these patients, and the diabetes may be brittle, although an insulin requirement about 40 units a day is uncommon. Diabetic complications such as retinopathy, glomerulosclerosis, and peripheral vascular disease are uncommon, perhaps because of the shorter duration of the diabetic state in patients with chronic pancreatitis. Diabetic ketoacidosis, however, is a distinct threat. Peripheral neuropathy is fairly common, probably because of the contributing factors of alcoholism and malnutrition.

Steatorrhea is common in chronic pancreatitis and often is disabling. Its presence signifies the destruction of at least 80% of the gland. Fecal fat losses in excess of 50% of the oral intake may result from a deficiency in pancreatic lipase. Weight loss and multiple nutritional deficiencies, particularly of the fat-soluble vitamins, result as a consequence of steatorrhea.

Chronic pancreatitis is usually not difficult to diagnose. The clinical history and the finding of pancreatic calcification in the presence of endocrine and/or exocrine pancreatic insufficiency are a sufficient basis for the diagnosis. The diagnosis is supported by tests of the pancreatic capacity to secrete enzymes, fluid, and bicarbonate. The secretin test, a measure of the ability of the pancreas to respond to an intravenous dose of secretin, is most commonly employed for this purpose. With a duodenal tube the baseline and serial levels of bicarconate concentration are measured.

Gross and microscopic examinations of the stool to detect excess quantities of fat are helpful in determining the presence of steatorrhea, but a 3-day quantitative fecal fat analysis is preferable. Steatorrhea resulting from chronic

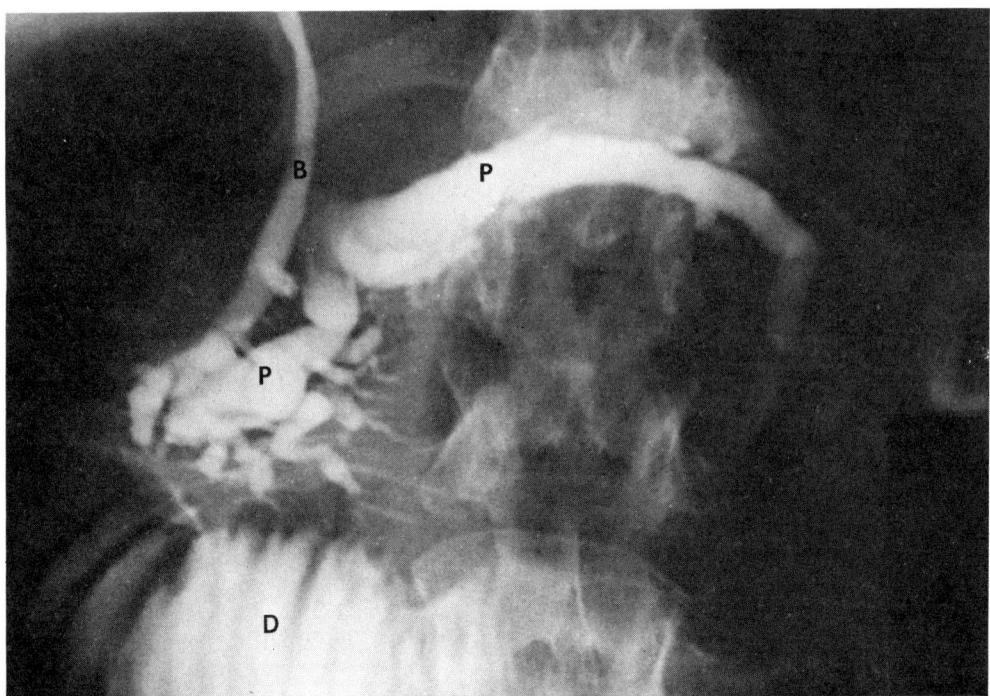

Fig. 182-2. Endoscopic retrograde cholangiopancreatography reveals marked dilation, irregularity, and "clubbing" of pancreatic ducts, changes found in chronic pancreatitis. *B*, Common bile duct; *D*, duodenum; *P*, main pancreatic duct. (Courtesy of Harvey Lefton, M.D.)

pancreatitis must be appropriately differentiated from that resulting from other causes. The D-xylose test, small bowel barium meal examination, and small bowel biopsy have normal results in cases of chronic pancreatitis and thus help to distinguish this steatorrhea from that produced by a mucosal disorder of the small intestine.

Selective angiography, endoscopic retrograde cholangiopancreatography, and selenomethionine Se 75 scintiscans of the pancreas may prove helpful in establishing the diagnosis (Fig. 182-2).

The treatment is directed to the endocrine and exocrine insufficiency. Diabetes mellitus should be treated appropriately. Steatorrhea should be treated with pancreatic extracts. Additional therapy with antacids or the H_2-receptor antagonist cimetidine may be helpful in protecting the pancreatic extracts because pancreatic enzymes are readily inactivated at a pH below 4.5. Vitamin supplements are indicated to correct any deficiencies. Satisfactory absorption and nutrition should be restored with the proper use of this therapy, but the caloric intake can be enhanced if necessary by adding easily absorbed medium-chain triglycerides to the diet.

Various surgical procedures have been employed in attempts to reestablish pancreatic drainage. These may be effective in cases in which a segmental obstruction of the pancreatic ducts can be demonstrated. In most cases, however, acinar destruction has occurred, prohibiting surgical correction.

Pain is frequently disabling in chronic pancreatitis. Because addiction is fairly common among these patients, a program of analgesia should be carefully planned. The value of neurosurgical procedures such as a dorsal root interruption or celiac axis ganglionectomy is debatable. More radical and dangerous surgery such as a subtotal pancreatectomy may have to be attempted in selected cases in an effort to control unremitting pain.

Tumors of the pancreas

Benign tumors of the exocrine pancreas may arise from acinar cells (adenomas and cystadenomas) or from supporting tissues (lipomas, neuromas, hemangiomas, fibromas, myxomas, and lymphangiomas). Benign tumors are rare and are not usually of clinical significance. Neoplasms may also arise in the endocrine pancreas. Gastrinomas and insulinomas are the most common of these, but glucagonomas, somatostatinomas, and VIP-secreting tumors also occur rarely. These may be benign or malignant. These endocrine tumors are not discussed in this chapter.

Carcinomas of the pancreas originate most commonly from ductal epithelial and occasionally from acinar tissue. Because of the inaccessibility of the pancreas and the insidious and nonspecific nature of symptoms related to carcinomas of the pancreas, the disease is rarely diagnosed early in its course. Pancreatic carcinomas are increasing in incidence and currently rank second to colonic carcinomas as the most common cause of death among carcinomas originating in the gastrointestinal tract.

The cause of carcinomas of the pancreas is unknown. Alcoholism, chronic pancreatitis, and diabetes mellitus have been mentioned as possible predisposing factors, but the evidence for these is inconclusive.

CLINICAL MANIFESTATIONS. The majority of patients with a pancreatic carcinoma have abdominal discomfort. The pain usually is not disabling, is nonspecific, and is confined to the epigastrium or right upper quadrant when the head of the pancreas is involved. When the tumor arises in the body or tail of the pancreas, the pain tends to be located in the midline or left upper quadrant. In its most characteristic form the pain radiates straight through to the back, is intensified when the patient is in the supine position, and is relieved by maneuvers that flex the spine, such as sitting up or lying on the side with the knees flexed.

Anorexia and weight loss are almost universal symptoms and may be extreme. Obstructive jaundice is present in at least 90% of patients with a carcinoma of the pancreatic head and is commonly the presenting complaint. Jaundice is a late manifestation of carcinomas of the body or tail of the pancreas and indicates the spread of the disease to the head of the pancreas or the liver.

Less common clinical symptoms and signs include fever and chills related to a biliary tract obstruction and/or tumor necrosis, nonbacterial thrombotic endocarditis, migratory thrombophlebitis, and psychiatric symptoms.

DIAGNOSIS. The diagnosis of a carcinoma of the head of the pancreas is strongly suggested by the appearance of relatively painless jaundice in an older patient along with a weight loss. Except for the jaundice and weight loss the results of the physical examination may be completely negative. Occasionally a distended gallbladder may be palpated (Courvoisier's sign). A metastatic spread to the liver results in a palpable enlargement of the organ, usually accompanied by irregularity and an increase in its consistency. Laboratory tests are helpful in confirming the presence of obstructive jaundice. Relatively high elevations of the levels of alkaline phosphatase, leucine aminopeptidase, 5'-nucleotidase, and γ-glutamyl transpeptidase in the presence of moderate elevations of serum transaminase values (serum glutamic-oxaloacetic transaminase and serum glutamic-pyruvic transaminase) of less than 300 units strongly suggest an obstructive process. There may be an impairment of glucose tolerance if there has been sufficient destruction of pancreatic islet cells.

The diagnosis is much more difficult to make in cases of carcinomas of the body or tail of the pancreas. The physical examination and routine laboratory studies are usually within normal limits until the process is advanced.

The conventional barium meal examination may reveal evidence of extrinsic pressure on the stomach and duodenal loop (Fig. 182-1). This is usually first manifested as a widening of the duodenal loop and an encroachment on the lumen of the duodenum. An extrinsic pressure or actual invasion of the greater curvature of the gastric antrum may also occur. Hypotonic duodenography may provide a more detailed picture of this area.

An increasing number of special studies that have become available during the last decade are helpful in detecting mass lesions of the pancreas. Angiographic visualization of the pancreas has been improved through the capability of introducing the contrast material into smaller arteries (superselective angiography) and through the use of magnification techniques. Characteristic features of carcinomas, such as the encasement of blood vessels, have been recognized.

An improved visualization of the biliary tree in cases of a suspected obstruction has resulted from a refinement of the techniques of percutaneous (Chiba fine needle) transhepatic cholangiography and endoscopic retrograde cholangiopancreatography.

Ultrasonography and computed tomography have been helpful in detecting mass lesions of the pancreas as well as in disclosing the presence of a dilated gallbladder or bile ducts. These relatively simple, noninvasive techniques are often employed early in the diagnostic process to confirm the suspected presence of obstructive jaundice or a pancreatic carcinoma.

Pancreatic scanning using selenomethionine has not proved sufficiently reliable in differentiating pancreatic carcinomas from pancreatitis and other nonneoplastic conditions.

MANAGEMENT. The abdomen should be surgically explored in suspected cases of carcinomas of the pancreas, especially when the head of the pancreas is thought to be involved. If there is no evidence of local or distant metastases, a radical pancreaticoduodenectomy (Whipple's operation) may be attempted in the hope of a cure. In the presence of metastatic spread, a palliative bypass procedure such as cholecystojejunostomy may be performed to relieve the obstructive jaundice and its attendant problems.

In patients with a carcinoma of the body and tail of the pancreas a curative operation is rarely performed because a metastatic spread of the tumor has almost invariably already taken place.

The medical management of patients with a carcinoma of the pancreas is aimed at the palliation of symptoms, such as the relief of pain, maintenance of nutrition, and treatment of complications. Chemotherapy and radiation have little or no influence on the primary lesion but may be helpful in the relief of pain.

The prognosis is extremely poor. Generaly the 5-year survival rate is below 2%. Most patients are dead within 1 year, regardless of the form of treatment. Patients with carcinomas that arise from the ampulla of Vater have a much better prognosis and a 5-year survival rate of up to 25%.

BIBLIOGRAPHY

Banks, P.A.: Acute pancreatitis, Gastroenterology **61**:382, 1971.
Bourke, J.B., and others: Drugs as associated factors in primary acute pancreatitis, Gut **18**:422, 1977.
Braganza, J.M., and others: A clinical evaluation of isotope scanning, ultrasonography and computerized tomography in pancreatic disease, Clin. Radiol. **29**:639, 1978.
Cohn, I.: Cancer of the pancreas: detection and diagnosis, Cancer **37**:582, 1976.
Rebet, A., and Balas, D.: Functional diagnosis of pancreatic disease. In Glass, G.B., editor: Progress in gastroenterology, vol. 3. New York, 1977, Grune & Stratton, Inc.
Sankaran, S., and Walt, A.J.: The natural and unnatural history of pancreatic pseudocysts, Br. J. Surg. **62**:37, 1975.
Sarles, H.: Chronic calcifying pancreatitis: chronic alcoholic pancreatitis, Gastroenterology **66**:604, 1974.

183 • DISEASES OF THE LIVER
Graham H. Jeffries

CLINICAL MANIFESTATIONS OF HEPATIC DISEASE
Jaundice

Jaundice (icterus) is a yellow discoloration of the skin or sclerae caused by an excessive level of bilirubin; this is usually detected when the serum level of bilirubin exceeds 2 to 3 mg/dl.

BILIRUBIN METABOLISM

Production. The major proportion of excreted bilirubin (80% to 90%) is derived from the catabolism of red cell hemoglobin by reticuloendothelial cells. Senescent red cells sequestered in the spleen are ingested by macrophages, and intracellular lysosomal enzymes separate iron and globin from the hemoglobin, open the tetrapyrrol ring, and catabolize the molecule through several intermediates (including biliverdin) to bilirubin. The color changes of a bruise reflect a similar degradation of hemoglobin by tissue macrophages. Small amounts of bilirubin are formed by the breakdown of other hemoproteins (myoglobin and cytochromes), particularly in the liver, or from hemoglobin synthesized by bone marrow cells but not incorporated into mature peripheral red cells.

Transport. The bilirubin released from reticuloendothelial cells is relatively nonpolar and poorly soluble in an aqueous solution; albumin, which has the capacity to bind two molecules of bilirubin on each protein molecule, is the major carrier of bilirubin in plasma and determines the distribution of the pigment. The high affinity between albumin and bilirubin limits the diffusion of bilirubin into cells (except in the liver) unless the plasma concentration exceeds the albumin binding capacity (see discussion of "Jaundice from impaired hepatic conjugation of bilirubin" later in this chapter). The albumin-bilirubin complex is not filtered in the glomeruli, and thus unconjugated pigment is not excreted in the urine.

Hepatic uptake. The uptake of bilirubin by liver cells is facilitated by the permeability of the hepatic sinusoids, which permits albumin-bilirubin to diffuse rapidly into Disse's space in contact with the liver cell membrane, and by binding proteins (Y and Z proteins), which concentrate bilirubin in the cytoplasm of liver cells; the displacement of bilirubin from albumin binding sites requires the presence of a high-affinity carrier protein at the liver cell membrane.

Hepatic conjugation. In the liver cells bilirubin is conjugated to form bilirubin diglucuronide (conjugated bilirubin) by a microsomal enzyme system, glucuronyl transferase in the presence of uridine diphosphate glucuronic acid; this reaction converts nonpolar bilirubin to a water-soluble organic anion that is excreted in bile. Conjugation is a prerequisite for the biliary secretion of bilirubin.

Hepatic secretion. The secretion of conjugated bilirubin into the bile canaliculi is an active process that is probably carrier mediated; this is normally the rate-limiting step in bilirubin excretion. Organic anions, including bilirubin and bile acids, are secreted into the bile canaliculi by independent mechanisms; in the Dubin-Johnson syndrome an impaired hepatic excretion of conjugated bilirubin and other organic anions is associated with a normal bile acid excretion. The rate of bilirubin secretion in bile nevertheless appears to be modulated by bile acid secretion.

Intestinal degradation. In the gut the conjugated bilirubin is deconjugated and converted to colorless urobilinogens by bacterial enzymes. The urobilinogen may be excreted in the stool or may be reabsorbed to undergo biliary or renal excretion.

PATHOPHYSIOLOGY OF JAUNDICE. Patients with jaundice can be divided into two groups. In cases of unconjugated hyperbilirubinemia there may be an excessive bilirubin production, an impaired hepatic uptake of bilirubin, or a depressed hepatic conjugation. Conjugated hyperbilirubinemia may result from the impaired hepatic excretion of bilirubin diglucuronide. The term "cholestasis" refers to abnormalities of hepatic excretion in which there are a reduced bile flow and an impaired hepatobiliary excretion; cholestatic jaundice results from intrahepatic lesions (intrahepatic cholestasis) or extrahepatic lesions obstructing the biliary system (extrahepatic cholestasis).

Jaundice from excessive bilirubin production. Increased red cell destruction *(hemolysis)* and ineffective erythropoiesis (as in cases of thalassemia and pernicious anemia) lead to excessive bilirubin production. The normal capacity of the liver to excrete bilirubin is such that the serum level of unconjugated bilirubin rarely exceeds 3 to 5 mg/dl in patients with chronic hemolytic disease. When acute or chronic liver disease reduces the hepatic excretion of conjugated bilirubin, an increased bilirubin load caused by hemolysis contributes to an increase in the serum level of conjugated bilirubin.

Jaundice from reduced hepatic uptake of bilirubin. In *Gilbert's disease* there is a reduced plasma clearance of unconjugated bilirubin resulting either from an impaired uptake at the liver cell membrane or from an altered transport within the cell; this is a common cause for mild unconjugated hyperbilirubinemia without other abnormalities of liver cell function. In some cases an increase in the bilirubin load (hemolysis) accentuates the patient's jaundice. Patients with a portal-systemic shunt may also exhibit mild unconjugated hyperbilirubinemia caused by a decreased plasma clearance of unconjugated bilirubin.

Jaundice from impaired hepatic conjugation of bilirubin. Unconjugated hyperbilirubinemia commonly occurs in the neonatal period, particularly in premature infants with a relatively immature transport and conjugating system for bilirubin. In the Crigler-Najjar syndrome a partial or complete lack of the enzyme systems for conjugating bilirubin leads to marked unconjugated hyperbilirubinemia. When the serum level of pigment exceeds the albumin binding capacity, diffusion of lipid-soluble bilirubin into the brain causes metabolic injury (kernicterus).

Jaundice from impaired excretion of conjugated bilirubin. In the Dubin-Johnson syndrome and Rotor's syndrome a metabolic defect in the hepatic transport of organic anions leads to conjugated hyperbilirubinemia. Patients with a liver cell injury, regardless of whether it is metabolic (such as hypoxia), toxic (such as carbon tetrachloride or ethanol toxicity), viral (such as hepatitis type A or B), or the result of other causes (such as bacterial endotoxin), commonly have jaundice caused by the impaired excretion of conjugated bilirubin. Damage to bile ductules within the portal triads (such as occurs in primary biliary cirrhosis) and infiltration of the liver (such as by a granuloma or neoplasm) also lead to intrahepatic cholestasis. An extrahepatic ductal obstruction may result from gallstones, a stricture, or a neoplasm; these are the more common causes of "surgical" obstructive jaundice (extrahepatic cholestasis).

Cutaneous manifestations

PRURITUS. Both intrahepatic and extrahepatic cholestasis are commonly associated with generalized itching; in some patients with chronic cholestasis (such as primary biliary cirrhosis), this symptom may precede the onset of jaundice, whereas patients with severe hepatocellular failure and deep jaundice may remain free of pruritus. This symptom may interfere with a patient's sleep and may lead to a severe skin excoriation with bleeding or infection. Although it has been suggested that retained bile acids cause the stimulation of skin receptors, the severity of pruritus is only weakly correlated with the concentration of bile acids in peripheral blood plasma or skin. The decrease in pruritus with cholestyramine therapy, which was formerly attributed to bile acid chelation with a lowering of plasma bile acid levels, may result from the chelation of some other agent that accumulates in patients with cholestasis.

SKIN RASHES. In patients with acute type B hepatitis a skin rash may precede or coincide with the episode of acute hepatitis; the rash is commonly an acute erythema with edema (hives) or may be maculopapular and purpuric, particularly on the legs. This rash results from vascular injury caused by circulating immune complexes and often coincides with arthralgias or overt acute arthritis.

PIGMENTATION. Chronic cholestasis with jaundice leads to an increase in the melanin pigmentation of the skin. In patients with primary or secondary hemochromatosis the skin may have a bronze or slate-gray color that varies with the deposition of melanin or iron; hypogonadism in these patients causes the skin to be soft in texture with a loss of axillary and pubic hair. Patients with porphyria cutanea tarda may have an increase in fine facial hair, particularly in the periorbital area; photosensitivity resulting from uroporphyrin retention may cause bullous skin lesions in areas exposed to the sun, along with secondary scarring and depigmentation.

SPIDER ANGIOMAS. Spider angiomas (vascular spiders) are arteriovenous anastomeses that vary in size from 1 to 10 mm in diameter, that are usually concentrated on the face, neck, upper thorax, and arms, and that typically have a pulsating central arteriole with radiating vessels. Although small spider angiomas may appear during the course of acute hepatitis, multiple large lesions are usually observed in patients with chronic progressive liver disease. Similar arteriovenous anastomoses have been demonstrated in the lungs. The pathogenesis of spider angiomas remains obscure. The appearance of small lesions during pregnancy suggests that they may be related to hormonal changes in chronic liver disease; alternatively, their development may be initiated by the same factors that cause palmar erythema and the increase in cardiac output in cirrhotic patients.

PALMAR ERYTHEMA. Erythema of the thenar and hypothenar eminences and the distal fingers is a common feature of chronic liver disease and is related to local vasodilation.

XANTHOMAS. The hepatic synthesis and secretion of a plasma high-density lipoprotein (lipoprotein X) containing cholesterol and phospholipid are greatly increased in patients with cholestasis. Deposits of lipoprotein in aggregates of macrophages in the skin are correlated with serum cholesterol levels in excess of 450 mg/dl. Flat yellow plaques (xanthelasma) are most common on the eyelids, in skin creases on the neck and palms, and in recent scars. Nodular xanthomas may develop over pressure areas.

NAIL CHANGES. Clubbing of the nails is relatively common in patients with chronic cholestasis; the pathogenesis is uncertain. White nails with a loss of lunulae are associated with hypoproteinemia in patients with chronic liver failure; local copper deposition in patients with Wilson's disease may rarely cause the lunulae to appear blue.

Oral manifestations

FETOR HEPATICUS. Fetor hepaticus is a sweetish, musty odor on the breath of patients with liver failure and/or an extensive portal systemic shunting of blood. The odor has been attributed to the excretion of mercaptans (methyl mercaptan and dimethylsulfide) that are produced by the bacterial degradation of methionine in the gut and that accumulate in the peripheral circulation because of an impaired hepatic detoxification or shunting past the liver.

LESIONS RESULTING FROM NUTRITIONAL DEFICIENCIES. Heavy alcohol ingestion is often accompanied by an inadequate diet; deficiencies of the B vitamins, vitamin C, folic acid, and zinc may cause oral lesions. Glossitis and cheilosis (resulting from B vitamin deficiency), a smooth tongue (folate deficiency), loosening of the teeth along with gingivitis and bleeding (vitamin C deficiency), and a crusting vesicular eruption around the mouth (zinc deficiency) are features that may accompany liver disease in alcoholic patients.

MUCOSAL BLEEDING. Depressed plasma levels of the clotting factors synthesized by the liver (along with a prolonged prothrombin time and partial thromboplastin time) result from a malabsorption of vitamin K in patients with obstructive jaundice or from an impaired hepatic protein synthesis in patients with liver failure. This may cause gingival bleeding or postoperative hemorrhage following the extraction of a tooth. Thrombocytopenia in patients with hypersplenism adds to the risk of bleeding, particularly when platelet function is depressed by aspirin.

Changes in liver size or consistency

Liver enlargement usually indicates liver disease and may reflect changes in the parenchymal cells (infiltration with fat or glycogen), intrahepatic or extrahepatic cholestasis, venous congestion (heart failure, constrictive pericarditis, or hepatic vein occlusion), diffuse inflammation (toxic and viral hepatitis), pyogenic or amebic abscess formation, a cellular infiltration that is either diffuse (macrophages in Gaucher's disease or hematopoietic cells in extramedullary hematopoiesis) or focal (granuloma or neoplasm), cyst formation (polycystic liver or hydatid disease), or fibrosis along with regeneration nodules (cirrhosis in alcoholics).

A small shrunken liver in patients with acute liver failure indicates massive or multilobular necrosis with collapse of the parenchyma; in patients with macronodular cirrhosis the liver is often shrunken and impalpable.

Hepatic tenderness suggests inflammation (acute hepatitis, an abscess, or cholangitis) or an acute stretching of the liver capsule (congestion or acute infiltration). Palpation is often helpful in detecting the induration associated with infiltration or fibrosis and the nodules associated with cirrhosis or a tumor; bimanual palpation may detect hepatic pulsation in patients with tricuspid insufficiency. Vascular bruits indicate arteriovenous fistulas, vascular neoplasms (particularly hepatomas), or an aortic compression caused by liver enlargement; the latter can be excluded from the diagnostic possibilities by positioning the patient. Friction rubs may be heard over superficial necrotic tumor nodules or in patients with acute perihepatitis.

Portal hypertension

Normally approximately 25% of the cardiac output of blood flows through the liver; the hepatic artery contributes approximately 0.5 L/min and the portal vein approximately 1 L/min. The pressure gradient across the sinusoidal bed between portal and hepatic veins fluctuates with the respiratory cycle between 0 and 5 mm Hg. In patients with portal hypertension this pressure gradient is increased in excess of 10 to 12 mm Hg either by an increase in the splanchnic blood flow or by an increase in the resistance to the blood flow through the liver.

PATHOGENESIS OF PORTAL HYPERTENSION

Conditions that increase splanchnic blood flow. Portal hypertension resulting from an increased splanchnic blood flow is relatively uncommon in the United States. Splenic, hepatic, or mesenteric arteriovenous fistulas may result from trauma or the rupture of congenital or acquired aneurysms. Massive splenomegaly is usually accompanied by an increase in the splenic blood flow; an increase in hepatic vascular resistance caused by a cellular infiltration of the hepatic sinusoids increases portal pressure in some patients with hematologic disorders (such as agnogenic myeloid metaplasia). Although arteriovenous shunts have been demonstrated in the splenic circulation of some patients with cirrhosis, changes in the splanchnic blood flow probably play a minor role in the pathogenesis of portal hypertension in these patients.

Conditions that increase hepatic vascular resistance. The lesions that may obstruct the liver's blood flow are clinically separable into the following four groups, each with different manifestations and prognoses.

Extrahepatic obstruction of the portal system. Portal vein thrombosis is usually a complication of an infection, inflammation, neoplasm, or clotting disorder. Umbilical sepsis in infancy may cause thrombosis of the portal vein at the porta hepatis. An intra-abdominal abscess complicating a ruptured appendix or diverticulum may lead to pylephlebitis. Acute hemorrhagic pancreatitis or neoplasms of the pancreas commonly cause thrombosis or an obstruction of the splenic vein; this may be confined to the splenic vein, causing localized splenic hypertension, or may extend to involve the portal vein. Portal vein thrombosis has been described as a complication of polycythemia vera, paroxysmal nocturnal hemoglobinuria, an antithrombin III deficiency, and the use of oral contraceptive hormones—conditions that increase the risk of venous thrombosis. In patients with established cirrhosis and portal hypertension, local venous stasis, hepatoma, or shunt surgery may be complicated by portal vein thrombosis.

Presinusoidal obstruction of portal vein radicles. Fibrosis of the portal triads in patients without cirrhosis can cause an obstruction in the portal venous system without increasing the hydrostatic pressure within the hepatic sinusoids. This fibrosis may be idiopathic in some patients with noncirrhotic portal hypertension or may be caused by schistosomiasis, chronic arsenic or vinyl chloride toxicity, congenital hepatic fibrosis, granulomatous disease (such as sarcoidosis), or neoplastic infiltration. In the absence of cirrhosis or hepatic infiltration, these patients usually maintain normal liver function.

Sinusoidal and postsinusoidal obstruction. Obstruction to the blood flow at the level of the sinusoidal bed and hepatic vein tributaries is the most common mechanism of portal hypertension in patients with cirrhosis. Fatty infiltration and inflammation contribute to reversible portal hypertension in patients with acute alcoholic hepatitis, but progressive fibrosis, particularly pericentrally in the hepatic lobule (central sclerosis), and nodular regeneration cause irreversible changes in blood flow. In patients with venoocclusive disease, toxic plant alkaloids initiate an inflammatory reaction around small tributaries of the hepatic veins and central veins, leading to subsequent fibrosis and thrombosis; a similar lesion may complicate radiation injury to the liver.

Hepatic venous obstruction (Budd-Chiari syndrome). The major hepatic veins may be occluded by congenital webs, by thrombosis, or by a neoplasm such as a hepatoma or lymphoma.

MANIFESTATIONS OF PORTAL HYPERTENSION

Portal-systemic venous collateral circulation. In response to the increased pressure gradient between the portal and systemic venous systems, venous collaterals are established in areas where these systems communicate. The most common and clinically significant collateral circulation is formed by anastomotic veins in and around the esophagus; a retrograde flow in the left gastric and gastroepiploic veins drains portal blood from the portal vein and spleen through gastric and esophageal varices into the azygos system. These collaterals may also communicate with bronchial veins in the mediastinum. In the falciform ligament, umbilical or paraumbilical veins drain from the left branch of the portal vein to the anterior abdominal wall at the umbilicus; the prominent collateral system radiating from the umbilicus to the epigastric, lateral thoracic, and saphenous veins is a *caput medusae*. The abdominal wall collaterals, which are best demonstrated when the patient is standing, must be distinguished from the ascending collaterals of an inferior vena caval obstruction. Turbulent blood flow at the umbilicus may establish a venous hum or palpable venous thrill. Hemorrhoidal vessels become more prominent as collaterals between the inferior mesenteric and the iliac venous systems. Spontaneous collaterals also develop between splenic and renal veins or in vascular adhesions between visceral and parietal areas of peritoneum.

Splenomegaly. Although portal hypertension leads to congestive splenomegaly, there is a poor correlation between the spleen's size and the severity of portal hypertension in patients with cirrhosis. The most significant problems relating to splenomegaly in patients with portal hypertension are an increased risk of traumatic rupture of the spleen and an increased splenic sequestration of blood cells contributing to anemia, leukopenia, and thrombocytopenia.

Ascites. Portal hypertension is the major factor determining the selective accumulation of fluid in the peritoneal cavity of patients with liver disease. The increased hydrostatic pressure in the splanchnic bed and in the relatively permeable hepatic sinusoids increases the transudation of lymph; when lymph formation exceeds the capacity of the lymphatic system to drain fluid from the abdomen, ascites accumulates. In the absence of sinusoidal congestion (as in patients with schistosomiasis or portal vein thrombosis), ascites is unusual; splanchnic congestion alone is insufficient to precipitate ascites. The lowered intravascular colloidal osmotic pressure in patients with hypoproteinemia contributes to the development of both ascites and peripheral edema. Patients with cirrhosis and ascites exhibit secondary hyperaldosteronism with increased rates of aldosterone secretion and excretion and elevated plasma hormone levels. The precise mechanism of the increased aldosterone secretion in these patients is not well defined, although it has been attributed to the splanchnic pooling of blood and a decrease in the systemic pool.

A right pleural effusion often accompanies tense ascites; this fluid has the same characteristics as the ascitic fluid and may result either from the direct leakage of ascitic fluid through the diaphragm or from the passage of lymph from the liver through the diaphragm.

Hepatic coma and precoma

Hepatic coma is a metabolic encephalopathy manifested by disturbances in higher integrative functions, fluctuating changes in the level of consciousness, psychiatric changes, impaired motor coordination along with increased reflexes, a flapping tremor and variable rigidity, and hyperventilation along with respiratory alkalosis. Electroencephalography shows that high-amplitude slow waves (2 to 3 cycles/sec) replace the normal α-waves. These neuropsychiatric abnormalities are observed in patients with metabolic encephalopathy from a variety of causes; patients with hepatic encephalopathy usually have overt clinical signs of liver disease and/or a major portal-systemic shunt (either spontaneous or surgically created). A marked hepatic fetor is usually present, particularly when portal-systemic shunting is a significant causal factor.

PATHOGENESIS OF HEPATIC COMA. A failure of the liver to detoxify exogenous substances such as depressant drugs or endogenous substances such as ammonia, coupled with a variable shunting of portal venous blood directly into the peripheral circulation, exposes the central nervous system to elevated blood levels of agents that are potentially toxic. Both clinical and experimental evidence suggests that ammonia may play a significant role in patients with chronic encephalopathy. Intestinal bacteria in the distal small bowel and colon generate ammonia by deamination of amino acids and hydrolysis of urea; a decrease in the rate of hepatic urea synthesis from ammonia increases the peripheral blood concentration of ammonia. The blood-brain barrier is relatively permeable to ammonia but limits the diffusion of ammonium ions; the pK of this weak alkali is such that a mild alkalosis reduces ionization and increases the ammonia diffusion. In experimental studies it has been shown that ammonia inhibits oxidative phosphorylation in the brain; this reversible metabolic change may be the biochemical basis for the disturbance of brain function.

In addition to ammonia, other products of bacterial metabolism can also accumulate and modify brain function; biogenic amines such as octopamine may act as false neurotransmitters.

In patients with liver disease, encephalopathy may also be precipitated by a variety of other metabolic stresses; those of particular clinical importance include the action of sedative agents or narcotics, disturbances of acid-base, fluid, and electrolyte balances (particularly hypokalemic alkalosis during diuretic therapy), infections, hypoxia, and hypoglycemia. Patients with cirrhosis may enter a deep coma following the administration of standard doses of a depressant drug, resulting in part from a decreased hepatic drug metabolism and in part from an increased brain sensitivity.

Impaired hepatic detoxification

The liver plays a central role in the detoxification and excretion of many endogenous and exogenous substances. Microsomal enzymes of the smooth endoplasmic reticulum participate in oxidative, hydrolytic, or conjugating reactions that modify organic substances and facilitate their excretion in either the bile or the urine. The activity of these enzyme systems may be genetically variable (for example, normal subjects may exhibit a slow or rapid acetylation of drugs) or may be stimulated by agents such as phenobarbital that induce hyperplasia of the smooth endoplasmic reticulum. The metabolism of individual compounds is influenced by hepatic blood flow, transport, and concentration in the liver cell ahd by enzyme activity; other agents that are similarly metabolized may competitively inhibit the metabolism of a given substance.

CHANGES IN DRUG METABOLISM IN LIVER DISEASE. The distribution and metabolism of drugs can be affected by several mechanisms in patients with acute or chronic liver disease. Hypoalbuminemia resulting from impaired plasma protein synthesis modifies the distribution and action of drugs by decreasing drug binding in plasma. A reduced hepatic blood flow or portal-systemic shunting reduces the plasma clearance of agents with a high rate of extraction during a single pass through the liver; conversely, agents with a low single-passage clearance are unaffected by changes in the hepatic blood flow. A decrease in the number of liver cells (cirrhosis) or the activity of liver cells (acute hepatitis) usually decreases the capacity for metabolizing drugs. Cholestasis in patients without liver cell damage is associated with a decrease in the hepatic excretion and enterohepatic circulation of many agents and thus modifies the route of their excretion without depressing their metabolism.

In alcoholic patients several variables may modify the action and metabolism of drugs. Chronic alcoholics usually have an increased central nervous system tolerance to sedative agents that parallels their tolerance to ethanol. When such a patient has elevated blood levels of ethanol, the metabolism of drugs is usually depressed, whereas chronic alcoholics withdrawn from ethanol usually exhibit an increased activity of hepatic microsomal enzymes along with an increased metabolism of drugs. Finally, in patients in whom alcoholism has caused acute or chronic liver disease the metabolism of drugs is again depressed.

Although the hepatic metabolism of exogenous agents usually produces nontoxic metabolites, this process is variable. Some drug metabolites such as propranolol metabolites remain therapeutically active, whereas others are hepatotoxic, such as the intermediates in the metabolism of acetaminophen (see discussion of "Toxic and drug-induced liver disease" later in this chapter).

CHANGES IN HORMONE METABOLISM. The endocrine abnormalities occurring in patients with liver disease may be only indirectly related to the liver disease or may result from changes in the distribution and metabolism of hormones by the liver.

Thyroid function in liver disease. There is an increased incidence of hypothyroidism and autoimmune thyroid disease in patients with idiopathic chronic active hepatitis and primary biliary cirrhosis. In alcoholic patients with liver disease there may be signs that suggest hyperthyroidism, such as a tremor, restlessness, hypermetabolism, tachycardia, and peripheral vasodilation; although altered levels of thyroid binding protein may modify the results of T_3 uptake tests, the serum thyroxine levels are usually normal.

Gonadal function in liver disease. *Hypogonadism* along with testicular atrophy, impotence, and gynecomastia is particularly common in patients with cirrhosis. Malnutrition causes an endocrine dysfunction, and ethanol directly inhibits spermatogenesis. In cases of hemochromatosis, an iron accumulation depresses the pituitary secretion of gonadotropin. Gynecomastia is associated with depressed levels of free testosterone and normal levels of estrogens. In women, chronic liver disease may suppress ovulation or lead to delayed menarche, oligomenorrhea, or amenorrhea.

Adrenal function in liver disease. A reduced plasma clearance of aldosterone contributes to the hyperaldosteronemia of patients with cirrhosis. Although liver disease may reduce the conjugation and excretion of glucocorticoids, normal regulatory mechanisms maintain normal plasma levels of free hormones.

Changes in nutrition and metabolism

MALNUTRITION. Malnutrition in patients with chronic liver disease may be caused by anorexia, a deficient diet, malabsorption, or increased catabolism. The diet of patients with alcoholic liver disease is often deficient in protein, folic and ascorbic acids, B vitamins, and minerals such as potassium, zinc, and magnesium; specific deficiencies in these patients may be accentuated by impaired utilization, such as the inhibition of folic acid utilization by ethanol, or by increased gastrointestinal or urinary losses of minerals. Chronic cholestasis increases the risk of a deficiency of the fat-soluble vitamins that require bile salt micelles for their intestinal absorption. In patients with liver failure the restriction of dietary protein for the control of hepatic encephalopathy accelerates muscle wasting and protein malnutrition.

CARBOHYDRATE METABOLISM. Because of the central role of the liver in regulating blood sugar levels by its uptake and conversion of monosaccharides to glycogen when carbohydrates are ingested and by the release of glucose from glycolysis or gluconeogenesis during fasting, it might be expected that liver disease would impair blood glucose homeostasis. Life-threatening hypoglycemia may complicate acute liver failure in patients with massive or multilobular hepatic necrosis (toxic or viral hepatitis with coma) or may be caused by the impaired gluconeogenesis occurring in alcoholics who drink after a period of fasting and in patients with Reye's syndrome or tetracycline toxicity. Hypoglycemia in patients with glycogen storage disease is the result of a genetically determined lack of the enzymes that control glycogenolysis. In some patients with a hepatocellular carcinoma (hepatoma), hypoglycemia results from a poor intake and glucose utilization by the neoplasm, whereas in others glycogen storage along with an impaired glucose release appears to play a major role.

Diabetes mellitus in patients with cirrhosis is either the coincidental occurrence of two common diseases or causally related (as in cases of hemochromatosis or chronic pancreatic insufficiency in the alcoholic with cirrhosis). Liver biopsies in diabetic patients usually demonstrate fatty infiltration, but in some diabetic patients the pathologic features of acute alcoholic hepatitis—pericentral fibrosis and alcoholic hyalin—have been described; these patients may be at risk for the development of cirrhosis. A glucose load in a cirrhotic patient often leads to hyperglycemia resulting from a delayed uptake of glucose; fasting glucose levels, however, are normal in nondiabetic patients.

NITROGEN METABOLISM. The functions of the liver in the metabolism of amino acids and proteins include the synthesis of nonessential amino acids, the synthesis of liver and plasma proteins, the catabolism of amino acids and proteins, and the conversion of ammonia to urea. The plasma levels of amino acids and proteins are regulated by hepatic synthesis, secretion, and uptake.

In patients with acute liver disease, impaired plasma protein synthesis is quickly reflected by a fall in the concentration of proteins that have a short half-life—the clotting factors—rather than those with a long half-life, such as albumin. A prolonged prothrombin time resulting from severe acute liver disease and impaired synthesis must be distinguished from a reduced level of synthesis resulting from the malabsorption of vitamin K associated with cholestasis; if the prothrombin time does not become normal after a parenteral vitamin K injection, the impaired synthesis is caused by liver failure. In comatose patients with acute hepatitis a fall in the level of blood urea nitrogen, an increase in the level of ammonia in the blood, and increased plasma and urinary levels of amino acids reflect the severe impairment of nitrogen metabolism. In patients with chronic liver disease a decrease in the concentration of plasma proteins synthesized by the liver may reflect protein malnutrition, depressed hepatic synthesis and secretion, or an expanded volume of distribution (with ascites). In stable patients with cirrhosis the reduced plasma protein synthesis is partially compensated for by a decreasing plasma protein catabolism.

FATTY ACID AND TRIGLYCERIDE METABOLISM. Fatty infiltration of the liver, evident histologically as membrane-bound triglyceride droplets in the parenchymal cells, either reflects an increase in stored triglyceride as in obese patients or results from derangements in liver cell metabolism. An excessive peripheral mobilization of triglyceride (in cases of uncontrolled diabetes mellitus) or impaired hepatic metabolism of fatty acids, derived from either the diet or fat depots (in cases of liver injury resulting from carbon tetrachloride, ethanol, or tetracycline), increases the hepatic level of triglyceride.

CHOLESTEROL, LIPOPROTEIN, AND BILE ACID METABOLISM. Cholesterol synthesis in the liver is regulated by the activity of the rate-limiting enzyme β-hydroxy-β-methylglutaric CoA-reductase; the concentration of the primary bile acid, chenodeoxycholic acid, returning to the liver from the gut as it undergoes enterohepatic recirculation, appears to modulate enzyme activity. Newly synthesized hepatic cholesterol is incorporated into liver cell membranes, converted to the primary bile acids (cholic acid and chenodeoxycholic acid), secreted into bile or utilized in the synthesis of plasma lipoproteins that are secreted by the liver.

The normal processes that regulate plasma lipoprotein synthesis and degradation are poorly understood; both genetic and dietary factors play a role in regulating plasma levels of both low-density and high-density lipoproteins. In patients with liver disease, cholestasis increases the hepatic synthesis and secretion of a high-density lipoprotein rich in cholesterol and phospholipid; the plasma remains clear despite markedly elevated cholesterol levels. Conversely, when hepatic synthesis is impaired, serum cholesterol and lipoprotein levels are depressed, and a reduced fraction of esterified cholesterol in the plasma reflects the decreased plasma levels of the enzyme lecithin cholesterol acyl transferase (see later discussion of "Enzymes reflecting hepatic synthesis"). The taurine and glycine conjugates of the primary bile acids, cholic and chenodeoxycholic acid, serve two important detergent functions in the enterohepatic circulation; in bile they form mixed micelles with phospholipid and solubilize cholesterol, and in the upper jejunum they form mixed micelles with long-chain fatty acids and monoglyceride and facilitate the intestinal absorption of fat and fat-soluble vitamins (A, D, and K). The role of altered bile acid and cholesterol secretion in the pathogenesis of cholesterol gallstones is discussed in detail in Chapter 184; the role of altered bile acid metabolism in the pathogenesis of malabsorption is discussed in Chapter 174. Normally there is a highly efficient clearance of bile acids from portal blood as it passes through the hepatic sinusoids; thus most of the bile acid pool is retained within the enterohepatic circulation, and peripheral blood levels are low, rising only transiently after meals. Cholestasis, liver cell dysfunction, and portal-systemic shunting each decrease the hepatic clearance of bile acids and elevate peripheral blood levels, particularly after meals. An increased concentration of bile acid in the peripheral blood is a very sensitive but nonspecific index of liver disease.

Hematologic abnormalities

ANEMIA. Chronic anemia in patients with liver disease is usually mild and results from a variable shortening of the survival of red blood cells caused by an accelerated splenic sequestration of cells coupled with a suppression of erythropoiesis. Peripheral blood cells are usually normochromic and normocytic but may have macrocytic indices; the reticulocyte count is usually low, and plasma haptoglobin levels are depressed because of both an increased red cell breakdown and a reduced protein synthesis. Factors other than protein depletion and ethanol that depress erythropoiesis in cases of liver disease remain undefined. In alcoholic patients folate deficiency causing severe anemia and megaloblastic erythropoiesis responds dramatically to folate therapy. Severe hemolytic anemia may be associated with hyperlipidemia in some patients with acute alcoholic hepatitis or is precipitated by acute viral hepatitis in patients with glucose-6-phosphate dehydrogenase deficiency; brisk hemolysis in patients with liver disease usually causes a dramatic increase in serum bilirubin levels. Acute viral hepatitis rarely may be complicated by aplastic anemia.

Acute bleeding is a life-threatening complication of ruptured esophageal varices. Recurrent blood loss is an obvious cause of iron deficiency anemia in patients with cirrhosis. Lesions other than esophageal varices—gastroesophageal tears, erosive gastritis, ulcer disease, and neoplasm—must be considered in the differential diagnosis of upper gastrointestinal bleeding in patients with cirrhosis.

LEUKOPENIA AND THROMBOCYTOPENIA. Hypersplenism in patients with cirrhosis often causes a modest reduction in peripheral white cells and platelets, but this reduction is rarely responsible for infection or bleeding. Thrombocytopenia coupled with altered platelet function and gastric erosions caused by the ingestion of aspirin in patients with portal hypertension increases the risk of massive gastric mucosal hemorrhage.

CLOTTING ABNORMALITIES. The increased risk of bleeding in patients with depressed synthesis and plasma concentrations of clotting proteins can usually be corrected by a prophylactic infusion of fresh-frozen plasma; patients with liver disease who are bleeding massively also require the appropriate replacement of clotting proteins with fresh blood or fresh-frozen plasma. In severe cases of acute liver disease (hepatitis with coma) or decompensated cirrhosis complicated by septicemia, disseminated intravascular coagulation is often a terminal complication.

Immunologic manifestations

In patients with acute type A or B viral hepatitis, serologic changes reflect the immune response to the viral agents (see later discussion of "Acute viral hepatitis").

In patients with chronic liver disease, particularly chronic active hepatitis, idiopathic cirrhosis, and primary biliary cirrhosis, polyclonal hypergammaglobulinemia is often accompanied by serologic abnormalities. In patients with chronic active hepatitis (especially hepatitis B negative), serologic tests for antinuclear antibody, rheumatoid factor, and antimitochondrial and smooth muscle antibodies as well as LE cell tests are often positive. In cases of primary biliary cirrhosis, increased plasma levels of IgM and immune complexes and positive results in tests for antimitochondrial antibodies are usual.

The role of immunologic mechanisms in the pathogenesis of these diseases of the liver is discussed in later sections describing individual diseases.

Circulatory and renal manifestations

Peripheral vasodilation, with a wide pulse pressure, and a precordial ejection systolic murmur are clinical signs of an increase in cardiac index that often accompanies liver failure. Vasoactive intestinal peptide, a duodenal hormone of the secretin group, may be responsible for these changes; with liver failure, the hormone escapes hepatic degradation, and peripheral blood levels increase.

Arterial oxygen saturation can be depressed in patients with cirrhosis and portal hypertension; when oxygen therapy does not correct this abnormality, the presence of vascular shunts that bypass pulmonary alveoli is suggested. These may be intrapulmonary arteriovenous shunts or portal-pulmonary shunts.

The total blood and plasma volumes are usually normal or slightly increased in patients with untreated cirrhosis.

Portal hypertension, however, increases the relative volume of blood in the splanchnic bed. With the onset of ascites the renal blood flow and glomerular filtration remain normal, but tubular reabsorption of sodium is maximally stimulated by high aldosterone levels, and the urine is low in volume, is concentrated, and has a low sodium and an increased potassium content. With progressive liver failure, patients with terminal liver disease and ascites usually exhibit a decreasing creatinine clearance along with progressive renal failure. This process is not a result of hypovolemia or decreased total renal blood flow but appears to be related to the intrarenal shunting of blood from the cortex to the medulla; the pathogenesis of this intrarenal circulatory change is unexplained. The term "hepatorenal syndrome" refers to this renal failure that complicates terminal liver disease.

CLINICAL AND LABORATORY ASSESSMENT OF PATIENTS
Assessment of liver function

The biochemical tests that are commonly performed in the evaluation of patients with liver disease do not provide a quantitative measure of liver function. These tests, however, are of value in establishing a differential diagnosis, in following the clinical course of patients with liver disease, and in determining their prognosis. In respect to any single liver disease the tests lack specificity (for example, elevations of the level of serum bilirubin are observed in patients with a wide range of liver diseases) and vary in their sensitivity (for example, jaundice develops in a minority of patients with acute viral hepatitis).

SERUM BILIRUBIN. In the van den Bergh reaction, formerly used to measure plasma levels of bilirubin, the amounts of diazopigment formed in the absence and presence of ethanol (direct and total reacting bilirubin) provided a measure of conjugated and total bilirubin concentrations. It is unfortunate that several of the methods that have been adapted for use by the autoanalyzer overestimate the levels of the conjugated fraction, particularly in patients with mild unconjugated hyperbilirubinemia.

In the absence of hemolysis an elevated serum bilirubin level is specific for liver disease but may result from impaired uptake or conjugation, parenchymal cell injury, or intrahepatic or extrahepatic cholestasis. Fractionation of the serum bilirubin level into conjugated and unconjugated fractions is of particular value in distinguishing patients with unconjugated hyperbilirubinemia caused by hemolysis or Gilbert's disease. Serial measurements of the total serum bilirubin are more accurate than the clinical evaluation of the degree of jaundice in following the course of icteric liver disease.

The serum bilirubin test is insensitive for liver disease. Many patients with acute hepatitis, cirrhosis, or extensive infiltrative disease may not have jaundice because of the high capacity of the liver to excrete conjugated bilirubin.

SERUM BILE ACIDS. Serum bile acid concentrations are measured by chromatographic and radioimmunoassay methods that are expensive and difficult to adapt for the routine clinical laboratory; these factors limit their clinical use. Fasting and/or postprandial levels of serum bile acids are usually elevated in patients with liver disease without jaundice; changes in the hepatic blood flow, parenchymal cell injury, or cholestasis reduces the hepatic clearance and excretion of bile acids. Serum bile acid measurements may be of particular value in the early detection of liver disease in patients exposed to potential hepatotoxins, such as occurs during methotrexate therapy for psoriasis; other liver tests have not been of value in detecting early progressive liver disease.

SULFOBROMOPHTHALEIN CLEARANCE. Sulfobromophthalein (BSP) is an organic anion that binds to albumin following intravenous injection and is subsequently concentrated by liver cells and secreted in bile partly as a glutathione conjugate. The plasma clearance of BSP, measured as the residual plasma concentration 30 or 45 minutes after an intravenous injection of the dye (5 mg/kg body weight), is a sensitive test for liver disease in patients without jaundice. The clinical value of this test has been offset by other diagnostic procedures and by the risk of local tissue necrosis if the agent is injected extravascularly, as well as by the rare occurrence of anaphylactic reactions.

SERUM ENZYMES

Enzymes reflecting liver cell injury. Enzymes present in high concentrations in liver cells are released with acute liver cell injury or necrosis; the levels of transaminases and lactic dehydrogenase are measured routinely, but many other enzymes have similar patterns of serum activity following acute liver injury. In patients with liver disease, serum transaminase levels in excess of 500 IU (normally less than 40 IU) indicate acute liver cell injury; values in a lower range are observed in patients with cholestasis and are of little value in a differential diagnosis. The serum glutamic-oxaloacetic transaminase may also originate from cardiac and skeletal muscle, as well as other sources. There is a poor correlation between the serum enzyme levels and the severity of liver cell necrosis revealed by a liver biopsy; the enzyme has a relatively short half-life in the blood, and the time of sampling may not coincide with the period of maximal liver cell injury.

Enzymes reflecting cholestasis. Cholestasis, regardless of whether it is intrahepatic or extrahepatic, causes an increase in the serum activity of alkaline phosphatase, 5'-nucleotidase, leucine aminopeptidase, and γ-glutamyl transpeptidase. An elevation of the level of serum alkaline phosphatase is not a specific sign of liver disease because this enzyme may also arise from bone (with increased osteoblastic activity), from the gut, from the placenta during pregnancy, and from certain tumor cells (such as carcinoma of the lung); the site of the origin of the increased serum enzyme can be analyzed by isoenzyme patterns or can be more simply determined by measuring enzymes that are liver specific, such as γ-glutamyl transpeptidase. The mechanism causing the enzyme level elevation in patients with cholestatis appears to be an increase in enzyme synthesis and release into the plasma rather than reduced excretion; thus there is no correlation between serum levels of conjugated bilirubin and elevated enzyme levels.

Enzymes reflecting hepatic synthesis. The enzyme lecithin-cholesterol acyl transferase, which determines esterification of cholesterol in plasma is synthesized by liver cells and secreted into the plasma. Depressed enzyme levels, as well as a reduced fraction of esterified cholesterol in the plasma, reflect an impaired hepatic protein synthesis in patients with liver failure. This enzyme is not measured routinely, but similar clinical information can be gained from other tests that measure protein synthesis in the liver (prothrombin time).

PLASMA PROTEINS

Albumin. Although a depressed level of serum albumin may reflect impaired hepatic protein synthesis, particularly in patients with chronic liver disease, other factors may also lower plasma levels; these include malnutrition, changes in the volume of distribution (with ascites), increased protein losses (with proteinuria, massive hemorrhage, or recurrent paracentesis), and hypercatabolism (with infections).

Globulins. The globulins are a large number of heterogeneous plasma proteins produced by the liver (α- and β-globulins) or by lymphoid cells (immunoglobulins). An electrophoretic or immunologic analysis of the concentration of individual globulins may be of diagnostic value. Lowered α_1-globulin levels occur in cases of α-1-antitrypsin deficiency, whereas extreme hypergammaglobulinemia occurs in patients with chronic active hepatitis.

Blood clotting factors. Depressed levels of blood clotting factors that are synthesized by the liver are reflected by changes in the prothrombin time. In patients with acute viral hepatitis a marked prolongation of the prothrombin time (greater than 20 seconds) is an early reflection of severe liver disease.

URINARY AND FECAL EXCRETION OF BILE PIGMENTS. In patients with unconjugated hyperbilirubinemia the urine remains free of conjugated bilirubin (that is, the jaundice is *acholuric*); the binding of lipid-soluble unconjugated bilirubin to albumin does not permit glomerular filtration. At low plasma levels, conjugated bilirubin is excreted in the urine and therefore a darkening of the urine is an early symptom of cholestasis.

An excessive bilirubin production by hemolysis or ineffective erythropoiesis increases pigment excretion and is quantitatively reflected by the 24-hour fecal excretion of urobilinogen. The urine may contain higher concentrations of urobilinogen in patients with increased fecal pigment or in patients with parenchymal liver disease and an impaired hepatic excretion of absorbed urobilinogen. Liver disease increases the urinary excretion of uroporphyrin and coproporphyrin, which are normally excreted in bile; in patients with the Dubin-Johnson syndrome there is a characteristic increase in the urinary excretion of coproporphyrin I.

Assessment for occult liver disease

Patients known to have a high risk for the development of liver disease may benefit from an early recognition of liver involvement before the onset of the clinical illness.

GENETICALLY DETERMINED DISEASES. In families with idiopathic hemochromatosis, those individuals most likely to be affected can be identified by HLA typing. Measurements of the serum levels of ferritin and iron and of the total iron-binding capacity provide evidence of excessive iron storage. The removal of excessive tissue iron by phlebotomy prevents parenchymal disease in the liver, endocrine system, and heart. Similarly, the early identification of patients with asymptomatic Wilson's disease by measurements of the plasma ceruloplasmin levels and the serum and urinary copper levels permits the use of chelation therapy and prevents progressive disease.

HEPATITIS B CARRIERS. With the advent of the routine serologic screening of blood donors for hepatitis B infection, many hepatitis B carriers have been identified. Patients without signs of liver disease and with repeatedly normal serum transaminase levels have normal liver biopsies. Those with elevated levels of serum transaminases and hypergammaglobulinemia require a liver biopsy to document or exclude a diagnosis of chronic active hepatitis.

TOXIC HEPATITIS. Patients who receive therapeutic agents that have a potential for causing liver disease not only should be informed of that risk but also if possible should be screened for the development of liver disease. In patients receiving isoniazid or methyldopa, a mild increase in the levels of serum transaminases precedes the onset of more severe, symptomatic, and potentially fatal acute hepatitis; high-risk patients receiving one of these agents should be screened with serial enzyme tests.

Not all patients with drug-related liver disease exhibit early changes demonstrated by the routine liver tests. In patients undergoing long-term methotrexate therapy for psoriasis, progressive hepatic fibrosis may develop that is not reflected by changes in the levels of serum enzymes; these patients require repeated liver biopsies at intervals of 6 to 12 months to prevent irreversible liver injury.

OCCUPATIONAL EXPOSURE TO POTENTIALLY TOXIC AGENTS. Occupational exposure to the vinyl chloride monomer in the manufacturing of polyvinylchloride is associated with an increased risk of hepatic fibrosis or an angiosarcoma of the liver. The most appropriate prophylactic measures against liver disease in these patients are environmental measures to prevent exposure; biochemical abnormalities may be absent during the period of exposure.

NEOPLASMS INVOLVING THE LIVER. The presence of metastatic disease in the liver may modify the patient's treatment and prognosis. The earliest biochemical changes preceding detectable liver enlargement are an increase in the levels of the serum enzymes associated with cholestasis (alkaline phosphatase, 5'-nucleotidase, and γ-glutamyl transpeptidase). Isotopic liver scanning and computed tomography of the liver are probably as sensitive as determinations of enzyme level elevations for establishing the presence of metastases in the liver; selective biopsies may be performed on lesions thus localized to provide a tissue diagnosis. The cost-benefit ratio for many of the relatively expensive scanning procedures used in the search for metastatic disease has not been established in prospective studies; such studies will be necessary to prevent the overuse of these procedures.

Assessment of the patient with jaundice

In the majority of patients with jaundice the correct diagnosis can be determined from the medical history and physical examination; confirmation of this diagnosis may require additional studies. In other patients the diagnosis can be based only on diagnostic tests.

Biochemical studies usually support the clinical data base in differentiating four groups of patients: (1) those with unconjugated hyperbilirubinemia, (2) those with acute liver cell injury (hepatitis), (3) those with chronic parenchymal liver disease (cirrhosis), and (4) those with intrahepatic or extrahepatic cholestasis. The further evaluation of each of these groups is discussed in the following sections.

UNCONJUGATED HYPERBILIRUBINEMIA. In adult patients hemolytic diseases and Gilbert's disease are the most common causes of unconjugated hyperbilirubinemia (see later discussion of "Disorders of bilirubin metabolism"). The patient with primary hemolytic disease usually is anemic and has an increased reticulocyte count and an increased fecal excretion of urobilinogen (see Chapter 67). Patients with Gilbert's disease exhibit fluctuating, mild jaundice with unconjugated hyperbilirubinemia but without anemia or other clinical or biochemical evidence of liver disease; they may need reassurance but require no further diagnostic studies.

ACUTE HEPATITIS. A diagnosis of acute drug-related or viral hepatitis is usually confirmed by a marked elevation of the levels of serum transaminases. A history of the use of a potentially toxic drug provides presumptive evidence of a drug-related illness; when the disorder is a hypersensitivity response, peripheral eosinophilia provides additional support for the diagnosis. The clinician usually must be satisfied with the patient's recovery following drug withdrawal; rechallenge with the drug to confirm the diagnosis unequivocally involves a high risk of death. In patients with viral hepatitis, serologic tests for hepatitis A antibody and the hepatitis B antigens may confirm the diagnosis (see later discussion of "Acute viral hepatitis"). A liver biopsy cannot differentiate between hepatitis caused by drugs or by viral agents; a needle biopsy is often of value, however, in the diagnosis of hepatitis with predominant cholestasis (see discussion of "Cholestasis").

CHRONIC PARENCHYMAL DISEASE (CIRRHOSIS). The cirrhotic patient with jaundice usually has other clinical signs of chronic liver disease and often exhibits other evidence of liver failure. When acute alcoholic hepatitis is responsible for jaundice with or without established cirrhosis, the ratio of the levels of serum transaminases in plasma (SGOT/SGPT) is usually in excess of 2:1. Ultrasonographic studies of the gallbladder, biliary tree, and pancreas are of value in excluding gallstones or an extrahepatic biliary obstruction from the diagnostic possibilities. A liver biopsy should be performed to confirm the diagnosis unless it is contraindicated by an increased risk of bleeding caused by a prolonged prothrombin time.

CHOLESTASIS. Biochemical tests are of minimal value in differentiating intrahepatic cholestasis from extrahepatic cholestasis. To document the cause of cholestasis the clinician must seek anatomic evidence of biliary tract obstruction. An ultrasonographic study of the biliary system usually documents the presence or absence of gallstones in the gallbladder and shows dilated intrahepatic and common bile ducts in patients with a complete extrahepatic obstruction of more than 10 days' duration. Computed tomography provides similar information about the biliary tree (at a higher cost) but gives a better definition of pancreatic lesions. In patients without evidence of a biliary tract obstruction, a liver biopsy can be performed with minimal risk of bile peritonitis; this may confirm the presence of an intrahepatic lesion or may suggest an extrahepatic obstruction when the portal triads are edematous and infiltrated with polymorphonuclear cells. Patients with evidence of a biliary obstruction (dilated ducts shown by ultrasonography) usually can be examined preoperatively by transhepatic (Chiba fine needle) and/or retrograde cholangiography.

DISEASES OF THE LIVER
Disorders of bilirubin metabolism

GILBERT'S DISEASE. Gilbert's disease is a familial disorder of bilirubin transport, probably is inherited as an autosomal dominant trait, and is the most common cause of chronic, mild, unconjugated hyperbilirubinemia in adults.

Pathogenesis. A decrease in the rate of clearance of labeled bilirubin from the plasma of patients with Gibert's disease suggests a hepatic uptake defect that requires a higher plasma level of unconjugated bilirubin to maintain the normal total bilirubin clearance. Compensated hemolysis accentuates the unconjugated hyperbilirubinemia in many patients. It has been reported that the activity of glucuronyl transferase is reduced in homogenates of liver obtained by a liver biopsy from patients with Gilbert's disease; it is possible that the same defect that impairs the bilirubin clearance from plasma also decreases the interaction between substrates and the enzyme system in vitro.

Clinical manifestations. Gilbert's disease is usually diagnosed in healthy young adults; if an intercurrent illness has led the patient to seek health care, the possibility of viral hepatitis if often considered. Concentrations of unconjugated bilirubin are usually less than 3 mg/dl (the normal level is less than 1 mg/dl) with exacerbations during febrile episodes or periods of fasting. Jaundice and unconjugated hyperbilirubinemia resolve completely when the subject is given a drug such as phenobarbital that stimulates hepatic microsomal drug metabolism.

Laboratory findings. The only laboratory abnormalities in patients with Gilbert's disease are an increase in unconjugated hyperbilirubinemia and possibly changes caused by mild compensated hemolysis: reticulocytosis and a lowered level of serum haptoglobin unaccompanied by anemia.

Differential diagnosis. Other causes for unconjugated hyperbilirubinemia must be considered; these include hemolytic disease, an excessive bilirubin production without hemolysis, an impaired hepatic uptake of bilirubin caused by drugs such as novobiocin, and parenchymal liver disease. Unconjugated bilirubinemia has been described during recovery from viral hepatitis (but may have resulted from coincidental Gilbert's disease) and also results from a delayed bilirubin clearance in cirrhotic patients with portacaval anastomoses.

Management. The mechanism causing jaundice should be explained to the patient, with reassurance concerning the benign nature of this disorder.

CRIGLER-NAJJAR SYNDROME. The Crigler-Najjar syndrome is a congenital, nonhemolytic, unconjugated hyperbilirubinemia associated with hepatic glucuronyl transferase deficiency.

Pathogenesis. The two types of Crigler-Najjar syndrome differ in their inheritance and in the severity of the metabolic defect. Patients with type I have an autosomal recessive defect that causes a complete lack of glucuronyl transferase activity in the liver; their serum bilirubin levels range from 25 to 31 mg/dl, and their bile is colorless. Patients with type II have an autosomal dominant defect causing a low level of hepatic glucuronyl transferase activity; their bilirubin levels are lower than those in patients with the type I defect, and the administration of phenobarbital decreases their jaundice by increasing hepatic conjugation and excretion of bilirubin.

Clinical manifestations. Patients with type I Crigler-Najjar syndrome usually die of severe kernicterus in infancy. Those with type II disease may have kernicterus in childhood but may also survive to adulthood without central nervous system damage. Deep acholuric jaundice may be the only clinical feature.

Differential diagnosis. There are no other causes for severe, chronic unconjugated hyperbilirubinemia in adults.

Management. Adult patients should receive genetic counseling with respect to the risk of transmitting the defect. Treatment with phenobarbital decreases jaundice in the adult but may require sedative doses. With infants, vigorous measures to prevent kernicterus may improve the chances of survival in patients with type II disease.

DUBIN-JOHNSON SYNDROME. The Dubin-Johnson syndrome is an autosomal recessive disorder of hepatic transport of conjugated bilirubin and other organic anions into bile.

Pathogenesis. Patients with the Dubin-Johnson syndrome have a normal hepatic uptake and conjugation of bilirubin but an impaired secretion of the conjugated pigment into the bile canaliculus; conjugated bilirubin returns to the plasma and is excreted in the urine. The transport defect is not confined to conjugated bilirubin; the biliary excretion of other organic anions, both endogenous (coproporphyrin I and metanephrine glucuronide) and exogenous (iopanoic acid [Telepaque], BSP, and indocyanine green), is also reduced. The striking black pigmentation of the liver that increases with the age of the patients with this syndrome has been attributed to the conversion of retained metanephrine glucuronide to melanin pigments. The impaired excretion of iodinated compounds, such as iopanoic acid, used in contrast roentgenography explains why the gallbladder is not seen on oral cholecystograms. The enterohepatic circulation of bile acids is normal in these patients, suggesting a dual transport mechanism for the organic constituents of bile.

Clinical manifestations. Patients with the Dubin-Johnson syndrome usually have mild jaundice that is often first noted during pregnancy when the excretion of bilirubin may be further impaired by increased hormone levels. Dark urine reflects the excretion of conjugated bilirubin. Unlike patients with cholestasis, these patients do not have pruritus, and the liver is normal in size. Intermittent and usually mild right upper quadrant discomfort has been described in some patients; this is unexplained.

Laboratory findings. Biochemical studies typically show mild to moderate elevations of conjugated bilirubin (usually lower than 10 mg/dl) with normal levels of serum alkaline phosphatase, transaminase, and serum proteins. Fasting and postprandial serum bile acid levels are normal. BSP excretion is atypical of patients with cholestasis; BSP retention is accompanied by a late increase in plasma BSP levels caused by the appearance of conjugated dye. There is a selective increase in the urinary excretion of coproporphyrin I that differs from the pattern of increased coproporphyrin III excretion in patients with cholestasis.

The diagnosis of the Dubin-Johnson syndrome is confirmed by the presence of dark pigment in the liver cells, particularly in the centrilobular areas.

Differential diagnosis. Intrahepatic or extrahepatic cholestasis can be differentiated from this syndrome by the elevation of the levels of serum enzymes, alkaline phosphatase, 5'-nucleotidase, or γ-glutamyl transpeptidase, by the presence of pruritus and elevated serum bile acid levels, and by the morphologic or anatomic lesions causing cholestasis.

Management. The patient should be educated and reassured about the benign nature of this syndrome. No treatment is indicated.

ROTOR'S SYNDROME. It was formerly thought that Rotor's syndrome was a variant of the Dubin-Johnson syndrome; there are, however, significant biochemical and morphologic differences. In patients with Rotor's syndrome the retention of conjugated bilirubin is not accompanied by hepatic pigmentation, oral cholecystography usually has normal results, and the urinary excretion of coproporphyrin I is not increased.

BENIGN RECURRENT INTRAHEPATIC CHOLESTASIS. Benign recurrent intrahepatic cholestasis is a rare, often familial disorder characterized by recurrent episodes of unexplained intrahepatic cholestasis. The first attack may occur during childhood, and the onset of each episode is usually acute and accompanied by variable nausea and vomiting; pruritus with dark urine and light stools accompanies the jaundice for periods of several months. A liver biopsy reveals the changes of intrahepatic cholestasis—bile stasis in dilated canaliculi—and mononuclear infiltration of the portal triads. Between attacks both liver function and hepatic morphology are normal.

Acute viral hepatitis

Viral hepatitis is an infectious disease caused by several hepatotropic viruses; the more common agents are the type A, B, and non-A, non-B viruses. Acute viral hepatitis (type A) was formerly called infectious hepatitis or short-incubation hepatitis. Type B hepatitis was previously called serum hepatitis, homologous serum jaundice, post-transfusion hepatitis, or long-incubation hepatitis. Type non-A, non-B hepatitis has been clinically recognized only recently with the development of serologic tests that exclude infections by the other agents.

ETIOLOGY. Type A hepatitis virus has been identified as a 27-nm particle present in the liver of infected marmosets and excreted in the stool of experimentally infected volunteers. Using the antigen recovered from infected marmosets (hepatitis A antigen, HAAg), serologic tests for the antibody to hepatitis A virus (anti-HA) are now commercially available.

Type B hepatitis virus is a deoxyribonucleic acid (DNA) virus with a particle size of 42 nm. The central DNA core has DNA polymerase activity and can be recognized immunologically as two separate antigens, hepatitis B core antigen (HB_cAg) and hepatitis B_e antigen (HB_eAg). Capsid antigen, designated as hepatitis B surface antigen (HB_sAg), has several distinct immunologic subtypes. In patients with acute type B hepatitis or in chronic carriers of HB_sAg, the hepatitis B antigens HB_cAg and HB_sAg have been identified by immunofluorescence methods in the nucleus and cytoplasm, respectively, of liver cells. A high concentration of particulate capsular antigen (HB_sAg) circulates in the blood with varying numbers of whole virus particles (Dane particles).

Type non-A, non-B hepatitis virus has been transmitted to chimpanzees, but the virus responsible for non-A, non-B hepatitis have not been characterized; serologic tests are being developed.

EPIDEMIOLOGY

Acute type A viral hepatitis. Hepatitis A may occur as a sporadic illness or in epidemic outbreaks. The virus is excreted in a high titer in the stool of acutely infected patients for a period of several days at the onset of the acute illness. Virus transmission is usually by the fecal-oral route. Epidemic outbreaks have been traced to contaminated drinking water and to the ingestion of contaminated shellfish that filter and concentrate the virus; the virus may not be inactivated by steaming bivalves. Male homosexual subjects have an increased risk of infection, and primate handlers have a high risk of infection from animals with an anicteric infection. Hepatitis A virus infection results in lasting immunity with high circulating titers of anti-HA antibody. In underdeveloped areas with poor sanitation, infection is most common in the young; in areas with optimal sanitation older age groups remain susceptible.

Acute type B viral hepatitis. The transmission of hepatitis B virus is usually related to the high titer of the virus that may be present in the blood of patients with acute or chronic illness or in healthy carriers. The following modes of transmission have been well documented.

Parenteral transmission. Epidemics of hepatitis B infection have been associated with the use of vaccines containing pooled human serum, such as with yellow fever vaccine during World War II, and the recurrent use of inadequately sterilized tattoo needles or syringes and needles, such as in early venereal disease clinics using intravenous arsenicals. Recipients of blood transfusions, particularly of multiple units obtained from paid donors, in the past were very likely to have an acute infection. With the routine use of sensitive screening tests for HB_sAg, the healthy carrier of the hepatitis B virus has been virtually eliminated from the donor pool, and the transmission of the hepatitis B virus by blood transfusion is now rare. There are certain blood fractions, however, that still contain significant titers of virus; pooled plasma, fibrinogen, and factor VIII concentrates may transmit infection. Parenteral drug abuse with shared, unsterilized needles is a major cause of infection in the young adult and adolescent population.

Vertical transmission. The risk of hepatitis B transmission from mother to infant is greatest when the mother has an acute hepatitis B infection during the last trimester of pregnancy or immediately after delivery; although HB_sAg has been detected in some samples of cord blood, the highest risk of infection appears to occur during delivery. Maternal hepatitis B carriers who have high titers of HB_sAg, who are HB_eAg positive, and who have previous children with serologic evidence of infection are most likely to transmit hepatitis B in subsequent pregnancies. The high incidence of the hepatitis B carrier state in several African and Asian populations may be related to the vertical transmission of the disease; the majority of infected infants become carriers.

Nonparenteral transmission. Many patients with a serologically documented hepatitis B infection do not have a history of parenteral exposure by a transfusion or needle. Although epidemiologic studies in a closed population of mentally defective children provided evidence for the nonparenteral transmission of hepatitis B, possibly by fecal-oral exposure, such transmission may require intimate contact. The familial clustering of hepatitis B infections may result in part from vertical transmission and in part from nonparenteral transmission. The possibility that the infection can be transmitted venereally is supported by the high incidence of hepatitis B infections among homosexual males (30% to 50% have either HB_sAg or anti-HB_s), but the incidence of infection among the spouses of HB_sAg-positive carriers is no greater than among family members.

Transmission by insect vectors. Although the transmission of the virus by insect vectors has not been proved, HB_{Ag} has been detected in homogenates of both mosquitoes and bedbugs collected in West Africa, and the antigen was shown to persist for several weeks in bedbugs that were either naturally or experimentally infected.

Nosocomial transmission. Surgeons, dental surgeons, and hospital personnel who have direct contact with blood (operating room, dialysis, and laboratory staff) have an increased risk of accidental parenteral exposure to the hepatitis B virus; the evidence of a past infection among these health care personnel demonstrates an incidence (16.8%) twice that in a matched population. Transmission from unrecognized carriers is probably more common in these personnel than that from patients with a known hepatitis infection. The relatively high rate of infection among health care personnel raises the question of whether hepatitis B might be transmitted to patients. On epidemiologic study concluded that an inhalation therapist with a severe exudative determatitis on both hands transmitted hepatitis B to two patients in an intensive care unit. There have also been well-documented outbreaks of hepatitis B among patients treated by oral surgeons who were subsequently found to be Hb_sAg positive. Serologic studies comparing the incidence of past hepatitis B infections among the patients of HB_sAg-positive and HB_sAg-negative surgeons provide no additional evidence of this hepatitis B transmission. The potential risk of hepatitis B transmission occurring during dental surgery may be reduced by the routine use of operating gloves.

Acute non-A, non-B viral hepatitis. Serologic studies of patients with posttransfusion hepatitis have documented the presence of transmissable agent(s) serologically distinct from hepatitis A and B viruses. Non-A, non-B infections have become the most common cause of posttransfusion hepatitis, particularly in patients receiving multiple units of blood. A chronic carrier state has been identified in one patient following an acute infection.

The sporadic occurrence of non-A, non-B hepatitis not associated with a transfusion or accidental inoculation is evidence of nonparenteral transmission; a recent epidemic of waterborne hepatitis serologically distinct from hepatitis A and B provides strong evidence for the fecal-oral transmission of another viral agent. The further characterization of non-A, non-B agents awaits the development of serologic methods to identify these viruses and their antibodies.

CLINICAL MANIFESTATIONS. The clinical manifestations of acute hepatitis resulting from viruses A, B, and non-A, non-B are similar. Differences in the incubation period following exposure have been well documented in experimental studies but usually cannot be defined in a clinical setting. Thus the diagnosis of the causative viral agent is usually based on serologic tests. The varying clinical pattern of infection with the hepatitis virus appears to be influenced by the age, nutrition, and immune status of the patient; the factors that affect the severity of the illness are not well defined.

The clinical spectrum of acute viral hepatitis includes the following typical and atypical patterns of the disease. The first three are typical patterns; the last two are atypical patterns.

1. Infection without clinical evidence of hepatitis
2. Anicteric hepatitis
3. Icteric hepatitis
4. Cholestatic viral hepatitis
5. Fulminant viral hepatitis

Infection without clinical evidence of hepatitis. Many subjects exposed to the hepatitis viruses remain well without evidence of liver disease. A transiently positive test for HB_sAg or a rising titer of antibodies to the hepatitis agents (anti-HA or anti-HB_s) provides immunologic evidence of infection. Serum transaminase levels may be increased for a variable period.

Anicteric hepatitis. Patients with anicteric hepatitis usually exhibit the prodromal symptoms of a viral illness (malaise, anorexia, nausea and vomiting, headache, and fever); abdominal discomfort may focus the physician's attention on a mildly enlarged tender liver. Although the patient remains anicteric, the urine may become dark because of the excretion of conjugated bilirubin. The symptomatic illness is usually of brief duration and coincides with the onset of elevated serum transaminase levels. Although patients with anicteric hepatitis usually recover completely, a significant percentage of those with a hepatitis B or non-A, non-B infection have late sequelae: chronic persistent hepatitis, chronic active hepatitis, or a chronic carrier state.

Icteric hepatitis. The *preicteric* or prodromal phase of icteric hepatitis may be abrupt in onset (usually in type A) or may develop insidiously (often in types B and non-A, non-B) with symptoms common to many viral illnesses. Fever is usually maximal at the onset of the illness and may persist until the onset of jaundice. Malaise, weakness, headache, and myalgia are relatively common, and gastrointestinal symptoms including nausea, vomiting, and anorexia along with right upper quadrant abdominal pain are prominent complaints; there may also be a striking loss of taste for cigarettes. During the preicteric period patients with a hepatitis B infection may exhibit the clinical manifestations of circulating immune complexes, which include maculopapular, urticarial, or petechial skin rashes, arthralgias, or acute arthritis. Late in the preicteric period hepatic enlargement and tenderness are usual, and the urine becomes dark before jaundice develops.

The *icteric phase* is one of increasing jaundice, with peak serum bilirubin levels usually less than 10 mg/dl within 10 to 14 days, followed by a slower decline to normal levels. The patient's symptoms usually improve within a few days of the onset of jaundice, although anorexia may persist for a longer period and pruritus increases in those with progressive cholestasis. The liver may remain enlarged through the icteric period, but tenderness usually declines during the early icteric phase. Splenomegaly may be noted during the acute illness.

The *convalescent phase* following the disappearance of jaundice may be brief but may extend over several months accompanied by complaints of malaise, early fatigue, particularly after an unaccustomed activity, and mild hepatic tenderness. During this period the levels of serum transaminases may remain mildly elevated.

Cholestatic viral hepatitis. Cholestatic viral hepatitis is a relatively uncommon clinical pattern of illness in which fairly typical icteric hepatitis passes into a more prolonged cholestatic phase with deep jaundice, marked pruritus, and prominent biochemical features of intrahepatic cholestasis. Despite the deep jaundice, which may persist over several weeks, the patient usually feels relatively well and does not appear to be seriously ill. Liver enlargement with minimal tenderness often persists during the period of jaundice. Diarrhea in these patients results from the cathartic action of fatty acids that are poorly absorbed with low intestinal concentration of bile acids.

Fulminant viral hepatitis. In patients with fulminant viral hepatitis (viral hepatitis with coma), extensive hepatic necrosis causes acute hepatic failure with coma and commonly leads to death. This is a rare complication of acute hepatitis (1% of icteric patients) caused by viruses A, B, or non-A, non-B. Clinically, the preicteric period may be brief and accompanied by severe abdominal pain, vomiting, and a high fever that persist despite bed rest. A sudden decrease in liver size, the early development of drowsiness, irritability, insomnia, or confusion, a marked prolongation of the prothrombin time that is not corrected by the parenteral administration of vitamin K, and signs of fluid retention are clinical features that suggest a fulminant course. The progression of hepatic failure leads to deepening hepatic encephalopathy accompanied by hyperventilation and respiratory alkalosis, convulsions (particularly in children), progressive stupor, and coma. Clinical problems that can be anticipated in these patients include hypoglycemia, severe bleeding caused by a deficiency in clotting factor synthesis, aspiration pneumonia or septicemia, lactic acidosis, cardiac arrhythmias or arrest, and renal failure.

LABORATORY FINDINGS. Liver cell damage and necrosis are reflected by an increase in serum levels of the transaminases; elevation of enzyme levels during recovery indicates persistent disease activity (see later discussions of "Chronic persistent hepatitis" and "Chronic active hepatitis"). In icteric patients, both conjugated and unconjugated serum bilirubin levels become elevated; the increase in conjugated bilirubin is caused by an impaired liver cell excretion of the conjugated pigment or intrahepatic cholestasis. Serum alkaline phosphatase levels rise during the icteric period and reach their peak values later than the peak values of transaminase; the most marked elevation occurs in patients with severe cholestasis. In patients with typical icteric hepatitis there may be a slight fall in serum albumin late in the clinical course. Hypoprothrombinemia indicates liver failure or a vitamin K deficiency in deeply jaundiced patients. During the recovery period a slight increase in serum γ-globulin levels is consistent with uncomplicated disease; marked elevations suggest the possibility of chronic active hepatitis.

Hematologic findings early in acute illness may include leukopenia along with relative lymphocytosis or the presence of atypical mononuclear cells. A mild anemia often develops during the course of the illness, resulting from a reduced bone marrow response to repeated blood drawing. Rarely the acute illness may be complicated by severe thrombocytopenia, hemolytic disease (particularly in patients with glucose-6-phosphate dehydrogenase deficiency), or aplastic anemia.

Serologic tests. In patients with acute type A hepatitis, anti-HA antibodies usually develop during the period of jaundice; the early immune response produces a high titer of IgM antibody followed by rising titers of IgG antibody. Patients with hepatitis B usually exhibit the viral antigens HB_sAg, HB_eAg, and DNA polymerase during the preicteric and early icteric phases. The hepatitis B antibodies anti-HB_s and anti-HB_e usually appear in the early icteric period when the antigens are cleared from the blood. In patients who recover but remain in a carrier state and in patients with chronic persistent or chronic active hepatitis, the hepatitis B antigens usually persist along with anti-HB_c but not anti-HB_s or anti-HB_e.

PATHOLOGY. In patients with typical viral hepatitis, regardless of whether it is asymptomatic, anicteric, or icteric, a liver biopsy shows evidence of parenchymal cell degeneration or necrosis, infiltration with inflammatory cells with proliferation of Kupffer's cells, and evidence of cell regeneration. Damaged parenchymal cells enlarge with ballooning of their cytoplasm or may undergo hyaline degeneration to form acidophilic bodies with pyknotic nuclei (Councilman's bodies); these degenerating cells are scattered focally throughout the liver lobule. Cell necrosis is usually balanced by cell regeneration that can be recognized by the presence of mitotic figures or multinucleated cells. Within the liver lobule, hyperplastic Kupffer's cells accumulate cell debris as an acid-fast pigment, lipofuscin, and foci of mononuclear cells collect at sites of cell necrosis.

In the portal tracts there are variable edema and an infiltration of inflammatory cells that are predominantly mononuclear. There may be evidence of ductular epithelial injury with cell vacuolation and later ductular proliferation. The inflammatory infiltrate expanding the portal triads usually persists into the later convalescent period when signs of parenchymal cell injury have resolved. A complete histologic recovery is the usual outcome.

Patients with cholestatic hepatitis usually exhibit varying degrees of parenchymal cell necrosis and inflammatory infiltration. In addition, the intrahepatic cholestasis is reflected histologically by the presence of bile plugs in dilated bile canaliculi, particularly in the central zones, and increased bile staining of parenchymal cells and Kupffer's cells.

In patients with fulminant hepatitis liver biopsies performed early in the acute illness usually show multilobular zones of necrosis with the collapse of the reticulum framework of the normal lobule. Autopsies have shown that massive necrosis leads to a shrunken bile-stained liver (acute yellow atrophy) with extensive areas of lobular collapse, few mononuclear inflammatory cells, and residual liver cells only in some areas adjacent to the preserved portal triads. In patients who survive fulminant hepatitis there is a complete regeneration of the normal lobular structure of the liver without fibrosis.

Some patients with typical icteric hepatitis, particularly those with a more prolonged course of severe disease, may have bridging or multilobular necrosis demonstrated by a liver biopsy rather than the typical focal necrosis. Clinically, these patients may recover without sequelae, or the disease may progress rapidly to fulminant hepatitis; in these patients chronic active hepatitis with progressive fibrosis and cirrhosis is more likely to develop than in patients with focal necrosis alone.

MANAGEMENT. There are no specific measures that significantly modify the course of typical acute viral hepatitis. The symptomatic patient usually feels better with bed rest, but progressive ambulation should be permitted as the patient improves and feels well. The patient should be encouraged to eat a normal diet of foods that appeal to him; specific restrictions are unnecessary. When anorexia or nausea is prolonged and the patient's caloric intake is not optimal, oral or intravenous supplements may be necessary. The majority of patients can be treated at home; hospitalization is indicated for high-risk patients—pregnant, diabetic, or elderly patients and those with complicating disease—and for those who are judged to be severely ill and are vomiting or have an elevated prothrombin time. Although corticosteroid therapy may accelerate the patient's biochemical improvement, the duration of the illness is not shortened, and a relapse appears to be more likely when the therapy ends; corticosteroid therapy is thus not indicated.

When the diagnosis has been established, further laboratory tests should be performed as necessary to monitor the patient's progress. When the patient is acutely ill, a daily measurement of the prothrombin time after a vitamin K injection (10 mg intramuscularly is of value in detecting a sudden deterioration in liver function. Measurements of the levels of serum bilirubin and enzymes at intervals of several days during the acute illness and at longer intervals during recovery provide objective data on the patient's course.

Drugs should be given cautiously to the acutely ill patient; the reduced activity of hepatic microsomal drug metabolizing enzymes may lead to a delayed plasma clearance of many sedative agents. Oxazepam (Serax) is an ideal sedative for patients with acute hepatitis because the volume of distribution, plasma binding, clearance, and excretion of this agent are not modified in acute hepatitis.

In patients with prominent cholestasis and severe itching, cholestyramine (up to 4 g three times a day) may provide symptomatic relief; this agent increases the malabsorption of fat-soluble vitamins and precipitates a vitamin K deficiency unless vitamin K is replaced parenterally.

Patients with fulminant hepatitis require intensive nursing care and support. A comatose patient requires a cuffed endotracheal tube and assisted ventilation, if necessary, to prevent aspiration and to ensure adequate ventilation. The continuous intravenous administration of glucose is necessary to provide calories and to prevent hypoglycemia in the absence of glycogen stores or gluconeogenesis. Bleeding may be controlled by infusions of fresh-frozen plasma to replace clotting factors, and measures to eliminate the ammonia production by intestinal bacteria should include cleansing enemas, the intragastric instillation of neomycin (4 to 6 g daily), and dietary protein elimination. Gastric neutralization achieved with antacids or intravenously administered cimetidine (300 mg every 6 hours) reduces the risk of massive bleeding from stress erosions in the stomach. Therapy with high doses of corticosteroids has been shown to increase the mortality of patients with severe viral hepatitis; the earlier use of these drugs was based on uncontrolled observations. Many measures have been proposed for the elimination of potential toxins normally removed by the liver, in the hope that this would reverse the coma and improve the survival rate; these measures include hemodialysis, plasmapheresis or an exchange transfusion, cross-perfusion with a human volunteer or primate, and charcoal hemoperfusion. Although these procedures may temporarily restore the patient's consciousness, they have not increased the survival rate of patients with fulminant hepatitis.

PROGNOSIS. The majority of patients recover completely from typical viral hepatitis. Some patients, however, have benign or serious sequelae. Early recovery from acute hepatitis may be followed by a relapse. A chronic carrier state without liver disease, chronic persistent hepatitis lasting for more than 6 months, or chronic active hepatitis may follow an acute infection with hepatitis B or non-A, non-B viruses.

Relapsing acute hepatitis. The relapse of acute hepatitis is usually milder than the initial episode but has similar clinical, laboratory, and pathologic features. The acute exacerbation may occur during the convalescent period or following complete clinical and biochemical recovery. The possibility that late relapses result from an infection by a different viral agent usually has not been excluded by serologic tests. At the onset of a relapse the patient usually notes a decrease in appetite with malaise and fatigue, and the liver again becomes enlarged and tender. The prognosis for full recovery following a relapse does not differ from that of the initial attack, and in the absence of clinical, biochemical, or histologic evidence of chronic active hepatitis the patient can be reassured.

Chronic hepatitis B carrier state. Following recovery from acute hepatitis B, regardless of whether it is asymptomatic, anicteric, or icteric, some patients fail to clear the hepatitis B antigens from the blood and remain carriers for a long period. The incidence of the chronic carrier state following infection is greatest in infancy and early childhood, possibly because of a greater immune tolerance, and in patients undergoing immunosuppressive therapy or long-term renal dialysis. The hepatitis B carrier may exhibit no clinical, biochemical, or pathologic evidence of liver disease, may be asymptomatic and have minor elevations of serum transaminase levels, or may have progressive chronic active hepatitis.

The major considerations in the management of the hepatitis B carrier are to define the presence or absence of progressive liver disease and to prevent the transmission of the disease. Patients with normal levels of serum enzymes demonstrated by repeated testing do not require further diagnostic assessment; liver biopsies do not show evidence of liver disease. Patients with elevated levels of serum transaminases may have chronic persistent hepatitis (a benign process) or chronic active hepatitis (a progressive disease); the latter is particularly likely if γ-globulin levels are elevated. A liver biopsy is indicated in patients with abnormal liver function to differentiate these disorders.

The hepatitis B carrier with a low titer of HB_sAg and a negative test result for HB_eAg with anti-HB_e probably has a low risk of transmitting the disease. The risk of the nonparenteral transmission of hepatitis is minimized with careful practice of personal hygiene. Some experimental studies have indicated that the use of interferon can terminate the carrier state, but this treatment is not currently clinically available.

Chronic persistent hepatitis. Chronic persistent hepatitis is a benign form of chronic hepatitis B or non-A, non-B that follows an acute infection. The patient may be asymptomatic or mildly symptomatic and may have lethargy, weakness, and mild hepatic tenderness; jaundice if present is mild, with a minimal, fluctuating elevation of serum transaminase levels and mild changes of acute hepatitis demonstrated by a liver biopsy. The disease often persists for months or years, but complete recovery is the final outcome. (Chronic active hepatitis is discussed in a later section.)

PROPHYLAXIS

General measures. Good personal hygiene is a major factor in reducing the fecal-oral transmission of the hepatitis viruses. Enteric precautions should be maintained with hospitalized patients who have acute hepatitis during the symptomatic period of early illness; the fecal excretion of hepatitis A virus does not extend into the later icteric phase (after 1 to 2 weeks of icterus) when the patient is recovering. Contact with infected blood should be avoided through the use of gloves, the careful disposal of needles, and the appropriate labeling and handling of blood specimens.

Prevention of transfusion-associated hepatitis. The use of sensitive tests for hepatitis B antigens has greatly reduced the incidence of posttransfusion hepatitis B. The risk of the transmission of hepatitis B virus by concentrates of antihemophilic globulin has been decreased experimentally by the addition of hepatitis B immune globulin (HBIG). Serologic tests to screen for carriers of non-A, non-B hepatitis are not yet available commercially; the risk of this infection may be decreased by excluding commercial donors and those with elevated serum transaminase levels.

Cleaning and sterilizing instruments and equipment. Instruments should be cleaned by a person wearing protective gloves and if possible should be sterilized by autoclaving before using again. When heat sterilization is not possible, such as with fiberoptic endoscopes, effective cold sterilizing procedures should be employed.

Prevention by passive immunization. Two preparations of γ-globulin are commercially available for hepatitis prophylaxis. Normal serum globulin (ISG) contains high titers of anti-HA and low titers (1:80) of anti-HB_s. Hepatitis B immune globulin (HBIG) prepared from specific immune sera has high titers of anti-HB_s. The recommendations of the U.S. Public Health Service for hepatitis prophylaxis are as follows.

Hepatitis A. Preexposure prophylaxis is recommended for travelers planning to visit tropical or developing countries; a single injection of 2 ml of ISG (in adults) is recommended for those staying less than 3 months and 5 ml for those staying 3 or more months, followed by repeated ISG injections at 4- to 6-month intervals. A similar schedule of ISG prophylaxis is recommended for those who handle recently imported primates.

Postexposure prophylaxis with ISG (0.02 ml/kg) is recommended within 2 weeks of exposure for those in close personal contact with a person who has hepatitis A, such as contact occurring within a household. Prophylaxis is of value for contacts within institutions when there is evidence of a hepatitis A outbreak; the risk of an institutional spread of the infection appears to be particularly high among those in contact with children under the age of 2 years who have anicteric infection.

Hepatitis B. Preexposure prophylaxis is recommended only in situations in which there may be repeated exposures and in which environmental measures to limit the risk of infection cannot be implemented; in these circumstances routine serologic monitoring for HB_sAg and anti-HB_s should be combined with ISG prophylaxis (0.05 ml/kg at 4-month intervals).

Postexposure prophylaxis with HBIG (0.05 ml/kg) within 7 days and repeated at 30 days is recommended following a single acute parenteral (needle) or oral exposure to a large inoculum. Infants of mothers who have acute hepatitis B during the last trimester or who are HB_sAg positive at the time of delivery may be protected with HBIG (0.13 ml/kg).

Passive immunization with γ-globulin may prevent infection in exposed individuals but more commonly suppresses the infection and leads to the development of subclinical hepatitis rather than icteric disease; the mild infection provides an active immunity. Prophylaxis for infants exposed to hepatitis B may reduce the risk of a chronic carrier state. The value of immune prophylaxis for non-A, non-B hepatitis has not yet been determined.

Active immunization. Vaccines for active immunization against hepatitis A and B are currently being developed.

HEPATITIS RESULTING FROM OTHER VIRAL AGENTS

Infectious mononucleosis. Patients with infectious mononucleosis usually have liver involvement. Jaundice is relatively uncommon but when it occurs is usually cholestatic unless there is brisk hemolysis, and the liver may be slightly enlarged and tender; biochemical signs of mild cholestasis (elevated levels of serum alkaline phosphatase, 5'-nucleotidase, and γ-glutamyl transpeptidase) commonly accompany a portal infiltration with mononuclear cells. The prognosis for complete recovery is excellent; no patients with infectious mononucleosis have had fulminant hepatitis or documented chronic liver disease.

Other viral infections in immunocompromised patients or neonates. *Congenital rubella* infections are commonly associated with an enlargement of the liver and spleen; the clinical pattern of liver disease ranges from cases of mild hepatitis along with minimal necrosis and inflammation to severe, fatal cases of giant cell hepatitis.

Herpes simplex (types 1 and 2) may cause severe hepatitis in patients with a generalized herpetic infection; in neonates the type 2 infection is more common, although either agent may be responsible for a generalized infection in malnourished or immunosuppressed patients. Diffuse hepatocellular necrosis may lead to liver failure.

Cytomegaloviruses are responsible for a spectrum of liver disease that varies with the age and susceptibility of the patient. The infection in healthy children or adults is usually subclinical. A neonatal infection may be mild and subclinical or may cause hepatomegaly with cholestatic jaundice. In adults the clinical syndrome of cytomegalic mononucleosis occurs spontaneously or follows a massive transfusion; the histologic picture is similar to that of viral hepatitis. In immunocompromised patients, hepatomegaly and liver dysfunction may accompany the more serious pulmonary infection.

Bacterial infection and liver disease

Gram-negative bacterial infection. Cholestatic jaundice is a relatively common complication of gram-negative sepsis in infants; an infection of the urinary tract is the most common source. In adults jaundice is a less common complication of a severe infection, which is usually intraabdominal and associated with septicemia. Pathologic changes in the liver include bile stasis with dilated bile canaliculi containing bile plugs, Kupffer's cell hyperplasia, and nonspecific cellular infiltration. The pathogenesis of cholestasis in patients with gram-negative sepsis may be related to the direct invasion of the liver by organisms or to the effects of bacterial toxins on the liver cell; experimental studies have shown that the endotoxins of *Escherichia coli* and *Salmonella enteritidis* reduce bile flow and organic anion excretion in isolated perfused rat livers.

Typhoid fever is accompanied by jaundice in up to 25% of the patients. The liver is usually enlarged and tender, and serum alkaline phosphatase and transaminase levels are moderately elevated (two to five times normal levels). Focal liver cell necrosis with marked mononuclear cell infiltration and Kupffer's cell hyperplasia is the usual hepatic lesion, which resolves within 2 weeks after the initiation of therapy; intrahepatic cholestasis may be mild.

Pneumococcal infection. Before antibiotics came into use, jaundice was reported as a complication in up to 30% of patients with lobar pneumonia; biochemical studies to determine the mechanism of this jaundice were not available at that time. In more recent clinical experience jaundice has been an uncommon feature of pneumococcal pneumonia. Cholestasis caused by hepatocellular injury is the most likely mechanism of jaundice, but the specific cause for this injury has not been determined; in some patients hemolysis may accentuate the jaundice.

Gonococcal infection. Gonococcal perihepatitis, causing the symptoms of right upper quadrant abdominal pain and guarding, may complicate gonococcal pelvic inflammatory disease in the female. Localized tenderness and a friction rub over the liver area are signs of local peritonitis. Liver tests may show a minimal elevation of the levels of serum transaminases without hyperbilirubinemia, and a liver biopsy demonstrates an acute inflammatory infiltration of the capsule and subcapsular liver parenchyma.

Spirochetal infection. A leptospiral infection may cause hepatocellular injury and jaundice. Usually jaundice in these patients is accentuated by a more severe renal lesion that limits the urinary excretion of conjugated bilirubin. The hepatic lesion is minimal and involves focal necrosis, Kupffer's cell hyperplasia, periportal infiltration, and cholestasis in deeply jaundiced patients.

Syphilis causes a diffuse hepatitis that may lead to pericellular fibrosis and cirrhosis in infants with congenital infection. Adults with early secondary syphilis may exhibit evidence of hepatitis with mild jaundice and elevated levels of serum enzymes; miliary granulomata and focal infiltrations with polymorphonuclear and mononuclear cells are the typical hepatic lesions.

Tuberculosis of the liver is discussed in the later section, "Granulomatous and infiltrative diseases."

Pyogenic liver abscess

A pyogenic liver abscess is a complication of cholangitis, portal pyemia, or septicemia. Biliary tract disease caused by an infection with gram-negative and anaerobic enteric organisms is now the most common recognized cause of acute liver abscesses; an infection extending from the biliary trees usually produces multiple lesions. Infections via the portal system, formerly a more common complication of umbilical sepsis in infancy or acute appendicitis, now have a lower incidence with the earlier diagnosis and therapy of the primary lesions; intra-abdominal sepsis may be followed by hepatic lesions, usually in the right lobe. Abscesses resulting from a staphylococcal infection may occur without a clinically detectable focus of the infection or may complicate an obvious focus at a distant site.

CLINICAL MANIFESTATIONS. The clinical features of a liver abscess are those of sepsis and a space-occupying lesion within the liver. The patient usually has fever and chills and polymorphonuclear leukocytosis with a shift to the left. Abdominal symptoms include anorexia, nausea, vomiting, and epigastric or right upper quadrant pain; these features may be of minimal diagnostic value in patients with preexisting abdominal disease. The right diaphragm is often elevated, and pleural effusion is caused by local inflammation. Jaundice may result from the predisposing biliary tract obstruction but is a late clinical manifestation of the liver abscess itself; it is associated with a high mortality. Hepatic enlargement and tenderness are commonly observed.

LABORATORY FINDINGS. In patients without biliary tract disease, liver tests often show only a minimal elevation of levels of serum alkaline phosphatase or transaminases; enzyme levels may remain normal. Hypoalbuminemia occurs commonly in these severely ill patients; both an impaired synthesis and an increased catabolism are its probable causes. Blood cultures have positive results in up to 50% of these patients. With isotope scanning of the liver, a focal area or areas of decreased uptake indicate the site of the hepatic lesion(s). A gallium scan may show a corresponding area of enhanced uptake. Ultrasonography or computed tomography may be of value in differentiating abscesses from solid space-occupying lesions.

DIAGNOSIS. Unless the clinician strongly suspects that the patient has a liver abscess, the lesion may not be diagnosed during life. This diagnosis must be considered in any patient with biliary tract disease complicated by sepsis and in patients with other foci of intra-abdominal sepsis that do not respond promptly to surgical drainage and antibiotic therapy. Pyogenic abscesses must be differentiated from amebic abscesses (see discussion of "Amebic liver abscess").

MANAGEMENT. Surgical drainage is the recommended treatment for pyogenic liver abscesses associated with biliary obstruction or some other intra-abdominal pathologic disorder. Conservative therapy using parenteral antibiotics may be appropriate for patients without another abdominal disease; a percutaneous needle aspiration of the abscess is of benefit in decompressing the abscess cavity and in providing pus for identification of the organism(s) by a Gram stain and aerobic and anaerobic cultures.

Toxic and drug-induced liver disease

Clinical and experimental evidence suggests that liver injury caused by toxic agents or drugs may be mediated by covalent binding of the agent or metabolite in the liver (toxicity) or by an immunologic reaction (hypersensitivity). Hepatotoxic reactions cause a predictable liver injury in both experimental animals and humans; the liver disease is related to the dose of the toxic agent or drug and is usually observed after a short latent period, such as occurs with carbon tetrachloride liver injury. Conversely, hypersensitivity reactions are uncommon and unpredictable and have not been observed in experimental animals; these reactions are unrelated to the drug dose, occur at variable intervals following exposure to the drug (decreasing with subsequent exposure), and may be accompanied by other signs of a hypersensitivity reaction, such as eosinophilia. These distinctions between hepatotoxic and hypersensitivity reactions have been blurred by an increasing knowledge of the hepatic metabolism of individual drugs. Individual variations in drug metabolism may be responsible for some hepatotoxic drug reactions that were formerly thought caused by hypersensitivity; that is, an individual "hypersensitivity" may be metabolic in some patients rather than immunologic.

TOXIC DRUG REACTIONS

Carbon tetrachloride. Carbon tetrachloride is a typical hepatotoxin that is metabolized by the liver to form toxic intermediates that bind to microsomal protein and cause liver cell necrosis. Its toxicity is increased by phenobarbital and ethanol, which increase the production of labile intermediates in the liver.

Carbon tetrachloride exposure by inhalation or ingestion usually occurs accidentally or as a suicide attempt. After an early period of variable central nervous depression with drowsiness, dizziness, headache, and nausea, there may be a period of 2 to 4 days before the onset of liver and renal disease. Jaundice and liver enlargement result from diffuse fatty degeneration and centrilobular necrosis; massive or bridging necrosis is relatively rare. The changes in liver function are similar to those caused by acute viral hepatitis with an extreme elevation of levels of serum transaminases in both anicteric and icteric patients. Although severe liver failure may cause death in hepatic coma during the first week of the illness, after that time renal failure is the dominant clinical problem. The supportive therapy for patients with fulminant viral hepatis is appropriate also for patients with severe toxic hepatitis; renal dialysis may be necessary for the management of acute renal failure. After a single exposure to carbon tetrachloride, survivors have normal liver function and structure, but repeated exposure (usually occupational) can cause hepatic fibrosis and cirrhosis.

Ethanol. Ethanol is a direct hepatotoxin in humans as well as experimental animals. The acute ingestion of intoxicating doses causes a fatty liver that may be accompanied by a minimal serum transaminase elevation. In baboons the chronic ingestion of ethanol with an adequate diet leads to the spectrum of pathologic changes that have been documented in alcoholic patients (see later discussion of "Alcoholic cirrhosis").

Acetaminophen. In recommended doses acetaminophen is a safe analgesic agent for healthy subjects; potentially toxic metabolites are rapidly conjugated with glutathione to form nontoxic compounds. With the ingestion of an excessive dose (usually in a suicide attempt), hepatic glutathione is depleted, and toxic metabolites that bind microsomal protein accumulate in the liver. A latent, asymptomatic period of up to 24 hours following the ingestion precedes evidence of severe liver cell necrosis that may cause fatal liver failure. With an early diagnosis of a suicidal overdosage, treatment with N-acetyl cysteine within 12 hours of ingestion protects against liver injury by providing a source of glutathione for drug detoxification.

Isoniazid. The high incidence (10% to 20%) of mild elevations of serum transaminase levels (usually less than 100 IU) among patients receiving isoniazid suggests that this agent is mildly hepatotoxic. Icteric liver disease occurring with the clinical, biochemical, and pathologic features that mimic acute viral hepatitis has been reported in approximately 1% of older patients receiving therapy with this drug. Severe isoniazid hepatitis was formerly thought to be a hypersensitivity (immunologic) reaction to the drug, but more recent metabolic studies in experimental animals document the formation of toxic metabolites, particularly when drug metabolism is stimulated by phenobarbital.

The minor elevations of serum transaminase levels during isoniazid therapy are usually transient and disappear with continued drug administration. Overt hepatitis is more common during the first 12 weeks of therapy but may be delayed; jaundice is usually preceded by anorexia, nausea, vomiting, and abdominal discomfort.

The prophylactic use of isoniazid should be restricted when possible to low-risk patients, those under the age of 35 who do not drink alcohol. When this agent is used in patients with a high risk of hepatitis, clinical and biochemical monitoring (SGOT tests at 2- to 4-week intervals) may provide earlier evidence of acute liver disease; severe, fatal hepatitis (occurring in 10% of icteric patients) may thus be reduced. Transient elevated levels of SGOT and SGPT occur in 10% to 20% of all patients taking isoniazid, however, and thus are not necessarily an indication for discontinuing this therapy.

Sex hormones. The synthetic androgens methyltestosterone and carbon 17 alkyl-substituted steroids cause a reversible, dose-related intrahepatic cholestasis. Clinical features include jaundice, a slight liver enlargement, and variable conjugated hyperbilirubinemia with elevated levels of alkaline phosphatase, 5'-nucleotidase, and γ-glutamyl transpeptidase. Liver biopsies show cholestasis without liver cell necrosis.

Prolonged therapy with anabolic steroids, usually in patients with aplastic anemia, has been associated with the development of peliosis hepatis, in which dilated sinusoids or blood-filled cystic spaces replace normal liver cords. In these patients liver enlargement usually precedes changes in liver function.

Intrahepatic cholestasis appearing in the third trimester of pregnancy and manifested as pruritus gravidarum or cholestatic jaundice with pruritus appears to result from an exaggeration of the mild biochemical cholestasis that is normal in late pregnancy. Patients with recurrent cholestasis of pregnancy have normal estrogen levels and normal hormone metabolism; following pregnancy liver function is normal unless they are challenged with exogenous estrogens. In these patients cholestatic jaundice may follow the administration of oral contraceptive hormones. The relation of oral contraceptive hormone therapy to the development of hepatic adenomas is discussed in the later section on "Neoplastic diseases."

HYPERSENSITIVITY DRUG REACTIONS

Chlorpromazine. Chlorpromazine is one of many drugs that may induce jaundice and intrahepatic cholestasis as the result of a sensitivity reaction. Up to 50% of patients taking this drug may exhibit minimal increases in levels of serum enzymes (alkaline phosphatase and transaminase), which may be caused by the binding of drug metabolites to proteins in the canalicular membrane. Cholestatic jaundice, occurring in 1% to 2% of treated patients, is often preceded by fever, skin rash, lymphadenopathy, and eosinophilia. A liver biopsy reveals intrahepatic cholestasis with minimal centrilobular cell necrosis and a portal infiltration of mononuclear cells and eosinophils. After the administration of the drug is discontinued, the jaundice usually subsides within a few weeks; rarely the condition may progress to a clinical picture of chronic intrahepatic cholestasis resembling primary biliary cirrhosis. With subsequent exposure to the drug there is usually a more rapid onset of recurrent liver disease.

The treatment of chlorpromazine jaundice includes the discontinuation of the drug, the parenteral administration of vitamin K to correct for its malabsorption, and the use of cholestyramine (up to 4 g with each meal) to reduce pruritus.

Fluorinated anesthetic agents. The use of halothane and methoxyflurane, particularly with repeated exposures, rarely is associated with acute hepatitis. Clinical and serologic studies have excluded hypoxia and acute viral hepatitis as causes of liver necrosis in many patients with this anesthetic exposure. Although metabolic injury remains a possible cause, the presence of an immunologic mechanism is supported by in vitro studies that demonstrate circulating antibodies in the patient's sera that bind to the surface membrane of liver cells from rabbits previously exposed to halothane. It is clinically observed that patients usually have an unexplained fever during the week after surgery, followed by anicteric hepatitis with a marked elevation of levels of serum transaminases or by hepatitis with jaundice. A liver biopsy reveals that liver cell necrosis is centrilobular in distribution and is accompanied by a mononuclear cell infiltration and Kupffer's cell hyperplasia. Massive necrosis with fulminant hepatitis is relatively common (50% of these patients). Patients with an unexplained fever or hepatic dysfunction following the use of fluorinated anesthetic agents should not be reexposed to these agents; a recurrent episode of drug hepatitis is more likely to be severe and fatal.

Methyldopa. Methyldopa may cause a drug-related acute hepatitis that resembles acute viral hepatitis. The onset of liver disease occurs usually within 4 weeks of the initiation of the therapy, and jaundice is often preceded by fever, malaise, anorexia, nausea, or vomiting and elevated serum transaminase levels. Early discontinuation of the drug before the onset of jaundice is usually followed by prompt recovery, but continued or recurrent drug therapy may lead to jaundice with massive liver necrosis and hepatic failure. Careful clinical follow-up with serum transaminase determinations during the first 8 weeks of therapy has been recommended to prevent severe acute liver disease.

Methyldopa therapy has also been associated with the development of chronic active hepatitis (see later discussion of "Chronic active hepatitis").

Fatty liver

The normal liver contains small amounts of fat (about 5% of its weight), which includes phospholipid, cholesterol and cholesterol esters, triglycerides, and fatty acids in cell membranes or in membrane-enclosed lipid droplets (liposomes) of stored fat or of lipoprotein. This normal lipid can be seen with a light microscope only when special lipid stains are used. As fat accumulates in the liver, the triglyceride content increases to up to 50% of liver weight, and large droplets of triglyceride distend the liver cells.

PATHOGENESIS. The mechansisms of triglyceride accumulation in the liver include (1) an increased amount of triglyceride or fatty acid presented to the liver either from the peripheral adipose tissue or from the diet, (2) an increased synthesis of fatty acid and triglyceride by the liver, and (3) a decreased hepatic oxidation of fatty acids or secretion of lipoprotein. These three mechanisms play varying roles in different clinical situations.

In cases of obesity the fatty liver reflects the general increases in triglyceride stores resulting from an excessive caloric intake. In cases of diabetes mellitus and starvation there is an increase in the mobilization of peripheral fat; the hepatic uptake of fatty acids in excess of oxidation and lipoprotein secretion leads to fatty liver. The fatty liver commonly present in alcoholics is caused by the hepatic accumulation of dietary or peripheral lipid when the hepatic oxidation of fatty acid is impaired by alcohol; the hepatic synthesis of fatty acid may also be increased. The severe derangement of protein metabolism in patients with protein malnutrition, in some patients with a toxic liver injury such as that caused by carbon tetrachloride, phosphorus poisoning, or tetracycline toxicity, or in patients with Reye's syndrome is accompanied by a fatty liver resulting from the impaired oxidation of fat and decreased lipoprotein synthesis and secretion.

CLINICAL MANIFESTATIONS AND LABORATORY FINDINGS. Enlargement of the liver is the most common clinical manifestation of fatty liver; associated hepatic tenderness varies with the rate of liver enlargement and the presence of inflammation or cell necrosis. Fatty liver often causes no impairment of liver function; a minor elevation of serum alkaline phosphatase or transaminase levels (less than twice the normal levels) is consistent with fatty liver but may reflect a toxic liver cell injury such as alcoholic hepatitis. When fatty liver is only one manifestation of a severe liver injury, patients exhibit features of hepatitis (see earlier discussions of "Carbon tetrachloride" and "Alcoholic hepatitis") or acute hepatic encephalopathy (fatty liver of pregnancy, tetracycline toxicity, or Reye's syndrome). Reye's syndrome is a fulminant illness in children (at a mean age of 11 years) that commonly follows an influenza B infection; the acute encephalopathy is caused in part by cerebral edema and in part by ammonia toxicity. In the liver there is histologic evidence of glycogen depletion, mitochondrial injury, and fatty infiltration; impaired gluconeogenesis and the depletion of glycogen precipitate hypoglycemia, the reduced levels of urea cycle enzymes impair urea synthesis and elevate the blood ammonia levels, and the cell membrane injury permits leakage of liver cell enzymes into the plasma.

MANAGEMENT AND PROGNOSIS. Fatty liver may be decreased by treatment of the underlying cause, including weight reduction, alcohol withdrawal, and improved diabetic control. Patients with liver failure require appropriate supportive care (see earlier discussion of "Fulminant viral hepatitis"). Milder degrees of fatty liver may persist for long periods without changes in liver structure. In patients with severe fatty liver, including diabetics, those with a short bowel syndrome or a jejunoileal bypass (as a treatment of massive obesity), and those undergoing long-term methotrexate therapy for psoriasis, histologic changes that mimic those occurring in alcoholic hepatitis (cell degeneration with hyaline inclusions and centrilobular fibrosis) sometimes progress to cirrhosis and liver failure; these changes are not revealed by liver function tests and require a liver biopsy for their early identification.

Liver disease resulting from hepatic congestion and/or decreased perfusion

CONGESTIVE HEART FAILURE. Right upper quadrant discomfort and liver enlargement and tenderness are common clinical features of heart failure; an expansile pulsation of the liver with corresponding pressure changes in the neck veins suggests tricuspid insufficiency. In patients with constrictive pericarditis an enlargement of the liver and spleen and abdominal distention with ascites sometimes mimic cirrhosis of the liver. The congested liver exhibits distended central veins and congested centrilobular sinusoids; the centrilobular liver cell necrosis is usually caused by decreased perfusion and hypoxia. Alterations in liver function include a mild elevation of enzyme levels or cholestasis; changes in the metabolism of drugs and protein synthesis may dramatically modify the patient's response to anticoagulant therapy.

SHOCK. Acute hypotension in patients with cardiovascular disease (such as occurs during open heart surgery or with cardiac arrest) followed by subsequent recovery is associated with hypoxic necrosis of centrilobular liver cells; this leads to a clinical and biochemical picture of acute hepatitis with a marked elevation of levels of serum transaminases followed by variable jaundice. With complete cardiovascular recovery, hepatic regeneration restores normal liver lobules; with repeated injury, centrilobular fibrosis replaces liver cells.

HEPATIC VEIN OCCLUSION. The causes of a hepatic venous obstruction (Budd-Chiari syndrome) include congenital webs, venous thrombosis (such as occurs in myeloproliferative disease, in paroxysmal nocturnal hemoglobinuria, and in pregnancy or with oral contraceptive use), neoplastic disease (such as a hepatoma or lymphoma), or endophlebitis with fibrosis complicating veno-occlusive disease and hepatic radiation therapy. An acute hepatic venous occlusion causes marked liver congestion, central zonal necrosis, and abdominal distention with a rapid accumulation of ascites. The clinical picture varies from an acute illness with dramatic abdominal pain, liver and abdominal enlargement, shock, and early death to a more chronic illness with features of portal hypertension including ascites, venous collaterals, and bleeding from esophageal varices. The diagnosis is supported by a centrilobular pattern of congestion and hemorrhagic necrosis revealed by a liver biopsy and is confirmed by roentgenographic studies of the inferior vena cava and hepatic veins. A liver scan often shows a diffuse decrease in the hepatic uptake of the isotope and a relative concentration of the isotope in the caudate lobe, which has an independent hepatic venous drainage into the inferior vena cava. The prognosis of a patient with the acute Budd-Chiari syndrome is poor; obstruction caused by congenital webs can be relieved surgically, but the removal of clots is usually unsuccessful. The relief of portal hypertension by a portacaval shunt may extend the life of some patients.

Chronic active hepatitis

Chronic active hepatitis is a chronic disease process resulting from varying causes in which a continued destruction of liver cells, usually in a periportal distribution, is associated with inflammation and a progressive fibrosis that replaces liver parenchyma and ultimately leads to cirrhosis.

ETIOLOGY. The important causative factors of chronic active hepatitis are infection by hepatitis B and non-A, non-B viruses, autoimmune liver injury, and hypersensitivity reactions to certain drugs (usually following recurrent or continued exposed to methyldopa, isoniazid, oxyphenisatin, and halothane). Patients with Wilson's disease and primary biliary cirrhosis may also have the clinical, biochemical, and pathologic features of chronic active hepatitis.

PATHOGENESIS. Humoral or cellular immunologic mechanisms or both probably play a major role in the pathogenesis of chronic active hepatitis, regardless of the primary cause. The evidence in support of an immunologic pathogenesis is as follows.

1. Patients with idiopathic or autoimmune chronic active hepatitis have an increased incidence of other diseases that may have an autoimmune basis, including Sjögren's syndrome, chronic thyroiditis, and pulmonary fibrosis. The higher incidence of the HLA-B8 antigen in these patients and an increased incidence of autoimmune diseases in close relatives suggest that genetic factors play some role.

2. Hypergammaglobulinemia in patients with chronic active hepatitis is often extreme, often parallels the disease activity, and is often accompanied by positive results on serologic tests for multiple autoantibodies that lack organ specificity; these include antinuclear, anti-DNA, antimitochondrial, and anti–smooth muscle antibodies as well as positive test results for LE cells. These immunologic phenomena are uncommon in patients with hepatitis B–related chronic active hepatitis.

3. Periportal areas adjacent to the liver lobule are heavily infiltrated with plasma cells and lymphocytes.

4. Immunologic phenomena that may play a specific role in liver cell injury have been reported to occur with chronic active hepatitis. Chronic active hepatitis in patients who are HB_sAg positive is associated with the localization of HB_sAg on the surface membrane of liver cells; liver cell injury may be caused by lymphocytes with Fc receptors that bind anti-HB_s and react with membrane-bound antigen. Specific lipoprotein antigen on the liver cell membrane has been suggested as the target for sensitized lymphocytes in cases of autoimmune chronic active hepatitis.

Although these immunologic phenomena provide an explanation for the chronic liver injury, the specific factors that regulate the development of the disease have not been determined.

CLINICAL MANIFESTATIONS. The clinical spectrum of chronic hepatitis is broad. A large proportion of patients with mild disease may remain well and asymptomatic, and in these the only evidence of a slowly progressive liver disease might be mild fluctuations in levels of serum transaminase and hyperglobulinemia; this asymptomatic course would explain the late development of cirrhosis many years after a hepatitis B infection. Alternatively, patients with a more active and rapidly progressive disease exhibit symptoms suggestive of an acute hepatitis of insidious onset; malaise, lethargy, anorexia, arthralgias, a low-grade fever, and right upper quadrant discomfort are relatively common. Jaundice with dark urine and pruritus is a feature of severe exacerbations. In young women with autoimmune disease, amenorrhea is common. The physical findings are related in part to hepatic inflammation (liver enlargement, tenderness, and cholestasis) and in part to chronic liver injury and/or cirrhosis (spider angiomas, splenomegaly, ascites, and collateral abdominal veins).

PATHOLOGY. In early chronic active hepatitis the normal lobular architecture of the liver is preserved. The portal areas are expanded and may be joined by fibrous septa, and the liver cell plates adjacent to the portal areas are disrupted; individual cells exhibit hyaline (piecemeal) necrosis, and other cells are separated from the normal cords by proliferating mesenchymal cells or acute and chronic inflammatory cells, particularly lymphocytes, plasma cells, and eosinophils. Regenerating liver cells form rosettes on the periphery of the lobule, and proliferation within the portal areas increases the number of bile ductules. Within the hepatic lobules, parenchymal cell necrosis and infiltration are minimal. Bile stasis may be noted in patients with jaundice.

As chronic active hepatitis progresses, the increasing fibrosis extending from portal areas into the lobule distorts the normal architecture, and regeneration nodules result in cirrhosis.

Either a spontaneous remission or treatment with corticosteroids decreases the parenchymal cell necrosis and inflammatory cell infiltration, leaving portal fibrosis or inactive cirrhosis.

DIFFERENTIAL DIAGNOSIS. A history of drug ingestion, evidence of a hepatitis B infection, or the potential exposure to non-A, non-B hepatitis through a transfusion, as well as high titers of autoantibodies, usually distinguishes patients with chronic active hepatitis caused by drugs, a hepatitis infection, or an autoimmune disease, respectively. The determination of the causal agent is of clinical importance because the cessation of drug therapy is usually followed by remission whereas patients with a hepatitis B infection are more likely to respond poorly to corticosteroid therapy.

In patients with prominent cholestasis, a high titer of antimitochondrial antibodies suggests a diagnosis of primary biliary cirrhosis; these patients are more likely to have a decreased number of smaller bile ducts as well as damage to larger bile ducts within the portal areas. In young patients Wilson's disease must be considered and excluded from diagnostic possibilities by measurements of serum ceruloplasmin and serum and urinary copper levels.

MANAGEMENT AND PROGNOSIS. Controlled clinical trials have shown that patients with severe chronic active hepatitis respond to treatment with prednisone or a combination of prednisone and azathioprine; 80% of symptomatic patients with severe biochemical changes (SGOT levels more than 10 times normal or five times normal along with γ-globulin levels twice the normal) treated with prednisone (60 mg daily initially, reduced to a maintenance dosage of 20 mg daily), or prednisone (30 mg daily initially, reduced to a maintenance dosage of 10 mg daily) and azathioprine (50 mg daily), have entered clinical, biochemical, and histologic remission. This remission is usually maintained by continued prednisone therapy, but slow withdrawal of drug therapy after 6 months of sustained remission is followed by a relapse in up to 50% of patients. A symptomatic and biochemical relapse requires further steroid therapy. Alternate-day prednisone therapy reduces the side effects of the treatment but appears to be less effective than daily doses of steroids in maintaining histologic remission.

Although symptomatic patients with severe autoimmune disease clearly benefit from drug therapy, the benefit of this treatment in patients who are asymptomatic and have less active disease remains uncertain; in patients with a slowly progressive disease the side effects of drug therapy may offset any benefit that results from a decrease in the disease activity.

In experimental studies the use of interferon in patients with a chronic hepatitis B infection led to a decrease in the titer of viral antigens and to improved liver function; further controlled studies of this therapy are indicated.

Cirrhosis of the liver

DEFINITION. In cirrhosis of the liver the normal lobular architecture of the liver is disrupted by fibrosis and regenerative nodules.

Etiology and classification. Cirrhosis is the end stage of chronic liver injury resulting from various causes, some of which are well defined whereas others are poorly understood. Despite the current limitations in our understanding of the mechanisms of cirrhosis, the following etiologic classification is most useful clinically:

I. Idiopathic or posthepatitic cirrhosis
II. Alcoholic cirrhosis
III. Metabolic cirrhosis
   A. Hemochromatosis
   B. Wilson's disease
   C. α-1-Antitrypsin deficiency
   D. Other metabolic disorders
IV. Biliary cirrhosis
   A. Primary
   B. Secondary
V. Congestive (cardiac) cirrhosis

Idiopathic or posthepatitic cirrhosis

Pathogenesis. The development of cirrhosis following hepatitis B or non-A, non-B infection has been well documented by serial liver biopsies. Bridging necrosis during the acute infection and chronic active hepatitis (regardless of the cause) are recognized precursor lesions. Many patients with established cirrhosis do not give a history of alcoholism or a preceding hepatitis infection and do not exhibit the features of chronic active liver disease; these patients with idiopathic cirrhosis may have the end stage of asymptomatic, undiagnosed chronic active hepatitis.

Pathology. The liver in patients with idiopathic or posthepatitic cirrhosis is more likely to have large irregular nodules and broad intervening bands of scarring (macronodular cirrhosis) than small regular nodules (micronodular cirrhosis); the liver is typically shrunken in patients with end-stage disease. In the earlier phase of active cirrhosis the microscopic features of chronic active hepatitis are present in addition to cirrhotic scarring and nodular regeneration. In the late stage, regenerative nodules often formed by double cords of liver cells are separated by dense fibrous bands containing proliferating bile ducts and sparse inflammatory cells.

Clinical manifestations. The clinical features of active idiopathic cirrhosis are those of chronic active hepatitis coupled with variable manifestations of the cirrhosis itself: portal hypertension with splenomegaly and hypersplenism, ascites, portal-systemic collaterals, and hepatic encephalopathy. Patients with compensated cirrhosis and normal liver function may show splenomegaly and hypersplenism;

patients with decompensated cirrhosis are more likely to have ascites and edema, bleeding from esophageal varices, or hepatic encephalopathy.

Management and prognosis. Patients with chronic active hepatitis and established posthepatitic cirrhosis may benefit from corticosteroid therapy (see earlier discussion of "Chronic active hepatitis"); the desired result of treatment is a compensated cirrhosis that is no longer progressive. The complications of cirrhosis require appropriate supportive therapy (see later discussion of "Management of complications of cirrhosis").

Alcoholic cirrhosis

Pathogenesis. The development of cirrhosis in chronic alcoholics is related to the amount of alcohol consumed and the duration of alcohol abuse; although undetermined factors may modify the development of liver disease in individual patients, cirrhosis is the usual outcome in those who have a liquor intake in excess of 1 pint a day for 15 years. Former hypotheses that various nutritional deficiencies associated with alcoholism are responsible for the development of cirrhosis are not supported by experimental studies with baboons; when carbohydrates were replaced by ethanol in an otherwise complete diet, these animals showed the pathologic spectrum of acute alcoholic hepatitis and cirrhosis occurring in patients who abuse alcohol. This evidence provides the strongest support for the current hypothesis that alcohol is a direct hepatotoxin.

Pathology. The earliest hepatic lesion observed following excessive alcohol consumption is a fatty liver without fibrosis or liver cell necrosis. With progressive injury the fatty liver may be accompanied by evidence of parenchymal cell injury; when examined with a light microscope, damaged cells exhibit eosinophilic inclusions (alcoholic hyalin) that correspond to collections of fibrillar material detected with electron microscopy. Cell organelles also exhibit degenerative changes. An infiltration with polymorphonuclear cells and early fibrosis, particularly within the lobule adjacent to the central veins, complete the pathologic picture of acute alcoholic hepatitis. Although the relationship of fatty liver, alcoholic hepatitis, and cirrhosis requires further clarification, the development of progressive scarring and cirrhosis following continued alcohol abuse is more rapid in patients who exhibit centrilobular fibrosis or sclerosis; indeed, patients with severe acute alcoholic hepatitis and central hyaline sclerosis progress rapidly to decompensated cirrhosis. End-stage cirrhosis in alcoholics is usually a micronodular cirrhosis with regular small regenerative nodules. The pathologic cause is manifested only in the lesions of continued alcoholic injury—fatty infiltration and alcoholic hyalin; these cellular changes may be nonspecific.

Clinical manifestations. The earliest indication of alcoholic liver disease is often an enlarged liver detected on a routine physical examination. Minor changes in serum enzyme levels reflect liver cell injury. The initial episodes of symptomatic hepatic decompensation accompanied by anorexia, nausea or vomiting, abdominal swelling, right upper quadrant abdominal pain, or jaundice are often precipitated by the superimposition of acute alcoholic hepatitis on hepatic fibrosis or cirrhosis from earlier injury. The patient with acute decompensation caused by alcoholic hepatitis is usually febrile, is often malnourished, and exhibits signs of both acute hepatitis and a more chronic liver disease, which may include an enlarged and tender liver, spider angiomas, gynecomastia, jaundice, ascites, and ethanol intoxication or withdrawal signs. Jaundice with conjugated hyperbilirubinemia, elevated levels of serum enzymes (with the SGOT level more than twice that of SGPT), and a prolonged prothrombin time reflect acute liver injury; in some patients cholestasis is predominant.

The clinical features of alcoholic cirrhosis without acute alcoholic hepatitis vary with the severity of the disease and its complications. A firm enlargement of the liver and spleen and normal results on routine tests of liver function are consistent with compensated alcoholic cirrhosis. Patients with decompensated cirrhosis usually exhibit signs of liver failure and have the complications of ascites, hepatic encephalopathy, and bleeding from esophageal varices as well as biochemical evidence of an impaired hepatic synthetic function (hypoproteinemia, prolonged prothrombin time, and an elevated level of ammonia in the blood).

Differential diagnosis. In patients with acute alcoholic hepatitis, sepsis and other causes of acute hepatitis must be considered. The causes of hepatic decompensation in patients with cirrhosis are discussed in subsequent sections on the management of portal hypertension, ascites, and encephalopathy. A percutaneous liver biopsy is of value in pathologically confirming the diagnosis of acute or chronic liver disease caused by alcohol and in assessing the prognosis of these patients.

Management and prognosis. Early withdrawal from alcohol is the only major factor that significantly modifies the course of alcoholic hepatitis and cirrhosis and prolongs the patient's survival. In patients with acute alcoholic hepatitis who stop drinking, the liver disease is reversible unless central hyaline sclerosis or cirrhosis is already present. Patients with end-stage cirrhosis and portal hypertension have irreversible lesions that progress despite the withdrawal from alcohol.

Nutritional support for the malnourished alcoholic patient should include oral protein supplements to restore the nitrogen balance (unless a high protein intake is contraindicated by the presence of hepatic encephalopathy), vitamin supplements to correct deficiencies of B vitamins, folic acid, and ascorbic acid, and supplements of potassium and trace metals such as zinc in patients with deficiencies.

Chlordiazepoxide (Librium) is recommended in the treatment of the manifestations of alcohol withdrawal; the parenterally administered doses should be adjusted to meet the individual needs of the patient.

The treatment of the complications of cirrhosis is discussed in sections on portal hypertension, ascites, and coma.

Metabolic cirrhosis

Hemochromatosis. Hemochromatosis results from an excessive deposition of iron in the liver and other organs. The disease may be genetically determined (idiopathic hemochromatosis) or may result from excessive iron absorption and storage in patients with diseases that modify iron metabolism, such as occurs with thalassemia or following portacaval shunting. The factors that cause an excessive intestinal absorption of iron in patients with either idiopathic hemochromatosis or secondary hemochromatosis are currently undetermined.

Idiopathic hemochromatosis is inherited as an autosomal defect that is either dominant with a varying expression or recessive; affected family members often have an HLA profile similar to that of the patient with the disease, and the incidence of the HLA-A3 gene is higher in patients with this disease.

PATHOLOGY. In patients with hemochromatosis, stored iron is increased from a normal level of 3 to 4 g to amounts in excess of 20 to 40 g; this excess iron is deposited in the parenchymal cells of many organs as well as in the reticuloendothelial system.

The earliest hepatic lesion in asymptomatic young relatives of patients with established hemochromatosis is an increase in both parenchymal and reticuloendothelial hepatic iron without fibrosis, Progressive iron overload leads to increasing portal fibrosis and the development of fibrous septa between lobules; a micronodular or occasional macronodular cirrhosis finally results. Parenchymal cells, Kupffer's cells, and the cells of proliferating bile ducts are heavily infiltrated with iron.

In the pancreas the iron deposits lead to fibrosis and degeneration of the islet cells. In the heart, infiltrated myocardial cells undergo degeneration with subsequent fibrosis. In the endocrine system, iron storage is particularly prominent in the thyroid, parathyroid, and anterior pituitary glands and in the zona glomerulosa of the adrenal gland; this storage does not lead to fibrosis. Testicular atrophy is associated with minimal iron deposition and probably results from pituitary dysfunction. Iron deposits in the chief cells of the gastric mucosa and in salivary glands do not impair secretion. In the larger joints the deposition of iron in the synovium is often accompanied by chondrocalcinosis, which may cause arthritic symptoms.

CLINICAL MANIFESTATIONS. Skin pigmentation, diabetes mellitus (usually insulin dependent), cirrhosis of the liver, hypogonadism, and cardiac arrhythmias or failure are the more common features of idiopathic hemochromatosis. Abdominal pain, usually in the right upper quadrant, is a prominent initial symptom. The liver is usually enlarged and firm, and splenomegaly is common. Liver function is well preserved in most patients; others exhibit a mild elevation of levels of serum transaminases (usually less than twice the normal level). Severe impairment of liver function is most often observed in patients with heart failure or with the late development of a hepatocellular carcinoma.

DIAGNOSIS. In patients with early or late hemochromatosis, excessive body iron stores are associated with a greatly increased saturation of serum transferrin (usually near 100%) and elevated serum levels of ferritin. A liver biopsy provides the most reliable evidence of the iron overload.

MANAGEMENT. Phlebotomy is the most effective means of removing iron from the body (250 mg iron/500 ml of blood); weekly phlebotomy is usually tolerated well by patients with idiopathic hemochromatosis; 1 to 2 years of treatment may be necessary to remove excess iron stores. When iron stores are depleted, the serum ferritin level usually falls below 3 μg/dl, the serum transferrin level rises and the iron saturation falls, and normal hemoglobin levels are no longer maintained. To maintain the depletion of iron stores, patients with idiopathic hemochromatosis require phlebotomy two to six times each year; their serum ferritin levels should be maintained below 20 μg/dl. In patients with secondary hemochromatosis and anemia, phlebotomy may not be possible; intravenous infusions of desferrioxamine are of minimal benefit.

Heart failure, diabetes mellitus, and other endocrine disorders require appropriate therapy.

PROGNOSIS. Without therapy patients with hemochromatosis in the past often died of cardiac complications. With phlebotomy, patients with established cirrhosis are more likely to live longer but have an increased incidence of hepatomas. It is probable that early treatment of the iron overload before the development of fibrosis or cirrhosis prevents all the later complications of hemochromatosis.

Wilson's disease. Wilson's disease is an autosomal recessive defect of copper metabolism. An excessive body accumulation of copper probably results from a decreased biliary excretion of the metal. The hepatic manifestations of established disease are chronic active hepatitis and cirrhosis. The liver contains an excessive amount of copper, usually more than 50 μg per gram of wetweight (the normal amount is 4 to 8 μg per gram). Nonhepatic manifestations of Wilson's disease include Kayser-Fleischer corneal rings, neurologic disease (causing tremor, rigidity, ataxia, and changes in mentation), acute hemolytic disease, renal tubular dysfunction, and bone demineralization.

The possibility of Wilson's disease should be considered in any young patient with chronic active hepatitis or cirrhosis of unknown cause. Kayser-Fleischer rings detected in a slit-lamp examination of the cornea and depressed serum levels of the copper protein ceruloplasmin are usually present. An elevated level of urinary copper excretion after a test dose of penicillamine or a direct measurement of hepatic copper content confirms the diagnosis. The treatment of Wilson's disease is penicillamine therapy (500 mg three times daily.)

α-1-Antitrypsin deficiency. The plasma protease inhibitor system, α-1-antitrypsin (the major α_1-globulin), is relatively deficient in patients with the Pi^{ZZ} phenotype (the normal phenotype is Pi^{MM}); these patients appear to have a defect in the hepatic secretion of α_1-globulin, which accumulates in membrane-bound vacuoles in the liver cells. Homozygous (Pi^{ZZ}) patients usually have cholestasis during their first year of life or progressive hepatomegaly and cirrhosis in later childhood. There is no specific therapy for this disorder; hepatic transplantation offers hope for the future.

Biliary cirrhosis

Primary biliary cirrhosis. Primary biliary cirrhosis, the cause of which has not been determined, is characterized clinically by chronic intrahepatic cholestasis and pathologically by chronic inflammation and fibrosis of portal triads with destruction of smaller bile ducts.

PATHOGENESIS. The current hypothesis is that primary biliary cirrhosis is an autoimmune disease in which small bile ducts are damaged or destroyed by immunologic mechanisms.

PATHOLOGY. The earliest hepatic lesions observed in biopsies of patients with mild asymptomatic cholestasis (an elevated level of serum alkaline phosphatase without jaundice) appear to be a mononuclear inflammatory reaction that expands the portal triads and an associated loss of smaller bile ducts or evidence of damage to the epithelium of larger bile ducts. The bile ducts may terminate in areas of heavy mononuclear cell infiltration or in granulomata. Initially the fibrosis is minimal, and the hepatic lobules are normal. As the disease progresses, piecemeal necrosis of liver cells adjacent to the portal areas disrupts liver cell plates, fibrosis extends to adjacent portal areas, and centrilobular cholestasis reflects the onset of jaundice. In the late stage of the disease a macronodular cirrhosis with prominent cholestasis is often present. Lipid-laden macrophages accumulate along the hepatic sinusoids in patients with extreme hyperlipidemia.

CLINICAL MANIFESTATIONS. The incidence of primary biliary cirrhosis is highest in women 40 to 60 years of age; males are rarely affected. Asymptomatic disease has been diagnosed by serologic tests and liver biopsies in patients with isolated elevations of the level of serum alkaline phosphatase; these patients often remain well without progression of their disease over long periods. Pruritus and jaundice are the most common presenting symptoms in patients with progressive disease. Chronic intrahepatic cholestasis leads to fat malabsorption with diarrhea in some patients, hypercholesterolemia with the development of xanthomas, and an increased risk of duodenal ulcer disease (probably related to a decreased duodenal neutralization of acid). In the early cholestatic phase of the illness the liver synthetic function is well preserved, and albumin levels remain normal. Later manifestations of cirrhosis in patients with a poor prognosis include the development of portal hypertension with bleeding from esophageal varices, ascites, and encephalopathy; these complications of cirrhosis are unusual presenting signs. Osteomalacia caused by malabsorption of vitamin D and of 25-hydroxycholecalciferol that is normally cycled through the enterohepatic circulation is a common cause of severe bone demineralization and pathologic fractures of the spine and ribs.

DIAGNOSIS. Primary biliary cirrhosis is usually associated with extremely high titers of antimitochondrial antibodies (lower titers are observed in patients with chronic active hepatitis). This serologic test combined with a liver biopsy is usually sufficient to establish the diagnosis in patients with prominent cholestasis. Transhepatic Chiba fine needle or endoscopic retrograde cholangiography is sometimes necessary to rule out an extrahepatic biliary tract obstruction in patients who may have gallstones.

MANAGEMENT. There is no specific treatment for primary biliary cirrhosis; these patients do not respond to corticosteroid or azathioprine therapy. The symptomatic and supportive treatment includes the use of oral cholestyramine (4 g up to three times a day) to relieve the itching and daily supplementary fat-soluble vitamins to prevent deficiencies of vitamins K, A, and D; the recommended daily oral dosages are 5 to 10 mg of vitamin K_1, 10,000 IU of vitamin A, and 100 to 200 μg of 25-hydroxycholecalciferol (vitamin D).

PROGNOSIS. The average life expectancy of symptomatic patients is 5 years after the onset of jaundice. Increasing jaundice and the complications of cirrhosis indicate a poor prognosis. Recent trials of penicillamine therapy designed to prevent the copper accumulation that might accelerate liver disease have shown that this agent is of minimal benefit.

Secondary biliary cirrhosis. An extrahepatic biliary obstruction with or without cholangitis leads to progressive portal fibrosis; true cirrhosis in these patients is rare. The clinical features are those of cholestatis with late hepatic failure and intermittent episodes of cholangitis. Pathologically, the early lesions are those of an extrahepatic obstruction with bile stasis, ductular proliferation, and the dilation of larger bile ducts. Bile infarcts and bile lakes, the foci of liver cells that have undergone necrosis with bile extravasation, are usually located at the periphery of lobules adjacent to the portal tracts. The portal tracts are edematous, have concentric fibrosis around bile ducts, and are infiltrated with mononuclear and polymorphonuclear cells. In cases of advanced secondary biliary cirrhosis, regenerative nodules are surrounded by condensed fibrous tissue containing proliferating bile ducts.

MANAGEMENT OF COMPLICATIONS OF CIRRHOSIS

Portal hypertension and upper gastrointestinal bleeding. The immediate management of patients with cirrhosis and massive upper gastrointestinal bleeding has four objectives: (1) to restore the circulating blood volume and to stabilize the patient, (2) to control the bleeding, (3) to define the site of bleeding, and (4) to anticipate and prevent or treat other complications of liver disease.

The patient usually requires intensive care monitoring and an immediate transfusion of whole blood. Measures that are effective in controlling bleeding, regardless of the bleeding site, include ice-water lavage of the stomach, intravenous infusions of vasopressin (Pitressin) (20 units over 10 minutes) to induce splanchnic constriction, and selective mesenteric artery infusions of vasopressin. Massive uncontrolled bleeding from esophageal or gastric varices may require the use of the Sengstaken-Blakemore esophageal tube; in inexperienced hands this method involves a high risk of esophageal erosion, esophageal perforation, and pulmonary aspiration. Patients with cirrhosis, portal hypertension, and esophageal varices may have bleeding from a variety of esophageal, gastric, and duodenal lesions. Bleeding is more likely to be from esophageal varices in patients whose cirrhosis is relatively compensated, whereas in patients with decompensated cirrhosis the bleeding commonly is from acute gastric erosions. Esophagogastroduodenoscopy provides the most accurate assessment of the bleeding site; alternatively, if the bleeding continues to be massive, selective arteriography with an injection of contrast dye may localize the site of the blood loss into the gut. Cirrhotic patients with massive bleeding are likely to develop ascites or hepatic coma; the measures for reducing these problems include the restriction of salt and measures that clear blood from the gastrointestinal tract and reduce bacterial action (see discussion of "Hepatic encephalopathy").

Measures aimed at reducing the risk of recurrent bleeding from esophageal varices have included drug therapy, sclerosis of the vessels by endoscopic or transhepatic injection, or surgical decompression of the portal system. A recent controlled clinical trial showed that propranolol therapy significantly decreased recurrent bleeding from esophageal varices in patients with alcoholic cirrhosis. Variceal occlusion provides only temporary benefit.

Surgical decompression of the portal system with a splenorenal, mesocaval, or portacaval anastomosis is usually effective in lowering the portal pressure and in the long-term control of variceal bleeding; patient survival may not be prolonged. These procedures have a high operative mortality in patients with hepatic decompensation and increase the risk of postoperative hepatic encephalopathy. The procedure of choice in low-risk patients may be a distal splenorenal shunt that selectively decompresses esophageal varices without significantly decreasing the mesenteric blood flow to the liver; progressive liver failure is less likely after this procedure. When evaluating patients for shunt surgery, it is necessary to demonstrate that the splenic, portal, and/or renal veins are patent by selective splenic arteriography or transhepatic or transsplenic portal venography. Measurements of the wedged hepatic venous pressure and the inferior vena cava pressure indicate the pressure gradient across the liver and differentiate a presinusoidal obstruction from cirrhosis.

Ascites. When ascites is present, it is important to determine the precipitating cause as well as to promote a safe diuresis. Causes for ascites other than liver disease must be considered, including heart failure, constrictive pericarditis, acute pancreatitis with a pancreaticoperitoneal fistula, bacterial peritonitis, and neoplastic infiltration of the peritoneal cavity. In patients with established cirrhosis and portal hypertension, ascites may be precipitated by bleeding (with an increase in secondary hyperaldosteronism), by an increase in salt intake, by peritoneal infection with enteric organisms or tubercle bacilli, by further hepatic decompensation, by the development of a hepatoma, or by thrombosis of hepatic or portal veins; the precipitating factor in the patient should be determined. An initial diagnostic paracentesis with examination of the ascitic fluid to detect bacteria, enzymes (LDH and amylase), malignant cells, and inflammatory cells is of particular value in the diagnosis of peritonitis and neoplastic disease. The following management program provides an effective and safe diuresis in most patients with cirrhosis and ascites:

1. The dietary sodium intake is restricted to less than 2 g daily; the fluid intake may also have to be restricted to 1000 ml daily in patients who exhibit a decrease in the serum sodium concentration below 130 mEq/L.
2. The diuretic program must provide aldosterone blockade to prevent severe hypokalemia. Initially over a period of several days an increase in the dosage of spironolactone from 100 mg to 400 mg daily is recommended; when the urinary sodium excretion exceeds that of potassium, the addition of hydrochlorothiazide (50 mg daily) or furosemide (40 mg daily) increases the sodium excretion without promoting potassium loss.
3. The weight loss in patients without peripheral edema should not exceed 0.5 kg daily; a more rapid diuresis at a rate that exceeds the rate of fluid mobilization from the peritoneal cavity increases the risk of hypovolemia.
4. Patients with severe hypoproteinemia should receive daily intravenous infusions of salt-poor albumin (25 to 50 g) to restore the plasma oncotic pressure and to maintain the plasma volume.
5. The patient's weight, renal function, serum electrolyte concentrations, and mental status should be monitored regularly to reduce complications of azotemia, electrolyte imbalances, and encephalopathy.

6. The goal of therapy should be not to eliminate all ascitic fluid but to reduce ascites and permit normal function.

Hepatic encephalopathy. In patients with cirrhosis, hepatic encephalopathy may be precipitated by gastrointestinal bleeding; by a fluid, electrolyte, or acid-base imbalance, particularly hypokalemic alkalosis or water intoxication; by infection; by the use of depressant drugs such as sedatives, tranquilizers, or narcotics; or by other metabolic insults including azotemia, hypoxia, hypoglycemia, and an increase in dietary protein intake. Precipitating causes should be identified and eliminated. In all patients with a chronic or intermittent hepatic encephalopathy, measures that lower the level of blood ammonia are of value in improving the patient's mental function; these measures include the restriction of dietary protein to a level that can be tolerated by the patient, enemas and cathartics to empty the colon, and orally administered neomycin or lactulose to reduce the formation and absorption of ammonia in the colon.

Granulomatous and infiltrative diseases

Hepatic granulomata have been described in association with a large number of local and systemic diseases. The most common causes of hepatic granulomata include sarcoidosis, pulmonary and miliary tuberculosis, histoplasmosis, brucellosis, primary biliary cirrhosis, Hodgkin's disease, and hypersensitivity reactions. The liver is usually enlarged and may be tender. The most common abnormalities in liver function are elevated levels of serum alkaline phosphatase and related enzymes; levels of serum transaminases are slightly elevated in patients with acute disease. The presence of hepatic granulomata is demonstrated by needle biopsy; the determination of the primary cause of hepatic granulomatous disease usually requires other clinical data, although the presence of caseating necrosis strongly suggests that miliary tuberculosis is the cause. Hepatic granulomata usually heal with fibrosis without long-term sequelae; rarely they may cause portal hypertension resulting from hepatic fibrosis.

Infiltrative disease of the liver such as that caused by metastatic carcinoma (see the following section), amyloidosis, or even fat also characteristically produces hepatic enlargement, possible tenderness, and elevations of the levels of serum alkaline phosphatase and related enzymes.

Neoplastic diseases

The liver may be involved in a variety of benign and malignant primary and metastatic neoplasms including carcinomas, lymphomas, hemangiomas, and angiosarcomas, the last of which may result from exposure to vinyl chloride. If large, a tumor produces hepatic enlargement sometimes accompanied by pain or tenderness. The mass may be demonstrated by means of radionuclide scanning, ultrasonography, computed tomography, or angiography. Malignant lesions often produce early and disproportionate elevations of the levels of serum alkaline phosphatase and related enzymes. Because of their clinical importance and incidence and the current interest in them, hepatic adenomas, primary carcinomas, and metastatic carcinomas are discussed in more detail below.

HEPATIC ADENOMAS. The development of large hepatic adenomas has been associated with the use of oral contraceptive steroids. Patients with these lesions may have abdominal pain, acute intraperitoneal bleeding and shock, or a palpable abdominal mass. The majority of these lesions have been resected, but conservative treatment with withdrawal from hormone therapy has led to a regression of the tumor in some patients. Hepatic adenomas occurring in patients not receiving oral contraceptive steroids are usually small and do not cause symptoms.

HEPATOCELLULAR CARCINOMA (HEPATOMA). The factors that predispose a patient to the development of primary carcinomas of the liver include cirrhosis (particularly hemochromatosis and idiopathic cirrhosis), chronic hepatitis B virus infection, and the exposure to high levels of aflatoxin in the diet. The high incidence of hepatitis B infections and the contamination of food with aflatoxin might contribute to the high incidence of hepatomas in certain populations in Asia and Africa.

The major clinical features of a hepatoma are sudden hepatic decompensation in a patient with previously stable cirrhosis (usually caused by a tumor invasion or thrombosis of portal or hepatic veins), gastrointestinal bleeding, the rapid development of ascites (often containing blood or malignant cells), sudden enlargement of the liver with local pain and a vascular bruit or friction rub, hypoglycemia, and increased plasma levels of α-fetoprotein. In patients without cirrhosis, a hepatic lobectomy or hepatic resection with transplantation occasionally provides a cure; in patients with cirrhosis, the development of a hepatoma usually leads to death; chemotherapy is of limited value in prolonging the patient's survival.

SECONDARY CARCINOMAS OF THE LIVER. The common primary carcinomas that metastasize to the liver are lesions of the lung, breast, and gastrointestinal tract (stomach, pancreas, and colon). The earliest clinical sign of hepatic involvement is usually mild cholestasis with an elevation of the levels of serum alkaline phosphatase, 5'-nucleotidase, and γ-glutamyl transpeptidase. Elevated levels of carcinoembryonic antigen indicate the presence of metastatic disease, and filling defects may be detected by liver scanning. Nodular hepatic enlargement and jaundice are later features of hepatic involvement. Rarely, metastatic deposits at the porta hepatis may cause extrahepatic cholestasis; this obstruction may be determined by transhepatic cholangiography and may be relieved by local radiotherapy.

BIBLIOGRAPHY

Davidson, C.S.: Liver pathophysiology: its relevance to human disease, Boston, 1970, Little, Brown & Co.

Scheuer, P.J.: Liver biopsy interpretation, ed. 3, London, 1980, Balliere, Tindall & Cassell, Ltd.

Schiff, L.: Diseases of the liver, ed. 4, Philadelphia, 1975, J.B. Lippincott Co.

Sherlock, S.: Diseases of the liver and biliary system, ed. 5, Oxford, England, 1975, Blackwell Scientific Publications.

184 • DISEASES OF THE BILIARY TRACT

Roger D. Soloway

Unparalleled recent progress in understanding the pathogenesis of the most common biliary tract disease, cholesterol cholelithiasis, the continued expansion of knowledge concerning bile secretion and the enterohepatic circulation of bile salts, and the development of endoscopic retrograde cholangiopancreatography, along with manometry and thin-needle cholangiography, have combined to clarify our understanding of biliary diseases and to underline their importance.

BILE SECRETION AND COMPOSITION

BIOCHEMISTRY. Cholesterol is an essential component of all biomembranes. Exogenous cholesterol originates in the diet and is a minor source of the cholesterol used. The liver is the major endogenous source of cholesterol; the small intestine and skin also contribute. The endogenous synthesis is in a complex balance with the intake and enterohepatic recirculation of cholesterol. The rate-limiting enzyme for cholesterol synthesis is hydroxymethylglutaryl-coenzyme A (HMG-CoA) reductase.

A knowledge of the characteristics of bile flow and composition is essential to an understanding of gallstone formation and dissolution. Bile salts are the major end product of cholesterol metabolism and are converted via a large number of intermediates only in the liver. The enzyme, 7-α-hydroxylase, which adds a hydroxyl group to the cholesterol molecule in the 7-α position of the steroid molecule, is the rate-limiting enzyme for bile acid synthesis and determines that the resultant compound can only be converted to bile acids.

Chenodeoxycholic acid (hydroxyl groups at the 3-α and 7-α positions on the sterol nucleus) and cholic acid (hydroxyl groups at the 3-α, 7-α, and 12-α positions) are the two primary bile acids produced by the liver from cholesterol. They are conjugated with taurine and glycine before their secretion into the bile; unconjugated bile acids are not excreted into the bile in appreciable quantities. Bile acids are reabsorbed from the jejunum and colon by passive transport and from the distal 100 cm of ileum by active transport. Most are reabsorbed unchanged and return to the liver via the portal vein, where they are efficiently taken up by the liver and resecreted into the bile. Bile acids entering the colon or otherwise exposed to bacteria undergo deconjugation and/or dehydroxylation. Thus some unconjugated primary bile acids return to the liver, where they are reconjugated before resecretion. Other primary bile acids are transformed by colonic bacterial dehydroxylation into secondary bile acids. Cholic acid is dehydroxylated at the 7-α position into deoxycholic acid, a major component of fecal bile acids. Deoxycholic acid is also extensively reabsorbed by passive diffusion and conjugated in the liver and excreted into the bile. In contrast, chenodeoxycholic acid is dehydroxylated into lithocholic acid, which is poorly reabsorbed and is the other principal fecal bile acid. These are the major steps in the enterohepatic circulation of bile acids that result in the preservation of 90% of the bile acids secreted each day.

Cholesterol and phospholipids require bile salts for their biliary secretion, and their secretion increases along with increasing bile salt secretion. At a high rate of bile salt secretion, bile is likely to be undersaturated with cholesterol.

PHYSICAL CHEMISTRY. Cholesterol is minimally soluble in water but is carried in bile micelles that are about 50 Å in diameter. Micelles are aggregates of phospholipids and bile salts that have their charged portions facing outward into the surrounding polar water environment and their nonpolar portions facing inward, creating a microenvironment suitable for the transport of nonpolar compounds such as cholesterol. Alone, bile salts form small micelles capable of solubilizing relatively small amounts of cholesterol. Phospholipids are insoluble in water, but when present in mixed micelles with bile salts, they greatly expand the micellar size, permitting the solubilization of a much greater quantity of cholesterol. The relationship of these three compounds can be plotted using triangular coordinates so that any point in the resultant triangular graph represents a mixture of these lipids. The use of in vitro mixtures of lipids has demonstrated the boundaries of a small micellar zone in which mixtures of cholesterol, bile salts, and phospholipids are transparent because all the compounds are in solution. Cholesterol does not precipitate from such solutions, even after standing for a long time. Mixtures supersaturated with cholesterol, even though initially clear, quickly demonstrate the formation of cholesterol crystals. The series of mixtures between the micellar and supersaturated zones delineates the metastable zone. In this zone the mixtures also develop cholesterol crystals, only slowly. Gallbladder bile samples taken from a control group and from patients with stones have conformed closely to the behavior of in vitro mixtures. Thus the formation of cholesterol microcrystals appears to follow closely the predictions developed from the in vitro systems. Additional factors, however, are probably operative in cholesterol stone formation.

Bilirubin, the end product of heme catabolism and the major component of pigment stones, is secreted into the bile at a rate of 300 mg daily after conjugation with glucuronic acid. Even though partial deconjugation occurs within the intestine, less than 10% of biliary bilirubin is reabsorbed unaltered for resecretion into the bile; the remainder is converted into various urobilinogens and stercobilinogens, which undergo a separate metabolism and excretion in urine or feces.

Little is known about the metabolism of the other components of pigment stones. Calcium is secreted into hepatic bile, perhaps as a cation for the anionic bile acids, and is also actively secreted by the gallbladder, especially in response to an obstruction. The mechanisms by which phosphate and carbonate are secreted into the bile are unknown, but because the pH of bile varies between 6.5 and 8, the concentration of these anions, which are significant components of some pigment stones, must be extremely small. Furthermore, the mechanism by which they reach high concentrations in stones is unknown.

PHYSIOLOGY. Bile salts are actively secreted into the canaliculus. The volume and electrolyte content of the canalicular flow are further modified as it passes through the ductular system. During fasting the gallbladder concentrates hepatic bile rapidly, at a rate of 16% of the volume present every hour. The average pressure in Oddi's sphincter during fasting is 20 to 30 mm Hg, which is greater than the pressure in the common duct. Some hepatic bile enters the intestine, but the bile salts are reabsorbed and resecreted into the bile. Because of this amplification process the gallbladder contains 80% to 95% of the bile acid pool after a 16-hour fast. In response to a meal containing fats or proteins, cholecystokinin, a polypeptide hormone, is released from cells in the intestinal wall, especially in the duodenum, and together with other hormones causes the relaxation of Oddi's sphincter and the coordinated contraction of the gallbladder. Over the following 2 to 3 hours the gallbladder remains contracted, and the bile acid pool circulates two to three times. The sphincter then returns to its resting level, and the gallbladder relaxes, again permitting a partial sequestration of the bile acid pool within the gallbladder before its release in response to the next meal.

The bile acid pool normally is 3 to 5 g. It circulates about eight to ten times daily. The fecal losses are balanced by the hepatic synthesis of about 300 to 500 mg daily. Thus at any time about 90% of the hepatic bile acids secreted are derived from recirculation. Because in humans the synthesis can replace only a 10% pool loss, efficient bile acid reabsorption is essential for preservation of the bile acid pool.

About 1 g of cholesterol is secreted by the liver each day, and 50% of this is reabsorbed. The conversion of cholesterol into bile salts enables more cholesterol to be excreted. These steps are the only means by which the body can excrete cholesterol. Phospholipids are hydrolyzed by pancreatic phospholipase, and the components are reabsorbed and synthesized into the triglycerides and phospholipids by the intestinal mucosal cells.

CHOLELITHIASIS AND CHOLECYSTITIS

DEFINITION. Cholelithiasis is the presence of gallstones within the gallbladder. Choledocholithiasis is the presence of stones in the common duct resulting from their passage from the gallbladder or their primary formation in the common duct. Intrahepatic stones may reflux into the intrahepatic ducts from the common duct or may form there primarily. In the United States stones rarely form outside the gallbladder, but this is common in the Orient. In postcholecystectomy patients in Western countries there is a rare but distinct incidence of choledocholithiasis.

Cholesterol stones

ETIOLOGY. Cholesterol stones are 50% to 99% cholesterol and are formed in the gallbladder when currently unclear factors permit the nidation of cholesterol and some calcium bilirubinate, followed by the growth of the stone through the addition of cholesterol crystals. The cholesterol concentration must exceed its solubility in bile for precipitation to occur; in addition, sufficient time must elapse. Except in rare instances hepatic bile does not contain cholesterol crystals, and in more than 98% of these cases cholesterol stones form only in the gallbladder. The growth of stones results from an imbalance occurring between that part of the day when bile contains excess cholesterol, causing precipitation, and that part of the day when bile is undersaturated with cholesterol, resulting in dissolution. The rates of these two processes in humans may not be equivalent, and therefore the balance in any individual cannot be calculated. Months to years are required for the formation of cholesterol stones.

EPIDEMIOLOGY. Approximately 20 million people in the United States have gallstones. Of these stones 75% are predominantly cholesterol and 25% predominantly pigment. The incidence of cholesterol stones is three times as high in females as in males; they are uncommon in patients before puberty and begin to become significantly more common after the age of 20, reaching a peak incidence in the eighth decade, an age at which the majority of the population has stones. The incidence and type of stones vary greatly among countries. Many European nations have an incidence comparable to that in the United States. Indian tribes throughout the United States and in parts of Latin America, where they have been studied, have an extraordinarily high incidence of gallstones, approaching 100% of the population in old age. In Bolivia 100% of the stones are of the cholesterol type. In contrast, among the Masai people in Africa, all types of gallstones are rare. In the Orient, pigment gallstones predominate except in urban Japan, where the westernization of the diet has been accompanied by a steady increase in cholesterol stones, which now equals the incidence in the United States (75%).

Obese patients are more likely to develop cholesterol stones because, like Indians, they have a higher secretion of biliary cholesterol and a lower secretion of bile acids. In obese patients the level of biliary cholesterol reverts to normal with a weight loss approaching the patient's ideal weight. In general, hypercholesterolemic patients do not have an increased secretion of biliary cholesterol and do not have an increased incidence of cholesterol stones.

PATHOGENESIS. The mechanism of the formation of supersaturated hepatic bile is still a matter of debate. Early attention focused on the increase in HMG-CoA reductase and the decrease in 7-α-hydroxylase in these patients as compared to a control group, suggesting that the cause of the biliary lipid abnormalities was an imbalance between the formation of cholesterol and bile acids. Further investigation disclosed that chenodeoxycholic acid could suppress the secretion of biliary cholesterol in less than 1 hour, indicating that this effect could occur without a change in the hepatic enzymatic content. It has been hypothesized that the types of bile acids being secreted determine at least in part the amount of cholesterol secreted into the bile and that the activity of HMG-CoA reductase and 7-α-hydroxylase results from this differential effect at the site of the formation of biliary micelles. The arrangement of lecithin and cholesterol within the micelle resembles the lipid structure of a membrane. Membranes in which micelle formation may occur include the canalicular microvilli and the microsomal and Golgi's membranes within the hepatocyte.

Although the secretion of bile supersaturated with cholesterol is a prerequisite for the formation of cholesterol stones, it is not a sufficient condition by itself for the formation of stones. Although the bile may remain lithogenic after cholecystectomy, cholesterol stones rarely form in the ducts and cholesterol crystals cannot be identified in the bile. Time is needed for the growth of a stone, and this is provided by sequestration within recesses in the gallbladder, especially if the gallbladder does not empty completely in response to a meal. Gallbladder mucus or desquamated epithelium together with small amounts of calcium bilirubinate provides an excellent nidus for stone formation. Many small nidi and microcrystals are probably evacuated by the gallbladder before a stone reaches a clinically significant size.

Chronic cholecystitis invariably accompanies chronic cholelithiasis, but it is unclear whether it is an initiating or a perpetuating feature in cholelithiasis because acalculous cholecystitis is observed in 5% of patients undergoing biliary tract surgery. Perhaps cholecystitis will be found to be an initiator, causing gallbladder obstruction resulting from edema and causing excessive mucus secretion. This would provide the nidus for the formation of a gallstone and the stasis needed for gallstone growth.

The operative incidence of cholelithiasis increases with the age of the patient; whether this occurs because over a longer time it is more likely that a random event will occur or because of the aging process is not clear. Females have an incidence of cholesterol cholelithiasis three times higher than that of males. Studies of pregnant women using real-time ultrasonography have demonstrated that during the third trimester the gallbladder is dilated and is less responsive to a standard contractile force. In addition, the increased levels of estrogens secreted at this time are associated with an increased cholesterol saturation and cholestasis. The incidence of cholelithiasis is higher in certain families. In addition, groups such as the American Indians have a dual biochemical defect, a higher hepatic secretion of cholesterol and a smaller bile salt pool with a lower secretion of bile salts. Obese patients also have this dual defect until their weight returns to the ideal range. The effects of diet on this disorder are being studied. Low-cholesterol, low-fat diets lower the level of cholesterol in bile by 20%, but the effects are complex because bile acid metabolism is also affected. Any disease reducing the conservation of circulating bile acids and therefore reducing the return of bile acids to the liver through the enterohepatic circulation results in a decreased secretion of bile acids into bile. In such diseases cholesterol secretion is virtually unchanged, and thus bile becomes supersaturated with cholesterol. Regional enteritis involving the terminal ileum, an ileojejunal bypass, cystic fibrosis, and small intestinal resection have been associated with a higher incidence of cholelithiasis caused by this mechanism. Various drugs have been implicated in the formation of stones, including oral contraceptives, estrogens, and clofibrate (a systemic cholesterol-lowering agent that increases the biliary secretion of cholesterol while decreasing the bile salt pool).

CLINICAL MANIFESTATIONS. One half of these patients may have gallstones for their entire adult life without the development of symptoms. Because of this long period of latency, it is not possible to know when the formation of symptomatic stones may have begun. Gallstones rarely cause symptoms in patients under the age of 20; the peak incidence occurs in patients 40 to 60 years of age.

Flatulence, bloating, eructation, fatty food intolerance, and nonspecific abdominal discomforts have been ascribed to cholelithiasis. Such symptoms are present with the same incidence in patients without stones, however, and these symptoms are not resolved by a cholecystectomy. The symptoms of cholelithiasis result from the passage or impaction of stones in the gallbladder or at Oddi's sphincter. The classic and most common symptom is pain caused by the impaction of stones in the ampulla of the gallbladder. Typically this occurs 4 to 6 hours after an evening meal and wakes the patient from sleep. The pain is steady, builds in intensity, lasts from 15 minutes to 6 hours, and may require the administration of narcotics for relief. It is usually terminated by the return of the stone to the body of the gallbladder. Typically such episodes are separated by symptom-free periods of months to years. Biliary pain is most commonly located in the epigastrium (28% of these patients) or subcostally in the right upper quadrant (22%) but also may be located any place within the abdomen, such as substernally (11%) or over the right or left lower rib cage or back (10%).

When pain occurs with each meal, it may be caused by the impaction of a stone in the cystic duct; the pain results from the contraction of the gallbladder behind the stone, increasing the gallbladder pressure. A similar syndrome may be caused by the impaction of a stone in Oddi's sphincter, but this condition is usually accompanied by constant pain, hyperamylasemia, and jaundice.

Stones that pass through the cystic duct and Oddi's sphincter without impaction do not cause further problems and are eliminated in the feces. However, severe pancreatitis may result from stone passage. Although pancreatitis that occurs because of passage of stones is not common, it is generally much more severe than alcoholic pancreatitis and more commonly leads to the formation of pseudocysts and pancreatic abscesses.

When an inflamed gallbladder attaches to the first or second portion of the duodenum, a fistula may result. Large gallstones can then pass into the intestine and become impacted at the ileocecal valve, the narrowest area between the fistula and the anus. This impaction may cause a progressive intestinal obstruction leading eventually to gallstone ileus.

In almost all cases of chronic cholecystitis in the United States, gallbladder bile and stones are not infected. When stones are infected, however, it is unlikely that they will become sterilized because of their labyrinthine structure. Thus any subsequent obstruction to a gallbladder containing infected stones often results in the development of an acute infection, causing bacteremia. Bacterial infection occurs more commonly in association with acute cholecystitis but is not necessary for its development.

When the bile is infected, cholangitis occurs following an obstruction of Oddi's sphincter. Once cholangitis develops, it is likely that there will be repeated episodes along with the subsequent passage of stones because of the persistent infection of the glands lining the ductular system. Stenosis of Oddi's sphincter may also result, leading to the formation of common duct and hepatic stones. Stones in these locations are associated with additional cholangitis and intrahepatic abscesses.

The chronic obstruction of the gallbladder neck by a stone or by fibrosis and/or swollen lymph nodes leads to the concentration of biliary calcium and to an increased secretion of calcium and mucus along with a resorption of biliary lipids. If the gallbladder continues to secrete, it may become very enlarged, a condition called hydrops that is more commonly visualized than palpated. This is the exception to Courvoisier's law that a palpable gallbladder in patients with obstructive jaundice indicates the likelihood of an obstructing tumor of the common duct rather than a stone. In cases of hydrops there is no evidence that the bile duct is obstructed because the levels of bilirubin and alkaline phosphatase are normal. If there is a significant secretion of calcium carbonate, the bile becomes radiopaque (so-called limy bile). If this condition is demonstrated on a plain film of the abdomen, it is proof that the gallbladder is chronically obstructed. Calcification in the wall of the gallbladder, called porcelain gallbladder, is an indication for cholecystectomy because such gallbladders are more susceptible to the development of a carcinoma.

LABORATORY FINDINGS AND DIAGNOSIS. Disease of the gallbladder is rarely associated with changes in the results of liver blood tests unless the bile duct is obstructed. Acute cholecystitis, however, may affect the liver surrounding the gallbladder bed, causing a rise in the levels of aminotransferases and alkaline phosphatase. This elevation occurs also if the gallbladder is intrahepatic in location. In cases of an obstruction of the bile duct or a postoperative stricture formation, the level of alkaline phosphatase is usually elevated, often with an elevated level of serum bilirubin.

Oral cholecystograms obtained following the administration of six iopanoic acid (Telepaque) tablets on 2 successive days allow for adequate visualization of more than 95% of normal gallbladders. Cholesterol stones, which are usually radiolucent, appear as filling defects in the opacified gallbladder. In 95% of the cases in which the gallbladder cannot be seen on the cholecystogram, this indicates the presence of gallbladder disease.

If the symptoms are typical of biliary pain and no stone is demonstrated, biliary drainage should be performed. Small stones and sludge can be demonstrated by the microscopic examination of bile collected through a duodenal tube following the administration of magnesium sulfate or cholecystokinin, which causes the gallbladder to contract. The presence of cholesterol crystals usually indicates the presence of a stone, sludge, or cholesterolosis. Cholesterol crystals occur in stacks; they are flat and rectangular with one corner commonly missing (resembling the state of Utah). The presence of these crystals can be confirmed by demonstrating birefringence using a polarizing light stage on the microscope.

An alternative method of diagnosis that avoids the use of radiation is an ultrasonographic examination of the gallbladder. This is as accurate as oral cholecystography; however, it does not allow an accurate measurement of the size of a stone and does not determine whether the patient may undergo medical dissolution because it cannot establish the gallbladder function.

In cases of severe abdominal pain, a failure of the gallbladder to concentrate intravenous technetium 99m PIPIDA, which is rapidly excreted into the biliary system, suggests the presence of acute cholecystitis or a blockage of the cystic duct.

Common duct stones cannot usually be effectively diagnosed by means of ultrasonography. In 20% of the cases of choledocholithiasis the common bile duct is not dilated, and in this situation either percutaneous transhepatic cholangiography (which may require 15 to 20 passes in a patient with a nondilated biliary tract) or endoscopic retrograde cholangiopancreatography is the procedure of choice. The contrast obtained in these procedures is so superior to that of intravenous cholangiography that the latter procedure is rapidly being abandoned.

MANAGEMENT. Cholecystectomy is currently the treatment of choice for symptomatic gallstones and is the standard against which all other treatments should be measured. The indications for cholecystectomy in patients with asymptomatic stones are debatable. The mortality of this procedure in patients younger than 60 years of age is about 0.5% to 1% in medical centers. The mortality and morbidity are higher if the surgeon is unfamiliar with the wide variety of vascular and biliary tree anomalies that occur in this region. The most common mistake is an inadvertent ligation or transection of the common bile duct. Nonetheless, a successful cholecystectomy results in a permanent cure in 95% of these patients, and there is also no measurable change in digestion.

Young patients may prefer an attempt at the medical dissolution of gallstones using chenodeoxycholic acid or its 7-β analog, ursodeoxycholic acid; this at present is an experimental approach. These bile acids act by reducing the cholesterol secretion into the bile and by increasing the size of the bile acid pool. Because of their possible teratogenicity, these drugs are not being administered to patients under 40 years of age, the group who would benefit most from this medication. These agents do not dissolve calcified cholesterol stones or stones in patients whose gallbladder cannot be visualized by oral cholecystography. The agents also have a reduced efficacy in patients with stones greater than 1 cm in diameter and in obese patients, and these agents do not dissolve radiolucent pigment stones. Thus dissolution occurs successfully in about 70% to 80% of cases after a 2-year course. In approximately 50% of these patients stones reform after this dissolution; it is not known what long-term regimen is needed for such patients.

Acute cholecystitis should be treated with an appropriate antibiotic coverage for intestinal flora, such as with ampicillin and gentamicin. Surgeons now tend to prefer performing a cholecystectomy promptly when the toxicity is controlled.

PREVENTION. Because heredity plays a major role in the formation of stones, there seems little that can be done to prevent stone formation. However, the maintenance of the patient's weight in the ideal range and the avoidance of prolonged fasts or drugs known to cause alterations in biliary lipid composition seem important. Eating frequent small meals and a snack just before bedtime to keep bile circulating for the longest possible time during the day should be helpful in keeping the bile undersaturated with cholesterol during the greatest portion of the day.

NEOPLASTIC DISEASE
Carcinoma of the gallbladder and extrahepatic biliary ducts

DEFINITION, ETIOLOGY, AND EPIDEMIOLOGY. Although other tumors may metastasize to the gallbladder, the predominant tumors are adenocarcinomas of the gallbladder and cholangiocarcinomas of the extrahepatic biliary ducts. The causes of these tumors are unknown. The incidence of gallbladder cancer is about 3:200,000 people in the United States. Bile duct cancer has a lower incidence. The incidence of gallbladder cancer is 3.4 times higher in females than in males, which parallels the incidence of gallstones. In contrast, the incidence of cancer of the biliary tract is equal in males and females. The incidence of cholelithiasis among patients with cancer of the gallbladder is at least 75%, whereas it is significantly less (32%) among those with biliary tract cancer. Patients in both groups have an average age of 63 to 65 years at the onset of the disease. In Japan the incidence of carcinoma is highest in patients with black stones (3.4%), intermediate in those with cholesterol stones (1%), and lowest in those with bilirubinate-palmitate stones (0.16%).

Cholangiocarcinomas have been associated with chronic intrahepatic cholangitis, hepatolithiasis, ulcerative colitis, and infections with *Opisthorchis sinensis*. The incidence of bile duct tumors is higher in patients with choledochocele after undergoing choledochoduodenostomy. One half of these tumors develop within 4 years of the operation, suggesting an interaction between biliary and intestinal components.

CLINICAL MANIFESTATIONS. Cancer of the gallbladder has been detected incidentally during elective cholecystectomy for gallstones, but unfortunately even these patients have a very poor survival rate. Patients with a clinically evident carcinoma usually have a palpable mass or right upper quadrant pain caused by peritoneal involvement. The disease is commonly unresectable. Cancer of the bile duct is usually detected at an earlier stage because even a slight growth causes a bile duct obstruction. Cancer of the left or right hepatic duct does not cause symptoms until it has reached a large size, since the complete obstruction of one duct does not cause jaundice because the unobstructed lobe can handle the increased biliary secretion. The level of alkaline phosphatase, however, may be very elevated. A tumor at the bifurcation of the left and right hepatic ducts, called a Klatskin tumor, causes early jaundice.

LABORATORY FINDINGS. Because of the bile duct obstruction, the level of alkaline phosphatase may be elevated as much as 20 to 40 times the normal level.

DIAGNOSIS. Ultrasonography may identify a gallbladder mass or a dilated intrahepatic duct. The diagnosis may be made with a fine-needle biopsy and/or with percutaneous fine-needle cholangiography or retrograde cholangiography. Fine-needle cholangiography is preferred for the diagnosis of intrahepatic lesions because percutaneous transhepatic catheters may be placed, depending on the patient, as a definitive procedure or as a decompressive measure before surgery, irradiation, or chemotherapy.

COURSE. Although bile duct tumors may be discovered at an early stage, patients with such tumors have a poor 5-year survival rate, and there is no evidence that radical surgical procedures extend the life expectancy. In patients with extensive disease the morbidity may be reduced by placement of percutaneous biliary catheters with multiple side-holes through the tumor. These tubes can eventually be clamped so that bile can drain internally from above to below the lesions and into the intestine. When bile can pass freely into the intestine, jaundice and pruritus can clear and the patient's appetite may increase. Various chemotherapeutic regimens have been tried without any striking success. Radiotherapy has been reported to increase the survival rate, but no controlled trials have been reported to date.

Carcinoma of the ampulla of Vater

Cancer arising from the ampulla of Vater is more common than cancer of the extrahepatic bile ducts but less common than cancer of the gallbladder. Patients with ampullary carcinoma usually have obstructive jaundice that must be differentiated from other types of extrahepatic obstruction such as that caused by carcinoma of the pancreas or the bile ducts, choledocholithiasis, a stricture of the common bile duct, and sclerosing cholangitis; this carcinoma must also be differentiated from intrahepatic cholestasis caused by drugs, primary biliary cirrhosis, and numerous other hepatic disorders. Ampullary carcinomas commonly produce occult blood in the feces but rarely bleed grossly. The diagnosis is probably best determined by endoscopic retrograde cholangiopancreatography (ERCP), which often permits a direct visualization of the lesion, and a biopsy, as well as roentgenographic visualization of the pancreatic and biliary ducts. If necessary, percutaneous fine-needle cholangiography, ultrasonography, or computed tomography may also be helpful in demonstrating dilated biliary ducts and an obstructing extrahepatic lesion. Patients with ampullary carcinoma have the best prognosis among those with biliary and pancreatic carcinomas; the 5-year survival rate after a radical pancreaticoduodenectomy (Whipple's procedure) may be as high as 25% to 50%.

BIBLIOGRAPHY
Cholelithiasis

Admirand, W.H., and Small, D.M.: The physicochemical basis of cholesterol gallstone formation in man, J. Clin. Invest. **47**:1043, 1968.

Bennion, L.J., and Grundy, S.M.: Effects of obesity and caloric intake on biliary lipid metabolism in man, J. Clin. Invest. **56**:996, 1975.

Bennion, L.J., and others: Effects of oral contraceptives on the gallbladder bile of normal women, N. Engl. J. Med. **294**:189, 1976.

Coyne, M.J., and others: Dietary cholesterol affects chenodeoxycholic acid action on biliary lipids, Gastroenterology **72**:927, 1977.

Danzinger, R.G., and others: Effect of oral chenodeoxycholic acid on bile acid kinetics and biliary lipid composition in women with cholelithiasis, J. Clin. Invest. **52**:2809, 1973.

Grundy, S.M., Metzger, A.L., and Adler, R.D.: Mechanisms of lithogenic bile formation in American Indian women with cholesterol gallstones, J. Clin. Invest. **51**:3026, 1972.

Holzbach, R.T., and others: Cholesterol solubility in bile: evidence that supersaturated bile is frequent in healthy man, J. Clin. Invest. **52**:1467, 1973.

Soloway, R.D., and Schoenfield, L.J.: Effects of meals and interruption of the enterohepatic circulation on flow, lipid composition and cholesterol saturation of bile in man after cholecystectomy, Am. J. Dig. Dis. **20**:99, 1975.

Wagner, C.I., Trotman, B.W., and Soloway, R.D.: Kinetic analysis of biliary lipid excretion in man and dog, J. Clin. Invest. **57**:473, 1976.

Carcinoma of the ampulla of Vater

Soloway, R.D., Balistreri, W.F., and Trotman, B.W.: The gallbladder and biliary tract. In Bouchier, I.A.D., editor: Recent advances in gastroenterology, ed. 4, New York, 1980, Churchill Livingstone Inc.

DENTAL CORRELATIONS

Barry H. Hendler, Barbara J. Steinberg, and Shirley Brown

The subject of gastrointestinal disorders may at first appear to have minimal significance for the dentist. However, careful consideration of the complete realm of these disorders reveals the important nature of this subject, particularly within the context of the thorough evaluation of the patient requesting dental treatment.

One such area involves drug interactions and altered drug metabolism. Corticosteroids, for example, which may be used to treat certain inflammatory disorders of the gastrointestinal tract, often react adversely with drugs commonly prescribed in dental practice and may cause generalized systemic reactions. Patients with chronic liver disease exhibit abnormal metabolism of many drugs, including lidocaine, penicillin, and tetracycline, and prolonged action of barbiturates. In addition, since blood coagulability is often impaired in chronic liver disease, special measures obviously must be taken with these patients in the surgical phases of dentistry. Patients with malabsorption problems may experience poor nutrition unrelated to masticatory insufficiency, and oral manifestations such as chronic ulcerations and stomatitis often accompany folic acid and vitamin B_{12} deficiency states. Since an overwhelming number of dentists are exposed to viral hepatitis, chronic carriers of the hepatitis B surface antigen must be identified in clinical practice, so that adequate precautions can be taken before treatment.

This discussion is organized in sequence, anatomically beginning with diseases of the esophagus and progressing to disorders of the stomach, intestines, liver, and pancreas. Nutritional disorders, including vitamin deficiencies, will be presented at the conclusion of this section.

DISEASES OF THE ESOPHAGUS

Although pathologic manifestations vary widely, the primary clinical symptom of all esophageal disorders is dysphagia. This symptom can have a number of etiologies, including the following:
1. Mechanical obstruction, such as a malignant esophageal tumor
2. Uncoordinated contraction reflex of the swallowing musculature because of neurologic disease
3. Plummer-Vinson syndrome, which results in muscular degeneration or stenosis
4. Collagen vascular disease (scleroderma or progressive systemic sclerosis), which causes increased rigidity of the esophageal wall
5. Infections, particularly *Candida* infections, which can cause retrosternal burning and esophageal spasm

From a diagnostic standpoint, the dentist should be aware that although patients frequently associate dysphagia with dental problems, this symptom usually indicates serious underlying systemic disease. Therefore, when all possible dental causes have been ruled out, diagnostic efforts should turn immediately to complete evaluation through medical consultation.

Plummer-Vinson syndrome occurs most frequently in women in the fourth and fifth decades. The primary cause of the syndrome is iron deficiency, and the main symptom, dysphagia, results from muscular degeneration in the esophagus and stenoses or webs of the esophageal mucosa.

In addition to dysphagia, Plummer-Vinson syndrome has many other clinical manifestations with significance in dental practice. Patients often have a thinned vermilion border of the lips, angular cheilitis, and reduced width of the mouth. The oral mucosa is thin, atrophic, inelastic, dry, and glazed, and the tongue often becomes red and painful and appears smooth because of loss of papillae. Patients are encouraged to eat a well-balanced diet, which at first consists of semiliquid or soft foods. Treatment of oral symptoms may include the use of viscous 2% lidocaine rinses to reduce pain and burning.

The atrophic mucosal changes of Plummer-Vinson syndrome appear to predispose these individuals to leukoplakia and, in some cases, oral and pharyngeal carcinoma. In a study of 250 patients with carcinoma of the mouth and upper respiratory tract, 70% had a history of Plummer-Vinson syndrome. The dentist should therefore observe these patients closely and be alert for ulcerative, hyperkeratotic, or other premalignant changes. A biopsy of suggestive lesions should be done and submitted for histologic examination.

Progressive systemic sclerosis (PSS, or scleroderma) is a chronic collagen vascular disease of possible autoimmune etiology. It is characterized by diffuse scleroses of the skin, gastrointestinal tract, heart muscle, lungs, and kidneys and most commonly affects women between the ages of 20 and 50. A recent study has shown that head and neck manifestations occur in 80% of scleroderma patients. These include dysphagia because of esophageal involvement; thinning and rigidity of the lips; narrowing of the oral aperture; loss of skin folds around the mouth, giving a masklike facies; hardness and rigidity of the tongue; and xerostomia, all of which may render speech extremely difficult. Restriction of mandibular movement sometimes occurs when the muscles of mastication are affected by the disease and become rigid. Dental roentgenograms commonly reveal a uniform thickening of the periodontal membrane space, especially around posterior teeth.

Progressive systemic sclerosis presents several problems unique to dentistry. Since the oral aperture may be narrowed and the face rigid, access to the teeth and periodontium is impaired. This may limit the scope of treatment and necessitate special prosthetic techniques. In addition, since these patients frequently suffer from sclerotic "clawing" of the hands (sclerodactyly) (Fig. 1), which

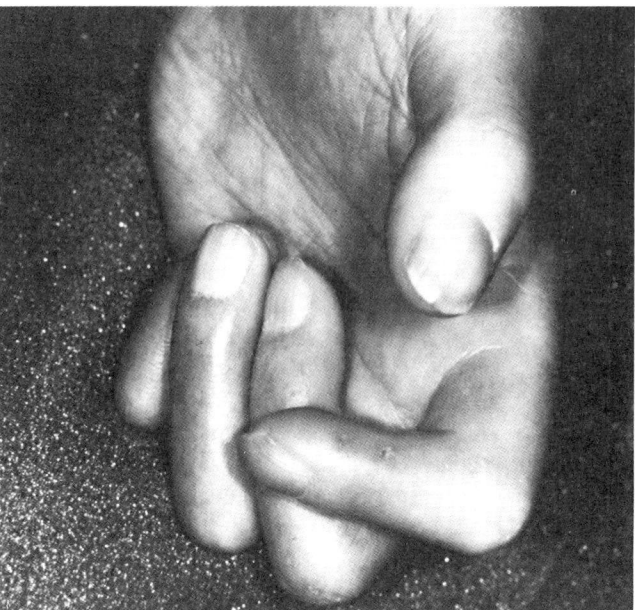

Fig. 1. Sclerodactyly in 55-year-old man with scleroderma.

diminishes manual dexterity, toothbrushing and flossing may be difficult or impossible. These patients therefore require constant comprehensive oral care and frequent professional oral prophylaxis.

Candida infections of the esophagus usually occur when the mouth and pharynx are also involved, a condition known as "candidal oropharyngoesophagitis." The disease is caused by an overgrowth of the hyphal form of *Candida albicans* and may occur in individuals with malignant disease or endocrine or immunologic disorders and in patients undergoing antibiotic, corticosteroid, or immunosuppressant therapy. These patients usually complain of chronic dysphagia, oropharyngeal soreness of varying intensity, and occasional retrosternal burning. The appearance of the candidal lesions is distinctive, characterized by soft, white, slightly elevated "curdlike" plaques that, when stripped from the tissue, leave a bleeding mucosal surface.

Treatment of candidal infections should be directed toward eliminating any systemic cause. Local palliative and supportive treatment may include rinsing with suspensions of nystatin in methylcellulose or administering nystatin oral tablets. The use of nystatin vaginal suppositories is often helpful when contact with the lesions over a longer time period is required.

ACID PEPTIC DISEASE

The dental patient with peptic ulcer disease requires special consideration in three general areas of treatment: drug therapy, stress management protocol, and oral surgery.

The dentist's knowledge of possible drug interactions or adverse drug effects often experienced by patients with acid peptic disease is vitally important. Aspirin, all aspirin-containing analgesics, phenylbutazone, and steroids must be strictly avoided, since they are known to excerbate peptic ulceration. Acetaminophen or any of its compounds (acetaminophen-codeine combinations) is therefore the analgesic of choice. Furthermore, patients with peptic ulcer disease are frequently treated with anticholinergic drugs and antacids, both of which may have some untoward effects for dental consideration. Anticholinergics may cause xerostomia with all of its attendant problems, and, since the caries rate may thus be elevated, patients taking anticholinergic drugs may benefit from a daily home regimen of fluoride applications. Antacids generally contain calcium, magnesium, or aluminum salts, which will bind to orally administered antibiotics, such as erythromycin and tetracycline. Because this binding action causes as much as an 80% decrease in the absorption of these antibiotics, they should not be taken within an hour of the antacid.

Since stress is known to contribute significantly to the severity of peptic ulcers, dental visits, as a rule, should be shortened and the use of presedation or conscious sedation (such as nitrous oxide) should be strongly considered during dental procedures.

Finally, people with peptic ulcers may have occult bleeding, leading to chronic anemia. For this reason the dentist should obtain a complete blood count, including hematocrit and hemoglobin levels, before extensive oral or periodontal surgery.

In oral diagnosis, the dentist can benefit from results of studies performed on a large number of hospitalized patients with and without peptic ulcer disease. The studies revealed that certain vascular formations of the lips occur more frequently and at an earlier age in patients with a history of peptic ulcer than in study groups without ulcers; however, the etiology of the formations is not clearly understood at this time. These vascular formations were seen more often in men than in women and were of three types:

1. *Microcherry.* This is a sharply circumscribed red dot, usually smaller than 1 mm in diameter. It is most commonly found on the inner surface of the lower lip but may be seen on the vermilion border and on the upper lip as well. Microcherries may occur singly, or there may be several that are widely separated.
2. *Glomerulus.* This formation is a 1- to 2-mm aggregate of tortuous, thin-walled red vessels that resembles the glomerulus of the kidney. When pressure is applied to the glomerulus, it blanches; as the pressure is released, it may pulsate.
3. *Venous lake.* This is a dilated portion of a submucosal vein that resembles a small varicosity. The venous lake is a single bluish mound that collapses on slight pressure and does not pulsate. It is often found at the inner surface of the labial commissures and less commonly along the vermilion border of the lip.

TUMORS AND VASCULAR AND INFLAMMATORY DISEASES OF THE GASTROINTESTINAL TRACT

This important group of gastrointestinal diseases has dental significance in two areas: oral diagnosis and physical evaluation of the dental patient. From the standpoint of oral diagnosis, the dentist should be conversant with the signs of each syndrome, ranging from fibrous tumors of the facial bones associated with Gardner's syndrome to the specific and nonspecific oral lesions of Crohn's disease. The dentist also should be aware that metastatic lesions of gastrointestinal tumors, such as gastric adenocarcinoma, can occur intraorally.

Proper dental management mandates that the dental practitioner fully understand the medical management of these patients or obtain medical consultation so that the side effects of medical treatment can be adequately differentiated from other systemic problems affecting oral health. Effects of common drug regimens, such as steroid therapy, can affect dental treatment, and, in many cases, drugs used in dentistry, such as aspirin compounds, are contraindicated for use in these patients.

Because chronic gastrointestinal bleeding is a hazard in many of these syndromes, patients may often be anemic and thrombocytopenic. They may also undergo changes in red and white blood cell counts secondary to the immunosuppressive drugs that are commonly used. As a general rule, therefore, the dentist should routinely obtain hematocrit and hemoglobin values and a complete blood cell count with differential before performing any oral surgical procedure.

TUMORS OF THE GUT
Adenocarcinoma of the stomach

Malignant gastric tumors can metastasize to the head and neck region as a tumor mass or manifest as hyperpigmentation of the dermis and oral mucosae. Only a few cases of metastatic oral lesions from gastric adenocarcinoma have been reported. Of clinical importance is the fact that metastatic lesions involving the oral or perioral structures may be the first evidence of malignant disease arising from a distant origin. These lesions may produce a variety of signs and symptoms, including swelling, pain, looseness of teeth, and paresthesia. In many cases, the patient is asymptomatic and the lesion is discovered during routine oral examination. Clinically, the oral malignant metastatic lesion may appear similar to a benign oral lesion, such as fibrous hyperplasia of the mucosa from ill-fitting dentures. It is clear, therefore, that after obtaining a careful medical history, a biopsy should be done on suggestive lesions.

The association between occult malignancy and acanthosis nigricans (focal or diffuse hyperpigmentation of the dermis) is well established. Greater than 50% of patients over 30 years of age who have acanthosis nigricans will eventually develop a malignancy, usually adenocarcinoma of the stomach. Acanthosis nigricans appears as velvety hyperpigmented, hyperkeratotic varicosities, usually in the skin folds of the neck, axillae, groin, anogenital regions, and other flexural surfaces. Oral manifestations occur in 30% to 40% of the patients, primarily on the tongue and lips. The papillae on the dorsum of the tongue become elongated and hypertrophic, producing deep furrows. The labial mucosa and vermilion border may become thickened and covered with papillomatous tumors and cracks. Papillomatous growths may also appear on the tongue, gingiva, and the buccal and palatal mucosa. In addition, leukoedema of the buccal mucosa may occur.

Adenocarcinoma of the colon and rectum

Although cases of metastatic adenocarcinoma in the head and neck region have been well documented, the number of such cases arising from a primary site in the colon and rectum are extremely rare. Moffat reported a lesion that began as a bony metastasis in the mandible with subsequent epulis formation. The patient appeared for treatment with a hard, ulcerated nodule (epulis) of 1.2 × 1 cm, arising from the alveolar margin.

Lee reported a case of adenocarcinoma of the colon with metastasis to the lip. The lesion was a single round, indurated pinkish gray nodule, 1 cm in diameter, at the vermilion border of the lower lip.

Cases of metastasis from the rectum to the parotid gland, palate, and gingiva, although extremely rare, have also been noted in the literature.

Gastrointestinal polyposis syndromes

Both Gardner's syndrome and Peutz-Jeghers syndrome, which are representative of this group of disorders, are generally identified via the family medical history, since they are both inherited as autosomal dominant conditions. Both syndromes demonstrate cutaneous, gastrointestinal, and orofacial manifestations.

In *Gardner's syndrome* epidermoid or sebaceous cysts of the skin may occur on the face, trunk, and extremities. Fibrous tumors of the skin—fibromas and desmoids—may also occur, the latter most notably seen on surgical scars of the abdomen. Multiple polyps of the colon and rectum with a high malignant potential are also characteristic of this syndrome, which generally develops during or after the second decade. Up to 15 years may elapse between the development of polyps and the onset of any malignant changes.

Manifestations in the head and neck region, in addition to the epidermoid cysts previously mentioned, include multiple asymptomatic osteomas that are scattered throughout the craniofacial skeleton (Fig. 2). These tumors generally appear at puberty and may involve the frontal bone, mandible, maxilla, and sinuses. The long bones may also show involvement. Odontomas, dentigerous cysts, bony exostoses, hypercementosis, supernumerary teeth, and permanent impacted teeth are other common oral findings associated with this syndrome.

Because of the high level of orofacial involvement in Gardner's syndrome, the dentist can have an important role in its diagnosis. Early diagnosis of the disease is essential, since malignancy rates in untreated individuals appear to be as high as 50% to 100%. Treatment usually involves surgery of the lower intestinal tract to remove the polypoid lesions and any adjacent normal tissue that is likely to undergo malignant transformation.

Like Gardner's syndrome, *Peutz-Jeghers syndrome* is characterized by intestinal polyposis, which may become symptomatic during or after the second decade. In this syndrome, however, the polyps rarely become malignant (less than 3%), and the skin and orofacial region are affected only by melanotic pigmentation. In about 50% of affected persons, who are usually dark complected, discrete brown or bluish black macules, ranging in size from 1 to 10 mm, are present on the skin. These macules are

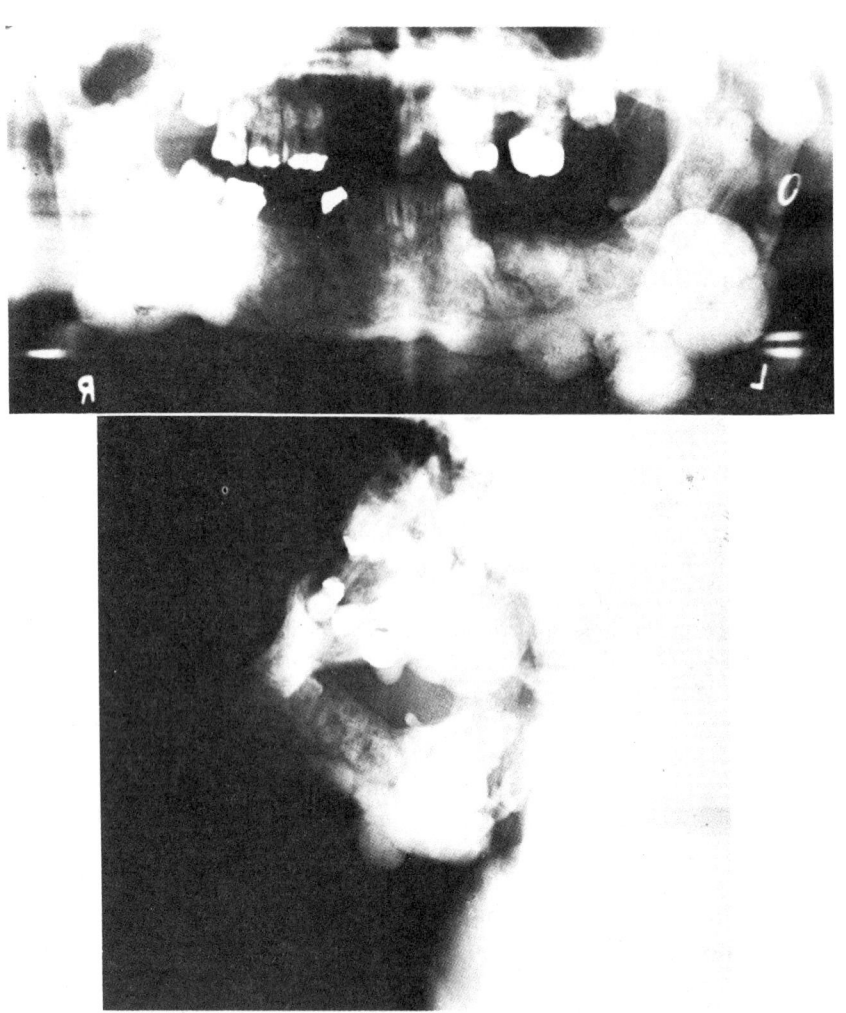

Fig. 2. Osteomas in 17-year-old man with Gardner's syndrome.

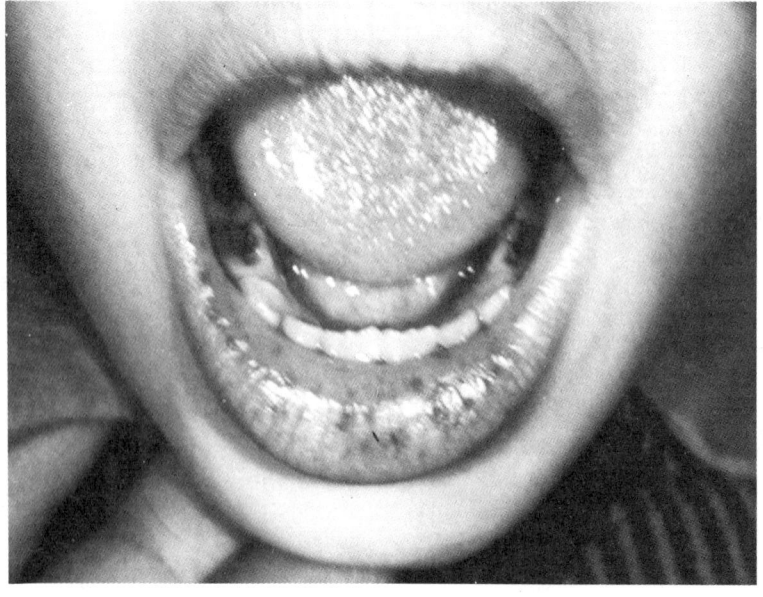

Fig. 3. Pigmentations in 9-year-old girl with Peutz-Jeghers syndrome.

seen most frequently about the perioral, perinasal, and periorbital orifices and may also occur on the hands, feet, and trunk. In the mouth, the buccal mucosa and lips are usually affected, and pigmentation may also occur on the palate, the gingiva, and, less often, the tongue. Intraoral lesions are round, oval, or irregular brown macules, 1 to 5 mm in diameter (Fig. 3).

Both mucosal and skin pigmentations first appear shortly after birth in individuals with Peutz-Jeghers syndrome. Since the skin pigmentations fade during adulthood, oral mucosal pigmentation remains the most constant feature of this syndrome. Dermabrasion for cosmetic treatment of the pigmented spots on the lips and oral mucosa occasionally has been attempted, with generally disappointing results. Recent studies indicate that the pigmentations can now be treated successfully with argon and ruby lasers.

VASCULAR DISEASE OF THE GUT
Hereditary hemorrhagic telangiectasia

Hereditary hemorrhagic telangiectasia (HHT) is a disorder of the capillaries and small blood vessels that is transmitted by simple autosomal dominant inheritance. A deficiency in elastic fibers results in abnormally thin vascular walls, vascular dilation, and spontaneous ruptures. These telangiectases, which occur on cutaneous, visceral, and mucosal surfaces, commonly appear before puberty or after menopause or the male climacteric. They appear as nonpulsating, red or purple, spiderlike or nodular lesions, and pressure will cause blanching that does not completely disappear.

Oral lesions of HHT develop most frequently on mucosal surfaces of the lips and on the tip and dorsum of the tongue, although the palate, gingiva, and buccal mucosa may also be affected. The early oral lesion is a cherry red macule, ranging from 1 to 3 mm in diameter. Biopsies are rarely indicated, since the syndrome is easily diagnosed from the pathognomonic skin and oral lesions and from the family history.

In addition to the obvious telangiectases, HHT is characterized by spontaneous bleeding, more frequently from mucous membranes than from the skin. The most common site of such bleeding in nearly all HHT patients is the nasal mucosa, with bleeding from oral telangiectases second in frequency to epistaxis. The gastric mucosa may also bleed chronically, as evidenced clinically by hematemesis and melena. The resultant anemia and thrombocytopenia may lead to facial pallor, fatigue, and generalized weakness.

Treatments to eliminate telangiectatic areas include x-irradiation and surgical excision. Aminocaproic acid may be applied topically for severe epistaxis. Estrogens have been administered systemically to reduce the frequency and severity of bleeding, with varying degrees of success. For good preventive treatment, a low-roughage diet and avoidance of drugs with erosive and anticoagulant properties, such as aspirin, are recommended for the patient with HHT, and living quarters should be well humidified to reduce irritation of the oral and nasal mucosae.

Although deaths from severe hemorrhage in HHT patients have been reported, the disease is seldom life threatening. The dentist should be aware that episodes of bleeding from oral lesions may occur in these individuals with or without traumatic insult. The patient with gingival telangiectases should be advised to brush the teeth gently to minimize trauma to the lesions. Hemorrhages, should they occur, may be controlled by applying direct pressure or by cauterizing accessible lesions.

Dental surgical procedures have been reported without postoperative complications. Because of the likelihood of anemia and thrombocytopenia from repeated bleeding episodes, it is imperative once again that invasive dental treatment be preceded by obtaining hemoglobin and hematocrit values and a platelet count in conjunction with medical consultation.

INFLAMMATORY BOWEL DISEASE

Some of the diseases included in this group have specific oral manifestations, which in certain cases are the initial signs of the disease.

Ulcerative colitis

In addition to gingivitis and oral candidiasis, four oral lesions occur frequently in patients with ulcerative colitis: recurrent aphthous ulcerations, pyoderma gangrenosum, pyostomatitis vegetans, and hemorrhagic ulcers of the oral mucosa and skin.

Recurrent aphthous ulcerations. Of patients with ulcerative colitis 4% to 20% exhibit aphthous ulcers that appear spontaneously and, in most cases, concurrently with other major symptoms of the disease. The ulcers are usually smaller than 10 mm in diameter and occur on the nonkeratinized mucosae of the lips, cheeks, oral vestibule, and margins of the tongue. They appear as round or oval ulcers surrounded by a bright red halo and covered by a grayish white, fibrinous exudate (Fig. 4). These painful lesions may persist for 4 to 14 days and generally heal without scarring. A very severe type of aphthous ulceration, referred to as "periadenitis mucosa necrotica recurrens," may accompany ulcerative colitis. These lesions are more painful and larger than those previously described, ranging as large as 30 mm in diameter. They appear as large necrotic areas with indurated borders surrounded by redness and edema (Fig. 5). Requiring between 10 and 40 days to heal, these lesions leave a fibrous retractile scar.

Pyoderma gangrenosum. Pyoderma gangrenosum is a severe, sometimes life-threatening complication of ulcerative colitis characterized by spreading ulcers of the extremities, abdomen, and perineum. The ulcers have a granulating base and deeply undermined edges and are surrounded by a striking blue-red areola. Very painful oral ulcerations

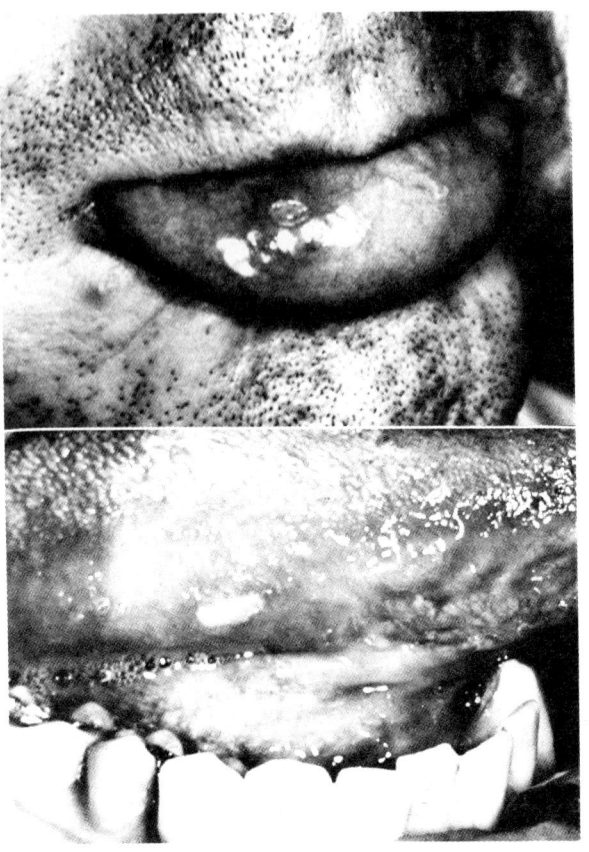

Fig. 4. Recurrent aphthous ulcerations associated with ulcerative colitis.

may also develop over the 4- to 8-week period when bowel symptoms are present. These irregularly shaped ulcerations of 10 to 20 mm in diameter have grayish bases and rolled margins.

Pyostomatitis vegetans. This unusual lesion of the oral mucous membranes seems to occur only in the individual with ulcerative colitis. Possibly the result of an autoimmune mechanism, the vegetative purulent lesions develop over a period of 6 to 8 weeks and tend to parallel the bowel symptoms in severity. They are usually sterile, resistant to local therapy, and best controlled by effectively treating the colitis. In addition to these lesions, the patient with pyostomatitis vegetans may have pyrexia and submandibular lymphadenopathy.

Hemorrhagic ulcers of oral mucosa and skin. Irregularly shaped hemorrhagic ulcers of various sizes may occur on the oral mucosa and skin of the cheeks and the inner aspect of the thighs, buttocks, and lower abdomen in patients with ulcerative colitis. The lesions develop within 1 to 3 days, starting as hemorrhagic bullae that subsequently burst to become ulcers.

The four types of oral lesions associated with ulcerative colitis generally do not respond to local treatment until the colitis is controlled by medical or surgical therapy. Local treatment consists of topical 2% viscous lidocaine application to relieve pain and topical steroids to reduce the severity of mucosal inflammation.

Crohn's disease

Crohn's disease, or regional enteritis, is characterized chiefly by granulomatous lesions of the intestinal tract that may fistulate onto the external surface of the abdomen.

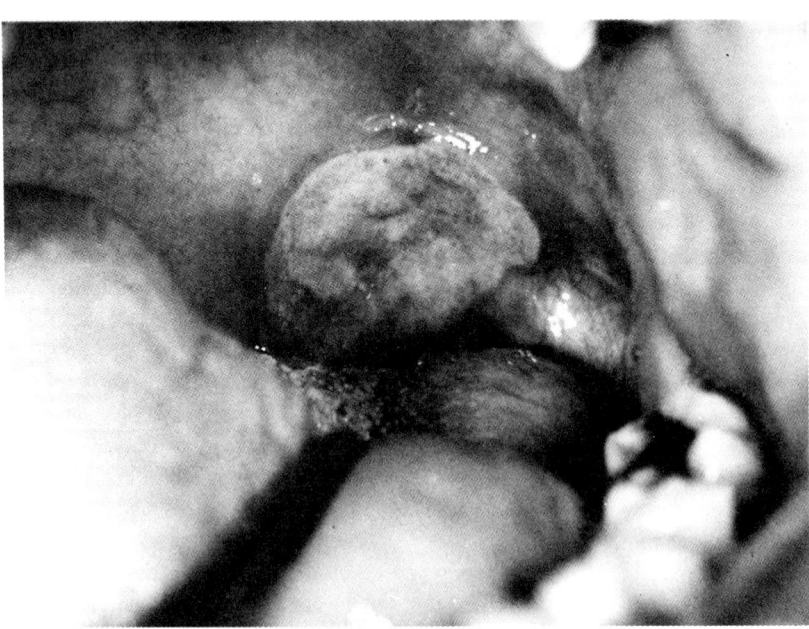

Fig. 5. Major aphthous ulcerations associated with ulcerative colitis.

The disease has no observed pattern of age or sex distribution and the cause is unknown.

Oral lesions have been found in approximately 6% to 20% of patients with Crohn's disease. They can occur at any time during the course of the disease and may be present before intestinal involvement is demonstrable. These lesions may recur in various forms and in different locations in the same patient and may or may not be correlated with the exacerbation and remission of intestinal symptoms. Oral lesions occur more commonly in patients with colonic disease than in those with disease confined to the small bowel. Patients with extraintestinal manifestations of Crohn's disease, such as skin and joint lesions, have a greater chance of developing oral lesions as well.

The oral lesions seen in patients with Crohn's disease are either "specific" or "nonspecific," as differentiated by clinical and histologic features. The specific oral lesions are histologically similar to the intestinal lesions of the disease. They most commonly occur in the mucobuccal fold or buccal mucosa, where they are described as having a lobulated, hypertrophic, fissured appearance, with or without linear ulcerations. The diffuse buccal lesions have a "cobblestone" appearance that is characteristic of Crohn's disease. Lesions on vestibular and retromolar mucosae are indurated and polypoid, often resembling denture granulomas (epulis fissuratum) (Fig. 6). Specific lesions of the gingiva, alveolar mucosa, and lips appear as areas of diffuse red swelling, sometimes accompanied by angular cheilitis.

Nonspecific lesions are the recurrent aphthous-type ulcers and are probably the most common oral lesions of Crohn's disease. The onset of these ulcers, which are generally widespread and severe, may be concurrent with bowel symptoms. The cause is not certain, but it is suspected that since measurably lower IgA secretion rates have been found in patients with active Crohn's disease, the oral mucous membranes may be more likely to undergo an immunologic reaction to exogenous oral antigens, resulting in these lesions.

The oral lesions generally regress when intestinal symptoms are brought under control. Local steroids may reduce inflammation in some patients, and 2% viscous lidocaine rinses are prescribed to reduce pain. Surgical excision of a severe lesion occasionally may be necessary.

A possible association between Crohn's disease and periodontal disease has been reported in the literature. Segal and Loewe reported altered neutrophil function and Koldkjaer and others reported enhanced lysozyme activity in patients with Crohn's disease. These two findings may also be seen in certain forms of rapid progressive periodontal disease. Further research in this area may provide new approaches to treating these conditions.

DISEASES OF THE LIVER

Diseases that affect the liver are of interest for several reasons. Obviously, the dental practitioner has the unique opportunity to function as primary diagnostician by using an accurate medical history or by recognizing the varied oral manifestations of hepatic disease or dysfunction. These manifestations run the gamut from fetor hepaticus, a sweetish musty odor on the breath of patients with liver failure or extensive portal systemic shunting of blood, to jaundice of the oral mucosa or sclera. In addition, enlargement of the parotid glands secondary to increased parotid

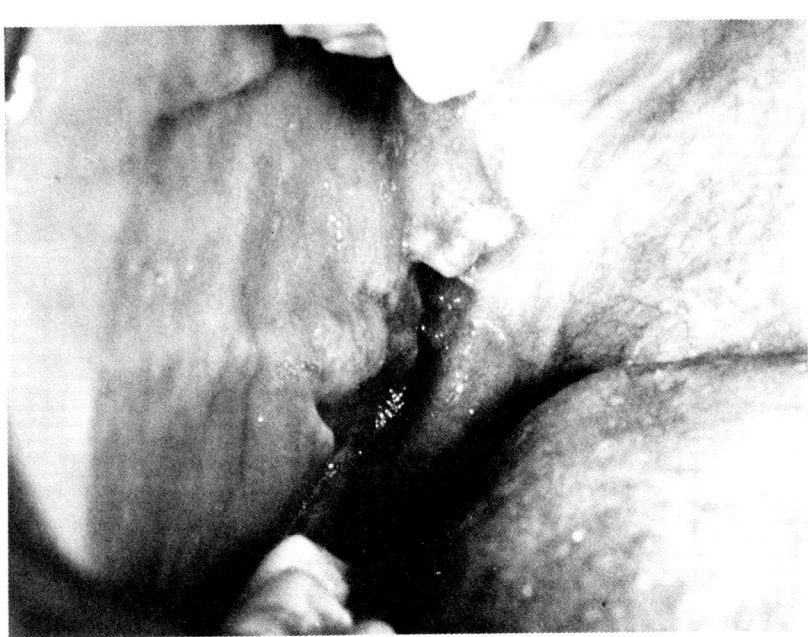

Fig. 6. Polypoid lesion in 14-year-old girl with Crohn's disease.

salivary flow in patients with alcoholic cirrhosis, lesions due to nutritional deficiency, and bleeding secondary to depressed plasma levels of clotting factors synthesized by the liver may be readily evident in patients having dental therapy. Also, since hepatitis virus is transmitted via blood and other body fluids through accidental needle punctures, open wound contact, accidental ingestion, or splashing of mucous membranes, a dentist and auxiliary personnel are at increased risk of exposure, making it mandatory to take specific and careful precautions when dealing with patients known to have contacted the virus.

Chronic liver disease

One of the characteristic features of chronic liver disease is multisystem involvement, and its occurrence is often quoted as evidence in favor of an autoimmune etiology. The dentist must therefore consider additional systemic possibilities when evaluating any patient whose history or physical evaluation suggests chronic liver involvement.

Foremost in the consideration of multisystem liver disease is the symptom of xerostomia associated with Sjögren's syndrome and the "sicca complex." Sjögren described the triad of keratoconjunctivitis sicca, xerostomia, and rheumatoid arthritis. Bloch later divided the syndrome into five groups, the fifth of which comprised those cases without arthritis having the sicca complex alone. Reports of concurrence of Sjögren's syndrome and autoimmune liver disease strongly suggest that the two disorders may be associated, and frequently patients with liver disease complain of dryness of the mouth and eyes. The literature confirms that nearly 40% of patients with chronic active hepatitis, primary biliary cirrhosis, or cryptogenic cirrhosis exhibit Sjögren's syndrome or the sicca complex. Xerostomia is obviously a result of salivary gland involvement, and a minor salivary gland biopsy is an invaluable diagnostic aid. Biopsy is easily achieved by local anesthetic infiltration in the mucosa of the lower lip to determine involvement of those minor salivary glands that would confirm the presence of Sjögren's syndrome. Histologically, glands show lymphoid infiltration, glandular atrophy, stromal fibrosis, and ductal changes. Involvement of the ductular epithelium is mainly hyperplastic.

Spontaneous or postsurgical bleeding

The dental literature is replete in discussion of various hereditary disorders of blood coagulation. These problems are well known and well documented, and detailed guidelines have been formulated for the prevention, diagnosis, and treatment of bleeding complications. There is less specific information, however, regarding acquired disorders of hemostasis, among which liver disease is probably the most frequent cause. Most experts agree that the prevention of postsurgical bleeding is directly related to a comprehensive bleeding history and preoperative screening tests of coagulation. If a patient has a history of significant liver disease as suggested by jaundice, alcoholism, and cirrhosis, a serious hemorrhagic disorder may be present, since most coagulation factors are produced in the liver. The prothrombin time (PT) will be prolonged, specifically in cases of factor VII deficiency and deficiencies of vitamin K. This is the most reliable test in assessing the coagulation phase in patients with possible liver disease. Since a large percentage of these patients also have a defect in platelet aggregation as a result of platelet destruction by the spleen, a partial thromboplastin time (PTT) is also indicated. A PTT measures the intrinsic clotting mechanism. This reflects the ability of blood within the intravascular compartment to coagulate in an area of trauma or injury. In addition to the PT and PTT, an assessment of platelet function through a platelet count and bleeding time is essential in the complete preliminary evaluation of a patient for coagulopathy. Also, since accelerated fibrinolysis may develop in patients with preexisting liver disease, it is important to be aware of this possible complication in any planned dental surgical intervention. This awareness is the only way to minimize postoperative bleeding in patients whose hemostatic abnormality arises during or after surgery.

The increased risk of bleeding in patients with depressed synthesis and plasma concentrations of clotting proteins can usually be corrected by prophylactic infusion of fresh frozen plasma. Patients with liver disease who are bleeding spontaneously will require appropriate replacement of clotting proteins with either fresh whole blood or fresh frozen plasma. All elective procedures should be performed in consultation with a hematologist. Patients with PTs less than 30% of control will usually bleed continuously postoperatively despite the use of local hemostatic agents, such as epinephrine, topical thrombin, suturing, or packing of surgical sites.

Viral hepatitis

Acute viral hepatitis is caused by at least three distinct viruses, types A, B, and non-A, non-B (NANB). These viruses each have distinct antigenic properties, but the clinical appearance of the disease is often indistinguishable. Type A hepatitis was formerly called infectious hepatitis, and type B was formerly termed serum hepatitis. NANB (type C) is a recently identified form that is essentially a diagnosis of exclusion when neither types A nor B can be serologically identified. Much confusion existed in the past because the mode of transmission of the various viral types was poorly understood. The classic idea that hepatitis B (long incubation) was transmitted parenterally and that hepatitis A was acquired by the fecal/oral route is no longer true. Hepatitis B has been shown to be transmitted parenterally, orally, and by sexual intercourse, and the hepatitis B surface antigen has been isolated in blood, as well as other body fluids, such as urine, sweat, saliva, nasopharyngeal secretions, semen, and breast milk. Hepatitis A is now known to be transmitted parenterally, as well as by the fecal/oral route; thus even though hepatitis A and B can be transmitted by either route, the fecal/oral route remains more common in type A and the parenteral route more common in type B.

Differentiating between the two forms of hepatitis is most important in order for the dentist to determine high-risk patients, that is, those who are carriers of hepatitis B. In an epidemiologic study of 1245 dentists, evidence of hepatitis B infection was reported to be 13.6%. However, among oral surgeons, the prevalence of hepatitis B is even greater. In a survey among 650 oral surgeons, the prevalence of hepatitis, as determined by serologic markers, was reported to be 29.3%. Current information dictates that a patient who has a history of hepatitis A may indeed be a carrier of hepatitis B. A patient who has fully recovered from hepatitis A is not infective. Therefore the positive identification of hepatitis A or B becomes extremely important to the dentist in determining which patients represent a danger to dental personnel and the other patients. The discovery of hepatitis B surface antigen (HB_sAg) made testing possible so that patients could be identified who are classified as chronic carriers. HB_sAg may be detected approximately 1 month before and 1 to 2 months after the development of the icteric or jaundiced phase of the disease.

The estimated lifetime risk of type B infection in the United States varies from almost 100% for the highest risk groups to approximately 5% for the population as a whole. An estimated 200,000 persons are infected each year. One fourth of them become ill with jaundice. More than 10,000 patients are hospitalized with hepatitis B each year, and an average of 250 die of fulminant disease. Between 6% and 10% of patients with type B infection become carriers. A carrier is defined as a person who is HB_sAg positive on at least two occasions, at least 6 months apart. The United States currently contains an estimated pool of 400,000 to 800,000 infectious carriers. A particularly high carrier rate is found in male homosexuals, patients with a history of lymphoma, persons with Down's syndrome, or patients receiving renal dialysis or immunosuppressive drugs. Also, patients should be considered as carriers of hepatitis B when, in addition to having a history of hepatitis, they abuse drugs or are in a generally debilitated state of health. Chronic active hepatitis develops in over 25% of carriers (100,000 to 200,000) and often progresses to cirrhosis. Furthermore, recent studies have demonstrated an association between the type B carrier state and the occurrence of liver cancer. It is estimated that 4000 persons die of hepatitis B–related liver cancer.

Saliva. HB_sAg has been detected in 76% of salivary samples from carriers and can be transmitted by kissing or in children by sharing food and toys.

Nasopharyngeal secretions. Nasopharyngeal secretions have been shown to be 40% antigen positive and may represent a source of potential transmission. Transmission by droplet spray, however, has not been adequately documented.

Semen. Semen was found to be positive in approximately 50% of carriers. Studies have shown increased evidence of hepatitis B among male homosexuals, prostitutes, and promiscuous individuals, suggesting a sexual mode of transmission.

Urine. The antigen has been detected in a small percentage of serum-positive patients, and this may be a source of infection, especially in incontinent individuals.

Feces. The presence of antigen in feces has not been adequately documented. Fecal transmission seldom occurs.

DENTAL MANAGEMENT. In dealing with the patient who has a history of hepatitis several categories need to be considered. The first category includes those patients with active hepatitis. Dental treatment of patients with active hepatitis is as follows:

1. Consultation
2. Emergency care only
3. Obtain preoperative PT and PTT
4. Hepatitis dental precautions
   a. Aseptic technique (using gloves, mask and gown).
   b. Minimize aerosol
   c. Sterilize and disinfect all instruments and equipment
   d. Minimize drugs metabolized in liver, such as local anesthetics, analgesics, sedatives (except phenobarbital), and antibiotics (especially ampicillin and tetracycline)

These patients should be treated on an emergency basis only, and if active hepatitis is suspected, medical consultation should be immediately obtained. If a patient has a past history of hepatitis, then it is important to categorize the type based on the medical history and consultation. If the patient has had type A and is recovered, then the patient may be treated as if he were normal and no precautions need be taken. If it has been determined that the patient has had type B and is recovered, then it must be determined if the patient is a chronic carrier (i.e., surface antigen positive). A radioimmunoassay test for HB_sAg must be performed. If the test is negative, then the patient can be treated as a normal patient. If the test is positive or the dentist is unable to determine or cannot obtain the test, then strict aseptic technique must be employed with active hepatitis precautions as above, involving the use of rubber gloves and a mask, the minimization of aerosol spray, and the scrubbing and sterilizing of all equipment after use. In addition, drugs that are metabolized by the liver should be minimized.

An equally glaring problem to the dental practitioner is the possible transmission of the disease from the dentist who is a chronic carrier to his or her patients. Rimland and others traced 55 cases of hepatitis B to an oral surgeon who was found to be an asymptomatic carrier. Although it is absolutely essential that a dentist with acute disease not see patients, a dentist who has been determined to be a carrier does not necessarily have to discontinue practice, unless it has been demonstrated that he or she is actively transmitting the disease. The risk of a carrier dentist infecting patients is greatly minimized if guidelines are followed that include sterilization, frequent hand washing, and the wearing of masks and gloves during patient treatment. Recently, another antigen, the e antigen, has been found in association with hepatitis B. This antigen is immunologically distinct from HB_sAg and core antigens and is a part of the B virus particle. The presence of e antigen and anti-e have been linked to the degree of infectivity of hepatitis. Approximately 50% of asymptomatic HB_sAg carriers have anti-e in their serum, whereas e antigen is found in the serum of 50% to 75% of patients with evidence of chronic hepatitis. It is likely that the presence of e antigen will prove helpful in identifying those individuals who are more likely to spread hepatitis B. Patients with anti-e–positive sera are not likely to develop or transmit hepatitis, whereas those e antigen–positive patients are.

IMMUNIZATION. It is generally accepted that if immune serum globulin (gamma globulin) is given soon after exposure to hepatitis A (within 1 to 2 weeks), illness is prevented or the symptoms are ameliorated in approximately 80% of cases. Prophylaxis against hepatitis B is somewhat less effective with hepatitis immunoglobulin (HBIG). Studies have shown that either immune serum globulin or hepatitis B immunoglobulin has an effectiveness in the range of 40% to 70% in preventing hepatitis B by postexposure injection. Current recommendations suggest the administration of hepatitis B immunoglobulin within 7 days of exposure followed by a second dose 25 to 30 days after the first.

It is obvious that the ultimate goal of hepatitis research has been achieved with the development of a vaccine to prevent the disease.

Hepatitis B vaccine. Hepatitis B virus vaccine is a suspension of inactivated, alum-absorbed, 22-nm surface antigen particles that have purified from human plasma by a combination of biophysical (ultracentrifugation) and biochemical procedures. Inactivation processes have been shown to inactivate type B virus and representative viruses from all known groups and thus should destroy any viruses potentially contaminating the vaccine. Hepatitis B virus vaccine contains 20 μ/ml of HB_sAg protein.

Field trials of the United States–manufactured vaccine have shown 80% to 95% efficacy in preventing infection or hepatitis among susceptible persons. Protection against illness was complete for persons who developed antibodies after vaccination but before exposure. Although the duration of protective effect of hepatitis B vaccine is unknown at present, available data suggest that immunity will last for about 5 years in patients who have received all three doses, after which time a single booster dose of vaccine might be necessary to maintain immunity.

Adverse reactions. Approximately half of all reported reactions were injection site soreness, which occurred somewhat more frequently among vaccine recipients. Other less common local reactions have included erythema, swelling, warmth, or induration. These signs and symptoms of local inflammation are generally well tolerated and usually subside within 2 days of vaccination.

Low-grade fever (less than 101° F) occurs occasionally and is usually confined to the 48-hour period following vaccination. Although uncommon, fever over 102° F has been reported.

Systemic complaints, including malaise, fatigue, headach, nausea, dizziness, myalgia, and arthralgia, are infrequent and have been limited to the first few days following vaccination. Rash has been reported rarely.

Indications. Hepatitis B vaccine is indicated for immunization against infection caused by all known subtypes of hepatitis B virus but will not prevent hepatitis caused by other agents, such as hepatitis A virus, NANB hepatitis viruses, or other viruses known to infect the liver.

Vaccination is recommended in persons 3 months of age or older, especially those who are at increased risk of infection with hepatitis B virus. Following are individuals at increased risk:

1. Health care personnel
    a. Dentists, all dental auxiliary personnel, and oral and maxillofacial surgeons
    b. Physicians and surgeons
    c. Nurses
    d. Paramedical personnel and custodial staff who may be exposed to the virus
    e. Laboratory personnel handling blood, blood products, and other patient specimens
    f. Dental, medical, and nursing students.
    g. Blood bank and plasma fractionation workers
2. Selected patients and patient contacts
    a. Patients and staff in hemodialysis units and hematology/oncology units
    b. Patients requiring frequent or large volume blood transfusions or clotting factor concentrates (such as persons with hemophilia or thalassemia)
    c. Clients (residents) and staff of institutions for the mentally handicapped
    d. Classroom contacts of deinstitutional mentally handicapped persons with persistent hepatitis B antigenemia
    e. Household and other intimate contacts of persons with persistent hepatitis B antigenemia
3. Populations with high incidence of the disease
4. Certain military and personnel
5. Morticians and embalmers
6. Persons at increased risk of the disease because of their sexual practices: persons who repeatedly contract sexually transmitted diseases, homosexually active males, and female prostitutes
7. Prisoners
8. Users of illicit injectable drugs

Table 1. Vaccine dosages for hepatitis B

Group	Initial dose	Dose at 1 month	Dose at 6 months
Younger children (3 months to 10 years of age)	0.5 ml	0.5 ml	0.5 ml
Adults and older children	1 ml	1 ml	1 ml
Dialysis and immunocompromised patients	2 ml*	2 ml*	2 ml*

*Two 1-ml doses given at different sites.

Vaccine dosage. Primary adult vaccination consists of three intramuscular doses of 1 ml of vaccine (20 µg) each. The second and third doses should be given 1 and 6 months, respectively, after the first. For patients undergoing hemodialysis or immunosuppressant therapy, three 2-ml doses should be used. For children under 10 years of age, three similarly spaced doses of 0.5 ml are sufficient. Vaccine doses administered at longer intervals than those stipulated provide equally satisfactory protection, but optimal protection is not conferred until after the third dose. Since hepatitis B virus vaccine is an inactivated (noninfective) product, it is presumed that there will be no interference with other simultaneously administered vaccines (Table 1).

DISEASES OF THE PANCREAS

Extensive investigation of the dental manifestations of patients with diseases of the pancreas has been limited. Nevertheless, two primary areas in which a basic understanding of pancreatic disease and its oral manifestations will be of invaluable benefit to both dentists and physicians. The first involves dental correlations of patients with cystic fibrosis, and the second focuses on the testing of parotid saliva in the diagnosis of pancreatic disorders.

Cystic fibrosis

Cystic fibrosis, fibrocystic disease of the pancreas, was first recognized in 1938 and is a genetically carried mendelian disease that occurs in approximately one out of every 2000 live births in whites. Pancreatic function may become severely impaired, thereby producing a malabsorption syndrome. The exocrine glands throughout the body are affected, leading to changes in secretions, which become viscid. Thickened mucus brings about obstructions of glands with consequent dilation, and manifestations are particularly evident in the pulmonary and digestive tracts. In children, mucous plugs occur in small airways and cause obstruction, with recurrent infection and eventually chronic bronchitis and bronchiectasis. The throat is often secondarily infected with streptococci, coagulase-positive staphylococci, pneumococci, and *Pseudomonas* organisms. Digestion is impaired, and therefore growth may be severely retarded. In the digestive tract, pancreatic secretions are insufficient, and newborns may develop intestinal obstructions because of luminal impaction of inspissated bile. Sweat glands, too, are often affected and the high sodium content of the secretions provides an important diagnostic tool.

ORAL MANIFESTATIONS. Patients with cystic fibrosis may show occlusion of the nasal cavity and maxillary sinus after recurrent infections. This results in chronic mouth breathing and a higher incidence of open bite malocclusions and a high palatal vault.

The submaxillary gland is usually enlarged and has been found to have highly turbid secretions. In the submaxillary saliva the values of total protein and many of the enzymes, as well as calcium and phosphorus, are elevated, whereas sodium chloride and potassium concentrations are within normal limits. With regard to minor salivary glands, eosinophilic plugs are frequently found in the ducts of the labial salivary glands. Weisman and others suggest that in reality, it is the secretion of the minor salivary glands scattered throughout the oral cavity in the buccal and labial mucosae, and hard and soft palates that have higher sodium values in patients with cystic fibrosis; these values, in fact, are considerably higher than those for parotid or submaxillary secretions.

Most salivary studies have involved the parotid gland and its relation to patients with cystic fibrosis. Several investigators have reported that patients with cystic fibrosis exhibited increased rates of flow of parotid saliva when the secretion was collected without stimulation. When the parotid secretion was reflexly stimulated, a higher flow rate was noted in one investigation. The results of two concurrent studies show that in a control group there was no significant difference in the resting state with a graded reflex stimulus of increasing intensity. There was a tendency for electrolyte levels of parotid saliva to be higher in a group of patients with cystic fibrosis than in a control group of comparable age and sex. Only in the case of inorganic phosphorus, however, was this elevation statistically significant. Also, the glycoproteins of parotid saliva were not found to be significantly altered either in amount or proportion in those patients.

The teeth of patients with cystic fibrosis are often discolored. The discoloration is more pronounced at the cervical and middle third of the clinical crown and is first seen at the cementoenamel junction where the enamel layer is thinnest. Tetracycline administration has often been implicated in this staining, since the drug has often been used to combat recurrent pulmonary infections. In addition to a relatively high prevalence of tetracycline discolorations, enamel defects have also been found in approximately 10% of these patients; however, the amount of dental caries has not been significantly elevated.

The possibility for delayed formation and consequent eruption of the teeth in patients with cystic fibrosis was suggested in light of the reported delay in other maturational processes. However, only an insignificant trend in dental age retardation was found in a study by Primosch when compared to chronologic age. A significant skeletal age retardation was noted but its deviation was not as severe as previously indicated. The magnitude of the skeletal age retardation over dental age supports the concept that skeletal development is more vulnerable than tooth formation. It is therefore doubtful, based on the findings of this study, that any evaluation of dental age in patients with cystic fibrosis will be of diagnostic value to the clinician.

DIAGNOSTIC TESTING FOR PANCREATIC DISORDERS BY EXAMINATION OF PAROTID SALIVA. Several results have been obtained from studies of parotid saliva in patients with pancreatic disorders, specifically chronic pancreatitis. First, the salivary output and the maximum bicarbonate concentration and amylase content in parotid saliva of patients with pancreatic disorders were significantly less than those of patients with nonpancreatic disorders. Second, an abnormal saliva test was found in 83% of patients with pancreatic disorders. Third, a comparison was made of the parotid saliva with the pancreozymin secretion test in regard to diagnostic reliability in both pancreatic and nonpancreatic disorders. These data indicated that an abnormal parotid saliva test was 88.6% accurate in diagnosing pancreatic disorders, whereas the positive pancreozymin secretion test was only 65.9% positive.

NUTRITIONAL DISORDERS
Julian Katz

Earlier in this century, certain significant diseases were shown to be states of nutritional deficiency. These readily recognized entities, such as scurvy, beriberi, and pernicious anemia, were cured by the administration of specific chemical substances that could be isolated and identified. This was an exciting time for nutritional research because curable diseases were being increasingly uncovered. For example, just 50 years ago many patients in psychiatric institutions in the United States had the curable and preventable illness pellagra. The availability and distribution of foods, education, and dietary fortification and enrichment eradicated this cause of mental disease. The physician or dentist today rarely sees the classic vitamin-deficiency diseases and considers nutritional problems concerns of those involved with public health and food technology. Educational, social, and economic failures are the major causes of clear-cut nutritional deficiencies. Yet obesity is a form of malnutrition, and certain diseases may be related to a chronic unsatisfactory diet. Diseases resulting from multifactorial causes, such as cardiovascular disease and bowel cancer, may also be related to an individual's susceptibility to certain foods and nutrients.

Nutritional disorders affect the entire body, although they may manifest initially in a limited area. The most common of these areas is the oral cavity, one of the most sensitive indicators of the body's nutritional status. The dentist is in a unique position to encounter early signs of nutritional deficiency among dental patients, since oral soft tissue changes are frequently significant in these metabolic derangements.

The components of good nutrition include carbohydrates, fats, proteins, amino acids, vitamins, water, and many elements that are required in small amounts. Carbohydrates are most quickly and easily digested by the body to meet its energy needs. Fats have twice the energy value of most other foods and are used in the transport and absorption of fat-soluble vitamins. Proteins provide the body with energy and are important constituents, through their component amino acids, of additional body proteins and an array of nitrogen-containing compounds needed by the body. Minerals form a part of many important compounds active in metabolism, and deficiencies in some of these essential minerals may have profound systemic effects. Vitamins are essential for the body to carry out many metabolic processes needed for growth and the maintenance of life. Water, which accounts for more than 60% of total body weight, is needed for the absorption and elimination of materials, for maintenance of body temperature, and as a medium in which many important chemical and physical reactions take place.

A state of chemical and physical equilibrium is maintained only when the necessary nutrients are supplied in suitable amounts. The specific requirement for any one substance is related to the overall composition of the diet and compensatory metabolic changes that can accommodate for quantitative fluctuation of each nutrient in the diet. When the limits of any nutritional requirement are violated because of either an inadequate or excessive supply, then the body's equilibrium can no longer be adequately maintained and clinical problems may occur.

Individuals may develop a nutritional deficiency when consuming an inadequate diet or when the absorption and utilization of ingested foods are satisfactory but other physical conditions increase the nutritional requirements.

General malnutrition

Primary malnutrition can be defined as undernutrition because of environmental lack of essential foodstuffs. It is especially prevalent in underdeveloped countries where the food supply is uncertain because of famine, drought, or other disasters or where nutritional education is limited and farming techniques are inadequate.

In secondary malnutrition, adequate food is available, but the individual is unable to make full use of it for other reasons.

Altered eating behaviors. Altered eating behaviors include the anorexia from chronic disorders such as advanced malignant disease, infection, renal failure, depression, and anorexia nervosa. Chronic anorexia with nutritional deficiency also is particularly common in alcoholics and can be induced by some drugs as an unwanted side effect. Food fads are common in adolescents and some dietary constituents may be proscribed by certain ethnic or religious practices. These can cause general malnutrition as well.

Obesity. Obesity is the most common form of malnutrition in the developed nations. The incidence of obesity in adults in North America may be 15% to 20%. Obesity is an excess of adipose tissue and is not the same as overweight, which is defined in terms of age, height, sex, and body frame tables. Adipose tissue can be evaluated practically with a caliper measurement of the skin fold thickness, but an individual who is 15% to 20% overweight can be considered obese.

Although an obese person ingests more calories than are required by the body for energy, the cause of obesity is not that obvious. Many obese people ingest no more or fewer calories than lean people. In few patients can well-defined causes of obesity be found, such as hypothalamic tumors, rare genetic disorders, and endocrine diseases. Most obesity, however, is related to psychologic, genetic, behavioral, and social factors. The fat cells of obese people contain more fat than those of lean subjects, and in cases of greater obesity there are more adipocytes in the body. The number of fat cells does not remain stable from childhood but actually may increase in adulthood.

Metabolic abnormalities are associated with obesity, apparently as the consequence of becoming obese. A relative resistance to the metabolic effects of insulin occurs, and the growth hormone response to various stimuli is blunted. The production of cortisol and the excretion of 17-hydroxysteroids are altered, and some studies have shown differences in the metabolism of thyroid hormones.

Epidemiologic studies show an association of certain diseases with obesity and an increased mortality in obese individuals. There are difficulties in interpreting these data, especially when several factors coexist. For example, although the incidence of arteriosclerotic coronary artery disease increases as weight increases, obesity alone does not seem to be associated with an increased risk of myocardial infarction. However, obesity does increase the incidence of angina and sudden death. When obese people achieve and maintain a desirable weight, the mortality falls.

The treatment of obesity is difficult. Over 90% of fat patients who successfully lose weight return to or surpass their initial weight within 5 years. Behavior modification is required. A diet reduced by 3500 to 7000 calories a week will provide a weekly loss of 1 to 2 pounds of adipose tissue. More drastic programs, such as fasting with protein supplements, result in a more rapid weight loss that may initially be due to loss of muscle mass with accompanying water, but these drastic diets rarely provide long-lasting weight loss. Physical activity is not very effective in losing weight, but moderate activity is usually accompanied by a decrease in caloric intake. The calories lost in 1 hour of vigorous tennis are about equal to those in a slice of cherry pie. Frequency of meals may be as important as diet composition; regular balanced meals are associated with weight control despite alterations in caloric intake. Most obese people eat little or no breakfast. Intestinal bypass surgery has been used for the treatment of morbid obesity, but there are considerable hazards associated with these procedures, such as electrolyte, vitamin, and mineral deficiencies and severe liver disease.

Disorders interfering with ingestion. Oropharyngeal disease is the cause of most ingestion disorders. Painful lesions, such as oral ulceration and glossopharyngeal neuralgia, neurologic syndromes interfering with the act of swallowing, such as bulbar palsy and myasthenia gravis, and mechanical obstruction from a neoplasm or esophageal stricture may all cause dysphagia, with reduced food intake leading to general malnutrition.

Problems of dental origin can certainly interfere with ingestion. These include poorly functioning partial or complete dentures, pain associated with periodontal disease, and decayed or poorly restored teeth. Masticatory insufficiency can also result from temporomandibular joint disease and occlusal abnormalities associated with maxillary and mandibular growth abnormalities, particularly those which cause severe prognathism, micrognathism, and apertognathia.

Defective absorption. A wide range of gastrointestinal disorders have been related to malabsorption of single or multiple dietary constituents. The most common of these are as follows:

1. Pancreatic failure and steatorrhea because of hepatobiliary disease. These are frequently associated with malabsorption of fat and fat-soluble vitamins such as retinol and calciferol.
2. Intestinal mucosal disorders, especially gluten-induced enteropathy and sprue. On occasion, these disorders present evidence of nutritional deficiency only, without symptoms of gastrointestinal disease.
3. Failure of special adaptive mechanisms for the absorption of individual dietary constituents, such as lack of intrinsic factor in vitamin B_{12} deficiency.
4. Rapid intestinal transmission of food after gastrectomy or vagotomy.
5. Bacterial colonization and overgrowth in various areas of the gut, resulting in steatorrhea.

Certain disorders may cause malabsorption through several different mechanisms. For example, regional ileitis or enteritis (Crohn's disease) leads to fat malabsorption by interfering with the recycling of bile salts, vitamin B_{12} deficiency by preventing specific ileal absorpiton of the vitamin B_{12} intrinsic factor complex, and general malabsorption of all nutrients if involvement of the gut is widespread.

Excessive loss of nutrients. Losses from the body for which intestinal absorption cannot compensate may lead to a deficiency in individual nutrients. Chronic blood loss, for example, is a major cause of iron deficiency, and protein-deficient states may result from severe proteinuria or from various enteropathies.

Increased requirements. During certain periods of life a more "normal" dietary intake may become inadequate in the face of increased requirements. Such relative malnutrition may arise in pregnancy and during periods of rapid growth in infancy and adolescence. Two mechanisms exist to offset the effects of some nutritional deficiencies, such as negative nitrogen balance. First, many nutrients exist in storage forms in the body, and these can be mobilized for a limited time to compensate for deficiencies in intake. Second, for certain deficiencies larger proportions of the individual nutrient can be absorbed from the diet.

Specific nutritional deficiencies

Energy is provided by dietary carbohydrates, fats, and proteins. One gram of carbohydrate yields 4 calories; 1 g of fat, 9 calories; and 1 g of protein, 4 calories. Ethanol has significant caloric value, providing 7 calories in 1 g. Energy requirements decline as adults grow older, but pregnancy and lactation require additional calories and protein. Carbohydrates, particularly plant foods, provide most of the calories in the diet, and fat provides highly concentrated energy. The body is not totally efficient in deriving energy from the three major nutrients, however, and there are individual differences in metabolic activity and physical activity. The following section is a discussion of essential nutrients and the effects of deficiency in each case, particularly as manifested in the oral cavity.

Proteins. Protein is a vital constituent of the diet, since it is the only source of essential amino acids, that is, those not produced by the body. Ingested protein is hydrolyzed in the intestine to the various component amino acids, which are subsequently absorbed by the bloodstream. Of the 20 amino acids found in food protein, only 8 (isoleucine, lysine, methionine, phenylalanine, tyrosine, threonine, tryptophan, and valine) are essential for adults, since they cannot be synthesized by the human body. During active growth in infancy histidine and arginine are also necessary in larger amounts and hence are considered by some to be semiessential amino acids. Since humans have no pool for storage of essential amino acids other than their own body protein, removal of just one of these essential amino acids can rapidly lower the level of protein synthesis. This is critical if it occurs during growth periods when metabolic demands require protein synthesis.

The effects of protein calorie deficiency in children may vary from mild growth retardation to general starvation or protein malnutrition (kwashiorkor). Infants in starvation characteristically remain alert, and reutilization of amino acids liberated from the child's own tissues allows synthesis of serum albumin to continue. In cases of protein malnutrition, generalized edema usually occurs because of a decrease in serum albumin. These individuals are characteristically lethargic and apathetic. Flaky dermatosis and pigmentary changes are also common.

Oral evidence of protein malnutrition includes edema of the tongue, with scalloping of the lateral margins from pressing against the teeth. The dorsum of the tongue may also appear smooth and erythematous, because of papillary atrophy. Angular cheilitis and fissuring around the lips may appear, in addition to changes in lip pigmentation that are particularly noticeable in dark-skinned individuals. Sialosis and xerostomia are other features of kwashiorkor and the resulting dry oral mucosa is particularly vulnerable to trauma and infection.

Fats. Two fatty acids, linoleic acid and linolenic acid, are essential dietary constituents that are necessary for the biosynthesis of prostaglandins. Although all other lipids can be manufactured in the body and thus are nonessential ingredients of the diet, their consumption does assist in the absorption of fat-soluble vitamins, such as retinol, calciferol, tocopherol, and vitamin K.

Prostaglandins are widely distributed in the tissues and are apparently synthesized from fatty acids stored within cellular membranes. Their mode of action is complex and includes a role in mediating the inflammatory response and in regulating a number of metabolic reactions. It is possible that prostaglandins act directly at several sites in the cell or indirectly by regulating the rate of cyclic AMP production. Deficiency of essential fatty acids is uncommon, virtually confined to infants being fed parenterally or on restricted diets. A dry, flaky dermatosis often develops. No oral manifestations of essential fatty acid deficiency have been documented in humans, although dentinogenesis has been altered in experimental animals.

Carbohydrates. Carbohydrates satisfy the major energy needs of the human body. The dietary switch from natural to refined carbohydrates in the United States has been widespread and may have significant effects on overall health status. High intake of sticky carbohydrate foods can increase caries incidence in the susceptible person.

Minerals. The essential need for any mineral can be determined by observing altered functions when the diet is deficient only in that element, demonstrating a response with the administration of the supplementary mineral, and then correlating the deficiency state with a low level of the mineral in blood or tissue. Minerals function as structural components of the skeleton and soft tissue and as solutes in body fluids.

Iron. Iron plays a vital role in cellular respiration. There are only 3 to 4 g of iron in the body. About 70% is in hemoglobin, both in circulating erythrocytes and in the normoblasts of the bone marrow. Twenty percent of the iron is in storage form (ferritin or hemosiderin) in the macrophages of the liver, spleen, and other organs. Another 5% of body iron is in the myoglobin of skeletal muscle, and a small, but functionally important, quantity is in iron-containing enzymes such as cytochromes A, B, and C; cytochrome oxidase catalase; peroxidase; and iron flavoproteins.

There are no excretory mechanisms for iron, although about 1 mg/day is lost passively through cell desquamation from the skin and intestines and through growth of nails and hair. In menstruating women fluid loss of around 30 ml further depletes iron by 0.5 mg daily, and additional deficits result from pregnancy and lactation. Children also have a high need for iron because of rapid growth and expansion of the blood volume.

The body iron content is thus determined almost entirely by absorption, the physiologic control of which is complex and mediated through events in the mucosal cells of the gastrointestinal tract. The average American diet contains 15 to 20 mg of iron per day of which the body requires around 10%. Since only about 5% to 10% of dietary iron is actually absorbed, this may be a marginal amount for individuals with a greater need for the substance. Although normal men and postmenopausal women need about 10 mg of iron in the diet daily, women with menstrual loss need about 18 mg/day, and an additional 1.5 mg/day of iron is needed during pregnancy for the tissues of the fetus and expansion of the maternal blood volume.

If iron is depleted through the chronic blood loss of certain diseases or if dietary iron absorption is impaired, a negative iron balance will result, and the pathologic tissue changes of iron deficiency will occur. Iron deficiency can cause changes in the tissues that are not related to the hematologic effects. In a large sample of patients with iron deficiency anemia, atrophic glossitis was found in 39% and angular cheilitis in 14%. These changes are due to tissue depletion of iron and may appear before the development of anemia. The severity of glossitis does not approach that seen in vitamin B_{12} or folic acid deficiency. In mild cases there is some discomfort and redness associated with flattening of the papillae around the margin of the tongue. In more severe cases there is redness and atrophy of the filiform and fungiform papillae. Angular cheilitis is a less specific abnormality and the absence of teeth and wearing ill-fitting dentures may favor its development.

Another result of iron deficiency is dysphagia due to postcricoid esophageal stricture, originally described by Kelly and Patterson in 1919. Plummer-Vinson syndrome occurs in about 7% of iron-deficient subjects and an esophageal web can be found in a number of such cases. The web consists of a fold of normal mucosa or a stricture with chronic inflammation of the muscle layers of the esophagus. The syndrome occurs most frequently in middle-aged women and is commonly accompanied by glossitis and angular cheilitis. In most cases glossitis improves quite rapidly after the commencement of iron replacement, with regeneration of the filiform papillae within 3 weeks. Angular cheilitis responds more slowly, probably because of concurrent infection.

Iodine. Iodine is needed for the production of thyroid hormones, thyroxine (T_4) and triiodothyronine (T_3). The adult human body contains about 40 mg of iodine, about half of which is located in the thyroid gland. Dietary sources include iodized salt, seafood, and foods grown in soil with adequate iodine content. Iodine deficiency may lead to goiter, a swelling of the thyroid gland due usually to iodine deficiency, which is endemic in regions away from the sea and where soil content of iodine is low. The decreased level of iodine causes the pituitary to release thyroid-stimulating hormone (TSH), which induces the thyroid to produce additional thyroid hormones. When this occurs over a significant length of time the gland gradually enlarges. The patient with a thyroid goiter may be hyperthyroid, hypothyroid, or euthyroid (normal functioning gland). Local pressure from thyroid swelling may lead to coughing, voice changes, and breathing difficulty.

The levels of circulating thyroid hormone, particularly T_3 and T_4, can be measured easily to determine the thyroid status of the patient. Children of parents with iodine deficiency may be born with cretinism (congenital hypothyroidism). The child may look normal at birth but eventually develops slowly and is small for his age, with a large tongue, late eruption of teeth, saddle depression of the nose, and possible mental retardation. Early administration of thyroid hormone can prevent these complications.

Since the metabolic rate is generally elevated in hyperthyroidism, administration of epinephrine to these individuals, such as in local anesthetics, should be avoided.

Calcium and phosphorus. Calcium and phosphorus are the most abundant minerals in the body. The bones and teeth can store about 99% of the body's calcium and 75% of the body's phosphorus, with the rest found in blood, soft tissue, and extracellular fluid. The main function of calcium is to provide rigidity and strength to bones and teeth. Since it is also necessary for proper muscle contraction, blood clotting, and nerve irritability, a low serum calcium level can lead to muscle cramps and tetany. Serum calcium is particularly important in maintaining viable cardiac muscle contractility. Phosphorus contributes to bone and teeth rigidity and plays a major role in the quick release of energy from adenosine triphosphate (ATP) and adenosine diphosphate (ADP) molecules. It is also an essential constituent of nucleic acids and nucleoproteins that are involved in DNA and RNA synthesis. Phosphorus aids in the absorption and metabolism of carbohydrates, such as glucose and glycogen, and, as a constituent of phospholipid, promotes emulsification and transportation of fats and fatty acids. Finally, phosphates have an important buffering function in blood and saliva.

Diseases associated with calcium and phosphorus deficiencies include osteoporosis, rickets, and osteomalacia. Osteoporosis is an abnormal rarefaction of bone resulting from failure of the osteoblasts to lay down bone matrix. The generalized form is associated with calcium and hormonal deficiencies, whereas the localized form is caused by disuse or immobilization. Rickets is a disturbance in normal mineralization of the osteoid matrix characterized by bending or distortion in bones. This is caused by a decreased absorption of calcium or phosphorus or both in calciferol-deficient children. Osteomalacia is an adult condition characterized by softening of the bone with pain and tenderness, which is caused by deficiency of calcium and phosphorus or of calciferol. Osteoporosis is treated with high-calcium diets, sex hormones, and fluorides. Rickets and osteomalacia are treated with calciferol and high-calcium diets.

Sodium and potassium. The greatest concentration of sodium in the body is in extracellular fluid. It is necessary for muscle contractility, nerve impulse conduction, maintaining equilibrium between the extracellular and intracellular fluid compartments, and maintaining the pH level of blood. The average daily intake of sodium in the United States is about 5 g, about five times the daily physiologic requirement. Excessive sweating can lead to salt depletion and result in symptoms of nausea, vomiting, cramps, exhaustion, or respiratory failure. Patients with severe vomiting and diarrhea can also develop rapid salt depletion.

Potassium is the main cation of the cell. Since it is present in many foods, a varied diet supplies an adequate amount of this mineral. Potassium deficiency results in muscle weakness and excess potassium can lead to cardiac irritability and arrhythmias. The most common causes of potassium deficiency are infectious or nutritional diarrhea and excess water loss from diuretic agents without potassium supplementation.

Magnesium. Magnesium is required for the proper action of enzymes responsible for energy transformation of phosphate bonds. The bones provide the body with magnesium stores; they contain around 70% of the magnesium in the average adult. Most vegetables contain useful amounts of the mineral, of which the average adult daily requirement is 300 to 350 mg. A greater amount of magnesium is required during pregnancy. Deficiency of this mineral can result in a condition similar to hypocalcemic tetany.

Copper. Copper is utilized in the body for the formation of hemoglobin and production of viable erythrocytes. No evidence of ill health resulting from dietary deficiency of copper has been reported.

Sulfur. Sulfur is present in all protein material but most abundantly in the amino acids methionine and cystine. It is also biologically active in the vitamins thiamine and biotin, in the cell as sulfate ion, such as chondroitin sulfate in bone and cartilage, and in the sulfhydryl (—SH) group of certain enzymes. Little is known regarding the sulfur requirement or deficiency in humans.

Fluoride. Fluoride has a more definite role in the prevention of caries; the safety and efficacy of fluoridated water have been demonstrated. Fluoride replaces some of the hydroxyl ions in hydroxyapatite, lessening the solubility of dental enamel. If excessive fluoride is ingested during tooth formation, mottled enamel occurs. A role for fluoride in preventing osteoporosis has not been established.

Trace elements. Zinc, manganese, molybdenum, cobalt, and selenium are needed by the body in small amounts. The balanced diet usually supplies these trace elements adequately. Little is known about their requirements or deficiency states in humans.

Vitamins. Vitamins may be defined as essential organic dietary factors that are incapable of being synthesized within the body. Although they are required by the body in relatively small amounts, their absence often results in pathologic conditions. The daily dietary allowance of vitamins recommended for adults is given in Table 2. Numerous vitamins exist and are classified as either water- or fat-soluble as follows:

Table 2. Recommended adult daily dietary allowance of vitamins

	Men	Women*
Fat-soluble vitamins		
Retinol (A)	5000 IU	4000 IU
Calciferol (D)	400 IU	400 IU
Tocopherol (E)	15 IU	12 IU
Water-soluble vitamins		
Ascorbic acid (C)	45 mg	45 mg
Niacin†	20 mg	14 mg
Riboflavin†	1.8 mg	1.4 mg
Thiamine†	1.5 mg	1.1 mg
Pyridoxine	2 mg	2 mg
B_{12}	3 μg	3 μg
Folic acid	400 μg	400 μg

*The allowances of all vitamins except calciferol are higher during pregnancy and lactation.
†The allowance decreases after age 22.

Fat-soluble vitamins	Water-soluble vitamins
Retinol (A)	Thiamine (B_1)
Calciferol (D)	Riboflavin (B_2)
Tocopherol (E)	Pyridoxine (B_6)
K	B_{12}
	Folic acid
	Pantothenic acid
	Biotin (H)
	Nicotinic acid (niacin)
	Ascorbic acid (C)

Retinol (vitamin A). Retinol is a long-chain, high molecular weight alcohol that is abundant in leafy green vegetables, animal fats, particularly certain fish liver oils, and milk. Carotenes, which form the yellow pigments of most fruits and vegetables, essentially consist of two molecules of retinol.

The main storage site of retinol is the liver, and sufficient reserves normally exist for as long as 1 year. For this reason there is no justification for including retinol in supplemental vitamin preparations if the individual is consuming a well-balanced diet.

Other than its action on the retina, where it serves as a precursor for rhodopsin (visual purple), the precise role that retinol plays in general metabolism is less clear. Retinol is essential for the maintenance of the structure and function of epithelial glandular tissue. There is a range of metabolic steps that appear to be influenced by retinol, in which epithelial cells are particularly sensitive. The effect of this vitamin on the membrane stability of plasma cells and lysosomes may account for its observed action in regulating keratinization. Endocrine function is also influenced by the availability of retinol, with thyroxine and steroid synthesis being sensitive to deficiencies. There may be some relationship between retinol and the vitamin B complex and ascorbic acid, since typical signs of vitamin B and ascorbic acid deficiency have occurred experimentally in animals under conditions of retinol deprivation.

In retinol deficiency the eyes are among the first sites to be affected; night blindness, xerophthalmia, and conjunctival ulcerations occur, in addition to photophobia and, in some cases, permanent blindness. The skin becomes dry and scaly because of an increase in keratinization. Since the body is unable to excrete large doses of the substance, disease states develop in individuals who have ingested excessive amounts. In hypervitaminosis A, alopecia, peeling of the skin, coarsened hair, and generalized bone pain occur.

Oral signs of retinol deficiency include increased keratinization of the oral mucosa and keratinization of formerly nonkeratinized tissues. The resultant hyperkeratotic areas may appear as white patches. Metaplasia of the salivary ductal epithelium has been reported, sometimes causing xerostomia and altered taste and smell. Although the relationship between retinol and enamel formation has been studied extensively, there is little convincing evidence that retinol causes any significant dental changes in humans.

Oral manifestations of hypervitaminosis A include atrophy of the oral mucosa, gingival inflammation, and scaling of the lips.

The keratin-decreasing property of retinol has been employed successfully in the management of certain hyperkeratotic lesions of the skin and oral mucosae.

Calciferol (vitamin D). Calciferol is the general name for a group of steroids possessing antirachitic activity. Their primary action is to increase the plasma calcium and phosphate concentration by stimulating intestinal absorption of these minerals and resorption of bone. Calciferol is thus utilized primarily in the absorption of calcium and phosphorus from the intestinal tract and in the formation and maintenance of the skeletal system and teeth. Fish liver oils are extremely rich in calciferol, as are all dairy products. Pasteurized milk is enriched to contain 400 IU of calciferol per quart, and many other foodstuffs, such as bread and cereals, are irradiated to increase their calciferol content. There is no evidence to suggest that increased calciferol intake has any beneficial action on the formation or eruption of teeth, nor does it render any caries protection. Calciferol deficiency leads to rickets in children and osteomalacia in adults.

RICKETS. Rickets usually appears during the first 24 months of life. The chief manifestations are seen in the bones, where defects in the mineralization of the organic matrix occur. Soft areas in the skull are frequently the earliest evidence of this disease. The rachitic child may have large prominent frontal bones, which give the head an enlarged appearance. Bowed legs and enlarged wrists and ankles are common signs of the disease, as are spontaneous fractures in severe cases.

In calciferol-sensitive rickets, a form of disease that responds to calciferol administration, there are surprisingly few oral manifestations. Since most of these children show no evidence of dentin or enamel hypoplasia, the level of calciferol does not seem to be critical in either amelogenesis or dentinogenesis. Calciferol-resistant rickets, a form of the disease that is due to renal tubular disorders, is usually more severe. These children reportedly develop dental abnormalities that include changes in the pulp horns and dentin. Eruption of the teeth may be delayed and roentgenographic signs, such as reduced density of the alveolar lamina dura and loss of crestal bone, are common.

OSTEOMALACIA (ADULT RICKETS). Osteomalacia, or adult calciferol deficiency, is almost nonexistent in the United States. The disease is characterized by an irregular increase in the thickness of the cortex and trabeculation of bones. These tissues are poorly calcified and contain fibrous bone marrow and islands of osteoid tissue. The diagnosis of calciferol deficiency may be confirmed by abnormally low serum calcium and phosphate and elevated alkaline phosphatase levels.

Tocopherol (vitamin E). Tocopherol is a fat-soluble vitamin and a component of grains, vegetable oils, and green vegetables. Diets lacking tocopherol have been known to produce thrombocytosis, hemolytic anemias, and dermatologic changes in children, particularly premature infants. Symptoms are far less notable in adults, but there may be alterations in the formation of erythrocytes. Dental or oral changes have not been noted in humans with tocopherol deficiency, although some minor alterations have been recorded in the periodontium and teeth of laboratory animals.

Vitamin K. Vitamin K is a water-soluble, heat-stable substance formed from phylloquinone and farnoquinone vitamin K_1 and K_2) and is required for hepatic synthesis of coagulation factors II (prothrombin), V, VII, IX (Christmas factor), and X (Stuart-Prower factor). Normal hepatic function and adequate dietary supplies of vitamin K are needed for successful production of these proteins. Phylloquinone is derived from leafy green vegetables, whereas farnoquinone is synthesized by intestinal bacteria.

Deficiency of vitamin K leads to inadequate production of the coagulation factors just listed and hence to significant hemorrhagic diathesis. In the adult, the most frequent cause of vitamin K deficiency is malabsorption, usually from steatorrhea or obstructive jaundice.

The oral manifestations of vitamin K deficiency include gingival bleeding and excessive postextraction hemorrhage. Therefore, to evaluate the magnitude of vitamin K deficiency in an individual before commencing a surgical procedure, a PT should be obtained. The surgical procedure should be postponed if the PT is less than 50% of control. Administration of intramuscular doses of vitamin K usually has a therapeutic effect in 8 to 12 hours, as reflected in a repeat PT that indicates adequate coagulability.

Vitamin B complex. Vitamin B complex is composed of many separate biologic factors; the exact chemical composition and significance in human nutrition are yet to be determined. The factors that make up the vitamin B complex are all water soluble but their solubility rates vary considerably. The clinically important B complex vitamins are thiamine (B_1), riboflavin (B_2), pyridoxine (B_6), folic acid, pantothenic acid, nicotinic acid (niacin), and biotin.

THIAMINE (VITAMIN B_1). The function of thiamine is to form the coenzyme thiamine pyrophosphate, which is required for oxidative decarboxylation of pyruvate and α-ketoglutarate. In thiamine deficiency, therefore, lactate and pyruvate build up and interfere with carbohydrate metabolism. This deficiency state is exacerbated by large amounts of carbohydrate in the diet. Affected individuals may become irritable and experience loss of appetite, nausea, and vomiting, in addition to chronic diarrhea and inflammatory lesions of the intestines. As the deficiency state worsens, cardiac dilation may occur, leading to congestive heart failure.

Preventive measures such as the enrichment of flour and other foods and the avoidance of polished rice as the primary food staple have limited the incidence of thiamine deficiency. This deficiency now occurs primarily in alcoholics. Disorders that prevent the ingestion and absorption of food and those which accelerate the metabolic rate can lead to a thiamine deficiency. Thiamine is lost in the urine in cases of profound diuresis, and glucose loading may provoke symptoms in individuals in whom thiamine stores are marginal. Few foods are rich in thiamine, but beans, nuts, whole grain, meats, fish, and eggs are good sources.

The syndromes caused by thiamine deficiency are beriberi, polyneuritis, Wernicke's encephalopathy, and Korsakoff's syndrome. The heart failure that occurs with a thiamine deficiency is a type of high-output failure occurring with clear lungs, an enlarged heart, a normal sinus rhythm, dependent edema, and an elevated venous pressure. Beriberi heart disease is associated with an insufficiency of other B vitamins when the diet has been grossly lacking in thiamine for over 4 months. The early symptoms of neuritic (dry) beriberi include numbness of the legs and paresthesias. Muscle weakness develops gradually and may cause quadriceps weakness along with a difficulty in rising from a squatting position. Paralysis occurs along with advanced polyneuritis. Wernicke's encephalopathy is characterized by apathy, confusion, occasionally delirium, and cerebellar ataxia. Eye signs are always present, including nystagmus and paralysis of the external rectus and other extraocular muscles. Patients with Korsakoff's syndrome have a defect in memory, particularly of recent events, as well as confabulation. The mortality of Wernicke's syndrome is quite high, but parenteral thiamine therapy and the institution of a good diet can lead to a complete recovery; however, the features of Korsakoff's syndrome may persist.

The oral lesions associated with thiamine deficiency are rarely severe enough for the patient to seek professional help. Some of these manifestations include hypersensitivity of the teeth and oral mucosa and enlargement of the fungiform papillae of the tongue. Small vesicles or ''cracks'' may appear in the vermilion border of the lips and commissures of the mouth. Therapeutic doses of approximately 100 mg daily are commonly administered to alcoholics and other thiamine-deficient individuals.

RIBOFLAVIN (VITAMIN B_2). Riboflavin is found within cells in combination with specific enzymes of cellular oxidation reactions. The biochemical role of riboflavin is to form the two flavoprotein coenzymes, flavin adenine dinucleotide and flavin mononucleotide. Riboflavin deficiency leads to the development of seborrheic dermatitis and corneal vascularization. Anemia may also develop and this may be related to disturbance of folate utilization, since the flavoprotein enzymes are involved in its metabolism.

Severe and varied lesions of the oral mucosa and circumoral tissues occur in riboflavin deficiency. Angular cheilosis, characterized by painful lesions in commissures of the mouth, is considered a specific manifestation of riboflavin deficiency, although it may also occur in deficiencies of pantothenic acid and pyridoxine hydrochloride. The pseudocheilotic areas associated with decreased vertical dimension and loss of intermaxillary space usually slant downward and outward, whereas the cheilotic lesions associated with ariboflavinosis are more horizontal. These fissures commonly become encrusted because of secondary infection. Glossitis is another reported effect of riboflavin deficiency, and enlargement of the fungiform papillae gives the dorsum of the tongue a granular appearance. There also may be complete atrophy of the filiform papillae. The vermilion border of the lips and, to a lesser extent, the buccal mucosa may acquire a purplish hue that resembles cyanosis. Individuals with chronic prolonged B complex deficiency have been known to develop bullous lichen planus and painful periodontitis.

PYRIDOXINE (VITAMIN B_6). Pyridoxine is a white crystalline substance that is soluble in water and alcohol. The three forms of the vitamin, all of which are derivatives of pyridine, are pyridoxine, pyridoxal, and pyridoxamine. The first is found in plants and the remaining two in animal products. Their wide distribution in nature makes dietary deficiency a rarity. The active forms of this vitamin are the coenzymes pyridoxal phosphate and pyridoxamine phosphate, which circulate in the plasma bound to albumin. They participate in several reactions of amino acid metabolism, including decarboxylation, transamination, and racemization. Pyridoxine may also be involved in antibody formation.

Clinical deficiency states of pyridoxine are most frequently associated with malnutrition secondary to alcoholism. Generalized dermatitis and neurologic disturbances, especially peripheral neuropathy, are common signs of deficiency. The oral changes in pyridoxine deficiency are relatively nonspecific and include angular cheilitis, glossitis, and generalized stomatitis. Papillary atrophy of the dorsum of the tongue may also develop. These oral changes are virtually identical to those found in iron deficiency, and it has been suggested that the oral changes of iron deficiency are related to coexisting changes in pyridoxine utilization. Simple deficiency states can be corrected with a daily dose of 50 to 150 mg of pyridoxine administered orally.

VITAMIN B_{12}. Vitamin B_{12} is the generic term for a group of cobalt-containing vitamins (cobalamins) that participate as coenzymes in a diverse group of metabolic reactions. Of the vast amount of biochemical work on their actions that has been conducted using bacteria, the two reactions proven to occur in humans are methylmalonate-succinate isomerization and methylation of homocysteine to cysteine, which occur in the synthesis and repair of DNA.

Vitamin B_{12} arises almost solely from bacterial sources; it is not found in plants and cannot be manufactured by higher animals. Humans are totally dependent on dietary vitamin B_{12}, the principal sources of which are animal products, especially meat, liver, kidney, egg yolk, and milk. Since the absorption rate is only 70%, 7 to 8 μg must be ingested daily to satisfy the metabolic requirement of 2 to 5 μg.

Vitamin B_{12} is stored in the liver in quantities sufficient to sustain requirements for many years. Successful absorption of dietary vitamin B_{12} from the gut depends on its binding to a gastric mucoprotein intrinsic factor (IF) secreted into normal gastric juice by the parietal cells. The B_{12}-IF complex so formed is carried down the small bowel and is absorbed in the ileum, where the mucosal cell membranes have specific receptors for this complex. Splitting of the complex occurs at the brush border of the cell and vitamin B_{12} is then absorbed. Most deficiency states are due to an absorptive defect, most frequently from lack of IF. This can result from primary gastric mucosal atrophy or gastrectomy.

Pernicious anemia is by far the most common effect of vitamin B_{12} deficiency, and the term should be reserved for this disease complex. The gastric mucosal lesion responsible for this disease is probably autoimmune, since these patients also have a high incidence of other organ-specific autoimmune disorders, such as Hashimoto's thyroiditis. In addition, there is a high incidence of antigastric parietal cell antibody and anti-intrinsic factor antibody in the sera of patients with pernicious anemia. Glossitis and stomatitis have long been observed in all forms of vitamin B_{12} deficiency. Glossitis occurs in 50% to 60% of patients with pernicious anemia and characteristically fluctuates in severity. Initially, an active inflammatory reaction occurs; the extreme tenderness, rawness, and edema usually interfere with eating. This inflammation regresses and is followed by progressive atrophy of the filiform and fungiform papillae. Recurrent oral ulceration without angular cheilitis is another feature of the disease.

Within 48 hours after specific B_{12} replacement therapy, the symptoms of pernicious anemia are often relieved, and regeneration of the tongue papillae may be evident within a week.

Since most defects are absorptive in nature, vitamin B_{12} replacement must be administered by injection. Initially, six to ten injections of 1000 μg of hydroxycobalamin is usually given in preference to cyanocobalamin, since the former is more efficiently retained. At the rate of one injection daily, this is usually sufficient to produce a therapeutic response and to reconstitute depleted body stores.

FOLIC ACID. This B complex vitamin is present in a wide variety of naturally occurring foodstuffs, especially liver, yeast, and green vegetables. Since folic acid is heat labile, large portions of food folate are lost during cooking. The daily requirement varies from 5 to 50 μg. Body stores are smaller than those of vitamin B_{12} and normal metabolism can only be sustained for a few months once folate is no longer included in the diet.

Dietary folate deficiency is especially common in alcoholics, the elderly, and the malnourished. Significant folic acid deficiency almost invariably occurs with malabsorption syndrome from widespread gastric mucosal disease, such as gluten enteropathy and tropical sprue. Increased body requirements of folic acid occur during pregnancy and in the presence of rapidly growing tumors or other processes characterized by rapid cell turnover. Antifolate cytotoxic drugs and anticonvulsant drugs, such as phenytoin, may also cause folate deficiency.

The clinical and hematologic effects of folic acid deficiency are virtually indistinguishable from those of vitamin B_{12} deficiency. The oral manifestations are also similar to those found in B_{12} deficiencies, with severe oral ulcerations as the predominant clinical sign. These lesions respond promptly to therapeutic folate administration. Oral therapy, usually consisting of 5 mg three times daily, is suitable for most patients, even those with malabsorption syndromes. Although vitamin B_{12} administration is harmless, folic acid should be administered to certain patients with caution. The potential hazards include precipitation of subacute combined degeneration of the spinal cord in patients who actually have vitamin B_{12} deficiency rather than folate deficiency and an increase in the growth rate of folate-dependent tumors. An accurate diagnosis of folic acid deficiency is thus vitally important.

Pantothenic acid. Pantothenic acid is utilized by the body in conjunction with folic acid and biotin. The body requires 10 to 15 mg daily of pantothenic acid for synthesis of coenzyme A. Deficiency of pantothenic acid in laboratory animals has produced adrenocortical deficiency, malformation and resorption of the roots of teeth, resorption of supporting tissues, and varying degrees of osteoporosis. It is not clear, however, whether deficiency syndromes exist in humans; there has been no clinical evidence that pantothenic acid deficiency in humans is associated with any particular lesion or syndrome.

Nicotinic acid (niacin). Lean meats, liver, potatoes, and vegetables are good sources of nicotinic acid. In general, animal tissues contain the vitamin in the form of the amide, whereas plants contain it in the form of acid. Nicotinic acid is converted by the body into its amide, nicotinamide, which is then used for the production of nicotinamide adenine dinucleotide (NAD) and nicotinamide adenine dinucleotide phosphate (NADP). As such, it is involved as an acceptor and donor in oxidation and reduction reactions.

Deficiency in nicotinic acid results in pellagra, a condition characterized by symmetric, red scaly dermatitis of the stocking and glove areas that may darken and subsequently desquamate. These lesions are aggravated by sunlight and heat and are often accompanied by diarrhea, numbness and burning sensations, vertigo, nervousness, progressive weakness, and anorexia. The prominent oral lesion of pellagra is generalized erythema of the mucosa with papillary atrophy of the tongue, which causes considerable discomfort. Fibrin-covered ulcerations may develop subsequently, the tongue may become fiery red, and shallow ulcerations may be noted on the dorsum and along the lateral margins. Secondary ulceronecrotic gingivostomatitis is also a finding in patients with pellagra, along with herpes labialis and angular cheilosis.

The treatment for pellagra consists of high therapeutic doses of niacinamide, usually 150 to 300 mg daily. Excess amounts do not cause serious side effects and are readily eliminated in the urine.

BIOTIN. Biotin functions as a coenzyme in carboxylation reactions. Egg white contains the substance avidin, which has a high binding affinity for biotin. Therefore when an individual ingests an abnormally large amount of raw egg whites, there is a tendency to bind the biotin from the diet and prevent its absorption. The only general effect of biotin deficiency known is a scaly dermatitis. Oral manifestations of biotin deficiency are infrequent and consist primarily of atrophy of the lingual papillae.

Ascorbic acid (Vitamin C). Ascorbic acid is a water-soluble vitamin found in citrus fruits and fresh vegetables, such as cabbage, cauliflower, and tomatoes. The ascorbic acid content of these foods varies considerably, depending on freshness and the method of storage. Comparatively little is lost in the usual cooking procedures. Ascorbic acid is a potent reducing agent and, together with dihydroascorbic acid, forms a redox system. Its primary function in humans is in the hydroxylation of proline.

In the extreme deficiency state, known as "scurvy," the collagen in connective tissue, osteoid, and dentin is functionally defective and leads to widespread clinical pathologic conditions of the supporting tissues of blood vessels, bones, and teeth. A hemorrhagic tendency due to capillary fragility is another characteristic effect, probably attributable to poor collagenous support of these vessels. Skin petechiae occur about the hair follicles and skin of the lower extremities and arms. Subperiosteal hemorrhages are characteristic findings and may be demonstrated on roentgenograms. Anemia often results, both from chronic bleeding and from hemolysis. Mild deficiency states of ascorbic acid are more common than scurvy, resulting from any condition that increases the metabolic demand in the absence of increased intake of the vitamin. Such imbalance may be manifested by impaired wound healing, hyperkeratosis, petechiae, and chronic gingivitis, with a tendency to hematoma formation.

In both mild ascorbic acid deficiency and scurvy, oral tissue pathologic conditions are significant. Gingivitis is one of the early manifestations, with bleeding at the gingival margins, swelling, and ulceration. As the deficiency becomes more acute, the gingiva becomes grossly inflamed and bleeds on the slightest pressure or probing. In this state the oral tissues are highly susceptible to secondary infection, particularly those caused by Vincent's organism *(Borrelia vincentii).* Local factors such as calculus, poor oral hygiene, and malocclusion further aggravate the effects of the deficiency state.

Recent studies now offer the first concrete evidence that subclinical ascorbic acid deficiency significantly increases susceptibility to periodontal disease. One report demonstrates that the periodontal tissues of animals fed a diet marginally deficient in ascorbic acid are more susceptible to breakdown when challenged by experimentally induced dental plaque than are control animals. In another report, a host defense factor was altered by an acute dietary deficiency of ascorbic acid. Animals fed diets with no ascorbic acid experienced an increase in the permeability of the gingival lining that could have contributed to the development of spontaneous scorbutic gingivitis.

A conclusive determination of the need for ascorbic acid intake above that required for general nutrition has not been made. It has also not been shown that ascorbic acid intake above that which is required for tissue saturation produces any preventive or therapeutic effects on the periodontium. At this time the requirement of ascorbic acid for wound healing and tissue repair is the only indication for its use in the treatment of oral lesions other than those associated with clinical scurvy. The usual therapeutic dose ranges from 300 to 500 mg daily, in divided doses.

Nutritional therapy

Patients in need of nutritional support require amino acids for protein synthesis and nonprotein calories to provide energy, as well as essential vitamins and minerals. If the gastrointestinal tract is functional, enteral feeding is preferable. Nutrition can be supplied with natural foods and with preparations in which nutritional components are added to produce a defined mixture. The available preparations generally provide 1 calorie/ml and serve as supplements and meal replacements. The carbohydrate source is usually corn syrup, sucrose, or lactose, but lactose-free products are best for patients with milk intolerance. When patients have problems with the digestion or absorption of fat, medium-chain triglycerides are a better source of calories than the usual long-chain triglycerides. Protein is usually derived from egg albumin, milk solids, and plant protein. Diets that supply amino acids and protein hydrolysates rather than intact proteins are termed "elemental diets." Elemental diets are used for nutritive support and therapeutic benefit in a variety of disorders, but the efficacy of these expensive diets has not been proved.

Parenteral nutrition involves the intravenous administration of protein nitrogen and calories, usually with a central superior vena cava catheter. Nonprotein calories must be administered for the synthesis of proteins; hypertonic dextrose is usually used. Fat may be equivalent to carbohydrates in its utilization for calories, and it also supplies essential fatty acids. Protein hydrolysates and crystalline amino acid mixtures are used as a source of nitrogen. Branched-chain amino acids have special properties and may be increasingly used in situations such as severe stress and liver failure in which they are less likely to provoke portal-systemic encephalopathy. The availability of synthetic amino acids makes it possible to vary the amino acid components of the solution. Parenteral hyperalimentation is effective in maintaining the nitrogen balance and promoting a weight gain and is used when enteral feeding cannot be used, in such conditions as enterocutaneous fistulas, a short bowel, and a prolonged ileus. Parenteral hyperalimentation has also been used in patients with renal failure, cancer, and extensive burns. Complications include sepsis and metabolic disorders such as hyperglycemia and deficiency states, particularly those involving trace elements. Vitamin deficiencies are rare because their replacement in the alimentation fluid is adequate. The home use of parenteral nutrition is becoming increasingly available.

Dietary goals. Dietary goals for the United States have been set by a congressional committee after consultation with many experts. The reaction from nutritional scientists, physicians, and the community has been widespread and diverse, and the value of dietary change remains controversial. There is no assurance that an altered diet provides protection from disease.

The first goal is to avoid becoming overweight. Moderation in caloric intake may be the single most important dietary practice the public could observe, but certainly many other risk factors are implicated in the probability of disease. Other goals are to increase the consumption of complex carbohydrates and to reduce the use of refined simple sugars. An advantage of this recommendation is that such a diet has a higher intake of dietary fiber, the nondigestible component of plant foods. High-fiber diets are epidemiologically associated with a lower incidence of colon cancer, diverticular disease, and hyperlipidemia. No firm evidence has implicated sugar as a cause of arteriosclerosis or diabetes, but controlled human studies have established that the incidence and prevalence of dental caries can be diminished by reducing sugar consumption.

Many studies have shown that blood lipid levels can be altered by reducing the amount of saturated fat in the diet. Whether this alteration can achieve the purpose of preventing arteriosclerotic heart disease is not certain. The association of a total fat intake with certain cancers also supports the goal of a reduction of the total fat in the diet rather than an increased intake of polyunsaturated fats. Obesity might also be effectively treated by decreasing the fat intake. A reduction in the consumption of cholesterol has also been proposed, yet dietary cholesterol may not be nearly as important as weight control and inherent metabolic processes in achieving beneficial lipid levels.

The goal to reduce the intake of salt has been set even though the optimal requirement for sodium has not been established. Sodium chloride may have an effect on the elevation of the blood pressure in some individuals, but many others are not susceptible.

To implement these goals most Americans would need to change their eating patterns. These recommendations are aimed at the prevention of diseases that have multiple causes but may involve an interaction with the diet. These goals should probably be recognized at this time as prudent, but tentative.

BIBLIOGRAPHY
Gastrointestinal disorders

Amato, A.E., and Small, E.W.: Oral manifestations of Gardner's syndrome: report of a case, J. Oral Surg. **28:**458, 1970.

Astacio, J.N., and Alfar, C.: Oral mucosa metastasis from gastric adenocarcinoma, Oral Surg. **28:**859, 1969.

Babin, R.W., Ceilley, R.I., and DeSanto, L.W.: Oral hyperpigmentation and occult malignancy: report of a case, J. Otolaryngol. 7:389, 1978.

Basu, M.K., and others: Oral manifestations of Crohn's disease, Gut 16:249, 1975.

Bernstein, M.L., and McDonald J.S.: Oral lesions in Crohn's disease: report of two cases and update of the literature, Oral Surg. 46:234, 1978.

Biedlingmaier, J.F., Blanchard, C.L., and Masi J.: Necrotizing sialometaplasia of the palate and adenocarcinoma of the esophagus, Ear Nose Throat J. 59:222, 1980.

Blacharsh, C.: Dental aspects of patients with cystic fibrosis: a preliminary clinical study, J. Am. Dent. Assoc. 95:106, 1977.

Caldwell, T.A., Schweber, S.J., and Lucchesi, F.J.: Resection of tongue lesion associated with hereditary telangiectasia (Osler-Weber-Rendu disease), J. Oral Surg. 28:299, 1970.

Carr, D.: Granulomatous cheilitis in Crohn's disease, Br. Med. J. 4:636, 1974.

Croft, C.B., and Wilkinson, A.R.: Ulceration of the mouth, pharynx, and larynx in Crohn's disease of the intestine, Br. J. Surg. 59:249, 1972.

Crumley, R.L.: Synchronous carcinomas of the parotid and colon, Ear Nose Throat J. 57:31, 1979.

Eccles, J.D., Erosion of teeth by gastric contents, Lancet, p. 479, 1978.

Eisenbud, L., Katzka, I., and Platt, N.: Oral manifestations of Crohn's disease, Oral Surg. 34:770, 1972.

Everett, F.G., and Hahn, C.R.: Hereditary hemorrhagic telangiectasia with gingival lesion, J. Periodontol. 47:295, 1976.

Ferguson, M.M., and others: Coeliac disease associated with recurrent aphthae, Gut 21:223, 1980.

Fraser, N.G., Kerr, N.W., and Donald D.: Oral lesions in dermatitis herpetiformis, Br. J. Dermatol. 89:439, 1973.

Gius, J.A., and others: Vascular formations of the lip and peptic ulcer, J.A.M.A. 183:725, 1963.

Glazer, R.I., Spatz, S.S., and Catone, G.A.: Viral hepatitis: a hazard to oral surgeons, J. Oral Surg. 31:504, 1973.

Golding, P.L., Smith, M., and Williams, R.: Multisystem involvement in chronic liver disease, Am. J. Med. 55:772, 1973.

Gorlin, R.J., and Goldman, H.M.: Thoma's oral pathology, ed. 6, St. Louis, 1970, The C.V. Mosby Co.

Harrison, P.V., Scott, D.G., and Cobden, I.: Buccal mucosa immunofluorescence in coeliac disease and dermatitis herpetiformis, Br. J. Dermatol. 102:687, 1980.

Hashimoto, K., and Pritzker, M.S.: Hereditary hemorrhagic telangiectasia: an electron microscopic study, Oral Surg., p. 751, 1972.

Hicks, K.A., and Dickie, W.R.: Amyloidosis: report of case presenting with macroglossia, Br. J. Plast. Surg. 26:274, 1973.

Howden, G.F.: Erosion as the presenting symptom in hiatus hernia, Br. Dent. J. 131:455, 1971.

Hurst, P.S., Lacey, J.H., and Crisp, A.H.: Teeth, vomiting and diet: a study of the dental characteristics of seventeen anorexia nervosa patients, Postgrad. Med. J. 53:298, 1977.

Jones, J.H., and Mason, D.K.: Oral manifestations of systemic disease, Philadelphia, 1980, W.B. Saunders Co.

Kakizaki, G., and others: A new diagnostic test for pancreatic disorders by examination of parotid saliva, Am. J. Gastroenterol. 65(5):437, 1976.

Keith, D.A.: Oral features of primary amyloidosis, Br. J. Oral Surg. 10:107, 1972.

Kelley, M.L., Jr.: Purulent mucocutaneous lesions associated with ulcerative colitis, Med. Radiogr. Photogr. 44:39, 1968.

Kutscher, A.H., and others: Parotid saliva in cystic fibrosis Am. J. Dis. Child. 110:643, 1965.

Lamster, I., and others: An association between Crohn's disease, periodontal disease and enhanced neutrophil function, J. Periodontol., p. 475, 1978.

Lee, B.M.: Metastasis of colon carcinoma to the lip, Arch. Dermatol. 105:608, 1972.

Levy, B., and Smith, W.K.: A jaw metastasis from the colon, Oral Surg., p. 769, 1974.

Little, J.W., and Falace, D.A.: Dental management of the medically compromised patient, St. Louis, 1980, The C.V. Mosby Co.

Lowe, N.J.: Peutz-Jeghers syndrome with pigmented oral papillomas, Arch. Dermatol. 3:503, 1975.

Lund, B.A., Moertel, C.G., and Gibelisco, J.A.: Metastasis of gastric adenocarcinoma to oral mucosa, Oral Surg. 25:805, 1968.

Lynch, M.A., editor: Burket's oral medicine, ed. 7, Philadelphia, 1977, J.B. Lippincott Co.

Mandel, I.D., and others: Parotid saliva in cystic fibrosis, Am. J. Dis. Child. 110:646, 1965.

Marmer, J., Barbero, G.J., and Sibinga, M.S.: The pattern of parotid gland secretion in cystic fibrosis of the pancreas, Gastroenterology 50:551, 1966.

Matthews, N., and others: Buccal biopsy in diagnosis of Crohn's disease, Lancet, p. 500, 1979.

Merck, Sharp, & Dohme, Division of Merck & Co., Inc., West Point, Pa. Package insert for Heptavax B, May 1982.

Moffat, D.A.: Metastatic adenocarcinoma of the rectum presenting as an epulis: a case report, Br. J. Oral Surg. 14:90, 1976.

Nugent, F.W., and Bulan, M.B.: Extracolonic manifestations of ulcerative colitis, Am. Fam. Phys. 5:68, 1972.

O'Brien, K.T., Saunders, D.R., and Templeton, F.E.: Chronic gastric erosions and oral aphthae case report, Dig. Dis. 17:447, 1972.

Ohsiro, T., and others: Treatment of pigmentation of the lips and oral mucosa in Peutz-Jeghers syndrome using ruby and argon lasers, Br. J. Plast. Surg. 33:346, 1980.

Pindborg, J.J.: Atlas of diseases of the oral mucosa, ed. 3, Philadelphia, 1980, W.B. Saunders Co.

Primosch, R.E.: Tetracycline discoloration, enamel defects, and dental caries in patients with cystic fibrosis, Oral Surg. 50(4):301, 1980.

Redding, S.W., Carr, R.F., and Foti, C.E.: Gardner's syndrome: report of a case, J. Oral Surg. 39:50, 1981.

Rimland, D., and others: Hepatitis B outbreak traced to an oral surgeon, N. Engl. J. Med. 296:953, 1977.

Ritter, S.B., and Petersen, G.: Esophageal cancer, hyperkeratosis and oral leukoplakia: follow-up family study, J.A.M.A. 236:1844, 1976.

Russotto, S.B., and Ship, I.I.: Oral manifestations of dermatitis herpetiformis, Oral Surg. 31:42, 1971.

Schwartz, H.C., and Olson, D.J.: Amyloidosis: a rational approach to diagnosis by intraoral biopsy, Oral Surg. 39:837, 1975.

Snyder, M.B., and Cawson, R.A.: Oral changes in Crohn's disease, J. Oral Surg. 34:594, 1976.

Stanback, J.S., and Peagler, F.D.: Primary amyloidosis, Oral Surg. 26:774, 1968.

Taylor, V.E., and Smith, C.J.: Oral manifestations of Crohn's disease without demonstrable gastrointestinal lesions, Oral Surg. 39:58, 1975.

Uthman, A.A.: Plummer-Vinson syndrome, Oral Surg. 20:449, 1965.

Walker, J.E.G.: Possible diagnostic test for Crohn's disease by use of buccal mucosa, Lancet, p. 759, 1978.

Weisman, R.A., and Calcaterra, T.C.: Head and neck manifestations of scleroderma, Ann. Otolaryngol. 87:332, 1978.

White, D.K., Hayes, R.C., and Benjamin R.N.: Loss of tooth structure associated with chronic regurgitation and vomiting, J. Am. Dent. Assoc. 97:833, 1978.

Wiesmann, U.N., Boat, T.F., and diSant'Agnese, P.A.: Sodium concentration in unstimulated parotid saliva and on oral mucosa in normal subjects and in patients with cystic fibrosis, J. Pediatr. 76:444, 1970.

Zambito, R.: Hospital dental practice: a manual, Garden City, N.Y., 1978, Medical Examination Publishing Co., Inc.

Nutritional disorders

Bigaouette, J., and Howard, L.: Nutrition-related disorders, Int. J. Dermatol. **16:**605, 1977.

Caddell, J.L.: Magnesium in the therapy of orofacial lesions of severe protein-calorie malnutrition, Br. J. Surg. **56:**826, 1969.

Delgado, H., and others: Nutritional status and the timing of deciduous tooth eruption, Am. J. Clin. Nutr. **28:**216, 1975.

Falconer, D.T.: Scurvy presenting with oral symptoms, Br. Dent. J. **146:**313, 1979.

Gigliotti, R., and others: Familial vitamin D refractory rickets, J. Am. Dent. Assoc. **82:**383, 1971.

Hjorting-Hansen, E., and Bertram, U.: Oral aspects of pernicious anemia, Br. Dent. J., p. 266, 1968.

Hood, J., Burns, C.A., and Hodges, R.E.: Sjögren's syndrome in scurvy, N. Engl. J. Med. **282:**1120, 1979.

Marks, S.C., Lindahl, R.L., and Bowden, J.W.: Dental and cephalometric findings in vitamin D resistant rickets, J. Dent. Child., p. 259, 1965.

Millard, H.D., and Gobetti, J.P.: Nonspecific stomatitis—a presenting sign in pernicious anemia, Oral Surg. **39:**562, 1975.

Nakamoto, T., and Mallek, H.M.: Significance of protein-energy malnutrition in dentistry: some suggestions for the profession, J. Am. Dent. Assoc. **100:**339, 1980.

Protein deficiency and tooth and salivary gland development, Nutr. Rev. **32:**24, 1974.

Sapiro, S.M.: Folic acid deficiency preceding nontropical sprue, J. Oral Med. **32:**106, 1977.

Soni, N.N., and Marks, S.C.: Microradiographic and polarized light study of dental tissues in vitamin D–resistant rickets, Oral Surg. **23:**755, 1967.

Section Fourteen

ENDOCRINOLOGY

edited by **Doris G. Bartuska**

---

185 • INTRODUCTION TO THE DISEASES OF THE ENDOCRINE SYSTEM AND THE MECHANISM OF ACTION OF HORMONES

Mary B. Dratman

Endocrine disorders are often slow in onset and subtle in presentation. They decrease longevity and erode the quality of life. Therefore identification and treatment of these disorders bring great benefit to the patient, as well as professional gratification to the physician. In recent years the chances of successfully treating previously unsuspected endocrinopathies have been greatly strengthened by the availability of sensitive techniques for measuring hormones and their metabolites. In addition to these biochemical procedures, a diversity of new imaging techniques make it possible to look inside the body and observe structural changes in even small endocrine glands. In spite of these advances, endocrine disorders often remain undiagnosed and therefore untreated for many years after their onset.

The material presented in this section is designed to deal with this dilemma. It emphasizes the great importance of physical diagnosis in endocrinology and stresses the features of the clinical presentation that signal the presence of early hormonal dysfunction. Throughout this section, attention is given to the important influence of genetic endowment, developmental processes, and previous life history on the clinical picture. An approach is thus provided for suspecting the presence of masked or unusual presentations of endocrine disorders. Great stress is also laid on the requirement for studying the patient with well-established chemical and imaging methods to substantiate the diagnosis.

In addition to establishing an organ-and-system-oriented approach to endocrine problems of patients in clinical practice, the responsiveness of endocrine systems is delineated at different stages of life and in patients with a variety of nonendocrine diseases. When appropriate, the basic role of hormones in maintaining health and defending against disease is considered. However, discussion of the biochemical mechanisms of endocrine functions and dysfunctions is necessarily limited. Therefore some current problems in basic endocrinology are mentioned to set the stage for the clinical discussions that follow.

CHANGING CONCEPTS OF THE NATURE AND DOMAIN OF ENDOCRINE SUBSTANCES. As a result of recent advances in the technology as well as the philosophy of hormone research, seemingly inviolate tenets of endocrinology have been subject to reexamination. Distinctions among different kinds of chemical messengers have become more tenuous. The endocrine gland can no longer be considered the sole source and guardian of its secretions. Nonendocrine cells such as neurons may produce hormones. Even individual cells dispersed among a variety of tissues may produce, store, or release such diverse information-transmitting substances as serotonin, norepinephrine, gastrointestinal peptides, calcitonin, glucagon, endorphins, and somatostatin. Whereas hormones were once thought to be disseminated only via the bloodstream, it is now evident that they travel by a variety of routes. Many do indeed reach their targets through the general circulation, but some are first secreted into a portal circulation and reach selected tissues in high concentration before they enter the mainstream. Some tissues receive high concentrations of hormones through innervation by neuroendocrine cells. For example, pituicytes in the neurohypophysis are rich in vasopressin delivered by nerve terminals from perikarya in the supraoptic and paraventricular nuclei. The effect of receiving a small quantity of hormone directly into the specialized extracellular space constituting a synaptic cleft or neuroeffector junction is far greater than the effect produced by receiving the hormone through the general circulation. The so-called parahormones may actually percolate from the hormone-synthesizing cell to an adjacent target cell, with the result that maximal concentrations are made available locally before there is any dilution whatsoever within the vascular compartment. This process is thought to operate, for example, among the different cells of the islets of Langerhans.

ROLE OF CELLULAR AND TISSUE RESPONSIVITY TO CHEMICAL MESSENGERS: IMPORTANCE OF THE RECEPTOR CONCEPT. Hormone effects are now known to be limited not only by their rate, route, and efficiency of dissemination and their half-life in extracellular fluids, but also by conditions prevailing at their cellular destination. The outer cell membrane is recognized to be functionally and morphologically complex. It acts as a responsive barrier to the passage of constituents to and from the extracellular fluid via its multiplicity of gates. It also bears specialized structures serving as recipients for and transducers of molecular information arriving at the surface of the cell. The most thoroughly studied hormone-sensing and information-transducing cell membrane structures, those linked to the ATP–cyclic AMP generating system, have become the prototype for the receptor concept. Receptors may be present in any part of the cell and are defined in terms of their special properties relevant to the molecules received. They are specific in that they differentiate (have discriminatory recognition sites) among closely related molecular species. At the same time they are capable of interacting with a wide variety of analogous substances that may block, feebly mimic, or occasionally produce even more potent effects than the reference ligands. Receptor capacity for a given class of compounds is limited, and the apparent kinetics of receptor-ligand interaction are susceptible to measurement and specification. It is now customary to define properties of hormones in terms of their "specific" binding, that is, their participation in limited-capacity, high-affinity binding interactions with proteins on or within cells or subcellular organelles. Old dogmas may be laid aside, but new ones take their place.

CELLULAR MECHANISMS OF HORMONE ACTION. Experiments based on the receptor concept have led to impressive ongoing discoveries of molecular mechanisms of peptide and steroid hormone action. According to present formulations, peptide hormones and biogenic amines are detained at the cell surface because of their size, water solubility, or spatial properties. There they encounter and bind to highly specialized regions of the plasma membrane (receptor regions), causing excitation of catalytic units at the cytoplasmic interface, culminating in a burst of intracellular second-messenger activity and a cascade of integrated molecular responses that acutely alter cellular function for self-limited periods.

Whereas peptide hormones are detained rather than excluded from entry into cells, the plasma membrane is thought to present no barrier to the passage of steroid hormones and their metabolites into the cell sap. They are either recognized and avidly bound by receptors in the cells, or they diffuse back out again. Changes in transcription, messenger ribonucleic acid (mRNA), and protein synthesis occur promptly following steroid hormone administration to adrenalectomized animals. These results are thought to stem from the formation of steroid hormone–receptor complexes in the cytoplasm of hormone-sensitive cells. When these complexes enter the nucleus, alterations in gene transcription result from still poorly understood effects of the steroid-receptor complexes on gene expression.

A number of different schemes involving receptor-ligand interactions have also been proposed to explain the mechanism of triiodothyronine (T_3) action. However, there is still considerable controversy regarding the site (nucleus, mitochondrion, or cell membrane) as well as the consequences of these putative receptor-T_3 binding interactions. If, as has been suggested, thyroid hormones are required amino acids, homologous with the parent amino acid tyrosine, they might be expected to participate in the formation of thyroxine-containing proteins (iodoproteins), iodomelanins, and so-called thyrocatecholamines. Entry of iodothyronines into such different pathways of metabolism and action might account for their diverse effects on growth, protein synthesis, and adrenergic nervous system function and would inevitably require the participation of many specific receptor-iodocompound interactions.

IMPORTANCE OF HORMONE METABOLISM IN DETERMINING ROUTES OF HORMONE ACTION. Some once confusing aspects of the actions of hormones have been clarified by recognizing that hormone actions and hormone metabolism are often highly interdependent processes. Not all hormone metabolites are generated in all tissues, and not all receptive tissues are responsive to the same metabolite. These principles have been most dramatically illustrated by recent observations relevant to testosterone action and to the actions of another steroid hormone, cholecalciferol. The latter molecule is either synthesized in the skin or derived from the diet (on which basis it was long considered to be a vitamin). It is then transported to several different tissues (such as liver and kidney), where it is differently metabolized and remetabolized by each of them; the metabolites are then transported once again to distant sites (bone, gut, and renal tubule), where they produce coordinated but different effects on calcium metabolism. The ultimate actions of these metabolites vary according to the state of the responding tissue and the presence or absence of other naturally occurring synergists and antagonists.

HORMONES AND THE NERVOUS SYSTEM. A serious new look is being taken at the functional consequences of hormone action in the nervous system. The recent discovery that a specific portion of a long-known pituitary hormone (β-lipotropin) exhibits the same amino acid sequence as a newly discovered putative neurotransmitter (the methionine enkephalin portion of β-endorphin, mediating endogenous morphinelike actions) has created a stir in the field of psychoneuroendocrine relationships. In addition, several recent observations suggest that not only biogenic amines but thyroid hormones, hypothalamic and gastrointestinal peptides, and steroid hormones are concentrated and metabolized within neurons and actively implicated in nervous system development and adult nervous system function. It therefore seems evident that further knowledge of the metabolism and fate of hormones in the brain, and their relationship to other chemical transformations occurring in the nervous system, may help to elucidate obscure aspects of the functions of both systems.

Ultimately, such knowledge will come to be crucial in the management of patients, not only as they require treatment for endocrine diseases, but also as they undergo hormonal changes in response to developmental, psychophysiologic, and aging processes throughout the course of their lives.

BIBLIOGRAPHY

Axelrod, J.: Relationships between catecholamines and other hormones, Recent Prog. Horm. Res. **31**:1, 1975.

Barker, J.I.: Peptides: roles in neuronal excitability, Physiol. Rev. **56**:435, 1976.

Cuatrecasas, P., and others: Hormone receptor complexes and their modulation of membrane function, Recent Prog. Horm. Res. **31**:37, 1975.

DeLuca, H.F.: Recent advances in the metabolism and function of vitamin D, Fed. Proc. **28**:1678, 1969.

Dratman, M.B.: On the mechanism of action of thyroxine, an amino acid analog of tyrosine, J. Theor. Biol. **46**:255, 1974.

Hoch, F.L.: Metabolic effects of thyroid hormones, Handbook Physiol. Sect. **7**(3):391, 1974.

Irvine, C.H.G.: A four compartment model of thyroxine metabolism. In Harland, W.A., and Orr, J.S., editors: Thyroid hormone metabolism, New York, 1975, Academic Press, Inc.

Kuhlenbeck, H.: The central nervous system of vertebrates: a general survey of its comparative anatomy with an introduction to the pertinent fundamental biologic and logical concepts, vols. 1-4, New York, 1967-1975, Academic Press, Inc.

Loh, H.H., and others: β-Endorphin is a potent analgesic agent, Proc. Natl. Acad. Sci. U.S.A. **73**:2895, 1976.

Oppenheimer, J.H.: Role of plasma proteins in the binding, distribution and metabolism of the thyroid hormone, N. Engl. J. Med. **278**:1153, 1968.

Sokoloff, L., and Kaufman, S.: Effects of thyroxine on amino acid incorporation into protein, Science **129**:569, 1959.

186 • HYPOTHALAMIC AND PITUITARY DISORDERS

Calvin Ezrin

ENDOCRINE HYPOTHALAMUS

The hypothalamic-pituitary relationship is the most important in neuroendocrinology. The hypothalamus, a complicated collection of nerve cells and fiber tracts, participates in the regulation of many autonomic functions and body rhythms. The hypothalamus also contains cells that combine neural and secretory activity. This portion is difficult to define anatomically, but since it produces hormones, it may accurately be designated as the "endocrine hypothalamus." The hormones it produces are delivered to the pituitary gland (Fig. 186-1). The endocrine hypothalamus is composed of cells that are typical neurons capable of being excited to conduct action potentials and releasing specific substances at their terminals. However, unlike typical neurons, which release neurotransmitters into synaptic clefts, neurosecretory cells release their products into perivascular spaces.

The first neurosecretory cells to be recognized were those of the supraoptic and paraventricular nuclei of the hypothalamus, whose cell bodies and axon processes color intensely with specific stains. Neurophysins, specific carrier proteins for vasopressin and oxytocin, are responsible for this intense staining. The axons of these neurons terminate in the posterior pituitary adjacent to capillaries. Depolarization of the axon terminal causes a release of hormone by a process called stimulation-secretion coupling, which occurs only in the presence of adequate calcium.

Many clinical and experimental observations have shown that anterior pituitary secretion is largely dependent on the hypothalamus. Certain neurons of the medial basal hypothalamus are believed to synthesize and secrete specific hypothalamic adenohypophysiotropic hormones, or regulatory factors, that stimulate or inhibit the secretion of anterior pituitary cells. Axons of these neurons terminate directly in the perivascular zone surrounding the primary capillary network of the pituitary portal circulation in the median eminence, from which they travel via the pituitary portal veins to the anterior lobe. Neurotransmitters, such as norepinephrine, 5-hydroxytryptamine, and acetylcholine, influence the secretion of hypothalamic-regulating hormones and factors and thus indirectly affect anterior pituitary function. One major exception to this rule is dopamine, which has a direct inhibitory action on the release of prolactin from the pituitary.

CONTROL OF ANTERIOR PITUITARY SECRETION

The adenohypophysis produces six distinct hormones: *thyrotropin* (thyroid-stimulating hormone), *corticotropin* (adrenocorticotropic hormone), two *gonadotropins* (follicle-stimulating hormone and luteinizing hormone), *prolactin,* and *somatotropin* (growth hormone). Morphologic studies have shown that the adenohypophysis contains at least five different cell types, each producing one or two closely related hormones. Thus the anterior pituitary may be regarded as a confederation of several relatively independent endocrine glands grouped together anatomically, probably to permit the hypothalamus to efficiently exert higher control. Consideration of the function of each of the anterior pituitary hormones and their regulation will lead to a better understanding of the entire endocrine system.

Thyrotropin, or thyroid-stimulating hormone (TSH)

The hypothalamic *thyrotropin-releasing hormone* (TRH) stimulates the release of TSH, which in turn acts on the thyroid to increase the output of its two hormones: tetraiodothyronine, or thyroxine (T_4), and triiodothyronine (T_3). The role of TRH in maintaining the narrow normal range of concentration of the circulating thyroid hormones is probably relatively minor. It seems to mediate thyroid activation that results from prolonged exposure to cold and

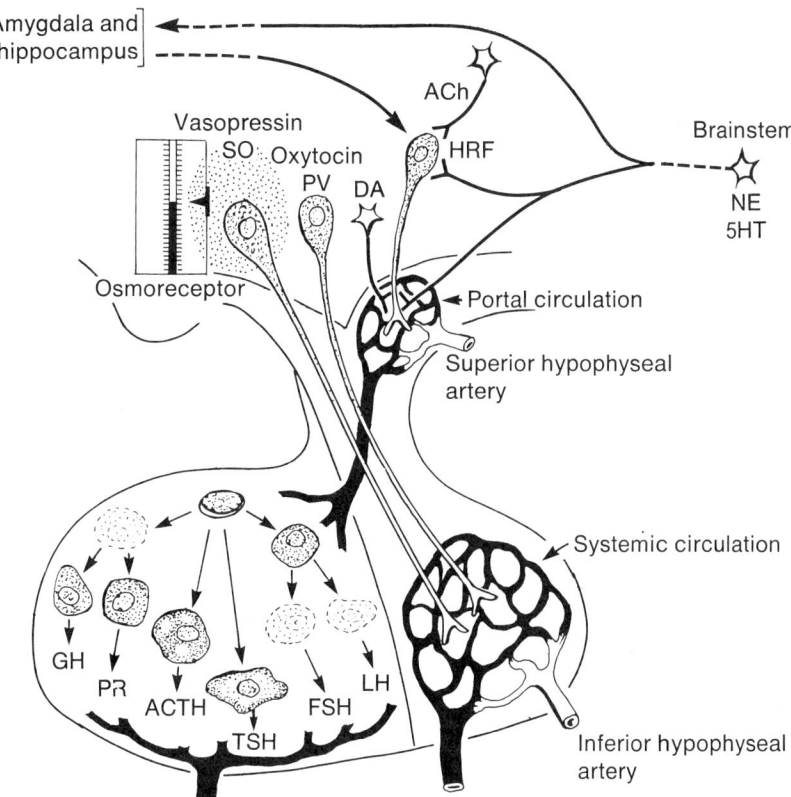

Fig. 186-1. "Endocrine hypothalamus" (see text). *SO*, supraoptic nuclei; *PV*, paraventricular nuclei; *HRF*, hypothalamic releasing factor; *DA*, dopamine; *NE*, norepinephrine; *5HT*, 5-hydroxytryptamine; *Ach*, acetylcholine; *GH*, growth hormone; *PR*, prolactin; *ACTH*, adrenocorticotropin; *TSH*, thyroid-stimulating hormone; *FSH*, follicle-stimulating hormone; *LH*, luteinizing hormone. (From Ezrin, C., Godden, J.O., and Volpé, R.: Systematic endocrinology, ed. 2, New York, 1979, Harper & Row, Publishers.)

also appears to be involved in the thyroid adaptation of the newborn to the relatively cold extrauterine environment. The increased serum T_4 level in the newborn represents a true hyperthyroid state that is self-correcting.

Hypothyroidism caused by thyroid insufficiency leads to increased secretion of TSH in an attempt to restore normal levels of circulating thyroid hormones. Increased serum TSH is the most sensitive test for primary hypothyroidism.

Corticotropin, or adrenocorticotropic hormone (ACTH)

ACTH, a polypeptide, regulates the growth and function of the adrenal cortex. It is especially important in the control of the production and release of glucocorticoid hormones such as cortisol, which is made by the zona fasciculata. The zona glomerulosa, which produces the important mineralocorticoid aldosterone, is largely controlled by the renin-angiotensin system. The production of sex steroids by the zona reticularis is governed by a mechanism that is still unclear. Cells containing ACTH account for no more than 10% of the anterior pituitary cell population. The pituitary "corticotroph" is the most basophilic and PAS-positive of all the pituitary cells. It undergoes a limited loss of granulation in a characteristic crescentic pattern under the influence of prolonged excessive levels of circulating cortisol, such as occurs in Cushing's syndrome, which may result from various causes (see Chapter 188). It seems that ACTH and β-lipotropin, a parent molecule of several polypeptide neurotransmitters, are both produced by the same basophil subtype. They probably share a common precursor.

The release of ACTH appears to be governed by at least three independent mechanisms:

1. *Negative feedback.* Cortisol, the principal adrenal glucocorticoid, inhibits ACTH release when its level rises higher than normal. If the cortisol level falls, ACTH secretion is stimulated through a negative feedback; the cortisol level rises again and turns off the ACTH.
2. *Diurnal rhythm.* In human beings ACTH secretion is maximal in the early morning hours with a gradual fall after 8 AM. Consequently, afternoon plasma cortisol levels (which closely reflect ACTH release) are only about one half of the 8 AM value. This diurnal rhythm may be abolished by certain central

nervous system lesions. It is also lost in Cushing's syndrome and may be absent in some emotionally depressed patients.

3. *A stress-activated mechanism.* Stressful stimuli, such as trauma, hypoglycemia, or pyrogens, increase the delivery of corticotropin-releasing factor (CRF) to the adenohypophysis. This stress mechanism, stimulating the corticotrophs, may override the negative feedback and diurnal rhythm control systems. The greater the stress, the more ACTH is secreted.

Gonadotropic hormones—follicle-stimulating hormone (FSH) and luteinizing hormone (LH)

Immunostaining reveals that FSH and LH arise from the same subtype of pituitary basophil cell. These gonadotropins play major roles in ovarian and testicular functions.

OVARIAN FUNCTION. FSH, a glycoprotein, enlarges a ripening ovarian follicle to the point of rupture. Under FSH influence the follicular cells secrete estrogen. Ovulation, in midcycle, results from an additional surge of secretion of another glycoprotein, LH. Both gonadotropins are released by a hypothalamic hormone designated gonadotropin-releasing hormone (GnRH) or luteinizing hormone-releasing hormone (LHRH or LRH). When the fertilized ovum is implanted, chorionic gonadotropin is secreted to maintain the corpus luteum beyond its normal life span of 2 weeks. Normal menstruation results from a falling level of progesterone.

The ovarian steroids, estrogen and progesterone, exert a negative feedback effect on both FSH and LH secretion. After physiologic ovarian failure (menopause) or destruction or removal of the ovaries, FSH and LH secretion rise considerably.

TESTICULAR FUNCTION. The gonadotropic control of testicular maturation and function is complex. FSH is necessary for the development of LH receptors to permit the full action of LH. FSH stimulates the production of androgen-binding protein, which transports testosterone into the seminiferous tubule where it helps to stimulate spermatogenesis. The testicular interstitial, or Leydig, cells are driven to produce testosterone by LH or, as it is known in the male, by interstitial cell–stimulating hormone (ICSH). In male patients with primary hypogonadism, as in females, the serum gonadotropin levels increase, suggesting that there is a negative feedback between the testes and the pituitary. When it is administered therapeutically, testosterone inhibits ICSH but not FSH. FSH secretion is probably normally inhibited by a nonsteroid substance (designated "inhibin") made by the tubules. In some aging men testosterone production falls and ICSH (LH) levels increase. Thus in men there may be a late menopause, but it has received little clinical attention because impotence and reduced performance in elderly men can usually be ascribed to other factors.

Prolactin

The recognition of prolactin as a separate human hormone was delayed for some time because of the considerable similarity in molecular structure of prolactin and growth hormone. These two hormones arise from separate subtypes of pituitary acidophils. Prolactin is one of the group of hormones necessary for sufficient breast development to permit milk secretion. When the breast has developed under the influence of estrogen, progesterone, and prolactin during pregnancy, milk secretion appears to depend on an additional postpartum pituitary secretion of prolactin. During the last trimester of pregnancy, when circulating levels of prolactin are high because of estrogen-induced prolactin cell hyperplasia, the breast is prevented from secreting milk by the accompanying increased levels of estrogen. Lactation ensues soon after delivery, which causes a rapid decrease in estrogen levels.

Breast-feeding raises serum prolactin levels and delays resumption of menses. Hyperprolactinemia may interfere with ovulation by decreasing the manufacture or release of GnRH. It may also decrease the responsiveness of the gonadotrophs to LRH or the ovaries to gonadotropins.

The manufacture and release of prolactin are under the control of a hypothalamic inhibitor, prolactin-inhibiting factor (PIF), which may be dopamine.

Somatotropin, or growth hormone

Somatotropin, a protein hormone consisting of 191 amino acids, is made by a subtype of acidophil cell. This hormone stimulates protein anabolism, releases free fatty acids by lipolysis, and induces hyperglycemia by interfering with glucose use. Radioimmunoassay shows that circulating levels of growth hormone fluctuate rapidly in response to nutritional and psychic events, to sleep, and to muscular exercise. The hypothalamic hormone somatostatin inhibits the release of growth hormone as well as several other hormones, including insulin, glucagon, and gastrin. Hyperglycemia inhibits the release of growth hormone, whereas hypoglycemia stimulates its output.

Some of the effects of growth hormone are mediated by serum peptides of hepatic origin, somatomedins, whose levels are dependent on growth hormone. To achieve normal adult body size in the first two decades of life, a person needs somatotropin. When a child lacks this hormone, growth is severely retarded. Growth hormone–deficient children respond to human growth hormone with a substantial increase in growth rate. Species specificity is seen in the clinical use of growth hormone and gonadotropins but not with any of the other pituitary hormones.

CLINICAL PITUITARY DISORDERS

The major disease processes involving the pituitary are tumor, infarct, and granuloma. In addition, congenital selective hypofunction may result from hypothalamic deficiency. Diseases of the pituitary may have many different presentations. Local compressive effects from expanding tumors and manifestations of endocrine imbalance are the most common events that bring a patient to clinical attention.

The optic chiasm and hypothalamus are the most important superior relations of the pituitary fossa. The pituitary gland lies above the sphenoid sinus, into which downward-growing pituitary tumors may project. The internal carotid arteries (as well as the third and sixth cranial nerves) are in the cavernous sinuses, which are lateral to the pituitary gland and may occasionally be compressed by pituitary tumors. Mistaking a carotid aneurysm for a pituitary tumor may lead to a fatal surgical outcome.

Hyperpituitary syndromes

Clinically significant pituitary hypersecretion usually results from tumors, some of which may not be readily apparent. Hyperplasia of specific cell types may result from target gland failure (such as primary hypothyroidism) or from alteration of normal hypothalamic regulatory mechanisms. Prolactin cell hyperplasia may result from suprahypophyseal lesions or drugs such as phenothiazines that interfere with the production and delivery of PIF to the pituitary.

ACROMEGALY. Acromegaly, the syndrome of adult growth hormone excess, and gigantism, its counterpart beginning in childhood, are the result of growth hormone–secreting tumors, some of which have an accompanying prolactin cell component. Acromegaly is characterized by enlargement of the extremities, coarsening of the facial features, and a high incidence of impaired sugar tolerance (Fig. 186-2). The pituitary tumor may reduce vision by compressing the visual pathway. Gigantism begins when the limb bones are still capable of further longitudinal growth. Pituitary giants may reach a height of 8 feet (240 cm) and weigh more than 300 pounds (135 kg). These individuals usually have some associated acromegalic features.

The symptoms and signs result from either local compression by the tumor or its metabolic effects. Headache, which may vary from mild to severe, is usually attributed to the expanding tumor pressing on the sensitive walls of the sella turcica; it may also be the result of hormonal influences. Pressure upward on the optic chiasm most commonly produces a bitemporal hemianopia, but other visual fields defects also occur.

The frequent association of diabetes mellitus with acromegaly indicates that somatotropin and insulin are antagonistic with respect to blood sugar levels. The bony and soft tissue overgrowth of acromegaly is an expression of the increased anabolism that characterizes this disorder. Hypermetabolism with heat intolerance and excessive perspiration is found in about one third of patients with acromegaly, whereas hyperthyroidism occurs in less than one twentieth of cases. Hyperparathyroidism may also accom-

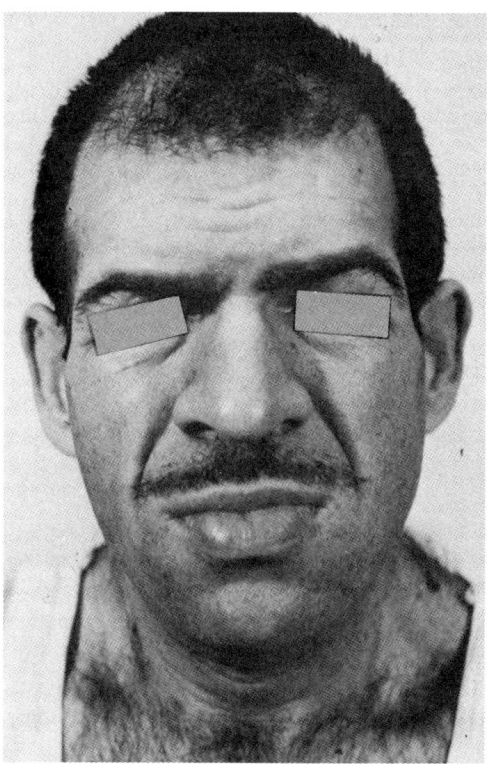

Fig. 186-2. This 36-year-old man had acromegaly owing to pituitary adenoma hypersecreting growth hormone (see text). (From Ezrin, C., Godden, J.O., and Volpé, R.: Systematic endocrinology, ed. 2, New York, 1979, Harper & Row, Publishers.)

pany acromegaly, sometimes as a feature of multiple endocrine adenomatosis, which may be familial and include pancreatic islet tumors. Some patients with acromegaly have galactorrhea, usually because the tumor consists of both prolactin- and growth hormone-producing cells.

Although conventional roentgenographic views of the sella turcica may sometimes miss a small adenoma causing acromegaly, this is usually disclosed by polytomography. Besides the usual finding of considerable sellar distortion, roentgenograms will often reveal enlargement of the accessory nasal sinuses, prognathism, thickening of the inner table of the skull, spinal osteoporosis, and tufting of the terminal phalanges. Increased thickness of the skin may be demonstrated by measuring the heel pad for the subcutaneous fat layer by roentgenography.

For the laboratory confirmation of acromegaly, circulating growth hormone levels should be measured by immunoassay. Normally the administration of glucose inhibits the secretion of growth hormone. In acromegaly this inhibition does not occur, and sustained elevations of growth hormone or even increased levels will be observed when the samples are taken during a glucose tolerance test. Impaired glucose tolerance is found in at least one third of patients with acromegaly, and one sixth have diabetes mellitus requiring treatment. Elevation of the fasting serum inorganic phosphate (greater than 4.5 mg/dl) is an indirect measure of growth hormone secretion. Often the administration of TRH leads to a rise in growth hormone levels in patients with acromegaly, a response not seen in normal subjects.

Until recently a transfrontal approach to pituitary tumors was the rule. However, both small and relatively large pituitary tumors may be more readily dealt with by a transsphenoidal approach, which has now become the preferred technique in most cases. Conventional high-voltage irradiation of the pituitary produces substantial benefit in more than one half of the patients so treated. Its main disadvantage is the long delay in controlling growth hormone excess; usually at least 6 months is required to achieve normal levels. High-energy particle radiation from a cyclotron, a more powerful treatment, has been successful in expert hands but is applicable only when the tumor is confined to the sella. A limited transsphenoidal removal of the adenoma is probably the best treatment for active acromegaly, even in the absence of chiasmal compression. A dopaminergic agent, bromocriptine (2-bromo-α-ergocriptine), has been used in the medical treatment of acromegaly. It blocks the release of growth hormone from the adenoma cells in some cases, but the doses required are higher than those needed to control hyperprolactinemia. Bromocriptine is useful while waiting for the delayed effects of conventional radiotherapy to appear.

CUSHING'S SYNDROME. Because most of the clinical features of Cushing's syndrome are a direct consequence of adrenocortical hyperfunction, it is discussed in Chapter 188.

PROLACTINOMA. Patients with prolactin-secreting tumors may have amenorrhea or galactorrhea. Because prolactin is antigonadotropic and to some extent antiandrogenic, prolactinoma should be considered in any man complaining of impotence. The tumors vary in size from microadenomas that do not distort the sellar outline to macroadenomas that may exert considerable pressure on surrounding structures. These tumors most often arise in the interior portions of the gland and by downward extension may erode the floor of the sella into the sphenoid sinus. Thus cerebrospinal rhinorrhea or meningitis may rarely be the presenting feature of such a tumor. Prolactinomas may not be associated with endocrine symptoms or signs in some patients and may be discovered on a skull roentgenogram taken for other reasons. Nonfunctioning pituitary tumors may induce excess prolactin secretion from the surrounding normal gland by interfering with the delivery of PIF. The final diagnosis of prolactinoma rests on the immunochemical demonstration of prolactin in tumor tissue supplemented by electron-microscopic identification of the cardinal features of the characteristic fine structure of this tumor.

Serum prolactin should be measured in every patient with prolonged amenorrhea, primary or secondary. Serum prolactin (normal upper limit in both sexes is 18 ng/ml) tends to be higher with larger tumors. Levels greater than 200 ng/ml are usually diagnostic of tumor. Intermediate levels may be caused by hyperplasia or tumor. In patients with normal sellar tomography and moderate prolactin excess, a failure to respond to TRH is strong evidence of tumor rather than hyperplasia. However, in some cases of prolactinoma there is a brisk response to TRH, perhaps from hyperplastic cells in the nontumorous portions of the gland.

Male patients usually do not have galactorrhea and only rarely show gynecomastia. Their most common symptom is impotence, sometimes with normal circulating levels of testosterone. In some cases of impotence with androgen deficiency, testosterone replacement does not help until the serum prolactin levels are lowered.

The antiprolactin drug bromocriptine has been very successful in reducing greatly elevated prolactin levels, sometimes to normal. In such cases the galactorrhea ceases, menses return, and fertility results. The usual effective dose is between 5 and 10 mg daily in two doses. The most prominent side effect is nausea, which diminishes as therapy is continued. Postural hypotension may also be troublesome, but it can be minimized by starting treatment with low doses such as 1.25 mg daily until tolerance is developed. Although there is no evidence that bromocriptine is teratogenic, the drug should be discontinued once pregnancy is diagnosed. Bromocriptine now seems to have significant antitumor effect, which is sometimes apparent shortly after treatment is begun. In most cases the prolactin level rises after therapy is withdrawn, but sometimes not to its former level.

Progressive tumor growth, particularly with optic chiasmal compression, is a clear indication for surgery. Most of these tumors, even those of considerable size, can be handled by a transsphenoidal approach. In patients with slow-growing tumors extending downward, resection may lead to complications of cerebrospinal fluid rhinorrhea or meningitis. In these cases a more conservative approach may be warranted, particularly in the elderly.

Resection of a microadenoma in an infertile woman may restore normal ovulatory cycles and remove the risk of aggravating tumor growth by the resulting estrogen excess of pregnancy. In a large series studying bromocriptine-treated infertile women with prolactinomas, several normal pregnancies resulted, with evidence of mild pituitary enlargement in some cases. These patients did not receive prepregnancy irradiation, which has been recommended as a means of inhibiting the estrogen-stimulated overgrowth of a prolactinoma in pregnancy. In no case was there sufficient growth of the tumor during pregnancy to warrant consideration of surgery. However, there have been instances of rapid advancement of tumors in pregnancy requiring decompression of the visual pathway or reinstitution of bromocriptine therapy in the last trimester, which seemed to produce an antitumor effect.

There is little experience with irradiation as the sole treatment of prolactinomas. Persistent hyperprolactinemia following tumor removal calls for either a course of irradiation or the use of bromocriptine.

THYROTROPIN-SECRETING ADENOMA. The uncommon diagnosis of a TSH-secreting pituitary adenoma can be considered when the serum TSH levels are elevated in association with increased serum T_4. If the serum TSH were measured routinely in patients with hyperthyroidism, more cases might be diagnosed. After treating the hyperthyroidism with antithyroid drugs and radioiodine, the pituitary tumor may be dealt with by surgery and, if necessary, postoperative irradiation.

Anterior pituitary insufficiency

The clinical picture in anterior pituitary insufficiency may vary greatly, depending on the patient's age at onset and the number of anterior pituitary hormones affected. Failure of a single anterior pituitary hormone may be the result of congenital hypothalamic deficit or, less commonly, selective pituitary failure. Hypogonadotropic hypogonadism with anosmia *(Kallman's syndrome)* is a relatively common example of a neurologic defect resulting in pituitary underactivity. These patients show delayed puberty and a eunuchoid habitus. Serum gonadotropin levels are low but respond to LRH, although sometimes only after repeated doses. Growth hormone lack is often caused by a hypothalamic defect. In some children with both growth hormone and TSH deficiency, a response to TRH indicates that the pituitary is not primarily at fault; the available stimuli for growth hormone do not act directly on the growth hormone cell (somatotroph), as does TRH on the thyrotroph.

It is remarkable how little anterior pituitary tissue is required to maintain normal endocrine equilibrium. Destruction of 50% of the adenohypophysis does not produce evidence of hypopituitarism. In patients with two thirds to three fourths of the anterior lobe lost, endocrine deficiency is only moderate. Severe hypopituitarism occurs only if 90% of the anterior pituitary is destroyed or separated from its hypothalamic connection.

Clinically, gonadotropic function appears to be most susceptible to factors that damage the pituitary. However, growth hormone secretion is often impaired in mild cases of pituitary insufficiency; sometimes it may be the only hormone affected. As insufficiency increases, evidence of thyroid and adrenocortical hypofunction also appears. Although hypopituitarism is more commonly chronic, a result of compression of the gland by tumor or granuloma, it may be acute after postpartum necrosis or after sudden pituitary failure associated with hemorrhage into a tumor ("pituitary apoplexy").

The pituitary gland is really a confederation of several relatively independent endocrine glands gathered together in close relation to the hypothalamus, which exerts considerable governing control. To encourage an organized approach to the clinical problems arising from insufficient pituitary function, each of the subglands of the pituitary should be considered separately in every case of pituitary disease.

GONADOTROPIC HORMONES (FSH AND LH). If gonadotropin (FSH and LH) production fails before sexual maturity, puberty does not take place. In growing males who lack androgenic hormone, the epiphyses remained unfused, and if the secretion of growth hormone is adequate, the long bones continue to grow. The arms and legs become disproportionately long, and the individual's arm span exceeds his height (normally they are equal). These eunuchoid patients may have osteoporosis, presumably because testicular androgens have not produced their protein anabolic effect. The penis remains small, the scrotum does not develop mature rugae, the testes are tiny, and the prostate is underdeveloped. These patients do not develop libido or become potent. Congenital absence of gonadotropin leads to poor gonadal development with hypoplastic testes, which are often undescended.

Girls with isolated hypogonadotropism have amenorrhea and poor sexual development. However, because pubic and axillary hair is also under the control of adrenal androgens, they do have a small amount of hair in these regions (if they have more severe disease with associated deficiency of corticotropin, pubic and axillary hair is completely absent). The epiphyses do not fuse at the normal time, and a eunuchoid habitus develops. Some patients have a partial congenital deficiency of hypothalamic stimulation of gonadotropic function, with sufficient basal output of estrogen to induce secondary sexual characteristics but no menses.

The manifestations are similar when gonadotropin deficiency develops in adult life, except that these patients do not have a eunuchoid habitus. Men have loss of libido and testicular atrophy. Pubic and axillary hair is decreased, and there is usually some loss of facial hair with decreased frequency of shaving. When testicular androgen production fails, hair may grow again on previously bald areas. In female patients secondary amenorrhea develops, usually with some regression of secondary sexual characteristics.

In general there are two types of hypogonadism. The first, caused by gonadal failure, is called primary hypogonadism. It is associated with elevated levels of pituitary gonadotropic secretion through failure of the normal negative feedback control of gonadal steroids on the pituitary. Secondary or hypogonadotropic hypogonadism is the result of pituitary or hypothalamic disease. GnRH is a 10–amino acid linear polypeptide that stimulates the release of both LH and FSH. Response to LRH ($100\mu g$ in a single intravenous injection) with a rise in serum LH and FSH indicates that the pituitary is not at fault; however, some patients with hypothalamic failure leading to hypogonadotropic hypogonadism respond only after a series of injections. In addition, some patients with only pituitary disease may be hypogonadotropic because of the failure of endogenous LRH to reach the gonadotrophs. In these cases relatively large doses of exogenous LRH may stimulate the gonadotrophs. Thus the response to hypothalamic releasing hormones is not always a reliable method of distinguishing between hypothalamic and pituitary pathology. A serum prolactin level should be determined in every patient with acquired hypogonadotropic hypogonadism because hyperprolactinemia can interfere with hypothalamic-pituitary-gonadal function in a variety of ways.

Male hypogonadism of testicular, pituitary, or hypothalamic origin may be treated by replacing the androgen, which may be given as an intramuscular compound such as testosterone propionate or testosterone enanthate. The usual replacement dose is 400 mg monthly. Oral androgens are available, but in some individuals these produce hepatocellular jaundice. The most useful oral agent is fluoxymesterone, a fluorinated derivative of methyltestosterone. A daily dose of 2 to 10 mg will usually suffice. To restore spermatogenesis requires the administration of human gonadotropic preparations containing both FSH and ICSH. Such treatment usually must continue at least 3 months to produce a full quantitative restoration of spermatogenesis.

In adult women sequential estrogen and progestational agents will restore secondary sexual characteristics and produce regular withdrawal menses. Infertility is treated by the sequential administration of human FSH followed by human chorionic gonadotropin, which induces ovulation. This treatment may be complicated by the production of ovarian cysts that may rupture and cause serious consequences. It may also produce multiple pregnancy.

Clomiphene citrate, an estrogen analog that blocks estrogen receptor sites, stimulates the hypothalamus to release LRH and thereby induces ovulation. An ovulatory response may be determined by careful basal body temperature readings or by the serum progesterone level, which rises greatly in the luteal phase.

THYROTROPIN. Pituitary hypothyroidism, resulting from a deficiency of thyrotropin (TSH), may produce all the characteristic signs of myxedema: lethargy, cold intolerance, bradycardia, excessive dryness, and myxedematous infiltration of the skin. Serum and T_3 resin uptake is decreased. The radioimmunoassay of TSH clearly distinguishes between primary myxedema and that arising from pituitary or hypothalamic failure. In primary hypothyroidism the serum TSH is usually substantially elevated. In "hypothalamic hypothyroidism" serum TSH is virtually undetectable until TRH is administered, following which there is a substantial rise in the serum TSH. In pituitary hypothyroidism TSH is usually undetectable before and after the administration of TRH. Thyrotropin deficiency rarely exists alone; it is usually accompanied by latent insufficiency of corticotropin and obvious hypogonadism.

CORTICOTROPIN. Lack of corticotropin (ACTH) is usually manifested by nausea, the earliest symptom of cortisol deficiency. Hypotension, loss of pubic and axillary hair in females (under adrenal androgen control), and hypoglycemia are other clues suggesting ACTH deficiency. These episodes of adrenal insufficiency are often precipitated by infection and other stress. Serum electrolyte levels are usually normal, although hyponatremia may sometimes be found, especially in patients who have been vomiting.

Most patients who have severe anterior pituitary insufficiency have pallor out of proportion to the moderate degree of anemia present. This pallor probably reflects a deficiency of the portion of the corticotropin molecule that has melanocyte-stimulating properties. Patients with primary adrenal insufficiency usually have increased pigmentation. These two conditions can be differentiated by the intravenous ACTH (Cortrosyn) test and the resultant response of plasma cortisol levels or of urinary excretion products of cortisol, that is, 17-hydroxycorticoids or urinary free cortisol (see Chapter 188). The ACTH reserve of the anterior pituitary can be assessed with metyrapone, which acts on the adrenal cortex by blocking the conversion of 11-desoxycortisol to cortisol and thus markedly reducing the normal cortisol inhibition of ACTH output. If the pituitary can respond by increasing its secretion of ACTH, urinary and plasma desoxycortisol increases along with 17-hydroxycorticoids derived from its metabolic degradation. In diseases of the endocrine hypothalamus, which affect the production of CRF, or pituitary disease, which involves the corticotrophs, there is not significant increase in desoxycortisol or 17-hydroxycorticoids.

Insulin-induced hypoglycemia has been used as a stress test of the responsiveness of the endocrine hypothalamus and the pituitary corticotrophs and somatotrophs. During hypoglycemia, plasma cortisol levels (a reflection of ACTH secretion) normally rise appreciably, as do growth hormone levels.

SOMATOTROPIN. If somatotropin is lacking, growth is severely retarded. If the patient is also hypogonadal with open epiphyses, slow growth will continue for several decades (Fig. 186-3).

Growth hormone seems to produce many of its effects through converting other factors into somatomedins, which are active growth-promoting substances. These polypeptides are made in the liver under the influence of growth hormone. Somatomedins are not found in the plasma of patients with hypopituitarism until after the administration of human growth hormone (HGH). The common problem of short stature is rarely caused by growth hormone deficiency. Fasting plasma growth hormone levels are frequently undetectable in normal children. Early experience suggests that the measurement of somatomedin-C by radioimmunoassay is a practical screening test for growth hormone deficiency. Other useful tests are vigorous exercise for 20 minutes to increase circulating growth hormone levels or the administration of estrogen, such as 20 μg of

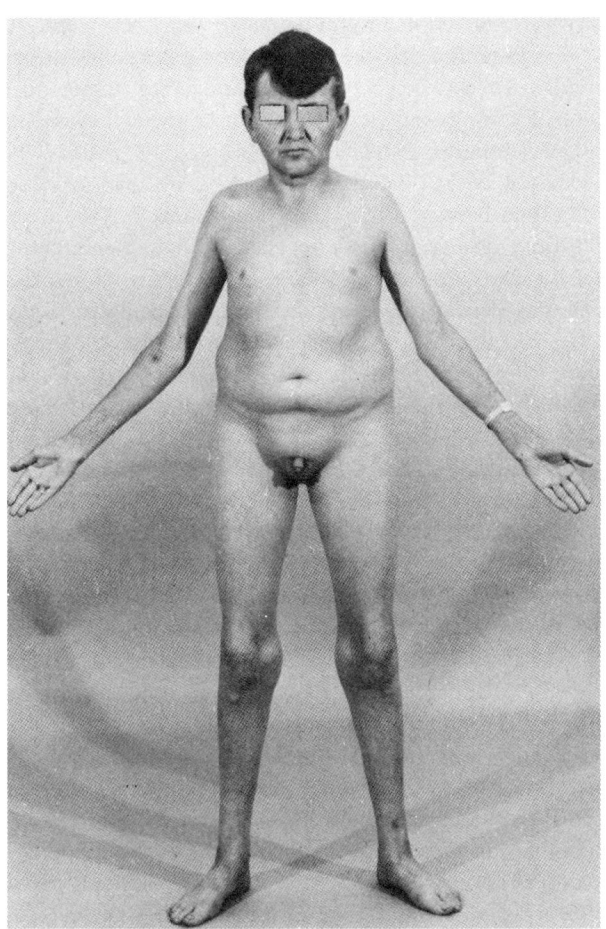

Fig. 186-3. This 47-year-old man with congenital pituitary dysplasia has deficient production of growth hormone, gonadotropins, and ACTH (see text). (From Ezrin, C., Godden, J.O., and Volpé, R.: Systematic endocrinology, ed. 2, New York, 1978, Harper & Row, Publishers.)

ethinyl estradiol daily for 3 days. If the clinical diagnosis of growth hormone deficiency is strongly suspected, the somatomedin-C level is below the normal range, or plasma growth hormone has failed to increase in response to screening tests, further definitive studies of growth hormone release are necessary. Administration of L-dopa, 10 mg/kg body weight by mouth, produces peak concentrations of more than 5 ng/ml of growth hormone in most normal children. Insulin-induced hypoglycemia to raise growth hormone levels can be used only with extreme caution, since prolonged reduction of blood sugar may cause permanent intellectual impairment or even death.

Failure of growth hormone response to various stimuli may be an early manifestation of progressive pituitary hypofunction. Usually the only other recognizable endocrine deficiency in these patients is hypogonadism.

Selective failure of growth hormone production has been reported in some members of certain families. These patients mature sexually somewhat later than usual, with androgenic hormone limiting further growth by inducing epiphyseal closure. Growth hormone–deficient children should be treated with HGH. 20 units weekly in two injections of 10 units. A successful response appears to be a growth rate of about 3 inches (7.5 cm) per year or at least a doubling of the pretreatment growth rate. The older, taller, and heavier the children and the more advanced their bone age, the less they respond to growth hormome treatment. Only HGH if effective in such patients. Some patients develop hormone-neutralizing antibodies that seem to decrease the effectiveness of therapy. A gradual onset of TSH deficiency develops in some patients during HGH treatment. The mechanism is unclear, but it may involve compensatory increases in the hypothalamic hormone somatostatin, which can block the response of TSH to TRH. Since thyroid insufficiency may decrease growth rate, the serum thyroxine levels should be determined about twice a year during HGH treatment. Glucocorticoid dosage in patients with multiple pituitary deficiencies should be kept as low as possible to minimize adverse effects on growth.

PROLACTIN. The sustained estrogen excess of pregnancy induces such a marked prolactin cell increase that at term the weight of the gland has nearly doubled. This enlarged pituitary seems especially vulnerable to ischemic infarction following severe postpartum hemorrhage. After postpartum shock sufficient to produce extensive pituitary necrosis, a woman does not lactate, presumably because of inadequate prolactin secretion. Such patients are deficient in other anterior pituitary hormones as well. Prolactin deficiency may be verified by the failure of TRH to induce a sharp increase in serum levels of prolactin.

General investigation of pituitary problems

VISUAL FIELD DEFECTS. Because the optic chiasm lies above the diaphragma sellae, an upward-extending pituitary tumor often produces a visual defect by pressure on this part of the visual pathway. This defect, usually a bitemporal hemianopia, results from compression of the crossing central fibers of the chiasm; the uncrossed lateral fibers are spared. A wide variety of visual field defects have been observed in such patients, but the usual earliest changes are enlargement of the blind spot, loss of color vision (especially for red), and a wedge-shaped area of decreased vision in the upper temporal quadrant that gradually enlarges to occupy the full temporal field. Most patients with extensive visual defect have primary optic atrophy. Although papilledema is rare, it may develop with large tumors that cause increased intracranial pressure. If the pressure in the visual pathway is relieved early enough, the visual fields may return to normal, often dramatically a few hours after surgery.

ROENTGENOGRAPHY OF PITUITARY TUMORS. An intrasellar tumor slowly expands the pituitary fossa and destroys or distorts the clinoid processes. Calcification in the suprasellar region is common in craniopharyngiomas, and thickening of the tuberculum sellae may result from a suprasellar meningioma. Computed tomography or air encephalography can show the degree to which the tumor has become suprasellar.

The subarachnoid space may expand into the pituitary fossa if there is a defect in the diaphragma sellae. The pituitary fossa thus may gradually enlarge. This enlargement may simulate a tumor, even producing a visual field defect by herniation of the optic chiasm and nerves into the sella. In these patients, even though the pituitary gland is compressed from above, there is usually no pituitary insufficiency. Computed comography can usually detect the presence of cerebrospinal fluid in the pituitary fossa, which is characteristic of the empty-sella syndrome. Pneumoencephalography also reveals considerable air in the pituitary fossa rather than the expected tumor tissue. This latter technique should probably be reserved for cases that cannot be diagnosed with computed tomography.

An aneurysm of the internal carotid artery may also expand the pituitary fossa from within. Carotid angiography may be required to exclude an aneurysm or meningioma.

Microadenomas within a nondistorted sella turcica on conventional roentgenography may be diagnosed with polytomographic techniques. Minimal bony roentgenographic changes can be detected in the floor and walls of the sella harboring a microadenoma. There is still much to be learned about normal variation in the roentgenographic anatomy with this technique. New high-resolution computed tomography scanners can detect some intrasellar microadenomas by either visualizing the tumor or showing a shift in the pituitary stalk.

Treatment of patients undergoing pituitary surgery

Before a patient with a pituitary tumor is operated on, accompanying adrenal or thyroid hypofunction must be treated. A typical protocol includes 100 mg of hydrocortisone intramuscularly 1 hour before surgery. Intraoperatively and postoperatively, 100 mg of hydrocortisone as the water-soluble hemisuccinate or phosphate in 1 L of glucose is given intravenously at a rate of approximately 100 ml per hour. The usual total dose is 300 mg over the first 24 hours. On subsequent days the glucocorticoid dosage can be reduced and given intramuscularly, 50 mg of hydrocortisone every 6 hours on the second day and 25 mg every 6 hours on the third day. By the fourth day the patient can be given hydrocortisone, 10 mg every 6 hours orally, and by the fifth day (if there have been no complications) maintenance with 20 to 30 mg of hydrocortisone in divided doses can be instituted.

The safest way to assess postoperative pituitary function is to compare serum thyroid hormone determinations with the preoperative values. If the operation has not produced hypothyroidism, pituitary resection has probably spared at least one fourth of the gland. If thyroid studies remain normal, adrenal steroid supplementation can probably be withdrawn, but this should be done cautiously, since selective corticotropin deficiency may be present.

It is essential that the patient with permanent hypopituitarism be convinced of the importance of proper treatment of the adrenal insufficiency accompanying anterior pituitary failure. Patients should obtain a Medic-Alert bracelet showing that they are taking hydrocortisone or prednisone because of pituitary insufficiency. Adjustment of steroid dosage to meet increased requirements during illness, stress, or surgery should be emphasized. The first symptom of relative adrenal insufficiency is nausea, which calls for a doubling of the usual steroid dosage until the situation is clarified. A portable injection kit of soluble hydrocortisone should be obtained for emergency use. Through such adjustments patients with pituitary insufficiency can lead vigorous lives.

Conditions simulating hypopituitarism

ANOREXIA NERVOSA. Because of superficial similarities and their respective clinical features, anorexia nervosa and adiposogenital dystrophy may be mistaken for organic pituitary disease. Anorexia nervosa is seen chiefly in psychoneurotic adolescent girls and is characterized by amenorrhea and extreme emaciation in the absence of any organic disease (Fig. 186-4). Until the patient is close to starvation, she remains active and hostile. When the syndrome is well developed, the body temperature is often subnormal and the pulse rate and blood pressure are low. Serum T_3 levels are reduced because of a decreased peripheral deiodination of T_4. An increase in reverse T_3 indicates a deflection of the normal peripheral disposal of T_4.

Amenorrhea is largely the result of hypothalamic dysfunction and may also be perpetuated by malnutrition. Resumption of normal menses usually does not occur until the patient's weight has returned to a sufficient level.

Effective treatment is based on the concept that the disorder is primarily psychiatric with secondary endocrine and metabolic manifestations. Psychotherapy to reduce conflict with the environment should be attempted only after extreme emaciation has been overcome, which sometimes requires duodenal or parenteral feeding. During the period of refeeding, the patient may become edematous. In general young patients respond more quickly with sympathetic, supportive handling. The older the patient and the longer she has had her symptoms, the more difficult and unsatisfactory is the treatment. There is an appreciable mortality rate in this condition from infection and suicide. Anorexia nervosa also occurs in males, although rarely.

ADIPOSOGENITAL DYSTROPHY. A more common form of emotionally engendered nutritional disturbance in males is adiposogenital dystrophy. It is seen in obese boys who have moderately delayed puberty. Less often, a similar clinical picture is produced by a tumor in the suprasellar region that causes hypogonadism and that by pressure on the hypothalamus produces hyperphagic obesity.

In the functional type of adiposogenital dystrophy the

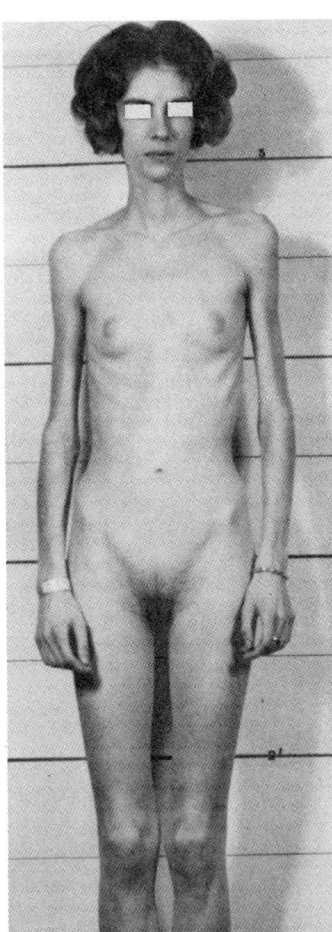

Fig. 186-4. Nineteen-year-old female with anorexia nervosa (see text). (From Ezrin, C., Godden, J.O., and Volpé, R.: Systematic endocrinology, ed. 2, New York, 1979, Harper & Row, Publishers.)

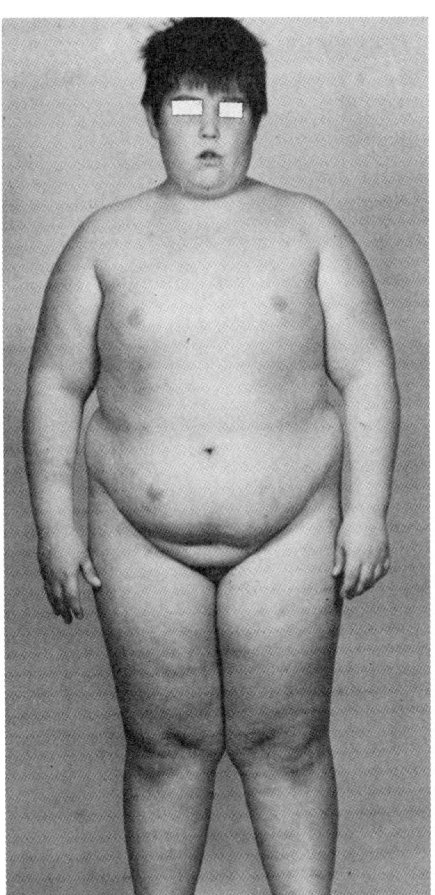

Fig. 186-5. Adiposogenital dystrophy in 16-year-old male (see text). (From Ezrin, C., Godden, J.O., and Volpé, R.: Systematic endocrinology, ed. 2, New York, 1979, Harper & Row, Publishers.)

obesity is usually associated with psychologic maladjustment. Evidence of thyroid or adrenal insufficiency should strongly suggest organic disease. In obese adolescent boys the genitalia often seem unduly small because the phallus is partly hidden by suprapubic fat (Fig. 186-5). They usually require only caloric restriction supplemented by a structured exercise program. Most of these boys later mature into normal fertile men, with the obesity often disappearing spontaneously.

Diseases of the posterior pituitary—diabetes insipidus

The antidiuretic hormone vasopressin is required to maintain the normal osmotic pressure of plasma. Increased plasma osmolality associated with dehydration stimulates "osmoreceptors" in the anterior hypothalamus, causing the neurohypophyseal terminals of the supraopticohypophyseal tract to release vasopressin into the general circulation. In the kidney vasopressin acts on the distal renal tubules and collecting ducts to increase reabsorption of water. Deficiency of or unresponsiveness to vasopressin causes diabetes insipidus, characterized by water diuresis and secondary polydipsia. It is usually associated with neurohypophyseal disease but also may arise from hypothalamic disorders.

ETIOLOGY. The known causes of diabetes insipidus can be divided into hereditary, traumatic (including postsurgical), inflammatory, and degenerative. A large number of cases appear to be idiopathic. Hereditary diabetes insipidus, a rare disorder, is thought to be caused by the failure of the supraoptic nuclei to develop sufficiently to produce adequate amounts of antidiuretic hormone. Another rare inherited variant, nephrogenic diabetes insipidus, results from the failure of the kidney to respond to vasopressin. With head injury the pituitary stalk may be torn without any associated skull fracture. Metastatic lesions in the hypothalamus or neurohypophysis may interfere with the production or delivery of vasopressin. Lithium and the antibiotic demeclocycline may produce a type of nephrogenic diabetes insipidus. A similar end-organ resistance to vasopressin accounts for the polyuria that may be seen with hypercalcemia and hypokalemia.

Chest and bone roentgenograms help diagnose sarcoid and eosinophilic granulomata, important causes of diabetes insipidus. The most useful diagnostic test is the serum osmolality, determined after 8 hours of fluid deprivation. Normal subjects successfully maintain their osmolality in spite of the challenge of dehydration. A random measurement of serum osmolality may give significant diagnostic information, since patients with psychogenic polydipsia may have a slight degree of water intoxication, whereas subjects with diabetes insipidus may be somewhat behind in their fluid replacement and therefore have a slightly higher than normal serum osmolality.

MANAGEMENT. A nasal spray of lysine-vasopressin may relieve polyuria for a few hours, but the limited effect of this therapy is a considerable drawback. The synthetic, long-acting vasopressin analog 1-deamino-8-D-arginine-vasopressin (DDAVP), given intranasally twice daily, provides good control of diuresis. This drug appears to be the treatment of choice. A less convenient therapy is the intramuscular administration of long-acting vasopressin in oil; 1 ml (containing 5 units) is usually given about three times a week.

In both nephrogenic and ordinary diabetes insipidus, thiazide diuretics paradoxically may act as antidiuretics. Additional potassium may be required to prevent hypokalemia in these patients. Vasopressin-responsive diabetes insipidus can also be treated with chlorpropamide, carbamazepine, or clofibrate, which either release small amounts of residual vasopressin or amplify the action of antidiuretic hormone at the renal level. The dosage of chlorpropamide varies from 125 to 500 mg daily. However, hypoglycemia may complicate this treatment, particularly in patients who have associated anterior pituitary disease.

Injudicious overtreatment resulting in too much water retention can be dangerous and sometimes fatal, particularly postoperatively with the production of serious cerebral edema.

PINEAL GLAND

The pineal gland may play a role in neuroendocrine control of the pituitary gland and in some circadian rhythms. There are important photic stimuli to the pineal gland; the visual information in the retina travels through the midbrain and reaches the pineal gland via sympathetic fibers. Darkness activates the sympathetic nerves and periods of light lead to a decrease in sympathetic activity. The pineal hormone, melatonin (5-methoxy-N-acetyl tryptamine), is produced during periods of darkness. The function of the pineal gland is unknown, but of clinical importance is the possibility of pineal calcification and tumor formation. Tumors that destroy the pineal gland can cause precocious puberty, and melatonin-synthesizing tumors may inhibit gonadal function.

BIBLIOGRAPHY

Bishop, P.M.: Clomiphene, Br. Med. Bull. **26**:22, 1970.
Blackwell, R.E., and Guillemin, R.: Hypothalamic control of adenohypophyseal secretions, Annu. Rev. Physiol. **35**:357, 1973.
Bloch, H.J., and Joplin, G.F.: Some aspects of radiological anatomy of the pituitary gland and its relationship to surrounding structures, Br. J. Radiol. **32**:527, 1959.
Crooke, A.C.: Induction of ovulation with gonadotropins, Br. Med. Bull. **26**:17, 1970.
Ezrin, C.: Hypophysis (pituitary gland), illustrated by Netter, F.H. In Endocrine system and selected metabolic diseases, Ciba Collection of Medical Illustrations **4(1)**:3, 1965. Ezrin, C., Kovacs, K., and Horvath, E.: Hyperprolactinemia: morphologic and clinical considerations, Med. Clin. North Am. **62**:393, 1978.
Ezrin, C., Horvath, E., and Kovacs, K.: Anatomy and cytology of the normal and abnormal pituitary gland. In De Groot, L.J., editor: Endocrinology, vol. 1, New York, 1979, Grune & Stratton, Inc.
Guyda, H.J., and others: Medical Research Council of Canada therapeutic trial of human growth hormone: first 5 years of therapy, Can. Med. Assoc. J. **112**:1301, 1975.
Hardy, J.: Transsphenoidal surgery of hypersecreting pituitary tumors. In Kohler, P.O. and Ross, G.T., editors: Diagnosis and treatment of pituitary tumors, New York, 1973, American Elsevier Publishers Inc.
Hershman, J.M.: Use of thyrotropin-releasing hormone in clinical medicine, Med. Clin. North Am. **62**:313, 1978.
Kreiger, D.T., Amarosa, K., and Linick, F.: Cyproheptadine-induced remission of Cushing's disease, N. Engl. J. Med. **293**:893, 1975.
Lawrence, A., Pinsky, S.M., and Goldfine, I.D.: Conventional radiation therapy in acromegaly: review and reassessment, Arch. Intern. Med. **128**:369, 1971.
McGregor, A.M., and others: Reduction in size of a pituitary tumor by bromocriptine therapy, N. Engl. J. Med. **300**:291, 1979.
Mortimer, C.H., and others: Gonadotropin releasing hormone therapy in hypogonadal males with hypothalamic pituitary dysfunction, Br. Med. J. **4**:617, 1974.
Robinson, A.G.: DDAVP in the treatment of central diabetes insipidus, N. Engl. J. Med. **294**:507, 1976.
Spark, R.E., Dickstein, G., and Pallotta, J.: Complete remission of acromegaly with medical treatment, J.A.M.A. **241**:573, 1979.
Tolis, G., and others: Pituitary hyperthyroidism, Am. J. Med. **64**:177, 1978.
Tyrrell, J.B., and others: Cushing's disease: selected transsphenoidal resection of pituitary microadenomas, N. Engl. J. Med. **298**:753, 1978.
Veldhuis, J.D., and Hammond, J.M.: Endocrine function after spontaneous infarction of the human pituitary: report, review, and reappraisal, Endocr. Rev. **1**:100, 1980.

187 • THE THYROID GLAND

Thomas F. Nikolai

ANATOMY

The thyroid gland (Fig. 187-1) is a relatively small structure lying low in the anterior neck. It is H or butterfly shaped, containing two lobes connected by an isthmus. The isthmus usually lies over the second and third rings of the trachea with the lobes lying along the anterolateral and lateral aspect of the trachea, although not infrequently it may be much lower in the neck and occasionally it may

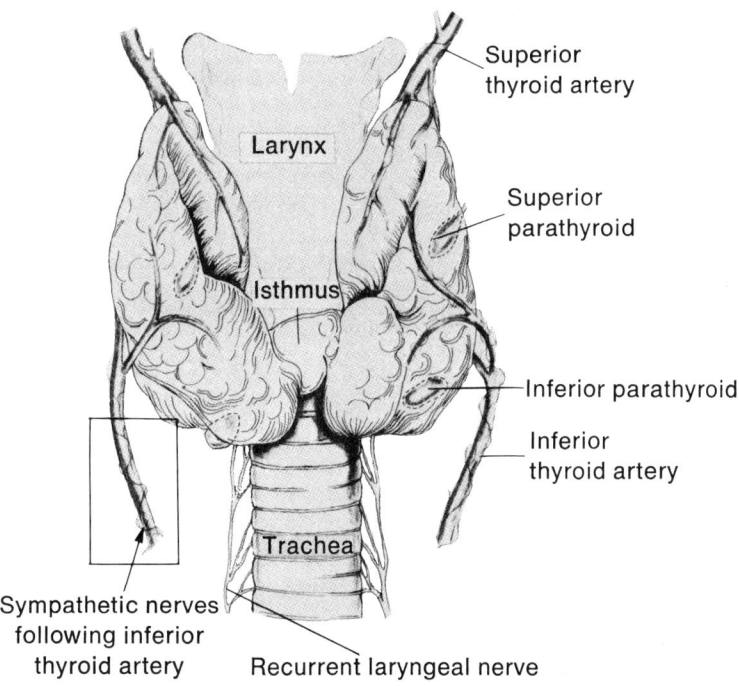

Fig. 187-1. Normal thyroid anatomy.

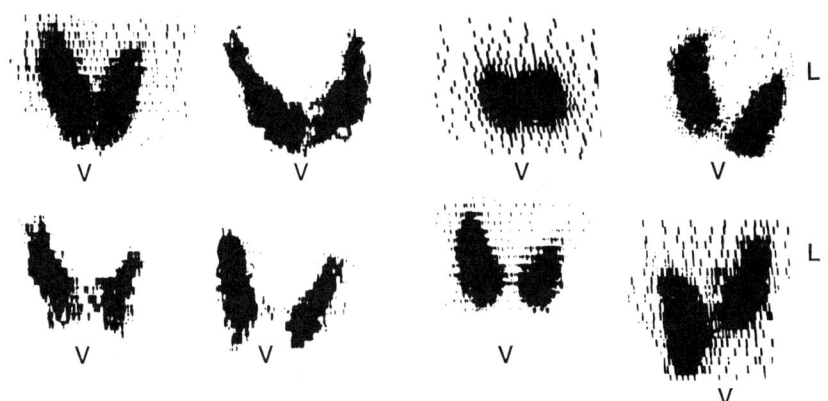

Fig. 187-2. Variation in size and shape of normal human thyroid by radioactive iodine (^{131}I) scanning.

be partially substernal. A pyramidal lobe juts upward from the isthmus in about 25% of individuals. The size of the thyroid is substantially smaller now than 20 to 30 years ago, probably as a result of the increase in iodine in the diet. In adults the thyroid weighs 16.7 ± 6.9 g, and the lobes measure 2 to 2.5 × 2 to 2.5 cm in width and thickness and 3.5 to 4 cm in height. The thyroid in females is larger than that in males by 5% to 10%. The child's thyroid weighs about 1.5 g at birth and reaches adult size by 15 to 19 years of age. There are minor differences in size and shape among normal thyroids (Fig. 187-2). The normal thyroid tissue is soft to slightly firm in consistency. Its surface is usually smooth, slightly lobulated, covered by a thin, fibrous capsule, and attached to adjacent structures by loose connective tissue.

The blood supply, which is extremely rich (4 to 6 ml/min per gram of thyroid tissue, about twice as much blood per gram as the kidney tissue receives), comes from the right and left superior thyroid arteries off the common carotid artery and the inferior thyroid arteries off the subclavian artery. Venous drainage occurs through the thyroid veins into the jugular system. An extensive lymphatic vascular system is also present. Innervation is supplied by the adrenergic and cholinergic autonomic nervous systems arising from the cervical sympathetic ganglia and following the arteries into the thyroid and the vagus nerves through the superior and inferior laryngeal nerves. The main function of the nerve supply of the thyroid is to regulate blood flow. The adrenergic fibers terminate at the basement membrane and may directly affect function of the follicular cell through the release of bioactive amines.

The four parathyroid glands (Fig. 187-1) lie on the back side of the thyroid, two near the superior poles and two near the inferior poles. They sometimes lie inside the capsule of the thyroid and occasionally are actually embedded within the thyroid tissue, not being visible on gross examination of the thyroid. The recurrent laryngeal nerve also lies on the posterior or medial posterior side of the thyroid lobes alongside the trachea, although its location may vary considerably.

HISTOLOGY

The lobes and isthmus of the thyroid are comprised of numerous lobules, each with its own blood, lymphatic, and nerve supply and each further divided into 20 to 40 follicles. Interspersed among the follicles are perifollicular light or "C" cells that produce calcitonin. They constitute only about 5% of the total cell population of the thyroid. Recently cells that produce somatostatin have been identified in the thyroid. The follicles are the main functional units, producing thyroxine (T_4) and triiodothyronine (T_3). They are spheroidal structures surrounded by follicle cells, about 200 to 300μm in size, and filled with pinkstaining colloid that is almost all stored thyroglobulin (TG). The size of the follicle and the amount of colloid present in each follicle are inversely related to the activity of the gland. The individual follicle cell tends to be small and cuboidal or somewhat flattened when less active and elongated from base to apex when stimulated. Electron microscopy has shown the relationship between the synthetic sequence of thyroid hormone and the anatomy of the follicle cell. Biosynthesis of noniodinated TG protein occurs in the ribosome. The TG then enters the ergastoplasmic vesicles and is transported to the Golgi apparatus where the carbohydrate moiety is added. Next it is transported in secretory droplets to the microvilli where it is released in the colloid.

CHEMISTRY

The thyroid gland's role in the body is the production of thyroid hormone in quantities sufficient to meet the needs of the whole organism. It produces two biologically active hormones: the iodothyronines (L-triiodothyronine[T_3] and L-thyroxine[T_4]) and the iodotyrosines (monoiodotyrosine[MIT] and diiodotyrosine[DIT]). The structures of these compounds and closely related compounds and metabolic products are shown in Fig. 187-3.

The iodothyronines are composed of two ether-linked benzene rings with a hydroxyl group at position 4' and an alanine side chain at position 1. T_4 has four iodine atoms. Deiodination at position 5 is the reaction that produces the majority of T_3. Tetrac (3,5,3',5'-tetraiodothyroacetic acid) and triac (3,5,3'-triiodothyroacetic acid) are produced by peripheral metabolism of thyroid hormones and have slight biologic activity, with more in some species than in others.

Another compound produced in the thyroid and containing three iodine atoms, 3,3',5'-triodothyronine (reverse T_3, RT_3), is metabolically inactive. Many similar compounds that have organic or halogen substitutions on the benzene ring or fatty acid substitutions for the end alanine have been synthesized and have biologic activity ranging from 1% to 617% of that of T_4.

Extrathyroidal iodine metabolism

Iodine is unique to the thyroid because it is the only substrate needed for hormone production that is not used by other tissues. Approximately 50μg of iodine is needed daily to maintain normal thyroid hormone biosynthesis. In recent years the iodine content of American diets has greatly increased so that the average person is ingesting 300 to 500 μg each day (much more in countries such as Japan where seafood is a major portion of the diet). Therefore iodine deficiency does not exist today in most of the world. Iodine is rapidly and efficiently absorbed from the gastrointestinal tract with little lost in the stool. The normal thyroid contains a large reserve (about 10 mg) of iodine, sufficient to provide iodine supplies for up to 6 months if none is ingested. Ninety-five percent of the thyroid iodine is present in colloid stores. In the plasma, iodine is present in two forms, as inorganic iodide not bound to serum proteins (1 to 1.5μg/dl) and as iodothyronines (T_4 and T_3) that are mainly bound to plasma proteins (4 to 8μg/dl) and are hormonally active.

The thyroid extracts iodine from the serum by an efficient trapping mechanism that normally concentrates iodide up to a 20:1 gradient between the thyroid and plasma. This trapping mechanism is stimulated by thyroid-stimulating hormone (TSH), is dependent on sodium, potassium, and magnesium ions, is blocked by thiocyanate, perchlorate, and iodides, and is slowed by hypopituitarism. Although iodide trapping also occurs to a much lesser extent in the salivary glands, stomach, breasts, and choroid plexus, iodothyronine synthesis does not occur in these tissues except for a minimal amount by mammary tissue. Most iodine not taken up by the thyroid, and that diffusing from the thyroid gland, is promptly lost in the urine. About the same amount of iodide absorbed is excreted in the urine each day except for 3% to 5% excreted in the stool, sweat, and expired air. Substantially more may be excreted by lactating women or in certain disease states such as those associated with heavy proteinuria or gastrointestinal malabsorption.

The kidney and the thyroid readily clear most of the ingested and recycled iodide from the serum. The renal clearance is about twice that of the thyroid.

Synthesis of thyroid hormones

The synthesis of thyroid hormones involves the uptake and use of iodine and amino acids to form the iodothyro-

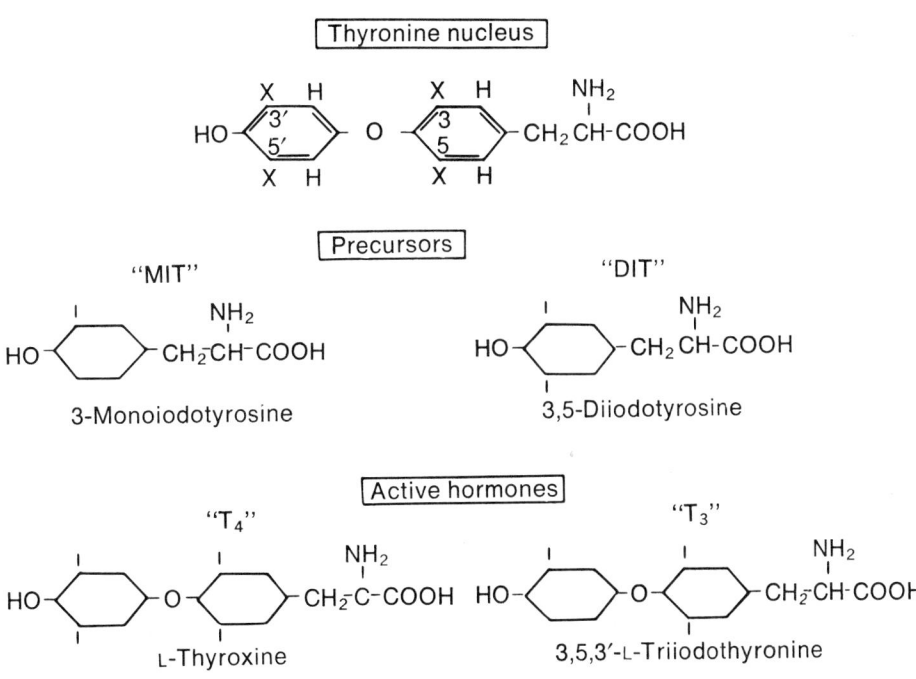

Fig. 187-3. Thyroid hormones and related compounds.

nines, T_4 and T_3, and the receptor protein TG. The sequence of synthesis of thyroid hormones is shown schematically in Fig. 187-4.

Iodine circulating in plasma is concentrated at the follicle cell surface by the iodide trapping mechanism against an electrical gradient and then is transported into the cell. The energy required to concentrate iodine is supplied by high-energy phosphate bonds. In the follicle cell the iodine is oxidized to a higher energy state by hydrogen peroxide derived from an ill-defined hydrogen peroxide–generating system that uses NADPH as a coenzyme. In this very reactive state the iodine readily reacts with the amino acid tyrosine, which is attached to TG, and the iodotyrosyl compounds MIT and DIT, which are formed under the influence of peroxidase enzyme. Whether the initial iodination of the tyrosine-TG complex occurs in the follicle cell lumen in the apex of the microvilli adjacent to the colloid or after exocytosis into the colloid is unknown. Oxidative coupling of MIT and DIT molecules attached to TG occurs to form T_3, T_4, and minute amounts of RT_3, probably catalyzed by the same peroxidase. TG at this point has approximately 120 molecules of MIT, DIT, T_3 and T_4 attached to it. The iodide trapping mechanism is influenced by multiple factors of which TSH seems to be the most important. TSH enhances iodide trapping by the thyroid, and hypophysectomy decreases it. Marked increases in the thyroid/plasma iodide ratio up to several hundred-fold have been reported in diffuse toxic goiter and in animal glands highly stimulated by TSH. Iodide trapping is inhibited by thiocyanate and perchlorate ions that in high concentrations also inhibit organic binding. The iodination of tyrosine is also stimulated by TSH and reduced by hypophy-

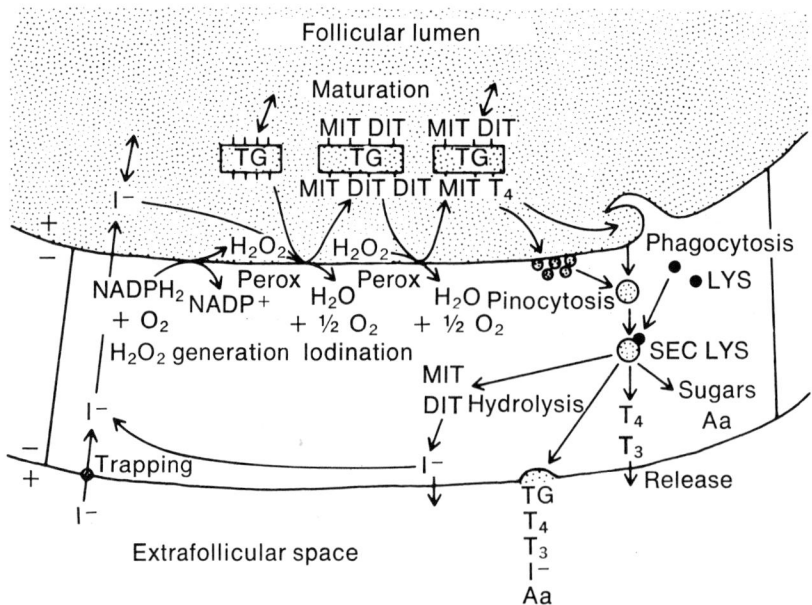

Fig. 187-4. Model of iodine metabolism in thyroid follicle. Follicular cell is shown facing follicular lumen *(stippled area)* and extracellular space *(lower part)*. Sequence of events shown has been largely documented. However, the possibility of active iodide transport at apex of cell or of intracellular iodination and the relative roles of pinocytosis versus phagocytosis and of diffusion versus secretion of thyroid hormones remain controversial. *Perox,* peroxidase; *TG,* thyroglobulin; *MIT,* monoiodotyrosine; *DIT,* diiodotyrosine; *LYS,* lysosome; *SEC LYS,* secondary lysosome; *Aa,* amino acids; + and −, electric charge of membranes (see text). (From Van Herle, A.J., and others. Reprinted by permission of the New England Journal of Medicine, **301,** 239, 1979.)

sectomy. The antithyroid drugs propylthiouracil and methimazole block iodination of tyrosine and also the coupling of MIT and DIT to form the iodotyrosines. An internal autoregulatory control of iodine metabolism called the Wolff-Chaikoff effect causes a block in the thyroid peroxidase system when excess iodide is present.

Storage and secretion of thyroid hormones

The colloid provides the organism with a large hormone reservoir that would last 3 to 4 months if no more thyroid hormone were made. If the thyroid is completely blocked by antithyroid agents, it takes as long as 2 weeks for any noticeable decrease in serum T_4 and an increase in TSH to occur. T_4 accounts for about 35% of the organic iodine content of the thyroid, and T_3 accounts for 5% to 8%. TG is the storage form of thyroid hormone. Secretion of thyroid hormone begins when colloid droplets are taken up by the follicular cell by phagocytosis. These colloid droplets are digested by proteases present in lysosomes. Once freed from TG, T_4, T_3, and RT_3 are secreted into the plasma and the MIT and DIT are deiodinated and recirculated. The TG molecule is broken down, first by reduction of disulfide bonds by glutathione and then by proteolysis. The iodine and tyrosine are reused in the metabolic cycle of the follicular cell. Microtubules are apparently involved in the secretory process, since inhibitors of these, namely colchicine and vincristine, block secretion of T_4 and T_3. Microsomal iodotyrosine dehalogenase is responsible for the separation of iodide from MIT and DIT and thus prevents these compounds from appearing in plasma. Very small amounts of TG leak out of the thyroid through the lymphatic system in normal individuals, and increased amounts occur in the plasma of patients with nontoxic goiter, hyperthyroidism, certain congenital goiters, thyroid malignancy, radiation thyroiditis, and subacute thyroiditis and from manipulation during thyroid surgery. Lysis of TG and secretion of T_4 and T_3 are inhibited by iodine and lithium.

There is little else in the colloid other than TG. TG is a 19S glycoprotein containing about 10% carbohydrate. It has a molecular weight of 660,000. Each TG molecule contains approximately 120 molecules of MIT (17% to 28%, DIT (24% to 42%), T_4(35%) and T_3(5% to 8%). Natural TG is distinctly heterogeneous between different species and to some extent even within the same animal species. Under the control of TSH, synthesis of TG occurs in the rough endoplasmic reticulum of the follicular cell, where the carbohydrate portion is also added. It then moves through the Golgi apparatus to the apex of the cell in the microvilli and into the colloid by exocytosis. A different iodoprotein has been found in very small quantities in normal thyroids and in larger quantities in thyroid disorders such as hyperthyroidism, nontoxic goiters, endemic goiter, and Hashimoto's thyroiditis. This protein has electrophoretic mobility similar to that of serum albumin. Congenital defects of TG synthesis lead to deficient thyroid hormone production and goiters.

Peripheral binding, metabolism, and physiologic effects of thyroid hormones

BINDING. On entering the blood, T_4 and T_3 are largely bound to the serum proteins thyroxine-binding globulin (TBG), thyroxine-binding prealbumin (TBPA), and thyroxine-binding albumin (TBA) in a reversible association. TBG and TBA bind both T_4 and T_3, but TBPA binds only T_4 (possibly a minor amount of T_3). Because of extensive binding of thyroid hormone by these proteins, the serum levels of thyroid hormone fluctuate with the levels of the proteins.

Both TBG and TBPA have only one binding site for T_4 on each molecule. Barbital, salicylate, penicillin, and 2,4-dinitrophenol inhibit thyroid hormone binding to TBPA. TBA poorly binds both T_4 and T_3. The functions of the thyroid-binding proteins are multiple. In combination with T_4 and T_3 they achieve a macromolecular size that results in little renal excretion of T_4 and T_3, providing a large metabolically inert reservoir, The interaction between thyroid-binding proteins and thyroid hormone is expressed by TBG and T_4 as follows:

$$T_4 + TBG \rightleftarrows T_4 - TBG$$

Since interaction strongly favors the bound form (T_4-TBG), only 0.02% to 0.03% of T_4 exists in a free form. Because T_3 has less affinity for TBG, 0.3% or about 10 times more than T_4, exists in free form. Only the free thyroid hormones are available to the peripheral tissues because the T_4-TBG complex is too large to leave the vascular system. Therefore the metabolic effects of thyroid hormone are due to the small amount of unbound or free hormone. As will be discussed later in the chapter, there are numerous factors and disease states that affect the concentration of thyroid-binding protein.

METABOLISM. T_4 and T_3 are deiodinated to inactive metabolites in the liver and kidney and probably in many other body tissues as well. It is generally agreed that the majority of T_3 in the blood comes from peripheral conversion of T_4 and that very little is synthesized within the thyroid itself. Since T_3 and RT_3 have more rapid clearance rates than T_4, their serum concentrations are much lower than that of T_4. Most T_3 and RT_3 is derived from extrathyroidal deiodination of T_4. Hypothyroid patients receiving T_4 replacement only and unable to produce any thyroid hormone of their own maintain near normal serum ratios of T_4, T_3 and RT_3, indicating indirectly that the amount of T_3 and RT_3 coming from the thyroid is relatively small.

Low T_3 syndrome. Abnormalities of peripheral T_4 and T_3 metabolism have been labeled the low T_3, reverse T_3, or sick euthyroid syndrome. The deiodination of T_4 to T_3 is depressed in certain situations, including total starvation, semistarvation (carbohydrate and protein but not lipid), acute infection, stress, many chronic diseases (pulmonary, cardiac, hepatic, renal, and neoplastic), and use of certain drugs. This results in decreased peripheral T_3 production and lowers the serum T_3 concentration frequently to subnormal levels. A gradual corresponding rise in the RT_3 concentration occurs as more T_4 is deiodinated through the T_4-to-RT_3 pathway. Not infrequently with this fall in serum T_3, the serum T_4 concentration slowly rises above normal, sometimes giving the false impression that the patient has hyperthyroidism. This phenomenon occurs within 36 to 48 hours of the start of acute starvation or illness and rapidly returns to normal with feeding or recovery.

This same change occurs in the full-term fetus and also is found in the cord blood at birth, probably related to immature deiodinating enzyme systems in the fetus and the neonate. Within a few hours after birth the serum T_3 rises by 200% to 400% and the T_4 by 25% to 50%, and the RT_3 declines very slightly, apparently as a result of a transient increase in TSH. A number of drugs block the conversion of T_4 to T_3. They include corticosteroids, propranolol, propylthiouracil, sodium iopanate, sodium ipodate, and amiodarone. Interestingly, corticosteroids, propranolol, and propylthiouracil are used for the treatment of severe thyrotoxicosis and thyrotoxic crisis, and this newly discovered effect of suppression of T_4-to-T_3 conversion contributes further to their pharmacologic effect. They also have other effects on thyroid function that will be discussed later.

The low serum T_3 concentration occurring at birth, from acute and chronic illness, and from starvation is probably a normal response of the organism to these states and leads to a decreased regulation of body metabolism. Since serum levels of hormones do not reflect their intracellular or nuclear concentration, the serum changes cannot be assumed to reflect what is happening at the cellular level where hormonal action is manifested.

ACTION OF THYROID HORMONES. It is impossible to relate all the effects of thyroid hormones to a single mechanism. At the present time their effects can best be explained by multiple mechanisms induced by the free thyroid hormone levels presented to the target tissues. Most of the metabolic effects of the thyroid hormones are due to T_3, since T_4 is primarily a prohormone. The free thyroid hormone diffuses easily into the extracellular fluid and enters the cells where it is reversibly bound to sites on the cell surface and to proteins within the cells.

Table 187-1 summarizes the possible mechanisms of action of thyroid hormone. The occupancy of nuclear binding receptors is a prerequisite for many of the actions of T_3. The T_3-occupied nuclear receptor promotes synthesis of messenger ribonucleic acid (mRNA), which is a rate-limiting factor in protein synthesis. Fasting decreases nuclear receptors for T_3, suggesting a physiologic downregulation of cellular metabolism. T_3 receptors are also located on the inner mitochondrial membrane in thyroid hormone–responsive tissues and are absent in tissues not responding to thyroid hormone such as brain and testes. With T_3 binding, uncoupling of oxidative phosphorylation,

Table 187-1. Sites and mechanisms of actions of thyroid hormones

Site	Action
Cell nucleus	Stimulated mRNA synthesis
	Increases target cell protein synthesis
Mitochondria	Increases α-glycerophosphate dehydrogenase
	Promotes uncoupling of oxidative phosphorylation
	Incraeases ATP generation
	Increases O_2 consumption
Cell membrane	Stimulates Na^+, K^+, ATPase ("sodium pump")
Adrenergic receptor pathway	Increases number of receptors
	Amplifies β-adrenergic sygnal
Tyrosine metabolic pathway	Modifies metabolic pathway
	Acts as precursor for alternate adrenergic neurotransmitters

increased oxygen consumption, and ATP generation occur in isolated mitochondrial vesicles.

It has been long noted clinically that many manifestations of hyperthyroidism resemble excessive adrenal medullary or epinephrine-like activity and that the β-adrenergic blocking agent propranolol blocks these effects. However, increased catecholamine secretion from the adrenal medulla is not present. The proposed mechanism of this effect of thyroid hormone is an increase in the number of β-adrenergic cellular receptors and/or an amplification of the β adrenergic signal at the cell membrane. Another possible mode of action of thyroid hormone is that it functions as amino acid analogs of tyrosine. These analogs enter into and modify metabolic pathways in tyrosine metabolism and act as precursors for alternate adrenergic neurotransmitters. In the nervous system, T_3 is concentrated in peripheral adrenergic nerves and in certain areas of the brain.

Many other effects on the body are noted in thyroid disease states and probably are the result of the actions already discussed. The actions and metabolism of other hormones, including 21-carbon corticosteroids, cortisol, aldosterone, epinephrine, parathyroid hormone, and glucagon, are modulated by T_3. Temperature regulation is also affected by thyroid hormone: myxedematous animals die readily with cold exposure. Growth retardation in hypothyroid children and animals is readily reversed by thyroid hormone. Hyperglycemia is produced by excessive thyroid hormone, and hyperthyroidism depletes liver and muscle glycogen. Marked hypercholesterolemia with increase in phospholipids and total lipids occurs in hypothyroidism. Vitamin deficiencies are sometimes associated with hyperthyroidism, probably owing to increased requirements. Osteoporosis and osteomalacia occur in long-standing hyperthyroidism as a result of increased bone resorption and decreased vitamin D–potentiated intestinal absorption of calcium.

ANTITHYROID AGENTS. Goitrogens are chemicals that inhibit thyroid hormone synthesis or release, leading to compensatory increases in TSH and thyroid enlargement. These chemicals occur naturally in certain foods such as cabbage, turnips, kohlrabi, and rutabagas, which are rarely eaten in quantities sufficient to cause a problem. They contain some thiocyanate and progoitrogens (thioglucosidases), that must be activated by intestinal bacteria.

The antithyroid agents generally encountered in clinical practice are those used to treat hyperthyroidism and drugs used for other purposes that also affect thyroid function. Drugs used in the treatment of hyperthyroidism manifest their effect in two ways. Monovalent anions such as thiocyanate and perchlorate block iodine trapping by the thyroid, which is overcome by excessive amounts of iodides. They are rarely used today because of significant toxic effects such as irreversible aplastic anemia.

The second group of drugs blocks intrathyroidal iodination of tyrosine and the coupling reaction. A wide variety of these agents are known, but the only two used in the United States are the thioureas, methimazole and propylthiouracil.

Drugs such as iodides and lithium that are commonly used for the treatment of other diseases may affect thyroid function. Iodides under certain conditions block intrathyroidal hormone synthesis and lead to thyroid enlargement and hypothyroidism. Goiters and hypothyroidism develop in 20% to 30% of patients undergoing long-term lithium therapy, owing to depression of hormone release from the thyroid.

THE THYROID IN PREGNANCY. The rise in estrogen level that occurs in the first month of pregnancy causes increased liver synthesis of TBG. This results in increased binding and concentrations of T_4 and T_3, although the free concentrations of both hormones remain essentially unchanged. These estrogen-induced effects return to normal or non-pregnant levels in 3 to 4 weeks after delivery.

The thyroid gland may increase in size by 25% to 50% during pregnancy, and occasionally a bruit is heard over it, reflecting increased blood flow. This effect is due to iodine deficiency caused by an increased renal iodide clearance in pregnancy. It is much less frequent in recent years owing to the increased amount of iodine in the American diet.

T_3, T_4, and TSH do not cross the placental barrier. Therefore thyroid failure in the mother or fetus is not prevented by transplacental transfer of T_4 and T_3. However, the thioureas do cross the placental barrier and can cause fetal hypothyroidism if administered in inappropriately high doses to the mother. The thyroid-stimulating immunoglobulin (TSI) present in Graves' disease also crosses the placental barrier and can be the cause of temporary hyperthyroidism in the fetus at birth (neonatal hyperthyroidism).

TESTS OF THYROID FUNCTION AND CONCENTRATION AND BINDING OF THYROID HORMONES

Several methods exist for measuring thyroid function. Careful clinical assessment for thyroid disease should precede thyroid testing except in specific circumstances where testing will uncover abnormalities that are not obvious clinically. There are several diseases of the thyroid affecting different measures of thyroid function, as well as frequently associated changes in peripheral binding and metabolism of thyroid hormones, and no one test can consistently measure all these changes. In addition, many drugs affect thyroid function and the thyroid tests. Interpretation of the test results should be made in light of these factors before a diagnosis is made and treatment is begun.

RADIOACTIVE IODINE UPTAKE. The radioactive iodine uptake (RAIU) test directly measures the accumulation of iodine by the thyroid. Two radioactive isotopes of iodine (^{131}I and ^{123}I) are now in common use. ^{123}I has the advantages of a shorter half-life and lower levels of radiation. The thyroid is unable to distinguish between stable iodine (^{127}I) and its radioactive isotopes. The RAIU test is used in the diagnosis of hypothyroidism, hyperthyroidism, thyrotoxicosis factitia, biosynthetic defects of the thyroid, and thyroiditis. In recent years new factors have appeared that have diminished the usefulness of this test. The improvement in the measurements of thyroid hormone concentrations by radioimmunoassay and the knowledge of the peripheral metabolism and binding of thyroid hormones give more precise information that the RAIU. Even more important, the increasing content of iodine in the diet, primarily owing to food preservatives, has caused a progressive decline in the normal value of the RAIU. The normal uptake of RAIU at 24 hours was 25% to 50% 15 to 20 years ago and now is only 10% to 25%, but this varies considerably in different areas of the United States and the world, primarily because of the differing dietary iodine content.

The RAIU is dependent on the daily iodine intake, the serum inorganic iodide concentration, the rate of iodine turnover in the thyroid, and the urinary clearance of iodine. When ^{131}I is used, the uptake is measured by scintillation counter over the thyroid at 24 hours. However, measurements at 2, 4, and 6 hours are sometimes useful, especially in hyperthyroidism. The value obtained is the percentage of the dose, administered orally or intravenously, that is counted in the thyroid. Each institution performing this test must establish its own range of normal values.

The RAIU is increased in 80% to 90% of the cases of hyperthyroidism. The uptake at 2, 4, or 6 hours frequently is more diagnostic of hyperthyroidism because the uptake, conversion, and excretion of iodine may be so rapid in this disease that the amount of isotope retained in the thyroid at 24 hours is less than at the shorter intervals. The RAIU is sometimes increased in the failing thyroid gland (Hashimoto's thyroiditis), in iodine deficiency, in pregnancy (relative iodine deficiency owing to increased renal iodine clearance), immediately after recovery from thyroiditis, in congenital intrathyroidal enzyme defects, and in nephrosis (as a result of excessive loss of thyroid-binding proteins). It is decreased or suppressed by elevated concentrations of inorganic iodine, in hypothyroidism, in thyroiditis, and by exogenous thyroid hormone intake. An increase in the inorganic iodide pool decreases the RAIU by a dilutional effect in the serum and by the inhibitory effects of increased intrathyroidal iodine, as discussed previously. Measurement of the 24-hour urinary iodine excretion can help establish the presence of excessive body iodide stores, since levels greater than 1 to 1.5 mg strongly suggest increased intake of iodine.

The RAIU used alone is a poor test for hypothyroidism, and this test must be combined with TSH stimulation to be of value. In thyroiditis (either subacute or lymphocytic) the RAIU may be quite variable depending on the degree to which the thyroid is affected by this disease. It is suppressed when exogenous thyroid is taken in physiologic or greater quantities unless autonomous thyroid function exists. Organic iodides such as those used in roentgenographic dye also suppress the RAIU for varying periods of time relative to their rates of deiodination and excretion. Dyes administered for renal studies are usually excreted in 3 to 5 days, whereas those used for cholecystography may persist from 3 weeks to 3 months.

Measurement of the 24-hour absolute iodine uptake (AIU) will make the RAIU much more sensitive, although it infrequently needs to be used. The AIU is calculated as follows:

$$\text{AIU} = \frac{\text{24-hour urinary iodide } (\mu g/24 \text{ hr}) \times \% \text{ RAIU}}{\% \text{ 24-hour urine RAI content}}$$

The normal thyroid takes up 70 to 75 μg of idine each day. Values greater than this tend to indicate hyperthyroidism and reduced values indicate hypothyroidism.

THYROID SCAN. The thyroid scan provides useful information concerning localization, size, shape, and uniformity of function of the thyroid. The thyroid gland is first labeled with a radioactive isotope (^{123}I or technetium 99). Following this a scanner makes a visual image or graphic representation of the uptake of the isotope in the thyroid tissue. The principal values of the thyroid scan are to provide (1) localization and function of nodules present within the thyroid and (2) localization of functioning thyroid tissue present in ectopic locations such as the lingual area, neck nodes, substernal area, and metastatic foci in bone, liver, lung, ovaries, and so forth.

Although most techniques are incapable of localizing areas of dysfunction less than 1 cm in size, a new technique called the pinhole thyroid scan gives resolution of functional areas as small as 2 to 3 mm.

THYROID ULTRASONOGRAPHY. The thyroid is easily and quickly identified by ultrasound techniques. Ultrasound usually cannot detect lesions smaller than 1 cm in diameter. Its predominant use is to distinguish solid nodules from cystic nodules; this can also be done by simple percutaneous needle aspiration. In addition, aspiration can provide cells for cytologic examination.

T_4 TEST. Several methods have been developed in the past 15 years to measure serum T_4 concentrations more precisely. These include column chromatography, competitive protein-binding analysis, and radioimmunoassays. Since the column chromatography method does not afford complete separation of T_4 when high concentrations of iodine are present, it has generally been discarded. The competitive protein-binding assay is much more precise because of the specificity of the interaction between T_4 and TBG that is the basis of the test procedure. However, because it requires 3 to 4 hours and several different steps, it has essentially been replaced by the radioimmunoassay for T_4, which is performed in one step in about 1½ hours. The normal values are 5 to 12 µg/dl. T_4 concentrations are increased in hyperthyroidism and elevated TBG states and decreased in hypothyroidism and low TBG states.

T_3 TEST. The T_3 assay procedure is quite similar to the T_4 radioimmunoassay. The normal values are 100 to 184 ng/dl. T_3 levels have been shown to decrease by about one third by 70 to 80 years of age. T_3 concentrations usually parallel T_4 changes in hypothyroidism and hyperthyroidism and with TBG change. As previously described, in the low T_3 syndrome T_3 levels decrease owing to a block in the peripheral T_4-to-T_3 metabolism. This may be caused by many acute and chronic illnesses and certain drugs. In T_3 thyrotoxicosis the thyroid gland overproduces only T_3, resulting in an elevated serum T_3 with a normal T_4 concentration.

FREE T_4 (FT_4) AND FREE T_3 (FT_3) TESTS. Since the free or unbound concentrations of T_4 and T_3 are correlated with their biologic effect, ways to measure the free levels have been sought. However, their concentrations are too low to be measured directly, and therefore an indirect dialysis method using radioactive-labeled T_4 or T_3 has been developed. Since the FT_4 test is relatively expensive and somewhat complicated and time consuming, its use in clinical medicine is not yet widespread. The FT_3 test is available only in research laboratories.

T_3 UPTAKE TEST. The T_3 uptake (T_3U) test measures the number of binding sites on the thyroid-binding proteins (TBG, TBPA, and TBA) that are unoccupied and serves as an index of the proportion of FT_4. Radioactive-labeled T_3 (T_3 ^{131}I) is added to a serum sample and allowed to saturate all the free binding sites present. An absorbent material such as a resin sponge is next added to take up the excess labeled T_3. The percentage of labeled T_3 attached to the absorbent material is calculated. T_3 uptake by the resin method gives normal values of 34% to 46%.

Excess binding sites are present in hypothyroidism because the T_4 is low and the TBG is less saturated. Therefore the T_3U is decreased, since more labeled T_3 can attach to TBG binding sites. The opposite occurs in hyperthyroidism. When elevated concentrations of TBG are present, as occurs in pregnant or estrogen-stimulated women, more unbound TBG sites are present and take up more labeled T_3, resulting in a low T_3U. Opposite changes occur with decreased TBG concentrations.

TBG TEST. Abnormalities in the concentration of TBG are frequently encountered in clinical practice, leading to substantial changes in the T_4, T_3, and T_3U test results. This can result in a false diagnosis of thyroid disease. The TBPA concentration is much less variable and rarely leads to abnormalities in these tests. Although a radioimmunoassay has been developed for TBG, the usual method of assay is to measure the T_4 binding capacity of this protein. There are many factors other than thyroid disease that can alter levels of TBG. They include the following:

Increase	Decrease
Estrogens	Chronic illness (diabetes, liver disease, renal disease, and so on)
Pregnancy	
Oral contraceptives	
Neonatal state	Androgens
Acute hepatitis	Other anabolic steroids
Genetic (X-chromosome linked)	Glucocorticoid (large dose)
Acute intermittent porphyria	Genetic (X-chromosome linked)
Idiopathic	Idiopathic
Fluorouracil	Starvation
Marijuana abuse	

The most common cause of low TBG is chronic disease states such as diabetes, mellitus, liver disease, and renal insufficiency. The usual cause of an increased TBG is a hyperestrogen state such as pregnancy, oral contraceptive therapy, or estrogen replacement therapy. However, it is rarely necessary in clinical practice to assess TBG binding capacity, since typical changes in the T_4 and T_3U occur from TBG increase or decrease. Simply stated, when hyperthyroidism or hypothyroidism is present, the T_4 and T_3U are elevated or depressed together, respectively. When TBG increase is present, a reciprocal change occurs (T_4 increases and T_3U decreases), and the reverse is true for TBG decrease (T_4 decreases and T_3U increases). Knowledge of these changes has resulted in the development of the free thyroxine index.

FREE THYROXINE INDEX. Since the free concentrations of T_4 and T_3 determine their biologic activity, their measurement is helpful, especially when abnormalities in the concentration of TBG are present as noted previously. Since the FT_4 method is expensive and cumbersome, an indirect method of calculating the free T_4 concentration called the free thyroxine index (FT_4I) has been developed. The FT_4I equals the product of the T_4 and T_3U. The normal values are 1.5 to 5.5. The FT_4I may be the easiest and cheapest measurement of the free T_4 level. Studies have shown that this index remains normal when the T_4 is elevated or decreased from TBG changes because of the reciprocal changes that occur in the T_3U. A similar calculation can be used to determine the free triiodothyronine index (FT_3I) from the product of the T_3 concentration and the T_3U.

TESTS THAT MEASURE THYROID-REGULATING FACTORS

TSH measurement and TRH stimulation test. The measurement of TSH or thyrotropin by radioimmunoassay is in common use in most medical centers and reflects the level of pituitary TSH stimulation of the thyroid. Normal TSH values are 0 to 8 $\mu U/ml$. The pituitary output of TSH responds inversely to the serum thyroid hormone levels and is stimulated by thyrotropin-releasing hormone (TRH) under negative feedback control through the hypothalamus and pituitary. There is no diurnal rhythm of TSH. High levels are seen in the neonate during the first 72 hours after birth and in primary hypothyroidism. In certain thyroid diseases such as lymphocytic thyroiditis, in goiter resulting from iodine excess or deficiency, or in the gland reduced in size by surgery or radioactive iodine therapy, elevations of serum TSH are present even when serum T_4 and T_3 concentrations are still normal because excess stimulation of the gland is required to maintain normal thyroid function. The TSH assay is useful to the clinician in three ways. First, it is helpful in distinguishing primary hypothyroidism (high levels of TSH) from pituitary or hypothalamic hypothyroidism (decreased levels) (Fig. 187-5). In this situation it has largely replaced the TSH stimulation test. Second, in primary hypothyroidism it is used to assess the adequacy of thyroid replacement, since elevated TSH levels should return to normal with proper replacement. Low TSH levels are also seen in hyperthyroidism except in the rare case of a TSH-producing pituitary tumor. It is debatable whether serum TSH levels should be measured in all cases of hyperthyroidism to spot this rare occurrence.

Lastly, the TSH assay is used to assess the response to TRH stimulation. TRH stimulation is helpful in (1) directly assessing pituitary TSH reserve; (2) detecting suppressed pituitary TSH resulting from excess serum thyroid hormone concentrations; and (3) differentiating between pituitary and hypothalamic hypothyroidism. From 200 to 500 μg of TRH is given intravenously, and the output of TSH is measured before and at different time intervals after the TRH is given. The maximal or peak response is usually seen between 20 and 40 minutes after TRH administration but can be delayed up to 60 minutes in hypothalamic disease. There is a gradual decline in the TSH response to TRH with age in men but not in women. Increased responses are seen in patients with hypothyroidism, and decreased responses are seen in hyperthyroidism. The TRH test's chief diagnostic value and use are in detecting states of thyroid hormone excess that suppress pi-

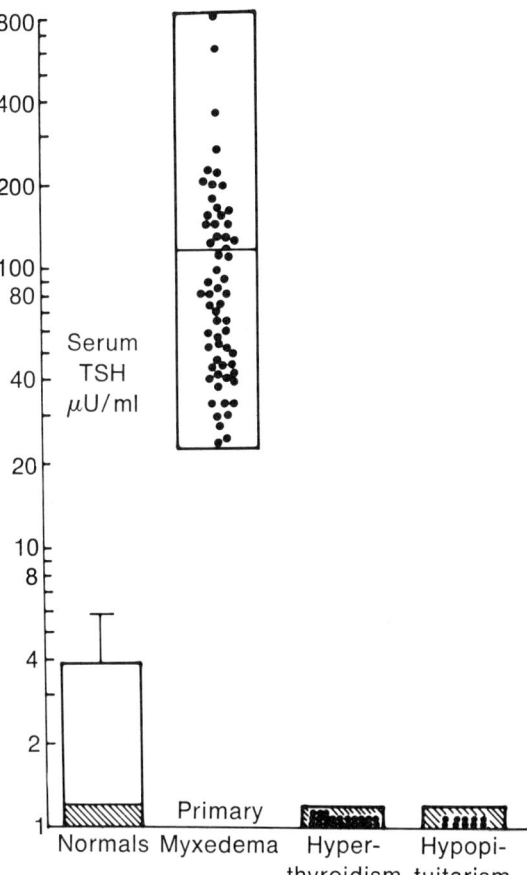

Fig. 187-5. Serum thyrotropin *(TSH)* in normal individuals (vertical bar shows standard deviation) and those with primary myxedema, hyperthyroidism, and hypothyroidism resulting from hypopituitarism. (From Hershman, J.M., and Pittman, J.A., Jr.: Ann. Intern. Med. 74:482, 1971.)

tuitary TSH. This test is very sensitive to slight increases in the T_4 and T_3 serum concentrations. Partial to complete suppression of the TSH response to TRH occurs with T_4 and T_3 levels within the normal range, although slightly in excess of what is normal for that individual. This test has largely replaced the T_3 suppression test because it is quickly performed and is safer.

TSH stimulation test. The TSH stimulation test detects the thyroid's ability to respond to TSH by an increase in the RAIU and the output of T_4 (and T_3). As usually performed, a 5- to 10-unit dose of TSH is injected intramuscularly after measurement of the RAIU, and the RAIU is measured again 24 hours later. The TSH stimulation dose is sometimes repeated 2 or 3 days in a row to ensure that maximal stimulation of the thyroid has occurred. The 1-day test dose is adequate in most instances. This test is useful in (1) detecting a decrease in thyroid reserve that occurs in the failing thyroid gland, (2) differentiating the suppressed thyroid resulting from increased concentrations of thyroid hormone from the damaged thyroid present in different forms of thyroiditis, and (3) differentiating primary hypothyroidism from pituitary and hypothalamic hypothyroidism caused by TSH deficiency. This test requires considerable time and may be dangerous in the elderly patient, and it is used much less frequently today because measurement of TSH and the TRH stimulation test give similar information as discussed previously.

T_3 suppression test. Thyroid hormone given in physiologic or pharmacologic quantities will completely suppress the normal thyroid by suppressing the hypothalamic pituitary axis, causing decreased TSH secretion. This can be measured by a decrease in the RAIU and the serum T_4 concentration (if T_3 is used to suppress). This phenomenon forms the basis of the thyroid suppression test in which 75 to 100 μg of T_3 is given orally for 7 to 10 days and the RAIU or the T_4 or both are measured before and after the T_3 is taken. Failure of suppression of the thyroid indicates autonomous function of the thyroid gland. This autonomy may be due to the thyroid stimulating immunoglobulin (TSI) present in Graves' disease or residing in the thyroid in nontoxic and toxic uninodular and multinodular goiter. The chief value of this test lies in its help in sorting out the different presentations of Graves' disease, such as the euthyroid form with exophthalmos, and in testing for the suppressability in nontoxic goiter. Since the TRH stimulation test gives similar information, the T_3 suppression test is used much less frequently today.

THYROID AUTOANTIBODIES. Five types of thyroid autoantibodies have been demonstrated: thyroglobulin antibody, microsomal antibody, colloid antibody, antinuclear antibody, and thyrotropin receptor antibody or TSI.

The two tests for these antibodies in general use are the antithyroglobulin and antimicrosomal methods. Low titers of antibodies occur in about 6% of normal individuals without evidence of thyroid disease. There is a gradual increase in frequency with age. A relatively high percentage of individuals with Graves' disease (35% to 50%), primary hypothyroidism (45% to 80%), and Hashimoto's thyroiditis (71% to 92%) have positive tests for thyroid autoantibodies, and these are all considered to be autoimmune thyroid diseases. The antimicrosomal antibodies are more likely to be present in higher concentration in all these diseases. Very high titers usually occur in patients with Hashimoto's thyroiditis and are probably diagnostic. Antibodies to the TSH receptor (TSI) stimulate the follicular cells in the same fashion as TSH. They will be discussed further under "Diffuse toxic goiter." The presence of thyroid autoantibodies must be interpreted in the light of the whole clinical picture; their presence alone is rarely meaningful unless other clinical or laboratory abnormalities of thyroid disease are present.

THYROID BIOPSY AND ASPIRATION CYTOLOGY. Thyroid tissue obtained by small open biopsy or percutaneous needle biopsy may be extremely valuable in establishing the correct diagnosis of a thyroid disorder. It is helpful in distinguishing between the different types of thyroiditis, between benign and malignant thyroid neoplasms, and between different types of nontoxic goiter.

The percutaneous needle biopsy is relatively easily done with the patient under local anesthesia. A Vim-Silverman-Franklin or True-Cut needle is used. The needle biopsy can be performed as an outpatient procedure and has a minimal morbidity risk. A small open biopsy can be done with the patient under local or general anesthesia and is generally better because a larger, more representative tissue specimen is obtained.

Aspiration of thyroid nodules suspected of harboring malignancy is being done with increasing frequency. The advocates of this procedure state that it has reliable diagnostic accuracy, does not spread cancer, and results in much less thyroid surgery. A small-gauge needle is passed into the nodule, and cells from the nodule are obtained by aspiration. The cells are classified by the cytologist as nonmalignant, malignant, or indeterminate. Patients with malignant or indeterminate cytology are subjected to thyroid surgery. The result is that two thirds of the patients who would ordinarily have had thyroid surgery are shown to have benign disease and are simply treated with thyroid suppression therapy.

CLINICAL ASSESSMENT OF THYROID FUNCTION

Thyroid disease is usually manifested by typical systemic symptoms and signs and/or by enlargement or irregularity of the thyroid gland with or without associated local neck symptoms. A carefully taken history and examination are the starting point of clinical assessment. Suspected or obvious thyroid disease can be substantiated by appropriately directed thyroid function studies.

Hypothyroidism

Hypothyroidism is a clinical disease state occurring when insufficient thyroid hormone is available to tissue sites of action. The severity of the hormone deficiency and the length of time it is present determine the extent of the clinical disease. Myxedema is a severe form of hypothyroidism. Cretinism results from severe hypothyroidism in the fetus or neonate.

ETIOLOGY. Hypothyroidism can be classified by age of onset and by etiology. Separation according to age is important because the clinical presentation varies substantially among the infant, the juvenile, and the adult. Hypothyroidism in the infant includes all cases in neonates until 4 to 5 years of age when brain development is complete. The juvenile period encompasses the 5- to 18-year age group until growth and sexual maturation are complete. All cases thereafter are classified as adult hypothyroidism. Endemic iodine deficiency, which previously was the most common cause of hypothyroidism in all age groups throughout the world, is still present in certain parts of the world but rarely occurs in the developed nations owing to iodine supplementation. The causes and incidence of hypothyroidism in the infant have been clearly established by mass screening of neonates. In 1977 the Newborn Screening Committee of the American Thyroid Association, after reviewing a number of screening studies, noted that 166 cases of permanent congenital hypothyroidism were found in 730,000 newborn infants for an incidence of 1 in 4400 births. About 85% of the affected infants had thyroid agenesis, about 10% had thyroid dysplasia with only a remnant of thyroid tissue in normal or ectopic location, and most of the rest had TSH deficiency owing to a sporadic or familial hypothalamic-pituitary disorder. In the same studies additional cases of decreased thyroid reserve in euthyroid infants manifested as low normal serum T_4 and elevated TSH concentrations were found. These averaged one case for every four or five cases of hypothyroidism. They are believed to represent mild defects in thyroid hormone synthesis or decreased tissue response to TSH or thyroxine. An occasional infant has hypothyroidism and goiter at birth as a result of maternal drug ingestion, usually methimazole or propylthiouracil taken for treatment of hyperthyroidism.

The causes of hypothyroidism are usually similar in the juvenile and the adult. The most frequent of these are idiopathic atrophy, chronic lymphocytic thyroiditis, and loss of tissue owing to thyroidectomy or radioactive iodine treatment. The incidence in juveniles is between 4 and 12 per 10,000. In adults the incidence is 5 to 8 cases per 1000 new patients seen. The causes are idiopathic atrophy or chronic lymphocytic thyroiditis in 60% to 70% and tissue loss from radioactive iodine therapy or thyroid surgery in about 30%. Between 50% and 80% of the patients with thyroid atrophy have significantly elevated thyroid antibody titers, suggesting that chronic lymphocytic thyroiditis is a factor in the thyroid failure. Less than 10% of cases are related to hypothalamic pituitary disease from Sheehan's syndrome, pituitary adenoma, craniopharyngioma, empty-sella syndrome, head trauma, and hypothalamic disease. TSH deficiency usually occurs in association with other pituitary hormone deficiencies. TRH deficiency as a cause of hypothyroidism is quite rare. It may occur as an isolated defect or in association with defects of other hypothalamic releasing hormones, secondary to intracranial neoplasms, serious head trauma, or central nervous system infection. Rare cases of hypothyroidism are due to ingestion of goitrogens (found in cabbage and some other vegetables). Iodine ingestion results in goiter and hypothyroidism in a few patients who do not escape the inhibitory effect of iodine on organic binding. Patients with chronic lymphocytic thyroiditis, Graves' disease, and radiation thyroiditis are more susceptible to this effect.

Females are more susceptible to almost all thyroid diseases. The neonatal screening programs have shown a 4:1 female to male preponderance. In juveniles and adults two to six females are affected for every male. Certain types of hypothyroidism such as that caused by chronic lymphocytic thyroiditis are inherited or occur with high frequency in some families. Peripheral resistance to thyroid hormone and intrathyroidal enzyme defects usually occur by autosomal recessive inheritance.

CLINICAL MANIFESTATIONS. At all ages the initial manifestations of hypothyroidism are very subtle and may be clinically nonevident or easily overlooked. The signs and symptoms listed below progress gradually in relation to the severity of the thyroid hormone deficiency.

General
Coarse or hoarse voice
Decreased growth (juvenile)
Weight gain (slight)
Psychomotor slowing
Hypokinesia
Somnolence
Cold sensitivity
Fluid retention
Mental retardation (infant)
Cretinoid facies (infant)

Skin and appendages
Decreased sweating
Decreased sebaceous activity
Thickened skin with hyperkeratosis
Coarse hair
Diffuse hair loss
Thick tongue

Cardiovascular
Bradycardia
Increased diastolic blood pressure
Narrow pulse pressure
Decreased cardiac output
Peripheral vasoconstriction
Enlarged heart

Respiratory
Hypoventilation

Gastrointestinal
Constipation
Decreased stooling rate
Abdominal distention
Increased gaseousness

Endocrine
Menorrhagia
Hypomenorrhea or amenorrhea
Decreased fertility
Impotence and oligospermia
Galactorrhea

Hematopoietic
Anemia

Neuromuscular
Weakness
Muscle cramps
Paresthesias
Peripheral neuropathy
Hypotonia
Ataxia
Incoordination

When thyroid hormone is withheld from athyreotic individuals, signs and symptoms of hypothyroidism may begin within 2 weeks and are present in all within 3 or 4 weeks. Frank myxedema is present within 6 to 8 weeks. Usually, however, the progression of hypothyroidism is much slower and more insidious so that the patient can seldom give an approximate date for the onset of symptoms. In patients with a history of previous radioactive iodine therapy or thyroid surgery or with fatigue, myalgias, arthralgias, weight gain, hypersomnolence, cold intolerance, hoarseness, constipation, normochromic and normocytic anemia, growth retardation, delayed puberty, menstrual abnormalities, and mental sluggishness, hypothyroidism should be suspected.

In infants typical characteristics gradually develop. These infants feed poorly, are lethargic and hypersomnolent, and move infrequently. Severe constipation and abdominal distention are almost always present. Hypoventilation, episodes of cyanosis, and choking are common. A large tongue may add to frequent respiratory difficulties. The skin is dry and coarse. An umbilical hernia is sometimes found. Carotenemia and prolonged icterus neonatorum occur. Hypothermia, bradycardia, and low pulse pressure are present. A goiter occurs if thyroid tissue and excess TSH are present. Within a few months of birth these signs and symptoms progress rapidly. Linear growth failure, delayed closure of the fontanelles, muscular hypotonia, and delayed relaxation of the deep tendon reflexes develop. All developmental stages are delayed. Intellectual retardation begins. The typical appearance of short stature with increased trunk-to-limb ratio; large head; broad, flat nose with widely set eyes; sparse, coarse hair; thick, dry skin; enlarged, protruding tongue; protuberant abdomen; and mental deficiency develops with time, resulting in the classic picture of cretinism.

In juveniles the principal features of hypothyroidism different from those found in adults are the development of growth retardation with increased trunk-to-limb ratio and delay in sexual maturation. These children become lethargic and less active. Although some mental sluggishness may develop, intellectual deterioration does not occur. When hypothyroidism is severe, linear growth and bone development essentially stop.

As hypothyroidism progresses at all ages, almost all areas of the body are affected with progression to full-blown myxedema (Fig. 187-6). This consists of mental sluggishness, sallow complexion, edematous-appearing facies, coarse voice with slow speech, and very dry, coarse skin. A goiter may or may not be present. If present it usually indicates excess TSH secretion and primary thyroid failure. The thyroid tissue that is present, whether of normal size or enlarged, is frequently substantially firmer than normal and bosselated, very suggestive of chronic lymphocytic thyroiditis. The speech is thick, slow, and sometimes slurred. The skin becomes dry, coarse, and cool. Marked pallor may develop as a result of associated anemia. Sweating and sebaceous activity are decreased. The lips appear puffy, pale, and dry. The pulse is slow and regular with decreased pulse pressure. Hypertension occasionally develops. Increased heart size may occur as a result of pericardial effusion. There may be abdominal distention, flatulence, and constipation, sometimes leading to fecal impaction. Mental sluggishness with poor memory, drowsiness, and personality changes gradually develops. Occasionally an organic psychosis (myxedema madness) results. Peripheral neuropathy, manifested by paresthesias and pain (usually have a burning character) in the extremities associated with ataxic gait, occurs. Although obese patients are often referred to endocrinologists for evaluation of possible hypothyroidism, not more than two thirds of hypothyroid patients gain weight and the weight gain is rarely more than 10 or 15 pounds.

Menstrual disorders sometimes occur in hypothyroid women. Most commonly, prolonged excessive bleeding results, but irregular menstrual periods, amenorrhea, and hypomenorrhea can also occur. Muscle aching and stiffness frequently occur. Galactorrhea with hyperprolactinemia is being reported with increasing frequency. Muscles sometimes appear hypertrophic and are quite firm and inelastic. Delayed relaxation of the deep tendon reflexes develops. Occasionally, if the diagnosis is overlooked for months, hypoventilation and extreme lethargy result. The patient must be stimulated to respond. Patients with severe myxedema eventually lapse into coma and die if untreated.

LABORATORY FINDINGS. The finding of a low T_4 level is common in all forms of hypothyroidism unless an elevated TBG concentration is present. In this instance the FT_4I ($T_4 \times T_3U$) will correct for the TBG change and show a low T_4. The FT_4 is also low. The level of protein-bound iodine (PBI) is usually low but may be normal or elevated if abnormal iodinated materials are present in the serum from exogenous sources or from diseases such as chronic lymphocytic thyroiditis in which abnormal iodinated proteins are released from the damaged thyroid into the blood.

The TSH should invariably be determined in hypothyroidism. In the majority of instances it is elevated, confirming primary hypothyroidism. If the TSH is normal or low (the radioimmunoassay for TSH, which is available in most laboratories, does not distinguish between normal and low values), pituitary or hypothalamic (secondary or tertiary) hypothyroidism must be considered.

The TRH stimulation test can distinguish between primary, secondary, and tertiary forms of hypothyroidism. In

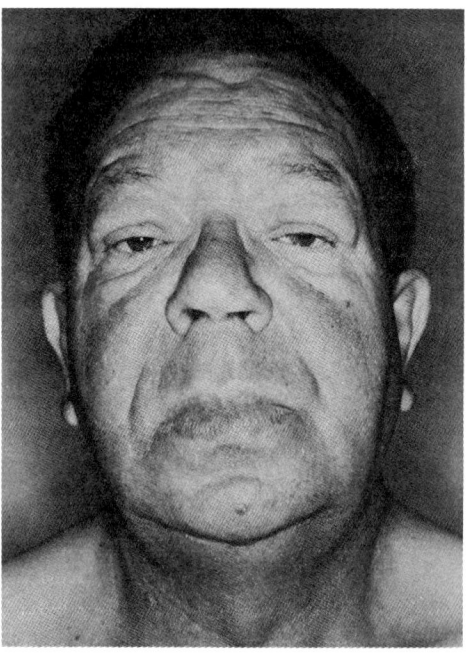

Fig. 187-6. Patient with classic features of myxedema. Note pale edematous appearance of facies with thick lips and puffy eyelids.

primary hypothyroidism the elevated serum TSH excessively responds to intravenously administered TRH (200 to 500 μg). In contrast, in pituitary hypothyroidism the normal or low serum TSH does not respond to TRH administration. In hypothalamic hypothyroidism the low or normal TSH responds normally, although sometimes sluggishly. The maximal response in the TSH may not occur until 1 hour after TRH administration, whereas normally the peak TSH response occurs at 20 to 30 minutes.

The RAIU test may be depressed to below 10% in hypothyroidism, but its diagnostic accuracy is not good enough to be used as a test for hypothyroidism. However, the RAIU does not respond to TSH stimulation in primary hypothyroidism because the thyroid is already being maximally stimulated by endogenous TSH. In pituitary TSH deficiency and hypothalamic TRH deficiency the RAIU responds to TSH stimulation and thus can be used to provide differentiation from primary hypothyroidism. However, in recent years, because of the availability of TRH and the ease of the TRH stimulation test, this test has largely replaced the TSH stimulation test in the diagnosis of hypothyroidism.

As previously noted, thyroid autoantibody titers are elevated in a high percentage of patients with idiopathic thyroid atrophy and in a higher percentage of patients with hypothyroidism and chronic lymphocytic thyroiditis. Other tests formerly used, the basal metabolic rate (BMR) and the Achilles reflex time, have been replaced by the more precise tests described above.

Anemia, which is usually normocytic and normochromic but occasionally macrocytic, occurs in about half of the advanced cases. When macrocytic anemia is present, the coexistence of pernicious anemia must also be considered. The serum cholesterol level is frequently elevated above 300 mg/dl, but this is of little diagnostic value because it is often elevated from other causes.

The electrocardiogram frequently shows bradycardia, low voltage, and inverted or low T waves. In severe myxedema, enzymes from muscle tissue such as creatinine phosphokinase (CPK), aldolase, and serum glutamicoxaloacetic transaminase (SGOT) may be elevated. Hyperprolactinemia, occasionally in the presence of galactorrhea, is not uncommon but is not usually measured. A low serum iron level, decreased iron binding capacity, elevated uric acid level, rapid sedimentation rate, and carotemia may be present. The serum proteins show minor changes such as slightly elevated β-globulin levels, slightly decreased albumin and γ-globulin levels, and slightly increased TBG binding capacity.

DIFFERENTIAL DIAGNOSIS. On occasion severe anemia, nephrotic syndrome, or Cushing's syndrome may have superficial resemblance to myxedema. In nephrosis the T_4 may be low because of abnormal metabolism of T_4 as well as excessive urinary excretion of TBG-T_4 complex. Measurement of the T_3 uptake, FT_4I, and TSH are needed for differentiation of these two diseases, and occasionally the TRH stimulation test may be necessary. Patients with neurasthenia and anorexia nervosa frequently are quite hypometabolic, and thyroid failure must be ruled out by multiple thyroid function tests. Liver disease also may cause hypometabolism and decreased or elevated serum proteins, resulting in decreased or elevated TBG levels and abnormal T_4 serum concentrations.

MANAGEMENT. Several preparations are available for replacement therapy in hypothyroidism. These medications include pure T_3, mixtures of T_3 and T_4, and pure T_4 (Table 187-2). They are all rapidly absorbed and are relatively inexpensive. They do not cause allergic reactions and have no side effects except hypermetabolic symptoms if excess amounts are given. Dosage requirements increase with body size, as noted in Table 187-2. Equivalent doses of the different preparations are also given in Table 187-2.

The need for thyroid hormone may decrease slightly with age and increase somewhat with stress and infection, although rarely is it necessary to adjust the dosage under these circumstances. The amount of thyroid hormone given to restore the euthyroid state varies among individuals but usually lies within the amounts noted in Table 187-2. The level at which replacement therapy should be started and the rate at which it should be increased vary depending on the severity and duration of the hypothyroidism and associated illnesses. Infants can be given a full replacement dose immediately. If a patient has had hypothyroidism for a short time and is young and healthy oth-

Table 187-2. Preparations of thyroid hormones

	Preparation	Composition	Equivalent dose	Usual daily requirement	Absorption (%)
T_3	L-Triiodothyronine	Pure T_3	25 μg	59–75 μg	85
	Desiccated thyroid	20–30 μ T_4, 7–11 μg T_3	60 mg	120–180 mg	50–70
T_3-T_4	Thyroglobulin	20–30 μg T_4, 7–11 μg T_3	60 mg	120–180 mg	50–75
combination	Synthetic liotrix (two products)	50 μg T_4 and 12.5 μg T_3; 60 μg T_4 and 15 μg T_3	1 tablet	2–3 tablets	70–80
T_4*	L-Thyroxine	Pure T_4	50–75 μg	120–200 μg	50–80

*Infants' and children's T_4 dosage should be calculated by body weight as follows:
0–1 yr: 9 μg/kg/day   6–10 yr: 4 μg/kg/day
1–5 yr: 5 μg/kg/day   11–20 yr: 3 μg/kg/day

erwise, replacement also can start at full dosage immediately. However, in those with hypothyroidism of moderate severity of many months' duration, initial dosage should be about one-fourth to one-third full dosage (50 to 75 μg of T_4) and increased by one fourth to one third at 10- to 14-day intervals until the euthyroid state is reached. In the elderly and those with associated serious disease, only about 25 μg of T_4 should be given initially and then the dosage should be increased by the same amount at 2- or 3-week intervals. The patient should be monitored carefully for aggravation of underlying disease or new problems each time before the dosage is increased.

Adequacy of replacement therapy is judged by several criteria. Although clinical judgment is very subjective, most clinicians continue to increase the amount of thyroid hormone until all signs and symptoms of the hypothyroid state have disappeared. More reliable criteria are the restoration of the T_4 to normal (usually 8 to 10 μg/dl) and suppression of the elevated TSH to normal.

In infants it is important to start thyroid replacement within the first few weeks of life to prevent mental retardation. Recent studies have demonstrated that if thyroid hormone is started by 3 months of age, mental retardation is unlikely. Retardation does occur and is progressive if treatment is delayed longer than 3 to 6 months. In the juvenile, treatment results in catch-up growth and normal physical and sexual development, although some decrease in stature may be the outcome if hypothyroidism has been present longer than 2 or 3 years.

In the past the most commonly used preparation of thyroid hormone was desiccated thyroid. Desiccated thyroid (thyroid extract) is an extract of animal thyroid gland and is standardized according to iodine content (0.2%). Thyroglobulin is a purified porcine protein whose biologic activity is measured by its ability to inhibit propylthiouracil-induced goiter in rats. It has been shown that the iodine content of these animal preparations varies considerably and does not reflect the T_4 and T_3 content well. In addition, the proportion of T_4 to T_3 varies among different batches of the extracted hormone.

When the synthetic T_3 and T_4 combinations became available, they were used frequently. However, there is no need to give T_3 and T_4 together, since there is substantial peripheral metabolism of T_4 to T_3 and steady serum T_4 and T_3 levels are easily maintained in the normal range throughout the day with adequate T_4 replacement alone. Furthermore, T_4 and T_3 combinations cause the serum T_3 level to peak substantially above normal each day between 2 and 8 hours after the daily dose is given. Thus it appears that the pure T_4 preparations are preferable for replacement therapy.

TRANSIENT HYPOTHYROIDISM. Transient hypothyroidism is not infrequent, and if it is unrecognized, lifelong thyroid replacement therapy may be given inappropriately. It occurs on recovery from subacute thyroiditis and following discontinuation of thyroid hormone that has been given to a patient with a normal thyroid gland for obesity, fatigue, or other reasons. Transient hypothyroidism can be the presenting feature of lymphocytic thyroiditis. It can also follow recovery from silent thyroiditis, a transient form of hyperthyroidism associated with lymphocytic thyroiditis (a postpartum association is common). The hypothyroidism in most of these patients is mild, and spontaneous recovery occurs within 6 to 8 weeks. Therefore patients with mild degrees of hypothyroidism should be observed for several months before instituting therapy or treatment should be limited to 3 to 6 months.

MYXEDEMA COMA. Myxedema coma is frequently fatal and must be treated promptly and aggressively. It usually occurs in elderly patients with prolonged hypothyroidism. Infection, cold exposure, trauma, and central nervous system depressants are frequent predisposing factors. Untreated hypopituitarism may mimic this condition. The clinical state varies from extreme lethargy, hypersomnolence, and impaired consciousness to deep coma. It is characterized by subnormal temperature (as much as 14° F [10° C] below normal at times), bradycardia, hypotension, and hypoventilation. Laboratory tests usually reveal a very low T_4 and FT_4I, elevated TSH, depressed arterial Po_2, and elevated Pco_2. Severe dilutional hyponatremia similar to the inappropriate ADH syndrome is not uncommon. Therapy should be started promptly with T_4 (500 μg intravenously) to replace the severe peripheral thyroid hormone deficit. Because relative adrenal insufficiency may be present owing to severe myxedema, hydrocortisone (100 mg intravenously) is given initially and repeated in doses of 25 to 50 mg every 6 hours thereafter. Hypertonic intravenous fluids and glucose are needed, but the fluids should be given judiciously to avoid fluid overload and resultant congestive heart failure. Assisted respiratory support with oxygen therapy is usually necessary. Further heat loss should be prevented by the use of blankets. Rapid rewarming should not be done. Intravenous T_4 (50 to 150 μg daily) should be continued until the patient is responding and can take it orally. The initial response to this type of treatment program begins within 24 hours with increase in body temperature and improvement in the vascular state.

Hyperthyroidism

Hyperthyroidism is a clinical hypermetabolic disorder produced by excessive secretion of thyroid hormone and its effect on peripheral tissues. The term "thyrotoxicosis" is frequently used interchangeably with hyperthyroidism, although technically thyrotoxicosis includes other states in which excessive thyroid hormone levels and action are present from sources other than the thyroid such as exogenous thyroid hormone intake. The following is a classification of thyrotoxicosis:

I. With elevated RAIU
  A. Diffuse toxic goiter (Graves' disease)
  B. Toxic multinodular goiter (Plummer's disease)
  C. Toxic uninodular goiter (toxic adenoma)
  D. Excess TSH production
    1. Pituitary tumor
    2. Autonomous pituitary function
    3. Excessive TRH secretion
  E. Tumor producing thyroid stimulators
    1. Hydatidiform mole and choriocarcinoma of uterus owing to excess human chorionic gonadotropin
    2. Embryonal carcinoma of testes
    3. Other malignancies
II. With suppressed RAIU
  A. Excess exogenous intake of thyroid hormone
    1. Factitious hyperthyroidism
    2. Iatrogenic hyperthyroidism
  B. Thyroiditis with transient hyperthyroidism
    1. Subacute thyroiditis
    2. Lymphocytic thyroiditis
  C. Iodide-induced hyperthyroidism (Jod-Basedow disease)
  D. Metastatic follicular carcinoma of the thyroid
  E. Struma ovarii

Diffuse toxic goiter, toxic multinodular goiter, toxic uninodular goiter, lymphocytic thyroiditis (a transient hyperthyroidism), and the thyrotoxicosis secondary to excessive exogenous intake of thyroid hormone given for thyroid suppression or replacement therapy account for 98% to 99% of all cases of hyperthyroidism. When there is a clinical impression or suspicion of hyperthyroidism, this should be substantiated by elevated serum T_4 and T_3 concentrations, a high T_3U, and elevated free thyroid indices (FT_4I and FT_3I). Hyperthyroidism is associated with an excess of both T_4 and T_3 except in three situations: (1) the occasional patient with T_3 hyperthyroidism, (2) hyperthyroidism associated with low T_3 syndrome, and (3) hyperthyroidism associated with low TBG. T_3 thyrotoxicosis with normal T_4 levels has been found in diffuse toxic goiter, toxic multinodular goiter, and toxic uninodular goiter. It appears that in some of these patients the onset of hyperthyroidism is first manifested by T_3 overproduction, but only after several weeks or months does excessive T_4 production occur. In one study T_4 and T_3 elevations were found in 87.5% of hyperthyroid patients, with the rest having only elevated T_4 levels. A normal serum T_3 concentration may be due to reduced peripheral T_4-to-T_3 conversion owing to associated acute and chronic illness. The TRH test may be used to help differentiate this form of hyperthyroidism from normal. Low TBG concentration, if present with hyperthyroidism, may result in normal T_4 and T_3 concentrations, but this association can be easily determined by noting a very high T_3U and elevated FTI.

Once the diagnosis of thyrotoxicosis appears established by the clinical impression and the finding of elevated serum concentrations of T_4 and T_3, the specific cause should be sought so that appropriate therapy can be given. An RAIU test should be performed in all patients except pregnant women to determine whether they have high or low RAIU, as outlined previously. Further differentiation will be outlined later as the individual disease entities are discussed.

CLINICAL MANIFESTATIONS. The severity of the illness caused by thyrotoxicosis is related to the severity and duration of the hormone excess, the age of the patient, and the presence or absence of other disease. Like hypothyroidism, hyperthyroidism affects almost all body systems, as listed below:

General
Weight loss
Irritability
Anxiety
Emotional lability
Hyperkinesia
Insomnia
Fatigue
Heat intolerance
Apathy
Decreased attention span
Psychosis

Skin and appendages
Onycholysis
Excessive diaphoresis
Increased sebaceous activity
Thinning of hair
Palmar erythema
Infiltrative dermopathy
Acropachy

Cardiovascular
Tachycardia
Increased systolic blood pressure
Wide pulse pressure
Increased cardiac output
Peripheral vasodilation
Systolic heart murmur

Pulmonary
Exertional dyspnea
Weakened respiratory muscles

Gastrointestinal
Increased stooling
Diarrhea
Nausea and vomiting
Anorexia
Polyphagia

Endocrine
Hypomenorrhea
Decreased fertility
Decreased potency and libido
Gynecomastia
Abnormal liver function

Hematopoietic
Decreased neutrophils
Increased lymphocytes

Neuromuscular
Weakness
Muscle wasting
Tremor
Hyperactive deep tendon reflexes

Optic
Infrequent blinking
Lid lag and retraction
Widened palpebral fissures
Decreased upward gaze
Photosensitivity
Proptosis
Increased tearing
Lid edema
Weakness of convergence
Infiltrative ophthalmopathy
Extraoculomotor paresis

The skin is warm, smooth, and thinned with loss of much of the keratin layer. Heat intolerance, excessive sweating, palmar erythema, fine soft hair, and onycholysis (Plummer's nails) frequently are present. Infiltrative dermopathy, commonly known as pretibial myxedema (Fig. 187-7), an infiltration of the skin and subcutaneous tissue with a mucopolysaccharide substance, occurs only in Graves' disease. It most commonly occurs in association

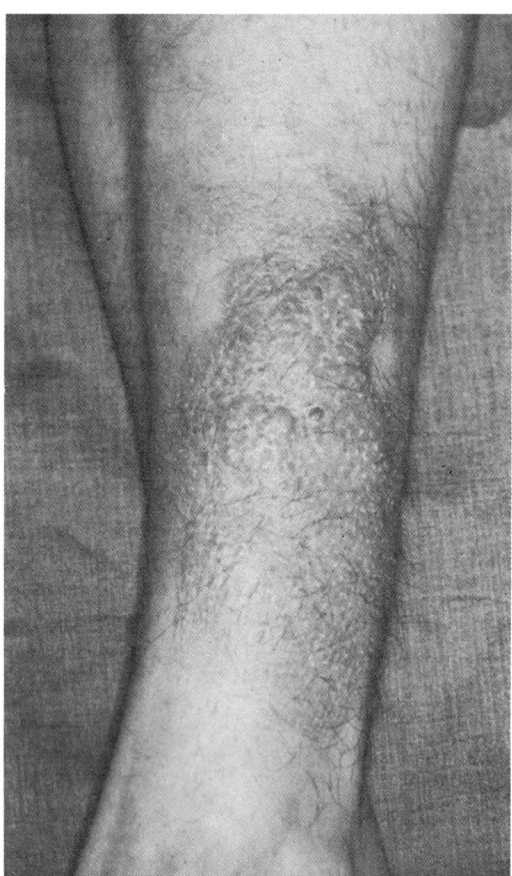

Fig. 187-7. Infiltrative dermopathy of Graves' disease, demonstrating typical plaque of pretibial myxedema.

with infiltrative ophthalmopathy. It is seen most often over the lower and middle one third of the pretibial areas, but it may also involve the ankles and feet and rarely the thighs and other parts of the body as well. Lesions appear as a painless, violaceous induration of the skin and subcutaneous tissue in irregular single or multiple plaques, most often in an asymmetric pattern. At times the skin changes are so mild that they are found only by careful inspection and palpation, and occasionally they are so severe that they resemble elephantiasis. Clubbing of the fingers with swelling and erythematous changes in the soft tissues at the base of the nails called thyroid acropachy develops occasionally in patients with Graves' disease, who usually also have infiltrative ophthalmopathy and dermopathy. Periosteal new bone formation may occur in association with these acral changes.

Optic manifestations. The characteristic eye changes (Fig. 187-8) that occur in thyrotoxicosis are referred to as an ophthalmopathy and are usually classified as (1) the benign (noninfiltrative) changes associated with most forms of thyrotoxicosis, and (2) the infiltrative forms seen only in Graves' disease. Forward protrusion or proptosis (exophthalmos) usually occurs only with Graves' disease. The noninfiltrative changes are generally related to increased

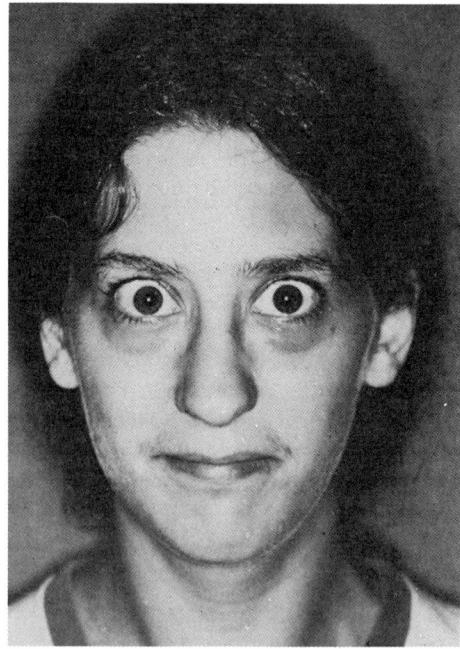

Fig. 187-8. Ophthalmopathy of Graves' disease. Patient has typical noninfiltrative changes (stare with marked upper and lower lid retraction).

adrenergic stimulation and consist of infrequent blinking (Stellwag's sign), widened palpebral fissures (Dalrymple's sign), lid lag (von Graefe's sign), decreased upward motion of the eye with associated decreased wrinkling of the forehead on upward gaze (Joffroy's sign), and weakness of convergence (Moöbius' sign). The severe infiltrative form is characterized by exophthalmos owing to increased retro-orbital edema and infiltration of fat, mucopolysaccharides, and fibrous tissue and to hypertrophic weakened extraocular muscles. Lid edema, diplopia, ophthalmoplegia, increased tearing, irritation, and photosensitivity accompany these infiltrative changes. Occasionally, visual impairment occurs owing to corneal ulceration, optic neuritis, retinal hemorrhage, and orbital or bulbar infection. These complications result from constant exposure of the cornea and from excessive traction on the optic nerve because of the severe proptosis.

Cardiovascular manifestations. The excess thyroid hormone causes a hyperdynamic cardiovascular response by direct stimulation of adenylate cyclase (cyclic AMP system) and by augmentation of adrenergic activity. This results in tachycardia even in the resting and sleeping states, widened pulse pressure, hyperdynamic precordial activity, increased cardiac output, peripheral vasodilation leading to prominent, bounding, peripheral arterial pulses, and warm erythematous extremities. Cardiac arrhythmias sometimes occur, especially in the elderly and in those with preexisting cardiac disease. The most common are atrial fibrillation that is poorly responsive to digitalis, premature ventricular contractions, and occasionally paroxysmal supraventricular tachycardia. Congestive heart failure may develop in the elderly and those with associated heart disease. Breathlessness is common, and occasionally mild hypoventilation results from weakness of respiratory muscles.

Gastrointestinal manifestations. Weight loss occurs in the majority of cases in spite of a marked increase in appetite and food intake. However, in about 10% no weight change is noted and in another 10% weight gain occurs. Severe thyrotoxicosis may result in anorexia, especially in the aged and in those with associated serious disease. Intestinal hypermotility with increased stooling is common. Frank diarrhea, nausea, vomiting, and abdominal pain may occur. In some cases the gastrointestinal symptoms predominate so that serious gastrointestinal disease is suspected. Occasionally hepatomegaly with abnormal liver function develops.

Neuromuscular and psychiatric manifestations. General manifestations include fatigue, increased irritability, increased emotional lability, restlessness, nervousness, and short attention span. Purposeless movements may be so severe at times that chorea is suspected. Speech may be very rapid. Teachers may note that affected children cannot concentrate and do poorly in schoolwork. Occasionally apathy, lethargy, and depression may predominate, and frank psychosis can occur. A fine tremor of the tongue, of the slightly closed lids, and of the fingers is usually present with hyperactive deep tendon reflexes. Muscle weakness occurs only after months of hyperthyroidism and is most prominent in the proximal muscles. Patients note difficulty in stair climbing, getting up from the squatting position, or holding the legs outstretched from a sitting position for more than 15 to 20 seconds (the healthy person can do this for up to 60 seconds). Muscle atrophy occurs in severely affected patients and frequently appears more severe than it actually is because of the associated subcutaneous fat atrophy from weight loss. Prolonged hyperthyroidism may lead to increased severity of osteoporosis or osteopenia already present and may result in compression fractures of vertebrae.

Genitourinary manifestations. Increased urinary frequency occurs as a result of increased renal blood flow and glomerular filtration. This is probably aggravated by nervousness and restlessness. Menstrual abnormalities, usually hypomenorrhea and occasionally amenorrhea, occur in about 50% of women. Infertility is common, especially in severe thyrotoxicosis. In men mild gynecomastia, decreased libido, and impotence have been reported.

DIFFUSE TOXIC GOITER (GRAVES' DISEASE). Diffuse toxic goiter or Graves' disease is the most common form of hyperthyroidism, accounting for 40% to 60% of all cases of thyrotoxicosis. It is characterized by a combination of (1) hyperthyroidism, (2) infiltrative ophthalmopathy, (3) infiltrative dermopathy, and (4) thyroid acropachy. Hyperthyroidism occurs alone in about 50% of the cases and with infiltrative ophthalmopathy in the other 50%. Infiltrative dermopathy develops in about 5% to 10% of patients with infiltrative ophthalmopathy. Thyroid acropachy occurs in 1% to 2%, usually those with infiltrative ophthalmopathy. About 5% to 10% of patients with infiltrative ophthalmopathy are euthyroid or hypothyroid when first seen. These patients usually have associated chronic lymphocytic thyroiditis that prevents the overstimulated thyroid from oversecreting thyroid hormone. The thyroid gland is symmetrically enlarged (30 to 80 g) in most cases of Graves' disease, but it is normal in about 10% and very large (over 100 g) in others. It is slightly firmer than normal and nontender. Vascularity is markedly increased so that a bruit is frequently heard over the thyroid. Microscopic examination shows marked hyperplasia and hypertrophy of the follicular epithelium. This disease occurs most often between the ages of 30 and 50 and affects females about seven times more frequently than males. There is an increased incidence in some families, suggesting autosomal recessive inheritance. Graves' disease is associated frequently with chronic lymphocytic thyroiditis and occasionally with rheumatoid arthritis, pernicious anemia, vitiligo, systemic lupus erythematosus, myasthenia gravis, premature menopause, and Addison's disease.

Etiology. The cause of Graves' disease is the body's production of an abnormal thyroid stimulator different from TSH. Severe physical or emotional trauma such as an automobile accident, death of a loved one, and divorce appears to be an inciting cause in about 50%. A marked increase in frequency occurred in Denmark during the German occupation in 1941 to 1945. A long-acting thyroid stimulator (LATS) is found in the blood of about 60% of patients with Graves' disease. This substance is characterized simply by its longer duration of action in stimulating the mouse thyroid compared to TSH. LATS is a 7S IgG immunoglobulin produced by B lymphocytes. It is capable of inducing thyroid hyperplasia and iodine accumulation in the thyroid independent of the pituitary gland. Before the discovery of LATS the pituitary gland and TSH were considered possible causes of Graves' disease. With the advent of the radioimmunoassay for TSH, TSH levels were found to be uniformly reduced in Graves' disease, further negating a pituitary role. Another IgG protein, LATS-protector (LATS-P), was subsequently found. It could stimulate only the human thyroid (not the mouse thyroid) but in addition prevented LATS from being neutralized in thyroid tissue assay systems. Subsequently, newly developed assay systems have shown multiple effects of these thyroid stimulating immunoglobulins (TSIs), as they are now called. These effects include (1) stimulation of endocytosis of colloid, which is a prerequisite for the release of thyroid hormone from follicular cells; (2) stimulation of the intrathyroidal adenylate–cylic AMP system; and (3) displacement of radioactive-labeled TSH from TSH cellular membrane receptors. Therefore at this time Graves' disease is believed to be an autoimmune disease caused by

TSIs, which are autoantibodies to TSH receptors on the follicular cell membrane and as such compete with TSH for these receptors. In addition, once TSIs attach to the receptors, they act exactly like TSH and activate the intracellular enzyme cascade system. Nearly all patients with diffuse toxic goiter have evidence of TSIs by these different assays.

The pathologic mechanism for stimulating B lymphocytes to start producing TSI is unknown. That it is a hereditary defect is suggested by (1) its strong concordance in monozygotic twins, (2) a frequent familial occurrence, (3) a frequent occurrence of other autoimmune disease in associated family members, and (4) the increased prevalence in those with HLA-B8 (whites and HLA-BW35 (Japanese) white cell antigens.

The natural history of Graves' disease was noted early in the twentieth century when effective treatment was unavailable. The severity of the hyperthyroidism was found to be variable with remissions and exacerbations and a tendency to resolve spontaneously in months or years. However, severe disability often resulted from the persistence of the hyperthyroidism, and death occurred in 10% to 20% of affected individuals. With the advent of effective treatment, death is infrequent and severe disability is unusual.

Diagnosis. The diagnosis is frequently obvious in the patient who has clinical hyperthyroidism with associated ophthalmopathy and pretibial myxedema or thyroid acropachy. In patients without other signs of Graves' disease, the presence of clinical hyperthyroidism with elevated serum levels of T_4 and T_3 and elevated RAIU is enough to confirm the diagnosis. The thyroid scan is usually not indicated in this disease but sometimes is helpful in differentiating diffuse toxic goiter from toxic multinodular goiter. The measurement of TSI or LATS is not routinely done but is indicated in diagnostic problems and probably will become routine as the TSI assay becomes readily available.

Management

Surgery. Except in a few centers, surgery is the treatment of choice only in selected patients, usually children and adolescents, especially if their hyperthyroidism is difficult to control with antithyroid drug therapy. The patient must be prepared with an antithyroid drug before surgery. Usually propylthiouracil or methimazole is administered for several weeks before surgery to render the patient euthyroid. Following this, inorganic iodine is given in addition for 7 to 10 days to reduce the marked vascularity of the gland caused by the thioureas. More recently propanoloalone given for 5 to 7 days before surgery has shown to be an effective means of controlling hyperthyroidism. During the surgical procedure 90% to 98% of the thyroid tissue is removed. Immediate postoperative complications include local hemorrhage, tracheal compression, and transient hypoparathyroidism. Permanent hypoparathyroidism and vocal cord paralysis owing to injury of the recurrent laryngeal nerve occur in less than 0.5% of patients. Permanent postoperative hypothyroidism occurs in 30% to 50% of patients with extensive thyroid resection. With less extensive thyroid resection, hypothyroidism is much less frequent but the incidence of postoperative recurrence of the hyperthyroidism, sometimes as long as 20 to 30 years later is substantially higher (15% to 20%).

Radioactive iodine. ^{131}I therapy is the most common mode of treatment given for Graves' disease in adults. It is contraindicated in children and adolescents and in pregnant women with hyperthyroidism. The main form of radiation from ^{131}I is the β-particle, which accounts for about 90% of its activity. Since these β-rays travel only about 2 mm within the thyroid gland, large doses can be directed to the thyroid gland without giving significant radiation to other structures. The usual dose is 5 to 15 mCi, which is generally calculated so that about 100 μCi is given per gram of thyroid tissue. The first effects of radioactive iodine begin to occur in about 1 month, and 80% of the patients achieve the euthyroid state within 2 to 3 months. The rest require more than one dose. The only significant adverse effect from radioactive iodine therapy is hypothyroidism; between 20% and 50% of patients are hypothyroid within 1 year. Those who do not become hypothyroid should be followed indefinitely because most follow-up studies have shown a 2% to 5% incidence of hypothyroidism per year after the first year.

There has been no evidence of other hazards from the effects of radiation on the body such as increased incidence of malignancy such as leukemia or of congenital abnormalities in the offspring of treated patients. Even in children, in whom other forms of radiation have been shown to be a major cause of thyroid carcinoma, the use of ^{131}I has not caused increased incidence of malignancies. The incidence of thyroid carcinoma is lower in patients treated with radioactive iodine than in the general population.

Thiourea therapy. Two drugs, propylthiouracil and methimazole, are used in the treatment of hyperthyroidism. These drugs ameliorate hyperthyroidism by inhibiting the peroxidase enzyme system, thus preventing oxidation of trapped iodine, iodination of tyrosines, and coupling of iodotyrosines. In addition, propylthiouracil but not methimazole inhibits the peripheral conversion of T_4 to T_3. The usual daily dosage of propylthiouracil is 400 to 600 mg in three or four divided doses. The equivalent dose of methimazole is about one-tenth that of propylthiouracil. Experience has shown that patients with severe hyperthyroidism may require larger doses, so starting daily doses of 800 to 1000 mg are sometimes used in severely ill patients. Clinical improvement with a fall in the T_4 and T_3 levels occurs within 2 or 3 weeks, and the majority of patients are rendered euthyroid within 6 to 8 weeks. The dosage is gradually reduced at that time. A maintenance dosage of 100 to 200 mg daily is usual. The thyroid gland also usually decreases in size with effective treatment. If it enlarges during therapy, progressive uncontrolled disease or the onset of hypothyroidism should be suspected. The main drawbacks of therapy with thioureas are their side effects and the length of time they must be given. Granulocytopenia occurs in less than 1% of patients, and leukocytosis, liver dysfunction, skin eruptions, arthralgias, myalgias, and lymphadenopathy occur in up to 5%. Initially, monthly monitoring of the T_4 white blood cell counts, and liver function tests is indicated. With control of the hyperthyroidism after 2 or 3 months, monitoring should take place every 2 or 3 months. Most physicians continue the thiourea therapy for 1 to 2 years. After discontinuation of the medication, the recurrence rate of the hyperthyroidism is about 50% to 60%, most often in the first 2 years. A recent report suggests that treatment can be discontinued after 3 or 4 months but the recurrence rate is higher. There is no method that predicts accurately whether a patient will have a recurrence when thiourea therapy is stopped. Recent investigations, however, suggest that the disappearance of TSI during thiourea therapy may indicate permanent remission. There is no evidence that antithyroid drugs alter the course of the disease, even though they suppress the production of thyroid hormone.

TOXIC MULTINODULAR GOITER. Toxic multinodular goiter is also known as Plummer's disease. It usually occurs in patients with long-standing nontoxic multinodular goiter resulting from autonomous or semiautonomous function of slowly growing nodules. It accounts for 10% to 20% of the cases of thyrotoxicosis and occurs most often in those over 50 years of age. The nodules probably synthesize thyroid hormone less efficiently than normal thyroid tissue so that substantially more nodular tissue must be present before overproduction and thyrotoxicosis occur. Usually 75 to 100 g or more of thyroid tissue is present when hyperthyroidism develops. The thyroid scan reveals localization of the iodine in the nodules with suppressed function in the intervening thyroid tissue. TSH stimulation activates the suppressed areas of function but stimulates the autonomous and semiautonomous functioning nodules only slightly or not at all because they have lost much of their responsiveness to TSH. Hyperthyroidism present in some patients with multinodular goiter may be a form of Graves' disease, since the thyroid tissue between the nodules is hyperplastic whereas the nodule tissue has large, relatively inactive follicles and does not accumulate iodine. The hyperthyroidism present with toxic multinodular goiter is usually mild, but because this disease occurs most often in patients over the age of 50 who frequently have other illnesses, severe disability can occur. It is much more frequent in women than in men. The symptoms and signs are similar to those seen in Graves' disease, but cardiac problems such as atrial fibrillation and congestive heart failure are much more common in this older age group. Infiltrative ophthalmopathy and dermopathy do not occur. The thyroid gland is quite nodular and varies greatly in size and contour.

Diagnosis. The elevation of the serum levels of T_4 and T_3 is usually mild, substantially less than in most cases of Graves' disease, and the RAIU may be elevated. The scan shows varying degrees or patchy areas of uptake. T_3 toxicosis, the low T_3 syndrome, and a low TBG sometimes confuse the laboratory studies. The TSH is suppressed, and TSIs are not present. In patients with only borderline elevation of T_4 and T_3 levels and in those with the low T_3 syndrome, TRH testing may be indicated. Lack of TSH response to TRH stimulation indicates excessive levels of thyroid hormone.

Management. The usual treatment recommended for elderly patients with toxic multinodular goiter is radioactive iodine. Because the RAIU is usually lower than in Graves' disease, substantially more radioactive iodine is needed. The average dose is at least 15 mCi and may be 30 mCi or more. Thyroidectomy is indicated if significant tracheal and esophageal obstruction is present or simply to debulk an extremely large goiter, which usually has considerable amounts of fibrous tissue. An occasional patient may choose thyroidectomy over radioactive iodine therapy for cosmetic reasons. The goiter rarely returns to normal size after radioactive iodine therapy. Thiourea therapy is used infrequently for this type of hyperthyroidism except as preparation for surgery or as interim therapy until radioactive iodine is effective.

TOXIC UNINODULAR GOITER. Toxic uninodular goiter is an autonomous functioning follicular adenoma of the thyroid that produces thyrotoxicosis, although in a rare instance it can be due to a follicular carcinoma. It causes 3% to 5% of the cases of thyrotoxicosis. It appears usually as a single nodule or rarely as two or three nodules. Hyperthyroidism seldom occurs while the autonomous functioning nodule is less than 2.5 to 3 cm, since nodules do not produce thyroid hormone as efficiently as normal tissue. TSH is suppressed and TSIs are not present in this disease. Slow progressive growth with increasing hormone production and suppression of normal thyroid tissue gradually occurs over many years.

Elevation of the serum T_4 and T_3 concentrations and the RAIU is usually present, although an occasional patient may have only T_3 toxicosis. The thyroid scan reveals uptake only in the nodule with suppression of the rest of the gland. TSH stimulation may occasionally be necessary to show areas of suppressed normal thyroid tissue. Radioactive iodine therapy (usually 20 to 30 mCi or more) and surgery (simple excision of the nodule) are equally effective treatments. After removal of the nodule by radioactive iodine therapy or surgery, the suppressed normal thyroid tissue will function again. A small residual nodule may remain after radioactive iodine treatment.

HYPERTHYROIDISM CAUSED BY EXCESS TSH. Excessive TSH production is an extremely rare cause of hyperthyroidism. It can be caused by a TSH-producing pituitary tumor or by excess pituitary production of TSH from autonomous function or from hypothalamic dysfunction causing excess TRH secretion. It is usually suspected only if the serum TSH is inadvertently found to be elevated or if visual field impairment or other signs and symptoms suggesting pituitary disease occur in a patient with hyperthyroidism. The presence of an elevated serum TSH concentration and the confirmation of the pituitary tumor and pituitary and hypothalamic dysfunction are necessary to confirm the diagnosis. The TSH level is normal or low in all other forms of hyperthyroidism.

HYPERTHYROIDISM CAUSED BY TUMORS. The clinical hyperthyroidism associated with choriocarcinoma or hydatidiform mole is rare and is generally mild in spite of sometimes greatly increased T_4 and T_3 concentrations. The presence of a high concentration of human chorionic gonadotropin (HCG), a weak thyroid stimulator, appears to be the cause of thyroid hyperfunction. Hyperthyroidism caused by other tumors producing thyroid stimulators is infrequent and poorly understood. Control of the tumor causes a reduction in the thyroid stimulators and cures the hyperthyroidism.

HYPERTHYROIDISM CAUSED BY THYROIDITIS. Subacute thyroiditis (to be discussed later in detail) is sometimes associated with transient hyperthyroidism owing to a release of substantial amounts of stored thyroid hormone from the damaged thyroid gland. The diagnosis is usually obvious; the patient has a firm, very tender, slightly enlarged thyroid with a mild to moderate degree of thyrotoxicosis. Subacute thyroiditis is frequently associated with a systemic illness manifested by malaise, diffuse aches and pains, and low-grade fever. It is sometimes preceded by a viral respiratory illness.

Lymphocytic thyroiditis with spontaneously resolving hyperthyroidism (silent thyroiditis) has been reported with increased frequency in recent years and now accounts for 10% to 20% of the cases of thyrotoxicosis. The thyroid gland is slightly enlarged in 50% of cases of lymphocytic thyroiditis and is usually firm and nontender. This disease is frequently confused with diffuse toxic goiter and is first suspected only when a suppressed RAIU is found. Percutaneous needle or open biopsy of the thyroid may be necessary to confirm the diagnosis. The hyperthyroidism usually lasts 6 to 12 weeks and requires treatment with sedatives, propranolol, or corticosteroids in patients with moderate or severe disease.

IODINE-INDUCED HYPERTHYROIDISM. Iodine-induced hyperthyroidism (Jod-Basedow disease) apparently was much more common when iodine prophylaxis was in vogue 20 or more years ago. Its present incidence is unknown. It usually occurs in a patient with a nontoxic multinodular goiter who has taken iodine for prophylaxis or treatment of other diseases or for roentgenographic studies. It has also been reported to occur in patients with a normal thyroid and those with other thyroid diseases. A disturbance or failure in the intrathyroidal control of iodine metabolism probably is the cause of this disease. It is usually transient, lasting 2 to 4 months. Iodine-induced hyperthyroidism should be suspected in any patient with hyperthyroidism and a depressed RAIU, and such patients should be questioned about recent inorganic or organic iodine intake. Excessive inorganic iodine intake or roentgenographic iodine-containing dyes may also depress the RAIU in patients with diffuse or toxic multinodular goiter. In this circumstance the suppressed RAIU becomes elevated within a few days after the inorganic iodine or renal roentgenographic dyes are excreted (although excretion may take up to 6 to 8 weeks to occur after cholecystographic contrast material is given). In contrast, the RAIU stays suppressed during the duration of the hyperthyroidism with Jod-Basedow disease. At times it may be necessary to measure the 24-hour urinary iodide concentration to determine whether excessive iodide ingestion is present. Levels greater than 2000 to 2500 μg confirm this.

THYROTOXICOSIS CAUSED BY EXOGENOUS THYROID HORMONE INTAKE

Thyrotoxicosis factitia. Thyrotoxicosis factitia is a form of thyrotoxicosis without hyperthyroidism. Thyrotoxicosis factitia owing to surreptitious self-administration of thyroid hormone is quite rare. It most often occurs in individuals with underlying psychiatric problems who have paramedical training and access to thyroid hormone. Most will vehemently deny intake of thyroid hormone. The diagnosis should be suspected in patients who meet the clinical criteria described previously and who have a suppressed uptake and a nonpalpable or small thyroid. TSH stimulation will produce function in the suppressed thyroid tissue.

Iatrogenic thyrotoxicosis. Iatrogenic thyrotoxicosis, which is usually mild, results when an excessive amount of thyroid hormone is administered to a patient with hypothyroidism or to a patient being given suppressive thyroid hormone therapy for a multinodular goiter that has developed some autonomous function. In a multinodular goiter the combination of the exogenous thyroid hormone intake and the persistent endogenous hormone production results in thyroid hormone excess and sometimes in mild thyrotoxic symptoms and signs. The diagnosis is usually obvious, and all that is needed is to stop administering thyroid hormone or reduce the amount given.

DIFFERENTIAL DIAGNOSIS OF THYROTOXICOSIS. Patients with psychoneurosis may have sweating, tremor, stare, tachycardia, weakness, fatigue, weight loss, and purposeless movements suggestive of thyrotoxicosis. Hypermetabolism associated with pheochromocytoma may produce severe sweating, tachycardia, tremor, and weight loss. Weight loss, fatigue, and other symptoms associated with occult malignancy, anemia, diabetes, hyperparathyroidism, cardiac disease, and myasthenia may suggest possible hyperthyroidism. Luft's syndrome, a rare abnormality caused by overgrowth and excessive function of skeletal muscle mitochondria, produces severe hypermetabolism and mimics hyperthyroidism. With many of these diseases there is an increased association of hyperthyroidism. In most instances, however, the available thyroid tests should easily prove or disprove the presence of hyperthyroidism.

SPECIAL ASPECTS OF HYPERTHYROIDISM

Hyperthyroidism in the infant, child, and adolescent. Neonatal hyperthyroidism is usually the result of transplacental transfer of TSI from the mother to the infant. Hyperthyroidism is present at birth and usually lasts for only 1 or 2 weeks until all the TSI has been metabolized and cleared from the neonate's blood. The mother almost always has a history of recent or remote Graves' disease.

Most other types of thyrotoxicosis seen during childhood and adolescence are due to Graves' disease. There is still controversy about the best mode of treatment. The majority of centers treat patients with thioureas initially, but a substantial number still recommend subtotal thyroidectomy. Radioactive iodine has been given as the initial treatment, but most physicians worry about its use because of the increased incidence of thyroid cancer in infants and children who have had head and neck irradiation. Children having toxic reactions to the thiourea compounds or not responding well to them are usually treated with subtotal thyroidectomy and occasionally with radioactive iodine.

Hyperthyroidism in pregnancy. Hyperthyroidism in pregnancy is almost always due to Graves' disease and is associated with an increased incidence of spontaneous abortion and stillbirths. Radioactive iodine should never be given to pregnant women because it crosses the placental barrier and the fetal thyroid concentrates iodine after the twelfth week of gestation. Propranolol also is contraindicated for treatment of hyperthyroidism because it may possibly cause intrauterine growth retardation, fetal distress, low Apgar scores, postnatal depression, hypoglycemia, bradycardia, and prolongation of labor. Subtotal thyroidectomy following preparation with thioureas is frequently done during the first half of pregnancy. Most physicians just use thioureas. Since these drugs cross the placenta and are accumulated by the fetal thyroid, substantially reduced doses are used, less than 300 mg of propylthiouracil each day to keep the T_4 level in the upper range of normal. T_4 and T_3 do not cross the placenta, so adding T_4 to the mother's treatment to prevent hypothyroidism in the infant does not work.

Thyrotoxic crisis. Thyrotoxic crisis (thyroid storm) is relatively rare and is precipitated in the hyperthyroid patient by infections, trauma, surgery, and withdrawal from antithyroid drugs (especially in patients with very large thyroids). It is a life-threatening condition manifested by marked restlessness, agitation, extreme tachycardia (130 to 160 beats/min), high fever (104° to 106° F [40° to 41° C]), prostration, dehydration, nausea, vomiting, diarrhea, delirium, and psychosis. Treatment must be instituted promptly as follows: (1) propylthiouracil, 800 to 1200 mg daily in four divided doses; (2) propranolol, 160 to 240 mg daily in four divided doses orally or 1 to 2 mg intravenously every 1 to 2 hours; (3) potassium iodide, 500 mg orally every 6 hours, or sodium iodide, 0.5 g by intravenous drip every 8 hours; (4) intravenous fluid therapy; (5) mechanical treatment of hyperthermia; *and* (6) corticosteroids in high doses if the patient does not show prompt response to the other treatment in 12 to 24 hours. Patients not responding to this regimen can be treated with peritoneal dialysis, exchange transfusion, or plasmapheresis to rapidly lower thyroid hormone levels.

Infiltrative ophthalmopathy. The course of infiltrative ophthalmopathy seen with Graves' disease is unpredictable. It usually occurs with hyperthyroidism but it can occur alone or before or within a few months or years after the hyperthyroidism. In the majority of cases it follows a relatively benign course with progressive proptosis over a period of months and then a slow, spontaneous remission over many weeks and months, sometimes leaving a small but significant residual proptosis. Although the benign, noninfiltrative eye changes disappear when the hyperthyroidism leaves, the severe changes generally follow an independent course. The typical presenting picture is bilateral, symmetric eye involvement with some restriction of extraocular muscle motion. However, in some cases the involvement may be unilateral or asymmetric, and the patient may be euthyroid or hypothyroid. At times a firm goiter is present. This indicates chronic lymphocytic thyroiditis, which is the cause of hypothyroidism or at least prevents hyperthyroidism as a result of the persisitent effect of TSI. Diagnostic evaluation includes tests to exclude the possibility of orbital tumor and other orbital disease and to confirm that Graves' disease is really present. Orbital roentgenography, tomography, computed tomography, or orbital ultrasonography can be used to check for orbital tumor. The presence of Graves' disease can be demonstrated in three ways. The first is the T_3 suppression test (previously discussed), which in most instances shows a nonsuppressible thyroid. The second, the TRH stimulation test, shows suppression of the hypothalamic pituitary function. Finally, the presence of TSI also supports the diagnosis of Graves' disease. However, in some cases of Graves' ophthalmopathy, one, two, or all of these tests may be normal.

The treatment of infiltrative ophthalmopathy depends on the severity of the ocular involvement. In most mild cases, sleeping with the head of the bed elevated and using thiazide diuretics will help reduce periorbital and lid edema. One percent methylcellulose drops in each eye as needed will help relieve the gritty sensation that many patients have. If diplopia is present, prism fitting will help correct the visual abnormality, but if it persists, extraocular muscle surgery may be necessary to restore binocular vision. When the corneas remain uncovered much of the time, tarsorrhaphy and/or section of Müller's muscle in the upper lid may be necessary to prevent recurrent corneal ulceration and orbital infection. Severe inflammatory changes can be treated with retrobulbar injections of corticosteroids or large oral doses of corticosteroids, which usually should be continued for several months. If this fails or if the proptosis is rapidly progressive and optic neuritis develops with visual loss, surgical orbital decompression is indicated. Supervoltage orbital radiotherapy is sometimes also effective if given within the first year after severe eye changes occur.

Nontoxic goiter

Nontoxic goiter is defined as any enlargement of the thyroid not associated with hypothyroidism or hyperthyroidism. The following is a classification of the causes of nontoxic goiter:

I. Nontoxic diffuse goiter
   A. Iodine deficiency
   B. Biosynthetic or enzymatic defects
   C. Goitrogens
   D. Thyroiditis
   E. Tissue resistance to thyroid hormone
II. Nontoxic multinodular goiter
   A. Long-standing nontoxic diffuse goiter
III. Nontoxic uninodular goiter
   A. Neoplasms
     1. Benign
     2. Malignant
   B. Cysts
   C. Thyroiditis
   D. Hemorrhage

This classification helps sort out the different goiters according to their physical characteristics, so that a logical diagnostic workup and treatment can be determined. The most frequent causes of nontoxic goiter are minor intrathyroidal biosynthetic defects, thyroiditis, neoplasms, cysts, and hemorrhage. The others are found relatively infrequently.

NONTOXIC DIFFUSE GOITER. Minor intrathyroidal biosynthetic defects in the thyroid comprise the majority of cases of nontoxic diffuse goiter. The exact cause of the minor intrathyroidal biosynthetic defect is unknown, but it appears to be sporadic and acquired in many patients and familial or hereditary in others. It is believed to represent a compensatory increase in thyroid size owing to minor degrees of decreased thyroid hormone synthesis, probably as a result of multiple causes such as minor intrathyroidal acquired enzyme defects. The slight decrease in serum thyroid hormone levels results in increased TSH stimulation of the thyroid. This returns thyroid hormone levels to normal but does not correct the underlying primary defect. Although increased TSH levels are not usually demonstrated, minor increases of TSH within the normal range are found and probably are sufficient to produce the thyroid enlargement. The role of TSH in initiating and maintaining the goiter is substantiated by the usual rapid regression of the goiter with suppressive doses of thyroid hormone, an action mediated only by suppression of TSH production. The exact intrathyroidal defect or defects are thought to be subtle and minor in degree. Whether they are acquired or congenital and why there is an extremely high female-to-male ratio (7 to 9:1) are unknown. Minor degrees of iodine deficiency and intake of weak goitrogens in drugs or food may further aggravate the intrathyroidal defect. Genetic factors probably play an important role, since similar goiters or other thyroid disease is found in 30% to 40% of these patients' relatives.

Although iodine deficiency is still common in some undeveloped areas of the world, it is no longer prevalent in North America owing to iodine salt supplementation for the past 60 to 70 years and to iodine compounds used to preserve foods in more recent years. Goitrogens in water, foods, and drugs occasionally cause minor outbreaks or isolated cases of goiter. It is not known whether ingestion of small amounts of weak goitrogens contributes to the generation of goiters in those with a genetic tendency, those with minor biosynthetic defects, or those with mild degrees of iodine deficiency. Established types of intrathyroidal enzyme defects are due to autosomal recessive inheritance. They occur most often in infants and children and frequently lead to hypothyroidism. Nontoxic diffuse goiter has also been reported in the rare syndrome of tissue resistance to thyroid hormones. Thyroiditis as the cause of goiter will be discussed as a separate entity later.

Diagnosis. The diagnosis of the types of nontoxic diffuse goiters discussed thus far is usually established by the history and physical findings. The RAIU and the serum concentrations of T_4, T_3, and TSH are normal except in the occasional patient whose defect is severe enough to cause hypothyroidism. Low titers of thyroid autoantibody may be present in some of these patients but do not help to clarify the diagnosis. Percutaneous needle or small open thyroid biopsy is helpful in establishing the pathologic diagnosis but is used infrequently, since the diagnosis is usually based on the clinical features. The use of sophisticated tests to check for intrathyroidal enzyme defects or for minor degrees of iodine deficiency is not indicated. The patient should be questioned about the use of drugs and foods that have goitrogenic activity, but this is rarely rewarding.

Management. Thyroid suppression is the principal mode of treatment of nontoxic diffuse goiters unless iodine deficiency or intake of goitrogens is found. Thyroid hormone in the form of T_4 (Table 187-2) is given in physiologic doses. It gradually suppresses TSH and thyroid hormone production and reduces the goiter to normal or near normal size within 2 to 6 months. Thyroid surgery is not indicated in this type of goiter except to help establish the diagnosis or reduce the bulk of very large goiters. Surgery should always be followed by thyroid suppression therapy, since removal of thyroid tissue only aggravates the defect and hyperplasia and regrowth of the residual thyroid tissue or frank hypothyroidism usually occurs with time. Iodine prophylaxis is not indicated unless iodine deficiency is established because it may induce Jod-Basedow disease or hypothyroidism.

Thyroiditis

ACUTE SUPPURATIVE THYROIDITIS. Acute thyroiditis is also known as suppurative or bacterial thyroiditis. The usual causative organisms are *Staphylococcus, Streptococcus,* and *Pneumococcus.* They gain entry to the thyroid from infected contiguous structures or from hematogenous spread from a distant focus. The onset is usually abrupt with fever, localied or diffuse swelling and pain radiating upward in the anterior lateral neck to the jaw and ear, localized erythema, increased heat, and painful swallowing. The condition is quite rare and must be differentiated from inflammation and infection from bacteria and fungi such as *Actinomyces,* usually in lymph nodes. Thyroid function studies are usually normal, but the thyroid scan shows decreased function in the suppurative area. Prompt antibiotic therapy causes rapid resolution in a few days, but an abscess can develop and surgical drainage may be necessary.

SUBACUTE THYROIDITIS (DE QUERVAIN'S THYROIDITIS). Subacute thyroiditis (de Quervain's, granulomatous, or giant cell thyroiditis) is a localized or diffuse, nonsuppurative inflammation of the thyroid characterized by multiple types of inflammatory cells (polymorphonuclear leukocytes and mononuclear cells), noncaseating granuloma formation with multinucleated giant cells, and disruption of thyroid follicles. The cause is considered to be an immunologic response to a viral infection, since it frequently occurs several weeks after a viral upper respiratory tract infection. This disorder is uncommon. There is a female predominance (3 to 4:1), and it occurs most often between the ages of 25 and 50 years.

The presenting complaint is usually a sore throat or earache of several weeks' duration, which is frequently misdiagnosed as pharyngitis or otitis media. The thyroid gland is usually diffusely enlarged with mild to severe localized tenderness, although there may be a localized area of enlargement and tenderness and infrequently a single nontender nodule. The thyroid tenderness may be exquisite, causing the patient to withdraw rapidly when thyroid palpation is attempted. In 10% to 20% of cases there are severe signs and symptoms of systemic disease and hyperthyroidism. These include fever, tachycardia, chills, sweats, malaise, severe dysphagia, and headache. The hyperthyroidism results from the release of excessive quantities of stored thyroid hormone from damaged thyroid follicles. Even in severe cases the diagnosis is frequently overlooked and the disease is misdiagnosed as fever of unknown origin (FUO), dental abscess, pharyngitis, otitis media, or influenza. The disease is self-limited, lasting 1 to 3 months. Other causes of tenderness in the thyroid area that may be confused with subacute thyroiditis include local hemorrhage into thyroid cysts, acute thyroiditis, acute inflammation or spasm of neck muscles, abscess of adjacent structures and lymph nodes, and tender carotid arteries. Laboratory studies are frequently normal in mild cases. In moderate or severe inflammation laboratory abnormalities may include (1) elevated sedimentation rate; (2) mild leukocytosis and occasionally mild anemia; (3) a depressed RAIU except in localized disease, in which the thyroid scan will show decreased uptake in the involved area; (4) elevated serum T_4 and T_3 concentrations in severely affected patients; and (5) the presence of low titers of thyroid autoantibodies in about 50% to 60% of patients. Thyroid biopsy may be needed in some cases, but the diagnosis is usually obvious on the basis of clinical criteria and laboratory studies.

Mild and moderate cases should be treated with analgesics such as aspirin and acetaminophen. The patient should be assured that the disease is self-limited and usually clears within 1 to 2 months. In severe cases, especially those with thyrotoxicosis, more potent antiinflammatory agents should be used. Corticosteroids provide prompt relief of symptoms and tenderness within 24 to 48 hours and should be continued for 3 to 4 weeks. The usual starting dose of prednisone is 30 to 50 mg daily, with gradual reduction by 5 to 10 mg every 4 to 7 days. About 10% of patients have a recurrence after 3 or 4 weeks of corticosteroids and require a second course of therapy. Following recovery from the moderate and severe episodes a transient hypothyroidism lasting 1 to 3 weeks may occur in 30% to 50% of patients. Thyroid damage leading to permanent hypothyroidism rarely develops in this disease.

CHRONIC LYMPHOCYTIC THYROIDITIS (HASHIMOTO'S THYROIDITIS). Chronic lymphocytic thyroiditis (Hashimoto's or autoimmune thyroiditis) is believed to be an autoimmune disease with development of multiple types of thyroid autoantibodies to thyroid proteins. It is a common disorder, accounting for over 90% of nontoxic diffuse goiter in children and over 50% in adults. It is far more frequent in women than in men and occurs most commonly between the ages of 20 and 50 years. A family history is present in over 70%, and Graves' disease is also common in affected families. There is an increased incidence of chronic lymphocytic thyroiditis in patients with other autoimmune disorders such as pernicious anemia, Addison's disease, rheumatoid arthritis, systemic lupus erythematosus, Sjögren's syndrome, and chronic hepatitis and in relatives of patients with these diseases. The pathologic changes in the thyroid vary from mild inflammation to total destruction and atrophy. Initially a focal or diffuse infiltration of lymphocytes occurs with gradual destruction of follicle cells and disruption of follicles. Intrafollicular macrophages appear in the disrupted follicles and fibrosis begins. Typical oxyphilic cytoplasmic changes occur in follicle cells, which are called Askanazy or Hürthle cells and are considered almost pathognomonic of the disease. With time, extensive fibrosis and destruction of thyroid follicles occur, not infrequently leading to hypothyroidism, thyroid atrophy, and nodularity of the remaining thyroid tissue.

The initial presentation is usually a small or medium-size, nontender (very slightly tender in about 10%), diffuse goiter that is slightly firmer than normal or rubbery in consistency. The goiter gradually enlarges over several years and becomes firmer, more bosselated, and somewhat nodular, but the nodules are usually of similar consistency and indistinct. About 20% of the patients initially have hypothyroidism. In children about 50% have spontaneous recovery after several months. A significant number of patients with lymphocytic (silent) thyroiditis have transient hypothyroidism. Occasionally, localized lymphadenopathy, vocal cord paralysis, and compression of the trachea and esophagus occur, especially with large goiter. In these cases malignancy must be ruled out by biopsy or surgical excision.

The diagnosis is established by the combination of clinical features and laboratory studies. The finding of a firm, diffusely enlarged thyroid is frequently the main criterion used to make the diagnosis. The T_4 and T_3 levels are usually normal, but the PBI may be elevated owing to the release of nonhormonal iodoproteins from the damaged thyroid follicles. In euthyroid patients, 10% to 20% have elevated baseline levels of TSH and up to 50% have lack of thyroid reserve shown by an excessive TSH response to TRH stimulation. The RAIU may be normal or increased, suggesting hyperthyroidism, but TSH stimulation does not increase the RAIU further. These responses to TRH and TSH stimulation indicate lack of thyroid reserve and an already maximally stimulated thyroid. Further confirmation of the diagnosis is made by the finding of high titers of thyroid antibodies; however, in 30% to 50% of patients antibody tests are negative or titers are low and thus nondiagnostic. Needle biopsy leads to definitive histologic diagnosis and should be used in problem cases or in index cases in families with a history of goiter. Differentiation of chronic lymphocytic thyroiditis from other types of diffuse goiter by clinical and laboratory tests without biopsy is accurate in only 70% to 80% of cases. However, further clarification of the diagnosis is unnecessary, since the treatment is the same, that is, suppressive doses of thyroid hormone. Differentiation from thyroid carcinoma is usually not difficult because thyroid carcinoma occurs as a single, hard nodule and chronic lymphocytic thyroiditis occurs as a firm, rubbery, diffusely enlarged thyroid.

SCLEROSING THYROIDITIS (REIDEL'S THYROIDITIS). Sclerosing thyroiditis (Reidel's thyroiditis) is an extremely rare form of thyroiditis characterized by extensive fibrosis and fixation of the thyroid to adjacent structures. It is often associated with mediastinal and retroperitoneal fibrosis and frequently causes symptoms by compression of adjacent structures such as the trachea, esophagus, and recurrent laryngeal nerves. The thyroid is slightly or moderately enlarged and nontender but strikingly hard and fixed, suggesting carcinoma. The presence of associated mediastinal and retinal peritoneal fibrosis should prompt suspicion of the disease. Biopsy is usually done to establish the diagnosis. Thyroid tests are usually normal, but hypothyroidism does occur. Surgery may be necessary to relieve local obstruction and nerve compression.

Adenomas

Adenomas of the thyroid are benign neoplasms classified according to their histologic characteristics (embryonal, fetal, microfollicular, macrofollicular, papillary cystadenoma, and Hürthle cell). They usually grow slowly and almost imperceptibly over years. They frequently have a well-developed capsule and do not invade blood vessels or the capsular structure. The rest of the thyroid is normal, unlike the thyroid in nontoxic multinodular goiter. Most follicular adenomas retain some ability to concentrate iodine and synthesize thyroid hormone. Hyperthyroidism may occur when the nodule is 2.5 to 3 cm or greater. Thyroid function tests are usually normal. The thyroid scan shows a cold area in the nonfunctioning adenomas and an increased uptake of iodine in the functioning nodules. The cold nodules require needle biopsy, aspiration cytology, or surgical excision to exclude malignancy. The presence of a functioning nodule is usually evidence against thyroid malignancy, since functioning follicular carcinomas of the thyroid rarely concentrate iodine well. The functioning nodules may simply be observed, but because they usually grow slowly with time, ablation with radioactive iodine or surgical excision should be done.

THYROID CYSTS. Thyroid cysts and hemorrhage into thyroid cysts or thyroid parenchyma account for the majority of the nonmalignant single nodules in the thyroid. These lesions usually arise from thyroid adenomas or from the nodules in nontoxic multinodular goiter. Some adenomas contain single or multiloculated cysts. Acute hemorrhage into the thyroid cyst or into the thyroid parenchyma probably occurs as the result of rupture of the fragile new blood vessels in these lesions. Hemorrhage into the thyroid usually causes the sudden onset of a painful thyroid mass that tends to resolve spontaneously in several weeks. Occasionally necrosis of the center of a malignant nodule occurs, leading to cyst formation. Sometimes a single asymptomatic thyroid nodule that is cold on the thyroid scan is found to be due to subacute or granulomatous thyroiditis on surgical biopsy.

Carcinoma of the thyroid

Thyroid cancer is rare and accounts for less than 1% of all malignancies. Its annual incidence is about 25 cases per million people. In autopsy series as many as 0.1% of thyroids are found to have small or microscopic papillary cancers that are of low-grade malignancy and questionable clinical significance. Malignant neoplasms of the thyroid are usually of four types: papillary or papillary-follicular, follicular, anaplastic, and medullary, although occasionally a primary lymphoma, lymphosarcoma, or sarcoma of the thyroid is found as well as metastatic malignancy from other areas of the body. The degree of malignancy varies considerably among these different thyroid tumors. Thyroid carcinomas usually occur as single nodules.

PAPILLARY CARCINOMA. Papillary and papillary-follicular carcinoma are considered to be the same kind of tumor. This relatively benign form of malignancy accounts for 50% or more of the cases of carcinoma of the thyroid and for nearly all the thyroid cancer that occurs in children and young adults. In recent years an epidemic of papillary carcinoma of the thyroid has occurred in young adults 5 to 20 years after they received radiotherapy of the head, neck, or chest for multiple reasons such as enlarged thymus, birthmarks, enlarged tonsils, and acne vulgaris. Papillary carcinoma usually occurs as an asymptomatic nodule in the normal thyroid and occasionally spreads to other areas of the thyroid or to the adjacent lymph nodes. It tends to be more malignant in those over 50 years of age. Distant metastases are unusual. The tumor may or may not be encapsulated. Histologic examination reveals masses of columnar epithelial cells arranged in papillary projections, with a significant number having some follicular structural features. These tumors do not accumulate radioactive iodine to any extent.

FOLLICULAR CARCINOMA. Follicular carcinoma accounts for about 25% of the cases of thyroid carcinoma. It generally occurs between 40 and 60 years of age. Its degree of malignancy varies considerably, but it is usually more malignant than the papillary type. It has a tendency for hematogenous spread via invasion of blood vessels to the lung, liver, and bone. The usual presentation is as a slow-growing, asymptomatic nodule in the thyroid like the papillary carcinoma, but occasionally metastatic lesions to bone or lung are found initially. Follicular carcinoma is generally more malignant in older people. The tumor is usually encapsulated and the histology varies greatly. At times histologic features appear completely benign to the pathologist and malignancy is proved only by the finding of distant metastases. These tumors sometimes accumulate radioactive iodine and synthesize thyroid hormone so that thyrotoxicosis occurs when bulky masses of the tumor are present, although this is rare.

ANAPLASTIC CARCINOMA. Anaplastic carcinoma of the thyroid accounts for about 10% of thyroid malignancies. It most often occurs over the age of 50 and is slightly more common in females. The malignancy usually is a rapidly growing lesion invading adjacent structures and metastasizing throughout the body. The tumors are unencapsulated and composed of anaplastic small or large cells with numerous mitoses. The clinical course is one of rapid growth of a neck mass that is sometimes painful and tender. Involvement of local structures occurs early in the course, causing hoarseness, tracheal obstruction, and difficulty in swallowing. There are also problems from distant metastases in brain, liver, and lung. The tumor mass is usually extremely hard and fixed. A rapid downhill course usually occurs, leading to death within 3 to 6 months.

MEDULLARY CARCINOMA. Medullary carcinoma arises from the C cells of the thyroid. It accounts for 5% to 10% of thyroid carcinoma and is more malignant than follicular carcinoma. It usually spreads by lymphatic channels within the thyroid to adjacent lymph nodes. It is sporadic in about half the cases and is caused by autosomal dominant inheritance in the rest. The hereditary variety, multiple endocrine neoplasia type IIA (MEN IIA, Sipple's syndrome), is associated with pheochromocytoma, parathyroid adenoma, carcinoid syndrome, and Cushing's syndrome. A syndrome called MEN IIB is similar to MEN IIA but also includes mucosal neuromas and marfanoid appearance. These tumors secrete calcitonin, which can be used to monitor results of treatment. C-cell hyperplasia precedes the appearance of the medullary carcinoma in the hereditary variety and can be detected by the finding of elevated baseline serum calcitonin concentrations or an excessive response of the serum calcitonin to pentagastrin or calcium infusion. Asymptomatic family members with occult medullary carcinoma or C-cell hyperplasia should be checked periodically with these tests. These tumors tend to be multicentric in the hereditary form but not in the sporadic variety. The finding of large amounts of amyloid material in histologic sections aids in the diagnosis.

DIAGNOSIS AND MANAGEMENT. The main concern in the patient with the single nodule is to determine if it represents thyroid cancer. There are certain clinical features and laboratory tests that help differentiate cancerous nodules from other lesions and point out those that are more likely to be carcinoma. Since most benign single nodules occur in those over the age of 40 and in women, the presence of a nodule in a patient of either sex under the age of 40 and in a man at any age makes carcinoma more likely. Also, anyone with a thyroid nodule and a history of irradiation of the head, neck, or chest in infancy or childhood should be considered to have carcinoma unless proved otherwise. Fixation of the thyroid, vocal cord paralysis, and enlarged anterior neck lymph nodes also increase the possibility of thyroid malignancy, as does nonfunction of the nodule on the thyroid scan. Some characteristics make a nodule less likely to be malignant. These include (1) presence in a multinodular gland (unless in a child); (2) thyroid cysts; (3) ability to concentrate iodine on the thyroid scan; (4) presence for years without growth; (5) nodules shown to be calcified on roentgenographic examination; and (6) benign classification on the basis of aspiration or needle biopsy cytology.

For years needle biopsy of thyroid nodules was believed to be contraindicated because of the chance of spreading cancer cells. However, in recent years needle biopsy and needle aspiration of single thyroid nodules have been increasingly reported and appear to be helpful in deciding if a nodule is malignant or benign. The tissue and cells obtained by these techniques are classified as benign, malignant, or indeterminant.

Treatment of the uninodular goiter consists of surgical excision of all nodules that fit the clinical criteria for increased malignancy or those classified as malignant or indeterminant by needle biopsy and aspiration. Either a near total thyroidectomy or removal of the lobe and isthmus is done unless there is local spread, which dictates more radical neck surgery to remove all cancerous tissue. If carcinoma is found and there is evidence of iodine accumulation, large doses (100 to 150 mCi) of ^{131}I are given except with the anaplastic and medullary varieties. Thyroid suppression therapy is also instituted postoperatively in maximal physiologic doses sufficient to keep the T_4 in the upper range of normal, to suppress the TSH to below normal, and to inhibit TSH response to TRH. In the patient with follicular carcinoma of the thyroid, large doses of ^{131}I are given postoperatively to ablate any remaining thyroid tissue and, if possible, to eradicate any residual malignancy. The long-term survival of those with papillary and follicular carcinoma of the thyroid is excellent and exceeds 80% at 10 years in most studies.

The primary mode of treatment of medullary carcinoma of the thyroid is total thyroidectomy. This is also done in family members documented to have increased levels of calcitonin and/or excessive calcitonin response to calcium or pentagastrin infusion, since they are usually found to have C-cell hyperplasia or occult carcinoma. Metastatic disease may respond to some types of chemotherapy.

Anaplastic carcinoma of the thyroid rarely responds to any form of treatment. Usually needle or open biopsy is done to establish the diagnosis, and postoperative radiotherapy may give short-term relief. Chemotherapy should be considered.

When a thyroid cyst is suspected, its presence can be confirmed by diagnostic ultrasonography or by aspiration, which also eliminates most of the mass and at the same time obtains cells for cytologic diagnosis. When a cyst is found, the patient is generally given thyroid suppression therapy and aspiration of the cyst is done at 1- to 3-month intervals. If recurrence of this cyst occurs after the third aspiration, surgical excision is carried out.

In women over the age of 40 who have nodules of the thyroid but do not have criteria for malignancy, thyroid suppression is begun and follow-up examinations are made at 3- to 6-month intervals. If there is evidence of growth of the lesion during suppression therapy, surgical excision is indicated.

BIBLIOGRAPHY

Brown, J., and others: Autoimmune thyroid diseases—Graves' and Hashimoto's, Ann. Intern. Med. **88:**379, 1978.

Caplan, R.H., and Kujak, R.: Thyroid uptake of radioactive iodine: a reevaluation, J.A.M.A. **215:**916, 1971.

Caplan, R.H., Pagliara, A.S., and Wickus, G.: Laboratory diagnosis of hyperthyroidism: a reappraisal, Postgrad. Med. **66:**75, 1979.

Chopra, I.J.: An assessment of daily production and significance of thyroidal secretion of 3,3'5'-triiodothyronine (reverse T_3) in man, J.Clin. Invest. **58:**32, 1976.

DeGroot, L.J.: Thyroid carcinoma, Med. Clin. North Am. **59:**1233, 1975.

Dratman, M.B.: The mechanism of thyroxine action. In Li, C.H., editor: Hormonal proteins and peptides, New York, 1978, Academic Press, Inc.

Grove, A.S., Jr.: Evaluation of exophthalmos, N. Engl. J. Med. **292:**1005, 1975.

Hamburger, J.I., Miller, J.M., and Kini, S.R.: Clinical-pathological evaluation of thyroid nodules—handbook and atlas, Detroit, 1979, Private publication.

Hamilton, C.R., Jr., and Maloof, F.: Unusual types of hyperthyroidism, Medicine **52:**195, 1973.

Haydar, N.A., and others: Severe hypermetabolism with primary abnormality of skeletal muscle mitochondria: functional and therapeutic effects of chloramphenicol treatment, Ann. Intern. Med. **74:**548, 1971.

Hollander, C.S., and others: Clinical and laboratory observations in cases of triiodothyronine toxicosis confirmed by radioimmunoassay, Lancet **1:**609, 1972.

Ingbar, S.H., and Woeber, K.A.: The thyroid gland. In Williams, R.C., editor: Textbook of endocrinology, ed. 5, Philadelphia, 1974, W.B. Saunders Co.

Mackin, J.F., Canary, J.J., and Pittman, C.S.: Thyroid storm and its management, N. Engl. J. Med. **291:**1396, 1974.

Miller, J.M.: Plummer's disease, Med. Clin. North Am. **59:**1203, 1975.

Mochizuky, Y., Mowafy, R., and Pasternack, B.: Weights of human thyroids in New York City, Health Phys. **9:**1299, 1963.

Nadler, N.J.: Iodination of thyroglobulin in the thyroid follicle. In Cassano, C., and Andreoli, M., editors: Current topics in thyroid research, New York, 1965, Academic Press, Inc.

Nikolai, T.F., and others: Lymphocytic thyroiditis with spontaneously resolving hyperthyroidism (silent thyroiditis), Arch. Intern. Med. **140:**478, 1980.

Royce, P.C.: Severely impaired consciousness in myxedema—a review, Am. J. Med. Sci. **261:**46, 1971.

Schimmel, M., and Utiger, R.D.: Thyroidal and peripheral production of thyroid hormones: review of recent findings and their clinical implications, Ann. Intern. Med. **87:**760, 1977.

Solomon, D.H., and others: Identification of subgroups of euthyroid Graves' ophthalmopathy, N. Engl. J. Med. **296:**181, 1977.

Sterling, K.: Thyroid hormone action at the cell level, N. Engl. J. Med. **300:**117, 173, 1979.

Van Herle, A.J., Vassart, G., and Dumont, J.E.: Control of thyroglobulin synthesis and secretion, N. Engl. J. Med. **301:**239, 307, 1979.

Volpé, R.: The role of autoimmunity in hypoendocrine and hyperendocrine function: with special emphasis on autoimmune thyroid disease, Ann. Intern. Med. **87:**86, 1977.

Werner, S.C., and Ingbar, S.H.: The thyroid, ed. 3, New York, 1971, Harper & Row, Publishers, Inc.

Zellmann, H.E.: Iatrogenic and factitious thyroidal disease, Med. Clin. North Am. **63:**329, 1979.

188 · THE ADRENAL CORTEX

Ernest M. Gold

STRUCTURE AND FUNCTION

The adrenal glands, weighing 3 to 5 g in the adult, are bilateral organs situated on the superior pole of each kidney. Each "suprarenal" gland is a composite of two tissues, an outer fatty layer, or *cortex,* which produces steroid hormones and comprises 80% of the gland, and an inner neural core, or *medulla,* which secretes catecholamines.

The hormones of the adrenal cortex, but not those of the medulla, are essential for the rapid vascular, muscular, and metabolic adaptations required for survival in normal individuals. While the cortex elaborates more than 25 different steroids, their principal biologic effects divide them into three groups: mineralocorticoids, glucocorticoids, and sex steroids. Each group arises from a histologically distinct zone of the adrenal cortex—the mineralocorticoids from the outermost *zone glomerulosa,* the glucocorticoids from the *zona fasciculata,* and the sex steroids from the inner *zone reticularis.*

BIOSYNTHESIS OF STEROID HORMONES. All steroid hormones are produced by the adrenal cortex or the gonads and arise from a common precursor, the circulating blood cholesterol. Cholesterol is transported to these tissues by a carrier (low-density) lipoprotein, and after cell entry the structure of cholesterol is progressively altered by a series of enzymes that produce each unique steroid hormone. The basic four-ringed structure of cholesterol remains intact and provides the "nucleus" typical of steroid hormones. Biosynthesis of steroids begins with the transport of cholesterol into the cell mitochondrion, where a small, six-carbon fatty acid chain is removed by a cleavage enzyme, thereby converting cholesterol to pregnenolone (Fig. 188-1). This is the critical, rate-limiting step in steroidogenesis influenced by all known hormones regulating steroid production such as adrenocorticotropic hormone (ACTH), angiotensin, and the gonadotropins. A single additional step—transposition of a hydrogen bond—converts pregnenolone to progesterone, a hormone in its own right as well as an important branch point for the further synthesis of all steroid hormones. For example, the addition of three hydroxyl groups to progesterone, each mediated by a specific hydroxylase, results in the production of cortisol (hydrocortisone), the principal glucocorticoid of man. Similarly, progesterone also is the substrate for another sequence of enzymes that leads to the biosynthesis of aldosterone, the most potent natural mineralocorticoid in man. Finally, a separate enzymatic sequence transforms progesterone into testosterone, which then can be converted to estradiol; these latter are the most important sex steroids in man. Since each enzymatic step is critical, inborn errors of enzyme deletion have two important consequences: omission of the final hormone product and accu-

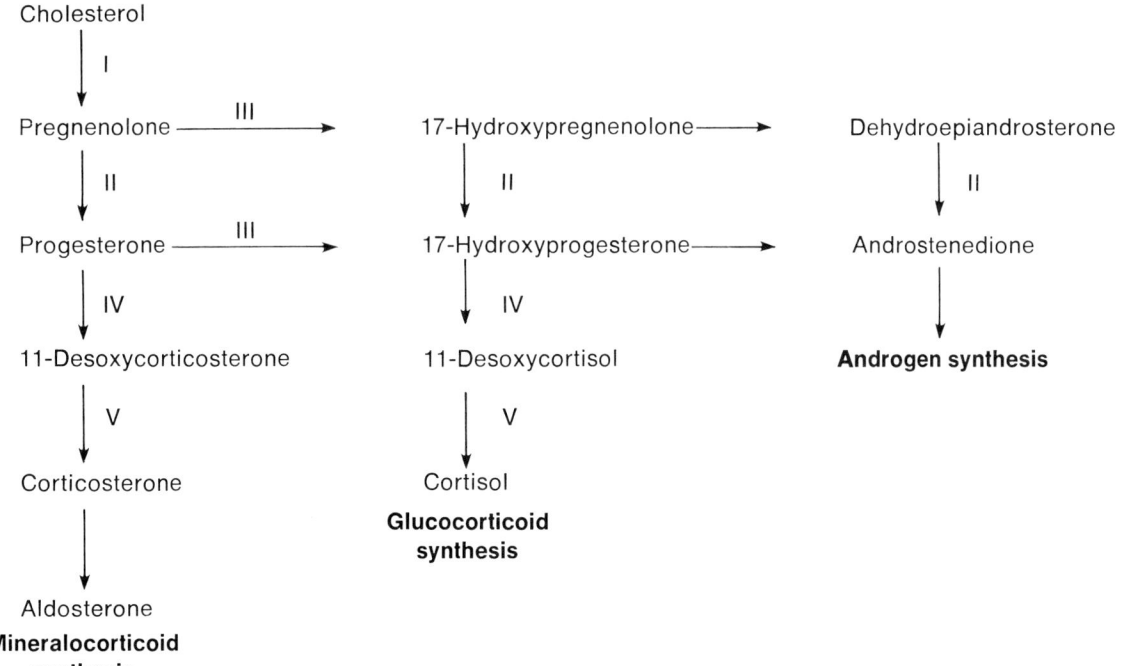

Fig. 188-1. Pathways of steroid biosynthesis. *I.* 10-Hydroxylase; *II,* 3-β-OH dehydrogenase; *III,* 17-α-hydroxylase; *IV.* 21-hydroxylase; *V,* 11-β-hydroxylase.

mulation of steroid precursors behind the deleted enzyme. Both of these consequences produce characteristic clinical syndromes that will be discussed further.

METABOLISM AND TRANSPORT. Once the hormone is synthesized, the adrenal cortex stores only small quantities of it. When released into the circulation, almost 90% of each steroid hormone becomes reversibly bound to a specific carrier protein. In the case of cortisol and aldosterone this transport globulin is termed "corticosteroid-binding globulin" (CBG), whereas "sex steroid-binding globulin" (SSBG) serves as the carrier for testosterone and estradiol. These transport globulins are produced by the liver, and their concentration in blood is independently influenced by several factors such as liver disease, which reduces production, or pregnancy and estrogen treatment, which increase production. However, only that critical fraction of each hormone that is unbound (or free) is sufficiently small to pass through capillary membranes and therefore become accessible to body cells.

The (free) steroid hormones can be metabolized and inactivated by many tissues, including red blood cells. The most important site, however, is the liver. Although the nuclear ring structure is never metabolized, enzymatic addition of a single hydrogen function or removal of a hydroxyl group can completely inactivate each steroid hormone. Since this can be accomplished at many sites on the molecule, as many as 40 different metabolites are excreted into the urine. The overall process is very efficient so that less than 1% of unmetabolized "free" cortisol escapes intact into the urine. The rate of degradation and the variety of steroid metabolites produced can be influenced by several conditions; for example, liver disease and hypothyroidism slow the removal of steroids from blood, whereas hyperthyroidism and certain drugs such as phenytoin accelerate metabolism.

CELLULAR ACTION. The free steroid molecule, dissociated from its transport protein and plasma, readily penetrates any cell membrane; however, only those cells bearing specific protein receptors in their cytoplasm that bind the hormone are responsive to the message it carries. Once bound, the steroid-receptor complex transmigrates through the nuclear membrane to specific deoxyribonucleic acid (DNA) receptor sites along the chromatin strands of selected nuclear chromosomes. Union with DNA initiates transcription of a new messenger ribonucleic acid (mRNA), which leaves the nucleus for ribosomal sites where translation of a specific new protein (for example, an enzyme) appears about 1 hour after cells are exposed to the steroid hormone. The specific protein(s) newly synthesized varies, of course, with each individual steroid as well as with each different target cell. In the case of glucocorticoids, for example, the hepatocyte responds to cortisol by synthesis of at least six new proteins, all of them enzymes involved in glucose metabolism. By contrast, the distal tubular cells of the kidney, the major site of aldosterone action, produce an intracellular protein that facilitates the transport of sodium from tubular urine back into the blood and simultaneously transports potassium from tubular blood into the urine.

PHYSIOLOGIC ACTION. Beyond the cellular level glucocorticoids influence almost every body tissue to bring about certain integrated physiologic adaptations (Table 188-1). Cortisol supports the responsiveness of arterial smooth muscle to normal pressor stimuli, thereby maintaining arterial pressure, cardiac output, and renal blood flow. The hormone also facilitates processes that sustain the blood sugar, such as the induction of hepatic enzymes that convert protein to glucose (gluconeogenesis); additionally, cortisol opposes the action of insulin on tissue uptake of glucose and amino acids, two effects frequently termed "catabolic" because synthesis of new protein and storage of fat are inhibited.

Taken together, the enhancement of cardiovascular function and mobilization of energy stores by cortisol have led to a view of the hormone's integrated contribution as "stress adaptation," the rapid preparation for "fight or flight." However, certain negative attributes also accompany cortisol action, particularly when the hormone is produced in excess for a sustained period. These detrimental features include suppression of the inflammatory response so that resistance to infection is lessened, inhibition of connective tissue growth so that wound healing is impaired and bone development is arrested, and, finally, suppression of immune surveillance so that normal antibody production is inhibited. This last effect assumes particular importance when potent synthetic glucocorticoids are used for an extended period in large doses to treat a variety of illnesses in man. Finally, glucocorticoids suppress pituitary synthesis of ACTH, the hormone that stimulates cortisol production, an important physiologic action of the hormone that is inseparable from its catabolic and anti-inflammatory actions.

By contrast, the actions of aldosterone are far more selective than those of cortisol. The principal physiologic effect of aldosterone is to maintain an effective circulating blood volume. This is accomplished chiefly by the retention of sodium, which, of course, increases not only blood volume but also extracellular fluid volume. The only other

Table 188-1. Major physiologic actions and aberrations of cortisol

Physiologic activity affected	Cortisol production rate	
	Decreased	Increased
Blood pressure	Hypotention	Hypertension
Renal function	Hyponatremia	Hypokalemia
Metabolism	Hypoglycemia	Hyperglycemia
Pituitary ACTH secretion	Increased	Decreased

major role of aldosterone is to enhance potassium excretion, a critical function because potassium is completely reabsorbed in the proximal renal tubule and must be secreted by active transport in the distal renal tubule. Both of these actions of aldosterone are accomplished by the hormone's effects on a single transport mechanism in distal tubular cells of the kidney. In this mechanism sodium is retained and potassium excreted by virtue of an aldosterone-sensitive action exchange enzyme "pump." Although this pump selectively retains sodium, it is less selective for potassium; hydrogen and ammonium ions may be excreted instead of potassium. These renal effects of aldosterone are shared by other mineralocorticoids, both endogenous and synthetic, and account for virtually all the clinical consequences of disorders of mineralocorticoid production observed in man.

PHYSIOLOGIC REGULATION. The adrenal cortex produces approximately 20 mg of cortisol each day, about the amount required to maintain adrenalectomized human adults. Cortisol production is entirely dependent on ACTH, and this pituitary hormone is in turn regulated by a specific hypothalamic neurohormone, corticotropin-releasing factor (CRF). Three separate mechanisms govern the pituitary secretion of ACTH. One of these is plasma (unbound) cortisol itself. As plasma levels rise, ACTH production falls—a classic negative feedback control system whereby cortisol directly suppresses pituitary ACTH cells and possibly hypothalamic CRF neurons as well. Superimposed on this continuous reciprocal pituitary-adrenal feedback interaction, CRF intermittently releases pituitary ACTH in response to two sets of neural signals received by the hypothalamus. One set of signals is time based, varying throughout the course of the day (circadian) so that cortisol secretion slows toward the end of each day as sleep approaches and rises once again in the early morning hours, even before wakening. The other mechanism that influences cortisol production is also mediated by hypothalamic CRF, triggered in response to a real or even threatened "stress," including trauma, illness, fright, and anesthesia. Physiologically, therefore, cortisol provides the brain with a potent, direct chemical link to almost every body cell, which allows it to quickly influence many vital processes such as blood pressure and glucose utilization. The failure of cortisol to increase under stress removes this supportive link and can result in sudden shock and even death.

Aldosterone production is regulated almost independently of the pituitary. The control mechanism for aldosterone secretion is located in the kidney, specifically in a group of specialized cells situated along the afferent glomerular arteriole, the juxtaglomerular (JG) cells. When arteriolar volume or pressure decreases, the JG cells promptly release a proteolytic enzyme, renin, into the circulation, which cleaves an α_2-globulin (angiotensinogen) from the liver to produce an inert decapeptide, angiotensin I. Angiotensin I is rapidly transformed to an active octapeptide, angiotensin II, by a "converting enzyme," a hydrolase commonly present in the vascular endothelium of the lungs and arteries. Angiotensin II has dual actions; it is the most potent, natural arteriolar vasoconstrictor, and it directly stimulates the glomerulosa cells of the adrenal cortex to produce aldosterone. Restoration of blood volume as a result of aldosterone-mediated sodium reabsorption thereby removes the stimulus for renin secretion by the JG cells. Thus aldosterone also is regulated by a negative feedback system whereby effective circulating blood volume is inversely related to aldosterone production. Conditions that reduce blood volume, such as hemorrhage, a low-salt diet, low serum protein levels, and some forms of heart failure, all result in renin release and increased aldosterone secretion. Some forms of hypertension, particularly those caused by excessive mineralocorticoids, decrease renin production and thereby also suppress both angiotensin II and aldosterone secretion.

GLUCOCORTICOID DEFICIENCY SYNDROMES (ADDISON'S DISEASE)

DEFINITION. The clinical syndrome of glucocorticoid deficiency in man is due to inadequate production of a single hormone, cortisol. When this results from lesions directly involving the adrenal cortex, the disorder is termed "primary adrenal failure" or Addison's disease. If, however, this is due to failure of ACTH to stimulate cortisol production, the resulting syndrome is termed "secondary adrenal failure."

Addison's disease is uncommon, with about 50 cases occurring in a population of 1 million. Although it may occur at all ages, it is more frequently found in women and usually occurs in young adults between the ages of 20 and 40. Diagnosis of this disease meant virtually certain death within several years until the 1940s, when this prognosis was dramatically reversed with the discovery and synthesis of the adrenal corticosteroids. Use of these agents then permitted the needed surgery on patients with Addison's disease and allowed for their normal survival.

PATHOGENESIS. Primary adrenocortical failure can be produced by any one of many disorders involving the adrenal cortex (Table 188-2). Tuberculosis was the most common cause early in this century but with current effective therapy is now an infrequent cause. The most frequent basis for Addison's disease currently is a disorder sometimes termed "idiopathic adrenal atrophy." The designation "idiopathic" is becoming less applicable in view of evidence that this is a destructive autoimmune disorder directed against an unknown adrenal antigen. This evidence includes (1) epidemiologic clustering of adrenal failure with other suspected autoimmune disorders such as insulin-deficient diabetes, hypothyroidism, and pernicious anemia: (2) demonstration of antibodies against adrenal tissue in the blood of newly diagnosed patients; (3) a common

Table 188-2. Causes of adrenal failure

Type	Cause
Primary adrenal failure (Addison's disease)	Idiopathic atrophy—autoimmune adrenalitis
	Infectious diseases—tuberculosis, overwhelming bacteremia
	Infiltrative diseases—amyloidosis, carcinoma
	Vascular disorders—hemorrhage, infarction
	Iatrogenic—surgical ablation
Secondary adrenal failure (ACTH deficiency)	Pituitary disorders—tumors, necrosis
	Hypothalamic disorders—tumors, trauma
	Iatrogenic—surgery, steroid therapy

HLA phenotype (DW3) in the majority of patients; (4) experimental induction of adrenalitis in rodents given adrenal tissue extracts; and (5) histologic adrenal lesions in man consistent with immunogenic disease, namely, lymphocytic infiltration and atrophy.

Secondary adrenocortical failure is caused by a variety of intrasellar lesions that destroy pituitary ACTH-producing cells; less frequently, it also results from brain lesions involving CRF neurons, thereby leading to failure of pituitary ACTH release. The most common cause of secondary adrenal failure seen today, and indeed the most common cause of glucocorticoid deficiency, is adrenocortical suppression of cortisol production following prolonged therapeutic use of synthetic glucorticoids.

Two important distinctions between primary and secondary adrenal failure are noteworthy and influence the associated clinical syndromes. (1) Addison's disease is commonly associated with loss of adrenal steroids other than cortisol, particularly aldosterone; by contrast, secondary adrenal failure is not associated with aldosterone deficiency. (2) Primary adrenal failure is accompanied by markedly elevated levels of plasma ACTH as a physiologic feedback consequence of cortisol deficiency; by definition, plasma ACTH is low or undetectable in secondary adrenal failure.

CLINICAL MANIFESTATIONS. Adrenal failure occurs as either an acute or a chronic syndrome.

The predominant feature of acute adrenal failure is hypotension. Sudden, unexpected shock may be the only finding that raises suspicion of the diagnosis. This commonly occurs during the course of a serious illness. When that illness is overwhelming bacteremia such as fulminant meningococcemia, in which the adrenal glands undergo hemorrhagic necrosis, it has been described as the Waterhouse-Friderichsen syndrome. More commonly, however, hypotension abruptly or early postoperatively precipitated by minor trauma or surgery may be the first indication of adrenal failure.

Chronic adrenal failure develops progressively over several years, the course being variable in duration and severity depending on the destructive process. During this period the cardinal features of the syndrome almost invariably occur in all patients. Weakness is a universal complaint, noted initially as easy fatigue but increasing in time to profound exhaustion that limits normal activity. Weight loss is also a regular occurrence, usually accompanied by poor appetite and sometimes by episodes of nausea and vomiting. Hypotension, particularly with upright posture, is regularly noted on examination. Occasionally this is symptomatic, with episodes of dizziness occurring after standing. In advanced cases a feeble pulse and small heart size are also found.

Hyperpigmentation is the single most characteristic physical finding of primary adrenal failure; it represents melanocyte stimulation induced by high levels of ACTH and thus is absent in secondary adrenal failure. The skin darkening is generalized but most intense over sun-exposed areas, sometimes described as a summer tan that never fades. Other involved areas, particularly in whites, include mucocutaneous junctions, which reveal bluish black mottling of the lips, the dentate margins of the gums, the buccal mucosa, the palate, and under the tongue. Similar speckled pigmentation is observed on the conjunctiva, nasal openings and vaginal and anal orifices. On the skin, freckles and moles become more intense, the nipple areolae darken, recent scars are heavily pigmented, the palmar and finger creases of the hand acquire pigmentation, linear pigment lines appear on the fingernails, and the extensor (pressure) surfaces of the extremities such as the elbows and knees acquire a dirty brown color.

Selected features sometimes present include hypoglycemia, salt craving, joint pains, and others equally nonspecific such as weakness, weight loss, and gastrointestinal complaints. However, when these are accompanied by low blood pressure and darkening of the skin, the syndrome of chronic adrenal failure should always be considered.

DIAGNOSIS. A number of routine laboratory tests reflect the profound metabolic disturbance resulting from glucocorticoid deficiency. These include elevations in serum potassium, calcium, and urea and a decrease in serum sodium and glucose. Eosinophilia, in excess of 4%, is noted in the white blood cell count. Although common, these alterations are not universal and, most important, are not specific.

Plasma cortisol or urinary cortisol metabolites are usually low although still within the normal range in almost one half of patients. Plasma ACTH is increased in virtually all cases of primary adrenal failure, often markedly, although such increases could also result from stress or illness.

The definitive procedure for the diagnosis of primary adrenal failure is the ACTH stimulation test. A variety of protocols for carrying out this test exist, varying in route of ACTH administration, sample collection time, and assay of cortisol in blood or urine. A simple screening procedure employs synthetic ACTH (cosyntropin) given as 0.25 mg intramuscularly, with measurement of plasma cortisol before and 30 minutes after injection; the increment in plasma cortisol should exceed 7 μg/dl, with an absolute value greater than 18 μg/dl. Regardless of ACTH dose and prolonged duration of administration, plasma cortisol levels in the addisonian patient will rarely rise above 20 μg/dl. A more discriminating version of the ACTH test employs 0.25 mg of cosyntropin intravenously over 4 hours; unlike the failure of cortisol to increase as expected with primary adrenal failure, prolonged ACTH administration results in some increase of cortisol, although subnormal, in patients with secondary adrenal failure.

The metyrapone test is used to establish the diagnosis of secondary adrenal failure. Metyrapone, a drug that blocks steroid 11-hydroxylation, interferes with cortisol biosynthesis and thereby elicits ACTH release in response to feedback demand. The drug-blocked adrenal gland responds to ACTH by increasing production of the cortisol precursor 11-desoxycortisol, which provides an index of both ACTH release and adrenal response. Several variants of the metyrapone test are available, perhaps the simplest being the oral administration of 750 mg of metyrapone every 4 hours for six doses; a significant rise (greater than 10 μg/dl) in plasma 11-desoxycortisol (compound S) excludes functional impairment of the adrenal gland and the release of pituitary ACTH and brain CRF. Therefore, to diagnose secondary adrenal failure with the metyrapone test, adrenal integrity must first be demonstrated separately by responsiveness to exogenous ACTH.

MANAGEMENT. All patients with adrenal failure, whether primary or secondary, require lifelong replacement therapy with cortisol.

Maintenance therapy for chronic adrenal failure commonly needs no more than 20 mg of hydrocortisone at breakfast and 10 mg taken in the late afternoon before dinner. Patients must be instructed to double this dose for several days during mild illness; when a disorder such as gastroenteritis prevents oral administration, it is imperative that patients obtain parenteral therapy from a physician. Many patients with primary adrenal failure also require mineralocorticoid replacement, the most common indications being hyperkalemia or hypotension. This is usually achieved by once daily (morning) administration of 0.1 mg of fludrocortisone (Florinef), a synthetic mineralocorticoid that is effective orally.

Acute adrenal failure requires substantially larger doses of hydrocortisone. A common protocol can be used either as treatment or for prophylaxis of addisonian crisis in patients scheduled for elective surgery. A day 1 regimen includes 100 mg of hydrocortisone given by bolus injection followed by 100 mg given intravenously every 8 hours (total dose 300 to 400 mg). On day 2, 50 mg of hydrocortisone is given intramuscularly every 6 hours; on day 3 this is reduced to 25 mg every 6 hours. By day 4, patients often can be given hydrocortisone orally in doses of 10 mg every 6 hours; by day 5, a maintenance regimen can be resumed.

GLUCOCORTICOID EXCESS SYNDROMES (CUSHING'S SYNDROME)

DEFINITION. The clinical conditions resulting from prolonged, excessive exposure to cortisol or its synthetic analogs are termed glucocorticoid excess syndromes. Cushing's syndrome and chronic hypercortisolism are common synonyms for these syndromes. The most common cause of Cushing's syndrome is iatrogenic, that is, caused by prescription of synthetic glucocorticoids such as prednisone and dexamethasone in large doses for treatment of a variety of chronic disorders.

PATHOGENESIS. The natural Cushing's syndrome is really a group of disorders that has in common one invariable feature—the sustained, excessive production of cortisol by the adrenal cortex. The syndrome usually indicates a tumor.

Pituitary Cushing's syndrome is the most common variant and accounts for two thirds of all cases of Cushing's syndrome. It is caused by excessive ACTH production, usually resulting from a small pituitary tumor found in two thirds of patients, the majority of whom are women of childbearing age. Why ACTH is overproduced in the other one third of patients without a demonstrable pituitary tumor remains unknown. Some believe that this represents a primary brain disorder mediated by excessive CRF secretion, which someday might be called *hypothalamic Cushing's syndrome*.

Adrenal Cushing's syndrome is caused by autonomous cortisol production by an adrenal tumor that is usually unilateral. Although this variant accounts for only 17% of all patients, it is common in children; adrenal cancer is the lesion in 65% of patients under the age of 15. In contrast to pituitary Cushing's syndrome, in which ACTH secretion is inappropriately normal or high and accompanied by adrenal hyperplasia, in the adrenal form pituitary ACTH is uniformly suppressed so that all normal adrenal tissue (including the contralateral adrenal gland) is completely atrophic.

Ectopic Cushing's syndrome is the result of autonomous ACTH production by one of more than 25 different extra-pituitary malignancies, the most common being lung cancer. This syndrome accounts for 15% of patients, and not surprisingly most are male and most are smokers. Plasma ACTH levels are markedly increased, and both adrenal glands are huge and hyperplastic.

CLINICAL MANIFESTATIONS. The three most common clinical features of Cushing's syndrome are obesity, hypertension, and a plethoric or red face (Table 188-3). Cortisol excess increases the sensitivity of the arterial system

Table 188-3. Clinical manifestations of Cushing's syndrome

Manifestation	Occurrence (%)
Obesity	90
Red face (plethora)	75
Hypertension	75
Hirsutism	65
Muscle weakness	60
Menstrual disorders	60
Acne	45
Bruising	40
Mental disorders	40
Backache (osteoporosis)	40

Table 188-4. Confirmatory measurements of Cushing's syndrome

Test procedure	Time	Plasma cortisol—upper limit (μg/dl)
Basal measurements	8 AM	30
	4 PM	15
Administration of dexamethasone, 1 mg	Midnight	
	8 AM following day	5

to neural and humoral pressor stimuli and results in hypertension. Protein synthesis slows as cortisol directs amino acids from muscle and connective tissues to the liver for conversion to glucose. Thus the extremities become thin and weak, bone structure becomes fragile and decalcified (osteoporosis), surface capillaries become fragile so that slight trauma causes hematomas, and separation of the subcutaneous skin produces the red truncal stripes (striae) seen with the typical syndrome. Glucose is poorly utilized because of insulin antagonism and becomes redistributed from muscle to adipose tissue, resulting in a round, cheeky face, prominent neck fat ("buffalo hump"), and increased abdominal girth or truncal obesity. Finally, as elevated insulin levels become insufficient to dispose of glucose, diabetes results. In women, particularly those with pituitary Cushing's syndrome, ACTH stimulates the zona reticularis to produce excessive androgens, resulting in acne and excessive facial and body hair (hirsutism).

The clinical spectrum is quite broad, however, and includes cases with the classical features as well as some unusual patients with no distinguishing features at all.

DIAGNOSIS. A systematic three-step approach to testing provides the least ambiguous and least expensive route for complete diagnosis of Cushing's syndrome. These three sequential steps are confirmation, differentiation, and localization.

Confirmation. Confirmation demands unequivocal demonstration of excessive cortisol production. In all cases, regardless of cause, cortisol secretion remains elevated throughout each day, uninfluenced by circadian time or even by many stressful stimuli. A useful outpatient screening protocol requires only three plasma cortisol measurements, taken in the morning, the evening, and the next morning following 1 mg of dexamethasone taken orally at midnight. All of these measurements will be abnormal in each of the three varieties of Cushing's syndrome (Table 188-4). Since plasma cortisol determinations are accurate and widely available, tedious urine collections for steroid measurements are no longer necessary. One urinary assay of considerable value, however, particularly in ambiguous cases, is the measurement of urinary free cortisol; excretion of free (unmetabolized) cortisol in excess of 100 μg daily is a common finding in all forms of Cushing's syndrome.

Differentiation. Once hypercortisolism is established, differentiation is directed toward the identification of one of the three variants of Cushing's syndrome–pituitary, adrenal, or ectopic. Plasma ACTH radioimmunoassay is the most useful measurement for this purpose.

Increased plasma cortisol with undetectable levels of plasma ACTH is diagnostic for the adrenal form; no further tests are necessary to establish this diagnosis. As might be expected, there is no increase in steroid production during the metyrapone test, and dexamethasone likewise fails to suppress autonomous tumor production of cortisol. By contrast, in the ectopic form, plasma ACTH levels are always above normal and are often markedly increased; plasma ACTH concentrations greater than 250 pg/ml almost always indicate an ectopic malignant source of ACTH production.

Normal ACTH levels in the presence of excessive plasma cortisol occur in only the pituitary form of Cushing's syndrome. Obviously, such normal levels of ACTH are inappropriate and clearly indicate pituitary insensitivity to physiologic negative feedback suppression. Clinically, this is confirmed by the low-dose dexamethasone suppression test, whereas the metyrapone test demonstrates that some pituitary control remains because cortisol blockade by this drug markedly increases both ACTH and steroidogenesis, a response characteristic only of the pituitary form. By contrast, metyrapone given to patients with the ectopic form, in whom ACTH is autonomously produced, results in no rise in ACTH or steroid production. The metyrapone test therefore nicely discriminates between the ectopic and pituitary forms of Cushing's syndrome, a distinction sometimes of crucial importance. This is particularly the case when ACTH levels are elevated, a situation found in about one half of patients with the pituitary form. Sine these ACTH elevations can overlap levels found in the ectopic syndrome, unequivocal differentiation becomes essential to any further management of such patients.

Localization. Once the variety of Cushing's syndrome has been established, localization defines the anatomic site of the lesion causing each syndrome, a lesion that in most cases is a tumor. For pituitary Cushing's syndrome, conventional skull roentgenograms for sella turcica size are often an initial procedure. However, fewer than 15% of pituitary tumors causing Cushing's syndrome are detected by this technique. Polytomography of the sella turcica and, more recently, computed tomography scan procedures represent a major diagnostic advance in the recognition of pituitary tumors. In the pituitary form detection of relatively minor deformities of the sella has made it possible to recognize microadenomas in almost two thirds of patients with this disorder.

Adrenal Cushing's syndrome is almost always an indication for surgery, and in such cases precise preoprative localization of the tumor is imperative. Since most of these lesions are unilateral, obviously the side to be operated on must be established before surgery. Noninvasive procedures such as computed tomography and ultrasonography of the adrenal areas are preferred for making this determination. In the case of ectopic Cushing's syndrome a routine chest roentgenogram will demonstrate a lung lesion in more than one half of such patients. If the chest film shows no evidence of lung cancer, a variety of specialized radiologic techniques may be required to examine the more than 25 different tissues where cancer can give rise to the ectopic form. Such a search can be particularly important, since about 10% of patients with this form have been cured by removal of circumscribed malignancies such as bronchial adenomas and medullary carcinomas of the thyroid.

MANAGEMENT. Three options are available for treatment of patients with Cushing's syndrome: surgery, irradiation, and drug therapy. The choice of optimal treatment is determined to a large extent by the specific cause of Cushing's syndrome.

Adrenal Cushing's syndrome is practically a mandate for adrenal surgery. Because the lesion is unilateral in the majority of cases, only one adrenal gland is removed. In most cases the suppressed contralateral adrenal gland regains normal function after several months. Most adrenal tumors are benign adenomas, but when found, adrenocortical carcinoma is often inoperable or is discovered at surgery to have metastasized. In such cases life expectancy is less than 2 years, but treatment with cortisol-blocking drugs such as mitotane (o,p'-DDD) can relieve some of the symptomatic consequences of hypercortisolism such as diabetes and hypokalemic alkalosis.

Irradiation of the pituitary area is obviously an option only for patients with pituitary Cushing's syndrome. This has been particularly useful for patients under 20 years of age and for some adults with only mild clinical symptoms. The major drawback of radiotherapy is the long lag period (18 months in some cases) before complete remission.

Drugs provide a second option for therapy and, although not definitive, are nonetheless useful adjuncts in the preoperative management of severely debilitated patients, as well as in those with inoperable or incompletely removed lesions and those awaiting remission after radiotherapy. Pharmacologic agents fall into two groups. The first group acts within the central nervous system to interfere with the neurohormonal (CRF) regulation of pituitary ACTH secretion. The two agents in this group are cyproheptadine, a serotonin antagonist, and bromocriptine, a dopamine agonist. Both of these drugs can be used only in the pituitary form; they have had some initial, although limited, success. A second group of drugs, applicable to all three varieties of Cushing's syndrome, acts directly on enzymes of the adrenal cortex to block the production of cortisol. The most widely used agents in this adrenal-active group are mitotane and metyrapone, both helpful in ameliorating Cushing's syndrome for several months without major toxicity.

The most notable recent advance in treatment has been the development of transsphenoidal pituitary microsurgery for the management of pituitary Cushing's syndrome in adults. Selective removal of pituitary microadenomas has been accomplished with negligible operative mortality and with restoration of normal ACTH production, including physiologic regulation.

MINERALOCORTICOID DEFICIENCY SYNDROMES

DEFINITION. Mineralocorticoid deficiency is synonymous with loss of aldosterone production. Since 1957, when the disorder was first described, fewer than 100 cases of selective deficiency of aldosterone have been reported; however, the frequency of these reports has notably increased within recent years.

PATHOGENESIS. Aldosterone deficiency most commonly is associated with loss of cortisol production in the course of primary adrenal failure resulting from destructive adrenocortical lesions. Isolated hypoaldosteronism is caused by inability of glomerulosa cells to synthesize the hormone, either as a result of inborn enzymatic defects or secondary to inadequate stimulation by angiotensin. Angiotensin failure is the most common basis for selective aldosterone deficiency and arises as a consequence of inadequate renin production by renal JG cells. JG cell destruction occurs during the course of chronic renal failure owing to a variety of tubulointerstitial lesions, most frequently in association with diabetic renal disease.

CLINICAL MANIFESTATIONS. Typically, selective hypoaldosteronism occurs in an elderly patient with chronic renal failure, hypertension, and diabetes. The only manifestation of mineralocorticoid deficiency in such a patient may be an electrolyte disorder. Hyperkalemia is usually present, with serum potassium sometimes approaching potentially lethal levels of 8 to 9 mEq/L. Hyperchloremic (metabolic) acidosis is common, occasionally accompanied by hyponatremia. The only clinical consequence of this electrolyte disturbance is the occasional occurrence of cardiac arrhythmias, including heart block and other conduction defects.

DIAGNOSIS. Serum aldosterone levels usually are below normal, and measurements of renin and angiotensin are also decreased. By contrast, in primary adrenal failure, plasma renin is usually elevated. The diagnosis of hyporeninemic hypoaldosteronism is confirmed by the demonstration that plasma renin fails to increase following salt deprivation or diuretic-induced volume depletion.

MANAGEMENT. Hyperkalemia is the most serious derangement resulting from mineralocorticoid deficiency. When serum potassium levels exceed 8 mEq/L, infusions of insulin given with glucose and saline are required to reduce these levels. For long-term treatment, satisfactory correction of mineralocorticoid deficiency can be obtained with 0.1 to 0.2 mg of fludrocortisone given orally each day.

MINERALOCORTICOID EXCESS SYNDROMES (ALDOSTERONISM)

DEFINITION. A clinical syndrome resulting from an excess of mineralocorticoids occurs as a result of overproduction of aldosterone, 11-desoxycorticosterone (DOC), or corticosterone. The steroid most commonly implicated is aldosterone; this syndrome is commonly termed primary aldosteronism or *Conn's syndrome*. Primary aldosteronism is the cause of hypertension in about 1% to 2% of all hypertensive patients, and it is the most frequent cause of curable hypertension.

The ingestion of enormous quantities of licorice extracts (glycyrrhizic acid) may result in hypertension, potassium depletion, and low plasma renin. There is also a familial disorder, *Liddle's syndrome,* in which there is excessive renal tubular absorption of sodium resulting in hypertension, potassium depletion with low plasm renin, and inhibition of aldosterone secretion.

PATHOGENESIS. Prolonged secretion of excessive aldosterone results from one of three lesions: (1) a solitary adrenocortical tumor, usually a benign adenoma; (2) bilateral adrenocortical hyperplasia; or (3) a tumor of the JG cells of the kidney, which autonomously produces renin. Rarely, mineralocorticoid excess is also caused by an adrenal tumor that secretes DOC or corticosterone, although when these unusual mineralocorticoids are involved, an inborn error in cortisol biosynthesis is the more common cause (see section on "Congenital adrenal hyperplasia"). The physiologic consequences of mineralocorticoid excess are identical for all three steroids.

Two principal actions of mineralocorticoids—sodium reabsorption and potassium excretion—account for the excess produced. These are the results of a coupled cation exchange process stimulated by mineralocorticoids acting on the distal renal tubule. Sodium retention leads to expansion of extracellular fluid, including an increase in effective circulating blood volume; together with enhanced arteriolar sensitivity to pressor stimuli, this accounts for the characteristic hypertension produced by an excess of mineralocorticoids. Remarkably, however, despite sustained exposure to mineralocorticoids, no edema develops. Volume expansion is limited to only about 10% in excess of normal; this is due to mineralocorticoid adaptation or an "escape" mechanism that occurs after about 7 to 10 days, in which further sodium reabsorption is attenuated as a result of proximal tubular rejection of additional sodium. Thus in the adapted patient further volume expansion is resisted, urinary sodium excretion returns to normal, and salt elimination becomes even more efficient than normal. Although the explanation of this escape mechanism remains unclear, a humoral factor seems implicated, and, in addition, normal heart, liver, and kidney functions are required. In contrast to primary aldosteronism, disorders of the heart, liver, and kidney are frequently accompanied by markedly enhanced proximal tubular sodium reabsorption, little or no urinary sodium excretion, unrestrained expansion of extracellular fluid volume, and resulting edema that can be massive. These conditions are commonly accompanied by huge increases in aldosterone production and are sometimes termed "secondary" aldosteronism, since aldosterone secretion is one of several mechanisms mobilized to compensate for a common pathologic association of edematous disorders, that is, a decrease in effective circulating blood volume.

The second major action of mineralocorticoids, potassium excretion, is closely linked to sodium retention. However, whereas sodium reabsorption is limited by an escape mechanism, depletion of total body potassium is progressive and may be profound. In addition to potassium, hydrogen ion is also exchanged for sodium, resulting in the alkalosis observed with mineralocorticoid excess syndromes. Potassium depletion is the most common basis for the symptomatic features that characterize mineralocorticoid excess syndromes.

CLINICAL MANIFESTATIONS. The physical appearance of patients with mineralocorticoid excess is entirely normal. The single universal finding present in all cases is diastolic hypertension, usually moderate in degree and sometimes accompanied by headaches and, on examination, possibly early hypertensive retinopathy and cardiomegaly without edema. The significant clues are a spectrum of symptoms attributable to potassium depletion that range from easy fatigue to profound weakness and even intermittent paralysis. Other muscle-related complaints include constipation, leg cramps, and even tetany, with the last resulting from the alkalosis that often accompanies hypokalemia. Other potassium-linked problems include renal insensitivity to antidiuretic hormone (ADH), sometimes manifest as polyuria, and impaired release of and impaired tissue sensitivity to insulin, occasionally resulting in diabetes mellitus.

It is important to recognize that the clinical features of mineralocorticoid excess can be modified by diet. For example, a diet unusually rich in potassium may obscure or even reverse virtually all the clinical manifestations in some mild cases; in most, however, failure to improve hypokalemia with potassium supplements may provide the first clue to primary aldosteronism. Similarly, salt restriction, a common therapy for hypertension, may not only lower blood pressure but even restore serum potassium to normal by reducing sodium available for distal tubular exchange with potassium.

Hypertension associated with hypokalemia is the most important hallmark of mineralocorticoid excess syndromes. In addition to dietary variables in sodium or potassium intake, the other common source of confusion is the treatment of hypertensive patients with diuretics, causing kaliuresis. Two features of diuretic therapy are noteworthy. Some agents, particularly thiazides, sometimes uncover the syndrome previously compensated by increased dietary potassium. More often, however, such patients do not have mineralocorticoid excess but represent merely the omission of supplemental potassium with thiazide diuretics; hypokalemia in such cases can be improved within 2 weeks by providing 80 to 100 mEq of supplemental potassium daily.

DIAGNOSIS. A mineralocorticoid excess syndrome should be considered in all patients with diastolic hypertension of unknown cause. Particular attention should be paid to the young or when hypertension is of recent onset or is associated with symptoms of potassium deficiency, diabetes, and disorders of sexual function.

Diagnosis ultimately requires a demonstration of the chronic, inappropriate, and excessive production of a specific mineralocorticoid and its tissue of origin. These objectives are commonly and most efficiently fulfilled by the sequence of confirmation, differentiation, and localization.

Confirmation. Mineralocorticoid hypertension is confirmed by the demonstration of (1) hypokalemia, (2) renin suppression, and (3) excessive mineralocorticoid production. Measurement of serum potassium is least costly and most readily available as an initial office screening procedure. In patients with a low serum potassium level (less than 3.5 mEq/L) the possibility of mineralocorticoid excess is reinforced by subsequent failure of hypokalemia to respond to average potassium supplementation (60 to 80 mEq daily). Restoration of normal serum potassium by salt restriction (10 to 20 mEq daily) or with spironolactone therapy (400 mg daily) also strongly suggests mineralocorticoid excess. Spironolactone, a synthetic mineralocorticoid antagonist, blocks distal tubular cation exchange and, most important, does so only if mineralocorticoids are produced. Thus hypertensive patients with normal serum potassium may be given 5 to 7 days of salt loading (200 to 300 mEq daily). If serum potassium falls, spironolactone treatment will reverse this decline, but only if a mineralocorticoid is being produced inappropriately, that is, during a period of high salt intake when such hormones should normally be suppressed.

Renin (and angiotensin II) suppression is an expected normal concomitant of volume expansion owing to excess mineralocorticoids. Therefore plasma renin activity (PRA) is uniformly low, even in random clinic samples, although this is most convincingly shown by demonstrating that PRA fails to respond after challenge by normal stimuli such as volume depletion or upright posture. This can be achieved in the office setting by several days of sodium restriction or a simple challenge test, such as an injection of 40 mg of furosemide followed by ambulation for 4 hours, after which a blood sample is obtained for PRA. Failure of PRA to increase in this context provides strong evidence for excessive mineralocorticoid production.

Finally, confirmation of the specific mineralocorticoid is required. This is always best accomplished in the presence of salt loading (when aldosterone normally is suppressed) after a high salt intake for several days and collection of a 24-hour urine sample or after infusion of intravenous saline and collection of blood samples; the suspected steroid is then determined. The first steroid to measure, of course, is aldosterone. High levels confirm the diagnosis of primary aldosteronism; low levels should lead to further analyses for DOC or corticosterone.

Differentiation. Differentiation is based on the recognition that each variety of mineralocorticoid excess, including primary aldosteronism, has several causes. In the case of primary aldosteronism, at least four variants have been identified. These include (1) glucocorticoid responsive hyperaldosteronism, in which an excess aldosterone production is suppressed by dexamethasone; (2) indeterminate hyperaldosteronism, in which aldosterone suppression occurs when another mineralocorticoid such as DOC or fludrocortisone is given; (3) bilateral hyperplasia, in which hypertension is unchanged by spironolactone therapy; and (4) an aldosterone-producing adenoma, in which aldosterone production is unresponsive to dexamethasone or fludrocortisone and blood pressure declines after 6 weeks of spironolactone therapy. This last variant is the most common cause.

Localization. Localization is important only in the case of an aldosterone-producing adenoma, the single form of primary aldosteronism appropriate for surgery. The principal objective is to establish the adenoma site preoperatively. This can be accomplished by noninvasive procedures such as computed tomography, ultrasonography, or nuclear scan techniques employing radioactive 19-iodocholesterol. However, since many of these tumors are very small, invasive procedures may be required, including arteriography or retrograde adrenal venography.

MANAGEMENT. Two forms of therapy are available for mineralocorticoid excess syndromes: surgery and drugs. Surgery is virtually a mandate when mineralocorticoids are being overproduced by a unilateral tumor. Postoperatively, several months may be required for return of renin production and recovery of aldosterone secretion by the contralateral adrenal. Tumor removal is followed by restoration of normal blood pressure in the majority of patients, although in about one third hypertension is lowered but persists. Spironolactone has been employed as a therapeutic alternative when surgery is contraindicated or refused; in limited follow-up studies successful control of hypertension has persisted for several years. The only other drugs employed for mineralocorticoid excess syndromes are the glucocorticoids, which specifically reverse those syndromes resulting from errors in cortisol biosynthesis.

CONGENITAL ADRENAL HYPERPLASIAS

DEFINITION. Adrenocortical hyperplasia during fetal development is a consequence of inborn errors in cortisol biosynthesis. Compensatory overproduction of ACTH by the fetus to overcome cortisol deficiency produces hyperplastic but inefficient adrenal cortices. Congenital adrenal hyperplasia (CAH), sometimes called the adrenogenital syndrome, was first described more than 100 years ago in association with anomalies of genital development. It is now appreciated that deletions of discrete enzymes produce these unique, often bizarre syndromes as a result of deficiencies and excesses of selective adrenocortical hormones. CAH occurs in about 1 of every 5000 births, indicating a current prevalence of 50,000 cases in the United States. The most common enzyme deletion is 21-hydroxylase deficiency.

PATHOGENESIS. CAH is the common result of deficiencies in any one of five enzyme systems that transform cholesterol to cortisol (Table 188-5). These enzymes, primarily hydroxylases, are only relatively specific so that a single enzyme such as 21-hydroxylase is essential not only for cortisol biosynthesis but also for aldosterone formation. Each enzyme deficiency is marked by consequences that uniquely identify the deficient step—steroid substrates *after* the block are decreased and steroid precursors *before* the block are increased.

The biologic implications of CAH depend entirely on the specific enzymatic step involved and the quantitative extent of the deficiency. All five of the common inborn errors share three features: (1) they are associated with varying degrees of (usually latent) cortisol deficiency; (2) they are accompanied by a compensatory increase in ACTH production, thereby producing adrenal hyperplasia; and (3) the biologically active precursors that accumulate produce diverse anatomic and physiologic aberrations responsible for the typical clinical manifestations of each syndrome. If the defects are quantitatively severe, these manifestations may be detected in the newborn. Subtle defects, however, may not become apparent until adult life in some patients.

Deficient or excessive androgen production is the usual cause for genital anomalies associated with CAH. When genetic males (46,XY) cannot produce testosterone, their genitalia do not differentiate from the basic female external phallus, a situation described as male pseudohermaphroditism. This occurs in three of the five CAH syndromes associated with deficient production of either 17-hydroxyprogesterone or its precursors, all essential for androgen production (Table 188-5). By contrast, the other two CAH syndromes are accompanied by excessive androgen production and therefore result in early masculinization of males or "precocious puberty." Genetic females (46,XX), on the other hand, are exposed to excess androgens in three of the five syndromes, thereby resulting in masculine-appearing genitalia (for example, clitoral hypertrophy) at birth. This condition, termed female pseudohermaphroditism, can result in mistaken sex identification and sometimes tragic gender maladjustments later in life. Midler degrees of the same enzyme deficiencies may not be recognized until adulthood, and in the female these may appear simply as hirsutism. Two of the five syndromes are associated with deficient androgen and estrogen production in genetic females, and despite normal external genitalia, such women do not mature sexually; they come to medical attention in adult life because of a failure to menstruate (primary amenorrhea) or because of infertility.

Deficient or excessive mineralocorticoid production is the other major clinical problem associated with CAH syndromes. Three of the five common enzymatic defects

Table 188-5. Congenital adrenal hyperplasia syndromes

Enzyme deficiency	Precursor steroid	Sodium balance*	Androgen excess†	Genitalia‡ Male§	Genitalia‡ Female‖
20-Hydroxylase	Cholesterol	—	—	F	F
3-βB-OH-dehydrogenase	Dehydroepiandrosterone (DHA)	—	Female only	F	M
18-β-Hydroxylase	Progesterone	+ (Corticosterone excess)	—	F	F
21-Hydroxylase	17-Hydroxyprogesterone	—	+	M	M
11-β-Hydroxylase	11-Desoxycortisol	+ (Desoxycorticosterone excess)	+	M	M

*—, Sodium loss; +, retention.
†—, Androgen deficiency; +, excess.
‡Development of female (F) or male (M) genitalia.
§Genetic male with (XY) sex chromosomes.
‖Genetic female with (XX) sex chromosomes.

cause deficient production of aldosterone as well as other potent mineralocorticoids. This results in failure to maintain sodium balance, a potentially lethal problem unless these "slat-losing" forms of CAH are appreciated early in infancy. The opposite situation, excessive mineralocorticoid production, occurs in the other two forms of CAH. In neither case is the responsible mineralocorticoid aldosterone, the normal end product of mineralocorticoid biosynthesis. In one case, 17-hydroxylase deficiency, huge amounts of the weak salt-retaining hormone, corticosterone, accumulate; in the other, 11-hydroxylase deficiency, excessive production of desoxycorticosterone, a potent mineralocorticoid, is responsible.

The occurrence of "adult-onset" CAH has also been described. It is still unclear if the late-onset form is acquired or is a mild form of the classic congenital type. Clinically, the onset of virilization is seen around the time of the menarche. Adult-onset CAH has many of the signs and symptoms of the polycystic ovarian syndrome, such as hirsutism, menstrual irregularity, and occasionally clitoral enlargement, and cannot be easily distinguished on physical examination.

Both the adrenal glands and gonads require some of the same enzymes for steroidogenesis, and in the mild forms of CAH it is probably necessary to stimulate the adrenal glands with ACTH and measure serum and urine steroid homrones to be certain of the abnormality.

There are several reports of hydroxysteroid dehydrogenase deficiency in older males in whom hypospadias was present at birth and gynecomastia developed at puberty.

CLINICAL MANIFESTATIONS. The distinctive clinical features of the CAH syndromes result from inappropriate production of both sex steroids and mineralocorticoids.

Genital abnormalities are the major clue to excessive androgen production infant girls. When this is accompanied by dehydration and hyponatremia, suggesting salt loss, 21-hydroxylase deficiency or the less common 3-β-OH-dehydrogenase deficiency syndrome should be suspected. However, virilized female children with hypertension and hypokalemia raise consideration of only one defect, 11-β-hydroxylase deficiency. Similarly, males with prematurely developed genitalia should be evaluated for salt-losing defects (21-hydroxylase deficiency), whereas if they retain excessive salt, 11-β-hydroxylase deficiency should be considered. Finally, a salt-losing syndrome in a phenotypic female may require determination of chromosomal sex to define a defect such as 20-hydroxylase deficiency.

In summary, the combination of sexual disorders with disorders of sodium and potassium balance should raise suspicion of CAH.

DIAGNOSIS. The precise diagnosis of the CAH syndromes involves determination of genetic sex by chromosomal studies and measurement of selected adrenocortical steroids to establish the enzymatic defect in cortisol biosynthesis. In the presence of appropriate clinical findings demonstration of unusual elevations in selected steroid precursors in blood or urine can be used to confirm the diagnosis with precision.

MANAGEMENT. The treatment of the CAH syndromes is much the same as that for adrenocortical failure. In all cases this involves lifelong replacement of cortisol in physiologic doses. In syndromes with mineralocorticoid deficiency, administration of fludrocortisone in daily maintenance doses is necessary. Genital ambiguities in the female are not reversible, and plastic surgery procedures are often required. Most important, cortisol not only provides replacement therapy but also suppresses excessive ACTH, ends further adrenal hyperplasia, and stops the overproduction of precursors responsible for all the physiologic aberrations associated with CAH.

BIBLIOGRAPHY

Besser, G.M., and Edwards, C.R.W.: Cushing's syndrome, Clin. Endocrinol. Metabol. **1**:451, 1972.

Biglieri, E.G., Stockigt, J.R., and Schambelan, M.: Adrenal mineralocorticoids causing hypertension, Am. J. Med. **52**:623, 1972.

Brook, C.G.D.: Congenital adrenal hyperplasia: pathology, diagnosis, and treatment. In James, V.H.T., editor: The adrenal gland, New York, 1979, Raven Press.

Burke, C.W., and Beardwell, C.G.: Cushing's syndrome, Q. J. Med. **42**:175, 1973.

Conn, J.W.: Primary aldosteronism: a new clinical syndrome, J. Lab. Clin. Med. **45**:3, 1955.

Crapo, L.: Cushing's syndrome: a review of diagnostic tests, Metabolism **28**:955, 1979.

Gold, E.M.: The Cushing syndromes: changing views of diagnosis and management, Ann. Intern. Med. **90**:829, 1979.

Grumbach, M.D., and others: Clinical disorders of adrenal function and puberty: an assessment of the role of the adrenal cortex in normal and abnormal puberty in man. In James, V.H.T., and others, editors: The endocrine function of the human adrenal cortex, London, 1978, Academic Press Inc.

Irvine, W.J., and Barnes, E.W.: Addison's disease, ovarian failure, and hypoparathyroidism. Clin. Endocrinol. **4**:379, 1975.

Irvine, W.J., Toft, A.D., and Feed, C.M.: Addison's disease. In James, V.H.T., editor: The adrenal gland, New York, 1979, Raven Press.

Jennings, A.S., Liddle, G.W., and Orth, D.N.: Results of treating childhood Cushing's disease with pituitary irradiation, N. Engl. J. Med. **297**:957, 1977.

Nerup, J.: Addison's disease—clinical studies: a sreport of 180 cases, Acta Endocrinol. **76**:127, 1974.

Newmark, S., and others: Partial 11- and 21-hydroxylase deficiencies in hirsute women, Am. J. Obstet. Gynecol. **127**:594, 1977.

Orth, D.N., and Liddle, G.W.: Rresults of treatment of 108 patients with Cushing's syndrome, N. Engl. J. Med. **285**:243, 1971.

Schambelan, M., Stockigt, J.R., and Biglieri, E.G.: Isolated hypoaldosteronism in adults: a renin-deficiency syndrome, N. Engl. J. Med. **287**:573, 1972.

Stockigt, J.R.: Mineralocorticoid excess. In James, V.H.T., editor: The adrenal gland, New York, 1979, Raven Press.

Thom, G.W.: The diagnosis and treatment of adrenal insufficiency, Springfield, Ill., 1951, Charles C Thomas, Publisher.

Tyrrell, J.B., and others: Cushing's disease: selective trans-sphenoidal resection of pituitary microadenomas, N. Engl. J. Med. **298**:753, 1978.

189 • PHEOCHROMOCYTOMA
Norman H. Ertel

Pheochromocytomas are chromaffin cell tumors derived from neuroectoderm. They are not common tumors; in 15,984 consecutive autopsies performed at one clinic, there were 15 cases with adrenal pheochromocytoma, an incidence of less than 0.1%. However, when patients with hypertension are screened for curable forms of this disease, 0.1% to 0.7% are found to have pheochromocytoma. Since hypertension, the most common chronic disease in the United States, affects 15% of the adult population, discovery of a curable form is most important.

Several important advances in the past decade have made the diagnosis and treatment of pheochromocytoma much easier: (1) the standardization and widespread use of accurate methods for the determination of urinary catecholamines and metabolites, as well as the recent development of sensitive and specific methods for measuring plasma catecholamines; (2) effective localization of tumors by selective adrenal angiography, ultrasound, and computed tomography (CT); and (3) widespread knowledge of proper preoperative and intraoperative care of patients, particularly the need for adrenergic blockade, attention to blood volume, and safe anesthetic agents.

PATHOLOGY. Pheochromocytomas are benign or malignant tumors composed of chromaffin cells that darken on exposure to chromium salts, are derived from neuroectoderm, and synthesize and secrete catecholamines. On electron microscopy both normal and neoplastic cells have characteristic granules that are similar to the chromaffin granules of the normal adrenal medulla. These electron-dense vesicles are about 100 to 300 nm in size and are key subcellular structures in the synthesis, storage, and secretion of the catecholamines. Although approximately 85% of the catecholamine in the normal adrenal medulla is epinephrine, norepinephrine secretion usually predominates in pheochromocytomas, possibly because tumor cells are not exposed to the high adrenal corticosteroid concentrations provided to the normal adrenal medulla by the portal blood supply from the adrenal cortex. The enzyme that converts norepinephrine to epinephrine, phenylethanolamine-N-methyltransferase (PNMT), is inducible by high levels of glucocorticoids. Less than 10% of pheochromocytomas are malignant. Histologic criteria, such as cellular atypia, increased mitotic figures, or invasion of blood vessels, are not helpful in predicting metastatic disease. However, malignant tumors are common in children, in large tumors, and in patients excreting large amounts of homovanillic acid (HVA), the urinary metabolite of dopamine. In nonfamilial cases about 80% of the tumors are located within the adrenal glands and are unilateral, about 10% are intraadrenal and bilateral, and about 10% are extra-adrenal. Fortunately, most extra-adrenal tumors (paragangliomas) are found within the abdomen, occurring either in the superior para-aortic area or at the bifurcation of the aorta. They are rarely found in the posterior mediastinum, neck, or bladder. Significant epinephrine secretion as determined by fractionation of urinary catecholamines greatly increases the likelihood of intra-adrenal tumor, although in rare instances intrathoracic pheochromocytomas have been able to secrete epinephrine. Intra-adrenal pheochromocytomas may range in size from less than 1 cm to palpable masses larger than the kidney and may weigh from 2 to 2000 g. However, the average tumor is usually less than 10 cm in diameter and weighs about 100 g.

FAMILIAL PHEOCHROMOCYTOMA. Pheochromocytoma is familial in up to 10% of patients. There are at least five syndromes (see following paragraphs), all characterized by an increased incidence of bilateral disease (more than 50% of cases). Adrenal medullary hyperplasia has been described both as a precursor of tumor and in association with early symptomatic disease. When genetic studies are adequately described, the familial disease is inherited as an autosomal dominant trait.

Simple familial pheochromocytoma. It is not known whether some of these families were unrecognized multiple endocrine neoplasia or adenoma (MEN or MEA) kindreds.

Multiple endocrine neoplasia type II (MEN II or IIA, Sipple's syndrome). The components of this syndrome include medullary carcinoma of the thyroid (MCT), pheochromocytoma or adrenal medullary hyperplasia, and parathyroid adenoma and hyperplasia. In a member of an affected family one or more of these manifestations may predominate. However, the other components may be present but asymptomatic. The early diagnosis of pheochromocytoma in such patients is particularly important, since the asymptomatic patient is still at risk for sudden death during a paroxysmal hypertension episode, particularly associated with surgery. As many as 30% of deaths in MEN II may be attributed to pheochromocytoma. Therefore screening of family members is important. In such patients total urinary catecholamines or catecholamine metabolites may be normal, and specific determination of urinary epinephrine may be necessary to make an early diagnosis.

Multiple endocrine neoplasia type III (MEN IIB or III, mucosal neuroma syndrome). Multiple endocrine neoplasia type III consists of multiple mucosal neuroma, MCT, and pheochromocytoma; hyperparathyroidism, is not found. In the 41 patients described up to 1975, oral neuromas occurring in the lips, tongue, and buccal mucosa were most common (37 patients). Additional findings are thickened eyelids and lips ("bumpy lips"), a marfanoid habitus, and a variety of gastrointestinal disturbances, including persistent diarrhea, constipation, and megacolon, related to diffuse intestinal ganglioneuromatosis. An interesting physical finding in all patients examined is thickening of the corneal nerves.

Pheochromocytoma and von Recklinghausen's neurofibromatosis. Less than 1% of patients with neurofibromatosis have pheochromocytoma, but about 5% of patients with pheochromocytoma have neurofibromatosis. However, the latter may be subtle, with multiple café au lait spots, isolated neurofibromas, or skeletal abnormalities.

Von Hippel-Lindau disease. Pheochromocytoma occurs in from 10% to 25% of patients with retinal-cerebellar hemangioblastomatosis and may be diagnosed only by roentgenographic techniques in a significant proportion of cases.

CLINICAL MANIFESTATIONS. Most patients with pheochromocytoma are detected as a result of screening patients with sustained hypertension or a history of paroxysms. The paroxysm is dramatic and the triad of severe headache, sweating, and palpitations occurs in the majority of attacks. Other common features of the paroxysm include pallor, nausea and vomiting, tremor, chest pain, epigastric pain, dyspnea, weakness, and severe anxiety (feelings of "impending doom"). Paroxysmal hypertension with return to normal blood pressure between attacks is present in only about 25% of patients. About 10% of patients have no demonstrable evidence of hypertension, and the remaining 65% have permanent hypertension. Of the patients with permanent hypertension, approximately 50% have had paroxysmal episodes but frequently are unaware of the significance of such symptoms. Only a minority of physicians recommend screening all newly diagnosed hypertensive patients for pheochromocytoma. The following clinical clues should call attention to the possibility of a potentially life-threatening tumor:

1. Patients with untreated essential hypertension have no change or a rise in blood pressure when they assume the standing position. A fall in blood pressure on standing is seen in the majority of patients with pheochromocytoma; this is thought to be a form of autonomic dysfunction secondary to circulating high catecholamine levels.
2. A history of hypertension, palpitations, or flushing during or after general anesthesia is suggestive of pheochromocytoma.
3. A paradoxical hypertensive response to the administration of antihypertensive drugs, such as methyldopa, reserpine, or guanethidine, should strongly suggest pheochromocytoma, since such drugs either displace catecholamines from storage sites or inhibit uptake at the sympathetic nerve endings.
4. Paroxysmal attacks provoked by a change in position, palpation of an abdominal mass, compression of the abdomen, or a hot or cold shower are of diagnostic value.
5. Even in patients without spontaneous or provoked paroxysms, the presence of unexplained sweating, fever, weight loss, or tachycardia, along with sustained hypertension, should suggest the possibility of pheochromocytoma.

When a paroxysm is provoked by micturition or swallowing, the presence of a pheochromocytoma in the bladder or posterior mediatinum, respectively, should be suspected. Physical signs, other than hypertension and those already noted, are uncommon. In patients whose pheochromocytoma is part of a familial MEN syndrome, the signs and symptoms of the associated disease, such as the enlarged thyroid and diarrhea associated with MCT, may predominate.

COURSE. Paroxysms may occur from once in several months to 25 times a day and last from 30 seconds to 1 week. They usually last less than 15 minutes but characteristically become more frequent with time. During a paroxysm the blood pressure often exceeds 250/150 and may be so high as to be unrecordable by the sphygmomanometer. Although patients with sustained hypertension may be susceptible to any of the complications of severe essential hypertension, including nephropathy, stroke, cardiac failure, or retinopathy, patients who are normotensive between paroxysms are relatively free of such disorders. Thus the latter group usually has normal fundi, whereas more than 50% of the patients with persistent hypertension have grade 3 or 4 hypertensive retinopathy. During the paroxysm the patient is in grave danger of sudden severe retinopathy, pulmonary edema with or without congestive heart failure, and cerebral hemorrhage. The paroxysmal form of the disease may evolve into sustained hypertension. Persistent rather than paroxysmal hypertension is seen more often in children and patients with malignant or multiple tumors. Pheochromocytoma occurring during pregnancy is unusually dangerous for both mother and child. It is frequently not recognized because the obstetrician may attribute the hypertension and other symptoms to toxemia of pregnancy. Although catastrophic episodes can occur at any time, shock, severe hyperpyrexia, arrhythmias, pulmonary edema, and cerebral hemorrhage are most frequently noted soon after delivery.

DIAGNOSIS. Measurement of urinary catecholamines and their major metabolites is the principal laboratory method for the diagnosis of pheochromocytoma. An abbreviated diagram of the biosynthesis and metabolism of the biologically active catecholamines is shown in Fig. 189-1. The major metabolites of norepinephrine are normetanephrine and vanillylmandelic acid (VMA); those of epinephrine are metanephrines and VMA; and the major one of dopamine is HVA. The most commonly used tests are for the urinary total catecholamines, metanephrines, and VMA. Any one of these tests will be elevated in more than 90% of patients with pheochromocytoma. A second assay will raise the yield to 95%. When a normal value is found in a patient who is thought to have this tumor on clinical grounds, further workup should include repeated assays, fractionation of total catecholamines (to epinephrine and norepinephrine) in the event that epinephrine secretion predominates, hourly collection of urine samples

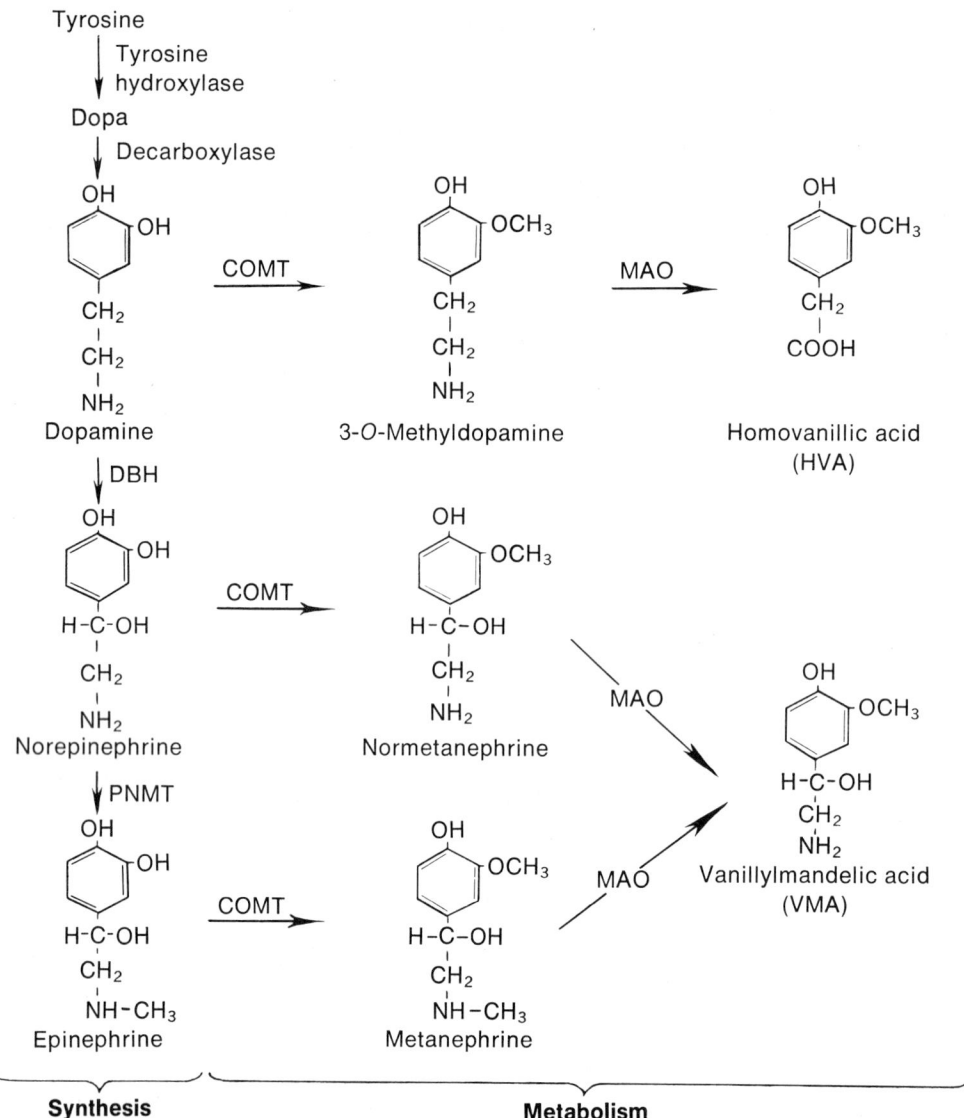

Fig. 189-1. Simplified scheme for biosynthesis and metabolism of major catecholamines. There are other routes of metabolism that are variably used, depending on tissue and species. *Dopa,* dihydroxyphenylalanine; *DBH,* dopamine-β-hydroxylase; *PNMT,* phenylethanolamine-*N*-methyltransferase; *COMT,* catechol-*O*-methyltransferase; *MAO,* monoamine oxidase.

during and immediately after an attack, or plasma catecholamine determinations. Normal values for 24-hour excretion of catecholamines and metabolites and a list of the drugs that interfere with determinations are shown in Table 189-1. Methyldopa (Aldomet) presents particular difficulties in the measurement of urinary catecholamines because it is frequently given to patients with hypertension and may lead to abnormally high results for a prolonged period after its discontinuance.

Recent studies suggest that plasma catecholamines may be as useful as, and possibly more useful than, urinary determinations in the diagnosis of pheochromocytoma (Fig. 189-2). In using plasma levels, the physician must be careful to eliminate other physiologic and pathologic causes of catecholamine elevation. Thus, although the upper limits for plasma norepinephrine and epinephrine in the resting, supine state are 400 and 70 ng/L, respectively, these values may be considerably elevated by cigarette smoking, exercise, hypoglycemia, or a stressful illness such as myocardial infarction or ketoacidosis. When these factors are eliminated, the plasma method has excellent diagnostic potential.

An abdominal flat-plate roentgenogram will locate the tumor in only 15% of patients, and less than 50% of tumors can be localized by intravenous pyelography with nephrotomography. The most important advance in the localization of both intra- and extra-adrenal pheochromocytomas has been the CT scan (Fig. 189-3). Since most pheochromocytomas are larger than 1 to 2 cm, they are usually defined by CT scan; it is currently recommended

Table 189-1. Urinary catecholamines and metabolites

Test	Normal range (mg/24 hr)	Interfering drugs*
Free catecholamines	<0.15	Methyldopa, L-dopa, isoproterenol, caffeine, theophylline
Norepinephrine	<0.07	
Epinephrine	+0.02	
Metanephrines Metanephrine Normetanephrine	<1.3	MAO (monoamine oxidase) inhibitors, caffeine, chlorpromazine, roentgenographic contrast media containing methylglucamine†
Vanillylmandelic acid (VMA)	<6.8	MAO inhibitors,† clofibrate,† nalidixic acid

*Cause a real or apparent increase in urinary values, except as indicated by †.
†Cause a real or apparent decrease in urinary values.

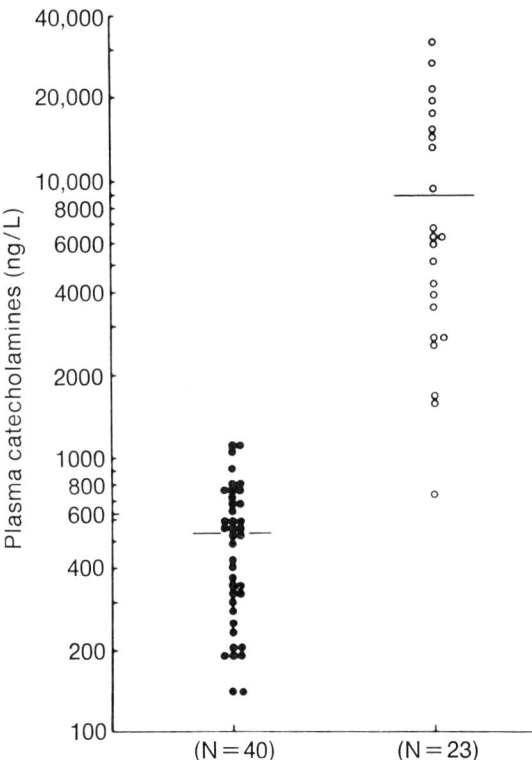

Fig. 189-2. Plasma catecholamines in 23 patients with proven pheochromocytoma and in 40 patients with suspected (but without) pheochromocytoma. (From Bravo, E.L., and others. Reprinted, by permission of the New England Journal of Medicine 301:682,1979.)

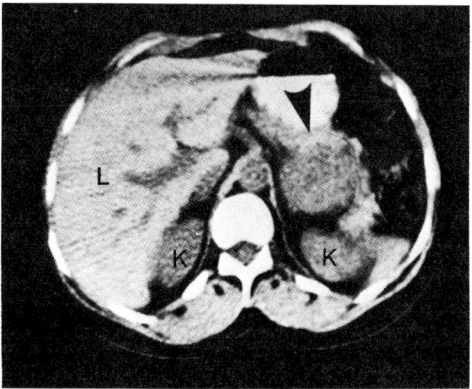

Fig. 189-3. CT scan showing large pheochromocytoma (arrow) anterior to left kidney. K, kidney; L, liver. (Courtesy of Marvin Kirschner, M.D., Newark Beth Israel Medical Center.)

that this be the initial roentgenographic procedure in the evaluation of patients with biochemical evidence of this tumor. Since some of the early scanners with slower scan times require bowel paralysis, it is important to warn the radiologist not to use glucagon for this purpose because glucagon may induce a hypertensive episode. Ultrasonography is also useful for the localization of pheochromocytoma (Fig. 189-4). Invasive procedures, such as aortography, selective adrenal arteriography, venography, and vena caval catheterization for plasma catecholamines, are hazardous and often misleading in the localization of tumors. Such procedures should be reserved for the patient who has had an unsuccessful exploration or who has recurrent disease. Such patients must be pretreated with phenoxybenzamine to prevent crisis.

Pharmacologic tests, such as a lowering of blood pressure with phentolamine or a rise in blood pressure with histamines, tyramine, or glucagon, were useful in the past but have little or no use at present. Phentolamine may be useful as both a diagnostic and therapeutic measure when a patient is seen in hypertensive crisis or with malignant hypertension.

MANAGEMENT. With the rare exception of patients with metastatic disease or those with severe illness preventing surgery, operative removal is the treatment of choice for pheochromocytoma. In the past such surgery was associated with mortality rates of up to 50%, mainly because of hypertensive crisis, congestive heart failure, and cardiac arrhythmias occurring during anesthesia or surgery. Fortunately, such complications have largely been eliminated by newer developments in preoperative and intraoperative management.

Medical therapy. Long-term medical therapy is always required in patients with functioning metastatic pheochromocytomas. In such patients, if malignancy is discovered at surgery, it is important to remove as much of the tumor as possible, since these tumors do not respond well

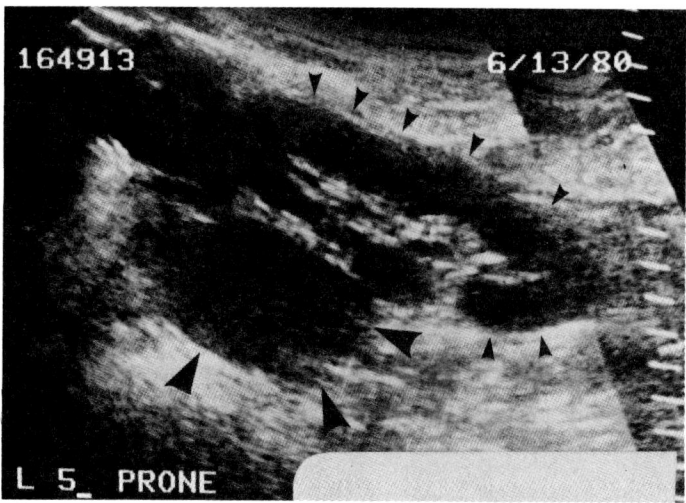

Fig. 189-4. Ultrasonogram demonstrating the same tumor *(large arrows)* near kidney *(small arrows)* as in Fig. 189-3.

to radiotherapy or the currently available cytotoxic agents. Malignant pheochromocytomas are frequently slow-growing; survival beyond 5 years is not unusual, although 50% of patients die within 2 years despite adequate adrenergic blockade. Long-term medical therapy may also be necessary in patients with major medical contraindications to surgery, such as severe cardiomyopathy or recent myocardial infarction. Phenoxybenzamine has been the agent of choice for long-term administration, but metyrosine may also prove to be an effective agent.

PHEOCHROMOCYTOMA IN PREGNANCY. Pheochromocytoma in pregnancy is rare but important to manage because in undiagnosed cases maternal mortality approaches 50%. Treatment includes adrenergic blockade and, if the pregnancy is near term, cesarean section with subsequent search for the tumor.

BIBLIOGRAPHY

Bravo, E.L., and others: Circulating and urinary catecholamines in pheochromocytoma, N. Engl. J. Med. **301**:682, 1979.

Engelman, K.: Pheochromocytoma, Clin. Endocrinol. Metabol. **6**:769, 1977.

Ertel, N.H., and Gutkin, M.: Pheochromocytoma. In Conn, H.F., and Conn, R.B., Jr., editors: Current diagnosis, Philadelphia, 1980, W.B. Saunders Co.

Ertel, N.H., and Modlinger, R.: Pheochromocytoma. In Conn, H.F., editor: Current therapy, Philadelphia, 1981, W.B. Saunders Co.

Khairi, M.R.A., and others: Mucosal neuroma, pheochromocytoma and medullary thyroid carcinoma: multiple endocrine neoplasia type 3, Medicine **54**:89, 1975.

Laursen, K., and Damgaard-Pedersen, K.: CT for pheochromocytoma diagnosis, Am. J. Radiol. **134**:277, 1980.

London, D.R.:Tumours secreting catecholamines. In Hunty, F.T.G., and Gardiner-Hill, H.: Modern trends in endocrinology, New York, 1972, Appleton-Century-Crofts.

Manger, W.M., and Gifford, R.W., Jr.: Pheochromocytoma, New York, 1977, Springer-Verlag, Inc.

190 • THE TESTES

Elaine German and **Leslie I. Rose**

EMBRYONIC DEVELOPMENT

Normal development of the testes and accessory sexual structures depends on (1) genetic determination—fertilization of the ovum by sperm carrying the Y chromosome, and (2) the activity of three testicular hormones—testosterone, dehydrotestosterone (DHT), and müllerian regression factor (MRF).

The primitive urogenital (UG) ridge, formed during the fourth to sixth weeks of fetal life, is capable of differentiation into either ovary or testis. Sex determination depends on the chromosomal composition of the primordial germ cells that migrate to the UG ridge from the yolk sac. Presence of a Y chromosome causes differentiation of testicular cords, which contain the precursors of Sertoli cells and sperm. Sertoli cells may produce MRF, which causes involution of the müllerian ducts, the precursors of female genital organs. Leydig cells, stimulated probably by chorionic gonadotropin, synthesize testosterone in the fetus at 7 to 8 weeks.

Testosterone, which is converted to DHT after it has entered the effector cell, is necessary for development and differentiation of the wolffian ducts into epididymis, vas deferens, seminal vesicles, and ejaculatory ducts. Development of male external genitalia also depends on testosterone activity. Fetal phallus, glans, and scrotal folds are identifiable by the ninth week, and testicular descent into the scrotum via the inguinal canal begins by the twelfth week.

At birth each testis measures 1.4 to 2 cm in length, 0.7

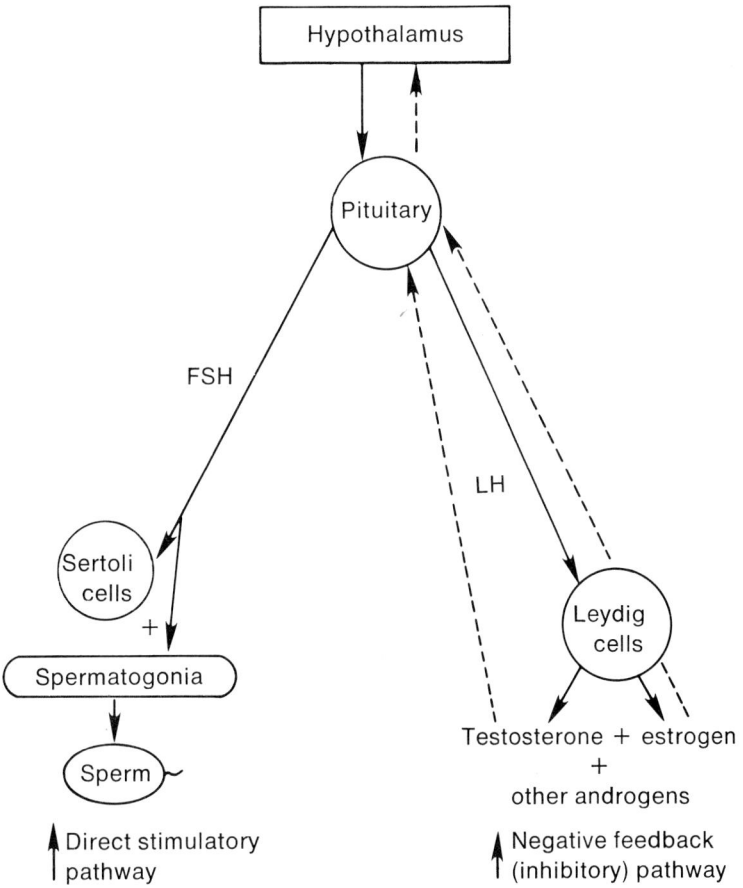

Fig. 190-1. Hypothalamic-pituitary-testicular feedback mechanisms (see text).

cm in width, and 1 cm in thickness and weighs approximately 0.5 g. Leydig cells become quiescent until puberty and hormone levels (gonadotropins, androgens, and estrogens) remain low throughout childhood. During adolescence the testis grows under the stimulation of pituitary FSH and locally produced androgens. The fully developed testis measures 3.5 to 5.5 cm in length, 2.1 to 3.2 cm in width, and 3 cm in anteroposterior diameter and weighs 15 to 20 g. Testes have two primary functions: production of sperm and secretion of androgens and estrogens.

Spermatogenesis and hormonal synthesis become active at puberty. This major event is controlled by the central nervous system (Fig. 190-1). Gonadotropin-releasing hormone (GnRH), a decapeptide synthesized in the hypothalamus, stimulates the release of two gonadotropin hormones produced by special cells in the pituitary: luteinizing hormone (LH), also called interstitial cell–stimulating hormone (ICSH), and follicle-stimulating hormone (FSH). LH stimulates the testicular Leydig cells to produce and secrete androgens and estrogens. FSH induces development and maturation of sperm in the seminiferous tubules.

If gonadal tissue does not develop (as in gonadal dysgenesis, genotypes XO, X isochromosome, and XY deleted) or if testosterone is not present or is inactive before differentiation of the genital ducts occurs, both internal and external genitalia will be female even though the genetic sex is male (XY). As is true with many other hormones, the androgens and estrogens produced as a result of gonadotropic stimulation act to suppress further gonadotropin release when certain systemic levels are reached (negative feedback).

Testosterone primarily inhibits LH, whereas estrogens appear to have more effect on FSH. In addition, a nonsteroidal substance produced by Sertoli cells called inhibin suppresses FSH secretion. All testicular hormones—testosterone, Δ^4 androstenedione, DHT, estradiol, and estrone—are synthesized from cholesterol. Approximately 7.5 mg of testosterone is produced daily by a normal man; 95% of this is made by the testes and the remaining 5% by the adrenal glands. Two thirds of estrogen production in the male is by the testes. The rest is by the adrenal glands and from conversion of testosterone and androstenedione to estrogen in peripheral tissues.

Abnormalities of the testes and testicular function can result from chromosome abnormalities, enzyme defects, end-organ hormone resistance, hormone deficiencies and excess, and unknown causes. These can be broadly classified under syndromes of *hypogonadism* (*decreased* androgen production and/or spermatogenesis) and *hypergonadism* (*increased* androgen production.) Hypogonadism occurs more frequently and is the more important group.

HYPOGONADISM

Primary hypogonadism may be present at birth as a genetic or embryologic defect or may occur at any time later in life as a result of infections, trauma, roentgen rays, or drugs. Secondary hypogonadism results from failure of the hypothalamus to elaborate GnRH or the pituitary to produce LH/FSH

I. Primary hypogonadism
   A. Developmental abnormalities
      1. Anorchia
      2. Cryptorchidism
      3. Klinefelter's syndrome
      4. Male Turner's syndrome
      5. Complete testicular feminization
      6. Incomplete testicular feminization (male pseudohermaphroditism)
         a. Reifenstein's syndrome
         b. Rosewater's syndrome
         c. Adrenal enzyme deficiency syndromes
         d. Testicular enzyme deficiency syndromes
      7. Sertoli-cell-only syndrome
      8. XYY karyotype
   B. Postpubertal abnormalities
      1. Varicoceles
      2. Spinal cord damage
      3. Infections
      4. Hypothyroidism and hyperthyroidism
      5. Malnutrition
      6. Heavy metal toxicity
      7. Drugs
      8. Myotonia dystrophica
      9. Physical factors
     10. Trauma
     11. Castration
II. Secondary hypogonadism
   A. Kallman's syndrome (isolated gonadotropin deficiency)
   B. Isolated LH (ICSH) deficiency (fertile eunuch)
   C. Panhypopituitarism
   D. Drugs
   E. Laurence-Moon-Biedl syndrome
   F. Stress
   G. Delayed puberty

The clinical picture of hypogonadism is related to the time at which androgen deficiency occurs. Prepubertal deficiency results in infantile genitalia, female axillary and pubic hair distribution, absence of acne and seborrhea, and absence of vocal changes. Growth continues at a slower rate and without the adolescent spurt. Since epiphyseal closure depends on sex steroids, these patients develop a eunuchoid habitus—long arms and legs and an arm span that is 2 inches (5 cm) greater than height. Gynecomastia, wide hips, and girdle obesity may also be present, and muscle mass is diminished.

Hypogonadism occurring after puberty usually produces less dramatic changes. However, in young men beard and hair growth may be diminished, genitalia may become smaller, and libido may be reduced or absent. Gynecomastia may occur; the voice remains deep. There may be fewer changes or none in older men.

Primary hypogonadism

DEVELOPMENTAL ABNORMALITIES

Anorchia (disappearing testis). Although phenotypically and genetically males, men with anorchia have small penises and no detectable gonadal tissue. Testes with androgen and MRF production must have been present in early fetal life to initiate male development and disappearance of female structures. However, for unknown reasons they are reabsorbed before complete development of external genitalia has occurred. Virilization at puberty does not occur; adrenal glands alone cannot produce sufficient testosterone. Lack of negative feedback causes elevated LH and FSH levels. Testosterone, given parenterally, is used in treatment to achieve maximal development of stature and secondary sexual characteristics.

Cryptorchidism. Failure of either one or both testes to descend into the scrotum occurs in about 10% of males at time of birth. However, by the time puberty has occurred, only 0.3% to 0.4% still have undescended testes. Unilateral cryptorchidism is five times more frequent than the bilateral form. The undescended testes lie within either the inguinal canal or the abdomen. These testes are very prone to malignant change (40 times more frequent than normally located testes) and are nonfunctional in their undescended positions. Orchiopexy is indicated at an early age to preserve testicular function and make observation for malignant changes feasible. Even after orchiopexy the previously undescended testis remains at increased risk for malignant change.

Bilateral cryptorchid testes result in a functionally castrated male if not corrected. They present the clinical picture of prepubertal hypogonadism.

Klinefelter's syndrome (seminiferous tubule dysgenesis). Klinefelter's syndrome is one of the most common genetic abnormalities, occurring in 1:500 newborn males. Classically, the chromosomal constitution is XXY, but multiple variants, including XY, exist. Moderate mental retardation and personality disorders are common. Testes are small and firm and histologically show hyalinization of the seminiferous tubules. Serum testosterone levels are low to low-normal, whereas gonadotropin levels are elevated.

Diabetes mellitus, chronic bronchitis, emphysema, autoimmune disorders, thyroid abnormalities, and malignancies occur frequently in these men.

Male Turner's syndrome (Noonan's syndrome). Males with male Turner's syndrome have the phenotypic appearance similar to females with Turner's syndrome (XO chromosome)—short stature, webbed neck, low-set ears, shieldlike chest, cubitus valgus, ptosis, ocular anomalies, mental retardation, cardiovascular anomalies, cryptorchidism and/or small fibrous testes, gynecomastia, and lymphedema of hands and feet. However, the chromosomal karyotype is usually XY. Treatment with testosterone is appropriate.

Complete testicular feminization. Individuals with complete testicular feminization have an XY karyotype but appear in adulthood as well-developed, often handsome women. The external genitalia are feminine, but the vagina is shallow and ends in a blind pouch. Axillary and pubic hair is absent.

The testes, which are prone to malignancy, are to be found in the labia majora, inguinal canal, or abdomen. Testosterone levels often are similar to those of normal males, indicating that the target tissues are unresponsive to androgens.

The testes should be removed as soon as the diagnosis is made. Since these individuals are psychologically and physically female, it is advisable to avoid all reference to male genetic sex and to inform parents and patient only of the need to remove abnormal gonadal tissue because of potential malignancy. Once the testes are removed, combination estrogen-progesterone therapy should be instituted.

Incomplete testicular feminization (male pseudohermaphroditism). Incomplete testicular feminization represents a number of conditions resulting from defective androgen synthesis or partial resistance of target tissues to androgens. Patients have an XY genotype with widely variable sexual abnormalities. Genitalia are often ambiguous because of hypospadias and failure of scrotal folds to fuse. Gynecomastia may also be present. If hypospadias is severe, individuals are usually reared as females, necessitating removal of the testes and treatment with estrogen at puberty; if mild, reconstructive surgery may be possible.

Reifenstein's syndrome. Reifenstein's syndrome is a hereditary sex-linked recessive testicular disorder. Individuals have hypospadias, gynecomastia, eunuchoidism and postpubertal testicular atrophy. The chromosomal constitution is normal.

Rosewater's syndrome. Rosewater's syndrome consists of familial hypogonadism and gynecomastia, probably caused by genetic mutation. Testosterone levels are normal; gonadotropin levels are normal or high. Estrogens are also elevated, resulting in gynecomastia.

A number of enzyme deficiencies in testes or adrenal glands resulting in defective androgen synthesis produce similar sexual abnormalities.

Adrenal enzyme deficiency syndromes. Adrenal enzyme deficiency syndromes resulting in hypogonadism include the following:

1. 3-β-Hydroxysteroid dehydrogenase deficiency produces mineralocorticoid and glucocorticoid defects, resulting in salt-losing patients with pseudohermaphroditism.
2. 17-Hydroxylase deficiency produces hypertension along with varying degrees of male pseudohermaphroditism because of deficits of androgens, estrogen, and cortisol. These patients also lack pubic and axillary hair.
3. A patient with C-21-hydroxylase deficiency virilizes early but usually has small testes and an abnormally pigmented scrotum (females are virilized).
4. C-11-hydroxylase deficiency results in mild sexual abnormalities in the male (females appear virilized) accompanied by hypertension owing to increased production of 11-deoxycorticosterone.

Testicular enzyme deficiency syndromes. The testicular enzyme deficiency syndromes resulting in hypogonadism include the following:

1. 17-β-Hydroxysteroid oxidoreductase deficiency results in impairment of androstenedione conversion to testosterone. Germinal elements are absent. Males have ambiguous genitalia, gynecomastia, and cryptorchidism.
2. Failure of conversion of testosterone to dehydrotestosterone in certain androgen target tissues results in hypospadias, but virilization occurs at puberty.

Sertoli-cell-only syndrome. Germinal cells are completely absent in the testes of patients with Sertoli-cell-only syndrome. Leydig cells are present and testosterone is produced, but levels are somewhat lower than normal. These men are virilized but infertile.

XYY karyotype. The XYY karyotype occurs with a frequency of 0.01% to 0.02% among males. Patients are tall and have pustular acne. Spermatogenesis may be impaired in spite of normal gonadotropin and testosterone levels.

POSTPUBERTAL ABNORMALITIES

Varicoceles. Varicoceles are often associated with decreased motility and number of sperm, thought to result from abnormal venous drainage or temperature control. Improvement occurs after surgical correction.

Spinal cord damage. Cord damage may cause elevated testicular temperature resulting in decreased sperm production. The ability to ejaculate is lost if lesions are located between the sixth thoracic and the third lumbar vertebrae.

Infections. Orchitis develops in 15% to 25% of males with parotitic mumps. Permanent damage to the seminiferous tubules may result if infection occurs during puberty or afterward. The full effect may not become apparent for 15 to 20 years.

Gonorrhea, leprosy, tuberculosis, brucellosis, syphilis, and disease caused by other organisms may also cause sufficient damage to produce infertility.

Hypothyroidism and hyperthyroidism. Oligospermia and low testosterone levels may occur in hypothyroidism. Severe hyperthyroidism may result in decreased sperm count and motility.

Malnutrition. Starvation, fad diets, chronic illness, or malignancy may produce decreased production of sperm and androgens because of malnutrition. Gonadotropin levels are also decreased.

Heavy metal toxicity. Testicular necrosis is caused by cadmium and to a lesser extent by bismuth, mercury, aluminum, platinum, lithium, silver, tin, nickel, uranium, boron, and lead.

Drugs. Methadone produces a 50% decrease in ejaculate volume, with low levels of prostatic and seminal vesicle fluid. Sperm motility is markedly reduced. Testosterone levels are also decreased. Various cytotoxic agents (alkylating agents, periwinkle, and alkaloids) inhibit spermatogenesis by direct toxic action on the germinal cells.

Myotonia dystrophica. Myotonia dystrophica is a genetic syndrome in which lenticular opacities, frontal baldness, and myotonia coexist with testicular atrophy. Testosterone levels are low and gonadotropins elevated. Patients with cystic fibrosis and other congenital conditions such as Laurence-Moon-Biedl syndrome (see section on "Secondary hypogonadism") also have failure of seminiferous tubule function.

Physical factors. Elevation of testicular temperature by 4° to 5° F (2° to 3° C) for only 30 minutes to 3 hours can cause diminished spermatogenesis. The temperature increase can result from fever, hot baths, and saunas. Very low temperatures, below 23° F ($-5°$ C), for prolonged periods can also cause impaired sperm production, probably as a result of diminished blood flow.

Damage to germinal cells will occur with a dose of 4000 to 6000 rad or greater from a source of 250-k V x-ray equipment. Genitals should be shielded during childhood, puberty, and adulthood when fertility is desired. People working with x-ray equipment and/or radioisotopes should also take precautions.

Men living at altitudes of 4270 feet (1280 M) or higher for more than 40 days have been found to have decreased sperm numbers and motility, as well as poor-quality semen. Space flight also alters spermatogenesis.

Some men in later years have diminished function of Leydig cells resulting in hot flashes, irritability, inability to concentrate, decreased libido with impotence, and depression, symptoms indicative of male climacteric. Interruption of vascular supply to the testes may be the cause.

Secondary hypogonadism

Decrease in the production or release of the gonadotropic hormones LH (also known as ICSH) and FSH will result in hypogonadism. The etiology may be in the hypothalamus, with decreased or ineffective secretion of GnRH, or because of a lesion in the pituitary itself. The absence of serum and urinary gonadotropins after the age of adolescence in patients with decreased gonadal function is diagnostic.

KALLMAN'S SYNDROME (ISOLATED GONADOTROPIN DEFICIENCY). Hypogonadism caused by decreased gonadotropins owing to hypothalamic dysfunction, associated with absence of sense of smell because of olfactory lobe agenesis, characterizes Kallman's syndrome. Other pituitary functions are intact. This syndrome occurs in both males and females. Patients are eunuchoid and may have midline abnormalities such as harelip and cleft palate. It may be associated with X-linked recessive or male limited-dominant inheritance or with no chromosomal abnormality.

ISOLATED LH (ICSH) DEFICIENCY (FERTILE EUNUCHS). Patients with isolated LH deficiency have gynecomastia and eunuchoid stature. LH and testosterone levels are decreased, but FSH secretion is normal. Spermatogenesis is feasible if testicular maturation is sufficient. Testosterone should be given. Human chorionic gonadotropin (HCG) may be given to promote full testicular development.

PANHYPOPITUITARISM. Failure of the pituitary to elaborate any of its tropic hormones (such as thyroid-stimulating, adrenocorticotropic, leutinizing/follicle-stimulating, and growth hormones) can result from tumors, histiocytosis, granulomata (such as tuberculoid and sarcoid), cysts, central nervous system infections, trauma, and vascular lesions or may be idiopathic. Hypothalamic lesions may lead to absent or diminished secretion of releasing hormones, also resulting in a drop of pituitary hormonal production. Patients with panhypopituitarism starting in childhood are short and have high-pitched voices and small external genitalia. They require lifelong replacement with thyroid hormone, cortisone, and testosterone. Adult hypopituitarism usually results from chromophobe adenomas but may also be related to trauma, metastatic tumors, infections, and so on. Involvement of the posterior pituitary with resultant diabetes insipidus may also occur.

DRUGS. Chlorpromazine, carbon tetrachloride, and estrogens all block gonadotropin secretion. This produces testicular hypofunction resulting in hypogonadism.

LAURENCE-MOON-BIEDL SYNDROME. Obesity, mental deficiency, hypogenitalism, retinitis pigmentosa, and polydactyly characterize the Laurence-Moon-Biedl syndrome, which is inherited as a recessive trait. Hypogonadism may be of either primary (testicular aplasia) or secondary (hypothalamic) origin. Patients with suspected secondary hypogonadism require complete evaluation of growth, thyroid, adrenal, and antidiuretic hormones.

STRESS. Major surgery, trauma, or burns and severe emotional stress may be sufficient to suppress gonadotropin secretion with a resultant drop in testosterone production.

DELAYED PUBERTY. Puberty, which occurs normally between 9 and 16 years of age, is occasionally delayed until ages 20 to 22. Slow development of the hypothalamus is believed to be responsible. Differentiation from hypogonadotropic eunuchoid patients is difficult. This disorder can be familial.

Evaluation and management

Patients with hypogonadism initially have developmental abnormalities, impotence, or infertility.

Important history will include age, occupation, past medical illness (especially tuberculosis, mumps, venereal disease, cryptorchidism, previous abdominal surgery, and hernia repair), smoking habits, ethanol use, medications, and sexual habits.

The physical examination should include special attention to body build, height, arm span, muscle development, hair distribution, external genitalia, sense of smell, palate, and lips.

Laboratory studies will depend on abnormalities found during the physical examination. Evaluation of the pituitary-hypothalamic-testicular axis requires determination of LH, FSH, and testosterone levels. Fertility evaluation requires sperm analysis.

Testosterone replacement should be given to patients with androgen deficiency. Long-acting parenteral preparations (testosterone cypionate, propionate, and so on) are recommended for patients under middle age when rapid prostatic enlargement will not produce problems with obstruction. Short-acting preparations (oral 17-α-methylated testosterone) are used in older men.

In patients who have germinal epithelium present in their testes, fertility may be possible if spermatogenesis and androgen production can be stimulated by exogenous gonadotropins. HCG, which acts like LH to stimulate Leydig cells, plus human menopausal gonadotropin, which, like FSH, stimulates spermatogenesis, may be effective. Therapy is protracted, expensive, and too often unsuccessful.

HYPERGONADISM

Hypergonadism in the male is caused by excess androgens. Children show all the manifestations of precocious puberty: growth of axillary and pubic hair, enlargement of phallus and testes, deepening of voice, acne, and so on. Testicular tumors and tumors in the region of the third ventricle (pinealoma, teratoma, astrocytoma, hamartoma, and craniopharyngioma) may be the cause. Familial precocious sexual development as well as hypergonadism from adrenal-androgen excess may also occur.

TESTICULAR TUMORS

Neoplasms of testes occur in approximately 1:100,000 normal men and are the most common tumors in the 24- to 35-year-old group. The frequency is much higher (1:2000) in cryptorchidism, even after surgical orchiopexy.

Testicular tumors in order of frequency are (1) seminoma; (2) teratocarcinoma; (3) embryonal carcinoma (chorioepithelioma and others); (4) teratoma; (5) interstitial cell (Leydig cell) tumor; (6) fibroma, lipoma, adrenoma, myxoma; and (7) unclassified neoplasms. Lymphomas, plasmacytomas, leukemia, and metastatic carcinomas may also occur. Embryonal carcinomas, particularly chorioepitheliomas and teratocarcinomas, may secrete gonadotropins, resulting in syndromes of hyperestrogenism. Interstitial cell tumors may produce hypergonadism, such as precocious puberty in children.

DIAGNOSIS. A mass is usually felt, although some tumors are so small that they can be identified only on multiple microscopic sections. Urinary excretion of 17-ketosteroids, estrogens, or gonadotropins is helpful in diagnosis when these are present. Serum α-fetoprotein may be elevated.

MANAGEMENT. Surgical removal combined with radiotherapy and chemotherapy has proved effective.

BIBLIOGRAPHY

Bunick, E.M., and Rose, L.I.: Testicular syndromes. I. Abnormalities of childhood and adolescence, Compr. Ther. **3**:62, 1977.

Bunick, E.M., and Rose, L.I.: Testicular syndromes. II. Adult abnormalities, Compr. Ther. **3**:69, 1977.

Ingbar, S., editor: Contemporary endocrinology I, New York, 1979, Plenum Publishing Co.

191 • THE OVARY

Leonore C. Huppert

The human ovary is a small, bilateral ovoid structure located on either side of the uterus adjacent to the lateral pelvic walls. The mature ovary measures approximately 2.5 to 5 cm in length, 1.5 to 3 cm in width, and 0.5 to 1.5 cm in thickness. The combined weight of both ovaries during the reproductive years is 10 to 20 g. Blood vessels and nerves enter the ovary via the mesovarium, a thin fold of tissue adherent to the posterior aspect of the broad ligament. In addition to the mesovarium, the ovary receives support from the infundibulopelvic and utero-ovarian ligaments.

HISTOLOGY AND EMBRYOLOGY

Histologically, the ovary is composed of follicles, which contain germ cells surrounded by specialized hormonally active tissue, and fibrous tissue stroma. Tissue that will eventually develop into an ovary is identifiable within the human embryo by 4 weeks after fertilization. At this stage in development the germ cells, containing the genetic information for the next generation, are located outside the embryo. During the next month of embryogenesis the germ cells migrate into the embryo and colonize the primitive ovary. The original 1000 to 2000 germ cells undergo rapid proliferation or mitosis to form about 600,000 oogonia by the end of the second month of intrauterine life. During the fourth month of gestation certain oogonia are transferred into primary oocytes by initiating the process of meiosis or reductional chromosomal division. These cells are arrested in an early stage of meiosis that will not be completed until many years later when the ovum is finally ovulated and fertilized. Because of continued mitosis and meiosis, at 5 months the ovary contains about 2 million oogonia and 5 million primary oocytes. Degeneration of both oogonia and primary oocytes takes place during the remainder of fetal life so that at birth the ovary contains approximately 2 million oocytes and no oogonia.

The developing primary oocyte becomes invested with a thin layer of flattened granulosa cells forming the primordial follicle. Certain primordial follicles further differentiate after birth into primary follicles, characterized by an increase in the number of granulosa cells and the development of a surrounding concentric arrangement of stromal cells destined to become the theca interna of the mature follicle. Follicular development up to this stage is independent of gonadotropin stimulation by the pituitary gland. Further follicular maturation, however, requires the action of gonadotropins.

FOLLICULAR GROWTH AND DEVELOPMENT

The ovaries steadily increase in size from birth until puberty. The prepubertal rise in gonadotropins permits further follicular maturation, with a resultant increase in ovarian estrogen (the most potent of which is estradiol [E_2]) production by the granulosa cells. The secondary, or graafian, follicle is characterized by increased numbers of granulosa cells surrounding a large, fluid-filled antral cavity into which the ovum projects. The concentrically arranged thecal cells surrounding the follicle further differentiate into theca interna and theca externa. The theca interna is very vascular and capable of hormone production.

In the pubertal female a number of follicles in each cycle, under the influence of cyclic gonadotropin stimulation from the pituitary gland, are stimulated to the stage of the graafian follicle. Further interaction between the ovary and the pituitary leads to the continued growth of usually two follicles. One of these tertiary follicles grows until it reaches a diameter of about 1 mm and then undergoes atresia. The follicle ultimately destined to ovulate reaches a diameter of 1.5 to 2 cm and migrates to the periphery of the ovary. Responding to the appropriate signal from the pituitary gland, ovulation takes place. Ovulation is not an explosive event but rather is characterized by a slow ooze of material from the follicle. The ovulatory process is thought to be mediated by prostaglandins whose levels increase within the follicle before rupture.

Immediately after release of the egg, follicular collapse and hemorrhage ensue. This is followed by hypertrophy of granulosa and theca interna cells. Morphologic and biochemical alterations in these cells lead to the formation of the corpus luteum, which replaces the original follicle. The granulosa cells, which previously were avascular, are penetrated by blood vessels. The corpus luteum is capable of both estrogen and progesterone production and has a self-limiting life span of approximately 12 to 14 days. As the corpus luteum regresses, it becomes fibrous and hyalinized. The remaining structure, called the corpus albicans, forms approximately 70 days after ovulation.

The postmenopausal years are heralded by a decline in the number of ova and follicles within the ovary. Ultimately, the combined processes of ovulation and atresia consume all remaining germ cells in the ovary, thus ending the endocrine and reproductive function of this organ. The postmenopausal ovary acquires a wrinkled surface appearance and shrinks to less than one third of its former active size.

ENDOCRINE EVENTS OF THE MENSTRUAL CYCLE

The adult menstrual cycle represents a delicate interaction of many components of the reproductive system. The ultimate target organ of the fluctuating hormone levels is the uterus, whose lining undergoes cyclic changes in response to the steroid hormones estrogen and progesterone, produced by the ovary. The ovary in turn produces its hormones and prepares an egg for ovulation under the influence of the pituitary gonadotropins follicle-stimulating hormone (FSH) and luteinizing hormone (LH). The regulation of gonadotropin secretion appears to be under the dual control of the hypothalamic hormone gonadotropin-releasing hormone (GnRH) and the local steroid hormone milieu.

Menstruation usually occurs every 25 to 30 days, although cycles of 21 to 42 days' duration may also be normal. The fixed portion of the menstrual cycle is the postovulatory phase, which usually lasts approximately 13 days. Variations in the length of the preovulatory phase therefore determine the overall length of the menstrual cycle.

A new menstrual cycle begins with the onset of menstruation when estrogen and progesterone levels are at a nadir (Fig. 191-1). The earliest hormonal event in the new cycle is an increase in pituitary FSH, which actually begins the day before the onset of menses. This hormone then stimulates the development of the graafian follicle. FSH specifically causes hyperplasia and hypertrophy of the granulosa cells and also induces more of its own receptors. There is also a rise in LH levels at the start of each cycle, which is probably necessary to maintain the low levels of steroidogenesis within the ovary. LH-stimulated androgenic steroid precursors from the theca interna diffuse into the avascular granulosa, where they are converted into estrogen. Continued follicular stimulation by FSH leads to the onset of significant estrogen production by the granulosa cells approximately 1 week before ovulation. This rise in estrogen enhances the FSH-mediated increase in FSH receptors and together with FSH induces LH receptors on the granulosa cells. An adequate complement of LH receptors is necessary to ensure normal ovulation and eventual

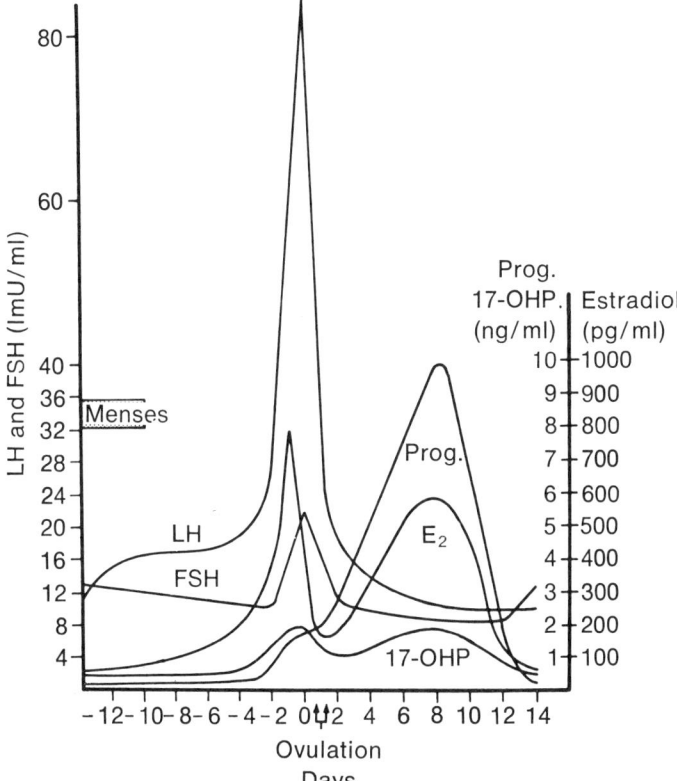

Fig. 191-1. Plasma hormone fluctuations during the human menstrual cycle. *LH,* luteinizing hormone; *FSH,* follicle-stimulating hormone; *Prog.,* progesterone; E_2, estradiol; *17-OHP,* 17-hydroxyprogesterone, (From Speroff, L., and VandeWiele, R.L.: Am. J. Obstet. Gynecol. **109:**234, 1971.)

corpus luteum formation. The ability of the granulosa to respond directly to LH during the immediate preovulatory period permits for the first time in the cycle the production of significant intrafollicular levels of progesterone.

As estrogen production by the ovary increases, the amount of FSH produced by the pituitary declines. The mechanism involved in this interaction is called negative feedback and is described in the next section. Before ovulation a large proportion of the estrogen being produced comes from those few follicles continuing to grow. The high local estrogen concentrations within these follicles augment their responsiveness to FSH by increasing their numbers and affinity to FSH receptors. The smaller follicles that produce significantly less estrogen, on the other hand, have a lesser response to FSH and eventually undergo atresia.

The rapid, late follicular rise in estrogen stimulates the release of a large burst of gonadotropin from the pituitary gland. The principal gonadotropin released at this time is LH, although a modest rise in FSH also occurs. Estrogen levels rapidly decline as LH levels start to rise. Ovum release occurs within 24 hours of the LH peak.

The newly formed corpus luteum produces large amounts of progesterone, with peak levels occurring 8 to 9 days after ovulation. Lesser but still significant amounts of estrogen are also produced. These high levels of estrogen and progesterone secretion by the ovary are responsible for maintaining FSH and LH production by the pituitary gland at a minimum. Even though LH levels are low at this time, some continued LH stimulation is necessary to support the corpus luteum for its normal life span. Unless pregnancy occurs, the corpus luteum starts to degenerate 9 to 11 days after ovulation. There is a rapid decline in progesterone and estrogen levels, which ultimately reach the point at which they can no longer maintain the endometrium, and menstruation ensues.

CONTROL MECHANISMS OF THE HYPOTHALAMIC-PITUITARY-OVARIAN AXIS

The interactions between the pituitary gland and ovary are controlled by negative and positive feedback mechanisms. The predominant mechanism throughout the cycle is the negative feedback effect of ovarian steroids on gonadotropin secretion. The most pronounced inhibitory effect is that of estrogen on FSH secretion, although low levels of estrogen may also inhibit tonic LH secretion. The midcycle LH surge, however, is controlled by positive feedback. The rapidly rising estrogen levels are fed back on the pituitary gland, leading to the large burst of LH release. Both the amount of estrogen produced and the duration of the estrogen peak appear to be important in activating the positive feedback mechanism.

In addition to the modulating action of steroid hormones on the pituitary gland, gonadotropin secretion also requires stimulation by GnRH. The pulsatile release of GnRH by the hypothalamus is essential for normal pituitary function. The response of the pituitary in terms of amount and ratio of gonadotropins, however, is dependent on the steroid milieu. An additional short negative feedback loop may also exist between the pituitary and the hypothalamus.

PITUITARY-OVARIAN RELATIONSHIPS FROM BIRTH TO MENOPAUSE

FSH and LH are first detected within the human fetal pituitary gland by 10 weeks of gestation. GnRH is also detectable within the fetal hypothalamus during the first trimester. Gonadotropin levels increase until midgestation, at which point they sharply decline and remain low until birth. The midpregnancy FSH surge is temporarily related to and may be responsible for the differentiation of oogonia to primary oocytes. The decline in gonadotropin levels probably is the result of negative feedback by high fetal estrogen levels derived from placental conversion of fetal and maternal precursor hormones. This interaction represents the first appearance of the negative feedback system.

Immediately after birth and delivery of the placenta, the precipitous drop in estrogen levels induces a surge of FSH in the neonate. By this time the hypothalamus and pituitary have acquired an exquisite sensitivity to the negative feedback effect of estrogen. The small amounts of estrogen produced by the ovary during childhood keep gonadotropins at a low level. Gonadotropin production starts to rise between the ages of 8 and 10, signaling the approach of puberty. Although the exact mechanism of the prepubertal gonadotropin rise is unknown, it is believed to be the result of a loss in sensitivity of the hypothalamus to negative feedback inhibition by estrogen. A characteristic nocturnal elevation of FSH and LH occurs during the peripubertal years and disappears once the adult pituitary-ovarian relationship establishes itself. Finally, before ovulatory cycles can occur, the hypothalamus and pituitary must develop their ability to respond in a positive manner to high levels of estrogen in order to produce the ovulatory surge of LH.

The approach of the menopause, on the other hand, is heralded by a small diminution in estrogen levels and a rise in FSH levels. This alteration is probably the consequence of decreased numbers of follicles present within the ovary, as well as of an impaired ability by the remaining follicles to produce estrogen. As estrogen levels further decline, the ability to generate a midcycle estrogen surge is lost and ovulation ceases. Cycles become more irregular and anovulatory bleeding occurs. Ultimately, estrogen levels decline to the point at which they are no longer sufficient to cause endometrial proliferation and the final menstrual flow or menopause occurs. As ovarian estrogen production ceases, gonadotropin levels continue to rise and finally reach stable postmenopausal values 1 to 3 years after the menopause. FSH levels are consistently higher than LH levels in postmenopausal women.

THE ABNORMAL OVARY

Ovarian disease may be divided into functional and neoplastic disorders.

Functional disorders—amenorrhea

Ovarian dysfunction often becomes apparent when the target organ, the endometrium, no longer functions appropriately. Thus amenorrhea (failure to menstruate) or abnormal uterine bleeding is often the clinical sign that prompts an investigation of ovarian function. Precocious or delayed pubertal development, as well as the premature onset of the menopause, also suggests a functional abnormality of the ovary. Although in some instances ovarian dysfunction is intrinsic to the ovary, failure of normal ovarian function more frequently results from improper stimulation. Infrequently, menstrual failure is caused by disease or absence of the uterus or abnormalities in the outflow tract.

PRIMARY AMENORRHEA. Extragonadal problems account for 40% of cases of primary amenorrhea. Outflow abnormalities include absence or obstruction of the vagina or cervix. Imperforate hymen is probably the most common cause of obstructed flow. Congenital absence of the vagina, aplasia of the vagina, and complete transverse vaginal septum are less frequent findings. Very rarely, severe cervical stenosis can prevent menstruation. Absence of the upper two thirds of the vagina together with absence of the uterus and fallopian tubes is classified as müllerian agenesis, also known as *Rokitansky-Kuster-Hauser syndrome*. A small, blind vaginal pouch is present in these patients. Ovarian function is completely normal, accounting for normal pubertal development.

Another group of patients with the same clinical picture, including blind vaginal pouch, absent uterus, and normal secondary sex characteristics, are those with *testicular feminization*. These patients, who are phenotypically female, are genetic males with an XY karyotype. They have normal testes producing normal male amounts of testosterone. The abnormality in this condition is an end-organ insensitivity to testosterone that prevents the formation of male internal and external genitalia. It is important to obtain a karyotype in all females with a blind vaginal pouch and absent uterus, since phenotype females with a Y chromosome in their karyotypes have a high risk of gonadal malignancy and should undergo gonadectomy. Vaginal dilation or reconstructive surgery is occasionally required to ensure a functioning vagina. In addition to absence of the uterus, amenorrhea may be the result of damage to the endometrium, rendering it unable to respond to normal cyclic stimulation. Intrauterine synechiae (scar tissue), a condition known as *Asherman's syndrome,* may be the result of overvigorous curettage after birth or at the time of abortion. The basal layer of endometrium from which subsequent endometrium regenerates becomes damaged, and no further proliferation, secretion, or menstruation will occur. Curettage for the purpose of removing the scar tissue followed by high-dose estrogen therapy occasionally results in endometrial regeneration. The endometrium can also become incompetent as a result of infection. This is exceedingly rare in the United States and may be due to tuberculosis or schistosomiasis.

Abnormal ovaries resulting from an abnormal sex chromosome complement account for approximately one third of cases of primary amenorrhea. The most common chromosomal abnormality is the absence of one X chromosome, producing a 45,XO karyotype and streak ovaries without ova or follicles. This condition, known as *Turner's syndrome,* is characterized by various somatic abnormalities, including short stature, webbed neck, shield chest, widely spaced nipples, an increased carrying angle of the arms, and occasionally coarctation of the aorta. Affected individuals fail to experience spontaneous puberty but do respond to hormone replacement therapy with breast development and menstruation. Occasionally, one individual may have multiple cell lines with different sex chromosome complements (for example, XO/XX and XO/XY). These mosaic conditions are also associated with streak gonads. Somatic abnormalities are much less frequent in these conditions than in pure Turner's syndrome. The presence of a Y chromosome in the karyotype of a phenotypic female dictates removal of the gonads because of an increased incidence of malignant degeneration.

SECONDARY AMENORRHEA. The ovary is less frequently a cause of secondary amenorrhea, or interruption of menstruation once it has already been established. One of the more common ovarian causes of secondary amenorrhea, however, is the *polycystic ovarian syndrome*. This condition, also known as the *Stein-Leventhal syndrome*, is characterized by amenorrhea, obesity, and hirsutism. Instead of the regular cyclic events of the normal menstrual cycle, hormones are produced in a steady state fashion. Typically, the ovary produces abnormal levels of weak androgenic hormones, which presumably interfere with the normal pituitary-ovarian feedback interaction. The pattern of gonadotropin secretion from the pituitary gland is characterized by low to low-normal levels of FSH and elevated LH levels. In addition to abnormal steroidogenesis within the ovary, there may also be a hypothalamic defect responsible for the elevated LH levels. The ovaries in this condition are enlarged and smooth, with no evidence of recent ovulatory activity. The smooth, shiny appearance of these ovaries is probably caused by anovulation rather than a consequence of the disease process itself. Patients with this condition are good candidates for the induction of ovulation with clomiphene citrate if they wish to conceive.

Rarely, women in the reproductive years may undergo premature menopause. Symptomatically and endocrinologically, this condition is indistinguishable from the normal physiologic event of the menopause. Occasionally, the cause of this premature menopause may be chromosomal mosaicism, which was mentioned earlier. A small number of patients who appear to be prematurely menopausal may have the *resistant ovary syndrome*. In this condition the ovary is refractory to gonadotropin stimulation. Little estrogen is produced and gonadotropin levels rise. Small follicles, however, are present, distinguishing this condition from the menopause.

The most common cause of secondary amenorrhea is an abnormality in the hypothalamic-pituitary axis leading to improper ovarian stimulation. Gonadotropin secretion from the pituitary may be compromised as a result of compression from intrinsic or extrinsic pituitary tumors or vascular lesions. Pituitary necrosis resulting from obstetric hemorrhage (Sheehan's syndrome) may also lead to amenorrhea. In these conditions surgery or hormonal replacement therapy is provided as needed.

Not infrequently, small pituitary tumors that produce abnormally large amounts of prolactin are identified. Patients with this condition often have amenorrhea and galactorrhea. Occasionally, no tumor can be demonstrated roentgenographically when prolactin levels are elevated. This suggests the presence of a tumor too small to be detected by current roentgenologic means or abnormal prolactin secretion caused by improper hypothalamic control. When prolactin levels are returned to normal, either surgically or medically with bromocriptine, menstruation will resume. Other hormonally active pituitary tumors such as those producing excess corticotropin (Cushing's disease) and abnormal amounts of growth hormone (acromegaly) may also interfere with menstrual function. A rare condition is the *empty-sella syndrome*, characterized by an enlarged sella turcica containing cerebrospinal fluid that displaces and compresses the pituitary gland.

Failure to uncover a pituitary disorder leads to the diagnosis of hypothalamic amenorrhea. Hypothalamic dysfunction is the most frequent cause of secondary amenorrhea. Essentially, it is a diagnosis of exclusion after uterine, ovarian, or pituitary abnormalities have been ruled out. No obvious endocrinopathy may be identified, but cyclic reproductive function ceases. Stress, extremes of weight, prior history of oral contraceptive use, and serious systemic illness are often associated factors. Induction of menstruation on a periodic basis with an oral progestogen is indicated to prevent continuous estrogen stimulation of the endometrium. Often patients with hypothalamic amenorrhea resume menstruation spontaneously.

DIAGNOSIS. Although the causes of amenorrhea are quite varied, the diagnostic approach to these patients is straightforward. Once the presence of anatomic abnormalities has been excluded, the administration of progesterone is indicated. Since progesterone will provoke menstruation only when the endometrium has been primed by estrogen, bleeding following withdrawal of progesterone rules out abnormalities of the outflow tract, uterus, and ovary other than polycystic ovarian disease. The measurement of serum androgens and an LH determination aid in the diagnosis of polycystic ovaries. The prolactin level must be determined in all patients to exclude a pituitary microadenoma.

If a patient does not bleed in response to progesterone, either she is hypoestrogenic because of ovarian, pituitary, or hypothalamic dysfunction or she has an unresponsive endometrium. The latter possibility may be discounted if the patient can be induced to bleed by combined estrogen and progesterone therapy. Further evaluation of the hypoestrogenic patient must include a determination of gonadotropin levels. Elevated gonadotropin levels indicate ovarian failure, and a karyotype should be ordered. Low or normal gonadotropin levels suggest pituitary or hypothalamic disease. A careful evaluation for pituitary tumor should be made in these patients. Periodic reevaluation for tumor is essential as long as the patient remains amenorrheic.

Ovarian neoplasm

Malignant ovarian tumors are a significant cause of morbidity and mortality in women. Of all diseases unique to women, cancer of the ovary ranks as the foremost cause of mortality. The chances of an ovarian neoplasm being malignant are lowest during the reproductive years. During these years true neoplasms must be distinguished from functioning cysts, which derive from the follicle or corpus luteum and often spontaneously regress. Ovarian neoplasms are rare in children, but if they should occur, the risk of malignancy is high. As women pass into the fifth and sixth decades of life, the risk of an ovarian neoplasm being malignant once again increases.

The most frequent presenting complaints in patients with ovarian neoplasms are abdominal swelling and discomfort. Often, however, ovarian neoplasms are asymptomatic and are detected only at the time of pelvic examination. The differential diagnosis of an enlarged ovary includes bowel lesions such as diverticulitis or carcinoma, an enlarged fallopian tube resulting from infection or ectopic pregnancy, or a pedunculated uterine leiomyoma. In young women laparoscopy is occasionally useful in distinguishing small, functional cysts from neoplastic tumors. In children or older women, however, the clinician usually proceeds directly to laparotomy. Findings at the time of surgery dictate either a conservative or a radical operative approach. Because ovarian carcinoma has usually metastasized by the time of diagnosis, surgery is frequently followed by chemotherapy.

Ovarian neoplasms are often classified according to their histologic type—60% to 70% of all ovarian neoplasms derive from the coelomic epithelium that surrounds each ovary; 15% to 20% of all neoplasms are of germ cell origin; another 5% to 10% derive from the stroma; and only 5% are metastatic in origin. Ovarian tumors may also be classified according to their degree of malignancy and if they are hormonally active.

BIBLIOGRAPHY

DiSaia, D.J., Morrow, C.P., and Townsend, D.E.: Synopsis of gynecologic oncology, New York, 1975, John Wiley & Sons, Inc.
Erickson, G.F.: Normal ovarian function, Clin. Obstet. Gynecol. **21**:31, 1978.
Givens, J.R.: Normal and abnormal androgen metabolism, Clin. Obstet. Gynecol. **21**:115, 1978.
Speroff, L., and VandeWiele, R.L.: Regulation of the human menstrual cycle, Am. J. Obstet. Gynecol. **109**:234, 1971.
Speroff, L., Glass, R.H., and Kase, N.G.: Clinical gynecologic endocrinology and infertility, ed. 2, Baltimore, 1978, The Williams & Wilkins Co.
Styne, D.M., and Grumbach, M.M.: Puberty in the male and female, its physiology and disorders. In Yen, S.S.C., and Jaffe, R.B., editors: Reproductive endocrinology: physiology, pathophysiology, and clinical management, Philadelphia, 1978, W.B. Saunders Co.
Winter, J.S.D., Faiman, C., and Rayes, F.I.: Normal and abnormal pubertal development, Clin. Obstet. Gynecol. **21**:67, 1968.
Yen, S.C.C.: The human menstrual cycle. In Yen, S.C.C., and Jaffe, R.B., editors: Reproductive endocrinology: physiology, pathophysiology, and clinical management, Philadelphia, 1978, W.B. Saunders Co.

192 • HUMORAL SYNDROMES ASSOCIATED WITH NEOPLASMS

Doris G. Bartuska

Clinical signs and symptoms resulting from hormonal production by nonendocrine cancers have been called paraneoplastic syndromes, humoral syndromes associated with cancer, or ectopic hormone syndromes. The availability of sensitive assay techniques has led to the elucidation of a wide variety of these syndromes. It is probable that all cancers elaborate humoral substances, but clinically only those that secrete biologically active materials are recognized. Examples of these "humors" include peptide hormones, precursors of peptide hormones, prostaglandins, fetal proteins, and enzymes. At least 21 hormones or their precursors have been shown to be produced by cancers, most of which are protein or peptide (see following list).

Humoral substances produced by nonendocrine neoplasms

Adrenocorticotropic hormone/melanocyte-stimulating hormone (ACTH/MSH); lipotropins
Gonadotropins (human chorionic gonadotropin, HCG)
Vasopressin (or antidiuretic hormone, ADH)
Parathyroid hormone (PTH)
Hypoglycemic producing factor
Erythropoietin
Gastrin and gastic peptides
Thyroid-stimulating hormone (TSH)
Hypophosphatemia-producing factor
Corticotropin-releasing hormone (CRH)
Calcitonin
Prolactin
Growth hormone
Kinins
Prostaglandins
Secretin
Glucagon
Human placental lactogen (HPL)
Somatomedins

Many of the symptoms and signs that appear in the patient with cancer are the result of endocrine or metabolic activities of the tumor itself. Several theories have been advanced to explain the phenomenon of humoral secretion by neoplasms. Cells contain genetic material coded with the same information; it is possible that gene derepression accompanies neoplastic transformation. Another hypothesis involves tissue dedifferentiation; this implies a return to more primitive gene expression and reversal of tumor tissue differentiation. Other investigators have provided evidence that specific types of tumors elaborate specific types of hormones and that the cells from the different tumors producing the same hormone are similar in morphologic, histochemical, and ultrastructural characteristics and in embryologic origin. A unified theory of polypeptide hormone production by these tumor cells suggests that they are caused by dysplasia of neural ectoderm. A common embryologic ancestry probably accounts for their shared endocrine potential. These cells have been designated APUD (amine precursor uptake and decarboxylation) cells to highlight their common ability to synthesize and store biogenic amines.

Current data suggest that all peptide hormones begin in the preprohormone form, which contains methionines, the universal codon for protein synthesis, plus a variable-length additional amino acid sequence. The preprohormone is degraded to the prohormone, which is generally biologically inactive. It is then enzymatically degraded to the bioactive hormone. After being secreted into the blood, it is degraded into the carboxy fragment, which is biologically inert, and the amino fragment, which may have biologic activity.

Physicians should be aware of these syndromes so that a correct diagnosis can be established. Humoral secretions by the neoplasm may precede other clinical evidence of the tumor by weeks or months. In addition, humoral production can be used to localize the tumor and to assess response to chemotherapy, surgery, or radiotherapy. The reappearance of the circulating ''humor'' can be used as a ''marker'' for recurrence of the neoplasm.

This chapter is concerned with some of the more common endocrine manifestations of malignancy.

Table 192-1 lists a spectrum of the endocrine syndromes associated with malignancy and the involved hormones. It has been estimated that one of these syndromes will be present in 15% to 50% of patients with cancer and that 75% of cancer patients will manifest some aspect of a paraneoplastic syndrome during their life span.

HYPERCALCEMIA AND NEOPLASMS

Hypercalcemia is the most common recognizable endocrine abnormality associated with neoplasia. Hypercalcemia occurs in about 0.3% of patients in a general hospital; of these about 20% have cancer and about 5% have hyperparathyroidism. It has been estimated that 10% to 20% of patients with cancer will have hypercalcemia at some time. It is often due to lysis of bone by metastases and is accompanied by normal or elevated phosphate levels, or it may develop because tumors elaborate ectopic PTH. These cancer patients have biochemical changes similar to those found in hyperparathyroidism, with hypophosphatemia as well as hypercalcemia. Other humoral substances, such as prostaglandins, calcitonin, osteoclast-activating factor, and vitamin D–like sterols elaborated by the tumor, may also influence the level of serum calcium.

Symptoms of hypercalcemia are subtle and nonspecific. The earliest manifestations are polyuria, nocturia, anorexia, nausea, vomiting, constipation, lethargy, weakness, dry mouth, or behavioral changes. Persistent progressive hypercalcemia results in severe dehydration, azotemia, mental confusion, coma, cardiovascular collapse, and death. The serum calcium level is usually between 12 and 16 mg/dl. Patients with primary hyperparathyroidism usually have only a modest elevation of serum calcium (up to 12 mg/dl). Hypercalcemia can be worsened by dehydration, immobilization, thiazide administration, adrenal insufficiency, hyperthyroidism, and vitamin D intake.

Table 192-1. Endocrine syndromes associated with malignancy

Syndrome	Hormone	Tumor sites
Hyperparathyroidism	PTH	Kidney, lung (squamous), ovary, many squamous sites
Cushing's	ACTH CRH	Lung (oat cell, bronchial adenoma), thymus, pancreas, thyroid (medullary), stomach, ovary
Inappropriate antidiuresis	ADH	Lung (oat cell)
Zollinger-Ellison	Gastrin	Pancreas (non–β-islet-cell adenomas)
Gynecomastia	Gonadotropins (HCG, α-, or β-subunits)	Lung (large cell), testes
Precocious puberty	Gonadotropins (HCG, α-, or β-subunits)	Liver, lung (bronchogenic), teratoma
Erythrocytosis	Erythropoietin	Cerebellum (hemangioblastoma), liver, uterus, kidney
Hypoglycemia	Uncertain	Retroperitoneal or intrathoracic fibrosarcomas, liver, adrenal glands
Galactorrhea	Prolactin	Kidney (hypernephroma)
Pigmentation	ACTH/MSH, lipotropin	Bronchus (oat cell)
Hyperthryoidism	Thyrotropin	Choriocarcinoma, testis, lung
Others	Serotonin, histamine, insulin, growth hormone, prostaglandins, kinins, secretin, HPL, gastric peptides	Various

Hypercalcemia is associated with nearly every type of malignancy. Breast cancer is the most common tumor associated with hypercalcemia; it is usually caused by local osteoclastic activity of the metastases to bone or prostaglandins. This is also common in myeloma, leukemia, and a variety of other tumors. On the other hand, bronchogenic (squamous cell) and renal carcinomas comprise about 60% of the tumors associated with the production of PTH or a PTH-like substance. This also appears to be the mechanism of production of hypercalcemia in squamous cell tumors of the head, neck and skin.

The differential diagnosis of primary hyperparathyroidism and the hypercalcemia of malignancy rarely presents a problem.

MANAGEMENT. Patients with hypercalcemia are usually dehydrated. *Hydration* is the most urgent objective and can be accomplished by giving intravenous isotonic saline (3 to 10 L/day) to correct the fluid depletion and induce a calcium diuresis. The amount of fluid and its composition are determined by the cardiopulmonary, renal, and electrolyte status of the patient. After initial volume repletion, forced diuresis with furosemide, 40 to 80 mg intravenously, results in appreciable calcium diuresis. Furosemide inhibits tubular reabsorption of sodium with a concomitant increase in excretion of calcium. Careful attention must be given to electrolyte losses and replacement. Thiazide diuretics are contraindicated because they may cause a decrease in urinary excretion of calcium.

Reversal of hypercalcemia and hypercalcuria can be achieved with *mithramycin* in doses considerably lower than those recommended for use in the treatment of tumors. This drug has a direct effect on bone by inhibiting resorption of calcium from bone. The recommended dose is 25 μg/kg body weight diluted in 1 L of 5% glucose in water and administered by slow intravenous infusion over 4 hours. Intravenous bolus injection has been used by some physicians. This causes reversal of hypercalcemia in 24 to 48 hours, and the effect may last several days. Additional therapy may be given in 2 or 3 days, and subsequent therapy at intervals of 1 week will maintain serum calcium at normal or near normal levels. Thrombocytopenia and abnormalities in clotting factors have been seen when the drug is used habitually, especially with the higher antitumor dosage.

Corticosteroids are effective in the treatment of hypercalcemia associated with myeloma and some breast cancers. They are less reliable in treating the hypercalcemia associated with other malignant neoplasms. Steroids may cause decreased bone resorption, decreased gastrointestinal absorption of calcium, and increased urinary excretion of calcium; they also have a direct action on bone by blocking the action of osteoclast-activating factor. Prednisone, 60 to 100 mg in divided doses orally, or hydrocortisone, 100 to 300 intravenously, every 24 hours has been used. The risks of regular steroid use are osteoporosis and the metabolic and electrolyte abnormalities of the cushingoid state.

Calcitonin (Calcimar) has a direct inhibitory action on bone and reduces osteoclastic resorption. Renal effects and gastrointestinal actions have also been described. Calcitonin lowers the elevated serum calcium of patients with carcinoma, multiple myeloma, and primary hyperparathyroidism. The recommended starting dose is 4 MRC (Medical Research Council) units/kg body weight every 12 hours subcutaneously or intramuscularly. The calcium lowering response occurs about 2 hours after the injection and lasts for 6 to 8 hours.

Neutral phosphates are effective, but the risk of ectopic calcifications must be recognized because phosphate combines with calcium and is deposited in bone and body tissues. Intravenous phosphate, 1.5 to 2 g, should be given slowly over 8 hours. Large amounts of phosphate given rapidly can cause hypocalcemia and shock and should be used only when other methods are not available.

When calcium is lowered to normal or near normal levels, oral phosphate 1 to 3 g/day, in divided doses is useful for regular use. A divided dose of 1.5 g daily is reliable, and the side effect of diarrhea that is seen with a larger dose of 3 g/day can be avoided.

Aspirin and indomethacin, which are prostaglandin synthetase inhibitors, have been used with some positive results.

Primary treatment of the tumor with surgery, irradiation, or cytotoxic agents will remove the source of PTH or other calcium-elevating substance and lower serum calcium. Adjunctive measures such as increasing body activity, avoiding immobilization, and providing hydration should be used whenever possible.

CUSHING'S SYNDROME

The secretion of large amounts of ACTH is associated with carcinoma of the lung (oat cell type). Lung cancer accounts for 60% of the cases; bronchial carcinoids, epithelial tumors of the thymus, medullary carcinoma of the thyroid, pancreatic tumor, pheochromocytoma, neuroblastoma, and other tumors may be other possible causes.

Tumors associated with this syndrome have also been associated with an increase in MSH; however, human β-MSH has been shown to be an artifact of extraction methods. Most purification methods split β-MSH from a larger peptide, which appears to be β-lipotropin (LPH). It has been found in more than 90% of tumor extracts from a variety of carcinomas and is elevated in 60% of patients with untreated lung cancer who do not have clinical Cushing's syndrome.

The clue to Cushing's syndrome is hypokalemic alkalosis. Any patient with a low serum potassium level, elevated blood sugar level, marked weakness, edema, hypertension, behavioral changes, and increased pigmentation should be studied. Confirmation is obtained by finding high levels of plasma cortisol with loss of the normal diurnal variation, increased urinary 17-hydroxycorticoids or free urinary cortisol, plasma ACTH greater than 200 pg/ml, and failure of suppression with exogenous glucocorticoids. Localization of occult tumors has been accomplished by finding elevated ACTH levels in selected venous samples.

Surgical removal of the tumor, irradiation, or chemotherapy results in remission of the symptoms resulting from cortisol excess. Treatment with metyrapone, an enzyme blocker, may be used as a temporary measure to reduce cortisol production. Mitotane also suppresses the synthesis of adrenal steroids but requires several weeks of treatment before it is effective.

INAPPROPRIATE ANTIDIURESIS

The continued secretion of antidiuretic hormone (ADH, or vasopressin) inappropriate to the body's needs leads to hyponatremia, overhydration, decreased serum osmolality, and concurrent inappropriately elevated urine osmolality. The resulting hypervolemia leads to irritability, drowsiness, lethargy, mental confusion, convulsions, and coma.

Treatment of this syndrome is directed against the tumor itself in the form of surgery, irradiation, or chemotherapy. Oversecretion of vasopressin is only associated with symptoms when excess water is given. Treatment consists of water restriction. Other forms of treatment include drugs that prevent the renal response to vasopressin, such as demeclocycline and lithium carbonate.

HYPOGLYCEMIA

Spontaneous hypoglycemia can occur in patients with nonpancreatic neoplasms. The majority of these are large, mesenchymal tumors such as retroperitoneal or intrathoracic fibrosarcomas, neurofibromas, hepatomas, and adrenocortical carcinomas. The symptoms include sweating, tachycardia, flushing, hunger, drowsiness, convulsions, and coma.

The cause of the hypoglycemia is uncertain. Suggested mechanisms include production of a nonsuppressible, insulin-like material (possibly somatomedin), excessive glucose use, and impaired gluconeogenesis. Surgical removal of the tumor alleviates the symptoms. When this is impossible, drug treatment has been tried; glucocorticoids in high doses have been used, as well as glucagon and streptozotocin. Continuous intravenous administration of 10% to 20% glucose can be used as an interim measure.

ECTOPIC GONADOTROPINS

Gynecomastia or precocious puberty results from the ectopic secretion of gonadotropins by neoplasms. These gonadotropins are similar to HCG. HCG-like material is present in normal tissue; however, there appear to be biochemical differences in the HCG that is elaborated with cancer. The ectopic production of the α- and β-subunits of HCG has also been described. The treatment includes surgery, irradiation, or chemotherapy directed at the tumor.

BIBLIOGRAPHY

Bartuska, D.: Humoral manifestations of neoplasms, Semin. Oncol. **2**:405, 1975.

Baylin, S.B., and Mendel, J.G.: Ectopic (inappropriate) hormone production by tumors: mechanisms involved and the biological and clinical implications, Endocr. Rev. **1**:45, 1980.

Odell, W.D., and Wolfson, A.R.: Humoral syndromes associated with cancer, Annu. Rev. Med. **29**:379, 1978.

Shnider, B., and Manalo, A.: Paraneoplastic syndromes: unusual manifestations of malignant disease, D.M. **25**:1, 1979.

193 • MINERAL METABOLISM AND METABOLIC BONE DISEASE

Howard Rasmussen

PHYSIOLOGY OF BONE

To understand the pathophysiology of the disease states discussed in this chapter, an understanding of both skeletal and mineral homeostasis is needed. One group of the diseases is disorders primarily of mineral homeostasis, another group is disorders primarily of skeletal homeostasis, and a third involves alterations in both. The last occurs because there is an intimate relationship between bone turnover and mineral metabolism. Before presenting a description of these three classes of bone disease, it is necessary to review briefly the structure and turnover of bone and the hormonal regulation of mineral metabolism.

Structure and turnover of bone

Bone is a tissue comprised of two components, an organic matrix made up largely of collagen and proteoglycans and a solid mineral phase. This mineral phase is not completely homogeneous but consists of several different types of calcium phosphate salts. The predominant one is small crystals of hydroxyapatite ($Ca_{10}[PO_4]_6[OH]_2$). There is a lesser content of amorphous calcium phosphate characterized by a lower calcium/phosphate ratio than that of crystalline hydroxyapatite. Regardless of which form exists in a particular region of bone, the essential fact is that matrix formation always precedes bone mineral deposition. This means that it is the amount and organization of the matrix that determine the size and shape of the bone. The mineral component is deposited in close apposition to the collagen fibrils. It is this intimate relationship that confers on bone its unique mechanical and tensile properties.

At the tissue level there are two types of bone, cortical and trabecular. The cortical bone forms the solid bone of the shafts of long bones and the tabular surfaces of the flat bones of the face, pelvis, and vertebrae. This bone is dense and solid except where it is penetrated by haversian canals. The trabecular or spongy bone fills the layer between the tables of flat bones and vertebrae and also the distal ends of the shafts of long bones. It is, as its name implies, a spongy lacework of tiny interlocking trabeculae.

There are two types of bone formation, endochondral and intramembranous. In the former, growth occurs on the surfaces of the vertebral bodies and at specialized epiphyseal plates at the end of long bones. At these sites the growth event is a proliferation of cartilage cells, which then lay down an extracellular organic matrix. The deposition of this new matrix actually extends the length of the bone. Following this phase the cartilage cells hypertrophy and partially resorb the previously elaborated matrix. The remaining matrix then undergoes calcification to form primary bone. Once formed, this primary bone undergoes successive remodeling cycles of resorption and redeposition of true bone (intramembranous bone).

At the periosteal surface of all long bones, as well as the bones of the face, the process of bone formation does not involve the formation of primary cartilaginous bone but occurs by direct bone deposition consisting of collagen synthesis, extracellular organization of the collagen into distinct lamellae, and mineralization of these lamellae. This type of bone formation is known as modeling, in contrast to remodeling (see discussion that follows). Since it continues at a slow rate throughout life, the total cortical diameter of the long bones increases slightly with age and the shape of the facial bones undergoes continued change. Although not usually influenced by changes in hormone concentration within the physiologic range, this bone is sensitive to excess amounts of growth hormone and parathyroid hormone. The former causes the rate of its formation to increase, accounting for the increase in glove and shoe size and the prognathism characteristic of acromegaly.

Cessation of longitudinal growth depends on the disappearance of the growth or epiphyseal plates. The rates of their maturation and growth vary independently, and both are under hormonal control. Thyroid hormone deficiency causes a delay in both, testosterone increases both, and growth hormone increases growth rate without altering maturation.

Once a human has reached adulthood the epiphyseal bone growth stops, but the skeleton continues to undergo constant remodeling throughout life. This remodeling is of two types: the haversian remodeling of cortical bone and the surface remodeling of trabecular bone. In the first type a group of bone-resorbing cells enters the cortical bone perpendicular to the long axis of the bone and then, after penetrating a variable distance, turns at right angles and cuts out a cylindric core of bone. This resorptive phase is followed by a quiescent phase and then a phase of new bone formation that fills or nearly refills the cylindric core except for a small canal, the haversian canal, containing blood vessels and nerve fibers. It is obvious that in this compact cortical bone, a remodeling sequence in one of these bone remodeling units (BMUs) must start with resorption of old bone followed by formation of new within the resorption cavity. Hence it is easy to appreciate that haversian remodeling is a sequential process involving activation of a group of cells to become *osteoclasts* that resorb bone, followed by a resorptive phase during which the osteoclasts remove old bone, followed by a reversal phase in which resorption has stopped and the bone surface is lined with mononuclear cells but no formation is occurring, followed by a phase of formation of new bone matrix by *osteoblasts,* followed finally by the mineralization of bone by *osteoid osteocytes.*

A clarifying comment concerning the processes of bone formation and resorption is necessary. As noted previously, the formation of either type of bone is a two-step process: (1) the elaboration of an organic matrix and (2) the subsequent mineralization of that matrix. However, when bone is resorbed, both matrix and mineral are removed simultaneously. Hence unmineralized bone, so-called osteoid, is a result of a failure of normal mineralization but does not occur as a consequence of the selective removal of the mineral from the matrix of old, previously mineralized bone.

Trabecular bone remodeling, a surface rather than an internal remodeling process, also follows this sequence of activation → resorption → reversal → formation → mineralization. The only difference, aside from the geometric one of internal versus surface remodeling, is that the process is more rapid in trabecular bone than in cortical bone.

After 20 to 25 years of age the constant remodeling of both trabecular and cortical bone is such that on average within each remodeling site, or BMU, the amount of bone removed during the resorption phase is not quite replaced during the phase of subsequent formation. This means there is a slow but progressive loss of skeletal mass at an annual rate of 0.5%. In men this continues at a more or less constant linear rate throughout life. In women, however, beginning at menopause (45 to 55 years of age), the net loss of bone is accelerated significantly for 4 to 7 years, so that in many women over 60 the mass of bone becomes critically reduced and vertebral and hip fractures are common. This condition, known as postmenopausal osteoporosis, will be discussed later in this chapter.

In a variety of other conditions changes in the rates of remodeling and the balance between resorption and formation can occur. The major hormones involved in regulating the various steps in bone remodeling are presented in Fig. 193-1.

To fully understand the remodeling process and the diseases associated with it, another of its features must be considered. This feature is its cellular basis. As previously mentioned, osteoclasts are responsible for resorption and

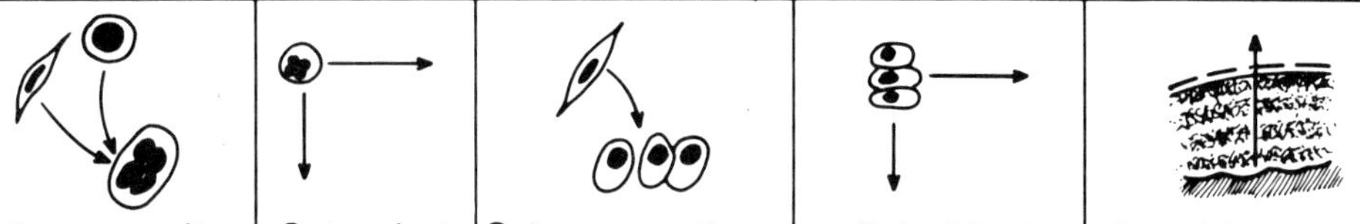

Phase	Activation	Resorption	Reversal	Formation	Mineralization
Cell or cellular event	Osteoprogenitor → Osteoclast	Osteoclast	Osteoprogenitor$_{II}$ → Osteoblast Osteoclast → ?	Osteoblast	Osteoid osteocyte
Control factors Positive	PTH↑ TH↑ Ca^{2+}↑ Paget's factor ↑	PTH↑ TH↑ Ca^{2+}↑ 1,25(OH)$_2$D$_3$↑	CT↑ Estrogen↑ Phosphate↑	Fluoride↑ Phosphate↑ 25(OH)D$_3$?	Phosphate↑ { 1,25(OH)$_2$D$_3$ { 24,25(OH)$_2$D$_3$ } ↑ 25(OH)D$_3$↑
Negative	CT↓ Estrogen ?↓	CT↓ EHDP↓ Fluoride↓	Cortisol↓ Immobilization↓ Age↓	Immobilization↓ Age↓ Cortisol↓ EHDP↓	Fluoride↓ EHDP↓

Fig. 193-1. Ionic and hormonal control of the bone remodeling process. Process is a sequential one of activation → resorption → reversal → formation → mineralization. Factors listed in lower half of the figure are thought to regulate the respective steps. *PTH*, parathyroid hormone; *TH*, thyroid hormone; *CT*, calcitonin; *EHDP*, disodium ethane-1 hydroxy-1 diphosphonate.

osteoblasts for bone formation. However, recent work has shown that these cells arise from separate precursor pools. Osteoclasts arise from bloodborne cells, probably a subclass of monocytes, and osteoblasts arise from bone tissue cells. In most situations in which an increase in the rate of activation of new BMUs occurs, there is a concomitant increase in both resorption and subsequent formation. For example, in most patients with mild hyperparathyroidism there is a significant increase in the rate of bone remodeling without a change in bone mass. This observation implies some type of close *coupling* between the number and activity of osteoclasts and the number and activity of the osteoblasts that will subsequently appear at a remodeling site. In other words, by some means not yet understood, the osteoclasts by their number and activity signal the osteoblast precursors to produce sufficient osteoblasts to replace the amount of bone previously removed.

The control of bone mineralization will be discussed after a consideration of the hormonal control of mineral metabolism.

Mineral metabolism

It is convenient to consider mineral metabolism in terms of two ions, calcium and phosphate; three organs, kidney, gut, and bone; and three hormones, vitamin D and its metabolites, parathyroid hormone (PTH), and calcitonin (CT). The first of these hormones is a group of sterols and the other two are peptides.

CALCIUM METABOLISM. There are two critical aspects of calcium metabolism. The first is that the plasma ionized calcium concentration is a major regulator of all types of cellular functions, the most notable of which is neuromuscular excitability. When this concentration falls, neuromuscular excitability increases and a condition of tetany with spontaneous contractions of the muscle may ensue. When full blown, the syndrome of tetany is characterized by muscle stiffness and cramps, carpal and/or pedal spasm, circumoral paresthesias, bronchospasm, laryngospasm, and, particularly in young children, grand mal seizures. Two useful clinical signs in the diagnosis of tetany are Chvostek's sign (contractions of the facial muscles in response to a light tapping of the facial nerve) and Trousseau's sign (carpal spasm induced by occluding the circulation to the forearm and hand with a blood pressure cuff). A lengthening of the QT$_c$ interval of the electrocardiogram is also a sign of hypocalcemia.

Hypercalcemia results in depressed neuromuscular excitability, anorexia, drowsiness, nausea, constipation, and often polyuria and polydipsia because of a direct effect of the high plasma calcium level on the concentrating ability of the kidney.

Because of calcium's many effects on cell function and its critical role in the maintenance of normal neuromuscular excitability, and elaborate system has been developed to maintain the plasma calcium concentration within a very narrow range of 9.5 to 10.5 mg/dl of total calcium or 3.8 to 4.8 mg/dl of ionized calcium. The difference between these values depends on the fact that approximately 60% of the serum calcium is bound, largely to albumin but also to a minor degree to organic anions. Only the ionized component of the serum calcium is biologically important in terms, for example, of neuromuscular excitability. However, in routine clinical practice it is usually the total calcium that is measured. In most cases when total calcium is increased or decreased, there is a corresponding increase or decrease in ionized calcium. However, there are conditions in which there is an increase or decrease in the total protein or anion content of the serum, and this is associated with an increase or decrease in total calcium but no change in ionized calcium.

The second feature of calcium metabolism is that the serum calcium concentration is maintained in spite of fluctuating demands of the skeleton. Therefore, even in periods of rapid skeletal growth, a fall in serum calcium concentration does not occur. It seems, in other words, that the growing skeleton communicates its need to the intestine.

A schematic representation of calcium metabolism is presented in Fig. 193-2. There is 1.5 to 2 kg of calcium in the average adult. Over 97% of this is in the skeleton, a small amount (5 to 10 g) is in the cells, and 1 to 2 g is in the plasma and extracellular fluids. In a normal young adult there is a constant exchange of calcium between the plasma and the bone, kidney, and intestine. When the daily dietary calcium intake is 1000 mg, there is a net absorption of approximately 250 mg and a total intestinal absorption of 400 mg because of an endogenous secretion of 150 mg. There is a net accretion of approximately 500 mg of calcium into new bone each day and a net removal of approximately 520 mg from old bone. The kidney filters 7000 mg daily and reabsorbs all but 250 mg, which is excreted into the urine. The bulk of the filtered calcium is reabsorbed in the proximal tubule, and this process is probably not regulated by hormones. The remainder, 700 to 1050 mg, is reabsorbed distally in a process controlled by PTH. A small amount of calcium is lost each day in shedding of the skin.

From a consideration of the data represented in Fig. 193-2, it is apparent that the intestine and kidney are of prime importance in determining that the organism maintain a normal or positive calcium balance. If the functions of these organs are integrated properly, a normal calcium balance can be maintained. The intestine normally absorbs only a small percentage of the ingested calcium. This percentage is obviously greater in growing children. The major hormone regulating this process of intestinal calcium absorption is the active metabolite of vitamin D, 1,25-dihydroxyvitamin D_3. However, since intestinal and renal adaptation to a low calcium intake is not completely efficient, individuals with a daily dietary intake of less than 300 mg may be in negative calcium balance, even though they absorb as much as 30% of the ingested amount. Furthermore, it is likely that the efficiency of this adaptation becomes poorer with advancing age. Under these circumstances the only source of calcium for the maintenance of a normal serum level is the calcium in bone mineral. Hence, dietary calcium lack leads to a progressive loss of bone mass.

PHOSPHATE METABOLISM. The normal adult contains approximately 1 kg of elemental phosphorus present as free inorganic phosphate ($HPO_4^=$, $H_2PO_4^-$, or $PO_4^{\equiv}$), as inorganic phosphate as part of the mineral lattice of bone mineral, or in a variety of organic phosphate esters ranging from deoxyribonucleic acid (DNA), ribonucleic acid (RNA), and adenosine triphosphate (ATP) to the glycolytic intermediates and phospholipid. Approximately 85% of the total is in bone, 0.008% in plasma and extracellular fluids, and the remainder in cells. As illustrated in Fig. 193-3, there is a constant turnover of phosphate in the body. A typical daily diet provides approximately 1000 mg of phosphate phosphorus. Between 65% and 80% is absorbed. The plasma and extracellular fluids contain only 800 mg. Following a normal meal, the plasma phosphate concentration of 2.8 to 4 mg/dl (as phosphorus) rises as much as 1 mg/dl. However, the kidney filters approximately 5000 mg each day, of which approximately 1000 mg is excreted and the remainder is reabsorbed. Reabsorption occurs in both the proximal and distal tubules and is inhibited at both sites by PTH. CT also inhibits proximal tubular reabsorption of phosphate. The effect of vitamin D

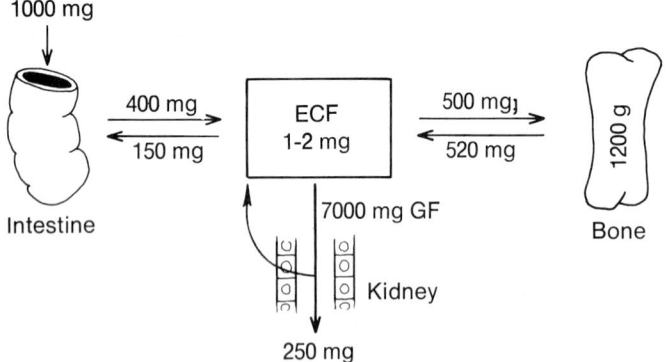

Fig. 193-2. Schematic representation of human calcium metabolism (see text). *ECF*, extracellular fluid; *GF*, glomerular filtration.

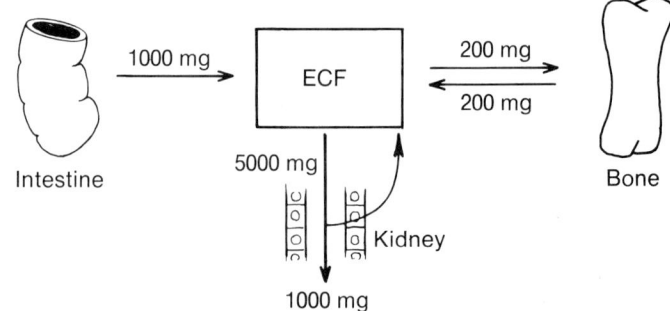

Fig. 193-3. Schematic representation of human phosphate metabolism (see text).

metabolites is controversial. There is evidence that 25-hydroxyvitamin D may stimulate proximal tubular phosphate reabsorption. Finally, there is the accretion of approximately 200 mg of phosphate into new bone each day and the removal of a slightly greater amount from the resorption of old bone.

A comparison of the scheme of calcium metabolism illustrated in Fig. 193-2 with that of phosphate metabolism shown in Fig. 193-3 reveals one important difference. The intestine plays the major role in determining the availability of the calcium ion. In the case of phosphate, the kidney plays the dominant role. This can be dramatically illustrated by the changes that occur in vitamin D deficiency. The active metabolite, $1,25(OH)_2D_3$, regulates the intestinal absorption of both calcium and phosphate. When the plasma concentration of $1,25(OH)_2D_3$ falls, the intestinal absorption of both ions decreases. However, calcium absorption may rapidly decrease to none and because of endogenous fecal excretion of calcium may lead to a net loss of calcium from the body. On the other hand, phosphate absorption, although it may diminish, will still lead to a net absorption of several hundred milligrams. Thus under most circumstances the plasma phosphate concentration is determined by the renal threshold for phosphate excretion (renal tubular maximum phosphate reabsorption/glomerular filtration rate, TmP/GFR), and not by the dietary intake. From this difference it is easy to see why phosphate accumulation and hyperphosphatemia commonly occur in chronic renal disease.

VITAMIN D METABOLISM. The natural source of vitamin D in humans is the skin, where under the influence of ultraviolet irradiation from the sun the provitamin 7-dehydrocholesterol is converted to vitamin D_3 (Fig. 193-4). This compound is biologically inert, at least in normal physiologic concentrations, and must undergo further metabolism before exerting its biologic effect. In city-dwellers who live in northern climates, work indoors, and go about fully clothed, the rate of vitamin D synthesis in the skin may be insufficient to supply the body's need. In this case what was once a hormone derived from skin becomes an essential dietary trace substance, a vitamin. This dietary need can be supplied by either synthetically prepared vitamin D_3 or vitamin D_2 (irradiated ergosterol). As far as is known, vitamin D_2 and vitamin D_3 are equipotent and are metabolized in the same way, although they have a difference in side chain structure.

Vitamin D_3 is considered a prohormone, not a hormone. It is normally made in the skin and either stored in adipose tissue or bound to a sterol-binding protein in the plasma. The first step in its metabolic conversion is to 25-hydroxyvitamin D_3 $(25[OH]D_3)$. This conversion takes place in the liver microsomes and is probably regulated by a number of factors. However, in general the higher the amount of D_3 made in the body, the higher the amount of

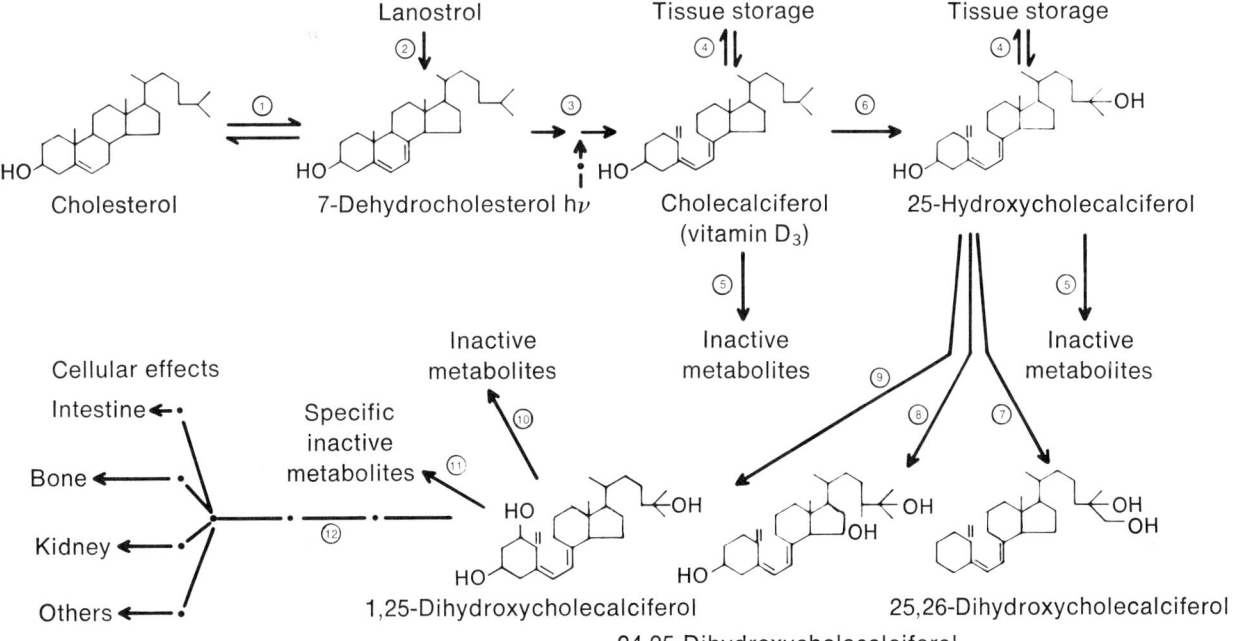

Fig. 193-4. Vitamin D metabolism. Vitamin can come from diet or be synthesized in skin from cholesterol. Cholesterol is converted first to 7-dehydrocholesterol *(1)*. This compound is activated by sunlight *(3)* and gives rise to vitamin D_3. Vitamin can be stored *(4)*, catabolized *(5)*, or converted in liver to 24-hydroxycholecalciferol (25-hydroxyvitamin D_3) *(6)*. This metabolite can be converted into one of three dihydroxymetabolites *(7, 8,* and *9)*. Little is known of $25.26(OH)_2D_3$. The $24.25(OH)_2D_3$ may have a function. The most studied and most active metabolite, $1.25 (OH)_2D_3$, is made in kidney. It acts on intestine, bone, and possibly kidney.

circulating 25 (OH)D_3. This compound is stored largely in the plasma, bound to the same sterol-binding protein as vitamin D_3. Its normal concentration in human plasma is 20 to 50 ng/ml. It has a direct action on bone by increasing bone resorption. It is less effective on a molar basis in this regard than is 1,25 (OH)$_2D_3$, but since it is present in considerably higher concentrations than 1,25(OH)$_2D_3$, it may play a physiologic role in regulating bone resorption. In addition, 25(OH)D_3 serves as the substrate for the further metabolic conversions to 1,25-dihydroxyvitamin D_3; 24,25-dihydroxyvitamin D_3; and 25,26-dihydroxyvitamin D_3 (Fig. 193-4). Very little work has been done on the biology and possible clinical relevance of 25,26(OH)$_2D_3$. Of the other two metabolites, 1,25(OH)$_2D_3$ is the more important and more fully studied and is used clinically. Both it and 24,25(OH)$_2D_3$ are made in the kidney mitochondria from 25(OH)D_3. There is evidence that 24,25(OH)$_2D_3$ is also made elsewhere, particularly in bone. However, the kidney appears to be the only source of 1,25(OH)$_2D_3$ in humans. The plasma concentration of 24,25(OH)$_2D_3$ is usually about one-tenth that of 25(OH)D_3, and little is known about the factors that regulate its synthesis. A striking fact about its metabolism is that its rate of catabolism is slow, with a turnover time of days rather than hours as is the case with 1,25(OH)$_2D_3$.

The renal biosynthesis of 1,25(OH)$_2D_3$ is highly regulated. Its concentration in normal human plasma is 35 to 60 pg/ml, or approximately 0.1% of the concentration of 25(OH)D_3. The major factors known to control its rate of synthesis are PTH and plasma phosphate. An increase in PTH or a fall in plasma phosphate will stimulate 1,25(OH)$_2D_3$ synthesis. However, other factors are obviously important because not all patients with primary hyperparathyroidism or acquired hypophosphatemia have high values of plasma 1,25(OH)$_2D_3$.

The intestine and bone are the major sites of action of 1,25(OH)$_2D_3$. Its major effect on the intestine is to stimulate the active absorption of both calcium and phosphate. Its effect on bone is to stimulate the resorption of bone, thereby liberating both calcium and phosphate from old bone. In addition to these well-established effects, it is clear that 1,25(OH)$_2D_3$ and the other metabolites of vitamin D have a direct action on muscle. A major sign of vitamin D deficiency is profound proximal muscle weakness.

The site(s) of action of 24,25(OH)$_2D_3$ is still a matter of controversy, but two effects of this metabolite may be of physiologic importance. It has been shown to suppress PTH secretion and stimulate bone mineralization. To understand the possible significance of these actions, it is necessary to consider the consequences of vitamin D deficiency.

The most dramatic result of vitamin D deficiency is the appearance of rickets and osteomalacia. These are failures of mineralization of endochrondal and membranous bone, respectively. As mentioned previously, bone formation is a two-step process of initial matrix formation followed by its mineralization; osteomalacia or rickets results from a delay in the mineralization process. In severe vitamin D deficiency the absolute rate of matrix synthesis also decreases, but there is always a greater relative decrease in the mineralization rate so that increasing amounts of unmineralized osteoid appear. There continue to be two schools of thought concerning the pathogenesis of the osteomalacia of vitamin D deficiency. One school holds that a deficiency of 1,25(OH)$_2D_3$ alone is sufficient to explain the process. In this view the two effects of 1,25(OH)$_2D_3$, that of increasing the absorption of calcium and phosphate from the gut and that of increasing the resorption of calcium and phosphate from old bone, are sufficient to raise the serum concentrations of calcium and phosphate to normal and thereby ensure the normal mineralization of bone. Thus the mineralization process proceeds normally as long as the ion product (Ca^{++} × HPO$_4^=$) in plasma is normal. The other school, while not disputing that 1,25(OH)$_2D_3$ exerts these effects, points out that there are conditions in which the mineral ion product and the plasma 1,25(OH)$_2D_3$ are normal, but the 25(OH)D_3 concentration is low and osteomalacia is seen. On the basis of this and other experimental data, they argue that 25(OH)D_3 or another vitamin D metabolite (possibly 24,25[OH]$_2D_3$) has a direct effect on the bone mineralization process.

PARATHYROID HORMONE (PTH) METABOLISM. PTH is a straight-chain polypeptide of 84 amino acids. It is unusual because it undergoes peripheral metabolism (Fig. 193-5), and this metabolic conversion leads to the appearance of multiple fragments in normal plasma. Not all of these are biologically active, and some of them may come from partial degradation of the native hormone in the gland before its release into the circulation. These multiple types of circulating fragments lead to considerable difficulty in making a direct correlation between immunoreactive PTH, that

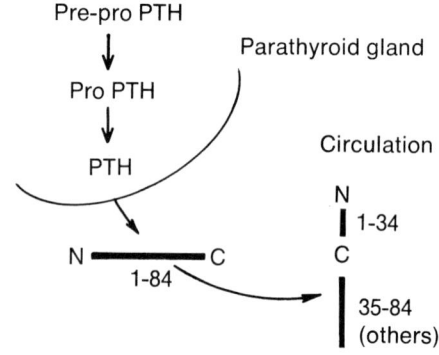

Fig. 193-5. Synthesis and metabolism of parathyroid hormone. Hormone is made as a larger precursor (pre-pro PTH) in parathyroid gland. This is processed (pro PTH) eventually to peptide containing 84 amino acid residues. This is the major secretory product of the gland. It is metabolized in periphery to N-terminal fragment (amino acids 1 to 34), which is biologically active, and C-terminal one, which is not.

measured by radioimmunoassay, and the biologically active hormone in plasma.

The major peripheral conversion is from the original molecule of 84 amino acids to a C-terminal fragment of amino acids 35 to 84 and an N-terminal fragment of amino acids 1 to 34. Both the parent 84 amino acid molecule and the N-terminal fragment are biologically active. It is not known with any certainty whether the conversion from the parent molecule to the N-terminal fragment is a necessary step before this hormone exerts its effects. Some believe that this is the case and that the 84 amino acid molecule is actually a prohormone. However, the data in support of this view are incomplete, and it remains possible that some of the physiologic effects, such as those on the kidney, are exerted by the N-terminal hormone and other effects, such as those on bone, by the 84 amino acid hormone. Alternatively, the peripheral conversion may represent a purely catabolic process and the pathway of hormone degradation. Against this view are the facts that synthetic human N-fragment possesses all the biologic actions of the 84 amino acid molecule and that peripheral conversion of the parent molecule to the N-terminal fragment is controlled by Ca^{++}. In any case there is very little N-terminal fragment normally present in plasma, and its half-life is a matter of minutes. On the other hand, there is considerably more of the 35 to 84 amino acid fragment and other C-terminal fragments derived from it. These are biologically inactive and persist for longer periods in the circulation.

Radioimmunoassay is a commonly used method of measuring the concentration of a hormone in plasma or serum. In theory this is a simple technique in which an antibody to the particular hormone is raised in a suitable animal. This antibody is then used as a reagent to measure the amount of the hormone in blood. The fact that PTH undergoes peripheral metabolism complicates matters and makes it difficult to develop an assay that measures the biologically active hormone in plasma. Different antibodies against the bovine 84 amino acid molecule recognize different antigenic determinants on this molecule, and when used in a radioimmunoassay they measure different mixtures of intact 84 amino acid molecule and C-terminal fragments. Hence, different assays give different absolute results on the same sample of plasma. Furthermore, since an absolute standard and human 84 amino acid molecules are not available, the standard employed in different assays is not the same. It is usually a serum from a patient or patients with hyperparathyroidism. To further complicate the issue, the kidney is a major site for the disposal of the C-terminal fragments. Hence, in chronic renal disease the level of immunoreactive PTH is high both because of phosphate retention and hypocalcemia leading to secondary hyperparathyroidism and because of a decreased rate of catabolism of C-terminal fragments.

PTH has two major functions: maintaining the plasma calcium concentration and regulating the rate of bone remodeling. There is a negative feedback relationship between the plasma calcium concentration and the rate of PTH secretion; a fall in calcium concentration causes a stimulation of secretion and a rise suppresses it. This basic control system is augmented by two other factors: catecholamines stimulate PTH secretion and $24,25(OH)_2D_3$ suppresses it. The physiologic significance of these subsidiary modulators is unknown.

The major effects of PTH are exerted on two organs, bone and kidney. The hormone acts on all bone cell types: preosteoclasts, osteoclasts, osteoblasts, and osteocytes. The physiologic consequences of its actions depend on the calcium balance of the organism. When dietary calcium is adequate, the actions of PTH on kidney (directly) and gut (indirectly) are the major factors in determining mineral homeostasis. In this case an increase in PTH does not lead to a net loss of bone mineral but only to an increase in the rate of bone remodeling. This occurs because PTH is a potent inducer of the activation step of the remodeling process (Fig. 193-1). However, in calcium deficiency states an increase in PTH leads to a net loss of bone mineral because, in addition to an enhanced rate of bone remodeling, there is an imbalance between bone resorption and subsequent formation. Under these circumstances the bone and kidney become the major organs determining plasma calcium concentration. Thus prolonged calcium deficiency leads to bone loss and the development of osteoporosis.

PTH exerts three major effects on the kidney at three anatomically distinct tubular sites. It inhibits proximal tubular phosphate reabsorption and also phosphate reabsorption at a late proximal site; it stimulates $1,25(OH)_2D_3$ synthesis at a proximal tubular site; and it stimulates the distal tubular reabsorption of calcium. Since $1,25(OH)_2D_3$ is the major hormonal regulator of intestinal calcium absorption, the PTH-mediated synthesis of $1,25(OH)_2D_3$ coordinates events in the intestine with those in the kidney. However, for the system to function correctly, the various renal tubular effects of PTH must be integrated. An imbalance between these renal effects can lead to hypercalciuria (excess urinary calcium excretion) and thereby to renal stones.

At the cellular level PTH has two effects. It increases the uptake of calcium, and it stimulates the enzyme adenylate cyclase. The latter effect is of practical significance because, as a consequence of cyclase activation in proximal renal tubular cells, the content of cyclic adenosine 3'5'-monophosphate (cyclic AMP) in the cell increases. Some of this leaks out of the cell across the luminal membrane and appears in the urine. Although other hormones such as vasopressin acting in other parts of the nephron also activate adenylate cyclase in their target cells, only in the case of PTH does this lead to an increase in the content of cyclic AMP in the urine. By measuring the creatinine clearance, the total urinary cyclic AMP, and the plasma cyclic AMP, it is possible to calculate the amount of cyclic

AMP filtered at the glomerulus and thus obtain a value known as the *nephrogenous cyclic AMP*. This is the total urinary cyclic AMP minus the filtered cyclic AMP It is reported in relation to renal mass, in terms of nmoles per 100 milliliters glomerular filtration rate (GFR). The normal values are 0.5 to 2.5 nmoles/100 ml GFR. They fall to 0 in hypoparathyroidism and range from 2.6 to 10 in hyperparathyroidism. The measurement of nephrogenous cyclic AMP is therefore an in vivo assay of biologically active PTH in man. It is a better discriminator between normal individuals and patients with hyperparathyroidism than are the usual radioimmunoassays for PTH. However, as will be discussed, there is another clinical condition that may be associated with hypercalcemia and high nephrogenous cyclic AMP: so-called humoral hypercalcemia of malignancy. By use of other tests this condition can be distinguished from primary hyperparathyroidism.

COORDINATE CONTROL OF MINERAL METABOLISM. To clarify the nature of the feedback system controlling the plasma calcium concentration, it is worthwhile to describe the physiologic consequences of calcium deficiency, PTH deficiency, phosphate deficiency, and vitamin D deficiency.

In the case of dietary calcium deficiency, the reduction in intestinal calcium absorption leads to a fall in the serum calcium concentration. This stimulates PTH secretion. The PTH acts on the distal nephron to increase the renal retention of calcium and on the proximal nephron to increase the synthesis of $1,25(OH)_2D_3$. The increased $1,25(OH)_2D_3$ acts on the intestine to stimulate intestinal calcium absorption, but this is relatively ineffective in cases of dietary calcium deficiency. In addition, the PTH and $1,25(OH)_2D_3$ act together to stimulate net removal of calcium from bone. By these direct or indirect effects on the three organs, PTH serves to maintain a normal serum calcium concentration at the expense of the net skeletal mineral balance. PTH also alters phosphate metabolism. At the level of both bone and intestine, the increased transfer of calcium into the extracellular fluids is accompanied by an increased transfer of phosphate. These effects would be expected to raise the serum phosphate concentration, but this does not occur. In fact, a slight fall in plasma phosphate concentration takes place because the increased circulating PTH blocks phosphate reabsorption in the proximal renal tubules.

In the case of a sudden PTH deficiency, the lack of effect of PTH on bone would reduce the delivery of both calcium and phosphate to the extracellular fluids. The loss of the renal effects would lead to an increase in renal calcium loss, a decrease in phosphate loss, and a decrease in $1,25(OH)_2D_3$ synthesis. A lack of the vitamin D hormone would lead to a decrease in the intestinal absorption of calcium and phosphate. Because of all these changes the serum calcium concentration would fall from its normal value of 9.5 to 10.5 mg/dl to the range of 5 to 6 mg/dl.

On the other hand, the plasma phosphate concentration would rise from 3 to 4.5 mg/dl to a value of 7 to 9 mg/dl. This would occur in spite of the delivery of less phosphate from bone intestine because of the profound change in the renal threshold (TmP/GFR) for phosphate excretion that occurs in the absence of PTH.

Phosphate deficiency from simple dietary lack is nearly unheard of, but if a low phosphate intake is combined with the administration of phosphate binders such as aluminum hydroxide (Amphojel), a state of phosphate deficiency results. It may also occur in patients with diabetic ketoacidosis or alcoholism, particularly during the treatment of these conditions. A deficiency of phosphate leads to a fall in plasma phosphate concentration. This stimulates the renal synthesis of $1,25(OH)_2D_3$ (independent of PTH action). The increased $1,25(OH)_2D_3$ stimulates intestinal calcium and phosphate absorption and the net removal of these ions from bone. These events cause a rise in the serum calcium concentration and hence a fall in PTH secretion. This leads to a decrease in the distal tubular reabsorption of calcium and thereby enhances the rate of disposal of calcium in the urine so that marked hypercalcemia does not occur. However, hypercalciuria is found because of the increased delivery of calcium from gut and bone. The excretion of phosphate in the urine declines to undetectable values because of both a lack of PTH effect on the proximal tubule and a direct effect of phosphate deficiency on the renal tubular phosphate transport system.

Vitamin D deficiency is the most complicated of the deficiency states discussed in this chapter. Deficiency of vitamin D does not have any immediate consequence because the body stores a considerable amount of this prohormone, which may be sufficient to supply the needs of the body for several months. Eventually, however, the concentration of $25(OH)D_3$ begins to fall. This leads to a decrease in bone resorption, which in turn causes a fall in the serum calcium concentration. As a result the rate of PTH secretion is increased, leading to the renal retention of calcium, an increase in the synthesis of $1,25(OH)_2D_3$, and an increase in renal phosphate loss. The biochemical findings at this point are a nearly normal plasma calcium concentration and a low plasma phosphate concentration. The low plasma phosphate and the $25(OH)D_3$ (or $24,25[OH]_2D_3$) levels lead to a decrease in the rate of bone mineralization so that osteomalacia develops. As the bone surface becomes increasingly covered with osteoid, less bone mineral is released. Furthermore, as the degree of vitamin D deficiency progresses, the plasma $1,25(OH)_2D_3$ level falls, leading to a decrease in intestinal calcium absorption and the plasma calcium concentration, and therefore to more severe secondary hyperparathyroidism. At this point the plasma calcium concentration is approximately 7 mg/dl and the phosphate concentration is 1.5 to 2 mg/dl. Profound muscle weakness develops, and the plasma alkaline phosphatase level rises.

The plasma alkaline phosphatase is derived from several organs, most notably liver and bone. Its concentration in blood increases in liver disease (particularly obstructive liver disease) and in a variety of metabolic bone diseases. Increased bone alkaline phosphatase activity occurs in bone diseases in which bone formation rates are high, such as Paget's disease and primary hyperparathyroidism, and in most states in which there is a mineralization defect, such as osteomalacia and vitamin D deficiency.

CALCITONIN (CT) METABOLISM. CT is a single-chain peptide hormone containing 32 amino acid residues. In contrast to PTH, the entire molecule of CT appears necessary for the hormone to exert its biologic effect. Also in contrast to PTH, there is no evidence that CT, once secreted, undergoes peripheral metabolism other than that of rapid degradation.

CT is secreted by the parenchymal or "C" cells of the human thyroid gland. These cells are distinct in function and embryologic origin from the classic cells that synthesize, store, and secrete thyroid hormones. The latter do not produce CT; the parenchymal cells produce CT but not thyroid hormones. Thus within the thyroid there are two distinct endocrine tissues.

As with PTH secretion, there is a feedback relationship between the secretion rate of CT and the plasma calcium concentration. However, in the case of CT secretion, the relationship is the opposite to that found with PTH. A rise in plasma calcium concentration is a stimulus to CT secretion, and a fall leads to a cessation of secretion. In addition, gastrin and possibly other gastrointestinal hormones enhance CT secretion. Following the ingestion of a meal containing calcium, there is an increase in secretion of CT before a detectable increase in plasma calcium concentration is observed.

One of the problems in defining the function of CT is that, in contrast to most other hormones, no clinical syndrome attributable to CT deficiency is yet known. Patients after total thyroidectomy do very well with only thyroid hormone replacement, and no significant changes in calcium or bone metabolism occur. A clinically recognizable syndrome in which CT excess is seen is medullary carcinoma. Even in these cases it is abnormalities other than the effect of CT on mineral metabolism that bring the patients to the attention of a physician. The most interesting speculation is that CT is a calcium storage hormone. Its secretion is stimulated by calcium ingestion, and its action on bone produces a net uptake of calcium by the skeleton during times of calcium surplus. It simultaneously minimizes any postprandial rise in plasma calcium concentration.

The target organs for CT are bone and kidney. In the kidney CT, like PTH, inhibits proximal tubular phosphate reabsorption, but unlike PTH it increases rather than decreases urinary calcium excretion. The effects on bone are of two types. The first is a rapid suppression of osteoclastic bone resorption and a shortening of osteoclast lifetime. The second, less rapid effect is a suppression of the activation of new bone remodeling units (BMUs). In this regard the effects of CT on bone remodeling are the opposite of those of PTH (Fig. 193-1).

In addition to acting on kidney and bone, CT also has the effect of increasing fluid and electrolyte secretion in the intestine. The physiologic significance of this is unknown.

PRIMARY DISORDERS OF MINERAL HOMEOSTASIS

A convenient way to classify the conditions in which the disorder of bone and mineral metabolism is one primarily of disturbed mineral metabolism is by the prominent pathophysiologic change seen in mineral metabolism. This section will consider conditions associated with hypercalcemia, primary hyperparathyroidism, hypocalcemia, hypoparathyroidism, pseudohypoparathyroidism, and medullary carcinoma.

Hypercalcemia

The following conditions are known to be manifested by hypercalcemia:

I. Neoplasia
   A. Local osteoclastic hypercalcemia
   B. Humoral hypercalcemia of malignancy
II. Hyperparathyroidism
   A. Primary idiopathic
   B. Primary familial
   C. Secondary
   D. Tertiary in renal disease
III. Drug therapy
   A. Vitamin D excess
   B. Vitamin A excess
   C. Thiazides
   D. Milk-alkali syndrome
IV. Other endocrinopathies
   A. Addison's disease
   B. Hyperthyroidism
   C. Pheochromocytoma
   D. Acromegaly
V. Possible increased sensitivity to vitamin D
   A. Sarcoidosis
   B. Chronic granulomatous disease of the lung
   C. Hypercalcemia of infancy
VI. Immobilization

Many of these are rare, and in some, such as thyrotoxicosis and Addison's disease, hypercalcemia is a secondary manifestation of a change in function of another major endocrine system. These are discussed elsewhere in the text. The major conditions to be discussed in this section include primary hyperparathyroidism, hypercalcemia of malignancy, hypercalcemia of immobilization, sarcoidosis, and vitamin D excess. First the signs and symptoms of hypercalcemia will be discussed, as well as an approach to its differential diagnosis and its treatment.

The reason for proceeding in this way is that regardless of cause, hypercalcemia is a potentially lethal condition that deserves immediate evaluation, particularly if the plasma calcium concentration is greater than 12 mg/dl. It is also a relatively common condition. Since the introduction of routine automated multiphasic screening, an incidence of hypercalcemia close to 2% has been noted.

CLINICAL MANIFESTATIONS. The diagnosis is commonly made by screening tests rather than by clinical history and physical examination because hypercalcemia is associated with a variety of common symptoms but few pathognomonic ones. Symptoms may include easy fatigability, anorexia, weight loss, nausea and vomiting, constipation, pruritus, subjective proximal muscle weakness, polyuria, and polydipsia. If the serum calcium concentration is greater than 12.5 mg/dl, hypercalcemia can lead to stupor, coma, acute toxic psychosis, and a variety of changes in affect or behavior. If polyuria occurs with anorexia and stupor, a state of progressive dehydration with prerenal azotemia can develop, and this will exaggerate the hypercalcemic state so that a rapid increase in plasma calcium concentration may occur over a few hours.

Hypercalcemic states may be categorized into *equilibrium* and *disequilibrium* types. In the former, such as in primary hyperparathyroidism, the plasma calcium concentration may be elevated but remains relatively stable. This is because the parathyroid gland still responds to a further rise in plasma calcium concentration by a decrease in secretion rate so that an equilibrium exists. In contrast, in patients with hypercalcemia of malignancy, a substance derived from the tumor is released into the bloodstream and causes a progressive increase in mobilization of calcium from the skeleton. However, regardless of the plasma calcium level, there is no feedback inhibition of the secretion of the hypercalcemic factor from the tumor, so a disequilibrium exists. This type of hypercalcemia is a greater threat because it may lead to a rapidly rising serum calcium concentration.

There are no specific findings on physical examination that are diagnostic of hypercalcemia. Depression of deep tendon reflexes and hypertension are commonly observed. Long-standing hypercalcemia may lead to corneal deposits of mineral crystals. It is usually necessary to perform a slit-lamp examination to detect them, but in extreme cases they may appear as *band keratopathy* visible with the use of an ophthalmoscope.

Hypercalcemia has a marked effect on the heart; sinus bradycardia, sinus arrhythmia, a shifting pacemaker, and varying degrees of heart block may occur. The effects of calcium on the heart can be objectively assessed by the measurement of the corrected QT interval (QT_c). This is shortened in hypercalcemia and prolonged in hypocalcemia. Hypercalcemia also produces a nonspecific, diffuse slowing in the electroencephalogram, but similar changes are seen in a variety of metabolic conditions.

DIAGNOSIS. The approach to the definitive diagnosis of the condition causing hypercalcemia depends on the degree of hypercalcemia. With plasma calcium concentrations greater than 12.5 to 13 mg/dl, immediate treatment of the hypercalcemia should be undertaken. Once the plasma calcium level has been lowered, definitive diagnostic procedures can be instituted. If, on the other hand, a patient with nonspecific symptoms is discovered by multiphasic screening to have a plasma calcium concentration between 10.6 and 12.5 mg/dl, a logical approach to the differential diagnosis can be followed (Fig. 193-6). The first step is that of establishing the validity of the measurement by repeating it. If two out of three consecutive measurements of fasting plasma calcium concentration are greater than 10.5 mg/dl, hypercalcemia exists. The next step, or one that can be carried out at the time of the collection of the second blood sample, is to obtain a spot urine sample for the simultaneous measurement of plasma and urine calcium, phosphate, and creatinine. From these data it is possible to calculate the TmP/GFR, a measure of the renal threshold for excretion. If this value is greater than 3.0, it virtually rules out humoral hypercalcemia of malignancy and primary hyperparathyroidism. If less than 2.7, it makes one of these two diagnoses very likely. Values between 2.7 and 3.0 are of borderline significance. Measurement of nephrogenous cyclic AMP can be obtained at the same time. If a high nephrogenous cyclic AMP is found in conjunction with either a low or borderline TmP/GFR, either primary hyperparathyroidism or humoral hypercalcemia of malignancy exists. A low nephrogenous cyclic AMP with a normal or high TmP/GFR rules out these conditions. In an occasional equivocal case, a patient may have a high normal nephrogenous cyclic AMP and a borderline TmP/GFR. In such a patient further diagnostic procedures are necessary. Other than these situations, the cause of the hypercalcemia can be separated into two broad categories: those characterized by normal or high TmP/GFR and low nephrogenous cyclic AMP and those with low TmP/GFR and high nephrogenous cyclic AMP.

The differentiation of patients with low nephrogenous cyclic AMP depends on a variety of types of information. A careful history of drug ingestion, particularly of calcium compounds, antacids, thiazide diuretics, and various forms of vitamin D, is essential. Also, a thorough search should be made for metastatic malignancy in bone, myeloma, lymphoma, or one of a variety of chronic pulmonary diseases, including sarcoidosis. Diagnostic procedures may include special roentgenographic examination such as bone scans, computed tomography scans for abnormal lymph nodes, and bone marrow biopsy. In addition, it may be necessary to measure the plasma concentrations of $25(OH)D_3$ and $1,25(OH)_2D_3$ to rule out vitamin D excess. Protein electrophoresis of serum or urine may assist in the diagnosis of multiple myeloma or sarcoidosis.

The differentiation between primary hyperparathyroid-

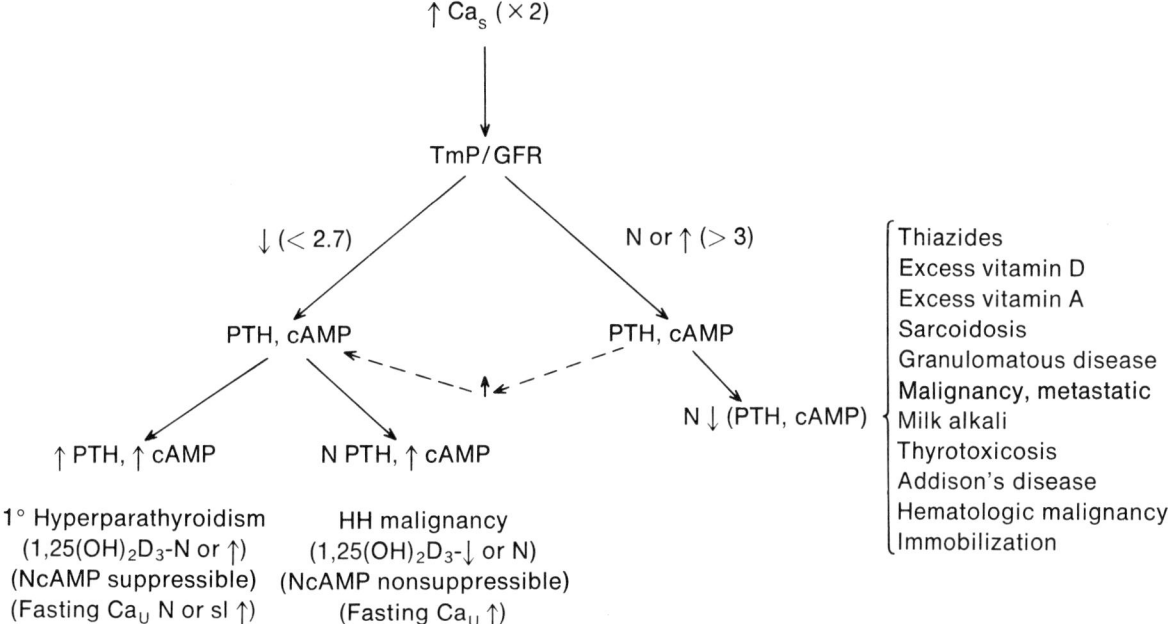

Fig. 193-6. Flow diagram of laboratory approach to differential diagnosis of hypercalcemia. Once presence of hypercalcemia is established, measurement of renal tubular maximum phosphate reabsorption/glomerular filtration rate (TmP/GFR), immunoreactive PTH, nephrogenous cyclic AMP, and in some cases plasma 1.25(OH)$_2$D$_3$ allows differentiation of various causes of hypercalcemia. *PTH,* parathyroid hormone; *cAMP,* cyclic AMP; *Ca$_s$,* serum calcium; *CA$_u$,* urinary calcium; *HH,* humoral hypercalcemia; *N,* normal; *NcAMP,* nephrogenous cyclic AMP.

ism and humoral hypercalcemia of malignancy is usually not difficult. In the majority of patients with the latter condition the presence of tumor is obvious by the time the hypercalcemia develops. In an occasional case difficulty may be encountered, but the diagnosis can usually be determined by the measurement of plasma immunoreactive PTH and 1,25 (OH)$_2$D$_3$ concentrations. These are usually high or high-normal in primary hyperparathyroidism and low or low-normal in humoral hypercalcemia of malignancy.

MANAGEMENT. The treatment of moderate hypercalcemia will be discussed in relation to the specific cause. However, severe hypercalcemia from any cause constitutes a medical emergency, and therapy aimed at reducing the serum calcium concentration should be instituted promptly. The first and most important step is prompt intravenous rehydration with normal saline. Once this has been accomplished, it is essential to evaluate the renal and cardiac status before proceeding further. If urine output is deemed adequate and cardiac function is normal, combined infusion of normal saline, 2 L every 6 hours, and furosemide, 40 mg every 6 hours, should be given. Since Ca^{++} and Na^+ reabsorption occurs predominantly in the proximal renal tubule, the effects of this therapy are to increase the filtered load of calcium. When proximal Na^+ reabsorption is blocked, Ca^{++} reabsorption is also inhibited so a marked calcium diuresis is produced. This therapy alone may lower the plasma calcium concentration by 1.5 to 2 mg/dl. However, it is difficult to maintain this form of therapy for more than few days because of the complicated problems with K^+ and Na^+ balances.

If the patient can take substances orally or as soon as he is able to do so, treatment with inorganic phosphate in doses of 0.25 to 0.5 g every 4 hours should be instituted. Before beginning this therapy, it is important to assess renal function and measure plasma phosphate. Most patients with severe hypercalcemia have low plasma phosphate concentrations. However, patients with hypercalcemia resulting from excess vitamin D have high levels of plasma phosphate. Phosphate therapy is contraindicated in this situation. Otherwise, in the typical patient with hypercalcemia who has normal renal function and a low plasma phosphate concentration, oral phosphate therapy is a safe and effective treatment that can be continued for days or weeks.

On the other hand, intravenous use of phosphate in the immediate treatment of hypercalcemia is highly controversial. Infusion of phosphate under these circumstances can lead to massive ectopic calcification, marked and rapidly developing hypocalcemia, and sudden death. This would seem to indicate that there is no place for this form of therapy in the treatment of hypercalcemia.

Although less widely used than several other agents, CT can be very effective in the treatment of acute hypercalcemia. This is particularly true if increased bone resorption contributes significantly to the hypercalcemia. CT treatment is especially effective when combined with oral phosphate therapy. Administration of 50 to 100 IU of CT intramuscularly or intravenously every 8 to 12 hours along with oral phosphate treatment is usually effective in controlling the hypercalcemia until a definitive diagnosis can be made and more specific therapy can be instituted.

Another class of drugs that may be employed is the glucocorticoids. They are particularly effective in treating the hypercalcemias of vitamin D excess, sarcoidosis, myeloma, and leukemias. Mithramycin, a potent antitumor agent, is also especially effective in the treatment of the hypercalcemia of malignancy. The use of these agents will be discussed in relation to specific conditions.

HYPERCALCEMIA OF MALIGNANCY. As its name implies, hypercalcemia of malignancy is the development of hypercalcemia in the setting of malignancy. In this syndrome hypercalcemia may develop either because of marked metastatic invasion of the bone or marrow cavity and thus a local stimulation of osteoclastic bone resorption or because of the production of a humoral factor by the tumor (not in bone), which acts on bone to stimulate bone resorption and inhibit bone formation. Hypercalcemia of malignancy is probably the most common cause of hypercalcemia in the hospital population (see Chapter 192).

PRIMARY HYPERPARATHYROIDISM

Definition. Primary hyperparathyroidism is a disorder of mineral and/or bone metabolism caused by increased and incompletely regulated secretion of PTH.

Etiology and pathology. The cause of primary hyperparathyroidism is unknown, but it is usually associated with either an adenoma of a single parathyroid gland (or rarely of two glands) or hyperplasia of all four glands. In very rare cases it is due to carcinoma of one of the glands. In contrast to the primary form, *secondary hyperparathyroidism* develops whenever prolonged hypocalcemia exists, as in chronic renal disease, states of calcium malabsorption, or vitamin D deficiency. Under these circumstances the hyperplastic glands of secondary hyperparathyroidism may become autonomous; that is, they then begin to behave like an adenoma. This *tertiary hyperparathyroidism* may be difficult to distinguish from the primary form. There is evidence that in certain patients with a long-standing renal leak of calcium, secondary hyperparathyroidism may eventually become primary because one of the four glands will undergo adenomatous transformation and secrete sufficient hormone to suppress the activity of the other glands.

The other feature of primary hyperparathyroidism, particularly that involving parathyroid hyperplasia, is its occurrence in the two syndromes of multiple endocrine neoplasia (MEN I and MEN II). In MEN I, parathyroid hyperfunction is found in conjunction with tumors of the pituitary gland and pancreatic islet cells. In these cases the hyperparathyroidism is often associated with recurrent peptic ulcer disease and gastric hypersecretion resulting from a gastrin-producing tumor in the pancreas or stomach (Zollinger-Ellison syndrome). In MEN II, hyperparathyroidism is associated with pheochromocytoma and medullary carcinoma of the thyroid. A subgroup of these patients may also have multiple neurofibromas. Both conditions appear to have autosomal dominant inheritance. Even so, there is a marked disparity in the time of appearance of the different types of tumors. Hyperparathyroidism may be the first manifestation of the syndrome or may appear years after one of the other endocrine tumors.

Another inherited form of primary hyperparathyroidism is familial hypocalciuric hypercalcemia (FHH), which is also known as familial benign hypercalcemia. This also occurs with an autosomal dominant pattern of inheritance, but it is not associated with other endocrine abnormalities.

Epidemiology. Primary hyperparathyroidism is more common in women. It is rare in children and young adults and has a peak incidence between 40 and 60 years of age. Multiparous women have a higher incidence than nulliparous ones. There do not appear to be any racial or geographic differences in incidence.

Pathogenesis. In discussing the pathogenesis of primary hyperparathyroidism, it is necessary to reemphasize that PTH acts on bone and kidney and that the primary consequence of excessive PTH is a rise in the serum calcium concentration. The second important aspect of the disease is that in nearly all circumstances, even though the adenoma or the hyperplastic glands secrete excessive amounts of the hormone, hormone secretion is still under feedback control. This means that patients with primary hyperparathyroidism have an equilibrium type of hypercalcemia. If a patient's serum calcium concentration is 12 mg/dl, it is possible to raise the calcium concentration by calcium infusion and thus show, by measuring nephrogenous cyclic AMP, a suppression of PTH secretion. This means that in the patient with hyperparathyroidism, overproduction of hormone results from one of two factors: (1) a change in the set point around which plasma calcium exerts its feedback control, or (2) an increase in parathyroid mass with a normal feedback control. In patients with adenomas both factors seem to be involved. In patients with primary hyperplasia the predominant factor appears to be an excessive amount of functioning tissue.

Regardless of whether the primary hyperparathyroidism is due to adenoma or hyperplasia, the disease will have one of the following presentations: (1) as mild hypercalcemia with marked hypercalciuria, usually renal stones, and very little bone disease; (2) as marked hypercalcemia with evident bone disease but with less marked hypercalciuria and no renal stones; (3) as moderate hypercalcemia without clinically evident bone or stone disease but with a variety of systemic complaints; or (4) as familial hypocalciuric hypercalcemia in which mild or occasionally marked hypercalcemia with hypocalciuria is found and no bone disease is evident.

The striking change in the hypercalciuric, stone-forming group is that moderate elevations of PTH and nephrogenous cyclic AMP are associated with significant elevations of plasma $1,25(OH)_2D_3$. Thus the effect of PTH on the renal synthesis of $1,25(OH)_2D_3$ appears to be the most important consequence of excessive PTH. It is the elevated $1,25(OH)_2D_3$ that is responsible for the increased intestinal absorption of calcium and the hypercalciuria that increases the risk of forming renal stones.

In patients with bone disease the major effects of PTH appear to be the action on bone and on the distal tubular reabsorption of calcium. In spite of plasma PTH levels similar to or even greater than those found in the stone-forming group, the plasma $1,25(OH)_2D_3$ is not elevated. Symptoms in these patients are a consequence of the hypercalcemia and of the bone disease, which on biopsy is characterized by a marked increase in bone remodeling and the appearance of marrow fibrosis and bone cysts resulting from accumulations and osteoclasts. It is a striking fact that resorptive activity is seen on the periosteal as well as the endosteal surfaces of long bones. The various changes give the condition its name, osteitis fibrosa cystica.

Patients with moderate hypercalcemia often have neither bone nor stone disease. These patients have a balanced organ response to PTH so that effects on kidney and bone are both moderate and the plasma $1,25(OH)_2D_3$ level is typically in the high-normal range. Symptoms in these individuals are a consequence of hypercalcemia. Patients in this category are often detected by multiphasic screening of a serum sample during a routine medical workup. This type of screening nearly always includes determination of the serum calcium concentration.

In the patients with hypocalciuric hyperparathyroidism the slightly increased amount of PTH affects the distal tubular reabsorption of calcium. This leads to hypercalcemia without an increase in plasma $1,25(OH)_2D_3$. Hence the rate of urinary excretion of calcium is low, usually less than 100 mg a day even when the serum calcium concentration and therefore the filtered load of calcium are high.

Clinical manifestations. As already discussed, the clinical manifestations of primary hyperparathyroidism depend on its type of presentation. However, in the absence of either recurrent renal calculi or some evidence of bone disease, the manifestations are protean in nature and reflect the effects of the hypercalcemia, the hypophosphatemia, and possibly the elevated PTH itself. The symptoms may range from vague abdominal pain, fatigability, headache, and emotional lability to severe debility, weight loss, anorexia, anemia, and an elevated erythrocyte sedimentation rate. Polydipsia and polyuria may occasionally be prominent. Conversely, proximal muscle weakness, aches and pain of the extremities, and abnormal fasciculations of the muscles, particularly the tongue, may be prominent. Rarely, glossal atrophy, sensory loss, and ataxia may be present. In other cases headache, hypertension, and pruritus may be the presenting signs. Bone tenderness can often be elicited even in patients without clinically or roentgenographically evident bone disease. The disease may occur as pseudogout or pancreatitis. It may also be discovered inadvertently during dental roentgenographic examination because of the loss of the lamina dura or because of a brown tumor or epulis of the jaw. If the hypercalcemia has been present for a long time, calcification in the cornea (band keratopathy) may be visible, but it is more often seen by slit-lamp examination.

Laboratory findings. The two most common biochemical changes in hyperparathyroidism are an increase in serum calcium concentration and a decrease in plasma phosphate concentration. The normal range of serum calcium concentration varies somewhat from laboratory to laboratory but is usually 9.5 to 10.5 mg/dl. Any patient who has three successive *fasting* values greater than 10.5 mg/dl should be considered to have hypercalcemia and be evaluated for the presence of hyperparathyroidism. Nearly all patients with this disease have persistent hypercalcemia. However, there is a small group of patients with so-called *normocalcemic hyperparathyroidism*. There are nearly always patients with hypercalciuria and elevated serum $1,25(OH)_2D_3$ values with or without renal stones. When followed, they show intermittent elevations of serum calcium concentration. They may present a particularly difficult diagnostic problem and must be clearly distinguished from patients with renal hypercalciuria and secondary hyperparathyroidism.

Although hypophosphatemia has been widely used as a sign of hyperparathyroidism, this test is less valuable than the measurement of serum calcium concentration because of the large number of factors that influence serum phosphate. However, the TmP/GFR (renal phosphate threshold) is of greater help and is usually below 2.7 in patients with primary hyperparathyroidism. Other findings may be mild metabolic acidosis, moderate anemia, and an elevated sedimentation rate. The measurement of urinary calcium excretion, although of great value in determining the type of hyperparathyroidism, is not of great help in the differential diagnosis because it can be low, normal, or high depending on the subtype of hyperparathyroidism.

Roentgenographic examination of the hands using highgrain industrial film may be of value in detecting subperiosteal erosions on the phalanges, but this sign is present only in a small minority of patients. A flat plate of the abdomen may reveal nephrocalcinosis, but this, too, is an uncommon manifestation of the disease. A rare finding currently is the presence of bone cysts (brown tumors).

The most definitive tests for the condition are either to measure plasma immunoreactive PTH (IPTH) or to measure plasma and urinary cyclic AMP and from these to estimate nephrogenous cyclic AMP. Each test has its advocates and each has its advantages and disadvantages. IPTH tests are more widely available commercially. The difficulty with IPTH measurements is their complexity. For one thing, PTH undergoes peripheral metabolism (Fig.

193-5), and therefore most assays measure a mixture of different PTH-derived peptides. Second, different antibodies detect a different spectrum of peptides. Third, different standards are employed by different laboratories. When carefully performed in a research laboratory, these tests measure high values in more than 95% of patients ultimately proven to have hyperparathyroidism. However, when they are performed by commercial firms, the percentage probably falls to less than 80% and a significant number of both false positive and false negative values are found. One difficulty with the nephrogenous cyclic AMP test is that it requires, in addition to a blood sample, a urine sample collected under a relatively standard set of conditions. In addition, an elevated nephrogenous cyclic AMP is also found in patients with humoral hypercalcemia of malignancy, which is also associated with hypercalcemia and a reduced TmP/GFR and must therefore be distinguished from primary hyperparathyroidism. Nevertheless, when the test is applied properly, nephrogenous cyclic AMP is found to be elevated in more than 97% of patients with primary hyperparathyroidism. Furthermore, in contrast to IPTH measurement, nephrogenous cyclic AMP measurements can distinguish between normal and low parathyroid function and can be used to measure rapid change in parathyroid function.

Differential diagnosis. An approach to the diagnosis in the patient with hypercalcemia has already been outlined. A difficult diagnostic choice is differentiating patients with primary hyperparathyroidism, renal stones, and intermittent hypercalcemia from those with renal calcium leak, renal stones, and secondary hyperparathyroidism. Another problem is differentiating between hypercalcemia without renal stones and humoral hypercalcemia of malignancy. Each of these is discussed later in the chapter.

Course. The course of hyperparathyroidism is quite variable. Some patients with moderate hypercalcemia (serum calcium concentration of about 11.5 mg/dl) without hypercalciuria have been followed for several years without significant change. Others, particularly those with bone disease, may have a rapidly progressive course with increasing hypercalcemia. Patients with hypercalciuria and stone disease nearly always continue to pass renal stones until treated. Patients with familial hypocalciuric hypercalcemia may be discovered at any age, and presumably in many the hypercalcemia has been present for years.

Management. There is at present no satisfactory medical treatment for hyperparathyroidism. Definitive therapy requires surgery. Attempts at developing methods for the preoperative localization of the tumor include selective venous catheterization with determination of IPTH, diagnostic ultrasound, and computed tomography. Since the latter two have only begun to develop a resolution sufficient to detect small tumors, their true value is still unknown. Selective catheterization is expensive, time consuming, and associated with some morbidity. It is reserved for patients in whom hyperparathyroidism persists after an initial unsuccessful parathyroid exploration.

The question of treatment versus observation is a perplexing one made more difficult by the increased incidence of mild hyperparathyroidism discovered as a result of widespread multiphasic screening. Treatment is safely deferred if the hypercalcemia is mild (serum calcium concentration of about 11.5 mg/dl) and the patient is asymptomatic, has no evidence of hypercalciuria or bone disease, and can return for regular evaluation. Otherwise, surgery is recommended.

Although it is a truism that all surgery should be performed only by qualified and experienced surgeons, this is particularly the case with parathyroid surgery. It is essential that the highest possible success rate be obtained at the initial procedure. This requires both surgical skill and a detailed knowledge of the anatomic variability in the location of the parathyroid glands. An essential determination is whether the disease is due to adenoma or hyperplasia. In theory this should be easy, but in practice it may be exceedingly difficult and requires close cooperation between the surgeon and the surgical pathologist. When a suspected adenoma is removed, biopsy of at least one other "normal" gland is necessary. If there is any question as to its anatomic structure, all four glands should be identified.

In cases of hyperplasia of all four glands, the surgical rule has been the removal of three and one half of the four glands. However, successful autotransplantation of parathyroid tissue into the forearm muscle is currently being explored as a way of managing this type of disease.

The one type of hyperparathyroidism in which surgery should not be done unless marked hypercalcemia develops is the familial hypocalciuric variety.

The major immediate postoperative complication is tetany caused by hypocalcemia. This is usually mild and can be managed by intravenous and oral calcium supplements, but if severe bone disease is present, it may be quite marked and administration of $1,25(OH)_2D_3$ in a dose of 1 to 3 μg a day along with oral calcium may be necessary.

There are no known measures by which to prevent hyperparathyroidism.

OTHER CAUSES OF HYPERCALCEMIA

Etiology. Hypercalcemia can arise from a variety of causes including excess vitamin D intake, sarcoidosis, immobilization, thiazide drug therapy, hyperthyroidism, and Addison's disease.

Pathogenesis. In sarcoidosis and vitamin D excess, hypercalcemia results from excessive intestinal absorption of calcium and excessive resorption of bone. In contrast to most other forms, this hypercalcemia is usually associated with a high TmP/GFR. Immobilization hypercalcemia is seen in young adults and children immobilized by spinal cord injuries or by casting of a large part of the body as a consequence of multiple fractures, such as those sustained in falls or auto accidents. The immobilization leads to a marked decrease in the rate of bone formation but continued resorption, so that a net loss of bone mineral occurs similar to that seen in hypercalcemia of malignancy. The hypercalcemia of thyrotoxicosis is also due largely to the increased net loss of calcium from bone. On the other hand, thiazide therapy leads to a stimulation of distal tubular reabsorption of calcium in the kidney (a PTH-like effect) and hence to renal hypercalcemia. Whether this can occur in an otherwise normal individual or is seen only in patients with impairment in the feedback control of PTH secretion continues to be a matter of controversy.

Clinical manifestations, laboratory findings, diagnosis, and management. The clinical manifestations of hypercalcemia are usually dominated by the underlying disease, but in the case of thiazide treatment the disorder is often found as a result of laboratory screening. The manifestations of hypercalcemia were described previously in the discussion of hypercalcemia of hyperparathyroidism.

In the cases under discussion (Fig. 193-6) hypercalcemia is usually found in association with a normal or high TmP/GFR, a normal IPTH, and a normal or low nephrogenous cyclic AMP. The serum $1,25(OH)_2D_3$ concentration is high in vitamin D excess, also high in sarcoidosis, and normal to low in thyrotoxicosis, immobilization hypercalcemia, and thiazide therapy.

The differential diagnosis of these states is usually not difficult, based on history, clinical manifestations, and laboratory findings.

The treatment of vitamin D excess and sarcoidosis is (1) cessation of vitamin D ingestion; (2) a low calcium diet; (3) glucocorticoids if necessary; and (4) maintenance of hydration. Thiazide hypercalcemia usually disappears with withdrawal of the drug, but patients with this condition should be evaluated for the possible presence of hyperparathyroidism. Specific treatment of thyrotoxicosis leads to a prompt fall in serum calcium. If this does not occur, the presence of associated hyperparathyroidism should be suspected. The most difficult of these conditions to treat is the hypercalcemia of immobilization. When initially discovered, it may be moderately severe and require rehydration and calcium diuresis. Maintenance therapy with CT and phosphate may be necessary. In some patients a 2-week course of high-dose glucocorticoid therapy has proved effective.

Hypocalcemia

Hypocalcemia, although less common than hypercalcemia, can also be life threatening. From the preceding discussion of the physiology of mineral metabolism, it is evident that hypocalcemia can develop (1) as a consequence of PTH deficiency or end-organ refractoriness to the actions of this hormone; (2) as a result of vitamin D deficiency; or (3) as a consequence of a marked increase in the serum phosphate concentration as seen in uremia, after chemotherapy for leukemia, or following phosphate infusion. Hypocalcemia may be seen in acute pancreatitis and in certain malignant states in which bone metastases stimulate a marked increase in osteoblastic activity. A condition of neonatal hypocalcemia is commonly seen in premature infants, those with diabetic mothers, and those with low birth weight for their gestational age.

The hallmark of hypocalcemia is tetany or increased neuromuscular irritability characterized by muscle twitching and cramps, carpopedal spasm, laryngeal stridor, and changes in the electrical and mechanical excitability of peripheral motor neurons. Hypocalcemia may also lead to increased CNS excitability and grand mal seizures. Seizures are common in young children and infants, occasionally seen in adolescents, and rare in adults. Hypocalcemia also leads to electrocardiographic changes, including an increase in the QT_c interval, particularly a prolongation of the ST segment.

Tetany can also occur because of hyperventilation and respiratory alkalosis without a change in the total serum calcium concentration (Table 193-1). Treatment of tetany of this type consists of having the subject rebreathe into a paper bag. However, true hypocalcemic tetany requires

Table 193-1. Differential diagnosis of tetany

Cause	Serum*				Urine nephrogenous cyclic AMP*
	Ca	P	pH	PTH	
Hypoparathyroidism	↓	↑	N	↓	↓
Mg deficiency	↓	N	N	↓	↓
Pseudohypoparathyroidism	↓	↑	N	↑	↓ N
Vitamin D deficiency	↓	↓	N	↑	↑
Alkalosis					
Respiratory	N	N	↑	N	↑ N
Metabolic	N	N	↑	N	N

*↓, Decreased; ↑, increased; N, normal.

prompt treatment to (1) overcome the patients' discomfort and fear; (2) prevent the occurrence of fatal laryngospasm; and (3) prevent the occurrence of seizure. Initial medical management consists of the intravenous infusion of calcium gluconate or chloride at a rate of 1 to 2 mg/kg intravenously over 15 to 20 minutes. A maintenance dose of 10 to 15 mg/kg every 6 to 12 hours will usually maintain a normal or low-normal serum calcium concentration until diagnosis and definitive treatment are begun.

Hypoparathyroidism

Hypoparathyroidism is the disorder of mineral metabolism resulting from the deficient secretion of parathyroid hormone.

ETIOLOGY. Hypoparathyroidism is rare but may arise from one of several causes. The most common is inadvertent removal of the parathyroid glands during thyroid surgery. An uncommon cause of hypoparathyroidism is hypomagnesemia resulting from a primary intestinal absorptive defect, from chronic alcoholism, or from severe Crohn's disease.

Idiopathic hypoparathyroidism is also rare. It may occur as an isolated entity, in association with agenesis of the thymus (DiGeorge's syndrome), or as a component of a multiple glandular failure. This familial syndrome is thought to be an autoimmune disease. It is manifested by chronic cutaneous, oral, and rarely intestinal moniliasis, parathyroid deficiency, adrenal deficiency, thyroid deficiency, pernicious anemia, and occasionally ovarian failure. Premature graying of hair and alopecia may also be seen. Not all of these manifestations appear in all affected individuals, and in any individual they may appear at wide intervals.

PATHOGENESIS. When PTH secretion falls, there is a loss of its effects on kidney and bone. This leads initially to a calcium diuresis and the removal of less calcium from bone. The plasma $1,25(OH)_2D_3$ level also falls so that less calcium is absorbed by the intestine. There is a rise in the TmP/GFR, leading to phosphate retention. These changes lead to a fall in the serum calcium concentration and a rise in the serum phosphate concentration. As the serum calcium concentration falls, the rate of urinary calcium excretion falls. The rate of bone remodeling also decreases.

CLINICAL MANIFESTATIONS. The presenting signs of hypoparathyroidism are those of tetany and/or a seizure disorder. In the condition with multiple glandular involvement, other signs and symptoms may appear that are related to the deficiencies of other glands. Because there is a strong association between parathyroid and adrenal insufficiency, weakness, hypotension, and the related symptoms of Addison's disease may be present. Before overt tetany appears, paresthesias and circumoral tingling may occur. Changes in affect, emotional lability, and impairment of memory may also be present. Cataracts are a consequence of chronic hypoparathyroidism, as is calcification of the basal ganglia. Enamel dysplasia and blunting of the roots of the teeth may occur if hypoparathyroidism is present at birth.

Complaints of numbness and tingling around the mouth or in the extremities or a history of severe muscle cramps should suggest latent tetany. Chvostek's and Trousseau's signs are positive. The former is a twitching of the facial muscles about the mouth and eyes in response to a tapping of the facial nerve at its point of origin anterior to the parotid gland. However, this sign may be positive in some normal subjects. Trousseau's sign is the induction of carpal spasm by inflating a blood pressure cuff above the systolic pressure and leaving it at that pressure for at least 1 minute.

LABORATORY FINDINGS AND DIAGNOSIS. The electrocardiogram may show a prolonged QT interval. The definitive diagnosis depends on the demonstration of hypocalcemia, an elevated TmP/GFR, a low nephrogenous cyclic AMP, and a low or normal IPTH. It is essential to measure the serum magnesium concentration because in rare cases the disease is due to primary magnesium deficiency. Under these circumstances PTH secretion is reduced even when hypocalcemia is present. Administration of magnesium leads to an increase in the rate of PTH secretion and restoration of a normal serum calcium. It is imperative to establish the presence or absence of hypomagnesemia before embarking on long-term treatment because hypomagnesemic patients require magnesium therapy rather than vitamin D and calcium.

COURSE. Hypoparathyroidism should always be treated. Without therapy the risk of sudden death exists. In addition, hypocalcemia is often associated with impaired affect or emotional lability.

MANAGEMENT. Treatment of chronic hypoparathyroidism is easy in theory but difficult in practice. The standard therapy is oral calcium, 1 to 2 g daily in the form of lactate or gluconate, and vitamin D_3, 40,000 to 100,000 units daily. This type of therapy renders patients asymptomatic. Therapy should be aimed at keeping the serum calcium concentration between 8.5 and 9 mg/dl. At higher values hypercalciuria develops because vitamin D does not increase distal tubular calcium reabsorption as does PTH. The problem with this treatment is that response is variable in the same patient. Most patients, particularly adolescents, have episodes of hypocalcemia and later ones of hypercalcemia while being maintained with the same dosage of vitamin D. The introduction of $1,25(OH)_2D_3$ as a therapeutic agent has improved this situation because it acts more quickly and has a shorter duration of action. Usually administration of 1 to 2 μg of this compound each day is adequate. However, in some patients this eventually may lead to hypercalcemia. In others or in the same patient at a later time, hypocalcemia may develop. Doses as high as 12 μg a day have been required during these periods. Regardless of the form of treatment, regular measurement of serum calcium concentration is a necessary part of proper management.

Pseudohypoparathyroidism

DEFINITION. Pseudohypoparathyroidism is a disorder of mineral metabolism in which there is end-organ unresponsiveness to the action of PTH. This unresponsiveness usually involves the kidney and not the bone, although clearly there are several different types. The changes in mineral metabolism are often associated with skeletal abnormalities, and in rare cases (so-called pseudo-pseudohypoparathyroidism) the latter appears without the former.

ETIOLOGY. Pseudohypoparathyroidism results either from a lack of PTH receptor in the appropriate end-organ or from a postreceptor defect that makes the target cell unresponsive to the action of the hormone. The condition is rare and is probably transmitted as a sex-linked dominant trait. The changes in stature are probably also attributable to an abnormal X chromosome.

PATHOGENESIS. In the completely unreactive type of pseudohypoparathyroidism the bones and kidneys are unresponsive to either endogenous or exogenous PTH. As a result the patients have the same changes in mineral metabolism as seen in those with hypoparathyroidism. However, assay of plasma IPTH gives a high rather than a normal or low value. In many patients it is clear that the bone and distal renal tubule are responsive to PTH when the proximal tubule is not. These patients also have hypocalcemia and hyperphosphatemia, but they may show signs of hyperparathyroid bone disease on roentgenography or biopsy.

CLINICAL MANIFESTATIONS. In addition to the signs and symptoms of hypocalcemia, patients with pseudohypoparathyroidism usually have short stature, mild obesity, shortening of one or more of the metacarpal or metatarsal bones, delayed dentition, and defective enamel formation or even complete aplasia of the teeth. Cataracts, calcification of the basal ganglia, soft tissue calcification, other skeletal abnormalities, and papilledema may all be seen.

DIAGNOSIS. The diagnosis is characterized by the biochemical findings of hypoparathyroidism in association with the constitutional changes of pseudohypoparathyroidism and with an elevated IPTH but a low nephrogenous cyclic AMP (Table 193-1). Confirmation of the diagnosis can be made by performing a PTH infusion and showing a lack of increase in both nephrogenous cyclic AMP and urinary phosphate excretion. However, a subtype of pseudohypoparathyroidism has been found to exhibit a fairly normal increase in cyclic AMP excretion in response to PTH infusion but a very small phosphaturic response.

MANAGEMENT. The treatment of pseudohypoparathyroidism is the same as that of hypoparathyroidism. However, control of hypocalcemia is usually easier, and smaller doses of the various forms of vitamin D are necessary. Evaluation of the long-term effects of the condition on bone mass has not been done.

Medullary carcinoma

DEFINITION. Medullary carcinoma is a syndrome produced by the overproduction of CT.

ETIOLOGY. Medullary carcinoma is caused by either hyperplasia or neoplasia of the parenchymal cells of the thyroid. It may occur as a sporadic tumor in older individuals, or it may be familial and be a part of the MEN II syndrome. In addition to medullary carcinoma, this syndrome includes hyperplasia or adenoma of the parathyroid glands, pheochromocytoma, multiple neuroma, and Cushing's syndrome. The condition is transmitted as an autosomal dominant trait. Any patient within a kindred may have any combination of the manifestations in any sequence. There is, however, a very high incidence of medullary carcinoma in affected families with MEN II. It is important to note that C-cell hyperplasia in the thyroid gland with high plasma calcitonin levels often precedes the appearance of carcinoma in the same gland.

PATHOGENESIS. Although high rates of CT secretion are the rule in medullary carcinoma, this rarely leads to hypocalcemia and tetany. The tumor may secrete histamine, prostaglandins, and serotonin as well as CT, which complicates interpretation of particular manifestations. Diarrhea is often a presenting complaint and may be due to the action of any combination of the secretory products.

CLINICAL MANIFESTATIONS. The presenting complaint may vary from a mass in the neck to severe and intractable diarrhea, facial flushing, cord compression from a neuroma, or other problems with gastrointestinal motility. A variety of other signs and symptoms may be present, depending on the associated endocrinopathy.

LABORATORY FINDINGS AND DIAGNOSIS. As noted previously, neither hypocalcemia nor hypophosphatemia is usually associated with medullary carcinoma. Laboratory diagnosis depends on the demonstration of elevated plasma CT by radioimmunoassay. In patients with a large tumor the fasting value may be abnormal, but in those with early disease an abnormality of secretion may be detected only by a provocative test. Two such tests are currently in use. An infusion of either calcium or pentagastrin is given, and CT levels are measured before and during the infusion. An abnormally large increase in plasma CT is indicative of the presence of either hyperplasia or carcinoma.

MANAGEMENT AND COURSE. Total thyroidectomy is indicated in any suspected case of medullary carcinoma. Once a kindred has been identified, it is essential to examine the younger members annually by means of a provocative test to identify the early appearance of the disease. If the disease is identified, early total thyroidectomy is required. If the affected gland demonstrates only C-cell hyperplasia, the chances are good that the disease will not recur. However, if carcinoma is present, recurrence is likely even after total thyroidectomy. The tumor usually spreads locally, is slow growing, and is not sensitive to chemotherapy or radiotherapy. The course may be indolent with recurrence years after a primary resection, or the tumor may spread widely and cause death within a few years.

DISORDERS OF SKELETAL AND MINERAL HOMEOSTASIS
Osteomalacia

The group of disorders characterized by vitamin D deficiency, inherited disorders of vitamin D metabolism, or association with chronic renal failure shows clinically detectable changes in mineral metabolism and skeletal abnormalities. In particular, they occur as one of the forms of osteomalacia.

DEFINITION. Osteomalacia is a defect in the mineralization of bone matrix leading to an accumulation of non-mineralized or poorly mineralized osteoid. Rickets, its counterpart in children, involves a failure of the mineralization of epiphyseal growth-plate cartilage.

ETIOLOGY. A wide number of conditions can lead to osteomalacia or rickets, as shown by the following outline:

I. Vitamin D deficiency
II. Vitamin D malabsorption
    A. Sprue syndrome
    B. Postgastrectomy—blind loop syndrome
    C. Small bowel resection or bypass
    D. Pancreatic insufficiency
    E. Exudative enteropathy
    F. Laxative abuse
    G. Bile salt deficiency
    H. Lactose intolerance
III. Impaired 25-hydroxylation (liver)
    A. Neonatal hepatitis
    B. Cirrhosis of liver
    C. Microsomal enzyme induction
        1. Phenytoin
        2. Barbiturates
        3. Glutethimide
IV. Impaired 1-hydroxylation (kidney)
    A. Genetic enzyme defect (vitamin D dependency)
    B. Chronic renal failure (CRF)
V. Phosphate depletion and hypophosphatemia
    A. Negative phosphorus balance
    B. Primary hypophosphatemia (vitamin D refractory)
    C. Metabolic acidosis
    D. Fanconi's syndrome
VI. Familial hypophosphatemic rickets
VII. Hypophosphatasia
VIII. Renal osteodystrophy

The majority of these conditions are related either to a deficiency or malabsorption of vitamin D or to an acquired alteration in its metabolism. In addition, phosphate deficiency, which is a common manifestation of vitamin D deficiency, may also lead to osteomalacia. Thus, diseases of the liver, kidney, or intestine can lead to altered vitamin D metabolism. One aspect of this metabolism not discussed previously is the enterohepatic circulation of the active forms of vitamin D. As a consequence of this circulation, in malabsorption syndromes even the vitamin D derived from the skin may be lost in the stool.

PATHOGENESIS. It is currently believed that $1,25(OH)_2D_3$ is the only active metabolite of vitamin D_3 and therefore that in cases of dietary lack, malabsorption, or phenytoin-induced catabolism of vitamin D, the major laboratory finding should be a reduction in serum $1,25(OH)_2D_3$ concentration. Some patients with these conditions do have low values, but many have normal or high values at a time when serum $25(OH)D_3$ values are low and both osseous and biochemical evidence indicates the presence of osteomalacia. Based on this information, it would seem that the several metabolites of vitamin D are all normally active. The possible roles of changes in the metabolism of different vitamin D metabolites in the pathogenesis of osteomalacia are shown in Fig. 193-7. In this scheme a deficiency of vitamin D_3 leads first to a decrease in the serum concentrations of $25(OH)D_3$, $24,25(OH)_2D_3$, and $1,25(OH)_2D_3$. These changes cause a decrease in bone resorption, bone mineralization, and intestinal calcium absorption. Both serum calcium and phosphate concentrations tend to fall. The fall in serum calcium concentration stimulates PTH secretion so that secondary hyperparathyroidism develops. This leads to a further fall in the serum phosphate concentration and so to a further delay in mineralization. It also leads to a stimulation of the renal production of $1,25(OH)_2D_3$ so that levels of this metabolite rise to the normal or even supranormal range. However, this alone is insufficient to enhance bone resorption, and it also causes a further fall in $25(OH)D_3$ levels. As the $25(OH)D_3$ is further depleted, the serum $1,25(OH)_2D_3$ concentration also falls.

Muscle weakness is also a prominent manifestation of these states. Its development is probably a consequence of phosphate deficiency and the deficiency of one or more metabolites of vitamin D. There is evidence that vitamin D and its metabolites act directly on muscle, but the metabolite involved and its precise function are unknown.

CLINICAL MANIFESTATIONS. Although the most dramatic effect of vitamin D deficiency is the development of osteomalacia, a striking presenting symptom is profound proximal muscle weakness. This leads to a characteristic waddling gait, an inability to climb stairs, and difficulty in rising from a sitting position. The weakness is often associated with bone pain and tenderness that may be diffuse. Latent tetany is commonly present, but overt tetany is uncommon in adults although frequent in children. If the cause is intestinal malabsorption, the signs and symptoms may range from marked steatorrhea with the passage of numerous, foul-smelling stools, bloating, and abdominal pain to minimal or no symptoms of gastrointestinal malfunction. In the latter cases measurement of stool fat and calcium absorption and/or intestinal mucosal biopsy may be necessary to establish the diagnosis. The signs and

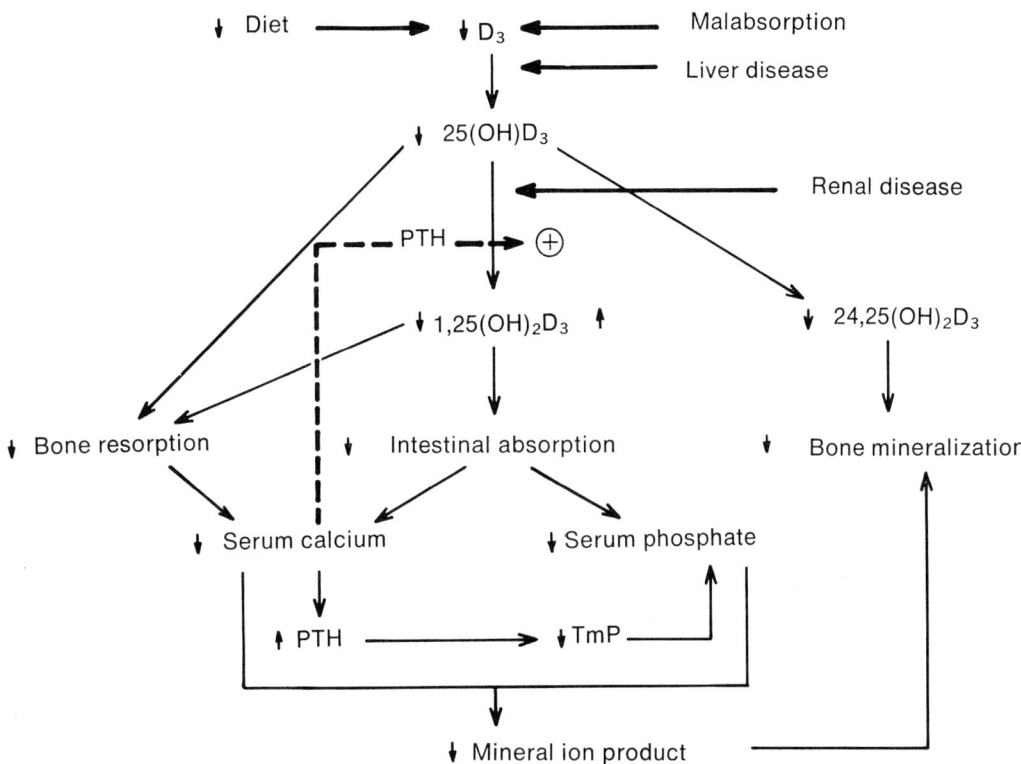

Fig. 193-7. Pathogenesis of osteomalacia of vitamin D deficiency (see text).

symptoms of renal osteodystrophy are discussed later in this chapter. Another occult cause is the ingestion of drugs such as phenytoin and phenobarbital, which induce nonspecific hepatic microsomal hydroxylases that increase the rate of vitamin D_3 catabolism. A careful history and the measurement of drug levels in plasma may be needed. Simple dietary lack of vitamin D as an explanation is rare in the United States but does occur in vegetarians, whose vitamin D intake may be quite low.

LABORATORY FINDINGS. Typically, adults with osteomalacia have a slightly reduced serum calcium concentration (7.5 to 8.5 mg/dl), a low serum phosphate concentration (1.5 to 2.5 mg/dl), an elevated alkaline phosphatase level (>120 IU), and reduced concentrations of $25(OH)D_3$ in the serum. The serum $1,25(OH)_2D_3$ level may be low, normal, or increased. Secondary hyperparathyroidism with elevated nephrogenous cyclic AMP, low TmP/GFR, and high IPTH is the rule. Although these are the usual findings, some patients early in their disease may have normal serum calcium and low phosphate levels, and others late in the course of the disease may have a normal or high serum phosphate concentration in spite of secondary hyperparathyroidism. Urinary calcium excretion is low, and if tested, intestinal calcium absorption is found to be reduced. Creatinine clearance is normal.

Roentgenographic examination usually reveals skeletal demineralization and in severe cases pseudofractures or Looser's zones, which are linear areas of undermineralization perpendicular to the long axis of the bones. They usually are symmetric and occur at the axillary margin of the scapula, interior arches of the femoral neck, pubic and ischial rami, ribs, and metatarsals.

DIAGNOSIS. In the typical case, diagnosis is easy once suspected. When it has been confirmed by clinical, laboratory, and roentgenographic examination, the problem becomes defining the cause of the altered metabolism of vitamin D. Such an evaluation includes a careful dietary history, a history of possible drug use, and a family history. Evaluation of renal, hepatic, and/or gastrointestinal function may be necessary. Often the history alone suggests the diagnostic approach to pursue. Rarely, biochemical vitamin D deficiency with muscle weakness occurs without apparent evidence of renal, hepatic, or intestinal disease. If dietary lack is clearly not involved, usually an occult malabsorption syndrome will be found.

COURSE. If left untreated, the deficiency progresses to severe and incapacitating weakness, skeletal pain, and debility.

MANAGEMENT. In most instances osteomalacia can be treated by increased oral doses of vitamin D_3. If malabsorption is present and can be corrected by a gluten-free diet or the administration of bile salts or pancreatic enzymes, the absorption of the vitamin will improve and doses in the range of 5000 to 10,000 units a day will be sufficient. Similar doses are usually effective in patients with the postgastrectomy blind loop syndrome. In these cases bacterial infection within the loop may be responsible for catabolism of vitamin D_3, and antibiotic therapy may be required in addition to vitamin D_3 administration. In some patients with a marked decrease in the amount of small bowel, for example, following resection for Chrohn's disease, larger doses of vitamin D may be required. In these cases the administration of the more polar $25(OH)D_3$ in doses of 50 to 75 μg a day may be more effective. In cases of phenytoin and/or phenobarbital ingestion in which continued administration is deemed necessary to control a seizure disorder, administration of 5000 to 10,000 units of vitamin D_3 a day is usually sufficient to prevent the development of vitamin D deficiency.

Inherited disorders of vitamin D metabolism

There are two clearly defined forms of inherited rickets and osteomalacia. The rarer is vitamin D–dependent rickets. It is inherited as an autosomal recessive trait and usually appears early in life with hypocalcemia, failure to thrive. muscle weakness, tetany, and seizures. Like vitamin D deficiency, it is characterized by hypocalcemia, variable serum phosphate concentrations, secondary hyperparathyroidism, and elevated alkaline phosphatase levels. However, in distinction to vitamin D deficiency, the serum $25(OH)D_3$ concentration is normal but the $1,25(OH)_2D_3$ level is low. Furthermore, vitamin D–dependent rickets fails to respond to small doses of vitamin D_3 but does respond to doses in the range of 5000 to 10,000 units a day or to small doses of $1,25(OH)_2D_3$ (1 to 2 μg a day). It is thought to be due to either deficiency of or an alteration in the renal enzyme (renal 1-α-hydroxylase) responsible for catalyzing the conversion of $25(OH)D_3$ to $1,25(OH)_2D_3$. If adequately treated, the rickets disappears and growth returns to normal.

The second condition, familial hypophosphatemic rickets or vitamin D–resistant rickets, is inherited as an X-linked dominant trait. It is characterized by a subnormal skeletal growth rate, marked hypophosphatemia, reduced TmP/GFR, and a variable reduction in the serum $1,25(OH)_2D_3$ concentration, with normal $25(OH)D_3$, normocalcemia, and no tetany or secondary hyperparathyroidism. On roentgenographic examination rickets may be seen, particularly in the epiphyses of the lower extremities, with a marked flaring of the distal ends of the femora. Bowing of the femora and tibiae is common, with varying degrees of torsion. The disease appears to be due to a disorder of renal tubular function resulting in a marked renal phosphate leak and, in spite of hypophosphatemia, an underproduction of $1,25(OH)_2D_3$ leading to intestinal malabsorption of calcium and phosphate. This condition is unresponsive to vitamin D_3 even in large doses but can be successfully treated with a combination of oral phosphate (0.25 to 0.75 g four times a day) and $1,25(OH)_2D_3$ (0.25 to 4 μg a day depending on the age and size of the patient and the severity of the disease). In many patients this program leads to a nearly complete healing of the rickets and the restoration of a nearly normal growth rate. However, to be effective, it must be continued throughout the entire growth period. The appropriate dose of $1,25(OH)_2D_3$ must be judged by giving amounts sufficient to prevent phosphate-induced secondary hyperparathyroidism but insufficient to produce hypercalciuria and its attendant risk of renal damage.

Although the manifestations of the disease lessen somewhat after cessation of skeletal growth and the serum alkaline phosphatase concentration returns to normal, most adults with this condition have persistent muscle and skeletal pains, fatigability, and moderate to marked osteomalacia on bone biopsy. These patients benefit significantly from combined phosphate and $1,25(OH)_2D_3$ therapy, but longterm studies of this therapy have not been reported.

Hypophosphatasia

Hypophosphatasia is a familial disease in which the skeletal deformities of rickets and osteomalacia develop in the presence of normal metabolism of vitamin D, parathyroid hormone, and bone mineral. It is inherited as an autosomal recessive trait. The disease may appear in infancy, childhood, or adulthood. The cardinal features of the disease are rickets and/or osteomalacia of variable severity with a low serum and bone alkaline phosphatase and the excretion of excessive amounts of phosphoethanolamine in the urine. On bone biopsy, rickets and osteomalacia are seen. The primary defect is thought to be a lack of the normal amount of alkaline phosphatase in bone matrix vesicles, leading to delay or inhibition of the nucleation of bone mineral crystals. There is no definitive treatment, but continuous high phosphate intake has been reported to lead to an improvement in some cases.

Renal osteodystrophy

DEFINITION. Renal osteodystrophy is the bone disease that develops in the setting of chronic renal failure. It includes a spectrum of osseous changes, ranging from almost pure osteomalacia on the one hand to nearly pure osteitis fibrosa cystica (that is, hyperparathyroid bone disease) on the other. It is associated with a variety of changes in mineral and vitamin D metabolism and parathyroid function.

PATHOGENESIS. Multiple factors are involved in the development of renal osteodystrophy. As renal function declines, a point is reached when phosphate clearance decreases. This leads to a rise in serum phosphate concentration, a decline in serum ionized calcium, and hence secondary hyperparathyroidism. The increase in IPTH leads to an increase in renal phosphate clearance so that for a time the serum phosphate may not rise significantly but secondary hyperparathyroidism with increased bone turnover may be evident. A further decline in renal function leads to progressive phosphate retention, hyperphosphatemia, and progressively more marked secondary hyperparathyroidism so that the total serum calcium concentration may be normal or high but ionized calcium is low. The excessive PTH produces progressively more marked osteitis fibrosa cystica. In addition, with renal failure the renal synthesis of $1,25(OH)_2D_3$ may decline, leading to a fall in serum $1,25(OH)_2D_3$ concentration and intestinal calcium absorption. In such cases hypocalcemia and secondary hyperparathyroidism develop. A third abnormality that commonly develops is metabolic acidosis, which may inhibit the calcification process in bone. However, although there are a number of factors that may play a pathogenic role in the development of osteodystrophy, there is no characteristic set of biochemical changes associated with a particular type of bone disease. Therefore, exactly why some patients manifest predominantly osteitis fibrosa cystica, others osteomalacia, and many a mixture of both is not clear. An additional poorly understood feature in many patients is a resistance to the actions of vitamin D.

CLINICAL MANIFESTATIONS. Eventually some type of bone disease appears in the majority of patients with chronic renal failure, whether treated conservatively or by chronic hemodialysis. The clinical presentation may include profound proximal muscle weakness similar to that seen in vitamin D deficiency, lethargy, fatigability, weight loss, anemia, pruritus, bone pain and tenderness, fractures, and soft tissue calcification. The presentation varies from patient to patient.

LABORATORY FINDINGS. The serum phosphate concentration is usually high, particularly in untreated cases, and is associated with a marked decrease in creatinine clearance. The serum calcium concentration may be low, normal, or high, but the ionized portion is usually low. However, if prolonged secondary hyperparathyroidism has been present, one or more of the hyperplastic glands may undergo an adenomatous transformation leading to the appearance of *tertiary* hyperparathyroidism with hypercalcemia. The serum $1,25(OH)_2D_3$ concentration is low to undetectable, and the $25(OH)D_3$ may also be moderately reduced. The alkaline phosphatase activity is usually increased. Elevated IPTH is the rule. However, there is no simple correlation between the elevation of IPTH and the degree of hyperparathyroidism. This is because PTH undergoes peripheral metabolism (Fig. 193-5). As a result, C-terminal, biologically inactive, but immunologically measurable peptides are generated. The kidney is a major site for the disposal of these peptides. In the case of progressive renal failure these inactive PTH fragments accumulate. Also, because with severe renal failure the measurement of nephrogenous cyclic AMP no longer is a valid indicator of parathyroid function, there is no way to accurately measure the amount of biologically active parathyroid hormone.

MANAGEMENT. Before any form of vitamin D therapy is given, it is essential to correct any underlying acidosis and to reduce the serum phosphate concentration to the normal range if possible. Measures to achieve this include a reduction in protein intake, hemodialysis, and the administration of nonabsorable antacids containing aluminum hydroxide, such as Basaljel. These bind dietary phosphate and hence decrease the intestinal absorption of phosphate. Until recently the only form of vitamin D available for treatment was vitamin D_3 itself. Its use gave variable results that were often complicated by hypercalcemia and soft tissue calcification. More recently, $1,25(OH)_2D_3$ and $25(OH)D_3$ have been employed. The results with each have been variable. Paradoxically, $1,25(OH)_2D_3$ is most effective in patients with predominantly osteitis fibrosa cystica, that is, severe secondary hyperparathyroidism. In these patients $1,25(OH)_2D_3$ administration leads to an increase in intestinal calcium absorption, a rise in serum calcium concentration, and a suppression of parathyroid function, resulting in an amelioration of the bone disease. Similar results have been reported following the administration of $25(OH)D_3$. When osteomalacia is a predominant feature of disease, $1,25(OH)_2D_3$ is less effective. It seems likely that some of these patients respond better to $25(OH)D_3$, but this has not been established. In some patients the bone disease appears to be resistant to treatment with any form of vitamin D. In others, regardless of the form of vitamin D therapy, severe hypercalcemia develops, and it may be necessary to carry out subtotal parathyroidectomy in such patients before any of these agents can be given.

The long-term management of this frequent and often debilitating complication of long-term hemodialysis is still far from ideal.

PRIMARY DISORDERS OF SKELETAL HOMEOSTASIS

The final group of conditions to be considered are those in which the predominant change is in the skeleton and the changes in mineral metabolism, parathyroid function, and vitamin D metabolism are a consequence of these primary osseous events. The most common of these is osteoporosis. Two uncommon inherited conditions, osteogenesis imperfecta and osteopetrosis, will be discussed only briefly. Paget's disease is discussed in Chapter 29.

Osteoporosis

DEFINITION. Osteoporosis is a condition characterized by a reduction in the total mass of calcified bone to a point at which a markedly increased risk of fracture develops.

ETIOLOGY. The syndrome develops from a number of causes, as outlined below. However, by far the most common is that seen in postmenopausal women.

I. Probable endocrine causes
   A. Postmenopausal osteoporosis
   B. Cushing's syndrome

C. Thyrotoxicosis
  D. Hypogonadism
  E. Hyperparathyroidism
  F. Diabetes
II. Dietary calcium deficiency
III. Inherited disorders of collagen metabolism
  A. Osteogenesis imperfecta
  B. Homocystinuria
  C. Ehlers-Danlos syndrome
  D. Marfan's syndrome
IV. Unknown
  A. Juvenile
  B. Senile
  C. Systemic mastocytosis
  D. Alcoholism
  E. Chronic liver disease
  F. Chronic obstructive pulmonary disease

PATHOGENESIS. In a few of the many causes just listed the pathogenesis of the disease is understood, but in many the factors responsible are unknown. In Cushing's syndrome or during prolonged glucocorticoid administration, a marked inhibition of bone formation associated with an inhibition of intestinal calcium absorption and mild secondary hyperparathyroidism may lead to a rapid loss of bone mass because of an increase in resorption and a decrease in formation. On the other hand, the factors involved in the development of juvenile osteoporosis or that seen in patients with alcoholism are unknown.

In the case of postmenopausal osteoporosis there has long been a debate as to whether the bone loss seen in women at or shortly after menopause is simply a consequence of the normal aging process or is a consequence of estrogen deficiency. Recent evidence supports the concept that estrogen deficiency plays a key role in the pathogenesis of osteoporosis (Fig. 193-8). The lack of estrogen appears to cause an increased sensitivity of bone osteoclasts to the action of PTH, and this leads to a decrease in the coupling of bone formation with resorption. A net shift of calcium from bone results in a suppression of parathyroid function, a decrease in plasma $1,25(OH)_2D_3$, an increase in TmP/GFR, and an increase in urinary calcium excretion. These changes occur in younger women following oophorectomy and in older women at the time of menopause. They are not seen in men, and they are prevented or reversed by the administration of estrogens.

CLINICAL MANIFESTATIONS. The usual finding in patients with osteoporosis is the sudden onset of back pain in the

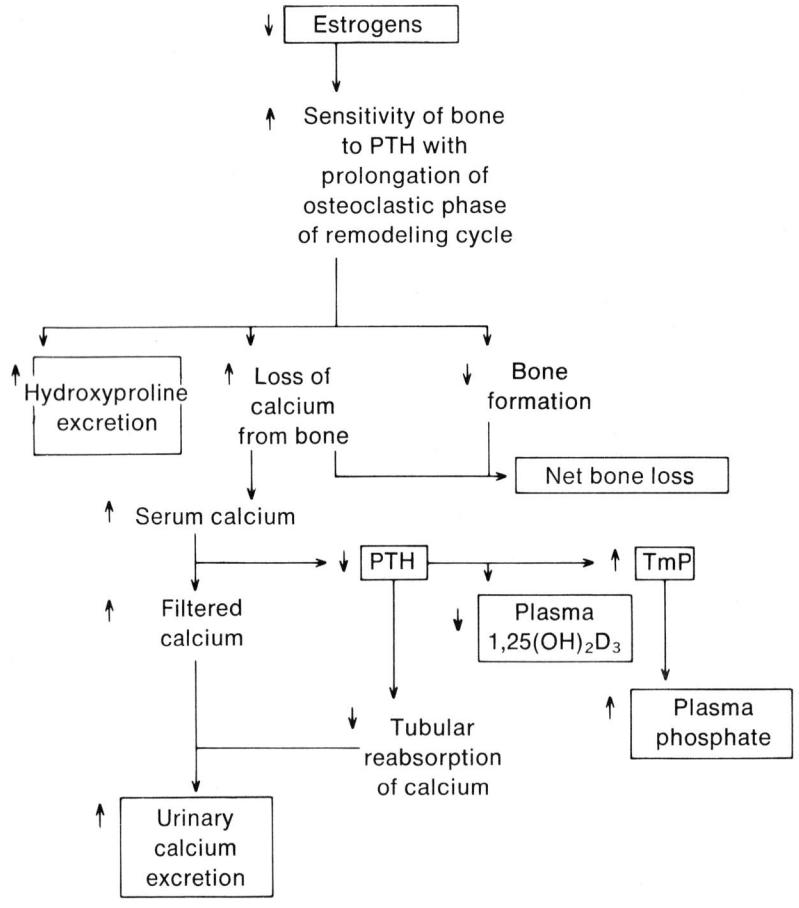

Fig. 193-8. Pathogenesis of postmenopausal osteoporosis (see text).

thoracic or lumbar spine brought on by physical activity. Roentgenography may reveal crush, wedge-shaped fractures of one or more vertebral bodies. The amount of pain varies enormously; some women have reduced stature and a history of chronic back pain, and others have a dramatic onset of severe pain. The pain following any fracture ameliorates with time but is usually followed by persistent dull, aching pain. Once osteoporosis has begun, the subject usually suffers multiple fractures over a period of several years. In some cases the disease is manifested by a Colles' fracture of the wrist or a femoral neck fracture after minimal trauma.

DIAGNOSIS. The diagnosis is usually relatively easy. It is necessary to rule out known endocrine causes. In an occasional older woman, hyperparathyroidism may be manifested by osteoporosis. The possibility of thyrotoxicosis, Cushing's syndrome, and diabetes should be considered. Vertebral fractures may occur in patients with myeloma, leukemia, or metastatic carcinoma. The laboratory findings depend on the stage of the disease but usually include increased urinary excretion of calcium and hydroxyproline.

COURSE. The course of osteoporosis is highly variable. One patient may have several fractures within a year, whereas others may have fractures separated by several years. However, the disease is usually progressive, and eventual loss of stature, persistent back pain, and kyphosis are common.

MANAGEMENT. At present there is no generally accepted specific therapy for osteoporosis once it has developed. General measures such as an adequate dietary intake of calcium, phosphate, and vitamin D, specific back exercises, and physical activity should be encouraged. Immobilization of the spine in a cast, brace, or corset is usually not helpful and may, in fact, accelerate the rate of bone loss. Various programs of calcium and vitamin D with or without fluorides, or a combination of estrogens and androgens, have been suggested but are not able to reverse the bone loss. Treatment with $1,25(OH)_2D_3$ has also been advocated, but its efficacy remains to be demonstrated. CT has been employed, but the results are highly variable. The distinction must be made between treatment given after the condition is clinically evident and prophylaxis given at the onset of menopause.

PREVENTION. The question of the prevention of osteoporosis has been the subject of considerable controversy. However, with the advent of more precise ways of estimating bone mass in patients by noninvasive means, considerable evidence has been gathered showing that administration of estrogens following surgically induced or natural menopause will prevent the loss of bone mineral and bone mass, as well as the other changes commonly seen. This evidence strongly suggests that estrogen prophylaxis can prevent or greatly reduce the occurrence of osteoporosis. However, there are several problems with the use of estrogens. First, if therapy is continued for several years and then stopped, the rate of bone loss promptly increases. The implication of this finding is that prophylaxis should be lifelong to be effective. Second, although all women show a phase of rapid bone loss in the immediate postmenopausal period, not all lose sufficient bone to lead to osteoporosis and fractures. It is not known what factors determine which women in a particular population will have clinically evident disease, nor is there any method currently available to identify the patients most likely to have the disease. Third, estrogen therapy is attended with several potentially serious side effects, in particular, a greater risk of thromboembolic disease and endometrial carcinoma. However, no careful evaluation of the relative risk or benefit of therapy versus no therapy has ever been made, even though the incidence of endometrial carcinoma and thromboembolic events is rare. Clinically significant osteoporosis is common, occurring in more than 25% of white women over the age of 60.

Osteogenesis imperfecta

Osteogenesis imperfecta is a disorder of collagen metabolism of unknown mechanism and variable severity. It is usually inherited as an autosomal dominant trait, and it is characterized by a propensity to fractures following minimal trauma, blue sclerae, and eventual deafness. The defect appears to be the inability of osteoblasts to make normal amounts of collagen. It may be very mild and the subject may have only a few fractures, or it may be severe with multiple, recurrent fractures and skeletal deformities. There is no specific therapy.

Osteopetrosis

Osteopetrosis is an extremely rare abnormality in which the normal process of bone remodeling is deficient because of abnormal osteoclasts that appear incapable of resorbing bone. Thus there is increasing bone density with time, leading to a reduction in the size of the marrow cavity, anemia, compression of cranial nerves, synostosis, and usually death in early childhood. There is no known treatment.

BIBLIOGRAPHY

Bijvoet, O.L.M.: Kidney function in calcium and phosphate metabolism. In Avioli, L.V., and Krane, S.M., editors: Metabolic bone disease, vol. 1, New York, 1977, Academic Press, Inc.

Broadus, A.E.: Nephrogenous cAMP as a parathyroid function test, Nephron **23**:136, 1979.

Broadus, A.E., and others: The importance of circulating 1,25-dihydroxyvitamin D in the pathogenesis of hypercalcemia and renal stone formation in primary hyperparathyroidism, N. Engl. J. Med. **302**:421, 1980.

Habener, J.F., and Potts, J.T., Jr.: Biosynthesis of parathyroid hormone, N. Engl. J. Med. **299**:580, 635, 1978.

Haussler, M.R., and McCain, T.A.: Basic and clinical concepts related to vitamin D metabolism and action, N. Engl. J. Med. **297**:974, 1977.

Lee, D:B.N., Zawada, E.T., and Kleeman, C.R.: The pathophysiology

and clinical aspects of hypercalcemic disorders, West J. Med. **129**:278, 1978.
Lloyd, H.M.: Primary hyperparathyroidism: an analysis of the role of the parathyroid tumor, Medicine **47**:53, 1968.
Mallette, L.E., and others: Primary hyperparathyroidism: clinical and biochemical features, Medicine **53**:127, 1974.
Marx, S.J., and others: Divalent cation metabolism: familial hypocalciuric hypercalcemia versus typical primary hyperparathyroidism, Am. J. Med. **65**:235, 1978.
Nordin, B.E.C.: Metabolic bone and stone disease, Baltimore, 1973, The Williams & Wilkins Co.
Pak, C.Y.C.: Calcium urolithiasis, New York, 1978, Plenum Publishing Corp.
Parfitt, A.M.: Equilibrium and disequilibrium hypercalcemia: new light on an old concept, Metab. Bone Dis. Rel. Res. **1**:279, 1979.
Rasmussen, H., and Bordier, P.: The physiological and cellular basis of metabolic bone disease, Baltimore, 1974, The Williams & Wilkins Co.
Rasmussen, H., and Bordier, P.: Vitamin D and bone, Metab. Bone Dis. Rel. Res. **1**:7, 1978.
Steward, A., and others: Biochemical evaluation of patients with malignancy associated hypercalcemia: evidence for humoral and non-humoral groups, N. Engl. J. Med. **303**:1377, 1980.

DENTAL CORRELATIONS

Barbara J. Steinberg and **Louis F. Rose**

DISORDERS OF PITUITARY

ORAL MANIFESTATIONS

Adult hyperpituitarism—acromegaly. The most striking feature in patients with acromegaly is the gradual proliferation of osseous and soft tissue of the acral parts of the body, especially the hands, feet, and face. The ears, nose, and lips are enlarged, which contributes to the typical coarse, acromegalic facial expression. Localized areas of hyperpigmentation are often seen along the nasolabial folds.

The tongue may enlarge disproportionately from the mouth, with marked papillary hypertrophy, and either protrude somewhat or develop indentations around the lateral margins from pressing against the teeth. The lingual enlargement appears to result in part from increased diameter of the muscle fibers, especially those in the anterior half, and from thickening of the epithelium and subepithelial connective tissue.

In acromegaly there is marked thickening of the cranium including the facial bones and paranasal sinuses, with pronounced bony ledging and massive frontal bossing.

The mandibular growth centers are stimulated in this disorder, especially the condyle. Exaggerated condylar growth causes a mesial shift in the occlusion and increased prominence of the chin. The width of the mandible is also increased. Recent studies indicate that a large proportion of acromegalic patients have an Angle Class III malocclusion with complete or partial crossbite. Overdevelopment of the mandible and pressure from the enlarged tongue on the alveolar processes can lead to a relative mandibular prognathism with flaring and spacing of the teeth. The size of the teeth is unchanged, but increased cementum deposition is a common finding.

Advanced periodontal disease is usually a feature of acromegaly, especially when the malocclusion is severe. Metabolic disturbance of the jaws and oral soft tissues may also contribute to periodontal breakdown.

An increase in the size of the larynx produces deepening of the voice.

Juvenile hyperpituitarism—gigantism. The clinical features of acromegaly rarely have been reported in children suffering from gigantism. It is commonly assumed that these changes do not occur while longitudinal growth is taking place. During puberty, the changes associated with hyperpituitarism are confined chiefly to the mandible and, to a lesser extent, the maxilla. These changes consist of thickening of the cortical bone of the mandible and enlargement of the paranasal sinuses. On occasion, periosteal ossifications are seen at the sites of muscle and tendon attachments.

The overdevelopment of the mandible and face begin to produce the pathognomonic facies of adult hyperpituitarism. Radiographically the bones are seen to be poorly calcified and have large trabeculae. Individuals with gigantism manifest accelerated dental development, including early eruption of the teeth. Mineralization of the teeth, however, is not affected by the excess in growth hormone.

DENTAL MANAGEMENT. Diabetes and hypertension are the significant complications most often associated with hyperpituitarism. The dentist must be familiar with the treatment and management of patients with these disorders. (Refer to appropriate sections in this text.)

Hypopituitarism

ORAL MANIFESTATIONS. There is a marked effect on both facial and dental development in children with hypopituitarism. Facial growth is disturbed, causing retardation of mandibular development, and this disproportionate growth leads to malocclusion with excessive crowding of the teeth. While the teeth are normal in size, the crowns are not always completely erupted and roots tend to be shortened. There is delayed and incomplete eruption of the teeth along with an even greater delay in skeletal development. The delay in dental development begins with overretained deciduous teeth with unresorbed roots. In addition, eruption of permanent teeth is delayed, with incomplete root formation and closure of the apical foramen.

When pituitary destruction occurs, regardless of the cause, there appears to be hypofunction of the salivary glands with resultant xerostomia. Decreased salivary flow increases the incidence of caries and periodontal disease.

DENTAL MANAGEMENT. Since these individuals experience a higher incidence of caries and gingival inflammation, frequent dental check-ups are important. Patients with destruction of the pituitary gland may be on maintenace replacement therapy, including steroids. It is therefore important for the dentist to understand the management of the patient on exogenous steroids (see section on adrenal cortex in this chapter).

DISORDERS OF THYROID GLAND
Hyperthyroidism

ORAL MANIFESTATIONS. The hyperthyroid patient presents with facial skin that is warm, moist, and often flushed. Excessive melanin pigmentation may occur on the skin and the patient's hair may be fine and friable.

Eye signs are a prominent feature of the condition and easily recognized by the dentist. These include infrequent blinking, dilated pupils, protrusion of the eyeballs (exophthalmos), and lid-lag caused by spasm of the muscles of the upper eyelid, which causes the sclera to be exposed above the corners when the patient is looking downward. In addition, weakness of the extrinsic muscles of the eyes occurs because of lymphocytic infiltration, which may cause squinting and double vision (diplopia).

Clinical examination of the thyroid may reveal a gland of normal dimension or enlargement as great as fourfold. Usually the gland is symmetrically involved and feels rather firm and lobulated. A systolic bruit may be heard over the thyroid as a result of engorgement of the gland's vascular supply.

Children with hyperthyroidism experience premature loss of deciduous teeth and early eruption of the permanent teeth, though the teeth and jaws are usually well formed and present no unusual irregularities. Infants born of hyperthyroid mothers have been reported to have several teeth erupted at birth.

There is a tendency toward osteoporosis of the alveolar bone in the hyperthryroid patient. These patients also appear to develop caries and periodontal disease at a rapid rate, possibly from consuming excessive amounts of sugars to satisfy increased caloric demands.

A few patients with hyperthyroidism have been found to have thyroid tissue in the tongue below the area of the embryonic thyroglossal duct. These patients should be evaluated by a physician for the presence of a normal thyroid gland before the mass is surgically removed.

DENTAL MANAGEMENT. In hyperthyroid individuals, emotional stress, infection, trauma, and surgery can precipitate a thyroid crisis or "storm," which may be fatal. Therefore palpation and inspection of the thyroid gland should be included in the routine head and neck examination performed by the dentist. If thyroid enlargement is noted, even in a patient who appears to be euthyroid, or if the dentists suspects hyperthyroidism, either from the medical history or from readily discernible clinical signs, the patient should be referred for medical consultation and management before dental treatment is begun. Once medical treatment has been instituted and the patient is euthyroid, there is no contraindication to dental treatment.

In the event of dental emergency in a hyperthyroid patient, such as an acute oral infection, the dentist must consult with the physician concerning management of the emergency. Often conservative treatment, consisting of antibiotics and analgesics, is advisable. If dental therapy must be rendered immediately, the controlled environment of a hospital operating room is optimum. Before any surgery the physician should bring the patient to a euthyroid state. Local anesthetics without epinephrine or other pressor amines should be used, if needed, since the myocardium in these patients is highly sensitive to epinephrine and its use can precipitate severe arrhythmias, tachycardia, and/or chest pain.

Many hyperthyroid patients take propylthiouracil to inhibit the excessive synthesis of thyroid hormone. Because this drug may cause agranulocytosis, hypoprothrombinemia, and bleeding, a complete blood count with differential and prothrombin time must be obtained before surgery.

The dentist should recognize the symptoms of thyroid storm and be able to manage this potentially fatal crisis. It has an abrupt onset with symptoms of extreme restlessness, nausea, vomiting, and abdominal pain. Shortly thereafter, fever, profuse sweating, tachycardia, pulmonary edema, and congestive heart failure develop. If the patient develops severe hypertension and becomes comatose, death may occur. Immediate treatment consists of large doses (600 to 1000 mg) of propylthiouracil, along with medication to diminish the metabolic effects of thyroid hormones. One of these, propranolol hydrochloride, is a β-adrenergic blocking agent and the drug of choice to reverse the cardiac and psychomotor effects of thyrotoxicosis when given intravenously at a rate of 1 mg/min until the crisis is controlled (usually 2 to 10 minutes), with the total dose not to exceed 10 mg. Proper treatment should also include general supportive measures such as replacement of fluids, glucose, electrolytes, and vitamin B complex and application of wet packs, cool air, and ice packs to control temperature.

Hypothyroidism

ORAL MANIFESTATIONS
Cretinism. The skin of the face is coarse, thick, dry, and wrinkled. The lips are enlarged, puffy, and pale, and the mouth frequently is held in a partially opened position, probably due in part to the increased size of the tongue.

The facial skeleton is irregularly affected, with the mandible disproportionately underdeveloped. The maxilla appears widened, due to a shortening of the base of the skull. The bridge of the nose is retracted and fontanelle closure is delayed, resulting in an unusually large head.

The gingiva is spongy, and both eruption and exfoliation of deciduous teeth are delayed. There is a high frequency of enamel hypoplasia in deciduous teeth; the permanent dentition is also hyperplastic, but to a lesser degree. Thus malocclusion is a relatively constant finding in cretinism because of the faulty patterns of growth and development. A widening of the dental arch with flaring and spacing of the teeth may be observed. An open bite, receding chin, and enlarged protruding tongue lead to mouth breathing, which eventually results in drying and breakdown of gingival tissues.

Juvenile myxedema. Juvenile myxedema has the same clinical picture as cretinism, but the symptoms are less severe. The oral changes consist of retardation of tooth eruption and defective formation of the jaws. There is delayed shedding of the primary teeth, which leads to retardation of secondary dentition development; that is, the completion of the roots of the permanent teeth slows and delays the eruption rate. The teeth are poorly formed and enamel hypoplasia is common. In the deciduous dentition the hypoplasis ia limited to those portions of teeth that mineralize in fetal life and infancy. In the permanent dentition, minor enamel hypoplasia dating from infancy and early childhood is found on incisors and first molars, but very rarely in premolars and second molars. In some seriously affected patients, dentin apposition is markedly delayed and the pulp chambers are larger than normal. The dental age of hypothyroid children is many years younger than their chronologic or bone age.

Adult myxedema. In adult hypothyroidism, the skin and lips are pale and their texture is dry and scaly. Even more striking, however, is the puffy, myxedematous appearance of the entire face, with the nose, ears, and lips especially enlarged. The hair is dry and brittle and the eyebrows thin or entirely absent.

Generalized swelling may affect the tongue, causing difficulty in speech and scalloping around the margins from constant pressure against the teeth. This swelling of the tongue, coupled with swelling of the vocal cords, produces a characteristic husky, low-pitched voice. Since dental development is complete before the onset of the condition, there is no effect on the teeth and supporting tissues. However, gingivitis and rampant caries frequently occur, due in part to mouth breathing that accompanies the tongue enlargement. Hypothyroidism has been associated with an impairment in the normal immune response, and patients may develop chronic mucocutaneous candidiasis.

DENTAL MANAGEMENT. The dentist may be the first person to suspect hypothyroidism by recognizing the typical orofacial changes. With early detection and medical management, permanent mental retardation can be avoided in very young individuals, as may the oral complications of delayed eruption of teeth, malocclusion, enlargement of the tongue, and skeletal retardation.

In general, there is probably no danger in providing dental care for the patient with mild symptoms of untreated hypothyroidism. However, there is still the slight risk that the patient will develop myxedema coma. This risk markedly increases in the elderly patient with very severe hypothyroidism, especially during the winter months.

A myxedema coma can be precipitated by infections, surgery and the use of CNS depressants. It is extremely important that the dentist be aware that the hypothyroid patient is hypersensitive to drugs. This is a result of the lowered metabolic rate and CNS depression. Extreme care should be exercised when administering analgesics, anesthetics, barbiturates, hypnotics, and tranquilizers. A standard adult dose of morphine or meperidine (Demerol), for example, is contraindicated in the hypothyroid patient since the cardiovascular system and kidneys may not be able to eliminate excess medication and thus cause prolonged CNS depression. It is prudent to seek medical evaluation and treatment before dental treatment. Emergency dental care for oral infections that can precipitate a crisis should be limited to conservative measures.

The dentist should be able to recognize and manage the initial stages of myxedema coma. The condition is characterized by hypothermia, bradycardia, severe hypotension, and epileptic seizures. Approximately 300 μg thyroxine should be administered intravenously and 100 to 200 μg given daily thereafter, with monitoring of the plasma thyroid hormone blood levels. Hypothermia is best treated by covering the patient with warm blankets and allowing endogenous body heat to raise the temperature gradually. Artificial respiration is necessary if patient shows signs of respiratory distress. If there is any suggestion of adrenal steroid insufficiency, 100 to 200 mg hydrocortisone should be given intravenously.

DISORDERS OF ADRENAL GLAND
Hyperadrenocorticism—Cushing's syndrome

ORAL MANIFESTATIONS. Patients with Cushing's syndrome develop a facial appearance that is a plethoric and round (moon face) with a ruddy color that simulates glowing health; Hirsutism and acne are also present. Overall-growth and development, including skeletal and dental age, are retarded in long-standing Cushing's syndrome. Osteoporosis, although rare, may occur in the jaws and gingival enlargement may evident.

A recent study revealed that there are alterations in oral sensation in some patients with Cushing's syndrome. Thresholds for light touch detection and two-point discrimination on the hands and in the mouth as well as oral and manual stereognosis were measured in patients with untreated Cushing's syndrome and in normal volunteers. Results indicated that patients with Cushing's syndrome displayed decreased two-point discrimination on the tongue and palate and decreased oral stereognosis.

DENTAL MANAGEMENT. The dentist should be aware that serious conditions may accompany Cushing's syndrome, including hypertension, heart failure, diabetes mellitus, osteoporosis, impaired healing, and emotional depression or psychosis. Evaluation and dental management of patients with these disorders are included in the appropriate sections of this text.

Hypoadrenocorticism—Addison's disease (primary adrenal insufficiency)

ORAL MANIFESTATIONS. An early manifestation of Addison's disease is an unusual pigmentation of the skin, especially at pressure points and on the oral mucous membranes. This results from stimulation of pituitary melanotrophic activity.

The oral pigmentations appear as irregular spots that may vary in color and intensity, ranging from pale brown to gray or even black. They occur most frequently on the cheek but may be found on the gingiva, palate, tongue, and lips.

Administration of corticosteroids is the usual treatment for Addison's disease and often leads to suppression of the individual's immune response. Consequently, patients receiving steroid therapy are more prone to developing gingival and periodontal disorders, chronic mucocutaneous candidiasis, and oral infections that may be difficult to treat with conventional therapy.

DENTAL MANAGEMENT. Dental management is the same as for the patient with secondary adrenal insufficiency. The latter condition is caused by the chronic administration of corticosteroids for a variety of reasons which can result in the suppression of endogenous steroid secretion.

Patients who are or have been taking steroids within the past year present two potential problems to the dentist: an increased susceptibility to infection and the possiblity of adrenal crisis.

Dental patients taking corticosteroids are at increased risk of developing severe dental infection, since corticosteroids alter the host's normal inflammatory response. The chance of infection can be minimized by employing atraumatic and aseptic technique and by adequate antimicrobial therapy. Some authors recommend that patients take bactericidal broad-spectrum antibiotics on the day of oral surgery and for 5 days thereafter.

Stress induced by infection, trauma, surgery, anesthesia, and the like may lead to adrenal crisis in any patient with primary or secondary adrenal insufficiency. In these patients there is adrenal atrophy with inhibition of the production of cortisol by suppression of the pituitary-adrenal feedback system. In time of physical or emotional stress there is an increased metabolic demand for corticoids. Since this demand cannot be met by the adrenal cortex, the dosage of exogenous corticoids must be increased. It is generally accepted that significant adrenal suppression will occur within 2 to 4 weeks of the daily administration of any corticosteroid, equivalent to 30 mg hydrocortisone. The patient continues to be at risk of experiencing adrenal crisis even if steroids were taken within 1 year, since this length of time is required for complete restoration of adrenal function. Consultation and close cooperation with the patient's physician are absolutely essential before initiating dental treatment in order to adjust the dosage of corticosteroids.

Patients who may incur minor stress, such as a routine restorative procedure, should have their steroid dosage increased to 75 to 100 mg hydrocortisone or its equivalent on the day of the procedure. This dose is generally tapered to the patient's daily dose over a period of a few days. Dental procedures that are likely to be very stressful require higher dosages and their procedures might best be performed in the hospital. In general, an intravenous infusion of 200 mg hydrocortisone and 150 mg cortisone is administered on the day of surgery and gradually tapered over a period of 5 to 7 days to the patient's usual dose.

Despite all precautions, an acute adrenal crisis may occur, and the dentist should be able to recognize and initially manage the condition. Signs and symptoms of crisis include hypotension, weakness, nausea, vomiting, headache, and fever. Immediate treatment consists of 100 mg hydrocortisone administered intravenously or intramuscularly. The patient should be transported to a medical facility as soon as possible.

PHEOCHROMOCYTOMA

ORAL MANIFESTATIONS. Multiple endocrine neoplasia (MEN) Type 2B is a designation that has been proposed for the combination of medullary thyroid carcinoma, parathyroid adenoma, pheochromocytoma, mucosal neuromas, and somatic abnormalities. Large, thick, nodular lips and thick, often everted upper eyelids form a distinct facies pathognomonic of this syndrome. Mucosal neuromas, which are microscopically composed of enlarged tortuous nerves, constitute a valuable clinical marker of the syndrome, since they are present in childhood and generally antedate clinical presentation of the thyroid and adrenal neoplasms. They produce a characteristic diffuse or nodular involvement of the anterior dorsum of the tongue, the lips, the buccal mucosa adjacent to the oral commissures, and occasionally the palate and mandible. They are asymptomatic and benign but may require surgical correction for esthetic reasons. The oral and labial neuromas usually appear in the first decade of life. Since mucosal neuromas may also be found in the conjunctiva, the dentist should examine this area.

MINERAL METABOLIC AND METABOLIC BONE DISEASE

Hyperparathyroidism
S. Gary Cohen

ORAL MANIFESTATIONS. The clinical signs and symptoms of hyperparathyroidism (HPTH) primarily reflect the pathophysiology of hypercalcemia. Whitlock summarizes them as "stones, bones, abdominal groans and psychic moans." However, an elevated serum calcium level may also be seen in sarcoidosis, vitamin D intoxication, multiple myeloma, and carcinoma of the lung. The serum calcium level in these diseases will be lowered by administration of 100 mg hydrocortisone per day (or its equivalent) given for 10 days, whereas calcium levels remain unchanged in hyperparathyroidism.

Bone and dental changes are late manifestations of hyperparathyroidism. Dependable radiographic changes only appear after a 30% loss of bony mineral content. In addition to increased serum calcium level, an elevated alkaline phosphatase level is a reflection of the amount of bony alteration. Alkaline phosphatase levels below 13 KA units rarely correlate with radiographic changes, while bony changes are evident with levels greater than 20 KA units.

A generalized osteoporosis with cortical resorption is the most common bone lesion. The dental radiographic signs include rarefactions, loss of trabeculation, goundglass appearance, total or partial loss of lamina dura, lytic lesions, and metastatic calcifications.

The rarefaction is secondary to the generalized osteoporosis. The finer trabeculae disappear later, leaving a coarser pattern. Small lytic lesions may occur that histologically prove to be giant cell tumors. The compact bone of the jaws may become thinned and eventually disappear. This may be evident as loss of the lower border of the mandible, the cortical margins of the inferior dental canal and floor of the antrum, and lamina dura. Spontaneous fractures may occur with the thinning of these areas of compact bone.

While the skeleton may undergo decalcification, fully developed teeth are not directly affected. However, in the presence of significant skeletal decalcification the teeth will appear more radiopaque.

The loss of lamina dura is neither pathognomonic nor a consistent sign of hyperparathyroidism. A similar loss of lamina dura may also be seen in Paget's disease, osteomalacia, fibrous dysplasia, sprue, and Cushing's and Addison's diseases. Various studies indicate lamina dura changes in only 40% to 50% of known hyperparathyroid patients.

The lesions of hyperparathyroidism are called brown tumors because they contain areas of old hemorrhage and clinically appear brown. As the tumor increases in size it may involve the cortex with resultant expansion. The cortex is eventually destroyed. Although the tumor rarely breaks through the periosteum, gingival swelling may result.

The brown tumor lesion contains an abundance of multinucleated giant cells, fibroblasts, and hemosiderin. This histologic appearance is also consistent with central giant cell tumor and giant cell reparative granuloma. Associated bone changes consist of a generalized osteitis fibrosa with patches of osteoclastic resorption on all bone surfaces. This is replaced by a vascular connective tissue that represents an abortive formation of coarse-fibered woven bone. This histologic picture may also be seen in fibrous dysplasia, giant cell reparative granuloma, osteomalacia, and Paget's disease.

All giant cell and osteoporotic lesions should be further investigated to rule out hyperparathyroidism. This should include a direct parathormone assay.

Other clinical manifestations of hyperparathyroidism include tooth mobility, malocclusion, and metastatic soft tissue calcifications. Increasing mobility and drifting of teeth with no apparent pathologic periodontal pocket formation may be seen. Periapical radiolucencies and root resorption may also be associated with this gradual loosening of the dentition. The teeth may be painful to percussion and mastilation. However, a positive thermal and electric pulp test response will be elicited. Splinting is a useful adjunct to prevent pain and further drifting. The splint should be maintained until adequate treatment of the hyperparathyroidism results in bone remineralization.

Malocclusion may result from the increased mobility and drifting of the dentition. Extreme demineralization and collapse of the temporomandibular and paratemporomandibular bones may also produce a malocclusion.

Metastatic calcifications, while rare, may occur in the oral mucosa and associated paraoral soft tissues including blood vessels. These calcifications are visible radiographically.

Since hyperparathyroidism may have a myriad of oral signs and symptoms the dentist is in an important position to recognize and diagnose this condition. Correlation of clinical, laboratory, radiographic, and histologie data is necessary for the definitive diagnosis. Early detection is imperative to circumvent potential irreversible kidney damage.

DENTAL MANAGEMENT. Generally, routine dental treatment involves no modifications unless there are associated medical complications present. In any phase of hyperparathyroidism prior to complete remineralization the dentist should take care to avoid latrogenic jaw fractures during surgical procedures.

Following corrective parathyroid surgery all bone lesions tend to regress spontaneously, although rather slowly at times. Recalcification of the skeleton takes place and serum calcium levels will return to normal. Surgical intervention of existing giant cell lesions is not necessary except to correct gross deformity or to extract displaced or resorbed teeth.

Hypoparathyroidism
S. Gary Cohen

Hypoparathyroidism is a metabolic abnormality characterized by hypocalcemia and consequent neuromuscular symptoms. Increased muscular and peripheral nerve irritability are often seen, causing a clinical picture that can be mistaken for a seizure disorder. These phenomena form the basis for the Chvostek's and Trousseau's signs. In frank tetany, painful muscular spasms occur that may involve oral and laryngeal musculature. Oral and dermatologic findings may precede the development of hypocalcemia. Soft tissue calcifications and ectopic development of true bone may occur, particularly in pseudohypoparathyroidism, as a result of the related hyperphosphatemia. An abnormal response to parathyroid hormone, ectopic calcifications, and other skeletal abnormalities may be indicative of idiopathic hypoparathyroidism, pseudohypoparathyroidism, pseudopseudohypoparathyroidism, basal ganglion calcification syndrome, basal cell nevus syndrome, Turner's syndrome, and Gardner's syndrome.

Aberrant developmental patterns may be seen if hypoparathyroidism occurs during tooth development (particularly ages 6 months to 3 years). Parathyroid hormone influences the eruption rate and affects both matrix formation and calcification. This may present as enamel hypoplasia, with single or parallel horizontal bands and poorly mineralized dentin. Malformed teeth, anodontia, short blunt root apices (particularly molars), elongated pulp chambers (often occluded by pulp stones even in primary teeth), multiple impacted teeth, and mandibular exostoses may be seen. Many of these developmental problems may be avoided with appropriately timed replacement therapy.

Acute or chronic hypoparathyroidism has no effect on erupted dentition. However, the maxilla and mandible may become abnormally dense despite a lowered serum calcium level. The trabeculae are increased in number and unusually well calcified. Surgically induced hypoparathyroidism does not cause oral problems except for occasional vague mouth discomfort that is relieved with normalization of serum calcium.

Idiopathic hypoparathyroidism may occur singly or as part of an autoimmune polyendocrinopathy syndrome that may consist of any combination of superficial mucocutaneous candidiasis, hypoadrenocorticism, keratoconjunctivitis, intestinal malabsorption, pernicious anemia, diabetes mellitus, thyroiditis, and mental retardation.

Acute and chronic oral candidiasis is the most consistent manifestation of the polyendocrinopathy syndrome. The enamel hypoplasia associated with the polyendocrinopathy syndrome is not solely the result of a lowered serum calcium but may be a manifestation of a more generalized ectodermal involvement.

Hypoparathyroidism should be included in any differential diagnosis of chronic or unresponsive candidiasis. Clinical and radiographic evaluation of the dentition (in children) may aid in the definitive diagnosis of a polyendocrinopathy syndrome. Early hormonal replacement may prevent the development of the more serious components of these syndromes.

Frequent oral evaluations are essential in the patient with any form of hypoparathyroidism. Hypoplastic teeth are caries prone; meticulous oral hygiene should be stressed. Periodic radiographic evaluations will aid in the detection of dentigerous cysts that may form at the sites of impacted teeth.

Before dental treatment the patient's serum calcium level should be monitored and should be above 8 mg/100 ml to prevent the possibility of cardiac arrhythmias, generalized convulsions, laryngospasm, or bronchospasm.

Hypophosphatasia

ORAL MANIFESTATIONS. Dental abnormalities have been described only in the juvenile type of hypophosphatasia, the first clinical symptom of which is often the premature loss of primary teeth. The teeth most frequently lost are the primary mandibular central and lateral incisors, followed by the maxillary incisors and, less commonly, the posterior teeth. Additional signs of juvenile hypophosphatasia are loss of alveolar bone, lack of periodontal attachment fibers, and reduced or complete absence of cementum.

Radiographic evidence of the disorder consists of enlarged pulp chambers and root canals, sometimes giving the tooth a "shell" appearance; reduction in the thickness of the dentin and irregular dentin formation with large dentinal tubules and many areas of interglobular dentin; enamel hypoplasia; and irregular calcifications and lesions in the alveolar bone. The histologic features of the jaw bones are similar to those of rickets and osteomalacia.

DENTAL MANAGEMENT. Involuntary twitching of the facial muscles may be an early sign of tetany caused by low serum calcium levels. The dentist should observe for this sign and refer the patient for medical management. Caution must be taken during dental procedures to avoid jaw fractures in hypocalcified areas. The oral manifestations of hypophosphatasia usually resolve with treatment of the disorder.

Osteomalacia

ORAL MANIFESTATIONS. While there seem to be no radiologic or chemical changes in the teeth of patients with osteomalacia, there are definite radiographic changes noted in the jawbones. There is evidence of generalized demineralization of bone with bony deformities containing excess osteoid and fibrous connective tissue and diminished or absent cortical bone shadows. These changes may affect the alveolar lamina dura, the outlines of the sinuses, the inferior dental canal, and the lower border of the mandible. In cancellous bone the trabeculae are thinner and may be absent on radiographs.

Other oral aspects of osteomalacia include loosening of the teeth and a predisposition of the weakened jawbones to fractures.

DENTAL MANAGEMENT. The dentist should observe for signs of tetany caused by low serum calcium levels, such as involuntary twitching of the muscles of the face. When performing dental procedures the dentist must exercise caution to avoid a jaw fracture. The jaw manifestations associated with osteomalacia generally respond to the treatment of the underlying deficiency.

Osteoporosis

ORAL MANIFESTATIONS. Alveolar bone is highly susceptible to osteoporosis, particularly in those patients in whom teeth have been lost and disuse atrophy has ensued. In the edentulous patient, especially one without a prosthetic replacement, disuse atrophy results in loss of normal trabeculation as well as general loss of contour of the alveolar process. The alveolar bone is often left devoid of its cortical layer and the residual ridges are sharp and covered with spicules from uneven resorption. In some cases so much alveolar bone is lost that the mandibular and maxillary ridges become flat. This loss of vertical dimension is manifested as a loss of facial height.

In addition, there are other local factors that may modify the bone density. Posttraumatic osteoporosis may occur, resulting from disuse and from interference with the blood supply. Immobilization of bone for long periods will invariably result in osteoporosis. Irradiation of bone, hyperemia of traumatic or inflammatory origin, and neurogenic disturbances, particularly those involving the sympathetic nervous system, may result secondarily in vascular changes that interfere with adequate nutrition to the involved bone, leading to osteoporosis.

The loss of bone substance in osteoporosis will weaken the mandible and make it more liable to fracture. This may occur during dental treatment or spontaneously.

The radiographic changes of osteoporosis consist of generalized increased radiolucency of the bone with fine, indistinct trabeculae and thinning of the cortex. The bone trabeculae that are resorbed are replaced with fatty marrow. In senile or postmenopausal osteoporosis the lamina dura of tooth sockets is said to be thinned but still discernible, whereas in the osteoporosis of Cushing's syndrome the lamina dura may be completely obliterated. In radiographs of osteoporotic jaws the teeth stand out sharply in contrast to the more lucent bone. Osteoporosis of the maxilla is accompanied by an increase in the size of the paranasal sinuses, often with marked thinning of the bone. In dentulous patients this results in the maxillary antrum extending deeply between the roots of the teeth. The canals in which the branches of the superior dental nerves usually run are lost and the nerves may be in the antral lining. In such cases, inflammation in the antrum is likely to cause referred pain in the maxillary teeth. The extension of the maxillary antrum weakens the bone and increases the likelihood of tuberosity fracture during extraction of maxillary molars.

DENTAL MANAGEMENT. The relationship between dietary calcium and phosphorus and alveolar bone resorption in edentulous patients has been under investigation. The results of studies comparing diets of subjects who had minimal bone resorption with diets of subjects who had severe alveolar bone loss indicate a direct cause-and-effect relationship between low calcium intake, calcium/phosphorus imbalance, and severe ridge resorption. In another study, the ingestion of calcium and vitamin D dietary supplements reduced the degree of postextraction alveolar bone resorption by 36%. Investigators administered 750 to 1000 mg calcium and 375 to 4000 IU vitamin D daily to patients who had a low calcium and/or a high phosphorous intake. They concluded that these dietary supplements helped increase the resistance of the alveolar bone to both mechanical and nutritional biochemical stresses.

The supporting mucosa in those individuals with osteoporosis who wear dentures may become sensitive to trauma from the denture base material. Therefore, denture bases should be lined with a soft reline material, extending over the entire support area, and the occlusion carefully balanced.

SEX HORMONAL ALTERATIONS
Ovaries

There are four periods of life during which there is an imbalance of female sex hormones. Puberty, menstruation, pregnancy, and menopause bring rapid changes in the sex hormone balance as the body accommodates to developmental and growth changes. These periods of imbalance may be times of early but definite tissue changes which are manifest in the mucous membranes of the oral cavity. Similar changes may be seen in women taking oral contraceptives. These changes are not necessarily the result of direct hormonal action on the tissues, but perhaps best explained as the effects of local traumatic factors on tissues conditioned to change by hormonal activity.

PUBERTY

Oral manifestations. During puberty there is a noticeable rise in the incidence of gingivitis associated with the commencement of sex hormone secretion. A nodular hyperplastic reaction of the gingiva occurs in areas where food debris, materia alba, plaque, and calculus are deposited. The inflamed tissues are deep red in color and may be lobulated, with ballooning distortion of the interdental papillae. Bleeding may occur during toothbrushing and mastication. Histologically, the tissue appearance is consistent with inflammatory hyperplasia.

Dental management. Local preventive care, including a vigorous program of good oral hygiene, is most important. Periodontal therapy may also be indicated in the individual with puberty gingivitis.

MENSTRUATION. Oral changes that may accompany the menses include swollen, erythematous gingival tissues, herpes labialis, aphthous ulcers, prolonged hemorrhage following oral surgery, and swelling of the salivary glands.

In some women, postoperative hemorrhage occurs more frequently during the menses than at other time. There are no significant hematologic findings accompanying this, other than a slight reduction in the platelet count and a slight increase in the clotting time.

Swelling of the salivary glands, particularly the parotid, occurs occasionally during menses. There is an associated increase in gynecologic complaints, though the cause is unclear.

Recurrent aphthous ulcerations occur in some women in a pattern that seems related to their menstrual cycle. The ulcers appear during the luteal phase of the cycle and heal following menstruation. Oral contraceptives, high doses of estrogens, and synthetic progesterones can help to resolve these lesions.

PREGNANCY

Oral manifestations. The popular notion that pregnancy causes tooth loss ("a tooth for every pregnancy") and that calcium is withdrawn in significant amounts from the maternal dentition to supply fetal requirements has no histologic, chemical, or radiographic evidence to support it. On the other hand, calcium is readily mobilized from bone to supply these demands, and demineralization of the alveolar processes is possible.

The relationship between dental caries and pregnancy is not well defined. The more comprehensive clinical studies suggest that pregnancy does not contribute directly to the carious process. It is most likely that when an increase in caries activity is noted, it can be attributed to an increase in local cariogenic factors.

Another condition that may influence the pregnant patient's teeth is acid erosion, which may be caused by repeated regurgitation of gastric contents associated with morning sickness or esophageal reflux.

Periodontal disease occurs in 50% to 100% of all pregnant women and is thus the most consistent oral manifestation. Gingival changes occur most frequently in association with poor oral higiene and local irritants, especially bacterial plaque. However, the hormonal and vascular changes that accompany pregnancy often exaggerate the inflammatory response to these local irritants. The high levels of progesterone, for example, have a direct effect on the microvasculature of the gingiva. Hormonal changes also disturb the nutrition, function, and metabolism of the cells in the supporting tissues of teeth. Gingival changes are most noticeable from the second month of gestation, readhing a maximum level in the eighth month. They occur earlier and more frequently in the anterior dental quadrants than in posterior areas.

Clinically, the appearance of inflamed gingiva during pregnancy is characterized by a fiery red color of the marginal gingiva and interdental papillae. The tissue is edematous, with a smooth, shiny surface texture, loss of resiliency, and a tendency to bleed easily. Hypertrophy of the interdental papillae may occur, with formation of pseudopockets.

In addition to generalized gingival changes, pregnancy may also give rise to single, tumorlike growths usually on the interdental papillae or other areas of frequent irritation. This localized area of gingival hypertrophy is referred to as a "pregnancy tumor," "epulis gravidarum," or "pregnancy granuloma." The last term is preferred since the histologic appearance is similar to the pyogenic granuloma. The reported frequency of pregnancy granuloma varies from 0 to 5%. The lesion occurs most frequently on the buccal aspect of the maxillary anterior region during the second trimester of gestation. It often undergoes rapid growth, although it seldom becomes larger than 2 cm in diameter. The pregnancy granuloma classically begins its development in an area afflicted by inflammatory gingivitis. Poor oral hygiene is invariably present, and often there are deposits of plaque and/or calculus on the teeth adjacent to the lesion. The gingiva becomes hyperplastic and enlarges in a nodular fashion to give rise to the clinical mass. The fully developed pregnancy granuloma is a sessile or pedunculated lesion that is usually painless. The color varies from purplish red to deep blue, depending on the vascularity of the lesion and the degree of venous stasis. The surface of the lesion may be ulcerated and covered by a yellowish exudate, and gentle manipulation of the mass easily induces hemorrhage. Bone destruction is rarely observed around pregnancy granulomas.

The majority of these lesions regress spontaneously several months after the termination of pregnancy. If chewing causes hemorrhage from the enlarged hyperemic gingival tissue or if ulceration has occurred, the growth should be removed surgically during pregnancy, ideally in the second trimester.

An additional oral finding that may be seen in the pregnant patient is generalized tooth mobility. This change is probably related to the degree of gingival disease and disturbance of the attachment apparatus, as well as to mineral changes in the lamina dura. This condition usually reverses after delivery.

Dental management. Dental evaluation of the pregnant patient, as all others, begins with a thorough medical history. The history should note any complications the patient has encountered in the pregnancy to date and record any previous miscarriage, recent cramping, spotting, or pernicious vomiting. If at all possible, the next step in management of the pregnant patient should be to contact the patient's obstetrician or physician to discuss the patient's medical status, her dental needs, and the proposed treatment plan. The most important objectives in planning dental treatment for the pregnant patient are to establish a healthy oral environment and to obtain optimum oral hygiene levels. These are achieved by means of a good preventive dental program consisting of nutritional counseling and rigorous plaque control measures in the dental office and at home.

The quality of the diet affects caries formation, pregnancy gingivitis, and oral infections. Diet is also important for the developing dentition during fetal gestation, since it influences chemical composition, eruption time, malocclusion, and susceptibility to caries.

A good plaque control program should be developed for the pregnant patient to minimize the exaggerated inflammatory response of the gingival tissues. This exaggerated tendency for gingival inflammation should be clearly explained to the patient so that acceptable oral hygiene techniques may be taught, reinforced, and monitored throughout the pregnancy. Scaling, polishing, and root planing may be performed whenever necessary.

Other than good plaque control, no elective dental care should be undertaken during the first trimester or last half of the third trimester. The first trimester is the period of organogenesis, when the fetus is very sensitive to environmental influences. In the last half of the third trimester there is the hazard of premature delivery, since the uterus is very sensitive to external stimuli. Prolonged chair time should be avoided, since supine hypotensive syndrome may occur. In a semireclining or supine position, the great vessels, particularly the inferior vena cava, are compressed by the gravid uterus. By interfering with venous return, this compression will cause hypotension, decreased cardiac output, and eventual loss of consciousness. Supine hypotensive syndrome can usually be reversed by turning the patient on her left side, thereby removing pressure on the vena cava and allowing blood to return from the lower extremities and pelvic area.

The second trimester is the safest period during which routine dental care can be provided. Even so, it is advisable to limit care to minimal treatment such as simple operative procedures. Emphasis should be placed on controlling active disease and eliminating potential problems that

Table 1. Drug use in pregnancy

Type of medication	"Safe" to use in pregnancy	Relatively safe (limited information)	Some risk associated	Contraindicated in pregnancy
Analgesics	Acetaminophen Meperidine Morphine Codeine	Percodan Hydromorphone	Salicylates Indomethacin	
Antibiotics	Ampicillin Erythromycin Isoniazid Miconazole Penicillin	Amikacin Amphotericin B Carbenicillin Cephalosporins Clindamycin Gentamicin Kanamycin Methicillin Nafcillin Oxacillin, dicloxacillin Tobramycin	Chloramphenicol Lincomycin Nitrofurantoin Streptomycin Sulfonamides Septra-Bactrim	Tetracycline
Anticoagulants	Heparin	Dipyridamole	Warfarin	
Antiemetics	Bendectin	Trimethobenzamide Hydroxyzine Prochlorperazine		
Bronchodilators	Aminophylline	Terbutaline Cromolyn sodium Beclomethasone		
Cardiac drugs	Digoxin Atropine Lidocaine	Procainamide Disopyramide Quinidine		
Cough preparations	Robitussin-DM, Robitussin-CF	Terpin hydrate		
Decongestants	Diphenhydramine Pseudoephedrine	Dimetapp Actifed All other over-the-counter preparations		
Local anesthetics	Lidocaine Mepivacaine			
Laxatives	Milk of magnesia	Metamucil Colace		
Sedatives	Barbiturates	Flurazepam	Diazepam Chlordiazepoxide	

could arise in late pregnancy. Extensive reconstructive procedures and major oral or periodontal surgery should be postponed until after delivery. Emergency dental care may be rendered at any time during pregnancy, after consultation with the patient's physician.

One controversial area in the treatment of the pregnant patient involves taking dental radiographs. Only serious dental emergencies require radiographic evaluation, especially during the first trimester when the developing fetus is particularly susceptible to the effects of radiation. Routine roentgenograms should be avoided and taken only when necessary therapy would otherwise be seriously compromised. The patient must wear a protective lead apron to reduce the amount of radiation emitted to the abdominal area. Excess scatter and secondary radiation can be avoided by periodic inspection of x-ray units to ensure proper beam collimation and filtration. High-speed film should be used to minimize exposure.

Another area of controversy involves drug therapy, since any drugs given to the pregnant patient can affect the fetus by diffusion across the placenta. Dentists should be particularly cautious when administering drugs of any kind to the pregnant patient (see Table 1). Most pharmaceutical houses caution against use of many of their products during pregnancy due to lack of well-controlled research on human subjects. In cases of pressing emergency, appropriate drug therapy can be instituted, but overprescribing should be avoided. It is fortunate that most of the drugs commonly used in dental practice can be given with relative safety. Nevertheless, documented consultation with the patient's physician before drug administration is recommended. It is considered safe practice to use local anesthetics with a vasoconstrictor (1:100,000). Analgesics, including acetaminophen and aspirin (excluding the third trimester, when bleeding problems can occur during or after delivery) are also safe. Antibiotics, including penicillin, cephalosporins, and erythromycin, also have relative safety in both mother and fetus.

There are certain drugs commonly prescribed by dentists that are known to cause complications in pregnancy and are therefore best avoided. These include: diazepam (Valium), chlordiazepoxide (Librium), flurazepam (Dalmane), meprobamate (Miltown), streptomycin, and tetracycline. It seems prudent to avoid use of nitrous oxide during organogenesis, and general anesthesia or intravenous sedation is to be generally avoided.

MENOPAUSE

Oral manifestations. During the menopausal years, women appear to experience an increase in oral symptoms which may result from endocrine disturbances (reduction in estrogen), vitamin deficiencies and various underlying psychologic factors. Menopausal women may experience flushing (hot flashes), sweating, headaches, and depression. They may also complain of a dry mouth because of decreased salivary secretion, as well as burning sensations of the mouth and tongue. Taste sensations may be altered, causing a frequent complaint of salty or "metallic" taste.

The gingival mucosa of menopausal women may undergo atrophy, in a manner similar to that of the vaginal mucosa. This gingival condition has been termed desquamative gingivitis and is noted for diminished surface keratinization and epithelial detachment from the subjacent connective tissue corium, with consequent bullous lesion formation and epithelial desquamation. The corium is then left exposed to the oral environment and undergoes a diffuse inflammatory response characterized by marked redness, shiny edema, hypersensitivity to tactile, chemical, and thermal stimuli, increased dryness, and burning pain.

Dental management. Many of the symptoms and complaints of the menopausal patient, such as abnormal taste sensations, glossodynia, and desquamative gingivitis, appear to resolve when dietary corrections and vitamin supplements are administered. Since low estrogen levels may also be responsible for these symptoms, many patients will respond favorably to estrogen supplement therapy. In addition, psychiatric treatment may be indicated for some patients, and it is most appropriate for the dentist to refer the menopausal patient for medical evaluation and treatment, to optimize the benefits of dental treatment.

ORAL CONTRACEPTIVES. The number of women taking oral contraceptives has reached an estimated 8 to 10 million in the United States and 50 million worldwide. As a result of such widespread use, many systemic and oral side effects have been detected.

Among the undesirable systemic effects associated with the use of oral contraceptives are an increased incidence of thromboembolic events, increased risk of myocardial infarction, and, in certain instances, a significant elevation in blood pressure.

Oral manifestations. One of the most common effects on the oral mucous membranes in those individuals taking oral contraceptives is gingival inflammation. Many such women have an exaggerated gingival inflammatory response to local irritants, characterized by fiery red, enlarged, and hemorrhagic gingival tissues. There are several mechanisms that may contribute to this exaggerated gingival response, including an alteration in the microvasculature caused by elevated serum levels of sex hormones. This results in increased vascular permeability and resultant edema of the perivascular tissue with a significant increase in gingival fluid. Recent investigation has shown that the addition of sex hormones to gingival tissue can cause a significant increase in the synthesis of prostaglandin E_2. Since E-type prostaglandins are potent mediators of inflammation, this may be another mechanism whereby sex hormones increase inflammation. Another factor under consideration is intake disruption of the gingival mast cells, liberating stores of histamine and proteolytic enzymes and thus aggravating the inflammation produced by local irritants.

Women taking oral contraceptives demonstrate a significant increase in the number of *Bacteroides* species in the gingival microflora. Increased female sex hormones substituting for the naphthoquinones required by certain *Bacteroides* species are most likely responsible for this rise. This suggests that estrogens and progesterone are capable of altering the subgingival microflora, thereby further mediating the increase in gingival inflammation observed in these individuals.

Although there appears to be no correlation between the severity of inflammation and the particular type of progesterone or estrogen in the various brands of oral contraceptives, there may be a direct relationship between the severity of inflammation or periodontal destruction and the duration of hormone therapy, which suggests that oral contraceptives may have a cumulative effect in altering host resistance. A radiographic change related to oral contraceptives is an increase in the number of punctate radiopaque areas in the mandible. The opacities are thought to result from a thickening of the endosteal plates of bone as a result of the parathyroid-stimulating effect of the estrogen in oral contraceptives. This effect is one of bone apposition, which could account for a denser and more radiopaque endosteum.

Measurable changes have been observed in the saliva of women taking sex hormones, including a decrease in concentrations of protein, sialic acid, hexosamine, fucose, hydrogen ion, and total electrolytes.

Since another side effect of oral contraceptives is spotty melanotic pigmentation of the skin, a relationship between the use of oral contraceptives and the occurrence of gingival melanosis in individuals with light complexions has been suggested.

The dental literature reports that women taking oral contraceptives have twofold to threefold increase in the incidence of localized osteitis following extraction of mandibular third molars. The higher incidence of osteitis in these patients may be attributed to the effects of oral contraceptives and estrogens on blood clotting factors. Since a patient's coagulation and fibrinolytic factors are cyclic when taking oral contraceptives, there may be a temporary shift, when fibrinolytic components are increased in relation to clotting factors. If this shift occurs while a patient is recovering from a third molar extraction, the loss of surgical clot may result. Another mechanism to be considered is the presence of tissue activators after teeth are removed, which may give rise to high fibrinolytic activity and consequent lysis of clots.

Dental management. The dentist should be aware of the systemic and oral side effects of oral contraceptives. A comprehensive medical history and assessment of vital signs, particularly blood pressure, are extremely important in these patients. Treatment of gingival inflammation exaggerated by oral contraceptives should include the establishment of an oral hygiene program and the elimination of all local predisposing factors. Periodontal surgery may be indicated if there is inadequate resolution after initial therapy (scaling, root planing, and curettage).

Testes

Gingival changes in pubertal males have been noted in association with increased secretion of both adrenal and testicular androgens. This may cause a diffuse gingival inflammatory lesion, which is exacerbated by local irritation.

There have been several reported cases of primary tumors of the testes exhibiting metastasis to the oral cavity. Metastatic lesions have appeared on the alveolar ridge, gingivobuccal sulci, alveolar mucosa, palate, and gingiva. In some instances the histologic appearance of the metastatic lesion is quite different from that of the primary testicular tumor.

KLINEFELTER'S SYNDROME. Patients with Klinefelter's syndrome have a slender face and marked malocclusion. Mandibular prognathism, a flat palate, and maxillary hypoplasia are commonly seen as well. A cleft palate may occur in the individual with an XXXXY karyotype.

TESTICULAR FEMINIZATION SYNDROME. Although 46, XY females have a generally female phenotype, the appearance of their teeth resembles that of a normal male. The large teeth in 46, XY females may be caused by modified endocrine function, or perhaps there is a gene (or genes) on the Y chromosome that increases the size of the teeth.

BIBLIOGRAPHY

Akinosi, J.O., Olumide, F., and Ogunbiyi, T.A.J.: Retrosternal parathyroid adenomas manifesting in the form of a giant-cell tumor of the mandible, Oral Surg. **39**:724, 1975.

Albers, D.D.: Conservative treatment of oral bony lesions of hyperparathyroidism, Oral Surg. **38**:209, 1974.

Alvesalo, L., and Varrela, J.: Permanent tooth sizes in 46, XY females, Am. J. Hum. Genet. **32**: 736, 1980.

Anneroth G., and Heimdahl, A.: Syndrome of multiple mucosal neurofibromas, pheochromocytoma and medullary thyroid carcinoma: report of a case, Int. J. Oral Surg. **7**:126, 1978.

Assif, D.: Dental changes in hypoparathyroidism, Isr. J. Den. Med. **26**:13, 1977.

Beck-Coon, R.J., and Beck-Coon, K.A.: Dental treatment in the pregnant or nursing patient, Gen. Dentistry, May-June 1982, p. 237.

Bonner, S.: Using the pill can affect the gingiva and periodontium, Dent. Student, January 1978, p. 54.

Brown, A.E., and others: Oral ulceration associated with hypothyroidism: report of a case, Oral Surg., **42**:216, 1978.

Casino, A.J., and others: Oral-facial manifestations of the multiple endocrine neoplasia syndrome, Oral Surg. May 1981, p. 516.

Catalanotto, F.A., and Henkin, R.I.: Manual and oral sensation in patients with Cushing's syndrome, J. Dent. Res. **56**:866, 1977.

Catellani, J.E., and others: Effect of oral contraceptive cycle on dry socket (localized alveolar osteitis), J. Am. Dent. Assoc. **101**:777, 1980.

Chapnick, P.: A review of hyperparathyroidism and an interesting case presenting with a giant cell lesion, Trans. Int. Conf. Oral/Surg. **4**:44, 1973.

Darzenta, N.C., and Giunta, J.L.: Radiographic changes of the mandible related to oral contraceptives, Oral Surg., March 1977, p. 478.

Delzer, D.D., and Provant, D.R., Jr.: Pregnancy and side effects of analgesics, Gen. Dentistry, January-February, 1981, p. 49.

Edler, R.J.: Dental and skeletal ages in hypopituitary patients, J. Dent. Res., October 1977, p. 1145.

El-Ashiry, G.M., and others: Comparative study of the influence of pregnancy and oral contraceptives on the gingivae, Oral Surg., October 1970, p. 472.

El Attar, T.M.A.: Prostaglandin E_2 in human gingiva in health and disease and its stimulation by female sex steroids, Prostaglandins **11**:650, 1976.

Fantasia, J.E., and Lie-chu, C.: A testicular tumor with gingival metastasis, Oral Surg. July 1979, p. 64.

Gorlin, R.J., and Goldman, H.M., editors: Thoma's Oral Pathology, ed. 6, vol. 1 and 2, St. Louis, 1970, The C.V. Mosby Co.

Greenberg, M.S., and others: Idiopathic hypoparathyroidism, chronic candidiasis, and dental hypoplasia, Oral Surg. **28**:42, 1969.

Hertz, R.S., Beckstead, P.C., and Brown, W.J.: Epithelial melanosis of the gingiva possibly resulting from the use of oral contraceptives, J. Am. Dent. Assoc. **100**:713, 1980.

Houston, J.B., and others: Radiography of secondary hyperparathyroidism, Oral Surg. **26**:746, 1968.

Jedrychowski, J.R., and Duperon, D.: Childhood hypophosphatasia with oral manifestations, J. Oral Med. **35**:18, 1979.

Jensen, J., Liljemark, W., and Bloomquist, C.: The effect of female sex hormones on subgingival plaque, J. Periodontol., October 1981, p. 599.

Jones, J.H., and Mason, D.K.: Oral manifestations of systemic disease, Philadelphia, W.B. Saunders Co., 1980.

Kalkwarf, K.L.: Effect of oral contraceptive therapy on gingival inflammation in humans, J. Periodontol., November 1978, p. 560.

Karolus, J.A.: A dental hygienist's approach to pregnancy and nutrition, Dent. Hyg., June 1980, p. 267.

Kennon, S., Tasch, E.G., and Arm, R.N.: Considerations in the management of patients taking oral contraceptives, J. Am. Dent. Assoc. **97**:641, 1978.

King, D.L.: Eruption rate of rat incisor after parathyroidectomy, J. Dent. Res. **55**:915, 1976.

Knight, G.M., and Wade, A.B.: The effects of hormonal contraceptives on the human periodontium, J. Periodont. Res. **9**:18, 1973.

Langer, A.: Prosthodontic failures in patients with systemic disorders, J. Oral Rehabil. **6**:13, 1979.

Little, J.A., and Falace, D.A.: Dental management of the medically compromised patient, St. Louis, 1980, The C.V. Mosby Co.

Lorio, G.P.: Effects of oral contraceptives on the oral structures: a review, Gen. Dentistry, March-April 1982, p. 140.

Lynch, M.A., editor: Burket's oral medicine, ed. 7, Philadelphia, J.B. Lippincott Co., 1977.

Magnusson, I., Ericson, T. and Hugoson, A.: The effect of oral contraceptives on the concentration of some salivary substances in women, Arch. Oral Biol. **20**:119, 1976.

Markovic, M., and Triscovic, D.: Some results of occlusal and metric analysis of acromegalic cases, p. 13.

Migita, H., and Ohno, A.: Oral bony lesion in a patient with medical history of hyperparathyroidism, Int. J. Oral Surg. **8**:67, 1979.

Miller, R.L., and others: The ultrastructure of oral neuromas in multiple mucosal neuromas, pheochromocytoma, medullary thyroid carcinoma syndrome, J. Oral Pathol., July 1977, p. 253.

Mueller, W.A., and Steinle, C.J.: Management of a hyperthyroid dental patient utilizing general anesthesia, Pediatr. Dentistry **3**:201.

Myllärniemi, S., and Perheentupa, J.: Oral findings in the autoimmune polyendocrinopathy–candidiasis syndrome (APECS) and other forms of hypoparathyroidism, Oral Surg. **45**:721, 1978.

Nelson, G., and others: Multiple endocrine neoplasia, type 2B, with medullary thyroid carcinoma: a diagnostic potential for dentistry, Pediatr. Dentistry **1**:125, 1979.

Nelson, J.F., Tsaknis, P.J., and Konzelman, J.L.: Dental changes in familial idiopathic hypoparathyroidism, J. Oral Med. **33**:115, 1978.

Nizel, A.E.: Nutrition in preventive dentistry: science and practice, ed. 2, Philadelphia, 1981, W.B. Saunders Co.

Ojanotko, A., Nienstedt, W., and Harri, M.P.: Metabolism of testosterone by human healthy and inflamed gingiva in vitro, Arch. Oral Biol. **25**:481, 1981.

Pankhurst, C.L., and others: The influence of oral contraceptive therapy on the periodontium—duration of drug therapy, J. Periodontol, October 1981, p. 617.

Pindborg, J.J.: Atlas of diseases of the oral mucosa, ed. 3, Philadelphia, 1980, W.B. Saunders Co.

Pisanty, S., and Garfunkel, A.: Familial hypoparathyroidism with candidiasis and mental retardation, Oral Surg. **44**:374, 1977.

Rosenberg, E.H., and Guralnick, W.C.: Hyperparathyroidism: a review of 220 proved cases, with special emphasis on findings in the jaws, Oral Surg. **26**:184, 1962.

Ruben, M.P.: Periodontosis: an analysis and clarification of its status as a disease entity, J. Periodontol. June 1979, p. 311.

Sedano, H.O., Sauk, J.J., Jr., and Gorlin, R.J.: Oral manifestations of inherited disorders, Boston, 1977, Butterworth Publishers, Inc.

Sutherland, K.J.G.: Medical conditions affecting dental treatment planning, Aust. Dent. J. **17**:169, 1972.

Sweet, J.B.: Pregnancy-associated dental problems, Contemp. OB/GYN **16**:33, 1980.

Sweet, J.B., and Butler, D.P.: Increased incidence of postoperative localized osteitis in mandibular third molar surgery associated with patients using oral contraceptives, Am. J. Obstet. Gynecol. **127**:518, 1977.

Terezhalmy, G.T., Feltman, R., and Bottomley, W.K.: Initial evidence of primary hyperparathyroidism presenting in the mouth: a case report, J. Oral Med. **33**:4, 1978.

Urbanska, D.K.: Care of the mouth and teeth, Nurs. Mirror, June 2, 1977, p. 29.

Vittek, J., and others: Concentration of circulating hormones and metabolism of androgens by human gingiva, J. Periodontol., May 1979, p. 254.

Walton, J.G., and Thompson, J.W.: Pharmacology for the dental practitioner, Br. Dent. J., Sept. 1969, p. 227.

Weir, J.C., Silberman, S.L., and Cohen, L.A.: Recurring oral pregnancy tumors, Obstet. Gynecol. **54**:358, 1979.

Whiteman, G.J., and Schneider, L.C.: Primary hyperparathyroidism detected by Gingival Biopsy, J. Periodontol. **49**:214, 1978.

Whitlock, R.I.H.: The jaw lesions associated with hyperparathyroidism, Trans. Int. Conf. Oral Surg. **3**:322, 1970.

Williamson-Lempesis, T.: The pregnant patient—problems, management and treatment, Dent. Assist., January-February 1979, p. 24.

Wittmann, A.L.: Macroglossia in acromegaly and hypothyroidism, Virchows Arch. (Pathol. Anat.), 1977, p. 352.

Yogge, J., and others: Changes in blood coagulation and fibrinolysis in women receiving oral contraceptives, Am. J. Obst. & Gynec., May 1969, Vol. 104, No. 1 87-98.

Yonaga, T.: Action of parathyroid hormone, with special reference to its anabolic effect on different kinds of tissues in rats, Bull. Tokyo Med. Dent. Univ. **25**:237-268, 1978.

Yudowsky, E.B.: The oral cavity as a diagnostic tool: pituitary and parathyroid dysfunction, So. Carolina Dent. J. **8**:25, Spring, 1978.

Yudowsky, E.B.: The oral cavity as a diagnostic tool: thyroid, adrenal, pancreas, and sex hormone dysfunction, So. Carolina Dent. J. **8**:28, Summer, 1978.

Section Fifteen
GENETICS AND METABOLISM
edited by **Doris G. Bartuska**

---

194 • HUMAN GENETICS
Kathleen Toomey

BASIC PRINCIPLES
Gene concept and single gene inheritance

The human genome is contained in the cellular component deoxyribonucleic acid (DNA), which is located within the nucleus of each cell, and in the as yet ill-defined "extranuclear" elements of inheritance. The DNA molecule is composed of two chains, with a repeating backbone of sugar-phosphate groups coiled and bound by the affinity of complementary attached base pairs (adenine-thymine and guanine-cytosine), the order of which determines the sequence of amino acids ultimately produced from any given segment of the molecule (Fig. 194-1). Each sequence of three base pairs, a codon, is capable of being transcribed into a complementary strand of messenger ribonucleic acid (mRNA), a molecule differing from DNA in sugar composition (ribose instead of deoxyribose) and in the substitution of uracil for thymine as a complement to adenine. The 20 amino acids are coded for by one or more of the 64 triplet possibilities, the so-called genetic code (Table 194-1). The mRNA transcription of the DNA code attaches to a ribosome located in the cytoplasm, where transfer RNA–amino acid complexes are assembled in line, peptide bonds are formed between amino acids, and a protein molecule is produced—the translation process (Fig. 194-2). The beginning and ending triplet condons are specialized messages of initiation and termination of the translation process. The protein products are enzymes, structural proteins, or regulator proteins. The entire process is undoubtedly under control mechanisms, many of which have yet to be elucidated. Certainly, one method of control is "feedback inhibition," in which the accumulation of the product itself turns off the process through interaction of the product with the gene itself or with some intermediary compounds.

Errors in the genetic code take the form of alterations in base composition. These may be point mutations in which a single base is changed or deletions of one or more bases from the sequence. As can be seen from Table 194-

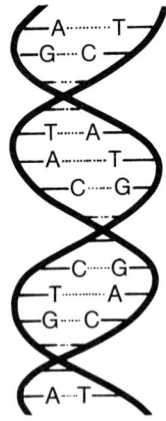

Fig. 194-1. Schematic representation of DNA molecule. Sugar (deoxyribose)-phosphate backbones in double helical configuration with *purines*, adenine, *A*, and guanine, *G*, attached by hydrogen bonds to *pyrimidines*, thymine, *T*, and cytosine, *C*, respectively. RNA molecule differs in sugar composition (ribose for deoxyribose) and one pyrimidine (uracil for thymine).

Table 194-1. The genetic code

Amino acid	DNA triplet codons
Alanine	CGA, CGG, CGT, CGC
Arginine	GCA, GCG, GCT, GCC, TCT, TCC
Asparagine	TTA, TTG
Aspartic acid	CTA, CTG
Cysteine	ACA, ACG
Glutamic acid	CTT, CTC
Glutamine	CTT, GTC
Glycine	CCA, CCG, CCT, CCC
Histidine	GTA, GTG,
Isoleucine	TAA, TAG, TAT
Leucine	AAT, AAC, GAA, GAG, GAT, GAC
Lysine	TTT, TTC
Methionine	TAC
Phenylalanine	AAA, AAG
Proline	GGA, GGG, GGT, GGC
Serine	AGA, AGG, AGT, AGC, TCA, TCG
Threonine	TGA, TGT, TGC, TGG
Tryptophan	ACC
Tyrosine	ATA, ATG
Valine	CAA, CAG, CAT, CAC
Chain end	ATT, ATC, ACT

1, there are potential mutations that will not alter the ultimate product. In general these involve the third member of the triplet; for example, glycine is coded for by DNA sequences CCA, CCG, CCT, or CCC. Arginine and leucine allow more room for error in being coded by six possible codons each, whereas the codes for methionine and tryptophan leave no room for error, having one specific codon each.

Depending on the position of the error, the new product may be clinically indistinguishable from the normal product and may or may not be ascertained biochemically. These are usually termed normal protein polymorphisms. A mutation may significantly alter the status of the protein product, making it less efficient or totally nonfunctional. Such changes are at the root of many of the inborn errors of metabolism or disorders involving a generalized alteration in a structural protein. Finally, a mutation may alter both the functional properties and the antigenicity of the product.

Errors in the genetic code also occur in the form of deletions of base pairs. Such errors result either in a "frameshift" of the code, if one or two bases are deleted, or in the deletion of an amino acid, if the deletion involves an entire triplet codon.

The human hemoglobins are replete with examples of each of these types of errors. Point mutations account for hemoglobins S, C, and E; frame-shifts for hemoglobins Tak, Wayne, and Cranston; and triplet deletions for hemoglobins Freiburg, Tochigi, Leiden, Lyon, and Tours. Elongation of the hemoglobin chain because of an error in the termination sequence accounts for hemoglobin Constant Spring and others.

MENDEL'S LAWS AND THE MEIOTIC PROCESS. During interphase the human genome is dispersed throughout the nucleus. During mitosis and meiosis the genome becomes recognizable as 22 distinct and identifiable chromosome pairs called autosomes and two sex chromosomes—XX in females and XY in males. These 46 chromosomes each contain hundreds or thousands of gene loci. The corresponding genes on two homologous (like) chromosomes are called alleles. If the two alleles are identical, they are said to be homozygous; if they are not alike, they are termed heterozygous alleles. Chromosomal behavior during meiosis explains the observations of Mendel that resulted in his laws of segregation and independent assortment. Further knowledge of chromosomal structure and behavior also explains apparent exceptions to these laws.

Each gamete contributes a haploid (n = 23) set of chromosomes to the zygote. This reduction of the chromosome number from the somatic diploid (2n) number of 46 is achieved by the process of meiosis. The meiotic process is preceded by a replication of the entire genome. Each chromosome is composed of two chromatids (sister chromatids), which in turn are each a single DNA, double helical structure. During the early stages of meiosis the DNA-protein threads condense, become visible, and align themselves into pairs of homologous chromosomes. This "synaptonemal complex" is thus composed of four chromatids (two homologous pairs of sister chromatids). They further condense, and exchanges of segments of DNA between homologous but *nonsister* chromatids take place. This is called chiasma formation. This process allows for crossing-over of DNA segments and further variation in the inheritance of combinations of genetic traits. By the end of the first meiotic division the paired chromosomes are aligned along the metaphase plate, chiasmata have disappeared, and one member of each pair of homologous chromosomes segregates randomly into one or the other of two daughter nuclei. The second meiotic division is a further division of each segregated chromosome without further replication of DNA. Thus each of four daughter nuclei receives a haploid set of chromosomes that have twice segregated at random into daughter nuclei. This process explains Mendel's law of segregation; that is, a parent transmits one and only one allele for a given trait via the germ cell to the offspring.

Mendel's law of independent assortment relies on the genes for traits studied being discontinuous and located on different chromosomes or very far apart on the same chromosome. Thus, when following the transmission of two or more such traits, the offspring will manifest combinations of traits in predictable ratios based on random segregation of chromosomes. The obvious exception to this law involves two traits, the loci for which are located close together on the same chromosome and are said to be "linked." The genes at such loci will not assort independently as predicted but at some other ratio that is nonetheless predictable on the basis of their distance apart on the chromosome (map unit distance). The closer two loci are, the more often they may be predicted to segregate together, and the farther apart they are, the more often they will be separated during the process of crossing-over. The assortment ratios of linked loci will not reach the randomness observed between unlinked genes.

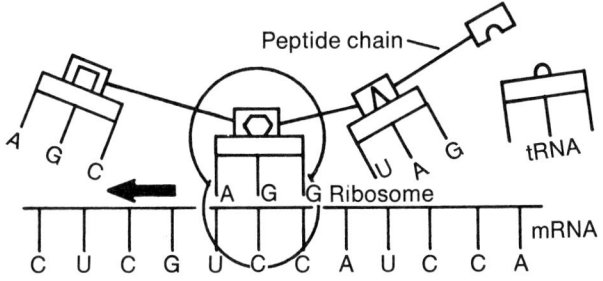

Fig. 194-2. Protein synthesis: mRNA chain is attached to ribosome in cytoplasm where amino acid—tRNA complexes are assembled as corresponding triplet is positioned at assembly sites. Peptide bond is formed between amino acids, tRNA separates from chian of amino acids, and protein molecule is released into cytoplasm. *A,* adenine; *G,* guanine; *C,* ctyosine; *U,* uracil.

Table 194-2. Mating possibilities: autosomal dominant (A) and recessive (a) allelic pairs

Mating type	Parental genotypes	Gametes	Genotypes of offspring
1	AA × AA	All A × all A	All AA
2	AA × Aa	All A × 1A:1a	1AA:1Aa
3	AA × aa	All A × all a	All Aa
4	Aa × Aa	1A:1a × 1A:1a	1AA:2Aa:1aa
5	Aa × aa	1A:1a × all a	1Aa:1aa
6	aa × aa	All a × all a	All aa

AUTOSOMAL DOMINANT INHERITANCE. The genotype of an individual is the composition of alleles at a given locus. One may or may not be able to ascertain this directly in the laboratory. In the case of hemoglobin it is possible to separate the products of each allele during hemoglobin electrophoresis and to know the genotype. If such precise determination cannot be made, we rely on other manifestations of gene expression. An individual's phenotype may be ascertained by enzyme activity, physical appearance, or a measure of some other biologic function. If an individual is heterozygous at a given locus, that trait manifesting itself phenotypically is said to be the dominant trait. The alternative allele is termed recessive. Only one allele for a dominant trait need be present for an individual to manifest that phenotype. For many dominant traits one cannot tell by examining the individual's phenotype whether they are homozygous or heterozygous at the locus.

For matings involving a given dominant trait, A, in one or both parents, five possibilities exist (mating types 1 to 5, Table 194-2). If dominant trait A is extremely common, most matings will be of genotypes 1 and 2. If, however, A is rare, most will be of type 5. If for some reason dominant trait A, although rare, results in a phenotype that causes mates to be attracted to each other, matings of types 1, 2, or 4 may be most frequent.

Autosomal dominant inheritance (the gene is located on 1 of the 22 autosomal pairs) is characterized by two additional features: males and females express the trait equally, and male-to-male transmission may be observed.

AUTOSOMAL RECESSIVE INHERITANCE. A recessive allele for a given characteristic segregates in the same manner as does a dominant allele. For a recessive allele to manifest itself fully, however, an individual is nearly always homozygous for the allele. Whereas physical examination may not reveal the heterozygous state of a recessive allele, some measure of biochemical activity may uncover a difference between either of the homozygous states (AA or aa) and the heterozygote, Aa, which is *phenotypically* indistinguishable from AA.*

---

*One can argue with the application of the word "phenotype." In general it has come to mean the physical and mental status of an individual determined by the usual means of examination and some laboratory aids. As more sophisticated means of examination become readily available, the definition of the word may change.

Most abnormal recessive genes are rare in the population, although all persons carry a certain number of them. While estimates vary, it is believed that we all carry one or two recessive alleles (in the heterozygous state) for traits that are lethal in the homozygous state. It is also thought that we all may carry another five or six that, when present in the double dose, are in some way deleterious to our well-being or reduce the "perfect functioning" of some body part or system. Although our knowledge is limited, it appears that genes that manifest as abnormal in the homozygous state (abnormal recessive genes), are genetic messages for enzymes or subunits of enzymes and that the *normal* message for an enzyme is most often the dominant allele. On the other hand, *abnormal* dominant alleles appear to involve structural proteins, which may account for the greater likelihood of an abnormal dominant gene being manifest in the heterozygous state as opposed to requiring laboratory aids. (There are, of course, exceptions to these generalizations.)

Matings involving the presence of a recessive allele, a, in one or both parents are shown in Table 194-2, matings 2 to 6. If the recessive allele is common, most matings will be of type 4, 5, or 6. If the recessive allele is lethal in the homozygous state, there will be virtually no matings of types 3, 5, and 6, and few (depending on the frequency of the gene in the population) of type 4; most matings involving a rare recessive gene will be of type 2.

PSEUDODOMINANCE. The inheritance of recessive gene (a) may be difficult to distinguish from dominant inheritance when it appears in both parent and child, as in matings 5 and 6. In the case of rare recessive genes, this may occur when a homozygous recessive individual mates with a relative who is a carrier of the same gene—mating 5. The resultant transmission from parent to child in this case is called pseudodominance.

HARDY-WEINBERG LAW. If the population incidence of the homozygous state for a recessive trait or disease is known, the frequency of carriers (heterozygotes) can be determined by applying the Hardy-Weinberg law. For any two alleles at a given locus, the frequency of genotypes AA, Aa, and aa will be equal to p^2, $2pq$, and q^2, respectively, where $p^2 + 2pq + q^2 = 1$, p equals the frequency of A and q equals the frequency of a in that population, and $p + q = 1$.

X-LINKED INHERITANCE. Just as the autosomes segregate randomly into daughter nuclei, so do the sex chromosomes. However, unlike gene pairs located on autosomes, genes located on the X chromosome will have two alleles in the 46,XX female and only one in the 46,XY male. There are not believed to be identical loci on the X and Y chromosomes. The male is said to be hemizygous for the locus, whereas a female may be homozygous or heterozygous. Because there is only one set of X chromosome loci in the male, his phenotype will behave as though he were homozygous for the alleles present on his X chromosome. Unlike autosomal inheritance, there will be a sex distribu-

Table 194-3. Mating possibilities: X-linked dominant (B) and recessive (b) allelic pairs

Mating type	Parental genotypes		Gametes		Genotypes of offspring	
	m	f	m	f	m	f
1	X^BY ×	X^BX^B	$1X^B:1Y$ ×	all X^B	All X^BY	All X^BX^B
2	X^BY ×	X^BX^b	$1X^B:1Y$ ×	$1X^B:1X^b$	$1X^BY:1X^bY$	$1X^BX^B:1X^BX^b$
3	X^BY ×	X^bX^b	$1X^B:1Y$ ×	all X^b	All X^bY	All X^BX^b
4	X^bY ×	X^BX^B	$1X^b:1Y$ ×	all X^B	All X^BY	All X^BX^b
5	X^bY ×	X^BX^b	$1X^b:1Y$ ×	$1X^B:1X^b$	$1X^BY:1X^bY$	$1X^BX^b:1X^bX^b$
6	X^bY ×	X^bX^b	$1X^b:1Y$ ×	all X^b	All X^bY	All X^bX^b

tion difference among the phenotypes for a given trait. Mating possibilities for dominant (B) and recessive (b) X-linked genes are given in Table 194-3.

It can be seen that if the *recessive* allele is lethal, there will be no matings of types 3, 4, 5, and 6, since females who are homozygous will be eliminated (3 and 6), as will hemizygous males (4, 5, and 6). Heterozygous females, however, will in general be phenotypically normal, and matings of types 1 and 2 will be most common.

On the other hand, if the *dominant* allele is lethal, the only mating that may occur is type 6.

If the X-linked trait in question is dominant but lethal only in the hemizygous X^BY or homozygous X^BX^B state, mating of types 1 to 4 will not occur and only matings of 5 and 6 will be seen. The heterozygous female for such a gene may or may not be phenotypically detectable.

LYON HYPOTHESIS. At about 16 days of gestational age in female embryos, a process known as random inactivation of the X chromosome occurs. On the average the X chromosome of maternal origin is inactivated in 50% of the cells.* This inactivated X chromosome can be detected in the interphase nucleus as a clump of darkly staining chromatin known as a Barr body. In most circumstances all but one X chromosome in a given cell are inactivated, and the total number of X chromosomes equals one plus the number of Barr bodies. Once either the maternal or paternal X chromosome is inactivated in a given nucleus, all daughter cells derived from that cell will have the same X chromosome inactivated. Since inactivation is a random process, the actual distribution of inactivated maternal and paternal X chromosomes fits a standard distribution curve such that there will be a few females at either end of the curve in whom a greater percentage of one or the other X chromosomes remains active. This is one explanation for a few heterozygous females manifesting an X-linked recessive trait. Two other explanations for such manifestation are homozygosity at the locus, such as may result from matings 4 or 6, and the presence of only one X chromosome in females with karyotypes 45,XO, who would behave at that locus as hemizygous males.

The key difference between X-linked inheritance and autosomal inheritance is the failure of father-to-son transmission in the case of X-linked traits. It may appear to have been transmitted from father to son if the mother is heterozygous at the locus for which the father is hemizygous, and the mother is phenotypically normal, whereas the father is not.

Y-LINKED (HOLANDRIC) INHERITANCE. There are undoubtedly genes on the Y chromosome that could be transmitted from father to son. Investigation into the presence of the HY antigen and a testis determining factor (Tdf) is now underway. The role of this or other male determining genes in sexual differentiation is not fully understood.

VARIABLE EXPRESSIVITY, INCOMPLETE PENETRANCE, AND AGE OF EXPRESSION. It must be remembered that the ability to detect the presence of a given gene depends on the availability of specific biochemical assays and the knowledge of the total spectrum of the gene's expression. The term "variable expressivity" refers to the phenomenon whereby a presumably identical gene possessed by two individuals is accompanied by apparently different manifestations. This is common among autosomal dominant genes. A grandparent and grandchild may clearly possess a certain dominant gene, yet the intervening parent (who must have transmitted the gene from parent to child) may show only some features of the trait or genetic disorder. If we are totally unable to detect evidence for the gene's expression in such an individual, or if this obligate person has not reached or did not live until the *age of expression* for the trait, the gene is said to demonstrate *incomplete penetrance*. As more is learned about genetic diseases and traits, previous cases of incomplete penetrance may be reclassified as new variation in expressivity.

MULTIPLE ALLELES. Thus far only two alternative alleles at any given locus have been considered. On occasion a locus will have multiple alleles. In that case the number of genotypes and phenotypes will depend on the number of different alleles and their respective dominance or recessivity. An example of this would be the locus for the ABO blood group in human beings where there are three possible alleles, which are of course only present two at a time.

CODOMINANCE. Codominance refers to the equal expression of two alleles at a given locus, whether they

---

*There is now evidence that a small portion of both X chromosomes is never inactivated.

are present in the homozygous or heterozygous state. In some cases this depends on the method of observation. The MN blood groups are the classic examples of codominance. When parents of types M and N are mated, their children may be M, N, or MN when studied immunologically. Electrophoretically, hemoglobins A and S (sickle cell hemoglobin) are codominant. Phenotypically, A is dominant and S recessive, since the homozygous SS genotype is required for a person to have sickle cell anemia. On the other hand, in the laboratory the S gene may be made to express itself in the heterozygous (AS) individual's blood cells (sickle cell trait). Under such conditions S acts as the dominant allele. The conditions under which observations have been made must always be considered when investigating the mode of inheritance of a given characteristic.

Chromosome structure and abnormalities

STRUCTURE AND NOMENCLATURE. The human chromosome complement is discussed and described as the chromosomes appear during or close to the metaphase portion of the mitotic process. It is at this time that the 22 autosomal pairs and two sex chromosomes are condensed and consist of two chromatids joined together at a dense construction known as the centromere (Fig. 194-3). Each chromosome consists of a short arm (p) and long arm (q).

By convention (Paris Conference, 1971) they are oriented with the short arm above and the long arm below the centromere, from largest to smallest, and grouped according to the relative lengths of the long and short arms.

Chromosomes 1, 2, and 3 belong to the A group, are the largest, and are *metacentric;* that is, the long and short arms are nearly equal in length. Chromosomes 4 and 5 (B group) are *submetacentric,* with the short arms easily recognizable. The C group consists of chromosomes 6 to 12 and the X chromosome. Before 1971 and the application of staining techniques that gave each chromosome a characteristic banding pattern, it was difficult to distinguish one since the C group are metacentric or submetacentric and larger than the *acrocentric* D group. This latter group consists of three chromosomes that often appear to have only a long arm and centromere. There may be a short arm of varying staining quality and additional polymorphic variants known as satellites. These structures are connected to the short arms of the acrocentric chromosomes by threadlike stalks of varying length. Satellites are singular or double and stain with varying intensity from person to person. The E (16 to 18) and F (19 to 20) groups of chromosomes are quite small but can be easily distinguished by their size, centromere location, and banding patterns. Chromosomes 21 and 22 (G group) are the smallest acrocentrics and like the D group may possess short arm and satellite

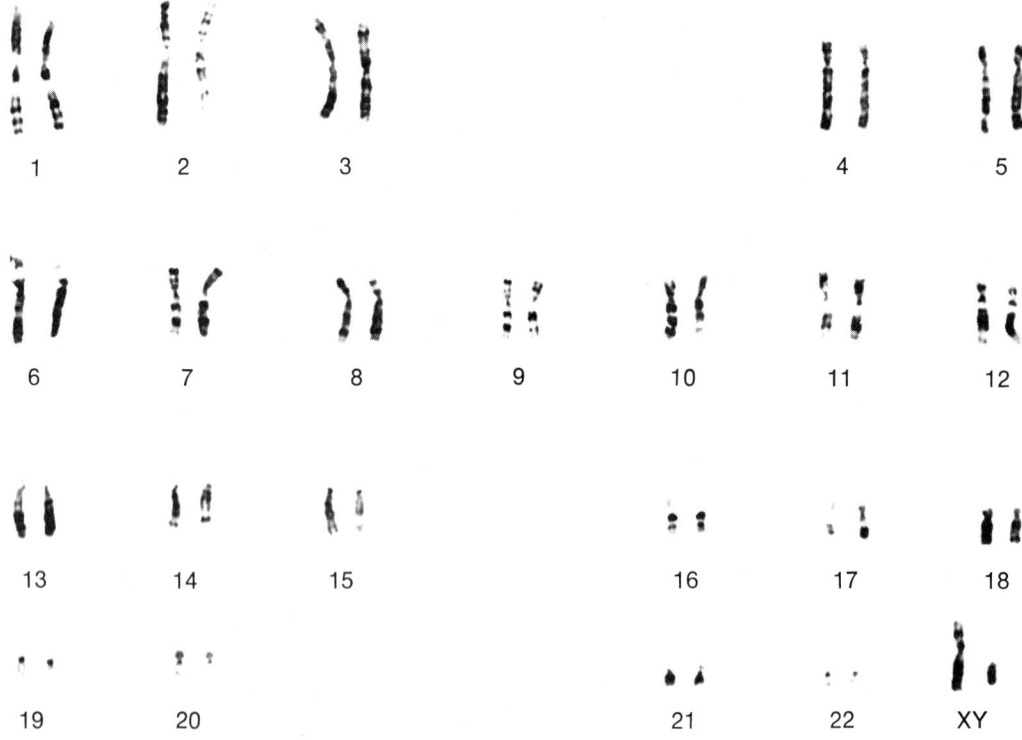

Fig. 194-3. Giemsa-banded male karyotype. Chromosomes are arranged in pairs from largest to smallest. Centromeres are positioned on drawn lines. *Metacentric* chromosomes have nearly equal long (q) and short (p) arms. The difference in length between q and p arms in *submetacentric* chromosomes is easily seen on inspection. In *acrocentric* chromosomes, there may be no p arm or only a very small one.

variants. The Y chromosome is often grouped with the G group based on size. It is, however, easily distinguishable from them by the more densely stained long arm and the more nearly parallel alignment of the long arms. Q-banding (discussed in the following) stains the Y chromosome a bright fluorescence, which is not shared with any other chromosome.

STAINING OF CHROMOSOMES. Chromosome preparations may be made from virtually any actively dividing cell line. Most commonly, peripheral blood, skin biopsies, bone marrow, and amniotic fluid fetal cells are used. The cells are allowed to grow and divide until a sufficient quantity are available for analysis. The time required to achieve this number is approximately 72 hours in the case of peripheral blood and 2 to 3 weeks in the case of fibroblast cultures derived from a skin biopsy or amniotic fluid aspirate. Bone marrow cells are already actively dividing cells. The culture is then treated with Colcemid for varying periods of time to halt the mitotic process at metaphase. Cells are then subjected to hypotonic treatment and fixation and dropped onto slides for staining.

With the introduction of a method for *consistently* reproducing a pattern of light and dark areas on chromosomes by Caspersson and Zech in 1968, it became necessary to standardize the nomenclature used in designating these areas (Fig. 194-4). Periodically, cytogeneticists update the first standardization, which was constructed during the Paris Conference in 1971. In general a routine preparation of banded metaphase chromosomes will not clearly show every band identified in the ideal preparation. A number of staining techniques have been devised that can be used to highlight areas of chromosomes not easily examined by the other techniques.

ABNORMALITIES. Abnormalities of the human chromosome complement involve either the number or the structure of chromosomes (Table 194-4).

The human karyotype is designated 46,XX or 46,XY. Chromosome number is followed by the sex chromosome complement, which is then followed by the appropriate designation for any variants or abnormalities. Errors in the *number* of chromosomes are either *aneuploidy* or *polyploidy*. Aneuploidy usually involves only one, but sometimes two, chromosomes that may be either missing (monosomy) or present in additional numbers (trisomy, tetrasomy, and so on). Aneuploidy may arise during meiosis in either the ovum or the sperm. Meiotic nondisjunction refers to the failure of a chromosome pair to segregate into daughter cells, with both members remaining in one cell and no member of the pair entering the second. In most cases the only surviving gamete will be that one with the extra chromosome. The fertilized product of a normal gamete and one that has had a nondisjunctional event is then said to be trisomic for the chromosome involved, such as trisomy 21. It is written 47,XX (or XY), +21. If both chromosomes 21 and 18 failed to segregate, the product would be 48,XX (or XY), +18,+21.

If nondisjunction occurs some time after fertilization or during mitosis, the result may be mosaicism for two or more cell lines, depending on the ability of the abnormal cell lines to reproduce. The karyotype may then appear 46,XX/47,XX,+21, indicating a female with two cell lines, one of which is trisomic for chromosome 21.

Nondisjunction may also involve the sex chromosomes. Resulting karyotypes may be 45,XO; 47,XXY; 47,XYY; and 47,XXX or mosaicism such as 45,XO/46,XX and 45,XO/46,XX/47,XXX.

Polyploidy refers to the presence of additional haploid (n) sets of chromosomes. There are 69 chromosomes in a triploid and 92 in a tetraploid cell. This may arise by retention of a polar body during meiosis (triploidy) or by failure of separation of dividing chromosomes into two separate nuclear membranes (tetraploidy.)

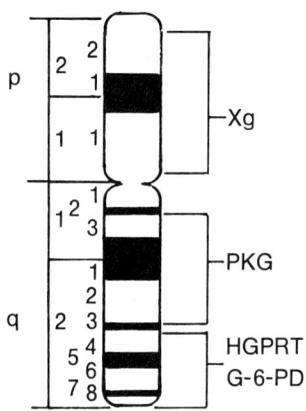

Fig. 194-4. Idealized banding pattern for X chromosome. Long, *q*, and short, *p*, arms are divided into large regions *1* and *2* by largest dark bands. Some longer chromosomes have three such regions. Both light and dark bands within each region are numbered consecutively from centromere distally. This system allows room for further band identification. A band is then designated by a notation including arm *(p* or *q)*, region *(1, 2, or 3)*, and band number (such as p 12, q 24). Notation to right indicates regional localization of loci for *Xg*, and enzymes *PGK, HGPRT*, and *G-6-PD*. Over 100 loci have been mapped to X chromosome.

Table 194-4. Chromosomal abnormalities

Type	Manifestations
Abnormalities of number	Aneuploidy—trisomy, monosomy, tetrasomy
	Mosaicism
	Fragments
	Polyploidy—triploid, tetraploid
Structural abnormalities	Deletions
	Inversions—paracentric, pericentric
	Rings
	Translocations (balanced or unbalanced)—robertsonian, reciprocal
	Isochromosomes—short arm, long arm

The most common *structural aberrations* of chromosomes are those involving one or more breaks on a single chromosome (deletions, inversions, rings, isochromosomes) and those involving breaks and/or fusions on two different chromosomes.

Deletions of a portion of a chromosome result from either one break, in which case the entire segment distal to the break is lost, or two breaks, in which case the proximal and distal chromosome parts may rejoin. In either case the cell is then monosomic for the lost fragment. If two breaks occur and the intervening segment is reversed in direction and rejoins at the breakpoints, an *inversion* results. If the breaks are both on the same side of the centromere, the inversion is paracentric. If the centromere is between the breakpoints, it is a pericentric inversion. In such aberrations one is usually unable to detect any deleted chromosome material. If two breaks occur near the ends of the long and short arms of a chromosome, the two deleted ends may join to form a *ring* chromosome. The amount of deleted material depends on the sites of the breaks, but it will involve the most distal ends of the chromosomes. Finally, if there is a horizontal break through the centromere of a chromosome, an *isochromosome* may form. One (rarely both) of the resulting fragments retains a functional amount of the centromere. The new structure will then consist of either two short arms or two long arms and is termed an isochromosome. The resulting nucleus will be trisomic for the remaining arm and monosomic for the lost arm.

Translocations between chromosomes may be either balanced, with no apparent loss of chromosome material, or unbalanced, in which there is deleted or trisomic material. Translocations resulting from the attachment of two acrocentric (13 to 15, 21 and 22) chromosomes at or near the centromere are termed robertsonian translocations, and those involving any other chromosome segments are termed reciprocal. The designation 45,XY,rob(14q21q) indicates that there are only 45 different structures in this male karyotype and that there has been a fusion of the long arms of chromosomes 14 and 21 without identifiable loss of chromosome material. (One assumes, however, that there is some loss of material in all rearrangements involving breaks. In many cases it appears to be clinically insignificant.) If a sperm from the "translocation carrier" contains the translocated chromosome (14q21q) as well as the paternal chromosome 21 and fertilizes an egg containing one 21 and one 14, the result is an unbalanced translocation and would be designated 46,XX, −14, +rob(14q21q). The zygote is trisomic for chromosome 21.

When fragments of chromosome arms are translocated, the karyotype nomenclature usually designates at what bands the breaks are thought to have occurred. For example, the karyotype 46,XY,rcp(3;13)(p24;q31) indicates that this is a male karyotype with a balanced reciprocal translocation. It arose when a fragment resulting from a break on the short arm (p) of chromosome 3 at band 24 attached to the long arm (q) of chromosome 13 at breakpoint 31, and the fragment of chromosome 13 from band q31 to the end of the long arm attached to breakpoint p24 of chromosome 3. As in the case of robertsonian translocations, such "balanced carriers" may form germ cells with "unbalanced" contents. The zygote may be normal, a balanced carrier, or an unbalanced carrier, being either trisomic for 3p beyond point 24 and monosomic for 13q beyond point 31, or monosomic for the 3p and trisomic for the 13q fragments.

Chromosome fragments resulting from a single break near the end of a chromosome arm are usually lost to subsequent generations of cells. However, the consistent presence of fragments has been reported in both normal and abnormal individuals. Occasionally, gaps and breaks without loss of material are found in preparations of human chromosomes. They may be related to inherent chromosome instability or the effects of drugs. The significance of such findings is under investigation. Several disorders have been described that are associated with increased chromosome instability. These are Bloom's syndrome, ataxia-telangiectasia, and Fanconi's anemia, which are quite dissimilar in their clinical picture. The highest degree of instability is seen in Bloom's syndrome, in which there is a 30% incidence of lymphoproliferative disease.

Multifactorial inheritance

Early eugenicists failed to outline the single gene mode of inheritance, undoubtedly because they selected traits that are not only determined by a number of different genes, or *polygenic,* but by nongenetic factors as well, or *multifactorial*. Most common traits of man, as well as a few common birth defects (congenital heart disease, dislocated hip, and cleft lip/palate) are inherited in this manner. It is supposed that everyone possesses a certain liability (number of genes) for a given multifactorial characteristic. An individual's liability may exceed the threshold beyond which the trait becomes evident, either on the basis of the number of genes alone or because some other factor (radiation, drug, virus, and so on) has pushed his liability beyond the threshold. Such traits are heritable, but to a lesser degree than traits determined by single genes. First-degree relatives of an only affected individual will share the trait 3% to 5% of the time. Unlike single gene inheritance, the greater the number of related individuals who share the trait, the greater is any other relative's liability over that of the general population. This liability depends on the number of relatives affected and their relationship to the person in question. Other factors are of varying importance for different multifactorial traits or disorders. For example, neural tube defects (spina bifida/anencephaly) have a higher incidence in populations of the British Isles than those of North America, cleft lip/palate is seen more frequently among Orientals than other groups, congenital dislocation of the hip affects females more often than males, and pyloric stenosis affects more males than females. For these latter two examples, if the proband is of the least often affected sex, his or her relatives are at a greater liability than if the proband is of the sex most often affected. Tables based on empiric data have been constructed for many of the traits and disorders and should be consulted on an individual basis.

CLINICAL GENETICS

Diagnosis of genetic disease requires an appreciation of the etiologic heterogeneity of seemingly similar disorders. Without this, errors in diagnosis may lead to erroneous counseling regarding prognosis, recurrence risks, and available therapeutic and reproductive options. Allowing an individual or family to be guided through the decision-making process with an accurate data base and assisting them in implementing *their* decision should be the goal of the genetic counseling team. As more individuals are trained in this process, genetic counseling will become a routine component in the practice of the medical arts.

Pedigree construction and analysis

The purposes of constructing the family history are (1) to determine the pattern of inheritance of a given trait of disease within any given family, *despite* the diagnosis; (2) to use the pattern of inheritance to narrow diagnostic possibilities; and (3) to determine other individuals at risk among extended family members.

The pedigree is constructed using the symbols depicted in Fig. 194-5. The individual who has come to attention is known as the proband and those seeking information are the consultands. The proband may or may not be the consultant. The sexes and ages of siblings, parents, grandparents, aunts, uncles, and cousins are indicated in the pedigree. If a pattern of abnormalities emerges from this investigation, it should be extended through appropriate family lines. Authors of a pedigree may designate affected individuals by their own symbols, although a few conventional symbols are indicated in the figure. Additional information includes occurrence of unexplained infertility, early childhood deaths, stillbirths, and miscarriages.

Often, simple examination of the pedigree will reveal a pattern of inheritance. It cannot be too strongly emphasized that all aspects of the condition in question must be considered before providing definitive information to the patient and family. Most common genetic disorders have been well described and their patterns of inheritance established; however, in any given family the possibility of a new variant, a previously unrecognized mode of inheritance of a given disorder, or nongenetic factors resulting in a phenocopy of a genetic disorder may be discovered.

CONSANGUINITY. Matings involving related individuals are termed consanguineous and are of particular interest when dealing with rare autosomal recessive diseases. You will recall that everyone "carries" at least one or two rare recessive "lethal" genes. These genes are derived from hundreds of possibilities, and the chance of any two unrelated individuals being carriers of the same recessive gene (heterozygotes) is the square of the frequency of carriers in the population. For even the most common of such genes, cystic fibrosis (CF), where the carrier frequency is 1 in 20 in the Caucasian population, the chance that two randomly mated persons share the CF gene is $(1/20)^2$, or $1/400$, and the chance that any random couple will have a child with CF is $1/400 \times 1/4 = 1/1600$. If two individuals are closely related and it is known that a common ancestor carries a specific recessive gene either through carrier testing or birth of an affected child, the related couple will be at a predictable increased risk of both being carriers. In the mating depicted in Fig. 194-6, first cousins whose grand-

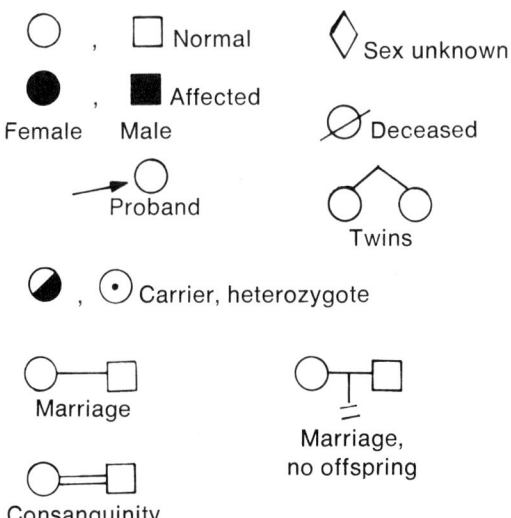

Fig.194-5. Pedigree symbols.

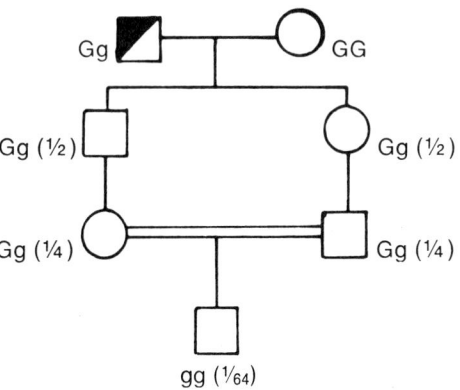

Fig. 194-6. Common grandfather in first-cousin mating is known to be heterozygote for recessive gene g. Mating is at 1/64 risk of producing child homozygous gg.

Table 194-5. Inbreeding coefficients of consanguineous matings

Mating	Inbreeding coefficient
Parent-child	1/4
Sibling-sibling	1/4
Uncle-niece	1/8
First cousin	1/16
Second cousin	1/64
First cousin once removed	1/32

father is known to be a carrier of a recessive lethal gene, g, each have a ¼ chance of also carrying the gene, and there is a 1/16 chance of both being carriers. Any given pregnancy is therefore at a (1/16 × ¼) = 1/64 risk of being homozygous for that gene, gg. The kinship coefficient of this mating is 1/16. The inbreeding coefficient of the offspring is the same, 1/16. The inbreeding coefficient of any product of a consanguineous union is the probability that two alleles at a given locus are identical by virtue of descent. Inbreeding coefficients for the most commonly encountered consanguineous matings are listed in Table 194-5. In Fig. 194-7 both common grandparents are assumed to be heterozygotes for the recessive gene, g, because of the birth of an affected child. The siblings of this child, who are themselves unaffected, have a ⅔ chance of being heterozygotes (two of the remaining three possibilities once the homozygous affected state is excluded). If there is no further consanguinity, the chance that both first cousins are heterozygotes is therefore (⅔ × ½)(⅔ × ½) = 1/9, and their risk of having an affected child is (1/9 × ¼) = 1/36.

Such calculations are necessary only when there is no means of carrier detection. If the diagnosis of an affected family member is known, it may be possible to determine the heterozygote state among unaffected relatives. It is always important to include carrier testing of the "obligate" heterozygotes in the family to eliminate the possibility of an unusual biochemical variant that may not be detected by the usual means.

ETHNICITY. The family history should also include information with regard to the ethnic origins of ancestors. There are now a number of genetic disorders known to occur in higher frequency among certain populations. An abbreviated list is found in Table 194-6. Such information is important both in searching for prospective disorders, especially when dealing with consanguineous matings, as well as in establishing diagnostic possibilities in individuals with rare diseases. Determination of such high-risk populations is also useful in implementing heterozygote detection programs. The prototype of such programs is the Tay-Sachs Disease–Carrier Screening Program. The desir-

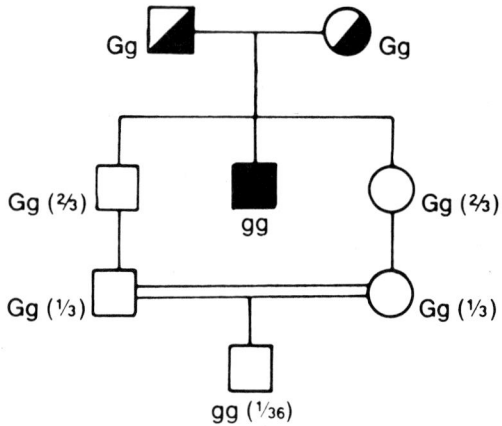

Fig. 194-7. Both common grandparents to first-cousin mating are known to be heterozygotes for g by virtue of affected child with gg genotype. Mating is at 1/36 risk of producing child homozygous gg.

Table 194-6. Genetic diseases demonstrating ethnic differences in frequency

Genetic disorder	Ethnic group with relatively high frequency
β-Thalassemia	Italians, Greeks
α-Thalassemia	Chinese
Adrenal hyperplasia	Eskimos
Tay-Sachs disease	Jews (Ashkenazi)
Familial dysautonomia	Jews (Ashkenazi)
Aspartyglycosaminuria	Finns
Neural tube defects	Irish

able criteria for such programs are met in this disease in the following ways:

1. An identifiable population is at high risk. Individuals of Eastern European (Ashkenazi) Jewish descent have a heterozygote frequency of approximately 1/27, compared to non-Ashkenazi Jews with a carrier frequency of 1/300.
2. Carrier detection is possible. The biochemical defect resulting in this lethal neurodegenerative disease is known to be a deficiency of the enzyme hexosaminidase A. Detection of the enzyme's activity may be performed on a blood sample or fibroblast cultures. Heterozygotes will demonstrate approximately 50% of normal activity.
3. Prenatal diagnosis is available via amniocentesis.

The ultimate fourth criterion, treatment, is not yet possible for this disease.

Clinical cytogenetic disorders

Generally, aberrations in the amount of chromosome material are associated with malformation syndromes of

Table 194-7. Incidence of chromosome abnormalities among live-born infants

Abnormality	Incidence
Trisomy 21	1:660
Trisomy 13	1:7000
Trisomy 18	1:7000
47,XXY	1:700 (males)
45,XO	1:2500-1:5000 (females)
47,XYY	1:700 (males)
47,XXX	1:2000-1:4000 (females)

varying complexity. Typically, chromosome abnormalities result in physical defects of many body parts, such that mental retardation, growth delay, congenital heart disease, renal abnormalities, and variations of development of ears, nose, fingers, and so on are noted with increased frequency in nearly every syndrome. Additionally, there are endless possibilities for deletions and trisomies such that it is practical to mention only the most commonly occurring (Table 194-7).

TRISOMY 21 (DOWN'S SYNDROME). Trisomy 21 is the most frequent autosomal trisomy among children, occurring in 1 in every 600 to 700 live births. Ninety-five percent of cases result from nondisjunction, whereas the other 5% are divided between mosaics and unbalanced translocations. Neonates with Down's syndrome may be recognized by a characteristic facial appearance consisting of flattened facial profile, flat nasal bridge, creases over the inner canthi of the eyes (epicanthal folds), small, low-set ears, increased folds of skin at the nape of the neck, hypoplastic irides (Brushfield's spots), hypotonia, and microcephaly. There may also be a single palmar crease, hypoplasia of the midphalanx of the fifth digit with an incurving of the fifth finger (clinodactyly), congenital heart disease (40%), and duodenal atresia (25%). There is an increased risk of childhood leukemia, and life expectancy is generally reduced depending on accompanying medical problems. Recurrent ear infections, as well as a probable congenital sensorineural hearing loss, result in hearing deficits.

There is an increased incidence of Down's syndrome and other aneuploidies with advanced maternal age. However, *all* infants with Down's syndrome should be karyotyped to rule out the possibility of translocation, in which case other family members (parents first, followed by others as necessary) should be studied. The recurrence risk for a chromosomally abnormal child after the birth of the first is 0.5% to 1% in the case of nondisjunction and may be 10% to 15% in the case of familial robertsonian translocations. If a parent is a carrier of a balanced translocation involving both chromosomes 21, the risk of recurrence for trisomy 21 is 100%. (The only gametes such a parent can produce have either no chromosome 21 or the translocation 21/21.)

TRISOMY 13 AND TRISOMY 18. Both trisomy 13 and 18 result in children with much more severe malformations than those with trisomy 21. There is a high frequency of severe congenital heart disease, neurologic and mental impairment, renal abnormalities, and growth retardation. Trisomy 13 can be distinguished by the presence of microphthalmia, polydactyly, and cleft lip/palate. Although infants with trisomy 18 may have these latter abnormalities, they are less frequent. More often they demonstrate prominent heels (rocker-bottom feet), flexion deformities of the fingers, small, round heads, and fingerprints (dermatoglyphics) consisting of 10 (or a majority) simple arch patterns. Life expectancy is severely reduced to weeks or months, although a number with only mild cardiac or renal anomalies may survive longer. Again, even though a diagnosis may be clinically obvious, karyotyping should be done to confirm the diagnosis and to rule out the presence of a translocation.

As already stated, the potential exists for many other clinical cytogenetic abnormalities. In general any individual with multiple malformations, especially if mental retardation is present, deserves a chromosome analysis. Syndromes accompanied by monosomy for a portion of chromosome material are usually more devastating than trisomy for the same material. Several chromosome abnormalities are seen almost exclusively in products of spontaneous abortion. No doubt these aberrations are associated with defects so severe as to interfere with even intrauterine survival.

ABNORMALITIES OF THE SEX CHROMOSOMES. Unlike aneuploidies of the autosomes, the phenotypic features of sex chromosome abnormalities are not as generally severe. Intelligence is often (if not usually) normal, and major disturbances of development concern the gonads. Many of the changes in physiognomy are secondary to malfunctioning ovaries or testes.

The most common sex chromosome abnormalities are Klinefelter's syndrome (47,XXY), Turner's syndrome (45,XO), males with 47,XYY constitution, and 47,XXX females.

Klinefelter's syndrome. Males with an additional X chromosome will have a positive buccal smear. Phenotypically, they are characterized by tall stature, decreased development of male secondary sex characteristics, a eunuchoid habitus, mild mental retardation, gynecomastia, and hypergonadotropic hypogonadism, with testicular atrophy demonstrating tubular sclerosis and Leydig cell hyperplasia on biopsy. Klinefelter's syndrome is often not suspected until adolescence or later, when the patient may be seen with a complaint of infertility.

Turner's syndrome. Among spontaneous abortuses of 12 weeks' gestation or less, 15% of chromosome abnormalities are 45,XO. This is indeed intriguing, since survivors with Turner's syndrome are certainly not severely physically nor mentally impaired. The phenotypic features of live-born girls with Turner's syndrome are lymphedema of hands and feet at birth (which later resolves), short stature in childhood and adolescence, and failure of development of secondary sex characteristics, with ovarian dysgenesis and usually infertility. Girls are also described as having a broad, "webbed" neck, an increased carrying angle of the arms (cubitus valgus), the appearance of widely spaced nipples and a "shield chest," multiple-pigmented nevi, and hyperconvex fingernails. Intellectually, girls with Turner's syndrome may exhibit a perceptual handicap but are not mentally retarded as a part of the syndrome. Coarctation of the aorta is seen in approximately 15%. It is interesting to speculate that the females known to have Turner's syndrome actually manifest a mild form of the more usual phenotype, which is so severe that it accounts for the large number of 45,XO karyotypes among abortuses. Such fetuses have been shown to have severe lymphedema, cystic hygromas, and hypoplastic left-heart syndrome, which is incompatible with life.

Mosaicism is common among girls with Turner's syndrome. The physical and developmental features vary depending on the exact chromosome constitution. Mosaics may be 45,XO/46,XX; 45,XO/46XX$_{iq}$; 45,XO/46XX$_{ip}$; and 45,XO/46,XY. A mosaic karyotype containing a 46,XY cell line is of particular importance. Dysgenetic gonads containing an XY cell line should be removed because of the high frequency of malignancy. Fertility has been reported in mosaics and rarely in a few females in whom only a 45,XO cell line could be detected.

Females with Turner's syndrome may be expected to attain an adult height of approximately 4 feet 10 inches. Hormonal replacement is begun sometime during the adolescent years. Timing of such therapy depends on both physical and psychologic parameters; however, discussion of the need for such therapy should begin with the parents during the early years.

XYY males and XXX females. The XYY male was originally detected among a group of incarcerated men and unfortunately came to be associated with a picture of a tall, aggressive, retarded male with severe acne. In fact, this karyotype is probably more common than previously appreciated and is associated with few if any physical or mental abnormalities and not with infertility.

The poly-X female may demonstrate mental deficiency (33%) and some minor dysmorphic features. XXX females may be fertile. The more X chromosomes there are in a male or female karyotype, the more severe are the physical abnormalities and the higher the incidence of mental retardation.

Single gene disorders

Those genetic diseases and variants that are inherited in the mendelian modes now number close to 3000. As it is not possible to adequately summarize all these disorders, several broad categories will be considered here. The reader is referred to more comprehensive reviews and to other chapters in this volume for further consideration.

LYSOSOMAL STORAGE DISEASE (LSD). Lysosomal enzymes (acid hydrolases) are responsible for the catabolism of various cellular materials. Their impaired function results in the accumulation of substrate within vacuoles, a process that may itself be toxic to the cell or that may result in accumulation of other cellular substances and limit cellular functioning in general. For any given enzyme deficiency, those tissues that engage in the highest rate of substrate turnover will be most severely affected by the alteration in biochemical activity, whereas other tissues will be affected to a lesser degree.

In general, lysosomal storage diseases are progressive, often fatal, and diagnosable biochemically or pathologically by the presence of stored material in characteristic configurations: myelin figures, "zebra bodies," Gaucher's cell, onionskin lesions, and so on.

AMINOACIDOPATHIES AND DISORDERS OF PURINE METABOLISM. Many of the disorders involving errors in amino acid metabolism are associated with mental retardation, seizure disorders, and failure to thrive in infancy. The nonspecificity of many of the symptoms has led to the use

Table 194-8. Signs and symptoms suggestive of some inborn errors of metabolism (all more common causes of the presenting finding must be ruled out)

Clinical sign or laboratory finding	Associated disorders
Failure to thrive	Almost all
Vomiting	Many
Diarrhea	Cystic fibrosis, galactosemia, Wolman's disease, congenital lactic acidosis
Jaundice	Galactosemia, Wolman's disease, Crigler-Najjar syndrome, carbamyl phosphate synthetase deficiency, hypothyroidism
Dislocated lens	Homocystinuria
Hypotonicity or hypertonicity	Almost all
Seizures	Amino acid disorders, glycogen storage disease
Coarse facial features	GM_1, GM_3, MPS, mucolipidosis II
Metabolic acidosis	Renal tubular acidosis, organic acid disorders
Hypoglycemia	Glycogen storage disease
Hyperammonemia	Urea cycle defects, hyperlysinemia
Thrombocytopenia	Organic acid disorders
Malodorous urine	Tyrosinemia, phenylketonuria (musty), maple syrup urine disease (maple sugar), methionine malabsorption (malts), isovaleric acidemia (cheesy)

Adapted from Burton, B.K., and Nadler, H.J.: Pediatrics **6**:398, 1978.

of the "amino acid screen" in infants and children with poorly defined illness. As astute practitioner will be able to clinically narrow the diagnostic possibilities. Table 194-8 lists the disorders to be suspected when one or more clinical signs or symptoms are particularly prominent.

Early recognition of an aminoacidopathy permits the prompt institution of an appropriate diet and in some cases the amelioration of the effects of the disorder. In addition, several aminoacidopathies are responsive to vitamin supplementation.

Phenylketonuria (PKU), the best-known disorder of amino acid metabolism, if untreated, is characterized by the development of mental retardation, seizures, eczema, and associated light pigmentation when compared to family members. PKU was the first inborn error of metabolism subjected to newborn screening attempts. Several states have now mandated the screening of every neonate for a panel of inborn errors of metabolism as well as congenital hypothyroidism. Optimally, disorders to be screened should be ascertained as early as possible and be amenable to some form of treatment.

A recently recognized problem is the case of the adult female who is no longer on a restricted diet and has a treated aminoacidopathy; most notable is PKU. During pregnancy the low phenylalanine diet must be reinstituted to prevent high levels of the amino acid crossing the placenta and affecting the fetus, even though there is very little likelihood of the fetus having the same genetic defect as the mother.

Not all of the inborn errors are necessarily manifested in infancy or childhood. Homocystinuria should be suspected in adults with dislocated lenses, early thromboembolic events, mild mental retardation, or schizophrenia. Renal calculi or disease may be present in cystinuria, hyperprolinemia, and cystinosis. An immunodeficiency state is associated with adenine deaminase deficiency and purine nucleoside phosphorylase deficiency. Hypoxanthine-guanine phosphoribosyltransferase (HGPRT) deficiency (Lesch-Nyhan syndrome) is associated with hyperuricemia, retardation, choreoathetosis, and self-destructive behavior. It is an X-linked disease.

HEMOGLOBINOPATHIES. Hemoglobin variants result from those mutations of the genetic code that have caused alterations in the amino acid sequence of one or more of the subunits of the hemoglobin molecule. The most common variants result from amino acid substitutions at a single point in the globin chain. Most of these variants have no clinical consequence and will usually only be detected if the substitution changes the electrophoretic properties of the molecule.

Clinically, five main types of hemoglobin disease are recognized: (1) unstable hemoglobins, usually owing to substitutions that affect the helical turns of the subunits, resulting in hemoglobin instability; (2) rapid hemoglobin oxidation, resulting in methemoglobinemia; (3) abnormal oxygen affinity, usually caused by inner chain substitutions; (4) sickle cell diseases, with instability of the red cell membrane; and (5) the thalassemias, in which there is diminished or absent synthesis of a hemoglobin chain. All of these mutations can be expressed in some way in the heterozygote state, although the homozygous state is required for severe clinical disease in the sickle cell anemias. Thalassemia pathology is more complex.

DISORDERS OF COAGULATION. The most common heritable disorders of coagulation are hemophilia A and B and von Willebrand's disease. Hemophilia A and B result from deficiencies of clotting factors VIII and IX, respectively, and are X linked. There is marked variability in the clinical pictures depending on the level of circulating factor. Males with up to 2% factor VIII levels are severely affected, those with 1% to 5% of normal are moderately affected, and those with 5% to 20% levels may encounter problems only with severe trauma or surgery. Because this is an X-linked gene, female carriers are subject to the effects of the Lyon hypothesis. About 70% of femal carriers have low levels of factor VIII (20% to 70% of normal) and may show mild symtoms. Unless a female has two affected sons, an affected brother and son, or an affected father, one cannot be certain that she is a carrier. An isolated case may represent a new mutation. Carrier testing is difficult and requires measurement not only of factor VIII but also of factor VIII–related antigen. These values must be plotted with well-established controls to determine the likelihood of any female being a carrier. In equivocal cases the entire family history must be analyzed and bayesian principles applied. By weighing the probabilities of various combinations of affected and unaffected relatives, a more precise "carrier" likelihood may be estimated.

Factor IX disease is similar to factor VIII deficiency in mode of inheritance and clinical manifestations. Carrier testing is less reliable than that for hemophilia A, and an in-depth family history is the best assessment of carrier probabilities.

Von Willebrand's disease is an autosomal dominant disorder in which there is an alteration in bleeding time. The von Willebrand factor is under autosomal control and serves as a substrate for an X-linked factor. Blood from a patient with hemophilia A will correct bleeding in a von Willebrand's patient; however, the reverse is not true. Diagnosis is made by demonstrating low factor VIII, decreased platelet adhesiveness, and prolonged bleeding time. An affected individual (male or female) is at 50% risk of passing the gene on to any given offspring.

Complex genetic syndromes

There are now recognized to be complex malformation syndromes inherited in an autosomal dominant, a recessive, or an X-linked manner in addition to those that result from chromosome abnormalities. The diagnosis of such syndromes is usually in the hands of the experienced dysmorphologist or clinical geneticist. Many believe it is only a matter of time before a new technique demonstrates the chromosome aberration or biochemical error responsible for these syndromes. Until then, counseling with regard to mode of inheritance must rely on data acquired from affected individuals and families.

In any given individual one defect or symptom may dominate the clinical picture. A search for other anomalies or symptoms may reveal that the dominant feature is not isolated but rather is only one component of a syndrome complex. Realizing the presence of such combinations allows the examiner to direct a search for related defects or symptoms. Accurate diagnosis is necessary to provide adequate management and counseling regarding recurrence risks.

The currently recommended terminology for patterns of morphologic defects includes the terms "sequence," "syndrome," "association," and "field defect."

A *sequence* refers to a given malformation and its secondary deformations. This term would apply, for example, to the former Pierre Robin syndrome (micrognathia and cleft palate). The primary malformation may be isolated or be accompanied by other malformations (with their secondary deformations) and therefore be part of a *malformation syndrome*. A group of anomalies (defects, primary malformations) that are thought to be pathogenetically and etiologically related is a syndrome. Syndromes are often of single gene inheritance or result from chromosome abnormalities. A few are caused by definite environmental agents such as alcohol, phenytoin, and rubella. An *association* is a nonrandom occurrence of several defects in more than one individual; however, no sequence or syndrome can be identified. For many patterns of malformation, association is a temporary designation until such time that a syndrome or sequence can be identified. A *field defect* is defined as the result of disturbed development in all or part of a morphogenic field. It differs from a sequence in that there are no disruptive forces at work and the primary defect no doubt traces back to an early germ layer.

Multifactorial disease

Most common diseases of man, as well as a few specific birth defects, of which cleft lip/palate is one, fall into the category of multifactorial inheritance. That is, the inheritance of the disease or trait is determined by the action of many genes (polygenic) interacting with a variety of environmental factors. Most traits that demonstrate continuous variation (height, weight, intelligence, and so on) in a population are multifactorial. Some seemingly discontinuous traits (one either does or does not possess the trait or the disease, such as diabetes, hypertension, or cleft lip/palate) may be considered to have a continuously distributed liability and a threshold for liability beyond which a specific trait is expressed.

The increased risk for relatives of an index case varies directly with the closeness of the relationship. In cleft lip/palate, which has a population incidence of 1:1000, first-degree relative risk is 40:1000, second-degree is 7:1000, and third-degree is 3:1000. In disorders in which there is an unequal sex distribution, relatives of the more rarely affected sex are at a greater risk. Such sex differences exist for pyloric stenosis (more males affected than females) and congenital dislocation of the hip (more females affected than males). The more severe the malformation (bilateral versus unilateral cleft lip), the greater the risk of recurrence, and the recurrence risk increases with increasing numbers of affected relatives. In general, after the birth of one affected individual, the risk for a second affected person is 3% to 5%; after two affected, 10%; and after three, 14%. It can be seen that a family with many affected individuals approaches the risks of single gene disorders (25% and 50%).

It is extremely important to eliminate the possibility that the individual possesses a complex malformation syndrome, of which the defect under consideration is only a part. Failure to do so may result in errors in counseling regarding recurrence risks or other associated features. For example, cleft lip/palate accompanied by lip pits or cysts is a dominantly inherited syndrome (van der Woude syndrome), and relatives without obvious clefts should be examined for the presence of lip pits to determine individuals at risk.

The human gene map, linkage, and association

It would appear that the clinician is investigating human genetics in very gross terms, whereas the DNA biochemists are experimenting on the smallest possible level. The final link between these two disciplines may soon be realized.

DNA sequencing, a relatively simple and elegant technique, will provide in time the exact order of nucleotide pairs on any given DNA segment. Such sequences may be known before the biochemical abnormality of a particular disease is recognized. The sequences may be able to tell us the mutation in the DNA code associated with a given disease. Until the entire DNA code can be quickly scanned for significant errors, potential error sites may be localized to specific chromosomes or parts of chromosomes by genetic linkage studies and somatic cell genetics. To date more than 150 loci have been localized to specific human autosomes, with over 100 of these pinpointed to the X chromosome. The loci may be quite biochemically specific (such as ABO blood group, various enzymes, and structural proteins) or as yet nonspecific, such as nailpatella syndrome (chromosome 9), testis determining factor (Y chromosome), and hereditary spherocytosis (chromosome 12). It is possible in a few instances to use linkage information in determining risk of disease, even though the specific biochemical abnormality of the disease in question is unknown. The genetic locus for the disease and the locus for a biochemical marker that can be measured must be closely linked. For example, the locus controlling the expression of blood types in tissues and fluids (saliva) other than blood, the secretor locus, has been used in the prenatal prediction of myotonic dystrophy (MD), an autosomal dominant disorder in which the specific metabolic error is unknown. By determining the genotypes of both parents with regard to secretor status and provided the mating is genetically informative, the secretor status of the fetus may be used to predict the likelihood of the occurrence of MD. (Informative refers to the arrangement of alleles for MD and secretor status in the parents. Ideally, the affected parent is a double heterozygote at the two loci.)

Not to be confused with linkage is association. Linkage refers to genes located on the same chromosome within some small distance of one another; association implies that there is a higher than random concurrence of a gene and a specific trait. Neither a direct causal relationship nor linkage is implied.

The HLA complex is located on chromosome 6. It can be said to be linked to the other loci on chromosome 6. Much confusion has arisen over the HLA-associated diseases. For the most part these are multifactorial diseases, and many are autoimmune diseases with familial aggregation. Five mechanisms of HLA disease associations have been considered: (1) HLA specificity at the cell surface acting as a receptor for a virus or pathogenic agent, (2) a weakening of immunologic tolerance occurring as a result of a cross-reaction of an HLA antigen with a viral or bacterial antigen, (3) linkage disequilibrium within the HLA locus itself, (4) mutations of genes linked to the HLA complex, and (5) immune response genes closely linked to the HLA locus that also demonstrate linkage disequilibrium. Mechanisms 1 and 5 are not mutually exclusive, and it may be that more than one of these will apply in various diseases.

Few genetic disorders are amenable to direct therapy at present. Ideally, endeavors such as recombinant DNA research will result in the ability to manufacture normal proteins to replace abnormal or missing gene products. Further investigation is under way to determine how these products can be packaged so as to arrive at their destination (central nervous system, bone marrow, kidney, liver, and so on) and still be physiologically active.

Prenatal diagnosis

Reference has been made to the availability of prenatal diagnostic studies for various genetic disorders. The most widely used techniques are fetal ultrasound and amniocentesis. Gray-scale and real-time ultrasound are routinely used to determine gestational age by measuring the fetal biparietal diameter, trunk and crown-rump length, and placenta size and location. In a pregnancy at risk the same instruments may be used to examine in greater detail the bony and dense soft tissue structures of the fetus. Meningoceles, occipital encephaloceles, anencephaly, absent kidneys, and anomalous limbs may be diagnosed in this manner. Amniocentesis in prenatal diagnosis involves the insertion of a needle into the amniotic cavity at the sixteenth to seventeenth week of gestation. Approximately 30 ml of fluid is removed under sterile conditions and referred to the genetics laboratory for appropriate analysis. A portion of the fluid may be separated and analyzed for α-1-fetoprotein (AFP), while the cell button (cells of fetal origin) is dispersed into flasks containing growth media. These cells are grown for approximately 2 to 3 weeks, by which time there is usually a sufficient number of actively dividing cells to perform a chromosome analysis or biochemical studies.

AFP is 100 times greater in concentration in fetal blood than adult blood. It was found to be elevated in the amniotic fluid of pregnancies affected with a variety of birth defects, including anencephaly, other open neural tube defects, congenital nephrosis, esophageal atresia, and omphalocele, as well as in fetal demise and twin pregnancies.

Fetoscopy (fetal visualization) and fetal blood sampling are as yet performed only in a limited number of centers. Fetal blood sampling has been used primarily in the diagnosis of hemophilia and the hemoglobinopathies. Fetoscopy may accompany fetal blood sampling or may be used alone to diagnose various structural malformations, such as polydactyly (as a sign of a more complex syndrome), cleft lip, and neural tube defects. Currently, fetal skin biopsy is being investigated as a means of diagnosing serious disorders via skin pathology.

Indications for prenatal counseling include:
1. Drug ingestion during gestation
2. Radiation exposure
3. Chemotherapy
4. Family history of nonmetabolic, nonchromosomal genetic disorder
5. More than two previous unexplained miscarriages
6. As part of infertility workup

Indications for amniocentesis in prenatal counseling include:
1. Advanced maternal age (woman over 35 years of age)
2. Previous child with trisomy or other aneuploidy
3. Previous child with multiple anomalies about which nothing more is known
4. Previous child with neural tube defect
5. Carrier X-linked disorder
6. Translocation carrier
7. Carrier of autosomal recessive disorder for which biochemical testing is available (ascertained through either previously affected child or voluntary screening program)

BIBLIOGRAPHY

Antenatal diagnosis, U.S. Department of Health and Human Services, Public Health Service, National Institutes of Health Pub. No. 79-1973, April 1979, Bethesda, Md.

Jackson, L.G., and Schimke, R.N.: Clinical genetics, a source book for physicians, New York, 1979, John Wiley & Sons, Inc.

McKusick, V.A.: Mendelian inheritance in man, ed. 5, Baltimore, 1978, The Johns Hopkins University Press.

Murphy, E.A., and Chase, G.A.: Principles of genetic counseling, Chicago, 1975, Year Book Medical Publishers.

Smith, D.W.: Recognizable patterns of human malformation, vol. VII, Major problems in clinical pediatrics, ed. 2, Philadelphia, 1976, W.B. Saunders Co.

Vogel, F., and Motulsky, A.G.: Human genetics, problems and approaches, New York, 1979, Springer-Verlag New York Inc.

195 • INHERITED METABOLIC DISORDERS

William A. Horton and **Robert D. Friedman**

The ramifications of a single mutant gene usually involve multiple organ systems. Since most genes code for proteins, the generalized nature of most genetic diseases is due to the widespread distribution of nearly all these proteins, whether they provide structural support or catalyze metabolic reactions. Thus in most cases, if a protein is absent or defective, all tissues in which that protein has a function may be damaged. In addition, if a metabolic pathway is blocked, all the cells in the body may be exposed to high levels of toxic precursor metabolites or deficiencies of vital end products. Hence genetic diseases cannot be broken down by organ systems but rather must be considered in broad categories. In this chapter disorders will be grouped according to whether they are of lysosomal storage, amino acid metabolism, nucleic acid metabolism, metal metabolism, or connective tissue.

DISORDERS OF LYSOSOMAL STORAGE
Glycosphingolipidoses

Glycosphingolipidoses are disorders of glycosphingolipid catabolism. The compounds are membrane lipids composed of a backbone of ceramide (sphingosine plus a long-chain fatty acid) to which various substances are attached. When the attached substance is a simple sugar or group of sugars, the compound is called a cerebroside. If it is a sialic (neuraminic) acid, the term "ganglioside" is used. When phosphocholine is attached, sphingomyelin is produced. Sphingomyelin and sulfatide (galactose and sulfate added in turn to ceramide) are the major lipids in myelinated nervous system membranes. Glycosphingolipids are normally degraded by the stepwise removal of the terminal sugar of other residue by lysosomal acid hydrolases (Fig. 195-1). When the pathway is blocked because of an enzyme deficiency, the precursor molecules accumulate in lysosomes causing enlargement, interruption of normal function, and eventually death of the cell. Clinically this is reflected by progressive neurologic deterioration with or without visceral involvement depending on the distribution of the stored glycosphingolipids, that is, cerebrosides in neuronal and extraneuronal tissues, gangliosides essentially in central nervous system gray matter, and sulfatides in central nervous system white matter. There is considerable variation in the age of onset and the rate of progression of disease even in disorders in which the same enzyme deficiency is found. This presumably reflects the degree of in vivo enzyme deficiency, which is not necessarily the same as that measured in vitro. In general there is no treatment for these disorders, but in many cases prenatal diagnosis is possible by measuring the activity of the enzyme in question in amniotic fluid cells. The major glycosphingolipidoses are labeled in Fig. 195-1 and listed in Table 195-1.

Two forms of *GM_1 gangliosidoses* (generalized gangliosidosis) are known. In the infantile form (type 1, *Landing's disease*) the initial manifestations are usually seen soon after birth. These include psychomotor degeneration, seizures, coarse facial features, enlargement of the tongue and aleveolar processes, corneal opacity, cherry-red spot of the retina, hepatosplenomegaly, and the bone changes of dysostosis multiplex (see "Mucopolysaccharidoses" later in this chapter). Death usually occurs by 2 years of age. The activity of the enzyme GM_1 β-galactosidase is reduced to between 1% and 5% of normal, and massive amounts of its substrate, GM_1 ganglioside, are found in the brain and viscera. Other galactose-containing substrates including mucopolysaccharides (glycosaminoglycans), polysaccharides, and glycoproteins are found in increased amounts in the liver, spleen, and bone.

In the less common juvenile (type 2) GM_1 gangliosidosis, development is normal during the first year. Progressive psychomotor deterioration accompanied by seizures, ataxia, and spasticity begins soon afterwards, and death usually ensues by 10 years of age. These children lack the retinal cherry-red spot, coarse facial features, and visceromegaly of type 1, and the bone changes are mild. The histologic features are similar to those of type 1 except that there is little visceral storage of the GM_1 ganglioside. GM_1 β-galactosidase activity is absent as with type 1, and the two disorders are thought to be allelic.

Tay-Sachs disease (GM_2 gangliosidosis I, infantile amaurotic idiocy) occurs primarily in Ashkenazi Jews, whose carrier rate for this autosomal recessive trait is approximately 1 in 30 persons. The disease is due to a deficiency in hexosaminidase A, one of the two main forms of the enzyme found in human tissues. GM_2 ganglioside is stored in the brain, but there is no visceral or bone involvement. The first symptoms of psychomotor deterioration appear at 6 to 9 months, and there is a rapid downhill course with blindness, deafness, seizures, and decerebrate rigidity over the next 2 to 3 years. Macrocephaly and a retinal cherry-red spot are commonly observed. Death occurs by 4 years of age.

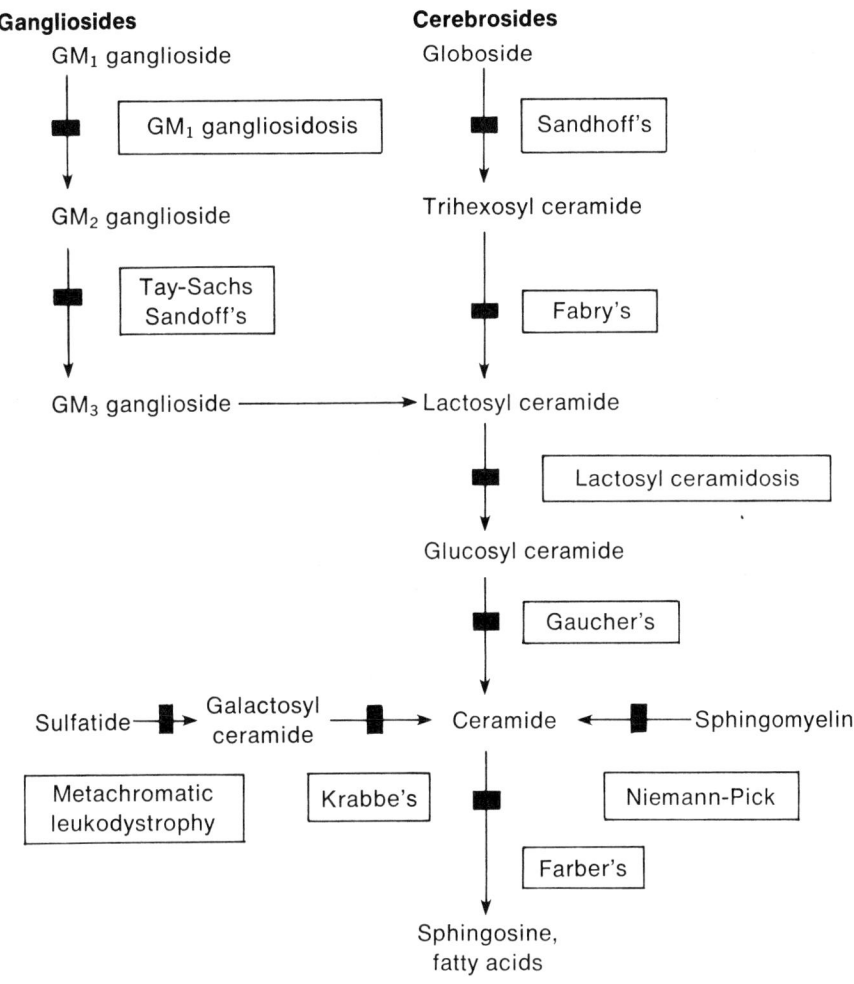

Fig. 195-1. Glycosphingolipid metabolism.

Table 195-1. Glycosphingolipidoses

Disorder	Common name	Inheritance*	Enzyme defect
GM_1 gangliosidosis	Landing's disease	AR	β-Galactosidase
GM_2 gangliosidosis I	Tay-Sachs disease	AR	Hexosaminidase A
GM_2 gangliosidosis II	Sandhoff's disease	AR	Hexosaminidase A, B
Trihexosyl ceramidosis	Fabry's disease	XL	α-Galactosidase
Lactosyl ceramidosis		AR	β-Galactosidase
Glucosyl ceramidosis	Gaucher's disease	AR	β-Glucosidase
Sphingomyelinosis	Niemann-Pick disease	AR	Sphingomyelinase
Sulfatide lipidosis	Metachromatic leukodystrophy	AR	Arylsulfatase A
Globoid cell leukodystrophy	Krabbe's disease	AR	β-Galactosidase
Lipogranulomatosis	Farber's disease	AR	Ceramidase

*AR, autosomal recessive; X-linked recessive.

GM_2 gangliosidosis II (Sandhoff's disease) is clinically almost identical to Tay-Sachs disease. It results from a deficiency of both hexosaminidases A and B. In addition to the storage of GM_2 ganglioside in the brain, these children also have accumulation of globoside in neuronal and visceral tissues; hexosaminidase B catalyzes the first step in globoside breakdown. This disorder has no particular ethnic predilection.

Trihexosyl ceramidosis (Fabry's disease, angiokeratoma corporis diffusum) has an X-linked inheritance; it is the only sphingolipidosis not transmitted as an autosomal recessive trait. In the hemizygous male, corneal opacities and burning pain in the lower extremities develop during early childhood. Raised red-purple skin lesions (angiokeratomas) distributed over the lower trunk and upper thighs usually appear during the second decade. Pinpoint angiokeratoma spots may also be seen on the lips and oral mucosa of some patients, but other tissues have not demonstrated well-developed clusters. Kidney failure is the most foreboding manifestation during adulthood, but cardiac disease may occur as well. Patients usually die in their forties. The clinical picture is variable in the heterozygote female; corneal lesions are often observed together with varying degrees of the other features. Trihexosyl ceramide is found in large amounts in nearly all tissues, as well as in the plasma and urine. This accumulation is due to a deficiency of trihexosyl α-galactosidase.

Lactosyl ceramidosis is a rare condition characterized by slowly progressive neurologic deterioration together with seizures and hepatosplenomegaly. Lactosyl ceramide is stored in lysosomes owing to deficiency of the specific β-galactosidase.

Gaucher's disease (glucosyl ceramidosis) is the most common of the sphingolipidoses. There are three distinct forms that differ in the age of onset and degree of central nervous system involvement. They are all characterized by varying degrees of marked splenomegaly, hepatomegaly, osteoporotic erosion of the skeleton, anemia, thrombocytopenia, and accumulation of lipid in cells of the reticuloendothelial system. Type 1, the adult or chronic nonneuronopathic type, is by far the most common and is seen primarily in Ashkenazi Jews. It appears during late childhood or early adulthood with splenomegaly, bone pain, and easy bruising. In adults the major problems are related to skeletal involvement (for example, pain and fractures) and hemorrhagic episodes. Lung involvement may predispose patients to pneumonia, a frequent cause of death, but the disease is compatible with a normal life span.

Knowledge of the type 1 form of Gaucher's disease is critical since the diagnostic signs and symptoms are usually not reported in early childhood, and the dentist may have the first opportunity to recognize this disorder. Gingival hemorrhage, epistaxis, hemoptysis, and pigmentation of the face, lips, neck, and hands are some of the characteristic signs, but the roentgenographic findings are often much more definitive. Areas of generalized osteoporosis and vacuolation with multiple irregular radiolucenies may appear Radiographically throughout the premolar and molar regions of the mandible and maxilla. Involvement of the mandible is probably more frequent than has been realized, and greater attention should be paid to oral radiographic findings. One complications of Gaucher's disease is hemorrhagic diathesis, which especially needs to be considered before oral surgical and/or periodontal intervention by the dentist.

Type 2, the acute neuronopathic or infantile form of Gaucher's disease, appears during infancy with loss of neurologic function, spasticity, and enlargement of the liver and spleen. Psychomotor deterioration progresses, and death usually ensues by 2 years of age. The even rarer type 3 juvenile or subacute neuronopathic form has many of the same features as type 2, but the course is more protracted. The onset is usually during the latter part of the first year, and death occurs near the end of the first decade.

The clinical features in all forms of Gaucher's disease result from the widespread deposition of glucosyl ceramide owing to a deficiency of glucocerebroside β-glucosidase (glucocerebrosidase). In contrast to most other glycosphingolipidoses, the degree of enzyme deficiency correlates with the severity of the disease. Patients with type 2 have less than 10% normal activity, those with type 3 about 15%, and those with type 1 up to 40%.

Sphingomyelin lipidosis (Niemann-Pick disease) is a group of disorders characterized by the storage of sphingomyelin and other lipids throughout the body. Although five types have been identified, over 80% of patients have type A. In this acute neuronopathic form, hepatosplenomegaly and central nervous system dysfunction are evident by 6 months of age. The cherry-red spot of the retina is often seen, as are anemia, thrombocytopenia, osteoporosis, and a brownish yellow discoloration of the skin. Death usually occurs by 3 years of age.

In type B, the chronic nonneuronopathic type, symptoms develop somewhat later and the course is more protracted. There is no neurologic impairment, but pulmonary infiltration is common. Type C, the chronic neuronopathic form, resembles type A, but the onset usually occurs during the second year and the children live to between 5 and 15 years of age. Type D is similar to type C, but all patients with type D have a common ancestry in Nova Scotia. The adult form, type E, has a later onset and mild chronic symptoms without neurologic involvement.

Pathologically there is an accumulation of sphingomyelin throughout the reticuloendothelial system in all types and in the brain in the neuronopathic forms. Cholesterol and other glycolipids may also be stored. A deficiency of sphingomyelinase has been demonstrated in types A, B, and C, but the defect remains unknown in types D and E.

Sulfatide lipidosis, often called *metachromatic leukodystrophy* (MLD), comprises three closely related disorders that are characterized by the accumulation of sulfur-containing glycosphingolipids. The most common is the late infantile form in which gait disturbance and incoordination develop during the second year. Seizures, spasticity, optic atrophy, incontinence, and dementia are seen subsequently, and death intervenes by 10 years of age. The juvenile form appears during the second decade with personality changes and mental deterioration. Many of the features of the infantile form eventually develop, and death usually comes during the thirties. The adult onset of psychosis and dementia with the late appearance of neurologic signs characterizes the very rare adult type of MLD.

In all three forms sulfatide is stored in the liver, gallbladder, kidney, peripheral nerves, and especially the central nervous system white matter. Histologically it is seen as metachromatically staining cytoplasmic inclusions. The urinary sediment also stains metachromatically. In addition, there is diffuse demyelination and gliosis in both the centreal and peripheral nervous systems. The sulfatide storage is due to a deficiency of arylsulfatase A, one of two lysosomal arylsulfatases. Interestingly, the other, arylsulfatase B, is deficient in the Maroteaux-Lamy syndrome (mucopolysaccharidosis type VI), which has clinical features quite distinct from MLD. There is also a condition known as multiple sulfatase deficiency (mucosulfatidoses) in which both arylsulfatases A and B and a microsomal arylsulfatase C are deficient. This condition has features of both MLD (late infantile form) and the mucopolysaccharidoses (see the following discussion).

Krabbe's disease (globoid cell leukodystrophy) affects primarily central nervous system white matter. The clinical picture is that of progressive psychomotor retardation, rigidity, seizures, and optic atrophy beginning between 4 and 6 months of age, with death occurring before 2 years of age. At autopsy almost total absence of myelin, severe gliosis, and the abundance of ''globoid cells'' are found in the cerebral white matter. The absence of activity of galactocerebroside β-galactosidase has been observed.

Farber's disease (lipogranulomatosis) is due to the deficiency of ceramidase. It is apparent during infancy and is manifested by hoarseness, painful and swollen joints, subcutaneous and periarticular nodules, growth retardation, pulmonary infiltration, and progressive neurologic dysfunction. The involved tissues show infiltration by macrophages and foam cells that form granulomas. There is also lipid storage in neurons.

Mucopolysaccharidoses

The mucopolysaccharidoses (MPS) are a heterogeneous group of disorders characterized by the widespread accumulation of mucopolysaccharides (glycosaminoglycans) throughout the body. Attached to a core protein, these substances normally comprise the so-called ground substance of connective tissue matrix. They consist of polymers of repeating disaccharide units composed of alternating uronic acid and hexosamine (often sulfated) residues. Four major mucopolysaccharides are found in human tissues: chondroitin sulfate (CS), dermatan sulfate (DS), heparan sulfate (HS), and keratan sulfate (KS). In normal tissues degradation of the polymers proceeds by the the sequential removal of the terminal residue by lysosomal exoglycosidases and sulfatases. If one of the enzymes is missing, degradation is blocked and the substance accumulates within the lysosomes. Since the enzymes are specific for particular residues that are frequently components of different mucopolysaccharides, more than one of these compounds often accumulates from such a block. There is, however, some partial breakdown of these polymers into smaller fragments by lysosomal endoglycosidases such as hyaluronidase; it is these fragments that are excreted in the urine.

The recognized mucopolysaccharidoses are listed in Table 195-2. Despite the variety of different enzyme deficiencies that are responsible for these disorders, there is a considerable overlap of clinical features. This is due to the ubiquitous nature of these substances in the body. The differences between the disorders, however, probably reflect in part the different distribution of the individual mucopolysaccharides (for example, KS is found predominantly in cartilage) and therefore the location of greatest

Table 195-2. Mucopolysaccharidoses

Designation	Eponym	Inheritance*	Urinary excretion†	Enzyme defect
MPS I H	Hurler	AR	DS, HS	α-L-Iduronidase
MPSI S‡	Scheie	AR	DS, HS	α-L-Iduronidase
MPS I H/S	Hurler-Scheie	AR	DS, HS	α-L-Iduronidase
MPS II severe	Hunter	XL	DS, HS	Iduronate sulfatase
MPS II mild	Hunter	XL	DS, HS	Iduronate sulfatase
MPS III A	Sanfilippo A	AR	HS	Heparan-N-sulfatase
MPS III B	Sanfilippo B	AR	HS	N-Acetyl-α-D-glucosaminidase
MPS III C	Sanfilippo C	AR	HS	a-Glucosaminidase
MPS IV	Morquio	AR	KS	Galactosamine-6-sulfate sulfatase
MPS V	Vacant			
MPS VI severe	Maroteaux-Lamy	AR	DS	Arylsulfatase B
MPS VI intermediate	Maroteaux-Lamy	AR	DS	Arylsulfatase B
MPS VI mild	Maroteaux-Lamy	AR	DS	Arylsulfatase B
MPS VII	Sly	AR	DS, HS	β-Glucuronidase
MPS VIII	DiFerrante	AR	KS, HS	Glucosamine-6-sulfate sulfatase

*AR, autosomal recessive; XL, X linked.
†DS, dermatan sulfate; HS, heparan sulfate; KS, keratan sulfate.
‡Scheie's syndrome was originally designated MPS V. When the defective enzyme was found to be the same as in Hurler's syndrome, the designation was changed to MPS I S.

tissue damage. Most patients with mucopolysaccharide storage disease exhibit varying degrees of coarsening of the facies, enlarged tongue, wide-spaced teeth, limitation of joint motion, and skeletal changes known as dysostosis, multiplex (enlarged or J-shaped sella turcica, widened ribs, beaking of the lumbar vertebrae, and short, broad, poorly modeled tubular bones of the limbs). Corneal clouding, mental retardation, and liver and spleen enlargement are common. Except for Hunter's syndrome (MPS II), which is X linked, all of these disorders are transmitted as autosomal recessive traits. Although there is no successful treatment for any of the conditions, prenatal diagnosis is available for most of them.

MPS I implies a deficiency of α-L-iduronidase and the resultant tissue storage and urinary excretion of DS and HS. Two clinical forms are recognized. *MPS I H, Hurler's syndrome,* is the prototype of the mucopolysaccharidoses. Large size, stiff joints, thoracolumbar kyphosis, and mild coarsening of facial features are noted between 6 and 12 months of age. During the second year, liver and spleen enlargement, corneal clouding, cardiac murmurs, macrocephaly, umbilical hernia, dwarfism, and grotesque facial features appear. Skeletal roentgenograms show the typical changes of dysostosis multiplex. Beyond 2 years of age mental and physical deterioration progresses, and death occurs between 6 and 10 years of age.

In the mild variety *MPS I S, Scheie's syndrome,* corneal clouding with retinal degeneration and glaucoma, clawhand, carpal tunnel syndrome, and frequently aortic regurgitation develop in midchildhood. The facies are moderately coarse and intelligence is normal. Life expectancy is well into adulthood and may be normal. Scheie's syndrome was originally designated MPS V, but when the enzyme defect was determined to be the same as in Hurler's syndrome, the designation was changed to MPS I S, leaving MPS V vacant. A few patients have been described with the biochemical features of MPS I and a clinical phenotype of intermediate severity. They are thought to be genetic compounds, having the combination of Hurler and Scheie genes at the α-L-iduronidase locus (MPS I H/S).

Mild and severe forms of *MPS II, Hunter's syndrome,* are recognized. Both are due to a deficiency of iduronate sulfatase and are X linked. Boys with the severe form closely resemble children with Hurler's syndrome except that they usually lack corneal clouding and tend to live into the second decade. In addition, deafness is more common. In mild Hunter's syndrome, survival is well into adulthood and intelligence is relatively well preserved.

MPS III, Sanfilippo's syndrome, is a phenotype consisting of severe mental retardation, mild to almost absent physical features of the mucopolysaccharidoses, minimal visceral and skeletal involvement, and excretion of HS in the urine. The screening test for mucopolysacchariduria may be borderline or even negative. Three distinct enzyme deficiencies that produce this phenotype have been identified (Table 195-2). They can be distinguished only by biochemical means. Sanfilippo A syndrome resulting from a deficiency of heparan-N-sulfatase is the most common.

The features of *MPS IV, Morquio's syndrome,* initially resemble those of the other mucopolysaccharidoses, but by midchildhood a distinct clinical picture emerges. It consists of corneal clouding, severe dwarfism, protruding chest with kyphoscoliosis, gait disturbance, genu valgum, and flat feet. Instability of the cervical spine owing to the combination of hypoplasia of the odontoid process and ligamentous laxity is common, as is aortic regurgitation. Intelligence is probably unaffected, and life expectancy is into the forties.

In general *MPS VI, Maroteaux-Lamy syndrome,* resembles Hurler's syndrome except for delayed onset, longer survival, normal intelligence, and the excretion of only DS. Three clinical forms are recognized. Striking dwarfism, corneal clouding, valvular heart disease, joint stiffness, and contractures, especially involving the hip and knee, characterize the severe form, which becomes apparent between 2 and 4 years of age. Odontoid hypoplasia may be a problem, and death usually supervenes in the third decade. The mild form is manifested by mild skeletal abnormalities, joint stiffness, corneal clouding, aortic stenosis, and survival into adulthood. As expected, the intermediate form shows a phenotype of intermediate severity, and it may represent a genetic compound between the severe and mild forms.

Recent reports have described a few patients with two additional mucopolysaccharide storage diseases. *MPS VII, Sly's syndrome,* is characterized by mental retardation, visceromegaly, dysostosis multiplex, and a deficiency of β-glucuronidase. Mild skeletal changes, mental retardation, ring-shaped metachromasia of lymphocytes, and a deficiency of glucosamine-6-sulfate sulfatase are found in *MPS VIII*.

A comprehensive survey of the oral manifestations of MPS IH and MPS II types has been provided by Gardner. Although basic metabolic disturbances are responsible for the variety of skeletal anomalies, it is not known whether these same factors act directly or indirectly to cause the involvement of intraoral and facial hard and soft tissues. Primary skeletal defects can possibly result in irregularities that interfere with the development of intraoral tissues and normal tooth eruption.

Those facial and intraoral findings associated primarily with MPS IH and MPS II can be subdivided into aberrations of teeth, the mandible, the temporomandibular joint, and the intraoral tissues.

TEETH

Occlusion. There is marked spacing of both the anterior and the posterior teeth, with the molars assuming a relatively more posterior position than normal. This spacing could be partly attributed to alveolar ridge hyperplasia and/

or the posterior position of the molars, which also exhibit distoangular tipping. In addition, an anterior open bite may be observed and has been associated with the presence of an enlarged, protruding tongue.

Size of teeth. There seems to be little reliable information regarding actual tooth size, although a tendency for bruxism leading to a marked generalized state of attrition may have been mistaken for reports of small teeth.

MANDIBLE

Size and anatomic relationships. The total distance around the arch of the mandible is greater than normal, which could account for the wide spacing of the teeth. The body of the mandible is vertically short, the rami are both short and narrow, and the angle of the mandible may be substantially increased, with the chin retruded in some cases. The gonions are extremely prominent, and a wide intergonial distance may give the false appearance of a massive lower jaw. The total area of the mandible is less than normal.

Lesions. There apparently is a greater tendency for lesions resembling dentigerous cysts radiographically, but that are actually dental follicles consisting of collagenous connective tissue.

TEMPOROMANDIBULAR JOINT. In addition to the shortening of the ramus, the neck of the condyles may be reduced in size. The condyles vary in the degree of abnormality. They may be absent, or just smaller than normal. Morphologic changes are usually bilateral and symmetric. Limitations in the motion of the temporomandibular joint are common in these disorders.

INTRAORAL TISSUES. The appearance of the gingiva ranges from normal to varying degrees of simple and hyperplastic gingivitis. It is possible that other nonmetabolic elements such as mouth breathing, oral hygiene, and intraoral irritants contribute to the gingival hyperplasia. Some confusion has developed regarding the cause-effect relationship of enlarged alveolar processes and hyperplastic gingiva. Both events need to be considered independently, since hyperplastic gingiva does not occur in all cases, but the alveolar processes are usually enlarged. Nevertheless, improved oral hygiene can only be beneficial.

Mucolipidoses

The mucolipidoses (ML) are a group of disorders characterized by lysosomal storage of mucopolysaccharides and glycosphingolipids in visceral, mesenchymal, and neuronal tissues. As a group they have many features of both the glycosphingolipidoses and the mucopolysaccharidoses, but they lack mucopolysacchariduria. All are quite rare and are thought to be inherited as autosomal recessive traits.

Mucolipidosis I is due to a deficiency of sialidase (neuraminidase). Pathologically there is an accumulation of sialic acid–containing substances. Two clinical forms have been observed. Sialidosis type 1, which is probably the same disorder that was previously termed the cherry-red spot–myoclonus syndrome, appears between 8 and 15 years of age with decreasing vision, retinal cherry-red spot, and progressive myoclonus. The children have normal intelligence and lack the typical features of lysosomal storage diseases. However, cytoplasmic inclusions, presumably enlarged lysosomes, have been observed on liver biopsy. The patients survive into adulthood. In sialidosis type 2 the phenotype is variable but resembles that seen in children with Hurler's syndrome, that is, corneal clouding, coarse facies, visceromegaly, short stature, joint stiffness, and the roentgenographic changes of dysostosis multiplex. The retinal cherry-red spot is found, and ataxia and mental retardation are common. The onset of this dysmorphic type may occur during the infantile or juvenile period.

Mucolipidosis II (I-cell disease) is characterized by the typical features of Hurler's syndrome, many of which are apparent at birth. The children usually die by 4 years of age. The name derives from the observation of cytoplasmic inclusions in cultured skin fibroblasts. In addition, there is a striking elevation of several lysosomal hydrolases in the plasma. The basic defect is thought to lie in the processing of these enzymes so that they are unable to be taken up by or retained within the lysosomes. Consequently, undegraded material accumulates in the lysosomes despite high levels of the lysosomal enzymes extracellularly. *Mucolipidosis III (pseudo-Hurler polydystrophy)* is closely related to ML II but has a later onset, less striking physical features, and a mild clinical course. The basic defect is thought to be the same as in ML II, but plasma levels of lysosomal enzymes are only moderately elevated.

Several patients have been described with early or even congenital corneal clouding and psychomotor retardation without substantial coarsening of facies or skeletal abnormalities. Electron microscopy shows many tissues containing peculiar membranous cytoplasmic bodies, which are thought to be lysosomes filled with stored gangliosides and hyaluronic acid. This condition, observed primarily in Ashkenazi Jews, has been designated *ML IV*. The basic defect is unknown.

Two other disorders resemble the mucolipidoses: *fucosidosis* and *mannosidosis*. The first occurs in two forms: fucosidosis type 1, which has a clinical picture very similar to Hurler's syndrome, and a milder type 2. Angiokeratomas of the skin similar to those seen in Fabry's disease occur in patients with the latter type. In both types, α-L-fucosidase is deficient and fucose-containing glycolipids are stored in lysosomes. The disorder is rare, and many of the patients have been Italian. Mannosidosis is more common but clinically similar to the infantile form of fucosidosis. Mannose-containing glycolipids are found in many tissues, and the enzyme α-D-mannosidase is deficient. Both fucosidosis and mannosidosis are autosomal recessive traits.

AMINOACIDOPATHIES

The aminoacidopathies result from deficient activity of enzymes that catalyse the normal interconversion and degradation of amino acids. In most cases the disease processes result from the toxic effects of substances that accumulate before the metabolic block. Sometimes, however, a deficiency of the product of the blocked reaction is responsible. In general these disorders are rare, are inherited as recessive traits, and may be diagnosed prenatally. Specific treatment is often possible.

Aromatic amino acid disorders

Disorders of aromatic amino acid metabolism are shown in Fig. 195-2. *Phenylketonuria (PKU)* is the most common aminoacidopathy, occurring at a rate of approximately 1 in 15,000 live births. It has an autosomal recessive inheritance and results from reduced activity of hepatic phenylalanine hydroxylase. Phenylalanine accumulates in the plasma, and its keto acid metabolites (such as phenylpyruvic acid) spill over into the urine. Infants are normal at birth, but if they are untreated, vomiting, poor growth, seizures, and mental retardation develop. Pigmentation is usually reduced because melanin is deficient, and eczema is common. The treatment consists of a diet low in phenylalanine. If instituted early and strictly adhered to, this allows normal development. The diet may be stopped after childhood, since the deleterious effects of high plasma phenylalanine levels seem to be directed primarily toward the developing nervous system. It should be restarted, however, in women planning pregnancy.

In addition to classic PKU, several variants have been identified. Some children have persistent mildly elevated plasma phenylalanine levels. Others show only a transient elevation in phenylalanine levels; this is thought to reflect immaturity of the normal hydroxylating enzyme system. Hyperphenylalaninemia can result from a defect in phenylalanine transaminase, an enzyme in an alternative disposal pathway. Normal development even without treatment can be expected in patients who have these variant conditions.

Recently some children with the characteristic features of PKU have been found to have progressive neurologic deterioration despite adequate dietary treatment. A deficiency in dihydropterine reductase has been identified. This enzyme is necessary for the synthesis of tetrahydrobiopterin, a cofactor for phenylalanine hydroxylase. No treatment is currently available for this autosomal recessive trait.

Disturbances of tyrosine metabolism occur in at least three conditions. Thirty percent of premature infants and 10% of term infants suffer from a transient elevation of tyrosine (and phenylalanine) in the neonatal period. This is thought to be due to immaturity of the enzyme parahydroxyphenylpyruvic acid oxidase. Treatment with high

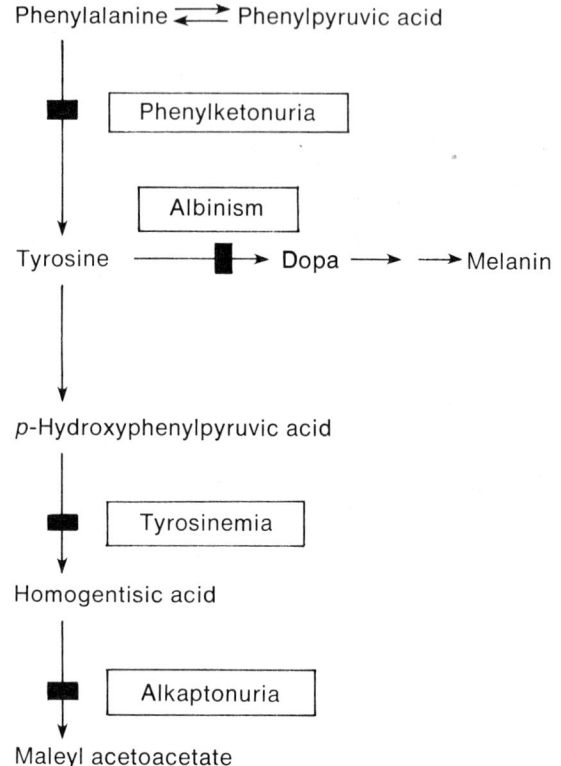

Fig. 195-2. Aromatic amino acid metabolism.

doses of vitamin C, a cofactor for this enzyme, is said to be curative. A deficiency of this enzyme occurs in *hereditary tyrosinemia*, a separate autosomal recessive disorder characterized by aberrant metabolism of carbohydrates, porphyrins, and methionine in addition to tyrosine. Although infants with this condition often die early from fulminant liver failure, they may survive into childhood but with progressive hepatic cirrhosis and kidney tubular dysfunction. Dietary restriction of phenylalanine and tyrosine may be of some benefit. At least one type of *oculocutaneous albinism* is due to the deficiency of tyrosinase, the enzyme that converts tyrosine to dopa in the first step in melanin synthesis. Affected individuals lack pigment in the skin, hair, and eyes and have an increased susceptibility to various skin cancers. This is an autosomal recessive trait.

Alkaptonuria is an autosomal recessive disorder that results from deficient activity of the enzyme homogentisic acid oxidase. The manifestations (degenerative arthritis of the spine, knees, hips, and shoulders) result from the deposition of blue-black ochronotic pigment (a polymer of homogentisic acid) in connective tissues, especially cartilage. The pigment can be seen in the cornea, nasal cartilage, and pinna.

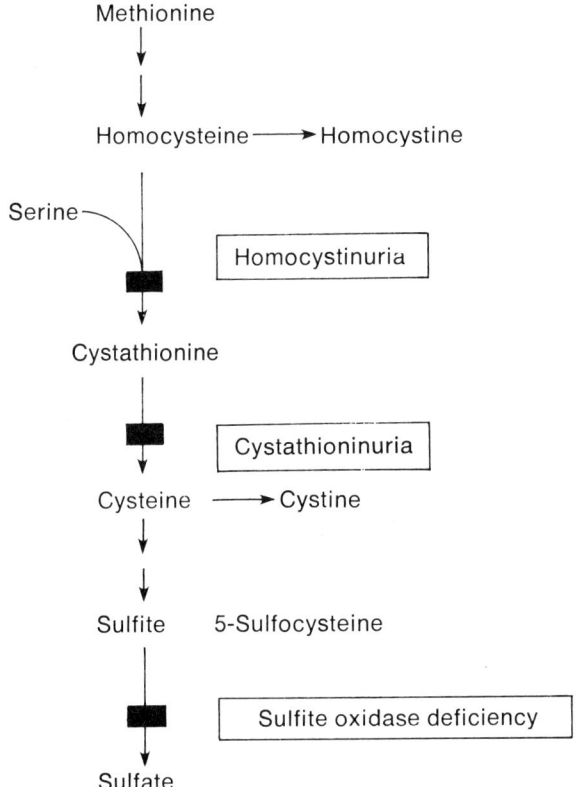

Fig. 195-3. Sulfur-containing amino acid metabolism.

Sulfur-containing amino acid disorders

Although the finding of homocystine in the urine occurs in several disorders, including the deficiency of N-5, 10-methylene tetrahydrofolate reductase and defects in the absorption and metabolism of vitamin B_{12}, the term "homocystinuria" usually refers to a specific autosomal recessive condition resulting from a deficiency of the enzyme cystathionine synthetase. The patients resemble those with Marfan's syndrome because of their tall stature, kyphoscoliosis, pectus excavatum, and dislocated lenses, but they lack joint laxity and valvular heart disease. Moreover, osteoporosis, mental retardation, and recurrent thromboembolic phenomena occur frequently in homocystinuria. The enzyme defect interferes with conversion of methionine to cystine and results in the accumulation of homocystine (Fig. 195-3). The majority of the clinical manifestations of homocystinuria are thought to result from the disruptive effects of homocystine on collagen cross-linking.

Cystathioninuria is another rare autosomal recessive disorder of sulfur-containing amino acids. It is due to the deficiency of cystathionase and is characterized by the presence of large amounts of cystathionine in the urine and plasma. The clinical features are variable, but most patients have some degree of mental and/or physical abnormalities. In most affected individuals the metabolic abnormalities are corrected by high doses of vitamin B_6.

Sulfite oxidase deficiency has been observed in a child with severe developmental delay, dislocated lenses, and the excretion of large amounts of the amino acid 5-sulfocysteine in the urine.

Branched-chain amino acid disorders

A number of disorders involve defective breakdown of branched-chain amino acids (Fig. 195-4). All are characterized by the accumulation of organic acids, but only maple syrup urine disease shows an excess of amino acids in the urine and plasma. Their clinical features are quite similar and include ketoacidosis (often with hyperammonemia), vomiting, flaccidity (sometimes spasticity), seizures, coma, leukopenia, thrombocytopenia, osteoporosis, and mental retardation. All are inherited as autosomal recessive traits, and prenatal diagnosis is available for many.

Maple syrup urine disease (MSUD) is the most common. It results from defective decarboxylation of the keto derivatives of leucine, isoleucine, and valine; these substances spill over into the urine imparting a distinctive odor. The infants usually become symptomatic and often die during the first week of life unless a diet restricted in these amino acids is imposed. In milder forms the symptoms occur episodically and survival is prolonged at least into childhood; one type shows a dramatic response to thiamine, the cofactor for the decarboxylase enzyme.

Propionic acidemia results from a deficiency of propionic acid decarboxylase. Usually infants have an overwhelming illness that follows protein feeding and is characterized by severe ketoacidosis, hyperammonemia, and hypoglycemia. The latter two metabolic derangements are thought to result from interference with ureagenesis and gluconeogenesis. In a few children, however, acidosis is intermittent and is brought on by acute infection or excessive dietary protein. Some patients show clinical improvement following the administration of biotin.

The conversion of methylmalonyl CoA to succinyl CoA requires the participation of two enzymes, methylmalonyl CoA racemase and methylmalonyl CoA mutase, and 5-deoxyadenosyl cobalamin, an active metabolite of vitamin B_{12}. *Methylmalonic acidemia* is due to a defect in this conversion; it can result from a deficiency of either enzyme or from failure to synthesize the B_{12} cofactor. As might be expected, the third type responds to treatment with high doses of vitamin B_{12}; the others are treated with protein restriction.

As noted in Fig. 195-4, several other defects in branched-chain amino acid degradation have been described. They are very rare, and genetic heterogeneity has been observed in most. They include isovaleric acidemia owing to isovaleryl CoA dehydrogenase deficiency, β-methylcrotonylglycinuria resulting from β-methylcrotonyl

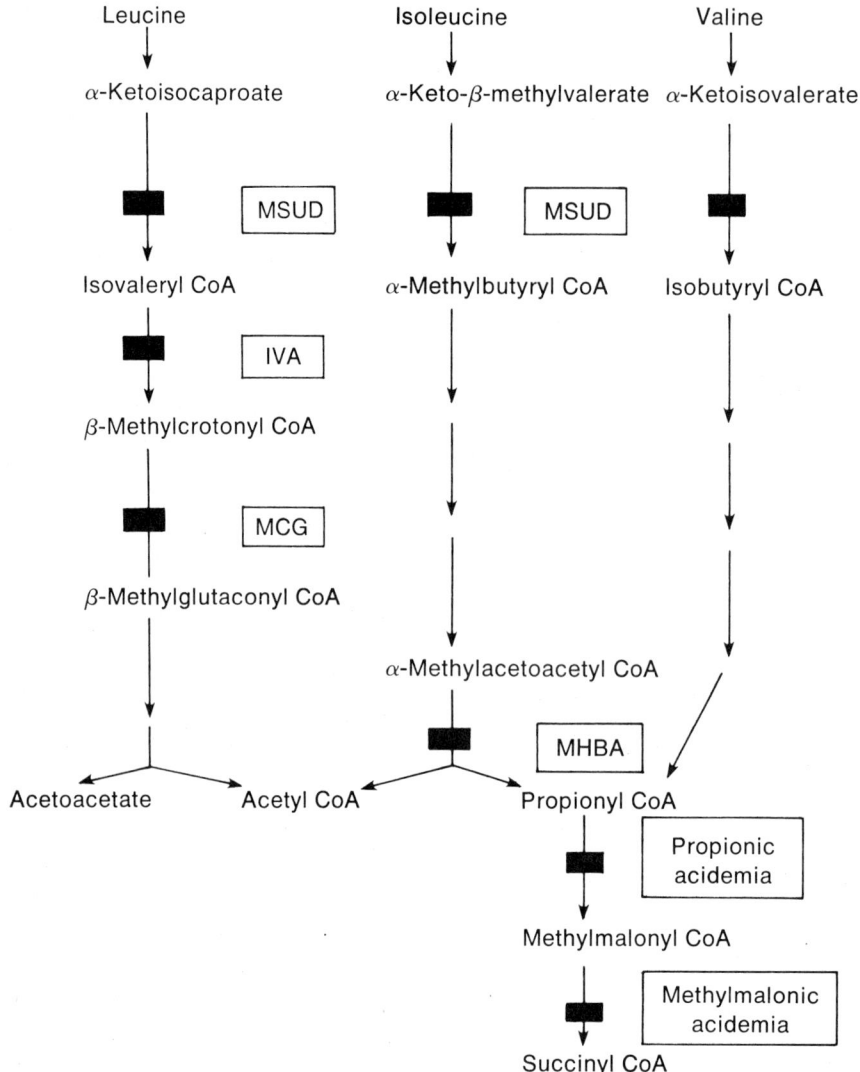

Fig. 195-4. Branched-chain amino acid metabolism. *MSUD*, maple syrup urine disease; *IVA*, isovaleric acidemia. *MCG*, methylcrotonylglycinuria; *MHBA*, methylhydroxybutyric and methylacetoacetic aciduria.

CoA carboxylase deficiency, and α-methyl-β hydroxybutyric and α-methylacetoacetic aciduria owing to α-methylacetoacetyl CoA β-ketothiolase deficiency.

UREA CYCLE DISORDERS

The urea cycle is responsible for removal of ammonia that results from protein degradation. Inherited deficiencies of five enzymes in this cycle have been identified (Fig. 195-5). Hyperammonemia is common to all disorders, but because of the cyclic nature of the system, the accumulation of urea cycle intermediates usually does not occur. In general all the syndromes exhibit neurologic dysfunction and protein intolerance; however, the severity may range from an overwhelming illness with seizures, stupor, and coma occurring after the beginning of milk feeding to episodic symptoms associated only with acute infections or high dietary protein intake. Mental retardation and hepatomegaly are common in these survivors, however. Frequent feeding of a high carbohydrate diet together with protein restriction is the only form of therapy currently available. The diagnosis is usually made by the assay of liver enzymes.

Argininosuccinic aciduria is the most common of the urea cycle disorders. It is due to a deficiency of the enzyme argininosuccinase. Three clinical forms have been established: a neonatal form with lethargy, seizures, and early death; an infantile form with vomiting, hepatomegaly, failure to thrive, and an onset during the first few weeks of life; and a chronic form with seizures, ataxia, mental retardation, and peculiar short, brittle, friable hair. All three are inherited as autosomal recessive traits and are probably allelic mutations.

The deficiency of ornithine transcarbamylase (OTCD) is an X-linked disorder that is lethal in boys. The features

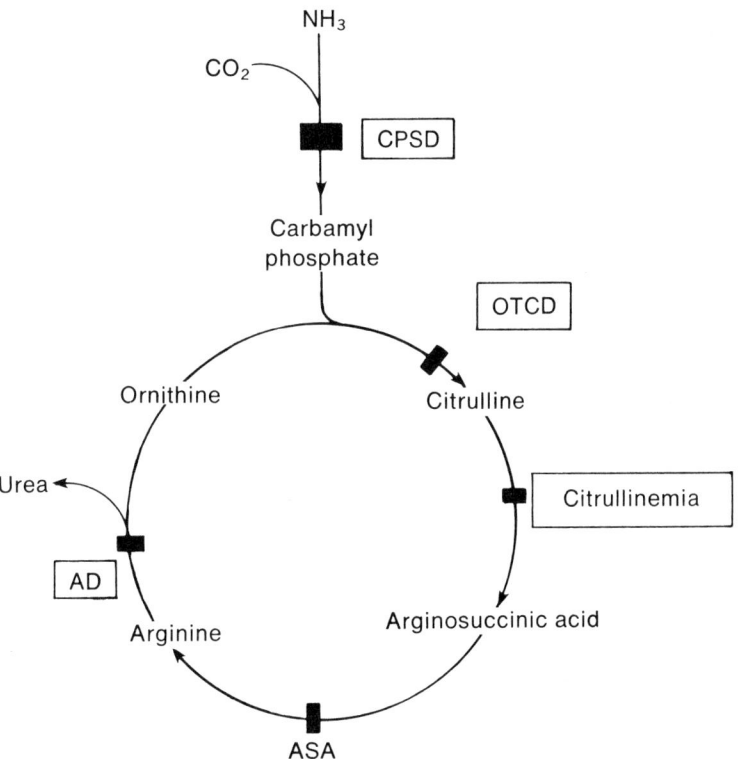

Fig. 195-5. Urea cycle. *CPSD*, carbamyl phosphate synthetase deficiency; *OTCD*, ornithine transcarbamylase deficiency; *ASA*, arginosuccinic aciduria; *AD*, arginase deficiency.

are variable in affected girls; some demonstrate the usual neurologic symptoms and others are essentially asymptomatic except during periods of stress or high protein intake.

At least three varieties of citrullinemia are recognized. The first is lethal in the neonatal period. Neurologic symptoms, hepatomegaly, and osteoporosis develop during the first year of life in the second. The third is apparently benign. They are due to a deficiency of argininosuccinic acid synthetase and have an autosomal recessive inheritance.

A few patients have been reported to have deficiencies of carbamyl phosphate synthetase and arginase. The first enzyme is responsible for trapping free ammonia and the other for cleaving urea from arginine to produce ornithine. Both deficiencies are autosomal recessive conditions.

Several biochemical defects in amino acid metabolism have been identified but appear to be of little clinical importance. In each case the precursors to the metabolic blocks accumulate in the blood and often are found in the urine. The disorders in this category include histidinemia owing to a lack of histidinase, hyperprolinemia owing to a deficiency of either proline oxidase or β-1-pyrroline-5-carboxylic acid dehydrogenase, hydroxyprolinemia resulting from the absence of hydroxyproline oxidase, and possibly lysinuria owing to a deficiency of lysine ketoglutarate reductase. All of these are autosomal recessive traits.

DISORDERS OF NUCLEIC ACID METABOLISM

The *Lesch-Nyhan syndrome* is an X-linked disorder of purine metabolism. Affected boys are normal at birth, but within a few months progressive choreoathetosis, spasticity, mental retardation, and a pecular tendency toward self-mutilation develop. Patients have increased production of uric acid and exhibit all the clinical features of gout including hyperuricemia, gouty arthritis, tophi, urinary tract stones, crystalluria, and nephropathy. Death usually comes during adolescence. The disorder is due to a deficiency of hypoxanthine-guanine phosphoribosyltransferase (HGPRT), the enzyme that normally catalyzes the transfer of 5-phosphoribosyl-1-pyrophosphate (PRPP) to guanine and hypoxanthine to form their respective ribonucleotides. The deficiency of HGPRT is associated with a high level of intracellular PRPP, which contributes to increased de novo purine synthesis and ultimately to increased uric acid production. Treatment with allopurinol reduces uric acid production and its sequelae but has little effect on the central nervous system abnormalities. Measurement of HGPRT activity in hair follicles (which are largely clonal in origin with regard to the X chromosome) has been successful for detecting carrier females.

Another disorder of purine metabolism is *xanthinuria*, an autosomal recessive disorder caused by a deficiency of xanthine oxidase. This enzyme is responsible for the last two steps in purine breakdown, the oxidation of hypoxanthine to xanthine and of xanthine to uric acid. In most patients the disorder is benign and is characterized by low levels of uric acid in the serum and urine and a high urinary excretion of hypoxanthine and xanthine. The latter may result in xanthine stones, in which case high fluid intake to maintain a large urinary volume is indicated.

Immune deficiency is associated with reduced activity of at least two enzymes involved in purine metabolism. In both cases the trait shows autosomal recessive inheritance and the mechanisms responsible for the immunodeficiency are not understood. Children with *adenosine deaminase deficiency* have profound lymphopenia and absent or very low levels of immunoglobulins, and in general they show evidence of combined B- and T-cell dysfunction. Some of these patients also have skeletal abnormalities resembling those seen in certain types of dwarfism, suggesting a common link between proliferating cartilage and lymphoid cells. If untreated, these children die of overwhelming infection; however, repeated transfusions with frozen red blood cells (as a source of the enzyme) or more recently histocompatibility-matched bone marrow transplantation has met with success in some patients.

Impaired immunity restricted primarily to T-lymphocyte dysfunction is associated with a deficiency of purine *nucleoside phosphorylase*. The infections tend to be less severe and most often involve viruses.

Orotic aciduria is an autosomal recessive disorder of pyrimidine metabolism. It is characterized by growth failure, hypochromic anemia associated with megaloblastic changes in the bone marrow, and the excessive urinary excretion of orotic acid. Two clinically identical forms can be distinguished biochemically. Type 1 results from the deficiency of two sequential enzymes involved in the conversion of orotic acid to uridine-5-phosphate. The enzymes are orotate phosphoribosyl transferase and orotidine 5'-phosphate decarboxylase. In type 2 only the decarboxylase is deficient. Both are inherited as autosomal recessive traits. Treatment with uridine results in hematologic remission, improvement in growth, and a decrease in urinary orotic acid excretion.

DISORDERS OF MINERAL METABOLISM

Wilson's disease is an autosomal recessive disorder of copper metabolism. The clinical manifestations usually develop during adolescence or early adulthood but may not appear until the forties. Nearly half the patients have neurologic symptoms such as spasticity, rigidity, dysarthria, tremor, and psychiatric disturbances, and about 40% have hepatic abnormalities such as hepatomegaly, cirrhosis, and hepatic failure. In addition, renal tubular dysfunction often develops during the course of the disease. Plasma levels of copper and its binding protein ceruloplasmin are low. In contrast, an excess of copper is found in the brain (especially in the basal ganglia), liver, kidney, and cornea (Kayser-Fleischer rings). The basic defect is unknown. If untreated, Wilson's disease is fatal, but therapy to reduce total body copper is often successful. The mainstay of treatment is penicillamine, which enhances urinary copper excretion.

Menkes' kinky hair syndrome is another disorder of copper metabolism. It is transmitted as an X-linked recessive trait and is characterized by sparse kinky hair that microscopically shows pili torti, progressive neurologic degeneration, metaphyseal irregularities of the long bones, hypothermia, and generalized arterial occlusive disease. Although the basic defect is not understood, many of the manifestations result from a deficiency of circulating copper. The connective tissue abnormalities probably reflect dysfunction of the copper-requiring enzyme lysyl oxidase, which is involved in cross-linking both elastin and collagen. Detection of carrier females may be possible by the identification of small patches of the abnormal scalp hair (pili torti).

Hemochromatosis is a disorder of iron metabolism. Although the precise mechanism is not understood, increased intestinal absorption of iron leads to the widespread accumulation of iron as hemosiderin. The liver, pancreas, heart, and pituitary and adrenal glands are especially involved. A bronze-tan pigmentation of the skin, hepatic cirrhosis, and diabetes mellitus form the classic clinical triad of the disease, and congestive heart failure, hypopituitarism, and arthritis often occur as well. The plasma iron level is increased and hemosiderin is present in the urine. The plasma iron-binding protein transferrin is reduced, while ferritin, the body's primary iron storage protein, is increased in the plasma. Because decades of increased iron absorption are required to accumulate enough iron to produce tissue damage, symptoms usually do not appear before 40 years of age. Moreover, the disease is clinically apparent less often in women because of their normal iron loss from menstruation and pregnancy. Treatment consists of repeated phlebotomy monitored by plasma ferritin levels.

Hemochromatosis is believed to be an autosomal recessive condition with partial expression in heterozygotes. The gene for hemochromatosis is closely linked to the HLA-A locus on chromosome number 6. This linkage makes it theoretically possible to identify affected individuals during the presymptomatic stage in certain families.

CONNECTIVE TISSUE DISORDERS

The so-called connective tissues of the body, including skin, bone, teeth, cartilage, ligament, tendon, fascia, joint capsule, sclera, and elements of the heart and blood vessels, are affected by many inherited disorders. In some conditions such as aminoacidopathies, connective tissue metabolism is altered as part of a generalized metabolic derangement. In other disorders such as mucopolysaccharidoses and mucolipidoses, it is disturbed by the lysosomal storage of material in connective tissue cells. In yet other situations primary defects in connective tissue metabolism have been identified or at least strongly suspected. Of those found, most have involved the biosynthesis of collagen, one of the three major components of connective tissue matrices. Collagen and the other two components, elastic fibers and mucopolysaccharides ("ground substance", glycosaminoglycans), are elaborated by a number of cells including fibroblasts, osteoblasts, odontoblasts, and chondroblasts.

Collagen is actually a heterogeneous group of similar fibrous proteins that provide tensile strength to connective tissues. Each has its own distinct composition and tissue distribution; that is, type 1 is found in skin, bone, tendon, fascia, and dentin, type II in cartilage, type III in blood vessel and skin, and type IV in basement membrane. However, they are thought to follow a common biosynthetic scheme (Fig. 195-6). After the initial synthesis of a precursor molecule (pro α-chain), many of the proline and lysine residues are hydroxylated and galactose and glucose may be added. Three pro α-chains are then folded together to form a triple helix (procollagen). As the molecule is secreted from the cell, short segments are removed from each end, leaving the rigid collagen monomer. Further alterations ultimately lead to extensive intramolecular and intermolecular cross-linking as the polymeric collagen fiber is formed. This series of posttranslational modifications is presumably required to ensure proper cross-linking, and therefore adequate strength, to the molecule. Defects identified in several of these steps are associated clinically with a "weakness" of connective tissues such as ligamentous laxity, the occurrence of hernias, and dislocation of joints. These features, however, are not very specific. Defects have also been observed in the synthesis of specific collagens, and to some extent the clinical picture can be correlated with tissue distribution of the collagens involved. Clinical abnormalities of connective tissues can result from abnormalities in other constituents such as elastin, but in these situations the disease process is not nearly as well understood.

Marfan's syndrome is the prototype of inherited connective tissue disorders. It is an autosomal dominant trait and occurs in all races. Tall stature with disproportionately long, thin limbs, especially distally (arachnodactyly), is the major skeletal feature, but dolichocephaly, pectus excavatum, pigeon breast, high-arched palate, and prognathism also occur. Laxity of joint capsules, ligaments, tendons, and fascia results in generalized joint hypermobility and kyphoscoliosis. The major ocular manifestations consist of myopia, retinual detachment, and ectopia lentis.

Nearly two thirds of patients with Marfan's syndrome have evidence of cardiovascular involvement. Areas receiving the greatest hemodynamic pulsatile stress, such as the aortic ring and ascending aorta, show the most damage. Usually aortic ring dilation occurs first, producing aortic regurgitation. It is soon followed by progressive widening of the ascending aorta, often accompanied by dissection and even rupture. Aortic dilation and its complications lead to death in 80% of patients dying of the syndrome. Mitral regurgitation owing to redundancy of the chordae tendineae is very common and may contribute to congestive heart failure. These patients have an increased susceptibility to bacterial endocarditis.

The phenotypic expression of Marfan's syndrome varies widely. Some patients exhibit the "classic findings" of the syndrome, whereas others are only very mildly affected. At the present time it is not clear if the syndrome is a single entity or several similar but distinct disorders. The basic defect remains unknown, although an abnormality in either collagen or elastin is suspected. Treatment consists of prophylactic antibiotics for dental extraction, hormonal induction of premature puberty to lessen the kyphoscoliosis, and possibly catecholamine-blocking agents such as propranolol to diminish left ventricular contractility and thus reduce the hemodynamic stress on the the ascending aorta.

The *Ehlers-Danlos (ED)* syndromes are a group of conditions characterized by hypermobility of joints, hyperextensibility of skin, and increased tissue friability. At least eight entities are recognized (Table 195-3). The

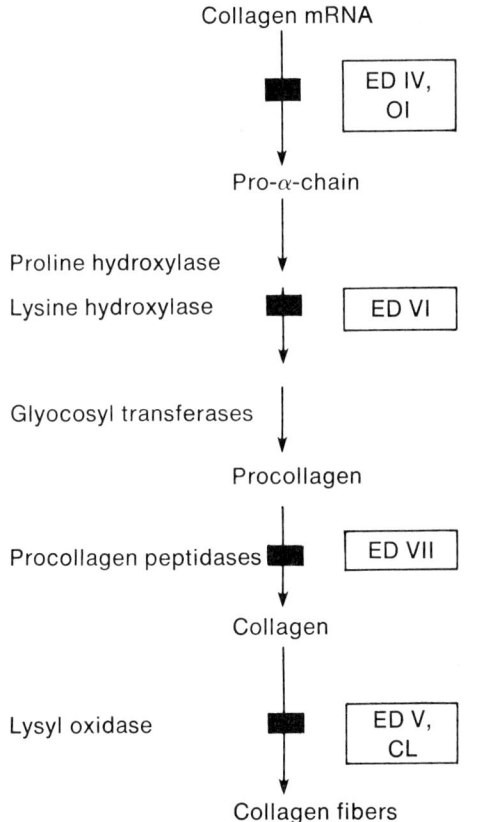

Fig. 195-6. Collagen synthesis. *ED,* Ehlers-Danlos; *OI,* osteogenesis imperfecta; *CL,* cutis laxa.

Table 195-3. Ehlers-Danlos syndromes

Classification	Type	Inheritance*	Clinical features	Basic defect
I	Gravis	AD	Generalized severe joint hypermobility, skin hyperextensibility, easy bruisability, molluscoid pseudotumors, subcutaneous spheroids, poor wound healing, premature rupture of fetal membranes	Unknown
II	Mitis	AD	Similar to ED I but milder, joint laxity limited to hands and feet, little cutaneous involvement and tissue friability	Unknown
III	Benign hypermobility	AD	Severe hypermobility of all joints	Unknown
IV	Arterial, ecchymotic, Sack's	AD/AR	Spontaneous rupture of large arteries, perforation of bowel, thin skin with prominent underlying veins	Reduced synthesis of type III collagen
V	X linked	XL	Marked hyperextensibility of skin, minimal joint hypermobility	Deficiency of lysyl oxidase
VI	Ocular	AR	Severe scoliosis, moderate joint involvement, ocular fragility with scleral rupture or retinal detachment or both	Deficiency of lysyl hydroxylase
VII	Arthrochalasis multiplex congenita	AR	Short stature, generalized joint hypermobility with multiple subluxations, abnormal facies	Deficiency of procollagen peptidase
VIII	Periodontal	AD	Mild to moderate skin hyperextensibility and joint hypermobility, marked skin friability, generalized periodontitis	Unknown

*AD, autosomal dominant; autosomal recessive; XL, X linked.

gravis type, ED I, is characterized by generalized severe joint hypermobility. Musculoskeletal deformities such as pes planus may occur. Skin hyperextensibility and easy bruising are severe, and the increased fragility leads to skin splitting and subsequent "cigarette-paper" scarring, particularly on the forehead, elbows, knees, and shins. Excessive bleeding after dental extraction is not uncommon. Varicose veins are frequent, as are molluscoid pseudotumors and subcutaneous calcified spheroids. Generalized tissue friability may complicate postsurgical or posttraumatic wound healing, as reflected by the premature rupture of fetal membranes.

The mitis type, ED II, resembles ED I but is milder. Joint laxity is often limited to the hands and feet, and cutaneous involvement is minimal. There is a slight tendency to bruising but little scar formation. Varicose veins are uncommon and tissue friability is rare. Severe hypermobility of all joints, usually without musculoskeletal deformities, characterized ED III, the benign hypermobility type. Skin changes are minimal. The arterial, ecchymotic, or Sack's type, ED IV, is the most malignant owing to the tendency to spontaneous rupture of large and intermediate arteries and bowel perforation. The skin is very thin and bruises easily; underlying veins are prominent, but stretchability is not a major feature.

The X-linked type, ED V, manifests only minimal joint hypermobility in contrast to marked hyperextensibility of the skin. Cutaneous bruisability and fragility are moderately increased. The ocular type, ED VI, is characterized by severe scoliosis and ocular fragility in addition to moderate joint and skin involvement. Corneoscleral rupture or retinal detachment may occur after minor trauma. Short stature and generalized joint hypermobility are characteristic of ED VII. Subluxations of hips, knees, elbows, and feet are common, and affected infants are floppy. Skin stretchability and bruisability are moderately increased. Abnormal facies, including hypertelorism, epicanthic folds, and scooped-out midfacies, may be part of the disorder. The major features of ED VIII include generalized severe periodontitis in addition to mild to moderate skin hyperextensibility and joint hypermobility and marked skin friability.

Dental abnormalities could serve as important diagnostic clues when associated with other features of Ehlers-Danlos syndrome. Both hard and soft oral tissues appear to be affected in this disorder. Excessive fragility of the mucous membranes and gingival tissues is apparent. Dental hard tissues findings include hypoplastic enamel and structural changes associated with the amelodentinal and cementodentinal junctions, irregular dentin formation, and an increased tendency to develop pulp stones. Several of these developmental pulpal aberrations result in the calcification of pulp tissue and/or malformed, stunted roots. Pulp stone masses appear to have a concentric pattern of formation and remain unattached to the surrounding chamber walls. There may be a direct developmental relationship to the degree of calcification of the dental papilla and deformation of the roots. In addition, reports in the literature have indicated that hypermobility of the temporomandibular joint can result in repeated jaw dislocations in some individuals.

The recognition of Ehlers-Danlos syndrome is especially important in treating dental or oral problems associated with bleeding or wound healing. It has therefore been suggested that all exodontia procedures be conducted in a hospital dental clinic and that special precautions be taken to prevent postoperative hemorrhage. In addition, great care should be exercised in placing sutures to minimize tissue tearing of mucoperiosteal flaps. It is possible to perform intraoral surgical procedures on patients with Ehlers-Danlos syndrome without any untoward effects.

A few cases of Ehlers-Danlos syndrome have been reported in association with severe destructive periodontitis. These associated findings must be considered as possibly emanating from other disorders with similar intraoral features, such as degenerative periodontal disease, neutropenia, hypophosphatasia, Papillon-LeFevre syndrome, and juvenile periodontosis.

Specific abnormalities in collagen biosynthesis have been identified in ED IV, V, VI, and VII. In ED IV, which seems to be inherited as an autosomal dominant trait in some families but in an autosomal recessive fashion in others, type III collagen synthesis is diminished. There is reduced activity of lysyl oxidase in ED V, lysyl hydroxylase in ED VI, and procollagen peptidase in ED VII. The basic defects have not been identified in ED I, II, III, and VIII.

The treatment varies according to the type. In general, patients should avoid trauma and wear protective padding over bony prominences. Particular care should be taken during surgical, dental, and obstetric procedures.

Cutis laxa is characterized by excessive loose skin over the entire body. The skin is extensible, but in contrast to the Ehler-Danlos syndromes it does not return to place on release, nor is there increased bruisability or friability. Joint hypermobility is usually not a feature. Both autosomal dominant and recessive forms are reported. Hernias, pulmonary emphysema, and diverticuli of the gastrointestinal and genitourinary tracts leading to early death occur in the recessive type, whereas in the dominant form involvement is limited to the skin. Recently an X-linked form was reported in which deficiency of lysyl oxidase, an enzyme important in cross-linking both collagen and elastin, was identified.

Osteogenesis imperfecta (OI) is a generalized disorder of the skeletal, ocular, cutaneous, otic, dental, and vascular tissues. The most characteristic feature is increased susceptibility to fractures that may result in deformities such as pseudarthroses, saber shins, marked bowing of the legs, and short stature. The fractures become less frequent following puberty. Radiologically the bones show severe generalized osteopenia with multiple fractures that heal with excessive callus formation. The vertebral bodies usually have the typical "codfish" appearance, and skull roentgenograms reveal multiple wormian bones. The face is usually triangular and the sclerae are frequently blue.

Table 195-4. OI syndromes

Type	Age at presentation	Inheritance*	Features
I	Newborn to adult	AD	Bone fragility, blue sclerae, deafness (dentinogenesis imperfecta uncommon)
II	Newborn	AR	Usually lethal in neonatal period
III	Newborn to childhood	AR	Progressive deformities of spine and limbs, normal sclerae, dentinogenesis imperfecta relatively common
IV	Newborn to adult	AD	Bone fragility, normal sclerae, dentinogenesis imperfecta (deafness uncommon)

*AD, autosomal dominant; AR, autosomal recessive.

The teeth are often yellow, brown, or opalescent and have a tendency to break easily (dentinogenesis imperfecta). The skin is thin and translucent. Joint laxity is increased. Beyond the second decade otosclerosis often leads to deafness.

The clinical severity varies considerably. At one end of the spectrum is a severe neonatal form characterized by multiple intrauterine fractures of the limbs and ribs and usually neonatal death. Some patients, however, are so mildly affected that they have only occasional fractures, blue sclerae, or mild deafness. The variability is probably due in part to genetic heterogeneity. A classification that divides OI into four types has recently been proposed (Table 195-4). A deficiency of type I collagen synthesis has been found in OI type II.

The division of osteogenesis imperfecta into at least four subtypes with different modes of inheritance and varied clinical features accentuates the need to fully characterize dental morphologic and biochemical findings associated with this disorder. Characteristics of dentinogenesis imperfecta have been found to vary both within and between families, and often such features have just not been investigated as thoroughly as other systemic factors in families with osteogenesis imperfecta.

Those characteristics of the teeth that need to be carefully scrutinized in all family members include coloration or tooth shade, brittleness of tooth enamel, and radiologic appearance of the pulp chamber and root canals. The precise incidence of all these variable dental features of dentinogenesis imperfecta associated with various forms of osteogenesis imperfecta has not been firmly established and needs to be further investigated.

Tooth coloration in both deciduous and adult dentitions ranges from a bluish brown to brown hue with an opalescent sheen. Crown morphology is variable, but bulbous crowns have been reported. The fragility of the tooth enamel, which occurs repeatedly and easily in most teeth, clearly differentiates dentinogenesis imperfecta from several intrinsic staining dental anomalies and other tooth-associated syndromes. Teeth tend to abrade very rapidly, especially deciduous teeth, so that often only stumps of crowns can be observed. Although the absence or obliteration of pulp chambers and root canals greatly enhances the diagnostic criteria, the expressivity of the gene seems to be somewhat variable. Thus large pulp chambers in primary teeth have been detected in family studies of a Brandywine triracial isolate with a form of dentinogenesis imperfecta.

Differential diagnosis includes such disorders as the coronal and radicular forms of dentin dysplasia, odontodysplasia, dentino-osseous dysplasia, branchioskeletogenital syndrome, pulpal dysplasia, and the ED VIII form of Ehlers-Danlos syndrome. Clinically, the dentin dysplasias are the most difficult to differentiate from dentinogenesis imperfecta. In the coronal form of dentin dysplasia there are few differences in the clinical characteristics compared to dentinogenesis imperfecta except for the persistence of a flame-shaped or thistle-shaped pulp chamber with normal root formation and spindly (thin) root canals. The radicular form of dentin dysplasia can be differentiated more easily because the teeth are colored normally and are lost by spontaneous exfoliation rather than extensive wear.

In odontodysplasia there are large segments of both dentitions that show hypoplasia and hypocalcification of enamel and dentin. Affected teeth are morphologically abnormal and their eruption schedule is usually delayed. The appearance of enlarged pulp chambers and the reduction in tooth density radiographically clearly differentiates odontodysplasia from dentinogenesis imperfecta.

Dentino-osseous dysplasia is more similar in clinical appearance to either the radicular form of dentin dysplasia or odontodysplasia than to dentinogenesis imperfecta. The teeth have a normal color but show short, abnormally formed roots. The thickened dense cortices of the long bones is peculiar to this disorder and account for the associated skeletal anomalies.

The branchioskeletogenital syndrome is characterized by anomalies associated with the first and second branchial arches, the skeleton including skull, vertebral column, and sternum, and penoscrotal hypospadias. This syndrome is included in the differential diagnostic series because there are multiple unerupted teeth with features that resemble the radicular form of dentin dysplasia. The maxilla is hypoplastic, giving the mandible a simulated prognathic appearance. There could be little likelihood of confusing this disorder with either dentinogenesis imperfecta or osteogenesis imperfecta.

In pulpal dysplasia, the principal dental characteristics are multiple pulp calcification extending into large root canals of both erupted and unerupted teeth. These pulp calcifications tend to partially obliterate the pulp chambers, but the disorder can be clearly differentiated from dentinogenesis imperfecta, in which there are completely obliterated pulp chambers and narrow obliterated root canals.

Similar tooth anomalies have not been reported in the Ehlers-Danlos syndrome. Recently, a few cases have been described in which there was an associated severe destructive periodontitis similar to that found in juvenile periodontosis or Papillon-LeFevre syndrome.

Therapy in OI is limited primarily to orthopedic surgical management of skeletal deformities. Immobilization may aggravate osteopenia and should be avoided.

Pseudoxanthoma elasticum (PXE) is a generalized connective tissue disorder that affects primarily the eyes, skin, and cardiovascular system. PXE has been tentatively classified into two autosomal dominant and two autosomal recessive types. The dominant type I is characterized by a subcutaneous yellow, raised rash over flexure sites, particularly the neck, axillae, groin, and cubital area, severe chorioretinitis, and complications of arterial degeneration (hypertension, angina pectoris, and intermittent claudication). Dominant type II is milder, showing only a macular rash, stretchable skin, retinal angioid streaks, myopia, high-arched palate, and blue sclerae. Recessive type I is manifested by skin changes similar to those of the dominant type I, plus angioid streaks and a predisposition to gastrointestinal hemorrhage. In the rare recessive type II there are not eye or vascular changes, but there is generalized lax skin infiltrated with degenerative elastic fibers. In general, PXE is thought to result from defective elastic fibers. There is no definitive treatment.

The dermatologic changes associated with this syndrome include an accentuation of perioral skin creases and folds, resulting in a somewhat flabby facial appearance. The inner surface of the lower lip becomes filled with multiple yellowish nodules similar to Fordyce granules. These nodules can also be seen in other mucosal areas such as the buccal, palatal, and tonsilar tissues and as elevations from many skin surfaces of the body. No special treatment is indicated, but diagnostic clarity regarding the intraoral findings is essential.

The *Winchester syndrome* is an autosomal recessive disorder characterized by coarse facial features, dwarfism, joint contractures, corneal opacities, osteoporosis, and carpal tunnel osteolysis. The destructive joint changes resemble rheumatoid arthritis. Although the basic defect is unknown, there is pathologic replacement of bone and cartilage by dense fibrous tissue, and structurally abnormal fibroblasts have been seen.

Clinical features of *fibrodysplasia ossificans progressiva*, an autosomal dominant disorder, include progressive ossification of fascia, tendons, ligaments, and aponeuroses. The process usually begins in childhood and leads to severe disability. Microdactyly, particularly of the first

Table 195-5. Partial list of chondrodystrophies

Disorder	Inheritance*	Age at diagnosis	Major clinical features	Oral manifestations	Complications
Achondroplasia	AD	Birth	Short limbs, bowed legs, stubby fingers, bulging forehead, sunken face	Malocclusion, overcrowding	Hydrocephalus (infant), lumbar spinal cord compression (adult)
Hypochondroplasia	AD	Childhood	Similar to achondroplasia but milder (may approach normality)	None	Usually none
Multiple epiphyseal dysplasia†	AD	Childhood to young adulthood	Short limbs (mild)	None	Precocious osteoarthritis‡
Spondyloepiphyseal dysplasia congenita	AD	Birth	Short trunk, barrel chest, myopia	Cleft palate	Subluxation of cervical spine owing to odontoid hypoplasia, retinal detachment, precocious osteoarthritis‡
Spondyloepiphyseal dysplasia tarda	XL	Childhood	Short trunk (mild)	None	Precocious osteoarthritis‡
Spondylometaphyseal dysplasia	AD	Infancy	Short trunk, barrel chest, bowed legs	None	Usually none
Metaphyseal chondrodysplasia, Schmid type	AD	Childhood	Short limbs, bowed legs	None	Usually none
Metaphyseal chondrodysplasia, McKusick type (cartilage-hair hypoplasia)	AR	Late infancy	Severe shortening of trunk and limbs, sparse blond hair, light complexion, immune deficiency	None	Squamous cell carcinoma of skin, complications of viral infections
Metatropic dwarfism	AR	Birth	Short limbs, severe progressive kyphoscoliosis, large joints, joint limitation	None	Usually none
Kniest syndrome	AD	Birth	Short limbs, kyphoscoliosis, large joints, contractures, myopia	Cleft palate	Retinal detachment, precocious osteoarthritis‡ with contractures
Pseudochondroplasia§	AD	Early childhood	Short trunk and limbs, ligamentous laxity, bowing of long bones (forearm)	None	Precocious osteoarthritis,‡ flexion contractures at knees
Diastrophic dwarfism	AR	Usually birth	Short limbs, kyphoscoliosis, joint contractures, clubfoot, hitchhiker thumb, cauliflower ear	Cleft palate	Precocious osteoarthritis‡ with contractures
Ellis–van Creveld syndrome	AR	Birth	Short limbs, polydactyly, congenital heart disease	Midline cleft upper lip; buccolabial frenula; natal, conical, and missing teeth	Usually none
Trichorhinophalangeal syndrome	AD	Childhood	Mild short stature, sparse hair, prominent nose, short hands	Malocclusion, supernumerary incisors	Usually none

*AD, autosomal dominant; XL, X-linked inheritance; AR, autosomal recessive.
†Two types: Fairbanks, which involves most epiphyses, and Ribbing, which is milder and often involves only capital femoral epiphyses.
‡Precocious arthritis involves weight-bearing joints, particularly the hips.
§Probably several types.

digits, is frequent, The basic defect remains unknown.

The combination of short stature, brachydactyly, limited joint mobility, myopia, and small spherical lenses that often dislocate characterizes the *Weill-Marchesani syndrome*. It is inherited as an autosomal recessive trait, although heterozygotes may have short stature.

The *chondrodystrophies* are a subgroup of connective tissue disorders that involve cartilage, especially cartilage growth (endochondral ossification). Since most of the skeleton develops embryologically and grows subsequently by this process, abnormalities are reflected by reduced skeletal growth, often with deformities. Membranous ossification may also be involved in the pathogenetic process. Although dwarfism usually dominates the clinical picture, extraskeletal problems are often present and abnormalities of dental development are common. There are over 75 recognized chondrodystrophies, most of which are very rare. The diagnosis rests on the combination of clinical, genetic, roentgenographic, and histologic features. The basic defects have not been identified in these disorders, except for the mucopolysaccharidoses and mucolipidoses in which lysosomal storage within chondrocytes is known to interfere with endochondral ossification and which are therefore considered chondrodystrophies. Likewise there is no treatment to stimulate skeletal growth. However, many of the nongrowth-related problems can be managed effectively. The salient features of several of these disorders are listed in Table 195-5.

BIBLIOGRAPHY

Aleck, K.A., and Shapiro, L.J.: Genetic-metabolic considerations in the sick neonate. Pediatr. Clin. North Am. **25**:431, 1978.

Barabas, A.P.: Ehlers-Danlos syndrome: associated with prematurity and premature rupture of foetal membranes; possible increase in incidence, Brit. Med. J. **2**:682, 1966.

Beasley, R.P., and Cohen, M.M., Jr.: A new presumably autosomal recessive form of the Ehlers-Danlos syndrome, Clin. Gen. **16**:19, 1979.

Bergsma, D.; Birth defects compendium, ed. 2, National Foundation–March of Dimes, New York, 1979, Alan R. Liss, Inc.

Bloskovics, M.E.: Phenylketonuria and other phenylalaninaemias. Clin. Endocrinol. Metabol. **3**:87, 1974.

Browne, W.G.; Oral pigmentation and root resorption in Gaucher's disease, J. Oral Surg. **35**:153, 1977.

Brustein, H.C., and Mautner, R.L.: Osteogenesis imperfecta, Oral Surg. **42**:42, 1976.

Cawson, R.A.: The oral changes in gargoylism, Proc.R. Soc. Med. **55**:1066, 1962.

Dorfman, A., and Matalon. R.: The mucopolysaccharidoses: a review, Proc. Natl. Acad. Sci. U.S.A. **73**:630, 1976.

Frimpter, G.W.: Aminoacidurias due to inherited disorders of metabolism (in two parts). N. Engl. J. Med. **289**:835, 895, 1973.

Gardner, D.G.: The oral manifestations of Hurler's syndrome, Oral Surg. **32**:46, 1971.

Gompertz. D.: Inborn errors of organic acid in metabolism. Clin. Endocrinol. Metabol. **3**:107, 1974.

Goodman, R.M., and Allison, M.L.: Chronic temporomandibular joint subluxation in Ehlers-Danlos syndrome: report of case, J. Oral Surg: **27**:659, 1969.

Gorlin, R.J., and Pindborg, J.J.: Syndromes of the head and neck, McGraw-Hill Book Co., Inc., p 275, New York, 1964.

Hirschorn. R., and Weissman,G.: Genetic disorders of lysosomes. Prog. Med. Genet. **1**:49, 1976.

Hoff, M.: Dental manifestations in Ehlers-Danlos syndrome, Oral Surg. **44**:864, 1977.

Horton. W.A.: Heritable connective tissue disorders. In Jackson, L.G., and Schimke, R.N., editors: Clinical genetics: a source book for physicians, New York, 1979, John Wiley & Sons, Inc.

Hughes, C.L.: Odontectomy in treatment of Ehlers-Danlos syndrome: report of case, J. Oral Surg. **28**:612, 1970.

Kelly, T.E.: The mucopolysaccharidoses and mucolipidoses, Clin. Orthop. **114**:116, 1976.

Lela, J., Polliack, A., and Ulmansky, M.: Involvement of the mandible in Gaucher's disease, Br. J. Oral Surg. **9**:246, 1972.

Linch, D.C., and Acton, C.H.C.: Ehlers-Danlos syndrome presenting with juvenile destructive periodontitis, Br. Dent. J. **147**:95, 1979.

McKusick, V.A.: Heritable disorders of connective tissue, ed. 4, St. Louis, 1972, The C. V. Mosby Co.

Michanowicz, A.E., Michanowicz, J.P., and Stein, G.M.: Gaucher's disease, report of a case, Oral Surg. **23**:36,1967.

Palmar, S.H.: Metabolic aspects of immunodeficiency disease. Semin. Hematol. **17**:30, 1980.

Pope, F.M.: Historical evidence for the genetic heterogeneity of pseudoxanthoma elasticum, Br. J. Dermatol. **92**:493, 1975.

Pope, F.M.: Two types of autosomal recessive pseudoxanthoma elasticum, Arch Dermatol. **110**:209,1974.

Prockop, D.J., and others: The biosynthesis of collagen and its disorders (in two parts), N. Engl. J. Med. **301**:13, 77, 1979.

Pyeritz, P.E., and McKusick, V.A.: The Marfan syndrome, diagnosis and management, N. Engl. J. Med. **300**:772, 1979.

Recant, B.S., and Lepman, J.S.: The Ehlers-Danlos syndrome: a case requiring oral surgery, Oral Surg. **28**:460, 1969.

Rimoin, D.L.: The chondrodystrophies, Adv. Hum. Genet. **5**:1, 1975.

Sass-Kortsak, A, and Bearn, A.: Hereditary disorders of copper metabolism. In. Stanbury, J.B., Wyngaarden, J.B., and Frederickson, D.S., editors: The metabolic basis of inherited disease, ed. 4, New York, 1978, McGraw-Hill Book Co.

Sillence, D.O., Serra, A., and Danks, D.M.: Genetic heterogeneity in osteogenesis imperfecta, J.Med. Genet. **16**:101, 1979.

Stewart, R.E., Hollister, D.W., and Rimoin, D.L.: A new variant of Ehlers-Danlos syndrome: an autosomal dominant disorder of fragile skin, abnormal scarring and generalized periodontitis, Birth Defects. **13**(3B):85, 1977.

Worth, H.M.: Hurler's syndrome; a study of radiologic appearances in the jaws, Oral Surg. **22**:21, 1966.

196 • THE PORPHYRIAS

Karl E. Anderson, Shigeru Sassa, and Attallah Kappas

The porphyrias are a group of inherited and acquired disorders characterized by abnormalities in the activities of specific enzymes of the heme biosynthetic pathway. Disturbances of porphyrin-heme biosynthesis can also be evoked by a wide variety of chemicals. Both the inherited and chemically induced porphyrias have provided valuable insights into the mechanisms by which cellular heme synthesis is controlled and the way in which heritable and environmental factors may disturb heme metabolism.

HEME BIOSYNTHETIC PATHWAY

Heme is probably synthesized in all aerobic cells because it is required for vital cellular hemoproteins, including mitochondrial respiratory cytochromes. More heme is made in the bone marrow and liver than in other organs. In the bone marrow, heme is utilized primarily to make hemoglobin, which is a transport protein for molecular oxygen, whereas in liver most newly formed heme is used for synthesis of cytochrome P-450. This cytochrome is a key component of the microsomal mixed-function oxidase system, which oxidizes a variety of drugs and endogenous steroids and utilizes both molecular oxygen and NADPH.

Porphyrins, porphyrinogens, and porphyrin precursors are intermediates in the heme biosynthetic pathway. Since the bone marrow and liver synthesize more heme than other tissues, it is not surprising that diseases of porphyrin metabolism should be expressed particularly in erythroid cells and in the liver. Thus the clinical porphyrias are commonly classified as being either erythropoietic or hepatic in origin, depending on whether excess intermediates are generated primarily from erythroid cells in the marrow or from hepatocytes.

The synthetic pathway for heme is illustrated in Fig. 196-1. The first and the last three enzymes in this sequence are mitochondrial, whereas the intermediate enzymes are found in the cytosol. The first enzyme of the pathway is a δ-aminolevulinic acid (ALA) synthase, which catalyzes the condensation of glycine and succinyl CoA to form ALA. This enzyme requires pyridoxal 5′-phosphate as a cofactor. ALA is a δ- rather than an α-amino acid and therefore does not participate in protein synthesis. It is, however, an obligate precursor for porphyrin and heme formation. Two moles of ALA are condensed to form a monopyrrole, porphobilinogen (PBG), by a cytosolic enzyme, ALA dehydratase. By the combined action of two other cytosolic enzymes, uroporphyrinogen (UROgen) I synthase and UROgen III cosynthase, four PBG molecules are then converted to a tetrapyrrole, UROgen III, in which one pyrrole is reversed, resulting in an asymmetric configuration. The symmetric (type I) isomers of UROgen and coproporphyrinogen (COPROgen) are normally produced in insignificant amounts, and there are no known heme compounds derived from these type I porphyrinogens.

The portion of the hime biosynthetic sequence in which UROgen III is metabolized to protoporphyrinogen (PROTOgen) IX is shown in Fig. 196-2. A cytosolic enzyme, UROgen decarboxylase, removes four carboxyl groups from four acetic acid side chains in a stepwise fashion, yielding COPROgen III (which contains four methyl groups rather than the four acetic acid groups). COPROgen III is oxidatively decarboxylated to PROTOgen IX by a mitochondrial enzyme, COPROgen oxidase. Thus PROTOgen IX contains two vinyl groups on rings A and B instead of the two propionic acid groups as in COPROgen III. PROTOgen oxidase then removes six hydrogen atoms to yield protoporphyrin (PROTO) IX. Finally, ferrous iron (Fe^{2+}) is inserted into PROTO IX by the action of ferrochelatase to form protoheme and thus heme. Outside the reducing environment of the cell, porphyrinogens are largely auto-oxidized to porphyrins and then excreted in urine or bile. Porphyrinogens are colorless and nonfluorescent, whereas porphyrins are aromatic compounds that are reddish and fluoresce bright red in ultraviolet light.

The rate of heme synthesis in the liver is thought to be controlled primarily by ALA synthase. ALA synthase activity in normal liver is very low; the level is sufficient to maintain the steady state of heme synthesis and concentrations of hepatic hemoproteins, but not to provide more ALA as is required when cytochrome P-450 formation in-

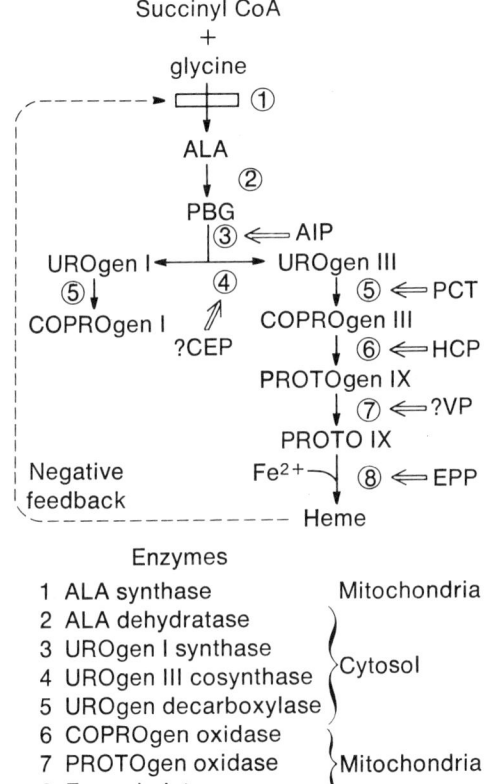

Fig. 196-1. Heme biosynthetic pathway showing chemical intermediates, enzymes and their subcellular locations, and enzymes that are primarily affected in human porphyrias. In porphyrias intermediates may accumulate in tissues and be excreted in urine or bile. Pattern of excretion of intermediates is largely determined by which of these enzymes is reduced in each type of porphyria. Excess UROgen, COPROgen, and PROTOgen are mostly auto-oxidized to corresponding porphyrins. ALA and PBG, which are porphyrin precursors, are excreted in urine, uroporphyrin in urine, coproporphyrin in urine and bile, and protoporphyrin only in bile. Biliary porphyrins may undergo enterohepatic circulation before they appear in stool. *AIP*, acute intermittent porphyria; *CEP*, congenital erythropoietic porphyria; *PCT*, porphyria cutanea tarda; *HCP*, hereditary coproporphyria; *VP*, variegate porphyria; *EPP*, erythropoietic protoporphyria; *ALA*, δ-aminolevulinic acid; *PBG*, porphobilinogen; *UROgen*, uroporphyrinogen; *COPROgen*, coproporphyrinogen; *PROTOgen*, protoporphyrinogen; *PROTO*, protoporphyrin.

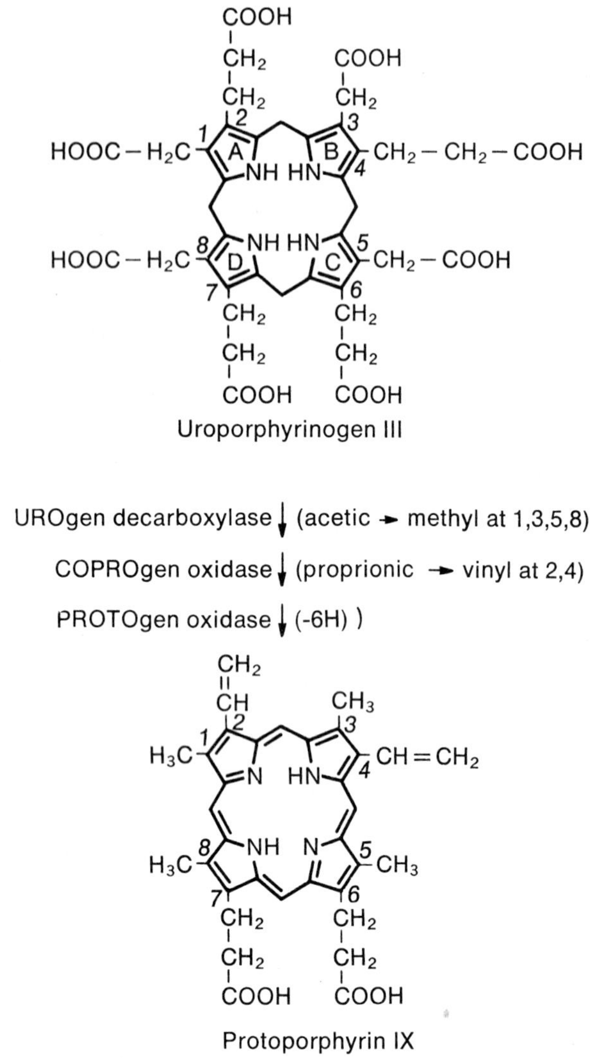

Fig. 196-2. Structure of uroporphyrinogen III and major chemical transformations whereby it is metabolized to protoporphyrin IX by the enzymes uroporphyrinogen decarboxylase, coproporphyrinogen oxidase, and protoporphyrinogen oxidase (see text).

creases. In response to various chemicals, drugs, and hormones, liver ALA synthase can be markedly induced (in experimental systems by 50-fold or more), indicating that this enzyme can greatly increase in amount when greater hepatic heme synthesis is required. Unlike ALA synthase, the activities of enzymes that convert ALA to heme are not rate limiting in the liver. The rate of turnover of ALA synthase is very rapid, which is a suitable characteristic for a rate-limiting enzyme. In livers of experimental animals the half-life of this enzyme is about 1 to 3 hours. This is considerably shorter than the average for mitochondrial proteins in general, which is about 5 days.

Hepatic ALA synthase is regulated by heme, the end product of the pathway, as indicated in Fig. 196-1. The enzyme can be inhibited by hemin at concentrations in the range of 5×10^{-6} molar. However, repression of synthesis of ALA synthase by hemin occurs at far lower concentrations, about 10^{-7} molar. Thus it appears that repression of enzyme synthesis rather than inhibition of activity is the principal regulatory action of hemin on ALA synthase in the liver.

Control of heme biosynthesis in erythroid cells appears to occur by a somewhat different mechanism than in the liver. Heme biosynthesis in erythroid cells is not necessarily regulated by ALA synthase but can also be controlled by ferrochelatase. Drugs and foreign chemicals that induce ALA synthase in the liver and produce hepatic porphyria experimentally do not induce this enzyme or stimulate porphyrinogenesis in erythroid cells.

Very little is known about the control of ALA synthase and heme biosynthesis in cell types other than liver and erythroid cells, but available evidence suggests that, as in the bone marrow, it may be different from the liver.

CLASSIFICATION AND DIAGNOSIS OF THE HUMAN PORPHYRIAS

Porphyrias are classified as either erythropoietic or hepatic depending on the primary organ in which overproduction of porphyrins or precursors takes place (Table 196-1). They are also characterized on the basis of clinical features and patterns of excretion of porphyrins and their precursors. As will be apparent, the two most important clinical features of the porphyrias are (1) neurovisceral manifestations in acute intermittent porphyria and other types of porphyria in which there is excess accumulation and excretion of porphyrin precursors (that is, ALA and PBG) and (2) cutaneous photosensitivity in those porphyrias in which excess porphyrins accumulate in blood and skin.

Because the human porphyrias differ greatly in their clinical manifestations and management, for proper therapy it is important to establish precisely which type of porphyria is present in a patient. In the inherited types it is important to study family members as well. For example, relatives of patients with the hereditary hepatic porphyrias should be screened, and those found to have clinically latent porphyria should be advised to avoid factors, including drugs such as barbiturates and sulfonamides, that can produce life-threatening neurologic attacks. Certain treatments for porphyria cutanea tarda (for example, phlebotomy and chloroquine) are not useful for other porphyrias. β-Carotene and sunscreens are useful for preventing photosensitivity mainly in erythropoietic protoporphyria.

Congenital erythropoietic porphyria

In humans congenital erythropoietic porphyria (CEP) is characterized biochemically by the excessive production and excretion in urine of type I isomers of uroporphyrin (URO) and coproporphyrin (COPRO). CEP is transmitted in an autosomal recessive fashion and is extremely rare. Only 60 authentic cases were reported up to 1978. The earliest sign of the disorder is massive excretion of URO,

Table 196-1. Classification and major features of the clinical porphyrias

Classification	Deficient enzyme	Autosomal inheritance	Major presenting symptoms*		Increased red cell porphyrins†	Excess excretion of ALA, PBG, porphyrins*†	
			Photo-sensitivity	Neuro-visceral		Urine	Stool
Erythropoietic							
Congenital erythropoietic porphyria	? UROgen III cosynthase	Recessive	+ (severe)	—	*URO I, COPRO I*	URO I, COPRO I	
Erythropoietic protoporphyria	Ferrochelatase	Dominant	+	—	*PROTO*	—	PROTO
Hepatic							
Acute intermittent porphyria	UROgen I synthase	Dominant	—	+	—	ALA, *PBG*	
Hereditary coproporphyria	COPROgen oxidase	Dominant	+	+	—	ALA, PBG, COPRO	*COPRO*
Variegate porphyria	? PROTOgen oxidase or ferrochelatase	Dominant	+	+	—	ALA, PBG, COPRO	COPRO, *PROTO*
Porphyria cutanea tarda	UROgen decarboxylase	‡	+	—	—	*URO*	*ISOCOPRO*

*+, Present; —, absent; UROgen, uroporphyrinogen; COPROgen, coproporphyrinogen; PROTOgen, protoporphyrinogen; URO, uroporphyrin; COPRO, coproporphyrin; PROTO, protoporphyrin; ALA, δ-aminolevulinic acid; PBG, porphobilinogen; ISOCOPRO, isocoproporphyrin.
†Findings of major diagnostic importance are italicized.
‡Dominant inheritance has been documented in some families but not others.

which may be evident in the neonate or young child as reddish or pink urine. CEP can also be recognized in utero by finding increased porphyrins in amniotic fluid. The disease appears to have no preferential population distribution.

CLINICAL MANIFESTATIONS. The major clinical characteristics are photosensitivity and hemolytic anemia, usually beginning in infancy. Reddish urine is also an early sign. The neurologic symptoms that characterize the hereditary hepatic porphyrias are not observed. Skin lesions resulting from photosensitivity are usually extensive and severe in children and adults with CEP. Vesicular and bullous skin lesions are present on the exposed portions of the body and occur more frequently in the summer months. Lesions may become infected and ulcerate, and this further promotes scarring and deformity. Severe deformities with loss of the nails, terminal phalanges, nasal and auricular tissue, and eyelids can occur. Hypertrichosis, hyperpigmentation, and hypopigmentation are very common. Both deciduous and permanent teeth may show brownish staining (erythrodontia) with intense red fluorescence under ultraviolet light, as is characteristic of porphyrins. Porphyrin deposited in the teeth and in bone is mainly URO, probably owing to its affinity for calcium phosphate.

Mild to severe hemolytic anemia is common, with associated erythroid hyperplasia in the bone marrow, reticulocytosis, circulating normoblasts, and increased fecal urobilinogen. Requirements for multiple transfusions have been reported, as has early death from anemia. The red cell life span is decreased, but it may be improved by splenectomy in some patients with CEP. The anemia of CEP may also result in part from ineffective erythropoiesis in the bone marrow. The bone marrow contains many fluorescent erythroblasts, and this porphyrin fluorescence is found principally in nuclei. Also, excess heme has been demonstrated in nuclei of bone marrow cells.

The mechanism of hemolysis in CEP is not fully understood. Photohemolysis of CEP red cells can be demonstrated in vitro, but the extent of hemolysis in vivo is not clearly correlated with exposure to light. Splenic destruction of porphyrin-laden erythrocytes is an important factor in the hemolytic process and explains why some patients with this disorder respond at least partially to splenectomy.

LABORATORY FINDINGS. Large amounts of URO and COPRO are excreted in urine, whereas ALA and PBG excretion is normal. The color of the urine varies from faint pink to dark red depending on the porphyrin content. The amount of COPRO is usually less than that of URO, which can sometimes reach 500 mg/day. Smaller amounts of the less carboxylated porphyrins (that is, 7-, 6-, and 5-carboxylated) are also excreted. Most of the urinary URO and COPRO is type I (Fig. 196-1), but smaller increases in type III URO and COPRO are also found. Feces contain large amounts of COPRO, less URO, but little or no increase in protoporphyrin (PROTO). Fecal COPRO is mainly type I. Plasma also contains URO and COPRO, whereas porphyrins are virtually undetectable in normal plasma. Circulating erythrocytes contain large amounts of URO I and lesser although still excessive concentrations of COPRO I. For reasons that are not clear, PROTO may increase and become the major porphyrin in erythrocytes in some patients with CEP.

UROgen III cosynthase is reported to be decreased to about one-tenth to one-third the normal level in erythrocytes. The basic abnormality may be a structural gene defect for UROgen III cosynthase. Other explanations are possible (including a regulatory mutation for a rate-limiting enzyme in the heme biosynthetic pathway for erythroid cells, or a structural gene mutation leading to hyperactive ALA synthase or UROgen I synthase), but no direct proof for such alternate mechanisms has been obtained.

MANAGEMENT. Therapy for this severe condition is difficult and often only marginally successful. Photopathic damage to the skin can result in scarring, and patients should be shielded from sunlight as much as possible. Sunscreens and β-carotene may be somewhat beneficial. Splenectomy may improve anemia in some patients with CEP.

Erythropoietic protoporphyria

Erythropoietic protoporphyria (EPP) is an inherited disease that is also characterized clinically by cutaneous photosensitivity, but this is generally much less severe than in CEP. Patients with EPP have marked increases in PROTO in erythrocytes, plasma, and feces but no increased porphyrins in urine. EPP is much more common than CEP, and more than 300 cases have been reported. EDP is an autosomal dominant disorder with a variable degree of clinical expression. In fact, it can be completely latent. In contrast to the hereditary hepatic porphyrias, which are also autosomal dominant disorders, latent EPP has not been found to be activated clinically by exposure to chemicals, drugs, or hormones.

CLINICAL MANIFESTATIONS. Signs and symptoms, usually beginning in childhood, follow exposure to sunlight. Burning and itching of the skin, often very soon after sun exposure, can be accompanied by edema and erythema. Vesicles and residual scarring are usually not prominent. Cholelithiasis can also be present, and liver function tests may be abnormal. Fluorescence of the teeth is not found. Hemolysis is usually absent or mild in EPP.

LABORATORY FINDINGS. Urine porphyrins and porphyrin precursors are normal. Increases of PROTO in erythrocytes and feces are striking, and significant amounts of PROTO are present in plasma. In EPP the increased erythrocyte PROTO is, for unknown reasons, not complexed with zinc, as it is in other conditions associated with excess red cell PROTO, such as lead poisoning and iron deficiency.

PROTO accumulation occurs in late normoblasts. Much of the porphyrin diffuses out of red cells into plasma as red cells mature, so that the PROTO level is much higher in reticulocytes than in mature red cells of patients with EPP. In contrast, in lead poisoning the increased erythrocyte zinc PROTO declines only slightly with cell aging. Therefore plasma PROTO is elevated in EPP but not in lead poisoning. Loss of PROTO from red cells in EPP has been estimated to be 40% of the total PROTO content of the circulating erythrocytes each day. This loss, combined with the additional loss from bone marrow normoblasts and reticulocytes, could readily account for most of the daily PROTO excretion in feces in this disorder without postulating a major extraerythropoietic source of PROTO formation, such as the liver. Nevertheless, there is evidence that excess PROTO may also be produced by the liver in EPP, and some have suggested renaming the disease "erythrohepatic protoporphyria."

Recent studies clearly indicate a deficiency in ferrochelatase in EPP, probably in all tissues. It is likely that this deficient enzyme becomes rate limiting for heme formation in erythroid cells in the marrow and possibly in the liver as well. Patients with clinically manifest EPP, as well as completely latent gene carriers of the EPP defect (with normal red cell porphyrins), can be identified by assessing ferrochelatase activity in cultured cells such as mitogen-stimulated lymphocytes. Latent gene carriers with normal erythrocyte porphyrins may also show minimal but definite increases in plasma porphyrins.

MANAGEMENT. Tolerance to sun exposure can be significantly increased by oral β-carotene in many patients with EPP. This treatment can produce a yellow or yellow-orange skin coloration, but it is seldom a major cosmetic problem. Liver dysfunction and considerable protoporphyrin deposition in the liver develop in a minority of patients with EPP. Other causes of liver disease should be sought and treated in such patients, and consideration should be given to cholestyramine therapy, which may increase fecal excretion of PROTO.

Acute intermittent porphyria

Acute intermittent porphyria (AIP), an autosomal dominant disease, is probably the most common type of the hereditary hepatic porphyrias (that is, AIP, hereditary coproporphyria, and variegate porphyria). In AIP the basic defect is an inherited deficiency of UROgen I synthase, the heme pathway enzyme that in the presence of UROgen III cosynthase metabolizes PBG to UROgen III (Fig. 196-1). Clinical manifestations rarely occur before puberty. AIP has been referred to as the Swedish type of porphyria, and it is perhaps most common in Scandinavia and the British Isles. The incidence of AIP was previously estimated on the basis of urinary ALA and PBG determinations to be 1.5 per 100,000 in Sweden. Since urinary ALA and PBG are not necessarily increased in a gene carrier of this disorder, this is clearly an underestimate. It was estimated more recently that the incidence of AIP in the population 15 years of age or older in Sweden is 7.7 per 100,000.

The highest incidence has been observed in Lapland (100 per 100,000), and all latent and expressed cases in that region appear to be related to a single family. Assays for erythrocyte UROgen I synthase can detect almost all gene carriers regardless of age or clinical severity. Such assays, when used to screen large numbers of relatives of AIP patients, may increase the apparent incidence of the gene carrier state for AIP by as much as 10-fold.

CLINICAL MANIFESTATIONS. The clinical symptoms of the three hereditary hepatic porphyrias are very similar, except that hereditary coproporphyria and variegate porphyria may be associated with photosensitivity, which does not occur in AIP. All symptoms in AIP can be related to neurologic disturbances involving especially the autonomic nervous system. Thus "neurovisceral" symptoms such as abdominal pain, vomiting, and constipation are thought to result from metabolic disturbances in autonomic nerves in the abdomen.

The severity of symptoms, frequency of acute episodes, and age at onset of the clinical expression of AIP are highly variable. In the great majority of gene carriers the disorder remains clinically latent throughout their lives. This and the fact that the degree of UROgen I synthase deficiency is not correlated with disease activity make it evident that additional factors including drug, nutritional, and hormonal influences are important in the clinical expression of AIP. Many drugs that are hazardous to patients with AIP cause the induction of ALA synthase in the liver.

Because the deficiency of UROgen I synthase is an autosomal dominant disorder, it is transmitted as commonly to males as to females. However, symptoms develop after puberty more frequently in women than in men, and they often occur in the luteal phase of the menstrual cycle and sometimes during pregnancy.

Acute episodes usually begin with abdominal pain. Because there is no peritoneal inflammation, the findings on physical examination are often not impressive. Ileus with rather diffuse small bowel dilation may be evident on a roentgenographic film of the abdomen. Leukocytosis and fever may be absent even when there is severe pain from AIP, although either or both may sometimes accompany an AIP attack. Hypertension and tachycardia occur frequently and are probably due to autonomic dysfunction. Peripheral neuropathy, mood changes, and other psychiatric manifestations can also occur in AIP. Other central nervous system complications may include seizures and hypothalamic involvement with inappropriate ADH secretion. Hyponatremia, which is not uncommon in patients with acute symptoms, may be caused by salt depletion from nausea and vomiting or by hemodilution owing to inappropriate ADH secretion. Neuropathy can progress over days or weeks and lead to muscle paralysis, quadriplegia, and death from respiratory paralysis. Such severe fatal attacks are quite rare unless porphyria is recognized late and the patient is treated with harmful medications before diagnosis. The mortality rate from AIP appears to be declining as better diagnostic methods become widely employed and as more relatives of known AIP patients are screened for the disease before the onset of symptoms.

Chronic symptoms including pain and depression occur between attacks in some patients with AIP. Management is difficult, and because AIP is characterized by acute rather than by long-term painful symptoms, other causes of pain should be sought carefully. Patients with AIP may have acute illnesses of other kinds, including appendicitis, and it should not be assumed that abdominal pain in a patient with AIP is always due to porphyria.

LABORATORY FINDINGS. UROgen I synthase deficiency is the primary genetic defect in AIP. Decreased UROgen I synthase activity has been described not only in the liver but also in erythrocytes, cultured skin fibroblasts, cultured amniotic cells, and mitogen-stimulated lymphocytes. This enzyme deficiency (about 50% of the normal level) is found regardless of the presence or absence of clinical symptoms. It is inherited as an autosomal dominant trait in families in which AIP appears, and the 50% of normal level of activity probably reflects the heterozygous state for the normal gene for this enzyme.

AIP is characterized also by the excretion of large amounts of ALA and PBG in urine. PBG is detected with Ehrlich's aldehyde reagent, with which it combines to form a complex with a reddish color (this is the Watson-Schwartz test). The PBG concentration in normal urine is too low to be detected by this method. When PBG excretion is markedly elevated, however, as in acute attacks of AIP, this test produces an intense reddish color. The original Watson-Schwartz test may give false positive results. Therefore a modified Watson-Schwartz test is commonly used in which extractions with both chloroform and butanol are carried out to distinguish the Ehrlich aldehyde complex with PBG from that with other compounds (especially urobilinogen). The PBG complex is not extractable with either of hese organic solvents. A preferable method, however, is the column chromatographic method of Mauzerall and Granick, which is specific for PBG and is also quantitative.

ALA in urine is usually increased in AIP but to a lesser degree than PBG is. Increased ALA in urine is less specific than PBG for the diagnosis of AIP, however, since ALA but not PBG may be increased in other conditions such as lead poisoning and hereditary tyrosinemia.

Urinary PBG may decrease during clinical remissions of AIP, but usually it remains increased for a prolonged period. Many gene carriers of AIP who have low UROgen I synthase activity in erythrocytes but never have symptoms excrete normal amounts of PBG throughout their lives, but some excrete very large amounts of ALA and PBG. Thus it is useful to measure and follow urine ALA and PBG excretion in AIP gene carriers, although this does not provide an absolute indication of when symptoms may occur.

Porphyrin concentrations may be increased in freshly voided urine from patients with AIP in remission and in relapse, presumably because of spontaneous cyclization of PBG to form porphyrins (especially URO). This nonenzymatic porphyrin formation is facilitated by prolonged storage of urine, an acidic urine pH, and light.

Both ALA and PBG have been detected in the plasma and cerebrospinal fluid of patients with AIP. ALA is chemically similar to γ-aminobutyric acid (GABA) and may interfere with normal GABA neutrotransmitter functions. It is not clear, however, that symptoms of AIP are caused by a direct effect of ALA on the central nervous system. Levels of ALA and PBG in cerebrospinal fluid are considerably lower than those in plasma in the acute porphyrias.

It seems improbable that gene carriers have differing levels of UROgen I synthase activity in their livers; it is therefore likely that decreased UROgen I synthase does not by itself determine clinical expression in AIP and that additional metabolic factors must also be involved.

Metabolic factors associated with clinical activation of AIP include the onset of puberty, hormonal variations in the menstrual cycle, exposure to a variety of drugs and environmental chemicals, changes in dietary carbohydrate or fat, and reduced caloric intake. Drugs known to be harmful to patients with acute intermittent porphyria, hereditary coproporphyria, and variegate porphyria include barbiturates, sulfonamides, meprobamate, glutethimide, methaqualone, anticonvulsants (phenytoin and others), griseofulvin, oral contraceptives, and alcohol. Narcotic analgesics (morphine and others), phenothiazines (chlorpromazine and others), chloral hydrate, aspirin, and penicillin are known to be safe for use by these patients. Information on the effect of most other drugs in these disorders is inadequate. Metabolites of gonadal and adrenal steroid hormones (such as androgens and progesterones) can induce ALA synthase. Estrogens and their metabolites appear to have less porphyrinogenic properties, and adrenal glucocorticoids have none.

Acute exacerbations of the hereditary hepatic porphyrias may occur after a reduced intake of calories and may be ameliorated by increases in carbohydrate ingestion or by infusions of large amounts of glucose. The salutary effect of glucose in the treatment of hereditary hepatic porphyrias has an experimental analogy, termed the "glucose effect," in the use of glucose to prevent chemically induced porphyria. Glucose administration can block the induction of hepatic ALA synthase by a number of porphyria-inducing drugs.

MANAGEMENT. When a diagnosis of AIP is established in an acutely ill patient, all drugs known to exacerbate the disease should be discontinued. An adequate caloric intake, preferably high in carbohydrates, should be ensured, if necessary by intravenous infusion of at least 300 g of glucose daily. In patients with hyponatremia owing to inappropriate ADH secretion, caution should be exercised to avoid a further excess in water in the form of intravenous solutions. Although glucose infusions in acute attacks of porphyria are not always beneficial, such treatment remains an important mode of therapy.

Pain is most effectively treated with morphine, meperidine, or codeine, and nausea with a phenothiazine such as chlorpromazine. The latter is often useful for sedation as well. Insomnia can be treated with chloral hydrate. Continued treatment between attacks is seldom needed, and there is no clear evidence that chlorpromazine or other drugs have a preventive action.

A more recently developed investigational treatment is intravenous hematin infusion. Hematin, which can be given only intravenously, appears to be effective in lowering urinary output of ALA and PBG. However, controlled studies of its potential clinical benefits have not been carried out.

Hereditary coproporphyria

Hereditary coproporphyria (HCP) is similar to AIP and variegate porphyria in its clinical symptoms. Unlike patients with AIP, however, those with HCP may also display cutaneous photosensitivity. Acute attacks of HCP are provoked by the same drugs that precipitate acute attacks of AIP. The disorder is inherited in an autosomal dominant fashion, the clinical expression and severity are quite variable, and as in AIP, latent carriers are common. HCP is generally less severe than AIP. As in AIP, acute attacks occur more commonly in females than in males.

LABORATORY FINDINGS. The predominant biochemical finding in clinically expressed HCP is marked elevation of COPRO III excretion in urine and stool. During acute attacks urinary ALA and PBG concentrations are also increased. In some patients with HCP greater than 95% of urinary porphyrins are COPRO, whereas in others URO is also increased to a degree similar to AIP. Feces contain large amounts of COPRO. Fecal PROTO may also be increased, but always much less than COPRO. Markedly elevated fecal "X porphyrin," a porphyrin-peptide complex, is not usually found in HCP.

GENE DEFECT. COPROgen oxidase has recently been shown to be approximately 50% deficient in patients with HCP. Since COPROgen oxidase is a mitochondrial enzyme, the enzyme assay must be carried out in cells other than circulating erythrocytes, and for this purpose cultured skin fibroblasts, cultured lymphocytes, and leukocytes have been employed. Activity of this enzyme is approximately one-half that in cells from normal subjects. The mode of inheritance is compatible with autosomal dominant transmission.

A 50% COPROgen oxidase deficiency in HCP still provides a level of activity for this enzyme that is far in excess of normal UROgen I synthase activity in the liver. Thus normally low activity of UROgen I synthase relative to that for COPROgen oxidase may explain the excessive excretion of ALA and PBF during acute attacks of HCP. As in AIP, attacks occur only when ALA synthase is increased by drugs, hormones, or other factors. Attacks occur less readily in HCP than in AIP, and HCP is a less severe disease, presumably because UROgen I synthase activity is normal in HCP whereas it is decreased by 50% in AIP.

A case of severe homozygous HCP has been described recently. In this patient's cells COPROgen oxidase activity was only 2% of normal, and it was 50% of normal in both parents. The patient excreted very large amounts of ALA and PBG in urine and COPRO in urine and feces. Perhaps the homozygous states in AIP, variegate porphyria, and EPP are incompatible with life.

Variegate porphyria

Variegate porphyria (VP) is another of the autosomal dominant types of hereditary hepatic porphyria. It is characterized by symptoms very similar to those of AIP and HCP. VP is sometimes called protocoproporphyria hereditaria or South African porphyria, since it is common in the white population in South Africa. It has also been found in other countries. The disease is called "variegate" porphyria because it can be manifested by an acute attack with neurovisceral symptoms or by cutaneous photosensitivity or both, and it can also be completely latent clinically. The neurovisceral symptoms are essentially the same as in AIP and HCP.

BIOCHEMICAL FINDINGS. Most patients with VP excrete large amounts of PROTO in feces, with lesser increases of COPRO, a pattern generally not observed in AIP, HCP, and porphyria cutanea tarda. As in HCP, urine PBG is elevated during acute attacks but it is often normal during remission of the disease. In AIP, in contrast, normal levels of urinary PBG are less common once the disorder has become clinically apparent.

Increased amounts of ether-insoluble, hydrophilic porphyrins are found in the feces of patients with VP. These compounds are collectively termed "X-porphyrin." They may also be found in excess in porphyria cutanea tarda and occasionally in AIP and HCP, and thus they may be of less help in the differential diagnosis of VP and porphyria cutanea tarda than was originally thought.

GENE DEFECT. The enzyme defect in VP is still unclear. The porphyrin excretion pattern (predominantly PROTO in feces) suggests that the biochemical defect may be at one of the terminal steps of the heme biosynthetic pathway. Evidence for a deficiency of PROTOgen oxidase or ferrochelatase has been put forward by different investigators. Either deficiency could result in excess protoporphyrin excretion.

Porphyria cutanea tarda

Porphyria cutanea tarda (PCT) is characterized by skin photosensitivity and excessive excretion of porphyrins in urine and feces. In contrast to the hereditary hepatic porphyrias (AIP, HCP, and VP), acute attacks of neurovisceral symptoms do not occur. Drugs known to precipitate acute attacks of hereditary hepatic porphyrias have no effect on PCT. Urine PBG is always normal, although occasionally mild elevations of ALA may occur.

PCT is probably the most common type of porphyria. It occurs widely, but the Bantu population of South Africa has a particularly high prevalence of the disease. The majority of patients with PCT are considered to have an acquired disorder. However, a hereditary form of the disease, with symptoms very similar to those of the acquired form, also occurs. Furthermore, a PCT-like syndrome can occur in normal subjects after exposure to certain chemicals, particularly halogenated hydrocarbons such as hexachlorobenzene, tetrachlorodibenzo[p]dioxin (TCDD), methyl chloride, and vinyl chloride.

CLINICAL MANIFESTATIONS. Skin lesions often begin with erythema and can progress to vesicular and bullous lesions that may eventually ulcerate. Chronic skin changes include hyperpigmentation, hypopigmentation, scarring, hypertrichosis, and sclerodermoid changes. Unlike EPP, the rapid development of painful erythema after exposure to light is usually not seen in PCT.

Liver dysfunction with or without cirrhosis is common among patients with PCT, and this is often, although not always, associated with excess alcohol intake. Liver biopsy frequently reveals siderosis, although not often to the degree found in hereditary hemochromatosis. The extent to which liver injury is essential to the development of PCT is unclear, but PCT is not found in the majority of patients with liver damage resulting from alcohol or other causes. Therefore an underlying constitutional abnormality, which could be either acquired or inherited, may produce PCT in some patients with liver dysfunction. Lupus erythematosus occurs in patients with PCT more often than in the normal population, but the reasons for this association are unknown.

Iron overload is another factor contributing to PCT. Its frequent occurrence has been well documented in a number of studies, and iron removal by repeated phlebotomy is known to be highly effective in the treatment of PCT. Although total iron-binding capacity in serum is usually normal, there is an increase in the saturation of serum transferrin with iron in most patients with PCT. The serum ferritin concentration may be a better index of iron overload and response to phlebotomy in PCT, but further experience is needed. Hepatic injury and iron excess may accentuate PCT when it is present in the latent form but are not sufficient in themselves to cause PCT.

PCT sometimes appears in men treated with estrogens for prostatic carcinoma and in women given estrogen-progestin combinations for birth control or estrogens alone for the treatment of menopausal symptoms. The time of onset of the PCT syndrome after beginning estrogen therapy is variable, ranging from a month to years. There are clearly individual determinants in the development of PCT after estrogen therapy, since it occurs in only a few individuals so treated.

Chloroquine administration to a patient with PCT results in acute hepatocellular damage, fever, malaise, nausea, and vomiting. This adverse reaction to chloroquine, which does not occur in nonporphyric individuals, is associated with a large amount of URO excreted in the urine. The apparent explanation is that chloroquine becomes concentrated in lysosomes and mitochondria where porphyrins also accumulate and forms a complex with the porphyrins. This is then released from hepatocytes and excreted in urine. The pathogenesis of the transitory liver cell injury is not understood but may result from release of proteolytic enzymes from lysosomes into the cytosol of hepatocytes.

LABORATORY FINDINGS. Urine porphyrins are increased in PCT. The main urinary porphyrins are URO, 7-carboxylic porphyrin with lesser increases of 6- and 5-carboxylic porphyrins, and COPRO. URO in urine is approximately 70% type I isomer, whereas the 7- and 6-carboxylic porphyrins are about 90% type III, and 5-carboxylic porphyrin and COPRO are about equally types I and III. The isomer distribution in the hepatic and fecal porphyrins is similar to that in the urinary porphyrins. The liver contains large amounts of porphyrins, but concentrations in erythrocytes and bone marrow are normal. As previously mentioned, urinary excretion of PBG is normal and urine ALA is normal or only slightly increased.

Fecal porphyrins are also increased and consist of COPRO, isocoproporphyrin, diethylisocoproporphyrin, and hydroxyisocoproporphyrin. The isocoproporphyrin series is normally present in stool in small amounts, but it is increased markedly in PCT as a result of the disorder's characteristic enzymatic defect in the liver. Isocoproporphyrin may also be found in urine. Ether-insoluble porphyrins ("X-porphyrin"), consisting of 7-carboxylic porphyrin–peptide complexes, are cometimes increased in PCT.

The laboratory diagnosis of PCT should include porphyrin analysis in both urine and feces. Erythropoietic porphyrias should be excluded by demonstrating that red cell porphyrin content is normal. The presence of large amounts of isocoproporphyrin in feces appears to be quite specific for PCT, although urine porphyrins should also be shown to have a pattern consistent with this disorder. Either thin-layer or high-pressure liquid chromatographic methods are most suitable for identification and quantitation of the individual porphyrins in urine and stool.

ENZYMATIC ABNORMALITY. Most cases of PCT are sporadic, and thus there is no history of the disease in other family members. Although well-documented cases of familial PCT are uncommon, it is suspected that there is a genetic or acquired predisposition even in sporadic cases.

Decreased UROgen decarboxylase activity has been reported in the livers of patients with PCT and in animals treated with hexachlorobenzene or TCDD. Hexachlorobenzene has no effect on UROgen decarboxylase activity in erythrocytes. On the other hand, decreased erythrocyte UROgen decarboxylase activity in patients with PCT and in about one half of their first-degree relatives has been reported by some workers but not others.

There appear in fact to be two (or more) distinct types of PCT, a sporadic type that is usually associated with hepatic injury owing to certain chemicals or alcohol, estrogen exposure, and/or hepatic siderosis, and a familial form that can occur in several members of the same family. The sporadic type, which appears to include the majority of patients with PCT, is characterized by decreased UROgen decarboxylase activity in the liver but probably not in erythrocytes. In familial PCT the deficiency of UROgen decarboxylase probably occurs in all cells and not just the liver. The mode of inheritance of erythrocyte UROgen decarboxylase deficiency in familial PCT is consistent with an autosomal dominant trait.

Porphyria associated with other disorders

HEREDITARY TYROSINEMIA. Hereditary tyrosinemia is an inborn error of metabolism characterized by hepatic cirrhosis in early childhood, renal tubular defects, and hypophosphatemic rickets. The derangement in tyrosine metabolism is associated with low activity of fumarylacetacetate hydrolase, the enzyme that catalyzes formation of succinylacetacetate from fumarylacetacetate. Some patients with tyrosinemia have symptoms similar to those in AIP, such as severe abdominal pain, nausea, vomiting, fever, hypertension, tachycardia, and pain and weakness in the lower extremities. As in AIP, urine ALA is increased; however, urine PBG is normal. Urine from patients with tyrosinemia also contains succinylacetone, a by-product of the deranged amino acid metabolism in this disorder and an extremely potent inhibitor of ALA dehydratase. ALA dehydratase activity is markedly reduced in erythrocytes and liver of patients with tyrosinemia. Production of succinylacetone therefore explains the excess urinary ALA excretion, which in turn may be related to the AIP-like symptoms in this disorder. The clinical symptoms of patients with tyrosinemia and elevated urinary excretion of ALA are remarkably similar to those observed in AIP or in lead poisoning. The prepubertal onset of symptoms and the normal levels of urinary PBG in tyrosinemia distinguish it from AIP. Lead poisoning can be excluded by measuring blood lead and erythrocyte protoporphyrin levels.

PORPHYRIA CUTANEA TARDA OCCURRING WITH OTHER DISORDERS. There have been several reports of skin blistering in patients undergoing hemodialysis for chronic renal failure. Most cases have been termed "pseudoporphyria" or "chronic bullous dermatosis of hemodialysis" because of the absence of elevated porphyrins in plasma, urine, or feces, but some have been associated with significant increases of porphyrins in urine, plasma, or blister fluid and a marked excess of isocoproporphyrin in feces. Photosensitizing chemicals derived from the dialysis system may be responsible.

PCT has been reported to occur in some patients with immunologic disorders such as systemic lupus erythematosus and Felty's syndrome. AIP also has been reported in association with systemic lupus erythematosus. The reasons for these associations have not been established.

Porphyrin-producing hepatocellular tumors occur rarely. Hepatocellular carcinomas have been reported to occur quite frequently in some series of patients with PCT, but presumably these are mostly complications of chronic liver disease or chemical exposure and are not porphyrin-producing tumors.

BIBLIOGRAPHY

Anderson, K.E., and others: Studies in porphyria VIII: relationship of the 5α-reductive metabolism of steroid hormones to clinical expression of the genetic defect in acute intermittent porphyria, Am. J. Med. **66**:644, 1979.

DeLeo, V.A., and others: Erythropoietic protoporphyria: 10 years experience, Am. J. Med. **60**:8, 1976.

Elder, G.H.: Differentiation of porphyria cutanea tarda symptomatica from other types of porphyria by measurement of isocoproporphyrin in feces, J. Clin. Pathol. **28**:601, 1975.

Grandchamp, B., Phung, N., and Nordmann, Y.: Homozygous case of hereditary coproporphyria, Lancet **2**:1348, 1977.

Lindblad, B., Lindstedt, S., and Steen, G.: On the enzymic defects in hereditary tyrosinemia, Proc. Natl. Acad. Sci. U.S.A. **74**:4641, 1977.

Meyer, U.A., and Schmid, R.: The porphyrias. In Stanbury, J.B., Wyngaarden, J.B., and Frederickson, D.S., editors: The metabolic basis of inherited disease, ed. 4, New York, 1978, McGraw-Hill Book Co.

Sassa, S., and Kappas, A.: Genetic, metabolic, and biochemical aspects of the porphyrias. In Harris, H., and Hirschorn, K.H., editors: Advances in human genetics, New York, 1981, Plenum Publishing Co.

Tschudy, D.P.: Porphyrin metabolism and the porphyrias. In Bondy, P.K., and Rosenberg, L.E., editors: Duncan's diseases of metabolism, ed. 7, Philadelphia, 1974, W.B. Saunders Co.

197 • METABOLIC AND DIRECT TOXIC EFFECTS OF ALCOHOL

Ralph Myerson

Alcohol exerts its effects on tissues and organs either directly by its action on enzymes and structural components of the cell or indirectly through changes induced during the metabolism of alcohol.

ALCOHOL METABOLISM

Alcohol is metabolized predominantly by the liver. The first step in its metabolism is its oxidation to acetaldehyde, and this reaction can be catalyzed by at least three different enzyme systems: alcohol dehydrogenase (ADH), catalase, and a microsomal ethanol oxidizing system (MEOS) (Fig. 197-1).

The central and major mechanism of alcohol oxidation is a reaction with the cytoplasmic enzyme ADH with nicotinamide adenine dinucleotide (NAD) as a cofactor. This reaction leads to the production of reduced NAD, NADH.

The enzyme catalase plays a negligible role in alcohol metabolism. Hydrogen peroxide is required, and again acetaldehyde is produced.

The third enzyme system, MEOS, is formed in the smooth endoplasmic reticulum of the hepatocyte. A number of drugs that are metabolized by the microsomal systems may show altered metabolism in alcoholics. Increased rates of metabolism of tolbutamide, warfarin, phenytoin, and certain sedative and anesthetic drugs have been reported in alcoholics during nondrinking periods. On the other hand, the metabolism of these drugs may be decreased when they are given concomitantly with alcohol. This may lead to drug intoxication. MEOS may serve as a

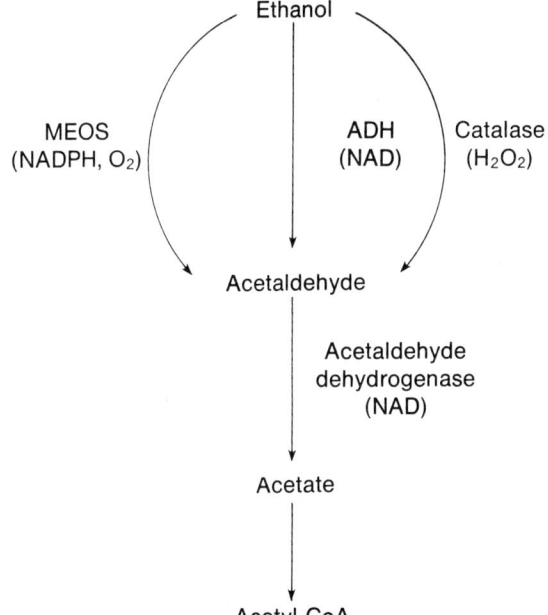

Fig. 197-1. Pathways in metabolism of alcohol. Ethanol is metabolized to acetaldehyde by three enzyme systems: (1) alcohol dehydrogenase (ADH) with nicotinamide adenine dinucleotide (NAD) as cofactor; (2) catalase in presence of H_2O_2; and (3) microsomal ethanol oxidizing system (MEOS) that requires presence of reduced nicotinamide adenine dinucleotide phosphate (NADPH) and O_2. Acetaldehyde is metabolized to acetate in presence of NAD. Acetate is then converted to acetyl coenzyme A (CoA).

reserve mechanism, acting in the presence of excess alcohol that ADH is incapable of metabolizing.

As already noted, the formation of acetaldehyde is the first step in the metabolism of alcohol. Acetaldehyde has been closely scrutinized for evidence that it is responsible for the toxic actions of alcohol. Acetaldehyde, however, is itself very rapidly metabolized into acetate by the enzyme acetaldehyde dehydrogenase. As a result of the speed of this reaction, only minute amounts of acetaldehyde accumulate in the blood—too little to produce toxicity. Disulfiram (Antabuse) blocks the action of the enzyme acetaldehyde dehydrogenase, allowing significant levels of acetaldehyde to accumulate if alcohol is consumed. The so-called aldehyde reaction results. This consists of intense flushing, sweating, and hypotension caused by vasodilitation. Disulfiram has been widely used as therapy to condition alcoholics against the use of alcohol. Acetaldehyde dehydrogenase also requires NAD as a substrate to accept hydrogen. This reaction, as well as the metabolism of ethanol to acetaldehyde, results in a depletion of NAD, an increase in NADH, and a change in the NAD/NADH ratio.

The final steps in alcohol metabolism involve the conversion of acetaldehyde to acetate and acetate to acetyl-CoA. The carbon skeleton of alcohol eventually becomes incorporated into a variety of metabolic products.

METABOLIC EFFECTS OF ALCOHOL

A variety of effects have been ascribed to the abnormalities produced by the metabolism of alcohol (see following outline). Some of these are the results in the change that occurs in the NAD/NADH ratio during alcohol metabolism. In essence, the excess NADH requires the presence of H receptors to restore NAD and the NAD/NADH ratio to normal.

Effects produced by alcohol metabolism

I. Carbohydrate metabolism
   A. Decrease in gluconeogenesis, producing hypoglycemia if glycogen depletion exists
   B. Inhibition of galactose metabolism
II. Protein metabolism
   A. Increased synthesis of lipoproteins (at high alcohol concentrations the opposite occurs)
   B. Decreased synthesis of albumin and other proteins
III. Lipid metabolism
   A. Increase in liver lipids (fatty liver)
   B. Increase in serum triglycerides
IV. Increase in lactate production
   A. Lactic acidosis
   B. Decrease in uric acid secretion and resultant hyperuricemia
V. Other effects
   A. Decreased serum levels of magnesium and phosphate
   B. Interference with citric acid cycle activity
   C. Increased catecholamine release
   D. Increased oxygen consumption

Some of these metabolic effects have clinical expressions that are of significance. A rare but serious effect is the development of *hypoglycemia* resulting from depression of gluconeogenesis by alcohol. This is manifest when there has been glycogen depletion by starvation.

The increase in NADH resulting from the metabolism of alcohol causes an increase in the reduction of pyruvate to lactate. The resultant *hyperlactacidemia* results in a decrease in urate excretion and *hyperuricemia*. Hyperlactacidemia may also result in an increase in urinary magnesium excretion and *hypomagnesemia*.

The profound effects of alcohol on lipid metabolism are apparently the result of several pathogenic mechanisms. Lipid accumulation in the liver is related primarily to increased hepatic lipid synthesis. The increase in NADH results in increased tissue levels of reduced metabolites, such as L-glycerophosphate, which provides the three-carbon skeleton for the synthesis of triglycerides. Mobilization of fat from peripheral deposits to the liver and decreased lipid oxidation in the liver by a decrease in the activity of the citric acid cycle are other mechanisms by which alcohol produces a *fatty liver*.

Alcoholism in nondiabetic patients can result in *ketoacidosis*. The typical history is one of heavy chronic alcohol intake and a recent binge of several days that is followed by anorexia, abdominal pain, and decreased food intake. There is subsequent vomiting, which leads to cessation of food and alcohol intake. The patients usually show symptoms 24 to 72 hours after their last alcoholic intake and are dehydrated and tachypneic and have mental obtundation. The blood sugar concentration is usually less than 400 mg/dl and indeed can be near normal. There is a metabolic acidosis caused primarily by hyperketonemia, low bicarbonate levels, and possible lactic acidosis.

Growth hormone and cortisol levels are high (much higher than in diabetic ketoacidosis and hyperosmolar coma), favoring augmented lipolysis. Insulin levels are low, and since peripheral ketone utilization is insulin dependent, this may explain the underutilization of ketone bodies. β-Hydroxybutyrate is elevated as much as five times higher than acetoacetate. In addition, plasma and urinary catecholamine levels are elevated when alcohol is withdrawn, and they stimulate adipose tissue lipolysis and further impair insulin secretion. These metabolic changes are exaggerated by the superimposition of starvation. It has been suggested that a genetic predisposition may be necessary for the development of this syndrome in chronic alcoholics.

These patients respond to small doses of insulin, glucose infusion, and small amounts of sodium bicarbonate. Careful attention is given to fluid and electrolyte replacement. The use of 5% glucose in the fluid therapy appears to be essential. A precipitating factor such as infection should be excluded, and appropriate treatment of alcohol withdrawal should be included.

DIRECT TOXIC EFFECTS OF ALCOHOL

Alcohol exerts direct effects on practically all organs and body systems, and many of these effects are expressed by clinical manifestations.

NERVOUS SYSTEM. Both the central and the peripheral nervous systems display a myriad of effects, both acute and chronic, that are directly or indirectly related to alcohol ingestion. The mechanisms of these effects are complex and hypothetical in most instances, but the evidence suggests that these manifestations are predominantly direct effects of alcohol.

There is evidence that alcohol affects a variety of nervous tissue parameters, including ion transfer across membranes, energy metabolism, the action potential of nerves, and neurotransmitter function and metabolism. Alcohol also has effects on neuroamine metabolism.

In addition to these direct effects of alcohol, there are indirect consequences of excessive alcohol intake, such as the propensity for trauma, infections, and vitamin and nutritional deficiency.

Acute effects of alcohol on the central nervous system include acute alcoholic intoxication, acute hallucinosis, and seizures ("rum fits"). Intoxication usually appears at blood alcohol levels of 100 to 200 mg/dl. With blood alcohol levels greater than 400 mg/dl, stupor and/or coma appear, and those greater than 500 mg/dl are often fatal. Seizures may also occur as a result of alcohol withdrawal, although delirium tremens is the most common of the withdrawal syndromes.

Chronic alcoholism may result in a slowly progressive process of global dementia. Other chronic processes include *cerebellar degeneration, central pontine myelolysis, Korsakoff's psychosis,* and *Marchiafava-Bignami disease. Wernicke's encephalopathy* is believed to be closely related to an associated deficiency in thiamine chloride.

Peripheral neurologic syndromes include alcoholic poly-neuritis and traumatic neuropathies, such as Saturday night palsy, which is secondary to radial nerve compression. Myopathy has also been described in alcoholics. The acute process may be severe enough to produce myoglobin-induced acute tubular necrosis of the kidney. In most instances overt manifestations of the myopathy are minimal or minor. Repeated bouts, however, may lead to a chronic disabling myopathy involving primarily proximal musculature.

In all central nervous disorders seen in alcoholics, the possibility of head trauma must be considered. Alcoholics have a propensity for skull fractures, cerebral contusions, and subdural hematomas.

LIVER. It has been demonstrated that in addition to effects exerted indirectly on the liver by the metabolism of alcohol, alcohol exerts a direct effect on the liver, readily producing demonstrable morphologic changes in both animals and human beings. When severe, these changes may give rise to overt clinical manifestations such as acute alcoholic hepatitis or the "fatty liver syndromes," including *Zieve syndrome* (severe hemolytic anemia and hyperlipidemia in alcoholic hepatitis). *Mallory's bodies* (intracytoplasmic eosinophilic clumps), cellular infiltration, and hepatocyte necrosis are the hallmarks of acute alcoholic hepatitis. Although clinically inapparent in most instances, this acute hepatitis may be manifest as a serious and possibly fatal clinical condition.

It is likely that repeated bouts of acute alcoholic hepatitis lead to the development of portal fibrosis and the picture of Laennec's cirrhosis. Other factors, however, obviously play important roles, since cirrhosis develops in only about 10% of chronic alcoholics. It is not clear what factors predispose to or prevent the development of cirrhosis, but genetic factors, androgen/estrogen imbalance, collagenase activity, heavy metals, and a host of others have been cited.

HEART—ALCOHOLIC MYOCARDIOPATHY. There is convincing clinical, laboratory, and experimental evidence to show that alcohol exerts a direct toxic effect on the myocardium. In vivo and in vitro experiments in human beings and animals have demonstrated that alcohol depresses myocardial function by decreasing myocardial contractility. Elevated end-diastolic ventricular pressure and cardiac failure result. Several factors contribute to these hemodynamic changes, including a loss of the inotropic effects of myocardial catecholamines and a decrease in oxidative enzymes. Mitochondrial changes are noted early after alcohol administration, followed by lipid accumulation and myofibrillar disruption. Changes in membrane permeability may be the basic mechanism causing these manifestations. Clinically, a low-output, chronic type of cardiac failure results, which may be difficult to differentiate from other cardiomyopathies.

In rare instances beriberi heart disease has been reported in alcoholics (occidental beriberi). This is a hyperkinetic, high-output failure, in contrast to the low-output cardiac failure characteristic of alcoholic cardiomyopathy.

HEMATOLOGIC EFFECTS. A variety of hematologic abnormalities have been described following excessive intake of alcohol. Many result from the complications of alcoholism—cirrhosis of the liver with hypersplenism, gastrointestinal bleeding, Zieve syndrome, and nutritional, folic acid, and vitamin deficiencies. However, evidence has shown that alcohol itself exerts a direct effect on the formed elements of the blood.

Reversible vacuolization of red blood cell and white blood cell precursors in the bone marrow has been noted. These changes resemble those seen with chloramphenicol toxicity. They occur in the absence of nutritional and vitamin deficiencies and have developed despite the concomitant administration of large doses of folic acid.

A reversible type of sideroblastic anemia associated with ringed sideroblasts in the iron-stained bone marrow has been reported following excessive ingestion of alcohol.

The changes can be reversed by treatment with parenteral administration of pyridoxal phosphate and are thought to result from the effects of alcohol on vitamin B_6 metabolism.

Stomatocytic changes of erythrocytes have been described in alcoholism and respond to withdrawal of alcohol.

Thrombocytopenia often accompanies acute alcoholic excess. There is usually a fairly rapid return to normal or near normal platelet counts following alcohol withdrawal. Leukopenia and reduced leukocyte bone marrow reserve have also been noted in alcoholics. This is probably related to the action of alcohol as a folate antagonist.

Alcohol has also been shown to produce a depression of leukocyte mobilization into areas of trauma in nutritionally normal individuals. A decrease in the bactericidal activity of serum in vitro has been reported to follow alcohol ingestion. These phenomena may help to explain the increased susceptibility of alcoholic individuals to infection.

GASTROINTESTINAL TRACT

Stomach. Alcoholic gastritis is an extremely common complication of alcohol ingestion and a frequent cause of hemorrhage. The evidence that alcohol is a secretagogue of gastric acid is not convincing. Most studies indicate that alcohol-induced damage to the gastric mucosa results from interference with the gastric mucosal barrier. This allows for back diffusion of hydrogen ions from the gastric lumen, with resultant histologic changes in the form of hemorrhage, edema, and cellular infiltration. The changes are variable and seem to be dependent on the concentration and amount of alcohol consumed. There is also evidence that nutritional status may play a role and that gastric mucus contributes a protective action.

Pancreas. The pancreas is a prime target for the effects of alcohol in certain individuals. Alcohol produces an increase in pancreatic secretion, apparently by stimulating the acid-secretin mechanism. Resection of the parietal cell mass abolishes the pancreatic response to alcohol.

There is also evidence that alcohol causes an increase in pancreatic duct pressure, apparently by a contraction of the sphincter of Oddi. The increased intrapancreatic pressure produced by a combination of increased pancreatic secretion and elevated intraductal pressure may be the cause of acinar rupture, leading to alcohol-induced pancreatitis.

Chronic pancreatitis is a common complication of alcoholism and may result from repeated attacks of acute pancreatitis. There is also evidence that qualitative and quantitative changes occur in pancreatic secretion following long-term use of alcohol. The role, if any, of these changes in the production of pancreatitis remains unsettled. Malnutrition may play a role in the pancreatic insufficiency seen in chronic alcoholics.

ENDOCRINE SYSTEM

Adrenal cortex. There are data indicating that the acute administration of alcohol results in an increase in adrenocortical function and a quantitative increase in the secretion of adrenocortical hormones. This appears to be dependent on the integrity of the pituitary-adrenal axis, since this response to alcohol does not occur in the hypophysectomized animal. This suggests that alcohol stimulates the release of ACTH. In human beings the data are controversial, but most studies report an increase in plasma cortisol levels following the acute administration of alcohol. There appears to be rough correlation between blood alcohol levels, degree of inebriation, and serum cortisol levels. Highest serum cortisol levels have been observed when subjects reported gastrointestinal symptoms. During the withdrawal phase, serum cortisol levels fall to prealcohol levels. Chronic alcoholics may not manifest an elevation of plasma cortisol after alcohol ingestion.

Increases in urinary catecholamines during long-term alcohol intake have been reported. Following withdrawal of alcohol, catecholamine excretion falls to normal. However, when higher blood levels were attained with free drinking and withdrawal symptoms ensued following alcohol withdrawal, catecholamine levels remained elevated, suggesting a relationship between withdrawal symptoms and catecholamines.

Withdrawal symptoms have been associated with a variety of other phenomena, including increased levels of serum cortisol, increased rate of fall of alcohol blood levels, magnesium deficiency, elevated spinal fluid lactate levels, and the presence of congeners in alcoholic beverages. Suffice it to say that no one concept has been found that satisfactorily explains the complex clinical picture of alcohol withdrawal.

There is increasing evidence that alcohol affects adrenal mineralocorticoid activity, as well as glucocorticoid activity. Increased aldosterone excretion and sodium retention have been reported following administration of alcohol.

Neurohypophysis. The diuretic effect of alcohol has been attributed to the inhibitory effect of alcohol on the secretion of antidiuretic hormone (ADH). On the other hand, water intoxication has been reported after heavy beer drinking, and inappropriate secretion of ADH has been postulated as a cause.

Alcohol also decreases uterine contractions by a central inhibition of oxytocin release from the neurohypophysis. Hypothalamic-pituitary suppression with low plasma gonadotropins has been demonstrated. Alcoholic men are also found to have high prolactin and estradiol levels.

Thyroid gland. No consistent effects of alcohol on thyroid function have been reported. Alcohol has been reported to result in an increase in the uptake of radioactive iodine by the thyroid gland. Other parameters of thyroid function are unchanged, except in the malnourished alcoholic who may have low thyroxine-binding globulin and therefore a low total thyroxine level and a high T_3 resin uptake.

Gonads. Chronic administration of alcohol to normal men and men with alcoholism but without evidence of liver disease results in a decrease in testosterone. This suppression is thought to be a direct effect on the testes. It is also known that alcohol accelerates the rate of testosterone degradation and decreases testosterone production. Men with alcoholism have an increase in sex steroid–binding globulin, which further reduces the amount of free biologically active testosterone. The gonadal abnormalities include infertility, sterility, gonadal atrophy, hypoandrogenism, and feminization.

BIBLIOGRAPHY

Israel, Y.: Cellular effects of alcohol: a review, Q. J. Stud. Alcohol **31**:293, 1970.

Isselbacher, K.J.: Metabolic and hepatic effects of alcohol, N. Engl. J. Med. **296**:612, 1977.

Lieber, C.S.: Metabolic derangement induced by alcohol, Annu. Rev. Med. **18**:35, 1967.

Mendelson, J.H.: Biologic concomitants of alcohol (in two parts), N. Engl. J. Med. **283**:24, 71, 1970.

Mendelson, J.H., and Mello, N.K.: Biologic concomitants of alcoholism, N. Engl. J. Med. **301**:912, 1979.

Myerson, R.M.: Metabolic aspects of alcohol and their biological significance, Med. Clin. North Am. **57**:925, 1973.

Rubin, E., and Lieber, C.S.: Fatty liver, alcoholic hepatitis and cirrhosis produced by alcohol in primates, N. Engl. J. Med. **290**:128, 1974.

198 • PATHOGENESIS AND DIAGNOSIS OF DIABETES MELLITUS

Oliver E. Owen, Charles R. Shuman, Guenther Boden, and **Robert D. Hoeldtke**

DEFINITION. Diabetes mellitus comprises several diseases that have different causes and mechanisms of transmission but share glucose intolerance as a cardinal clinical feature. Current evidence supporting the view that multiple causes are responsible for this common serious metabolic disorder includes the following: (1) glucose intolerance is associated with over 30 distinct disorders; (2) clinical presentation among patients varies from the thin, ketosis-prone, insulin-dependent diabetic patient to the obese, hyperglycemic, ketone-resistant diabetic patient; (3) genetic and immune studies show that diabetic patients have varying profiles (4) inheritance of glucose intolerance differs among the various types of diabetic patients; (5) the incidence of glucose intolerance and the clinical features of diabetes mellitus vary among ethnic groups; and (6) therapeutic responses are different among the various disorders of glucose intolerance. It has become evident that age is a poor criterion in classifying diabetes as insulin-dependent ketosis-prone or as non-insulin-dependent ketosis-resistant.

The precise prevalence of diabetes mellitus in the general population is unknown. However, it is certainly the most common metabolic disorder encountered in clinical medicine, affecting 2% to 5% of the American population.

There are several broad categories of glucose intolerance, and some of these are listed in Table 198-1. This chapter focuses primarily on type I (insulin-dependent diabetes mellitus, IDDM) and type II (non-insulin-dependent diabetes mellitus, NIDDM) diabetes (National Diabetes Data Group classification).

ETIOLOGY. Causes for various metabolic disorders leading to the clinical diagnosis of diabetes mellitus are many. Therefore the subtypes of diabetes are discussed separately.

Type I—insulin-dependent diabetes mellitus. Patients with IDDM comprise several subsets. Genetic determinants of certain serologically demonstrable glycoprotein antigens on human lymphocytes (HLA) have an increased prevalence in patients with IDDM. These HLA haplotypes are controlled by gene alleles, one derived from each parent, and are located on chromosome 6 at five loci: A, B, C, D, and DR. There is an increased frequency of IDDM with certain gene alleles, including A1, A2, B8, B15, B18, CW3, DW3, and DW4, and a decreased incidence of IDDM with gene alleles AW32, B5, B7, BW35, D2, and DRW2. Individuals with both B8 and B15 HLA haplotypes (a double dose of diabetes-linked genes) have an even greater predisposition to diabetes mellitus. Although the frequency of IDDM is linked to the presence or absence of these genetically determined cell surface antigens of lymphocytes, they are not direct markers or the only determinants for diabetes mellitus. Furthermore, within the subsets of patients with IDDM the HLA haplotypes vary. For example, in patients with IDDM between the ages of 12 and 15 years there is a particularly strong association with allele DW4, whereas in all ages allele DW3 induces a susceptibility to IDDM. Different HLA haplotypes are associated with IDDM among various races.

The association of various IDDM subsets and HLA antigens has offered some insight into the genetic nature of these disorders. However, the exact modes of transfer of IDDM in heterogeneous patient populations have not been defined. Suggested mechanisms for the genetic transfer of IDDM, including autosomal dominance with varying degrees of expression (penetration), recessive and polygenic, are poorly understood and are complicated by environmental factors. This is borne out by studies of monozygotic twins in which one twin was affected with diabetes mellitus. If genetic mechanisms alone dictated the development of glucose intolerance, the presence of diabetes in one twin should be temporally related to the development of diabetes in the other twin. Studies have shown, however, that a maximum of only 50% of monozygotic twins 40 years or younger are concordant for IDDM. This is in contrast to obese monozygotic twins with NIDDM that developed after 50 years of age. In this latter group of twins concord-

Table 198-1. Conditions with glucose intolerance

Category	Characteristics	Category	Characteristics
Diabetes mellitus			
Type I: insulin-dependent diabetes mellitus (IDDM)	Dependent on exogenous insulin to maintain life		Usually occurs in association with symptoms referable to the primary disease such as pancreatic insufficiency, endocrinopathies, and drug reactions
	Ketosis-prone		
	Endogenous insulinopenia		
	Usually occurs under 40 years of age but can occur at any age	Gestational diabetes mellitus (GDM)	Glucose intolerance developing during pregnancy
	Associated with certain HLA types and abnormal autoimmune reactions, including islet cell antibodies		Associated with increased perinatal risk and fetal mortality
			Hormonal interplay and insulin resistance partly responsible
Type II: non-insulin-dependent diabetes mellitus (NIDDM)	Not usually dependent on exogenous insulin to maintain life; however, under stress exogenous insulin may be needed transiently to prevent excessive catabolism		Requires reclassification after termination of pregnancy
		Impaired glucose tolerance (IGT)	Usually asymptomatic
			Impaired glucose tolerance but not gross enough to be diagnostic of diabetes mellitus
	Obesity common trait		Occurs in association with endocrinopathies, hepatic disease, drug reactions, certain genetic disorders, malignancy, and stress
	Ketosis-resistant		
	Endogenous insulinopenia to hyperinsulinemia		
	Usually occurs past 40 years of age but can occur at younger age		Increased susceptibility to atherosclerosis and neuropathic diseases
	Strong inheritance tendency		
	Not associated with HLA types or autoimmune reaction		May decompensate to overt diabetes at an annual rate of 4% to 5%
	Insulin receptor or postreceptor defects present		
Secondary diabetes mellitus	Includes a variety of diseases that result in glucose intolerance severe enough to meet the diagnostic criteria of diabetes mellitus		

ance is the rule. Thus, at least in the twins studied, environmental factors seem to play a role in precipitating IDDM.

Viral infections have been shown to precede the development of IDDM. There is a particularly strong relationship between coxsackievirus (group B), mumps, rubella, and cytomegalovirus infections and the development of IDDM. Further evidence for the importance of viral infections is offered by the observation that the onset of IDDM is primarily seasonal, with the highest incidence occurring in fall and winter when viral infections are peaking. In addition, coxsackievirus and cytomegalovirus have been isolated from infected pancreases of diabetic patients in whom catastrophic catabolism has resulted in death.

There is general agreement that immunologic mechanisms contribute to the development of two types of IDDM. In these subsets both humoral and cell-mediated immunities are involved in β-cell destruction. In the more common form of IDDM (type Ia), which is possibly initiated by viral infection, there is subsequent development of complement-fixing IgG antibodies directed against islet cells. These antibody titers decrease or disappear with the progression of the disease. In the other form of IDDM (type Ib), which occurs in patients with autoimmune polyendocrinopathies, serum titers of islet cell antibodies are present before or at the time IDDM develops, and they persist indefinitely. Type Ib diabetes usually has a more gradual onset and tends to occur in patients between the ages of 20 and 50 years. In addition to complement-fixing IgG islet cell antibodies, patients with IDDM have circulating lymphocytes with cytolytic activity directed toward β-cells.

Chemicals from the environment may also cause injury to β-cells. Such injury may predispose β-cells to latent viral infections and subsequent humoral and cell-mediated immune destruction. Further investigation into what initiates humoral and cellular immune responses and how these responses can be controlled is of the utmost importance for developing appropriate therapeutic approaches to some forms of IDDM.

Type II—non-insulin-dependent diabetes mellitus. NIDDM also probably comprises several subsets, the causes of which are unknown. The outcomes are manifested by hyperglycemia and other metabolic derangements common to diabetes mellitus. The presence of genetic determinants is evidenced by family aggregation of diabetes, which appears to be inherited as an autosomal dominant disease. Concordance for diabetes is the rule in monozygotic twins. The onset of carbohydrate intolerance occurs after 40 years of age; however, type II diabetes can occur in adolescents or young adults. HLA haplotypes and autoimmune responses have no relevance in NIDDM. Environmental factors play a role in inducing glucose intolerance; about 60% to 90% of patients with NIDDM form a subset characterized by obesity. In these patients glucose tolerance is improved with weight control. Among these obese patients receptor or postreceptor site defects or both are present.

INSULIN RESISTANCE. Because of the recent developments pertaining to insulin-resistant states, primarily in type II diabetes mellitus, these disorders will be presented.

Insulin resistance is present when the usual hypoglycemic response to insulin is absent. The recognition and amplitude of insulin-resistant states have undergone major expansions in recent years. It is now known that insulin resistance can occur independent of glucose intolerance. Insulin resistance can sometimes be present with euglycemic states if supernormal concentrations of insulin are achieved through adequate β-cell secretory capacity. On the other hand, persistent hyperglycemia may be present even though pharmacologic doses of exogenous insulin are administered. Thus the spectrum of causes and factors in insulin resistance or insensitivity is wide. To discern the cause of insulin resistance, it is important to recognize that the first step in the action of insulin is binding to receptor molecules on the plasma membrane. Therefore for convenience the mechanism of insulin resistance can be categorized as being before (prereceptor), during (receptor), or after (postreceptor) the hormone-receptor interaction.

One cause of prereceptor insulin resistance is the presence of anti-insulin antibodies to injected animal (or human) insulin preparations, which impairs access of insulin to its receptor. IgG anti-insulin antibodies develop in nearly all insulin-dependent patients, but in less than 1 in 1000 patients do anti-insulin antibody titers and affinity become sufficient to cause resistance. Most commonly, antibody-mediated insulin resistance develops in a patient who has been previously exposed to exogenous insulin that was discontinued and then subsequently given again. The repeated challenge with insulin induces a reaction similar to the anamnestic responses observed to other antigens. Some anti-insulin antibody–resistant diabetic patients have malignant lesions, especially sarcomas. Substantial antibody titers to insulin can be detected by modifications of the radioimmunoassay techniques for measuring insulin in serum or plasma. However, the relationship between antiinsulin antibody titers and degrees of insulin resistance is only qualitative.

Another cause for prereceptor insulin resistance is the secretion of an abnormal insulin molecule that has defective binding to insulin receptors and has lost most of its biologic activity. This type of insulin abnormality is rare. Yet another form of insulin resistance, which may occur in insulin-dependent diabetic patients, is a nonimmune phenomenon related to reduced bioavailability of insulin following subcutaneous injection. This phenomenon is thought to be due to local destruction of insulin situated in a subcutaneous depot. Recent investigations suggest that this is probably due to protease enzymes that catabolize depot insulin.

Obesity is the most common and best studied factor associated with insulin resistance. The insulin resistance is a heterogeneous disorder not related to the degree of obesity. In mildly hyperinsulinemic resistant patients with NIDDM, the concentration of insulin receptors on the plasma membrane is reduced and the insulin resistance is primarily due to the decrease in insulin receptors. In markedly hyperinsulinemic resistant obese patients with NIDDM, in addition to reduced insulin receptors, a postreceptor defect is present. However, the receptor impairment seems to be the major cause of insulin resistance. Fortunately, the loss of receptors is reversible with weight reduction and the insulin response usually returns toward normal.

Other forms of insulin resistance occur in three syndromes recently recognized. One of these syndromes, known as type B, is an autoimmune disease characterized by hyperglycemia, acanthosis nigricans, diminished binding of insulin to receptor owing to the presence of circulating antireceptor antibodies, and several accompanying disorders such as lupus erythematosus, Sjögren's syndrome, and ataxia-telangiectasia. Antireceptor antibody titer may fall dramatically with time or after immunosuppressive therapy.

Another syndrome, known as type A, occurs in females and is usually characterized by hyperglycemia, acanthosis nigricans, and polycystic ovaries. Testosterone concentrations are increased, and various degrees of virilization have been observed. The concentration of insulin receptors on circulating monocytes is reduced, and the receptor defect is not improved by dietary restriction as it is in obesity. In addition, some of these patients seem to have a postreceptor defect.

The third syndrome is characterized by familial occurrence of insulin resistance together with acanthosis nigricans, acral hypertrophy, and muscle cramps. Ovarian dysfunction may occur in females, whereas testicular function may be normal in males. Fasting euglycemia or hyperglycemia may be present, but patients are resistant to the hypoglycemic response to intravenously administered insulin. Endogenous hyperinsulinemia is present, and insulin receptors on circulating monocytes are reduced in concentration.

Endocrinopathies such as Cushing's disease or syndrome, pheochromocytoma, acromegaly, thyrotoxicosis, and profound type IV or V hyperlipidemia are associated with increased insulin requirements for diabetic control. Glucocorticoid excess is associated with reduced affinity of insulin receptors. In practice, however, increased insulin requirements are usually not seen in patients taking less than the equivalent of 20 mg of prednisone daily. Epinephrine induces peripheral and hepatic insulin insensitivity through its β-adrenergic receptor, which impairs tissue responses to increased plasma insulin concentrations. Whether the catecholamine effect is mediated through altered insulin sensitivity, heightened cyclic AMP levels, or a postreceptor site mechanism is unclear. Medical or surgical management of hyperthyroidism, Cushing's disease, and acromegaly is indicated before good control of carbohydrate disturbances can be obtained.

Diabetic lipoatrophy is an insulin-resistant state characterized by the lack of subcutaneous fat, hyperlipidemia, and an elevated metabolic rate. Sometimes it is associated with acanthosis nigricans and autoimmune disorders. This rare and complex disease may or may not be associated with circulating anti-insulin receptor antibodies, altered insulin-binding to receptors because of reduced insulin receptor concentration, or insulin affinity. Unfortunately, therapy is limited primarily to dietary manipulations and exogenous insulin administration.

ISLETS OF LANGERHANS. The islets of Langerhans contain β-, α-, and δ-cells that have specific functions. Normal β-cells synthesize, store, and secrete insulin. Insul secretion is stimulated primarily by an increase in blood glucose, although other substrates and upper gastrointestinal tract hormones augment secretion. Insulin is released from storage granules following interaction of glucose and glucose receptor on the β-cell surface, intracellular metabolism of glucose, or both. There are three phases of insulin secretion: (1) a rapid secretory burst of insulin from storage granules influenced by calcium-dependent contraction of intracellular microfilamentous structures (2 to 10 units/hr); (2) a second phase of insulin secretion with a more gradual release of stored insulin and newly synthesized insulin (1 to 2 units/hr); (3) and a third phase of persistent insulin secretion needed to control release of endogenous fuel stores during food deprivation (0.5 to 1 unit/hr).

Insulin is the cardinal hormone promoting substrate uptake, synthesis, and storage. Its anticatabolic and anabolic effects on the metabolism of carbohydrates, fats, and proteins are most readily demonstrated in liver, muscle, and adipose tissue, and these effects are listed in Table 198-2.

Table 198-2. Insulin action

	Anticatabolic effects	Anabolic effects
Liver	Decreased glycogenolysis, gluconeogenesis, and ketogenesis	Increased glycogen synthesis and fatty acid synthesis
Adipose tissue	Decreased lipolysis	Increased glycerol synthesis and fatty acid synthesis
Muscle	Decreased protein catabolism and amino acid output	Increased amino acid uptake, protein synthesis, and glycogen synthesis

Normal α-cells synthesize, store, and secrete *glucagon*. Glucagon secretion is stimulated primarily by a decrease in blood glucose concentration or by increases in blood amino acid concentrations. It is released by exocytosis from storage granules in the α-cells of the islets of Langerhans. Plasma glucagon concentration is increased during ketotic states seen in starvation, alcoholism, and diabetes mellitus (type I), and it is decreased during physiologic hyperglycemia such as that following glucose ingestion.

Glucagon is a hormone responsive to cellular nutritional needs. It promotes hepatic gluconeogenesis, glycogenolysis, and ketogenesis. It may promote peripheral proteolysis and lipolysis, wlhhough this is questionable. In the presence of insulin deficiency, the hyperglycemia and hyperketonemic effects of glucagon are exaggerated.

Glucagon secretion is increased in diabetes mellitus (IDDM and NIDDM). Hyperglycemia fails to suppress glucagon secretion and hypoglycemia fails to elicit glucagon secretion in both IDDM and NIDDM. However, insulin replacement therapy normalizes glucagon responses in IDDM but not in NIDDM.

Somatostatin is synthesized, stored, and secreted by cells throughout the body as well as by the δ-cells of the islets of Langerhans. Pancreatic somatostatin secretion is stimulated by nutrients and gastrointestinal hormones (glucose, amino acids, pancreozymin-cholecystokinin, and secretin). Somatostatin in pharmacologic quantities administered via peripheral veins diminishes gastric emptying, gallbladder mobility, and pancreatic exocrine secretion. It also decreases insulin, glucagon, HC1, pepsin, gastrin, motilin, secretin, and gut glucagon secretions. Furthermore, somatostatin diminishes splanchnic blood flow and absorption of glucose and triglycerides. It has been postulated that the net effect of somatostatin on food and hormone metabolism is regulation of the influx of nutrients from the gut. Its altered behavior, if any, in diabetic states has not been defined.

Pancreatic polypeptide hormone is another hormone secreted by the pancreas of humans. The cells containing and secreting pancreatic polypeptide hormone are located in the paraduodenal area of the pancreas, predominantly in the exocrine parenchyma rather than in the islets. The gastrointestinal tract is important in mediating the secretory response of pancreatic polypeptide hormone, which is large and biphasic after ingestion of a mixed meal. Fasting, exercise, and acute hypoglycemia all stimulate its secretion. The physiologic effects of pancreatic polypeptide are unknown, but it may be important in curtailing postprandial pancreatic bicarbonate secretion, and it may affect the brain satiety center during the postprandial period. Basal plasma concentrations of pancreatic polypeptide hormone are elevated in IDDM and NIDDM. The significance of these alterations is unknown.

PATHOPHYSIOLOGY AND CLINICAL MANIFESTATIONS. Diabetes mellitus is recognized in its mild form by glucose intolerance and in its severe form by generalized tissue catabolism. Although diabetes mellitus is a heterogeneous group of disorders, in general there are an absolute or relative primary insufficiency of insulin and frequently excessive secondary amounts of insulin counterregulatory hormones, that is, glucagon, cortisol, catecholamines, and growth hormone. The most important function of insulin is to regulate fuel homeostasis. The chronic manifestations of insulin insufficiency are continuous hyperglycemia, hyperlipidemia, and hyperkinetic amino acid fluxes. These abnormal metabolic events are eventually accompanied by atherosclerotic and microangiopathic cardiovascular disease, neuropathies, nephropathy, arthropathies, dermopathies, and cataracts. The acute manifestations of severe insulin insufficiency result in hyperglycemic-hyperketotic syndromes.

The symptoms of overt type I diabetes (IDDM) are abrupt in onset and almost invariably include polyuria, poly-dypsia, polyphagia, and rapid weight loss. Less severe forms of type I diabetes may have more subtle symptoms such as mild thirst, pruritus, weight loss, and fatigue. The symptoms of type II diabetes (NIDDM) are less pronounced; nonetheless, thirst, pruritus, and fatigue are frequent complaints. Obesity is present in 60% to 90% of patients with type II diabetes.

In IDDM (type I) there is partial to total absence of insulin secretion. If this state persists, diabetic ketoacidosis develops with its array of abnormal metabolites, electrolyte and acid-base derangements, and the secretion of stress hormones. This severe form of insulin deficiency is a life-threatening metabolic disorder characterized by a lack of reciprocity among the rates of hepatic glycogenolysis, gluconeogenesis, and ketogenesis, resulting in inappropriately elevated hepatic production rates of glucose and ketone bodies and subsequently hyperglycemia and hyperketonemia. This, coupled with increased free fatty acid mobilization from adipose tissue and concurrent proteolysis, floods the bloodstream with an overabundance of fuels that compete as oxidative substrates. The major hormonal abnormality is an insufficient quantity of circulating insulin to restrain unwarranted catabolism. The insulin deficiency is made worse by excessive glucagon secretion. Hyperglucagonemia coupled with hypoinsulinemia accelerates the unneeded production of glucose from glycogenolysis and gluconeogenesis and of ketone bodies (β-hydroxybutyric acid, acetoacetic acid, and acetone) from free fatty acids. Hyperglycemia produces an osmotic diuresis, resulting in volume depletion that augments catecholamine release. Epinephrine in conjunction with glucagon synergistically promotes gluconeogenesis, glycogenolysis, and ketogenesis in the liver. In addition, epinephrine diminishes residual insulin secretion, and glucagon depletes hepatic malonyl CoA concentrations and may increase hepatic carnitine concentrations. This facilitates fatty acylcarnitine translocation across the mitochondrium so that free fatty acids undergo β oxidation for ketone body synthesis. Increased ketone body production coupled with diminished ketone body oxidation results in marked hyperketonemia that induces massive ketonuria, accentuating loss of body water. The release of other stress hormones (cortisol and growth hormone) may also contribute to the late development of diabetic ketoacidosis, since these hormones also exhibit anti-insulin activity. The mechanisms responsible for the maintenance of hyperglycemia and hyperketonemia in established diabetic ketoacidosis may be different than those that initiated the inappropriate and excess hepatic production of glucose and ketone bodies. For example, depressed rates of glucose and ketone body disposal coupled with heightened renal retrieval of glucose and ketone bodies during volume depletion may be partially responsible for the persistent or progressive hyperglycemia and hyperketonemia. Even though glucose and ketone bodies have no maximal renal tubular reabsorption rates during diabetic ketoacidosis, glycosuria and ketonuria occur because less than 100% of these filtered compounds are reabsorbed by the renal tubules. Massive renal glucose and ketone body wastage owing to induced osmotic diuresis is accompanied by large losses of sodium, potassium, calcium, phosphate, ammonium, and other ions in the urine. Severe losses of water and electrolytes combined with marked acidemia produce cardiovascular collapse and death.

In NIDDM (type II) the basal serum insulin concentration is normal or elevated. Stimulated insulin secretion is variable but usually sluggish. The insulin secretory defect is limited to the initial secretory burst. Perhaps this is due to altered β-cell glucose receptors or increased α-adrenergic activity or prostaglandin activity. In addition to the delayed secretion of insulin, some subsets of NIDDM have insulin resistance in target tissues (muscle, liver, and adipose tissue).

TESTS AND DIAGNOSTIC CRITERIA. Venous blood should

be collected in a tube containing sodium fluoride to prevent in vitro glucose metabolism before analysis. If Dextrostix is used, fresh whole blood is obtained by finger prick. Plasma or serum is preferred over whole blood for glucose determinations because less interference with equipment occurs and plasma or serum is independent of hematocrit differences. Glucose is present in the water component of blood. Water comprises about 70% of red blood cells and about 93% of plasma. Thus plasma or serum contains approximately 12% to 15% more glucose than does whole blood. For example, if normal venous whole blood has a glucose concentration of 100 mg/dl, the plasma or serum glucose concentration should be 115 mg/dl.

There is lack of unanimity concerning the concentration values of plasma or serum (or blood) glucose needed to identify diabetes mellitus. However, the current National Diabetes Data Group recommends the following:

Fasting plasma glucose	>140 mg/dl
2-Hour plasma glucose	>200 mg/dl
With one intervening value	>200 mg/dl

These values are used as criteria in the interpretation of the oral glucose tolerance test (OGTT). They may be helpful in the evaluation of "spot" and plasma or serum glucose determinations. An OGTT is unnecessary if the fasting plasma or serum glucose is elevated on two occasions or if a high fasting plasma or serum glucose level is associated with glycosuria and/or ketonuria, family history of diabetes, or other clinical concomitants.

When needed, the OGTT must be performed following 3 days of normal activity and an unrestricted diet containing no less than 150 g of carbohydrate daily. A glucose load for the nonpregnant adult is 75 g (1.75 g/kg body weight for children up to a maximum of 75 g). This is midway between the load of 50 g used in Europe and 100 g used in the United States. The patients are studied after a 10- to 12-hour overnight fast. The diluted glucose solution (in 300 ml) is ingested as a flavored beverage 5 minutes after a fasting blood sample is obtained, and subsequent samples are drawn at 30-minute intervals for 2 hours following the start of the drink. Certain drugs such as anovulatory agents, phenytoin, glucocorticoids, and diuretic agents may induce glucose intolerance and should be discontinued, if possible, 2 weeks before the test. Acute conditions such as cerebrovascular accident, myocardial infarction, postoperative phase, postictal phase, and thyrotoxicosis may disturb glucose tolerance. Although lesser degrees of glucose intolerance (borderline curves) cannot be ignored, serial testing has shown that some individuals will revert to normal, others will show no significant change in the degree of intolerance, and a small percentage will manifest deterioration.

Gestational diabetes mellitus (GDM) represents a special problem in which diagnostic criteria are more stringent. For pregnant subjects the glucose load is 100 g and plasma glucose concentrations must be determined after fasting and at 1, 2, and 3 hours after glucose ingestion. Two or more of the following values must be met or exceeded to diagnose GDM: fasting plasma glucose, 105 mg/dl; 1-hour plasma glucose, 190 mg/dl; 2-hour plasma glucose, 165 mg/dl; and 3-hour plasma glucose, 145 mg/dl. These strict criteria are used because obstetric risks are increased even with mild degrees of glucose intolerance. Glucose intolerance during pregnancy increases neonatal morbidity and is predictive of the risk of subsequent diabetes mellitus. The diabetogenicity of pregnancy may become apparent early in gestation or during the second or third trimester and frequently, but not always, necessitates the use of insulin.

BIBLIOGRAPHY

Bottazzo, G.F., and others: Evidence for a primary autoimmune type of diabetes mellitus, Br. Med. J. **2**:1253, 1978.

Bottazzo, G.F., and others: Complement-fixing islet-cell antibodies in type-I diabetes; possible monitors of active beta-cell damage, Lancet **1**:668, 1980.

Craighead, J.E.: Current views on the etiology of insulin-dependent diabetes mellitus, N. Engl. J. Med. **229**:1439, 1978.

Flier, J.S., Kahn, C.R., and Roth, J.: Receptors, antireceptor antibodies and mechanisms of insulin resistance, N. Engl. J. Med. **300**:413, 1979.

Kolterman, O.G., and others: Mechanisms of insulin resistance in human obesity: evidence for receptor and postreceptor defects. J. Clin. Invest. **65**:1272, 1980.

Miles, J.M., and others: Effects of acute insulin deficiency on glucose amd ketone body turnover in man: evidence for the primary of overproduction of glucose and ketone bodies in the genesis of diabetic ketoacidosis, Diabetes **29**:926, 1980.

National Diabetes Data Group: Classification and diagnosis of diabetes mellitus and other categories of glucose intolerance, Diabetes **28**:1039, 1979.

Owen, O.E., and others: Human splanchnic metabolism during diabetic ketoacidosis, Metabolism **26**:381, 1977.

Owen, O.E., and others: Effects of therapy on the nature and quantity of fuels oxidized during diabetic ketoacidosis, Diabetes **29**:365, 1980.

Unger, R.H., Dobbs, R.E., and Orci, L.: Insulin, glucagon, and somatostatin secretion in the regulation of metabolism, Annu. Rev. Physiol. **40**:307, 1978.

199 • TREATMENT OF DIABETES MELLITUS

Harry Gottlieb

The concentration of blood glucose reflects a balance between glucose absorption, production, and utilization. Insulin promotes anabolic processes such as hepatic glycogen synthesis, amino acid incorporation into protein, and fat deposition. Glucagon and other hormones such as epinephrine, glucocorticoids, and growth hormone stimulate glocose production, lipolysis, and gluconeogenesis.

Insulin release is stimulated by glucose, amino acids, ketones, free fatty acids, and gastrointestinal hormones and inhibited by somatostatin, epinephrine, and low blood glucose.

During feeding, increased insulin and decreased glucagon secretion contribute to diminished glucose release and favor glycogen synthesis. During fasting most of these metabolic processes are reversed—blood insulin falls and glucagon rises. These changes are typified by increased gluconeogenesis, glycogenolysis, and lipolysis.

The relationship beteen hyperglycemia (and its pathophysiologic and biochemical consequences) and the acute and chronic complications of diabetes mellitus remains a subject of debate among diabetologists. It is clear that hyperglycemia directly or as a result of insulin deficiency can be associated with increased intracellular concentrations of sorbitol (such as in the lens of the eye), elaboration of minor hemoglobin components (such as Hb A_{IC}), increase in platelet aggregation, and changes in basement membranes. Although no available prospective study provides irrefutable proof, convincing data suggest that persistent hyperglycemia may be the requisite milieu or at least the "trigger" to set into motion the chain of events responsible for the development of microvascular and macrovascular changes associated with the complications of diabetes mellitus. In addition to possible long-term benefits, good control is important in preventing diabetic ketoacidosis, inhibiting bacterial infection, accelerating wound healing, decreasing perinatal morbidity and mortality, and promoting normal growth and development in the young diabetic.

A normal fasting blood glucose level and a 2-hour postprandial serum or plasma glucose level of 150 mg/dl or lower are typically strived for in the diabetic patient. These glucose levels, however, must be consistent with the patient's ability to function productively. Although these levels may be routinely achieved in the patient with maturity-onset diabetes, they are more difficult to obtain in the ketosis-prone, hypoinsulinemic (type I) diabetic patient. However, it must be recognized that the use of multiple injections of regular insulin cannot duplicate the constant endogenous spurts that normal β-cell insulin secretion provides. Only the perfection of a glucose electrode or transplants of β-cells or of a total pancreas can provide this type of control (that is, immediate response to minimal increases or decreases in blood glucose with bursts of insulin or glucagon release).

DIET

Diet remains the cornerstone of diabetic therapy. The objectives are to promote proper growth and development in children, to provide proper nutrition with a balance of protein, carbohydrate, and fat (saturated and unsaturated), and to normalize weight. In addition, the diet proportions during the day must be tailored to the type of insulin used and to the individual's activity in order to normalize blood sugars while preventing hypoglycemia.

The following principles are of utmost importance in diet treatment:

1. Approach the diet to be used as a prescription. In using the exchange diet lists advocated by the American Diabetes Association and the American Dietetic Association, the prescriber *must* be familiar with the contents of those lists. A team approach, using the individual expertise of physician, dietitian, and nurse and enlisting other family members when appropriate, can provide the best possible background for diet education and subsequent patient compliance.
2. Obtain a dietary history, including height, weight, type of work, food preferences, and activity patterns, including exercise.
3. Individualize the diet prescription.

Calculate the ideal weight of the patient as follows: women—100 pounds for the first 5 feet of height, 5 pounds for each additional inch; men—106 pounds for the first 5 feet of height, 6 pounds for each additional inch. Subtract 10% for a small frame and add 10% for a large frame. The total calories required are the basal calories of the patient plus activity needs. Basal calories are 10 calories for each pound of ideal body weight. Add 30% of basal calories to the diet prescription for a sedentary individual, 50% of basal calories for an individual engaging in moderate activity, and 100% of basal calories for strenuous activity. Add or subtract 3500 calories from the diet for the patient to gain or lose 1 pound. Therefore, subtract 500 calories a day from the total caloric prescription for the patient to lose 1 pound a week, and add 500 calories a day to the diet prescription to gain 1 pound a week. The current recommended distribution for the diet components of the American Diabetes Association are carbohydrate, 45% to 55% of the total calories; fat, 30% to 35%; and protein, 15% to 20%. Most insulin-dependent diabetic patients taking intermediate-acting insulin (see Table 199-1) do well on a distribution of breakfast, 20% of the total daily calories; lunch, 30%; midafternoon snack, 10%; dinner, 30%; and evening snack, 10%. Some active young diabetic patients also require a midmorning snack. It is recommended at present that the diet have 10% of the calories as saturated fats and include high-fiber foods in the food selection. It should be clear that, although total carbohydrate intake has been increased, simple sugars are restricted.

The diet should be flexible and understandable to both patient and physician. Weight loss alone in the obese patient may decrease insulin requirements. Efficacy of the diet will be determined by whether the patient achieves the intended result of proper growth and development and normalization of weight in a normal work or school setting without hyperglycemia or hypoglycemia.

Table 199-1. Insulin preparations

Type and preparation	Proinsulin (ppm)	Peak (hr)	Duration (hr)	Type and preparation	Proinsulin (ppm)	Peak (hr)	Duration (hr)
Rapid-acting				Lente			
Regular				Lente Iletin I (Lilly)*	<50	6-12	24
Iletin I (Lilly)*	<50	2-4	5-7	Lente Iletin II (Lilly)†‡	<10	6-12	24
Iletin II (Lilly)†‡	<10	2-4	5-7	Lente Insulin Suspension (Squibb)			
Insulin Regular Injection (Squibb)				Improved‡	<25	6-12	24
Improved†	<25	2-4	5-7	Purified‡	<10	6-12	24
Purified†	<10	2-4	5-7	Monotard (Novo)†	<1	6-12	24
Actrapid (Novo)†	<1	2-4	5-7	Lentard (Novo)*	<1	6-12	24
Velosulin (Nordisk)†	<10	2-4	5-7	Long-acting			
Semilente				Protamine zinc			
Iletin I (Lilly)*	<50	2-4	12-16	Protamine Zinc Iletin I (Lilly)*	<50	14-24	36+
Semilente Insulin Suspension (Squibb)‡	<25	2-4	12-16	Protamine Zinc Iletin II (Lilly)†‡	<10	14-24	36+
Semitard (Novo)†	<1	2-4	12-16	Protamine Zinc Insulin Suspension (Squibb)‡	<25	14-24	36+
Intermediate-acting				Ultralente			
NPH				Ultralente Iletin (Lilly)*	<50	18-24	36+
NPH Iletin I (Lilly)*	<50	6-12	24	Ultralente Insulin Suspension (Squibb)‡	<25	18-24	36+
NPH Iletin II (Lilly)†‡	<10	6-12	24	Ultratard (Novo)‡	<1	18-24	36+
Isophane Insulin Suspension (Squibb)							
Improved‡	<25	6-12	24				
Purified‡	<10	6-12	24				
Protaphane (Novo)†	<1	6-12	24				
Mixtard (Nordisk)†§	<10	4-8	24				
Insulatard NPH (Nordisk)†	<10	6-12	24				

*Available as beef-pork insulin preparation.
†Available as pork insulin preparation.
‡Available as beef insulin preparation.
§Combination of 30% Velosulin and 70% Insulatard.

ORAL HYPOGLYCEMIC AGENTS

While diet therapy remains the foundation of all treatment of diabetic patients, some require drugs in addition to diet to normalize their blood sugar. This may be a result of the patient's inability to comply fully with the diet or the patient's hypoinsulinemia, for which diet therapy alone cannot compensate. In the controversial multicentered University Group Data Project study sponsored by the National Institutes of Health, the investigators concluded that tolbutamide was no more effective than diet alone in the treatment of diabetes and that patients so treated had a significant increase in cardiac-related deaths. This controversy is now dormant after heated debate in the early 1970s. Many physicians continue to use the sulfonyl-ureas in the treatment of certain patients who have maturity-onset diabetes with residual β-cell secreting capacity, believing them to be safe drugs. Although several studies indicate that even in those patients in whom the drugs are effective initially there is a 25% secondary failure rate, some patients are able to use these drugs for long periods. There are no available hard data that show these drugs to be harmful in patients who maintain normal fasting glucose levels and 2-hour postprandial plasma glucose levels less than 150 mg/dl.

Drugs currently used in the United States are tolbutamide (Orinase), acetohexamide (Dymelor), tolazamide (Tolinase), and chlorpropamide (Diabinese); glibenclamide (glyburide) is used abroad. The sulfonylureas act by stimulating insulin secretion. Recent studies demonstrate that these agents also promote their biologic effect by increasing insulin receptor numbers and affinity in adipose tissue, skeletal muscle, and liver cells. Tolbutamide, with a duration of 6 hours, and glibenclamide, 6 to 8 hours, are short acting. Tolazamide, lasting about 10 hours, and acetohexamide, acting about 12 to 14 hours, are intermediate-acting sulfonylureas, whereas chlorpropamide is long acting, up to 72 hours. All sulfonylureas are metabolized in the liver except chlorpropamide, which is excreted unchanged by the kidney. Glyburide is excreted in the urine and feces. Tolazamide and particularly acetohexamide have metabolites with hypoglycemic action. In addition, chlorpropamide has antidiuretic and disulfiram-like effects.

Hypoglycemic reactions with sulfonylureas, although less common than with insulin, can be quite severe and last for several days, particularly with long-acting chlorpropamide in patients with renal insufficiency. For reasons of metabolism and excretion, sulfonylureas are contraindicated in patients with hepatic and renal insufficiency. In using sulfonylureas, special attention must be given to drug interactions, as with acetylsalicylic acid, phenytoin, propranolol, barbiturates, ethanol, clofibrate, phenylbutazone, and acetaminophen, all of which may potentiate or inhibit the hypoglycemic activity of sulfonylureas.

The daily dosage range of these drugs is as follows: tolbutamide, 0.5 to 3 g; acetohexamide, 0.25 to 1.5 g; tolazamide, 0.1 to 1 g; chlorpropamide, 0.1 to 0.5 g; and glibenclamide, 2.5 to 20 mg. The starting dose of tolbutamide is 0.5 g twice daily, and there is rarely any advantage in using more than 1.5 g/day.

The other class of oral hypoglycemic drugs is the biguanides. These drugs presumably act by decreasing glucose uptake from the gastrointestinal tract and inhibiting gluconeogenesis. Because these drugs are associated with lactic acidosis, they are no longer used in the United States.

Sulfonylureas are used with diet in the treatment of some patients with maturity-onset diabetes. They are not prescribed for patients with the hypoinsulinemic, juvenile type (type I) diabetes nor by most physicians during pregnancy or major surgery. Even in patients controlled with these agents, control can be lost with infection and severe emotional stress. Once oral agents become ineffective, they should be discontinued while better control is sought with insulin therapy.

INSULIN THERAPY

The object of diabetic management is to keep the patient symptom free and prevent complications while the individual pursues a normal life-style. Since there appears to be a positive relationship between control and complications, normalization of intermediary metabolism is recommended. Although an appropriate diet is the most important part of diabetic management, insulin is the most important medication for the hypoinsulinemic (type I) patient.

Insulin is used primarily for the hypoinsulinemic, ketosis-prone diabetic patient. It is also used for the insulin-resistant, overweight patient who does not comply with the prescribed diet. Insulin treatment may be initiated for short periods in some patients during pregnancy, severe infection, and stress. At present, single-peak and monocomponent beef, pork, and beef-pork mixtures of insulin are available. Single-peak insulin is purified by a molecular sieve and yields a single peak on gel chromatography. Monocomponent insulin is single-peak insulin that has been purified further and is less likely to produce insulin allergy or resistance. Monocomponent insulin is more expensive and at this time is recommended for newly diagnosed diabetic patients, previously diagnosed diabetic patients who are insulin resistant or have insulin allergy, patients with lipoatrophy, and patients who receive insulin temporarily in stress situations. Short-acting insulins (regular and semilente), intermediate-acting insulins (NPH and lente), and long-acting insulins (protamine zinc and ultralente) are available in single-peak and monocomponent forms. One monocomponent, highly purified preparation has a proinsulin level (an indication of impurities) of less than 0.001%; other insulins have less than 0.0001% proinsulin. As with any change in insulin therapy, some patients changing to highly purified insulin or to a different type of insulin may require a decrease of insulin dose by 10% to 20%. The time actions of the currently used insulins are listed in Table 199-1.

In stabilizing a new adult diabetic patient, one may begin with 10 to 20 units of an intermediate-acting insulin, NPH or lente, using the blood sugar level as a guide. The morning dose of insulin is usually not increased by more than 5 to 10 units/day except in acute situations. Some physicians use a "sliding scale" of insulin therapy based on urine glucose. Generally for 4+ glycosuria, 20 units of regular insulin is given; for 3+, 15 units; 2+, 10 units; and 1+, 5 units. It is desirable that a double-voided urine sample be obtained; the bladder should be emptied on arising and the urine specimen obtained approximately 30 minutes later. This second urine specimen reflects current metabolic activity more closely, but it still has the disadvantage of relying on a urinary glucose threshold, which varies from individual to individual and from time to time. A comparison of a blood sugar and a simultaneous urine sugar provides a rough assessment of the renal handling of glucose.

Using another approach, the patient may be given multiple doses of regular insulin (before meals and at bedtime or later if necessary). If the patient refuses multiple doses of regular insulin and once the blood sugar levels have stabilized, two thirds to three fourths of the total dose of regular insulin may be given as an intermediate-acting insulin before breakfast. Regular insulin is added to this dose in the same syringe if there is morning postprandial hyperglycemia. The majority of type I diabetic patients are controlled by injections of both short- and intermediate-acting insulins given at 8 AM and 5 to 6 PM daily. When the morning dose of intermediate-acting insulin exceeds 40 units, it may be necessary to split the dose because wide swings in blood sugar may occur, resulting in a low sugar level at peak insulin action followed by reactive hyperglycemia (called the Somogyi effect), which is caused by the action of counterregulatory hormones (catecholamines, glucagon, cortisol, and growth hormone). Usually two thirds of the total insulin dose is given in the morning and one third in the afternoon. Increasing numbers of type I diabetic patients are using multiple doses of regular insulin with self-monitoring of blood glucose in an attempt to achieve better control. Glucose monitoring at home is done by placing a drop of blood obtained by a finger prick on a glucose oxidase reagent strip that develops a color corresponding to the blood glucose level. The intensity of the color is read from a sensitive color chart or in a reflectance meter. Much evidence is accumulating that suggests that good metabolic control can delay or prevent microvascular complications in patients with diabetes. The level of glycosylated hemoglobin (Hb A_{ic}) can also be used to monitor control. It is normally 3% to 6% of the total hemoglobin but is elevated when diabetes is out of control. It rarely exceeds 15%. Since Hb A_{ic} is present during the life of the red blood cell, it can be used as a reflection of glucose control over a prolonged period.

Insulin management in special situations

SURGERY. With minor procedures under local anesthesia there is no change in the oral hypoglycemic or insulin regimen. With major procedures a variety of methods are used, including the following.

An intravenous drip of 1000 ml of 5% glucose in water is started preoperatively. One third to one half of the usual morning intermediate insulin dose is administered preoperatively and the remainder postoperatively, or regular insulin is given as needed postoperatively. One practice is to use a low-dose continuous infusion of regular insulin during surgery. The drip consists of 100 units of regular insulin added to 500 ml of 0.5 normal saline solution. Albumin or blood is not used in the insulin drip. One hundred milliliters of infusion mixture is allowed to run through the tubing rapidly before connecting it to the patient to minimize adherence of insulin to the bottle or tubing. A bolus of 2 to 4 units of regular insulin is given intravenously, and a continuous drip of 2 to 3 units of regular insulin is then continued every hour. Blood sugar levels are measured every ½ hour, and the dose of the insulin drip is raised or lowered as needed. In this way intraoperative hypoglycemia is avoided, and a smoother postoperative course is ensured.

The patient should have a full *liquid exchange diet* (equal calories of carbohydrate, protein, and fat composition). If only a clear liquid diet can be retained, the diet can be isocaloric and purely carbohydrate in content. If persistent vomiting occurs, the physician should be notified.

INFECTIONS AND EXERCISE. Infections increase the need for insulin, and exercise decreases the need. Therefore the insulin dose should be raised in response to infections and lowered with increase in exercise.

HYPOGLYCEMIA. The patient must be instructed to be aware of untoward symptoms at the time of peak insulin action. Short-acting insulins are more likely to produce catecholamine-type symptoms of tachycardia, hunger, circumoral pallor, and sweating. The longer-acting insulins are more likely to yield psychiatric, neurologic, or central nervous system symptoms such as bizarre behavior, lethargy, nausea, vomiting, stupor, or coma. Hypoglycemic symptoms are myriad but usually are repeated in a given individual. The importance of eating on time, including snacks, and making allowances for extreme activity needs to be emphasized and recommendations should be individualized. The insulin-dependent patient should be instructed to have sugar or hard candy available if hypoglycemic symptoms occur. Concentrated glucose preparations such as Glutose are also available.

INSULIN ALLERGY. Allergic reactions may occur within 15 to 20 minutes, or a delayed reaction may occur at least 4 hours after an injection; both can be local or systemic. The local reaction is manifested by swelling, redness, or hives, and it usually subsides after a week. If it persists, monocomponent insulin should be substituted if that insulin has not been used previously. If anaphylactoid or vasculitis (systemic) type reactions occur in a patient who is insulin dependent, desensitization to insulin can be tried. The patient should not receive insulin for at least 12 hours before the attempted desensitization procedure. Epinephrine 1:1000 should be available to be given in doses of 0.1 to 0.3 ml subcutaneously if needed. Insulin is given at ½-hour intervals in increasing doses of 0.001, 0.002, 0.004, 0.01, 0.02, 0.04, 0.1, 0.2, 0.5, 1, 2, 4, and 8 units of regular insulin as long as there are no untoward reactions. The first three insulin doses are given intradermally, and the remainder may be given subcutaneously.

LIPOATROPHY. Lipoatrophy is an indication for monocomponent insulin, and improvement can be seen when insulin is injected directly into the atrophic area.

INSULIN RESISTANCE. Insulin antibodies of the IgG type may appear within 6 to 8 weeks after the initiation of insulin therapy but do not necessarily result in resistance. Resistance had been defined as a need for more than 200 units of insulin a day. Realistically, it should refer to any diabetic patient taking more insulin than a nondiabetic person requires to maintain normoglycemia (40 to 50 units/day). For the majority of these patients, switching to monocomponent insulin in a decreased dose will ameliorate the condition. For others, corticosteroids may be needed. It is clear that the category of insulin resistance covers a myriad of entities. Some of these are receptor abnormalities, such as obesity with decreased insulin receptors, and receptor and postreceptor antibody states.

Although insulin remains the cornerstone of drug therapy for the hypoinsulinemic diabetic patient, advances in the type of insulin to be used and in methods of insulin delivery are at various stages of development. It is hoped that the availability of monocomponent insulin will eliminate a majority of insulin antibodies, allergic reactions and lipoatrophy in new diabetic patients. When DNA replication techniques are applied to mass production procedures, unlimited human insulin will be available.

Portable open-loop insulin devices preprogrammed to provide continuous basal low-dose insulin infusion and insulin boluses before meals and at bedtime are available. For most patients these devices have no advantage over multiple-dose regular insulin regimens. Their use in the treatment of type I diabetes is limited by their lack of response to changing blood glucose concentrations. On the horizon is improved insulin delivery mimicking normal β-cell secretion. This awaits the availability of a portable closed loop system with an implantable glucose electrode that can release insulin in response to changing blood sugar concentrations or the successful transplantation of β-cells or the entire pancreas.

DIABETIC KETOACIDOSIS

Diabetic ketoacidosis (DKA) is the ultimate result of extreme insulin deficiency and glucagon excess. Increased insulin need may be precipitated by infection, stress, or as the result of the contrainsulin effects of glucagon, catecholamines, steroids, and growth hormone. The resultant hypoinsulinemia causes increased glucose production by the liver and decreased end-organ utilization. The increasing hyperglycemia produces glycosuria and associated water and electrolyte loss as a result of solute diuresis. The decreased insulin and increased glucagon outputs result in increasing lipolysis, gluconeogenesis, and increased activity of carnitine acyltransferase. This enzyme system controls the transfer of fatty acids to the mitochondria for β oxidation and ketogenesis. Thus there is increased production of β-hydroxybutyric acid, acetoacetic acid, and other strong organic ketogenic acids. With the increased production of these acids by the liver, ketoacidosis is eventually produced when use of ketones by peripheral tissues is exceeded by their supply, and the renal and respiratory compensatory mechanisms that were brought into play eventually fail to maintain a normal pH.

The time interval from the onset of hyperglycemia to the development of DKA is variable. The signs and symptoms most commonly seen are polyuria, polydipsia, polyphagia, weakness, weight loss, signs of dehydration (sunken eyeballs, decreased skin turgor, and dry mucous membranes), tachycardia, hypotension, vomiting, Kussmaul respirations, flaccid reflexes, abdominal tenderness and distention, lipemia retinalis, fever, depressed sensorium, and finally coma. The degree of obtundation seems to correlate more closely with the hyperosmolality present than with the height of the blood sugar level or degree of acidosis.

DKA must be suspected in any diabetic patient with a changing sensorium. Hypoglycemic coma, lactic acidosis, alcoholic ketoacidosis, and drug intoxication (such as with salicylates or ethylene glycol) must be part of the differential diagnosis. Initial studies usually include a complete blood count, a urinalysis, and a capillary glucose test using a glucose oxidase reagent strip for a rapid rough estimate of the blood sugar. In addition, a blood sugar determination, serum acetone with dilutions, serum electrolytes (sodium, potassium, carbon dioxide, and chloride), blood urea nitrogen, serum calcium and phosphorus, arterial blood gas (for pH, PCO_2, and PO_2), electrocardiogram, chest roentgenogram, and cultures from blood, urine, stool, or other indicated sites are essential. Bacterial infection is the most common documented precipitating factor in DKA, but usually the specific cause is obscure. Therefore a careful history and a meticulous physical examination are important in directing studies and treatment. It is very useful to use a flow sheet that includes all laboratory data, intake and output of fluids, serum ketones, urinary glucose and ketones, insulin therapy, and electrolyte replacement. Blood sugar and electrolytes should be checked hourly after the onset of therapy, serum acetone approximately every 2 hours, and blood gases every 4 hours depending on the clinical response.

Successful treatment of DKA requires normalization of the metabolic state, replacement of fluid and electrolyte deficits, and treatment of the initiating cause, such as infection, acute myocardial infarction, or pancreatitis. Individualization of patient treatment with careful monitoring by the physician remains the key to decreased mortality.

Most medical centers currently use continuous low-dose intravenous insulin infusions in the treatment of DKA. It is clear that nearly maximal insulin effect is achieved with plasma insulin levels of 20 to 200 μU/ml. In most cases plasma insulin levels within that range will result in a decrease in blood sugar of 70 to 100 mg/dl/hr. These plasma levels can be achieved with infusion of regular insulin at a rate of 2 to 10 units/hr. These plasma insulin levels can also be achieved by giving an intramuscular injection of 10 units of regular insulin initially and then 5 units of regular insulin hourly intramuscularly. Intramuscular treatment is not recommended in severe DKA, since there is marked dehydration and decreased tissue perfusion with resultant decreased uptake of intramuscularly or subcutaneously injected insulin.

These low-dose regimens result in less hypoglycemia and hypokalemia. Since continuous low-dose regimens are not 100% effective, it is recommended that 10 units of regular insulin by intravenous bolus be administered, followed by 10 units of regular insulin in each hour by continuous infusion initially. The dose is then increased or decreased depending on the effect on blood sugar. The solution usually contains 100 units of regular insulin in 500 ml of normal saline, and 100 ml of this solution is allowed to run through the tubing before connecting it to the patient. More concentrated insulin solutions are made when larger hourly insulin doses are infused. Once acidosis and dehydration are corrected, regular insulin may be given subcutaneously.

Fluid therapy is promptly instituted with normal saline to increase intravascular volume. The first 1 or 2 L can usually be given rapidly in the first hour while monitoring the patient's cardiovascular status. Since the water deficit is usually more marked than the electrolyte deficit, a switch is made to half-normal saline after 1 or 2 L of normal saline, depending on the severity of dehydration, intravascular volume depletion, and hypotension. The last is usually corrected by normal saline solution, except in critical clinical situations such as concomitant gram-negative bacillary bacteremia or an acute myocardial infarction. Rarely, volume expanders such as albumin must be used. At the onset of therapy, gastric contents are aspirated to prevent aspiration by the patient and the nasogastric tube is removed. Intake and output are monitored throughout therapy. A central venous line may be necessary to monitor fluid therapy. When the blood sugar level drops to 250 mg/dl, 5% glucose in water, normal saline, or half-normal saline, depending on the clinical situation, is added to the fluid therapy.

Total body potassium depletion is always present initially in DKA. Intravascular volume contraction and potassium shift from inside cells to the extracellular fluid give falsely high values of serum potassium at the onset of therapy for the ketoacidotic state. Serum potassium usually reaches its low point 2 to 4 hours after the onset of therapy as a direct result of rehydration and potassium shift into cells. During the time the ketoacidotic state is being reversed, potassium is driven into the cell in exchange for hydrogen and sodium. If sodium bicarbomate is used in therapy, it will further increase potassium influx into the cell and decrease the serum value even more. With pH levels at 7.1 or below, sodium bicarbonate is usually given intravenously; this is of debatable value because the increase in blood pH shifts the oxyhemoglobin dissociation curve and will decrease delivery of oxygen to tissues. If the serum potassium level is low at the onset of therapy (below 3 mEq/dl), replacement potassium therapy is initiated immediately in the form of chloride or phosphate salts (40 mEq/L of intravenous solution). If serum potassium is 4 mEq/L or higher, one may wait 1 or 2 hours before introducing potassium therapy.

Phosphate deficit is usually present at the onset of therapy. Repletion of phosphate may be part of potassium replacement given as potassium phosphate. Initial serum calcium and phosphorus levels must be measured, and further monitoring of these levels is important if phosphate therapy is initiated. If phosphorus levels become elevated, phosphate complexing with calcium could be disastrous by producing interstitial calcifications and hypocalcemia that could result in arrhythmias and respiratory paralysis. Phosphorus levels below 1 mg/dl should be treated judiciously. Once the patient can accept oral feeding, adequate phosphorus can be provided in the diet to make up the deficit.

In summary, DKA is a medical emergency that requires urgent attention, with therapy directed to correcting the metabolic deficits, to expanding intravascular volume to increase tissue perfusion, and finally to treating any identifiable precipitating cause.

HYPERGLYCEMIC, HYPEROSMOLAR, NONKETOTIC COMA

Although hyperglycemic, hyperosmolar, nonketotic coma can occur in any type of diabetic patient, it usually occurs in those with diet- or oral agent–controlled maturity-onset (type II) diabetes and rarely occurs in children. The absence of significant ketosis in combination with the hyperglycemia is related to the presence of enough insulin secretion to inhibit lipolysis. There is severe osmotic diuresis with loss of water and electrolytes; water is lost in excess of electrolytes. Water loss is severe and serum osmolalities are elevated above 350 mOsm/kg water. Sodium levels routinely are greater than normal, sometimes in the range of 170 to 180 mEq/L. High sodium levels signify extreme dehydration and volume contraction. The plasma glucose level may be very high, usually 600 to 1000 mg/dl or higher. With increasingly high osmolalities, neurologic signs appear, ranging from lethargy and confusion to coma. Hemoconcentration may precipitate thrombotic events. Although there is the typical diabetic triad of polyuria, polydipsia, and polyphagia at the onset, eventually central nervous system stimulation of the thirst mechanism is impaired as the succeeding events of progressive dehydration, volume contraction, and coma ensue.

The treatment is intravascular volume expansion. Initially normal saline solution is given. The first 2 L is given in 2 to 3 hours. Subsequent to these initial intravenous fluids and as the intravascular fluid space is expanded, half-normal saline solution is substituted. As the blood glucose approaches 250 mg/dl, 5% dextrose can be used in saline, half-normal saline, or water as required by the clinical situation. Electrolytes must be replaced, as in diabetic ketoacidosis. Either a small amount of insulin or no insulin is necessary for the treatment of these patients. Low-dose continuous insulin infusions in the range of 0.5 to 2 units of regular insulin in each hour have been used initially. A central venous pressure line is needed to monitor fluid therapy. It is important to treat the precipitating cause if identifiable. Infection, dialysis (because of the large amounts of glucose infused), and drug therapy with thiazides, intravenous phenytoin, high-dose corticosteroids, and propranolol (which impair insulin secretion or glucose disposal) have been implicated as factors precipitating hyperglycemic, hyperosmolar, nonketotic coma.

ALCOHOLIC KETOACIDOSIS

Alcoholic ketoacidosis occurs in the chronic ethanol abuser who has had decreased ethanol intake for several days. Since vomiting is a frequent associated symptom, food and alcohol intake is limited. Alcohol levels are usually low at the time of admission to the hospital. In contrast, alcoholic hypoglycemia is generally associated with high ethanol levels and is due to inhibition of gluconeogenesis. Blood sugars in alcoholic ketoacidosis are usually less than 400 mg/dl, and plasma insulin levels are decreased. The β-hydroxybutyrate/acetoacetate ratio is often 2 to 2½ times higher than in diabetic ketoacidosis. Acidosis is usually not profound, and these patients generally respond to small doses of insulin and dextrose infusion (see Chapter 197).

COMBINED KETOACIDOSIS AND LACTIC ACIDOSIS

The combination of ketoacidosis and lactic acidosis exists in states such as anoxic states and shock that predispose diabetic patients to lactic acidosis. If extreme metabolic acidosis is present with hyperglycemia and negative serum acetone, lactic acidosis should be suspected. β-Hydroxybutyric acid is not measured by the nitroprusside reagent Acetest, which is the most commonly used qualitative reagent to measure plasma or serum ketones. Although these reagent strips do measure acetoacetic acid and acetone, β-hydroxybutyric acid production is favored in lactic acidosis. Serum lactate and pyruvate levels should be obtained for diagnostic purposes. Treatment of the primary disease producing the lactic acidosis, in addition to the treatment of the diabetic ketoacidosis, is of prime importance. Phenformin, no longer used in the United States, has been implicated in several reports in the ketoacidosis–lactic acidosis syndrome.

DIABETES IN PREGNANCY

Insulin requirements usually decrease in the first trimester, level off during the first part of the second trimester, and increase in the second half of pregnancy. Insulin requirements decrease early in the pregnancy as a result of the demand of the fetus for glucose and amino acids from the maternal circulation in the first half of the pregnancy. The elaboration of significant amounts of human placental lactogen, increased free cortisol, and increased insulin degradation by the placenta in the second half of pregnancy increase insulin requirements. Generally, by the third trimester most women who were insulin dependent before pregnancy will require a morning and late afternoon dose of both intermediate insulin (lente or NPH) and short-acting insulin (semilente or regular).

During pregnancy, fasting blood sugars should be kept to less than 100 mg/dl without the development of hypoglycemia; this correlates with increased fetal survival and decreased perinatal morbidity. It is important to be aware of the rise in insulin requirements coincident with the increasing elaboration of placental contrainsulin factors. Failure to make immediate and sometimes dramatic insulin dose adjustments could lead to diabetic ketoacidosis in the mother and almost certain fetal death. Starvation ketosis itself may adversely affect the fetus and must be differentiated from diabetic ketoacidosis to determine the proper therapeutic approach.

Dietary management is as important in the pregnant as in the nonpregnant state. There is one major difference in the goal of the diet prescription in the pregnant diabetic woman; no attempt is made to normalize maternal weight in order to avoid starvation ketosis. Instead, it is best to aim for a weight gain of 24 to 26 pounds during the pregnancy. A diet of 16 calories for each pound of body weight is prescribed. The distribution of total calories into carbohydrate, protein, and fat is individualized for each patient. The diet of the pregnant diabetic patient, as recommended by the American Diabetes Association in 1979, should include 50% to 60% of the total calories in the form of carbohydrate and 12% to 20% in the form of protein. The remaining calories are supplied as fats; 10% of the total calories should be in the form of polyunsaturated fatty acids.

When feasible, delivery is attempted vaginally. In patients whose obstetric or medical circumstances dictate early delivery, cesarean section may be required. Fetal well-being during pregnancy is monitored by estriol determinations, human placental lactogen levels, stress tests, nonstress tests, amniocentesis, and ultrasound. When it is important to consider early delivery, the lecithin/sphingomyelin ratio is determined. This ratio can be a factor in the decision to delay delivery when the ratio is less than 2.5 and the other parameters of fetal and maternal well-being are stable. However, a major fall (one third) in insulin requirements, maternal toxemia, or fetal distress may force immediate delivery even with lower lecithin/sphingomyelin ratios.

Delivery requires the recognition prospectively of the postpartum loss of contrainsulin factors mentioned previously. To compensate for this a low-dose continuous regular insulin drip of ½ to 2 units per hour following a 1- to 2-unit bolus injection may be administered. There is usually a postpartum decrease in insulin requirements (there may even be a total loss of insulin need for as long as 10 days). This phenomenon is thought to result from inhibition of growth hormone by human placental lactogen during gestation.

In summary, management of the pregnant diabetic woman requires a team approach involving an internist, an obstetrician, and a pediatrician, who pay careful attention to the unique pathophysiologic demands of the fetus and mother during pregnancy and tailor insulin, dietary, obstetric, and delivery decisions to meet these demands.

BIBLIOGRAPHY

Felig, P.: Diabetes mellitus, In Burrow, G.N., and Ferris, T.F., editors: Medical complications during pregnancy, Philadelphia, 1975, W.B. Saunders Co.

Galloway, J.A., and Bressler, R.: Insulin treatment in diabetes mellitus, Med. Clin. North Am. **62**:663, 1978.

Gerich, J.E.: Potential future modes of therapy in diabetes mellitus, Minn. Med. **62**:46, 1979.

Gliedman, M.L., and others: Long term effects of pancreatic transplant function in patients with advanced juvenile onset diabetes, Diabetic Care **1**:1, 1978.

Kidson, W., and others: Treatment of severe diabetes mellitus by insulin infusion, Br. Med. J. **2**:691, 1974.

Krall, L.P., and Chabot, V.A.: Oral hypoglycemic agent update, Med. Clin. North Am. **62**:681, 1978.

Kreisberg, R.A.: Diabetic ketoacidosis, Ann. Intern. Med. **88**:681, 1978.

Matas, A.J., and Sutherland, E.R.: Current states of islet and pancreatic transplantation in diabetes, Diabetes **25**:785, 1976.

Ney, D., and Hollingsworth, D.R.: Nutritional management of pregnancy complicated by diabetes, Diabetes Care **4**:647, 1981.

Page, M.M., and others, Treatment of diabetic coma with continuous low dose infusion of insulin, Br. Med. J. **2**:687, 1974.

Santiago, J.F., and others: Open loop and closed loop devices for blood glucose control in normal and diabetic subjects, Diabetes **28**:71, 1979.

Semple, P.F., White, C., and Manderson, W.F.: Continuous intravenous infusion of small doses of insulin in treatment of diabetic ketoacidosis, Br. Med. J. **2**:694, 1974.

Skyler, J.S., and Cahill, G.F., Jr., editors: Symposium on diabetes mellitus (in three parts), Am. J. Med. **70**:101, 325, 579, 1981.

200 • CHRONIC COMPLICATIONS OF DIABETES MELLITUS

Robert L. Lavine

With the discovery of insulin and with improved therapy patients having diabetes mellitus are living longer. With increased longevity the occurrence of chronic complications of this disease has become a major concern. These chronic complications correlate in large part with the duration of the disordered carbohydrate metabolism; whether they also correlate with the degree of metabolic abnormality remains debatable. An in-depth discussion of this controversy is beyond the scope of this chapter. However, one common bias is that there is a correlation—the worse the control of the diabetic state or the worse the metabolic abnormality, the worse the complication and the earlier it is seen in the course of the diabetes. Data are accruing to support this viewpoint. The purpose of this chapter is to describe the various chronic complications of diabetes mellitus in order to give the reader an overview of the widespread and varied systemic involvement that can occur in this disease.

ARTERIOSCLEROTIC COMPLICATIONS

Arteriosclerotic complications occur at least twice as frequently in diabetic patients as in nondiabetic patients. Diabetes mellitus seems to accelerate the arteriosclerotic process, but how it does this is unknown. It is likely that the severe and widespread arteriosclerotic involvement in the diabetic patient differs from arteriosclerosis in the nondiabetic patient only in degree and severity and does not represent an arteriosclerotic process unique to diabetes mellitus. Arteriosclerosis observed in diabetic patients occurs at an earlier age, is more diffuse, involves smaller arteries as well as larger ones, progresses at a more rapid rate, is as common in women (even in premenopausal women) as in men, demonstrates an increased incidence of medial sclerosis of the arteries (the pathogenic significance of which is unknown), and is associated with a poorer prognosis. Major arteriosclerotic complications occur in the coronary arteries, cerebral arteries, and peripheral arteries.

Coronary artery disease

Coronary artery disease results from accumulation of fat and cholesterol deposits in the media of the coronary arteries. These deposits may coalesce to become plaques (atheroma), which can become calcified and fibrotic and lead to narrowing and obstruction of the vessel. The plaques may also ulcerate, resulting in thrombus formation that can cause partial or complete occlusion of the vessel. Complete occlusion leads to myocardial ischemia, which results in myocardial infarction with loss of heart tissue. Partial occlusion may result in the exertional chest pain of angina pectoris.

In diabetic patients the incidence of coronary artery disease is greater than in nondiabetic individuals, and survival after myocardial infarction, especially long-term survival, is shorter. As in the nondiabetic patient, most diabetic patients with myocardial infarction have a crushing, burning, substernal chest pain that may radiate down the arms and up the neck. This pain is associated with profound fatigue, nausea, and sweating. However, 10% of diabetic patients have little or no pain during a myocardial infarction. There may be a higher incidence of ventricular tachyarrhythmias following myocardial infarction in diabetic patients; however, the course is no different than in nondiabetic patients, except that the myocardial infarction will deteriorate diabetic control or may cause diabetes in a previously nondiabetic patient. Whereas hypoglycemia must be avoided because it may precipitate arrhythmias, control of the diabetes must continue during and after infarction because the elevation of free fatty acids that accompanies uncontrolled diabetes may adversely affect myocardial function.

Cerebrovascular disease

As a result of arteriosclerotic involvement of the cerebral arteries, thrombotic cerebrovascular accidents (CVAs) are frequently observed in diabetic patients. The CVA syndromes are similar to those observed in nondiabetic patients; however, there seems to be a higher incidence of CVAs involving the branches of the vertebrobasilar system of the brain. In evaluating a diabetic patient with a CVA, it must be kept in mind that hypoglycemia and hyperosmolar, hyperglycemic, nonketotic coma can produce similar neurologic dysfunction that will be reversed with appropriate treatment. However, when these disorders have been ruled out, treatment of a CVA is similar to that rendered to nondiabetic patients plus treatment of the diabetes.

Peripheral vascular disease

Seventy percent of all non-trauma-induced amputations in the United States are the result of diabetes mellitus. Involvement of peripheral arteries by the accelerated arteriosclerosis of diabetes leads to claudication (exertional muscle pain caused by muscle ischemia when blood flow is adequate at rest but inadequate with exercise) or loss of the extremity when blood flow is totally inadequate. Peripheral pulses are usually absent. In 20% of diabetic patients, however, palpable pulses are present, but signs of peripheral vascular disease are observed. This results from involvement of smaller arteries without significant large arterial involvement. Since small arteries as well as large arteries are affected in diabetes, it is common to first see small distal areas (tip of a toe or heel) involved before large areas (foot or leg). In the nondiabetic patient large areas (foot or leg) are usually involved at the outset because large arteries are mainly affected. Why peripheral vascular disease is symptomatically a disease of the lower extremities in both diabetic and nondiabetic patients is unknown. However, it may be related to the higher pressures normally observed in lower extremity arteries than those of the upper extremities.

Although surgical removal of atheromatous plaques and occlusions (endarterectomy) or the use of bypass procedures is of help in nondiabetic peripheral vascular disease these procedures are less likely to help the diabetic patient because the arteriosclerotic process is more diffuse and also involves smaller arteries. However, in selected cases arteriography and endarterectomy or bypass is worth considering. Unfortunately, amputation is frequently the only procedure feasible.

THE "DIABETIC FOOT"

The "diabetic foot" is the complex result of several processes, ending in foot ulceration, infection, gangrene, and tissue loss and leading to loss of locomotion. A deficiency in the blood flow that maintains tissue survival, caused by peripheral vascular disease, plays an important role. Another process involves thickening of the basement membrane of the microscopic vessels, the arterioles. Diabetic peripheral neuropathy (see "Neuropathy" later in this chapter), which causes decreased sensation and foot deformity and thereby leads to trauma, also plays a role. Finally, a fourth pathologic process, infection, may turn this condition into an emergency.

In all patients it is important to make a clinical judgment as to whether the foot lesion has resulted predominantly from ischemia or neuropathy. Despite the knowledge that both conditions are present to some degree and that almost all are complicated by infection, this differentiation is important, since healing can occur when the lesion is primarily neuropathic, whereas the prognosis is extremely bad when the lesion is predominantly ischemic. A patient with decreased sensation in the feet who has little pain despite an infected foot lesion and who has loss of position and vibratory senses, wasting of the interosseous muscles of the feet, loss of the ankle jerk, and a warm foot with good pulses has a predominantly neuropathic lesion. This patient has a good chance of healing and therefore must be treated aggressively. If osteomyelitis is present, the prognosis becomes poor. A patient with a painful lesion, with or without absent pulses, who exhibits dependent rubor, a cool foot, and poor venous filling (in the absence of varicose veins) and who also has other evidence of ischemia, such as thickened nails and hair loss on the foot and leg, has a much poorer prognosis for healing.

The objectives of treatment are to heal the foot lesion and preserve tissue. If this is not feasible, amputation will be necessary. All patients with significant foot lesions should be hospitalized and treated with bed rest, antibiotics (after appropriate cultures), local therapy with whirlpool, debridement, and drainage. The last two procedures must be done in an extremely conservative fashion in the patient with a predominantly vascular lesion, since the ability to heal this type of lesion is questionable. Roentgenograms are helpful to determine whether osteomyelitis is present or not. However, films must be interpreted cautiously, since neuropathy can produce osteoporotic "washed out" bones and may be confused with osteomyelitis. If healing cannot be accomplished, adequate amputation must be carried out. Finally, diabetes must be well controlled to maximize the patient's ability to heal and combat the infection.

An important aspect to consider when discussing the "diabetic foot" is prevention. Many of the events that lead to eventual amputation are preventable. Therefore the patient must be educated regarding proper care and attention to the feet.

EYE COMPLICATIONS—CATARACTS AND RETINOPATHY

A leading cause of blindness in the United States is diabetes mellitus. Uncontrolled diabetes may be accompanied by reversible blurred vision, which may become worse as diabetes is initially controlled. This is caused by swelling of the lens, a result of the accumulation of fructose and sorbitol that increases the osmolality within the lens. If this process continues or is frequent, lens protein is denatured and cataracts form. Two types of cataracts are seen: (1) metabolic or juvenile cataracts, which may be observed in children and young adults who have grossly uncontrolled diabetes, and (2) senile cataracts, which are more common than metabolic cataracts. These cataracts are similar to the senile cataracts of nondiabetic patients but tend to occur at a younger age.

A major eye problem is diabetic retinopathy. This problem is typically observed 10 to 15 years after the onset of diabetes. Diabetic retinopathy is classified into three categories:

1. Background retinopathy consists of microaneurysms, intraretinal hemorrhages (blot, dot, and flame hemorrhages), retinal edema, and hard, waxy exudates.
2. Maculopathy consists of hard exudates, edema, and less often hemorrhage in the macula yielding a marked deficit in visual acuity.
3. Proliferative retinopathy (malignant retinopathy) consists of new blood vessel formation, glial scars, and preretinal and vitreous hemorrhages that lead to vitreous opacity and retinal detachment. Sixty percent of the patients discovered to have this form of diabetic retinopathy will be blind in that eye within 5 years, whereas patients having only background retinopathy will not become blind unless maculopathy or proliferative retinopathy supervenes.

The cause of diabetic retinopathy is thought to be related to retinal ischemia resulting from the metabolic abnormalities of the diabetic state. The increased blood coagulability, increased blood viscosity, increased red cell clumping, and increased platelet adhesiveness that are present in diabetes can reduce blood flow in the retinal capillaries and cause ischemia. In addition, the elevated levels of hemoglobin A_{IC} observed in diabetes may add to the ischemia, since this hemoglobin less readily gives up oxygen to the tissues. It is postulated that ischemic areas of the retina release a blood vessel–stimulating factor leading to new blood vessel formation not only in the retina but also in the anterior chamber of the eye and iris. Repeated hemorrhage into the anterior chamber can lead to glaucoma.

No treatment is indicated for background retinopathy at present except for diabetic control. Therapy using the xenon arc or the argon laser has been demonstrated to be beneficial in proliferative retinopathy and maculopathy and is now the treatment of choice. Vitrectomy may have a place in treatment; however, more experience is necessary. Pituitary ablation is not now indicated in most cases.

NEPHROPATHY

Diabetic nephropathy is a clinical syndrome of progressive renal dysfunction leading to hypertension, varying degrees of the nephrotic syndrome, and renal failure. Although most patients having diabetes for 20 years will have some histopathologic evidence of diabetic renal involvement, only 50% of patients will have the clinical syndrome, usually observed 10 to 15 years after the onset of diabetes.

Typically, proteinuria is the first manifestation of the syndrome; this increases with time. Later, progressive renal failure is evidence by increasing urea nitrogen and creatinine levels. By the time the patient is excreting a significant amount of protein (2 to 3 g/24 hr), life expectancy is decreased to 6 years. When urea nitrogen and creatinine are elevated, life expectany drops to 3 years. During this latter period hypertension appears or becomes severe and difficult to control. This not only increases the renal damage but also markedly increases the retinal deterioration; almost all patients with nephropathy have retinopathy.

Death is inevitable unless dialysis and renal transplantation are employed. Although in the past many centers would not accept diabetic patients for either long-term dialysis or renal transplant programs because of poor results, fortunately this is changing. Chronic renal failure from diabetic nephropathy is the most common renal disease treated in many renal failure treatment centers.

None of the histopathologic changes observed in the kidneys of diabetic patients is specific for diabetes mellitus. However, the widespread changes and the variety of lesions observed strongly suggest diabetes. Typical lesions include glomerular capillary basement membrane thickening, along with deposits of basement membrane–like material in the mesangial areas (diffuse glomerulosclerosis), thickening of the arteriolar basement membrane (arteriolosclerosis), nodular accumulations of basement membrane–like material in the mesangium, the so-called Kimmelstiel-Wilson lesion (nodular glomerulosclerosis), and cellular infiltrates and scarring of the renal interstitum (interstitial disease). Other common lesions include the capsular drop and hyaline cap ("exudative lesions") and glycogen deposition in the renal tubules. Usually all the lesions are present to varying degrees. However, the lesion that seems to correlate best with the clinical picture is the lesion of diffuse glomerulosclerosis.

In addition to proper therapy for diabetes, treatment consists of finding and treating any other entity that will cause deterioration of renal function, such as hypertension, urinary infection, urinary obstruction, and nephrotoxic drugs. As renal function deteriorates, the patient should be evaluated for entrance into renal dialysis and transplantation programs as well as for the appropriate time to place an access ateriovenous fistula. When terminal renal failure appears, insulin requirements may need to be drastically reduced; however, usually some insulin is necessary.

NEUROPATHY

The nervous system is affected by diabetes mellitus in many ways. Diabetic neuropathy refers to abnormalities of the function of peripheral nerves (and certain cranial nerves) in diabetes mellitus. Although diabetic neuropathy can be the presenting symptom of diabetes mellitus, more typically the clinical signs of the neuropathies are observed about 10 years after the onset of the disease. The neuropathies can be classified according to the nervous tissue element involved.

Peripheral neuropathy

Peripheral neuropathy is a metabolic disorder of the peripheral nerves possibly caused by increased sorbitol and decreased myo-inositol levels in the nerve fibers. This leads to a decrease in the conduction velocity of the nerve impulse. This disorder affects the distal segments of the nerves before the proximal segments and affects the nerves in the lower extremities to a greater degree than those of the upper extremities. The dysfunction results in a "stocking-glove" distribution of the symptoms and signs. Both motor and sensory functions are affected, resulting in numbness, dysesthesia, loss of position and vibratory sensation, muscle wasting, and deformity of the foot. Peripheral neuropathy leads to two serious problems: (1) trauma to the feet and trauma to and deterioration of joints (Charcot's joint), with ultimate production of the "diabetic foot" and loss of locomotion; and (2) incapacitating pain syndrome. This syndrome is associated with depression, weight loss, and markedly uncontrolled diabetes.

Mononeuropathy

Mononeuropathy is caused by infarcts of a single nerve or different single nerves (mononeuropathy multiplex). The onset is relatively rapid and is accompanied by loss of motor and sensory function of the involved nerve. There may be severe pain in the distribution of the nerve and a positive Tinel's sign (shooting pain along the nerve when percussed). If this process occurs in the cranial nerves of the eye (nerves III, IV, or VI), it is termed cranial neuropathy. Cranial neuropathy most frequently involves the third cranial nerve. Symptoms include ophthalmoplegia, ptosis, unilateral headache, and a dilated pupil with a spared pupillary light reflex. The major condition to be considered in the differential diagnosis is aneurysm of the circle of Willis. However, third nerve palsy caused by aneurysm is usually associated with loss of the pupillary light reflex.

The prognosis of diabetic mononeuropathy of both types is good, with gradual improvement over 4 to 6 weeks. Treatment consists of physical therapy and splinting. An eye patch for cranial neuropathy is helpful.

Radiculopathy

Radiculopathy is caused by infarction of the nerve root. This yields a sensory syndrome whose symptoms and signs are present in the distribution of the nerve root. Patients complain of pain in a root distribution, which may be aggravated with coughing or straining. A classic presentation is intercostal neuritis. Certain cases of upper abdominal pain in the diabetic patient result from involvement of the lower thoracic nerve roots. This must be kept in mind when evaluating a diabetic patient with abdominal pain.

Amyotrophy

Amyotrophy is characterized by asymmetric wasting and weakness of the muscles of the pelvic girdle. There may be pain and loss of reflexes or occasionally increased reflexes. Fasciculations are sometimes observed. In contrast to the other neuropathies, this type of neuropathy is usually seen in middle-aged or older men who have diabetes of recent onset or newly diagnosed diabetes.

The cause of this lesion is disputed. Some consider it to be secondary to infarction of the lumbar plexus, whereas others consider it to be secondary to a metabolic abnormality of the nerve terminals. Although biopsy is usually unnecessary, muscle biopsy reveals noninflammatory degeneration of single muscle fibers. Electromyography reveals changes of denervation but no evidence of primary muscle disease.

Autonomic neuropathy

Any autonomic function can be affected by diabetes mellitus. Patients with autonomic neuropathy usually have had long-term diabetes with other major complications. The role of autonomic neuropathy in the morbidity and mortality of diabetes mellitus is being more widely appreciated. The various autonomic neuropathies are listed in the following outline. Treatment is mainly symptomatic. However, metoclopramide has been successfully used in Europe for gastroparesis, and broad-spectrum, nonabsorbable antibiotics may be helpful in treating some cases of diabetic diarrhea.

Types of autonomic neuropathy
I. Pupillary abnormalities
II. Cardiovascular abnormalities
   A. Persistent tachycardia
   B. Persistent bradycardia
   C. Cardiac denervation syndrome (loss of sympathetic and parasympathetic nerve function)
   D. Abnormalities in Valsalva's maneuver
   E. Abnormal beat-to-beat variation
   F. Postural hypotension
III. Gastrointestinal abnormalities
   A. Esophageal motility disorders
   B. Gastroparesis (gastric atony)
   C. Gallbladder motility abnormalities
   D. "Diabetic diarrhea"
   E. Colonic motility problems (constipation, "megacolon")
IV. Genitourinary abnormalities
   A. Atonic bladder
   B. Impotence
   C. Retrograde ejaculation
V. Abnormalities of sweat gland and sebaceous gland function
   A. Hyperhidrosis
   B. Hypohidrosis
   C. Deficient sebum production

Diabetic pseudotabes

The term "diabetic pseudotabes" is sometimes used to denote a disorder caused by the signs and symptoms of the various diabetic neuropathies, which together resemble the disorder tabes dorsalis. It does not denote another form of diabetic neuropathy. Diagnosis rests with evaluation of serum and spinal fluid serologic tests for syphilis. The level of spinal fluid protein is not of diagnostic help, since elevated levels are observed in diabetic neuropathy.

DERMOPATHY

Patients with diabetic dermopathy may have pigmented atrophic lesions over the shins ("shin spots"). These lesions are thought to be related to trauma. Another chronic skin manifestation of diabetes is necrobiosis lipoidica diabeticorum. This lesion is usually observed in young diabetic women whose diabetes started in childhood. Typically, these lesions are noted on the anterior shin (the process is usually bilateral, but not symmetric). The lesions have a pink to tan border and a waxy-looking and waxy-feeling depressed central area in which telangiectatic vessels are observed. Histologically, the lesions reveal necrosis and loss of the subcutaneous fat, capillaries with thick basement membranes, and granuloma formation.

Both dermopathy and necrobiosis are usually of no medical consequence. However, necrobiosis may be a cosmetic problem and does respond to intralesional injection of corticosteroids. This lesion occasionally ulcerates and requires skin grafting.

BIBLIOGRAPHY

Balodimos, M.C.: Diabetic nephropathy. In Marble, A., and others, editors: Joslin's diabetic mellitus, ed. 11, Philadelphia, 1971, Lea & Febiger.

Bradley, W.E., editor: Aspects of autonomic neuropathy, Ann. Intern. Med. **92**:293, 1980.

Bunick, E.M., and Lavine, R.L.: The role of hyperglycemia in the development of complications in the diabetic patient. In Coodley, E.L., and others: Internal medicine update: 1979-1980, New York, 1979, Grune & Stratton, Inc.

Jarrett, J.: Diabetes and the heart: coronary heart disease, Clin. Endocrinol. Metabol. **6**:389, 1977.

Kohner, E.M., and Oakley, N.W.: Diabetic retinopathy, Metabolism **24**:1085, 1975.

Levin, M.E.: The diabetic foot, J. Am. Podiatry Assoc. **66**:825, 1976.

Pirart, J.: Diabetes mellitus and its degenerative complications: a prospective study of 4400 patients observed between 1947 and 1973, Diabetes Care **1**:168, 252, 1978.

Ward, J.D.: Diabetic neuropathy. Clin. Endocrinol. Metabol. **1**:809, 1972.

West, K.M., editor: Symposium of epidemiology of diabetes and its macrovascular complications, Diabetes Care **2**:63, 1979.

201 • HYPOGLYCEMIA AND HYPOGLYCEMIC DISORDERS

Clinton W. Young and John H. Karam

Symptomatic hypoglycemia occurs when the central nervous system is deprived of sufficient glucose to meet its metabolic needs. It is usually seen when the blood glucose level drops below 40 mg/dl.

PATHOPHYSIOLOGY. Numerous mechanisms serve to maintain blood glucose within a narrow range (80 to 100 mg/dl). The postprandial rise in blood glucose stimulates the pancreatic β-cells to secrete insulin, which promotes the uptake of glucose into adipose tissue, muscle, and the liver, thus normalizing the blood glucose level within 2 hours. Overstimulation of the β-cells postprandially, as a result of accelerated glucose absorption after rapid gastric emptying, may result in a too rapid disposal of ingested glucose and consequent hypoglycemia 2 to 5 hours after eating (postprandial or reactive hypoglycemia).

By 5 to 8 hours after eating (the postabsorptive state), circulating nutrients of exogenous origin have returned to premeal levels. At this time glucose must arise endogenously from hepatic glycogenolysis and gluconeogenesis to provide sufficient fuel for proper functioning of the central nervous system. An adequate rate of hepatic glucose production depends primarily on an appropriate decline in circulating insulin levels with fasting and, to a lesser extent, on a rise in glucagon, growth hormone, and cortisol levels. These hormonal changes program the hepatic enzymatic steps necessary for glycogenolysis and gluconeogenesis. Any condition that impairs hepatic glucose production (for example, hyperinsulinism; deficiency of cortisol, glucagon, or growth hormone; severe hepatic parenchymal disease; or hepatic enzymatic deficiencies) may result in fasting hypoglycemia.

The causes of hypoglycemia are outlined as follows:

Insulin reaction
Postprandial (reactive) hypoglycemia
    Early hypoglycemia (alimentary)
        Gastrectomy
        Increased vagal tone (functional)
    Late hypoglycemia (occult diabetes)
Fasting hypoglycemia
    Without hyperinsulinism
        Endocrine or enzymatic disorders
        Severe hepatic dysfunction
        Extrahepatic tumors
    With hyperinsulinism
        Pancreatic β-cell tumor
        Surreptitious administration of insulin or sulfonylureas (factitious hypoglycemia)
Alcohol hypoglycemia

ETIOLOGY

Insulin reaction. Insulin reaction, the most commonly seen hypoglycemic disorder, results from insulin overdosage in the diabetic patient. This usually occurs when the patient fails to eat adequately or engages in strenuous physical activity without an appropriate reduction in insulin dosage.

Postprandial (reactive) hypoglycemia. Postprandial hypoglycemia may be classified as early (within 2 to 3 hours of a meal) or late (3 to 5 hours after eating). Early, or alimentary, hypoglycemia occurs when there is a rapid discharge of ingested carbohydrate into the small bowel, followed by rapid glucose absorption and hyperinsulinism. It may be seen after gastrointestinal surgery, particularly in association with the "dumping syndrome" after gastrectomy; more commonly it is functional and may result from overactivity of the parasympathetic nervous system mediated via the vagus nerves. Late hypoglycemia (occult diabetes) is caused by a delay in early insulin release, which results in exaggeration of the initial hyperglycemia during a glucose tolerance test. An exaggerated insulin response to this hyperglycemia produces late hypoglycemia.

Fasting hypoglycemia. Fasting hypoglycemia may occur spontaneously in certain endocrine diseases (such as hypopituitarism, Addison's disease, or myxedema), in disorders causing severe hepatic dysfunction, or as a consequence of inborn metabolic diseases of childhood such as glycogen storage disease. These conditions are usually obvious, with hypoglycemia being only a secondary feature. When fasting hypoglycemia is a primary manifestation in an adult with a clinically apparent endocrine or hepatic disorder, the principal causes are (1) hyperinsulinism owing to either pancreatic β-cell tumors or surreptitious administration of insulin or sulfonylureas; and (2) non-insulin-producing extrahepatic tumors.

Alcohol hypoglycemia. Alcohol hypoglycemia may occur after a period of fasting or within several hours after drinking ethanol in combination with mixes containing sugar. In either case the blood ethanol level may be considerably below legal standards for being "under the influence."

CLINICAL MANIFESTATIONS. Regardless of the cause of hypoglycemia, it is characterized by Whipple's triad, which comprises (1) a history of hypoglycemia symptoms; (2) an associated blood glucose level of 40 mg/dl or less; and (3) immediate recovery following administration of glucose.

Acute hypoglycemia. A precipitous fall in blood glucose to hypoglycemic levels is often heralded by symptoms of adrenergic discharge (sweating, palpitations, anxiety, and tremulousness). Syncope or convulsions may also occur. These symptoms and signs are more commonly associated with an insulin reaction or postprandial reactive hypoglycemia than with fasting hypoglycemia.

Subacute and chronic hypoglycemia. Neuroglycopenic symptoms are the principal manifestation of slowly developing hypoglycemia. They evidence a lack of glucose in the central nervous system and can include blurred vision or diplopia, headache, feelings of detachment, slurred speech, and weakness. Personality and mental changes vary from anxiety to psychotic behavior. These symptoms and signs are more commonly associated with the disorders producing fasting hypoglycemia.

MANAGEMENT. Prolonged hypoglycemia may cause permanent brain damage, convulsions, and death. Prompt recognition and treatment are therefore mandatory. If the patient is conscious and able to swallow, sugar, glucose, candy, or orange juice should be given. If the patient is unconscious, the danger of aspiration necessitates reliance on one of two methods: the intravenous administration of 20 to 50 ml of 50% dextrose over 1 to 2 minutes (the treatment of choice) or the intravenous or intramuscular administration of 1 mg glucagon if the hepatic glycogen reserve is adequate. When consciousness is restored, oral feeding may begin.

Prevention of recurrent hypoglycemic attacks depends on proper diagnosis and management of the underlying disorder.

POSTPRANDIAL (REACTIVE) HYPOGLYCEMIA

Postgastrectomy alimentary hypoglycemia. Treatment of postgastrectomy alimentary hypoglycemia involves more frequent feedings with small portions of rapidly assimilated carbohydrate and larger portions of slowly absorbed fat and protein. Occasionally, anticholinergic drugs such as propantheline (15 mg orally four times daily) may be useful in reducing vagal overactivity.

Functional alimentary hypoglycemia. Early alimentary-type reactive hypoglycemia in a patient who has not undergone surgery is classified as functional. It is most often associated with chronic fatigue, anxiety, irritability, weakness, poor concentration, decreased libido, headaches, hunger after meals, and tremulousness. However, most patients with these symptoms do not have hypoglycemia. Furthermore, even in those with documented early hypoglycemia, it is likely to be only a secondary manifestion of their nervous imbalance, with consequent vagal overactivity causing increased gastric emptying and early hyperinsulinism.

Indiscriminate use and overinterpretation of glucose tolerance tests have led to an unfortunate tendency to overdiagnose functional hypoglycemia. As many as one third or more of normal subjects have hypoglycemia with or without symptoms during a 5-hour glucose tolerance test; thus the nonspecificity of this test makes it a highly unreliable tool for evaluating patients with suspected episodes of postprandial hypoglycemia. Accordingly, to increase diagnostic reliability, hypoglycemia should be documented at the time of a spontaneous symptomatic episode during routine daily activity. Personality evaluation suggestive of hyperkinetic compulsive behavior in thin, anxious patients, particularly women, will support this diagnosis in those with a compatible history.

With documented functional postprandial hypoglycemia, there is no harm and occasional benefit in reducing or eliminating the content of refined sugars in the patient's diet while increasing the frequency and reducing the size of meals. However, it should not be expected that these maneuvers will cure the neurasthenia, since the reflex response to hypoglycemia is only one component of a generalized primary nervous hyperactivity. Supportive counseling and mild sedation should be the mainstays of therapy, with dietary manipulation only an adjunct. Oral anticholinergic drugs have helped in certain advanced cases.

Late hypoglycemia (occult diabetes). Patients with late hypoglycemia are usually quite different from those with early hypoglycemia. They are more phlegmatic and often obese and frequently have a family history of diabetes mellitus. In obese patients treatment is directed at reduction to ideal weight. These patients often respond to reduced carbohydrate intake with multiple, spaced, small feedings that are high in protein. They should be considered early diabetic patients and advised to have periodic medical evaluations.

HYPOGLYCEMIA CAUSED BY PANCREATIC β-CELL TUMORS. Fasting hypoglycemia in an otherwise healthy adult is most commonly due to an adenoma of the islets of Langerhans (insulinoma). Ninety percent of such tumors are single and benign, but multiple adenomas can occur, as well as malignancies with functional metastases. (β-Cell hyperplasia as a cause of fasting hypoglycemia is not well documented in adults.) Adenomas may be familial and have been found in conjunction with tumors of the parathyroid glands and the pituitary gland (multiple endocrine adenomatosis, type 1).

Clinical diagnosis. The signs and symptoms of tumor-related hypoglycemia are those of subacute or chronic hypoglycemia. Permanent and irreversible brain damage may occur. Delayed diagnosis has often resulted in prolonged psychiatric care or treatment for psychomotor epilepsy. In chronic cases obesity can result as a consequence of overeating to relieve symptoms. These often develop in the early morning or after missing a meal, and they occasionally occur after exercise. Typically they begin with evidence of glucose lack in the central nervous system. Sweating and palpitations may not occur with subacute hypoglycemia until a profound degree of hypoglycemia develops.

Laboratory diagnosis. β-Cell tumors do not reduce secretion in the presence of hypoglycemia, and a serum insulin level of 15 μU/ml or more with a concomitant blood glucose value below 40 mg/dl suggests an insulinoma. Other causes of hyperinsulinemic hypoglycemia must be considered, however, such as surreptitious administration of insulin or sulfonylureas.

PROLONGED FAST. Demonstration of hypoglycemia with inappropriate fasting hyperinsulinism during a prolonged, hospital-supervised fast remains the most reliable diagnostic maneuver for insulinoma. In normal men the blood glucose value will not fall below 55 mg/dl during a 72-hour fast; in some normal women, however, the value may fall to as low as 22 mg/dl and lower limits have not been established. (These women remain asymptomatic despite this degree of hypoglycemia, probably because ketogenesis is able to provide sufficient fuel for the central nervous system.) Ratios of insulin (in microunits per milliliter) to glucose (in milligrams per deciliter) are therefore essential. Nonobese, normal subjects maintain a ratio of less than 0.3. Obese subjects may have an elevated ratio, but hypoglycemia does not occur. Virtually 100% of patients with insulinomas have an abnormal insulin-to-glucose ratio during prolonged fasting.

ORAL GLUCOSE TOLERANCE TESTING. Oral glucose tolerance testing has *not* been a valuable diagnostic tool because the variable responsiveness of insulinomas to glucose gives confusing results. Most insulinomas respond poorly to glucose, and a diabetic oral glucose tolerance curve results. In the rare tumors that release insulin in response to glucose, a "flat" curve may be seen. However, "flat" curves are also seen in normal subjects.

STIMULATION TESTS. Demonstration of an exaggerated insulin response to intravenous tolbutamide (insulin level >200 μU/ml within 15 minutes) or glucagon (insulin level >135 μU/ml) may be helpful in documenting insulinoma. However, this response is seen in only 50% to 80% of patients with insulinomas and many false positive results occur (for example, in obesity or hepatic disease). In addition, these tests may produce prolonged, hazardous hypoglycemia in patients with insulinomas.

SUPPRESSION TEST. Suppression of C-peptide during insulin-induced hypoglycemia is the basis of a recently developed diagnostic test for insulinoma. This small peptide, connecting the A and B chains of insulin, is released in equimolar quantities with endogenous insulin and thus reflects endogenous insulin secretion, which cannot be directly monitored during insulin infusion. Whereas in normal subjects C-peptide levels will be suppressed to 50% or less of baseline levels during hypoglycemia induced by 0.1 unit of insulin/kg body weight/hr, absence of suppression suggests the presence of an autonomous insulin-secreting tumor.

ROENTGENOGRAPHY. Pancreatic arteriography can occassionally locate tumors preoperatively; however, because of the small size of β-cell adenomas (1 cm or less in most cases), the accuracy rate is only 50% and the false positive rate is about 5%. Computed tomography has not proved helpful because of its inability to distinguish small tumors within the pancreas. Pancreatic vein catheterization with insulin assay is currently being studied as a means of localizing insulinomas.

DOCUMENTATION OF FACTITIOUS HYPOGLYCEMIA. Surreptitious insulin or sulfonylurea administration may be difficult to prove. A suspicion of self-induced hypoglycemia is strengthened if the patient is associated with the health professions or has access to insulin or sulfonylurea drugs taken by a diabetic family member. The triad of hypoglycemia, high immunoreactive insulin, and suppressed plasma C-peptide immunoreactivity is pathognomonic of exogenous insulin administration. Demonstration of circulating antibodies to insulin supports this diagnosis in suspected cases. When sulfonylurea abuse is suspected, a chemical test of the plasma to detect the presence of these drugs will distinguish factitious hypoglycemia from insulinoma.

Management

SURGICAL MEASURES. Surgery is the treatment of choice, preferably by an experienced surgeon who is capable of mobilizing the pancreas and adequately exploring the posterior surface of the head and body, as well as the tail. Blood glucose should be monitored throughout surgery, and 10% dextrose in water should be infused at a rate of 100 ml/hr or faster. In cases in which the diagnosis has been established but no ademoma is located, subtotal pancreatectomy is usually indicated, including the entire body and tail of the pancreas. Total pancreatectomy is seldom required in view of the efficacy of long-term therapy with diazoxide in most patients. Recent development of the "closed loop" artificial pancreas permits monitoring of plasma glucose and infusion of dextrose. This not only protects against hypoglycemia but also aids in determining whether all insulin-secreting tumors have been removed, at which time the dextrose infusion is stopped and blood glucose rises.

DIET AND CHEMOTHERAPY. In patients with inoperable functioning islet cell carcinoma or in patients in whom subtotal removal of the pancreas has failed to produce a cure, reliance on frequent feedings is necessary. Since most tumors are not responsive to glucose, carbohydrate feedings every 2 to 3 hours will usually prevent hypoglycemia, although obesity may become a problem. Glucagon should be available for emergency use. Certain drugs, such as diazoxide (300 to 600 mg daily orally), have been useful. (To control the sodium retention characteristic of diazoxide, thiazides should be given). Streptozotocin, a cytotoxic drug, has been found to be especially useful in decreasing insulin secretion in islet cell carcinomas, and effective doses have been achieved without the undue renal toxicity that characterized early experience with the drug.

Prognosis. When insulinoma is diagnosed early and cured surgically, complete recovery is likely–although brain damage following severe hypoglycemia is not reversible. A significant increase in the survival rate has been shown in streptozotocin-treated patients with islet cell carcinoma, with reduction in tumor mass as well as decreased hyperinsulinism.

HYPOGLYCEMIA CAUSED BY EXTRAPANCREATIC TUMORS

Hypoglycemia may rarely be caused by extrapancreatic tumors, including mesenchymal tumors (retroperitoneal sarcomas, hepatomas, and adrenocortical carcinomas) and miscellaneous epithelial-type tumors. They are frequently large and readily palpated or visualized on urograms.

Laboratory diagnosis depends on the demonstration of fasting hypoglycemia associated with serum insulin levels generally below 10 μU/ml. None of these tumors has ever been reported to release immunoreactive insulin, and the mechanism of their hypoglycemic effect remains obscure.

The prognosis is generally poor, and surgical removal should be attempted when feasible. Dietary management of the hypoglycemia is the mainstay of medical treatment, since diazoxide is usually ineffective.

ALCOHOL HYPOGLYCEMIA

Fasting hypoglycemia after alcohol ingestion. After 18 to 24 hours of fasting, hepatic glycogen reserves become depleted and continued hepatic glucose production becomes totally dependent on gluconeogenesis. Under these circumstances a blood concentration of ethanol as low as 45 mg/dl (considerably below most states' legal "under the influence" level of 100 mg/dl) can produce profound hypoglycemia by blocking gluconeogenesis. Neuroglycopenic symptoms in a patient whose breath smells of alcohol may be mistaken for alcoholic stupor. Adequate food intake during alcohol ingestion prevents this type of hypoglycemia.

Reactive hypoglycemia after alcohol ingestion. When soft drinks containing sugar are used as mixers to dilute alcohol in beverages (gin and tonic, rum and cola), insulin release appears to be greater than when the soft drink alone is ingested, and there is a greater tendency for a late hypoglycemic overswing 3 to 4 hours later. This can be prevented by a avoiding the use of sugar mixers while drinking alcohol or ensuring supplementary food intake to provide sustained absorption.

BIBLIOGRAPHY

Cryer, P.E.: Glucose counterregulation in man. Diabetes **30**:261, 1981.

Daggett, P.R., and others: Is preoperative localisation of insulinomas necessary? Lancet **1**:483, 1981.

Fajans, S.S., and Floyd, J.C., Jr.: Fasting hypoglycemia in adults. N. Engl. J. Med. **294**:766, 1976.

Horwitz, D.L., and Rubenstein. A.H.: Insulin suppression. Lancet **2**:1021, 1974.

Isselbacher, K.J.: Metabolic and hepatic effects of alcohol, N. Engl. J. Med. **296**:612, 1977.

Johnson, D.D., and others: Reactive hypoglycemia. J.A.M.A. **243**:1151, 1980.

Jordan, R.M., Kammer, H., and Riddle, M.R.: Sulfonylurea-induced factitious hypoglycemia: a growing problem, Arch. Intern. Med. **137**:390, 1977.

Karam, J.H., and others: Feedback-controlled dextrose infusion during surgical management of insulinomas, Am. J. Med. **66**:675, 1979.

LeQuesne, L.P., and others: The management of insulin tumours of the pancreas. Br. J. Surg. **66**:373, 1979.

Scarlett, J.A., and others: Factitious hypoglycemia: diagnosis by measurement of serum C-peptide immunoreactivity and insulin-binding antibodies, N. Engl. J. Med. **297**:1029, 1977.

Service, F.J., and others: Insulinoma: clinical and diagnostic features in 60 consecutive cases, Mayo Clin. Proc. **51**:417, 1976.

Yager, J.., and Young, R.T.: Non-hypoglycemia is an epidemic condition, N. Engl. J. Med. **291**:907, 1974.

202 • DISORDERS OF LIPOPROTEIN METABOLISM

David M. Capuzzi

A wealth of evidence assembled over the past 20 years indicates an association between elevations of plasma lipid levels (hyperlipidemia) and the premature development of atherosclerotic coronary heart disease (CHD). Plasma lipoproteins function as water-soluble vehicles that transport lipids in the bloodstream. Hyperlipidemia can be explained dynamically as resulting from an increased rate of synthesis and/or a decreased rate of clearance of the circulating lipoproteins. All the major plasma lipids are transported in the circulation bound noncovalently to proteins, and a rise in circulating lipid levels is always associated with an elevation of plasma lipoproteins. Several prospective large-scale survey studies have provided evidence linking elevations of serum cholesterol and triglycerides with the accelerated development of atherosclerotic vascular disease. Some forms of hyperlipidemia are associated with episodes of acute pancreatitis. Significant elevations of plasma lipids can lead to deposits of lipids in the skin and tendons called xanthomas. Rational treatment of elevated lipoprotein levels (hyperlipoproteinemia) requires some understanding of the structure and function of lipoproteins and their dynamic interactions in vivo. Over the past decade there have been dramatic advances in delineating the formation and metabolism of lipoproteins and in defining the pathophysiology and inheritance of lipoprotein disorders. The application of this growing information should bring about significant improvements in diagnostic and therapeutic approaches. For routine clinical purposes emphasis has been placed on determinations of plasma or serum levels of lipids, particularly cholesterol and triglycerides, and on estimates of elevations of specific lipoprotein classes by electrophoretic methods. Operational separations by such means have been useful for the broad classification of several phenotypic disorders of lipid transport, but the various types of hyperlipoproteinemia are heterogeneous in origin and represent the result of complex interactions of environmental and genetic factors. The five general types of hyperlipoproteinemia are numbered types I, II, III, IV, or V, depending on which plasma lipoprotein class is elevated. A given type of hyperlipoproteinemia may reflect a number of underlying metabolic abnormalities, and conversely a specific disease of lipoprotein transport can display different phenotypic patterns on lipoprotein electrophoretic analysis.

In recent years the emphasis in studies of lipoprotein pathophysiology has shifted to monitoring the circulating levels, kinetics, and disposal sites for metabolic removal of the apoprotein moieties of the circulating lipoproteins. These investigations have led to the discovery of a number of apolipoprotein abnormalities. In addition, the development of specific radioimmunoassays for determination of plasma apolipoprotein levels ensures that such apoprotein measurements will inevitably be widely applied for more definitive delineation of specific lipoprotein disturbances.

PLASMA LIPOPROTEINS

The circulating lipoproteins are classified by their density characteristics, by ultracentrifugal flotation, and by their electrophoretic mobility. The plasma lipoproteins contain small amounts of carbohydrates covalently bound to the apoproteins in addition to a large complement of noncovalently bound lipid. Nonpolar lipids such as triglyceride and cholesterol esters form the oily core of the lipoprotein molecule, whereas unesterified cholesterol, phospholipids, and apoproteins comprise the surface components. Four major classes of plasma lipoproteins can be separated by ultracentrifugal and electrophoretic means (Table 202-1 and Fig. 202-1). The larger and lighter lipoproteins contain a higher percentage of lipid, especially triglyceride, and a lower percentage of protein than the smaller and denser lipoproteins. In order of decreasing size and increasing density are the chylomicrons, very low-density lipoproteins (VLDL), low-density lipoproteins (LDL), and high-density lipoproteins (HDL). By ultracentrifugal analysis, these lipoprotein families can be classified according to density (d) and Svedberg flotation constant (S_f) rates as follows: chylomicrons: $d < 1.006$, $S_f > 400$; VLDL: $d < 1.006$, S_f 20 to 400; LDL: $1.006 < d < 1.063$, S_f 0 to 20, and HDL: $1.063 < d < 1.21$. After electrophoretic separation of lipoproteins on paper or agarose gel, chylomicrons remain at the origin, VLDL has pre-β-mobility, LDL has β-mobility, and HDL has α-mobility. Each major lipoprotein class contains a complement of each major lipid class, but the proportions differ. Whereas lipoprotein triglycerides represent transport cargo in the triglyceride-rich lipoproteins (chylomicrons and VLDL), the other lipids probably serve to stabilize the structure of the circulating aggregate and to facilitate its solubility in plasma.

PLASMA APOLIPOPROTEINS

Several methods have been developed for the preparation, isolation, and characterization of the apolipoproteins.

Table 202-1. The plasma lipoproteins

Lipoprotein class	Density (d)	Electrophoretic mobility	Apoprotein content	Lipid composition
Chylomicrons	d < 1.006	Remain at origin	Apo C* Apo B* Apo A-I Apo A-II	Triglycerides (85%-95%) Cholesterol (about 5%) Phospholipids (about 5%) Protein (1%-2%)
Very-low-density lipoproteins (VLDL)	d < 1.006	Pre-β	Apo B* Apo C* Apo E Apo A-I Apo A-II	Trigiycerides (55%-75%) Cholesterol (about 10%) Phospholipids (about 15%) Protein (5%-10%)
Low-density lipoproteins (LDL)	1.006 < d < 1.063	β	Apo B* Apo C Apo E	Triglycerides (10%-15%) Cholesterol (50%) Phospholipids (15%-20%) Protein (20%)
High-density lipoproteins (HDL)	1.063 < d < 1.21	α	Apo A-I* Apo A-II* Apo C Apo E	Triglycerides (5%) Cholesterol (20%) Phospholipids (25%) Protein (50%)

*Indicates major apoprotein components.

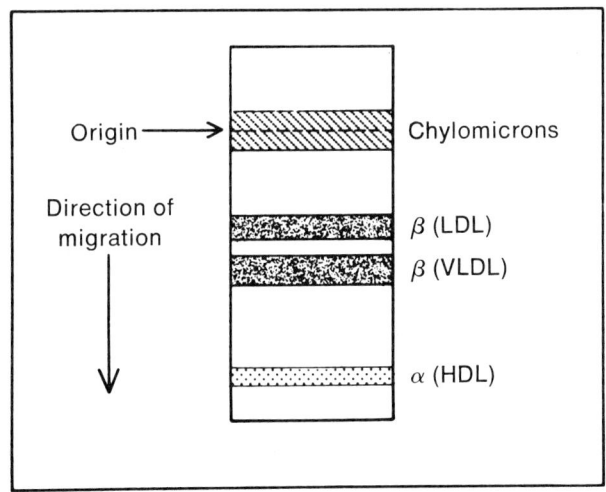

Fig. 202-1. Electrophoretic mobility of plasma lipoproteins.

A number of these apolipoproteins have been sequenced. As is evident from Table 202-1, each plasma lipoprotein density class contains a characteristic distribution of apoproteins, and many of these apoproteins are present in more than one lipoprotein density class. The A apoproteins (apo A-1 and apo A-II) are the major apoproteins of human HDL. Apo A-I and apo A-II are also present in small amounts in chylomicrons and in trace amounts in VLDL. Apo A-I is an activator of the enzyme lecithin: cholesterol acyltransferase (LCAT), which catalyzes the transfer of a fatty acyl moiety from the position 2 of lecithin to the position 3 of cholesterol in HDL and thereby forms cholesterol esters in plasma.

Apoprotein B (apo B), the major apoprotein of human LDL, constitutes more than 95% of the LDL apoproteins and about 25% of the total LDL mass. Apo B is also a major apoprotein constituent of chylomicrons and VLDL and appears to be a requirement for the cellular secretion of these lipoproteins.

A group of small-molecular-weight apoproteins (molecular weight 10,000 or less), termed the C apoproteins and collectively designated apo C, consists of at least three distinct proteins: apo C-I, apo C-II, and PO C-III. The C apoproteins constitute the major protein moieties of chylomicrons and VLDL and are also present in small amounts in HDL and in trace amounts in LDL. Apo C-II is the specific cofactor necessary for triglyceride hydrolysis by lipoprotein lipases of extrahepatic origin and hence plays a crucial role in the metabolism of triglyceride-rich lipoproteins.

The arginine-rich apoprotein, or apo E, is found in small amounts in both VLDL and HDL, with a total plasma level of about 10 mg/dl in the human. Apo E levels are dramatically elevated in the unusual β-VLDL isolated from subjects with type III hyperlipoproteinemia. Apo E enrichment also occurs in abnormal lipoproteins (β-VLDL and HDL_c) isolated from cholesterol-fed animals. Further separation of apo E into constituents (E-I, E-II, and E-III) can be accomplished by isoelectric focusing. Other apolipoproteins (apo D, apo A-III, and apo F) have also been recently identified.

DYNAMICS OF LIPID TRANSPORT BY LIPOPROTEINS

The various circulating lipoproteins are all interrelated, and lipid transport in the plasma must be considered as a complex metabolic process regulated by a variety of dietary and hormonal controls. Triglycerides are quantitatively the major lipids transported in plasma, since 70 to 150 g of triglyceride enters and leaves the plasma daily, while approximately 1 g of cholesterol or phospholipid traverses the plasma compartment. In addition to triglyceride transport, the plasma lipoproteins may also remove cholesterol esters from tissues, provide cholesterol for membrane and steroid hormone synthesis, and transport carotenoids and fat-soluble vitamins. It is likely that the plasma lipoproteins and apolipoproteins have other significant, although as yet unknown, functions.

Chylomicrons are synthesized by the intestinal mucosal cells following a triglyceride-containing meal. The fatty acids and monoglycerides derived from the intraluminal action of pancreatic lipase on exogenous long-chain glycerides are emulsified by bile salts to form micellar aggregates that are absorbed by jejunal mucosal cells and reesterified to triglycerides intracellularly. Chylomicrons are thus formed with triglycerides as their major constituent (90% to 95%) and with minor amounts of other lipids and apoproteins (1% to 2%). These particles (800 to 5000 Å in diameter) are secreted into the intestinal lymphatics and reach the bloodstream via the thoracic duct.

Apo B constitutes 20% and apo C 70% to 90% of the apoprotein complement of chylomicrons. Since only minor amounts of the C apoproteins are synthesized in intestinal mucosal cells, their presence in the lymph is largely due to a transfer of apo C from lipoproteins of hepatic origin. The intestinal mucosa produces VLDL and HDL both in the fasting state and during lipid absorption. In abetalipoproteinemia apo B is completely absent from the plasma. Apparently because of an absence of apo B synthesis, intracellular glycerides accumulate in the intestine and liver, and the plasma is devoid of chylomicrons, VLDL, and LDL.

Endogenous triglyceride is generated mainly in the hepatic parenchymal cells from fatty acids that are mobilized from adipose tissue depots or synthesized de novo from carbohydrate precursors. The triglyceride cargo is packaged with apoproteins at the junctions of smooth and rough endoplasmic reticulum and secreted from the Golgi vesicles into the hepatic sinusoids as VLDL. Triglyceride forms the major component (55% to 75% by weight) of VLDL. The apoprotein portion of VLDL is comprised mainly of apo B (40%) and apo C (40% to 60%). A number of factors, such as increased intake of calories and carbohydrates, excessive intake of alcohol, and rises in cir-

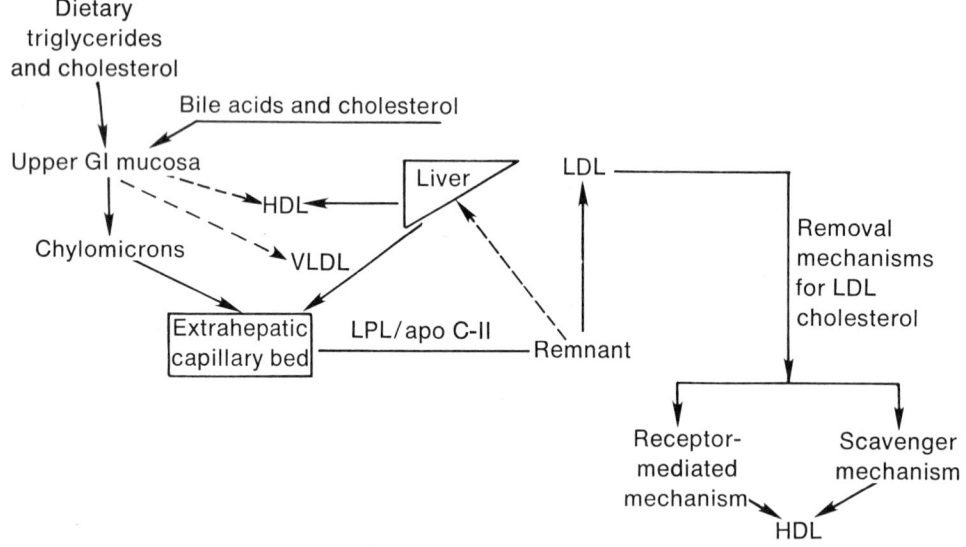

Fig. 202-2. Formation and degradation of plasma lipoproteins. After ingestion of triglycerides and cholesterol from diet, bile acids, biliary cholesterol, and pancreatic lipase enter upper intestinal lumen. Chylomicrons and to lesser extent VLDL and HDL are also produced by upper intestinal mucosal cells. VLDL and HDL are synthesized and secreted into bloodstream by liver as their quantitatively major source. Triglycerides of chylomicrons and VLDL are removed in extrahepatic capillary beds, mainly of adipose tissues and muscle, after hydrolysis by LPL, activated by its apo C-II cofactor. Triglyceride-depleted remnants thereby formed are then further metabolized to LDL by lipolytic and remodeling processes that may involve both LPL and hepatic triglyceride lipase. Extrahepatic tissues remove and catabolize LDL as source of cholesterol both by specific, receptor-mediated, endocytotic, high-affinity uptake process and by nonspecific, low-affinity, scavenger mechanism. It is speculated that HDL and LCAT subsequently remove cellular cholesterol from extrahepatic tissues and return sterol to liver for excretion.

culating insulin levels, stimulate the production of VLDL.

The concept has emerged that the triglyceride-rich lipoproteins (chylomicrons and VLDL) share common removal mechanisms, with distinct and sequential extrahepatic and hepatic stages in the degradation of both lipoprotein classes. The production and removal of the circulating lipoproteins are shown schematically in Fig. 202-2. Accordingly, depletion of the surface constituents and core triglycerides of these particles occurs at the endothelial surfaces of extra-hepatic capillaries (mainly in adipose tissues, muscle, and heart) by the actions of lipoprotein lipases (LPL). This enzyme system is activated by the apo C-II of chylomicrons and VLDL and catalyzes the hydrolysis of triglyceride to fatty acids and glycerol, which enter extrahepatic cells for oxidation and energy production or for reesterification and energy storage. As triglycerides are removed from the glyceride-laden particles, HDL and LCAT interact in concerted fashion to remove the surface components (phospholipids, unesterified cholesterol, and apo C) and thereby remodel the chylomicrons or VLDL substrate so that LPL can continue to split the triglyceride core. The lecithin phospholipids and free cholesterol that are transferred to HDL interact with the LCAT enzyme to form esterified cholesterol and lysolecithins. HDL and LCAT, secretory products of the liver, may remove cholesterol both from the surfaces of triglyceride-rich lipoproteins during hydrolysis and from the cell membranes of extrahepatic tissues, thereby providing a return transport system for cholesterol excretion by the liver.

The progressive hydrolysis of chylomicrons or VLDL results in smaller and denser particles called "remnants" or "intermediate density" lipoproteins (IDL), which then undergo hepatic removal. These triglyceride-rich remnants are enriched in apo B and cholesterol esters. Chylomicron remnants are taken up by the hepatocyte as a unit by a saturable receptor-mediated process and metabolized, but the disposal of VLDL remnants is less well understood. Present evidence suggests that VLDL remnants are removed by hepatocytes and that at least a portion of the remnant VLDL reenters the circulation as LDL after the action of a triglyceride lipase on the hepatocyte cell surface. Whether the conversion of VLDL to LDL occurs totally in the liver, partially in peripheral tissues, or at both sites is unknown. The relative extent of pathways for complete hepatic degradation of the VLDL remnant versus conversion of the remnant to LDL may be an important determinant of circulating LDL levels in different animal species.

LDL arises as a catabolic end product of VLDL degradation. Whether LDL can also be synthesized and secreted de novo by the liver is unclear. LDL appears to be removed from the plasma by both hepatic and extrahepatic tissues, where it provides cholesterol for membrane synthesis. The specific tissue sites for LDL disposal in the human are undefined. Tissue culture studies of both hepatocytes and nonhepatic cells such as fibroblasts and arterial smooth muscle cells have demonstrated the presence of specific surface receptors that bind and lead to the catabolism of labeled LDL. Consequent to binding of LDL to the cell surface receptor, the LDL is internalized with degradation of its apoprotein and cholesterol ester components. The generation of free cholesterol within the cell inhibits hydroxymethylglutaryl CoA reductase, the rate-limiting enzyme for cholesterol synthesis. Failure to bind or internalize LDL by such cells because of deficiency or absence of high-affinity LDL receptors may account for the elevated LDL levels found in subjects with familial forms of hypercholesterolemia.

HDL precursors appear to arise from three sources: (1) direct secretion by the liver into the plasma; (2) secretion by the intestinal mucosal cells into the lymph; and (3) formation from the surface components of chylomicrons. Newly secreted HDL is discoidal and has a somewhat different composition than the spherical HDL found in normal plasma. The intestine also releases a discoidal HDL, rich in apoproteins and lecithin but poor in cholesterol. During the conversion of chylomicrons to remnants, chylomicron surface components are transferred to HDL, and the free cholesterol of HDL is esterified by LCAT. Precursor discoidal HDL is thereby transformed into spherical HDL. The cholesterol esters formed during this process can transfer from HDL to VLDL and then to LDL. The lysolecithin formed by the LCAT reaction is removed by binding to plasma albumin. Patients lacking LCAT have little or no cholesterol esters, and their HDL remains discoidal. Nascent HDL may also be formed by the association of apo A-I and phospholipids released during chylomicron metabolism.

Very little is known about the fate of circulating HDL in the human. Because of the accumulation of cholesterol esters in the tissues of patients with HDL deficiency (Tangier disease), it has been suggested that HDL may be required for the transport of cholesterol from peripheral tissues to removal and excretory sites in the liver. Net transfer of free cholesterol from membranes of cultivated cells has been shown to occur when the culture medium contains LCAT. HDL also reduces the binding and uptake of LDL by cultured aortic smooth muscle cells, a phenomenon postulated to explain the inverse relation found between plasma HDL levels and the incidence of CHD. HDL binds to human fibroblasts in culture, but not to high-affinity binding sites. Binding is followed by uptake and degradation at rates consistent with a process of adsorptive endocytosis. Evidence suggests that the liver plays an important role in HDL removal consistent with its function as the major site of cholesterol excretion.

It is clear from the preceding that the plasma lipoproteins are undergoing constant change because of metabolic interactions and exchanges among themselves and the cells of the organism as they circulate. Because of lipid and apoprotein transfers, all the plasma lipoproteins are interrelated in a state of dynamic equilibrium. Both enzymatic and nonenzymatic interactions occur among the lipoprotein components, and the plasma half-lives of the apoprotein constituents of a given lipoprotein class are heterogeneous. Knowledge of the molecular events involved in lipid transport should lead to improved methods for diagnosis and therapy, but measurement of fasting lipid and sometimes lipoprotein levels is still the conventional approach to evaluation of the hyperlipidemias. Apolipoprotein measurements and perhaps even binding and enzymatic assays of various sorts will in time become more feasible, permitting more specifically tailored therapy.

PATHOPHYSIOLOGY OF LIPID TRANSPORT

Because of their molecular complexity and the multiplicity of steps in production and catabolism, the regulation of plasma lipoprotein levels is more complicated than that of most other plasma proteins. Rates of lipoprotein synthesis may be altered by factors that influence the availability of lipids, the formation of the apoproteins, coupling of lipids to apoproteins, or secretion of the nascent lipoproteins. In addition, degradation of the plasma lipoproteins involves removal of the various apolipoproteins from the circulation by diverse tissues and rapid intermolecular exchanges among lipoprotein constituents.

Hyperlipoproteinemia may result from an inherited genetic disorder of lipoprotein metabolism or may stem from other underlying diseases or environmental factors. The value of determinations of fasting lipid and even lipoprotein levels to define abnormalities in lipid transport is limited because they provide only static measurements in a dynamic system. Such measurements are not likely to detect the subtle but significant abnormalities in lipoprotein composition or homeostasis that are present in various disease states. Nonetheless, fasting lipid and lipoprotein levels have been determined in a sufficient number of subjects to define acceptable ranges for various populations.

The major pathophysiologic abnormalities that cause the various forms of hyperlipoproteinemia include overproduction of triglyceride-rich lipoproteins and defective or delayed clearance of triglyceride-rich lipoproteins, of triglyceride-rich lipoprotein remnants, or of LDL.

Overproduction of triglyceride-rich lipoproteins

Both in normal individuals and in those who are hypertriglyceridemic, there is a postprandial rise in plasma triglyceride levels representing the transport of dietary fat as chylomicrons. These particles normally disappear very rapidly from the circulation, with half-lives of less than 1 hour. In the postabsorptive state, fatty acids derived from depot fat or formed by lipogenesis from carbohydrate are esterified with glycerol to form triglycerides that are destined for transport as VLDL. The fate of fatty acids within the hepatocyte appears to be under hormonal control. Glucagon excess and insulin deficiency favor the partition pathway of fatty acids toward mitochondrial oxidation and away from esterification to triglycerides.

Insulin appears to have a direct positive effect on hepatic triglyceride and VLDL production, and considerable positive correlation in human subjects exists between circulating insulin levels, triglyceride production rates, and plasma triglyceride concentrations. In many conditions insulin resistance and consequent hyperinsulinism are associated with VLDL overproduction. Obesity is the prime example. Other such conditions include pregnancy, therapy with estrogens or glucocorticoids, chronic renal failure with significant azotemia, and acromegaly. Implicit in this association is the hypothesis that the insulin resistance is selective for extrahepatic tissues, whereas the liver remains sensitive to insulin. Direct proof of this selective resistance is lacking at present. Another, less widely accepted concept proposes that the hypertriglyceridemia itself causes insulin resistance and hyperinsulinemia.

Nephrosis and alcoholism are other states that lead to increased endogenous VLDL production not necessarily involving insulin. In the nephrotic syndrome, compensatory hepatic hyperplasia in response to albumin loss can result in stimulation of VLDL generation. Excessive intake of alcohol can enhance hepatic esterification, impair the hepatic oxidation of fatty acids, and increase the export of VLDL. Enhanced production of VLDL can also be a feature of familial hypertriglyceridemia, a monogenic, heritable disorder. The combination of an acquired form of VLDL hypersecretion with a familial form often leads to massive hypertriglyceridemia and even fasting chylomicronemia because of the readily saturable removal mechanisms for triglyceride-rich lipoproteins.

Delayed clearance of triglyceride-rich lipoproteins

The primary destinations of the triglyceride that enters the plasma in chylomicrons and VLDL are the adipose tissues and skeletal muscles. Present in these tissues and in lung, heart, mammary tissues, and perhaps vascular endothelium is the enzyme LPL. LPL in adipose tissue is insulin sensitive. After a fatty meal and the increase in insulin secretion that accompanies eating, the triglyceride cargo of chylomicrons and VLDL is hydrolyzed to fatty acids, which enter the adipocytes and become reesterified to triglyceride for energy storage. In the fasting state, diminished levels of plasma insulin activate the hormone-sensitive lipase of adipocytes to hydrolyze the stored triglycerides to fatty acids, which can be used by most tissues of the body for energy. Other hormones, such as catecholamines released from terminals of the autonomic nervous system, glucagon, growth hormone, and thyroid hormones, have either direct or permissive effects on mobilization of fatty acids from the adipose tissues.

In a variety of conditions, deficiencies in LPL activity may lead to accumulation of chylomicrons and/or VLDL in the bloodstream. the estimated half-life of VLDL triglycerides in the human usually ranges from 2 to 4 hours. Since insulin stimulates LPL production or activity, insulin deficiency in uncontrolled diabetes mellitus can interfere with triglyceride clearance from plasma and result in elevated levels of chylomicrons and/or VLDL. Replenishment with insulin corrects the LPL abnormality and, provided another cause of hypertriglyceridemia is not concurrently present, should result in a reduction of VLDL levels. Since LPL activity is also reduced in hypothyroid patients, plasma triglyceride levels rise despite low free fatty acid (FFA) levels in such patients. Treatment with thyroid hormone corrects the abnormality in lipoprotein clearance in this instance. In patients with chronic renal failure and uremia, the presence of a toxic metabolite may interfere with LPL activity and provide an additional mechanism for the hypertriglyceridemia often seen in this condition. A primary defect in LPL activity can result from an inherited absence of LPL in adipose tissues of affected subjects. This rare genetic abnormality is inherited as an autosomal recessive condition. A more recently described defect is the absence of the apo C-II activator of LPL.

Defective catabolism of triglyceride-rich lipoprotein remnants

Following partial extrahepatic removal of apo C, phospholipids, and triglycerides from chylomicrons and large VLDL, a partially degraded lipoprotein remnant is formed. Its destination is the liver, where further triglyceride is removed, probably by hepatic triglyceride lipase. Some cholesterol and surface protein are also removed, resulting in the formation of LDL, a cholesterol-rich lipoprotein with an apoprotein complement composed mainly of apo B, along with some apo C and apo E. When triglyceride-rich lipoprotein remnants accumulate in plasma ("remnant removal disease," "broad β disease," or type III hyperlipoproteinemia), they distribute in the density range less than 1.019, with the flotation characteristics of VLDL and LDL, and migrate on electrophoresis between the β and pre-β regions, forming a "broad β band." Patients with inherited type III hyperlipoproteinemia have a deficiency of apo E-III despite an enrichment in total apo E. Since about 1% of the population is homozygous for deficient apo E and yet the vast majority of homozygotes are not hyperlipidemic, an additional defect is considered necessary to lead to the hyperlipidemia found in this condition. Although hyperlipidemia is usually not expressed until early adulthood, a pediatric form of the disease has recently been discovered. Remnant accumulation apparently results in broad β disease from a defect in the later stages of chylomicron and VLDL catabolism. The remnants become readily deposited within the walls of muscular arteries throughout the body and are very atherogenic. Tissue culture studies have demonstrated uptake of remnants by monolayers of fibroblasts or arterial smooth muscle cells.

The broad β pattern can rarely be seen on an acquired basis. Conditions that have been associated on occasion with remnant accumulation include hypothyroidism, systemic lupus erythematosus with lupus nephritis, diabetic ketoacidosis, and liver disease. Treatment in the acquired forms of the condition is directed toward treatment of the underlying disorder.

Defective catabolism of LDL

The fate of LDL has been examined in more detail than that of the other lipoproteins. LDL as it normally arises from triglyceride-rich lipoprotein remnants appears to conserve the apo B entirely, even as the other apoproteins originally associated with circulating VLDL have been removed. With its rich complement of cholesterol and cholesterol esters, LDL appears to provide a circulating sterol reservoir for use in membrane biosynthesis by extrahepatic tissues. In normal human subjects, the biologic half-life of LDL protein varies between 2.25 and 3.58 days, and the rate of LDL catabolism appears to be an important determinant of plasma LDL levels. One of the metabolic abnormalities identified in subjects having familial hypercholesterolemia with elevated LDL levels is a defect in the removal of LDL from the circulation with a consequent prolongation of the LDL half-life. Skin fibroblasts grown in culture from patients with the autosomal dominant form of this disorder may have one of several distinct mutations resulting in the absence (homozygotes) or deficiency (heterozygotes) of receptor binding sites for LDL apo B. The LDL receptor does not appear to have absolute specificity for apo B, since the same receptor can also "recognize" and bind HDL_c, a lipoprotein devoid of apo B, that is isolated from the plasma of hypercholesterolemic animals. HDL_c contains apo E, and an apo E receptor has been identified in the liver. Defective removal of circulating LDL by extrahepatic receptors may account for the elevations of LDL observed in many patients with familial hypercholesterolemia who have deficient LDL receptors. Elevated LDL levels can also be associated with familial combined hyperlipidemia, a genetic form of hyperlipoproteinemia with apparently normal LDL receptors. The mechanism of the LDL elevations seen in this condition is unknown.

Alterations in circulating LDL can stem from dietary or drug interventions or may reflect other underlying conditions. Elevated LDL levels can result from diets high in cholesterol and saturated fat, and conversely, LDL levels can be lowered by institution of a diet low in cholesterol and enriched with polyunsaturated fatty acids. Certain plasma lipid-lowering agents such as bile acid–binding resins and D-thyroxine appear to lower circulating LDL levels by an increase in LDL catabolism.

Patients with hypothyroidism have increased LDL levels resulting from defective LDL removal, a defect that is corrected by the administration of thyroid hormone. Hypothyroidism also markedly exaggerates the lipid and lipoprotein abnormalities of type III hyperlipoproteinemia. In the nephrotic syndrome raised LDL levels are associated with normal fractional catabolic rates of LDL and may be caused by hepatic overproduction of VLDL, the precursor of LDL. LDL elevations are frequently observed in patients with acute intermittent porphyria, anorexia nervosa, ateliotic dwarfism, and various forms of dysproteinemia, but the mechanisms for such elevations remain unclear.

Liver disease and lipoprotein metabolism

Because of the central function of the liver in lipoprotein biosynthesis and its less well-defined role in lipoprotein metabolism, changes in lipoprotein levels and composition are not unusual in various liver diseases. Cholesterol and phospholipids are excreted as such in bile by the hepatic parenchymal cells. Cholesterol is also converted into the bile acids cholic acid and chenodeoxycholic acid, a large proportion of which undergoes enterohepatic recirculation following biliary secretion. Cholesterol for biliary disposal may be derived from the surface of triglyceride-rich lipoproteins via the LCAT-HDL system, from lipoprotein remnants during the hepatic processing of remnant to LDL, or from LDL itself.

Obstruction of bile flow can result in an interaction between refluxed bile acid and plasma constituents, with formation of an abnormal lipoprotein termed "lipoprotein X" that is composed mainly of phospholipids, free cholesterol, albumin, and apo C. Various combinations of HDL and LCAT deficiency can be observed in hepatocellular diseases, presumably consequent to their decreased production by the liver. The resultant declines in "normal" HDL production may lead to diminished plasma levels of cholesterol esters and to increases in free cholesterol and phospholipids in plasma. Insufficient apo A-I is transferred to HDL in the course of reaction with LCAT, leading to abnormal electrophoretic mobility. Since HDL and LCAT are involved in the catabolism of chylomicrons and VLDL, these triglyceride-rich lipoproteins cannot be degraded normally, and remnant lipoproteins that cannot undergo adequate hepatic clearance accumulate in the plasma. Hypertriglyceridemia results, since the triglyceride core of these particles cannot be replaced by cholesterol esters and their polar surface components cannot be depleted.

CLASSIFICATION OF HYPERLIPOPROTEINEMIA

Based on separation of plasma lipoproteins by electrophoresis (Fig. 202-3), the hyperlipoproteinemias have been classified phenotypically into five types, each of which represents a heterogeneous group of primary and secondary abnormalities. About one in five subjects with plasma lipid elevations has an inherited genetic disorder of lipoprotein metabolism. Classification by typing is solely morphologic and does not elucidate the genetic or pathophysiologic mechanisms responsible for the disorder. A

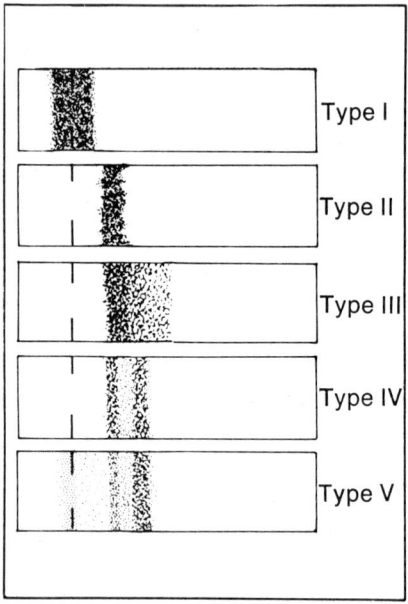

Fig. 202-3. Major lipoprotein phenotypes on paper electrophoresis.

single disorder may lead to different lipoprotein patterns, and a single pattern may result from a variety of mechanisms. Each type results from an increased plasma concentration of chylomicrons, VLDL (pre-β lipoproteins), and/or LDL (β lipoproteins) in postabsorptive plasma, that is, 12 to 14 hours after the last meal. The types are numbered in sequential fashion, depending on which lipoprotein class is elevated in concentration, as the electrophoretic pattern, stained with a lipid stain, is read from left to right. In type I, the presence of chylomicrons is indicated by a band at the origin. The next band on the electrophoretic medium is the β band, and an increase in its intensity leads to a type II pattern, indicating an elevated level of LDL. Type II has been further subdivided into two patterns: type IIA, in which LDL alone is elevated, and type IIB, in which both LDL and VLDL are elevated. In type III hyperlipoproteinemia a broad β band diffusely extends from the β to the pre-β region of the electrophoretic strip, indicating the presence of VLDL remnants in the plasma. An increased intensity of the pre-β band denotes the presence of increased circulating levels of VLDL and a type IV pattern. The type V pattern, in which there is stainable lipoprotein at the origin and an increased pre-β band, indicates the presence of chylomicrons and an excess of pre-β lipoproteins.

Genetic hyperlipoproteinemias

The familial hyperlipoproteinemias consist of six disorders, each apparently inherited by a single-gene mechanism.

FAMILIAL LPL DEFICIENCY. Familial LPL deficiency is an autosomal recessive condition characterized by an inability to dispose of exogenous triglyceride resulting in massive chylomicronemia and a type I lipoprotein pattern. The manifestations are evident during childhood and include bouts of abdominal colic from pancreatitis, eruptive xanthomas, and hepatosplenomegaly. Improvement occurs with limitation of dietary fat intake. There is a major increase in serum triglyceride levels, and the circulating triglyceride/cholesterol ratio exceeds 5:1. LPL activity in the adipose tissues of affected subjects appears to be deficient or absent, and LPL cannot be released into the plasma by injection of heparin.

FAMILIAL HYPERCHOLESTEROLEMIA. Familial hypercholesterolemia is an autosomal dominant disorder associated with elevated plasma LDL levels and a type II lipoprotein pattern. Affected individuals show cutaneous and tendinous xanthomas and strikingly premature CHD that begins in childhood in homozygotes. Subjects with a double dose of the mutant gene are affected more seriously and at earlier ages than the heterozygotes, whose heart disease usually becomes manifest around 30 years of age. The basic molecular defect appears to be a deficiency in cell surface receptors involved in the catabolism of LDL.

FAMILIAL REMNANT REMOVAL DISEASE. This condition is probably a dominant disorder characterized by the presence of lipoproteins of abnormal composition in the plasma. The most typical of these is β-VLDL, which has a higher cholesterol/triglyceride ratio and a different apoprotein content than the normal α-VLDL. This lipoprotein is visualized on the electrophoretic strip as the broad β band or type III pattern. Symptoms include premature coronary and peripheral arteriosclerosis and characteristic palmar xanthomas, usually detected in adulthood. Cholesterol and triglyceride levels are elevated to roughly the same degree. The underlying defect is unclear but involves a defect in the clearance of triglyceride-rich lipoprotein remnants.

FAMILIAL HYPERTRIGLYCERIDEMIA. Familial hypertriglyceridemia appears to be an autosomal dominant lipoprotein abnormality that results in elevated plasma VLDL levels and a type IV lipoprotein pattern. Affected individuals are usually detected in early adulthood and usually display associated obesity, glucose intolerance, hyperuricemia, and some predisposition to CHD. Hepatosplenomegaly and eruptive xanthomas may be found, but only in florid cases of the disorder. Circulating triglyceride levels are always increased, whereas cholesterol levels are normal or mildly raised. Patients with familial hypertriglyceridemia can undergo a change from a type IV to a type V lipoprotein pattern when their lipoprotein removal mechanisms are challenged by estrogen administration, by excessive intake of alcohol or carbohydrate, or by insulin deficiency. The basic biochemical defect in this disorder remains undefined.

FAMILIAL TYPE V HYPERLIPOPROTEINEMIA. The familial type V disorder shows massive triglyceride elevations resulting from both increased VLDL levels and persistent chylomicrons that fail to clear normally unless fat is removed from the diet. This disease may represent an unusually severe form of familial hypertriglyceridemia or a different genetic abnormality that is generally not expressed before early adulthood. Abdominal colic, pancreatitis, and eruptive xanthomas may occur, but these manifestations respond to restriction of calories and dietary fat. In contrast to type I abnormalities, LPL activity appears in plasma after heparin injection. Despite this phenomenon, the overall functional capacity for clearance of triglyceride-rich lipoproteins may be impaired. Intensely staining bands appear at both the origin and pre-β regions of the electrophoretic strip. The triglyceride/cholesterol ratio usually exceeds 5:1. The nature of the underlying defect is unknown.

FAMILIAL COMBINED HYPERLIPIDEMIA. Familial combined hyperlipidemia is the most recently delineated familial lipoprotein disorder and appears to have autosomal dominant inheritance. Affected subjects have elevated plasma levels of VLDL and/or LDL and can show type IIA, IIB, or IV lipoprotein patterns on electrophoresis. They also are predisposed to the premature development of CHD. Overproduction of VLDL is postulated to occur in this condition, but the basic biochemical defect is not understood.

EVALUATION OF PATIENTS
Clinical assessment

Various underlying conditions and a variety of diseases or environmental factors can lead to the development of a given abnormal lipoprotein pattern. Some patterns are more common with certain underlying factors than others. Generally, however, any of the following may cause or be associated with secondary hyperlipidemia: alcohol, estrogen, or glucocorticoid intake, pregnancy, hypothyroidism, nephrotic syndrome, chronic renal disease, obstructive or parenchymal liver disease, pancreatitis, anorexia nervosa, acute intermittent porphyria, obesity, poorly controlled diabetes mellitus, glycogen storage diseases, and dysproteinemias such as multiple myeloma or macroglobulinemia. Such conditions can usually be diagnosed by an adequate history and physical examination and by the use of simple screening tests. Routine studies should include a urinalysis for detection of proteinuria or glycosuria, 2-hour postprandial serum glucose level, serum T_4 level, serum creatinine and BUN levels, serum bilirubin, alkaline phosphatase, and transaminase levels. Further tests would be dictated by suggestive findings obtained during the history or physical examination. A patient may have both a primary and a secondary cause for hyperlipidemia, such as LPL deficiency in combination with alcoholism. A given individual may also have more than one secondary cause for hyperlipidemia, such as obesity and uncontrolled diabetes mellitus. Diagnosis and management are aimed first at detection and removal of underlying causes. Thereafter, persistence of an abnormal lipoprotein pattern or plasma lipid elevation is managed by dietary means and at times with adjunctive drug therapy.

The clinical clues that lead to a suspicion of hyperlipidemia include a family history of or the presence of premature coronary or peripheral arterial disease, xanthomas, premature corneal arcus, and the occurrence of frequent bouts of acute pancreatitis. The presence of any of these would constitute a clear indication for determination of plasma or serum lipid levels; however, a case can be made for lipid determinations as part of any health care evaluation. Relatives, particularly children of hyperlipidemic adults, should have a set of fasting serum triglyceride and cholesterol determinations, since the earlier institution of indicated corrective measures is more apt to be beneficial. Determination of serum lipid concentrations should also be combined with an assessment of potential cardiovascular risk. Other clear-cut risk factors that appear to accelerate the development of atherosclerosis must be identified during the patient evaluation. Such factors include hypertension, cigarette smoking, diabetes mellitus, severe emotional stress, obesity greater than 30% above ideal body weight, sedentary life-style, and hyperuricemia. Other risks have been identified, but they do not appear to have the same impact as these factors. Therefore therapy must be directed to alteration not only of hyperlipidemia but also of the other correctable risk factors.

In history taking, particular attention should be paid to assessment of the patient's intake of alcohol, exposure to hormonal preparations, and ingestion of dietary elements. Although severe degrees of hyperlipidemia are invariably the result of a metabolic abnormality or stem from another disease, mild elevations of plasma lipids frequently occur in subjects who ingest large quantities of calories, cholesterol, or animal fat. The hyperlipidemia in such individuals is likely to respond readily to dietary measures.

The physical examination should include a careful examination of the eye for the presence of a premature corneal arcus–a whitish, crescentic deposit of cholesterol crystals in the cornea that suggests elevations in LDL when seen in younger patients. A number of lipoprotein disorders are associated with observable patterns of lipid accumulation in the skin or tendons called xanthomas. Thickenings of the extensor tendons of the hands or feet and particularly of the Achilles tendons are seen in individuals with familial hypercholesterolemia. Eruptive xanthomas are crops of yellowish papules, each with a reddish base, that characteristically occur on extensor surfaces of the body when triglyceride levels are greatly elevated. They can appear and disappear within a few days as the fat content of the diet is altered and usually indicate hyperchylomicronemia. Eruptive xanthomas are common in patients with type I or type V lipoprotein patterns.

Except for the eruptive and palpebral xanthomas, the occurrence of xanthomas usually is limited to the primary genetic forms of hyperlipoproteinemia. Tuberous xanthomas often begin as lesions that initially resemble eruptive xanthomas but have a redder base and coalesce to form larger accumulations. These can occur in familial hyperlipoproteinemias having types II, III, or IV patterns. Planar xanthomas, yellowish or whitish discolorations of the palmar or interdigital creases, occur in remnant removal disease (type III) and at times in biliary cirrhosis. Xanthelasma, or xanthoma in or around eyelids, may be associated with LDL elevations, but in about one half of the subjects with this skin lesion no currently definable lipoprotein disorder can be detected. Patients with triglyceride levels greater than 2000 mg/dl may display lipemia retinalis, a whitish appearance of retinal arterioles and venules that results from altered reflection of light from the column of blood in these vessels. Hepatosplenomegaly in patients with hyperchylomicronemia appears to be related to engorgement with triglyceride by reticuloendothelial cells, which occurs when normal removal mechanisms are overloaded or fail. Foam cells, or fat-laden macrophages, can be observed in bone marrow specimens from such patients. Attacks of abdominal pain are usually the result of acute pancreatitis, caused perhaps by pancreatic microinfarcts secondary to impedance of the capillary circulation by chylomicrons. Serum amylase levels may be normal in patients having pancreatitis associated with hypertriglyceridemia.

Plasma lipid and lipoprotein sampling

LDL and to a lesser extent VLDL have long been recognized as having atherogenic potential. Patients with elevations of LDL and/or VLDL have an increased risk of accelerated premature coronary atherosclerosis. Premature coronary and peripheral vascular disease is often associated with prolonged exposure to LDL in the circulation. Recent studies suggest that HDL confers protection against the development of premature atherosclerosis. Thus an inverse relation has been generally observed between plasma HDL cholesterol levels and the incidence of myocardial infarction. HDL cholesterol can be measured in the supernatant fraction of serum after removal of chylomicrons, VLDL, and LDL by heparin and manganese precipitation. Normal levels of HDL cholesterol in adults range from about 40 to 80 mg/dl, with higher levels providing supposed protection against coronary artery disease (CAD). It is important to remember that some factors with potential untoward effects can also be associated with high HDL levels. These include estrogen intake, overindulgence in alcohol, and poisoning with polychlorinated pesticides. Premenopausal females generally have higher HDL cholesterol levels than males of similar ages. Chronic renal failure can lower circulating HDL levels and exercise can raise them. When the serum triglycerides are not elevated, the correlation between total cholesterol and LDL levels is so great that measurements of HDL cholesterol levels for the most part are unnecessary.

Measurements of total cholesterol and triglyceride levels in plasma or serum should be carried out after a 12- to 14-hour fast, with visual examination of the serum specimen as well. The patient should be on his customary diet for several days before sampling but should avoid intake of alcohol for at least 3 days beforehand. The patient ideally should be ambulatory, since acute illness, stresses, and trauma can affect plasma lipoprotein levels in either direction. The presence of turbid or lactescent serum in a fasting specimen is always abnormal and usually indicates the presence of triglyceride levels greater than 500 mg/dl. Opalescence may also occur at lower triglyceride levels, particularly if chylomicrons are present. Refrigerated serum will begin to display lactescence at triglyceride levels between 200 and 250 mg/dl because chylomicrons and VLDL aggregate at lower temperatures, producing larger particles that scatter light to a greater degree. The refrigerated sample can also be tentatively used to identify the abnormal lipoprotein pattern, since chylomicrons float to the surface of the sample, whereas VLDL particles do not. Thus a floating layer of fat over clear serum is indicative of isolated chylomicronemia (type I pattern). Patients with type IV pattern will demonstrate evenly distributed opalescence. Elevations of chylomicrons and VLDL (type V) appear as a creamy layer superimposed over a lactescent infranatant. Remnant removal abnormalities (type III) usually present a uniformly turbid serum specimen but can on occasion reveal a floating creamy layer if chylomicron remnants are also present. Hypercholesterolemia without triglyceride elevations does not impart turbidity to serum. The combination of elevated cholesterol with normal triglyceride levels almost always indicates a type II pattern with elevated LDL, except for the rare instances of isolated HDL elevations. Measurements of cholesterol but not triglycerides can be carried out on plasma or serum of nonfasting patients, since LDL levels do not vary only greatly in relation to meals. Firm diagnosis of type III disorders requires the use of ultracentrifugal flotation at serum density to demonstrate the presence of the VLDL remnant that has B mobility on electrophoresis but pre-β density on ultracentrifugation.

Because serum cholesterol and triglyceride levels vary among populations with differing life-styles and increase with age, ideally a subject's levels should be compared with values obtained from normal subjects from the same population in the same age range. An approximation of the upper limit of acceptability of serum cholesterol concentration in an adult under 65 years of age would be 200 mg/dl plus the person's age in years. For the serum triglycerides the upper acceptable limit would be 200 to 250 mg/dl. Such levels are not labeled "normal" because at present an accurate definition of what constitutes normal levels cannot be made. The association between preexisting serum cholesterol levels and the later development of CAD is linear without a plateau or breakpoint. Assessment of associated risk factors also influences the decision of whether a given set of serum lipid levels is acceptable. It is easy to advocate vigorous therapy for severe degrees of hyperlipidemia, but it is difficult to apply specific rules to the management of the modest elevations of serum lipids that are more commonly seen in clinical practice. Sound judgment is often required to decide whether or not to treat. The institution of dietary and/or drug therapy is apt to be long-term, and interventions that do not require radical alterations in life-style are more likely to meet with positive patient compliance.

MANAGEMENT OF HYPERLIPIDEMIA

Dietary management, which includes both caloric restriction and limitation of saturated fat, cholesterol, and alcohol intake, remains the keystone of therapy in hyperlipidemia. Even when drug therapy is employed, the effects of diet and drugs are synergistic and sound dietary principles must be followed. Evidence suggests that a prudent diet coupled with a sensible exercise program can lower serum lipid and lipoprotein levels and perhaps diminish carciovascular risk. Definitive proof that dietary or drug interventions can decelerate or reverse atherosclerosis is lacking. The likelihood is that, although the great majority of individuals will benefit to some degree from such interventions, some will not. Effective therapeutic interventions will require more specific delineation of the metabolic lipoprotein abnormalities present, as well as a more basic understanding of the means to reverse these abnormalities than is presently available.

Since weight reduction alone can lower serum lipid levels in some subjects, the attainment and maintenance of ideal body weight should be the initial therapeutic goal and may be sufficient to correct the hyperlipoproteinemia. Present evidence suggests that severe obesity probably reduces life expectancy and increases the risk of vascular complications. Dietary restriction can improve most hyperlipoproteinemias, with the exception of hyperbetalipoproteinemia, in which optimal diet alone rarely achieves greater than a 20% lowering of serum cholesterol levels. A given therapeutic regimen with diet or drug usually requires a trial of 6 to 8 weeks to determine whether it is beneficial.

In the case of LPL deficiency or other defects in the removal of triglyceride-rich lipoproteins, the therapeutic aim should be to lower chylomicron levels sufficiently to prevent attacks of pancreatitis and triglyceride deposition in the skin, liver, and spleen. This goal can be achieved by simple restriction of fat intake to 25 or 30 g/day. Dietary substitution of short or medium-chain triglycerides for the long-chain variety can be made with commercially available powdered or oil preparations. When diminished LPL activity is caused by a deficiency of insulin or thyroxine, administration of the deficient hormone is indicated. When LPL activity is impaired by the intake of alcohol or high doses of estrogens or glucocorticoids, the causative agent should be discontinued.

To lower serum cholesterol levels in patients, regardless of whether the pattern is type IIA, IIB, III, or even IV, a diet low in cholesterol and saturated fat should be instituted. Populations consuming diets rich in cholesterol and saturated fat generally have higher serum cholesterol levels and a higher prevalence of atherosclerosis than those on a low-fat diet. Considerable controversy exists concerning the effects of dietary cholesterol intake on circulating cholesterol levels. There is individual variation in the cholesterol levels reached in response to a given dietary intake of the sterol. However, cholesterol levels generally correlate in linear fashion with dietary cholesterol as intake increases in the 0 to 600 mg/day range. When the dietary cholesterol exceeds 600 mg/day, the serum concentration usually rises no further, perhaps because of inhibition of hepatic cholesterol synthesis by a negative feedback mechanism. However, even when serum cholesterol levels reach a plateau, there is evidence in animals and probably in the human that a more atherogenic cholesterol-rich lipoprotein accumulates in the circulation. Therefore dietary cholesterol intake should be limited to 300 mg/day. The intake of saturated fat should be reduced with replacement by polyunsaturated fat to achieve a polyunsaturated/saturated fat ratio of 2:1 To follow a low-cholesterol, low-saturated-fat diet requires limited intake of meat (especially beef and pork), egg yolks, dairy products (except soft margarine, skimmed milk, or cottage cheese), commercial pastries, candy and chocolates, and coconut oil products. The ingestion of organ meats (brain, kidneys, and sweetbreads) must be particularly curtailed. The diet should be supplemented with polyunsaturated oils such as corn oil or safflower oil.

The evidence linking serum triglyceride elevations to premature atherogenesis is available but is less convincing than is the case for hypercholesterolemia. Thus mild to modest rises in serum triglycerides caused by VLDL elevations have usually been linked to premature CAD only when serum cholesterol levels are also raised. However, measures should be instituted to lower significant elevations of serum triglycerides, particularly when these elevations exceed 350 mg/dl. Weight reduction through caloric restriction is by far the most important therapeutic measure. Although it is probably wise to limit the intake of simple refined sugars, overall restriction of carbohydrate as a percentage of daily dietary calories is not indicated, contrary to previous concepts. In fact an increase in poorly digested and unabsorbed plant polysaccharides in the form of dietary fiber may well have a beneficial effect on lipid and carbohydrate metabolism. Intake of alcohol must be severely curtailed in most subjects with triglyceride elevations, some of whom may be unusually sensitive in their serum triglyceride responses to even minimal amounts.

Drug therapy

When dietary means do not sufficiently reduce levels of cholesterol and/or triglycerides, drug therapy can be instituted as the diet is continued. Anticipated benefits from drug administration must be carefully weighed against the problems of long-term intake. Factors to be considered in this decision include estimation of cardiovascular risk, expense and toxicity of the drug, age of the patient, and likelihood of patient compliance. Drugs that lower LDL and hence serum cholesterol levels include sitosterols, anionic exchange resins, nicotinic acid, D-thyroxine, and probucol. Sitosterols are plant sterols that interfere with absorption of dietary cholesterol, and in doses of 6 g before each meal, produce a mild cholesterol-lowering effect. Sitosterols are essentially free of adverse side effects. Certain anionic exchange resins bind bile acids, interfere with the enterohepatic circulation of bile acids, and thereby increase the catabolism and biliary excretion of cholesterol. The resins appear to enhance the hepatic removal of LDL cholesterol from the circulation. The hypolipidemic resins that are effective include colestipol hydrochloride (15 to 30 g/day) and cholestyramine resin (12 to 24 g/day). The shortcomings involved with the use of these agents include the inconvenience of mixing the powder with a liquid, poor palatability, frequent gastrointestinal side effects, malabsorption of fat-soluble vitamins, and binding of other acidic drugs by the resins.

Nicotinic acid, used in gradually increasing doses to a maintenance level of between 3 and 6 g/day, appears to reduce the production and plasma levels of VLDL. Nicotinic acid may impair hepatic production of VLDL by an inhibition of FFA mobilization from adipose tissue stores and consequent deficiency of substrate for hepatic triglyceride synthesis. Since LDL is the product of VLDL catabolism, within days LDL levels also fall. This drug is associated with pruritus and cutaneous flushing that occurs within 1 to 2 hours after intake, but tachyphylaxis to these effects develops in most patients even as the dose is increased. More troublesome but reversible side effects include glucose intolerance, hyperuricemia, and plasma elevations of liver enzymes. The drug may also potentiate the postural hypotensive effects of antihypertensive agents. D-thyroxine, the dextrorotatory isomer of thyroxine, lowers circulating LDL and cholesterol levels probably by enhancing the catabolism of LDL. The dose of D-thyroxine must be raised slowly over many weeks until a daily maintenance dose of 4 to 6 mg is reached. Since this agent is potentially cardiotoxic by precipitating arrhythmias in patients with coronary atherosclerosis, its use should be confined to young patients who are free of evident coronary artery disease. Other side effects include abnormal liver function tests, glucose intolerance, and neutropenia. Probucol, another agent with hypocholesterolemic activity, is used in divided doses of from 0.5 to 1 g/day. Probucol can produce a variety of mild adverse effects, the most common of which are abdominal discomfort, diarrhea, nausea, and headache. The mechanism of action of this drug is unknown.

Drugs used primarily to lower serum triglyceride levels include nicotinic acid and clofibrate. Some hormonal agents with anabolic or progestational activity can promote triglyceride clearance in some patients but have not been uniformly effective. Clofibrate (Atromid S), the agent most widely used to treat hypertriglyceridemia, is a branched-chain fatty acid ester used in a total dose of 1.5 to 2 g/day. This agent has a variety of effects on lipid and lipoprotein metabolism in the body, but the mechanism of its hypolipidemic effect is unclear and controversial. Most evidence suggests that this drug acts by a stimulation of removal mechanisms for circulating VLDL. Although clofibrate is usually well tolerated by patients, some of its adverse effects are nausea, diarrhea, skin rash, reversibly abnormal liver function tests, weight gain, and ectopic ventricular beats. Two recently completed large-scale studies have raised questions about the long-term use of clofibrate and have suggested that the drug may be cardiotoxic and perhaps even tumorigenic in some patients. Thus its use has been curtailed until further studies clarify these questions. Nevertheless, clofibrate remains a very effective agent in reducing serum triglyceride levels and is particularly useful in the management of remnant removal disorders.

Innovative forms of therapy

Because of the serious nature of familial hypercholesterolemia, unusual and somewhat daring modalities of treatment have been tried in resistant cases with mixed success. Surgical bypass of the distal ileum to prevent bile acid recycling and to cause body cholesterol depletion has been unsuccessful in homozygotes but has reduced serum cholesterol levels in heterozygotes. End-to-side portacaval anastomosis in a homozygous patient caused a profound reduction in plasma LDL and cholesterol levels. Disappearance of or improvement in angina pectoris and reversal of coronary artery narrowing have been reported with both surgical approaches, but at present these procedures must be considered as experimental since little is known about their long-term effects. Other unconventional therapies that have caused rapid reduction of plasma cholesterol in homozygotes with familial hypercholesterolemia have included intravenous hyperalimentation and plasma exchange. The intravenous administration of high-caloric solutions that contain glucose, amino acids, and vitamins has a cholesterol-lowering action, the mechanism of which is unknown. Repeated plasma exchanges with use of a continuous-flow blood cell separator effectively diminishes plasma cholesterol levels and can be instituted on an outpatient basis.

. . .

The causal associations among various specific forms of hyperlipoproteinemia and the predisposition to premature atherogenesis, episodic acute pancreatitis, and xanthoma formation have been confirmed in a variety of studies. The importance of lowering plasma lipid levels to control bouts of abdominal pain and xanthomas has been amply demonstrated. However, definitive proof for the deceleration or reversal of atherosclerosis by reduction of plasma lipid and lipoprotein levels, which is the most common present indication for the treatment of hyperlipidemia, is lacking. The answers to several key questions remain elusive. At what age must plasma lipoproteins be lowered to prevent atherosclerosis? How vigorously should moderate degrees of hyperlipidemia be treated? How does one rationally determine the optimal treatment approach in a specific patient given the present state of knowledge? How can one feasibly monitor the effect of therapy on the progression of the atherosclerotic process? Are fasting plasma lipid or lipoprotein measurements adequate parameters to serve as guidelines to therapy?

According to most specialists in the field, the close association between hyperlipidemia and coronary disease justifies efforts to control plasma lipid levels, particularly LDL cholesterol levels. However, a sensible preventive strategy for approaching this problem begins with the identification of all positive risk factors in a given patient and a concerted attempt to modify individual life-styles as indicated to improve the risk profile of the patient. Relatives of patients with familial hyperlipoproteinemias or premature atherosclerosis, especially offspring, should be screened by plasma lipid measurements. Such screening is particularly important in cases of familial hypercholesterolemia, in which the diagnosis can be made in infants by sampling umbilical cord blood. Thus dietary modification can be introduced early and is more likely to be effective. The majority of patients with hyperlipidemia display mild to modest plasma lipid elevations. Dietary therapy and life-style modification should suffice in these cases. Increased intake of plant products and foods containing polyunsaturated fats and a regular exercise program are important positive measures. Decreased intake of calories, refined sugar, cholesterol, saturated fat, salt, and alcohol, elimination of cigarette smoking, avoidance of oral contraceptives, and amelioration of stress comprise a preventive regimen that can improve the quality of life of most patients.

FAMILIAL LIPOPROTEIN DEFICIENCY DISORDERS
Abetalipoproteinemia

Abetalipoproteinemia is inherited as an autosomal recessive trait and is considered an inborn error of metabolism characterized by the absence of measurable circulating apoprotein B. Since apo B is undetectable, the plasma of subjects with this disorder lacks chylomicrons, VLDL, and LDL. Fat malabsorption is present from birth, and jejunal mucosal cells are extensively vacuolated with lipids, particularly triglycerides. There is severe malabsorption of the fat-soluble vitamins A, D, and K. Although hepatic enlargement and liver function abnormalities are usually absent, light microscopic examination reveals extensive engorgement of the hepatocytes with lipid but no gross distortion of liver architecture. Vacuolization of both mucosal and hepatic cells is thought to be a consequence of the defect of apo B production. Because of the effects of the plasma lipoprotein abnormality on plasma membrane structure and function, the red blood cells have abnormal, notched surfaces with thorny projections. These crenated erythrocytes are termed acanthocytes.

The neurologic manifestations of abetalipoproteinemia are devastating and involve extensive segmental demyelinization of a number of nerve pathways. The areas principally disturbed include the dorsal root ganglia, posterior columns, spinocerebellar axis, and corticospinal tracts. Thus there is loss of position and vibratory sense with ataxia, incoordination, tremor, hypotonia, nystagmus, and abnormal reflexes. Visual difficulties caused by progressive retinal pigmentary changes lead to night blindness, a possible consequence of defective carotenoid transport.

Levels of all the major plasma lipids are strikingly diminished in this condition. Triglyceride levels are usually below levels that can be confidently measured by conventional techniques. There is marked hypocholesterolemia, and virtually all the plasma cholesterol in abetalipoproteinemia is associated with HDL.

Hypobetalipoproteinemia

Hypobetalipoproteinemia is considered to be distinct from classic abetalipoproteinemia. There is a decreased concentration rather than an absence of plasma VLDL and LDL, accompanied by low levels of circulating cholesterol and triglycerides. Evidently this condition can rarely occur as a genetically determined abnormality but is more commonly acquired as a result of severe debilitating diseases or malabsorption syndromes. In the familial form the mutations involved appear to differ from those that cause abetalipoproteinemia; apoprotein B can be synthesized, although at a lower than normal rate. Chylomicrons can be formed and some absorption of fat occurs. The clinical manifestations of familial hypobetalipoproteinemia can simulate those found in abetalipoproteinemia but are generally much milder.

Tangier disease

Tangier disease, a rare, genetically determined disorder, is names after the Chesapeake Bay island home of the first discovered cases. The condition is characterized by a marked deficiency or absence of normal HDL and an accumulation of cholesterol esters, particularly in reticuloendothelial tissues but also in other body tissues. The nature of the fundamental biochemical defect in Tangier disease remains unclear. An abnormal HDL, termed HDL_T, has been described and differs in some respects from normal HDL when subjected to a variety of physicochemical measures. The small quantities of HDL in plasma differ quantitatively and qualitatively from normal HDL, particularly in apoprotein content and composition. Plasma concentrations of both apo A-I and apo A-II are greatly reduced, and the small amount of apo A-I present is recovered in the density greater than 1.21 g/ml plasma fraction. Tangier disease appears to be an autosomal recessive disorder that affects the relative rate of synthesis and/or catabolism of individual HDL apoproteins. The apo A-I synthesized in this condition may be abnormal. Because of these alterations, cholesterol esters accumulate in tissues, especially in the liver, spleen, lymph nodes, thymus, skin, and intestinal and rectal mucosa.

The tonsils are hyperplastic and have a peculiar orange or yellowish gray discoloration, making it possible to detect the condition through examination of the oropharynx. When the tonsils have been excised, residual tags of mucosa that have the same discoloration will reveal the diagnosis on careful examination. The combination of low plasma cholesterol, with normal or elevated triglyceride levels, and enlarged, lobulated, orange-yellow tonsils and adenoids is diagnostic of this disorder. The pathognomonic color and striations of the tonsils result from stored cholesterol esters in tonsillar foam cells. Biopsy of the rectal mucosa also reveals foamy histiocytes throughout the mucosa and submucosa. Focal findings of lipid-laden cells have also been observed in kidneys, heart valves, testes, and corneas.

Besides the tonsillar findings, clinical manifestations include hepatosplenomegaly, lymphadenopathy, and a subtle or overt peripheral neuropathy in the form of mononeuritis multiplex. The neurologic findings may be sensory, motor, or mixed, and transient or permanent with variable symptoms and signs. Because of the limited number of subjects with Tangier disease and their relatively normal longevity, the vascular consequences of this condition are uncertain, but they do not seem to include premature cardiovascular disease. Whether cholesterol esters are deposited at an accelerated rate in the lining of blood vessels is unknown.

Familial LCAT deficiency

Familial deficiency of lecithin: cholesterol acyltransferase (LCAT) is a rare inborn error of lipoprotein metabolism that was first discovered in a Norwegian family. The primary defect results in a lack of LCAT enzyme activity in plasma. LCAT catalyzes the plasma transfer of fatty acids from the 2 position of lecithin to cholesterol, with the formation of lysolecithin and cholesterol esters. Lecithin-rich HDL is the preferred lipoprotein substrate. Absence of this enzyme results in a number of plasma lipoprotein abnormalities. As expected, circulating lipoproteins in this condition contain relatively large amounts of lecithin and unesterified cholesterol. The absolute plasma levels of HDL and cholesterol esters are very low. The HDL particles are unusually heterogeneous, with disk-shaped and very small globular structures. Absence of LCAT action on HDL leads to accumulations of unesterified cholesterol in plasma and tissues, whereas absence of the esters causes the abnormal sizes and shapes of the HDL particles. VLDL migrates abnormally slowly on electrophoresis because of a low content of apo C-II and apo C-III. VLDL concentrations are usually elevated, but their content of cholesterol esters is low. The LDL particles are also abnormally large and contain mainly lecithin and unesterified cholesterol similar to the lipoprotein X isolated from patients with obstructive jaundice.

Histopathologic specimens from subjects with LCAT deficiency reveal lipid-laden foam cells in the bone marrow, kidney, spleen, and arteries. Foam cells are found in the bone marrow and spleen of affected patients; those that appear light blue after Giemsa staining are termed "sea-blue histiocytes." Clinical findings include proteinuria, anemia, hyperlipidemia, and corneal arcus. The proteinuria that is consistently found may be caused by lipid accumulation in the glomerular tufts, and renal involvement can progress to the point of kidney failure. The erythrocytes are abnormal in both shape and composition. They contain excessive amounts of unesterified cholesterol and lecithin and show abnormal configurations similar to those seen in patients with obstructive jaundice or Mediterranean anemia. Many of these erythrocytes are "target cells," that is, cells with a peripheral rim and a center spot of red staining material. Anemia develops, probably from a combination of increased destruction and decreased formation of erythrocytes. Accumulation of lipid in bone marrow foam cells may interfere in some way with erythrogenesis. The important role of LCAT in the remodeling of VLDL during triglyceride removal by LPL is illustrated by the elevations of VLDL triglyceride levels observed with LCAT deficiency. Premature atherosclerotic changes occur in the large and small arteries of patients with familial LCAT deficiency. The corneal opacities reflect deposition of free cholesterol in the corneas. These clinical abnormalities lend support to the postulated role of LCAT in the clearance of plasma triglycerides and particularly in the transport of cholesterol from the peripheral tissues to the liver.

Although the lipoprotein deficiency disorders are rare, they illustrate the multiple, far-flung consequences of genetic deletion of a structural or regulatory protein involved in the complex cycle of lipoprotein formation and removal. The features of these inherited disorders also suggest that plasma lipoproteins serve other crucial physiologic needs in addition to transport of triglyceride for energy flux in the body.

BIBLIOGRAPHY

Bierman, E.L.: Hyperlipoproteinemia, current concepts, Kalamazoo, Mich., 1976, The Upjohn Co. (Scope Publication).

Brown, M.S., and Goldstein, J.L.: Familial hypercholesterolemia: genetic, biochemical, and pathophysiologic considerations, Adv. Intern. Med. **20**:273, 1975.

Brown, M.S., Dana, S.E., and Goldstein, J.L.: Regulation of 3-hydroxy-3-methylglutaryl Co A reductase activity in cultured human fibroblasts, J. Biol. Chem. **249**:789, 1974.

Buchwald, H., Moore, R.B., and Varco, R.L.: Ten years clinical experience with partial ileal bypass in management of the hyperlipidemias, Ann. Surg. **180**:384, 1974.

Cameron, J.L., and others: Acute pancreatitis and hyperlipemia, evidence for a persistent defect in lipid metabolism, Am. J. Med. **56**:482, 1974.

Committee of Principal Investigators: A cooperative trial in the primary prevention of ischaemic heart disease using clofibrate, Br. Heart J. **40**:1069, 1978.

Coronary Drug Project Research Group: Clofibrate and niacin in coronary heart disease, J.A.M.A. **231**:360, 1975.

Eisenberg, S., and Levy, R.I.: Lipoprotein metabolism, Adv. Lipid Res. **13**:1, 1975.

Frederickson, D.S.: It's time to be practical, Circulation **51**:209, 1975.

Frederickson, D.S., Goldstein, J.L., and Brown, M.S.: The familial hyperlipoproteinemias. In Stanbury, J.B., Wyngaarden, J.B., and Frederickson, D.S., editors: The metabolic basis of inherited disease, ed. 4, New York, 1978, McGraw-Hill Book Co.

Frederickson, D.S., Levy, R.I., and Lees, R.S.: Fat transport in lipoproteins—an integrated approach to mechanisms and disorders, N. Engl. J. Med. **276**:32, 94, 148, 215, 273, 1967.

Gjone, E., Norum, K.R., and Glomset, J.A.: Familial lecithin: cholesterol acyltransferase deficiency. In Stanbury, J.B., Wyngaarden, J.B., and Frederickson, D.S., editors: The metabolic basis of inherited disease, ed. 4, New York, 1978, McGraw-Hill Book Co.

Havel, R.J., Eder, H.A., and Bragdon, J.H.: The distribution and chemical composition of ultracentrifugally separated lipoproteins in human serum, J. Clin. Invest. **34**:1345, 1955.

Herbert, P.N., Gotto, A.M., and Frederickson, D.S.: Familial lipoprotein deficiency. In Stanbury, J.B., Wyngaarden, J.B., and Frederickson, D.S., editors: The metabolic basis of inherited disease, ed. 4, New York, 1978, McGraw-Hill Book Co.

Langer, T., Strober, W., and Levy, R.I.: The metabolism of low density lipoprotein in familial type II hyperlipoproteinemia, J. Clin. Invest. **51**:1528, 1972.

Lees, R.S., and Wilson, D.E.: The treatment of hyperlipidemia, N. Engl. J. Med. **284**:186, 1971.

Margolis, S., and Capuzzi, D.M.: Serum lipoprotein synthesis and metabolism. In Nelson, G.J., editor: Blood lipids and lipoproteins, New York, 1972, John Wiley & Sons, Inc.

Morgaaroth, J., Levy, R.I., and Frederickson, D.S.: The biochemical, clinical, and genetic features of type III hyperlipoproteinemia, Ann. Intern. Med. **82**:158, 1975.

Starzl, T.E., and others: Follow-up of patient with portacaval shunt for the treatment of hyperlipidemia, Lancet **2**:714, 1974.

DENTAL CORRELATIONS

DIABETES MELLITUS
Terry S. Gotthelf and Louis F. Rose

ORAL MANIFESTATIONS. One of the initial findings in the oral examination of the patient with uncontrolled diabetes is dry, cracked lips and cheilosis. The appearance of the oral mucosa may range from slightly red to inflamed, edematous, and ulcerated. Examination of the tongue reveals enlarged and hyperemic fungiform papillae and atrophied filiform papillae. Decreased salivary flow has also been noted. The oral signs and symptoms of a diabetic patient can range from minimal to severe and involve the complete spectrum of dental complaints. Symptoms include xerostomia, painless swelling of the salivary glands with decreased salivary flow, inflamed, painful, hemorrhagic gingiva, alterations in the fungiform and filiform papillae of the tongue, glossodynia, dry cracked lips, cheilosis, loss of alveolar bone, tooth mobility, and odontalgia.

A frequent complaint of the uncontrolled diabetic individual is xerostomia. Dehydration of the oral tissues (from systemic dehydration) as well as neuropathy may contribute to symptoms of generalized tenderness, altered taste, and burning sensations. Dehydration may also relate to reported alterations in salivary flow, which may, in turn, relate to the altered oral flora reported in the insulin-dependent diabetic. The subgingival flora is composed mainly of *Capnocytophaga* and other gram-negative organisms including *Fusobacterium* and *Campylobacter* and occasionally *Actinobacillus actinomycetemcomitans*.

The manifestations of the periodontal tissues have received the most attention in the dental literature. The gingival response of the uncontrolled diabetic to plaque accumulation is usually accentuated, resulting in hyperplastic, erythematous gingiva. Other gingival findings frequently noted include acute fulminating gingival abscesses and granular subgingival proliferations. Radiographic findings include widening of the periodontal ligament and excessive alveolar bone loss resulting in extreme tooth mobility and early tooth loss.

By the mid 1960s, most investigators agreed that even controlled diabetic patients have a higher prevalence and greater severity of peridontal disease than nondiabetic individuals. Significant differences in the severity of periodontal disease exist between diabetic and nondiabetic subjects, even when such variable factors as the degree of plaque, age of patient, and brushing frequency are controlled.

Oral infection such as periapical or periodontal abscesses or periodontal disease has been demonstrated to affect insulin requirements in diabetic patients. It has been noted that patients with active periodontal disease required a decrease in insulin dosage after appropriate periodontal treatment was carried out. Infections in general tend to make control of diabetes more difficult, and infection and inflammation often increase insulin requirements in previously stable diabetic patients. Other studies have demonstrated a positive correlation between impaired glucose tolerance and the presence of periodontal disease as well as to a decreased healing response to oral prophylaxis.

The gingival response of healthy individuals to plaque includes a change in vascular topography and function, the accumulation of inflammatory cells, and decreased vascular permeability and exudate formation. The gingiva of the diabetic patient reveals a decreased vascular response to irritation, an impaired response of inflammatory cells, and a thickened basement lamina in the gingival microvessels that may limit the permeability of these vessels.

Microvascular changes observed in other tissues, such as skeletal muscle or kidney tissue, are also found in gingival tissue. These changes include a disruption of the normally flattened endothelial wall lining cells and the presence of varying amounts of periodic acid Schiff (PAS)–positive infiltrate subendothelially as a basement membrane thickening. This material has been reported to be glycogen and is not thought to be related to the degree of severity or the duration of diabetes. The altered thickness of the capillary basement lamina in the diabetic individual is thought to affect the permeability of these vessels and may relate to the decreased resistance of the diabetic to infection.

Histologic examination of biopsy material from the oral cavity shows splitting and the opening of the basement membrane and the deposition of a micropolysaccharide substance in the basement membrane of small blood vessels of diabetic and many prediabetic individuals. The result is narrowing of the lamina of gingival arterioles and degenerative changes within the vessel wall. The presence of this "obliterative endarteritis" in gingival submucosa suggests that local blood supply to the tissue is impaired, resulting in poor tissue nutrition. This may decrease the resilience of these tissues and explain the poor level of healing observed in diabetic patients. Almost all studies of the small blood vessels of diabetic gingiva report significant differences between diabetic and nondiabetic persons. These changes were studied extensively for some time in the hope of discovering a tool for the early detection and diagnosis of diabetes.

The compromised response of the diabetic patient to oral bacterial infection has also been studied immunologically. Many studies have concerned themselves with polymorphonuclear (PMN) leukocyte deficiency as a cause of the increased susceptibility of the diabetic to infection. Hyperglycemia alone has been shown to decrease phagocytosis, diapedesis, and intracellular bactericidal activity of PMN leukocytes. Diabetic patients have been found to have PMN leukocytes that respond poorly to chemotactic stimuli. Poch found that following mechanical irritation, the diabetic gingival crevice contained fewer PMN leukocytes than were found in controls. Many of these findings are also noted in nondiabetic relatives of diabetic individuals. Impairments in chemotaxis may be due to various biochemical alterations in metabolism. For example, some diabetic persons demonstrate an increased level of free fatty acids. Palmitic acid, a saturated fatty acid, has been found to completely inhibit chemotaxis in high doses and to cause a marked inhibition of chemotaxis in concentrations close to those found in diabetics. This defect could be related to the increased susceptibility of the diabetic individual to infection and facilitate the development of periodontal disease in diabetic persons.

DENTAL MANAGEMENT. The diabetic patient who is well controlled and not medically compromised in any other way (i.e., hypertension or coronary heart disease) can receive indicated dental therapy without any alteration of the proposed treatment. The diabetic patient who is brittle or uncontrolled or who has serious underlying organic disease needs to have treatment altered in order to delay elective dental care or surgical procedures until blood glucose has been adequately regulated. The patient's physician should be consulted and become a partner in the management of the patient during the pre- and postoperative period.

When the diabetic patient is being treated it is best to schedule appointments when insulin is not at peak effect, usually in the mid-morning following the patient's normal insulin dose and breakfast. There is no contraindication to the use of local anesthetics with or without vasoconstrictor in the diabetic patient, though outpatient general anesthesia is usually not undertaken. On occasion, light sedation with oral or intravenous barbiturates may be used safely. In addition to routine postoperative instructions, the patient must be encouraged to maintain normal caloric intake even though soft foods or a liquid diet is required because of impaired masticatory function.

There appears to be general agreement that healing is delayed in uncontrolled diabetics and that they are more prone to infections following oral surgical procedures. Infection may present special problems in these individuals since fever will increase the metabolic rate and decrease the effectiveness of insulin. Prophylactic antibiotic coverage is not recommended for routine dental or surgical procedures in the well-controlled diabetic individual, but if infection exists or if the patient is poorly controlled, then antibiotics are so indicated.

Since infection from the oral cavity can cause complications in regulation and control of the diabetes, it is incumbent upon any treating dentist to be aggressive in eliminating oral infection. The patient must be committed to an optimal oral hygiene program as well as to frequent dental visits, especially because the incidence and severity of periodontal disease in these patients is so high.

Again, it is important that patients being treated with insulin follow their diet closely. If they fail to eat normally but continue to take their regular insulin dosage, a hypoglycemic reaction may occur because of excesses (insulin shock). The dentist must be prepared to deal with this emergency should it occur in the office. The treatment of choice for the conscious patient who is cooperative and demonstrates clinical symptoms of hypoglycemia is the administration of a high-carbohydrate beverage, such as orange juice, cola, ginger ale, or a glucose drink such as Glucola. A 6- to 12-ounce portion of a cola soft drink contains 20 to 40 g of glucose. The patient will respond almost immediately and should be observed until vital signs are stable and all signs and symptoms of hypoglycemia have disappeared. In the unconscious individual 50% dextrose in water (30 to 50 ml) should be administered intravenously at once. Within 3 to 5 minutes after injection the patient should regain consciousness. Another drug that can be administered is glucagon, 1 mg intramuscularly. The patient will respond to the glucagon within 5 to 10 minutes after the injection. However since 50% dextrose is faster acting it is the treatment of choice. Any patient who has experienced periods of unconsciousness should not be permitted to go home but rather should be taken to a hospital for further evaluation and treatment. In addition to the above, management of the unconscious patient includes airway maintenance, oxygen administration, and monitoring of vital signs.

In conclusion, it is imperative that the dentist ascertain a comprehensive medical history from the known or suspected diabetic patient. The severity of the disease and degree of control must be established before making the decision whether dental care should be rendered at that particular time.

BIBLIOGRAPHY

Belting, E., and others: The influence of diabetes mellitus on the severity of periodontal disease, J. Periodont. **35:**476, 1964.

Cohen, D.W., and others: Diabetes mellitus and periodontal disease: 2 year longitudinal observations, J. Periodont. **41:**709, 1969.

Finestone, A., and Boorujy, S.: Diabetes and periodontal disease, Diabetes **16:**336, 1967.

Goldman, H., and Cohen, D.W.: Periodontal therapy, ed 5, St. Louis, 1973, The C.V. Mosby Co., pp. 278–279.

Harrison, T.R.: Principles of internal medicine, ed. 8, New York, 1977, McGraw-Hill, Inc.

Malamed, S.F.: Handbook of medical emergencies in the dental office, St. Louis, 1978, The C.V. Mosby Co.

Pay, I., and others: The response of young diabetics to periodontal treatment, J. Periodont. **48:**806, 1974.

Rose, L.F., and Hendler, B.H.: Medical emergencies in dental practice, Chicago, 1981, Quintessence Publishing Co. Inc.

Saadoun, A.P.: Diabetes and periodontal disease: a review and update (abstract), J. Western Soc. Periodontol. **28**(4):116, 1980.

Scopp, I.: Periodontics and diabetes, N.Y. J. Dent. **47:**9, 1977.

Williams, R.C., and Mehan, C.J.: Periodontal disease and diabetes in young adults, J.A.M.A. **172:**776, 1960.

DISORDERS OF LIPOPROTEIN METABOLISM
Barbara J. Steinberg
Barry H. Hendler

Fabry-Anderson syndrome

ORAL MANIFESTATIONS. Angiokeratomas, which are small blood-filled cavities, occur in the oral mucosa. They are maroon or blue black, flat or slightly elevated, and a few millimeters in diameter. The lips (most prominently the lower lip) are involved near the mucosa-skin junction. Although rare, the mucosa near the soft palate, the buccal mucosa, the gingiva, and the facial skin may also be affected. The tongue, however, is not an observed site for these vascularities. The histologic picture reveals variable dilation of superficial mucosal and cutaneous blood vessels.

DENTAL MANAGEMENT. The dentist should exercise caution when manipulating affected oral tissues to minimize hemorrhage. In the event that hemorrhage cannot be avoided, accessible angiokeratomas respond well to electrocoagulation and to topical application of 50% trichloroacetic acid.

Since the renal, cardiovascular, and nervous systems may be affected by this disease, referral, to these sections of this text is suggested for effective dental management.

Gaucher's disease

ORAL MANIFESTATIONS. Yellow pigmentation occurring on the face, lips, conjunctivae, and oral mucosa is an important sign. Additional changes occur in the jaws, where the radiograph may reverse irregular osteoporotic defects with gradual expansion, thinning of the cortex, and resorption of dental roots, especially in the molar region.

DENTAL MANAGEMENT. Since extraction of teeth from affected regions of the jaws may result in hemorrhage, and since any oral peridontal surgical procedure may be further complicated by the attendant pancytopenia, the dentist must be prepared to employ precautionary measures for hemostasis. These include a complete blood count, prothrombin time (PT), partial thromboplastin time (PTT), bleeding time, and platelet count preoperatively, as well as a consultation with the patient's physician.

Urbach-Wiethe disease

ORAL MANIFESTATIONS. Granular and/or nodular deposits in the skin and mucous membranes are pathognomonic of Urbach-Wiethe disease. In the head and neck region lesions may be found in the facial skin, larynx, oral mucous membranes, and pharynx. When the yellow waxy nodules that occur on the face become confluent, fissuring may then occur, especially around the eyes and lips, giving the face an appearance that is typical of the disease. Laryngeal involvement produces hoarseness and dysphasia that are noted in even early childhood. Lesions of the oral mucosa vary in appearance from solitary dots to confluent plaques and from whitish to yellowish white, according to the age of the patient. In general, the older the patient, the more indurated the plaques. The lower lip assumes a cobblestone appearance and the tongue may become firm and lose its papillae. There is also evidence of macroglossia, and the tongue seems to be bound to the floor of the mouth, probably secondary to infiltration of the lingual frenum. When the buccal mucosa is involved stenosis of the parotid ducts can occur with subsequent parotitis. Teeth may fail to develop or they may be hypoplastic. The skin papules and mucosal plaques contain abundant lipids, especially cholesterol (66%) and phospholipids (27%).

Type V hyperlipoproteinemia

ORAL MANIFESTATIONS. Patients with type V hyperlipoproteinemia have with a chief complaint of xerostomia. Salivary scans indicate that focal inflammatory, infiltrative, or obstructive lesions of the major salivary glands may be present.

DENTAL MANAGEMENT. Parotid biopsy confirms the diagnosis. Patients complaining of xerostomia should be given a salivary stimulating agent to provide symptomatic relief.

ALCOHOLISM
Barbara J. Steinberg
Barry H. Hendler

ORAL MANIFESTATIONS. Oral abnormalities secondary to alcoholism generally occur from neglect of oral hygiene, from fatty infiltration of the salivary glands, and from moderate to severe nutritional deficiencies. Alcoholic individuals also experience an increased risk of developing carcinoma of the oral cavity, pharynx, larynx, and esophagus.

As a result of poor oral hygiene, alcoholic patients frequently have a coated tongue and gross deposits of plaque and calculus on the teeth. They have an increased rate of chronic, advanced, generalized periodontitis with inflamed gingival tissues, as evidenced by loss of gingival stippling, punched-out, interdental papillae, and deep periodontal pockets with advanced loss of alveolar bone. Alcoholics tend to have more missing teeth than nonalcoholic, age-matched control groups, although the DMF profile of alcoholics as a whole is similar to the general population.

Some chronic alcoholics have enlargement of the major salivary glands, especially the parotid glands. This asymptomatic swelling usually occurs bilaterally. Salivary flow may increase or remain unaffected. Histologically, fatty deposits infiltrate the salivary glands as a result of generalized disturbance in lipid metabolism.

Nutritional deficiencies, which are very often encountered in the alcoholic patient, also cause significant oral change. The most common deficiency states involve the B-

Table 1. Drug interactions with alcohol

Drug	Interaction	Prevention
Anticoagulants oral (coumarin derivatives)	Inhibited anticoagulant effect with chronic alcohol use; enhanced anticoagulant effect with acute intoxication	Restrict alcohol intake to small amounts
Antihistamines	Enhanced CNS depression	Prohibit or sharply curtail alcohol use
Aspirin or another salicylate	Gastrointestinal bleeding	Prohibit alcohol use in patients taking salicylates regularly
Barbiturates	Enhanced activity of each drug with acute intoxication; sedative effect diminished with chronic alcohol use	Prohibit or sharply curtail alcohol use during administration
Chloral betaine (Beta-Chlor), chloral hydrate (Kessodrate, Noctec, Somnos)	CNS depression; tachycardia; vasodilation	Prohibit or sharply curtail alcohol use during administration; cardiac patients on long-term therapy should not take alcohol
Chlordiazepoxide (Libritabs), or chlordiazepoxide HCl (A-poxide, Librium, Sk-Lygen, Tenax)	In some patients, enhanced CNS depression	Inform patients of this effect, especially regarding operation of hazardous equipment or motor vehicles
Cyclobenzaprine HCl (Flexeril)	Enhanced effects of alcohol	Inform patients of this effect, especially regarding operation of hazardous equipment or motor vehicles
Diazepam (Valium)	Increased diazepam-induced sedation with high blood levels of alcohol	Instruct patients concerning excessive alcohol use while taking diazepam
Guanethidine sulfate (Ismelin)	Enhanced orthostatic hypotension from alcohol's vasodilating effect	Warn patients about this effect; limit alcohol intake in patients prone to orthostatic hypotension
Hypnotics (nonbarbiturate)	Enhanced CNS depression	Prohibit alcohol use
Insulin	Hypoglycemia (dose related)	If necessary, reduce insulin dosage during periods of substantial intake
Lorazepam (Ativan)	Potentiated CNS depressant effects	Inform patients of this effect, especially regarding operation of hazardous equipment or motor vehicles
MAO inhibitors	Sedation; with tyramine-containing alcoholic beverages, hypertensive crisis	If patient becomes sedated, prohibit alcohol; tyramine-containing alcoholic beverages must not be taken
Meprobamate (Equanil, Kesso-Bamate, Meprospan, Miltown, SK-Bamate)	Enhanced CNS depression; impairment of motor skills	Warn patients that meprobamate may increase alcohol's intoxicating effects
Metronidazole (Flagyl)	Acute alcohol intolerance (contradictory information in literature)	Prohibit alcohol use until true significance of interaction is resolved
Narcotics	Enhanced CNS depression	Prohibit or sharply curtail alcohol use
Nitroglycerin (Cardabid, Nitro-Bid, Nitroglyn, Nitrospan, Nitrostat)	Hypotension	Pending further evaluation of this interaction, warn patients to use alcohol with caution
Phenothiazines	CNS depression; sedation	Prohibit alcohol use
Phenytoin (Dilantin); phenytoin sodium (Dilantin)	Enhanced anticonvulsant metabolism with chronic alcohol use; seizures in epileptic persons previously controlled with phenytoin	Observe patients for decreased anticonvulsant effect; adjust dosage if necessary
Propoxyphene HCl (Darvon, Dolene, SK-65); propoxyphene napsylate (Darvon-N)	Enhanced respiratory and CNS depression (dose related)	Warn patients taking therapeutic doses against excessive alcohol use
Sulfonylureas (hypoglycemics)	Enhanced hypoglycemic effect, especially in fasting patients; flushing, sweating, and tachycardia; accelerated sulfonylurea metabolism in patients who regularly consume large amounts of alcohol	Prohibit alcohol use
Tricyclic antidepressants	CNS depression and sedation	Prohibit alcohol use
Tranquilizers, minor	Enhanced CNS depression	Prohibit or sharply curtail alcohol use
Valproic acid (Depakene)	Potentiated CNS depressant effects	Prohibit or sharply curtail alcohol use during administration; inform patients of this effect, especially regarding operation of hazardous equipment or motor vehicles

complex vitamins, specifically thiamin, niacin, riboflavin, pyridoxine, and folic acid. Thiamin deficiency produces hyperesthesia of the oral mucosa, burning tongue, and loss or diminution of taste perception. Niacin deficiency causes an inflamed and erythematous tongue with papillary atrophy, hyperemia of the buccal mucosa, and generalized oral erosions. A deficiency in riboflavin causes macerated lesions at the corners of the mouth (angular cheilosis), which may become infected with bacteria or *Candida,* a condition known as angular cheilitis. Riboflavin deficiency may also result in glossitis and generalized erythema of the oral mucosa as well as redness of the conjunctiva and burning and excessive dryness of the eyes. Pyridoxine deficiency is evidenced by cheilosis, conjunctivitis, and glossitis. The patient who is deficient in folic acid has extreme pallor of the skin and complains of burning of the tongue and oral mucosa. The tongue appears red and swollen, with enlarged papillae and numerous small vesicular lesions. Angular cheilosis, gingivitis, and diffuse painful ulcerations, particularly of the palate, tongue, and buccal mucosa, are also common findings.

DENTAL MANAGEMENT. The alcoholic patient presents challenges in almost every aspect of dental treatment, including hematologic complications, increased susceptibility to infection, impaired wound healing, alcohol-drug interactions, and psychologic disturbances.

Pancytopenia, iron deficiency anemia, and abnormalities in both function and number of platelets, leading to hemorrhagic diathesis, may occur secondary to alcohol consumption and/or subsequent liver disease. Certain basic diagnostic laboratory studies should be obtained. These include a complete blood count and differential, platelet count, prothrombin time, partial thromboplastin time, and bleeding time. In addition, consultation with the patient's physician is advisable before providing dental care.

Alcoholic individuals are frequently susceptible to infection due to suppression of immune mechanisms. The alcoholic patient with severe systemic infection of unknown origin should be examined to rule out an oral focus. Antibiotic therapy is certainly a strong consideration when performing any dental surgery.

The relationship between alcohol and abnormal wound healing should also be recognized. A dose-related increase in postoperative healing time often occurs in the alcoholic patient because of interference with the proper formation and deposition of collagen.

Alcohol-drug interactions are of particular importance in dental therapy (Table 1). For example, alcohol combined with salicylates can predispose to delayed clot formation and possible postoperative hemorrhage. The dentist should inform the alcoholic patient when alcohol is contraindicated with drugs that are being prescribed, while making a concerted effort to select drugs with minimal interaction potential.

Patients who are known or suspected alcoholics should be completely detoxified before performing any elective dental surgery because the stress of the procedure may precipitate severe, life-threatening withdrawal symptoms. During the period of detoxification, electrolyte imbalances, blood disorders, and liver disease should be evaluated and treated. Patients undergoing therapy for delirium tremens may have depressed gag and cough reflexes, rendering them more likely to aspirate oral and gastric secretions.

Alcoholism presents a variety of psychosocial, nutritional, and clinical problems. Lack of motivation to maintain good oral hygiene severely limits the long-term efficacy of caries control, advanced restorative dentistry, and periodontal therapy in alcoholic patients. In addition to the necessary dental care, the dental practitioner can provide nutritional counseling and encouragement to the alcoholic patient. Optimized dietary intake will have a remarkable impact on the alcoholic's health, and an awareness of the psychosocial factors affecting the patient's perception of dental treatment will permit a more effective approach to the patient and his illness.

PORPHYRIA
Barbara J. Steinberg
Barry H. Hendler

ORAL MANIFESTATIONS. In patients with erythropoietic uroporphyria, there may be calcium phosphate deposits in the dentin and enamel. This imparts a reddish brown or pink color to the deciduous and permanent teeth known as erythrodontin. The porphyrin deposits may occur in discrete bands, evidence of exacerbations of the disease during tooth formation. Affected teeth fluoresce bright scarlet under ultraviolet light. Advanced local periodontal changes and atrophic cheilitis may also occur.

In the hepatic form of porphyria, painful bullous lesions may erupt following oral manipulation. These oral lesions are histologically similar to the cutaneous lesions that appear in individuals with this disorder.

DENTAL MANAGEMENT. Drugs known to cause acute exacerbations of porphyria must be avoided. It is mandatory, for example, that no barbiturates, either oral or intravenous, and no barbiturate-based anesthetics be administered to such patients. To do so could precipitate a serious crisis with lower motor neuron paralysis that may not appear for some days after the administration of the drug.

The dentist should exercise great care in manipulating oral tissues to prevent the occurrence of bullous lesions.

BIBLIOGRAPHY

Aznar, J., and others: Study of the lipids in the skin lesions in Urbach-Wiethe disease, Short Communication, Amsterdam, 1977, Elsevier/North-Holland Biomedical Press.

Becker, C.E.: Review of pharmacologic and toxicologic effects of alcohol, J. Am. Dent. Assoc. **99**:494, 1979.

Bergenholtz, A., Hofer, P.A., and Ohman, J.: Oral, pharyngeal and laryngeal manifestations in Urbach-Wiethe disease, Ann. Clin. Res. **9**:1, 1977.

Browne, W.G.: Oral pigmentation and root resorption in Gaucher's disease, J. Oral Surg. **35**:153, 1977.

Gorlin, R.J., and Sedano, H.O.: Stomatologic aspects of cutaneous diseases, J. Dermatol. Surg. Oncol. **5**(3):180, 1979.

Green, J.B., and Trowbridge, A.A.: Hematologic and oncologic implications of alcoholism, Postgrad. Med. **61**(5):149, 1977.

Hillman, R.W., and Kissin, B.: Oral cytologic patterns and nutritional status: some relationships in alcoholic subjects, Oral Surg., **38**: 34, 1980.

Reinertsen, J.L., and others: Sicca-like syndrome in type V hyperlipoproteinemia, Arthritis Rheum. **23**(1):114, 1980.

Ritter, F.N.: Salivary gland involvement in systemic diseases, Otolaryngol. Clin. North Am. **10**(2):371, 1977.

Schuckit, M.A.: Overview of alcoholism, J. Am. Dent. Assoc. **99**:489, 1979.

Smith, K.G.: Alcoholism—a nutritional approach, Dent. Hyg. **50**:263, 1976.

Young, W.G., Pihlstrom, B.L., and Sauk, J.J., Jr.: Granulomatous gingivitis in Anderson-Fabry disease, J. Periodont., **51**: 95, 1980.

Section Sixteen
CRANIOFACIAL MALFORMATIONS
edited by **Louis F. Rose**

203 • MALFORMATIONS OF THE CRANIOFACIAL COMPLEX: AN OVERVIEW

Ray E. Stewart

Congenital malformations are those present at birth. They are not uncommon in humans. In fact, various sources report that between 3% and 7% of live-born infants have some developmental anomaly requiring treatment, and it is generally accepted that 15% to 20% of cases of neonatal death are a result of congenital malformations.

These figures are conservative in that they do not include anomalies that do not become apparent until the child is older nor do they include the high frequency of developmental disorders observed on examination of the products of spontaneous abortion. Since many abortions go unnoticed because they occur very early in gestation, before the formation of a clinically recognizable embryo or fetus, the true magnitude of congenital malformations is almost certainly much larger than the available statistical data would indicate.

Malformations of the face and cranium constitute a special category of congenital malformations and are among the most significant of all birth defects relative to the impact and potential for the influence of the individual's physiologic, psychologic, and social adaption to his environment. It has been said, "The face of man is his window to the world." The face contains the organs of sight, smell, taste, hearing, and speech—all of which allow him to receive stimuli and react to the various elements of his environment.

Although individually, specific structural craniofacial malformations may be quite rare, collectively, they are among the most prevalent of all birth defects. Approximately 15 of every 1000 births are affected by congenital craniofacial malformations. It can be seen in Fig. 203-1 that only structural malformations involving the limbs are more common.

Approximately 65% of all congenital craniofacial malformations involve clefts of the primary or secondary pal-

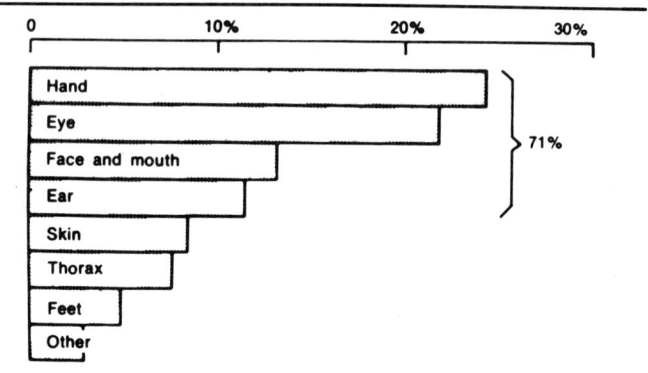

Fig. 203-1. Distribution of congenital malformations according to organ or system affected. (After Smith, D.W.: Recognizable patterns of human malformations, ed. 2, Philadelphia, 1976, W.B. Saunders Co.)

Table 203-1. Incidence of selected craniofacial malformations

Malformation	Incidence
Cleft palate	1:2000
Cleft lip with or without cleft palate	1:800
Anencephaly	1:2000
Hydrocephaly	1:1000
Craniosynostosis	
Apert's syndrome	1:160,000
Crouzon's disease	1:30,000
Treacher Collins syndrome	1:10,000
Oculoauriculovertebral (OAC) syndrome (includes hemifacial microsomia and Goldenhar's syndrome)	1:3500

ate. Such statistics are meaningless unless translated into some terms that give relevance to the scope and magnitude of the problem. Nearly 20,000 infants are born in the United States each year who will require extensive and costly treatment of their congenital craniofacial malformations. Table 203-1 gives estimated incidences for selected craniofacial anomalies as they occur in the United States.

DEFINITIONS AND NOMENCLATURE

Craniofacial malformations are a heterogeneous group of development and acquired abnormalities affecting various structures and tissues of the head, face, and neck. They may occur singly or in combination and can be described by a variety of terms and definitions, which, if used improperly, can lead to erroneous concepts and conclusions. To avoid this possibility, it is appropriate to review a number of terms and definitions that will be used throughout the remainder of this chapter.

For a trait or structure to be considered anomalous or abnormal, it is necessary to define and conceptualize what is "normal." *Normal* is usually defined as a quantitative trait that is within 2 standard deviations of the *mean* as measured for a given population. To arrive at this mean requires some knowledge of the range of variation of the size, shape, and relationships of the various elements of the traits or structures being measured, in this case the craniofacial complex. It also requires some consideration of epidemiologic issues, such as incidence and prevalence, as well as the physical, emotional, and psychosocial impact caused by these abnormalities.

The assessment of the clinical phenotype and a determination of whether it is *normal* or *abnormal* has until recently been a very subjective procedure requiring a good deal of experience and the ability of an examiner to "gestalt" a patient. More recently, a number of standards have been developed for the measurement of the size and shape of relative positions of a variety of craniofacial structures; these standards enable the examiner to evaluate patients and to compare clinical findings and measurements. In this way the examiner is better able to make a valid assessment of whether the size or placement or relationship of one structure to another is "significantly different from normal," thereby qualifying the trait as a malformation or anomaly.

The nomenclature in the field of congenital malformations has proved to be somewhat of a problem because of the lack of standardization of terms and definitions between clinicians and basic scientists. A recent conference held at the National Institutes of Health has proposed several general categories for developmental abnormalities in an attempt to facilitate some standardization in this area:

malformation A primary structural abnormality that results from a localized defect in morphogenesis; for example, cleft lip

deformation An alteration in shape or structure of a previously normal part; for example, torticollis

anomalad or malformation complex A malformation together with its subsequently derived structural changes; for example, Pierre Robin syndrome

malformation syndrome a recognized pattern of malformations presumably having the same etiology and currently not interpreted as a consequence of a localized defect in morphogenesis; for example, Down's syndrome

ETIOLOGY OF CRANIOFACIAL MALFORMATIONS

Malformations of the craniofacial complex can be classified as acquired or congenital. *Acquired* malformations generally appear after the time of birth and can be categorized into three major types based on etiology: (1) trauma, (2) infection, and (3) neoplastic lesions.

Malformations that have a traumatic etiology are relatively common in all age groups and often require extensive reconstructive and rehabilitative treatment procedures.

Malformations secondary to infectious processes have in the large part been eliminated by the use of antibiotics and public health measures. There are a significant number of cases seen each year that have an infectious origin, the most common of which is osteomyelitis, which can lead to malformation particularly in the growing child.

Neoplastic lesions are quite rare in children; however, when they occur, they are often highly malignant and very aggressive, requiring extensive resection and thereby leaving significant malformations. Although acquired malformations comprise a significant portion of the total problem, they will not be considered further in this discussion, which will concentrate on congenital craniofacial malformations.

Congenital malformations are generally considered to fall in three primary categories: (1) genetic, (2) environmental or teratogenic, and (3) multifactorial, which combines genetic and environmental etiologic factors.

Those malformations derived primarily from genetic defects fall into two major categories. The first consists of those caused by aberrations of chromosome structure and number, including translocations, deletions, inversions, and polyploidy. Individuals who have some type of chromosomal abnormality generally have multiple congenital malformations that often cluster to form consistent patterns of malformation referred to as a syndrome. An example of this is *Down's syndrome,* which results from an extra chromosome number 21 and gives rise to a constellation of abnormalities, many of which involve various craniofacial structures.

The true incidence of cytogenetic abnormalities leading to aberrant morphogenesis is higher than one would suspect based on the number of living individuals with detectable chromosomal malformations responsible for a particular pattern of malformation. Various studies have revealed that approximately one in five, or 20%, of conceptions does not reach term and is spontaneously aborted. Since many abortions probably occur very early in development, prior to the formation of a recognizable embryo, an accurate estimate of the incidence of congenital abnormalities in products of conception would certainly be far greater than the observed statistical information. Some researchers have found an incidence of significant errors in morphogenesis in excess of 50% when examining products of spontaneous abortion. Of this group approximately 50% (or 25% of the total) had detectable chromosomal abnormalities.

The second major category of heritable disorders that give rise to malformations affecting the craniofacial complex are the single gene disorders. Single gene disorders are characterized by the presence of a pattern of mendelian transmission of genetic traits that are located on the autosomes or sex chromosomes. The patterns of transmission follow a dominant or recessive pattern, depending on the tendency of the trait to be expressed in either the heterozygous or homozygous state. Recent investigations indicate that certain traits may also be inherited by genes outside the nucleus known as extranuclear or cytoplasmic DNA.

Although we know that a particular trait or malformation is determined by a single gene and is transmitted in a dominant or recessive pattern, we may not know the specific molecular defect that gives rise to a particular anomaly. An example of this is seen in *Treacher Collins syndrome*, which is inherited as an autosomal dominant trait and results in a typical cluster of craniofacial malformations, including malar and zygomatic hypoplasia, antimongoloid slant to the palpebral fissures, hypoplastic external ears, micrognathia, and other less consistent features. In spite of our ability to identify this syndrome clinically, we are as yet entirely in the dark with regard to the molecular defect or structural protein abnormality that gives rise to these malformations.

In only a few cases have we been able to determine the precise molecular event and subsequent abnormality of protein structure that cause clinically recognizable syndromes or malformation complexes. An example of this is seen in one variety of *Ehlers-Danlos syndrome*, which is a heterogeneous group of heritable connective tissue disorders characterized by stretchy skin, hypermobile joints, easy bruisability, and peculiar scarring. These patients may also exhibit certain consistent craniofacial malformations, which may be either a direct or a secondary result of the basic molecular defect in collagen that gives rise to this clinical entity. In the case of Ehlers-Danlos type V a mutation gives rise to a structural defect in the enzyme lysyl-hydroxylase that prevents the normal synthesis and organization of collagen. Individuals with this basic collagen defect characteristically have certain craniofacial features that are rather remarkable. In addition to the extremely stretchable skin, the presence of bony protuberances from the base of the occiput (known as occipital horns) and the susceptibility to marked periodontitis are characteristics of this variety of Ehlers-Danlos syndrome.

Similarly, the basic molecular defect is known in many of the hereditary inborn areas of metabolism that show consistent alterations in craniofacial morphology. An example of this is *mucopolysaccharidosis type I* or *Hurler's syndrome*. This syndrome is an autosomal recessive disorder caused by a gene mutation that gives rise to a defect in the degradative enzyme α-L-iduronidase. The clinical features of Hurler's syndrome are easily distinguished and include developmental abnormalities of the craniofacial structures such that a "gargoylelike" facial appearance is invariably described. In addition, the alveolar mucosa is extremely dense and thickened in the maxillary palatal region, and there is severe disruption of normal central nervous system development, resulting in marked mental retardation. On roentgen examination numerous changes are noted in the craniofacial skeleton, including a pathognomonic change in the cranial base involving the sphenoid bone described as a "J-shaped" sella turcica.

The second major category of factors giving rise to congenital malformations affecting the craniofacial complex are environmental or teratogenic factors. Environmental substances or teratogens capable of causing structural defects from disruptions of the normal morphogenetic processes can be classified into several major categories:

1. Mutagenetic substances, which cause a structural mutation in the DNA molecule by insertion or deletion of one or more bases, giving rise to a gene that codes for a faulty protein or loses its normal control functions
2. Inhibitors of protein synthesis, which cause alterations in the normal translation and transcription of DNA to RNA and subsequent disruption of amino acid sequencing
3. Extremes in body temperature, for example, hypothermia and hyperthermia
4. Radiation, which may result in mutation, cell death, or alteration of cell function (carcinogenesis)
5. Infectious agents, including microorganisms, which can cause disruptions in normal morphogenesis
6. Chemicals and other environmental pollutants, which can lead to mutagenesis or carcinogenesis
7. Maternal metabolic disorders, which can cause disruptive influences on the normal fetal metabolism
8. Various forms of interaction of any of these environmental agents with each other, with the genetic makeup determining susceptibility, and with the time at which the fetus is exposed.

This discussion will focus on those agents known to impose abnormal influences on craniofacial growth and development. As with any teratogen, the effect of the agent on a particular tissue or organ system is directly related to the stage of development of the organism at the time of exposure, to the duration of the exposure, and to the dose or concentration of the particular agent. Congenital malformations resulting from abnormal morphogenesis are generally thought to have their origin before normal development would have proceeded beyond the stage of arrest represented by the malformation. It should not be construed, however, that something happened at a particular time in development. Rather, it can be said with certainty that a problem existed before a particular time of development. Errors in morphogenesis that occur before 23 days of gestation usually do not permit the organism to survive and are therefore seldom seen clinically. Exceptions include conjoined twins, which represent a partial or complete duplication of Hensen's node and the primitive streak, which is initiated before 16 days of gestation. Similarly, the holoprosencephalic malformation complex appears to be a defect in the differentiation of precordal mesoderm, which is thought to develop before 23 days of gestation.

Several well-recognized clinical entities are caused by exposure to various environmental agents or teratogens and include malformations of the craniofacial complex as primary features.

Rubella syndrome

Maternal infection with rubella virus during the first trimester of pregnancy may result in generalized growth deficiency with microcephaly and congenital deafness as a result of damage to the eighth cranial nerve. Various ophthalmologic abnormalities, including glaucoma, corneal opacity, microphthalmia, and strabismus, also occur. Occasionally, large anterior fontanelles, late eruption of teeth, and morphologic abnormalities of teeth have been noted. Defects of the central nervous system may lead to to mental deficiency, with 60% of patients having IQs below 90 and 20% of patients having IQs below 70.

Aminopterin and methotrexate syndrome

Aminopterin is a folic acid antagonist and has been used as an agent to induce abortion during the first trimester of pregnancy. Methotrexate, which is the methyl derivative of aminopterin, is used as a chemotherapeutic agent. The pattern of malformations that develops from exposure to these folic acid antagonists includes severe hypoplasia of the frontal, parietal, temporal, and occipital bones with wide fontanelles and occasional synostosis of the lambdoidal and coronal sutures. Often noted is a broad nasal bridge, shallow superorbital ridges, proptosis, and micrognathia. Low-set ears and epicanthal folds are common, as are various orthopedic and limb reduction abnormalities.

Fetal warfarin syndrome

Developmental abnormalities have been associated with exposure to warfarin derivatives such as coumadin in

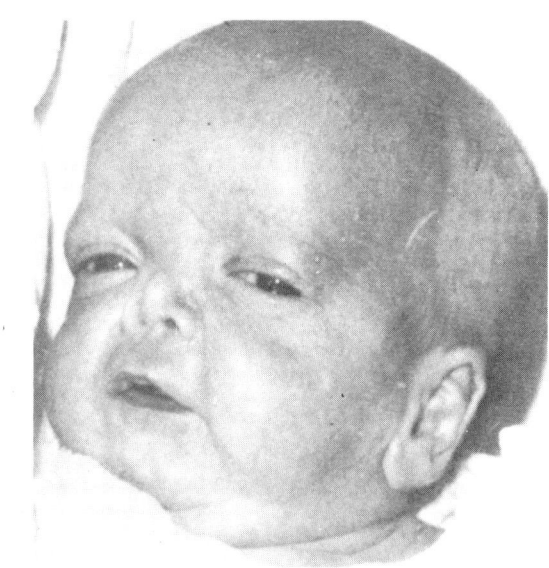

Fig. 203-2. Fetal warfarin syndrome. Note flat nasal bridge and nasal hypoplasia. (Courtesy of D.W. Smith, M.D.)

mothers who were being treated with anticoagulants because they had prosthetic heart valves. In addition to the developmental and intellectual deficiency reported in all of these patients, certain craniofacial abnormalities appear to characterize the teratogenic effects of these drugs. Most prominent of these features is hypoplasia of the nose with a very flat nasal bridge (Fig. 203-2). Stipled mineralization at various epiphyseal growth centers is commonly noted.

Fetal phenytoin syndrome

Phenytoin has resulted in a combination of abnormalities that consist of prenatal onset growth retardation, mild to moderate mental retardation, and craniofacial abnormalities consisting of wide anterior fontanelles, orbital hypertelorism, broad and depressed nasal bridge, low-set hypoplastic ears, and broad alveolar ridges with occasional cleft lip and cleft palate.

Fetal alcohol syndrome

A pattern of malformations has been described in children born to women who were severe chronic alcoholics before and during their pregnancies. These include prenatal and postnatal growth deficiency, microcephaly with reduced IQ, fine motor dysfunction, and various craniofacial abnormalities, which characteristically include short palpebral fissures, maxillary hypoplasia, ptosis, strabismus, and cleft palate (Fig. 203-3).

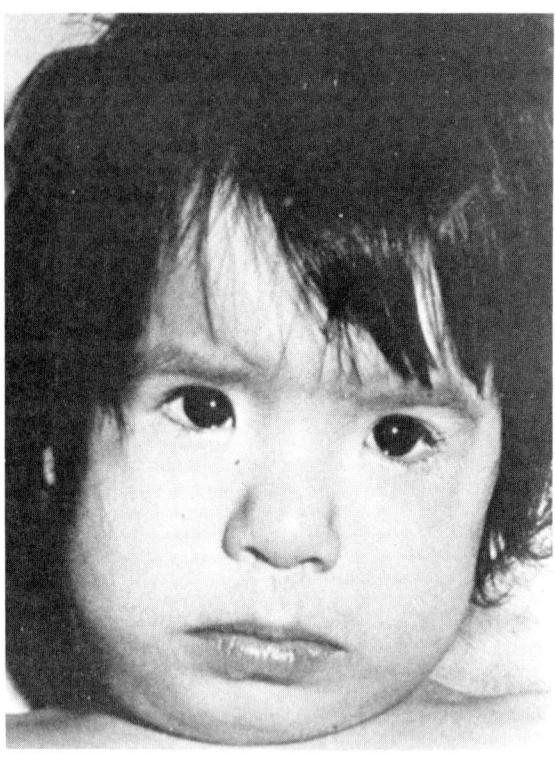

Fig. 203-3. Fetal alcohol syndrome. Note short palpebral fissures, maxillary hypoplasia, and ptosis. (Courtesy of K. Jones, M.D.)

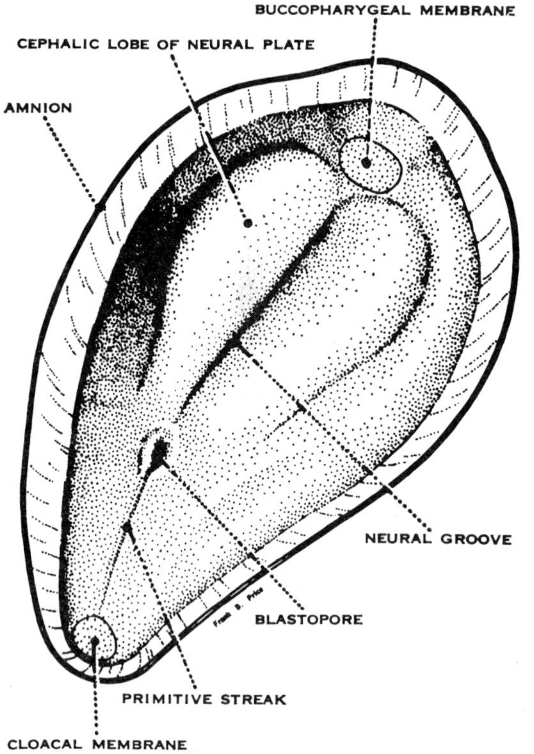

Fig. 203-4. Early embryo showing bilaminar disc with differentiation of Hensen's node, notochord, and prechordal plate. (From Patton.)

PRENATAL CRANIOFACIAL DEVELOPMENT

To appreciate the origin and natural history of abnormalities that occur in craniofacial development, a brief review of normal embryology and morphogenesis of this region is appropriate.

Development of the embryo commences at fertilization and proceeds sequentially through the stages of cleavage, blastocyst formation, formation of the extraembryonic membranes, and development of the presomite embryo. By 14 days of gestation the early presomite embryo has formed a circular bilaminar disc containing the ectodermal and endodermal components of the prechordal plate, primitive streak, Hensen's node, notochordal process, and cloacal membrane (Fig. 203-4). Certain specific developmental processes occur in the region of Hensen's node that eventually give rise to many of the primordia of the craniofacial complex.

The third primary germ layer, the mesoderm, appears during the third week of development and converts the bilaminar germ disk into a trilaminar structure. The three primary germ layers serve as a basis for the differentiating tissues and organ systems. From the ectoderm develops the cutaneous and neural elements of the embryo; from the mesoderm arises cardiovascular structures, bones, muscles, and connective tissue; and from the endoderm develops the lining epithelium of the gut between the pharynx and the anus, as well as the secretory cells of the liver and pancreas and the lining epithelium of the respiratory system.

Development of the ectoderm into its cutaneous and neural portions occurs by a proliferation of ectodermal cells that make up the neural plate. The neural plate overlies the notochord along the midline axis, which, through differential proliferation, gives rise to the neural tube. From this region arises a very important group of ectodermally derived cells commonly referred to as *neural crest cells* (Fig. 203-5).

Morphogenesis during the early embryonic stage, which involves the differentiation of various cell types and the development of primordia of various structures and organs in the craniofacial complex, is controlled primarily by intrinsic genetic factors. These factors probably have direct control over the critical process of neural crest cell migration, which involves the movement of cells to certain specific locations in the developing embryo, beginning during the gastrula stage. Similarly, intrinsic genetic factors probably exert the primary control in the early interaction or induction that occurs between adjacent cell groups and tissue types. Induction is an essential determinant of later stages of embryonic development and is a

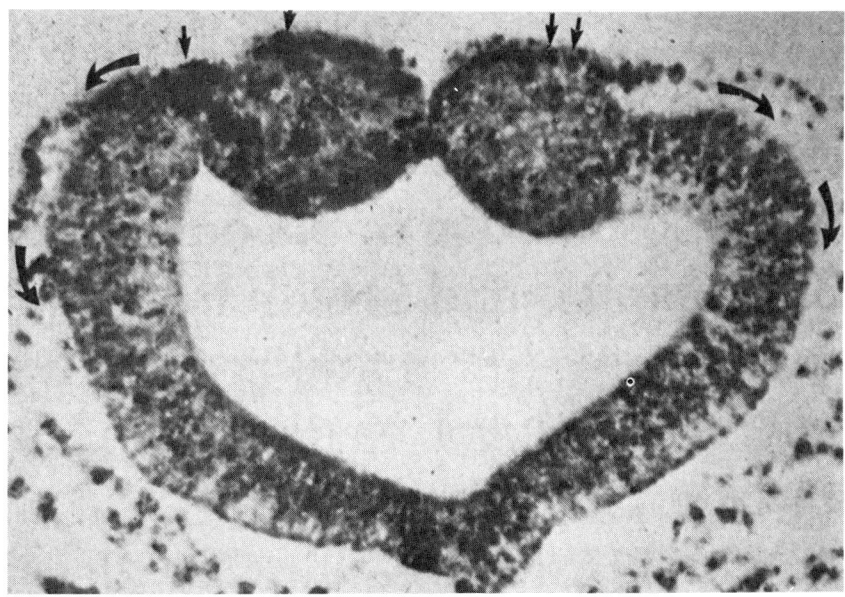

Fig. 203-5. Cross section through neural tube showing origin and migration paths of neural crest cells.

process by which certain cell groups mediate and direct the differentiation of adjacent groups. An example of this phenomenon exists in the early development of the neural tube and vertebral column. Induction occurs between a condensation of cells along the primitive streak of the gastrula (the notochord) and adjacent tissues to form somites, which are the structures from which the greater part of the axial skeleton and musculature will develop.

In the early somite stage (21 to 31 days) the cranial portion of the embryo develops the first of several ectodermally bound mesenchymal elevations known as the facial processes and pharyngeal arches. These facial processes are the first signs of development of the face and viscerocranium. As successive arches appear, the pericardium is progressively displaced from the caudal margin of the stomodeum.

At approximately 24 to 26 days of gestation the branchial arches appear. The first pharyngeal arch appears caudal to the stomodeum and is divided by a branchial cleft, which separates the mandibular and maxillary processes. Caudal to the mandibular process of the first arch the prominent second (hyoid) arch and the narrower second branchial cleft appear. The otic placode is an ectodermal thickening that appears just dorsal to the second branchial arch. It is the precursor of the membranous middle ear derivatives.

The role of neural crest cells in the development of skeletal and connective tissue derivatives of the craniofacial complex has been well documented (Fig. 203-7). These cells emanate from a condensation of ectodermal cells at the junction between the neural plate and surface ectoderm and are classified by their relationship to the de-

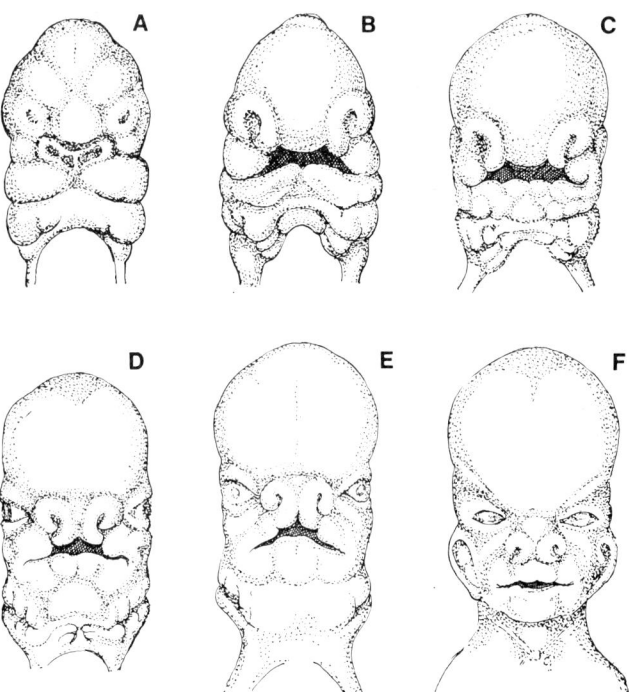

Fig. 203-6. Sequential development of the human face from 4 through 8 weeks of gestation.

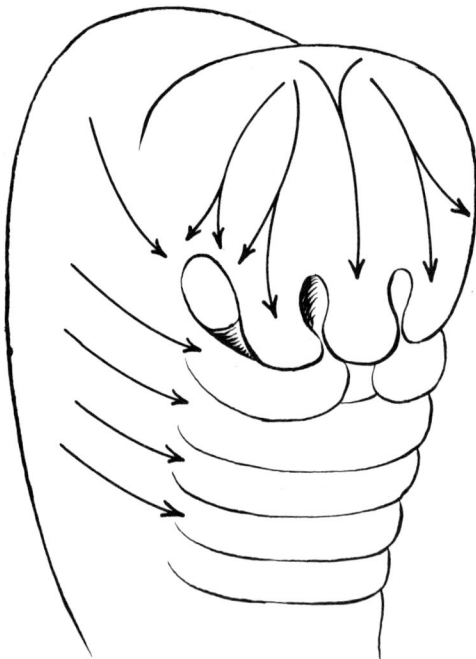

Fig. 203-7. Migration of neural crest cells into specific regions of developing face is critical for normal developmental processes to occur. Interference with this process or failure of this process to occur leads to a number of well-recognized dysmorphic entities.

veloping otic capsule as preotic (cephalic to otic capsule) and postotic (caudal to otic capsule). Experimental evidence indicates that the postotic cells migrate lateroventrally into the facial region. There they interact with local cells and environment to stimulate differentiation of a variety of tissues, including bone, connective tissue, and cartilaginous derivatives. Available information indicates that the preotic neural crest cells migrate anteriorly into the midface region. The source of the inductive influence that acts to produce and control differentiation leading to the development of specific craniofacial structures is not well understood. It seems certain, however, that cell interaction and localization are most likely determined by various cell surface antigens or markers.

Development of the viscerocranium is marked by a breakdown of the oropharyngeal membrane, thereby establishing continuity between the stomodeum and the primitive pharynx. The maxillary process grows medially and ventrally toward the stomodeum from the dorsal end of the first arch. The stomodeum is bounded cranially by the frontal bulge of the forebrain, laterally by the maxillary processes, and caudally by the mandibular processes, which approach each other and fuse at the midline to form the primitive lower jaw and lip.

Bilateral ectodermal thickenings called olfactory placodes appear above the lateral angles of the stomodeum. Proliferation of the mesenchyme near each placode causes the elevation of a horseshoe-shaped area of surrounding ectoderm. The margins of the placode are termed the medial and lateral nasal folds. The nasal folds, together with the intervening convex frontal area, constitute the frontonasal process.

The control factors that operate in the embryonic period during differentiation of the chondrocranium continue to be strongly genetically determined and are subject to minimal environmental influence. After initial differentiation of specific cell types, the growth of the desmocranium and viscerocranium appears to be subject to diminishing intrinsic genetic determinants, whereas the influence of epigenetic and local environmental factors becomes stronger.

Clinical as well as experimental data emphasize a close relationship between normal development of the craniofacial complex and the presence and the condition of all the primordia of head and neck structures. Good examples of these relationships are those existing between eye and orbit. If there is no eye primordium, there will be no orbit. If there is only a single eye primordium, a single orbit will develop. If two eye primordia lie close together, as in the holoprosencephaly malformation complex, two contiguous orbits will develop. If there is abnormal width between these primordia, the orbits also will develop with abnormal space between, as in hypertelorism. An abnormally large eye results in large orbits, whereas a small eye primordia (microphthalmia) results in small orbits. These observations provide evidence that the development of bony orbits with respect to their number, position, and size depends entirely on the presence, number, position, and size of the globe itself.

A similar interactive developmental relationship exists for many other parts of the embryonic skull where adjacent structures determine the presence, position, and form of neighboring parts. It is therefore logical to assume that these adjacent structures exert powerful morphogenetic influences on one another, and since the development of the skull normally proceeds in a genetically determined, species-specific pattern, we may class these influences in the category of "local epigenetic factors."

At approximately 45 days of gestation the occipital sclerotomal mesenchyme (occipital somites) concentrates around the notochord underlying the developing hindbrain. From this region the mesenchymal concentration extends cephalad, forming the posterior portion of a floor for the developing brain. Conversion of this undifferentiated mesenchyme into cartilage constitutes the beginning of the chondrocranium or cranial base (Fig. 203-8).

The initially separate cartilaginous centers of cranial base fuse into a single, irregular cranial base. The early establishment of the blood vessels, cranial nerves, and spinal cord between the developing brain and its extracranial contacts before chondrification determines the presence and location of the numerous perforations or foramina.

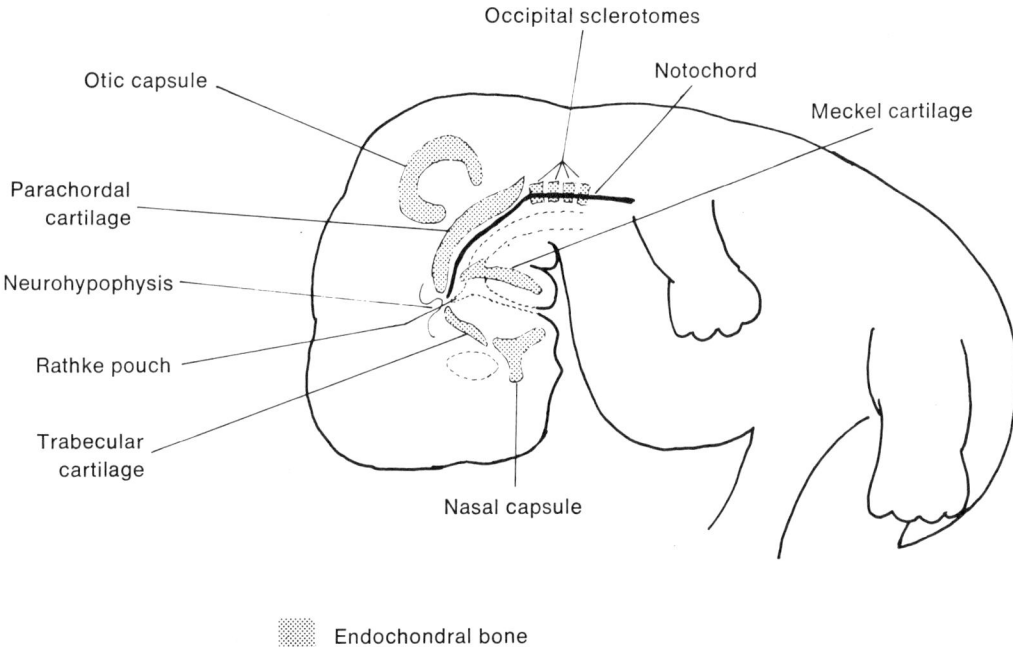

Fig. 203-8. Early development of cranial base occurs with several separate concentrations of mesenchymal cells that differentiate into cartilagenous centers, which eventually merge to form discrete elements such as the ethmoid, sphenoid, and occipital bones.

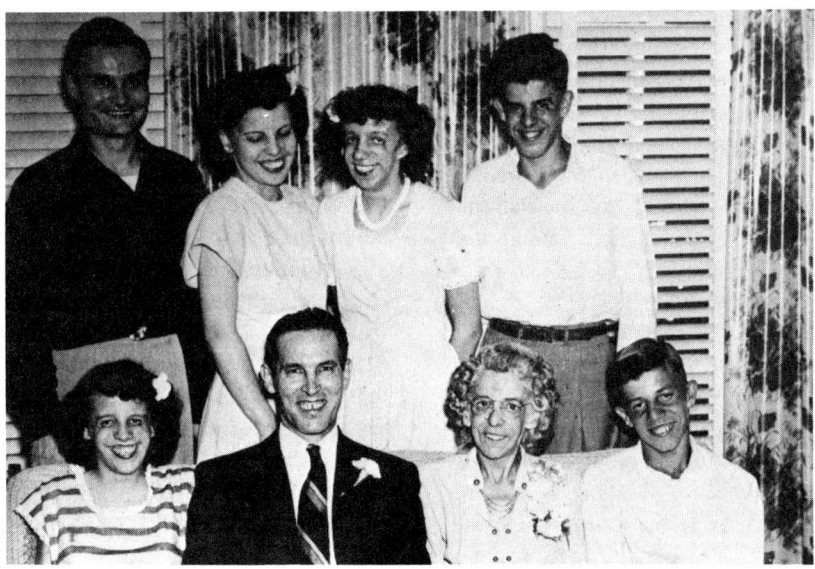

Fig. 203-9. Family portrait demonstrating autosomal dominant segregation and extensive variability of clinical features of Treacher-Collins syndrome. From top left, persons carrying the gene and affected are nos. 3 and 4; in the bottom row nos. 1, 3 (mother), and 4 are affected.

Almost simultaneously with the formation of the chondrocranium and cranial base, the differentiation of the desmocranium or cranial vault begins.

The mesenchyme, which gives rise to the cranial vault, is first arranged as a capsular membrane around the developing brain. The membrane later subdivides into two layers, an inner endomeninges and an outer ectomeninges.

Several primary and secondary ossification centers develop in the outer layer of the ectomeninges to form the individual islands of calvarial bone. These centers of ossification increase rapidly in size and soon take the shape of the calvarial bones to be formed in these areas, that is, the frontal bones, parietal bones, interparietal (squamous) portion of the occipital bone, and squamous portions of the temporal bones. As the ossification centers grow, the quantity of interposed condensed mesenchyme decreases. The narrow strips of connective tissue that remain between the bones become the sutures; the membranous layer of mesenchyme covering the bones forms the periosteum. Until this time, genetic factors determining cell differentiation have played the predominant role in craniofacial development.

During the late embryonic period, development of the face and viscerocranium is characterized mainly by changes in proportion and relative position of individual structures. Intrinsic genetic factors become less and less important, whereas epigenetic factors increase in influence. The forebrain continues to expand, and the eyes, initially directed laterally, gradually become directed anteriorly. The nasal fossae are at first widely separated, but gradually come together. The primitive nasal septum becomes thinned, and the medial nasal folds fuse. At the same time a transverse groove appears, defining the upper limit of the external nose and separating it from the frontal prominence. The primitive external ear, which develops around the margins of the first ectodermal groove, is at first caudal to the developing face but gradually assumes a more cephalic orientation and eventually passes the level of the mouth.

At approximately 60 days of gestation the embryo has acquired all of its basic morphologic characteristics and enters the fetal period. The expansion of the cranium that occurs from the fetal period onward takes place as a result of a combination of interstitial growth, endochondral growth, and expansion at the sutures or translational growth. The cartilage remnants of the chondrocranium that persist between the bones of the cranial base are known as synchondroses and contribute variably to cranial elongation and lateral expansion during active growth.

In addition to growth changes that occur at the basilar synchondroses, the cranial base undergoes selective appositional remodeling by resorption and deposition. This process is mediated by activity on the part of the bone-forming cells, the osteoblasts, as well as the bone-destroying cells, the osteoclasts. Remodeling of bone allows preexisting spaces in the skull, such as the brain cavity and the orbits, to grow in size and enables new cavities, such as the paranasal sinuses, to be formed. Marked resorption also occurs in the floors of the cranial fossae, deepening these endocranial compartments. This deepening process is aided by the bodily displacement of the floors of the fossae as a result of sutural expansion of the lateral walls of the neurocranium.

During the early stages of the fetal period the initial centers of ossification in the facial region also begin to develop and enlarge intramembranously within the condensed mesenchyme of the embryonic facial processes.

PATHOGENESIS AND CLASSIFICATION OF CRANIOFACIAL MALFORMATIONS

The complex embryologic processes just outlined are essential for normal craniofacial development and are never more evident than when an abnormality occurs, resulting in what is commonly referred to as "an experiment in nature." Numerous examples exist in which errors in morphogenesis result in significant structural alterations in the head and face. For example, a number of aberrations in normal craniofacial growth have been attributed to abnormalities or deficiencies in the initial formation, migration, and differentiation of cranial neural crest cells. Neural crest abnormalities can be divided into two broad pathogenetic categories: those resulting from defects in neural crest cell migration and those from defects in differentiation.

Deficiencies in the number of neural crest cells are frequently reflected in deficient development of facial derivatives and are often accompanied by structural defects in the forebrain and eyes. Experiments that artificially reduce the number of neural crest cells in avian embryos through the extirpation of small wedges of the neural folds just prior to crest cell migration result in characteristic brain-eye-face malformations. Removal of tissue from the anterior or preotic crest tissues results in facial defects involving the frontonasal process, whereas defects or derivatives of the maxillary processes and visceral arches are more commonly seen when postotic tissue is removed. Similar defects have been produced in mice by irradiating specific areas of the anterior neural crests, thereby producing cell death limited to that region. The number of migrating cells is substantially reduced, resulting in median facial clefts and other frontonasal deficiency defects. The mass of the neural plate itself is concomitantly reduced and presumably accounts for the associated brain and eye defects.

A recognized pattern of human malformation results from deficiencies in the number of derivatives of neural crest cells. There is a spectrum of brain-eye-face malformations in which the most consistent feature is a failure of fusion of the cerebral hemispheres called holoprosencephaly. This group of malformation syndromes is discussed in detail under midface malformations.

Defects of the viscerocranium may occur sporadically or as part of several genetic disorders. Among the more noteworthy anomalies are the "scooped-out" facial appearance resulting from maxillary hypoplasia and a depressed nasal bridge in achondroplasia, Down's syndrome (trisomy 21), and anhydrotic ectodermal dysplasia. In mandibulofacial dysostosis (Treacher Collins syndrome) the sunken appearance of the midface occurs secondary to severe malar hypoplasia and hypoplasia or absence of the zygomatic bones.

The extensive evidence of the role and importance of the neural crest cells in normal craniofacial development provides strong support for the role of classic genetic mechanisms involving DNA translation, transcription, and protein synthesis as a basic mechanism in craniofacial growth. The normal development of the craniofacial complex is organized and guided by an orderly and sequential activation and deactivation of specific genes at specific times. It is well known that under normal conditions only a small portion of the total genetic material is activated at any particular time, whereas the majority of the genome remains quiescent. Normal development also depends on the inductive effect of embryonic tissues on one another. The phenotypic characteristics of a differentiated cell will therefore depend both on its genotype and on the type and degree of gene repression and environmental factors present in the course of differentiation. Disturbances in normal growth and development may result from several pathogenetic mechanisms, including defective genes or mutations producing abnormal structural proteins; abnormal amounts of genetic material, as in the case on aneuploidy or polyploidy; and disturbances of the inductive patterns of embryonic tissues. A large number of craniofacial malformation syndromes can be classified into subgroups based on these pathogenetic mechanisms, location of anatomic defect, and structures or organs involved. It is convenient to refer to the following major groups of malformations: (1) otocraniofacial syndromes; (2) craniosynostosis syndromes; (3) midface syndromes, including holoprosencephalic malformation complex and frontonasal dysplasia malformation complex; (4) craniofacial clefts; and (5) clefts of the primary and secondary palate.

Otocraniofacial syndromes

The heterogeneous group of otocraniofacial malformation syndromes has been referred to by various terms, such as branchial arch syndromes, branchial arch dysplasias, first arch syndromes, first and second branchial arch syndromes, and hemifacial microsomia. All of these terms are oversimplifications and leave the erroneous impression that only branchial arch derivatives of the face are dysmorphically involved. In many cases, however, cardiac, renal, and extracranial skeletal anomalies occur and must be considered as much a part of the syndromes as structures derived from branchial arch components.

This group of malformations will be considered under two primary subheadings; the first will include those entities that have *bilateral symmetric* facial involvement, and the second will include those entities that have *unilateral* or *bilateral asymmetric* facial malformations.

SYNDROMES WITH BILATERAL SYMMETRIC FACIAL INVOLVEMENT. The most common of the bilateral symmetric otocraniofacial syndromes is *Treacher Collins syndrome,* or mandibulofacial dysostosis. This syndrome is inherited as an autosomal dominant gene with complete penetrance but variable expressivity. The gene does seem to have some lethal effects prenatally, since fetal wastage is more common in families carrying this gene.

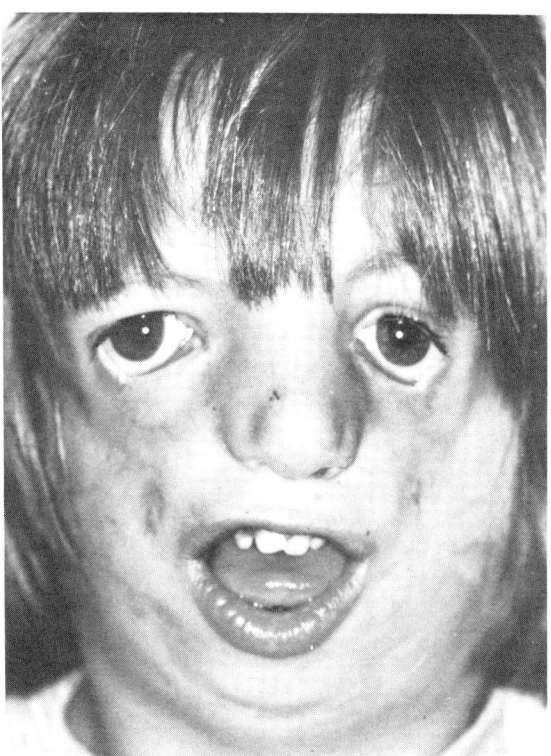

Fig. 203-10. Treacher Collins syndrome. Note the typical microtia, antimongoloid slant of palpebral fissures, malar and zygomatic hypoplasia, micrognathia, and defects of the lower eyelids.

The major features of this syndrome seen in virtually all cases include malar and zygomatic hypoplasia, antimongoloid slant of the palpebral fissures, eyelid colobomas, and external ear abnormalities (Fig. 203-10). The eyelid colobomas occur most frequently in the outer third of the lower eyelid (75%), and there is often a deficiency of the eyelashes medial to the coloboma (50%). This malformation is related to the severity of outer canthal displacement. Approximately 25% of affected individuals have an unusual "tongue-shaped" extension of hair that extends downward and forward from the temporal region onto the cheek.

Ear tags and preauricular pits occur between the tragus of the ear and the angle of the mouth in over half of the cases. The external ear is frequently deformed, being large and floppy in some cases and microtic or hypoplastic, crumpled and anteriorly displaced in others. Approximately 30% of patients have absence of the external auditory meatus, which is frequently accompanied by malformations of the middle ear ossicles, compounding the problems of conductive deafness. Tomographic examination of the temporal bones is essential in all patients with Treacher Collins syndrome with extensive ear involvement or suspected of a conductive hearing loss to fully evaluate the status of the middle ear structures.

The body of mandible is frequently hypoplastic and the

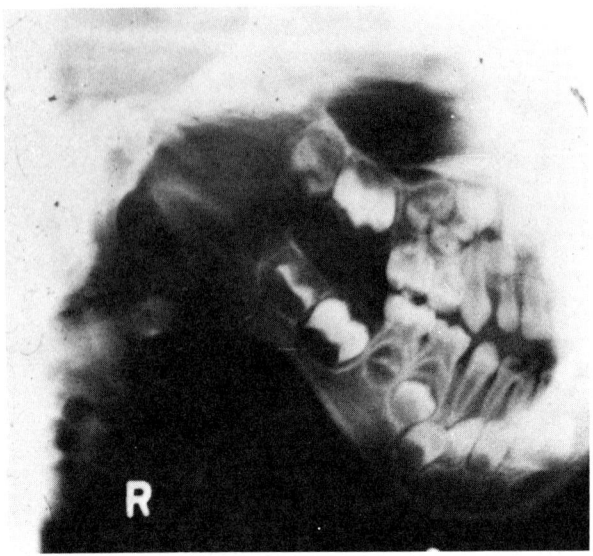

Fig. 203-11. Radiograph illustrating marked mandibular hypoplasia and typical "antigonial notch" in lower border of mandible.

chin severely retruded. Radiographs show a characteristic curvature (antigonial notch) in the lower border of the mandible and often reveals hypoplasia of the coronoid and condylar processes, although they are invariably present (Fig. 203-11). Cleft palate is found in approximately 30% of patients. A high frequency of dental malocclusion results from the discrepancy in jaw and tooth size and the gross dysmorphology of the mandible.

Mental retardation has often been reported in the literature but in many cases may have been attributable to hearing loss rather than actual intellectual deficiency. Other defects that have been described as being associated with Treacher Collins syndrome but that occur less frequently include ventricular septal defects and other cardiac malformations.

There are two other recognizable syndromes that are bilaterally symmetric and share many clinical features with Treacher Collins syndrome. These syndromes and their primary features are presented in Table 203-2.

SYNDROMES WITH ASYMMETRIC INVOLVEMENT. The subgroup of otocraniofacial syndromes characterized by asymmetric involvement of craniofacial structures includes mainly branchial arch derivatives. Affected individuals commonly have asymmetric involvement of ears, mouth, and jaws. The ascending portions of the mandible are with hypoplasia of ramus and condyle. The majority of reported cases have been sporadic. In those few families with multiple occurrences, reports concerning the mode of inheritance are conflicting. Several reports of successive generations have been published, as well as studies of affected siblings of normal parents. It appears that autosomal dominant, autosomal recessive, and multifactorial modes of inheritance are all possible.

Overall this group of malformations appears to occur with a relatively high frequency. It has been estimated that 1 in 3500 live-born infants is affected.

Of the variants that have been described among the asymmetric otocraniofacial disorders, two comprise the vast majority of reported cases. Although there are many transitional forms between these two entities, which in fact may represent a spectrum of the same syndrome, it is convenient to discuss them separately as Goldenhar's syndrome (oculoauriculovertebral dysplasia) and hemifacial microsomia.

The Goldenhar variant is distinguished from hemifacial microsomia primarily by the presence of epibulbar dermoid cysts, which occur at the limbus or corneal margin of the lower outer quadrant (Fig. 203-12). These lesions are usually milky white to yellow in color and have a solid, smooth surface. They are often difficult to detect and may appear only as small white streaks or specks. The ocular defects generally occur bilaterally; however, approximately 30% of patients have unilateral lesions.

The Goldenhar and hemifacial microsomia variants are marked by striking facial asymmetry and dysmorphogenesis resulting largely from the hypoplasia and displacement of the external ear structures; maxillary, temporal, and malar bone hypoplasia; and hypoplasia of the mandibular ramus and condyle (Fig. 203-13). Approximately 40% of patients have bilateral involvement; however, one side is nearly always more severe than the other. Interestingly, the right side is involved most severely in approximately 62% of cases. Malformation of the external ear varies widely, from complete aplasia to large, hypoplastic pinnae that may be displaced anteriorly and inferiorly. Ear involvement may occur bilaterally, especially in the Goldenhar variant, but is usually asymmetric. Supernumerary ear tags occur frequently on the cheek between the tragus and the angle of the mouth. These structures are most commonly seen in patients who have concomitant macrostomia. Preauricular pits are often found in the same areas. Conductive hearing loss resulting from middle ear abnormalities or the absence of an external auditory meatus is noted in approximately 50% of cases. An important clinical consideration is the significant correlation between external ear abnormalities and hearing loss caused by hypoplasia of the ossicles.

Eyelid colobomas are also a common finding in Goldenhar's syndrome, with defects in the upper lid occurring in 50% to 60% of patients who have epibulbar dermoids (Fig. 203-12). The defect most generally occurs in the medial third of the upper lid. Microphthalmia may also be present in severely involved cases and, when present, is usually accompanied by mental retardation.

There is a wide range of dysplastic involvement of the mandibular condyle and ramus on the affected side. Microtia occurs in over 70% of patients with mandibular hypoplasia. Approximately 30% of patients with agenesis of

Table 203-2. Otocraniofacial syndromes with bilateral symmetric involvement

Syndrome	Clinical features	Etiology
Treacher Collins syndrome	Mandibulofacial dysostosis, occasionally other extracranial anomalies (heart)	Autosomal dominant
Nager acrofacial dysostosis	Mandibulofacial dysostosis, preaxial upper limb reductions, other anomalies	Sporadic; possibly autosomal recessive
Wildervanck-Smith syndrome	Mandibulofacial dysostosis, preaxial and postaxial upper and lower limb deficiency, other anomalies	Unknown; sporadic to date

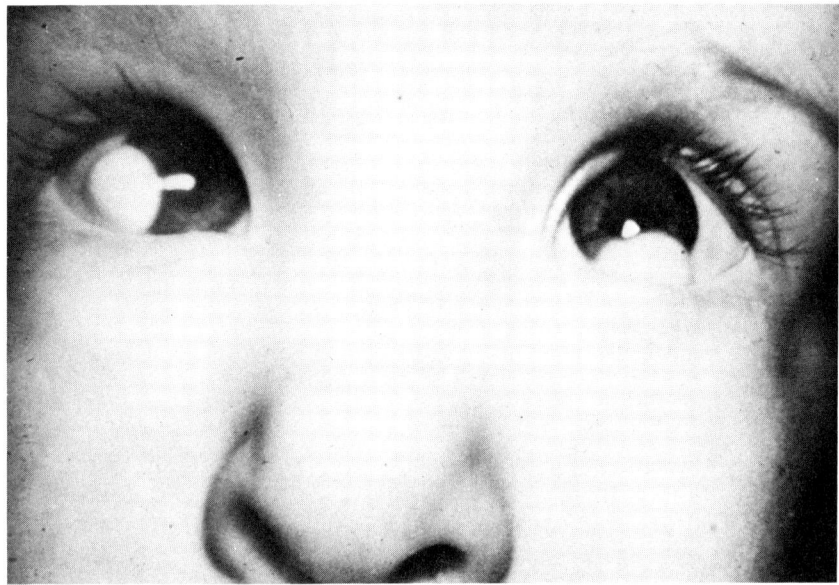

Fig. 203-12. Epibulbar dermoid cyst of eye frequently seen in Goldenhar's syndrome.

the ramus have associated macrostomia on the affected side. There is frequent failure of development of the parotid gland, as well as hypoplasia of various muscles, including the masseter, temporalis, and pterygoid muscles and muscles of facial expression.

The severity of malocclusion that characterizes this syndrome is proportional to the degree of hypoplasia of the maxilla and mandible. Close assessment of these features is essential, particularly when planning a coordinated surgical-orthodontic reconstruction for affected individuals. It is also noteworthy that in most cases the facial asymmetry tends to become more pronounced with increasing age. This is probably the result of an imbalance in growth rates between the normal and the affected sides of the face that tends to accentuate the asymmetry.

Extracranial abnormalities have been observed in many patients. Anomalies of the axial skeleton, particularly in the cervical region, are seen in approximately 50% of patients. The most common findings include occipitalization of the atlas, cuneiform vertebrae, and complete or partial fusion of cervical vertebrae. Less frequently observed are supernumerary vertebrae, hemivertebrae, spina bifida occulta, and anomalous ribs. Clubfoot has been observed in approximately 20% of cases.

Approximately 50% of patients have some type of congenital heart disease, ranging from ventricular septal defect and patent ductus arteriosus to tetralogy of Fallot. Pulmonary agenesis or hypoplasia has been noted in several cases, with the lung missing on the same side as the facial abnormalities.

The etiology and pathogenesis of these unilateral asymmetric anomalies have recently been duplicated experimentally in laboratory animals by interfering with differentiating tissues in the region of the ear and jaw. This disruption is caused by an expanding hematoma produced during a critical period in stapedial artery complex development. The severity of the facial malformations is directly related to the degree of local destruction and disruption caused by the hematoma.

With respect to confirmation of a diagnosis and subsequent genetic counseling in cases of otocraniofacial syndromes, it is fair to say that one should evaluate each pa-

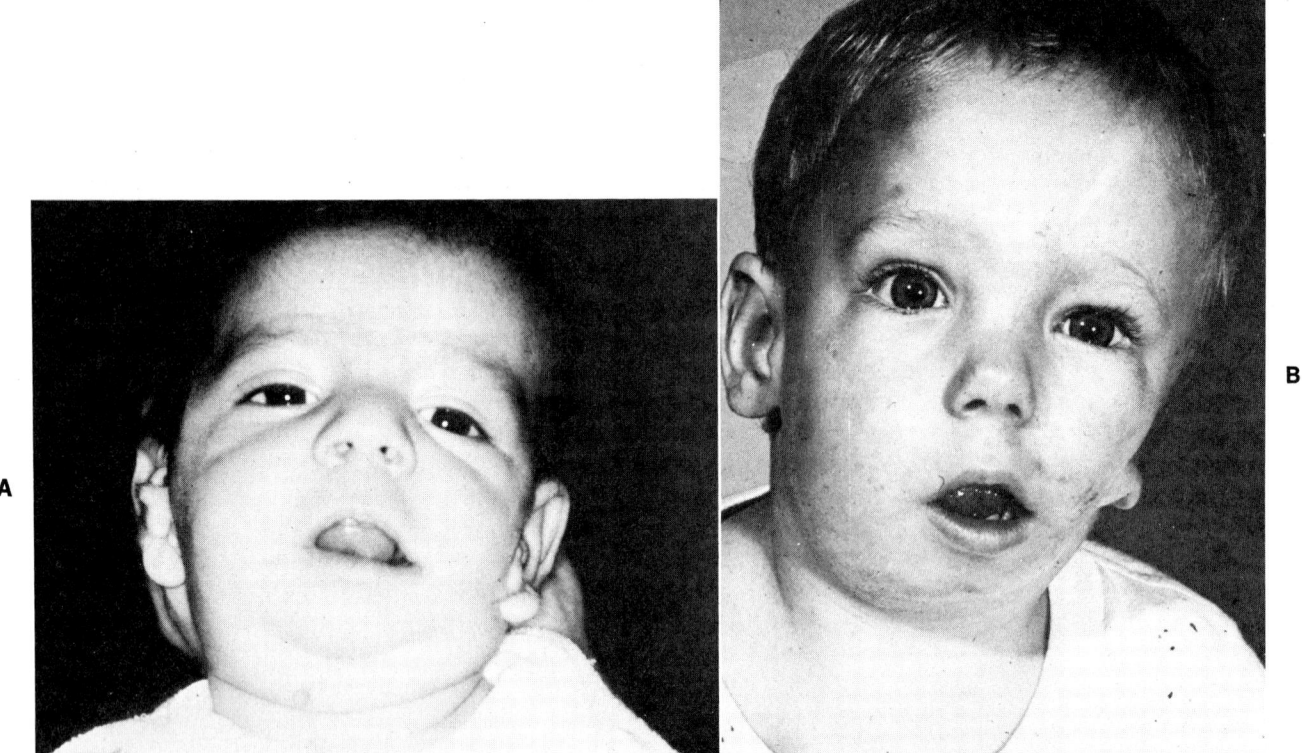

Fig. 203-13. **A,** Goldenhar's syndrome. Note asymmetric involvement of facial structures. **B,** Hemifacial microsomia. That more pronounced asymmetry and lack of dermoid cysts differentiate this from Goldenhar's syndrome is controversial.

tient and family individually, bearing in mind the extensive variability of expression characteristic of this group of malformations. Although familial occurrence of Goldenhar's syndrome has been encountered, the vast majority of cases are sporadic. Since autosomal inheritance has been reported, the importance of recognizing minimal manifestations in family members of affected individuals cannot be overemphasized and is extremely important for accurate genetic counseling. For the purposes of genetic counseling, a thorough evaluation of the skeletal, cardiac, and other extracranial systems should also be carried out on all patients and their first-degree relatives whenever possible. The presence of single minor anomalies, such as preauricular tags, pits, or hypoplastic ear, or isolated skeletal, cardiac, or renal anomalies in relatives has genetic significance and should be considered when an attempt is made to establish risk of recurrence.

Craniosynostosis syndromes

Premature fusion of cranial sutures, or craniosynostosis, is a nonspecific abnormality that may occur as an isolated finding or in conjunction with other abnormalities and is a feature of several recognizable syndromes. Whether an isolated clinical finding or a part of a syndrome, craniosynostosis consists of an arrest of growth in one or more of the cranial sutures brought on by a premature fusion of the cranial bones and subsequent limitation of expansive growth normally accommodated by that suture. Although the underlying cause is not known, it is clear that premature fusion can be precipitated by several mechanisms, including abnormal cranial base morphology, intrauterine crowding with fetal head constraint, and abnormal brain development. It should be remembered that the development of the neurocranium is, in large part, influenced by the development of the underlying brain.

At birth the size of the normal cranium is approximately 65% of its adult size, and by 5 years it reaches approximately 90% of adult size. The adult width of the cranium is attained during the first or second year of life. In the newborn infant, several fontanelles, or "soft spots," are present between the bones of the cranium. These fontanelles close at various times, but under normal circumstances all have been reduced to sutures by approximately the eighteenth month. The sutures themselves have regular margins with very little interlocking and interdigitation, as is typical of an adult suture. The metopic suture, which separates the right and left halves of the frontal bone, is the first to fuse and does so at approximately 2 years of age. The other sutures close gradually over a period of time following completion of brain growth and normally remain patent well into the second decade of life. An important concept, and one that is frequently over-

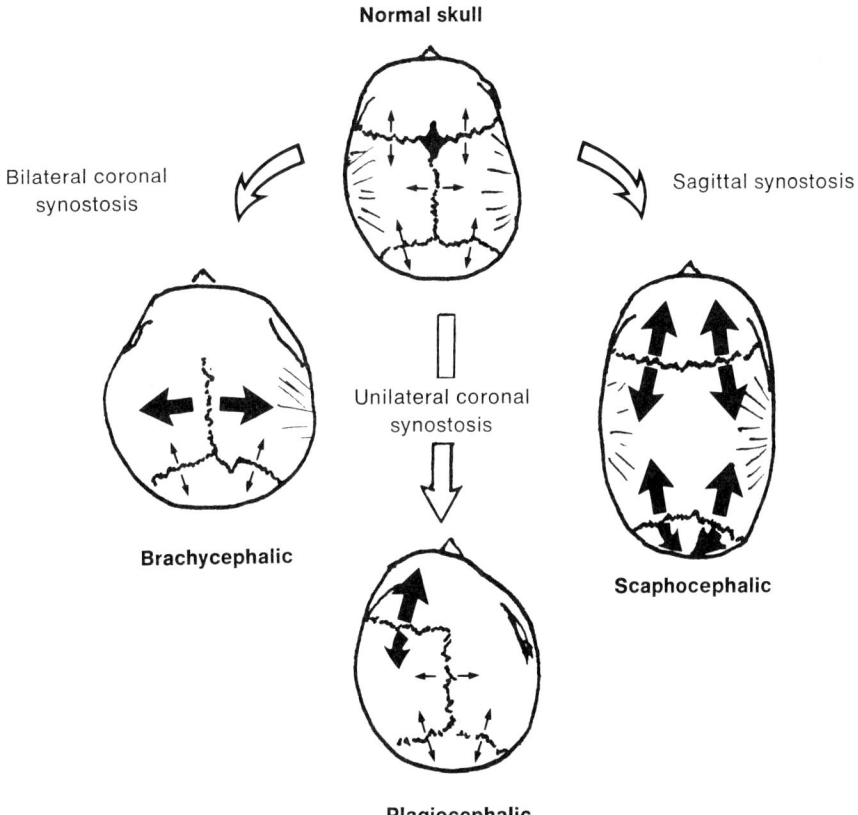

Fig. 203-14. Head shapes resulting from premature fusion of various sutures singly or in combination.

looked, is that the cranial sutures "grow" in response to the expanding brain, which acts to separate the bones of the calvarium and displace or "translate" them in an outward direction. This movement in response to the enlarging brain mass causes tension at the sutures, which respond by depositing new bone at the sutural margins, effectively causing the cranial bones to enlarge. If this expansion is too rapid, as in hydrocephalus, the sutures may become very wide and distended, since the separation has been too rapid for bone deposition to keep up. The overall increase in cranial volume accomplished by an outward drifting of the cranial bones is also accompanied by remodeling of the inside and outside of the cranial table, allowing the cranial bones to assume their respective shapes. Premature fusion of one or more cranial sutures results in an arrest of growth of the cranium in one dimension, with compensatory growth occurring in a direction of less resistance accomodated by sutures that remain patent. This redirected growth leads to the alterations in the size, shape, and contour of the skull. Fig. 203-14 illustrates the effects of premature synostosis of selected sutures and the typical patterns of subsequent cranial distortion. Based on an assessment of head shape, and astute clinician is frequently able to predict not only craniosynostosis but more specifically which of the cranial sutures have been prematurely fused.

In addition to the direct effects on skull shape, a number of secondary effects occur as a result of the altered cranial growth through craniosynostosis. Specifically, the proptosis, or exorbitism, frequently observed in these patients results from reduced size of the orbit and its inability to accommodate the globe. This condition is a result of the increased intracranial pressure on the cranial base causing an anterior displacement of the greater wings of the sphenoid from their normal position in the middle cranial fossa, thereby impinging on and restricting normal growth of the bony orbit. Similarly, the effects of the increased intracranial pressure cause a downward and forward displacement of the ethmoid plate, which results in the hypertelorism frequently seen in patients with craniosynostosis.

The severe distortion of the cranial base that often accompanies untreated craniosynostosis leads to a characteristic restricted growth in the maxilla frequently reflected by a reduced size of the nasopharynx and restricted capacity for air exchange.

An important feature exhibited in many of the craniosynostosis syndromes is a tendency for increasing severity in the craniofacial disproportion and deformity with increasing age and growth. Without treatment or surgical intervention little improvement should be expected because of the marked disproportion of growth potential at the various craniofacial growth centers.

The classification and nosology of the craniosynostosis syndromes have been the subject of considerable confusion and misconception. The craniosynostosis syndromes should never be classified on the basis of which sutures are prematurely fused or the severity of cranial deformity or mental retardation that may accompany these syndromes. It is clear that different sutures may be affected in different patients with the same syndrome, and there is great variability in the clinical expression of these disorders.

The primary concern, once it has been established that a suture is prematurely closed, is related to the risk of central nervous system damage created by the increased intracranial pressure and adverse cosmetic sequelae frequently observed in these conditions. Rarely is there evidence of brain damage secondary to increased intracranial pressure when the sagittal suture alone is involved. The risk of permanent damage to the central nervous system is significantly higher when the coronal or lambdoidal sutures are involved. Once craniosynostosis is diagnosed, consideration of craniectomy is indicated to relieve both the cosmetic and the functional problems that may ensue. Delays in treatment only cause the deformity to become exaggerated and reduce the potential for resumption of normal growth once the fused suture is reconstructed. In the case of synostosis of an isolated sagittal suture the urgency of surgery to avoid complications of the central nervous system is reduced, but surgery remains a definite consideration if for no other reason than cosmetic improvement.

A large number of syndromes with associated craniosynostosis have been described. Only the most common are detailed, including Apert's syndrome (Fig. 203-15), Carpenter's syndrome (Fig. 203-16), Crouzon's disease (Fig. 203-17), Pfeiffer's syndrome (Fig. 203-18), and Saethre-Chotzen syndrome (Fig. 203-19) (see also Table 3.)

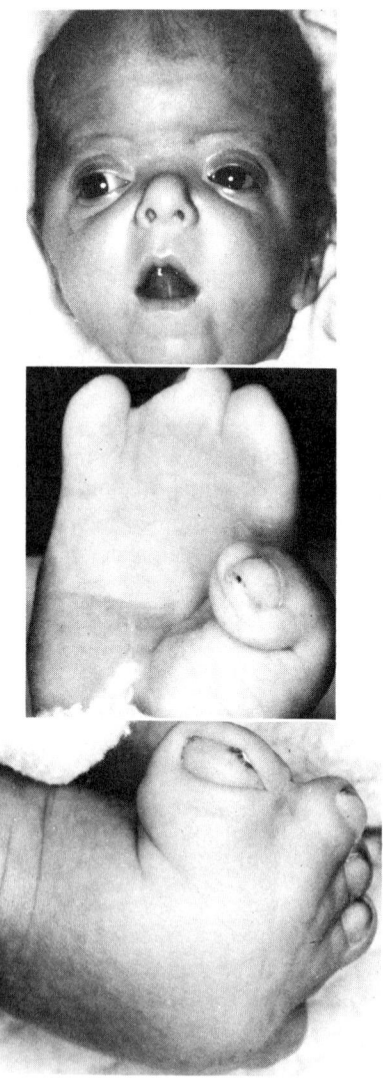

Fig. 203-15. Apert's syndrome.

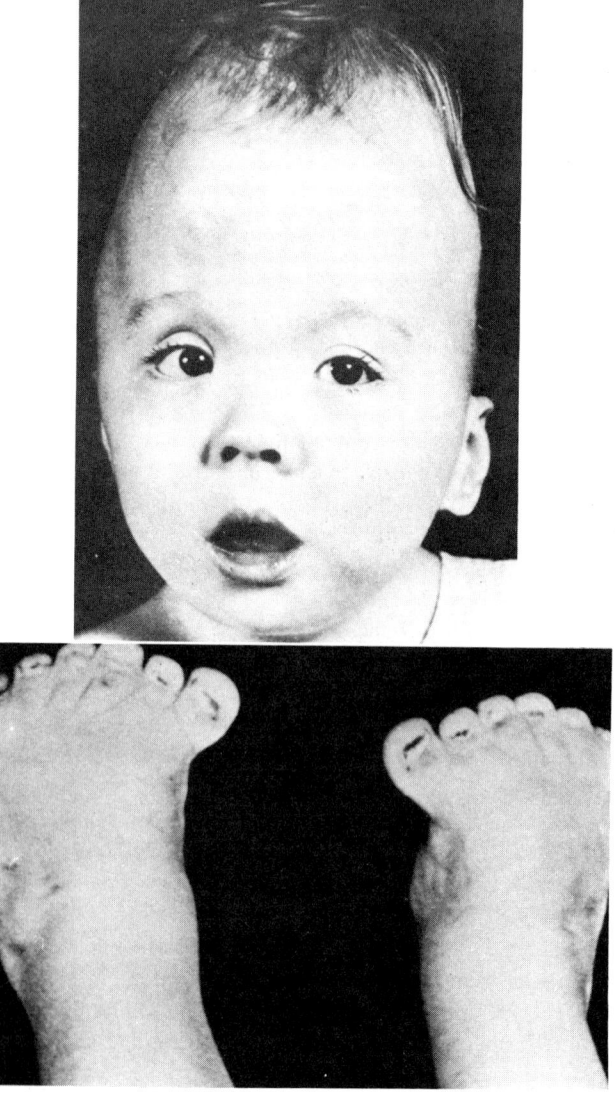

Fig. 203-16. Carpenter's syndrome.

203 • Malformations of the craniofacial complex: an overview 1315

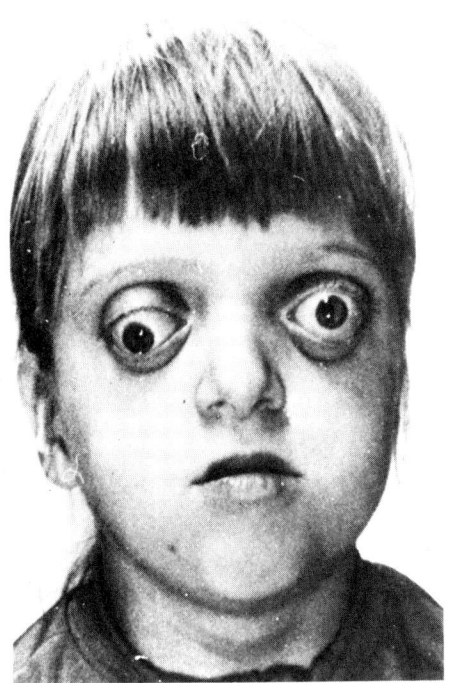

Fig. 203-17. Crouzon's disease.

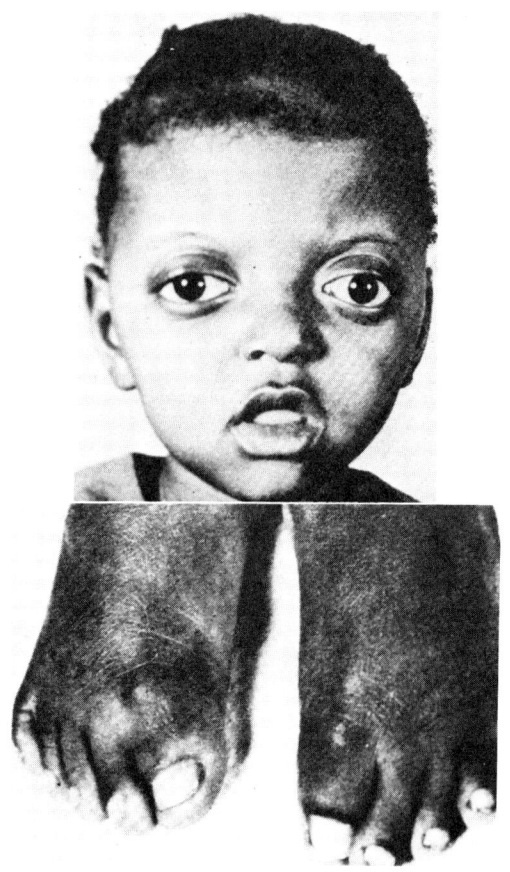

Fig. 203-18. Pfeiffer's syndrome.

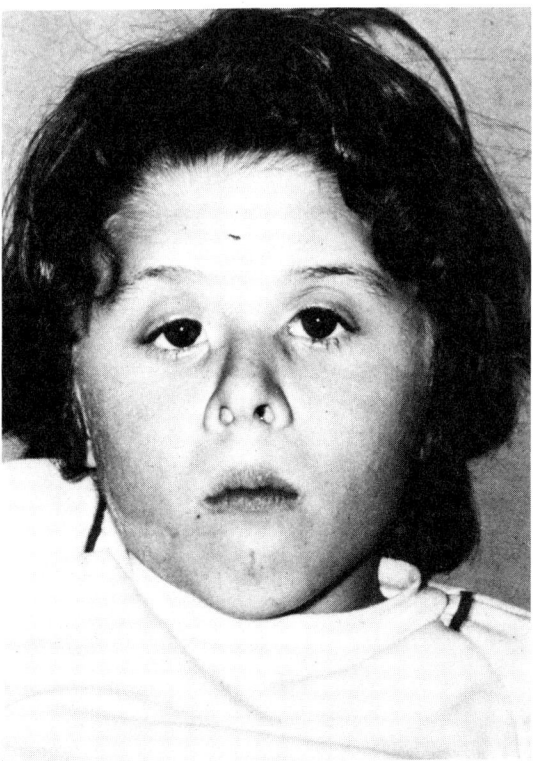

Fig. 203-19. Saethre-Chotzen syndrome.

Table 203-3. Craniosynostosis syndromes

Syndrome	Clinical features	Frequency of craniosynostosis	Inheritance
Apert syndrome (acrocephalosyndactyly) (Fig. 203-15)	Craniosynostosis; proptosis; down-slanting palpebral fissures; strabismus; orbital hypertelorism; midface deficiency; high-arched palate; symmetric syndactyly of hands and feet involving second, third, and fourth digits	Almost all cases	Autosomal dominant
Carpenter's syndrome (acrocephalopolysyndactyly) (Fig. 203-16)	Craniosynostosis; mental deficiency; preaxial polysyndactyly of feet; variable soft tissue syndactyly with brachymesophalangy of hands; displaced patellae; congenital heart defects; short stature; obesity	All reported cases	Autosomal recessive
Crouzon's disease (craniofacial dysostosis) (Fig 203-17)	Craniosynostosis; shallow orbits with proptosis; strabismus; midface deficiency	Almost all cases	Autosomal dominant
Pfeiffer's syndrome (Fig. 203-18)	Craniosynostosis; proptosis; strabismus; ocular hypertelorism; down-slanting palpebral fissures; midface deficiency; broad thumbs and great toes; mild and variable cutaneous syndactyly of fingers and toes	All known cases	Autosomal dominant
Saethre-Chotzen syndrome (acrocephalosyndactyly type 3) (Fig. 203-19)	Craniosynostosis; facial asymmetry; low-set frontal hairline; ptosis; deviated septum; variable brachydactyly and cutaneous syndactyly, especially of second and third fingers; normal thumbs and toes	All known cases	Autosomal dominant

Midface syndromes

Malformation syndromes affecting primarily the midline structures of the face and cranium may be divided into two major categories: the holoprosencephalic malformation complex and the frontonasal dysplasia malformation complex.

HOLOPROSENCEPHALIC MALFORMATION COMPLEX. The holoprosencephalic malformation complex is marked by malformations that result from defective neural plate formation or neural crest cell death, leading to deficient volume of frontonasal mesenchyme with subsequent absence or malformation of the various midface structures. Designating this group of malformations as the holoprosencephaly malformation complex denotes the fact that the developing prosencephalon develops abnormally, or holistically, when proper cleavage does not appear. Normally the prosencephalon divides sagittally to produce the cerebral hemispheres, horizontally into the olfactory and optic bulbs, and transversely into the telencephalon and diencephalon. There is an intimate relationship between the prosencephalon and various midfacial structures. The severity of anomalous facial development reflects and is accompanied by equally significant abnormalities in the brain.

The basic pathogenetic mechanism of the holoprosencephalic malformation complex lies in the faulty interaction between the notochord, the neuroectoderm of the developing brain, and the oral plate. Normally the notochord arises just caudal to the optic plates. If the notochord is abnormally short and assumes a caudally displaced position, abnormalities occur in the development of the neuroectoderm at the cephalic extension, including the entire frontonasal process of the developing embryo. The net result is a failure of the optic placodes to become separated, giving rise to the hypoteloric deformities that characterize this malformation complex.

The role of heredity in holoprosencephaly is not entirely clear, the majority of cases being sporadic with no positive family history. This anomaly is frequently seen in trisomy-13 syndrome and is an occasional feature in the short-arm 18 deletion syndrome. An autosomal recessive mode of inheritance is apparent in several kindreds where the malformation occurs in siblings born to normal parents.

The prognosis for central nervous system function in individuals manifesting these types of facial defects is very poor. Patients with the more severe form of this complex usually do not survive beyond a few hours or days. Pa-

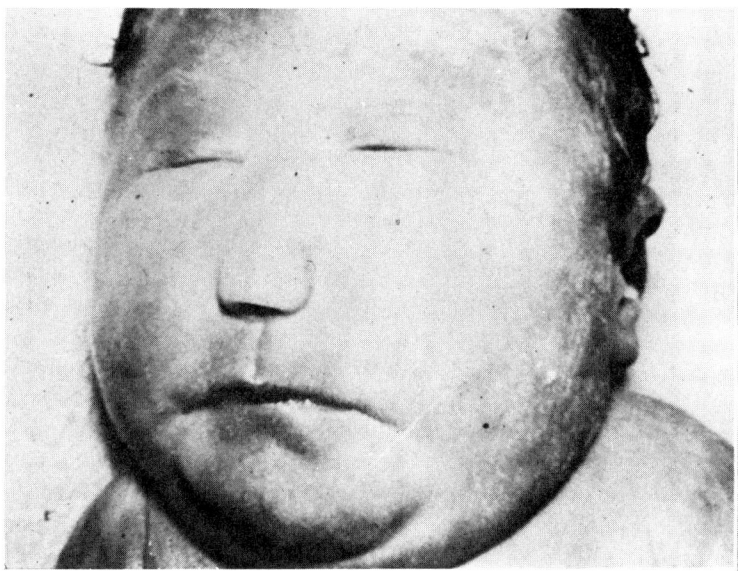

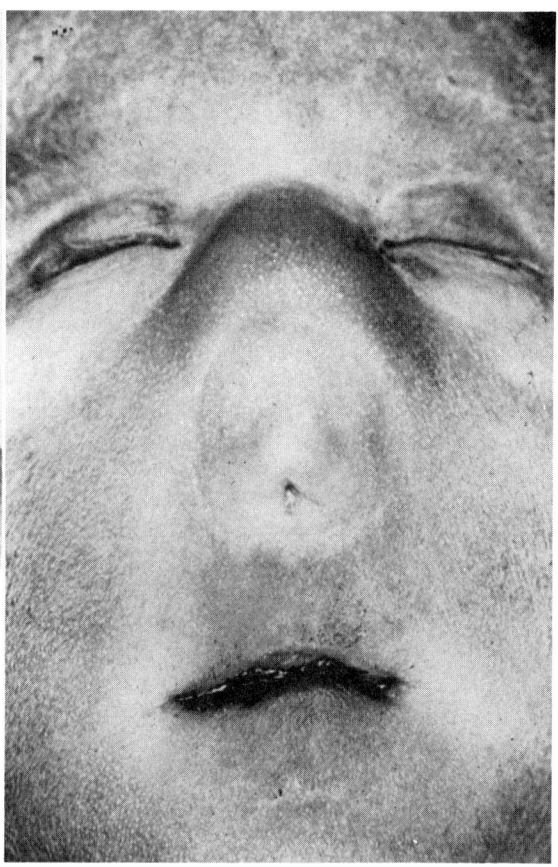

Fig. 203-20. Holoprosencephalic malformation complex consists of several patterns of malformation that have a common pathogenesis but represent a spectrum of severity in clinical features.

tients with the less severe forms may have extended life expectancies; however, uniformly there are severe developmental and intellectual anomalies.

Several facial anomalies are associated with holoprosencephaly and have been classified into five subtypes according to the faciocerebral relationships. In effect this classification represents a transition through varying degrees of severity of the holoprosencephalic malformation complex (Fig. 203-20).

Cyclopia. Cyclopia consists of; a single or partially divided eye in a single orbit, absence of the nose or presence of a proboscis, and severe microcephaly with no division between the anterior lobes of the brain (alobar holoprosencephaly).

Ethmocephaly. Ethmocephaly consists of: severe hypotelorism with separate and distinct orbits; there may be absence of the nose, or a proboscis and severe microcephaly and accompany alobar holoprosencephaly.

Cebocephaly. In cebocephaly there is severe hypertelorism with separate orbits, a proboscis-like nose, and severe microcephaly, most commonly with alobar holoprosencephaly.

Median cleft lip. In median cleft lip there is orbital hypertelorism with separate orbits, a hypoplastic nose, premaxillary agenesis and absence of the median portion of the upper lip, and usually alobar holoproscencephaly.

Median cleft lip with premaxillary hypoplasia. The major characteristics of median cleft lip with premaxillary hypoplasia are orbital hypotelorism with separate orbits, a median cleft of the upper lip with hypoplastic premaxilla, hypoplastic and flattened nose, and microcephaly with partial formation of interhemispheric fissure (semilobar holoprosencephaly).

FRONTONASAL DYSPLASIA MALFORMATION COMPLEX. The frontonasal dysplasia malformation complex is characterized by a group of facial defects that are related and possibly transitional forms encompassing common pathogenetic phenomena. Various defects such as ocular hypertelorism, broad nasal root, V-shaped widows peak hairline, median clefts of the nose and/or lip, cranium bifidum occultum, and varying degrees of cleft lip with or without cleft palate may be seen singly or in combination. The term "frontonasal dysplasia" (Fig. 203-21) has been suggested and proposed classification of frontonasal malformations subdivided by the location of the defects, that is as follows: (1) upper face region, (2) midcephalic borderline region, and (3) lower and lateral face region.

Embryologically the frontonasal dysplasia malformation complex differs from the holoprosencephalic complex in that the amount of tissue in the midface is nearly normal and occasionally exists in excess. The defects that occur in this condition are thought to be a result of a failure in development of the nasal capsule, thereby allowing the brain to develop caudally and occupy the space normally assumed by the nasal capsule. This caudal displacement of the brain produces cranium bifidum occultum and also results in an arrest in the normal development of various

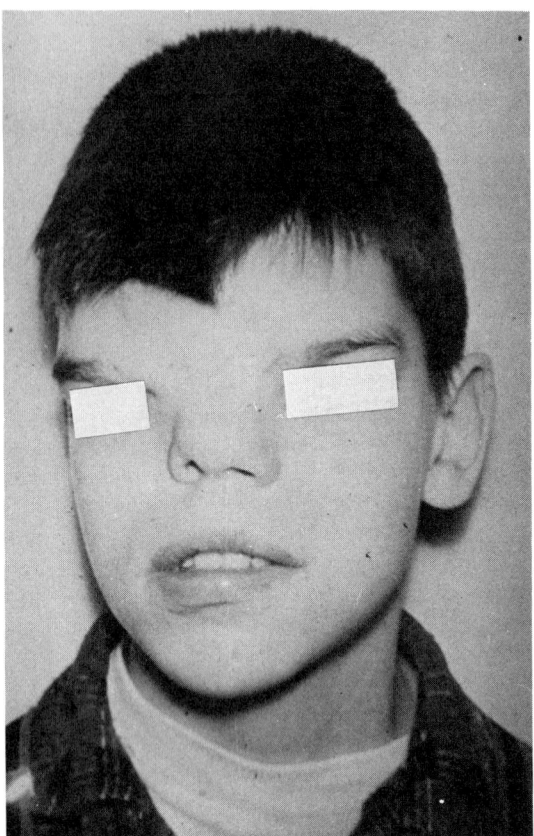

Fig. 203-21. Frontonasal dysplasia. Note hypertelorism that is distinguishing feature of this malformation complex.

facial structures such as hypertelorism, lack of formation of the nasal tip with occasional clefting of the nose, and occasionally midline notching or clefting of the upper lip. The widow's peak hair pattern frequently results and is directly related to the orbital hypertelorism wherein the two periocular fields of hair growth suppression are more laterally displaced than usual.

Mental retardation is occasionally present but is much less common than in holoprosencephaly. When the orbital hypertelorism is severe and the craniofacial malformations are accompanied by extracephalic anomalies, the probability of mental deficiency is increased. In less severe forms of hypertelorism and in the absence of extraencephalic anomalies, the probability of mental deficiency is greatly reduced.

Radiographic examination frequently reveals anterior cranium bifidum and obliteration of the frontal sinuses. There is frequently an accompanying anterior encephalocele, and occasionally midline lipomas or teratomas may be associated with the condition.

Almost all reported cases of frontonasal dysplasia have been sporadic; however, the condition has been observed in multiple individuals in some kindreds, suggesting the possibility of dominant inheritance, with the majority of cases representing fresh mutations. Polygenic inheritance is also a possibility.

Craniofacial clefts

Of all the craniofacial anomalies, none is more noticeable than facial clefts. The morphogenesis of craniofacial clefts is thought to be largely caused by a combination of events leading to a lack of fusion between normally joined parts or by a lack of normal development and penetration of mesodermal tissue in the cleft areas.

Although several systems for classifying craniofacial clefts have been proposed, the Tessier system will be used herein. Before this system of classification was developed, craniofacial clefts were referred to as cleft lip, cleft palate, oblique facial cleft including naso-ocular clefts, and oro-ocular clefts, oroaural or transverse facial clefts, and mandibular clefts. The drawback to this system of classification is that it fails to include or discriminate between many major cleft types such as those observed in the Treacher Collins syndrome.

The Tessier classification is based on not only the soft tissue or surface anatomy of the clefts but also on the structural malformations of the underlying bony structures observed at the time of reconstructive plastic surgery. The correlation of the clinical appearance with surgical anatomy makes the system uniquely informative and practical.

The clefts are numbered 0 through 14 (Fig. 203-22). The orbit is regarded as an important landmark, since it is considered to be part of both the cranium and the face. The clefts that are directed cephalad, or "northbound," extend through the upper eyelid and are considered mainly "cranial" in nature. The caudally directed, or "southbound," clefts pass through the lower eyelid to become "facial." The combination of northbound and southbound clefts may be combined to form "craniofacial" clefts. When this occurs the clefts consistently follow a well-defined course. Thus the following combinations can be seen clinically: 0-14, 1-13, 2-12, 3-11, and 4-10.

Keeping this cleft extension concept in mind encourages the clinician to look up and down the entire facial axis for malformations. An examination conducted in this manner will often reveal subtle and unexpected malformations (Fig. 203-23). For example, the common cleft lip is a part of clefts 1, 2, and 3. This fact should alert the clinician to carefully inspect the more cephalic structures with care to rule out involvement of peripheral facial and cranial structures. An example is the combination of a common bilateral cleft lip with a porcine-type nose frequently associated with a short frontal process of the maxilla. These two features are also part of cleft 3. On close examination a slight medial canthal dystopia and excessive tearing, indicative of a blocked lacrimal apparatus, are frequently observed, indicating a defect or cleft extending from the lip to the nose and then to the orbit.

The extent of involvement of the soft and bony tissue is variable from patient to patient. As a general rule, facial clefts located between the midline and the infraorbital foramen have proportionally less bony deformation when compared to those found lateral to the foramen.

203 • Malformations of the craniofacial complex: an overview 1319

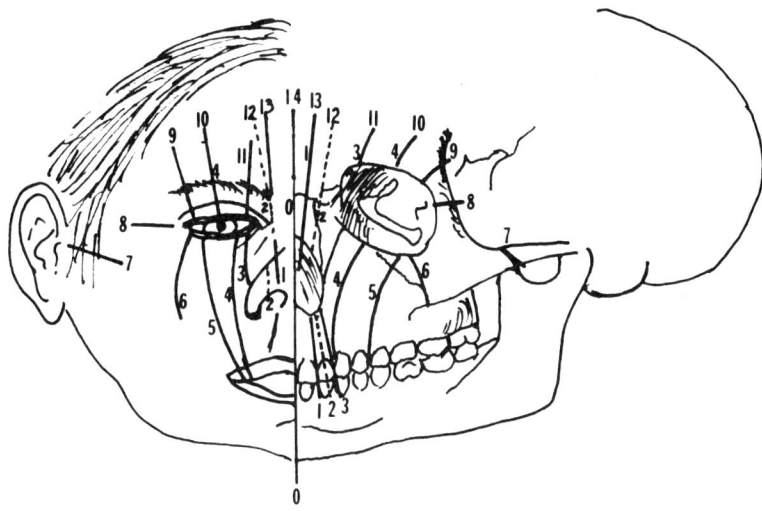

Fig. 203-22. Tessier classification of craniofacial clefts showing soft tissue and skeletal structures involved in various types of clefts.

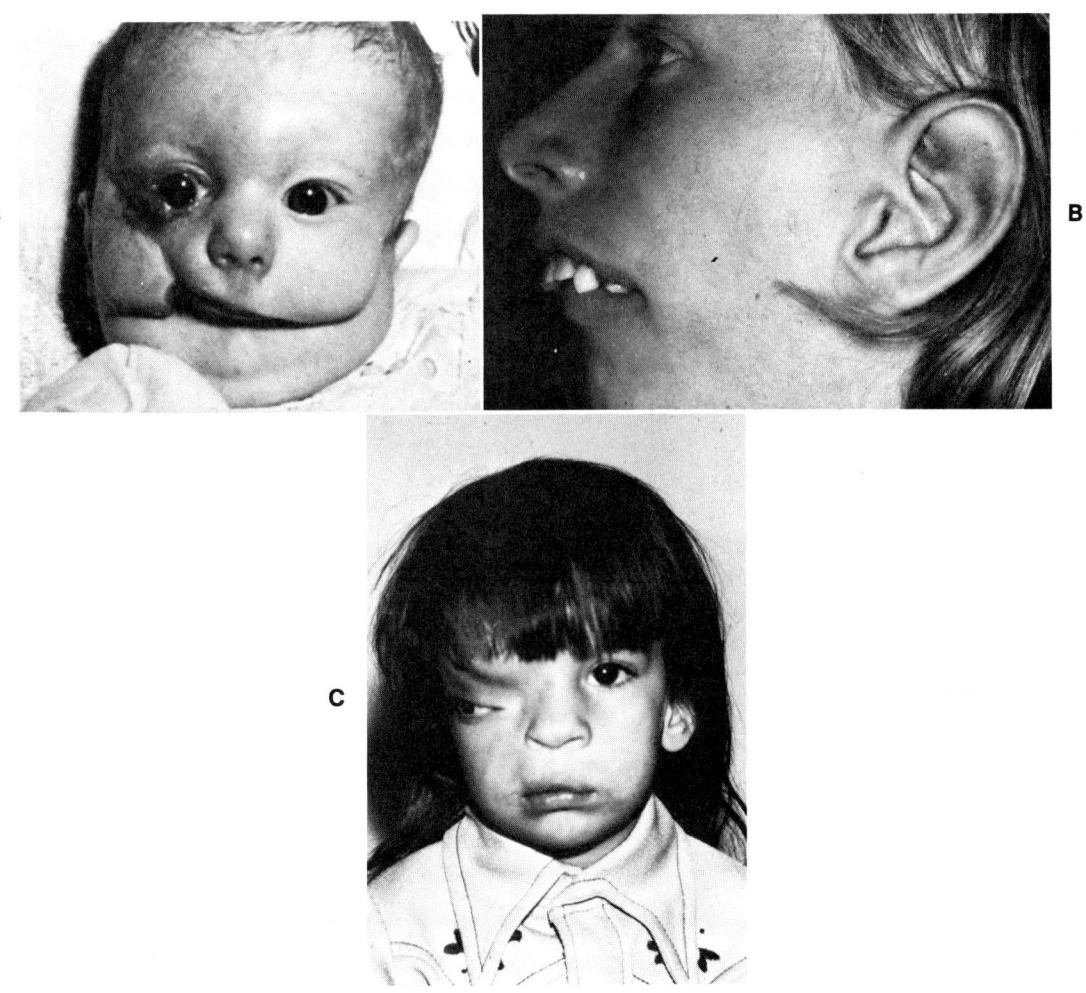

Fig. 203-23. A, Craniofacial cleft 2-12 by Tessier classification. **B,** 3-11 craniofacial cleft. **C,** 4 facial cleft. (Courtesy of H. Kawamoto, M.D.)

Clefts of the primary and secondary palates

The most common craniofacial abnormalities to confront the physician and dentist are clefts involving the primary and secondary palates. The primary and secondary palates are developmentally distinct structures and undergo development at times separated by approximately 3 to 4 weeks in early gestation. Because of the variable nature and timing of developmental mechanisms, these malformations will be discussed separately even though they frequently appear together in patients.

CLEFTS OF THE PRIMARY PALATE. Clefts of the primary palate (Fig. 203-24), including the structures and tissues of the lips and circumoral musculature, the premaxillary segment of the alveolus, and the hard palate posterior to the nasopalatine foramina, are among the most frequently encountered facial malformations. These clefts vary widely in their position and severity from unilateral incomplete clefts to bilateral complete clefts resulting in communication between the oral and nasal cavity. In the most severe cases of bilateral cleft lip the defect extends through the lip and alveolus, resulting in a median mass of tissue connected to the nasal septum by a vomer stock and separated widely from the lateral segments.

The incidence of clefts in the primary palate varies with respect to sex and racial background. These clefts are most commonly seen in males, with an incidence of approximately 1 per 1000 births in white populations, 2 per 1000 births in Oriental populations and 0.5 per 1000 births in black populations. Human fetuses and newborn infants affected with clefts of the primary palate show statistically significant increases in the width of the face, particularly the maxilla.

The mechanisms by which clefting of the primary palate occur are not clearly understood and are somewhat controversial because of the paucity of human embryos that have been examined in this early stage of development. The controversy surrounding this subject centers on how the primary palate is formed from the developing embryonic facial processes. There is general agreement that the development of the primary palate and that of the nose are closely related in that the invagination of the nasal cavity requires the proper coalescence of the surrounding facial processes to form the primary palate. The precise method by which the primary palate forms, however, is not widely agreed on, with two distinct mechanisms hypothesized. On the one hand a *fusion* of epithelial surfaces occurs between two facial processes that are approaching each other in a particular plane in space, forming a distinct and continuous structure that becomes the primary palate. The alternate hypothesis is not based on the process of fusion between facial processes but rather on a *mergence* of mesoderm that flows into a continuous band of mesenchyme known as the isthmus, which is in the primary palate region. According to this hypothesis, the mergence of facial elevations brought about by the migration of mesoderm into these areas would possibly trap epithelium between them and form a seam that would serve to partially separate the median and nasal maxillary processes. In most cases this epithelial seam degenerates and permits a more complete confluence of the adjacent mesenchyme and disappearance of the grooves or seams. If these seams persist, the penetration and mergence of mesodermal masses in those regions might be inhibited, resulting in an eventual rupture or dehiscence of these elements observed clinically as clefting.

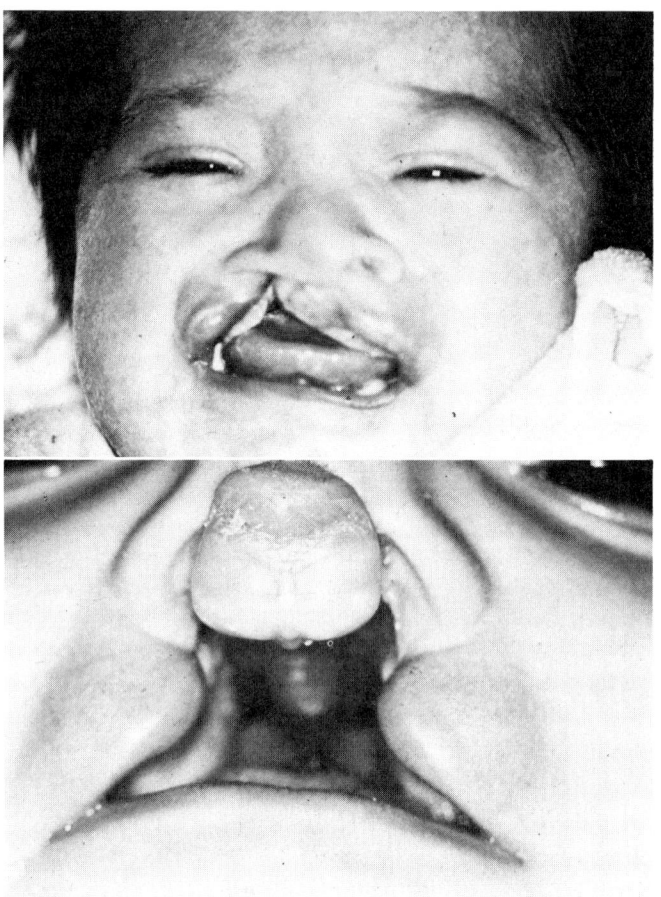

Fig. 203-24. Clefts of primary palate. **A,** Unilateral incomplete. **B,** Bilateral complete.

Most people working in the area of cleft formation have adopted the "mergence" hypothesis, which accounts for nearly all of the various forms of facial clefting clinically observed. Those few cases that do not fit this line of reasoning by virtue of the cleft not being located in areas where mergence would occur between facial processes can be accounted for by other mechanisms, such as the formation of amniotic adhesions to various regions of the face giving rise to the bizarre clefts that do not correspond to the usual lines of coalescence of the facial processes.

Clefts of the secondary palate are frequently seen in association with clefts of the primary palate and are thought to be a direct result of interference with normal palatal development imposed by the presence of the cleft of the primary palate. The clefts of the secondary palate are probably related to the inability of the palatal shell to elevate and meet at the midline at the appropriate time.

ISOLATED CLEFTS OF THE SECONDARY PALATE. Isolated clefts of the secondary palate can include complete or partial clefts of both the hard and soft palate from the incisive foramen posteriorly to the uvula (Fig. 203-25). Clefts of the secondary palate are formed in an embryologically distinct manner from those clefts that occur in association with clefts of the primary palate. Development of the palate posterior to the incisive foramen occurs at much later time developmentally than formation of the primary palate. The palatal shells first make their appearance during the fifth week of development and become enlarged and eventually elevate to fuse at the midline in an anterior to posterior direction; this fusion is finally completed at approximately the twelfth week of intrauterine life. This relatively long span of time provides a rather extended period during which various environmental and genetic factors can have adverse effects of palatal development and result in the cleft phenomenon.

The frequency with which isolated clefts of the secondary palate are observed is of interest in that the lack of variability between racial subgroups and in most cases the lack of a clearly demonstrable hereditary pattern suggest that genetic factors do not play as important a role as in clefts of the primary palate.

The submucous cleft palate, which is characterized by an intact epithelial lining of the entire palate but an absence of muscular and osseous tissues within those palatal elements, is apparently the result of a failure of proper mesodermal migration into the developing palate and represents a microform of the cleft palate. Similarly, bifid uvula may also represent a minor expression of the basic defect leading to isolated cleft palate (Fig. 203-26).

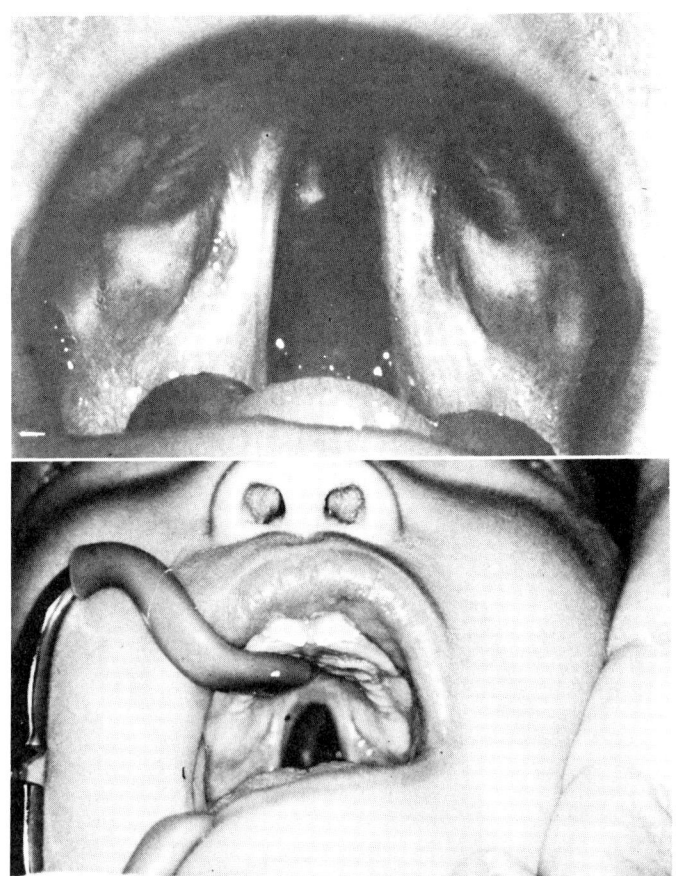

Fig. 203-25. Isolated cleft palate. **A,** Complete; **B,** incomplete.

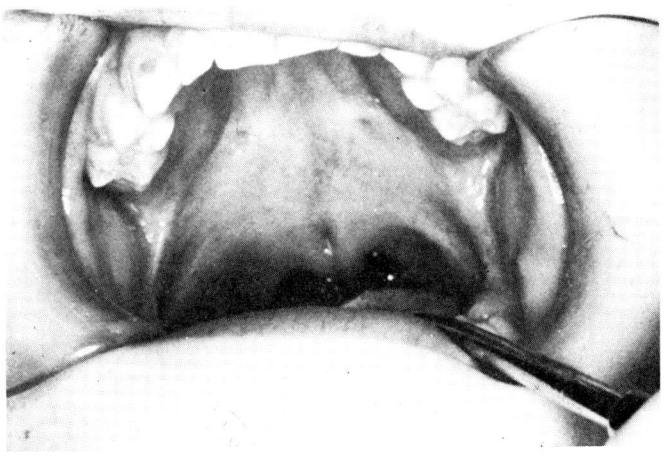

Fig. 203-26. Bifid uvula and submucous cleft palate.

BIBLIOGRAPHY

Clarren, S., and Smith, D.W.: Congenital deformities, Pediatr. Clin. North Am. **24:**665, 1977.

Clifford, E.: Psychosocial aspects of orofacial anomalies: speculations in search of data. In Orofacial anomalies: clinical and research implications, ASHA Reports #8, 1973.

Cohen, M.M., Jr.: An etiologic and nosologic overview of craniosynostosis syndromes, Birth Defects **11:**137, 1975.

Cohen, M.M., Jr., and others: Frontonasal dysplasia (median cleft face syndrome): comments on etiology and pathogenesis, Birth Defects **7:**117, 1971.

DeMeyer, W.: The median cleft face syndrome. Differential diagnosis of cranial bifidum occultum, hypertelorism, and median cleft nose, lip and palate, Neurology **17:**961, 1967.

DeMeyer, W., Zeman, W., and Palmer, C.A.: The face predicts the brain: diagnostic significance of median facial anomalies for holoprosencephaly (arrhinencephaly), Pediatrics **34:**256, 1964.

Di Saia, P.J.: Pregnancy and delivery of a patient with a Starr-Edwards mitral valve prosthesis: report of a case, Obstet. Gynecol. **28**:469, 1966.

Enlow D.E.: The human face: an account of the postnatal growth and development of the craniofacial skeleton, New York, 1968, Harper & Row, Publishers.

Fedrick, J.: Epilepsy and pregnancy: a report from the Oxford Record Linkage Study, Br. Med. J. **2**:442, 1973.

Gorlin, R.J., Pindborg, J.J., and Cohen, M.M., Jr.: Syndromes of the head and neck, ed. 2, New York, 1976, McGraw-Hill Book Co.

Gregg, N.: Congenital cataract following German measles in the mother, Trans. Ophthalmol. Soc. Aust. **3**:35, 1941.

Hardy, J.B.: Clinical and development aspects of congenital rubella, Arch. Otolaryngol. **98**:230, 1973.

Holmes, L.B., and others: Mental retardation—an atlas of diseases with associated physical abnormalities, New York, 1972, Macmillan, Inc.

Johnston, M.C.: Morphogenesis and malformation of face and brain, Birth Defects **11**:1, 1975.

Jones, K.L., and others: Pattern of malformation in offspring of chronic alcoholic mothers, Lancet **1**:1267, 1973.

Jones, K.L., and others: A pattern of craniofacial and limb defects secondary to aberrant tissue bands, J. Pediatr. **84**:90, 1974.

Kawamoto, H.K.: The kaleidoscopic world of craniofacial clefts: order out of chaos (Tessier Classifications), Clin. Plast. Surg. **3**:529, 1976.

Lindsay, W.K.: The epidemiology of usual facial clefts in Ontario, Canada. In Longacre, J. J., editor: Craniofacial anomalies: pathogenesis and repair, Philadelphia, 1968, J.B. Lippincott Co.

Kerber, I.J., Warr, O.S., and Richardson, C.: Pregnancy in a patient with a prosthetic mitral valve associated with the fetal anomaly attributed to warfarin sodium, J.A.M.A. **203**:223, 1968.

Lenz, W.: Chemicals and malformations in man. In Fishbein, M., editor: Congenital malformations, New York, 1964, International Medical Congress.

Mazzola, R.F.: Congenital malformations in the frontonasal area: their pathogenesis and classification, Clin. Plast. Surg. **3**:573, 1976.

Meadow, S.R.: Anticonvulsant drugs and congenital abnormalities, Lancet **2**:1296, 1968.

Meskin, L.N., Gorlin, R.J., and Isaacson, R.J.: Abnormal morphology of the soft palate. 1. The prevalence of cleft uvula, Cleft Palate J. **1**:342, 1964.

Millard, D.R.: Cleft craft. I. The unilateral deformity, Boston, 1976, Little, Brown and Co.

Monson, R.R., and others: Diphenylhydantoin and selected congenital malformations, N. Engl. J. Med. **289**:1049, 1973.

Poswillo, D.: Observations of fetal posture and causal mechanisms of congenital deformity of palate, mandible, and limbs, J. Dent. Res. **45**:584, 1966.

Poswillo, D.: The pathogenesis of the first and second branchial arch syndrome, Oral Surg. **35**:302, 1973.

Pourtois, M.: Influence of cleft lip upon palatal closure in Ajax mice, Cleft Palate J. **4**:120, 1967.

Pruzansky, S.: Clinical investigation of the experiments in nature. In Orofacial anomalies: clincial and research impliciations, ASHA Reports #8, 1973.

Ross, R.B., and Johnston, M.C.: Cleft lip and palate, Baltimore, 1972, The Williams & Wilkins Co.

Sedano, H.O., and others: Frontonasal dysplasia, J. Pediatr. **76**:906, 1970.

Shepard, T.: Catalog of teratogenic agents, ed. 2, Baltimore, 1976, The Johns Hopkins University Press.

Singh, R.P., and Carr, D.H.: Anatomic findings in human abortions of known chromosomal constitutions, Obstet. Gynecol. **29**:806, 1967.

Smith, D.W.: Classification, nomenclature, and naming of morphologic defects, J. Pediatr. **87**:162, 1975.

Smith, D.W.: Recognizable patterns of human malformation, ed. 2, Philadelphia, 1976, W.B. Saunders Co.

Speidel, B.D., and Meadow, S.R.: Maternal epilepsy and abnormalities of the fetus and newborn, Lancet **2**:839, 1972.

Stewart, J.M., Ott, J.E., and LaGace, R.: Submucous cleft palate: prevalance in a school population, Cleft Palate J. **9**:246, 1972.

Stewart, R.E.: Craniofacial malformations clinical and genetic considerations, Pediatr. Clin. North Am. **25**:485, 1978.

Tessier, P.: The definitive plastic surgical treatment of the severe facial deformities of craniofacial dysostosis, Crouzon's and Apert's diseases, Plast. Reconstr. Surg. **48**:419, 1971.

Thiersch, J.B.: Therapeutic abortions with a folic acid antagonist, 4-aminopteroylglutamic acid (4-amino P.G.A.) administered by the oral route, Am. J. Obstet. Gynecol. **63**:1298, 1952.

Trasler, D.G., and Fraser, F.C.: Role of the tongue in producing cleft palate in mice with spontaneous cleft lip, Dev. Biol. **6**:45, 1963.

van der Klaauw, C.J.: Size and position of the functional components of the skull: a contribution to the knowledge of the architecture of the skull, based on data in the literature (conclusion), Arch. Neerl. Zool. **9**:369, 1952.

van Limborgh, J.: A new view on the control of the morphogenesis of the skull, Acta Morphol. Neerl. Scand. **8**:143, 1970.

Warkany, J.: Congenital malformations, Chicago, 1971, Year Book Medical Publishers, Inc.

Wilson, J.G.: Current status of teratology; general principles and mechanisms derived from animal studies. In Wilson, J.G., and Fraser, F.C., editors: Handbook of teratology, vol. 1, New York, 1977, Plenum Press.

Wilson, J.G., and Fraser, F.C., editors: Handbook of teratology, vol. 1 and 2, New York, 1977, Plenum Press.

INDEX

A

A apoproteins, 1281
A locus antigens, 643
AA; see Amyloid A
Abdomen
 abscesses in; see Abscesses, intra-abdominal
 actinomycosis and, 247
 aortic aneurysms and, 565, 567
 aortography and; see Aortography
 bloating and, 960-961; see also Distention
 evaluation of, 12-13, 694
 guarding and, 950
 pain in; see Pain
 paracentesis and, 1044
 roentgenograms of, 1025, 1026; see also Roentgenograms
 ultrasonography and, 969-971
Abdominal angina, 1020
Abdominoperineal resection, 1031, 1041
Abducens nucleus lesions, 766
Abetalipoproteinemia, 1291-1292
Ablative procedures, 444
ABO systems, 348-349
Abortion, spontaneous, 127, 218
Abscesses
 anaerobes and, 249-251
 anal, 1030, 1031
 brain, 139, 191-194, 579, 844
 drainage of, 192, 193, 199
 gingival, diabetes and, 1294
 granulomatous, 357
 intra-abdominal, 1047
  appendiceal, 1015-1016
  Crohn's disease and, 1012
  of intestines, 1007, 1012, 1017, 1019
  of liver; see Liver, abscesses of
  of pancreas, 1054
  of spleen, 398
  ultrasound and, 970
 lung, 698-700
  anaerobic organisms and, 178
  dental care and, 746
  hydatid cysts and, 294
  nontuberculous mycobacteria and, 261
 pelvic, 218
 periapical, diabetes and, 1294
 perinephric, 199
 periodontal, 421, 1294
 peritonsillar, 224, 225
 radiation enteritis and, 1019
 surgical drainage of, 250
 thyroid, 1149
 tubo-ovarian, 218
 Welch's, 253
Absence seizures, 781, 783
Absorption, 940-949
 defective, 1103
 disorders of, 998-1005
 physiology of, 998-999, 1004
Abuse of drugs; see Drug abuse
ABVD therapy; see Doxorubicin, bleomycin, vinblastine, and imidazole carboxamide
Acalculia, 759

Acanthamoeba, 283
Acanthocytes, 315, 806, 1292
Acanthosis nigricans, 887-888
 Bloom's syndrome and, 882
 internal malignancy and, 913, 1035, 1093
ACB; see Antibody-coated bacteria
Access, hemodialysis, 640, 641, 1274
Accessory conduction pathway, 500-501
Accessory ribs, 737
ACE; see Angiotensin-converting enzyme, serum
Acetaldehyde, 776, 1256
Acetaminophen
 allergy and, 28
 aspirin sensitivity and, 24
 dialysis and, 641
 Epstein-Barr virus and, 134
 hyponatremia and, 594
 liver and, 1062, 1075
 osteoarthritis and, 85
 peptic ulcers and, 1092
 pregnancy and, 1212, 1213
 renal disease and, 625, 670
 sulfonylureas and, 1267
 thyroiditis and, 1149
Acetanilid, 329
Acetazolamide
 edema and, 597
 Friedreich's ataxia and, 806
 gout and, 92
 metabolic alkalosis and, 600
 neutropenia and, 360
 pseudotumor cerebri and, 848
Acetohexamide, 1266, 1267
Acetophenetidin, 329
Acetylcholine
 asthma and, 705
 gastric secretion and, 943, 944
 insecticide poisoning and, 754
 myasthenia gravis and, 855
Acetylcysteine, 697, 1075
Acetyl-para-aminophenol, 629
Acetylsalicylic acid; see Aspirin
N_2-Acetylsulfanilamide, 330
ACh; see Acetylcholine
Achalasia, 962, 976-979, 981
Achilles tendinitis, 52
Achlorhydria, 318, 1033, 1035
Achondroplasia, 1245, 1308
Acid; see also Acid-base disorders
 in corrosive agents, ingestion of, 985
 esophagus and, 962, 983
 mucosal barrier to, 943, 996
 poisoning from, 754
 in stomach, 942, 943
  control of, 743
  lack of; see Achlorhydria
  ulcers and, 987-998; see also Digestive system, acid-peptic diseases of
  vomitus and, 957
  Zollinger-Ellison syndrome and, 994-995
 teeth erosion and, 1211
 urine and, 316, 593, 649, 655
Acid back-diffusion, mucosal barrier to, 943, 996

Acid maltase deficiency, 858
Acid peptic disease, 987-998; see also Digestive system, acid peptic diseases of
Acid phosphatase, 397, 435, 660
Acidaminococcus, 249
Acid-base disorders, 588, 593-603; see also Acidosis; Alkalosis; Kidney diseases
 compensation of, 603
 diagnosis of, 602
 homeostasis and kidney in, 592-593
 mixed, 601-603
Acid-fast stains, 119, 1047
Acidification of urine, 593, 655; see also Aciduria
Acidophilus tablets, 908
Acidosis
 biguanides and, 1267
 chronic renal failure and, 636
 glucose-6-phosphate dehydrogenase deficiency and, 330
 ketoacidosis and; see Ketoacidosis
 metabolic, 599-600, 636
 potassium secretion and, 593
 renal tubular, 622-623
 respiratory, 600-601
Acid-peptic diseases, 987-998; see also Digestive system, acid-peptic diseases of
Aciduria, 1238; see also Acidification of urine
 kidney stones and, 649
 megaloblastic anemia and, 316
Acini of pancreas, 1049
Acne, 887, 897
Acoustic neuroma, 795, 844
Acrocentric D chromosomes, 1220
Acrocephalopolysyndactyly, 1314, 1316
Acrocephalosyndactyly, 1314, 1315, 1316
Acrocyanosis, 63
Acrodermatitis enteropathica, 894-895
Acrofacial dysostosis, Nager, 1311
Acrolentiginous melanoma, 918
Acromegaly, 1119-1120
 amenorrhea and, 1177
 dental correlations in, 1204
 skin disorders and, 886
Acropachy, thyroid, 1142, 1143
Acrosclerosis, 58, 903-904
Acylamide, 853
Acrylic, allergy to, 30
Acrylic bite splints, 874
Acrylic extensions, 873
ACTH; see Adrenocorticotropic hormone
Actifed, 1212
Actin, 454
Actinic keratosis, 914, 918
Actinobacillus actinomycete-comitans, 1294
Actinomyces, 247, 250, 305
 endocarditis and, 302
 mycetoma and, 277
 oral infection and, 305
 in pneumonia, 171
Actinomyces israelii, 247, 305
Actinomycin D, 440, 449, 450
Actinomycosis, 247, 305; see also *Actinomyces*

1323

Action potentials, sensory, 806
Acute intermittent porphyria, 854, 888, 1249, 1250-1252
Acute necrotizing ulcerative gingivitis, 302, 307, 862
Acute tubular necrosis, 624-635, 645
Acyanotic heart lesions, 502-506
Acycloguanosine
  cytomegalovirus and, 131
  herpes simplex and, 129
  varicella-zoster and, 130
Acyclovir, 299
Acyl CoA, 534
ADA deficiency; see Adenosine deaminase deficiency
Adamkiewicz, artery of, 835
Addiction; see Alcoholism; Drug abuse
Addison's disease, 1122, 1155-1157; see also Cortisol
  dentistry and, 1207
  hypercalcemia and, 1194
  skin disorders of, 886-887
  tests for, 1156-1157
ADE; see Encephalomyelitis, acute disseminated
Adenine arabinoside, 127, 129, 154, 826
Adenine deaminase deficiency, 1227
Adenitis, 148
Adenocarcinoma; see also Carcinomas
  of anus, 1042
  of colon, 1039-1041, 1093
  of esophagus, 1032-1033
  of gallbladder, 1089
  of lung, 447
  of rectum, 1093
  of small bowel, 1037
  of stomach, 1035-1036, 1093
Adenohypophysis; see Pituitary gland, anterior
Adenoids, 143, 1292
Adenoma sebaceum, 784, 869, 880-881
Adenomas
  aldosterone-producing, 1161
  bronchial, 743
  of liver, 1084
  multiple endocrine, 994, 1164, 1192
  of pancreas, 1056, 1278-1279
  of parathyroid gland, 879, 1192
  polyps and, 1033, 1038
  renal, 656
  sebaceous, 913
  of small bowel, 1037
  of thyroid, 1145, 1150
  thyrotropin-secreting, 1121
Adenopathy; see also Lymph nodes, enlarged; Lymphadenopathy
  erythema nodosum and, 925
  histoplasmosis and, 274
  Hodgkin's disease and, 389
  infectious mononucleosis and, 132
  inguinal, 1
  lymphogranuloma venereum and, 216
  sarcoidosis and, 76, 78, 716, 717
  syphilis and, 266
Adenosine arabinoside, 130, 927
Adenosine deaminase deficiency, 33, 1240
Adenosine diphosphate
  myocardial infarction and, 534
  phosphorus and, 1105
  platelet aggregation and, 400
Adenosine monophosphate, cyclic; see Cyclic adenosine monophosphate
Adenosine triphosphate
  asthma and, 705
  myocardial infarction and, 534
  phosphate metabolism and, 1184

Adenosine triphosphate—cont'd
  phosphorus and, 1105
  receptor concept and, 1115
Adenovillous polyps, 1038
Adenoviruses, 123
  exanthems and, 148
  gastroenteritis and, 149, 150
  respiratory infections and, 140, 143, 172, 177
  vaccine for, 143-144, 148
Adenyl cyclase, 704, 705, 706
Adenylate cyclase, 1187
ADH; see Antidiuretic hormone
ADH catalase; see Alcohol dehydrogenase catalase
Adhesions, violin-string, 231
Adhesive capsulitis, 101
Adipose tissue, 79, 1103; see also Obesity
Adiposogenital dystrophy, 1124-1125
Administration route, 157
ADP; see Adenosine diphosphate
Adrenal cortex, 1153-1163
  adrenocorticotropic hormone and; see Corticosteroids
  alcohol and, 1258
  congenital hyperplasia and, 1162-1163
  dentistry and, 1206-1207
  function of, 1153-1155
  and glucocorticoids; see also Glucocorticoids
    deficiency syndromes in, 1155-1157; see also Addison's disease
    excess syndromes in, 1157-1159; see also Cushing's syndrome
  and mineralocorticoids; see also Mineralocorticoids
    deficiency syndromes in, 1159-1160
    excess syndromes in, 1160-1162; see also Aldosteronism
  skin disorders and, 887
  structure of, 1153-1155
Adrenal glands
  congenital hyperplasias of, 1162-1163
  cortex of; see Adrenal cortex
  corticosteroids and; see Corticosteroids
  Cushing's syndrome and; see Cushing's syndrome
  dentistry and, 1207
  enzyme deficiency and, hypogonadism in, 1171
  idiopathic atrophy of, 1155-1156
  insufficiency of, 1122, 1155-1157; see also Addison's disease
    anterior pituitary insufficiency and, 1122
    dentistry and, 1207
    malabsorption and, 1004
    skin disorders of, 886-887
  liver disease and, 1062
  medullary hyperplasia of, 1164-1168
  mineralocorticoids and; see Mineralocorticoids
  pheochromocytoma and, 1164-1168
  removal of, 444, 448
  tests for, 1156, 1157, 1158, 1159, 1161, 1163
Adrenalectomy
  breast cancer and, 448
  medical, 444
  neoplasia and, 444
Adrenergics
  as agonists
    asthma and, 24, 704, 705, 706, 707
    chronic obstructive pulmonary disease and, 693
    respiratory failure and, 711
  alpha, hypertension and, 473, 474
  beta, 19; see also Beta-adrenergic blockers
  hypertension and, 467, 472, 473, 474

Adrenergics—cont'd
  thyroid hormones and, 1132
Adrenocorticosteroids; see Corticosteroids
Adrenocorticotropic hormone, 93, 1117-1118
  alcohol and, 1258
  biosynthesis and, 1153
  cortisol and, 1154
  Crohn's disease and, 1014
  deficiency of, 1122, 1156-1157, 1162-1163
  ectopic secretion of, 435, 437
  excess of, 1157-1159
  heart rate and, 458
  metyrapone test and, 1157, 1158
  multiple sclerosis and, 801
  neoplasms and, 1179, 1180-1181
    renal cell, 657
    Zollinger-Ellison syndrome and, 994
  releasing factor for, 1118, 1155, 1157, 1159
  side effects of, 1010-1011
  stimulation tests for, 1122, 1156-1157
  ulcerative colitis and, 1010-1011
Adrenogenital syndrome, 1162-1163
Adrenoleukodystrophy, 802
Adriamycin; see Doxorubicin
Adson maneuver, 100
Adult respiratory distress syndrome, 477, 708-709
  bacteremia and, 240
  right-to-left shunts and, 682
  Rocky Mountain spotted fever and, 211
  septic shock and, 240
Advanced life support, 540
Adventitious lung sounds, 12, 685
Adynamic ileus, 1024, 1025, 1026
Aerophagia, 960
Aerosolized tantalum powder, 689
AEt, 385, 386
Affect, 763
Afibrinogenemia, 429
Aflatoxins, 432, 656, 1084
AFP; see Alpha-fetoprotein
African trypanosomiasis, 286-287
Afterload, 454, 457, 458, 460
Agammaglobulinemia, 31, 33
Agar diffusion test, 155
Agar dilution test, 155
Agenesis
  müllerian, 1176
  renal, 649
  of thymus, 1196
  thyroid, 1137
Agglutinin disease, cold, 418
Agglutinin tests; see Hemagglutinin tests; Microhemagglutination tests
Agnogenic myeloid metaplasia, 374-376
Agnosia, 759, 763, 770, 771
Agranulocytosis, 358-361
Agraphesthesia, 759
Agraphia, 759
AHF; see Antihemophilic factor
AIHA; see Autoimmune disease, hemolytic anemias in
AIP; see Acute intermittent porphyria
Air bronchograms, 702-703
Air embolism, 688, 701
Air pollution, 691, 738; see also Environment
Airway; see also Airway obstruction
  artificial, 711
  syncope and, 864
Airway obstruction, 680, 690, 693, 694; see also Respiratory diseases
  bronchi and; see Bronchi, obstruction of
  dental care in bronchitis and, 745
  drug abuse and, 863

Airway obstruction—cont'd
 intraluminal, 710
 lung cancer and, 740
 supportive care and, 445
 upper, 713
Airway resistance, 680
AIU; see Iodine uptake, absolute
Akinetic mutism, 764
Akineton; see Biperiden
AL chains; see Amyloid light chains
ALA; see δ-Aminolevulinic acid
ALA synthase; see δ-Aminolevulinic acid synthase
Albinism, oculocutaneous, 1236
Albright's syndrome, 104, 879
Albumin, 350
 ascites and, 1045, 1083
 bilirubin and, 1057
 hepatitis and, 1071
 liver disease and, 1065, 1071
 nephrotic syndrome and, 612-613
 organ preservation and, 644
 posthemorrhagic anemia and, 323
 prerenal azotemia and, 632
 pseudomembranous enterocolitis and, 1018
 radiolabeled, 352, 492, 687, 966
 right ventricular infarction and, 536
 salt-poor, ascites and, 1083
 serum; see Serum, albumin in
 thyroxine-binding, 1131, 1134
 in urine, 605, 912
Albuterol, 706
Alcohol
 abuse of; see Alcoholism
 antihypertensives and, 574
 body fluid osmolality and, 596
 bruxism and, 861
 calories in, 1104
 carbon tetrachloride and, 1075
 cardiomyopathy and, 520
 cephalosporins and, 165
 coronary artery disease and, 527
 dietary restriction of, 92
 drug interactions with, 1297, 1298
 encephalopathies and, 768
 esophagitis and, 982
 in fetal alcohol syndrome, 1303, 1304
 folate deficiency and, 316, 317
 gastrointestinal disease and, 943, 958, 994, 996, 1001
 gout and, 91
 griseofulvin and, 279
 hematologic effects of, 1257-1258
 hemolysis and, 342
 Hodgkin's disease and, 387
 hypernatremia and, 595
 hypoglycemia and, 1270, 1277, 1279
 hypoparathyroidism and, 1196
 hypothermia and, 756
 ileal mucosa and, 317
 lipoproteins and, 1284, 1287, 1288, 1289
 liver disease and, 1059, 1063, 1075, 1080-1081
 metabolic encephalopathies and, 768
 metabolism of, 1255-1256
 metronidazole and, 170
 neoplasia and, 446, 659
 nephropathy and, 629, 630
 neutrophils and, 356-357
 nutritional deficiencies and, 1001, 1059, 1062-1063, 1080
 osteoporosis and, 1202
 pancreatitis and, 1051, 1055, 1258
 phosphate deficiency and, 1188

Alcohol—cont'd
 porphyria and, 854, 888, 1252, 1254
 premalignant lesions and, 919
 procarbazine and, 443
 seizures and, 786, 787
 sulfonylureas and, 1267
 thrombocytopenia and, 400, 401
 toxic effect of, 1255-1259
 tremor and, 816
Alcohol dehydrogenase catalase, 1255
Alcoholism, 775-776; see also Alcohol
 cirrhosis and, 1080-1081
 dentistry and, 862-864, 1296-1298
 drug detoxification and, 1062
 esophageal disorders and, 982
 folate deficiency and, 316, 317, 1109
 hemolysis and, 343
 ketoacidosis and, 1270-1271
 malabsorption and, 1001; see also Alcohol, nutritional deficiencies and
 myopathies and, 859
 neuropathy and, 849, 853, 1257
 oral manifestations of, 1296-1298
 parotid gland enlargement and, 1097-1098
 pyridoxine deficiency and, 1109
 thiamine and, 1108
 withdrawal and, 776, 784, 786, 787, 1080, 1257, 1258, 1298
Aldehyde reaction, 1256
Aldolase, 60, 65, 853
Aldomet; see Methyldopa
Aldosterone, 1153, 1154, 1155, 1162-1163
 blood pressure and, 467, 468
 cirrhosis and ascites and, 1061, 1062
 deficiency of, 1156, 1159-1160
 excess of, 468, 469, 470, 474, 1160-1162
 heart failure and, 461
 heart rate and, 458
 hyporeninemic hypoaldosteronism and, 623
 potassium and, 593, 597, 598
 sodium reabsorption and, 592
 triiodothyronine and, 1132
Aldosteronism, 468, 469, 474, 1160-1162
 blood pressure and, 468, 470, 474
 cirrhosis and ascites and, 1061, 1062
Alexander's disease, 803
ALG; see Antilymphocyte globulin
Alkali; see also Alkalosis
 in corrosive agents, ingestion of, 985, 986
 kidney stones and, 649
 poisoning from, 754
 renal failure in myeloma and, 618
 renal tubular acidosis and, 623
Alkaline phosphatase
 bone, 1189
 gallbladder disease and, 1088
 hyperparathyroidism and, 1208
 leukocyte, polycythemia vera and, 353
 liver disease and, 1065, 1066, 1068, 1071
 neoplastic biliary disease and, 1089
 Paget's disease and, 87
 placental tumors and, 435
 plasma, 1189
 temporal arteritis and, 75
Alkaloids, vinca; see Vinca alkaloids
Alkalosis
 metabolic, 600, 967
 penicillins and, 164
 potassium secretion and, 593
 respiratory, 601
Alkaptonuria, 1236
Alkylating agents, 440, 442-443; see also specific agent
 amyloidosis and, 617

Alkylating agents—cont'd
 as carcinogens, 432
 carcinoid tumors and, 450
 histiocytosis and, 398
 hypogonadism and, 1172
 leukemias and, 364, 366, 370, 371, 372
 myeloid metaplasia and, 376
 myeloma and, 382, 618
 neutropenia and, 358
 ovarian carcinoma and, 449
 in thrombocythemia, 374
 Waldenström's macroglobulinemia and, 383, 618
ALL; see Lymphoblastic leukemias, acute
Alleles, 1217-1219
Allergens, 19
 drugs and, 28
 hypersensitivity pneumonitis and, 727
 rhinitis and, 20
Allergy
 angiitis and, 66, 67
 angioedema and, 25-26
 aspergillosis and, 277, 705
 asthma and, 23-25, 704, 705, 728
 atopy and, 19-25; see also Atopy
 contact dermatitis and, 27
 diarrhea and, 954
 drug, 27-30
  anaphylactic shock and, 576
  angioedema and, 25, 26
  contrast materials in, 606; see also Contrast agents
  insulin in, 1268
  Schönlein-Henoch purpura and, 70
 ear pain and, 867
 food; see Food allergy
 immunology and, 15-19, 31-34
 interstitial nephritis and, 620
 to pollens, immunotherapy in, 22
 pulmonary vasculitides and, 719
 rhinitis and, 20, 22-23
 serum sickness and, 26-27
 transfusions and, 351
 urticaria and, 25-26
Allodermanyssus sanguineus, 211
Allogeneic leukocyte transfusion, 263
Alloimmune anemia, 337
Allopurinol
 gout and, 92
 kidney stones and, 648
 Lesch-Nyhan syndrome and, 1239
 leukemias and, 368, 372
 6-mercaptopurine and, 441
 multiple myeloma and, 382
 nephropathy and, 622, 624, 625
 thiazide-induced hyperuricemia and, 472
 tumor cell breakdown and, 447
Alopecia
 acrodermatitis enteropathica and, 895
 lupus erythematosus and, 55
 sarcoidosis and, 910
 syphilis and, 268
Alpha chain, beta-thalassemia and, 336
Alpha fetoprotein, 435, 809, 1229
Alpha globulins
 deficiency of, 1082
 liver disease and, 1065
 nephrotic syndrome and, 612
Alpha rays, 749
Alpha-adrenergic blockade, 473, 474
Alpha-l-antiprotease deficiency, 694
Alpha-l-antitrypsin, 172, 693, 694, 1082
Alpha-L-fucosidase deficiency, 1235

Alpha-hemolytic streptococci, 222; see also Streptococci
7-Alpha-hydroxylase, 1085
17-Alpha-hydroxylase deficiency, 1162, 1163
Alpha-L-iduronidase, 1233, 1234, 1302
Alpha-D-mannosidase deficiency, 1235
Alpha-methylacetoacetic aciduria, 1238
17-Alpha-methylated testosterone, 1173
Alpha-methyl-beta-hydroxybutyric aciduria, 1237-1238
Alphamethyldopa; see Methyldopa
Alpha-methyl-para-tyrosine, 812
Alpha-thalassemias, 336
Alport's syndrome, 611-612
ALS; see Amyotrophic lateral sclerosis
Alternaria, 727
Altitudes, hypoxemia and, 681-682
Aluminum antacids, 633, 992; see also Aluminum hydroxide; Antacids
Aluminum carbonate, 639
Aluminum hydroxide
  esophagitis and, 985
  phosphate deficiency and, 1188
  renal failure and, 639
  renal osteodystrophy and, 1201
Alveolar bone
  histiocytosis X and, 425
  osteoporosis and, 115, 1205, 1210
Alveolar cell carcinomas, 59
Alveolar gas; see also Carbon dioxide tension, arterial; Oxygen tension
  composition of, 673, 681
  exchange of, 673, 674-676, 682, 708, 711; see also Ventilation, alveolar
Alveolar hypoventilation, 682, 708, 711; see also Ventilation, alveolar
Alveolar macrophages, 172, 686
Alveolar-arterial oxygen tension difference, 673, 681
Alveoli, 672, 685; see also Alveolar gas
Alzheimer's disease, 774, 846
Amalgam, allergy to, 30
Amalgam tattoos, 919
Amantadine
  influenza and, 132
  parkinsonism and, 815, 870
  spasmodic torticollis and, 820
  viruses and, 154
Amaurosis fugax, 836
Amaurotic idiocy, infantile, 1230-1231; see also Tay-Sachs disease
Ambilhar; see Niridazole
Amblyopia, nutritional, 850
Amebiasis, 189, 203, 281-283
Ameboma, 282, 283
Amenorrhea
  adrenal hyperplasia and, 1162
  functional, 1176-1177
  prolactinoma and, 1120
American Society for Dentistry for the Handicapped, 872
American trypanosomiasis, 286, 287
Ames' assay, 433
Amicar; see ε-Aminocaproic acid
Amides, allergy to, 30
Amikacin, 161, 166
  anaerobic infections and, 250
  bacterial meningitis and, 190
  gram-negative bacillary bacteremia and, 241
  pregnancy and, 1212
Amiloride
  edema and, 597
  hyperkalemia and, 598
  hypertension and, 472

Amine precursor uptake decarboxylation cells, 941, 994, 1179
Amines, 1115, 1205
Amino acids; see also Proteins
  branched-chain, 1237-1238
  calcitonin and, 1189
  deoxyribonucleic acid and, 1216
  essential, 1104
  gastric secretion and, 943, 944, 947
  liver disease and, 1062-1063
  metabolic disorders and, 587-590, 1226-1227, 1236-1238
  parathyroid hormone and, 1187
  parenteral nutrition and, 445
Aminoacidopathies, 1226-1227, 1236-1238
γ-Aminobutyric acid, 817, 1252
ε-Aminocaproic acid, 429
  epistaxis and, 1095
  fibrinolytic states and, 413
  hemophilia and, 410, 428
  liver disease and, 411
  platelet transfusion and, 426
  polycythemia vera and, 419
  sickle cell disease and, 618
  subarachnoid hemorrhage and, 840
  thrombasthenia and, 426
  von Willebrand's disease and, 427
Aminoglutethimide, 444
Aminoglycosides, 161, 165-167; see also specific agent
  abdominal abscess and, 1047
  administration route for, 157, 159
  anaerobic infections and, 250
  bacteremia and, 241
  bactericidal activity of, 156
  bronchiectasis and, 697
  chancroid and, 239
  dosages of, 157-158
  endocarditis and, 184
  enterococci and, 227
  excretion of, 158
  listeriosis and, 246
  meningitis and, 190
  myasthenia gravis and, 856
  neoplasia and, 446
  nephritis and, 619, 620
  pancreatitis and, 1053
  parenteral, failure of, 159
  peritonitis and, 1047
  for *Pseudomonas,* 177, 306
  renal insufficiency and, 158
  site of infection and, 157, 159
  toxicity of, 158, 625, 627, 628, 630, 631
  in tuberculosis, 259
  viridans streptococci and, 228
δ-Aminolevulinic acid, 1248, 1252, 1254
δ-Aminolevulinic acid synthase, 1247
Aminophylline, 706, 728, 1212
Aminopterin syndrome, 1303
Aminopyrine, 23, 329, 360
Aminorex, 496
Aminosalicylate, 627, 1010
Aminosalicylate sodium, 627
p-Aminosalicylic acid
  drug-induced disease and, 329, 721, 722
  globoid cell leukodystrophy and, 802
  hemolysis and, 329, 342
  ileal mucosa and, 317
  lung disease and, 259, 721, 722
  malabsorption and, 1002
  thrombocytopenia and, 400
  in tuberculosis, 259
2-Amino-5-sulfanilythiazole, 330
Aminotransferase elevation, 1088

Amiodarone, 1131
Amipaque; see Metrizamide
Amitriptyline
  headache and, 789
  hyponatremia and, 594
  lung disease and, 722
  neurologic effects of, 779
  parkinsonism and, 815
  salivary flow and, 870
AML; see Leukemias, acute myelogenous
Ammonia
  fatty liver and, 1077
  hepatic coma and, 1061
  inhalational lung disease and, 729
  in saliva, 666, 667
  spirits of, 576, 864
  urea cycle disorders and, 1238
Ammonium chloride, 600, 777, 779
Amnesias, 759, 763, 770, 772, 836
Amniocentesis, 1229
Amoeba, 139
Amorphosynthesis, 759
Amoxicillin, 160, 164
  diarrhea from, 1018
  gonococcal infections and, 232
  Haemophilus influenzae and, 236
  lung abscess and, 699
  renal disease and, 670
  urinary tract infection and, 197, 198
AMP, cyclic; see Cyclic adenosine monophosphate
Amphetamines
  abuse of, 862
  cerebrovascular accident and, 829
  Gilles de la Tourette's syndrome and, 822
  guanethidine and, 472
  hypertension and, 469
  toxicity of, 625, 626, 629, 777
Amphojel; see Aluminum hydroxide
Amphotericin B, 278
  aspergillosis and, 276
  blastomycosis and, 275
  Candida and, 276, 308, 422, 929, 985
  chromomycosis and, 277
  coccidioidomycosis and, 275
  cryptococcosis and, 276
  drug fever and, 159
  endocarditis and, 184
  with flucytosine, 278
  histoplasmosis and, 275, 307
  intertrigo and, 929
  monilial infection and, 299
  mucormycosis and, 277
  Naegleria meningoencephalitis and, 283
  neoplasia and, 446
  pregnancy and, 1212
  renal tubular acidosis and, 623
  sporotrichosis and, 81, 276
  toxic nephropathy and, 625, 627, 628, 630
Ampicillin, 159, 160, 163
  anaerobic infections and, 250
  asthma and, 728
  bacteremia and, 208, 241
  bronchiectasis and, 697
  bronchitis and, 693
  cholecystitis and, 1089
  diarrhea from, 1018
  endocarditis and, 185
  enteric fever and, 202, 208
  enterococci and, 227
  gonococcal infections and, 232, 302
  Haemophilus influenzae and, 176, 236
  hepatitis and, 1099
  listeriosis and, 246

Ampicillin—cont'd
  lung abscess and, 699
  meningitis and, 190
  pancreatitis and, 1053
  pregnancy and, 1212
  renal disease and, 627, 629, 670
  respiratory failure and, 711
  shigellosis and, 202, 206
  toxic nephropathy and, 627, 629
  urinary tract infection and, 197, 198
Amprolium, 728
Ampulla of Vater carcinoma, 1089
Amputations, 253, 1273
  clostridial infection and, 253
  diabetes mellitus and, 1273
Amyl nitrite, 748
Amylase, 954, 1049, 1052, 1102
Amyloid, 617, 719 see also Amyloidosis
Amyloid A, 385, 386
Amyloid fibrils, 385, 386
Amyloid light chains, 385-386
Amyloidosis, 385-387
  cardiomyopathies and, 523
  dentistry and, 423-424
  lung and, 719
  malabsorption and, 1003
  Mediterranean fever and, 1048
  myeloma and, 422, 899
  neuropathy and, 854
  purpura and, 406
  reactive systemic, 385
  renal lesions and, 617
Amyotrophic lateral sclerosis, 803-804, 868, 869
Amyotrophy, 803-804, 860-861, 1275
ANA; see Antinuclear antibodies
Anabolic steroids
  liver disease and, 1076
  multiple myeloma and, 382
  osteoporosis and, 89
  renal failure and, 639
  thyroxine binding globulin and, 1134
Anaerobic bacteria, 249-254; see also Anaerobic cocci
  clostridial, 251-254
  cultures for, 250
  nonsporeforming, 249-251, 253
  pneumonia and, 172, 177-178
Anaerobic cocci, 177, 228, 230-235, 249, 303; see also Anaerobic bacteria
Analgesics; see also specific agent
  abuse of, 778
  avascular necrosis and, 104
  bursitis and, 98
  dermatomyositis and, 905
  disc disease and, 860
  drug-induced hemolysis and, 329
  for facial pain of cerebrovascular accident, 872
  hemophilia and, 428
  hepatitis and, 1099
  herpangina and, 301
  herpes simplex and, 129, 927
  hyperthyroidism and, 1205
  hypothyroidism and, 1206
  influenza and, 141
  kidney stones and, 649
  lumbar puncture headache and, 790
  mumps and, 140
  neutropenia and, 360
  Paget's disease and, 87-88
  peptic ulcers and, 1092
  phlebitis and, 495
  pregnancy and, 1212, 1213
  renal disease and, 670
    nephritis in, 619, 621

Analgesics—cont'd
  renal disease and—cont'd
    nephropathy in, 625, 627, 629
  in respiratory disease, 745, 746
  rotator cuff tears and, 101
  shock and, 575
  sickle cell anemia and, 417
  tendinitis and, 99
  thrombocytopenia and, 426
  thrombocytosis and, 426
  Trichinella spiralis and, 203
  urinary tract neoplasms and, 658
  varicella-zoster and, 130
Anaphylactoid purpura; see Schönlein-Henoch purpura
Anaphylatoxin, 17
Anaphylaxis, 17, 28, 29, 476, 478
  dentistry and, 30, 576
  eosinophilic chemotactic factor of, 372, 705
  management of, 29
  purpura and; see Schönlein-Henoch purpura
  slow-reacting substance of, 18, 372, 705
  transfusion reactions and, 351
Anasarca, 612
Anastomoses; see also Cardiac shunts
  of aorta to pulmonary artery, side-to-side, 507
  of bowel
    Crohn's disease and, 1015
    diverticulosis and, 1018
    esophageal disorders and, 982, 985-986
    megacolon and, 1026
    neoplasms and, 1041
    and rectal stump, 1026
    ulcerative colitis and, 1011
  mesocaval, 1083
  portacaval, 1083
  splenorenal, 1083
  between subclavian artery and pulmonary artery, 507
  Waterston, 507
Anatomy
  of coronary artery, 524-526
  of esophagus, 972-974
  of perianal region, 1029-1030
  of peritoneum, 1043
  of thyroid gland, 1126-1128
Ancylostoma, 172, 291, 721
Ancylostoma braziliense, 291
Ancylostoma duodenale, 172, 291
Andrade amyloidosis, 854
Androgenic steroids
  multiple myeloma and, 382
  thrombocytopenia and, 402
  for tumors, 444
Androgens, 1169, 1170
  anemia and, 320, 321, 322, 361
  angioedema and, 26
  bone marrow and, 361, 1203
  cholestasis and, 1076
  congenital adrenal hyperplasia and, 1162
  dialysis and, 642
  hereditary hemorrhagic telangiectasia and, 1024
  hypergonadism and, 1173
  hypogonadism and, 1122, 1170-1173
  myeloid metaplasia and, 376
  osteoporosis and, 1203
  paroxysmal nocturnal hemoglobinuria and, 342
  porphyria and, 1252
  receptors for, 443
  renal cell carcinomas and, 658
  synthesis of, 1153
  thyroxine binding globulin and, 1134
Androstenedione, 1153

Andy Gump caricature, 36
ANE; see Encephalomyelitis, acute necrotizing
Anemias, 310-351
  alloimmune, 337
  aplastic, 319-320
    chloramphenicol and, 168, 169
    dentistry and, 415
    idiopathic, 319
    neutropenia and, 358
    platelet production and, 401
    sickle cell anemia and, 332
  blood banking and, 346-351
  cardiomyopathies and, 523
  of chronic disease, 324, 325-326, 667
  colorectal carcinoma and, 1040
  Cooley's, 334-335
  Crohn's disease and, 1015
  dentistry and, 414-420
  diagnosis in, 310, 311, 312, 313-315
  Diamond-Blackfan, 318, 319
  endocarditis and, 182
  enzyme deficiency and, 418
  Fanconi's, 168, 318, 319, 624
  gastric carcinoma and, 1035
  gastric polyps and, 1034
  gastrointestinal bleeding and, 958, 1092
  heavy-chain disease and, 384
  hemochromatosis in, 345-346
  hemoglobin pigment abnormalities in, 343-344
  hemolytic, 326-343; see also Hemolytic anemia
  hexokinase deficiency, 418
  histiocytic medullary reticulosis and, 398
  history and, 312-313
  Hodgkin's disease and, 387
  hypersplenism and, 396
  hypochromic microcytic, 323-325
  hypoplastic, 319-320
  iron deficiency; see Iron deficiency anemia
  iron metabolism disorders in, 311, 345-356, 1240
  lead poisoning and, 753
  leukemias and, 364, 366, 368, 371
  liver disease and, 1063-1064
  lupus erythematosus and, 56
  malaria and, 280
  megaloblastic, 316-318, 358
  multiple myeloma and, 379
  myeloid metaplasia and, 375
  myelophthisic, 322-323
  pernicious; see Pernicious anemia
  physical examination and, 312-313
  posthemorrhagic, 323
  pyridoxine-responsive, 325
  red cell destruction, 326-343
    acquired, 337-343
    congenital, 326-343; see also Hemolytic anemia, congenital
  red cell production, 311-326
    bone marrow failure and, 318-323
    chronic disease and, 324, 325-326
    hypochromic microcytic, 323-325
    iron deficiency; see Iron deficiency anemia
    megaloblastic, 316-318, 358
    myelophthisic, 322-323
    pathology of, 311-312
    posthemorrhagic, 323
    refractory, 320
    sideroblastic, 308-309, 1257-1258
  refractory, 320-321
  renal failure and, 636, 639
  sickle cell; see Sickle cell disease
  sideroblastic, 308-309, 1257-1258
  spur cell, 343

Anemias—cont'd
  transfusions and, 346-351
  ulcerative colitis and, 1008
  Waldenström's macroglobulinemia and, 382
Anergy, 257, 911
Anesthetics
  alveolar hypoventilation and, 682
  angina and, 583
  anorectal disorders and, 1031
  antihypertensives and, 574
  arrhythmia and, 585
  Candida and, 929
  catecholamines with, coronary heart disease and, 583
  diabetes insipidus and, 621
  drug abusers and, 863
  hemolysis and, 342
  hemophilia and, 427
  hyperpyrexia and, 858
  hypertension and, 574
  hypothyroidism and, 1206
  liver toxicity and, 1076
  local; *see* Local anesthetics
  malignant hyperthermia and, 875
  nephritis and, 620, 621
  nephropathy and, 625, 627, 628, 629, 630, 631
  pericarditis and, 550
  pheochromocytoma and, 1165
  pregnancy and, 1213
  in renal disease, 669-670
  in respiratory disease, 745, 747
  seizures and, 866
  sickle cell anemia and, 417
  thrombocytopenia and, 426
  topical
    epidermolysis bullosa dystrophica and, 878
    erythema migrans and, 938
    erythema multiforme and, 924
    herpes simplex and, 129
    lichen planus and, 939
    oral ulcers from chemotherapy and, 451
    pemphigoid and, 935
    pemphigus and, 933
    psoriasis and, 937
    radiation stomatitis and, 919
    Reiter's syndrome and, 908
    scalded skin syndrome and, 932
    ulcerative stomatitis and, 415
  von Willebrand's disease and, 426
Aneuploidy, 1221
Aneurysms, 565-567
  aortic, 470, 559, 560
  Charcot-Bouchard, 838
  circle of Willis, 839, 1275
  fusiform, 839
  Kawasaki disease and, 147
  mediastinal, 735-736
  mycotic, 181
  popliteal artery, 567
  subarachnoid, 839-840
  syphilitic, 269
  ventricular, 536-537
Angel dust, 778-779
Angel wings, 725
Angiitis, allergic, 66, 67; *see also* Vasculitis
Angina; *see also* Angina pectoris
  abdominal, 1020
  dentistry and, 583
  intestinal, 949, 951, 989
  Prinzmetal's variant, 533
  unstable, 532
  Vincent's, 224

Angina pectoris, 527-533; *see also* Angina
  effort-induced, 529
  electrocardiogram and, 484
  with normal coronary arteries, 533
  postprandial, 949
Angiocardiography, 488-489, 536
Angioedema, 17, 25-26, 351
Angiofibromatous hamartoma, 880
Angiography
  aortic dissection and, 562
  arterial occlusion and, 569
  cerebral, 564-565, 761
  coronary, 489, 530-531
  gastrointestinal, 771-772, 959, 1021
  neurologic diseases and, 761
  of pancreas, 1057, 1278
  pulmonary, 489, 492, 493, 689-690
  renal, 606, 607, 657, 661-662
  spinal, 762
Angioid streaks, 87, 884
Angiokeratoma corporis diffusum, 668, 911-912, 1231-1232
Angiokeratomas, 911-912, 1231-1232
  dentistry and, 668, 1296
  of palate, 912
Angiolipomas, renal, 656
Angiomas
  dentistry and, 869, 872, 881-882
  encephalotrigeminal, 810, 881-882
  hemorrhage from, 882
  of jaw, Sturge-Weber syndrome and, 869
  spider, 863, 894, 896, 1059
Angiomatosis, craniofacial, 881-882
Angioneurotic edema, 17, 25-26, 30, 351
Angio-osteohypertrophy, 881-882
Angiosarcomas of liver, 1084
Angiotensin, 1155
  aldosterone deficiency and, 1159
  blood pressure and, 467, 468
  heart failure and, 462
  heart rate and, 458
  inhibitors of, 467, 1161
  renal artery stenosis and, 661
  shock and, 477
  toxemia of pregnancy and, 665
Angiotensin-converting enzyme, serum, 77-78, 717, 718
Angular cheilitis, 276, 1298
  iron deficiency and, 1105
  Plummer-Vinson syndrome and, 1091, 1105
  protein malnutrition and, 1104
  pyridoxine deficiency and, 1109
  vitamin B_{12} deficiency and, 1109
Angular cheilosis; *see also* Cheilosis
  niacin deficiency and, 1110
  psoriasis and, 937
  riboflavin deficiency and, 1108
Anhydrotic ectodermal dysplasia, 876-877, 1308
Aniline dyes, 659
Anionic exchange resins, 1290
Anisakiasis, 291
Anisakis marina, 291
Ankle, 77, 102
Ankylosing spondylitis, 48-50, 737-738
  inflammatory bowel disease and, 1006, 1008
  pulmonary fibrosis and, 716
  valvular disease and, 580
Ankylosis; *see also* Ankylosing spondylitis
  fibrous, intermaxillary fixation and, 106
  juvenile rheumatoid arthritis and, 106
  of temporomandibular joint, 107, 861
Ann Arbor staging, 388-389
Annular pancreas, 1050

Anodontia, anhydrotic ectodermal dysplasia and, 877
Anomalad, 1301
Anomalies
  cardiovascular, 497-509; *see also* Congenital heart disease
  Ebstein's, 507-508, 554
  Pelger-Huët-like, 321
  renal, 649-650
  ureteral, 650-651
  of urethra, 651
  of urinary bladder, 651
Anopheles mosquito, 279
Anorchia, 1170
Anorectal disorders, 1029-1031; *see also* Anus
Anorexia, 496, 961, 1102, 1124, 1125
Anorexia nervosa, 1124, 1125
Anosognosia, 759
Anovulatory drugs; *see* Oral contraceptives
Anserine bursitis, 99
Antabuse; *see* Disulfiram
Antacids
  acidosis and, 633
  aluminum, 633, 992; *see also* Aluminum hydroxide
  calcium and, 1190
  dialysis and, 642
  digestive system pain and, 950, 975, 996
    peptic ulcers and, 987, 988, 989, 991-992, 993, 994, 1092
    stress erosions and, 996
  electrical injury and, 752
  in esophageal disorders, 62, 736, 981, 985
  gaseousness and, 961
  gastrointestinal bleeding, 959
  hepatitis and, 1072
  hiatus hernia and, 736
  low-salt, 992
  pancreatitis and, 1053, 1056
  renal osteodystrophy and, 1201
Antagonism of antimicrobials, 156; *see also* Antimicrobials
Antegrade pyelography, 607; *see also* Pyelography
Anterior descending coronary arteries, 524
Anterior horn cell disease, 803-804
Anterior inferior cerebellar artery syndrome, 833
Anterior spinal artery syndrome, 835-836
Anthracycline antibiotics, 366, 367, 440, 441
Anthralin, 937
Anthrax, 245, 305
Anti-acetylcholine receptor antibody, 19
Anti-alpha-adrenergic agents, 450
Antianthrax serum, 305
Antiarrhythmic agents, 585; *see also* specific agent
Antiasthmatics, 705, 706, 707; *see also* Asthma
Antibiotics; *see also* Antimicrobials; specific agent
  abscesses and
    abdominal, 1047
    liver, 1075
    lung, 699-700
  acute necrotizing ulcerative gingivitis and, 302
  adult respiratory distress syndrome and, 709
  anaerobic infections and, 251
  aneurysm resection and, 567
  antacids and, 1092
  anthracycline, 366, 367, 440, 441
  antitumor, 441, 446
  aplastic anemia and, 416
  appendicitis and, 1016
  bacterial endocarditis and, 301-302

Antibiotics—cont'd
bowel obstruction and, 1026
bronchiectasis and, 697
bronchitis and, 691, 693
bullae and, 701
bursitis and, 98
Candida and, 307, 929, 1092
caustic ingestion and, 985
cavernous sinus thrombosis and, 303
congenital heart disease and, 579
corticosteroids and, 1207
cystic fibrosis and, 700
diabetes and, 1273, 1275, 1295
dialysis and, 641
diarrhea from, 1018
diphtheria and, 248
diverticulosis and, 1018
endocarditis and, 183, 184, 185, 506, 581
erythema multiforme and, 30, 924
glomerulonephritis and, 610
gonococcal stomatitis and, 302
gram-negative oral lesions and, 306
hemolysis from, 329
hepatitis and, 1099
histiocytosis and, 398
hyperthyroidism and, 1205
interstitial nephritis and, 619
intestinal ulcer and, 1019
ischemic colitis and, 1021
leukemias and, 366, 367, 368, 372
lupus erythematosus and, 111
Lyell's disease and, 932
mediastinitis and, 105, 734
mitral valve prolapse and, 511
in mouthwash, 451
multiple myeloma and, 422
neoplasia and, 441, 446
nephrotic syndrome and, 613
neutropenia and, 360, 361
neutrophil dysfunction and, 420
nongonococcal septic arthritis and, 80
obstructive uropathy and, 656
oral ulcers and, 415, 421, 422
for osteomyelitis, 82, 116, 222
Paget's disease and, 114
pancreatitis and, 1053
pemphigus and, 933, 934
pericarditis and, 553, 586
pregnancy and, 1212, 1213
prosthetic valves and, 515
pulmonary fibrosis and, 714
radiation and, 750, 1019
regimens for, 162-163
renal disease and, 613, 617, 634, 639, 670
toxic nephropathy in, 624, 625, 626, 627, 628-629, 631
uremic stomatitis and, 667
respiratory failure and, 711
sarcoidosis and, 718
scleroderma and, 1004
septic shock and, 478
sickle cell anemia and, 417
silicosis and, 724
sinusitis and, 790
skin infections and, 219
specimen contamination and, 124
splenectomy and, 395
sprue and, 1001-1002
staphylococcal enterocolitis and, 220
superinfections and, 142
before surgery, 251
Sydenham's chorea and, 818, 819
thrombocytopenia and, 425

Antibiotics—cont'd
thrush and, 276
toxic shock syndrome and, 298
ulcerative stomatitis and, 415
upper respiratory infections and, 145
varicella-zoster and, 130
vitamin K deficiency and, 411
Whipple's disease and, 1003
Antibodies, 15, 16; *see also* Immunology
antigastric parietal cell, 996, 1109
anti-glomerular basement membrane, 608, 610
anti-HA, 1069, 1071
anti-IgA, 351
anti-intrinsic factor, 1109
antileukocyte, 351
antimitochondrial, 1082
antineutrophil, 359
antinuclear; *see* Antinuclear antibodies
anti-PL^{A1}, 404
antiplatelet, 19, 403
anti-red cell, 19
anti-Rh$_o$, 349
antisalivary-duct, 37
antithyroid, 19, 903; *see also* Thyrotropin receptor antibody
antitoxoplasma, 65
antitreponemal, 271
autoantibodies in, 54, 1136, 1139; *see also* Autoimmune disease
blocking, 19
blood groups and, 348-349
colloid, 1136
colon, 1006
Donath-Landsteiner, 340
to factor VIII, 409, 411, 428
to factor IX, 428
glomerulonephritis and, 608, 610
Haemophilus influenzae and, 236
hemophilia and, 428
hepatitis, 1069, 1071
herpes simplex and, 128
heterophil, 132
immunoglobulin G, 338, 1260
insulin resistance and, 19, 1261
islet cell, 1260
against lipids, 266
measurement of, 31; *see also* Antibody testing
microsomal, 1136
parainfluenza viruses and, 143
parietal cell, 996, 1109
PM-1, 65
production defects of, 32-33
to streptolysin O, 223
teichoic acid, 220
testing and; *see* Antibody testing
thyroglobulin, 1136
thyroid, 1136, 1139
thyrotropin receptor; *see* Thyrotropin receptor antibody
varicella and, 129
warts and, 927
Antibody testing, 31; *see also* Antibody titers
urinary tract infection and, 196, 197
viruses and, 119, 124, 138, 143
Antibody titers, 31, 119, 124, 138
Antibody-coated bacteria, 196, 197
Anticholinergics
chronic obstructive pulmonary disease and, 693
diarrheas and, 954
diverticulosis and, 1017
dystonia musculorum deformans and, 821
encephalopathies and, 768

Anticholinergics—cont'd
esophageal reflux and, 982
esophageal spasm and, 981
gaseousness and, 961
gastric dilation and, 997
gastric secretion and, 943
hypoglycemia and, 1277
irritable bowel syndrome and, 1027, 1029
jaw spasm and, 821
megacolon and, 1027
multiple sclerosis and, 801
parkinsonism and, 813, 870
peptic ulcers and, 991, 1092
phenothiazine intoxication and, 779
in respiratory disease, 711, 745, 746
respiratory failure and, 711
torsion dystonias and, 820, 821
Zollinger-Ellison syndrome and, 995
Anticholinesterases, 856, 874, 976
Anticoagulants
alcohol and, 1297
aortic stenosis and, 515
aspirin and, 426
cerebrovascular disease and, 586, 832
coagulation disorders and, 411, 413-414
countershock and, 550
dentistry and, 429-430, 577-578
dialysis and, 640, 641
Dressler's syndrome and, 537
emboli and, 492-494, 568
fetal warfarin syndrome and, 1303
gastrointestinal bleeding and, 958
hemopericardium and, 553
intra-articular bleeding and, 104-105
lupus erythematosus and, 412
mitral stenosis and, 513
myocardial infarction and, 537
paroxysmal nocturnal hemoglobinuria and, 342
phlebitis and, 495
pregnancy and, 1212
pulmonary hypertension and, 497
Reiter's syndrome and, 908
venous thrombosis and, 663, 841
Anticonvulsants
alcohol withdrawal seizures and, 776
anesthesia and, 866
cysticercosis and, 293
dentistry and, 864-867
folate deficiency and, 1109
lupuslike syndrome and, 57
Ménière's syndrome and, 793
meningitis and, 190
nephritis and, 619, 620
nephropathy and, 625, 627, 631
neuropathy and, 853
neutropenia and, 360
perinatal virus and, 127
porphyrias and, 889, 1252
side effects of, 865
toxemia of pregnancy and, 665
trigeminal neuralgia and, 791
Anti-D immune globulin, 349
Antidepressants
abuse of, 862, 863
dementia and, 775
hemolysis and, 342
herpes zoster neuropathy and, 855
neurologic effects of, 779
tricyclic
alcohol and, 1297
fibrositis and, 97
guanethidine and, 472
neurologic effects of, 779

Antidepressants—cont'd
  tricyclic—cont'd
    non-REM sleep and, 96
    parkinsonism and, 813
    procarbazine and, 443
    salivary flow and, 870
    seizures and, 787
    sudden death and, 538
Antidiarrhea agents, 1029; see also specific agent
Antidiuresis, inappropriate, 135, 594, 595, 740, 1179, 1181
Antidiuretic hormone; see also Vasopressin
  alcohol and, 1258
  diabetes insipidus and, 621, 622, 1125
  ectopic secretion of, 435, 437
  heart failure and, 461
  hypernatremia and, 595
  inappropriate secretion of, 594, 595, 740
    encephalitis and, 135
    malignancy and, 740, 1179, 1181
  mineralocorticoid excess and, 1160
  neoplasms and, 1179, 1181
  renal mechanisms and, 591, 592, 594
  vascular control and, 458-459
Anti-DNA, 19
Anti-e, 1100
Antiemetics, 1212
Antiepileptics; see Anticonvulsants
Antiestrogens, 448
Antifibrinolytic agents, 421
Antifreeze; see Ethylene glycol
Anti-gamma-globulin antibody, 19
Antigastric parietal cell antibody, 996, 1109
Antigen drifts, 140
Antigen shifts, 140
Antigen-antibody complexes, 18, 27; see also Antibodies; Antigens
Antigens, 15, 119, 124; see also Immunology
  A locus, 643
  in antigen-antibody complexes, 19, 27
  B locus, 643
  B lymphocyte and, 11; see also Bone marrow–derived cells
  capsid, 132, 133, 1068
  carcinoembryonic, 435, 1010, 1040, 1041
  D locus, 643
  e, 126
  early, 132, 133
  Epstein-Barr virus-associated nuclear, 132, 133
  fetal, 435
  hepatitis, 347, 1068, 1071, 1091, 1098, 1099
  histocompatibility; see Histocompatibility antigens; Human lymphocyte antigens
  human lymphocyte; see Human lymphocyte antigens
  HY, 1219
  influenza and, 140
  KI, 186
  leukemia-associated, 365
  M protein, 609
  oncofetal, 434-435
  outer membrane, 186
  parainfluenza viruses and, 142
  pituitary, 727
  Rh, 349
  thymic dependent, 16; see also Thymus-derived cells
  thymic independent, 16
  tumor-specific, 444; see also specific antigen
Anti-glomerular basement membrane antibodies, 608, 610
Antigout medications, 91, 92, 93, 109
Anti-HA antibody, 1069, 1071

Antihemophilic factor, 428
Antihistamines; see also specific agent
  abuse of, 863
  alcohol and, 1297
  anaphylaxis and, 29
  angioedema and, 26
  asthma and, 728
  chronic obstructive pulmonary disease and, 693
  dentistry and, 746
  erythema multiforme and, 924
  fish poisoning and, 200
  hemolysis and, 342
  mastocystosis and, 910
  Ménière's syndrome and, 793
  parkinsonism and, 813
  rhinitis and, 22, 23
  salivary flow and, 870
  seizures and, 787
  serum sickness and, 27
  transfusion reactions and, 351
  urticaria and, 26
Antihypertensives, 472-475; see also specific agent
  amphetamine intoxication and, 777
  glomerulonephritis and, 610
  headache and, 789
  postural hypotension and, 780
  renal artery stenosis and, 662
  renal failure and, 639
  scleroderma and, 62, 616
  shock and, 476
  side effects and interactions of, 574, 575
  toxemia of pregnancy and, 665
Anti-inflammatory drugs; see also specific agent
  adhesive capsulitis and, 101
  anemia and, 312
  ankylosing spondylitis and, 50
  asthma and, 704
  avascular necrosis and, 104
  bursitis and, 98
  costochondritis and, 100, 737
  in crystal deposition disease, 95
  fibrositis and, 97
  gastritis and, 996
  gastrointestinal bleeding and, 958
  gout and, 93
  interstitial nephritis and, 619
  lupus erythematosus and, 57
  myofascial dysfunction and, 109, 875
  nephropathy and, 621, 625, 626, 627, 629
  neutropenia and, 360
  and osteoarthritis, 85, 86, 107
  osteochondritis and, 737
  otalgia and, 867
  Paget's disease and, 87-88
  pericarditis and, 551, 553, 555
  platelet aggregation and, 405
  pseudogout and, 95
  psoriatic arthritis and, 51
  pulmonary hyperosteoarthropathy and, 103
  Reiter's syndrome and, 53
  relapsing polychondritis and, 103
  rheumatoid arthritis and, 42, 46, 47, 106
  rotator cuff tears and, 101
  sensitivity to, 23-24
  tendinitis and, 99
  ulcers and, 988, 991
Anti-insulin antibody, 19, 1261
Anti-intrinsic factor antibody, 1109
Antileukocyte antibodies, 351
Antilymphocyte globulin, 644
Antimalarials; see also specific agent
  ankylosing spondylitis and, 50

Antimalarials—cont'd
  hemolysis and, 329
  lupus erythematosus and, 57
  rheumatoid arthritis and, 42
Antimetabolites, 287, 398, 440-441
Antimicrobials, 155-171; see also Antibiotics
  anaerobic infections and, 250-251
  bacteriostatic versus bactericidal activity in, 156
  doses of, 158, 160-161
  duration of therapy of, 158
  failure of therapy with, 159
  pharmacology of, 157-158
  regimens for, 162-163, 183
  review of, 159-171; see also specific agent
  site of infection and, 156-157
  susceptibility and, 155
  toxicity of, 158
Antimitochondrial antibodies, 1082
Antimony, 296, 628
Antineoplastic drugs; see Chemotherapy
Antineutrophil antibodies, 359
Antinuclear antibodies, 19, 1136
  lupus erythematosus and, 54, 56, 57
  rheumatoid arthritis and, 37, 44, 45
  systemic sclerosis and, 60, 903
Anti-PL^{A1} antibodies, 404
Antiplatelet agents
  cerebral infarction and, 832
  in Raynaud's phenomenon, 61
  thrombotic thrombocytopenic purpura and, 404
  transient ischemic attack and, 837
Antiplatelet antibody, 19, 403
α-l-Antiprotease deficiency, 694
Antipruritics, 130, 893
Antipyretics; see also specific agent
  chills and, 118
  fever and, 118, 208
  hemolysis and, 329
  influenza and, 141
Antipyrine, 329
Antirabies serum, equine, 153
Anti-red cell antibody, 19
Antireflux operations, 982
Antirenin drugs, 616
Anti-Rh$_o$ antibodies, 349
Antisalivary-duct antibody, 37
Antiseptics, 225, 893
Antiserum, 26-27
Antispasmodics
  gaseousness and, 961
  pseudomembranous enterocolitis and, 1018
  radiation enteritis and, 1019
Antithymocyte globulin, 361
Antithyroid agents, 1132; see also specific agent
  Graves' disease and, 1144-1145
  neutropenia and, 360, 361
Antithyroid antibody, 19, 903; see also Thyrotropin receptor antibody
Antitoxin
  botulism and, 204
  clostridial polyvalent, 253
  diphtheria, 248
  tetanus, 252
Antitoxoplasma antibodies, 65
Antitreponemal antibodies, 271
α-l-Antitrypsin, 172, 693, 694, 1082
Antituberculous agents, 258, 259-260; see also specific agent
  nontuberculous mycobacteria and, 261
  peritonitis and, 1047
  toxic nephropathy and, 624, 627, 628
Antitumor antibiotics, 441, 446

Antiviral agents, 122, 153-154; see also specific agent
Anton's syndrome, 832
Antral polyp prolapse, 1034
Antrectomy, 996
Anturane; see Sulfinpyrazone
ANUG; see Acute necrotizing ulcerative gingivitis
Anuria, 610, 630
Anus, 947-948
  disorders of, 1029-1031, 1042
Aorta, 555-563
  anatomy of, 555-556
  aneurysms of, 470, 557-560
  angiography of, 120, 489, 607
  ascending, 555-556, 558-559
  branches of, 564-571
  coarctation of, 340, 474, 505, 557, 573
  congenital anomalies of, 556-557
  dental correlations in disease of, 586-587
  dissection of, 560-562
  distal, 564-571
  fistula between esophagus and, 1032
  inflammation of, 48, 563
  Marfan's syndrome and, 1241
  regurgitation into, 515-516, 561
  stenosis of; see Aortic stenosis
  syphilis and, 179, 268-269, 563
  truncus arteriosus and, 505
Aortic arch, 559, 562-563
Aortic bodies, 677
Aortic knob, calcified, 561
Aortic regurgitation, 515-516, 561
Aortic root enlargement, 561
Aortic stenosis, 505-506, 514-515, 518, 522
Aorticopulmonary window, 505
Aortitis, 48, 563
Aorto-esophageal fistula, 1032
Aortofemoral bypass grafting, 570
Aortography, 120, 489, 607
Aortoiliac disease, 569
Apallic state, 764
Apert's syndromes, 1314, 1316
Aphasias, 763, 770, 771, 772
  Broca's, 757, 758, 772
  conduction, 772
  Wernicke's, 759, 772
Aphthous ulcers
  Crohn's disease and, 1097
  menstruation and, 1211
  ulcerative colitis and, 892, 1095
Apical impulse, presystolic, 470
Aplasia
  bone marrow, 169, 319, 320, 358; see also Bone marrow
  tooth, rubella and, 300
Aplastic anemia, 319-320
  chloramphenicol and, 168, 169
  dentistry and, 415
  neutropenia and, 358
  platelet production and, 401
  sickle cell anemia and, 332
Aplastic crisis, 332
Apnea, 766
  sleep, 769-770
Apneustic breathing, 766
Apolipoproteins, plasma, 1280-1281
Apomorphine, 956
Apoplexy, pituitary, 838, 1121
Apoproteins, 1280-1281, 1292
A-poxide; see Chlordiazepoxide
Appendix, 947, 948
  abscess of, 1015-1016
  inflammation of, 232, 951, 1015-1016

Appendix—cont'd
  removal of, 1016
Apperception, 772
Apraxia, 758, 759, 763, 770, 771
APUD cells; see Amine precursor uptake decarboxylation cells
Apudomas, 941, 994
Arabinosyl cytosine; see Cytosine arabinoside
Arabinosyl hypoxanthine, 154
Ara-C; see Cytosine arabinoside
Arachnia, 171
Arachnoiditis, progressive adhesive, 194
Aralen; see Chloroquine
ARAS; see Ascending reticular activating system
Arboviruses, 135, 825
ARDS; see Adult respiratory distress syndrome
Areflexia, detrusor, 799
Arenaviruses, 123
Areola, 11
ARF; see Renal failure, acute; Rheumatic fever, acute
Arfonad; see Trimethaphan
Argentaffinomas, 948
Arginase deficiency, 1239
Arginine hydrochloride, 600
Argininosuccinic acid synthetase deficiency, 1239
Argon lasers, 1095, 1274
Argyll Robertson pupil, 269
Arm, disorders of upper, 98, 100
Arnold-Chiari malformations, 807, 811
Aromatic amino acid disorders, 1236
Aromatic spirits of ammonia, 576, 864
Arrhythmias, 541-550
  bradycardias and, 546-548
  cardiomyopathy and, 519
  cardioversion and, 549-550
  chronic obstructive pulmonary disease and, 692
  dentistry and, 584-585
  drugs for, 585; see also specific drug
  Ebstein's anomaly and, 508
  heart block and, 546-548
  heart failure and, 571
  induced, 540
  mitral valve prolapse and, 511
  myocardial infarction and, 536
  normal conduction and, 541-542
  normal rhythm and, 541-542
  pediatric, 500-501
  sudden death and, 538-540
  supraventricular, 500, 508
  tachycardias and, 542-546
  transposition of great arteries and, 508
  ventricular ectopic beats and, 548
  Wolff-Parkinson-White syndrome and, 548-549
Arsenicals
  Bowen's disease and, 914
  as carcinogen, 432
  poisoning from, 754, 853
  portal hypertension and, 1060
  toxic nephropathy and, 627, 628
  trypanosomiasis and, 287
ART; see Automated Reagin Test
Artane; see Trihexyphenidyl
Arterial blood gases, 599-603, 673-676
  asthma and, 24, 706
  atelectasis and, 702
  carbon dioxide in; see Carbon dioxide tension, arterial
  congenital heart lesions and, 506
  hypercapnia and, 681
  hypoxemia and, 676, 681-682, 683

Arterial blood gases—cont'd
  initial evaluation of, 681
  oxygen in; see Oxygen tension, arterial
  pH and, 462, 592, 599
  respiratory failure and, 710
Arterial disease, atherosclerotic, 564-571
Arterial insufficiency, acute, 567-568
Arterial reconstruction, 569
Arteries; see Blood vessels; specific artery
Arteriography; see Angiography
Arterioles, vasoconstriction of, 683
Arteriosclerosis; see also Atherosclerosis
  aneurysms and, 559
  diabetes mellitus and, 1272-1273
  malabsorption and, 1003
  parkinsonism and, 814
Arteriovenous fistulas, 840; see also Arteriovenous malformations; Shunts
  access, 640, 641, 1274
  hemolysis and, 340
Arteriovenous malformations, 840; see also Arteriovenous fistulas
  angiography and, 971
  intestines and, 1022-1023
Arteritis; see also Endarteritis; Vasculitis
  cerebral hemorrhage and, 838
  collagen vascular disease and, 841
  coronary, 147
  dentistry and, 872
  giant cell, 69, 74-75
    headache in, 789-790
    management of, 69-70
    Takayasu's, 69, 70, 563; see also Pulseless disease
    temporal, 68, 69, 74-75, 789-790, 841
  Kawasaki disease and, 147
  ophthalmic, 69
Arthralgia, 28
Arthritis
  acute migratory, 229
  Behçet's syndrome and, 110, 907
  colitic, 1007
  enteric, 53
  gouty, of temporomandibular joint, 108-109; see also Gout
  infectious, 79-82
    fungal, 81
    gonococcal, 231, 232
    Haemophilus influenzae and, 236
    nongonococcal, 79-81
    rat-bite fever and, 272
    streptococcal, 226
    of temporomandibular joint, 108
    tuberculosis and, 81, 256
    viruses and, 81-82
  Jaccoud's, 229
  Lyme disease and, 297, 298, 925, 926
  meningococcemia and, 235
  psoriatic, 50-52, 106-107, 937
  reactive, 52, 53
  Reiter's syndrome and, 907
  rheumatoid; see Rheumatoid arthritis
  terminology and, 35
Arthrocentesis, 81
Arthropathy, 86, 94; see also Arthritis
Arthroplasty, 42
Artificial airway, 711
Artificial saliva, 911, 919
Arylhydrocarbon hydroxylase, 433
Arylsulfatase, 18, 802, 1233
ASA; see Aspirin
Asbestos, 432, 725-726, 1047
Asbestos bodies, 726
Asbestosis, 726; see also Asbestos

ASc, 385, 386
Ascariasis, 290, 721
Ascaris lumbricoides, 172, 290
Ascending reticular activating system, 764-765
Aschoff's bodies, 228
Ascites, 1044-1046
 colorectal carcinoma and, 1040
 heart failure and, 461
 management of, 1083-1084
 pancreatic, 1045, 1054
 portal hypertension and, 1061
 ultrasound and, 970-971
Ascorbic acid, 1106, 1110-1111
 hemolysis and, 330
 liver diseases and, 1059, 1080
 methemoglobinemias and, 344
 oxalate and, 648
 phencyclidine intoxication and, 779
 purpura and, 406
 urinary tract infection and, 198
 vitamin A and, 1107
Aseptic meningitis; *see* Meningitis, aseptic
Asherman's syndrome, 1176
Ashman's phenomenon, 544
Asian influenza, 154
Askanazy cells, 1150
Ask-Upmark kidney, 650
ASO titer, 223
Asparaginase, 366, 442, 1051
Aspergilloma, 705
Aspergillosis, 276-277, 446, 451, 705; *see also Aspergillus*
Aspergillus, 172, 179, 182, 276-277, 727
 allergic bronchopulmonary aspergillosis and, 705
 bronchiectasis and, 696
 bronchoscopy and, 689
 leukemia and, 421
Aspergillus clavatus, 727
Aspergillus fumigatus, 705, 727
Aspiration
 of lung, 689, 746
 nasogastric; *see* Nasogastric suction
 of pancreas, 969
 pneumonia after, 172, 177-178, 698-700, 746
 of thyroid, 1136
 transtracheal, 176
Aspiration pneumonia syndrome, 172, 177-178, 698-700, 746
Aspirin
 alcohol and, 1297
 anemia and, 312
 angioedema and, 26
 antihypertensives and, 574
 arthritis and, 42, 46, 47, 51, 106
 asthma and, 23-24, 704
 bleeding disorders and, 399
 cerebral infarction and, 832
 chills and, 118
 Dressler's syndrome and, 537
 Epstein-Barr virus and, 134
 fever and, 118
 fibrositis and, 97
 gastritis and, 943, 996
 gastrointestinal bleeding and, 958, 1093
 hemolysis and, 329
 hemophilia and, 428
 hereditary hemorrhagic telangiectasia and, 1095
 hypercalcemia and, 1180
 in Jarisch-Herxheimer reaction, 272
 Kawasaki disease and, 148
 lung disease and, 721
 Lyme disease and, 298

Aspirin—cont'd
 mastocytosis and, 909
 myofascial pain dysfunction and, 109
 nasal polyps and, 23-24
 oral bleeding and, 426
 osteoarthritis and, 85
 osteochondritis and, 737
 otalgia and, 867
 peptic ulcers and, 1092
 pericarditis and, 551
 platelet function and, 353, 400, 405, 908
 porphyria and, 1252
 pregnancy and, 1213
 in Raynaud's phenomenon, 61
 renal disease and, 621, 625, 627, 670
 rheumatic fever and, 230
 sensitivity to, 23
 shock and, 575
 sulfonylureas and, 1267
 in systemic sclerosis, 62
 thrombocytopenia and, 400, 426, 1059, 1064
 thrombocytosis and, 404, 426
 thrombotic thrombocytopenic purpura and, 404
 thyroiditis and, 1149
 transient ischemic attack and, 837
 ulcers and, 988, 991
 urinary tract neoplasms and, 658
 urticaria and, 25
Association cortex, 771
Associations, genetic, 1228-1229
Astereognosis, 759
Asterixis, 766
Asteroid bodies, 911
Asthma, 704-707
 allergy and, 23-25, 704, 705
 aspirin sensitivity and, 23-24, 26
 dentistry and, 747
 granulomatosis and, 67
 lung disease and, 704, 719
 nasal polyps and, 23, 26
 occupational, 728
 prevention of, 25
 respiratory failure and, 708, 710-711
Astiban; *see* Stibocaptate
Astrocytic tumors, 843-844
Astrovirus, 149, 150
Asymmetric hypertrophy of heart, 179, 517-520
Asymptomatic bacteriuria, 195, 197-198
Asymptomatic bruit, 565
Atabrine; *see* Quinacrine
Ataxia
 cerebellar, 130, 137, 138, 1076
 Friedreich's, 805-806
 gait, 759
 homolateral, 835
 progressive hereditary, 805-807
 Sanger Brown, 806
 telangiectasia and, 33, 809-810, 869, 882; *see also* Telangiectasia
Ataxia-telangiectasia, 33, 809-810; *see also* Telangiectasia
 Bloom's syndrome and, 882
 dentistry and, 869
Atelectasis, 685-686, 702-703, 740
Atenolol, 472
Atheroma, 1272
Atherosclerosis; *see also* Arteriosclerosis
 aneurysms and, 565
 aortic arch syndrome and, 562
 arterial disease and, 564-571
 cardiovascular disease and
  angina pectoris and, 528
  myocardial infarction and, 533
  sudden death and, 538, 539

Atherosclerosis—cont'd
 dentistry and, 583, 586
 hyperlipidemia and, 1280, 1288; *see also* Lipoprotein metabolism disorders
 renal artery stenosis and, 660
Athlete's foot, 928
Ativan; *see* Lorazepam
Atlantoaxial joint subluxation, 45
ATN; *see* Nephropathy, toxic
Atopognosia, 759
Atopy, 19-25
 asthma and, 23-25, 704, 705
 dermatitis of anus and, 1030
 eczema and, 20
 immunoglobulin E antibodies and, 19-20
 tests for, 21-22
ATP; *see* Adenosine triphosphate
Atransferrinemia, 325
Atresia, 506-507
Atrial extrastimulus technique, 547
Atrial fibrillation, 512, 513, 522, 543-544
Atrial flutter, 543-544
Atrial hypertrophy, electrocardiogram and, 500
Atrial myxomas, 182, 513, 516, 842
Atrial overdrive pacing, 547
Atrial pressures, 552
Atrial septal defect
 anomalous pulmonary venous return and, 503
 ostium primum, 504
 ostium secundum, 503
 transposition of great arteries and, 508
Atrial tachycardia, 542-543, 692
Atrioventricular block, 547-548
Atrioventricular canal, 504
Atrioventricular junctional tachycardia, 545
Atrioventricular node, 479, 541
Atromid S; *see* Clofibrate
Atrophic papulosis, malignant, 893-894, 1003
Atrophy
 dorsal interosseous, 36
 Fazio-Londe, 804
 gastric, 996-997
 hemifacial, scleroderma and, 903
 infantile muscular, 804
 peroneal muscle, 805, 855
 pontocerebellar, 812
 spinal, 804-805
 Sudeck's, 100
 of tongue, syphilis and, 303
Atropine, *see also* Atropine-like drugs
 carotid sinus syncope and, 781
 hypotension and, 584
 insecticide poisoning and, 754
 mastocytosis and, 909
 neurologic effects, 779
 parietal cells and, 943
 pregnancy and, 1212
 respiratory disease and, 745, 746
 sick sinus syndrome and, 547
 vasovagal syncope and, 576, 577
Atropine-like drugs, 765, 1014
Attention span testing, 773
Au 198; *see* Radioactive gold
Audiometry tests, 9, 795
Auer's bodies, 365
Auerbach's plexus, 942, 973, 978, 1027
Aura, 781, 783, 865
Aural calcification, 103
Aural symptoms with dental conditions, 867-868
Auranofin, 42
Aureobasidium pullulans, 727
Auscultation, 7, 12, 684-685
Auspitz sign, 936
Austin-Flint murmur, 516

Autoantibodies, 54, 1136, 1139; *see also* Autoimmune disease
   lupus erythematosus and, 54
   thyroid, 1136, 1139
Autoerythrocyte sensitization, 406
Autohemolysis test, 329
Autoimmune disease, 19
   esophageal disorders and, 1091
   hemolytic anemias in, 338-340, 406; *see also* Hemolytic anemia
   liver and, 1078, 1098
   lupus erythematosus and, 53; *see also* Lupus erythematosus
   monocytosis and, 362
   neutropenia and, 359
   peritonitis and, 1048
   pernicious anemia and, 317
   systemic sclerosis and, 58; *see also* Systemic sclerosis
   thyroid, 1062, 1149-1150
   tumors and, 438
Autoimmune polyendocrinopathy syndrome, 1209
Autologous clot injection, 959
Autologous transfusion, 347
Automated cell separators, 346-347
Automated Reagin Test, 271
Automaticity, 479, 542
Autonomic nervous system; *see also* Sympathetic nervous system
   cardiac output and, 458
   diabetes mellitus and, 1275
   dysregulation of, 467
Autoregulation, 458, 459
Autosomal dominant inheritance, 1218
Autosomal recessive inheritance, 1218
Autosomes, 1217
Autosplenectomy, 395
AV node; *see* Atrioventricular node
Avascular necrosis, 104
Avidin, 1110
AVM; *see* Arteriovenous malformations
Axillae
   acanthosis nigricans in, 887
   evaluation of, 11; *see also* Adenopathy
   neoplastic involvement and, 448
Axonal neuropathy, 852
Axostyle, 284
Azaribine, 901
Azathioprim, oral candidiasis and, 307
Azathioprine
   autoimmune hemolytic anemia and, 339
   Crohn's disease and, 1014
   hepatitis and, 1079
   lung disease and, 722
   lupus erythematosus and, 57
   multiple sclerosis and, 801
   pancreatitis and, 1051
   pemphigus and, 932, 934
   polyarteritis nodosa and, 616
   relapsing polychondritis and, 103
   renal transplantation and, 644
   rheumatoid arthritis and, 42
   sarcoidosis and, 78
   Schönlein-Henoch purpura and, 616
   scleroderma and, 903
   ulcerative colitis and, 1011
   Wegener's granulomatosis and, 73
Azlocillin, 164
Azotemia, 630, 632-633, 638
   chronic renal failure and, 638
   prerenal, 631, 632-633
   systemic sclerosis and, 60
Azulfidine; *see* Salicylazosulfapyridine

B

B apoproteins, 1281, 1292
B cells; *see* Bone marrow-derived cells
B_{12} cofactor, 1237
B locus antigens, 643
B lymphocytes; *see* Bone marrow-derived cells
B virus particle, 1100
Babesia, 288, 343
Babesiosis, 288, 343
Babinski's sign, 14
   frontal lobe lesions and, 757
   multiple sclerosis and, 799
   subacute combined degeneration and, 851
Bacampicillin, 163
Bacille Calmette Guérin, 260-261, 445
   leprosy and, 263
   in leukemias, 368
   in melanomas, 450, 918
   mycosis fungoides and, 901
Bacilli; *see* Gram-negative bacilli; *see* Gram-positive bacilli
Bacillus anthracis, 171, 245, 305
Bacillus cereus, 201, 202, 205, 953
Bacillus subtilis, 728
Bacitracin
   streptococcal impetigo and, 226
   toxic nephropathy and, 627, 628
   ulcerative stomatitis and, 415
Back, 98, 102
Backwash ileitis, 1006
Baclofen, 800, 804
Bacteremia; *see also* Septicemia
   antimicrobials and, 156
   cholecystitis and, 1088
   endocarditis and, 180, 181, 182, 301
   gonococcal, 231
   gram-negative bacillary, 239-241
   Haemophilus influenzae and, 236
   osteomyelitis and, 221
   plague and, 242
   pneumococcal pneumonia and, 173
   Salmonella, 202, 208
   staphylococcal, 220
   streptococcal, 175, 226, 227, 241, 581
   tularemia and, 243
   urinary tract infection and, 196, 197
Bacteria, 155-274
   acrodermatitis enteropathica and, 895
   agents against, 155-171; *see also* Antibiotics; Antimicrobials
   anaerobic; *see* Anaerobic bacteria
   central nervous system and, 186-195; *see also* Central nervous system, bacterial infections of
   Chlamydiae in, 214-216
   dentistry and, 301-306
   diabetic ketoacidosis and, 1269
   diarrhea and, 953
   donor blood and, 351
   endocarditis and; *see* Endocarditis
   folic acid deficiency and, 415
   foodborne disease and, 199-209
   gram-negative bacilli in, 235-245; *see also* Gram-negative bacilli
   gram-negative cocci in, 230-235
   gram-positive bacilli in, 245-249
   gram-positive cocci in, 218-230; *see also* Gram-positive cocci
   leukemias and, 371, 421
   leukemoid reactions and, 362
   liver disease and, 1074
   malabsorption and, 1003
   meningitis and, 139, 186-191
   mycobacteria in, 254-264

Bacteria—cont'd
   mycoplasmas in, 217-218
   neutrophils and, 356-359
   oral, endocarditis and, 581
   overgrowth of, in digestive tract, 62, 947, 1103
   perinephric abscess and, 199
   pneumonia and, 171-178, 729; *see also* Pneumonia
   prostatitis and, 198
   pyuria and, 590
   rickettsiae in, 209-214
   spirochetes in, 264-274; *see also* Spirochetes
   temporomandibular joint asthma and, 108
   thyroiditis and, 1149
   toxins of; *see* Toxins, bacterial
   urinary tract and, 195-199
   waterborne disease and, 199-209
Bacterial spores, 727
Bacterial toxins; *see* Toxins, bacterial
Bactericidal activity, 156
Bacteriology, 119, 258
Bacteriostatic activity, 156
Bacteriuria
   asymptomatic, 195, 197-198
   in pregnancy, 666
   urinary tract infections and, 195-199
Bacteroides, 172, 177-178, 179, 249, 250, 253
   drugs for, 167
   endocarditis and, 179, 302
   oral contraceptives and, 1214
   in pneumonia, 172, 177-178
Bacteroides asaccharolyticus, 249
Bacteroides fragilis, 177-178, 249, 250
   abscesses and
      abdominal, 1047
      lung, 699
      pancreatic, 1054
   bacteremia and, 239, 241
   drugs for, 163, 165, 167, 168, 169, 170
   in pneumonia, 177-178
Bacteroides melaninogenicus, 249, 699
Bacteroides thetaiotaomicron, 249
BAER; *see* Brainstem auditory evoked response
Bagassosis, 727
Baker's cyst, 84, 567
Baking soda; *see* Sodium bicarbonate
BAL; *see* Dimercaprol
Balanitis circinate, 52
Balkan nephropathy, 658
Balloon pumping, 532
Balloon septostomy, 508
Bamboo spine, 49, 50, 737
Bancroftian filariasis, 292, 921
Band cells, 356
Band keratopathy, 1190
Banti's syndrome, 396
BAO; *see* Basal acid output
Bárány's test, 792
Barbital, 1131
Barbiturates
   abuse of, 862
   alcohol and, 776, 1297
   allergy and, 28
   cocaine intoxication and, 778
   coma and, 764
   coumarins and, 414
   cyclophosphamide and, 442
   diabetes and, 1295
   erythema multiforme and, 30, 923
   heart medication and, 572
   hemolysis and, 342
   hyponatremia and, 594
   hypothyroidism and, 1206

Barbiturates—cont'd
  liver disease and, 1090
  osteomalacia and, 1198, 1199, 1200
  porphyria and, 854, 889, 1248, 1252, 1298
  pregnancy and, 1212
  in respiratory disease, 746, 747
  seizures and, 866, 867
  sulfonylureas and, 1267
  Sydenham's chorea and, 819
  toxicity of, 777
Barium
  in enemas
    bowel obstruction and, 1026
    colorectal carcinoma and, 1040, 1041
    Crohn's disease and, 1012, 1013
    diverticulosis and, 1017
    ischemic colitis and, 1021, 1022, 1023
    large bowel neoplasms and, 1038, 1039
    ulcerative colitis and, 1008, 1009, 1010
  esophageal disease and, 983, 1032, 1033
  gastric carcinoma and, 1035
  gastric polyps and, 1034
  hypokalemia and, 597
  inspissated, bowel obstruction and, 1026
  pancreatic carcinoma and, 1056-1057
  ulcers and, 989, 990
Barognosis, 771
Baroreceptors, 467, 477
Barotrauma, 709
Barr body, 1219
Barrel chest, 694
Barrett's esophagus, 983, 1032
Bartholin's glands, 231
Basal acid output, 944
Basal cell carcinoma
  of anus, 1031
  of face, 883
  of mouth, 918, 919
  of skin, 915-916
Basal cell nevus syndrome, 883, 1209
Basal ganglia, 759, 812-824
  calcification of, 1209
  chorea and, 774, 816-818
  essential tremor and, 815-816
  Gilles de la Tourette's syndrome and, 821
  orthostatic hypotension and, 823-824
  parkinsonism and, 812-815
  torsion dystonias and, 819-821
  Wilson's disease and, 822-823
Basal ganglion calcification syndrome, 1209
Basaljel, 1201
Basic life support, 540
Basilar artery syndromes, 833-835
Basilar atelectasis, 702
Basilar impression, 811
Basilar invagination, 811
Basophils, 17, 315, 369
Basosquamous cell carcinoma, 916
Bassen-Kornzweig syndrome, 1291-1292
BCB; see Brilliant cresyl blue
BCG; see Bacille Calmette Guérin
BCNU, 442
  cyclophosphamide, vinblastine, procarbazine, and prednisone, 390, 391
  Hodgkin's disease and, 390, 391
  lung disease and, 722
B-complex vitamins; see Vitamins, B complex
BCVPP therapy; see BCNU, cyclophosphamide, vinblastine, procarbazine, and prednisone
Bechterew's disease, 48
Becker muscular dystrophy, 857
Beclomethasone, 707, 1212

Bedsonia, 214
Beef tapeworm, 293, 294
Beefy red tongue, 414
Behavior, 763
Behçet's syndrome, 110-111
  aseptic meningoencephalitis and, 139
  dentistry and, 110-111
  differential diagnosis of, 189
  Reiter's syndrome and, 110
  skin lesions of, 906-907
Belching, excessive, 960-961
Bell's palsy, 138
Belladonna, 450
Belsey's procedure, 985
Benadryl; see Diphenhydramine
Bence Jones proteins, 379, 380, 605
Bendectin, 1212
Bendroflumethiazide, 472
Benedikt's syndrome, 833
Benemid; see Probenecid
Benzathine penicillin, 160, 163
  endocarditis and, 582
  erysipeloid and, 246
  impetigo and, 226
  pharyngitis and, 225
  rheumatic fever and, 230
  syphilis and, 271, 272
Benzene
  as carcinogen, 432
  leukemias and, 364, 369
  myelofibrosis and, 374
Benzidene test, 959
Benzimidazole, 287
Benzodiazepines; see also specific agent
  alcohol withdrawal and, 776
  cocaine intoxication and, 778
  essential tremor and, 816
  Hunting's chorea and, 818
  side effects of, 871
  toxicity of, 777
Benztropine, 815, 821, 870
Benzyl penicillin, 159, 163
Berger's disease, 611
Beriberi, 1108
  alcohol and, 1257
  cardiomyopathies and, 523
  peripheral neuropathy and, 849
Bernard-Soulier syndrome, 405
Bernstein test, 961-962, 983
Berry aneurysms, 839
Beryllium, 627, 628
Beta lactam antibiotic, penicillinase-resistant, 303
Beta rays, 749
Beta-adrenergic agonists, asthma and, 24, 705, 706, 707
Beta-adrenergic blockers; see also specific agent
  angina pectoris and, 531
  asthma and, 706, 748
  heart failure and, 464
  hypertension and, 467, 472, 473
  pheochromocytoma and, 1164, 1168
  pulmonary edema and, 710
  Raynaud's phenomenon and, 63
  tetanus and, 252
  thyrotoxicosis and, 1205
  toxemia of pregnancy and, 665
Beta-carotene; see Carotenes
Beta-cells
  hyperplasia of, 1278
  tumors of, 1278-1279
Beta-Chlor; see Chloral betaine
Betadine; see Povidone-iodine

Beta-endorphin, 1115
Beta-galactosidase, 802
Beta-glucuronidase deficiency, 1233, 1234
Beta-hemolytic streptococci, 175, 222; see also Streptococci
Beta-hydroxy-beta-methylglutaric CoA-reductase, 1063
11-Beta-hydroxylase deficiency, 1162, 1163
3-Beta-hydroxysteroid dehydrogenase deficiency, 1171
17-Beta-hydroxysteroid oxidoreductase deficiency, 1171
Beta-lipoprotein deficiency, 999, 1292
Beta-lipotropin, 1115
Betamethasone, 939
Beta-monoglyceride, 998-999
3-Beta-OH-dehydrogenase deficiency, 1162, 1163
Beta-1-pyrroline-5-carboxylic acid dehydrogenase deficiency, 1239
Beta-thalassemias, 334-337, 418-419
Betazole, 993
Betel nuts, 432
Bethanechol, 801, 985
Bezoars, 998
Bezold-von Jarish reflex, 535
Bicarbonate, 599
  acidosis and, 600, 601
  alkalosis and, 600, 601
  calcium, in mouthrinses, 908
  methyl alcohol poisoning and, 777
  in pancreatic juice, 1050
  in plasma, 592
  in saliva, 1102
  tubular reabsorption of, 592
Bicarbonate sodium; see Sodium bicarbonate
Bicarbonate-carbonic acid system, 599
Bicipital tendinitis, 99
Bicuspid valves, aortic stenosis and, 514
Bifid uvula, 1321
Bifidobacterium, 249
Biguanides, 1267
Bile, 945-946, 1085-1086; see also Bile acids; Bile salts
  hepatic supersaturated, 1087
  limy, 1088
  pancreatitis and, 1051
  radiopaque, 1088
  secretion of, 1085-1086
  in vomitus, 957
Bile acid-binding resins, 1285
Bile acids, 940, 946
  liver diseases and, 1063
  low density lipoproteins and, 1285
  pool of, 1086
  serum, 1065
  synthesis of, 1085
Bile ascites, 1045-1046
Bile ducts
  blockage of; see Cholestasis
  common, stones in, 950, 1086, 1088
  extrahepatic, 1058, 1089
  inflammation of, 105, 1088, 1089
Bile micelles, 1085
Bile peritonitis, 1046
Bile pigments, 1065-1066
Bile salts, 1085, 1086
  absorption and, 998, 999
  Crohn's disease and, 1012
  osteomalacia and, 1199
Bilharziasis, 294-297
Biliary catheters, percutaneous, 1089

Biliary cirrhosis, 889-890, 1082; see also Cirrhosis
Biliary colic, 950-951, 988, 1087-1088
Biliary tract, 1085-1090
  bile and; see Bile
  cholecystitis and, 1086-1089
  cholelithiasis and, 1086-1090
  cholestatic jaundice and, 967
  computed tomography and, 971
  decompression of, 968
  diagnosis and, 967-969, 970, 971
  drainage of, 1088
  endoprostheses and, 968
  liver abscesses and, 1074
  malnutrition and, 1103
  neoplasms and, 445, 1089
  pain and; see Biliary colic
  pancreatitis and, 1051, 1052
  sclerosing cholangitis and, 105, 1089
  ultrasound and, 970
Bilirubin, 1086
  conjugated, 1058, 1064, 1068
  hepatitis and, 1070, 1071
  jaundice and, 1058
  metabolism of, 1057-1058, 1067-1068
  serum, 1064, 1070, 1071
  unconjugated, 338, 1064, 1066, 1067
Bilirubin diglucuronide, 945-946
Billroth II procedure, 993, 1004
Biofeedback, 867
Biogenic amines, 1115
Biopsy, 434
  bone, osteomyelitis and, 222
  bone marrow, 313
    aplastic anemia and, 320
    leukemias and, 369
    multiple myeloma and, 380
    myeloid metaplasia and, 375
    thrombocytopenia and, 402
  brain, 128, 135, 136, 137
  cartilage and, 103
  donovanosis and, 238
  of esophagus, 1032
  of fetal skin, 1229
  fever of unknown origin and, 120
  gastric, 963
  lip and, 37
  of liver, 965
    cholestasis and, 1067
    granulomatous disease and, 1084
    hepatitis and, 126, 1071
    sarcoidosis and, 77, 718
  lung
    cancer and, 740-741
    open, 689
    pulmonary fibrosis and, 714
    sarcoidosis and, 718
    transbronchial, 689, 718
  lymph node, 31, 689; see also Mediastinoscopy
  lymphoma and, 424
  microbial diseases and, 118
  of muscle, 65, 875
  oral
    amyloidosis and, 423
    candidiasis and, 34
    erythema multiforme and, 924
    Kaposi's sarcoma and, 922
    lichen planus and, 939
    pemphigoid and, 935
    pemphigus and, 933
    pemphigus vegetans and, 934

Biopsy—cont'd
  oral—cont'd
    psoriasis and, 937
    sarcoidosis and, 114, 911
    stomach carcinoma and, 1093
    thrombotic thrombocytopenic purpura and, 425
  of pancreas, 969
  of peripheral nerve, 852
  of peritoneum, 1044
  pleural
    effusions and, 732
    malignant mesothelioma and, 726
    sarcoidosis and, 716
    thoracentesis and, 688
  rectal
    amyloidosis and, 386
    Crohn's disease and, 1013
    ulcerative colitis and, 1007, 1008
  renal, 72, 608, 638
  of salivary gland, 1098
  skin, 139, 211, 1229
  of small bowel, 384, 964
  of synovium, 81, 94
  of temporal artery, 68, 69, 75
  of thyroid, 1136, 1152
  transbronchial, 689, 718
Biotin, 1106, 1110, 1237
Biperiden, 870
Bird fancier's lung, 727
Birth control pills; see Oral contraceptives
Bisacodyl, 1002
Bismuth, 612, 627, 630
Bite splints, 867, 873; see also Splints
Bitemporal hemianopia, 1119, 1123
BL; see Burkitt's lymphoma
Blackwater fever, 280
Bladder, urinary
  anomalies of, 651
  catheters for, 199, 568, 633, 656
  multiple sclerosis and, 799
  neoplasms of, 449, 659
  urinary tract infection and, 196
Blalock-Taussig operation, 507
Blast cells, 366, 374
Blastomyces dermatitidis, 275
Blastomycosis, 275
Bleach, 828
Blebs, 686, 700, 701
Bleeding; see also Coagulation; Hemostatic disorders
  afibrinogenemia and, 429
  anemia and, 323
    aplastic, 320, 415
    iron deficiency, 324, 325
  from angiomas, 882
  cerebral, 829, 830, 838-839, 841; see also Cerebrovascular accident
  cystitis and, 143
  drug abuse and, postsurgical, 862
  Ehlers-Danlos syndrome and, 1243
  endocarditis and, 181
  gastric leiomyomas and, 1034
  gastrointestinal; see Digestive system, bleeding and
  Gaucher's disease and, 425, 1232
  gingival, 427
    aplastic anemia and, 415
    Gaucher's disease and, 1232
    hemophilia and, 427
    leukemia and, 420
    macroglobulinemia and, 423
    telangiectasia and, 894

Bleeding—cont'd
  gingival—cont'd
    thrombocytopenia and, 425
    uremia and, 667
    vitamin K and, 1108
    von Willebrand's disease and, 426
  hereditary hemorrhagic telangiectasia and, 1095
  hypersplenism and, 396
  hypertension and, 575
  intramedullary, 840
  intraperitoneal, 971
  Kaposi's sarcoma and, 920-922
  leukemias and, 368, 420
  in lipoprotein metabolism disorders, 1296
  liver disease and postsurgical, 1098
  lupus erythematosus and, 112
  menstruation and, postoperative, 1210
  multiple myeloma and, 379, 422-423
  neoplasia and, 446
  of newborn, 411
  from nose, 407, 894
  oral
    anticoagulant therapy and, 429, 430
    aspirin and, 426
    chemotherapy and, 451
    disseminated intravascular coagulopathy and, 429
    hemophilia and, 427, 428
    multiple myeloma and, 422, 423
    thrombocytosis and, 426
  Paget's disease and, 114
  parenchymal, 829, 838-839
  polycythemia vera and, 419
  pulmonary, 611, 720-721
  rectal, 1007
  into renal cyst, 651
  rhinitis and, 269
  shock and, 476
  spinal cord, 840
  subarachnoid, 790, 839-840
  subdural, 192, 844
  subhyaloid, 765, 839
  systemic sclerosis and, 112
  telangiectasia and, 894, 1023-1024; see also Osler-Weber-Rendu disease
  thrombasthenia and, 426
  thrombocythemia and, 374
  into thyroid, 1150
  transfusions and; see Blood transfusions
  vertigo and, 793-794
  vitamin K and, 1108
  Waldenström's macroglobulinemia and, 383
Bleeding diathesis, 383, 1232, 1298
Bleeding disorders; see Hemostatic disorders
Bleeding profile, 416, 419
Bleeding time, 106, 1098
Blenoxane; see Bleomycin
Bleomycin, 440, 441
  carcinoma and, 449
  Hodgkin's disease and, 390, 391
  lung disease and, 722
  malignant effusions and, 445
  mycosis fungoides and, 901
  oral ulcers and, 450
BLFD; see Bucco-linguo-facial dyskinesia
Blindness; see also Vision
  diabetes mellitus and, 1273
  functional, 759
  optokinetic nystagmus and, 759
  temporal arteritis and, 75
  trachoma and, 214
  vitamin A and, 1107

Bloating, abdominal, 960-961; see also Distention
Bloch-Sulzberger syndrome, 810
Blocking antibodies, 19
β-Blocking drugs; see Beta-adrenergic blockers
Blood; see also Circulation
    banking of, 346-351
    cells of; see Red blood cells; White blood cells
    clotting of; see Coagulation
    compatibility of, 348-349
    loss of; see Bleeding
    malaria and, 280
    myelophthisis and, 322
    to peritoneum, 1043
    pH of, 462, 592, 599
    proteins in, 17
    splanchnic flow of, 948-949
    in stools, 957, 959-960, 988, 996
    to thyroid, 1127
    transfusions of; see Blood transfusions
    venous, in anticoagulation therapy, 430; see also Veins
    volume of; see Blood volume
Blood banking, 346-351
Blood cell count
    fever of unknown origin and, 120
    lymphomas and, 424
    microbial diseases and, 118, 119
    red; see Red blood cells
    white, 32, 310
        in cerebrospinal fluid, 135
        infectious mononucleosis and, 132
        leukemias and, 364, 369, 371
        leukemoid reactions and, 361
        leukocytosis and, 361
        pleural effusion and, 731
Blood cells; see Red blood cells; White blood cells
Blood chemistries, 313; see also Serum
Blood clotting factors; see Blood component therapy; Clotting factors
Blood component therapy, 311, 346, 350, 1098; see also Transfusions
Blood cultures, 182, 184, 188; see also Cultures
Blood dyscrasias; see specific disease
Blood factors; see Clotting factors
Blood gases, arterial; see Arterial blood gases
Blood group, 348-349
    Duffy, 280
    gastric carcinoma and, 1035
    MN, 1220
Blood pool labeling, 489, 521, 530
Blood pressure, 465-467; see also Hypertension; Hypotension
    coronary artery disease and, 527
    cortisol and, 1154
    elevated, 465-475; see also Hypertension
    myocardial infarction and, 534
    myocardial ischemia and, 528
    pheochromocytoma and, 1165
    variations in, 466
Blood proteins, circulating, 17
Blood sampling, fetal, 1229
Blood smear, peripheral; see Peripheral blood smears
Blood transfusions, 315, 345-351; see also Transfusions
    anemia and, 321, 323
    azotemia and, 632
    cirrhosis complications and, 1082
    cold agglutinin disease and, 339
    Crohn's disease and, 1015
    cytomegalovirus and, 130

Blood—cont'd
    disseminated intravascular coagulation and, 413
    in hematologic disorders, 311
    hepatitis and, 1068, 1069, 1073
    iron excess and, 345
    liver disease and, 1098
    pancreatitis and, 1053
    perinatal virus and, 127
    pregnancy and, 127
    principles of, 346-351
    reactions to, 351
        anemia and, 337
        ataxia-telangiectasia and, 809
        immunodeficiency diseases and, 34
    spherocytosis and, 329
    temperature of, 350
    thalassemias and, 337
    ulcers and, 993-994
Blood urea nitrogen, 604
    acute renal failure and, 630
    heart failure and, 462
    lupus erythematosus and, 55
    obstructive uropathy and, 655-656
    pregnancy and, 664
Blood values, 313; see also Serum
Blood vessels; see also Cardiovascular diseases; Veins; specific vessel
    antigen-antibody complexes and, 27, 66
    electrical injury and, 751
    pulmonary; see Pulmonary vessels
    systemic sclerosis and, 59
Blood volume
    aldosterone and, 1154
    liver disease and, 1064
    posthemorrhagic anemia and, 323
    septic shock and, 240
Bloom's syndrome, 882-883, 1222
Blue bloater, 710
Blue nevus, 918-919
Blumer's shelf, 1035, 1040
BMUs; see Bone remodeling units
Bobbing, ocular, 833
Bochdalek, foramen of, 736
Body plethysmography, 679
Body temperature
    evaluation of; see Fever
    and pressure saturated with water vapor, 673
    reduced, 118, 756
    regulation of, 755
Boeck's sarcoid, 910-911; see also Sarcoidosis
Bohr effect, 331
Bombesin, 941
Bone
    alveolar; see Alveolar bone
    biopsy of, osteomyelitis and, 222; see also Biopsy, bone marrow
    congenital syphilis and, 269-270
    cranial, dental infection and, 303
    disrupted blood supply to, 104
    eosinophilic granuloma of, 397
    Gardner's syndrome and, 1093
    Gaucher's disease and, 397
    mastocystosis and, 910
    metabolic disease of, 1181-1204
        dentistry and, 1207-1210
        mineral homeostasis and, 1189-1198, 1207-1210
        physiology in, 1181-1189
        skeletal homeostasis and, 1198-1203
    modeling of, 1182, 1183, 1203
    multiple myeloma and, 379
    osteomyelitis and; see Osteomyelitis
    pain in, 88, 89, 374

Bone—cont'd
    physiology of, 1181-1189
    remodeling of, 1182-1183, 1203, 1308
    sarcoidosis of, 77, 78, 911; see also Sarcoidosis
    scans of
        cancer staging and, 436
        osteomyelitis and, 222
        Paget's disease and, 86-87
    sickle cell anemia and, 416-417
    streptococcal infection of, 226
    structure of, 1181-1183
    tuberculosis in, 256
    turnover of, 1181-1183
Bone alkaline phosphatase, 1189
Bone marrow
    aplasia of, 169, 318, 319-320, 358
    aspiration of, 313
    biopsy of; see Biopsy, bone marrow
    chloramphenicol and, 169
    erythropoietin and, 313
    failure of, 318-323, 326
    fibrosis of, 374-376
    heavy-chain disease and, 384
    hypersplenism and, 396
    hypoplasia of, 358
    infiltrative disorders of, 358; see also specific disease
    leukemias and, 365, 369
    multiple myeloma and, 380, 381
    myeloid metaplasia and, 375
    neutropenia and, 361
    suppression of
        drug-related, 401
        iatrogenic, 401
        oral ulcers and, 450-451
    thrombocytopenia and, 401, 402
    transit time through, 356
    transplants of, 33, 58, 319, 320, 1240
        in leukemias, 368
        paroxysmal nocturnal hemoglobinuria and, 342
        Wiskott-Aldrich syndrome and, 33
        Waldenstöm's macroglobulinemia and, 383
Bone marrow–derived cells, 15-16, 376
    defects in, 32-33
    disorders of, 31, 376-387; see also Plasma cell disorders
    evaluation of, 31-32
    function of, 377
    infectious mononucleosis and, 132
    lymphocytic leukemias and, 371
    markers of, 365
    non-Hodgkin's lymphoma and, 392
    pneumonia and, 173
Bone remodeling units, 1182, 1183
Bony orbit, development of, 1306
Bordetella, 237, 238
Bordetella bronchiseptica, 237
Bordetella parapertussis, 237
Bordetella pertussis, 237
Bordet-Gengou culture, 237, 238
Bornholm disease, 730
Borrelia vincentii, 1110
Bossing, frontal, 877
Botulism, 201, 204, 209, 856
Bouchard's nodes, 83, 84
Bougienage, 979
Bourneville's disease, 810; see also Tuberous sclerosis Bourneville-Pringle syndrome, 668, 880-881
Boutonniére deformities of hand, 36, 37
Bovine tuberculosis, 304
Bowel; see Intestines

Bowen's disease, 914, 1031
Bowman's capsule, 590
Boyle's law, 679
Brachial plexus, 100, 860-861
Bradycardia-hypotension syndrome, 534
Bradycardias, 546-548
   definition of, 542
   myocardial infarction and, 435
Bradykinesia
   Huntington's chorea and, 817
   parkinsonism and, 812, 813
Brain; see also Neurologic diseases
   abscesses of, 139, 191-194, 579, 844
   angiography of, 564-565, 761
   biopsy of, 128, 135, 136, 137
   circulation of, 829-835
      angiography of, 564-565, 761
      heart failure and, 462
      syndromes of, 832-835
   congenital cytomegalovirus and, 125
   cysticercosis and, 293
   emboli of; see Cerebrovascular accident
   hemispheres of; see Cerebral hemispheres
   hemorrhage into, 830, 838-839; see also Cerebrovascular accident
   herniation of, 767, 846
   infarction of, 830-835
      hypertensive encephalopathy and, 841
      myocardial infarction and, 536
      vertigo and, 793-794
   ischemia of; see Cerebral ischemia
   radiation injury and, 749, 750
   scans of; see Brain scans; Computed tomography, brain and
   tumors of, 843-848
      benign, 843
      intracerebral hemorrhage and, 838
      parkinsonism and, 814
      supratentorial, 767, 845
Brain scans, 761
   abscess and, 192
   cerebral infarction and, 832
   computed tomography and; see Computed tomography, brain and
   herpes simplex encephalitis and, 136
Brain stones, 880
Brainstem
   anatomy of, 834
   consciousness and, 763
   encephalomyelitis and, 801
   lesions of, 760
   reflexes and, 14
Brainstem auditory evoked response, 762, 795
Branched-chain amino acid disorders, 1236-1237
Branchial arch dysplasias, 1309
Branchial arch syndrome, 1309
Branchial clefts, 1305
Branchioskeletogenital syndrome, 1244
Breasts
   cancer of, 435, 448
   evaluation of, 11
Breath sounds, 12, 684-685
Breslow classification of melanoma, 918
Brilliant cresyl blue, 331
Brill-Zinsser disease, 210, 212-213
Broad beta disease, 1285
Broca's aphasia, 757, 772
Bromides, 777, 922, 924
2-Bromo-alpha-ergocriptine; see Bromocriptine
Bromocriptine
   acromegaly and, 1120
   amenorrhea and, 1177
   Cushing's syndrome and, 1159
   parkinsonism and, 815

Bromocriptine—cont'd
   prolactinoma and, 1120-1121
Bromphenol-impregnated protein indicator, 604
Brompton's solution, 446
Bronchi, 672
   adenoma of, 743
   allergic aspergillosis of, 277, 705
   angiography of, 689-690
   aortic dissection and, 561
   biopsy of, 689, 718
   breath sounds and, 685
   carcinoma of, 686
   circulation of, 674
   constriction of, 23-25; see also Asthma
   cysts of, 701, 735
   dilation of; see Bronchiectasis; Bronchodilators
   epithelium of, 739
   hyperirritable, 24
   hyperreactivity of, to cooling, 23
   inflammation of; see Bronchitis, chronic
   obstruction of, 713
      aspiration and, 178
      atelectasis and, 702, 703
      supportive care and, 445
   smoking and, 738, 739; see also smoking
   study of; see Bronchography; Bronschoscopy
   tumors of, 738-742
Bronchial asthma; see Asthma
Bronchiectasis, 696-698
   cystic fibrosis and, 700, 1101
   dental care in, 746
   sputum and, 686
Bronchiectasis sicca, 697
Bronchioles
   epithelial, necrosis of, 141
   inflammation of
      echoviruses and, 144
      parainfluenza viruses and, 142
      respiratory syncytial virus and, 141, 142
Bronchitis, chronic, 691-693
   bullae and, 700
   chronic obstructive pulmonary disease and, 710-711
   cystic fibrosis and, 1101
   dental care and, 745-746
   lung cancer and, 742
   pneumonia and, 173
Bronchoalveolar carcinoma, 686; see also Lung, malignancies of
Bronchoconstriction, 23-25; see also Asthma
Bronchodilators, 24
   asthma and, 24, 705, 706, 728
   atelectasis and, 703
   bronchiectasis and, 697
   chronic obstructive pulmonary disease and, 693
   fish poisoning and, 200
   pregnancy and, 1212
   respiratory failure and, 711
   smoke inhalation and, 729
Bronchogenic carcinoma; see Lung malignancies of
Bronchogenic cysts, 701, 735
Bronchography, 689, 697, 702-703
Bronchopneumonia; see also Pneumonia
   bronchiectasis and, 698
   measles and, 145
   respiratory syncytial virus and, 142
Bronchopulmonary aspergillosis, allergic, 277, 705
Bronchoscopy, 688-689
   bronchiectasis and, 698
   endocarditis and, 185
   lung cancer and, 740

Bronzing of skin, 345, 878, 890
Broth test, 155
Brown tumors, 1193, 1208
Brucella, 243-245, 362
Brucella abortus, 243, 244
Brucella canis, 243-244
Brucella melitensis, 243, 244
Brucella suis, 243, 244
Brucellosis, 243-245, 362
Brugia malayi, 292
Bruits
   asymptomatic, 565
   hepatic changes and, 1059
   hyperthyroidism and systolic, 1205
   renal artery stenosis and, 661
Brunner's gland hyperplasia, 1037
Brushfield's spots, 1225
Bruton-type X-linked agammaglobulinemia, 32
Bruxism, nocturnal, 861
BSB clearance; see Sulfobromophthalein clearance
BTPS; see Body temperature and pressure saturated with water vapor
Bubo, 242, 266
Bubonic plague, 242
Buccal mucosa, 9
   Behçet's disease and, 907
   Crohn's disease and, 1097
   dermatitis herpetiformis and, 893
   lichen planus and, 938
   melanotic macule of, 919
   Peutz-Jeghers syndrome and, 1095
   pseudoxanthoma elasticum and, 884
   riboflavin deficiency and, 1108
Bucco-linguo-facial dyskinesia, 870
Budd-Chiari syndrome, 1045, 1060, 1077-1078
Buerger's disease, 69, 570
Buffers, 592-593, 599
Bulbar palsy, 760, 803
Bulbar telangiectases, 809
Bulk agents; see Hydrophilic bulk agents
Bullae, 700-701
   chest roentgenograms and, 686
   dermatitis herpetiformis and, 893
   diabetes and, 885
   dialysis and, 1255
   emphysema and, 694, 700-701, 724, 747
   epidermolysis bullosa dystrophica and, 877
   head-foot-and-mouth disease and, 300
   impetigo, 219
   myringitis and, 217
   pemphigoid and, 935
   porphyria and, 1298
   toxic epidermal necrolysis and, 306
Bull-neck appearance, 248
Bullosis diabeticorum, 885
Bullous dermatosis of hemodialysis, 1255
Bullous emphysema, 694, 700-701, 724, 747
Bullous impetigo, 219
Bullous myringitis, 217
Bullous pemphigoid, 935
Bumpy lips, 1164
BUN; see Blood urea nitrogen
Burkitt's lymphoma, 131, 132, 300
Burns, 166
Burr cells, 315
Bursitis, 52, 98-99
Busulfan, 442
   leukemias and, 370
   lung disease and, 722
   myeloid metaplasia and, 376
   thrombocytopenia and, 400
   thrombocytosis and, 404
   toxicity of, 370

Butazolidin; see Phenylbutazone
Butterfly lesions, 54, 55, 578, 882
Butyrophenones, 871
Bypass procedures
 aneurysm of sinus of Valsalva and, 558
 aortofemoral, 570
 arthritis and, 53
 coronary artery, 532
 diabetes mellitus and, 1273
 femoropopliteal, 570
 intestinal, 1103
  Crohn's disease and, 1015
  of distal ileum, 1291
  jejunal, 53, 1077
  occlusive vascular disease of gut and, 1020
 of superficial temporal artery to middle cerebral artery, 837

C

^{14}C; see Carbon, radioactive
C apoproteins, 1281
C cells, 1128, 1151, 1189, 1197
C3 complement, 46
Cabot rings, 315, 333
Cachexia, 438
CAD; see Coronary heart disease
Cadaver donors, 644
Cadmium
 as carcinogen, 432
 inhalational lung disease and, 729
 interstitial nephritis and, 619, 620
 toxic nephropathy and, 627
Café au lait spots, 808, 878, 879, 882
Café coronary, 713
Caffeine
 coronary artery disease and, 527
 gastric secretion and, 943, 944
 nephropathy and, 621
 seizures and, 786
 toxicity of, 777
 ulcers and, 991
 urinary catecholamines and, 1168
CAH; see Congenital adrenal hyperplasias
Caisson disease, 104
Calcaneal bursitis, 52
Calcaneal spurs, 102
Calciferol; see Vitamins, D
Calcification
 aortic aneurysm and, 566
 aural, 103
 basal ganglion, 1209; see also Basal ganglia
 of cartilage, 94, 95
 chest roentgenograms and, 685
 histoplasmosis and, 274
 hyperparathyroidism and, 1208
 intracerebral, 125, 126, 810, 880, 881
 in pancreas, 1055
 pericardial, 551, 552
 scleroderma and, 904
 silicosis and, 724
 Sturge-Weber syndrome and, 810, 881
 tendinitis and, 99
 viral infection and, 125, 126
Calcimar; see Calcitonin
Calcinosis
 cartilage and, 94, 95
 dermatomyositis and, 905-906
 diphosphonates and probenecid in, 62
 in Raynaud's phenomenon, sclerodactyly, and telangiectasia syndrome, 58, 60, 904
 systemic sclerosis and, 58, 60, 904
Calcinosis cutis, 904
Calcitonin, 1128
 C-cell hyperplasia and, 1151, 1152, 1197

Calcitonin—cont'd
 ectopic secretion of, 435
 fibrous dysplasia and, 104
 hypercalcemia and, 445, 1180, 1189, 1191-1192, 1195
 medullary carcinoma and, 1197
 metabolism of, 1189
 osteoporosis and, 89, 1203
 Paget's disease and, 88
 phosphate metabolism and, 1184
 serum, 1151, 1152, 1197
Calcium
 antagonists to, 465, 532, 533
 calcitonin and, 445, 1180, 1189, 1191-1192, 1195
 cardiac cells and, 479
 C-cell hyperplasia and, 1151, 1152, 1197
 deficiency of; see Hypocalcemia
 diabetic ketoacidosis and, 1270
 dialysis and, 642
 dietary deficiency of, 1188-1189
 excess of; see Hypercalcemia
 excretion of, 647, 648
 fluoride poisoning and, 754
 gastric secretion and, 943, 944, 1004
 hyperkalemia and, 599
 kidney stones and, 646-648
 metabolism of, 1183-1184
 multiple myeloma and, 382
 neuromuscular blockade and, 167
 osteoporosis and, 89, 1202, 1203, 1210
 pancreatitis and, 1052
 after parathyroid gland removal, 1194
 parathyroid hormone and, 1187
 plasma, 1183-1184, 1189-1196
 pregnancy and, 1211
 in renal cyst, 651
 renal failure and, 636, 639
 respiratory paralysis and, 169
 sarcoidosis and, 717
 serum, 1183-1184, 1189-1196
  hyperparathyroidism and, 1207-1208
  hypoparathyroidism and, 1209
  kidney stones and, 648
  neoplasms and, 1179-1180
  osteomalacia and, 1198, 1199
 renal failure and, 636
 whole blood transfusions and, 350, 351
Calcium antagonists, 465, 532, 533
Calcium bicarbonate mouthrinses, 908
Calcium carbonate, 991-992, 1088
Calcium chloride, 1196
Calcium gluconate
 hyperkalemia and, 633
 hypoparathyroidism and, 1196
 lead poisoning and, 753
 tetany and, 1196
Calcium hydroxyapatite crystals, 95
Calcium lactate, 633, 1196
Calcium oxalate nephrolithiasis, 648
Calcium pyrophosphate crystal disease, 94
Calcium pyrophosphate dihydrate crystals, 94-95
Calculi
 cholesterol, 1086-1089
 in common bile duct, 950, 1086, 1089
 kidney; see Kidney stones
California encephalitis, 135, 825
Caloric tests, 766, 792
Calories, 1104
Calymmatobacterium granulomatis, 238
Campylobacter, 202
 diabetes and, 1294
 diarrhea and, 202, 953
 Reiter's syndrome and, 907

Campylobacter fetus, 202
Canaliculus, 1086
Cancers, 431; see also Carcinomas; Neoplasia
 chemotherapy for; see Chemotherapy
 radiation for; see Radiation
Candida, 33, 276, 278, 279, 929-930
 acrodermatitis enteropathica and, 895
 cancer chemotherapy and, 451
 diabetes and, 885
 dysphagia and, 1091, 1092
 in endocarditis, 179, 181
 in esophagitis, 307, 985, 1092
 folic acid deficiency and, 415
 Hodgkin's disease and, 424
 immunodeficiency diseases and, 31
 leukemia and, 421-422
 myeloperoxidase deficiency and, 357
 neoplasia and, 446
 odynophagia and, 975
 oral; see Oral candidiasis
 in pneumonia, 172
 psoriasis and, 937-938
 renal disease and, 897
 sarcoidosis and, 911
Candida albicans, 276; see also *Candida*
 anal disorders and, 1030
 esophagitis and, 307, 985
 Hailey-Hailey disease and, 934
 oral lesions of; see Oral candidiasis
 skin lesions and, 929-930
Candidiasis; see *Candida*
Candle guttering, 810
Cannabis, 778, 1134
Cannibalism, 828
Cannon's law, 976
CAPD; see Peritoneal dialysis, chronic ambulatory
Capillaria philippinensis, 1003
Capillariasis, 1003
Capillaries
 hydrostatic pressure of pleural, 730
 permeability of subperitoneal, 1044
 pulmonary; see Pulmonary capillaries
Caplan's syndrome, 715
Capnocytophagia, 302, 1294
Capreomycin, 259-260, 627, 628
Capsid, 121
Capsid antigen, 1068
Capsulitis, adhesive, 101
Captopril
 heart failure and, 465
 hypertension and, 474
 with renal crisis, 62
 renal failure and, 639
 scleroderma and, 62, 616
Caput medusae, 1060
Carbamazepine
 dental care and, 866
 diabetes insipidus and, 1126
 dystonia musculorum deformans and, 821
 epilepsy and, 786
 erythema multiforme and, 30
 herpes zoster neuropathy and, 855
 hyponatremia and, 594
 trigeminal neuralgia and, 791
Carbamyl phosphate synthetase deficiency, 1239
Carbenicillin, 160, 164
 bacteremia and, 241
 lung abscess and, 699
 meningitis and, 190
 neoplasia and, 446
 neutropenia and, 361
 oral lesions and, 241, 306, 421
 pneumonia and, 177

Carbenicillin—cont'd
  pregnancy and, 1212
  Pseudomonas oral lesions and, 241, 306
  renal disease and, 670
  toxic nephropathy and, 625
Carbenicillin indanyl sodium, 160, 164, 198
Carbenoxolone, 600
Carbocaine, 866
Carbodopa, 814
Carbohydrates, 1102
  absorption of, 1004-1005
  calories in, 1104
  deficiencies of, 1104
  diabetes mellitus and, 1261
  irritable bowel disease and, 1028
  liver disease and, 1062
  Norwalk-like agents and, 150
  nutritional therapy and, 1111
  rotaviruses and, 150
Carbolic acid, 927, 928
Carbon, radioactive, 1005
Carbon 17 alkyl-substituted steroids, 1076
Carbon dioxide, 708, 960-961; *see also* Carbon dioxide tension, arterial
Carbon dioxide snow, 882
Carbon dioxide tension, arterial, 673; *see also* Arterial blood gases
  acidosis and, 600, 601
  alkalosis and , 600, 601
  asthma and, 24, 706
  atelectasis and, 592, 702
  heart failure and, 462
  hypoxemia and, 602, 603, 681-682
    mixed acid-base disorders and, 601-603
  pulmonary capillary blood flow and, 674-676
  respiratory failure and, 707, 708, 710, 712
  ventilation-perfusion abnormalities and, 674-676
Carbon monoxide
  carboxyhemoglobinemia and, 344
  diffusing capacity of, 676
  polycythemia and, 354
Carbon monoxide transfer factor, 676
Carbon tetrachloride
  hypogonadism and, 1172
  liver toxicity and, 1063, 1075, 1077
  toxic nephropathy and, 627, 629, 630, 631
Carbonic acid system, 599; *see also* Bicarbonate
Carbonic anhydrase, 592
Carboxyhemoglobin, 344
Carboxylesterase, 1049
Carboxypeptidase A and B, 1050
Carbuncles, 219
Carcinoembryonic antigen, 435, 1010, 1040, 1041
Carcinogenesis, 431-434
Carcinoid tumors, 450
  bronchial adenoma and, 743
  of large bowel, 1042
  malabsorption and, 1004
  of small bowel, 1037-1038
  syndrome of, 450, 743, 1037-1038
Carcinomas; *see also* Adenocarcinoma; Neoplasia
  alveolar cell, 59
  of ampulla of Vater, 1089
  anorectal, 1031
  of anus, 1031, 1042
  basal cell; *see* Basal cell carcinoma
  of biliary ducts, 445, 1089
  of bladder, 449, 659
  of breast, 435, 448
  bronchoalveolar, 686
  bronchogenic; *see* Lung, malignancies of
  of cervix, 433, 449

Carcinomas—cont'd
  of colon, 1039-1041, 1093
    management of, 448
    Streptococcus bovis and, 228
    ulcerative colitis and, 1008, 1009, 1010
  diffuse; *see* Carcinomatosis
  epidermoid; *see* Epidermoid carcinoma
  of esophagus, 447, 979, 1032-1033
  of gallbladder, 1089
  of gastrointestinal tract, 1035-1036
    carcinoembryonic antigen and, 435
    iron deficiency anemia and, 324
    management of, 447-448
    polyps and, 1033
    remnants and, 997
    Streptococcus bovis and, 228
    ulcers and, 989, 993
  head and neck, 449
  of liver; *see* Liver, neoplasms of
  of lung; *see* Lung, malignancies of
  meningitis and, 139
  of mouth, 918, 919
  neuropathies and, 855
  of ovary, 449, 1045, 1177-1178
  of pancrease; *see* pancreas, carcinomas of
  of prostate, 449, 659-660
  of rectum, 448, 1031, 1039-1041
  renal cell, 449, 656-658
  second primary site of, 919
  of small bowel, 445, 1013-1014, 1037-1038
  squamous cell, 416, 447, 915, 919
  testicular, 435, 449, 1173
  of thyroid; *see* Thyroid, carcinoma of
Carcinomatosis
  hemolysis and, 341
  lymphangitic, of lung, 743-744
  meningeal, 139, 845
  secondary peritoneal, 1047
Carcinosarcoma, embryonal, 658
Cardabid; *see* Nitroglycerin
Cardiac arrhythmias; *see* Arrhythmias
Cardiac care unit, 537
Cardiac catheterization, 487-489
  angiocardiography and, 488-489
  aortic stenosis and, 515
  in congenital heart disease, 501-502
  constrictive pericarditis and, 552
  heart failure and, 462-463
  mitral regurgitation and, 511
  mitral stenosis and, 513
  pulmonary hypertension and, 496-497
  right-sided, 488
  treatment and, 502
Cardiac cell polarity, 479
Cardiac glycosides; *see also* specific agent
  digitalis in; *see* Digitalis
  pregnancy and, 1212
  silicosis and, 724
Cardiac murmurs; *see* Murmurs, cardiac
Cardiac output, 457, 458, 467, 461, 528
Cardiac pain, dental correlations in, 582-583
Cardiac pulmonary edema, 708, 710
Cardiac shunts, 191, 353; *see also* Anastomoses
Cardiac syncope, 780
Cardiac tamponade, 553, 554, 555
  amebiasis and, 283
  heart failure and, 453-454, 461
  shock and, 476
Cardiogenic shock, 477, 576
Cardiology, 479-489
  cardiac catheterization in; *see* Cardiac catheterization
  echocardiography in, 485-487; *see also* Echocardiography

Cardiology—cont'd
  electrocardiography in, 479-495; *see also* Electrocardiograms
  nuclear cardiology in, 489
Cardiomyopathies, 517-524
  arrhythmia and, 585
  classification of, 517
  congestive heart failure and, 453
  dentistry and, 582
  effusive pericarditis and, 554
  idiopathic
    dilated congestive, 520-522
    hypertrophic, 517-520
    restrictive, 522
  metabolic, 523
  nutritional, 523
  secondary, 522-523
  terminology and, 517
Cardiopulmonary bypass; *see* Bypass procedures
Cardiopulmonary resuscitation, 540, 583-584, 752
Cardiovascular diseases, 452-587
  aorta and, 586-587; *see also* Aorta
    distal and aortic branches in, 564-571
    thoracic, 555-563
  arrhythmias in, 541-550; *see also* Arrhythmias
  cardiomyopathies in, 517-524, 582; *see also* Cardiomyopathies
  congenital heart disease in, 497-509, 578-579; *see also* Congenital heart disease
  congenital rubella and, 126
  congestive heart failure in, 452-465, 571-572; *see also* Heart failure
  coronary, 524-541, 582-584; *see also* Coronary heart disease
  dentistry and, 571-587
    aorta and, 586-587
    arrhythmia and, 584-585
    cardiomyopathy and, 582
    congenital heart disease and, 578-579
    congestive heart failure and, 571-572
    coronary heart disease and, 582-584
    hypertension and, 572-575
    pericarditis and, 585-587
    pulmonary embolism and, 577-578
    pulmonary hypertension and, 578
    shock and, 575-577
    valvular disease and, 579-582
  diagnosis in, 479-489; *see also* Cardiology
  hypertension in, 465-475, 572-575; *see also* Hypertension, portal
  hyperthyroidism and, 1142-1143
  Marfan's syndrome and, 1241
  normal function and, 454-459
  pericarditis in, 550-555, 585-587; *see also* Pericarditis
  physiologic response to, 459-460
  pulmonary embolism in, 489-494, 577-578; *see also* Pulmonary emboli
  pulmonary hypertension in, 496-497, 578; *see also* Pulmonary hypertension
  relapsing polychondritis and, 102-103
  shock in, 475-479, 575-577
  sickle cell anemia and, 332
  syphilis and, 265, 268-269
  thrombophlebitis and, 494-495
  valvular, 340, 510-517, 579-582
Cardioversion, 546, 549-550
Carditis, 229, 230; *see also* Endocarditis; Pericarditis
Caries
  congenital heart disease and, 579
  drug abuse and, 862
  immunodeficiency disease and, 34

Caries—cont'd
  pregnancy and, 1211
Carmustine; see BCNU
Carnitine deficiency myopathy, 859
Carotenes, 888, 1106, 1248, 1250
Carotid artery
  endarterectomy of, 565
  evaluation of, 10-11, 872
    phonoangiography in, 565
  hypertrophic cardiomyopathy and, 519
  pain from pressure on, 791-792
  stenosis in, 564
  valvular disease and, 580
Carotid bodies, 677
Carotid sinus, 547, 780-781
Carotid sinus syncope, 586-587, 780-781
Carotidynia, 791-792
Carpal tunnel syndrome, 60, 98
Carpenter's syndrome, 1314, 1316
Carpometacarpal joint, 84
Carriers, 1223-1224
  alpha-thalassemia and, 336
  hemoglobinopathies and, 331
  hepatitis, 1091, 1099-1100
  of sickle cell trait, 334
  testing for, 1224
  translocation, 1222
Cartilage, 94, 95, 103
Carvallo's sign, 516
Cascara, 589
Caseation necrosis, 254
Casoni's test, 294
Casts
  hyaline, 605
  red blood cell, 588, 605, 610
Catalepsy, 764
Catamenial pneumothorax, 733
Cataplexy, 769
Catapres; see Clonidine
Cataracts, 750, 1273
Catatonic stupor, 764
Catecholamine-blocking agents, 1241
Catecholamines; see also specific agent
  with anesthetics, coronary heart disease and, 583
  arrhythmias and, 585
  biosynthesis of, 1166
  blood pressure and, 468
  heart rate and, 458
  metabolism of, 1166
  parathyroid hormone and, 1187
  peripheral vascular resistance and, 460
  pheochromocytoma and, 1164-1168
  shock and, 477
  syncope and, 864
  urinary, 1166, 1168, 1258
Catechol-O-methyltransferase, 1166
Cathartic colon, 956
Cathartics, 1002
Catheters
  bacteremia and, 241
  cardiac; see Cardiac catheterization
  percutaneous biliary, 967, 968, 1089
  Swan-Ganz, 478, 708
  of urinary bladder, 199, 568, 633, 656
Cation exchange resins, hyperkalemia and, 599, 634; see also Sodium polystyrene sulfonate
Cat-scratch fever, 151, 300-301
Causalgia, 100
Caustic agents, ingestion of, 985-986
Cautery
  angiokeratoma corporis diffusum and, 912
  chemical, hemophilia and, 428

Cautery—cont'd
  Reiter's syndrome and, 908
  snare, 1034, 1038, 1040; see also Electrocoagulation
Cavernous hemangiomas, giant, 341
Cavernous sinus thrombosis, 303-304, 873
Cavitron, 578
C3b, 16
CBG; see Corticosteroid-binding globulin
CCK-PZ; see Cholecystokinin, pancreozymin and
CCNU; see Lomustine
CDLE; see Lupus erythematosus, chronic discoid
CE; see California encephalitis
CEA; see Carcinoembryonic antigen
Cebocephaly, 1317
Cecostomy, decompression, 1011
Cecum, 947, 1011, 1019
Cefaclor, 160, 165
Cefamandole, 160, 165, 176
Cefazolin, 160, 164
  bacteremia and, 241
  cellulitis and, 226
  endocarditis and, 183
  lung abscess and, 699
Cefoperazone, 160, 165, 241
Cefotaxime, 160, 165, 241
Cefoxitin, 160, 165, 232, 699
Cefsulodin, 165
Ceftazidime, 165
Ceftizoxime, 165
Ceftriaxone, 165
Celiac axis, occlusive disease of, 1020
Celiac disease, 941, 999, 1001
Cell count; see Blood cell count
Cell cycles, 439, 440, 442, 443
Cell rests, 844
Cell separators, automated, 346
Cell-kill hypotheses, 439
Cell-mediated immunity, 19, 27, 377; see also Bone marrow–derived cells; Immune system; Thymus-derived cells
  chronic mucocutaneous candidiasis and, 307
  classification and, 33
  dentistry and, 30
  Hodgkin's disease and, 387
  polymyositis and, 64
  tuberculosis and, 254
  vascular damage and, 66
  viruses and, 122
Cellular acidosis, 539
Cellular fluid osmolality, 593
Cellular immunity; see Cell-mediated immunity
Cellulase, 998
Cellulitis, 219
  clostridial, 252-253, 254
  facial, sickle cell anemia and, 417
  Haemophilus influenzae and, 236
  staphylococcal, 226
  streptococcal, 226
Cellulose phosphate, 648
Centers for Disease Control, 134, 138, 232
Central core disease, 859
Central cyanosis, 571, 578
Central nervous system; see also Brain; Neurologic diseases
  alveolar hypoventilation and, 682
  bacterial infections of, 186-195, 303, 868
  Behçet's syndrome and, 110-111
  coma and; see Coma
  craniosynostosis syndromes and, 1314
  heredofamilial diseases of, 801-810
  intoxications and, 775-779
  multiple sclerosis and, 796-801
  schistosomiasis and, 296

Central nervous system—cont'd
  sickle cell anemia and, 332
  syphilis and, 265, 268, 269
  tumors of, 843-848; see also Brain, tumors of
  vertigo and, 793-794
  viral infections of; see Viral diseases of central nervous system
Central pontine myelolysis, 1257
Central sleep apnea, 708, 711
Central terminal of Wilson, 480
Central transtentorial herniation, 767
Central venous pressure, 478, 571
Centromere, 1220
CEP; see Porphyrias, congenital erythropoietic
Cephalexin, 157, 160, 165
  lung abscess and, 699
  staphylococcal infections and, 221
  urinary tract infection and, 197, 198
Cephaloridine, 164-165, 627, 628
Cephalosporins, 160, 164-165
  abdominal abscess and, 1047
  allergy and, 28
  with aminoglycosides, 166, 176-177, 241
  anaerobes and, 250
  bacteremia and, 241
  bactericidal activity of, 156
  cellulitis and, 226
  chancroid and, 239
  diarrhea from, 1018
  dosages of, 158
  drug fever and, 159
  endocarditis and, 183, 184
  enterococci and, 228
  erysipeloid and, 246
  excretion of, 158
  gram-negative oral lesions and, 306
  hemolysis and, 342
  leukopenia and, 29
  lung abscess and, 699
  meningitis and, 190
  neoplasia and, 446
  nephropathy and, 625, 627, 628
  and osteomyelitis, 116, 222
  pancreatitis and, 1053
  pneumonia and, 175, 176-177
  pregnancy and, 1212, 1213
  renal insufficiency and, 158
  staphylococci and, 175, 183, 184, 221
  streptococci and, 183, 227, 228
Cephalothin, 160, 164
  aminoglycosides and, 166
  bacteremia and, 241
  cellulitis and, 226
  clostridial infection and, 253
  endocarditis and, 183
  excretion of, 158
  lung abscess and, 699
  nephropathy and, 624, 627
  neutropenia and, 361
  pneumonia and, 176
  site of infection and, 157
  staphylococci and, 183, 221
Cephapirin, 160, 164
Cephradine, 160, 165, 197, 198
Ceramidase deficiency, 1231, 1233
Ceramide, 1230
Ceramide glucose accumulation, 396
Ceramidetrihexosidase, 911
Cercariae, 295
Cerebellar arteries, syndromes of, 833, 834
Cerebellar ataxia, 130, 137, 138, 759
Cerebellum
  astrocytomas of, 843-844
  ataxia and, 130, 137, 138, 759
  cortical degeneration and, 850

Cerebellum—cont'd
　hemangioblastoma of, 809
　lesions of, 354, 759-760, 1257
Cerebral abscesses, 139, 191-194, 844; see also
　　Brain
Cerebral angiography, 564-565, 761
Cerebral arteries, syndromes of, 832-833
Cerebral calcifications; see Calcification, intracerebral
Cerebral circulation, 829-835
　angiography of, 564-565, 761
　heart failure and, 462
　malformations in, dental implications of, 869, 872
　syncope and, 864
Cerebral cortex; see Cortex, cerebral
Cerebral emboli, 511, 830-835
Cerebral hemispheres
　aphasic right, 771
　cognition and, 770
　computed tomography and, 757, 758
　consciousness and, 763
　lesions of, 765
　　diffuse, 773-775
　　focal, 770-773
　　unconsciousness and, 765
Cerebral hemorrhage, 829, 830, 838-839, 841;
　　see also Cerebrovascular accident
Cerebral herniation, 767, 846
Cerebral infarction, 830-835
　dentistry and, 873
　hypertensive encephalopathy and, 841
　myocardial infarction and, 536
Cerebral ischemia, 829; see also Cerebrovascular
　　accident
　aortic arch syndrome and, 563
　transient, 563, 564, 586, 836-838
Cerebral syndrome, radiation and, 749, 750
Cerebrosidase, 802
Cerebroside, 1230
Cerebrospinal fluid; see also Lumbar puncture
　antimicrobials in, 156
　craniosynostosis syndromes and, 1313, 1314
　cryptococcosis and, 275
　leptospirosis and, 273
　listeriosis and, 245
　meningitis and, 186, 187, 188, 825
　multiple sclerosis and, 800
　syphilis and, 268, 269
　tuberculosis and, 257
　unconsciousness and, 768
　viral disease of central nervous system and, 135, 137
Cerebrospinal fluid shunts, 187
Cerebrospinal pleocytosis, 188
Cerebrovascular accident, 564-565, 829, 830-835
　brain tumor and, 846
　dentistry and, 586-587, 871-873
　diabetes mellitus and, 1272-1273
　hemichorea and, 818
　mitral valve prolapse and, 511
Ceruloplasmin, 1066, 1081-1082
Cerveau isolé, 764
Cervical lymphadenitis, tuberculous, 256, 304
Cervical lymphadenopathy, 69; see also Lymphadenopathy
　cat-scratch disease and, 300
　diptheria and, 305
　leukemia and, 420
　sarcoidosis and, 113
Cervical myelopathy, spondylitic, 860
Cervical nodes, 256, 304; see also Adenopathy;
　　Cervical lymphadenopathy

Cervical ribs, 101
Cervical spine, 36, 38, 39, 860; see also Spine
Cervical tension state, 100
Cervicofacial actinomycosis, 305
Cervix, 215, 433, 449
Cesarean section, 127, 1168
Cestodes, 292-294, 317
CF; see Complement fixation
CGD; see Granulomatous diseases
Chagas' disease, 287
　achalasia and, 977
　beta-thalassemia and, 336
　megacolon and, 1027
Chamberlain's line, 811
Chancre, 266, 267
　oral, primary syphilis and, 302-303
　trypanosomal, 287
Chancroid, 238-239
Chaotic atrial tachycardia, 542-543
Charcoal, 627
Charcot joints, 86, 94, 1275
Charcot-Bouchard aneurysms, 838
Charcot-Marie-Tooth disease, 805, 855
Chédiak-Higashi syndrome, 357, 397, 420
Cheeks
　erythema of, 147
　mucosa of; see Buccal mucosa
　tuberous sclerosis and, 880
Cheese washer's lung, 727
Cheilitis, angular; see Angular cheilitis
Cheilosis
　angular; see Angular cheilosis
　diabetes and, 1294
　malabsorption and, 1000
　pyridoxine deficiency and, 1298
　riboflavin deficiency and, 1298
Chelating agents
　blood transfusions and, 337
　heavy metal poisoning and, 627
　iron, 322, 346
　multiple myeloma and, 382
　scleroderma and, 903
　Waldenström's macroglobulinemia and, 383
　Wilson's disease and, 823
Chemical cautery, 428
Chemical mediators, 18, 25, 27; see also specific
　　mediator
Chemical messengers, 1114-1115
Chemicals
　aplastic anemia and, 318, 319
　aspiration pneumonitis and, 178
　diabetes mellitus and, 1260-1261
　in food, poisoning from, 200
　hemolysis from, 342
　injuries from, 752-755
　leukemias and, 364
　nasal congestion and, 20
Chemistries, serum, 313; see also Serum
Chemoreceptors, 711
Chemosurgery, 883, 915
Chemotaxis, 15, 356-357
Chemotherapy, 439-443; see also Cytotoxic
　　agents
　antituberculous; see Antituberculous agents
　antiviral, 122, 153-154; see also specific agent
　aplastic anemia and, 319, 320
　Bowen's disease and, 914
　combination; see Combination chemotherapy
　dentistry and, 450-451, 919
　gastric neoplasm and, 1036, 1037
　influenza vaccine and, 153
　in insulinomas, 1279
　Kaposi's sarcoma and, 922
　large bowel neoplasms and, 1041

Chemotherapy—cont'd
　in leukemias, 366-367, 421
　lung cancer and, 742
　lymphomas and, 424
　macroglobulinemia and, 423
　meningitis prophylaxis and, 190, 191
　mesothelioma and, 1047
　myeloma and, 422, 618, 918
　nephroblastoma and, 658
　nephropathy and, 622, 625
　neurologic complications of, 847, 853
　in non-Hodgkin's lymphoma, 393
　oral candidiasis and, 307
　prostatic carcinoma and, 660
　radiation pneumonitis and, 722
　shock and, 575
　small bowel neoplasms and, 1037, 1038
　thrombocytopenia and, 400, 401
　tumor growth fractions and, 439
　Waldenström's macroglobulinemia and, 383
Chenodeoxycholic acid, 1063, 1085
　cholelithiasis and, 1089
Cherry-red spot–myoclonus syndrome, 1235
Chest; see also Thorax
　myofascial syndromes and, 98
　pain in
　　angina and, 527-533
　　aortic dissection and, 560
　　cardiomyopathy and, 521, 522
　　dental correlations, 582-583
　　myocardial infarction and, 534
　　pericarditis and, 550-551
　rheumatic disorders of, 100-101
　roentgenograms of, 685-686; see also Roentgenograms
　　acute respiratory distress syndrome and, 709
　　atelectasis and, 702
　　bronchitis and, 692
　　bullae and, 700
　　in congenital heart diseae, 501
　　emphysema and, 694, 695
　　hyperlucent airspaces in, 686
　　lung abscess and, 699
　　lung cancer and, 739, 740
　　perfusion scan and, 687
　　pleural effusion and, 731
　　pneumonia and, 173, 174, 217
　　pulmonary embolism and, 491
　　sarcoidosis and, 76, 78
　　solitary pulmonary nodule and, 685, 743, 744
　silent, asthma and, 706
　wall of, 12, 685, 737-738
Chest bellows disease, 712
Cheyne-Stokes respiration, 766
Chiasma formation, 1217
Chiba needle, 968
Chicken raiser's disease, 727
Chickenpox; see Varicella
Chief cells, 942, 943
Chief complaint, 5
Children; see also Infants; Newborn
　adenoviruses and, 143
　arthritis and, 43-47
　cat-scratch fever and, 151
　central nervous system disease and, 135, 137-138
　congenital heart disease in; see Congenital
　　heart disease
　cytomegalovirus and, 131
　dermatomyositis of, 65
　eczema in, 20
　encephalitis and, 135
　erythema infectiosum and, 147

Children—cont'd
 hyperthyroidism in, 1147, 1205
 hypothyroidism and, 1136-1138, 1140
 influenza and, 140
 iron deficiency anemia and, 324
 Kawasaki disease and, 147
 parainfluenza viruses and, 142
 respiratory syncytial virus and, 141
 rotaviruses and, 149-150
 varicella and, 129
Chills, 118
Chin, recession of, 36
Chinese restaurant syndrome, 200
Chlamydia psittaci, 216
 Chlamydia trachomatis, 214-216
 drugs for, 162, 167
 nongonococcal urethritis and, 232
 oral infection with, 302
Chlamydiae, 172, 214-216, 232
 drugs for, 168
 in pneumonia, 172
 Reiter's syndrome and, 52, 907
Chloral betaine, 1297
Chloral hydrate, 819, 1252, 1297
Chlorambucil, 442
 Kaposi's sarcoma, 922
 leukemias and, 371
 Waldenström's macroglobulinemia and, 383
Chloramines, 342
Chloramphenicol, 161, 168-169
 abdominal abscess and, 1047
 administration route for, 157
 anaerobic infections and, 178, 250
 anthrax and, 245
 arthritis and, 80
 bacteriostatic activity of, 156
 bone marrow toxicity and, 319
 brain abscess and, 192, 193
 cavernous sinus thrombosis and, 303
 donovanosis and, 238
 enteric fever and, 192, 208
 erysipeloid and, 246
 excretion of, 158
 gray baby syndrome and, 158
 Haemophilus influenzae and, 176, 236
 hemolysis and, 329
 leukemias and, 364
 listeriosis and, 246
 liver and, 158
 lung abscess and, 699
 meningitis and, 190
 methotrexate and, 440
 neutropenia and, 360
 plague and, 242
 pneumonia and, 176
 pregnancy and, 1212
 rickettsial diseases and, 210
 Rocky Mountain spotted fever and, 211
 Salmonella and, 108
 sideroblastic anemia and, 321
 site of infection and, 156
 subdural empyema and, 193
 thrombocytopenia and, 400, 401
 tularemia and, 243
Chlordiazepoxide
 alcohol and, 776, 1080-1081, 1297
 lung disease and, 722
 pregnancy and, 1212, 1213
 respiratory alkalosis and, 601
 side effects of, 871
 toxicity of, 777
Chlorhexidine, 302, 421, 866
Chloride
 cystic fibrosis and, 700

Chloride—cont'd
 metabolic alkalosis and, 600
 respiratory acidosis and, 601
Chlorinated hydrocarbons, 888
Chlorinated insecticides, 754
Chlorine, 729
Chloroma, 898
Chloromethyl ethers, 432
Chloromycetin, 415
Chloroquine
 amebic abscess and, 283
 hemolysis and, 329
 juvenile rheumatoid arthritis and, 40
 lupus erythematosus and, 903
 malaria and, 281
 porphyria and, 888, 1248, 1254
 resistance to, 281
 rheumatoid arthritis and, 42
 urine and, 588
Chlorothiazide, 472
Chlorpheniramine maleate, 22
Chlorpromazine
 guanethidine and, 472
 hypogonadism and, 1172
 liver toxicity and, 1076
 neutropenia and, 360
 non-REM sleep and, 96
 pheochromocytoma tests and, 471
 porphyria and, 1252
 proteinuria and, 590
 side effects of, 871
 urinary catecholamines and, 1168
Chlorpropamide
 diabetes insipidus and, 1126
 diabetes mellitus and, 1266, 1267
 hemolysis and, 342
 hyponatremia and, 594
 lung disease and, 721, 722
Chlortetracycline, 168, 421
Chlorthalidone, 472, 597, 1051
Chlor-Trimeton; *see* Chlorpheniramine maleate
Cholangiocarcinomas, 1089
Cholangiography, transhepatic, 967, 968, 1089
Cholangiopancreatography, endoscopic retrograde; *see* Endoscopic retrograde cholangiopancreatography
Cholangitis, 105, 1088, 1089
Cholecalciferol metabolism, 1115
Cholecystectomy
 cholelithiasis and, 1089
 enteric fever and, 208
Cholecystitis, 1086-1089
 biliary tract imaging and, 969
 pain and, 950, 988
 spherocytosis and, 328
Cholecystojejunostomy, 1057
Cholecystokinin, 1086
 cholesterol stones and, 1088
 irritable bowel disease and, 1027
 pancreozymin and, 941, 946, 1050
Choledochoduodenostomy, 1089
Choledocholithiasis, 950, 1086, 1089
Cholelithiasis, 1086-1089
 cholangiography and, 967, 968
 Crohn's disease and, 1012
 endoscopic retrograde cannulation and, 968-969
 formation and dissolution of, 1085
 gallbladder carcinoma and, 1089
 pain and, 950
 spherocytosis and, 328
 ultrasound and, 970
Cholera, 201, 204-205, 209
 diarrhea and, 953

Cholera—cont'd
 malabsorption and, 1003
 pancreatic, 1049
 vaccine for, 205
Cholestasis, 1087
 enzymes and, 1065
 extrahepatic, 1058
 hepatitis and, 1070
 intrahepatic, 1058, 1068
 jaundice and, 168, 1067
 sex hormones and, 1076
 term of, 1058
Cholesterol, 1153, 1162, 1280; *see also* Hypercholesterolemia
 accumulation of, 397, 1286
 bile and, 946
 cholelithiasis and, 1086-1089
 coronary artery disease and, 527, 528
 dietary, 1111
 familial hypercholesterolemia and, 1287
 familial lecithin:cholesterol acyltransferase deficiency and, 1292-1293
 familial remnant removal disease and, 1287
 generation of free, 1283
 hyperlipidemia and, 1280
 lipoproteins and, 1285, 1288
 liver disease and, 1063, 1065, 1286
 measurement of total, 1288-1289
 pleural effusion and, 731
 synthesis of, 1085-1086
 Tangier disease and, 1292
 transport of, 1282-1286
Cholesterol crystals, 1085
Cholesterol stones, 1086-1089
Cholesterolosis, 1088
Cholestyramine
 biliary cirrhosis and, 1082
 chlorpromazine jaundice and, 1076
 Crohn's disease and, 1014
 hepatitis and, 1072
 hyperlipidemias and, 1290
 hyperoxaluria and, 648
 malabsorption and, 1002
 porphyria and, 1250
 pruritus and, 1058
 pseudomembranous enterocolitis and, 1018
Cholic acid, 1063, 1085
Choline chloride, 817
Cholinergics
 achalasia and, 976, 979
 asthma and, 705
 esophageal spasm and, 980
 esophagitis and, 985
 irritable bowel syndrome and, 1027
 obstructive uropathy and, 656
Cholinesterase inhibitor-type insecticides, 754
Choretic diarrhea, 952, 953
Chondrocalcinosis, 94, 95
Chondrocranium, formation of, 1306, 1307, 1308
Chondrodynia costosternalis, 103
Chondrodystrophies, 1245, 1246
Chondroitin sulfate, 1233
Chondromatosis of temporomandibular joint, synovial, 108
Chondrometaplasia of temporomandibular joint, 108
CHOP; *see* Cyclophosphamide, hydroxydaunomycin, Oncovin, and prednisone
Chordae tendineae, ruptured, 510
Chorea, 774, 816-818
 Huntington's, 774, 816-818
 Sydenham's, 119, 818-819
Choriocarcinoma 735, 1146

Chorionic gonadotropin, human; *see* Human chorionic gonadotropin
Chorioretinitis, 125, 154, 285, 286
Christmas disease, 410
Chromaffin cell tumors, 1164
Chromatography, column, 1251
Chrome, allergy to nickel in, 30
Chromium
  as carcinogen, 432
  radiolabeled, 313
    half-life activity of, 328
    hemolytic anemia and, 328
    red cell mass measurement and, 352
Chromomycosis, 272
Chromosome fragments, 1222
Chromosomes
  abnormalities of, 498, 1220-1222, 1225, 1301-1302
  errors in number of, 1221
  leukemias and, 369, 370
  marker, 364
  meiosis and, 1217
  Philadelphia, 369, 370
  ring, 1221, 1222
  sex, 1217
    abnormalities of, 1171, 1222, 1224-1226
    X, 856-857, 1218-1219, 1221
    Y, 1168, 1219, 1223
  staining of, 1221
  structure of, 1220-1222
  submetacentric, 1220
Chronic discoid lupus erythematosus, 57, 111, 902
Chronic obstructive pulmonary disease, 684, 690-695
  entities in, 680
  Haemophilus influenzae pneumonia and, 176
  hypercapnia and, 681
  respiratory failure and, 708, 710-711
Churg-Strauss syndrome, 719
Chvostek's sign, 1183, 1196, 1208
C-21-hydroxylase deficiency, 1171
Chylomicronemia, 1284, 1288, 1289
Chylomicrons, 998, 1281, 1282, 1283
  accumulation of, 1003, 1288, 1289
  catabolism defect of, 1285
  measurement of, 1289
  plasma concentration of, 1284, 1286, 1288, 1289
  synthesis of, 1282
Chylothorax, 731
Chylous ascites, 1046
Chyluria, 292
Chyme, 940, 946
Chymotrypsin, 1050
Chymotrypsinogen, 945
Cicatricial pemphigoid, 935
CIE; *see* Counter immunoelectrophoresis
Cigarette smoking; *see* Smoking
Ciguatera fish poisoning, 200
Cimetidine
  endocrine tumors and, 450
  in esophageal disorders
    of hypomotility, 62
    of inflammations, 985
    from systemic diseases, 981
  in gastrointestinal disorders
    of bleeding, 959
    of electrical injury, 752
    of gastritis, 996
    parietal cells and, 943
    of peptic ulcers, 987, 991, 992, 993, 994
    prophylactic use in, 994
    of stress erosions, 996
    Zollinger-Ellison syndrome and, 995

Cimetidine—cont'd
  hepatitis and, 1072
  pancreatitis and, 1053, 1056
  toxic nephropathy and, 625
Cinnamon oil, allergy to, 30
Circle of Willis aneurysm, 839, 1275
Circulation, 458-459; *see also* Blood; Cardiovascular diseases; Hemodynamics
  capillaries and; *see* Capillaries
  cerebral, 829-835; *see also* Brain
    angiography of, 564-565, 761
    heart failure and, 462
  collateral, portal-systemic venous, 1060
  coronary; *see* Coronary arteries
  enterohepatic, 940, 946, 999
  hyperdynamic, 470
  liver disease and, 1064
  neurogenic mechanisms for, 458
  renal; *see* Kidney, blood flow through
  shock and, 475-479
  splanchnic, 948-949, 1043, 1060, 1061
Circumflex coronary arteries, 524
Circumoral fibrosis, 112
Circumoral pallor, 224
Cirrhosis
  alcoholic, 1080-1081
  ascites and, 1045, 1061-1062
  biliary, 889, 1082
  complications of, 1083,1084
  hyperlipidemia and, 889-890
  idiopathic, 1079-1080
  iron excess and, 345
  jaundice and, 1067
  Laennec's, 1257
  macronodular, 1079
  metabolic, 1081-1082
  micronodular, 1079
  neutropenia and, 359
  posthepatitic, 1079-1080
  systemic sclerosis and, 60
Cisplatin, 440, 443
  in cancer, 447, 449
  hemolysis and, 342
  toxic nephropathy and, 626, 627, 628
Cisternography, isotopic, 775
Citrate, toxic effects of, 350, 351
Citrate sodium, 600
Citrullinemia, 1239
Clark's melanoma staging, 918
Clasp-knife phenomenon, 812
Claudication
  arterial insufficiency and, 568
  diabetes mellitus and, 1273
  masseter, 75
Clawhand, 877, 903, 1091
Clear cell tumors of kidney, 657
Clefts
  craniofacial, 1318, 1319
  facial, 1318
  of lip, 1228, 1317, 1318
  of nose, 1317, 1318
  of palates, 1228, 1320-1321
Clindamycin, 161, 167-168
  and abscesses, 699, 1047
  anaerobic infections and, 178, 250
  bacteremia and, 241
  bacteriostatic activity of, 156
  diarrhea from, 1018
  erysipeloid and, 246
  excretion of, 158
  liver and, 158
  meningitis and, 190
  parenteral, failure of, 159
  pregnancy and, 1212

Clindamycin—cont'd
  in renal disease, 670
  streptococci and, 227
Clinoril; *see* Sulindac
CLL; *see* Lymphocytic leukemia, chronic
Cloacal exstrophy, 651
Cloacogenic carcinoma of anus, 1031
Clofazimine, 263
Clofibrate
  cholesterol stones and, 1087
  diabetes insipidus and, 1126
  hyperlipidemias and, 1291
  platelets and, 406
  sulfonylureas and, 1267
  urinary catecholamines and, 1168
Clomiphene citrate
  amenorrhea and, 1177
  female hypogonadism and, 1122
  ovarian overstimulation syndrome and, 1045
Clonidine
  Gilles de la Tourette's syndrome and, 822
  hypertension and, 472-473, 474, 475
  renal failure and, 639
  side effects of, 574
  toxemia of pregnancy and, 665
Closed-loop bowel obstruction, 1024
Clostridial infection, 251-254, 343, 1003; *see also* specific species
Clostridium botulinum, 201, 204, 856
Clostridium difficile, 167, 168, 251, 1018
Clostridium histolyticum, 251, 252
Clostridium novyi, 251, 252
Clostridium perfringens, 201, 251, 252, 253, 953
Clostridium septicum, 251, 252
Clostridium sordellii, 251
Clostridium tetani, 251
Clotrimazole, 279
  fungal infections and, 928
  oral candidiasis and, 308
  pruritus and, 885
Clotting factors; *see also* Blood component therapy; Coagulation
  V, 411,429
  VII, 411, 429, 1098
  VIII
    abnormalities of, 407
    antibodies to, 409, 411, 428
    assays for, 410
    concentrates of, 105, 410, 411, 1069
    deficiency of, 409-410, 1227
    disseminated intravascular coagulation and, 413
    sickle cell disease and von Willebrand's disease and, 618
  IX
    antibodies to, hemophilia and, 428
    deficiency of, 410
    dentistry and, 428-429
    disease of, 1227
  X, 411, 429
  XI, 411
    dentistry and, 429
  XII
    deficiency of, 411
    septic shock and, 240
  XIII, 411
  coumarins and, 414
  dentistry and, 428-429
  Hageman; *see* Clotting factors, XII
  hemarthrosis and, 105
  leukemias and, 368
  liver diseases and, 1059, 1063, 1064, 1065, 1098

Clotting factors—cont'd
　topical spraying of, 963
　vitamin K and, 1107
Cloxacillin, 157, 221, 670
Clubbing
　of fingers and toes, 103, 181, 578, 683-684
　hereditary, 684
　of pancreatic ducts, 1055
Cluster headache, 789
CM; see Capreomycin
CMC; see Critical micellar concentration
CML; see Leukemias, chronic myelogenous
C-MOPP; see Cyclophosphamide, vincristine, procarbazine, and prednisone
CMV; see Cytomegalovirus
CNS; see Central nervous system
CO; see Carbon monoxide
CO_2; see Carbon dioxide
CO diffusing capacity; see Carbon monoxide, diffusing capacity of
Coagulase, 218
Coagulation, 408; see also Clotting factors
　disorders of, 408-414, 1227
　　acquired, 411-413
　　inherited, 409-410
　　liver disease and, 1064
　　disseminated intravascular; see Disseminated intravascular coagulation
　　drugs to prevent; see Anticoagulants
　mechanism of, 408-414
　tests for, 408-409
　thrombophlebitis and, 495
Coagulation factors; see Clotting factors
Coagulopathy, 402; see also Disseminated intravascular coagulation
Coal macule, 725
Coal workers pneumoconiosis, 725
Coarctation of aorta, 340, 474, 505, 557, 573
Coast of Maine appearance, 879
Cobalamins, 1109
Cobalt prostheses, allergy to, 30
Cobblestone appearance
　of buccal lesions, 1097
　of intestinal surface, 1011, 1012
　of skin, 88
Cocaine
　abuse of, 778, 862
　neoplasia and, 446
Cocarboxylase, 849
Cocci, anaerobic, 177, 230-235, 249, 303; see also Gram-positive cocci
Coccidioides, 278
Coccidioides immitis, 172, 275
Coccidioidomycosis, 81, 139, 275, 278, 1003
Cockayne's syndrome, 882
Coconut cake rectum, 290
Codeine
　irritable bowel disease and, 1029
　lumbar puncture headache and, 790
　mastocytosis and, 909, 910
　peptic ulcers and, 1092
　porphyria and, 1252
　pregnancy and, 1212
Codfish vertebrae, 89, 1243
Codominance, 1219-1220
Codon, 1216
Coenzyme A, 1110
Coffee, 527; see also Caffeine
Coffee worker's lung, 727
Cogentin; see Benztropine
Cognition, 763, 770-775
Coin lesions, 744
Colace; see Dioctyl sodium sulfosuccinate
Colcemid, 1221

Colchicine
　amyloidosis and, 386
　Behçet's syndrome and, 111
　gout and, 92, 93
　ileal mucosa and, 317
　malabsorption and, 1002
　paroxysmal polyserositis and, 1048
　sarcoidosis and, 78
　systemic sclerosis and, 61
　thyroid hormones and, 1130
Cold agglutinin syndromes, 339-340, 418
Cold shock, 240, 476
Cold-reacting autoimmune hemolytic anemias, 339-340
Colds, common, 141, 144
Coldsore, recurrent, 299
Colectomy
　Crohn's disease and, 1015
　diverticulosis and, 1018
　polyposis syndromes and, 1042
　ulcerative colitis and, 1011
Colestipol hydrochloride, 1290
Colic
　biliary, 950-951, 988, 1087-1088
　esophageal, 979
　lead, 753
　mastocytoma and, 909
　renal, 951
Colistin, 169, 627, 628
Colitic arthritis, 1007
Colitis
　amebic, 282
　ischemic, 1021, 1022, 1023
　lymphogranuloma venereum and, 216
　pseudomembranous enterocolitis and, 1018
　spastic, 1027
　transmural, 1011; see also Crohn's disease
　ulcerative; see Ulcerative colitis
Collagen
　bone and, 1181
　Ehlers-Danlos syndrome and 407, 1241-1243, 1302
　gingival, 865
　metabolism disorder of, 1203
　microfibrillar; see Microfibrillar collagen
　sprue and, 1002
　synthesis of, 1241-1246
　systemic sclerosis and, 58
　vascular diseases and
　　esophageal motility disorders and, 981-982, 1091
　　pregnancy and, 666
　　renal lesions in, 615-617
Collateral circulation, portal, 1060
Collins' solution, 644
Colloidal volume expander, 958; see also Volume expanders
Colloids, 350
　antibody to, 1136
　osmotic pressure and, 730, 1044
　pancreatitis and, 1053
　radiolabeled, 727, 966
　in third ventricular cyst, 844
　in volume expanders, 958; see also Volume expanders
Colobomas, 1309, 1310
Colocynth, 1002
Colon, 947-948; see also Intestines, large
　adenocarcinoma of, 1093; see also Carcinoma of colon
　carcinoma of; see Carcinomas of colon
　colostomy and; see Colostomy
　contractile patterns of, 1027
　dentistry and polyps of, 1093-1095

Colon—cont'd
　diagnosis and; see Colonoscopy
　diverticular disease of, 324, 951, 1017-1018, 1021; see also Diverticulitis
　esophageal anastomoses and, 982, 985-986
　excision of; see Colectomy
　and ileum, anastomosis between, 1015
　inflammation of; see Colitis
　irritable, 1005, 1027
　lactose intolerance and, 1005, 1028
　mechanical obstruction of, 1024-1026
　megacolon and, 1007, 1008, 1011, 1026-1027
　motility of, 948
　neoplasms of, 228, 1038-1042, 1093; see also Carcinomas of colon
　pacemakers of, 1027
　and rectal stump, anastomosis between, 1026
　resection of; see Colectomy
　sigmoid; see Sigmoid colon
Colon antibodies, 1006
Colon cutoff sign, 1052
Colonic interposition, 982, 986
Colonoscopy, 965
　Crohn's disease and, 1013
　diverticulosis and, 1017
　large bowel neoplasms and, 1038, 1040
　ulcerative colitis and, 1009, 1010
Colony-stimulating factors, 355-356, 360, 362
Colorectal cancer; see Carcinomas of colon
Colostomy
　diverticulosis and, 1018
　ischemic colitis and, 1021
　large bowel neoplasms and, 1041
　radiation enteritis and, 1019
Coma, 763-764
　central neurogenic hyperventilation and, 766
　diabetes mellitus and, 1270
　electrical injury and, 751
　hepatic, 1061, 1084
　myxedema, 1138, 1140, 1206
　patient examination in, 765-766
　viral hepatitis and, 1070
Coma vigil, 764
Combination chemotherapy, 443
　histiocytic medullary reticulosis and, 398
　Hodgkin's disease and, 391
　in leukemias, 367, 368
　in non-Hodgkin's lymphoma, 393
　testicular carcinoma and, 449
　toxic effects of, 391
　in tuberculosis, 260
Combined systems disease, 33-34, 808, 851
Commissurotomy, 112, 514
Common bile duct stones, 950, 1086, 1088
Common colds, 141, 144
Compatibility, blood, 348-349
Complement, 17; see also Complement fixation
　defects in, 31
　evaluation of, 32
　glomerulonephritis and, 609, 610, 613, 614
　hemorrhagic lung disease and, 720
　lymphocytic system and, 16, 1260
　pathways of, 17, 18
　pneumonia and, 173
　pulmonary fibrosis and, 713
　pulmonary vasculitides and, 719
　serum levels of, 27
　viruses and, 122, 124; see also Complement fixation
Complement fixation, 112
　adenoviruses and, 148
　coronaviruses and, 144
　cytomegalovirus and, 131
　measles and, 146

Complement fixation—cont'd
  parainfluenza viruses and, 142, 143
  rubella and, 146
  toxoplasmosis and, 186
  varicella and, 129, 130
Complete blood count; see Blood cell count
Compliance
  chronic obstructive pulmonary disease and, 692-693, 694
  of large arteries, 460
  static, 693, 694
Component therapy, blood, 311, 346, 350, 1098; see also Transfusions
Composite resin, allergy to, 30
Compression from tumors, 436, 445
Computed digital angiography, 761
Computed tomography
  brain and
    abscesses of, 192
    averaging and, 762
    cerebral hemispheres and, 184, 185
    hemorrhage of, 839
    herpes simplex encephalitis and, 136
    hydrocephalus and, 775
    infarction of, 831-832
    pseudotumor cerebri and, 848
    seizures and, 785
    tumor of, 846-847
    unconsciousness and, 768
    white matter diseases and, 796
  cancer staging and, 436
  cholestasis and, 1067
  digestive system and, 971
  fever of unknown origin and, 120
  kidneys and, 607
  of lung, 686
  multiple sclerosis and, 800
  neurologic diseases and, 761, 762; see also Computed tomography, brain and
  venous thrombosis and, 841
COMT; see Catechol-O-methyltransferase
Concanavalin A, 16, 32
Conceptualization, 771
Conchoid bodies, 911
Concussion, labyrinthine, 793
Conduction
  of body heat, 755
  of heart, 541-542
    accessory pathway of, in children, 500-501
    block of, 500, 546-548
    multiple sclerosis and, 797
Conduction aphasia, 772
Conductive hearing loss, 795
Conduit surgery, 509
Condyle, shaving of, 107
Condylomata lata, 267, 268, 269, 1030
Condylotomy, 107
Congenital adrenal hyperplasias, 1162-1163
Congenital heart disease, 497-509
  and acyanotic lesions, 502-506
  alveolar hypoxemia and, 682
  arrhythmias and, 500-501
  bicuspid valves with aortic stenosis in, 514
  cardiac catheterization in, 501-502
  cardiomyopathy and, 518
  chest roentgenogram in, 501
  cyanotic, 506-509, 578
  dentistry and, 578-579
  electrocardiogram and, 499-500
  endocarditis and, 179, 301
  familial patterns of, 498
  hemodynamics of, 498-499
  myocardial failure in, 508-509
  noninvasive studies of, 502

Congenital heart disease—cont'd
  of pericardium, 555
  surgery for, 509
  tricuspid valve disease and, 516
Congenital hemolytic anemias; see Hemolytic anemia, congenital
Congenital hemolytic jaundice, 328-329
Congenital hip dislocation, 1228
Congenital infection, 122, 125-127, 1073-1074
Congenital malformations of head and neck; see Craniofacial malformations
Congenital myopathies, 859
Congenital neutropenia, 359-360
Congenital pancreatic abnormalities, 1050-1051
Congenital platelet disorders, 401, 405
Congenital rubella, 125, 126, 127, 1073
Congenital skin diseases, 876-884
Congenital syphilis, 265, 269-270, 303
Congenital toxoplasmosis, 285, 286
Congenital urinary tract malformations, 649-651, 654, 655
Congestive cardiomyopathies; see Cardiomyopathies
Congestive heart failure; see Heart failure, congestive
Congestive shock, 476-477
Conjugate horizontal nystagmus on lateral gaze, 760
Conjunctiva
  evaluation of, 8
  inflammations of; see Conjunctivitis
  pigmentation on, Gaucher's disease and, 1296
  sulfonamides in, 215
  vitamin A and ulcers of, 1107
Conjunctivitis, 926
  adenoviruses and, 140, 143, 148
  Behçet's disease and, 907
  congenital herpes simplex and, 127
  gonococcal, 230
  pyrodoxine deficiency and, 1298
  Reiter's syndrome and, 52, 907
  trypanosomiasis and, 287
Conn's syndrome, 470, 573, 1160; see also Aldosteronism
Connective tissue disorders, 1240-1246
  drug-induced, 57
  hemolytic anemia and, 338
  mixed, pulmonary fibrosis and, 716
  skin lesions of, 902-908
  terminology and, 35
Consanguinity, 1223-1224
Consciousness
  alterations in, 762-769
  dehydration and, 596
Constipation, 955-956, 1026
Consumption coagulopathy, 412
Contact allergy, oral, 30
Contact dermatitis, 27
Contamination
  of donor blood, 351
  of specimens for viral isolation, 124
  in surgery, 251
Continuous positive airway pressure, 733
Contraceptives, oral; see Oral contraceptives
Contractility, 454, 457, 458, 459
Contractures, 101, 877, 903, 1091
Contrast agents; see also Iodides
  allergy to, 25, 27, 606
  angiocardiography and, 488
  kidney roentgenograms and, 605-606
  nephropathy and, 625, 628, 630, 631
  pulmonary embolism and, 492
  renal failure in myeloma and, 617
Conus artery, 524

Convection, heat, 755
Convergence nystagmus, 760
Convulsions; see Seizures
Cooley's anemia, 334-335
Cooley facies, thalassemia and, 418
Coombs' test, 339, 340
Coordination, 14
COP therapy; see Cyclophosphamide, vincristine, and prednisone
COPD; see Chronic obstructive pulmonary disease
Cope's needle, 1044
Copper
  deficiency of, 1106
  Hodgkin's disease and, 387
  interstitial nephritis and, 619
  liver disease and, 1066, 1081-1082
  metabolism disorders of, 822-823, 1066, 1081-1082, 1240
  nephropathy and, 627, 628
  Wilson's disease and, 822-823, 1066, 1081-1082, 1240
COPRO; see Coproporphyrin
COPROgen; see Coproporphyrinogen
COPROgen oxidase; see Coproporphyrinogen oxidase
Coprolalia, 821
Coproporphyria, 888, 889, 1252-1253
Coproporphyrin
  I, 1068
  III, 753
  urinary, 1066
Coproporphyrinogen, 1247, 1248, 1249, 1252
Coproporphyrinogen oxidase, 1252
Cor pulmonale, 692, 693, 695, 696
Coracidium, 293
Cording factor, 254
Core biopsy, 320
Cork dust, 727
Corkscrew esophagus, 979, 980
Cornea
  arcus of, premature, 1288
  evaluation of, 8
  herpes simplex and, 154
Coronary arteries
  anatomy of, 524-525
  angiography of, 488-489, 530-531
  disease of; see Coronary heart disease
  percutaneous dilation of, 532
  resistance and, 525-526
  right, dominance of, 524
  vasodilation of, 528, 982; see also Vasodilators
Coronary arteritis, 147
Coronary care unit, 536
Coronary heart disease, 524-541; see also Coronary arteries
  anatomy in, 524-526
  aneurysms in, 147
  angina pectoris in, 527-533
  bypass grafting for, 532
  congenital anomalies in, 525
  dentistry and, 582-584
  diabetes mellitus and, 1272
  epidemiology and, 526-527
  heart failure and, 462
  inflammation in, 147
  mitral regurgitation and, 510
  myocardial perfusion in, 524-526
  occlusions in, 524-530; see also Myocardial infarction
  prevention of, 526-527
  small vessel, 453
  sudden death and, 538-540
  ventricular fibrillation and, 585

Coronary venous system, 525
Coronaviruses, 123, 140, 144, 149, 150
Corpus albicans, 1174
Corpus luteum, 1174, 1175
Corrected reticulocyte count, 313
Corrigan pulse, 580
Corrosive agent ingestion, 985
Cortex
  adrenal; *see* Adrenal cortex
  cerebral
    association, 771
    blindness and, 759
    consciousness and, 763
    degeneration of, 850
    language-processing, 771-772
    lesions of pathways of, 759
    parietal, cognition and, 771
    prefrontal, 772
    primary receptive, 771
    sensory loss and, 758
Cortication, 774
Corticosteroid-binding globulin, 1154
Corticosteroids; *see also* Steroids
  Addison's disease and, 1207
  adhesive capsulitis and, 101
  adult respiratory distress syndrome and, 709
  allergies and, 30, 478
  anemia and, 320, 321, 416
  ankylosing spondylitis and, 50
  arteritis and, 69, 563, 790
  arthritis and, 38, 42, 51, 80, 106, 906
  asthma and, 24
  autoimmune neutropenia and, 359
  avascular necrosis and, 54, 104
  Behçet's syndrome and, 111
  bone marrow failure and, 54, 361
  brain abscess and, 193
  brain hemorrhage and, 839
  bronchitis and, 693
  brucellosis and, 244
  bursitis and, 98
  calcaneal spurs and, 102
  candidiasis and, 1092
  carpal tunnel syndrome and, 98
  caustic ingestion and, 985
  celiac disease and, 1001
  cellular immunity and, 32
  Chédiak-Higashi syndrome and, 357
  cirrhosis and, 1080
  contrast agent allergy and, 606
  costochondritis and, 100
  cryptococcosis and, 275-276
  in crystal deposition disease, 95
  dermatitis herpetiformis and, 893
  dermatomyositis and, 905
  diabetic coma and, 1270
  Dressler's syndrome and, 537
  drug interactions and, 1090
  dysphagia and, 976
  endocrine tumors and, 450
  enteric fever and, 208
  Epstein-Barr virus and, 134
  erythema multiforme and, 924
  erythema nodosum and, 925
  fever and, 118
  fibrofatty nodules and, 102
  fibrositis and, 97
  gastritis and, 996
  gastroenteritis and, 1003
  gout and, 93
  Graves' ophthalmopathy and, 1148
  in hematologic disorders, 310
  hepatitis and, 1072, 1079
  herpes zoster and, 927
Corticosteroids—cont'd
  histiocytosis and, 398
  hypercalcemia and, 445, 1180
  hyperpigmentation and, 887
  hypertension and, 469
  insulin resistance and, 1268
  in leukemias, 366, 367, 371
  lichen planus and, 938
  lipoid nephrosis and, 613
  lupus erythematosus and, 57, 903
  Lyell's disease and, 932
  mediastinal masses and, 735
  meningococcemia and, 234
  meralgia paresthetica and, 98
  mucormycosis and, 277
  multiple myeloma and, 382
  mumps and, 140
  myasthenia gravis and, 856
  mycosis fungoides and, 901
  myeloid metaplasia and, 376
  necrobiosis lipoidica diabeticorum and, 886, 1276
  nephritis and, 620
  neutrophils and, 357, 361
  nocardiosis and, 247
  oral candidiasis and, 307
  pancreatitis and, 1051
  paroxysmal nocturnal hemoglobinuria and, 342
  pemphigoid and, 935
  pemphigus and, 932, 933, 934
  pericarditis and, 551, 552, 553
  peripheral polyneuropathies and, 779
  pertussis and, 238
  pneumocystosis and, 287, 288
  pneumonia and, 721
  polyarteritis nodosa and, 616
  polymyalgia rheumatica and, 858
  polymyositis and, 64, 65
  porphyrias and, 1252
  pseudogout and, 95
  psoriasis and, 51, 937
  pulmonary fibrosis and, 714
  pulmonary hyperosteoarthropathy and, 104
  pulmonary infiltrates and, 363
  purpura and, 406
  radiation pneumonitis and, 722
  reflex sympathetic dystrophy and, 100
  Reiter's syndrome and, 53, 907, 908
  relapsing polychondritis and, 103
  respiratory failure and, 711
  rheumatic fever and, 229-230
  rhinitis and, 22
  sarcoidosis and, 78, 911
  Schönlein-Henoch purpura and, 70, 616
  scleroderma and, 62, 903
  serum sickness and, 27
  strongyloidiasis and, 291
  subdural empyema and, 193
  synovial cysts and, 102
  tendinitis and, 99
  thrombocytopenia and, 402, 403
  thrush and, 176
  thyroiditis and, 1146, 1149
  thyrotoxic crisis and, 1147
  thyroxine-to-triiodothyronine conversion and, 1131
  toxoplasmosis and, 286
  transfusion reactions and, 351
  after transplants, dental management and, 669
  trichinosis and, 203, 292
  triiodothyronine and, 1132
  in tuberculosis, 260
  tumor supportive care and, 445
  ulcerative colitis and, 1011
Corticosteroids—cont'd
  in vasculitides, 69
  Waldenström's macroglobulinemia and, 383
  Weber-Christian disease and, 79
  Wegener's granulomatosis and, 73
  white cell transfusions and, 347
Corticosterone, 1153, 1160, 1161, 1162, 1163; *see also* Cortisone
Corticotropin; *see* Adrenocorticotropic hormone
Corticotropin-releasing factor, 1118, 1155, 1157, 1159
Cortisol; *see also* Hydrocortisone
  action of, 1154
  adrenocorticotropic hormone and, 1117, 1153, 1155
  catabolic effects of, 1154
  deficiency of, 1122, 1155, 1162; *see also* Addison's disease
  excess of, 1157-1159
  obesity and, 1103
  plasma alcohol and, 1258
  production of, 1153
  in replacement therapy, 1157, 1163
  suppression of, 1156, 1159, 1162
  triiodothyronine and, 1132
Cortisone, 1031, 1207; *see also* Corticosterone
Cortrosyn; *see* Cosyntropin
Corynebacterium, 167, 247, 302, 445
Corynebacterium diphtheriae, 167, 247
Corynebacterium parvum, 445
Coryza, measles and, 145; *see also* Common colds
Costen's syndrome, 100, 867
Costochondral osteochondritis, 100, 737
Costochondritis, 100
Costoclavicular syndrome, 101
Cosyntropin, 1122, 1156
Co-trimoxazole, 161, 170
Cough
  asthma and, 705
  smoker's, 691, 745; *see also* Smoking
  suppressants of, 693
Cough preparations, pregnancy and, 1212
Coumadin; *see* Warfarin
Coumarins
  alcohol and, 1297
  coagulation disorders and, 414
  dentistry and, 429-430, 577
  griseofulvin and, 279
  paroxysmal nocturnal hemoglobinuria and, 342
  vitamin K deficiency and, 411
Councilman's bodies, 1071
Counter immunoelectrophoresis, 188, 189
Counter-pulsation devices, intra-aortic, 532
Countershock, 546, 549
Courvoisier's law, 1088
Courvoisier's sign, 1056
Cowdry type A intranuclear inclusions, 136
Coxiella, 209-210, 213
Coxiella burnetii, 172, 182, 213
Coxsackieviruses
  Bornholm disease and, 730
  cardiomyopathy and, 520
  central nervous system disease and, 135, 136
  dentistry and, 300, 301
  neonatal, 126
  pericarditis and, 586
  respiratory infections and, 144, 172
CPA; *see* Carotid artery, phonoangiography of
CPAP; *see* Continuous positive airway pressure
CPE; *see* Cytopathic effect
C-peptide suppression test, 1278
CPK; *see* Creatine phosphokinase
CPM; *see* Myelinolysis, central pontine

CPPD; *see* Calcium pyrophosphate dihydrate crystals
^{51}Cr; *see* Chromium, radiolabeled
Cramps, heat, 755
Cranial arteritis, 68, 69, 74-75, 789-790, 841
Cranial nerves
　brainstem lesions and, 760
　diabetes mellitus and, 1275
　evaluation of, 13-14, 586
　neuropathies and; *see* Neuropathies
　pneumococcal meningitis and, 187
　trigeminal neuralgia and, 790-791
Cranial sutures, premature fusion of, 1312-1315
Cranial vault, development of, 1307
Craniectomy, 1314
Craniofacial angiomatosis, 881-882
Craniofacial clefts, 1318, 1319
Craniofacial dysostosis, 1314, 1315, 1316
Craniofacial malformations, 1300-1322
　acquired, 1301
　classification of, 1308-1321; *see also* Craniofacial malformations, pathogenesis and classification of
　congenital, 1301-1303
　definitions in, 1301
　etiology of, 1301-1303
　incidence of, 1300-1301
　nomenclature in, 1301
　pathogenesis and classification of, 1308-1321
　　clefts of primary and secondary palates in, 1320-1321
　　craniofacial clefts in, 1318, 1319
　　craniosynostosis syndromes in, 1312-1315
　　midface syndromes in, 1316-1318
　　otocraniofacial syndromes in, 1309-1312
　prenatal development in, 1304-1308
Craniofacial mucormycosis, 277
Craniofacial structures, standards of measurement for, 1301; *see also* Cranium
Craniosynostosis syndrome, 1312-1315
Craniovertebral junction abnormalities, 810-811
Cranium
　dental infection and, 303
　development of, 1306, 1307, 1308
　malformations of; *see* Craniofacial malformations
　measurements of, 1301
　thickening of, acromegaly and, 1204
Cranium bifidum occultum, 1317
C-reactive protein, 46
Creatine phosphokinase
　malignant hyperthermia and, 875
　myocardial infarction and, 535
　neuromuscular disorders and, 853, 857
　polymyositis and, 65
Creatinine
　clearance of, 603
　　dialysis and, 642
　　glomerulonephritis and, 610
　　liver disease and, 1064
　　renal failure and, 631, 632, 635, 638, 640
　plasma, 604
　pregnancy and, 664
　serum, 462, 630
Creeping eruption, 291
Crepitation, 249
Crepitus, 253
Crescents, 609, 610, 611, 616, 618
Cretinism, 1105, 1136, 1138, 1205-1206
Creutzfeldt-Jakob disease, 774, 828, 868
CRF; *see* Corticotropin-releasing factor; Renal failure, chronic
Cricopharyngeal disorders, 975, 976
Cricopharyngeus muscle, 973

Crigler-Najjar syndrome, 1058, 1067-1068
Critical micellar concentration, 998
Crohn's disease, 892, 1006, 1008, 1011-1015
　anal fistulas and, 1031
　dentistry and, 1096-1097
　hypoparathyroidism and, 1196
　malnutrition and, 1103
　obstruction management and, 1026
　reactive arthritis and, 53
　skin lesions and, 892-893
Cromolyn sodium, 25, 704, 706-707, 1212
Cronkhite-Canada syndrome, 891
Cross-linkage, 440, 441, 442, 443
Cross-match tests, 349
Cross-modality reference, 771
Croup, 142, 145
Crouzon's disease, 1314, 1315, 1316
CRST syndrome; *see* Calcinosis in Raynaud's phenomenon, sclerodactyly, and telangiectasia syndrome
Cryoglobulinemia
　kidney diseases and, 618
　Lyme disease and, 297
　multiple myeloma and, 899
　purpura and, 407
　vasculitis and, 1022
Cryoprecipitate
　disseminated intravascular coagulation and, 413
　factor deficiencies and, 429
　von Willebrand's disease and, 408, 427
Cryopreservation, 347
Crypt, intestinal, 945, 1007
Cryptococcosis, 275-276, 278
　aseptic meningoencephalitis and, 139
　Hodgkin's disease and, 387
　and meningitis, immunodeficiency diseases and, 31
　neoplasia and, 446
Cryptococcus neoformans, 172, 275
Cryptorchidism, 882, 1170
Cryptostroma corticale, 727
Crystal deposition disease, 95; *see also* Gout
Crystal nidus, 646
Crystalloids, 350, 535
CS; *see* Chondroitin sulfate; Cycloserine
CSF; *see* Cerebrospinal fluid
CT; *see* Calcitonin; Computed tomography
CTD; *see* Connective tissue disorders
C-terminal fragment, 1187
Cullen's sign, 1051
Cultures, 119
　anaerobic, 250
　bone marrow, 319
　Bordetella and, 237, 238
　endocarditis and, 182, 184
　media for, 119
　meningitis and, 188, 189
　throat, 224
　viral, 123-124
　　central nervous system disease and, 139
　　mumps and, 138
　　varicella zoster and, 138
Cuprimine; *see* Penicillamine
Cuprophan, 641
Curare, 252, 871
Curare-like drugs, 167
Curling's ulcer, 996
Currant jelly sputum, 176
Cushing's disease, 1177, 1262; *see also* Cushing's syndrome
Cushing's syndrome, 1120, 1157-1159
　adrenocorticotropic hormone release and, 1118
　dentistry and, 1206-1207

Cushing's syndrome—cont'd
　ectopic, 1157, 1158, 1159
　hypertension and, 470-471, 474, 573
　insulin resistance and, 1262
　neoplasms and, 1179, 1180-1181
　osteoporosis of, 1210
　purpura and, 406
　skin disorders of, 887
　tests for, 1158-1159
Cushing's ulcer, 996
Cushion defects, endocardial, 503-504
Cutaneous anthrax, 245; *see also* Skin diseases
Cutaneous diphtheria, 248
Cutaneous larva migrans, 291
Cutaneous lesions, 876-939; *see also* Mucocutaneous infections; Skin diseases
Cutaneous metastases, 912-913
Cutaneous thrush, 276
Cutis laxa, 1243
Cutis marmorata, 887
Cutis verticis gyrata, 878, 886
CVA; *see* Cerebrovascular accident
CWP; *see* Coal workers pneumoconiosis
Cyanide, 768
Cyanocobalamin, 1109
　Crohn's disease and, 1015
　in hematologic disorders, 310
　refractory anemia and, 321
　subacute combined degeneration and, 851
　in therapy, 318
Cyanosis, 683
　central, 571, 578
　in congenital heart lesions, 502, 506-509
　methemoglobinemia and, 343, 344
　peripheral, 571
Cyclic adenosine monophosphate
　asthma and, 704, 705, 706
　diarrhea and, 940-941, 952
　esophageal sphincter and, 974
　nephrogenous, 1188
　　hypercalcemia and, 1190, 1193, 1194
　　hyperparathyroidism and, 1192-1193
　　hypoparathyroidism and, 1196
　　parathyroid hormone and, 1187-1188
Cyclic AMP; *see* Cyclic adenosine monophosphate
Cyclic guanidine monophosphate, 704, 705
Cyclic neutropenia, 360
Cyclobenzaprine hydrochloride, 1297
Cyclo-oxygenase, 400, 405
Cyclophosphamide, 442
　anemia and, 322, 339
　in cancer, 447, 448, 449
　doxorubicin toxicity and, 441
　Hodgkin's disease and, 390, 391
　hydroxydaunomycin, Oncovin, and prednisone, 393, 394
　in leukemias, 366, 367
　lipoid nephrosis and, 613
　lung diseases induced by, 722
　lupus erythematosus and, 57, 615
　multiple myeloma and, 382
　multiple sclerosis and, 801
　in non-Hodgkin's lymphoma, 393
　pemphigus and, 932, 934
　polyarteritis nodosa and, 616
　relapsing polychondritis and, 103
　renal transplantation and, 644
　in sarcomas, 450
　thrombocytopenia and, 400
　in vasculitides, 69
　vincristine
　　and prednisone, 393
　　procarbazine, and prednisone, 393

Cyclophosphamide—cont'd
  Waldenström's macroglobulinemia and, 383
  Wegener's granulomatosis and, 69, 72, 616, 720
Cyclopia, 1317
Cycloserine, 259
Cyclosporin A, 644
Cycrimine, 870
Cypionate, 1173
Cyproheptadine
  carcinoid tumors and, 450
  Cushing's syndrome and, 1159
Cystadenoma
  bronchial, 743
  of pancreas, 1056
Cystathionine synthetase deficiency, 1237
Cystathioniuria, 1237
Cystenterostomy, 1054
Cystic fibrosis, 696, 700, 1050-1051
  bronchiectasis and, 696
  dentistry and, 747, 1101-1102
  malabsorption and, 1001
Cystic medial necrosis, 558, 560
Cysticercosis, 293
Cysticercus, 292, 293
Cystine in urine, 1227
Cystine kidney stones, 646, 649
Cystinosis, 1227
Cystinuria, 1227
Cystitis, 143, 195
Cystourethrogram, 650
Cysts
  Baker's, 84, 567
  bronchogenic, 735
  chest roentgenograms and, 686
  dentigerous, 891, 1093
  dermoid, 735, 1310, 1311
  of gallbladder; see Cholecystitis
  giardiasis and, 284
  in head and neck, Gardner's syndrome and, 1093
  hydatid, 294
  of jaw, 668, 883
  of kidney, 651-653
  of liver, 282
  of lung, 700, 701, 747
  mesenteric, 1049
  ovarian, 1177, 1178
  of pancreas, 700, 1050-1051
  pericardial, 555
  pneumocystosis and, 287
  popliteal, 84
  punched-out, 910
  of spleen, 398
  synovial, 101-102
  thyroid, 1150
Cytidine analogs, 367
Cytochrome P-450, 1247
Cytogenetic disorders, clinical, 1224-1226
Cytology
  ascites and, 1045
  of esophagus, 1032
  gastric neoplasm and, 1036, 1037
  herpes simplex and, 299
  of sputum, 686-687
Cytomegalovirus, 130-131, 134, 135, 826
  blood transfusion and, 348
  chorioretinitis and, 154
  cold agglutinin syndromes and, 339
  congenital, 125-126, 127
  dentistry and, 300
  drug abuse and, 863
  hepatitis and, 1074
  immunodeficiency diseases and, 31

Cytomegalovirus—cont'd
  interferon and, 154
  Kaposi's sarcoma and, 922
  renal transplantation and, 645
  vaccine for, 131
Cytonuclear dissociation, 316
Cytopathic effect, 124
Cytopenia, 322
Cytoplasmic inclusions, eosinophilic, 146
Cytoreduction, 366
Cytosine arabinoside
  as cell cycle-specific agent, 440
  in leukemias, 366, 367
  myeloid metaplasia and, 376
  thrombocytopenia and, 400
Cytotoxic agents, 439-443; see also Chemotherapy
  acquired anticoagulants and, 411
  amyloidosis and, 386
  antifolate, 1109
  cadaver donors and, 644
  in cancer, 448, 449, 1047
  dermatomyositis and, 113
  histiocytosis and, 398
  in Hodgkin's disease, 390, 391
  lung disease and, 722
  lupus nephritis and, 615
  mucormycosis and, 277
  neutropenia and, 358, 360
  in non-Hodgkin's lymphoma, 393
  systemic sclerosis and, 61
  Wegener's granulomatosis and, 72, 113
Cytotoxic factors, 15
Cytotoxic reactions, 18
Cytotoxicity testing, 22
Cytoxan; see Cyclophosphamide

D

D$_{LCO}$; see Carbon monoxide, diffusing capacity of
D cells, 943
D locus antigens, 643
Da Nang lung, 708; see also Adult respiratory distress syndrome
Dacarbazine, 442-443
  action of, 440, 442-443
  Hodgkin's disease and, 390
  melanomas and, 450, 918
Dacryocyte, 315
Dactinomycin, 441, 450
Dactylitis, sickle cell, 332
Dakin's fluid, 828
Dalrymple's sign, 1142
Danazol, 26
Dane particles, 1068
Dantrolene sodium, 858, 875
Dapsone
  dermatitis herpetiformis and, 893, 1002
  Hailey-Hailey disease and, 935
  hemolysis and, 330
  in leprosy, 263
  psoriasis and, 937
Darier's sign, 909
Darier-Roussy sarcoid, 911
Darkfield microscopy, 264, 270-271
Darvon; see Propoxyphene
Darvon-N; see Propoxyphene napsylate
Daunorubicin, 441
  with cytosine arabinoside, 440
  in leukemias, 366, 367, 368
  urine and, 588
Db; see Decibels
DBH; see Dopamine-β-hydroxylase
DDAVP; see l-Deamino-8-D-arginine-vasopressin

DDS; see Diaminodiphenylsulfone
DDT, 754
Dead space, anatomic, 673
Deafness
  congenital disease and, 125-126, 270
  nephritis and, 611
  syphilis and, 270
  vancomycin and, 167
l-Deamino-8-D-arginine-vasopressin, 1126
Death
  coxsackievirus B and, 126
  cytomegalovirus and, 131
  herpes simplex and, 128
  influenza and, 140-141
  Kawasaki disease and, 147
  lymphocytic choriomeningitis virus and, 138
  measles encephalitis and, 138
  sudden, 538-540
  varicella and, 126, 130
  viral gastroenteritis and, 149
  viral respiratory infections and, 140
De Bakey's aortic dissection categorization, 561, 562
Debridement
  acute necrotizing ulcerative gingivitis and, 302
  anaerobic infections and, 250
  clostridia and, 253
  diabetic foot and, 1273
Decarboxylase, 814, 1166
Decayed, missing, and filled teeth, 579
Decerebrate patients, facial muscles and, 870, 871
Decibels, 794
Decoding process, 772
Decompression
  of biliary tract, 968
  of bowel, 1011, 1026
  microvascular, 791
Decongestants
  atelectasis and, 703
  bronchiectasis and, 697
  pregnancy and, 1212
  sinusitis and, 790
Decorticate posture, 766
Decortication, 774
Deep tendon reflexes, 14, 761
Defecation reflex, 948
Defibrillation, arrhythmias and, 585
Defibrination syndrome, 412
Deficiency states, dental correlations in, 414-420
Deformation, definition of, 1301
Degenerative diseases
  of central nervous system, 803-805, 868-869
  of heart, 179
  of joints, 83, 107
  of vertebrae, 860
  vitamin B$_{12}$ deficiency and, 849, 850, 851
Deglutition, 942, 973
  cerebrovascular accident and, 872
  difficulty with, 974
  pain and, 975
Deglycerolization, 347
Degos' disease, 893-894, 1003
Dehydration, 129, 150, 596-597, 707, 957; see also Fluids
Dehydroepiandrosterone, 1153, 1162
3-β-OH-Dehydrogenase deficiency, 1162, 1163
Dehydrotestosterone, 1168
Déjà vu, 783
Dejerine-Roussy syndrome, 832
Dejerine-Sottas disease, 855
Delayed hypersensitivity, 15, 19, 32; see also Skin tests
Deletions, 1217, 1222

Delirium, 763, 764
Delirium tremens, 776, 1298
Delta sign, 841
Delta sleep, 769
Delta wave, 500
Delta-aminolevulinic acid, 1247, 1252, 1254
Delta-cells, 1049
Deltoid muscle, myofascial syndromes and, 98
D'emblee mycosis fungoides, 901
Demeclocycline, 168
    antidiuresis from neoplasms and, 1181
    diabetes insipidus and, 621, 1125
    hypernatremia and, 595
    hyponatremia and, 445
    toxic nephropathy and, 625, 626
Dementia, 763
    brain tumor and, 845
    Creutzfeldt-Jakob disease and, 828
    Huntington's chorea and, 817
    multi-infarct, 835
    parkinsonism and, 813
Demethylchlortetracycline, 168, 625, 629
Demineralization, osteoporosis and, 115
Demyelinating diseases, 796-801, 852, 868-869
Denervation, 820, 852, 976
Dental abnormalities, Ehlers-Danlos syndrome and, 1242-1243
Dental amalgam, allergy to, 30
Dental appliances, removable, radiopaque markers for, 866
Dental caries, 34, 1211
Dental health questionnaire, 1, 2-3
Dental hygiene, 178
Dental precautions for hepatitis, 1099
Dental prostheses, 30, 415
Dental pulp, dysplasia of, 1244
Dental radiation dose, 751
Dental radiographs; *see* Radiographs, dental
Dental restoration, hemophilia and, 427
Dentigerous cysts, 891, 1093
Dentin
    dentinogenesis imperfecta and, 1244
    Ehlers-Danlos syndrome and, 1242
    vitamin C and, 1110
    vitamin D and, 1107
Dentinogenesis imperfecta, 1243-1244
Dentino-osseous dysplasia, dentinogenesis imperfecta and, 1244
Dentoalveolar infection, congenital heart disease and, 579
Denture stomatitis, oral candidiasis and, 307
Dentures
    anhydrotic ectodermal dysplasia and, 877
    cerebrovascular disease and, 587
    malnutrition and, 1103
    osteoporosis and, 1210
    Paget's disease and, 114
    pemphigoid and, 935
Deoxycholic acid, 1085
Deoxycorticosterone
    aldosteronism and, 1160, 1161
    congenital adrenal hyperplasia and, 1162, 1163
    hypertension and, 1171
    hypokalemia and, 597
    in steroid synthesis, 1153
11-Deoxycortisol, 1153, 1157, 1162
2-Deoxyglucose, 154
Deoxyhemoglobin S, 332
Deoxyribonuclease, 223, 945, 1050
Deoxyribonucleic acid, 1216
    autoimmunity and, 19
    phosphate metabolism and, 1184
    radiation and, 749
    scission of strands of, 440, 441

Deoxyribonucleic acid—cont'd
    sequencing of, 1228-1229
    steroids and, 1154
    synthesis of
        chemotherapy and, 440, 441, 442, 443
        megaloblastic anemia and, 316
        vidarabine and, 154
        viruses and, 121, 123, 127, 143, 154
Depakene; *see* Valproic acid
Depen; *see* Penicillamine
Depolarization, 479-480
Depolymerization, 440, 442
Depot insulin, 1261
Depressant drugs, 775-777, 1061, 1084
Depression
    dementia and, 775
    drugs producing; *see* Depressant drugs; specific agent
    drugs for treatment of; *see* Antidepressants
    sleep and, 770
    sleep disturbance with, 861-862
de Quervain's disease, 99
de Quervain's thyroiditis, 1149
Dermacentor andersoni, 210
Dermacentor variabilis, 210
Dermatan sulfate, 1233
Dermatitis; *see also* Dermatomyositis
    anal, 1030
    contact, 27
    Duhring's disease and, 892-893, 1002
    exfoliative, malignant lymphoma and, 900
    pemphigus and, 933
    schistosomiasis and, 295
Dermatitis herpetiformis, 892-893, 1002
Dermatitis vegetans, 933
Dermatologic syndromes; *see* Skin diseases
Dermatomyositis, 64-65, 858, 904-906; *see also* Dermatitis
    cancer detection and, 434
    dentistry and, 112-113
    esophageal disorders and, 975, 981
    pulmonary fibrosis and, 716
Dermatopathic lymphadenopathy, 900
Dermatophytes, 279, 885, 928-929
Dermatosis papulosa nigra, 913
Dermoid cysts, 735, 1310, 1311
Dermopathy; *see* Skin diseases
Desensitization to insulin, 1268
Desferrioxamine, 320, 337, 1081
Desiccated thyroid, 1139, 1140
Desipramine, 779
Desmoids, 891
Desoxycorticosterone; *see* Deoxycorticosterone
11-Desoxycortisol, 1153, 1157, 1162
Desquamative gingivitis, 937, 1213
Detergents, 342
Detrusor reflex function, 799
Development
    mandibular malposition and, 861
    prenatal, 1304-1308
Devil's grip, 144, 730
Dexamethasone
    aldosteronism and, 1161
    cerebral hemorrhage and, 839
    Cushing's syndrome and, 1157, 1158
    meningitis and, 191
    pseudotumor cerebri and, 848
    in suppression tests, 1158
    for tumors, 444
Dextran
    gastrointestinal bleeding and, 958
    platelet adhesion and, 405, 406
    septic shock and, 240
    and starch, 350
Dextroamphetamine, 769

Dextropropoxyphene, 23
Dextrose
    alcoholic ketoacidosis and, 1271
    dialysis and, 641
    hyperglycemic, hyperosmolar, nonketotic coma and, 1270
    hypoglycemia and, 1277, 1295
    pancreatic insulinomas and, 1279
    status epilepticus and, 787, 867
Dextrostix, 1264
Dextro-thyroxine, 1285, 1290; *see also* Thyroxine
DHL; *see* Lymphomas, diffuse
DHT; *see* Dehydrotestosterone
Diabetes insipidus, 1125-1126
    Hand-Schüller-Christian disease and, 719
    hypernatremia and, 595
    nephrogenic, 621-622
Diabetes mellitus, 1259-1276
    access arteriovenous fistula and, 1274
    acromegaly and, 1119
    arterial insufficiency and, 569
    bronze, 345, 890
    catabolism and, 1263
    chronic complications of, 1272-1276
    cirrhosis and, 1062
    coronary artery disease and, 527
    dentistry and, 1294-1295
    diagnosis of, 1259-1264
    esophageal disorders and, 982
    fatty liver and, 1077
    foot in, 1273, 1275
    gestational, 1261, 1264
    glucose-6-phosphate dehydrogenase deficiency and coma of, 330
    hemochromatosis and, 345, 890
    hyperpituitarism and, 1204
    ketoacidosis and, 1269-1270, 1271
    lichen planus and, 939
    lipoatrophy of, 1262, 1268
    malabsorption and, 1003-1004
    nephropathy and, 617, 1274
    neuropathy of, 853, 1274-1275
    occult, 1278
    oral candidiasis and, 307
    oral dysesthesias and, 874
    oral manifestations of, 1294-1295
    pancreatitis and, 1055
    pathogenesis of, 1259-1264
    pseudotabes of, 1276
    renal lesions and, 617
    retinopathy and, 1273-1274
    skin disorders of, 884-886
    treatment of, 1264-1272
    xanthomas and, 890
Diabinese; *see* Chlorpropamide
Dialogue medical history, 1, 4
Dialysate, 640-641, 642
Dialysis, 640-642
    complications of, 642
    dental management and, 668-669
    diabetic nephropathy and, 617, 1274
    glomerulonephritis and, 610, 611, 612
    hyperglycemic, hyperosmolar, nonketotic coma and, 1270
    hyperkalemia and, 634
    indications for, 635
    interstitial nephritis and, 620
    obstructive uropathy and, 656
    in oliguria, 633, 634
    peritoneal; *see* Peritoneal dialysis
    polycystic disease and, 652
    pregnancy and, 664
    preparing and initiating, 639-640

Dialysis—cont'd
  renal amyloidosis and, 617
  renal failure and, 632, 633, 634
    chronic, 635, 638, 639-640
    in myeloma, 618
  scleroderma and, 616
  sickle cell disease and, 618
  skin disorders and, 897, 1255
  toxic nephropathy and, 627, 629
  vascular access and, 640, 641, 1274
Dialyzers, 641
Diaminodiphenylsulfone, 330
cis-Diamminedichloroplatinum; see Cisplatin
Diamond-Blackfan anemia, 318, 319
Diaper rash, 929
Diaphorase, 343, 344
Diaphragm, 672
  disease of, 736-737
  excursion of, 736
  paralysis of, 736
Diarrhea, 940, 952-954
  acrodermatitis enteropathica and, 895
  antibiotic-induced, 1018
    clindamycin and, 168
    lincomycin and, 168
    tetracycline and, 27
  cholera and, 205
  Crohn's disease and, 1011
  giardiasis and, 284
  irritable bowel disease and, 1028, 1029
  nonocclusive vascular disease of gut and, 1021
  Norwalk-like agents and, 150
  osmotic, 952, 954
  polyposis syndromes and, 1042
  radiation enteritis and, 1019
  rotaviruses and, 150
  serotonin-related, 450
  ulcerative colitis and, 1007
  Zollinger-Ellison syndrome and, 995
Diascopy, purpura and, 425
Diathesis, bleeding, 383
Diatrizoate, 605
Diazepam
  alcohol and, 1297
  amyotrophic lateral sclerosis and, 804
  facial muscle rigidity and, 870
  lysergic acid diethylamide overdose and, 778
  multiple sclerosis and, 801
  muscle contraction headache and, 789
  myofascial pain dysfunction and, 109
  phencyclidine intoxication and, 779
  pregnancy and, 1212, 1213
  renal disease and, 670
  seizures and, 866
  side effects of, 871
  status epilepticus and, 787, 867
  tetanus and, 252
  torsion dystonias and, 820
  toxemia of pregnancy and, 665
  toxicity of, 777
  withdrawal symptoms and, 863
Diazoxide
  endocrine tumors and, 450
  hypertension and, 473-474
  in insulinomas, 1279
  pulmonary hypertension and, 497
  toxemia of pregnancy and, 665
DIC; see Disseminated intravascular coagulation
Dicloxacillin, 160, 164
  pregnancy and, 1212
  renal disease and, 670
  site of infection and, 157
  staphylococcal infections and, 221
Diencephalic region, 763

Diet; see also Nutrition
  calcium in, 1184
  and diabetes mellitus, 1265, 1268, 1271
  disorders of; see Nutrition, deficiencies in
  elemental, 1111
  elimination, 26
  fiber content in, 1028
  heart failure and, 464
  hypertension and, 471
  in insulinomas, 1279
  iron deficiency anemia and, 324
  ketogenic, 806
  lipoprotein abnormalities and, 1289-1290
  low-residue, 1014
  mineralocorticoid excess and, 1160
  nutritional therapy and, 1111
  obesity and, 1103
  in oliguria, 633
  phosphates in, 1184
  pregnancy and, 1211
  renal failure and, 639
  tumors and, 446
  ulcers and, 991
  vitamin D and, 1185
Diethylcarbamazine, 290, 292
Diethylenetriamine penta-acetic acid; see DTPA
Diethylstilbestrol
  acanthosis nigricans and, 887
  cancer and, 432, 444, 449
DiFerrante syndrome, 1233, 1234
Differential white cell counts, 361; see also
    Blood cell count, white
Diffuse lung disease, dental care in, 747; see also
    Lung
Diffuse scleroderma, 904
Diffusion; see also Diffusion capacity
  alveolar hypoxemia and, 682
  alveolar-capillary gas transfer and, 676
  respiratory failure and, 708
Diffusion capacity, 676, 694; see also Diffusion
DiGeorge's syndrome, 33, 1196
Digestion and absorption, 940-949, 998-1005;
    see also Digestive system; Intestines
Digestive enzymes, 945
Digestive system, 940-1113; see also Intestines
  absorption in, 940-949, 998-999
  acid-peptic diseases of, 987-998
    bezoars and, 998
    dental care and, 1092
    diverticula and, 998
    gastric dilation in, 997
    gastritis in, 996-997; see also Gastritis
    gastroesophageal reflux disease in, 982-985
    pyloric stenosis in, 997-998
    stress erosions in, 995-996
    ulcer disease in, 987-994; see also Ulcers
    volvulus in, 998
    Zollinger-Ellison syndrome in, 994-995
  alcohol and, 1258
  anorectal disorders in, 1029-1031
  anthrax and, 245
  biliary tract disease and, 1085-1090; see also
    Biliary tract
  bleeding and, 957-960
    angiography and, 971, 972
    cirrhosis and, 1083
    colorectal carcinoma and, 1040
    Crohn's disease and, 1011
    diverticulosis and, 1017
    endoscopy and, 963
    large bowel neoplasms and, 1038
    polyposis syndromes and, 1042
    small bowel tumors and, 1037
    telangiectasia and, 1023-1024

Digestive system—cont'd
  bleeding and —cont'd
    ulcers and, 988, 990, 993-994, 1092
  calcitonin and, 1189
  cancer of; see Carcinomas of gastrointestinal
    tract
  cutaneous lesions and, 891-895
  dentistry and, 1090-1113
    acid peptic disease in, 1092
    esophageal diseases in, 1091-1092
    inflammatory diseases in, 1092-1093, 1095-1097
    liver diseases in, 1097-1101
    nutritional disorders in, 1102-1111
    pancreatic diseases in, 1101-1102
    tumors in, 1092-1095
  diagnosis and, 748, 949-961
    angiography in, 959, 971-972, 1021, 1023
    colon in, 964-965; see also Colonoscopy
    computed tomography in, 971
    esophagus in, 961-962
    hepatobiliary tree in, 967-969
    liver in, 965-967
    pancreas in, 968, 969
    prophylactic regimens for, 185
    small bowel in, 964
    stomach in, 962-964
    ultrasound in, 969-971
  esophagus in, 972-987, 1091-1092; see also
    Esophagus
  functional bowel disease in, 1027-1029
  gram-negative bacillary bacteremia and, 239
  heart failure and, 461
  histology of, 941
  hyperthyroidism and, 1143
  inflammatory intestinal diseases in, 1005-1020;
    see also Intestines, inflammations of
    dental care and, 1092-1093, 1095-1097
  Kaposi's sarcoma and, 921
  larva migrans and, 290, 721
  liver disease and, 1057-1085, 1097-1101; see
    also Liver
  malabsorption syndrome in, 998-1005
  mesenteric diseases in, 1043-1049
  obstruction of, 445, 951, 993, 1024-1027
  pancreatic disease and, 1049-1057, 1101-1102; see also Pancreas
  peritoneal diseases in, 1043-1049; see also
    Peritoneum
  polyposis syndromes and, 1042-1043; see also
    Polyposis syndromes
  psychophysiologic reaction and, 1027
  radiation and, 750
  staphylococci in syndromes of, 220
  structure and function of, 940-949
  symptoms and, 949-961
    bleeding in, 957-960; see also Digestive
      system, bleeding and
    constipation in, 955-956
    diarrhea in, 952-954; see also Diarrhea
    gaseousness in, 960-961
    nausea and vomiting in, 956-957
    pain in, 950-952
  systemic sclerosis and, 60, 61
  tuberculosis and, 257
  tumors of, 1031-1043
    colonic, 448, 1038-1042
      ulcerative colitis and, 1008, 1009, 1010
    dental care and, 1092-1095
    esophageal, 447, 979, 1031-1033
    gastric, 447-448, 1033-1037, 1192
    polyposis syndromes in, 1042-1043; see
      also Polyposis syndromes
    rectal, 1038-1042

Digestive system—cont'd
  tumors of—cont'd
    small bowel, 445, 1013-1014, 1037-1038
  vascular diseases of, 951, 1020-1024
    dental care and, 1092-1093, 1095
  viral infections of, 122, 130
Digital angiography, computed, 761
Digital chancres, 265
Digital pallor, 62-63, 906
Digitalis
  allergy and, 28
  anomalous pulmonary venous return and, 503
  arrhythmias and, 572
  atrial fibrillation and, 544, 545, 1142
  atrial flutter and, 544
  atrioventricular junctional tachycardia and, 545
  cardiomyopathy and, 62, 520, 522
  congestive heart failure and, 464, 502, 509, 584
  countershock and, 550
  electrocardiogram and, 484
  endocardial cushion defects and, 504
  intoxication from, 546
  mitral regurgitation and, 511
  myocardial infarction and, 584
  nonparoxysmal atrial tachycardia and, 542
  pancreatitis and, 1053
  preexcitation patterns and, 501
  respiratory failure and, 711
  sudden death and, 538
  supraventricular tachycardia and, 500
  tricuspid regurgitation and, 517
  Wolff-Parkinson-White syndrome and, 548, 549
Digitalization, 464
Digitoxin, 511
Digits; see also Fingers; Hands
  chancre of, 265
  contractures of, scleroderma and, 903
  necrosis of, 62-63, 906
Digoxin
  cor pulmonale and, 693
  heart failure and, 464, 584
  mitral regurgitation and, 511
  mitral stenosis and, 513
  pregnancy and, 1212
DiGuglielmo syndrome, 322
Dihydropterine reductase deficiency, 1236
Dihydroxyphenylalanine, 1166
1,25-Dihydroxyvitamin D_3, 1186
  calcium and, 648, 1184
  hyperparathyroidism and, 1193
  hypoparathyroidism and, 1196
  osteomalacia and, 1198, 1199, 1200, 1201
  osteoporosis and, 1202, 1203
  parathyroid hormone and, 1187, 1193, 1196
  phosphate and, 1185
  renal osteodystrophy and, 1201
  rickets and, 1200
24,25-Dihydroxyvitamin D_3, 1186, 1187, 1198, 1199
25,26-Dihydroxyvitamin D_3, 1186
Diiodohydroxyquin, 203, 283
Diiodotyrosine, 1128, 1129-1130
Dilantin; see Phenytoin
Diloxanide furoate, 283
Dimercaprol
  heavy metal toxicity and, 627, 752, 753, 754, 853
  hemolysis and, 330
Dimetapp, 1212
Dimethyl sulfoxide, 386, 903
N,N'-(2,6-Dimethylphenylcarbamoylmethyl) iminodiacetic acid; see HIDA

Dimethyltriazenoimidazolecarboxamide; see Dacarbazine
Dinitrochlorobenzene, 32, 927
2,4-Dinitrophenol, 1131
Dioctyl sodium sulfosuccinate, 1212
DIP; see Distal interphalangeal joints
Diphenhydramine
  acute herpetic gingivostomatitis and, 299
  allergic reactions and, 22, 30, 576
  drug reactions and, 29
  oral ulcers and, 415, 451, 876
  pemphigus and, 933
  phenothiazine intoxication and, 779
  pregnancy and, 1212
  radiation stomatitis and, 919
  Reiter's syndrome and, 908
  scalded skin syndrome and, 932
  urticaria and, 26
Diphenoxylate, 953, 1014, 1029
2,3-Diphosphoglycerate, 325
Diphosphonates, 62, 88
Diphtheria, 247-249
  dentistry and, 305
  differential diagnosis of, 224
  neuropathy and, 855
  pseudomembrane of oral mucosa in, 305
  vaccines for, 238, 248, 252
Diphtheria antitoxin, 248
Diphtheria toxoid, 248
Diphtheria-pertussis-tetanus vaccines, 238, 248, 252
Diphtheria-tetanus vaccine, 248
Diphyllobothriasis, 293
Diphyllobothrium latum, 293, 317
Diplegia, spastic, 146
Diplococci, 108, 691
Diplococcus pneumoniae, 691
Diploid cell vaccine, human, 153
Diplopia, 760
Dipstick test, 588, 589-590, 604
Dipyridamole
  cerebral infarction and, 832
  platelet aggregation and, 353, 405, 406
  pregnancy and, 1212
  in Raynaud's phenomenon, 61
  thrombocytosis and, 404
  thrombotic thrombocytopenic purpura and, 404
  transient ischemic attack and, 837
Disappearing testis, 1170
Disc disease, 48, 50, 860
Disc edema, 798
Discoid lupus erythematosus, chronic, 57
  dentistry and, 111
Diseases; see also Syndromes
  Addison's; see Addison's disease
  Alexander's, 803
  Alzheimer's, 774, 846
  Bechterew's, 48
  Behçet's; see Behçet's syndrome
  Berger's, 611
  Bornholm, 730
  Bourneville's, 810
  Bowen's, 914, 1031
  Buerger's, 69, 570
  Caisson, 104
  calcium pyrophosphate crystal, 94
  central core, 859
  Chagas', 287, 977, 1027
  Charcot joint, 86
  Charcot-Marie-Tooth, 805, 855
  chest bellows, 712
  Christmas, 410
  combined system, 33-34, 808, 851
  Creutzfeldt-Jakob, 774, 828, 868

Diseases—cont'd
  Crohn's; see Crohn's disease
  Crouzon's, 1314, 1315, 1316
  crystal deposition, 95
  Cushing's, 1177, 1262; see also Cushing's syndrome
  Degos', 893-894, 1003
  DeQuervain's, 99
  Fabry's, 911-912, 1231-1232
  Farber's, 1231, 1233
  Forestier's, 86
  Gaucher's; see Gaucher's disease
  Gilbert's, 1058, 1066, 1067
  Graves'; see Graves' disease
  Gunther's, 888; see also Porphyrias, congenital erythropoietic
  Hailey-Hailey, 934-935
  Hallervorden-Spatz, 775
  Hand-Schüller-Christian, 397, 425, 718
  heavy chain, 384
  Heerfordt's, 77, 113, 717, 910, 911
  Hirschsprung's, 1026
  Hodgkin's; see Hodgkin's disease
  Huntington's, 774, 816-818
  I-cell, 1235
  intermittent, 53
  Jod-Basedow, 1146
  Kawasaki, 68, 69, 142-148
  Kohlmeier-Dagos, 893-894, 1003
  Krabbe's, 802, 1231, 1233
  Kugelberg-Welander, 804-805
  Landing's, 1230, 1231
  Legg-Calvé-Perthes, 104
  Legionnaires', 177, 216
  Letterer-Siwe, 397, 718
  Lou Gehrig's, 803-804
  Lyell's, 931-932
  Lyme; see Lyme disease
  maple syrup urine, 1237, 1238
  Marchiafava-Bignami, 1257
  Marie-Strümpell, 48
  McArdle's, 858
  Menetrier's, 997
  Ménière's, 793, 795
  minimal lesion, 613
  Moyamoya, 843
  Niemann-Pick; see Niemann-Pick disease
  nil, 613
  Osler-Weber-Rendu; see Osler-Weber-Rendu disease
  Paget's, 86-88, 114-115
  Parkinson's, 812-815
  Pelizaeus-Merzbacher, 802
  periodic, 53
  Peyronie's, 105
  Pick's, 774
  Plummer's, 1145
  Pompe's, 522
  Pott's, 81, 256
  pulseless; see Pulseless disease
  Quincke's, 580
  Raynaud's, 63-64, 496, 683, 981; see also Raynaud's phenomenon
  Refsum's, 806, 855
  Sandhoff's, 1231
  Schilder's, 802
  sickle cell; see Sickle cell disease
  Sjögren's, 893
  Still's, 43, 45-46
  Stokes-Adams, 500, 780
  storage-pool, 405
  Sutton's, 110
  Takayasu's; see Pulseless disease
  Tangier, 1292

Diseases—cont'd
  Tay-Sachs, 358, 1224, 1230-1231
  Thomsen's, 859
  Urbach-Wiethe, 1296
  von Gierke's, 890
  von Hippel-Lindau, 809, 1165
  von Recklinghausen's; see von Recklinghausen's disease
  von Willebrand's, 407-408, 410, 1227
    dentistry and, 426-427
    sickle cell trait and, 334
  Weber-Christian, 78-79
  Weil's, 273
  Werdnig-Hoffmann, 804
  Wernicke's; see Wernicke's encephalopathy
  Whipple's, 941, 1002-1003
  Wilson's, 822-823, 1066, 1081-1082, 1240
    hemolysis in, 342
    juvenile parkinsonism and, 812
Dislocation, 1228, 1241
Disodium cromoglycate, 721, 728
Disopyramide
  pregnancy and, 1212
  side effects of, 585
  ventricular fibrillation and, 546
Disorientation, right-left, 759
Disseminated encephalomyelitis, acute, 801, 827
Disseminated intravascular coagulation, 412-413
  dentistry and, 429
  fulminant meningococcemia and, 234
  hemolysis and, 341
  oral bleeding and, 421
  platelet destruction and, 404
  septic shock and, 240
Disseminated vasculitis, 29
Disseminated zoster, 927
Dissemination
  of candidiasis, 276
  of coccidioidomycosis, 275
  of herpes zoster, 927
  of histiocytosis, 397
  of histoplasmosis, 274
  multiple sclerosis and, 796
  visceral, varicella and, 130
Distal interphalangeal joints, 51
Distention, 960-961
  accommodation to, 963
  ascites and, 1044
  bowel obstruction and, 1024, 1025
  colorectal carcinoma and, 1040
  functional bowel disease and, 1027, 1028
  gastric dilation and, 997
  jugular venous, 580
Disulfiram, 1256
DIT; see Diiodotyrosine
Diuresis
  osmotic, 595, 1270; see also Diruetics
  postobstructive, 655
  renal failure and, 632, 635
Diuretics, 597
  aortic dissection and, 562
  ascites and, 1046, 1084
  blood urea nitrogen and, 462
  bromide intoxication and, 777
  calcium and, 1190, 1191
  cardiomyopathy and, 62, 520, 522
  cor pulmonale and, 693
  electrolyte imbalance and, 572
  glomerulonephritis and, 610
  Graves' ophthalmopathy and, 1147
  guanethidine and, 472
  heart failure and, 464, 465
  hepatic coma and, 1061
  hypercalcemia and, 1180, 1191

Diuretics—cont'd
  hyperkalemia and, 598, 599
  hypernatremia and, 596, 597
  hypertension and, 467, 472, 473, 474, 475
  hypokalemia and, 598
  hyponatremia and, 595
  hyporeninemic hypoaldosteronism and, 623
  hypoxia and, 696
  interstitial nephritis and, 619
  kidney stones and, 647, 648
  lithium overdose and, 779
  loop, 572, 574
  Ménière's syndrome and, 793
  metabolic alkalosis and, 600
  mineralocorticoid excess and, 1161
  mitral regurgitation and, 511
  mitral stenosis and, 513
  myoglobinuria and, 860
  nephrotic syndrome and, 613
  neutropenia and, 360
  obstructive uropathy and, 655
  pancreatitis and, 1053
  pickwickian syndrome and, 712
  postural hypotension and, 780
  potassium-sparing; see Potassium-sparing diuretics
  pseudotumor cerebri and, 848
  pulmonary edema and, 465
  renal failure and, 637, 639
  sickle cell disease and, 618
  sudden death and, 538
  thiazide; see Thiazides
  toxic nephropathy and, 624, 625, 626, 627, 629
  transfusions and, 318
  tricuspid regurgitation and, 517
  tumor supportive care and, 445
Diurnal rhythm, 1117-1118
Diverticula
  of esophagus, 736, 975, 976
  gastric, 998
  intestinal, 324, 1017-1018; see also Diverticulitis
  urethral, 651
  Zenker's, 736, 975, 976
Diverticulitis, 324, 951, 1017-1018, 1021
Diverticulosis, 1017-1018
Dizziness; see Vertigo
DKA; see Diabetes mellitus, ketoacidosis and
D-L antibody; see Donath-Landsteiner antibody
DMD; see Duchenne muscular dystrophy
DMF; see Decayed, missing, and filled teeth
DML; see Lymphomas, diffuse
DNA; see Deoxyribonucleic acid
DNase; see Deoxyribonuclease
Dobutamine, 465
DOC; see Deoxycorticosterone
Dolene; see Propoxyphene
Doll's head reflex, 766
Dominant traits, 1218, 1219
Donath-Landsteiner antibody, 340
Donors
  of blood, 347, 348-349
  renal transplantation and, 643-644
Donovan bodies, 238
Donovanosis, 238, 239
Dopa, 1166
L-Dopa; see Levodopa
Dopamine, 1165, 1166
  agonists of, 815
  heart failure and, 465
  meningococcemia and, 234
  Parkinson's disease and, 812
  pericardial tamponade and, 555

Dopamine—cont'd
  pulmonary emboli and, 494
  shock and, 240, 478
Dopamine receptor agonists, 815
Dopamine-β-hydroxylase, 468, 820, 1166
Doppler ultrasound; see Ultrasonography
Dorsal interosseous muscle atrophy, 36
Double kidney, 650
Double product, 528
Double-refractile bodies, 605, 612, 912
Down's facies, 578
Down's syndrome, 1221, 1225
  craniofacial malformations and, 1301, 1308
Downbeat nystagmus, 760, 811
Doxorubicin, 441
  bleomycin, vinblastine, and imidazole carboxamide, 390, 391
  and cancer, 447-449
  cardiotoxicity of, 441
  endocrine tumors and, 450
  Hodgkin's disease and, 390, 391
  in leukemias, 366, 367
  in non-Hodgkin's lymphoma, 392, 393
  in sarcomas, 450
  thrombocytopenia and, 400
  urine and, 588
Doxycycline, 161, 168
  administration route for, 157
  excretion of, 158
  renal disease and, 670
DPDLL; see Lymphomas, diffuse
2,3-DPG; see 2,3-Diphosphoglycerate
DPT vaccine; see Diphtheria-pertussis-tetanus vaccines
Drainage
  abscesses and, 192, 193, 199
  diabetic foot and, 1273
  postural, 697
  subdural empyema and, 193
Drepanocyte, 315
Dressler's syndrome, 537
Drop attack, 836
Droplike psoriasis, 936
Drug abuse, 775-779
  dentistry and, 862-864
  endocarditis and, 181
  Mediterranean fever and, 1048
  multiple drugs and, 863
  toxic nephropathy and, 629
Drug fever, 28
  antimicrobial agents and, 159
Drugs; see also specific drug
  abuse of; see Drug abuse
  allergy to, 27-30
    anaphylactic shock and, 576
    angioedema and, 25, 26
    Schönlein-Henoch purpura and, 70
    asthma from, 704
  calcium and, 1190, 1191
  as carcinogenic agents, 432
  cardiomyopathy and, 520-521
  connective tissue disease from, 57
  Fanconi's syndrome and, 624
  gastrointestinal bleeding and, 958
  hemolysis from, 329-330, 342
  hepatic detoxification and, 1061-1062
  interactions of
    with alcohol, 1297, 1298
    dentistry and, 1090
    sulfonylureas and, 1267
  lung disease from, 721-722
  lupus from, 57
  malabsorption and, 1002
  neurologic effects of, 779

Drugs—cont'd
  neuropathies from, 853
  neutropenia from, 360
  overdose of, alveolar hypoventilation and, 682
  pericarditis and reactions to, 550
  platelet disorders and, 400-401, 402, 405-406
  pregnancy and, 1212, 1213
  shock and, 476
  sudden death and, 538
  Sydenham's chorea and intoxication from, 819
  testes and, 1172
  thrombocytopenia and, 400-401, 402, 403-404
  toxicity of, 775-779, 819; see also specific drug
    chorea and, 819
  urticaria and, 25, 26
  withdrawal seizures and, 787
Dry bronchiectasis, 697
Dry pleurisy, 255
Dry skin, 876-877
Drying agents in respiratory disease, 746
DS; see Dermatan sulfate
dT vaccine; see Diphtheria-tetanus vaccine
DTIC; see Dacarbazine
DTPA, 964
DTs; see Delirium tremens
Dubin-Johnson syndrome, 1058, 1068
Duchenne muscular dystrophy, 856-857
Duck embryo vaccine, 153
Ductus arteriosus, patent, 499, 504-505
  cyanotic heart lesions and, 506, 683
  transposition of great arteries and, 508
Duffy blood group systems, 280
DUL; see Lymphomas, diffuse
Dumping syndrome, 944, 946, 993; see also Postgastrectomy syndrome
  hypoglycemia and, 1277
  malabsorption and, 1004
Duncan's syndrome, 133
Duodenoscope, 964
Duodenum
  structure and function of, 945
  study of, 964
  ulcer of, 987-994
Duplication
  of Hensen's node, 1303
  of kidneys, 650
  of primitive streak, 1303
Dupuytren's contracture, 101
Dust in lung disease, 723, 727
Dwarfism, 882, 1245
DWDLL; see Lymphomas, diffuse
Dyclone; see Dyclonine
Dyclonine, 415, 451, 876
Dyes, 28, 659, 704; see also Contrast agents
Dymelor; see Acetohexamide
Dynamic compliance, 693
Dynamic compression of airway, 690
Dysarthria, 760, 835
Dysarthria–clumsy hand syndrome, 835
Dysconjugate gaze, 760
Dyscrasias, blood; see specific disease
Dysentery, 206
Dysesthesia, 667, 872
Dysfibrinogenemias, 411
Dysgenesis, seminiferous tubule, 1170
Dysgeusia, 666
Dyskinesia, 870
Dysmyelinating diseases, 796, 801-803
Dysostosis
  craniofacial, 1314, 1315, 1316
  Nager acrofacial, 1311
Dysostosis multiplex, 1234
Dysphagia, 961, 974, 975-976

Dysphagia—cont'd
  bulbar palsy and, 760
  dentistry and, 1091
  iron deficiency and, 1105
  malnutrition and, 1103
  sideropenic, 416
Dysplasia
  anhydrotic ectodermal, 876-877
  branchial arch, 1309
  dentin, 1244
  fibromuscular, 842
  fibrous, 104, 115-116
  frontonasal, 1317-1318
  multiple epiphyseal, 1245
  oculoauriculovertebral, 1300, 1310-1312
  polyostotic, 116
  pulpal, 1244
  refractive anemia and, 321
  renal, 650
  thyroid, 1137
Dyspnea
  heart failure and, 460
  mitral regurgitation and, 510
  mitral stenosis and, 512
  noncardiac causes of, 463
  paroxysmal nocturnal, 461
  at rest, pulmonary embolism and, 490-491
  thoracentesis and, 687
Dystonia musculorum deformans, 820-821
Dystonias, torsion, 819-821
Dystrophy
  adiposogenital, 1124-1125
  muscular, 856-858, 975
  myotonic, 859
  reflex sympathetic, 100

E
E_2; see Estradiol
e antigen, 126, 1100
E apoproteins, 1281
EA; see Early antigens
EACA; see ϵ-Aminocaproic acid
Early antigens, 132, 133
Ears; see also Deafness; Hearing loss
  brain abscess and, 191
  calcification and, 103
  evaluation of, 9
  labyrinthine diseases and, 792-793
  leprosy and, 262, 304
  otitis and, 193, 217, 795
  otocraniofacial syndromes and, 1309, 1310
  ototoxic drugs and, 158, 166
  pain in, dental conditions and, 867-868
  relapsing polychondritis and, 102, 103
Eastern equine encephalitis, 135, 825
Eating behaviors, altered, 1102-1103
EBNA; see Epstein-Barr virus-associated nuclear antigen
Ebstein's anomaly, 507-508, 554
EBV; see Epstein-Barr virus
EC cells, 943
Eccentric ventricular hypertrophy, 459
Ecchymoses, purpura and, 402-403
ECF; see Extracellular fluid
ECF-A; see Eosinophil chemotactic factor of anaphylaxis
ECG; see Electrocardiograms
Echinococcosis, 294, 398
Echinococcus granulosus, 172, 294
Echinococcus multilocularis, 294
Echocardiography, 485-487
  aortic regurgitation and, 516
  aortic stenosis and, 515
  cardiomyopathy and, 519, 521

Echocardiography—cont'd
  congenital heart disease and, 502
  heart failure and, 462
  mitral regurgitation and, 511
  mitral stenosis and, 513, 514
  mitral valve prolapse and, 511
  pulmonary hypertension and, 496
  two-dimensional, 487
Echoviruses
  cardiomyopathy and, 520
  central nervous sytem disease and, 135, 136
  in pneumonia, 172
  respiratory infections and, 144
ECL cells, 943
Eclampsia, 665-666
ECM; see Erythema chronicum migrans
ECMO; see Extracorporeal membrane oxygenator
Ecthyma gangrenosum, 240
Ectoderm, development of, 1304
Ectodermal dysplasia, anhydrotic, 876-877
Ectopic adrenocorticotropic hormone, 435, 437
Ectopic beat, 542
Ectopic Cushing's syndrome, 1157, 1158, 1159
Ectopic endometrium, 733
Ectopic focus, 500
Ectopic gonadotropins, 1181
Ectopic hormone syndromes, 1178
Ectopic islet cell tissue, 1037
Ectopic kidney, 650
Ectopic pancreas, 1035, 1037, 1050
Ectopic polypeptides, 435
Ectopic thyroid, 1137, 1146
Eczema, 20, 926
Eczema herpeticum, 926
ED syndromes; see Ehlers-Danlos syndromes
Edema
  angioneurotic, 30, 351
  disc, 798, 846
  examination of, 13
  heart failure and, 460; see also Heart failure
  kidney function and, 597
    focal glomerulosclerosis and, 614
    nephrotic syndrome and, 612-613
    site of injury and, 588
  laryngeal, 17, 25-26, 351
  peripheral, 461
  phalangeal, 51
  pulmonary; see Pulmonary edema
  of tongue, 667
  toxemia of pregnancy and, 665
  of uvula, 667
Edetate, 753
Edrophonium, 856
EDTA, 627
EEE; see Eastern equine encephalitis
EEG; see Electroencephalogram
Effort independence of expiratory flow, 679
Effusions
  malignant, 445, 688, 731, 732
  pericardial, 60, 553-555
  pleural; see Pleural effusions
Eggs, allergy to, 153
Eggshell calcification, 724
Ehlers-Danlos syndromes, 407, 1241-1243, 1302
Ehrlich's aldehyde reagent, 1251
Eisenmenger's complex, 504
Eisenmenger's syndrome, 504
Ejection click
  aortic stenosis and, 505
  coarctation of aorta and, 505
  hypertension and, 470
  pulmonary stenosis and, 506
Ejection fraction, 530, 540
Elastase, 945, 1050

Elastic recoil of lung, 691
Elastotic skin, 914
Elavil; *see* Amitryptyline
Elbow, disorders of, 84, 98, 101-102
Electrical axis, 482-483
Electrical injury, 751-752
Electrocardiograms, 479-485
   abnormalities of, 484-485
   angina pectoris and, 529, 530
   cardiomyopathy and, 519, 521, 522
   chronic obstructive pulmonary disease and, 692, 694
   conduction defects and, 542; *see also* specific defect
   in congenital heart disease, 499-500
   electrophysiology in, 479-480
   endocardial cushion defects and, 504
   heart failure and, 462
   lead systems and, 480, 481
   mitral regurgitation and, 510-511
   mitral stenosis and, 513
   mitral valve prolapse and, 511
   myocardial infarction and, 535-536
   normal, 480-484
   pericarditis and, 551
   pulmonary embolism and, 491
   recording of, 480
   renal failure and, 632
   tricuspid stenosis and, 516
Electrocardioversion, synchronous, 584, 585
Electrocoagulation; *see also* Snare-cautery
   angiokeratomas and, 1296
   hereditary hemorrhagic telangiectasia and, 1024
   intestinal ulcer and, 1019
Electrodissection, 882
Electroencephalogram, 762
   barbiturate intoxication and, 777
   brain tumor and, 847
   cerebral infarction and, 832
   epilepsy and, 783
   herpes simplex encephalitis and, 136
   parkinsonism and, 814
   sleep disorders and, 769
   unconsciousness and, 768
Electrolytes; *see also* specific electrolyte
   disturbances of, 588, 593-603; *see also* Kidney diseases
      bowel obstruction and, 1024
      mineralocorticoid deficiency and, 1159
      vomiting and, 957
   replacement of; *see also* specific agent
      hyperglycemic hyperosmolar, nonketotic coma and, 1270
      staphylococcal enterocolitis and, 220
      thyrotoxicosis and, 1205
      viral gastroenteritis and, 150
Electromagnetic ionizing radiation, 749
Electromyography, 762
   botulism and, 204
   neuromuscular disorders and, 852-853
   polymyositis and, 65
Electron microscopy, 122, 124
   cytomegalovirus and, 131
   Norwalk-like agents and, 150
   rotaviruses and, 150
   viral gastroenteritis and, 149, 150
Electronystagmography, 792
Electrophoresis; *see also* Immunoelectrophoresis
   hemoglobin, 333
   plasma lipoproteins and, 1281
   protein
      heavy-chain disease and, 384
      multiple myeloma and, 380

Electrophoresis—cont'd
   protein—cont'd
      normal, 378
      Waldenström's macroglobulinemia and, 383
Electrophysiology, 800, 852-853
Electrosurgery, hemophilia and, 428
Elek test, 248
Elemental diets, 1111
Elephantiasis, 292, 921
Elfin facies, 578
Elimination diet, 26
Ellis-van Creveld syndrome, 1245
Elongation factor, 248
EM pathway; *see* Embden-Meyerhof pathway
EMB; *see* Ethambutol
Embden-Meyerhof pathway, 418
Embolectomy, 494
Emboli
   acute arterial insufficiency and, 568
   air, 688, 701
   cerebral, 511, 830-831
   congenital heart disease and, 579
   congestive heart failure and, 463
   endocarditis and, 180, 181
   myocardial infarction and, 536
   pulmonary; *see* Pulmonary emboli
   removal of, 494
   septic, 180, 181, 489
Embryology, 1304-1308
Embryonal carcinosarcoma, 658
Emesis; *see* Vomiting
EMG; *see* Electromyography
Emodin, 589
Emotion, 763, 772
Emotional incontinence, 835
Emphysema, 690, 693-695, 700-701
   bullous, 694, 700-701, 724
   dentistry and, 747
   centrilobular, 693, 694
   coal workers' pneumoconiosis and, 725
   dentistry and, 746, 747
   lung cancer and, 740, 742
   panacinar, 700
   panlobular, 693, 694, 700
Empty-sella syndrome, 1124, 1177
Empyema
   lung abscess and, 699, 700
   subdural, 193
   tuberculous, 255
En coup de sabre, 903
Enamel
   hypoplastic
      anhydrotic ectodermal dysplasia and, 877
      Ehlers-Danlos syndrome and, 1242
      epidermolysis bullosa dystrophica and, 878
      hemolytic disease of newborn and, 418
      hypothyroidism and, 1206
      rubella and, 300
      tuberous sclerosis and, 881
      osteogenesis imperfecta and, 1244
      scleroderma and, 903
Encephale isolé, 764
Encephalitis, 135, 825-826; *see also* Encephalomyelitis; Encephalopathy
   brain abscess and, 192
   California, 138, 825
   Eastern equine, 135, 825
   enteroviruses and, 137
   evaluation of, 139
   herpes simplex, 128, 135, 825-826
      empiric therapy versus brain biopsy in, 136
      neonatal, 126, 135
      vidarabine and, 154
   measles and, 138, 145

Encephalitis—cont'd
   mumps and, 137
   parkinsonism and, 812
   rabies and, 139
   St. Louis, 135, 825
   toxoplasmosis and, 285
   trypanosomiasis and, 287
   varicella and, 138
   Venezuelan equine, 135
   von Economo's, 812
   Western equine, 135
Encephalitis lethargica, 812
Encephalomyelitis; *see also* Encephalitis; Encephalopathy
   acute
      disseminated, 801, 827
      necrotizing, 801
   postvaccinal, 801, 827
Encephalopathy; *see also* Encephalitis; Encephalomyelitis
   hepatic, 1061, 1084
   hypertensive, 469, 841
   lead poisoning and, 753
   metabolic, unconsciousness and, 768
   subacute spongiform, 828
   Wernicke's; *see* Wernicke's encephalopathy
Encephalotrigeminal angiomatosis, 810, 881-882
Endarterectomy, 565, 1273
Endarteritis
   differential diagnosis of, 179
   Salmonella, 208
   syphilis and, 265, 269
End-capillary oxygen tensions, 676
Endobronchial tuberculosis, 255
Endocardial cushion defects, 503-504
Endocardial fibroelastosis, 516, 522
Endocarditis, 178-185
   aortic regurgitation and, 515
   dentistry and, 180, 185, 579, 581-582
   bacterial endocarditis in, 301-302
   erysipeloid and, 246
   glomerulonephritis with, 611
   Haemophilus influenzae and, 236
   Löffler's, 522; *see also* Löffler's syndrome
   pulmonic regurgitation and, 517
   Q fever, 213
   Salmonella, 208
   streptococci and, 227, 228
Endocardium
   cardiomyopathies and, 522
   congestive heart failure and, 453
   cushion defects of, 503-504
   fibroelastosis of, 516, 522
   inflammation of; *see* Endocarditis
Endocrine diseases, 1114-1215; *see also* Endocrine system
   adrenal cortex in, 1153-1163, 1206-1207; *see also* Adrenal cortex; Adrenal glands
   dentistry and, 1204-1215
      adrenal gland and, 1206-1207
      metabolic bone disease and, 1207-1210
      mineral metabolism and, 1207-1210
      pheochromocytoma and, 1207
      pituitary gland and, 1204-1205
      sex hormonal alterations and, 1210-1214
      thyroid gland and, 1205-1206
   hormone action in, 1114-1116; *see also* Hormones
   humoral syndromes with neoplasms in, 1178-1181
   hypothalamic disorders in, 1116-1126, 1204-1205
      anterior pituitary and, 1116-1118
      clinical disorders and, 1118-1126

Endocrine diseases—cont'd
  hypothalamic disorders in—cont'd
    pineal gland and, 1126
  malabsorption and, 1003-1004
  metabolic bone disease and, 1181-1204, 1207-1210; see also Bone, metabolic disease of
  mineral metabolism in, 1181-1204, 1207-1210; see also Mineral metabolism
  neoplasms and, 443-444, 450, 1178-1181; see also Multiple endocrine neoplasias
  oral candidiasis and, 307
  ovary in, 1173-1178; see also Ovary
  pheochromocytoma in, 1164-1168, 1207
  skin disorders and, 884-891
  testes in, 1168-1173; see also Testes
  thyroid gland in, 1126-1152, 1205-1206; see also Thyroid
Endocrine neoplasia, multiple; see Multiple endocrine neoplasias
Endocrine system
  alcohol and, 1258-1259
  blood pressure and, 467-468
  circulation and, 458
  diseases of; see Endocrine diseases
  hypothalamus in, 1116-1126; see also Pituitary gland
  pancreas and, 1049-1050; see also Pancreas
  renal failure and, 637
Endodontics, hemophilia and, 427
Endogenous vasoactive substances, 477
Endometriosis, 733
Endometrium, 449, 733, 1176
Endomyocardial fibrosis, 516, 522
Endorphins, 241, 1115
Endoscopic retrograde cholangiopancreatography, 968-969
  ampullary carcinomas and, 1089
  choledocholithiasis and, 1089
  pancreatitis and, 1055
Endoscopy, 962-963; see also Endoscopic retrograde cholangiopancreatography
  colorectal carcinoma and, 1040
  esophageal carcinoma and, 1032
  gastric neoplasm and, 1036, 1037
  gastrointestinal bleeding and, 959
  ulcers and, 989
Endotoxin, septic shock and, 240; see also Toxins, bacterial
Enemas, 251, 634, 1026; see also Barium in enemas
  bowel obstruction and, 1026
  cation exchange resins and, 634
Enflurane, 627, 629
Enkephalin, 941
ENL; see Erythema nodosum leprosum
Entamoeba histolytica, 281, 282, 283
  diarrhea and, 953
  drugs for, 170
  pleural effusion and, 731
Enteric bacilli; see also specific species
  arthritis and, 53, 80
  leukemia and, 421
  peritonitis and, 1047
Enteric fever, 202, 207-208
Enteritis, 1002, 1018-1019; see also Crohn's disease; Intestines
Enterobacter; see also Enterobacteriaceae
  drugs for, 163, 164, 165, 166
  leukemia and, 421
  oral lesions and, 306
  in pneumonia, 171
Enterobacteriaceae, 171, 250, 253; see also specific genus

Enterobacteriaceae—cont'd
  abdominal abscess and, 1047
  bacteremia and, 239
  drugs for, 163, 164, 165, 166
Enterobiasis, 289-290, 1030
Enterobius vermicularis, 289-290, 1030
Enterococci, 227-228, 249; see also Streptococci
  endocarditis and, 181, 227, 228
Enterocolitis, 220, 1018; see also Intestines
Enterogastric reflux, 964
Enteroglucagon, 941
Enterohepatic circulation, 940, 946, 999
Enteropathy, gluten, 1001
Enterotoxins, 201, 218
Enteroviruses; see also Viral diseases
  central nervous sytem disease and, 135, 136-137
  exanthems and, 148-149
  respiratory infections and, 140, 144
Environment
  asthma and, 25, 704, 728
  carcinogenesis and, 431-433, 659
  craniofacial malformations and, 1302-1303
  injuries from, 749-756, 847
  liver disease and, 1066
  lung disease and, 691, 723-730, 738
  dental care in, 747-748
Enzymes
  asthma and, 705, 706
  deficiency of
    congenital adrenal hyperplasia and, 1162, 1163
    congenital hemolytic anemia and, 329-331, 418
    dentistry and, 418
    sexual abnormalities and, 1171
  digestive, 945
  in heme biosynthetic pathway, 1247
  in leukemias, 366
  lipolytic, 218, 945, 1049
  lysosomal, 17, 18, 90
  methemoglobinemia and, 344
  muscle, 65
  neuromuscular disorders and, 853
  nucleolytic, 1050
  pancreatic; see Pancreatic enzymes
  proteolytic, 694; see also specific enzyme
  serum, 1065; see also specific enzyme
  viruses and, 125
Eosinophil chemotactic factor, 18
  of anaphylaxis, 372, 705
Eosinophil and eosinophilic syndromes; see Eosinophilic diseases
Eosinophilia, 21, 362-363, 372-373
  allergic granulomatosis and, 67
  asthma and, 24
  drug allergy and, 29
  drug fever and, 28
  parasitic infections and, 119, 289, 372
  pleural fluid, 732
Eosinophilic cytoplasmic inclusions, 146
Eosinophilic diseases, 372-373; see also Eosinophilia; Eosinophilic granuloma
  gastroenteritis and, 1003
  leukemia and, 363, 369
  lung and, 362-363, 372-373, 721
Eosinophilic granuloma, 718-719; see also Granulomas
  of bone, 397
  diabetes insipidus and, 1126
Eosinophils; see also Eosinophilia; Eosinophilic diseases
  life span of, 362

Eosinophils—cont'd
  in nasal secretions, 21
  normal, 362, 372
  precursors of, 362
Ependymomas, 844
Ephedrine, 575, 781, 824
Ephelis, oral cavity and, 919
Epibulbar dermoid cysts, 1310, 1311
Epicondylitis, lateral, 99-100
Epidemic parotitis, 301
Epidermal necrolysis, toxic, 306, 931-932
Epidermoid carcinoma, 915
  of anus, 1031, 1042
  of esophagus, 1032
  of lung, 447
Epidermolysin, 932
Epidermolysis bullosa dystrophica, 877-878
Epidermolytic toxins, 218
Epidermophyton, 279, 928-929
Epidermophyton floccosum, 928, 929
Epididymitis, 215, 256
Epidural infections, 139, 191-194
Epidural spinal cord compression, 445
Epigenetic factors, local, 1306
Epiglottitis, 236
Epilepsia partialis continua, 782
Epilepsy, 781-787; see also Seizures
  adenoma sebaceum, and mental deficiency, triad of, 880
  dentistry and, 864-867
  vertigo and, 794
Epiloia, 880
Epinephrine, 1165, 1166, 1168
  allergic reactions and, 26, 29, 30, 478, 576
  antihypertensives and, 574
  arrhythmias and, 585
  asthma and, 706
  coronary heart disease and, 583
  heart rate and, 458
  hypertension and, 574, 575
  hyperthyroidism and, 1105, 1205
  insulin desensitization and, 1268
  insulin resistance and, 1262
  neutrophils and, 356
  platelet aggregation and, 400
  propranolol and, 583
  prothrombin time and, 1098
  respiratory alkalosis and, 601
  shock and, 477
  syncope and, 864
  transfusion reactions and, 351
  tremor and syncope with, 27
  triiodothyronine and, 1132
  urticaria and, 26
Epiphyseal dysplasia, multiple, 1245
Epiphyseal plates, 1182
Epispadia, 651
Epistaxis
  Gaucher's disease and, 1232
  hereditary hemorrhagic telangiectasia and, 1095
  von Willebrand's disease and, 407
  Weber-Osler-Rendu disease and, 894
Epithelial cells, 142, 941
Epithelial polyps of large bowel, 1038
Epithelium, bronchial, smoking and, 738, 739
EPP; see Erythropoietic protoporphyria
Epsilon-aminocaproic acid
  epistaxis and, 1095
  fibrinolytic states and, 413
  hemophilia and, 410, 428
  liver disease and, 411
  platelet transfusion and, 426
  polycythemia vera and, 419

Epsilon-aminocaproic acid—cont'd
  sickle cell disease and, 618
  subarachnoid hemorrhage and, 840
  thrombasthenia and, 426
  von Willebrand's disease and, 427
Epstein-Barr virus, 131-134, 135, 387
  and atypical pneumonia syndrome, 177
  cold agglutinin syndromes and, 339
  dentistry and, 300
  neoplasia and, 433
  in pneumonia, 172
Epstein-Barr virus–associated nuclear antigen, 132, 133
Epulis fissuratum, 919
Epulis gravidarum, 1211
Equanil; see Meprobamate
Equations, Fick and Henderson-Hasselbalch, 708
Equine antirabies serum, 153
ER; see Estrogen receptors
Erb's point, 516
ERCP; see Endoscopic retrograde cholangiopancreatography
Ergosterol, irradiated, 1185
Ergotamine tartrate, 788
Ergots, 63, 625
Eructations, 960-961
Eruptions; see also Rash; Skin diseases
  heliotrope, 904
  xanthomas and, 885, 890
Erysipelas, streptococcal, 226
Erysipeloid, 246
Erysipelothrix rhusiopathiae, 246
Erythema, 922-926; see also specific erythema
  cat-scratch fever and, 151
  of cheeks, 147
  Kawasaki disease and, 147
  liver diseases and, 896, 1059
  of oropharynx, 69
  rheumatoid arthritis and, 36
  tuberculous, nodular gingivitis and, 304
Erythema chronicum migrans, 297, 298, 925-926
Erythema contusiformis, 925
Erythema gyratum repens, 912-913
Erythema infectiosum, 147
Erythema marginatum, 229
Erythema migrans, 938; see also Geographic tongue
Erythema multiforme, 28-29, 30, 110, 922-924
Erythema nodosum, 28, 924-925
  sarcoidosis and, 77, 78, 910
  subcutaneous nodules and, 79
  ulcerative colitis and, 1007
Erythema nodosum leprosum, 263
Erythermalgia, 897-898
Erythroblastosis fetalis, 337-338, 418
Erythrocyte sedimentation rate, 118, 119, 120
  ankylosing spondylitis and, 49
  arthritis and, 37, 46, 51
  Behçet's disease and, 907
  fever of unknown origin and, 120
  Hodgkin's disease and, 387
  Kawasaki disease and, 148
  lupus erythematosus and, 56
  midline granuloma and, 73
  osteomyelitis and, 82
  polymyalgia rheumatica and, 75
  Reiter's syndrome and, 52
  sarcoidosis and, 77
  systemic sclerosis and, 60
  temporal arteritis and, 75, 790
  Waldenström's macroglobulinemia and, 383
  Wegener's granulomatosis and, 71, 73
Erythrocytes; see Red blood cells
Erythrocythemia, 352; see also Polycythemia
Erythrocytosis with malignancy, 1179

Erythroderma, exfoliative, 937
Erythrodontia, prophyrias and, 889
Erythrodontin, 1298
Erythrogenic toxin, 223
Erythroid cells, heme biosynthesis in, 1248
Erythroleukemia, 316
Erythromelalgia, 897-898
Erythromycin, 161, 167, 168
  actinomycosis and, 247
  allergy and, 28
  antacids and, 1092
  antrhax and, 245
  arthritis and, 80
  bacteriostatic activity of, 156
  bronchitis and, 693
  Campylobacter fetus and, 202
  Chlamydia and, 214, 215, 216
  diphtheria and, 248
  endocarditis and, 185, 581, 582
  erysipeloid and, 246
  excretion of, 158
  gonococci and, 232
  impetigo and, 219, 226
  injection of, 157
  Legionnaires' disease and, 177
  listeriosis and, 246
  liver and, 158
  mycoplasmas and, 218
  oral streptococci and, 302
  pertussis and, 238
  pharyngitis and, 225
  pneumococci and, 175
  pneumonia and, 175, 217
  pregnancy and, 1212, 1213
  renal disease and, 667, 670
  site of infection and, 157
  streptococci and, 225, 226, 227
  syphilis and, 272
Erythromycin stearate, 215
Erythroplasia of Queyrate, 914
Erythropoiesis
  disorders of, 311-326; see also Anemias, red cell production
  ineffective, 312
  normal, 311-312
  polycythemia in, 352-355
  transfusions and, 342, 346-351
Erythropoietic coproporphyria, 888
Erythropoietic porphyrias, 888, 1248-1250
Erythropoietic protoporphyria, 888, 1249, 1250
Erythropoietin, 311-312, 352
  aplastic anemia and, 319, 320
  bone marrow and, 313
  increased production of, 353
Escherichia coli, 201, 202, 205, 249
  asparaginase and, 442
  bacteremia and, 239
  diarrhea and, 952, 953
  disseminated intravascular coagulation and, 412
  drugs for, 159, 162, 163, 164, 165, 166, 169, 170, 171
  enterotoxigenic, 201
  immunodeficiency diseases and, 31
  leukemias and, 368, 421
  liver disease and, 1074
  malabsorption and, 1003
  neoplasia and, 446
  oral lesions of, 306
  in pneumonia, 171, 172
  schistosomiasis and, 296
  strongyloidiasis and, 291
Esophageal colic, 979
Esophageal mucosa, scarring of, 877
Esophageal myotomy, 976, 979, 981, 982

Esophageal reflux, 950, 962, 982-985, 988-989
Esophageal web, 1105
Esophagitis
  from infectious diseases, 307, 985
  from physical agents, 985-986
  reflux, 950, 962, 982-985, 988-989
Esophagogastrostomy, 982
Esophagoscopy, 962, 983
Esophagus, 942, 972-987
  anatomy and physiology of, 972-974
  Barrett's, 983, 1032
  corkscrew, 979, 980
  dentistry and, 1091-1092
  diagnosis and, 961-962, 973-974, 982-983, 1032
  diverticula of, 736, 975, 976
  eructations and, 960
  fibrosis of, 983
  gastrostomy and, 982
  hiatus hernia and, 982-985
  inflammation of; see Esophagitis
  laceration of, 986-987
  manometry and, 962
  mediastinal masses and, 736
  motility disorders of, 975-982
    management of, 62
    smooth muscle, 976-981
    striated muscle, 975-976
    studies of, 973-974
    systemic diseases and, 981-982
  mucosal scarring and, 877
  myotomy of, 976, 979, 981, 982
  neoplasms of, 1031-1033
    achalasia and, 979
    dentistry and, 1091
    management of, 447
  perforation of, 734, 986-987
  reflux and, 950, 982-985, 988-989
  tests for, 961-962
  spasm of, 975
    diffuse, 979-981
    manometry and, 962
    pain and, 950
  strictures of
    caustic ingestion and, 985
    dysphagia and, 1105
    esophagitis and, 983
  swallowing and, 973-975
  symptoms and, 974-975
  systemic sclerosis and, 60, 61
  varices of, 1060
    achalasia and, 979
    management of, 1083
    rupture of, 1063
    schistosomiasis and, 296
  web of, 1105
ESR; see Erythrocyte sedimentation rate
Esterase inhibitor, 17, 26
Estradiol, 1153, 1174, 1175
Estrogen analogs, 444; see also Estrogens
Estrogen receptors, 443, 448
Estrogens
  amenorrhea and, 1177
  aphthous ulcerations and, 1211
  as carcinogens, 432
  cholesterol stones and, 1087
  ear pain and, 867
  esophageal reflux and, 982
  hereditary hemorrhagic telangiectasia and, 407, 894, 1024, 1095
  hypogonadism and, 1172
  lipoproteins and, 1284, 1287, 1288, 1290
  luteinizing hormones and, 1169
  menopause and, 1213

Estrogens—cont'd
  menstrual cycle and, 1174-1175
  negative feedback effect of, 1176
  osteoporosis and, 89, 1202, 1203
  ovary and, 1174, 1176
  pancreatitis and, 1051
  porphyrias and, 888, 1252, 1253-1254
  premature menopause and, 1177
  receptors for, 443, 448
  subgingival microflora and, 1214
  testicular feminization and, 1171
  thrombocytopenia and, 400, 401
  thyroxine-binding globulin and, 1132, 1134
  and tumor therapy, 444, 448, 656
    in breast carcinoma, 448
  Weber-Osler-Rendu disease and, 407, 894, 1024, 1095
État lacunaire, 829, 835
ETH; see Ethionamide
Ethacrynic acid, 597
  aminoglycosides and, 166
  gout and, 92
  heart failure and, 465
  hypertension and, 472
  kidney stones and, 647
  pancreatitis and, 1051
  renal failure and, 639
  sickle cell disease and, 618
Ethambutol, 121, 259, 261
Ethanol; see Alcohol
Ethchlorvynol, 722
Ether, 908
Ethionamide, 259
Ethmocephaly, 1317
Ethnicity, 1224
Ethosuximide
  dental care and, 866
  epilepsy and, 786
  Sydenham's chorea and, 819
Ethrane; see Enflurane
Ethyl alcohol; see Alcohol
Ethylene glycol
  oxalate and, 621, 648
  toxic nephropathy and, 627, 629, 631
Ethylsuccinate, 215
Etidronate disodium, 88
Etiocholanolone, 356
Eton-Lambert syndrome, 856
Eubacterium, 249
Eunuchs, fertile, 1172
Euthyroid syndrome, 1131
Evaluation of patient, 1-14
Evans' syndrome, 403
Evaporation, 755
Eventration of diaphragm, 736
Ewald tube, 989
Ewing's sarcoma, 449, 450
Examination, physical, 7-14
Exanthem subitum, 147
Exanthems, viral, 145-149
  measles and, 300
  varicella-zoster and, 129-130
Exchange diet, liquid, 1268
Exhange resins, 599, 634, 1290; see also Sodium polystyrene sulfonate
Exchange transfusions
  hemolytic disease of newborn and, 338
  purpura and, 404, 617
  sickle cell anemia and, 334
Excursion, diaphragmatic, 736
Exercise
  asthma and, 23, 704
  cardiac output and, 461
  insulin and, 1268
  march hemoglobinuria and, 341

Exercise—cont'd
  proteinuria and, 589
  tests and, 502, 530, 679
Exfoliation, tooth, 299-300
Exfoliative cytology, 1032, 1036, 1037; see also Cytology
Exfoliative dermatitis, 900
Exfoliative erythroderma, 937
Exocrine pancreas, 1049-1050
Exophthalmos, 719, 1142
Exostoses, body, 1093
Exotoxins, 247, 248, 253; see also Toxins, bacterial
Expectorants, 693
Expiration, 672-673
Expiratory flow, effort independence of, 679
Exploring electrode, 480
Exstrophy, cloacal, 651
External ears, 9
Extinction, 759
Extracardiac conduit with valve, 509
Extracellular fluid
  bicarbonate and, 592; see also Bicarbonate
  blood pressure and, 467, 468
  osmolality of, 591, 593
  potassium and, 593, 597
  renal failure and, 636
  sodium and, 592, 594-595
Extracorporeal membrane oxygenator, 709
Extracranial arteries, 564
Extracranial headache, 788
Extraction, tooth
  hemophilia and, 427-428
  midline granuloma and, 113
Extrahepatic biliary ducts, 1058, 1089
Extraintestinal amebiasis, 282, 283
Extralobar sequestration, 736
Extramedullary hematopoiesis, 396
Extranodal disease, 389, 394
Extraocular movements, 8
Extrapancreatic tumors, hypoglycemia from, 1279
Extrapyramidal lesions, 759; see also Basal ganglia
Extrasystolic rhythms in children, 500
Extrathyroidal iodine metabolism, 1128
Extravascular fluid reabsorption, 477
Extremities; see also Leg
  arterial insufficiency and, 569
  evaluation of, 13
  lower; see Leg
  popliteal aneurysms and, 567
Extrinsic asthma, 23-25, 704, 705; see also Asthma
Exudates, pleural, 731
  ascites and, 1044-1045
  pleural effusions and, 687-688
Eyes; see also Vision
  Acanthamoeba and, 283
  albinism and, 1236
  Behçet's syndrome and, 110
  Chlamydia and, 214, 215
  development of, 1306
  diabetes mellitus and, 1273-1274
  evaluation of, 8-9
  hypertension and, 469, 470
  hyperthyroidism and, 1142, 1143, 1147-1148, 1205
  lacrimal gland inflammation and, 36
  neurologic disorders and, 766, 833, 857-858
    brain infarction and, 564, 833
    brainstem lesions and, 760
    coma and, 765, 766

Eyes—cont'd
  neurologic disorders and—cont'd
    frontal lobe lesions in, 757
    headache in, 790
    multiple sclerosis in, 798
    parietal lobe lesions and, 759
    parkinsonism in, 814
  ophthalmia neonatorum and, 230
  pemphigoid and, 935
  pemphigus and, 935
  proptosis and, 1142, 1147
  relapsing polychondritis and, 102
  retina of; see Retina
  sarcoidosis and, 77, 78
  toxoplasmosis and, 284, 285
  trypanosomiasis and, 287
  tularemia and, 243
  viruses and, 122, 126, 128
  Waldenström's macroglobulinemias and, 382
  Wegener's granulomatosis and, 71

F

Fab fragment, 16, 377
Fabry's disease, 911-912, 1231-1232
  orofacial abnormalities and, 668
Fabry-Anderson syndrome, 1296
Face
  asymmetry of, neurofibromatosis and, 879
  basal cell carcinomas of, 883
  cellulitis of, sickle cell anemia and, 417
  craniofacial malformations of, 1300-1322; see also Craniofacial malformations
  development of, 1305-1306, 1308
  pigmentation on, Gaucher's disease and, 1296
Facial clefts, 1318
Facial muscle function, 873-874
Facial myokymia, 799
Facial nerve paralysis, tuberculoid leprosy and, 305
Facial neuralgia, atypical, 791
Facial nevus, 810
Facial pain, 790-791
  cerebrovascular accident and, 872
  multiple sclerosis and, 868
  peripheral neuropathy and, 874
Facial palsy, zoster and, 118
Facies
  Cooley, 418
  Down's, 578
  elfin, 578
  leonine, 304
  moon, 887
Facioscapulohumeral muscular dystrophy, 857
Factors of blood; see Clotting factors
Fainting; see Syncope
Falciparum malaria, 139; see also Malaria
Fallopian tube
  abscesses of, 218
  inflammation of, 218, 231, 232
  pregnancy and, 232
  removal of, 449
  scarring of, 256
Fallot, tetralogy of, 507
False aneurysms, 565
False lumen, 562
FAMA; see Fluorescent antibody to membrane antigen test
Familial central nervous system disease, dentistry and, 868-869
Family history, 7
FANA; see Fluorescent antibody stains for antinuclear antibodies
Fanconi's anemia, 318, 319
  tetracyclines and, 168

Fanconi's anemia—cont'd
  toxic nephropathy and, 624
Farber's disease, 1231, 1233
Farmer's lung, 727
Fasciculations, 761
Fasciculus, medial longitudinal, 766
  syndromes of, 760, 766, 798, 833
Fasciitis, 58, 102
Fasting hypoglycemia, 1277
Fat cells, 1103
Fat necrosis, subcutaneous nodular, 913
Fatigue
  heart failure and, 461
  mitral regurgitation and, 510
Fats, 1102; see also Fatty acids; Lipids
  absorption of, 998, 999-1000
    disorders of, 999-1004
  calories in, 1104
  deficiency of, 1104
  metabolism of, Norwalk-like agents and, 150
  nutritional therapy and, 1111
  polyunsaturated, 1290
  stool, 1000, 1055
  vitamins soluble in; see Fat-soluble vitamins; Vitamins
Fat-soluble vitamins; see also Vitamins
  Crohn's disease and, 1015
  fat absorption and, 998, 1000, 1104
  liver disease and, 1063
Fatty acids, 998, 999, 1104, 1284, 1285
  diabetes and, 1295
  digestion and, 947
  free, 998, 999, 1284, 1285
  hemolysis and, 342
  liver disease and, 1063
  multiple sclerosis and, 797
Fatty liver, 1063, 1077, 1080, 1256, 1257
Fava beans, 330
Favism, 330
Fazio-Londe atrophy, 804
Fc fragment, 16, 377
FDP; see Fibrinogen-fibrin degradation products
^{59}Fe; see Iron 59
Febrile convulsions, 147; see also Seizures
Febrile illnesses, proteinuria and, 589; see also Fever
Febrile transfusion reactions, 351
Fecaliths, 1015-1016
Feces; see also Constipation; Diarrhea
  bile pigments in, 1065
  blood in, 957, 959-960, 988, 996
  fat in, 1000, 1005
  fever of unknown origin and, 120
  fluid loss and, 596
  hepatitis and, 1099
  impaction of, 955, 1025, 1026
  leukocytes and, 203
  porphyrins in, 1253, 1254
  softeners of, 442, 446, 537; see also Hydrophilic bulk agents
Feculent vomitus, 957
Feedback mechanisms
  adrenocorticotropic hormone and, 1117
  hypothalamic-pituitary-ovarian, 1175
  hypothalamic-pituitary-testicular, 1169
Feet; see Foot
FEF_{25-75}; see Flow rate between 25% and 75% of vital capacity
Felty's syndrome, 36
  dental management of, 106
  hypersplenism and, 396
  neutropenia and, 359
Female genitalia; see Genitalia
Female puberty, oral manifestations of, 1210

Female sex hormones; see Estrogens; Progesterones
Feminization, testicular, 1171, 1176
Femoral cutaneous nerve compression, 98
Femoral occlusion, superficial, 570
Femoropopliteal bypass, 570
Femur, bowing of, 87
Fenoprofen, 42, 627, 629
Fernandez reaction, 262
Ferritin, serum, 313
  hemochromatosis and, 345
  liver disease and, 1066, 1081
Ferrochelatase deficiency, 1250
Ferrokinetics, 313; see also Iron
Ferrous sulfate
  hookworm and, 291
  iron deficiency anemia and, 325, 416
  nephropathy and, 628
Ferruginous bodies, 726
Fertile eunuchs, 1172
Fetal alcohol syndrome, 1303, 1304
Fetal antigens, 435
Fetal circulation, persistent, 499
Fetal hemoglobin, 336, 337, 498
Fetal phenytoin syndrome, 1303
Fetal warfarin syndrome, 1303
α-Fetoprotein, 435, 809, 1229
Fetor hepaticus, 1059, 1097
Fetoscopy, 1229
Fetus
  blood sampling from, 1229
  circulation of, 498, 499
  growth retardation of, 125
  hematopoietic function and, 396
  position of, 774
  rubella and, 146
  skin biopsy of, 1229
  sulfonamides and, 169-170
  transfusions for, 338
  ultrasound of, 1229
  viral infections of, 125-127
$FEV_{1.0}$; see Forced expiratory volume in 1 second
$FEV_{3.0}$; see Forced expiratory volume in 3 seconds
Fever, 118, 119-121
  babesiosis and, 288
  blackwater, 280
  convulsions and, 147; see also Seizures
  drug, 28, 159
  drugs for; see Antipyretics
  endocarditis and, 180
  foodborne bacterial illnesses and, 202
  Haverhill, 272
  Katayama, 295
  malaria and, 280
  Mediterranean, 385, 1048
  myeloid metaplasia and, 374
  postpartum, 218
  proteinuria and, 589
  rat-bite, 272-273
  Rocky Mountain spotted, 210-211, 213
    disseminated intravascular coagulation and, 412
    meningoencephalitis and, 139
  roseola and, 147
  sore throat, and adenopathy, triad of, 132
  transfusions and, 351
  typhoid; see Typhoid fever
  of unknown origin, 119-121
  uveoparotid, 910, 911
  valvular disease and, 580
  waterborne bacteria illnesses and, 202
Fever blister, recurrent, 299
FFA; see Free fatty acids

FHH; see Hypercalcemia, familial hypocalciuric
Fiber
  in diet, 1028
  muscle, 852
  Rosenthal, 803
Fiber-type disproportion, congenital, 859
Fiberoptic bronchoscope, 688-689; see also Bronchoscopy
Fiberoptic endoscope, 962; see also Endoscopy
Fiberoptic sigmoidoscopy, 965; see also Sigmoidoscopy
Fibrillary astrocytoma, 844
Fibrillation
  atrial, 543-544
    cardiomyopathy and, 522
    mitral stenosis and, 512, 513
  ventricular
    coronary artery disease and, 585
    sudden death and, 538
Fibrin
  deficiency of, 411
  disseminated intravascular coagulation and, 412
  formation of, 408
  thrombin, and venous blood, anticoagulant therapy and, 430
Fibrin stabilization deficiency, 411
Fibrinogen, 409
  afibrinogenemia and, 429
  deficiency of, 411
  disseminated intravascular coagulation and, 412, 413
  fibrinolytic states and, 413
  hepatitis and, 1069
  liver disease and, 411
  malignant atrophic papulosis and, 894
  radioiodinated, phlebitis and, 495
Fibrinogen-fibrin degradation products, 412, 413
Fibrinoid leukodystrophy, 803
Fibrinolytic states, 413
Fibrinopurulent pneumonia, 177
Fibroblast proliferation, 58
Fibrocystic disease of pancreas, 1101-1102
Fibrodysplasia ossificans progressiva, 1244-1246
Fibroelastosis, endocardial, 516, 522
Fibrofatty nodules, 102
Fibrolytic agents, 111
Fibroma molluscum, 878
Fibromas, 880, 1056
Fibromuscular dysplasia, 842
Fibromyalgia, 42, 96
Fibromyositis, 96
Fibrosclerosis, multifocal, 105
Fibrosing mediastinitis, 105
Fibrosing syndromes, 105
Fibrosis, 105
  of bone marrow, 374-376
  circumoral, systemic sclerosis and, 112
  congenital viral infection and, 125
  cystic; see Cystic fibrosis
  endocardial, 516, 522
  of esophagus, 983
  of intestines, 1011, 1019
  of joint capsule, 48
  of liver, 1059, 1060, 1078, 1079-1084
  of lungs
    asbestos and, 726
    coal workers' pneumoconiosis and, 725
    diffuse diseases and, 713-716
    radiation, 722
  mediastinal, 105, 555
  mesenteric, 1048
  myelophthisis and, 322
  of pancreas, 1055

Fibrosis—cont'd
  pericarditis and, 551
  of portal triads, 1060
  renal artery stenosis and, 660
  retroperitoneal, 105
  syndromes of, 105
  systemic sclerosis and, 58, 61
Fibrositis, 96-97
Fibrous ankylosis, intermaxillary fixation and, 106
Fibrous dysplasia, 104, 115-116
Fibrous papules, 880
Fick equation, 708
Field changes, oral dysplasias and, 919
Field defects, 1228
Field irradiation, 390
Fifth cranial nerve, trigeminal neuralgia and, 791
Fifth disease, 147
Filariasis, 292, 921
Filtration fraction, 664
Fingers; see also Digits; Hands
  agnosia and, 759
  clubbing of, 103, 181, 578, 683-684
  sausage appearance of, 51
  trigger, 99
First arch syndromes, 1309
Fish poisoning, 200
Fish tapeworm, 293, 317
Fissures, anal, 1031
Fistulas
  anal, 1101, 1031
  aortoesophageal, 1032
  arteriovenous, 840; see also Arteriovenous malformations; Shunts
    access, 640, 641, 1274
    hemolysis and, 340
  cholelithiasis and, 1088
  enterocutaneous, 1012
  mumps and, 301
  radiation enteritis and, 1019
  tracheoesophageal, 1032
Fitzgerald factor deficiency, 411
Fitz-Hugh–Curtis syndrome, 231
Five Ps mnemonic, 567
Fixation, intermaxillary, rheumatoid arthritis and, 106
Flagyl; see Metronidazole
Flank pain, 662, 663
Flank strip, 1044
Flat feet, 102
Flatulence, 960-961, 1028; see also Distention
Flavin adenine dinucleotide, 1108
Flavin mononucleotide, 1108
Fleas, 242, 293
  typhus fever and, 212-213, 214
Fletcher factor deficiency, 411
Flexeril; see Cyclobenzaprine hydrochloride
Flexor tenosynovitis, 99
Flora of skin and mucous membranes, 249-250
Florinef; see Fludrocortisone
Flow murmurs, 504; see also Murmurs, cardiac
Flow rate between 25% and 75% of vital capacity, 677, 678
Flucytosine, 278
  with amphotericin B, 278
  candidiasis and, 276
  chromomycosis and, 277
  cryptococcosis and, 276
  endocarditis and, 184
  renal insufficiency and, 158
Fludrocortisone
  Addison's disease and, 1157
  congenital adrenal hyperplasias and, 1163
  hyperkalemia and, 599

Fludrocortisone—cont'd
  mineralocorticoid deficiency and, 1160
  orthostatic hypotension and, 824
  primary aldosteronism and, 1161
Fluids; see also specific fluid
  in diabetic ketoacidosis, 1269-1270
  extracellular; see Extracellular fluid
  herpes simplex and, 129
  kidney stones and, 649
  in oliguria, 633
  parenteral alimentation and, 1015
  pericardial tamponade and, 555
  pH of; see pH
  routes of loss of, 596
  status epilepticus and, 867
Flukes, 294-297
Fluorescent antibody to membrane antigen test, 130
Fluorescent antibody stains, 119
  for antinuclear antibodies, 56, 57
  in syphilis, 271
  toxoplasmosis and, 286
Fluoride
  anticholinergics and, 1092
  excessive, 1106
  halogen sensitivity and, 893
  mouthwashes and, 876
  multiple myeloma and, 382
  osteoporosis and, 89
  poisoning from, 754
  radiation damage to teeth and, 919
  sickle cell anemia and, 417
Fluorinated anesthetics, 1076; see also specific agent
Fluorinated insecticides, 754
Fluoromar; see Fluroxene
5-Fluorouracil, 440-441
  actinic keratoses and, 914
  cancer and
    bladder, 449
    breast, 448
    colorectal, 448
    gastric, 448
    pancreatic, 448
    prostatic, 449
  endocrine tumors and, 450
  Kaposi's sarcoma and, 922
  malignant effusions and, 445
  thyroxine binding globulin and, 1134
Fluoxymesterone, 1122
Flurazepam, 777, 1212, 1213
Fluroxene, 627, 629
FMF; see Fever, Mediterranean
Foam cells, 721, 1288, 1293
Focal emphysema, 725
Focal encephalitis, 192
Focal glomerulosclerosis, 614
Focal hemispheric lesions, 770-773
Focal motor seizures, 766, 781, 782-783
Focal neurologic signs
  brain abscess and, 192
  brain tumor and, 845
  metabolic encephalopathy and, 768
Fogarty catheter, 568
Folate, 315, 1106, 1109-1110; see also Folic acid
  deficiency of
    liver disease and, 1059, 1062, 1063
    malabsorption and, 1000
    megaloblastic anemia and, 316
  metabolism of, 286, 316
  polycythemia and, 354
  red cell, 318
  refractory anemia and, 321

Folate—cont'd
  Reiter's syndrome and, 908
  sprue and, 1001-1002
  in therapy, 318
Folate-dependent tumors, 1110
Folic acid, 318, 1106, 1109-1110; see also Folate
  anemia and
    pernicious, 853
    sickle cell, 334
    sideroblastic, 322
  antagonists of, 366, 440, 1303; see also Methotrexate
  deficiency of, 1109-1110
    dentistry and, 415, 1091, 1109-1110, 1298
    liver diseases and, 1059, 1062, 1063, 1080
    neutropenia and, 358
    renal failure and, 636, 639
    spherocytosis and, 329
    sulfasalazine and, 1010
Folic acid analogs, 366, 440; see also Methotrexate
Folic acid antagonists, 366, 440, 1303; see also Methotrexate
Folinic acid; see Leucovorin
Follicle-stimulating hormone, 1118
  deficiency of, 1121-1122
  feedback mechanisms and, 1169, 1175
  female hypogonadism and, 1122
  menopause and, 1176
  menstrual cycle and, 1174-1175
Follicular carcinoma of thyroid, 1146, 1151
Fontane procedure, 507
Fontanelles, 1312
Food allergy
  angioedema and, 25, 26
  diarrhea and, 954
  eczema and, 20
  eggs and, 153
  malabsorption and, 1003
  Schönlein-Henoch purpura and, 70
  tests for, 22
  urticaria and, 25, 26
Food fads, 1102-1103
Food poisoning, 200, 220
Foodborne and waterborne diseases, 199-209
  botulism in, 204, 209
  cholera in, 204-205, 209
  salmonelloses in, 206-208, 209
  shigellosis in, 205-206, 209
Foot; see also Toes
  diabetic, 1273, 1275
  flat, 102
  rheumatic disorders of, 84, 102
  tarsal tunnel syndrome and, 98
  tenderness of, 52
Foramina of Bochdalek and Morgagni, 736
Forced expiratory vital capacity, 677-679, 706
Forced expiratory volume
  in 1 second, 678, 679, 684, 690, 692, 706
  in 3 seconds, 678, 679
Forced inspiratory oxygen, 709, 710
Forced vital capacity; see Forced expiratory vital capacity
Foreign bodies, intracranial, 187
Forestier's disease, 86
Formaldehyde, 777
Formalin, 294
Formic acid, 777
Fossa ovalis, 503
Fourth ventricle, 807
Foville's syndrome, 833
Fracture
  mandibular, sleep apnea syndrome and, 861

Fracture—cont'd
  pathologic, 88, 89, 379
  of teeth, 906
  of vertebral bodies, 1203
Frameshifts, 1217
Francisella tularensis, 171, 243, 244, 305
Franklin modification of Vim-Silverman needle, 608
Frank-Starling law, 454, 456, 457, 458, 1044; *see also* Starling's law
FRC; *see* Functional residual capacity
Free fatty acids, 998, 999, 1284, 1285
Free monomer, allergy to, 30
Free thyroxine index, 1134-1135, 1141
Free thyroxine tests, 1134
Free triiodothyronine test, 1134
Freezing of blood, 347; *see also* Frozen red blood cells; Plasma, fresh-frozen
Fremitus, vocal, 684
Fresh-frozen plasma; *see* Plasma, fresh-frozen
Friction rubs
  hepatic changes and, 1059
  pericarditis and, 551
  pleuritis and, 730
Friedländer's pneumonia, 176
Friedreich's ataxia, 805-806
Frog, mumps and, 301
Frontal bossing, 877
Frontal lobe lesions, 757-758
Frontal sinuses, obliteration of, 1318
Frontonasal dysplasia malformation complex, 1317-1318
Frontonasal process, 1306
Frost, uremic, 896
Frozen plasma; *see* Plasma, fresh-frozen
Frozen red blood cells, 347, 1240
Frozen shoulder, 101
Fructokinase deficiency, 858
FSH; *see* Follicle-stimulating hormone
FSH muscular dystrophy; *see* Facioscapulohumeral muscular dystrophy
FT_3; *see* Free triiodothyronine test
FT_4; *see* Free thyroxine tests
FTI; *see* Free thyroxine index
5-FU; *see* 5-Fluorouracil
α-L-Fucosidase deficiency, 1235
Fucosidosis, 1235
Functional blindness, 759
Functional bowel disease, 951, 989, 1027-1029
Functional marrow inadequacy, 326; *see also* Bone marrow
Functional residual capacity, 679, 709, 712
Fundoplication, 982
Fungal diseases, 274-278, 451; *see also* specific fungus
  anemia and, 322
  arthritis and, 81
  aspergillosis in, 176-177, 446, 705
  blastomycosis in, 275
  brucellosis and, 243-245, 362
  candidiasis in; *see* Candida
  chromomycosis in, 277
  coccidioidomycosis in, 275; *see also* Coccidioidomycosis
  cryptococcosis in, 275-276; *see also* Cryptococcosis
  Cushing's syndrome and, 887
  dentistry and, 306-308
  diabetes and, 885
  endocarditis and, 179, 181, 182, 184
  esophagitis and, 985
  histoplasmosis in, 274-275, 278
  Hodgkin's disease and, 387, 424
  immunodeficiency diseases and, 31

Fungal diseases—cont'd
  leukemias and, 368, 421
  meningitis in, 189
  meningoencephalitis and, 139
  mucormycosis in, 277, 308, 446, 451, 727
  mycetoma in, 247, 277
  neoplasia and, 446, 901-902
  paracoccidioidomycosis in, 278
  pneumonitis and, 727
  of skin, 928-929
  sporotrichosis in, 81, 276
  treatment of, 278-279
Fungus ball, 277
Funnel chest, 737
FUO; *see* Fever of unknown origin
Furacin; *see* Nitrofurazone
Furadantin; *see* Nitrofurantoin
Furazolidone, 330
Furosemide, 597
  aminoglycosides and, 166
  aortic dissection and, 562
  ascites and, 1083
  gout and, 92
  heart failure and, 464, 465
  hypercalcemia and, 1180, 1191
  hypernatremia and, 596
  hypertension and, 472
  hypertonic saline and, 595
  kidney stones and, 647
  with mannitol, cisplatin and, 443
  mineralocorticoid excess and, 1161
  pancreatitis and, 1051
  pigment nephrotoxicity and, 629
  prerenal azotemia and, 633
  pseudotumor cerebri and, 848
  pyuria and, 590
  renal failure and, 639
  sickle cell disease and, 618
  side effects and interactions of, 574
  toxic nephropathy and, 624, 625, 626, 627, 628, 629
  transfusion reactions and, 351
Furoxone; *see* Furazolidone
Furrier's lung, 727
Furuncles, 218, 219, 306
Fusobacterium, 177, 249
  dentistry and, 303
  diabetes and, 1294
  endocarditis and, 302
  lung abscess and, 699
  in pneumonia, 177
  uremic stomatitis and, 667
Fusobacterium nucleatum, 249
Fusospirochetal infections, 302; *see also* specific genus
FVC; *see* Forced expiratory vital capacity

G

G cells; *see* Gastrin-producing cells
GABA; *see* Gamma-aminobutyric acid
Gaisböck's syndrome, 355
Gait, 759, 813
Galactorrhea, 1120, 1179
Galactose, 947
β-Galactosidase, 802
Gallbladder
  carcinoma of, 1089
  digestion and, 945-946
  inflammation of; *see* Cholecystitis
  pain and, 950, 988, 1087-1088
  porcelain, 1088
  removal of; *see* Cholecystectomy
  stones in; *see* Cholelithiasis
  study of, 967, 968, 970, 1088-1089

Gallbladder hydrops, 1088
Gallium scanning
  hepatic imaging and, 967
  Hodgkin's disease and, 389
  osteomyelitis and, 222
Gallstone ileus, 1088
Gallstones; *see* Cholelithiasis
Gamma globulins, 32; *see also* Immunoglobulins, G
  agammaglobulinemia and, 31, 33
  antibody against, 19
  contraindications to, 34
  dentistry and, 34
  hepatitis and, 1073
  hypogammaglobulinemia and, 31, 32
  leukemias and, 372
  liver disease and, 1078
  measles and, 145-146
  purpura and, 407
  replacement of, 33
  scleroderma and, 903
Gamma rays, 489, 749
Gamma-aminobutyric acid, 817, 1252
Gamma-beta-thalassemia, 335
Gamma-glutamyl transpeptidase, 1065, 1066, 1068
Gamma-hemolytic streptococci, 222; *see also* Streptococci
Ganglia, 101-102
  basal; *see* Basal ganglia
  myenteric, 1026
  neuralgia and, 791
  sphenopalatine, 791
  vascular disease of gut and, 1021
Ganglionic blockade, 1021
Ganglioside, 1230
Gangliosidoses, 1230-1231
Gangrene, gas, 252-253, 254
Gantrisin; *see* Sulfisoxazole
Gardner's syndrome, 1042, 1093, 1094, 1209
Gargoylelike appearance, 1302
Gas
  arterial; *see* Arterial blood gases
  clostridial cellulitis and, 253
  exchange area of, 672
  inhaled, lung disease and, 728-730
  intestinal, 1028; *see also* Distention
  in mediastinum, 735
Gas gangrene, 252-253, 254
Gaseousness, 960-961; *see also* Distention
Gasoline poisoning, 754-755
Gastrectomy
  gastric carcinoma and, 1036
  gastritis and, 996
  hypoglycemia after, 1277
  leiomyomas and, 1035
  malabsorption and, 1004
  malnutrition and, 1103
  steatorrhea and, 999
  stress erosions and, 996
  vagotomy with, 993
  Zollinger-Ellison syndrome and, 995
Gastric acid, 942, 943, 1035
  control of, 944
  ulcers and, 987
  Zollinger-Ellison syndrome and, 994-995
Gastric analysis, 1035
Gastric atrophy, 996-997
Gastric biopsy, 963
Gastric carcinoma; *see* Carcinomas of gastrointestinal tract
Gastric contents, 943-944
  analysis of, 1035
  emptying of, 944-945, 963-964

Gastric contents—cont'd
　hyperparathyroidism and, 1192
Gastric dilation, acute, 997; see also Distention
Gastric diverticula, 998
Gastric hypersecretion, hyperparathyroidism and, 1192
Gastric inhibitory polypeptide, 941
Gastric leiomyomas, 1034
Gastric lesions, diagnosis of, 962-964
Gastric motility studies, 963-964
Gastric polyps, 1033-1034
Gastric remnants, 997
Gastric secretion, 943-944; see also Gastric contents
Gastric suction; see Nasogastric suction
Gastric ulcer, 987, 989, 993; see also Ulcers
Gastric varices, 1060, 1083
Gastric volvulus, 998
Gastrin, 941, 943
　achalasia and, 976-977
　calcitonin and, 1189
　esophageal spasm and, 980
　gastric secretion and, 943, 944
　irritable bowel disease and, 1027
　pancreatic secretion and, 1049
　reflux disease and, 982
　ulcers and, 989
　Zollinger-Ellison syndrome and, 994-995
Gastrinoma, 954, 994-995, 1049, 1056
Gastrin-producing cells, 943, 994, 995
Gastritis, 996-997
　acid back-diffusion and, 943
　alcoholic, 1258
　carcinoma and, 1035
Gastroenteritis; see also Gastritis
　eosinophilic, 1003
　malabsorption and, 1003
　Salmonella, 202, 206-207
　viral, 149-151, 1003
Gastroesophageal reflux disease, 950, 962, 982-985, 988-989
Gastroesophageal scintigram, 962
Gastrointestinal polyposis syndromes; see Polyposis syndromes
Gastrointestinal series; see Barium
Gastrointestinal system; see Digestive system; Intestines; Stomach
Gastrojejunostomy, 993, 1015
Gastropathy, 997
Gastroscopy, 1034
Gated blood pool scanning, 521, 530
Gaucher's cells, 397
Gaucher's disease, 1231, 1232
　dentistry and, 425, 1296
　lung and, 721
　myelophthisic anemia and, 322
　neutropenia and, 358
　reticuloendothelial system and, 396-397
Gaviscon; see Aluminum hydroxide
Gaze, dysconjugate, 760
Gd, 329
Gd Mediterranean, 329
GdA+ and GdA−, 329
GdB+, 329
GDM; see Diabetes mellitus, gestational
Gegenhalten, 758
Gelatin sponge, 959
Gelfoam; see Gelatin sponge
Gene concept, 1216-1220; see also Genetics and metabolism
Gene map, 1228-1229
General anesthetics; see Anesthetics
Genetic code, 1216-1217
Genetic counseling, 1223-1224

Genetic counseling—cont'd
　otocraniofacial syndromes and, 1311-1312
　thalassemias and, 337
Genetics and metabolism, 1216-1293
　alcohol in, 1255-1259; see also Alcohol
　allergy and, 20; see also Allergy
　aminoacidopathies in, 1226-1227, 1236-1238
　blood pressure and, 468
　in carcinogenesis, 433
　chromosome structure and abnormalities in, 1220-1222; see also Chromosomes
　clinical genetics in, 1223-1229
　complex syndromes in, 1227-1228
　craniofacial malformations and, 1301-1302, 1309
　dentistry and, 1294-1299
　diabetes mellitus in, 1259-1276; see also Diabetes mellitus
　gene concept in, 1216-1220
　hypoglycemia in, 1276-1280; see also Hypoglycemia
　inflammatory bowel disease and, 1006
　inherited metabolic disorders in, 1230-1246
　iron excess and, 345
　lipoprotein disorders in, 1280-1293; see also Lipoprotein metabolism disorders
　liver disease and, 1066, 1081
　lupus erythematosus and, 54
　lysosomal storage disorders in, 396, 397, 1226, 1230-1235
　medullary cystic disease and, 653
　multifactorial inheritance in, 1222-1223
　polycystic kidney disease and, 470, 651-653
　porphyrias in, 1246-1255; see also Porphyrias
　renal transplantation and, 643-644
　single gene inheritance in, 1216-1220
　skin disorders and, 877, 878, 880, 882, 883, 884
　vitamin D metabolism and, 1200
Genitalia; see also Genitourinary tract
　Behçet's syndrome and, 110, 907
　Chlamydia and, 214, 216
　congenital adrenal hyperplasia and anomalies of, 1162
　herpetic lesions of, 128, 926
　male, 1168-1173
　　evaluation of, 13
　　Reiter's syndrome and, 907
　　syphilis and, 265, 266
　　tuberculosis in, 256
　mycoplasmas and, 218
　tuberculosis in, 256
　venereal ulcerative lesions of, 266
Genitourinary tract; see also Urinary tract
　bacteremia and, 239
　endocarditis and, 180, 181
　hyperthyroidism and, 1143
　prophylactic regimens and, 185
　tumor management and, 449; see also specific tumor
Gentamicin, 161, 166
　abdominal abscess and, 1047
　anaerobic infections and, 250
　bacteremia and, 241
　cholecystitis and, 1089
　donovanosis and, 238
　endocarditis and, 121, 183, 184, 185
　gram-negative oral lesions and, 306
　labyrinth dysfunction and, 792
　meningitis and, 190
　nephritis and, 619
　nephropathy and, 624, 626, 627, 628
　neutropenia and, 361
　oral ulcers and, 306, 421

Gentamicin—cont'd
　pancreatitis and, 1053
　pneumonia and, 176
　pregnancy and, 1212
Gentian violet, 276
Geographic tongue, 908, 937, 938
Germ cell tumors, 435
German measles; see Rubella
Germinal tumors of mediastinum, 735
Gerstmann's syndrome, 759
GFR; see Glomerular filtration, rate of
GH; see Growth hormone
Ghon complex, 258
Giant bullae, 701; see also Bullae
Giant cavernous hemangiomas, 341
Giant cell arteritides; see Arteritis, giant cell
Giant cell granulomata, 75, 254
Giant cell pneumonia, 146
Giant cell thyroiditis, 1149
Giant cells, multinucleated
　herpes simplex and, 128
　measles and, 146
　perinatal viruses and, 126
　varicella-zoster and, 129
Giant hairy nevus, 917
Giantism, 1119-1120
Giardia lamblia, 203, 283-284
　diarrhea and, 953
　drugs for, 170
　immunodeficiency diseases and, 31, 32
　malabsorption and, 1003
Giardiasis; see *Giardia lamblia*
Gibbus formation, 256
Giemsa stain, 130
Gigantism, 1204
Gilbert's disease, 1058, 1066, 1067
Gilles de la Tourette's syndrome, 821-822
Gingiva
　acute herpetic gingivostomatitis and, 298
　biopsy of, 423, 425
　bleeding from; see Bleeding, gingival
　diabetes mellitus and, 1294
　Ehlers-Danlos syndrome and, 1242
　Epstein-Barr virus and, 300
　evaluation of, 9
　hyperplasia of; see Gingival hyperplasia
　inflammation of; see Gingivitis; Gingivostomatitis
　kidney disease and ulcers of, 667
　lichen planus and, 938
　melanotic macule of, 919
　mucopolysaccharidoses and, 1235
　oral contraceptives and, 1214
　pemphigoid and, 935
　scleroderma and, 903
　tuberous sclerosis and, 869, 880
Gingival hyperplasia
　leukemia and, 898
　mucopolysaccharidoses and, 1235
　phenytoin and, 865-866, 880, 882
　pregnancy and, 1211
　tuberous sclerosis and, 869, 880
　Wegener's granulomatosis and, 113
Gingivitis
　acute necrotizing ulcerative, 302, 307, 862
　desquamative, 937, 1213
　neutrophil dysfunction and, 420
　oral contraceptives and, 1213
　pregnancy and, 1211, 1212
　puberty and, 1210, 1214
　tuberculous erythematous nodular, 304
　vitamin C and, 1110
　Wegener's granulomatosis and, 113, 906
Gingivostomatitis, 128, 926

Gingivostomatitis—cont'd
  herpes simplex and, 128, 298-299, 926
  niacin deficiency and, 1110
GIP; see Gastric inhibitory polypeptide
Glanzmann's thrombasthenia, 426
Glaucoma, diabetes and, 1274
Glibenclamide, 1266, 1267
Glioblastoma multiforme, 844
Gliomas, orbital, 878-879
Global amnesia, transient, 772, 836
Global cyanosis, 683
Globin synthesis defect, 325
Globoid cell leukodystrophy, 802, 1231, 1233
Globoside accumulation, 1231
α-Globulin, 612, 1065, 1082
γ-Globulin; see Gamma globulins
Globulins; see also Immune globulin; Immunoglobulins
  alpha, 612, 1065, 1082
  antilymphocyte, 644
  antithymocyte, 361
  gamma; see Gamma globulins
  hepatitis and, 1071, 1073
  hyperimmune human, 238
  liver disease and, 1065, 1078, 1082
  mumps and, 138
  pertussis and, 238
  sex steroid–binding, 1154
  thyroxine-binding, 1131
  transport, 1154
  in urine, 605
Globus hystericus, 974
Glomerular filtration, 590-591; see also Glomeruli
  rate of, 603
    chronic renal failure and, 636, 638
    obstructive uropathy and, 655
    pregnancy and, 663-664
Glomeruli, 590; see also Glomerular filtration
  capillary basement membrane of, 611
  disease of; see also Glomerulonephritis
    biopsy and, 608
    nephrotic syndrome from, 613-614
      primary, 608-614
      toxic nephropathy and, 626
  hyalinization of, 614
  of lips, 1092
Glomerulonephritis, 608-614; see also Nephritis
  with bacterial endocarditis, 611
  chronic, 614
  focal, 611
  hemolysis and, 341
  impetigo, 225
  interstitial nephritis and, 620
  membranoproliferative, 613-614
  mesangiocapillary, 613-614
  poststreptococcal, 609-610
  pregnancy and, 664
  proliferative, 614
  rapidly progressive, 610
  renal vein thrombosis and, 662
  streptococcal pharyngitis and, 225
  syphilis and, 266
  with ventriculoatrial shunt infection, 611
  Wegener's granulomatosis and, 70
Glomerulosclerosis, focal, 614
Glomerulus of lips, 1092
Glossitis
  acrodermatitis enteropathica and, 895
  erythema migrans and, 938
  iron deficiency and, 1105
  syphilitic, 303, 919
  vitamin deficiency and, 1298
    B_{12}, 1109

Glossitis—cont'd
  vitamin deficiency and—cont'd
    pyridoxine, 1109, 1298
    riboflavin, 1108
Glossitis migrans, 908, 937, 938
Glossodynia, 1294
Glossopharyngeal neuralgia, 791
Glucagon, 1262, 1263
  diabetic ketoacidosis and, 1269
  diverticulosis and, 1017
  fatty acids and, 1284
  formation of, 945, 1049
  glucagonoma and, 913
  and hypoglycemia, 1277, 1279, 1295
    from neoplasms, 1181
  pheochromocytoma and, 1167
  triiodothyronine and, 1132
  Zollinger-Ellison syndrome and, 994
Glucagonoma syndrome, 913
Glucocerebrosidase deficiency, 396, 721
Glucocerebroside β-glucosidase deficiency, 1232
Glucocorticoids, 1153, 1154
  deficiency syndromes of; see Addison's disease
  excess of, 1157-1159, 1262
  hypercalcemia and, 1192, 1195
  hypoglycemia from neoplasms and, 1181
  lipoproteins and, 1284, 1287, 1290
  mineralocorticoid excess and, 1162
  osteoporosis and, 1202
  pituitary deficiencies and, 1123
  porphyria and, 1252
  receptors for, 443
  synthesis of, 1153
  synthetic, 1156
  thyroxine-binding globulin and, 1134
Glucola, 1295
Gluconeogenesis, 1154, 1276
Glucosamine-6-sulfate sulfatase deficiency, 1233, 1234
Glucose; see also Hyperglycemia; Hypoglycemia
  alcohol and, 1256
    withdrawal from, 776
  body fluid osmolality and, 596
  body heat and, 755
  in cerebrospinal fluid, 135
  cholera and, 205
  coma and, 765
  dehydration and, 597
  diabetes mellitus and, 1268
  dialysis and, 641
  digestion and, 947
  hepatitis and, 1072
  hyperkalemia and, 599, 634
  hypernatremia and, 595, 596
  hypertonic; see Hypertonic glucose
  hypoglycemia and, 1268, 1276-1279
  hypokalemia and, 597
  hyponatremia and, 594
  intolerance for, 1260, 1261, 1264, 1278
  in oliguria, 633
  porphyria and, 1252
  syncope and, 781
  thyrotoxicosis and, 1205
  in urine, tests for, 604
  viral gastroenteritis and, 150
Glucose oxidase-impregnated dipstick, 604
Glucose tolerance, 1260
  insulin resistance and, 1261
  tests for, 1264, 1277, 1278
Glucose-6-phosphate dehydrogenase deficiency, 329-331, 357
  dentistry and, 418
Glucosyl ceramidosis, 1231, 1232
β-Glucuronidase deficiency, 1233, 1234

Glucuronyl transferase, 1067
Glue sniffing, 853
Glutamic-oxaloacetic transaminase, 535, 853, 1065; see also Serum, transaminases in
γ-Glutamyl transpeptidase, 1065, 1066, 1068
Glutathione, 329
Gluten enteropathy, 1001, 1103, 1109
Gluten-free diet, 1001
Glutethimide
  osteomalacia and, 1198
  porphyria and, 1252
  pupillary reflexes and, 765
  toxicity of, 777
Gluteus spasm, 98
Glutose; see Glucose
Glyburide; see Glibenclamide
Glycerine, 876
Glycerol, 347
Glycogen absorption, 1004
Glycogen storage disease, 522, 858
Glycogenolysis, 1276
Glycogenosis, 858
Glycols, 625, 627, 629, 631
Glycoproteins, 405
Glycosaminoglycans
  accumulation of, 1233
  relapsing polychondritis and, 102
  urates and, 90
Glycosphingolipidoses, 1230-1235
Glycosphingolipids, 1231, 1232
Glycyrrhizic acid, 1160
GM_1 gangliosidoses, 1230, 1231
GM_2 gangliosidoses, 1230-1231; see also Tay-Sachs disease
GMP; see Guanidine monophosphate
Gnosis, 771
GnRH; see Gonadotropin-releasing hormone
Goblet cells, intestinal, 945, 1007
Goiter
  diffuse
    lymphocytic thyroiditis and, 1150
    nontoxic, 1148-1149
    toxic, 1143-1145
  iodine deficiency and, 1105
  mediastinal, 735
  multinodular, 1145
  nontoxic, 1148-1149
    diffuse, 1148-1149
    multinodular, 1145
    uninodular, 1145
  toxic, 1143-1145
  uninodular, 1145
Goitrogens, 1132, 1148
Gold; see also Gold salts
  ankylosing spondylitis and, 50
  nephrotic syndrome and, 612, 613
  psoriatic arthritis and, 51
  radioactive, 727, 966
  rheumatoid arthritis and, 42, 46, 47
  toxicity to, 42, 624, 625, 626, 627
Gold salts; see also Gold
  neutropenia and, 360
  rheumatoid arthritis and, 106
  thrombocytopenia and, 401
Goldenhar's syndrome, 1300, 1310-1312
Gonadal hormones, porphyria and, 1252; see also Sex hormones; specific hormone
Gonadotropic hormones; see Gonadotropins
Gonadotropin-releasing hormone, 1118, 1169, 1174, 1175
Gonadotropins, 1118
  deficiency of, 1121-1122, 1172
  ectopic, neoplasms and, 1181

Gonadotropins—cont'd
  feedback mechanism and, 1175
  follicular development and, 1173
  human chorionic; see Human chorionic gonadotropin
  human menopausal, 1045, 1173
  male hypogonadism and, 1122
  menopause and, 1176, 1177
  menstrual cycle and, 1174-1175
  renal cell carcinoma and, 657
Gonads, 1062, 1259; see also Ovary; Testes
Gonococci, 230-233
  arthritis and, 108, 231, 232
  blood borne lesions and, 232
  Chlamydiae and, 214, 215
  drugs and, 162, 170
  endocarditis and, 184
  liver disease and, 1074
  oral lesions of, 302
  Reiter's syndrome and, 53
  stomatitis and, 302
  syphilis and, 265
Gonorrhea; see Gonococci
Goodpasture's syndrome, 611, 720
Gottron's papules, 905
Gout, 89-94
  psoriatic arthritis and, 51
  renal failure and, 622
  of temporomandibular joint, 108-109
Gower's sign, 852
G-6-PD deficiency; see Glucose-6-phosphate dehydrogenase deficiency
Graafian follicle, 1174
Graft nonfunction, 558, 645; see also Bypass procedures; Heterograft, porcine
Graft-versus-host disease, 19, 34, 58
Gram stains, 119
  meningitis and, 188, 189
  pneumococcal pneumonia and, 173
  pyogenic arthritis and, 80
  urethritis and, 215
  viruses and, 144
Gram-negative bacilli, 235-245
  abdominal abscess and, 1047
  arthritis and, 79, 80
  bacteremia and, 239-241
  brucellosis in, 243-245, 362
  chancroid in, 238-239
  chemotherapy and, 451
  disseminated intravascular coagulation and, 412
  donovanosis in, 238
  granuloma inguinale and, 238
  Haemophilus influenzae in, 235-237; see also *Haemophilus influenzae*
  immunodeficiency diseases and, 31
  leukemias and, 368, 421
  oral lesions of, 306
  osteomyelitis and, 82
  pertussis in, 143, 208, 237-238
  plague in, 242
  pneumonia and, 176-177
  Pseudomonas pseudomallei in, 171
  red cell injury and, 343
  tularemia in, 242-243
Gram-negative bacteria; see also Gram-negative bacilli; Gram-negative cocci
  granulomatous disease and, 239, 357
  liver disease and, 2074
  neoplasia and, 446
Gram-negative cocci, 108, 230-235
Gram-positive bacilli, 245-249
  actinomycosis in, 247; see also *Actinomyces*
  anthrax in, 245

Gram-positive bacilli—cont'd
  diphtheria in, 247-249
  erysipeloid in, 246, 247
  listeriosis in, 246; see also Listeriosis
  nocardiosis in, 171, 247, 645
Gram-positive cocci, 218-222
  abdominal abscess and, 1047
  dentistry and, 303
  red cell injury and, 343
  rheumatic fever and, 225, 228-230; see also Rheumatic fever
  staphylococcal infections and, 218-222
  streptococcal infections and, 222-230
Grand mal seizures, 781, 783; see also Seizures
Granular cell tumors of kidney, 657
Granulocytes
  precursor cells of, 356
  production of, 320, 355
  splenomegaly and, 396
  transfusions of
    aplastic anemia and, 320
    leukemias and, 368
    neutrophil dysfunction and, 420
Granulocytic leukemias; see Leukemias, myelogenous
Granulocytic precursor cells, 356
Granulocytopoiesis, ineffective, 320
Granuloma annulare, 885
Granuloma inguinale, 238, 239
Granulomas; see also Granulomatosis; Granulomatous diseases
  anisakiasis and, 291
  arteritis and, 841-842
  brucellosis and, 244
  Crohn's disease and, 1011
  diabetes insipidus and, 1126
  diabetes mellitus and, 885
  eosinophilic; see Eosinophilic granuloma
  giant cell, sarcoidosis and, 75
  leprosy and, 261
  of liver, 1084
  macrophages and, 66
  mediastinitis and, 735
  midline, 70, 73-74, 113
  nontuberculous mycobacteria and, 261
  peritonitis and, 1047, 1048
  pneumonitis and, 727
  pregnancy, 1211
  sarcoidosis and, 75, 716-717, 1126
  schistosomiasis and, 296
  swimming pool, 261
  thyroiditis and, 1149
  tuberculosis and, 254, 304, 1047, 1048
  veneral, 238-239, 265-266, 268
Granulomatosis; see also Granulomas; Granulomatous diseases
  lymphomatoid
    cellular infiltrates and, 67-69
    cutaneous lesions of, 906
    management of, 69
    vasculitis and, 66, 67
  Wegener's; see Wegener's granulomatosis
Granulomatous diseases, 35-117; see also Granulomas; Granulomatosis
  ankylosing spondylitis and, 48-50; see also Ankylosing spondylitis
  avascular necrosis in, 104
  Behçet's syndrome and, 110-111
  chondrometaplasia of temporomandibular joint and, 108
  dentistry and, 117; see also specific disease
  dermatomyositis and, 64-65; see also Dermatomyositis
    dentistry and, 112-113

Granulomatous diseases—cont'd
  fibrosing syndromes in, 105
  and fibrous dysplasia, 104, 115-116
  and gout, 51, 89-94, 108, 622
  hemarthrosis in, 104-105, 409-410
  hypertrophic osteoarthropathy in, 103-104
  infectious arthritis in, 79-82; see also Arthritis, infectious
  intermittent rheumatic diseases in, 53
  lupus erythematosus and, 53-58
    dentistry and, 111-112
  microbicidal activity and, 357
  midline granuloma in, 70, 73-74
    dentistry and, 113
  myofascial pain dysfunction syndrome of temporomandibular joint and, 109-110
  nonarticular rheumatism in, 96-102
  and osteoarthritis, 83-86, 107, 860
  and osteomyelitis, 82-83, 116-117; see also Osteomyelitis
  and osteoporosis, 88-89; see also Osteoporosis
    dentistry and, 115
  and Paget's disease, 86-88, 114-115
  polymyalgia rheumatica in, 69, 74-75, 858
  polymyositis and, 64-65; see also Polymyositis
    dentistry and, 112-113
  pseudogout in, 89, 94-95
  and psoriatic arthritis, 50-52, 106
  Raynaud's phenomenon and, 62-64; see also Raynaud's phenomenon
  and Reiter's syndrome, 52-53, 110; see also Reiter's syndrome
  relapsing polychondritis in, 102-103
  rheumatoid arthritis in, 35-43; see also Rheumatoid arthritis
    dentistry and, 105-106
    juvenile, 43-47
  sarcoidosis in, 75-78, 113-114
  Schönlein-Henoch purpura and, 70
  septic arthritis of temporomandibular joint and, 108
  synovial chondromatosis of temporomandibular joint and, 108
  systemic sclerosis and, 58-62, 112
  temporal arteritis in, 74-75
  terminology and, 35
  vasculitis, 45, 66-70, 1022
  Weber-Christian disease in, 78-79
  Wegener's granulomatosis and, 70-73, 113; see also Wegener's granulomatosis
Grape cells, 380
Grasping reflex, 758
Graves' disease, 1141-1142, 1143-1145
  children and, 1147
  infiltrative ophthalmopathy of, 1142, 1143, 1147-1148
  pregnancy and, 1147
Gray baby syndrome, 158, 169
Great arteries, transposition of, 508
Grenz-ray therapy
  Hailey-Hailey disease and, 935
  psoriasis and, 937
Griseofulvin, 279, 888, 928, 929, 1252
Grönblad-Strandberg syndrome, 884; see also Pseudoxanthoma elasticum
Growth fraction of tumor, 439
Growth hormone, 1118, 1122-1123
Growth plates of bone, 1182
Growth retardation, intrauterine, 125
GSH; see Glutathione
GTP; see Guanidine triphosphate
Guaiac test, 959
Guanethidine
  alcohol and, 1297

Guanethidine—cont'd
  hypertension and, 472, 473, 474
  pheochromocytoma and, 1165
  in Raynaud's phenomenon, 61, 64
  renal insufficiency and, 475, 639
  side effects and interactions of, 574
Guanidine
  asthma and, 704, 705
  botulism and, 204
  neuromuscular junction disorders and, 856
Guanidine monophosphate, 704, 705
Guanidine triphosphate, 705
Guanyl cyclase, 705
Guarding, abdominal, 950
Guillain-Barré syndrome, 854-855
  cytomegalovirus and, 131
  infectious mononucleosis and, 133
  mumps and, 137
  mycoplasmal pneumonia and, 217
  respiratory failure and, 712
  swine influenza vaccine and, 153
  varicella and, 138
Guinea pig kidney, heterophil antibody response and, 132
Gumma, 265-266, 268, 303
Gums; see Gingiva
Gunther's disease, 888; see also Porphyrias, congenital erythropoietic
Guttate psoriasis, 936
Guttering, candle, 810
Gynecomastia, 1179

H

Haemophilus ducreyi, 238
Haemophilus influenzae, 235-237
  arthritis and, 79
  bronchiectasis and, 696
  bronchitis and, 691
  disseminated intravascular coagulation and, 412
  drugs for, 159, 162, 163, 165, 169
  in endocarditis, 179
  immunodeficiency diseases and, 31, 32, 33
  influenza and, 141
  leukemias and, 371
  lung abscess and, 698
  meningitis and, 186, 188, 190
  multiple myeloma and, 379
  pneumonia and, 171, 172, 173, 175-176
  respiratory failure and, 711
  splenectomy and, 329, 395
  vaccine for, 236
Hageman factor
  deficiency of, 411
  septic shock and, 240
Hailey-Hailey disease, 934-935
Hairy nevus, giant, 917
Half-life, 158, 328
Hallervorden-Spatz disease, 775
Hallopeau-type pemphigus vegetans, 933
Hallucinations, hypnagogic, 769
Hallucinosis, alcoholic, 776
Halogenated hydrocarbons, 1253
Halogens, sensitivity to, 893
Haloperidol
  Huntington's chorea and, 774, 817
  parkinsonism and, 815
  phencyclidine intoxication and, 779
  side effects of, 871
  Sydenham's chorea and, 819
  torsion dystonias and, 820, 821
Haloprogin, 279
Halothane
  arrhythmias and, 585

Halothane—cont'd
  liver toxicity and, 1076, 1078
  malignant hyperpyrexia and, 858
  mastocystosis and, 910
  muscle biopsy and, 875
Hamartoma
  angiofibromatous, 880
  gastrointestinal polyposis syndromes and, 1042
  of large bowel, 1038
  of lung, 743
  renal, 656
Hamman-Rich syndrome, 715
Hand-foot-and-mouth disease, 148, 300
Hand-foot syndrome, 332
Hands; see also Digits; Fingers
  carpal tunnel syndrome and, 98
  clawhand and, 877, 903, 1091
  multiple sclerosis and, 798
  osteoarthritis and, 83, 84
  rheumatic disorders of, 101-102
Hand-Schüller-Christian disease, 397, 425, 718
Hangover, 776
Haptoglobin, 45, 657
Hardy-Weinberg law, 1218
Hashimoto's thyroiditis, 1149-1150
Haverhill fever, 272
Hawley appliance, 109
Hb; see Hemoglobins
HB$_s$Ag; see Hepatitis B surface antigen
HBDH; see Hydroxybutyric dehydrogenase
HBIG; see Hepatitis B immune globulin
HCG; see Human chorionic gonadotropin
HCP; see Coproporphyria
HDL; see High-density lipoproteins
HDN; see Hemolytic disease of newborn
HE; see Elliptocytosis, hereditary
Head
  craniofacial malformations of, 1300-1322; see also Craniofacial malformations
  enlargement of, 803; see also Hydrocephalus
  evaluation of, 8, 11
  Gardner's syndrome and cysts of, 1093
  intention tremors of, 870
  myofascial syndromes and, 97
  and neck
    cancer of, 449, 751
    non-Hodgkin's lymphoma and, 393
    rheumatic disorders of, 100
  shapes of, 1313
  trauma to
    coma and, 765
    epilepsy and, 784
    labyrinth and, 793
Headache, 788-790
  brain abscess and, 192
  brain tumors and, 845-846
  lower half, 791
  mastocystosis and, 910·
  tension, 100
  vomiting, and papilledema, triad of, 846
Hearing loss, 794-795; see also Deafness
  aminoglycosides and, 166
  central, 795
  congenital cytomegalovirus and, 125-126
  tests for, 9
Heart; see also Cardiovascular diseases
  alcohol and, 1257
  arrhythmias of; see Arrhythmias
  catheterization of; see Cardiac catheterization
  conduction of, 541-542
  disease of
    cardiomyopathies and; see Cardiomyopathies

Heart—cont'd
  disease of—cont'd
    congenital; see Congenital heart disease
    coronary; see Coronary heart disease
    endocarditis and, 179; see also Endocarditis
    portal hypertension and, 1045
    sickle cell anemia and, 332
    valvular, 340, 510-517
    vascular disease of gut and, 1021
  emboli and, 568; see also Myocardial infarction
  emphysema and, 694
  evaluation of, 12; see also Cardiology; Heart sounds; Pulse
  failure of; see Heart failure
  hypercalcemia and, 1190
  hypertrophy of, 517, 518; see also Cardiomyopathies
  Lyme disease and, 297
  murmurs and; see Murmurs, cardiac
  myocardial diseases and; see Cardiomyopathies; Myocardial infarction
  output of; see Cardiac output
  pulmonary edema and, 708, 710
  rate of; see Pulse
  rheumatic fever and, 229, 230
  rhythm of, 541-542; see also Arrhythmias
  shunts and; see Anastomoses; Cardiac shunts
  study of; see Cardiology
  surgery of, 301, 551, 558-559
  systemic sclerosis and, 60
  tamponade and; see Cardiac tamponade
Heart block, 500, 546-548
Heart failure
  biventricular, 692
  bronchitis and, 692
  congestive, 452-465
    cardiac catheterization and, 502
    congenital, 508-509
    course of, 463
    definition of, 452
    dentistry and, 571-572
    diagnosis of, 463
    endocarditis and, 181, 185
    epidemiology of, 454
    etiology of, 452-454
    high-output, 454
    hypertension and, 470
    laboratory findings and, 462-463
    liver disease and, 1077
    management of, 463-465
    normal cardiovascular function in, 454-459
    pathophysiology of, 459-463
    portal hypertension and, 1045
    prognosis in, 463
    signs and symptoms of, 460-462
    thiamine and, 1108
  endocarditis and, 181, 185
  hypertrophic cardiomyopathy and, 517
  portal hypertension and, 1045
  pulmonary edema and, 710
  pulmonary embolism and, 491
  rheumatic fever and, 230
  shock and, 476-477, 478
Heart medication, dental management and, 571-572
Heart murmurs; see Murmurs, cardiac
Heart rate; see Pulse
Heart sounds, 7
  angina pectoris and, 529
  aortic regurgitation and, 516
  aortic stenosis and, 514
  cardiomyopathy and, 521
  mitral regurgitation and, 510

Heart sounds—cont'd
   mitral stenosis and, 512-513
   myocardial infarction and, 534
   pulmonary hypertension and, 696
Heart surgery, open, 301, 551, 558-559
Heart valves
   disease of, 340, 510-517; see also Valvular heart disease
   prosthetic; see Prosthetic valves
Heartburn, 950, 974-975
   reflux disease and, 982
   ulcer pain and, 988-989
Heat
   body; see Body temperature
   otalgia and, 867
Heat cramps, 755
Heat exhaustion, 755
Heat pyrexia, 755
Heat stroke, 755
Heat syncope, 755
Heater probe, 963
Heat-labile nicotinamide-adenine dinucleotide, 235
Heat-stable hematin, 235
Heavy chains, 16, 377, 384
Heavy metals
   interstitial nephritis and, 619, 620
   Raynaud's phenomenon and, 63
   renal cell carcinomas and, 656
   toxicity of, 200, 752-754
      hemolysis and, 342
      metabolic encephalopathies and, 768
      nephropathy and, 624, 626, 627-628, 630, 631
      neuropathy and, 853
      testes and, 1172
Heba agent, 171
Heberden's nodes, 83, 84
Hecht's pneumonia, 146
Heel, 52, 102
Heerfordt's disease, 77, 717
   sarcoidosis and, 113, 910, 911
Heimlich maneuver, 713
Heliotrope rash, 64, 904
Helium dilution method, 679
Heller's myotomy, 979
Helminthic diseases, 289-297; see also Parasites
   cestodes in, 292-294, 317
   eosinophilia and, 119, 289, 372
   nematodes in, 289-292
   trematodes in, 294-297
Helper factor, 15-16
Helper T cells, 15
Hemadsorption, 124
Hemagglutinin tests, 118, 119, 124, 273-274; see also Microhemagglutination test
   influenza and, 140
   measles and, 146
   parainfluenza viruses and, 142, 143
   rubella and, 146
Hemangioblastomas, 809, 1165
Hemangiomas
   giant cavernous, 341
   of liver, 1084
   of pancreas, 1056
   retinal, 809
   of small bowel, 1037
Hemangiomatosis, orofacial, 872
Hemangiopericytomas, renal, 656
Hemarthroses
   hemophilia and, 409-410, 427
   rheumatic diseases and, 104-105
Hematemesis, 957, 975
   gastritis and, 996

Hematemesis—cont'd
   Mallory-Weiss syndrome and, 987
   ulcers and, 988
Hematin, 235, 1252
Hematochezia, 957
Hematocrit, 311, 352, 353, 354
Hematologic disorders, 310-430
   anemias in; see Anemias
   blood banking and, 346-351
   blood valves and, 311, 313
   dentistry and, 414-430
      amyloidosis and, 423-424
      anemias and, 414-420
      anticoagulant therapy and, 429-430
      deficiency states and, 414-420
      disseminated intravascular coagulopathy and, 429
      factor deficiencies and, 428-429
      Gaucher's disease and, 425
      hemophilia and, 427-428
      histiocytosis X and, 425
      leukemia and, 420-422
      lymphoma and, 424
      macroglobulinemia and, 423
      multiple myeloma and, 422-423
      neutrophil dysfunction syndromes and, 420
      platelet disorders and, 425-426
      von Willebrand's disease and, 426-427
   drug allergy and, 29
   hemochromatosis in, 345-346; see also Hemochromatosis
   hemoglobin pigment, 343-344; see also Hemoglobins
   hemostatic disorders in, 399-414; see also Hemostatic disorders
   liver disease and, 1063-1064
   oral candidiasis and, 307
   polycythemia and, 352-355; see also Polycythemia
   primary, 310
   radiation and, 749-750
   secondary, 310
   skin diseases and, 897-902
   transfusion therapy and, 346-351
   tumors and, 437-438
      fusospirochetal infections and, 302
      laboratory investigation of, 310
      myelophthisic anemia and, 322
   white blood cell in, 355-399; see also White blood cell, disorders of
Hematologic values, 311, 313
Hematomas
   of aorta, dissecting, 560
   hemophilia and, 410, 427
   subdural, 192, 844
   vitamin C and, 1110
Hematomyelia, 840
Hematopoiesis; see also Erythropoiesis
   anemias and
      aplastic, 319
      megaloblastic, 316
      sickle cell, 332
   extramedullary, 396
   neutrophils and, 355-356
   radiation and, 749-750
Hematopoietic crisis, 332
Hematoxylin bodies, 54
Hematuria, 908-909; see also Hemoglobinuria
   bladder neoplasms and, 659
   glomerulonephritis and, 611, 612, 614
   nephrolithiasis and, 646
   polycystic kidney disease and, 652
   renal cell carcinoma and, 657
   renal vein thrombosis and, 663

Hematuria—cont'd
   sickle cell disease and, 618
   toxic nephropathy and, 625, 626
   urothelial tumors and, 659
Heme biosynthesis, 1247-1248
   disturbances of, 321, 1246-1255
Hemianopia, bitemporal, 1119, 1123
Hemiballism, 818
Hemichorea, 818
Hemicrania, 789
Hemidiaphragm, 736
Hemifacial atrophy, 903
Hemifacial microsomia, 1300, 1309, 1310-1312
Hemiplegia, dental implications of, 872; see also Cerebral vascular accident
Hemispheres, cerebral; see Cerebral hemispheres
Hemizygous male, 1218, 1219
Hemoccult test, 960
Hemochromatosis, 345-346, 890, 1240
   cardiomyopathies and, 523
   cirrhosis and, 1081
Hemodialysis; see Dialysis
Hemodynamics; see also Circulation
   arrhythmia and, 584
   of congenital heart disease, 498-499, 501
   hypertension and, 470
   myocardial infarction and, 537-538
   positive end-expiratory pressure and, 709
Hemoglobinemia, 327
Hemoglobinopathies, 331-334, 1227; see also Hemoglobins; Sickle cell disease
Hemoglobins, 311
   A, 331, 337
   A_2, 331
   anemias and; see also Anemias
      iron deficiency, 325
      posthemorrhagic, 323
      sickle cell, 331-332, 334; see also Sickle cell disease
   Barts, 336
   Chesapeake, 354
   destruction of, 327; see also Hemolysis
   disorders of, 331-344, 1227
   electrophoresis of, 315, 333
   fetal, 331, 498
      beta-thalassemias and, 336
      hereditary persistence of, 337
   free, in blood plasma, 327
   genetic code errors and, 1217
   H, 336
   hemoglobinopathies and, 331-332, 1227; see also Sickle cell disease
   Lepore, 335
   M, 344
   oxygen transport and, 707
   polycythemia and, 352, 353, 354
   S, 331-332, 334, 1220; see also Sickle cell disease
   synthesis of, 888
   toxic nephropathy and, 627, 631
   unstable, 1227
   Waldenström's macroglobulinemia and, 382
Hemoglobinuria, 327
   march, 341
   paroxysmal 319, 340, 341-342, 358
Hemolysins, 218
Hemolysis, 326-343; see also Hemolytic anemia
   acquired abnormalities and, 337-343
      chemicals in, 342
      drugs in, 29, 329-330, 342
      infections in, 218, 222, 343
      metabolic causes in, 343
      poisons in, 342
      pregnancy and, 340

Hemolysis—cont'd
  acquired abnormalities and—cont'd
    toxins in, 342; see also Toxins
    transfusions and, 351
  congenital disorders of, 328-337; see also Hemolytic anemia, congenital
  immune, 29, 329-330, 332-335, 342
  intravascular, 327; see also Disseminated intravascular coagulation
  march hemoglobinuria and, 341
  streptococci and, 222-223; see also Streptococci
  uremia and, 340, 404, 617
Hemolytic anemia, 326-343; see also Hemolysis
  autoimmune, 338-340, 406; see also Autoimmune disease
  babesiosis and, 288
  cardiovascular anomalies and, 340
  causes of, 327-328
  congenital, 328-337
    enzyme defects in, 329-331
    hemoglobin disorders in, 331-340
    membrane defects in, 328-329
  from drugs, 29, 329-330, 342
  glucose-6-phosphate dehydrogenase deficiency and, 330
  immunogenic, 337-340, 342
  microangiopathic, 340-341
  of newborn, 337-338, 418
  paroxysmal nocturnal hemoglobinuria and, 319, 341-342, 358
  perinatal viruses and, 126
  porphyria and, 1249
  thrombocytosis and, 405
  traumatic, 340-341
Hemolytic crisis, 332
Hemolytic disease of newborn, 337-338, 418
Hemolytic jaundice, congenital, 328-329
Hemolytic syndrome, postpartum, 341
Hemolytic transfusion reaction, 351
Hemolytic uremic syndrome, 340, 404, 617
Hemopericardium, 553, 554
Hemophilia
  A, 409-410, 579
  B, 410, 1227
  dentistry and, 428-429
  dentistry and, 427-428
  hemarthrosis and, 104
Hemoptysis
  bronchiectasis and, 697
  Gaucher's disease and, 1232
  hemorrhagic lung disease and, 720
  lung cysts and, 701
  pulmonary perfusion and, 674
  tuberculosis and, 255
Hemorrhage; see Bleeding
Hemorrhagic cystitis, 143
Hemorrhagic diathesis, 383, 1232, 1298
Hemorrhagic disease of newborn, 411
Hemorrhagic infarction of brain, 830, 838-839
Hemorrhagic lung disease, diffuse, 611, 720-721
Hemorrhagic rhinitis, 269
Hemorrhagic sarcoma, Kaposi's, 920-922
Hemorrhagic telangiectasia, hereditary; see Osler-Weber-Rendu disease
Hemorrhoidal plexus, 948
Hemorrhoids, 948, 1030-1031, 1060; see also Varices
Hemosiderin, 720
Hemosiderosis, pulmonary, 720-721
Hemostasis, 399
Hemostatic agents, 426
Hemostatic disorders, 399-414
  coagulation mechanism in, 408-414

Hemostatic disorders—cont'd
  hemostasis and, 399
  history and, 399
  laboratory investigation of, 310
  platelet disorders in, 400-408; see also Platelets, disorders of
  uremia and, 667
  vascular disorders in, 400-408
Henderson-Hasselbalch equation, 708
Henle's loop, 590, 591
Henoch-Schönlein purpura; see Schönlein-Henoch purpura
Hensen's node, duplication of, 1303
Heparan-N-sulfatase deficiency, 1233, 1234
Heparan sulfate, 1233
Heparin
  adult respiratory distress syndrome and, 709
  cerebral infarction and, 832
  coagulation disorders and, 413-414
  dentistry and, 429, 430, 577, 578
  dialysate and, 640, 641
  disseminated intravascular coagulation and, 413, 446
  hypertriglyceridemia and, 1287
  leukemias and, 368
  lung abscess and, 700
  mastocytosis and, 909
  meningitis and, 190
  meningococcemia and, 234
  myocardial infarction and, 537
  paroxysmal nocturnal hemoglobinuria and, 342
  phlebitis and, 495
  pregnancy and, 1212
  pulmonary emboli and, 490, 492, 494, 536
  thrombocytopenia and, 401
  thrombocytosis and, 405
  transient ischemic attack and, 837
Hepatic abscesses; see Liver, abscesses of
Hepatic angle, obliteration of, 1044
Hepatic bile, supersaturated, 1087
Hepatic coma and precoma, 1061, 1084
Hepatic diseases; see Liver
Hepatic encephalopathy, 1061, 1084
Hepatic flexure, 947
Hepatic porphyrias, 888, 1253
Hepatic pulsation, 1059
Hepatic schistosomiasis, 296
Hepatic vein obstruction, 1045, 1060, 1077-1078
Hepatitis
  A; see Hepatitis A
  acute
    jaundice and, 1066-1067
    relapsing, 1072
    viral, 1068-1073
  alcoholic, 1257
  anicteric, 1070
  B; see Hepatitis B
  blood transfusions and, 347
  carriers of, 1091, 1099-1100
  chronic, 1073, 1078-1079
  dental precautions for, 1099
  dialysis and, 641
  drug abuse and, 863
  glucose-6-phosphate dehydrogenase deficiency and, 330
  icteric, 1070
  individuals at risk for, 1100
  isoniazid toxicity and, 259
  non-A, non-B, 1068-1073
    chronic active, 1078-1079
    cirrhosis and, 1079
    dentistry and, 1098-1101
  syphilis and, 268
  toxic, 1066, 1075-1076

Hepatitis A, 203, 1068-1073; see also Hepatitis
  dentistry and, 1098-1101
  gastroenteritis and, 149
Hepatitis B, 1066, 1068-1073; see also Hepatitis
  arthritis and, 81
  chronic active, 1078-1079
  cirrhosis and, 1079
  dentistry and, 1098-1101
  drug abuse and, 863
  immunodeficiency diseases and, 31
  neonatal, 126
  renal transplants and, 669
Hepatitis B carriers, 1066, 1069, 1073
Hepatitis B immune globulin, 1073, 1100
Hepatitis B surface antigen, 1091, 1098, 1099
Hepatitis B vaccine, 1100-1101
Hepatitis-associated antigen, 347, 1068, 1071
Hepatobiliary tree, 967-969, 1103; see also Liver, diagnosis and
Hepatocellular carcinoma, 1084
Hepatojugular reflux, 461, 463
Hepatolenticular degeneration, 822-823; see also Wilson's disease
Hepatomas, 1084
  alpha-fetoprotein and, 435
  hemochromatosis and, 1081
  polycythemia and, 354
Hepatomegaly, 1059
  congenital cytomegalovirus and, 125
  heart failure and, 461
  infectious mononucleosis in, 132
  sickle cell anemia and, 333
Hepatorenal syndrome, 1064
Hepatotoxic reactions, 1075-1076
Herbicides, 853
Hereditary coproporphyria, 889
Hereditary hemorrhagic telangiectasia; see Osler-Weber-Rendu disease
Hernias, 1241
  cerebral, 767, 846
  hiatus, 736, 982-985
  mesenteric, 1049
  pain and, 951, 989
Heroin
  abuse of, 778, 862, 863
  lung disease and, 722
  toxic nephropathy and, 625, 627, 629
Herpangina, 144, 148, 301
Herpes labialis
  erythema multiforme and, 30
  niacin deficiency and, 1110
  recurrent, 299
Herpes simplex, 128, 134, 926; see also Herpesviruses
  autopsy of brain tissue and, 135
  cancer chemotherapy and, 451
  central nervous system disease and, 135-136
  Chlamydia trachomatis and, 215
  corneal ulcers and, 154
  dentistry and, 298-299
  encephalitis and, 128, 135, 825-826
    empiric therapy versus brain biopsy in, 136
    neonatal, 126, 135
    vidarabine and, 154
  erythema multiforme and, 30
  esophagitis and, 985
  hepatitis and, 1074
  humoral antibodies and, 128
  immunodeficiency diseases and, 31
  interferon and, 154
  neonatal, 126, 127, 154
  neoplasia and, 433
  pericarditis and, 586
  recurrent, 299

Herpes simplex—cont'd
 T-lymphocyte disorders and, 34
 vaccine for, 129
Herpes zoster, 129-130, 134, 826, 927; see also
    Herpesviruses; Varicella
 cancer chemotherapy and, 451
 central nervous system disease and, 135, 138
 dentistry and, 299-300
 disseminated, 927
 Hodgkin's disease and, 387, 424
 immunodeficiency diseases and, 31
 interferon and, 154
 lymphocytic leukemia and, 899
 multiple myeloma and, 379
 neuropathy and, 855
 vaccine for, 130
 vidarabine and, 154
Herpesviruses, 127-134; see also Herpes simplex;
    Herpes zoster
 chancroid and, 239
 clinical manifestations of, 123
 disseminated intravascular coagulation and, 412
 gingivostomatitis and, 298-299
 immunodeficiency diseases and, 31
 lipid envelope of, 127
 odynophagia and, 975
 renal transplantation and, 645
 sialadenitis and, 299
 vidarabine and, 154
Herpetic whitlow, 926
Hetacillin, 163
Heterograft, porcine, 511, 514, 515
Heterophil antibodies, 132
Heterozygotes, 1218, 1219
 hemoglobinopathies and, 331
  sickle cell trait in, 334
  thalassemias in, 335, 336, 337
Hexachlorobenzene, 888, 1253, 1254
Hexachlorophene, 828
Hexamethonium, 722
n-Hexane, 853
Hexokinase deficiency anemia, 418
Hexosaminidase A deficiency, 1224, 1230
Hexosaminidase B deficiency, 1230-1231
Hexose-monophosphate shunt deficiencies, 329-331
HGH; see Growth hormone
HGPRT deficiency; see Hypoxanthine-guanine
   phosphoribosyltransferase deficiency
5-HIAA; see 5-Hydroxyindoleacetic acid
Hiatus hernia, 736, 982-985
Hiatus leukemicus, 365
Hibitane; see Chlorhexidine
HIDA, 964, 969
High-density lipoproteins, 1280-1292
 coronary artery disease and, 526
 liver disease and, 1286
 myocardial infarction and, 1288
 Tangier disease and, 1292
Hilar adenopathy; see also Adenopathy
 erythema nodosum and, 925
 and histoplasmosis, 274
 Hodgkin's disease and, 389
 sarcoidosis and, 76, 78, 716, 717
Hilar shadows, 740
Hill's procedure, 985
Hip
 congenital dislocation of, 1228
 osteoarthritis of, 84
Hippuran iodine 131; see Iodine-labeled orthoiodohippuric acid
Hirschsprung's disease, 1026
Hirsutism, 1162

His bundle, 479, 541-542
His-Purkinje system, 480
Histalog; see Betazole
Histaminase, 18
Histamine, 318
 asthma and, 705
 gastric secretion and, 943, 944, 993
 headache and, 789
 mastocystosis and, 910
 pheochromocytoma and, 1167
 receptor blockade and; see Cimetidine
 release of, 17, 25, 26
 urticaria pigmentosa and, 26
Histamine headache, 789
Histamine H_2-receptor blockers; see Cimetidine
Histidinemia, 1239
Histiocytes, 719; see also Histiocytosis
 sea-blue, 1293
Histiocytic lymphoma, diffuse, 392, 393
Histiocytic medullary reticulosis, 398
Histiocytosis
 disseminated, 397, 718-719
 idiopathic, 397-398
 lipochrome, 357
 localized, 397
 malignant, 398
Histiocytosis X, 397, 425, 718-719
Histocompatibility antigens; see also Human
    lymphocyte antigens
 ankylosing spondylitis and, 48, 49
 inflammatory bowel disease and, 1006, 1008
 juvenile rheumatoid arthritis and, 43
 multiple sclerosis and, 796
 psoriatic spondylitis and, 50, 51
 Reiter's syndrome and, 52, 53
 renal transplantation and, 643-644
 Wegener's granulomatosis and, 72
Histology
 cancer detection and, 434
 herpesviruses and, 136, 138
 of ovary, 1173-1174
 of thyroid gland, 1128
 tuberculosis and, 258
 varicella-zoster and, 138
Histoplasma, 179, 182, 307
Histoplasma capsulatum, 172, 274-275
Histoplasmosis, 179, 182, 274-275, 278
 dentistry and, 306-307
History of patient, 1, 4, 5-9, 434
Hives, 25-26
HK deficiency; see Hexokinase deficiency anemia
HLA; see Human lymphocyte antigens
HMG-CoA; see Hydroxymethylglutaryl CoA reductase
HMP deficiencies; see Hexose-monophosphate
    shunt deficiencies
H2N2 influenza, 154
Hodgkin's disease, 387-391
 dentistry and, 424
 meningitis and, 187
 myelofibrosis and, 322
 skin lesions of, 900
 staging of, 388-389
 zoster and, 129
Holandric inheritance, 1219
Hollenhorst plaques, 836
Holoprosencephalic malformation complex, 1303, 1316-1317
Holoprosencephaly, 1308
Holt-Oram syndrome, 498
Homans' sign, 495
Homeostasis
 insulin and, 1263
 mineral

Homeostasis—cont'd
 mineral—cont'd
  primary disorders of, 1189-1198
  and skeletal homeostasis, disorders of, 1198-1201
 skeletal
  disorders of, 1198-1201
  and mineral homeostasis, disorders of, 1198-1201
  primary, disorders of, 1201-1203
Homocystinuria, 842, 1227, 1237
Homogentisic acid oxidase deficiency, 1236
Homolateral ataxia syndrome, 835
Homosexuality
 cytomegalovirus and, 131
 hepatitis and, 1069
 Kaposi's sarcoma and, 922
Homovanillic acid, 1164, 1165, 1166
Homozygous individual, 334-337, 1218, 1219
Honeycomb lung, 726
Hookworm, 291, 1003
Horizontal eye movements, 766
Hormones, 1114-1116; see also Endocrine diseases; specific hormone
 antibodies and, 19
 binding of, 1115
 cellular mechanisms of, 1115
 in hypothyroidism, 1139-1140
 liver disease and, 1062
 Marfan's syndrome and, 1241
 neoplasms and, 443-444, 659, 1178-1181
 pancreatic enzymes and, 1051, 1056
 renal failure and, 636, 637
 sex; see Sex hormones
 syndromes of ectopic, 1178
 thyroid; see Thyroid hormones
 Turner's syndrome and, 1226
Horn cell disease, anterior, 803-804
Horner's syndrome, 833
 atypical facial pain and, 791
 cluster headache and, 789
 pupillary reflexes and, 765
Horse antitoxin, 204
Horse red blood cells, heterophil antibodies to, 132
Horse serum, 25, 26
Horseshoe kidney, 650
Horton's headache, 789
Hospice concept, 47
Host, immunocompromised, 159
Host systems for viral isolation, 123
Housemaid's knee, 99
Howell-Jolly bodies, 315, 333, 395
HPFH; see Fetal hemoglobin
HPTH; see Hyperparathyroidism
HS; see Heparan sulfate; Spherocytosis, hereditary
HSV; see Herpes simplex
Human albumin, radiolabeled, 352, 492, 687, 966
Human chorionic gonadotropin
 hyperthyroidism and, 1146
 hypogonadism and, 1122, 1172, 1173
 neoplasms and, 435, 1179, 1180
Human diploid cell vaccine, 153
Human follicle-stimulating hormone; see Follicle-stimulating hormone
Human genetics; see Genetics and metabolism
Human globulin, hyperimmune, 238
Human growth hormone; see Growth hormone
Human lymphocyte antigens, 1229, 1259; see
    also Histocompatibility antigens
 ankylosing spondylitis and, 48, 49, 737
 granulocytes compatible with, 446

Human lymphocyte antigens—cont'd
  liver disease and, 1066, 1081
  multiple sclerosis and, 796
  platelets matched to, 320, 446
  psoriatic spondylitis and, 50, 51
  Reiter's syndrome and, 52, 53
  Wegener's granulomatosis and, 72
Human menopausal gonadotropin, 1045, 1173
Human rabies immune globulin, 153
Human serum albumin aggregated, radiolabeled, 352, 492, 687, 966
Humatin; see Paromomycin
Humidifiers, 25
Humoral immunity, 15, 122, 376; see also Immune system
Humoral syndromes with neoplasms, 1178-1181
Hunchback deformity, 256
Hung-up reflex, 818
Hunt's syndrome, 130, 138
Hunter's syndrome, 1233, 1234
Huntington's chorea, 774, 816-818
Hurler's syndrome, 1233, 1234, 1302
Hürthle cells, 1150
Hutchinsonian triad, 270, 303
Hutchinson's plaques, 910
Hutchinson's teeth, 270
HVA; see Homovanillic acid
HY antigen, 1219
Hyaline casts, 605
Hyalinization, 829
Hyalinosis, 614
Hyaluronidase, 223
  diphtheria and, 248
Hydatid disease, 294
Hydatid sand, 294
Hydatidiform mole, 1146
Hydralazine
  cardiomyopathy and, 522
  disseminated vasculitis and, 29
  heart failure and, 465
  hypertension and, 473, 474, 475, 497
  lung disease and, 722
  lupuslike syndrome and, 57
  mitral regurgitation and, 511
  pericarditis and, 550
  renal failure and, 62, 639
  in scleroderma, 62
  side effects of, 574
  syncope and, 578
  toxemia of pregnancy and, 665
  urticaria and, 25
Hydration, 129, 150, 596-597, 707, 957; see also Fluids
Hydraulic suction biopsy tube, 964
Hydrocarbons
  halogenated, 1253
  porphyria cutanea tarda and, 888
  renal cell carcinomas and, 656
  toxic nephropathy and, 625, 627, 629
Hydrocephalus
  Arnold-Chiari malformations and, 811
  fibrinoid leukodystrophy and, 803
  normal pressure, 775
  otitic, 848
  tumors and, 845
Hydrochloric acid
  dilute, metabolic alkalosis and, 600
  in stomach, 942, 943
    control of, 944
    lack of; see Achlorhydria
    ulcers and, 987-988; see also Digestive system, acid-peptic diseases of
    vomitus and, 957
  Zollinger-Ellison syndrome and, 994-995
Hydrochloroquine, 46

Hydrochlorothiazide, 472, 597, 1083
Hydrocortisone, 1153; see also Cortisol
  adrenal crisis and, 1207
  with aminoglutethimide, 444
  anaphylactic shock and, 576
  hypercalcemia and, 1180
  myxedema coma and, 1140, 1206
  and pituitary insufficiency, 1124
    after surgery, 1124
  serum calcium and, 1208
Hydrogen in intestines, 960
Hydrogen ion concentration; see pH
Hydrogen peroxide; see Peroxide
Hydromorphone, 446, 1212
Hydronephrosis, 653, 655
Hydrophilic bulk agents, 954, 956
  diverticulosis and, 1017
  irritable bowel disease and, 1028
  radiation enteritis and, 1019
Hydrophobia, 139
Hydrops, gallbladder, 1088
Hydrops fetalis
  with hemoglobin Bart's, 336
  hemolytic disease of newborn and, 338
Hydroxyapatite, 1181
β-Hydroxy-beta-methylglutaryl CoA-reductase, 1063
Hydroxybutyric dehydrogenase, 535
Hydroxychloroquine, 42, 57, 903
25-Hydroxycholecalciferol, 1082; see also Vitamins, D_3
Hydroxycobalamin, 318, 1109
Hydroxydaunomycin; see Doxorubicin
Hydroxyethyl starch, 347
5-Hydroxyindoleacetic acid
  bronchial adenoma and, 743
  carcinoid syndrome and, 1038
  migraine and, 788
7-α-Hydroxylase, 1085
C-11-Hydroxylase deficiency, 1171
11-β-Hydroxylase deficiency, 1162, 1163
17-Hydroxylase deficiency, 1171
17-β-Hydroxylase deficiency, 1162, 1163
20-Hydroxylase deficiency, 1162, 1163
21-Hydroxylase deficiency, 1162, 1163
Hydroxymethylglutaryl CoA reductase, 1085, 1283
17-Hydroxypregnanolone, 1153
17-Hydroxyprogesterone, 1153, 1162, 1175
Hydroxyproline, urinary, 60, 78, 87
Hydroxyprolinemia, 1239
Hydroxypropranolol, 531
3-β-Hydroxysteroid dehydrogenase deficiency, 1171
17-β-Hydroxysteroid oxidoreductase deficiency, 1171
17-Hydroxysteroids, obesity and, 1103; see also specific steroid
5-Hydroxytryptamine; see Serotonin
Hydroxyurea, 443
  leukemias and, 368, 370
  myeloid metaplasia and, 376
  renal cell tumors and, 449
  thrombocytosis and, 404
25-Hydroxyvitamin D, 1185
25-Hydroxyvitamin D_3, 1185-1186
  osteomalacia and, 1198, 1199, 1200
  renal osteodystrophy and, 1201
Hydroxyzine
  angioedema and, 26
  drug reactions and, 29
  pregnancy and, 1212
  urticaria and, 26
Hyperabduction syndrome, 101

Hyperadrenocorticism, dentistry and, 1206-1207; see also Adrenal cortex
Hyperaldosteronism; see Aldosteronism
Hyperalimentation, parenteral, 1111
  acrodermatitis enteropathica and, 895
  Crohn's disease and, 1015
  hypercholesterolemia and, 1291
  in oliguria, 633
Hyperammonemia, 1238
Hyperbaric oxygen, 116, 253
Hyperbilirubinemia, unconjugated, 1066, 1067
Hypercalcemia, 1183, 1189-1196; see also Calcium; Hypercalciuria
  disequilibrium types of, 1190
  equilibrium types of, 1190
  familial hypocalciuric, 1192
  hyperparathyroidism and, 1192, 1207
  kidney stones and, 646-648
  neoplasms and, 657, 1179-1180, 1192
  nephropathy and, 622
  supportive care and, 445
  thiazide-induced, 472
Hypercalciuria, 647-648, 1187; see also Hypercalcemia
  hyperparathyroidism and, 1192, 1193, 1194
  idiopathic, 647
Hypercapnia, 681, 710; see also Carbon dioxide tension, arterial
Hypercarbia, respiratory failure and, 708, 709
Hypercementosis, 1093
Hypercholesterolemia, 397, 1285, 1286; see also Cholesterol
  coronary artery disease and, 526
  familial, 1287
Hyperchylomicronemia, 1003, 1288, 1289
Hypercortisolism, 1157-1159; see also Cushing's syndrome
Hyperdynamic circulation, 470; see also Hemodynamics
Hypereosinophilic syndromes, 363, 373; see also Eosinophilia
Hypergammaglobulinemia, 903, 1078; see also Gamma globulins
Hyperglycemia; see also Glucose
  coronary artery disease and, 527
  diabetes mellitus and, 1261, 1262, 1263
  hyperosmolar, and nonketotic coma, 1270
  thiazide-induced, 472
Hypergonadism, 1173
Hyperimmune globulin, 138, 238; see also Immune globulin
Hyperinfective syndrome, 291
Hyperinflation, lung, 694
Hyperinsulinism, 1284
Hyperirritable bronchi, 24
Hyperkalemia, 597, 598-599; see also Potassium
  periodic paralysis and, 858
  renal failure and, 633-634
  in vitro, 598, 599
Hyperkeratosis, 888, 1110
Hyperlactacidemia, 1256
Hyperlipidemia, 1280-1291; see also Lipoprotein metabolism disorders
  coronary artery disease and, 526
  familial combined, 1287
  management of, 1289-1291
  pancreatitis and, 1051, 1052
  skin disorders of, 889-890
Hyperlipoproteinemia
  classification of, 1280, 1286-1287
  genetic, 1287
  pathophysiology of, 1284-1286
  skin disorders of, 889-890
  type III, 1285

Hyperlipoproteinemia—cont'd
    type V familial, 1287, 1296
Hyperlucent airspaces, 686
Hypernatremia, 595-596; see also Sodium
Hypernephroma, 354, 656-658
Hyperosmolar, hyperglycemic, nonketotic coma, 1270, 1272
Hyperostosis, 50, 86, 880-881
Hyperoxaluria, 620-621, 648
Hyperparathyroidism, 1187
    dentistry and, 668, 1207-1208
    kidney stones and, 647
    with malignancy, 1179
    normocalcemic, 1193
    osteoporosis and, 115
    pancreatitis and, 1051
    primary, hypercalcemia of, 1192-1194
    renal failure and, 636, 638
    secondary, 1192
    tertiary, 1192, 1201
Hyperphenylalaninemia, 1236
Hyperphosphatemia, 1185; see also Phosphates
Hyperpigmentation, 886, 1156; see also Pigmentation
Hyperpituitary syndromes, 1119-1121, 1204
Hyperplasias
    of adrenal cortex, 887, 1162-1163
    of adrenal medulla, 1164
    of Brunner's gland, 1037
    β-cell, 1278
    gingival; see Gingival hyperplasia
    of large bowel polyps, 1038
    of lymphoid tissues, 134; see also Adenopathy; Lymphadenopathy
    of parathyroid gland, 1192
    sinusitis and, 21
Hyperpnea, 766
Hyperprolactinemia, 1118
Hyperprolinemia, 1227, 1239
Hyperpyrexia, malignant, 858; see also Fever
Hyperreflexia, detrusor, 799
Hypersensitivity; see also Allergy
    anaphylaxis and, 18; see also Anaphylaxis
    angiitis of lung and, 719
    aspirin and, 23
    cephalosporins and, 165
    delayed, 15, 19, 32; see also Skin tests
    denervation, 976
    immediate reactions in, 18
    liver and, 1075, 1076, 1078
    nephropathy and, 624, 628, 629
    nitrofurantoin and, 17
    penicillins and, 164
    pneumonitis and, 723, 727-728
    to rifampin, 259
    spectinomycin and, 170
    sulfonamides and, 169
    vasculitides and, 69
Hypersensitivity skin tests; see Skin tests
Hypersomnia–sleep apnea syndrome, 769
Hypersplenism; see Splenomegaly
Hypertelorism, 1313, 1317, 1318
Hypertension, 465-475
    amyloidosis and, 617
    angiokeratoma corporis diffusum and, 912
    benign intracranial, 779, 790, 848
    cardiomyopathy and, 518, 522-523
    cerebrovascular disease and, 829
    classification of, 469
    clinical manifestations of, 469-470
    complications of, 475
    congestive heart failure and, 454, 571
    coronary artery disease and, 527
    Cushing's syndrome and, 1157, 1158

Hypertension—cont'd
    definition of, 466-467
    dentistry and, 572
    drugs for; see Antihypertensives
    emergencies and, 474
    encephalopathy and, 469, 841
    headache and, 789
    hypercalcemia and, 622
    hyperpituitarism and, 1204
    intracranial, 779, 790, 848
    kidney injury and, 469, 471, 474, 475, 573, 588, 660-662
        glomerulonephritis in, 610, 614
        glomerulosclerosis in, 614
        obstructive uropathy in, 655
        polycystic disease in, 652
        renal failure in, 637, 639
    labile, 466
    laboratory findings in, 470, 471
    malignant, 60, 341, 469, 616
    management of, 471-475
    mineralocorticoid excess and, 1160
    pheochromocytoma and, 1164-1168
    portal, 1060-1061
        ascites and, 1045
        cirrhosis and, 1083
        splenomegaly and, 394
    pulmonary; see Pulmonary hypertension
    after renal transplantation, 645
    renovascular; see Hypertension, kidney injury and
    scleroderma and, 60, 616
    secondary, clinical findings of, 572, 573
    toxemia of pregnancy and, 665-666
    valvular disease and, 580
Hypertensive emergencies, 474
Hypertensive encephalopathy, 469, 841
Hypertensive headache, 789
Hyperthermia, malignant, 858, 875; see also Fever
Hyperthyroidism, 1140-1148
    in adolescents, 1147
    cardiomyopathies and, 523
    in child, 1147
    dentistry and, 1205
    epinephrine hazard and, 1105
    from excess thyrotropin-stimulating hormone, 1145-1146
    hypercalcemia and, 1194
    in infant, 1132, 1147
    iodine-induced, 1146
    liver disease and, 1062
    malabsorption and, 1004
    in pregnancy, 1147
    secondary hypertension and, 573
    skin disorders of, 886
    testes and, 1171
    tests for, 1141, 1143-1144, 1145, 1146, 1147
    from thyroiditis, 1146
    transient, 1141
    from tumors, 1146, 1179
Hypertonic dehydration, 596-597
Hypertonic glucose
    dialysis and, 641
    hyperkalemia and, 634
    in oliguria, 633
Hypertonic saline
    hydatid cysts and, 294
    hyperkalemia and, 599
    hyponatremia and, 595
    hypotonic dehydration and, 597
Hypertrichosis, 878, 882, 912
Hypertrichosis lanuginosa, 912

Hypertriglyceridemia, 91, 1284, 1286, 1287; see also Triglycerides
Hypertrophic cardiomyopathy, 517-520, 522
Hypertrophic cervicitis, 215
Hypertrophic gastritis, 997
Hypertrophic gingiva; see Gingival hyperplasia
Hypertrophic neuropathy, 855
Hypertrophic osteoarthropathy, 103-104
Hypertrophic pyloric stenosis, 997
Hyperuricemia; see also Uric acid
    alcohol and, 1256
    asymptomatic, 93
    and gout, 89-90, 91-92, 109
    polycystic kidney disease and, 652
    thiazide-induced, 472
Hyperuricosuria; see Uric acid, kidney and
Hyperventilation, 673, 781
    coma and, 766
    dizziness and, 794
    respiratory alkalosis and, 601
    subdural empyema and, 193
    syncope and, 781, 794
Hyperventilation syndrome, 781, 794
Hyperviscosity, serum
    cerebrovascular disease and, 842
    multiple myeloma and, 380
    plasma exchange and, 346
    Waldenström's macroglobulinemia and, 382, 383
Hyperviscosity syndromes, 346, 423, 842
Hypervitaminosis A, 1107
Hypnagogic hallucinations, 769
Hypnotics
    alcohol and, 1297
    drug abuse and, 862-864
    hypothyroidism and, 1206
    iatrogenic sleep disorders and, 770
Hypoadrenalism, 307, 1207; see also Adrenal glands
Hypoalbuminemia, 612-613, 1045; see also Albumin
Hypoaldosteronism, 623, 1159-1160; see also Aldosterone
Hypobetalipoproteinemia, 999, 1292; see also Lipoproteins
Hypocalcemia, 1105-1106, 1183, 1195-1196; see also Calcium
    hypoparathyroidism and, 1209
    malabsorption and, 1000
    neonatal, 1195
    renal failure and, 636
Hypocalciuric hypercalcemia, familial, 1192
Hypochlorhydria, 1035
Hypocholesterolemia, 1292
Hypochondroplasia, 1245
Hypochromic anemias, 323-325
Hypogammaglobulinemia, 31, 32
Hypoglycemia, 1276-1280
    alcohol and, 1256, 1270
    cerebrovascular accident and, 1272
    dentistry and, 1295
    fasting, 1277
    insulin and, 1123, 1268
    liver disease and, 1062
    neoplasms and, 1179, 1181
    plasma cortisol and, 1122
    syncope and, 781, 864
Hypoglycemic agents; see also Insulin
    neutropenia and, 360
    oral, 1266-1267, 1279, 1297
Hypoglycorrhachia, 189
Hypogonadism, 1170-1173
    hypogonadotropic, 1121-1122
    liver disease and, 1062

Hypogonadism—cont'd
  primary, 1121
  secondary, 1121-1122, 1172
Hypoinsulinemia, oral agents and, 1266, 1267
Hypokalemia, 597-598, 1106; see also Potassium
  hypertension with, 1161
  nephropathy and, 622
  penicillins and, 164
  periodic paralysis and, 858
Hypomagnesemia, 1106
  alcohol and, 1256
  hypoparathyroidism and, 1196
  malabsorption and, 1000
Hyponatremia, 594-595, 1106; see also Sodium
  body fluid osmolality and, 596
  steatorrhea and, 1000
  supportive care and, 445
Hypoparathyroidism, 1188, 1196-1197
  dentistry and, 1208-1209
  malabsorption and, 1004
  oral candidiasis and, 307
  parkinsonism and, 814
Hypopharynx, 942
Hypophosphatasia, 1200, 1209
Hypophosphatemia, 1186, 1188, 1193; see also Phosphates
  hemolysis and, 343
  osteomalacia and, 1198, 1199, 1200
  rickets and, 1200
Hypophysectomy, 444, 448
Hypopituitarism; see also Pituitary gland
  conditions simulating, 1124
  dentistry and, 1204-1205
Hypoplasia
  bone marrow, 358; see also Bone marrow
  congenital syphilis and, 303
  enamel; see Enamel, hypoplastic
  renal, 649-650
Hypoplastic anemia, 319-320
Hypoplastic crisis, 332
Hypoproteinemia, 999-1000
Hyporeninemic hypoaldosteronism, 623
Hyposensitization, 22-23; see also Immunotherapy
Hypospadias, 651
  Bloom's syndrome and, 882
  hypogonadism and, 1171
Hyposplenism, 395
Hypotension
  arrhythmias and, 584
  hypertension and, 572, 574
  ischemia and, 829
  mastocystosis and, 910
  postural, 780
    idiopathic, 823-824
    parkinsonism and, 814
  pregnancy and, 1212
  shock and, 475-479
Hypotensive syndrome, supine, 1212
Hypothalamic-pituitary-ovarian axis, 1175
Hypothalamic-pituitary-testicular feedback mechanisms, 1169
Hypothalamus, 1116-1126; see also Pituitary gland
  amenorrhea and, 1177
  anterior pituitary secretion and, 1116-1118
  clinical disorders and, 1118-1126
  coma and, 765
  Cushing's syndrome and, 1157
  endocrine, 1116, 1117
  hypogonadism and, 1172
  hypothyroidism and, 1122
  pineal gland and, 1126
Hypothermia, 118, 756

Hypotheses, Lyon, 1219
Hypothyroidism, 1136-1140
  cardiomyopathy and, 521, 523
  dentistry and, 1205-1206
  hypothalamic, 1122
  liver disease and, 1062
  myopathy and, 858
  pituitary, 1122
  radiation and, 750
  skin disorders of, 886
  testes and, 1171
  tests for, 1133-1136
  thyroid-stimulating hormone and, 1117
  transient, 1140
Hypotonic dehydration, 597
Hypotonic paralysis, 757
Hypotonic solution, 596, 618
Hypoventilation, 673, 682, 708, 711; see also Ventilation, alveolar
Hypovolemia, 631, 1024; see also Hypovolemic shock
Hypovolemic shock, 476
  dentistry and, 575
  gastrointestinal bleeding and, 957-958
  transfusion reactions and, 351
Hypoxanthine-guanine phosphoribosyltransferase deficiency, 1227, 1239
Hypoxemia, 708, 709, 710, 711, 712; see also Hypoxia
  arterial, 681-682, 683
  exercise-induced, 679
  respiratory failure and, 708
Hypoxia, 708; see also Hypoxemia
  oxygen therapy and, 729, 730
  polycythemia and, 353-354
  pulmonary hypertension and, 696
  respiratory failure and, 708
  sudden death and, 539
Hysterectomy, 253, 449

I
^{125}I; see Iodine 125
^{131}I; see Iodine 131
IAA; see Anemias, aplastic, idiopathic
IAHA; see Immune adherence hemagglutination
Ibuprofen
  rheumatoid arthritis and, 42, 46, 106
  sensitivity to, 932
I-cell disease, 1235
Ice-water lavage, 1083
Ichthyosis, 882, 900, 912
ICSH; see Interstitial cell-stimulating hormone
Ictal automatism, 783
Icterus; see Jaundice
IDDM; see Insulin-dependent diabetes mellitus
Identification, patient, 5
Idiopathic cold agglutinin disease, chronic, 339
Idiopathic hypoparathyroidism, 1209
Idiopathic pulmonary fibrosis, 713-715
Idiopathic pulmonary hemosiderosis, 720-721
Idiopathic recurrent polyneuropathy, 855
Idiopathic skeletal hyperostosis, diffuse, 50, 86
Idiopathic thrombocytopenic purpura, 402-404
Idiopathic thrombocytopenic purpura-like syndromes, 403
Idiosyncratic reactions, 27
IDL; see Intermediate density lipoproteins
Idoxuridine, 129, 154, 299
Iduronate sulfatase deficiency, 1233, 1234
α-L-Iduronidase, 1233, 1234, 1302
IF; see Intrinsic factor
IFA test; see Indirect fluorescent antibody test
Ig; see Immunoglobulins
IGT; see Impaired glucose tolerance

Ileal effluent, excessive, 952
Ileitis
  backwash, 1006
  regional; see also Crohn's disease
    malnutrition and, 1103
    skin disorders of, 892
Ileojejunitis, diffuse, 1003
Ileorectal anastomosis
  Crohn's disease and, 1015
  diverticulosis and, 1018
  ulcerative colitis and, 1011
Ileostomy
  Crohn's disease and, 1015
  inflammation of stoma of, 1015
  ulcerative colitis and, 1011
Ileum, 945
  backwash ileitis and, 1006
  bypass of, 1291
  and colon, anastomosis between, 1015
  Crohn's disease and; see Crohn's disease
  excessive effluent from, 952
  ileostomy and, 1011, 1015
  malabsorption and, 1003
  and rectum, anastomosis between
    Crohn's disease and, 1015
    diverticulosis and, 1018
    ulcerative colitis and, 1011
  segmental removal of, 1012, 1015
Ileus, 1024-1026, 1088
Illness, evaluation of, 5
IM; see Infectious mononucleosis
Imidazoles, 278, 308, 390, 391; see also Dacarbazine
Imipramine
  cataplexy and, 769
  fibrositis and, 97
  lung disease and, 722
  neurologic effects of, 779
  parkinsonism and, 815
  salivary flow and, 870
Immediate hypersensitivity reactions, 18; see also Anaphylaxis
Immobilization, 1194
Immune adherence hemagglutination, 130
Immune complexes, 19
  in blood vessel walls, 19, 66, 67, 341, 719
  circulating, 27
  hemorrhagic lung disease and, 720
  hypersensitivity vasculitis and, 67, 341
  lupus erythematosus and, 53, 54, 615
  nephritis and, 27, 615
  pulmonary fibrosis and, 713, 714
  pulmonary vasculitides and, 719
  Schönlein-Henoch purpura and, 616; see also Schönlein-Henoch purpura
  toxic nephropathy and, 624, 626
  Wegener's granulomatosis and, 70
Immune deficiencies; see Immunodeficiency
Immune factors in carcinogenesis, 433-434
Immune globulin; see also Immunoglobulins
  anti-D, 349
  hepatitis and, 1073, 1100
  human rabies, 153
  measles and, 138, 147, 152
  mumps and, 138
  pertussis and, 238
  Rh, 349
  zoster, 127, 130, 138
Immune hemolysis, 29, 329-330, 332-335, 342
Immune suppression of hematopoiesis, 319
Immune system, 376; see also Autoimmune disease; Immunology
  cell-mediated; see Cell-mediated immunity
  combination reactions in, 19

Immune system—cont'd
  endocarditis and, 180
  evaluation of, 31-32
  Hodgkin's disease and, 387
  insulin-dependent diabetes mellitus and, 1259
  Lyme disease and, 298
  pernicious anemia and, 317
  sarcoidosis and, 76, 718
  syphilis and, 266
  toxoplasmosis and, 275
  trypanosomiasis and, 287
  types of reactions in, 18-19
  viruses and, 121-122
Immunization; *see also* Vaccines
  hepatitis and, 1073, 1100-1101
  meningitis and, 190, 191
  neonatal viruses and, 127
  varicella and, 130
Immunoassays; *see* Radioimmunoassay
Immunoblastic sarcoma, 392
Immunocompromised host, 159
Immunocyte dyscrasias with amyloidosis, 385
Immunodeficiency, 31-34
  classification of, 32
  common variable, 33
  graft-versus-host disease and, 19
  management of, 34
  non-Hodgkin's lymphoma and, 391
  with thymoma, 33
Immunoelectrophoresis, 188, 189, 378, 380
Immunofluorescence, 124
  adenoviruses and, 143
  cytomegalovirus and, 131
  herpes simplex and, 128, 136
  influenza and, 141
  measles and, 146
  parainfluenza viruses and, 143
  rabies and, 139, 153
  respiratory syncytial virus and, 141
  varicella-zoster and, 138
Immunoglobulins, 16-17; *see also* Globulins; Immune globulin
  A, 16, 17, 31
    anaphylactoid reactions and, 348
    Crohn's disease and, 1907
    deficiency of, 32
    gingival hyperplasia and, 865
    heavy-chain disease and, 384
    malignant atrophic papulosis and, 894
    multiple myeloma and, 381
    nephropathy and, 611
    sarcoidosis and, 911
    secretory, 941-942
    transfusion reactions and, 351
    Bloom's syndrome and, 882
  D, 16, 17, 381
  deficiencies of, 32-33
  dermatitis herpetiformis and, 893
  E, 16, 17
    allergy and, 19-20
    angioedema and, 25, 26
    asthma and, 23, 704, 705
    immunologic reactions and, 18
    Kawasaki disease and, 148
    multiple myeloma and, 381
    serum level of, 21, 24
    serum sickness and, 27
    urticaria and, 25, 26
  excessive or abnormal, 376-387
  G, 16; *see also* Gamma globulins
    blood compatibility and, 349
    deficiency of, 32
    essential cryoglobulinemia, 618
    gout and, 90

Immunoglobulins—cont'd
  G—cont'd
    heavy-chain disease and, 384
    hemolytic disease of newborn and, 338
    hemorrhagic lung disease and, 720
    hepatitis and, 1071
    immunologic reactions and, 18
    infectious mononucleosis and, 132, 133
    insulin-dependent diabetes mellitus and, 1260
    multiple myeloma and, 381
    multiple sclerosis and, 797
    nephrotic syndrome and, 613
    normal, 31
    pulmonary fibrosis and, 713
    rheumatoid arthritis and, 36
    sarcoidosis and, 911
    serum sickness and, 27
  glomerulonephritis and, 610, 611
  gout and, 90
  hemorrhagic lung disease and, 720
  iodine 125-radiolabeled, 124
  on lymphocytes, 16
  M, 16, 377
    blood compatibility and, 348
    deficiency of, 32
    disorders of, 376-387
    elevated, 32
    essential cryoglobulinemia and, 618
    glomerular basement membrane and, 618
    heavy-chain disease and, 384
    hepatitis and, 1071
    immunologic reactions and, 18
    infectious mononucleosis and, 132, 133
    Lyme disease and, 297
    multiple myeloma and, 381
    neonatal viruses and, 127
    rubella and, 146
    sarcoidosis and, 911
    in serum, 379
    serum sickness and, 27
    toxoplasmosis and, 286
    trypanosomiasis and,•287
    viruses and, 124
    Waldenström's macroglobulinemia and, 383
  multiple myeloma and, 381
  nephrotic syndrome and, 613
  pneumonia and, 173
  pulmonary fibrosis and, 713, 714
  serum level of, 31
  structure of, 377
  thyroid-stimulating; *see* Thyrotropin receptor antibody
Immunohemolytic anemias, 29, 329-330, 337-340, 342
Immunologic reactions; *see* Immune system; Immunology
Immunology, 15-34; *see also* Immune system
  angioedema and, 25-26
  atopic disease and, 19-24
  contact dermatitis and, 27
  digestive system and, 941-942, 997
  drug allergy and, 27-30, 329-330, 342
  idiopathic thrombocytopenic purpura and, 400, 402
  immunodeficiency diseases and, 31-34; *see also* Immunodeficiency
  inflammatory bowel disease and, 1006
  liver disease and, 1064, 1078
  principles of, 15-19
  relapsing polychondritis and, 102
  serum sickness and, 26-27
  urticaria and, 25-26
Immunoreactive parathyroid hormone, 1193-1194, 1196

Immunosuppressives
  acquired anticoagulants and, 411
  arthritis and, 42, 52
  Behçet's syndrome and, 111
  Candida and, 307, 929, 1092
  as carcinogens, 432, 434
  gastrointestinal bleeding and, 1093
  glomerulonephritis and, 610
  hemorrhagic lung disease and, 720
  hepatitis and, 1099
  herpesvirus and, 827
  Kaposi's sarcoma and, 922
  listeriosis and, 246
  lupus erythematosus and, 57
  pemphigoid and, 935
  pemphigus and, 932, 933, 934
  polymyositis and, 65
  premalignant lesions and, 919
  pulmonary fibrosis and, 713, 714
  relapsing polychondritis and, 103
  renal transplantation and, 644, 669
  strongyloidiasis and, 291
  thrombotic thrombocytopenic purpura and, 617
  toxoplasmosis and, 285, 286
  ulcerative colitis and, 1011
Immunotherapy, 22-23
  allergic rhinitis and, 22
  asthma and, 25
  gastric neoplasms and, 1036
  in leprosy, 263
  in leukemias, 368
  in neoplasia, 444-445, 1036
Impactions, 955, 1025, 1026
Impaired glucose tolerance, 1260; *see also* Glucose tolerance
Impedance, 460
Impedance phlebography, 495
Impetigo, 219-220
  staphylococcal, 225-226
  streptococcal, 223, 225-226
Implants, radioactive, 1047
Impotence, 823, 1120
Impulse transmission, 797
Inappropriate antidiuretic hormone secretion, 594, 595, 740
  encephalitis and, 135
  malignancy and, 740, 1179, 1181
Inborn errors of metabolism, 1226-1227, 1236-1238
  craniofacial malformations and, 1302
  lipoprotein deficiency disorders and, 1291-1293
Inbreeding coefficients, 1224
Incisura, 767
Inclusion bodies, 315
  Chédiak-Higashi syndrome and, 397
  herpes simplex and, 128, 136, 299
  idiopathic orthostatic hypotension and, 823
Incomplete penetrance, 1219
Incontinentia pigmenti, 810, 869
Inderal; *see* Propranolol
Indirect fluorescent antibody test, 286; *see also* Fluorescent antibody stains
Indium 111 and DTPA, 964
Indocin; *see* Indomethacin
Indomethacin
  ankylosing spondylitis and, 50, 737
  asthma and, 704
  coumarins and, 414
  gastritis and, 996
  gout and, 93
  and hypercalcemia, 445, 657, 1180
  hyponatremia and, 594
  nephropathy and, 621, 625, 627, 629

Indomethacin—cont'd
  neutropenia and, 360
  osteoarthritis and, 85
  patent ductus arteriosus and, 557
  pericarditis and, 551
  platelet function and, 405
  pregnancy and, 1212
  pseudogout and, 95
  relapsing polychondritis and, 103
  rheumatoid arthritis and, 42, 46, 106
  secretory diarrhea and, 954
  sensitivity to, 23
  tendinitis and, 99
  ulcers and, 988
Inert gas dilution method, 679
Infantile muscular atrophy, 804
Infantile polycystic disease, 652-653
Infantile reflexes, 586
Infants; see also Children; Newborn
  adenoviruses and, 143
  botulism and, 201, 204
  chlamydial ophthalmia neonatorum and, 215
  genital mycoplasmas and, 218
  gonococcal conjunctivitis and, 230
  hyperthyroidism in, 1147
  hypothyroidism and, 1136-1138, 1140
  muscular atrophy and, 804
  parainfluenza viruses and, 142
  polycystic disease of, 652-653
  premature, 499, 503
  respiratory syncytial virus and, 141
  roseola and, 147
  rotaviruses and, 150
  Staphylococcus aureus pneumonia and, 175
Infarction
  of brain, 830-835
    hypertensive encephalopathy and, 469, 841
    vertigo and, 793-794
  myocardial; see Myocardial infarction
  omental, 1049
  paronychial, 906
  sickle cell anemia and, 332
  of spinal cord, 835-836
  splenic, 398
Infarctive crisis, 332
Infections; see also Microbial diseases
  abortion and, 218
  alcoholism and, 1298
  arthritis and; see Arthritis, infectious
  bacterial; see Bacteria
  candidal; see *Candida*
  of central nervous system, precautions for, 868
  Chédiak-Higashi syndrome and, 397
  demyelinating diseases and, 868
  dentoalveolar, congenital heart disease and, 579
  drug abuse and, 863
  dysphagia and, 1091, 1092
  emboli and, 180, 489, 579
  endocarditis and, 178-185, 301-302; see also Endocarditis
  epidural, 139, 191-194
  esophagitis and, 985
  fungal; see Fungal diseases
  glucose-6-phosphate dehydrogenase deficiency and, 330
  hemolysis from, 343
  Hodgkin's disease and, 387, 424
  hyposplenism and, 395
  immunodeficiency diseases and, 31
  inflammatory bowel disease and, 1005-1006
  insulin management and, 1268
  interstitial nephritis and, 619, 620
  leukemias and, 368, 371, 421

Infections—cont'd
  leukemoid reactions and, 361
  liver disease and, 1068-1075
  monocytosis and, 362
  mucocutaneous; see Mucocutaneous infections
  multiple myeloma and, 379, 422
  neonatal; see Newborn
  neoplasia and, 446
  neuropathies and, 854-855
  neutropenia and, 359
  neutrophil levels and, 361
  obstructive uropathy and, 654, 656
  oral, diabetes and, 1294
  pancreatitis and, 1051
  parameningeal, 139, 189, 191-194
  perinatal, 125-127; see also Newborn
  of peritoneum, 1046-1047
  renal failure and, 634
  renal transplantation and, 645
  site of, antimicrobial activity at, 156-157
  skin, 926-931; see also specific infection
  after splenectomy, 395
  streptococcal; see Streptococci
  subdural, 139
  of testes, 1171
  urinary tract, 195-199
    endocarditis and, 180
    pregnancy and, 664, 666
    schistosomiasis and, 296
  viral causes of, 122; see also Viral diseases
Infectious arthritis; see Arthritis, infectious
Infectious mononucleosis, 131, 132
  blood transfusions and, 348
  dentistry and, 300
  hepatitis and, 1073
  Hodgkin's disease and, 387
  neutropenia and, 359
Infectious mononucleosis–like syndrome, 131, 133
Infectious rhinitis, 21, 23
Inferior mesenteric artery occlusion, 1020
Inferior quadrantanopsias, 759
Inferior vena cava, 494, 1045
Infertility, 1120, 1162
Infiltrates
  leukemic, 421
  mycosis fungoides and, 901-902
  thrombocytopenia and, 426
Infiltrative dermopathy of Graves' disease, 1141-1142, 1143
Infiltrative diseases of liver, 1084
Inflammation; see also specific inflammation
  amebiasis and, 282
  of appendix, 232, 951, 1015-1016
  of ileostomy stoma, 1015
  of intestines, 1005-1020
    antibiotic-induced diarrhea in, 1018
    appendicitis and appendiceal abscess in, 232, 951, 1015-1016
    colitis in; see Colitis
    dentistry and, 1092-1093, 1095-1097
    diverticular colon disease in, 324, 1017-1018
    inflammatory bowel disease in, 1005-1015
    malabsorption and, 1002
    pseudomembranous enterocolitis and, 1018
    radiation enteritis in, 1002, 1018-1019
    staphylococcal, 220
    ulcer in, 1019
  of iris; see Iritis
  of lung; see Pneumonia; Pneumonitis
  of lymph nodes; see Lymph nodes; Lymphadenitis
  of mediastinum, 105, 734-735

Inflammation—cont'd
  mesenteric, 1048-1049
  myopathies and, 858
  of pancreas; see Pancreatitis
  pelvic, 215, 218, 231, 232
  of pericardium; see Pericarditis
  of peritoneum; see Peritonitis
  of pharynx; see Pharyngitis
  of pleura, 255, 730-731
  of synovia, 36, 81, 99, 231
  systemic sclerosis and, 58
  of veins; see Phlebitis; Thrombophlebitis
  of vessels; see Vasculitis
Inflammatory bowel disease, 1005-1015
  comparisons in, 1008
  Crohn's disease in, 1011-1015; see also Crohn's disease
  dentistry and, 1095-1097
  ulcerative colitis and, 1007-1011; see also Ulcerative colitis
Inflammatory myopathies, dentistry and, 874-875
Influenza, 135, 140-141
  amantadine and, 154
  disseminated intravascular coagulation and, 412
  neutropenia and, 359
  pneumonia and, 171, 172, 175
  septic arthritis of temporomandibular joint and, 108
  swine, 140
  vaccines for, 152-153
Influenza A and B viruses, 172
Information processing, 770-773
Information source, 5
Infranodal conduction, 541-542
Infraspinatus, 98
Infratentorial lesions, 767-768, 845
Ingestion of foods, disorders of, 1103; see also Dysphagia
Inguinal adenopathy, 216
INH; see Isoniazid
Inhalants
  abuse of, 862, 863
  hypertension and, 574
  renal disease and, 670
  in respiratory disease, 745
Inhalation
  anthrax and, 245
  Q fever and, 213
  of steroids, 707
Inhalation challenge test, 22
Inhalational lung disease, 728-730
Inheritance; see also Chromosomes; Genetics and metabolism
  multifactorial, 1222-1223
  patterns of, 1223-1224
  single gene, 1216-1220
    dystrophies of, 856-857
Inhibin, 1118
Inhibition, zone size of, 155
Injections, 157
Injuries; see Trauma
Innominate artery, 563
Inoculation herpes, 926
Inotropic agents, 464, 465, 478 see also Digitalis; specific agent
Insecticides, 754, 853
Insomnias, 769-770
Inspection, 7, 12, 684-685
Inspiration, 672, 681-682
Inspiratory muscle fatigue, 684
Inspiratory noise, 684
Instinctive behavior, 763
Insulin, 1261

INDEX 1373

Insulin—cont'd
  action of, 1262
  administration of, 1267-1269
    devices for, 1269
    in intravenous drip, 618, 621, 1268
    preparations for, 1266
    surreptitious, 1279
  alcohol and, 1256, 1271, 1297
  allergy to, 1268
  anabolic effects of, 1262
  chronic renal failure and, 637, 639
  deficiency of, 1263, 1269
  desensitization to, 1268
  diabetes dependent on, 1259-1261
  diuretics and, 472
  fatty acids and, 1284
  formation of, 945, 1049
  growth hormone and, 1123
  hyperglycemic, hyperosmolar, nonketotic coma and, 1270
  hyperkalemia and, 599, 634
  hypoglycemia and, 1123, 1276, 1277, 1279
  hypokalemia and, 597
  islet cell tumors and; see Insulinomas
  ketoacidosis and, 600, 1269, 1271
  lipoproteins and, 1284, 1287, 1289
  monocompetent, 1267, 1268
  obesity and, 1103
  pancreatitis and, 1055
  peridontal disease and, 1294
  pregnancy and, 1271
  reaction to, 1276, 1277
  receptors for, 19, 1261
  renal failure and, 637
  resistance to, 1261, 1268, 1284
  secretion of, 1262
  single-peak, 1267
  syncope and, 781
  vascular complications of diabetes and, 527
  xanthomas and, 890
  Zollinger-Ellison syndrome and, 994
Insulin drip, 1268, 1271
Insulin molecule, abnormal, 1261
Insulin reaction, 1276, 1277
Insulin receptor, 19, 1261
Insulin resistance, 1261, 1268, 1284
Insulin-dependent diabetes mellitus, 1259-1261
Insulin-induced hypoglycemia, 1123
Insulinomas, 994, 1056, 1278-1279
  malignant, 450
  placental proteins and, 435
Intensive care unit, 537
Intention tremors, 799, 870
Intercostal muscles, 100, 672
Intercostal nerves, 100, 1043, 1275
Interdental massage, 866
Interferon, 15, 110, 145
  cytomegalovirus and, 131
  hepatitis and, 1073, 1079
  herpes simplex and, 129
  in neoplasia, 445
  varicella-zoster and, 130
Intermaxillary fixation, 106
Intermediate density lipoproteins, 1283
Intermittent atrioventricular block, 547
Intermittent disease, 53
Intermittent porphyria, acute, 854, 888, 1249, 1250-1252
Intermittent positive-pressure breathing; see also Mechanical ventilation
  asthma and, 706
  chronic obstructive pulmonary disease and, 693
  pancreatitis and, 1053

Intermittent positive-pressure breathing—cont'd
  respiratory failure and, 711, 712
Internal mammary artery grafts, 532
Internuclear ophthalmoplegia, 833
  brainstem lesions and, 760
  coma and, 766
  multiple sclerosis and, 798
Interstitial cell-stimulating hormone, 1118, 1169
Interstitial keratitis, 270
Interstitial lung diseases
  cytomegalovirus and, 131
  drugs and, 722
  infiltrate in, 685
  pneumonitis and, 64, 715, 721
  of unknown cause, 716-719
Interstitial nephritis, 619-621
Interstitial nephropathy, 619, 626
Intertrigo, 929
Intervertebral disc syndrome, 50, 860
Interview approach to history, 6, 7
Intestinal angina, 949, 951, 989
Intestinal bypass surgery; see Bypass procedures, intestinal
Intestinal lymphangiectasia, 999, 1003
Intestinal lymphoma, 1002, 1041
Intestinal villi, 945
Intestines; see also Digestive system
  abscesses of, 1007, 1012, 1017, 1019; see also Abscesses, intra-abdominal
  amebiasis and, 203, 281-283
  angina and, 949, 951, 989
  bacterial overgrowth and, 62, 947
  bypass surgery and; see Bypass procedures, intestinal
  colitis in; see Colitis
  decompression of, 1011, 1026
  diverticula of, 324, 1017-1018
  enteritis and 220, 1002, 1018-1019
  functional disease of, 1027-1029
  gas in, 1028; see also Distention
  inflammations of, 1005-1020
    antibiotic-induced diarrhea in, 1018
    appendicitis and appendiceal abscess in, 232, 951, 1015-1016
    colitis in; see Colitis
    dentistry and, 1092-1093, 1095-1097
    diverticular colon disease in, 324, 1017-1018
    inflammatory bowel disease in, 1005-1015
    malabsorption and, 1002
    pseudomembranous enterocolitis and, 1018
    radiation enteritis and, 1002, 1018-1019
    staphylococcal, 220
    ulcer in, 1019
  irritable, 1005, 1027
  ischemic syndromes of, 1029-1024
  large, 746-747; see also Colon
    decompression of, 1011, 1026
    diagnosis and, 964-965; see also Colonoscopy
    fibrosis of, 1011, 1019
    inflammatory disease of; see Intestines, inflammations of
    mechanical cleansing of, 251, 965; see also Enemas
    megacolon of, 1007, 1008, 1011, 1026-1027
    motility of, 948, 1026-1029
    neoplasms of, 1038-1042
    obstructions of, 445, 951, 1024-1027
    ulcer of, 1019
  lymphomas of, 1002, 1037, 1041
  malabsorption and, 998-1005; see also Nutrition

Intestines—cont'd
  malabsorption and—cont'd
    Crohn's disease and, 1012
    lymphangiectasis and, 999, 1003
    lymphoma and, 1002
  motility disorders of, 1026-1029
  obstruction of, 445, 951, 1024-1027
  polyps of, 1037, 1038, 1039, 1042-1043
    carcinoma and, 1039
    Peutz-Jeghers syndrome and, 891
    syndrome of, 1042-1043
  preparation of, for colonoscopy, 965
  pseudo-obstruction of, 981
  resection of
    diverticulosis and, 1018
    ischemic colitis and, 1021
    large bowel neoplasms and, 1041
    malabsorption and, 1002
    occlusive vascular disease and, 1020
    steatorrhea and, 999
    venous thrombosis and, 1022
  sigmoidoscopy and; see Sigmoidoscopy
  small, 945-947
    absorption in, 946-947
    biopsy of, 384, 964
    carcinomas of, Crohn's disease and, 1013-1014
    diagnosis and, 964
    digestion in, 946-947
    ischemia of, 1003
    malabsorption and, 1002, 1003
    motility and, 946-947
    neoplasms of, 445, 1013-1014, 1037-1038
    obstructions of, 445, 1024-1027
    polyps in, 1037
    resection of, 1001
    roentgenograms of, 1012, 1013
    ulcers and, 987
  strangulation of, 1024-1025
  ulcer of; see Ulcers, intestinal
  villi of, 945
Intimal tear, 560
Intoxication, 775-779, 1257; see also Alcoholism
Intra-abdominal abscess; see Abscesses, intra-abdominal
Intra-aortic balloon pumping, 532
Intra-articular steroids, 106, 107
Intracellular parasites, 31
Intracerebral hemorrhage, 829, 830, 838-839, 841; see also Brain; Cerebrovascular accident
Intracerebral mucormycosis, 308
Intracranial calcifications, 125, 126, 810, 880, 881
Intracranial foreign bodies, 187
Intracranial headache, 788
Intracranial hypertension, benign, 779, 790, 848
Intracranial pressure, 846, 1313, 1314; see also Cerebrospinal fluid; Intracranial hypertension, benign
Intracytoplasmic inclusion bodies, 823
Intraepidermal vesicles, 129
Intraepithelial vesicles, 299
Intrahepatic cholestasis, 1058, 1068 see also Bile ducts
Intramedullary hemorrhage, 840
Intramedullary spinal cord tumors, 807
Intramuscular injections, 157
Intranasal challenge, provocative, 21, 22
Intranuclear inclusions, 128, 136
Intraparenchymal infiltrate, 685
Intraperitoneal bleeding, 971
Intraperitoneal fluids, ultrasound and, 970-971
Intraperitoneal transfusions, 338

Intrapulmonary cysts, 700, 701
Intrasellar pituitary tumor, 1123-1124
Intrauterine growth retardation, 125
Intrauterine synechiae, 1176
Intrauterine transfusions, hydrops fetalis and, 338
Intravascular coagulation, disseminated; see Disseminated intravascular coagulation
Intravascular hemolysis, 327, 341; see also Disseminated intravascular coagulation
Intravascular volume, 476, 478, 1270; see also Volume expanders
Intravenous fluids; see Fluids
Intravenous hyperalimentation; see Hyperalimentation
Intravenous injection, 157
Intravenous pyelography, 196, 656
Intravenous urography, 606, 661, 663
Intraventricular septum, rupture of, 536
Intrinsic asthma, 704; see also Asthma
Intrinsic factor, 317, 940, 942, 943, 1109
  antibodies to, 19
  malnutrition and, 1103, 1109
Intussusception
  large bowel neoplasms and, 1038, 1041
  management of, 1026
  polyposis syndromes and, 1042
Inulin clearance, 603
Invagination, basilar, 811
Inversions, chromosomal, 1222
Involuntary ventilation, 711; see also Ventilation
Iodide trapping, 1128, 1130
Iodides
  anaphylactoid reaction and, 27
  contrast material and; see Contrast agents
  erythema multiforme and, 922
  erythema nodosum and, 924
  thyroid function and, 1132
  thyrotoxic crisis and, 1147
  trapping of, 1128, 1130
  urticaria and, 25
Iodine
  deficiency of, 1105, 1132, 1148
  extrathyroidal metabolism of, 1128
  Graves' disease and, 1144
  halogen sensitivity and, 893
  hydatid cysts and, 294
  hyperthyroidism and, 1146
  hypothyroidism and, 1137
  radioactive; see Radioactive iodine
  thyroid hormone storage and, 1130
Iodine 125, 124, 448
Iodine 131
  albumin labeled with, red cell mass measurement and, 353
  hepatic imaging and, 966
  ovarian disease and, 1045
Iodine uptake, absolute, 1133
Iodine-labeled orthoiodohippuric acid, 607-608
Iodothyronines, 1128, 1129
Ionizing radiation; see Radiation
IPF; see Idiopathic pulmonary fibrosis
IPTH; see Immunoreactive parathyroid hormone
Iridocyclitis, 45, 47
Iris, 923
Iritis
  Behçet's disease and, 907
  juvenile rheumatoid arthritis and, 45, 47
  Reiter's syndrome and, 52
Iron
  absorption of, 1105
  deficiency of, 1104-1105; see also Iron deficiency anemia
    anemia of chronic disease and, 326

Iron—cont'd
  deficiency of—cont'd
    diet and, 313
    malabsorption and, 1000
    Plummer-Vinson syndrome and, 1091, 1105
    renal failure and, 636, 639
    thrombocytosis and, 404-405
  deposition of, in body tissues, 345; see also Iron loading
  excess; see also Iron loading
    dietary, 345
    liver disease and, 1059, 1066, 1081
    in lung tissue, 720
    mitochondria and, 321
  metabolism of, 324
    disorder of, 311, 345-346, 1240
    hypochromic anemia and, 325
    sideroblastic anemia and, 321
  in therapy; see Iron therapy
Iron 59, 313-315
Iron deficiency anemia, 315, 323-325; see also Iron, deficiency of
  chronic disease and, 326
  colorectal carcinoma and, 1040
  dentistry and, 416
  gastric carcinoma and, 1035
  gastric polyps and, 1034
  gastrointestinal bleeding and, 960
  hemorrhagic lung disease and, 720
  hookworm and, 291
Iron loading; see also Iron, excess
  blood transfusions and, 337
  porphyria and, 1253
  sideroblastic anemia and, 321-322
Iron therapy, 310
  anemia and, 315-316, 325
  dialysis and, 642
  hemochromatosis and, 345
  paroxysmal nocturnal hemoglobinuria and, 342
  polycythemia and, 354
  postgastrectomy syndrome and, 1004
  Reiter's syndrome and, 908
  teeth staining and, 668
Iron-chelating agents
  hemochromatosis and, 346
  sideroblastic anemia and, 322
Irradiated ergosterol, 1185
Irradiation; see Radiation
Irreversible shock, 478
Irritable bowel or colon, 1005, 1027, 1028
Ischemia
  arrhythmia and, 585
  of bowel, 1020-1024
  cerebral, 829; see also Cerebrovascular accident
    aortic arch syndrome and, 563
    transient, 563, 564, 586, 836-838
  dentistry and, 586-587
  in diabetes, 1273, 1274
  myocardial; see Myocardial ischemia
  popliteal aneurysms and, 567
  renal, 631, 660-662
  spinal cord, 556
Ischemic syndromes of bowel, 1020-1024
Ischial bursitis, 99
ISG; see Immune globulin
Islet cell tumors; see Insulinomas
Islets of Langerhans, 1049, 1262-1263; see also Pancreas
  antibodies to cells of, 1260
  ectopic tissue of, 1037
  tumors and; see Insulinomas
Ismelin; see Guanethidine
Isoagglutinin titers, 290

Isochromosome, 1221, 1222
Isoflow, volume of, 692
Isoimmune anemia, 337
Isolated gonadotropin deficiency, 1172
Isolated luteinizing hormone deficiency, 1172
Isolation, 123, 124, 127
Isoleucine, 1237, 1238
Isomorphic phenomenon, 936, 937
Isoniazid
  anemia and, 321, 325, 329
  excretion of, 158
  hemolysis and, 329
  hepatitis and, 1066, 1075-1076, 1078
  Huntington's chorea and, 817
  lung disease and, 721, 722
  lupuslike syndrome and, 57
  neuropathy and, 779, 853
  nontuberculous mycobacteria and, 261
  phenytoin and, 786
  pregnancy and, 1212
  silicosis and, 725
  tuberculosis and, 121, 258, 259, 260
Isophendylate, 761
Isopropyl oil, 432
Isoproterenol
  heart failure and, 465
  pericardial tamponade and, 555
  pulmonary hypertension and, 497
  sick sinus syndrome and, 547
  urinary catecholamines and, 1168
Isosorbide dinitrate, 531
Isospora belli, 1003
Isotonic dehydration, 596
Isotonic lever system, 457
Isotonic saline; see Normal saline
Isotope brain scan; see Brain scans
Isotope cisternography, 775
Isotopic renogram, 608
Isovaleric acidemia, 1237
Isovolemic exchange transfusion, 334
ITP; see Idiopathic thrombocytopenic purpura
Ivy method, 106
Ixodes dammini, 297
Ixodidae, 210, 297, 925

J

Jaccoud's arthritis, 229
Jacksonian seizures, 781, 782-783
Jalap, 1002
Jamshuti needle, 965
Janeway's lesions, 180, 181
Jarisch-Herxheimer reaction, 266, 272
Jaundice, 1058
  acholuric, 1065
  assessment of, 1066-1067
  biliary tract imaging and, 969
  bilirubin metabolism and, 1058
  cholestatic
    erythromycin and, 168
    extrahepatic obstruction and, 967
    vitamin K and, 411
  colorectal carcinoma and, 1040
  congenital hemolytic, 328-329
  cytomegalovirus and, 125
  gastrointestinal disorders and, 961
  glucose-6-phosphate dehydrogenase deficiency and, 330
  hepatitis and, 1070
  of oral mucosa or sclera, 1097
  pancreatic carcinoma and, 1056
Jaw
  abnormal involuntary movements of, 870-871
  actinomycosis and lumpy, 305

Jaw—cont'd
  cysts of, 668, 883
  Epstein-Barr virus and, 300
  fibrous dysplasia of, 115-116
  Gaucher's disease and, 425
  histiocytosis X and, 425
  intention tremors of, 870
  lymphoma and, 424
  metastasis of renal tumors to, 668
  multiple myeloma and, 422-423
  osteomalacia and, 1209
  osteomyelitis of, 116-117, 417
  osteonecrosis of, herpes zoster and, 299-300
  osteoporosis of, 1210
  Paget's disease of, 114-115
  pain and, 583, 869
  sickle cell anemia and, 416-417
  spasms of, 821
  Sturge-Weber syndrome and angiomas of, 869
  tuberculous osteomyelitis of, 304
JC virus, 828
Jejunocolic bypass, 53, 1077
Jejunoileal bypass, 1077
Jejunum, 945
  bypass surgery of, 53, 1077
  ulcer of, 987
Jerk nystagmus, 760
JG cells; *see* Juxtaglomerular cells
Jimsonweed poisoning, 818
Job's syndrome, 357
Jock itch, 929
Jod-Basedow disease, 1146
Joffroy's sign, 1142
Joints
  ankylosing spondylitis and, 48
  atlantoaxial, 45
  bloody effusion into, 104
  Charcot's, 86, 94, 1275
  degenerative disease of, 83, 107
  dislocation of, 1241
  interphalangeal, 51
  lupus erythematosus and, 54
  metacarpophalangeal, 36, 37
  peripheral, evaluation of, 13
  popliteal artery aneurysm and, 567
  rheumatoid process and, 36, 37
  sickle cell anemia and, 333
  streptococcal infection of, 226
  temporomandibular; *see* Temporomandibular joints
  tuberculosis of, 81, 256
Jones' criteria, 229, 580
JP; *see* Juvenile periodontitis
JRA; *see* Juvenile rheumatoid arthritis
J-shaped sella turcica, 1302
Judkins' technique, 531
Jugular veins, 10, 463, 552, 580
Juvenile cataracts, 1273
Juvenile hyperpituitarism, dentistry and, 1204
Juvenile myxedema, dentistry and, 1206
Juvenile periodontitis, neutrophil dysfunction and, 420
Juvenile periodontosis, connective tissue disorders and, 1243, 1244
Juvenile polyposis, 1037, 1038, 1042-1043
Juvenile progressive spinal muscular atrophy, 804-805
Juvenile rheumatoid arthritis, 43-47
  differential diagnosis and, 47
  drug treatment of, 46
  pauciarticular, 45
  polyarticular, 43-45
  subgroups of, 44

Juvenile rheumatoid arthritis—cont'd
  temporomandibular joint in, 106
Juxtaglomerular cells, 1155, 1159

K

K 1 antigen, 186
K complexes, 769
Kallikrein, 450, 468
Kallman's syndrome, 1121, 1172
Kanamycin, 161, 165-166
  labyrinth and, 792
  nephropathy and, 627, 628
  plague and, 242
  pregnancy and, 1212
  in tuberculosis, 260
Kaolin/pectin, diphenhydramine and dyclonine with, 415
Kaposi's sarcoma, 863, 920-922
Kartagener's syndrome, 691, 696
Karyotypes, 1171, 1220, 1221
Kasabach-Merritt syndrome, 341
Katayama fever, 295
Kato thick smear, 296
Kawasaki disease, 68, 69, 147-148
Kayexalate; *see* Sodium polystyrene sulfonate
Kayser-Fleischer ring, 822, 823
Kemadrin; *see* Procyclidine
Keratan sulfate, 1233
Keratinization of oral mucosa, 1107
Keratitis, 270, 907
Keratoconjunctivitis, 127, 143, 926
Keratocysts, odontogenic, 883
Keratoderma blenorrhagicum, 52, 907
Keratopathy, band, 1190
Keratosis, 913, 914
Kerion, 928
Kerley's lines, 462
Kernicterus, 1058, 1067
Kernig's sign, 839
Kernohan's notch, 767
Kerosene poisoning, 754-755
Kesso-Bamate; *see* Meprobamate
Kessodrate; *see* Chloral hydrate
Ketamine, convulsions and, 866
Ketoacidosis, 599-600
  alcohol and, 1256, 1270-1271
  diabetic, 1269-1270, 1271
  lactic acidosis and, 1271
Ketoconazole, 278, 928, 929
  acrodermatitis enteropathica and, 895
  candidiasis and, 276, 308, 929, 938
  coccidioidomycosis and, 275
  histoplasmosis and, 275
Ketogenic diets, 806
Ketones, 598; *see also* Ketoacidosis
Ketosis, starvation, 1271; *see also* Ketoacidosis
Kidney, 590-593
  aldosterone and, 1155
  angiography of, 606, 607, 657, 661-662
  antimicrobials and, 158
    aminoglycoside, 166
    cephaloridine and, 164-165
    methenamine hippurate in, 171
    methenamine mandelate in, 171
    nalidixic acid in, 161, 171
    nitrofurantoin in, 171
    sulfonamide, 169
  biopsy of, 72, 608, 638
  blood flow through, 592; *see also* Renal artery; Renal vein
    heart failure and, 461-462
    obstructive uropathy and, 655
    pregnancy and, 663-664

Kidney—cont'd
  blood flow through—cont'd
    shock and, 477, 478
  blood pressure and, 467, 468; *see also* Hypertension, kidney injury and
  calcitonin and, 1189
  clearance measurements for, 603-604; *see also* specific test
  clinical assessment of, 603-605
  concentrating ability of, 604
  cortisol and, 1154
  diabetes mellitus and, 617, 1274
  disease of; *see* Kidney diseases
  diuretics and; *see* Diuretics
  double, 650
  fluid loss and, 596
  heart failure and, 462
  liver disease and, 1064
  medullary sponge, 653
  parathyroid hormone and, 1187
  potassium and, 593
  scans of, 607-608
  sodium and, 591-592
  systemic sclerosis and, 60
  tests for; *see* Tests for kidney disease
  transplantation of; *see* Renal transplantation
  ultrasound of, 607
  water handled by, 591-592
Kidney diseases, 588-666; *see also* Kidney; Nephropathy
  acid-base metabolism disturbances in, 593-603; *see also* Acidosis; Alkalosis
    homeostasis and, 592-593
  anomalies in, orofacial abnormalities and, 668
  cutaneous signs of, 896-897
  cysts and cystic diseases in, 470, 651-653
  dentistry and, 666-671
  diabetes insipidus and, 621-622
  dialysis in; *see* Dialysis
  electrolyte disturbances in, 593-603
  endocarditis and, 181
  fluid disturbances in, 593-603
  glucose-6-phosphate dehydrogenase deficiency and, 330
  hematuria in, 588-589; *see also* Hematuria
  hypertension and; *see* Hypertension, kidney injury and
  hyporeninemic hypoaldosteronism in, 623
  interstitial nephritis in, 619-621
  ischemia in, 631
    hypertension and, 660-662
  kidney structure and function in, 590-593; *see also* Kidney
  liver disease and, 1064
  malformations in, 649-651
    orofacial abnormalities and, 668
  neoplasms in, 449, 656-659
    diagnosis and, 607, 608
    jaw metastasis and, 668
  nephrolithiasis in; *see* Kidney stones
  nephropathy in; *see* Nephropathy
  obstructive uropathy in, 653-656; *see also* Obstructive uropathy
  oral manifestations of, 666-668
  osteodystrophy and, 636-637, 639, 1200-1201
  pain in, 951
  in pregnancy, 663-666
  primary glomerular disease in, 608-614
  proteinuria in, 589-590; *see also* Proteinuria
  pyuria in, 590
  renal failure in; *see* Renal failure
  renal tubular acidosis in, 622-623
  sickle cell anemia and, 333

Kidney diseases—cont'd
  site of injury in, 588
  systemic disease and, 615-619
    lupus erythematosus and, 55
    systemic sclerosis and, 60
    tuberculosis in, 256
    Wegener's granulomatosis in, 71
  tests for, 603-608, 632-633
  transplantation in; *see* Renal transplantation
  vascular disorders in, 660-663
Kidney stones, 646-649
  Crohn's disease and, 1012
  inhibitors of, 646
  obstructive uropathy and, 656
  uric acid, 92, 94, 648
Killer cells, 15, 154
Killip classification, 535
Kinetics
  neutrophil, 355-356
  tumor cell, 439
Kinins, 17, 18
  sodium reabsorption and, 592
Kissing disease, 132
Klatskin tumor, 1089
Klebsiella, 238; *see also Klebsiella-Enterobacter*
  leukemia and, 421
  lung abscess and, 698, 700
  oral lesions of, 306
  pneumonia and, 176
Klebsiella pneumoniae, 171, 172, 173, 176
Klebsiella-Enterobacter; *see also Klebsiella*
  bacteremia and, 239
  disseminated intravascular coagulation and, 412
  drugs for, 164, 165, 166, 170, 171
  immunodeficiency diseases and, 31
  neoplasia and, 446
Kleine-Levin syndrome, 770
Klinefelter's syndrome, 1170, 1214, 1224
Klippel-Feil syndrome, 811
Klippel-Trenaunay syndrome, 881, 882
KM; *see* Kanamycin
Knees, 84, 567
Kniest syndrome, 1245
Koebner phenomenon, 936, 937
Köhlmeier-Degos disease, 893-894, 1003
Koilonychia, iron deficiency anemia and, 416
Koplik's spots, 145, 146, 300
Korotkoff sounds, 466
Korsakoff's psychosis, 772, 849-850, 1108, 1257
  thalamus lesions and, 759
Kostman's syndrome, 360
Krabbe's disease, 802, 1231, 1233
Krukenberg's tumor, 1035
KS; *see* Keratan sulfate
Kugelberg-Welander disease, 804-805
Kupffer's cells
  hepatitis and, 1071
  hyperplasia of, 1074, 1076
  iron in, 1081
Kuru, 828
Kussmaul's sign, pericarditis and, 585
Kussmaul respirations, 1269
Kveim test, 77, 718, 911
Kwashiorkor, 1104
Kynex; *see* Sulfamethoxypyridazine
Kyphoscoliosis, 712, 737
Kyphosis, 48, 50, 737

L

Labyrinthine diseases, 792-793
Lacrimal gland inflammation, 36
Lactase deficiency, 947, 1004-1005, 1027, 1028

Lactate, intracellular, 534
Lactated Ringer's solution, 205, 350
Lactation, 1118
Lactic acid; *see also* Lactic acidosis
  alcohol and, 1256
  hyperuricemia and, 90
  respiratory alkalosis and, 601
Lactic acidosis, 600, 1267, 1271
Lactic dehydrogenase
  liver disease and, 1065
  myocardial infarction and, 535
  neuromuscular disorders and, 853
  pleural effusion and, 731
    polymyositis and, 65
    renal cell carcinoma and, 657
Lactobacillus, 249, 302
Lactoferrin, 172, 356
Lactose intolerance, 1004-1005, 1028
Lactosyl ceramidosis, 1231, 1232
Lactulose, 1084
Lacunar cells, 388
Lacunar syndromes, 835
Laennec's cirrhosis, 1257
Lamina dura, hyperparathyroidism and, 1208
Lamina propria, 941, 973
Lancefield's group D enterococci, 181
Landing's disease, 1230, 1231
Langhans' giant cells, 76, 254
Language-processing cortex, 771-772
LAP score; *see* Leukocyte alkaline phosphatase score
Laparoscopy, 966
Laparotomy
  exploratory, 120
  Hodgkin's disease and, 389
  ovarian neoplasms and, 1178
Laplace's law, 460, 565, 1017
Large intestines; *see* Intestines, large
Larva migrans, 721
Laryngeal nerve, recurrent, 1127, 1128
Laryngotracheobronchitis, 142, 143
Larynx
  acromegaly and, 1204
  edema of, 17, 25-26, 351
  parainfluenza viruses and, 142, 143
  tuberculosis of, 256
Laser
  diabetic retinopathy and, 1274
  for gastrointestinal hemorrhage, 963
  hereditary hemorrhagic telangiectasia and, 1024
  skin pigmentations and, 1095
Latency, viral, 121
Lateral leads, 483
Lateral medullary syndrome, 835
Lateral pterygoid muscle pain, 109
Lateral sclerosis, amyotrophic, 803-804
Lateropulsion, 813
Latex fixation test, 77
LATS; *see* Long-acting thyroid stimulator
LATS-P; *see* Long-acting thyroid stimulator-protector
Laurence-Moon-Bordet-Biedl syndrome, 498, 1172
Laws
  Boyle's, 679
  Cannon's, 976
  Courvoisier's, 1088
  Frank-Starling, 454, 456, 457, 458; *see also* Laws, Starling's ascites and, 1044
  Hardy-Weinberg, 1218
  Laplace's, 460, 565, 1017
  Mendel's, 1217
  Ohm's, 751

Laws—cont'd
  Starling's, 688; *see also* Laws, Frank-Starling
    respiratory failure and, 709, 710
Laxatives; *see also* specific agent
  abuse of, 956, 1027
  diarrhea and, 954
  hypokalemia and, 597
  myocardial infarction and, 537
  pregnancy and, 1212
  urine and, 589
Lazy leukocyte syndrome, 357, 420
LCAT; *see* Lecithin: cholesterol acyltransferase
LCM; *see* Lymphocytic choriomeningitis virus
LD Hodgkin's disease; *see* Lymphocyte depletion Hodgkin's disease
LDH; *see* Lactic dehydrogenase
LDL; *see* Low-density lipoproteins
LE; *see* Lupus erythematosus
LE cell; *see* Lupus erythematosus cell
Lead
  gout and, 91, 622
  interstitial nephritis and, 619, 620
  poisoning from, 325, 753, 853
  toxic nephropathy and, 624, 625, 627, 630, 631
  urinary, 753
Lead colic, 753
Lead line on teeth, 753
Lead sulfide on teeth, 753
Learned behavior, 763
Lecithin, 817, 946
Lecithin: cholesterol acyltransferase, 1281, 1282, 1283, 1286
  deficiency of
    familial, 1292-1293
    liver disease and, 1063, 1065, 1286
Lecithin/sphingomyelin ratio, 1271
Left atrial hypertrophy, 500
Left ventricle; *see also* Ventricles
  aneurysmectomy and, 540
  ejection fraction of, 459, 488-489
  end-diastolic pressure and, 459
  enlargement of; *see also* Ventricular hypertrophy
    aortic regurgitation and, 515
    aortic stenosis and, 514
    cardiomyopathy and, 521-522
    electrocardiogram and, 500
  failure of, 459, 470, 534
  outflow resistance and, 460
Left ventricular failure, 459, 470, 534
Left-to-right shunts, 501, 502-505
Leg; *see also* Extremities
  bursitis in, 99
  external rotation of, 766
  myofascial syndromes and, 98
  rheumatic disorders of, 102
  ulcerations of, 333
Legg-Calvé-Perthes disease, 104
Legionella pneumophilia, 167, 171, 172, 177
Legionnaires' disease, 171, 172, 177
  differential diagnosis of, 217
  drugs for, 167
  psittacosis and, 216
Leiomyomas
  of esophagus, 1031-1032
  of large bowel, 1039
  renal, 656
  of small bowel, 1037
  of stomach, 1034
Leiomyosarcomas, 1037, 1042
Leishmaniasis, 343
Lens, evaluation of, 8
Lentigo, oral cavity and, 919

Lentigo maligna, 916
Leonine facies, 262, 304
Lepromatous leprosy, 262, 304-305; see also Leprosy
Lepromin skin test, 262
Leprosy, 261-263, 264
    dentistry and, 304-305
    neuropathy and, 855
Leptomeninges, 186
Leptospira icterohaemorrhagiae, 273
Leptospira interrogans, 273
Leptospirosis, 273-274
Leriche's syndrome, 569-570
Lesch-Nyhan syndrome, 316, 1227, 1239
Leser-Trélat sign, 912, 913
Letterer-Siwe disease, 397, 718
Leucine, defective decarboxylation and, 1237, 1238
Leucine aminopeptidase, 1065
Leucovorin, 286, 440
Leukapheresis, 346, 368
Leukemia-associated antigens, 365
Leukemias, 363-372
    acute, 363, 364-369
        lymphoblastic, 364, 365, 366-367
        myeloblastic, 353
        myelogenous, 364, 365, 366, 367-368
        oral lesions of, 306
        undifferentiated, 365
    basophilic, 369
    chronic
        blastic transformation and, 370
        lymphocytic, 370-372
        myelogenous, 363, 365, 366, 369-370
        neutrophilic, 362
    dentistry and, 420-422
    eosinophilic, 363, 369
    granulocytic, 373
    meningitis and, 368
    minimal residual disease and, 363
    myelogenous, 373
        acute, 364, 365, 366, 367-368
        chloroma and, 898
        chronic, 363, 365, 366, 369-370
    neutropenia and, 358
    neutrophilic, chronic, 362
    radiation and, 750
    remission of, 366
    skin lesions of, 898-899
    viruses and, 131, 433
Leukemic cells, 364, 368
Leukemic infiltrates, oral signs of, 421
Leukemids, 899
Leukemoid reactions, 361-362
Leukocyte alkaline phosphatase, 353, 369
Leukocyte alkaline phosphatase score, 369
Leukocytes, 358
    alcohol and, 1258
    cerebrospinal fluid, 32
    evaluation of, 32
    fecal, 203
    increase in; *see* Leukocytosis
    lazy, syndrome of, 357, 420
    normal, 358
        fewer than; *see* Leukopenia
    polymorphonuclear; *see* Polymorphonuclear leukocytes
    transfusions of, 347, 361
        bacteremia and, 241
        in leprosy, 263
        leukemias and, 368
        multiple myeloma and, 382
    viremia in, 145
Leukocytosis, 32

Leukocytosis—cont'd
    amebic liver abscess and, 282
    appendicitis and, 1016
    bacterial infection and, 119
    chronic idiopathic, 362
    diverticulosis and, 1017
    eosinophilic; *see* Eosinophilia
    infectious mononucleosis and, 132
    Kawasaki disease and, 148
    nongonococcal septic arthritis and, 80
    Norwalk-like agents and, 150
    pleural fluid, 731-732
    polycythemia vera and, 353
    rat-bite fever and, 272
    reactive, 361
Leukodystrophy
    fibrinoid, 803
    globoid cell, 802, 1231, 1233
    metachromatic, 801-802, 1231, 1232-1233
    sudanophilic, 802
Leukoencephalpathy, progressive multifocal, 828, 868
Leukoerythroblastic peripheral blood changes, 322
Leukopenia
    bacteremia and, 241
    cytomegalovirus and, 300
    drug allergy and, 29
    liver disease and, 1064
    lupus erythematosus and, 56, 111
    penicillins and, 164
    refractory anemia and, 320, 321
    splenomegaly and, 396
Leukoplakia, 303
Levamisole
    mycosis fungoides and, 901
    Reiter's syndrome and, 908
    tumors and, 445
Levarterenol bitartrate, 29
Levator ani, 948
LeVeen shunt, 1046
Levodopa
    chorea and, 816
    dystonia musculorum deformans and, 821
    Gilles de la Tourette's syndrome and, 822
    growth hormone and, 1123
    immune hemolysis and, 342
    oropharyngeal dysphagia and, 976
    parkinsonism and, 814-815
    postural hypotension and, 780, 824
    side effects of, 871
    urinary catecholamines and, 1168
Levorphanol, 446
Levo-thyroxine, 1139; *see also* Thyroxine
Levo-triiodothyronine, 1139; *see also* Triiodothyronine
Lewis substance, 1035
Lewy bodies, 824
Leydig cells, 1168, 1169
LGV; *see* Lymphogranuloma venereum
LH; *see* Luteinizing hormone
Lhermitte's sign, 799
L'homme rouge, 900
LHRH; *see* Luteinizing hormone-releasing hormone
Librium; *see* Chlordiazepoxide
Libritabs; *see* Chlordiazepoxide
Lichen planus, 939-940
    anal disorders and, 1030
    chronic discoid lupus erythematosus and, 111
    premalignant lesions and, 919
    riboflavin deficiency and, 1109
Lichenoid amyloid, 386
Licorice, 598, 600, 1160

Liddle's syndrome, 1160
Lidocaine
    acute herpetic gingivostomatitis and, 299
    allergy and, 28
    antidepressant overdose and, 779
    arrhythmias and, 500, 548, 585
    liver disease and, 1090
    multiple sclerosis and, 869
    myocardial infarction and, 537
    and oral lesions, 299, 876
        of Crohn's disease, 1097
        of Plummer-Vinson syndrome, 1091
        of radiation stomatitis, 919
        of Reiter's syndrome, 908
        of ulcerative colitis, 1096
    pregnancy and, 1212
    seizures and, 787, 866
Lids, evaluation of, 8
Life support, advanced, 540
Ligament of Treitz, 957, 958
Ligamentous laxity, 1241
Ligation
    of internal hemorrhoids, 1031
    patent ductus arteriosus and, 557
Light chains, 16, 377
    amyloid, 385-386
    multiple myeloma and, 380, 382
Lightning injury, 751-752
Limb; *see* Extremities; Leg
Limb-girdle muscular dystrophy, 857
Limbic system, 763
Limulus lysate assay, 188, 189
Lincomycin, 156, 158, 167, 168
    pregnancy and, 1212
Linear atelectasis, 702
Linear subcutaneous bands, 906
Lingual nerve, dysesthesia of, 667
Linitis plastica, 1035
Linkage, 1228-1229
Linoleic acid, 1104
Linolenic acid, 1104
Lioresal; *see* Baclofen
Liotrix, synthetic, 1139
LIP; *see* Lymphocytic interstitial pneumonitis
Lip; *see* Lips
Lipase, 1049, 1052
Lipemia retinalis, 1288
Lipid envelope, 121, 127
Lipid storage diseases, 358, 859
Lipid-laden cells, 1289, 1292
Lipidoses, 396-397, 582
    sulfatide, 801-802, 1231, 1232-1233
Lipids; *see also* Fats
    antibodies against, 266, 271
    coronary artery disease and, 526
    in diet, 998, 999
    excess; *see* Hyperlipidemia
    mesenteric inflammatory disease and, 1048
    pancreatitis and, 1052
    plasma, 1288-1289
    transport of, 1282-1286
    in urine, 612
Lipiduria, 612
Lipoatrophy, diabetic, 1262, 1268
Lipochrome histiocytosis, 357
Lipfuscin, 1071
Lipogranulomatosis, 1231, 1233
Lipoid nephrosis, 613
Lipolytic enzymes, 218, 945, 1049
Lipomas
    of large bowel, 1039
    mediastinal, 735
    of pancreas, 1056
β-Lipoprotein deficiency, 999, 1292

Lipoprotein lipases, 1283, 1284-1285
  familial, deficiency of, 1286-1287
  inherited absence of, 1285
Lipoprotein metabolism disorders, 1280-1293; see also Hyperlipidemia; Lipoproteins
  classification in, 1286-1287
  dentistry and, 1296
  evaluation in, 1287-1289
  familial lipoprotein deficiency disorders in, 1291-1293
  hyperlipidemia in; see Hyperlipidemia
  lipid transport in, 1282-1286
  liver disease and, 1286
  plasma apolipoproteins in, 1280-1281
  plasma lipoproteins in, 1280, 1282, 1288-1289
  skin disorders of, 889-890
Lipoprotein remnants, 1283, 1285
Lipoprotein X, 1286
Lipoproteins
  cholestasis and, 1059
  deficiency of, 999, 1291-1293
  excess; see Hyperlipoproteinemia
  high-density; see High-density lipoproteins
  intermediate density, 1283
  lipid transport by, 1282-1286
  liver disease and, 1063
  low-density; see Low-density lipoproteins
  metabolism disorders of; see Lipoprotein metabolism disorders
  plasma, 1280, 1282, 1288-1289
    degradation of, 1282
    electrophoretic mobility of, 1281
    formation of, 1282
    sampling of, 1288-1289
  triglyceride-rich, 1284-1285
  very-low-density, 1280-1292
    defect in catabolism of, 1285
    increased plasma concentration of, 1286
Lipoteichoic acid, 223
β-Lipotropin, 1115
Lips
  acanthosis nigricans and, 888, 1093
  actinic keratosis of, 918
  acute herpetic gingivostomatitis and, 298, 299
  Behçet's disease and, 907
  biopsy of, 37
  bumpy, 1164
  chronic discoid lupus erythematosus and, 111
  cleft, 1228, 1317, 1318
  cobblestone appearance of, Urbach-Wiethe disease and, 1296
  evaluation of, 9
  fibrous growth on, tuberous sclerosis and, 880
  furuncles of, 306
  Gaucher's disease and, 1296
  lichen planus and, 938
  melanotic macule of, 919
  neurofibromas and, 879
  paresthesia of, Epstein-Barr virus and, 300
  Peutz-Jeghers syndrome and, 1095
  Plummer-Vinson syndrome and, 1091, 1105
  protein malnutrition and, 1104
  scleroderma and, 112, 903
  telangiectasia and, 894, 1095
  tubercular lesions of, 304
  vascular formations of, 1092
  vitamin deficiencies and, 1108
Liquid exchange diet, 1268
Liquid nitrogen, 927, 928
Listeria; see Listeriosis
Listeria monocytogenes, 246
  in endocarditis, 179
  immunodeficiency diseases and, 31
  meningitis and, 186, 187
Listeriosis, 246
  aseptic meningoencephalitis and, 139
  endocarditis and, 179
  Hodgkin's disease and, 387
  renal transplantation and, 645
Lithiasis; see Calculi
Lithium
  antidiuresis from neoplasms and, 1181
  cluster headache and, 789
  colony-stimulating factor and, 361
  diabetes insipidus and, 621, 1125
  hypernatremia and, 595
  neurologic effects of, 779
  renal tubular acidosis and, 623
  thyroid function and, 1130, 1132
  toxic nephropathy and, 625, 627, 629
Lithocholic acid, 1085
Liver, 1057-1085
  abscesses of, 1074-1075
    amebic, 282, 283
    appendicitis and, 1016
    hydatid cysts and, 294
    radionuclide imaging and, 967
  adenomas of, 1084
  alcohol and; see Alcohol, liver disease and
  amebiasis and, 282, 283
  antimicrobials and, 158
  ascites and, 1044
  bacterial disease of, 1074
  bilirubin metabolism and, 1057-1058
    disorders of, 1067-1068
  biopsy of; see Biopsy of liver
  black pigmentation of, 1068
  blood transfusions and, 350
  carcinoma and, 1084
    renal cell, 657
  changes in size or consistency of, 1059; see also Hepatomegaly
  cholecystitis and, 1088
  cirrhosis of; see Cirrhosis
  coagulation disorders and, 411
  congestion of, 1077-1078
  dentistry and, 1097-1101
  detoxification in, 1061-1062
  diagnosis and, 965-967, 1064-1067
    alkaline phosphatase and, 1065, 1066, 1068, 1071
    angiography in, 971
    carcinoembryonic antigen and, 435
    cardiac index and, 1064
    computed tomography in, 971
    fever of unknown origin in, 120
    microbial disease in, 119
    radionuclide imaging in, 966-967, 1078
    serum enzymes and, 1065
    ultrasound in, 970
  drug-induced disease and, 1075-1076, 1090
  enlargement of; see Hepatomegaly
  enzymes and, 1065
  examination of, 13
  fatty, 1063, 1077
    alcohol and, 1080, 1256, 1257
  fibrosis of; see Fibrosis of liver
  glucose production in, 1276
  granulomas and, 1084
  heart failure and, 462
  heme synthesis and, 1247-1248
  hepatomas of; see Hepatomas
  hydatid cysts and, 294
  hyperlipidemia and, 889-890
  infiltrations in, 1084
  inflammation of; see Hepatitis
  isoniazid toxicity and, 259, 260
  lipoprotein metabolism and, 1286
Liver—cont'd
  malnutrition and, 1103
  neoplasms of, 1066, 1084
    carcinoembryonic antigen and, 435
    radionuclide imaging and, 966-967
    renal cell carcinoma and, 657
  pain and, 951
    ulcer, 989
  perfusion of
    decreased, 1045, 1060, 1077-1078
    vascular resistance and, 1060
  porphyria and, 888, 1253
  schistosomiasis and, 296
  sickle cell anemia and, 333
  skin disorders and, 896, 1058-1059
  steroid metabolism and, 1154
  structure and function of, 945-946
  symptoms and, 1057-1064; see also Jaundice
  systemic sclerosis and, 60
  tenderness of, 1059
  toxic disease of, 1075-1076
  transplantation and, 34
  ulcerative colitis and, 1008
  Weil's disease and, 273
Liver function tests, 1064-1065
Liver palms, 896, 1059
Liver scans, 966-967, 1078
Liver transplants, 34
Local anesthetics
  adhesive capsulitis and, 101
  allergy to, 29-30
  arrhythmias and, 585
  coronary heart disease and, 583
  costochondritis and, 100
  diabetes and, 1295
  fibrositis and, 97
  hemolysis and, 342
  hemophilia and, 427
  hepatitis and, 1099
  herpangina and, 301
  hypertension and, 574
  hyperthyroidism and, 1105, 1205
  kidney disease and, 669-670
  multiple sclerosis and, 869
  myofascial pain dysfunction and, 109
  pregnancy and, 1212, 1213
  thoracic outlet syndromes and, 101
Local epigenetic factors, 1306
Locked-in syndrome, 764, 833
Locus minoris resistentiae, 299
Löffgren's syndrome, 77, 78, 716, 925
Löffler's syndrome, 372, 721
  cardiomyopathies and, 522
  eosinophilia and, 362
  pleural effusion and, 732
Lomustine, 442, 918
Long-acting thyroid stimulator, 19, 1143
Long-acting thyroid stimulator-protector, 1143
Longitudinal system, 454
Long-term memory, 773
Loop diuretics, 572, 574; see also Diuretics
Looser's zones, 1199
Loperamide, 1014, 1029
Lorazepam, 871, 1297
Lou Gehrig's disease, 803-804, 868, 869
Louis-Bar syndrome, 882
Louse-borne typhus fever, 212, 213-214
Lover's heel, 52
Low-density lipoproteins, 1280-1292
  defective catabolism of, 1285-1286
  increased plasma concentration of, 1286
Lower back stiffness, 48
Lower extremities; see Extremities; Leg
Lower half headache, 791

Lower nephron nephrosis, 630
Lown grading, 540
Low-residue diet, 1014
Low-salt antacids, 992
Low-triiodothyronine syndrome, 1131
LP Hodgkin's disease; *see* Lymphocyte predominance Hodgkin's disease
LPL; *see* Lipoprotein lipases
LRH; *see* Luteinizing hormone-releasing hormone
LSD; *see* Lysergic acid diethylamide; Lysosomal storage disease
LTA; *see* Lipoteichoic acid
Lues, meningovascular, 842; *see also* Syphilis
Luft's syndrome, 1146-1147
Lumbar disc syndrome, 48, 50, 860
Lumbar puncture, 762; *see also* Cerebrospinal fluid
  brain tumor and, 847
  headache from, 790
  seizures and, 785
Lumbosacral canal stenosis, 860
Lumbosacral spondylosis, 860
Lumpy jaw, 305
Lung; *see also* Respiratory diseases
  abscess of, 698-700
    anaerobic, 178
    dentistry and, 746
    hydatid cysts and, 294
  atelectasis of; *see* Atelectasis
  benign tumors of, 743
  biopsy of; *see* Biopsy, lung
  brain abscesses and, 191
  categorization of disease of, 680
  cysts of, 700, 701, 747
  diffuse disease of, 713-723
    dentistry and, 747
    drug-induced, 721-722
    eosinophilic, 363, 372-373, 721
    familial, 721
    fibrosis in, 713-716, 722, 725, 726
    hemorrhagic, 611, 720-721
    hemosiderosis in, 720-721
    interstitial, of unknown cause, 716-719; *see also* Interstitial lung diseases
    radiation pneumonitis in, 722
    relapsing polychondritis in, 102-103
    vasculitides in, 719-720
  edema of; *see* Pulmonary edema
  elastic recoil of, 691
  emboli in; *see* Pulmonary emboli
  evaluation of, 12, 685
  fibrosis of; *see* Fibrosis of lungs
  fluid loss and, 596
  histoplasmosis and, 179, 183, 274-275, 278
  honeycomb, 726
  hyperinflation of, 694
  infiltrates in; *see* Pulmonary infiltrates
  inflammations of; *see* Pneumonia; Pneumonitis
  influenza and, 141
  interstitial disease of; *see* Interstitial lung diseases
  lymphangitis carcinomatosis of, 743-744
  malignancies of, 738-742
    asbestos and, 727
    ectopic Cushing's syndrome and, 1157, 1159
    histology and, 434
    infiltrates in, 740
    lymphangitic carcinomatosis in, 743-744
    management of, 447
    metastatic, 743-744
    middle lobe syndrome and, 703
    primary, 738-742

Lung—cont'd
  parenchymal disease of, 171, 685, 696
    congestive heart failure and, 454
    emboli and, 490
    emphysema and, 694
    sarcoidosis and, 717
    pneumocystosis and, 287-288; *see also Pneumocystis; Pneumocystis carinii*
  quiet zone of, 680
  resection of; *see* Thoracotomy
  scanning of, 687
    pulmonary embolism and, 492, 493, 687
  shock, 240, 477, 708; *see also* Adult respiratory distress syndrome
  sickle cell anemia and, 332
  sounds of, 12, 685
  systemic sclerosis and, 59, 60
  tomograms of, 686
  tumors of, 685, 738-744; *see also* Lung, malignancies of
  unilateral hyperlucent, 686
  volumes and capacities of, 677, 680
  Wegener's granulomatosis and, 71
Lung scans, 686
  pulmonary embolism and, 492, 493, 687
Lung sounds, 12, 684-685
Lung water, 708-709
Lung white-out, 709
Lupus anticoagulant, 412
Lupus band test, 54
Lupus erythematosus
  Bloom's syndrome and, 882
  chronic discoid, 57, 111
  cutaneous lesions of, 902-903
  dentistry and, 111-112
  drug-induced, 57
  endocarditis and, 182
  systemic, 53-58
    aplastic anemia and, 319
    cutaneous lesions of, 902-903
    dentistry and, 111-112
    esophageal motility disorders and, 981
    hypertension and, 474
    intestinal vasculitis and, 1022
    neuropathy and, 854
    pregnancy and, 666
    pulmonary fibrosis and, 715
    renal lesions and, 615
Lupus erythematosus cell, 54, 56, 57
Lupus pernio, 716, 910
Luteinizing hormone, 1118, 1169, 1170
  deficiency of, 1121-1122, 1172
  feedback mechanisms and, 1175
  menopause and, 1176
  menstrual cycle and, 1174-1175
  ovarian dysfunction and, 1177
Luteinizing hormone-releasing hormone, 1118
LVH; *see* Left ventricle, enlargement of
Lye, 754, 985, 986
Lyell's disease, 931-932
Lyme disease, 297-298
  arthritis in, 82
  erythema chronicum migrans and, 925, 926
Lymph, 1044
Lymph node syndrome, mucocutaneous, 69
Lymph nodes; *see also* Lymphadenopathy
  biopsies of, 31, 689; *see also* Mediastinoscopy
  enlarged; *see also* Adenopathy; Lymphadenopathy
    infectious mononucleosis and, 132
    lymphocytic leukemias and, 371
    mediastinal, 735
    varicella-zoster and, 130
  filariasis and, 292

Lymph nodes—cont'd
  inflammation of; *see* Lymphadenitis
  of neck, superficial, 9-10
  resected, 151, 918
  toxoplasmosis and, 285
Lymphadenitis; *see also* Adenopathy; Lymphadenopathy
  chronic granulomatous disease and, 357
  nontuberculous mycobacteria and, 261
  plague and, 242
  tuberculous, 255, 304
Lymphadenopathy; *see also* Adenopathy; Lymph nodes
  acute necrotizing ulcerative gingivitis and, 302
  cancer detection and, 434
  cat-scratch fever and, 151
  cervical; *see* Cervical lymphadenopathy
  chronic granulomatous disease and, 357
  Hodgkin's disease and, 388-390
  mycosis fungoides and, 900
  plague and, 242
  sickle cell anemia and, 333
  syphilis and, 267
  trypanosomiasis and, 287
Lymphangiectasia, 941, 999
Lymphangiography, 120, 389, 390
Lymphangiomas of pancreas, 1056
Lymphangitic carcinomatosis of lung, 743-744
Lymphatic transport disorders, 1003
Lymphoblastic leukemias, acute, 363, 364, 365, 366-367
Lymphoblastic lymphoma, 392
Lymphocyte depletion Hodgkin's disease, 388
Lymphocyte predominance Hodgkin's disease, 388
Lymphocytes, 15-16, 371
  atypical, 119, 132
  B; *see* Bone marrow–derived cells
  bronchiolitis and, 141
  Hodgkin's disease and, 388
  immune system and, 376
  increase in, 371-372
  influenza and, 141
  interferon and, 154
  lymphocytic leukemia and, 363, 370-372, 898
  lymphomas and, 392, 393
  meningitis and, 825
  multiple sclerosis and, 797
  non-Hodgkin's lymphoma and, 392
  normal count of, 371
  pneumonitis and, 715
  thyroiditis and; *see* Lymphocytic thyroiditis
Lymphocytic choriomeningitis virus, 138
Lymphocytic interstitial pneumonitis, 715
Lymphocytic leukemia, chronic, 363, 370-372, 898
Lymphocytic lymphomas, 392, 393
Lymphocytic thyroiditis, 1141
  chronic, 1149-1150
  Graves' disease and, 1143
  with hyperthyroidism, 1146
Lymphogranuloma venereum, 216, 302
Lymphoid hyperplasia, 134
Lymphokines, 15, 27, 32
Lymphomas
  Burkitt's, 131, 132, 300, 393
  Crohn's disease and, 1012
  dentistry and, 424
  differential diagnosis in, 195
  diffuse, 392, 393
  Hodgkin's disease and; *see* Hodgkin's disease
  intestinal, 1002, 1037, 1041
  of liver, 1084
  lung and, 743

Lymphomas—cont'd
  lymphoblastic, 392
  lymphocytic, 392, 393
  malabsorption and, 1002
  meningitis and, 139
  nodular, 392, 393
  non-Hodgkin's, 391-394
    dentistry and, 424
    neutropenia and, 358
  skin lesions of, 899-900
  of stomach, 1036-1037
Lymphomatoid granulomatosis
  cellular infiltrates and, 67-69
  cutaneous lesions of, 906
  management of, 69
  vasculitis and, 67-69
Lymphomatous meningitis, 139
Lymphoproliferative disorders; see also specific disorder
  lung and, 743
  warm-reacting autoimmune hemolytic anemia and, 338
Lyon hypothesis, 1219
Lysergic acid diethylamide, 778, 829, 862
Lysine, 600, 1239
Lysine-vasopressin nasal spray, 1126
Lysinuria, 1239
Lysis, host cell, 143
Lysolecithin, 1051
Lysosomal enzymes, 17, 18, 90
Lysosomal storage disease, 396, 397, 1226, 1230-1235
  Chédiak-Higashi syndrome and, 397
  Gaucher's disease and, 396
Lysozyme, 172
Lysyl oxidase, 1240, 1243
Lysyl-hydroxylase structural defect, 1302

M

M protein, 223, 377
M protein antigen, 609
Macleod's syndrome, 686
Macroamylasemia, 1053
Macrocytosis, 316, 317-318
Macrodantin; see Nitrofurantoin
Macroglobulinemia, 382-384, 423, 618
Macroglobulins, increased, 382; see also Macroglobulinemia
Macroglossia
  amyloidosis and, 422, 423
  neurofibromatosis and, 869, 879
  Urbach-Wiethe disease and, 1296
Macrophage inhibition factor, 32
Macrophages, 17
  alveolar, 172, 686
  hemosiderin-laden, lung disease and, 720
  inhibiting factor for, 32
  interferons and, 154
  production of, 355
  T cells and, 15
Macropsia, 783
Macroscopic slide agglutination test, 273-274
Macular sparing, 759
Macules
  cherry red, telangiectasia and, 1095
  coal, 725
  lanceotate leaf-shaped, 880
  melanotic, 919
  pigmented, Peutz-Jeghers syndrome and, 1093-1095
  syphilis and, 303
Maculopathy, 1274
Maculourticarial erythema multiforme, 923
Maduromycosis, 277

Magnesium
  alcohol and, 1256
  in antacids, 992
  Crohn's disease and, 1015
  deficiency of; see Hypomagnesemia
  hypoparathyroidism and, 1196
  malabsorption and, 1000
  pancreatitis and, 1052
Magnesium hydroxide, 415, 451, 1212
Magnesium sulfate, 665, 1088
Main en lorgnette, 51
Malabsorption, 998-1005; see also Nutrition
  acrodermatitis enteropathica and, 895
  Crohn's disease and, 1012
  cystic fibrosis and, 1101
  folic acid deficiency and, 1109, 1110
  lymphangiectasia and, 999, 1003
  lymphoma and, 1002
Malar hypoplasia, 1309, 1310
Malaria, 279-281
  blood transfusions and, 347, 348
  disseminated intravascular coagulation and, 412
  meningoencephalitis and, 139
  ring form of, 281
Malayan filariasis, 292
Male genitalia, 1168-1173; see also Genitalia
  evaluation of, 13
  tuberculosis in, 256
Male karyotype, 1220
Male pseudohermaphroditism, 1171
Male puberty, oral manifestations of, 1214
Male Turner's syndrome, 1170-1171
Malformation complex, 1301
Malformation syndrome, 1228, 1301
Malformations
  Arnold-Chiari, 807, 811
  arteriovenous; see Arteriovenous malformations
  craniofacial, 1300-1322; see also Craniofacial malformations
  definition of, 1301
  normal standards and, 1301
  or urinary tract, 649-651, 654, 655
  viruses and congenital, 125
Malignancy; see also Neoplasia
  cutaneous signs of, 912-913
  endocrine syndrome with, 1179
  hematologic, 302, 322
  hypercalcemia of, 657, 1179-1180, 1192
  of lung; see Lung, malignancies of
  of mast cells, 26
  middle lobe syndrome and, 703
  oral candidiasis and, 307
  polymyositis and, 64-65
  pulmonary embolism and, 490
  after renal transplantation, 645
  skin neoplasms and, 914-922
  of testes, hypogonadism and, 1170, 1171
Malignant acanthosis, 887-888
Malignant atrophic papulosis, 893-894; see also Degos' disease
Malignant effusions, 445, 688, 731, 732
Malignant hyperpyrexia, 858
Malignant hypertension, 469
  hemolysis and, 341
  systemic sclerosis and, 60, 616
Malignant hyperthermia, 858, 875
Malignant melanomas of mouth, 919
Malignant mesothelioma, pleural, 726-727, 734
Malignant pleural effusion, 445, 688, 731, 732
Malignant retinopathy, 1274
Mallory's bodies, 1257
Mallory-Weiss syndrome, 986-987

Mallory-Weiss tears, 958, 959
Malnutrition, 1102-1104; see also Nutrition
  alcoholism and, 1001, 1059, 1062-1063, 1080
  testes and, 1172
Malocclusion
  acromegaly and, 1204
  hyperparathyroidism and, 1208
  Klinefelter's syndrome and, 1214
  thalassemia and, 418
Malposition of mandible, developmental, 861
Malt worker's lung, 727
Maltase deficiency, acid, 858
Maltese crosses, 605, 612, 912
Mammary artery, grafts of internal, 532
Mammography, 434
Mandible
  fracture of, sleep apnea syndrome and, 861
  Gaucher's disease and, 1232
  hyperpituitarism and, 1204
  malformations of, 1302, 1308, 1309-1310, 1311
  malposition of, 861
  mucopolysaccharidoses and, 1235
  neurofibromatosis and, 879
  osteoporosis and, 115, 1210
  Paget's disease and, 114
  prognathism of, 878
  retrognathism of, 861
Mandibulofacial dysostosis, 1302, 1308, 1309-1310, 1311
Mannitol
  body fluid osmolality and, 596
  brain abscess and, 193
  cerebral hemorrhage and, 839
  cisplatin and, 443
  hypernatremia and, 595
  hyponatremia and, 594
  lumbar puncture and, 847
  meningitis and, 190
  myoglobinuria and, 860
  pigment nephrotoxicity and, 629
  prerenal azotemia and, 632
  in renal ischemia, 631
  sickle cell disease and, 618
  subdural empyema and, 193
  transfusion reactions and, 351
α-D-Mannosidase deficiency, 1235
Mannosidosis, 1235
Manometry of esophagus, 962
Mantle, cortical, 763
Mantoux test, 257, 260
MAO; see Maximal acid output; Monoamine oxidase
Maple bark disease, 727
Maple syrup urine disease, 1237, 1238
March hemoglobinuria, 341
Marche à petits pas, 835
Marchiafava-Bignami disease, 1257
Marchiafava-Micheli syndrome, 341-342
Marcus Gunn's pupillary sign, 798
Marfan's habitus, 581
Marfan's syndrome, 1241
  aneurysms of sinuses of Valsalva and, 558
  aortic dissection and, 560
  endocarditis and, 179
Marie-Strümpell disease, 48
Marijuana
  abuse of, 778
  contaminated, 863
  thyroxine-binding globulin and, 1134
Marker chromosomes, 364
Maroteaux-Lamy syndrome, 1233, 1234
Marrow, bone; see Bone marrow
Masklike facies, 1091

Masseter claudication, 75
Mast cells, 25, 26
　asthma and, 704, 705, 706
　immunoglobulin E and, 17
　malabsorption and, 1004
　malignancy of, 26
Mastectomy, 448
Mastication, 873-874
　insufficiency of, 872, 1103
Mastocytoma, 909
Mastocytosis, 26, 909-910
Mastoiditis, 191, 192
MAT; see Multifocal atrial tachycardia
Maternal viremia, 125
Mating possibilities, 1218, 1219
Matulane; see Procarbazine
Mauzerall and Granick column chromatography, 1251
Maxilla
　craniosynostosis syndromes and, 1313
　drug abuse and trauma to, 862
　epidermolysis bullosa dystrophica and, 878
　myofascial pain dysfunction and, 109
　neurofibromatosis and, 879
　nocturnal bruxism and, 861; see also Night guards
　osteoporosis of, 1210
　otocraniofacial syndromes and, 1310
　Paget's disease and, 114
Maxillary sinus, 277
Maxillofacial trauma, drug abuse and, 862
Maximal acid output, 944
Maximal flow rates at 25%-75% of forced expiratory vital capacity, 679
MB; see Methylene blue
MBC; see Minimal bactericidal concentration
MC Hodgkin's disease; see Mixed cellularity Hodgkin's disease
McArdle's disease, 858
McBurney's point, 1016
MCH; see Mean corpuscular hemoglobin
MCHC; see Mean corpuscular hemoglobin concentration
MCT; see Medium-chain triglycerides; Medullary carcinoma of thyroid
MCV; see Mean corpuscular volume
MEA; see Multiple endocrine neoplasias
Mean corpuscular hemoglobin, 313
Mean corpuscular hemoglobin concentration, 313, 328
Mean corpuscular volume, 313, 316, 318, 333
Measles, 145-146
　atypical, 145, 146
　central nervous system disease and, 135, 138
　dentistry and, 108, 300
　pneumonia and, 172
　subacute sclerosing panencephalitis and, 828
　vaccines for, 138, 145-146, 152
Measles virus vaccine, 152
Measles-mumps-rubella vaccine, 138
Meatus, evaluation of, 9
Mebendazole
　ascariasis and, 290
　cysticercosis and, 293
　enterobiasis and, 290
　hookworm and, 291
　hydatid cysts and, 294
　trichuriasis and, 290
Mecamylamine, 722
Mechanical ventilation; see also Intermittent positive-pressure breathing
　emphysema and, 695
　hypersensitivity pneumonitis and, 728
　perinatal virus and, 127

Mechanical ventilation—cont'd
　pneumothorax and, 733
　respiratory failure and, 709, 710
Mechlorethamine, 442
　Hodgkin's disease and, 390
　Kaposi's sarcoma and, 922
　malignant effusions and, 445
　mycosis fungoides and, 901
　neuropathy and, 853
　thrombocytopenia and, 400
　vincristine, prednisone, and procarbazine, 390, 391
Mecholyl; see Methacholine
Meckel's diverticulum, 324
Meclofenamic acid, 42
Media for culture, 119
Medial longitudinal fasciculus, 766
　syndrome of, 760, 766, 833; see also Internuclear ophthalmoplegia
Medial medullary syndrome, 835
Medial pontine syndromes, 833
Median cleft lip, 1317
Mediastinitis, 734-735
　fibrosing, 105, 555
Mediastinoscopy, 689, 718, 741
Mediastinotomy, 689
Mediastinum
　adenopathy of, 389
　aortic dissection and, 561
　disease of, 734-736
　fibrosis of, 105, 555
　incision in, 689
　inflammation of, 105, 734-735
　lung cancer and, 741
　lung cysts and, 701
　sarcoidosis and, 76, 78, 716, 717, 718
　transposition of great arteries and, 508
Medical history, 5-9
　dialogue, 1, 4
Medic-Alert bracelet, 1124
Medications; see Drugs; specific drug
Mediterranean fever, familial, 385, 1048
Medium-chain triglycerides, 999; see also Triglycerides
　lymphangiectasia and, 1003
　radiation enteritis and, 1002
Medroxyprogesterone, 712
Medulla, syndromes of, 835
Medullary bone lesions, fibrous dysplasia of jaws and, 115
Medullary carcinoma of thyroid, 1151, 1197-1198
　calcitonin and, 1189
　hyperparathyroidism and, 1192
　Sipple's syndrome and, 1164
Medullary cystic disease, 398, 653
Medullary sponge kidney, 653
Medulloblastoma, 844
Mees' lines, 853
Mefenamic acid
　asthma and, 704
　hemolysis and, 342
　nephropathy and, 621
　sensitivity to, 23
Megacolon, 1026-1027
　ulcerative colitis and, 1007, 1008, 1011
Megakaryocytes, 400, 401-402, 404
Megalencephaly, 803
Megaloblastic anemia, 316-318, 358
Megaloblasts, 316-318, 321, 358
Megalourethra, 651
Mega-syndromes, 287
Meglumine diatrizoate, 605; see also Contrast agents

Meglumine iothalamate, 605; see also Contrast agents
Meigs' syndrome, 731, 1045
Meiosis, 1217, 1221
Meissner's plexus, 942, 973
Melanin, 345, 1042, 1059
Melanocyte-stimulating hormone, 886, 1179, 1180
Melanocytic nevus, 917
Melanoma, malignant, 916-918
　of anus, 103, 1042
　management of, 450, 918
　of mouth, 919
Melanosis, oral cavity and, 919, 1214
Melanosis coli, 954
Melanosis-polyposis, 891, 958, 1042
Melanotic macule in oral cavity, 919
Melatonin, 1126
Melena, 957, 988, 996
Mellaril; see Thioridazine
Melphalan; see L-Phenylalanine mustard
Membrane potentials, 479
Membranoproliferative glomerulonephritis, 613-614
Membranous nephropathy, 613
Memory, 772, 773
MEN; see Multiple endocrine neoplasias
Mendel's laws, 1217
Menetrier's disease, 997
Mengheni needle, 965
Ménière's disease, 793, 795
Meningeal carcinomatosis, 139, 845
Meningiomas, 844
Meningitis; see also Meningoencephalitis
　aseptic, 134, 824-825
　　bacterial meningitis and, 188, 189
　　enteroviruses and, 136, 137, 144
　　evaluation of, 139
　　herpes simplex virus and, 128, 135
　　Kawasaki disease and, 147
　　lymphocytic choriomeningitis virus and, 138
　　mumps and, 137
　　varicella and, 138
　bacterial, 139, 186-191
　carcinomatous, 139, 845
　chemoprophylaxis and, 190, 191
　coccidiodomycosis and, 275
　cryptococcosis and, 275
　differential diagnosis of, 189
　echoviruses and, 144
　Haemophilus influenzae and, 236
　headache in, 790
　leptospirosis and, 273
　leukemic, 368
　lymphomatous, 139
　meningococcal, 234
　plague and, 242
　syphilitic, 139, 268, 269, 842
　tuberculous, 139, 189, 255, 256-257, 260
Meningitis-cerebritis syndrome, 187
Meningococcemia; see also Meningococci
　acute fulminant, 234
　disseminated intravascular coagulation and, 412
　without meningitis, 234
Meningococci, 233-235; see also Meningococcemia
　drugs for, 168
　endocarditis and, 184
　immunodeficiency diseases and, 31
　meningitis and, 186, 187
　splenectomy and, 329, 395
　vaccine for, 233

Meningoencephalitis, 134, 139, 824; *see also* Meningitis
  amebic, 283
  Lyme disease and, 297
  syphilis and, 139, 268, 269, 842
Menkes' kinky hair syndrome, 1240
Menopausal gonadotropins, human, 1045, 1173
Menopause, 1176, 1177, 1213
Menorrhagia, 407
Menstrual cycle, 1174-1175
  iron deficiency anemia and, 324
  oral changes and, 1210-1211
  pneumothorax and, 733
Mental nerve, neuropathy of, 417
Mental retardation
  cytomegalovirus and, 125
  epilepsy, and adenoma sebaceum, triad of, 880
  hypogonadism and, 1170
  rubella and, 126, 146
Mental status evaluation, 14, 773
Mentation, 762, 845
MEOS; *see* Microsomal ethanol oxidizing system
Meperidine
  abuse of, 778
  diverticulosis and, 1017
  hypothyroidism and, 1206
  mastocystosis and, 910
  myocardial infarction and, 537
  neoplasia and, 446
  pancreatitis and, 1053
  porphyria and, 1252
  pregnancy and, 1212
Mephenesin, 722
Mephenytoin, 722
Mepivacaine, 1212
Meprobamate, 1213, 1252, 1297
Meprospan; *see* Meprobamate
Meralgia paresthetica, 98
6-Mercaptopurine, 366, 367, 441, 616
Mercury
  allergy to, 30
  nephrotic syndrome and, 613
  neutropenia and, 360
  poisoning from, 753-754
  toxicity of, 30
    nephropathy and, 624, 625, 627, 630, 631
Merozoites, 280
Mesangial lesions, 54
Mesenteric artery, 1020
Mesenteric cysts, 1049
Mesenteric inflammatory disease, 1048-1049
Mesenteric tumors, 1049
Mesenteric vein thrombosis, 1021-1022
Mesentery, 941, 1043-1049
Mesocaval anastomosis, 1083
Mesoderm, development of, 1304
Mesotheliomas
  asbestos and, 432, 726
  malignant, 726-727, 734
  pleura and, 730, 734
  primary, 1047
Mesovarium, 1173
Messenger ribonucleic acid, 1216
  hormone action and, 1115, 1131, 1154
Mestinon; *see* Pyridostigmine
Metabolic acidosis, 599-600, 636
Metabolic alkalosis, 600, 957
Metabolic disorders
  cardiomyopathies and, 523
  cataracts and, 1273
  encephalopathies in, 768
  hemolysis from, 343

Metabolic disorders—cont'd
  inherited, 1230-1246; *see also* Genetics and metabolism
  myopathies and, 858
  neuropathies and, 853-854
  neutropenia and, 359
  renal lesions and, 617-619
  skin disorders of, 884-891
  supportive care and, 445
  vomiting and, 957
Metabolism, 1216-1293; *see also* Genetics and metabolism
  acid-base disturbances in, 588, 593-603; *see also* Kidney diseases
  alcohol and, 1255-1256
  of aromatic amino acids, 1236
  of bilirubin, 1057-1058
  blood pressure and, 467-468
  bone disease and; *see* Bone, metabolic disease of
  of calcitonin, 1189
  of calcium, 1183-1184
  of collagen, disorders of, 1203
  cortisol and, 1154
  disorders of; *see* Metabolic disorders
  fainting and, 780
  folate, 316
  glycosphingolipid, 1231
  hormone, 1115; *see also* Hormones
  inborn errors of, 1226-1227, 1236-1238
    craniofacial malformations and, 1302
    lipoprotein deficiency disorders and, 1291-1293
  of iodine, extrathyroidal, 1128
  of lipoproteins; *see* Lipoprotein metabolism disorders
  mineral, 1183-1189
    corrdinate control of, 1188-1189
    disorders of; *see* Mineral metabolism, disorders of
  parathyroid hormone, 1186-1188
  phosphate, 1184-1185
  potassium, 468, 597-599
    blood pressure and, 468
  sodium, 593-597, 1044
  of thyroid hormones, 1131-1132
  vitamin B_{12}, 317
  vitamin D, 1185-1186, 1200
  of water, kidney and, 593-597
Metabolites, urinary, 1166, 1168
Metacarpophalangeal joint subluxation, 36
Metacentric chromosomes, 1220
Metachromasia, 801
Metachromatic leukodystrophy, 801-802, 1231, 1232-1233
Metals, heavy; *see* Heavy metals
Metamucil; *see* Psyllium muciloid
Metamyelocytes, 356
Metanephrine, 1165, 1166, 1168
Metanephrine glucuronide, 1068
Metaphyseal chondrodysplasia, 1245
Metaplasia
  myeloid; *see* Myeloid metaplasia
  of synovial membrane, 108
Metaproterenol, 706
Metastases
  brain tumor and, 844
  central nervous system and, 847-848
  cutaneous, 912-913
  hepatic, 435
  lung malignancy and, 741, 742, 743-744
  to mouth, 1093, 1214
  myelophthisic anemia and, 322

Metastases—cont'd
  to peritoneum, 1047
  of renal tumors to jaw, 668
Metastatic calcifications, hyperparathyroidism and, 1208
Metastatic infection, 206, 220
Metatropic dwarfism, 1245
Methacholine
  achalasia and, 976, 977
  asthma and, 705
  bronchoconstriction and, 24
  esophageal spasm and, 980
Methacholine challenge test, 705
Methacycline, 168
Methadone
  hypogonadism and, 1172
  lung disease and, 722
  opiate withdrawal and, 778
  withdrawal symptoms and, 863
Methane gas, 960-961
Methantheline, 801
Methaqualone, 777, 1252
Methemoglobinemia, 343-344, 1227
Methenamine hippurate, 161, 171
Methenamine mandelate, 161, 171, 198
Methicillin, 160, 164
  administration route for, 157
  endocarditis and, 183, 184
  nephritis and, 619
  nephropathy and, 624, 625, 626, 627, 629
  neutropenia and, 360
  pregnancy and, 1212
  renal disease and, 670
  site of infection, 157
  staphylococci and, 183, 184, 221
  vasculitis and, 29
Methimazole, 1132
  Graves' disease and, 1144-1145
  hypothyroidism at birth and, 1137
  neutropenia and, 360
  thyroid hormone synthesis and, 1130
Methionine, 198
Methotrexate, 440
  cancer and, 447, 448, 450
  dermatomyositis and, 113
  DNA synthesis and, 440
  folate deficiency and, 316
  hepatitis and, 1066
  intrathecal, 366
  Kaposi's sarcoma and, 922
  in leukemias, 366
  with leukovorin rescue, 450
  lung disease and, 427, 447, 721, 722
  mycosis fungoides and, 901
  pemphigus and, 932, 934
  polymyositis and, 65
  psoriasis and, 52, 937, 938
  oral ulcers and, 450
  sarcomas and, 450, 922
  serum bile acids and, 1065
  thrombocytopenia and, 400
  toxicity of, 625, 847, 1077
Methotrexate syndrome, 1303
Methoxyflurane
  diabetes insipidus and, 621-622
  hypernatremia and, 595
  liver toxicity and, 1076
  nephritis and, 620, 621
  nephropathy and, 625, 627, 628, 629, 630
  oxalate and, 648
8-Methoxypsoralen, 937
Methyl alcohol; *see also* Alcohol
  metabolic encephalopathies and, 768

Methyl alcohol—cont'd
  poisoning from, 776-777
  toxic nephropathy and, 630
Methyl chloride, 1253
Methyl lomustine, 442, 918
α-Methylacetoacetic aciduria, 1238
17-α-Methylated testosterone, 1173
α-Methyl-beta-hydroxybutyric aciduria, 1237-1238
Methyl-CCNU; see Methyl lomustine
Methylcellulose, 1017, 1092, 1147
Methylcrotonylglycinuria, 1237
Methyldopa
  heart failure and, 464
  hemolysis and, 29, 342
  hepatitis and, 1066, 1076, 1078
  hydralazine and, 472
  hypertension and, 472, 473, 474, 475
  lung disease and, 722
  parkinsonism and, 812, 814-815
  pheochromocytoma and, 1165
  in Raynaud's phenomenon, 61, 64
  renal failure and, 62, 639
  in scleroderma, 62
  side effects of, 574
  thrombocytopenia and, 401
  toxemia of pregnancy and, 665
  urine and, 588, 1166, 1168
3-o-Methyldopamine, 1166
Methylene blue, 150, 331, 344
Methylglucamine, 1168
Methylmalonic acidemia, 1237, 1238
α-Methyl-para-tyrosine, 812
Methylphenidate, 769, 777
Methylprednisolone
  bronchitis and, 693
  lupus erythematosus and, 57, 615
  rejection reactions and, 645
  septic shock and, 241
Methyltestosterone, 1076
Methylthiouracil, 722
Methylxanthines, 705, 706
Methysergide
  carcinoid tumors and, 450
  headache and, 788, 789
  nephropathy and, 625, 627, 629
  Raynaud's phenomenon and, 63
  retroperitoneal fibrosis and, 105
Metoclopramide, 964
  diabetic gastroparesis and, 1275
  esophageal disorders and, 62, 981-982, 985
Metolazone, 472, 597, 639
Metopirone; see Metyrapone
Metoprolol, 472, 473, 474, 531
Metrazol; see Pentylenetetrazol
Metrizamide, 761, 762
Metrizoate, 605; see also Contrast agents
Metronidazole, 161, 170
  abscesses and, 192, 283, 1047
  acute necrotizing ulcerative gingivitis and, 302
  alcohol and, 1297
  amebiasis and, 203, 283
  anaerobic infections and, 250
  anal fistulas and, 1031
  giardiasis and, 203, 284, 1003
  perineal fistulas and, 1014
  trichomoniasis and, 286
  urine and, 588
Metyrapone, 1122, 1157, 1158, 1159, 1181
Metyrapone tests, 1157, 1158
Mezlocillin, 160, 164, 241
MG; see Myasthenia gravis
β-MG; see β-Monoglyceride

MHA-TP; see Microhemagglutination test
MI; see Myocardial infarction
MIC; see Minimal inhibitory concentration
Micelles, 998, 999, 1085
Miconazole, 278, 928
  candidiasis and, 276, 308
  histoplasmosis and, 307
  pregnancy and, 1212
  pruritus and, 885
Miconazole nitrate gel, 308
Microangiopathic hemolysis, 340-341
Microatelectasis, 702
Microbial diseases, 118-309
  antimicrobials and, 155-171; see also Antimicrobials
  bacterial diseases in, 155-274, 301-306; see also Bacteria
  dentistry and, 298-308
    bacteria and, 301-306
    fungi, and, 306-308
    viruses and, 298-301
  diagnosis of, 118-119
  fever and; see also Fever
    chills in, 118
    unknown origin of, 119-121
  fungi in, 174-178, 306-308; see also Fungal diseases
  helminthic, 289-297; see also Helminthic diseases
  laboratory evaluation of, 118-119
  Lyme disease in, 82, 297-298, 925-926
  management of, 119
  protozoal, 279-289; see also Protozoal diseases
  resistance in, 159
  toxic shock syndrome in, 298
  viral diseases in, 121-155, 298-301; see also Viral diseases
Microbicidal activity, defects in, 347
Microcephaly, 125
Microcherry, 1092
Microcytic hypochromic anemias, 323-325
Microfibrillar collagen
  gingival bleeding and, 421
  hemophilia and, 427, 428
  platelet transfusion and, 426
  polycythemia vera and, 419
  on skin and mucous membranes, 249
  subgingival, oral contraceptives and, 1214
  thrombocytosis and, 426
  von Willebrand's disease and, 427
Micrognathia, 45
Micrographia, 813
Microhemagglutination test, 118, 119; see also Hemagglutinin tests
  in leptospirosis, 273-274
  for *Treponema pallidum*, 271
Micropolyspora faeni, 727
Micropsia, 783
Microscopic agglutination test; see Microhemagglutination test
Microscopy, 118-119
  darkfield, 264, 270-271
  electron, 122, 124
    cytomegalovirus and, 131
    Norwalk-like agents and, 150
    rotaviruses and, 150
    viral gastroenteritis and, 149, 150
  fever of unknown origin and, 120
  of urinary sediment, 604-605, 616
Microsomal antibody, 1136
Microsomal ethanol oxidizing system, 1255
Microsomia, hemifacial, 1300, 1309, 1310-1312
Microsporum, 279, 928-929

Microsporum canis, 928, 929
Microstomia, 112
Microsurgery, pituitary, 1159
Microvascular decompression, 791
Micturition syncope, 780
Midbrain lesion, 765
Middle ear structures, 5
Middle lobe syndrome, 703
Midface syndromes, 1316-1318
Midline cerebellar lesions, 759
Midline granuloma, 70, 73-74, 113
MIF; see Migration inhibition factor
Migraine, 788-789, 794
Migraine equivalent, 794
Migration inhibition factor, 15
Migratory arthritis, 229
Migratory thrombophlebitis, 495, 913
Miliary sarcoid, 910
Miliary tuberculosis, 255, 257
Milk of magnesia; see Magnesium hydroxide
Milk secretion, 1118
Milk-alkali syndrome, 992
Milkmaid's grasp, 816
Millard-Gubler syndrome, 833
Miltown; see Meprobamate
Milwaukee shoulder, 95
Mineral metabolism, 1183-1189
  coordinate control of, 1188-1189
  disorders of, 1181-1204
    inherited, 1240
    dentistry and, 1207-1210
    physiology and, 1181-1189
    primary homeostatic, 1189-1198
    and skeletal homeostatic disorders, 1198-1201
Mineralocorticoids, 1153, 1155
  blood pressure and, 468
  deficiency of, syndromes of, 1159-1160
  excess of
    congenital adrenal hyperplasia and, 1162
    syndromes of, 1160-1162; see also Aldosteronism
  hyperkalemia and, 599
  hypokalemia and, 598
  hyporeninemic hypoaldosteronism and, 623
  replacement of, 1157
  synthesis of, 1153
Minerals, 1102
  deficiencies of, 1104-1106
  heavy; see Heavy metals
  metabolism of; see Mineral metabolism
Minimal bactericidal concentration, 155
Minimal inhibitory concentration, 155
Minimal lesion disease, 613
Minireovirus, 149, 150
Minnesota Tongue Stent, 871
Minocycline, 168, 261
Minoxidil
  hypertension and, 473, 474, 475
  renal failure and, 639
  scleroderma and, 616
  toxemia of pregnancy and, 665
Minute ventilation, 673
Minute volume, 673
Miricidium, 295
MIT; see Monoiodotyrosine
Mites, 211
Mithramycin, 441
  hypercalcemia and, 445, 1180, 1192
  multiple myeloma and, 382
Mitochondrial iron accumulation, 321
Mitogenic factors, 15
Mitomycin C, 440, 441, 448

Mitosis, nondisjunction during, 1221
Mitotane, 1159, 1181
Mitral valve
　calcified anulus of, 510, 511
　myxomatous degeneration of leaflets of, 510, 511
　prolapse of, 179, 301, 511, 842
　regurgitation and, 488, 510-511
　replaced, 511
　stenosis of, 512-514
Mitsuda reaction, 262
Mixed cellularity Hodgkin's disease, 388
Mixed connective tissue disease, 35, 906
Mixed venous oxygen, 708, 709
Miyagawanella, 214
ML; *see* Mucolipidoses
MLD; *see* Metachromatic leukodystrophy
MLF; *see* Medial longitudinal fasciculus
MLG; *see* Midline granuloma
MMM; *see* Myeloid metaplasia
M-mode echo; *see* Motion mode echocardiography
MMR vaccine; *see* Measles-mumps-rubella vaccine
MN blood groups, 1220
Mobitz blocks, 546
Möbius sign, 1142
Modeling of bone, 1182; *see also* Bone
Mohs chemosurgery, 883, 915
Moist inspired oxygen tension, 673
Molars, mulberry, 303
Moles, hydatidiform, 1146
Mollaret's recurrent meningitis, 189
Molluscum contagiosum, 927-928
Monilia infections; *see Candida*
Monoamine oxidase, 1166
Monoamine oxidase inhibitors, 574, 824, 1168, 1297
Monoclonal immunoglobulins; *see* Immunoglobulins, M
Monocomponent insulin, 1267, 1268
Monocytes, 362, 899
Monocytosis, 362, 899
β-Monoglyceride, 998-999
Monoiodotyrosine, 1128, 1129-1130
Monomer, allergy to free, 30
Mononeuropathy, diabetic, 1275
Mononuclear pleocytosis, 128
Mononucleosis, infectious; *see* Infectious mononucleosis
Monosodium glutamate, 200
Monosodium urate crystals, 92, 93
Monosomy, 1221
Moon facies, 887, 1206
MOPP therapy; *see* Mechlorethamine, vincristine, prednisone, and procarbazine
Morgagni, rectal columns of, 948, 1029
Morgagni's foramen, herniation through, 736
Moria, 772
Morphea, 903
Morpheiform basal cell carcinoma, 916
Morphine
　abuse of, 778
　aortic dissection and, 562
　heart failure and, 464
　hyponatremia and, 594
　hypothyroidism and, 1206
　mastocytosis and, 909
　myocardial infarction and, 537, 583
　neoplasia and, 446
　porphyria and, 1252
　pregnancy and, 1212
　pulmonary edema and, 465
　tetralogy of Fallot and, 507

Morphine—cont'd
　urticaria and, 25
Morphogenesis, 1304-1308
Morquio's syndrome, 1233, 1234
Morular cells, 380
Mosaicism, 1221, 1225-1226
Mosquitos, 279-280, 825; *see also* Malaria
Mothballs, 330
Motilin, 941
Motion-mode echocardiography, 486
Motor neuron disease, 802-804, 852
Motor system, 851
　coma and, 765-766
　neuropathies and, 802-804, 852
　testing of, 14, 773
Motrin; *see* Ibuprofen
Mott cells, 380
Mouth; *see also* Teeth; Tongue
　Addison's disease and, 1207
　bacteremia and, 180
　bacteria in, 180, 302, 581
　Behçet's disease and, 110, 111, 907
　biopsy of; *see* Biopsy, oral
　bleeding from; *see* Bleeding, oral
　breath sounds at, 684-685
　buccal mucosa and; *see* Buccal mucosa
　cancer chemotherapy and, 450-451
　candidiasis and, 34, 307-308, 1209
　cerebrovascular accident and, 586
　Cushing's syndrome and, 1206
　diphtheria pseudomembrane and, 305
　drug allergy and, 29-30
　evaluation of, 9, 11
　immunodeficiency disease and, 34
　jaundice of mucosa of, 1097
　jaw spasm and, 821
　keratinization in, 1107
　leukemia and, 421-422
　liver diseases and, 1059
　lupus erythematosus and, 55, 111, 902
　malabsorption and, 1000
　midline granuloma and, 113
　multiple myeloma and, 422
　neoplasia of, 918-919
　　basal cell carcinomas in, 918, 919
　　malignant melanomas in, 919
　　metastatic, 1093, 1214
　　radiation doses and, 751
　oropharynx and; *see* Oropharynx
　palatal ulcer of, 55; *see also* Palate
　pemphigus and, 932-933
　pemphigus vegetans and, 934
　pericarditis and, 586
　pernicious anemia and, 414
　psoriasis and, 937
　Reiter's syndrome and, 52, 110, 908
　sarcoidosis and, 113, 114
　Sjögren's syndrome and, 36
　skin graft and, 935
　systemic sclerosis and, 119, 903
　thiamine deficiency and, 1108
　thrombocytopenia and, 571
　ulcerative colitis and, 1007, 1095, 1096
　urate crystals in tissues of, 667
　viruses and, 122, 128
　Wegener's granulomatosis and, 71, 72, 113
Mouth breathing, 684-685
Mouthrinses, 451, 876; *see also* Oral hygiene; Peroxide
　acrodermatitis enteropathica and, 895
　dermatitis herpetiformis and, 893
　erythema multiforme and, 924
　gingival bleeding and, 425
　herpangina and, 301

Mouthrinses—cont'd
　lichen planus and, 939
　oral candidiasis and, 451
　pemphigus and, 933
　Reiter's syndrome and, 908
　scrofulosis and, 304
　ulcerative stomatitis and, 415
Moxalactam, 160, 165, 190, 241
Moyamoya disease, 843
MPS; *see* Mucopolysaccharidoses
MRF; *see* Müllerian regression factor
mRNA; *see* Messenger ribonucleic acid
MSH; *see* Melanocyte-stimulating hormone
MSUD; *see* Maple syrup urine disease
Mucilloid bulk agents; *see* Hydrophilic bulk agents
Mucocutaneous infections; *see also* Mucocutaneous lymph node syndrome; Mucous membranes
　candidiasis and, 33, 307, 929-930; *see also Candida*
　herpes simplex and, 128
Mucocutaneous lymph node syndrome, 69, 147
Mucolipidoses, 1235
Mucolytic agents, 703
Mucopolysaccharides, 886, 1233-1234
Mucopolysaccharidoses, 1233-1234
　craniofacial malformations and, 1302
　oral manifestations of, 1234-1235
Mucor, 277, 308, 727; *see also* Mucormycosis
Mucor stolonifer, 727
Mucormycosis, 277, 308, 446, 451; *see also*
Mucosa; *see also* Mucous membranes
　acid back-diffusion and, 943, 996
　bleeding from, 1059
　buccal; *see* Buccal mucosa; Mouth
　esophageal, scarring of, 877
　malabsorption and, 941, 999, 1001-1003
　pigmentation on, Gaucher's disease and, 1296
Mucosal disease, 941, 999, 1001-1003
Mucosal neuroma syndrome, 1164, 1207
Mucosal pemphigoid, benign, 935
Mucosulfatidoses, 1233
Mucous cells, 942, 943, 945
Mucous membrane pemphigoid, benign, 935
Mucous membranes; *see also* Mucosa
　Ehlers-Danlos syndrome and, 1242
　infections of, 122; *see also* Mucocutaneous infections
　syphilis and, 267, 268, 303
　Urbach-Wiethe disease and, 1296
　viruses and, 122
Mucous patches, syphilis and, 303
Mucous plugs, 710; *see also* Mucoviscidosis
Mucoviscidosis, 696, 700, 1050-1051, 1101-1102
Mulberry cells, 912
Mulberry molars, 303
Müllerian agenesis, 1176
Müllerian regression factor, 1168
Multifactorial disease, 1228
Multifactorial inheritance, 1222-1223
Multifocal atrial tachycardia, 542-543, 692
Multifocal demyelination, 798
Multifocal fibrosclerosis, 105
Multifocal leukoencephalopathy, progressive, 828, 868
Multi-infarct dementia, 835
Multimodal information processing, 771-772
Multinodular goiter, 1145
Multinucleated cells
　giant; *see* Giant cells, multinucleated
　herpes simplex and, 128, 299
Multiple alleles, 1219

INDEX 1385

Multiple endocrine neoplasias, 879, 1164
   dentistry and, 1207
   hyperparathyroidism and, 1192
   medullary carcinoma and, 1151, 1164, 1197-1198
   Zollinger-Ellison syndrome and, 994
Multiple epiphyseal dysplasia, 1245
Multiple myeloma, 378-382
   dentistry and, 422-423
   kidney disease and, 617-618
   neutropenia and, 358
   skin lesions of, 899
Multiple sclerosis, 794, 796-801, 868-869
Multiple sulfatase deficiency, 1233
Multipurpose biopsy tube, 964
Multivalent antitoxin, 204
Multivitamins, 633
Mumps, 139-140
   aseptic meningitis and, 135
   central nervous system disease and, 135, 137-138
   dentistry and, 301
   orchitis and, 1171
   sarcoidosis and, 911
   vaccine for, 137, 138, 152
Murine typhus fever, 212-213, 214
Murmurs, cardiac, 580
   of aortic regurgitation, 516, 561
   aortic stenosis and, 505, 514
   cardiomyopathy and, 519
   coarctation of aorta and, 505
   Ebstein's anomaly and, 508
   endocarditis and, 180
   hypertension and, 470
   mitral prolapse and, 511
   mitral regurgitation and, 510
   palpable, 12
   patent ductus arteriosus and, 504, 505
   pulmonary stenosis and, 506
   tetralogy of Fallot and, 507
   tricuspid atresia and, 506
   valvular disease and, 580
   ventricular septal defects and, 504
Muscle contraction headache, 789
Muscle diseases of heart; *see* Cardiomyopathies
Muscle enzymes, 65
Muscle pain; *see* Muscles, pain in
Muscle relaxants, 109, 867
Muscles, 851; *see also* specific muscle
   atrophy of
      dorsal interosseous, 36
      infantile muscular, 804
      peroneal, 804, 855
      spinal, 804-805
   biopsy of, 65, 875
   contractions of, 851; *see also* Contractility
   electrical injury and, 751
   degenerative neurological disease and, 802-804, 852; *see also* specific disease
   dentistry and, 873-875
   headache and, 789
   lesions of, 761, 856-860; *see also* Myopathies
   myofascial pain dysfunction syndrome and, 109
   neuromuscular disorders and; *see* Neuromuscular disorders
   pain in
      fibrositis and, 96
      influenza vaccines and, 152
      intercostal, 100
      leptospirosis and, 273
      myofascial pain dysfunction and, 109
      trapezius and, 98
      trichinosis and, 292

Muscles—cont'd
   parkinsonism and, 812, 813
   of respiration, 672-673
   systemic sclerosis and, 59-60
   tetanus and, 252
   weakness of, 856-858, 975
      enteroviruses and, 137
      polymyositis and, 64
      vitamin D deficiency and, 1198
Muscular atrophies, progressive spinal, 804-805
Muscular dystrophies, 856-858, 975
Muscularis externa, 941
Muscularis mucosae, 941, 973
Mushroom poisoning, 200
Mushroom worker's lung, 727
Musset's sign, 580
Mustard's operation, 508
Mustargen; *see* Mechlorethamine
Mutations, 1216-1217
Mutism, akinetic, 764
Mutton fat precipitates, 910
Myalgia; *see* Muscles, pain in
Myasthenia gravis, 855-856
   aminoglycosides and, 167
   dentistry and, 874
   oropharyngeal dysphagia and, 975
Myasthenic syndrome, 856
Mycetoma, 247, 277
Mycobacteria, 254-264
   atypical, 261
   brucellosis and, 244
   leprosy in, 261-263, 264
   monocytes and, 362
   nontuberculous infections in, 261-263, 264
   in pneumonia, 172
   scrofula and, 81, 261, 304
   tuberculosis in, 254-261; *see also* Tuberculosis
      arthritis of, 81
      Hodgkin's disease and, 387
      pneumonia and, 172
      silicosis and, 724
Mycobacterium avium-intracellulare complex, 261
Mycobacterium bovis, 254, 256, 261
Mycobacterium chelonei, 261
Mycobacterium fortuitum, 261
Mycobacterium intracellularis, 81
Mycobacterium kansasii, 81, 261
Mycobacterium leprae, 261-262
Mycobacterium marinum, 81, 261
Mycobacterium scrofulaceum, 81, 261, 304
Mycobacterium simiae, 261
Mycobacterium szulgai, 261
Mycobacterium tuberculosis; see Mycobacteria, tuberculosis in
Mycobacterium ulcerans, 261
Mycobacterium xenopi, 261
Mycoplasma, 217-218; *see also Mycoplasma pneumoniae*
   bronchitis and, 691
   drugs for, 162, 167, 168
   Reiter's syndrome and, 52, 907
   urogenital infections and, 217, 218
Mycoplasma hominis, 217, 218
Mycoplasma pneumoniae, 177
   cold agglutinin syndromes and, 339
   drugs for, 162, 167
   erythema multiforme and, 922
   lung abscess and, 698
   in pneumonia, 172
   psittacosis and, 216
Mycosis fungoides, 900-902
Mycostatin; *see* Nystatin
Mycotic infections; *see* Fungal diseases

Mydriatics, 924
Myectomy, 520
Myelinolysis, central pontine, 1257
Myelitis, 824
   differential diagnosis of, 194
   transverse, 138, 194
Myeloblastic leukemia, acute, 353
Myeloblasts, 353, 356
Myelocytes, 356
Myelodysplastic syndromes, 320-321, 341
Myelofibrosis
   acute, 376
   idiopathic, 358
   with myeloid metaplasia, 374-376
   pericarditis and, 586
   secondary forms of, 322-323
Myelogenous leukemia; *see* Leukemias, myelogenous
Myelography, 762
Myeloid metaplasia
   agnogenic, 374-376
   leukemias and, 370
   myelofibrosis with, 374-376
   pericarditis and, 586
Myeloma kidney, 379
Myelomas, 378-382
   multiple; *see* Multiple myeloma
Myelomeningocele, 811
Myeloneuropathy, drug abuse, 863
Myelopathy, 138, 194, 860
Myeloperoxidase, 357, 898
Myelophthisis, 322-323
Myeloproliferative disease, 373-376, 404, 406
Myenteric ganglion cells, congenital absence of, 1026
Myenteric plexus, 942, 974, 1007
Myleran; *see* Busulfan
Myocardial infarction
   acute, 533-538
      aortic dissection and, 560, 561
      electrocardiograms and, 484, 485
   cardiac catheterization and, 488
   dentistry and, 583, 584
   digitalis and, 584
   Killip classification of, 535
   nuclear cardiology and, 530, 536
   pericarditis after, 550
   pulmonary embolism and, 490
   sudden death and, 539, 540
   unstable angina and, 532
Myocardial ischemia, 528-529; *see also* Angina pectoris
   cardiomyopathies and, 522-523
   infarction and, 533
   pericarditis and, 550
   transient, 484-485, 528
Myocardial perfusion, 489, 524-526
Myocarditis, 235, 248, 453
Myocardium
   alcoholism and, 1257
   congenital heart disease and, 508-509
   congestive heart failure and, 453
   granulomatous disease of, 717
   infarction of; *see* Myocardial infarction
   inflammation of, 235, 248, 453
   ischemia of; *see* Myocardial ischemia
   mechanics of, 454-458
   perfusion of, 489, 524-526
   pericarditis and, 552, 554
   trypanosomiasis and, 287
   ultrastructure of, 454, 455
Myochrysine; *see* Gold
Myoclonus
   coma and, 766

Myoclonus—cont'd
  Creutzfeldt-Jakob disease and, 828
  palatal, 833
  penicillins and, 164
Myoedema, 858
Myofascial dysfunction, oral, 107, 109-110, 874-875
  dermatomyositis and, 905
Myofascial syndromes, 97-98
Myofasciitis, 96, 97-98
Myofibrils, 454
Myoglobin, 588, 627, 631, 859-860
  synthesis of, 888
Myokymia, facial, 799
Myomonitor, 870
Myonecrosis, 252
Myopathies, 852, 856-860
  alcoholics and, 1257
  centronuclear, 859
  congenital, 859
  inflammatory, 858, 874-875
  myotubular, 859
  nemaline, 859
  ocular, 857-858
Myophosphorylase deficiency, 858
Myosin, 454
Myotomy
  cardiomyopathy and, 520
  cricopharyngeal, 976
  esophageal disorders and, 976, 979, 981, 982
  Heller's, 979
Myotonia congenita, 859
Myotonic disorders, 859, 1172
Myotonic dystrophy, 859, 1172
Myotubular myopathy, 859
Myringitis, bullous, 217
Mysoline; *see* Primidone
Myxedema, 1136, 1137, 1138, 1139
  ascites and, 1045
  coma and, 1138, 1140, 1206
  dentistry and, 1206
  juvenile, hypothyroidism and, 1206
  pretibial, 886
  skin lesions of, 886
  thyrotropin deficiency and, 1122
  xanthomatosis in, 890
Myxedema coma, 1138, 1140, 1206
Myxomas
  atrial, 182, 513, 516, 842
  of pancreas, 1056

N

NAD; *see* Nicotinamide adenine dinucleotide
NADase; *see* Nicotinamide-adenine dinucleotidase
NADH; *see* Nicotinamide adenine dinucleotide, reduced
Nadolol, 472, 474
NADP; *see* Nicotinamide adenine dinucleotide phosphate
NADPH; *see* Nicotinamide adenine dinucleotide phosphate, reduced
Naegleria, 283
Nafcillin, 160, 164
  abscesses and, 192, 700
  cellulitis and, 226
  endocarditis and, 183
  excretion of, 158
  liver and, 157, 158
  meningitis and, 190
  neutropenia and, 360
  pneumonia and, 175
  pregnancy and, 1212
  site of infection and, 157

Nafcillin—cont'd
  staphylococci and, 175, 183, 221
Nager acrofacial dysostosis, 1311
Nail changes, 51, 937, 1059
Naked tubercle, 911
Naked viruses, 121
Nalidixic acid, 161, 171
  hemolysis and, 329
  pseudotumor cerebri and, 848
  urinary catecholamines and, 1168
  urinary tract infection and, 198
Naloxone, 241, 682, 778
Nandrolone, 376, 639
Naphthalene, 330
Naprosyn; *see* Naproxen
Naproxen
  nephropathy and, 627, 629
  platelet function and, 405
  rheumatoid arthritis and, 42, 46
Narcan; *see* Naloxone
Narcolepsy, 769
Narcotic analgesics, porphyrias and, 1252
Narcotics; *see also* Opiates; specific agent
  addiction to, 778-779
    dentistry and, 862-874
    Mediterranean fever and, 1048
  alcohol and, 1297
  allergy and, 28
  arrhythmias and, 585
  cholelithiasis and, 1088
  hepatic coma and, 1061, 1084
  megacolon and, 1027
  in respiratory disease, 746, 747
  sickle cell anemia and, 334
Nasal capsule, failure in development of, 1317
Nasal cavity infection, 21
Nasal congestion, 20-23, 73, 269
Nasal polyps, aspirin sensitivity, and asthma, triad of, 23, 26
Nasal prongs, 710
Nasal septum, perforation of, 73
Nasogastric suction
  bleeding and, 958, 959
  bowel obstruction and, 1026
  gastric dilation and, 997
  pancreatitis and, 1053
  ulcers and, 989, 993
Nasopharynx
  carcinoma of, 131, 132
  craniosynostosis syndromes and, 1313
  meningococcal disease and, 234
  secretions from, hepatitis and, 1099
Natal infections, 125-127, 1073-1074; *see also* Newborn
National Council on Radiation Protection and Measurement, 751
Natriuretic hormone, 592
Nausea and vomiting, 956-957; *see also* Vomiting
  gastric carcinoma and, 1035
  peptic ulcers and, 988
  radiation enteritis and, 1019
NBT dye test; *see* Nitroblue tetrazolium dye test
NCRP; *see* National Council on Radiation Protection and Measurement
NCV; *see* Nerve conduction velocity
Nebulized acetylcysteine, 697
Nebulizers, contaminated, 176
Necator americanus, 291
Neck
  cancer of, 449
  craniofacial malformations of, 1300-1322; *see also* Craniofacial malformations
  cysts in, Gardner's syndrome in, 1093

Neck—cont'd
  evaluation of, 9-11
  lymph nodes of, 10; *see also* Lymph nodes
  lymphoma and, 424
    non-Hodgkin's, 394
  myofascial syndromes and, 97
  radiation doses for, 751
  relapsing polychondritis and, 102
  rheumatic disorders of, 100
Neck vein distention, 571
Necrobiosis lipoidica diabeticorum, 885-886, 1276
Necrolysis, toxic epidermal, 306, 931-932
Necrosis
  aortic aneurysms and, 558
  aortic dissection and, 560
  avascular, 104
  of bronchiolar epithelium, 141
  caseation, 254
  congenital viral infection and, 125
  cystic medial, 558, 560
  of digits, 62-63, 906
  encephalomyelopathy and, 801
  fat, 913
  gas gangrene, 252, 253
  Legionnaire's disease and, 177
  pituitary, 1123
  radiation, 847
  tubular, 624-630, 645
    renal failure and, 630-635
  vasculitis and, 66-67, 69
Necrotizing encephalomyelopathy, 801
Necrotizing ulcerative gingivitis, acute, 307, 862
Necrotizing vasculitis, systemic, 66-67, 69
Needle aspiration, 689, 969
Needle biopsy
  of kidney, 608
  of liver, 965
  of peritoneum, 1044
  of thyroid, 1136, 1152
Needle pericardiocentesis, 555
Negative feedback, 1117, 1169, 1176
Negative pleural space pressure, 730
Neisseria, 171, 186, 230-233; *see also* Gonococci
Neisseria gonorrhoeae; *see* Gonococci
Neisseria meningitidis, 162, 171, 186, 230, 233
Nemaline myopathy, 859
Nematodes, 289-292
Neocortex, 763
Neomycin, 161, 165-166
  and bacitracin, ulcerative stomatitis and, 415
  hepatic disease and, 1072, 1084
  ileal mucosa and, 317
  labyrinth and, 792
  malabsorption and, 1002
  nephropathy and, 627, 628
Neonate; *see* Newborn
Neoplasia, 431-451; *see also* Carcinomas; Malignancy; Tumors
  of biliary tract, 445, 1089
  of bladder, 449, 659
  brain abscess and, 192
  carcinogenesis and, 431-434
  central nervous sytem and, 843-848; *see also* Brain, tumors of
  clinical manifestations of, 436-438
  Cushing's syndrome and, 1179, 1180-1181
  dentistry and, 450-451
  detection of, 434
  diagnosis of, 434-436
  ectopic gonadotropins and, 1181
  endometrial, 449
  of esophagus; *see* Esophagus, neoplasms of

Neoplasia—cont'd
 gastrointestinal; see Carcinomas of gastrointestinal tract
 humoral syndromes with, 1178-1181
 hypercalcemia and, 657, 1179-1180, 1192
 hypoglycemia and, 1179, 1181
 inappropriate antidiuresis and, 740, 1179, 1181
 leukemoid reactions and, 362
 liver and; see Liver, neoplasms of
 metronidazole and, 170
 of mouth, 918-919
 multiple endocrine; see Multiple endocrine neoplasias
 neurogenic, 1053
 neutropenia and, 358
 ovarian, 449, 1045, 1177-1178
 overview of, 431-438
 of peritoneum, 726-727, 1047
 of rib cage, 737
 of skin, 913-922
 staging and, 435-436
 supportive care and, 445-447
 systemic therapy for, 438-447; see also Chemotherapy
  combined modality approaches in, 438
  complications of, 438
  disseminated neoplasia and, 439-447
  localized neoplasia and, 438
  natural products for, 441-442
  regional, 438
  specific neoplasms in, 447-450
 of testes, 435, 449, 1173
 of upper airways, midline granuloma and, 73
 of urinary tract, 656-660
Neostigmine, 167, 169, 856
Nephrectomy
 glomerulonephritis and, 611
 hemorrhagic lung disease and, 720
 renal cell carcinomas and, 657-658
 scleroderma and, 616
 urothelial tumors and, 659
Nephritic syndrome, 609-612
Nephritis; see also Glomerulonephritis
 drug allergy and, 29
 hereditary, 611-612
 immune complex, 27
 interstitial, 619-621
 lupus, 615
 penicillins and, 164
Nephroblastoma, 658
Nephrocalcinosis, 622, 646
Nephrogenic diabetes insipidus, 621-622
Nephrogenous cyclic adenosine monophosphate; see Cyclic adenosine monophosphate, nephrogenous
Nephrogram, 606
Nephrolithiasis; see Kidney stones
Nephronophthisis, 653
Nephrons, 590
Nephropathy; see also Kidney stones
 analgesic abuse and, 621
 Balkan, 658
 diabetic, 617, 1274
 hypercalcemic, 622
 hypokalemic, 622
 interstitial, 619, 626
 membranous, 613
 nephrotoxic, 630; see also Nephrotoxicity
 reflux, 651
 toxic, 624-630, 631
 uric acid, 622
 vasomotor, 630, 631
Nephrosclerosis, malignant, 469

Nephrosis, lipoid, 613
Nephrotic syndrome, 612-614
 ascites and, 1045
 diabetes mellitus and, 1274
 drug abuse and, 863
 malaria and, 280
 mercury poisoning and, 754
 pleural effusion and, 731
 pregnancy and, 664-665
 sickle cell anemia and, 333
 site of injury and, 588
 syphilis and, 266
 tumors and, 438
Nephrotomography, 606
Nephrotoxic nephropathy, 630
Nephrotoxicity, 158, 624-630, 631
 aminoglycosides and, 166
 polymyxins and, 169
Nerve conduction velocity, 797, 852
Nerve deafness, 270, 611; see also Deafness
Nerve root lesions, 761
Nerves; see also Nervous system; Neurologic diseases; specific nerve
 cranial; see Cranial nerves
 denervation and, 820, 852, 976
 dentistry and, 873-875
 entrapments of, 60, 98
 inflammation of; see Neuritis
 intercostal, 100, 1043, 1275
 motor; see Motor system
 pain and; see Neuralgia
 peripheral; see Neuropathies, peripheral; Peripheral nerves
 of peritoneum, 1043
 sensory, 14, 851
  neuropathies and, 853, 854, 855
 spinal, 860, 1043
 of thyroid, 1127
 vagus; see Vagus nerve
Nervous system; see also Nerves; Neurologic diseases
 alcohol and, 1257
 blood pressure and, 467
 central; see Central nervous system
 digestion and, 942
 hormones and, 1115-1116
 lupus erythematosus and, 55
 sympathetic; see Autonomic nervous system; Sympathetic nervous system
 systemic sclerosis and, 60
Netilmicin, 166
Neumann-type pemphigus vegetans, 933
Neural crest, abnormalities of, 1308
Neural crest cells, 1304, 1305, 1306
 death of, 1316
 deficiencies in number of derivatives of, 1308
Neural plate formation, defective, 1316
Neuralgia
 atypical facial, 791
 brachial plexus and, 860-861
 glossopharyngeal, 791
 postherpetic, 927
 trigeminal; see Trigeminal neuralgia
Neuraminidase, 140, 1235
Neuritis
 Behçet's disease and, 907
 intercostal, 100, 1275
 optic, 798
 retrobulbar, 798
Neurocutaneous syndromes, 808-810
Neuroectoderm, 1164
Neurofibromatosis, 808-809, 878-880
 dentistry and, 869
 hyperparathyroidism and, 1192

Neurofibromatosis—cont'd
 lungs and, 721
 pheochromocytoma and, 1164-1165
 tumors and, 844
Neurohypophysis; see Pituitary gland
Neuroleptics, 342
Neurologic complications; see also Neuropathies
 of abetalipoproteinemia, 1292
 of aminoglycosides, 167
 of brain abscess, 192
 of brain tumor, 845
 of cancer therapy, 847, 853
 endocarditis and, 181
 Lyme disease and, 297, 298
 spinal abscess and, 194
 of thoracic aortic dissection, 561
 of tumors, 437, 845
Neurologic diseases, 757-875; see also Nerves; Nervous system; Neurologic complications
 of basal ganglia, 812-824
  chorea and, 816-818
  essential tremor and, 815-816
  Gilles de la Tourette's syndrome and, 821-822
  orthostatic hypotension and, 823-824
  parkinsonism and, 812-815
  torsion dystonias and, 819-821
  Wilson's disease and, 822-823
 cognition disorders in, 770-775
 consciousness alterations in, 762-769
 of craniovertebral junction, 810-811
 degenerative, 803-805, 868-870
 demyelinating, 796-801, 852, 868-870
 dentistry and, 861-875
  abnormal involuntary jaw movements in, 870-871
  alcoholism and, 862-864
  degenerative diseases in, 868-870
  demyelinating diseases in, 868-870
  drug abuse and, 862-864
  epilepsy and, 864-867
  heredofamilial diseases in, 868-870
  inflammatory myopathies in, 874-875
  malignant hyperthermia and, 875
  myasthenia gravis in, 874
  neuromuscular disease in, 873-874
  odontogenic dizziness and, 867-868
  otomandibular syndrome and, 867-868
  peripheral neuropathy in, 874
  sleep disorders in, 861-862
  stroke in, 871-873
  syncope in, 864
  temporomandibular joint dysfunction and, 867-868
  tremors in, 870-871
 diagnosis of, 13-14, 761-762
 dizziness in, 792-794, 836
 dysmyelinating, 796, 801-803
 epilepsy in, 781-787, 864-867; see also Seizures
 eyes and; see Eyes, neurologic disorders and
 face pain in, 790-791
 headache and, 788-790
 hearing loss in, 794-795
 heredofamilial, 801-810, 868-870
 intoxications in, 775-779, 862-864
 lesions in, 757-761
 neuromuscular disorders and; see Neuromuscular disorders
 neuropathies and; see Neuropathies
 nutritional, 849-851, 853
 pseudotumor cerebri and, 779, 790, 848
 sleep disorders in, 769-770, 861-862

Neurologic diseases—cont'd
    syncope in, 780-781, 864; see also Syncope
    tests for, 761-762
    tumors and, 843-848
    vascular, 829-843; see also Vascular diseases of central nervous system
    viral; see Viral diseases of central nervous system
Neuromas
    acoustic, 795, 844
    heel, 102
    mucosal, pheochromocytoma and, 1207
    of pancreas, 1056
Neuromuscular disorders, 851-861
    alveolar hypoventilation and, 682
    dentistry and, 873-874
    hyperthyroidism and, 1143
    hypocalcemia and, 1195
    muscles and, 856-860
    neuromuscular junction and, 761, 855-856
    pathophysiology of, 852-853
    peripheral neuropathies in, 853-855; see also Neuropathies, peripheral
    respiratory failure and, 712
    signs and symptoms of, 852
    spine and, 860
    structure and function and, 851-852
Neuromuscular junction disorders, 761, 855-856
Neuronal degeneration of substantia nigra, 812
Neuropathies, 852; see also Cranial nerves; Neurologic complications
    alcoholics and, 849, 853, 1257
    antimitotic drugs and, 853
    arthropathy and, 86
    diabetic, 1273, 1274-1275
    drug-related, 779, 853
    entrapment, 60
    hereditary, 855
    hypertrophic, 855
    idiopathic recurrent, 855
    mental nerve, 417
    peripheral, 853-855; see also Peripheral nerves
        dentistry and, 874
        diabetes mellitus and, 1273, 1275
        drug-related, 779, 853
        lead poisoning and, 753
        malabsorption and, 1000
        vitamin deficit and, 317, 849
    vitamin B_{12}, 317
Neurophysins, 1116
Neuroreceptors, 711
Neurosecretory cells, 1116
Neurosyphilis, 269
Neurotoxicity, 169, 200
Neurotransmitters, thyroid hormones and, 1132; see also specific neurotransmitter
Neurotropic viruses, 824-828; see also Viral diseases of central nervous system
Neutral phosphates, 1180, 1191
Neutralization, 124, 130, 131
Neutropenia, 356-357, 358-361
    chronic idiopathic, 360
    congenital, 359-360
    cyclic, 360
    drug-induced, 360
    management of, 361
    oral ulcers and, 420, 450-451
Neutrophil counts, 358
Neutrophil dysfunction syndromes, 356-357, 420
Neutrophil releasing factor, 356
Neutrophilic leukemia, chronic, 362
Neutrophils, 358
    circulating, 356

Neutrophils—cont'd
    disorders of, 355-363, 420, 450-451
    half-life of, 356
    kinetics of, 355-356
    marginal, 356
    segmented, 356
Nevi
    basal cell, syndrome of, 1209
    facial, 810
    melanomas and, 917
    neurofibromatosis and, 878
    oral, 918-919, 1209
    syndromes of, 883, 1209
Nevoid basal cell carcinoma syndrome, 883
Nevoid basalioma syndrome, 883
Nevus flammeus, 881-882
Newborn; see also Infants
    glucose-6-phosphate dehydrogenase deficiency and, 330
    hemolytic disease of, 337-338, 418
    hemorrhagic disease of, 411
    hyperthyroidism of, 1132
    hypocalcemia of, 1195
    listeriosis and, 246
    scalded skin syndrome and, 219, 110, 932
    streptococci and, 227
    sulfonamides and, 170
    triiodothyronine and, 1131
    viral infections of, 125-127, 1073-1074
NGSA; see Nongonococcal septic arthritis
NGU; see Nongonococcal urethritis
NHL; see Non-Hogkin's lymphoma
Niacin, 1106, 1110
    acanthosis nigricans and, 887
    deficiency of, 850, 1298
    hyperlipidemias and, 1290
Niacinamide, 1110
Nickel, 30, 432
Niclosamide, 294
Nicotinamide adenine dinucleotide, 1110
    alcohol and, 1255, 1256
    Haemophilus influenzae and, 235
    reduced, 1255, 1256
Nicotinamide adenine dinucleotide phosphate, 1110
    reduced, 1129
        oxidase, granulomatous disease and, 357
        thyroid hormone synthesis and, 1129
Nicotinamide-adenine dinucleotidase, 223
Nicotine; see also Smoking
    coronary artery disease and, 526
    esophageal reflux and, 982, 985
    stomatitis and, 919
Nicotinic acid; see Niacin
NIDDM; see Non-insulin-dependent diabetes mellitus
Niemann-Pick disease, 1231, 1232
    lung and, 721
    neutropenia and, 358
    reticuloendothelial system and, 396-397
Nifedipine, 465, 532, 533
Nifurtimox, 287
Night blindness, 1107
Night guards
    cerebrovascular accident and, 873
    myofascial pain dysfunction and, 109
    nocturnal bruxism and, 861
    parkinsonism and, 870
    peripheral neuropathy and, 874
Night sweats, 255
Nikolsky's sign, 220, 877
    Lyell's disease and, 931
    pemphigus and, 933

Nikolsky's sign—cont'd
    scalded skin syndrome and, 932
Nil disease, 613
Nipple, 11
Niridazole, 296
Nissen's procedure, 985
Nitrates; see also Nitroglycerin
    angina pectoris and, 531, 532
    as carcinogens, 432
    cardiomyopathy and, 522
    heart failure and, 465
    myocardial infarction and, 537
Nitrazine paper, 198
Nitrites, 862, 863, 981
Nitro-Bid; see Nitroglycerin
Nitroblue tetrazolium dye test, 357
Nitrofurans, 330
Nitrofurantoin, 161, 170-171
    hemolysis and, 330
    lung disease and, 721, 722
    neuropathy and, 779, 853
    peripheral polyneuropathies and, 779, 853
    pregnancy and, 1212
    urinary concentrations of, 157
    urinary tract infection and, 197, 198, 199
Nitrofurazone, 330
Nitrogen
    gastrointestinal gas and, 960-961
    liquid, 927, 928
    liver disease and, 1062-1063
Nitrogen mustard; see Mechlorethamine
Nitrogen oxides, 697, 729
Nitroglycerin; see also Nitrates
    alcohol and, 1297
    angina pectoris and, 531, 532, 583
    esophageal spasm and, 981
    myocardial infarction and, 474, 537
Nitroglyn; see Nitroglycerin
Nitroimadazoles, 283
Nitroprusside
    aortic dissection and, 562
    cyanide in fetus and, 665
    heart failure and, 464, 465
    hypertension and, 474
    myocardial infarction and, 537
    pulmonary edema and, 465
    in shock, 478
    in urine test, 649
Nitrosamines, 656
Nitrosoureas, 440, 442
    carcinoma and, 447, 448
    metastatic melanoma and, 918
    mycosis fungoides and, 901
    neutropenia and, 358
    thrombocytopenia and, 400
Nitrospan; see Nitroglycerin
Nitrostat; see Nitroglycerin
Nitrous oxide
    abuse of, 853, 862, 863
    for sedation
        arrhythmias and, 585
        in epileptic, 866
        facial muscle rigidity and, 870
        hypertension and, 574
        pregnancy and, 1213
        renal disease and, 670
        in respiratory disease, 746, 747
        sickle cell anemia and, 417
        stress of dental visits and, 1092
Nizoral; see Ketoconazole
NLL; see Nodular lymphocytic lymphoma
Nocardia, 171, 247, 645
Nocardiosis, 247; see also *Nocardia*

Noctec; *see* Chloral hydrate
Nocturnal bruxism, 861
Nocturnal dyspnea, paroxysmal, 461
Nocturnal hemoglobinuria, paroxysmal, 319, 341-342, 358
Nodal tachycardia, 545
Nodes; *see also* Lymph nodes; Nodules
 Bouchard's, 83, 84
 Heberden's, 83, 84
 Hodgkin's disease and, 388
 lymphoma and, 424
 of neck, 9-10
 Osler's, 180, 181
 Schmorl's, 89
Nodular fat necrosis, 913
Nodular gingivitis, tuberculous erythematous, 304
Nodular lymphocytic lymphoma, 392, 393
Nodular lymphomas, 392, 393
Nodular melanoma, 917
Nodular sclerosis Hodgkin's disease, 388
Nodules; *see also* Nodes
 fibrofatty, 102
 in liver, 1059, 1079-1084; *see also* Cirrhosis
 lung cancer and, 740
 oral leprosy and, 304-305
 rheumatoid, 229, 906
 silicotic, 724
 solitary
  malignant lymphoma and, 900
  pulmonary, 685, 743, 744
 subcutaneous; *see* Subcutaneous nodules
 in Weber-Christian disease, 79
Nonallergic asthma, 704; *see also* Asthma
Nonarticular rheumatism, 96-102
Nonfluent aphasia, 758
Nongonococcal pelvic inflammatory disease, 215
Nongonococcal septic arthritis, 79-81; *see also* Arthritis, infectious
Nongonococcal urethritis, 214, 218
Non-Hodgkin's lymphoma, 358, 391-394, 424
Non-insulin-dependent diabetes mellitus, 1261-1262, 1263
Nonocclusive vascular disease of gut, 1020-1021
Nonparoxysmal atrial tachycardia, 542
Nonparoxysmal atrioventricular junctional tachycardia, 545
Nonparoxysmal ventricular tachycardia, 545
Non-rapid eye movement sleep, 769
Non-REM; *see* Non-rapid eye movement sleep
Nonspecific pericarditis, 550
Nonspecific urethritis, 214, 217
Nonsteroidal anti-inflammatory agents; *see* Anti-inflammatory drugs
Nontoxic goiter, 1148-1149
Nontuberculous mycobacterial infections, 261-263, 264
Noonan's syndrome, 1170-1171
Norepinephrine, 1165, 1166, 1168
 heart failure and, 465
 heart rate and, 458
 pheochromocytoma and, 1164
 reserpine and, 575
 shock and, 477
Normal, definitions of, 1301
Normal pressure hydrocephalus, 775
Normal saline; *see also* Saline
 hypercalcemia and, 1180, 1191
 hyponatremia and, 595
 hypotonic dehydration and, 597
 septic shock and, 240
Normetanephrine, 1166, 1168
Normokalemic periodic paralysis, 858

Normotensive individuals, 466
Norwalk-like agents, 149, 150
Nose
 bleeding from; *see* Epistaxis
 clefts of, 1317, 1318
 evaluation of, 9
 infection and, 21
 midline granuloma and, 73
Nose drops, 21, 23
Nosocomial transmission, 172, 176-177, 1069
Notching of ribs, 737
Notochord, abnormal, 1316
Novobiocin, 1067
Novocaine; *see* Procaine hydrochloride
NPC; *see* Nasopharynx, carcinoma of
NPH; *see* Normal pressure hydrocephalus
NS Hodgkin's disease; *see* Nodular sclerosis Hodgkin's disease
NSAIDs; *see* Anti-inflammatory drugs
NSU; *see* Nonspecific urethritis
N-terminal fragment, 1187
Nuclear cardiology, 489
Nuclear inclusion bodies, 299
Nucleated red blood cells, 315; *see also* Red blood cells
Nucleic acid
 metabolism disorders of, 1239-1240
 of viruses, 122, 123
Nucleocapsid proteins, 140
Nucleolytic enzymes, 1050
Nucleoside phosphorylase deficiency, 33, 1240
5′-Nucleotidase, 1065, 1066, 1068
Null cells, 16, 361, 392
Nutrients, 1103-1104
Nutrition, 1102-1111; *see also* Diet, Malnutrition
 amblyopia and, 850
 cardiomyopathies and, 523
 deficiencies in, 1104-1111
  liver diseases and, 1059, 1062-1063, 1080
  nervous system and, 849-851, 853
  peripheral neuropathies and, 853
 therapy for, 1111
 tumors and, 446
 in oliguria, 633
Nystagmus
 brainstem lesions and, 760
 downbeat, 769, 811
 evaluation of, 8
 intention tremor, and scanning speech, triad of, 799
 parietal lobe lesions and, 759
 positional vertigo and, 794
Nystatin, 279, 929, 938
 acrodermatitis enteropathica and, 895
 in anemia with ulcerative stomatitis, 415
 for candidiasis, 276, 299, 308; *see also* Oral candidiasis
  cancer chemotherapy and, 451
  in leukemic oral ulcers, 421-422
  oropharyngoesophagitis and, 1092
 in psoriasis, 938
 in esophagitis, 985, 1092
 tetracycline with, 451

O

O₂; *see* Oxygen
Oat cell lung carcinoma, 434, 447
Obesity, 1103, 1111
 cholesterol stones and, 1087
 coronary artery disease and, 527
 Cushing's syndrome and, 1157, 1158
 hypoventilation and, 712
 insulin resistance and, 1261

Obesity—cont'd
 non-insulin-dependent diabetes mellitus and, 1261
Obesity-hypoventilation syndrome, 712
Obliterative endarteritis, 1294
Obstipation, 1025, 1026, 1028
Obstruction
 of airway; *see* Airway obstruction
 biliary tract; *see* Biliary tract
 of bronchi; *see* Bronchi, obstruction of
 gastric, 1024-1027
  polyps and, 1034
  ulcers and, 993
 of hepatic vein, 1045, 1060, 1077-1078
 of inferior vena cava and hepatic vein, 1045
 of intestines; *see* Intestines, obstruction of
 of portal vein, 1060
 from tumors, 416, 445, 654, 660
 of urinary tract, 606, 653-656; *see also* Obstructive uropathy
Obstructive emphysema, 740; *see also* Emphysema
Obstructive jaundice; *see* Jaundice
Obstructive sleep apnea, 708, 711
Obstructive uropathy, 653-656
 functional, 654
 prostatic carcinoma and, 660
 tests for, 606, 633
 toxic nephropathy and, 627
Obstructive ventilatory disorders, 680, 740, 863; *see also* Airway obstruction
Obtundation, 764, 766
Obtuse marginal artery, 524
Occipital horns, 1302
Occipital lobe lesions, 759
Occlusal appliances, 109, 861; *see also* Night guards
Occlusion; *see also* specific disease
 atherosclerotic, aortic arch syndrome and, 562
 femoral, 570
 mucopolysaccharidoses and, 1234-1235
 thrombotic, 568; *see also* Emboli; Thrombi
 vascular disease of gut and, 951, 1020-1024
Occult blood in stool, 957, 959-960
Occult diabetes, 1278
Occupational disease; *see* Environment
Ochronotic pigment deposition, 1236
Octopamine, 1061
Ocular bobbing, 833
Ocular myopathy, 857-858
Oculoauriculovertebral dysplasia, 1300, 1310-1312
Oculocephalic reflex, 766
Oculocutaneous albinism, 1236
Oculogenital syndrome, 215
Oculoglandular tularemia, 243
Oculogyric crises, 814
Oculopharyngeal dystrophy, 857-858
Oculoplethysmography, 564
Oddi's sphincter stenosis, 1088
Odontalgia, diabetes mellitus and, 1294
Odontodysplasia, 305, 1244
Odontodysplasia leprosa, 305
Odontogenic dizziness, 794, 867-868
Odontogenic keratocysts, 883
Odontomas, 891, 1093
Odynophagia, 950, 975
OGTT; *see* Oral glucose tolerance test
1,25(OH)₂D₃; *see* 1,25-Dihydroxyvitamin D₃
24,25(OH)₂D₃; *see* 24,25-Dihydroxyvitamin D₃
25(OH)D₃; *see* 25-Hydroxyvitamin D₃
25,26(OH)₂D₃; *see* 25,26-Dihydroxyvitamin D₃
3-β-OH-dehydrogenase deficiency, 1162, 1163

Ohm's law, 751
17-OHP; *see* 17-Hydroxyprogesterone
OI; *see* Osteogenesis imperfecta
Oil retention enema, 1026
OKN; *see* Optokinetic nystagmus
Olecranon bursitis, 98
Olfactory placodes, 1306
Oligoclonal bands, 797
Oligodendroglioma, 843
Oligodontia, 877
Oligohydramnios, 649
Oligomeganephronia, 650
Oligosaccharidases, deficiency or absence of, 1004
Oliguria
   glomerulonephritis and, 610, 611
   management of, 633-634
   protracted, 634
   renal failure and
      acute, 630, 631-632, 633-634
      chronic, 636
Olivopontocerebellar atrophy, 806
OM antigens; *see* Outer membrane antigens
Omentectomy, partial, 449
Omentum, diseases of, 449, 1048-1049
Oncofetal antigens, 434-435
Oncology; *see* Neoplasia
Oncosphere, 294
Oncotic pressure, glomerular capillary, 591
Oncovin; *see* Vincristine
One and one-half syndrome, 833
Onion bulb formation, 806
Onycholysis, 886, 1141
Onychomycosis, 276, 929
Onychopathy, uremic, 897
Oocysts, 285, 286
Oocytes, 1174, 1175
Oogonia, 1174, 1175
Oophorectomy, 444, 448
Open heart surgery, 301, 551, 558-559
Open lung biopsy, 689
Open pleural biopsy, 726
Opera-glass hand, 51
OPG; *see* Oculoplethysmography
Ophthalmia neonatorum, 230
Ophthalmic arteritis, 69
Ophthalmic artery, carotid disease and, 564
Ophthalmic vein, dental infections and, 303
Ophthalmopathy, 1142, 1143, 1147-1148
Ophthalmoplegia plus, 857
Ophthalmoplegias, internuclear, 760, 766, 798
Ophthalmoscopic examination, 8-9; *see also* Eyes
Opiate derivatives, 862
Opiates; *see also* Narcotics
   abuse of, 778
   anal fissures and, 1031
   arrhythmias and, 585
   carcinoid tumors and, 450
   diarrhea and, 953
   encephalopathies and, 768
   heart medication and, 572
   intoxication with, 682
   pupillary reflexes and, 765
Opisthotonos, 252
Opsonization, 16
Optic fundi, 470; *see also* Eyes
Optic neuritis, 798
Optokinetic nystagmus, 759
Ora serrata, 973
Orabase, 876
Oral biopsy; *see* Biopsy, oral
Oral bleeding; *see* Bleeding, oral

Oral candidiasis, 276, 307-308, 1209; *see also* *Candida*
   acrodermatitis enteropathica and, 895
   cancer chemotherapy and, 451
   in esophagitis, 985, 1092
   herpetic gingivostomatitis and, 299
   leukemia and, 421-422
   lymphoma and, 424
   odonyophagia and, 975
   in polyendocrinopathy syndrome, 1209
   in psoriasis, 938
   T-lymphocyte disorders and, 34
Oral contraceptives
   aphthous ulcerations and, 1211
   Candida and, 276, 307, 929
   cerebrovascular disease and, 843
   cholesterol stones and, 1087
   coronary artery disease and, 527
   erythema nodosum and, 924
   folic acid deficiency and, 415
   hemolysis and, 341
   hepatic adenomas and, 1084
   hypertension and, 469, 475, 496
   liver disease and, 1076, 1077
   lupus erythematosus and, 57
   lupuslike syndrome and, 57
   mesenteric venous thrombosis and, 1021
   migraine and, 788
   oral manifestations of, 1213-1214
   porphyria and, 1252, 1254
   pseudotumor cerebri and, 790, 848
   pulmonary embolism and, 490
   Raynaud's phenomenon and, 63
   rifampin and, 259
   thyroxine-binding globulin and, 1134
   venous thrombosis and, 841
   von Willebrand's disease and, 407
Oral diseases; *see* Mouth
Oral glucose tolerance test, 1264; *see also* Glucose tolerance
Oral hygiene; *see also* Mouthrinses
   aplastic anemia and, 415
   cerebrovascular accident and, 873
   gingival hyperplasia and, 866
   oral lesions and, 876
Oral hypoglycemic agents, 628, 1266-1267, 1279
   alcohol and, 1297
Oral prostheses, cerebrovascular accident and, 873
Oral surgery, hemophilia and, 428
Oral ulcers; *see also* Mouth
   cancer chemotherapy and, 450
   immunodeficiency disease and, 34
   leukemia and, 421-422
   tuberculosis and, 304
   ulcerative colitis and, 1095, 1096
Orbit, 105, 1306
Orbital glioma syndrome, 878-879
Orchiectomy, 444, 449
Orchiopexy, 1170
Orchitis, 140, 1171
Organ preservation, 644; *see also* Renal transplantation; Transplantation
Organic dust, 727
Organic iodides; *see* Iodides
Orinase; *see* Tolbutamide
Ornithine transcarbamylase deficiency, 1238-1239
Ornithosis, 216
Orofacial abnormalities, renal abnormalities and, 668; *see also* Craniofacial malformations

Orofacial hemangiomatosis, 872
Orofacial pain, peripheral neuropathy and, 874
Orofacial tuberculosis, 304
Oromandibular dystonia, 821
Oropharyngoesophagitis, candidal, 1092; *see also* Oral candidiasis
Oropharynx
   dysphagia and, 974, 975-976
   erythema of, 69
   malnutrition and, 1103
   pneumonia and, 177, 178
Orotic aciduria, 316, 1240
Orthodontia, hemophilia and, 427
Orthoiodohippuric acid, iodine-labeled, 607
Orthomyxoviruses, 123
Orthopedic injuries, 490; *see also* Dislocation; Fracture; Subluxation
Orthophosphates, 648
Orthopnea, 460-461
   dentistry and, 745, 746, 748
   mitral stenosis and, 512
Orthostatic hypotension, 780
   antihypertensives and, 574, 575
   idiopathic, 824
   parkinsonism and, 814
   syncope and, 864
Orthostatic proteinuria, 589, 605
Osler's nodes, 180, 181
Osler-Weber-Rendu disease, 894, 1095; *see also* Telangiectasia
   gastrointestinal bleeding and, 958, 959
   intestines and, 1023-1024
   purpura and, 407
Osmolality
   of cellular fluid, 593
   effective, 596
   of extracellular fluid, 591, 593
   serum, 596, 1126
   of urine, 591, 595
Osmotic diarrhea, 952, 954
Osmotic diuresis, 595, 1270
Osmotic diuretics, 597; *see also* Diuresis; Diuretics
Osmotic fragility test, 328-329
Osmotic pressure, 730, 1044
Osteitis, oral contraceptives and, 1214
Osteitis deformans, 86-88, 114-115
Osteitis fibrosa cystica, 667, 1193, 1200
Osteoarthritis, 83-86, 107, 860
Osteoarthropathy, hypertrophic, 103
Osteoarthrosis, 83
Osteoblasts, 1182, 1183
Osteochondritis, costochondral, 100, 737
Osteoclastomas of jaws, 668
Osteoclasts, 1182, 1183
Osteocytes, osteoid, 1182, 1183
Osteodystrophy, renal, 636-637, 639, 1200-1201
   oral manifestations of, 667
Osteogenesis imperfecta, 407, 1203, 1243
Osteogenic sarcoma, 449-450
Osteoid osteocytes, 1182, 1183
Osteomalacia, 1106, 1186, 1188, 1198-1200
   biliary cirrhosis and, 1082
   dentistry and, 1209-1210
   hypophosphatasia and, 1200
   renal osteodystrophy and, 1200
   vitamin D and, 1107
Osteomas, 891, 1042, 1093
Osteomyelitis, 82-83
   acute, 221-222
   amyloid deposits and, 385
   bacteremia and, 236
   chronic, 82, 221

Osteomyelitis—cont'd
  contiguous focus of infection and, 221
  fungal infections and, 81
  of jaws, 116-117, 304, 417
  nongonococcal septic arthritis and, 80, 81
  of skull, 193
  staphylococcal, 221-222
  streptococcal, 226
  tuberculosis and, 81, 304
Osteonecrosis, 104, 299-300
Osteopetrosis, 1203
Osteoporosis, 88-89, 1201-1203
  of alveolar bone, hyperthyroidism and, 1205
  classification of, 88
  dentistry and, 115, 1210
  hyperparathyroidism and, 1208
  intra-articular steroids and, 106
  of jaw, 422, 425
  mineral deficiency and, 1105-1106
  multiple myeloma and, 379, 422
  nongonococcal septic arthritis and, 80
  postmenopausal, 1182, 1202
  tuberculosis and, 81
Osteosclerosis, 374, 375
Ostium primum atrial septal defect, 504
Ostium secundum atrial septal defect, 503
Otalgia, 867
OTCD deficiency; *see* Ornithine transcarbamylase deficiency
Otic suppuration, 191
Otitic hydrocephalus, 848
Otitis, 795
  brain abscesses and, 191
  mycoplasmas and, 217
  subdural empyema and, 193
Otitis media, 795
Otocraniofacial syndrome, 1309-1312
Otomandibular syndrome, 867-868
Otosclerosis, 795
Otoscopic examination, 9
Ototoxicity, 158, 166; *see also* Hearing loss
Outer cell membrane, 1114-1115
Outer membrane antigens, 186
Ovarian follicles, 1174
Ovarian overstimulation syndrome, 1045
Ovary, 1173-1178
  carcinoma of, 449, 1045, 1177-1178
  disease of, 1176-1178
    abscess in, 218
    ascites in, 1045
    neoplasms in, 449, 1045, 1177-1178
  ectopic thyroid in, 1146
  embryology of, 1173-1174
  follicular growth and development and, 1174
  gonadotropic hormones and, 1118
  oral manifestations and, 1210-1214
  polycystic, 1177
Overbite, thalassemia and, 418
Overlap syndrome, 66, 67
  pulmonary fibrosis and, 716, 719
  skin disorders of, 906
Overweight, 1103; *see also* Obesity
Ovulation, 1174, 1175
Oxacillin, 160, 164
  cellulitis and, 226
  endocarditis and, 183
  pregnancy and, 1212
  renal disease and, 670
  site of infection and, 157
  staphylococci and, 183, 221
Oxalate, urinary, 620-621, 648
Oxazepam, 670, 1072
Oxidizing mouthwashes, 425; *see also* Peroxide

Oxolinic acid, 161, 171
Oxygen
  arterial, tension of; *see* Oxygen tension, arterial
  carboxyhemoglobinemia and, 344
  heart failure and, 461
  myocardial demands for, 528, 583
  nitrous oxide and; *see also* Nitrous oxide
  in therapy; *see also* Oxygen therapy
  toxicity of, 729-730
  transport of, 707-708
Oxygen affinity, 331, 1227
Oxygen dissociation curve, 331, 676, 682, 707
  hemoglobin mutants and, 354
Oxygen saturation of hemoglobin, 707
Oxygen tension, 676; *see also* Arterial blood gases
  arterial, 673
    alveolar gas composition and, 673
    atelectasis and, 702
    heart failure and, 462
    initial evaluation of, 681
    liver disease and, 1064
    mean, 673
    polycythemia and, 353, 354
    pulmonary capillary blood flow and, 674, 675
    pulmonary embolism and, 491, 492
    respiratory failure and, 707, 708, 709, 710
    ventilation-perfusion abnormalities and, 676
  asthma and, 24, 706, 707
  end-capillary, 676
  fetal blood and, 498
  hypoxemia and, 681-682
  inspiration and, 681-682
  moist inspired, 673
  respiratory failure and, 707, 708, 709, 710
Oxygen therapy
  arrhythmias and, 584, 585
  arterial hypoxemia and, 682
  asbestosis and, 726
  asthma and, 706, 707
  bronchitis and, 693
  emphysema and, 695
  heart failure and, 464
  hyperbaric, 116, 253
  hypoglycemia and, 1295
  hypoxia and, 682, 696
  ischemia and, 587
  lung disease from, 722
  malignant hyperpyrexia and, 858
  myocardial infarction and, 537
  myxedema coma and, 1140
  nitrous oxide and; *see* Nitrous oxide
  pancreatitis and, 1053
  pneumonitis and, 728
  pulmonary edema and, 465
  pulmonary emboli and, 494
  pulmonary fibrosis and, 714
  pulmonary hypertension and, 497
  respiratory acidosis and, 601
  in respiratory disease, 746
  respiratory failure and, 710, 711
  in seizures, 866
  silicosis and, 724
  smoke inhalation and, 729
  tetralogy of Fallot and, 507
  vasovagal syncope and, 576
Oxyhemoglobin dissociation curves, 331, 676, 682, 707
  hemoglobin mutants and, 354
Oxyphenbutazone, 93
Oxyphenisatin, 1078

Oxytetracycline, 168
Oxytocin, 594, 1258
Ozone, 729

P

^{32}P; *see* Radioactive phosphorus
P_{50}, 331, 707
P_{CO_2}; *see* Carbon dioxide tension, arterial
P_{IO_2}; *see* Moist inspired oxygen tension
P_{O_2}; *see* Oxygen tension
P_{VO_2}; *see* Mixed venous oxygen
P component, 386
P wave, 482, 483
PA; *see* Pernicious anemia
Pa_{CO_2}; *see* Carbon dioxide tension, arterial
Pa_{O_2}; *see* Oxygen tension, arterial
$P(A-a)_{O_2}$; *see* Alveolar-arterial oxygen tension difference
PABA, actinic keratosis of lips and, 918
Pacemaker cells, 479
Pacemakers
  atrioventricular block and, 548
  in children, 500, 501
  of colon, 1027
  dental equipment and, 585
  of heart, 541
  in stomach, 944
  subsidiary, 547
  temporary transvenous, 537
Packed red blood cells, 318, 342
Paget's disease, 86-88, 114-115
Pagitane; *see* Cycrimine
PAH clearance; *see* Para-aminohippurate clearance
Pain
  abdominal, 950-952
  anorectal disorders and, 1029, 1031
  appendicitis and, 1016
  arterial insufficiency and, 568
  ascites and, 1046
  biliary, 950-951, 988, 1087-1088
  in bone, 88, 89, 374
  bowel obstruction and, 1024, 1025
  cardiac, dentistry and, 582-583
  chest; *see* Chest, pain in
  colic in; *see* Colic
  colorectal carcinoma and, 1040
  diverticular disease of colon and, 1017
  in ear, dentistry and, 867-868
  evaluation of, 14
  facial, 790-791
    cerebrovascular accident and, 872
    multiple sclerosis and, 868
    peripheral neuropathy and, 874
  fibrositis and, 96
  flank, 662, 663
  functional bowel disease and, 1027, 1028
  gastric carcinoma and, 1035
  gastrointestinal polyposis syndromes and, 1042
  jaw, dentistry and, 869
  large bowel neoplasms and, 1042
  lupus erythematosus and, 54
  multiple myeloma and, 379
  muscle; *see* Muscles, pain in
  pancreatic carcinoma and, 1056, 1057
  pancreatitis and, 950, 989, 1051, 1053, 1055, 1056
  pelvic girdle, 48
  peptic ulcers and, 988
  peripheral neuropathy and, 1275
  peritoneum and, 1043, 1046-1049
  porphyria and, 1251
  sickle cell anemia and, 332

Pain—cont'd
  small bowel neoplasms and, 1037
  spinal epidural abscess and, 194
  supportive care for, 446
  on swallowing, 975
  throat, 132, 791
  vascular disease of gut and, 1020, 1201
Painful stimuli, 763
Palate
  angiokeratoma of, 912
  cleft, 1228, 1320-1321
  evaluation of, 9
  lichen planus and, 938
  midline granuloma and, 73
  myoclonus and, 833
  non-Hodgkin's lymphoma of, 424
  soft, rubella and spots on, 300
  ulcer of, 55
Pallor
  circumoral, 224
  digital, 62-63, 906
  heart failure and, 461
Palmar erythema, 896, 1059
Palmar fascia contracture, 101
Palmar flappings, 766
Palmar-plantar subungual-mucosal melanoma, 918
Palmoplantar pustulosis, 937
Palpation, 7
  of abdomen, 12-13
  of heart, 12
  of thorax, 12, 684
Palpebral xanthomas, 889
Palsy, 269; see also Paralysis
  Bell's 138
  bulbar, 760, 803
  facial, 130, 138
  supranuclear, 774-775
Pamaquine, 329
Panacinar emphysema, 693, 694, 700
Pancoast's syndrome, 739
Pancreas, 1049-1057
  abscess of, 1054
  alcohol and, 1051, 1055, 1258
  annular, 1050
  arteriography of, 1278
  artificial, 1279
  ascites and, 1045, 1054
  biopsy of, 969
  carcinomas of, 1056-1057
    ascites and, 1045
    diagnosis of, 968, 969, 971
    malabsorption and, 1001
    management of, 448
    oncofetal antigen and, 435
  cholera and, 954, 1049
  congenital anomalies of, 1050-1051
  dentistry and diseases of, 1101-1102
  diagnosis and, 968, 969
  ectopic, 1035, 1037, 1050
  endoscopic retrograde cannulation and; see Endoscopic retrograde cholangiopancreatography
  enzymes of; see Pancreatic enzymes
  exocrine, 1049-1050
  fibrosis of, 1055
  inflammation of; see Pancreatitis
  islet cell tumors of, 450, 994, 1056, 1278-1279
  malabsorption and, 1001
  needle aspiration of, 969
  pseudocysts of, 970, 1045, 1054
  replacement therapy and, 1051, 1056
  resection of, 1279

Pancreas—cont'd
  resection of—cont'd
    malabsorption and, 1001
    radical, 1057, 1089
    subtotal, 1056
  structure and function of, 945-946
  tumors of, 1056-1057; see also Pancreas, carcinomas of
    hyperparathyroidism and, 1192
    islet cell, 450, 994, 1056, 1278-1279
    Zollinger-Ellison syndrome and; see Zollinger-Ellison syndrome
  ultrasound and, 970
Pancreatectomy, 1279
  malabsorption and, 1001
  radical, 1057, 1089
  subtotal, 1056
Pancreatic ascites, 1045, 1054
Pancreatic beta-cell tumors, 450, 994, 1056, 1278-1279
Pancreatic cholera, 965, 1049
Pancreatic enzymes, 1049-1050
  malabsorption and, 1001, 1004
  osteomalacia and, 1199
Pancreatic extracts in replacement therapy, 1051, 1055
Pancreatic phospholipase, 1086
Pancreatic polypeptide, 945, 1049, 1263
Pancreaticoduodenectomy, radical, 1057, 1089
Pancreatitis
  acute, 1051-1055
  ascites and, 1045, 1054
  cholelithiasis and, 1088
  chronic, 1055-1056
    malabsorption and, 1001
    saliva tests and, 1102
    xanthoma disseminatum and, 890
  computed tomography and, 971
  hyperlipidemia and, 1280
  pain and, 950, 989, 1051, 1053, 1055, 1056
  pleural effusion and, 732
  ultrasound and, 970
Pancreozymin secretion test, 1102
Pancytopenia, 320, 323, 398
Panencephalitis, subacute sclerosing, 138, 828
Paneth's cells, 945
Panhypopituitarism, 1172
Panlobular emphysema, 693, 694, 700
Panniculitis, 78, 79, 1048
Pantopaque; see Isophendylate
Pantothenic acid, 1106, 1110
PAO; see Peak acid output
PAP; see Pulmonary artery pressure
Papain, 998
Papanicolaou smears, 434
Papillae, 416, 1029
Papillary carcinoma of thyroid, 1151
Papillary muscle, rupture of, 536
Papillary tumors of bladder, 659
Papilledema, 798, 846
Papillon-LeFevre syndrome, 1243, 1244
Papovaviruses, 123, 828, 1030
Pappenheimer bodies, 333
Paprika splitter's lung, 727
Papules, 303, 880, 905
Papulosis, malignant atrophic, 893-894, 1003
Para-aminobenzenes, 28
Para-aminobenzoic acid, 30, 903
Para-aminohippurate clearance, 604
Para-aminosalicylate
  drug-induced disease and, 329, 721, 722
  globoid cell leukodystrophy and, 802
  hemolysis and, 329, 342
  ileal mucosa and, 317

Para-aminosalicylate—cont'd
  lung disease and, 259, 721, 722
  malabsorption and, 1002
  thrombocytopenia and, 400
  in tuberculosis, 259
Paracentesis, 446, 1044
Paracoccidioidomycosis, 278
Paradoxic embolization, congenital heart disease and, 579
Paradoxical pulse
  pericardial tamponade and, 553, 554, 705-706
  pericarditis and, 585
Paragangliomas, 1164
Parainfluenza viruses, 140, 142-143, 172, 177
Paraisopropyl iminodiacetic acid, 969
Paraldehyde, 776, 787
Paralysis; see also Palsy
  enteroviruses and, 137
  facial nerve, tuberculoid leprosy and, 305
  frontal lobe lesions and, 757
  hypotonic, 757
  multiple sclerosis and, 798-799
  periodic, 858
  poliovirus vaccines and, 151; see also Poliomyelitis
  respiratory, 169, 204
  shellfish poisoning and, 200
  sleep, 769
  spinal epidural abscess and, 194
  syringomyelia and, 807
Paralysis agitans; see Parkinsonism
Paralytic aneurysms, 839
Paralytic ileus, 1024-1026
Parameningeal infections, 139, 189, 191-194
Paramethadione, 627
Paramyxoviruses, 123, 140, 141-143, 177
Paranasal sinuses, 73
Paraneoplastic syndromes, 437-438, 855, 1178
Paraparesis, spastic, 799, 807
Paraproteins, 435
Parapsoriasis en plaques, 900
Parasites; see also Helminthic diseases
  diarrhea and, 953
  eosinophilia and, 372
  immunodeficiency diseases and, 31
  intracellular, 31
  malabsorption and, 1003
Parasomnias, 770
Parasystole, 542, 545
Parathyroid glands, 1127, 1128; see also Hyperparathyroidism; Hypoparathyroidism; Parathyroid hormone
  adenomas of, 879, 1192
  autotransplantation and, 1194
  failure to develop, 33
  hyperplasia of, 1192
  removal of, 639, 1194, 1201
Parathyroid hormone; see also Parathyroid glands
  calcium metabolism and, 1184, 1195
  deficiency of, 1188, 1196-1197; see also Hypoparathyroidism
    hypocalcemia and, 1195
  ectopic, 1179-1180
  end-organ unresponsiveness to, 1197
  immunoreactive, 1193-1194, 1196
  kidney stones and, 647, 648
  metabolism of, 1186-1188
  phosphate metabolism and, 1184
  primary hyperparathyroidism and, 1192-1194
  renal failure and, 636, 637
  triiodothyronine and, 1132
  vitamin D and, 1186
Parathyroidectomy, 639, 1194, 1201
Paratonia, 758, 767

Paratrigeminal neuralgia, 791
Parenchymal disease, 690
　chronic liver; see Cirrhosis
　pulmonary, 171, 685, 696
　　congestive heart failure and, 454
　　emboli and, 490
　　emphysema and, 694
　　sarcoidosis and, 717
　　renal, secondary hypertension and, 573
Parenchymal hemorrhage, cerebral, 829, 838
Parenteral hyperalimentation; see Hyperalimentation, parenteral
Parenteral nutrition, 1111
Paresis, 269; see also Palsy; Paralysis
Paresthesias
　of lip, Epstein-Barr virus and, 300
　multiple sclerosis and, 799
　osteomyelitis of mandible and, 116
　vitamin B_{12} deficiency and, 808
Parietal capillary hydrostatic pressure, 730
Parietal cells, 942, 943
　antibodies to, 997
　gastritis and, 996
　Zollinger-Ellison syndrome and, 994
Parietal cortex, 771
Parietal lobe lesions, 758-759
Parietal pleura, 730
Parinaud's syndrome, 760
Parkinsonism, 812-815
　essential tremor and, 815
　facial muscles and, 870-871
　iatrogenic, 812
　idiopathic, 812-815
Parlodel; see Bromocriptine
Paromomycin, 283, 294
Paronychial infarctions, 906
Parotid ducts, stenosis of, 1296
Parotid glands
　antiparkinsonism drugs and, 871
　cystic fibrosis and, 1101
　enlargement of
　　alcoholic cirrhosis and, 1097-1098, 1296
　　sarcoidosis and, 113
　　herpangina and, 301
　　mumps and, 137, 139, 307, 1171
Parotid saliva, diagnostic tests of, 1101, 1102
Parotitis; see also Parotid glands
　antiparkinsonism drugs and, 871
　herpangina and, 301
　mumps and, 137, 139, 307, 1171
Paroxysmal atrial fibrillation, 549
Paroxysmal atrial flutter, 543, 549
Paroxysmal atrial tachycardia, 542
Paroxysmal atrioventricular junctional tachycardia, 545
Paroxysmal cold hemoglobinuria, 340
Paroxysmal hemicrania, chronic, 789
Paroxysmal nocturnal dyspnea, 461
Paroxysmal nocturnal hemoglobinuria, 319, 341-342, 358
Paroxysmal polyserositis, 1048
Paroxysmal supraventricular tachycardia, 548-549
Paroxysmal syndromes, 799
Paroxysmal ventricular tachycardia, 545-546
Paroxysmal vertigo, 794
Parrot, pseudoparalysis of, 270
Partial pressure
　of carbon dioxide in arteries; see Carbon dioxide tension, arterial
　of oxygen; see Oxygen tension
Partial seizures, 781, 782-783, 866
Partial thromboplastin time, 409, 430, 1098
Particulate ionizing radiation, 749

Passovoy factor deficiency, 411
Pasteurella multocida, 171
Pasteurella pestis, 242
Pastia's lines, 224
Patches
　mucous, secondary syphilis and, 303
　Peyer's, 207, 941
　Shagreen, 880
Patent ductus arteriosus, 489, 504-505, 556-557
　cyanosis and, 506, 683
　transposition of great arteries and, 508
Pathologic fractures, 88, 89, 379
Pathologic reflexes, 14
Pathways, 17, 18
Patient identification, 5
PBG; see Porphobilinogen
PBI; see Protein-bound iodine
PCC; see Prothrombin complex concentrate
PCH; see Paroxysmal cold hemoglobinuria
PCP; see Phencyclidine
PCT; see Porphyria cutanea tarda
PCWP; see Pulmonary capillary wedge pressure
Peak acid output, 944
Peak expiratory flow rate, 679, 692
Pectinate line, 1029
Pectoral muscles, 98, 101
Pectus carinatum, 737
Pectus excavatum, 737
Pediatrics; see Children
Pedigrees, 1223-1224
PEFR; see Peak expiratory flow rate
Peg-shaped teeth, anhydrotic ectodermal dysplasia and, 877
Pelger-Huët-like anomaly, 321
Peliosis hepatis, 1076
Pelizaeus-Merzbacher disease, 802
Pellagra, 850, 1110
Pelvic abscesses, 218
Pelvic actinomycosis, 247
Pelvic girdle pain, 48
Pelvic inflammatory disease, 215, 218, 231, 232
Pelvicrural contraction, 774
Pemoline, sleep disorders and, 769
Pemphigoid, 932, 935
Pemphigus, 932-935
Pemphigus erythematosus, 934
Pemphigus foliaceus, 934
Pemphigus vegetans, 933-934
Pemphigus vulgaris, 932-933
Pencil-in-cup deformity, 51
Penicillamine
　biliary cirrhosis and, 1082
　cystine kidney stones and, 649
　heavy metal toxicity and, 753, 754
　lead neuropathy and, 853
　lupuslike syndrome and, 57
　nephrotic syndrome and, 612, 613
　rheumatoid arthritis and, 42, 46
　scleroderma and, 61, 903
　toxic nephropathy and, 624, 625, 626, 629
　Wilson's disease and, 823, 1082, 1240
Penicillin analogs, 590
Penicillin G, 159-163
　abscesses and, 192, 225
　aqueous, 159, 160
　benzathine, 246
　endocarditis and, 181, 183, 185, 581
　erysipeloid and, 246
　injection of, 157
　leptospirosis and, 274
　listeriosis and, 246
　nephropathy and, 627, 629
　pneumonia and, 175
　renal disease and, 670

Penicillin G—cont'd
　rheumatic fever and, 230
　staphylococci and, 183, 221
　subdural empyema and, 193
　syphilis and, 271, 272
Penicillin homologues, 625
Penicillin V, 160, 163
　actinomycosis and, 247
　anthrax and, 245
　endocarditis and, 185, 581
　pharyngitis and, 225
　pneumonia and, 175
　rat-bite fever and, 272
　renal disease and, 670
Penicillinase-producing gonococcus, 232
Penicillinase-resistant beta lactam antibiotic, 303
Penicillinase-resistant penicillin, 220, 221
　bacteremia and, 220
　brain abscess and, 192
　bronchiectasis and, 697
　endocarditis and, 183, 184
　enterocolitis and, 220
　pneumonia and, 175
　semisynthetic, 226
　skin diseases and, 219
Penicillinase-sensitive penicillins, 159-163; see also Penicillins
Penicillins, 159-164
　abscesses and
　　abdominal, 1047
　　cerebral epidural, 193
　　lung, 699
　acute necrotizing ulcerative gingivitis and, 302
　allergy and, 27-28, 170, 576
　with aminoglycosides, 121, 166, 176, 227, 228
　anaerobes and, 178, 228, 250
　bactericidal activity of, 156
　benzathine; see Benzathine penicillin
　benzyl; see Penicillin G
　cavernous sinus thrombosis and, 303
　cervicofacial actinomycosis and, 305
　Chlamydia trachomatis and, 214
　clostridia and, 253
　diphtheria and, 248
　dosages of, 158
　drug fever and, 159
　endocarditis and, 121, 184
　enterococci and, 227
　environmental contamination and, 29
　erysipeloid and, 246
　erythema multiforme and, 922
　erythema nodosum and, 28
　excretion and, 158
　G; see Penicillin G
　gonococci and, 215, 232
　hemolysis and, 29, 342
　hypokalemia and, 598
　impetigo and, 226
　leukopenia and, 29
　listeriosis and, 246
　liver disease and, 1090
　lung disease and, 178, 699, 721, 722
　Lyme disease and, 298
　meningitis and, 189, 190
　nephritis and, 619, 620
　nephropathy and, 624, 625, 626, 627, 629
　oral streptococci and, 302
　oral ulcers and, 421
　osteomyelitis and, 222
　penicillinase-resistant; see Penicillinase-resistant penicillin
　phenoxymethyl, 160, 163
　platelet function and, 406

Penicillins—cont'd
  pneumonia and, 175, 218, 234
  porphyria and, 1252
  pregnancy and, 1212, 1213
  with probenecid, 232
  procaine; see Procaine penicillin
  prophylactic, endocarditis and, 581, 582
  proteinuria and, 590
  rat-bite fever and, 272, 273
  renal disease and, 670
  renal insufficiency and, 159
  rheumatic fever and, 230
  shock and, 476, 478
  site of infection and, 156
  splenectomy and, 395
  streptococci and, 175, 225, 226, 227, 228
  and streptomycin, 302, 581
  syphilis and, 264, 265, 268, 272
  tetanus and, 252
  thrombocytopenia and, 29
  thyroid hormone binding and, 1131
  toxic nephropathy and, 626
  uremic stomatitis and, 667
  urethritis and, 215
  urticaria and, 20
  V; see Penicillin V
  vasculitis and, 29
  Whipple's disease and, 1003
Penicillium caseii, 727
Penis; see also Genitalia
  evaluation of, 13
  Reiter's syndrome and, 907
  syphilis and, 266, 267
  tuberculosis and, 256
Pentagastrin, 944
  C-cell hyperplasia and, 1151, 1152, 1197
  ulcers and, 993
Pentamidine, 288
Pentaquine, 329
Pentazocine, 23, 1017
Penthrane; see Methoxyflurane
Pentobarbital, 777
Pentylenetetrazol, 762
Pepsin, 942
Pepsinogen, 940, 942, 943
Peptic acid diseases, 987-998; see also Digestive system, acid-peptic diseases of; Ulcers
Peptide hormones, 943, 944, 1115
Peptococcus, 249, 699
Peptostreptococcus, 249, 302, 699
Perception, focal hemispheric lesions and, 771
Perchlorate, iodine trapping and, 1132
Percodan, 862, 1212
Percussion, 7, 12, 13, 684
Percutaneous aspiration, 689, 969
Percutaneous cholangiography, 968, 1088, 1089
Percutaneous coronary dilation, 532
Perforation
  of appendix, 1016
  in diverticulosis, 1017
  of esophagus, 734, 986-987
  of peptic ulcer, 988, 993, 1052
Perfusion
  myocardial, 489, 524-526
  pulmonary, 673-674; see also Pulmonary vessels
    pulmonary embolism and, 492, 493
    scanning and, 687
  tissue, congestive heart failure and, 452
Periadenitis mucosa necrotica recurrens, 1095
Perianal area; see also Anus
  fistulas in, 1011
  pinworms and, 290
  thrush and, 276

Periapical abscesses, diabetes and, 1294
Periarteritis nodosa, 363, 666
Peribronchiolar infiltrate, lymphocytic, 141
Pericardial calcification, 551, 552
Pericardial cysts, 555
Pericardial effusion, 553-555
  lax, 553, 554, 555
  systemic sclerosis and, 60
Pericardial friction rub, 551
Pericardial knock, 552
Pericardial sclerosing agents, 555
Pericardial tamponade, 553, 554, 555
  amebiasis and, 283
  heart failure and, 453-454, 461
  shock and, 476
Pericardial window technique, 555
Pericardiectomy, 551, 553, 555
Pericardiocentesis, 555
Pericarditis, 550-555
  acute, 550-551
  constrictive, 1045, 1077
  dentistry and, 585-587
  diffuse, 550
  effusive, 553-555
  effusive-constrictive, 555
  focal, 550
  idiopathic, 550
  juvenile rheumatoid arthritis and, 47
  meningococcemia and, 235
  myocardial infarction and, 536
  nonspecific, 550
  systemic sclerosis and, 60
Pericardium, 550
  calcification of, 551, 552
  congenital defects of, 555
  congestive heart failure and, 453-454
  cysts of, 555
  effusions of; see Pericardial effusion
  excision of; see Pericardiectomy
  inflammations of; see Pericarditis
  primary tumors of, 555
  tuberculosis in, 256, 260
Pericemental anesthesia, 426
Perifollicular light cells, 1128; see also C cells
Perihepatitis, 231
Perinatal infections, 125-127, 1073-1074; see also Newborn
Perinephric abscess, 199
Periodic alternating nystagmus, 760
Periodic disease, 53
Periodic paralysis, 858
Periodontal abscesses, 421, 1294
Periodontal disease
  acromegaly and, 1204
  bacteremia and, 180
  diabetes and, 1294
  immunodeficiency disease and, 34
  malnutrition and, 1103
  neutrophil dysfunction and, 420
  pregnancy and, 1211
  vitamin C and, 1110-1111
Periodontal ligament spaces, 112
Periodontal membrane lesions, 115
Periodontal therapy, hemophilia and, 427
Periodontitis
  alcoholism and, 1296
  Ehlers-Danlos syndrome and, 1243, 1302
  juvenile, neutrophil dysfunction and, 420
  riboflavin deficiency and, 1109
Periodontosis, juvenile, 420, 1243, 1244
Perioral rhagades, congenital syphilis and, 303
Peripheral blood smears, 310, 313-315
  glucose-6-phosphate dehydrogenase deficiency and, 331
  leukoerythroblastic changes in, 322

Peripheral blood smears—cont'd
  myeloid metaplasia and, 375
  myelophthisis and, 322
  sickle cell anemia and, 333
  spherocytosis and, 328
Peripheral cyanosis, cardiac decompensation and, 571
Peripheral edema, 461; see also Edema
Peripheral joints, 13
Peripheral nerves
  biopsy of, 852
  compression of, supportive care and, 445
  leprosy and, 261, 263
  lesions of, 761
  neuropathies of; see Neuropathies, peripheral
Peripheral vascular system
  central venous pressure and, 571
  diabetes mellitus and, 1273
  evaluation of, 13
  resistance in, 460
    hypertension with increased, 467
Peripheral vertigo, 792
Peristalsis
  esophagus and, 973-974
    absence of, 976, 981
  failure of, 1024-1026
Peritoneal dialysis, 640-641, 642
  chronic ambulatory, 641
  diabetic nephropathy and, 617
  interstitial nephritis and, 620
  preparing and initiating, 639-640
  renal failure and, 635
Peritoneal fluid, 1043, 1044, 1047
Peritoneal lavage, 971
Peritoneal lymphatics, 1043
Peritoneal membrane, 1043
Peritoneal vasculitis, 1048
Peritoneoscopy, 966, 1044
Peritoneum, 1043-1049
  biopsy of, 1044
  bleeding in, 971
  dialysis and; see Peritoneal dialysis
  inflammation of; see Peritonitis
  mesothelioma of, 726
  neoplasia of, 726-727, 1047
  transfusions and, 338
  tuberculosis and, 256, 1046-1047
  ultrasound and, 256
Peritonitis
  appendicitis and, 1015-1016
  bile, 1046
  colorectal carcinoma and, 1040
  diverticulosis and, 1017
  granulomatous, 1047, 1048
  nonocclusive vascular disease of gut and, 1021
  pain and, 951
  peritoneal dialysis and, 641
  practolol and, 105
  tuberculous, 1046-1047
Peritonsillar abscess, 224, 225
Periwinkle alkaloids; see Vinca alkaloids
Perleche, 307, 895
Permeability of capillaries, 1044
Pernicious anemia, 317, 851, 1109
  dentistry and, 414-415
  neuropathy and, 853
  neutropenia and, 359
  vitamin B_{12} deficiency and, 808
Peroneal muscular atrophy, 805, 855
Peroxidase, 1129
Peroxide, 876
  acute necrotizing ulcerative gingivitis and, 302, 357
  chronic granulomatous disease and, 357

Peroxide—cont'd
  pemphigoid and, 935
  pemphigus and, 933
  Reiter's syndrome and, 908
Persantine; see Dipyridamole
Persistent fetal circulation, 499
Perspiration, 596, 755
Pertinent negatives, 5
Pertussis, 143, 237-238, 248, 252
Pes planus, 102
Pessaries, 308
PET: see Positron emission tomography
Petechiae
  cytomegalovirus and, 125
  endocarditis and, 181
  idiopathic thrombocytopenic purpura and, 402-403
  vitamin C and, 1110
Petit mal seizures, 781, 783
Petroleum poisoning, 754-755
Peutz-Jeghers syndrome, 891, 1042
  dentistry and, 1093-1095
  gastrointestinal bleeding and, 958
Peyer's patches, 207, 941
Peyronie's disease, 105
Pfeiffer's syndrome, 1314, 1315, 1316
pH
  antimicrobials and, 157
  of blood, 592, 599
    heart failure and, 462
  of body fluids, 599
    esophageal, 962, 983
    gastric, 943
    pleural effusion and, 731
  of urine, 592-593, 604
    renal tubular acidosis and, 623
pH probe test, 962
Phagocytosis, 17, 356
  antibodies and, 16
  defects in, 357
Phakomatoses, 808-810, 869, 872
Phalanges
  disappearance of, 60
  sausage-like swelling of, 51
  subluxation and, 36
Phalen's sign, 98
Pharmacology of antimicrobials, 157-158; see also Drugs
Pharyngeal arches, 1305
Pharyngeal pouches, 33
Pharyngitis
  antibiotics and, 144
  aplastic anemia and, 415
  dermatomyositis and, 905
  gonococcal, 231
  mycoplasmas and, 217
  streptococcal, 175, 223-225, 228
  viral, 224
    adenovirus in, 143, 148
    infectious mononucleosis and, 132
Pharyngoconjunctival fever, 143
Pharynx
  diphtheria and, 248
  evaluation of, 9
  inflammation of; see Pharyngitis
  Wegener's granulomatosis and, 71
Phenacetin
  glucose-6-phosphate dehydrogenase deficiency and, 418
  hemolysis and, 329, 342
  nephropathy and, 621, 625, 627, 629
  renal disease and, 670
  urinary tract neoplasms and, 658
  urine and, 588, 590

Phenazopyridine, 589
Phencyclidine, 778-779, 862
Phenformin, 1051
Phenindione, 589, 624, 629
Phenobarbital
  carbon tetrachloride and, 1075
  Crigler-Najjar syndrome and, 1067
  epilepsy and, 786, 787, 866
  Gilbert's disease and, 1067
  hepatic detoxification and, 1061
  hepatitis and, 1099
  isoniazid and, 1076
  osteomalacia and, 1199
  for prophylactic control of seizures, 866
  respiratory alkalosis and, 601
  Sydenham's chorea and, 819
  toxemia of pregnancy and, 665
  toxicity of, 777
Phenol, 908
Phenolphthalein, 588, 922-923
Phenomena
  Ashman's, 544
  clasp-knife, 812
  isomorphic, 936, 937
  Koebner, 936, 937
  Raynaud's; see Raynaud's phenomenon
Phenothiazines; see also specific agent
  alcohol and, 776, 1297
  carcinoid tumors and, 450
  depressant withdrawal and, 777
  Huntington's chorea and, 774, 817
  hypothermia and, 756
  lupuslike syndrome and, 57
  megacolon and, 1027
  neoplasia and, 446
  neurologic effects of, 779
  neutropenia and, 360
  parkinsonism and, 815
  phencyclidine intoxication and, 779
  porphyria and, 1252
  postural hypotension and, 780
  prolactin and, 1119
  pseudotumor cerebri and, 848
  seizures and, 787
  side effects of, 871
  sudden death and, 538
  Sydenham's chorea and, 819
  torsion dystonias and, 820, 821
  urine and, 588, 589
Phenotypes, 1218
Phenoxybenzamine
  carcinoid tumors and, 450
  hypertension and, 473, 474
  pheochromocytoma and, 1167, 1168
Phenoxymethyl penicillin, 160, 163
Phentolamine, 450, 473, 474, 1167
Phenylalanine, 1227, 1236
L-Phenylalanine mustard, 442
  lung disease and, 722
  multiple myeloma and, 382
  myeloid metaplasia and, 376
  thrombocythemia and, 374
  Waldenström's macroglobulinemia and, 383
Phenylbutazone
  alkylosing spondylitis and, 50, 737
  aplastic anemia and, 908
  coumarins and, 414
  erythema multiforme and, 30
  gastritis and, 996
  gout and, 93
  nephropathy and, 621, 627
  neutropenia and, 360, 361
  peptic ulcers and, 1092
  pseudogout and, 95

Phenylbutazone—cont'd
  rheumatoid arthritis and, 106
  sulfonylureas and, 1267
  thrombocytopenia and, 400, 401
  ulcers and, 988
Phenylephrine, 575, 824, 864
Phenylethanolamine-N-methyltransferase, 1164, 1166
Phenylhydrazine, 330
Phenylketonuria, 1227, 1236
Phenytoin
  alcohol and, 1255, 1297
  dental care and, 866
  depressant withdrawal and, 777
  endocrine tumors and, 450
  epilepsy and, 785, 786, 787, 867
  erythema multiforme and, 922
  in fetal phenytoin syndrome, 1303
  folate deficiency and, 316, 1109
  folic acid deficiency and, 415
  gingival hyperplasia and, 765, 865-866, 880, 882
  hemolysis and, 342
  hyperglycemic, hyperosmolar, nonketotic coma and, 1270
  hypernatremia and, 595
  isoniazid and, 259
  lung disease and, 722
  methotrexate and, 440
  myasthenia gravis and, 855
  myotonic dystrophy and, 859
  nephropathy and, 625, 627
  neuropathy and, 853, 855
  neutropenia and, 360
  nystagmus and, 760
  osteomalacia and, 1198, 1199, 1200
  periodontal disease and, 765, 865-866, 880, 882
  porphyria and, 1252
  status epilepticus and, 867
  steroid metabolism and, 1154
  sulfonylureas and, 1267
  Sydenham's chorea and, 819
  toxic nephropathy and, 626
  trigeminal neuralgia and, 791
  urine and, 588
  ventricular tachycardia and, 500
Pheochromocytoma, 469, 471, 474, 1164-1168
  dentistry and, 1207
  familial, 1164-1165
  hyperparathyroidism and, 1192
  neurofibromatosis and, 879
  secondary hypertension and, 573
Philadelphia chromosome, 369, 370
Phlebitis, 494-495; see also Thrombophlebitis
  pulmonary embolism and, 490
  vancomycin and, 167
Phlebography, 495, 663
Phlebotomies
  hemochromatosis and, 345, 346, 1066, 1081
  polycythemia vera and, 353, 354
  porphyria and, 888, 1253
  renal failure and, 633
  renal vein, 663
Phonoangiography, carotid, 565
Phosphatase; see Acid phosphatase; Alkaline phosphatase
Phosphates
  antacids and, 992
  deficiency of; see Hypophosphatemia
  diabetic ketoacidosis and, 1270
  function of, 1105
  hypercalcemia and, 1180, 1191, 1195
  hypocalcemia and, 1195

Phosphates—cont'd
  kidney stones and, 648
  metabolism of, 1184-1185
  myocardial infarction and, 534
  renal failure and, 636, 639
  renal osteodystrophy and, 1200
  rickets and, 1200
Phosphodiesterase, 405, 705, 706
Phospholipase, 18, 342, 1049, 1086
Phospholipids, 1085, 1086
  liver disease and, 1286
  phosphate metabolism and, 1184
  phosphorus and, 1105
  transport of, 1282
Phosphoribosylpyrophosphate, 1239
Phosphorus
  deficiency of, 1105-1106
  liver toxicity and, 1077
  osteoporosis and, 1210
  radioactive; see Radioactive phosphorus
Photic stimuli, 1126
Photochemotherapy, 338, 937
Photophobia, 895, 907, 1107; see also Photosensitivity
Photosensitivity, 29; see also Photophobia
  liver diseases and, 1059
  porphyria and, 888, 1249, 1250, 1252, 1253
  tetracyclines and, 168
Phototherapy, 338; see also Photochemotherapy
Phrenic nerves, 1043
Phycomycetes, leukemia and, 421
Physical examination, 7-14, 434
Physiology
  of absorption, 998-999, 1004
  of bone, 1181-1189
  of carbohydrate absorption, 1004
  of peritoneum, 1043
Physostigmine, 779, 806, 817
Phytobezoars, 998
Phytohemagglutinin, 16, 32
Pick's disease, 774
Pickwickian syndrome, 712
Picornaviruses, 123, 140, 144, 149
PID; see Pelvic inflammatory disease
PIE syndrome; see Pulmonary infiltrates with eosinophilia
Pierre Robin syndrome, 1228
PIF; see Prolactin-inhibiting factor
Pigeon breast, 737
Pigeon breeder's lung, 727
Pigmentation; see also Pigments
  adrenal failure and, 886, 1156
  gastrointestinal polyposis syndromes and, 1042
  Gaucher's disease and, 1232, 1296
  hemochromatosis and, 345
  liver diseases and, 1059, 1068
  neurofibromatosis and, 878-879
  oat cell lung carcinoma and, 1179
  ochronotic, 1236
  oral, Addison's disease and, 1207
  Peutz-Jeghers syndrome and, 891, 1093-1095
  scleroderma and, 59, 903, 904
Pigments; see also Pigmentation
  stones and, 1086
  toxic nephropathy and, 627, 629, 631
Pineal gland, 1126
Pink puffer, 694
Pinworms, 289-290, 1030
Piperacillin, 160, 164, 241
Piperazine, 728
PIPIDA; see Paraisopropyl iminodiacetic acid
Pitressin; see Vasopressin
Pitting, tooth, 300
Pituitary antigens, 727

Pituitary apoplexy, 838, 1121
Pituitary gland; see also Hypothalamus
  adrenocorticotropic hormone and; see Adrenocorticotropic hormone
  anterior
    insufficiency of, 1121-1123
    secretion of, 1116-1118
  antigens and, 727
  disorders of, 1116-1126
    cerebral hemorrhage and, 838, 1121
    Cushing's syndrome and, 1157, 1158, 1159
    dentistry and, 1204-1205
    endocrine hypothalamus and, 1116, 1117
    hypothyroidism and, 1122
    pineal gland and, 1126
    prolactin deficiency and, 1123
    tumors in; see Pituitary gland, tumors of
  feedback mechanisms and, 1169, 1175
  posterior, 1116
    alcohol and, 1258
    diseases of, 1125-1126
  surgery of, 444, 448, 1120, 1124, 1159
  tumors of
    amenorrhea and, 1177
    hyperparathyroidism and, 1192
    roentgenography of, 1123-1124
    thyroid-stimulating hormone and, 1145-1146
Pituitary snuff taker's lung, 727
Pityrosporum orbiculare, 887
PK deficiency; see Pyruvate kinase deficiency
PKU; see Phenylketonuria
PL^{A1}, 400
Placenta, 16, 125, 434-435
Placental alkaline phosphatase, 435
Placental proteins, 435
Placodes, olfactory, 1306
Plague, 242
Plane xanthomas, 890, 896
Plant alkaloids; see Vinca alkaloids
Plantar fasciitis, 102
Plantar melanoma, 918
Plaquenil; see Hydrochloroquine
Plaques
  acanthosis nigricans and, 888
  asbestos and, 726
  candidal oropharyngoesophagitis and, 1092
  of demyelination, 797
  Hollenhorst, 836
  Hutchinson's, 910
  lichen planus and, 938
  mycosis fungoides and, 900-901
  pleural, 726
  pregnancy and, 1212
  sarcoidosis and, 910
Plasma
  alkaline phosphatase in, 1189
  antimicrobials in, 157-158
  apolipoproteins in, 1280-1281
  bicarbonate in, 592
  calcium in, 1183-1184, 1189-1196
  catecholamines in, 1166, 1168
  ceruloplasmin in, 1066, 1081
  cortisol in, 1258
  creatinine in, 604
  cryoglobulins in; see Cryoglobulinemia
  fresh-frozen, 350
    anticoagulants and, 577
    factor deficiencies and, 429
    hepatitis and, 1072
    liver disease and, 1064, 1098
    von Willebrand's disease and, 427
  lipids in, 1288-1289
  lipoproteins in, 1280, 1282, 1288-1289

Plasma—cont'd
  lipoproteins in—cont'd
    degradation of, 1282
    electrophoretic mobility of, 1281
    formation of, 1282
    sampling of, 1288-1289
  organ preservation and, 644
  proteins in
    abnormal, 605
    abnormal tubular reabsorption and, 605
    anaphylactic reactions to, 351
    liver disease and, 1062-1063, 1065
    transfusions and, 350
    urinary tests and, 605
  renal, 590
  renin activity and, 598, 1161; see also Renin
  shock and loss of, 476
  transfusions of, 350; see also Plasmapheresis
    disseminated intravascular coagulation and, 413
    exchange, 404, 428, 1291
    factor XIII deficiency and, 411
    fresh-frozen; see Plasma, fresh-frozen
    gastrointestinal bleeding and, 958
    hemophilia and, 410, 428
    incompatibility and, 348
    liver disease and, 411
    pooled, hepatitis and, 1069
    posthemorrhagic anemia and, 323
    proteins in, 350
    substitutes for, 350
    vitamin K deficiency and, 411
  volume of, 311, 354, 1064; see also Volume expanders
Plasma cell disorders, 376-387
  amyloidosis in, 385-387; see also Amyloidosis
  heavy-chain disease in, 384
  multiple myeloma in, 378-382; see also Multiple myeloma
  Waldenström's macroglobulinemia in, 382-384, 618
Plasma cell tumor, multiple myeloma and, 422
Plasma exchange, 404, 428, 1291
Plasma fibrinogen, malignant atrophic papulosis and, 894
Plasma immunoreactive parathyroid hormone, 1193-1194, 1196
Plasma lipid sampling, 1288-1289
Plasma protein derivative, 350
Plasma protein solution, 350
Plasma renin activity; see also Renin
  hyperkalemia and, 598
  hypokalemia and, 598
  mineralocorticoid excess and, 467, 468, 1161
Plasma volume, 311, 354, 1064; see also Volume expanders
Plasmacytosis, atypical, 382
Plasmanate, 632
Plasmapheresis, 347
  acquired anticoagulants and, 411
  cryoglobulinemia with kidney disease and, 618
  glomerulonephritis and, 610
  hemorrhagic lung disease and, 720
  lupus erythematosus and, 57, 615
  myasthenia gravis and, 856
  polyneuropathy and, 855
  posttransfusion purpura and, 404
  Refsum's disease and, 855
  and renal failure, 618
  thrombotic thrombocytopenic purpura and, 617
  Waldenström's macroglobulinemia and, 383, 618
Plasmodia, 279, 280, 281
  drugs for, 169

Plasmodia—cont'd
  red cell injury and, 343
Plasmodium falciparum, 169, 279, 280, 281
Plasmodium malariae, 280, 281
Plasmodium ovale, 280
Plasmodium vivax, 280, 281
Platelet activating factor, 18
Platelet count; *see also* Platelets
  aplastic anemia and, 416
  elevation of, 373-374, 404-405; *see also* Thrombocytosis
  Gaucher's disease and, 425
  liver disease and, 1098
Platelet granules, deficiency of, 405
Platelet-associated antigen PL^{A1}, 404
Plateletpheresis, 346, 404
Platelets
  adherence of, 400, 405
  aggregation of, 400
    aspirin and, 106, 353, 400, 405
    disorder of, 405, 1098
  disorders of, 400-408
    congenital, 401, 405
    dentistry and, 425-426
    distribution, 404
    liver disease and, 1098
    purpura and, 898; *see also* Purpura
    qualitative, 405-406
  normal, 400
  release reaction to, 400
  size of, 403
  splenomegaly and, 396
  thrombocytopenia and, 400-404, 1098; *see also* Thrombocytopenia
  transfusions of, 347, 350
    aplastic anemia and, 320
    Bernard-Soulier syndrome and, 405
    disseminated intravascular coagulation and, 413
    leukemias and, 368
    liver disease and, 411
    neoplasia and, 446
    perinatal virus and, 127
    storage-pool disease and, 405
    thrombasthenia and, 405
    thrombocytopenia and, 402, 425, 426
    von Willebrand's disease and, 407
Platinum, 704
Platybasia, 811
PLB; *see* Pursed lip breathing
Pleocytosis, 128, 188
Plerocercoid, 293
Plethora, 1157, 1158
Plethysmography, 679
Pleura
  biopsy of
    effusions and, 732
    malignant mesothelioma and, 727
    sarcoidosis and, 716
    thoracentesis and, 688
  diseases of, 730-734
    asbestos and, 726
    coxsackieviruses and, 144
    effusions in; *see* Pleural effusions
    inflammations in, 255, 730-731
    mesothelioma in, 726
    tumors in, 734
Pleural cavity, 730
Pleural effusions, 731-733
  aortic dissection and, 561
  ascites and, 1061
  chest roentgenograms and, 686
  heart failure and, 461
  lung cancer and, 740

Pleural effusions—cont'd
  lupus erythematosus and, 715
  pneumonia and, 173, 175
  rheumatoid arthritis and, 715
  sarcoidosis and, 716
  thoracentesis and, 687-688
  tuberculous, 255, 260
Pleural fluid, 730
  analysis of, 688
  eosinophilia and, 732
  leukocytosis and, 731-732
  osmotic pressure of, 730
  ultrasound and, 687
Pleural friction rub, 730
Pleural plaques, 726
Pleurisy, 255, 730
Pleuritis, 255, 730-731
Pleurodynia, epidemic, 144
Pleuroscopy, 732
Plexuses
  brachial, 100, 101, 860-861
  destruction of, 978, 1027
  of digestive system, 942, 948, 973, 974
Plicae circulares, 945
PLT; *see* Psittacosis-lymphogranuloma-trachoma
Plummer's disease, 1145
Plummer's nails, 1141
Plummer-Vinson syndrome, 416, 1091, 1105
PM-1 antibodies, 65
PMF; *see* Progressive massive fibrosis
PMN leukocytes; *see* Polymorphonuclear leukocytes
PMR; *see* Polymyalgia rheumatica
Pneumatic dilation of esophagus, 979, 981
Pneumococcal vaccine
  nephrotic syndrome and, 613
  polyvalent, 175
  sickle cell anemia and, 334
  splenectomy and, 329, 337
Pneumococcemia, 241, 395
Pneumococci
  bacteremia and, 241, 395
  cystic fibrosis and, 1101
  disseminated intravascular coagulation, 412
  endocarditis and, 184
  influenza and, 141
  leukemias and, 371
  liver disease and, 1074
  meningitis and, 186, 187
  multiple myeloma and, 379
  pneumonia and, 173-176
  septic arthritis of temporomandibular joint and, 108
  splenectomy and, 329, 337
  thyroiditis and, 1149
  vaccine for, 175, 329, 334, 337, 613
Pneumoconiosis, 723, 725
Pneumocystis, 287-288
  bronchoscopy and, 689
  drugs for, 170, 172
Pneumocystis carinii
  drugs for, 170
  Hodgkin's disease and, 387
  immunodeficiency diseases and, 31
  leukemias and, 368
  lymphangitic tumor and, 744
  neoplasia and, 446
  in pneumonia, 172
  renal transplantation and, 645
Pneumocystosis, 287-288; *see also Pneumocystis; Pneumocystis carinii*
Pneumoencephalography, 761
Pneumomediastinum, 735
Pneumonectomy, 687

Pneumonia; *see also* Bronchopneumonia
  aspergillosis and, 276, 705
  aspiration, 172, 177-178, 698-700, 746
  atelectasis and, 703; *see also* Atelectasis
  bacterial, 171-178, 729
  blastomycosis and, 275
  bronchiectasis and, 698
  bronchography and, 689
  Chlamydia and, 216
  coccidioidomycosis and, 275
  cryptococcosis and, 275
  eosinophilic, chronic, 721
  etiologic agents of, 171-172
  fibrinopurulent, 177
  giant cell, 146
  Haemophilus influenzae and, 236
  Hecht's, 146
  meningococcal, 234-235
  mycoplasmal, 217
  plague and, 242
  psittacosis and, 216
  streptococcal, 175, 177, 226
  syndromes of, 173-178, 698-700
  tuberculous, 255
  tularemia and, 243
  viral
    adenoviruses in, 143
    amantadine and, 154
    cytomegalovirus in, 131
    differential diagnosis of, 217
    influenza in, 140
    measles in, 145, 146
    parainfluenza viruses in, 142
    respiratory syncytial virus in, 141, 142
    varicella in, 130
Pneumonitis
  aspiration and, 178
  cat-scratch fever and, 151
  hypersensitivity, 723, 727-728
  interstitial, 64, 715, 721
  Q fever and, 213
  radiation, 722
Pneumothorax, 687, 733-734
PNH; *see* Paroxysmal nocturnal hemoglobinuria
PNMT; *see* Phenylethanolamine-*N*-methyltransferase
Podagra, 90, 91, 92
Podophyllin, 927, 1002, 1030
Podophyllotoxins, 447
Poikiloderma atrophicans vasculare, 905
Poikilodermatomyositis, 905
Point mutations, 1216
Poison ivy, 27
Poisons, 752-755
  food, 200, 220
  hemolysis from, 342
  jimsonweed, 819
  lead; *see* Lead
Poker spine, 48
Pokeweed mitogen, 16
Poliomyelitis, 135, 137, 144, 826
  vaccines for, 151-152
Poliosis, 880
Polioviruses, 135, 137, 144, 826
  in pneumonia, 172
  vaccines for, 151-152
Pollens, 22
Pollution, air, 691, 738; *see also* Environment
Polyarteritis nodosa, 66-67, 841
  hypertension and, 474
  intestinal vasculitis and, 1022
  lung and, 719
  neuropathy and, 854
  renal lesions and, 616

Polyarteritis nodosa-like syndrome, 29
Polyarthritis
  erythema nodosum with, 910
  gout and, 91
  indolent, 36
  juvenile chronic, 43
  sarcoidosis and, 77, 78, 910
Polyarticular juvenile rheumatoid arthritis, 43-45
Polychondritis, relapsing, 102-103
Polycystic kidneys, 470, 651-653
Polycystic ovaries, 1177
Polycythemia, 352-355; see also Polycythemia vera
  benign, 354
  cerebrovascular disease and, 842
  congestive heart failure and, 571
  familial, 354
  with malignancy, 1179
  relative, 354-355
  secondary, 352, 353-354
Polycythemia vera, 352-353; see also Polycythemia
  dentistry and, 419
  malabsorption and, 1003
  phlebotomy and, 353, 354
  skin disorders of, 897-898
  thrombocytosis and, 404
Polydystrophy, pseudo-Hurler, 1235
Polyendocrinopathy syndrome, autoimmune, 1209
Polyfructosan clearance, 603
Polygenic traits, 1222
Polymorphonuclear leukocytes, 17, 32
  bacterial infections and, 144
  deficiency of, diabetes and, 1294-1295
  disorders of, 31, 318
  influenza and, 141
  pneumonia and, 173
Polymyalgia rheumatica, 74-75, 858
  dentistry and, 874-875
  temporal arteritis and, 69
Polymyositis, 64-65, 1175
  dentistry and, 112-113
  oropharyngeal dysphagia and, 975
  pulmonary fibrosis and, 716
Polymyxin B, 909
Polymyxins, 169
  bactericidal activity of, 156
  excretion of, 158
  mastocytosis and, 909
  renal toxicity and, 158, 627, 628
Polyneuritis, thiamine and, 1108
Polyneuropathy; see also Neuropathies
  alcoholic, 849, 853, 1257
  drug-related, 779, 853
  idiopathic recurrent, 855
Polyostotic dysplasia, 116
Polyostotic osteitis deformans of jaws, 114-115
Polypeptide chains, 16; see also Heavy chains
Polypeptides, 16
  ectopic, 435
  gastric inhibitory, 941
  pancreatic, 945, 1049, 1263
  vasoactive intestinal; see Vasoactive intestinal polypeptide
Polyploidy, 1221
Polypoidal melanoma, 917
Polyposis, juvenile, 1042-1043; see also Polyposis syndromes
Polyposis coli, familial, 1042
Polyposis syndromes, 1042-1043; see also Polyps
  colorectal carcinoma and, 1039
  dentistry and, 1093-1095

Polyposis syndromes—cont'd
  gastrointestinal bleeding and, 891
  large bowel and, 1038, 1039, 1042-1043
  small bowel and, 1037
Polyps; see also Polyposis syndromes
  adenovillous, 1038
  esophagus and, 1032
  Gardner's syndrome and, 891
  gastric, 1033-1034
  of large bowel, 1038, 1039, 1042-1043
    carcinoma and, 1039
    dentistry and, 1093-1095
    syndromes of, 1042-1043
  in small bowel, 891, 1037
Polyradiculoneuropathy, acute idiopathic postinfectious, 854-855; see also Guillain-Barré syndrome
Polyribose ribitol phosphate, 186, 235, 236
Polyserositis, familial paroxysmal, 1048
Polysomnography, 769
Polystyrene sulfonate sodium, 599, 634, 639
Polysynaptic eye movements, 757
Polyunsaturated fat, 1290
Polyuria, 621-622
Polyvinylchloride, 1066
Pompe's disease, 522
Ponstel; see Mefenamic acid
Pontine astrocytoma, 844
Pontine lesions, 833
  alcoholism and, 1257
  astrocytoma and, 844
  gaze center and, 766
  pupillary reflexes and, 765
Pontine paramedian reticular formation lesions, 757-758, 833
Pontocerebellar atrophy, 812
Pontomedullary respiratory center lesion, 766
Popcorn calcifications, 685
Popliteal artery aneurysms, 567
Popliteal cyst, 84
Porcelain gallbladder, 1088
Porcine heterografts, 511, 514, 515
Pork tapeworm, 293, 294
Porphobilinogen, 1247, 1248, 1252, 1253
Porphyria cutanea tarda, 888-889, 1253-1254
  with other disorders, 1254-1255
Porphyria variegata, 888, 1253
Porphyrias, 888-889, 1246-1255
  acute intermittent, 888, 1249, 1250-1252
    neuropathy and, 854
  classification and diagnosis of, 1248-1255
  congenital erythropoietic, 888, 1248-1250
  dentistry and, 1298-1299
  hepatic, 888, 1253
  with other disorders, 1254-1255
  variegate, 888, 1253
Porphyrin
  deposits of, in teeth, 1298
  in feces, 1253, 1254
  pyridoxine-responsive anemia and, 325
  in urine, 1252, 1253, 1254
    lead poisoning and, 753
Portacaval anastomosis, 1081, 1083, 1291
Portal hypertension, 1060-1061
  ascites and, 1044, 1045
  cirrhosis and, 1083
  splenomegaly and, 394
Portal venous system, 1043
  collateral circulation and, 1060
  obstruction of, 1060
  pressure in, ascites and, 1044, 1045; see also Portal hypertension
  surgical decompression of, 1083

Port-wine stain, 881-882
Positional vertigo, 794
Positive end-expiratory pressure, 709, 733
Positron emission tomography, 761
Postcardiotomy syndrome, 550
Postconcussion headache, 789
Postencephalitic parkinsonism, 812
Posterior fossa lesions, 767-768
Posterior inferior cerebellar artery syndrome, 835
Posterior pituitary; see Pituitary gland, posterior
Posterior spinal artery syndrome, 836
Postgastrectomy syndrome, 993, 1004, 1199-1200; see also Dumping syndrome
Postgonococcal urethritis, 215, 218
Posthemiplegic chorea, 818
Posthemorrhagic anemia, 323
Postherpetic neuralgia, 927
Postinfectious encephalitis, 134, 827; see also Encephalitis
Postinfectious polyradiculoneuropathy, acute idiopathic, 854-855; see also Guillain-Barré syndrome
Postmenopausal osteoporosis, 1182, 1202
Postmyocardial infarction syndrome, 550
Postnatal infections, 125-127; see also Newborn
Postobstructive diuresis, 655
Postoperative atelectasis, 703
Postoperative hemorrhage, menstruation and, 1210
Postoperative infection, 251
Postoperative trauma, oral candidiasis and, 307
Postpartum aspiration pneumonia, dental care and, 746
Postpartum patients; see also Pregnancy
  cardiomyopathy and, 521
  fever of, 218, 226-227
  hemolytic syndrome of, 341
  renal failure and, 664
Postperfusion syndrome, 131
Postphlebitic syndrome, 495
Postprandial angina pectoris, 949
Postprandial hypoglycemia, 1277-1278
Postprandial syndrome, 993
Postpubertal testicular abnormalities, 1171-1172
Postreceptor insulin resistance, 1261
Postsplenectomy sepsis, 395
Poststreptococcal glomerulonephritis, 609-610
Posttransfusion hepatitis, 1068, 1069, 1073
Posttransfusion purpura, 404
Posttraumatic headache, 789
Postural drainage, 697, 699
Postural hypotension; see Orthostatic hypotension
Postvaccinal encephalomyelitis, 801, 827
Potash, sulfurated, 823
Potassium
  alcoholic cirrhosis and, 1080
  aldosterone and, 1155
  bicarbonate and, 592
  blood pressure and, 468
  cardiac cells and, 479
  congenital adrenal hyperplasia and, 1163
  deficit of; see Hypokalemia
  diabetes insipidus and, 1126
  for diabetic ketoacidosis, 1270
  dietary, renal failure and, 639
  diuretics and, 472
    potassium-sparing; see Potassium-sparing diuretics
  excess of; see Hyperkalemia
  heart rate and, 458
  metabolic alkalosis and, 600
  metabolism of, 597-599
    blood pressure and, 468
  mineralocorticoids and, 1160

Potassium—cont'd
  periodic paralyses and, 858
  pseudomembranous enterocolitis and, 1018
  respiratory acidosis and, 601
  supplements of, 598
    diuretics and, 465, 472
      mineralocorticoid excess and, 1161
    renal tubular acidosis and, 623
    whole blood transfusions and, 350
Potassium chloride, 205, 1022, 1270
Potassium iodide, 276, 625, 1147
Potassium phosphate salts, 1270
Potassium sulfide, 823
Potassium-sparing diuretics, 597
  hyperkalemia and, 598
  hypokalemia and, 598
  metabolic alkalosis and, 600
  renal failure and, 639
  side effects and interactions of, 574
Pott's disease, 81, 256
Povidone-iodine, 421, 422, 451, 828
Poxviruses, 123, 927
PPD; see Purified protein derivative
PPRF lesions; see Pontine paramedian reticular formation lesions
PR; see Progesterone receptors
PR intervals, 483
PRA; see Plasma renin activity
Practolol peritonitis, 105
Prazosin
  heart failure and, 465
  hypertension and, 473, 474, 475
  Raynaud's phenomenon and, 64
  renal failure and, 639
  side effects of, 574
  toxemia of pregnancy and, 665
Prealbumin, thyroxine-binding, 1131
Pre-B cells, 365
Precocious puberty, 1162, 1179
Prednisone
  angioedema and, 26
  arteritis and, 69, 75, 616, 790
  breast carcinoma and, 449
  bronchitis and, 693
  brucellosis and, 245
  cluster headaches and, 789
  Crohn's disease and, 1014
  Cushing's syndrome and, 1157
  dermatomyositis and, 905
  drug reactions and, 29
  glomerulonephritis and, 610
  hemolytic anemia and, 339
  hepatitis and, 1079
  Hodgkin's disease and, 390, 391
  hypercalcemia and, 1180
  hypercalciuria with sarcoidosis and, 647
  insulin resistance and, 1262
  in leukemias, 366, 370, 371
  lipoid nephrosis and, 613
  lupus erythematosus and, 57, 615
  Lyme disease and, 298
  multiple myeloma and, 382
  multiple sclerosis and, 801
  in non-Hodgkin's lymphoma, 392, 393
  osteomyelitis of jaws and, 116
  pituitary insufficiency and, 1124
  polyarteritis nodosa and, 616
  polymyalgia rheumatica and, 75
  polymyositis and, 65
  pseudotumor cerebri and, 848
  renal transplantation and, 644
  rheumatic fever and, 230
  rheumatoid arthritis and, 42
  sarcoidosis and, 78, 647

Prednisone—cont'd
  serum sickness and, 27
  thrombocytopenic purpura and, 403
  thyroiditis and, 1149
  for tumors, 444
  ulcerative colitis and, 1010
  urticaria and, 26
  visceral larva migrans and, 290
  Wegener's granulomatosis and, 73
Preeclampsia, 664, 665
Preexcitation patterns in children, 500-501
Prefrontal cortex, 772
Pregnancy; see also Postpartum patients
  anemia and, 324, 333
  aortic dissection, 560
  bacteriuria in, 196
  bromocriptine and, 1120-1121
  cerebrovascular disease and, 842-843
  cholestasis and, 1076
  cytomegalovirus and, 130
  diabetes and, 1271
  drugs in, 1212, 1213
  hemolysis and, 340
  hyperthyroidism in, 1147
  insulin and, 1267
  oral manifestations of, 1211-1213
  oral radiology and, 751
  pheochromocytoma and, 1165, 1168
  primary herpetic gingivostomatitis and, 299
  prolactinoma and, 1120
  pulmonary embolism and, 490
  renal disease in, 663-666
  rubella and, 146, 152
  syphilis and, 265, 269
  tetracyclines and, 168, 232
  thyroid in, 1132
  tubal, 232
  urinary tract infection and, 196, 197
  vaccines and, 152, 153
  von Willebrand's disease and, 407
Pregnancy granuloma, 1211
Pregnancy tumor, 1211
Pregnenolone, 1153
Preleukemic syndromes, 320-321, 322
Preload, 454, 457, 458
Premalignant skin lesions, 914, 919
Premature beats, 538, 540, 542
Premature infant, 307, 499, 503
Premature ventricular contraction, 538, 540, 542
Premaxillary hypoplasia, median cleft lip with, 1317
Prenatal counseling, 1229
Prenatal craniofacial development, 1304-1308
Prenatal diagnosis, 1229
Prepatellar bursitis, 99
Preprohormone, 1179
Prereceptor insulin resistance, 1261
Preretinal subhyaloid hemorrhages, 839
Presbyesophagus, 982
Present illness, evaluation of, 5
Pressor amines, hyperthyroidism and, 1205
Pressors, 574, 575
Pressure syringe, thrombocytopenia and, 426
Pressures; see specific pressure
Presystolic apical impulse, 470
Pretibial myxedema, 886
Primaquine, 281, 329, 588
Primary adrenal failure, 1155, 1156
Primary adrenal insufficiency; see Addison's disease
Primary airway disease, 690
Primary aldosteronism, 1160
  blood pressure and, 468, 470, 474
Primary alveolar hypoventilation, 708, 711

Primary amyloidosis, 854
Primary encephalitis, 134
Primary glomerular disease, 608-614
Primary muscle diseases of heart, 517-524; see also Cardiomyopathies
Primary orthostatic hypotension, 823
Primary osteoarthritis, 83-85, 107
Primary pulmonary hypertension, 496-497, 578, 696
Primary receptive cortex, 771
Primary refractory anemia, 320-321
Primary tumors of pericardium, 555
Primidone, 786, 866
Primitive reflexes, 758
Primitive streak, duplication of, 1303
Prinzmetal's variant angina, 533
Proaminopeptidase, 945
Probenecid
  in calcinosis, 62
  enteric fever and, excretion of, 158
  gonococcal infections and, 232
  gout and, 91
  hemolysis and, 330
  nephropathy and, 625, 627
  nephrotic syndrome and, 612
  thiazide-induced hyperuricemia and, 472
Probucol, 1290
Procainamide
  cardiomyopathy and, 522
  disseminated vasculitis and, 29
  lung disease and, 722
  lupuslike syndrome and, 57
  myasthenia gravis and, 856
  myotonic dystrophy and, 859
  oropharyngeal dysphagia and, 976
  pancreatitis and, 1051
  pericarditis and, 550
  pregnancy and, 1212
  side effects of, 585
  sudden death and, 538
  ventricular arrhythmias and, 500, 538, 546
Procaine hydrochloride, 869
Procaine penicillin; see also Penicillins
  anthrax and, 245
  diphtheria and, 248
  endocarditis and, 183, 185
  gonococcal stomatitis and, 302
  rat-bite fever and, 272
Procaine penicillin G, 159-163; see also Penicillin G
Procarbazine, 440, 443
  Hodgkin's disease and, 390, 391
  lung disease and, 447, 722
  mycosis fungoides and, 901
  non-Hodgkin's lymphoma and, 393
Procarboxypeptidase, 945
Procercoid, 293
Prochlorperazine, 1212
Procollagen, 1241
Proctectomy, 1011, 1015, 1042
Proctitis, gonococcal, 231
Proctocolectomy, 1011, 1015, 1042
Proctosigmoiditis, 1006, 1010
Procyclidine, 870
Prodrome, 781, 783, 865
Progestational agents, renal cell tumors and, 449; see also specific agent
Progesterone receptors, 443
Progesterones, 1153, 1162, 1174, 1175
  amenorrhea and, 1177
  aphthous ulcerations and, 1211
  endometrial cancer and, 449
  esophageal reflux and, 982
  and estrogen therapy, 1171, 1177

Progesterones—cont'd
  porphyria and, 1252
  renal cell tumors and, 449
  respiratory alkalosis and, 601
  subgingival microflora and, 1214
  testicular feminization and, 1171
Progestins, 368, 444
Progestogens, 658, 1177
Prognathism, mandibular, 878
Progesssive bulbar palsy, 803
Progressive hereditary ataxia syndromes, 805-807
Progressive massive fibrosis, 725
Progressive multifocal leukoencephalopathy, 828, 868
Progressive primary tuberculosis, 255
Progressive spinal muscular atrophies, 804-805
Progressive supranuclear palsy, 774-775
Progressive systemic sclerosis; see also Systemic sclerosis
  dental care and, 1091-1092
  pulmonary fibrosis and, 715
  renal lesions in, 615-616
  scleroderma and, 903-904
Prohormone, 1179
Prolactin, 1118
  amenorrhea and, 1177
  blood pressure and, 468
  deficiency of, 1123
  tumors and, 1120-1121
Prolactin-inhibiting factor, 1118
Prolactinoma, 1120-1121
Prolapse, mitral valve, 179, 301, 511, 842
Proliferative disorders, reticuloendothelial, 397-398
Proliferative glomerulonephritis, 614
Proliferative retinopathy, 1274
Proline, excess of, 1226, 1239
Proline oxidase deficiency, 1239
Promizole; see Thiazolsulfone
Promyelocytes, 356
Propantheline, 801, 1277
Properdin pathway, 17
Propionate, 1173
Propionibacterium, 249
Propionic acid decarboxylase deficiency, 1237, 1238
Propionic acidemia, 1237, 1238
Propoxyphene
  alcohol and, 1297
  aspirin sensitivity and, 24
  lung disease and, 722
  nephropathy and, 621
Propoxyphene napsylate, 1297
Propranolol
  angina pectoris and, 531, 532
  antidepressant overdose and, 779
  aortic dissection and, 562
  asthma and, 706, 748
  atrial fibrillation and, 544, 545
  atrial flutter and, 544
  atrioventricular junctional tachycardia and, 545
  cardiomyopathy and, 520
  epinephrine and, 583
  esophageal varices and, 1083
  hepatic metabolism and, 1062
  hydralazine and, 473
  hyperglycemic, hyperosmolar, nonketotic coma and, 1270
  hypertension and, 472, 473
  hyperthyroidism and, 1144, 1147
  Marfan's syndrome and, 1241
  migraine and, 788
  mitral prolapse and, 511

Propranolol—cont'd
  mitral stenosis and, 513
  multiple sclerosis and, 800
  renal insufficiency and, 62, 475, 625, 639
  scleroderma and, 62, 616
  sick sinus syndrome and, 547
  side effects of, 531, 574, 585
  sulfonylureas and, 1267
  supraventricular tachycardia and, 500
  tetanus and, 252
  tetralogy of Fallot and, 507
  thyroid hormone and, 1132
  thyroiditis and, 1146
  thyrotoxic crisis and, 1147
  thyrotoxicosis and, 1205
  thyroxine-to-triiodothyronine conversion and, 1131
  toxic nephropathy and, 625
  tremor and, 816
Proprioception, 14
Proptosis, 1142, 1147, 1313
Propulsive gait, 813
Propyliodone oil suspension, 689
Propylthiouracil, 1132
  Graves' disease and, 1144-1145
  hyperthyroidism and, 1205
  hypothyroidism at birth and, 1137
  lung disease and, 722
  neutropenia and, 360
  pregnancy and, 1147
  thyroid hormone synthesis and, 1130
  thyrotoxic crisis and, 1147
  thyroxine-to-triiodothyronine conversion and, 1131
  vitamin K deficiency and, 411
Prorenin, 467, 468
Prosencephalon, abnormal development of, 1316
Prostaglandin inhibitors, 445
Prostaglandins
  aspirin-induced asthma and, 24
  blood pressure and, 468
  cytoprotective properties of, 943
  diarrhea and, 954
  fats and, 1104
  gastritis and, 996
  inflammatory bowel disease and, 1006
  inhibitors of, 445
  multiple sclerosis and, 797
  nephropathy and, 629
  ovulation and, 1174, 1175
  renal cell carcinoma and, 657
  sodium reabsorption and, 592
Prostate
  carcinoma of, 449, 659-660
  examination of, 13
  inflammation of, 198
Prostatitis, 198
Prostheses; see also Prosthetic valves
  for aortic arch replacement, 559
  cobalt, allergy to, 30
  in esophagus, 1032
  pernicious anemia and dental, 415
Prosthetic valves
  aortic stenosis and, 506, 515
  endocarditis and, 179, 181-182, 184, 301, 302
  hemolysis and, 340
  mitral regurgitation and, 511
  mitral stenosis and, 514
Prostigmin; see Neostigmine
Protamine, 414, 641
Protein capsid, 127, 129
Protein electrophoresis, 378, 380, 383, 384
Protein malnutrition, 1104
Protein polymorphisms, normal, 1217

Protein-bound iodine, 1138, 1150
Proteins; see also Amino acids
  amyloidosis and, 385-386
  antimicrobials and, 157
  ascitic fluid and, 1044
  Bence Jones, 379, 380, 605
  blood, 17, 999-1000
  calories in, 1104
  in cerebrospinal fluid, 135
  deficiencies of, 115, 1104
  in diet, 1102
    alcoholic cirrhosis and, 1080
    nephrotic syndrome and, 613
    renal failure and, 639
  electrophoresis and, 378, 380, 383, 384
  influenza and, 140
  liver disease and, 1063, 1065
  M, 223, 377
  multiple myeloma and, 380
  normal urinary, 589; see also Proteinuria
  nucleocapsid, 140
  nutritional therapy and, 1111
  placental, tumors and, 435
  plasma; see Plasma, proteins in
  synthesis of, 1059, 1217
  Tamm-Horsfall, 605
  Y, 1058
  Z, 1058
Proteinuria, 589-590
  assessment of, 605
  focal glomerulosclerosis and, 614
  glomerulonephritis and, 611, 612, 614
  nephrolithiasis and, 646
  nephropathy and, 626, 1274
  nephrotic syndrome and, 612-613
  orthostatic, 589, 605
  pregnancy and, 664, 666
  renal vein thrombosis and, 662, 663
  systemic sclerosis and, 60
Proteoglycans, 90, 1181
Proteolytic enzymes, 694, 1049-1050; see also specific enzyme
Proteus
  bacteremia and, 239
  disseminated intravascular coagulation and, 412
  drugs for, 163, 164, 165, 166, 169, 170, 171
  immunodeficiency diseases and, 31
  leukemia and, 421
  oral lesions of, 306
  in pneumonia, 171
  struvite stones and, 648
Proteus mirabilis, 159, 163, 164, 165
Prothrombin, deficiency of, 411
Prothrombin complex concentrate, 428, 429
Prothrombin time, 409
  anticoagulant therapy and, 430
  coumarins and, 414
  heart failure and, 462
  liver disease and, 1063, 1065, 1072, 1098
  pulmonary embolism and, 492
  vitamin K and, 1108
PROTO; see Protoporphyrin
Protocoproporphyria hereditaria, 1253
PROTOgen; see Protoporphyrinogen
Protoporphyria, erythropoietic, 888, 1249, 1250
Protoporphyrin, 1247, 1250, 1253
Protoporphyrinogen, 1247
Protozoal diseases, 279-289
  amebiasis in, 189, 203, 281-283
  babesiosis in, 288, 343
  diarrhea and, 953
  giardiasis in, 283-284; see also *Giardia lamblia*

Protozoal diseases—cont'd
  Hodgkin's disease and, 387
  immunodeficiency diseases and, 31
  leishmaniasis in, 343
  malaria and, 279-281; see also Malaria
  pneumocystosis in, 287-288; see also Pneumocystis; Pneumocystis carinii
  red cell injury and, 343
  toxoplasmosis in, 284-286; see also Toxoplasmosis
  trichomoniasis in, 170, 286
  trypanosomiasis in, 287, 1027
Provitamin 7-dehydrocholesterol, 1185
Provocative intranasal challenge, 21, 22
PRP; see Polyribose ribitol phosphate
PRPP; see Phosphoribosylpyrophosphate
Pruritus
  anal, 1030
  biliary disease and, 896
  diabetes and, 885
  drugs for, 130, 885, 893
  Hodgkin's disease and, 912
  leukemia and, 899
  liver diseases and, 1058
  polycythemia vera and, 897
Pseudoacanthosis nigricans, 887
Pseudoachondroplasia, 1245
Pseudobulbar palsy, 835
Pseudochylous ascites, 1046
Pseudochylous pleural effusions, 731
Pseudocysts, pancreatic, 970, 1045, 1054
Pseudodominance, 1218
Pseudoephedrine, 1212
Pseudogout, 89, 94-95
Pseudohermaphroditism, 1162, 1171
Pseudo-Hurler polydystrophy, 1235
Pseudohydrocephaly, 879
Pseudohyperkalemia, 598
Pseudohypertrophy of muscle, 852
Pseudohypoparathyroidism, 1197, 1209
Pseudomembrane, 220, 305, 938, 1018
Pseudomembranous enterocolitis, 220, 1018
Pseudomonas; see also *Pseudomonas aeruginosa*
  bacteremia and, 239, 240, 241
  cystic fibrosis and, 700, 1101
  disseminated intravascular coagulation and, 412
  drugs for, 164
  endocarditis and, 181
  immunodeficiency diseases and, 31
  inflammatory bowel disease and, 1006
  leukemias and, 368, 421
  lung abscess and, 698
  oral lesions of, 306
  pneumonia and, 172
  smoke inhalation and, 729
Pseudomonas aeruginosa; see also *Pseudomonas*
  bronchiectasis and, 696, 697
  drugs for, 163, 164, 165, 166, 169
  neoplasia and, 446
  neutropenia and, 361
  nongonococcal septic arthritis and, 80
  oral lesions of, 306
  osteomyelitis and, 82
  in pneumonia, 171, 172
Pseudomonas pseudomallei, 171
Pseudo-obstruction of intestines, 981
Pseudoparalysis of Parrot, 270
Pseudopolycythemia, 355
Pseudopolyps, 1007, 1038
Pseudoporphyria, 1255
Pseudo-pseudohypoparathyroidism, 1197, 1209
Pseudoremission, 370
Pseudoscleroderma, 58

Pseudotabes, diabetic, 1276
Pseudotumor cerebri, 779, 790, 848
Pseudotumors, 105, 410, 427
  cerebral, 779, 790, 848
Pseudoxanthoma elasticum, 407, 884, 1244
Psittacosis, 214, 216, 217
Psittacosis-lymphogranuloma-trachoma, 214
Psoas muscle shadow obliteration, 1044
Psoas sign, 1016
Psoriasiform lesions, Reiter's syndrome and, 110, 907, 908
Psoriasis, 936-938
  anal disorders and, 1030
  arthritis and, 50-52, 106-107
  basal cell carcinoma and, 916
  guttate, 936
PSS; see Progressive systemic sclerosis
Psychiatric manifestations of hyperthyroidism, 1143
Psychologic factors
  in asthma, 23
  inflammatory bowel disease and, 1006-1007
  neoplasia and, 447
Psychomotor seizures, 781, 782, 783
Psychoneuroendocrine relationships, 1115
Psychophysiologic gastrointestinal reaction, 1027
Psychoses, Korsakoff's, 759, 849-850, 1257
Psyllium muciloid, 1212
Psyllium seed, 954, 956, 1017
PT; see Prothrombin time
Pterygoid muscle, 97, 98, 109
PTH; see Parathyroid hormone
PTT; see Partial thromboplastin time
Puberty
  delayed, 1172
  female, oral manifestations of, 1210
  male, oral manifestations of, 1214
  precocious, 1162, 1179
Puddle sign, 1044
Puerperium; see Postpartum patients
Pull-through anastomosis of bowel, 1026
Pulmonary artery; see also Pulmonary vessels
  hypertension of, mitral stenosis and, 512
  pressure in, 489, 674
  side-to-side anastomosis of ascending aorta to, 507
  stenosis of, 506
  and subclavian artery, anastomosis between, 507
Pulmonary artery pressure, 489, 674
Pulmonary capillaries
  blood flow through, 674
  pressure in, 478, 488, 709, 710
  red blood cell passage through, 676
  surface area of alveolar interface of, 672
Pulmonary capillary wedge pressure, 478, 488, 709, 710
Pulmonary disease; see Lung; Respiratory diseases
Pulmonary edema, 460, 710
  acute, treatment of, 572
  bacteremia and, 240
  cardiac, 708, 710
  myocardial infarction and, 536
  neurogenic, 708, 710
  pulmonary embolism and, 491
  sputum and, 686
  thoracentesis and, 688
Pulmonary emboli, 489-494
  angiography and, 689-690
  congestive heart failure and, 463
  dentistry and, 577
  multiple, 490
  radionuclide scans and, 492, 493, 687

Pulmonary emboli—cont'd
  removal of, 494
  saddling of, 489-490
Pulmonary fibrosis, 713-716, 722, 725, 726
Pulmonary function, 672-673
  asthma and, 24
  polymyositis and, 65
Pulmonary hemorrhage, 611, 720-721
Pulmonary hemosiderosis, 720-721
Pulmonary hypertension, 696
  alveolar hypoxemia and, 682
  mitral stenosis and, 512
  primary, 496-497, 578, 696
  pulmonic regurgitation and, 517
  tricuspid regurgitation and, 516, 517
Pulmonary infiltrates
  cancer and, 740
  drugs and, 722
  with eosinophilia, 363, 372-373, 721
Pulmonary nodule, solitary, 685, 743, 744
  chest roentgenograms and, 685, 743, 744
Pulmonary parenchymal disease; see Lung, parenchymal disease of
Pulmonary performance; see Pulmonary function
Pulmonary perfusion, 673-674; see also Pulmonary vessels
  scanning and, 492, 493, 687
Pulmonary sequestration, 696
Pulmonary/systemic flow ratio, 503, 504
Pulmonary tumors, 685, 738-744; see also Lung, malignancies of
Pulmonary valve, 503, 504, 673-674
  disease of, 516-517
    atresia in, 507
    obstruction in, cyanotic heart lesions and, 506-507
    regurgitation in, 517
    stenosis in, 506, 517
Pulmonary vascular resistance, 499, 503, 674
Pulmonary vasculitides, 719-720
Pulmonary vein, 503, 696
Pulmonary vessels, 673-674
  angiography of, 488, 689-690
  pulmonary embolism and, 492, 493
  capillaries and; see Pulmonary capillaries
  congestive heart failure and, 454
  hypertension and; see Pulmonary hypertension
  inflammations of, 719-720
  pulmonary artery in; see Pulmonary artery
  pulmonary vein in, 503, 696
  resistance and, 499, 503, 674
  roentgenograms and, 501
  vasculitis of, 719-720
Pulmonic valve; see Pulmonary valve
Pulp chambers, osteogenesis imperfecta and, 1244
Pulp stones, Ehlers-Danlos syndrome and, 1242
Pulpal dysplasia, 1244
Pulse
  cardiac dysfunction and, 459
  carotid, valvular disease and, 580
  control of, 458-459
  Corrigan, valvular disease and, 580
  paradoxical
    pericardial tamponade and, 553, 554, 705-706
    pericarditis and, 585
  peripheral, evaluation of, 13
  water-hammer, 516, 580
Pulse pressure, 505, 516; see also Blood pressure
Pulse therapy, 57
Pulseless disease, 68, 69, 563, 841
  vasculitis and, 1022
Pulsion diverticula, 736

Pulsus alternans, 463
Pulsus paradoxus, 553, 554, 705-706
Punch biopsy, sarcoidosis and, 114
Punched-out lesions, 379, 380, 422
Pupils
  Argyll Robertson, 269
  brainstem lesions and, 760
  coma and, 765
  evaluation of, 8
  intracranial pressure and, 846
  multiple sclerosis and, 798
Pure red cell aplasia, 319
Purified protein derivative, 32, 81, 257, 260
Purine analogs, 366
Purine antagonists, 441
Purine nucleoside phosphorylase deficiency, 1227
Purines, 92, 1226-1227, 1239
Purkinje fibers, 542
Purkinje network, 477
Purpura
  aplastic anemia and, 415
  intestinal vasculitis and, 1022
  oral, thrombocytopenia and, 571
  platelet abnormalities and, 898
  posttransfusion, 404
  Schönlein-Henoch, 70, 406-407, 616
  thrombocytopenic; see Thrombocytopenic purpura
Purpura simplex, 407
Pursed lip breathing, 684
Purulent sputum, 686
Pustules, 907, 937
Putrid vomitus, 957
PVC, see Premature ventricular contraction
PVR; see Pulmonary vascular resistance
PXE; see Pseudoxanthoma elasticum
Pyelography, 196, 606, 607, 656
Pyelonephritis, 195, 196, 199, 666
Pyloric stenosis, 997-998, 1228
Pyloroplasty, 993, 996
Pylorus
  antral polyp prolapse into, 1034
  stenosis of, 997-998, 1228
  surgery of, 993, 996
Pyoderma, streptococcal, 223, 225-226
Pyoderma gangrenosum, 892
  rheumatoid arthritis and, 906
  ulcerative colitis and, 892, 895, 1007, 1095-1096
Pyoderma vegetans, 933
Pyostomatitis vegetans, 892, 934, 1007
  ulcerative colitis and, 1095, 1096
Pyramidal tract, 803, 805
Pyrantel pamoate, 290, 291
Pyrazinamide, 92, 259, 321
Pyrexia, heat, 755; see also Fever
Pyridostigmine, 856
Pyridoxal phosphate, 321, 779, 1258
Pyridoxine, 1106, 1109
  anemia and, 325, 321, 416
  cystathioninuria and, 1237
  deficiency of, 416, 1298
  hyperoxaluria and, 648
  isoniazid toxicity and, 259
  neuropathy and, 779, 853
  Wilson's disease and, 823
Pyridoxine-responsive anemia, 325
Pyrimethamine, 281, 286
Pyrimidine antagonists, 440
Pyrimidine nucleoside analog, 366
Pyrophosphate arthropathy, 94
Pyrosis, 950, 974-975
  ulcer pain and, 988-989

β-1-Pyrroline-5-carboxylic acid dehydrogenase deficiency, 1239
Pyuria, 590
  sterile, 256, 258
PZA; see Pyrazinamide

Q

Q fever, 213, 217
Q wave, 480, 483, 484
QRS complex, 482, 483, 484
QS complex, 482
QT intervals, 483-484
Quadrantanopsias, 759
Quarantine, 242
Quartan malaria, 280
Questionnaire, dental health, 1, 2-3
Queyrat, erythroplasia of, 914
Quiescent phase of tumors, 439
Quiet zone of lung, 680
Quinacrine
  cestodes and, 294
  effusions and, 445
  giardiasis and, 284
  hemolysis and, 329
  lupus erythematosus and, 903
  mesothelioma and, 734
  peritoneal carcinomatosis and, 1047
Quincke's disease, 580
Quinidine
  atrial fibrillation and, 544
  atrial flutter and, 544
  cardiomyopathy and, 522
  ectopic foci and, 500
  electrocardiogram and, 483-484
  hemolysis and, 330, 342
  intoxication and, 546
  pregnancy and, 1212
  side effects of, 585
  sudden death and, 538
  thrombocytopenia and, 29, 400, 403
  ventricular tachycardia and, 546
Quinine
  hemolysis and, 329, 342
  malaria and, 281
  myasthenia gravis and, 856
  myotonic dystrophy and, 859
  oropharyngeal dysphagia and, 976
  thrombocytopenia and, 29, 400, 403
  urine and, 588
  urticaria and, 25
Quinocide, 329
Quinsy, 224
Quinton tube, 964

R

R; see Respiratory exchange ratio; Roentgen
R wave, 480-482, 483
  myocardial infarction and, 484, 485
Rabbit syndrome, 871
Rabies, 135, 138-139, 826
  antitoxin and, 26
  human immune globulin for, 153
  vaccines for, 153, 827
Rabies antitoxin, 26
Rabies immune globulin, human, 153
Rad, 749
Radiation, 749
  aplastic anemia and, 318, 319
  ataxia-telangiectasia and, 809
  atelectasis and, 702
  of body heat, 755
  cancer and, 438-439

Radiation—cont'd
  cancer and—cont'd
    bladder, 448, 659
    breast, 448
    cervical, 449
    disseminated, 439
    endometrial, 449
    esophageal, 447, 1032, 1033
    gastric, 1036
    head and neck, 449
    large bowel, 448, 1041
    lung, 447, 742
    ovarian, 449
    pancreatic, 448
    prostatic, 449, 660
    renal cell, 658
    small bowel, 1037
    testicular, 449
  carcinogenesis and, 432
  Cushing's syndrome and, 1159
  dental dose of, 751
  dental evaluation before, 919
  enteritis after, 1002, 1018-1019
  esophagitis and, 986
  Hodgkin's disease and, 390
  injury from, 749-751, 847
    enteritis in, 1002, 1018-1019
    pneumonitis and fibrosis in, 722
    spinal cord lesions in, 847
  Kaposi's sarcoma and, 922
  leukemias and, 364, 369, 371
  lymphomas and, 424
  mesothelioma and, 1047
  midline granuloma and, 74
  multiple myeloma and, 422
  myelofibrosis and, 374
  nephroblastoma and, 658
  neurologic complications of, 847
  neutropenia and, 358
  non-Hodgkin's lymphoma and, 391, 394
  oral candidiasis and, 307
  oral dysplasia and, 919
  osteomyelitis of jaws and, 116
  of pituitary, 1120
  prolactinomas and, 1120, 1121
  in sarcomas, 450
  solid tumors and, 750
  thrombocytopenia and, 401
Radiation dose, dental, 751
Radiation enteritis, 1002, 1018-1019
Radiation stomatitis, 919
Radicular pain, 194
Radiculitis, 137
Radiculopathy, diabetic, 1275
Radioactive carbon, 1005
Radioactive colloids, 727, 966
Radioactive gold, 727, 966
Radioactive implants, 1047
Radioactive iodine
  adenomas of thyroid and, 1150
  albumin and, 352
  with fibrinogen, phlebitis and, 495
  Graves' disease and, 1144, 1147
  hepatic imaging and, 966
  immunoglobulin labeling and, 124
  orthoiodohippuric acid labeling and, 607-608
  ovarian disease and, 1045
  pancreatic carcinoma and, 448
  pretibial myxedema and, 886
  thyroid carcinoma and, 1152
  thyroid scan and, 1133
  toxic goiter and, 1145
  uptake of, 1133

Radioactive iodine—cont'd
  uptake of—cont'd
    hypothyroidism and, 1139
    thyroid-stimulating hormone test and, 1135
    triiodothyronine suppression test and, 1136
Radioactive iron, 313-315
Radioactive phosphorus, 353, 374, 404, 734
Radioactive xenon, 492, 687
Radioallergosorbent test, 21
Radiographs, dental
  basal cell carcinoma of face and, 883
  chronic renal failure and, 667-668
  diabetes and, 1294
  fibrous dysplasia of jaws and, 115
  Gaucher's disease and, 425, 1232
  oral contraceptives and, 1214
  osteoporosis and, 115
  otocraniofacial syndromes and, 1310
  Paget's disease of jaws and, 114
  pregnancy and, 1213
  psoriatic arthritis of temporomandidular joint and, 106-107
  scleroderma and, 1091
  sickle cell anemia and, 417
  synovial chondromatosis of temporomandibular joint and, 108
  systemic sclerosis and, 112
  thalassemia and, 418
  tuberculous osteomyelitis and, 304
Radioimmunoassay
  of parathyroid hormone, 1187
  for thyroxine, 1134
  for triiodothyronine, 1134
  viruses and, 124
Radioisotope imaging of kidney, 607-608, 661
Radioisotopes, cardiac disease and, 489
Radiolabeled albumin, 352, 492, 687, 966
Radiolabeled chromium, 313, 328, 352
Radiolabeled colloids, 727, 966
Radionuclide scanning; *see* Scans
Radiopaque contrast agents; *see* Contrast agents
Radiopaque markers, 866
Radiotherapy; *see* Radiation
Raeder's syndrome, 791
Ragocytes, 37
RAIU; *see* Radioactive iodine, uptake of
Ramsay Hunt syndrome, 806
Ramus intermedius, 524
Rana, mumps and, 301
Random inactivation of X chromosome, 1219
Ranula, mumps and, 301
Rapid eye movement sleep, 769, 861
Rapid Plasma Reagin test, 271
Rappaport classification, 392
Rarefaction, hyperparathyroidism and, 1208
Rash; *see also* Eruptions; Skin diseases
  adenovirus and, 148
  allergic, 28
  bacteremia and, 231
  butterfly, 54, 55, 578
  cat-scratch fever and, 151
  cytomegalovirus and, 125
  desquamative, 69
  erythema infectiosum and, 147
  heliotrope, 64, 904
  liver diseases and, 1058-1059
  lupus erythematosus and, 54
  Lyme disease and, 297
  measles and, 145
  meningitis and, 187
  meningococcemia and, 234
  Rocky Mountain spotted fever and, 211
  roseola and, 147

Rash—cont'd
  scarlet fever and, 224
  typhus fever and, 212
  varicella-zoster and, 129-130
Raspberry tongue, 224
RAST; *see* Radioallergosorbent test
Rat plague, 242
Rat-bite fever, 272-273
Raynaud's disease, 63-64; *see also* Raynaud's phenomenon
  cyanosis and, 683
  esophageal motility disorders and, 981
  pulmonary hypertension and, 496
Raynaud's phenomenon, 55, 62-64, 100; *see also* Raynaud's disease
  acrosclerosis and, 903, 904
  Buerger's disease and, 570
  coronary, 522-523
  esophageal motility disorders and, 981
  mycoplasmal pneumonia and, 217
  polymyositis and, 64
  primary pulmonary hypertension and, 578
  systemic sclerosis and, 58, 59, 61, 112, 903, 904
  treatment of, 61-62
  Waldenström's macroglobulinemia and, 382, 383
Rays, radiation, 749; *see also* Radiation
  cardiac disease and, 489
RBC; *see* Red blood cells
RE cells; *see* Reticuloendothelial cells
RE system; *see* Reticuloendothelial system
Reactive arthritis, 52, 53
Reagin, 17
Reagin antibodies, 704, 705; *see also* Immunoglobulins, E
Rebound congestion, 21
Rebound tenderness, 13, 951, 1043
Receptive relaxation, 963
Receptor-ligand interaction, 1115
Receptors
  hormones and, 1114-1115
  insulin, 1261
  lymphocytes and, 16
Recessive alleles, 1218, 1219
Reciprocal translocations, 1222
Recognition, cortex and, 771
Recording of physical examination, 8
Recrudescent typhus, 210, 212-213
Recruitment, hearing loss and, 795
Rectal columns of Morgagni, 948, 1029
Rectal probe thermocouples, 756
Rectal shelf, 1035, 1040
Rectal stump and colon, anastomosis between, 1026
Rectal swabs, 137
Rectal valves, 948
Rectum, 947-948
  biopsy of; *see* Biopsy, rectal
  bleeding from, 1007
  carcinoma of, 448, 1031, 1039-1041, 1093
  evaluation of, 13
  and ileum, anastomosis between, 1015, 1018
  megacolon surgery and, 1026
  neoplasms of, 448, 1031, 1038-1042, 1093
  polyps of, dental correlations and, 1093-1095; *see also* Polyps of large bowel
  prolapse of, 1038
  ulcer of, 1019
  ulcerative colitis and, 1011
Recurrent aphthous ulcers, 1095, 1097; *see also* Aphthous ulcers
Recurrent laryngeal nerve, 1127, 1128

Recurrent meningitis, Mollaret's, 189
Recurrent polyneuropathy, idiopathic, 855
Red blood cell casts, 588, 605, 610
Red blood cells
  adenosine deaminase deficiency and, 1240
  aging of, 327
  aplasia of, pure, 319
  in casts, 588, 605, 610
  in cerebrospinal fluid, 135
  cyanosis and, 683
  destruction of; *see* Hemolysis
  destruction disorders of, 326-343
    acquired, 337-343
    congenital hemolytic anemias in, 328-337; *see also* Hemolytic anemia, congenital
  folate and, 318
  fragmentation syndromes of, 340-341
  hemoglobin degradation and, 327
  histiocytic medullary reticulosis and, 398
  horse, heterophil antibodies to, 132
  incompatibility between, 348
  increased number of, 352-355; *see also* Polycythemia
  indices for, 313, 324
  malaria and, 280
  mass of, 352
  pleural effusion and, 731
  production of; *see* Erythropoiesis
  pulmonary capillaries and, 676
  removal of, 327
  in renal failure, 636
  sedimentation rate and; *see* Erythrocyte sedimentation rate
  sensitization to, purpura and, 406; *see also* Purpura
  sheep, 16, 32 132
  splenomegaly and, 396
  survival of, 313, 326, 328
  tear-shaped, 375
  transfusions of, 350
    chronic disease anemia and, 326
    frozen, 347, 1240
    paroxysmal nocturnal hemoglobinuria and, 342
    in pernicious anemia, 318
  in urine; *see* Hematuria
Reduviid bug, 286
Reed-Sternberg cell, 387
Reflex behavior, 772
Reflex sympathetic dystrophy, 100
Reflexes, 14
  Bezold-von Jarisch, 535
  brainstem, 14
  coma and, 765-766
  deep tendon, 14, 761
  defecation, 948
  detrusor, 799
  hung-up, 818
  infantile, cerebrovascular disease and, 586
  primitive, 758
  superficial, 14
Reflux
  enterogastric, 964
  esophageal, 950, 962, 982-985, 988-989
  hepatojugular, 461, 463
  vesicoureteral, 196, 197, 650-651
Reflux esophagitis, 950, 962, 982-985, 988-989
Refractory anemia, primary, 320-321
Refusum's disease, 806, 855
Regan isoenzyme, 435
Regional enteritis; *see* Crohn's disease
Regional examination, 11
Regional ileitis, malnutrition and, 1103

Regional lymphadenitis; *see* Adenopathy; Lymphadenitis; Lymphadenopathy
Regurgitation, 956-957
 aortic, 515-516, 561
 mitral, 488, 510-511
 nocturnal, 975, 977
 pulmonic, 517
 tricuspid, 516-517
Reid index, 691
Reidel's thyroiditis, 105, 1150
Reifenstein's syndrome, 1171
Reiter's cells, 52
Reiter's syndrome, 52-53
 chlamydial urethritis and, 215
 dentistry and, 110, 668
 gonococcal arthritis and, 232
 orofacial abnormalities and, 668
 skin lesions of, 907-908
Rejection reactions, 341, 644-645; *see also* Renal transplantation; Transplantation
Relapses
 pancreatitis and, 1055
 urinary tract infection and, 195-199
Relapsing acute pancreatitis, 1055
Relapsing polychondritis, 102-103
Release reaction of platelets, 400
REM sleep; *see* Rapid eye movement sleep
Remissions
 arthritis and, 42, 51
 of leukemias, 366
 multiple sclerosis and, 800
Remnant removal disease, 1285, 1287
Remodeling of bone, 1182-1183, 1203, 1308
Renal agenesis, 649
Renal angiography, 606, 607, 657, 661-662
Renal anomalies, 649-650
Renal artery
 reconstruction of, 662
 stenosis of, 470, 660-662
  angiography and, 607
  radioisotope imaging and, 608
Renal biopsy, 72, 608, 638
Renal blood flow, 592; *see also* Renal artery; Renal vein
 heart failure and, 462
 obstructive uropathy and, 655
 pregnancy and, 663-664
 shock and, 477, 478
Renal cell carcinomas, 449, 656-658
Renal colic, 951
Renal cysts, 651-653
Renal disease; *see* Kidney diseases
Renal dysplasia, 650
Renal factors, blood pressure and, 467, 468; *see also* Hypertension, kidney injury and
Renal failure; *see also* Uremia
 acute, 630-635
  pregnancy and, 664
  toxic nephropathy and, 625-626
 chronic, 635-640
  anemia and, 667
  dental radiographs and, 667-668
  toxic nephropathy and, 626
 contrast agent allergy and, 606
 dialysis for, 640-642; *see also* Dialysis
 focal glomerulosclerosis and, 614
 glomerulonephritis and, 610, 611, 614
 hemolysis and, 343
 leukemias and, 368
 malaria and, 280
 multiple myeloma and, 380
 nephrotic syndrome and, 613
 obstructive uropathy and, 655
 postpartum, 664

Renal failure—cont'd
 radioisotope imaging and, 608
 transplantation for; *see* Renal transplantation
 Weil's disease and, 273
Renal hypoplasia, 649-650
Renal ischemia, 631, 660-662
Renal neoplasms, 449, 656-659
 computed tomography and, 607
 radioisotope imaging and, 608
 ultrasound and, 607
Renal osteitis fibrosa cystica, 667
Renal osteodystrophy, 636-637, 639, 1200-1201
 oral manifestations of, 667
Renal parenchymal disease, secondary hypertension and, 573
Renal pelvis, tumors of, 658-659
Renal phosphate clearance, 1200
Renal scans, 607-608, 661
Renal transplantation, 643-646
 amyloidosis and, 617
 chronic renal failure and, 635, 638, 639-640
 complications of, 644-645
 cytomegalovirus and, 130, 131
 dentistry and, 667, 669
 diabetic nephropathy and, 617, 1274
 glomerulonephritis and, 610, 612, 614
 hemolysis after, 341
 interstitial nephritis and, 620
 myeloma and, 618
 outcome of, 646
 patient selection and preparation for, 643-644
 polycystic disease and, 652
 preparing for, and initiating, 639-640
 procedures for, 644
 radioisotope imaging and, 608
 scleroderma and, 616
 sickle cell disease and, 618
Renal tubular acidosis, 622-623
Renal tubular defects, oral manifestations of rickets and, 668
Renal tubular maximum phosphate reabsorption/glomerular filtration rate, 1185
 hypercalcemia and, 1190, 1193, 1194, 1195
 hypoparathyroidism and, 1196
Renal tubules; *see* Tubules, renal
Renal ultrasonography, 607
Renal vein
 phlebography of, 663
 renin concentration in, 607, 661-662
 thrombosis of, 662-663
  angiography and, 607
  venography of, 606, 607, 661-662
Rendu-Osler-Weber disease; *see* Osler-Weber-Rendu disease
Renin
 blood pressure and, 467, 468
 heart failure and, 462
 hyporeninemic hypoaldosteronism and, 623
 mineralocorticoid excess and, 1161
 peripheral vascular resistance and, 460
 plasma; *see* Renin activity, plasma
 renal artery stenosis and, 661
 renal cell carcinoma and, 657
 renal vein, 661
  angiography and, 607, 661-662
Renin activity, plasma; *see also* Renin
 hyperkalemia and, 598
 hypokalemia and, 598
 mineralocorticoid excess and, 467, 468, 1161
Renin-angiotensin system, 467, 468; *see also* Renin
Renography, radioisotope, 607-608, 661
Renovascular hypertension; *see* Hypertension, kidney injury and

Reovirus, 123, 203
Replacement therapy; *see* Hormones
Replication of tumor, 439
RES; *see* Reticuloendothelial system
Resection; *see also* Surgery
 abdominoperineal, 1031, 1041
 aneurysm, 566-567
 of intestines; *see* Intestines, resection of
 lymph nodes and, 151, 918
 of pancreas; *see* Pancreas, resection of
 thoracotomy and; *see* Thoracotomy
Reserpine
 heart failure and, 464
 Huntington's chorea and, 774
 hydralazine and, 473
 hypertension and, 473, 474
 lung disease and, 722
 parkinsonism and, 812
 pheochromocytoma and, 1165
 in Raynaud's phenomenon, 61, 64
 side effects and interactions of, 574, 575, 871
Reserpine derivatives, side effects of, 871
Reset osmostat syndrome, 594
Residual bladder urine, 656
Residual volume, 677
Resin, composite, 30
Resistance
 airway, 680
 microbial, 159
 vascular pulmonary, 499, 503, 674
Resistant ovary syndrome, 1177
Resonant percussion note, 684
Respirations, 672-673; *see also* Respiratory diseases
 abnormal, with normal lungs, 711-712
 Cheyne-Stokes, 766
 coma and, 766
 dyspnea and; *see* Dyspnea
 Kussmaul, 1269
Respiratory acidosis, 600-601
Respiratory alkalosis, 601
Respiratory burst, 356
Respiratory center, 676-677, 711, 766
Respiratory depressants, dental care and, 746
Respiratory diseases, 672-748; *see also* Lung
 actinomycosis and, 247
 adult respiratory distress syndrome in; *see* Adult respiratory distress syndrome
 asthma in, 704-707; *see also* Asthma
 atelectasis and, 702-703; *see also* Atelectasis
 bronchiectasis in, 696-698; *see also* Bronchiectasis
 bronchitis in, 691-693; *see also* Bronchitis, chronic
 of chest wall, 737-738
 coccidioidomycosis and, 275
 cor pulmonale in, 696; *see also* Cor pulmonale
 cystic fibrosis in, 700; *see also* Cystic fibrosis
 definitions of, 672
 dentistry and, 744-748
 diagnosis of, 683-690
  angiography in, 489, 492, 493, 689-690
 of diaphragm, 736-737
 diffuse lung diseases in, 713-723; *see also* Lung, diffuse disease of
 emphysema in, 690, 693-695, 700-701; *see also* Emphysema
 environmental, 691, 723-730, 738
  dental care and, 747-748
 eosinophilia and, 362-363, 372-373, 721
 helminthic disease and, 290, 291
 and histoplasmosis, 274
 Kaposi's sarcoma and, 921
 lung abscess in; *see* Lung, abscess of

Respiratory diseases—cont'd
    lung cysts in, 700, 701
    of mediastinum, 734-736
    mucormycosis and, 277
    nontuberculous mycobacteria and, 261
    obstructive, drug abuse and, 863
    physiology and, 672-683; see also Pulmonary function
    of pleura, 730-734; see also Pleura
    pulmonary hypertension and, 696; see also Pulmonary hypertension
    respiratory failure in, 707-713; see also Respiratory failure
    sarcoidosis and, 76
    schistosomiasis and, 296
    sickle cell anemia and, 332
    tuberculosis in, 255-256; see also Tuberculosis
    tumors in, 738-744
        benign, 743
        bronchial adenoma in, 743
        lymphoma in, 743
        lymphoproliferative disorders in, 743
        metastatic, 743-744
        primary malignant, 738-742
        solitary nodule in, 685, 743, 744
    viral, 122, 140-145, 217; see also Pneumonia, viral
    Wegener's granulomatosis and, 70
Respiratory distress syndrome, adult; see Adult respiratory distress syndrome
Respiratory exchange ratio, 673
Respiratory failure, 707-713
    acute, 708, 710, 711
    chronic, 708, 710-711
    classification of, 708
    Legionnaires' disease and, 177
    normal lungs and, 708, 711-713
    paralysis and, 169, 204
Respiratory impairment, dental care and, 745
Respiratory isolation; see Isolation
Respiratory stimulants, syncope and, 864
Respiratory syncytial virus, 140, 141-142, 171, 177
Rest pain, 568
Resting membrane potential, 479
Resting phase of tumor development, 439
Restrictive cardiomyopathies, 522, 523, 552
Restrictive ventilatory disorders, 680
Resuscitation, 540, 583-584, 752
Retardation, mental; see Mental retardation
Retching, severe, 957; see also Vomiting
Reticular activating system, 763, 764-765, 769
Reticular formation lesions, pontine paramedian, 833
Reticulocyte count, 310, 313, 328
Reticulocytes, 311
    count of; see Reticulocyte count
    hemolytic anemia and, 328
Reticuloendothelial cells, 394, 397
Reticuloendothelial system, 324
    chronic stimulation of, 378
    diseases of, 394-399
Reticulosis, histiocytic medullary, 398
Retina
    cytomegalovirus and, 125, 154
    diabetes mellitus and, 1273-1274
    hypertension and, 470
    inflammation of, 125, 126, 285, 286
    medullary cystic disease and, 653
    pheochromocytoma and, 1165
    pseudoxanthoma elasticum and, 884
    toxemia of pregnancy and, 665
    toxoplasmosis and, 285, 286
    von Hippel-Lindau disease and, 809

Retinal hemangiomas, 809
Retinal sheen, 665
Retinal-cerebellar hemangioblastomatosis, 1165
Retinochoroiditis, 125, 154, 285, 286
Retinol; see Vitamins, A
Retinopathy
    diabetes mellitus and, 1273-1274
    hypertensive, 469
    malignant, 1274
    medullary cystic disease and, 653
Retractile mesenteritis, 1048
Retraction nystagmus, 760
Retrobulbar neuritis, 798
Retrognathism, mandibular, 861
Retrograde amnesia, 772
Retrograde aortic dissection, 561
Retrograde cholangiopancreatography; see Endoscopic retrograde cholangiopancreatography
Retrograde pyelography, 606
Retroperitoneal fibrosis, 105
Retropulsion, 813
Reverse triiodothyronine; see 3,3′,5′-Triiodothyronine
Review of systems, 5-7
Rewarming after hypothermia, 756
Reye's syndrome, 827, 1077
    infectious mononucleosis and, 133
    influenza and, 141
    varicella and, 130, 138
RF; see Rheumatoid factor
Rh systems, 348, 349
    hemolytic disease and, 337-338
Rhabdomyosarcoma, embryonal, 449, 450
Rhabdovirus, 123
Rhagades, 270, 303
Rheumatic diseases, 35-117
    ankylosing spondylitis and, 48-50; see also Ankylosing spondylitis
    aortic regurgitation and, 515
    aortic stenosis and, 514
    avascular necrosis in, 104
    Behçet's syndrome and, 110-111
    chondrometaplasia of temporomandibular joint and, 108
    dentistry and, 105-117; see also specific disease
    dermatomyositis and, 64-65; see also Dermatomyositis
        dentistry and, 112-113
    fibrosing syndromes in, 105
    and fibrous dysplasia, 104, 115-116
    and gout, 51, 89-94, 622
        of temporomandibular joint, 108
    hemarthrosis in, 104-105, 409-410
    hypertrophic osteoarthropathy in, 103-104
    infectious arthritis in, 79-82; see also Arthritis, infectious
        temporomandibular joint and, 108
    intermittent, 53
    lupus erythematosus and, 53-58, 111-112
    microbicidal activity and, 357
    midline granuloma in, 70, 73-74, 113
    myofascial pain dysfunction syndrome of temporomandibular joint and, 109-110
    nonarticular rheumatism in, 96-102
    and osteoarthritis, 83-86, 860
        of temporomandibular joint, 107
    and osteomyelitis, 82-83; see also Osteomyelitis
        of jaws, 116-117
    and osteoporosis, 88-89; see also Osteoporosis
        dentistry and, 115

Rheumatic diseases—cont'd
    and Paget's disease, 86-88
        of jaws, 114-115
    polymyalgia rheumatica in, 69, 74-75, 858
    polymyositis and, 64-65; see also Polymyositis
        dentistry and, 112-113
    pseudogout and, 89, 94-95
    psoriatic arthritis and, 50-52
        temporomandibular joint and, 106
    Raynaud's phenomenon and, 62-64; see also Raynaud's phenomenon
    and Reiter's syndrome, 52-53; see also Reiter's syndrome
        dentistry and, 110
    relapsing polychondritis in, 102-103
    rheumatoid arthritis and, 35-43; see also Rheumatoid arthritis
        dentistry and, 105-106
        juvenile, 43-47
    sarcoidosis and, 75-78
        dentistry and, 113-114
    Schönlein-Henoch purpura and, 70
    systemic sclerosis and, 58-62
        dentistry and, 112
    temporal arteritis in, 74-75
    terminology and, 35
    tumors and, 437
    vasculitis and, 45, 66-70, 1022
    Weber-Christian disease in, 78-79
    Wegener's granulomatosis and, 70-73; see also Wegener's granulomatosis
        dentistry and, 113
Rheumatic fever
    acute, 225, 228-230
    dentistry and, 579-580, 582
    endocarditis and, 179, 182
    mitral regurgitation and, 510
    mitral stenosis and, 512
    oral streptococci and, 302
    Sydenham's chorea and, 818
Rheumatism, 96-102; see also Rheumatic diseases
Rheumatoid arthritis, 35-43
    amyloid deposits and, 385
    clinical manifestations of, 36
    dentistry and, 105-106
    diagnosis and, 38
    esophageal motility disorders and, 981
    hospitalization for, 43
    joint involvement and, 37
    juvenile, 43-47
        temporomandibular joint in, 106
    laboratory findings in, 37-38
    management and, 38-42
    neutropenia and, 359
    occupational therapy in, 42
    pathogenesis of, 35-36
    physical therapy in, 42
    prognosis and, 43
    psychosocial-sexual problems and, 42
    pulmonary fibrosis and, 715-716
    skin disorders of, 906
    surgery and, 42-43
Rheumatoid factor, 19, 36
    endocarditis and, 182
    psoriatic arthritis of temporomandibular joint and, 107
    rheumatoid arthritis and, 37, 43, 46
    scleroderma and, 903
Rheumatoid nodules, subcutaneous, 36
Rheumatoid spondylitis, 48
Rheumatoid vasculitis, 45, 1022
Rhinitis, 20-23, 73, 269
Rhinitis medicamentosum, 21, 23

Rhinorrhea, 72
Rhinoviruses, 140, 144, 172
Rhizopus, 277
Rhodopsin, 1107
Rhonchi, 24, 141
Rhythm of heart, 541-542; *see also* Arrhythmias
Rib lesions, 100, 101, 737
Riboflavin, 1106, 1108-1109, 1298
Ribonuclease, 945, 1050
Ribonucleic acid
  bladder neoplasms and, 659
  chemotherapy and, 440, 441, 443
  messenger; *see* Messenger ribonucleic acid
  phosphate metabolism and, 1184
  viruses and, 121, 123, 140
    measles in, 145
    mumps in, 139
    picornaviruses in, 144
Ribs, 737
  cervical, 101
  costochondritis and, 100
Rickets, 1106, 1107, 1186, 1198
  familial hypophosphatcmic, 1200
  hypophosphatasia and, 1200
  vitamin D-dependent, 1200
  vitamin D-resistant, 668, 1200
Rickettsia, 168, 209-214
Rickettsia akari, 211
Rickettsia australis, 209, 210
Rickettsia conorii, 209, 210
Rickettsia mooseri, 212
Rickettsia prowazekii, 212
Rickettsia quintana, 210
Rickettsia rickettsii, 209, 210-211
Rickettsia sibirica, 209, 210
Rickettsia typhi, 212
Rickettsialpox, 211-212, 213
Riedel's thyroiditis, 105, 1150
RIF; *see* Rifampin
Rifampin
  administration route for, 157
  endocarditis and, 184
  excretion of, 158
  in leprosy, 263
  meningitis and, 191, 236-237
  nephritis and, 619, 620
  nephropathy and, 624, 627, 628
  nontuberculous mycobacteria and, 261
  site of infection and, 156
  thrombocytopenia and, 400
  in tuberculosis, 258, 259
  urine and, 589
Right atrial hypertrophy, 500
Right atrial pressure, 552
Right coronary artery dominance, 524
Right hemisphere, aphasic, 771
Right lower lobe atelectasis, 702
Right middle lobe syndrome, 703
Right ventricle
  failure of, 459
    bronchitis and, 692
    mitral stenosis and, 512
    pulmonary emboli and, 490
    pulmonary hypertension and, 696
  hypertrophy of, 496, 499, 500
  infarction of, 536
  pressure in, 552
    end-diastolic, 459
Right-left disorientation, 759
Right-sided heart failure, 470
Right-to-left shunts, 506, 682
Rigidity, 812, 813, 870
Ring chromosome, 1221, 1222
Ring form of malaria, 281

Ringed sideroblasts, 322, 325
Ringer's lactate, 205, 350
Rings
  Cabot's, 315, 333
  Kayser-Fleischer, 822, 823
Ringworm, 928
Rinne test, 9, 795
Risk factors, dental care in respiratory disease and, 745, 746, 747, 748
Ristocetin, 400, 405, 407, 408
Ristocetin cofactor, 407, 408
Risus sardonicus, 252
RMSF; *see* Rocky Mountain spotted fever
RNA; *see* Ribonucleic acid
RNA viruses, 123, 140
Robertsonian translocations, 1222
Robitussin-CF, 1212
Robitussin-DM, 1212
Rochalimaea, 209-210
Rochalimaea quintana, 209, 210
Rocky Mountain spotted fever, 210-211, 213
  disseminated intravascular coagulation and, 412
  meningoencephalitis and, 139
Rodent mites, 212
Rodent ulcer, 916
Roentgen, 749
Roentgenograms
  acromegaly and, 1119
  avascular necrosis and, 104
  bowel obstruction and, 1025, 1026
  chest; *see* Chest, roentgenograms of
  in congenital heart disease, 501
  dental; *see* Radiographs, dental
  diffuse idiopathic skeletal hyperostosis and, 86
  fever of unknown origin and, 120
  fibrous dysplasia and, 105
  gout and, 92
  heart failure and, 462
  hemarthroses and, 105
  of kidneys, 605-608
  mastocystosis and, 910
  meningitis and, 188
  microbial disease and, 119
  mitral stenosis and, 513
  multiple myeloma and, 379, 380
  myeloid metaplasia and, 375
  obstructive uropathy and, 656
  and osteoarthritis, 84, 107
  osteomalacia and, 1199
  osteomyelitis and, 82, 221-222
  Paget's disease and, 87
  pancreatic tumors and, 1278-1279
  pancreatitis and, 1052
  peritoneal disease and, 1043-1044
  of pituitary tumors, 1123-1124
  in pseudogout, 94-95
  pulmonary hypertension and, 496, 497
  rheumatoid arthritis and, 106
  scleroderma and, 903, 904
  skull, 761, 769
  syringomyelia and, 807
  tuberculosis and, 258
Rokitansky-Kuster-Hauser syndrome, 1176
Romaña's sign, 287
Romberg's sign, 805
Root pain, spinal, 194
Rooting reflex, 758
Ropes test, 37
Rose bengal sodium iodine 131, 966
Rose spots, 207
Rosenthal fibers, 803
Roseola, 147
Rosettes with sheep red blood cells, 16, 32, 132

Rosewater's syndrome, 1171
Rotator cuff injury, 95, 101
Rotatory nystagmus, 760
Rotaviruses, 149-150
Roth's spots, 180, 181
Rotor's syndrome, 1058, 1068
Roundworms, 289-292
Roussy-Lévy syndrome, 806
Roving eye movements, 766
RPR test; *see* Rapid Plasma Reagin test
R-S cell; *see* Reed-Sternberg cell
RSV; *see* Respiratory syncytial virus
RT_3; *see* $3,3',5'$-Triiodothyronine
RTA; *see* Renal tubular acidosis
Rubber dam, 747
Rubella, 146-147
  congenital, 125, 126, 127, 1073
  dentistry and, 300
  hepatitis and, 1073
  polyarthritis and, 81-82
  vaccine for, 126, 127, 152
Rubella syndrome, 1303
Rubella virus, congenital, 125, 126, 127, 1073
Rubella virus vaccine, 152
Rubeola, 145-146, 300
Rubin tube, 964
Ruby lasers, 1095
Rugger-jersey spine, 637
Rukavina primary amyloidosis, 854
Rum fits, 776
Rumpel-Leede sign, 224
Runyon classification, 261
Rupture
  of chordae tendineae, 510
  of esophageal varices, 1063
  of spleen, 134, 398
Russell's bodies, 380
RV; *see* Residual volume
RV infarction; *see* Right ventricle, infarction of
RVH; *see* Right ventricle, hypertrophy of
Rye classification, 387

S

S_f; *see* Svedberg flotation constant
S_{O_2}; *see* Oxygen saturation of hemoglobin
S_3 gallop, 710
S wave, 482, 483
SA node, 479
SAA; *see* Serum, amyloid A in, 386
SAARD; *see* Slow-acting antirheumatic drugs
Saber shins, 270
Saber stroke, 903
Sabin-Feldman dye test, 286
Sack's type of Ehlers-Danlos syndromes, 1242
Sacral sparing, 760
Saddle deformity, 102
Saddle nose, 877
Saethre-Chotzen syndrome, 1314, 1315, 1316
St. Louis encephalitis, 135, 825
St. Vitus' dance, 229
Sal-eze, 876
Salicylates; *see also* Aspirin; specific drug
  alcohol and, 1297, 1298
  ankylosing spondylitis and, 738
  asthma and, 704
  coumarins and, 414
  erythema multiforme and, 923
  gout and, 92
  hepatitis arthralgia and, 81
  lung disease and, 721, 722
  lupus erythematosus and, 57
  methotrexate and, 440
  nephropathy and, 621
  pregnancy and, 1212

Salicylates—cont'd
  psoriatic arthritis of temporomandibular joint and, 107
  pulmonary hyperosteoarthropathy and, 103
  respiratory alkalosis and, 601
  rheumatic fever and, 229-230
  sarcoidosis and, 78
  sensitivity to, 23-24
  thyroid hormone binding and, 1131
  vitamin K deficiency and, 411
Salicylazosulfapyridine, 330
Salicylic acid, 927
Saline, 350; see also Salt; Sodium; Sodium chloride
  anaphylaxis and, 29
  gastrointestinal bleeding and, 958
  hypertonic; see Hypertonic saline
  isotonic; see Normal saline
  posthemorrhagic anemia and, 323
  prerenal azotemia and, 632
  right ventricular infarction and, 536
  shock and, 240, 478
  ulcerative stomatitis and, 415
Saliva
  ammonia in, 666, 667
  anticholinergics and, 870
  anticholinesterases and, 874
  artificial, 114, 911, 919
  diabetes and, 1294
  diagnostic tests of, 1101, 1102
  hepatitis and, 1099
  oral contraceptives and, 1214
  urea in, 666, 667
Salivart, 876
Salivary glands
  biopsy of, 1098
  cystic fibrosis and, 1101
  cytomegalovirus and, 300
  enlargement of, 1211, 1296
  Epstein-Barr virus and, 300
  hyperlipoproteinemia and, 1296
  hypopituitarism and, 1204
  mumps and, 301
  sarcoidosis and, 114, 911
  Sjögren's syndrome and, 36
  tuberculosis of, 304
Salmonella, 202, 206-208
  diarrhea and, 953
  drugs for, 159, 163, 169
  endocarditis and, 179
  liver disease and, 1074
  osteomyelitis and, 82
  in pneumonia, 171
  reactive arthritis and, 53
  Reiter's syndrome and, 907
  schistosomiasis and, 296
  sickle cell anemia and, 333
Salmonella choleraesuis, 208
Salmonella enteritidis, 206, 1074
Salmonella heidelberg, 206
Salmonella newport, 206
Salmonella paratyphi, 207
Salmonella typhi, 207
Salmonella typhimurium, 206, 208
Salpingitis, 217, 231, 232
Salpingo-oophorectomy, 449
Salt; see also Saline; Sodium; Sodium chloride
  congential adrenal hyperplasias and, 1163
  heat syndromes and, 755
  hyponatremia and, 595
  mineralocorticoid excess and, 1161
  postural hypotension and, 780
Salt-and-pepper appearance of skull, 637
Salt-poor albumin, 1083

Salvage therapy, 390-391
Sanctuaries, 366
Sandhoff's disease, 1231
Sanfilippo's syndrome, 1233, 1234
Sanger Brown spinal ataxia, 806
Sansert; see Methysergide
Saphenous vein grafts, 532
Saralasin, 661
Sarcoidosis, 75-78, 716-718, 910-911
  cardiomyopathies and, 522-523
  cutaneous lesions of, 911
  dentistry and, 113-114
  diabetes insipidus and, 1126
  hypercalcemia and, 1194
  kidney disease and, 618
  meningoencephalitis and, 139
Sarcolemma, 454
Sarcomas
  immunoblastic, 392
  Kaposi's, 863, 920-922
  management of, 449-450
  osteogenic, 449-450
Sarcomeres, 454, 456
Satellism, 235
Satellite bubo, 266
Satellite lesions, intertrigo and, 929
Saturated potassium iodide, 276; see also Potassium iodide
SCA; see Sickle cell disease
Scalded skin syndrome, 219, 220, 932
Scalene muscles, 672
  myofascial syndromes and, 98, 100, 101
Scalenus anticus syndrome, 100, 101
Scanning speech, nystagmus, and intention tremor, triad of, 799
Scans; see also Radioactive iodine
  blood pool, 489, 521, 530
  bone, 86-87, 222, 436
  brain, 761
    abscess and, 192
    cerebral infarction and, 831-832
    computed tomography and; see Computed tomography, brain and
    diffuse cerebellar lesions in, 759
    herpes simplex encephalitis and, 136
  cancer staging and, 436
  enterogastric reflux and, 962
  fever of unknown origin and, 120
  gallium, 222, 389, 967
  gastroesophageal, 962
  hepatic, 966-967
  lung, 492, 493, 687
  microbial disease and, 119
  myocardial infarction, 527-528, 530
  renal, 607-608, 661
  technetium 99m; see also Technetium 99m labeling
    angina pectoris and, 530
    myocardial infarction and, 535
    renal, 607-608
    thyroid and, 1133
  thallium 201, 489
    angina pectoris and, 530
    cardiomyopathy and, 521
    myocardial infarction and, 536
    thrombophlebitis and, 495
  thyroid, 1133
Scarlet fever, 224
SCD; see Subacute combined degeneration
Schaumann bodies, 911
Scheie's syndrome, 1233, 1234
Schick test, 249
Schilder's disease, 802
Schilling test, 318

Schistocyte, 315
Schistosoma haematobium, 294, 295, 296
  carcinoma and, 432, 659
Schistosoma japonicum, 294, 295, 296
Schistosoma mansoni, 294, 295, 296
Schistosomiasis, 294-297; see also *Schistosoma haematobium*
  diarrhea and, 953
  hepatic, 296
  pneumonia and, 172
Schistosomula, 295
Schizogony, 279, 280
Schizonts, 280
Schmorl's nodes, 89
Schönlein-Henoch purpura, 70, 406-407
  intestinal vasculitis and, 1022
  renal lesions in, 616
Schuffner's dots, 281
Schwartzman reaction, 234
Sciatica, 50, 84
Scintigraphy; see Scans
Sclera, 8, 1097
Sclerodactyly
  acrosclerosis and, 903
  Raynaud's phenomenon and, 63
  systemic sclerosis and, 58, 60, 61, 903
Scleroderma, 58-62, 903-904
  cardiomyopathies and, 522-523
  dentistry and, 1091-1092
  esophageal disorders and, 981, 982
  malabsorption and, 1004
  pregnancy and, 666
  pulmonary fibrosis and, 715
  renal lesions in, 615-616
Sclerodermatomyositis, 905
Sclerosing agents
  angiokeratoma corporis diffusum and, 912
  angiomas and, 882
  esophageal and gastric bleeding and, 959
  hemorrhoids and, 1031
  intestinal ulcer and, 1019
  intraperitoneal, 446
  pericardial effusion and, 555
  telangiectasia and, 894
Sclerosing cholangitis, 105, 1089
Sclerosing mediastinitis, 735
Sclerosing panencephalitis, subacute, 138, 828
Sclerosing thyroiditis, 1150
Sclerosis
  amyotrophic lateral, 803-804, 868, 869
  basal cell carcinoma and, 916
  chemically induced, 58; see also Sclerosing agents
  multiple, 794, 796-801, 868-869
  progressive systemic; see Systemic sclerosis
  systemic; see Systemic sclerosis
  tuberous, 721, 810, 869, 880-881
Scolex, 292, 294
Scoliosis, 712, 737
Scombroid fish poisoning, 200
Scopolamine, 745, 746
Scrofula, 256
Scrofulosis, 304
Scrotum, 13
Scurvy, 406, 1110
Sea-blue histiocytes, 1293
Sebaceous adenomas, 913
Seborrhea, 813-814, 913, 1030
Secondary adrenal failure, 1155, 1156
Secondary aldosteronism, 1160
Secondary cardiomyopathies, 522-523
Secondary osteoarthritis of temporomandibular joint, 107
Second-degree atrioventricular block, 547

Secretin, 941, 946
  pancreatic secretion and, 1050
  test for, 995, 1055
Secretor locus, 1229
Secretory component, 17
Secretory immunoglobulin A, 941–942
Sectional tray technique, 112
Sedation, 670; *see also* Nitrous oxide; Sedatives
Sedatives; *see also* specific agent
  abuse of, 862, 863
  alcoholics and, 1062
  alveolar hypoventilation and, 682
  angina and, 583
  bronchitis and, 693
  cerebrovascular disease and, 586
  dementia and, 775
  diabetes and, 1295
  heart medication and, 571-572, 574
  hepatic coma and, 1061, 1084
  hepatitis and, 1099
  metabolic encephalopathies and, 768
  overdose of, 708, 710, 711, 712
  pregnancy and, 1212
  in respiratory disease, 745, 746, 747
  respiratory failure and, 708, 710, 711, 712
  tremor and, 816
  vasovagal syncope and, 577
Sediment in urine, 604-605, 616
Sedimentation rate, erythrocyte; *see* Erythrocyte sedimentation rate
Seesaw nystagmus, 760
Segmented neutrophils, 356
Seizures, 781-787
  absence, 781, 783
  alcohol withdrawal and, 776
  brain tumor and, 845
  coma and, 765, 766
  cytomegalovirus and, 125
  drugs for; *see* Anticonvulsants
  encephalitis and, 135
  fainting and, 780
  febrile, 147
  generalized, 781, 782, 783
  idiopathic, 781, 782, 783
  management of, 866-867
  metronidazole and, 170
  neurofibromatosis and, 879
  parietal lobe lesions and, 759
  penicillins and, 164
  roseola and, 147
  subdural empyema and, 193
  tetanus and, 252
Self-associated rheumatoid factor complexes, 36
Sella turcica, J-shaped, 1032
Semen, hepatitis and, 1099
Semicoma, 764
Seminiferous tubule dysgenesis, 1170
Seminomas, 449, 735
Semistupor, 764
Semustine; *see* Methyl lomustine
Senear-Usher syndrome, 934
Sengstaken-Blakemore tube, 959, 1083
Senile cataracts, 1273
Senile keratosis, 914
Senile tremor, 815-816, 870
Sensitivity; *see* Allergy; Hypersensitivity
Sensitization, 28, 406; *see also* Autoimmune disease
Sensorineural hearing loss, 795
Sensory action potentials, 806
Sensory loss, 758, 760
Sensory nerves, 14, 851
  disorders of, 758, 759, 852, 855
Sentinel loop, 1052

Sentinel polyp of large bowel, 1038
Sepsis; *see* Infections
Septal defects
  atrial, 503, 504, 508
  ventricular, 504
    cardiac catheterization and, 488
    rupture and, 536
    tetralogy of Fallot and, 507
    transposition of great arteries and, 508
Septal hypertrophy, asymmetric, 179, 517-520
Septal Q waves, 483
Septic arthritis, 79-82; *see also* Infections
  fungal, 81
  gonococcal, 231, 232
  Haemophilus influenzae and, 236
  nongonococcal, 79-81
  rat-bite fever and, 272
  streptococcal, 226
  of temporomandibular joint, 108
  tuberculosis and, 81, 256
  viruses and, 81-82
Septic emboli, 180, 489, 579
Septic shock, 118, 476, 478; *see also* Septicemia
  dentistry and, 575
  gram-negative bacilli and, 239-240
Septicemia; *see also* Bacteremia
  Clostridium perfringens and, 253
  disseminated intravascular coagulation and, 412
  plague and, 242
  streptococcal, 226
Septostomy, balloon, 508
Septra-Bactrim, 1212
Sequences, 1228
Sequestration, pulmonary, 696, 736
Sequestration syndrome, 332
Sequoiasis, 727
SER; *see* Somatosensory evoked response
Serax; *see* Oxazepam
Serine esterase, 17
Serology, 119; *see also* Serum
  for amebae, 282
  central nervous system disease and, 139
  fever of unknown origin and, 120
  hepatitis and, 1071
  for rheumatoid factor, 182
  in syphilis, 271, 903
  in toxoplasmosis, 285-286
  viruses and, 124
    lymphocytic choriomeningitis and, 138
    mumps and, 138
    neonatal, 127
Serositis, 54
Serotonin, 18, 941, 942
  bronchial adenoma and, 743
  carcinoid syndrome and, 450, 743, 1038
  migraine and, 788
  Zollinger-Ellison syndrome and, 994
Serotonin antagonists, 450, 743, 1038
Serous otitis, 795
Serpasil; *see* Reserpine
Serratia, 80
  drugs for, 164, 165
  oral lesions of, 306
  in pneumonia, 171
Sertoli cells, 1168, 1169, 1171
Sertoli-cell-only syndrome, 1171
Serum, 313; *see also* Serology
  acid phosphatase in, 397, 435, 660
  albumin in; *see also* Albumin
    liver disease and, 1065, 1071
    radiolabeling of, 352, 492, 687, 966
  alkaline phosphatase in; *see* Alkaline phosphatase

Serum—cont'd
  amylase in, 945, 1049, 1052
  amyloid A in, 386
  angiotensin-converting enzyme in, 77, 717, 718
  antianthrax, 305
  antimicrobials and, 157-158
  bile acids in, 1065
  bilirubin in, 1064, 1070, 1071
  calcitonin in, 1151, 1152, 1197
  calcium in, 1183-1184, 1189-1196
    hyperparathyroidism and, 1207-1208
    hypoparathyroidism and, 1209
    kidney stones and, 648
    neoplasms and, 1179-1180
    osteomalacia and, 1198, 1199
    renal failure and, 636
  ceruloplasmin in, 1066, 1081-1082
  creatinine in, 462, 630; *see also* Creatinine
  enzymes in, 1065; *see also* specific enzyme
  ferritin in, 313
    hemochromatosis and, 345
    liver disease and, 1066, 1081
  folate in, 318; *see also* Folate
  gamma-glutamyl transpeptidase in, 1065, 1066, 1068
  gastrin in, 989, 995; *see also* Gastrin
  globulins in; *see* Globulins
  glutamic-oxaloacetic transaminase in; *see also* Serum, transaminases in
    liver disease and, 1065
    myocardial infarction and, 535
    neuromuscular disorders and, 853
  horse, 25, 26
  hyperviscosity of; *see* Hyperviscosity, serum
  iron in; *see* Iron
  lactic dehydrogenase in; *see* Lactic dehydrogenase
  leucine aminopeptidase in, 1065
  lipase in, 1052
  lipids in; *see* Lipids
  5'-nucleotidase in, 1065, 1066, 1068
  osmolality of, 596, 1126
  phosphate in; *see* Phosphates
  potassium in; *see* Potassium
  sodium in; *see* Sodium
  thyrotropin in, 1135
  thyroxine in, 1134, 1136, 1141
  transaminases in
    jaundice and, 1067
    liver disease and, 1065, 1071, 1072
    myocardial infarction and, 535
    neuromuscular disorders and, 853
  transferrin in, 1081
  triiodothyronine in, 1134, 1141
  unconsciousness and tests of, 768
  urate levels in, 89-90
  vitamin B_{12} in, 353
Serum sickness, 26-27
Sex chromosomes, 1217, 1221, 1225
Sex determination, 1168
Sex hormones, 1169; *see also* specific hormone
  cholestasis and, 1076
  oral manifestations of, 1210-1214
  porphyria and, 1252
Sex steroid–binding globulin, 1154
Sex steroids, 1153; *see also* specific steroid
Sézary syndrome, 901
SGOT; *see* Serum, glutamic-oxaloacetic transaminase in
SH; *see* Sulfhemoglobinemia
Shagreen patches, 880
Shaving of condyle, 107
Sheehan's syndrome, 1177

Sheep red blood cells, 16, 32, 132
Shellfish poisoning, 200
Shields for oral radiation, 751
Shigella, 202, 205-206, 209
    diarrhea and, 952-953
    drugs for, 163
    malabsorption and, 1003
    Reiter's syndrome and, 52, 53, 907
Shigella boydii, 205
Shigella dysenteriae, 205, 206
Shigella flexneri, 205
Shigella sonnei, 205, 206
Shin splints, 102
Shin spots, diabetic, 885, 1276
Shingles; see Herpes zoster
Shiny skin, scleroderma and, 903
Shock, 475-479
    anaphylaxis and, 28, 29, 476, 478
        dentistry and, 576
    cardiogenic, dentistry and, 576
    cold, 240, 476
    compensatory mechanisms and, 477
    dentistry and, 575-577
    hypovolemic, 476
        dentistry and, 575
        gastrointestinal bleeding and, 597-598
        transfusion reactions and, 351
    irreversible, 478
    Legionnaires' disease and, 177
    liver disease and, 1077
    in microbial diseases, 118; see also Septic shock
    myocardial infarction and, 536
    septic; see Septic shock
    spinal, 836
    warm, 240, 476
Shock kidney, 630
Shock lung, 240, 477, 708; see also Adult respiratory distress syndrome
    bacteremia and, 240
Shohl's solution; see Sodium citrate
Short bowel syndrome, 1077
Short-arm 18 deletion syndrome, 1316
Short-term memory, 772-773
Shoulder disorders, 100, 537
    frozen, 101
    Milwaukee, 95
    myofascial syndromes and, 98
    osteoarthritis and, 84
Shoulder-hand syndrome, 100, 537
Shoulder-pad sign, 386
Shunts; see also Anastomoses
    cardiac, 191, 353
    cerebrospinal fluid, 182
    glomerulonephritis with infection of, 611
    left-to-right, congenital, 501, 502-505
    LeVeen, 1046
    right-to-left, 506, 682
    signs and symptoms of, 499
Shy-Drager syndrome, 814, 823
SIADH; see Syndromes of inappropriate antidiuretic hormone secretion
Sialadenitis, 299, 300
Sialadenotropism, 300
Sialidase deficiency, 1235
Sialidosis, 1235
Sialorrhea, 870, 876
Sicca complex, 1098
Sick euthyroid syndrome, 1131
Sick sinus syndrome, 501, 546-547
Sickle cell disease, 332-334, 1227
    cerebrovascular disease and, 842
    crises and, 332
    dactylitis and, 332

Sickle cell disease—cont'd
    dentistry and, 416-417
    endocarditis and, 182
    hyposplenism and, 395
    kidney diseases and, 618
    pneumococcal pneumonia and, 175
    skin disorders of, 898
Sickle cell hemoglobin, 331-332, 334, 1220; see also Sickle cell disease
Sickle cell trait, 331, 334, 1220
Sideroblastic anemia, 308-309, 1257
Sideroblasts, ringed, 322, 325
Sideropenic dysphagia, 416
Side-to-side anastomosis of ascending aorta to pulmonary artery, 507
Sigmoid colon
    resection of, in diverticulosis, 1018
    study of; see Sigmoidoscopy
    ulcer of, 1019
    volvulus of, 1026
Sigmoidoscopy, 965
    antibiotic-induced diarrhea and, 1018
    colorectal carcinoma and, 1040
    Crohn's disease and, 1012
    fever of unknown origin and, 120
    large bowel neoplasms and, 1038
    radiation enteritis and, 1019
    ulcerative colitis and, 1008
Signs
    Auspitz, 936
    Babinski's; see Babinski's sign
    Carvallo's, 516
    Chvostek's, 1183, 1196, 1208
    colon cutoff, 1052
    Courvoisier's, 1056
    Cullen's, 1051
    Dalrymple's, 1142
    Darier's, 909
    delta, 841
    focal neurologic, 192, 768, 845
    frontal release, 758
    Gower's, 852
    Homans', 495
    Joffroy's, 1142
    Kernig's, 839
    Kussmaul's, 585
    Leser-Trélat, 912, 913
    Lhermitte's, 799
    Marcus Gunn's pupillary, 798
    Möbius', 1142
    Musset's, 580
    Nikolsky's, 220, 877
        Lyell's disease and, 931
        pemphigus and, 933
        scalded skin syndrome and, 932
    Phalen's, 98
    psoas, 1016
    puddle, 1044
    pyramidal tract, 803
    Romaña's, 287
    Romberg's, 805
    Rumpel-Leede, 224
    shoulder-pad, 386
    splenic flexure cutoff, 1021
    Stellwag's, 1142
    string, 1012
    swinging flashlight, 798
    Tinel's, 98, 1275
    Trousseau's, 1183, 1196, 1208
    Turner's, 1051
    Uhthoff's, 798
    von Graefe's, 1142
    Wimberger's, 270
Silent carrier alpha-thalassemia, 336

Silent chest, 706
Silicon, 723; see also Silicosis
Silicosis, 723-725
Silver, nephropathy and, 627, 628
Silver nitrate, 233, 908
Silver syndrome, 879
Sinemet; see Levodopa
Single gene disorders, 1226-1227, 1302
Single gene inheritance, 1216-1220
Single-peak insulin, 1267
Sinoatrial block, 546
Sinoatrial conduction, 541
Sinus arrest, 547
Sinus bradycardia, 546-547
Sinus node, 541
    disorders of, in children, 501
    tests of, 547
Sinus rhythm, normal, 542
Sinus tachycardia, 542
Sinus thrombosis, cavernous, 303-304
Sinuses
    infection and, 21
        brain abscesses and, 191, 192
        dental infection and, 303-304
        headache from, 790
        subdural empyema and, 193
    paranasal, midline granuloma and, 73
    of Valsalva, aneurymsms of, 558
Sinusitis; see Sinuses, infection and
Sipple's syndrome, 879, 1151, 1164
Sisomicin, 166
Sitophilus granarius, 727
Sitosterols, 1290
Situs inversus, 696
Sitz baths, 1031
Sjögren's syndrome, 36-37
    dermatitis herpetiformis and, 893
    insulin resistance and, 1261
    juvenile rheumatoid arthritis and, 45
    liver disease and, 1098
    macroglobulinemia and, 423
    pulmonary fibrosis and, 716
    sarcoidosis and, 77
SK-65; see Propoxyphene
SK-Bamate; see Meprobamate
Skeletal homeostasis, disorders of, 1198-1203
    primary, 1201-1203
    systemic sclerosis and, 59-60
Skeletal hyperostosis, diffuse idiopathic, 50, 86
Skeletal mass, loss of, 1182
Skene's glands, 231
Skin, 8; see also Skin diseases
    biopsy of, 139, 211, 1229
    bronze, 345, 878, 890
    cancer detection and, 434
    dry, 876-877
    elastotic, 914
    fluid loss and, 596
    premalignant lesions of, 914
Skin diseases, 876-939; see also Rash
    angiokeratoma corporis diffusum and, 911-912, 1231-1232
        orofacial abnormalities and, 668
    anorectal, 1030
    anthrax and, 245
    arterial insufficiency and, 568
    congenital, 876-884
    connective tissue disorders and, 902-908
    contact dermatitis and, 27
    dermatomyositis and, 64
    diabetes mellitus and, 885, 1276
    diphtheria and, 248
    endocrine disorders and, 884-891
    erythemas and, 922-926; see also Erythema

Skin diseases—cont'd
  Fabry's disease and, 911-912, 1231-1232
    orofacial abnormalities and, 668
  gastrointestinal disorders and, 891-895
  Graves' disease and, 1141-1142, 1143
  hematologic disorders and, 897-902
  hypersensitivity vasculitis and, 67
  hyperthyroidism and, 1141-1142
  infections and, 926-931; see also specific infection
  internal malignancy and, 912-913
  larva migrans and, 291
  leprosy and, 262
  lichen planus and, 938, 1030
  liver disease and, 896, 1058-1059
  Lyell's disease and, 931-932
  mastocytosis and, 909-910
  metabolic disorders and, 884-891
  necrobiosis lipoidica diabeticorum and, 1276
  neoplasms and, 438, 913-922
  neurocutaneous, 808-810
  nontuberculous mycobacteria and, 261
  pemphigoid and, 932, 935
  pemphigus and, 932-935
  porphyria and, 1249, 1253
  psoriasis and, 936-938; see also Psoriasis
  radiation and, 750
  rash in; see Rash
  renal disorders and, 896-897
  sarcoidosis and, 76-77, 910-911; see also Sarcoidosis
  scleroderma and, 903
  staphylococcal, 219-220
  streptococcal, 223, 225-226
  syphilis and, 267
  systemic sclerosis and, 59, 61
  thrush and, 276
  toxic epidermal necrolysis and, 931-932
  ulcerative colitis and, 1095, 1096
  Urbach-Wiethe disease and, 1296
  viral causes of, 122; see also Rash
    herpes simplex in, 126, 128
    varicella in, 130
    varicella-zoster in, 126, 129-130
Skin graft, 935, 1276
Skin tests, 21-22
  cat-scratch fever and, 151
  delayed hypersensitivity, 32
  fever of unknown origin and, 120
  and histoplasmosis, 274
  Kveim, 75, 718, 911
  lepromin, 262
  microbial disease and, 119
  tuberculin, 81, 257, 260
Skipper hypotheses, 439
SK-Lygen; see Chlordiazepoxide
Skull
  development of, 1306
  fractures of, abscess and, 191, 192
  Hand-Schüller-Christian disease and, 719
  osteomyelitis of, cerebral epidural abscess and, 193
  roentgenogram of, 761, 769
  salt-and-pepper appearance of, 637
  shape of, 1313
Slapped cheeks, 147
SLE; see Lupus erythematosus, systemic; St. Louis encephalitis
Sleep
  cerebral frequencies and, 769
  dentistry and, 861-862
  fibrositis and, 96
  paroxysmal nocturnal hemoglobinuria and, 341
Sleep apneas, 708, 711, 769-770, 861

Sleep paralysis, 769
Sleep spindles, 769
Sleeping pills; see Sedatives
Sleeping sickness, 286, 814
Slow virus infection, 828, 868
Slow-acting antirheumatic drugs, 46, 47
Slow-reacting substance of anaphylaxis, 18, 372, 705
Sluder's sphenopalatine ganglion neuralgia, 791
Sly's syndrome, 1233, 1234
SM; see Streptomycin
Small cell carcinoma of lung, 434, 447
Small intestines; see Intestines, small
Small vessel coronary artery disease, 453
Smallpox vaccine, 827
Smears; see Gram stains; Peripheral blood smears
Smoke inhalation, 729
Smoker's cough, 691, 745
Smoking; see also Nicotine
  asbestos and, 727
  Buerger's disease and, 570
  cancer and, 432
    bladder, 659
    lung, 727, 738, 739
    prostatic, 659
  chronic obstructive pulmonary disease and, 691, 692, 693, 694
  coronary artery disease and, 526
  esophagitis and, 982, 985
  oral candidiasis and, 307, 308
  polycythemia and, 354-355
  premalignant lesions and, 919
  thromboangiitis obliterans and, 69
  ulcers and, 988, 991
Snails, 295
Snare-cautery, 1034, 1038, 1040
SNI; see Subtotal nodal irradiation
Snout reflex, 758
Snuff, 919
Soap, antiseptic, 225
Social history, 7, 432
Social Security Administration, 691
Sodium; see also Saline; Salt; Sodium chloride
  blood pressure and, 468
  body fluid osmolality and, 596
  bromide intoxication and, 777
  cardiac cells and, 479
  congenital adrenal hyperplasia and, 1163
  cystic fibrosis and, 700
  deficiency of; see Hyponatremia
  dehydration and, 597
  dietary, 1111
    renal failure and, 639
    restriction of, 471, 612, 1161
  digestion and, 947
  excess of, 595-596
  heart failure and, 464
  hyperglycemic, hyperosmolar, nonketotic coma and, 1270
  liver disease and, 1064
  metabolism of, 593-597, 1044
  mineralocorticoids and, 1160
  tubular reabsorption of, 592
Sodium acetate, 205
Sodium aurothioglucose, 42
Sodium aurothiomalate, 42
Sodium bicarbonate
  alcohol and, 1256
  antacids and, 991
  cholera and, 205
  diabetic ketoacidosis and, 1270
  hyperkalemia and, 599, 633-634
  lithium overdose and, 779
  meningococcemia and, 234

Sodium bicarbonate—cont'd
  metabolic acidosis and, 639
  in mouth care, 876
    for herpetic gingivostomatitis, 299
    for Reiter's syndrome, 908
    for ulcerative stomatitis, 415
  multiple sclerosis and, 797-798
  pigment nephrotoxicity and, 629
  pseudomembranous enterocolitis and, 1018
  renal failure and, 633-634
  renal tubular acidosis and, 623
  sickle cell disease and, 618
  whole blood transfusions and, 350
Sodium carbonate, 754
Sodium chloride; see also Saline; Salt; Sodium
  cholera and, 205
  heat syndromes and, 755
  orthostatic hypotension and, 824
Sodium citrate, 600
Sodium diatrizoate, 605; see also Contrast agents
Sodium fluoride, 89
Sodium hydroxide, 754, 985, 986
Sodium iodide, 1147
Sodium iodide 131, rose bengal, 966
Sodium iopanate, 1131
Sodium ipodate, 1131
Sodium nitroprusside; see Nitroprusside
Sodium polystyrene sulfonate
  hyperkalemia and, 599, 634
  hyporeninemic hypoaldosteronism and, 623
  renal failure and, 639
Sodium salicylate; see Salicylates
Soft palate, spots on, 300
Soft tissues
  clostridial infections and, 252-253, 254
  Gardner's syndrome and, 1042
  of mouth, urate crystals in, 667
  rheumatism and, 96-102
  sausagelike swelling of, 51
Solar elastotic skin, 914
Solar keratosis, 914
Solganal; see Gold
Solitary pulmonary nodule, 685, 743, 744
  chest roentgenograms and, 685, 743, 744
  malignant lymphoma and, 900
Soluble-antigen complement fixation test, 286
Solvents, organic, 853
Somatognosia, 771
Somatomedin-C, 1122, 1123
Somatomedins, 1118, 1122, 1123, 1181
Somatosensory evoked response, 762
Somatostatin, 942, 943, 1118, 1262
  endocrine pancreas and, 1049
  formation of, 945
  thyroid and, 1128
Somatotropin; see Growth hormone
Somnos; see Chloral hydrate
Somogyi effect, 1267
Sones' coronary angiography, 631
Sorbitol, 634
Soret band, 888
Sound waves, 794
South African porphyria, 1253
Spasmodic torticollis, 819-820
Spasms; see also Spasticity
  of esophagus; see Esophagus, spasm of
  torsion, 820-821
  torticollis and, 819-820
Spastic colitis, 1005, 1027, 1028
  lactose intolerance and, 1005, 1028
Spastic diplegia, 146
Spastic paraparesis, 799, 807
Spasticity; see also Spasms
  of colon, 1005, 1027

Spasticity—cont'd
  congenital cytomegalovirus and, 125
  frontal lobe lesions and, 757
  multiple sclerosis and, 799
  rubella and, 146
  syringomyelia and, 807
Specific binding of hormones, 1115
Specific gravity of urine, 604
Spectinomycin, 170, 232
Spectrum of activity, 155
Speech, cerebrovascular accident and, 872
Spermatogenesis, 1169
Sphenopalatine ganglion neuralgia, 791
Spherocyte, 315, 328-329
Spherocytosis, hereditary, 328-329
Sphingomyelin, 397, 1230, 1231, 1232
Sphingomyelin lipidosis, 1231, 1232
Sphingomyelinase deficiency, 397, 721
Sphygmomanometric examinations; see also Blood pressure
  atherosclerosis and, 583
  hypertension and, 572-575
Spider angiomas, 863, 894, 896, 1059
Spinal artery syndrome, 835-836
Spinal ataxia, 805, 806
Spinal cord disorders, 760-761, 860
  compression in
    Klippel-Feil syndrome and, 811
    radicular pain and, 194
    supportive care and, 445
  developmental abnormalities in, 320-321, 341
  diabetes mellitus and, 1275
  folic acid deficiency and, 1110
  Friedreich's ataxia and, 805
  hemorrhage in, 840
  infarction in, 835-836
  inflammation in, 136
  intramedullary tumors in, 807
  ischemia in, 556
  radiation-induced, 847
  Sanger Brown ataxia and, 806
  testes and, 1171
  tumors and, 807, 860
Spinal fluid; see Cerebrospinal fluid
Spinal nerves, 1043
Spinal roots, disorders of, 860
Spinal shock, 836
Spindle cell tumors of kidney, 657
Spine; see also Vertebrae
  angiography and, 762
  ankylosing spondylosis and; see Spondylitis, ankylosing
  bamboo, 49, 50, 737
  cervical
    spondylosis of, 860
    subluxation of, 36, 38, 39
  computed tomography and, 762
  dysplasias and, 1245
  epidural abscess and, 193-194
  evaluation of, 13
  kyphoscoliosis and, 712, 737
  kyphosis and, 48, 50, 737
  osteoarthritis and, 84
  progressive muscular atrophies and, 804-805
  roentgenograms of, 761-762
  rugger-jersey, 637
  Sanger Brown ataxia and, 806
  thoracic, 737
    ankylosing spondylitis and, 48, 50
    tuberculosis of, 256, 257
    vitamin B_{12} deficiency and, 851
Spinhaler, 707
Spiramycin, 728
Spirillary rat-bite fever, 272-273

Spirillum minus, 272
Spirochetes, 264-274
  congenital syphilis and, 303
  leptospirosis in, 273-274
  liver disease and, 1074
  rat-bite fever in, 272-273
  syphilis in, 264-272; *see also* Syphilis
Spirometers, 678, 679
Spironolactone, 597
  ascites and, 1083
  heart failure and, 465
  hyperkalemia and, 598
  hypertension and, 472
  hypokalemia and, 598
  kidney stones and, 647
  mineralocorticoid excess and, 1161, 1162
  renal failure and, 639
  renal tubular acidosis and, 623
  side effects and interactions of, 574
Splanchnic blood flow, 948-949, 1043, 1060, 1061
Splanchnic lymph drainage, 1044
Spleen, 394-399
  abscesses of, 398
  absence of, 395
  cysts of, 398
  enlarged; *see* Splenomegaly
  examination of, 13
  function of, 395
  infarction of, 398
  removal of; *see* Splenectomy
  rupture of, 134, 398
  small, 395
  space-occupying lesions of, 398
  tumors of, 398
Splenectomy, 395
  anemia and, 320, 339
  infection after, 395
  porphyrias and, 888
  spherocytosis and, 329
  thalassemia and, 337
  thrombocytopenic purpura and, 403, 404
  thrombocytosis and, 404
Splenic flexure, 947
Splenic flexure cutoff sign, 1021
Splenomegaly, 395-396
  endocarditis and, 181
  evaluation of, 395
  idiopathic, 395
  infectious mononucleosis and, 132
  malaria and, 280
  myeloid metaplasia and, 374
  neutropenia and, 359
  polycythemia vera and, 353
  portal hypertension and, 1060-1061
  sickle cell anemia and, 333
  thrombocytosis and, 404
Splenorenal anastomosis, 1083
Splinter hemorrhages, 181
Splints
  cerebrovascular accident and, 873
  hyperparathyroidism and, 1208
  night; *see* Night guards
  pemphigoid and, 935
  temporomandibular joint dysfunction and, 867, 873
  ulcerative stomatitis and, 415
Split papules, secondary syphilis and, 303
Spondylitic cervical myelopathy, 860
Spondylitis, ankylosing, 48-50, 737-738
  inflammatory bowel disease and, 1006, 1008
  pulmonary fibrosis and, 716
  valvular disease and, 580
Spondyloepiphyseal dysplasia congenita, 1245

Spondyloepiphyseal dysplasia tarda, 1245
Spondylometaphyseal dysplasia, 1245
Spondylosis, 84, 860
Sponge kidney, medullary, 653
Spongiform encephalopathies, subacute, 828
Spongy degeneration of white matter, 802-803
Spontaneous abortion, 127, 218
Spontaneous pneumothorax, 733
Spores, 727
Sporocyst, 295
Sporogony, 279-280
Sporothrix schenckii, 276
Sporotrichosis, 81, 276
Sporozoites, 280, 287
Spreading factor, 248
Sprengel's deformity, 811
Sprue
  celiac, 999, 1001
  collagenous, 1002
  tropical, 1001-1002, 1103, 1109
Spur cell anemia, 343
Spur cells, 315, 343
Spurious polycythemia, 354
Spurs, calcaneal, 102
Sputum, 686
  blood in; *see* Hemoptysis
  bronchiectasis and, 697
  bronchitis and, 692
  Klebsiella pneumoniae and, 176
  lung cancer and, 740
  purulent, 686
  tuberculosis and, 258
Squamous cells
  and carcinoma, 915
    of lung, 447
    of mouth, 919
    Plummer-Vinson syndrome and, 416
  in sputum, 686
SRS-A; *see* Slow-reacting substance of anaphylaxis
SSBG; *see* Sex steroid–binding globulin
SSPE; *see* Subacute sclerosing panencephalitis
SSSS; *see* Staphylococcal scalded skin syndrome
ST segment, 482, 483, 484, 485
Staging
  of Hodgkin's disease, 388-389
  of melanomas, 918
  of non-Hodgkin's lymphoma, 392-393
  of tumors, 435-436
Stagnant loop syndrome, 947
Staining of teeth, 168, 668, 889, 1101
Staining anomalies, osteogenesis imperfecta and, 1244
Stains; *see also* specific stain
  of chromosomes, 1221
  histologic; *see* Histology
  immunofluorescent; *see* Immunofluorescence
  microbial diseases and, 119
STA-MCA bypass; *see* Superficial temporal artery to middle cerebral artery bypass
Standard temperature and pressure of dry gas, 673
Staphylococcal scalded skin syndrome, 219, 220, 932
Staphylococci, 218-222; *see also Staphylococcus aureus*
  bronchiectasis and, 697
  cavernous sinus thrombosis and, 303
  cellulitis and, 226
  cystic fibrosis and, 1101
  diarrhea and, 953
  disseminated intravascular coagulation and, 412
  endocarditis and, 179, 184, 302

Staphylococci—cont'd
  glomerulonephritis and, 611
  Hailey-Hailey disease and, 934
  impetigo and, 225-226
  liver abscess and, 1074
  malabsorption and, 1003
  oral lesions of, 306
  scalded skin syndrome and, 219, 220, 932
  septic arthritis of temporomandibular joint and, 108
  thyroiditis and, 1149
Staphylococcus albus, 116, 611
Staphylococcus aureus, 218-222; *see also* Staphylococci
  abscesses and, 698, 700, 1054
  arthritis and, 79, 80
  Chédiak-Higashi syndrome and, 397
  cystic fibrosis and, 700
  diabetes and, 885
  drugs for, 159, 162, 164, 166, 167, 168
  endocarditis and, 175, 179, 181, 183
  food poisoning and, 201
  glomerulonephritis and, 611
  granulomatous disease and, 357
  Haemophilus influenzae and, 235
  immunodeficiency diseases and, 31
  influenza and, 141, 235
  leukemias and, 368
  meningitis and, 187
  microbial resistance and, 159
  midline granuloma and, 73
  neutropenia and, 361
  oral lesions of, 306
  and osteomyelitis, 82, 116
  pneumonia and, 171, 172, 173, 175
  scalded skin syndrome and, 219, 220, 932
  smoke inhalation and, 729
  superinfection and, 1018
  toxic shock syndrome and, 298
Staphylococcus epidermidis
  drugs for, 159, 164, 167
  in endocarditis, 179
  in meningitis, 187
Staphylococcus marcescens, 166
Starch absorption, 1004
Starling's law; *see also* Frank-Starling law
  respiratory failure and, 709, 710
  thoracentesis and, 688
Starvation ketosis, 1271
Static compliance, 693, 694
Status asthmaticus, 705, 708, 710-711
Status epilepticus, 787, 867
Steatorrhea, 999-1005, 1103
  hyperoxaluria and, 621
  pancreatitis and, 1055
  vitamin K deficiency and, 411
Stein-Leventhal syndrome, 1177
Stellwag's sign, 1142
Stem cells, 352, 355, 373
Stenosis
  anal, 1031
  aortic, 505-506, 514-515
    cardiomyopathy and, 518, 522
  in carotid artery, 564
  lumbosacral canal, 860
  mitral, 512-514
  of Oddi's sphincter, 1088
  pulmonic, 506, 517
  pyloric, 997-998, 1228
  renal artery; *see* Renal artery, stenosis of
  tricuspid, 516
  urethral, 651
Stents, 871
Stereognosis, 14, 771

Stereotactic thalamotomy, 815, 821
Sterile pustules, 907
Sterility, 139, 750
Sternal abnormalities, 737
Sternocleidomastoid muscle, 672
Steroids, 1115; *see also* Corticosteroids; specific steroid
  acanthosis nigricans and, 888
  acne from, 887, 897
  acquired anticoagulants and, 411
  Addison's disease and, 1207
  adult respiratory distress syndrome and, 709, 710
  anabolic; *see* Anabolic steroids
  anaphylaxis and, 29
  androgenic, 382, 402, 444
  anemias and, 322, 416
  aspergillosis and, 705
  asthma and, 24, 705, 707, 728
  biosynthesis of, 1153-1154
  cholestasis and, 1076
  chronic discoid lupus erythematosus and, 111
  in contact dermatitis, 27
  Crohn's disease oral lesions and, 1097
  cysticercosis and, 293
  demyelinating diseases and, 800, 801
  dermatitis herpetiformis and, 893
  dermatomyositis and, 113
  in enemas, 1019
  epidermolysis bullosa dystrophica and, 877
  erythema multiforme and, 924
  glomerulonephritis and, 610, 613, 614
  gold-induced thrombocytopenia and, 404
  hemolysis and, 342
  hemorrhagic lung disease and, 720
  hypersensitivity pneumonitis and, 728
  hypopituitarism and, 1205
  idiopathic recurrent polyneuropathy and, 855
  ileojejunitis and, 1003
  ileostomy stoma inflammation and, 1015
  intra-articular; 106, 107
  intralesional, 937, 938, 939
  juvenile rheumatoid arthritis and, 46, 47
  Kawasaki disease and, 148
  Kveim test and, 718
  lichen planus and, 939
  listeriosis and, 246
  in Löffler's syndrome, 372
  long term, hazards of, 908
  lumbar puncture and, 847
  lupus erythematosus and, 111-112, 615
  lymphangitic tumor and, 744
  membranous nephropathy and, 613
  menstrual cycle and, 1174
  multiple myeloma and, 422
  multiple sclerosis and, 800, 801
  by nasal spray, 22
  oral contraceptive; *see* Oral contraceptives
  osteoarthritis and, 85, 107
  osteoporosis and, 115
  pemphigoid and, 935
  pemphigus and, 933
  pemphigus vegetans and, 934
  peptic ulcers and, 1092
  peritoneal vasculitis and, 1048
  pituitary insufficiency and, 1124
  polymyalgia rheumatica and, 75
  porphyria and, 1252
  pseudotumor cerebri and, 848
  pulmonary fibrosis and, 713
  in pulmonary infiltrates, 373
  radiation and, 722, 847
  receptors for, 444, 1115
  rejection reactions and, 645

Steroids—cont'd
  retroperitoneal fibrosis and, 105
  rheumatic fever and, 230
  rhinitis and, 23
  sarcoidosis and, 114, 718, 911
  septic shock and, 241
  sex, 1153; *see also* specific steroid
  shock and, 575
  side effects of, 1010-1011
  smoke inhalation and, 729
  systemic sclerosis and, 61
  thrombocytopenia and, 426
  thrombotic thrombocytopenic purpura and, 404, 617
  tuberculous peritonitis and, 1047
  ulcerative colitis oral lesions and, 1096
  ulcers and, 988
  varicella-zoster and, 130
  visceral larva migrans and, 290
  vitamin A and, 1107
  Weber-Osler-Rendu disease and, 894
Stevens-Johnson syndrome, 29, 923, 924
  mycoplasmal pneumonia and, 217
  sulfonamides and, 170
Stibocaptate, 296
Stibophen, 342
Still's disease, 43, 45-46
Stimulants, 769, 777, 864
Stimulation-secretion coupling, 1116
Stocking-glove symptoms, 1275
Stokes-Adams disease, 500, 780
Stomach, 942-945
  acid in; *see* Gastric acid
  alcohol and, 1258
  atrophy of, 996-997
  biopsy of, 963
  carcinoma of, 1035-1036, 1093
    management of, 447-448
  diagnosis and, 962-964
  dilation of, acute, 997
  diverticula of, 998
  emptying of
    measurement of, 963-964
    rate of, 994-995
  excision of; *see* Gastrectomy
  fluid analysis and, 1035
  gastric inhibitory polypeptide and, 941
  inflammation of; *see* Gastritis
  leiomyomas of, 1034
  motility phenomena of, 963
  neoplasms of, 447-448, 1033-1037
    hyperparathyroidism and, 1192
  non-Hodgkin's lymphoma and, 394
  polyps in, 1033-1034
  remnants and, 997
  secretion in, 943-944, 1192
  suction of, 958, 959
  ulcer of, 987
    malignancy and, 989, 993
  varices and, 1060, 1083
  volvulus and, 998
Stomatitis
  acrodermatitis enteropathica and, 895
  aphthous, 892, 1095, 1097, 1211; *see also* Aphthous ulcers; Gingivostomatitis
  aplastic anemia and, 415
  candidiasis and, 307
  dermatomyositis and, 113, 905
  erythema migrans and, 938
  gonococcal, 302
  measles and, 300
  neutrophil dysfunction and, 420
  nicotine, 919
  pernicious anemia and, 415

Stomatitis—cont'd
 pyridoxine deficiency and, 1109
 radiation, 919
 uremic, 666-667
 vitamin B_{12} deficiency and, 1109
Stomatocyte, 315
Stones; see Calculi
Stool softeners, 442, 446, 537
Stools; see Feces
Storage-pool disease, 405
STPD; see Standard temperature and pressure of dry gas
Strabismus, 8
Strangulation
 of anal hemorrhoids, 1031
 of bowel, 1024-1025
Strawberry tongue, 224
Streaks, angioid, 87, 884
Strep throat, 223-225
Streptobacillary rat-bite fever, 272
Streptobacillus moniliformis, 272
Streptococci, 222-230; see also specific species
 anaerobic bacteria and, 177, 228, 249
 bacteremia and, 175, 226, 227, 241
 cavernous sinus thrombosis and, 303
 cystic fibrosis and, 1101
 disseminated intravascular coagulation and, 412
 endocarditis and, 179, 181, 183, 302
 glomerulonephritis and, 609-610, 611
 group A, 223-227
  beta-hemolytic, 31, 145, 175, 582
  drugs for, 159, 162, 582
  in endocarditis, 179
  leukemias and, 371
  multiple myeloma and, 379
 group B, 227
 group G, 227
 hypersensitivity to, 70, 406
 microaerophilic, 228
  lung abscess and, 699
  pneumonia and, 177
 nonhemolytic, 222
 osteomyelitis of jaws and, 116
 pancreatic abscess and, 1054
 partial hemolysis and, 222
 pharyngitis and, 175
 pneumonia and, 175, 177, 226
 rheumatic fever and, 580
 Schönlein-Henoch purpura and, 70, 406
 septic arthritis of temporomandibular joint and, 108
 thyroiditis and, 1149
Streptococcus agalactiae, 227
Streptococcus bovis, 227, 228
 endocarditis and, 179, 181
Streptococcus equinus, 227, 228
 endocarditis and, 181
Streptococcus faecalis, 227
Streptococcus milleri, 228
Streptococcus mitior, 228
Streptococcus mutans, 228
Streptococcus pneumoniae, 171, 172, 173
 arthritis and, 80
 bronchiectasis and, 696
 drugs for, 159, 162
 hypogammaglobulinemia and, 32, 33
 immunodeficiency diseases and, 31
 in meningitis, 186
 in pneumonia, 171, 175
 postsplenectomy sepsis and, 395
 respiratory failure and, 711
 sickle cell anemia and, 333

Streptococcus pyogenes, 175, 223-227
 arthritis and, 80
 bronchiectasis and, 696
 in pneumonia, 171, 175
Streptococcus salivarius, 228
Streptococcus sanguis, 228
Streptococcus viridans, 581, 586
Streptokinase, 223, 494
Streptolysin O, 223
Streptolysin S, 223
Streptomycin, 161, 165
 brucellosis and, 245
 endocarditis and, 121, 183, 184, 581
 labyrinth, 792
 nephropathy and, 627, 628
 oral streptococci and, 302
 plague and, 242
 pregnancy and, 1212, 1213
 rat-bite fever and, 273
 in tuberculosis, 259
 tularemia and, 243
Streptozocin, 442
 endocrine tumors and, 450
 hypoglycemia from neoplasms and, 1181
 insulinomas and, 1279
 nephropathy and, 627
 in pancreatic carcinoma, 448
Streptozotocin; see Streptozocin
Streptozyme test, 225
Stress
 adrenocorticotropic hormone and, 1118
 hypogonadism and, 1172
 irritable bowel disease and, 1028
Stress erosions, 995-996
Stress polycythemia, 352, 354, 355
Stress test exercises, 530
Stretch receptors, 467
Strictures
 of bowel, 1019, 1021
 of esophagus, 983, 985
 obstructive uropathy and, 654
 radiation enteritis and, 1019
String sign, 1012
Stroke; see Cerebrovascular accidents
Stroke volume, 457, 458, 515-516
Strongyloides, 291, 292
 diarrhea and, 953
 eosinophilia and, 372, 721
 malabsorption and, 1003
 in pneumonia, 172
Strongyloides stercoralis, 291, 292
 malabsorption and, 1003
 in pneumonia, 172
Struma ovarii, 1045, 1146
Struvite kidney stones, 646, 648
Stupor, 763-764
Sturge-Weber syndrome, 810, 881-882
 dentistry and, 869, 872
Subacute combined degeneration, 33, 808, 851
Subacute sclerosing panencephalitis, 138, 828
Subacute spongiform encephalopathies, 828
Subacute thyroiditis, 1149
Subarachnoid hemorrhage, 790, 839-840
Subclavian artery
 compression of, 100, 101
 and pulmonary artery, anastomosis between, 507
 subclavian steal syndrome and, 563, 793, 837
Subclavian steal syndrome, 563, 793, 837
Subclavian vein compression, 100, 101
Subcutaneous bands, linear, 906
Subcutaneous nodules; see also Nodules
 fat, malignancy and, 913
 rheumatic fever and, 229

Subcutaneous nodules—cont'd
 Weber-Christian disease and, 79
Subdeltoid bursitis, 98-99
Subdural empyema, 193
Subdural hematomas, 192, 844
Subdural infections, 139
Suberosis, 727
Subgingival microflora, oral contraceptives and, 1214
Subhyaloid hemorrhages, 765, 839
Subluxation, 36, 38, 39, 45
Submandibular gland, mumps and, 301
Submaxillary gland, cystic fibrosis and, 1101
Submetacentric chromosomes, 1220
Submucosa, 941, 973
Submucous cleft palate, 1321
Submucous plexus, 942
Subscapularis muscle, 98
Substantia nigra, neuronal degeneration of, 812
Subtotal nodal irradiation, 390
Subungual fibromas, 880
Subungual-mucosal melanoma, palmar-plantar, 918
Succinylacetone, 1254
Succinylcholine, 858, 871
Succession splash, 997
Suck reflex, 758
Suction; see Aspiration
Subanophilic leukodystrophy, 802
Sudden death, 538-540
Sudden infant death syndrome, 538
Sudeck's atrophy, 100
Sulfa drugs, malaria and, 281; see also specific sulfa drug
Sulfacetamide, 330
Sulfadiazine, 169
 malaria and, 281
 nephropathy and, 627
 plague and, 242
 toxoplasmosis and, 286
Sulfadimethoxine, 169
Sulfadoxine, 281
Sulfamethoxazone, 161, 169
 nephropathy and, 627, 628
 pneumocystosis and, 288
 and trimethoprim, 446, 1212
Sulfamethoxypyridazine, 169, 330
Sulfanilamide, 329, 588
Sulfapyridine
 dermatitis herpetiformis and, 893, 1002
 hemolysis and, 330
 nephropathy and, 627
 pemphigoid and, 935
Sulfasalazine, 1010, 1014, 1031
Sulfasuxidine, 169
Sulfatase deficiency, multiple, 1233
Sulfate, 598
Sulfathiazole, 627
Sulfatide, 1230
Sulfatide lipidosis, 1231, 1232-1233
Sulfhemoglobinemia, 344
Sulfinpyrazone, 93, 405, 837
Sulfisoxazole, 161, 169
 chancroid and, 239
 hemolysis and, 330
 lymphogranuloma venereum and, 216
 rheumatic fever and, 230
 urinary tract infection and, 197, 198
Sulfite oxidase deficiency, 1237
Sulfobromophthalein clearance, 1065, 1068
Sulfonamides, 161, 169-170; see also specific agent
 allergy and, 28, 170
 bacteriostatic activity of, 156

Sulfonamides—cont'd
 Chlamydia and, 214, 215, 216
 disseminated vasculitis and, 29
 erythema multiforme and, 922
 erythema nodosum and, 28, 924
 excretion of, 158
 glucose-6-phosphate dehydrogenase deficiency and, 418
 hemolysis and, 329-330
 kernicterus and, 158
 leukopenia and, 29
 listeriosis and, 246
 lung disease and, 721, 722
 lupus erythematosus and, 57
 lupuslike syndrome and, 57
 methotrexate and, 440
 nephritis and, 619, 620
 nephropathy and, 624, 625, 626, 627, 629, 630
 neutropenia and, 360, 361
 nocardiosis and, 247
 pancreatitis and, 1051
 plague and, 242
 porphyria and, 854, 889, 1248, 1252
 pregnancy and, 1212
 proteinuria and, 590
 renal insufficiency and, 158
 site of infection and, 156
 sunburn and, 29
 thrombocytopenia and, 400, 401
 urinary tract infection and, 197
 urticaria and, 25
Sulfones, 330, 893
Sulfonylureas
 alcohol and, 1297
 diabetes mellitus and, 1266-1267
 surreptitious administration of, 1279
Sulfosalicylic acid, 590
Sulfoxone, 330
Sulfur, 247, 1106, 1237
Sulfur colloid, technetium 99m, 966
Sulfur dioxide, 729
Sulfur oxide exposure, 697
Sulfurated potash, 823
Sulindac
 gout and, 93
 hypersensitivity to, 932
 nephropathy and, 621
 rheumatoid arthritis and, 42
Sunlight sensitivity, 882
Sunscreen
 actinic keratosis and, 918
 lupus erythematosus and, 57
 porphyria and, 888, 1248, 1250
Superficial femoral occlusion, 570
Superficial pain, 14
Superficial reflexes, 14
Superficial temporal artery to middle cerebral artery bypass, 837
Superinfection, 1018
Superior cerebellar artery syndrome, 833
Superior mesenteric artery, occlusive disease of, 1020
Superior quadrantanopsias, 759
Superior vena caval syndrome, 735
 lung cancer and, 739
 mediastinoscopy and, 689
 supportive care and, 445
Supernumerary teeth, 891, 1093
Supine hypotensive syndrome, 1212
Suppressor T cells, 15, 797
Suppurative otitis, 191, 795
Suppurative thyroiditis, acute, 1149
Supranuclear palsy, progressive, 774-775

Suprasellar pituitary tumor, 1124
Supraspinatus muscle, 98
Supratentorial tumors, 767, 845
Supraventricular arrhythmias, 500, 508, 585
Suramin, 287
Surgery; see also Resection; specific procedure
 ablative procedures in, 444
 abscesses and, 193, 199, 250
 anaerobic infection and, 251
 aneurysm of sinus of Valsalva and, 558
 aortic aneurysms and, 560
 aortic dissection and, 562
 bacteremia and, 180
 for cancer, 438-439; see also specific procedure
 coarctation of aorta and, 557
 for congenital heart disease, 509
 contaminated, 251
 Cushing's syndrome and, 1159
 emboli and, 490, 568
 endocarditis and, 184
 esophageal reflux and, 982
 gastrointestinal tract, 185
 genitourinary, 185, 199
 hemophilia and, 428
 insulin management and, 1268
 mineralocorticoid excess and, 1161
 open heart, 301, 551, 558-559
 osteomyelitis and, 222
 pheochromocytoma and, 1167
 pituitary, 444, 448, 1120, 1124, 1159
 subdural empyema and, 193
 sympathectomy and, 64, 569
 thoracotomy in; see Thoracotomy
 in tuberculosis, 260
Susceptibility, 155
Sutton's disease, 110
Sutures, 184, 1312-1315
Svedberg flotation constant, 1280
Swallowing, 942, 973
 difficulty in, 961, 974, 975-976
  bulbar palsy and, 760
  cerebrovascular accident and, 872
 pain on, 975
Swan-Ganz catheter, 478, 708
Swan-neck deformities, 36, 37
Sweating, 596, 755
Swelling; see Edema
Swimmers' itch, 295
Swimming pool granuloma, 261
Swine influenza, 140
Swinging flashlight sign, 798
Swyer-James syndrome, 686
Sydenham's chorea, 229, 818-819
Sylvatic plague, 242
Symmetrel; see Amantadine
Symmetric hypertrophy of heart, 518
Sympathectomy, 64, 569, 903
Sympathetic dystrophy, reflex, 100
Sympathetic nervous system; see also Autonomic nervous system
 blood pressure and, 467
 peritoneum and, 1043
 surgery of, 64, 569
Sympatholytics, 464
Sympathomimetics
 carotid sinus syncope and, 781
 heart failure and, 464
 procarbazine and, 443
 Raynaud's phenomenon and, 63
 septic shock and, 241
Syncope, 780-781
 carotid sinus, cerebrovascular disease and, 587
 dentistry and, 576-577, 864

Syncope—cont'd
 heat, 755
 metronidazole and, 170
 vasodepressor, sudden death and, 538
 vasovagal, 576-577, 780
Syncytia, 141
Syndactyly, 882
Syndesmophytes, 48, 50
Syndromes; see also Diseases
 adrenal enzyme deficiency, 1171
 adrenogenital, 1162-1163
 adult respiratory distress; see Adult respiratory distress syndrome
 Albright's, 104, 879
 Alport's, 611-612
 aminopterin, 1303
 amnestic, 759, 763, 770, 772, 836
 of angioedema, asthma, and nasal polyps, 23, 26
 of anterior inferior cerebellar artery, 833-835
 of anterior spinal artery, 835-836
 Anton's, 832
 aortic arch, 562-563
 Apert's, 1314, 1316
 Asherman's, 1176
 ataxia telangiectasia, 869
 autoimmune polyendocrinopathy, 1209
 Banti's, 396
 basal cell nevus, 883, 1209
 basal ganglion calcification, 1209
 of basilar artery system, 833-835
 Bassen-Kornzweig, 1291-1292
 Behçet's; see Behçet's syndrome
 Benedikt's, 833
 Bernard-Soulier, 405
 Bloch-Sulzberger, 810
 Bloom's, 882-883, 1222
 Bourneville-Pringle, 668, 880-881
 bradykinetic, Huntington's chorea and, 817
 branchial arch, 1309
 branchioskeletogenital, 1244
 Budd-Chiari, 1045, 1060, 1077-1078
 Caplan's, 715
 carcinoid, 450, 743, 1037-1038
 carpal tunnel, 60, 98
 of cerebellar arteries, 833, 834
 of cerebral arteries, 749, 750, 832-833
 Chédiak-Higashi, 357, 397, 420
 cherry-red spot–myoclonus, 1235
 Chinese restaurant, 200
 Churg-Strauss, 719
 Cockayne's, 882
 cold agglutinin, 339-340
 colitis, 216
 common cold, 144
 congenital rubella, 125
 Conn's, 470, 1160; see also Aldosteronism
  secondary hypertension and, 573
 Costen's, 100, 867
 costoclavicular, 101
 craniosynostosis, 1312-1315
 Crigler-Najjar, 1058, 1067-1068
 Cronkhite-Canada, 891
 croup, 142
 CRST; see Calcinosis in Raynaud's phenomenon, sclerodactyly, and telangiectasia syndrome
 Cushing's; see Cushing's syndrome
 defibrination, 412
 of Dejerine-Roussy, 832
 DiFerrante, 1233, 1234
 DiGeorge's, 33, 1196
 DiGuglielmo, 322

Syndromes—cont'd
  Down's, 1221, 1225
    craniofacial malformations and, 1301, 1308
  Dressler's, 537
  Dubin-Johnson, 1058, 1068
  dumping, 944, 946, 993; see also Syndromes, postgastrectomy
    hypoglycemia and, 1277
    malabsorption and, 1004
  Duncan's, 133
  dysarthria–clumsy hand, 835
  Eaton-Lambert, 856
  Ehlers-Danlos, 1241-1243, 1302
    dental abnormalities in, 1242-1243
    purpura and, 407
  Eisenmenger's, 504
  Ellis-van Creveld, 1245
  empty-sella, 1124, 1177
  encephalomyelitis and, 801
  of endocarditis, 181-182
  Evans', 403
  Fabry's; see Fabry's disease
  Fabry-Anderson, 1296
  Fanconi's, 168, 318, 319, 624
  Felty's, 36, 106, 359, 396
  fetal
    alcohol, 1303, 1304
    phenytoin, 1303
    warfarin, 1303
  fibromyalgia, 38
  fibrosin, 105
  Fitz-Hugh–Curtis, 231
  Foville's, 833
  Gaisböck's, 354
  Gardner's, 891, 1042, 1093, 1094, 1209
  gastrointestinal polyposis, 1093-1095; see also Polyps
  Gerstmann's, 759
  Gilles de la Tourette's, 821-822
  glucagonoma, 913
  glucocorticoid deficiency; see Addison's disease
  glucocorticoid excess, 1157-1159
  Goldenhar's, 1300, 1310-1312
  Goodpasture's, 611, 720
  gray baby, 158, 169
  Grönblad-Strandberg, 884
  Guillain-Barré; see Guillain-Barré syndrome
  Hamman-Rich, 715
  hand-foot, 332
  heat, 755
  Heerfordt's; see Heerfordt's disease
  hemolytic uremic, 340, 617
  hepatorenal, 1064
  Holt-Oram, 498
  of homolateral ataxia, 835
  Horner's; see Horner's syndrome
  Hunt's, 130, 138
  Hunter's, 1233, 1234
  Hurler's, 1233, 1234, 1302
  hyperabduction, 101
  hypereosinophilic, 363, 373
  hyperpituitary, 1119-1121
  hypersomnia–sleep apnea, 769
  hyperventilation, 781, 794
  hyperviscosity, 346, 423, 842
  idiopathic thrombocytopenic purpura–like, 403
  of inappropriate antidiuretic hormone secretion, 594, 595, 740
    encephalitis and, 135
    malignancy and, 740, 1179, 1181
  infectious mononucleosis–like, 131
  of insulin resistance, 1261
  intervertebral disc, 50

Syndromes—cont'd
  irritable bowel, 1027-1029
    lactose intolerance and, 1005, 1028
  ischemic bowel, 1020-1024
  Job's, 357
  Kallman's, 1121, 1172
  Kartagener's, 691, 696
  Kasabach-Merritt, 341
  Kleine-Levin, 770
  Klinefelter's, 1170, 1214, 1225
  Klippel-Feil, 811
  Klippel-Trenaunay, 881, 882
  Kniest, 1245
  Korsakoff's, 772, 849–850, 1108, 1257
    thalamus lesions and, 759
  Kostman's, 360
  lacunar, 835
  lateral medullary, 835
  Laurence-Moon-Bordet-Biedl, 498, 1172
  lazy leukocyte, 357, 420
  Leriche's, 569-570
  Lesch-Nyhan, 316, 1227, 1239
  Liddle's, 1160
  locked-in, 764, 833
  Löffgren's, 77, 78, 716, 925
  Löffler's; see Löffler's syndrome
  Louis-Bar, 882
  Luft's, 1146-1147
  lumbar disc, 48, 50
  Macleod's, 686
  malabsorption, 998-1005
    Crohn's disease and, 1012
    cystic fibrosis and, 1101
    folic acid deficiency and, 1109, 1110
  malformation, 1227-1228, 1301
  Mallory-Weiss, 986-987
  Marchiafava-Micheli, 341-342
  Marfan's, 179, 558, 560, 1241
  Maroteaux-Lamy, 1233, 1234
  medial
    longitudinal fasciculus, 760, 766, 833; see also Internuclear ophthalmoplegia
    medullary, 835
    pontine, 833
  Meigs', 731, 1045
  Ménière's, 793, 795
  meningitis-cerebritis, 187
  Menkes' kinky hair, 1240
  methotrexate, 1303
  middle lobe, 703
  midface, 1316-1318
  milk-alkali, 992
  Millard-Gubler, 833
  mineralocorticoid deficiency, 1159-1160
  mineralocorticoid excess, 1160-1162; see also Aldosteronism
  Morquio's, 1233, 1234
  mucocutaneous lymph node, 69, 147
  mucosal neuroma, 1164
  multiple endocrine adenomatosis; see Multiple endocrine neoplasias
  muscle pain amplification, 96
  myasthenic, 856
  myelodysplastic, 320-321, 341
  myofascial, 97-98
    dermatomyositis and, 905
    of temporomandibular joint, 107, 109-110
  nephritic, 609-612
  nephrotic; see Nephrotic syndrome
  neurocutaneous, 808-810
  neutropenic, chronic idiopathic, 360
  neutrophil dysfunction, 356-357, 420
  nevoid, 883
  Noonan's, 1170-1171

Syndromes—cont'd
  obesity-hypoventilation, 712
  oculogenital, 215
  one and one-half, 833
  orbital glioma, 878-879
  Osler-Weber-Rendu; see Osler-Weber-Rendu disease
  osteogenesis imperfecta, 1242
  otocraniofacial, 1309-1312
  otomandibular, 867-868
  ovarian overstimulation, 1045
  overlap, 66, 67
    pulmonary fibrosis and, 716, 719
    skin disorders and, 906
  Pancoast's, 739
  Papillon-LeFevre, 1243, 1244
  Parinaud's, 760
  paroxysmal, 799
  pectoralis minor, 101
  Peutz-Jeghers, 891, 1042
    dentistry and, 1093-1095
    gastrointestinal bleeding and, 958
  Pfeiffer's, 1314, 1315, 1316
  pickwickian, 712
  Pierre Robin, 1228
  Plummer-Vinson, 416, 1091, 1105
  pneumonia, 173-178, 698-700; see also Pneumonia
  polyarteritis nodosa–like, 29
  polycystic ovarian, 1177
  polymyalgia rheumatica, 69
  polyposis; see Polyposis syndromes
  postcardiotomy, 550
  of posterior inferior cerebellar artery, 835
  of posterior spinal artery, 836
  postgastrectomy, 993, 1004, 1199-1200; see also Syndromes, dumping
  postgonococcal urethritis, 215, 218
  postmyocardial infarction, 550
  postpartum hemolytic, 341
  postperfusion, 131
  postphlebitic, 495
  postprandial, 993; see also Syndromes, dumping; Syndromes, postgastrectomy
  preleukemic, 320-321
  of progressive hereditary ataxia, 805-807
  pulmonary infiltration with eosinophilia, 363, 721
  rabbit, 871
  Raeder's, 791
  Ramsay Hunt, 806
  Raynaud's; see Raynaud's disease
  red cell fragmentation, 340-341
  Reifenstein's, 1171
  Reiter's; see Reiter's syndrome
  reset osmostat, 594
  resistant ovary, 1177
  respiratory distress; see Adult respiratory distress syndrome
  reverse triiodothyronine, 1131
  Reye's; see Reye's syndrome
  right middle lobe, 703
  Rokitansky-Kuster-Hauser, 1176
  Rosewater's, 1171
  Rotor's, 1058, 1068
  Roussy-Lévy, 806
  rubella, 1303
  Saethre-Chotzen, 1314, 1315, 1316
  Sanfilippo's, 1233, 1234
  scalded skin, staphylococcal, 219, 220, 932
  scalenus anticus, 100, 101
  Scheie's, 1233, 1234
  Senear-Usher, 934
  septic shock; see Septic shock

Syndromes—cont'd
  sequestration, 332
  Sertoli-cell-only, 1171
  serum sickness, 26-27
  Sézary, 901
  Sheehan's, 1177
  short bowel, 1077
  short-arm 18 deletion, 1316
  shoulder-hand, 100, 537
  Shy-Drager, 814, 823
  sick euthyroid, 1131
  sick sinus, 501, 546-547
  Silver, 879
  Sipple's, 879, 1151, 1164
  Sjögren's; see Sjögren's syndrome
  sleep apnea, 711, 769-770, 861
  Sly's, 1233, 1234
  stagnant loop, 947
  Stein-Leventhal, 1177
  Stevens-Johnson, 29, 923, 924
    mycoplasmal pneumonia and, 217
    sulfonamides and, 170
  Stokes-Adams, 500, 780
  Sturge-Weber, 810, 881-882, 869, 872
  subclavian steal, 563, 793, 837
  sudden infant death, 538
  superior cerebellar artery, 833
  superior vena caval; see Superior vena caval syndrome
  supine hypotensive, pregnancy and, 1212
  Swyer-James, 686
  tardive dyskinesia and, 871
  tarsal tunnel, 98
  temporomandibular, 100
  testicular enzyme deficiency, 1171
  testicular feminization, 1214
  thalassemic, 334-337
  Thibierge-Weisenbach, 904
  thoracic outlet, 100-101
  Tietze's, 100, 737
  Torre's, 913
  Tourette's, 821
  Treacher Collins, 1302, 1308, 1309-1310, 1311
  trichorhinophalangeal, 1245
  triiodothyronine, low, 1131
  trisomy-13, 1316
  tumor cachexia, 438
  tumor lysis, 446
  Turner's, 1176-1177, 1225-1226
    coarctation of aorta and, 505
    dentistry and, 1209
    male, 1170-1171
  uremic; see Uremia
  urethral, 214
  van der Woude, 1228
  of vertebral arteries, 835
  von Hippel-Lindau, 872
  Wallenberg's, 793, 835, 872
  Waterhouse-Friderichsen, 234, 1156
  watery diarrhea, 954
  Weber's, 833
  Weill-Marchesani, 1246
  Wildervanck-Smith, 1311
  Winchester, 1244
  Wiskott-Aldrich, 33
  Wolff-Parkinson-White, 543, 544, 548-549
    in children, 500-501
  Zieve, 1257
  Zollinger-Ellison; see Zollinger-Ellison syndrome
Synechiae, intrauterine, 1176
Synergism, 156
Synovectomy, 42
Synovia; see Synovium
Synovial chondromatosis of temporomandibular joint, 108
Synovial fluid
  gout and, 92
  pseudogout and, 94, 95
  Reiter's syndrome and, 52
  rheumatoid arthritis and, 37-38
    juvenile, 46-47
Synovial membrane, metaplasia of, 108
Synovitis, tuberculous, 81; see also Tenosynovitis
Synovium
  biopsy of, 81, 94
  cysts of, 101-102
  excision of, 42
  fluid in; see Synovial fluid
  inflammation of, 81; see also Tenosynovitis
Synthetic liotrix, 1139
Syphilis, 264-272
  blood transfusions and, 347
  congenital, 265, 269-270
  dentistry and, 302-303
  epidemiology and, 264
  glossitis and, 919
  gonococcal infections and, 233
  late, 268-269
  latent, 268
  liver disease and, 1074
  meningoencephalitis and, 139, 268, 269, 842
  nonvenereal transmission of, 265
  primary, 266-267
  secondary, 267-268
  tests for, 270-271
  valvular disease and, 179, 563, 580
Syringomyelia, 807-808, 869
Systemic lupus erythematosus; see Lupus erythematosus, systemic
Systemic necrotizing vasculitis, 66-67, 69
Systemic sclerosis, 58-62, 903-904
  cardiomyopathies and, 522-523
  dentistry and, 112, 1091-1092
  esophageal, 981, 982
  malabsorption and, 1004
  pregnancy and, 666
  progressive, 615-616, 715, 903-904
    dentistry and, 1091-1092
  pulmonary fibrosis and, 715
  renal lesions and, 615-616
Systems, review of, 5-7
Systolic bruit, 1205
Systolic clicks, 511

T

T_3; see Triiodothyronine
T_4; see Thyroxine
T cells; see Thymus-derived cells
T lymphocytes; see Thymus-derived cells
T system; see Tubular system of muscle fiber
T wave, 482, 483
  influenza and, 141
  ischemic heart disease and, 484, 485
  myocardial infarction and, 484, 485
Tabes dorsalis, 269; see also Syphilis
  diabetic pseudotabes and, 1276
Tachycardia, 542-546
  chronic obstructive pulmonary disease and, 692
  congestive heart failure and, 571
  dentistry and, 584-585
  influenza and, 141
  pediatric, 500
  Wolff-Parkinson-White syndrome and, 549
Tachycardia-bradycardia, 547
Tachyphemia, 813
Tachypnea, 460, 580
Taenia coli, 948
Taenia saginata, 293, 294
Taenia solium, 293, 294
Tagamet; see Cimetidine
Takayasu's arteritis, 68, 69, 70, 563
Takayasu's disease, 841; see also Pulseless disease
  vasculitis and, 1022
Talc, 445, 734
Tamm-Horsfall protein, 605
Tamoxifen, 444
Tamponade; see Pericardial tamponade
Tampons, 298
Tangier disease, 1292
Tantalum powder, aerosolized, 689
TAO; see Thromboangiitis obliterans
Tapeworms, 292-294, 317
Tar, 907, 937
Tardive dyskinesias, 870, 871
Target cell, 315, 395
Target lesion, 28, 923, 924
Tarsal tunnel syndrome, 98
Tartar emetic, 296
Tartrate-inhibitable acid phosphatase, 435
Tartrazine, 24, 704
Taste abnormalities, 872
Tatlock agent, 171
Tattoos, amalgam, 919
Tay-Sachs disease, 1230-1231
  neutropenia and, 358
  screening program and, 1224
TBA; see Thyroxine-binding albumin
TBG; see Thyroxine-binding globulin
TBPA; see Thyroxine-binding prealbumin
^{99m}Tc labeling; see Technetium 99m labeling
TCBS agar; see Thiosulfate citrate bile salts sucrose agar
TCDD; see Tetrachlorodibenzo [p] dioxin
TDF; see Testis determining factor
TDI; see Toluene-di-isocyanate
Technetium 99m labeling
  bone scans and, 222
  of diethylenetriamine penta-acetic acid, 607
  of dimercaptosuccinic acid, 608
  gastroesophgeal scintigrams and, 962
  of glucoheptonate, 608
  of HIDA, 964, 969
  of human albumin microspheres, perfusion scan and, 687
  nuclear cardiology and, 489, 530, 535
  of PIPIDA, 969
  of pyrophosphate, 489, 530, 535
  of sulfur colloid, 966, 983
  thyroid scan and, 1133
Teeth
  cardiac pain and, 583
  congenital syphilis and, 303
  cystic fibrosis and, 1101-1102
  enamel of; see Enamel
  Epstein-Barr virus and, 300
  evaluation of, 9
  extraction of, 113, 427-428
  fracture of, 906
  hemolytic disease of newborn and, 418
  herpes zoster and, 299-300
  hexokinase deficiency anemia and, 418
  histiocytosis X and, 425
  Hutchinson's, 270
  hyperparathyroidism and, 1208
  hyperthyroidism and, 1205
  hypoparathyroidism and, 1209
  hypophosphatasia and, 1209

Teeth—cont'd
  hypopituitarism and, 1204
  hypothyroidism and, 1205-1206
  lead line on, 753
  leprosy and, 305
  mucopolysaccharidoses and, 1234-1235
  osteogenesis imperfecta and, 1243-1244
  Paget's disease and, 114
  pantothenic acid deficiency and, 1110
  pitting of, 300
  porphyrias and, 889, 1298
  pregnancy and, 1211
  radiation damage and, 919
  rickets and, 1107
  rubella and, 300
  staining of, 168, 418, 668, 753, 889, 1101
  supernumerary, 891, 1093
  testicular feminization syndrome and, 1214
  tetracyclines and, 168
  thalassemia and, 418
  thiamine deficiency and, 1108
  tuberous sclerosis and, 881
  unerupted, 891
  Urbach-Wiethe disease and, 1296
  vitamin C and, 1110
Tegretol; see Carbamazepine
Teichoic acid antibody, 220
Telangiectasia, 33, 809-810; see also Osler-Weber-Rendu disease
  ataxia, 869, 882
  hereditary, 894, 1023-1024, 1095
  mastocytosis and, 909
  on mucous membranes, 407
  spider, 863, 894, 896, 1059
  systemic sclerosis and, 58, 60, 904
Telangiectasia macularis eruptiva perstans, 909
Telescoped sediment, 616
Temperature; see also Fever
  multiple sclerosis and, 797
  regulation abnormalities of, 755-756
  testicular, 1172
Temporal arteritis, 68, 69, 74-75, 789-790, 841; see also Arteritis
Temporal artery to cerebral artery bypass, 837
Temporal artery biopsy, 68, 69, 75
Temporal hypoplasia, otocraniofacial syndromes and, 1310
Temporal lobe
  lesions of, 759
  seizures and, 781, 782, 783
Temporalis muscle pain, 109
Temporomandibular joint syndrome, 100, 874-875; see also Temporomandibular joints
  ears and, 867-868
Temporomandibular joints, 100, 874-875
  ankylosis of, 48, 861
  arthritis of, 36
    gouty, 108-109
    juvenile rheumatoid, 45, 47
    psoriatic, 106-107
    rheumatoid, 105-106
    septic, 108
  chondrometaplasia of, 108
  dermatomyositis and, 905
  Ehlers-Danlos syndrome and, 1242
  hemarthrosis of, 427
  mucopolysaccharidoses and, 1235
  osteoarthritis of, 107
  otalgia and, 867-868
  psoriasis and, 106-107, 937
  synovial chondromatosis of, 108
  urate crystals in, 667
Tenax; see Chlordiazepoxide

Tendinitis, 52, 99-100
Tendinous xanthomas, 889
Tendon reflexes, deep, 14, 761
Tennis elbow, 99-100
Tenosynovitis, 81
  arthritis and
    gonococcal, 231
    rheumatoid, 36
  flexor, 99
Tensilon; see Edrophonium
Tension headache, 100, 789
Tension pneumothorax, 733
Tentorium cerebelli, 767
Teratogens, 1302-1303
Teratomas of mediastinum, 735
Terbutaline, 693, 706, 1212
Terpin hydrate, 1212
Tertian malaria, 280
Tessier system of cleft classification, 1318, 1319
Test; see Tests
Testes, 1168-1173
  developmental abnormalities of, 1170-1171, 1176
  embryonic development of, 1168-1170
  evaluation of, 13
  feedback mechanisms and, 1169
  genetics and, 1219
  gonadotropic hormones and, 1118
  oral manifestations of changes in, 1214
  tumors of, 449, 1173
    alpha-fetoprotein and, 435
    oral metastasis of, 1214
Testicular enzyme deficiency syndromes, 1171
Testicular feminization, 1171, 1176, 1214
Testicular-pituitary-hypothalamic feedback mechanisms, 1169
Testis determining factor, 1219
Testosterone, 1153, 1162
  alcohol and, 1259
  17-alpha-methylated, 1173
  hypogonadism and, 1122, 1171, 1172, 1173
  myeloid metaplasia and, 376
  renal failure and, 639
  testicular development and, 1168, 1169
Testosterone enanthate, 1122
Testosterone propionate, 1122
Tests; see also specific test
  for Addison's disease, 1156-1157
  for adrenal function, 1156, 1157, 1158, 1159, 1161, 1163
  adrenocorticotropic hormone stimulation, 1122, 1156-1157
  agar diffusion, 155
  agar dilution, 155
  antibody-coated bacteria, 196, 197
  for antimicrobial susceptibility, 155
  for atopic disease, 21-22
  audiometry, 9, 795
  autohemolysis, 329
  Bárány's, 792
  for blood coagulation, 408, 409, 410
  broth, 155
  Brucella agglutination, 244
  caloric, 792
  Casoni's, 294
  for central nervous system disease, 139, 761-762
  complement fixation; see Complement fixation
  Coombs', 339, 340
  Cortrosyn; see Tests, adrenocorticotropic hormone stimulation
  C-peptide suppression, 1278
  cross-match, 349

Tests—cont'd
  for Cushing's syndrome, 1158-1159
  for cytomegalovirus, 131
  darkfield microscopy, 264, 270-271
  dexamethasone suppression, 1158
  for diabetes mellitus, 1264, 1278
  for digestive system disorders, 961-972; see also Digestive system, diagnosis and
  electron microscopy; see Electron microscopy
  Elek, 248
  erythrocyte sedimentation rate; see Erythrocyte sedimentation rate
  for factor VIII, 410
  for fever of unknown origin, 120
  fluorescent antibody; see Fluorescent antibody stains
  glucose tolerance, 1264, 1277, 1278
  guaiac, 959
  hearing, 9, 795
  hemagglutin; see Hemagglutin in tests; Microhemagglutination test
  of hematologic disorders, 310
  IgM-fluorescent antibody, 286
  for immunity, 31-32
  for infectious mononucleosis, 132, 133
  for influenza, 141
  for kidney disease, 588, 589-590, 603-608, 633, 638-639
    nitroprusside screening in, 649
    prerenal azotemia in, 632-633
    urinalysis in; see Urinalysis
  Kveim, 77, 718, 911
  latex fixation, 77
  liver function, 1064-1065
  lupus band, 54
  macroscopic slide agglutination, 273-274
  for malabsorption of fats, 1000-1001
  Mantoux, 257, 260
  metyrapone, 1157, 1158
  microbial diseases and, 118-119; see also specific test
  microhemagglutination, 118, 119; see also Hemagglutinin tests
    leptospirosis and, 273-274
    for Treponema pallidum, 271
  for mumps, 138
  nitroblue tetrazolium dye, 357
  for occult blood in stool, 959-960
  osmotic fragility, 328-329
  for pheochromocytoma, 1165, 1168
  for platelet function, 106
  for rabies, 139, 153
  radioallergosorbent, 21
  radioimmunoassay in; see Radioimmunoassay
  Rapid Plasma Reagin, 271
  for respiratory syncytial virus, 142
  for rheumatoid factor, 182
  Rinne, 9, 795
  Ropes, 37
  Sabin-Feldman dye, 286
  Schick, 248
  Schilling, 318
  secretin, 995, 1055
  serologic; see Serology
  of sinus node function, 547
  skin; see Skin tests
  streptozyme, 225
  stress, 530
  for syphilis, 270-271
  of thyroid function, 1133-1136
  thyrotropin-releasing hormone; see Thyrotropin-releasing hormone in tests
  unconsciousness and, 768-769
  urinalysis in; see Urinalysis

Tests—cont'd
  urinary sediment, 604-605, 616
  urinary tract obstruction, 633, 655-656
  for varicella-zoster, 130
  Venereal Disease Research Laboratories, 268, 269, 271
  for viral diseases, 122-125; see also specific test
    gastroenteritis in, 149
  vitamin B_{12} absorption, 318
  Watson-Schwartz, 1251
  Weber's, 9, 795
  Weill-Felix, 210
  Widal's, 207
  D-xylose, 150
Tetanic muscle contractions, 751; see also Tetany
Tetanus, 251-252, 253-254
Tetanus antitoxin, 26, 27, 252
Tetanus toxoid, 252
Tetany, 1183, 1195-1196, 1209
  osteomalacia and, 1209
Tetrac, 1128
Tetrachlorodibenzo [p] dioxin, 1253, 1254
Tetrachloroethylene, 627, 629
Tetracyclines, 161, 168
  actinomycosis and, 247
  alcoholism and, 1062, 1077
  allergy and, 28
  antacids and, 992, 1092
  anthrax and, 245
  bacteriostatic activity of, 156
  bronchiectasis and, 697
  bronchitis and, 693
  brucellosis and, 245
  chancroid and, 239
  Chlamydia and, 214, 215-216
  cholera and, 201, 205
  diarrhea with, 27
  donovanosis and, 238
  erysipeloid and, 246
  excretion of, 158
  gonococcal infections and, 232, 302
  hepatitis and, 1099
  injection of, 157
  in intestinal bacterial overgrowth, 62
  leptospirosis and, 274
  listeriosis and, 246
  liver disease and, 1090
  Lyme disease and, 298
  malignant effusions and, 445
  mesothelioma and, 734
  methotrexate and, 440
  mycoplasmas and, 217, 218
  nephropathy and, 624, 625, 627, 629
  nontuberculous mycobacteria and, 261
  oral ulcers and, 451
  pancreatitis and, 1051
  periodontal disease and, 158
  plague and, 242
  pneumothorax and, 734
  pregnancy and, 1212
  pseudotumor cerebri and, 848
  rat-bite fever and, 272
  Reiter's syndrome and, 53, 908
  renal disease and, 158, 670
  respiratory failure and, 711
  rickettsial diseases and, 210, 212, 213
  Rocky Mountain spotted fever and, 211
  shigellosis and, 202, 206
  streptococcal infections and, 225
  sunburn and, 29
  syphilis and, 272
  teeth staining and, 158, 668, 1101
  tetanus and, 252

Tetracyclines—cont'd
  tularemia and, 243
  urinary tract infection and, 197
  Whipple's disease and, 1003
  Yersinia enterocolitica and, 202
3,5,3',5'-Tetraiodothyroacetic acid; see Tetrac
Tetraiodothyronine, 1116-1117
Tetralogy of Fallot, 507
Tetraploidy, 1221
Tetrasomy, 1221
TG; see Thyroglobulin
Thalamotomy, stereotactic, 815, 821
Thalamus; see also Thalamotomy, stereotactic
  hemorrhage of, 766
  lesions of, 759
Thalassemia trait, 324
Thalassemias, 334-337, 1227
  dentistry and, 418-419
  globin synthesis and, 325
  iron metabolism and, 324, 1081
Thalidomide, 263
Thallium
  nephropathy and, 627, 628
  poisoning from, 754
  in scanning, 489, 521, 530, 536
Thayer-Martin selective medium, 230, 232
Theca externa, 1174
Theca interna, 1174
Theo-Dur; see Theophyllines
Theophyllines
  asthma and, 24, 706, 707
  chronic obstructive pulmonary disease and, 693
  pickwickian syndrome and, 712
  platelet function and, 406
  respiratory failure and, 711
  urinary catecholamines and, 1168
Thermoactinomyces vulgaris, 727
Thiabendazole
  larva migrans and, 290, 291
  strongyloidiasis and, 292, 1003
  trichinosis and, 203, 291
Thiamine
  alcoholism and, 776, 1257
  deficiency of, 772, 849
    mouth and, 1298
  in maple syrup urine disease, 1237
  nutrition and, 1106, 1108
Thiazides, 597
  calcium and, 1190, 1191
    hypercalcemia in, 1179, 1189, 1194
  diabetes insipidus and, 1126
  diazoxide and, 1279
  gout and, 91
  Graves' ophthalmopathy and, 1147
  heart failure and, 465
  hyperglycemic, hyperosmolar, nonketotic coma and, 1270
  hypertension and, 472, 474, 475
  hyperuricemia and, 90
  kidney stones and, 647, 648
  lung disease and, 722
  mineralocorticoid excess and, 1161
  nephrotic syndrome and, 613
  neutropenia and, 360
  pancreatitis and, 1051
  renal insufficiency and, 475
  sedatives and, 572
  side effects and interactions of, 574
  sunburn and, 29
  thrombocytopenia and, 400, 401
  toxic nephropathy and, 625, 626, 627, 629
Thiazolsulfone, 330
Thibierge-Weisenbach syndrome, 904

Thiocyanate, 1132
Thioguanine, 366, 367, 370, 441
Thiopental, 665
Thioridazine, 871
Thiosulfate citrate bile salts sucrose agar, 205
ThioTEPA, 445
Thiouracils, 57
Thioureas, 1144-1145, 1147
Third nerve lesions, 765
Third ventricle, colloid cyst of, 844
Thirst mechanism, defective, 596
Thomsen's disease, 859
Thoracentesis, 687-688
Thoracic aorta; see Aorta
Thoracic outlet syndrome, 100-101
Thoracic seminomas of mediastinum, 735
Thoracic spinal abnormalities, 737; see also Spine
  ankylosing spondylitis and, 48, 50
Thoracoplasty, 712
Thoracostomy, tube, 733
Thoracotomy
  lung cancer and, 741, 742
  lung cysts and, 744
  patent ductus arteriosus and, 557
  scans and, 687
  solitary pulmonary nodule and, 744
  Wegener's granulomatosis and, 72
Thorax
  abnormalities of, 511
  evaluation of, 12, 684-685
  thoracoplasty and, 712
  thoracostomy and, 733
  thoracotomy and; see Thoracotomy
Thorazine, 342
Threshold effect, 749
Thrills, 12
Throat cultures, 224
Throat pack, epidermolysis bullosa dystrophica and, 878
Throat pain, 132, 791
Throat swabs, 137
Thrombasthenia, 405, 426
Thrombectomy, 1020
Thrombi, 568, 840-841; see also Emboli; Thrombophlebitis; Thrombosis
  disseminated; see Disseminated intravascular coagulation
  endocarditis and, 182
  infected, 489
  myocardial infarction and, 536; see also Myocardial infarction
  occlusive vascular disease of gut and, 1020
  in pulmonary artery, 489-494
  pulmonary emboli and, 490; see also Pulmonary emboli
  venography and, 607
Thrombin
  anticoagulant therapy and, 430
  gingival bleeding and, 421
  hemophilia and, 427
  polycythemia and, 419
  prothrombin time and, 1098
Thrombin time, 409, 414
Thromboangiitis obliterans, 69, 570
Thrombocythemia, essential, 373-374; see also Thrombocytosis
Thrombocytopenia, 400-404
  anemia and, 320, 321
  cytomegalovirus and, 300
  dentistry and, 425-426
  drug allergy and, 29
  Gaucher's disease and, 425
  leukemia and, 420

Thrombocytopenia—cont'd
  liver disease and, 411, 1064
  lupus erythematosus and, 112
  perinatal viruses and, 126
  purpura and; see Thrombocytopenic purpura
Thrombocytopenic purpura, 425, 898
  idiopathic, 402-403
  oral purpuras and, 571
  thrombotic, 404, 937
    cerebrovascular disease and, 842
    dentistry and, 425
    hemolysis and, 340
Thrombocytopoiesis, ineffective, 320-321
Thrombocytosis, 373-374, 404-405
  dentistry and, 426
  Kawasaki disease and, 148
  polycythemia vera and, 353
Thromboembolism; see Emboli; Thrombi; Thrombophlebitis
Thrombophlebitis, 491, 494-495; see also Phlebitis
  cephalosporins and, 165
  dentistry and, 577
  migratory, 495, 913
  tetracyclines and, 168
  ulcerative colitis and, 1008
Thromboplastin time, partial, 409, 430
Thrombosis, 840-841; see also Thrombi
  cavernous sinus, 303-304, 873
  cerebral infarction and, 831, 873
  of deep veins, 491; see also Phlebitis; Thrombophlebitis
  intestines and, 1021-1022
  malignant atrophic papulosis and, 894
  mesenteric venous, 1021-1022
  paroxysmal nocturnal hemoglobinuria and, 341
  polycythemia vera and, 419
  portal vein, 1060
  renal vein, 607, 662-663
Thrombotic thrombocytopenic purpura; see Thrombocytopenic purpura, thrombotic
Thromboxane A_2, 400, 405
Thrombus; see Thrombi; Thrombophlebitis
Thrush; see Oral candidiasis
Thumb-printing, 1021
Thymic dependent and independent antigens, 16; see also Thymus-derived cells
Thymomas, 33, 735
Thymus
  agenesis of, 1196
  failure of, to develop, 33
  neoplasms of, 33, 735
  transplantation of, 33
Thymus-derived cell markers, 365
Thymus-derived cell subsets, 32
Thymus-derived cells, 15-16, 376
  disorders of, 31, 33, 34
  evaluation of, 32
  infectious mononucleosis and, 132
  lymphomas and, 392
  pneumonia and, 172-173
  sarcoidosis and, 718
Thyroacropachy, 1142, 1143
Thyroglobulin, 1128, 1129, 1130, 1139
Thyroglobulin antibody, 1136
Thyroid, 1126-1152; see also Hyperthyroidism; Hypothyroidism
  abscess of, 1149
  adenomas of, 1145, 1150
  agenesis of, 1137
  alcohol and, 1258
  anatomy of, 1126-1128
  aspiration cytology of, 1136
  biopsy of, 1136, 1152

Thyroid—cont'd
  biosynthetic defect of, 1148
  carcinoma of, 1150-1152
    follicular, 1146, 1151
    medullary; see Medullary carcinoma of thyroid
    metastatic, 1146
    multiple endocrine neoplasia and, 879
  cardiomyopathies and, 523
  chemistry of, 1128-1132
  clinical assessment of, 10, 1136-1152
  cysts of, 1150
  dentistry and, 1205-1206
  desiccated, 1139, 1140
  dysplasia of, 1137
  ectopic, 1137, 1146
  enzyme defects and, 1148
  goiter in; see Goiter
  hemorrhage in, 1150
  histology of, 1128
  hormones of; see Thyroid hormones
  human growth hormone treatment and, 1123
  hyperthyroidism and, 1140-1148; see also Hyperthyroidism
  hypothyroidism and, 1136-1140; see also Hypothyroidism
  liver disease and, 1062
  in pregnancy, 1132
  scan of, 1133
  skin disorders and, 886
  surgery of, 1144-1150, 1152, 1197
  tests and, 1133-1136, 1152
  thyroiditis in; see Thyroiditis
  thyrotoxicosis and; see Thyrotoxicosis
  ultrasound and, 1134
Thyroid acropachy, 1142, 1143
Thyroid autoantibodies, 1136, 1139
Thyroid binding tests, 1133-1136
Thyroid concentration tests, 1133-1136
Thyroid extract, 1139, 1140
Thyroid hormones
  cretinism and, 1105
  excessive administration of, 1146
  lipoproteins and, 1284, 1285
  lymphocytic thyroiditis and, 1150; see also Lymphocytic thyroiditis
  metabolism of, 1131-1132
  nontoxic diffuse goiter and, 1148; see also Goiter
  peripheral binding of, 1131-1132
  physiologic effects of, 1131-1132
  self-administration of, 1146
  storage and secretion of, 1130
  synthesis of, 1128-1130
  tests for, 1133-1136, 1152
  thyroid carcinoma and, 1152
  thyrotoxicosis from exogenous uptake of, 1146
Thyroid shields, 751
Thyroid stimulator, abnormal, 19, 1143
Thyroid storm, 1147, 1205
Thyroidectomy, 1144-1150, 1152, 1197
Thyroiditis, 1149-1150
  hyperthyroidism from, 1146
  lymphocytic; see Lymphocytic thyroiditis
  Riedel's, 105, 1150
Thyroid-stimulating hormone, 1116-1117, 1128, 1130, 1135
  acromegaly and, 1120
  adenoma and, 1121
  antibodies and; see Thyrotropin receptor antibody
  deficiency of, 1122-1137
  hormone releasing; see Thyrotropin-releasing hormone

Thyroid-stimulating hormone—cont'd
  hypothyroidism and, 1138, 1139, 1145-1146
  measurement of, 1135-1136
  synthesis of thyroglobulin and, 1130
Thyroid-stimulating hormone stimulation test, 1135-1136
Thyroid-stimulating immunoglobulin; see Thyrotropin receptor antibody
Thyrotoxic crisis, 1147, 1205
Thyrotoxicosis
  cardiomyopathies and, 523
  classification of, 1140-1141
  dentistry and, 1205
  diagnosis of, 1141, 1146-1147
  from exogenous thyroid hormone uptake, 1146
  Graves' disease and, 1143-1145
  iatrogenic, 1146
  toxic goiter and, 1145
Thyrotoxicosis factitia, 1146
Thyrotropin; see Thyroid-stimulating hormone
Thyrotropin receptor antibody, 19, 1133, 1136, 1144
  Graves' ophthalmopathy and, 1147
  transplacental transfer of, 1147
Thyrotropin-releasing hormone, 1116, 1135
  in tests, 1135-1136
  hypothyroidism and, 1138-1139
Thyrotropin-secreting adenoma, 1121
Thyroxine, 1116, 1128, 1129
  binding of, 1131
  hyperlipidemias and, 1290
  hyperthyroidism and, 1141
  hypothyroidism and, 1138, 1139, 1140, 1141
  replacement therapy in, 1139-1140
  index of free, 1134-1135
  iodine and, 1105
  lipoprotein lipase deficiency and, 1289
  liver disease and, 1062
  low-density lipoproteins and, 1285
  metabolism of, 1131
  myxedema coma and, 1206
  nontoxic diffuse goiter and, 1148
  serum, hyperthyroidism and, 1141
  storage of, 1130
  synthesis of, 1129
  tests for, 1134
  vitamin A and, 1107
D-Thyroxine, 1139, 1285, 1290; see also Thyroxine
Thyroxine-binding albumin, 1131, 1134
Thyroxine-binding globulin, 1131
Thyroxine-binding prealbumin, 1131
TIA; see Transient cerebral ischemia
Tibia, bowing of, 87
Tibial nerve entrapment, 98
Tic, 821
Tic douloureux, 790-791, 799
  multiple sclerosis and, 868
  tuberculoid leprosy and, 305
Ticarcillin, 160, 164
  and aminoglycosides, 177, 241
  bacteremia and, 241
  neoplasia and, 446
  nephropathy and, 625
  pneumonia and, 177
Tick-borne rickettsioses, 210-211
Tick-borne typhus, 210-211; see also Rocky Mountain spotted fever
Ticks
  babesiosis and, 288
  erythema chronicum migrans and, 925
  Lyme disease and, 297
  rickettsioses and, 210-211
Tics, 821

Tidal volume, 673
Tietze's syndrome, 100, 737
Tinea infections, 279, 928-929
Tinel's sign, 98, 1275
Tissue adhesives, 963
Tissue culture isolation, 123
Titers, antibody; see Antibody testing
TLC; see Total lung capacity
TMJ; see Temporomandibular joints
TmP/GFR; see Renal tubular maximum phosphate reabsorption/glomerular filtration rate
TNI; see Total nodal irradiation
TNM classification; see Tumor-node-metastases anatomic classification
Tobacco; see Smoking
Tobramycin, 161, 166
  and ampicillin, 241
  anaerobic infections and, 250
  bacteremia and, 241
  and cephalothin, 241
  meningitis and, 190
  nephritis and, 619
  nephropathy and, 627, 628
  pregnancy and, 1212
Tocopherol; see Vitamins, E
Toes; see also Foot
  clubbing of, 103, 181, 683-684
  sausagelike swelling of, 51
  tarsal tunnel syndrome and, 98
Tofranil; see Imipramine
Togavirus, 123
Tolazamide, 1266, 1267
Tolazoline, 61
Tolbutamide, 590, 1255, 1266, 1267
Tolectin; see Tolmetin
Tolinase; see Tolazamide
Tolmetin, 42, 46, 47
Tolnaftate, 279
Toluene, 623
Toluene-di-isocyanate, 704
Tomography, computed; see Computed tomography
Tongue
  acanthosis nigricans and, 888, 1093
  acromegaly and, 1204
  actinomycosis of, 305
  beefy red, 414
  Behçet's disease and, 907
  chronic discoid lupus erythematosus and, 111
  dermatitis herpetiformis and, 893
  dermatomyositis and, 112, 113, 905-906
  diabetes mellitus and, 1294
  edema of, 667
  evaluation of, 9
  folic acid deficiency and, 415, 1298
  geographic, 908, 937, 938
  inflammation of; see Glossitis
  iron deficiency and, 1105
  lichen planus and, 938
  malabsorption and, 1000
  myxedema and, 1206
  neuralgia and, 791
  neurofibromas and, 879
  nicotinic acid deficiency and, 1110
  Plummer-Vinson syndrome and, 1091, 1105
  protein malnutrition and, 1104
  psoriasis and, 937
  pyridoxine deficiency and, 1109
  raspberry, 224
  riboflavin deficiency and, 1108
  strawberry, 224
  syphilis and atrophy of, 303
  systemic sclerosis and, 112

Tongue—cont'd
  telangiectasia and, 894, 1095
  thiamine deficiency and, 1108
  thyroid tissue in, 1205
  tuberous sclerosis and, 880
  Urbach-Wiethe disease and, 1296
  vitamin B_{12} deficiency and, 1109
Tonic-clonic seizures, 783; see also Seizures
Tonicity, effective, 596
Tonsillectomy, 185
Tonsillitis, 144
Tonsils
  adenoviruses and, 143
  antibiotics for infection of, 144
  evaluation of, 9
  orange-yellow, 1292
  pharyngitis and, 224
  removal of, 185
Tooth; see Teeth
Tophi, 92, 93
Torre's syndrome, 913
Torsade des pointes, 546
Torsion, 998, 1049
Torsion dystonias, 819-821
Torticollis, spasmodic, 819-820
Total iron-binding capacity, 1066
Total lung capacity, 677, 726
Total nodal irradiation, 390, 393
Total oral radiation dose, 751
Total parenteral nutrition; see Hyperalimentation, parenteral
Total serum osmolality, 596
Total ventilation versus alveolar ventilation, 673
Tourette's syndrome, 821-822
Toxemia of pregnancy, 665-666
Toxic epidermal necrolysis, 306, 931-932
Toxic goiter, 1143-1145
Toxic liver disease, 1066
Toxic megacolon, 1007, 1008, 1011, 1027
Toxic nephropathy, 624-630, 631
Toxic neuropathies, 853-854
Toxic shock syndrome, 298
Toxicity
  of drugs, 775-779; see also specific drug
    antimicrobials in, 158
    heart medications in, 572
  of mercury, 30
Toxins
  bacterial, 201, 205
    of diphtheria, 247, 248
    Escherichia coli and, 201
    group A streptococci and, 223
    Staphylococcus aureus in, 218
  Clostridium perfringens and, 253
  Fanconi's syndrome and, 624
  hemolysis from, 342
  shock and, 476
Toxocara canis, 290, 372, 721
Toxocara cati, 290, 372
Toxoids, 248, 252
Toxoplasma gondii, 172, 284, 285, 286
Toxoplasmosis, 284-286
  aseptic meningoencephalitis and, 139
  immunodeficiency diseases and, 31
  pneumonia and, 172
  red cell injury and, 343
TPN; see Hyperalimentation
Trabeculation, decreased, 115
Trace elements, 1106
Trachea
  aortic dissection and, 561
  evaluation of, 10
  inflammation of, 217
  obstruction of, 713

Tracheobronchitis, 217
Tracheoesophageal fistula, 1032
Tracheostomy, 713
Trachoma, 214
Trachoma-inclusion conjunctivitis, 214
Traction diverticula, 736
Traction headache, 790
Tractotomy, 872
Tram lines, 810, 881
Tranquilizers; see also specific agent
  abuse of, 862, 873
  alcohol and, 1297
  anal pruritus and, 1030
  asthma and, 706
  chorea and, 816
  Gilles de la Tourette's syndrome and, 821
  hemolysis and, 342
  hepatic coma and, 1084
  Huntington's chorea and, 817
  hypothyroidism and, 1206
  respiratory failure and, 712
  Sydenham's chorea and, 819
  torsion dystonias and, 820
  tremor and, 812, 813, 815, 816
  ulcers and, 994
  vertigo and, 793
Transaminases, serum; see Serum, transaminases in
Transbronchial biopsy, 689, 718
Transcutaneous nerve stimulation, 855
Transfer factor, 15
  Behçet's syndrome and, 111
  candidiasis and, 33
  in leprosy, 263
  tumors and, 445
  Wiskott-Aldrich syndrome and, 33
Transfer ribonucleic acid, 1216
Transferrin, 1081
Transfusions, 310-311, 345-351
  aplastic anemia and, 416
  autologous, 347
  blood; see Blood transfusions
  blood component, 310-311, 346, 350
  clotting factors and; see Clotting factors
  emergency, 349
  erythropoiesis suppressed by, 342
  exchange; see Exchange transfusions
  factor VIII after, 408
  granulocyte
    aplastic anemia and, 320
    leukemias and, 368
    neoplasia and, 446
    neutrophil dysfunction and, 420
  hepatitis and, 1068, 1069, 1073
  intraperitoneal, 338
  intrauterine, 338
  leukocyte, 342, 357
    bacteremia and, 241
    in leprosy, 263
    leukemias and, 368
    multiple myeloma and, 382
  perinatal virus and, 127
  plasma; see Plasma, transfusions of
  platelet; see Platelets, transfusions of
  purpura after, 404
  red blood cells and; see Red blood cells, transfusions of
  white cell, 342, 361; see also Transfusions, granulocyte; Transfusions, leukocyte
Transgrow, 232
Transhepatic cholangiography, 967, 968, 1089
Transient cerebral ischemia, 563, 564, 836-838
  dentistry and, 586, 871
Transient global amnesia, 772, 836
Transient hyperthyroidism, 1141

Transient hypothyroidism, 1140
Transient ischemic attacks, 563, 564, 836-838
  dentistry and, 586, 871
Transient myocardial ischemia, 484-485, 528; see also Angina pectoris
Transitional cell tumors of urinary tract, 658-659
Transketolase, 849, 850
Translocation carriers, 1222
Translocations, 1221, 1222
Transmural colitis, 1011; see also Crohn's disease
Transplantation
  of bone marrow; see Bone marrow, transplants of
  cytomegalovirus and, 130, 131
  graft-versus-host disease and, 19
  liver, 34
  renal; see Renal transplantation
  of thymus, 33
Transport globulins, 1154
Transposition of great vessels, 508
Transsphenoidal pituitary microsurgery, 1120, 1124, 1159
Transtentorial herniation, 767
Transthoracic liver biopsy, 965
Transtracheal aspiration, 176
Transudates, 688, 731, 1044
Transverse myelitis, 138, 194
Transverse myelopathy, 138, 194
Transverse tubules, 454
Trapezius muscle pain, 98
Trauma
  coma and, 765
  from environment; see Environment, injuries from
  esophageal rupture and, 986
  to head, 765, 784, 793
  headache after, 789
  labyrinthopathy and, 793
  maxillofacial, drug abuse and, 862
  osteomyelitis and, 221
  postoperative, oral candidiasis and, 307
  rotator cuff tears and, 95, 101
  wounds and, 201, 253
Traumatic hemolytic anemias, 340-341
Traumatic wet lung, 708-709; see also Adult respiratory distress syndrome
Travenol needle, 608
Treacher Collins syndrome, 1302, 1308, 1309-1310, 1311
Treitz, ligament of, 957, 958
Trematodes, 294-297
Tremors
  alcohol abuse and, 776
  essential, 815-816
  familial, 815-816
  jaws and facial muscles and, 870-871
  multiple sclerosis and, 799
  parkinsonism and, 812; see also Parkinsonism
Trendelenburg position, 576
Treponema carateum, 264
Treponema pallidum, 264, 265, 267, 268, 271, 303; see also Syphilis
  drugs for, 167, 168
Treponema pertenue, 264
TRH; see Thyrotropin-releasing hormone
Triac, 1128
Triamterene, 597
  folate deficiency and, 316
  heart failure and, 465
  hyperkalemia and, 598
  hypertension and, 472
  renal failure and, 639
  side effects and interactions of, 574

TRIC; see Trachoma-inclusion conjunctivitis
Trichinella spiralis, 172, 203, 292, 858
Trichinosis, 203, 292
  dentistry and, 875
  eosinophilia and, 372
  myopathy and, 858
  pneumonia and, 172
Trichloroacetic acid, 927, 1296
Trichloroethylene, 626, 627, 629
Trichobezoars, 998
Trichomonas vaginalis, 170, 286
Trichomoniasis, 170, 286
Trichophyton, 279
  anal disorders and, 1030
  Cushing's syndrome and, 887
  sarcoidosis and, 911
  skin infections and, 911, 928-929
Trichophyton mentagrophytes, 928, 929
Trichophyton rubrum, 887, 928, 929
Trichorhinophalangeal syndrome, 1245
Trichuriasis, 290
Trichuris trichura, 290
Tricuspid valve, 516-517
  atresia of, 506-507
  drug addiction and, 181
  Ebstein's anomaly of, 507-508
  liver disease and, 1077
  regurgitation of, 516-517
  septal defects and, 504
Tricyclic antidepressants; see Antidepressants, tricyclic
Triethylenethiophosphoramide, 659
Trifluoperazine, 871
Trigeminal nerve; see also Trigeminal neuralgia
  lesions of, 760
  peripheral neuropathy of, 874
Trigeminal neuralgia, 790-791, 799
  multiple sclerosis and, 799, 868
  tuberculoid leprosy and, 305
Trigger fingers, 99
Triggered automaticity, 542
Triglyceride-rich lipoproteins, 1284-1285
Triglycerides
  accumulation of, 91, 1284, 1286, 1287
  ascites and, 1046
  deficient, 1292
  in diet, 998, 999
  digestion and, 947
  hyperlipidemia and, 1280
  hypertriglyceridemia and, 91, 1284, 1286, 1287
  levels of, 1280
  lipoprotein lipase deficiency and, 1287
  in lipoproteins, disorders of, 1284-1285
  liver disease and, 1063, 1077
  measurement of total, 1288-1289
  medium-chain; see Medium-chain triglycerides
  remnant removal disease and, 1287
  synthesis of, 1282
  transport of, 1282
  xanthomas and, 890
Trihexosyl ceramidosis, 1231-1232
Trihexyphenidyl, 815, 820, 821, 870
Triiodinated meglumine diatrizoate, 605; see also Contrast agents
Triiodinated sodium diatrizoate, 605; see also Contrast agents
3,5,3'-Triiodothyroacetic acid; see Triac
Triiodothyronine, 1116, 1128, 1129
  action of, 1115, 1131-1132
  binding of, 1131
  hyperthyroidism and, 1141
  in hypothyroidism replacement therapy, 1139-1140

Triiodothyronine—cont'd
  iodine and, 1105
  metabolism of, 1131
  storage of, 1130
  syndrome of low, 1131
  synthesis of, 1129
  tests of, 1134, 1136
3,3',5'-Triiodothyronine, 1128
  metabolism of, 1131
  storage of, 1130
  syndrome of, 1131
L-Triiodothyronine, 1139; see also Triiodothyronine
Triiodothyronine suppression test, 1136
Triiodothyronine uptake test, 1134
Trimethadione, 360, 612, 613, 627
Trimethaphan, 473, 474, 562
Trimethobenzamide, 1212
Trimethoprim, 161, 170
  folate deficiency and, 316
  sulfamethoxazole with, 161, 170
    bronchitis and, 693
    enteric fever and, 208
    Haemophilus influenzae and, 236
    leukemic infections and, 368
    neoplasia and, 446
    nephropathy and, 628
    plague and, 242
    pneumocystosis and, 288
    prostatitis and, 198
    shigellosis and, 206
    urinary tract infection and, 197, 198, 199
Trinitrotoluene, 330
Triorthocresylphosphate, 853
Triploidy, 1221
Trismus, 252
Trisomies, 1221, 1225
  10, 882
  13, 1316
  21, 1301, 1308
Trisulfapyrimidines, 169
Trochanteric bursitis, 99
Trophozoite, 282, 284, 287
Tropical pulmonary eosinophilia, 373
Tropical sprue, 1001-1002
Trousseau's sign, 1183, 1196, 1208
Truncal ataxia, 759
Truncus arteriosus, 505
Trypanosoma brucei, 286
Trypanosoma cruzi, 286, 1027
Trypanosomiasis, 286-287, 1027
Trypsin, 1050
Trypsinogen, 945
Tsetse fly, 286
TSI; see Thyrotropin receptor antibody
TSS; see Toxic shock syndrome
T-strain mycoplasma, 217; see also *Ureaplasma urealyticum*
TT; see Thrombin time
TTP; see Thrombocytopenic purpura, thrombotic
T_3U; see Triiodothyronine uptake test
Tubal abscesses, 218
Tubal pregnancy, 232
Tubal scarring, 256
Tube thoracostomy, 733
Tuberculin skin test, 81, 257, 260
Tuberculoid leprosy, 262, 305
Tuberculosis, 254-261
  anemia and, 322
  arthritis and, 81
  dentistry and, 304
  drugs for; see Antituberculous agents
  Hodgkin's disease and, 387
  immunodeficiency diseases and, 31

Tuberculosis—cont'd
  liver and, 1084
  meningitis and, 139, 189, 255, 256-257, 260
  neutropenia and, 358
  peritonitis and, 1046-1047
  pleural effusion and, 688, 731
  silicosis and, 724
  vaccine for, 260-261
Tuberous sclerosis, 721, 810, 880-881
  café au lait spots and, 879
  dentistry and, 869
  lung and, 721
Tuberous xanthomas, 889
D-Tubocurarine, 574
Tubo-ovarian abscesses, 218
Tubular graft for aortic aneurysms, 558
Tubular system of muscle fiber, 851-852
  of myocardium, 454
Tubules, renal, 590
  disorder or disease of, 619, 622-623
    renal failure and, 630-635
    after renal transplantation, 645
    toxic nephropathy and, 624-630, 631
  potassium secretion and, 593
  and reabsorption
    of bicarbonate, 592
    of phosphate; see Renal tubular maximum phosphate reabsorption/glomerular filtration rate
    of sodium, 592
Tubulovillous polyps, 1038
Tularemia, 242-243, 305
Tumor cachexia syndrome, 438
Tumor cell
  kinetics of, 439
  in marrow, myelofibrosis and, 322
Tumor lysis syndrome, 446
Tumor markers, 434-435
Tumor-node-metastases anatomic classification, 436
Tumors; see also Neoplasia; specific tumor
  aldosteronism and, 1160, 1161
  anorectal, 1031
  brain; see Brain, tumors of
  brown, 1193, 1208
  carcinoid; see Carcinoid tumors
  of cardiovascular structures, 488, 555
  cell kinetics and, 439
  central nervous system and, 843-848; see also Brain, tumors of
  chromaffin cell, 1164
  compression by, 436, 445
  Cushing's syndrome and, 1157, 1158, 1159
  diagnosis of, 434-435
  of diaphragm, 736-737
  of digestive system, 1031-1043; see also Digestive system, tumors of
  endocrine, 443-444, 450, 1178-1181; see also Multiple endocrine neoplasias
  eosinophilia and, 363
  epilepsy and, 784
  of esophagus, dental care and, 1091
  folate-dependent, 1110
  genitourinary, management of, 449; see also specific tumor
  germ cell, 435
  headache and, 790
  hepatic; see Hepatomas; Liver, neoplasms of
  hyperthyroidism from, 1146
  islet cell; see Insulinomas
  of kidneys, 658-659
    jaw metastases and, 668
  Klatskin, 1089
  Krukenberg's, 1035

Tumors—cont'd
  of lung, 685, 738-744; see also Lung, malignancies of
  lung abscess and, 698
  malignant mesothelioma and, 726-727
  of mediastinum, 735
  mesenteric, 1049
  monocytosis and, 362
  mycosis fungoides and, 446, 901-902
  myeloma, 378-382; see also Multiple myeloma
  obstruction and, 436, 445
    uropathy and, 654, 660
  organ function and, 437
  of pancreas; see Pancreas, tumors of
  paraneoplastic syndromes and, 437-438
  pituitary; see Pituitary gland, tumors of
  plasma cell, multiple myeloma and, 422
  pleural, 734
  polycythemia and, 354
  pregnancy and, 1211
  preoperative devascularization of, 971
  radiation and; see Radiation
  of renal pelvis and upper ureters, 658-659
  secretion and, 437
  spinal cord, 860
  of spleen, 398
  staging of, 435-436; see also Staging
  supportive care and, 445
  testicular, 435, 449, 1173, 1214
  Wilms', 658
Tumor-specific antigens, 444; see also specific antigen
Turbinaire Decadron, 22
Turkey raiser's disease, 727
Turner's sign, 1051
Turner's syndrome, 1176-1177, 1225-1226
  coarctation of aorta and, 505
  dentistry and, 1209
  male, 1170-1171
Tympanic membrane, 9
Typhoid fever, 202, 207-208
  liver disease and, 1074
  neutropenia and, 359
Typhoidal tularemia, 243
Typhus, 210-213, 214; see also Rocky Mountain spotted fever
Tyramine, 443, 788, 824, 1167
Tyrosine, 1166, 1236, 1254
  metabolism of, 1132
  thyroid hormone and, 1129, 1132
Tyrosinemia, 1236, 1254

U

U wave, 482, 483
UG ridge; see Urogenital ridge
Uhthoff's sign, 798
Ulcerative colitis, 1005-1006, 1007-1011
  Behçet's syndrome, 110
  colorectal carcinoma and, 1039
  dentistry and, 1095-1096
  ischemic colitis and, 1021
  reactive arthritis and, 53
  skin disorders of, 892
  surgery for, 1011
Ulcerative gingivitis, acute necrotizing, 302, 307, 862
Ulcerative stomatitis, anemia and, 415
Ulceroglandular tularemia, 243
Ulcers
  amebiasis and, 282
  aphthous; see Aphthous ulcers
  Curling's, 995
  Cushing's, 995
  of genitalia, 266

Ulcers—cont'd
  of gingiva, 302, 307, 667, 862
  hyperparathyroidism and, 1192
  intestinal, 1019; see also Ulcerative colitis
    amebiasis and, 282
    Crohn's disease and, 1011
  oral; see Oral ulcers; Mouth
  peptic, 987-994
    dental care and, 1092
    pain and, 950
    perforation of, 988, 993, 1052
    surgery and, 993-994
  rodent, 916
  of skin, ulcerative colitis and, 1095, 1096
  systemic sclerosis and, 59, 61
  tularemia and, 243
Ultrasonography
  abdominal, 969-971
  arterial insufficiency and, 569
  cancer staging and, 436
  carotid artery system and, 872
  cholestasis and, 1067
  fetal, 1229
  fever of unknown origin and, 120
  of kidney, 607
  of lung, 687
  myofascial pain dysfunction and, 109
  obstructive uropathy and, 656
  pancreatitis and, 1052
  pheochromocytoma and, 1167, 1168
  phlebography and, 495
  thyroid, 1134
Ultraviolet light, 937
Umbilicus, turbulent blood flow at, 1060
Uncal herniation, 767
Unconsciousness, 762-769
Undecylenic acid, 279
Unilateral hyperlucent lung, 686
Uninodular goiter, toxic, 1145
Unresponsiveness, 762-769
  hysterical, 764
Unstable angina, 532
Unstable hemoglobins, 1227
Upper airway; see also Respiratory diseases
  neoplasms of, 73
  obstruction of; see Airway obstruction
Upper arm disorders, 98, 100
Upper brainstem, 763
Upper gastrointestinal series; see Barium
Uracil mustard, 404
Uranium, 432, 619, 627, 630
Urate, 89-90, 92, 93, 667
Urbach-Wiethe disease, 1296
Urban plague, 242
Urea
  body fluid osmolality and, 596
  disorders of, 1238-1239
  hypernatremia and, 595
  in saliva, 666, 667
Ureaplasma urealyticum, 214, 217, 218, 232
Urease inhibitors, 648
Uremia, 632, 635-640; see also Renal failure
  glomerulonephritis and, 610
  glucose-6-phosphate dehydrogenase deficiency and, 330
  in hemolytic-uremic syndrome, 340, 617
  neuropathies of, 853-854
  oral manifestations of, 666-667
  platelet function and, 406
  skin disorders of, 896-897
  stomatitis of, 666-667
  term of, 635
  toxins in, 636
Uremic frost, 896

INDEX 1423

Ureteral orifice, cystoscopy and, 650
Ureters
　anomalies of, 650-651
　cystoscopy and, 650
　obstruction of, supportive care and, 445; see also Uropathy, obstructive
　tumors of upper, 658-659
Urethral anomalies, 651
Urethral syndrome, 214
Urethritis
　chlamydial, 214-215
　gonococcal, 214, 215, 231
　mycoplasmas and, 217, 218
　nonspecific, 214, 217, 218
　postgonococcal, 215, 218
　Reiter's syndrome and, 52
Uric acid
　excess of; see Hyperuricemia
　kidney and
　　nephropathy of, 622, 625
　　stones in, 92, 94, 648
　Lesch-Nyhan syndrome and, 1239
　lithiasis, 968-969
　gout and, 92, 94
Uricosuric agents, 472, 622
Uridine, 1240
Urinalysis, 604-605; see also Urine
　fever of unknown origin and, 120
　microbial diseases and, 118, 119
　obstructive uropathy and, 655-656
Urinary bladder; see Bladder, urinary
Urinary tract; see also Genitourinary tract
　bacterial infection of, 195-199
　endocarditis and infections of, 180
　malformations of, 649-651
　neoplasms of, 656-660
　obstruction of; see Obstructive uropathy
　pregnancy and, 664, 666
　pyelography and, 196, 606, 607, 656
　reinfection of, 195, 196, 197, 198-199
　schistosomiasis and, 296
　sickle cell anemia and, 333
Urine; see also Urinalysis
　acidification of, 593, 655; see also Aciduria
　　obstructive uropathy and, 655
　albumin in, 605, 912
　alkalinization of, 649
　antimicrobial concentrations in, 157
　anuria and, 610, 630
　asymptomatic abnormalities of, 609
　bacteria in; see Bacteriuria
　bile pigments in, 1065-1066
　blood in; see Hematuria; Hemoglobinurias
　catecholamines in, 1166, 1168, 1258
　chyle in, 292
　concentration of, 591, 655
　copper in, 1066, 1082
　coproporphyrin in, 1066
　cystathione in, 1237
　cystine in, 1227
　1,25-dihydroxyvitamin D_3 in, 647
　dilution of, 591
　excessive, 621
　falsely appearing to contain blood, 588
　glucose in, 604
　hepatitis and, 1099
　homogentisic acid in, 1236
　hydroxyproline, 60, 78, 87
　lead levels in, 753
　lipids in, 612
　lysine in, 1239
　metabolites in, 1166, 1168
　myoglobin in, 588, 627, 631, 859-860
　osmolality of, 591, 595

Urine—cont'd
　oxalates in, 620-621, 648
　pH of, 592-593, 604
　　renal tubular acidosis and, 623
　porphyrin in, 1252, 1253, 1254
　　lead poisoning and, 753
　residual, 656
　sediment in, 604-605
　　telescoped, 616
　tests of, 604-605; see also Urinalysis
　uric acid in; see Uric acid, kidney and
　urinary tract infection and, 196
　white cells in, 588, 590, 626
　xanthines in, 1239-1240
URO; see Uroporphyrin
Urobilinogen, 1058
　fecal, 1065
Urogenital ridge, 1168
UROgens; see Uroporphyrinogens
Urography, 606, 661, 663
Urokinase, 494
Urolithiasis, 646-649; see also Kidney stones
Uromucoid, 605
Uropathy, obstructive, 653-656
　prostatic carcinoma and, 660
　tests for, 606, 633
　toxic nephropathy and, 627
Uroporphyrin
　excessive, 1248-1249, 1252
　urinary, 1066
Uroporphyrinogens, 1247, 1248
　deficiency of, 1250-1252
Urothelial tumors of kidney, 658-659
Ursodeoxycholic acid, 1089
Urticaria, 25-26, 909
　hepatitis B and, 896
Urticaria pigmentosa, 26, 909
Useless hand, 798
Uterine myonecrosis, 253
Uterine tube; see Fallopian tube
Uveitis
　ankylosing spondylitis and, 48, 50
　Behçet's disease and, 907
　sarcoidosis and, 716, 910
Uveoparotid fever, 910, 911; see also Heerfordt's disease
Uvula
　bifid, 1321
　edema of, 667

V

$V_{max 25\%-75\%}$; see Maximal flow rates at 25%-75% forced expiratory vital capacity
V factor, 235
V̇a/Q̇c; see Ventilation-perfusion ratio
Vaccines, 151-153
　adenoviruses and, 143, 148
　Bacille Calmette Guérin; see Bacille Calmette Guérin
　for bacterial meningitis, 191
　cholera and, 205
　cytomegalovirus and, 131
　diphtheria-pertussis-tetanus, 238, 249, 252
　diphtheria-tetanus, 248
　enteric fever and, 208
　Haemophilus influenzae, 236
　hepatitis B, 1100-1101
　herpes simplex, 129
　human diploid cell, 153
　influenza and, 152-153
　measles, 138, 145-146, 152
　measles-mumps-rubella, 138
　for meningococcal disease, 233
　for mumps, 137, 138, 152

Vaccines—cont'd
　pertussis, 237, 238, 248, 252
　pneumococcal
　　nephrotic syndrome and, 613
　　polyvalent, 175
　　sickle cell anemia and, 334
　　splenectomy and, 329, 337
　postvaccinal encephalomyelitis and, 827
　rabies, 153, 827
　rubella, 126, 127, 152
　for tuberculosis, 260-261
　tularemia, 243
　typhus fever and, 212
　varicella-zoster and, 130
Vaccinia, 918
Vacuformed splint, 415
Vaginal moniliasis, 276, 929
Vaginitis, 230
Vagotomy, 993, 996, 1103
Vagus nerve
　asthma and, 705
　division of, 993, 996
　gastric secretion and, 943
　pancreatic secretion and, 1050
　receptors innervated by, 677
Vail's vidian neuralgia, 791
Valine, 1237, 1238
Valium; see Diazepam
Valproic acid, 786, 1297
Valsalva, aneurysms of sinuses of, 558
Valsalva's maneuver, 461, 823
Valved conduits, 509
Valvular heart disease, 510-517; see also specific valve
　arrhythmias and, 584
　congestive heart failure and, 453
　dentistry and, 579-582
　endocarditis and, 301
　hemolysis and, 340
　rheumatic, 179, 180
Van Allen primary amyloidosis, 854
van der Woude syndrome, 1228
Vancomycin, 161, 167
　administration route for, 157
　arthritis and, 81
　bactericidal activity of, 156
　cellulitis and, 226
　drug fever and, 159
　endocarditis and, 183, 184, 185, 581
　enterococci and, 227
　enterocolitis and, 220, 1018
　excretion of, 158
　meningitis and, 190
　pneumonia and, 175
　renal insufficiency and, 158
　staphylococcal infections and, 175, 183, 184, 200, 221
　streptococci and, 183, 227, 228, 302
Vanillylmandelic acid, 1165, 1166, 1168
Vapors, inhaled, 728-730
Variable expressivity, 1219
Variant angina, Prinzmetal's, 533
Varicella, 129-130, 134, 135, 826
　central nervous system disease and, 135, 138
　dentistry and, 299
　herpes zoster and; see Herpes zoster
　interferon and, 154
　lesions of, 927
　neonatal, 126, 127
　neuropathy and, 855
　in pneumonia, 172
　rickettsialpox and, 212
　vaccine for, 130
Varicella-zoster; see Herpes zoster

Varices, 1060
  achalasia and, 979
  in anus, 948, 1030-1031, 1060
  bleeding, management of, 1083
  bronchiectasis and, 697
  rupture of, 1063
  schistosomiasis and, 296
Varicoceles, 659, 1171
Varicosities; see Varices
Variegate porphyria, 888, 1253
Vasa vasorum, 265, 269
Vascular bruits; see Bruits
Vascular capacitance, 476
Vascular congestion, ulcerative colitis and, 1007; see also Erythema
Vascular diseases
  of central nervous system, 829-843
    brain infarction and, 830-835
    cerebral circulation and, 829-835
    cerebral hemorrhage and, 830, 838-839; see also Cerebrovascular accident
    hypertensive encephalopathy and, 469, 841
    spinal cord hemorrhage and, 840
    spinal cord infarction and, 835-836
    subarachnoid hemorrhage and, 839-840
    transient ischemic attacks and, 836-838
    uncommon, 841-843
    venous thrombosis and, 840-841
  of gastrointestinal tract, 951, 1020-1024
    dental care and, 1092-1093, 1095
  inflammations in; see Vasculitis
  of kidney, 660-663
  platelet disorders and, 400-408
  purpuras and; see Purpura
  systemic sclerosis and, 58-59
  thromboangiitis obliterans and, 69
  toxic nephropathy and, 626
  vertigo and, 793-794
Vascular formations of lips, 1092
Vascular headache, 788-789, 794
Vascular resistance, pulmonary, 499, 503, 674
Vascular spiders, 896, 1059
Vascular stasis, pulmonary embolism and, 577
Vascular system
  disease of; see Vascular diseases
  heart and; see Cardiovascular diseases
  peripheral; see Peripheral vascular system
Vasculitis, 18, 66-70
  Behçet's disease and, 110, 906-907
  classification of, 66
  congenital viral infection and, 125
  dermatomyositis and, 65
  disseminated, 29; see also Disseminated intravascular coagulation
  endocarditis and, 180
  gastrointestinal tract and, 1022
  hemolysis and, 341
  hypersensitivity; see also Schönlein-Henoch purpura
    intestines and, 1022
    management of, 69
  hypertension and, 474
  lupus erythematosus and, 54; see also Lupus erythematosus
  meningoencephalitis and, 139
  overlap; see Overlap syndrome
  peritoneal, 1048
  pulmonary, 719-720
  purpura and, 406; see also Purpura
  rheumatoid, 45, 906
  systemic necrotizing, 66-67, 69
  trypanosomiasis, 287
Vasoactive intestinal polypeptide, 941
  diarrhea and, 954

Vasoactive intestinal polypeptide—cont'd
  esophageal sphincter and, 974
  production of, 1049
  Zollinger-Ellison syndrome and, 994
Vasoactive substances, endogenous, 477
Vasoconstriction, cyanosis and, 683; see also specific disease
Vasoconstrictors; see also Vasopressin
  anaphylaxis and, 29
  arrhythmias and, 585
  diabetes and, 1295
  intestinal ischemia and, 1020
  with local anesthetics, coronary heart disease and, 583
  migraine and, 788
  monoamine oxidase inhibitors and, 574
  pregnancy and, 1213
  renal disease and, 669-670
  sickle cell anemia and, 417
  syncope and, 864
Vasodepressor syncope, 538; see also Syncope
Vasodilation, pulmonary edema and, 465; see also specific disease
Vasodilators
  cardiomyopathy and, 522
  esophageal reflux and, 982
  heart failure and, 464, 465
  hypertension and, 473, 474, 475
  nonocclusive vascular disease of gut and, 1021
  in Raynaud's phenomenon, 61
  scleroderma and, 616, 903
  in shock, 478
Vasomotor nephropathy, 630, 631
Vasomotor rhinitis, 20-21, 23
Vaso-occlusive crisis, 332
Vasopressin; see also Antidiuretic hormone
  cirrhosis and, 1083
  diabetes insipidus and, 622, 1125-1126
  diverticulosis and, 1018
  gastritis and, 996
  gastrointestinal bleeding and, 972, 987
  neoplasms and, 1179, 1181
  renal concentrating ability and, 604
  shock and, 477
  stress erosions and, 996
  varices and, 959, 1083
  vascular control and, 458-459
Vasopressors; see Vasoconstrictors; Vasopressin
Vasospasm, 842
Vasovagal syncope, 576-577, 780; see also Syncope
VC; see Vital capacity
VCA; see Viral capsid antigen
VDRL test; see Venereal Disease Research Laboratories test
VEBs; see Ventricular ectopic beats
Vectors; see specific vector
VEE; see Venezuelan equine encephalitis
Vegetarians, 317
Vegetations, 179, 892, 1007
Veillonella, 249, 302
Veins; see also Blood vessels; specific vein
  collateral circulation of portal-systemic, 1060
  coronary, 525
  dental infection and, 303
  endothelial damage of, 494; see also Thrombophlebitis
  grafts of saphenous, 532
  inflammation of; see Phlebitis; Thrombophlebitis
  jugular, 10, 552, 580
  phlebography and, 495, 663
  portal; see Portal venous system
  pressure in, 478, 552

Veins—cont'd
  pulmonary, 503, 696
  renal; see Renal vein
  respiratory failure and, 708
  thrombosis of, 840-841; see also Thrombi; Thrombosis
    intestines and, 1021-1022
  vena cavae in; see Vena cavae
Velban; see Vinblastine
Vena cavae
  portal hypertension and, 1045
  pulmonary emboli and, 494
  superior, syndrome of; see Superior vena caval syndrome
Venereal Disease Research Laboratories test, 268, 269, 271
Venereal diseases; see specific disease
Venezuelan equine encephalitis, 135
Venous admixture, 708
Venous blood, fibrin, and thrombin, 430
Venous lake, 1092
Venous pressure, 478, 552
Venous stasis, 494, 495; see also Phlebitis; Thrombophlebitis
Ventilation, 677, 711; see also Respirations; Respiratory diseases; Ventilation-perfusion ratio
  abnormal, normal lungs and, 711-712
  alveolar, 673, 674-676
    and arterial carbon dioxide tension, 673
    diminished, 682, 708, 711
    distribution of, 674
    pulmonary capillary blood flow and, 674
    total ventilation versus, 673
  artificial; see Mechanical ventilation
  chemical drive to, 677
  control of, 676-677, 711, 766
  respiratory acidosis and, 601
  scanning and, 687
    pulmonary embolism and, 492, 493, 687
  total versus alveolar, 673
Ventilation scan, 687
  pulmonary embolism and, 492, 493, 687
Ventilation-perfusion ratio, 674-676
  arterial carbon dioxide tension and, 674-676
  arterial oxygen tension and, 676
  mismatch of, 682
  respiratory failure and, 708, 709, 710, 711, 712
Ventricles
  aneurysm of, 536-537, 540
  dilation of, 459
  ectopic beats and, 541, 545, 548
  ejection fraction and, 459, 488-489
  failure of; see Left ventricular failure; Right ventricle, failure of
  fibrillation of, 538, 585
  hypertrophy of; see Ventricular hypertrophy
  left; see Left ventricle
  pressure in; see Ventricular pressures
  radiographic visualization of, 488-489
  right; see Right ventricle
  septal defects of; see Ventricular septal defects
  tachycardia and, 500, 545-546
  wall of, 536
Ventricular aneurysmectomy, left, 540
Ventricular ectopic beats, 541, 545, 548
Ventricular ejection fraction, 459, 488-489
Ventricular failure; see Left ventricular failure; Right ventricle, failure of
Ventricular fibrillation, 538, 585
Ventricular hypertrophy
  cardiac dysfunction and, 459-460
  eccentric, 459

Ventricular hypertrophy—cont'd
  electrocardiograms and, 499, 500
  left; see Left ventricle, enlargement of
  pulmonary hypertension and, 496
Ventricular pressures
  filling, 460
  pericarditis and, 552
Ventricular septal defects, 504
  cardiac catheterization and, 488
  rupture in, 536
  tetralogy of Fallot and, 507
  transposition of great arteries and, 508
Ventricular tachycardia, 545-546
  in children, 500
Ventricular wall, rupture of, 536
Ventriculoatrial shunt infection, 611
Ventriculography, 488-489
Venturi masks, 710
VER; see Visual evoked response
Verapamil
  angina pectoris and, 532, 533
  atrial fibrillation and, 544, 545
  atrial flutter and, 544
  atrioventricular junctional tachycardia and, 545
  cardiomyopathy and, 520
  supraventricular tachycardia and, 500
Verbal conceptual level, 772
Verbal stimuli, 763
Verdoperoxidase, 898; see also Myeloperoxidase
Verres needle, 966
Verrucae, 927
Verrucous plaques, 888
Versenate; see Edetate
Vertebrae; see also Spine
  codfish, 89, 1243
  disc disease of, 48, 50, 860
  squaring of, 50
  subluxation of, 36
  thoracic; see Thoracic spinal abnormalities
Vertebral artery syndromes, 84, 835
Vertebral bodies, fractures of, 1203
Vertebral osteoarthritis, degenerative, 860
Vertebral osteomyelitis, 221
Vertebrobasilar artery insufficiency, 793
Vertical nystagmus, 760
Vertigo, 792-794
  odontogenic, 867-868
  transient ischemic attacks and, 836
Very-low-density lipoproteins; see Lipoproteins, very-low-density
Vesicles
  herpes simplex and, 126, 128, 299
  lichen planus and, 938
  varicella-zoster and, 126, 129-130, 138
Vesicoureteral reflux, 196, 197, 650
Vesicular breath sounds, 685
Vesiculobullous lesions, 895, 923
Vessels; see Arteries; Blood vessels; Veins
Vestibular damage, 159, 166; see also Hearing loss
Vibration in evaluation, 14
Vibrio, 201, 202, 204
  brucellosis and, 244
  diarrhea and, 953
Vibrio cholerae, 201, 204
Vibrio parahaemolyticus, 202, 953
Vidarabine, 154
  herpes simplex and, 129, 299
    encephalitis and, 136
  zoster and, 138
Vidian neuralgia, Vail's, 791
Villi, intestinal, 945
Villoglandular polyps, mixed, 1038
Villous adenomas of large bowel, 1038

Vim-Silverman needle, 965, 1044
  Franklin modification of, 608
Vinblastine, 440, 442
  histiocytosis and, 398
  Hodgkin's disease and, 390, 391
  hyponatremia and, 594
  Kaposi's sarcoma and, 922
  testicular carcinoma and, 449
Vinca alkaloids, 440, 441-442; see also Vinblastine; Vincristine
  hepatic veins and, 1060
  histiocytosis and, 398
  hypogonadism and, 1172
  in leukemias, 366
  in lung carcinoma, 447, 448
  neuropathy and, 853
Vincent's angina, 224
  uremic stomatitis and, 667
  vitamin C and, 1110
Vincristine, 440, 442
  carcinoma and
    breast, 448
    oat cell lung, 447
    testicular, 449
  Chédiak-Higashi syndrome and, 357
  Hodgkin's disease and, 390
  hyponatremia and, 594
  in leukemias, 366, 370, 421
  in non-Hodgkin's lymphoma, 392, 393
  oral ulcers and, 450
  in sarcomas, 450
  thyroid hormones and, 1130
  toxicity of, 847
Vindesine, 447
Vinyl chloride
  as carcinogen, 432, 1066, 1084
  liver disease and, 432, 1066, 1084
  porphyria and, 1253
  portal hypertension and, 1060
Violin-string adhesions, 231
VIP; see Vasoactive intestinal polypeptide
Vipoma, 954
Viral capsid antigen, 132, 133
Viral diseases, 121-155
  agents against, 153-154
  and arthritis, 81-82, 108
  bone marrow failure and, 319
  cardiomyopathy and, 520
  cat-scratch fever in, 151
  of central nervous system, 122, 134-139, 824-828
    amyotrophic lateral sclerosis in, 803
    encephalitis in, 139
  classification of, 122, 123
  dentistry and, 298-301
  diabetes mellitus and, 1260
  diarrhea and, 952, 953
  disseminated intravascular coagulation and, 412
  enteric; see Enteroviruses
  Epstein-Barr virus and; see Epstein-Barr virus
  exanthems in, 129-130, 145-149
  of fetus and newborn, 125-127, 1073-1074
  fever of unknown origin and, 120
  gastroenteritis in, 149-151
    malabsorption and, 1003
  hepatitis in, 1068; 1073, 1098-1101; see also Hepatitis
  herpesviruses in, 127-134; see also Herpes simplex; Herpes zoster; Herpesviruses
  Hodgkin's disease and, 387, 424
  immunodeficiency diseases and, 31
  inflammatory bowel disease and, 1006
  influenza and, 140; see also Influenza

Viral diseases—cont'd
  interferon and, 154; see also Interferon
  laboratory diagnosis of, 122-125, 139
    hemagglutinin in; see Hemagglutinin tests
  leukemias and, 364
  lipid envelope and, 121, 127
  lupus erythematosus and, 54
  multiple myeloma and, 378-379
  multiple sclerosis and, 797
  mumps in, 139-140; see also Mumps
  neutropenia and, 359
  oncogenesis and, 433, 656, 659
  oral ulcers and, 451
  Paget's disease and, 86
  pancreatitis and, 1051
  pharyngitides in; see Pharyngitis, viral
  prostatic carcinoma and, 659
  renal cell carcinoma and, 656
  respiratory, 122, 140-145; see also Pneumonia, viral
  of skin, 926-928
  smallpox in, 827
  thyroiditis and, 1149
  transmission of, 121, 125
  vaccines for, 151-153; see also Vaccines
  viremia in; see Viremia
Virchow's node, 1035
Viremia
  Herpes simplex and, 128
  maternal, 125
  measles and, 145
  rubella virus vaccine and, 152
Viridans streptococci, 228
Virions, 121
Virulence factors, 249
Viruses; see Viral diseases
Visceral angiography, 971-972
Visceral larva migrans, 290-291, 721
Visceral pleura, 730
Visceral scleroderma, 904
Visceral varicella, 130
Vision, 8-9; see also Eyes
  agnosia and, 771
  cytomegalovirus and, 125
  multiple sclerosis and, 798
  occipital lobe lesions and, 759
  pituitary tumors and, 1123
  visual evoked response and, 762, 800
Visual association agnosia, 771
Visual evoked response, 762, 800
Visual fields
  evaluation of, 8
  pituitary tumors and, 1123
Visual object agnosia, 771
Vital capacity, 677
  asbestosis and, 726
  chest bellows disease and, 712
  forced expiratory, 677-679
Vital signs, 8, 11; see also specific vital sign
  syncope and, 864
Vitamin D-dependent rickets, 1200
Vitamin D-resistant rickets, 668, 1200
Vitamin K-dependent factor concentrates, 410, 411
Vitamins, 1102, 1106-1111
  A, 1106-1107
    abetalipoproteinemia and, 1292
    Crohn's disease and, 1015
    excessive, 1107
    fat absorption and, 998, 1000, 1104
    hypercalcemia and excess of, 1189
    kidney stones and, 647
    liver disease and, 1063, 1082
    pseudotumor cerebri and, 790, 848

Vitamins—cont'd
B
deficiency of, 849, 850, 851
liver diseases and, 1059, 1080
thyrotoxicosis and, 1205
B_1; see Thiamine
B_2, 1106, 1108-1109, 1298
B_6; see Pyridoxine
B_{12}, 1106, 1109
absorption of, 318, 940
anemia and, 315
combined system disease and, 33-34, 808, 851
Crohn's disease and, 1012, 1015
gastritis and, 996
malabsorption and, 1000, 1001
malnutrition and, 1103, 1109
megaloblastic anemia and, 316-318
metabolism and, 317
in methylmalonic acidemia, 1237
neuropathy and, 853
neutropenia and, 358
oral manifestations of deficiency of, 1091, 1109
pernicious anemia and; see Pernicious anemia
polycythemia vera and, 353
Reiter's syndrome and, 908
renal failure and, 636, 637, 639
sprue and, 1001
subacute combined degeneration and, 851
tapeworm and, 293
in therapy, 318
B complex, 1106, 1108-1110
alcoholism and, 1296-1298
vitamin A and, 1107
C; see Ascorbic acid
D, 1106, 1107, 1188
abetalipoproteinemia and, 1292
calcium and, 1179, 1180, 1190, 1191, 1194, 1195
Crohn's disease and, 1015
dialysis and, 642
enterohepatic circulation of, 1198
fat absorption and, 998, 1000, 1104
hypercalcemia and, 1179, 1189, 1194
hypocalcemia and, 1195
inherited disorders and, 1200
kidney stones and, 647-648
liver disease and, 1063, 1082
metabolism of, 1185-1186, 1200
multiple myeloma and, 382
osteomalacia and, 1186, 1198-1201
osteoporosis and, 89, 1203, 1210
postgastrectomy syndrome and, 1004
renal failure and, 636, 637, 639
rickets and, 1186
sarcoidosis and, 717
toxic nephropathy and, 627
D_2, 1185
D_3, 1185-1186; see also 1,25-Dihydroxyvitamin D_3
deficiency of, 1198
hypoparathyroidism and, 1196
osteomalacia and, 1199-1200
deficiencies of, 849-851; see also specific vitamin
alcoholism and, 1296-1298
liver disease and, 1059, 1062-1063, 1080
E, 1106, 1107
Crohn's disease and, 1015
fat absorption and, 998, 1104
pseudoxanthoma elasticum and, 884

Vitamins—cont'd
epidermolysis bullosa dystrophica and, 877
fat absorption and, 998, 1000
fat-soluble; see Fat-soluble vitamins; specific vitamin
K, 1106, 1107-1108
antagonists to, 414
biliary cirrhosis and, 1082
chlorpromazine jaundice and, 1076
cholestyramine and, 1072
coumarins and, 414, 577
Crohn's disease and, 1015
deficiency of, 411
dental surgery hemorrhage and, 862
fat absorption and, 998, 1000, 1104
heart failure and, 462
hemolysis and, 330
liver diseases and, 1059, 1063, 1072, 1082, 1098
nephrotic syndrome and, 613
Reiter's syndrome and, 908
supplements of
biliary cirrhosis and, 1082
osteoporosis and, 89
pancreatitis and, 1056
postgastrectomy syndrome and, 1004
total parenteral nutrition and, 446
Vitreous opacification, 907
VLDL; see Lipoproteins, very-low-density
Vocal fremitus, 684
Voice sounds, 9, 12, 684
Volume depletion states, 596-597
Volume expanders; see also Plasma volume
anaphylaxis and, 29
gastrointestinal bleeding and, 958
hyperglycemic, hyperosmolar, nonketotic coma and, 1270
posthemorrhagic anemia and, 323
shock and, 478
Voluntary ventilation, 711; see also Respirations; Ventilation
Volvulus, 998, 1026
Vomiting, 956-957
bowel obstruction and, 1024, 1025
esophageal rupture and, 986
gastric carcinoma and, 1035
hematemesis and; see Hematemesis
nonocclusive vascular disease of gout and, 1021
Norwalk-like agents and, 150
papilledema, and headache, triad of, 846
peptic ulcers and, 988
radiation enteritis and, 1019
Vomiting center, 956
Vomitus, analysis of, 956-957
Von Economo's encephalitis, 812
Von Gierke's disease, 890
von Graefe's sign, 1142
Von Hippel-Lindau disease, 809, 872, 1165
von Recklinghausen's disease, 808-809, 878-880
hyperparathyroidism and, 1192
lung and, 721
pheochromocytoma and, 1164-1165
tumors and, 844
Von Willebrand's disease, 407-408, 410, 1227
dentistry and, 426-427
sickle cell trait and, 334
Von Zumbusch psoriasis, 937
VP; see Variegate porphyria
VP 16, 447
Vulvovaginitis, 230

W

Waldenström's macroglobulinemia, 382-384
dentistry and, 423
kidney disease and, 618
Waldeyer's ring, 424
Wallenberg's syndrome, 793, 835, 872
Warfarin
alcohol and, 1255
cerebral infarction and, 832
dentistry and, 577
dialysis and, 641
in fetal warfarin syndrome, 1303
mitral stenosis and, 513
phenytoin and, 786
pregnancy and, 1212
pulmonary emboli and, 492
rifampin and, 259
thrombocytosis and, 405
transient ischemic attack and, 837
Warm shock, 240, 476
Warming, hypothermia and, 756
Warm-reacting autoimmune hemolytic anemias, 338-339
Warts, 927
anal, 1030
Wash-in, 687
Washing soda, poisoning from, 754
Washout, 687
Water; see also Fluids
diseases carried in, 199-209; see also Foodborne and waterborne diseases
excessive loss of, 595-596
hyponatremia and, 593-594; see also Hyponatremia
lung, 708-709; see also Adult respiratory distress syndrome
metabolism of, kidney and, 593-597
nutrition and, 1102
reduced intake of, 129, 150, 596-597, 707, 957
Water brash, 975
Waterborne diseases, 199-209; see also Foodborne and waterborne diseases
Water-hammer pulse, 516, 580
Waterhouse-Friderichsen syndrome, 234, 1156
Water-Pik, 876
Waterston anastomosis, 507
Watery diarrhea syndrome, 954
Watson-Schwartz tests, 1251
WBCs; see White blood cells
Weaver's bottom, 99
Weber's syndrome, 833
Weber's test, 9, 795
Weber-Christian disease, 78-79
Webs, 1077
WEE; see Western equine encephalitis
Wegener's granulomatosis, 70-73
cutaneous lesions of, 906
dentistry and, 113
lung and, 719-720
management of, 69
midline granuloma and, 74
renal lesions in, 616
vasculitis and, 69
Weight, diabetes mellitus and, 1265; see also Obesity
Weil's disease, 273
Weil-Felix reaction, 210
Weill-Marchesani syndrome, 1246
Welch's abscess, 253
Wenckebach sinoatrial block, 546
Werdnig-Hoffman disease, 804
Wernicke's aphasia, 759, 772

Wernicke's encephalopathy, 849-850, 1108, 1257
 thalamus lesions and, 759
Western equine encephalitis, 135, 825
WG; see Wegener's granulomatosis
Wheat weevil disease, 727
Wheezing, 23, 141, 685
Whipple's disease, 941, 1002-1003
Whipple's operation, 1057, 1089
Whipple's triad, 1277
Whipworm, 290
White blood cells
 in cerebrospinal fluid, 135
 count of; see Blood cell count, white
 disorders of, 355-399
  eosinophil, and eosinophilic syndrome; see Eosinophilic diseases
  Hodgkin's disease in, 387-391; see also Hodgkin's disease
  leukemias and, 363-372; see also Leukemias
  myeloproliferative, 373-376, 404, 406
  neutrophil, 355-363
  non-Hodgkin's lymphomas in, 358, 391-394
  plasma cell disorders and, 376-387; see also Plasma cell disorders
  reticuloendothelial system in, 394-399
  spleen and, 134, 394-399
 transfusions of, 347, 361; see also Transfusions, granulocyte; Transfusions, leukocyte
 in urine, 590
  site of injury and, 588
  toxic nephropathy and, 626
White matter, diseases of, 796-804, 852
White-out, lung, 709
Whitlow, herpetic, 926
Whole blood transfusions; see Blood transfusions
Whooping cough, 143, 237-238, 248, 252
Wickham's striae, 938
Widal's test, 207
Widow's peak hair pattern, 1317, 1318
Wiga, 172
Wildervanck-Smith syndrome, 1311
Willis, aneurysm of circle of, 839, 1275
Wilms' tumor, 658
Wilson, central terminal of, 480
Wilson's disease, 822-823, 1066, 1081-1082, 1240
 hemolysis in, 342
 juvenile parkinsonism and, 812
Wimberger's sign, 270
Winchester syndrome, 1244
Wire looping, 54, 615
Wiskott-Aldrich syndrome, 33

Withdrawal
 from alcohol, 776, 784, 787, 1080, 1257, 1258, 1298
 opiate, 778
Withdrawal seizures, 784, 786, 787
Witzelsucht, 772
Wolff-Chaikoff effect, 1130
Wolff-Parkinson-White syndrome, 543, 544, 548-549
 in children, 500-501
Wood pulp worker's disease, 727
Wounds, 204, 252, 253; see also Trauma
WPW syndrome; see Wolff-Parkinson-White syndrome
Wright's stain, 238
Wrist, disorders of, 84, 101-102
Writer's cramp, 821
Wuchereria bancrofti, 292

X

X bodies, 719
X chromosomes; see also X-linked inheritance
 banding pattern for, 1221
 random inactivation of, 1219
X factor, 235
X porphyrin, 1252, 1253
Xanthelasma, 889
Xanthine oxidase inhibitors, 472
Xanthines
 chronic obstructive pulmonary disease and, 693
 in urine, 1239-1240
Xanthomas
 biliary disease and, 896
 diabetes and, 885
 hyperlipidemia and, 889-890, 1280, 1287, 1288
 liver diseases and, 1059
 multiple myeloma and, 899
 palpebral, 889
 plane, 890, 896
 tuberous, 889
Xenon arc, 1274
Xenon 133 ventilation scan, 492, 687
Xeroderma pigmentosum, 433
Xerosis, 885, 1107
Xerostomia
 anticholinergics and, 1092
 diabetes mellitus and, 1294
 hyperlipoproteinemia and, 1296
 liver disease and, 1098
 management of, 876
 opiate-induced, 862
 radiation and, 919
 sarcoidosis and, 113, 114, 911
 scleroderma and, 1091

X-linked immunodeficiency, 32
X-linked inheritance, 877, 1218-1219
 dystrophies of, 856-857
X-rays, 749, 1172; see also Roentgenograms
XXX females, 1226
Xylocaine; see Lidocaine
D-Xylose absorption, 150
XYY karyotype, 1171, 1226

Y

Y chromosome, 1168, 1219
Y proteins, 1058
Yeast infections; see *Candida; Candida albicans*
Yellow dye, 704
Yellow nail syndrome, 696
Yersinia, 202
 brucellosis and, 244
 diarrhea and, 953
 erythema nodosum and, 924
 malabsorption and, 1003
 plague and, 242
 pneumonia and, 172
 Reiter's syndrome and, 52, 907
Yersinia enterocolitica, 202, 953
Yersinia pestis, 172, 242
Y-linked inheritance, 1219

Z

Z line, 973
Z proteins, 1058
Zarontin; see Ethosuximide
Zenker's diverticulum, 736, 975, 976
Zieve syndrome, 1257
ZIG; see Zoster immune globulin
Zinc
 acrodermatitis enteropathica and, 894-895
 Candida and, 929
 hemolysis and, 342
 liver disease and, 1059, 1080
 Reiter's syndrome and, 908
Zinc chloride paste fixation, 918
Zinc oxide, 918
Zollinger-Ellison syndrome, 994-995
 gastric folds and, 997
 hyperparathyroidism and, 1192
 malabsorption and, 1001, 1004
 with malignancy, 1179
Zona fasciculata, 1153
Zona glomerulosa, 1153
Zona reticularis, 1153
Zoster; see Herpes zoster; Varicella
Zoster immune globulin, 127, 130, 138
Zygomatic hypoplasia, 1309
Zymogens, 1050